USING THIS BOOK

This book is a comprehensive and integrated product. Each part of the book presents select content in detail. To take full advantage of all content you will need to move between the various parts of the book. You may use the book as an easy reference to look up something specific in any single section, or you may use parts of several sections across the text to develop a full plan of care. Consider these examples.

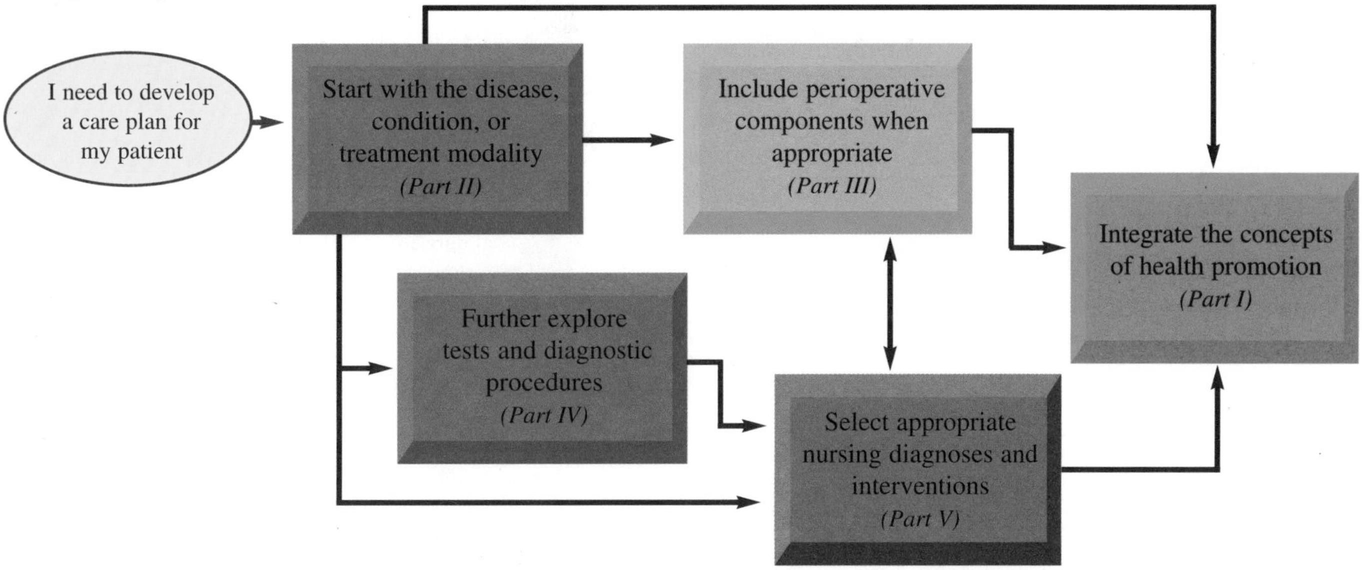
I need to develop a care plan for my patient
Start with the disease, condition, or treatment modality (Part II)
Include perioperative components when appropriate (Part III)
Integrate the concepts of health promotion (Part I)
Further explore tests and diagnostic procedures (Part IV)
Select appropriate nursing diagnoses and interventions (Part V)

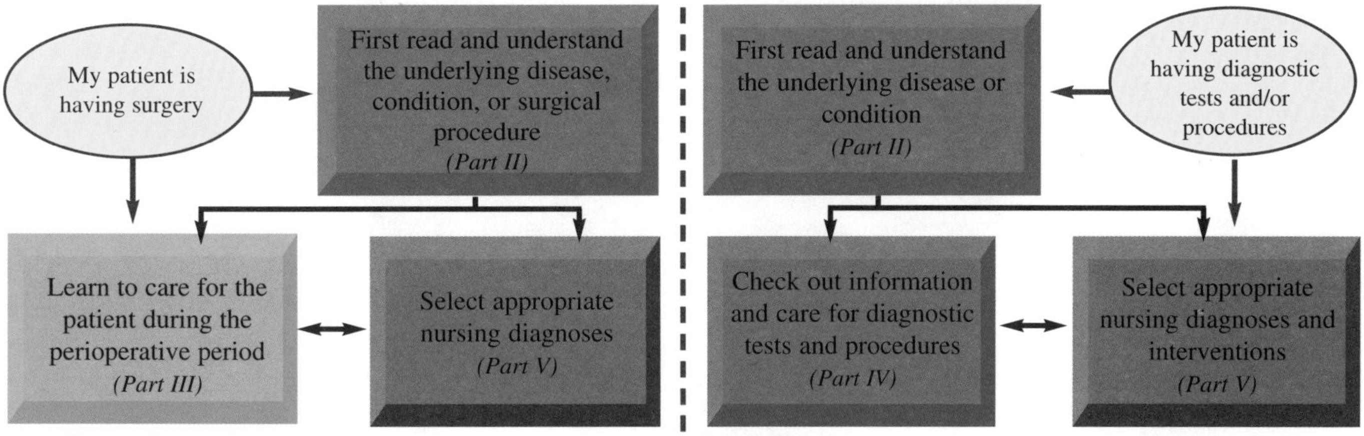
My patient is having surgery
First read and understand the underlying disease, condition, or surgical procedure (Part II)
Learn to care for the patient during the perioperative period (Part III)
Select appropriate nursing diagnoses (Part V)
My patient is having diagnostic tests and/or procedures
First read and understand the underlying disease or condition (Part II)
Check out information and care for diagnostic tests and procedures (Part IV)
Select appropriate nursing diagnoses and interventions (Part V)

Teach me about health promotion, prevention, and alternative modalities

Part I

1. What is Health?
2. *Healthy People 2010*
3. National Health Promotion Priorities
4. Preventive Care Guidelines
5. *Canadian Health Guidelines*
6. Alternative Therapies
7. Complementary Therapies
8. Health Education Strategies

Teach me about diseases, conditions, and treatment modalities

Part II

Body system anatomy and physiology
Normal assessment findings

For each disease or condition

1. Overview of a select disease, condition, or treatment modality
2. Diagnostic studies and findings
3. Multidisciplinary plan
4. Nursing assessment
5. Nursing care with rationales, NANDA diagnoses, and NIC interventions
6. Patient education/continuum of care plan
7. Collaborative interventions and related nursing care
8. Evaluation of outcomes and treatment modalities

Teach me about nursing diagnoses

Part III

For each health pattern

Nursing diagnosis
Definition
Related factors and defining characteristics
Expected outcomes
Nursing interventions with rationales

Mosby's

Clinical Nursing

5th Edition

Mosby's Clinical Nursing

5th Edition

JUNE M. THOMPSON, RN, DR.PH
Former Director of Nursing Research, Education, and Standards
University Hospital
University of New Mexico Health Sciences Center
Albuquerque, New Mexico

GERTRUDE K. MCFARLAND, RN, DNSC, FAAN
Health Scientist Administrator
Nursing Research Study Section
Center for Scientific Review
National Institutes of Health
Bethesda, Maryland

JANE E. HIRSCH, RN, MS
Director of Nursing and Patient Care Services
UCSF Medical Center
University of California, San Francisco
San Francisco, California

SUSAN M. TUCKER, RN, MSN, PHN, CNAA
Healthcare Consultant
Santa Rosa, California

Mosby

St. Louis London Philadelphia Sydney Toronto

Mosby

Vice President, Publishing Director: Sally Schrefer
Executive Editor: Darlene Como
Developmental Editor: Barbara Watts
Project Manager: John Rogers
Project Specialist: Cheryl A. Abbott
Designer and Cover Art: Kathi Gosche

Fifth Edition

NOTICE

Pharmacology is an ever-changing field. Standard safety precautions must be followed, but as new research and clinical experience broaden our knowledge, changes in treatment and drug therapy may become necessary or appropriate. Readers are advised to check the most current product information provided by the manufacturer of each drug to be administered to verify the recommended dose, the method and duration of administration, and contraindications. It is the responsibility of the licensed prescriber, relying on experience and knowledge of the patient, to determine dosages and the best treatment for each individual patient. Neither the publisher nor the editor assumes any liability for any injury and/or damage to persons or property arising from this publication.

Mosby, Inc.
11830 Westline Industrial Drive
St. Louis, Missouri 63146

Printed in the United States of America

International Standard Book Number 0-323-01195-0

1 05 GW/RRD-W 9 8 7 6 5 4 3 2 1

Contributors

Rubi Agana-Defensor, RN, MS*
Nurse Consultant
National Institutes of Health
Bethesda, Maryland
Chapter 11

Anne Elizabeth Belcher, RN, PhD, AOCN, FAAN
Professor and Director of Undergraduate Programs
Department of Nursing
College of Health Professions
Thomas Jefferson University
Philadelphia, Pennsylvania
Chapter 17

Sarah Bernstein, RN, MS, AOCN*
Oncology Research Nurse Specialist
National Cancer Institute
National Naval Hospital
Bethesda, Maryland
Chapter 18

Kathleen Calitri Brown, RN, MN, CETN
ET Nurse Coordinator
The Emory Clinic
Atlanta, Georgia
Chapter 14

Victor G. Campbell, RN, PhD
Professor, Nursing
Mount Carmel College of Nursing
Columbus, Ohio
Chapter 5

Louise Dulaney Canada, RN, MSN, CRNO*
Clinical Research Nurse
Clinical Center Nursing Department
National Institutes of Health
Bethesda, Maryland
Chapter 11

Shelley A. Carroll, RN, MSN, CNOR
Clinical Nurse III, Perioperative
UCSF Medical Center
University of California, San Francisco
San Francisco, California
Chapter 21

Nikky Chahon, RN
Assistant Nurse Manager
Medical ICU
University of California, Davis, Medical Center
Sacramento, California
Chapter 22

*The opinions expressed herein are those of the authors and do not necessarily reflect those of the U.S. Department of Health and Human Services or the National Institutes of Health.

Joyce E. Dains, RN, Dr.PH, JD, FNP, CS
Assistant Professor
Baylor College of Medicine
Houston, Texas
Chapter 7

Sheila Gleeson, RN, BSN
Practice Manager
Surgery Faculty Practice
UCSF Medical Center
San Francisco, California
Chapter 21

Mikel Gray, PhD, CUNP, CCCN, FAAN
Nurse Practitioner and Associate Professor
Department of Urology and School of Nursing
University of Virginia
Charlottesville, Virginia
Chapter 14

Deanna E. Grimes, Dr.PH, RN, CS, FAAN
Associate Professor
University of Texas Health Science Center
School of Nursing
Houston, Texas
Chapter 15

Kevin A. Grimes, BS
MD-MPH Candidate
University of Texas Health Science Center
Houston, Texas
Chapter 15

Debra A. Hagler, RN, MS, CS, CCRN
Clinical Associate Professor
Arizona State University College of Nursing
Tempe, Arizona
Chapter 4

Kim Hart, RN, MS, ANP
Graduate Research Assistant
School of Nursing
Northern Illinois University
DeKalb, Illinois
Chapter 19

James Hill, BSN, RN
Clinical Resource Nurse
Surgical Intensive Care Unit
University of California, Davis Medical Center
Sacramento, California
Chapter 22

Jane E. Hirsch, RN, MS
Director of Nursing and Patient Care Services
UCSF Medical Center
University of California, San Francisco
San Francisco, California

MARY G. HIRSCH, RN, MSN, CETN
Reimbursement Consultant
Health Care Economics
TYCO Mallinckrodt
St. Louis, Missouri
Chapter 10

BRIGID IDE, RN, MS
Director, Performance Improvement
UCSF Medical Center
Assistant Clinical Professor
University of California, San Francisco, School of Nursing
San Francisco, California
Chapter 3

JOAN LABARR, RN, BSN
Assistant Manager
Medical ICU
University of California, Davis, Medical Center
Sacramento, California
Chapter 22

PRISCILLA LEMONE, RN, DSN, FAAN
Associate Professor
Sinclair School of Nursing
University of Missouri, Columbia
Columbia, Missouri
Chapter 23

ROXANNE W. MCDANIEL, RN, PHD
Associate Professor
Sinclair School of Nursing
University of Missouri, Columbia
Columbia, Missouri
Chapter 23

GERTRUDE K. MCFARLAND, RN, DNSC, FAAN*
Health Scientist Administrator
Nursing Research Study Section
Center for Scientific Review
National Institutes of Health
Bethesda, Maryland
Chapter 20

CHRISTINE MIASKOWSKI, RN, PHD, FAAN
Professor and Chair
Department of Physiological Nursing
University of California, San Francisco
San Francisco, California
Chapter 16

MARSHA A. MILLER, RN, MED, CNOR
Manager, Global Education and Training
Advanced Sterilization Products
Irvine, California
Chapter 21

LEONA A. MOURAD, RN, MSN, BSED, ONC
Associate Professor Emerita
Ohio State University
Columbus, Ohio
Chapter 6

LYNN NOLAND, RN, PHD, NP
Assistant Professor of Nursing, Nephrology
Nurse Practitioner
University of Virginia School of Nursing
Charlottesville, Virginia
Chapter 13

ROBERT J. O'MALLEY, RNC, MS, NP
Trauma Nurse Practitioner and Clinical Faculty
University of California, Davis, Medical Center
Sacramento, California;
Assistant Clinical Professor
University of California
San Francisco, California;
Private Practice Nurse Practitioner
Obstetrics and Gynecology
Rancho Cordova, California
Chapter 12

ANN M. O'MARA, RN, PHD, MPH, AOCN*
Cancer Prevention Fellow
National Institutes of Health
National Cancer Institute
Bethesda, Maryland
Chapter 18

PEGGY L. PAYNE, RN, BSN, MN, DSN
Nursing Instructor
Department of Veteran Affairs
W.G. Hefner Medical Center
Salisbury, North Carolina
Chapter 23

BARBARA A. SIGLER, RN, MNED
Technical Publications Editor
Oncology Nursing Press
Former Clinical Nurse Specialist
University of Pittsburgh
Department of Otolaryngology
Pittsburgh, Pennsylvania
Chapter 9

SARAH C. SMITH, RN, MA, CRNO
Advanced Practice Nurse
University of Iowa Health Care
Department of Ophthalmology
Iowa City, Iowa
Chapter 8

MOLLY SOLARES, RN
Nurse Consultant
Swinton
Yorkshire, England;
Former Endocrine Specialist
Division of Endochrinology
Harbor—UCLA Research and Education Institute
Torrance, California
Chapter 11

CYNTHIA SONG-MAYEDA, RN, CDE, PHN
Diabetes—Endocrine Nursing Care Specialist
Harbor—UCLA Medical Center
Torrance, California
Chapter 11

June M. Thompson, RN, Dr.PH
Former Director of Nursing Research, Education, and Standards
University Hospital
University of New Mexico Health Sciences Center
Albuquerque, New Mexico

Gayle A. Traver, RN, MSN
Associate Professor of Nursing and Assistant Professor of Clinical Medicine
University of Arizona
Tucson, Arizona
Chapter 4

Susan M. Tucker, RN, MSN, PHN, CNAA
Healthcare Consultant
Santa Rosa, California
Chapters 2, 12

Georgia Griffith Whitley, RN, EdD
Professor Emerita
Northern Illinois University
School of Nursing
DeKalb, Illinois
Chapter 19

Carolyn M. Zack, BSMT (ASCP), MPH
Infection Control Practitioner
Memorial Hermann Hospital
Houston, Texas
Chapter 15

Reviewers

Donna L. Cramer, BS, BA, RN
Clinical Analyst
Capital Service Area Information Technology
Kaiser Permanente Medical Center
Sacramento, California

Darcy Folzenlogen, MD
Assistant Professor of Internal Medicine
Chairman, Clinical Affairs Council, Department of Medicine
Assistant Director, Internal Medicine Residency Program
University of Missouri, Columbia
Columbia, Missouri

Sue Baird Holmes, MS, RN, ONC
Clinical Nurse Specialist—Orthopedics
St. Joseph's Hospital
Milwaukee, Wisconsin

Robert Keisling, MD
Medical Director for Mental Health
Unity Healthcare
Washington, DC

Kathryn A. King, RPh, PhD
Pharmacist II
University of Missouri Health Sciences Center Pharmacy
University of Missouri, Columbia
Columbia, Missouri

Kimberly A. Litton, RN, MS, CS, CCRN
Clinical Nurse Specialist/Educator
Harris Methodist Health System
Fort Worth, Texas

Carol Lynn Mandle, PhD, RN, CS-FNP
Associate Professor Boston College School of Nursing
Co-Director, Medical Symptoms Reduction Clinic Programs
Mind Body Medical Institute and Beth Israel Deaconess Medical Center
Harvard Medical School
Boston, Massachusetts

Jamie S. Myers, RN, MN, ACCN
Oncology Clinical Nurse Specialist and Head Nurse
Research Medical Center
Kansas City, Missouri

June Hart Romero, PhD, NP-C
Director, MSN Program
Cleveland State University
Cleveland, Ohio

Meg Shea, RN, MS, CS, PNP
Pediatric Nurse Practitioner
Washington University School of Medicine
Department of Pediatric
St. Louis Children's Hospital
St. Louis, Missouri

Sue G. Thacker, RNC, PhD
Professor
Wytheville Community College
Wytheville, Virginia

Preface

In 1986 as the first edition of this work was published, we wrote

> This text has evolved as a result of the demand by professional nurses from across the United States and Canada. Nurses said there was a need to clarify nursing practice—to "put it all together" in one book. They said, "Put together the nursing theories; nursing process, including nursing diagnoses and physiology, and pathophysiology. Use those theory bases and an interdisciplinary health care approach to develop a contemporary and comprehensive text that reflects the potential scope of professional nursing practice."

That was 16 years ago, and during this time and four subsequent editions, this succinct reference and text remains broad in scope and intensive in content. In each edition of the text, we have continued to grow and to adapt with the changes in health care, nursing science, medical research, patient needs, and care modalities.

The first edition of this text was written following the standards of the American Nurses Association's guidelines, *Standards of Nursing Practice*[1] and *Nursing: A Social Policy Statement.*[2] These important documents were among the first to delineate the scope of professional clinical nursing practice and to establish standards integrating the art and science of nursing. During the subsequent 20 years, these time tested standards were revised by the ANA in 1998 as the *Standards of Clinical Nursing Practice,* second edition.[3]

As with the first edition of *Clinical Nursing,* the American Nurses Association's *Standards of Clinical Nursing Practice* serves as the core for approach and organization. The "standards" and relevant nursing actions follow:

- **Standard 1** *Assessment:* Collect patient health data
- **Standard 2** *Diagnosis:* Analyze assessment data to determine diagnoses
- **Standard 3** *Outcome Identification:* Identify expected outcomes individualized to the patient
- **Standard 4** *Planning:* Develop a plan of care that prescribes interventions to attain expected outcomes
- **Standard 5** *Implementation:* Implement interventions identified in the plan of care
- **Standard 6** *Evaluation:* Evaluate the patient's progress toward attainment of outcomes

The standards provide the framework for implementing standard-based nursing care. *Clinical Nursing,* fifth edition, uses these nursing standards and interdisciplinary methods and interventions to provide guidance for comprehensive patient care and outcome evaluation. *Clinical Nursing,* fifth edition, provides clear and detailed information synthesizing disease processes, including anatomy and physiology, pathophysiology, nursing diagnoses, interventions and evaluation, using the North American Nursing Diagnoses (NANDA) taxonomy and the Nursing Interventions Classification (NIC) as well as interdisciplinary care details, outcome evaluation parameters, and continuity of care guides.

Mosby's Clinical Nursing, fifth edition, has been carefully developed and designed so that the user, either student or clinician, may quickly and easily access the detailed information required to provide care or receive quick clinical consultation.

PART I HEALTH INITIATIVES AND ALTERNATIVE MODALITIES

This section is new to *Clinical Nursing,* fifth edition. Health promotion and complementary and alternative therapies are important considerations in today's health system. Nurses have unique opportunities to implement interventions to promote health and wellness. The health promotion chapter details the United States *Healthy People 2010* and the Canadian *Health Promotion Strategies for Promoting the Health of Individuals and Families.* The chapter on alternative therapies provides descriptive information about the many alternative therapies that are being reported more frequently. By understanding these therapies, the nurse is in a better position to consider the blending of treatment modalities.

PART II CLINICAL NURSING PRACTICE

This section provides the comprehensive clinical care details for 18 body systems. Following these chapters, the section concludes with a chapter on mental health disorders in the elderly. Each chapter has consistent formatting for easy access and reference, and each begins with a review of anatomy and physiology. This is followed by a detailed and standardized presentation of each disease or disorder including:

- **Pathophysiology, Diagnostic Studies and Findings** and **Normal** and **Abnormal Findings.**
- **Multidisciplinary Plan,** including surgery, medications, and general management as appropriate.
- **Nursing Care** encompassing the appropriate detailing of the significant **Patient Problems and Nursing Diagnoses.** Each patient problem is stated according to the Nursing Intervention Classification (NIC) terminology. Following each NIC statement is the bolded NANDA nursing diagnoses, appropriate interventions, and rationale. For easy reference, the rationale appear in *italics.* The **NIC statements** are identified with a special icon NIC. For each nursing diagnosis and intervention, there is a discussion of **Evaluation/Patient Outcomes.**
- **Older adult variations** highlighted with a unique icon.
- **Patient Education/Continuum of Care Plan** discussions with a special icon for easy identification.
- **Emergency Alert** boxes listing appropriate assessment and intervention details.

---

[1]American Nurses Association: *Standards of nursing practice,* Washington, DC, 1973, The Association.

[2]American Nurses Association: *Nursing: a social policy statement,* Kansas City, 1980, The Association.

[3]American Nurses Association: *Standards of clinical nursing practice,* ed 2, Washington, DC, 1998, The Association.

- ***Healthy People 2010*** boxes highlighting major health promotion and disease prevention goals and objectives.

PART III Perioperative Nursing

This section discusses patient care before, during, and after surgery. Preparation for surgery focuses on the immediate preoperative period, asepsis, positioning the patient, and a detailed discussion of anesthesia, potential perioperative complications, and nursing care of the postanesthesia patient.

PART IV Diagnostic Studies and Laboratory Values

This section provides a handy reference to more than 160 common diagnostic studies and laboratory tests. Where appropriate, nursing care is discussed.

PART V Nursing Diagnoses, Outcomes, and Interventions

This rich reference section includes **Definitions, Related Factors, Defining Characteristics,** and **Expected Patient Outcomes** for each of the NANDA Nursing Diagnoses. The NANDA Nursing Diagnoses are the latest 2001-2002 release. The nursing interventions include NIC terminology with appropriate rationale.

The first edition of this textbook was reported to provide a comprehensive standard for clinical nursing practice. Sixteen years later, this comprehensive text is now referenced as the "gold standard" for clinical nursing practice and is the best clinical consultant you will ever have.

We hope you find this comprehensive volume rich with content, easy to use, and an authoritative reference as you plan and provide care for your patients.

June M. Thompson
Gertrude K. McFarland
Jane E. Hirsch
Susan M. Tucker

Acknowledgments

Each time this large and complex text is revised, we realize the never-ending dedication and hard work by all involved.

To each of the contributors, we thank you for your careful preparation of the manuscript, your careful review of content, and for your patience with the process of publishing a text of this magnitude and complexity.

Our heartfelt thanks are also extended to Sally Schrefer, Vice President, Publishing Director, for her overall leadership. In past editions, Sally has directly managed the revision of this text and, in part, is responsible for its fine quality today. Thanks go to Darlene Como, Executive Editor, who assisted us with planning and executing this edition. Darlene's experience and long publishing history was just the touch of excellence we needed to plan this new comprehensive edition. We also thank Barb Watts, our Developmental Editor, for her endless persistence, careful editing, problem solving, gentle nudging, and long hours of work to ensure that this text published according to schedule; Cheryl Abbott, Project Specialist, for her coordination of production, attention to detail, careful editing, and her unending patience; John Rogers, Project Manager, for his involvement and oversight to make sure that this text was developed and published just as it was planned.

In addition, we would like to thank all those who have supported us during this long revision process. To the nurses, students, faculty, sales reps, bookstore managers, and all those who take the time to know this edition and who take the time to see the depth and breadth of the content, we appreciate your commitment. Our thanks also go to all those colleagues who put this textbook to use while planning and providing care.

A personal thank you is extended by Gertrude McFarland to her husband, Al McFarland, and her mother, Emma Ramseier, for their loving support throughout the project.

Contents in Brief

Contents

PART I

HEALTH INITIATIVES AND ALTERNATIVE MODALITIES

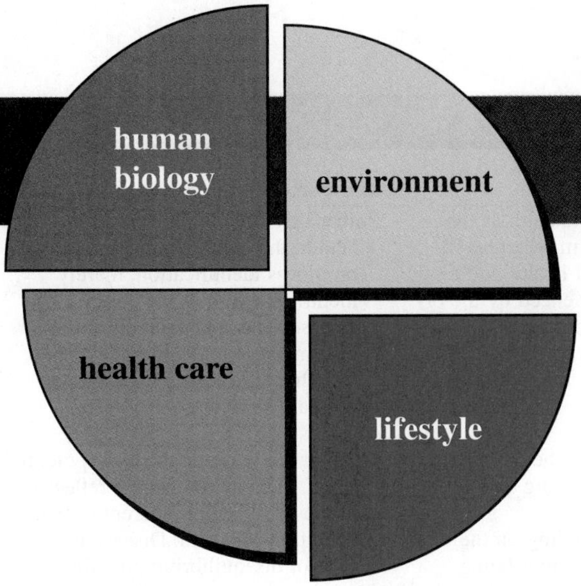

1

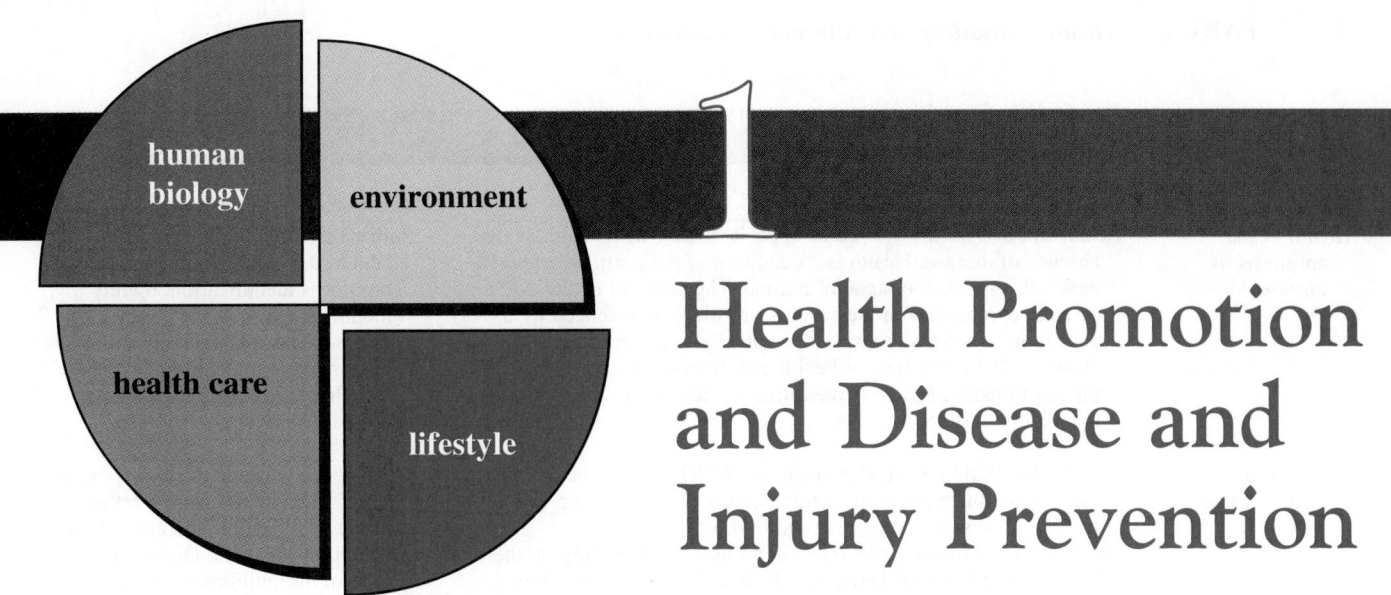

Health Promotion and Disease and Injury Prevention

June M. Thompson

Health, wellness, high-level wellness, screening, patient teaching, compliance, and the like are all terms health-care professionals use daily while caring for patients, clients, families, and groups of individuals. Throughout this text, reference is made to screening, health promotion, and related patient teaching. For years, individuals and families have learned to depend on personal health-care providers to "guide them" to health, "counsel them" to maintain wellness, and be available to provide them care and consultation when needed. Times have changed in this complex health-care environment. It is now vital that health-care professionals actively work with all consumers of health-care services to screen their current health status, to teach them how and when to care for themselves, and to empower them to assume responsibility for their own health status monitoring. This is a tall assignment and certainly one that is not simple or straightforward. One can be dying and still be well, one can be healthy and still be sick, one can be informed and still hurt himself or herself, one can have information and still be noncompliant, and one can be noncompliant and still be healthy. Indeed health, health promotion, wellness, disease prevention, and injury prevention are complex topics. This chapter takes a factual approach regarding the state of the nations and screening guidelines but also explores the topics of compliance and personal health promotion.

Definitions of Health

What Is Health?

What is health? Is it the absence of disease? A total balance of body, mind, and spirit? Having a chronic disease under control? Or being within the perfect height-weight category for your gender and age? Health may be a reference for disease or it may be a panacea. Arnold and Breen[8] provide an interesting and succinct analysis of the concepts of health. Many ways to conceptualize health are reported, and as each of these is viewed in its unique aspects, one may see a vast variety of concepts. Health may be the antithesis of disease, a balanced state, growth, functionality, goodness of fit, wholeness, a sense of well-being, transcendence, or empowerment. All of these are summarized in Table 1-1.

Measures of Health

Historically and still in many national data sources, measures of health status have been based primarily on mortality data. Researchers assume that a low age-adjusted death rate and high life expectancy reflect good health in a population. Currently, a higher proportion of the population lives to old age than ever before, and this group suffers from various chronic and disabling illnesses. Therefore using mortality data as the index for health is no longer adequate. Researchers continue to fine-tune quality-of-life assessment tools and indicators of and for health. Numerous health risk appraisal tools are now being used to investigate illness and injury risk as measures of the quality of life for persons with chronic and/or terminal illnesses. These are helpful in that even though an individual may have a chronic or terminal illness, he or she may be experiencing a high quality of life and thus "health."

Levels of Health Prevention

Useful concepts of health prevention developed by Leavell and Clark[13] are the three levels of prevention. These levels—primary, secondary, and tertiary—facilitate goals for prevention regardless of an individual's disease state or condition (see Table 1-2, p. 6).

Primary prevention keeps the disease process from becoming established by eliminating causes of disease or increasing resistance to disease. Interventions include health promotion and specific targeted disease prevention such as nutrition and immunizations. *Secondary prevention* interrupts the disease process before it becomes symptomatic. Interventions include early diagnosis and rapid intervention to prevent permanent sequelae. *Tertiary prevention* limits the physical and social consequences of symptomatic disease (see Table 1-2). Interventions include limiting disability and ensuring appropriate and prompt

Table 1-1 Imaging Health: Health as . . .

Model	Overview	Limitations and/or Assumptions
Health as the antithesis of disease	Health and disease are viewed as opposite states, with health as the absence of disease. Health is a condition of the norm, whereas illness falls outside the range of normal. The states of health and disease are expressions of the success or failure experienced by the organism in its efforts to respond adaptively to environmental changes. The conditions of health and disease are expressions of bipolar thinking. Health is measured by morbidity and mortality data (Dubos, 1965).	Rather than defining the components of health, the medical model, relying on illness identification, merely identifies health as the absence of disease. Thus parameters for being healthy are not identified, except for what falls within the range of normal.
Health as a balanced state	In 1947 the World Health Organization (WHO) defined health as a state of complete physical, mental, and social well-being and not merely the absence of disease and infirmity. Dunn (1961) augmented the WHO definition by expanding on the idea of complete well-being, in which well-being implies being well not only in the body and mind but also within the family and community and having a compatible work interest. Dunn was able to move beyond the interrelatedness of wellness of the body, mind, and environment to define high-level wellness. High-level wellness for the individual is defined as an integrated method of functioning that is oriented toward maximizing the potential of which the individual is capable. Oriental medicine is also based on a principle of health as a balance. Balance is found through the harmony of yin and yang. The forces of yin and yang are described as active/passive; masculine/feminine; stimulating/nurturing; and heavenly/earthy. Energy balance is possible through the interrelatedness of these seemingly opposite forces working together. Ayurveda, which originated in India, defines the trinity of life as body, mind, and spiritual awareness (Fugh-Berman, 1996). To a practitioner of Ayurveda, imbalances in doshas—physiologic principles, or bodily humors—can cause specific diseases. Various foods and emotions are believed to cause imbalances. The image of health as a balanced state is also incorporated in epidemiology, which provides an important framework for the clarification of the term *health. Epidemiology* is the study of patterns of health; the patterns of disease, disability, and death; and other problems in populations or persons (Leavell and Clark, 1965). A major goal of epidemiology is to identify aggregates, or subpopulations, in the community at high risk for disease. Once identified, preventive efforts are directed at the aggregates in hope that these interventions will benefit the population. In this model, health is identified along a continuum of health-illness-death. The origins of health and illness are indicative of other processes before the human body is affected. Key to the processes are the interactions of conditions in the environment, factors of the agent for disease, and predisposing genetic forces.	The balance between the host, potential agent, and environment is reflective of the equilibrium inherent in the condition of health. Disease is a state of disequilibrium, or "dis-ease," and health is a state of balance, or equilibrium. Equilibrium is achieved through the interaction of the multiple factors and forces that influence and contribute to health. The balance of health is reflected in the nature and intensity of these interactions. Physical, physiologic, social, cultural, spiritual, political, and economic forces interact and contribute to the unique picture of health for each individual, family, and community, as well as the image of health for populations of persons, families, groups, and community. Health is a balance along a goal-directed continuum within the context of the environment.
Health as growth	Developmental theorists such as Dewey, Piaget, Elkind, Erikson, Duvall, and Havinghurst created the foundations for health as	Established norms are used to measure growth at each developmental stage.

Modified from Gorin and Arnold.[8]

Bertalanffy LV: *General system theory,* New York, 1968, George Braziller.
Dubos R: *Man adapting,* New Haven, Conn, 1965, Yale University Press.
Dunn H: *High-level wellness,* Arlington, Va, 1961, Beatty.
Fugh-Berman A: *Alternative medicine: what works,* Tucson, Ariz, 1996, Odonian Press.
Lalonde M: *A new perspective on the health of Canadians,* Ottawa, 1974, Government of Canada.
Leavell HR, Clark EG: *Preventive medicine for the doctor in his community: an epidemiological approach,* New York, 1965, McGraw-Hill.
Robertson A, Minkler M: New health promotion movement, *Health Educ Q* 21(3):295, 1994.
Seedhouse D: Well-being: Health promotion's red herring, *Health Promotion Int* 10(1):61, 1995.
U.S. Office of Alternative Medicine, National Institutes of Health: *Alternative medicine: expanding medical horizons: a report to the National Institutes of Health on alternative medical systems and practices in the U.S.,* Washington, DC, 1994, The Office.
Wheeler RJ: The theoretical and empirical structure of general well-being, *Soc Indicators Res* 24:71, 1991.
World Health Organization: Constitution of the World Health Organization, *Chronicle World Health Org* 1(1-2):29, 1947.

Model	Overview	Limitations and/or Assumptions
	growth. Health is viewed as the successful fulfillment of certain tasks appropriate to particular life stages. Health as growth is seen as an ongoing process that occurs continuously and systematically throughout the life span. Growth is viewed as progressive. Health is seen as being intimately determined by individual lifestyle and behavior choices. Interventions at critical life stages are believed to be the most effective and foster optimal growth. When using this framework, the concept of aging takes on healthy dimensions. Instead of viewing "old age" as the final, end stage of life with anticipated decline, dependency, and potential helplessness, old age may be viewed as a time of final goal attainment. From this broad viewpoint, aging is recognized as being a complex cultural issue that cannot be defined from biologic parameters alone. While there may be altered physical abilities and changing expectations, aging persons retain the capacity for full participation in life. The process of aging is viewed as a process of life.	An established pattern of expected progression through life stages is viewed as both desirable and anticipated. The movement from one stage of growth to another is predicated on some of the life skills and tasks accomplished at an earlier stage. The "failure" to achieve certain developmental skills during a particular stage may be viewed as retarding growth into the next stage.
Health as functionality	Health is viewed as the capacity to fulfill critical life functions. Functionality is viewed as the ability to carry out a given task. Healthy functioning is relevant for individuals, families, and communities. For the *individual,* it includes physiologic and psychologic functioning. Physiologic functions include digestion, hydration, sleep, elimination, and circulation. Psychologic functioning encompasses behavior, communication, and emotional development. Likewise, *families* have functions to fulfill, including the capacity to nurture their members through physical, emotional, educational, and social supportive activities. *Communities* function to provide their membership with resources to sustain themselves.	When a person's family, group, or community functioning capacity is limited, health is altered and adaptation is necessary to adjust to the environment and to fulfill functions. From this perspective, disability is viewed as a "different" ability that requires an altered environment so that a person can achieve vital life functions.
Health as goodness of fit	Human biology, environment, health care, and lifestyle have been identified as the four major determinants of health (Lalonde, 1974). Although lifestyle and personal health habits are only one fourth of the determinants, they are of special importance because these are about making choices. Individuals, families, groups, and communities choose options that set into motion the unique interaction of factors and forces that have the potential to produce health or illness. Examples that affect Americans most are unintentional injuries, cardiovascular disease, and cancer.	No one single factor alone is a determinant of an individual's health. Instead, health is shaped by the interlocking of these forces. The U.S. *Healthy People 2010* uses this model as the foundation for its objectives and interventions.
Health as wholeness	The holistic nature of health is central to healing and complementary health-care delivery. Every aspect of a human being, family, or community is linked, and interacting comes from systems theory (Bertalanffy, 1968). Humans are constructed of subsystems that work together, as well as a subsystem of the family and community, which also are interacting parts of each other. Each system is a subsystem while simultaneously a super system. Boundaries define each system and allow, through their regulation, the flow of input and output that maintains energy and enables growth.	In this framework, health can be viewed as the integrity and unity of system function. Supporting the integrity of the human system is the focus for promoting and maintaining health.
Health as sense of well-being	Although the actual structure of general well-being is not clearly understood, it is thought to include the following contributors: emotions, beliefs, temperaments, behaviors, situations, experiences, and health (Wheeler, 1991). Although a sense of well-being is a personal experience, there is some consensus that it includes three components: life satisfaction, positive affect, and negative affect (Seedhouse, 1995).	Well-being may be experienced many ways. Often, humor and laughter have been shown to affect both neurologic and physiologic transmissions in the body. It can reduce tension and frustration and startle a person out of complacency.

Continued

Table 1-1 Imaging Health: Health as . . . cont'd

Model	Overview	Limitations and/or Assumptions
Health as transcendence	Viewing health as transcendence is to see the human potential for growth and development as limitless. Any boundaries of the mind and body are believed to be self-imposed. According to this framework, humans are constantly evolving, as are new tools and modalities of treatment. Health is seen as a process of self-discovery. Understanding on a cognitive level is not necessary for an intervention to be therapeutic. Health is seen as being interrelated with the larger universe, integrating emotional and spiritual factors. The process of "body-mind-spirit" is understood as a unified whole that has great potential for experiencing, altering, and expressing health. Spirituality generally can be defined as "one's inward sense of something greater than the individual self or the meaning one perceives that transcends the immediate circumstances" (U.S. Office of Alternative Medicine, 1994). This "spiritual" nature of health is experienced as fully as any of the "physical" components.	The perceived meaning that one attaches to an experience or an event is recognized as having an integral connection to one's overall health experience. These perceived meanings affect both the choices and the impact of health interventions.
Health as empowerment	A strong link between individuals' or communities' sense of power and the level of health they experience has been identified (Robertson and Minkler, 1994). Being in control and having power over self is linked to health, whereas powerlessness has been identified as a broad-based risk factor for the development of disease. The empowerment process as a health promotion intervention strategy has been correlated with improving the health of individuals and, more important, communities. Self-care and feeling in control to direct one's own life course depend on knowledge and skills. Self-determination and self-care are the essence of health when health is viewed as power.	Empowered health is based on the belief that individuals possess numerous and diverse self-care abilities. What individuals need is certain skills of self-care to feel in control and to direct their own life course.

Modified from Gorin and Arnold.[8]

Bertalanffy LV: *General system theory,* New York, 1968, George Braziller.
Dubos R: *Man adapting,* New Haven, Conn, 1965, Yale University Press.
Dunn H: *High-level wellness,* Arlington, Va, 1961, Beatty.
Fugh-Berman A: *Alternative medicine: what works,* Tucson, Ariz, 1996, Odonian Press.
Lalonde M: *A new perspective on the health of Canadians,* Ottawa, 1974, Government of Canada.
Leavell HR, Clark EG: *Preventive medicine for the doctor in his community: an epidemiological approach,* New York, 1965, McGraw-Hill.
Robertson A, Minkler M: New health promotion movement, *Health Educ Q* 21(3):295, 1994.
Seedhouse D: Well-being: Health promotion's red herring, *Health Promotion Int* 10(1):61, 1995.
U.S. Office of Alternative Medicine, National Institutes of Health: *Alternative medicine: expanding medical horizons: a report to the National Institutes of Health on alternative medical systems and practices in the U.S.,* Washington, DC, 1994, The Office.
Wheeler RJ: The theoretical and empirical structure of general well-being, *Soc Indicators Res* 24:71, 1991.
World Health Organization: Constitution of the World Health Organization, *Chronicle World Health Org* 1(1-2):29, 1947.

Table 1-2 Levels of Health Promotion and Disease Prevention

		Interventions	
Stages of Disease	**Level of Prevention**	**Overview**	**Examples**
Predisease	Primary prevention	Health promotion and specific disease prevention	Immunizations Adequate nutrition Adequate exercise
Latent disease	Secondary prevention	Presymptomatic diagnosis and treatment	Diagnostic screening: cancer screening, cardiovascular screening, periodic examinations
Symptomatic disease	Tertiary prevention	Intervention for early symptomatic disease and/or rehabilitation for late symptomatic disease	Appropriate therapies for chronic diseases to limit impairment. This includes early treatment for such findings as hyperlipidemia, hypertension, obesity, and diabetes mellitus. It also includes early rehabilitation for injury and serious illnesses such as stroke, joint replacement, hip fractures, and head injuries

Modified from Leavell and Clark.[13]

rehabilitation. Over the past few decades, significant efforts have been made to identify and implement strategies to improve health at all three prevention levels. In the United States two of the most significant national agendas are *Healthy People 2010* and the *U.S. Preventive Services Task Force.* In Canada, *Perspectives on the Health of Canadians* has set the agenda.

UNITED STATES

Health Initiatives for the Nation's Health: Year 2010

The year 1979 serves as the cornerstone for the nation's *Healthy People* agenda. It was in that year that *Healthy People: The Surgeon General's Report on Health Promotion and Disease Prevention* was published. This comprehensive report provided challenges to prevent and reduce major illnesses such as heart disease, cancer, strokes, and both unintentional and intentional injuries. The focus has been on *primary* and *secondary prevention.* By 1990 the review of the accomplishments was not as significant as the developing awakening and synergy of the health-care agencies, health-care providers, and public toward learning about health and building strategies to reduce and prevent illness and injury. The commitment of these individuals and groups has been so strong that *Healthy People 2000: National Health Promotion and Disease Prevention Objectives* and now *Healthy People 2010* have evolved and drive the health-care agenda for the nation. These guide health promotion efforts and provide health targets against which program initiatives, client, community, and national health-care outcomes may be measured.

Healthy People 2010 is about improving the health of individuals, communities, and the nation. The structure of *Healthy People 2010* has two overarching goals for the nation, specifically: (1) increase years of healthy life and (2) eliminate health disparities. Within this structure, there are enabling goals and related focus areas. This is summarized in FIG. 1-1.

The *Healthy People 2010* goals and objectives are reported in Table 1-3. Toward this end, the 2010 agenda will monitor 28 focus areas that include 467 detailed objectives. Many of the objectives focus on interventions designed to reduce or eliminate illness, disability, and premature death among individuals and communities. These objectives are summarized in Table 1-4, on p. 9, and are further detailed in the appropriate chapters throughout this text.

Healthy People 2010 uses a systems model framework to understand the multifactor components of health and well-being. This model uses the holistic approach of the individual's *biologic* and *behavioral makeup* and the *physical* and *social environments* in which the individual lives as the core determinants of health. Influencing these core determinants are the policies and interventions of health care, as well as the access to quality health-care issues. The systems model approach demonstrates the interdependence these various factors have with each other. Table 1-5, on p. 9, provides the details of this model, as well as many of the factors that affect each component

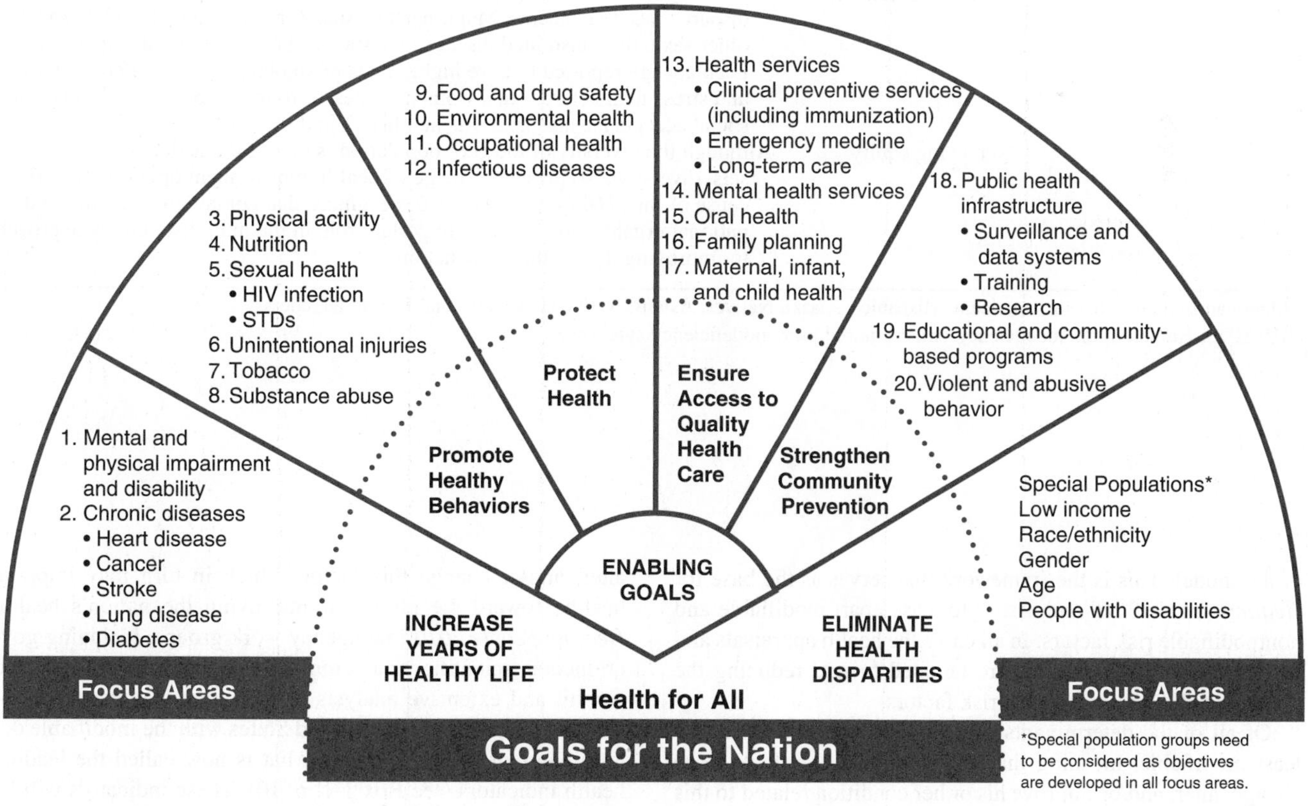

1. Mental and physical impairment and disability
2. Chronic diseases
• Heart disease
• Cancer
• Stroke
• Lung disease
• Diabetes
3. Physical activity
4. Nutrition
5. Sexual health
• HIV infection
• STDs
6. Unintentional injuries
7. Tobacco
8. Substance abuse
9. Food and drug safety
10. Environmental health
11. Occupational health
12. Infectious diseases
13. Health services
• Clinical preventive services (including immunization)
• Emergency medicine
• Long-term care
14. Mental health services
15. Oral health
16. Family planning
17. Maternal, infant, and child health
18. Public health infrastructure
• Surveillance and data systems
• Training
• Research
19. Educational and community-based programs
20. Violent and abusive behavior
Special Populations*
Low income
Race/ethnicity
Gender
Age
People with disabilities
Promote Healthy Behaviors
Protect Health
Ensure Access to Quality Health Care
Strengthen Community Prevention
ENABLING GOALS
INCREASE YEARS OF HEALTHY LIFE
ELIMINATE HEALTH DISPARITIES
Focus Areas
Health for All
Focus Areas
Goals for the Nation
*Special population groups need to be considered as objectives are developed in all focus areas.

FIG. 1-1

Overview of *Healthy People 2010*.

Table 1-3 *Healthy People 2010:* Goals

Goals	Indicators	Details
Increase quality and years of healthy life	Life expectancy	Life expectancy in the United States is currently 77 years. Individuals age 65 years can expect to live an average of 18 more years. Individuals age 75 years can expect to live 11 more years. The major opportunities for improvement include gender, racial, and socioeconomic group differences.
	Quality of life	This reflects a general sense of happiness and satisfaction with our lives and environment. Quality of life includes health, recreation, culture, rights, values, beliefs, aspirations, and the conditions that support a life containing these elements.
	Achieving a longer and healthier life	An increase in life expectancy and quality of life during the next 10 years may be achieved by assisting individuals to gain the knowledge, motivation, and opportunities needed to make informed decisions about their health. Groups of lower socioeconomic levels are in greatest need of these strategies.
Eliminate health disparities	Gender	Men currently have a life expectancy that is 6 years less than that of women. In addition, men have higher death rates for each of the 10 leading causes of death. Even though women outlive men in the United States, women have shown an increased death rate over the past decade in areas where men have experienced improvement, such as lung cancer.
	Race and ethnicity	Current knowledge of the biologic and genetic characteristics of the nation's major racial and ethnic groups* does not explain the observed health discrepancies when these groups are compared with the white, non-Hispanic population in the United States.
	Income and education	Inequalities in income and education underlie many health disparities in the United States.
	Disability	An estimated 21% of the U.S. population has a documented activity limitation that is classified as a disability. These individuals tend to report more anxiety, pain, sleeplessness, and days of depression of vitality than do people without activity limitations. They also report lower rates of physical activity and higher rates of obesity.
	Rural localities	Twenty-five percent of Americans live in rural areas of fewer than 2500 residents. These individuals have a higher incidence of and death rate from injury, heart disease, cancer, and diabetes than their urban counterparts.
	Sexual orientation	The U.S. gay and lesbian population is composed of a diverse community with disparate health concerns. Major health issues for gay men include HIV/AIDS, other sexually transmitted diseases, substance abuse, depression, and suicide. Lesbians are reported to have higher rates of smoking, obesity, alcohol abuse, and stress than heterosexual women. Issues surrounding personal, family, and social acceptance also affect mental health and personal safety.
	Achieving equity	Although the diversity of the U.S. population is one of the nation's greatest assets, diversity also presents a range of health improvement opportunities. Because of this, *Healthy People 2010* recognizes that communities, states, and national organizations play an important role in the multidisciplinary approach to improving the health of the nation.

*American Indians, African-Americans, Hispanics, Alaska Natives, Asians, Native Hawaiians, and Pacific Islanders.
HIV/AIDS, Human immunodeficiency virus/acquired immunodeficiency syndrome.

of the model. This is the framework that serves as the base for *Healthy People 2010* and assists to tease apart modifiable and nonmodifiable risk factors. In all cases the health appraisals and related prevention strategies are targeted toward reducing the risks related to the modifiable risk factors.

Of all of the determinants of health, human biology is the least modifiable, meaning that the individual can do little to change, alter, and/or improve his or her condition related to this element. The rest of the determinants may be modified, meaning that the individual or community may take steps to improve, alter, and/or change this factor, which in turn may improve health. Toward the efforts of improving the nation's health, *Healthy People 2010* interagency work groups, including governmental, scientific, and community services, have conducted careful and extensive analysis to index the leading causes of death and disability in the United States with the modifiable determinants of health to create what is now called the leading health indicators (see Box 1-1, p. 10). These indicators will be tracked and will serve as the targets for programmatic and individual primary prevention interventions.

Table 1-4 ***Healthy People 2010* Focus Areas and the Chapter in Clinical Nursing Where Additional Information Is Found**

Healthy People 2010 Focus Areas	Clinical Nursing Chapter
Arthritis, Osteoporosis, and Chronic Back Conditions	6, Musculoskeletal System
Cancer	18, Neoplasia
Chronic Kidney Disease	13, Renal System
Diabetes	11, Endocrine and Metabolic Systems
Educational and Community-Based Programs	1, Health Promotion and Disease and Injury Prevention
Family Planning	12, Female Reproductive System
Food Safety	10, Gastrointestinal System
Health Communication	1, Health Promotion and Disease and Injury Prevention
Heart Disease and Stroke	3, Cardiovascular System
HIV	15, Infectious Diseases
Immunization and Infectious Diseases	15, Infectious Diseases
Injury and Violence Prevention	1, Health Promotion
Maternal, Infant, and Child Health	12, Female Reproductive System
Mental Health and Mental Disorders	19, Mental Health
Nutrition and Overweight	3, Gastrointestinal System
Oral Health	9, Ears, Nose, and Throat
Physical Activity and Fitness	3, Cardiovascular System
Respiratory Diseases	4, Respiratory System
Sexually Transmitted Diseases	15, Infectious Diseases
Substance Use	19, Mental Health
Tobacco Use	4, Respiratory System
Vision and Hearing	8, The Eye; 9, Ear, Nose, and Throat

Table 1-5 **Determinants of Health**

Individual Factors		Environmental Factors		Health Systems Factors	
Biology	Behaviors	Social	Physical	Policies and Interventions	Access to Quality Health Care
Genetic makeup Family history Physical health Mental health Age	Diet Physical activity Smoking Stress Alcohol Use of illicit drugs Injury or violence Exposure to toxins	Interactions with family, friends, co-workers, and others The workplace, places of worship, schools Housing Public transportation Absence of violence in the community	Atmosphere and air Ozone Radiation Toxins Irritants Infectious agents Physical hazards	Health promotion campaigns Policies and laws Disease prevention services	Availability of health information Availability of timely health-care services Availability of appropriate health-care services

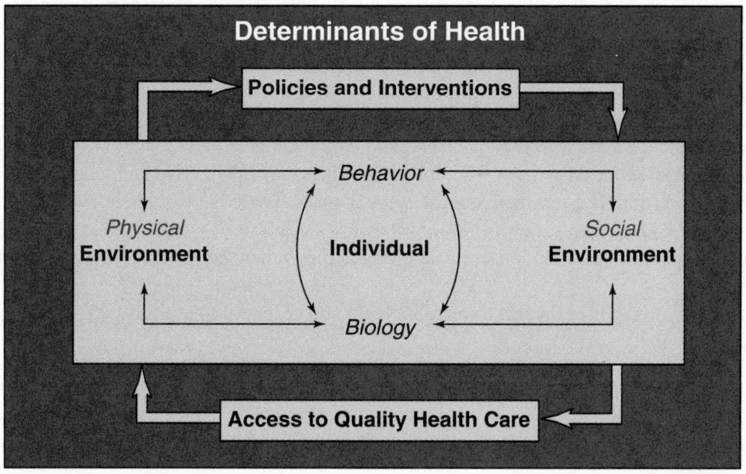

HEALTHY PEOPLE 2010 LEADING HEALTH INDICATORS — Box 1-1

- Physical activity
- Overweight and obesity
- Tobacco use
- Substance abuse
- Responsible sexual behavior
- Mental health
- Injury and violence
- Environmental quality
- Immunizations
- Access to health care

Table 1-6 Health Screening Recommendations

General for All Ages

Periodic hypertension screening
Periodic coronary artery disease screening
Periodic height and weight screening
Periodic vision screening
Periodic hearing screening
Periodic oral health screening
Use of and pattern of alcohol use
Use of and pattern of tobacco use
General periodic mental health screening: Dementia, depression, anxiety, behavioral problems, eating disorders, adjustment disorders, grieving, suicide risk
General periodic assault and abuse screening: Sexual abuse and assault, domestic violence, elder abuse and/or neglect

Age (years)	Women	Men
20-29	Cervical cancer screening* Rubella susceptibility screening† Breast self-examination Screening during pregnancy§	Testicular cancer self-examination
30-39	Cervical cancer screening* Breast self-examination Screening during pregnancy§	Testicular cancer self-examination
40-49	Cervical cancer screening* Breast examination, annually Mammogram, annually Screening during pregnancy§	Testicular cancer self-examination Hypercholesterolemia Digital rectal examination (men at high risk)
50-59	Cervical cancer screening* Breast examination, annually Mammogram, annually Colorectal cancer screening	Digital rectal examination Testicular cancer self-examination Hypercholesterolemia Prostate-specific antigen (PSA) test‡
60-69	Cervical cancer screening* Hypercholesterolemia Mammogram, annually Breast examination, annually Colorectal cancer screening	Digital rectal examination Testicular cancer self-examination Hypercholesterolemia PSA test‡
70-79	Cervical cancer screening* Colorectal cancer screening	Digital rectal examination Testicular cancer self-examination PSA test‡
80 and older	Cervical cancer screening* Colorectal cancer screening	Digital rectal examination Testicular cancer self-examination

Data from U.S. Preventive Health Service, American Cancer Society, and American Heart Association.

*A Papanicolaou (Pap) test is recommended for all women who are or have been sexually active and who have a cervix. Pap smears should begin with the onset of sexual activity and should be repeated at least every 3 years. There is insufficient evidence to recommend for or against an upper age limit for testing.

†Rubella susceptibility screening by history of vaccination or by serology is recommended for all women of childbearing age at their first clinical visit.

‡American Cancer Society recommendation. Offer the test to men 50 years and older who have a life expectancy of at least 10 years and to younger men with high prostate cancer risk.

§Screening during pregnancy:
- Iron deficiency anemia screening
- Hepatitis B screening (HBV) during first prenatal visit
- Serologic screening for syphilis
- Urine culture for asymptomatic bacteriuria
- D blood typing and antibody screening are recommended during first prenatal visit

U.S. Preventive Services Task Force Health Screening

The U.S. Preventive Services Task Force began in 1984 as a government-appointed expert panel charged with the task of developing recommendations for primary care providers on the appropriate content for periodic health examinations and screenings to ensure early diagnosis of health problems *(secondary prevention).* The initial work of the task force was completed over a 5-year period and consisted of a systematic review of almost 2500 published papers reporting the results of relevant clinical research. The group's initial work was completed in 1989. Since that time, the task force has continued to review scientific data and continues to make recommendations regarding the clinical effectiveness of more than 170 preventive services, including screening tests, counseling interventions, immunizations, and chemoprophylactic regimens. The most recent work of the task force, *Guide to Clinical Preventive Services,* was published in 1996. In addition to the ongoing work of the task force, national organizations, societies, and associations also establish guidelines for health screening and related secondary prevention. An overview of the current guidelines is summarized in Table 1-6.

CANADA

Perspectives on the Health of Canadians

The governments of the provinces and the federal government of Canada have also long recognized that good physical health and mental health are necessary for good quality of life. Reported in the founding document, *A New Perspective on the Health of Canadians* (1974), good health is the bedrock on which social progress is built. This perspectives document outlined the "Health Field Concept," comprising four main elements for health. Similar to *Healthy People 2010,* these are as follows:

Human biology
The environment
Lifestyle
Health-care organizations

The innovative Canadian framework and document published over a quarter century ago has provided impetus to national and international health initiatives in knowledge development, health promotion, health protection, and health care.

Today the Health Promotion and Programs Branch (HPPB) of Health Canada plays a national role in helping to improve the physical and mental health and well-being of Canadians. The HPPB has developed the *Framework for Action* national strategy that charts the course for Canada's Health Promotion and Programs Branch initiatives until 2002. Core to the initiatives are a range of interrelated social, economic, behavioral, physical, and biologic factors, as well as the health-care system itself. These determinants of health are reported in Box 1-2. They serve as the foundation for improving the health of Canadians and decreasing the inequities in the health status among various Canadian population groups. Most recently, the Federal, Provincial, and Territorial Advisory Committee on Population Health and Health Canada published *Toward a Healthy Future.*[10] This landmark public policy report examines in detail the health status of Canadians and details the major factors, or "determinants," that influence health status. Table 1-7 summarizes the findings and sets the stage for prevention strategies.

The illness and injury prevention strategies for Canada use a population health approach. The two main goals for Canada are as follows:

CANADA: DETERMINANTS OF HEALTH — Box 1-2

Social and economic environment	Personal resources and coping
The physical environment	Health knowledge
Health services	Lifestyle behaviors

From Federal, Provincial, and Territorial Ministers of Health: *Toward a healthy future: second report on the health of Canadians,* Health Canada. © Minister of Public Works and Government Services Canada, 2001.[11]

Table 1-7 Health Status of Canadians: Highlights

How healthy are Canadians?	Canada ranks in the top three developed countries in the world in terms of measures of life expectancy, self-rated health, and mortality rates. Life expectancy in Canada has reached a new high: 75.7 years for men and 81.4 years for women. Most recent immigrants to Canada are in good health, and the great majority of older citizens enjoy independence and good health. In 1966 Canada's infant mortality rate dropped below 6:1000 live births. The United Nations ranks Canada first in the world on its Human Development Index. That standing drops to tenth when the Human Poverty Index for industrialized countries is applied.

From Federal, Provincial, and Territorial Ministers of Health: *Toward a healthy future: second report on the health of Canadians,* Health Canada. © Minister of Public Works and Government Services Canada, 2001.[11]

Continued

Table 1-7 Health Status of Canadians: Highlights—cont'd

Factors That Affect Health	Details
Gender and age	Men are more likely to die prematurely than women. Causes are cardiovascular disease, injury, cancer, and suicide. Although women live longer than men, they are more likely to suffer from depression, stress overload, chronic conditions such as allergies and arthritis, and injuries and death from family violence. While cancer deaths have decreased in men, they remain steady in women, mainly as a result of increases in lung cancer mortality. Teenage girls are more likely to smoke than adolescent boys. Unintentional injuries are the leading cause of death among children and youth. Boys are injured at a higher rate than girls. Rates of physical activity drop quickly as age increases, and males are more active than females in every age group.
Income and income distribution	Only 47% of Canadians in the lowest income bracket rate their health as very good or excellent, compared with 73% of Canadians in the highest income group. Low-income Canadians are more likely to die earlier and to suffer more illness than Canadians with higher incomes, regardless of age, sex, race, or place of residence. As income increases, there is less sickness, longer life expectancies, and improved health. In 1995 almost 50% of single-parent, mother-led families were in low-income situations. A greater proportion of Aboriginal families are experiencing problems with housing and food affordability than Canadian families as a whole. In 1995 44% of the Aboriginal population lived in low-income situations. The distribution of income in the society is thought to be a more important determinant of health than the total amount of income earned by society members. Overall, inequities in income distribution remained relatively constant in Canada between 1985 and 1995. Changes in income distribution are closely related to changes in employment and wages. Although women are making progress in the workplace, they still earn less than men.
Social environment	By and large, Canadians are a caring people. They offer important buffers in times of stress. Family violence has a devastating effect on the health of women and children. In 1996 family members were accused in 24% of all assaults against children. In 1997 about 40% of female homicide victims were killed by a man with whom they had experienced an intimate relationship. Although the incidence of violent youth crime has decreased in recent years, it remains much higher than it was a decade ago.
Education and literacy	Canadians with low literacy skills are more likely to be unemployed and poor, to suffer poorer health, and to die earlier than Canadians with high levels of literacy. In 1994-1995 about 17% of Canadians scored in the lowest prose literacy category. In 1995 Canada had twice the proportion of citizens who lacked adequate literacy skills as Sweden, the number one ranked country on this index. People with higher levels of education have better access to healthy physical environments and are better able to prepare their children for school than people with lower levels of education. These individuals also smoke less, are more physically active, and have access to healthier foods.
Physical environment	The prevalence of childhood asthma has increased sharply over the past two decades, especially in children from birth to age 6 years. Major contaminants (especially for poor children) are airborne and environmental toxins and tobacco smoke. In 1996 many Canadians faced a housing affordability crisis. Often more than 30% of total income would be spent on housing. As many as 200,000 Canadians were estimated to be homeless, including increasing numbers of women and children, Aboriginal people, adolescents, and persons with mental illness. Climate changes and lack of adequate food may have a particularly negative effect on Aboriginal people.
Personal health practices	Tobacco use accounts for at last one fourth of all deaths of adults between ages 35 and 84 years. Smoking rates have increased substantially among young people, particularly among young women. Smoking rates among Aboriginal people are double the overall rate for Canada. Multiple risk-taking and unsafe sex practices remain high among young people, particularly among young men. Multiple drug use has increased among high school students. The proportion of new AIDS cases attributed to men who have sex with men declined steadily from nearly 80% in the 1980s to just over 50% in 1997. In contrast, 20% of adult AIDS cases in 1997 were attributed to injection drug use, compared with 2% before 1990.
Health services	Disease and injury prevention activities in areas such as immunizations and the use of mammography are showing positive results. Advances in the treatment of HIV/AIDS and other diseases are improving the length and quality of life of people living with life-threatening diseases.

From Federal, Provincial, and Territorial Ministers of Health: *Toward a healthy future: second report on the health of Canadians,* Health Canada. © Minister of Public Works and Government Services Canada, 2001.[11]

Factors That Affect Health	Details
	The annual growth rate of Canada's insured health-care expenditures fell from 11.1% (between 1975 and 1991) to 2.5% (between 1991 and 1996).
	There has been a substantial decline in the average length of stay in hospitals. This has shifted care into the community and home, thus increasing the financial, physical, and emotional burden placed on families, especially women.
	In 1998 29% of Canadians rated Canada's health-care system as "excellent" or "very good," down from 61% in 1991.
	Access to universally insured care remains largely unrelated to income; however, many low- and moderate-income Canadians have limited or no access to health services such as eye care, dentistry, mental health counseling, and prescription drugs.
Biology and genetics	Studies in neurobiology confirm that when optimal conditions for a child's development are provided in the investment phase (between conception and age 5 years), the brain develops in ways that have positive outcomes for life.
	Aging is not synonymous with poor health. Active living and lifelong learning are important for maintaining health and cognitive ability.

From Federal, Provincial, and Territorial Ministers of Health: *Toward a healthy future: second report on the health of Canadians,* Health Canada. © Minister of Public Works and Government Services Canada, 2001.[11]

Table 1-8 Canada: Priorities for Action

Strategic Directions for Improving the Health of All Canadians	Implications
1. Positive, supportive living and working conditions in all communities	A thriving and sustainable economy with meaningful work for all
	An adequate income for all Canadians and a reduction in the number of families living in poverty
	A more equitable distribution of income
	Healthy working conditions
	Educational, literacy, and lifelong learning opportunities for all
	Supportive friendships and social support networks in all communities
2. A safe, high-quality physical environment	A healthy and sustainable environment for all with access to good-quality air, water, and food and freedom from exposure to harmful toxins
	Suitable, adequate, and affordable housing
	Safe, well-designed communities
3. Opportunities for healthy development and support for individual choices that enhance health and foster independence	Healthy child development
	Healthy life choice decisions
	Enhanced independence for those who require assistance with activities of daily living
4. Appropriate and affordable health services that are accessible to all	Continue a commitment to a health service system based on the principles of universality, accessibility, comprehensiveness, portability, and public administration
	Improve access to services that have been proven cost-effective but are not consistently or uniformly available
	Decrease utilization of services, technologies, and medications that evidence indicates are inappropriate
	Improve service integration and effectiveness and increase accountability for improving health outcomes
5. Reductions in preventable illness, injury, and premature death	Reduce health problems that take a significant toll on the health of Canadians and for which effective prevention or intervention strategies are available
	Initial focus on priorities currently being addressed by several provinces and territories and the federal government

From Federal, Provincial, and Territorial Ministers of Health: *Toward a healthy future: second report on the health of Canadians,* Health Canada. © Minister of Public Works and Government Services Canada, 2001.[11]

Strengthen the underlying and interrelated conditions in the environment so that all Canadians can enjoy optimum surroundings for healthy living

Reduce inequities in the underlying conditions that put some Canadians at a disadvantage for attaining and maintaining optimum health and well-being

To actualize these goals, the Advisory Committee on Population Health (ACPH) has established three broad priority areas for action. Within each of the priority areas are objectives around which program evaluation strategies may be developed. The APCH plans are detailed in Table 1-8.

HEALTH BELIEFS AND HEALTH EDUCATION TEACHING AND LEARNING

Like the concepts of health, many models guide the successful implementation of health education. Regardless of one's country of origin, the strategies for teaching must begin with where the individual and/or family is at the time teaching is needed. Often the needs for health teaching may not occur at the same time as the patient's readiness to learn. The U.S. Preventive Services Task Force provides select strategies for health education and counseling. Although these recommendations, reported in Box 1-3, must be individualized, they provide a succinct review of some handy teaching and learning principles.

What actually motivates individuals to learn and comply with what they have learned is a complex issue. Knowledge and compliance are two very distinct issues. Often an individual has information about what may or may not alter his or her health and yet may or may not implement the strategies. Green and Kreuter[9] define health education as any combination of learning experiences designed to facilitate voluntary adaptations of behavior conductive to health. This notion has its roots in the health belief model, which was developed in the 1950s by social psychologists at the U.S. Public Health Services to describe why people did not participate in programs to detect or prevent disease. The health belief model is still used today to assist and provide health-care professionals with a strategy to investigate an individual's beliefs about personal health and related potentials for health education. The model consists of four main components: individual perceptions or beliefs of susceptibility to the disease, perceived seriousness of the disease, perceived benefits of using the information or changing one's behaviors, and perceived barriers to acting. Influencing these four perceptions are personal factors, knowledge, overall motivation, and assistance from health-care professionals. FIG. 1-2 presents a capsule view of the model.

The four main components of the health belief model touch on main perceptions that are thought to drive individuals' decisions about learning and complying with their own knowledge. As a health-care professional, the nurse is frequently challenged to assist the patient to modify knowledge and behavior. Often, because of financial or personnel constraints, patients are given educational handouts, offered printed materials, or forced to watch a video, attend a class, or meet with a certain

STRATEGIES FOR HEALTH EDUCATION AND COUNSELING — Box 1-3

1. Frame the teaching to match the patient's perception.
2. Fully inform patients of the purposes and expected effects of interventions and when to expect these effects.
3. Suggest small changes rather than large ones.
4. Be specific.
5. Be aware that it is sometimes easier to add new behaviors than to eliminate established behaviors.
6. Link new behaviors to old behaviors.
7. Use the power of the profession and your relationship with the patient.
8. Get explicit commitments from the patient.
9. Use a combination of strategies.
10. Involve other health-care professionals with whom the patient has a relationship.
11. Refer.
12. Monitor progress through follow-up.

Modified from U.S. Preventive Services Task Force.[19]

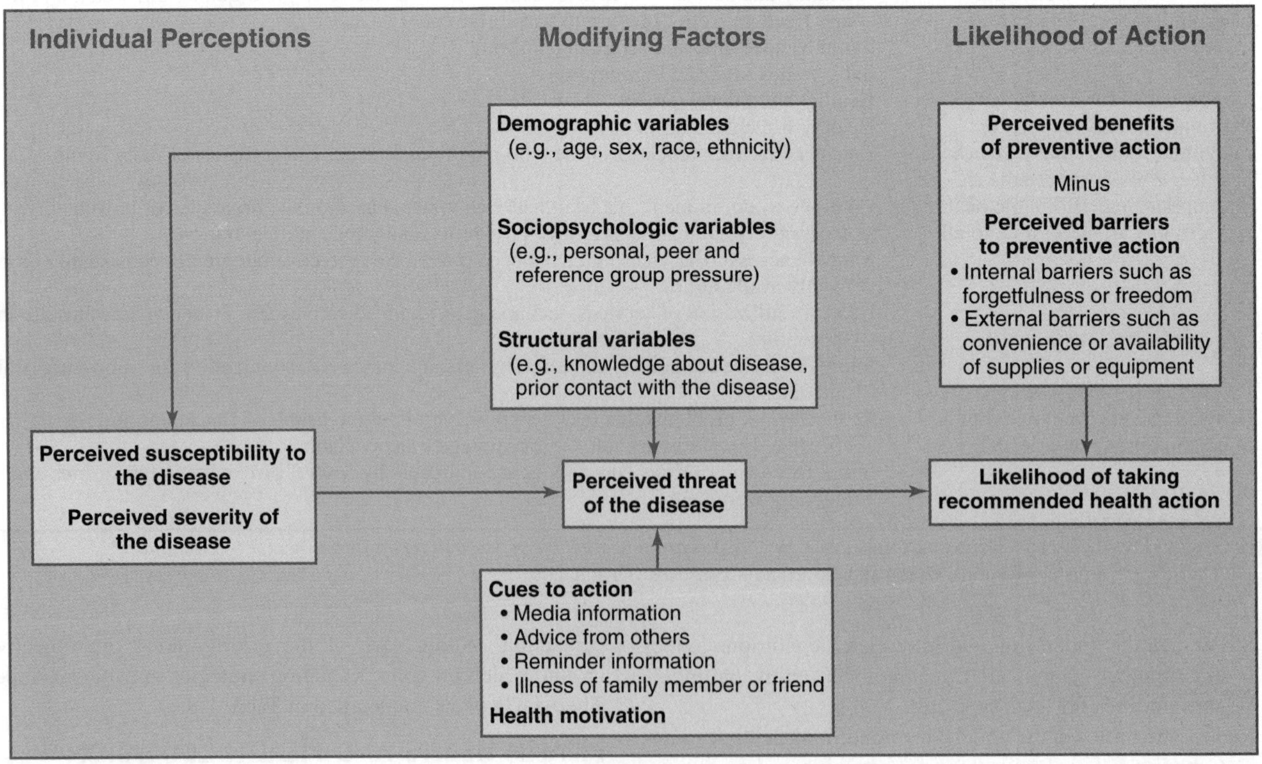

FIG. 1-2
Health belief model.

type of educator to "learn what must be learned." Many times an educational method is chosen to meet the needs of the health-care providers and/or facility and not the carefully evaluated needs of the individual or family. If the nurse or other health-care provider is to be successful in teaching or helping to modify an individual's health-care habits and beliefs, he or she must first fully understand the beliefs, personal perceptions, and motivations of the patient and family. The health belief model is one such tool that shows the many components that must be carefully evaluated and considered when planning educational strategies. In addition, social learning theory, recently renamed social cognitive theory,[3] provides solid groundwork for the nurse to understand how the patient and/or family perceive health and possible compliance with health education information. Box 1-4 details questions that may assist in constructing effective educational and motivational interventions.

Linking the principles of the health belief model and social cognitive theory, it appears clear that health education is complex, and patient learning and compliance are even more complex. Based on the theoretic models presented, the guidelines outlined in Table 1-9 may be useful in assessing the individual and the family before determining strategies for health education.

DETERMINANTS FOR EDUCATION SUCCESS FROM THE CONCEPTS OF SOCIAL COGNITIVE THEORY — Box 1-4

1. What is the nature of the physical and social environment in which the behavior occurs?
2. What are the characteristics of the situation in which the behavior occurs?
3. What factors tend to reinforce existing behaviors? What rewards or praise would help a person make behavioral changes?
4. Are there appropriate social models in the environment from whom the person might learn new behaviors vicariously?
5. What opportunities exist for the person to manage personal rewards?
6. Does the person have the skills or capabilities needed to make changes?
7. What does the person expect to happen as a result of these changes?
8. What does the person value as outcomes to practicing new behaviors?
9. Will the person be able to monitor his or her behavior and control the reinforcers in the environment?
10. Does the person believe in a personal sense of competence to achieve new behaviors?
11. In what ways will the environment be influenced by the person's new behaviors?

Data from Edelman and Mandle.[7]

Table 1-9 Guiding Principles for Health Education

Determinants for Educational Success: Social Cognitive Theory	Health Belief Model	Implications for Education
What is the nature of the physical and social environment in which the behavior occurs?	Demographic, sociopsychologic, and/or structural variables may affect education. Perceived barriers may prevent education from occurring.	Every person operates within an environment, and the variables of the environment affect how and when he or she is ready to learn. Getting to know the patient and his or her family will provide clues as to the timing and nature of appropriate education. Culture and/or family position may be important factors. Just as important may be finances, stress, available time, and related life events.
What are the characteristics of the situation in which the behavior occurs?	Perceived susceptibility and seriousness may affect how one views a problem. Peer and/or group pressure may either help or hinder one's ability to learn. Often cues to action by others play an important part.	Whether one is ready to learn or, even more important, comply with what is known may depend on the situation in which the person finds himself or herself. Often peers, family, and the situation are important variables that must be considered. Try to align education opportunities with people and situations that the patient and/or family values. This may mean involving another health-care provider or group.
What factors tend to reinforce existing behaviors?	Perceived benefits of preventive action minus perceived barriers often result in compliance with knowledge.	Even if a patient has knowledge, whether there is compliance with what is known often depends on the weighing of benefits versus barriers. In addition, often limitations of supplies and equipment, for example, may affect one's ability to comply with what is known. Take the time to get to know the patient and family and learn what is important and how to reinforce.
What rewards or praise would help a person make behavioral changes?	Cues to action appropriate to one's demographic and sociopsychologic variables are often important reinforcers.	Rewards and praise are often important reinforcers for compliance with what is known. Learn to keep these appropriate to the situation and the patient.

Continued

Table 1-9 Guiding Principles for Health Education—cont'd

Determinants for Educational Success: Social Cognitive Theory	Health Belief Model	Implications for Education
Are there appropriate social models in the environment from whom the person might learn new behaviors vicariously?	Cues to action from the media, influential others, peers, and other persons may often positively influence a person's choices and behaviors.	Try to identify positive role models and individuals or groups to whom the patient and/or family will positively relate. Often if the patient does not feel alone, compliance will improve. Similarly, identify educational models that are closest to the patient's values and beliefs.
What opportunities exist for the person to manage personal rewards? Does the person have the skills or capabilities needed to make changes?	Personal knowledge and skill are modifiable factors that will assist the person to manage his or her own health.	In addition to one's perceptions of the importance of health education and compliance of new behavior, if the patient feels powerful through knowledge, skill, or both, there is greater opportunity for compliance with what has been taught.
What does the person value as outcomes to practicing new behaviors?	Perceived susceptibility to the disease, perceived seriousness of the problem or potential problem, and perceived benefits are integral to implementing knowledge and improving one's health status.	Even if a patient has knowledge about some aspect of health, whether he or she implements the knowledge to decrease risk or enhance health often depends on his or her perceptions of risk and benefit. Perceptions are often the most difficult factor to modify and are often independent of knowledge. Trust is one important component of perception modification. Take time to get to know the patient and family.
Will the person be able to monitor his or her behavior and control the reinforcers in the environment?	Reinforcement is often a cue to action that may be learned or provided by an outside person or group. An outside person or group may influence either positively or negatively.	Having guideposts and guides along the path is often helpful to modifying health. If the patient or family does not quite meet the expectations of others, it is often important to have a coach to continue to positively reinforce and guide.
Does the person believe in a personal sense of competence to achieve new behaviors?	Demographic, sociopsychologic, and structural variables are all modifiable. Knowledge and confidence in self along with support from others and cues to action are important.	Each patient is different; personal factors, knowledge, and support from others may be important factors related to the sense of competence to achieve new or different health behaviors.
In what ways will the environment be influenced by the person's new behaviors?	Perceived susceptibility, perceived seriousness, and knowledge are all important factors related to how a person or group may modify health or health risk behavior.	Often negative health behaviors may affect more than just the patient or the patient's family. Negative health behaviors such as alcohol, tobacco, obesity, and lack of mental health support may have negative social and economic impacts. On the other hand, positive health behaviors will improve society's overall health status.

SUMMARY

Health and health care are integral to each individual and family and are a significant component of each nation's agenda. In the United States, *Healthy People 2010* provides foundational strategies to improve the health of individuals, the environment, and communities. The U.S. Preventive Services Task Force and national associations and organizations have published guidelines for secondary prevention screening. In Canada the Federal, Provincial, and Territorial Advisory Committee on Population Health and Health Canada have established national and regional priorities to improve health. Now it is the challenge of nursing to do the following:

- Understand the various models and concepts of health
- Use the national priorities for the improvement of health
- Follow the recommendations for secondary prevention
- Make and take the time to understand the educational needs of those we serve and to individualize health education strategies

When all of these interrelated components are addressed, the health of individuals of all nations will be improved.

REFERENCES

1. American Cancer Society, Inc: *www.cancer.org,* 2000.
2. American Heart Association, Inc: *www.americanheart.org,* 1999.
3. Bandura A: *Social foundations of thought and action,* Englewod Cliffs, NJ, 1986, Prentice-Hall.
4. Bertalanffy LV: *General systems theory,* New York, 1968, George Braziller.
5. Dubos R: *Man adapting,* New Haven, Conn, 1965, Yale University Press.
6. Dunn H: *High-level wellness,* Arlington, Va, 1961, Beatty.
7. Edelman CL, Mandle CL: *Health promotion throughout the life-span,* ed 4, St. Louis, 1998, Mosby.
8. Gorin SS, Arnold J: *Health promotion handbook,* St. Louis, 1998, Mosby.

9. Green L, Kreuter M: Health promotion as a public health strategy for the 1990s, *Annu Rev Public Health* 11:319, 1990.
10. Deleted in proofs.
11. Federal, Provincial, and Territorial Ministers of Health: Toward a healthy future: second report on the health of Canadians, Health Canada. *www.hc-sc.gc.ca/hppb/phdd/report/toward,* 2001.
12. Jekel J et al: *Epidemiology, biostatistics, and preventive medicine,* Philadelphia, 1996, WB Saunders.
13. Leavell HR, Clark EG: *Preventive medicine for the doctor in the community,* ed 3, New York, 1965, McGraw-Hill.
14. Office of Disease Prevention and Health Promotion, Office of Public Health and Science, Office of the Secretary: *Healthy people 2000,* Washington, DC, 2000, U.S. Department of Health and Human Services.
15. Parcel GS, Baronowski T: Social learning theory and health education, *Health Educ* 12(3):14, 1981.
16. Rosenstock IM: Historical origins of the health belief model, *Health Educ Monogr* 2(4):328, 1974.
17. Timmreci TC et al: Health education and health promotion: a look at the jungle of supportive fields, philosophies and theoretical foundations, *Health Educ* 18(6):23, 1987.
18. U.S. Department of Health and Human Services: *Healthy People 2010* (conference edition, in two volumes), Washington, DC, January 2000, The Department.
19. U.S. Preventive Services Task Force: *Guide to clinical preventive services,* ed 2, Baltimore, 1996, Williams & Wilkins.

2

Complementary and Alternative Medicine and Contemporary Nursing Practice

Susan M. Tucker

This chapter describes a broad array of complementary and alternative therapies in use today. Considering the variety of therapies available and the popularity of some forms of complementary and alternative medicine (CAM), it is important for nurses to be aware of the therapies their patients may be using. With this knowledge, nurses can work with their patients to use these therapies to complement those "mainstream" therapies being carried out by the nurse and the multidisciplinary health care team. The pursuit of health, orientation to wellness, and treatment of illness have stimulated curiosity about the utility of well-established ancient and historic medical systems that continue to offer support and treatment for the individual. Since the onset of time there have been healers and their patients. Although complementary and alternative medicine (CAM) therapies represent a new discovery for numerous individuals, many of these traditions are hundreds or thousands of years old and have been used by people in all parts of the world. What appears to many of us now as an alternative has actually been a part of mainstream medical care in the culture of origin.[5,9]

For eons the interrelationship between health and illness and the person within his or her environment has been the cornerstone of the healing arts. Until the last two or three centuries, therapies were predominantly what we would now call alternative medicine, with emphasis on herbal, energetic, and spiritual aspects of healing. Just a short century ago Florence Nightingale, focusing on the environment, wrote about the major concepts of ventilation with fresh air, warmth, light, diet, cleanliness, and noise. Since then modern nursing theorists have shared their views, concepts, and theories about the paradigm of nursing, the person, health, and the environment. These theories have been clustered into concepts related to the art and science of humanistic nursing, interpersonal relationships, systems, and energy fields.[4] These concepts are aligned with the theories on which CAM therapies are based because of their holistic approach, that is, they consider the whole person, including physical, mental, emotional, and spiritual aspects.

Since the dawn of the scientific method the healing arts diverged into two distinct directions: mainstream (allopathic) and alternative medicine. Allopathy presented itself as the scientific branch of medicine, rendering the practices of competing sects of medicine, such as homeopathic, botanical, and hydropathic medicine, to be quackery. Allopathic medicine eliminated the competition by establishing licensing laws in the late 1800s that excluded nonallopathic practitioners. In addition, the American Medical Association, in an effort to identify weak and inadequate medical schools, commissioned Abraham Flexner to write the famous Flexner report of 1910, which effectively nearly eliminated nonallopathic medical schools in the United States. Since that time, modern scientific medicine has prevailed and flourished.[8]

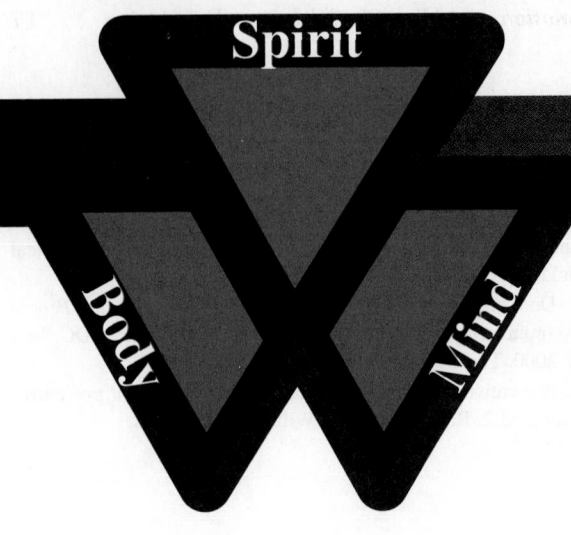

However, since the advent of "modern (Western) medicine," some individuals continued to practice alternative methods and to train others. Patients often preferred nontraditional therapies to mainstream medicine, and many alternative therapies became a discreet enterprise, going underground. During the 1970s a consumer movement and social phenomena occurred, focusing on the use of natural products and alternative/complementary medicine. Some individuals mistrusted institutions and new technologies and saw conventional medicine as an impersonal and profit-motivated system. At present, allopathic or mainstream medicine is playing catch-up with regard to its understanding of the uses of complementary and alternative therapies.

In 1992 the Office of Alternative Medicine (OAM) was established within the National Institutes of Health (NIH) Office of the Director to coordinate the evaluation of alternative medical treatment modalities through research projects and other initiatives within the NIH. In 1998 Congress established the National Center for Complementary and Alternative Medicine (NCCAM) at the NIH to stimulate, develop, and support research on CAM for the benefit of the public. The NCCAM is an advocate for quality science, rigorous and relevant research, and open and objective inquiry into which practices work, which do not, and why. Its overriding mission is to give the American public reliable information about the safety and effectiveness of CAM practices.[7] A large body of knowledge has been published about most CAM therapies and, with the recent and planned increases in funding, additional research will generate more well-designed studies. Health practitioners are becoming more aware of the possibility that a balance of allopathic and alternative medicine therapies can be more effective in treating the whole person within the context of the environment than traditional mainstream medicine alone.

Complementary therapies are those used *in addition* to conventional (traditional Western or allopathic) medicine. Alternative therapies can include the same interventions as complementary therapies but are used as *a replacement* for allopathic medical care. A published survey shows that the number of Americans using an alternative therapy rose from about 33% in 1990 to more than 42% in 1997.[2] People in this study reported using the following therapies most often: herbal medicine, massage, megavitamins, self-help groups, folk remedies, energy healing, and homeopathy. It is estimated that about half of the U.S. population uses one or more forms of CAM. By 1997 visits to CAM professionals exceeded total visits to all U.S. primary care physicians,[2] and the majority of medical schools currently offer elective courses in CAM or include CAM topics in required courses.[7]

The major categories of CAM are mind-body interventions, bioelectromagnetic applications, alternative systems of medical practice, community-based health-care practices, pharmacologic and biologic treatments, diet and nutrition, and unclassified methods. Under each of these major categories there are several CAM therapies, which are described later. It is important to remember that the use of complementary and alternative medicine does not preclude the use of mainstream medical therapies. In essence, the use of these therapies is not mutually exclusive with mainstream medicine, and in fact the patient may have a better outcome when a combination of therapies is used.[8]

CAM is employed more often than we are aware of in the patient population served by nurses. Various forms of CAM are practiced by nurses who offer therapies in relaxation, imagery, massage, and therapeutic touch to their patients.[1] The nurse may be in the best position to solicit the patient's input regarding the patient's use of CAM therapies and to assist in determining the appropriate integration of these therapies into the patient's plan of care.

MAJOR CATEGORIES AND THERAPIES OF COMPLEMENTARY AND ALTERNATIVE MEDICINE

MIND-BODY INTERVENTIONS

Mind-body interventions are therapies that emphasize using the mind or brain in conjunction with the body to assist the healing process.

Art Therapy. Art therapy involves the use of art media to lead an individual toward neutralization of conflict through sublimation or as a vehicle to moderate symbolic speech and to move the individual toward verbalization of inner conflicts. Art therapy is often used when traditional forms of verbal psychotherapy have failed or been rejected by an individual and when individuals have difficulty expressing feelings or use verbalization as a defense mechanism.[8]

Biofeedback. Biofeedback is a therapy in which sensors are placed on the body for the purpose of measuring muscle responses, heart rate, sweat responses, or neural activity. Information is provided by visual-auditory or body–muscle cell activation for the purpose of teaching to either increase or decrease physiologic activity to improve health problems, for example, pain, anxiety, or high blood pressure.[10]

Dance/Movement Therapy. Dance/movement therapy is a movement-based technique that aids in promoting feeling and awareness. The goal is to integrate body, mind, and self-esteem. This therapy uses different parts of the body, such as fingers, wrists, and arms, to respond to music.[10]

Hypnotherapy. Selective attention is used in hypnotherapy to induce a specific altered state (trance) for memory retrieval, relaxation, or suggestion. This therapy is often used to alter habits (e.g., smoking/obesity); treat biologic mechanisms, such as hypertension or cardiac arrhythmias; deal with the symptoms of a disease; alter an individual's reaction to disease; and affect an illness and its course through the body.[8]

Interactive Guided Imagery. The focus of interactive guided imagery is on the target visual stimulus to produce a specific physiologic change that can promote healing. Imagery is effective in almost all of the major physiologic systems of the body, including respiration, heart rate, blood pressure, metabolic rates in cells, gastrointestinal mobility and secretion, sexual function, cortisol levels, blood lipids, and immune responsiveness.[8]

Meditation. Meditation is an intentional self-regulation of posture, concentration, contemplation, and visualization to attenuate stress reactivity, affect neuroendocrine function, enhance a sense of control or self-efficacy, and prevent relapse for disorders such as chronic pain and anxiety.[8]

Music Therapy.
The use of music, either in an active or in a passive mode, can be effective in helping individuals improve receptive communication, express or communicate feelings, reduce stress, enhance relaxation or pain management, improve perceptual-motor coordination, and improve socialization. Other types of vibratory sounds can be used, mainly to reduce stress, anxiety, and pain.[10]

Neurolinguistic Programming.
Neurolinguistic programming is the study of the structure of subjective experience, or how we make sense of our experiences and construct our mental world. The intent is to give individuals more choices in their own frames of reference. It can be used for various psychosomatic conditions, behavior modification treatment, or stress management.[8]

Poetry Therapy.
Poetry therapy is also called *bibliotherapy* and is the intentional use of poetry and other forms of literature for healing and personal growth. This therapy enables individuals to express what they may be unable to say in other ways and is used within individual, marital, and family psychotherapy formats.[8]

Relaxation Therapies.
The relaxation therapies include lighter levels of altered states of consciousness through indirect or direct refocusing techniques, conscious breathing, and body awareness. These techniques are applicable for the stresses of everyday living, particularly stress disorders (e.g., anxiety and panic disorders), adjustment disorders, and addictions. Relaxation is also used for chronic illnesses of all kinds, including headache, irritable bowel syndrome, peptic ulcer disease, inflammatory bowel disease, hypertension, arrhythmias, coronary artery disease, and musculoskeletal pain/joint disorders.[8]

Spiritual Healing and Prayer.
Prayers are offered to a higher being or authority for the purpose of reducing stress, promoting healing, or arresting disease. Spiritual healing may be practiced by the individual patient, by groups, or by others with or without the patient's knowledge.[10]

Yoga.
Yoga involves the integration of posture and controlled breathing, relaxation, and/or meditation. *Hatha yoga* involves physical exercise, breathing practices, and movement designed to have a salutary effect on posture, flexibility, and strength for the ultimate purpose of preparing the body to remain still for long periods of meditation. *Raja yoga* includes all of the other forms of yoga practice. The practitioner is instructed to follow moral directives, physical exercises, breathing exercises, meditation, devotion, and service to others to facilitate religious awakening. Yoga techniques have been effective in regulating heart rate, blood pressure, circulation, and digestion, as well as in healing chronic back pain, menstrual problems, carpal tunnel syndrome, and respiratory disease.[8]

Bioelectromagnetic Applications

Diathermy.
Diathermy refers to the use of high-frequency electrical currents as a form of physical therapy and in surgical procedures. The three forms of diathermy used by physical therapists are short-wave, ultrasound, and microwave.[10]

Light Therapy.
Natural light or light of specified wavelengths is used to treat disease. This may include ultraviolet light, colored light, or low-intensity laser light. The eye is generally the initial entry point for the light because of its direct connection to the brain through the retinal hypothalamic pathway, which affects the autonomic nervous system and endocrine function. It has been used primarily for attention deficit disorders, cataracts, conjunctivitis, headaches, head trauma, hyperactivity, lazy eye, macular degeneration, migraine, night blindness, poor eyesight, stroke, and vision disorders. Secondarily, light therapy has been effective in treating eczema, fever, psoriasis, addictions, allergies, anxiety, autism, bronchitis, childbirth, glaucoma, insomnia, muscle spasm, premenstrual syndrome, stress, and strep throat. Light therapy complements many other treatments for these and other conditions.[8,10]

Magnetic Field Therapy.
Magnets are placed directly on the skin, stimulating living cells and increasing blood flow by ionic currents created from polarities on the magnets. Trigger points for magnets are acupuncture points where the action of the magnets serves to activate the tendinomuscular system to readily and widely transmit electrical stimuli. Magnets also increase tissue oxygen perfusion by decreasing vascular resistance, decreasing nerve cell firing, and stimulating various cellular structures (e.g., changes in calcium channels, sodium-potassium pump, RNA/DNA production, conversion of ATP to ADP, removal of oxygen and water from the cell, and stimulation of cyclic AMP). Common physiologic responses include vasodilation, analgesia, antiinflammatory action, spasmolytic activity, accelerated healing, and antiedema activity.[8,10]

Neuroelectric Therapy.
Transcranial, cranial neuroelectric, or transcutaneous electric nerve stimulation (TENS) was initially used in the 1950s to treat insomnia. In a typical TENS session, surface electrodes are placed in the mastoid region (behind the ear) and, similar to electroacupuncture, stimulated using a low-amperage, low-frequency alternating current. The action may stimulate endogenous neurotransmitters, such as endorphins, that produce symptomatic relief.[10]

Alternative Systems of Medical Practice

Oriental Medical Practices.
Oriental medical practices refer to ancient forms of medicine that focus on prevention and secondarily treat disease, with an emphasis on maintaining balance through the body by stimulating a constant, smooth-flowing Qi energy. Herbs, acupuncture, massage, diet, and exercise are also used.[8]

Acupressure.
In acupressure, manual pressure is applied at specific points on the body located along channels of energy. *Shiatsu* is a Japanese form of acupressure involving finger pressure at specific points on the body, mainly for the purpose of balancing energy in the body. The major focus is on prevention, that is, keeping the body healthy, but this technique is also used to relieve common ailments and tensions, including sinus problems, shoulder and neck pain, back spasm, chronic fatigue, fibromyalgia, muscular tension, temporomandibular joint syndrome, and general aches and pains.[8]

Acupuncture. Thin needles are inserted superficially on the skin at locations throughout the body. Points are located along meridians or channels of energy. Heat can also be applied by burning (moxibustion) or electric current (electroacupuncture). Healing is proposed by the restoration of a balance of energy flow called "Qi." Another explanation suggests that the stimulation activates endorphin receptors. Acupuncture is highly effective in treating both acute and chronic pain associated with multiple causes. In addition, common conditions are effectively treated, including sinusitis, allergies, tinnitus, sore throats, high blood pressure, gastroesophageal reflex, hyperacidity and peptic ulcer disease, constipation, diarrhea, spastic colon, urinary incontinence, bladder and kidney infection, premenstrual syndrome (PMS), infertility, dysmenorrhea, memory problems, sensory disturbances, depression, anxiety, and other psychologic disorders.[8,10]

Traditional Chinese Herbal Medicine. Herbs are used to treat various health conditions, including chronic or acute pain, allergies, menopausal issues, arthritis, stress, fatigue, and digestive disorders. Herbs are also used to promote optimal well-being and prevent disease by strengthening resistance and the immune system.[8]

Tai Chi. Tai chi is a technique that uses slow, purposeful, motor-physical movements of the body for the purpose of control to increase outer body mass strength and achieve a more balanced physiologic and psychologic state. Tai chi has positive effects on the respiratory, cardiovascular, and cerebral functions in both children and older adults, including reducing the incidence of falls in older people.[8,10]

Qi Gong. Qi Gong is a form of Chinese exercise-stimulation therapy that proposes to improve health by redirecting mental focus, breathing, coordination, and relaxation. The goal is to rebalance the body's own healing capacities by activating proposed electrical or energetic currents that flow along meridians located throughout the body. These meridians do not follow conventional nerve or muscle pathways. In Chinese medical training and practice this therapy includes "external Qi," which is energy transmitted from one person to another for the purpose of healing. Qi Gong has been effective in the management of chronic illness (e.g., hypertension, asthma, allergies, chronic fatigue, fibromyalgia, diabetes, arthritis), wellness promotion, stress management, terminal illness as palliation, gastrointestinal conditions, musculoskeletal pains and sports injuries, tension headaches, colds and flu, and tinnitus.[8,10]

PROFESSIONALIZED HEALTH-CARE SYSTEMS

Ayurveda. Ayurveda is a major health-care system that emphasizes a preventive approach to health, focusing on an inner state of harmony and spiritual realization for self-healing. It includes special types of diets, herbs, and mineral parts and changes based on a system of constitutional categories in lifestyle. Enemas and purgation are used to cleanse the body of excess toxins. Ayurveda emphasizes lifestyle analysis and change as the most significant aspects of the healing process.[10]

Homeopathy. Homeopathy is a form of treatment in which substances (minerals, plant extracts, chemicals, or disease-producing germs) that in sufficient doses would produce a set of illness symptoms in healthy individuals are given in microdoses to produce a "cure" of those same symptoms. The symptom is not thought to be part of the illness but rather part of a curative process. Homeopathy works by activating the self-healing capacity of the individual.[10]

Naturopathic Medicine. The basic philosophic premise of naturopathic medicine is that there is an inherent healing power in nature and in every human being.[9] This major health system includes practices that emphasize diet, nutrition, homeopathy, and various mind-body therapies. Emphasis is placed on self-healing and treatment through changes in lifestyle and the use of prevention techniques that promote health. Naturopathic doctors (ND) are licensed in about one quarter of all states in the United States.[9,10]

COMMUNITY-BASED HEALTH-CARE PRACTICES

Traditional Medicine in Latin America. Traditional Latin American medicine is an ethnomedical system representing many healing practices throughout Latin America. In Mexico it is known as *curanderismo.* This system of medicine combines various theoretical elements into a holistic approach to illness. The etiology of illness is framed in terms of imbalance, which can be between hot and cold in the body, between parts of the body, between patients and the social environment, or between patients and the spiritual realm. These illnesses can be treated by curanderismo and biomedicine, but only the *curandero* can treat supernatural ailments. This system has been used to treat susto (fear), believed to cause the soul to become dislodged from the body, resulting in illness; empacho, a gastrointestinal disorder believed to be caused by blockage in the stomach or intestine; and mal de ojo (evil eye), characterized by fever, irritability, headache, and weeping, generally affecting children.[8]

Native American Medicine. Therapies used by many Native American Indian tribes include their own healing herbs and ceremonies that use components with a spiritual emphasis. This type of medicine is the opposite of science and focuses on the *heart of spirit* and the acknowledgment that the spirit, mind, and emotions all have interplay with the environment. An individual's connection to Nature and Mother Earth and communion with the spirit world is either in or out of harmony. The unique energies of the eight directions of the medicine wheel, as well as the sky, sun, moon, and earth, all play an integral part in Native American cosmology. Symptoms of illness are seen as connected with the spirit, and energy is then used as a catalyst to help patients come back into harmony.[8,10]

There are several forms of therapy, which include the following: sweat lodge ceremony to heal; sacred pipe; sacred sage, sweet grass, cedar, and other herbs, wafted over the patient with the use of a feather; herbs used in a tea, eaten, used in a bath, or burned with the smoke inhaled; rattles to break up blocks of dead or jammed energy; and drums to align the person's spirit with the heartbeat of Mother Earth. All diseases have been treated with the use of Native American medicine, which does not preclude the use of additional mainstream medical therapies. This medicine is a safe modality when performed by the medicine person, who is an essential part of helping patients return to a state of harmony. It should not be attempted by individuals who do not have the education or training needed.[8]

Shamanism. Personal healing, transformation, and regeneration through access to a "higher power" forms the foundation of shamanic healing. Sickness, disease, and illness are indicators that the individual is out of balance and in disharmony within the essential nature. Success can be achieved if people are, first, willing to take responsibility for the creation of the disease and, second, open to nonphysical realities of life and willing to engage with their inner spirit and their higher selves. This type of healing has been effective for sexual dysfunction, chronic fatigue syndrome, mental health concerns, and obesity and other eating disorders.[8]

MANUAL HEALING METHODS

Chiropractic. Chiropractic relies on adjustment of the spinal column to improve health or arrest disease through both stimulation and body manipulation. Treatment is achieved by applying controlled and directed forces to adjust the affected joint to alter, restore, and preserve musculoskeletal function and alleviate symptoms.[8] Doctors of chiropractic (DC) are licensed to perform this technique.

Osteopathic Medicine. Osteopathic medicine is founded on basic principles of body unity, self-regulation, and the interrelationship of structure and function. Disease indicates a breakdown in the body's capacity for self-regulation. Osteopathic physicians, or Doctors of Osteopathy (DOs), use palpatory diagnosis and osteopathic manipulation to treat related somatic problems; however, they are complete and licensed physicians who can practice in all areas of medicine and surgery, with the majority holding hospital staff privileges.[8]

Massage Therapy. Massage therapy relies on soft tissue manipulation through stroking, kneading, friction, and vibration to improve health and provide comfort.

Bodywork

Alexander Technique. The Alexander technique is a bodywork technique in which rebalancing of "postural sets" (i.e., physical alignment) is taught by mentally focusing on the way correct alignments should look and feel and through verbal and tactile guidance by the practitioner.[8]

Aston-Patterning. Aston-Patterning is a bodywork technique to accommodate asymmetry and individual uniqueness of the human body to match human function to the environment. Appropriate alignment of the body provides the human structure with its most optimal support and adds the dynamic quality that facilitates motion. Alignment can be threatened by accidents, illnesses, or surgeries, and movement patterns are taught to include the asymmetric pattern rather than allowing a tension pattern to develop. This technique has been applied to fitness training and ergonomic and product design.[8]

Bowen Technique. The Bowen technique is a system of gentle but powerful soft tissue mobilizations using the thumbs and fingers over muscles, tendons, nerves, and fascia to restore the self-healing mechanism of the body. This technique has been used for conditions affecting the musculoskeletal system, including back, neck, hip, and shoulder pain.[8]

Craniosacral Therapy. Craniosacral therapy is a form of gentle manual manipulation used for diagnosis and for making corrections in a system made up of cerebrospinal fluid, cranial and dural membranes, cranial bones, and sacrum. This system is proposed to be dynamic with its own physiologic frequency. Through touch and pressure, tension is supposed to be reduced and cranial rhythms normalized, leading to improvement in health and disease.[8]

FeldenKrais Method. The FeldenKrais method is a bodywork technique in which its founder used the integration of physics, judo, and yoga. The practitioner directs sequences of movement using verbal or hands-on techniques or teaches a system of self-directed exercises to treat physical impairments through the learning of new movement patterns.[8]

Hellerwork Structural Integration. The Hellerwork structural integration is a bodywork technique that consists of deep pressure on soft tissues to improve alignment, movement reeducation to avoid unnecessary stress on the body structure, and dialogue with a practitioner to enhance the individual's awareness of how attitude affects structure and movement pattern.[8]

Pilates Method. The Pilates method is a gentle but focused exercise-based system that tones, stretches, and strengthens the body in a non-impact balanced system of body-mind exercise and mobilizes the body to move with maximum efficiency and minimum effort. Classes include mat work and use of equipment designed to provide resistance against tensioned springs to isolate and develop specific muscle groups. This method can achieve an improvement of body alignment and breathing, increased body awareness, and efficient and graceful movement.

Bonnie Prudden Myotherapy. Bonnie Prudden Myotherapy is a method of applying manual pressure on muscles with the fingers, knuckles, and elbows to defuse trigger points and relax muscle spasm, improve circulation, and alleviate pain.[8]

Polarity Therapy. In polarity therapy there is a hands-on manipulation of bone, soft tissue, and energy points, with vegetarian, nutritional, and attitudinal counseling. Specific stretching exercises using sound and movement remove energy blockages and restore the individual to balance and optimal health.[8]

Reflexology. Reflexology is a bodywork technique that uses reflex points on the hands and feet. Pressure is applied at points that correspond to various body parts with the intention of eliminating blockages thought to produce pain or disease. The goal is to bring the body into balance.[10]

Reiki. Reiki is based on the Japanese word meaning "universal life force energy." The practitioner serves as a conduit for healing energy directed into the body or energy field of the recipient without physical contact with the body.[10]

Rolfing Structural Integration. Rolfing is a bodywork technique that involves the myofascia. The body is realigned by using the hands to apply a deep pressure and friction that allows more efficient posture, movement, and the release of emotions from the body.[10]

Rosen Method. In the Rosen method movement exercises are designed to move all of the joints in the body through their available range of motion and expand the chest to free up breathing capacity.[8]

Therapeutic Touch. Therapeutic touch is a body energy field technique in which hands are passed over the body without actually touching to recreate and change proposed "energy imbalances" for restoring innate healing forces. Verbal interaction between patient and therapist helps to maximize effects.[10]

Trager Approach. The Trager approach is a bodywork technique in which the practitioner enters a meditative state and guides the client through gentle, light, rhythmic nonintrusive movements. Mentastics, or movement education, exercises using self-healing movements are taught to the clients.[8]

Pharmacologic and Biologic Treatments

Antineoplastons. Antineoplastons are naturally occurring peptides, amino acid derivatives, and carboxylic acids proposed to control neoplastic cell growth using the patient's own biochemical defense system, which works jointly with the immune system.[10]

Chelation Therapy. Chelation therapy involves the intravenous infusion of a chelating agent—synthetic amino acid ethylenediaminetetraacetic acid (EDTA)—of metal, toxins, lead, mercury, nickel, copper, cadmium, and plaque for the purpose of treating certain diseases (e.g., cardiovascular). Ancillary treatments include the use of vitamins, changes in diet, and exercise.[10]

Enzyme Therapy. Enzyme therapy involves the use of enzymes to catalyze chemical reactions. Enzymes can accelerate the progress of inflammation necessary for healing, with some products useful in cases of trauma, acute and chronic inflammation, emboli, thrombosis, viral infections, and cancer. Proteolytic enzymes are used for wound debridement (i.e., collagenase, fibrinolysin; desoxyribonuclease [Elase]). Other enzymes are used to digest fibrin or blood clots (i.e., streptokinase), and others are used as chemotherapeutic agents.[8]

Flower Essences. Derived from a flower, tree, bush, or water source, these essences are used to address spiritual, mental, and emotional as well as physical problems.[8]

Herbal Medicine. Herbal medicine is the use of medicinal products containing as active ingredients exclusively plant material and/or vegetable drug preparations used to treat various health conditions. Herbal medicine (phytotherapy) is a major form of treatment for more than 70% of the world's population[6,8] (see Tables 2-1 and 2-2).

Hyperthermia. Hyperthermia involves the use of various heating methods, such as electromagnetic therapy, to produce temperature elevations of a few degrees in cells and tissues, leading to a proposed antitumor effect. This is often used in conjunction with radiotherapy or chemotherapy for cancer treatment.[10]

Immunoaugmentative Therapy. Immunoaugmentative therapy, a cancer treatment, proposes that cancer cells can be arrested by the use of four different blood proteins. This approach is also proposed to restore the immune system and can be used as an adjunctive therapy.[10]

Phytotherapy. Phytotherapy involves the use of plants for medicinal purposes (same as herbal medicine).[6]

Table 2-1 Safe or Effective Herbs Determined by Non-U.S. Regulatory Authorities

Common Name	Effects	Examples of Uses
Aloe	Antiinflammatory Acceleration of wound healing Alkalinization of digestive juices	Minor burns Wound healing Gastrointestinal (GI) disorders
Astralagus	Stimulant of immune system	Cancer
Bilberry	Improvement of microcirculation in eyes Mild antiinflammatory	Myopia Retinal problems GI disorders
Cat's claw	Stimulant of immune system Antioxidant Antiinflammatory Lowering of blood pressure	Cancer GI disorders Hypertension Infections
Chamomile	Antiinflammatory Antispasmodic Antiinfective	Inflammatory disease of GI and upper respiratory tracts Inflammation of skin and mucous membranes GI spasms

From Lewis, Heitkemper, and Dirksen.[3]

Continued

Table 2-1 Safe or Effective Herbs Determined by Non-U.S. Regulatory Authorities—cont'd

Common Name	Effects	Examples of Uses
Dong quai	Antispasmodic Vasodilation Balancing effects of estrogen Mild sedative effect	Menstrual cramps Premenstrual syndrome Menstrual irregularities Hot flashes Vaginal dryness
Echinacea	Stimulant of immune system Antiinflammatory Antibacterial	Upper respiratory tract infection Allergic rhinitis Wound healing
Feverfew	Antiinflammatory Inhibition of serotonin and prostaglandins Vasodilator	Migraine headaches Arthritis
Garlic	Lowering of lipids Inhibition of platelet aggregation Antibacterial	Elevated cholesterol levels Hypertension Diabetes Infections
Ginger	Antiemetic	Nausea and vomiting Motion sickness
Gingko biloba	Memory improvement Increasing blood flow Antioxidant Increased metabolism efficiency	Alzheimer's disease Dementia Eye disease Heart disease Poor circulation Varicose veins Anxiety Age-related diseases
Ginseng	Increased physical endurance "Balancing" of body Resistance to stress	Fatigue Headaches Decreased libido Hot flashes
Goldenseal	Antiinflammatory Antibacterial Laxative	Respiratory and GI infections Gallbladder inflammation Cirrhosis of liver
Hawthorn	Increased O_2 utilization by heart Lowering of cholesterol Peripheral vasodilator	Angina Coronary artery disease
Milk thistle	Stimulation of production of new liver cells Protection of liver from damage	Liver disease
St. John's Wort (hypericum)	Inhibition of monoamine oxidase (MAO) and serotonin reuptake Antiviral Antibacterial WARNING: Avoid foods containing tyramine, such as aged cheese, red wine.	Mild to moderate depression Viral infections Wound healing
Saw palmetto	Prevention of conversion of testosterone to dihydrotestosterone (needed for prostate cell multiplication) Balancing of sex hormones	Benign prostatic hyperplasia Urinary problems
Valerian	Minor tranquilizer Central nervous system (CNS) depression	Sleep disorders Restlessness

From Lewis, Heitkemper, and Dirksen.[3]

Table 2-2 Unsafe Herbs

Common Name	Use/Effect	Comments
Borage	Diuretic Antidiarrheal	Contains toxic pyrrolizidine alkaloids
Calamus	Fever Digestive aid	Contains varying amounts of carcinogenic *cis*-isoasarone; Indian type most toxic; North American type nontoxic
Chaparral	Anticancer	No proven efficacy; may induce severe liver toxicity
Coltsfoot	Antitussive Demulcent	Contains carcinogenic pyrrolizidine alkaloids

Common Name	Use/Effect	Comments
Comfrey	Wound healing	Contains large number of toxic pyrrolizidine alkaloids; may induce veno-occlusive disease
Ephedra (Ma Huang)	CNS stimulant Anorectic Bronchodilator Cardiac stimulation	Unsafe for people with hypertension, diabetes, or thyroid disease; avoid consumption with caffeine
Germander	Anorectic	Causes hepatotoxicity because of diterpenoid derivatives
Life root	Menstrual flow stimulant	Hepatotoxic; contains toxic pyrrolizidine alkaloids
Pokeroot	Antirheumatic Anticancer	May be fatal in children
Sassafras	Stimulant Antispasmodic Antirheumatic	Volatile oil contains carcinogenic safrole

Diet and Nutrition in the Prevention and Treatment of Disease

Macronutrients. Proteins, fats, and carbohydrates are macronutrients. These nutrients can help to improve almost every acute and chronic disease.[8]

Micronutrients. Vitamins and minerals are micronutrients. In the presence of inadequate nutrient intake the provision of supplemental vitamins and minerals, as well as intake above the recommended daily allowance (RDA) of some nutrients (megavitamins), can reduce the risk of illness.[8]

Oxidative Stress. In oxidative stress the use of antioxidant intake in the diet may provide both preventive and therapeutic advantage and reduce the damaging effects of free radicals on cellular constituents.[8]

Orthomolecular Medicine. Orthomolecular medicine is a therapeutic approach that uses naturally occurring substances within the body, such as proteins, fat, and water, that promote restoration, balance, or both by using vitamins, minerals, or other forms of nutrition to subsequently treat disease, promote healing, or both.[10]

Nutritional Oncology and Integrative Cancer Care

Bristol Cancer Help Center Diet. The Bristol Cancer Help Center (BCHC) diet is a stringent diet of raw and partly cooked vegetables with proteins from soy. It is claimed to enhance the quality of life and attitude toward illness in cancer patients.[10]

Other Diagnostic and Treatment Methods

Applied Kinesiology. This form of treatment uses nutrition, physical manipulation, vitamins, diets, and exercise for the purpose of restoring and energizing the body. Weak muscles are proposed to be a source of dysfunctional health.[8]

Aromatherapy. Aromatherapy is a form of herbal medicine that uses various oils from plants. The route of administration can be through absorption in the skin or inhalation. The action of antiviral and antibacterial agents is proposed to aid healing. The aromatic biochemical structures of certain herbs are thought to act in areas of the brain related to past experiences and emotions (e.g., limbic system).[10]

Biologic Dentistry. Alternative or complementary dentistry may also be called environmental, biocompatible, or holistic dentistry. The concern is about the effect that dentistry may have on the overall health of an individual. The mouth is treated as a part of the human body, and dental care and dental health cannot be separated from the body and its influence on systemic health. When amalgams that contain mercury are replaced with nonmercury restoratives, the patient becomes "mercury free."[8]

Colon Hydrotherapy. Colon hydrotherapy is an extended and more complete form of an enema, as well as a safe and effective method of removing waste from the large intestine without using drugs. Colon hydrotherapy is used to treat constipation or impaction, as preparation for diagnostic studies of the large intestine (barium enema, sigmoidoscopy, or colonoscopy), and as preparation for or after surgery. The procedure is also used for bowel training for paraplegics or quadriplegics, those with arthritis, and patients who have suspected autointoxication or intestinal toxemia.[8]

Color Therapy. With color therapy the wavelengths of the energy of light are used to assist the body in self-healing. This is often employed as a complementary treatment for seasonal affective disorder, depression, and stress.[8]

Detoxification Therapy. Cleansing of the body through nutritional action, centering on gastrointestinal function, characterizes detoxification therapy. It is used to assist in the transition from an unhealthy lifestyle to a healthier one by an improved selection of nutrients and elimination of some modern-day abuses, specifically, *s*ugar, *n*icotine, *a*lcohol, *c*affeine, and *c*hemicals, often referred to SNACCs.[8]

Environmental Medicine. Environmental medicine involves a practice of medicine in which the major focus is on cause-and-effect relationships in health. Evaluations are made of such factors as eating and living habits and types of air breathed. Testing in the patient's own environment is performed to determine what precipitators are present that may be related to disease or other health problems. A treatment protocol is developed from this information.[10]

Fasting. Fasting involves the elimination of foods with the addition of fluids such as mineral water, herbal and fruit teas, broth, and fruit juices for a limited period of time as a component of detoxification. This therapy requires the supervision of a health professional experienced in this form of therapy.[8]

Juice Therapy. In juice therapy, concentrated nutritional elixirs of fruit extracts and vegetables are used for nutritional maintenance, illness prevention, detoxification, and adjunctive treatment of allergies, digestive disorders, rheumatoid arthritis, skin diseases, and other conditions such as hypotension and hypertension, bronchitis, obesity, and insomnia.[8]

Iridology. Iridology is the process of identifying certain problems or abnormalities occurring in the human body through indications shown in the iris of the eye, well before the appearance of clinical symptoms. This is also referred to as *iris diagnosis.*[8]

Quartz Crystal Therapy. Quartz crystal therapy involves placement of a four- or six-sided quartz crystal over a chakra, or major energy station, of the body such as the brow, throat, heart, stomach, abdomen, base of the spine, or near the skull to act as a destressor and to support the immune system.[8]

Complementary and alternative therapies increasingly are being used within the context of mainstream medicine. It is important for nurses to have knowledge of CAM, to inquire about CAM therapies patients may be using, and to incorporate appropriate therapies into the plan of care of the patient. This chapter provides an overview of numerous CAM therapies that will assist the nurse to address the needs of the whole patient.

References

1. Caudell KA: Complementary and alternative therapies. In Lewis SM, Heitkemper MM, Dirksen SR, editors: *Medical-surgical nursing,* ed 5, St. Louis, 2000, Mosby.
2. Eisenberg DM et al: Trends in alternative medicine use in the United States, 1990-1997: results of a follow-up national survey, *JAMA* 280(18):1569, 1998.
3. Lewis SM, Heitkemper MM, Dirksen SR, editors: *Medical-surgical nursing,* St. Louis, 2000, Mosby.
4. Marriner A: *Nursing theorists and their work,* St. Louis, 1986, Mosby.
5. Micozzi MS: *Fundamentals of complementary and alternative medicine,* New York, 1996, Churchill Livingstone.
6. Mills S, Bone K: *Principles and practice of phytotherapy,* London, 2000, Churchill Livingstone.
7. National Center for Complementary and Alternative Medicine, Washington DC, 2000, National Institutes of Health, *http://nccam.nih.gov.nccam.*
8. Novey DW: *Complementary/alternative medicine,* St. Louis, 2000, Mosby.
9. Pizzorno JE, Murray MT: *Textbook of natural medicine,* ed 2, London, 1999, Churchill Livingstone.
10. Spencer JW, Jacobs, JJ: *Complementary/alternative medicine,* St. Louis, 2000, Mosby.

PART II

CLINICAL NURSING PRACTICE

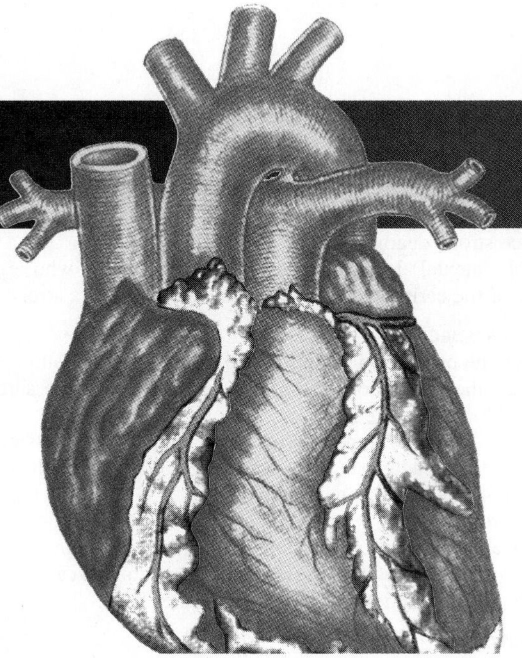

3 Cardiovascular System

Brigid Ide

Overview

Despite recent advances in medicine and surgery, cardiovascular disorders continue to be a principal cause of morbidity and mortality in the United States. In the day-to-day care of patients, nurses deal with cardiovascular disorders in terms of their physical signs and symptoms and appropriate therapeutic interventions. However, they must also consider the socioeconomic and emotional effect of these disorders on the patient and family.

During the past 30 years, progress has been made in prevention, diagnosis, treatment, and rehabilitation. Yet, despite a demonstrated decrease in cardiac mortality, more people die from cardiovascular disease than from all other causes of death combined. Almost 60 million Americans have some form of cardiovascular disease, at an estimated cost of $1 billion. Additional costs incurred through job-related losses are difficult to determine.

Cardiac disease can be divided into those acquired during life and congenital defects.

Major acquired cardiovascular disorders, which cause approximately 1 million deaths per year, include hypertension (high blood pressure), myocardial infarction (heart attack), congestive heart failure, cerebrovascular accident (stroke), and rheumatic heart disease.

High blood pressure, known as the silent killer, is a major factor contributing to heart attacks and strokes. Studies have estimated that one in four adults has high blood pressure.[4] Among African-Americans the prevalence is 30% or greater. Research is now focusing on early detection because studies have identified high blood pressure in children as young as age 4 years.[4]

Heart attacks are the number one cause of death in the United States.[4] About 6 million Americans are treated for heart attacks, or angina pectoris, each year. Major research has been undertaken to identify factors, such as occupation, sex, age, dietary habits, serum lipoprotein levels, and activity levels, that may be linked to many underlying diseases that contribute to death by heart attack.[52] In recent years, health professionals and community organizations have made major efforts to inform the public about risk factors and early warning signals of heart attacks and strokes. Because fewer than half of cardiac deaths occur in hospitals, organizations such as the American Heart Association and the American Red Cross have initiated programs to teach the public the basic techniques of cardiopulmonary resuscitation (CPR). Legislation is now under way to remove barriers to the use of "smart defibrillators" and encourage public access to defibrillation. An encouraging shift in mortality may be credited to increased public awareness and education; the death rate from heart attack declined 31.4% from 1982 to 1992.[3,4]

Congestive heart failure is a consequence of myocardial dysfunction. Although often controllable with drugs, it remains the major form of chronic cardiac disability. It is also one of the most expensive in terms of medical and nursing services, repeated hospital and nursing home services, drug costs, and job disability.

Stroke, which is the third leading cause of death, occurs most often as a result of high blood pressure. Approximately 3 million Americans have had strokes, even though strokes can usually be prevented.[4]

Rheumatic heart disease occurs in both children and adults and results from rheumatic fever, which is preventable. Although the incidence of rheumatic fever has declined, it is still a problem in urban populations where preventive measures and timely access to affordable health care are inadequate. About 1.9% of deaths in the United States are associated with rheumatic heart disease.[4]

Congenital cardiovascular malformations are the principal cause of death for children age 5 years and younger. About 1 in 300 live-born infants has some form of heart defect. However, since the advent of heart surgery, death from congenital heart disease has declined, and although the severity (and therefore the medical and surgical care) of these disorders varies, most children survive to adulthood. The growing number of these adults is a challenge to caregivers, particularly because they are at greater risk if faced with concomitant acquired cardiovascular disorders.

HEALTHY PEOPLE 2010

HEALTH STATUS—HEART DISEASE AND STROKE

Goal: Improve cardiovascular health and quality of life through the prevention, detection, and treatment of risk factors; early identification and treatment of heart attacks and strokes; and prevention of recurrent cardiovascular events.

HEART DISEASE
- Reduce coronary heart disease deaths.
- (Developmental) Increase the proportion of adults age 20 years and older who are aware of the early warning symptoms and signs of a heart attack and the importance of accessing rapid emergency care by calling 911.
- (Developmental) Increase the proportion of eligible patients with heart attacks who receive artery-opening therapy within an hour of symptom onset.
- (Developmental) Increase the proportion of adults age 20 years and older who call 911 and administer cardiopulmonary resuscitation (CPR) when they witness an out-of-hospital cardiac arrest.
- (Developmental) Increase the proportion of persons with witnessed out-of-hospital cardiac arrest who are eligible and receive their first therapeutic electrical shock within 6 minutes after collapse recognition.
- Reduce hospitalizations of older adults with heart failure as the principal diagnosis.

STROKE
- Reduce stroke deaths.
- (Developmental) Increase the proportion of adults who are aware of the early warning symptoms and signs of a stroke.

BLOOD PRESSURE
- Reduce the proportion of adults with high blood pressure.
- Increase the proportion of adults with high blood pressure whose blood pressure is under control.
- Increase the proportion of adults with high blood pressure who are taking action (e.g., losing weight, increasing physical activity, and reducing sodium intake) to help control their blood pressure.
- Increase the proportion of adults who have had their blood pressure measured within the preceding 2 years and can state whether their blood pressure was normal or high.

CHOLESTEROL
- Reduce the mean total blood cholesterol levels among adults.
- Reduce the proportion of adults with high total blood cholesterol levels.
- Increase the proportion of adults who have had their blood cholesterol checked within the preceding 5 years.
- (Developmental) Increase the proportion of persons with coronary heart disease who have their LDL-cholesterol level treated to a goal of less than or equal to 100 mg/dl.

Modified from U.S. Department of Health and Human Services: *Healthy people 2010* (conference edition, in two volumes), Washington, DC, January 2000.

NOTE: *Developmental* indicates that criteria for measurement and strategies to improve health have not as yet been specified.

HEALTHY PEOPLE 2010

HEALTH STATUS—PHYSICAL ACTIVITY IN ADULTS

Goal: Improve health, fitness, and quality of life through daily physical activity.

HEALTHY ACTIVITY IN ADULTS
- Reduce the proportion of adults who engage in no leisure-time physical activity.
- Increase the proportion of adults who engage regularly, preferably daily, in moderate physical activity for at least 30 minutes per day.
- Increase the proportion of adults who engage in vigorous physical activity that promotes the development and maintenance of cardiorespiratory fitness 3 or more days per week for 20 or more minutes per occasion.

MUSCULAR STRENGTH/ENDURANCE AND FLEXIBILITY
- Increase the proportion of adults who perform physical activities that enhance and maintain muscular strength and endurance.
- Increase the proportion of adults who perform physical activities that enhance and maintain flexibility.

PHYSICAL ACTIVITY IN CHILDREN AND ADOLESCENTS
- Increase the proportion of adolescents who engage in moderate physical activity for at least 30 minutes on 5 or more of the previous 7 days.
- Increase the proportion of adolescents who engage in vigorous physical activity that promotes cardiorespiratory fitness 3 or more days per week for 20 or more minutes per occasion.
- Increase the proportion of the nation's public and private schools that require daily physical education for all students.
- Increase the proportion of adolescents who participate in daily school physical education.
- Increase the proportion of adolescents who spend at least 50% of school physical education class time being physically active.
- Increase the proportion of children and adolescents who view television 2 or fewer hours per day.

ACCESS
- (Developmental) Increase the proportion of the Nation's public and private schools that provide access to their physical activity spaces and facilities for all persons outside of normal school hours (i.e., before and after the school day, on weekends, and during summer and other vacations).
- Increase the proportion of worksites offering employer-sponsored physical activity and fitness programs.
- Increase the proportion of trips made by walking.
- Increase the proportion of trips made by bicycling.

Modified from U.S. Department of Health and Human Services: *Healthy people 2010* (conference edition, in two volumes), Washington, DC, January 2000.

NOTE: *Developmental* indicates that criteria for measurement and strategies to improve health have not as yet been specified.

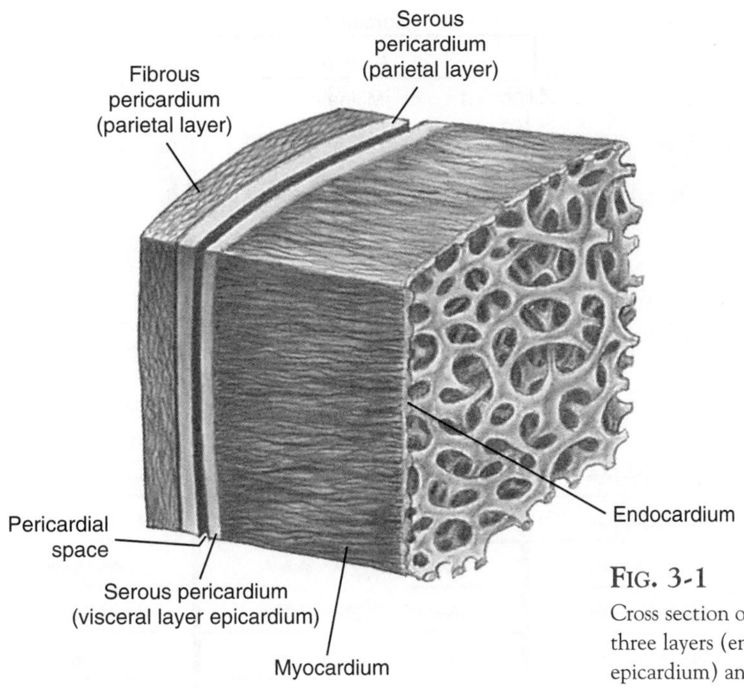

FIG. 3-1
Cross section of cardiac muscle showing its three layers (endocardium, myocardium, and epicardium) and pericardium.

ANATOMY, PHYSIOLOGY, AND RELATED PATHOPHYSIOLOGY

The heart is a hollow muscular organ weighing between 250 and 350 g. It is within the thoracic cavity in the mediastinal space, with two thirds extending to the left of the midline. It is flanked by the lungs and protected anteriorly by the sternum and ribs and posteriorly by the vertebral column.

Layers of the Heart

Cardiac muscle has three layers (FIG. 3-1). The epicardium, the outer layer, covers the surface of the heart and extends to the great vessels. The myocardium, the middle layer, is responsible for the major pumping action of the ventricles. The endocardium, the innermost layer, is a thin layer of endothelium and a thin layer of underlying connective tissue. The endocardium lines the inner chambers of the heart, valves, chordae tendineae, and papillary muscles. It is continuous with the blood vessels that enter and leave the heart. Cardiac muscle cells are made of striated muscle fibrils consisting of contractile elements known as myofibrils. The fibrils are grouped together in a band and are arranged in parallel rows extending from one end of a cell to the other (FIG. 3-2). A membrane junction, the intercalated disk, connects cell to cell.

Pericardium

The heart is enclosed in a double-walled fibroserous sac, the pericardium. The inner layer (visceral pericardium), made of fibrous elastic connective tissue, covers the entire surface of the heart and is the outermost layer of the heart wall (epicardium) (see FIG. 3-1).

The outer layer (parietal pericardium) is made of strong, elastic, fibrous connective tissue lined with smooth, translucent serous membrane. It is attached inferiorly to the diaphragm and laterally to the pleura of the lung. Superiorly the parietal pericardium attaches to the larger blood vessels (aorta, pulmonary artery, and superior vena cava), but not to the heart itself. This results in a potential space known as the pericardial cavity.

The space between the visceral and parietal layers contains 10 to 30 ml of clear, lymphlike fluid that helps maintain the smooth, easy motion of the heart during contraction and expansion. The pericardial cavity can hold 300 ml of fluid without interference in cardiac function. It can hold up to 1 L in some chronic disease states. The degree to which pericardial fluid compromises cardiac function depends more on the rate of rise in intrapericardial volume than on the amount. During rapid filling, as little as 100 ml may cause acute tamponade,[12] but patients who have slowly developing pericardial effusions can hold up to 1 L of fluid without hampering heart function. The rate of filling is also more important than the amount in the relationship between intrapericardial fluid volume and intrapericardial pressure. Normal pressure is 2 to 5 mm Hg. A sudden increase in pressure may occur if fluid rapidly fills the pericardial space, regardless of the amount of fluid.

The pericardium shields against infection and trauma and aids cardiac function by helping with the free pumping motion of the heart.

Chambers of the Heart

The heart is a four-chambered organ but functions as a two-sided pump (FIG. 3-3). The right side is a low-pressure system pumping venous or deoxygenated blood to the lung. The left side is a higher-pressure system pumping arterial or oxygenated blood to the systemic circulation.

Right Atrium. The right atrium (RA) is a thin-walled muscle that acts as a receiving chamber. It receives systemic venous blood from the superior vena cava (SVC), which drains the upper part of the body, and from the inferior vena cava (IVC), which drains blood from the lower extremities.

The coronary sinus, which drains venous blood from the myocardial circulation, also empties into the RA just above the

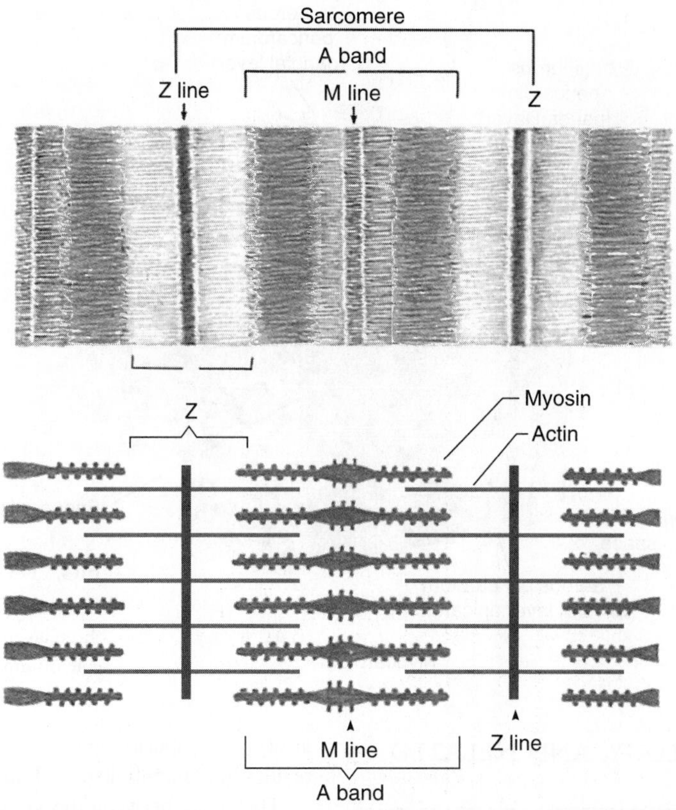

FIG. 3-2
Histologic representation of myocardial tissue showing arrangement of myofibrils in relaxed state.

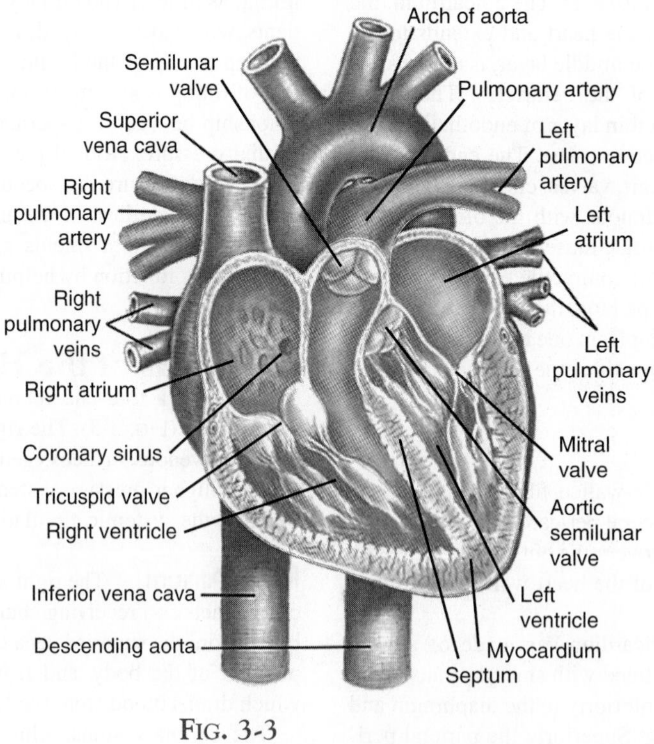

FIG. 3-3
Frontal schematic view of heart.

tricuspid valve. The pressure exerted during normal filling of the RA is 0 to 7 mm Hg and varies with respiration. During inspiration, RA pressure drops below the pressure in veins outside the chest cavity. Because blood flows from an area of high pressure to an area of lower pressure, blood flow to the RA occurs mainly during inspiration.

Oxygen saturation of blood in the RA varies, depending on the place of entry into the RA (IVC, 80%; SVC, 70%; coronary sinus, 30%), but the combined oxygen saturation of RA mixed venous blood is about 75%, or 40 mm Hg.

Right Ventricle. The right ventricle (RV) is normally the most anterior chamber of the heart, lying directly beneath the sternum. The RV functions as both an inflow and an outflow tract. The inflow tract includes the tricuspid area and the criss-cross muscular bands (trabeculations) that make up the inner surface of the ventricle. The outflow tract is commonly referred to as the infundibulum.

During diastole, blood enters the RV through the tricuspid valve and is ejected into the pulmonary circulation through the pulmonic valve into the main pulmonary artery. Because of low resistance in the pulmonary circulation, systolic or ejection pressures of the RV are also low. RV pressures range from 20 to 25/0 to 5 mm Hg. RV oxygen saturation is similar to that in the RA.

Left Atrium. The left atrium (LA), the most posterior cardiac structure, receives oxygenated blood from the lungs via the right and left pulmonary veins. The wall of the LA is slightly thicker than that of the RA and exerts a filling pressure of 5 to 10 mm Hg with little breathing variation. The arterial oxygen saturation is 98% (95 mm Hg).

Left Ventricle. The left ventricle (LV) lies posterior and to the left of the RV. It is ellipsoid, with a wall made of thick muscular tissue measuring 8 to 16 mm, two to three times thicker than the wall of the RV. This increased muscle mass is necessary to generate enough pressure to move blood into the circulation. LV pressure is normally 100 to 120/0 to 10 mm Hg with oxygen saturation of 95%. The inflow tract is funnel shaped, formed by the mitral valve annulus, the two mitral leaflets, and the chordae tendineae. The outflow tract is surrounded by the anterior mitral leaflet, the interventricular septum, and the left ventricular free wall. During systole, blood is propelled above and to the right across the aortic valve into the aorta.

Cardiac Valves

The heart's efficiency as a pump depends on the integrity of the cardiac valves (FIG. 3-4). Their sole purpose is to ensure one-way, forward blood flow.

Atrioventricular Valves. The two atrioventricular (AV) valves are similar in function but differ in several anatomic details. They are positioned along the AV groove, which separates the atria from the ventricles.

The tricuspid (right side) and mitral (left side) apparatus is composed of the annulus fibrosus, the valvular tissue (leaflets) to which the chordae tendineae are attached, and the papillary muscles connecting the chordae to the floor of the ventricular wall. This arrangement allows the leaflets to balloon upward during ventricular systole, but it prevents eversion of the cusps into the atria. These components are considered as a single unit because disruption of any one element can result in serious hemodynamic dysfunction.

The tricuspid valve is larger and thinner than the mitral valve and has three separate leaflets: anterior, posterior, and septal. Competence of the anterior and posterior leaflets depends on RV lateral wall function. The septal leaflet attaches to portions of the interventricular septum and sits close to the AV node.

The mitral valve is composed of two cusps: anterior and posterior. The anterior leaflet has a wide range of motion. It descends deep into the LV during diastole and rises quickly in systole to meet the posterior leaflet. The posterior leaflet is smaller and more restricted in its motion. The orifice is normally 4 to 6 cm^2 in adults.

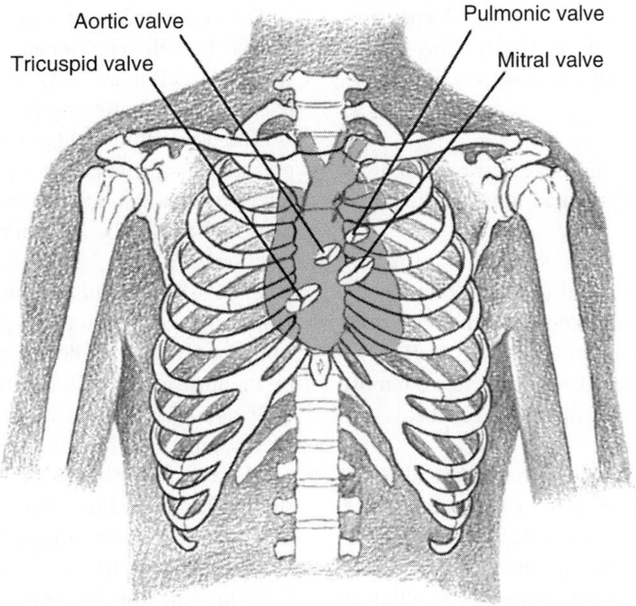

FIG. 3-4
Anatomic position of cardiac valves.

Semilunar Valves.
The two semilunar valves are the aortic and the pulmonic. They are smaller than the AV valves and are similar to each other except that the aortic cusps tend to be thicker. The semilunar valves sit above the outflow tracts of their respective ventricles. Each is composed of a fibrous supporting ring called the annulus and three fibrous valve cusps. The normal valve orifice is 2.6 to 3.5 cm^2.

Coronary Circulation
The right and left coronary arteries, which arise from the aorta just above and behind the aortic valve, supply blood to the myocardium.

Right Coronary Artery.
The right coronary artery (RCA) arises from the right aortic sinus of Valsalva and branches out along the AV groove to supply the anterior portion of the RV. In 90% of persons the RCA curves posteriorly within the AV groove and supplies the posterior septum, the posterior left papillary muscle, and the sinus and AV nodes.

Left Coronary Artery.
The left coronary artery (LCA) arises from the left aortic sinus of Valsalva. It begins as a common artery referred to as the left main artery and then divides into the left anterior descending (LAD) artery and the circumflex artery. The LAD artery descends along the anterior interventricular sulcus to nourish a large portion of the anterior left ventricular wall, including the anterior septum, the anterior papillary muscle, and the apical portion of the myocardium.

The left circumflex (LCX) artery extends from the left main coronary artery along a groove between the LA and LV. In some persons the circumflex artery supplies the inferior and posterior portions of the LV. This is known as left coronary dominance.

Cardiac Veins.
Three main divisions of cardiac veins comprise the venous circulation and closely parallel the coronary arteries. These include the thebesian veins, most of which empty into the atria; the anterior cardiac veins, which empty into the RA; and the coronary sinus, a short vein lying on the posterior side of the heart. Most venous circulation drains into the coronary sinus, which receives blood from the deeper myocardium and empties into the RA at the coronary sinus ostium between the tricuspid valve and the opening of the IVC.

Conduction
A special system transmits and coordinates electrical impulses throughout the heart. It consists of atypical muscle fibers and has the following characteristics.

Impulse Formation.
The sinoatrial (SA), or sinus, node gives rise to a self-generating impulse known as the heartbeat. The SA node is at the border of the SVC and the RA. It is the dominant pacemaker of the heart because it generates the most frequent electrical impulses at a rate of 60 to 100 beats per minute (FIG. 3-5, *A*).

The SA node is supplied primarily by the proximal RCA (60%) and the LCX artery and is innervated by sympathetic and parasympathetic nerve fibers. If the sinus node is depressed, escape ectopic beats from other inherent pacemakers in the AV node or ventricle appear and can assume pacemaker function at rates of 40 to 60 beats per minute. In addition, rapid impulses in other areas of the heart may produce atrial, junctional, or ventricular tachycardias. These can occur when an ischemic myocardium causes an alteration in the heart's conductivity, producing what are called reentry pathways.

Conduction Pathways.
The normal sinus impulse is transmitted through the heart by a highly specialized network of fibers known as the conduction system. When the impulse reaches the ventricles, stimulation of the myocardium causes depolarization of the cells, and contraction occurs.

The conduction system is made up of the AV node, bundle of His, and right and left bundle branches. The AV node filters atrial impulses as they pass through to the ventricles. It can initiate its own impulse, but usually at lower rates (40 to 60 beats per minute). It is generally supplied by the RCA and is also innervated by the autonomic nervous system (FIG. 3-5, *B*).

The bundle of His provides infranodal conduction traversing the two sides of the intraventricular system, where it divides into the right and left bundle branches. The bundle branches end in a fine network of conductive tissue called the Purkinje fibers. These fibers extend to the papillary muscles and lateral walls of the ventricles. The His bundle and its branches are supplied by the proximal branches of the LAD coronary artery (FIG. 3-5, *C*).

Electrophysiology.
Transmission of the electrical impulse or action potential of the myocardium is preceded by a series of sequential ionic changes across the cardiac cell membrane, which results in depolarization and subsequent contraction of the myocardium. These events correspond in time to the mechanical events described later. After depolarization the cells return for recovery to a resting state called repolarization, diastole, or relaxation.

A resting (polarized) cell has a net charge of −90 mV. Potassium is the predominant intracellular cation, and sodium is the predominant extracellular cation. The difference in concentrations of these ions results in a resting state of electrical potential commonly referred to as the resting membrane potential (RMP).

On initiation of an electrical stimulus, sodium ions move across the cell membrane, converting the net electrical force within the cell to a positive charge. The cell is then depolarized, resulting in a shortening of the cell.

The electrical potential created by this ionic movement progresses through adjacent regions of the cell membrane and is referred to as the action potential. FIG. 3-6 illustrates the five phases of the cardiac action potential and its relationship to the electrocardiogram.

Phase 0 represents the depolarization of the cell, with the rapid influx of sodium causing a reversal of the ionic charge (the inner surface of the cell becomes positive). This is depicted by the upstroke of the action potential curve (see FIG. 3-6, *A*).

Phase 1 is the brief rapid change toward the repolarization process, during which the membrane potential returns to 0 mV.

Phase 2 is a plateau or stabilization period caused by the slow influx of sodium and the slow exit of potassium. During this period, calcium ions enter the cell through slow calcium channels, triggering the release of large quantities of calcium. Calcium functions in the process of cellular contraction.

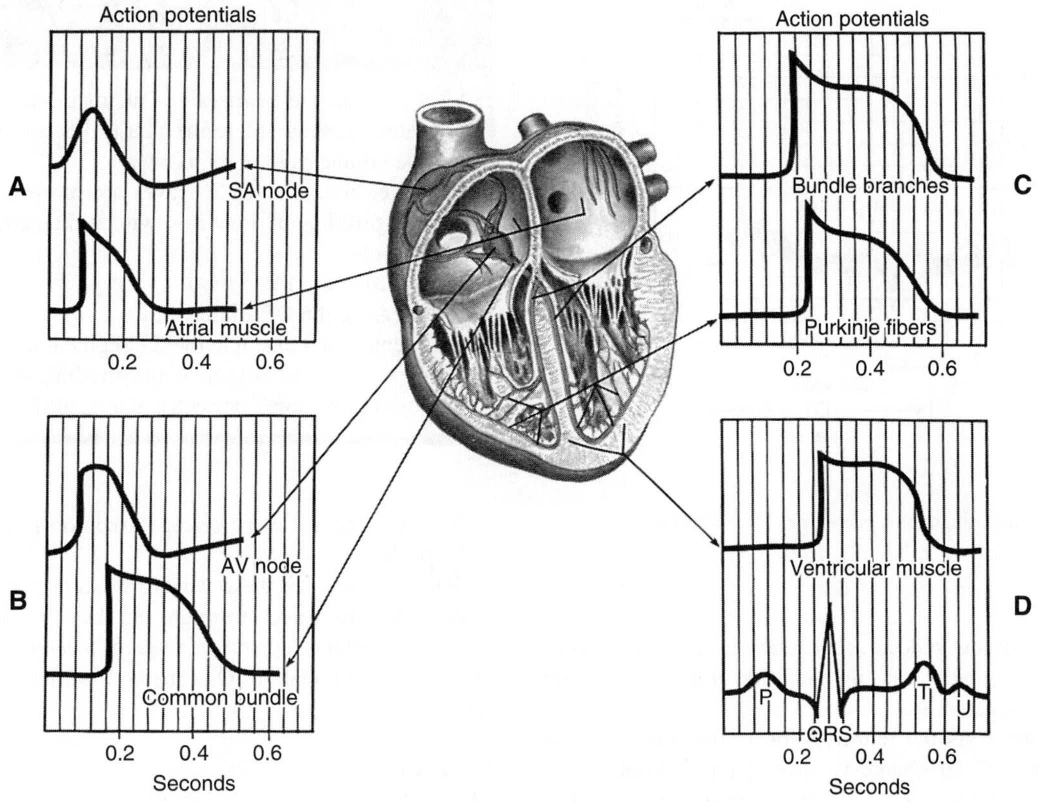

FIG. 3-5

Heart with normal conduction pathways and transmembrane action potential of **A,** SA node; **B,** AV node; **C,** bundle branches; and **D,** ventricular muscle.

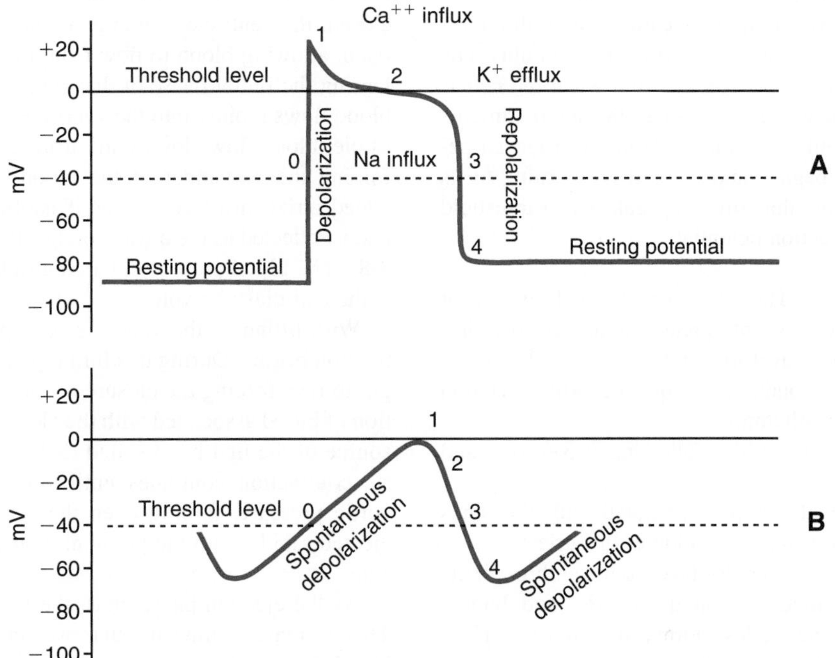

FIG. 3-6

Cardiac action potentials. **A,** Action potential phases 0 to 4 of nonpacemaker cardiac cells. **B,** Action potential of pacemaker cell.

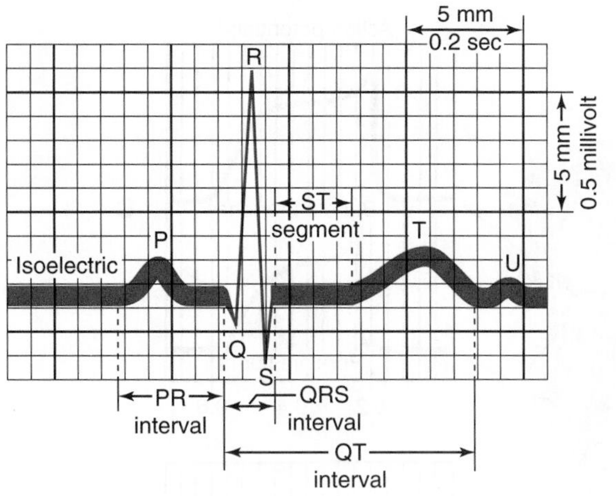

FIG. 3-7
Normal electrocardiographic waveform. (From Tucker et al.[99])

SYSTEMATIC APPROACH TO ECG INTERPRETATION

1. Calculate the heart rate. Calculate atrial (P waves) rate. Calculate the ventricular (QRS complexes) rate.
2. Determine rhythm regularity.
3. Determine whether P waves are present. Determine the position of P waves with relation to the QRS complex.
4. Measure the PR interval.
5. Measure the QRS interval.
6. Identify and examine the ST segment and T wave.
7. Determine the origin of the rhythm. Is it of sinus, atrial, junctional, or ventricular origin?

Phase 3 represents sudden acceleration in repolarization as potassium leaves rapidly, causing the inside of the cell to move toward a more negative state.

Phase 4 represents the return to the resting phase during which the intracellular charge is once again electronegative, leading to the initiation of the action potential (phase 0). Any excess sodium is eliminated from the cell in exchange for potassium that left the cell during phases 2 and 3.

Throughout these phases the cardiac cell goes through a series of refractory periods during which the cell is incapable of accepting another stimulus and responding with a full action potential. An absolute refractory period occurs during depolarization and at the beginning of repolarization (phases 0, 1, and 2). During this period, excitation of the cardiac cell will not result in another impulse, no matter how strong the stimulus. The relative refractory period represents the time when the cell is once again electronegative. A stronger-than-threshold stimulus can initiate another impulse. A vulnerable or supernormal period occurs as phase 4 begins, and the cell is returning to its resting potential. During this time a weaker-than-threshold stimulus can initiate an action potential.

Electrocardiogram. The electromechanical events of the heart can be recorded and interpreted on an electrocardiogram (ECG). The various waveforms in FIG. 3-7 have been correlated with the normal conduction sequence. Any deviation from normal indicates dysrhythmia.

The cardiac cycle includes the following waveforms and time intervals:

P wave: The electrical activity associated with the sinus node impulse and its depolarization of the atria

PR interval: The time the impulse takes to travel through the atria to the AV node, the bundle of His and bundle branches, and the ventricles; normal duration is 0.12 to 0.20 seconds

QRS complex: Electrical depolarization and contraction of the ventricles

ST segment: The period between the completion of depolarization and the repolarization of the ventricles

T wave: The recovery or repolarization phase of the ventricles

Intervals between these waveforms reflect the time an impulse takes to travel through the heart. Identification of rhythms, normal or otherwise, requires a careful systematic approach to interpretation. One method is described in the box above.

Cardiac Cycle

The cardiac cycle is divided into two phases: systole and diastole. Systole is the time interval during which blood is ejected from the ventricles. Diastole is the time interval during which the ventricles are relaxed and filling with blood from the atria. Diastole is discussed first because filling pressures often predict the effectiveness of systolic ejection.

As described previously, the atria are reservoirs for blood entering the heart. During diastole the semilunar valves are closed, the ventricles are at rest, and the AV valves are forced open, allowing blood to flow from the atria into the ventricles. During the initial phase of diastole, approximately 70% of the blood flows rapidly into the ventricles. In the second half of diastole, blood flow slows until atrial contraction is accelerated, forcing the remainder of the blood into the ventricles. This added atrial thrust completes diastolic filling of the ventricle and is reflected as the a wave on the atrial pressure tracing (FIG. 3-8). The blood present in the ventricles at the end of diastole is the end-diastolic volume.

With filling of the ventricles complete, isovolumetric contraction begins. During this initial phase, systolic pressures begin to rise, forcing the closure of the AV valves. The deceleration of blood associated with the closure of the AV valves is the source of the first heart sound (S_1) (see FIG. 3-8). Isovolumetric contraction continues until ventricular pressure exceeds aortic pressure, forcing open the semilunar valves. Blood is ejected rapidly into the pulmonary artery and aorta on the left side.

As the ejection phase ends, the ventricular muscle relaxes. This decreases intraventricular pressures and causes reversal of blood flow in the aorta, which forces the semilunar valves to close. Ventricular relaxation with closure of the semilunar valves is the source of the second heart sound (S_2, reflected by a dicrotic notch on the pressure waveform of the aorta; see FIG. 3-8).

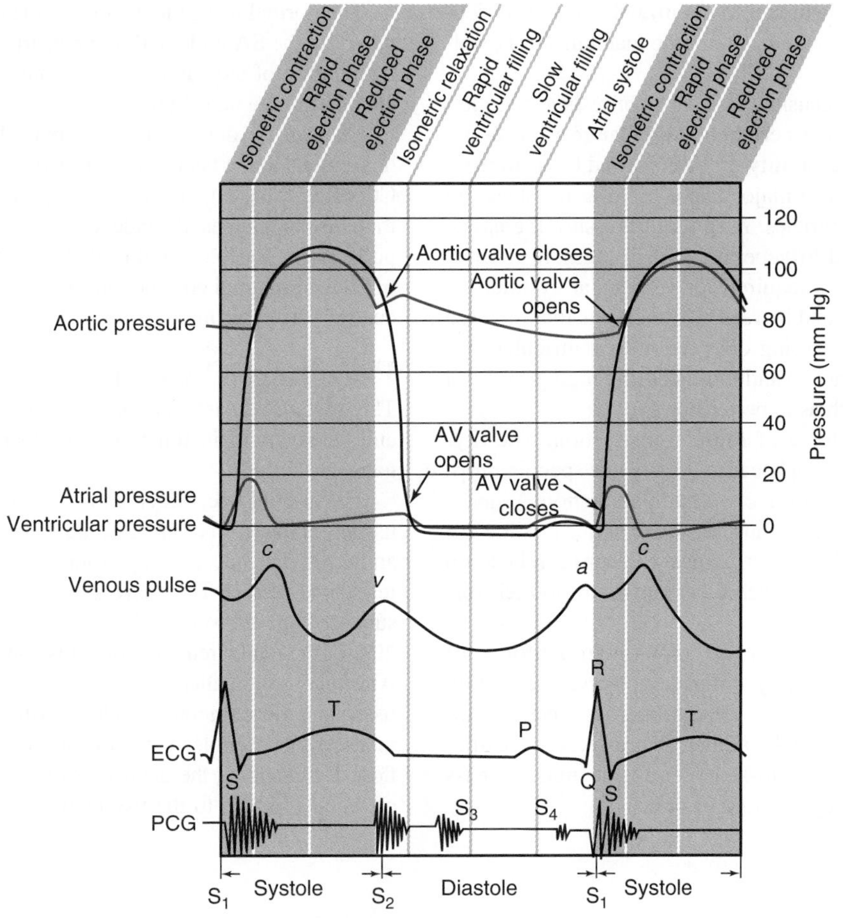

FIG. 3-8

Left ventricular pressure pulses correlated in time with ventricular volume, heart sounds, and electrocardiogram. (From Guzzetta and Dossey.[44])

After the semilunar valves close, ventricular wall tension or pressure falls rapidly. On the atrial pressure tracing the v wave reflects the period in which the ventricles are relaxing and blood is entering the atrium. The downsloping after the v wave is the signal that ventricular relaxation is complete. As ventricular pressure falls below atrial pressure, the AV valves once again open and the cycle is repeated.

Factors Affecting Cardiac Function

A basic function of the heart is to transport oxygen and other nutrients to various parts of the body via the circulation and to return carbon dioxide and the waste products of metabolism to the lungs for excretion. The circulating volume varies according to the tissue cells' need. Any increase in the work of the cells causes an increase in blood flow and thus increases the work of the heart and myocardial oxygen consumption (MVo_2).

The heart's function is governed by the closely integrated working of three major factors: intrinsic properties of the heart; extrinsic factors, including the nervous system, blood volume, and venous return; and peripheral circulation.

Cardiac function is based on the adequacy of the cardiac output (CO), which is the amount of blood pumped from the left ventricle per minute. CO is calculated by multiplying the amount of blood ejected from one ventricle with one heartbeat (stroke volume [SV]) by the heart rate (HR): CO = SV × HR. In a normal 70-kg (150-pound) adult at rest, the CO is 5 L/min. The main factors affecting CO are preload (filling of the heart during diastole), afterload (the resistance against which the heart must pump), contractility of the heart muscle, and heart rate.

Preload is the degree of fiber stretch that occurs as a result of load or tension placed on the muscle before contraction. The term *load* refers to the quantity of blood and the term *tension* to the pressure the blood exerts in the left ventricle at the end of diastole (filling) just before systole (ejection). This is commonly referred to as left ventricular end-diastolic pressure (LVEDP).

The ability of the muscle fibers to stretch in response to increasing loads of incoming blood (venous return) is related to the Frank-Starling principle, which states that the greater the presystolic fiber stretch (within physiologic limits), the stronger is the ventricular contraction. In other words, the more the ventricle fills with blood during diastole, the greater is the quantity of blood it will pump during systole. Preload is a major determinant of myocardial oxygen consumption.

Afterload is the resistance to blood flow as it leaves the ventricles. Afterload is a function of both arterial pressure and left ventricular size. Any increase in vascular resistance (pressure against which the heart is forced to pump) will cause ventricular contractility to increase in an attempt to maintain stroke volume and CO.

The principal factors causing impedance or resistance to left ventricular outflow are the peripheral vascular resistance and the compliance and distensibility of the aorta and large arteries. Pressure in the arteries is a major factor offering resistance to blood flow from the ventricles. As arterial pressure increases, more energy is required to generate enough pressure to eject blood. As more energy is required for ventricular systole, the myocardial oxygen demand increases. Conditions that increase afterload include those causing obstruction to ventricular outflow (such as aortic stenosis) and those causing high peripheral vascular resistance (such as hypertension).

Contractility is the force of muscle contraction. The myocardium is a unique muscle because it has some specific properties that contribute to its effective pumping action. When a stimulus is applied to heart muscle, the myofibrils slide together and overlap, and contraction occurs. During relaxation the filaments pull away from each other and return to their former positions.

The rate (chronotropic force) and force (inotropic force) of contraction can be increased by sympathetic nerve stimulation or administration of drugs with these properties, such as isoproterenol, epinephrine, and dopamine. Depressed contractility is generally the result of a loss of contractile muscle mass through injury, disease, dysrhythmias, or drugs.

The normal heart rate is 60 to 100 beats per minute. It is initiated by the SA node within the heart, but other factors such as stimulation of the autonomic nervous system can greatly influence heart rate and rhythm.

CO can be depressed or increased, directly changing the heart rate. With a heart rate of less than 40 beats per minute, the CO often falls, impairing cardiac performance. With low rates there is an increased tendency for dysrhythmias. With rapid pulse rates, diastole is reduced. This reduces time for both ventricular filling and coronary artery perfusion, both of which occur primarily during diastole.

Peripheral Vascular System

The vascular system is composed of the arteries, capillaries, and veins. Its main function is to distribute blood to body organs and tissues.

The arterial tree, which carries oxygenated blood to all body tissues, is made up of arteries, arterioles, and capillaries. Arteries are easily distended, high-pressure conduits (FIG. 3-9) known as resistance vessels. They have a high elastic fiber content that can support high pressure and hold large volumes of blood. About 20% of the total circulating blood is contained within the arteries. Arterioles are smaller branches whose walls contain less elastic tissue and more smooth muscle. Constriction or dilation of the lumens of the arterioles is the major control of pressure and blood flow. By changing the diameter of the blood vessels, the volume of blood supplied to the tissues may be increased or decreased.

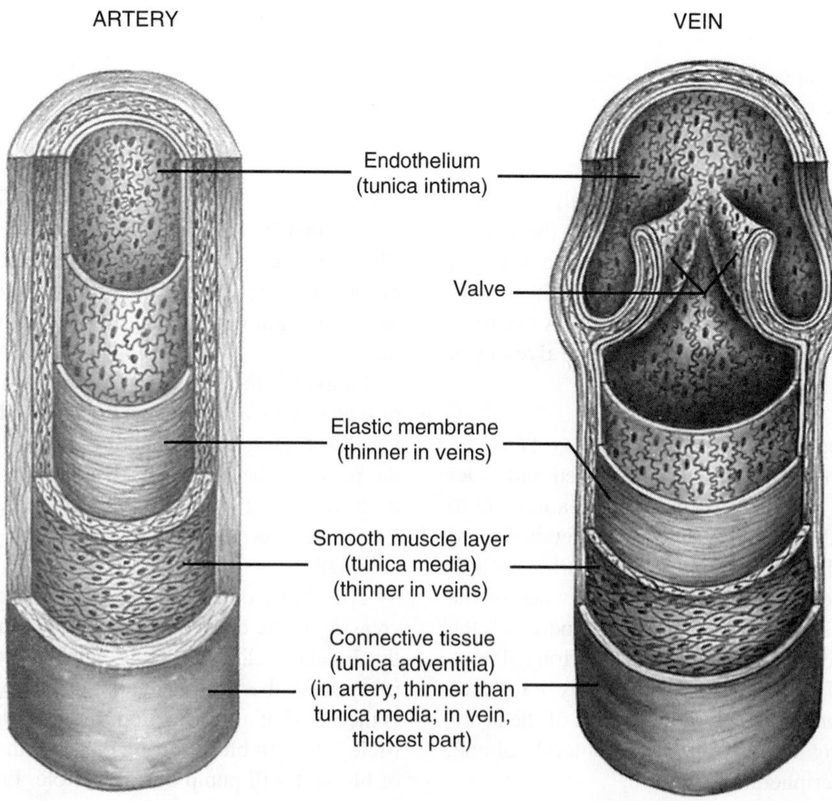

FIG. 3-9

Cross sections of artery and vein showing the three layers: tunica intima, tunica media, and tunica adventitia. Note difference in wall thickness between artery and vein.

Arteries and arterioles respond to the autonomic nervous system and to chemical stimulation. Nerve impulses from reflex centers in the brain may constrict or dilate the vessels. Chemical substances may alter the size of a blood vessel by acting directly on the vessel or by stimulating sensory receptors, thus beginning reflex control. Temperature can also alter the size of the blood vessels.

Capillaries are microscopic (0.1 mm), inelastic endothelial vessels. The large capillary bed is permeable to the molecules that are exchanged between blood cells and tissue cells (FIG. 3-10). The vital exchange of oxygen, nutrients, and metabolic waste products between blood and interstitial fluid occurs here. Blood flow through the capillaries is regulated by the demand for oxygen by cells. The precapillary sphincter helps control blood flow through the capillary bed, allowing blood into the tissue when more oxygen is needed.

The capillaries also respond to nervous control such as sympathetic stimulation, which causes constriction. However, local capillary response is mainly the result of humoral factors, that is, chemicals from tissue metabolism or chemical substances in the blood. Such chemical substances include histamine, which dilates, and catecholamines such as epinephrine, which constrict. Oxygen and pH can also influence local blood flow.

The venous system of venules and veins returns blood to the heart. Venules, the exchange vessels, are small, thin tubules that join to form veins. They collect blood from the capillary bed. Veins are thin, elastic vessels that can store large amounts of blood. Thus they are referred to as capacitance vessels (see FIG. 3-10). They hold 60% to 70% of a body's total blood volume and change as tissue needs change. Veins contain valves at varying intervals that maintain forward blood flow to the heart (venous return) and prevent reflux. Venous blood flow is influenced by arterial flow, skeletal muscle contractions, changes in thoracic and abdominal pressure, and right atrial pressure.

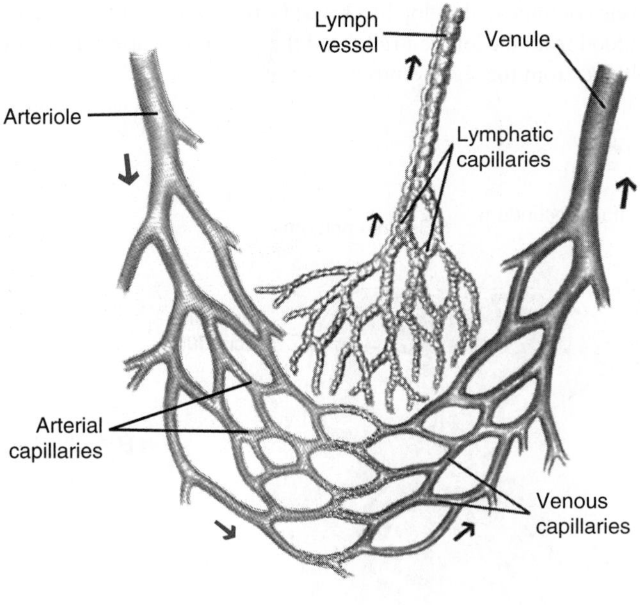

FIG. 3-10
Microcirculation involving blood, interstitial fluid, oxygen, and nutrients.

Neural Control of the Cardiovascular System

The heart and blood vessels are innervated by divisions of the autonomic nervous system.

Heart. The heart can begin its own impulse through the SA node. This is known as automaticity. It is influenced by both divisions of the autonomic nervous system. Sympathetic fibers innervate the heart through nerves arising from the cervical and upper thoracic ganglia of the sympathetic trunks and by the parasympathetic fibers arising in the vagal branches. Combined, they form the cardiac plexuses located close to the arch of the aorta.[95] From these plexuses, nerve fibers accompany the right and left coronary arteries to enter the heart. The fibers then extend to the SA node, AV node, and atrial myocardium.

Sympathetic cardiac nerves, or accelerator nerves, increase the heart rate when activated. Parasympathetic nerves, or vagus fibers, slow the heart rate by decreasing conduction through the AV node. Sympathetic system action is effected through the release of epinephrine. The parasympathetic effects are caused by the vagal release of acetylcholine. Pain, exercise, temperature, emotions, and drugs may also activate this autonomic receptor system.

Blood Vessels. Arteries and arterioles are also under the control of the sympathetic nerves. Contraction and relaxation of the muscle fibers of the blood vessels control the diameter of the vessels. The muscles are supplied by vasoconstrictor fibers, which constrict the vascular smooth muscle, and vasodilator fibers, which relax it. Vascular reflexes, helped by the action of chemical substances in the blood, regulate the diameter of vessels to distribute blood properly to tissues in response to their needs.

Baroreceptors. Baroreceptor cells are in the carotid sinus and aortic arch. Stimulation by stretch or pressure slows the vasomotor center, resulting in vasodilation. As more impulses go to the heart, stimulating parasympathetic fibers, the heartbeat slows and the arterioles and venules dilate.

Chemoreceptors. Vasomotor chemoreceptors are in the aortic arch and carotid bodies. They are very sensitive to lowered $Pa{O_2}$, raised $P{CO_2}$, and lowered pH. When stimulated, the chemoreceptors send impulses to the vasoconstrictor centers in the medulla, causing vasoconstriction of arterioles and the venous reservoir.

Arterial Blood Pressure

Arterial blood pressure is a measure of the pressure blood exerts within the blood vessels. This pressure depends largely on the work of the heart (cardiac output), blood volume, and peripheral resistance, including the elasticity of arterial walls.

Peripheral resistance is the resistance to blood flow caused by the force created by the aorta, arteries, and arterioles. The amount of pressure on the blood is highest in the aorta (120 mm Hg) and becomes lower in arteries (80 mm Hg), arterioles (55 mm Hg), capillaries (30 mm Hg), and veins (20 mm Hg).[43] This pressure difference (gradient) determines blood flow because blood flows naturally from high pressure to low. Other factors include blood viscosity and the size and patency of the vessel lumen.

The vascular tone of the arteries and arterioles allows them to constrict or dilate, influencing the resistance to flow. For example, the greater the resistance in the arteriole, the less is the blood flow to capillaries. Therefore more blood remains in the arteries, creating a higher arterial pressure.

Blood viscosity depends on red blood cells and protein molecules in the blood. Greater pressure is needed to propel viscous, or thick, fluid. Altered blood protein levels or reduced red blood cell levels, as in anemia or hemorrhage, reduce peripheral resistance and arterial pressure.

Measurement of Arterial Pressure.

Arterial pressure may be measured directly or indirectly. Direct measurement is done by placing a catheter, attached to a recording monitor, into the artery. Indirect measurement is performed with a stethoscope and a blood pressure cuff.

Fetal Development

From the onset of gestation the developing embryo undergoes rapid cellular diffusion, forming tissues that will later become the heart. By the third week a primitive single-tubular structure made up of two layers of germ cells is formed. The mesoderm contributes to the pericardial wall (epicardium) and myocardium, and within this layer a single longitudinal tube is formed that will eventually become the endocardium.

The tube's position permits it to accommodate rapid growth. During the first 28 days the primitive cardiac tube grows and bends to the side, twisting into a loop. At this stage the cardiac structures are developing and identifiable: the sinuatrium, which connects the atria with the primitive ventricle; the conus cordis, which will later become the outflow tract for the ventricles; and the truncus arteriosus, which later divides into the aorta and pulmonary artery.

From the fourth through the eighth weeks, transition to a four-chambered heart occurs. A midline groove forms at the apex of the ventricular loop, beginning the division between the right and left sides. Blood flow remains undivided and continuously enters the atria and sinus venosus and leaves via the truncus arteriosus.

Atria.

Atrial development begins from the common AV canal. Two tissue bundles, the endocardial cushions, arise from the AV canal, forming a dorsal (back) and ventral side. By the sixth week these tissues merge in the center of the heart, dividing the AV canal into left and right channels and developing what will later be the tricuspid and mitral valves.

Atrial septation develops from the septum primum, which grows toward the AV canal and endocardial cushions. An intercommunication between the left and right atria, called the foramen primum, remains (FIG. 3-11, *A*). As atrial division continues, a second atrial septum (septum secundum) is established in the center and to the right of the septum primum. The septum primum continues to fuse with the endocardial cushions, obliterating the foramen primum (FIG. 3-11, *B*). However, the lower portion remains as a flap valve that prevents blood flow from reversing. Throughout fetal life, blood flow is directed right to left through the foramen ovale, supplying oxygen to the left side of the heart and fetal structures (FIG. 3-12). The foramen ovale closes shortly after birth.

Ventricles.

Septation of the ventricles takes place during the second month of fetal development. Rapid growth occurs from the apex of the common ventricle upward toward the expanding endocardial cushions and AV canal. This upward-growing muscular tissue does not merge with the cushions. Thus an interventricular communication is created that exists until the tissues from the endocardial cushion and conus ridges of the truncus arteriosus grow downward and eventually obliterate it. The upper portion of the septum thins out into a fibrous sheet referred to as the membranous portion of the septum, while the lower portion remains muscular.

Great Vessels and Cardiac Valves.

The truncus arteriosus, which is initially a single undivided tubular structure, undergoes its own partitioning process. The conus ridges in the ventricular septum fuse and divide the truncus into a left and a right side, forming the aorta and pulmonary artery. These vessels continue to develop in a spiral fashion, so the aorta receives blood from the left ventricle, and the pulmonary artery receives blood from the right ventricle.

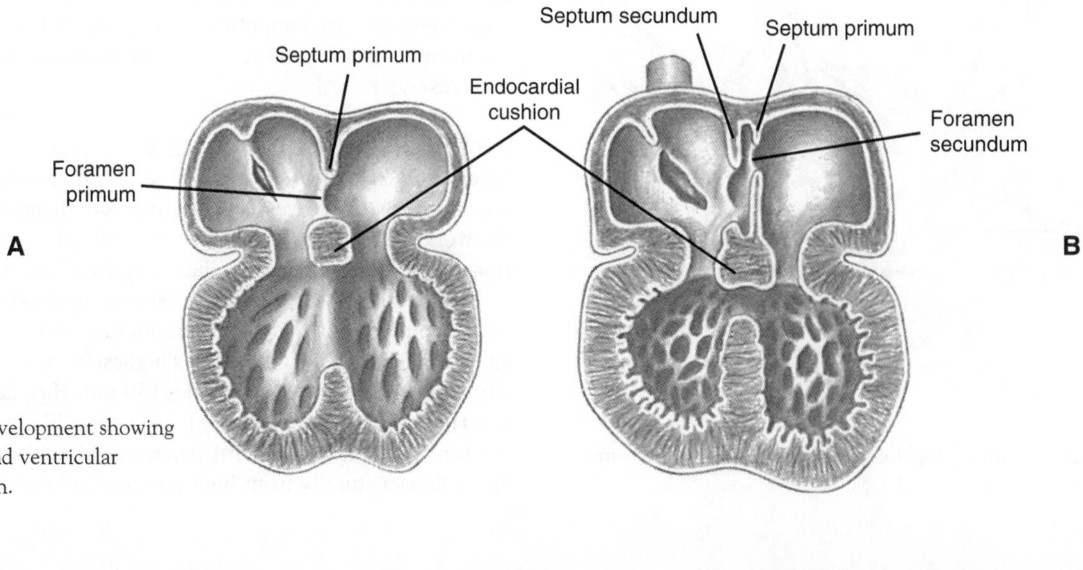

FIG. 3-11
Chamber development showing atrial (**A**) and ventricular (**B**) septation.

Embryonic connective tissue grows outward from the endocardial tissue of each conus ridge to form the three cusps of the aortic and pulmonic valves. Meanwhile, the mitral and tricuspid valves are being formed by the proliferation and thinning of the tissues that project from the endocardial tissues and outer walls of the AV canal. The papillary muscles and chordae tendineae arise from alteration of the muscular tissues of the inner surface of the ventricles.

Fetal Circulation. Fetal circulation differs dramatically from that after birth. The developing fetus secures oxygen and nutrients through the placenta, where an interchange of gases, foods, and wastes occurs between fetal and maternal blood. The fetal blood receives oxygen and nutritive substances by diffusion and gives up waste products. The fetus is connected to the placenta by the umbilical cord, which contains two umbilical arteries and one umbilical vein.

Because the lungs are nonfunctional during fetal life, their blood supply is limited. However, three structures exist during fetal life to ensure circulation within the heart. These are the foramen ovale in the interatrial septum, which allows the blood in the right atrium to pass directly into the left atrium; the ductus arteriosus, which connects the pulmonary artery directly with the aorta; and the ductus venosus, which allows blood to pass directly to the inferior vena cava.

The heart begins to beat in about the fourth week of fetal life. Fetal circulation of blood is similar to that in adults with the exception of the heart, lungs, and placenta. Blood reaches the placenta via the umbilical arteries. Within the placenta, blood passes through the capillaries of the villi and then returns to the fetus by way of the umbilical vein to the liver. Most of the blood is shunted directly to the inferior vena cava by way of the ductus venosus; the remainder is directed into the liver.

Circulation within the heart is a mixture of oxygenated blood received from the ductus venosus and deoxygenated blood returning from the alimentary canal, liver, and lower extremities, as well as from the coronary arteries, upper extremities, and superior vena cava. Blood enters the right atrium via the inferior vena cava and is shunted directly to the left atrium through the foramen ovale, bypassing most of the right ventricle and lungs. Blood that does enter the right ventricle is pumped to the pulmonary artery, where it divides. A portion goes directly to the lung, and the remainder is shunted through the narrow ductus arteriosus to the descending aorta. Blood entering the left atrium mixes with a small amount of blood received from the pulmonary veins and passes into the left ventricle. From there it is pumped through the aorta and into the general circulation.

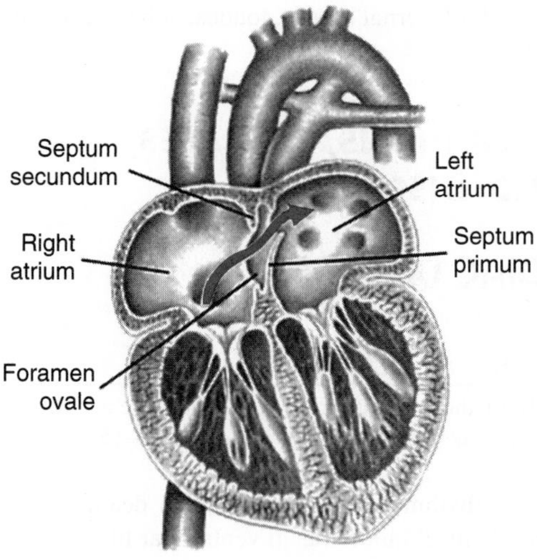

FIG. 3-12
Blood flow being directed through foramen ovale.

Circulatory Changes at Birth. With the first inspiration at birth the lungs expand and begin functioning. Placental circulation ceases, and the connection with the placenta ends with the cutting of the umbilical cord, causing several major changes. During fetal life the lungs have a high vascular resistance. As a result, the blood ejected from the right ventricle into the pulmonary artery is shunted via the ductus arteriosus into the descending aorta. With the first breath the alveoli expand, the pulmonary vascular resistance drops rapidly, and pulmonary blood flow increases. Simultaneously, the loss of placental blood flow causes the right atrial pressure to drop. The combination of decreased pulmonary vascular resistance, increased pulmonary blood flow, and decreased right atrial pressure causes the left atrial pressure to rise above the right atrial pressure. The foramen ovale then closes, and the increase in oxygen saturation following the changes in pulmonary vascular resistance stimulates constriction and eventual closure of the ductus arteriosus.

NORMAL FINDINGS*

The assessment of any patient begins with careful attention to the patient's chief complaint. The problem, whether chest pain, palpitations, or shortness of breath, should guide the direction of questioning. Questions regarding the problem may be organized into seven categories: Location, quality, quantity, precipitating factors, aggravating factors, duration, and associated symptoms.

History

Cardiovascular Risk Factor Profile (see p. 56)

Past medical history and general health status: Congenital heart disease; childhood disease (rheumatic fever, scarlet fever); coronary artery disease; vascular disorders; bleeding disorders; hypertension; kidney disease; diabetes; hyperlipidemia; heart murmurs; allergies; genetic disorders (e.g., Marfan's syndrome)

Family history: Age, sex, and health of parents, siblings, and children, and cause of death for deceased members; data regarding history of hypertension, heart disease, diabetes, elevated lipid levels, sudden deaths

Sociocultural: Culture, ethnicity, and religion; alcohol consumption; economic situation

Occupation: Type of employment; physical and emotional demands; environmental or occupational hazards (actual, potential) (e.g., chemical exposures, dust)

Activity level: Exercise: amount, frequency, intensity; sexual behavior: frequency, recent changes, problems or presence of symptoms (e.g., chest pain, shortness of breath during or after intercourse); sports: type (e.g., competitive versus leisure), contact (e.g., football, soccer)

*⭘ = Older adult.

Sleep: Number of pillows used; presence of paroxysmal nocturnal dyspnea; number of times up to urinate
Nutrition: Fluid and dietary restriction; any recent weight increases or decreases
Dental history: Major problems; last dental visit; knowledge regarding antibiotic prophylaxis if pertinent
Medications: Prescription and nonprescription drugs; contraceptives; regular use of street drugs (e.g., cocaine, crack)
Smoking history: Type: cigarettes, cigars, pipe, chewing tobacco, snuff; duration; frequency
Female history: Birth control measures: intrauterine devices, diaphragm, sponge/foam, male contraception; hormone therapy: type and years used; pregnancies: para, gravida, any related complications; menopause: age, types of hormone replacement therapy
Psychosocial: Perception of illness; response to health problems; patterns of coping or adaptation; understanding of current and past health problems
Support system: Marital status; primary support system

Physical Examination

General appearance: Level of consciousness (alert, oriented); respiratory rate and pattern (passive breathing 12 to 20 respirations per minute, respiratory/pulse rate ratio 1:4, no shortness of breath or dyspnea); nutritional state (well nourished); weight and height normal
Blood pressure: Systolic 100 to 140 mm Hg (tends to be 5 to 15 mm Hg higher in right arm); diastolic 60 to 90 mm Hg; pulse pressure 30 to 40 mm Hg; older adult: maximum systolic pressure 160 mm Hg; with standing, there may be systolic drop of 10 to 15 mm Hg and diastolic drop of 5 mm Hg
Arterial pulse (heart rate): 60 to 90 beats per minute; older adult: slows with age because of increase in vagal tone; wide range (40 to 100 beats per minute); occasional ectopic beats may be felt; rhythm (regular); amplitude and contour (upstroke full, strong, rounded, brisk); symmetric response (equal on right and left); timing (equal for all arterial pulsations, e.g., brachial, femoral); auscultation (no murmurs or bruits); amplitude:

4^+ = Strong, bounding (normal)
3^+ = Easily palpable
2^+ = Difficult to palpate
1^+ = Diminished, weak, thready
0 = Absent

⭘ Amplitude and contour (upstroke more rapid, smooth)
Jugular venous pressure (JVP) (Fig. 3-13): Should not exceed 3 cm (1 inch) above level of sternal angle with head of client elevated to 30 to 45 degrees
Jugular pulsations: Undulations; movement with inspiration; increase or decrease with change in body position

Wave pulsations (see Fig. 3-8)

a wave: First positive wave visualized; coincides with S_1; represents right atrial contraction and retrograde transmission of pressure pulse to jugular veins
x descent: First negative "trough" undulation; occurs between S_1 and S_2; results from right atrial diastole, plus the effects of the tricuspid valve being pulled down during ventricular systole
v wave: Third positive wave; coincides with S_2; continued atrial filling

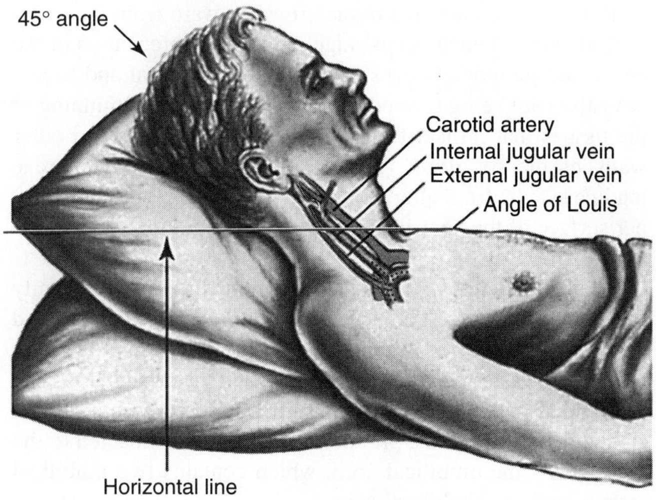

Fig. 3-13
Inspection of external jugular venous pressure.

y descent: Represents fall in right atrial pressure from peak of v wave after tricuspid valve opening and occurs during period of rapid atrial emptying in early diastole
Precordium (Fig. 3-14: Point of maximum impulse (PMI) 5 to 7 cm left of midsternal border at fifth intercostal space (ICS) and 1 to 2 cm (⅓ to ½ inch) in diameter; palpable areas: aortic area—at second ICS to right of sternal border, pulmonic area—at second ICS to left of sternal border, apex—at fifth ICS 5 to 7 cm to left of sternal border; precordial motion symmetric, even with respiration
Heart sounds (see Fig. 3-8): First heart sound (S_1) closing of AV valves; components are tricuspid first heart sound (T_1), located at fifth ICS and left lower sternal border (LLSB), and mitral (M_1), located in apical area at fifth ICS and 5 to 7 cm left of sternal border; loudest at apical area; normal splitting heard at LLSB, fifth ICS; S_2 closure of semilunar valves; components are aortic (A_2), located at second ICS to right of sternal border, and pulmonic (P_2), located at second ICS to left of sternal border; loudest at base; normal splitting heard at P_2

Conditions, Diseases, and Disorders

CARDIAC DISEASES

Cardiac Dysrhythmias

A dysrhythmia is a disorder of the heart rate and rhythm caused by a conduction system disturbance (Fig. 3-15).

Cardiac dysrhythmias can cause sudden death resulting from electromechanical failure (as in ventricular fibrillation) or from impaired cardiac function.

Early recognition and treatment are needed because dysrhythmias such as premature ventricular ectopic beats may

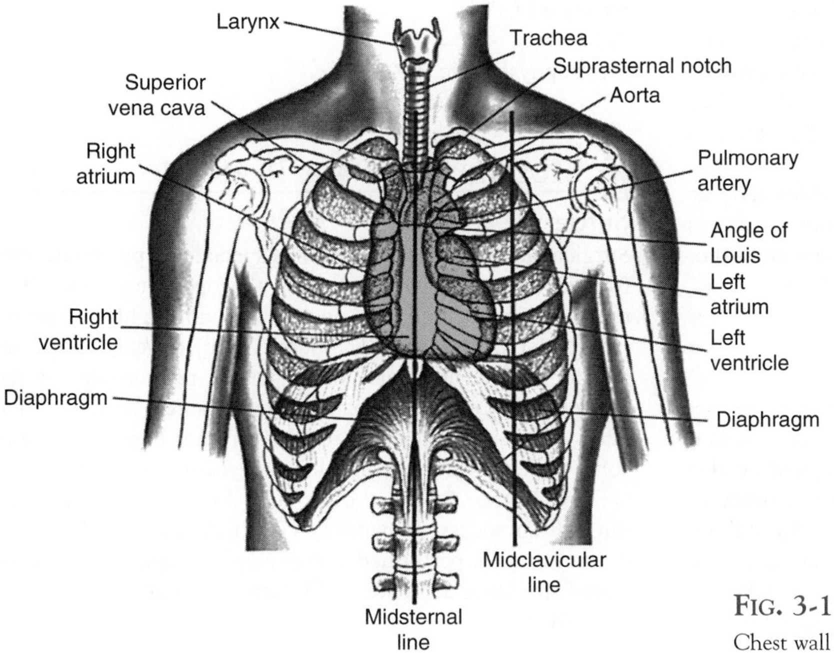

FIG. 3-14
Chest wall landmarks for inspection, percussion, and palpation.

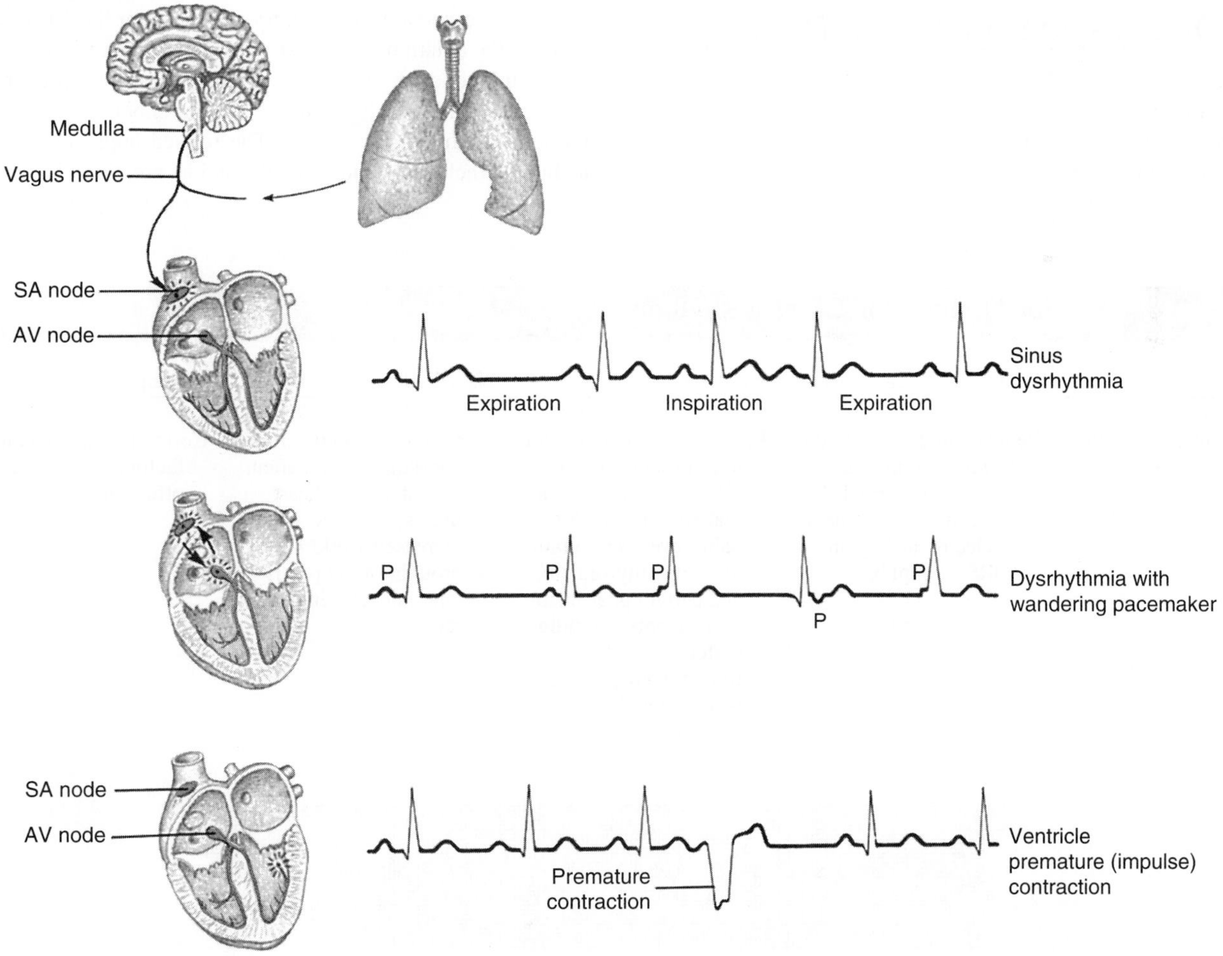

FIG. 3-15
Cardiac dysrhythmias. (From Canobbio.[15])

spontaneously become frequent or multifocal. For example, in a patient with myocardial ischemia the ectopic beat may convert to ventricular tachycardia or ventricular fibrillation without warning. About 60% of deaths from acute myocardial infarction occur within the first hour, generally before the victim can reach a hospital.

Careful continuous ECG monitoring now enables early detection and prompt treatment of potentially serious dysrhythmias. However, proper treatment involves diagnosis and a thorough understanding of the underlying etiologic factors.

PATHOPHYSIOLOGY

Cardiac dysrhythmias may be classified into abnormalities of impulse formation (sinus, atrial, ventricular), impulse conduction, or a combination.[10] Dysrhythmias may also be described on the basis of rate (bradydysrhythmia, tachydysrhythmia) or seriousness (minor, life threatening). Dysrhythmias may occur as a result of a primary cardiac disorder, as a secondary response to a systemic problem, or as a complication of drug toxicity or electrolyte imbalance.

Each of the major dysrhythmias is described in the section on nursing assessment.

DIAGNOSTIC STUDIES AND FINDINGS

ECG
See Table 3-1
24-hour ambulatory ECG
Cardiac event recorder
Exercise ECG
Tilt table
Electrophysiologic (EP) studies

MULTIDISCIPLINARY PLAN

Surgery

Surgical ablation, or resection, is a specialized procedure performed by direct visualization in the operating room. It is rarely performed and only on patients with highly refractory ventricular tachycardia. The surgical objective is to excise, isolate, or interrupt heart tissue that is responsible for the tachycardia. Cardiac sympathectomy, a radical treatment that alters adrenergic influences to the heart, has been effective in some patients whose ventricular tachycardia includes a long QT syndrome. Surgical correction for tachydysrhythmias through an accessory pathway (Wolff-Parkinson-White syndrome) may be performed during surgical repair for an associated structural defect (e.g., Ebstein's anomaly of the tricuspid valve).

Interventional Therapy

Catheter Ablation Therapy. The development of better energy delivery systems has made the 1990s the era of nonsurgical interventional procedures for drug-refractory tachydysrhythmias, especially supraventricular tachycardia.[53] The object of catheter ablation is to destroy arrhythmogenic myocardial tissue and conduction tissue by delivering electrical energy in the form of a direct high-energy current shock or, more commonly, radiofrequency energy. The refined application of this technique includes AV junctional ablation, ablation of accessory

Text continued on p. 53.

Table 3-1 Specific Findings for Cardiac Rhythms

Rhythm	Characteristics	Etiology	Clinical Significance	Management
Sinus origin				
Sinus tachycardia (FIG. 3-16)	Regular rhythm; rate 100-180 beats/min (higher in infants); normal P wave; normal segment of electrocardiogram (QRS) complex	Rate increase may be normal response to exercise, emotion, or abnormal stressors such as pain, fever, pump failure, hyperthyroidism, and certain pharmacologic agents, including caffeine, nitrates, atropine, epinephrine, isoproterenol, and nicotine	May have hemodynamic consequence in patient with damaged heart that is unable to sustain increased workloads brought on by persistent increases in heart rate	Correcting underlying factors; discontinuing offending drugs

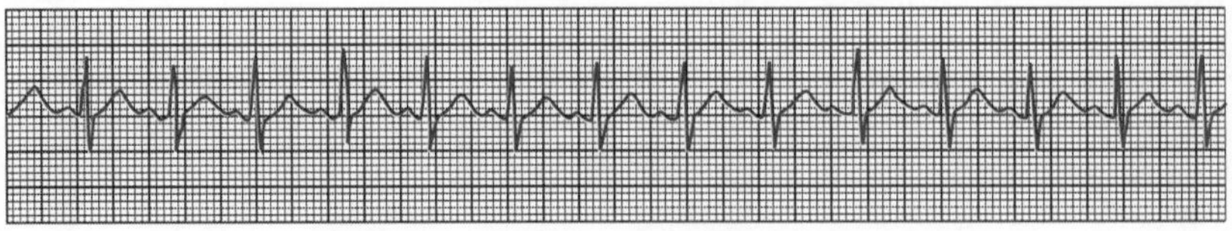

FIG. 3-16
Sinus tachycardia. (From Andreoli et al.[5])

Rhythm	Characteristics	Etiology	Clinical Significance	Management
Sinus bradycardia (FIG. 3-17)	Regular rhythm; rate less than 60 beats/min; normal P wave; normal PR interval; normal QRS complex	Rate decrease may be normal response to sleep or in well-conditioned athlete; abnormal drops in rate may be caused by diminished blood flow to SA node, vagal stimulation, hypothyroidism, increased intracranial pressure, or pharmacologic agents such as digoxin, propranolol, quinidine, beta-blockers, amiodarone, or procainamide	None unless associated with signs of impaired cardiac output; symptoms: dizziness, syncope, chest pain	Correcting underlying cause; atropine 0.5-1 mg IV; transcutaneous or transvenous pacing

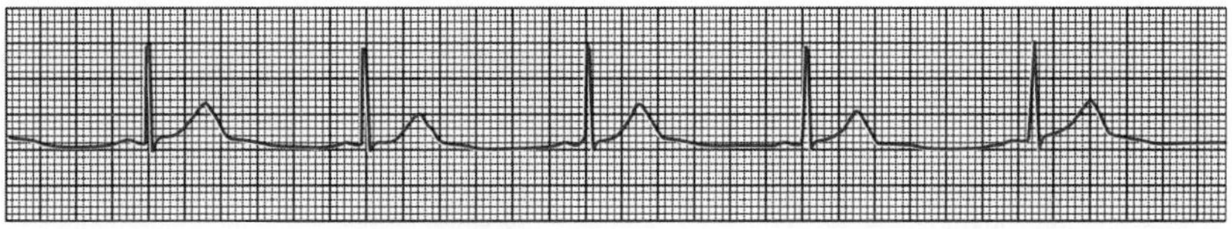

FIG. 3-17
Sinus bradycardia. (From Andreoli et al.[5])

Rhythm	Characteristics	Etiology	Clinical Significance	Management
Sinus dysrhythmia (FIG. 3-18)	Irregular rhythm; may be phasic with respiration, slowing during inspiration and increasing with expiration; rate 60-100 beats/min; normal PR interval; normal QRS complex	Sinus rhythm with cyclic variation caused by vagal impulses that influence rhythm during respiration; occurs commonly in children, young adults, and the elderly; usually disappears as heart rate increases	None unless heart rate decreases; symptoms: dizziness with decreased rate	None indicated unless heart rate decreases and symptoms occur

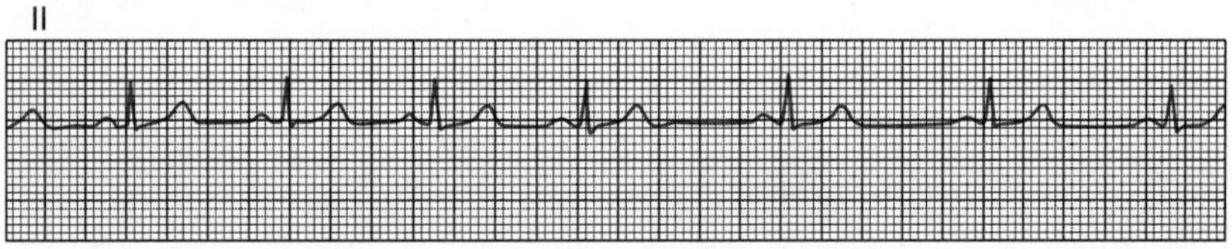

FIG. 3-18
Sinus dysrhythmia. (Copyright Mary H. Boureau Conover, Santa Cruz, Calif; from Conover.[19])

Continued

Table 3-1 Specific Findings for Cardiac Rhythms—cont'd

Rhythm	Characteristics	Etiology	Clinical Significance	Management
Atrial origin				
Atrial premature contractions (APCs, PACs) (FIG. 3-19)	Irregular rhythm owing to ectopic beats followed by incomplete compensatory pause; rate normal or increased depending on number of ectopic beats; P wave present but different from normal underlying sinus beat; PR interval may be shorter or longer than normal sinus beat; normal QRS complex	May be precipitated in healthy persons by anxiety, fatigue, caffeine, smoking, and alcohol; observed in patients with ischemia or organic heart disease and those receiving digoxin	May indicate atrial strain or hypoxia; frequent PACs (more than 6/min) reflect atrial irritability and often mark onset of atrial fibrillation	Correcting underlying cause; usually not treated; for frequent PACs, treat with class 1-A antidysrhythmic drugs

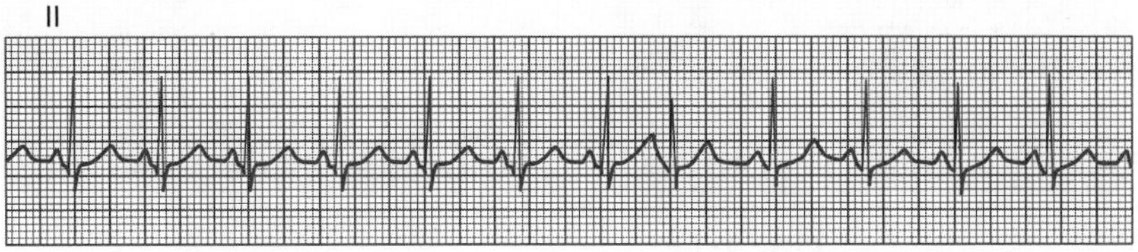

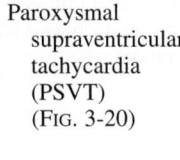

FIG. 3-19
Atrial premature contractions (APCs, PACs). (From Conover.[21])

Paroxysmal supraventricular tachycardia (PSVT) (FIG. 3-20)	Sudden, rapid onset of tachycardia with stimulus originating above AV node; regular rhythm; rate 150-250 beats/min; P wave uniform, may or may not be buried in preceding T wave; PR interval may vary, often difficult to measure; normal QRS complex	Begins and ends spontaneously or precipitated by excitement, fatigue, caffeine, smoking, or alcohol	Usually no significant impairment; patient complains of palpitations and shortness of breath; if persistent or occurring in patients with preexisting organic heart disease, may cause decrease in cardiac output and/or blood pressure, resulting in pump failure or shock	Performing vagal stimulation with carotid sinus massage; using Valsalva maneuver to stimulate baroreceptors (may be used in conjunction with carotid sinus massage); decreasing ventricular response with medication to block AV conduction; sedation to reduce sympathetic stimulation; adenosine 6-12 mg IV push rapidly; verapamil 5-10 mg IV push; propanolol (Inderal) slowly IV in 1-mg increments up to 4 mg (contraindicated in patients with heart failure); cardioversion if resistant to preceding; for chronic control of recurrent PSVT: disopyramide, flecainide, propafenone, sotalol hydrochloride

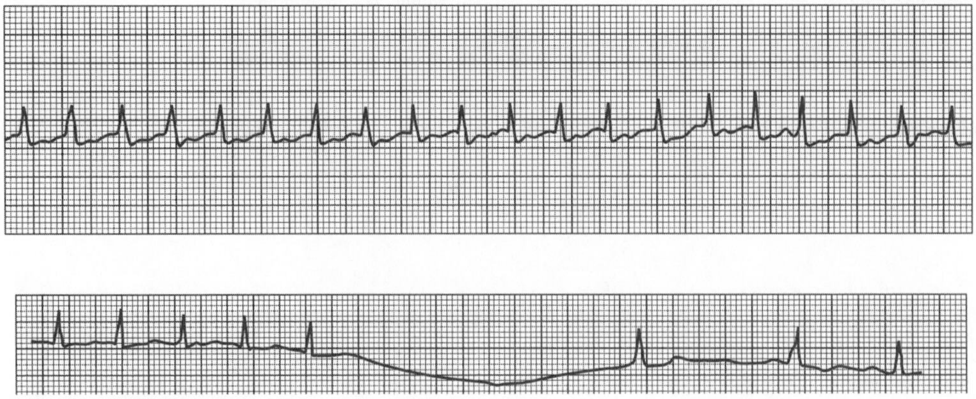

FIG. 3-20
Paroxysmal supraventricular tachycardia (PSVT). (From Andreoli et al.[5])

Rhythm	Characteristics	Etiology	Clinical Significance	Management
Atrial flutter (AF) (FIG. 3-21)	Rhythm may be regular or irregular; rate: atrial 250-350 beats/min, characterized by an identical morphology in any single lead, after accounting for QRS and ST segment and T waves; sawtooth flutter waves are seen in leads II, III, aVF; ventricular rate depends on AV conduction, may occur at 2:1, 3:1, or 4:1 ratio; PR interval not measurable; normal QRS complex	The underlying mechanism in two thirds of patients is a reentry arrhythmia located in the right atrium (type I, flutter); seen in patients with organic heart disorders such as coronary heart disease and valvular heart disease	Patient complains of palpitations, which may be associated with heart failure, and chest pain, particularly in presence of rapid ventricular rates	Cardioversion; digoxin if cardioversion is not used or is unsuccessful; ibutilide for rapid conversion; procainamide in acute phase; for chronic control of recurrent AF may also use disopyramide, flecainide

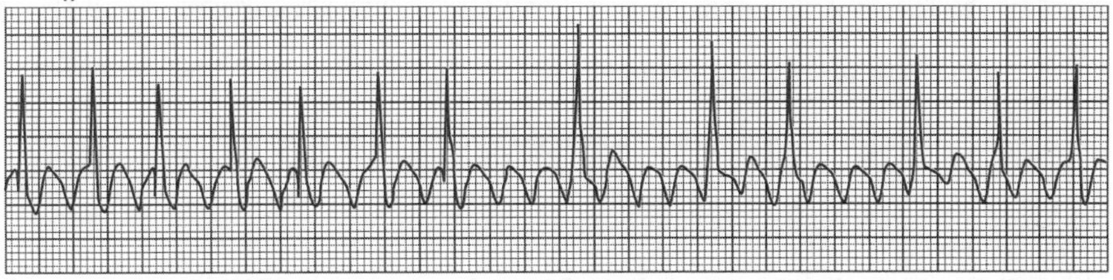

FIG. 3-21
Atrial flutter (AF). (From Conover.[21])

Rhythm	Characteristics	Etiology	Clinical Significance	Management
Atrial fibrillation (FIG. 3-22)	Rhythm irregular; rate: atrial more than 350 beats/min; absence of uniform atrial depolarization produces undulations (f waves) of inconsistent morphology; ventricular varies according to AV conduction; may range from 50 to 150 beats/min	Results from multiple atrial foci discharging almost simultaneously; atria never uniformly depolarize; reflects organic heart disease; may also occur with digitalis toxicity	With rapid ventricular rates, cardiac output may be impaired, resulting in heart failure, angina, and shock If atrial fibrillation is episodic, patient may form atrial thrombus that could embolize, causing target organ damage (e.g., CVA)	Determination of underlying cause and whether acute or chronic; cardioversion for rapid ventricular response; digoxin if cardioversion is not used; ibutilide for rapid conversion; procainamide; verapamil in acute phase; for chronic management of recurrent atrial fibrillation; disopyramide, propafenone, sotalol, amiodarone, quinidine Oral anticoagulants: warfarin

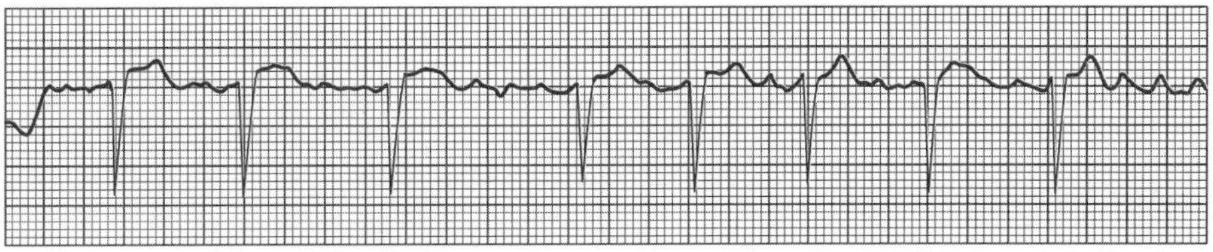

FIG. 3-22
Atrial fibrillation. (From Conover.[21])

Continued

Table 3-1 Specific Findings for Cardiac Rhythms—cont'd

Rhythm	Characteristics	Etiology	Clinical Significance	Management
Junctional rhythms Junctional escape rhythm (nodal) (FIG. 3-23)	Regular rhythm; rate 40-60 beats/min; P wave abnormal, may occur before, during, or after QRS complex, may be inverted in leads II, III, and augmented V lead (aVF); QRS complex usually normal	Occurs when sinus node is suppressed and atria fail to depolarize AV junction; may be the result of digitalis toxicity, vagal stimulation, or ischemic damage to SA node	Usually none; transient; if condition persists, slow rates may allow foci with rapid rates to take over; may also produce symptoms of diminished cardiac output	Treatment or correction of underlying cause if persistent or if symptoms occur; pacemaker rarely indicated
Premature junctional contractions (FIG. 3-24)	Rhythm regular except for junctional beat; rate normal; P wave as described for junctional escape rhythm; PR interval shortened when P wave precedes QRS complex; QRS complex usually normal	Results from increased automaticity of AV junction, causing ectopic focus in AV node to discharge before onset of impulse from sinus node; cause of ectopic beats: ischemia or digitalis toxicity	Usually none; frequency reflects junctional irritability	None indicated

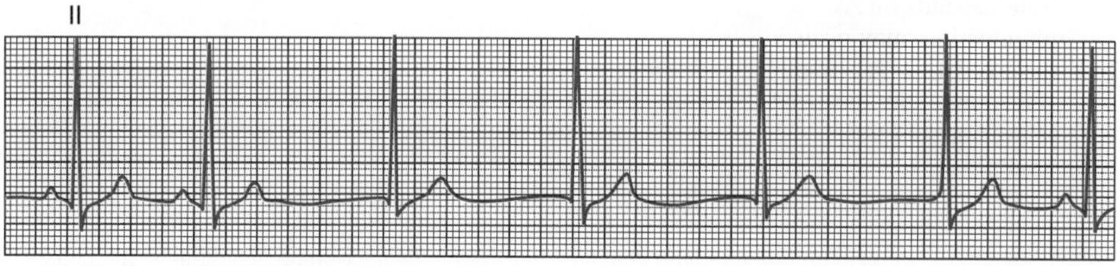

FIG. 3-23
Junctional escape rhythm (nodal). (From Conover.[21])

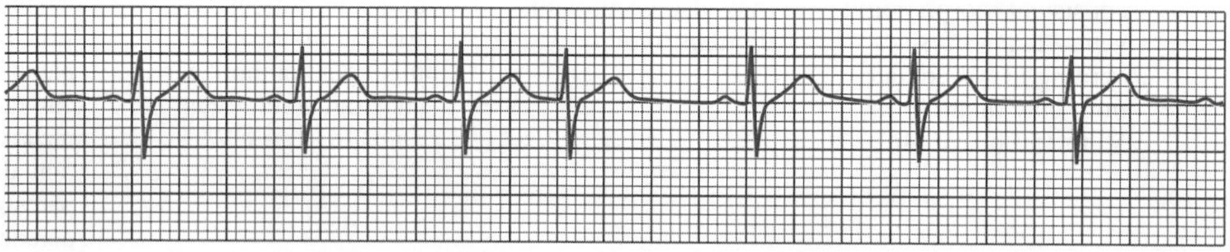

FIG. 3-24
Premature junctional contractions. (From Conover.[21])

Rhythm	Characteristics	Etiology	Clinical Significance	Management
Ventricular dysrhythmias				
Premature ventricular contractions (PVCs) (FIG. 3-25)	Rhythm irregular owing to ectopic beats followed by full compensatory pause; rate normal or increased depending on number of ectopic beats; P wave absent in ectopic beat; PR interval absent; QRS complex widened and distorted; T wave is in opposition to R wave; morphology varies depending on ectopic focus	Caused by irritable focus within ventricle, commonly associated with myocardial infarction; other causes include hypoxia, hypocalcemia, and acidosis	PVCs occurring frequently (more than 8/min) or in pairs indicate increased ventricular irritability	Aimed at suppression of PVCs; if frequent, IV bolus of lidocaine (50-100 mg) followed by continuous IV infusion; additional antidysrhythmic agents in classes I and II may be given; infrequent PVCs require no treatment

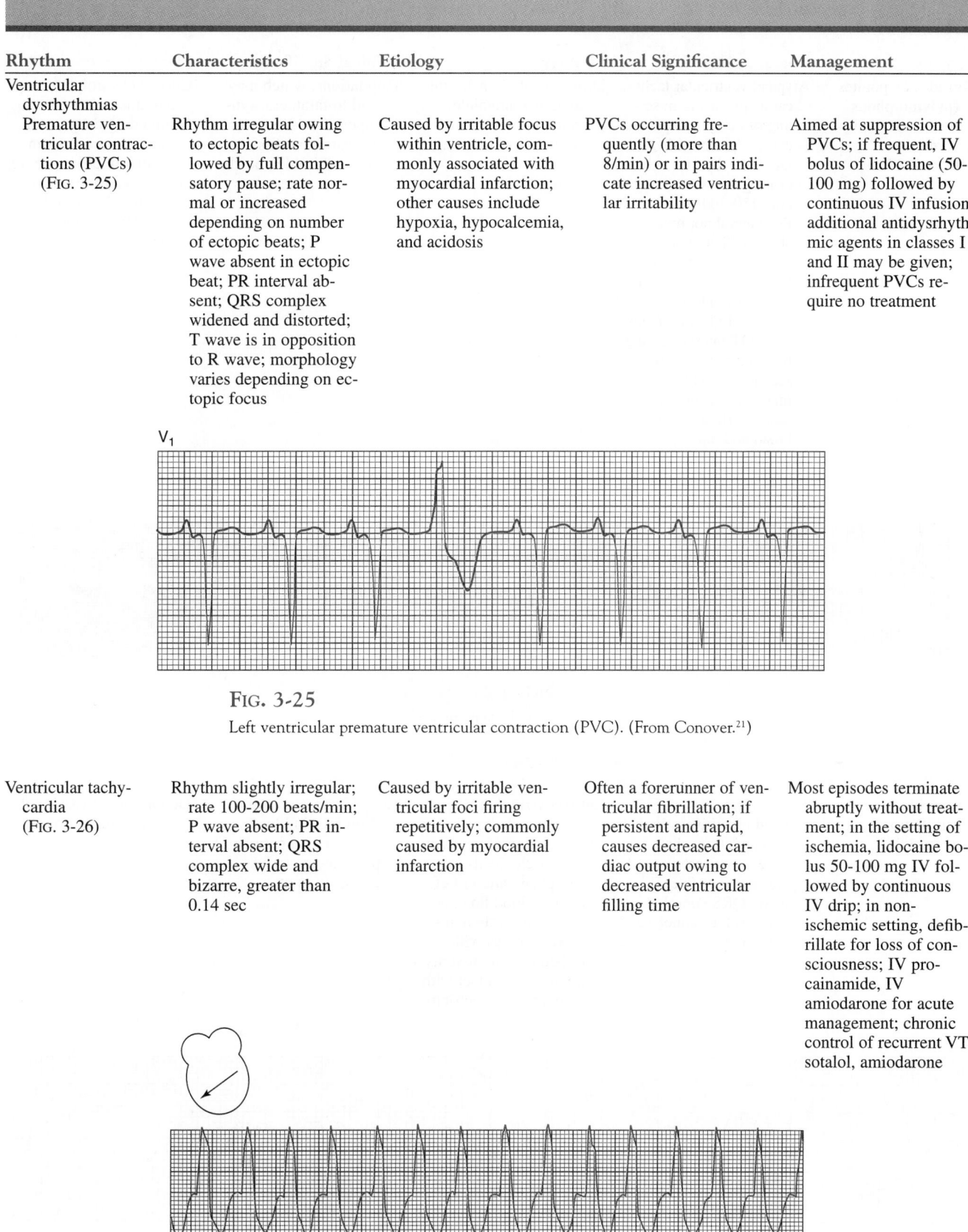

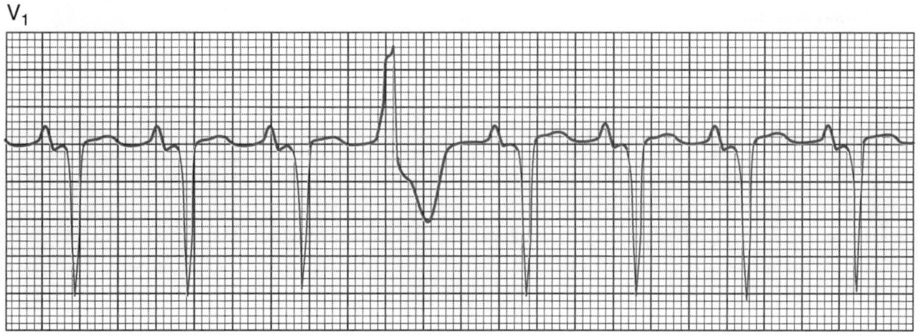

FIG. 3-25
Left ventricular premature ventricular contraction (PVC). (From Conover.[21])

Rhythm	Characteristics	Etiology	Clinical Significance	Management
Ventricular tachycardia (FIG. 3-26)	Rhythm slightly irregular; rate 100-200 beats/min; P wave absent; PR interval absent; QRS complex wide and bizarre, greater than 0.14 sec	Caused by irritable ventricular foci firing repetitively; commonly caused by myocardial infarction	Often a forerunner of ventricular fibrillation; if persistent and rapid, causes decreased cardiac output owing to decreased ventricular filling time	Most episodes terminate abruptly without treatment; in the setting of ischemia, lidocaine bolus 50-100 mg IV followed by continuous IV drip; in nonischemic setting, defibrillate for loss of consciousness; IV procainamide, IV amiodarone for acute management; chronic control of recurrent VT; sotalol, amiodarone

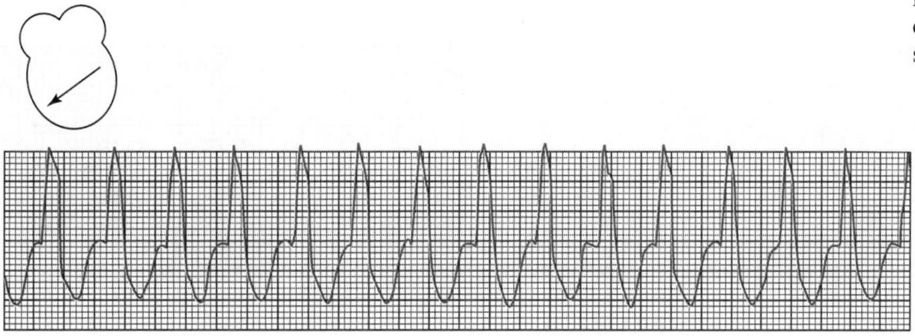

FIG. 3-26
Ventricular tachycardia (VT). (From Conover.[21])

Continued

Table 3-1 Specific Findings for Cardiac Rhythms—cont'd

Rhythm	Characteristics	Etiology	Clinical Significance	Management
Torsades de pointes (polymorphous ventricular tachycardia) (FIG. 3-27)	Atypical ventricular tachycardia occurring in setting of delayed depolarization (prolonged QT interval); rhythm regular or irregular; ventricular rate, 150-300 beats/min; PR interval not measurable; QRS complex wide and bizarre in configuration lasting >0.12 sec; amplitude and direction of QRS complex vary; QT interval during baseline rhythm >0.46 sec or >33% of baseline; T wave during baseline rhythm very broad and flat	Drug toxicity (e.g., quinidine, procainamide, amiodarone); electrolyte imbalance (e.g., hypokalemia, hypomagnesemia)	Palpitations, which may lead to faintness, syncope; often forerunner of ventricular fibrillation and sudden death	Correct electrolytes; stop administration of offending drugs; temporary overdrive ventricular or atrial pacing; IV magnesium sulfate: IV push 2 g over 1-2 min, IV infusion 1-2 g for 4-6 h
Ventricular fibrillation (FIG. 3-28)	Rhythm irregular; rate: rapid repetitive waves or undulations that have no uniformity and are coarse or fine; P wave, QRS complex, and T wave cannot be identified	Lethal dysrhythmia resulting from electrical stimulation of ventricular muscle; leads to abrupt cessation of effective blood flow; occurs in severely damaged hearts as with ischemia, drug toxicity, trauma, or contact with high-voltage electricity	Loss of consciousness; decreases in blood pressure and peripheral pulse owing to loss of cardiac output	Defibrillation; cardiopulmonary resuscitation

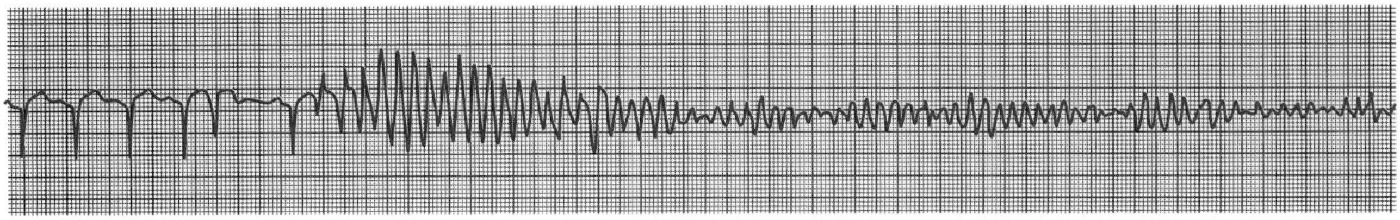

FIG. 3-27
Torsade de pointes.

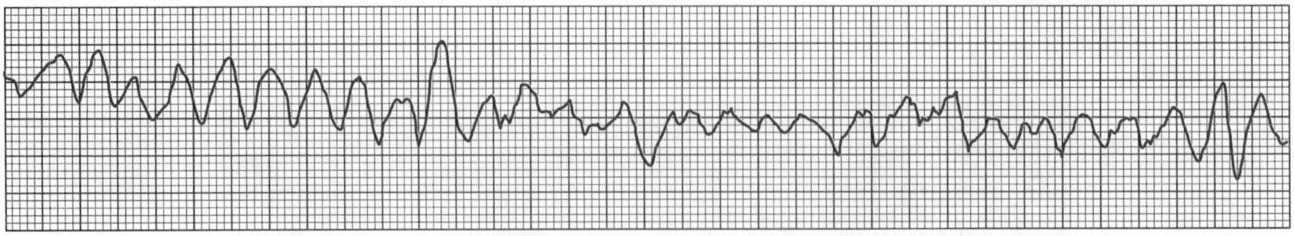

FIG. 3-28
Ventricular fibrillation. (From Conover.[21])

Rhythm	Characteristics	Etiology	Clinical Significance	Management
Conduction disturbances				
First-degree AV heart block (FIG. 3-29)	Rhythm regular; rate normal; P wave normal; PR interval prolonged to greater than 0.2 sec; QRS complex normal	Represents delay in impulse conduction through AV node; occurs as result of increased vagal tone, digoxin administration, or congenital anomalies	No associated symptoms	None indicated; digoxin discontinued if causative factor

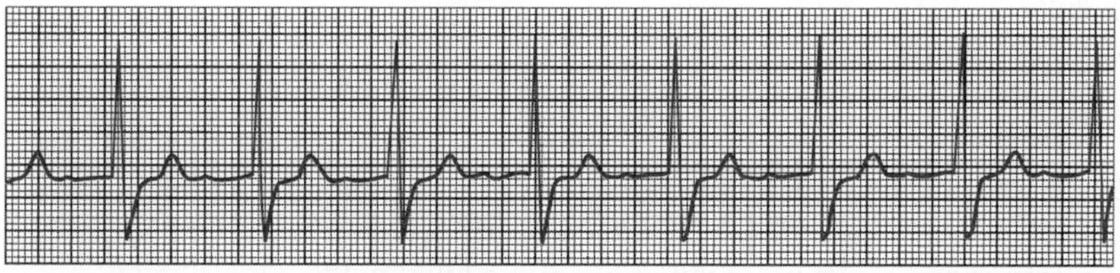

FIG. 3-29
First-degree AV block. (From Conover.[21])

Rhythm	Characteristics	Etiology	Clinical Significance	Management
Second-degree AV heart block Mobitz type I (Wenckebach phenomenon) (FIG. 3-30)	Rhythm: atrial regular, ventricular irregular; rate: atrial greater than ventricular; P wave: multiple P waves before QRS complex; PR interval: progressive prolongation of PR interval until one impulse is completely blocked; QRS complex normal: RR interval becomes progressively shortened until one QRS complex is dropped	Represents progressive decrease in conduction velocity involving AV node and proximal bundle of His; occurs as result of coronary artery disease, digitalis toxicity, rheumatic fever, viral infections, or inferior wall myocardial infarction	No associated symptoms if ventricular rate is adequately maintained	None usually indicated; elimination or correction of underlying cause

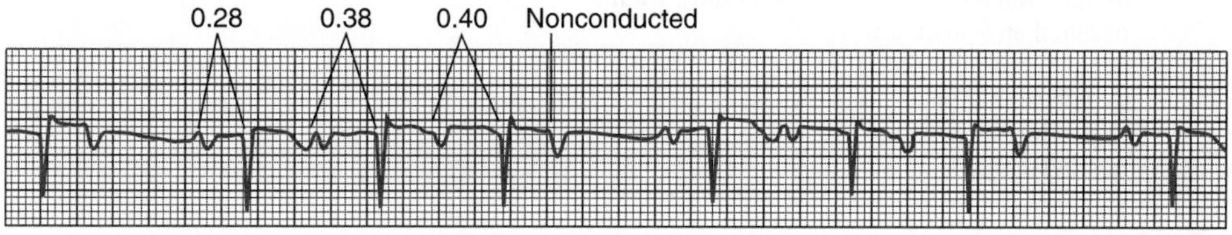

FIG. 3-30
Mobitz type I. (From Conover.[21])

Continued

Table 3-1 Specific Findings for Cardiac Rhythms—cont'd

Rhythm	Characteristics	Etiology	Clinical Significance	Management
Mobitz type II (FIG. 3-31)	Rhythm: atrial regular, ventricular varies; rate: atrial slow to normal; ventricular may be slow, usually half or one-third atrial rate; P wave normal, occurring in multiples before QRS complex; PR interval normal or slightly prolonged, always constant; QRS complex normal or slightly prolonged	Represents block of impulse below level of AV node and within His-Purkinje system; occurs as result of ischemia, digitalis or quinidine toxicity, anterior wall myocardial infarction	No associated symptoms if ventricular rate is adequately maintained; if rate is slow, cardiac output may be impaired, causing dizziness and weakness	Correction or elimination of underlying cause; tends to be recurrent, may progress to complete heart block; transcutaneous or transvenous demand pacing may be required

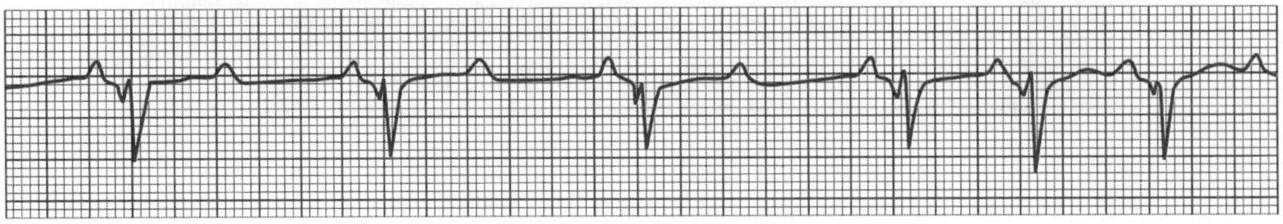

FIG. 3-31
Mobitz type II. (From Conover.[21])

Rhythm	Characteristics	Etiology	Clinical Significance	Management
Third-degree AV block (complete heart block) (FIG. 3-32)	Rhythm: atrial and ventricular regular but act independent of each other; rate: atrial 60-90 beats/min, ventricular 30-40 beats/min; P wave normal but occurs in greater frequency than QRS complex; PR interval: no relationship with QRS complex, therefore never constant; QRS complex normal if ventricular depolarization initiated by junctional escape pacemaker, widened if depolarization initiated by ventricular pacemaker low in conduction system	Represents failure of AV node to conduct impulse to ventricles; block may occur at any point in conduction system at or below level of AV node; occurs as result of coronary artery disease, degenerative fibrosis of conduction system, congenital anomalies, myocarditis, drug toxicity (digitalis, quinidine, procainamide, verapamil), trauma	Patient may tolerate slow heart rate with no sequelae; symptoms associated with low cardiac output owing to slow ventricular rates; include syncope and signs of ventricular failure	If without symptoms, observe on telemetry With symptoms, evaluate need for transcutaneous or transvenous pacing while waiting for permanent pacemaker insertion

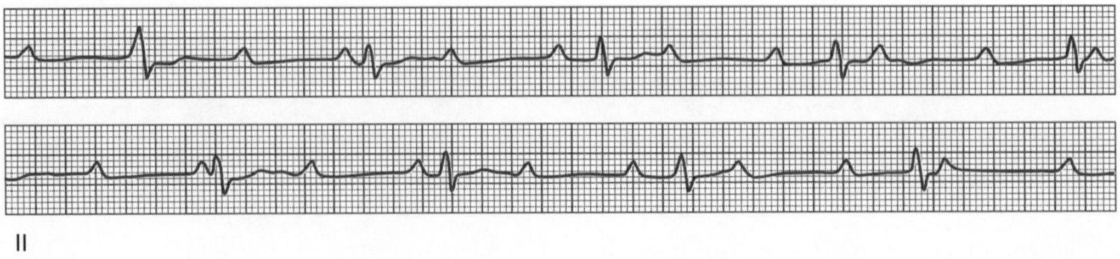

FIG. 3-32
Third-degree AV block. (From Andreoli et al.[5])

pathways, AV nodal reentry, and atrial tachycardias or flutters.[26,91] Treatment of ventricular tachycardia (VT) with catheter ablation is limited to only those patients with focal-origin VT without structural heart disease.

Medications

The following information is based on the Vaughn-Williams Classification and Pharmacology of Antiarrhythmic Drugs:

Antidysrhythmic drugs: Class I-A—Potent local anesthetic drugs that affect nerves, as well as myocardial fibers; decreases conduction velocity by retarding influx of sodium and reducing maximum rate of depolarizing action potential

Quinidine

Indications: Suppresses atrial, junctional, or ventricular ectopy, VT, and paroxysmal atrial tachycardia; may be used to convert atrial fibrillation or flutter to sinus rhythm or to maintain sinus rhythm after cardioversion

Usual dosage: 200-400 mg PO q4-6h

Onset of action: 15 min with peak activity in 2-4 h

Therapeutic blood levels: 2-6 mg/ml

Toxic signs: Widened QRS, prolonged QT bundle branch block, complete heart block, VT, asystole

Sustained-release preparations: Quinidex, 300 mg q8-12h; Quinaglute, 324 mg q8-12h; Cardioquin, 275 mg q6h

Procainamide (Pronestyl)

Indications: Similar to quinidine; suppresses ventricular ectopy; may be less effective in controlling atrial dysrhythmias

Usual dosage: 250-750 mg PO q4-6h; 100 mg PO q5-15 min for total of 1 g IV

Peak action: Within 30 min if PO

Therapeutic blood levels: 4-8 mg/ml

Sustained-release preparations: Procan SR, 500-1000 mg PO q6h

Disopyramide phosphate (Norpace)

Indications: Suppresses or prevents ventricular dysrhythmias; not particularly effective in treating atrial dysrhythmias

Usual dosage: 400-800 mg/day PO in four doses with loading dose of 200 mg

Peak action: 2-4 h

Therapeutic blood levels: 2-4 mg/ml

Antidysrhythmic agents: Class I-B—Reduces rapid upstroke and shortens action potential duration

Lidocaine (Xylocaine)

Indications and actions: Controls ventricular dysrhythmias by depressing automaticity in Purkinje network and increasing excitability threshold of ventricles

Usual dosage: 50-100 mg (1-2 mg/kg) by IV bolus followed by 1.5-4 mg/min

Mexiletine

Indications: Local anesthetic whose electrophysiologic properties closely resemble those of lidocaine; used in management of ventricular dysrhythmias

Usual dosage: IV loading 10-15 mg/min (200-300 mg over 30 min), maintenance 250-500 mg q12h; PO loading 100-400 mg, maintenance 200-300 mg q8h

Onset of action: IV 5 min; PO 1-2 h

Therapeutic blood levels: 0.5-2 mg/ml

Tocainide (Tonocard)

Indications and actions: Class I antidysrhythmic similar to lidocaine given for control of ventricular dysrhythmias; decreases excitability of myocardial cells

Usual dosage: Loading 400-600 mg PO q8h, maintenance 1200-1800 mg in divided doses over 8 h

Onset of action: 1½ h

Therapeutic blood levels: 6-12 mg/ml

Antidysrhythmic agents: Class I-C—Significantly reduces rapid upstroke, primarily slows conduction and minimally prolongs refractoriness

Flecainide (Tambocor)

Indications: Ventricular arrhythmias, supraventricular tachycardia

Usual dosage: 100-200 mg PO q12h

Propafenone (Rhythmol)

Indications: VT

Usual dosage: 150-300 mg PO tid

Onset of action: 45-90 sec

Duration of action: 20 min

Therapeutic blood levels: 1.5-5 mg/ml

Antidysrhythmic drugs: Class II—Controls dysrhythmias by blocking sympathetic stimulation, which shortens phase 4 depolarization of action potential

Propranolol (Inderal)

Indications and actions: Controls supraventricular tachycardia resulting from reentry mechanism; used to control ventricular response to atrial fibrillation and flutter by depressing AV nodal conduction

Usual dosage: 10-80 mg PO qid; 0.5-1 mg IV push slowly to control heart rate

Onset of action: 1-1½ h with PO dose

Therapeutic blood levels: Not determined

Atenolol

Usual dosage: 50-100 mg/day PO

Pindolol

Usual dosage: 10-60 mg bid PO

Antidysrhythmic drugs: Class III—Acts directly on myocardium, prolonging action potential

Amiodarone

Indications: Effective in treatment and prevention of wide variety of atrial and ventricular dysrhythmias

Usual dosage: 200-800 mg/day; loading dose 800-1200 mg/d PO for 1 wk

Onset of action: 4-8 h

Bretylium tosylate (Bretylol)

Indications: Life-threatening ventricular dysrhythmias; not recommended to treat asymptomatic ventricular ectopic beats

Usual dosage: 5-10 mg/kg IV push up to total of 30 mg/kg; may repeat in 15-30 min; slow continuous infusion 5-10 mg/kg q6-8h

Sotalol

Indications: Nonselective beta-blocker with some class IV qualities; used in treatment of ventricular arrhythmias and atrial tachycardia

Usual dosage: 80-160 mg PO bid

Antidysrhythmic drugs: Class IV—Inhibits calcium transport into cells, depresses activity of the SA and AV nodes, prolongs conduction in AV node, and increases AV node refractoriness

Verapamil (Calan, Isoptin)

Indications: Reentrant paroxysmal supraventricular tachydysrhythmias; suppresses AV junctional tachycardia and controls ventricular response to atrial fibrillation and flutter

Usual dosage: 5-10 mg (0.1 mg/kg) IV or 40-80 mg PO q6-8h

Peak action: IV 3-5 min; PO 3-4 h

Diltiazem (Cardizem)

Indications: Same as verapamil

Usual dosage: 0.25 mg/kg bolus over 2 min (approximately 20 mg); infusion rate at 10 mg/h for 24 h

Unclassified agents

Adenosine (Adenocard) A naturally occurring nucleoside used in the treatment of supraventricular tachycardias

Indications: Decreases AV node conduction and interrupts AV reentry pathways

Usual dosage: 6 mg through central IV access, 12 mg peripheral IV × 2 at 5- to 10-min intervals given as IV bolus to convert paroxysmal supraventricular tachycardias to normal sinus rhythm

Ibutilide

Indications: Acute termination of recent-onset atrial fibrillation or flutter

Usual dosage: IV 1 mg given over 10 min; may repeat once

General Management

Cardiac monitoring: Continuous electrocardiographic monitoring provides most efficient and reliable method of detecting dysrhythmias

Electrical countershock: Treatment of choice for tachydysrhythmias that produce a change in the level of consciousness; also used if the arrhythmia produces a decrease in cardiac output or if it is resistant to pharmacologic interventions

Cardioversion: Synchronized discharge of electrical impulse used to convert atrial fibrillation, atrial flutter, or supraventricular tachycardia to sinus rhythm

Defibrillation: Emergency procedure that is unsynchronized; used in treatment of ventricular fibrillation

Cardiac pacemakers: Battery-operated electrical devices used to initiate and control heart rate; may be used as temporary assistive devices or implanted permanently; have various modalities that are selected on the basis of rhythm disturbance; most common indication for pacemaker implantation is bradydysrhythmias, but recent advances in technology have broadened their use to treatment of suppressing supraventricular dysrhythmias otherwise resistant to drug therapy

Automatic implantable cardioverter defibrillator (ICD): Device capable of detecting the presence of ventricular tachydysrhythmias and then delivering electrical countershock via cardioversion or defibrillation within 15 to 20 sec (further discussion on p. 119)

Manage contributing factors: Control or treat underlying causes of dysrhythmia, including thyroid imbalance, adrenal abnormality, recent cardiac surgery, fever, or anxiety disorder (panic attacks)

Diet: Restrictions usually directed to underlying disease process; patients with diagnosed supraventricular tachydysrhythmias instructed to avoid using stimulants such as caffeine, which is found in coffee, certain teas, soft drinks, and chocolate

Smoking: Use of nicotine contraindicated because of its effect on ventricular threshold, which may be the basis for dysrhythmias that could precipitate fatal rhythms

Activity: Restrictions based on the ability to reproduce the rhythm; characteristics of dysrhythmia (usually ventricular) determined by exercise stress testing

NURSING CARE

Nursing Assessment

General

Presence of palpitations, dizziness, lightheadedness, chest pain, syncope

Degree of anxiety, level of understanding, and fears associated with dysrhythmias and treatment to determine source of anxiety

Physical Examination

Continuous cardiac monitoring with evaluation of heart rate and rhythm

Skin: Pallor, diaphoresis

Arterial pulse: Normal with ectopy, tachycardia, bradycardia

Hypotension

Mental status: Confusion, agitation, anxiety

Embolic sequelae reflected in target organ damage

Drug History

Names, dosages of current antidysrhythmic agents

Laboratory values: Electrolyte imbalance; therapeutic levels of drug; thyroid imbalance

Use of artificial stimulants: Caffeine, nicotine, diet pills, decongestants, illicit drugs

Potential Complications

Sequelae from sustained hypotension; end-organ damage from embolic events

Patient Problems/Nursing Diagnoses & Interventions

NIC Coping Assistance

Anxiety related to threat of death secondary to sympathetic stimulation and altered heart action

- Provide continual explanations for the various monitoring devices in use; use short, simple explanations.
- Offer reassurance during periods of heightened anxiety.
- Administer sedation as ordered *to reduce anxiety and to promote rest.*

- Provide referrals for continued supportive counseling *to deal with fears and anxieties.*

NIC Tissue Perfusion Management

Decreased cardiac output related to electrical factors (alteration in rate, rhythm, and conduction)

- Monitor vital signs frequently, according to policy and patient's condition.
- Initiate prompt treatment of life-threatening dysrhythmias per protocol: cardiopulmonary resuscitation (CPR), electrical cardioversion, appropriate drug therapy, and preparation for pacemaker insertion.
- Monitor and record changes in ECG tracings *to use as baseline.*
- Notify physician promptly if any decrease in cardiac output occurs as evidenced by disturbance in rate, respirations, blood pressure, or mental status.
- Administer antidysrhythmic agents as ordered; monitor serum blood levels as guide for dosage *to maintain therapeutic drug levels and avoid drug toxicity;* use caution to avoid drug interactions.
- Administer oxygen therapy *to increase cardiac oxygenation.*

Patient Education/Continuum of Care Plan

Instruction for a patient with a cardiac dysrhythmia begins with the initial phase of care, whether in a coronary care unit or in an outpatient setting. Include the following points:

1. Offer a brief explanation of the disease etiology, rhythm disturbances, and associated symptoms.
2. Explain any diagnostic or therapeutic procedures that are planned or anticipated.
3. Explain the monitoring equipment that may be used.
4. Outline dietary restrictions that may be prescribed: need to avoid caffeine, nicotine, over-the-counter diet pills, and decongestants.
5. Give instructions regarding drug therapy and its purpose, desired effects, dosage, and side effects to report to the physician.
6. Explain need for and method of taking pulse.
7. Emphasize need for follow-up care: pacemaker check, ICD check, drug levels.
8. Provide documentation of dysrhythmia (ECG strip) for patient to carry and medical alert card describing medications, device, etc., in case of emergency.
9. Advise family to learn CPR for high-risk dysrhythmias.

Evaluation/Patient Outcomes

Coping Assistance: Anxiety level is reduced. Patient demonstrates decreased anxiety. Patient appears relaxed, with decreased tension. Patient verbalizes fear and asks questions.

Tissue Perfusion Management: Heart returns to baseline rhythm. ECG tracing reflects baseline rhythm. Blood pressure and heart rate are within normal limits. There is no ectopy. Cardiac output is adequate to maintain cerebral perfusion. Patient is alert and has no dizziness, syncopal episodes, or chest pains. Vital signs are stable. Peripheral perfusion is good.

Coronary Artery Disease

Coronary artery disease (CAD) is a disorder of the coronary arteries that disrupts blood supply to the myocardium.

Permanent disruption of blood flow causes myocardial dysfunction and necrosis, which may lead to a cascade of complications, including sudden death (Fig. 3-33). The rate and severity of CAD vary considerably among world populations. Serious study of the natural history of CAD began in 1948 with the Framingham Heart Study under the auspices of the National Heart Lung and Blood Institute.[52] The data collected in these early studies established certain factors related to the incidence and progression of coronary atherosclerotic disease. These include age, sex, hypertension, lipid levels, obesity, smoking, sedentary life-style, diabetes, and psychosocial factors (see box on p. 56). Rarely is a single factor solely responsible for the occurrence of CAD. More commonly, several risk factors play a role.

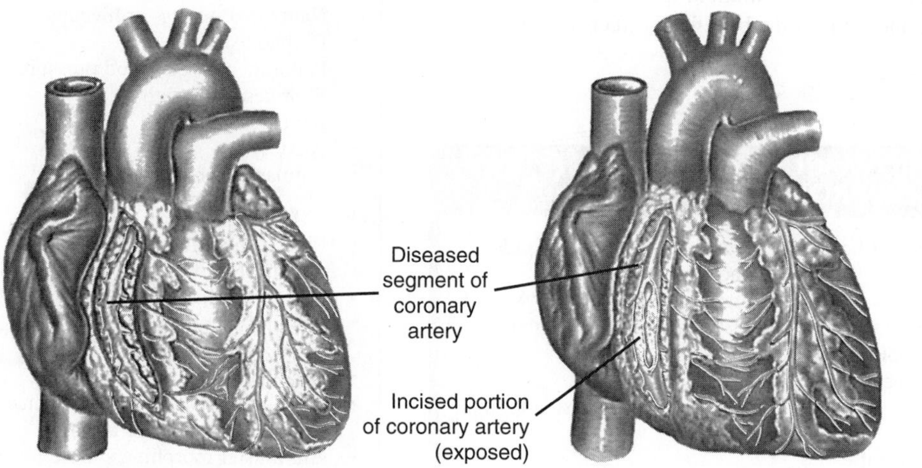

Fig. 3-33
Coronary artery disease. (From Canobbio.[15])

Age and Sex. The incidence of CAD increases with age, with men having a higher incidence of CAD than women. Deaths are reported to be five times as frequent for men as for women in the 35- to 40-year-old age group. After menopause, the risk in women approaches the same level as that for men. The delay in onset in women is thought to be due to premenopausal exposure to endogenous ovarian estrogen. Women who do develop a myocardial infarction have a higher risk of death and complications than do men. About four out of five people who die of heart attacks are age 65 years or older. CAD in persons younger than age 30 years is usually linked to hyperlipidemia, hypertension, and smoking.

Hypertension. Although systolic hypertension is closely linked to cardiovascular disease, elevated systolic and diastolic pressures are associated with ischemic heart disease. Systolic pressures greater than 140 mm Hg or diastolic pressures greater than 90 mm Hg are considered a high-risk factor for heart attacks, particularly in younger persons.[51] Left ventricular hypertrophy results from chronic pressure loads on the ventricle and represents a form of target organ damage that especially contributes to CAD.

Lipid Levels. Of the various types of circulating lipoproteins, cholesterol and triglycerides are most commonly linked to CAD. Increased levels of blood cholesterol, a by-product of metabolism, raise the risk of CAD. In the presence of other risk factors (e.g., high blood pressure or smoking), the risk rises even more. Total serum concentrations of 200 mg/dl in middle-age adults indicate a relatively low risk of CAD; rates of 200 to 240 mg/dl indicate moderate and increasing risk; and levels greater than 240 mg/dl double the risk.[6] It is estimated that more than 27% of the U.S. population falls into this category.

Hyperlipidemia may be a primary disorder or may occur as a result of diabetes, myxedema, or alcoholism. Lipoproteins are broken down and measured separately to determine levels of those persons who are atherogenic. Low-density lipids (LDLs) carry a high percentage of cholesterol in plasma and, in high levels, help produce atheromas. Elevated LDL cholesterol is a major predisposing factor in CAD. Oxidized LDL impairs the functional response of vascular smooth muscle, reduces endothelium-dependent vasodilation, generates an inflammatory response, and inhibits the beneficial effects of nitric oxide on platelets. Optimal serum LDL levels are 120 mg/dl or less for those with no CAD. Levels less than 100 mg/dl are recommended for patients with CAD.

High-density lipids (HDLs) are mostly protein and carry a smaller percentage of cholesterol, thereby helping to remove lipids from the cell through liver metabolism. Studies show that the ratio of HDLs to LDLs is lower in patients with CAD and that a high ratio of HDLs helps reduce vascular disease. HDLs are formed through exercise, fat-controlled diets, and estrogens.[10]

Obesity. Studies have shown that obese people (those who are more than 30% over their ideal weight) are more likely to develop CAD because obesity influences blood pressure and blood cholesterol. Obesity also can lead to diabetes.[4]

Smoking. Cigarette smoking is now clearly linked to heart disease. New studies show that smokers' risk of heart attack is more than twice that of nonsmokers.[4] Primarily through adrenergic stimulation, nicotine contributes to increases in heart rate, stroke volume, cardiac output, and blood pressure. Nicotine also causes peripheral vasoconstriction and, in persons with decreased blood flow, enhances ischemic changes. Cigarette smoking has also been demonstrated to have adverse effects on

CARDIOVASCULAR RISK FACTOR PROFILE

Family history of heart disease	Elevated serum level of lipids and fats
Sex	Diabetes mellitus
Males (35-55 years)	Physical inactivity; sedentary lifestyle
Females (>50 years or after menopause)	Stress
Hypertension	For women <50 years: smoking
Smoking	
Overweight/obesity	

From Tucker et al.[99]

! EMERGENCY ALERT

CHEST PAIN WITH MYOCARDIAL INFARCTION

Pain described as intense crushing, pressure, or heaviness in the chest, frequently accompanied by an impending sense of doom. Pain may be localized in the substernal area with radiation to the jaw and left arm. Myocardial infarction is localized ischemia of an area of the heart muscle. Rapid identification of the culprit coronary artery and rapid treatment are imperative. Time is muscle.

Assessment

- PQRST pain assessment:
  - P—Provoking
  - Q—Quality
  - R—Radiating
  - S—Severity
  - T—Time
- Nausea, vomiting, or hiccups
- Diaphoresis
- Pallor, decreased blood pressure
- Shortness of breath
- Increased pulse
- Anxiety
- Jugular venous distention

Interventions

- Place patient in comfortable position.
- Administer oxygen by nasal cannula (3 to 5 L).
- Obtain 12-lead ECG.
- Administer nitroglycerin (sublingual or IV as ordered), ASA, or beta-blockers.
- Establish IV at keep-open rate.
- Obtain blood samples for cardiac enzymes.
- Monitor oxygen saturation.
- Administer morphine sulfate for pain as ordered.
- Prepare for reperfusion therapy (thrombolytic or catheter-based intervention).

the lipid profile. When paired with the use of oral contraceptives, smoking is considered to increase the risk for CAD by a factor of 10. Smoking decreases the threshold for ventricular fibrillation because it interferes with oxygen binding to hemoglobin, thus slowing the diffusion of oxygen into mitochondria. Nonsmokers may be exposed to increased risk of CAD by passive, or secondhand, smoke.

Sedentary Lifestyle. Although the positive effects of exercise on the risk of CAD are difficult to assess, studies show that people who exercise heavily are at a decreased risk of having CAD. Inactivity is associated with decreases in HDLs.

Psychosocial Factors. A type A personality is more characteristic of persons in whom CAD will develop. This type of person is usually aggressive, competitive, and rushed. When the type A personality is combined with other risk factors, such as older age, high lipid levels, and smoking, the risk of heart disease may increase.

Other Risk Factors. Other factors also linked to CAD include diabetes and genetic factors. Diabetes, both type 1 and type 2, is a powerful risk factor for CAD. Diabetes accentuates the progression of atherosclerosis, and by age 55 years, almost 35% of men and women with type 1 diabetes die of CAD. The role of heredity is also unclear. Apparently a tendency toward hypertension, hyperlipidemia, and diabetes exists in some families. Whether the tendency is inherited or simply the result of lifestyle patterns is unknown. Oral contraceptives have been linked to CAD when taken by women age 45 years or younger. This finding results from studies that show high serum cholesterol and triglyceride levels in women taking oral contraceptives.[28]

PATHOPHYSIOLOGY

Atherosclerosis, the basic underlying disease affecting coronary lumen size, is marked by changes in the intimal lining of the arteries. It begins as an irregular thickening process producing fatty streaks. This becomes a more severe form, combining large amounts of lipids with collagen to produce fibroblasts that lead to fibrous atherosclerotic plaques.

The severity of the disease is measured by the degree of obstruction within each artery and the number of vessels involved. Obstructions exceeding 75% of the lumen of one or more of the three coronary arteries increase the risk of death. The annual death rate of persons with one-vessel disease is 1% to 3%. Three-vessel disease increases the risk to 10% to 15%. Among people with 75% obstruction of the left main artery, however, the annual death rate is 30% to 40%.

Myocardial Perfusion

The basic physiologic changes resulting from the atherosclerotic process are problems of myocardial oxygen supply and demand. When myocardial oxygen demand exceeds the supply provided by the coronary arteries, ischemia results. Myocardial metabolism is oxygen dependent (aerobic), extracting up to 80% of the oxygen from the coronary blood supply. Blood flow to the myocardium occurs mainly during diastole. Factors influencing supply include cardiac output, intramyocardial tension, aortic pressure, and coronary artery resistance. Coronary blood flow can be increased by raising the cardiac output and aortic pressure and lowering coronary artery resistance and intramyocardial tension.

Factors determining myocardial oxygen demand are heart rate, myocardial wall tension, and contractile state of the myocardium. As the heart rate increases, so does the demand for oxygen to the myocardial cells. Myocardial wall tension occurs during contraction and is influenced by ventricular and systolic (arterial) pressure. Myocardial contractility is stimulated by the release of catecholamines or sympathetic stimulation. These increase wall tension and thus energy or oxygen demands.

Myocardial ischemia is the result of impaired myocardial perfusion. Coronary atherosclerotic heart disease is the most common cause of myocardial ischemia. Obstruction varies in degree and may be well tolerated as long as myocardial oxygen demand is low. As the demand increases and the obstruction persists or advances, ischemia results. Coronary blood vessel distribution is also important in providing oxygen to the myocardium. The coronary arteries sit on the epicardial surface of the heart. Blood travels in toward the endocardium. The inner subendocardial layers of the myocardium therefore are particularly at risk for ischemia. Increases in heart rate and wall tension can reduce flow to the endocardium.

The coronary arteries also supply major conduction structures within the myocardium. The right coronary artery (RCA) supplies the sinus node in 55% to 60% of persons. In the remainder it is supplied by a branch of the circumflex artery. The RCA also supplies the AV node in 85% of persons. In the remaining 15% of persons the AV node is supplied by the left coronary artery (LCA). The septum is supplied mainly by the left anterior descending (LAD) artery, although part of the posterior wall is supplied by the RCA. An obstruction of any of the major arteries or their branches results in ischemia to the portion of myocardium supplied by that vessel. Obstruction of the LAD results in ischemic changes of the anterior wall of the ventricle. RCA obstruction results in infarction and ischemia of the right ventricle and the inferior wall of the left ventricle. The degree of obstruction and number of coronary arteries involved influence how serious the disease will be. CAD is described in terms of single-, double-, or triple-vessel disease. When a major obstruction occurs in the first branch of the LCA or the left main artery before bifurcation, the risk for a major infarction and death rises. This is called left main disease.

The major signs of ischemia are chest pain and ECG changes. Other symptoms result from compromised cardiac function.

Angina Pectoris

The term *angina pectoris,* which means chest pain, is used to describe pain as a symptom of myocardial ischemia. Myocardial ischemia is the result of an imbalance between myocardial oxygen supply and demand. It occurs most often with coronary atherosclerosis but can also occur in patients with normal coronary arteries. For example, patients with aortic stenosis, hypertension, and hypertrophic cardiomyopathy may have symptoms of angina pectoris. In these patients, myocardial work is increased, and perfusion of the hypertrophied muscle is inadequate. This results in myocardial ischemia despite normal coronary arteries.

Various terms have been used to describe the many types of angina. They are described here.

Stable angina pectoris is marked by predictable chest discomfort caused by effort, with or without radiation, that lasts from a few seconds to 15 minutes. It is generally relieved by rest and the removal of provoking factors or by sublingual vasodilators.

Unstable angina pectoris is marked by a change in a previous pattern of stable angina, that is, it comes on more easily, lasts longer, or is more frequent. It may occur at rest and may indicate progression of the underlying disease. Various names used to describe this syndrome include crescendo angina, preinfarction angina, and angina decubitus.

Variant (Prinzmetal's) angina is marked by chest pain that occurs at rest and is often linked to ST elevations on the ECG. The underlying cause is thought to be coronary artery spasm. Unlike stable angina, variant angina is caused by a sudden reduction in coronary blood flow brought on by the spasm and not by increased myocardial oxygen demand.

Anginal equivalents are symptoms other than chest pain that indicate myocardial ischemia and serve as angina surrogates. They include dyspnea, diaphoresis, and fatigue. Anginal equivalents are consistent within the same patient but vary from person to person and are most common in the elderly.

Acute Coronary Syndromes

Acute coronary syndromes are a cluster of clinical situations that include unstable angina, non–Q-wave infarction, and Q-wave infarction. They represent varying patterns of injury, resulting from the rupture of a "vulnerable" atherosclerotic plaque. Plaque rupture promotes platelet activation and thrombus generation, ultimately leading to thrombus formation and myocardial necrosis.

Myocardial Infarction

Myocardial infarction (MI) is the development of ischemia and necrosis of myocardial tissue. It results from a sudden decrease in coronary perfusion or an increase in myocardial oxygen demand without adequate coronary perfusion.

Two types of infarction have been described. Non–Q-wave (formerly known as subendocardial) infarction is generally confined to small areas of the myocardium. It is usually within the subendocardial wall of the left ventricle, the ventricular septum, or the papillary muscles and does not result in the development of a Q wave on the 12-lead ECG. A true Q-wave infarction (formerly known as a transmural or full-thickness infarction) is widespread myocardial necrosis, extending from the endocardium to the epicardium (FIG. 3-34). This damage is reflected on the 12-lead ECG with the appearance of Q waves in the leads reflecting electrical activation over the area of damage.

Myocardial tissue death is usually preceded by sudden occlusion of a major coronary artery. Coronary thrombosis is the most common cause of infarction, but other factors may be responsible. These include coronary artery spasm, platelet aggregation and embolism from a mural thrombus, a thrombus on a prosthetic mitral or aortic valve, or a dislodged calcium plaque from a calcified aortic or mitral valve.

Persistent cellular ischemia interferes with myocardial tissue metabolism, causing a rapid development of permanent cell damage. At first there are three zones of tissue damage. The first is a central area of necrotic myocardial cells, capillaries, and connective tissue. Surrounding this tissue is a second zone of "injured" cells that are potentially viable if enough circulation is quickly restored. The third zone, characterized by ischemia, is also viable and can be expected to recover unless the ischemia persists or worsens. The severity or extension of an MI often depends on the fate of the injured and ischemic zones. Ischemia may progress to necrosis if untreated. Because the infarction process may take up to 6 hours to complete, restoration of adequate myocardial perfusion is important to limit necrosis.

DIAGNOSTIC STUDIES AND FINDINGS

See Diagnostic Studies and Findings table.

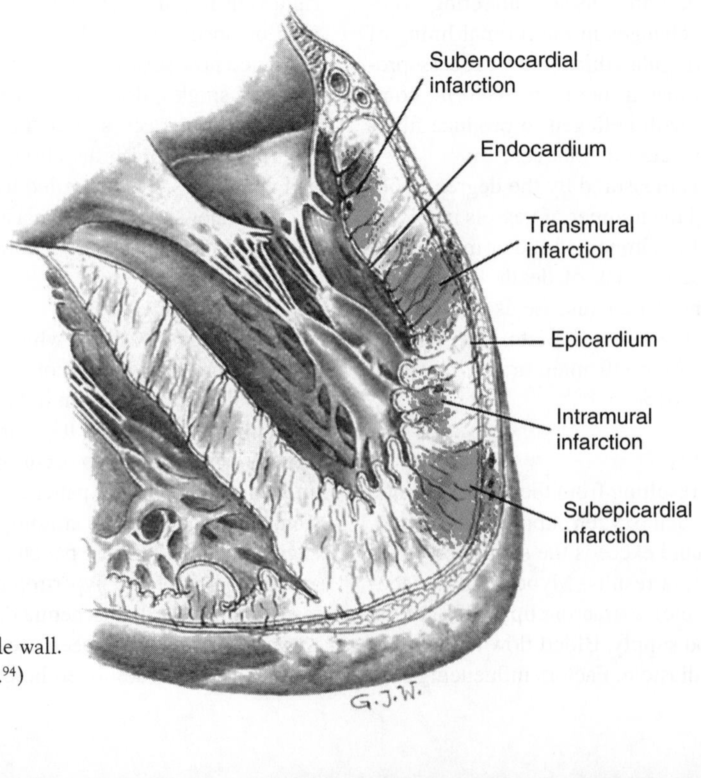

FIG. 3-34
Location of infarctions in ventricle wall. (From Thelan, Urden, and Davie.[94])

Diagnostic Studies and Findings

Study	Stable Angina Pectoris	Variant (Prinzmetal's) Angina	Unstable Angina Pectoris	Myocardial Infarction
ECG	Changes usually seen during anginal episodes; 50%-70% of patients have normal ECG during pain-free episodes; ischemia determined by horizontal ST segment or downsloping with depression of 1 mm; T wave inversion represents impaired depolarization caused by ischemia	Ischemia appears as ST elevation during anginal attack but regresses as pain subsides; ECG changes may be seen before patient complains of chest pain or may be recorded in absence of pain; AV conduction defects may occur, particularly when RCA is involved, and include Mobitz type II and compete AV block; ventricular irritability such as premature ventricular contractions, ventricular tachycardia, or fibrillation can occur, particularly during ischemic attack	Ischemia determined by horizontal ST segment or downsloping with depression of 1 mm; T wave inversion represents impaired repolarization caused by ischemia; ventricular irritability such as premature ventricular contractions, ventricular tachycardia, or fibrillation	Changes are evolutionary and indicate progression of infarction; in acute stage, ST elevations with subsequent T wave inversion and Q wave formation; Q waves indicate necrosis and are considered pathologic if they are 0.04 sec or greater in duration, 0.4 mm or greater in depth, or present in leads that do not normally have Q waves; ST elevations reflect myocardial injury that interferes with polarization of cells are seen in leads facing injured area, and return to normal (isoelectric) within days; ST elevations beyond 4-6 wk should raise suspicion of ventricular aneurysm; infarction location determined by identifying leads that demonstrate characteristic ECG changes; such leads are those with positive terminals that face injured site of heart; reciprocal changes, seen in leads that face *opposite* surface of damaged heart, are absence of Q wave, increase in R wave amplitude, depressed ST segment, upright tall T wave; RVMI: ST elevation in right precordial leads (V_3R to V_6R); V_4R may be most sensitive and predictive
Laboratory tests				
Enzymes	No elevation; checked to rule out MI	No elevation; checked to rule out MI	No elevation; checked to rule out MI	See table on p. 60
Complete blood count (CBC)	No elevation; checked to rule out anemia-induced angina	No elevation; checked to rule out anemia-induced angina	No elevation; check to rule out anemia-induced angina	May see slight elevation of white blood count (WBC) and erythrocyte sedimentation rate (ESR).
Glucose	No elevation	No elevation	No elevation	Transiently elevated owing to adrenergic response
Lipid levels (triglycerides, cholesterol, high- and low-density lipids)	Checked to determine any lipoprotein abnormalities	Checked to determine any lipoprotein abnormalities	Checked to determine any lipoprotein abnormalities	Checked to determine any lipoprotein abnormalities
Exercise stress test (EST)	Chest pain; horizontal ST segment or downsloping of 1 mm or more; failure of systolic blood pressure to rise or drop; ST elevations	Normal stress test done to differentiate between variant and classic angina; ST elevation with or without associated chest pain occasionally develops	As in stable angina pectoris; should not be done until patient has been stable and pain free for 24 h	Not done in presence of documented MI; low-level test may be performed before discharge from hospital
Thallium-201 scintigraphy	Ischemic areas appear as "cold" areas, reflecting reduced thallium uptake; when ischemia relieved, "cold" areas show normal thallium uptake		Similar to stable angina pectoris	Similar to stable angina pectoris; used to confirm diagnosis; with decreased blood flow an area of decreased activity is visualized

Continued

Diagnostic Studies and Findings—cont'd

Study	Stable Angina Pectoris	Variant (Prinzmetal's) Angina	Unstable Angina Pectoris	Myocardial Infarction
Radionuclide blood pool imaging with technetium-99m				Confirms myocardial damage by localizing and permitting estimation of size of transmural infarction; must be done within 2-6 days after acute infarction; determines wall motion abnormalities; permits estimation of ventricular function by determining ejection fractions
Cardiac catheterization and coronary angiography	Determines number and location of obstructive lesions, condition of artery distal to obstructive lesion, and ventricular function	Distinguishes spasm in normal coronary arteries from those with severe obstructive lesions; intravenous injection or ergonovine maleate provokes coronary artery spasm in patients with variant angina	As in stable angina pectoris	Generally not performed as diagnostic procedure during acute period; performed as part of percutaneous angioplasty

Enzyme Laboratory Test for Myocardial Infarction

Serum Marker	Positive Level	Begins to Rise (Hours)	Peak (Hours)*	Return to Normal (Days)
CK-MB	0-5μg/L	4-6	10-24	2-3
Troponin T (aTnT)	0.1-0.2 μg/L	3-5	10-24	5-14
Troponin I (aTnI)	1.5-3.1 μg/L	3-5	14-18	5-9
Myoglobin	Serum levels double with q2 h serial samples	2-3	3-15	0.5-1

CK-MB, Creatine kinase, myocardial-bound.

*Lack of standardized upper reference levels account for variations in values.

Multidisciplinary Plan

Surgery

Coronary artery bypass grafting (CABG): Only direct method of increasing myocardial coronary blood flow; provides symptomatic relief in 80% of patients with significant angina and has low operative mortality

Indications: Persistent angina that is refractory to medical therapy or a catheter-based intervention, high-risk coronary anatomy (left main stenosis), and significant obstructive lesions in all three coronary arteries (p. 120 describes care of patients undergoing open-heart surgery)

Interventional Catheter-Based Therapy

Percutaneous transluminal coronary angioplasty (PTCA): Attempts to restore luminal patency by compressing atheromatous plaques with balloon inflation inside the vessel. The deployment of a stent may further ensure long-term patency.

Atherectomy: Interventional devices to revascularize stenotic coronary arteries include directional atherectomy, rotational atherectomy, and laser angioplasty. These devices may be used alone or in combination with balloon angioplasty for access to more complex lesions and prevention of restenosis (see p. 135).

Enhanced External Counterpulsation (EECP)

EECP is a noninvasive method for alleviating myocardial ischemia by increasing aortic blood pressure during diastole and reducing pressure in systole. This is done by sequential pneumatic compression and decompression of the lower limbs and buttocks through the inflation and deflation of a series of large cuffs that are wrapped around the patient's lower body. The physiologic rationale of EECP is based on augmented perfusion to the myocardium during diastole and reduction of myocardial oxygen consumption (MVO_2) during systole. It is hypothesized that it aids in the development of collateral coronary blood vessels. The therapy is generally delivered in a course of 35 1-hour sessions administered five times a week. Research supports the reduction in anginal symptoms for 4 to 7 years after therapy in patients with angina refractory to conventional medical management.[64] Further investigations are currently under way to define the role of this therapy in chronic stable angina.

Experimental Interventions

Medical/molecular bypass or therapeutic angiogenesis: The transfer of genetically engineered growth factors to stimulate endothelial cell growth and development of collateral blood vessels. One such angiogenic substance is referred to as vascular endothelial growth factor (VEGF)[36,49] and is currently under investigation for patients with New York Heart Association (NYHA) functional class III/IV refractory angina.

Transmyocardial revascularization (TMR): Laser beams are used to drill channels in ischemic areas of the myocardium. Originally the procedure involved open heart surgery. It is now experimentally performed percutaneously with the arterial insertion of a fiberoptic laser catheter and is referred to as percutaneous myocardial revascularization (PMR).[77] Several tiny holes are formed in the left ventricular wall, allowing increased blood flow to the myocardium. Although the channels tend to occlude, early relief of angina is achieved. This palliative procedure is reserved for patients with severe disease refractory to conventional therapy.

Medications

Thrombolytics (intravenous thrombolysis): Pharmacologic reperfusion therapy used in the treatment of acute transmural MI; purpose is to interrupt the evolution of myocardial ischemia to necrosis and to limit infarction size; most improvement of ischemic area can be achieved if therapy is initiated within 4-6 h of onset of infarction (p. 137 describes care of patients undergoing thrombolytic therapy)

Indications: Recommended in all patients with MI demonstrated by ST segment elevation (>1 mm in two contiguous leads) or new left bundle branch block who present within 12 h of the onset of symptoms

Vasodilators

Nitrates

Intravenous nitroglycerin: Start continuous controlled infusion of 10-20 μg/min and increase by 5 μg/min every 5-10 min to control symptoms or decrease mean arterial blood pressure

Short-acting nitrates: Sublingual nitroglycerin (0.4-0.6 mg); isosorbide dinitrate (5 mg) PO

Duration of action: 30 min–2 h

Long-acting oral nitrates: Isosorbide dinitrate, 10-20 mg qid

Topical 2% nitroglycerin ointment, 1-2 inches q4-6h

Duration of action: Up to 6 h or longer

Beta-adrenergic blocking agents

Propranolol (Inderal)

Usual dosage: 10-20 mg PO tid or qid; IV 1 mg/min not exceeding 3-5 mg

Metoprolol (Lopressor)]

Indications: Early treatment for MI

Usual dosage: IV bolus 5 mg q2-3 min, then 50 mg PO q6 for 48h, maintenance dose 100 mg/day; increase as needed to max of 450 mg/day

Nadolol (Corgard)

Indications: Treatment of angina and hypertension

Usual dosage: 40-80 mg PO up to 240 mg/day as necessary

Duration of action: About 20-24 h

Timolol (Blocadren)

Indications: Reduction of mortality and reinfarction after MI; hypertension

Usual dosage: 20-60 mg bid PO

Atenolol (Tenormin)

Indications: Approved for use of hypertension but may have potential use in treating angina and reducing infarction size

Usual dosage: 50-100 mg/day PO

Angiotensin-converting enzyme (ACE) inhibitors: Reduces mortality after MI by preventing progressive ventricular enlargement, thereby preventing complications such as congestive heart failure; also thought to prevent future infarctions

Captopril (Capoten)

Usual dosage: 6.25-100 mg tid PO

Enalapril maleate (Vasotec)

Usual dosage: 2.5-20 mg bid PO

Calcium channel blockers: Calcium channel blockers have not proven beneficial in the treatment or prevention of acute MI; they are useful in the treatment of some angina, hypertension, and arrhythmia management

Nifedipine (Procardia)

Indications: Angina pectoris caused by coronary artery spasm, chronic stable angina pectoris

Usual dosage: 10 mg PO; sublingual 10-40 mg q8h (not to exceed 180 mg)

Verapamil (Calan, Isoptin)

Indications: Treatment of angina pectoris and coronary artery spasm

Usual dosage: 80-160 mg PO q8h (not to exceed 480 mg/day); IV 0.075-0.15 mg/kg (not to exceed 15 mg/30 min)

Diltiazem (Cardizem)

Indications: Treatment of variant angina

Usual dosage: Initially 30 mg PO qid, increasing gradually to 80 mg tid (total 240 mg/day)

Antihyperlipidemic agents: Interfere with reabsorption of cholesterol and lower triglyceride levels; HMC-CoA reductase inhibitors reduce cholesterol synthesis and lower LDL cholesterol; two subtypes of these drugs called statins are available; natural or fermentation–derived statins are lovastatin, pravastatin, and simvastatin (dosages listed below); synthetic statins are also available and include atorvastatin and fluvastatin; all are oral agents

Simvastatin (Zocor)

Usual dosage: 5-40 mg qhs

Pravastatin (Pravachol)

Usual dosage: 20-40 mg qhs

Lovastatin (Mevacor)

Usual dosage: 10-80 mg/day with meals

The following agents interfere with the absorption of cholesterol and triglycerides:

Cholestyramine (Questran)

Usual dosage: 4-8 g bid

Neomycin sulfate

Usual dosage: 0.5-2 g/day

Clofibrate (Atromid-S)

Usual dosage: 500 mg tid

Gemfibrozil (Lopid)

Usual dosage: 600 mg bid

Niacin (nicotinic acid)

Usual dosage: 1-2 g tid with meals

Anticoagulants

Heparin

Indications: Unfractionated intravenous heparin in acute-setting MI to aid lysis of existing clot and prevent thrombus formation; adjunctive therapy for patients undergoing reperfusion therapy with alteplase; low-molecular-weight heparin for patients with non-ST elevation MI; exact dosages and indications in the setting of acute MI remain under current clinical investigation

Usual IV dosage: Unfractionated heparin dose is a weight-adjusted bolus of 70 U/kg followed by 15 U/kg/h as a continuous infusion to maintain a PTT 1.5 to 2 times normal or a range of 50-75 sec

Usual subcutaneous unfractionated dosage: Enoxaparin 1 mg/kg bid; therapeutic levels not monitored with standard bleeding parameters

Antiplatelet/Platelet-blocking agents

Aspirin (acetylsalicylic acid, ASA)

Indications: Used in setting of acute coronary artery thrombosis and in the prevention of further atherogenesis; because of beneficial effects, used in patients with acute coronary syndromes and MI

Usual dosage: 325-1300 mg/day PO

Ticlopidine (Ticlid)

Indications: Inhibits platelet aggregation 24-48 h after administration; reduces vascular death in MI patients with unstable angina; neutropenia is a serious side effect when treatment is continued more than 2 wk

Usual dosage: 250 mg/bid with food PO

Clopidogrel (Plavix)

Indications: Also inhibits platelets but without the neutropenic side effects

Usual dosage: 75 mg/day PO

Abciximab (ReoPro)

Glycoprotein IIb/IIIa receptor antagonist that deactivates platelets

Indications: Catheter-based coronary revascularization procedures in which there is a threat to abrupt vessel closure

Usual dosage: 0.25 mg/kg IV bolus administered at the start of the procedure, followed by a continuous infusion of 0.125 μg/kg/min for 12 h

Magnesium sulfate

Indications: Correction of documented magnesium (and/or potassium) deficits; treatment of torsades de pointes type of VT associated with a prolonged QT interval; data to support standard magnesium administration in the setting of an acute MI not available

Usual dosage: 2 g over 1-2 min, followed by an infusion of 3-20 mg/min

General Management

Cardiovascular monitoring: Used to assess and monitor for signs of life-threatening complications associated with severe myocardial ischemia and necrosis, including dysrhythmias, heart failure, extension of MI, cardiogenic shock (p. 126, ventricular or papillary muscle rupture, and ventricular aneurysm; complications occur within first 3 to 5 days in half of patients with acute MI; early detection depends on careful and frequent continuous monitoring of various hemodynamic parameters and clinical status that reflect left ventricular function: arterial pressure, pulmonary artery pressure (PAP), pulmonary capillary wedge pressure (PCWP).

ECG: Used to determine serial changes reflective of myocardial ischemia, injury, or extension of MI and to detect changes in heart rhythms.

Intraaortic balloon counterpulsation (IABP): Used mainly in patients with acute MI to protect ischemic myocardium by decreasing preload, afterload, and myocardial oxygen demand; diastolic pressure is supported, thus improving coronary perfusion and cardiac output; most successful in patients who are treated less than 6 hours after infarction, are undergoing their first MI, and have no aortic insufficiency (p. 130 describes specific care).

Admission to coronary care unit (CCU) or coronary observation unit: Indicated for patients with unstable acute coronary syndromes, MI monitoring, and treatment.

Admission diet: Depends on clinical status; during acute phase, patient may be permitted nothing by mouth (NPO).

Discharge diet: Depends on several factors, including cholesterol and triglyceride levels, total body weight, and clinical status; American Heart Association suggests diet of reduced saturated fats and cholesterol, restriction of sodium, and limiting total caloric consumption to maintain ideal body weight.[5]

Activity: Bed rest with bedside commode until the patient is 24 hours without chest pain, progressing to monitored activity and return to activities of daily living (ADLs); progressive cardiac rehabilitation recommended 4 weeks after discharge.

Oxygenation: Patients evaluated early for hypoxemia, which may result from ventilation/perfusion abnormalities; providing additional inspired oxygen to patient in absence of hypoxemia does not ensure increased oxygen delivery to myocardium. Arterial oxygen saturation by pulse oximetry should be measured on admission to coronary care unit; if normal, oxygen therapy may be omitted; hypoxemic patients should receive oxygen therapy as required; intermittent or continuous pulse oximetry and arterial blood gas determinations as indicated by clinical picture to monitor effectiveness of therapy.

NURSING CARE

NURSING ASSESSMENT

See Assessment Considerations table.

Assessment Considerations

Area of Concern	Stable Angina Pectoris	Variant (Prinzmetal's) Angina	Unstable Angina Pectoris	Myocardial Infarction
Chest pain				
Quality	Aching, sharp, tingling, or burning sensation or pressure	Similar to stable angina pectoris	Similar to stable angina pectoris but may be more severe	Crushing, squeezing, stabbing, oppressive sensation or as if heavy object is sitting on chest
Location and radiation	Substernal with radiation to left shoulder, down inner aspect of left arm or both arms; neck, jaw, and scapula may be additional sites of radiation	Similar to stable angina pectoris	Similar to stable angina pectoris	Substernal with radiation to left shoulder, down inner aspect of left arm or both arms; neck, jaw, and scapula may be additional sites of radiation
Precipitating factors	Onset classically associated with exercise or activities that increase myocardial oxygen demand, e.g., physical exercise, heavy lifting, emotional stress, cold temperatures	Onset at rest; pain is cyclic, often occurring during sleep	Pain may be brought on with less than usual exertion; may occur at rest	May occur at rest or during exertion
Duration and alleviating factors	3-15 min; relieved by rest, stopping pain-inducing activities, taking sublingual nitroglycerin (NTG) tablet	Characteristically, pain intensifies quickly, tends to last longer than angina, and subsides with exercise	Prolonged and not usually as quickly relieved by rest or taking NTG	Described as continuous, lasting more than 30 min, unrelieved by rest, position change, or taking NTG tablets
Associated signs and symptoms	During anginal attack, dyspnea, anxiety, diaphoresis, cool clammy skin	Similar to stable angina pectoris	Similar to stable angina pectoris but symptoms may be more prominent and may persist; may be associated with nausea	Anxiety, restlessness, weakness, associated profuse diaphoresis, dyspnea, dizziness; signs of vasomotor response including nausea, vomiting, faintness, and cold clammy skin; hiccups and other gastrointestinal distress may be present; low-grade temperature elevations common for first 24-48 h but may last several days (this is inflammatory response to myocardial tissue damage)

Continued

Assessment Considerations—cont'd

Area of Concern	Stable Angina Pectoris	Variant (Prinzmetal's) Angina	Unstable Angina Pectoris	Myocardial Infarction
Physical examination	Normal during asymptomatic periods; during anginal attacks, increased heart rate, pulsus alternans, and transient abnormal findings including precordial bulge and atrial and ventricular gallops (S_3, S_4)	Similar to stable angina pectoris	Similar to stable angina pectoris; may also demonstrate irregular pulse, hypertension, or signs of left ventricular dysfunction	May be unremarkable unless signs of ventricular failure or cardiogenic shock are present; blood pressure normal, elevated, or decreased (initially elevated when pain is present but usually decreases for first few days); respirations: Cheyne-Stokes respiration owing to central nervous system hypoperfusion or opiate therapy; initial tachypnea returns to normal once pain subsides; heart sounds: S_3, S_4 gallops indicative of ventricular dysfunction; systolic murmurs reflecting papillary muscle dysfunction; diminished heart sounds and pericardial friction rub may occur; with left ventricular dysfunction: pulmonary rales, decreased urine output, increased amplitude of a wave in jugular vein; with right ventricular dysfunction: increased jugular venous distention, peripheral edema, liver tenderness; pulse often within normal limits; bradycardia present with inferior wall MI; tachycardia with rates greater than 100 beats/min may reflect compromised ventricle

Potential Complications

Arrhythmias; heart failure; cardiogenic shock; papillary muscle or ventricular septal rupture; ventricular aneurysm and/or clot formation; pericarditis; ventricular rupture

! EMERGENCY ALERT

CARDIAC ARREST

Complete cessation of systemic circulation; patient is unconscious, apneic, pale, or cyanotic; pulses are absent

Assessment

- Airway patency
- Breathing effectiveness, chest rise and fall, spontaneous respiration
- Circulation: Are femoral or carotid pulses present?

Interventions

- Perform basic life support.
- Call emergency medical services (EMS).
- Clear airway using jaw-thrust or chin-lift maneuver.
- Suction patient and remove foreign body if present.
- Assist ventilations using mouth-to-mouth or bag-valve-mask assistance.
- Administer high-flow oxygen by mask (10-15 L).
- Perform external cardiac compressions, 80-100/min, at 15:2 compression/breath ratio.
- Prepare for in-hospital defibrillation and emergency care.

Patient Problems/Nursing Diagnoses & Interventions

NIC Physical Comfort Promotion

Acute pain (chest) related to imbalance of myocardial oxygen supply and demand

Acute care

- Assess and record description of pain and response to prescribed interventions.
- Assess baseline and 12-lead ECG with pain and after intervention.
- Assess and report signs of decreased cardiac output: decreased blood pressure, increased heart rate, decreased urine output, fatigue, and cool clammy skin.
- Assess for signs and symptoms of fear and anxiety: verbalizations, restlessness, insomnia, irritability, facial expression, and noncompliance.
- Stop angina-inducing activity.
- Maintain bed rest *to reduce myocardial oxygen demand.*
- Administer drug therapy as ordered *to relieve pain;* assess and record response.
- Administer oxygen therapy as ordered *to increase oxygen supply to myocardium.*
- Obtain 12-lead ECG *to document ischemia during chest pain episode.*
- Monitor vital signs frequently throughout episode of chest pain.
- Avoid activities and stimulants that increase vasoconstriction.

Convalescent care

- Administer long-acting nitrates and beta-blockers as ordered.
- Encourage activities commensurate with patient's physical abilities and anginal threshold.

NIC Tissue Perfusion Management

Decreased cardiac output related to loss of myocardial contractility

Acute care

- Maintain bed rest *to reduce myocardial oxygen demand.*
- Monitor ECG for dysrhythmias and alterations.
- Maintain IV as ordered with 5% glucose in water for drug administration.
- Administer drug therapy as ordered.
- Auscultate breath sounds and heart tones every 1 to 4 hours.
- Monitor vital signs and hemodynamic parameters as indicated: arterial pressure, pulmonary artery pressure, PCWP, and central venous pressure (CVP) *to detect signs and symptoms of myocardial dysfunction.*

Convalescent care

- Monitor for early complications: hypotension, dysrhythmias, heart failure, and heart rupture.
- Begin progressive ambulation as patient's condition stabilizes.
- Restrict sodium intake as ordered.
- Monitor intake and output closely *to detect and prevent circulatory overload.*

NIC Coping Assistance

Anxiety related to perceived or actual threat to biologic integrity

- Offer reassurance during episodes of pain.
- Initiate comfort measures such as a quiet, restful environment and relaxation techniques.
- Administer sedation as ordered.
- Stay with patient as much as possible.
- Use a calm, reassuring voice.
- Allow family members to assist patient if possible.
- Explain all procedures and routine care as they occur.
- Encourage expression of feelings.

NIC Activity and Exercise Management

Activity intolerance related to imbalance of oxygen supply and demand

Acute care

- Maintain bed rest *to reduce myocardial workload and increase oxygenation.*
- Increase activities as ordered, using ECG changes, heart rate, blood pressure, and patient's clinical status (e.g., complicated versus uncomplicated MI) as guidelines. Bed or tub baths cause fewer hemodynamic and postural changes than showers. Backrubs may have a soothing effect.
- Allow patient out of bed for toileting because this does not seem to have adverse effects.
- Perform passive range-of-motion (ROM) exercise *to prevent thromboembolism,* progressing to active ROM exercises.

Convalescent care

- Begin phase I rehabilitation; refer to Patient Education/Continuum of Care Plan.
- Teach necessity for increasing activity gradually at home while continuing periods of rest.

Patient Education/Continuum of Care Plan

1. Explain the disease process, risk factors involved, methods of modification, associated symptoms, and actions to take when the symptoms occur. Associated complications are irregular heartbeats, chest pain, and shortness of breath.
2. Explain the name, purpose, side effects, and method of administration of all drugs.
3. Explain activity allowances and limitations, including the patient's return to work, resumption of sexual activity, and need to avoid or modify activity after heavy meals and alcohol consumption and in periods of emotional stress or extremes of temperatures.
4. Refer the patient to a rehabilitation program to assist with a progressive increase in activity levels.
5. Teach the patient to avoid foods high in sodium, saturated fats, and triglycerides. Teach good nutritional habits and alternative ways of seasoning food to avoid cooking with salt and salt products.
6. Explain importance of controlling any coexisting condition that may aggravate recovery, such as hypertension, obesity, and diabetes.

PHASES OF CARDIAC REHABILITATION

Phase I: Inpatient activities; anywhere from 4 to 16 stages; patient should be at 3-5 metabolic equivalents of tasks (METs) at discharge
Phase II: Begins with discharge and continues until healing has been completed; patient is evaluated with a stress test that is symptom limited
Phase III: Begins 4-6 wk after MI or surgery; training phase; patient exercises 2-5 times a week under supervision for usually 12 wk; patient should be able to perform at 10 METs or greater at the end of this phase
Phase IV: A maintenance phase of indefinite length; begins at the end of the training phase and continues for another 3-6 months (some believe it continues for the patient's lifetime); patient maintains level of training by exercising 2-3 times a week; stress tests usually done at yearly intervals to measure effectiveness and amend exercise prescription

Modified from Guzzetta and Dassey.[44]

Evaluation/Patient Outcomes

Physical Comfort Promotion: Patient is free from chest pain. Patient verbalizes absence of pain. Blood pressure and heart rate are within normal limits. Patient engages in hospital routines and activities without pain. Patient appears relaxed and expresses a sense of calm.

Tissue Perfusion Management: Cardiac output is improved or maintained. ECG, vital signs, and urine output are within normal limits.

Coping Assistance: Anxiety level is reduced. Patient appears relaxed.

Activity and Exercise Management: Activity level is improved. Patient verbalizes ability to perform ADLs without difficulty. ECG, blood pressure, and heart rate are within acceptable limits.

Congestive Heart Failure

Congestive heart failure (CHF) is a complex clinical syndrome that results from the heart's inability to increase cardiac output sufficiently to meet the body's metabolic demands (Fig. 3-35).

Congestive heart failure occurs as a result of myocardial damage. It is estimated that 3 million Americans suffer from CHF and that up to 35,000 will die from this chronic disorder.[1]

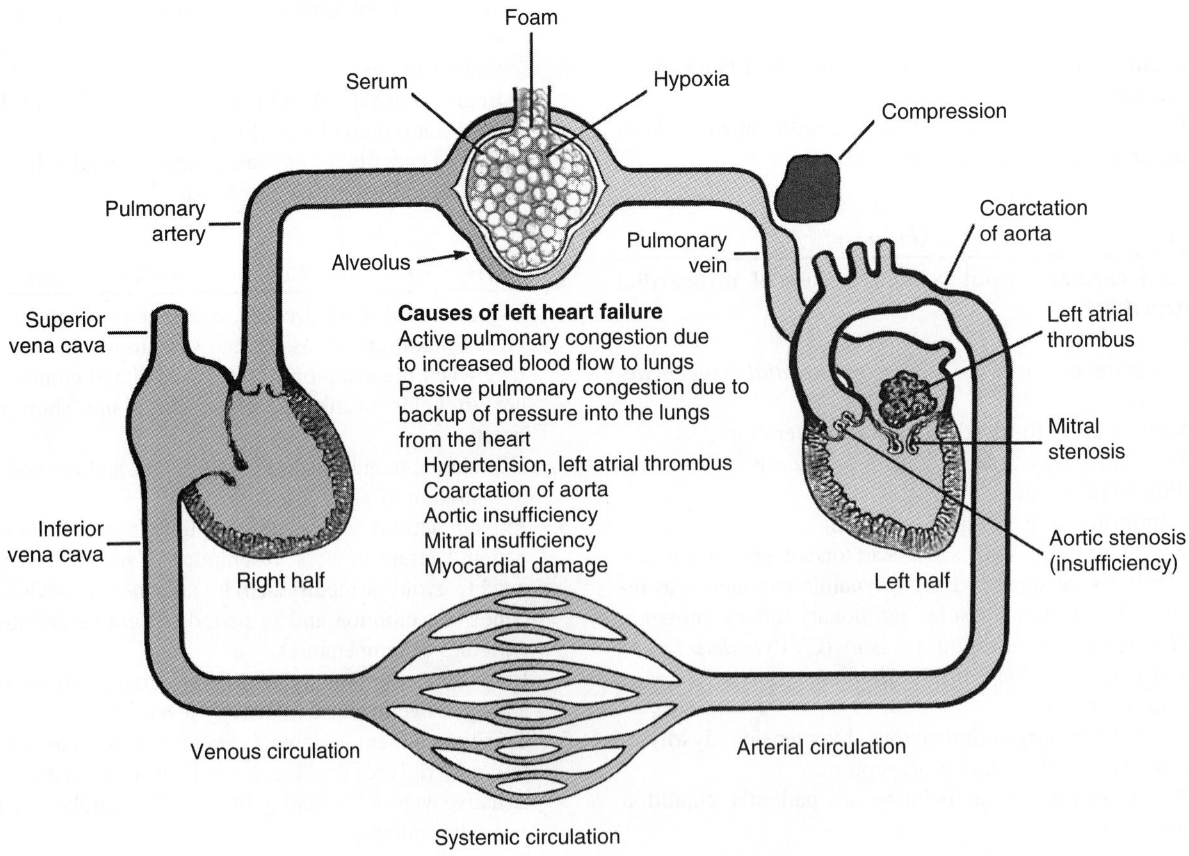

Fig. 3-35
Congestive heart failure. (From Canobbio.[15])

PATHOPHYSIOLOGY

The underlying causes of CHF vary, but the ultimate result is the heart's inability to act as an effective pump. Decreased myocardial contractility may result from a primary disorder or an excessive workload placed on the heart, such as systemic hypertension or a valvular disorder. Causes of primary myocardial disorders and disorders that increase the heart's workload are summarized as follows:

- Causes of decreased myocardial contractility
  - Coronary artery disease
  - Myocarditis
  - Cardiomyopathies
    - Dilated
    - Restrictive
    - Hypertrophic
  - Infiltrative diseases
    - Amyloidosis
    - Tumors
    - Sarcoidosis
  - Collagen-vascular diseases
    - Systemic lupus erythematosus
    - Scleroderma
  - Iatrogenic factors: Drugs such as beta-blockers, calcium antagonists, alcohol
- Causes of increased myocardial workload
  - Hypertension
  - Pulmonary hypertension
  - Valvular heart disease
    - Aortic or pulmonic stenosis
    - Mitral, tricuspid, or aortic insufficiency
  - Intracardiac shunting
  - High-output states
    - Anemia
    - Hyperthyroidism
    - Beriberi
    - Arteriovenous fistula

Disorders that interfere with the normal stretch of the ventricle, thereby decreasing ventricular filling, cause a drop in cardiac output. Pericardial tamponade and constrictive pericarditis are examples. Persistent tachydysrhythmias reduce ventricular filling time, and marked bradydysrhythmias greatly reduce cardiac output because the ventricles cannot augment the stroke volume. Loss of coordinated atrial contraction, as occurs in atrial fibrillation, can decrease cardiac output, probably because of loss of the atrial "kick" that contributes to normal ventricular filling.

The primary dysfunction in CHF is decreased myocardial contractility. However, secondary changes in preload and afterload also contribute to heart failure. Heart failure can be divided into left- and right-sided ventricular failure; these two types can occur independently or together.

Left Ventricular Heart Failure

Any sustained elevation in left ventricular end-diastolic pressure (LVEDP) increases left atrial pressure. This is transmitted to the pulmonary vascular bed and is manifest as an increase in PCWP. If the PCWP exceeds the colloid osmotic pressure of the pulmonary capillaries, transudation of fluid into the interstitial spaces and eventually into alveolar spaces will occur. This leads to hypoxia (resulting from poor oxygen exchange) and clinically to dyspnea, cough, orthopnea, and paroxysmal nocturnal dyspnea.

Right Ventricular Heart Failure

Right-sided heart failure may occur as a primary disorder of the right ventricle, as in tricuspid regurgitation, in right ventricular myocardial infarction (RVMI), or as a result of cor pulmonale. Persistent elevation of LVEDP eventually leads to right-sided failure marked by venous congestion in the systemic circulation. Distended neck veins, hepatomegaly, and dependent edema occur.

DIAGNOSTIC STUDIES AND FINDINGS

Electrolytes: Hyponatremia owing to water retention; urinary sodium loss in response to diuretics; hypokalemia from excessive use of diuretics or as secondary manifestation of aldosteronism; hypochloremia as a result of diuretic therapy; metabolic acidosis or alkalosis

Blood chemistry: Blood urea nitrogen (BUN) and creatinine increase with decreased glomerular filtration; liver function values (serum glutamate oxaloacetate transaminase [SGOT], bilirubin, alkaline phosphatase) mildly increased from passive liver engorgement; can also prolong prothrombin time; glucose levels can be elevated because of stress

Arterial blood gases: Hypoxemia; decreased oxygen saturation; (early) mild respiratory alkalosis; (late) hypercarbia, hypoxia

Urine studies: Urine output decreased; metabolic acidosis or alkalosis; specific gravity 1.010: excessive fluid intake, 1.035: decreased fluid intake; proteinuria; glucosuria

Pulmonary function tests: Reduced vital capacity; reduced total lung capacity; increased residual volume

Chest x-ray (FIGS. 3-36 and 3-37): Increased pulmonary congestion: redistribution of pulmonary blood flow, interstitial edema (intraseptal edema—Kerley-B lines; perivascular edema), alveolar edema, pleural effusion; (early) little or no change in size or contour of cardiac silhouette; (late) increased cardiothoracic ratio

ECG: Changes reflect primary disorders as well as chronic changes from compensation of heart failure: left ventricular hypertrophy (LVH), right ventricular hypertrophy (RVH), atrial hypertrophy, tachycardia, dysrhythmias; frequently, atrial fibrillation and ventricular tachycardia present; VT is the cause of death in 50% of patients with end-stage heart failure

Echocardiogram (FIG. 3-38): Increased or decreased ventricular chambers or structures reflect primary disorder; left ventricular failure: increased LVEDP (5.6 cm), decreased wall motion; two-dimensional echocardiography with Doppler flow studies provides an estimate of left ventricular ejection fraction (LVEF), which is the most important measurement in the assessment of heart failure; measuring LVEF is the primary method for distinguishing patients with systolic dysfunction from those with other causes of heart failure, including diastolic dysfunction; also used to predict prognosis based

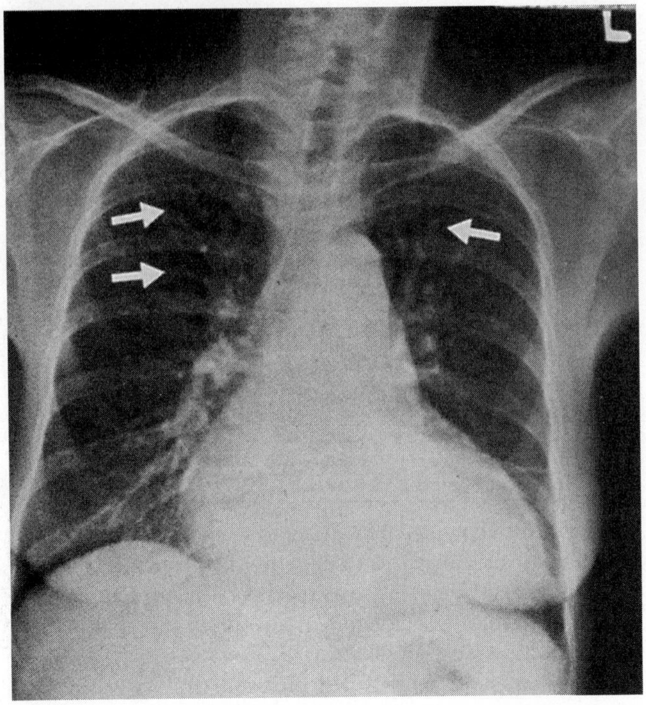

FIG. 3-36
Pulmonary congestion. Upper lobe distention *(arrows)*. Enlarged cardiac silhouette. (Courtesy Batra P, Department of Radiology, UCLA School of Medicine, Los Angeles. From Michaelson CR, editor: *Congestive heart failure*, St. Louis, 1983, Mosby.)

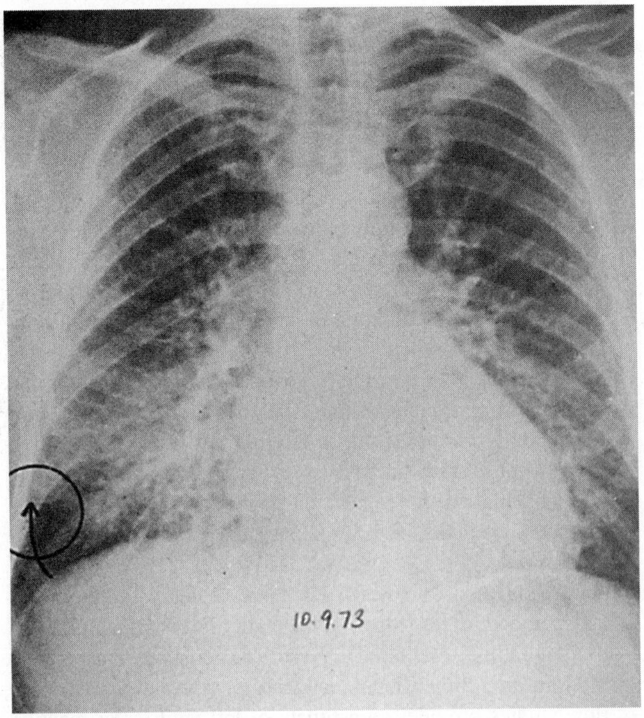

FIG. 3-37
Interstitial edema. Hilar areas are blurred and hazy. Cardiac silhouette is enlarged. Fluid collected within intralobular septa of lungs is visible as Kerley-B lines *(arrow)*. (Courtesy Batra P, Department of Radiology, UCLA School of Medicine, Los Angeles.)

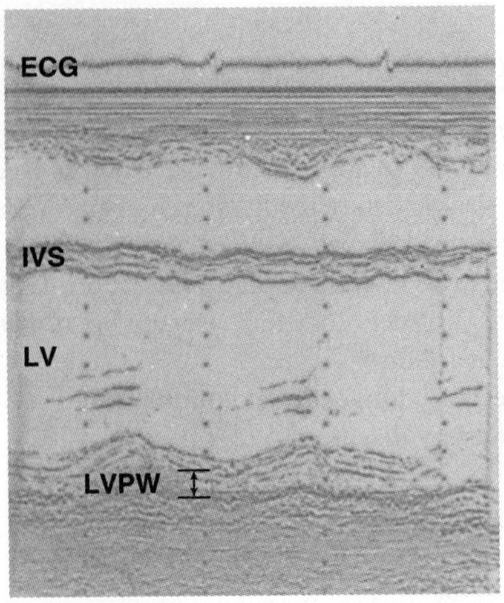

FIG. 3-38
Patient with dilated left ventricle (6.7 cm) and normal intraventricular septum (1 cm). (Courtesy Non Invasive Labs, Division of Cardiology, UCLA School of Medicine, Los Angeles.)

on etiology and determine response to therapeutic interventions

Radionuclide angiography (scintigraphy): Nuclear cardiac images can be acquired using a special high count–rate camera that images an intravenous tracer element (e.g., technetium 99m) injected into the patient's bloodstream; images can calculate left and right ventricular ejection fractions and determine adequacy of myocardial perfusion; a useful but high-cost alternative to an echocardiogram for determining ejection fraction in patients with congestive heart failure

Hemodynamic monitoring (right heart catheterization): Left ventricular failure: elevated PCWP and pulmonary artery diastolic pressure (PADP), decreased cardiac output, decreased ejection fractions; right ventricular failure: elevated pulmonary artery pressure (PAP), right ventricular pressure, and right atrial pressure (RAP)

MULTIDISCIPLINARY PLAN

Surgery

Directed by underlying condition; mortality is greater among patients with left ventricular dysfunction

Coronary revascularization

Dynamic cardiomyoplasty

Cardiac transplantation may be considered as an option for end-stage myocardial dysfunction

Medications

Diuretics: Reduce sodium retention by inhibiting the reabsorption of sodium or chloride at specific sites in the renal tubules

Thiazide diuretics (hydrochlorothiazide): May be used for mild volume overload

Usual oral dosage: 25-50 mg

Loop diuretics: Used for more severe volume overload or persistent edema despite thiazide diuretics
Usual oral dosage:
Furosemide (Lasix): 10-40 mg qd to 240 mg bid
Bumetanide (Bumex): 0.5-1.0 mg qd to 10 mg qd
Ethacrynic acid (Edecrin): 50 mg qd to 200 mg bid
Potassium-sparing diuretics: May be more effective than oral potassium supplements at maintaining total body potassium stores
Usual oral dosage
Spironolactone (Aldactone): 25 mg qd to 200 mg bid
Amiloride (Midamor): 5-40 mg qd
Thiazide-related diuretic (metolazone): Potent diuretic used for refractory volume overload despite increased doses of loop diuretics
Usual oral dosage: 2.5-20 mg qd

Angiotensin-converting enzyme (ACE) inhibitors: Should be used in patients with left ventricular dysfunction as a primary afterload-reducing agent; shown to reduce mortality and improve functional class
Usual oral dosage:
Captopril (Capoten): 6.25-100 mg tid
Enalapril (Vasotec): 2.5-20 mg bid
Lisinopril (Prinivil): 5-40 mg qd
Quinapril (Accupril): 5-20 mg bid
Side effects: Hypotension, hyperkalemia, renal insufficiency, cough

Angiotensin II type I receptor antagonists: Provide greater blockade from the effects of angiotensin without increasing bradykinin levels
Usual oral dosage: Losartan: 25-100 mg qd

Digoxin: Increased cardiac contractility and cardiac output; shown to improve physical function and decrease symptoms of heart failure in some studies
Usual oral dosage: 0.125-0.25 mg qd

Vasodilators
Hydralazine/isosorbide dinitrate: Alternative in patients with contraindications or intolerance of ACE inhibitors or refractory hypertension or congestive heart failure
Usual oral dosage: Hydralazine: 10-100 mg tid
Side effects: Headache, nausea, dizziness, lupuslike syndrome
Usual oral dosage: Isosorbide dinitrate: 10-80 mg tid
Side effects: Headache, hypotension, flushing

Beta-blocker therapy: To down-regulate the sympathetic nervous system; prescribed for stable NYHA class II or III heart failure due to left ventricular systolic dysfunction unless patients are intolerant or have contraindications to such therapy; beta-blockers are used in conjunction with diuretic and ACE inhibitors
Vasodilator–beta-blockers: Agents that combine the properties of both classes of drugs
Carvedilol: 12.5-25 mg PO bid

Intravenous inotropic therapy: To increase renal blood flow and facilitate diuresis in patients with severe heart failure
Dobutamine: Direct-acting synthetic beta-1 agonist, also with beta-2 agonist activity; increases contractility, cardiac output
Usual dosage: 2-15 mg/kg/min; in stable patient, may be used in home care setting infused through a long-term central venous port as a bridge to cardiac transplantation
Dopamine: Direct and indirect agonist at alpha-, beta-, and dopaminergic receptors; response varies according to dosage
Usual dosage: 2-10 mg/kg/min
Milrinone: phosphodiesterase inhibitor; increases contractility and peripheral vasodilation
Usual dosage: 0.375-0.75 mg/kg/min
Amrinone-phosphodiesterase inhibitor: Increases contractility and peripheral vasodilation
Usual dosage: 0.75 mg/kg bolus, then 5-20 μg/kg/min

General Management

IABP: Counterpulsation device that assists failing heart by decreasing afterload and increasing coronary artery perfusion (p. 130 gives further discussion); used only for temporary relief of the failing left ventricle
Hemodynamic monitoring (PAP, PCWP, SVR, CO/CI): Initiated as a direct means of assessing hemodynamic status of heart and effectiveness of treatment; also assists in direction of therapy (see p. 126)
Ventricular assist devices (VAD), right or left: Mechanical devices that decrease work of the myocardium while maintaining systemic pressure; positioned outside the body or implanted into the abdomen, VAD works as an artificial pump to maintain circulation so the heart can rest and recover; it is a longer-term support for the failing heart and is used as a bridge to transplantation
ECG: Used to assess for strain, hypertrophy, ischemia, and dysrhythmias
Bed rest: Head of bed elevated to 45 degrees to reduce myocardial oxygen demand and decrease circulating volume returning to the heart; ambulation as soon as patient can tolerate to prevent or reverse physical deconditioning
Restriction of sodium and water: Daily measurement of weight to detect early fluid retention
Sodium-restricted diet: 4 g is "no added salt" and 2 g is all salt eliminated from cooking
Oxygen therapy: Initiated if patient is hypoxic

NURSING CARE

NURSING ASSESSMENT

General Complaints

Dyspnea owing to increased pulmonary venous and interstitial pressures; variations; dyspnea on exertion (DOE), orthopnea, paroxysmal nocturnal dyspnea (PND)
Fatigue: Moderate to severe, owing to diminished cardiac output
Skin: Pallor, diaphoresis
Gastrointestinal symptoms resulting from splanchnic congestion: Anorexia, nausea, vomiting, abdominal distention, right upper quadrant pain

Physical Examination

Assess and monitor blood pressure, apical pulse, heart rate, respirations, heart and lung sounds every 4 hours or as indicated to detect early signs and symptoms of decreased cardiac output.

Assess and monitor for changes in respiratory function to detect signs and symptoms of impaired ventilation or perfusion: restlessness, confusion, somnolence, hypoxia, and hypercapnia.

Assess and monitor increased or decreased jugular venous distention; assess and monitor intake and output to detect signs of fluid retention.

Auscultate heart sounds and breath sounds every 1 to 2 hours to detect increased congestion and response to treatment.

Assess for decreased cardiac output: fatigue, tachycardia, pulsus alternans, weak thready pulse, hypotension, narrowed pulse pressure, pallor, diaphoresis, cool and clammy skin, altered mental status, dizziness, syncope, decreased urine output.

Assess for increased PCWP: rapid labored respiration, cough, frothy or blood-tinged sputum, moist rales on pulmonary auscultation, left ventricular S_3 and systolic murmur at apex on cardiac auscultation, precordial movement—displaced apical impulse and palpable thrills.

Assess for increased right atrial pressure: weight gain, elevated jugular venous pressure (rise in a and v waves), hepatojugular reflex, precordial movement (right ventricular impulse along lower left sternal border or subxiphoid); on auscultation, right ventricular S_3 heard best at lower left sternal border; presence of systolic murmur, hepatomegaly, splenomegaly, peripheral edema, dilation of peripheral veins.

Observe daily for signs of malnutrition: dry body weight 20% less than ideal weight for age, height, and body size; decreased triceps skinfold measurements; stomatitis; anorexia; increasing fatigue and weakness; decreased serum albumin, transferrin, and BUN levels.

Assess and monitor for signs of activity intolerance.

Check blood pressure, heart rate, and respiration before and after activity because orthostatic hypotension can result from prolonged periods of bed rest.

Monitor skin integrity, noting color, texture, temperature, and signs of redness, scaling, breaks, or ulcerations.

Potential Complications

Arrhythmias; pleural effusions; venous thromboembolism; ascites; iatrogenic complications as a result of pharmacotherapeutics

Patient Problems/Nursing Diagnoses & Interventions

NIC Tissue Perfusion Management

Decreased cardiac output related to mechanical factors (preload, afterload, contractility)

- Maintain bed rest *to conserve energy and decrease oxygen demand.* Elevate head of bed 30 to 60 degrees. Lean patient forward on padded over-bed table *to facilitate ventilation and decrease workload of breathing.*
- Monitor hemodynamic parameters as ordered *to evaluate patient's clinical status and response to therapy.* Blood pressure and arterial pressures reflect tissue perfusion. Pulmonary artery pressure, PCWP, and cardiac output reflect LVEDP and myocardial contractility.
- Administer drug therapy as ordered. Monitor for signs of drug toxicity.
- Monitor EGG rate and rhythm *to detect early dysrhythmias.*
- Limit IV fluids as ordered *to prevent circulatory overload.*
- Restrict activities as indicated. Plan care *to prevent fatigue,* which increases oxygen demand.
- Provide rest periods between procedures.

Impaired skin integrity related to altered circulation, metabolic state, and immobility

- If patient is on bed rest, turn and reposition every 2 to 4 hours *to relieve pressure areas and improve circulation, muscle tone, and joint mobility.*
- Administer skin care daily. Massage bony pressure areas *to increase tissue perfusion to affected areas. To avoid causing skin excoriations, do not massage reddened areas.*
- Anticipate and initiate preventive measures for a patient considered at high risk for skin breakdown: a cachectic, debilitated, or edematous patient who is immobile.
- Use alternative preventive measures *to ensure skin integrity as indicated:* air pressure bed, alternating pressure mattress, sheepskin.
- Prevent and eliminate pressure and friction. Position pillows or other supports between pressure areas *to prevent friction, abrasions, and rubbing of two skin areas.*
- Keep skin dry when diaphoretic *because moisture contributes to skin breakdown and infection.*
- Initiate aggressive decubitus care at first sign of reddened areas, tissue breakdown, or ulceration *because decubiti can develop in a matter of hours.*

NIC Respiratory Management

Impaired gas exchange related to elevated alveolar-capillary membrane changes caused by increased pulmonary capillary pressure

- Monitor arterial blood gas *to identify hypoxemia and hypercapnia.*
- Administer oxygen therapy as ordered, via nasal prongs, mask, or positive-pressure device.
- Administer morphine sulfate IV per protocol *to reduce hyperventilation.*
- Elevate head of bed *to enhance ventilation.*
- Auscultate breath sounds every hour *to detect increases in congestion and determine adequacy of ventilatory effort.*
- Prepare for intubation and assisted ventilation if required.
- Explain all procedures and modalities briefly to patient *to prevent hyperventilation resulting from fear or anxiety.*

NIC Fluid and Nutritional Support

Excess fluid volume related to increased systemic venous congestion or right ventricular failure

- Maintain patent IV for drug administration.
- Administer rapid-acting diuretics as ordered to *decrease circulating volume.*
- Restrict sodium and fluid intake *to control sodium reabsorption.*

- Weigh patient daily (same time of day, same amount of clothing) *to determine fluid loss or retention.*
- Monitor intake and output; report output of less than 30 ml/h.
- Monitor serum electrolytes, especially sodium and potassium.

Imbalanced nutrition: less than body requirements, related to impaired absorption of nutrients secondary to low cardiac output, increased catabolic rate, and increased myocardial demands

- Weigh patient daily: on rising, after voiding, with same clothing, *to obtain consistent and accurate body weight.*
- Maintain diet as ordered. Do not force patient to eat, but offer small, frequent meals, tempt appetite with food preferences compatible with diet restrictions and cultural values, and supplement with high-calorie feedings as indicated *to maintain minimum required caloric intake.*
- Administer antiemetics and analgesics before meals *to ensure patient's comfort and improve appetite.*
- Initiate caloric count if patient's nutritional status fails to improve. Obtain dietary consultation *to evaluate nutritional status and assist patient in selection of foods.*

NIC Activity and Exercise Management

Activity intolerance related to weakness secondary to decreased cardiac output

- Identify factors known *to cause fatigue.* Restrict or limit activities as indicated *to promote energy conservation.*
- Space treatment and procedures *to allow for periods of uninterrupted rest.*
- Implement measures that will improve activity tolerance by minimizing fatigue *to limit or reduce energy expenditure.*

NIC Patient Education

Deficient knowledge related to lack of information

- Identify and address barriers to learning.
- Instruct patient regarding congestive heart failure, in-hospital treatment plan, and measures *to reduce exacerbations.*

Patient Education/Continuum of Care Plan

Instruction is directed toward long-term maintenance of the therapeutic program.

1. Describe the disease process, the underlying cause, and any precipitating factors.
2. Discuss with the patient the need to report symptoms of increased failure to physician: dyspnea on exertion, cough, paroxysmal nocturnal dyspnea, and decreased exercise tolerance.
3. Explain to the patient the need to limit strenuous physical activity and avoid fatigue.
4. Explain to the patient the need to limit the intake of salt in the diet and avoid foods that have a high sodium content; instruct the patient in label reading. Provide information about alternative ways to season food.
5. Discuss with the patient the need to weigh daily in the morning before the first meal with the same scale and wearing the same clothing and to report weight gain of more than 2 pounds in 24 hours.
6. Ensure that the patient can name and describe methods of administering drugs and their potential side effects.
7. Instruct the patient to avoid alcoholic beverages and refrain from inhaling passive cigarette smoke.
8. Emphasize and reevaluate patient compliance with medical regimen as an important variable for future referral for cardiac transplantation.
9. Perform home care monitoring as indicated, especially for outpatient IV inotropic support.

Evaluation/Patient Outcomes

Tissue Perfusion Management: Ventricular function is improved. Heart rate and PCWP are decreased. Cardiac output is increased. Mental status is improved. Urine output is increased. Skin integrity is maintained. Skin: intact, warm, dry; signs of healing over areas of breakdown.

Respiratory Management: Gas exchange is improved. Lung sounds are clear. Anxiety level is diminished. Orthopnea and dyspnea are reduced. Hypoxemia and hypercarbia are absent. Respirations are improved.

Fluid and Nutritional Support: Nutritional status is improved. Dry body weight is normal or improved for age and body build. Fluid overload is decreased. Patient achieves dry weight. Jugular venous distention is decreased. Breath sounds are improved. Peripheral edema is decreased.

Activity and Exercise Management: Energy and exercise tolerance is adequate. Patient verbalizes strategies to obtain enough rest and minimize fatigue.

Patient Education: Knowledge level is increased. Patient verbalizes knowledge regarding importance of daily weight, taking prescribed medication, activity allowances and limitations, and dietary restrictions. Anxiety level is decreased. Patient appears relaxed. Patient demonstrates ability to rest and sleep without complaints. Patient verbalizes fears regarding disease process, asking appropriate questions.

Shock (Hypovolemic, Vasogenic, Cardiogenic)

Shock is an abnormal physical state that is the first phase of the body's alarm reaction to stress (Fig. 3-39).

Shock occurs most commonly as an extreme syndrome linked to abnormal cellular metabolism, which in most cases is caused by inadequate tissue perfusion. If shock is untreated, circulatory collapse and impaired cellular metabolism develop, eventually leading to death.

Pathophysiology

Various methods of classifying shock have been used. The following three categories based on causes are commonly used in the clinical setting:

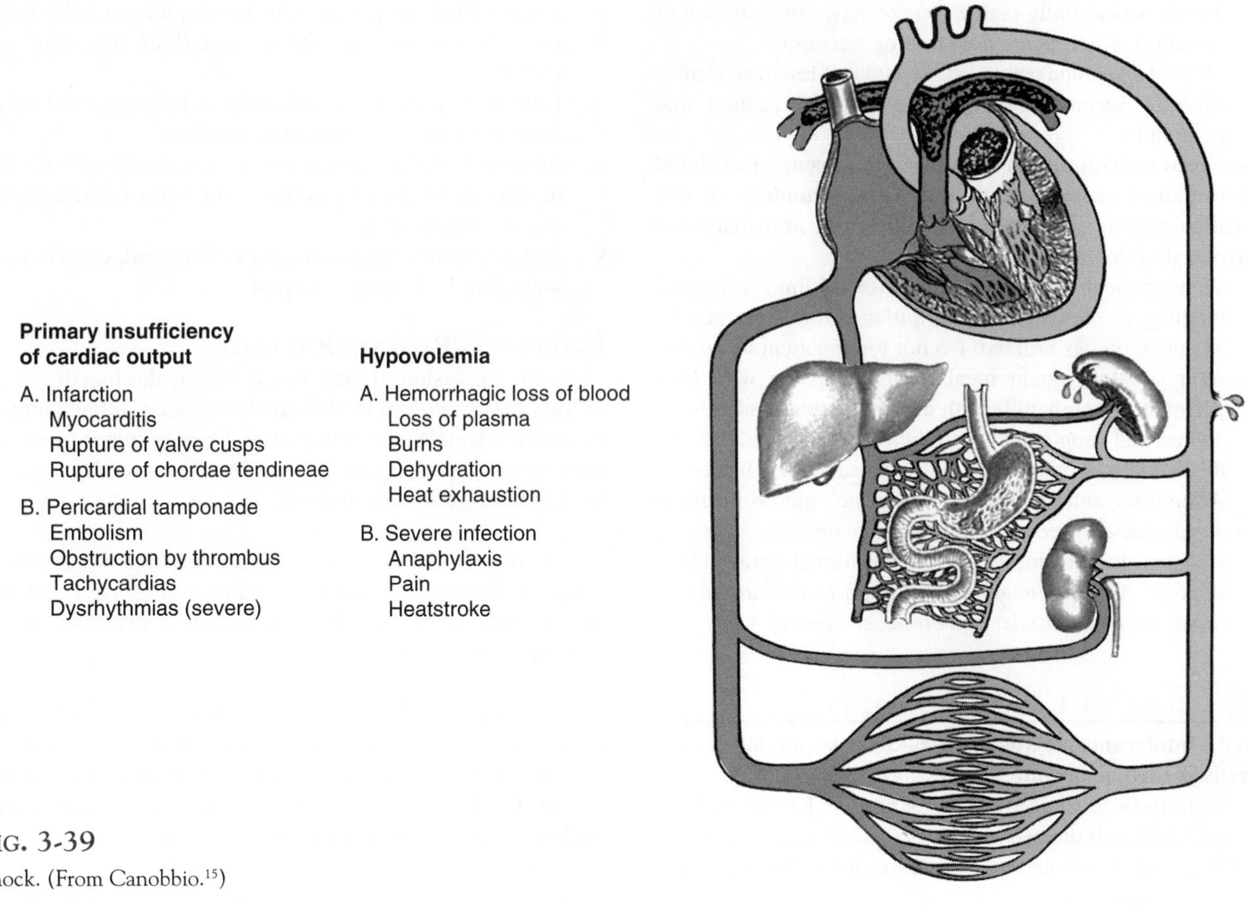

FIG. 3-39
Shock. (From Canobbio.[15])

Hypovolemic
- Loss of blood volume (hemorrhage)
- Loss of plasma volume (dehydration)

Vasogenic
- Sepsis
- Immune mediated (anaphylaxis)
- Deep anesthesia effects

Cardiogenic
- Acute MI
- Other causes (pulmonary emboli, cardiac surgery, tamponade)

Hypovolemic Shock

Hypovolemic shock, or "cold" shock, results from a decrease in intravascular volume and generally occurs when there is also a deficit involving at least 15% of the total blood volume. Hypovolemia is the most common cause of hypotension in critically ill patients, particularly in the postoperative phase.

Hypovolemic shock may be caused by excessive loss of plasma volume, as occurs in burns or pancreatitis, when extracellular fluid is sequestered in injured or inflamed tissue cells. Severe dehydration and hypovolemia may also be caused by diabetic ketoacidosis, extreme vomiting, or diarrhea. The most common cause of hypovolemic shock, however, is excessive blood loss through damage to a major blood vessel or organ such as the kidney, spleen, or liver; through injury or disease of the gastrointestinal system, such as rupture of esophageal varices; or through ruptured aneurysms.

The severity of hypovolemic shock is related to the amount and rate of volume loss. If volume is replaced quickly, the shock state can be easily reversed. If low aortic pressures last longer than 60 minutes, the process may be irreversible.

The major hemodynamic changes linked to fluid loss are low cardiac output, increased systemic vascular resistance, and decreased central venous pressure. The patient usually has cool clammy skin, increased heart and respiratory rates, and decreased urine output, owing to compensatory vasoconstriction. The blood pressure may be normal or low, particularly in the early phase of cold shock.

Vasogenic Shock

Unlike hypovolemic shock, which leads to vasoconstriction, vasogenic shock results in massive vasodilation from an increase in total vascular capacity. Circulating volume is lost because of venous pooling, increased capillary permeability, and third spacing of fluid. If intravascular volume is not replaced, hypovolemia occurs. Whereas a patient with hypovolemia has cold extremities as a result of vasoconstriction, a patient with vasogenic shock has warm extremities, giving rise to the term *warm shock.* Warm shock is present in 30% to 50% of patients in the early phase of septic shock.

Sepsis is the most common form of vasogenic shock, but it may also occur as a result of other factors, including food allergies and anaphylactic reactions to drugs and insect stings.

Septic shock is commonly related to the release of bacterial endotoxins after a gram-negative bacterial infection. The organisms most often found in septic shock are the gram-negative bacteria *Escherichia coli, Klebsiella, Enterobacter, Pseudomonas, Serratia, Proteus,* and *Bacteroides fragilis;* the gram-positive bacteria *Stapylococcus, Pneumococcus,* and alpha or beta streptococcus; and the fungus *Candida.* Many are a part of the natural body flora or are commonly present in hospitals. The microbes linked to the highest death rate are *Proteus, Pseudomonas, Candida,* and *B. fragilis.* Although patients in critical care units are the most likely to acquire infections in the hospital, patients in general hospital units are also vulnerable. Patients particularly susceptible to septic shock are the elderly, immunosuppressed patients, patients who have indwelling catheters (urinary, intravenous, or intracardiac) or urinary tract infection, patients who have had surgery of the digestive or urinary tract, and patients who have undergone manipulative instrumentation.

Although deaths from septic shock have decreased since the 1960s, the death rate continues to be as high as 50%. This is the result of several factors, the most striking of which are the changing pattern of microbial resistance to antimicrobial agents[12] and the rapidly changing nature of microbes.

Certain hemodynamic changes have been recognized as probable causes of septic shock. In early phases a hyperdynamic state exists in which the cardiac output, stroke volume, and heart rate are increased and the systemic vascular resistance and central venous pressure are decreased. The patient appears warm, dry, and flushed because of generalized vasodilation and venous pooling. This state is probably caused by the effects of various substances released by exotoxins or from the injured or infected tissue.

The circulatory changes combined with the decreased systemic vascular resistance may stimulate a sympathetic response. This causes the increased heart rate and maintenance of normal blood pressure that occur during this warm shock phase.

If hyperdynamic shock continues, the increase in capillary leaking increases hypovolemia to the point that the process converts to a hypodynamic phase known as the cold phase of septic shock. In this state the systemic vascular resistance increases, cardiac output drops, and the patient appears cold, pale, and clammy. The cause of this change is related to ineffective circulating blood volume, sympathetic vasoconstriction, and pump failure.

In anaphylactic reactions from drugs, insect stings, or food allergies, the mechanism involved is an antibody-antigen interaction that provokes the release of chemicals such as histamine. These mediators act mainly on the vascular membranes and smooth muscles. Histamine release causes veins and arterioles to dilate, decreasing cardiac output and arterial pressure. Histamine also increases capillary permeability, causing fluid to escape from the intravascular compartment into the interstitial space. The result is volume depletion; however, while plasma water is removed from the capillaries, the red blood cells remain and the hemoglobin levels and hematocrit values rise. The immediate reactions in anaphylaxis are pharyngeal and laryngeal edema, probably because of the effects of histamines, and bronchoconstriction, with the immediate threat of death from asphyxiation.

Deep anesthesia can cause severe depression of the vasomotor centers of the brain, which may result in vasomotor collapse and venous pooling. These responses decrease venous return to the heart and diminish cardiac output.

Cardiogenic Shock

Cardiogenic shock occurs when the heart cannot maintain enough output to meet the body's demands (FIG. 3-40). MI is the most common cause of cardiogenic shock, but it also may result from various other cardiac disorders, such as acute myocarditis, end-stage cardiomyopathy (dilated, hypertrophic, or restrictive), valvular heart disease (ruptured papillary muscle), cardiac tamponade, acute ventricular septal defect, and prolonged cardiopulmonary bypass. Other causes include pulmonary embolism and tension pneumothorax. The major feature of cardiogenic shock is inadequate tissue perfusion and oxygen delivery, resulting from a severely impaired ventricle.

The incidence of cardiogenic shock resulting from MI is 10% to 15%, with a mortality rate exceeding 80%. The higher mortality rates are seen in hospitals without facilities for IABP, high-risk angioplasty, and surgical revascularization. Accordingly, current therapies focus on early aggressive intervention to reduce ischemia and limit permanent myocardial damage.

In patients with MI, shock develops as a result of abnormal reflexes arising from the ischemic myocardium. The inability to increase systemic vascular resistance makes it difficult to maintain an adequate arterial pressure. This leads to hypoperfusion of an already ischemic myocardium, causing further insufficiency of the left ventricle's pumping action. Failure of the left ventricle to generate enough energy to pump blood into the systemic circulation further decreases perfusion and myocardial oxygen supply.

Cardiogenic shock has been linked to the destruction of 40% or more of the left ventricular muscle. The mechanism of cardiogenic shock is complex, with a vicious cycle of changes that lead rapidly to further deterioration of cardiac function. If left untreated, the reduction in tissue blood flow and oxygen delivery to the myocardium results in circulatory collapse, impaired cellular metabolism, and eventual death.

Compensatory Mechanisms of Shock

A number of compensatory mechanisms are activated when arterial pressure and tissue perfusion are reduced. These mechanisms are controlled by the sympathetic nervous system and the release of endogenous vasoconstrictors and hormonal substances.[80]

Baroreceptors. A reduction in mean arterial pressure and pulse pressure is sensed by baroreceptors in the carotid sinus and aortic arch. By secreting epinephrine and norepinephrine, they produce a generalized sympathetic stimulation, resulting in increased peripheral vascular resistance, arterial pressure, and myocardial contractility.

Fluid Shifts. The major endogenous vasoactive substances released during shock are catecholamines and vasopressin, which augment sympathetic activity when activated further. The release of these substances also reduces vascular capacity,

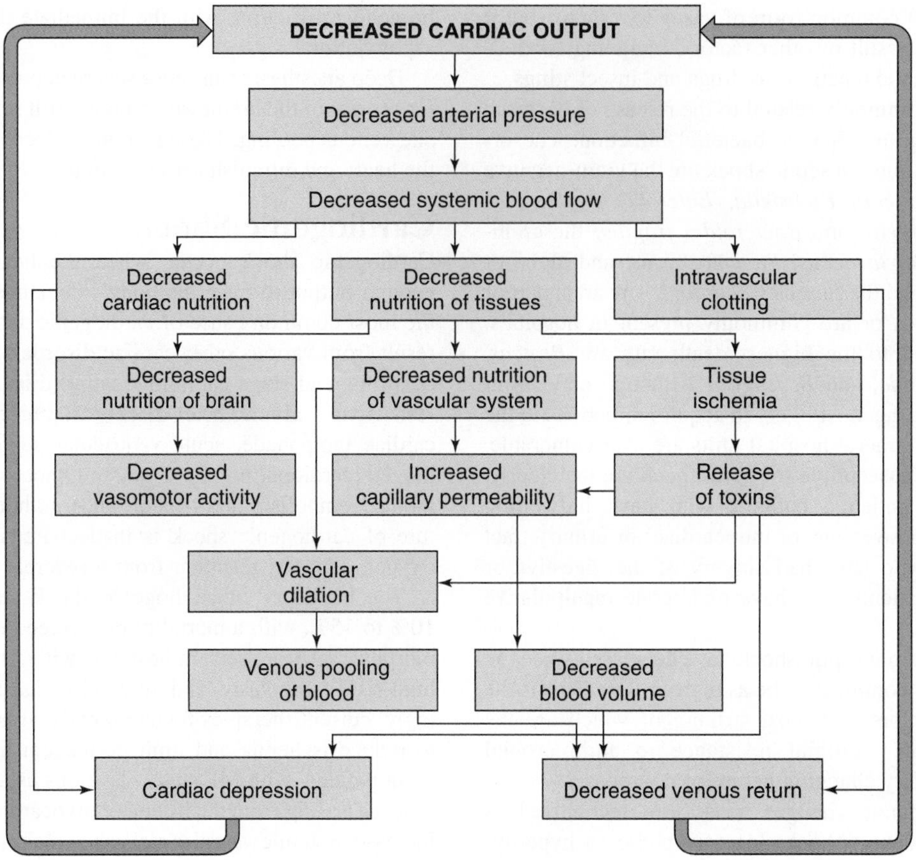

FIG. 3-40

Different types of feedback that can lead to progression of shock. (Modified from Guyton.[43])

which eases the osmotic movement of interstitial fluid into the vascular compartments to restore blood volume.

Renin-Angiotensin-Aldosterone System. When renal ischemia occurs, the renin-angiotensin-aldosterone system is activated to help maintain blood pressure and intravascular volume. Reducing renal perfusion pressure results in the release of renin, which in time is converted to angiotensin II, a powerful vasoconstrictor. Angiotensin II stimulates the release of aldosterone, which enhances sodium and water reabsorption by the renal tubules to help maintain intravascular volume.

Antidiuretic Hormone. The release of antidiuretic hormone (ADH) from the posterior pituitary gland in response to hypotension plays a role in volume regulation during circulatory shock. ADH enhances reabsorption of sodium and water by increasing permeability of the renal tubules.

Progressive Shock

If the compensatory mechanisms cannot restore effective perfusion to vital organs, circulatory function deteriorates further, leading to a cycle of changes that decrease cardiac output. FIG. 3-40 illustrates some of the changes that contribute to decreased cardiac output and circulatory collapse.

Cell Deterioration. As shock becomes severe, local changes in cellular metabolism occur. Prolonged tissue ischemia results in incomplete oxidation at the cellular level, diminishing mitochondrial activity. Adenosine triphosphate (ATP) stores then begin to be used, and the cells resort to anaerobic metabolism of glucose to provide energy. This process of glycolysis produces lactic acid, which builds up in the blood. The effects of an acidic pH include depressed myocardial function and a decreased vascular response to epinephrine and norepinephrine, leading to vasomotor collapse late in shock.[10,27]

Another significant cellular change resulting from continued ischemia is the release of vasoactive metabolites into the circulation. Substances such as bradykinin, histamine, serotonin, and prostaglandins, along with decreased vascular tone, lead to increases in venous pooling and capillary permeability. Excessive vasodilation then decreases venous return and cardiac filling. The increased permeability of the capillaries allows large quantities of fluid to escape into the interstitial spaces.

Organ and Tissue Changes

As the shock syndrome becomes severe, generalized organ deterioration begins.

Renal Function. Although reduced renal perfusion activates certain compensatory mechanisms, in the early phases of shock, prolonged decreased renal blood flow leads to ischemia and acute tubular necrosis. This is marked by fluid, electrolyte, and metabolic disturbances.

Pulmonary Function. Ischemia of the pulmonary circulation in the early phases of shock can damage pulmonary function to cause adult respiratory distress syndrome. Damage to the pulmonary capillary endothelial cells increases capillary permeability. This leads to interstitial and alveolar edema that impairs gas exchange. The resulting hypoxemia and respiratory acidosis further reduce tissue oxygen delivery and organ function.

Gastrointestinal Function. Ischemic damage to the digestive tract causes a loss of the protective mucosal covering in the intestine. This can lead to intestinal damage and necrosis by digestive enzymes. It may also account for the release of bacteria and toxins into the bloodstream, causing sepsis and further circulatory problems.

The reticuloendothelial system may also be damaged during shock, impairing the patient's ability to withstand infection.

Intravascular Clotting. As the products of cell deterioration begin to accumulate in the capillaries and vasodilation occurs, blood flow becomes sluggish. The stagnation, along with local chemical changes in the capillaries, leads to blood aggregation and intravascular clotting. The formation of microemboli enhances tissue ischemia by further decreasing blood flow through the capillaries. This hypercoagulability response may occur as an early compensatory mechanism, particularly with hemorrhage. In the late stages of shock, however, a reversal in clotting occurs, leading to a hypocoagulability state. This results from loss of clotting factors through bleeding or decreased production caused by poor tissue perfusion. It may also be the result of a consumption of clotting factors that occurs in disseminated intravascular coagulation.

Myocardial Depression. Except with cardiogenic shock, the major cardiac effects of shock occur in the late stage and are by far the most important factors in the deterioration caused by shock. As arterial pressure continues to drop, so does coronary blood flow. This leads to depressed myocardial function and a further reduction in cardiac output. Myocardial contractility is depressed further by the combined effects of toxins, acidosis, and tissue hypoxia that results from cell deterioration. Thus circulatory failure is a syndrome that involves all systems, and it is usually the deterioration of heart function that makes shock irreversible.

Diagnostic Studies and Findings

Hematocrit: Decreased; however, in hypovolemia, may be increased because of intravascular fluid shift

Hemoglobin: Decreased in hemorrhage

White blood cell count with differential: Increased; leukopenia in gram-negative sepsis; leukocytosis with increased neutrophils in all forms of shock

Erythrocyte sedimentation rate: Increased in response to tissue injury

Cultures: Blood (obtain two to four cultures before initiation of antibiotic therapy), urine, and sputum: positive growth of an organism

Serum electrolytes: Sodium: increased during diuretic phase of acute tubular necrosis, decreased with administration of hypotonic fluid after fluid loss; potassium: increased with cellular death during oliguric phase, in acidosis, and after transfusion reactions

Serum chemistry: BUN, creatinine: increased, reflecting impaired renal function; lactate levels: increased; glucose levels: increased in early shock, reflecting release of liver glycogen stores in response to catecholamines

Prothrombin time (PT), partial thromboplastin time (PTT): Prolonged

Platelets: Thrombocytopenia is present in over half the patients with septic shock

Arterial blood gases: Respiratory alkalosis; metabolic acidosis

Urine studies: Specific gravity: increased in response to action of antidiuretic hormone and during oliguric phase; osmolality: high during oliguric phase; sodium: decreased

ECG (12-lead continuous monitoring): To determine changes in heart rate and rhythm and ischemic changes

Chest x-ray: To determine pulmonary status and rule out other causes of shock state: early—normal; late—shows signs of pulmonary congestion

Hemodynamic monitoring (pulmonary artery pressure, PCWP, cardiac output): To provide information regarding serial changes in left ventricular function in response to specific treatments, such as fluid replacement and vasoactive agents

Echocardiography: Noninvasive method of sorting out etiology of shock; also provides information on regional and global systolic wall function, valvular integrity, and presence or absence of pericardial effusion

Multidisciplinary Plan

Medications

Fluid-Volume Regulation. Except with patients in cardiogenic shock, restoration of intravascular volume is the most significant therapeutic intervention, particularly in the early phases of therapy.

Volume replacement should be initiated rapidly with 3 to 5 L of saline solution or other volume expanders over a 30- to 60-minute period. Ringer's lactate provides effective intravascular expansion and is the usual fluid of choice; however, a buffered solution with lactate may be used for severe shock.

Regulation of fluids should be based on hemodynamic response to the rapid fluid infusion. Careful monitoring of mean arterial pressure, PCWP, pulmonary artery end-diastolic pressure (PAEDP), or central venous pressure, and urine output guides fluid replacement.

Blood plasma expanders should be given after the initial volume deficit is corrected. With massive hemorrhage, replacement should be with whole blood if the hematocrit value is less than 30%. If the hematocrit value is greater than 30%, plasma expanders may be given. Packed cells are used if the right atrial pressure or PCWP is elevated and in cases such as cardiogenic shock in which myocardial dysfunction limits the amount and speed of fluid replacement.

In a patient in shock after acute MI, volume deficits may occur and fluid replacement may be necessary to restore a depressed cardiac output to normal. Continuous monitoring of the

PCWP is the most precise method of determining volume deficits. If the PCWP is below the desired level of 15 to 18 mm Hg, fluid replacement may be given to increase cardiac output (Starling's law). The PCWP should be kept below 18 mm Hg to prevent pulmonary congestion.

If the PCWP of a patient in shock is elevated, fluid replacement is contraindicated and diuretics may be necessary to return the PCWP to therapeutic range. Diuretics are generally given only to patients in cardiogenic shock with an elevated PCWP. They reduce preload through their effect on venous capacitance and decrease total circulating fluid.

Maintenance of Adequate Hemodynamic State.

In shock, myocardial dysfunction develops as a result of workload, limited coronary blood flow, and decreased myocardial oxygenation. Sympathomimetic agents are used to maintain an adequate hemodynamic state. The effects of these agents are mediated through the action of alpha- and beta-adrenergic receptors. Alpha-receptors in the smooth muscle of the vascular bed cause vasoconstriction, thereby increasing peripheral resistance and venous return. In contrast, beta-1 receptors are located in the myocardium, arteries, and lungs. Myocardial beta-1 receptors act to increase heart rate and contractility, whereas activation of beta-2 receptors causes vasodilation.

The various adrenergic drugs differ with respect to their relative peripheral and myocardial effects. The rationale for selecting any drug depends on the specific vascular bed on which the drug acts and the desired cardiovascular effect. In cardiogenic shock, for example, drugs with positive inotropic and vasoconstrictor properties are used to increase cardiac output by augmenting myocardial contractility and to improve blood flow to vital organs by increasing total vascular resistance. Dopamine, norepinephrine, and epinephrine, which have both constrictor and inotropic properties, are commonly used in the treatment of cardiogenic shock.

The following agents are most commonly used in the treatment of patients with shock.

ADRENERGIC DRUGS. Dopamine (Intropin) is one of the most widely used drugs in the treatment of shock. Its effects depend on the dose used and on the adrenergic state of the patient's physiology. In low doses (0.5 to 2 mg/kg/min), it activates the dopaminergic receptors and produces dilation of renal and mesenteric blood vessels. Urine output increases commensurate with increased renal blood flow and a reduction in sodium retention triggered by its natriuretic properties. In higher doses (2 to 5 mg/kg/min), dopamine activates both the dopaminergic and beta-1 receptors and improves cardiac output by increasing cardiac contractility. At 5 to 10 mg/kg/min the drug affects primarily beta-1 receptors. At therapeutic levels (10 to 15 mg/kg/min), dopamine increases cardiac output and blood pressure by alpha and beta activation. In doses greater than 20 mg/kg/min, there is a pure alpha effect on vasomotor tone. Infusions should be started with low doses (3 to 5 mg/kg/min), increasing slowly until optimum arterial pressure is achieved.

Dobutamine (Dobutrex) is used primarily for its inotropic effect. It stimulates beta-1 receptors to increase myocardial contractility and stroke volume, resulting in improved cardiac output. Because dobutamine has minimal beta-2 and alpha effects, it produces little change in blood pressure and heart rate; however, systolic blood pressure may be increased because of increased cardiac output. Coronary blood flow and MVO_2 are also increased because of increased myocardial contractility. Infusions begin at 2 to 5 mg/kg/min, with therapeutic doses between 2.5 and 10 mg/kg/min.

Milrinone is a nonglycoside that also is used primarily for its inotropic effect. It inhibits phosphodiesterase (PDE) II activity, which increases myocardial contractility and vasodilation. Infusion begins at 0.375 to 0.75 μg/kg/min.

Epinephrine is a potent alpha and beta catecholamine causing vasoconstriction of the splanchnic and renal beds. Although it does increase cardiac output, its effects on peripheral resistance do not favor redistribution of blood flow to vital organs. It is also considered less advantageous than other adrenergic drugs because it increases automaticity, which can initiate serious dysrhythmias.

Norepinephrine has both alpha and beta actions. It increases myocardial contractility by stimulating beta-1 receptors and causes arteriovenous constriction by stimulating alpha-receptors. Thus norepinephrine increases systemic arterial pressure by increasing the cardiac output and peripheral vascular resistance. Once again the actual hemodynamic effects depend on the dose employed. With small doses the beta effect predominates, causing slight increases in blood pressure and cardiac output. With very high doses, norepinephrine produces significant vasoconstriction, causing an increased systemic resistance and blood pressure. However, the cardiac output may fall despite the positive inotropic effect. The usual starting dose is 2 to 8 mg/min. Norepinephrine should be administered through an indwelling catheter placed in a large vein because it is known to cause tissue necrosis with extravasation. The disadvantage of this drug is its vasoconstricting effect on the kidneys, which can result in impaired renal perfusion and oliguria.

Isoproterenol (Isuprel) is a pure beta agonist that augments myocardial contractility and heart rate with beta-1 properties and causes peripheral vasodilation through beta-2 activation. Cardiac output is always increased, but blood pressure response is less predictable. If the systemic blood vessels are too relaxed, blood pressure can fall despite tachycardia. Substantial increase in myocardial oxygen consumption occurs with this drug, which can exacerbate myocardial ischemia in a patient with cardiogenic shock.

CARDIAC GLYCOSIDES. The role of digitalis in the treatment of shock is questionable. It has been noted that inotropic drugs such as digoxin become less effective as the degree of left ventricular failure increases. As an inotropic agent for the treatment of severe or cardiogenic shock, digitalis is relatively weak when compared with the sympathomimetic drugs. Furthermore, because of the impaired renal function, acidosis, and hypoxia occurring in shock states, the patient is predisposed to digitalis-induced dysrhythmias.[27]

VASODILATORS. Vasodilator therapy is generally limited to patients with failing ventricular function, and its use is still debated in the routine treatment of cardiogenic shock. However, it may be of use for patients with severe hypotension whose severe vasoconstriction continues despite volume replacement. Excessive vasoconstriction, which occurs initially as a compensatory response to hypoperfusion, can reduce blood flow and oxygen delivery, as well as cause such a loss of intravascular volume that it leads to further reduction of cardiac output. The rationale for using vasodilator therapy in shock is to break this progressive positive-feedback cycle.

Vasodilator agents improve left ventricular function by decreasing myocardial oxygen demand through the reduction of preload and afterload. These drugs have no direct inotropic action on the heart. The increased cardiac output produced by vasodilators is caused by the changes in preload and afterload.

Arterial vasodilators are used to decrease peripheral vascular resistance, which then decreases resistance to left ventricular ejection and therefore afterload. Venodilators are used to increase venous capacitance, causing a decrease in venous return that decreases PCWP and preload.

The potential role of vasodilator therapy in cardiogenic shock merits further study. Although inappropriate as a single form of therapy, the use of vasodilators combined with external counterpulsation and other inotropic agents appears to be effective in providing efficient ventricular function. Nitroprusside and phentolamine are the vasodilator agents most commonly used in the treatment of cardiogenic shock.

ANTIHYPERTENSIVE AGENTS. Nitroprusside (Nipride, Nitropress) causes both arterial and venous dilation, thereby decreasing venous return and left ventricular filling (decreased preload), as well as resistance to left ventricular ejection (decreased afterload). The drug is administered intravenously with an initial dose of 0.5 to 10 mg/kg/min, which is increased in increments of 5 to 10 mg/kg/min every 5 minutes or until an improvement in hemodynamics is observed. Fluid replacement may be required if filling pressures drop excessively. Fluid volumes should be determined before administration of these agents. In hypovolemic patients, massive vasodilation only worsens the clinical picture by further decreasing venous return.

ALPHA-ADRENERGIC BLOCKING AGENTS. Phentolamine mesylate (Regitine) inhibits vasoconstriction by blocking alpha-adrenergic receptors. It lowers arterial pressure, thereby decreasing afterload. The drug is given intravenously at a dosage of 0.1 to 2 mg/min.

General Management

IABP: Counterpulsation is the most frequently used method of mechanically assisting circulation after profound cardiovascular collapse. Counterpulsation augments aortic pressure during diastole with subsequent reduction of afterload, thus effectively reducing the work of the myocardium and improving coronary blood flow. It can be used for short-term support. A catheter with a 10- to 50-cc balloon is inserted into the femoral artery and positioned in the thoracic aorta just distal to the left subclavian artery. With the ECG used for synchronization, the balloon is inflated during diastole and deflated during systole.

Ventricular assist device (VAD): VADs support failing left, right, or both ventricles. VADs approximate normal hemodynamic parameters, supporting circulation for several days to months.

Oxygenation: Ventilation/perfusion ratios should be determined early to ensure adequate ventilation. Oxygen exchange may be impaired in patients with shock, especially if cardiac output is decreased. Oxygen therapy should be given from the onset of treatment to maintain an arterial PO_2 of at least 80 mm Hg. Intubation may be indicated if arterial blood gases show worsening hypoxemia despite high oxygen concentrations. The indications for mechanical ventilation are a PaO_2 of less than 50 mm Hg while the patient is receiving oxygen concentrations of 50%, a vital capacity of less than 15 ml/kg body weight, a PCO_2 of greater than 45 mm Hg, and an arterial pH of less than 7.25.

Hemodynamic monitoring: For diagnostic information and to evaluate the patient outcome of ongoing therapy, arterial pressures, pulmonary artery pressure, pulmonary artery diastolic pressures, and PCWP should be monitored initially every 5 to 10 minutes. A cardiac index of less than 2 L/min reflects a shock state.

Nutrition: Patients in shock should receive nothing by mouth, but care must be taken to provide nutrition, preferably with total parenteral nutrition.

Acid-base balance: Frequent monitoring of acid-base balance is necessary to avert profound acidosis. Intravenous administration of sodium bicarbonate may be necessary to maintain or correct the pH to 7.35.

Renal function: Hourly urine output measurements with frequent checks are necessary to determine adequate kidney perfusion. Urine output of less than 30 ml/h reflects inadequate renal perfusion. Elevated serum blood urea nitrogen and creatinine levels reflect renal dysfunction.

Activity: Efforts should be made to minimize energy expenditure. The patient should be maintained on complete bed rest in a supine position. Reverse Trendelenberg may be necessary to support blood pressure.

NURSING CARE

NURSING ASSESSMENT

Assess for signs and symptoms indicative of altered tissue perfusion: cool skin temperature, pale or cyanotic color, decreased arterial pulses, altered mental status, decreased blood pressure, tachycardia, decreased urine output, thirst.

Assess and monitor for signs and symptoms indicative of decreased cardiac output: fatigue, skin pallor, diaphoresis, oliguria, anuria, hypotension, tachycardia.

Monitor hemodynamic parameters as ordered to evaluate patient's clinical status and response to therapy: blood pressure, arterial pressure, pulmonary artery pressure, PCWP.

Monitor and calculate cardiac output (CO) and cardiac index (CI) to evaluate cardiac function.

Assess for signs and symptoms of fluid volume deficit: hypotension and decreased venous filling, pulse volume, and pressure.

Assess skin for increased temperature, color, and turgor.

Assess and monitor respiratory pattern, noting rate, rhythm, and use of accessory muscles.
Monitor arterial blood gas levels, and venous oxygen saturation (SvO_2) if pulmonary artery catheter is in place.
Assess for signs of increased congestion.
Assess for signs of early malnutrition; monitor laboratory values daily.
Assess for signs of fear and anxiety; determine source of fears.
Assess for signs and symptoms of systemic infection.
See Assessment Considerations table.

Assessment Considerations

Area of Concern	Hypovolemic Shock	Cardiogenic Shock	Vasogenic Shock
General appearance	Anxiety, restlessness	Anxiety, restlessness	Anxiety, vertigo, restlessness
Level of consciousness	Lethargy, stupor, or coma	Lethargy, stupor, or coma	Lethargy, stupor, or coma
Temperature	Increased or decreased	Increased	Increased or decreased
Heart rate	Increased, pulse thready	Increased, pulse thready	Increased, pulse thready
Auscultation		S_3, S_4; murmurs	
Blood pressure			
Early	Pulse pressure decreased; diastolic pressure increased	Pulse pressure decreased; diastolic pressure increased	Normal; pulse pressure decreased
Late	Systolic pressure decreased	Systolic pressure decreased	Systolic pressure decreased
Skin temperature and texture	Cool, moist, clammy, pale	Cool, moist, clammy, pale, cyanosis	Early: warm, dry; late: cool, moist, clammy; color: pale, cyanosis (late)
Capillary refill time	Decreased	Decreased	Decreased
Peripheral pulses	Absent or diminished	Absent or diminished	Absent or diminished (late)
Jugular venous distention	Absent or flat	Elevated	Early: flat; late: elevated
Hemodynamic findings			
Central venous pressure	Decreased	Increased	Decreased
Pulmonary capillary wedge pressure	Decreased	Increased	Decreased
Cardiac output	Decreased	Decreased	Increased or decreased
Peripheral vascular resistance	Decreased	Increased	Decreased or normal; late: increased
Pulmonary function			
Respiratory rate	Increased; shallow or Cheyne-Stokes respirations	Increased; late: Cheyne-Stokes respirations, apnea	Increased; late: Cheyne-Stokes respirations
Auscultation	Early: clear; late: rales	Rales	Early: clear; late: rales
Acid-base changes			
Early	Respiratory alkalosis	Respiratory alkalosis	Respiratory alkalosis
Late	Metabolic (lactic) acidosis	Metabolic (lactic) acidosis	Metabolic (lactic) acidosis
Urine output			
Early	Decreased (<20 ml/mm)	Decreased (<20 ml/mm)	Decreased (<20 ml/mm)
Late	Anuria	Anuria	Anuria
Urine sodium concentration	Decreased	Decreased	Decreased
Urine osmolality	Increased	Increased	Increased

! EMERGENCY ALERT

CARDIOGENIC SHOCK

Cardiogenic shock occurs when systolic blood pressure falls below 90 mm Hg during an acute MI; this leads to pump failure. The heart cannot contact effectively and is unable to pump enough blood. Cardiogenic shock occurs in about 15% of patients with acute MI; 85% to 90% of these patients do not survive.

Assessment

- Signs of MI
- Decreased peripheral pulses
- Increased but shallow respirations
- Decreased blood pressure
- Altered level of consciousness, anxiety, or restlessness
- Clammy skin
- Decreased urinary output
- Acute metabolic acidosis
- ECG changes

Interventions

- Administer high-flow oxygen (10-15 L).
- Obtain IV access.
- Prepare to administer inotropic agents and vasodilators.
- IABP

Potential Complications

Target organ damage from prolonged hypotension; adult respiratory distress syndrome and long-term respiratory compromise; iatrogenic effects of pharmacotherapeutics, devices, and immobility; infection; skin breakdown

Patient Problems/Nursing Diagnoses & Interventions

NIC Tissue Perfusion Management

Deficient fluid volume related to hemorrhage and fluid loss

- Administer fluids as ordered.
- Monitor hemodynamic parameters, including PCWP, heart rate, urine output, and central venous pressure.
- Maintain patient's core temperature by covering patient with blankets as needed.
- Maintain accurate intake and output record.
- Monitor electrolytes.
- Measure all-body fluid loss; estimate loss in dressings.

Decreased cardiac output related to mechanical factors (preload, afterload, contractility)

- Maintain bed rest *to conserve energy and decrease oxygen demand.*
- Calculate systemic vascular resistance as ordered *to determine left ventricular afterload.*
- Evaluate cardiovascular response to drug therapy.
- Administer sympathomimetic and vasodilator drugs as ordered *to increase myocardial contractility and reduce systemic vascular resistance (SVR).*
- Administer plasma volume expanders as ordered.
- Restrict activities as indicated.
- Plan care to prevent fatigue, which increases oxygen demand.
- Initiate IABP or VAD as ordered *to decrease cardiac workload and increase coronary perfusion.*
- Measure intake and output every 1 to 2 hours.
- Monitor indices of renal function: BUN and creatinine levels.

Ineffective tissue perfusion (renal, cerebral, cardiopulmonary, and peripheral) related to decreased cardiac output (CO)

- Maintain complete bed rest *to minimize metabolic needs.*
- Maintain flat position or position that *facilitates or improves circulation.*
- Keep patient warm *to minimize metabolic needs.*
- Measure intake and output every 1 to 2 hours or as indicated *to evaluate renal function.*
- Administer parenteral therapy, blood products, and volume expanders as ordered and in accordance with hemodynamic parameters.
- Check blood pressure and peripheral pulses every 1 to 2 hours as ordered *to assess tissue perfusion.*
- Apply support measures *to control bleeding as indicated:* pressure dressings, shock trousers.

NIC Respiratory Management

Impaired gas exchange related to perceived threat to or change in health status

- Report if SVO_2 is less than 60%.
- Administer oxygen as ordered via mask or through endotracheal tube.
- Auscultate breath sounds every hour *for increasing pulmonary congestion and atelectasis.*
- Prepare for intubation and assisted ventilation as indicated.
- Review serial chest x-rays as ordered.

NIC Nutritional Support

Imbalanced nutrition: less than body requirements, related to depleted glycogen stores

- Record weight on admission *to establish baseline.*
- Weigh daily at same time of day, using same scale.
- Begin tube feedings, intralipids, and total parenteral nutrition as ordered.

NIC Coping Assistance

Anxiety related to fear

- Explain all procedures and treatments.
- Remain with patient *to offer reassurance.*
- Maintain as quiet and calm an atmosphere as possible.
- Allow family to be with patient as condition permits.
- Encourage expressions of feelings.
- Maintain calm and reassuring manner; stay with patient *to provide sense of security.*

Patient Education/Continuum of Care Plan

Explain all procedures and treatments as they occur. Refer to the primary disorder for specific teaching protocol.

Evaluation/Patient Outcomes

Tissue Perfusion Management: Tissue perfusion is improved. Patient is alert, oriented, and normotensive; urine output is normal; skin is warm and dry; peripheral pulse palpable. Cardiac output 4 to 5 L/min. Patient is normotensive. PCWP is 10 to 15 mm Hg. Fluid volume is restored.

Respiratory Management: Gas exchange is improved. PaO_2 is 80 to 100 mm Hg. PCO_2 is 35 to 45 mm Hg. Lungs are clear. Patient verbalizes that breathing is easier.

Nutritional Support: Nutritional status is maintained or improved. Weight remains stable or increases. Albumin and tranferrin levels are within normal limits. Nitrogen balance is maintained.

Coping Assistance: Anxiety is decreased. Patient verbalizes fears and asks questions. Patient appears relaxed and is resting quietly.

CARDIOMYOPATHY

The term *cardiomyopathy* is applied to diseases that affect the myocardium, resulting in enlargement or ventricular dysfunction (FIG. 3-41).

In the past three decades great advances in the understanding of this complex disorder have been made. There are three main types of cardiomyopathy, classified according to the pathophysiologic process resulting in myocardial dysfunction: dilated, hypertrophic, and restrictive. The etiologic factors contributing to cardiomyopathy are frequently unknown (idiopathic) but can be summarized in the following categories:

- Primary myocardial disease
  - Ischemic (coronary artery disease)
- Endocardial fibroelastosis
- Familial cardiomyopathies

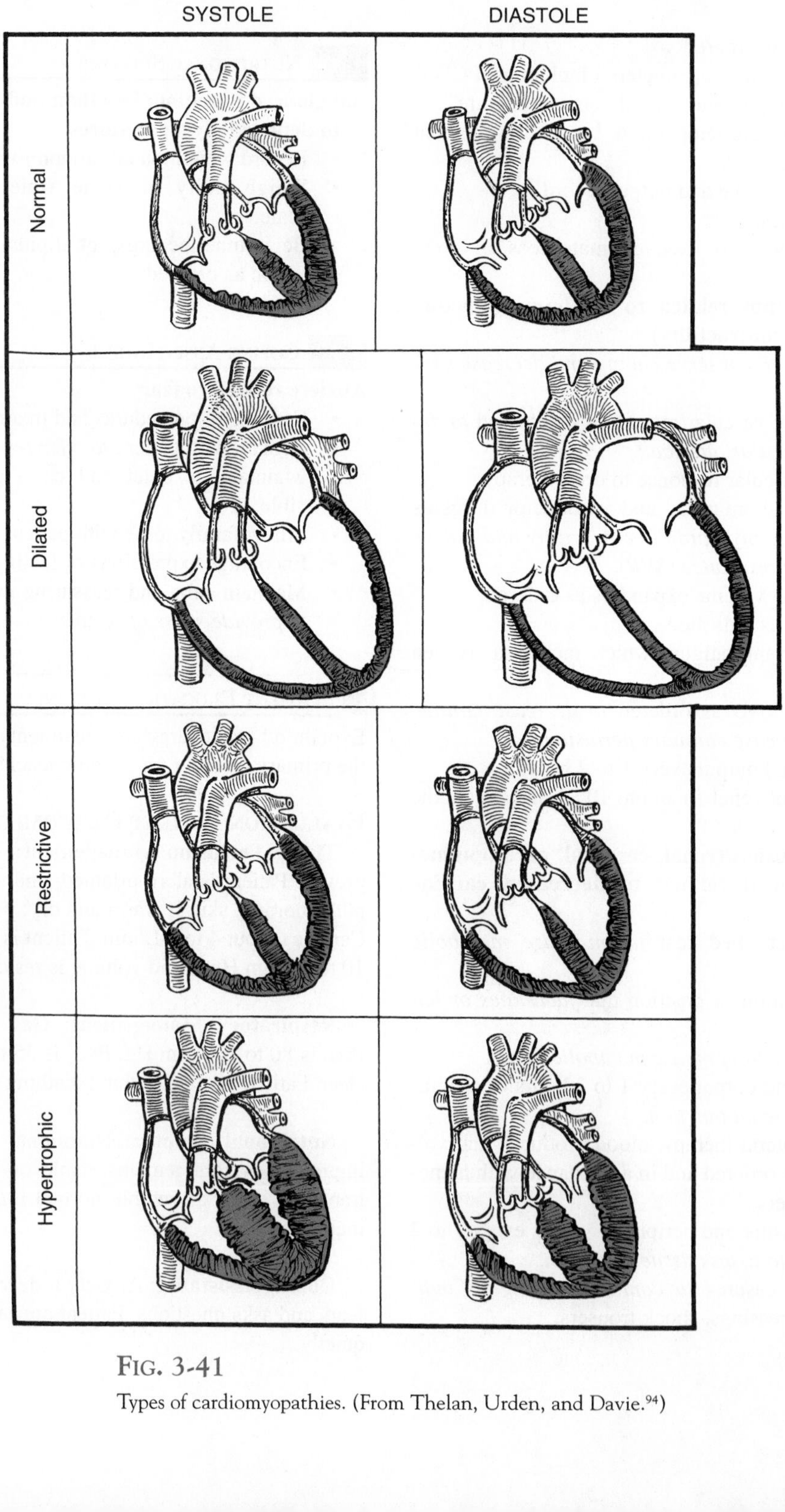

FIG. 3-41
Types of cardiomyopathies. (From Thelan, Urden, and Davie.[94])

- Metabolic storage diseases
  - Pompe's disease (glycogen)
  - Fabry's disease (glycolipid)
- Muscular dystrophies
- Friedreich's ataxia
- Sickle cell anemia

Inflammatory disorders
- Infections
  - Viral (such as coxsackievirus, rubella, human immunodeficiency virus [HIV])
  - Rickettsial (typhus, Q fever)
  - Bacterial (streptococcal)
  - Spirochetal (leptospirosis, syphilis)
  - Fungal (histoplasmosis, coccidioidomycosis)
  - Parasitic (Chagas' disease, schistosomiasis)
- Noninfectious (collagen)
  - Rheumatic heart disease
  - Scleroderma
  - Systemic lupus erythematosus
  - Polyarteritis
  - Löffler's disease
  - Dermatomyositis

Infiltrative disorders
- Sarcoidosis
- Amyloidosis
- Neoplastic disease

Metabolic disorders
- Endocrine disorders
  - Thyrotoxicosis
  - Myxedema
- Nutritional disorders
  - Starvation, malnutrition
  - Beriberi

Toxic agents
- Alcohol
- Carbon monoxide
- Arsenic
- Immunosuppressive drugs (doxorubicin)
- Cocaine

Miscellaneous
- Postpartum
- Radiation

PATHOPHYSIOLOGY

Hypertrophic Cardiomyopathy

Hypertrophic cardiomyopathy (HCM) is the form of myocardial disease whose pathophysiologic, etiologic, and clinical features continue to receive the widest attention. As a result, it has acquired an extensive list of identifying terms that generally describe features of the disease not present in all cases. These include idiopathic hypertrophic subaortic stenosis (IHSS), asymmetric septal hypertrophy (ASH), and hypertrophic obstructive cardiomyopathy (HOCM).

Hypertrophic cardiomyopathy is marked by a distinctive pattern of hypertrophy, with thickening of the interventricular septum when compared with the free wall of the left ventricle (FIG. 3-42). The overgrowth of muscle mass makes the ventricular walls rigid, increasing resistance as blood enters from the left atrium. Obstruction of left ventricular outflow is another characteristic. Consequently, left ventricular ejection is impeded throughout systole. Contributing to outflow obstruction is the obstruction caused by apposition of the anterior mitral leaflet against the hypertrophied septum during midsystole. Left ventricular function in hypertrophic cardiomyopathy is usually supranormal, but later in the disease extensive myocardial fibrosis may occur, resulting in impaired left ventricular function. Systolic motion of the anterior mitral leaflet has been used to determine the severity of outflow obstruction.[10] Elevated systolic pressure gradients occur in the range of 70% to 90% of left ventricular volumes.[68] Failure occurs as resistance to diastolic filling increases because of a stiff, noncompliant left ventricle.

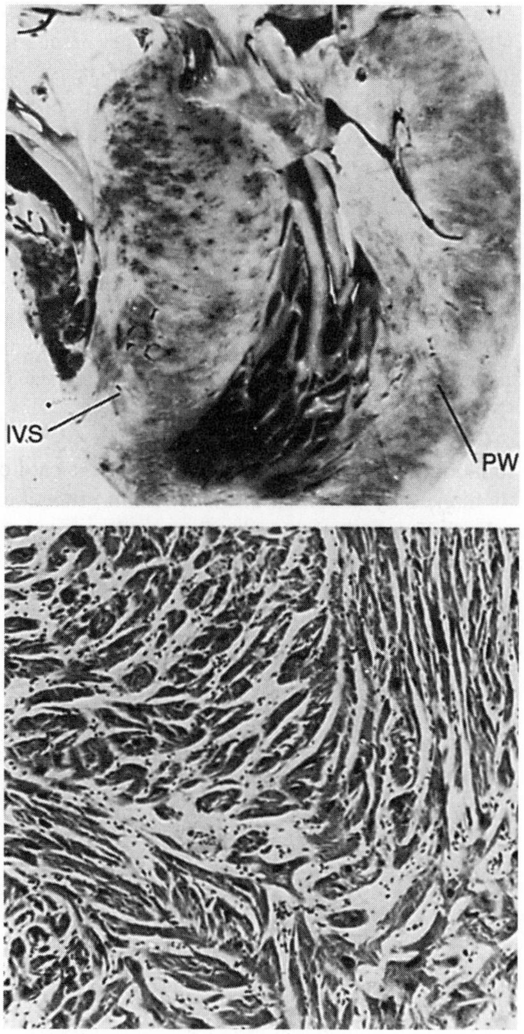

FIG. 3-42

Heart with hypertrophic cardiomyopathy. Interventricular septum, *IVS*, is thicker than posterior wall, *PW.* Histologic section (lower illustration) shows marked disorganization of myocardium that is especially prominent in septum. (Hematoxylin and eosin, × 50.) (From Bulkley BH: Advances in cardiac pathology. In Hurst JW, editor: *The heart, update I*, New York, 1979, McGraw-Hill.)

These hearts show massive overgrowth of myocardial tissue with small ventricular cavities. The atria are also hypertrophied and dilated, reflecting the high resistance to ventricular filling.

Histologically the heart muscle may show myocardial fiber disarray (see FIG. 3-42). First described in 1958 by Donald Teare, this form of hypertrophic cardiomyopathy is thought to reflect a genetic defect that results in abnormal heart structure. This feature is not limited to hypertrophic cardiomyopathy; similar disorganization has been seen in some cases of acquired or congenital heart disease.

Dilated Cardiomyopathy

The most common form of cardiomyopathy is marked by gross dilation of the heart, interference with systolic function, and damage to myofibrils. Dilated cardiomyopathy is marked by impaired systolic function (ejection fractions of 15% to 20% are common), which leads to increased end-diastolic and end-systolic volumes.

The heart has a globular shape with enlargement, and dilation of all four chambers (FIG. 3-43). Although the heart may weigh up to 700 g (normal is 350 g), the wall thickness may be normal or decreased. Left ventricular filling pressures are generally higher as a result of poor contractile function. The cardiac valves are basically normal, as are the coronary arteries. Endocardial thrombi are common, particularly in the ventricular apex. Histologic examination reveals nonspecific changes, including cell hypertrophy and extensive interstitial and perivascular fibrosis. The cause of this disorder is not clear, but it has been linked to various factors that predispose to the development of cardiomyopathy, including alcohol, pregnancy, infections, and toxic agents.

Restrictive Cardiomyopathy

A less common form of cardiomyopathy, restrictive cardiomyopathy, is marked by abnormal diastolic (filling) function and excessively rigid ventricular walls. Contractility is relatively unimpaired with normal systolic emptying of the ventricles. Hemodynamically, this group of cardiomyopathies resembles constrictive pericarditis.

The abnormal diastolic filling occurs as a result of infiltration of the endocardium or myocardium with fibroelastic tissue similar to that seen in Löffler's endocarditis, endomyocardial fibrosis, and amyloidosis.

DIAGNOSTIC STUDIES AND FINDINGS

See Diagnostic Studies and Findings table.

MULTIDISCIPLINARY PLAN

Surgery

Septalmyotomy-myectomy: For patient with hypertrophic cardiomyopathy who has intractable symptoms and severe obstruction; hypertrophied septum is excised, which diminishes left ventricular gradient and mitral regurgitation; procedure improves symptoms but has not been reported to prolong life

Excision of fibrotic endocardium: Successful in limited number of cases of restrictive cardiomyopathy; procedure apparently decreases ventricular filling pressures and increases cardiac output

Cardiac transplantation: Increasingly becoming the treatment of choice for dilated cardiomyopathy refractory to medical therapy, but requires careful evaluation of patient and family (p. 124 describes care of patient after transplantation)

Other surgical interventions: Essentially nonexistent; valve replacement considered in individual cases but generally not favored

Medications

Hypertrophic cardiomyopathy: Goals of drug therapy are to decrease ventricular contractility and increase ventricular volume and left ventricular outflow without vasodilation

Type IA antidysrhythmics

Disopyramide (Norpace)

Indications: Negative inotropic drug demonstrated to significantly decrease left ventricular pressure gradient; currently drug of choice in treatment of obstructive hypertrophic cardiomyopathy

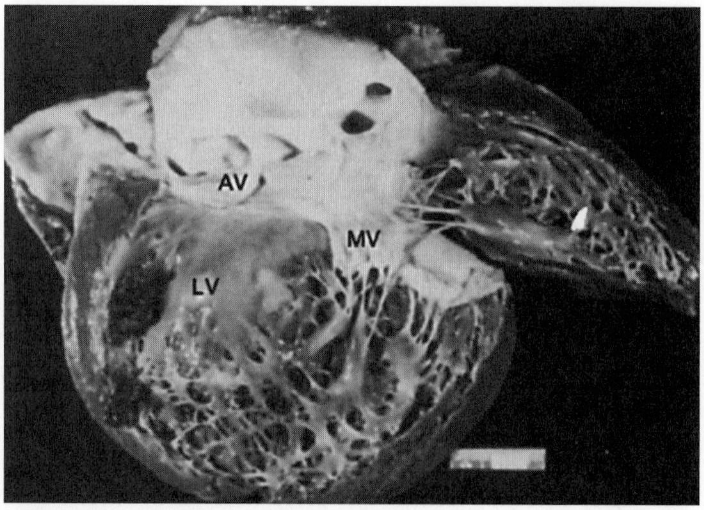

FIG. 3-43

Heart with idiopathic dilated congestive cardiomyopathy. Opened left ventricle, *LV*, has dilated and globular configuration. Aortic valves, *AV*, and mitral valves, *MV*, are normal. (From Kaye.[54])

Diagnostic Studies and Findings

Study	Hypertrophic Cardiomyopathy	Dilated Cardiomyopathy	Restrictive Cardiomyopathy
Chest x-ray	Enlarged cardiac silhouette (mild to moderate)	Enlarged cardiac silhouette; prominence of left ventricle (LV) (moderate to marked); pleural effusions	Cardiac enlargement (mild)
ECG (24-h ambulatory monitor)	LV hypertrophy; ST segment and T wave changes; Q waves may be seen in inferior and precordial leads; atrial and ventricular dysrhythmias	LV hypertrophy; sinus tachycardia; atrial and ventricular dysrhythmias; ST segment and T wave changes; conduction disturbances	Low-voltage conduction disturbances
Echocardiogram	Narrow LV outflow tract; abnormal thickened septum; systolic anterior motion of mitral valve; decreased internal dimension of LV; LV hypertrophy	LV dilation; abnormal diastolic mitral valve motion; enlarged atria; decreased ejection fraction (15%-20%)	Increased LV wall thickness and mass; small or normal LV cavity; normal systolic function; pericardial effusion
Radionuclide studies	Hyperdynamic systolic function; technetium shows decreased LV volume; thallium-201 shows increased muscle mass, ischemia; gated blood pool imaging evaluates size and motion of septum and LV	LV dilation and hypokinesis; decreased ejection fraction	Myocardial infiltration; small or normal LV cavity; normal systolic function; computed tomography and MRI define pericardial thickness
Cardiac catheterization	Decreased LV compliance; mitral regurgitation; hyperdynamic systolic function; LV outflow obstruction	LV enlargement and dysfunction; mitral and tricuspid regurgitation; elevated diastolic filling pressures; decreased cardiac output	Decreased LV compliance; normal systolic function; elevated diastolic filling process
Endomyocardial biopsy		To identify specific etiologies (e.g., sarcoidosis, myocarditis)	To detect eosinophil infiltration

Usual dosage: 600-800 mg/d PO

Beta-adrenergic blocking agents: Propranolol (Inderal), metoprolol (Lopressor)

Indications: Negative inotropic effects on myocardial contractility and thus is believed to prevent increase in outflow obstruction, decrease myocardial oxygen consumption, and exert antidysrhythmic actions; may be used in combination with Norpace for optimizing therapy

Calcium channel blockers: Verapamil (Calan)

Indications: Has been shown to decrease left ventricular outflow obstruction and increase exercise tolerance; however, the vasodilatory effects may lead to worsening obstruction thus should be used with caution

Usual dosage: 80-160 mg q8h PO (not to exceed 480 mg/d)

Dilated cardiomyopathy: Cannot be halted or reversed by any pharmacologic agent; pharmacologic interventions directed largely by symptoms of congestive heart failure or dysrhythmias

Restrictive cardiomyopathy: Pharmacologic agents directed by underlying disorder; digitalis and diuretics often employed to treat dysrhythmias and signs of failure, but their effectiveness is limited

General Management

Hemodynamic monitoring: Initiated as means of assessing left ventricular function and cardiac output

IABP: Used to sustain severely depressed ventricular function

Ventricular assist device: Bridge to cardiac transplantation for end-stage ventricular failure

Atrioventricular sequential pacing: Capable of reducing or abolishing obstructive pressure gradient in hypertrophic cardiomyopathy by pacing right side of ventricular septum, widening left ventricular outflow tract

Internal cardiac defibrillator (ICD): May be used in hypertrophic cardiomyopathy with ventricular tachycardia or fibrillation

Cardiac monitoring: Used to determine presence of atrial or ventricular dysrhythmias or conduction defects and to assess effectiveness of antidysrhythmic agents

Cardioversion: Used in treatment of atrial fibrillation with rapid ventricular response

Restriction of sodium and fluid intake

Oxygen therapy

NURSING CARE

Nursing Assessment

Observe for signs and symptoms of decreased left ventricular functioning: chest pain, syncope, peripheral constriction, and cyanosis.

Assess and monitor patient's tolerance to activities, noting which activities aggravate symptoms.

Observe for signs of decreased ventricular function and fluid retention: increased adventitious lung sounds, presence of S_3, shortness of breath, cough, peripheral edema, increased venous filling.

See Assessment Considerations table.

Assessment Considerations

Area of Concern	Hypertrophic Cardiomyopathy	Dilated Cardiomyopathy	Restrictive Cardiomyopathy
General complaints	Dyspnea; shortness of breath; angina pectoris; fatigue; palpitations; syncope (may be exertional)	Dyspnea; fatigue; complaints associated with biventricular failure; palpitations	Dyspnea; fatigue; complaints associated with right ventricular failure
Arterial pressure		Normal or low systolic; narrowed pulse pressure	Narrowed pulse pressure
Arterial pulse	Brisk carotid upstroke; pulsus bisferiens	Low amplitude and volume; pulsus alternans	
Jugular venous pressure	Dominant a wave	Distended; prominent a and v waves	Distended
Palpation	Apical systolic thrill and heave	Apical impulse displaced laterally; parasternal impulses and heaves; pulsatile liver	Apical impulse difficult to palpate
Auscultation	Systolic murmur heard best at apex and at lower left sternal border, increasing in intensity with Valsalva maneuver; S_4 gallop	Murmurs of mitral and tricuspid regurgitation; S_3 and S_4 gallops; pulmonary crackles	Murmurs of mitral regurgitation; S_3 and S_4 gallops, heart sounds distant

Potential Complications

Hypertrophic cardiomyopathy

Arrhythmias, atrial fibrillation, supraventricular tachycardias

Abnormal response to exercise: Sudden cardiac death has been reported with moderate to severe exercise

Dilated cardiomyopathy

See section on congestive heart failure (p. 66)

Restricted cardiomyopathy

See section on congestive heart failure (p. 66)

Patient Problems/Nursing Diagnoses & Interventions

NIC Tissue Perfusion Management

Decreased cardiac output related to mechanical factors (preload, afterload, or contractility)

- Encourage appropriate activity levels based on clinical condition and disease state.
- Limit self-care activities *to conserve energy and decrease oxygen demand.*
- Monitor arterial pressure, PCWP, cardiac output, and ECG as indicated.
- Administer drugs as ordered.
- Limit and monitor IV fluids as ordered.

Convalescent care

- Progressively increase activity level as indicated by improvement in patient status.
- Monitor vital signs and report any changes in heart rate or blood pressure.
- Teach patient and family the importance of monitoring vital signs and how to check blood pressure and pulse accurately.

NIC Coping Assistance

Ineffective coping related to inability to deal with multiple stressors and progressive deterioration of health status

- Determine baseline knowledge of disease.
- Answer all questions about disease and future health.
- Encourage discussion of feelings of hopelessness and fears.
- Assist patient to participate in decision-making process with regard to any adjustments in lifestyle.
- Provide patient education and instructions for home care.
- Include family or significant other in care.
- Encourage family to learn cardiopulmonary resuscitation.

NIC Activity and Exercise Management

Activity intolerance related to diminished cardiac reserve

- Coordinate care to promote rest and *to ensure periods of uninterrupted rest.*
- Increase activities gradually; assist as necessary.
- Instruct patient in energy conservation methods *to limit or reduce energy expenditure.*

NIC Electrolyte and Acid-Base Management

Excess fluid volume related to increased levels of aldosterone, sodium retention, and antidiuretic hormone (secondary to right or left ventricular dysfunction)

- Maintain patent IV line for drug administration.
- Administer diuretics as ordered *to decrease circulating volume.*
- Restrict sodium and fluid intake.
- Weigh patient daily (same time of day, same amount of clothing) *to determine fluid loss or retention.*
- Monitor intake and output.
- Monitor serum electrolytes, especially sodium and potassium.

Other related nursing diagnoses: Impaired gas exchange related to elevated pulmonary capillary pressure; imbalanced nutrition: less than body requirements, related to impaired absorption of nutrients; acute pain (chest) related to myocardial ischemia

PATIENT EDUCATION/CONTINUUM OF CARE PLAN

1. Describe the nature and type of cardiomyopathy.
2. Explain the prognosis and the limitations of the disease on lifestyle, especially important because many patients were considered "healthy" before diagnosis was made.
3. Explain the signs and symptoms to report to the physician.
4. Describe activity allowances and limitations; explain the importance of avoiding isometric exercises; explain the importance of resting when feeling fatigued.
5. Explain dietary and fluid restrictions.
6. Explain the name, purpose, dosage, and side effects of prescribed medications; warn against the effects of abruptly stopping propranolol.
7. Explain the need for daily weighing when ordered and reporting increase of more than 2 pounds in a 24-hour period.
8. Discuss the importance of follow-up appointment.
9. Provide referrals for community support services.

EVALUATION/PATIENT OUTCOMES

Tissue Perfusion Management: Ventricular volume is optimized; outflow obstruction is decreased. Cardiac output is increased and LVEDP is decreased. Fatigue, dyspnea, and angina are relieved. Patient loses excess fluid weight. Dyspnea and shortness of breath are relieved.

Coping Assistance: Patient copes effectively with diagnosis. Patient follows up with medical therapy. Patient reports taking medications. Patient verbalizes feeling less anxious and fearful.

Activity and Exercise Management: Patient exhibits tolerance to ADL and to an increasing level of activity. Patient is normotensive; heart rate is within 10 to 20 beats per minute of resting rate; reports no symptoms of activity intolerance.

Electrolyte and Acid-Base Management: Electrolytes are normal with diuretic therapy. Dry weight is established and maintained.

VALVULAR HEART DISEASE

Valvular heart disease (VHD) is an acquired or congenital disorder of a cardiac valve, marked by stenosis and obstructed blood flow or by valvular breakdown and regurgitation of blood (FIG. 3-44).

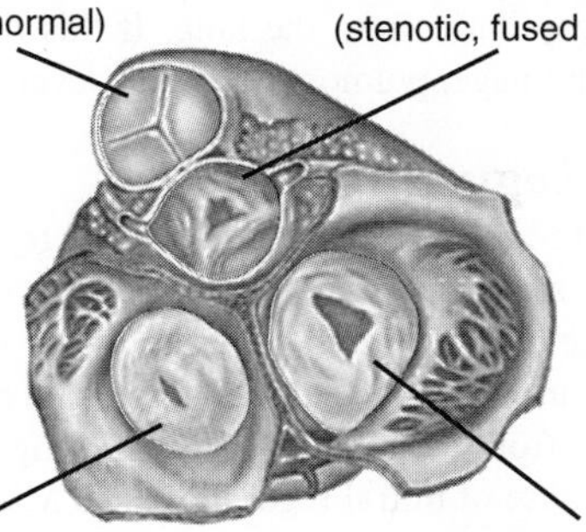

FIG. 3-44
Valvular heart disease. (From Canobbio.[15])

With the introduction of antibiotic therapy and with improved diagnostic procedures, the incidence of VHD has declined over the past three decades. It is most commonly a chronic illness, and symptoms requiring therapy may take years to develop. VHD may also occur as an acute illness after trauma, MI, or endocarditis.

PATHOPHYSIOLOGY

The etiology of VHD can be classified into congenital and acquired disorders.

Congenital disorders include bicuspid aortic valve and pulmonary stenosis. Although not usually classified as VHD, tricuspid and pulmonary atresia, mitral valve prolapse, and Ebstein's anomaly are all defects involving valve function.

Rheumatic fever and endocarditis account for the greatest number of cases of acquired VHD.[4,10] Other disorders such as Marfan's syndrome, cardiomyopathy, MI, myxomatous degeneration of the mitral valve, and trauma can also lead to valve dysfunction.

Cardiac valves are unidirectional, ensuring efficient flow of blood throughout the heart as well as the pulmonary and systemic circulation. Valve disorders occur when the integrity of the valve leaflets or the surrounding structures are disrupted.

Two basic valve abnormalities exist: stenosis and regurgitation. In stenosis the valve opening narrows as a result of thickening and rigidity of the valve leaflets. Stenosis blocks the flow of blood across the valve, increasing the pressure gradient. In regurgitation (insufficiency, incompetency), calcification, scarring, and retraction of the leaflets or adjacent structures lead to an incomplete valve closure that results in reversed blood flow.

Mixed lesions producing both stenosis and regurgitation can occur. In addition, more than one valve may be affected.

Mitral Stenosis

The most common cause of mitral stenosis is rheumatic valvulitis that leads to fibrotic thickening and fusion of the valve commissures. Scarring of the free margins of the leaflets occurs with shortening and thickening of the chordae tendineae, which may lead to the regurgitation often seen with mitral stenosis.

The normal mitral valve opening is 4 to 6 cm^2. When this opening is reduced, flow across the valve is blocked, increasing the pressure gradient needed to eject blood from the left atrium to the left ventricle. The pressure gradient rises to maintain cardiac output. When the mitral orifice is decreased to 2 cm^2, cardiac output drops and symptoms appear with exertion. As the disease progresses, the mean left atrial pressure rises, causing the left atrial chamber to enlarge. The increased left atrial pressure is reflected in the pulmonary capillaries and pulmonary artery. As pulmonary capillary pressure rises, fluid flows back across the alveolar membrane, eventually exceeding oncotic pressure of the plasma proteins in the blood and forcing fluid out of the capillaries into the lung. If this fluid cannot be removed by drainage, pulmonary edema develops.

Mitral Regurgitation

Rheumatic fever, the usual cause of mitral regurgitation, causes thickening, scarring, rigidity, and calcification of the valve leaflets. The commissures become fused with the chordae tendineae, causing the leaflets to shorten and retract, which prevents them from complete closure during systole. A nonrheumatic cause of mitral regurgitation is MI, which causes dilation of the left ventricle and displacement of the papillary muscles. Papillary muscle dysfunction may also occur as a result of rupture or fibrosis caused by ischemia, infarction, and ventricular aneurysm at the base of a papillary muscle. In addition, annular dilation may lead to an incomplete mitral apparatus. The most common cause is left ventricular dilation resulting from aortic regurgitation, coronary artery disease, or dilated cardiomyopathy.

As the mitral valve disorder progresses, the reverse flow to the left atrium causes left atrial pressure to rise. This pressure is reflected in the pulmonary veins, leading to leakage of fluid into the lungs.

The increase in left atrial pressure causes atrial dilation and enlargement. The left ventricle becomes hypertrophied because it must deal with the larger volume of blood that is lost to the left atrium during systole.

MITRAL VALVE PROLAPSE

Mitral valve prolapse (MVP) is the superior systolic displacement of the mitral leaflets. It has become one of the most commonly found disorders involving the mitral valve. It is reported that as many as 15% of otherwise healthy young persons will demonstrate some normal superior systolic displacement of the mitral leaflets. However, excessive valvuloventricular disproportion reflects a primary connective tissue abnormality of the mitral leaflets, the annulus, and chordae tendineae. This abnormality is referred to as MVP (FIG. 3-45).

Clinical findings depend on the degree to which the leaflets prolapse in the atrium. If the mitral leaflets prolapse to such an extent that the contact between the two leaflets is impaired, mitral regurgitation will result.

Aortic Stenosis

The most common cause of aortic stenosis is congenital bicuspid valve. This defect occurs in 1% of the population, more often in males (3:1).

The normal aortic valve opening measures 2.6 to 3.5 cm^2. Valve narrowing results from calcification of the leaflets. Calcification may extend into the aortic wall or onto the anterior leaflet of the mitral valve, which accounts for the mitral disease commonly occurring with aortic stenosis. Calcification may also extend into the conduction system, leading to conduction defects. As the disease progresses, calcification makes the valve inflexible, reducing the opening to a small slit.

As the aortic valve opening decreases, left ventricular pressure rises to create enough pressure to eject a normal stroke volume and propel flow across the valve into the aorta. This obstruction to left ventricular outflow leads to a pressure gradient between the aorta and left ventricle during systole. To maintain flow across the narrowed opening, wall thickness gradually increases in the pressure-overloaded left ventricle, leading to hypertrophy. In time the flow across the valve becomes fixed and cardiac output does not increase in response to demand.

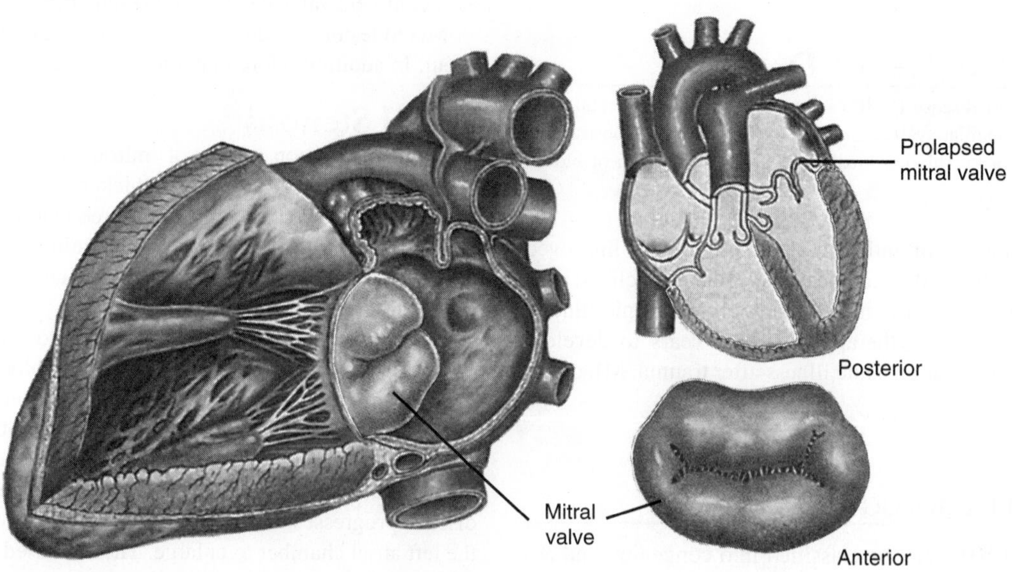

FIG. 3-45
Mitral valve prolapse. (From Canobbio.[15])

During exercise the increased flow to extremities with fixed cardiac output causes a decreased cerebral and coronary blood flow, resulting in dizziness or syncope and chest pain.

As the LVEDP rises, left atrial pressure rises, and eventually pulmonary congestion appears with signs and symptoms of congestive heart failure.

The course of aortic stenosis depends on the size of the valve opening and the left ventricle.

The onset of symptoms of heart failure indicates moderate to severe disease, and death often occurs less than 5 years after symptoms appear. Sudden death is linked to severe aortic stenosis (0.5 to 0.6 cm^2).

Aortic Regurgitation

Rheumatic fever, syphilis, connective tissue disorder, and infective endocarditis are common causes of aortic valve disorders.

The basic hemodynamic problem in aortic regurgitation is a volume-overloaded left ventricle. Blood ejected during normal systole reenters the left ventricle in diastole. To compensate for this volume, the left ventricle must produce a higher stroke volume by increasing the systolic pressure, resulting in eventual hypertrophy of the left ventricle.

With time, LVEDP and left atrial pressure increase. As myocardial contractility diminishes and failure takes place, mitral regurgitation may occur as a result of the malpositioning of papillary muscles.

Diagnostic Studies and Findings

See Diagnostic Studies and Findings table.

Multidisciplinary Plan

Surgery

Indicated when medical therapy no longer alleviates clinical symptoms or when there is diagnostic evidence of progressive myocardial dysfunction (such as progressive enlargement of heart)

Valvotomy: Surgical splitting of fused commissures or thickened leaflets

Valvular annuloplasty: Reparative procedure of valve ring, chordae, or papillary muscle performed primarily for mitral and tricuspid regurgitation

Valve replacement: Replacement of stenotic or incompetent valve with bioprosthetic or mechanical valve; commonly used valves include pynolite tilting disks, porcine heterografts, homografts, autografts, pericardial valves, and ball-in-cage valves

Medications

Guided by patient's clinical signs and symptoms or echocardiographic evidence of increasing left atrial or left ventricular size or increased regurgitation

ACE inhibitors, afterload reduction for a volume-loaded left atrium or left ventricle

Digitalis and diuretics for heart failure (see p. 68)

Dysrhythmia management (see p. 44)

Anticoagulants for patients in atrial fibrillation who are at risk for systemic or pulmonary embolization; warfarin sodium (Coumadin) in doses titrated to maintain prothrombin time at two times control or International Normalized Ratio (INR) of 1.5-2.5

Antibiotic prophylaxis before any procedure that increases risk of endocarditis (Table 3-2)

Diagnostic Studies and Findings

Study	Mitral Stenosis	Mitral Regurgitation	Aortic Stenosis	Aortic Regurgitation
ECG	LA enlargement; notched P wave (P mitrale); RV hypertrophy; atrial fibrillation (in 40%-50% of cases)	LA enlargement; LV hypertrophy; atrial fibrillation	LV hypertrophy; conduction defects; first-degree AV block, left bundle branch block	LV hypertrophy
Chest x-ray	LA and RV enlargement; pulmonary venous congestion; interstitial pulmonary edema	LA and LV enlargement; pulmonary vascular congestion	Poststenotic aortic dilation; aortic valve calcification	Aortic valve calcification; LV enlargement; dilation of ascending aorta
Echocardiogram	Decreased excursion of leaflets; diminished E to F slope; stenotic valve is thickened	LA enlargement; hyperdynamic LV	Nonrestricted movement of aortic valve; thickening of LV wall	LV dilation; diastolic fluttering of anterior leaflet
Radionuclide studies	To determine resting and exercise ejection fraction	To determine resting and exercise ejection fraction	To determine resting and exercise ejection fraction	To determine resting and exercise ejection fraction
Cardiac catheterization	Pressure across mitral valve increased; LA pressure increased; PCWP increased; low cardiac output	LVEDP increased; LAP increased; angiography with contrast media performed to quantify regurgitation	Pressure gradient in systole across aortic valve; LVEDP increased	Pulse pressure increased; LVEDP increased; LAP increased; angiography with contrast media performed to quantify regurgitation

General Management

Cardioversion: Indicated for patients with mitral stenosis in atrial fibrillation to decrease risk of emboli

Dictated by severity of valvular disorder (see pp. 68 and 53 for supportive care of patients in heart failure or with dysrhythmias)

Diet therapy: Sodium restriction for patients with mild to moderate signs of pulmonary congestion

Balloon valvuloplasty: Nonsurgical procedure used in treatment of calcific mitral valvular stenosis, the procedure involves passing a balloon-tipped catheter under fluoroscopy across the stenotic valve; once in place, the balloon is inflated repeatedly until the valve gradient is relieved. Procedure is of limited value in aortic or tricuspid stenosis and of no value with bioprosthetic valves.

Table 3-2 Recommended Antibiotic Coverage for Endocarditis Prophylaxis in the Adult

Patient		Regimen
STANDARD REGIMEN FOR DENTAL/ORAL/UPPER RESPIRATORY TRACT PROCEDURES		
At risk (includes patients with prosthetic heart valves and other high-risk patients)	1 h before procedure	Amoxicillin 2.0 g orally.
Amoxicillin/penicillin allergy	1 h before procedure	Clindamycin 600 mg orally, cephalaxin or cefadroxel 2.0 g orally or azithromycin 500 mg orally
Unable to take oral medications	30 min before procedure	Ampicillin 2.0 g IV or IM
	6 h after initial dose	Ampicillin 1.0 g IV or IM
Amoxicillin/penicillin allergy	30 min before procedure	Clindamycin 600 mg IV or cefazolin 1.0 g IV
STANDARD REGIMEN FOR GENITOURINARY/GASTROINTESTINAL PROCEDURES		
At high risk	30 min before procedure	Ampicillin 2.0 g IV (or IM) *plus* gentamicin 1.5 mg/kg IV (or IM) not to exceed 120 mg
	6 h after initial dose	Amoxicillin 1.0 g orally, IM or IV
Amoxicillin/ampicillin/penicillin allergy	1 h before procedure	Vancomycin 1.0 g IV administered over 1 h *plus* gentamicin 1.5 mg/kg IV (or IM) not to exceed 120 mg
At moderate risk	30 min before procedure	Amoxicillin 3.0 g orally, ampicillin 2.0 g IV, or vancomycin 1.0 g IV

Modified from Prevention of bacterial endocarditis: recommendations by the American Heart Association, *JAMA* 227:1794, 1997.

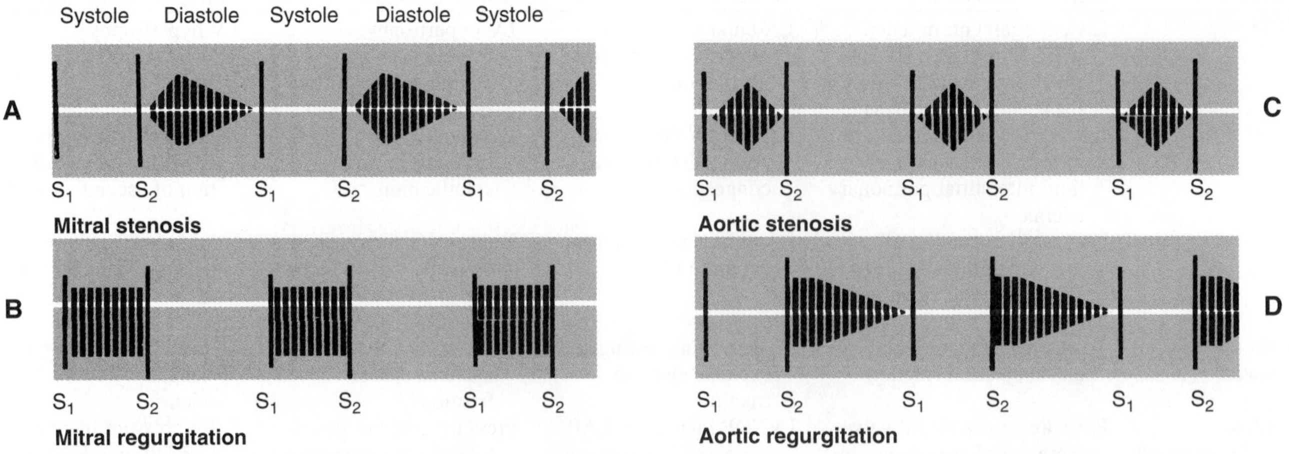

FIG. 3-46

Auscultation of valvular heart disease murmurs. **A,** Mitral stenosis. **B,** Mitral regurgitation. **C,** Aortic stenosis. **D,** Aortic regurgitation. (From Guzzetta and Dossey.[44])

NURSING CARE

NURSING ASSESSMENT

Establish baseline assessment of cardiovascular status to evaluate disease process and response to therapy
Monitor vital signs every 4 to 8 hours or as indicated.
Monitor nutrition with dietary sodium and fluid restrictions.
Monitor intake and output to determine response to therapy.
Monitor electrolyte levels, blood chemistry findings, hemoglobin level, and hematocrit.
See Assessment Considerations table.

POTENTIAL COMPLICATIONS

Thromboembolism; endocarditis; acute aortic dissection; congestive heart failure; arrhythmias; syncope

PATIENT PROBLEMS/NURSING DIAGNOSES & INTERVENTIONS

NIC TISSUE PERFUSION MANAGEMENT

Decreased cardiac output related to mechanical factors (preload, afterload)

Excess fluid volume (risk for) related to cardiac decompensation

- Administer medications as ordered.
- Limit or modify activities during acute phase *to conserve energy and decrease myocardial oxygen demand.*
- Monitor and record ECG rate and rhythm; observe and record dysrhythmia.
- Assess for signs and symptoms of fluid volume excess: weight gain, increased jugular venous pressure, lung congestion.
- Administer diuretic and vasodilator therapy as ordered.
- Weigh patient daily (same time of day, same amount of clothing) to detect fluid retention.

Other related nursing diagnoses: Ineffective tissue perfusion related to interruption of arterial blood flow secondary to embolism; activity intolerance related to cardiac decompensation; anxiety related to altered heart function

PATIENT EDUCATION/CONTINUUM OF CARE PLAN

1. Assess the patient's level of knowledge and teach the patient about the disease, including etiology, medications, diet restrictions, exercise levels, and possible complications.
2. Assist the patient during diagnostic work-up and assist with the decision for medical or surgical treatment.
3. Include the patient's family in the teaching and decision-making process.
4. Ensure that the patient knows the name, dosage, and purpose of medications.
5. Discuss with the patient the disease process and associated symptoms to report to the physician.

Assessment Considerations

Area of Concern	Mitral Stenosis	Mitral Regurgitation	Aortic Stenosis	Aortic Regurgitation
General complaints	Fatigue; dyspnea on exertion; palpitations; hemoptysis; hoarseness; orthopnea; paroxysmal nocturnal dyspnea	Dyspnea; fatigue; exercise intolerance; orthopnea; palpitations	Fatigue; dyspnea; orthopnea; angina pectoris; dizziness; syncope	Dyspnea on exertion; palpitations; orthopnea; exertional chest pain
Physical examination	Resting tachycardia; irregular pulse; jugular venous distention increased in presence of RV failure; prominent a wave in presence of pulmonary hypertension (absent in atrial fibrillation)	Irregular pulse; sharp upstroke of arterial pulse; jugular venous distention increased in presence of RV failure; prominent a wave in presence of increased RV pressure	Early: normal blood pressure; late: systolic pressure decreased; narrow pulse pressure; carotid pulse slow with small pulse volume	Arterial pulsations; bounding pulse with rapid rise and fall (water-hammer pulse); widened pulse pressure; head bobbing (Musset's sign); skin warm, damp, and flushed
Palpation	Diastolic thrill at apex	Apical impulse forceful and displaced downward and to left	Systolic thrill palpable at base of heart; apical pulse strong and sustained throughout systole	Diastolic thrill along left sternal border; laterally displaced apical impulse; systolic thrill in jugular notch and along carotid arteries
Auscultation (FIG. 3-46)	Loud S_1; opening snap; low snap; low-pitched, rumbling diastolic murmur	Diminished or absent S_1; wide splitting of S_2; S_3, S_4 heard in severe regurgitation; holosystolic murmur heard best at apex	Diminished or absent A_2; crescendo-decrescendo harsh systolic murmur heard best at base (second intercostal space to right of sternum); aortic ejection sound	Decrescendo diastolic murmur (blowing), high pitched and heard best at base (second intercostal space to right of sternum); systolic ejection murmur heard best at base

6. Discuss activity allowances and limitations.
7. Expain diet and fluid restrictions.
8. Explain to the patient antibiotic prophylaxis to prevent infectious endocarditis (see Table 3-2, p. 88).
9. Explain the importance of notifying the dentist, urologist, and gynecologist of valvular heart disease.
10. Provide a female patient with instruction regarding contraception and risk associated with pregnancy.
11. Discuss with the patient the need to maintain good oral hygiene, daily care, and regular visits to dentist.
12. Discuss importance of ongoing medical care.

EVALUATION/PATIENT OUTCOMES

Tissue Perfusion Management: Cardiac output is maintained. Lungs are clear. Patient reports improvement of symptoms. Heart rate is within acceptable limits. Fluid balance is regained. Baseline weight is achieved. There is no peripheral edema or sign of fluid overload.

PERICARDITIS

Pericarditis is an inflammatory process involving the parietal and visceral layer of the pericardium and outer myocardium (FIG. 3-47).

Pericarditis may occur by itself or as a complication of another disease. Acute pericarditis, which can occur within 2 weeks of the offending condition, lasts up to 6 weeks. There may be effusion or tamponade (see box on p. 91). Chronic pericarditis may follow acute pericarditis and may last up to 6 months.

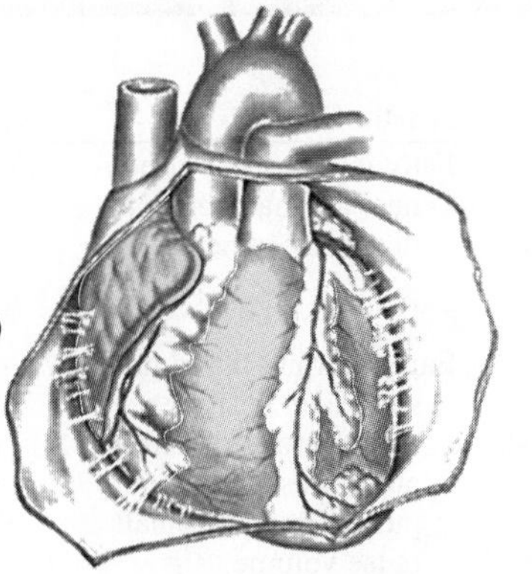

FIG. 3-47
Pericarditis. (From Canobbio.[15])

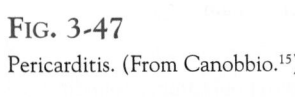

PATHOPHYSIOLOGY

Because of the closeness of the pericardium to the pleura, lung, sternum, diaphragm, and myocardium, pericarditis may be the result of a number of disease states. The most common cause, however, is viral, which generally has a good prognosis. The causes of pericarditis can be summarized as follows:

- Viral (idiopathic): Organism may never be isolated
- Infectious
  - Bacterial
  - Tuberculous
  - Fungal
- After myocardial infarction
  - Dressler's syndrome
  - Postmyocardial infarction syndrome
- After cardiac surgery (postpericardiotomy syndrome or Dressler's syndrome)
- Neoplastic diseases
- Chemotherapy
- Radiotherapy
- Uremia
- Trauma, blunt or penetrating
- Connective tissue diseases
  - Systemic lupus erythematosus
  - Rheumatoid arthritis
  - Scleroderma
  - Dermatomyositis

Inflammation may occur by direct extension or by irritation. Under normal conditions the pericardial sac contains up to 50 ml of clear, serouslike fluid. When an injury occurs, an exudate of fibrin, white blood cells, and endothelial cells is released, covering the parietal and visceral layers of pericardium. Friction between the layers causes irritation and inflammation of the surrounding pleura and tissues. This may remain in one region of the heart or be widespread. Acute pericarditis may be "dry" and fibrinous or obstruct the heart's venous and lymphatic drainage, causing seepage into the pericardial sac, which creates pericardial effusion.[10]

Serofibrinous exudates occur in varying amounts from 100 ml to 3 L and may appear straw colored or turbid with fibrin strands. The exudate of pyogenic pericarditis is purulent. The characteristics of pericardial exudate fluid are summarized in Table 3-3.

A slowly developing effusion of a moderate amount (350 to 500 ml) may not alter the cardiovascular dynamics. How-

Table 3-3 Characteristics of Pericardial Fluid

Characteristic	Normal Fluid	Exudate Effusion
Appearance	Clear	Clear or turbid with fibrin shreds; straw or amber color; may appear hemorrhagic because of red blood cells; may be purulent
Volume	50 ml	>100 ml (up to 3 L)
Specific gravity	<1.015	>1.015 (usually 1.017)
Total protein	<2 g/dl	>3 g/dl
Seromucin clot	Negative	Positive
Coagulation	Uncommon	Usual
Cells	Few	Few
Glucose	Nearly equal to plasma glucose	Nearly equal to plasma glucose
Culture	Negative	Negative

ever, a rapidly accumulating effusion, regardless of amount, can interfere with diastolic filling and lead to cardiac tamponade (FIG. 3-48).

Chronic pericarditis can occur in various forms, including chronic pericardial effusion and constrictive or adhesive pericarditis. Chronic effusion may lead to constrictive effusion.

Constrictive pericarditis is marked by pericardial thickening and scarring of the parietal or visceral pericardium. The layers adhere to each other, blocking out the pericardial space. This eventually involves the surface of the myocardium, causing the pericardium to become useless. In some cases the pericardium calcifies.

As the pericardium becomes scarred and rigid, normal diastolic filling of the heart is impeded. In severe cases, left ventricular end-diastolic volume may be less than stroke volume. This causes the stroke volume to be reduced with a subsequent drop in cardiac output. The normal tachycardia is unable to improve the cardiac output because of constriction of the myocardium.

Constrictive pericarditis usually occurs in all four chambers but may be limited to certain areas such as the right ventricle, pulmonary artery, or aortic root. When all chambers are involved, left and right ventricular diastolic pressure and atrial pressures become equal. As stroke volume diminishes, left and right filling pressures rise. When this is combined with reduced cardiac output, systemic and pulmonary congestion results.

DIAGNOSTIC STUDIES AND FINDINGS

Blood studies: Elevated white blood cells (WBCs), erythrocyte sedimentation rate (ESR)

Viral serology studies: Elevated titers—performed during acute and convalescent periods

Blood and urine cultures: Identification of organism in infectious process

ECG

Acute pericarditis

Stage I (FIG. 3-49) ST-T segment elevation in left ventricular leads V_5, V_6, I, II, aV_L, and aV_F during first few days; PR interval depression

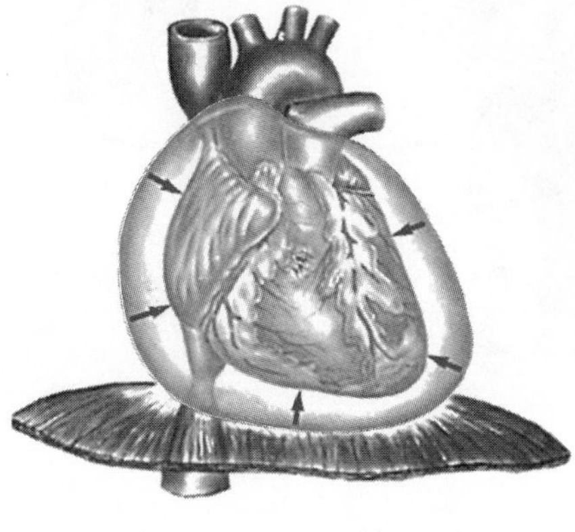

FIG. 3-48

Hemopericardium and cardiac tamponade. (From Canobbio.[15])

Stage II Return of ST segment to baseline; PR interval depression may persist

Stage III T wave inversions

Stage IV Normalization of T waves

Low-voltage QRS complexes in presence of pericardial effusion

Atrial dysrhythmias

Constrictive pericarditis: Wide P wave in leads I, II, and V_6; Q waves deep and wide; T waves flattened or inverted; low QRS voltage

Chest x-ray

Cardiac silhouette: Enlargement depends on underlying disease or amount of pericardial effusion (enlarges with 250 ml of more of accumulated fluid) (FIG. 3-50)

Acute pericarditis: Normal if pericardial fluid less than 250 ml

Constrictive pericarditis: Normal or small; enlargement occurs as a result of pericardial thickening or effusion; calcification of pericardium; pleural effusion

Echocardiogram: Confirms accumulation of free fluid in pericardial sac; as fluid accumulates, separation of pericardial and epicardial echoes occurs, resulting in echo-free space; minimum of 20 ml detected; evaluates ventricular function; in constrictive pericarditis demonstrates reduced motion of posterior wall of left ventricle; abnormal movement of interventricular septum characterized by flattening in systole and paradoxic movement in diastole; two separate echoes representing visceral and parietal pericardium separated by clear space of 1 mm throughout cardiac cycle

Radionuclide blood pool scanning (technetium-labeled macroaggregated albumin and thallium): Demonstrates shadow of pericardial effusion outside cardiac chambers; seen as abnormal space between heart and liver or heart and lungs

Magnetic resonance imaging (MRI): Visualizes pericardium; can define thickened pericardium differentiating acute from chronic

CARDIAC TAMPONADE

Cardiac tamponade is an acute cardiac compression caused when fluid accumulates within the pericardial sac and exerts increased pressure around the heart (FIG. 3-49). Normally the sac holds 30 to 50 ml of fluid. Fluid or blood can fill the pericardial space slowly or rapidly, depending on inflammatory vs. traumatic etiologies. Ultimately, the result of this excessive extracardiac volume is restricted blood flow in and out of the ventricles, causing decreased cardiac output. Pulsus paradoxus, an important hemodynamic feature of tamponade, is a measurable fall in systemic blood pressure of 10 mm Hg or more during inspiration. Hypotension and shock are the inevitable manifestations of severe tamponade. Medical management of this life-threatening problem is frequently emergent and occasionally resuscitative. Needle aspiration of pericardial fluid or blood (pericardiocentesis) is the only nonsurgical method to rapidly decompress the pericardial space. Hemodynamic improvement is immediate. Subsequently, medical care must be directed at the inciting cause of fluid accumulation (e.g., postoperative bleeding, traumatic injury, pericarditis, malignancy).

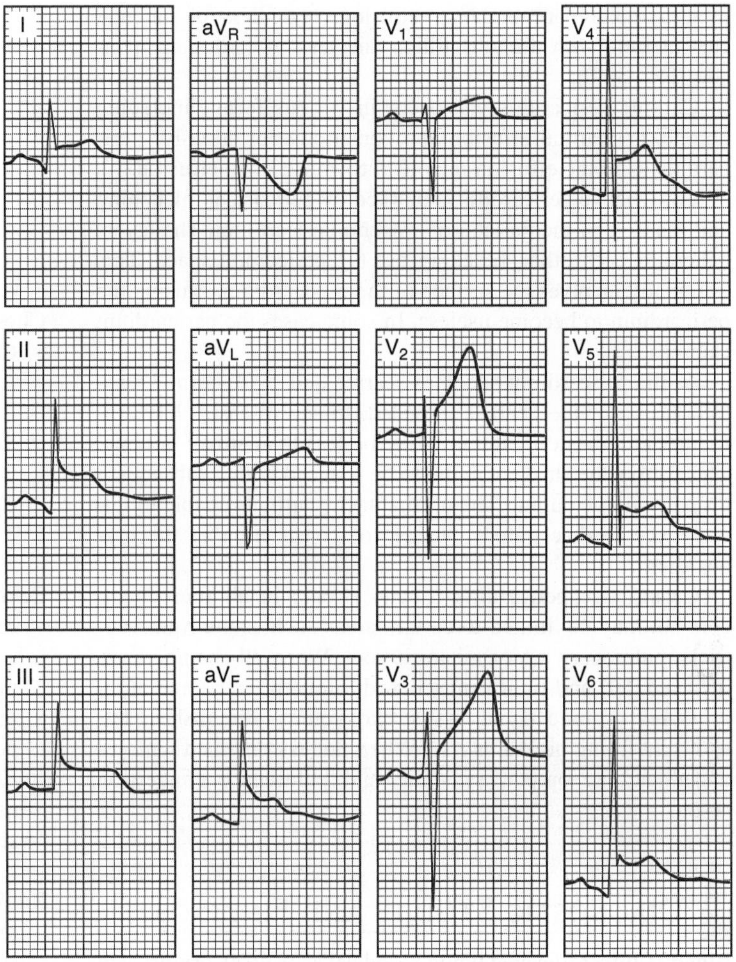

FIG. 3-49
In acute pericarditis, ST segment elevation is typically upward and concave in leads I, II, aV_f, and V_4 to V_6. (From Guzzetta and Dossey.[44])

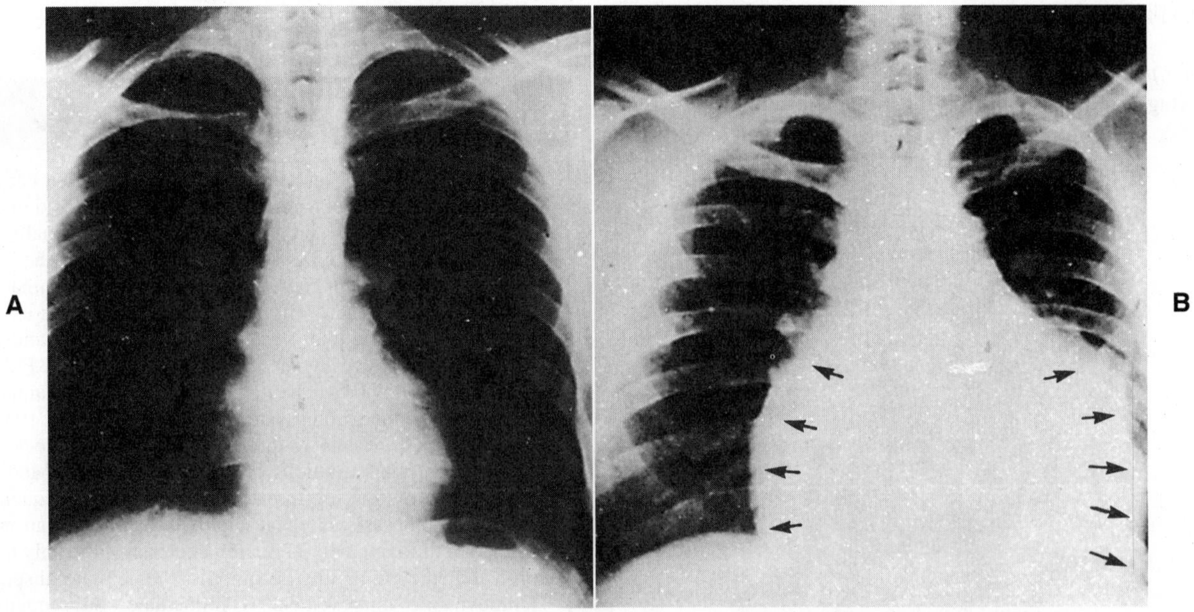

FIG. 3-50
A, Normal chest x-ray. **B,** With pericardial effusion, cardiac silhouette is enlarged and has globular shape *(arrows)*. (From Guzzetta and Dossey.[44])

Cardiac catheterization: Demonstrates characteristic pericardial shadow outside opacified cardiac chambers, which are increased by pericardial thickening or fluid accumulation

Constrictive pericarditis: Increased left and right atrial pressures; loss of respiratory variation of right atrial pressure curve; elevated pulmonary artery systolic pressure (35 to 40 mm Hg); elevated diastolic pressures equal in all four chambers, rarely differing by more than 5 mm Hg at rest or during exercise; cardiac output normal in early stages, later decreased (<2.3 L/min/m^2); ejection fraction normal or decreased

MULTIDISCIPLINARY PLAN

Surgery

Pericardiocentesis: Removal of pericardial fluid or blood by aspiration through needle or catheter inserted into parietal pericardium; indicated when persistent or large effusions are compromising left ventricular function; a small catheter can be left in place in the pericardium to allow for continuous drainage into a sterile collection reservoir

Pericardial window: Open pericardial drainage implemented for acute suppurative and chronic effusions; has certain advantages over pericardiocentesis: multiple aspirations can be avoided, pericardial tissue can be obtained for culture, pericardium can be visualized, and clots and fibrin deposits can be removed

Pericardiectomy: Surgical removal of visceral and parietal pericardium; has excellent long-term benefits and low operative mortality; best results when myocardial fibrosis and ventricular atrophy are not far advanced and when total or near-total pericardiectomy is performed; if hemodynamic improvement is not seen immediately, elevated pressures and abnormal waveforms continue for several weeks owing to atrophy of ventricles that have been immobilized for long periods; thus early pericardiectomy is encouraged before dense fibrosis and myocardial atrophy occur; postoperative care similar to that of any cardiac surgical patient (p. 120)

Medications

Acute pericarditis

Antiinflammatory agents for symptomatic relief of chest pain, fever, and malaise in absence of clinical signs of cardiac tamponade

Analgesic-antipyretics: Aspirin

Usual dosage: 600-900 mg qid PO

Nonsteroidal antiinflammatory drugs (NSAIDs): Indomethacin (Indocin)

Usual dosage: Divided doses beginning with 25 mg qid to maximum of 200 mg/day PO

Precautions: Patients should be instructed to take medicine on a full stomach

Corticosteroids

Indications: Considered in treatment of moderate to severe cases in recurring pericarditis and effusion

Constrictive pericarditis: Pharmacologic agents aimed at specific cause; for example, patients with known or suspected tuberculosis should receive antituberculous therapy before and after pericardiectomy

General Management

Electrocardiography: Performed to rule out MI when cardiac tamponade is suspected and if patient demonstrates signs of cardiac decompensation

Hemodynamic monitoring: Indicated if cardiac tamponade is evident (see box, p. 91); for patients with constrictive pericarditis, closer monitoring of right atrial and pulmonary arterial pressures and cardiac output; after pericardiectomy, elevated pressures may continue for several weeks or months

Acute pericarditis: Activity limited during acute period, with modification of all activities for 2 weeks to allow inflammatory reaction of the pericardium to resolve; regular diet; encourage fluids during febrile period; discontinue oral anticoagulants; give IV heparin if anticoagulation is necessary; pain relief with NSAIDs or, in severe cases, a short course of corticosteroids

Constrictive pericarditis: Bed rest with activity limitations before pericardiectomy; extent of limitation dictated by degree of hemodynamic compromise and symptoms

NURSING CARE

NURSING ASSESSMENT

Assess quality of chest pain to distinguish pericardial pain from myocardial ischemia.

Assess for signs of fear and anxiety: restlessness, facial expressions.

Assess for signs of cardiac tamponade (p. 91): narrowing pulse pressure and pulsus paradoxus to detect early signs of increasing intrapericardial pressure and development of tamponade.

Auscultate heart sounds for presence of pericardial friction rub (may be distant).

See Assessment Considerations table.

POTENTIAL COMPLICATIONS

Cardiac tamponade; development of hemopericardium

PATIENT PROBLEMS/NURSING DIAGNOSES & INTERVENTIONS

NIC TISSUE PERFUSION MANAGEMENT

Decreased cardiac output related to reduced ventricular filling

- Monitor vital signs *to detect evidence of ventricular decompensation.*
- Prepare for pericardiocentesis or pericardiectomy as indicated by clinical status.
- Place on cardiac monitor, checking rhythm every 1 to 2 hours.

NIC PSYCHOLOGIC COMFORT PROMOTION

Anxiety related to actual or perceived threat to biologic integrity

- Provide supportive care *to ensure sense of trust and comfort.*

Assessment Considerations

Area of Concern	Acute Pericarditis	Constrictive Pericarditis
General complaints	Chest pain: Location retrosternal or precordial radiating to neck and back, sudden pleuritic-like pain that worsens with deep inspiration, movement, or lying down and is relieved by sitting up or leaning forward; sharp, deep, persistent ache; tachypnea; shallow breathing; dyspnea in presence of pleural effusion or owing to impaired cardiac filling from compression of heart; restlessness; anxiety; malaise; dysphagia	Exertional dyspnea; fatigue; orthopnea; palpitations; paroxysmal nocturnal dyspnea; cough; pericardial edema
Physical examination	Low-grade temperature (30°C [102°F]); may be associated with diaphoresis and chills; auscultation: pericardial friction rub—best heard with patient leaning forward, heard in second, third, or fourth intercostal space to left of sternal border or at apex, loudest during inspiration, varies in intensity (grade 4-5), may be transient, triphasic consisting of presystolic, systolic, and diastolic components, scratchy, grating	Afebrile; elevated jugular venous pressure with presence of Kussmaul's sign (increased distention during inspiration); arterial pressure normal or slightly reduced; diffuse precordial movement; decreased amplitude; absence of localized apical impulse; paradoxic pulse (rarely exceeds 15 mm Hg); auscultation: quiet, distant heart sounds, pericardial knock—early diastolic sound, accentuated with inspiration and heard best along lower left sternal border; clinical signs of elevated venous pressure: peripheral edema, hepatomegaly, ascites

- Explain disease process and procedures as they are implemented.
- Ensure quiet environment *to reduce external stimuli.*
- Maintain family contact.

NIC PHYSICAL COMFORT PROMOTION

Acute pain related to pericardial inflammation

- Administer pain medication as ordered *to relieve pericardial chest pain.*
- Encourage bed rest with head of bed elevated or in position of comfort.
- Instruct patient to lean forward on over-bed table *to reduce pain.*

PATIENT EDUCATION/CONTINUUM OF CARE PLAN

1. Explain the underlying cause and disease process.
2. Explain signs and symptoms of recurring inflammation to the patient, and tell the patient to notify the physician if they occur.
3. Explain the purpose, method of administration, and side effects of medications.

EVALUATION/PATIENT OUTCOMES

Tissue Perfusion Management: Cardiac output is maintained. Patient demonstrates hemodynamic stability; blood pressure and pulse rate are maintained at baseline. Heart and breath sounds are normal. Absence of pulsus paradoxus. ECG is normal. There is no friction rub. White blood cell count and sedimentation rate are normal.

Psychologic Comfort Promotion: Patient demonstrates decreased anxiety. Patient verbalizes relief of pain. Patient demonstrates ability to rest and sleep without complaint. Patient appears relaxed.

Physical Comfort Promotion: Patient is free of chest pain. Patient verbalizes no chest discomfort. Patient tolerates routine activities and procedures without complaining of pain or shortness of breath.

ENDOCARDITIS

Endocarditis is an inflammatory process involving the endothelial layer of the heart, including the cardiac valves and septal defects, if present (FIG. 3-51).

The designations *acute* and *subacute* were used previously to classify patients with infective endocarditis (IE) and were based on the progression of untreated infection. Acute endocarditis has a rapid onset (days to weeks). Patients have a toxic febrile illness with major cardiac symptoms, including congestive heart failure, valvular insufficiency, and cardiac conduction abnormalities. In contrast, subacute endocarditis is an indolent, chronic illness (weeks to months) with less specific symptoms: weight loss, malaise, fever, and heart murmur. Patients with subacute endocarditis can also have Osler nodes, Janeway lesions, splenomegaly, and hematuria.

The incidence of IE is not known. In one report the frequency was about 0.16 to 5.4 cases per 1000 hospital admissions.[10] Endocarditis primarily involves older adults, with a mean age of 55 years. Men are affected more often by a ratio of 2:1 to 5:1 in several series.[22]

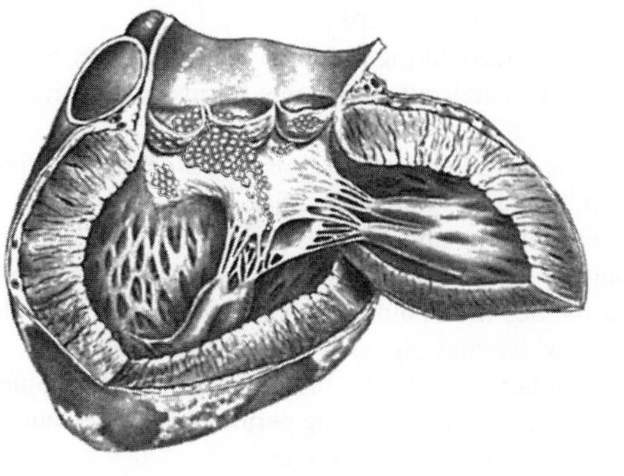

FIG. 3-51
Endocarditis. (From Canobbio.[15])

Persons at risk for IE include patients who have a history of rheumatic heart disease, valvular heart disease, or congenital heart defects; who have prosthetic heart valves or arteriovenous shunts for dialysis; or who are intravenous drug users. Previously, rheumatic valvular heart disease was the most common predisposing factor; now mitral valve prolapse (MVP) with regurgitation is the most common underlying cardiac defect predisposing to IE.

PATHOPHYSIOLOGY

Endocarditis can be linked to a number of organisms. Diagnosis and treatment depend on isolating the organism.

Streptococcal strains account for 50% to 60% of all subacute bacterial endocarditis (SBE) cases. These low-virulence bacteria generally affect already damaged valves. *Streptococcus viridans,* the most commonly implicated alpha-hemolytic organism, is found in the mouth and upper respiratory tract.

Staphylococcus aureus, which affects normal valves, is responsible for 25% of cases of IE. It is associated with a mortality rate ranging from 45% to 73%. Less common enterococcal strains *(Staphylococcus faecalis)* have increasingly been seen in IE. *Enterococcus* is found in the gastrointestinal and genitourinary tracts as well as the oral cavity. It occurs often in elderly patients, particularly men undergoing urologic procedures, and has been reported in women of childbearing age. *Staphylococcus epidermidis* is commonly seen in endocarditis after prosthetic valve replacement.

Other known pathogens linked to endocarditis include gram-negative organisms, fungi, and yeast. Endocarditis caused by gram-negative cocci and bacilli *(Serratia marcescens, Klebsiella, Pseudomonas)* occurs in the elderly and in mainline drug abusers. The increase in incidence of endocarditis caused by fungi *(Candida, Aspergillus)* may be linked to the increase in IV drug abuse and the widespread use of antimicrobial and corticosteroid therapies. Fungal vegetations tend to be large and to embolize in major blood vessels, particularly in the legs.

Endocarditis generally begins as a transient bacteremia (or fungemia) introduced into the circulation through several portals of entry (Table 3-4). Bacteria more commonly settle on cardiac structures that have already been damaged. The valves are especially susceptible. Patients with unrepaired ventricular septal defects, coarctation of the aorta, patent ductus arteriosus, and unrepaired tetralogy of Fallot are also susceptible. Infected structures are often those in which turbulent blood flow is forced across an area of high pressure to low pressure. Trauma to the endothelial surface of the low-pressure side of the damaged site causes local clotting. As a result, an aggregation of platelets and fibrin thrombi forms on the injured structure. During the active phase of the infection these thrombi can foster the growth of microorganisms.

The pathogenesis of endocarditis is related to the adherence of infected thrombi to cardiac structures, which, in the case of the valves, can lead to scarring and retraction of the leaflets. The destruction may be sufficient to cause erosion of the leaflets and perforation, leading to valvular insufficiency. The infectious process may also spread to the annulus, creating

Table 3-4 Possible Ports of Entry and Factors Predisposing to Bacteremia

Port of Entry	Infecting Organism
Oral cavity	*Streptococcus, Staphylococcus epidermidis*
Extractions, teeth cleaning, periodontal disease (abscesses), periodontal operations, use of unwaxed dental floss, oral irrigation, bridgework	
Upper respiratory tract	*Staphylococcus aureus, Streptococcus, Haemophilus* species, *Streptococcus pneumoniae, Staphylococcus epidermidis*
Tonsilloadenoidectomy, orotracheal intubation, bronchoscopy (rigid tubes), pneumonia	
Gastrointestinal tract	Gram-negative rods, *Enterobacter, Escherichia coli, Klebsiella*
Barium enema, sigmoidoscopy, colonoscopy, percutaneous biopsy of liver	
Genitourinary system	*E. coli,* gram-negative bacilli, *Enterococcus*
Catheterization, urethrotomy, transurethral prostatectomy, retropubic prostatectomy, cystoscopy	
Female reproductive system	*E. coli*
Delivery, abortion (therapeutic, illegal), intrauterine devices	
Skin	*Staphyloccocus aureus, Staphyloccocus epidermidis*
Furuncles, acne (infected, squeezed), skin piercing, tattoos, acupuncture	
Other sources of infection	
Pacemaker (transvenous), prolonged use of polyethylene catheter (atrial), hemodialysis (arteriovenous cannulas), infection (hematogenous osteomyelitis, Q fever, meningococcemia)	

abscesses, or rupture the chordae tendineae. Mycotic aneurysms may result from septic embolization, which develops in the aorta, cerebral arteries, sinus of Valsalva, ligated ductus arteriosus, and smaller arterial vessels (of the lung, kidney, or spleen).

DIAGNOSTIC STUDIES AND FINDINGS

Complete blood count (CBC): Anemia; elevated sedimentation rate; leukocytosis; thrombocytopenia

Blood cultures (4 to 6 cultures from different venipuncture sites within 6 to 72 hours before therapy started): Identification of causative organism

Urine: Proteinuria; red blood cell or leukocyte casts; microhematuria

Rheumatoid factor: Positive in 50% of patients with infection of 6 weeks duration

Blood chemistry: Elevated BUN and creatinine values in patients with renal complications

Echocardiogram (transesophageal echocardiogram): Presence of vegetations or abscesses; involvement of damage to cardiac valves; ventricular function; hemodynamic changes such as regurgitation

ECG: Early infection—normal; late infection—conduction defects; atrial fibrillation, flutter

Radionuclide studies: Gallium-67 citrate may accumulate in areas of inflammation

MULTIDISCIPLINARY PLAN

Surgery

Valvuloplasty by debridement or valvectomy with or without valve replacement; surgical removal of vegetations and thrombi not indicated unless uncontrollable sepsis occurs, and then combined with long-term antimicrobial therapy; if infectious process is fulminant and resistant to antimicrobial therapy, excision of vegetations, unroofing of abscesses, and valve replacement recommended; presence of congestive heart failure is a major indication for surgery, increasing the mortality rate to a range of 9% to 14%[10]

Medications

Antibiotics: Long-term IV antibiotic therapy inhibits bacterial growth; because appropriate therapy depends on isolation of infecting organism, serial blood cultures are required before initiation of therapy; initiation of antibiotic therapy is guided by patients' clinical state and the type of valve that is infected (native or prosthetic): for patients who have been ill for weeks or months, delaying therapy until culture results are available will not endanger patient, but treatment for an acutely ill patient should begin immediately; therapy usually continues 4-6 weeks with parenteral administration as recommended route; culture-negative endocarditis is uncommon (5%-10%), and most often occurs in patients who have recently received broad-spectrum antibiotics; for these patients and those with fulminating acute IE, a combination of IV vancomycin and low-dose gentamycin should be instituted

Analgesic-antipyretics (salicyates) given for elevated temperature

General Management

Rest: Encouraged during acute phase; patient may require prolonged hospitalization or home intravenous therapy lasting several weeks

Vital signs: Checked every 4 to 8 hours, decreasing frequency as indicated by improved clinical condition

ECG telemetry monitoring: For patients with acute infection to monitor for abnormalities or progression of conduction abnormalities (heart blocks or intraventricular conduction delays), which may signal progression of disease.

Diet: Regular; patient may require high-caloric supplemental feedings; force fluids during periods of elevated temperature if there is no ventricular failure

Monitor parenteral therapy for rate and amount of infusion; check regularly for localized signs of inflammation, phlebitis; assess antibiotic drug levels to avoid toxic effects, while optimizing treatment; evaluate patient's aptitude for home parenteral antibiotic therapy

NURSING CARE

NURSING ASSESSMENT

General

Determine whether IE is acute or chronic:

- Acute: High-grade fever (39° to 40° C [102° to 104° F])
- Chronic: Low-grade fever (less than 39.4° C [103° F]), weakness, malaise, weight loss, anorexia, arthralgia, sweats, headache, dyspnea

Assess patient for signs of progressive weight loss or malnutrition: dry weight below normal for age and height, fatigue, decreased triceps skinfold measurements.

Assess for dehydration: diaphoresis, poor skin turgor, dry mucous membranes; monitor laboratory reports.

Assess for signs of embolization (cerebral, systemic, peripheral):

- Cerebroneurologic checks: Neurologic changes (behavioral changes, aphasia, paralysis, seizures)
- Splenic: Assess for splenomegaly, tender or painful abdomen
- Renal: Decreased urine output may reflect embolism or infarction
- Pulmonary: Auscultate lung sounds and check oxygen saturation
- Peripheral: Petechiae in conjunctivae, palate, buccal mucosa, and extremities; splinter hemorrhages (linear, dark red streaks on nail beds); Osler's nodes (small, tender, raised nodules frequently found on finger and toe pads); Janeway's lesions (nontender, flat, erythematous maculae on palms and soles); splenomegaly; Roth's spots (retinal hemorrhages with white centers)

Auscultation

Murmurs not present in early phase of infection may become apparent if valvular damage occurs, or existing murmurs may change in intensity.

POTENTIAL COMPLICATIONS

Cardiac complications: Abscesses, valvular dysfunction (p. 85), heart failure (p. 66), conduction system disturbances

Embolization: Cerebral, renal, splenic, coronary

Mycotic aneurysms
Glomerulonephritis
Central nervous system (CNS) abscess

Patient Problems/Nursing Diagnoses & Interventions

NIC Tissue Perfusion Management

Ineffective tissue perfusion related to embolism

- Report any physical changes indicative of embolism to physician immediately.
- Administer anticoagulant therapy as ordered.
- Instruct patient about need to continue with anticoagulants, if ordered, *to prevent further embolic episodes.*
- Obtain and monitor arterial blood gases as ordered.

NIC Nutritional Support

Imbalanced nutrition: less than body requirements, related to biologic factors (fever, infection)

- Weigh patient daily *to determine weight loss and need for supplemental feedings.* Decrease frequency as weight stabilizes.
- Monitor daily caloric intake as indicated by patient's appetite and food intake.
- Offer high-calorie, high-protein supplemental feedings *to ensure adequate intake of daily nutrients during anorexic periods.*
- Ensure patient comfort during mealtime *to stimulate appetite.*
- Encourage patient participation in food selections.

NIC Thermoregulation

Hyperthermia (elevated body temperature) related to infectious process

- Obtain temperature every 4 to 8 hours as indicated.
- Monitor fluid intake and output, noting water loss through perspiration.
- Encourage fluid intake as tolerated *to maintain fluid balance.*
- Administer antipyretics as ordered.

Patient Education/Continuum of Care Plan

1. Provide instruction regarding the disease process and the purpose and method of treatment.
2. Coordinate outpatient parenteral antibiotic management with home care nurse, home care pharmacy, and infectious disease specialist.
3. Teach patient care requirements of long-term IV antibiotic therapy; review care of IV site and signs of infection and inflammation to report to nurse or physician; discuss care of antibiotic infusion; permit time for return demonstration.
4. Explain precipitating risk factors that can lead to bacteremia and reinfection: poor oral hygiene, dental work (gum cleaning or treatment, extractions), gastrointestinal or genitourinary procedures, vaginal deliveries, furuncles, staphylococcal infections, surgical procedures.
5. Encourage regular follow-up care with a physician.
6. Explain to the patient the need for good oral hygiene and regular dental care.
7. Explain and reinforce the need for antibiotic prophylaxis before procedures that predispose to bacteremia (see Table 3-2 on p. 88 for specific recommendations).

Evaluation/Patient Outcomes

Tissue Perfusion Management: Tissue perfusion is maintained. Patient is alert and oriented. No signs of embolism present. Lung sounds are clear, and urine output is normal.

Nutritional Support: Patient reports feeling less fatigued and has improved appetite, weight gain, and absence of sweats and headache. Nutritional status is improved and maintained. Baseline or normal body weight is regained. Usual activities are resumed.

Thermoregulation: There is absence of inflammatory processes. Temperature, blood cultures, white blood cell count, and other laboratory findings are normal. Patient's sense of well-being is improved.

Myocarditis

Myocarditis is an inflammatory process of the heart caused by an infectious agent.

Endocarditis and pericarditis are also inflammatory diseases of the heart, but myocarditis specifically involves the myocytes, interstitium, and vascular elements. The prevalence and incidence of viral myocarditis in the general population are unknown, but approximately 5% of a population infected with a virus (e.g., influenza) may experience some form of cardiac involvement associated with the acute illness.

Pathophysiology

Myocarditis characteristically develops several weeks after the initial systemic infection, suggesting involvement of an immunologic mechanism. The physiologic end point of severe myocarditis is dilated cardiomyopathy, presumably a consequence of viral-mediated immunologic cardiac damage.[10] Virtually any infectious agent may produce cardiac inflammation, viruses being the most common. Myocarditis may also be caused by allergic reactions and pharmacologic agents.

The clinical consequences of myocarditis depend on the size and number of myocardial lesions, which are usually randomly distributed in the heart. Clinical expression ranges from often asymptomatic and unrecognized cases to acute, and sometimes fatal, congestive heart failure. Dysrhythmias, particularly ventricular, may be the only sign of otherwise unrecognized myocarditis. Specifically, 17% to 21% of sudden deaths not attributed to accidents or violence can be linked to myocarditis.

Signs and symptoms of cardiovascular disease are usually absent but, depending on the severity of disease, may include fatigue, dyspnea, palpitations, chest pain, and tachycardia. Histologic findings are usually nonspecific, but the hallmark of myocarditis is an inflammatory myocardial infiltrate with associated evidence of myocardial damage.[10]

ETIOLOGIES OF MYOCARDITIS

VIRAL
Coxsackievirus (A and B)
Influenza
Cytomegalovirus
Hepatitis
Mumps
Herpes simplex
Rabies
Epstein-Barr virus
Human immunodeficiency virus
Echovirus

RICKETTSIAL
Q fever
Rocky Mountain spotted fever
Scrub typhus

FUNGAL
Candidiasis
Histoplasmosis
Aspergillus

PROTOZOAL AND METAZOAL
Trypanosomiasis
Toxoplasmosis
Malaria
Schistosomiasis
Trichinosis

BACTERIAL
Diphtheria
Tuberculosis
Legionella
Brucella
Clostridium
Salmonella/Shigella
Meningococcus
Yersinia

SPIROCHETAL
Borrelia (Lyme disease)

DIAGNOSTIC STUDIES AND FINDINGS

ECG: Usually nonspecific ST segment and T wave abnormalities

Chest x-ray: Enlarged cardiac silhouette; pulmonary congestion in severe cases

Echocardiogram: Left ventricular wall motion abnormalities; increased wall thickness or late-stage dilation; left ventricular thrombi

Radionuclide scanning: Inflammatory and necrotic changes characteristic of myocarditis

Viral serology studies: Culture stool, throat, blood, myocardium, pericardial fluid; distinct increase in virus-neutralizing antibody, complement fixation, and hemagglutination inhibition titers

Endomyocardial biopsy: To confirm diagnosis; however, a negative biopsy does not exclude myocarditis

MULTIDISCIPLINARY PLAN

Surgery
None for primary disease; cardiac transplant if myocarditis results in end-stage dilated cardiomyopathy

Medications
Diuretics, digoxin, ACE inhibitors for heart failure management
Antidysrhythmic therapy
Immunosuppressant therapy (use in acute disease is controversial)
- Corticosteroids
- Cyclosporine
- NSAIDs
- Anticoagulation (with caution in setting of thrombus)

General Management
Focus on systemic manifestations (heart failure, dysrhythmias).
Bed rest: Restrict activity during acute phase of disease because exercise may intensify myocardial damage.

NURSING CARE

NURSING ASSESSMENT
Assess for signs of congestive heart failure and dysrhythmia frequently during acute phase. See CHF Assessment on p. 69.

POTENTIAL COMPLICATIONS
Cardiogenic shock; conduction abnormalities (heart blocks) leading to Stokes-Adams attacks; ventricular arrhythmias; sudden death; development of chronic congestive heart failure

PATIENT PROBLEMS/NURSING DIAGNOSES & INTERVENTIONS
See Patient Problems/Nursing Diagnoses & Interventions listed for congestive heart failure, p. 70.

NIC TISSUE PERFUSION MANAGEMENT

Ineffective tissue perfusion related to inflammatory myocardial lesions, dysrhythmias
- Maintain bed rest.

NIC COPING ASSISTANCE

Anxiety/fear related to sick role restriction/risk of death in previously healthy individual
Ineffective denial related to absence of disabling symptoms and lack of cardiovascular disease
- Provide for quiet environment, access to significant others, rest time.
- Explain procedures, changes, medications to enhance self-control.
- Explain risks associated with sudden death during exertional activity.
- Outline long-term consequences of myocardial damage if not recognized early.

PATIENT EDUCATION/CONTINUUM OF CARE PLAN

1. Monitor patient's cardiac status, medication tolerance, compliance.
2. Perform cardiac rehabilitation if patient's pre-illness activity level has been compromised by prolonged bed rest, symptoms.
3. Monitor medication regimen/heart failure management routine by telephone.
4. Assess patient and family for cardiac transplant candidacy.

EVALUATION/PATIENT OUTCOMES
See section on congestive heart failure on p. 66.

Tissue Perfusion Management: Cardiac output is maintained. Vital signs are stable. Urine output is adequate. Dysrhythmia is under control.

Coping Assistance: Patient's anxiety is minimized in acute care environment. Patient verbalizes understanding of procedures, medications. Patient seeks support of significant others. Patient shows increased level of cooperation.

CONGENITAL HEART DISEASE

A congenital heart disorder is any structural or functional abnormality or defect of the heart or great vessels existing from birth.

Congenital heart disease is a specialty of pediatrics. However, because of advances in medical and surgical management, persons with congenital defects are now living longer and are being treated as adults. Although the incidence of congenital heart disease has decreased over the decades, it continues to occur at a rate of 5 to 8 per 1000 live births.[4]

PATHOPHYSIOLOGY

In most cases the cause for the congenital defect cannot be determined. However, various factors are believed to contribute to these malformations.

Genetics. Several studies have demonstrated prevalence rates among siblings and blood relatives to be 1.5% to 5%,[79] suggesting a genetic link in the etiology of cardiac malformations. This genetic link could become important as more children with congenital heart disease reach adulthood and are therefore capable of bearing offspring. This growing population of procreating adults with congenital heart disease offers geneticists a closer look at the inheritance of heart defects. Certain chromosomal abnormalities, including Turner syndrome and Down syndrome, have been linked to heart defects.

Environmental Factors. Although difficult to prove as isolated causes, environmental factors along with genetic factors have been linked to heart defects. Factors include pollution, smoking, and alcohol use by the mother.

Teratogens. Use of certain drugs such as alcohol and warfarin and exposure to viruses such as rubella during fetal development have been shown to cause not only heart defects but also widespread injury to the embryo.

Altitude. Altitude may cause the ductus arteriosus to fail to close after birth.

Common Defects in Which Prolonged Survival Occurs

Patent Ductus Arteriosus (FIG. 3-52). The ductus arteriosus is a vascular connection that during fetal life directs

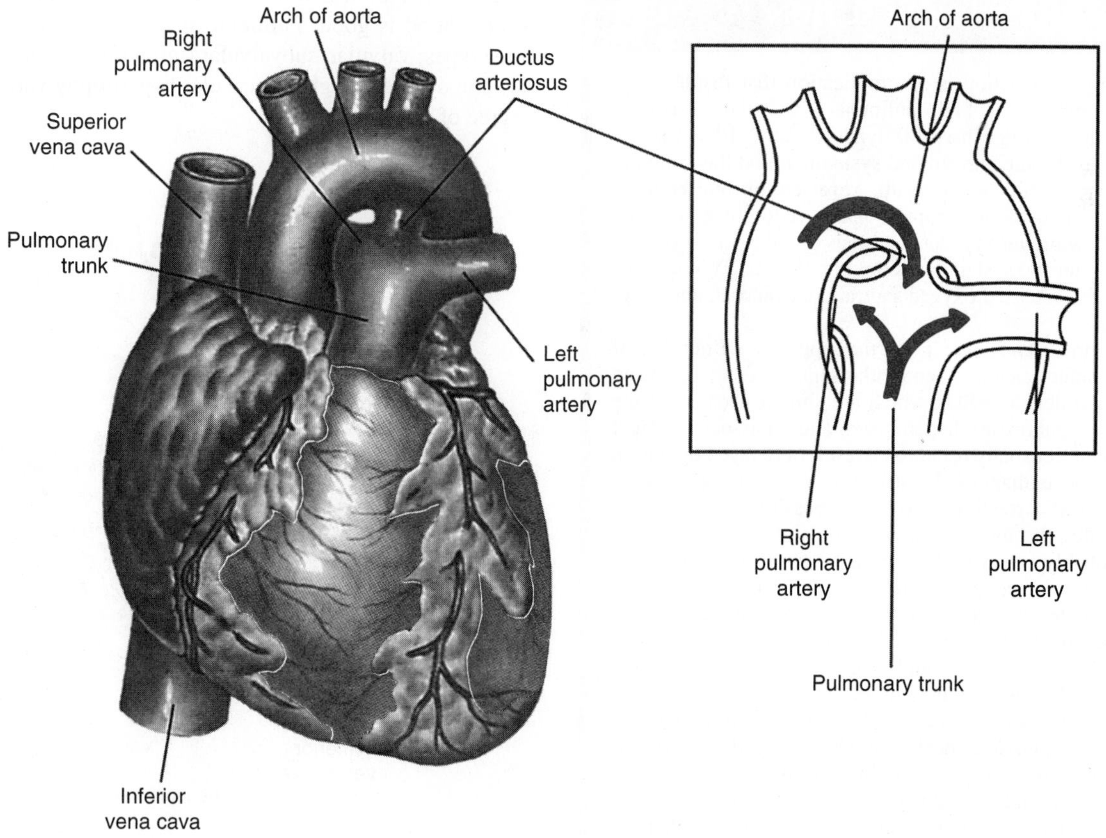

FIG. 3-52
Patent ductus arteriosus. (From Canobbio.[15])

blood flow from the pulmonary artery to the aorta, bypassing the lungs. Functional closure of the ductus arteriosus occurs after birth. In some cases, it takes 6 months to several years before complete closure. If the ductus remains patent, the direction of blood flow is reversed from left to right because of high systemic pressure in the aorta. Blood is shunted through the ductus arteriosus to the pulmonary artery during both systole and diastole. This raises pressure in the pulmonary circulation and increases the pressure against which the right ventricle must work. Consequently, a large ductus arteriosus with unrestricted flow could eventually lead to pulmonary vascular disease and Eisenmenger's complex (see box below).

Atrial Septal Defect (FIG. 3-53). An atrial septal defect is an abnormal opening between the right and left atria, causing blood to be shunted from left to right. There are two common forms. In ostium secundum, the more common of the two, the defect is in the middle of the septal wall near the fossa ovalis. Ostium primum results from failure of fusion of the left portions of the endocardial cushions occurring low in the atrial position. An associated cleft (separation) is present in the anterior mitral valve leaflet, which can lead to mitral regurgitation. Again, this defect occurs more frequently in females, and it is not uncommon that a child may escape diagnosis until early adult life.

Ventricular Septal Defect (FIG. 3-54). A ventricular septal defect is an abnormal opening between the right and left ventricles. It varies in size (7 mm to 3 cm in diameter) and occurs in either the upper or lower portion of the ventricular septum. The size of the defect determines the extent of the shunt from left to right ventricle. The larger the shunt, the greater is the volume of blood ejected into the right ventricle and lungs. Therefore large defects cause a volume overload for both ventricles. Large defects can also lead to an increase in pulmonary vascular resistance, producing pulmonary hypertension. If this occurs, the shunt may be reversed from right to left, causing systemic cyanosis and Eisenmenger's syndrome, which renders the case inoperable.

EISENMENGER'S REACTION

Eisenmenger's reaction is a complication that results from the development of high pulmonary vascular resistance (PVR) that is greater than 800 dynes-sec/cm^{-5}. PVR rises in response to chronic unrestricted systemic blood flow into the pulmonary circuit. As a result, reversed or bidirectional shunts occur at the aorticopulmonary, ventricular, or atrial levels, allowing unoxygenated venous blood to cross the defect and enter the systemic arterial circulation. PVR is associated with decreased oxygen saturation, cyanosis, and polycythemia.

The term *Eisenmenger's reaction* applies to a number of shunting defects, such as ventricular septal defect (VSD) and atrial septal defect (ASD), which are similar because of the presence of pulmonary hypertension and an associated right to left shunt. It usually occurs as a result of delayed operation and may be undiagnosed until adolescence or adulthood, when surgical correction is no longer possible.

Clinically, the most common complaint is effort intolerance, probably because of decreased arterial oxygen saturation. In later stages, symptoms are more commonly caused by right ventricular failure. Other common features include cyanosis, with clubbing, and polycythemia.

Most patients survive and live reasonably active lives throughout the fourth and fifth decades. Sudden death, presumably from dysrhythmias, is the most common cause of death. Other causes of death include heart failure and pulmonary infarction from arterial thrombosis.

Survival into adulthood is possible. Patent ductus arteriosus occurs more often in girls and can be linked to other defects such as ventricular septal defect and coarctation of the aorta.

Tetralogy of Fallot (FIG. 3-55). Tetralogy of Fallot is an anomaly marked by four defects: ventricular septal defect, right ventricular outflow obstruction (pulmonic stenosis), deviation (dextroposition) of the aorta so it overrides the ventricular septum, and right ventricular hypertrophy. It is the most common cyanotic lesion in which survival to adulthood is expected. The severity of symptoms depends on the size of the ventricular septal defect, the degree of pulmonic stenosis, and the position of the aorta. Right ventricular outflow is obstructed, resulting in hypertrophy of the right ventricle and a right-to-left shunt. This produces decreased systemic arterial oxygen saturation, cyanosis, reduced pulmonary blood flow, and, in some cases, a hypoplastic pulmonary artery.

Pulmonic Valvular Stenosis (FIG. 3-56). Congenital pulmonic valvular stenosis may occur by itself, with other defects such as atrial or ventricular septal defect, or as part of tetralogy of Fallot. If it occurs by itself, the chance of survival to adulthood is good. Pulmonic stenosis may occur as one of three types: valvular, subvalvular (infundibular), or supravalvular. The degree of right ventricular hypertrophy varies with the degree of obstruction.

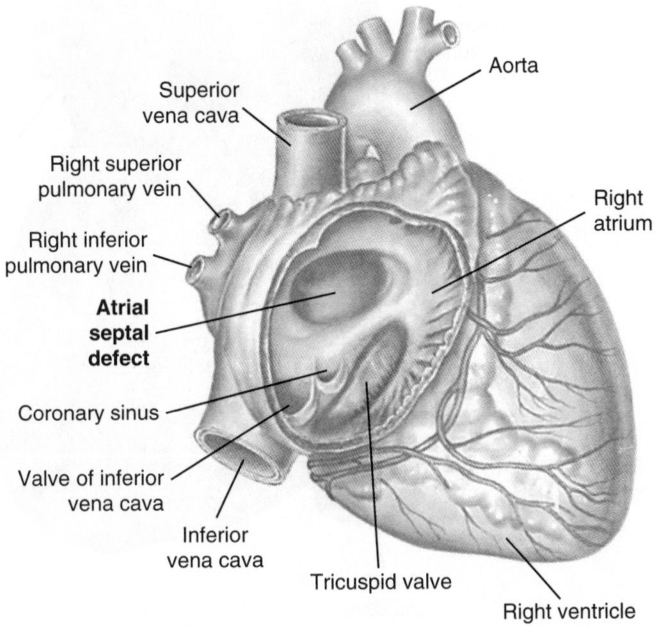

FIG. 3-53
Atrial septal defect. (From Canobbio.[15])

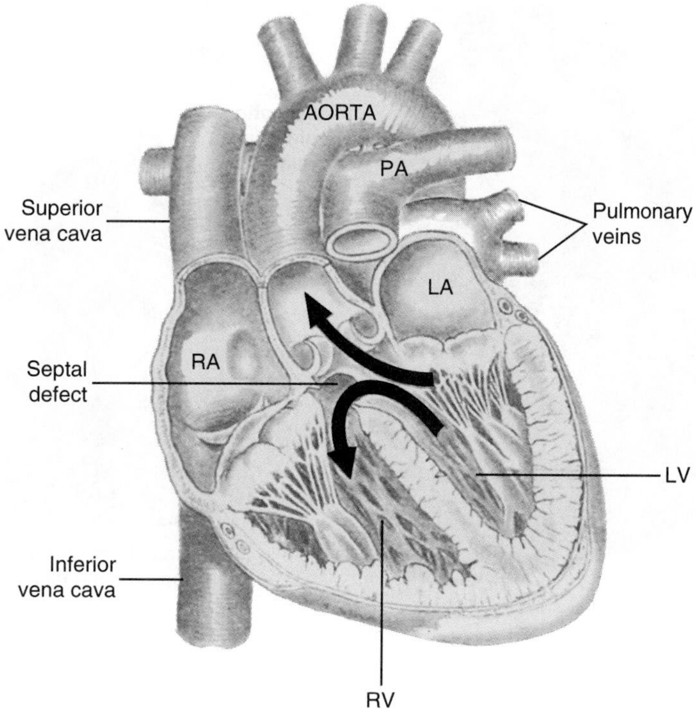

FIG. 3-54
Ventricular septal defect. (From Canobbio.[15])

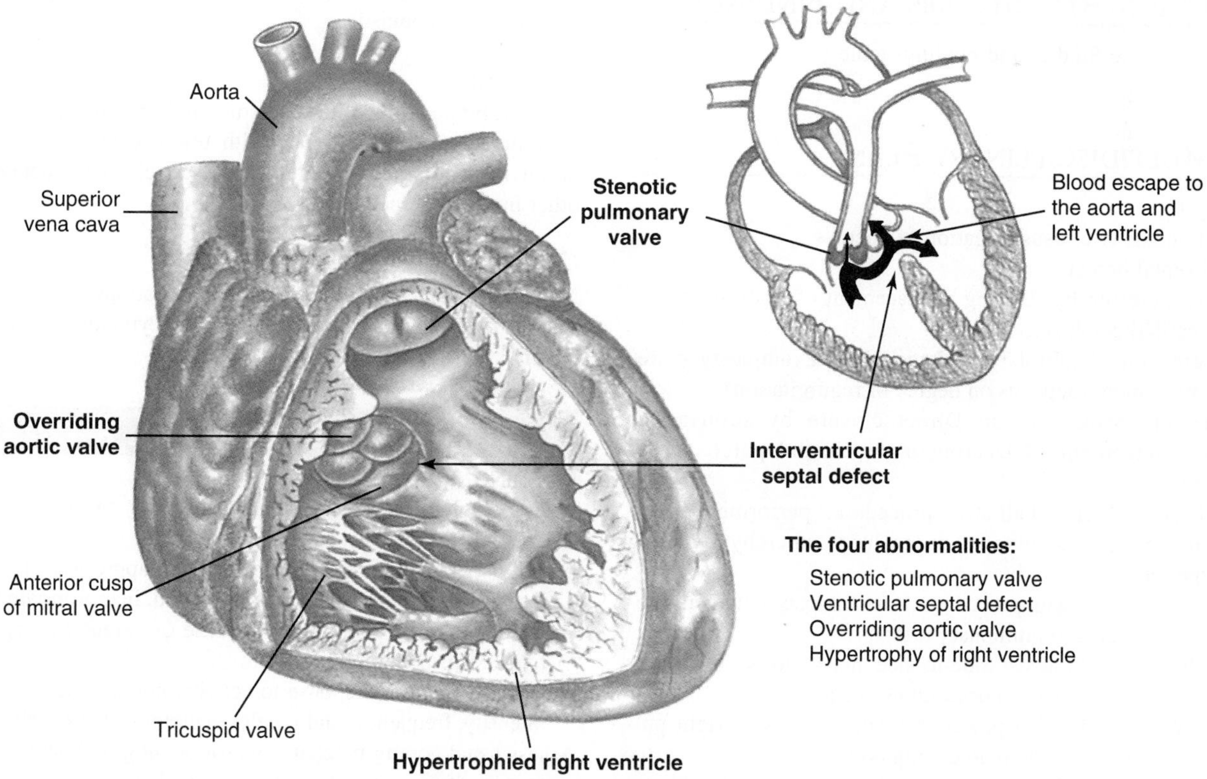

FIG. 3-55
Tetralogy of Fallot. (From Canobbio.[15])

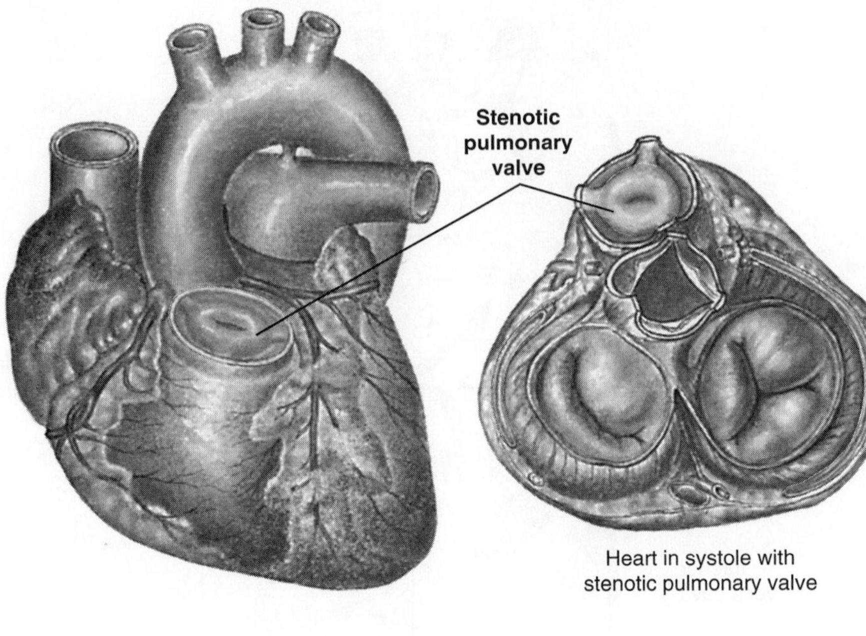

FIG. 3-56
Pulmonic valvular stenosis. (From Canobbio.[15])

DIAGNOSTIC STUDIES AND FINDINGS

See Diagnostic Studies and Findings table.

MULTIDISCIPLINARY PLAN

Surgery

Patent ductus arteriosus: Ligation of ductus
Atrial septal defect
- Direct closure by suturing or placement of Dacron or pericardial patch across defect
- Correction of mitral regurgitation by valvuloplasty or replacement (depends on degree of regurgitation)

Ventricular septal defect: Direct closure by suturing or with placement of Dacron or pericardial patch across defect
Tetralogy of Fallot: Palliative procedures performed on infants to enhance blood flow to lungs, thereby reducing hypoxia
- Blalock-Taussig procedure: Anastomosis between subclavian and pulmonary arteries
- Potts' anastomosis: Side-to-side anastomosis of left pulmonary artery to descending aorta
- Waterston-Cooley procedure: Anastomosis of right pulmonary artery to ascending aorta

Pulmonic stenosis: Valvotomy; resection of excess infundibular muscle; valve replacement
Corrective surgery: Intracardiac repair of ventricular septal defect and pulmonic stenosis; contraindicated if pulmonary artery is hypoplastic

Medications

Dictated by patient's clinical picture and presence of ventricular failure and dysrhythmias; with few exceptions, antibiotic prophylaxis for infective endocarditis is given for dental and other invasive procedures

General Management

Nonspecific unless indicated by complications such as heart failure, dysrhythmias, or effects of polycythemia in cyanotic patient

NURSING CARE

NURSING ASSESSMENT

Assess level of anxiety; determine primary cause to identify any misconceptions, fears, and concerns.
Assess usual level of activity; determine if appropriate for medical condition; may be overly restricted, inappropriate to degree of cardiac impairment because of parental overprotectiveness or patient's own fears.
Assess and monitor response to activity, noting type of activity, intensity, frequency, and type of symptoms that develop.
Assess usual coping mechanisms for dealing with stress to determine if they are adequate to control anxiety.
See Assessment Considerations table.

Diagnostic Studies and Findings

Study	Patent Ductus Arteriosus	Atrial Septal Defect	Ventricular Septal Defect	Tetralogy of Fallot	Pulmonic Stenosis
ECG	Normal (small ductus); left ventricular hypertrophy (LVH); PR interval may be prolonged; atrial fibrillation in adults	Normal; right ventricular hypertrophy (RVH); right bundle branch block; PR interval may be prolonged; left axis deviation (ostium primum); normal or right axis (ostium secundum)	Normal if defect is small; if moderate to large, LVH; LVH/RVH in presence of pulmonary hypertension	RVH	Normal if stenosis is mild; if moderate to severe, RVH and right axis deviation; if severe, right atrial hypertrophy (RAH)
Chest x-ray	Normal; with moderate to large shunt, enlarged cardiac silhouette with enlarged LA, LV, and pulmonary artery (PA); enlarged aorta; enlarged pulmonary trunk and increased pulmonary flow	Enlarged RA, RV, PA; increased pulmonary vascular markings; LA, LV, and aortic knob may be small	Mild LVH with small shunt; with large shunt, increased LV, dilation of PA, increased pulmonary vascular markings, enlarged LA	Small cardiac silhouette; small PA; prominent aorta (may arch to right in 25% of cases)	Enlarged RV and PA; if severe, decreased peripheral pulmonary vascular markings
Echocardiogram/ transesophageal echocardiogram (TEE)	Enlarged LA and LV owing to left-to-right shunt; TEE may be necessary to visualize ductus	With ostium secundum, enlarged RV, paradoxic movement of septum during systole; with ostium primum, mitral valve displaced inferiorly and anteriorly	Large shunt; enlarged RA and RV; for smaller defects, bubble contrast through peripheral IV can be visualized crossing defect, especially during Valsalva's maneuver	Overriding aorta visualized; pulmonary stenosis visualized with degree of obstruction; enlarged ventricular septum (septal motion remains normal)	Normal if stenosis is mild; if moderate to severe, enlarged RA and RV, possible tricuspid regurgitation
Laboratory tests	No specific findings	No specific findings	No specific findings unless patient is cyanotic, then increased hematocrit value and hemoglobin level and decreased arterial oxygen saturation	Increased hematocrit value; degree depends on amount of deoxygenated systemic blood	No specific findings
Cardiac catheterization	Left-to-right shunt; increased pulmonary blood flow; increased oxygen saturation in PA; intracardiac pressures normal; RV and PA pressures may be slightly elevated	Left-to-right shunt at atrial level; increased oxygen saturation in RA; RA pressure usually normal; mitral regurgitation	Left-to-right shunt (LV to RV); study determines degree of shunt; increased pulmonary blood flow, oxygen saturation in RV, and systolic pressure in RV and PA	RV outflow obstruction; increased RV pressure; RV to LV shunt; decreased PA pressure as catheter crosses obstruction	Increased RA pressure, which determines systolic pressure gradient between RV and PA
Magnetic resonance imaging (MRI)/ angiography	Angiography capability to image anatomy of ductus and flow without contrast			Images anatomy of pulmonary arteries without contrast of invasive catheter	

Assessment Considerations

Area of Concern	Patent Ductus Arteriosus	Atrial Septal Defect	Ventricular Septal Defect	Tetralogy of Fallot	Pulmonic Stenosis
Physical examination	Small shunt: asymptomatic, increased respiratory infections, small for age; large shunt: exertional dyspnea, decreased exercise tolerance	Small shunt: asymptomatic; moderate to large shunt: exertional dyspnea, decreased exercise tolerance, palpitations	Small to moderate shunt: asymptomatic, exertional dyspnea; large shunt: failure **in infancy,** growth failure, feeding difficulties	**In infancy:** paroxysmal attacks of dyspnea with loss of consciousness ("blue" spells), small for age; **in later childhood:** cyanosis with clubbing of fingers and toes; **in adulthood** (after palliation): exertional dyspnea, cyanosis with clubbing	Asymptomatic during childhood; exertional dyspnea; decreased exercise tolerance
Palpation	Neck vessels dilated and pulsating	Left parasternal lift	Large shunt: left parasternal lift	Precordial prominence; parasternal heave	Left parasternal heave; subxiphoid pulsation
Auscultation	Systolic pressure normal; diastolic pressure low; wide pulse pressure; harsh, loud, continuous murmur in first, second, and third intercostal spaces (ICS) at lower sternal border (LSB); machinery-like murmur best heard when patient is lying down, becoming fainter when patient is standing	Soft-blowing systolic murmur at second ICS at LSB	Small shunt: holosystolic at third, fourth, and fifth ICS, systolic thrill; large shunt: holosystolic murmur at third, fourth, and fifth ICS, splitting of S_2 during expiration, widening during inspiration, systolic ejection sound at second ICS at LSB	Single S_2; systolic ejection murmur at third ICS, may radiate upward to left side of neck	S_1 normal; early systolic ejection click heard at base; midsystolic murmur at second and third ICS at LSB, radiates to suprasternal notch and to left side of neck; S_2 widely split

Potential Complications

Endocarditis; arrhythmias; congestive heart failure

Patient Problems/Nursing Diagnoses & Interventions

NIC Patient Education

Deficient knowledge related to lack of understanding or information misinterpretation

- Instruct patient and family on type of defect and how to manage at home; provide referral services for assistance with home care.
- For adult patients, provide detailed explanation of defect, surgical interventions, and treatments as dictated by defect.

NIC Coping Assistance

Anxiety related to actual or perceived threat to biologic integrity

- Encourage verbalization of feelings.
- Elicit questions and concerns of patient.
- Assist the patient to deal realistically with anxiety, providing alternative methods for dealing with anxiety.
- Refer the patient to long-term counseling if necessary.

NIC Activity and Exercise Management

Risk for activity intolerance related to lack of mobility or progressive decrease in cardiac reserve

- Develop exercise prescription in accordance with patient's cardiac anomaly and compensatory mechanisms.

Patient Education/Continuum of Care Plan

1. Instruct the patient and family concerning the primary defect and any surgical procedures that have occurred. Explain the associated signs and symptoms and describe what is normal and abnormal.
2. Explain activity allowances and limitations, including schooling, sports, and occupation.
3. For adolescents and adults, provide counseling on issues concerning genetics, marriage, contraception, and childbearing.

4. Explain dietary restrictions as indicated.
5. Explain the need to prevent endocarditis (p. 97)

Evaluation/Patient Outcomes

Patient Education: Level of knowledge is increased. Patient and family verbalize knowledge regarding defect, prescribed care, medication, need for return visits, and endocarditis prophylaxis.

Coping Assistance: Anxiety is decreased. Patient and family verbalize reduction in anxiety level and demonstrate appropriate behavior in self-care management.

Activity and Exercise Management: Optimum level of activity is maintained. Patient engages in activities appropriate to clinical status; verbalizes absence of fatigue, weakness.

VASCULAR DISEASES

Systemic Hypertension

An intermittent or sustained elevation in systolic or diastolic blood pressure, hypertension is a major cause of cerebrovascular accident (stroke), cardiac disease, and renal failure (Fig. 3-57).

An estimated 60 million Americans have hypertension, and an additional 25 million have borderline hypertension. Half of those affected are unaware of it. Among African-Americans, hypertension is estimated to be higher than in whites, appears earlier, and results in higher risks of mortality and morbidity from stroke and heart failure. Death rates from cardiovascular disease are 45% higher for black men than for white men and 67% higher for black women than for white women.[4,74] Current guidelines define persons with blood pressures less than 130/85 mm Hg as normal; those with systolic blood pressure (SBP) between 130 and 139 mm Hg and diastolic blood pressure (DBP) between 85 and 89 mm Hg are defined as high normal (Table 3-5).

In the elderly, systolic hypertension results from a loss of arterial compliance, reduced cardiac output and left ventricular ejection rate, and increased resistance of the larger arteries.[109] After age 50 years, systemic vascular resistance increases at a rate of 1% per year.[100,109] For persons ages 65 to 74 years, isolated systolic hypertension (SBP >140 mm Hg and DPB >90 mm Hg) affects 10.3% of the male population and 11.8% of the female population. The results of clinical trials demonstrate significant cardiovascular benefit in treating hypertension.[103]

Although there is no way of predicting in whom high blood pressure will develop, hypertension can be detected easily. Therefore the major emphasis in the control of hypertension should be on early detection and effective treatment.

Table 3-5 Classification of Initial Blood Pressure for Adults Age 18 Years and Older

Category	Systolic (mm Hg)	Diastolic (mm Hg)
Normal	<130	<85
High normal	130-139	85-89
Hypertension: Average of two determinations/two visits		
Stage 1 (mild)	140-159	90-99
Stage 2 (moderate)	160-179	100-109
Stage 3 (severe)q	≥180	110-119
Stage 4 (very severe)	≥210	≥120

Modified from National Institutes of Health and National Heart, Lung, and Blood Institute.[50]

Pathophysiology

Primary (essential) hypertension is the most common form, accounting for 90% of all cases. It is an abnormal state in which excessive neurohumoral stimulation results in increased arterial tone. The cause is unknown, but certain risk factors have been identified. These include family history, age group, race, obesity, stress, cigarette smoking, and a diet high in salt and saturated fats. Although there is a strong family relationship with predisposition for hypertension, the search for genetic determinants is handicapped by the absence of a genetic marker to predict the disease before the blood pressure rises.

Secondary hypertension refers to elevated blood pressure that is related to some underlying disease. The most common causes include the following:

- Renal parenchymal disorders
  - Pyelonephritis
  - Glomerulonephritis
  - Hydronephrosis
  - Polycystic kidney
  - Juxtaglomerular (renin-producing) tumors
  - After kidney transplant
- Renal artery disease
  - Artherosclerosis
  - Arthritis
  - Embolism
  - Aneurysm
  - Diabetic nephrosclerosis

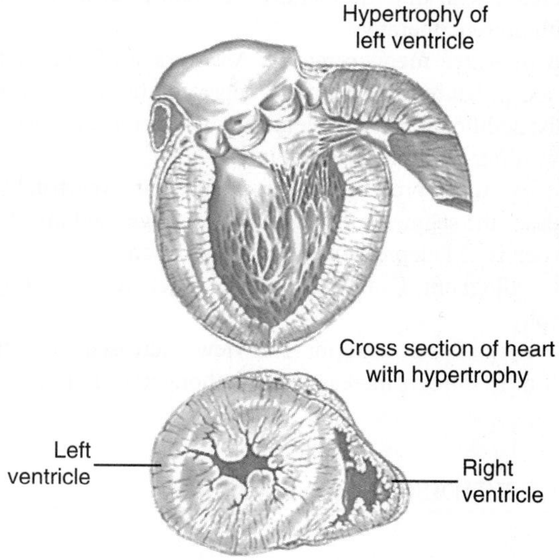

Fig. 3-57
Hypertension. (From Canobbio.[15])

Endocrine and metabolic disorders
- Pheochromocytoma
- Cushing's syndrome
- Aldosteronism (primary)
- Hypercalcemia
- Acromegaly
- Myxedema
- Oral contraceptives
- Chronic licorice ingestion

CNS disorders
- Increased intracranial pressure
- Brain tumor
- Neurogenic; psychogenic
- Polyneuritis (porphyria)

Coarctation of aorta

The pathogenesis of hypertension is complex because various homeostatic mechanisms contribute to the maintenance of normal arterial pressure.

Cardiac output (stroke volume times heart rate) and peripheral vascular resistance determine arterial pressure. Increases in blood volume (high-output states), heart rate, or arterial vasoconstriction that cause an increase in peripheral resistance can lead to hypertension.

Stimulation and production of high plasma levels of renin (a proteolytic enzyme produced by juxtaglomerular cells) contribute to a complex relationship between extracellular fluid and pressure, leading to sympathetic activation and elevated arterial pressure. FIG. 3-58 outlines the conversion of renin to angiotensin I and II.

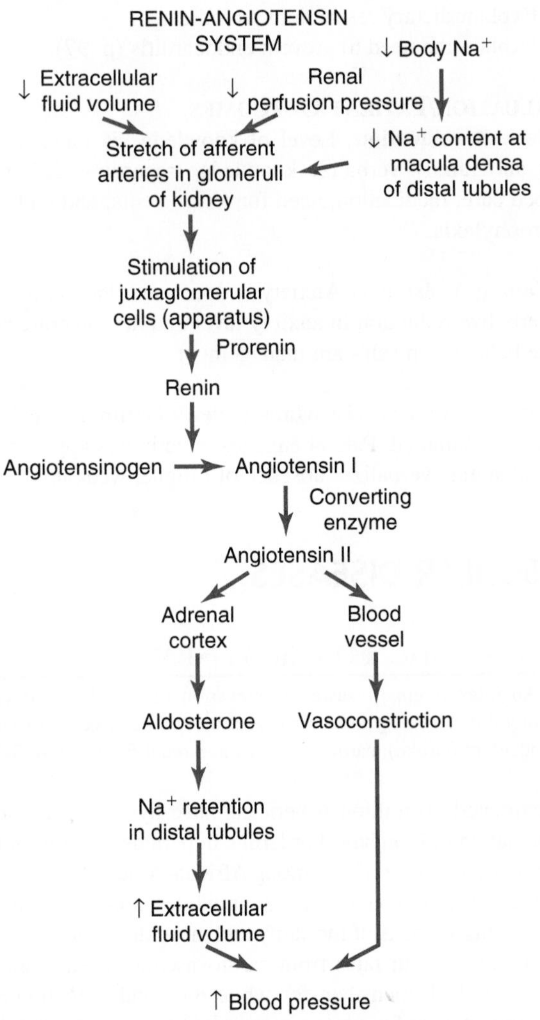

FIG. 3-58

Complex relationship between extracellular fluid volume and pressure as mediated by renal hormonal mechanisms. These involve production of renin and angiotensin. Angiotensin is a potent vasoconstrictor that stimulates aldosterone synthesis, resulting in sodium retention and increased volume. (From Kaye.[54])

DIAGNOSTIC STUDIES AND FINDINGS

Urine studies including microscopic examination: Proteinuria, hematuria

Blood chemistry: BUN 20 mg/dl; creatinine 1.5 mg/dl; potassium 5 mEq/L in renal failure; 3.5 mEq/L in primary aldosteronism and with diuretic administration; cholesterol and lipid levels elevated in hyperlipidemia; uric acid level may increase with diuretic therapy; calcium level may increase with diuretic therapy

Blood pressure measurements: An average of two or more blood pressure measurements separated by 2-minute intervals; additional measurements are obtained if first two readings differ by more than 5 mm Hg

ECG: Evaluates presence of left ventricular hypertrophy (increases the segment of ECG [QRS] voltage) and myocardial ischemia: ST depression, T wave inversion

Echocardiogram: Evaluates presence of left ventricular hypertrophy

Chest x-ray: Posteroanterior (PA) view: Increased convexity of left heart border; increased cardiothoracic (CT) ratio

MULTIDISCIPLINARY PLAN

Surgery

None for primary hypertension (see Chapter 13 for surgical interventions for renal disorders)

Medications

Oral

Dosages may vary based on patient response and practitioner practice.

Diuretics

Thiazides (partial listing)
- Chlorothiazide (Diuril) (250-1000 mg/day)
- Hydrochlorothiazide (Esidrix, HydroDIURIL) (50-100 mg/day)
- Bendroflumethiazide (Naturetin) (2.5-10 mg/day)

Thiazide-like diuretics
- Chlorthalidone (Hygroton, Thalitone) (12.5-50 mg/day)
- Metolazone (Diulo, Zaroxolyn) (0.5-2.5 mg/day)

Loop diuretics
- Furosemide (Lasix) (10-120 mg/day dosed bid or qid)
- Ethacrynic acid (Edecrin) (25-50 mg/day)
- Bumetanide (Bumex (0.5-2.0 mg/day)

Potassium-sparing diuretics
Spironolactone (Aldactone) (25-50 mg/day or bid)
Triamterene (Dyrenium) (25-150 mg/day)
Amiloride (Midamor) (5-10 mg/day)

Beta-adrenergic blocking agents
Propranolol (Inderal) (40-160 mg/day or bid)
Metroprolol tartrate (Lopressor) (50-200 mg/day or bid)
Pindolol (Visken) (10-60 mg/day)
Atenolol (Tenormin) (50-100 mg/day)
Timolol maleate (Blocadren) (20-40 mg/day)
Nadolol (Corgard) (80-320 mg/day)
Labetolol (Normodyne) (100-200 mg/day but can go as high as 1200 mg/day)

Alpha-2 agonists: CNS acting agents
Methyldopa (Aldomet) (125-250 mg/day or bid; can be dosed as high as 2000 mg/day)
Clonidine (Catapres) (0.1-0.6 mg/day)
Guanethidine (Ismelin) (range 10-200 mg/day)
Prazosin (Minipress) (1-2 mg/day or bid; can be dosed up to 20 mg/day)
Trazosin (Hytrin) (1-5 mg/day; can be dosed up to 20 mg/day)

Peripheral antagonists (partial listing): Guanethidine (Ismelin) (10-50 mg/day up to 150 mg/day)

ACE inhibitors (partial listing)
Captopril (Capoten) (25-150 mg tid)
Enalapril (Vasotec) (2.5-40 mg qd)
Lisinopril (Zestril) (5.0-40 mg qd)
Quinapril (Accupril) (5.0-80 mg qd)
Benazepril (Lotensin) (10-40 mg qd)

Calcium antagonists (partial listing)
Diltiazem (Cardizem) (90-360 mg)
Verapamil (Calan, Isoptin) (80-480 mg)
Nifedipine (Procardia) (30-120 mg)

Vasodilators
Hydralazine (Apresoline) (12.5-50 mg/day bid or tid)
Minoxidil (Loniten) (2.5-10 mg/bid or tid)
Sodium nitroprusside (Nipride) (0.5-10 mg/kg/min IV)
Diazoxide (Hyperstat) (300 mg by rapid IV bolus) rarely used

General Management

The stepped-care approach (FIG. 3-59) in the treatment of high blood pressure (based on recommendations of the National Joint Committee (JNCIV)[50] on Detection, Evaluation and Treatment of High Blood Pressure) is an individualized, systematic approach to treatment:

Step 1: Lifestyle modification, including weight reduction, regular physical activity; limit alcohol intake, reduce sodium intake, and undertake smoking cessation.

Step 2: Begin with small doses of a single agent, then advance the dosages until blood pressure control is achieved; thiazide diuretics or beta-blockers are suggested as initial treatment. Continue lifestyle modification.

Step 3: If response to single agent is inadequate, increase the drug dose or add another agent from a different class of drugs.

Step 4: If response is still inadequate, add a second or third agent from a different class.

Cardiac monitoring for hypertensive crisis

! EMERGENCY ALERT

HYPERTENSIVE CRISIS

Diastolic blood pressure above 120 mm Hg; must determine and treat underlying cause

ASSESSMENT

- Rule out renal artery stenosis, drug overdose, drug withdrawal, cocaine use, hyperthyroidism, pheochromocytoma, primary aldosteronism.

INTERVENTIONS

- Continuous noninvasive or invasive blood pressure monitoring during therapy.
- Assess end-organ function such as urine output and perfusion.
- Obtain urinalysis, electrolytes, creatinine, uric acid.
- Obtain ECG.
- Obtain chest x-ray.
- Administer high-flow oxygen by mask (10-15 L).
- Obtain IV access.
- To lower blood pressures, administer medications that are appropriate for the cause (e.g., sodium nitroprusside, lasix, alpha- and beta-blocking agents, ACE inhibitors).

Continuous blood pressure monitoring for hypertensive crisis

Dietary management
Sodium restriction: May range from mild to rigid restriction depending on degree of hypertension; JNC IV recommended dietary restriction to 2 to 3 g/day
Alcohol: Limit intake to 2 ounces 100-proof whiskey, 8 ounces wine, 24 ounces beer per day
Caffeine: Restrict intake
Cholesterol, lipids, saturated fats: Reduce intake

Weight control: Recommend weight loss of 5% or more in obese patient

Exercise
Regular aerobic exercise appropriate for age and health status
Refer to cardiac rehabilitation for prescribed exercise program
Avoid isometric exercises

Stress reduction and management

Monitor blood pressure on regular basis; frequency determined by blood pressure elevations

NURSING CARE

NURSING ASSESSMENT

Symptoms

Mild to moderate hypertension: Asymptomatic

Moderate to severe hypertension: Headaches, dizziness, fatigue, vertigo, palpitations

Severe hypertension: Throbbing suboccipital headache (may be present when patient awakens in morning, disappearing spontaneously after several hours); epistaxis

Physical Examination

Blood pressure: Mild, moderate, severe, very severe as described in Table 3-5 on p.90.

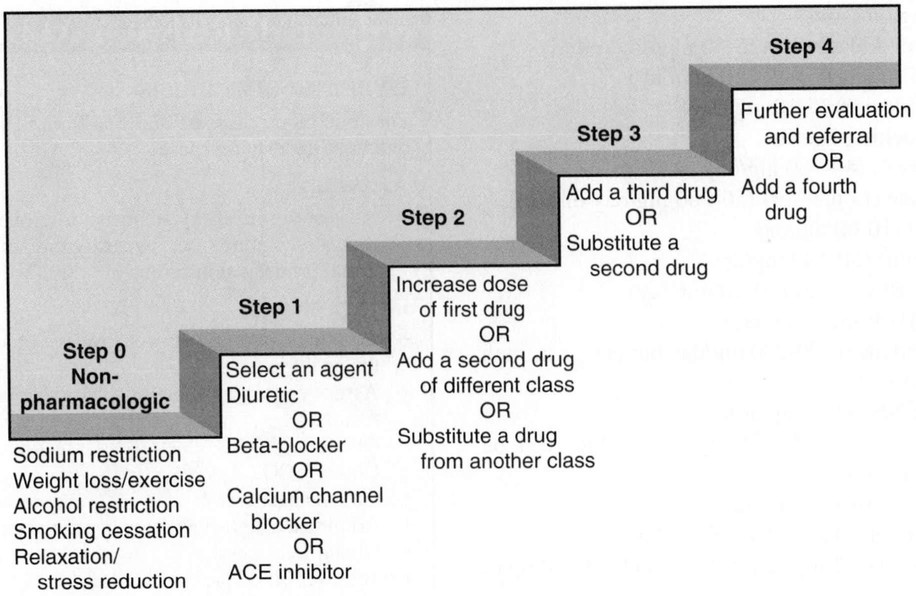

FIG. 3-59

Stepped-care approach in treatment of high blood pressure. (From Canobbio.[15])

Pulse: Tachycardia; bounding; femoral delay as compared with radial or brachial pulsation

Precordium: Displaced but forceful apical impulse; ventricular heave (apical lift)

Auscultation: Bruits over carotid and femoral areas; accentuated S_2 at base; apical systolic murmur; audible S_4; early diastolic blowing murmur (right and left sternal borders and intercostal spaces)

Optic fundi: Retinal changes: grade I—minimal arteriolar narrowing or irregularity; grade II—marked arteriolar narrowing and irregularity with focal tortuosity or spasm; grade III—marked arteriolar narrowing and irregularity with generalized tortuosity, flame-shaped hemorrhages, cotton-wool exudates; grade IV—same as grade III, plus papilledema

Assess quality of pain and presence of associated symptoms such as nausea, vomiting, and epistaxis.

Assess and monitor level of consciousness. Check neurologic signs every hour during hypertensive crisis. Notify physician of any sudden changes in mentation, pupillary response, or movement of extremities.

Assess factors that will influence the patient's ability to adhere to the therapeutic plan: financial status, age, culture, health status, occupation.

Assess the patient's attitudes and feelings toward prescribed health-care regimen; explore factors that may be influencing patient's ability to adhere to the treatment plan.

POTENTIAL COMPLICATIONS

MI; left ventricular hypertrophy; congestive heart failure; cerebral vascular accidents; peripheral arterial insufficiency, neuropathy; retinopathy; kidney damage, with and without renal failure; premature mortality

PATIENT PROBLEMS/NURSING DIAGNOSES & INTERVENTIONS

NIC PHYSICAL AND PSYCHOLOGIC COMFORT PROMOTION

Acute and/or chronic pain (headache) related to increased cerebrovascular pressure

- Initiate measures to relieve pain and reduce external stimuli:
  - Maintain a quiet environment with reduced lighting.
  - Limit activities.
  - Avoid sudden jarring motion.
  - Limit visitors.
  - Use additional comfort measures such as cold packs and position changes.
- Administer pain relievers and antiemetics as ordered.
- Assist with ambulation because patient may experience dizziness.

NIC TISSUE PERFUSION MANAGEMENT

Ineffective tissue perfusion (cerebral, renal, vascular) related to increased peripheral vascular resistance

- Maintain seizure precautions as indicated; maintain quiet environment.
- Monitor arterial pressures as indicated; use same arm for blood pressure; use Doppler sensor, if indicated.
- Monitor parenteral fluids with medications as ordered.
- Administer medications as ordered.
- Measure intake and output; check output, noting amount and color of urine; measure specific gravity.
- Keep NPO if nausea or vomiting is present.

NIC BEHAVIORAL THERAPY

Noncompliance related to side effects of prescribed treatment and conflict with sociocultural influences

- Review behaviors that place patient at risk for cardiovascular event. Identify and clarify any misconceptions the patient has regarding disease state.
- Design a program that is compatible with the patient's habits, lifestyle, and personality. Include the patient in program design.
- Provide opportunities to discuss feelings toward recommended lifestyle changes.
- Explore alternative measures to increase compliant behaviors, such as contracting, self-monitoring, behavior modification, shaping behavior, and support groups.

PATIENT EDUCATION/CONTINUUM OF CARE PLAN

1. Instruct the patient and family about high blood pressure, factors that contribute to increasing blood pressure, influencing factors.
2. Instruct patient on home blood pressure monitoring, interpretation of results, and actions to take if significant change occurs. Permit time for practice using home equipment. If patient is unable to perform blood pressure monitoring at home, provide information and referrals to have regular blood pressure checks. Refer to home health agency as necessary.
3. Explain diet therapy, including sodium, calorie, and fat restrictions as ordered; include the rationale in explanation. Discuss the importance of restricting alcohol.
4. Explain the role of regular exercise in blood pressure regulation and weight control.
5. Explain the relationship between stress and hypertension, factors that produce stress, and methods to modify stress.
6. Explain antihypertensive therapy, including name, rationale, dosage, and side effects of all prescribed medications.
7. Discuss the importance of not smoking or using tobacco products.

EVALUATION/PATIENT OUTCOMES

Physical and Psychologic Comfort Promotion: Patient has no complaints of headache or dizziness.

Tissue Perfusion Management: Tissue perfusion is improved. Blood pressure is within acceptable limits. Laboratory values are within normal limits.

Behavioral Therapy: Patient complies with therapeutic plan. Patient is normotensive, reports taking medication, loses weight, and has no symptoms.

PRIMARY PULMONARY HYPERTENSION

Primary pulmonary hypertension (PPH) is a rare vascular abnormality of the pulmonary arterial system.

The cause is unknown, and the diagnosis is made only after thorough investigation of all possible etiologic factors (thromboembolism, congenital or immunologic abnormalities, collagen-vascular disease, drug ingestion, etc.). In 1981 the National Institutes of Health defined PPH as a disorder by hemodynamic criteria with the mean pulmonary artery pressure over 25 mm Hg at rest or 30 mm Hg during exercise.

The prevalence and incidence of PPH shows a 3:1 predisposition for females[35] and tends to be diagnosed between ages 21 and 40 years. There is some evidence of genetic transmission and links to liver disease. Despite the overall incidence of PPH being rare, mortality rates of 80% within 5 years of clinical diagnosis make this vascular disease the focus of intense investigation.

PATHOPHYSIOLOGY

Many pathologic mechanisms have been postulated to describe the morphologic changes in the pulmonary vascular bed of patients with PPH. The plexogenic pulmonary arteriopathy characteristically seen in PPH may be the result of intense vasoconstriction, secondary to marked vasoreactivity and spasm, with resultant fibrosis and necrosis of the muscular pulmonary arteries. Plexiform or distorted vessels develop subsequently. Eventually these diseased vessels are destroyed, and the remaining vessels in this shrinking pulmonary arterial bed suffer a permanent increase in pulmonary vascular resistance.

Signs and symptoms include exertional dyspnea, syncope, chest pain, weakness, fatigue, palpitations, hoarseness (from enlarged pulmonary trunk pressing on recurrent laryngeal nerve), cough, and sometimes hemoptysis. On physical examination, there is a large a wave in the jugular venous pulse (tricuspid valve closure against a hypertensive right ventricle), a left parasternal heave (enlarged right ventricle), a systolic pulsation in the second left interspace, and a loud second heart sound (pulmonary valve closure). In advanced disease, right ventricular failure is closely linked to mortality, so careful assessment of tricuspid and pulmonary valve function is important. The systolic murmur of tricuspid regurgitation or the diastolic murmur (Graham-Steell murmur) of hypertensive pulmonary regurgitation must be closely followed.

DIAGNOSTIC STUDIES AND FINDINGS

Chest x-ray: Cardiomegaly, prominent central pulmonary arteries, marked tapering of peripheral arteries, right atrial and right ventricular enlargement

ECG: Right ventricular hypertrophy, right atrial enlargement, right axis deviation

Two-dimensional echocardiogram: Right atrial and right ventricular enlargement/hypertrophy, right ventricular free wall motion, position and motion of ventricular septum, presence of intraatrial shunt (atrial septal defect or patent foramen ovale); permits estimate of right ventricular systolic pressure

Cardiac catheterization: Pulmonary artery flotation catheter is the diagnostic gold standard and is used to measure pulmonary artery pressures and response to vasoactive agents; pulmonary arteriography can be used to rule out thromboembolic disease but has been associated with some mortality

Computed tomography (CT) scan: Contrast study of the thorax can define pulmonary artery anatomy and identify thrombus with lower risk than invasive catheterization

Ventilation/perfusion (V/Q) lung scan: Nuclear contrast study to delineate pulmonary blood flow, identify areas of hypoperfusion possibly secondary to thrombus

MULTIDISCIPLINARY PLAN

Surgery

Heart-lung or, more commonly, single lung transplant is the surgical intervention of choice. Currently, donor availability is a major obstacle for most PPH patients awaiting transplant. One-year survival after lung or heart-lung transplant still does not surpass 70% in most institutions, and major complications such as obliterative bronchiolitis significantly affect recipients' quality of life.

Medications

Pulmonary vasodilators: Effective only in patients with PPH who exhibit pulmonary reactivity rather than fixed pulmonary vascular resistance; caution must be used to avoid systemic hypotension because the agents are given in very large dosages titrated to individual patient tolerance

Nifedipine (Procardia)

Verapamil (Calan, Isoptin)

Diltiazam (Cardizem)

Prostacycline (Epoprostenol, Flolan) (continuous IV infusion through a permanent central venous catheter)

Oxygen (pulmonary vasodilator at higher concentrations) if patients are hypoxemic

Anticoagulation: Coumadin—may improve prognosis in some patients with PPH, especially if intrapulmonary emboli or thrombus is identified (titrated to INR range of 2-3)

Right heart failure management (as appropriate): Digoxin and diuretics

General Management

Medical management is directed at decreasing resistance to pulmonary blood flow and improving circulatory response to right ventricular pressure overload.

Activity restrictions: Patients with PPH must avoid all strenuous, heavy isometric exercise, including lifting, pushing, or pulling. No sudden, start-stop exercise, which requires sudden peripheral vasodilation with increased cardiac output is allowed; this can trigger syncope and often death (especially in patients with significantly elevated, fixed pulmonary vascular resistance).

Pregnancy/contraception: Because many patients diagnosed with PPH are young women, advice must be given to avoid pregnancy because it carries a 50% maternal mortality. Caution must also be taken with the use of oral contraceptives (containing estrogen) because these may increase pulmonary vascular resistance, as well as predispose to thrombogenesis.

Altitude/air travel: Patients with PPH should be cautioned against traveling or living at high altitudes (greater than 2000 ft) because of decreased concentrations of oxygen secondary to lower atmospheric pressure (predisposing to increased vasoconstriction).

Preventive measures: Advise annual flu and pneumonia vaccines.

Heart failure management: Low-salt diet, daily weighing.

NURSING CARE

NURSING ASSESSMENT

Assess for dyspnea, fatigue, syncope, chest pain, palpitations.

Determine level of right heart failure.

Assess activity level and exercise tolerance.

Assess home situation and patient's attitudes and feelings toward prescribed therapies.

POTENTIAL COMPLICATIONS

Pulmonary microemboli, supraventricular tachycardia, decompensation from severe right heart failure

PATIENT PROBLEMS/NURSING DIAGNOSES & INTERVENTIONS

NIC TISSUE PERFUSION MANAGEMENT

Impaired gas exchange related to ventilation/perfusion mismatch secondary to pulmonary vascular disease

Decreased cardiac output related to fixed pulmonary vascular resistance and systemic vasodilation secondary to isometric activity, vasodilatory medications, dehydration

- Optimize pulmonary vasodilator therapy while monitoring for hypotension and increase in symptoms.
- Titrate oxygen therapy as prescribed.
- Increase activity gradually, evaluating tolerance.
- Instruct patient to avoid exposure to community-acquired viruses and to obtain flu and pneumonia vaccines.
- Instruct patient to notify physician at early signs of respiratory infection, new cough, or hemoptysis.
- Assess blood pressure and vital signs frequently while titrating vasoactive medications; have patient keep home blood pressure diary.
- Instruct patient regarding activity restrictions *to avoid syncope.*
- Maintain adequate hydration in setting of hot weather, fever, diarrhea.
- Instruct patient on low-salt diet, and obtain daily weights *to assess subtle signs of right heart failure.*

NIC PSYCHOLOGIC COMFORT PROMOTION

Anxiety/fear related to poor prognosis, fear of death; syncopal episode secondary to lack of information, lack of perceived control

- Instruct patient on activity guidelines, emphasizing control over adverse symptoms.
- Provide information/explanation regarding procedures, monitoring equipment.
- Provide access for patient to PPH or lung transplant support group.
- Provide supportive/grief counseling in setting of life-threatening condition; provide information regarding advanced directive, chaplain services when appropriate.

- Provide access or timely referral to regional lung or heart/lung transplant program.

Patient Education/Continuum of Care Plan

1. Instruct patient on home blood pressure monitoring when appropriate.
2. Provide access to home IV prostacyclin therapy where available. Ensure that patient is able to manage drug therapy at home. Secure partner in learning about the drug and IV management.
3. Teach patient management of central IV line.
4. Instruct patient to monitor for fluid accumulation (heart failure) by assessing weights, evaluating swelling, and avoiding salts.
5. Monitor anticoagulation where appropriate to maintain INR 2-3.

Evaluation/Patient Outcomes

Tissue Perfusion Management: Patient tolerates therapeutic doses of vasodilator therapy Patient demonstrates increased exercise tolerance, decreased breathlessness, and absence of syncope. Patient demonstrates understanding of risky behaviors. Patient understands the risks of isometrics, pregnancy, traveling to high altitudes.

Psychologic Comfort Promotion: Patient expresses understanding of severity of disease Patient is able to channel physical reserve to adaptive behaviors such as expression of grief, arrangement for home/family support, and inquiring about potential therapeutic options.

Acute Arterial Insufficiency

Arterial insufficiency is a sudden decrease in the arterial supply to an extremity (Fig. 3-60).

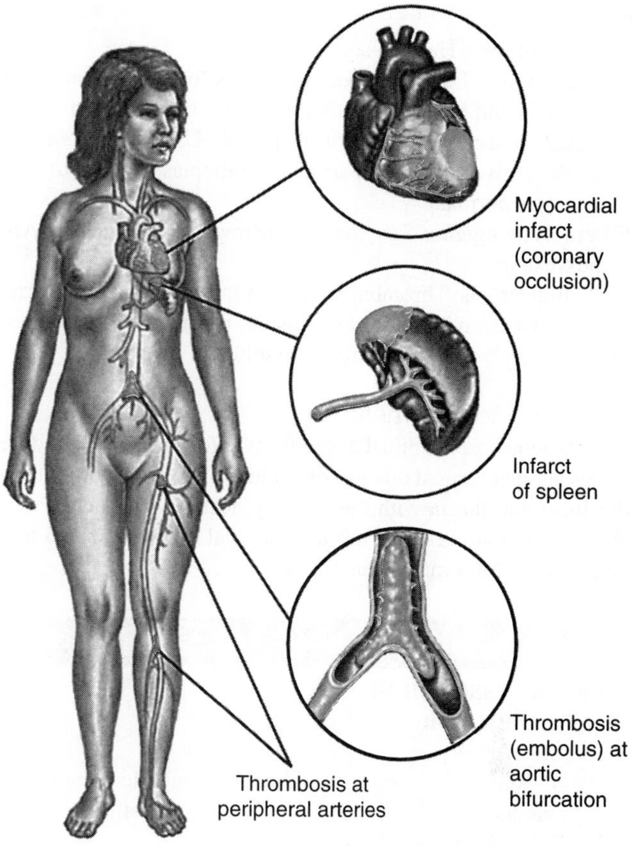

Fig. 3-60
Acute arterial insufficiency. (From Canobbio.[15])

Classified as an acute disorder, obstruction of any major artery produces symptoms. The most common causes of acute arterial insufficiency are embolism, thrombosis, and trauma. Cardiac disorders are the main source of thrombi on the left side of the heart. The legs are most commonly involved. The femoral artery is most often affected (46%), followed by the popliteal tibial tree (11%) and the iliac arteries (8%).[90] Acute arterial obstruction may also occur as a result of injury produced by compression, shearing, or laceration of a vessel. Furthermore, severe hypothermia may produce sudden severe vasoconstriction.

Pathophysiology

Once dislodged, an embolus may travel throughout the systemic circulation, lodging in an arterial branch and stagnating flow in the distal circulation. This leads to the formation of a soft coagulum proximal and distal to the area of stagnant blood flow. The result is the formation of a secondary thrombus, which extends along the arterial wall and progressively compromises collateral circulation. Without adequate collateral circulation the distal tissues are deprived of oxygenation, a situation that leads to ischemia, pain, and paresthesia in the affected area. With prolonged ischemia, cellular damage occurs, leading to muscle necrosis.

Diagnostic Studies and Findings

Doppler ultrasonography: Abnormal blood flow pattern proximal to occlusion; "pistol shot" sound characterizes absence of diastolic flow component; ankle/brachial index of 0.25 reflects severe ischemia and impending gangrene

Echocardiography: Determines whether heart is source of emboli; transesophageal echo if high suspicion, or question right-to-left shunt, such as patent foramen ovale

Arteriography: Determines location of obstruction and character of arterial circulation proximal and distal to obstruction

Multidisciplinary Plan

Surgery

Embolectomy: Embolus can be removed directly via femoral arteriotomy using soft balloon-tipped catheter known as a Fogarty catheter; catheter is passed distal to occlusion, carefully inflated, and withdrawn

Amputation of limb: For severe advanced ischemia

Medications

Anticoagulants: Heparin sodium

Indications: Initiated once diagnosis of embolization is made and before operative treatment is performed

Usual dosage: Loading, 5000-10,000 U IV; maintenance dose given to keep partial thromboplastin time to two times normal

Fibrinolytic agents: Streptokinase (Streptase), urokinase (Abbokinase)

Indications: Thrombolytic agents instilled by intra-arterial infusion into site of occlusion; method of action is fibrinolysis causing fibrin dissolution

General Management

Percutaneous transluminal angioplasty: Nonsurgical procedure involving mechanical dilation of occluded artery performed under local anesthesia with fluoroscopy; lesions considered suitable are stenotic vessels with intraluminal diameter of 2.5 mm and length of not more than 10 cm

NURSING CARE

NURSING ASSESSMENT

Peripheral Extremity

Moderate obstruction

Pain: Sudden in onset; numbness; "embolic syndrome" characterized by five Ps: pain, pallor, paresthesia, pulselessness, and paralysis

Temperature: Decreased

Skin: Pale yellow color

Pulses: Absence of distal arterial pulsations of affected extremity

Poor capillary filling

Severe obstruction: Leg muscle (gastrocnemius) becomes firm; dorsiflexion of foot produces pain

Mesenteric Artery Occlusion

Abdominal cramping, diarrhea with food intake

Weight loss from eating aversion (fear of food syndrome)

Assess arterial pulses distal to occlusion every 1 to 2 hours to determine arterial blood flow patterns.

Assess quality and degree of pain to determine if acute or chronic. Provide for position of most comfort.

POTENTIAL COMPLICATIONS

Loss of limb or infarction of target organ with specific organ-related sequelae; compartment syndrome

PATIENT PROBLEMS/NURSING DIAGNOSES & INTERVENTIONS

NIC TISSUE PERFUSION MANAGEMENT

Ineffective tissue perfusion related to interruption of arterial flow

- Evaluate signs of further ischemia by checking the color and temperature of the extremity, the presence or absence of sensation, and the level of motor deficit.
- Provide bed rest during acute periods.
- Administer anticoagulants as ordered *to prevent enlargement of thrombus and further embolization.*
- Monitor partial thromboplastin time (PTT), hemoglobin (Hgb), and hematocrit (Hct) daily or as indicated *to maintain therapeutic range and avoid hemorrhagic complications.*
- Keep extremities below level of heart *to maintain optimum gravitational flow.*

NIC PHYSICAL COMFORT PROMOTION

Acute and/or chronic pain related to peripheral ischemia

- Maintain bed rest during acute phase.
- Do not raise knee gatch, elevate extremity, or allow hips to be maintained in prolonged flexion *because these procedures can interfere with arterial circulation.*
- Administer analgesics as ordered.
- Protect affected extremity by using a bed cradle, cotton blankets, or sheepskin.
- Provide regular active and passive range of motion exercises unless contraindicated.

Other related nursing diagnosis: Anxiety related to threat or change in health status (possible loss of limb)

PATIENT EDUCATION/CONTINUUM OF CARE PLAN

1. Instruct the patient and family about the disease process, possible causes, and therapeutic modalities.
2. At discharge, explain anticoagulant therapy and the need for follow-up monitoring with clotting studies.
3. Explain to the patient and family how to avoid situations that cause blood pooling or interruption of blood flow: crossing legs, smoking, sitting, or standing for extended periods.

EVALUATION/PATIENT OUTCOMES

Tissue Perfusion Management: Peripheral perfusion is improved. Distal and proximal pulses are present. Extremity has normal color. Normal motor function returns in affected extremity.

Physical Comfort Promotion: Pain is relieved or reduced to a tolerable level.

CHRONIC ARTERIAL INSUFFICIENCY

Chronic arterial insufficiency is inadequate blood flow in arteries. It is caused by occlusive atherosclerotic plaques or emboli, damaged or diseased vessels, aneurysms, hypercoagulability states, or heavy use of tobacco (FIG. 3-61).

Atherosclerosis obliterans is the primary cause of chronic arterial insufficiency. Other causes, although rare, may lead to arterial insufficiency of the legs. These include thromboangiitis obliterans (Buerger's disease), cystic degeneration of the popliteal artery, popliteal entrapment, and some connective tissue disorders. A progressive ischemic syndrome, arteriosclerosis obliterans is more common in men, and the incidence rises with age and in women after menopause. It is a diffuse process but is generally confined to short segments of arteries near bifurcations and origins. The aortoiliac and femoropopliteal areas are common sites.

Pathophysiology

Progressive narrowing of the arterial tree by atherosclerotic plaques gives rise to collateral vessels that tend to ensure adequate blood supply and prevent peripheral ischemia. However, the effectiveness of these collateral pathways is limited by their small size and high resistance, as well as by the extent of occlusive disease. Progressive occlusion leads to hypoperfusion and ischemia. These are related directly to the number of occlusions and to the adequacy of collateral vessels. The arms and legs are the most vulnerable to ischemia.

Diagnostic Studies and Findings

Doppler ultrasonography: Quantitates degree of ischemia; ankle/branchial index: arterial pressure less than pressure in brachial artery; normal: 0.9, severe: 0.5 or less

Plethysmography: Evaluates blood flow and determines degree to which peripheral circulation is decreased

Transcutaneous Po_2 ($TcPo_2$): Assesses cutaneous oxygen delivery and oxygen demand

EMERGENCY ALERT

AORTIC ANEURYSM/DISSECTION

An aortic aneurysm/dissection occurs when the intimal layer of the aorta tears and blood leaks between the intimal and medial layers. This may occlude the major vessels that branch off the aorta, including the myocardial, cerebral, or mesenteric vessels. Rupture of the dissection can cause pericardial tamponade, exsanguination, and shock.

Assessment

- Excruciating/tearing chest pain
- Pain: Center of chest, radiating to back or abdomen; may mimic myocardial infarction, back pain, or ulcer
- Hypertension
- Dyspnea
- Orthopnea
- Diaphoresis, pallor
- Apprehension
- Syncope
- Tachycardia
- Absence of major arterial pulse, unilateral
- Bilateral pressure difference
- Pulsation at sternoclavicular joint

Interventions

- Place patient in high-Fowler's position.
- Administer high-flow oxygen (10-12 L).
- Obtain IV access.
- Anticipate nipride and inderal drips.
- Prepare patient for angiography or surgery.
- Provide support and reassurance.

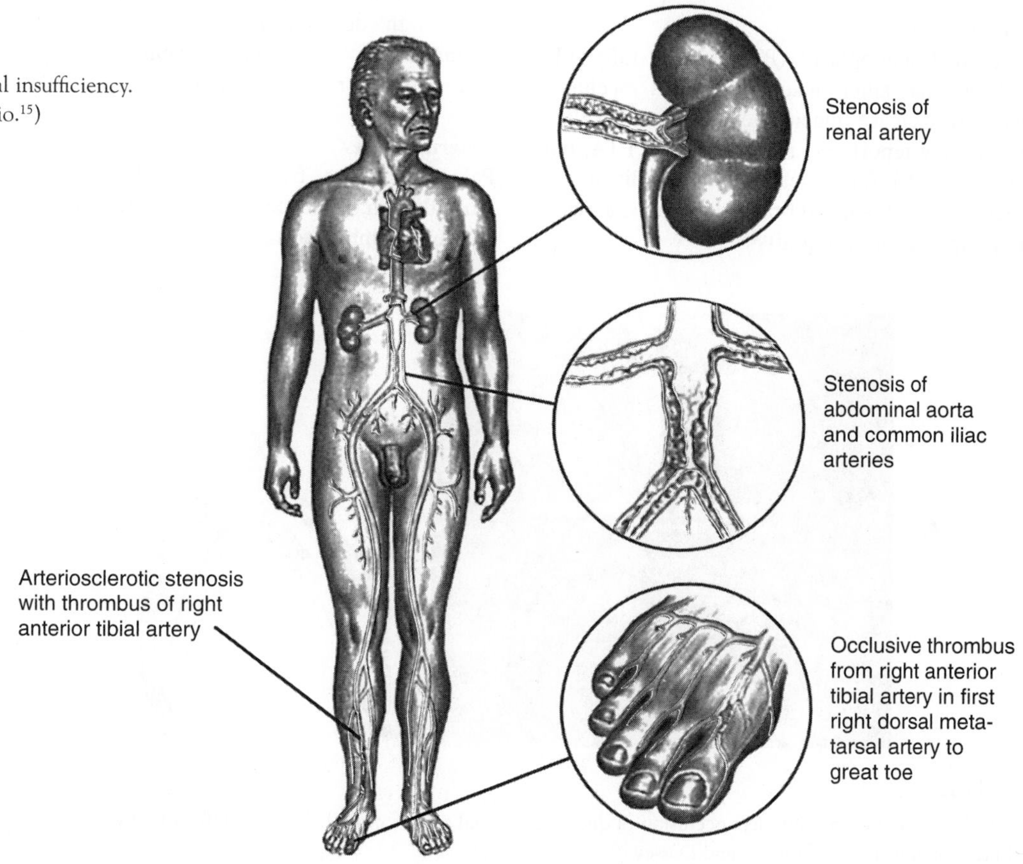

Fig. 3-61
Chronic arterial insufficiency. (From Canobbio.[15])

Multidisciplinary Plan

Surgery

Percutaneous transluminal angioplasty (PTA): Mechanically enlarges diameter of stenotic artery

Endovascular stenting: A percutaneous technique whereby a Dacron stenting graft is deployed into a diseased aortic aneurysm through the use of an endoscope; blood flow is restored, sparing the patient the traditional open surgical grafting procedure

Arterial revascularization, reconstruction: Performed to restore unimpeded pulsatile blood flow, usually beginning with proximal segments (aortoiliac-femoral)

- Endarterectomy: Removal of atheromatous intima from artery
- Bypass graft surgery: Use of Dacron conduit to deliver blood from aorta to femoral vessels, bypassing diseased segments (Fig. 3-62)
- Femoropopliteal reconstruction: Femoropopliteal bypass
- Profundoplasty: Local endarterectomy of proximal profunda femoris artery

Lumbar sympathectomy: Removal of second and third lumbar ganglia; performed to improve blood flow to skin

Amputation of limb: For severe, irreversible ischemia (gangrene)

Medications

Anticoagulants, vasodilators, and antiplatelets have been used but tend to be unhelpful or only palliative. Pentoxifylline (Trental) decreases blood viscosity, improves tissue oxygen delivery, and is used to increase claudication distance.

General Management

Peripheral transluminal angioplasty (PTA): With inflatable balloon-tipped catheter, atheromatous plaque is mechanically compressed to increase lumen patency; vessels of iliac or femoral arteries are reported to respond best to PTA, but success has been reported for vessels of aorta, popliteal, superior mesenteric, subclavian, and brachial systems, as well as stenoses in peripheral arterial grafts[29]

Laser thermal angioplasty (LTA): A new, experimental method of obliterating the atheromatous plaque by heat vaporization; with a fiberoptic catheter, energy from laser source is applied to occlusive lesion; often performed in conjunction with PTA

Risk reduction program: Aimed at weight reduction for the obese patient, smoking cessation, and a low-cholesterol, low–saturated fat diet; evaluation and control of diabetes and hyperlipidemia should be carried out to slow progression of atherosclerotic process

Daily foot care: Inspection; cleaning; use of cotton socks; attention to nails, corns, calluses

Regular walking program: Walking to point of claudication several times a day may improve patient's walking distance; improvement may be due to development of increased collateral arterial flow, progressive adaptation to discomfort or gait modification, metabolic changes in the muscles, or redistribution of blood flow to the muscles[109]

NURSING CARE

Nursing Assessment

Peripheral Tissue Perfusion

Mild to moderate obstruction: Intermittent claudication—calf pain, fatigue induced by walking and relieved by rest; pain in thigh and buttocks (foot rarely involved)

Severe obstruction: Ischemic rest pain—continuous burning pain confined to toes, aggravated by elevation and improved by dependence; occurs at rest and improved with walking; may occur at night, interfering with sleep

- Observe skin color changes (pallor) and venous filling with elevation and dependency procedures to estimate the degree of ischemia

Edema of affected extremity: Sensory changes—numbness of toes, foot, or lower portion of leg; paresthesia

Arterial Pulses

Palpation: Ranges from slightly reduced to absent

Auscultation: Presence of bruits are rest and after exercise; sites are abdominal aorta and iliac and femoral arteries

A

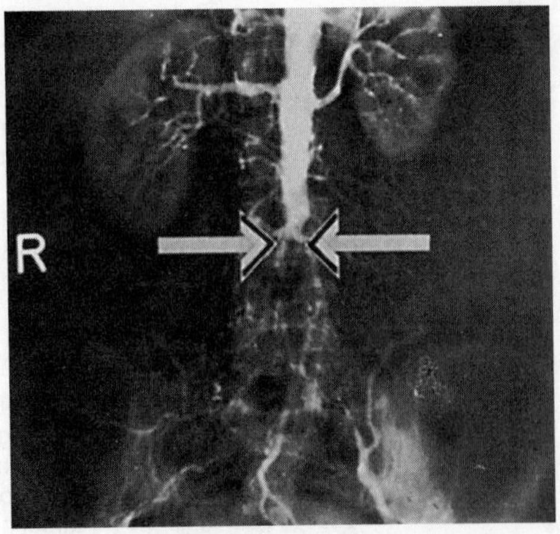

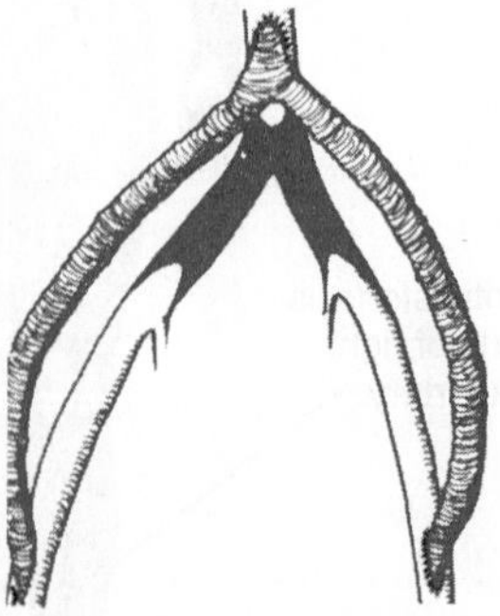

B

Fig. 3-62

A, Arteriogram depicting complete occlusion of distal abdominal aorta *(arrows)*. **B,** Aortobifemoral bypass graft using synthetic conduit. (From Guzzetta and Dossey.[44])

Skin, Nails, Hair
Ulcerations; glossy, cold, smooth skin; pallor, increasing with elevation of extremity; atrophic nails; hair loss; delayed capillary refill time (greater than 3 seconds)

Sexual Function
Impotence in men (reflects decrease in arterial blood flow to branch of internal iliac artery, which may interfere with penile erections)

Potential Complications
Organ damage from downstream chronic ischemia; development of acute arterial insufficiency

Patient Problems/Nursing Diagnoses & Interventions

NIC Tissue Perfusion Management

Ineffective peripheral tissue perfusion (chronic) related to interruption of arterial flow
- Avoid procedures or bed positions that interfere with gravitational blood flow (arterial flow is downward), such as elevating affected extremity or using knee gatch.
- Protect the affected extremity: place bed cradle over affected areas; avoid use of heating devices on lower extremities.
- Instruct the patient to avoid nicotine *because it causes both small and larger vessels to constrict and damage intimal cells.*

NIC Skin/Wound Management

Impaired skin integrity (actual and risk for) related to impaired circulation
- Provide daily skin care *to prevent fissures and infection.*
- Ensure that skin is thoroughly dried.
- Treat ulcerations as they occur.
- Administer soaks, medications, and dressings as ordered.
- Avoid using adhesive tape directly on skin.
- Avoid use of tight, constricting socks or hose; use cotton or wool socks that are proper length and size.

NIC Physical Comfort Promotion

Acute and/or chronic pain related to peripheral ischemia
- Assist the patient to identify activities that precipitate or aggravate pain *to define a baseline for activity intolerance.*
- Provide position of most comfort.
- Frequent, small position changes may be helpful during periods of restlessness brought on by pain.
- Instruct the patient on methods to relieve pain: standing or dangling at bedside *to obtain relief from ischemic pain.*
- Begin a slow, progressive exercise program.

Patient Education/Continuum of Care Plan

1. Provide information regarding the disease process and precipitating risk factors.
2. Explain the importance of daily skin care. Tell the patient to wash with mild soap, dry well, and apply lanolin-based lotions.
3. Clean small cuts or abrasions with soap and water; report cuts or skin breaks that do not begin to heal within 2 to 3 days.
4. Nails, corns, and calluses should be managed professionally. Encourage the patient to wear well-fitted, hard-soled shoes.
5. Discuss a daily progressive walking program with the patient: walk until pain increases, stop and stand still to decrease pain, then continue walking.
6. Explain the need to avoid the use of nicotine.
7. Provide weight counseling for obese patients.
8. Explain the need for a low-cholesterol, low-fat diet.
9. Instruct the patient to avoid crossing the legs and sitting or standing for long periods.

Evaluation/Patient Outcomes

Tissue Perfusion Management: Peripheral perfusion is improved. Pulses are present, equal, and bilateral. Skin color is normal; skin is warm to touch.

Skin/Wound Management: Skin integrity is maintained. Skin shows no signs of ulcerations. Skin color and temperature are normal.

Physical Comfort Promotion: Patient reports relief of pain (claudication). Comfort level is achieved. Patient verbalizes absence or control of pain. Patient demonstrates use of variety of strategies to reduce pain level.

Raynaud's Disease

Raynaud's disease is a disorder of small cutaneous arteries, most frequently involving the fingers; it is marked by episodic vasospasm.

Raynaud's disease may occur by itself or may follow other disorders. By itself it occurs more commonly in young women, is often triggered by emotional stress and cold, and involves both hands.

Pathophysiology

Raynaud's disease involves three phases. First, severe constriction of cutaneous vessels results in blanching of the fingers. The vessels then dilate, slowing blood flow. This allows hemoglobin to release more oxygen into the tissues. During this ischemic phase the fingers are first white and then cyanotic, numb, and cold. This phase is followed by a reactive hyperemic phase during which the fingers become red and the patient has throbbing pain. Because attacks are often triggered by stress and cold, the disease may be related to vasoconstriction caused by the release of catecholamines. The attacks may last a few minutes or, in severe cases, several hours.

In severe cases, progressive ischemia with trophic skin changes may lead to recurring infection and gangrene. However, Raynaud's disease is rare and is most often seen in mild form.

Diagnostic Studies and Findings

Digital plethysmography: Abnormal perfusion pressure and pulsatile contour

Peripheral arteriography: Visualization of distal arteries of hands

Multidisciplinary Plan

Surgery

Sympathectomy
Lumbar ganglionectomy for relief of symptoms involving feet
Ganglionectomy for relief of symptoms involving hands
Amputation of terminal phalanges (very rare)

Medications

Calcium channel blockers
Nifedipine Immediate Release (other agents in this group have no proven efficacy)
Usual dosage: 10-30 mg tid PO
Alpha-1–adrenergic antagonists
Prazosin (other agents in this group have no proven efficacy)
Usual dosage: 1 mg PO
Topical agents: Nitroglycerin ointment applied tid to affected digits may reduce symptoms.

General Management

Avoidance of exposure to irritants such as cold, mechanical or chemical injury, and stressful situations

NURSING CARE

Nursing Assessment

Hands and Fingers
Initially blanched and numb after exposure to cold or stress; then fingers become cyanotic; this is followed by change in color to red; trophic changes (ulcerations, chronic paronychia) may occur in long-standing disease

Assess for aggravating factors leading to vasospasm.

Potential Complications

None

Patient Problems/Nursing Diagnoses & Interventions

NIC Tissue Perfusion Management

Ineffective peripheral tissue perfusion related to vasoconstriction; acute and/or chronic pain related to ischemia

- Remove aggravating factors when possible; for example, provide warmth to fingers, encourage the patient to stop smoking.
- Assist the patient to modify stressful situations that may aggravate vasospasm.
- Instruct the patient as to the cause of the pain.
- Avoid exposure to cold, mechanical and chemical irritants, or other stressful factors.

Patient Education/Continuum of Care Plan

1. Discuss with the patient how to avoid exposure to cold temperatures and the need to wear gloves or mittens when handling cold items or in cold weather.
2. Explain to the patient the need to avoid smoking.
3. Explain the need to avoid stressful situations. Teach ways to deal with stress, such as relaxation techniques.
4. Explain the purpose, side effects, and dosage of medications.

Evaluation/Patient Outcomes

Tissue Perfusion Management: Circulation in hands and fingers is improved. There is no pain. Color is normal and skin is warm. Skin integrity is maintained.

Venous Thrombosis

Venous thrombosis is an abnormal vascular condition; a thrombus develops within a blood vessel (Fig. 3-63).

Deep venous thrombosis (DVT) is the most common venous disorder. The greatest incidence is in those having surgery (30% to 60%), with the development of pulmonary embolism estimated to be 7.3% to 54%, and deaths estimated to be 200,000 per year.[15] Patients undergoing spinal or pelvic surgery are at highest risk. Increased frequency of DVT is seen with advanced age, immobility, and malignancy. Previous DVT is a substantial risk for recurrence in hospitalized patients. The following terms are commonly used to describe venous disorders that reflect thrombus formation or inflammation:

Phlebitis: Inflammation of vein
Phlebothrombosis (venous thrombosis): Intraluminal thrombus with minimal or no inflammation; have greater tendency to embolize
Thromboembolism: Thrombus dislodgment and migration
Thrombophlebitis: Acute condition marked by thrombus and inflammation in deep or superficial veins

Pathophysiology

The triad of stasis, intimal damage, and hypercoagulability is responsible for most venous thrombosis. Venous stasis occurs in persons who are inactive for a time because of bed rest or immobilization of the lower extremities. Thrombus formation results from a reduction of flow-induced dilution and a decrease in natural circulating anticoagulants (antithrombin III, platelet factor IV, and some prostaglandins).[90] Stasis caused by reduced flow increases the contact between platelets and coagulation factors that enhance platelet aggregation.

Intimal damage may occur as a result of internal or external trauma, such as IV therapy. Endothelial damage leads to exposure of the subintimal collagen membrane, which promotes platelet adherence, and activation of intrinsic coagulation factors, which contribute to thrombus formation.

Hypercoagulability reflects an alteration in coagulability. This occurs in some patients with disorders such as polycythemias and anemias, excessive estrogen or steroid use, or malignancies.

Once formed, the thrombus begins an inflammatory process leading to fibrosis. The enlarging thrombus eventually occludes the lumen of the vein or detaches and migrates to the systemic circulation.

Frequent sites for venous thrombus formation are the soleal and gastrocnemius venous sinuses and the larger veins. Throm-

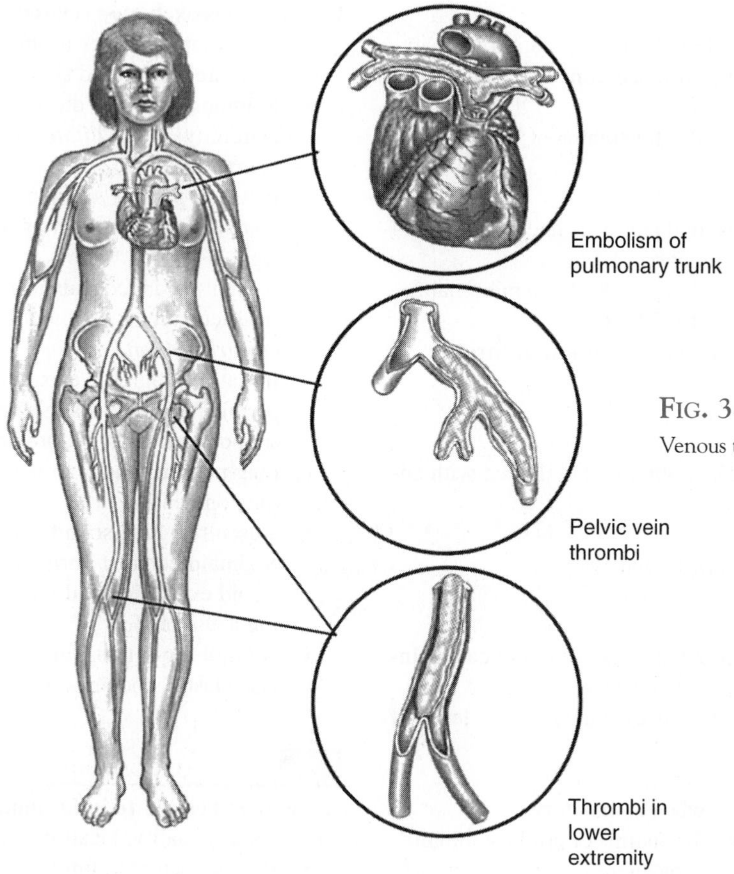

FIG. 3-63

Venous thrombosis. (From Canobbio.[15])

bosis of these veins is linked to increased risk of clotting. Thrombosis in subcutaneous veins rarely leads to pulmonary embolism.

DIAGNOSTIC STUDIES AND FINDINGS

Plethysmography: Shows decreased circulation distal to affected area

Doppler ultrasonography: Identifies reduced blood flow to specific area; shows obstruction to venous flow

Venography: Angiographically confirms diagnosis; shows filling defects

MRI: Noninvasive test with improved specificity and sensitivity for diagnosis

^{125}I fibrinogen scan: Defines location of clot and any emboli that may have dislodged

MULTIDISCIPLINARY PLAN

Surgery

Rarely indicated

Techniques used for deep vein thrombophlebitis necessitating venous interruption: ligation or clipping

Iliofemoral thrombectomy: May be considered for patients with acute iliofemoral thrombosis and compromised arterial perfusion that fail to respond to conventional therapy

Procedures to prevent distal embolization

- Extravascular vena cava interruption: Application of a partitioning clip around the vein; used prophylactically for patients who are considered at high risk for embolization and are undergoing abdominal surgery for another reason
- Intracaval filters (Mobin-Uddin umbrella, Kimray-Greenfield filter): Interrruption devices inserted into right internal jugular vein and advanced to vena cava via catheter; once in place, devices permit continuous venous flow while filtering clots, thus preventing further embolization

Medications

Prophylaxis: A significant reduction in the incidence of deep vein thrombosis can be achieved when patients at risk are given appropriate prophylaxis

Heparin sodium (unfractionated heparin)

Usual dosage: 5000 U SQ 8-12 h

Low molecular weight heparin (LMWH) (Enoxaparin)

Usual dosage: 30 mg SQ bid

Anticoagulant therapy

Heparin sodium

Indications: Initially administered IV to augment fibrinolytic activity and aid in thrombolysis

Usual dosage: 30-70 U/kg followed by infusion of 1000 U/h or 1.5 U/kg/min

LMWH: Enoxaparin: usual dosage: 1 mg/kg SQ bid

Warfarin

Indications: Given after initial anticoagulation to maintain prothrombin time to twice control level or INR 1.5-2.5; usually for 3 mon

Fibrinolytic agents: Controversial for treatment of deep vein thrombosis

Streptokinase (Streptase)

Indications: Produces total clot lysis and restores normal venous valve function

Usual dosage: IV initially 250,000 IU/30 min; maintenance 100,000 IU/h for 24-72 h

Antiplatelet agents (oral) (used in prevention of thrombus)

Aspirin (ASA)

Usual dosage: 325 mg/day

Dipyridamole (Persantine)

Usual dosage: 800 mg/day; 400 mg/day if used with anticoagulants

Ticlopidine (Ticlid)

Usual dose: 250 mg bid with food

General Management

Prophylaxis when heparin prophylaxis is contraindicated: Intermittent pneumatic compression devices

Bed rest with elevation of affected extremity above level of right atrium

Warm, moist heat

Custom-fitted elastic stockings when ambulatory

Monitoring the partial thromboplastin time or prothrombin time while patient is receiving anticoagulant therapy

NURSING CARE

Nursing Assessment

Assess circulation of affected extremity and check pulses in all extremities.

Observe for signs of pulmonary embolism: chest pain, dyspnea, tachypnea.

Lower Extremity (Deep Veins)

Calf pain and tenderness; Homans' sign (calf pain on dorsiflexion of foot); dilated superficial veins; edema of involved extremity (30% to 50% of deep vein thromboses may be clinically silent); pain and tenderness over involved vein (e.g., groin); increased size compared with unaffected side

Upper Extremity (Superficial Veins)

Redness, warmth, and tenderness over affected vein; veins visible and palpable

Potential Complications

Pulmonary embolism: Migration of the deep vein thrombosis into the pulmonary circulation; can be serious and life-threatening

Patient Problems/Nursing Diagnoses & Interventions

NIC Tissue Perfusion Management

Ineffective tissue perfusion related to interruption of venous flow

Impaired gas exchange related to embolization of thrombus

- Use Doppler sensor if pulses seem absent.
- Measure and record size of affected limb every day.
- Maintain bed rest during acute phase; elevate affected extremity *to facilitate venous circulation toward the heart.*
- Instruct patient to avoid positions that restrict venous blood flow, such as use of knee gatch or crossing legs.
- Administer anticoagulant and fibrolytic therapy as ordered.
- Instruct patient to avoid use of nicotine *to prevent further constriction and damage to intimal cells.*
- Initiate a progressive exercise program as ordered. Never permit patient to dangle legs. Instruct patient to apply support stockings before ambulating, avoid standing for long periods, and alternate position by standing on toes, then on heels.
- Auscultate lung sounds every 8 hours or as indicated.
- Maintain bed rest during acute period.
- Avoid exercising and massage of affected extremity during acute phase.
- Administer anticoagulant therapy as ordered.
- Use elastic stockings during periods of ambulation.

NIC Physical Comfort Promotion

Acute pain related to inflammatory process

- Assess quality, location, and intensity of pain.
- Provide bed rest; limit self-care activities.
- Elevate affected limb above level of right atrium.
- Do not use knee gatch.
- Administer analgesics as ordered.
- Apply warm, moist compresses as ordered.
- Measure calf or thigh or both daily and record.
- Use elastic stockings/pneumatic compression devices as ordered.

Patient Education/Continuum of Care Plan

1. Discuss with the patient and family the nature of the disorder and methods of preventing recurrence.
2. The patient must understand the need to avoid constrictive clothing and crossing legs when sitting.
3. The patient and family must understand the need for skin care.
4. Explain the value of rest periods with legs raised.
5. Explain the need to lose weight if the patient is obese.
6. Discuss with the patient the need to avoid use of nicotine and oral contraceptives.
7. Explain the need for a regular or moderate exercise program.
8. Explain anticoagulant therapy and precautions and stress need for follow-up.

Evaluation/Patient Outcomes

Tissue Perfusion Management: Tissue perfusion is improved. Swelling and redness are reduced. Patient exhibits no signs of respiratory distress. Arterial blood gases (ABGs) are within normal limits. Respirations are at baseline. Lungs are clear. Chest x-ray is normal.

Physical Comfort Promotion: Comfort level is achieved. Patient verbalizes absence or control of pain. Patient demonstrates appropriate strategies to reduce pain.

COLLABORATIVE INTERVENTIONS AND RELATED NURSING CARE

IMPLANTABLE CARDIOVERTER DEFIBRILLATOR

Description and Rationale

The automatic implantable cardioverter defibrillator (ICD) is a self-contained system capable of identifying and treating life-threatening ventricular dysrhythmias. Originally designed to correct ventricular fibrillation, ICD units now also have the ability to identify and treat ventricular tachycardia.

The ICD continuously monitors and analyzes the patient's heart rate and waveform configuration. Most ICDs also function as backup pacemakers. In rapid ventricular tachycardia and ventricular fibrillation, electrical countershock is delivered directly to the heart via a transcardiac electrode attached to the ICD generator. The generator is powered by lithium-silver vanadium oxide batteries, which last 3 to 6 years depending on the model and frequency of activation. The lead system is designed to sense, pace, and defibrillate.

ICDs are currently implanted almost exclusively using a transvenous approach. Subclavian or cephalic veins are most often used for access. The dominant lead is positioned in the RV. A second transvenous coil to complete the shock circuit can be placed in the superior vena cava, or the generator itself can be used. The generator is implanted in a subcutaneous or submuscular pocket located in the pectoral area or upper abdomen.

Patients for whom the ICD is indicated include those who have survived sudden cardiac death not associated with acute MI and whose dysrhythmias are not controlled with antidysrhythmic therapy, those who have had more than one cardiac arrest but whose dysrhythmia cannot be induced during electrophysiologic testing, and those with sustained ventricular tachycardia not controlled with conventional antidysrhythmic agents.

Cautions

Avoidance of strong magnetic fields is necessary because they can activate or deactivate the ICD device.

Preprocedural Care

Initiate preoperative instruction for the patient and family, including information about the ICD device, its benefits and risks, the implantation procedure, and postoperative care. Include discussion regarding surgical approaches that may be used and routine postoperative procedures and equipment. Most patients can return to a telemetry nursing unit and do not require intensive care postoperatively.

Ensure that written informed consent is obtained.

Obtain baseline data as ordered: ECG (baseline rhythm), vital signs, and laboratory work.

Perform skin preparation of chest and abdomen.

Permit nothing by mouth (NPO).

Acknowledge preoperative anxiety and fears of discomfort associated with shocks and possible malfunction of the device.

MULTIDISCIPLINARY PLAN

Surgery

Approach for implantation is determined by various clinical circumstances, but most ICDs are placed in a manner similar to transvenous pacemaker placements. Devices can also be placed during open heart surgery.

Medications

Antidysrhythmics are carefully selected to avoid interfering with defibrillation threshold.

General Management

Continuous ECG monitoring during and after implantation, observing for inappropriate shocks during sinus rhythm or patient's preestablished rhythm

Diet as ordered

Intravenous therapy as ordered

Activity level determined by clinical status: patients can be discharged the day after their procedure and resume ADLs

Pain management as needed

NURSING CARE

NURSING ASSESSMENT

Observe functioning of device if arrhythmia occurs
- Failure to sense and discharge
- Sudden death

ECG rhythm
- Appropriate discharge for ventricular tachycardia/ventricular fibrillation
- Transient episodes of supraventricular dysrhythmias, nonsustained ventricular tachycardia
- False-positive discharges of shocks in the presence of normal sinus rhythm; spurious shocks may be caused by fractured leads or by miscounting of the heart rate because of oversensing

Infection of the pulse generator pocket site: Redness, swelling, heat, fluid collection or drainage, skin irritation or breakdown

Learning needs: Assess level of understanding, encouraging the patient to verbalize subjective feelings and perceptions

Pain management: Assess level of discomfort

POTENTIAL COMPLICATIONS

Pneumothorax during ICD placement; cardiac tamponade; infection

PATIENT PROBLEMS/NURSING DIAGNOSES & INTERVENTIONS

NIC COPING ASSISTANCE

Fear related to anticipated shock, possible battery failure, and death
- Provide information *to correct distorted perceptions.*
- Assist the patient to identify sources of fear.
- Assist the patient to cope with fears.

- Review strategies to cope with unpredictability of the dysrhythmias and discomfort from the shocks.
- Offer a brief description of the shock, including symptoms that may accompany it.
- Review the signs and symptoms of battery failure or device malfunction and interventions to take if suspected.
- Refer to ICD support group.

Other related nursing diagnosis: Decreased cardiac output related to recurrent ventricular dysrhythmias

Patient Education/Continuum of Care Plan

1. Explain to the patient and family the purpose and basic function of the ICD device. Describe benefits and limitations.
2. Describe the ICD device, discussing the signs and symptoms of defibrillation discharge.
3. Describe the signs and symptoms of ICD malfunction, such as inappropriate shocks or loss of consciousness, and the need to notify physician if suspected.
4. Explain the need for regular follow-up magnet testing to predict the end of generator life. Describe the use of the transtelephonic system if available.
5. Explain the signs and symptoms of wound or pocket infection, and instruct the patient or family to report any fever or drainage to the physician.
6. Explain to the patient the need to protect the implantation site and to avoid constricting clothing such as belts and girdles.
7. Describe activity allowances and limitations. Explain that most former activities may be resumed. If the patient has had loss of consciousness with the arrhythmia, driving is not usually permitted until the patient has been 1 year without an event. Explain to the patient that this precaution is because of the underlying arrhythmia, not the ICD. Sexual activity can be resumed without danger to patient or partner.
8. Discuss the need to avoid strong magnetic fields that may activate or deactivate the ICD unit, such as areas around radio or television transmitting towers and use of diathermy motors. Instruct the patient not to touch spark plugs of a running motor, as on a lawn mower or car.
9. Assure the patient that normal household appliances such as microwave ovens will not interfere with the ICD unit.
10. Assure the patient that if the unit discharges during physical contact with another person, that person may feel a slight muscular contraction but will not be harmed.
11. Explain the need to carry ICD identification card and wear medical alert bracelet at all times.
12. Direct patient to ICD support group when available, if appropriate.

Evaluation/Patient Outcomes

Coping Assistance: Fear level is reduced. Patient is able to verbalize specific fears and concerns regarding ICD unit. Patient verbalizes comfort with ICD unit and asks appropriate questions regarding home maintenance hemodynamic monitoring. ICD unit functions properly with appropriate discharge response during magnet testing.

Cardiac Surgery

Cardiac surgeries include coronary artery bypass graft, valve surgeries, repair of septal defects, ventricular aneurysm resection, mapping, congenital defect repairs.

Description and Rationale

Surgical intervention for cardiac disorders may be employed as a corrective measure in congenital heart disease or as an alternative treatment modality when a patient's clinical course becomes refractory to medical management.

Cardiac surgery may be broadly classified as an open or a closed procedure. Open-heart techniques were made possible with the development of the cardiopulmonary bypass machine (extracorporeal circulation) in the early 1950s. Since that time, advances in myocardial preservation, in preoperative and postoperative support devices, and in pharmacology have contributed to improved mortality and morbidity rates and to a greater number of operative procedures for cardiac disorders.

Procedures for Acquired Disorders

Coronary artery bypass graft (CABG) surgery: Myocardial revascularization for coronary artery disease; aimed at relief of unstable angina pectoris; Figs. 3-64 and 3-65 show a saphenous vein used as a graft to the coronary artery; because of the need at times for multiple grafts or repeat CABG surgeries, arterial grafts using the internal mammary arteries, the gastric-epiploic artery, and radial arteries have been used with success

Valve surgery: Valvulotomy (commissurotomy), valvuloplasty (repair of valve), replacement with prosthetic valve, Ross procedure (pulmonary autograft implanted in aortic valve location, homograft used to replace pulmonary valve)

Resection of ventricular aneurysm: Resection of nonviable myocardium

Septal defects: Closure of atrial or ventricular septal defect by direct suturing or placement of Dacron patch across defect

Antidysrhythmia surgery: Mapped (directed endocardial resection), and aneurysmectomy

Procedures for Congenital Defects

Closure of patent ductus arteriosus

Closure of atrial or ventricular septal defect

Repair of coarctation of aorta

Repair of tetralogy of Fallot

Fontan or modified Fontan procedure for tricuspid atresia and single ventricle

Mustard procedure or arterial switch for transposition of great vessels

Rastelli (valved-conduit) repair for severe pulmonary stenosis (or pulmonary atresia) and ventricular septal defect

Contraindications

Contraindications to cardiac surgery include severe bleeding disorders and acute (recent) cerebrovascular accident (stroke).

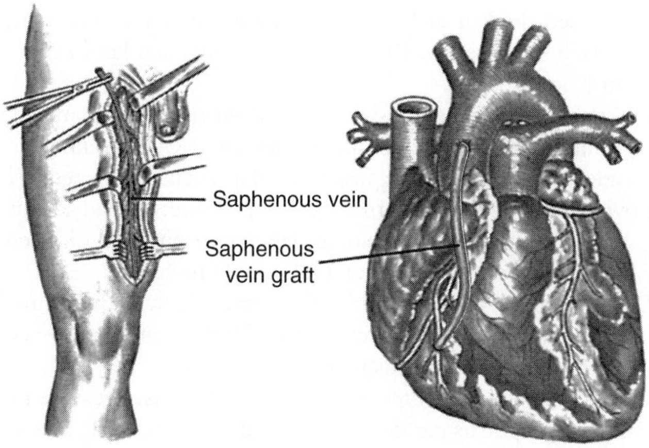

FIG. 3-64
Coronary artery bypass graft using saphenous vein. (From Thelan, Urden and Davie..[94])

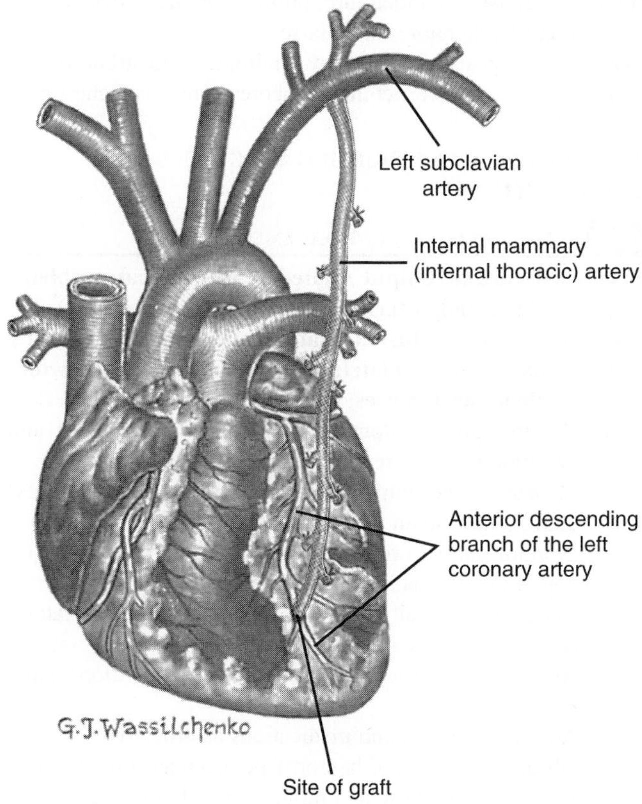

FIG. 3-65
Coronary artery bypass graft using internal mammary artery. (From Thelan, Urden and Davie.[94])

Cautions

Cardiac surgery may be performed with added risk in the presence of pulmonary hypertension, in patients with an active infectious process, in refractory ventricular failure, in the immediate peri-infarction or postinfarction period.

Preprocedural Care

Understand the type of lesion and associated risks.
Initiate preoperative instruction for the patient and family, including information about the operative procedure and postoperative care: routine procedures of the intensive care unit (suctioning, coughing, turning, monitoring of vital signs); various tubes (endotracheal, chest, gastrointestinal, urinary catheter, intravenous); equipment (respirators, monitors); pain management; level of consciousness and emotional response; and visitor policies.
Ensure that written informed consent is obtained.
Obtain baseline data: chest x-ray; ECG; laboratory work; complete blood count, blood type and crossmatch, electrolytes, serum chemistries, and urinalysis; weight; height; and vital signs.
Perform skin preparation: chest, legs for vein harvesting.
Hold or modify preoperative medications:
- Digoxin: may be discontinued 24 to 36 hours before surgery.
- Antiplatelets: Instruct patient not to take these up to 1 week before surgery.
- Anticoagulants: Discontinue warfarin; initiate heparin therapy in hospital before surgery.
- Antidysrhythmics, antihypertensives: In most cases continue until 24 to 48 hours before surgery.

Initiate pulmonary preparation by instructing the patient to stop smoking, teaching the patient methods for coughing and deep breathing, and using an incentive spirometer.
Assess preoperative anxiety, offering reassurance and support.
Assist with insertion of pulmonary artery balloon flotation catheter, if ordered, before surgery.
Administer preoperative sedation.
Permit nothing by mouth for 12 hours before procedure.

Multidisciplinary Plan

Surgery

Cardiopulmonary bypass machine (extracorporeal circulation; heart-lung machine): Assumes function of heart and lungs, providing bloodless operative field; procedure involves cannulation of great vessels, allowing drainage of unoxygenated blood that is emptied into venous reservoir; blood is then passed to oxygenator, where it is fully saturated; to reduce tissue oxygen requirements, temperature of blood circulating in extracorporeal unit is lowered; cold blood is returned to patient, reducing total body temperature and slowing metabolic processes; myocardial preservation is required while the heart is arrested and includes coronary perfusion, topical cooling (profound hypothermia), and cold cardioplegia arrest

Medications

Preoperative management: Maintenance of medical management plan to provide inotropic support, dysrhythmia management, hypertension control, and fluid and electrolyte balance
Postoperative management: Based on clinical symptoms, complications, and progress of patient
- Parenteral fluids administered based on postoperative hemodynamic parameters
  - Volume expanders (Hespan, albumin)
  - Blood replacement (packed cells, fresh frozen plasma)
- Inotropic support administered to maintain blood pressure and increase cardiac output
  - Dopamine
  - Dobutamine

Vasodilator therapy administered to improve circulation and venous return during high catecholamine surgery immediately postoperatively
Nipride
Nitroglycerin

General Management

Intraaortic balloon pump: Used when severe ventricular dysfunction occurs as patient is removed from bypass; provides circulatory support to failing myocardium
Hemodynamic monitoring: Arterial, left atrial, pulmonary artery, and pulmonary capillary wedge pressures; cardiac output, cardiac index, and systemic vascular resistance measurements may be required
Ventricular assist devices: For severe ventricular dysfunction or inability to wean patient from cardiopulmonary bypass support
ECG monitoring: Continuous evaluation of heart rate, rhythm
Pacemakers: Temporary epicardial wires for backup if intrinsic pacemakers fail
Immediate postoperative measures
Assisted mechanical ventilation
Suctioning
Chest tubes
Diet therapy: Sodium and fluid restrictions on basis of patient's clinical status
Pulmonary toilet: Encourage coughing, deep breathing, and use of incentive spirometry
Physical therapy: Exercises and early ambulation

NURSING CARE

Nursing Assessment

Level of Consciousness

Early: Arousable
Late: Alert and oriented
Pupils: May be small, but reactive to light
Sensory-motor function: As patient awakens, moves all extremities; shivering may occur during rewarming

Respiratory Function

Early
Atelectasis; diminished breath sounds at base
Monitor respirations, observing rate and quality as the patient is weaned from the respirator
Late: Clear with full aeration; arterial blood gases normal

Cardiovascular System

Monitor pulmonary artery pressure, PCWP, mixed venous oxygen saturation (SVo_2), and arterial pressures every 15 minutes during the immediate postoperative period, decreasing frequency as the clinical status stabilizes.
Monitor vital signs every 1 to 2 hours in immediate postoperative period.

Potential Complications

Pleural effusions: Diminished breath sounds at the bases, low-grade fever, shallow respiration; positive E to A egophony
Atelectasis
Monitor respirations, lung sounds, skin color, use of accessory muscles, and arterial blood gases to determine lung expansion and detect diminished sounds that may be due to increased fluid or atelectasis; auscultate chest for diminished breath sounds, initially every 1 to 2 hours and later every 4 to 6 hours.
Fluid shifts: Monitor for signs of fluid volume excess; monitor filling pressures: right atrial pressure (RAP), pulmonary artery diastolic pressure, inspect for dependent edema and JVD
Low cardiac output: Narrow pulse pressure; thready, rapid pulse; decreased urine output; labored respiration; disorientation; increased PCWP and left atrial pressure
Dysrhythmias: Atrial fibrillation and flutter; junctional rhythms; heart block; ventricular rhythms: premature ventricular contractions, tachycardia, fibrillation
Cardiac tamponade: Hypotension; narrowed pulse pressure (10 mm Hg); pulsus paradoxus; widened mediastinal shadow on chest x-ray; increased venous pressure
Bleeding: Profuse chest tube drainage at least 250 ml/h; hypotension; disorientation; prolonged prothrombin time and partial thromboplastin time; decreased platelet levels
Infection: Elevated temperature; purulent drainage from suture sites; chills; diaphoresis; malaise
Pericarditis or postpericardiotomy syndrome: Pericardial friction rub; low-grade fever; chills; diaphoresis; malaise; chest pain

Patient Problems/Nursing Diagnoses & Interventions

NIC Tissue Perfusion Management

Decreased cardiac output related to mechanical problems (altered preload, afterload, contractility, heart rate)
Ineffective tissue perfusion related to hemorrhage resulting from disruption in platelet function and clotting factors or surgical anastomoses

- Obtain cardiac output and calculate cardiac index and systemic vascular resistance as indicated.
- Measure urine output every hour; report output of less than 30 ml/h in an adult patient.
- Monitor and record ECG ratio and rhythm every 4 to 6 hours; initiate pacing as indicated.
- Check peripheral perfusion: pulses, skin temperature, color.
- Auscultate chest for heart sounds *to detect gallops, murmurs, or rubs.*
- Administer fluids and medications as ordered.
- Observe for signs of hemorrhage: decreased blood pressure, disorientation, and falling hemoglobin level.
- Measure chest tube drainage every 30 to 60 minutes.
- Report output in excess of 150 ml/h for an adult or 5 ml/kg/h for a child.
- Check hemoglobin, hematocrit, and clotting studies on the patient's arrival in the intensive care unit and every 2 to 4 hours as ordered.
- Administer drugs as ordered.
- Administer blood and blood products as ordered.

NIC Respiratory Management

Ineffective breathing pattern related to decreased lung expansion, incision pain, or anxiety

- Reposition the patient from one side to the other during the immediate postoperative period t*o encourage lung expansion.*

- Assist and encourage the patient to cough and deep breathe, and use incentive spirometry.
- Administer pain medications before coughing procedure; individualize pain management as needed, such as patient-controlled analgesia or epidural anesthesia.
- Obtain serial chest x-rays *to check for progressive or resolving atelectasis and pleural effusions.*

NIC **Electrolyte and Acid-Base Management**

Excess fluid volume related to postoperative expanded extracellular fluid volume and to postoperative sodium and water retention

- During rewarming, check right atrial pressure, left atrial pressure, and pulmonary artery pressure every 5 minutes until stable, then every 30 to 60 minutes.
- Titrate parenteral fluids according to hemodynamic parameters per protocol.
- Measure output every hour. Check specific gravity as ordered.
- Limit fluid intake as ordered.
- Monitor electrolyte, hemoglobin, and hematocrit values.
- Weigh daily as indicated by clinical picture.

NIC **Physical Comfort Promotion**

Acute pain related to surgical incisions and operative and postoperative procedures

- Provide pain medications as prescribed *to keep patient comfortable.*
- Encourage early activity and ambulation.
- Teach splinting *to decrease pain when coughing.*

NIC **Coping Assistance**

Anxiety related to actual or perceived threat to biologic integrity

Preoperative

- Provide adequate instruction, answering questions and offering reassurance.
- Explain the method of communication to be used after the operation while the patient is intubated.

Postoperative

- Implement measures that will reduce level of anxiety.
- Orient the patient to time, situation, and location.
- Inform the patient that the surgery is over.
- Assist with communication.
- Anticipate needs if possible.
- Provide pain management as necessary.
- Allow family support and participation.
- Provide reassurance of daily progress.
- Encourage verbalization of fears and questions regarding the operation, recovery, and discharge.
- Begin postoperative instruction.

NIC **Patient Education**

Deficient knowledge related to lack of information

- Identify any barriers to learning.
- Inform patient and family of what to expect before, during, and after surgery.
- Provide patient with trajectory of care up to and including discharge.
- Present information early and often using written and audiovisual techniques.

Patient Education/Continuum of Care Plan

General

1. Review the surgical procedure, emphasizing any precautions or complications that may be associated with it.
2. Clarify what action(s) should be taken if symptoms of infection, bleeding, heart failure, or dysrhythmias develop.
3. Review diet and fluid restrictions.
4. Review discharge medication, including purpose, dosages, side effects, and need for specific follow-up laboratory studies as indicated.
5. Discuss activity allowances or limitations. Refer patient to cardiac rehabilitation for progressive ambulation.
6. Discuss the importance of avoiding fatigue and resting.
7. Discuss care of incisions and symptoms of wound infection to report to the physician.

After valve replacement

1. Discuss the importance of anticoagulation therapy.
2. Discuss the importance of reporting signs of endocarditis (p. 97).
3. Discuss the importance of prophylactic antibiotic therapy before procedures that predispose to bacteremia (p. 88).
4. Provide medical alert card for artificial valve or anticoagulation therapy.

Evaluation/Patient Outcomes

Tissue Perfusion Management: Hemodynamic and electromechanical stability is achieved; cardiac output is adequate. Blood pressure, pulmonary artery pressure, and cardiac output are within acceptable range. There is no dysrhythmia. ECG findings are within acceptable limits. Hematologic hemostasis is achieved. Hematocrit and hemoglobin level are within normal limits. A progressive decline in chest drainage occurs.

Respiratory Management: Oxygenation, ventilation, and lung perfusion are adequate. PaO_2 and PCO_2 are within normal limits. There is no dyspnea or tachypnea. Lungs are clear on auscultation and radiography.

Electrolyte and Acid-Base Management: Intake and output are balanced. Weight is wtihin normal limits.

Physical Comfort Promotion: Patient is comfortable. Pain does not interfere with ambulation or activities.

Coping Assistance: Anxiety is reduced, absent, or decreased. Patient demonstrates appropriate behavior patterns: asks questions and participates in self-care.

Patient Education: Patient has knowledge and understanding of primary cardiac disorder, surgical procedure performed, and discharge instructions. Patient is able to describe specific action to take regarding diet, medications, and care of incisions(s). Patient is able to describe activity allowances and limitations.

Cardiac Transplantation

Description and Rationale

Cardiac transplantation has evolved rapidly during the past 20 years, yet it was first performed in 1905 when Carrel and Guthrie transplanted the heart of one dog to another. However, it was not until 1967, when Christian Barnard performed the first human cardiac transplantation, that serious interest was stimulated. Because early survival rates were poor, transplantations continued to be performed on a limited basis. Since the introduction of the immunosuppressant agent cyclosporine in 1980, the number of centers performing heart transplantations has grown steadily.

From 1982 to 1995 there were 34,326 heart transplants performed worldwide in 271 centers.[48] The primary indication for cardiac transplantation is end-stage heart disease that is refractory to medical and surgical interventions. Survival rates are reported to be 80% at 1 year, 70% at 3 years, and 40% at 10 years.[48] Infection and organ rejection continue to be the most common medical complications and the primary causes of death in long-term follow-up. However, as survival time increases, other medical problems are being identified, and these have contributed to the increased morbidity and mortality of patients over time.

Infection remains a major cause of morbidity and mortality for long-term, immunosuppressed transplant recipients, although the incidence and severity of infections decrease after the first year. Bacteria and viruses account for more than 80% of infections after transplantation. The most common bacterial infections early after transplantation are nosocomial, due to infected intravascular lines/catheters or gram-negative pneumonias. The most common site of infection is the lung, accounting for up to one third of all infections. Other sites include the urinary tract, mediastinum, and retina.

Infection/Rejection

Bacterial infections *(Escherichia coli, Pseudomonas)* make up 66% of all infections in the transplant recipient; 17% are viruses (cytomegalovirus, herpes simplex, herpes zoster); 12% are fungal *(Candida, Aspergillus, Cryptococcus);* and 5% are protozoal.[102]

Rejection of the transplanted heart remains the primary lifelong threat to the recipient. Cardiac rejection can occur as an acute episode or a chronic condition. The risk of acute rejection is highest in the first days and weeks after transplantation while the immunosuppressant therapy is being adjusted. Although rejection rates decrease with each year of survival, the recipient is always at risk if therapy is interrupted or stopped. Immunosuppression is the only safeguard against acute rejection.

Graft atherosclerosis, or chronic rejection, has been reported to occur in approximately 35% to 40% of patients who survive 5 years after transplantation. The incidence among patients who had coronary artery disease before receiving the transplant is similar to that among patients with pretransplant cardiomyopathy. Furthermore, because the donor heart has been denervated, patients who develop diffuse occlusive coronary artery disease do not present clinically with angina pectoris. Thus, if not monitored carefully, they can die suddenly or develop ventricular failure.

Malignancies, particularly lymphomas of the histiocyte type, have been reported.[89] Their occurrence is thought to be associated with immunosuppression therapy, particularly including antithymocyte globulin in addition to cyclosporine. Other reported malignancies include epithelial tumors of the skin and leukemia.

Other late complications associated with lifelong immunosuppression in long-term survivors include osteoporosis (18.2%), spinal disorders (8.8%), and visual problems (14.3%).[25,34]

The quality of life after cardiac transplantation has also been evaluated. It is currently estimated that between 32% and 50% of heart transplant recipients return to work, although nearly 60% report that they are able to do so.[34] Lough and associates[66] reported that an average of 3.7 years after surgery 89% of heart recipients perceived their quality of life as good to excellent, and 82% reported satisfaction with life as good to very satisfactory. Factors associated with negative life change were reported to be financial status, physical appearance, and sexual function. All recipients were bothered by the side effects associated with immunosuppression therapy, but these were found to have little effect on their evaluation of quality of life and life satisfaction.

With respect to immunosuppression, increased understanding of immune suppression and the introduction of various immunosuppressive agents have made organ transplantation a viable treatment modality. Since the late 1960s a variety of nonselective immunosuppressive agents had been used in transplantations, but these were associated with impairment of the immune system, leaving the host vulnerable to any number of infections. With the introduction of cyclosporine, morbidity and mortality figures have been significantly reduced.

The primary goal of immunosuppressive therapy is to prevent rejection of the foreign graft (heart), yet retain the host's natural immune system, which protects against infections.

The immune system is a complex response mechanism. Its purpose is to destroy any tissue invasion or foreign material to maintain hemostasis. There are two primary types of immune response: humoral and cell-mediated. Both are derived from lymphocytes.

Multidisciplinary Plan

Surgery

Heart transplantation procedures:

Orthotopic: Recipient's heart is excised, leaving the posterior walls of the atria, and is replaced with donor heart

Heterotopic "piggyback": Donor heart is placed in right chest adjacent to the recipient's heart; anastomosis of the two hearts permits blood to pass through one or both hearts

Medications

Various immunosuppressant agents are available. Maintenance immunosuppression protocols for cardiac transplant patients vary but can include the following:

Cyclosporine (Sandimmune): Naturally occurring polypeptide antibiotic produced by fungi; inhibits T cell lymphocyte proliferation and activity, which is responsible for tissue graft rejection

Azathioprine (Imuran): Antimetabolite that produces immunosuppression by inhibiting purine and DNA synthesis

Antithymocyte globulin (ATG): Reduces T lymphocytes; used to prevent rejection, or as an adjunct to immunosuppression therapy during rejection episodes

Orthoclone (OKT3): Monoclonal antibody similar to antithyroglobulin (ATG); reduces T cell function; used to prevent graft rejection

Corticosteroids: Antiinflammatory agents used to suppress both T and B lymphocyte function and to reverse capillary permeability, vasodilation, and edema; may be used as part of maintenance program to prevent rejection or as adjunct therapy when there is evidence of rejection

- Prednisone (Meticorten, Deltasone): Used as maintenance therapy
- Methylprednisolone (Medrol, Depo-Medrol, Solu-Medrol): Used when there is evidence of rejection
- Pravastatin (HMG-CoA reduction inhibitor): Used to treat hypercholesterolemia to minimize graft atherosclerosis; found to have immunosuppressant qualities[61]

General Management

ECG changes: Reflect lack of autonomic innervation of heart that occurs as a result of denervation when donor heart is removed

- Heart rate: Resting heart rate generally higher (90-100 beats per minute); response to metabolic demands such as fever or exercise in a denervated patient is one in which heart rate changes gradually; as a result of these changes, response to drugs whose effect on the heart is mediated by autonomic nervous system is also altered
- Rhythm: Normal sinus but without respiratory variation
- P wave: Transplant procedure generally involves retaining posterior portion of recipient's atria, which includes SA node; therefore second P wave is visible

Endomyocardial biopsy: After first year, endomyocardial biopsies are performed on an interval basis, depending on recipient's clinical status

Diet: Low saturated fat and cholesterol; moderate decrease in sodium intake

Laboratory studies: Regular monitoring to detect adverse reactions to immunosuppressive therapy: complete blood count (CBC), serum BUN and creatinine, liver function tests (SGOT, SGPT, LDH), glucose, urinalysis

Serum cholesterol: Triglycerides; high-density, low-density lipoproteins (HDL, LDL); magnesium; potassium

Lymphocyte count; T cell studies—while receiving ATG or OKT_3

Cyclosporine levels

NURSING CARE

Nursing Assessment

Acute rejection

- Mild or early rejection: Generally no symptoms associated; to detect early rejection, diagnosis is done with endocardial muscle biopsy

Severe rejection

- Weakness, fatigue, malaise
- Anorexia
- Nausea, vomiting
- Decreased urine output
- Weight gain
- Peripheral edema
- Distended neck veins
- Increased jugular venous pulsations and decreased perfusion: Cool pale skin, diminished pulses, diaphoresis, confusion, restlessness
- Pulmonary venous congestion: Dyspnea on exertion, cough, tachypnea
- Development of S3 and S4

ECG: Using conventional immunosuppression; 20% decrease in QRS voltage; right axis shift; atrial dysrhythmias (e.g., PAC, atrial fibrillation, atrial flutter [with cyclosporine these ECG changes may not be seen])

Chest x-ray: Increased cardiothoracic ratio (cardiomegaly)

Echocardiogram: Thickening of left ventricle; decreased left ventricular function; decreased contractility

Endomyocardial biopsy (EMB): Changes in lymphocytes; finding varies according to degree of rejection

- Mild—Occasional white blood cells
- Severe—Extensive perivascular infiltration of lymphocytes, interstitial edema, and myocyte necrosis
- Increased CPK-MB, SGOT, LDH

Infection: Usual signs and symptoms of infection often absent in immunosuppressed patient

- Fever—Low grade; baseline temperature may be lower than before transplant, so elevation to 37.2° C (99° F) may be significant
- Malaise

Compliance: Assess and evaluate patient for understanding and cognitive appraisal of prescribed lifelong therapy

Potential Complications

Rejection and infection as identified above; hypertension; hyperlipidemia; osteoporosis; malignancy; biliary disease

Patient Problems/Nursing Diagnoses & Interventions

NIC Risk Management

Risk for injury: rejection, related to noncompliance with prescribed medical regimen

Risk for infection related to immunosuppressive drug therapy

- Encourage discussion regarding changes in lifestyle that have been positive or negative.
- Anticipate and allow questions regarding prescribed therapy.
- Take temperature every 4 hours.
- Obtain cultures as indicated: sputum, throat, urine, any suspicious drainage sites in wounds.
- Obtain and assess complete blood count and chest x-ray as indicated. NOTE: Laboratory values may be altered because of steroids.
- Minimize or avoid use of invasive procedures that increase risk of infection: IV, indwelling catheters.

- Change IV tubings, bags, and dressings daily using aseptic technique.
- Avoid placing patient in room with other patient who is at risk for infection *to avoid potential cross-contamination;* initiate reverse isolation for staff and family.
- Minimize number of visitors.
- Restrict visitors who show signs of infections, such as colds, herpes simplex.
- Administer antibiotic therapy as ordered.

NIC TISSUE PERFUSION MANAGEMENT

Decreased cardiac output related to severe rejection

- Auscultate heart sounds, assessing for presence of S_3 and S_4.
- Auscultate chest for lung sounds, assessing for signs of increased pulmonary congestion.
- Weigh daily.
- Prepare patient for endomyocardial biopsy.
- Administer immunosuppressive therapy as ordered.

Other related nursing diagnosis: Ineffective coping related to threat of disease process and inadequate coping resources

PATIENT EDUCATION/CONTINUUM OF CARE PLAN

1. Discuss and review signs and symptoms of rejection. Emphasize the importance of keeping scheduled endomyocardial biopsy appointments because there are usually no signs of early rejection and appearance of symptoms is associated with moderate to severe rejection.
2. Discuss and review the need to take medications lifelong and the need to take them exactly as prescribed. Caution the patient never to stop taking medication. Review medications, checking dosage, method of administration, and side effects.
3. Discuss signs and symptoms of infection to report: elevation of baseline temperature; early signs of sore throat, cold, or flu; and cuts and lesions that do not heal.
4. Discuss the need to reduce the risk of infection by avoiding individuals with infections or contagious diseases, avoiding large crowds, and wearing a face mask when traveling in crowded areas.
5. Discuss the importance of lifelong follow-up: clinic visits, endomyocardical biopsy appointments, and periodic stress tests, radionuclide studies, and cardiac catheterization.
6. Discuss activities, allowances, and limitations. Tell the patient to check with the physician before engaging in strenuous or competitive activities or sports.

EVALUATION/PATIENT OUTCOMES

Risk Management: There is no infection. The patient maintains baseline temperature. There is no sign of infection: Complete blood count, urinalysis, and cultures are within normal limits. Patient complies with therapeutic regimen. Serum drug levels are maintained. Patient keeps follow-up appointments and offers questions and concerns appropriately.

Tissue Perfusion Management: There are no signs of rejection on biopsy. There are no new changes in endomyocardial biopsy results. There are no clinical signs of rejection.

HEMODYNAMIC MONITORING

Description and Rationale

Monitoring to assess a patient's circulatory status may be done by indirect (noninvasive) or direct (invasive) methods. Indirect methods include arterial pressure monitoring by sphygmomanometer and stethoscope, heart rate monitoring by chest electrode replacement, and cardiac monitoring. Direct methods are indicated by the term *hemodynamic monitoring.*

Hemodynamic monitoring is a technique that permits close examination of cardiac function in acutely ill patients. Used primarily in critical care units, hemodynamic monitoring permits rapid identification of complications of MI, guides the diagnosis and management of patients with low cardiac output, and helps to differentiate pulmonary disease from left ventricular failure.[44]

With use of a balloon-tipped, flow-directed catheter to provide continuous monitoring of the pulmonary artery pressure and PCWP, myocardial function can be evaluated in terms of preload, afterload, and contractility. From these parameters, the LVEDP can be estimated. Other possible measurements include cardiac output and venous oxygen saturation. Hemodynamic monitoring also provides a direct means of assessing the patient's progress and response to fluid and drug management and permits careful titration of specific therapies.

Pulmonary Artery Pressure and Pulmonary Capillary Wedge Pressure. Although the LVEDP is the major determinant of left ventricular function, it cannot be measured at the bedside. However, the LVEDP can be reflected by the pressure in the pulmonary capillaries and by the pulmonary artery pressure at the end of diastole. The catheter, which is introduced percutaneously or by cutdown, is passed through the right side of the heart into the pulmonary artery (FIG. 3-66). There the balloon is inflated, occluding the artery. With the balloon inflated, the catheter is wedged in a distal branch of the capillaries (FIG. 3-67). The pressure recorded reflects left atrial pressure, which corresponds to the LVEDP and is called the pulmonary capillary wedge pressure (PCWP).

Intraarterial Pressure (Arterial Line). Direct continuous monitoring of systemic arterial pressure is made possible by placement of an indwelling catheter, connected to a transducer and monitor, into a major artery. Central artery pressures, although more accurate, are used less frequently. The radial artery is the most common site for placement. The line also facilitates obtaining blood samples to measure arterial blood gases.

Cardiac Output. The cardiac output, the volume of blood the heart pumps per minute, can be measured using a cal-

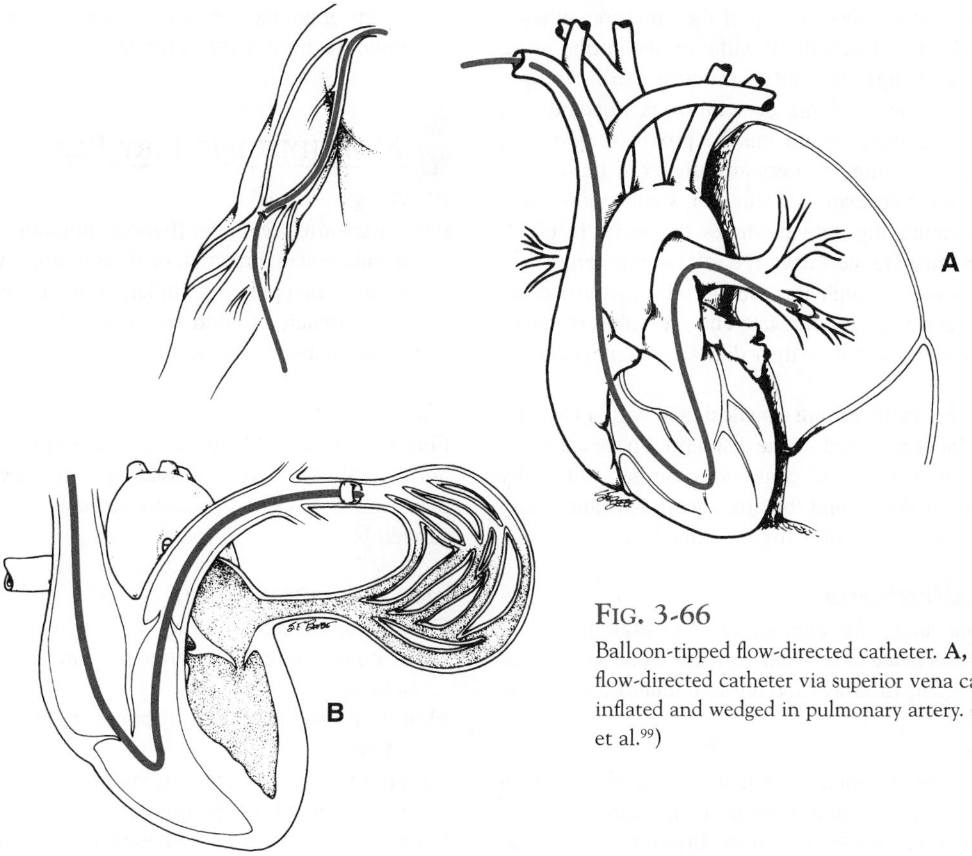

FIG. 3-66
Balloon-tipped flow-directed catheter. **A,** Placement of flow-directed catheter via superior vena cava. **B,** Balloon inflated and wedged in pulmonary artery. (From Tucker et al.[99])

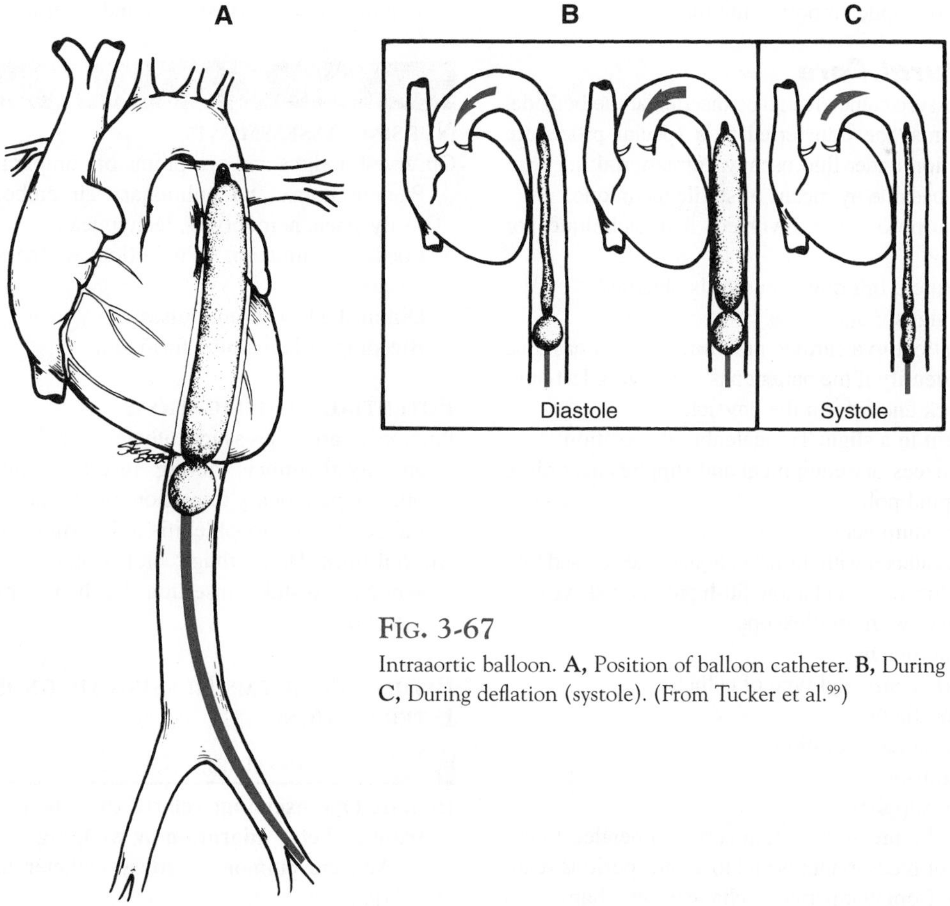

FIG. 3-67
Intraaortic balloon. **A,** Position of balloon catheter. **B,** During inflation (diastole). **C,** During deflation (systole). (From Tucker et al.[99])

ibrated thermistor located near the tip of the pressure catheter. Based on the Fick principle, a thermodilution technique using blood temperature changes is used to produce cardiac output determinations. A known volume of solution is injected at a specific rate into the right atrium via the proximal port of a three- or four-lumen pulmonary pressure catheter. Although the original practice was to use an iced solution, studies now show that room temperature injectate produces the same results.[85] The temperature-sensitive thermister records the temperature of the blood as it passes through the catheter. The difference in temperature between the iced injectate and the blood is calculated, and the cardiac output is then digitally displayed by a special computer.

Pulmonary artery catheters are also designed with a Doppler ultrasound transducer mounted on the distal tip. These catheters can measure instantaneous and continuous cardiac output by measuring average velocity and the cross-sectional pulmonary artery area. The cardiac output is digitally displayed.

Contraindications

Use of the radial artery for monitoring is contraindicated in the presence of inadequate circulation. Relative contraindications include severe bleeding disorders and severe immunosuppression.

Cautions

Patients with left bundle branch block should be observed for the development of right bundle branch block during insertion and while the flotation catheter is in place. Insertion of the flotation catheter in a patient with right-sided endocarditis may cause dislodgment of septic emboli to the lung.

Preprocedural Care

1. Pulmonary pressure catheters can be inserted at the bedside, or the patient may be transferred to a special procedure room for insertion under fluoroscopy. Intraarterial lines are inserted at the bedside by means of sterile technique.
2. Explain the purpose, risks involved, and techniques of insertion.
3. Ensure that written, informed consent is obtained.
4. Measure vital signs.
5. Connect the patient to a cardiac monitor; obtain a baseline rhythm strip. Identify if the patient has underlying left bundle branch block and inform the physician.
6. Place the patient in a slight Trendelenburg's position.
7. Assemble the necessary equipment and supplies according to routine hospital policies:
   - Monitoring equipment
     - Pressure catheter with flush solution, related closed tubing, stopcocks, and a low-flush pressurized system
     - Transducer with oscilloscope
   - Insertion equipment
     - Appropriate size and type of catheter
     - Local anesthetic
     - Skin preparation solution
     - Sterile gloves
     - Dressing supplies
8. Calibration of the pressure system is recommended to ensure accuracy of measurements and to avoid spurious readings resulting from temperature changes, or changes in transducer level. Calibrate the pressure monitor according to the manufacturer's directions; for PAP readings, calibrate the transducer to the level of the right atrium.

MULTIDISCIPLINARY PLAN

Surgery

Pulmonary artery catheter (balloon flotation): Inserted via jugular, subclavian, brachial, or right femoral vein by cutdown or percutaneous puncture under local anesthesia

Arterial catheter: Inserted via radial, brachial, or femoral artery by percutaneous method

Medications

Flushing system: Continuous microdrip of solution (usually normal saline), kept in closed system under pressure greater than patient's systolic pressure (usually 300 mm Hg) by pressurized bag

General Management

Continuous ECG monitoring

Chest x-ray immediately after placement of pulmonary artery catheter

Monitoring and recording of pressures every 1 to 2 hours or as ordered

Calibration of transducer and monitoring every 12 to 24 hours or as specified by manufacturer

Maintaining patency of catheters with continuous pressurized flushing device

Maintaining sterility of system and insertion sites

NURSING CARE

NURSING ASSESSMENT

Observe for signs and symptoms of complications:

- Pneumothorax and pulmonary air embolism: Chest pain, dyspnea, hemoptysis, tachypnea
- Local inflammation or infection: Redness, swelling, drainage, fever
- Diminished or absent pulses
- Bleeding or hematoma formation

POTENTIAL COMPLICATIONS

Pulmonary artery pressure catheters (Table 3-6): Pneumothorax and dysrhythmias during insertion; pulmonary air embolism; pulmonary infarction; pulmonary artery perforation; infection; thrombophlebitis at insertion site

Arterial lines: Hemorrhage; clot formation; diminished or absent pulse distal to insertion site; hematoma at insertion site; infection

PATIENT PROBLEMS/NURSING DIAGNOSES & INTERVENTIONS

NIC TISSUE PERFUSION MANAGEMENT

Impaired gas exchange related to embolization of thrombus from catheter migration or wedging

- Manage pulmonary artery catheter *to prevent balloon rupture:*
  - Inflate balloon for 3 seconds only.

Table 3-6 Problems Observed in Pressure Waveforms

Observation	Etiologic Factors	Interventions
Loss of waveform on oscilloscope	Displacement of catheter	Reposition patient: notify physician
Loss of PAP; PCWP is displayed on monitor	Self-wedging	Instruct patient to cough Obtain x-ray examination
Loss of PWP	Displaced into PAP; balloon rupture	Use diastolic of PAP
Decreased amplitude of waveform (damped waveform)	Damping due to: Clot in catheter tip Air bubbles Kinking of catheter Occluded catheter Tip against artery wall	Flush lines; *do not force if resistance is met* Check all connections for air leaks: flush air bubbles Notify physician Reposition patient; have patient cough
Loss of PCWP; no resistance with inflation	Rupture of balloon	Seal off balloon lumen; *do not allow any injection of air*
Air bubbles in pressure lines Damping of waveform Inaccurate reading	Air leak in system	Check that all connections are secure
Artifacts and inadequate pressure readings	Respiratory interference from handling of pressure equipment during readings	Record pressure at end exhalation using printed waveform
	Inaccurate calibration of equipment	Check for possible interference with tubing during readings
	Faulty equipment	Check electrical system for grounding Check calibration of and level to RA of transducer Check all equipment for proper functioning

From Tucker et al.[99]

Ensure balloon is deflated after wedge pressure measurement (passive air expulsion).

Observe waveform for signs of self-wedge or damped tracing.

Secure and label catheter and injection ports *to avoid confusion of lines.*

Monitor oxygen saturation as ordered *to identify fall in arterial* $Pa{O_2}$.

Administer oxygen therapy as ordered.

Check patency of lines, tubes, and connections.

Never use force to flush or irrigate a line that is resistant.

NIC RISK MANAGEMENT

Risk for infection related to contamination

- Take measures to prevent infection:
  - Maintain sterile technique during insertion.
  - Change flushing solution every day, IV tubing and transducer every 72 hours.
  - Clean site with antiseptic solution and change occlusive dressing every 72 hours (or when occlusive seal is interrupted).

NIC COPING ASSISTANCE

Anxiety related to perceived threat or change in health status

- Provide continuous explanation of procedure.
- Offer frequent reassurance, encouraging verbalization and questions regarding progress.
- Allow family and significant others to visit

NORMAL RANGES OF HEMODYNAMIC PARAMETERS

Right atrial pressure	2-6 mm Hg (mean pressure)
Right ventricular pressure	Systolic: 20-30 mm Hg Diastolic: 0-5 mm Hg End-diastolic: 2-6 mm Hg
Pulmonary artery pressure (PAP)	Systolic: 20-30 mm Hg End-diastolic: 8-12 mm Hg Mean: 10-20 mm Hg
Pulmonary arterial wedge pressure (PAWP)	4-12 mm Hg (mean pressure)
Arterial pressure (intraarterial)	Peak systolic: 100-140 mm Hg End-diastolic: 60-80 mm Hg Mean: 70-90 mm Hg
Cardiac output (CO)	4-8 L/min
Cardiac index (CO/body surface area)	2.5-4 L/min
Systemic vascular resistance (SVR)	800-1200 dynes/sec/cm^{-5} or 10-25 Wood units
Pulmonary vascular resistance (PVR)	20-120 dynes/sec/cm^{-5} or 0.25-1.5 Wood units

PATIENT EDUCATION/CONTINUUM OF CARE PLAN

1. Explain to the patient and family the purpose of the procedure, as cited in preprocedural care.
2. Explain to the patient not to move the insertion area.

Evaluation/Patient Outcomes

Tissue Perfusion Management: Lung aeration and perfusion are normal. Chest x-ray is normal. Pressure lines are patent. Waveform is normal.

Risk Management: There is no infection. Patient is afebrile.

Coping Assistance: Anxiety is reduced. Patient verbalizes absence of anxiety or decrease in anxiety level.

Intraaortic Balloon Pumping

Description and Rationale

An intraaortic balloon pump (IABP) is a mechanical device that provides circulatory assistance to the failing myocardium. Using the principles of counterpulsation, the balloon inflates with diastole and deflates during systole.

A tightly wrapped sausage-shaped balloon incorporated into a 9 Fr catheter is inserted through the common femoral artery and passed upward into the aorta. It lies in the descending aorta just distal to the left subclavian artery (see Fig. 3-67). Externally the catheter is connected to a power console that has ECG input. Helium gas is used to inflate the balloon.

The IABP is used in the treatment of cardiogenic shock in low–cardiac output states, after cardiopulmonary bypass, in drug-resistant dysrhythmias caused by ischemia, and in unstable angina. The effect of counterpulsation on left ventricular function is produced by diastolic augmentation and afterload reduction.

The first phase of balloon pumping (Fig. 3-68), with diastolic augmentations, occurs when the balloon inflates during diastole. This displaces the blood remaining in the aorta after ventricular ejection back into the aortic root. The increased blood in the aortic root results in an elevation of diastolic pressure, increasing coronary blood flow and perfusion.

Afterload reduction, the second phase of balloon pumping, occurs when the balloon deflates during systole. With balloon deflation, blood flow is encouraged forward out of the left ventricle. This produces decreased myocardial wall tension during diastole (decreased resistance), decreased myocardial oxygen consumption, and improved left ventricular output.

Contraindications

Contraindications to IABP include severe aortic regurgitation, aortic dissection, abdominal aortic aneurysm, and terminal illness.

Cautions

The cannulated extremity should not be flexed or bent.

Preprocedural Care

1. Explain procedure, insertion technique, equipment to be used, and sensations that may be felt.
2. Ensure that written informed consent from the patient or family is obtained.
3. Prepare the patient:
   a. Assess and record peripheral circulation, checking pulses and noting color and warmth of extremities; vital signs, including heart and breath sounds; hemodynamic status (arterial pressure, pulmonary artery pressure, PCWP, cardiac output); and level of awareness (mentation).

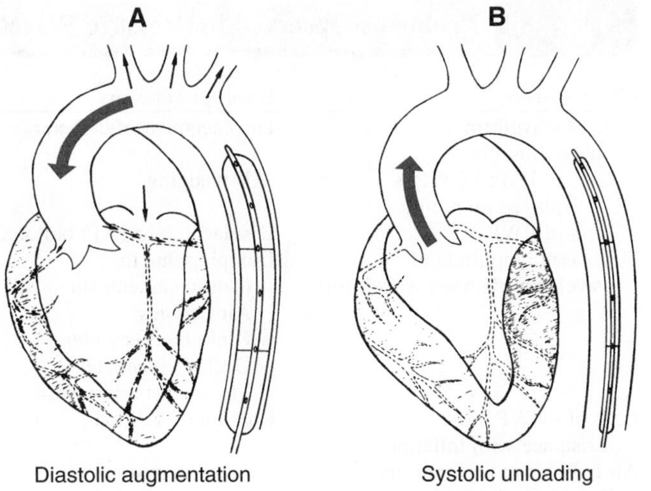

Fig. 3-68

Two phases of balloon pumping. **A,** Balloon inflation occurs from closure of aortic valve to end of diastole. Inflation causes retrograde flow of blood in aorta, increasing coronary perfusion pressure without increasing myocardial work on oxygen demand. Inflation also causes antegrade flow, increasing mean arterial pressure, renal flow, and cerebral flow. **B,** Balloon deflation occurs from just before opening of aortic valve to closure of aortic valve. Deflation encourages antegrade flow, decreasing afterload or resistance to left ventricular ejection. Deflation also decreases oxygen required by left ventricle, shortens systolic ejection, and increases stroke volume. (Copyright Cydney R. Michaelson, Los Angeles. From Michaelson CR, editor: *Congestive heart failure*, St. Louis, 1983, Mosby).

   b. Obtain baseline laboratory data (clotting studies, hemoglobin, hematocrit, white blood cell count, and platelets).
   c. Obtain baseline ECG rate and rhythm.
   d. Prepare groin area.

Multidisciplinary Plan

Medications

Local anesthetic agents: Lidocaine (Xylocaine)

General Management

Continuous monitoring during and after insertion, including ECG, arterial pressure, pulmonary artery pressure, cardiac output
Diet as ordered
Intravenous therapy as ordered
Oxygen therapy as indicated
Bed rest; turning every 2 hours with assistance

NURSING CARE

Nursing Assessment

Cannulated Extremity

Normal: Decreased pulse volume and contour
Complications at insertion site:
Infection: Fever, local tenderness, swelling, purulent drainage
Bleeding, hematoma: Ecchymosis, swelling

Ischemia or arterial thrombus formation and dislodgment:
Diminished or absent pulses, numbness, pallor, pain.
Assess skin color, temperature, and pulses, which are indicators of peripheral tissue perfusion.
Monitor peripheral extremities for decreased perfusion every 1 to 2 hours.

POTENTIAL COMPLICATIONS

General
- Aortic dissection, perforation: Sudden, severe, sharp pain in abdomen and back; hypotension; tachycardia; decreased hematocrit value
- Thrombocytopenia: Bleeding; decreased platelet count (fewer than 150,000/ml)

Machine console and equipment
- Balloon synchronization: Inflation (augmentation) at dicrotic notch of aortic waveform; deflation at end of diastole
- Complications: Catheter kinking; malposition; balloon rupture

PATIENT PROBLEMS/NURSING DIAGNOSES & INTERVENTIONS

NIC TISSUE PERFUSION MANAGEMENT

Ineffective tissue perfusion related to interruption of arterial flow
- Provide protection to cannulated extremity.
- Perform passive range-of-motion exercises every 4 hours.
- Avoid bending extremity; use leg immobilizer if necessary.
- Provide skin care every 2 to 4 hours.

NIC COPING ASSISTANCE

Anxiety related to perceived health status
- Provide continued explanations of procedure and treatments.
- Offer frequent reassurance, encouraging verbalization and questions regarding progress.
- Allow family and significant others to visit patient when feasible.

PATIENT EDUCATION/CONTINUUM OF CARE PLAN

1. Explain to the patient and family the purpose of the procedure, as cited in preprocedural care.
2. Explain to the patient the importance of stability at the insertion site and the need for some mobility restrictions. Describe the use of the knee immobilizer to restrict knee flexion/groin flexion.

EVALUATION/PATIENT OUTCOMES

Tissue Perfusion Management: Perfusion of cannulated extremity is adequate. Extremity is warm. Capillary filling time is normal. Pulses are palpable. Color is normal. Mobility of extremity is normal.

Coping Assistance: Patient and family understand the use of the IABP and need for bed rest. Questions are answered.

PACEMAKER

Description and Rationale

Pacemakers are battery-operated generators that initiate and control the heart rate by delivering an electrical impulse via an electrode to the myocardium. Implantation of myocardial electrodes is initiated when a patient has symptomatic AV block. However, since the development of pacemakers in 1960, their use has expanded to include treatment of symptomatic brachydysrhythmias from other causes and refractory tachydysrhythmias.

Pacemaker implantation may be performed for temporary or long-term pacing. Temporary cardiac pacing is most commonly used for hemodynamic or life support purposes. The therapeutic indications include prophylactic pacing for symptomatic complete heart block, symptomatic bradydysrhythmias, particularly in the setting of acute MI, and as an emergency measure for malfunction of an implanted permanent pacemaker. In addition to control of heart rate, temporary pacing is often used in the electrophysiologic laboratory to evaluate cardiac dysrhythmias and to interrupt refractory tachydysrhythmias (e.g., supraventricular tachydysrhythmias, ventricular tachycardia).

Permanent cardiac pacing is indicated in the presence of symptomatic bradydysrhythmias.

Based on a universal code, pacemakers are described using a five-letter code, designating their characteristics. The position of the letters represent, in the following order, (1) chamber paced, (2) chamber sensed, (3) pacemaker's response to sensing, (4) programmability, and (5) antiarrhythmia function. For example, a pacemaker programmed with VVI capability paces the ventricle (V), senses in the ventricle (V), and is inhibited by the patient's own intrinsic impulse (I); there is no programmability and no arrhythmia function. Table 3-7 gives a full description of the universally accepted code combinations.

Table 3-7 The NASPE/BPEG Generic (NBG) Code

Position	I	II	III	IV	V
Category	Chamber(s) paced O = None A = Atrium V = Ventricle D = (A + V)	Chamber(s) sensed O = None A = Atrium V = Ventricle D = Dual (A + V)	Response to sensing O = None T = Triggered I = Inhibited D = Dual (T + I)	Programmability, rate modulation O = None P = Simple programmable M = Multiprogrammable C = Communicating R = Rate modulation	Antitachyarrhythmia function(s) O = None P = Pacing S = Shock D = Dual (P + S)

From Bernstein et al.[8]
Manufacturers' designation only: S, single (A or V); S, single (A or V).
NOTE: Positions I through III are used exclusively for antibradyarrhythmia function.

There are three primary characteristics of pacing:

Asynchronous or fixed rate pacing, in which rate and rhythm of pacemaker beats are unaffected by spontaneous beats. This type of pacing is rarely used.

Demand pacing discharges (fires) only when patient's intrinsic heart rate drops below a preset rate. This pacing requires synchrony with the patient's own rhythm.

Synchronous pacing, in which a sensing circuit is used to detect atrial and ventricular activity.

Overdrive pacing is a fourth type of pacing in which the pacemaker fires at a rate much faster than the patient's own heart rate in an effort to gain control of the heart rhythm. This is usually employed to treat a tachycardia. When the overdrive pacing ceases, the patient's intrinsic tachycardia cycle is broken and, hopefully, the sinus node recovers control of the heart rhythm.

Contraindications

Permanent pacemaker implantation is contraindicated for patients with active infections. Potential contraindications include the presence of any poorly controlled supraventricular tachycardia.

Cautions

Safety from electrical hazards should be ensured. Older pacemakers are sensitive to microwaves.

Preprocedural Care

1. Initiate preoperative instruction for the patient and family, including purpose and indications for pacemaker implantation, benefits and associated risks, information regarding method of insertion, type and mode of pacemaker to be used, and postoperative care, including need for routine 24-hour ECG monitoring and need to restrict activities for 4 to 6 hours.
2. Ensure that written informed consent is obtained.
3. Perform skin preparation.
4. Obtain baseline vital signs and ECG.
5. Permit nothing by mouth (NPO) 6 to 8 hours before procedure.
6. Initiate intravenous line.
7. Check functioning of external generator (for a temporary unit).

MULTIDISCIPLINARY PLAN

Surgery

Method of implantation depends on whether pacing will be temporary or permanent.

Temporary

Transvenous approach: Most common technique for temporary pacing; catheter electrode is passed into right ventricle via peripheral vein (brachial, femoral, subclavian, or internal jugular); electrode is connected to external pulse generator that can be set manually for pacing mode (FIG. 3-69)

Transthoracic approach: Used primarily with open heart surgery; pacing wires are threaded onto the exposed epicardium; at the close of the operation, the wires are passed through the chest wall and attached to a pulse generator

Transcutaneous approach: Adhesive pads are capable of delivering pacing stimuli through the skin

Permanent

Transvenous pacing: Catheter electrode is passed into right ventricle and attached to small, sealed, battery-operated pulse generator planted subcutaneously in shoulder or upper left quadrant (FIG. 3-70)

Epicardial pacing: Performed less frequently; electrode is sutured to epicardial surface of right ventricle; procedure requires an open chest approach

Medications

Preoperative: Mild sedation, tranquilizers

Intraoperative:

Local anesthesia, used for temporary and long-term transvenous pacing

General anesthesia, used for transthoracic approach

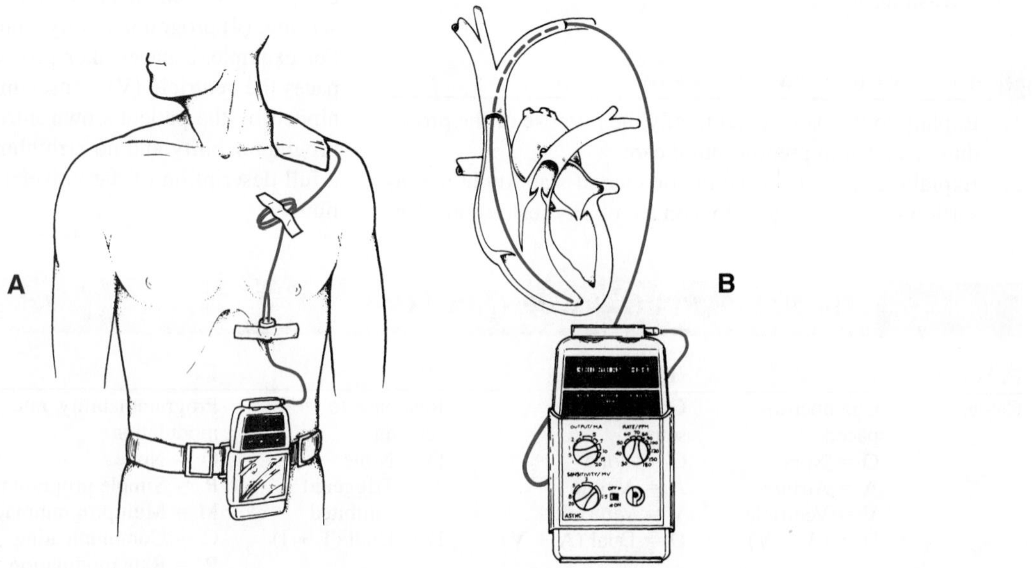

FIG. 3-69

A, Temporary external pacemaker. **B,** Temporary pacemaker unit, transvenous approach. (From Tucker et al.[99])

General Management

Cardiac monitoring: ECG pattern observed for rate, pacemaker response, signs of pacemaker failure, dysrhythmias

Pacemaker unit

Pulse generator: Self-contained device consisting of electronic circuit and power source of lithium batteries; device is hermetically sealed for protection from biologic environment; lithium-powered pacemakers can last 8 to 10 years before battery change is required

Pacing leads: Pulse generators use either unipolar or bipolar leads, and most generators are programmable to both; with unipolar leads, electrode (negative terminal) is at distal tip of catheter touching endocardium or myocardium, the pulse generator is the positive terminal; with bipolar lead, two electrodes are located at distal tip of catheter; current flows from pulse generator through distal electrodes into heart, where it stimulates myocardial contraction

Bed rest for 4 h after implantation, keeping arm closest to insertion site below level of shoulder

Range-of-motion exercises to affected extremity when ordered after third postoperative day.

NURSING CARE

Nursing Assessment

General

Level of anxiety, level of understanding, and fears associated with pacemaker implantation.

Cardiac rhythm and physical response to pacing.

Quality and source of pain.

Level of knowledge.

Pacemaker failure

Clinical symptoms: Syncope, hypotension, bradycardia, pallor, shortness of breath, chest muscle spasm, hiccups

ECG rhythm: Loss of pacemaker artifact, change in paced QRS complex, decreased amplitude of pacemaker artifact, competition between patient's underlying rhythm and paced beats, dysrhythmias

Infection at incision site: Redness, swelling, heat, fluid collection and drainage, skin breakdown, soreness

Dysrhythmias: Premature ventricular beats, ventricular tachycardia, patient complains of palpitations

Potential Complications

Pericardial friction rub; dysrhythmias; perforation of the ventricular wall or septum; local infection and phlebitis; pneumothorax; cardiac tamponade

Patient Problems/Nursing Diagnoses & Interventions

NIC Coping Assistance

Anxiety related to perceived or actual change in health status, role functioning

- Provide explanation and rationale for pacemaker, gauging the patient's reactions.
- Anticipate and allow the patient's questions regarding changes in lifestyle, cautions, and concerns over pacemaker management.

NIC Tissue Perfusion Management

Decreased cardiac output related to electrical alterations in rate, rhythm, and conduction

- Monitor vital signs every 4 hours after insertion.
- Analyze ECG rhythm strip every 4 hours for 24 hours after insertion.
- If temporary pacing: Inspect pacing circuit at least every 8 hours and with any indication of pacing failure, ECG rhythm change, or change in blood pressure or level of consciousness.

NIC Physical Comfort Management

Acute pain related to incision and physical mobility of affected arm

- Administer pain medication as ordered.

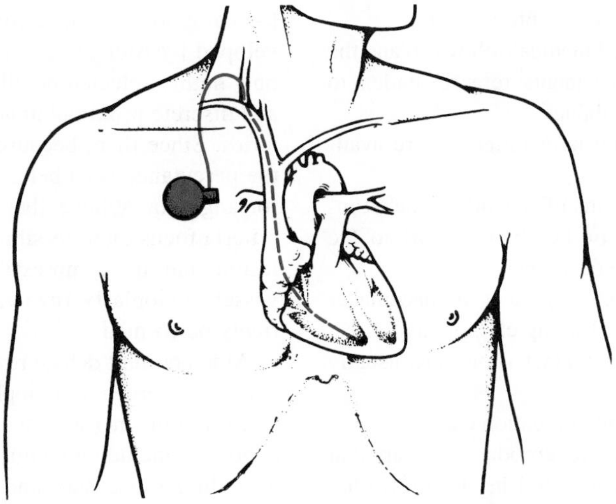

FIG. 3-70

Permanent pacemaker. (From Tucker et al.[99])

- Encourage range-of-motion exercises to affected shoulder 72 hours after insertion or as ordered.

NIC Patient Education

Deficient knowledge related to lack of information about pacemaker implantation

- Correct any misconceptions regarding pacemaker function.
- Initiate patient education program, providing audiovisual presentations and pamphlets.
- Provide follow-up.

Patient Education/Continuum of Care Plan

1. Discuss with the patient and family the purpose, rationale, and basic function of the permanent pacemaker.
2. Describe the type of pacemaker and the pacemaker's set rate. Instruct the patient on pulse rate and rhythm checking, emphasizing that pulse rate monitoring in lithium pacemakers must be done once a week or when symptoms occur.
3. Describe the signs and symptoms of pacemaker failure, including dizziness, weakness, light-headedness, and drop in pacemaker's set rate. Discuss actions to take if pacemaker malfunction is suspected, including calling for a pacemaker check via transtelephonic monitoring and notifying the physician or pacemaker clinic.
4. Describe activity allowances and limitations. Tell the patient to avoid driving for the first 4 weeks after insertion. Encourage the patient to resume normal daily activities and recreational interests, except competitive contact sports, which can increase the risk of lead dislodgment.
5. Discuss the need to avoid and protect against hazards from high-output electrical generators such as diathermy motors, welding equipment, and radar. Close contact with cell phones is not recommended. A distance of 6 inches from the device should be maintained. Metal detectors in airports, and hand-held detectors should be avoided as well. Most household electrical devices (such as microwave ovens and blow dryers) are considered safe, but review symptoms that may reflect electromagnetic interference and the action to take if symptoms occur.
6. Explain the need for continued medical follow-up and the need for periodic battery replacements; refer the patient to a pacemaker clinic where available.
7. Describe the use of telephone transmitters where available.
8. Explain the signs and symptoms of wound or pocket infection; instruct the patient or family to report to the physician if fever or drainage develops.
9. Explain to the patient the need to protect the pacemaker site and the need to avoid constricting clothing and direct contact or blows to the site; contact sports are usually contraindicated.
10. Explain the need to carry an identification card.
11. Reassure a female patient in her reproductive years that pregnancy is not contraindicated. Tell her to inform her physician of the desired pregnancy before conception so the pacemaker program can be checked and adapted to rate changes commonly associated with pregnancy.

Evaluation/Patient Outcomes

Tissue Perfusion Management: Cardiac output is maintained. Patient remains normotensive. Skin is warm and dry. Patient verbalizes no chest discomfort and rests quietly. Vital signs remain stable. Patient is free of infection. Patient is afebrile. Incisional site is clean with no swelling or redness. Pacemaker functions properly. Patient is normotensive and without dizziness, syncope, palpitations, chest pain, shortness of breath, or fatigue. Heart rate is acceptable. A temporary pacemaker fires at preset rate, sensing mechanism is visualized, and pacemaker artifact is visualized on ECG. A permanent pacemaker fires at appropriate rate, and pacemaker artifact is visualized on ECG.

Physical Comfort Management: Patient verbalizes comfort.

Coping Assistance: Anxiety level is reduced. Patient demonstrates reduced anxiety level and appears relaxed and less tense. Patient verbalizes feeling less fearful and asks appropriate questions.

Patient Education: Patient verbalizes understanding of procedures. Misconceptions are corrected.

INTERVENTIONAL TECHNIQUES FOR CORONARY ARTERY REVASCULARIZATION

Percutaneous Transluminal Coronary Angioplasty

Description and Rationale

Percutaneous transluminal coronary angioplasty (PTCA) is an invasive, nonsurgical, therapeutic procedure that restores arterial luminal patency, thereby relieving myocardial ischemia by compressing atheromatous plaques. PTCA has evolved over the past two decades as an extension of peripheral balloon angioplasty. Intracoronary transluminal dilation, first developed by Andreas Gruntzig in 1977, was at first used only on a highly selected population of patients with stable angina and discrete proximal noncalcified lesions of the coronary arteries. Since then, because of advances and modifications of the percutaneous catheter, the selection criteria of candidates for angioplasty have also widened. Current patient selection criteria focus on accessibility, complexity, and location of the lesion and its compressibility. Both single- and multiple-vessel angioplasty involving complex lesions are now routinely performed.

Much current debate revolves around the treatment of acute MI with emergency angioplasty in lieu of thrombolytic therapy. There are distinct advantages to this aggressive interventional approach, including an improved 5-year mortality rate[110]; however, limitations surround the emergency availability of the catheterization laboratory. Thus this approach is reserved for larger cardiac specialty centers. The procedure, which is technically similar to a standard cardiac catheterization, involves passing a balloon-tipped catheter into a stenosed coronary artery, where the balloon is then inflated and deflated using a handhold syringe or pressure-controlled device (FIG. 3-71). Successful dilation is usually accompanied by reduction in the systolic gradient across the stenosis; however, the gradient may not be abolished, and the inflation-deflation cycle may have to be repeated several times until the post-angioplasty arteriogram demonstrates improved luminal diameter. Successful PTCA is defined as an increase of at least 20% in lumen size, but resultant flow is graded using criteria named after a series of angiographic research projects called the "Thrombosis in Myocardial Infarction" (TIMI) trials. TIMI 0 reflects complete occlusion. TIMI 1 means there is penetration of the obstruction by contrast but no distal perfusion, TIMI 2 flow means there is perfusion of the entire artery but with delayed flow, and TIMI 3 flow means there is full perfusion and normal flow.[97]

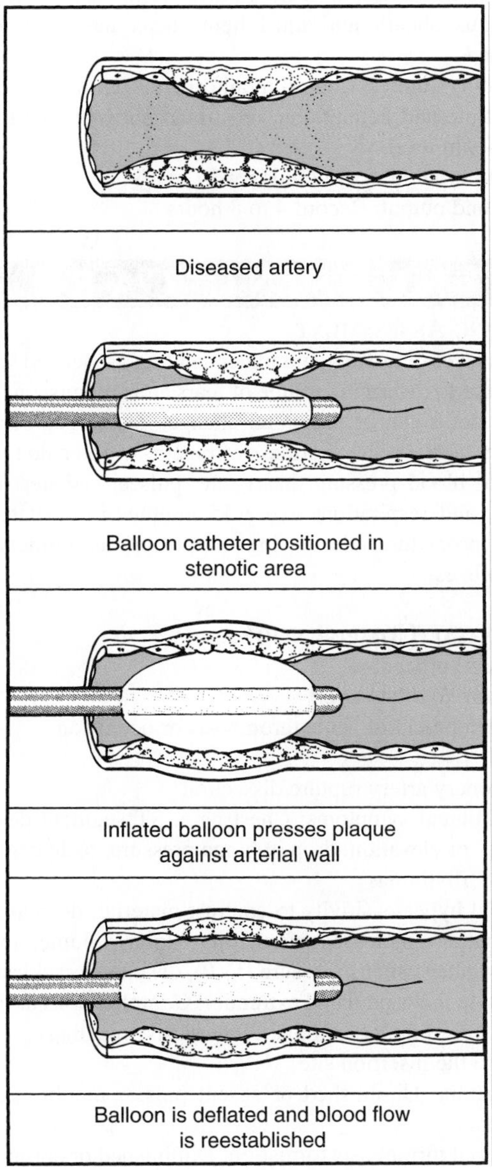

FIG. 3-71
Coronary angioplasty procedure. (From Canobbio.[15])

Currently, primary success rates are being achieved in 85% to 90% of patients undergoing PTCA. Symptomatic relief is being achieved in 80%, and long-term follow-up shows continued lumen patency and symptomatic improvement from 6 months to 2 years.[55] The restenosis rate, however, is currently 30%, which is the major driving force behind the development of new interventional devices.[55]

The angioplasty procedure involves using a two-catheter system. First, a guiding sheath is introduced percutaneously via the femoral or brachial artery cutdown. After the guiding catheter is at the orifice of the stenosed coronary artery, a second double-lumen dilation catheter is inserted and advanced under fluoroscopy until the balloon straddles the lesion. Pressure is applied at 5 to 10 atmospheres for 30 seconds or longer at a time, depending on patient tolerance or ischemia. After angioplasty the deflation catheter is removed, leaving the sheath in place.

Arteriograms are performed before and after the procedure, using the guiding catheter in the angiographic catheter. This allows evaluation of the results and decisions regarding the need for further dilation.

Directional Coronary Atherectomy (DCA). DCA reduces stenosis by removing atheromatous material rather than by compressing the plaque or stretching the arterial wall. DCA is most appropriate for lesions in medium to large coronary arteries, especially in the proximal and middle portion of the vessel. Highly eccentric lesions are appropriate for DCA. The safety is comparable to PTCA, and restenosis rates are modestly better. The device consists of a catheter-mounted cylindrical metallic housing with a central rotating blade.[39] The blade shaves off atherosclerotic plaque and deposits it in the nose cone of the housing so it can be extracted.

Rotational Atherectomy (Rotablator). The Rotablator device is an elliptical brass burr coated with diamond chips that is attached to a flexible, high-speed rotating shaft.[39] The plaque is micro-abraded, and the debris is flushed into the distal coronary circulation. Particles should be small enough to pass through the distal vascular bed. This device is best used in small coronary arteries with tortuous anatomy, diffuse disease, or distal stenoses. It is particularly useful with heavily calcified lesions. Acute success rates are good, but size limitations may necessitate adjunctive PTCA for optimal result.

Laser Angioplasty. Short pulses of laser energy are delivered through a catheter consisting of concentric bundles of optical fibers. Indications for laser angioplasty are long, diffuse, calcified, ostial, and vein graft lesions, as well as totally occluded vessels. Capable of increasing lumen size, laser ablation is often combined with PTCA to gain access for balloon insertion over a guide wire.

Coronary Stents. Designed to reduce restenosis and prevent acute occlusion resulting from angioplasty. A stent can maintain dissected vessel patency by compressing the intimal flap against the vessel wall. Several types of stents are commercially available. A major complication of stent placement is acute thrombosis in the first several weeks, before endothelialization of the stent occurs. Pharmacologic intervention in this area is aggressive. Antiplatelet inhibitors called glycoprotein IIb/IIIa inhibitors have revolutionized the procedure because of their profound reduction in post-procedure artery closure. Any form of anticoagulation can lead to vascular complications related to bleeding and thus prolonged hospitalizations. Drug dosage and administration strategies to minimize bleeding while protecting against stent thrombosis have been developed based on large prospective clinical trials.

Indications

Chronic stable angina; unstable angina; acute MI; clinical features that make bypass surgery unacceptable

Contraindications

Left main coronary artery disease

Preprocedural Care

1. Initiate preprocedural instruction for patient and family.
2. Ensure that written informed consent for PTCA or interventional revascularization is obtained. (Cardiothoracic surgical team should be available for emergency CABG in the event of serious complications.)
3. Obtain baseline data for PTCA: complete blood count; coagulation studies; electrolyte, BUN, and creatinine levels; blood type and crossmatch; ECG; chest x-ray; vital signs.
4. Perform skin preparation of both right and left groin areas.
5. Permit nothing by mouth (NPO) for at least 8 hours before procedure.
6. Establish a patent intravenous line.
7. Administer medications as ordered.
8. Administer preoperative sedatives as ordered.

Multidisciplinary Plan

Medications

Before procedure
- Antiplatelet agents: Aspirin, 325 mg chewable before procedure to decrease risk of platelet adhesion[96]
- Clopidogrel (Plavix) 300 mg PO
- Heparin 5000-10,000 units IV bolus
- Beta-blockers may be held

During procedure (options)
- Heparin infusion
- Glycoprotein IIb/IIIa inhibitor: Abciximab (ReoPro), eptifibatide (Integrelin), or tirofiban (Aggrastat) by continuous intravenous drip
- Intracoronary IV nitroglycerin, 100-300 mg/min; sublingual nifedipine, 10 mg; or both to prevent coronary artery spasm as catheter is introduced
- Thrombolytic agents as necessary

After procedure
- Immediate
  - Heparin infusion, 800-1200 U/h; tapered doses for 12-24 h to prevent coronary thrombosis from possible intimal tear
  - Complete infusions of abciximab, eptifibatide, or tirofiban
- Long-term options
  - Aspirin PO for 6 months; dosage will vary; 60 mg/day (baby aspirin); 325 mg PO qid or bid
  - For those who cannot tolerate aspirin:
  - Ticlopidine, 250 mg PO bid (high risk of neutropenia, must monitor blood tests)
  - Clopidogrel, 75 mg PO daily
  - Dipyridamole, 75 mg PO tid for 3 months

General Management

Cardiac monitoring: ECG pattern observed for changes in ST segment of the ECG in the leads that reflect the dilated coronary artery; monitor rate, dysrhythmias

Continuous blood pressure: Observed during and after procedure

Intraaortic balloon pump: Must be available on standby during procedure

Bed rest for first 6 to 8 hours after removal of arterial and venous sheath and until hemostasis has been reestablished

Laboratory studies: Careful monitoring of partial thromboplastin time and hemoglobin creatinine phosphokinase (CPK), troponin levels

Diet: As ordered; force fluids for 24 hours

Intake and output: Record 4 to 8 hours

NURSING CARE

Nursing Assessment

Assess level of anxiety and understanding associated with procedure to determine source of fears and any misconceptions.

Assess for signs of ischemia: changes in ST segment, chest pain, tachycardia, shortness of breath, hypotension.

Monitor blood pressure, heart rate, pulses, catheter insertion site, and respirations every 15 minutes immediately after the procedure, decreasing frequency as clinical status stabilizes.

Potential Complications

Related to procedure
- Failure to dilate artery
- Development of acute thrombosis or occlusion
- MI
- Coronary artery rupture/dissection
  - Clinical symptoms: Chest pain, ST segment depression or elevation, drop in blood pressure, tachycardia, dysrhythmias
- Renal hypersensitivity to contrast material, decreased urine output, increased circulating blood volume, increased jugular venous pressure (JVP), dyspnea, crackles

Related to the cannulated extremity: Complications at insertion site: bleeding, hematoma, ecchymosis, swelling

Distal to the insertion site
- Ischemia: Diminished or absent pulses, numbness, pallor, pain
- Arterial thrombosis formation: Diminished or absent pulses, numbness, pain, swelling, pale skin

PATIENT PROBLEMS/NURSING DIAGNOSES & INTERVENTIONS

NIC TISSUE PERFUSION MANAGEMENT

Decreased cardiac output related to myocardial ischemia or electrical instability (dysrhythmias)

Ineffective tissue perfusion related to thrombus formation

- Obtain baseline 12-lead ECG and compare to ECG ischemic pattern during angioplasty.
- Administer medications as ordered: IV nitroglycerin *to decrease incidence of coronary spasm and antiplatelet agents to reduce risk of restenosis.*
- Maintain bed rest in flat position until arterial sheaths are removed.
- Instruct the patient to keep the catheterized extremity immobile and extended *to decrease risk of bleeding.*
- After the catheter sheaths are removed, maintain pressure and monitor in accordance with hospital policy: sand bags, mechanical pressure devices, manual pressure, or closure devices.
- Adjust heparin according to coagulation studies, reporting prolonged partial thromboplastin time or abnormal results to the physician.
- Administer antiplatelet agents as ordered *to reduce risk of restenosis.*

NIC COPING ASSISTANCE

Anxiety (preoperative) related to perceived and actual threat to biologic integrity

- Provide explanations and description of procedure, including sensation to be experienced.
- Provide an opportunity for questions.
- Assist the patient to explore fears and discuss feelings.
- Provide the patient with an opportunity to meet the catheterization staff and visit the laboratory.

PATIENT EDUCATION/CONTINUUM OF CARE PLAN

Before procedure

1. Explain to the patient and family the purpose and indications for PTCA, its benefits, and associated risks.
2. Describe the procedure, explaining its similarity to cardiac catheterization; it may last 2 to 5 hours. Review sensations to be experienced, such as pressure during insertion of catheter; explain that there may be chest discomfort with actual balloon inflation.
3. Explain and review postprocedure routines: that the affected leg must be kept immobile immediately after the procedure, that patient will remain on bed rest for up to 8 hours, and that discharge home is usually within 24 hours.

After procedure

1. Reinforce explanation of procedure and postprocedure results.
2. Describe activity allowances and limitations. Explain that, unless contraindicated by postprocedure status, the patient may resume work within a week after discharge.
3. Instruct patient to be aware of late bleeding or hematoma at the puncture site, need to hold pressure if bleeding occurs, and need to notify the cardiologist immediately.
3. Discuss the importance of avoiding nicotine, which is associated with an increased incidence of restenosis after PTCA.
4. Discuss the need to modify or continue to modify coronary risk factors.
5. Discuss the importance of continued follow-up.
6. Review medications, discussing dosage, method of administration, and side effects.
7. Discuss the need to modify or continue to modify coronary risk factors.

EVALUATION/PATIENT OUTCOMES

Tissue Perfusion Management: Cardiac output is maintained. Patient remains normotensive. Skin is warm and dry. Patient verbalizes having no chest pain or discomfort. Vital signs remain stable. Tissue perfusion is maintained. Pulses distal to cannulation site are palpable. Extremities are warm and dry. Coagulation studies are within normal limits.

Coping Assistance: Anxiety level is reduced. Patient appears relaxed. Patient verbalizes less fearfully and asks appropriate questions. Misconceptions are corrected.

THROMBOLYTIC THERAPY FOR ACUTE MI

Description and Rationale

Long-term survival after MI depends on maintaining ventricular function. However, only in the past decade have investigators actively sought interventions to retard myocardial necrosis. Thrombolytic therapy has emerged as a successful modality in the treatment of acute MI; its use is based on studies that examined the role of coronary thrombosis as the precipitating factor of MIs and on studies that demonstrated how clot lysis and reperfusion of an infarct-related vessel can reduce infarct size and preserve myocardial function.[38] In the acute stage of MI (first 6 hours), abrupt coronary occlusion in the setting of an already narrowed coronary artery is caused by intracoronary thrombosis.[38] Total coronary occlusion from intraluminal thrombosis occurs in 80% to 90% of patients with transmural infarctions, and subtotal occlusion occurs in 15% to 20% of patients.[38,45]

Intracoronary infusion of thrombolytic agents, first reported by Rentrop et al,[82] achieves clot lysis, restores coronary blood flow, and limits myocardial ischemia. However, the extent to which thrombolytic therapy salvages myocardial function is time dependent. Time from onset of clinical symptoms to initiation of intracoronary thrombolysis is the strongest predictor of achieving coronary reperfusion. It is now generally accepted that thrombolytic therapy initiated within the first 4 to 6 hours for patients with an evolving acute MI can reduce in-hospital and 1-year mortality rates.

Thrombolytic Agents. Thrombogenesis, the result of a complex interplay of coagulation factors, begins with platelet aggregation and adhesion. Prothrombin is then converted to thrombin, which contributes to the conversion of fibrinogen to fibrin. Fibrin stabilizes platelet aggregation, forming a hemostatic plug. The development of fibrin-specific thrombolytic agents has been the key to the dissolution of coronary thrombi. Lysis of thrombi results from two actions: invasion of the injury site by leukocytes and activation of the fibrinolytic system. Normally the fibrinolytic system, which involves plasminogen activators, converts plasminogen, a circulating proenzyme, to plasmin. Plasmin, the proteolytic enzyme responsible for clot lysis, degrades fibrin into soluble fragments that are removed in the microcirculation. This system is inadequate to dissolve the fibrin mass of a large thrombus. However, the introduction of exogenous plasminogen activators produces more plasmin, which depletes circulating fibrinogen and generates high titers of fibrinogen degradation products (FDPs), which promote lysis. Exogenous plasminogen activators also destroy coagulation factors V and VIII, causing a systemic lytic state that increases the risk of bleeding.[98,109]

Streptokinase. Streptokinase (SK, Streptase, Kabikinase), a synthetic protein, is derived from group C-hemolytic streptococci. It forms an activator complex with plasminogen to activate the fibrinolytic process.[98] In addition, SK depletes fibrinogen levels and other coagulation factors such as V and VIII, predisposing the patient to bleeding. Furthermore, because SK is a bacterial protein with antigenicity, it can lead to a variety of allergic reactions.

Tissue Plasminogen Activator (Activase). Tissue plasminogen activator (t-PA) is a naturally occurring human enzyme present in endothelium, circulating blood, and human tissue. Unlike SK, which activates plasminogen systemically, t-PA is fibrin specific, activating plasminogen only after binding to the plasminogen bound to fibrin contained in the thrombus.[18] Thus t-PA is a clot-specific agent; because it produces relatively little circulating plasmin, it does not deplete other clotting factors, and therefore it theoretically reduces the risk of bleeding. Several third-generation plasminogen activators are now under investigation.

Recent international clinical studies suggest that rapidly administered t-PA with heparin is currently the most effective thrombolytic therapy for early reperfusion after an MI.[42] It has a small survival benefit but a large financial cost when compared with streptokinase, as well as a higher risk of intracerebral hemorrhage. Most hospitals have developed protocols that outline the most appropriate drug given specific clinical presentations.

The American College of Cardiology and the American Heart Association published a consensus, evidence-based document, "Guidelines for the Management of Patients With Acute Myocardial Infarction."[1] Included in their document are recommendations on thrombolytic therapy, which are as follows:

Indications:

1. Patients with ST segment elevation (greater than 0.1 mV, two or more contiguous leads), time to therapy 12 hours or less. Time of symptom onset is defined as the beginning of continuous, persistent discomfort. The earlier the therapy begins, the better is the reperfusion outcome.
2. Patients with bundle branch block that could obscure ST segment analysis and a presentation suggesting acute MI.
3. Patients who are age 75 years with ST segment elevation also show benefit, but have a higher risk of complications from thrombolytics. When blood pressure is greater than 180 mm Hg systolic and/or greater than 110 mm Hg diastolic, an attempt to lower blood pressure first is recommended.

Contraindications

- Active internal bleeding
- History of cerebrovascular event
- Intracranial neoplasm, aneurysm
- Suspected aortic dissection

Relative contraindications

- Major surgery (within 10 day)
- Recent gastrointestinal or genitourinary bleeding (within 2-4 wk)
- Recent trauma
- Traumatic cardiopulmonary resuscitation (CPR)
- Uncontrolled hypertension (>180/110 mm Hg)
- Current use of anticoagulants with INR in the therapeutic range
- Prior exposure to streptokinase
- Pregnancy
- Chronic severe hypertension

Preprocedural Nursing Care

Initiate preprocedural explanation of procedure to patient and family.

- Instruct patient and family about purpose and indications for thrombolytic therapy, its benefits, and associated risks.
- Explain and review procedures and routines associated with procedure: Monitoring in critical care unit, heart rhythm problems, and bleeding; explain need for bed rest during and after administration and for frequent blood sampling to monitor clotting times.
- Instruct patient to inform nurse if chest pain develops.

Consents are required to perform cardiac catheterization, angioplasty, and CABG surgery.

Obtain baseline laboratory data to determine hemostatic status and degree of myocardial injury: CBC with platelets, PT, fibrinogen and fibrin split-product levels, CPK-MB, troponin levels, BUN, creatinine.

Obtain diagnostic data such as 12-lead ECG, chest x-ray; obtain vital signs and perform clinical assessment.

Administer medication as ordered.

Prepare for cardiac catheterization if indicated.

Establish at least two patent IV lines.

Multidisciplinary Plan

Medications

Streptokinase

IV: 1.5 million units infused over 30-60 min; infusion may be initiated in emergency room or coronary care unit; heparin 6 h after SK and when activated partial thromboplastin time is less than 2 times control or about 70 sec.

Half-life: A half-life during which serum levels can be detected is 18 min and enzymatic action persists 18-80 min; enzymatic action on coagulation system persists up to 24 h

Side effects: Hypotension, reported in 15% of patients, may occur during rapid bolus infusion; allergic reactions reported in 5% of patients and include fever, flushing, rash, periorbital swelling, and bronchospasms; anaphylaxis is rare

Anistreplase (APSAC): Anisoylated plasminogen-streptokinase activator complex is a second-generation agent consisting of streptokinase bound in vitro to plasminogen, resulting in a much more stable enzyme complex and a longer half-life, permitting the agent to be administered as a single bolus

Usual dosage: IV, 30 units over 5 min

Half-life: 95 min

Tissue plasminogen activator (t-PA)

Usual dosage: 15 mg IV bolus, then 0.75 mg/kg over 30 min up to 50 mg, then 0.5 mg/kg up to 35 mg over the next 1 h with IV heparin 5000 U bolus followed by IV infusion of 1000 U/h (1200 U/h in patients >80 kg)

Half-life: 5-7 min

Side effect: Bleeding

Heparin: As outlined above

General Management

Cardiac monitoring: ECG pattern observed in patient for signs of reperfusion: resolution of preprocedure ECG changes; dysrhythmias

Hemodynamic monitoring: Pulmonary artery pressure and PCWP as indicated

Bed rest with commode: Until patient is pain free 24 hours

Diet: As ordered

Laboratory studies: Careful monitoring during and after thrombolysis: serum fibrinogen levels (will be less than 50 mg/dl after infusion of thrombolytic agent, returning to baseline within 24 h of completion of thrombolytic infusion); partial thromboplastin time; hemoglobin; creatinine phosphokinase (CPK-MB), troponin levels

NURSING CARE

Nursing Assessment

Myocardial ischemia: Assessment as described with acute MI

Assess and record level of comfort, including patient's verbal and nonverbal expressions. Compare with preprocedural chest pain complaints.

Reperfusion: Develops within 30 to 60 minutes of administration of thrombolytic therapy; abrupt cessation of chest discomfort; rapid fall in ST elevation; appearance of reperfusion dysrhythmias (may not be accurate indicator of reperfusion): sinus bradycardia and atrioventricular block with hypotension; accelerated idioventricular rhythm; ventricular ectopy; early peaking of CPK-MB levels within 12 hours after onset of symptoms

Assess and record changes in ECG tracing during and after thrombolytic therapy to determine any changes in baseline cardiac rate or appearance of reperfusion dysrhythmias.

Monitor vital signs frequently according to protocol and the patient's condition.

Bleeding and hemorrhage:

Assess for signs of bleeding: swelling, pain, or discoloration at puncture sites; petechiae; hematoma; flank pain indicating retroperitoneal bleeding; signs of internal bleeding or hemorrhage: tachycardia, tachypnea, hypotension, coolness of skin, pallor, thirst, restlessness, hematuria, occult blood in emesis or stool.

Monitor blood pressure, heart rate, and respiratory rate every 15 minutes during first hour, decreasing frequency as condition stabilizes.

Assess for changes in neurologic status, complaints of headache, or evidence of gastrointestinal bleeding such as occult blood in emesis or stool or hematuria for up to 24 hours after thrombolytic infusion.

Recurrent ischemia or infarction

Related to reocclusion, which has been reported to occur in 20% to 40% of patients after successful recanalization[39,45]

Chest pain

ECG: ST-T wave changes

Dysrhythmias

Skin cool, clammy, diaphoretic

Hypotension, tachycardia

Patient Problems/Nursing Diagnoses & Interventions

NIC Tissue Perfusion Management

Deficient fluid volume related to bleeding or hemorrhage secondary to thrombolysis-induced coagulopathy

Decreased cardiac output related to reperfusion dysrhythmias

Ineffective tissue perfusion (cerebral, renal, or gastrointestinal) related to thrombolytic drug-induced coagulopathy

- Inspect puncture sites every 15 minutes.
- Apply manual pressure when removing catheters and after venipunctures *to control superficial bleeding.*
- Monitor coagulation values until hemostasis has been reestablished.
- Avoid any interruption of vascular integrity after fibrinolytic therapy.
- Avoid venous or arterial punctures.
- Use heparin lock for blood sampling and IV access.
- Administer antidysrhythmic medications as ordered.
- Notify the physician promptly of any signs of decreased cardiac output as evidenced by changes in heart rate, blood pressure, and mental status.
- Initiate prompt treatment for life-threatening dysrhythmias per protocol: CPR, drug therapy, and preparation for pacemaker insertion.
- Report any abrupt change from baseline to determine need for change in or discontinuation of thrombolytic or anticoagulation therapy.

NIC PHYSICAL COMFORT PROMOTION

Acute pain (chest) related to decreased myocardial oxygen supply secondary to reocclusion of coronary artery

- Record any activity that preceded onset of pain to determine etiology.
- Maintain bed rest to reduce myocardial oxygen demand.
- Obtain 12-lead ECG to document recurrent ischemia.
- Administer drug therapy as ordered to relieve pain; assess and record response.
- Prepare for possible cardiac catheterization, repeat thrombolysis, PTCA, or CABG.

EVALUATION/PATIENT OUTCOMES

Tissue Perfusion Management: There is no evidence of bleeding. Hemostasis is reestablished. Coagulation studies are within acceptable limits. There are no overt or covert signs of bleeding: No hematomas or petechiae. Vital signs are within normal limits. Patient is alert and oriented. Cardiac output is maintained. ECG remains stable; dysrhythmias are absent. Vital signs are stable.

Physical Comfort Promotion: Comfort level is achieved. Patient verbalizes absence of chest discomfort or pain. Patient is able to resume previous activity level without complaints of pain.

PATIENT EDUCATION/CONTINUUM OF CARE PLAN

Before procedure

1. Explain to the patient and family about purpose and indications for thrombolytic therapy, its benefits, and associated risks.
2. Explain and review procedures and routines associated with the procedure: monitoring in the coronary care unit for heart rhythm problems and bleeding, need for bed rest during and after administration of thrombolytic therapy, and need for frequent blood sampling to monitor clotting times.
3. Inform the patient to notify a nurse if chest pain develops.

After procedure

1. Review the explanation of the procedure and postprocedure results.
2. Discuss with the patient the need to report any signs of bleeding: bruising, bleeding gums, hematuria, or tarry stools.
3. Instruct the patient to report pain relief or new onset of pain.
4. Discuss activity allowances and limitations.
5. Discuss the need to modify or continue to modify coronary risk factors.
6. Discuss the importance of continued follow-up. Explain that coronary angiography may be necessary to evaluate the patency of coronary arteries.
7. Review medications, discussing dosage, method of administration, and side effects.

REFERENCES

1. American College of Cardiology/American Heart Association Task Force. 1999 Update: ACC/AHA guidelines for the management of patients with acute myocardial infarction: executive summary and recommendations, *Circulation* 100(9):1016, 1999.
2. American Heart Association: Recommendation for prophylaxis of infective endocarditis, *JAMA* 277:1794, 1997.
3. American Heart Association: Standards and guidelines for cardiopulmonary resuscitation and emergency cardiac care, *JAMA* 225:2841, 1986.
4. American Heart Association: Heart and stroke facts—1995, Dallas, 1995, National Center.
5. Andreoli K et al: *Comprehensive cardiac care,* ed 2, St. Louis, 1987, Mosby.
6. Ball M, Mann J: *Lipids and heart disease: a guide for the primary care team,* ed 2, Oxford, 1994, Oxford University Press.
7. Belloni FL: The local control of coronary blood flow, *Cardiovasc Res* 13:63, 1979.
8. Bernstein AD et al: *PACE* 10 July/Aug, 1987.
9. Blake S: The clinical diagnosis of constrictive pericarditis, *Am Heart J* 106:432, 1983.
10. Braunwald E, editor: *Heart disease: A textbook of cardiovascular medicine,* ed 4, Philadelphia, 1992, WB Saunders.
11. Brown KK: Surgical therapy of chronic heart failure and severe ventricular function, *Crit Care Nurs Q* 18:45, 1995.
12. Brown WJ: A classification of microorganisms frequently causing sepsis, *Heart Lung* 5:397, 1976.
13. Calafiore AM et al: Coronary revascularization—the radial artery: new interest for an old condition, *J Cardiovasc Surg* 10:140, 1995.
14. Califf RM, Bengtson GR: Cardiogenic shock, *N Engl J Med* 330(24):1724, 1994.
15. Canobbio M: *Cardiovascular disorders,* St. Louis, 1990, Mosby.
16. Canobbio M: Eisenmenger syndrome, *Nurs Clin North Am* 19:573, 1984.
17. Cohn LH: Aortic valve prostheses, *Cardiol Rev* 2:219, 1994.
18. Collen D et al: Coronary thrombolysis with recombinant human tissue-type plasminogen activator: A prospective randomized, placebo controlled trial, *Circulation* 70:1012, 1984.
19. Conover MB: *Cardiac arrhythmias: exercises in pattern interpretation,* ed 2, St. Louis, 1978, Mosby.
20. Conover MB: *Exercises in diagnosing ECG tracings,* ed 3, St. Louis, Mosby.
21. Conover MB: *Understanding electrocardiology: physiological and interpretative concepts,* ed 3, St. Louis, 1980, Mosby.
22. Dajani AS et al: Prevention of endocarditis: recommendations by the American Heart Association, *JAMA* 264:299, 1990.
23. Dalen JE, Alpert JS: Natural history of pulmonary embolism, *Prog Cardiovasc Dis* 17:259, 1975.
24. D'Alonzo GE et al: Survival in patients with primary pulmonary hypertension, *Ann Intern Med* 115:3343, 1991.
25. De Campli WM et al: Characteristics of patients surviving more than 10 years after cardiac transplantation, *J Thorac Cardiovasc Surg* 109:1103, 1995.
26. Deshpande S et al: Catheter ablation in supraventricular tachyarrhythmias, *J Interventional Cardiol* 8:59, 1993.
27. Dole WP, O'Rourke RA: Pathophysiology and management of cardiogenic shock, *Curr Probl Cardiol* 8:1, 1983.
28. Douglas PS, editor: *Cardiovascular health and diseases in women,* Philadelphia, 1993, WB Saunders.

29. Doyle B: Nursing challenge: the patients with end-stage renal failure. In Kerr LS, editor: *Cardiac critical care,* Rockville, Md, 1988, Aspen.
30. Doyle JE: Treatment modalities in peripheral vascular disease, *Nurs Clin North Am* 58:139, 1983.
31. Earp JK: The gastroepiploic arteries as alternative coronary artery bypass conduits, *Crit Care Nurs* 14(1):24, 1994.
32. English MA: Dynamic cardiomyoplasty, *Crit Care Nurs Q* 18:56, 1995.
33. Essop R: Transesophageal echocardiography in infective endocarditis: the standard for the 1990's? *Am Heart J* 120:402, 1995.
34. Evans RW: Socioeconomic aspects of heart transplantation, *Curr Opin Cardiol* 10:169, 1995.
35. Fuster V et al: Primary pulmonary hypertension: natural history and importance of thrombosis, *Circulation* 70(4):580, 1984.
36. Futterman L, Lembert L: VEGF and TMR revascularization in the next millenium, *Am J Crit Care* 8(5):349, 1999
37. Gallego-Alvarez M, Obrien M: Right gastroepiploic artery conduit use in myocardial revascularization, *AORN J* 60:763, 1994.
38. GISSI trial: Effectiveness of intravenous thrombolytic treatment in acute myocardial infarction, *Lancet* 1:397, 1986.
39. Gist HC, Messobian HD, Ziskind AA: New interventional techniques for coronary revascularization, *Heart Dis Stroke* 2:198, 1993.
40. Goldberger E: *Textbook of clinical cardiology,* St. Louis, 1982, Mosby.
41. Groer MW, Shekleton ME: *Basic pathophysiology: a conceptual approach,* St. Louis, 1983, Mosby.
42. GUSTO Investigators: Global utilization of streptokinase and tissue plasminogen activator for occluded coronary arteries, *N Engl J Med* 329:673, 1993.
43. Guyton AC: *Textbook of medical physiology,* ed 8, Philadelphia, 1980, WB Saunders.
44. Guzzetta CE, Dossey BM: Cardiovascular nursing: bodymind tapestry, St. Louis, 1984, Mosby.
45. Habib GB: Current status of thrombolysis in acute myocardial infarction. II. Optimal utilization of thrombolysis in clinical subsets, *Chest* 107:528, 1995.
46. Harris L et al: The cardiovascular effects of caffeine on postmyocardial infarction, *Circulation* 72(suppl 3):116, 1985.
47. Hirman JA: Nursing assessment/nursing diagnosis in patients with peripheral vascular disease, *Nurs Clin North Am* 21:219, 1986.
48. Hosenpled JD, Norvick RS, Bennett LE et al: The Registry of the International Society for Heart and Lung Transplantation: thirteenth official report 1996, *J Heart Lung Transplant* 15:655, 1996.
49. Isner JM: Vascular endothelial growth factor: gene therapy and therapeutic angiogenesis (abstract), *Am J Cardiol* 82(suppl 10A):63S, 1998.
50. National Institutes of Health, National Heart, Lung, and Blood Institute: *The sixth report of the Joint National Committee on Prevention, Detection, Evaluation, and Treatment of High Blood Pressure,* NIH Publication #98-4080, pp. 1-70, 1997.
51. Joint National Committee: The fifth report of the Joint National Committee on Detection, Evaluation/Patient Outcomes and Treatment of High Blood Pressure, *Arch Intern Med* 153:154, 1993.
52. Kannel WB, McGee D, Gordon T: A general cardiovascular risk profile: the Framingham study, *Am J Cardiol* 38:46, 1976.
53. Kaushik RR: Surgery for cardiac arrhythmia, *J Interventional Cardiol* 8:83, 1995.
54. Kaye D, editor: *Infective endocarditis,* ed 2, New York, 1992, Raven Press.
55. Kent KM: Transluminal coronary angioplasty. In Rackey CE, editor: Advances in critical care cardiology, *Cardiovasc Clin* 16:53, 1986.
56. Kinney MR et al, editors: *AACN's clinical reference for critical care nurses,* New York, 1981, McGraw-Hill.
57. Kirchhoff KT: An examination of the physiologic basis for "coronary precautions," *Heart Lung* 15:874, 1981.
58. Kistner RL et al: Incidence of pulmonary embolism and thrombophlebitis of lower extremities, *Am J Surg* 124:169, 1972.
59. Kline-Rogers E, Martin J, Smith D: New era of reperfusion in acute myocardial infarction, *Crit Care Nurse* 19(1):21, 1999.
60. Kloner RA, Braunwald E: Effects of calcium antagonist on infarcting myocardium, *Am J Cardiol* 30:59(3):84B, 1987.
61. Kobashigawa JA et al: Effect of pravastatin on outcomes after cardiac transplantation, *N Engl J Med* 333(10):621, 1995.
62. Konstam MA, Dracup K: *Heart failure: evaluation/patient outcomes and care of patients with left ventricular systolic dysfunction, clinical practice guidelines,* 1994, U.S. Department Health and Human Services Pub. No. 94-061.
63. Lai WT, Huycke EC, Sung RJ: Supraventricular tachyarrhythmias: mechanism, types, and management, *Postgrad Med J* 83:209, 1988.
64. Lawson WE et al: Enhanced external counterpulsation: review of US clinical research to date, *CVR&R* 18:25, 1997.
65. LeFrock JL et al: Transient bacteremia associated with nasotracheal suctioning, *JAMA* 236:1610, 1977.
66. Lough ME: Quality of life issues following heart transplantation, *Prog Cardiovasc Nurs* 1:17, 1986.
67. Manapat ARE et al: Gastroepiploic and inferior epigastric arteries for coronary artery bypass: early results and evolving applications, *Circulation* 90(2):144, 1994.
68. Maron BJ et al: Management of hypertrophic cardiomyopathy, *Heart Dis Stroke* 2:203, 1993.
69. Moroney DA, Reedy JE: Understanding ventricular assist devices: a self-study guide, *J Cardiovasc Nurs* 8:1, 1994.
70. Mueller HS: Role of intra-aortic counterpulsation in cardiogenic shock and acute myocardial infarction, *Cardiology* 84:168, 1994.
71. Muirhead J: Heart and heart-lung transplantation, *Crit Care Nurs Clin North Am* 4(1):97, 1992.
72. Nagelhout J: Pharmacologic treatment of heart failure, *Nurs Clin North Am* 26:401, 1991.
73. Noel DK et al: Challenging concerns for patients with automatic implantable cardioverter defibrillators, *Focus Crit Care* 13:50, 1986.
74. Otten MW: The effect of known risk factors on excess mortality of black adults in US, *JAMA* 263:845, 1990.
75. Parker MJ, Cohen JN, editors: Consensus recommendations for the management of chronic heart failure, *Am J Cardiol* 83(2A), 1999.
76. Parsonnet V, Furman S, Symth N: A revised code for pacemaker identification: pacemaker study group, *Circulation* 64:60A, 1981.
77. Patterson S et al: Percutaneous myocardial revascularization: new treatment options for patients with angina, *Crit Care Nurse* 19(5):27, 1999.
78. Perez MM, Pintos Diaz G: Arteriosclerosis obliterans of the lower limbs, *Cardiovasc Rev* 4:1357, 1983.
79. Perloff JK: *Clinical recognition of congenital heart disease,* Philadelphia, 1994, WB Saunders.

80. Perry AG, Potter PA: *Shock: comprehensive nursing management,* St. Louis, 1983, Mosby.
81. Rao AK, TIMI Investigators: Thrombolysis in myocardial infarction trial (phase I): effect of intravenous tissue plasminogen activator and streptokinase on plasma fibrinogen and the fibrinolytic system, *Circulation* 72(3):416, 1985.
82. Rentrop KP et al: Effects of intracoronary streptokinase and intracoronary nitroglycerin infusion on coronary angiographic patterns and mortality in patients with acute myocardial infarction, *N Engl J Med* 311:1457, 1984.
83. Rubin LT et al: Treatment of primary pulmonary hypertension with continuous intravenous prostacyclin, *Ann Intern Med* 112:485, 1990.
84. Schneider JR: Effects of caffeine ingestion on heart rate, blood pressure, myocardial oxygen consumption, and cardiac rhythm in acute myocardial infarction patients, *Heart Lung* 16:167, 1987.
85. Shellock FG, Riedinger MS: Reproducibility and accuracy of using room temperature vs. ice temperature for thermodilution cardiac output determination, *Heart Lung* 12:175, 1983.
86. Shinn AE, Joseph D: Concepts of intra-aortic balloon counterpulsation, *J Cardiovasc Nurs* 8:45, 1994.
87. Silva J: Anaerobic infections, *Heart Lung* 5:406, 1976.
88. Skidmore-Roth L: *Mosby's 1996 drug reference,* St. Louis, 1996, Mosby.
89. Sklarin NT, Dutcher JP, Wiernik PH: Lymphomas following cardiac transplantation, *Am J Hematol* 37(2):105, 1991.
90. Spittell JA, editor: *Contemporary issues in peripheral vascular disease,* Philadelphia, 1992, FA Davis.
91. Steinberg JS et al: Radiofrequency catheter ablation of atrial flutter: procedural success and long term outcome, *Am Heart J* 130:85, 1995.
92. Swearingen PL, Sommers MS, Miller K: *Manual of critical care: applying nursing diagnoses to adult critical illness.* St. Louis, 1988, Mosby.
93. Tavilla G et al: Complete arterial myocardial revascularization using right gastroepiploic artery and both internal thoracic arteries as pedicled grafts, *J Cardiovasc Surg* 36(3):257, 1995.
94. Thelan L, Urden L, Davie J: *Textbook of critical care: diagnosis and management,* St. Louis, 1990, Mosby.
95. Thibodeau GA, Patton KT: *Anatomy and physiology,* ed 3, St. Louis, 1996, Mosby.
96. Tilkian AG, Daily EK: *Cardiovascular procedures: diagnostic techniques and therapeutic procedures,* St. Louis, 1986, Mosby.
97. TIMI Study Groups: The thrombolysis in myocardial infarction (TIMI) trial: phase I findings, *N Engl J Med* 312:932, 1985.
98. Topol EJ, editor: *Textbook of interventional cardiology,* ed 2, Philadelphia, 1994, WB Saunders.
99. Tucker SM et al: *Patient care standards: collaborative practice planning guides,* ed 6, St. Louis, 1996, Mosby.
100. Uber LA, Umber WF: Hypertensive crisis in 1990's, *Crit Care Nurs Q* 16:27, 1993.
101. Urban N: Integrating hemodynamic parameters with clinical decision making, *Crit Care Nurse* 6:48, 1986.
102. Vaska PL: Common infections in heart transplant patients, *Am J Crit Care* 2:145, 1993.
103. Wang WWT: Hypertension update: highlights from 1993 National Report, *Prog Cardiovasc Nurs* 8:13, 1993.
104. Wilkerson JT, editor: *Treatment of heart diseases,* New York, 1992, Gower.
105. Wilkerson JT, Cohn JN, editors: *Cardiovascular medicine,* New York, 1995, Churchill Livingstone.
106. Winslow EH: Cardiovascular consequences of bed rest, *Heart Lung* 14:236, 1985.
107. Wirsing P, Andriopoulous A, Botticher R: Arterial embolectomies in the upper extremity after acute occlusion, *J Cardiovasc Surg* 24:40, 1983.
108. Wit AL, Rosen MR: Pathophysiologic mechanisms of cardiac arrhythmias. *Am Heart J* 106:798, 1983.
109. Wood S et al: *Cardiac nursing,* ed 3, Philadelphia, 1995, JB Lippincott.
110. Zijlstra F et al: Long term benefit of primary angioplasty as compared with thrombolytic therapy for acute myocardial infarction, *N Engl J Med* 341(19):1413, 1999.

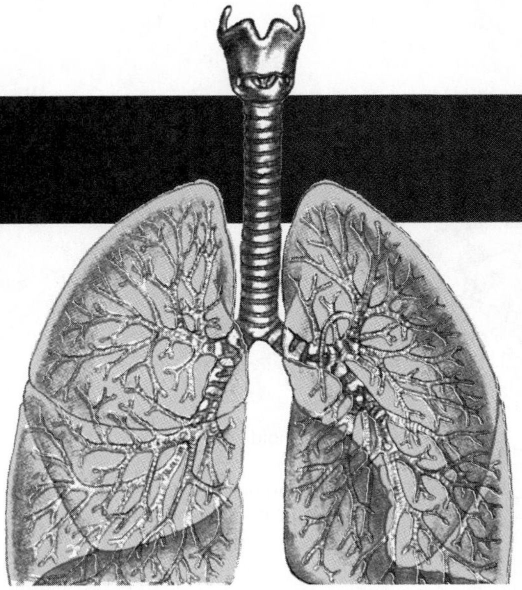

4 Respiratory System

Debra A. Hagler
Gayle A. Traver

OVERVIEW

The major functions of the pulmonary system are ventilation, gas exchange, and lung defense. Ventilation is a major component of the gas exchange function but is also a measure of the mechanical function of the lung. Gas exchange is the transfer of oxygen and carbon dioxide between the external environment and the blood. Oxygen is transported to cells where it is required for energy (adenosine triphosphate [ATP]) production via the citric acid cycle and oxidative phosphorylation. Carbon dioxide and water are metabolic by-products. This cellular use of oxygen and production of carbon dioxide is termed *cellular respiration.* The third function, lung defense, prevents the entry of noxious substances and microorganisms into the lung and subsequently into the body.

Smoking is the single most common cause of respiratory problems in adults. It is the major cause of chronic bronchitis, emphysema, and lung cancer in the United States. Environmental factors have become more important over the last several decades as by-products of industrialization and urbanization have polluted the air. Small particles of inhaled air pollutants may cause disease. Major air pollutants include sulfur dioxide and sulfur trioxide, nitrogen dioxide, carbon monoxide, chlorine, ammonia, hydrocarbons, silica, cobalt, asbestos, and coal dust. These chemicals also cause smog and haze, which affect crop growth. Other factors influencing the incidence of respiratory problems include genetic predispositions (asthma, cystic fibrosis) and acute infectious disease.

The following sections discuss the physiologic factors contributing to the major functions of the pulmonary system: ventilation, diffusion, perfusion, lung defense, and control of ventilation. Abnormalities of these factors are discussed in relation to specific disease states.

ANATOMY, PHYSIOLOGY, AND RELATED PATHOPHYSIOLOGY[21,23,40]

The anatomy of the respiratory system is discussed from a functional perspective within each of the following levels:

1. Ventilation: The movement of air from outside to inside the body and its distribution within the tracheobronchial system to the gas exchange units of the lungs.
2. Diffusion: The movement of oxygen and carbon dioxide across the alveolar-capillary membrane to the blood in the pulmonary capillaries.
3. Perfusion: The movement of blood through the pulmonary and arterial circulations and the distribution and exchange of oxygen and carbon dioxide.
4. Defense mechanism: The regulation of the internal environment, involving mechanical barriers, cough, and immune function.
5. Control of breathing: The regulation of ventilation to maintain adequate gas exchange, usually in accordance with changing metabolic demands or other special needs. Ventilation is the process that moves air from outside the body to the gas exchange units of the lungs. There must be enough force to overcome the resistance in the respiratory system so that air will be drawn into the tracheobronchial tree. The volume of air that enters is determined by the mechanical properties of the lung parenchyma, airways, and chest wall.

Chest Wall

The sternum forms the anterior border of the thorax. The posterior portion is formed by 12 thoracic vertebrae, and the lateral boundaries by 12 pairs of ribs that connect to the vertebrae. The first seven ribs also connect anteriorly to the sternum by the costal cartilages (FIG. 4-1). The bottom of the thoracic cage is formed by the diaphragm.

The diaphragm is the main muscle of inspiration (FIG. 4-2). During deep inspiration the diaphragm contracts and moves downward. This contraction, which occurs because of stimulation by the phrenic nerve, forces two major movements to promote ventilation. The first raises the lower ribs upward and laterally, increasing the transverse and lateral intrathoracic space. The second action forces the abdominal contents downward.

In addition to the diaphragm, the chest wall muscles that contribute to normal inspiration are the external intercostal and parasternal muscles. With increased inspiratory effort, the

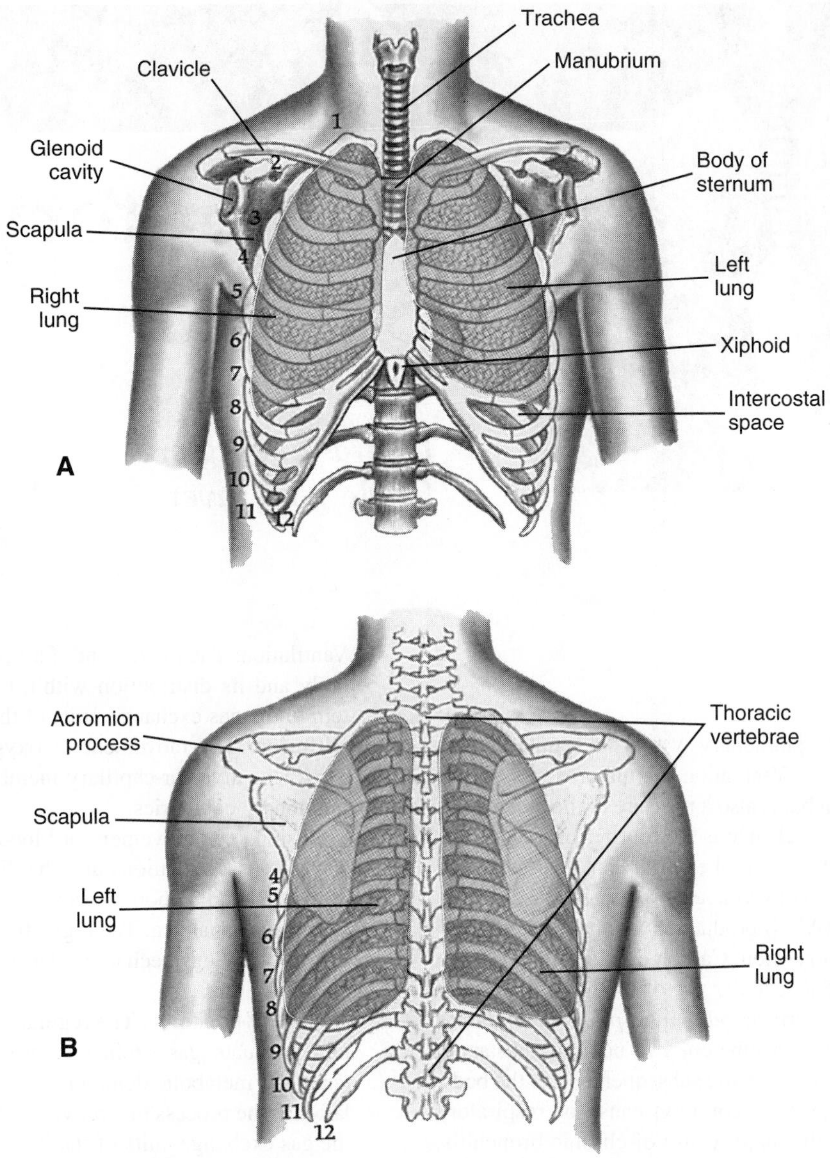

FIG. 4-1
Structures of chest wall. **A,** Anterior view. **B,** Posterior view.

accessory muscles raise the first two ribs, stabilize the chest wall, and raise the sternum.

Normal relaxed expiration requires no muscle force. Forced expiration is assisted by contraction of the abdominal and internal intercostal muscles.

Thoracic Cavity

The main structures of the thoracic cavity include the pleura, pleural space, mediastinum, and lungs. The lungs occupy most of the thoracic cavity. The right lung has three lobes and accounts for slightly over half of the ventilation; the left lung has two lobes and is smaller than the right lung. FIG. 4-3 details this anatomy.

The pleura is a two-layered protective membrane. The first layer is the parietal pleura, which lines the thoracic cavity on the chest wall side. The second is the visceral or pulmonary pleura, which covers each lung. Although each is given a separate name, the pleurae are continuous with one another and form one closed sac. Between the two pleurae is a potential space, the pleural space, which contains a serous lubricant film that allows one pleural surface to slip over the other. The intrapleural space also maintains a subatmospheric pressure.

The mediastinum is the region between the right and left lungs; it is also covered by parietal pleura. The mediastinum is bordered by the sternum on the front and the thoracic vertebrae on the back. The heart, contained in its own pericardial sac, is in the middle of the mediastinum. Also in the mediastinum are the great vessels that enter and leave the heart, the bifurcation of the trachea, the mainstem bronchi, most of the esophagus, the thymus gland, lymph nodes, and various nerves.

Upper Airway

The upper airway, consisting of the nose, pharynx, larynx, and extrathoracic trachea (FIG. 4-4), has three major functions:

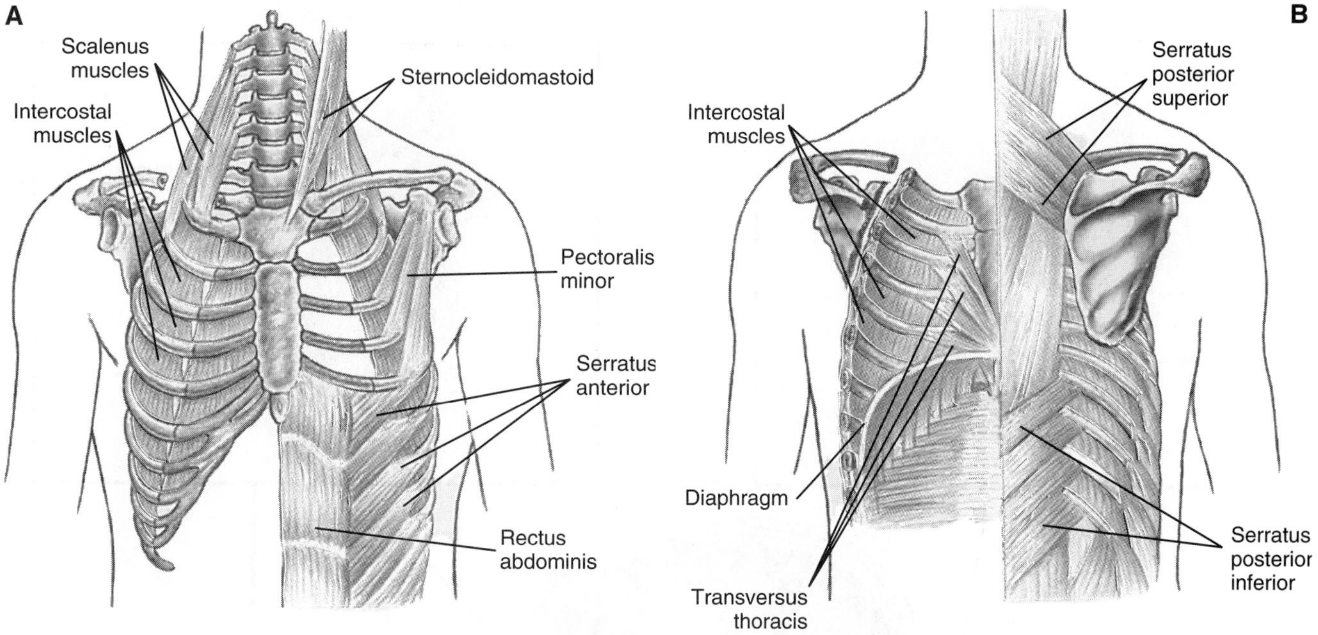

FIG. 4-2

Muscles of ventilation. **A,** Anterior view. **B,** Posterior view.

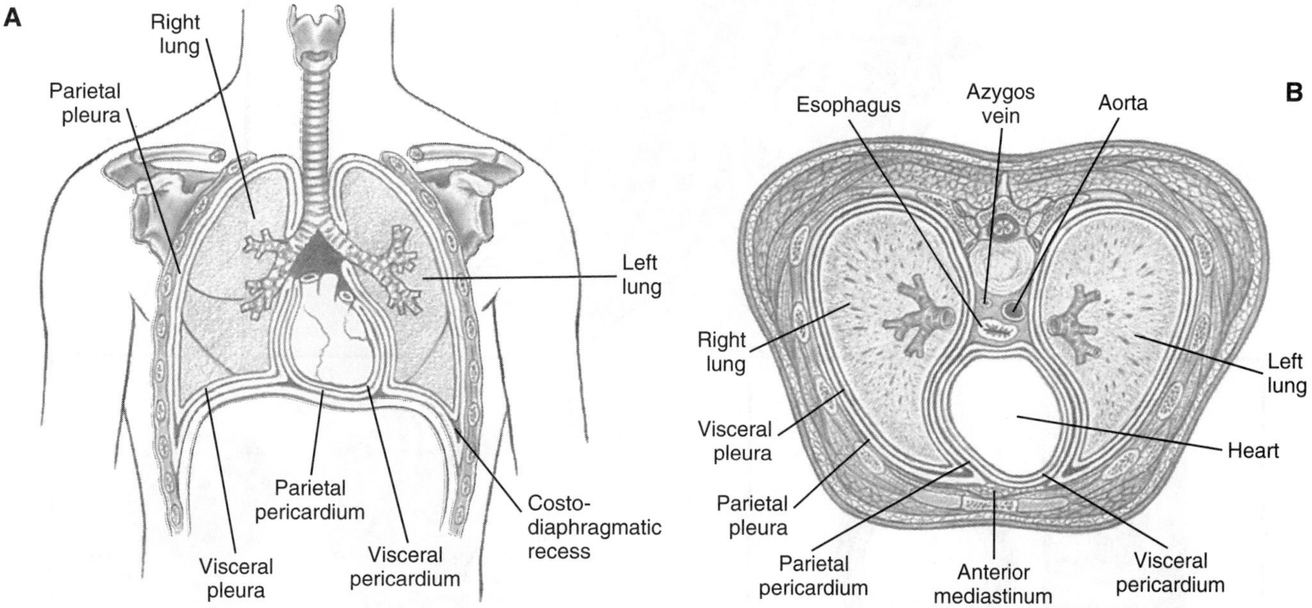

FIG. 4-3

Chest cavity-related structures. **A,** Anterior view. **B,** Cross section.

1. To conduct air to the lower airway
2. To protect the lower airway from foreign substances
3. To warm, filter, and humidify inspired air

The structure of the nose provides maximum contact between inspired air and the nasal mucosa. By the time inspired air reaches the bronchi, it is 100% water vapor saturated and has reached body temperature; large particles have been filtered out.

The major functions of the larynx are phonation and prevention of aspiration of foreign material. The larynx has many irritant receptors that respond by stimulating a cough reflex.

Lower Airway

The lower airway is made up of the trachea, mainstem bronchi, lobar bronchi, segmental bronchi, subsegmental bronchi, terminal bronchioles, and gas exchange units (FIG. 4-5).

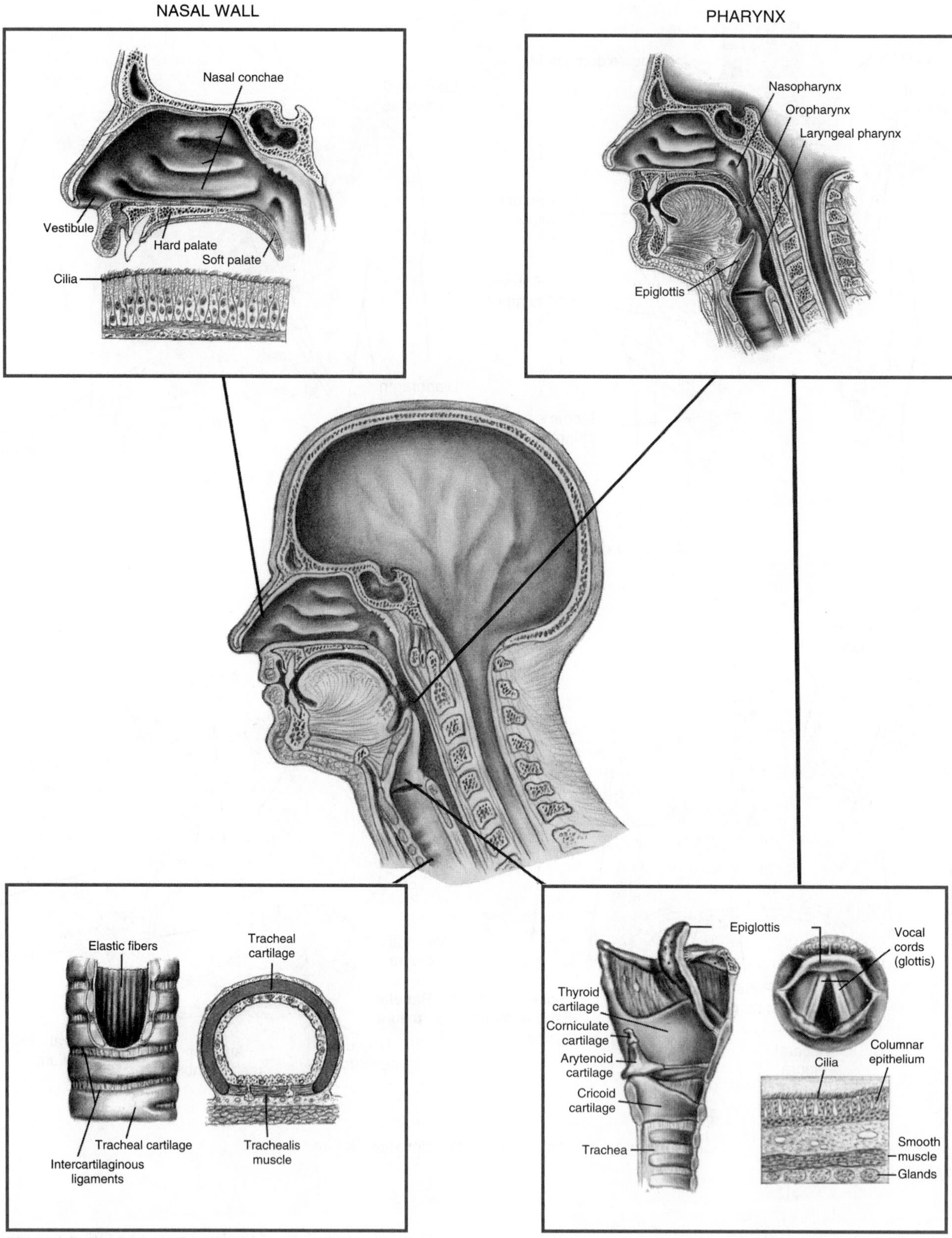

FIG. 4-4
Structures of upper airway.

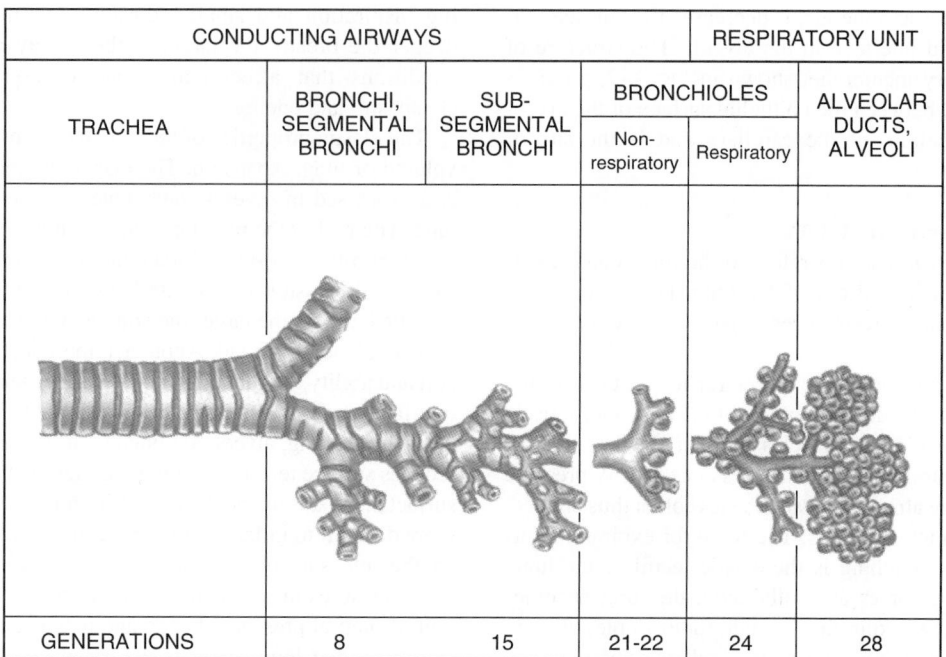

CONDUCTING AIRWAYS				RESPIRATORY UNIT	
TRACHEA	BRONCHI, SEGMENTAL BRONCHI	SUB-SEGMENTAL BRONCHI	BRONCHIOLES: Non-respiratory	BRONCHIOLES: Respiratory	ALVEOLAR DUCTS, ALVEOLI
GENERATIONS	8	15	21-22	24	28

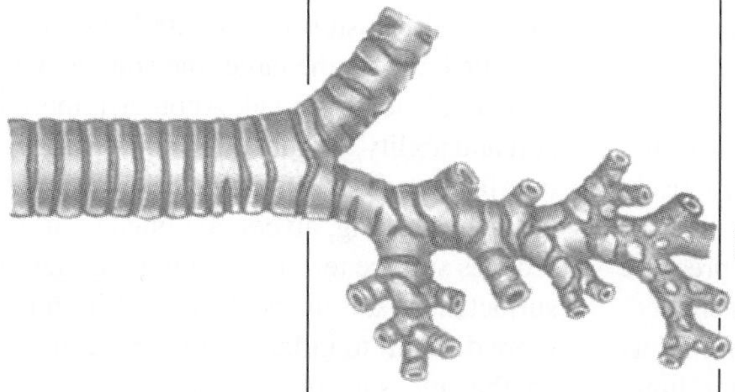

FIG. 4-5
Lower airway branches.

Between the trachea and the gas exchange units the airway branches 23 to 26 times (23 to 26 generations). Down to the level of the terminal bronchioles, air passages are conducting airways only. At the level of the respiratory bronchioles, gas exchange begins.

The trachea, which is 2 to 2.5 cm wide and 11 to 12 cm long, is supported by C-shaped rings of cartilage. It extends from the larynx to the major carina, where it divides into the right and left mainstem bronchi. The mainstem bronchi further divide into smaller and smaller bronchi to supply the lobes, segments, and subsegments of each lung. The trachea and bronchi are lined by ciliated columnar epithelium, mucus-producing goblet cells, and mucous glands. There are also bands of smooth muscle that control airway lumen diameter. All of these airways contain cartilage. In the bronchi there are plates of cartilage (as opposed to the C-shaped rings in the trachea), that become fewer in number as the airway grows smaller.

The smaller airways are called bronchioles or small airways. The bronchioles do not contain cartilage or mucous glands. Cilia and goblet cells are still present, as is smooth muscle. The first several branches of bronchioles conduct air just like the bronchi. The last bronchiole of the conducting type is called the terminal bronchiole. The next generations are respiratory bronchioles; alveoli begin to appear in their walls, and in addition to conducting gas between the lung and the atmosphere, these airways also participate in gas exchange. The most distal section of the lower respiratory tract consists of the terminal respiratory units (acini), which include the respiratory bronchioles, alveolar ducts, alveolar sacs, and terminal air sacs, called alveoli. An acinus is the site of gas exchange. FIG. 4-6 shows the cluster arrangement of these units. Note the intertwining of alveoli and capillary plexus.

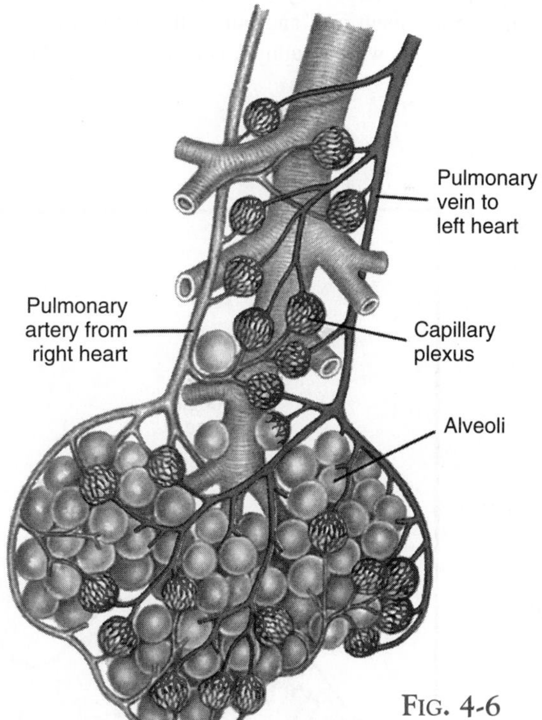

FIG. 4-6
Terminal respiratory units.

The membrane surface of the terminal respiratory units is a flattened, one-cell-thick epithelial surface, the type I cell, where gas exchange takes place. The type II cell of the alveolar epithelium is the repair cell and secretes the lipoprotein substance called surfactant. Surfactant forms a thin layer between the surface of the alveoli and the air; it decreases the surface tension of the air-liquid interface in the alveoli. The structure of the alveolar-capillary membrane, shown in FIG. 4-7, provides for intimate contact between the epithelial surface of the alveolus and the endothelium of the capillary and is the site of gas exchange.

Process of Ventilation

The term *pulmonary mechanics* refers to the forces and resistances to moving air in and out of the lung. Decreases in the forces or increases in the resistances impair ventilation.

The Forces. The ventilatory forces for inspiration are the inspiratory muscles, the diaphragm, and the chest wall muscle groups. When the inspiratory muscles contract, the thorax is enlarged and intrapleural and alveolar pressures fall. A pressure gradient between the atmosphere and the alveoli is thus created, and air is "pulled into" the lungs. The force for expiration during normal relaxed breathing is the elastic recoil of the lung. Once the expanding forces are withdrawn, the lung becomes smaller. When a forced expiration (cough, for example) or more rapid expiration is required, the abdominal muscles contract, pushing the abdominal contents against the diaphragm and increasing expiratory force.

The Resistances. The basic resistances to ventilation are airways resistance (the caliber of the airway lumen) and the lung's elastic properties. The airway caliber has a major impact on the rate of air movement into and out of the lung. Airway caliber normally changes with breathing, becoming larger during inspiration and smaller during expiration. Similarly, the deeper the breath, the larger is the airway caliber. Abnormal conditions that affect caliber are excessive mucus, bronchospasm, and edema.

The elastic properties of the lung have a major impact on the volume of lung expansion. The elastic properties are measured and expressed in several ways. One is the elastic recoil of the lung. The higher the recoil pressure, that is, the greater the pressure that must be used to inflate the lung, the stiffer is the lung. The recoil pressure varies with lung volume. As an analogy, for a single balloon, the larger the volume of the balloon, the greater is its tendency to recoil. Another important factor affecting recoil and ability to inflate the lung is surface tension. At a fluid/air interface, surface tension makes it difficult to inflate small "bubbles." In the lung, alveoli are lined with surfactant. This material reduces surface tension, making it easier to inflate alveoli. When surfactant is absent or decreased in amount, the lung is much more difficult to inflate and lung recoil increases. Compliance is another measure of the elastic properties of the lung. Compliance measures the amount of volume change accomplished per unit of pleural pressure change and is thus a measure of distensibility. When lung recoil is increased, the lung is stiffer and more difficult to inflate, and lung compliance is usually reduced (less volume change per unit of pleural pressure change). Conversely, decreased recoil means that the lung is easier to inflate and compliance is usually increased.

Although the elastic properties of the lung receive more attention, the chest wall also exhibits elastic properties. The stiffness of the chest wall affects the volume of air drawn into the lung with inspiration.

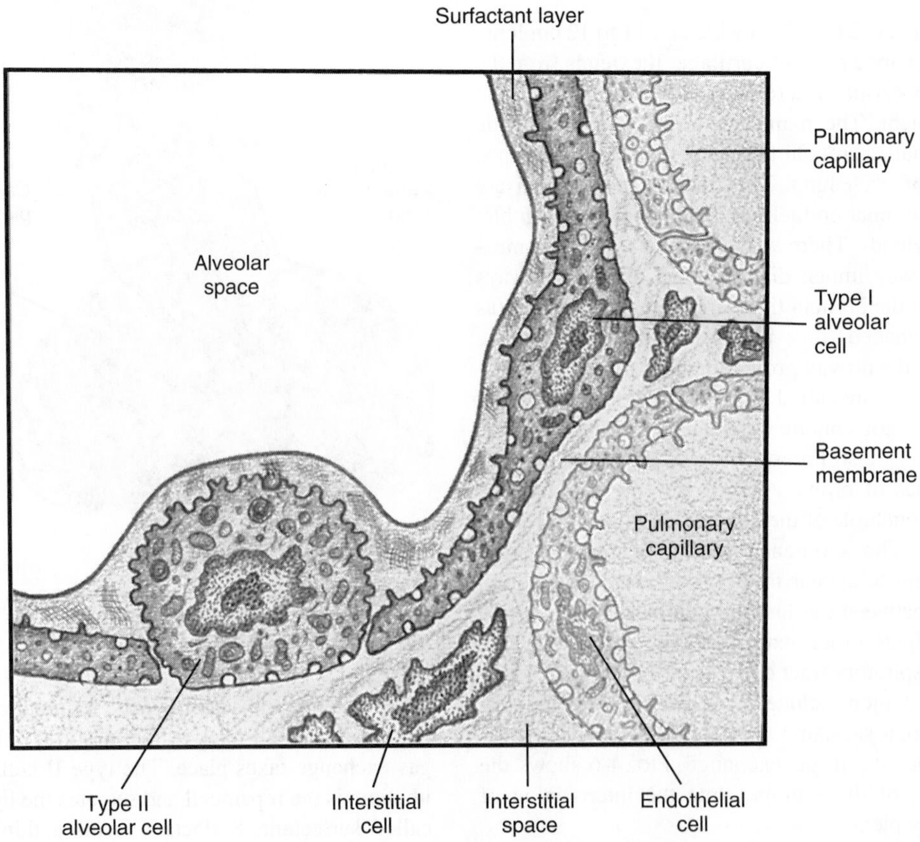

FIG. 4-7 Alveolar-capillary membrane.

Gas Exchange

The requirements for gas exchange are ventilation of alveoli, perfusion of the lung, diffusion of gases between the alveoli and capillaries, and matching of the distribution of gas and blood in the lung.

Ventilation.

The normal volume of gas that enters the lung per minute is about 7.5 L in an adult. However, not all of that gas reaches alveoli. Some of it remains in the conducting airways, the anatomic dead space. The amount of ventilation available for gas exchange is about 5 L/min.

Perfusion.

The major purpose of the pulmonary circulation is to deliver blood in a thin film to the alveoli so that gas exchange can occur. The pulmonary vascular system is a high volume–low pressure system. This means that a large amount of blood flows through the lungs and that the capillary resistance to that blood flow is very low.

Blood from the right ventricle of the heart is pumped into the right and left pulmonary arteries, which branch into the alveolar capillaries. At the alveolar-capillary membrane the blood picks up oxygen and loses carbon dioxide. After being oxygenated the blood flows into the four pulmonary veins, which return it to the left atrium of the heart. Under normal resting conditions only a portion of the pulmonary capillaries is actively perfused. As cardiac output increases, pulmonary arterial pressure remains fairly constant because of two mechanisms:

1. Recruitment of previously unperfused capillaries, which decreases pulmonary vascular resistance and thus permits increased blood flow through the vessels.
2. Capillary dilation, which directly increases the capillary size and decreases the resistance to flow.

Both of these mechanisms can adjust to an increase in cardiac output. A malfunction of these mechanisms could lead to pulmonary hypertension. The pulmonary artery catheter is commonly used to measure the pulmonary arterial pressure in critically ill persons. Pulmonary artery pressures may also be measured during cardiac catheterization.

Diffusion.

Once the air reaches the surface of the alveoli, the oxygen must cross the alveolar-capillary membrane and enter the pulmonary capillary system. Similarly, the carbon dioxide must cross the alveolar-capillary membrane to be exhaled form the lungs. Diffusion of the gases oxygen and carbon dioxide is a constant process, with both gases moving across the membrane simultaneously.

The process of diffusion depends on the thickness of the respiratory membrane, the surface area of the membrane, the diffusion coefficients of the gases, and the partial pressure differences of the gases being diffused. Any changes in the alveolar membrane or the interstitial spaces between the alveoli and the capillary can affect the rate of gas diffusion.

The process of gas exchange between the air in the alveoli and the blood in the lung capillaries occurs because of a difference in the partial pressures of the gases. FIG. 4-8 shows the partial pressures. Each gas diffuses from an area of high partial pressure to an area of low partial pressure. When the concentration of oxygen is altered, as occurs during oxygen therapy, the partial pressures of the gases are also altered (FIG. 4-9).

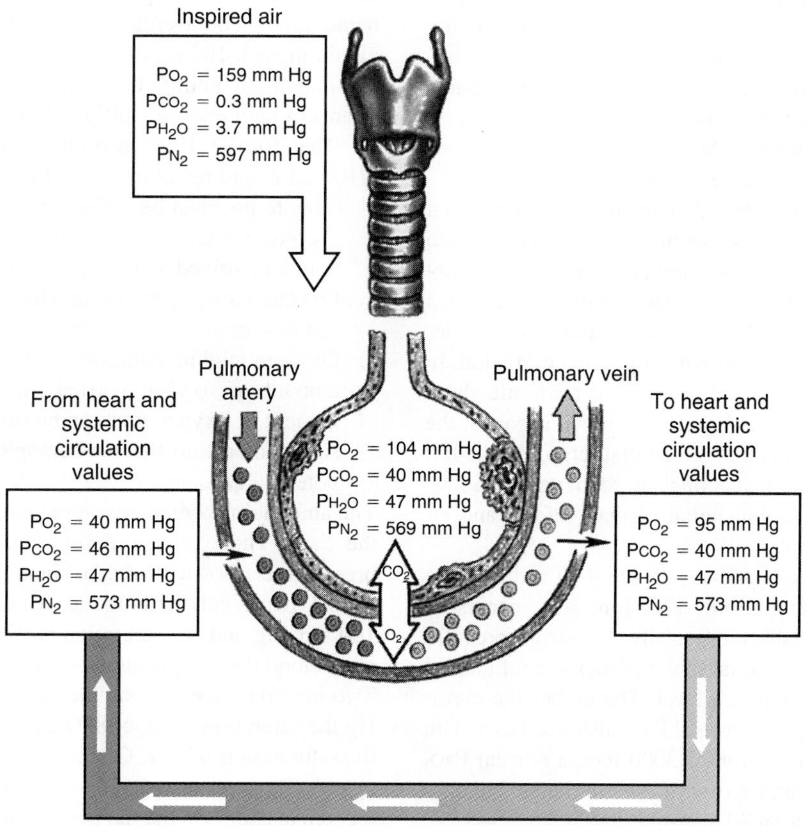

FIG. 4-8
Partial pressure of respiratory gases in normal respiration.

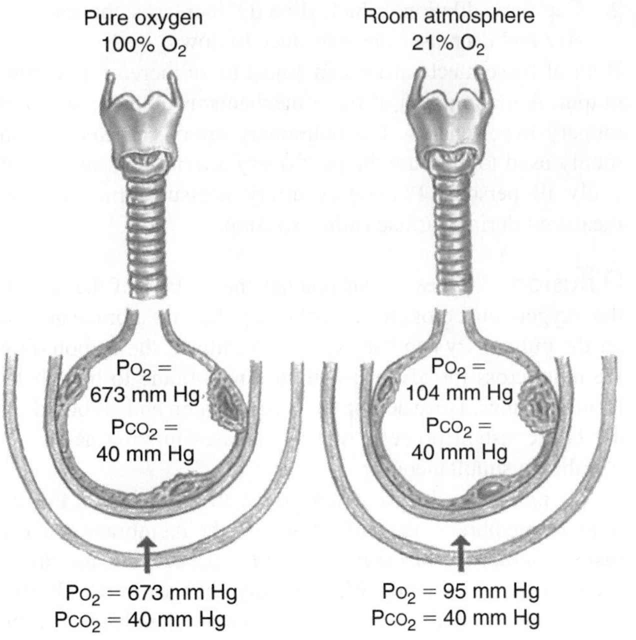

FIG. 4-9

Effect of varying oxygen concentration.

Common Alterations in Ventilation/Perfusion Matching. Efficient gas exchange requires a matching of ventilation (V) and perfusion (Q) in each alveolar-capillary unit. In the normal lung, ventilation and perfusion are quite well matched, with an average ventilation/perfusion ratio (V/Q) of 0.8.

When there is more blood than air entering an area of lung, that part of the lung has a high V/Q ratio. *Dead space* is the term used to describe lung where there is air but a complete absence of blood. In the normal lung the airways are dead space; approximately one third of every breath is dead space. A disease state such as a pulmonary embolus, where a pulmonary arterial vessel is blocked, also creates dead space.

Where there is less air than blood in an area of the lung, that area has a low V/Q ratio. Because the blood does not come into contact with a ventilated alveolus, there is decreased oxygenation of that blood. Low V/Q occurs in various diseases and is a common cause of hypoxemia. *Shunt* is the term used to describe the complete absence of air with continued perfusion. In the normal person there is a small amount of anatomic shunt (about 2% to 5% of the cardiac output); this blood is part of the bronchial and cardiac circulation—blood that returns to the left side of the heart without "contacting" a ventilated alveolus. Disease conditions such as congenital cardiac defects and atelectasis can result in shunt.

The arterial blood gases (ABGs) (Table 4-1) indicate the effectiveness of the ventilation, diffusion, and perfusion processes. Blood gas variables, especially the partial pressure of oxygen dissolved in the arterial blood (Pao_2), are influenced by elevation in comparison to sea level. The higher the elevation, the lower is the Pao_2. The normal Pao_2 also decreases with age. For example, at an elevation of 3000 feet, a normal Pao_2 would be about 75 to 80 mm Hg for a 40-year-old man, but only about 65 to 70 mm Hg for an 80-year-old man.

Table 4-1 Normal Values for Arterial Blood Gases (at Sea Level)

Pao_2	90 ± 10 mm Hg
O_2 saturation	97% ± 2%
$Paco_2$	40 ± 3 mm Hg
pH	7.4 ± 0.03
Bicarbonate	22-26 mEq/L

Gas Transport

After the diffusion of gases at the alveolar level, the gases must be transported to the tissues for use. The following describes how oxygen and carbon dioxide are carried in the blood and the importance of hemoglobin. The cardiac chapter describes how the gases are then transported to the tissues.

Oxygen. Oxygen in the blood is carried two ways: dissolved in the liquid part of the blood plasma and in chemical combination with hemoglobin. Most oxygen is transported in the second manner.

The amount of dissolved oxygen carried in the plasma is directly proportional to the partial pressure of oxygen. There is 0.003 ml of oxygen dissolved in each 100 ml of blood for each 1 mm Hg partial pressure of oxygen. Thus at an ideal Pao_2 of 100 mm Hg, only 0.3 ml of oxygen would be carried per 100 ml of plasma.

Most oxygen in the body is transported to the cells in combination with hemoglobin. Oxygen combines loosely and reversibly with the heme portion of hemoglobin. When the Po_2 is low, as in the tissue capillaries, the oxygen is released from the hemoglobin. The average individual has about 15 g of hemoglobin in each 100 ml of blood. Each gram of hemoglobin has the maximum ability to combine with 1.34 ml of oxygen. Grams of hemoglobin multiplied by 1.34 yields oxygen capacity. Therefore at 100% saturation, a hemoglobin level of 15 g/100 ml would result in 20.1 ml of oxygen.

Three terms must be differentiated:

1. Oxygen content is the total amount of oxygen carried in both a dissolved and a combined state per 100 ml of blood.
2. Oxygen capacity is the maximum amount of oxygen that can be carried.
3. Oxyhemoglobin saturation is the relationship between the amount of oxygen carried on the hemoglobin and the amount of oxygen that can be carried. For example, a 90% saturation means that the hemoglobin is carrying 90% of its potential capacity.

The amount of oxygen combined with hemoglobin depends on the Pao_2. The oxyhemoglobin saturation at different partial pressures is shown in the oxyhemoglobin dissociation curve (FIG. 4-10). When the blood leaves the lungs, the Pao_2 is about 100 mm Hg and the saturation is 97.5%. In normal mixed venous blood the $P\bar{v}o_2$ is about 40 mm Hg with a 75% saturation. Two important areas along the curve are (1) at a Po_2 of 55 mm Hg the saturation is about 88% and (2) at a Po_2 of 100 mm Hg the saturation is 97.5%. On the steep portion of the curve, large changes in saturation occur with relatively small changes in oxygen tension. On the flat portion of the curve, the changes are

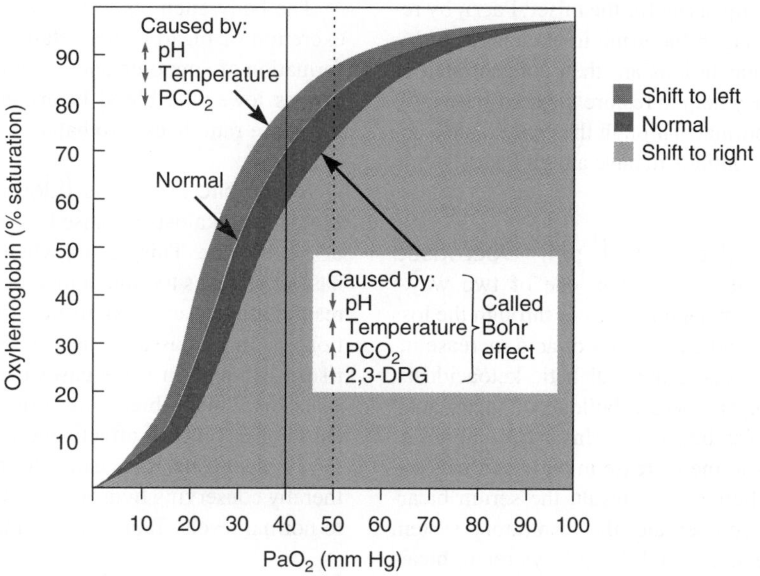

FIG. 4-10
Oxyhemoglobin dissociation curve. (From Lewis, et. al.[20a])

much smaller. For example, a change in Po_2 from 100 to 55 mm Hg decreases saturation by only 10%.

Various changes in the blood can also cause changes in the oxyhemoglobin dissociation curve (see FIG. 4-10). Shifts to the right are produced by a decrease in pH, a rise in Pco_2, and an increase in body temperature. A dissociation curve shift to the right means that the hemoglobin's bond to oxygen is weakened and that higher gas pressure is needed for binding. The advantage of a right shift is that oxygen escapes hemoglobin more easily and is more available to the tissues.

Shifts to the left are produced by an increase in pH, a decrease in Pco_2, and a decrease in body temperature. When there is a shift to the left, the affinity of hemoglobin for oxygen is increased. The hemoglobin binds the oxygen more firmly than normal, and although less pressure is needed to bind the two, it is more difficult to separate them at the cellular level. Normally the curve shifts to the left to help pick up oxygen in the lung. In disease states, with an abnormal shift to the left, tissues may be hypoxic because the oxygen remains bound to hemoglobin instead of being released for tissue use.

Carbon Dioxide. Carbon dioxide transport must be understood clearly because the amount of carbon dioxide in transit helps determine the acid-base balance of the body. Carbon dioxide is carried in various forms. The majority (70%) is carried as a bicarbonate (HCO_3^-), with a lesser amount carried in dissolved forms as carbonic acid (H_2CO_3) and as carbamino compounds. One such carbamino compound is reduced hemoglobin.

Acid-Base Balance and Blood Gases

For body cells to function best, body fluids and blood must remain within a specific, narrow acid-base range (pH). Deviations of body pH outside this narrow range interfere with cellular metabolism and can cause cell death. Interactions of substances in the body should produce a hydrogen ion concentration sufficient to maintain a blood pH of 7.35 to 7.45. (pH is the negative log of the hydrogen ion concentration; as the concentration of hydrogen ion increases, the pH falls and vice versa.) This normal acid-base balance is maintained by respiratory and kidney function. The acid-base balance is evaluated using the HCO_3^- carbonic acid system. The respiratory system determines the carbon dioxide concentration, thereby regulating the hydrogen ion concentration. Increased amounts of carbon dioxide lead to increased amounts of carbonic acid and more hydrogen ion. The renal system uses buffering mechanisms to regulate bicarbonate concentrations.

Blood pH depends on the ratio of bicarbonate to carbon dioxide. As long as that ratio is 20:1, the pH is 7.4. If the blood pH falls below that level, acidemia occurs; an elevated pH defines alkalemia.

Acid-base imbalances are classified according to whether the person is acidemic or alkalemic and by the causative mechanism, either respiratory or metabolic. A respiratory mechanism is one in which the primary change causing the acid-base disorder is a change in the arterial carbon dioxide tension. A metabolic mechanism is one in which the primary change is the addition of an acid other than carbonic acid or a change in bicarbonate.

Acidosis States

Respiratory Acidosis (Decreased pH, Increased $Paco_2$). Respiratory acidosis is the result of alveolar hypoventilation. This may occur in response to cardiopulmonary, neuromuscular, skeletal, or airway diseases; to acute infections; or to the actions of drugs such as narcotics or sedatives. The partial pressure of arterial carbon dioxide increases, and pH drops.

The body attempts to compensate for the raised $PaCO_2$ by removing excess hydrogen ions in the urine in exchange for bicarbonate ions. The bicarbonate ions are then concentrated in the blood plasma, where they help to restore the acid-base ratio and thus return the pH to normal. Through the process of compensation, the patient may continue to have a high $PaCO_2$, while the pH returns to normal.

Metabolic Acidosis (Decreased pH, Decreased HCO_3^-). Metabolic acidosis is caused in one of two ways: through the increase of fixed metabolic acids or through the loss of bicarbonate in the body fluids. Examples of acid increase include salicylate poisoning, renal failure, diabetic ketoacidosis, and circulatory failure that produces a buildup of lactic acid. Persistent diarrhea causes bicarbonate loss. In such situations of acidosis the body responds to the increase in body acids by using bicarbonate ions as a buffer. As a result, the serum bicarbonate levels are low. To compensate, the respiratory system increases ventilation immediately, and the kidneys retain bicarbonate eventually. Table 4-2 summarizes this process.

Alkalosis States

Respiratory Alkalosis (Elevated pH, Decreased $PaCO_2$). Respiratory alkalosis occurs when excess amounts of carbon dioxide are exhaled. Alveolar hyperventilation removes carbon dioxide from the blood, decreasing the $PaCO_2$ and elevating the pH. Hyperventilation from anxiety is perhaps the best example. Other causes of alkalosis include brain injury or brain tumors, response to increased ventilatory drive, and hyperventilation with a mechanical ventilator.

The body attempts to compensate by increasing the kidney excretion of bicarbonate, retaining chloride, and reducing the formation of ammonia and excretion of acid salts. These mechanisms lower the blood bicarbonate level and thus bring the acid-base ratio back into balance.

Metabolic Alkalosis (Elevated pH, Elevated HCO_3). Metabolic alkalosis is caused by an increase in the body's level of bicarbonate. This occurs when the patient ingests too much base or receives too much bicarbonate during cardiopulmonary resuscitation. Acid loss results from vomiting or gastric suctioning. In all cases the acid-base ratio is altered and the pH rises. Although in some cases the respiratory system compensates by slowing breathing, this compensation is unusual because of the normal effectiveness of ventilatory drive. The kidneys respond by increasing the removal of bicarbonate ions, thereby conserving hydrogen ions. As a result, the pH decreases to normal levels. Table 4-3 summarizes these processes.

Lung Defense Mechanisms

Lung defenses include both nonspecific and specific mechanisms of protection. Nonspecific mechanisms work to prevent the entry of any foreign substance or particle. Nonspecific mechanisms of lung defense include mucociliary clearance, cough, and macrophage clearance.

Mucociliary Clearance. Conducting airways are coated by a layer of mucus, which traps inhaled particles. Ciliary movement transports the particles and mucus to the pharynx, where the mucus is swallowed without conscious awareness.

Table 4-2 Summary of the Acidosis Process

$$CO_2 + H_2O <=> H_2CO_3 <=> H^+ + HCO_3^-$$

	Initial Cause	Compensation
Respiratory acidosis	↑PCO_2	Kidneys Elimination of H^- HCO_3^- conserved (the higher the PCO_2, the more HCO_3^- reabsorbed)
Metabolic acidosis	↓Base ↑Fixed acids	Lungs Elimination of CO_2 Kidneys Conserve HCO_3^- (the lower the HCO_3^-, the more HCO_3^- conserved)

From Harper.[14a]
*Movement to the right refers to moving from the left side of the equation above to the right side, therefore decreasing CO_2 production.

Table 4-3 Summary of the Alkalosis Process

$$CO_2 + H_2O <=> H_2CO_3 <=> H^+ + HCO_3^-$$

	Initial Cause	Compensation
Respiratory alkalosis	↓PCO_2	Kidneys Conservation of H^- HCO_3^- excretion (the lower the PCO_2, the less HCO_3^- reabsorbed)
Metabolic alkalosis	↑Base ↓Fixed acids	Kidneys Conserve H^+ by excreting HCO_3^- (the higher the plasma HCO_3^-, the greater the HCO_3^- excretion) Lungs (in severe alkalosis) ↓Ventilation to ↑PCO_2

Cough. Chemical or mechanical stimulation of the irritant receptors in the airway initiates a cough reflex. The high velocity created during a cough expels noxious materials and mucus.

Macrophage Clearance. Macrophages are specialized leukocytes that defend against particles that reach the alveolar level. Particles are either engulfed or transported out of the area by the macrophages.

Adaptive Immunity. Specific, or adaptive, lung defense mechanisms protect against particular types of antigenic substances or, in some instances, may initiate an injury response on the part of the lung. Specific mechanisms include immunoglobulins, cellular components, and classic activation of complement. In the process of normal aging, some adaptive lung defenses become less effective. Elderly persons are therefore increasingly vulnerable to respiratory infections.

Control of Breathing

The central respiratory centers are found in the medulla and pons. In addition, a less well-delineated area in the medulla contains chemoreceptors. These are referred to as the central chemoreceptors. Their major stimulus is pH change; they are depressed by hypoxia. The central respiratory centers also receive input from the cerebral cortex and the periphery. Voluntary breath holding is an example of higher cerebral input. Peripheral inputs include mechanical stimulation (irritant receptors in airways, J receptors in lung) and carotid body chemoreceptor response to PaO_2, $PaCO_2$, and pH.

To briefly summarize a complicated system, the greatest influence on the central nervous system's ventilation control comes from the concentration of carbon dioxide in the fluid around the central chemoreceptors. Carbon dioxide leads to the production of hydrogen ion that is a potent stimulus to the central chemoreceptors and results in an increase in the depth and rate of breathing. Sensory input comes from the peripheral chemoreceptors, mechanical receptors, and higher cortical centers; this input modifies the output of the respiratory centers to maintain acid-base balance, meet gas exchange needs (e.g., exercise), and provide for voluntary control (e.g., breath holding).

NORMAL FINDINGS*[18,35]

General appearance: Appears relaxed; breathing is quiet and easy without apparent effort; facial expressions and limb movements are relaxed

Breathing pattern: Pattern is smooth and regular; may have occasional sighing respirations; breathing is quiet and passive with symmetric chest expansion; abdomen bulges slightly with inhalation

⭘ Calcification at rib articulation points may decrease chest expansion

Respiratory rate: 12 to 20 respirations/minutes

Skin: Oral mucous membranes are pink; no cyanosis or pallor present

Palpation of skin and chest wall reveals smooth skin and a stable chest wall; no crepitations, masses, or painful areas

Nails: Angulation between base of nail and finger; no thickening of distal finger width; no clubbing

Chest wall configuration (FIG. 4-11)**:** Symmetric, bilateral muscle development; anteroposterior (A-P) to transverse

*⭘ = Older adult.

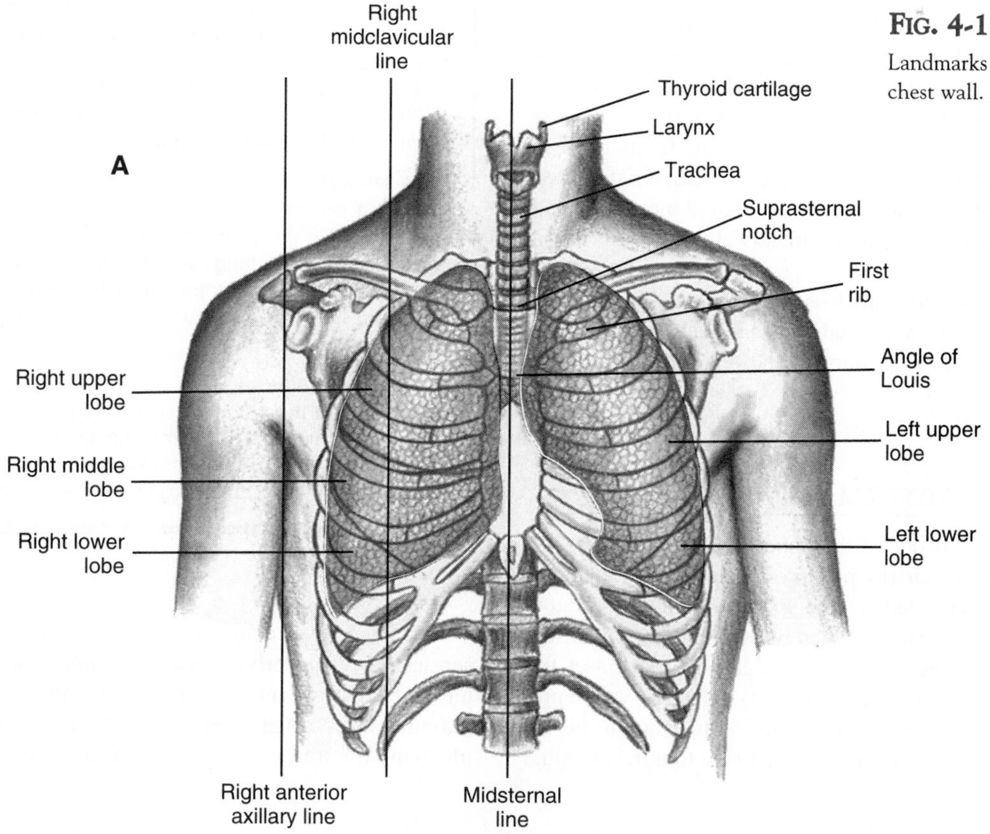

FIG. 4-11 Landmarks and structures of chest wall. **A,** Anterior view.

Continued

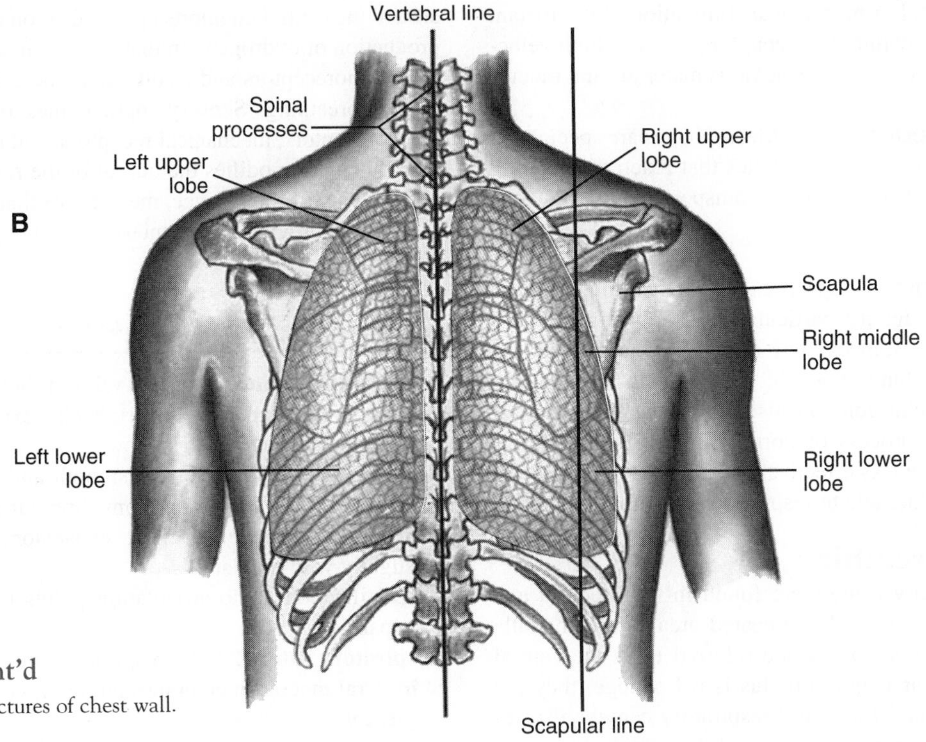

FIG. 4-11—cont'd
Landmarks and structures of chest wall.
B, Posterior view.

ratio is 1:2 to 5:7; straight spinal processes; downward and equal slope of ribs

- Kyphosis is a common finding in elderly persons; a decrease in intervertebral disk space size may cause a slight increase in the A-P/transverse ratio

Tracheal position: Midline and straight; directly above the suprasternal notch

- Trachea may be slightly deviated if kyphoscoliosis is present

Vocal fremitus: Bilaterally equal mild sensation; more intense vibratory feeling in upper posterior wall medial to scapula, decreases toward lung periphery; see box at right

Percussion: Resonance heard throughout lung fields; see FIG. 4-12 and Table 4-4 for percussion tone characteristics; percussion of diaphragmatic excursion should measure 4 to 6 cm; inhaled position is approximately at tenth posterior rib level

Auscultation: Quiet breathing heard throughout all lung fields; FIG. 4-13 shows normal sounds heard in each lung field, and Table 4-5 describes the normal and abnormal breath and voice sounds

OVERVIEW OF VOCAL FREMITUS

Vocal fremitus is the sensation of sound vibrations produced when the patient speaks.

The examiner may feel for these vibrations by placing the extended hand gently on the chest wall. The spoken voice produces low-frequency vibrations through the vocal cords, the airways, and the pleura. These vibrations are felt and compared bilaterally.

The examiner instructs the patient to say "one-two-three" or "how-now-brown-cow." As these words are spoken, the examiner feels for the vibrations.

ABNORMAL RESPONSES

Increased Fremitus

An increase in the vibratory sensation is felt when there is consolidation of the lung caused by fluid-filled or solid structures, which would transmit the vibrations better than air-filled lungs. This occurs, for example, with pneumonia or a tumor of the lung.

Decreased Fremitus

A decrease in the vibratory sensation is felt when more air than normal is blocked or trapped in the lungs or pleural space; vibrations of the spoken voice are decreased. This occurs, for example, with emphysema or a pneumothorax.

COMMON ABNORMAL FINDINGS

Cough. Cough is one of the important body reflexes. It is intended to maintain airway patency by eliminating materials accumulated or deposited on the mucosa of the respiratory tract, such as tracheobronchial secretions, blood, aspirated substances, and other foreign bodies. Cough of recent onset frequently is caused by an acute respiratory infection. A nonproductive cough may be the result of inflammation of the respiratory mucosa, bronchoconstriction, tumor, or other causes.

The intensity of cough has no relationship to the severity or seriousness of underlying bronchopulmonary disease. It is not unusual for a patient with serious pulmonary disease to have minimal or no cough. On the other hand, a mild viral infection involving the trachea or the bronchi may cause a troublesome cough.

Table 4-4 Percussion Tones

Type of Tone	Intensity	Pitch	Duration	Quality
Resonant	Loud	Low	Long	Hollow
Flat	Soft	High	Short	Extremely dull
Dull	Medium	Medium-high	Medium	Thudlike
Tympanic	Loud	High	Medium	Drumlike
Hyperresonant*	Very loud	Very low	Longer	Booming

*Hyperresonance is abnormal sound heard during percussion in adults. It represents air trapping such as occurs in obstructive lung diseases.

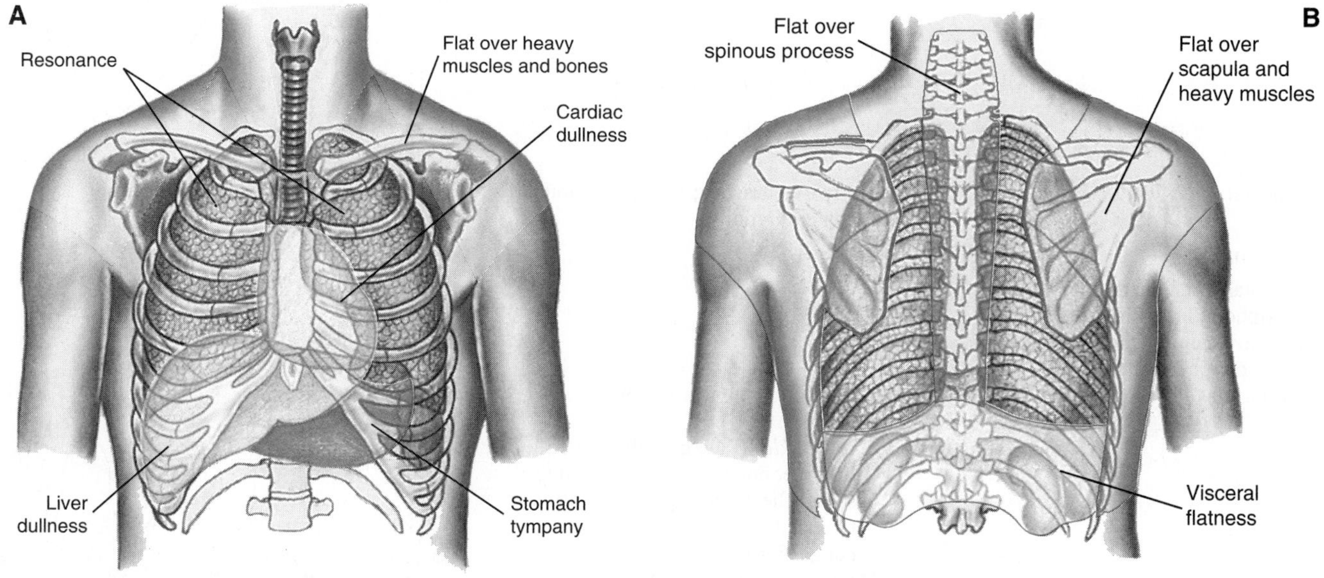

FIG. 4-12
Percussion tones. **A,** Anterior view. **B,** Posterior view.

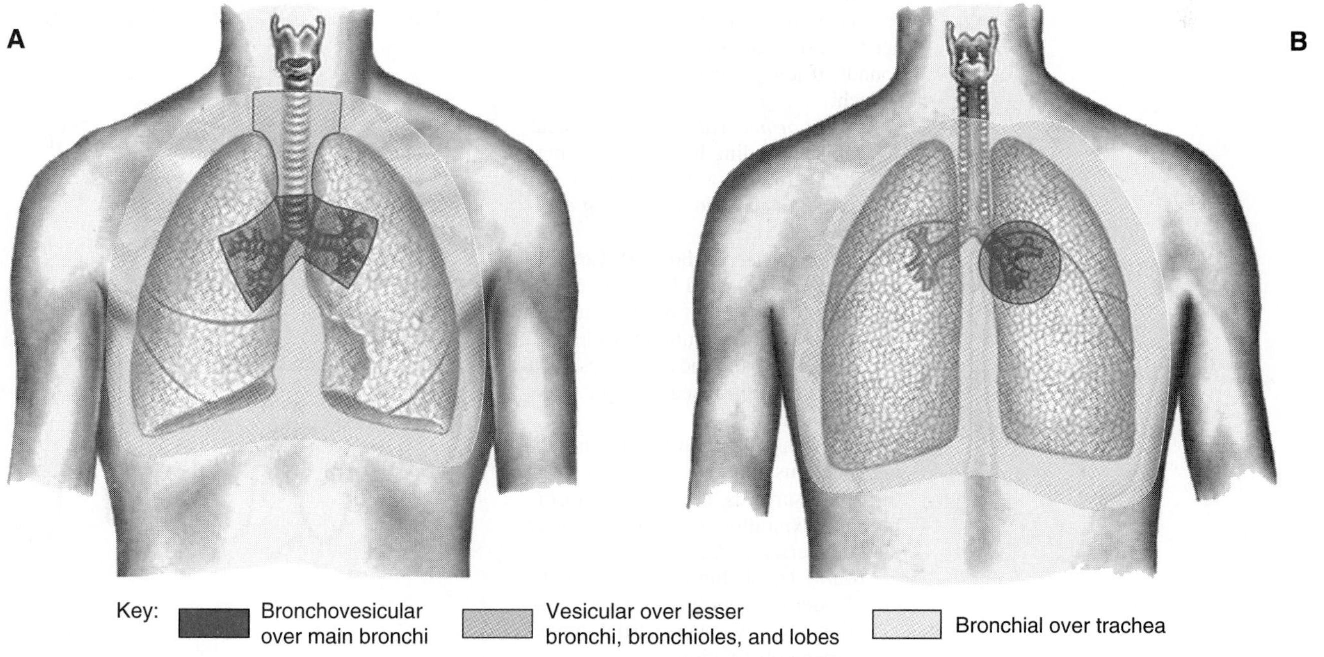

FIG. 4-13
Normal auscultatory sounds. **A,** Anterior view. **B,** Posterior view.

Table 4-5 Breath and Voice Sounds: Normal and Abnormal

Breath and Voice Sounds	Characteristics	Findings
NORMAL		
Vesicular	Heard over most of lung fields; low pitch; soft and short expirations (see FIG. 4-13)	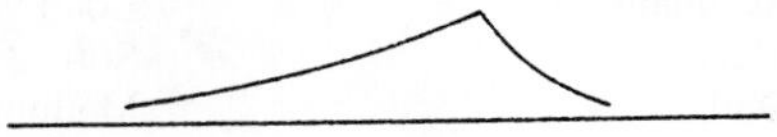 Low pitch, soft expirations
Bronchovesicular	Heard over main bronchus area and over upper right posterior lung field; medium pitch; expiration equals inspiration	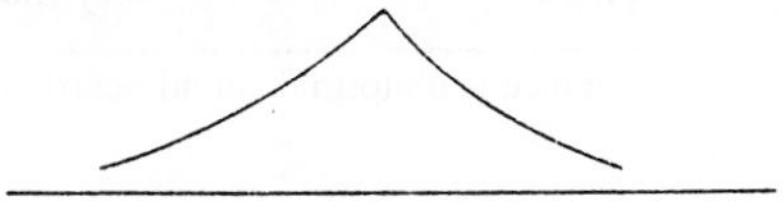 Medium pitch, medium expirations
Bronchial	Heard only over trachea; high pitch; loud and long expirations	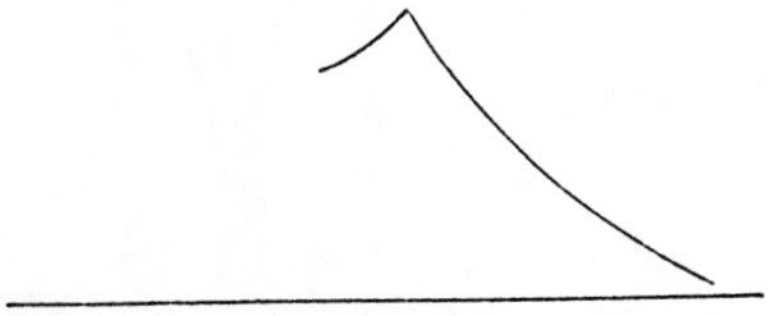 High pitch, loud expirations
ABNORMAL		
Bronchial when heard over peripheral lung fields		
Bronchovesicular when heard over peripheral lung fields		
Adventitious	Crackles: discrete, noncontinuous sounds	
	Fine crackles (rales): High-pitched, discrete, noncontinuous crackling sounds heard during end of inspiration (indicates inflammation or congestion)	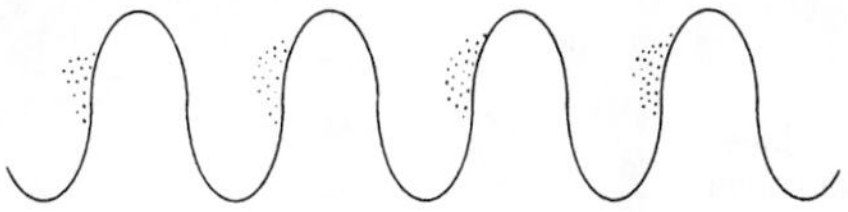
	Medium crackles (rales): Lower, moister sound heard during midstage of inspiration; not cleared by a cough	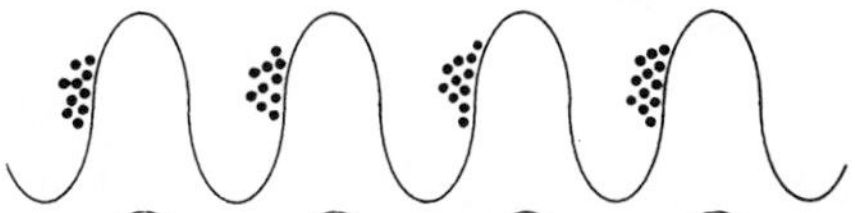
	Coarse crackles (rales): Loud, bubbly noise heard during inspiration; not cleared by a cough	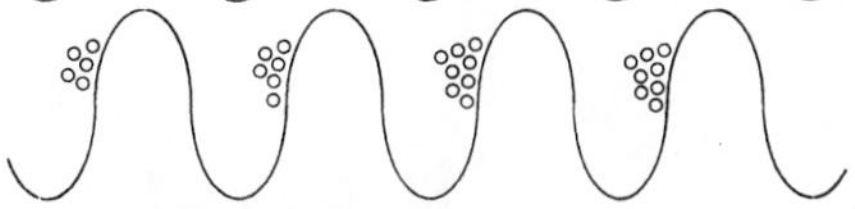
	Wheezes: Continuous musical sounds; if low pitched, may be called rhonchi	
	Sibilant or musical wheeze: Musical noise sounding like a squeak; may be heard during inspiration or expiration; usually louder during expiration	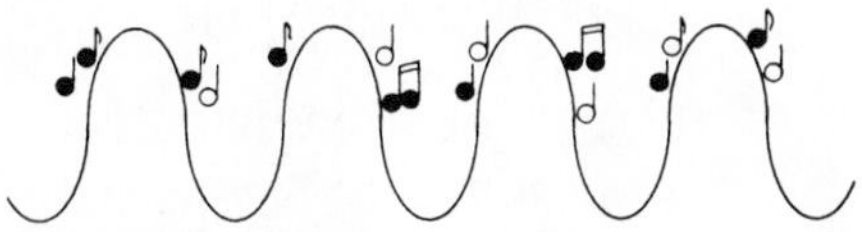
	Sonorous wheeze (rhonchi): Loud, low, coarse sound like a snore heard at any point of inspiration or expiration; coughing may clear sound (usually means mucus accumulation in trachea or large bronchi)	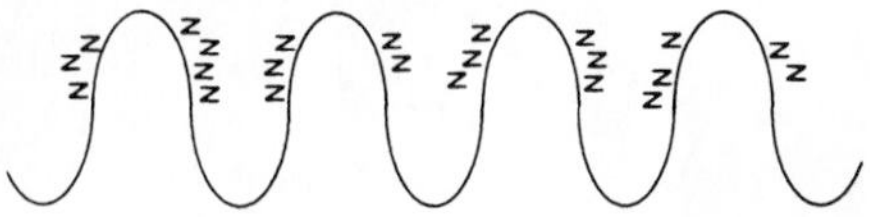
	Pleural friction rub: Dry, rubbing, or grating sound, usually due to inflammation of pleural surfaces; heard during inspiration or expiration; loudest over lower lateral anterior surface	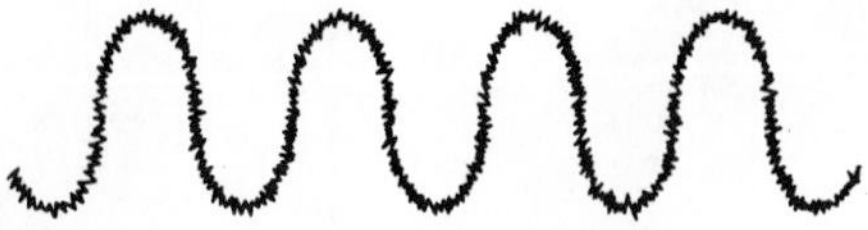
	Stridor: Harsh, high-pitched sound; louder on inspiration than expiration (usually means partial upper airway obstruction)	

Breath and Voice Sounds	Characteristics	Findings
Resonance of spoken voice	*Bronchophony:* Using diaphragm of stethoscope, listen to posterior chest as patient says "ninety-nine	Negative response: Muffled "nin-nin" sound heard Positive response: Clear, loud, "ninety-nine" response heard because lung tissues is consolidated
	Whispered pectoriloquy: Listen to posterior chest as patient whispers "one, two, three"	Negative response: Muffled sounds heard Positive response: Clear "one, two, three" is heard because of lung consolidation
	Egophony: Listen to posterior chest as the patient says "e-e-e"	Negative response: Muffled "e-e-e" sound heard Positive response: Sound of "e" changes to "a-a-a" sound because of consolidation

Expectoration. Expectoration is the act of coughing up and spitting material raised from the lower respiratory tract. Sputum consists of secretions formed continuously by the mucous glands and the goblet cells of the tracheobronchial tree.

In pathologic conditions, increased tracheobronchial secretions may result from stimulation of normal secretory cells or an increase in the number of these cells. In acute situations, increased sputum production is the result of transient stimulation of mucous glands and goblet cells. In addition to mucus, expectorated material may contain other fluids from various sites in the respiratory tract, including the alveoli. It may contain white blood cells accumulated for the purpose of fighting infection, necrotic material, blood, aspirated vomitus, or other foreign material.

The gross appearance of sputum may suggest the underlying condition. Normal sputum is a scant amount of clear to white thin mucus. Yellow sputum generally indicates the presence of large numbers of white blood cells, which are the major component of pus. Green discoloration signifies the production of an enzyme from stagnant pus. Red or brownish sputum is usually due to the presence of red blood cells.

Labored Breathing. When breathing requires a greater than usual effort, as in partial airway obstruction with mucus, or when needs for ventilation increase, as with intense exercise or a high fever, the normal relaxed respiratory effort becomes labored. Nasal flaring and open mouth breathing are efforts to increase the rate of airflow into the lungs. Shoulder and neck muscles are used to further expand the chest. Intercostal retractions are seen when an extremely negative pressure is created in the chest by forced attempts at deep inspiration. Abdominal muscles are contracted to increase the rate and force of exhalation, which allow for inspirations to occur more frequently.

Dyspnea. Dyspnea is a shortness of breath or difficulty breathing. The awareness of breathing may range in intensity from mild discomfort to extreme distress. Dyspnea, like pain, is a subjective sign likely to be influenced by the patient's reaction, sensitivity, and emotional state. Dyspnea involves both a physiologic and a cognitive component. Mild to moderate hypoxemia does not cause the sensation of dyspnea, although severe hypoxemia may. Dyspnea does not cause hypoxemia either, although pathologic processes may result in simultaneous dyspnea and hypoxemia.

Dyspnea is usually a result of impaired mechanical function and occurs under numerous clinical conditions. Some basic causes are increased airway resistance, as in upper airway obstruction, asthma, and airway obstructive diseases; reduced pulmonary compliance as a result of pulmonary fibrosis, congestion, edema, and various other parenchymal lung diseases; mechanical interference with lung expansion because of massive pleural effusion or pneumothorax; and abnormality of chest wall and respiratory muscles, resulting in inefficient respiratory efforts.

The circumstance in which the symptom occurs has diagnostic importance. Breathlessness may occur with certain body positions. Orthopnea refers to dyspnea relieved by sitting up. Paroxysmal nocturnal dyspnea is the sudden onset of shortness of breath during the night that occurs in cardiac patients. The cause is thought to be transient pulmonary edema as a result of intravascular reabsorption of peripheral edema fluid.

A recent increase in dyspnea in a patient with chronic respiratory disease indicates an acute event. This may result from increased airway resistance, as with bronchospasm, secretions, and infection, or reduced pulmonary compliance, as with pulmonary congestion or edema.

Hemoptysis. Hemoptysis is the expectoration of blood from the respiratory tract below the pharynx. The three major conditions causing hemoptysis are infection, neoplasm, and cardiovascular disease. Common infectious causes of hemoptysis are pneumonia, tuberculosis, bronchiectasis, and lung abscess. Bronchogenic carcinoma is the neoplastic disease that most commonly causes hemoptysis. Hemoptysis is a symptom of certain cardiovascular diseases, such as pulmonary embolism, congestive heart failure, and mitral stenosis.

Chest Pain. Chest pain of pulmonary origin can derive from the chest wall, parietal pleura, or visceral pleura. The thoracic wall is the most common source of chest pain; skin, muscles, nerves, and bones may cause pain. The lung parenchyma is insensitive to painful stimuli; however, the parietal layer of the pleura is very pain sensitive. Pathologic processes involving the parietal pleura commonly cause either a dull, poorly localized chest pain or a sharp pleuritic pain that is aggravated by deep breathing and chest wall movement.

Pain with pneumonia and the other inflammatory diseases of the lung, as well as the pain of pulmonary embolism, is due to pleural reaction. In lung cancer, chest pain is frequently indicative of pleural reaction or chest wall invasion. Pulmonary arterial hypertension sometimes causes chest pain because of increased tension in the arterial walls or strain on the right side of the heart muscle.

CONDITIONS, DISEASES, AND DISORDERS

INFECTIOUS DISEASES OF THE LUNG

This section will concentrate on two of the common infectious problems: acute bronchitis and pneumonia. The pneumonia section will discuss both community acquired and nosocomial pneumonias. The common contagious diseases (e.g., tuberculosis) and fungal diseases are covered in Chapter 15.

ACUTE BRONCHITIS

Acute bronchitis is an inflammation of the bronchi, trachea, or both that results from irritation or infection (FIG. 4-14).

Acute bronchitic infections may occur in otherwise healthy people or may occur as exacerbations in persons with underlying chronic lung disease. These acute airway infections are most common in the winter and are usually viral (common agents include respiratory syncytial virus, rhinoviruses, adenovirus, and influenza) in etiology, although bacterial causes also occur (*Streptococcus pneumoniae, Hemophilus influenzae*). Exposure to toxic environmental agents such as fumes from strong acids or ammonia can also cause an acute bronchitic response (Table 4-6).

In the healthy individual the acute inflammatory process usually resolves without pharmacologic therapy. If the patient already has a chronic pulmonary or cardiovascular disease, acute bronchitis may become serious. Pneumonia is the most common complication.

PATHOPHYSIOLOGY

Congestion of the bronchial mucous membranes is the earliest physiologic change. This is followed by desquamation or shedding of the submucosa. The congestion and shedding process causes submucosal edema with leukocyte infiltration. This process interferes with the normal function of the ciliated bronchial epithelium and the phagocytes. The result is a sticky or mucopurulent exudate that stays in the bronchi until coughed out.

The impaired function of the mucociliary escalator system may allow a secondary bacterial infection. At the beginning of the disease process the sputum of a patient with acute bronchitis is normally mucoid. If the sputum becomes mucopurulent or purulent, a superimposed bacterial infection is suspected.

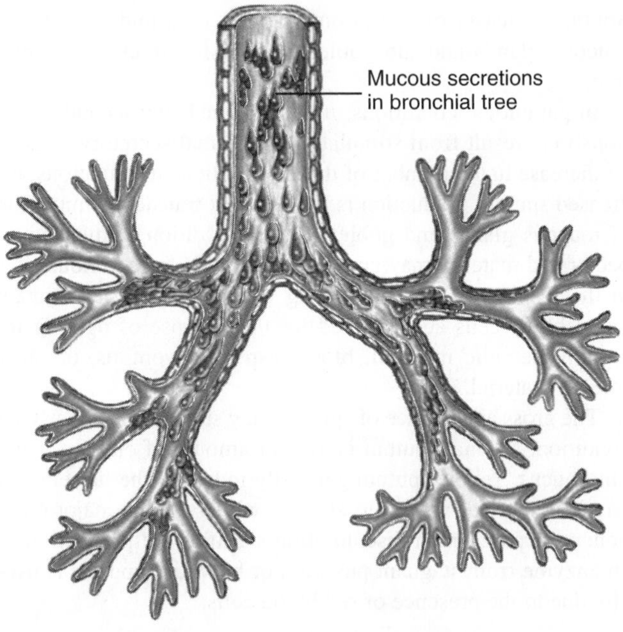

FIG. 4-14
Acute bronchitis. (From Wilson and Thompson.[41])

Table 4-6 Noninfectious Agents Commonly Causing Acute Bronchitis and Pneumonitis

Product	Industry	Injury
Aldehydes (acrylaldehyde, formaldehyde, and acetaldehydes)	Plastic, rubber, textiles, resins, disinfectant	Bronchitis, asthma
Ammonia	Fertilizer, explosives, refrigeration	Tracheobronchitis, pulmonary edema
Chlorine and hydrochloric acid	Bleaches, disinfectants, plastics, refining, dye making, organic chemical synthesis	Tracheobronchitis, pulmonary edema
Nitrogen dioxide	Fertilizer, dyes, explosives, farming, rockets, arc welding	Tracheobronchitis, pulmonary edema, bronchiolitis obliterans
Ozone	Arc welding, sewage and water treatment	Tracheobronchitis
Phosgene	Chemical industry, dyes, insecticides	Tracheobronchitis, pulmonary edema
Sulfur dioxide	Bleaching, smelting, paper manufacture, refrigeration	Tracheobronchitis, pulmonary edema (rare)

From Cherniack.[9]

Acute bronchitic infections may also increase bronchial hyperreactivity.

Diagnostic Studies and Findings

Clinical examination: Cough initially dry and nonproductive but may produce mucoid sputum within a few days of onset; often preceded by symptoms of an upper respiratory infection (runny nose, sneezing, sore throat, malaise); fever (38.3° to 38.9° C [101° to 102° F]) if cause is bacterial; midsternal chest pain (raw sensation), scattered crackles and rhonchi; if patient already has chronic lung disease, sputum may change from clear and thin to thick and tenacious or purulent.

Chest roentgenogram: Normal chest film.

Multidisciplinary Plan

The goals of the treatment plan are to provide supportive therapy during the course of the self-limited disease and to prevent secondary infections.

Medications

Antitussive agents

Nonnarcotic cough suppressants: Many agents available such as dextromethorphan (Romilar, Benylin CM, Pertussin, Congespirin), 10-20 mg or 30 mg q6-8h; often reserved for bedtime use to help rest; if used too frequently will become ineffective.

Narcotic cough suppressants: Use with extreme caution in patients with chronic lung disease.

Hydrocodone bitartrate (Codone, Dicodid, Hycodan), 5-10 mg tid or qid

Codeine phosphate (tablets and in mixture form in numerous syrups), 10-20 mg q4-6h

Bronchodilators: Beta-2 agonists (e.g., Albuterol) by aerosol (metered dose inhaler or small volume nebulizer).

Antiinfective agents: Most cases of bronchitis are viral, so antibacterial medications are not effective.

Antibiotics: Used when superimposed respiratory infection is suspected on basis of clinical evidence such as purulent sputum, high fever, and ill-appearing patient; antibiotics also indicated for patients with chronic obstructive lung disease. Usually a broad-spectrum antibiotic is used, such as a macrolide (Biaxin) in younger adults, while a drug such as Bactrim would be used in those over age 60 years.

Antipyretic-analgesics: To reduce fever and relieve malaise.

Antiinflammatories: Corticosteroids may be administered when there is persistent cough and intermittent wheeze as a response to the airway inflammation.

General Management

Increase in fluid intake to maintain hydration

Steam or mist vaporizer to humidify inspired air

Rest to conserve energy

Culture of sputum if sputum becomes purulent or patient's illness becomes progressively worse

Chest roentgenogram is not indicated unless symptoms indicate progression of disease

NURSING CARE

Nursing Assessment

Because acute bronchitis is generally a self-limited disease, assessment is important to identify complications, superimposed infections, or adverse effects of therapy.

Respiratory status: Cough, characteristics and duration, and sputum production are often the only symptoms; may complain of chest wall soreness due to coughing; others, as follows, should be reported because they may indicate progression:

Musical and/or sonorous wheeze (rhonchi); crackles; dyspnea; chest tightness (often associated with wheeze); pleuritic chest wall pain; fever

Potential Complications

Pneumonia, exacerbation of airway obstructive disease

Patient Problems/Nursing Diagnoses & Interventions

NIC Respiratory Management

Ineffective airway clearance related to mucopurulent sputum and airway inflammation

- Assess patient to identify inability to move secretions. If inability is identified, assist with appropriate measures (coughing, positioning, liquifying secretions, and so on).
- If chest wall soreness, use towel to splint chest.
- Provide adequate hydration to avoid viscous secretions.
- Assess for signs and symptoms of infection, fever, dyspnea, and change in sputum color, amount, or odor.
- Obtain sputum for culture and sensitivity.
- Protect patient from known sources of secondary infection.

Patient Education/Continuum of Care Plan

1. Teach patient measures to treat episode, symptoms of progression, and how to access health-care delivery system if symptoms progress.
2. Teach elderly or those with comorbid conditions to request annual influenza vaccine.

Evaluation/Patient Outcomes

Respiratory Management: Airways are patent. Breathing occurs without cough or substernal tightness. Breath sounds are clear. Secondary infection is prevented. Temperature and white blood cell (WBC) count within normal limits. Sputum expectorated effectively, appears clear to white, volume decreasing. Fatigue is minimized. Cough is decreased. Sufficient sleep/rest is obtained.

Pneumonia[42]

Pneumonia is an inflammatory process of the respiratory bronchioles and the alveolar spaces that is caused by infection.

The clinical definition of pneumonia includes evidence of consolidation on the chest x-ray, fever (>38.3° C), elevated WBC count, and purulent secretions. Pneumonia may be caused by bacteria, viruses, *Mycoplasma pneumoniae* (often referred to as "atypical pneumonia"), fungi, and parasites. Pneumonia is often classified as community acquired (CAP) or nosocomial (acquired after 48 hours in the hospital).

Estimates indicate that there are 4 million cases of CAP every year; approximately 20% of these require hospitalization. Although no causative organism can be identified in 50% of cases, the most common organism identified is *S. pneumoniae.* The emergence of drug-resistant strains of *S. pneumoniae* is cause for concern. Other common causes of CAP are *M. pneumoniae* and *H. influenzae.* Uncommon pathogens that have gained a certain amount of public notoriety are *Legionella* and the hantavirus. CAP occurs most often during the winter and early spring and in persons age 60 years or older. The following co-existing conditions also put persons at increased risk to develop pneumonia: chronic obstructive pulmonary disease (COPD), diabetes, chronic liver disease, congestive heart failure, chronic renal failure, malnourishment, and altered mental state.

Persons most at risk for nosocomial (hospital-acquired) pneumonia are the very young or very old, those with cardiopulmonary disease, immunosuppression, decreased level of consciousness, or after chest/abdominal surgery. The most common causative organisms in hospital-acquired pneumonias are *S. aureus, P. aeruginosa,* and *Enterobacter.* As with CAP, the emergence of drug-resistant strains (e.g., MRSA) is a matter of concern. Nosocomial infections are often caused by anaerobic organisms, which cause necrosis of lung tissue that can progress to lung abscess and bronchopleural fistula. Pathogens such as *Pneumocystis carinii,* which are associated with immunosuppression, were discussed in Chapter 2.

Additional terms, related to cause or distribution, are often used to describe a pneumonia. A common one is *aspiration pneumonia,* the term used to describe a pneumonia resulting from the inspiration of substances into the lower airways. Usually the patient is in an altered state of consciousness because of a seizure, drugs, alcohol, anesthesia, acute infection, or shock. Aspiration may also occur when the anatomy is altered by esophageal stricture, tracheal fistula, or a nasogastric tube or when neuromuscular disease impairs the swallowing mechanism. The development of pneumonia may be caused by foreign body aspiration with airway obstruction or aspiration of body substances such as saliva or gastric contents. Even when bacteria are not present, these substances irritate the epithelial lining of the lung, resulting in an extensive inflammatory response. *Lobar pneumonia* refers to consolidation of an entire lobe (FIG. 4-15). *Bronchopneumonia* involves the airway and alveoli and results in a patchy distribution of infectious areas around and involving the bronchi. A chest roentgenogram of bronchopneumonia shows patchy segmental or subsegmental infiltration in one or more dependent lobes. Mycoplasmal and viral pneumonias produce the *"atypical" pneumonia.* The chest roentgenogram demonstrates variable findings; a defined area of consolidation is often lacking.

PATHOPHYSIOLOGY

The introduction of the infecting agent is usually by inhalation of droplet nuclei but may also occur with aspiration of oral pharyngeal contents. The specific pathologic picture depends on the etiologic agent. *S. pneumoniae* is the organism best studied; it is marked by an intraalveolar suppurative exudate with consolidation. In the atypical pneumonias there is usually an acute bronchiolitis or damage to the cilia; inflammatory cells invade the interstitium and alveoli. Regardless of the specific etiologic agent, the pneumonias result in decreased ventilation to the involved area with resulting low V/Q and hypoxemia.

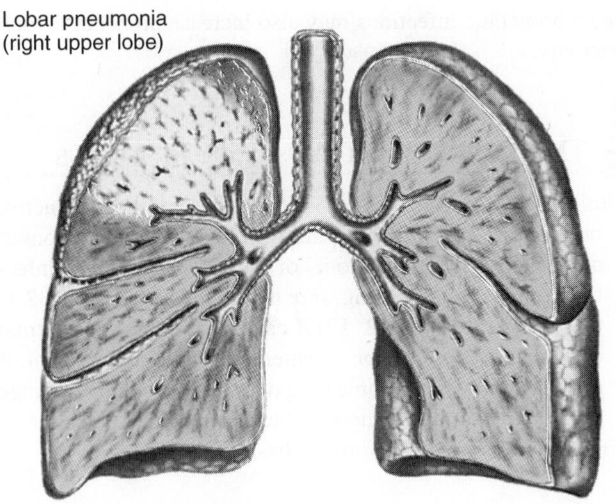

Pneumococcal pneumonia

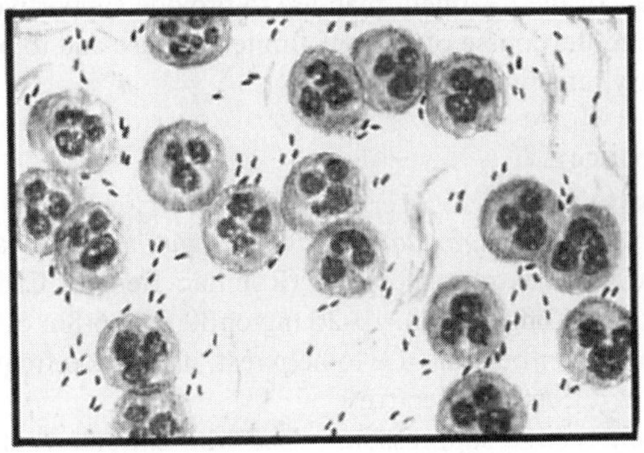

Purulent sputum with pneumococci and polymorphonuclear leukocytes

FIG. 4-15
Pneumonia. (From Wilson and Thompson.[41])

DIAGNOSTIC STUDIES AND FINDINGS

Typical Pneumonia (Bacterial, Usually *S. pneumoniae*)

Clinical appearance: Fever and chills, pleuritic chest pain, cough, sputum
Chest auscultation: Crackles, may be areas of decreased breath sounds, dullness if large consolidated areas
Laboratory findings: Leukocytosis with left shift (increased polymorphonuclear leukocytes [PMNs] and band cells)
Chest roentgenogram: Lobar consolidation (FIG. 4-16)

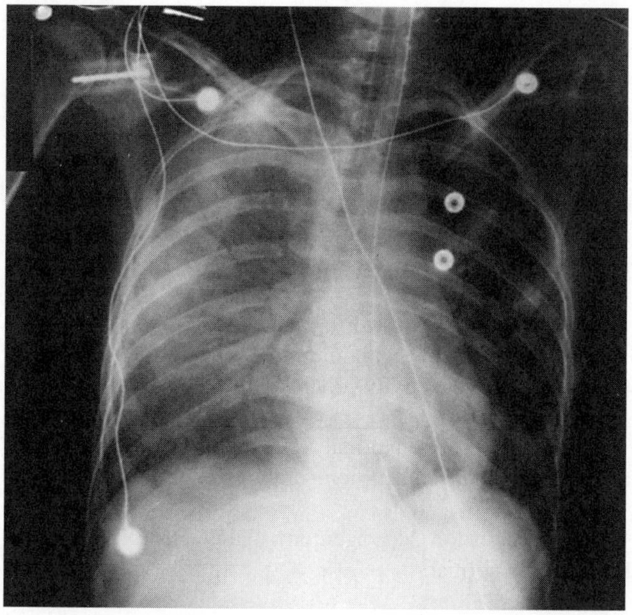

FIG. 4-16

Chest roentgenogram of patient with pneumonia. Note infiltrate of right middle and lower zones with air bronchogram seen; right heart border not obliterated. Also note monitor electrodes, gown snaps, endotracheal tube, and ventilator tubing. (Courtesy R. Keith Wilson, MD, Baylor College of Medicine, Houston, Tex.)

Atypical Pneumonia (*Mycoplasma pneumoniae*)

Clinical appearance: Patient usually young, dry cough, malaise, moderate fever

Chest auscultation: Few to no findings on chest auscultation

Laboratory findings: WBC often normal

Chest roentgenogram: Highly variable, diffuse infiltrates

Typical and Atypical Pneumonia

Cultures: In all patients requiring hospitalization for pneumonia, an attempt is made to obtain sputum or bronchial secretions for culture and sensitivity. Other special studies may also be indicated, such as special stains (e.g., acid-fast stain for tuberculosis), viral cultures, or polymerase chain reaction. If an adequate expectorated sputum sample cannot be obtained, bronchial secretions may be obtained by fiberoptic bronchoscopy or suction. Blood cultures may also be used to identify the organism.

Blood gases: Hypoxemia (decreased Pa_{O_2}); usually hyperventilation (decreased Pa_{CO_2}), but in the presence of other comorbid conditions, may see hypoventilation (elevated Pa_{CO_2}).

MULTIDISCIPLINARY PLAN

Medications

Antiinfective agents specific to cultured organisms; if complications such as abscess are present, antiinfective therapy is for much longer duration

General Management

Oxygenation: Oxygen usually by nasal cannula if patient has Pa_{O_2} less than 60 mm Hg

General supportive measures: Hydration, antipyretics, etc.

NURSING CARE

NURSING ASSESSMENT

Respiratory status: Tachypnea; retractions; labored breathing; dyspnea; nasal flaring; crackles; rhonchi with large airway secretions; pleural friction rub; diminished breath sounds over area of consolidation; labored or irregular breathing; breathing tiring for patient; percussion tone dull over area of consolidation; monitor oxygenation by pulse oximetry arterial blood gases; hypoxemia will also contribute to tachycardia, restlessness, confusion; may see cyanosis

Cough and sputum: Amount and productivity of cough; color, consistency, odor, and amount of sputum; fatigue related to coughing; chest wall pain contributing to decreased cough effort; cough effectiveness/ease of expectoration

Gas exchange: Hospitalized patient usually hypoxemic and hyperventilating; if patient seriously ill, monitor for decreased pH and Pa_{O_2} and increased Pa_{CO_2} (O_2 <60, CO_2 >50 on room air)

Laboratory values: Evidence of elevated leukocyte count with left shift (increased neutrophils); inability to mount an elevated WBC count is a poor prognostic sign, as is a very high WBC count (>30,000 or <4000 = poor prognostic sign); anemia (hemoglobin <9 g), serum creatinine over 1.2 are poor prognostic signs because they indicate underlying chronic illness

Temperature: Monitor for elevation

Hydration state: Intake and output; tissue turgor; liquidity of sputum; electrolytes

POTENTIAL COMPLICATIONS

Pleural effusion, atelectasis, empyema, lung abscess, meningitis, and sepsis

PATIENT PROBLEMS/NURSING DIAGNOSES & INTERVENTIONS

NIC RESPIRATORY MANAGEMENT

Ineffective airway clearance related to mucopurulent sputum, impaired mucociliary function, pain with deep breathing and cough

Impaired gas exchange related to impaired V/Q relationships (low V/Q and shunt)

Ineffective breathing pattern related to pleuritic pain, and increased ventilatory drive

Impaired oral mucous membrane related to mouth breathing and infectious condition

- Assist with cough: teach effective techniques, assist to splint chest wall with coughing if painful.
- If patient unable to clear airway, suction.
- Promptly administer bronchodilators per protocol to *dilate airways;* observe for therapeutic response and side effects.
- Provide hydration to *liquify secretions and replace fluids.*

- Administer mucolytics and expectorants *to liquify secretions and promote expectoration.*
- Position *to facilitate use of accessory muscle ventilation* (head of bed in semi-Fowler's position or patient sitting and leaning forward on overbed table).
- Assist with mouth care, especially after respiratory treatments and before meals.
- In patients with copious secretions or lung abscess, position *to facilitate drainage of involved area* (postural drainage with/without percussion and vibration, see p. 205).
- If necessary and with physician consultation, administer oxygen by nasal cannula or Venturi mask to maintain Pao_2 above 60 mm Hg.

NIC ACTIVITY AND EXERCISE MANAGEMENT

Risk for activity intolerance related to hypoxemia, increased work of breathing
Fatigue related to infection, increased metabolic demands, frequent cough

- Provide for rest periods.
- Encourage gradual increase of activities as tolerated.
- Monitor oxygen during exercise to determine if supplemental oxygen is needed.
- If patient is seriously ill and maintained on bed rest, encourage or provide active or passive range of motion *to maintain adequate muscle tone.*

NIC RISK MANAGEMENT

Risk for imbalanced body temperature caused by infection
Risk for infection related to ineffective airway clearance (secondary infection)

- Monitor temperature and give antipyretics as indicated.
- Monitor for signs of superimposed infection, progression.
- Provide airway care as above.
- Help patient choose foods that are easy to chew and swallow.
- Assist by cutting and feeding if patient tires easily.

NIC TISSUE PERFUSION MANAGEMENT

Risk for deficient fluid volume as a result of increased insensible loss, decreased intake

- Monitor intake and output (I and O).
- Evaluate skin turgor and buccal mucosa for fluid deficit.

PATIENT EDUCATION/CONTINUUM OF CARE PLAN

1. Teach appropriate airway care measures.
2. Teach patient medications: how to take, when to take, how long to take, possible side effects.
3. Teach signs of worsening infection, complications, and means of contacting care provider if needed.
4. Ensure patient has follow-up appointment.

EVALUATION/PATIENT OUTCOMES

Respiratory Management: Airway is patent. Cough and sputum production have at least decreased if not disappeared. (For many, cough may be present for several weeks.) If sputum is still present, color has cleared and amount is decreasing. Breath sounds are present in all lung fields; adventitial sounds (rhonchi, crackles) are absent or at least decreased. Chest roentenogram demonstrates clearing. Blood gases are within normal range for the individual. (Note that patients are often discharged from hospital before complete clearing, return of blood gases to normal; patients with underlying COPD may require a month post–hospital stay to return to baseline.)

Activity and Exercise Management: Activities of daily living are accomplished with minimal fatigue. Patient states importance of gradual activity progression.

Risk Management: Normal weight is maintained; patient is eating a well-balanced diet; temperature is normal.

Tissue Perfusion Management: Fluid intake is adequate; skin turgor is normal.

ATELECTASIS[4]

Atelectasis is a condition in which all or part of the normally aerated and expanded lung collapses because of the absence of air in the alveoli.

Atelectasis is a common complication of thoracic or upper abdominal surgery or prolonged bed rest. Regional hypoventilation leads to alveolar collapse and bronchial obstruction with mucus. Atelectasis may also be caused by complete obstruction of an airway or compression of the lung tissue from hemothorax, pneumothorax, or tumor. High-level oxygen therapy may cause absorption atelectasis.

PATHOPHYSIOLOGY

Atelectasis that results from hypoventilation may progress from minor to extensive respiratory compromise. In airway blockage the extent of atelectasis depends on the site and rapidity of the blockage. If the mainstem bronchus to one lung is blocked, that entire lung becomes atelectatic and respiratory compromise is great. If only a small bronchiole becomes slowly blocked because of a buildup of secretions, symptoms may be minor and the respiratory system is able to compensate.

When airway blockage occurs, the gas distal to the obstruction is absorbed into the circulation because the oxygen tension in the pulmonary capillaries is lower than the oxygen tension in the alveoli. The higher the oxygen concentration (FIo_2) of the inspired air at the time of the blockage, the faster is the alveolar collapse. Alveolar collapse results in hypoxemia unless lung compensatory mechanisms transfer blood flow to unaffected areas of the lung.

DIAGNOSTIC STUDIES AND FINDINGS

Arterial blood gases: Pao_2 less than 80 mm Hg; $Paco_2$ may be normal, low as a result of hyperventilation with hypoxemia, or elevated as a result of underlying disease

Serial chest roentgenograms: Airless area visualized; trachea and heart in mediastinum deviated toward atelectatic area; diaphragm elevated on affected side; rib spaces narrowed

MULTIDISCIPLINARY PLAN

The ultimate treatment plan for atelectasis is effective management of the underlying cause

Bronchoscopy: May be performed to remove retained secretions or possible foreign bodies when atelectasis is not relieved by suction, coughing and deep breathing, or postural drainage

Thoracostomy with chest tube placement: Performed to relieve atelectasis caused by compression such as hemothorax or pneumothorax

Medications

Bronchodilators given by nebulizer: Albuterol, metaproterenol sulfate (Alupent)

Mucolytic agents such a *N*-acetylcysteine given by nebulizer if sputum is thick

Antiinfective agents (use is controversial): Broad-spectrum antibiotic (e.g., penicillin or ampicillin) given as soon as symptoms are noted; drug may be modified appropriately if specific pathogen is isolated from bronchial secretions

NURSING CARE

NURSING ASSESSMENT

Respiratory status: Tachypnea; dyspnea; retractions; nasal flaring; crackles, diminished breath sounds over affected area; percussion tones dull or flat over affected area if the atelectatic area is large.

Laboratory values: Pulse oximetry every 4 hours, or continuously for hypoxemic patients; maintain Spo_2 >93% or as ordered

Arterial blood gases: Report increases or decreases of more than 10 mm Hg in $Paco_2$ and Pao_2

Cardiovascular status: Electrocardiogram for dysrhythmias resulting from alterations in blood gases

Infection: Body temperature, which may increase as a result of secondary infection or ineffective treatment

POTENTIAL COMPLICATIONS

Hypoxia: Restlessness; confusion; tachycardia; hypertension early; hypotension late; cyanosis

Bronchopulmonary infection: Temperature elevation; sputum color changes, purulence

PATIENT PROBLEMS/NURSING DIAGNOSES & INTERVENTIONS

NIC RESPIRATORY MANAGEMENT

Impaired gas exchange related to alveolar collapse
Ineffective airway clearance related to bronchial obstruction
Preventive measures

- Teach patient and family deep breathing and cough techniques preoperatively.
- After surgery or during periods of bed rest, encourage deep breathing and coughing hourly; reposition patient every 1 to 2 hours. After surgery, position patient with pillow along incision site to function as a splint.
- Use incentive spirometry to *encourage deep breathing.*
- Control pain, while avoiding excessive doses of sedatives, which depress cough reflex and respirations.
- Begin ambulation as soon and as often as tolerated.
- Liquify secretions by humidifying inspired air and maintaining body hydration.

If lobar atelectasis is present, add:

- Position patient with the uninvolved side in a dependent position *to promote drainage of the affected area* (postural drainage).
- Perform percussion and vibration over affected area *to mobilize secretions and reexpand lung* (see p. 205 for technique).

PATIENT EDUCATION/CONTINUUM OF CARE PLAN

1. Teach patient and family to continue deep breathing and cough techniques at home.
2. Teach splinting of incisions and pain control measures that allow for deep breathing and coughing effectively.
3. Teach correct use of the incentive spirometer, to continue every 1 to 2 hours while awake for 48 hours postoperatively, or until risk of atelectasis has decreased.

EVALUATION/PATIENT OUTCOMES

Respiratory Management: Airway is patent. No signs of respiratory distress are noted. Breath sounds are clear throughout. Chest x-ray is clear. Gas exchange is effective. Arterial blood gases are within normal limits.

PLEURAL DISEASES[3,27,31,37]

The pleural space normally contains only a few milliliters of lubricating fluid. If the pleural space fills with air or liquid, the lung cannot fully expand in the thoracic cavity. Pleural effusion, empyema, pneumothorax, and hemothorax are all problems related to unusual accumulations in the pleural space.

PLEURAL EFFUSION

A pleural effusion develops when excess nonpurulent fluid accumulates in the pleural space between the visceral and parietal pleurae (FIG. 4-17).

Pleural effusion is not a disease but generally occurs as a secondary problem when lymphatic drainage or capillary membrane permeability is altered.

PATHOPHYSIOLOGY

The viscera and parietal pleurae form a continuous sac, lining the lung and the chest wall. Normally only a potential space containing less than 10 ml of fluid separates these surfaces. Fluid continuously moves in and out of the pleural space because of a balance between hydrostatic pressures, colloidal

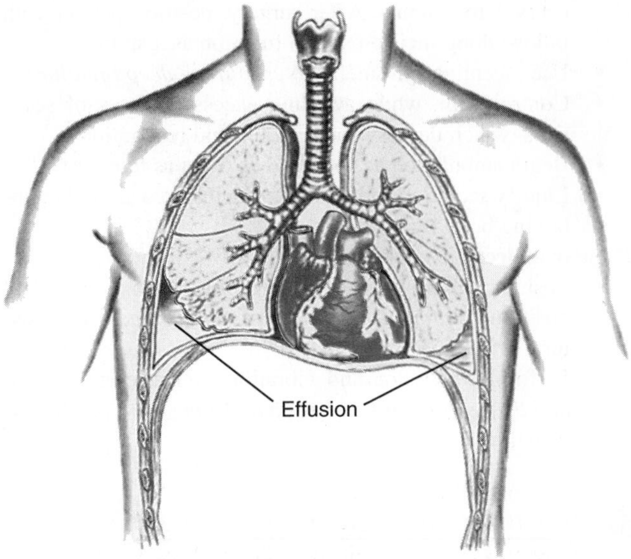

FIG. 4-17
Pleural effusion. (From Wilson and Thompson.[41])

osmotic pressures, and the membrane characteristics of capillaries and pleurae. An alteration in this balance can lead to the formation of an effusion.

Pleural effusions may be divided into two categories: transudates and exudates. The distinction between transudate and exudate is based on the protein content of aspirated fluid.

Transudates accumulate as a result of a disturbance in fluid pressures. Increased capillary pressure in heart failure and reduced plasma oncotic pressure in certain kidney or liver diseases are known causes of transudate accumulation. Transudate fluid is clear or pale yellow, has a specific gravity of 1.015 or less, and has a protein content that is either normal or less than 3 g/dl.

Exudates result from a disease of the pleural surface or an obstruction in the lymphatic system that inhibits the drainage of proteins. Exudates are often associated with infection. The fluid is dark yellow or amber, with a specific gravity greater than 1.016, a protein content greater than 3 g/dl, and an increased WBC count. If the effusion is grossly purulent, it is called an empyema. A bloody effusion without history of chest trauma suggests malignancy or pulmonary embolism.

DIAGNOSTIC STUDIES AND FINDINGS

Chest roentgenogram: Effusions typically located at a dependent area of the pleural space; moderate amount of fluid (250 to 300 ml) must accumulate to be seen on upright posterior-anterior, decubitus, or lateral chest roentgenogram; effusion seen as dense opacity (FIG. 4-18); large effusions may obliterate a hemithorax

Thoracentesis: For pleural fluid analysis; stain, culture, and sensitivity of pleural fluid; cytologic examination of pleural fluid for evaluation of potential neoplastic involvement

Pleural biopsy with tissue analysis: Indicated when fluid analysis fails to establish cause

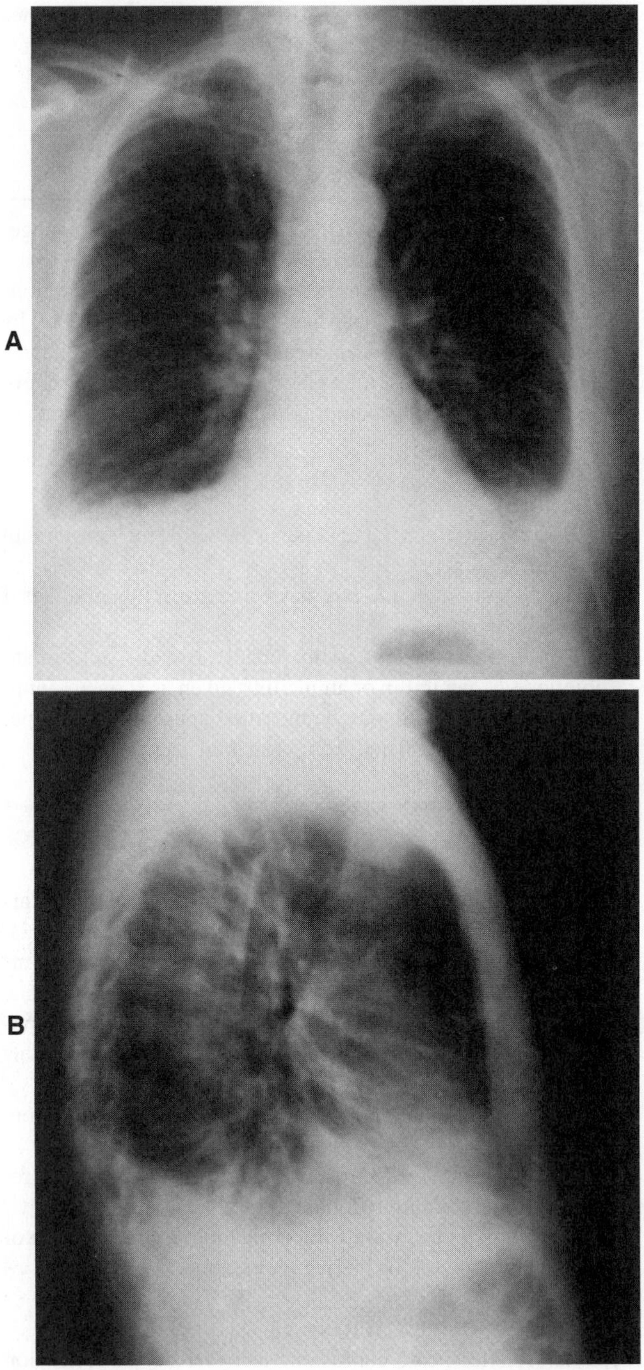

FIG. 4-18
Chest roentgenogram of patient with pleural effusion. **A,** PA view: note obliteration of costophrenic angles bilaterally; pulmonary vasculature appears normal. **B,** Lateral view: note lack of costophrenic angles. (Courtesy R. Keith Wilson, MD, Baylor College of Medicine, Houston, Tex.)

MULTIDISCIPLINARY PLAN

Treatment of pleural effusion depends on the etiology and clinical consequences. The following discussion refers to the general treatment of effusion. Refer also to the section of the text dealing with the cause of the effusion, such as renal failure or congestive heart failure.

Thoracentesis: To drain excess fluid from pleural space and relieve dyspnea or hypoxemia

Thoracostomy: Tube may be connected to underwater seal drainage system and left in place if accumulation of fluids is large and compromising respiratory function

If pleural effusion is caused by malignancy, tube may be inserted to drain fluid and left in place to provide insertion point for medications and therapeutic techniques such as pleurodesis

Medications

Antibiotics: Administered if effusion is thought to be caused by infectious process

General Management

Treatment of underlying disease or problem causing effusion

NURSING CARE

NURSING ASSESSMENT

Respiratory status: Respiratory distress: nasal flaring; tachypnea; decreased chest wall movement; dyspnea; restlessness; tachycardia; decreased breath sounds; paradoxic breathing; dullness to percussion, which shifts with change in position; decreased or absent breath sounds over affected area; egophony above effusion site; dyspnea if effusion has occurred rapidly; if effusion is large, intercostal bulging or decreased chest wall movement during breathing, pleuritic chest pain with respiration

POTENTIAL COMPLICATIONS

Dyspnea: Rapid lung reexpansion by thoracentesis may cause a brief sensation of severe dyspnea

Pneumothorax: Complication of thoracentesis—diminished or absent breath sounds on the side punctured, dyspnea, decreased oxygen saturation

Bronchopulmonary infection: Fever; sputum color change or purulence

Reaccumulation of fluid: If underlying cause not resolved, signs of effusion recur

PATIENT PROBLEMS/NURSING DIAGNOSES & INTERVENTIONS

NIC RESPIRATORY MANAGEMENT

Impaired gas exchange related to alveolar collapse secondary to pleural fluid accumulation

- Maintain oxygen saturation >93% or as ordered.
- Encourage incentive spirometry *to prevent further atelectasis.*
- Turn patient frequently *to promote chest drainage and minimize local atelectasis.*
- Assist with thoracentesis procedure and monitor patient's response after procedure.
- If chest tube is in place, assess and provide care as indicated on pp. 210-213.

PATIENT EDUCATION/CONTINUUM OF CARE PLAN

1. Teach the patient about the thoracentesis or thoracostomy procedures. If the patient will return home with chest drainage, teach care of the tube site, drainage apparatus, and signs of complications.
2. Teach the importance of deep breathing and coughing to keep the lungs aerated and to prevent further atelectasis or pulmonary infection.
3. If the pleural effusion is a recurrent problem, teach signs of reaccumulation for the patient to report.

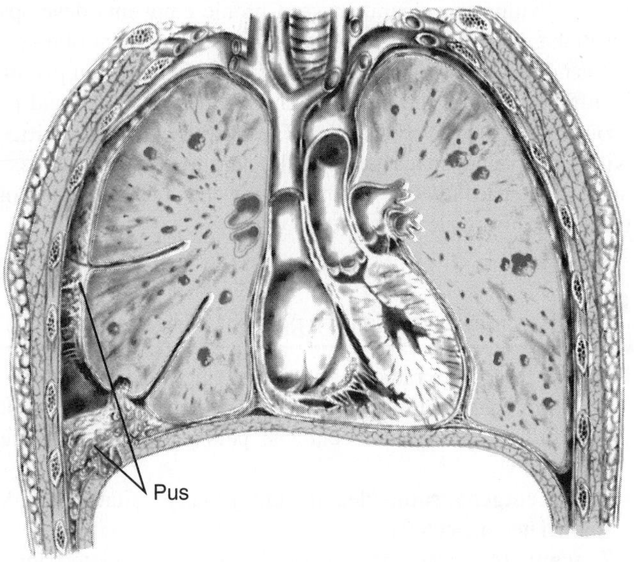

FIG. 4-19
Empyema. (From Wilson and Thompson.[41])

EVALUATION/PATIENT OUTCOMES

Respiratory Management: Gas exchange is optimal. Blood gases are within normal limits. Minimal fluid remains in pleural space. Chest roentgenogram shows no evidence of fluid accumulation. Breath sounds are clear and bilaterally equal; percussion tone is resonant over all lung fields.

EMPYEMA

Empyema is the accumulation of infected fluid or pus in the pleural space (FIG. 4-19).

The accumulation of purulent exudate in the pleural cavity may occur in several ways. The most common cause is direct extension from an adjacent structure, as occurs in pneumonia, tuberculosis, pulmonary abscess, or esophageal rupture. Exudate accumulation may also occur from direct contamination, such as that caused by penetrating chest wounds or chest surgery. Empyema is an uncommon but serious disorder that usually occurs in debilitated patients.

PATHOPHYSIOLOGY

Empyema may affect a small area of pleural space or involve the entire pleural cavity. In the acute stage the affected area appears inflamed and has a thin layer of exudate with a low leukocyte count. If untreated, the exudate thickens and pus may accumulate. The pleura may thicken, and adhesions can occur, causing the exudate to be loculated in pockets rather than freely moving within the pleural space. Chronic empyema develops when there are recurrent infections or when treatment of a previous infection was incomplete. Treatment of chronic empyema is difficult because the pleura often becomes thickened and fibrous, decreasing ventilation. The multiloculated cavities within the pleural space are difficult to drain of the purulent exudate. The space filled by empyema prevents lung expansion in the area, causing atelectasis.

Diagnostic Studies and Findings

History: Recent thoracic or abdominal surgery; blunt or penetrating chest trauma; esophageal fistula; lung infections; aspiration; recent thoracentesis; persistent fever despite antibiotics

Chest roentgenogram: Pleural fluid, usually unilateral, with associated atelectasis

CT scan: To verify location of material and related lung pathology

Thoracentesis: Purulent pleural exudate obtained

Laboratory examination of pleural exudates: Odor and general appearance; specific gravity; cell count; Gram's stain; aerobic and anaerobic cultures (NOTE: When materials are sent for culture, all air must be expressed from syringe and sample must be quickly transported to laboratory for anaerobic evaluation.)

Multidisciplinary Plan

Surgery

Thoracentesis: To drain empyema if area is small and localized; also done under guidance of computerized tomography when drainage is loculated or technically difficult to reach

Thoracic drainage: Closed drainage system; a large-diameter tube is usually required and connected to closed system under water-seal drainage

Intrapleural aspiration and instillation of medications: Chest tube or small pigtail catheter may be used to aspirate pleural drainage and as vehicle for instillation of antibiotics and fibrinolytic enzymes

Thoracotomy: May be necessary for patients not effectively treated by tube drainage system; area with empyema is resected, and thickened membrane is stripped by process called decortication to permit reexpansion of lung

Medications

Antiinfective agents: Antibiotic therapy based initially on results of Gram's stain; alterations made if necessary when culture results are available

Fibrinolytic agents (intrapleural): Urokinase, streptokinase instilled into the chest tube to dissolve fibrin clots that form pockets in the pleural cavity

NURSING CARE

Nursing Assessment

Respiratory status: Nasal flaring; tachypnea, dyspnea; restlessness, tachycardia, decreased chest wall movement; decreased breath sounds; paradoxical breathing; dull percussion tone; decreased vocal fremitus; pleural friction rub; localized chest pain; decreased oxygen saturation

Characteristics of drainage from pleural cavity: Amount, odor, and color of drainage; specimens sent periodically to laboratory for analysis and culture

Bronchopulmonary infection: Fever, elevated WBC count; sputum specimen for culture and sensitivity

Potential Complication

Sepsis: Increased or decreased WBC count, fever or hypothermia, hypotension, tachycardia, restlessness, decreased urine output

Patient Problems/Nursing Diagnoses & Interventions

NIC Respiratory Management

Impaired gas exchange related to inflammation and alveolar collapse

Ineffective breathing pattern related to lung compression

- Encourage deep breathing, coughing, and use of incentive spirometer.
- Monitor for signs of increasing atelectasis resulting from decreased ventilation.
- Maintain patient in position that facilitates easy ventilation, such as semi-Fowler's position.
- Turn patient frequently *to prevent pooling of secretions within lungs and pleural space* and *to promote drainage of empyema via chest drainage tube.*
- Provide analgesics, if needed, *to promote effective cough and deep breathing.*

Patient Education/Continuum of Care Plan

1. Teach the patient the importance of positioning to facilitate the ventilatory effort.
2. Teach the patient the importance of deep breathing and coughing to keep the lungs aerated and prevent further complications.
3. Prepare the patient for thoracentesis or the insertion of chest tubes.
4. If the patient is to go home with a chest tube left in place for drainage, teach care techniques (such as aseptic dressing change).
5. Teach the patient and family about empyema; inform them that the healing process may be slow and that repeated treatments, drainage, irrigation, and chest roentgenograms may be necessary.
6. Teach the patient and family symptoms of recurrent empyema to report

Evaluation/Patient Outcomes

Respiratory Management: Breath sounds are clear and bilaterally equal; percussion tone is resonant over all lung fields. Blood gases are within normal limits. Chest roentgenogram shows no evidence of purulent material in the pleural space.

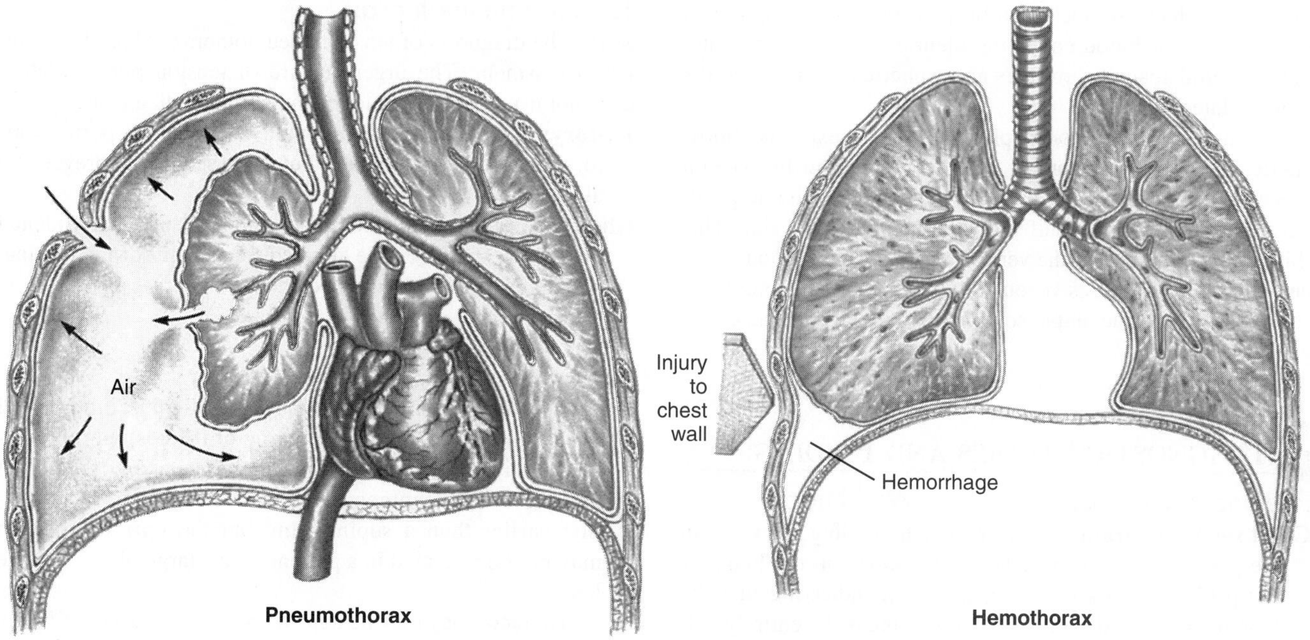

FIG. 4-20
Pneumothorax and hemothorax. (From Wilson and Thompson.[41])

PNEUMOTHORAX AND HEMOTHORAX

The presence of air in the pleural space between the parietal and visceral pleurae is a pneumothorax.

The presence of blood in the pleural space is a hemothorax (FIG. 4-20). If both air and blood are trapped in the pleural space, the term *hemopneumothorax* is used.

A pneumothorax may be caused by trauma or surgery, or it may occur spontaneously. A penetrating injury to the chest wall can permit air to enter the pleural space directly. An injury to a rib may tear the lung surface. Iatrogenic causes of pneumothorax include thoracentesis or subclavian venipuncture that penetrates the pleural surface as well as application of positive pressure ventilation, which may tear the lung surface internally, and laparoscopy. In each case, air may gather in the pleural space, resulting in a pneumothorax.

A spontaneous pneumothorax occurs suddenly without injury and may or may not be the result of underlying pulmonary disease. Pulmonary diseases such as emphysema, pneumonia, and neoplasms weaken lung tissue, so a spontaneous pneumothorax may occur. In apparently healthy persons, usually tall men between ages 20 and 40 years, a subpleural bleb rupture during Valsalva's maneuver allows air to leak into the pleural space.

PATHOPHYSIOLOGY

The pleural space normally maintains a negative pressure, which facilitates lung expansion during ventilation. When there is penetration into the pleural space by an object external to the chest wall (such as a knife or needle) or by an

! EMERGENCY ALERT

MASSIVE PNEUMOTHORAX OR HEMOTHORAX

A pneumothorax occurs when injury to the lung results in an accumulation of air in the pleural space that leads to partial or total collapse of the lung. An open wound to the chest wall produces an open pneumothorax where air enters through the wound and trachea. A tension pneumothorax is a life-threatening situation where the pressure increase is significant and air cannot escape, resulting in total collapse of the affected lung, mediastinal shift, and complete cardiovascular compromise. A hemothorax refers to the accumulation of blood in the pleural space.

ASSESSMENT

- Dyspnea, tachypnea, tachycardia
- Chest pain
- Decreased or absent breath sounds on the affected side
- Hyperresonance (pneumothorax)
- Dullness (hemothorax)
- Open, sucking chest wound (open pneumothorax)
- Hypotension, distended neck veins, and tracheal shift plus rapidly worsening vital signs (tension pneumothorax)

INTERVENTIONS

- Maintain airway, breathing, and circulation
  - Administer high-flow O_2 by mask (10-15 L)
  - Prepare for chest tube insertion
  - Obtain IV access
  - If open pneumothorax: Cover wound with sterile, nonporous dressing and tape on three sides; one side is left open to vent excess pressure.
  - If tension pneumothorax: Perform needle thoracentesis if chest tube insertion is not immediately available
  - If hemothorax: Prepare for blood administration, autotransfusion
- Prepare patient for possible corrective surgical intervention

internal mechanism (such as a broken rib or bleb rupture of the lung), air or blood enters the pleural space. The pressure in the pleural space approaches atmospheric pressure, and the lung deflates.

In tension pneumothorax, pleural pressure exceeds atmospheric pressure as air continues to accumulate in the pleural space. As the pleural space pressure increases and the lung collapses, the mediastinum shifts toward the unaffected side. This shift causes pressure on the venae cavae returning blood to the heart and thus decreases venous return. Tension pneumothorax compromises cardiac output so severely that it creates an emergency situation.

Diagnostic Studies and Findings

Pneumothorax—Closed (Chest Wall Intact)

Chest roentgenogram: The characteristic finding shows air in the pleural cavity without lateral markings on the lungs. A sharp pleural margin is seen medially, indicating that the lung has collapsed (Fig. 4-21). If the lung is not entirely collapsed, this margin may be subtle and better identified on an upright expiratory film.

Pneumothorax—Open (Chest Wall Not Intact)

History: Penetrating injury or invasive procedure of the chest wall.

Chest roentgenogram: Complete lung collapse on the affected side; soft tissue swelling or chest wall defect may be visible.

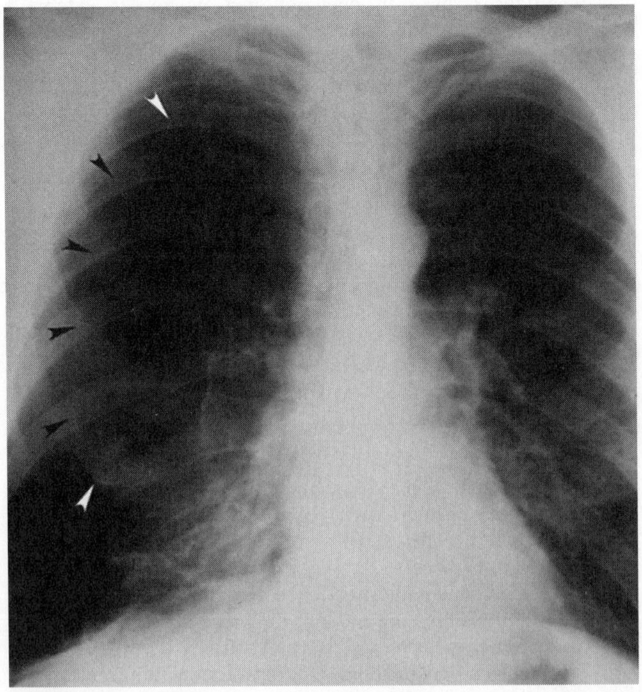

Fig. 4-21
Chest roentgenogram of patient with pneumothorax. Note narrowing of pleural edge at arrow point and lack of lung markings beyond pleural line. (Courtesy R. Keith Wilson, MD, Baylor College of Medicine, Houston, Tex.)

Tension Pneumothorax

NOTE: The diagnosis of tension pneumothorax is based on clinical assessment. The urgent nature of tension pneumothorax does not usually allow time for radiographic diagnosis.

History: Injury to the chest wall or lung that permits air to enter the pleural space but then seals off, preventing air escape.

Chest roentgenogram: Complete lung collapse and widened intercostal spaces on the affected side; a shift of mediastinal structures toward the unaffected side.

Hemothorax

History: Chest trauma.

Chest roentgenogram: A minimum of 250 ml of intrapleural fluid will collect before a blunting of the costophrenic angle is visible on an upright chest roentgenogram. An upright chest roentgenogram will show pleural collection earlier than a supine film, but the upright position may not be tolerated in a patient with a large blood volume loss.

Thoracoscopy may be done to explore the extent of injury causing hemothorax.

Computed tomography is used to differentiate hemothorax from intrapulmonary or extrapleural conditions.

Multidisciplinary Plan

Surgery

Tube thoracostomy (chest tube): This technique is used to treat most types of pneumothorax or hemothorax. The exception is a small, spontaneous pneumothorax in an otherwise healthy individual, which might be monitored without treatment. The chest tube is inserted in the fifth and sixth intercostal space at the midaxillary line. The axillary site is effective, while avoiding the cosmetic defect produced when anterior sites are used. If the distal end of the tube is positioned posteriorly and toward the apex of the lung, it can effectively remove air and fluid. Tubes vary in size from a small pigtail catheter for air removal to a large-bore tube for drainage of blood. A Heimlich valve may be attached to the chest tube to allow for continued removal of air from the pleura without the need for a large chest drainage apparatus. See pp. 210-213 for discussion of chest tubes.

Pleurodesis: Recurrent spontaneous pneumothorax is treated by pleurodesis, instillation of a sclerosing agent into the pleural space. Inflammation caused by the instilled agent creates fibrous adhesions that seal the pleural layers together, preventing future pneumothorax on the treated side.

Needle thoracostomy: Tension pneumothorax requires immediate and specific medical intervention. The building pressure in the pleural space must be reversed rapidly. The most effective way to release the pressure is needle thoracostomy, insertion of a large-bore needle (16 to 18 gauge) anteriorly at the midclavicular line between the second and third intercostal spaces. Once the needle is inserted, the patient's condition should improve remarkably. Tube thoracostomy is then required.

Thoracotomy: A hemothorax may require thoracotomy for repair of injury. Indications for this procedure include initial thoracostomy tube drainage greater than 1500 ml of blood, a persistent bleeding rate greater than 500 ml/h, an increasing hemothorax seen on chest roentgenogram, and an unstable hypotensive state despite adequate blood replacement.

Medications

Intravenous fluids and blood are aggressively replaced in hemothorax to restore the circulating blood volume.

Vasopressors are generally avoided for treatment of hypotension with pleural accumulations, as hemothorax responds rapidly to blood volume replacement and tension pneumothorax responds rapidly to decompression by needle thoracostomy.

Narcotic analgesics may be given for pain.

Antiinfectives are given to prevent infection in penetrating chest injuries.

General Management

Oxygenation: Provide oxygen to maintain adequate blood gas levels

Open pneumothorax: Entrance wound into the chest wall should be immediately covered by petrolatum jelly gauze or other sterile occlusive dressing; three sides of the gauze or dressing should be taped; the fourth is left open to permit escape of excessive pressure; if the wound is completely sealed off, tension pneumothorax may result. The respiratory status of the patient is monitored continuously until stabilized.

NURSING CARE

NURSING ASSESSMENT

Respiratory Status

Closed pneumothorax: Shortness of breath and chest pain in 50% of cases; patient may appear acutely ill with cyanosis and tachypnea or may appear to be healthy; the difference in the clinical signs depends on the size of the pneumothorax; breath sounds are generally diminished; percussion tones are hyperresonant over involved area; approximately 25% of patients have subcutaneous emphysema; in addition, the patient may demonstrate syncope and Hamman's sign (a crunching sound with each heartbeat resulting from mediastinal air accumulation)

Open pneumothorax: Penetration of the chest wall, a sucking sound on inspiration as the chest wall rises, subcutaneous emphysema, and varying signs of respiratory distress, depending on the size of the pneumothorax

Tension pneumothorax: As the positive pressure on the affected side increases, the clinical signs will become more severe; these include neck vein distention resulting from pressure on the superior vena cava, dyspnea, deviated trachea toward the unaffected side, cyanosis, distant heart sounds, subcutaneous emphysema, absence of breath sounds on the affected side, hyperresonance on percussion of the affected side, hypotension, and tachycardia

Hemothorax: Tachycardia, hypotension, pallor, anxiety, dullness on chest percussion, decreased or absent breath sounds, flat neck veins; the severity of the hemothorax may be determined by the amount of blood accumulation: less than 300 ml is considered minor and may not cause significant clinical signs; 300 to 1400 ml is moderate; and over 1400 ml is severe

Chest tube drainage: Assess function of drainage system and amount and characteristics of drainage; see p. 210 for further nursing care of the patient with chest tubes

Anxiety: Fear, air hunger, pain, confusion, particularly during and after acute event

POTENTIAL COMPLICATIONS

Hypoxia: Restlessness, confusion, tachycardia, cyanosis

Decreased cardiac output: Blood pressure, heart rate, auscultation quality, tissue perfusion, urinary output, jugular venous distention with tension pneumothorax, flat jugular veins with hemothorax

Atelectasis from pulmonary compression: Decreased breath sounds, crackles in affected area

PATIENT PROBLEMS/NURSING DIAGNOSES & INTERVENTIONS

NIC RESPIRATORY MANAGEMENT

Impaired gas exchange related to alveolar compression by pleural collection

- Administer oxygen to maintain oxygen saturation at 93% or as ordered.
- Assist with chest tube insertion if indicated.
- Provide chest tube care consistent with the guidelines presented.
- Encourage deep breathing and coughing, incentive spirometry every 1 to 2 hours *to promote lung reexpansion.*
- Reposition patient every 1 to 2 hours *to promote drainage of pleural fluids into chest tube.*
- Protect patient from known sources of secondary infection.
- Identify contributing factors such as airway clearance or obstruction problem or weakness that may contribute to the patient's respiratory distress.

NIC PHYSICAL COMFORT PROMOTION

Acute pain related to chest trauma or pleural puncture

- Teach patient to splint area of chest tube insertion or injury with a pillow *to decrease discomfort when coughing.*
- Provide analgesia as needed *to promote effective ventilation and coughing.*
- Maintain patient positioning to facilitate comfortable ventilation, such as semi-Fowler's position.

NIC PSYCHOLOGIC COMFORT PROMOTION

Anxiety related to sudden respiratory distress episode

- Give brief and clear explanations during the respiratory crisis and treatment.
- Assess patient's level of concern related to the present health state.
- Provide feedback to patient on progress, emphasizing each level of improvement.

PATIENT EDUCATION/CONTINUUM OF CARE PLAN

1. Teach the patient and family about the chest tubes, their purpose and function, and the care that must be taken during their use.
2. Teach the patient to splint the site and use pain medications as needed to allow effective ventilation and cough.
3. Teach importance of regular medical reevaluations after the pneumothorax.

EVALUATION/PATIENT OUTCOMES

Respiratory Management: Blood gas values are within normal limits Clear breath sounds are heard in all areas. Chest roentgenograms show full lung expansion with no evidence of pneumothorax or hemothorax. Vital signs normalize.

Physical Comfort Promotion: Pain is controlled at a level allowing for effective ventilation and cough. Patient describes a reduction in level of anxiety.

Psychologic Comfort Promotion: Concerns are expressed by patient, and appropriate clarification and education and feedback are demonstrated.

AIRWAYS OBSTRUCTIVE DISEASE

The term *airways obstructive disease* refers to a group of diseases, all of which are characterized by airway narrowing (obstruction) and slowing of forced expiration.

The diseases most commonly included are asthma, chronic obstructive bronchitis, and emphysema. Cystic fibrosis (CF) is also an airways obstructive disease. The term *chronic obstructive pulmonary disease (COPD)* is a general term for chronic obstructive bronchitis and emphysema, diseases with irreversible airways obstruction. In asthma the airway obstruction is completely or at least partially reversible. All three of these airways obstructive diseases (asthma, chronic obstructive bronchitis, and emphysema) can coexist in the same patient. (See FIG. 4-22 for

FIG. 4-22

Pathogenesis of airways obstructive diseases. The figure demonstrates the interaction between environmental and personal susceptibility factors in the development of airways obstructive disease. The *shaded lines* trace the development of each disease.

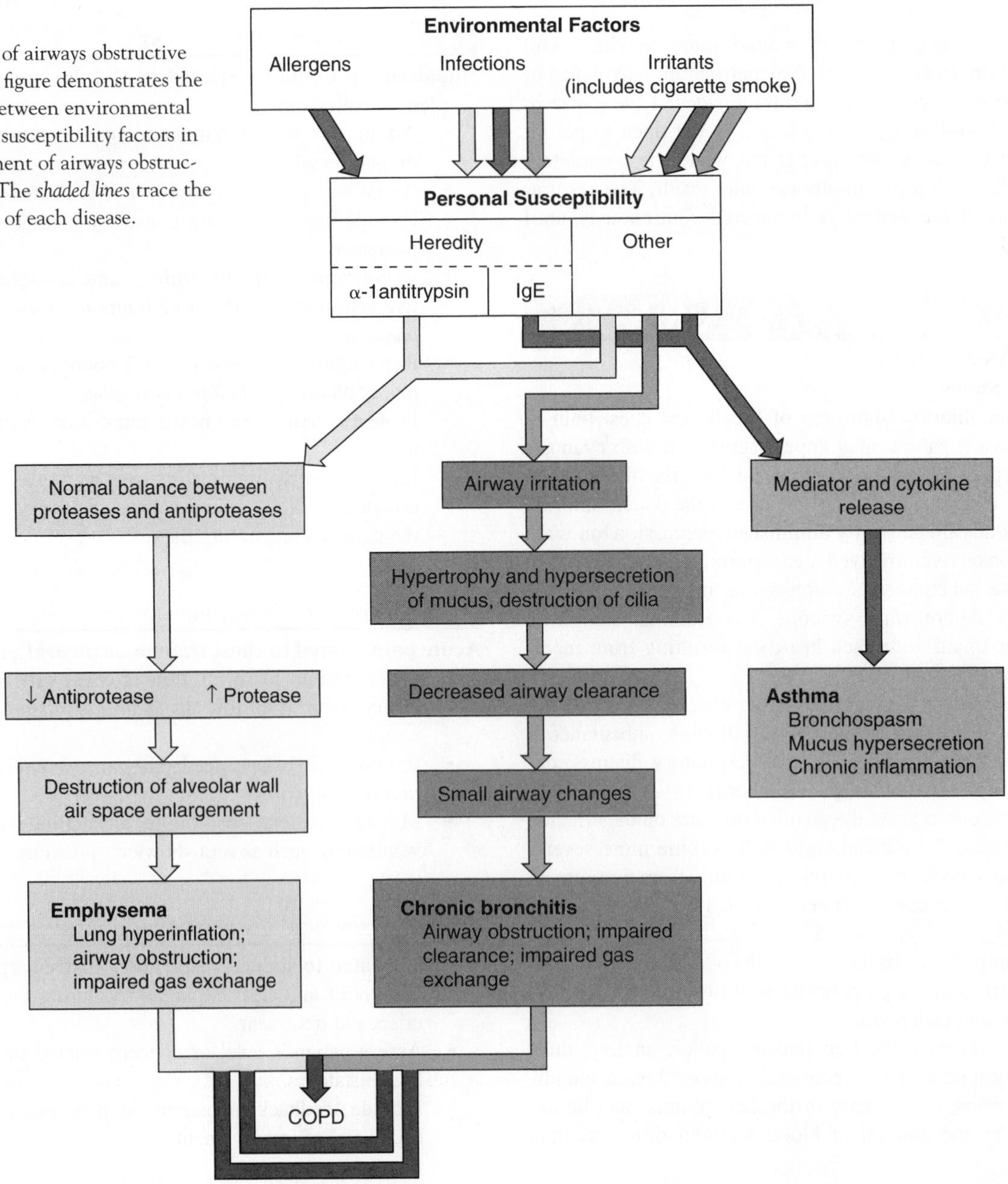

an overview of the relationships between the major airways obstructive diseases.) CF is an inherited disease and, although previously thought of as a disease of childhood, is now increasingly becoming a disease of adults. It is also important to recognize that patients with CF may also have asthma. The health care professional must identify the sources of obstruction for each individual so that maximal therapeutic benefit can be attained.

COPD: Chronic Bronchitis and Emphysema[1,7,22,34,39]

COPD is a major cause of death and disability in the United States. An estimated 14 million people in the United States have COPD. While the mortality rates for other diseases are decreasing, the mortality rate for COPD is increasing, making it the fourth leading cause of death in the United States. Both chronic bronchitis and emphysema (and most patients with COPD have a component of both) are usually associated with a significant smoking history. Chronic bronchitis (chronic obstructive bronchitis) is characterized by excessive mucus secretion and cough. Prolonged exposure to irritants such as cigarette smoke not only increases mucus production and impairs clearance, but also results in the irreversible narrowing of the small airways. Emphysema refers to abnormal enlargement of the distal air spaces and destruction of the lung distal to the terminal bronchiole. The result is a loss of lung recoil that is reflected in increased lung compliance and the loss of small airway support with subsequent airway narrowing. The destruction of alveolar walls also means that there is a loss of gas exchange surface. In both of these diseases there is persistent, irreversible, progressive airways obstruction. The development of chronic bronchitis or emphysema is determined by interaction of the individual's genetic vulnerability and environmental factors. The prevalence of chronic bronchitis and emphysema remains greater in men than in women, possibly because of smoking history and choice of occupation, but the prevalence in women is increasing as the rates of smoking among women increase. Most persons who develop COPD have smoked at least a pack a day for a minimum of 20 years. Because of the insidious nature of these diseases, symptoms that make a person seek health care are not usually experienced until the person is in the fifth or sixth decade of life.

Pathophysiology

Chronic Bronchitis

One of the earliest changes in chronic bronchitis is the increase in size and number of mucus-secreting glands and cells. In addition, there may be hypertrophy of the smooth muscle and squamous metaplasia. The net result is increased amounts of mucus and narrowing of bronchioles and small bronchi. The major change is chronic neutrophilic inflammation of the small airways that progresses to fibrosis and structural narrowing of the airways (Fig. 4-23). In addition, many persons with chronic bronchitis also have episodic bronchoconstriction that adds to the airway obstruction. The narrowing results in an increased work of breathing, air trapping, and gas exchange abnormalities related to V/Q mismatching.

HEALTHY PEOPLE 2010

Health Status—Tobacco Use

Goal: Reduce illness, disability, and death related to tobacco use and exposure to secondhand smoke.

Tobacco Use in Population Groups

- Reduce the proportion of children and adolescents who have dental caries in their primary or permanent teeth.
- Reduce tobacco use by adolescents.
- (Developmental) Reduce initiation of tobacco use among children and adolescents.
- Increase the average age of first use of tobacco products by adolescents and young adults.
- Increase smoking cessation attempts by adult smokers.
- Increase smoking cessation during pregnancy.
- Increase tobacco use cessation attempts by adolescent smokers.
- Increase insurance coverage for evidence-based treatment for nicotine dependency.

Exposure to Secondhand Smoke

- Reduce the proportion of children who are regularly exposed to tobacco smoke at home.
- Reduce the proportion of nonsmokers exposed to environmental tobacco smoke.
- Increase smoke-free and tobacco-free environments in schools, including all school facilities, property, vehicles, and school events.
- Increase the proportion of worksites with formal smoking policies that prohibit smoking or limit it to separately ventilated areas.
- Establish laws on smoke-free indoor air that prohibit smoking or limit it to separately ventilated areas in public places and worksites.

Social and Environmental Changes

- Reduce the illegal buy rate among minors through enforcement of laws prohibiting the sale of tobacco products to minors.
- Objective: Jurisdictions with a 5% or less illegal buy rate among minors.
- Increase the number of states and the District of Columbia that suspend or revoke state retail licenses for violations of laws prohibiting the sale of tobacco to minors.
- Increase adolescents' disapproval of smoking.
- (Developmental) Increase the number of tribes, territories, and states and the District of Columbia with comprehensive, evidence-based tobacco control programs.
- Eliminate laws that preempt stronger tobacco control laws.
- (Developmental) Reduce the toxicity of tobacco products by establishing a regulatory structure to monitor toxicity.
- Increase the average federal and state tax on tobacco products.

Modified from U.S. Department of Health and Human Services: *Healthy people 2010* (conference edition, in two volumes), Washington, DC, January 2000.

NOTE: *Developmental* indicates that criteria for measurement and strategies to improve health have not as yet been specified.

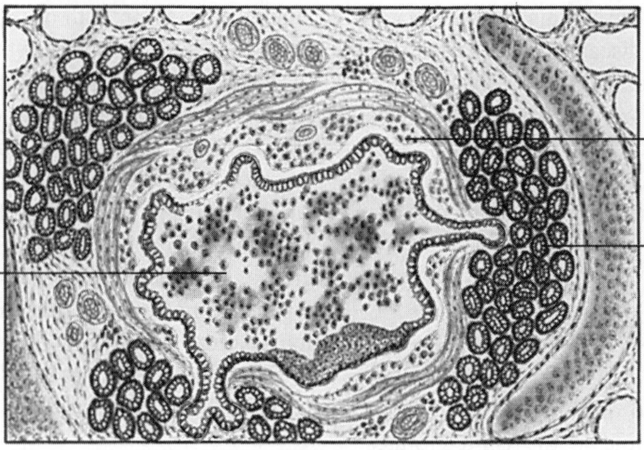

FIG. 4-23
Chronic bronchitis.
(From Wilson and Thompson.[41])

Emphysema

The main defect underlying emphysema is the derangement of lung elastin by proteases. Protease and antiprotease activity is normally in balance to prevent lung destruction. Stimuli such as cigarette smoking appear to increase protease activity, making the person susceptible to lung destruction. One of the antiproteases is alpha-1 antitrypsin. Some individuals have a genetic abnormality (referred to as the PiZZ type) and do not produce alpha-1 antitrypsin. These persons often develop severe emphysema in early adulthood. Alpha-1 antitrypsin deficiency is relatively rare and accounts for less than 1% of cases of emphysema.

The lungs of the patient with emphysema are very large and hyperinflated because of the loss of recoil with destruction of the terminal respiratory units (FIG. 4-24). As recoil is lost, the lung becomes more easily distended and compliance is increased. Some patients with emphysema develop bullae. Bullae are areas of destruction that become severely hyperinflated because of a ball-valve effect; air gets in but cannot get out. (Bullae look like large, thin-walled, empty balloons.) Bullous emphysema is frequently seen in alpha-1 antitrypsin deficiency. Two important physiologic consequences of emphysema are air trapping and decreased gas exchange. The air trapping is caused by a loss of elastic recoil and airways obstruction. The decreased gas exchange is a result of the loss of gas exchange surface and the uneven distribution of ventilation and perfusion

DIAGNOSTIC STUDIES AND FINDINGS

Chronic bronchitis and emphysema are typically "silent" for years before the patient has even minimal symptoms. When symptoms appear, usually at age 50 to 60 years, diagnostic studies evaluating the shortness of breath and cough are generally performed.

Pulmonary function: Pulmonary function tests (PFTs) are the physiologic basis of the diagnosis and are also used to assess the course of disease and to evaluate treatment effects. The routine measures are forced vital capacity (FVC), forced expiratory volume in 1 second (FEV_1), and FEV_1/FVC. (Table 4-7).

Gas exchange: Arterial blood gas measurements are indicated when the FEV_1 falls to less than 50% of predicted. The PaO_2

Table 4-7 COPD: Tests of Lung Function

Pulmonary Function Test	Findings in COPD
FEV_1	Decreased, less than 70% predicted; may fall as much as 50 to 75 ml/year
FVC	Usually decreased
FEV_1/FVC ratio	Decreased, <70%; this measure is hallmark of obstruction
Total lung capacity (TLC)	Increased, especially in emphysema because of decreased lung recoil
Residual volume (RV)	Increased, because of air trapping and decreased lung recoil
Airway resistance	Increased, especially on expiration
Functional residual capacity (FRC)	Increased
Diffusion capacity	Decreased in emphysema because of destruction of lung

! EMERGENCY ALERT

ACUTE CO_2 RETENTION

During an acute exacerbation (because of a variety of conditions—pneumonia, heart failure, etc.), patients with COPD may develop acute CO_2 retention and acidemia. Symptoms include hypersomnolence, confusion, and asterixis. The patient may not be hypoxemic by pulse oximetry if oxygen is being administered and often does not appear to be in respiratory distress. Immediate nursing intervention involves waking the patient and encouraging deep breaths; the patient must be stimulated to stay awake and breathing until blood gas measurements can be obtained to verify the condition. Oxygen is administered to maintain an oxygen saturation around 90%; high saturation (>93%) may actually be detrimental. Stimulating the patient can often reverse the acute acidemia and avoid the need for mechanical ventilation.

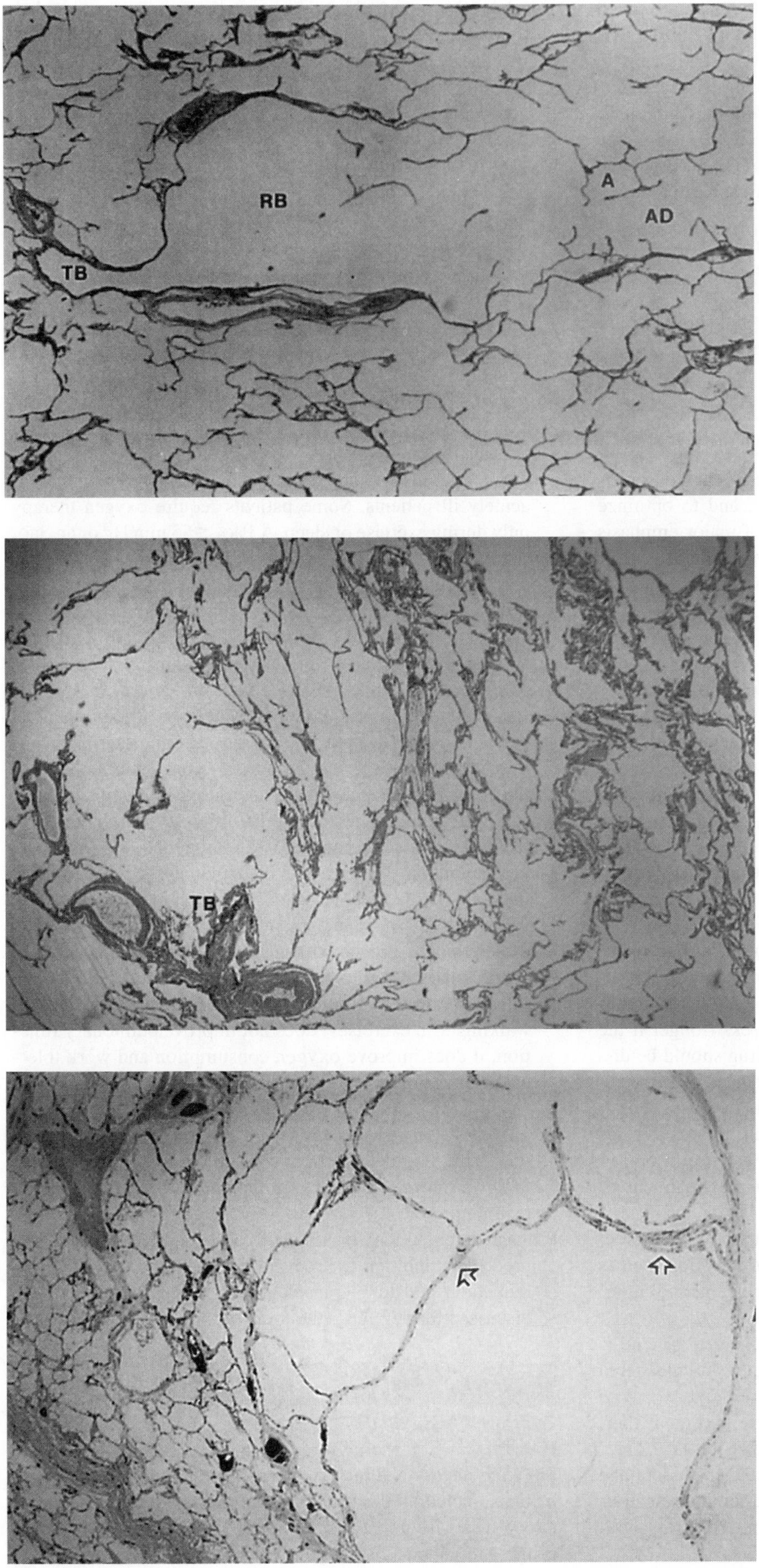

FIG. 4-24

A, Centriacinar emphysema showing distention of respiratory bronchioleas while alveoli remain normal in size. **B,** Panacinar emphysema showing destruction of both proximal and distal portions of the lung acinus resulting in enlarged air spaces that cannot be identified as respiratory bronchloles, alveolar ducts, or alveolar sacs. **C,** Distal acinar emphysema with enlarged subpleural acini and associated fine fibrosis. (Original magnification × 19.) (From Murray and Nadel.[23])

is decreased. The $Paco_2$ is not increased until late, advanced disease (the $Paco_2$ is usually not elevated until the FEV_1 is less than 1 L).

Chest roentgenogram: Findings are a big lung with flattened diaphragms and increased anteroposterior (A-P) diameter; in emphysema, vascular markings may be decreased and bullae may be present. Computed tomography (CT) scans of the lung may be done to visualize bullae if surgical intervention is being considered.

Laboratory values: Hemoglobin and hematocrit may be elevated if the patient is chronically hypoxemic.

ECG: May show atrial arrhythmias; tall, symmetric P waves in leads II, III, and AVF; vertical QRS axis; and signs of right ventricular hypertrophy late in the disease.

MULTIDISCIPLINARY PLAN

The goals of care are to treat promptly or prevent acute exacerbations, to slow the progress of the disease, and to optimize functional status and quality of life. Areas of major emphasis are smoking cessation, identification and treatment of any reversible airway obstruction, and pulmonary rehabilitation.

Medications

Bronchodilators

Inhaled anticholinergics (ipratropium): 2-3 puffs 3-4 times a day.

Inhaled beta agonists (e.g., albuterol, metaproterenol): Short-acting agents are prescribed as needed for shortness of breath, usually 2 puffs up to 4-5 times in 24 h; long-acting beta agonists (salmeterol) may also be used, 2 puffs bid.

Methylxanthines (theophylline): These drugs are not used as frequently as in the past; therapeutic levels are usually maintained at levels of 8-12 mg/L.

Corticosteroids: Although controversy about their chronic use in COPD continues, both inhaled and oral corticosteroids have been used in the chronic treatment of COPD. If no objective improvement is evident after 2 weeks (longer if the original trial is on inhaled steroids), the drug should be discontinued. If the drug is maintained, the inhaled form is preferred. If oral corticosteroids are required, the lowest possible dose with therapeutic effect is used. Intravenous steroids may be used during acute exacerbations. The use of oral or parenteral corticosteroids is common in the treatment of acute exacerbations of COPD.

Antibiotics: Broad-spectrum antibiotics are used to treat infectious exacerbations (should be evidence of infection such as fever, leukocytosis, etc). In chronic management, antibiotics are begun without culture reports.

Influenza and pneumococcal vaccines: Influenza vaccine is administered yearly. Pneumococcal vaccine is administered every 6 years in this population.

Alpha-1 antitrypsin therapy: Antitrypsin replacement therapy is available for persons who are homozygotes (PiZZ) for the deficiency. The drug is used in younger middle-age adults who have already demonstrated emphysematous changes. The drug is very expensive and requires intravenous administration.

Psychoactive agents: If antidepressants (tricyclics) are needed, they are administered with caution to avoid depression of ventilatory drive; for management of anxiety, benzodiazepines are the drugs of choice.

General Management

Oxygen: Continuous oxygen therapy, usually via nasal cannula, is indicated for patients who are unable to maintain a Pao_2 of 55 mm Hg while at rest and breathing room air. The flow rate should be adjusted to maintain a resting Pao_2 close to 60 mm Hg. Flow rates of 1 to 3 L/min are usually sufficient. Because patients with chronic bronchitis and emphysema may have chronic hypercapnia, they are considered to be sensitive to increased arterial oxygen. This means that their ventilatory drive may be suppressed by increasing the Pao_2 to high levels. Care must be taken to closely monitor oxygen administration. When flows are increased, the increments are usually small to avoid over-oxygenating. Use of the Venturi mask allows more precise oxygen administration in acutely ill patients. Some patients require oxygen therapy only during exercise or sleep. A $Pao_2 \leq 55$ mm Hg or an $Sao_2 \leq 88\%$ during these times indicates oxygen need.

Chest physiotherapy: Breathing techniques are taught to control dyspnea. Cough techniques are taught to improve airway clearance. Percussion and postural drainage are used only for patients with large amounts of sputum production (see p. 205 for techniques).

Mechanical ventilation: In the treatment of COPD, mechanical ventilation is used both in acute and chronic settings. Noninvasive mechanical ventilation via a mask may be used to improve gas exchange during an exacerbation or in the home setting for patients with severe chronic carbon dioxide retention. In the acute care setting, intubation and mechanical ventilation may be necessary if supplemental oxygen cannot maintain the Pao_2 above 40 to 50 mm Hg with a pH greater than 7.25. If a patient with severe airways obstructive disease requires surgery with general anesthesia, mechanical ventilation is likely to be required postoperatively.

Physical training: Although physical training (bicycling, walking, arm exercises) does not improve pulmonary function, it does improve oxygen consumption and work tolerance. In addition, there are often psychosocial benefits to training, with an improvement in dyspnea tolerance, improved sense of well-being, and generally improved quality of life. Exercise training is often included in a rehabilitation program that involves patient education, breathing techniques, etc.

Surgical intervention: In selected cases, surgical treatment is used for emphysema. Procedures include bullectomy, lung reduction, and lung transplantation. These procedures are discussed further under the topic of thoracic surgery.

NURSING CARE

NURSING ASSESSMENT

History

Smoking history and history of exposure to known respiratory irritants, including duration of each; history of previous respiratory diseases, infections, allergies, etc.; history of chronic cough and characteristics of cough; family history of respiratory diseases; description of activity tolerance, including fatigue and dyspnea

Current therapy: Careful and complete history of current respiratory-related medications, as well as use of over-the-counter medications and inhalers; observe and evaluate use of inhalers

History of use of oxygen: Include when initiated, delivery device, liter flow, when used, and therapeutic response

Home (usually night time) ventilation is used only in selected cases. If used, note when it was initiated, ventilator settings, when the modality is used, and therapeutic response,

Respiratory Status

Observed symptoms of impaired mechanical function include dyspnea, cough, sputum production, use of accessory muscles (note if inspiratory, expiratory, or both), pursed lip exhalation, tripod posture, and barrel chest; observe for a paradoxical inward movement of the lower chest with inspiration (usually associated with severe hyperinflation). For changes in the ventilatory pattern with activity, stress should be noted. Auscultory findings in COPD include prolonged expiratory phase, decreased breath sounds, wheeze—sonorous and musical—and hyperresonance (especially in emphysema). Pulsus paradoxus may be present during periods of respiratory distress. Pulmonary function studies should be reviewed if available, especially FEV_1 level (Table 4-8).

Gas exchange is best assessed by arterial blood gases. Oximetry is also used to follow oxygenation. Observed symptoms are often nonspecific.

Symptoms of severe hypoxemia include restlessness, tachycardia, confusion, hypotension, cyanosis, and dysrhythmias. Signs and symptoms of chronic hypoxemia include fatigue, poor memory, problems concentrating, and morning headache. If the Pao_2 is less than 55 mm Hg chronically, a secondary erythrocytosis may be seen. Symptoms of an acute rise in $Paco_2$ include asterixis and mental status changes (the changes are variable, some become somnolent, some become combative). Chronic changes in $Paco_2$ often do not cause symptoms but may be detected from changes in electrolytes: an increase in carbon dioxide and a decrease in chloride levels. (Note that other problems such as metabolic alkalosis may cause similar changes in electrolytes.)

Other Assessment Data

Nutritional status, specifically, being overweight or underweight or having decreased dietary and fluid intake, and depression

Potential Complications

Pneumonia: Signs and symptoms of infection—increased cough and sputum, purulent sputum, elevated temperature, elevated WBC count, pleuritic chest wall pain

Cor pulmonale and heart failure: Pedal edema, elevated jugular venous pressure, hepatic engorgement (see section on cor pulmonale)

Respiratory failure: Severe hypoxemia, acute hypercapnia with acidemia

Table 4-8 Relationship between FEV_1 and ADLs

FEV_1 (L)	Activity Response
>3	Normal value for adult
2-1.5	Complaints of dyspnea on exertion such as carrying packages or climbing stairs
About 1	Breathlessness when trying to perform ADLs such as cooking, cleaning, bathing, dressing, walking Subject to complications of carbon dioxide retention and cor pulmonale
<0.75	Individual unable to work, usually housebound

Data from Fries and Ehrlich.[11a]

Pneumothorax: Acute chest wall pain, shortness of breath

Pulmonary emboli: Acute chest wall pain, shortness of breath, signs of right-sided heart failure

Patient Problems/Nursing Diagnoses & Interventions

NIC Respiratory Management

Ineffective breathing pattern related to airway obstruction, hyperinflation

Impaired gas exchange related to ventilation/perfusion mismatch

Ineffective airway clearance related to increased mucus production, decreased cough effectiveness

- Maintain position that facilitates ventilation (usually sitting, tripod).
- Administer bronchodilators as ordered; teach correct inhaler technique.
- Assure adequate fluid intake *to aid in sputum expectoration.*
- Cough techniques: Perform after bronchodilator treatments.
- Perform postural drainage, if ordered, at least 1 hour after meals and after bronchodilator treatments.
- Conserve energy; avoid increasing O_2 demands; ensure rest periods.
- Administer oxygen as ordered.
- Monitor changes in auscultation findings.
- Monitor blood gas status (symptoms, oximetry, arterial blood gases [ABGs]). Report increases in $Paco_2$ and decreases in Pao_2 of more than 10 mm Hg; any Pao_2 below 50 mm Hg or pH less than 7.3 should be reported.
- Avoid depressing ventilation by excessive sedation, sleeping medications, etc.

NIC Activity and Exercise Management

Activity intolerance related to impaired gas exchange and shortness of breath

Impaired physical mobility related to shortness of breath and deconditioning

- Assess and document activities that cause patient to tire easily and become short of breath.

- Encourage use of adaptive breathing techniques during activity *to decrease dyspnea.*
- Assist patient to space activities *to provide periods of rest during and between activities to prolong endurance.*
- Encourage gradual increase of activities as tolerated *to increase muscle mass.*
- Problem-solve with patient to determine methods of conserving energy while still performing ADLs (e.g., using stool to sit while in the bathroom shaving).
- Evaluate during activity for possible increased oxygen need during exercise.

NIC NUTRITION SUPPORT

Imbalanced nutrition: less than body requirements, related to dyspnea, disease process

Imbalanced nutrition: more than body requirements, related to excessive intake and decreased mobility

- Assess dietary intake.
- If overweight, help plan diet with lower caloric intake.
- If underweight:
  - Plan smaller, more frequent meals.
  - Increase caloric value without increasing bulk.
- Assist patient to choose foods that are easy to chew and swallow; assist by cutting and feeding if patient tires easily. Medications, sputum, and shortness of breath may cause anorexia, nausea, and vomiting.

PATIENT EDUCATION/CONTINUUM OF CARE PLAN

1. Preventive measures include providing information about the detrimental effects of smoking, resources for smoking cessation programs, support groups, and encouraging patient/family to use resources for smoking cessation. Patient/family must know specific care techniques, including:
   a. Proper use of inhalers
   b. Appropriate cough techniques
   c. Controlled breathing techniques
   d. Home oxygen use if indicated
2. Education needs also include understanding of medications: when to take, what they do, symptoms for which the patient should obtain emergency care or contact care provider (e.g., morning headache, new pedal edema, confusion, purulent sputum), ways to adapt/pace lifestyle so as to maintain quality of life (e.g., exercise program, energy conservation).

EVALUATION/PATIENT OUTCOMES

Respiratory Management: Sputum and cough are absent or minimal. Sputum, if present, should be clear or white. No rhonchi on auscultation. Chest roentgenogram shows no infiltrates.

Lung function improved after exacerbation; FEV_1 and FVC are at patient's usual level. Dyspnea is reduced; patient is able to speak in complete sentences.

PaO_2 is greater than 60 mm Hg. $PaCO_2$ is normal for patient; pH is in normal range. (Note that following hospitalization for an acute exacerbation it may require 1 month for the patient's blood gases to return to baseline.)

Patient can demonstrate breathing techniques, cough techniques, inhaler techniques. Knows home medications: what they are and schedule for use. Can state when to use prn inhalers. Understands home oxygen therapy: how to maintain equipment and flow rate changes with exercise and sleep if ordered. Understands when to call care provider.

Activity and Exercise Management: Able to perform ADLs; can describe how will pace activities; uses controlled breathing pattern while walking; has plan for exercise at home.

Nutrition Support: Able to state modifications in diet: meal scheduling and food selection; weight stabilized (if losing).

ASTHMA[25]

Asthma, a chronic inflammatory disease of the airways, is defined by several physiologic characteristics. These are inflammation, hyperresponsive airways, and airways obstruction that is reversible either spontaneously or with treatment.

The inflammation results in episodic, recurrent symptoms of wheeze, dyspnea, chest tightness, and cough. The symptoms are often worse at night. *Status asthmaticus* is the term used to describe an asthma exacerbation that does not respond on usual therapy.

Asthma affects more than 10 million people in the United States, and the prevalence is increasing. In those under age 20 years, the prevalence is about 5%; in adults the prevalence rate is about 3.4%. Hospitalization rates and health care costs are also increasing, as are mortality rates. In 1988 more than 4500 persons died from asthma in the United States. Certain risk factors for mortality have been identified. Prevalence and mortality rates are significantly higher in African-Americans than in whites. Also, patients with asthma who have had a prior episode of respiratory failure during an asthmatic attack are at greater risk. The most important factor contributing to mortality is inadequate treatment.

In recognition of the increasing asthma problem, a National Asthma Education Program (NAEP) was initiated by the National Institutes of Health. Experts from a variety of health-care disciplines and care consumers reviewed the current literature and current practice and published asthma guidelines. In 1997 the revised Guidelines for the Diagnosis and Management of Asthma[25] were published. Additional publications have included a Clinicians Guide, Guidelines for the Diagnosis and Management of Asthma during Pregnancy, and Diagnosis and Management of Asthma in the Elderly. The purpose of the NAEP is to educate health-care professionals and consumers so as to improve the management of asthma and thus reduce morbidity and mortality.

PATHOPHYSIOLOGY

Airway inflammation and bronchial hyperreactivity are the hallmarks of asthma (FIG. 4-25). The origin of these changes can be related to allergy in the majority of cases. The allergic reaction is one of immediate hypersensitivity mediated by IgE. The reaction of an aeroallergen and IgE causes mast cells to de-

HEALTHY PEOPLE 2010

Health Status—Respiratory Disease

Goal: Promote respiratory health through better prevention, detection, treatment, and education.

Asthma

- Reduce deaths of persons with asthma.
- Reduce hospitalization for persons with asthma.
- Reduce hospital emergency department visits for persons with asthma.
- Reduce activity limitations among persons with asthma.
- (Developmental) Reduce the number of school or work days missed as a result of asthma by persons with asthma.
- Increase the proportion of persons with asthma who receive formal patient education, including information about community and self-help resources, as an essential part of the management of their condition.
- (Developmental) Increase the proportion of persons with asthma who receive appropriate asthma care according to the NAEPP Guidelines.
- (Developmental) Establish a surveillance system of at least 15 states for tracking asthma death, illness, and disability; impact of occupational and environmental factors on asthma; access to medical care; and asthma management.

Chronic Obstructive Pulmonaroy Disease

- Reduce the proportion of adults whose activity is limited because of chronic lung and breathing problems.
- Reduce deaths from chronic obstructive pulmonary disease (COPD) among adults.

Obstructive Sleep Apnea

- (Developmental) Increase the proportion of persons with symptoms of obstructive sleep apnea whose condition is medically managed.
- (Developmental) Reduce the proportion of vehicular crashes caused by persons with excessive sleepiness.

Modified from U.S. Department of Health and Human Services: *Healthy people 2010* (conference edition, in two volumes), Washington, DC, January 2000.

NOTE: *Developmental* indicates that criteria for measurement and strategies to improve health have not as yet been specified.

granulate with the release of mediators. Many of these mediators can directly cause bronchospasm. Others stimulate cytokine production and the influx of inflammatory cells. The chronic inflammation contributes to the bronchial hyperreactivity. The mediators and inflammation also contribute to mucus hypersecretion and airway edema. In addition to allergens, other stimuli, such as infections, chemical irritants, and physical exercise, may precipitate a hyperreactive response. One of the chemical irritants that may exacerbate asthma symptoms is reflux of stomach contents: GERD, gastroesophageal reflux disease. Certain occupational exposures may also cause an allergic response and asthma; in this circumstance the diagnosis *occupational asthma* is often used.

All of these factors (bronchospasm, inflammation, edema, hypersecretion) lead to airways obstruction. Air trapping occurs, and the FRC increases. As a result of the increased effort required and the overinflation, the patient uses the accessory muscles of respiration. Gas exchange abnormalities occur because of ventilation/perfusion mismatching. There is hypoxemia, but the patient is usually able to hyperventilate. In severe exacerbations, when the FEV_1 falls to *very* low values, hypoventilation (increases $PaCO_2$) may occur.

Diagnostic Studies and Findings

Pulmonary function: Decrease in peak expiratory flow (PEF) and FEV_1 with exacerbations. In mild disease these measurements may be near 80% of predicted; as the severity of disease worsens, so does the fall in FEV_1 and PEF. Increased variability in flows between morning and evening measures is usually present, and there is at least a 10% to 12% increase in FEV_1 postbronchodilator administration. The FEV_1/FVC ratio is decreased during attacks, and FRC is increased. (See Tables 4-9 and 4-10 for classifying asthma severity.)

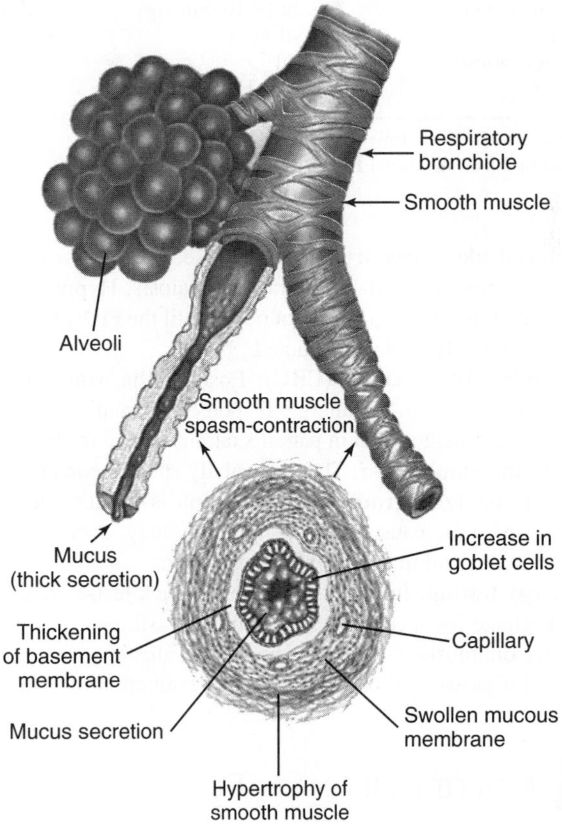

FIG. 4-25

In bronchial asthma the bronchiole is obstructed by muscle spasm, edema of the mucosa, inflammation, and thick secretions. (From Wilson and Thompson.[41])

Table 4-9 Classification of Asthma Severity

Severity Level	Symptoms	Pulmonary Function
Mild, intermittent	Less than twice a week and only last a short time; asymptomatic between exacerbation; nighttime symptoms less than twice a month	FEV_1 or PEF 80% of predicted or higher
Mild, persistent	More symptoms than mild but not daily; nighttime symptoms occur more than twice a month	FEV_1 or PEF 80% of predicted or greater
Moderate, persistent	Symptoms occur daily and require daily use of bronchodilators; exacerbations occur two or more times a week and may last days; nighttime symptoms occur several times a week	FEV_1 or PEF 60%-80% of predicted
Severe, persistent	Continual symptoms that limit activity; frequent exacerbations and frequent nighttime symptoms	FEV_1 or PEF less than 60% of predicted

Modified from National Heart, Lung, and Blood Institute.[25]

Table 4-10 Signs and Symptoms of Asthma Severity

Signs/Symptoms	Mild	Moderate	Severe
Shortness of breath (SOB)	SOB walking; able to speak in sentences; can lie down	SOB speaking; prefers to sit	SOB at rest; sits upright
Alertness	May be agitated	Usually agitated	Usually agitated
Respiratory rate	Increased	Increased	Over 30/min
Pulse rate	Less than 100	100-120	Over 120
Use of accessory muscles/retractions	Not present	Common	Usual
Wheeze	Often only end expiratory	Obvious throughout all of expiration	Usually loud, heard during both inspiration and expiration
Pulsus paradoxus	Absent (<10 mm Hg)	May be present; if yes, 10-25 mm Hg	Often present at levels over 25 mm Hg
PEF	80% of best	50%-80% of best	Less than 50%
Oxygenation*	Normal	Po_2 >60; saturation ≥90 mm Hg	Po_2 <60; saturation ≤90 mm Hg
CO_2*	<42 mm Hg	<42 mm Hg	>42 mm Hg

*ABGs are usually only needed in severe exacerbations.
Modified from National Heart, Lung, and Blood Institute.[25]

Arterial blood gases: Pao_2 is decreased; there is usually hyperventilation with a respiratory alkalosis. Hypoventilation with a rise in $Paco_2$ does not occur until the FEV_1 falls to approximately 25% of predicted.

Complete blood count (CBC): Eosinophilia, which is often associated with the allergic response, is usually seen. (May not see eosinophilia in patients taking oral steroids.)

Sputum examination: There is usually sputum eosinophilia.

Chest roentgenogram: The radiograph is usually clear. Hyperinflation caused by air trapping may occur in acute episodes and in persistent, chronic cases.

Allergy testing: Immediate skin tests (prick tests) are done to evaluate for specific allergic causes of asthma.

Other diagnostic tests: IgE antibodies; evaluation of esophageal pH if gastric reflux is a possibility; evaluation of sinuses.

MULTIDISCIPLINARY PLAN

The goals of therapy are to prevent asthma attacks, maintain normal or near-normal pulmonary function, prevent side effects from medications, prevent symptoms, and maintain normal activity levels. Asthma is a chronic illness and is treated as a problem that can be controlled rather than cured. Most important,

! EMERGENCY ALERT

ASTHMA

The patient with asthma who is in severe distress can progress to respiratory arrest. The signs and symptoms of impending respiratory arrest in the asthma patient with a severe exacerbation are drowsiness or confusion; the respiratory pattern demonstrates a paradoxical pattern (related to impending respiratory muscle fatigue and severe hyperinflation). The patient's airways are now so obstructed that the wheeze disappears. The pulse slows and may become bradycardic. The pulsus paradoxus that was present when the patient was struggling to breathe disappears because of the severe respiratory muscle fatigue. The drowsiness and lack of wheeze must not be interpreted to mean that the patient is improved. At this stage, blood gases often demonstrate hypoventilation (elevated $Paco_2$) and acidemia. These patients are cared for in the intensive care unit (ICU) with increased amounts of pharmacologic intervention, including continuous bronchodilator aerosols, intubation, and mechanical ventilation.

Table 4-11 Asthma Therapy by Disease Severity

Severity Level	Quick Relief	Long-Term Control
Mild, intermittent	Short-acting bronchodilator, 2 puffs as needed; if more than 2/wk, add long-term control	None needed
Mild, persistent	Short-acting bronchodilator; if daily, increase control medications	Inhaled corticosteroid (low dose) or cromolyn or nedocromil; may add leukotriene modifier or theophylline as an alternative
Moderate, persistent	As for mild, persistent	Inhaled corticosteroid (medium dose) and long-acting beta agonist inhaler
Severe, persistent	As for mild, persistent	High-dose inhaled corticosteroid, long-acting bronchodilator, *and* oral corticosteroids

Modified from National Heart, Lung, and Blood Institute.[25]

however, is the goal of preventing symptoms and the potential for long-term airway changes.

Medications

Pharmacologic therapy for asthma includes medications used for "quick relief" and those for "long-term control." The quick relief medications are short-acting beta-2 agonist inhaled bronchodilators (e.g., metaproterenol, albuterol). In addition, systemic corticosteroids (e.g., prednisone), given for a brief time during an acute exacerbation, are considered to be in the quick relief category. Long-term medications include the antiinflammatories (corticosteroids, cromolyn sodium and nedocromil, leukotriene modifier), and long-acting bronchodilators, either beta agonists or theophylline. The use of the drugs is determined by the severity of the disease. Those with mild severity are treated at home; moderate to severe asthma exacerbations often require hospitalization. Table 4-11 presents the chronic pharmacologic therapy by asthma severity.

When exacerbations require hospital admission, the intensity of the pharmacologic therapy is increased. Aerosolized bronchodilators are given every 20 minutes for three doses and then every 1 to 4 hours as needed; in addition, injected beta-2 agonists may be given (these drugs are usually not given to adults over age 40 years because of the danger of cardiac side effects). Anticholinergics (ipratropium bromide) are frequently given with the beta-agonist bronchodilator. Corticosteroid dose is also increased (up to 120 to 180 mg/day) for 48 hours followed by doses of 60 to 80 mg/day.

General Management

Oxygenation: Humidified oxygen is administered during moderate to severe acute exacerbations, usually by nasal cannula, to maintain $Pa{O_2}$ in the 60 to 70 mm Hg range; oxygen saturation should be ≥93%.

Fluid and electrolyte therapy: Fluids are given to maintain water balance (insensible loss increased with rapid respiratory rate and intake often decreased because of shortness of breath).

Environment: Avoid exposure to triggers; maintain calm environment.

Immunotherapy: Desensitization is used in patients for whom allergen avoidance is not possible; allergens most likely to be involved are house dust mite, cat dander, and alternaria (a mold). (Immunotherapy is not done during acute exacerbations.)

NURSING CARE

NURSING ASSESSMENT

History: Known family or personal history of allergy, infantile eczema

Past asthma history, including severity and treatment (previous episodes of asthma, history of recent severe attack, previous hospitalization for asthma, need for systemic steroids, episode of respiratory failure)

Medications: Careful and complete history of current respiratory-related medications, as well as most recent dose and time taken before hospital arrival

Respiratory status: In addition to the major assessment presented in Tables 4-9 and 4-10:

Airway clearance: Presence of cough/sputum, purulent sputum

Hypoxemia: Assessed by pulse oximetry or ABGs; symptoms such as tachycardia, restlessness are part of the asthma exacerbation and may be present without hypoxemia

Hydration: Intake and output to monitor hydration; presence of diaphoresis

Psychosocial status: Anxiety, agitation, fear of suffocation

POTENTIAL COMPLICATIONS

Respiratory infection; respiratory failure

PATIENT PROBLEMS/NURSING DIAGNOSES & INTERVENTIONS

NIC RESPIRATORY MANAGEMENT

Ineffective breathing pattern related to airways obstruction, anxiety, fatigue

Impaired gas exchange related to ventilation/perfusion mismatch

Ineffective airway clearance related to airways obstruction and excessive mucus production

- Administer bronchodilator medications as ordered.
- Monitor peak flow response to therapy.
- Maintain patient positioning *to facilitate ventilation* (i.e., sitting and leaning forward on overbed table).
- Encourage patient to use adaptive breathing techniques *to prolong expiratory time.*
- Maintain oxygen therapy as needed.

- Assist patient in pulmonary hygiene routines that *facilitate mucus expectoration and minimize risk of secondary infections.*
- Identify contributing factors such as allergens in immediate environment or other irritants that may exacerbate condition.
- Cover pillows with allergen-proof covers *to eliminate dust and other irritants.*
- Assist patient to space activities to provide periods of rest in between and prevent increasing ventilatory demands.

NIC RISK MANAGEMENT

Risk for infection related to steroid therapy and ineffective airway clearance

- Instruct patient in use of spacer device with inhaled steroid *to prevent oral deposition.*
- Instruct patient using inhaled corticosteroids to perform thorough mouth washing after each use *to prevent mouth irritation and oral candidiasis.*
- Assess mouth and oral mucosa for presence of mouth irritation *to prevent possible mouth infection secondary to inhaled corticosteroids.*
- Assess for secondary respiratory infection resulting from retained secretions.
- Monitor results of CBC and report abnormal leukocyte level.
- Support patient in altering environment *to decrease antigen, irritant exposure.*
- Provide immunization (influenza, pneumococcal) if appropriate or information about obtaining an immunization.
- Provide patient education related to decreasing risk for infection for long-term control.

PATIENT EDUCATION/CONTINUUM OF CARE PLAN

1. Work with patient and physician to develop plan of care for chronic care; include guidelines for self-management (teaching patient when to increase medications, etc.)
2. Educate patient about current approach to therapy and his or her role in management.
3. Teach patient how to use peak flow (PF) meter.
4. Teach patient how to monitor disease (symptoms and peak flows).
5. Instruct in use of inhalers and spacers.
6. Assess with patient or family home and environmental triggers that may exacerbate asthma episode.
7. Provide education regarding need to avoid contact with irritant allergens.
8. Be sure that appointment is made and that patient/family understand the importance of a follow-up visit within 7 to 10 days of discharge from an emergency department or hospital stay.

EVALUATION/PATIENT OUTCOMES

Respiratory Management: FEV_1 and PF are at least 80% of predicted (or at 80% of patient's best). Airways are clear, breath sounds are clear. Blood gas values are within normal limits.

Risk Management: WBC and differential normal; afebrile. Patient and family have sufficient information to comply with discharge regimen. Includes ability to discuss medications (purpose, side effects, route, and schedule) and plan for long-term follow-up maintenance; demonstrate correct use of PF meter and interpretation of results; state what to do if an exacerbation occurs; state time of next scheduled visit.

CYSTIC FIBROSIS[14,43]

Cystic fibrosis (CF) is an autosomal recessive disorder of the exocrine glands that causes those glands to produce abnormally thick secretions of mucus (FIG. 4-26).

In the United States, CF is the most common cause of life-threatening pulmonary disease of Caucasians during childhood and adolescence. The disease incidence in the United States is 1 in 3500 live births. Today CF is a disease of both children and adults. The median survival is 31 years, and over 35% of patients are adults. One in 25 persons in the United States carries the CF gene. The disease is least prevalent in African-Americans, Native Americans, and persons of Asian ancestry. Males and females are equally affected.

Although CF is a widespread multisystem disease, the progressive pulmonary infections are the most important clinical problem and are responsible for over 90% of the mortality. Advances in the treatment of the respiratory components of the disease have been important in improving the prognosis, but maximum success cannot be achieved unless all involved systems as well as psychologic aspects are also managed. There is no known cure for CF, but much has been done to lengthen the survival of patients. In 1989 a CF gene was identified. Since then it has been determined that multiple mutations of the gene are involved. The specific genetic mutation(s) are associated with varying levels of disease severity. Future therapy may involve genetic manipulation to prevent the disease.

PATHOPHYSIOLOGY

CF (mucoviscidosis) is a disease of altered ion transport. The defect alters the characteristics of secreted mucus, but exactly how this defect affects the various organ systems involved in CF is not completely clear. It is known that the exocrine glands secrete a thick, sticky mucus rather than the usual dilute mucus. CF affects many organ systems (see FIG. 4-26). In the adult, the most important complication of this genetic disorder is pulmonary involvement (FIG. 4-27).

Pulmonary System

Thick mucus causes plugging of the ducts of the mucus glands and accumulation of dried, thick secretions in the airway. This environment makes the airways, including the sinuses, more likely to be infected. The predominant organism infecting the airway in adults with CF is *Pseudomona aeruginosa;* this organism is not common in patients with other types of lung disease. As infections become more frequent and the airway is continually inflamed, airway obstruction progresses (because of inflammation, secretions, changes in the airway wall), and bronchiectasis results. Bronchiectasis is a destruc-

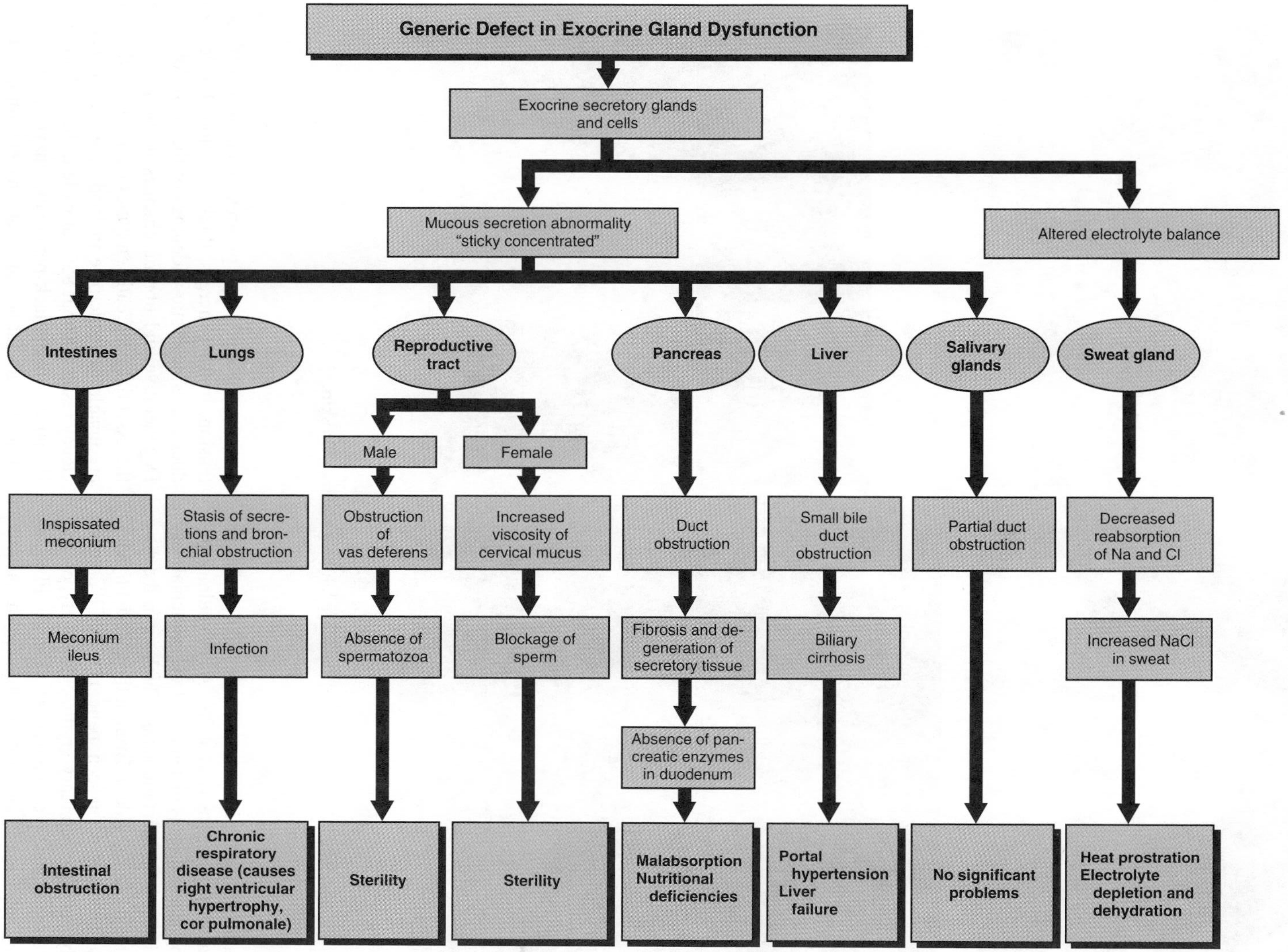

FIG. 4-26
Pathogenesis of CF. (From Wilson and Thompson.[41])

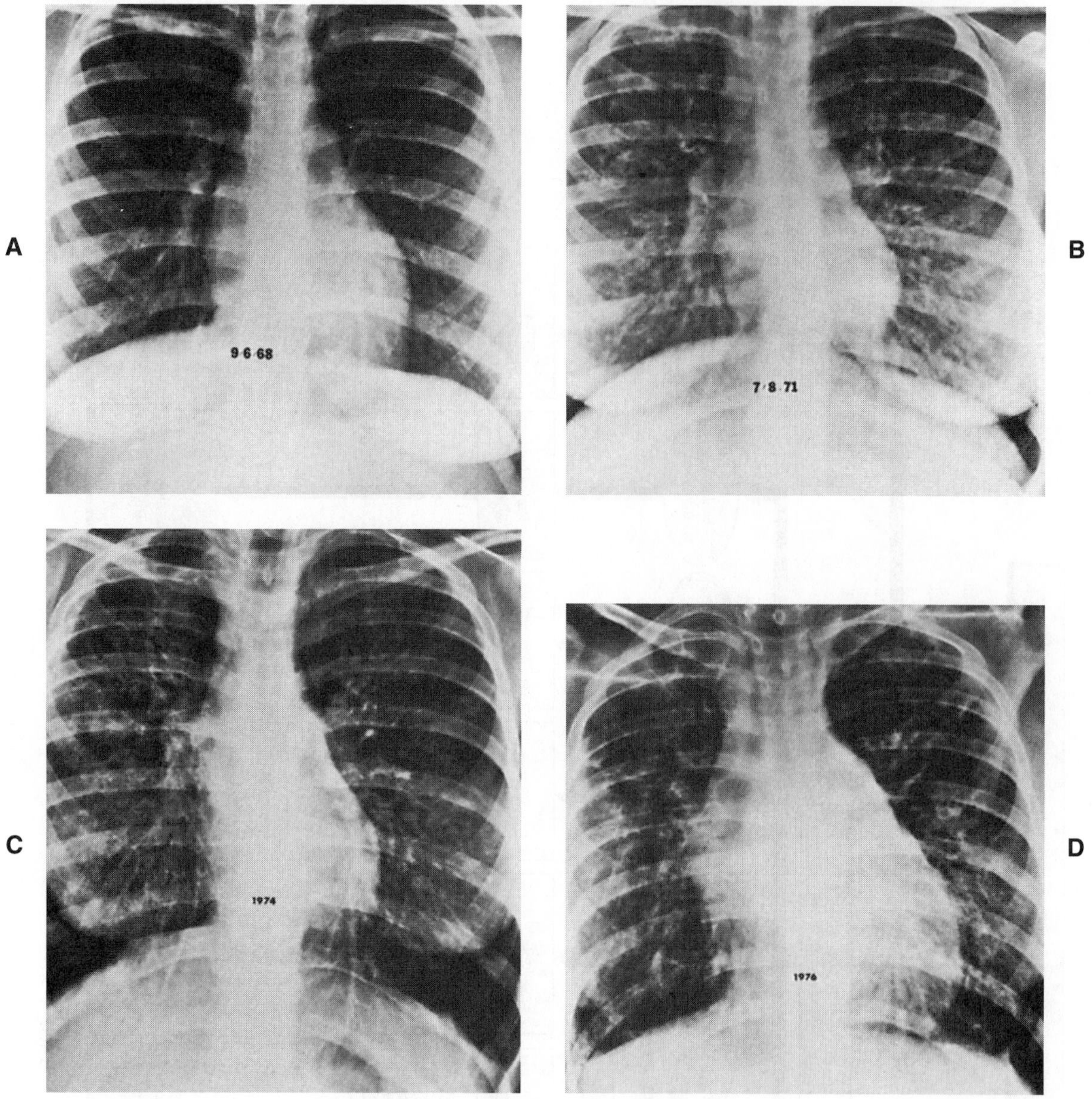

FIG. 4-27
CF, adult onset. (From Groskin.[12])

tion of the airway wall; the wall becomes floppy and contributes to even more stasis of secretions (FIG. 4-28). As the pulmonary involvement progresses, there is distention of the bronchial vessels, especially in the bronchiectatic areas. Clubbing of the digits (fingers and toes) is also evident. Even in those patients with mild disease, hypoxemia is often seen; patients with CF do not, however, usually develop secondary erythrocytosis. Hypercapnia develops late in the course of the disease when the FEV_1 is very low. Airway infection is an ongoing problem in patients with CF. About 80% of adults with CF have *P. aeruginosa.* Other infecting organisms are *Burkholderia cepacia* and aspergillus. The development of drug resistance is common.

Gastrointestinal System

The involvement of the exocrine pancreas contributes to intestinal absorption problems; in addition, there is liver involvement that in adults may progress to cirrhosis with portal hypertension. In the pancreas, thick secretions block the pancreatic ducts, causing cystic widenings of the small lobes of the acini. Degenerative and fibrotic changes in the pancreas result, and the essential pancreatic enzymes (trypsin, amylase, and lipase) are unable to participate in food digestion. Pancreatic insufficiency results. About 85% of patients have abnormal digestion. Because patients lack pancreatic enzymes, they cannot digest fat nor absorb fat-soluble vitamins, etc. Impaired digestion and absorption with increased dietary need (related to chronic infections, etc.) and decreased intake result in weight loss and failure to thrive.

Endocrine System

About three fourths of patients age 30 years have diabetes mellitus (called CFRD: CF-related diabetes).

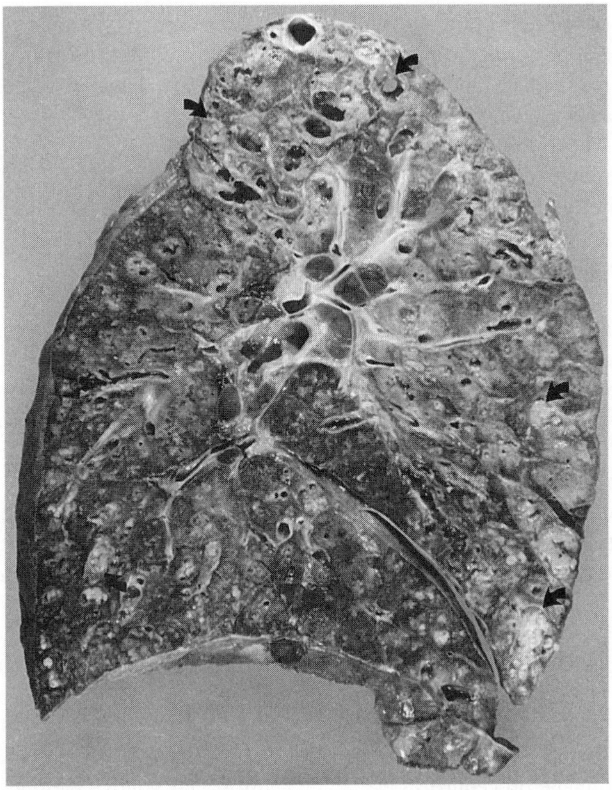

FIG. 4-28
Severe bronchiectasis in CF. Many of the dilated airways are filled with purulent mucus. (From Murray and Nadel.[23])

Reproductive System

CF involvement of the reproductive system also causes special problems for adult patients. Males are usually aspermic. Females ovulate but because of obstruction of the fallopian tubes often have fertility problems.

DIAGNOSTIC STUDIES AND FINDINGS

CF may be diagnosed at any age from infancy to adulthood. Diagnosis is based on clinical presentation and is confirmed by an elevated sweat chloride level, the most consistent diagnostic test available, although even this has a 2% false-positive and false-negative rate. A sweat chloride concentration greater than 60 mEq/L is considered diagnostic in adults.

History: Frequent pulmonary infections; history of siblings or other family members with CF; in infants, mother often notes that baby "tastes salty"; nutrition history: appetite; percentages of carbohydrate, fat, and protein in diet

Systems review

Appearance: Often thin, appears malnourished, fingers clubbed

Lung: Crackles, repeated infections

GI function: Insufficient absorption producing bulky, foul-smelling, pale, watery stools (large volumes of fat excreted in the stool [steatorrhea] suggestive of CF); jaundice; enlarged liver; enlarged spleen; ascites; evidence of intestinal obstruction, fecal impaction, or rectal prolapse

Laboratory tests: Abnormal liver function findings; elevated glucose level (diabetes); decreased serum sodium, chloride; examination of duodenal secretions, blood, or stool for presence of enzymes; absence of enzymes suggestive of potential CF; albumin level and prealbumin low; stool examination for fat; fat absorption tests conducted for 3 days to calculate ratio of fat in oral intake to fat in stool; culture and sensitivity of sputum

ABGs: Mild hypoxemia; increased Pa_{CO_2} not seen until late stages of pulmonary involvement

Chest roentgenogram: Evidence of bronchiectasis suggestive of CF (see FIG. 4-27); most commonly in upper lobes

MULTIDISCIPLINARY PLAN

Therapy for patients with CF is aimed at slowing progression of the bronchiectasis, improving absorption and thus nutritional status, and preventing/treating other complications. In the adult CF patient, emphasis must also be placed on psychosocial issues related to the role in the family and community. Death is most commonly caused by cardiac and respiratory insufficiency.

Surgery

Bilateral double lung transplantation (usually without heart transplantation) may be an option; may also be a living donor transplant (two donors each donate a lobe)

Invasive Therapies

Bronchial artery embolization for massive hemoptysis

Medications

Because of the many organs often involved and the variety of medications taken, care must be taken to check for drug interactions.

Antiinfective agents: May be prescribed only at time of illness and infection or prophylactically; if prescribed for infection, antibiotic of choice depends on organism and sensitivity. Antibiotics given orally, IV, or aerosolized. Oral antibiotics specific for *P. aeruginosa* are the fluoroquinolones. The sulfa drugs (trimethoprim-sulfamethoxazole) and chloramphenicol may be administered orally or parenterally and are used for *B. Cepacia.* Parenteral antibiotics for *P. aeruginosa* are the beta-lactams (e.g., piperacillin, cephalosporins, and aminoglycosides (tobramycin); tobramycin is also administered by aerosol. Some CF patients have long-term, indwelling catheters and use IV antibiotics in the home setting. Also, present approaches to therapy include specialized sensitivity tests to ascertain which combination of drugs would be most helpful.

Mucolytics: Dornase alfa (Pulmozyme) (usually referred to as DNAse): Given daily by aerosol to hydrolyze DNA in sputum, decreasing sputum viscosity and elasticity.

Corticosteroids: May benefit those patients with an asthmatic component in burst doses; role in chronic therapy of CF is unclear.

Bronchodilators: Not used in all patients.

Beta agonists (e.g., albuterol)

Metered aerosol 1-2 puffs q4-6h; (dosage by small-volume nebulizer varies with the specific beta agonist) often administered with drainage procedure.

Theophylline PO or IV: When used must be monitored because drug clearance is highly variable among CF patients; many require higher dosage to reach therapeutic level.

Digestive agents: Pancreatic enzymes are administered to assist in digestion of carbohydrates, fats, and proteins.

Enteric coated: 500 lipase units/kg with meals (taken in split dose during meal—one third at beginning, at midpoint, and at end); 20 lipase units/kg with snacks (when nonenteric-coated preparations are used, the dose may be doubled) (NOTE: Be very sure of the "activity" of the preparation used; there are wide variations.)

Contraindication: Hypersensitivity to pork or beef

Common side effects: Nausea, diarrhea, vomiting, anorexia

Histamine blockers (H_2): Neutralize gastric acids that deactivate enzyme supplements; used when patient responds poorly to enzyme supplements

Immunizations: Routine immunizations against pneumococcal pneumonia and influenza recommended as preventive measures.

General Management

Oxygen: May be indicated for persons unable to maintain adequate oxygen levels; oxygen concentrations should be as low as possible while maintaining adequate Pao_2 level

Aerosol therapy: May be used intermittently in conjunction with physiotherapy, drainage maneuvers

Diet: Sufficient calories; increased work of breathing may increase energy expenditure by 150%; at least 40% of calories should be from fat; many adults may require enteral feeding

Physical therapy: Airway clearance techniques—significant priority of daily health maintenance for the patient with CF; techniques used 1 to 2 times a day in stable disease, increased to 4 times or more daily during acute illness; may include postural drainage, percussion, use of flutter valve, percussion vests, forced expiratory technique, and others.

NURSING CARE

NURSING ASSESSMENT

Respiratory status

Examination: Barrel chest; use of accessory muscles, retractions, decreased chest wall movement, tachypnea; dull percussion tone over consolidation or areas of atelectasis; clubbing of fingers and toes

Breath sounds: Crackles; decreased or unequal breath sounds; sonorous wheeze (rhonchus) with excessive large airway secretions

Sputum: Productive cough with thick, often purulent sputum; report if hemoptysis

Pulmonary function: Decreased vital capacity; decreased FEV_1, decreased FEV_1/FVC

Gas exchange: Decreased O_2 saturation, hypoxemia (decreased Pao_2); symptoms may include headache, tachycardia, dizziness, changes in mental status; hypercapnia in late stages ($Paco_2 > 42$); usually no symptoms if chronic; if acute may see confusion, somnolence, asterixis

Nutritional status: Weight, dietary intake, tolerance of meals (e.g., fatty stools)

Psychosocial status: Support systems; networking with CF resource groups; ADLs; self-esteem; interaction with peers; sexuality; body image; vocational history

POTENTIAL COMPLICATIONS

Complications of pulmonary involvement include pneumothorax, major episodes of hemoptysis, cor pulmonale, and heart failure. Respiratory and cardiac complications tend to become severe with increasing age.

PATIENT PROBLEMS/NURSING DIAGNOSES & INTERVENTIONS

NIC RESPIRATORY MANAGEMENT

Ineffective airway clearance related to tracheobronchial obstruction

Ineffective breathing pattern related to tracheobronchial obstruction

Impaired gas exchange related to alveolar-capillary membrane changes

- Carefully and frequently auscultate chest for quality of breath sounds and adventitious sounds. Note cough and sputum characteristics.
- Provide hydration to replace fluids.
- Assist with airway clearance measures, including end-expiratory cough, drainage, forced expiratory technique (FET) coughing, autodrainage as indicated/ordered.
- Promptly administer mucolytics and expectorants as ordered. Observe for therapeutic response and side effects.
- Administer aerosol and perform airway clearance measures at least 1 hour before meals; provide oral hygiene after treatment.

- Maintain patient positioning *to facilitate use of accessory muscles of ventilation* (tripod position).
- Encourage patient to use adaptive breathing techniques *to decrease work of breathing.*
- Protect patient from known sources of secondary infection or respiratory irritants such as smoking.
- Assess patient to identify signs, such as restlessness, confusion, and irritability, that may indicate body's response to altered blood gas states.
- If patient is very ill, monitor ABGs. Report increases or decreases of more than 5 to 10 mm Hg in $Paco_2$ and Pao_2.
- Administer oxygen as ordered and monitor to maintain Pao_2 of 60 to 70 mm Hg, saturation >90%.
- Venturi mask may be used if needed. If adequate blood gas levels cannot be maintained, noninvasive positive pressure ventilation (NPPV) may be used; intubation and mechanical ventilation may be required.
- If patient is very ill, monitor electrocardiogram and cardiac status for arrhythmias resulting from alterations in blood gas levels.
- Monitor and record kidney functioning and urinary output, which may be affected by chronic tissue hypoxia and alterations in metabolism.
- Monitor serum electrolyte levels, which may change owing to alterations in oxygenation and metabolism.
- Carefully monitor body temperature. Elevations in temperature increase tissue demands for oxygen.

NIC Nutrition Support

Imbalanced nutrition: less than body requirements, related to increased caloric needs and impaired nutrient absorption

Delayed growth and development related to impaired absorption and chronic illness

- Assess nutritional status by weighing, monitoring intake and output.
- Provide balanced diet; fat is no longer restricted as in past; in fact, fat is a good source of calories.
- Be sure that enzymes are taken with meals and snacks.
- Provide vitamin supplementation of fat-soluble vitamins (A, D, E, K).
- Provide small, frequent feedings in patients who are dyspneic.
- Monitor for signs and symptoms of malnutrition.
- Assess stool; note odor, color, amount, frequency, and consistency.
- Observe for signs of intestinal obstruction.
- Administer stool softener as ordered and report results.
- Monitor invasive methods of nutritional supplementation; ensure adequate intake without interfering with airway care treatments; dressings as indicated, etc.

NIC Coping Assistance

Ineffective coping related to chronic illness

Ineffective role performance

Sexual dysfunction

Risk for activity intolerance

- Assess patient's understanding of present and chronic disease state.
- Determine patient's ability to cooperate with health-care providers in interventions such as breathing techniques, drainage maneuvers, exercise progression, enzyme therapy.
- Determine if referral needed for discussion of genetics; note impact on marriage, childbearing.
- Discuss impact of disease on role functions of adulthood.
- Assist patient to develop appropriate coping strategies based on personal strengths and past experience.
- Assist patient to participate in care.
- Encourage patient to maintain program of regular exercise.

Patient Education/Continuum of Care Plan

CF patients require extensive education because long-term compliance with complicated therapy, including frequent hospitalizations (periodic "tune-ups"), is necessary.

1. Teach patient about disease process, multisystem involvement, and genetic basis.
2. Teach patient airway clearance techniques.
3. Instruct patient about diet and use of pharmacologic interventions to ensure adequate nutrition.
4. Instruct patient regarding need for continued surveillance and long-term follow-up.
5. Provide information regarding sources of counseling (role development, marriage, vocational opportunities).

Evaluation/Patient Outcomes

Respiratory Management: Airway is patent. Breathing occurs without tiring patient. Chest auscultation demonstrates that adventitial sounds are at patient's baseline (may always have crackles). Patient demonstrates modified breathing techniques that facilitate dyspnea control. Patient understands and uses respiratory medications appropriately; patient understands importance of daily airway clearance and performs on a regular basis. Oxygenation is adequate. Pao_2 is maintained >60 mm Hg; saturation >90%.

Nutrition Support: Patient understands need for enzyme replacement; takes replacement therapy; is able to maintain weight (should be normal); and takes vitamin supplements.

Coping Assistance: Patient understands disease and therapy; is actively involved in own therapy; returns for regularly scheduled visits; is progressing through normal developmental stages for adults; can discuss issues related to childbearing.

Interstitial Lung Disease[19,30]

Interstitial lung disease (ILD) is a general term used to describe those diseases that involve the supporting structures of the lung, those structures found in the interstitium (connective tissue, alveolar septa, lymphatic space).

These diseases usually involve an inflammatory response with the development of fibrosis. Some of the interstitial diseases have known causes, while others do not. The pneumoconioses are interstitial lung diseases caused by inhalation of mineral dusts (silicosis, asbestosis). Other known causes of interstitial lung disease include lung radiation, responses to certain drugs such as bleomycin, and interstitial involvement by tumor. There are also many interstitial lung diseases for which there is no known etiology. Examples include idiopathic pulmonary fibrosis (IPF), sarcoidosis, venoocclusive disease of the lung, and ILD associated with collagen vascular disease (rheumatoid arthritis and rheumatoid lung); *Hamman-Rich syndrome* was the name historically used to describe a very aggressive form of idiopathic fibrosis.

Some interstitial diseases respond to treatment, but many do not. For the pneumoconioses the major aim is prevention by reducing or eliminating exposure. Some interstitial diseases have a chronic, prolonged course, while others have a very rapid, fulminant course. Some, such as sarcoidosis, are more common among younger to middle-age adults, while some, such as IPF, are more common among persons in their 50s and 60s; IPF is also more common in men. This section will present the pathophysiology and diagnostic findings of interstitial pulmonary fibrosis with emphasis on IPF.

Pathophysiology

Although the specific mechanism of injury varies among the different ILDs, the end result is an inflammatory reaction in the lung, an influx of inflammatory cells into the interstitium of the lung, and the development of lung fibrosis.

Idiopathic Pulmonary Fibrosis

There are subtypes of idiopathic pulmonary fibrosis (IPF), the most common of which is the usual interstitial pneumonia (UIP). The onset is usually insidious. There is initially an inflammatory change but over time remodeling of the lung parenchyma occurs. The disease is usually patchy, with areas of normal lung, areas demonstrating inflammation but not fibrosis, and areas of extensive fibrosis (Fig. 4-29). In IPF the precipitating event in lung scarring is unknown. The entire process is thought to be an excessive immune response; the lung is trying to heal itself but instead overresponds, resulting in extensive scarring. Even with treatment, mortality is 59% to 70%.[19]

Sarcoidosis

Sarcoidosis is another interstitial disease without a known etiology. The initial lung lesion is hilar lymphadenopathy. The pathologic change is one of noncaseating granuloma formation. Some of the granulomas regress, and others progress to fibrotic changes. There is no good way to predict which patients will progress to chronic interstitial pulmonary disease. The disease, which can affect multiple organs (eyes, heart, skin, spleen), is related to impaired cellular immunity; these patients are usually anergic—they do not react to any delayed hypersensitivity skin tests (e.g., TB, mumps).

Hypersensitivity Pneumonitis

This disease (also called *allergic alveolitis*) has a known etiology; it is a specific reaction to an inhaled antigen. Examples are Farmer's lung, caused by an antigen in moldy hay, and bird fancier's lung, caused by an antigen in bird products. Acutely the person will have fever, chills, cough, and dyspnea; the reaction will begin several hours after exposure and is usually self-limited. With continued exposure a chronic form of the disease with fibrotic changes in the lung occurs.

Progression of ILD

In all of these examples, progression of the disease results in a restrictive pulmonary disease. The changes in pulmonary function tests [PFTs] are more variable in hypersensitivity pneumonitis. The inflammation and scarring result in a stiff lung; there is increased recoil and decreased compliance. Lung volumes (total lung capacity [TLC], residual volume [RV], vital capacity [VC]) are reduced, especially in IPF. There is no slowing of expiration because the defect is in the lung parenchyma, not the airway. The FEV_1 will be reduced but proportionately to the FVC; the FEV_1/FVC ratio is normal. The dramatic symptom of pulmonary fibrosis is dyspnea. The patient has a relatively rapid respiratory rate; the expiratory time is short.

Gas exchange is also affected. Early in the disease gas exchange is maintained. The patient's arterial oxygenation is adequate at rest, but the patient often has to hyperventilate (low $Paco_2$) to maintain the Pao_2. With exercise the level of oxygenation often falls dramatically. Because the alveoli are filled with debris, these patients are much more difficult to oxygenate than are patients who have diseases such as COPD. At end-stage disease, hypoventilation (CO_2 retention) may occur.

Diagnostic Studies and Findings

History: An extensive history is taken to rule out any possibility of immune suppression (e.g., HIV), inhalation exposure (e.g., birds, drugs, workplace), or presence of a collagen-vascular disease (e.g., lupus, arthritis); various conditions are capable of producing the roentgenographic picture seen in IPF, and many known diseases can produce inflammation and fibrosis. For example, in allergic alveolitis the history will demonstrate the presumed antigen and further tests will confirm it. Occupational exposure will make one suspect pneumoconiosis. The diagnosis of IPF is one of exclusion—other reasons for developing fibrosis must be excluded.

Clinical examination (symptoms often absent in early disease): Findings include rapid respiratory rate, short expiratory time, and crackles on auscultation. Clubbing is common in IPF and asbestosis; it is not usually seen in sarcoidosis and is variable in hypersensitivity pneumonitis.

Chest roentgenogram: Films reveal increased interstitial markings (pattern varies with different etiologies of the fibrosis), bilateral patchy infiltrates, and decreased lung volumes. Obtaining old films is helpful to determine the time of onset and progression of the changes. A high-resolution CT scan is often required to visualize the presence and/or extent of the changes.

Pulmonary function studies: Studies show decreased lung volumes (TLC, RV, VC). FEV_1/FVC is normal (FEV_1 will be decreased proportionate to the decrease in VC). Diffusion capacity of the lung for carbon monoxide (DLco) is decreased. ABGs often demonstrate hyperventilation; Pao_2 is usually maintained at rest in early disease. Rest and exercise pulse oximetry (or ABGs) often demonstrates a fall in oxygenation with exercise.

Bronchoscopy: Bronchoscopy with bronchoalveolar lavage (BAL) and/or transbronchial biopsy is per-

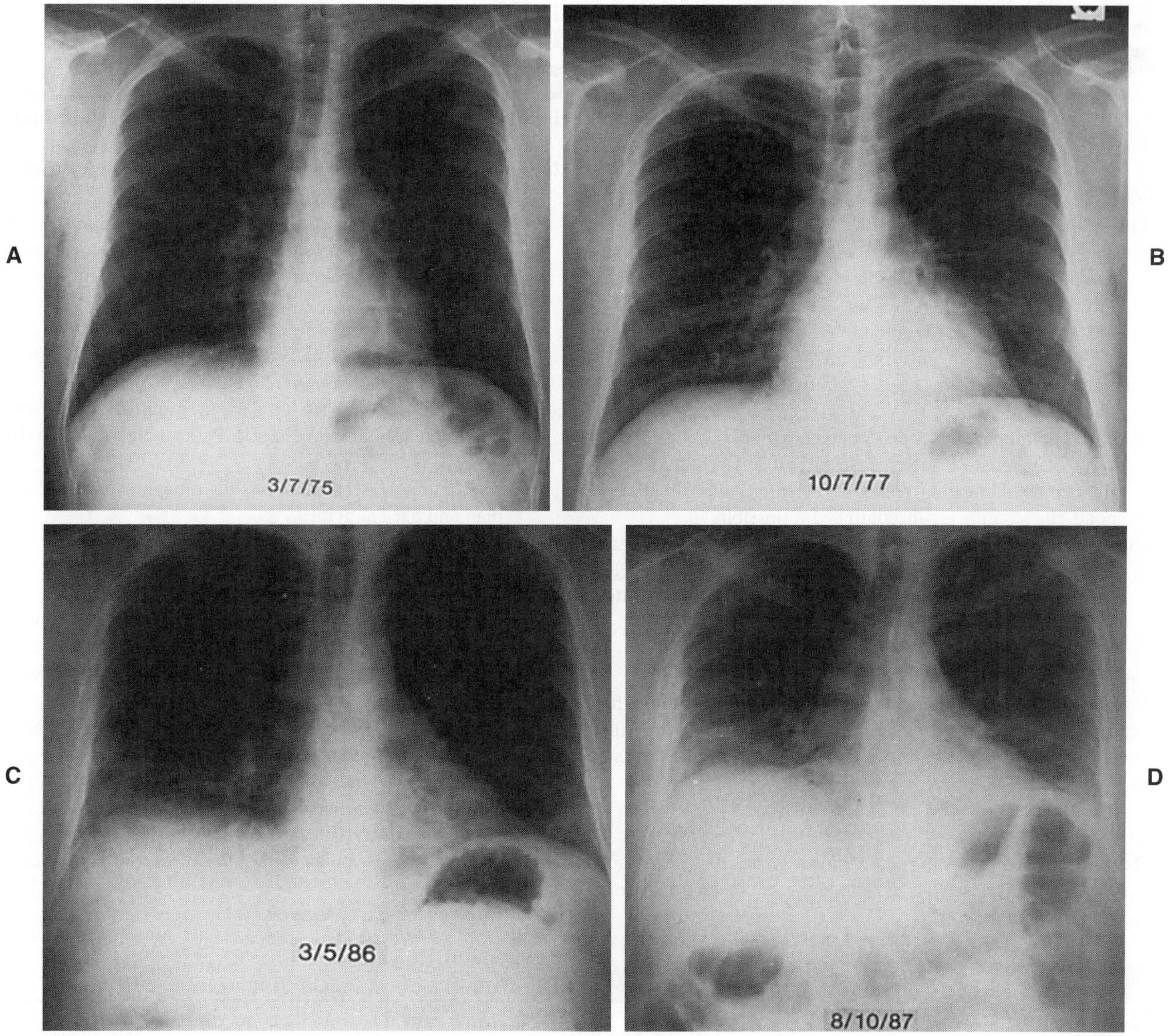

FIG. 4-29

These serial chest roentgenograms were made in a patient with idiopathic pulmonary fibrosis. **A,** Posteroanterior roentgenogram of the chest obtained at the time of onset of breathlessness with exercise and mild cough. The chest appears normal. **B,** Follow-up film reveals progressive loss of lung volume and bibasilar, predominantly reticular, infiltrates. The patient had stopped regular exercise because of breathlessness with exertion. **C,** Progressive changes are evident, with severe loss of lung volume. Predominantly in the lower lung zone, diffuse, bilateral, coarse reticular infiltrates are seen, typically of the roentgenographic appearance of the mid to late stage of pulmonary fibrosis. **D,** Continued disease progression with evidence of honeycombing and pulmonary hypertension. Open lung biopsy reveals usual interstitial pneumonitis with extensive fibrosis and histologic honeycombing. Treatment with corticosteroids and cyclophosphamide (Cytoxan) was started, but the patient experienced a progressive decline in functional status and died 6 months following lung transplantation. (From Murray and Nadel.[23])

formed to obtain a sample of the inflammatory cells in the alveoli (BAL) or an actual piece of lung tissue (biopsy). The presence of an infectious process must be ruled out; cultures from the bronchoscopy will facilitate this process.

Lung biopsy: A thoracoscopic or open lung biopsy may be done to obtain a sample of lung tissue. The so-called "gold standard," the study to which other results are compared, is the open lung biopsy. The tissue is cultured, pathologic changes are described, and if indicated, various stains and immunochemical studies can be performed to help identify the cause and extent of the process.

Other tests: In sarcoid, skin tests are performed to determine if the patient is anergic. In hypersensitivity pneumonitis titers of antibody to the offending antigen can be identified. If collagen vascular disease is suspected, rheumatoid factor and other identifiers will be tested.

MULTIDISCIPLINARY PLAN

Surgery

Lung transplantation has been used in IPF; both single- and double-lung procedures have been performed.

Medications

Antiinflammatory agents: The antiinflammatory medications have variable effects, but are usually instituted in persons with progressive fibrotic disease. Therapy is usually begun with corticosteroids and then may go on to include cytotoxic agents. Patients must be monitored closely for side effects and evaluated for benefit of the therapy.

Corticosteroids: Prednisone is given in relatively large doses (60 mg/day) initially; if there is a therapeutic response (improved pulmonary function, roentgenographic changes), the dose is tapered to a lower dose to reduce side effects but maintain the therapeutic response. In patients who do not respond, the steroids are discontinued if possible.

Cytotoxic agents such as cyclophosphamide (Cytoxan), azathioprine (Immuran), or methotrexate: May be used in IPF; recently cyclosporine has also been used. Dosages are individualized and monitored by leukocyte count.

General Management

If an etiologic agent is identified, terminating or controlling the exposure is the treatment of choice (e.g., if disorder is drug induced, stop the drug; if Farmer's lung, reduce/control exposure to moldy hay).

Oxygen Therapy

Oxygen by cannula; may require flows greater than 5 L/min (LPM) with exercise (some patients use special oxygen-conserving cannulas).

NURSING CARE

NURSING ASSESSMENT

Respiratory status: Tachypnea, use of accessory muscles with inspiration, dyspnea, short expiratory phase; crackles (note that crackles are usually present); dry, nonproductive cough; clinical indicators of potential hypoxemia include tachycardia, tachypnea, restlessness, cyanosis, impaired judgment (tachycardia may be present without hypoxemia)

Pulmonary function studies: Reduced in VC and FEV_1; changes in oxygenation with exercise (pulmonary function studies will assist nurse to evaluate/set goals for patient's activity, tolerance level)

WBC count: Monitored to follow response and determine dosage of immunosuppressive therapy

Cardiovascular status: Assess for signs and symptoms of cor pulmonale (see p. 189)

Infection: Assess for signs of infection in lung and elsewhere; may not demonstrate usual febrile response or high WBC count because of immunosuppressive therapy

Anxiety: Fear, air hunger

Other: Assess for side effects of the specific drugs used

POTENTIAL COMPLICATIONS

Cor pulmonale, severe hypoxemia

PATIENT PROBLEMS/NURSING DIAGNOSES & INTERVENTIONS

NIC RESPIRATORY MANAGEMENT

Ineffective breathing pattern related to decreased compliance, increased ventilatory drive

Impaired gas exchange related to alveolar-capillary membrane changes, low V/Q

- Position *to improve efficiency of the accessory muscles of inspiration* (tripod position); note that position can also be maintained during walking by having patient push a cart, wheelchair, etc.
- Time activities *to provide rest periods.*
- Administer oxygen as ordered *to maintain Pao_2;* flow rates usually increased with activity.
- In collaboration with physician, monitor ABGs; report increases or decreases in Pao_2 or $Paco_2$ >5 to 10 mm Hg.
- Avoid unnecessary increases in oxygen consumption; plan and pace activities.

NIC RISK MANAGEMENT

Risk for infection because of altered immunologic status

- If appropriate, modify environment *to reduce/eliminate airborne exposure.*
- Ensure that appropriate immunizations (influenza, pneumococcal pneumonia, etc.) are received.
- Teach patient/family to avoid exposure to infections.
- Monitor for signs and symptoms of infection: changes in amount, characteristics of sputum; febrile response (will frequently be less than usual); WBC response; pain; cuts that do not heal.
- Monitor for response to cytotoxic drugs

PATIENT EDUCATION/CONTINUUM OF CARE PLAN

1. Teach patient and family about disease.
2. Teach about drugs, monitoring, and side effects.
3. If patient is taking cytotoxic drugs, ensure patient understands need for close follow-up and routine blood work.
4. If patient has a fulminant type of pulmonary fibrosis (IPF of the rapidly progressive type), determine if they have discussed end-of-life decision making.

EVALUATION/PATIENT OUTCOMES

Respiratory Management: Breathing pattern is optimal for patient's level of pulmonary function; as patient's condition progresses moderate to severe dyspnea may be constantly present. Gas exchange is adequate. Pao_2 is maintained at >60 mm Hg at rest and >55 mm Hg with exercise. Patient has methods to conserve energy.

Risk Management: Has received pneumococcal and influenza vaccines as indicated. Infection is not present. Patient can relate signs and symptoms of infection/knows when to seek emergency care. Patient has schedule for routine blood work. Environmental exposure is decreased/eliminated.

PULMONARY HYPERTENSION AND COR PULMONALE[15,29,38]

Pulmonary hypertension is defined as an increase in the main pulmonary artery pressure at rest or during exercise.

Cor pulmonale is a condition of hypertrophy and dilation of the right ventricle of the heart resulting from a disease process that affects the function or structure of the lung or its vasculature.

The pressure in the pulmonary artery exceeds 30/18 mm Hg at rest. Pulmonary hypertension occurs most often secondary to a pulmonary disorder.

A rare and severe form of pulmonary hypertension is primary pulmonary hypertension, which usually affects women age 20 to 40 years (FIG. 4-30). Primary pulmonary hypertension develops for yet unknown reasons, but recently has been linked to the use of the antiobesity drugs fenfluramine and dexfenfluramine. Other factors thought to be related to the development of primary pulmonary hypertension are oral contraceptive use, elevated catecholamines, and hepatic dysfunction.

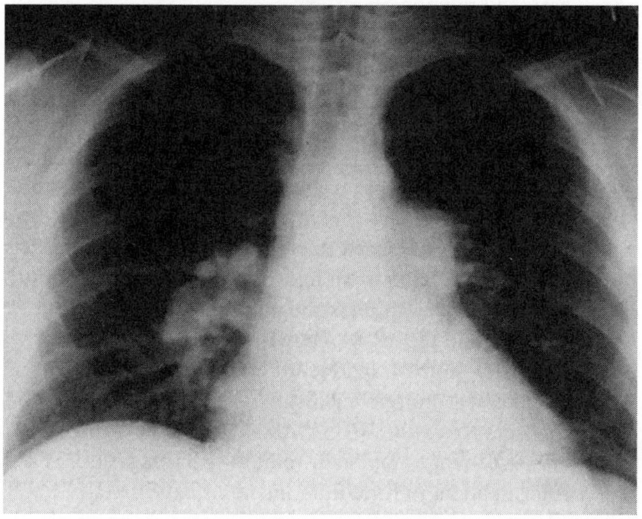

FIG. 4-30
Chest roentgenogram from a patient with primary pulmonary hypertension. (From Murray and Nadel.[23])

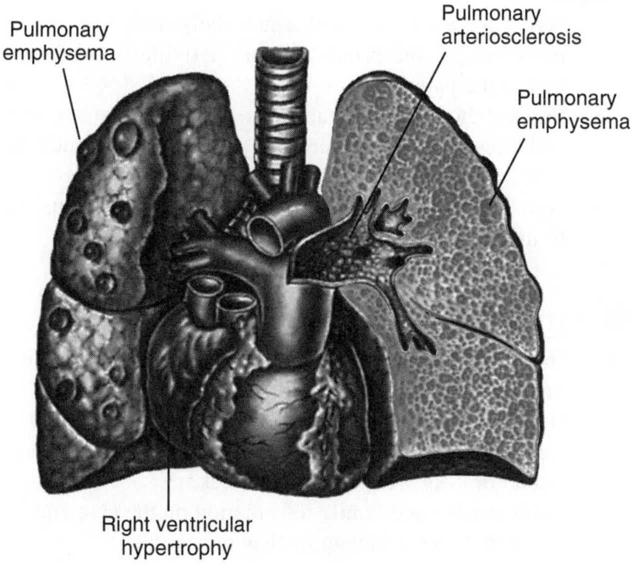

FIG. 4-31
Cor pulmonale secondary to emphysema. (From Wilson and Thompson.[41])

Cor pulmonale occurs as a secondary process after a primary pulmonary disease. COPD accounts for the majority of cases of cor pulmonale in the United States (FIG. 4-31). Other disorders leading to cor pulmonale are vascular diseases such as chronic thromboembolism, restrictive lung diseases such as pulmonary interstitial fibrosis, and chest wall disorders such as kyphoscoliosis.

PATHOPHYSIOLOGY

The pulmonary circulation is normally a low-pressure, low-resistance system. There are three primary factors in the development of cor pulmonale and secondary pulmonary hypertension: (1) reduction in the size of the pulmonary vascular bed as a result of destruction of pulmonary capillaries or loss of large amounts of lung tissue; (2) increased resistance in the pulmonary vascular bed from damage to the lining of pulmonary vessels; and (3) pulmonary vasoconstriction and elevation of pressure in the pulmonary artery because of local hypoxia in underventilated areas of the lung. FIG. 4-32 shows the pathogenesis of cor pulmonale.

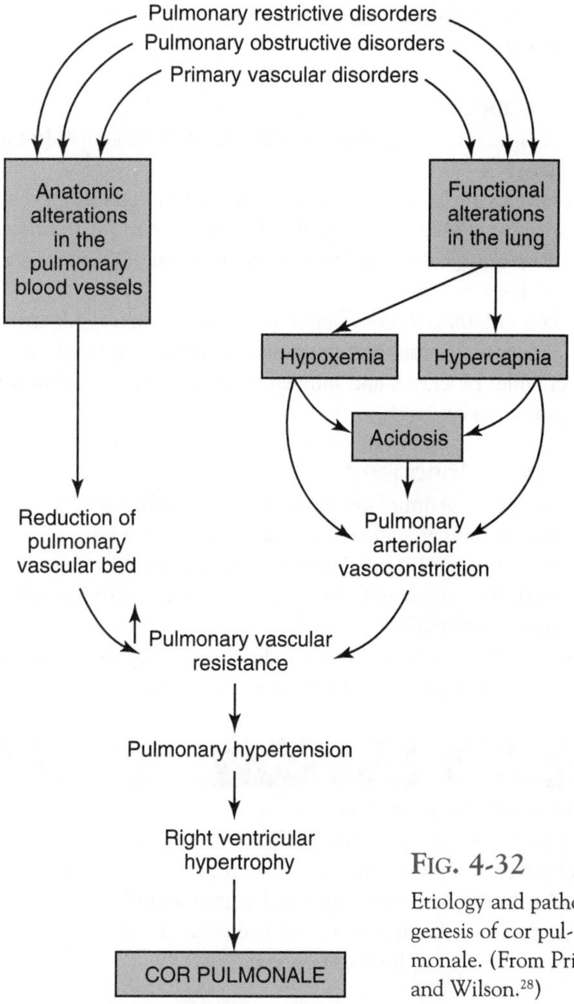

FIG. 4-32
Etiology and pathogenesis of cor pulmonale. (From Price and Wilson.[28])

Diagnostic Studies and Findings

Arterial blood gases: Decreased Pao_2 in range of 40 to 60 mm Hg; $Paco_2$ varies with underlying disease
Chest roentgenogram: Enlarged pulmonary arteries, right ventricular hypertrophy
Echocardiogram: Right ventricular enlargement
Electrocardiogram: Dysrhythmias resulting from hypoxia; right bundle-branch block; right axis deviation; right ventricular hypertrophy
Complete blood count: Elevated hemoglobin level and hematocrit value (erythrocytosis) resulting from chronic hypoxia
Cardiac catheterization or pulmonary artery catheter placement: Pulmonary artery systolic pressure above 30 mm Hg; diastolic pressure above 18 mm Hg

Multidisciplinary Plan

The underlying pulmonary and cardiac diseases must be treated as well. (See Chapter 3 for cardiac disease guidelines.)

Surgery

Lung transplantation or heart-lung transplantation may be done for primary pulmonary hypertension. See p. 213 for further information about transplantation.

Pulmonary thromboendarterectomy may be done to treat severe chronic thromboembolic pulmonary hypertension. Cardiopulmonary bypass is required during surgery.

Medications

Anticoagulants: To prevent occlusion of damaged pulmonary vessels
Diuretics: Initial diuresis can lower pulmonary artery pressure by decreasing total blood volume; careful monitoring of serum electrolyte levels needed when administering diuretics
Bronchodilators: Recommended to improve airway obstruction
In primary pulmonary hypertension, prostacyclines, calcium channel blockers, and inhaled nitric oxide are used to dilate pulmonary vessels.

General Management

Oxygenation: Administered as needed to achieve 93% to 95% arterial oxygen saturation or arterial oxygen tension greater than 60 mm Hg; providing adequate inspired oxygen is the most effective way to promote pulmonary vasodilation
Sodium-restricted diet
Therapeutic phlebotomy: To reduce erythrocytosis and blood viscosity; used when hematocrit is >58%

NURSING CARE

Nursing Assessment

Evidence of chronic lung diseases; dyspnea; tachycardia; tachypnea cough; cyanosis; wheezing; distended neck veins; loud split S2; gallop rhythm and occasional murmur resulting from functional insufficiency of tricuspid and pulmonic valves; dependent edema; liver enlargement

Patient Problems/Nursing Diagnoses & Interventions

Nursing diagnoses and care should be directed toward the primary disease state. In addition, the following diagnoses and care strategies are specific for cor pulmonale and pulmonary hypertension.

NIC Respiratory Management

Impaired gas exchange related to V/Q mismatch

- Monitor oxygen saturation and ABG studies. Administer oxygen to maintain oxygen saturation between 90% and 95%.
- If patient has chronic hypercapnia, keep oxygen saturation at 90% to 93%. Avoid saturations >95% to prevent depression of the ventilatory drive.
- Maintain bed rest during acute episodes to conserve energy and pulmonary effort.
- Monitor electrocardiogram and cardiac status for dysrhythmias resulting from alterations in blood gas levels.

NIC Tissue Perfusion Management

Decreased cardiac output related to pulmonary vascular narrowing
Excess fluid volume related to right ventricular failure

- Carefully monitor systemic hypotensive effects of vasodilators given to relax the pulmonary vessels.
- Monitor and record weight daily.
- Carefully monitor and record intake and output.
- Administer diuretic medications in collaboration with physician.
- Assist patient to maintain sodium-restricted diet.
- Assist patient to limit fluid intake, if excessive.
- Monitor serum electrolytes, which may change owing to administration of diuretics.

NIC Activity and Exercise Management

Fatigue

- Assist patient to identify which daily activities use the most energy, and prioritize those activities most important to the patient.
- Support the patient in learning to accept help to complete activities that require increased energy and in identifying resources for help.
- Assist the patient to identify ways to complete usual activities that save energy.

Patient Education/Continuum of Care Plan

The primary education is directed toward patient's primary disease; refer to patient education for the appropriate disease.

1. Teach importance of restricting salt and fluid intake.
2. Teach patient to weigh daily and report greater than a 2-pound or 1-kg weight gain per week.
3. Provide patient and family information on the care and use of oxygen devices, including cleaning.
4. Emphasize that oxygen ordered for continuous use must be worn for a least 22 of 24 hours to avoid pulmonary vasoconstriction and increasing right heart failure.

EVALUATION/PATIENT OUTCOMES

Also see patient outcomes for the underlying disease state.

Respiratory Management: Optimum gas exchange. Blood gas values are within normal limits for patient's chronic condition.

Tissue Perfusion Management: Cardiac output is adequate to maintain cerebral function, renal function, activity level. Fluid and electrolyte balance is restored. There is no evidence of fluid retention; serum electrolyte levels are within normal limits.

Activity and Exercise Management: Patient identifies resources and energy-saving strategies. Fatigue is managed at a level acceptable to the patient.

PULMONARY EDEMA

Pulmonary edema is the accumulation of serous fluid in the interstitial lung tissue and alveoli.

Pulmonary edema may be described as cardiogenic or noncardiogenic. Cardiogenic pulmonary edema results from increased hydrostatic pressure caused by left ventricular failure. See the section on congestive heart failure (in Chapter 3) for further discussion of cardiogenic pulmonary edema.

Noncardiogenic pulmonary edema results from increased capillary permeability, such as occurs with adult respiratory distress syndrome (ARDS), or from decreased colloid osmotic pressure, such as occurs in nephritis or hepatic failure. See the discussion of ARDS (pp. 195-196) for further description of noncardiogenic pulmonary edema.

When interstitial lung spaces are engorged with fluid, the fluid moves across alveolar capillary membranes into the alveoli. If fluid accumulates faster than it can be cleared, acute pulmonary edema interferes with oxygen diffusion, resulting in acute respiratory failure. See the discussion of acute respiratory failure in this chapter.

PULMONARY EMBOLISM AND PULMONARY INFARCTION[11,17,33]

Pulmonary embolism is the blockage of a pulmonary artery by thrombus, fat, air, or foreign matter.

The blockage obstructs blood flow through an area of the lung (FIG. 4-33). The most common type of pulmonary embolus, a dislodged thrombus, will be discussed.

Pulmonary embolism is the third most common cardiovascular disease in the United States. Overall, predisposing factors are most often surgery/trauma (43%), idiopathic (40%), heart disease (12%), or neoplastic disease (4%). Patients who suffer a massive pulmonary embolism often die within the first 24 hours. Resolution of smaller emboli usually occurs in 7 to 10 days with supportive treatment. Pulmonary infarction is an uncommon and serious complication of pulmonary embolism, resulting in a localized area of lung ischemic necrosis distal to the area of embolus.

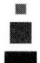

PATHOPHYSIOLOGY

Three factors (Virchow's triad) are related to the development of a venous thrombus: venous stasis, injury to the vein wall, and increased blood coagulability. Pulmonary embolism usually occurs in patients with risk factors for deep venous thrombosis, including the following:

Thombophlebitis	Elderly
Major surgery	Chronic illness
Use of estrogens	Congestive heart failure
Obesity	Pregnancy/recent childbirth
Smoking	Venous insufficiency
Leg trauma	Immobilization from fracture
Myocardial infarction	Polycythemia vera

Persons with a previous episode of thrombus development or a family history of clots are at increased risk for pulmonary embolus.

The most common sites for thrombus formation are the deep veins of the legs, especially the iliac, femoral, and popliteal veins, and the pelvic veins. The thrombus breaks loose and travels with the flow of blood, where it lodges in a pulmonary artery or arteriole. The ischemic chest pain that results is often severe, manifested as either pleuritic pain or substernal pain similar to myocardial infarction.

A pulmonary embolism produces an area of the lung that is ventilated but underperfused. This results in an increase in physiologic dead space ventilation. Reflex bronchoconstriction

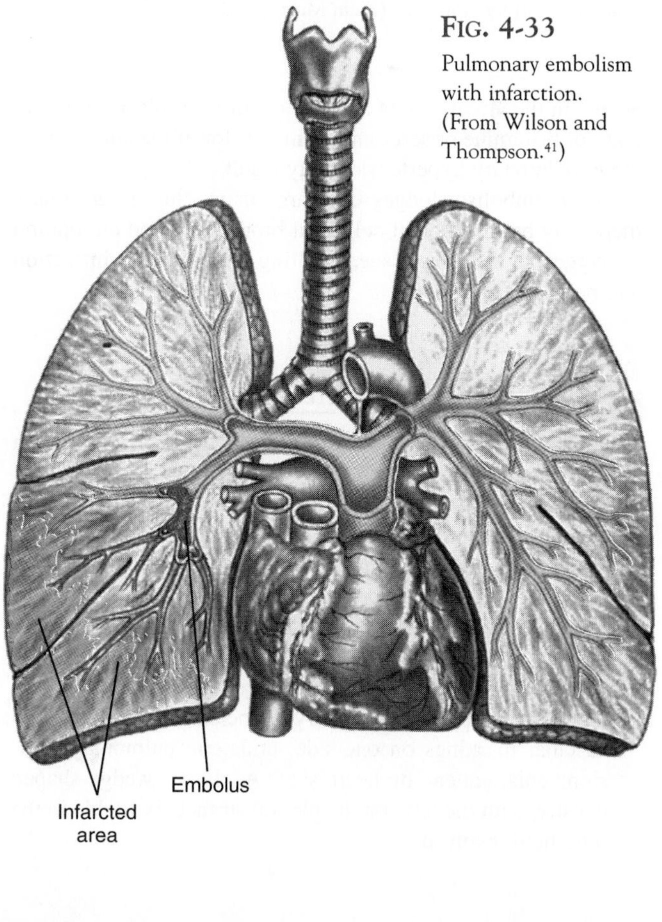

FIG. 4-33 Pulmonary embolism with infarction. (From Wilson and Thompson.[41])

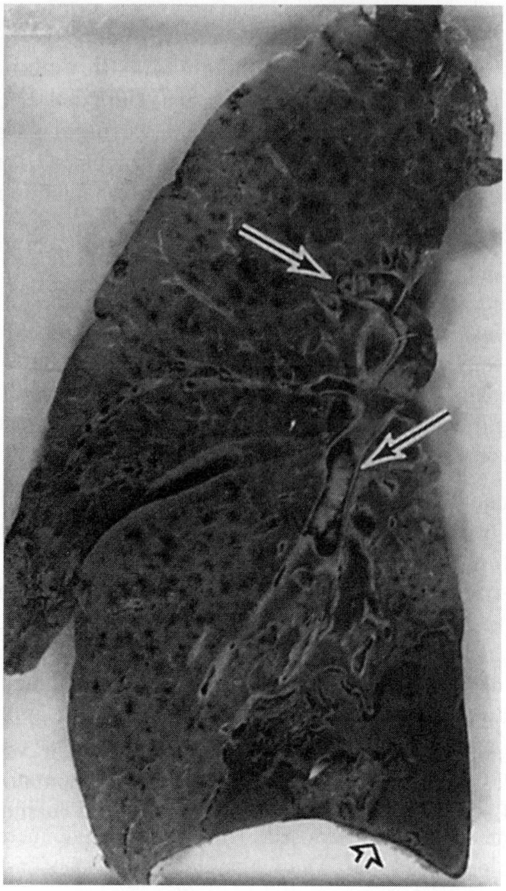

FIG. 4-34

Large emboli *(closed arrows)* are present in the upper and lower lobe pulmonary artery branches. (From Murray and Nadel.[23])

EMERGENCY ALERT

PULMONARY EMBOLUS

Often confusing and very difficult to diagnose. A pulmonary infarction results from a detached venous thrombus that forms an embolus that then lodges in a branch of the pulmonary artery, tachypnea, causing a partial or total occlusion.

ASSESSMENT

- Symptoms often nonspecific, may mimic myocardial infarction
- SOB, tachypnea, tachycardia
- Angina-like chest pain, pallor, or cyanosis
- Anxiety
- Decreased blood pressure
- Wheezes, rales on auscultation
- Abnormal ECG possible
- Elevated temperature

INTERVENTIONS

- Obtain ABGs, chest radiograph, ECG.
- Obtain ventilation/perfusion (VQ) scan.
- Maintain airway, breathing, and circulation.
- Administer high-flow oxygen by mask.
- Obtain IV access.
- Administer analgesia.
- Consider bronchodilators.
- Monitor clotting times and prepare to anticoagulate with heparin.
- Thrombolytic therapy and/or surgical interventions may be considered.

occurs in the affected area and is thought to result from the release of histamine or serotonin from the clot. If the embolism is large, pulmonary hypertension may result.

If the embolism lodges in a large or medium-sized artery, there may be insufficient collateral bronchial blood circulation to oxygenate the lung tissue, resulting in pulmonary infarction and necrosis (FIG. 4-34).

DIAGNOSTIC STUDIES AND FINDINGS

Blood gases: Pao_2 is less than 60 mm Hg. Hyperventilation leads to $Paco_2$ <40 mm Hg.

Electrocardiogram: The following classic signs help to differentiate pulmonary embolism from myocardial infarction: ST segment depression, right axis deviation, incomplete or complete right bundle-branch block, tall peaked P waves, S wave in lead I, Q wave in lead III, and T wave inversion in V_1-V_2.

Chest roentgenogram: Unilateral diaphragm elevation, enlarged main pulmonary artery associated with decreased vascular markings on one side, unilateral pulmonary effusion, enlargement of heart size. A classic wedge-shaped density, with the base on the pleural surface, is visible in the lung field involved.

Ventilation/perfusion (V/Q) scans: Significant diagnostic findings reveal a perfusion deficiency (FIG. 4-35). Results are generally reported as either a high or low probability that the V/Q mismatch pattern is typical of pulmonary embolus.

Pulmonary angiography: A highly specific but invasive diagnostic procedure. Criteria to diagnose pulmonary embolus are intraarterial filling defects and complete obstruction of a pulmonary artery branch.

Spiral CT scan: Shows presence of clot in pulmonary vessels.

Noninvasive ultrasonography: Evidence of residual clot in the leg veins is presumptive for a diagnosis of embolus.

MULTIDISCIPLINARY PLAN

Surgery

Indicated for removal of a massive embolus, requires cardiopulmonary bypass. Surgical embolectomy may also be done to remove multiple small clots that are causing pulmonary hypertension.

Surgical prevention: An umbrella filter may be surgically placed in the inferior vena cava. The filter strains blood returning from the lower body and prevents the progress of emboli toward the right heart and lungs.

Medications

Heparin: Does not directly lead to clot lysis; instead, heparin halts clot propagation, enabling natural fibrinolytic mechanisms to remove the clot. Heparin is administered by con-

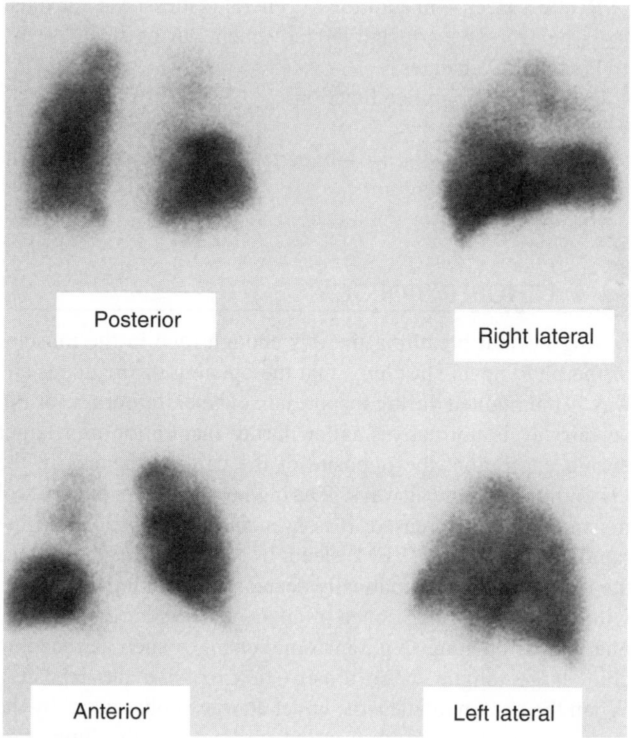

FIG. 4-35

Lung perfusion scan showing pulmonary embolism. Note decreased perfusion of right upper lobe indicative of pulmonary embolism. (Courtesy R. Keith Wilson, MD, Baylor College of Medicine, Houston, Tex.)

tinuous intravenous infusion due to the short half-life. Continuous infusion: 18-20 U/kg/h to start, adjusted as necessary to keep partial thromboplastin time (PTT) 2 to 3 times the control values. The drug is generally continued until warfarin (Coumadin) elevates the prothrombin time (PT) therapeutically. Should a severe bleeding event occur secondary to the use of heparin, or rapid reversal be needed, diluted protamine sulfate may be given intravenously.

Warfarin: Should be started as soon as oral therapy is possible to decrease the length of time heparin is required. Warfarin levels are monitored by PT and also reported as an international normalized ratio (INR). When INR levels reach 2.0-3.0 on warfarin, heparin is discontinued. Warfarin may be used for 6 months to life, depending on the cause of the embolus and likelihood of recurrence. Oral dose: 2.5-10 mg daily, titrated to PT level.

Fibrinolytic enzymes: Fibrinolytic therapy may be used in massive pulmonary embolus associated with hemodynamic instability. Examples of fibrinolytic enzymes are streptokinase, urokinase, and recombinant tissue-type plasminogen activator (rt-PA).

Low molecular weight heparins: Derived from separating heparins into fraction components; are used subcutaneously for thrombus prophylaxis.

General Management

Oxygen therapy: Administer oxygen by mask or cannula to maintain blood gas levels

Leg compression devices: Decrease venous stasis in the legs; used for prevention of venous thrombus, not used on a leg when thrombus is already present

NURSING CARE

Nursing Assessment

Respiratory status: Dyspnea, tachypnea, pleuritic pain, apprehension, restlessness, confusion, cough, unexplained hemoptysis, sweats, localized crackles, pleural friction rub, tachycardia, cyanosis, low-grade fever, thrombophlebitis

Potential Complications

Cor pulmonale, pulmonary hypertension, atelectasis

Patient Problems/Nursing Diagnoses & Interventions

NIC Respiratory Management

Impaired gas exchange related to ventilation/perfusion abnormalities

- Administer oxygen to maintain SpO_2 >93% or as ordered.
- Monitor ABGs; report increases or decreases in $Paco_2$ and Pao_2 of more than 5 to 10 mm Hg.
- Identify contributing factors such as airway clearance problem, postoperative pain, or weakness.
- Monitor ECG and cardiac status for arrhythmias secondary to alterations in blood gas levels.
- As long as patient is in respiratory distress, maintain bed rest; proceed with ambulation as soon as tolerated after anticoagulation attained.
- Position patient *to facilitate easy ventilation,* such as semi-Fowler's position.
- Encourage patient to space activities *to provide periods of rest in-between.*

NIC Physical Comfort Promotion

Acute pain related to ischemia

- Administer analgesics as needed to relieve pain and promote effective ventilation.

NIC Drug Management

See Patient Education/Continuum of Care Plan.

Patient Education/Continuum of Care Plan

1. Teach preventive measures to all patients preoperatively. Initiate early mobility postoperatively when condition allows.
2. Teach prevention strategies to persons at risk for venous pooling, such as avoiding prolonged sitting or standing, crossing legs, or tight clothing.
3. Teach patient and family about safe use of anticoagulants, including the need for ongoing monitoring of coagulation times.
4. Teach patient and family to monitor for signs of excess anticoagulation such as blood in urine, red or tarry stool, hemoptysis, or excessive bruising.

5. Teach patient to avoid physical trauma by avoiding contact sports, wearing safety belts while anticoagulated.
6. Teach patient and family to inform all health-care providers, including dentists and phlebotomists, of anticoagulated status.

Evaluation/Patient Outcomes

Respiratory Management: Blood gas values are within normal limits for patient. Respirations are relaxed. Chest roentgenogram or lung scan shows no evidence of pulmonary embolism.

Physical Comfort Promotion: Chest discomfort is relieved.

Drug Management: Patient and family are to discuss medications (purpose, side effects, route, and schedule), dietary therapy regimen, activity progression regimen, and plan for follow-up anticoagulant monitoring.

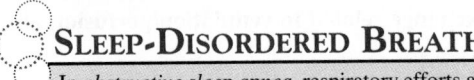

Sleep-Disordered Breathing[2,26,32]

In *obstructive sleep apnea,* respiratory efforts are made, but there is no airflow because the upper airway is obstructed. The term *central sleep apnea* refers to the loss of ventilatory drive during sleep, resulting in periodic apnea.

Sleep-disordered breathing encompasses several diagnoses, but the most common is obstructive sleep apnea. Others include snoring, central sleep apnea (Cheyne-Stokes respirations is one type of central apnea), and primary alveolar hypoventilation syndrome (Ondine's curse). Some patients have mixed apnea, an episode of central apnea followed by an obstructive apnea. In primary alveolar hypoventilation the individual has a decreased drive to breathe during sleep with decreased ventilation (hypopnea). Patients with neuromuscular diseases such as amyotrophic lateral sclerosis may also develop hypoventilation at night related to the effect of position and decreased drive on respiratory muscle function.

Persons with sleep apnea (obstructive or central) have episodes when they do not breathe during sleep. Although many persons have some brief periods with no breathing during sleep, the occurrence of more than five apneic episodes per hour is abnormal. (To be called apnea, the episode of absence of airflow must last at least 10 seconds.) In addition, many patients have periods of hypopnea (extremely shallow breathing). These periods of apnea and hypopnea are often associated with significant hypoxemia. The diagnosis is more prevalent among men than among women, and it is uncommon in premenopausal women. Sleep apnea is also associated with older age groups, obesity (approximately 50% of persons with obstructive sleep apnea are obese), and snoring. In the general population it is estimated that 1% to 4% of adults have obstructive sleep apnea.

Clinical symptoms associated with obstructive sleep apnea include the following:

Loud snoring—the bed partner is often forced to sleep in another room because of the noise
Daytime hypersomnolence—may be so severe that the person will fall asleep while driving a car
Restless sleep—in addition to general restlessness, may also be excessive arm and leg movement during sleep
Personality changes
Diminished cognitive function
Impotence
Cardiovascular disease—hypertension, arrhythmias, congestive heart failure

Pathophysiology

During normal breathing there is enough tone in the muscles of the pharyngeal structures that the opening of the upper airway is maintained during inspiration. (The extrathoracic or upper airway is normally smaller during inspiration and larger during expiration, the opposite of the caliber changes in the lower, intrathoracic airways.) During normal sleep, pharyngeal muscle tone is decreased; it is even further decreased during rapid eye movement (REM) sleep. In patients with sleep apnea the muscle tone is dramatically decreased. In addition, patients with obstructive sleep apnea often have a smaller than normal pharyngeal opening (e.g., anatomic changes such as receding chin, large tongue, large tonsils, or excessive fat deposits). When the person inhales, the upper airway is obstructed by the tongue or soft palate, preventing airflow into the lung even though respiratory efforts are made. There are frequently snoring noises, and an abrupt "snort" when the obstruction is broken and the patient inhales. During apneic periods the patient's arterial oxygen level can drop dramatically and the $PaCO_2$ rises. When the obstruction is only partial, the patient has an hypopneic episode. Hypopnea can also result in hypoxemia and hypercapnia during the episode. If untreated, nighttime hypoxemia can lead to pulmonary hypertension and right heart failure.

In addition to the blood gas changes, these episodes lead to fragmented sleep. The altered blood gas levels cause an arousal—awakening. As a result, the person never progresses to the deeper sleep phases. They will also have daytime hypersomnolence because of the fragmentation of sleep at night.

Diagnostic Studies and Findings

Clinical history: Sleep history (e.g., hours of usual sleep, time retiring, awakening, sense of "refreshment" after sleep), presence of snoring, observed apnea, daytime hypersomnolence (answers to some questions require the presence of a bed partner); drug and alcohol use

Physical examination: Demonstrates small pharynx, large tongue, receding chin, and other jaw malformations

Polysomnography (PSG; a sleep study): The patient is monitored during sleep; monitoring includes electroencephalogram so that the stages of sleep can be identified, ECG, chest movements, nasal air flow, and pulse oximetry; the sleep study includes monitoring at baseline to identify the problem and then with interventions to ensure that oxygenation is maintained and that the apneic and hypopneic periods are abolished or at least reduced to normal levels.

Multidisciplinary Plan

Surgery

Tracheostomy (the tracheostomy is closed during the day and opened at night to bypass the upper airway obstruction); uvulopalatopharyngoplasty, which widens the posterior pharynx and may be done using a laser technique

Medications

Respiratory stimulants may be used in patients with central sleep apnea; (e.g., medroxyprogsterone, acetazolamide, and theophylline); hypnotics are avoided

General Management

Oxygen: Via nasal cannula during sleep or via continuous positive airway pressure (CPAP) apparatus (for most, CPAP corrects the hypoxemia and supplemental oxygen is not needed)

CPAP: Applied via a nasal mask or nasal pillows, though in some patients, a full face mask may be used; some patients, especially those who require high pressures (>15 cm H_2O), may not tolerate a continuous pressure, so bilevel devices may be applied; bilevel devices are also used to treat central sleep apnea

Appliances: To reposition the mandible (move it anteriorly)

Weight loss: Weight loss has not been a very successful approach to care

NURSING CARE

Nursing Assessment

Clinical history: Sleep pattern, daytime somnolence, falling asleep with driving, sleepiness during daytime activities; question family and patient regarding snoring, apnea; if previously diagnosed, ascertain usual home therapy (CPAP or other device)

Clinical observation: Observe the patient during sleep for snoring, apnea, excessive limb movements

Oxygenation: Monitor pulse oximetry at night (often requires continuous recording so periodic episodes are not missed)

Potential Complications

Chronic hypoxemia, right-sided heart failure, chronic hypercapnea

Patient Problems/Nursing Diagnoses & Interventions

NIC Self-Care Facilitation

Disturbed sleep pattern
Sleep deprivation related to frequent arousals
Imbalanced nutrition: more than body requirements

- Avoid drugs that would impair sleep (e.g., coffee, alcohol).
- Assist patient in developing good sleep hygiene.
- Obtain dietary consultation.
- Assist patient with dietary selections.
- Encourage patient in weight reduction efforts.

NIC Respiratory Management

Ineffective breathing pattern related to upper airway obstruction, obesity
Impaired gas exchange related to apneic and hypopneic periods, obesity

- Apply CPAP or bilevel apparatus as ordered during sleep.
- Encourage patient adherence to use of ventilatory device; discuss reasons why patient does/does not use equipment.
- If tracheotomized, be sure tracheostomy tube is unplugged while patient is sleeping.
- Perform tracheostomy care.
- Administer oxygen as ordered.

Patient Education/Continuum of Care Plan

1. Teach patient about importance of weight loss if obese.
2. Teach patient good sleep hygiene measures.
3. Teach patient about use of ventilatory device and how to obtain help when at home.
4. Teach patient about signs and symptoms of inadequate sleep and when to seek help.
5. Teach patient about oxygen therapy if ordered.

Evaluation/Patient Outcomes

Self-Care Facilitation: Patient demonstrates weight loss and change in eating habits, food selection. Patient avoids drugs, activities that would interfere with sleep. Patient is able to describe major points of good sleep hygiene.

Respiratory Management: Compliant with use of ventilatory device. Tracheostomy tube clean, no skin breakdown. Respiratory pattern during sleep void of apneic, hypopneic episode. Oxygenation maintained at saturation >90% during sleep. Decrease in daytime hypersomnolence.

Acute Respiratory Failure[6,10,33]

Acute respiratory failure is not a disease but an acute onset of inadequate gas exchange secondary to another condition or disease process.

Respiratory failure is manifested by a Pao_2 less than 60 mm Hg. Acute respiratory failure may be present during exacerbation of chronic respiratory conditions, such as a pneumonia superimposed on emphysema, or as a result of an acute situation, such as postoperative airway obstruction or trauma. Respiratory failure is generally considered in two categories: hypoxemic respiratory failure and ventilatory respiratory failure.

Pathophysiology

Hypoxemic Respiratory Failure

Hypoxemic respiratory failure is manifested by a Pao_2 less than 60 mm Hg on room air, with either a normal or low $Paco_2$. The low Pao_2 stimulates respiratory efforts, resulting in hyperventilation and lowering of the $Paco_2$ until fatigue sets in. Examples

EMERGENCY ALERT

CARBON MONOXIDE (CO) POISONING

CO poisoning is often associated with smoke inhalation from fires, engine exhaust, and faulty home heating systems. CO's affinity is 200 times greater than oxygen for hemoglobin. Hypoxia results from the reduced oxygen-carrying capacity of the blood, impaired release of oxygen to the tissue, and impaired cellular respiration.

ASSESSMENT

Mild

- Throbbing headache, nausea/vomiting
- Impaired function of complex tasks

Moderate

- Irritability, weakness, visual changes
- Palpitations
- Loss of dexterity, decreased mentation

Severe

- Tachycardia, tachypnea, collapse, syncope

Life-Threatening

- Coma, seizures, Cheyne-Stokes respirations
- Cherry-red mucous membranes

INTERVENTIONS

- Maintain airway, breathing, and circulation.
- Obtain IV access.
- Monitor cardiac status.
- Administer high-flow oxygen (10 to 15 L) by tight-fitting mask for 4 h or until $HbCO_2$ <5%.
- Consider hyperbaric oxygen therapy.
- Monitor ABGs using measured, rather than calculated, Sao_2. Pulse oximetry is not accurate when CO is bound to hemoglobin and will read falsely high

of diseases associated with hypoxemic respiratory failure include the following:

1. Increased pulmonary capillary pressure with edema
   a. Left ventricular heart failure
   b. Fluid volume excess
2. Lung parenchymal injury
   a. Lung infections
   b. Near drowning
   c. Chemical or smoke inhalation
   d. Liquid aspiration

Hypoxemic respiratory failure results from areas of low V/Q, including areas of shunt (a complete lack of ventilation with continued blood flow). The more extensive the areas of shunt, the less is the response to supplemental oxygen. If severe hypoxemia (Pao_2 40 mm Hg) cannot be corrected, a metabolic acidosis will result from increased anaerobic metabolism. Cardiac output and alveolar ventilation increase, if possible, to compensate for the hypoxemia.

A particularly severe and deadly form of acute respiratory failure is **acute respiratory distress syndrome (ARDS).** A direct lung injury, such as those already listed, or an indirect injury from sepsis, pulmonary embolus, shock, or disseminated intravascular coagulation (DIC) may lead to the inflammatory-immune responses that produce ARDS. Development of ARDS involves a combination of tissue injury, release of toxic cellular substances, and sustained inflammatory responses with capillary leak and loss of alveolar surfactant. Pulmonary vasoconstriction and microemboli formation caused by the release of chemical mediators lead to acute pulmonary hypertension. The pulmonary edema present with ARDS is a noncardiogenic form of pulmonary edema related to increased capillary permeability rather than fluid overload (FIG. 4-36). Despite aggressive research on new therapies, mortality for ARDS remains high.

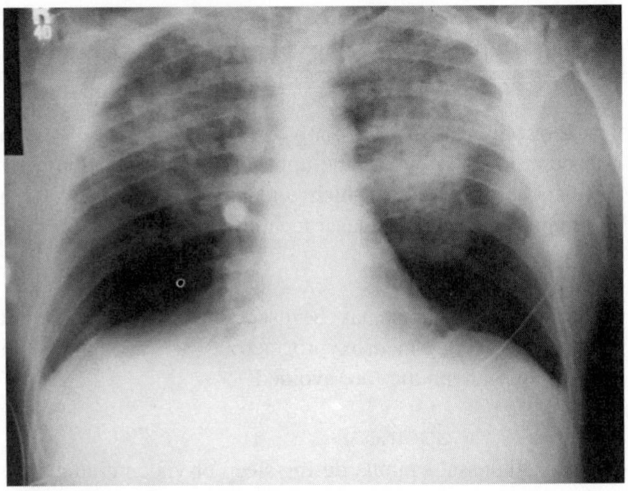

FIG. 4-36

Chest roentgenogram of patient with ARDS. Heart is normal size; note diffuse infiltrates in upper and middle zones of lungs. (Courtesy R. Keith Wilson, MD, Baylor College of Medicine, Houston, Tex.)

EMERGENCY ALERT

SMOKE/TOXIC INHALATION

Occurs when a person has inhaled a noxious gas that was a product of combustion.

ASSESSMENT

- Obtain history, including duration of exposure, if patient was in a confined area, and the material that was burning
- Burning pain to throat and/or chest
- Upper airway irritation
- Singed facial/nasal hairs, facial burns
- Carbonaceous sputum
- Auscultate for rales, rhonchi, wheezes
- Dyspnea, restlessness, cough, hoarseness
- Signs of pulmonary edema

INTERVENTIONS

- Maintain airway, breathing, and circulation.
- Administer high-flow, humidified oxygen by mask (10 to 15 L).
- Obtain IV access.
- Monitor ABGs and/or O_2 saturation.
- Admit and observe.
- Prepare to intubate emergently as needed.
- Encourage coughing, deep breathing, and raising of sputum.

Ventilatory Respiratory Failure

Ventilatory respiratory failure is manifested by a $Paco_2$ acutely elevated over 50 mm Hg, with a Pao_2 less than 60 mm Hg on room air. Ventilation, the actual movement of air between the environment and the alveolar/capillary membrane, is inadequate. Acute alveolar hypoventilation results from either pulmonary disease or central nervous system (CNS)/neuromuscular dysfunction and leads to respiratory acidosis. Examples of diseases and disorders that cause ventilatory respiratory failure include the following:

1. CNS respiratory center depression
   a. Drug effects, particularly narcotics
   b. CNS lesions or infections
2. Inability to generate effective respiratory muscle contraction
   a. Guillain-Barré syndrome
   b. Multiple sclerosis
   c. Spinal cord injury
   d. Myasthenia gravis
   e. Muscular dystrophies
   f. Poliomyelitis
   g. Tetanus
3. Obstructive and restrictive pulmonary disorders
   a. Asthma
   b. Chronic bronchitis
   c. Emphysema
   d. Massive obesity
   e. Severe kyphoscoliosis

The primary problem in ventilatory respiratory failure is the inability to generate enough alveolar ventilation, although right-to-left shunting and V/Q mismatch may also contribute to the hypoxemia with hypercarbia.

Respiratory failure from CNS depression most commonly follows an overdose of opiates, alcohol, tricyclic antidepressants, barbiturates, or other sedative drugs. After the body takes in large quantities of any of these drugs, stimulation of the respiratory center is depressed and the rate of breathing is lowered, with little change in tidal volume. The depressed respiratory center does not respond to the rising $Paco_2$.

The main respiratory difficulty for patients with a neuromuscular disease is the inability to generate enough force for ventilation and for deep breathing or coughing. Maintaining clear airways and preventing respiratory failure is a continual challenge, particularly when the neuromuscular disease is degenerative over time.

When $Paco_2$ elevates acutely, there is generally insufficient bicarbonate present to buffer the pH, so the arterial pH decreases, causing respiratory acidemia. When chronic hypercapnea is exacerbated by an acute condition, the arterial pH may not be as low as expected because of some previous bicarbonate buffering of the chronic respiratory acidosis.

DIAGNOSTIC STUDIES AND FINDINGS

Arterial blood gases

Hypoxemic respiratory failure: Pao_2 below 60 mm Hg; initially normal to low $Paco_2$ may rise; pH increased early secondary to hyperventilation, but as condition worsens, pH decreases

ARDS: Hypoxemia with a Pao_2/FIO_2 ratio <200

Ventilatory failure: Pao_2 below 60 mm Hg and $Paco_2$ over 50 mm Hg

Lactic acid levels: May be increased in tissue hypoxia

Chest roentgenogram: Findings relate to the specific disease process causing the respiratory failure. Common findings are infiltrates and areas of poor ventilation.

Early diagnostic radiographic changes in ARDS include thickened or blurred margins of the bronchi or vessels with progression to "whited out" areas of infiltrates; Fig. 4-36 shows diffuse and hazy blurred appearance throughout the lung fields

Pulmonary capillary wedge pressure (PCWP): In ARDS, low to normal pressure seen, less than 18 mm Hg

MULTIDISCIPLINARY PLAN

The plan is focused in three areas:

1. Supportive, to provide adequate oxygenation and mechanical ventilation to reverse the hypoxemia and expand the distal gas exchange units so as to prevent further airway and alveolar collapse
2. Therapeutic, to treat the systemic responses caused by alterations in pulmonary function
3. Curative, to identify and treat the underlying disease, when possible

Oxygenation/Mechanical Ventilation

Oxygenation support via mask may be used in the early stages of acute respiratory failure. Continuous pulse oximetry is generally used to monitor oxygen saturation. If hypoxemia persists despite maximal oxygen support, intubation and mechanical ventilation are indicated to support oxygenation and ventilation. In ventilatory failure, a trial of noninvasive positive pressure ventilation via a specially fitted mask may be indicated for alert patients with an underlying disease that is likely to improve rapidly, or for patients who decline to be intubated. When indicated, the patient is intubated and mechanically ventilated.

Medications

There are no specific drugs to treat acute respiratory failure. Drugs used are primarily supportive of other therapeutic measures, such as mechanical ventilation, or to treat the underlying disease causing acute respiratory failure.

General Management

Fluid and electrolyte therapy: Fluids are monitored carefully to optimize cardiac output. PCWP is much more reliable than the central venous pressure (CVP) when trying to determine the quantity of fluids to be administered. In most situations, maintenance of the PCWP at 10 to 15 mm Hg provides adequate, but not excessive, intravascular volumes.

Nutritional support: Either enteral feedings via a small feeding tube or hyperalimentation should be undertaken from the onset to prevent wasting of respiratory muscles

NURSING CARE

NURSING ASSESSMENT

Respiratory status: Signs and symptoms vary with the underlying cause of the respiratory failure

Respiratory distress: Dyspnea, tachypnea, nasal flaring, chest wall retractions, decreased chest wall movement,

labored breathing, depressed respirations, tachycardia, hypotension
Breath sounds: Crackles, wheeze, decreased, bilaterally unequal
Breathing pattern: Labored, irregular
Cough with or without sputum production
Pulmonary function: Decreased VC
Hypoxia: Restlessness, confusion, impaired motor function, hypotension, cyanosis, tachycardia
Hypercapnia: Headache, dizziness, confusion, unconsciousness, twitching, hypertension, sweating, flushed face

Laboratory values: Decreased Pao_2 and pH, increased or decreased $Paco_2$, increased lactic acid levels

Psychosocial status: Restlessness, lethargy, fear of suffocation, fear of breathing control by ventilator, fear of unknown, level of family support, ability to communicate

Potential Complications

Dysrhythmias secondary to blood pH alterations and hypoxemia; assess for pulse rate and regularity, changes in ECG rhythm

Patient Problems/Nursing Diagnoses & Interventions[10]

NIC Respiratory Management

Ineffective airway clearance related to lack of effective cough secondary to neuromuscular disease or altered secretions

Ineffective breathing pattern related to decreased lung compliance

Impaired gas exchange related to ventilation/perfusion mismatch

Impaired spontaneous ventilation

Risk for aspiration related to dyspnea, use of artificial airway, or positive pressure ventilation

- Monitor pulse oximetry. Provide supplemental oxygen to maintain Spo_2 90% to 93%. If Spo_2 >92%, consider decreasing administered oxygen *to decrease potential for oxygen toxicity.*
- Monitor ABGs; report increases or decreases of $Paco_2$ and Pao_2 of more than 5 to 10 mm Hg.
- Identify contributing factors such as decreased airway clearance or obstruction problem, pain, decreased level of consciousness, or weakness.
- Maintain patient position to facilitate ventilation in semi-Fowler's position or tripod position with arms supported *to maximize breathing potential for patient breathing spontaneously.*
- In collaboration with physician, prepare for and institute mechanical ventilation when patient cannot maintain adequate blood gas levels or demonstrates tiring with breathing efforts.
- When patient is receiving mechanical ventilation, provide care and monitoring consistent with the guidelines presented on pp. 211 to 213.
- Prevent physiologic factors that promote restlessness or anxiety such as pain, uncomfortable positioning, or full bladder. Restlessness increases oxygen consumption and CO_2 production. Administer treatments or medications *to relieve discomfort.*
- Avoid hyperthermia, which increases oxygen demand.
- Enhance patient's ability to rest between specified activities *to decrease oxygen demand.*
- Assist patient to perform ADLs or provide all ADLs as necessary during acute phase.
- Avoid triggering gag mechanism when performing mouth care.
- Observe amount of oral secretions present and patient's ability to swallow secretions effectively.
- Suction trachea and oropharynx when necessary *to remove secretions and maintain patent airway.*
- For patients with reduced level of consciousness, ensure that head of bed is elevated, unless contraindicated.

NIC Nutrition Support

Imbalanced nutrition: less than body requirements, related to increased calorie requirements of labored breathing

- Maintain tube feedings or hyperalimentation.
- Carbohydrate breakdown increases production of carbon dioxide. Consult nutritional support professional regarding products relatively lower in carbohydrates.

NIC Tissue Perfusion Management

Risk for deficient fluid volume related to gastrointestinal hemorrhage secondary to physiologic stress

- Monitor serial hemoglobin and hematocrit; check all stools, emesis, and nasogastric aspirate for presence of blood; observe changes in vital signs or abdominal girth.
- Initiate prevention measures; for example, minimize activities for uninterrupted periods of time, maintain calm and restful environment, encourage patient to participate in care as tolerated, explain all therapy before administering, incorporate family into care.
- Provide enteral feedings, if tolerated, *to maintain gut mucosal integrity.*
- Administer gastric acid blockers as ordered.

Risk for infection related to equipment and bypass of normal defenses

- Good handwashing before and after patient or equipment contact.
- Use sterile procedures and sterile equipment when entering the lower airway.
- Tracheobronchial suction only when required by presence of secretions that the patient cannot clear, but as often as needed *to maintain effective ventilation.* Avoid routinely scheduled suction times, since each suctioning episode has potential for causing hypoxemia, traumatizing tissue, introducing bacteria, and increasing patient discomfort.

NIC Communication Enhancement

Impaired verbal communication related to significant dyspnea or support devices

- Suggest an alternative method of communication appropriate to the patient's comprehension and motor ability, such as letter/word board, paper and pencil, sign language, head motions, mouthing words.

- If patient is intubated, assure patient that the inability to speak is temporary and will return as soon as the endotracheal tube is removed.
- Observe for signs of frustration or patient withdrawal secondary to the inability to speak.
- Teach family members appropriate methods to communicate with patient. Encourage them to use a method that the patient and family agree on.

Patient Education/Continuum of Care Plan

1. Teaching includes the present disease process as well as the underlying disorder that triggered acute respiratory failure.
2. During the critical phase, neuromuscular blocking agents and sedatives may be used to allow effective mechanical ventilation. Teach the family appropriate ways *to reorient and communicate with the patient.*
3. Teach the patient/family the purpose of procedures and equipment used *to promote oxygenation and prevent complications of immobility.*

Evaluation/Patient Outcomes

Respiratory Management: Tissue oxygenation is adequate. Blood gases, pulse oximetry are within normal limits. Signs of hypoxia or hypercapnia are resolved. Breath sounds are clear in all areas. Breathing pattern is comfortable and unlabored. Aspiration is avoided. Breath sounds are clear. Absence of fever. No evidence of acute aspiration on chest roentgenogram. Immune defenses are maintained. Temperature, WBC within normal limits. Sputum clear to white. Absence of infiltrates on chest roentgenogram.

Nutrition Support: Nutritional level is maintained. Weight stabilizes. Serum electrolytes, serum albumin are normal.

Tissue Perfusion Management: Fluid volume balance is achieved. Vital signs, PCWP are normal. Urine output is adequate. Hematocrit is within normal limits.

Communication Enhancement: Communication is facilitated. Patient uses alternative methods to express needs and concerns to family and caregivers.

Collaborative Interventions and Related Nursing Care

Oxygen Therapy

Description and Rationale

The ultimate goal of oxygen therapy is to provide sufficient amounts of oxygen to the tissues so that normal metabolism can occur. Clinically the goal is to provide oxygen at the lowest fractional inspired oxygen (FIO_2) to maintain a PaO_2 of at least 60 mm Hg. Therapy is indicated when the patient is unable to maintain an adequate PaO_2 by his or her own spontaneous respirations.

Hypoxemia may be caused by a variety of factors. Following are the most common:

Reduced alveolar oxygen: Results from either low ambient oxygen or hypoventilation; the PaO_2 falls by approximately the same amount the $PaCO_2$ rises (assuming no change in inspired oxygen).

Ventilation/perfusion ratio imbalance: Decreased or absent alveolar ventilation in relation to capillary blood flow (low V/Q); anatomic shunting that occurs secondary to congenital defects, disease, or trauma. Low V/Q is the most common cause of hypoxemia and is seen in pneumonia, airway obstructive diseases, pulmonary fibrosis, heart failure, etc. The PaO_2 falls while the $PaCO_2$ is usually low or normal. The worse the V/Q matching, the more difficult it is to oxygenate the patient.

Impaired alveolar-capillary diffusion: Occurs secondary to pathologic changes such as fibrosis, increased connective tissue, interstitial edema, or loss of gas exchange area. Clinically, diffusion is generally not a problem at rest until far advanced disease; it can be a problem during exercise.

Contraindications/Cautions

Following are risks and precautions regarding the use of therapeutic oxygen:

1. Oxygen-induced hypoventilation: When the arterial carbon dioxide tension is greater than 50 mm Hg, the risk of oxygen-induced hypoventilation increases. It is therefore advised, especially for patients with chronic lung diseases, to maintain oxygen therapy so the arterial oxygen tension remains about 60 to 65 mm Hg. To prevent induced hypoventilation, use low concentrations of oxygen if the patient is not mechanically ventilated. It is equally important, however, to adequately oxygenate the patient.
2. Atelectasis: The collapse of alveoli may occur secondary to high concentrations of oxygen in inspired air. To prevent this complication, if possible, limit the duration of 100% inspired oxygen to no more than 20 minutes.
3. Oxygen toxicity: Although it is not clear exactly what FIO_2 causes oxygen toxicity, it is most probable than an FIO_2 of over 50% administered for longer than 24 hours increases the risk.

Description of Equipment

Oxygen therapy equipment may be divided into two major types: low-flow and high-flow systems.

Low-flow systems do not supply all of the inspired gases that the patient breathes. This means that the patient breathes some room air along with the oxygen. For the system to be effective, the patient must be able to maintain a normal tidal volume, have a regular ventilatory pattern, and be able to cooperate. As the patient's ventilatory pattern changes, so does the concentration of inspired oxygen. Examples of low-flow systems include nasal cannula, simple oxygen mask, partial rebreathing mask with reservoir bag, and nonrebreathing mask with reservoir bag.

High-flow systems supply all gases at a preset FIO_2. These systems are generally not affected by changes in ventilatory pattern. The Venturi mask is the most common example of the high-flow system. Another example is a mechanical ventilator.

Table 4-12 summarizes the major types of oxygen therapy systems, their benefits, problems, and precautions.

Table 4-12 Oxygen Therapy Systems

Type of System	Description	Flow Rate (L/min)*	Approximate Oxygen Concentration Delivered (%)	Benefits	Problems	Nursing Care
LOW-FLOW SYSTEMS						
Nasal cannula		1 2 3 4 5 6	22-24 26-28 28-32 32-36 36-40 40-44 (concentration delivered varies with patient's respiratory rate and volume)	Comfortable, convenient method of delivering concentration of oxygen ranging from 22%-44%. Major advantages of this method are low cost of equipment, allowance for patient mobility, ability to deliver oxygen and still permit patient to eat and talk, and lack of necessity for humidification of inspired gas mixture. Practical system for long-term therapy. Mouth breathing will not affect concentration of delivered oxygen.	Nasal, cheek, and ear irritation. Unable to deliver oxygen concentration over 44%. Assumes a stable breathing pattern. Equipment may not be used if patient has nasal problem or if unable to tolerate nasal prongs. Patient must be able to cooperate to keep prongs in place.	Evaluate for pressure areas over ears and cheek areas. Liter flow above 6 L/min will *not* increase the FIO_2.
Simple face mask		6 6-7 >7	40 50 60-70	If patient's ventilatory needs exceed flow of gas, holes on sides of mask allow for entry of room air. Permits higher oxygen delivery than nasal cannula. System does not tend to dry out mucous membranes of nose or mouth.	Mask must be removed for coughing or eating. Should be operated at flow >5 L/min. Face mask may increase anxiety in some patients. Not practical for long-term therapy. May feel hot and confining for some patients.	Do not operate at flow less than 5-6 L/min (will not flush out accumulated CO_2). Should not be used for patients with chronic lung diseases. Equipment should be removed and cleaned several times each day.
Partial rebreathing mask with reservoir bag	Masks similar to simple face mask with addition of a reservoir oxygen bag; the purpose of the rebreathing mask is to increase FIO_2 by inhaling from a reservoir; some rebreathing of CO_2	10-12	60	The bag makes possible delivery of oxygen concentration between 40% and 60% provided that the reservoir is kept full by a continuous flow of oxygen.	Must be removed for eating and coughing. Bag may kink or twist. Impractical for long-term therapy.	Must maintain flow sufficient to keep reservoir bag from completely deflating during inspiration. FIO_2 may decrease if poor mask fit allows room air entry. All other functions as with simple mask.

Nonrebreathing mask with reservoir bag	Similar to rebreathing bag, but this mask has one-way expiratory valve that prevents rebreathing of expired gases.	12-15	90	Effective as short-term therapy. May deliver oxygen concentration up to 90%.	Impractical for long-term therapy. Must be removed for eating and coughing.	Check mask for leaks around face: FIO_2 may decrease if mask is not tight fitting. All other functions as with simple mask.
HIGH-FLOW SYSTEMS						
Venturi mask	Works on Bernoulli principle of air entrainment: for each liter of oxygen that passes through a fixed orifice, a fixed proportion of room air will be entrained; by varying size of orifice and flow of oxygen, precise FIO_2 is maintained.	Varies with equipment used	24 28 31 35 40 50	Delivers exact concentration. FIO_2 remains constant regardless of the patient's ventilatory pattern.	May irritate face skin. Interferes with eating and drinking. If greater than 50% concentration is desired, must switch to different oxygen delivery system.	All other functions as with simple face mask. NOTE: Check that flow rates properly set for ordered oxygen concentration.
Transtracheal oxygen catheter	Small, percutaneous tracheal catheter secured by a neck chain.	¼-4 L/min		Avoids nasal drying and facial/ear irritation. May be concealed by clothing. Decreased liter flow of oxygen required compared to nasal cannula.	Requires regular cleaning. May be prone to more frequent lower respiratory infections. May develop mucous balls.	Varies with phase of therapy. Catheter cleaned in place while tract immature. Catheter removed for cleaning after tract mature, usually twice daily.

*Normal breathing patterns are assumed.

Preprocedural Nursing Care

Assessment of Need for Supplemental Oxygen

Although signs and symptoms may make one suspect that a patient is hypoxemic, pulse oximetry or ABG measurements are needed. The major indicator for oxygen therapy is a Pao_2 <60 (Sao_2 <90) in someone who was previously healthy and is acutely ill; in someone with chronic illness or in whom home oxygen is being considered, a Pao_2 ≤55 or Sao_2 <88% indicates the need for oxygen.

Clinical signs and symptoms vary with the underlying cause of the hypoxemia, and many may also result from various other problems such as anxiety or heart failure. Commonly cited symptoms include the following:

Tachypnea
Dyspnea (*do not* equate dyspnea with hypoxemia)
Tachycardia
Cardiac dysrhythmias
Decreased concentration
Headache
Confusion
Anxiety
Impaired judgment

NURSING CARE

Nursing Assessment

Respiratory status: Observe for response to oxygen, change in signs and symptoms listed in preprocedural assessment

Mucosal hydration: Oxygen can be drying; assess nasal and mucous membranes

Skin integrity: Skin irritation, reaction to device being used to administer oxygen

Safety: While oxygen is in use, prohibit smoking in the area. If the patient is to have home oxygen, assess the following:

- Home environment: Architectural factors that would affect type of home equipment (e.g., stairs, distance between bedroom and living area) (see box on home oxygen systems)
- Usual activity level at home: Does patient go out on a regular basis? Seldom? Never?
- What is the flow rate needed at rest, exercise?

Potential Complications

Oxygen toxicity; ventilatory depression; mucosal drying; skin irritation

Patient Problems/Nursing Diagnoses & Interventions

NIC Respiratory Management

Impaired gas exchange related to altered oxygen supply, hypovention, or low V/Q

- Assess patient *to identify signs such as restlessness, confusion, and irritability,* which may indicate the body's response to altered blood gas states.
- In collaboration with physician, monitor ABGs; report increases or decreases of $Paco_2$ of more than 5 to 10 mm Hg.
- In collaboration with physician consultation, administer oxygen *to maintain Pao_2 above 60 mm Hg.*
- Assess patient *to determine which oxygen therapy system is best to maintain the required Pao_2 level.*
- Monitor ECG and cardiac status for arrhythmias secondary to alterations in blood gases.

HOME OXYGEN SYSTEMS

Stationary System

Concentrator

Advantages:	Allows flows up to 5 L/min*
	Continuous source of oxygen, won't "run out"
Disadvantages:	Adds to electric bill
	Generates heat
	Some noise

Liquid oxygen

Advantages:	No additional electrical expense
	Flows up to 6 L/min*
	Quiet
Disadvantages:	Requires frequent delivery
	Fills require removing unit from home—difficult if stairs
	Often not available in remote areas

Portable Unit

Compressed gas: E cylinder with usual gauges, lasts 5 h at 2 L/min; E cylinder requires cart on wheels; usually requires refilling by DME supplier; for some patients can use with conserving device, pulse flow (allows use of smaller lighter tank that many patients can carry).

Liquid unit: Patient can fill from stationary unit (requires liquid stationary unit); highest flow usually 6 L/min; compared to E cylinder with standard gauges, lighter for same amount of oxygen; some patients can carry without cart; cart also available

Conserving Devices

Pulse flow units: Several types available, essentially provide oxygen when patient inhaling, not while exhaling; patient must be tested to ensure that triggers device and that flows sufficient (often not effective if patient requires continuous flows ≥4 L/min)

Conserving cannulas: Special oxygen cannulas with incorporated reservoir; often allow better oxygenation at equivalent flows; patient must be tested to evaluate effectiveness.

*If flows >6 L/min, two systems are required.

- Provide humidification with liter flows greater than 2 L/min or in low-humidity environments.
- Provide saline nasal spray *to prevent drying of nasal mucosa.*
- Ensure that oxygen therapy is not interrupted when patient is out of bed, up about, during sleep.
- Monitor SpO_2 to determine if oxygen needs to be increased with activity.
- If humidifier is used, clean on a regular basis.
- Assure tubing, delivery device periodically changed.

Patient Education/Continuum of Care Plan

1. Discuss desired outcomes (immediate and long-term) of oxygen therapy with patient and family; be sure that patient understands why oxygen therapy does not necessarily abolish dyspnea.
2. Instruct patient regarding importance of using oxygen as ordered (e.g., not removing with activity).
3. Teach necessary safety precautions to patient and visitors.
4. For patients going home on chronic oxygen therapy, additional patient education includes the following:

a. Expand patient's knowledge about safety precautions the patient must follow outside the hospital setting but do not create unfounded fears (e.g., if there is a candle on the table in a restaurant, the patient's oxygen will *not* blow up—a common misunderstanding).
b. Teach patient about amount of oxygen to use—liter flow at rest, with exercise, and during sleep.
c. Ensure that patient understands operation and care of home oxygen equipment or that arrangements have been made for further education in the home.
d. Discuss with patient ways of adapting chronic oxygen therapy to home use—for example, how to place portable oxygen unit in the car, ability to travel, ability to participate in out-of-home activities.

EVALUATION/PATIENT OUTCOMES

Respiratory Management: ABGs, pulse oximetry improved—$Pa{O_2} > 60$ mm Hg at rest and exercise. Mentation improved. No morning headache. Patient compliant with oxygen therapy.

BREATHING TECHNIQUES

The following are some breathing techniques that may be taught to the patient to facilitate effective ventilation:

Abdominal or diaphragmatic breathing
Deep breathing and coughing
Incentive spirometry

These are useful and specific measures to increase the volume of air entering the lungs, as well as being expelled from the lungs. These techniques are discussed according to indications and procedural techniques.

ABDOMINAL/DIAPHRAGMATIC BREATHING

Indications

Patients with chronic and acute obstructive ventilatory disorders may be taught to use a prolonged expiratory time, with slow inspiration. The longer, slow expiration allows better emptying of the lung, with the diaphragm attaining a higher and thus more efficient position. A forced expiration only contributes to narrowing of the airways. In classic "abdominal breathing" the patient is encouraged to limit movement of the upper chest wall and to emphasize movement of the abdomen with breathing. NOTE: The abdominal pattern may be detrimental in patient with severe hyperinflation because of advanced obstructive disease (the lung is so hyperinflated that upper chest muscles must be used); the pattern of slow, prolonged exhalation and slow deep inhalations is also detrimental in patients with restrictive disease.

Procedural Guidelines

1. Assist patient to attain position of comfort, usually sitting or in semi-Fowler's position in bed. Abdominal muscles should be relaxed and knees and hips flexed.
2. Instruct patient to inhale slowly. As patient inhales, the focus should be to pull the diaphragm down and to relax the abdominal wall, allowing the abdomen to bulge outward. If a hand is placed on the patient's abdomen, the hand should rise. In traditional diaphragmatic breathing, upper chest movement should be minimal. Note that in patients who are severely hyperinflated, upper chest movement is usually necessary to maintain ventilation and should not be discouraged.
3. Instruct patient to pause slightly after a slow and even inspiration and then, using a pursed-lip technique, to exhale quietly and naturally.
4. Explain the expiration should last two to three times longer than inspiration.
5. Have patient practice the diaphragmatic breathing technique so that it can be used easily at times of stress, increased respiratory distress.

PURSED-LIP BREATHING

Indications

This technique is used to control expiration and to facilitate emptying of the lung in patients with obstructive diseases. The technique probably decreases the dynamic compression of airways and thus keeps them open longer. Many patients, especially those with emphysema, do pursed-lip breathing spontaneously, without instruction.

Procedural Guidelines

1. Assist patient to a position of comfort.
2. Instruct patient to inhale and to pause slightly at end of inspiration.
3. Instruct patient to exhale slowly through pursed lips; a blowing effect occurs.
4. Explain that exhalation should be slow and purposeful.
5. Have patient practice technique for use at times of stress, increased respiratory rate (maintaining adequate expiration will decrease hyperinflation and dyspnea at times of stress).

DEEP BREATHING AND COUGHING

Indications

Patients having upper abdominal or thoracic surgery are at very high risk for the development of postoperative pulmonary complications, especially atelectasis and pneumonia. Patients with pneumonia and those who are immobilized are also susceptible to secretion retention and atelectasis. Deep breathing and coughing are used to expand underventilated alveoli and to prevent retention of secretions.

Procedural Guidelines

1. Position patient to facilitate deep inspiration and coughing in a sitting or semi-Fowler's position if possible.
2. Instruct patient to take a slow, deep inspiration. Placing one's hands on the lateral chest and telling the patient to "push my hands out" will help the patient feel the chest motion you are trying to accomplish. The patient should do a breath hold (to a count of 5) at the peak of inspiration. (The term *sustained maximal inspiration [SMI]* describes the slow deep breath and breath hold.) Another means to attain the slow deep inspiration is to ask the patient to yawn; this maneuver is often easier and more "natural" for a patient than are techniques using equipment (e.g., incentive

spirometry). If the patient is postoperative, pain medications may need to be administered 20 to 30 minutes before initiating the procedure.
3. After several deep breaths, instruct the patient to cough if there has not been a spontaneous cough. (Often effective deep breathing will stimulate a cough.) See the following for cough techniques; provide the patient with tissues to collect expelled sputum.
4. Splinting, if required to reduce pain, may be accomplished in several ways. An abdominal incision can be splinted by a pillow and hand pressure over the incision. A sternotomy is splinted by a pillow "hugged" to the chest. A lateral thoracotomy incision is splinted by hand pressure over the incision area or by a towel wrapped around the chest.

INCENTIVE SPIROMETRY

Indications

The incentive spirometer may be used to encourage deep breathing. It provides visual feedback to encourage the patient's efforts; it does not "make" the person breathe deeply. Incentive spirometry does not replace other deep breathing and coughing interventions. Most incentive spirometers are of the volume type, although some are of the flow design. In the volume type there is a measure of how much air the person inhaled. A marker is placed at the desired volume to provide a goal for the patient.

Procedural Guidelines

1. Position patient in semi-Fowler's position if possible.
2. Instruct patient to seal mouth around mouthpiece and to inhale slowly after a normal exhalation. Be sure the patient is inhaling from the mouthpiece and not around it, not through the nose.
3. Instruct patient to hold the deep breath for a few seconds before exhaling.
4. The incentive spirometry should be used at least every 2 to 3 hours during the postoperative period until the patient is ambulatory and initiates effective deep breathing and coughing without assistance.

Evaluation

All of the breathing techniques have similar evaluation criteria. Optimum movement of air in and out of lungs occurs. In patients with acute disease, there is no evidence of dyspnea or hypoxemia. In patients with chronic disease, patient is able to control dyspnea level at times of stress and is at usual best in terms of dyspnea and hypoxemia. Patient is able to ask for splinting assistance or splints self during deep breathing and coughing exercises.

AIRWAY MAINTENANCE[10,27,33]

Interventions

Airway maintenance procedures include cough techniques; postural drainage; percussion and vibration; orotracheal, nasotracheal, or endotracheal suctioning; oropharyngeal or nasopharyngeal airways; endotracheal intubation; and tracheostomy.

Clinical Assessment General to Airway Maintenance Procedures

Restlessness, labored breathing
Wheezing, stridor, noisy respirations
Rhonchi over large airways, decreased breath sounds
Retractions: Intercostal, suprasternal, supraclavicular
Mouth breathing, nasal flaring
Tachycardia
Decreased oxygen saturation

Preprocedural Nursing Care

General Teaching for Airway Maintenance Procedures

If the patient requires airway maintenance procedures in an emergency, teaching may be limited to a very simple and rapid explanation. Additional information can be provided after the airway is safely secured.

NONINVASIVE TECHNIQUES

COUGH TECHNIQUES

Indications

Cough techniques are taught to improve cough effectiveness and maintain airway clearance. Many types of patients need assistance with cough: those who are postoperative, those with inability to take a deep breath (neuromuscular disease, pain), those who are unable to generate rapid expiratory flows (airways obstructive diseases).

Procedural Guidelines

Several cough techniques can be used, as follows:
1. In the normal cough the individual inhales to a large inspiratory volume and then performs several "coughs," each with less air in the lung (cascade cough). Patients should be instructed to cough in a similar manner. Have the patient inhale deeply, hold the breath for several seconds, and then perform several coughs before inhaling again.
2. For the patient with easily collapsible airways, an open glottic technique is used. This type of cough has been called huff coughing or forced expiratory technique (FET) cough. The same maneuver is followed as described for normal cough. The difference is that the repeated expiratory maneuvers are performed without glottic closure/opening; therefore there is no cough noise. Again, several forced expiratory maneuvers should be done on the one deep breath before the patient inhales again. The huff cough may not result in expectoration, but it usually stimulates a natural cough; because secretions have been moved mouthward by the "huffing," the natural cough becomes effective. The huff cough is also effective in postoperative patients.
3. A type of cough used in patients with bronchiectatic types of disease is the end-expiratory cough. The patient inhales deeply, does a short breath hold, and breathes out slowly through pursed lips. Just before the next inhalation, a short cough is done, exhaling the air remaining in the lung. The cough should be performed after most of the air has been exhaled. Several end-expiratory cough maneuvers will often move secretions to a point in the airway where they can be expectorated using a normal cough maneuver.

4. The augmented cough is a modification of the Heimlich maneuver. This maneuver has several variations and is used in patients who are unable to produce sufficient expiratory force during a cough maneuver. Patients with chest wall pain/discomfort often attempt to refrain from coughing or cough with less force. Wrapping a towel around the chest and pulling it snugly during the forced expiratory maneuver often contributes to expiratory force and reduces pain. The abdominal thrust maneuver is used in patients with neuromuscular disease who are unable to generate sufficient abdominal pressure to produce an effective cough. (Examples are tetraplegics, paraplegics with loss of abdominal muscles, and those with amyotrophic lateral sclerosis or muscular dystrophy.) The patient is instructed to take a deep breath (in neuromuscular disease, positive pressure delivered by a self-inflating bag or mechanical device may be used to accomplish a deep breath; a technique of "breath stacking" is often used—several inhalations without exhaling in order to achieve a maximal inspiration); then as the patient attempts to cough, abruptly compress the abdomen with an in-and-up motion. (The caregiver's hand is placed on the abdominal wall throughout the inspiratory and expiratory maneuver so the action is one of compressing, not hitting.)

Mechanical Devices to Improve Cough Effectiveness

In those patients (usually those with neuromuscular disease) who are unable to generate sufficient inspiratory volumes and expiratory flows, mechanical devices have been used to assist in the expectoration of sputum. Some of these devices (IPV) are discussed as alternatives to postural drainage.

One device specifically for cough is the "coughalator" (In-exsufflator). This device delivers air under positive pressure. Once the patient has taken a deep breath, the patient is switched (either automatically or manually) to exhalation and a negative pressure is applied to the airway. The larger pressure gradients on both inspiration and expiration result in a deeper breath and a more forceful expiration than the patient would be able to take unassisted. Inspiratory pressures used with the device are usually in the +25 to +30 cm H_2O range and the expiratory pressures are −40 cm H_2O. The patient uses the device for three or four breaths, coughs, and then relaxes. The procedure is then repeated. Care is taken not to hyperventilate the patient. In addition to assisting cough, many neuromuscular patients use this device at home to help them take periodic deep breaths.

Postural Drainage, Percussion, and Vibration

Postural drainage, percussion, and vibration are effective methods for loosening and moving secretions when patients are unable to maintain airway clearance. The techniques are most helpful for patients who raise copious amounts of sputum (>30 ml/day) and are frequently used in the chronic management of cystic fibrosis and bronchiectasis. These techniques may also be used in other patients when airway clearance is a problem, but the effectiveness must be evaluated individually. Postural drainage with percussion and vibration has also been demonstrated to be effective in reinflating atelectatic lung. Treatments are usually done after an aerosolized bronchodilator.

Contraindications/Cautions

1. Patients with significant hemoptysis
2. Patients in whom a head-down position is contraindicated (e.g., those with head injury)
3. Patients with bleeding disorders
4. Patients with rib fractures, or predisposition to pathologic fractures
5. Patients in whom the techniques cause increased dyspnea, wheezing

Procedural Guidelines

Postural drainage consists of specific positioning of the patient so that the different segments of the lung are drained by gravity. The postural drainage treatment may be done to drain all areas or may concentrate on one or two positions (e.g., to concentrate on a left lower lobe atelectasis). Each position is maintained for at least 5 minutes. (Postural drainage positions are depicted in Fig. 4-37). The figure demonstrates all positions, but it is common that emphasis is placed on three or four lower lobe positions (those for the basal segments) and two upper lobe positions. After each position the patient should do several deep breaths with prolonged exhalation and end-expiratory cough, followed by a cascade cough.

If positioning and coughing are not effective, percussion and vibration may be added. The percussion and vibrations are done over the areas being drained (see Fig. 4-37), these techniques

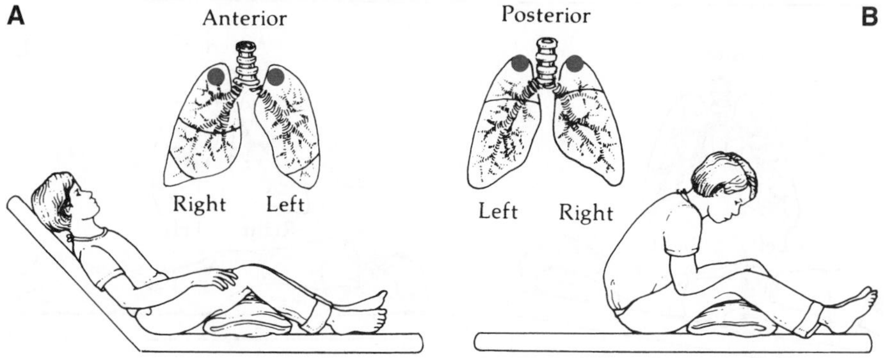

Fig. 4-37

Positions for postural drainage. **A,** Anterior apical segment; sitting. **B,** Posterior apical segment; sitting. (From Hirsch and Hannock.[16])

Continued

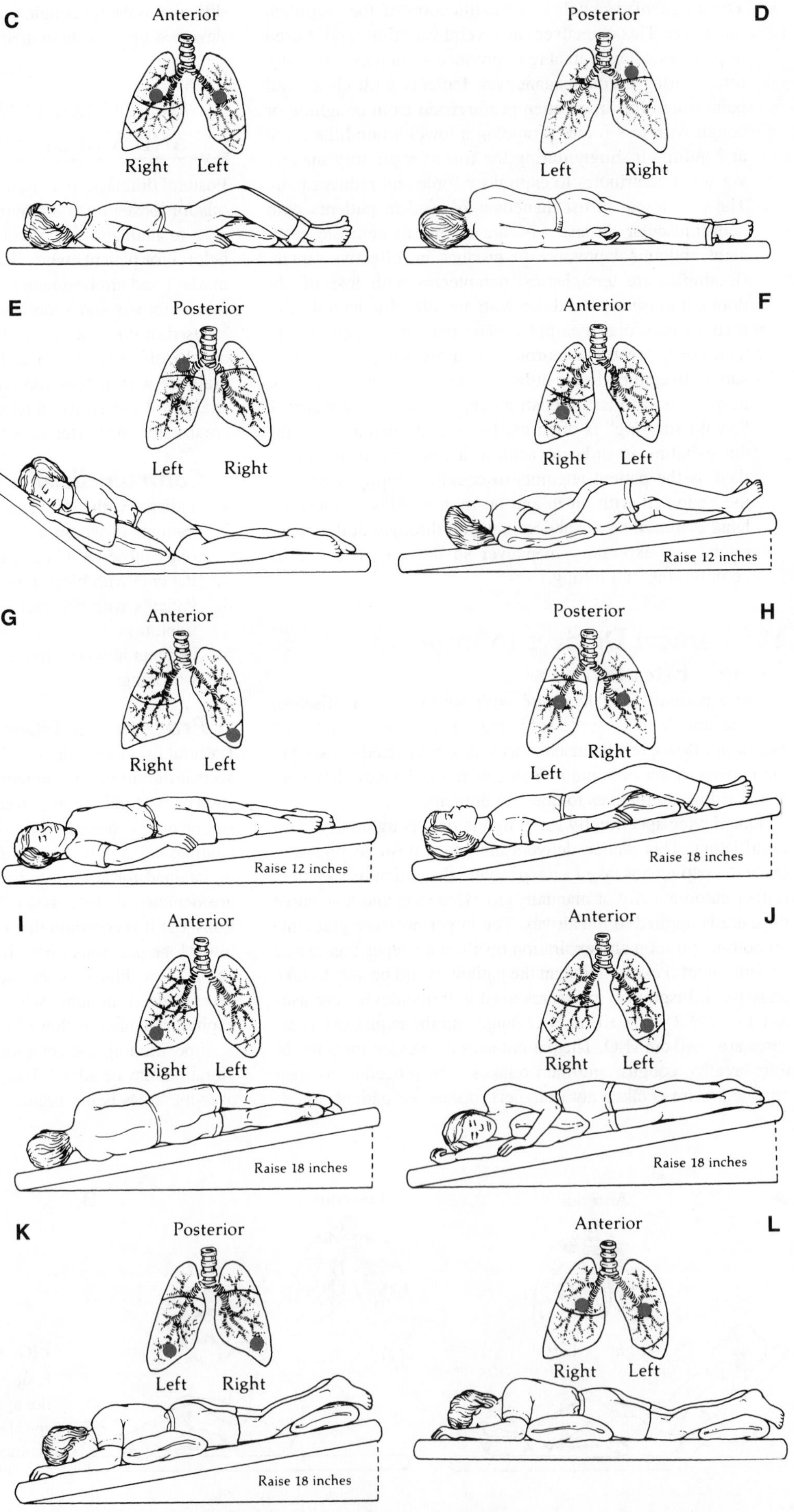

FIG. 4-37, cont'd
Positions for postural drainage. **C,** Anterior segment; lying flat on back. **D,** Right posterior segment; lying on left side. **E,** Left posterior segment; lying on right side. **F,** Right middle lobe; lying on left side. **G,** Left lingula, lying on right side. **H,** Anterior segments; lying on back. **I,** Right lateral segment; lying on left side. **J,** Left lateral segment; lying on right side. **K,** Posterior segments; lying on stomach. **L,** Superior segments; lying on stomach. (From Hirsch and Hannock.[16])

should always be done over ribs, not over the sternum, over vertebral bodies, or below the ribs.

To percuss, cup the hands and rhythmically strike the chest wall. The percussion is usually done over one thin layer of clothing. A hollow, deep sound indicates the technique is being performed correctly; there should not be a slapping sound. The area being drained is percussed for 1 to 3 minutes. In many settings, plastic cups are used instead of the hands. The purpose of the percussion is to transmit vibration through the chest wall; the percussion does not need to be forceful!

Following the percussion, the hand is flattened and applied to the chest wall (same area that was percussed). Have the patient take a deep breath. As the patient does a prolonged exhalation, vibrate and compress the chest wall. Vibration is usually repeated for two to three breaths. If the vibration does not stimulate a productive cough, have the patient cough voluntarily. If necessary, repeat the percussion and vibration before moving to the next position.

Alternatives to Postural Drainage With Percussion and Vibration[20]

Various techniques have been developed as an alternative to postural drainage with percussion and vibration. Their purpose is to make therapy for patients easier, especially in the home setting, and to avoid some of the side effects of standard postural drainage with percussion and vibration. Some of those more commonly used are discussed here. Additional techniques that are used more extensively in CF populations are autogenic drainage (a combination of breathing techniques and FET coughing) and positive expiratory pressure therapy (similar to the flutter valve).

Flutter Valve

The flutter valve is a small handheld device. The patient takes a slow deep breath and then exhales through the flutter valve. The flutter creates a vibrating column of air in the airway, similar to the sensation as with percussion and vibration. When the patient is using the device correctly, a vibration should be felt inside the chest. After a few normal exhalations, the patient exhales more forcefully. The maneuver often stimulates a spontaneous cough. Studies have demonstrated that the technique is beneficial in CF, and it has also been used for patients with bronchiectasis. Many patients have been able to replace postural drainage with daily use of the flutter valve. When the technique is effective, patients appreciate the simplicity of treatments, the ability to use the technique while away from home, and the fact that they do not require assistance from others.

High-Frequency Chest Oscillation

The high-frequency chest oscillation technique has been used to replace postural drainage in patients with CF and bronchiectasis. The technique can be used in the hospital or at home. The procedure is carried out with the patient in a sitting position. A vest is put on the patient; the vest is attached to a device that creates high-frequency vibration of the chest wall. Several different frequencies are used to optimize airway clearance. Treatments require about 15 minutes (less time than full postural drainage). After each change in frequency, the patient is requested to cough.

Intrapulmonary Percussive Ventilation (IPV)

IPV is a mechanical device that has been used for patients with CF, bronchiectasis, atelectasis, and neuromuscular disease. The device generates an oscillating pressure. Air is delivered to the patient in short bursts (15 to 25/slow inhalation). Because the inspired oscillating gas flow is delivered under pressure, the results are a deep breath, enlargement of the airways, and vibration of the airways. The vibration tends to move secretions mouthward. The device is used with a mouthpiece or mask, or it can be attached directly to a tracheostomy tube or endotracheal tube. With this device the bronchodilator aerosol is delivered as part of the treatment rather than separately.

Evaluation

Evaluation of all the noninvasive home devices/techniques used to improve airway clearance is similar. The chest should be auscultated and the patient assessed immediately after the technique and again within an hour. Often the techniques "move" secretions, but they are not expectorated until 30 to 60 minutes after treatment. Other goals are as follows:

- Improvement in adventitial breath sounds
- Sputum is produced
- Breathing patterns are effective without dyspnea; respiratory rate and rhythm are adequate
- Gas exchange is adequate; ABGs are within acceptable range
- Therapy does not overly tire the patient

Invasive Techniques

Orotracheal, Nasotracheal, or Endotracheal Suctioning[33]

Indications

Signs of respiratory distress
Noisy, wet breathing
Auscultated rhonchi
Ineffective cough effort

Contraindications

Tight wheeze with bronchospasm or croup

Procedural Guidelines

1. If possible, position patient in semi-Fowler's position.
2. Use sterile, gloved technique.
3. Use smallest catheter size possible to remove secretions.
4. Monitor baseline Spo_2 and heart rate.
5. Hyperoxygenate patient and hyperinflate before suctioning procedure, or ask the patient to breathe deeply. If orotracheal or nasotracheal suction approach is used, maintain oxygen cannula or mask on during procedure.
6. Lubricate catheter tip with sterile saline solution or water before procedure. Use water-soluble gel lubricant only for nasotracheal approach.
7. Do not apply suction while catheter is being inserted.

8. Insert and advance catheter. If resistance is met, withdraw catheter 0.5 cm.
9. Apply suction for 5 to 10 seconds interval while gently rotating and withdrawing catheter.
10. Administer oxygen and hyperinflate between suctioning passes. Monitor Spo_2 and heart rate for changes after each pass. Allow patient to recover to baseline or $Spo_2 >90\%$ before making another suction pass.
11. Note and record amount and character of sputum.
12. Note and record patient's response to suctioning procedure.
13. Discard catheter after each treatment.
14. Change vacuum container and tubing every day.

Closed Suction Systems

Closed, in-line suction catheter systems are available for use with endotracheal or tracheostomy tubes. Advantages include the ability to maintain positive pressures and hyperoxygenate via a mechanical ventilator during suctioning, as well as elimination of the nurse's exposure to sputum.

Potential Complications

Wheezing or stridor during or after procedure indicating bronchospasm or laryngospasm (if noted, administer oxygen and contact physician)
Traumatic airway ulceration with hemorrhage
Infection
Hypoxemia
Cardiac dysrhythmias

Oropharyngeal or Nasopharyngeal Airways

Indications

Potential or actual upper airway obstruction owing to altered levels of consciousness, resulting in relaxation of the tongue against the hypopharynx
Trauma-induced upper airway obstruction

Procedural Guidelines

1. Determine type of airway according to individual patient needs.
   a. Oropharyngeal airway (poorly tolerated in awake patients, causes gagging): Length should be from front teeth to the mandibular angle of jaw.
   b. Nasopharyngeal airway: May be indicated if patient has associated mouth injury; the width should be slightly narrower than the nares' diameter.
2. Insertion techniques
   a. Oropharyngeal airway: Approaching from the side of the mouth, insert airway upside down (with distal end pointing up), then rotate the airway over the tongue 180 degrees; the flange of the airway should be securely positioned outside the teeth.
   b. Nasopharyngeal airway: Elevating the tip of the nose, the airway should be inserted in anatomic line with the nasal passage. Use water-soluble gel as a lubricant.
3. Position patient on side to facilitate drainage.
4. Remove and clean oral airway at least every 6 to 8 hours; observe for ulcerations of mucous membranes.
5. Remove and clean nasal airway every 12 to 24 hours; rotate to other nare; observe for ulcerations of mucous membranes.
6. Carefully observe position of airway at least every hour; suction if needed via the airway.
7. Provide mouth and nose care at least every 2 hours.
8. Airway removal: Observe patient's level of consciousness and presence of gag and swallow reflexes; when patient is awake, instruct him or her to push oral airway out with tongue; carefully observe patient for adequate airway maintenance after removal.

Potential Complications

Aspiration of secretions not prevented; suction must be available
May cause awake patient to gag
May become clogged or dislodged, so that the tube becomes an obstruction
Bleeding or infection secondary to trauma of insertion
Ulceration of nares or pharynx after prolonged insertion

Endotracheal Intubation

Indications

Airway obstruction not resolved with use of a simple oral or nasal airway
Prevention of pulmonary aspiration in an unconscious patient
Access to remove tracheobronchial secretions
Route to provide mechanical ventilation

Procedural Guidelines

1. Assemble all equipment before attempting intubation procedure.
2. Check the cuff on endotracheal tube for leakage.
3. Assist to position patient in the sniffing position; this should bring the mouth, larynx, and trachea in line.
4. Before intubation, explain the procedure and ensure that any dentures or mouth appliances have been removed.
5. Before intubation, hyperventilate patient using self-inflating bag with supplemental 100% oxygen.
6. If intubation attempt is prolonged, interrupt the procedure and oxygenate the patient. Monitor Spo_2 and ECG throughout intubation procedure.
7. Once the endotracheal tube is in place, assist to determine proper endotracheal tube placement; this is done by considering the following:
   a. Correct placement: Bilateral lung inflation, breath sounds heard equally throughout all lobes. Obtain a chest roentgenogram after insertion to ascertain exact positioning of tube.
   b. Incorrect placement:
      (1) Esophagus: Absence of breath sounds, respiratory distress, cyanosis; if these are noted, the endotracheal tube should be removed and reinserted.
      (2) Right mainstem bronchus or carina: The endotracheal tube has been inserted too far; clinical signs include unilateral breath

sounds on the right and coughing; if this is noted and confirmed by radiographic examination, the endotracheal tube should be retracted slightly and resecured; reassessment should indicate proper placement.

8. Once the endotracheal tube is in correct position, tape it securely to avoid movement.
9. If patient cannot cooperate with maintaining tube placement, use soft wrist restraints to prevent self-extubation with potential laryngeal injury.
10. Monitor tube placement and patency at least every hour; this assessment should include the following:
    a. Tube position
    b. Tube patency
    c. Lung inflation
    d. Respiratory distress, need for suctioning
11. Provide ongoing care for patients with endotracheal tube in place:
    a. Provide mouth care every 2 hours.
    b. Clean nares and around endotracheal tube at least every 6 to 8 hours.
    c. Reposition and retape oral endotracheal tube at least daily.
12. If tube has cuff, use minimal occlusive volume technique to maintain the airway seal; record the amount of air inserted to inflate the cuff; monitor cuff pressures each shift; attempt to maintain pressures <20 mm Hg to avoid tracheal pressure injury.
13. Use bite block or oral airway if the patient bites the endotracheal tube.
14. While intubated, patient should receive oxygen (100% humidification).
15. If patient is awake, provide writing materials for communication or agree on use of sign language/communication board. Remind patient that ability to speak returns after tube removal.
16. Extubation: Should be attempted only in a controlled environment, with staff available who can reintubate, if necessary.
    a. Assess patient's ability to breathe on own and protect airway before extubation.
    b. Determine that patient is able to maintain spontaneous respiratory rate and tidal volume sufficient to maintain stable blood gas values.
    c. Carefully suction endotracheal tube and pharynx above endotracheal cuff before deflating cuff for extubation.
    d. Immediately after extubation, assess for signs of respiratory distress or laryngeal spasm, such as dyspnea, noisy breathing, use of abdominal or accessory muscles, restlessness, irritability, tachycardia, tachypnea, decreased Pao_2, or increased $Paco_2$;if these are noted, consult physician immediately and prepare for reinsertion of endotracheal tube.
    e. Teach patient that throat discomfort from the endotracheal tube generally resolves in 24 to 48 hours.

Potential Complications

Delay of oxygenation or ventilation during intubation procedure

Placement of endotracheal tube into right mainstem bronchus, resulting in unilateral aeration with potential for pneumothorax on right side, atelectasis on left side

Ulceration of trachea or tracheoesophageal fistula

Mucous plugs or other blockage of endotracheal tube may lead to hypoxia and respiratory distress

Unplanned extubation by combative patient or secondary to poorly secured tube requires immediate airway and ventilatory assessment by the nurse, as well as potential need for oral airway, patient positioning, and ventilation by Ambu-bag with supplemental oxygen

Pulmonary aspiration of secretions secondary to poorly inflated cuff, inadequate suctioning before cuff deflation, or too small noncuffed endotracheal tube used

Potential laryngospasm or laryngeal edema after intubation or extubation

NURSING CARE

Nursing Assessment

Ability to maintain patent airway

Chest auscultation: Bilaterally equal breath sounds, presence of adventitial sounds, ease of respiration

Gas exchange: Oximetry, ABGs

Sputum production, ease of expectoration

Potential Complications

Increased shortness of breath, increased wheeze

Airway trauma (varies with technique used)

Hypoxemia

Dysrhythmias

Patient Problems/Nursing Diagnoses & Interventions

NIC Respiratory Management

Ineffective airway clearance related to increased tracheobronchial secretions, decreased cough effectiveness, foreign body, or decreased level of consciousness

Impaired gas exchange

Risk for aspiration related to excessive oral secretions and presence of tube in airway

- Maintain oxygenation during airway care procedure.
- Select appropriate airway technique to maintain airway patency; must consider risk/benefit ratio for individual (see procedures for specific techniques).
- Encourage frequent position changes.
- Using sterile technique, suction as needed to maintain airway.
- If patient has oral endotracheal tube in place, teach him or her to avoid biting the tube. If necessary, provide oropharyngeal airway or bite block *to prevent biting on the endotracheal tube.*
- If swallowing reflex is diminished, elevate head of bed when performing mouth care.
- Avoid triggering gag mechanism when performing mouth care.
- Avoid scheduled airway care measures after meals.
- Ensure adequate humidification and fluid intake.

- For patients with reduced level of consciousness, ensure head of bed is elevated t*o prevent gastric regurgitation and aspiration,* unless contraindicated.
- Position patients with reduced level of consciousness laterally *to allow drainage of oral secretions out of mouth,* unless position is contraindicated.

NIC COMMUNICATION ENHANCEMENT

Impaired verbal communication related to dyspnea or presence of artificial airway

- Teach family how to support patient and use an alternative means, if necessary, of communication, such as letter board, pencil and paper, signing, or mouthing words.
- Provide frequent information about procedures before the patient is surprised or becomes anxious.
- Provide emotional support for the difficulty of communication and frustration that can occur for patient, family, and health-care providers.
- Teach patient/family how to participate in airway care techniques.

EVALUATION/PATIENT OUTCOMES

Respiratory Management: Airway is patent. Breath sounds are clear and bilaterally equal. Rhonchi are decreased. Breathing is easy. Blood gas values are within normal limits for patient. Pulmonary aspiration did not occur. Temperature and respiratory rate are within normal limits. Lung fields are clear on chest radiograph.

Communication Enhancement: Patient is able to communicate needs and concerns to staff and family. Family interacts with patient using a method acceptable to both patient and family. Patient/family understands use of selected technique.

CHEST TUBES AND CHEST DRAINAGE SYSTEMS

Description and Rationale

Chest tubes, with attached drainage systems, are placed in the pleural cavity to drain fluid, blood, or air from the pleural cavity and to reestablish a negative pressure that will facilitate expansion of the lung. Chest tubes may be inserted postoperatively, as an emergency procedure after chest trauma, or therapeutically as a disease treatment modality. Chest tubes are also used to drain the mediastinum after cardiac surgery. Following are chest tube insertion sites for different pleural collections:

Pneumothorax: Usually in second and third intercostal spaces (anterior or lateral)

Hemothorax: Usually in seventh, eighth, or ninth intercostal space (posterolateral)

Thoracotomy: One tube generally inserted in second or third intercostal space (anterior) and another in lower posterior axillary line

Mediastinal: Generally two tubes, inserted below xiphoid process

Chest tubes are removed when radiographic examination determines that the lung is reexpanded and the drainage is minimal.

Cautions

Chest tubes are inserted by a physician and sutured into place. Cautions specific to chest tubes and drainage systems include the following:

Sterility must be maintained so as not to introduce infection into the pleural cavity.

The system must remain patent: The tubing must not become blocked; if this occurs, a tension pneumothorax may result.

If the drainage tubing becomes dislodged from the patient chest tube or a drainage bottle breaks, reestablish drainage with a sterile system immediately.

If the chest tube becomes dislodged from the patient's chest, the patient should exhale forcefully, and the chest wall incision should be quickly covered with a petrolatum jelly gauze (see Pneumothorax, p. 167.)

Preprocedural Nursing Care

Carefully assess patient's preprocedural condition, including respiratory rate and quality. Note evidence of dyspnea, labored breathing, tachypnea, tachycardia, quality and distribution of breath sounds, mediastinal shift, subcutaneous emphysema, and crepitus. Teach the patient the purpose and goal of chest drainage. Set up drainage equipment appropriately for the type of system being used, most commonly disposable three-chamber units (FIG. 4-38) or three-bottle systems. Some sys-

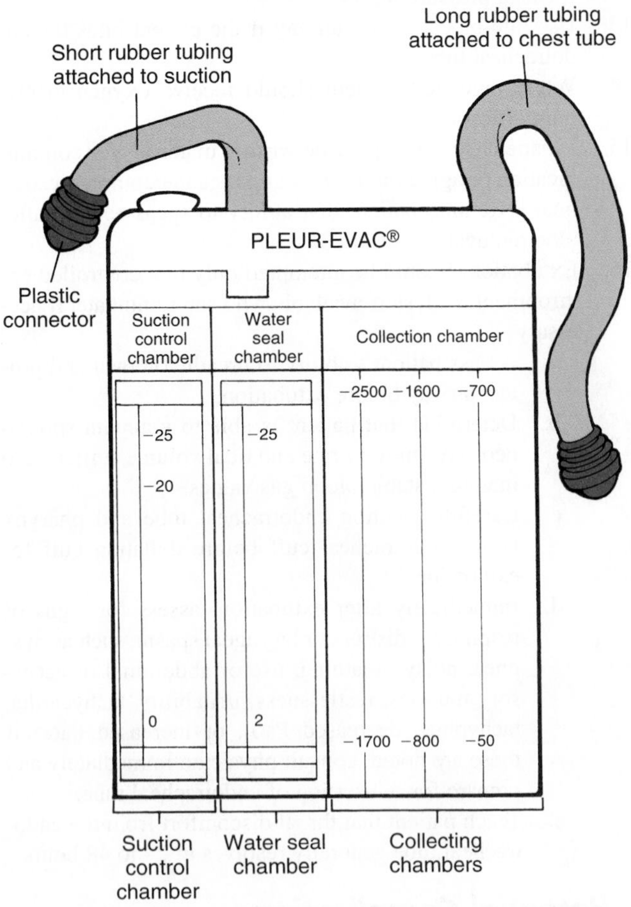

FIG. 4-38
Commercial chest drainage system.

tems provide access to collected blood for autotransfusion back to the patient, either with or without additional processing of the collected blood.

Removal of Chest Tubes

Chest tubes may be removed after the lung has been reinflated. Indications for removal are usually confirmed by chest radiographic examination. Removal of either pleural or mediastinal chest tubes is associated with significant discomfort. Analgesics should be administered before tube removal. Removal procedures include the following:

1. Place patient in semi-Fowler's position or on side.
2. Physician instructs patient to take a deep breath and hold it.
3. The chest tube suture is clipped, and the tube is quickly removed.
4. An occlusive dressing or petrolatum jelly gauze is placed over the chest wall wound.
5. Patient is instructed to breathe normally, and the dressing is taped securely.

NURSING CARE

NURSING ASSESSMENT

Accumulation of air in the pleural space (can occur before tube inserted, after tube in place, or after tube removal): Dyspnea, tachypnea, tachycardia, anxiety, and restlessness; decreased or absent breath sounds on affected side; tracheal shift; increased subcutaneous emphysema; decreased oxygen saturation

Drainage system function:

- Water in the water seal chamber should fluctuate slightly with respirations; indicates that tube is patent
- Continuous bubbling in the water seal chamber suggests an air leak in the drainage system (or a massive pleural air leak)
- Intermittent bubbling in the water seal chamber is expected until the pleural air leak is resolved
- Note drainage volume, color, consistency

POTENTIAL COMPLICATION

Infection, elevated WBC count, increased temperature, evidence of purulent drainage through chest tube or around site

PATIENT PROBLEMS, NURSING DIAGNOSES & INTERVENTIONS

NIC RESPIRATORY MANAGEMENT

Impaired gas exchange related to decreased lung expansion from pleural accumulation

- Maintain patency of chest tubes by keeping a continuous drainage path without kinks or dependent loops.
- Always keep chest tube drainage system lower than the patient's chest.
- Ensure that all tubing connections are securely attached and taped.
- Assist patient to cough, deep breathe, and change position at least every 2 hours *to promote drainage of accumulated fluid.*
- Observe special positioning if indicated because of special technique or surgery.

NIC PHYSICAL COMFORT PROMOTION

Acute pain related to chest tube placement and surgical incision

- Assist patient to splint areas of chest tube insertion and incision with a pillow or folded towel.
- Provide analgesia as needed *to promote effective ventilation.*

EVALUATION/PATIENT OUTCOMES

Respiratory Management: Breath sounds are clear bilaterally. Roentgenograms confirm lung reexpansion. Blood gases are within normal limits for patient.

Physical Comfort Promotion: Patient is able to breathe deeply without pain.

MECHANICAL VENTILATION

Description and Rationale

Mechanical support of ventilation is indicated for patients who are unable to maintain adequate ventilation on their own. The following description of ventilatory devices is a brief overview of those that are used outside the setting of the intensive care unit. For more information on these devices or a discussion of the ventilatory techniques used for critically ill patients, the reader is referred to specialty texts for more information. The terminology of ventilatory devices is presented in Table 4-13.

Patient-machine interfaces are presented in Table 4-14.

Patient populations who may require non–intensive care unit (ICU) mechanical ventilatory assistance are as follows:

- Patients who require a prolonged weaning period after mechanical ventilation for acute respiratory failure. These patients are often transferred to non-ICU settings that specialize in chronic ventilation and weaning. Patient is usually tracheotomized. Usual ventilator is a volume ventilator or bilevel device.
- Patients with chronic obstructive lung disease with an acute exacerbation that causes acute CO_2 retention. Noninvasive ventilation with bilevel or volume device may be instituted to avoid the need for intubation. Patients in this category require very close assessment and care to avoid intubation.
- Selected patients who have severe chronic respiratory disease with significant chronic CO_2 retention. Institution of ventilatory assistance during sleep may stabilize the CO_2 level, decrease fatigue, and improve daytime function. This type of assistance may be used for long periods in the home setting. A noninvasive approach (mask) is used; the usual device is bilevel assistance, although a volume ventilator may also be used.
- Patients with neuromuscular disease who have absent/significantly impaired inspiratory muscle strength. Some require only nighttime ventilation, while others may require continuous assistance. The device is usually bilevel or a volume ventilator. The patient/machine interface may be via a mask or via tracheostomy tube.
- Patients with obstructive sleep apnea (see p. 194). CPAP device is used during sleep. If the patient requires high pressures, a bilevel device may improve tolerance.

Table 4-13 Ventilator Terminology

Term	Definition/Description
Major Categories of Ventilation	
Positive pressure ventilation	Positive pressure is applied to the inspired air. The device is connected to the airway via a mouthpiece, mask, tracheal tube. Air is essentially "pushed" into the lung. Most of the devices used today to assist ventilation are of the positive pressure type.
Negative pressure ventilation	Negative pressure is applied around the thorax during inspiration. The negative pressure pulls the chest wall outward and air flows into the lung. There is nothing connected to the airway. The iron lung is a negative pressure device.
Terms Used in Positive Pressure Ventilation	
Intermittent positive pressure	Positive pressure applied during inspiration; expiration is passive
Positive end-expiratory pressure (PEEP)	Positive pressure is applied at end expiration instead of allowing the airway pressure to fall to atmospheric pressure
Continuous positive airway pressure (CPAP)	A continuous pressure is applied over the airway during spontaneous breathing. Instead of inspiration and expiration varying over and under a baseline of "0" pressure, they now vary over and under a preset positive pressure (see text for further discussion)
Types of Positive Pressure Ventilators Used in the Non-ICU Setting	
Volume cycled ventilator	The equipment allows the delivery of a specific tidal volume to the patient. The amount of pressure required may vary from breath to breath. Small volume ventilators with internal battery packs are available for home use.
Pressure cycled ventilator	A predetermined inspiratory pressure is set. The ventilator delivers gas to the patient until that pressure is met. The volume actually delivered with each breath may vary.
Bilevel ventilation	Differing amounts of positive pressure are applied to the airway during inspiration (inspiratory pressure) and expiration (expiratory pressure or PEEP); a greater amount of airway pressure is applied during inspiration with little or no pressure applied during expiration; the bilevel device uses "pressure support," a type of pressure cycling.

Table 4-14 Patient-Machine Interfaces: Home Setting

Tracheostomy tube	Usually reserved for those who require continuous ventilation or who are completely unable to protect the airway. See pp. 210-211 on care of patient with artificial airway.
Nasal mask, nasal pillows	Used with both bilevel and volume ventilator; appropriate size must be determined; patients often have two different styles to alternate, relieve pressure areas. Addition of heated humidification often improves tolerance. Different types of headgear, used to keep mask in place, are also available.
Full face mask	Used when adequate seal/ventilation not possible with one of the nasal masks or pillows; used with both bilevel and volume ventilator. Use mask with special emergency disconnect devices and safety valve so that patient can breathe if power failure to ventilatory device occurs.

Preprocedural Nursing Care

1. Review with physician/chart reason patient requires ventilatory assistance:
   Obstructive sleep apnea, inspiratory muscle weakness, chronic CO_2 retention, acute CO_2 retention in patient with chronic lung disease (remember this list does not include problems usually found in the ICU).
2. Is ventilation to be continuous or nighttime?
3. Nighttime Spo_2 or ABGs; daytime Spo_2 or ABGs.
4. Does patient/family understand reason for instituting ventilatory assistance?
5. Review the type of device ordered for the patient.

Procedural Guidelines

1. In noninvasive techniques, assist with application of patient-machine interface.
2. If invasive (tracheostomy), a cuffed tube is usually used; inflate cuff when patient on ventilator (see sections on tracheostomy, suctioning).
3. Pressure/volume (volume ventilator would not be used for sleep apnea) must be appropriate for goals. If obstructive sleep apnea, need enough pressure to abolish significant apneas and hypopneas. If for chronic disease with inadequate ventilation, need enough pressure difference/volume to allow adequate tidal ventilation.
4. Observe for good chest expansion, in synchrony with the ventilator.
5. Observe that snoring is abolished.
6. Observe that paradoxical respirations and use of accessory muscles on inspiration are abolished.
7. Observe that apneas are abolished; automatic rate may be required if there is central apnea or respiratory muscle paralysis.
8. Measure ABGs and or Spo_2 during ventilation to demonstrate improvement.
9. Make sure equipment is functioning properly: rise and fall in pressure; cycling between inspiration and expiration; no kinks in the tubing.

HINTS FOR APPLYING NASAL MASKS IN NONEMERGENCY SITUATIONS

1. Be sure patient was measured for appropriate mask size.
2. Allow patient to hold mask and breathe through it before it is connected to machine.
3. While patient is holding mask, connect to ventilatory device; may start at lower pressures than goal for initial session.
4. When patient is comfortable, attach to headgear; remember with bilevel device, a small leak will be tolerated.
5. As patient relaxes, is comfortable; pressure is increased to level desired.
6. Patient may tolerate better with humidification.

EVALUATION/PATIENT OUTCOMES

Gas exchange improved/stabilized (ABGs, oximetry)
Improvement in daytime energy level
Decreased fatigue
Decreased dyspnea

THORACIC SURGERY[8,36]

Thoracotomy

Thoracotomy refers to a surgical incision of the chest wall. An exploratory thoracotomy may be performed to obtain a biopsy specimen or locate a source of bleeding. During the procedure the ribs are spread and the pleura is opened. Closed chest drainage is generally required postoperatively.

Pneumonectomy

Pneumonectomy refers to surgical removal of an entire lung. The surgeon severs and sutures off the main arteries, veins, and the mainstem bronchus at the bifurcation. The major indication for pneumonectomy is removal of lung cancer that has not spread beyond a single lung. Closed chest drainage is not used postoperatively, so that the thoracic cavity on the affected side will fill with serous exudates and eventually consolidate. The phrenic nerve on the affected side may be severed to elevate the diaphragm, which also assists to fill the empty thoracic space.

Lobectomy, Segmental Resection, and Wedge Resection

When less than an entire lung is removed, the procedure name refers to the amount of tissue removed. For example, a lobectomy refers to removal of a single lung lobe. Indications for these procedures include isolated tumor or injury or unresponsive cyst, tuberculosis, or abscess. A wedge resection may also be done for diagnostic biopsy. Closed chest drainage is used after partial lung removal. The remaining lung tissue on the operative side expands to fill the chest cavity, so breath sounds will be heard over the area where tissue was removed.

Decortication

Decortication refers to the stripping off of a thick fibrous membrane that may develop over the visceral pleura secondary to empyema or the prolonged presence of blood or fluid in the pleural space. Closed chest drainage is required postoperatively.

Lung Reduction

Lung reduction surgery is a therapeutic intervention in a highly select group of patients with emphysema. The principles are that a reduction of lung volume will (1) decrease the tension of the respiratory muscles and therefore decrease dyspnea and (2) allow normal lung that was previously compressed to expand and thus improve gas exchange. Two approaches are used. In one, a midline sternotomy is performed and both lungs "trimmed." Strips of bovine pericardium are usually used to help seal the cut surface of the lung and prevent large postoperative air leaks. In the other procedure a laser beam is used to trim the lung, usually through multiple thorascopic incisions.

Lung Transplant

Lung transplantation originally required a heart-lung transplantation. Today, lung transplantation without transplanting the heart is possible. Depending on the recipient's underlying pulmonary pathology, a heart-lung, single-lung, or double-lung transplantation can be done.

Heart-lung transplantations are done for patients with primary pulmonary hypertension and for cardiac defects associated with pulmonary hypertension (Eisenmenger's syndrome). Heart-lung transplantations are done via a midline sternotomy incision.

Double-lung and double single-lung transplantation (in other words, a right and left lung are transplanted; the trachea is native to the recipient) is the procedure done in patients with CF. Because of the risk of infection if one native lung were left, single-lung transplantation is avoided. The double-lung transplantation is usually the procedure of choice in younger candidates. The double-lung transplantation is usually done via a clam shell incision (anteriorly, from side to side at the lower thoracic border). Some surgeons also prefer the double-lung transplantation for patients with emphysema.

The single-lung transplantation is done for patients with interstitial fibrosis. Some surgeons also use this approach for patients with emphysema. This procedure allows more persons to receive a transplant, a consideration when donors are not always available. A lateral thoracotomy incision is usually used. In single-lung transplantation, one must always remember that the native lung with its disease is still present. The aim is for the native lung to essentially shut down, with blood flow and ventilation going to the new lung (FIG. 4-39).

Whenever a lung is transplanted, consideration is given not only to blood type and HLA typing but also to the size of the donor and recipient. (If the lung is too small, it may not fill the thorax; if the transplanted lung is too large, it may be difficult to fully inflate it.) Lung transplantation patients receive immunosuppressive medication, as do other transplantation patients. Another specific consideration in lung transplantation involves problems with airway clearance. The donor lung has no cough reflex (the lung is denervated), and the bronchial arteries are not attached to the recipient's systemic circulation. Mucus tends to be more tenacious, and mucociliary clearance is often impaired; coupling this finding with loss of the cough reflex

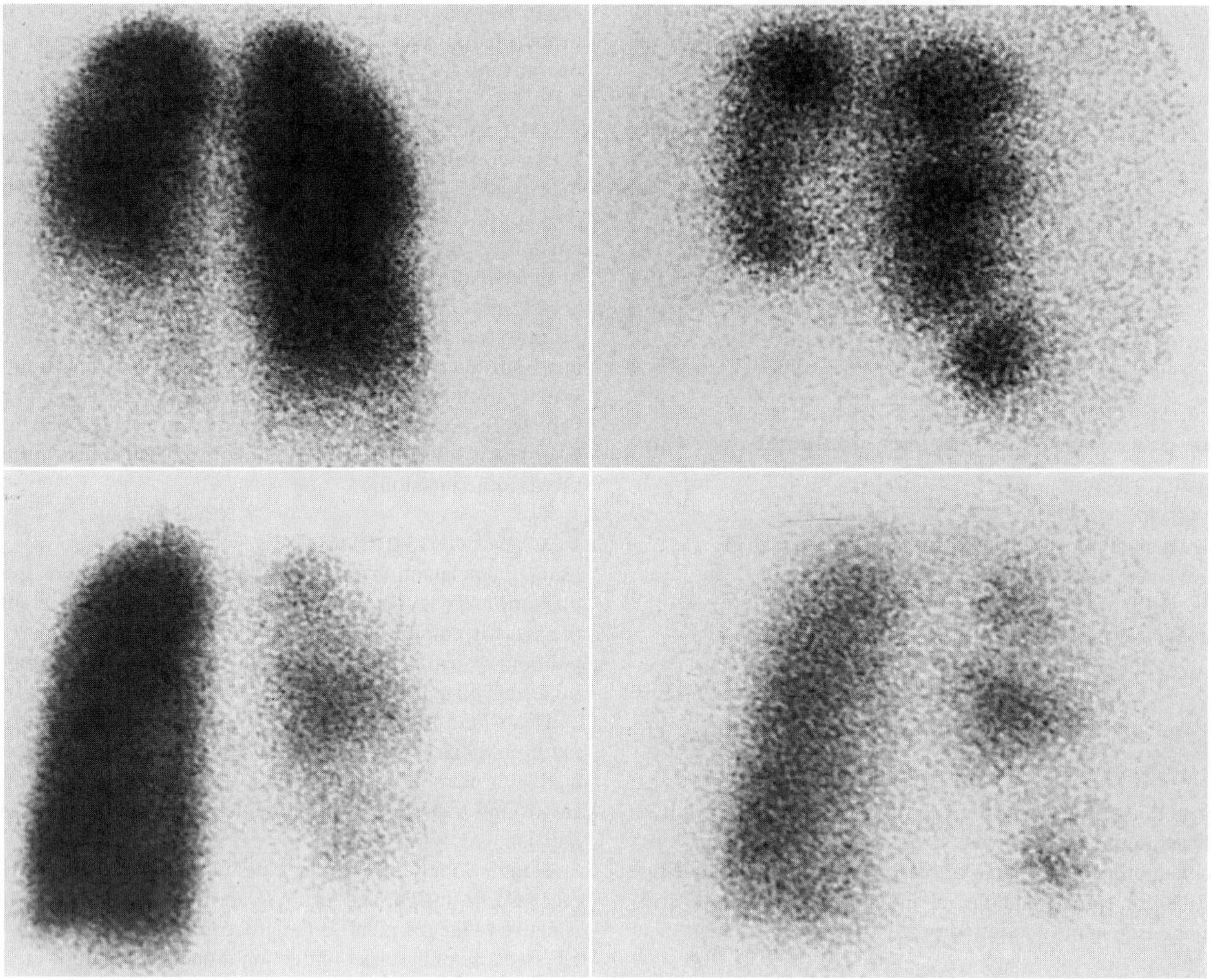

FIG. 4-39

Ventilation-perfusion lung scans obtained before and after single lung transplantation in a patient with severe obstructive pulmonary disease and pulmonary hypertension. The preoperative perfusion (**A**) and ventilation (**B**) scans show matched abnormalities. After transplantation, perfusion (**C**) and ventilation (**D**) shift strongly to the transplanted lung. Perfusion shifts are typically more prominent than ventilation shifts, especially in patients with pulmonary hypertension in the remaining lung. (From Murray and Nadel.[23])

means that nursing care and patient teaching regarding airway clearance are of prime importance. Patients are taught to voluntarily cough several times a day, and most are taught to do postural drainage every day.

Impaired bronchial circulation after lung transplant may allow strictures to develop at the bronchial anastamosis. Strictures are treated with bronchial stent placement via fiberoptic bronchoscopy.

Both acute and chronic rejection can be more difficult to diagnose in lung transplantation than in heart transplantations. It is often difficult to differentiate a pulmonary infection because of immunosuppression from rejection. The patient may be unaware of subtle changes in lung function. Thus patients do daily monitoring of spirometry (FEV_1 and FVC); a fall in FEV_1 or FVC is a signal to contact their caregivers. Bronchoscopy with biopsy may identify the cause of the fall in function, but patients are often treated for both infection (antibiotics) and rejection (corticosteroids) simultaneously. Chronic rejection in lung transplantation results in bronchiolitis obliterans with severe airways obstruction.

Contraindications/Cautions

The following are potential complications of thoracic surgery:

- Respiratory insufficiency
- Tension pneumothorax
- Atelectasis
- Bronchopleural fistula
- Pulmonary edema
- Subcutaneous emphysema
- Diaphragm paralysis
- Infection

Preprocedural Nursing Care

Carefully determine preoperative status of patient, including the following:

- Baseline pulmonary function studies

ECG
ABGs
Electrolytes
Other existing health problems
Current respiratory status: Amount and extent of dyspnea, cough, sputum production, and respiratory distress
General nutrition and hydration state

Provide preoperative teaching to include the following:
Need to stop smoking preoperatively
Coughing and deep breathing techniques
Overview of equipment and procedures that will most likely occur postoperatively
Listen preoperatively to patient and family questions and concerns; provide information and clarification when indicated.
Assure patient that pain medication will be available postoperatively to assist with discomfort.
Teach patient the need for postoperative ROM and leg exercises, early ambulation.

NURSING CARE

POSTOPERATIVE NURSING ASSESSMENT

Respiratory status: Dyspnea, tachypnea, restlessness, inadequate chest expansion, stridor, shallow respirations, crackles, rhonchi, decreased tidal volume, cough effectiveness, sputum characteristics, mediastinal shift, paradoxical motion, SpO_2, ABG results

Chest tube drainage: Characteristics of drainage, function of closed drainage system, presence of air leak
Pain: Pain with activities of turning, coughing, deep breathing, and ROM
Fluid and electrolyte balance: Vital signs, electrolytes, adequate urinary output

POTENTIAL COMPLICATIONS

Infection: Increased WBC count, fever, purulent drainage or sputum, redness around incision area, decreased breath sounds, crackles, rhonchi
Hemorrhage: Tachycardia, hypotension, decreased or absent breath sounds, dullness to percussion, hemoptysis, increased sanguinous drainage with clots from chest tubes

PATIENT PROBLEMS/NURSING DIAGNOSES & INTERVENTIONS

NIC RESPIRATORY MANAGEMENT

Ineffective airway clearance related to increased tracheobronchial secretions, muscle weakness, pain

Impaired gas exchange related to pleural fluid accumulation, hypoventilation

- Maintain patent airway by suctioning and positioning; if patient has endotracheal tube, see p. 208 for additional strategies.
- See closed-chest drainage system, p. 210, for additional strategies.
- Encourage coughing and deep breathing and use of incentive spirometry on a regular basis until patient is able to maintain procedure by self; observe and record response.
- Facilitate patient rest between activities.

NIC IMMOBILITY MANAGEMENT

Impaired physical mobility related to incisional pain and chest tubes

- Place a call button for the patient to reach conveniently without straining.
- The patient is at risk for developing stiffness and ankylosis of the shoulder on the side with the chest tubes; encourage and assist ROM activities for that shoulder on a regular schedule.
- Encourage passive and active ROM of the legs *to decrease the potential for thrombosis.*
- Administer analgesics as ordered *to manage pain and promote mobility.*
- Ambulate patient as soon as possible and in accordance with patient's ability to tolerate ambulation.

EVALUATION/PATIENT OUTCOMES

Evaluation criteria are based on the individual procedure performed and the underlying disease state.

Respiratory Management: Airways are patent. Breath sounds are clear. ABGs are within acceptable range.

Immobility Management: ROM of the affected shoulder is maintained. Breathing pattern is effective without severe pain. Patient is able to increase activity.

REFERENCES

1. ACCP/AACVPR Evidence-Based Guidelines: pulmonary rehabilitation, *Chest* 112:1363, 1997.
2. Bootzin RR, et al: Sleep disorders, *Compr Ther* 21:401, 1995.
3. Bouros D et al: Intrapleural urokinase versus normal saline in the treatment of complicated parapneumonic effusions and empyema, *Am J Respir Crit Care Med* 159:37, 1999.
4. Brooks-Brunn J: Validation of a predictive model for postoperative pulmonary complications, *Heart Lung* 27(3):151, 1998.
5. Campisi P, Voitk AJ: Outpatient treatment of spontaneous pneumothorax in a community hospital using a Heimlich flutter valve: a case series, *J Emerg Med* 15(1):115, 1997.
6. Celikel T et al: Comparison of noninvasive positive pressure ventilation with standard medical therapy in hypercapnic acute respiratory failure, *Chest* 114(6):1636, 1998.
7. Celli BR: Standards for the optimal management of COPD: a summary, *Chest* 113(4):283S, 1998.
8. Cerfolio RJ et al: A prospective algorithm for the management of air leaks after pulmonary resection, *Ann Thorac Surg* 66:1726, 1998.
9. Cherniack RM: Current therapy of respiratory disease, ed 2, Philadelphia, 1986, BC Decker.
10. Chulay M, Guzzetta C, Dossey B: *AACN handbook of critical care nursing,* Stamford, CT, 1997, Appleton & Lange.
11. Collins LM: Deep venous thrombosis, *Nurse Pract Forum* 9(3):163, 1998.

11a. Fries JF, Ehrlich GE: *Prognosis: contemporary outcomes of disease,* Bowie, Md, 1981, Charles Press.

12. Groskin SA: *Heitzman's the lung: radiologic-pathologic correlations,* St. Louis, 1993, Mosby.
13. Guenter CA, Welch MH: *Pulmonary medicine,* Philadelphia, 1997, JB Lippincott.

14. Hamer L, Parker HW: Treatment of cystic fibrosis in adults, *Am Fam Physician* 54(4):1291, 1996.
14a. Harper RW: *A guide to respiratory care: physiology and clinical approaches,* Philadelphia, 1981, JB Lippincott.
15. Higgenbottom T, Stenmark K, Simonneau G: Treatments for severe pulmonary hypertension, *Lancet* 353:338, 1999.
16. Hirsch J, Hannock L: *Mosby's manual of clinical nursing practice,* St. Louis, 1981, Mosby.
17. Ihnat DM et al: Treatment of patients with venous thromboembolism and malignant disease: should vena cava filter placement be routine? *J Vasc Surg* 28:800, 1998.
18. Jarvis C: *Physical examination and health assessment* ed 3, Philadelphia, 2000, WB Saunders.
19. Katzenstein AA, Myers J: Idiopathic pulmonary fibrosis, *Am J Respir Crit Care Med* 157:1301, 1998.
20. Langenderfer B: Alternatives to percussion and postural drainage, *J Cardiopul Rehabil* 18:283, 1998.
20a. Lewis SM, Collier IC, Heitkemper MM: *Medical-surgical nursing: assessment and management of clinical problems,* ed 5, St. Louis, 2000, Mosby.
21. McCance KL, Huether SE: *Pathophysiology: the biologic basis for disease in adults and children,* ed 2, St. Louis, 1994, Mosby.
22. Morse CJ: Lung volume reduction surgery: a review, *Crit Care Nurs Q* 21(1):1, 1998.
23. Murray JF, Nadel JA: *Textbook of respiratory medicine,* Philadelphia, 1994, WB Saunders.
24. NANDA: NANDA nursing diagnoses: definitions and classifications, 1999-2000, Philadelphia, 1999, The Association.
25. National Heart, Lung, and Blood Institute: Guidelines for the diagnosis and management of asthma, Bethesda, MD, 1997, U.S. Department of Health and Human Services, National Institute of Health, Pub. No. 97-4051A. Retrieved 1/2000 on the World Wide Web: *http://www.nhlbi.nih.gov/guidelines/asthma/asthgdl. htm.*
26. Noureddine SN: Sleep apnea: a challenge in critical care, *Heart Lung,* 25:1, 1996.
27. Pettinicchi TA: Trouble shooting chest tubes, *Nursing 98,* March 58-59, 1998.
28. Price SA, Wilson LM: *Pathophysiology: clinical concepts of disease processes,* ed 5, St. Louis, 1996, Mosby.
28a. Rakel RE: *Conn's current therapy,* Philadelphia, 1987, WB Saunders.
29. Ricciardi MJ, Rubenfire M: How to manage secondary pulmonary hypertension: recognizing and treating cor pulmonale and chronic thromboembolism, *Postgrad Med* 105(2):183, 1999.
30. Ryu JH, Colby TV, Hartman TE: Idiopathic pulmonary fibrosis: current concepts. *Mayo Clin Proc* 73(11):1085, 1998.
31. Samuel JR: Management of recurrent spontaneous pneumothorax and recurrent symptomatic pleural effusion with chest tube pleurodesis, *Crit Care Nurs* 17(1):28, 1997.
32. Teran-Santos J, Jimenez-Gomez A, Crodero-Guevara J: The association between sleep apnea and the risk of traffic accidents, *N Engl J Med* 340(11):847, 1999.
33. Thelan LA et al: *Critical care nursing: diagnosis and management,* ed 3, St. Louis, 1998, Mosby.
34. The National Lung Health Education Program: Strategies in preserving lung health and preventing COPD and associated diseases, *Chest* 113(2):123S, 1998.
35. Thompson JM, Wilson SF: *Health assessment for nursing practice,* St. Louis, 1996, Mosby.
36. Tovar EA et al: One day admission for a lung lobectomy: an incidental result of a clinical pathway, *Ann Thorac Surg* 65:803, 1998.
37. Velmahos GC et al: Predicting the need for thorascopic evacuation of residual traumatic hemothorax: chest radiograph is insufficient, *J Trauma* 46(1):65, 1999.
38. Wallace LS: Pulmonary hypertension: a deadly threat, *RN* 61(10):48, 1998.
39. Weg JG, Haas CF: Long-term oxygen therapy for COPD: improving longevity and quality of life in hypoxemic patients, *Postgrad Med* 103(4):143, 1998.
40. West J: *Respiratory physiology: the essentials,* Baltimore, 1979, Williams & Wilkins.
41. Wilson SF, Thompson JM: *Mosby's clinical nursing series: respiratory disorders,* St. Louis, 1990, Mosby.
42. Yagan MB: Hospital-acquired pneumonia and its management, *Crit Care Nurs Q* 20(3):36, 1997.
43. Yankaskas JR, Knowles MR, editors: *Cystic fibrosis in the adult,* Philadelphia, 1999, Lippincott-Raven.

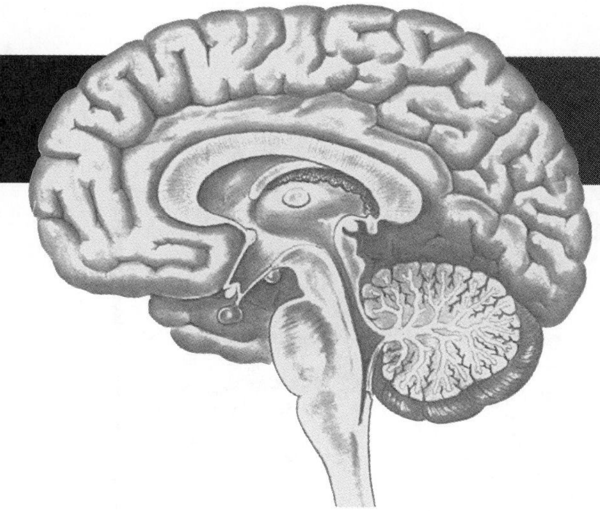

5 Neurologic System

Victor G. Campbell

Overview

The human nervous system consists of complex structures and processes that control the various functions of the body. Because these functions are integrative, the physiologic and psychologic ramifications of a neurologic dysfunction can be devastating.

Anatomy, Physiology, and Related Pathophysiology

The nervous system is divided into two fairly distinct structural categories: the central nervous system (CNS), which consists of the brain and spinal cord, and the peripheral nervous system (PNS), which is made up of 12 pairs of cranial nerves, 31 pairs of spinal nerves, and the sympathetic and parasympathetic subdivisions of the autonomic nervous system. Functionally, the central and peripheral nervous systems are interdependent because each is made of millions of shared neurons and neuroglia cells. The neuron is the basic unit of the nervous system. The neuroglia cells support the neuron.

Neuroglia Cells

About 40% of the structures of the brain and spinal cord are neuroglia cells. These cells protect, support, and nourish the cell bodies and processes of the neurons. There are four distinct types of neuroglia cells: astrocyte, ependyma, microglia, and oligodendroglia (Fig. 5-1). Unlike neurons, neuroglia cells can divide and multiply by mitosis, therefore they are a main source for nervous system tumors.

Astrocyte cells (astroglia) look like stars because of the many processes extending from their cell bodies. Their functions include helping to conduct impulses, supply nutrition, store information, support the neuronal structures, and maintain the blood-brain barrier.

Ependymal cells are found within the epithelial lining of the cerebral ventricles, the choroid plexuses, and the spinal cord's central canal. Their main function is to help produce cerebrospinal fluid.

Microglia are stationary cells scattered throughout the CNS, mainly in white matter. The function of microglia is phagocytosis, during which the microglia become mobile and ingest and digest tissue debris.

Oligodendroglia cells synthesize a lipid-protein complex that forms myelin sheaths around the axonal projections of neurons in the CNS. Functions of the myelin sheath include holding nerve fibers together, providing insulation, promoting ionic flow, and transmitting nerve impulses (termed *saltatory conduction*).

Neurons

Neurons (Fig. 5-2) have properties of excitation and electrical-chemical conductivity. In the CNS, groups of neurons are called nuclei; in the peripheral nervous system they are called ganglia.

Cytologic Features. The neuron is made of a cell body, or perikaryon; prosections, called dendrites; and an axon. The nerve cell body is the gray matter of the nervous system. Each neuron contains only one centrally located nucleus. The nucleus is a large, double-membraned structure containing deoxyribonucleic acid (DNA). Inside the nucleus is a single nucleolus containing ribonucleic acid (RNA). Surrounding the nucleus is granular cytoplasm containing many organelles, including Nissl bodies, mitochondria, the Golgi complex, neurofilaments, and microtubules. Nissl bodies help to synthesize protein. Mitochondria are rod-shaped organelles that regulate the cell's respiratory metabolism. The Golgi complex, located in the cytoplasm, condenses and store substances needed to transmit impulses. Dense neurofilaments are made of structures called neurotubules or microtubules. Together they form the neurofibril, which is involved in axoplasmic transport with cells.

Processes. Extending from the cell body is a long, smooth projection called the axon, or axis cylinder (Fig. 5-2). The axon originates from the neuron's cell body at a point called the axon hillock. The myelin around the axon protects and insulates it. Axons, which carry efferent impulses away from cell bodies, form the white matter of the CNS. Terminal branches

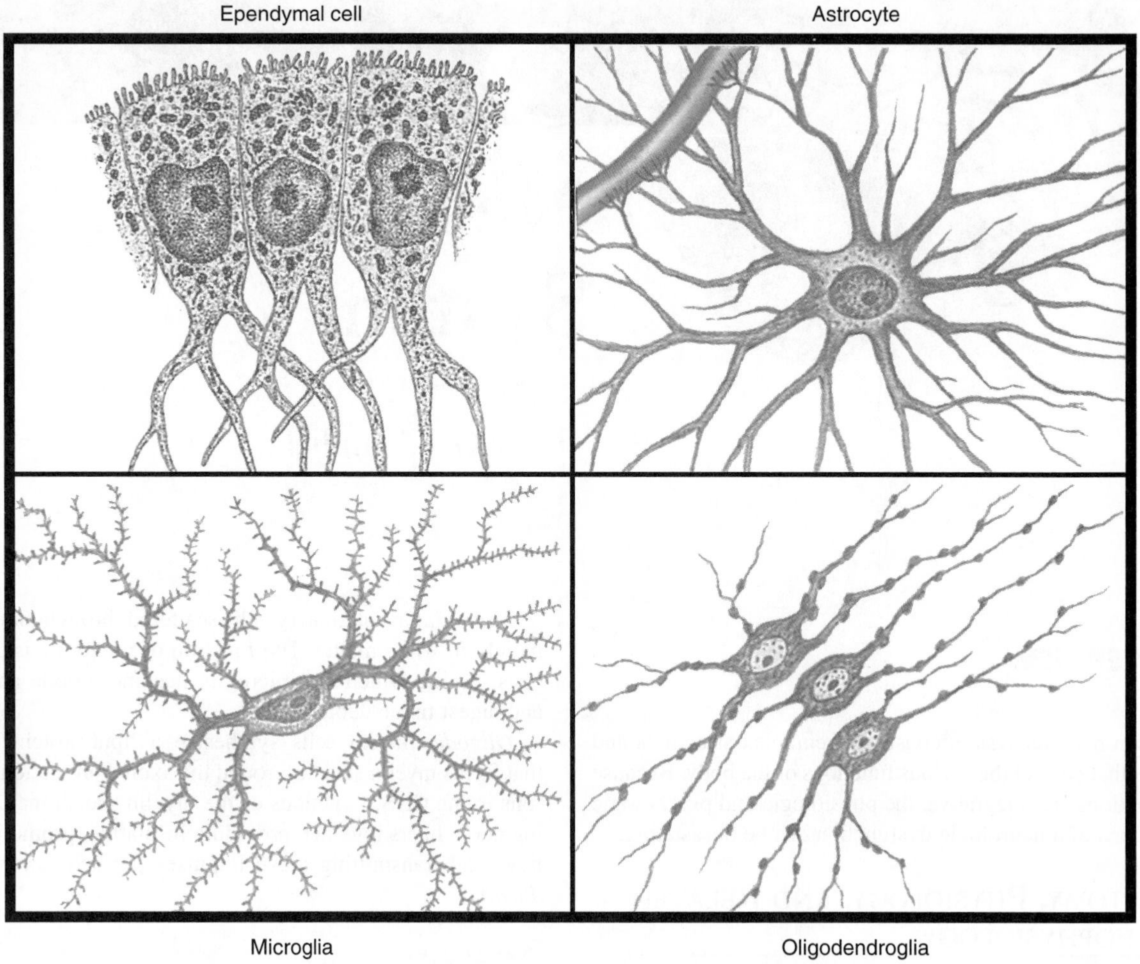

FIG. 5-1
Types of neuroglia cells.

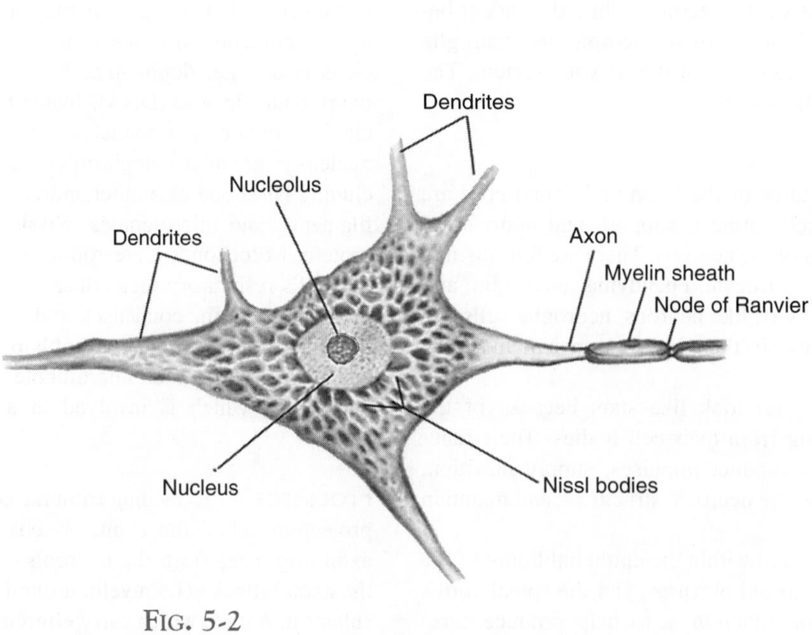

FIG. 5-2
Diagram of neuron with composite parts. (From Rudy.[11])

of the axon are called terminal filaments, or boutons (axon telodendria).

Extending from the cell body to the immediate surrounding areas are short receptive processes, or dendrites. The branchlike dendrites have no myelin sheath and lie with the cell body in the gray matter. The dendritic branches increase the surface area from which neuronal impulses can be picked up. Dendrites transmit afferent impulses toward the cell body. Rootlike terminal endings of the dendrite, or dendritic spines, help to transmit synapses.

Classification. Structurally, neurons can be subdivided according to the number of processes and the axon lengths (FIG. 5-3).

Unipolar neurons have only one process or pole, which divides close to the cell body. One branch of this division, called the peripheral process, carries afferent impulses toward the cell body. The other branch, the central process, conducts efferent impulses away from the body. *Bipolar* neurons have two processes: one axon and one dendrite. Bipolar neurons are found in the spinal ganglia, the nasal mucous membrane, and the rod and cone cells of the retina. *Multipolar* neurons make up most of the CNS, including all association (internuncial) and motor neurons. Multipolar neurons consist of a cell body, one long projection, and one or more shorter branches.

Neurons can also be classified by the axon length. Subdivisions within this classification are Golgi type I and Golgi type II cells (see FIG. 5-3). *Golgi type I* neurons are large and have long axons. They are found in the long fiber tracts located in the cerebral cortex, cerebellum, and spinal cord. *Golgi type II* neurons are small cells found between larger neurons that establish complex circuits in the nervous system. These neurons are found throughout the brain and spinal cord. Golgi type II neurons have short axons that branch repeatedly and end near the cell body.

Functionally, the neurons are classified as afferent, internuncial (association), or efferent (see FIG. 5-3). *Afferent* (sensory) neurons conduct impulses to the CNS. *Internuncial* (association) neurons are in the CNS and conduct afferent and efferent impulses. *Efferent* (motor) neurons transmit impulses to effector organs and tissue.

Nerves

In the peripheral nervous system the neuron carries impulses to and from the CNS via the chainlike grouping of neuron cell fibers into nerves (FIG. 5-4). (The term *nerve* applies only to cell fibers in the peripheral nervous system. In the CNS these are called *fiber tracts.*)

The axon is the part of the nerve that conducts impulses. The myelin sheath around the axon insulates, protects, and nourishes

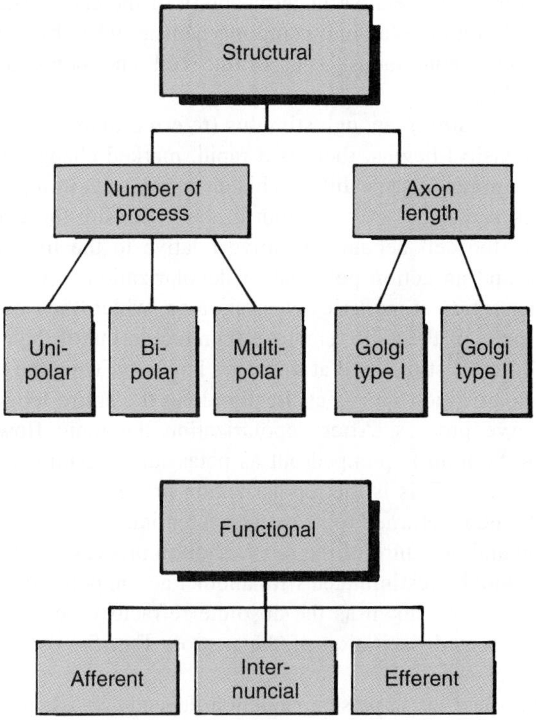

FIG. 5-3
Structural and functional neuron classification.

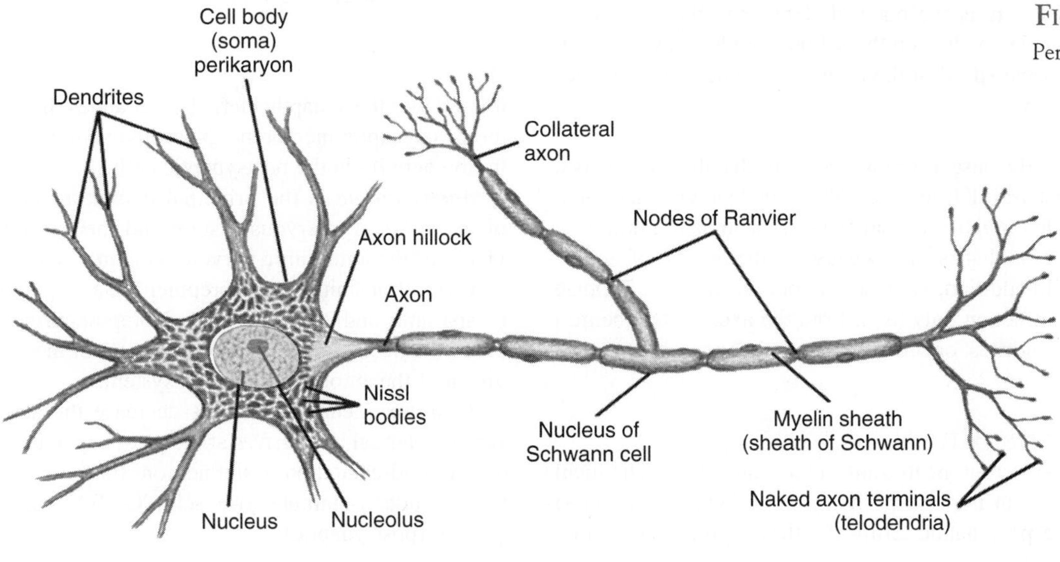

FIG. 5-4
Peripheral nerve.

the axon. Periodic interruptions of the myelin sheath are called *nodes of Ranvier.* These nodes allow action potentials to skip from node to node, increasing impulse conduction.

The nerve fibers in the peripheral nervous system are classified according to their function: afferent, internuncial (association), or efferent.

Nerve Impulse. Nerve fibers are charged (polarized) in their resting state. In this state the inside of the cell membrane has a negative charge in relation to the outside. There is a high concentration of sodium (Na^+) outside the cell and a high concentration of potassium (K^+) in the cell. This results in unequal electrical charges across the cell membrane. This difference is the result of the relative impermeability of the cell to sodium and the sodium-potassium pump mechanism, whereby sodium is pumped continuously out of the cell and potassium is pumped in.

When a strong enough stimulus (referred to as the threshold intensity) begins, there is a rapid, marked change in the cell membrane permeability. This change results in a gain of sodium and a loss of potassium in the cell. With the gain of sodium the cell becomes positive relative to the interstitial space, and an action potential or depolarization results. The depolarization stimulus excites one area, which then excites other parts of the cell membrane (conduction) until the entire membrane is stimulated at the same intensity. Thus the wave of depolarization moves cyclically along the entire length of the nerve process. After depolarization the ionic flow reverses. Sodium is pumped out as potassium is pumped back into the cell. This is the repolarization process, whereby the membrane is returned to its resting potential. During depolarization and one third of the repolarization process the neuron cell cannot be restimulated with another action potential. This time interval, known as the absolute refractory period, prevents repeated excitation of the neuron. FIG. 5-5 illustrates this process.

The speed of impulse conduction depends on whether the nerve has a myelin sheath. In the unmyelinated nerve the action potential must travel the entire length of the nerve fiber. In myelinated nerves the axon is exposed only at the nodes of Ranvier; therefore the action potential is not transmitted along the entire axon membrane. Instead the action potential "skips" discontinuously, from one node of Ranvier to the next. With this node-to-node conduction the action potential travels faster. This increases the speed of the impulses and decreases the demand for energy.

Synapse. Because neurons occur in chainlike pathways, impulses must travel from one cell to another via functional junctions called *synapses.* Actual synaptic transmission is a chemical process that occurs because of the release of neurotransmitters. In addition, synapses are polarized so the impulse flows in one direction only (e.g., from the axon of one neuron to the axon, dendrites, or cell body of another neuron in a pathway) (FIG. 5-6).

Neurotransmitters

At least 30 different neurotransmitters can affect chemical transmission of an impulse at the synapse. When an impulse stimulates the presynaptic terminals, they secrete neurotransmitters into the synaptic cleft. This changes the permeability of the postsynaptic membrane. Neurotransmitters either excite or inhibit activity in the postsynaptic cell.

Acetylcholine is the principal excitatory neurotransmitter of the voluntary nervous system and the parasympathetic division of the autonomic nervous system. Other central excitatory neurotransmitters are norepinephrine, dopamine, serotonin, L-aspartate, and glutamic acid. Norepinephrine is the major postsynaptic excitatory neurotransmitter in the sympathetic division of the autonomic nervous system.

Inhibitory neurotransmitters decrease the amplitude of the action potential as it arrives at the presynaptic terminals and decreases end-excitation of the neuron. Inhibitory neurotransmitters include γ-aminobutyric acid (GABA) (presynaptic) and glycine (postsynaptic).

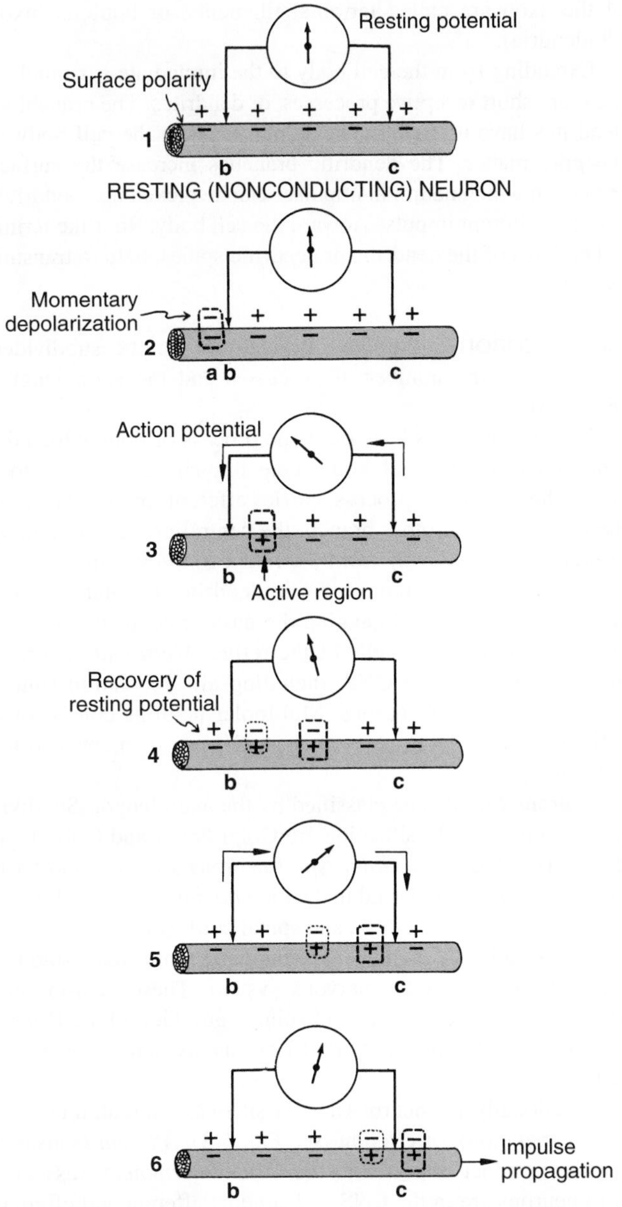

FIG. 5-5
Stages in impulse propagation. (From Schottelius and Schottelius.[11a])

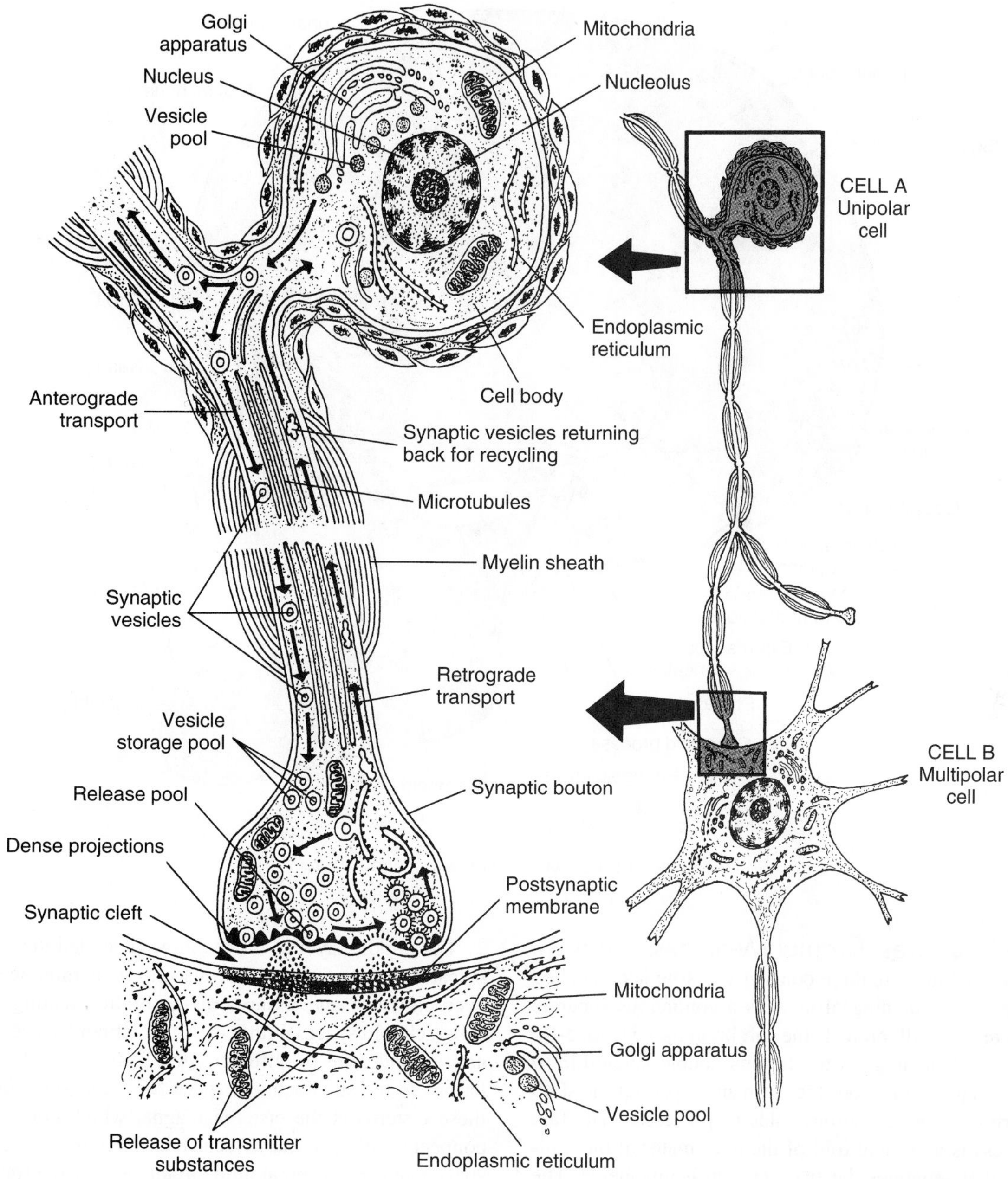

FIG. 5-6

Functional relationship between two neurons in pathway. Electrical impulse travels along axon of first neuron to synapse. Chemical transmitter is secreted into synaptic space to depolarize membrane (dendrite or cell body) of next neuron in pathway. *Cell A* represents unipolar cell; *cell B* represents multipolar cell.

Central Nervous System

Protective Structure: Skull. The brain is protected by the bony structure of the skull (FIG. 5-7). The skull is divided into two primary sections: the cranium and the skeleton of the face. The cranial portion of the skull is made up of eight relatively flat and irregular bones joined together by a series of fixed joints called sutures. These bones are composed of three layers: The solid *outer table,* the spongy middle *diploe,* and the solid *inner table.* The inner table of the skull forms a cavity filled with ridges and convolutions that are custom designed for holding the brain. This internal cavity has three major regions: the anterior fossa, the middle fossa, and the posterior fossa. The anterior fossa contains the frontal lobes; the middle fossa contains the temporal, parietal, and occipital lobes; and the posterior fossa contains the brainstem and cerebellum.

At the base of the skull in the inferoanterior portion of the occipital bone is a large oval opening called the foramen magnum. At the foramen magnum the brain and spinal cord become continuous. Also at the base of the skull is a series of openings (called foramina) for the entrance and exit of paired cranial nerves and cerebral blood vessels.

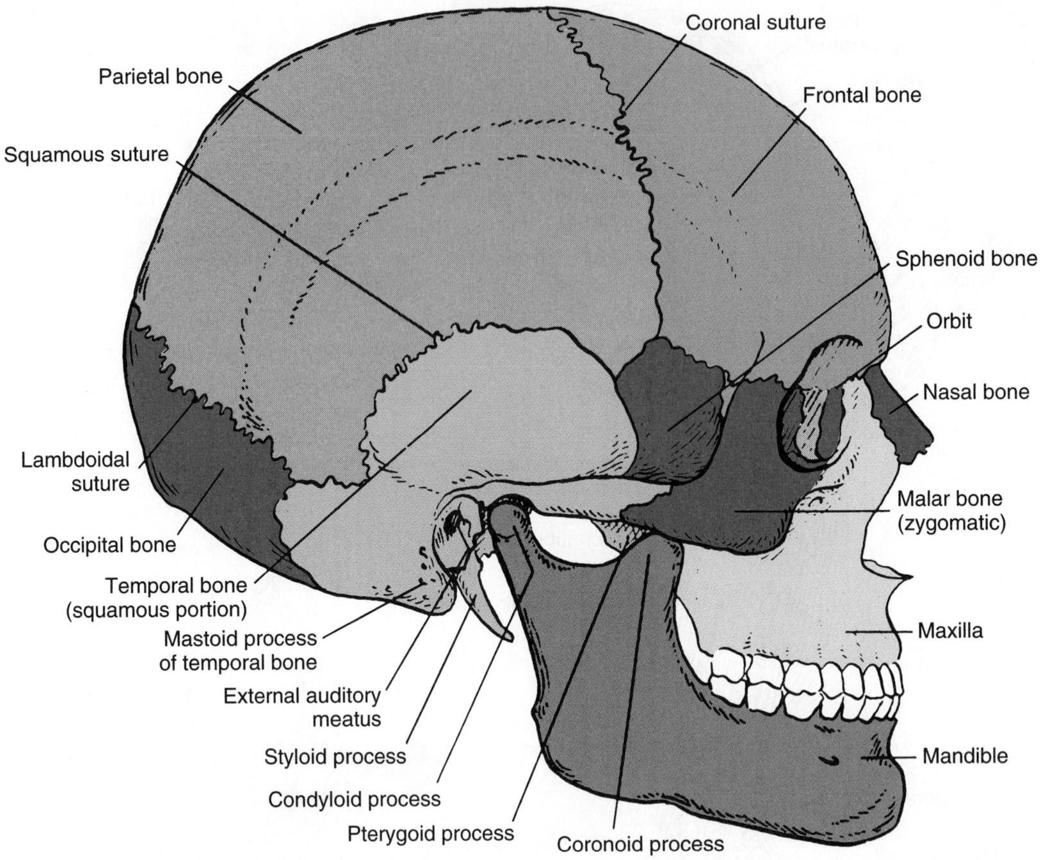

FIG. 5-7

Lateral view of skull. (From Thibodeau and Patton.[15])

Protective Structures: Cranial Meninges. Between the skull and the brain are three connective tissue layers called the meninges. Each meningeal layer is a continuous separate sheet that, like the skull, protects the soft brain tissue (FIG. 5-8).

The outermost meninge is the fibrous double-layered *dura mater.* The dura mater envelops the brain and separates the skull into compartments by its various folds or processes. The falx cerebri process is a vertical fold of the dura mater at the midsagittal line that separates the two cerebral hemispheres. The tentorium cerebelli is a horizontal double fold of dura that supports the temporal and occipital lobes and separates the cerebral hemispheres from the brainstem and the cerebellum. (The tentorium provides an important line of division. Structures above the tentorium are called supratentorial, and those below it are called infratentorial.) The falx cerebelli separates the two hemispheres of the cerebellum.

The cranial dura mater differs significantly from spinal dura mater in the following ways: the cranial dura is attached firmly, but the spinal dura is not attached to the vertebrae; cranial dura is made of two layers, periosteal and meningeal, but the spinal dura has only one meningeal layer; and the cranial dura separates in places and forms venous sinuses, which the one-layer spinal dura does not.

Between the dura mater and the middle meningeal layer is a narrow serous cavity called the subdural space. Vessels within the subdural space have few support structures and therefore are easily injured.

The middle layer of the meninges is called the arachnoid. It is made of a two-layered, fibrous, elastic membrane that crosses over the folds and fissures of the brain, creating the spongy subarachnoid space. Within the subarachnoid space are cerebral arteries and veins of different sizes. At the base of the brain, dilations in the subarachnoid space form cisterns. The largest of these cisterns is the cisterna magna, which communicates or connects with the fourth ventricle. It is in the subarachnoid space that cerebrospinal fluid circulates over the surfaces of the brain.

The innermost layer of meninges is called the pia mater. The pia mater is rich in small blood vessels, which supply the brain with a large volume of blood. It is also in direct contact with the external surface of the brain tissue. The arachnoid and pia membranes are collectively called the leptomeninges.

Brain

Next to the pia mater is the brain. The brain (encephalon) is divided into three major anatomic areas: The cerebrum, the cerebellum, and the brainstem.

Cerebrum. The cerebrum is the largest anatomic portion of the brain and is covered with several layers of gray cells that make up the cerebral cortex. It consists of cerebral hemispheres, the rhinencephalon, the internal capsule and basal ganglia, and the diencephalon (i.e., thalamus and hy-

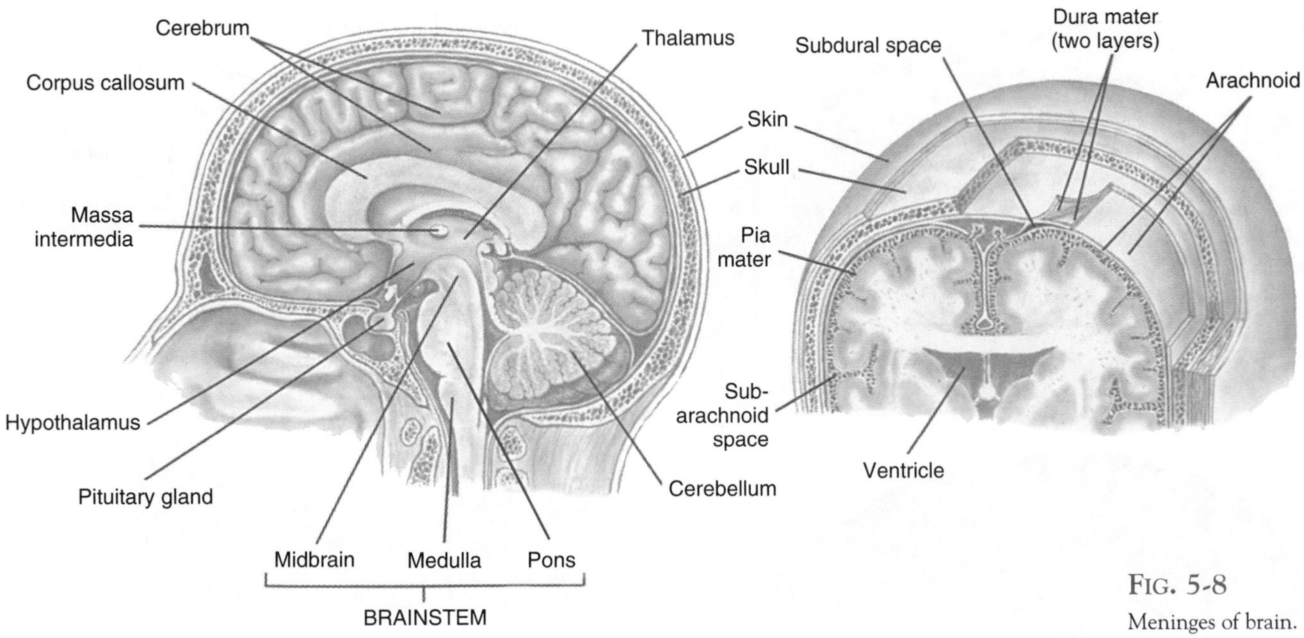

FIG. 5-8
Meninges of brain.

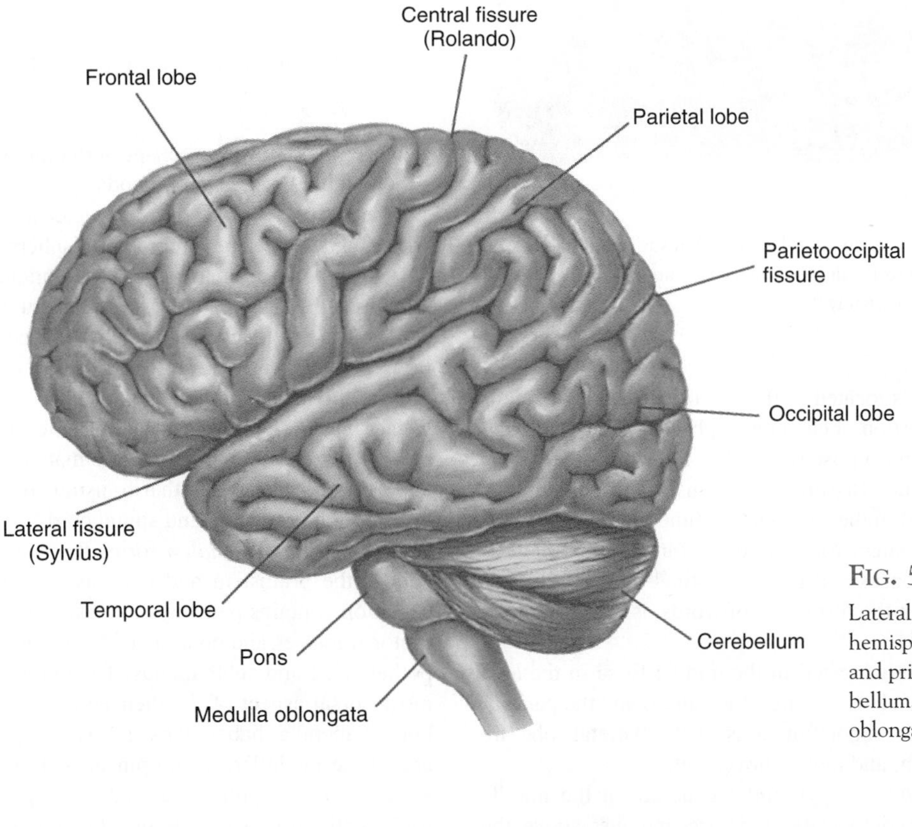

FIG. 5-9
Lateral view of cerebral hemisphere (showing lobes and principal fissures), cerebellum, pons, and medulla oblongata. (From Rudy.[11])

pothalamus). The cerebrum is divided lengthwise into symmetric right and left sides by the longitudinal fissure. Each half is called a lateral cerebral hemisphere. The hemispheres are joined lengthwise by a large tract of white commissural fibers, the corpus callosum, that serves as the communication link between the hemispheres. The major folds of the cortex divide each lateral hemisphere into four lobes, or cerebral hemispheres, which are named for the overlying cranial bones: frontal, parietal, occipital, and temporal (FIG. 5-9).

Certain areas of the cerebral cortex are responsible for specific functions of the cerebrum. Probably the best-known classification of these areas is *Brodmann's map.* On the basis of histologic studies, Brodmann developed a map of 46 different areas of the cerebral cortex (FIG. 5-10) and classified them as primary function areas or association areas.

Primary function areas are those in which movement or the perception of movement occurs. *Association areas* surround the primary function areas. They provide higher levels of integration (i.e., memory, learning) for sensory experiences.

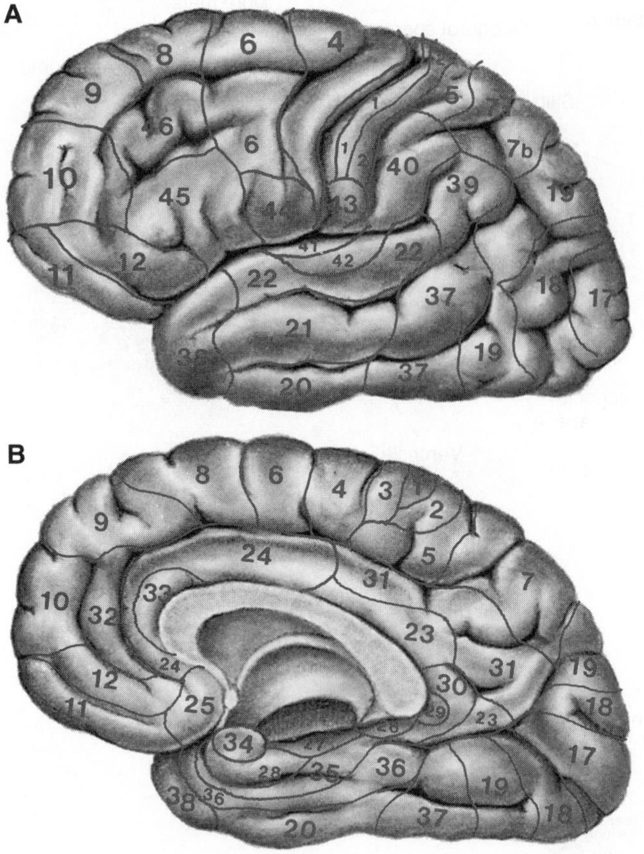

FIG. 5-10
Cytoarchitectural map of the lateral and medial surface of the human cortex according to Brodmann's map. **A,** Lateral surface. **B,** Medial surface. (From Rudy.[11])

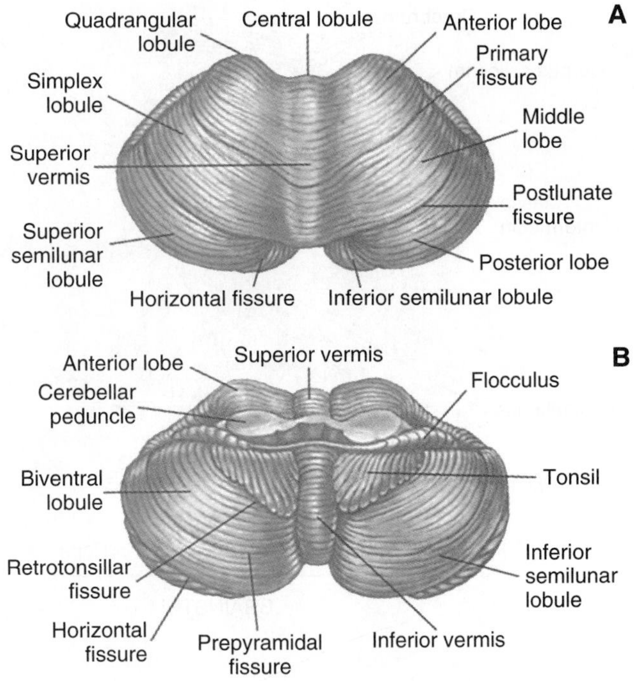

FIG. 5-11
Cerebellum. **A,** Superior surface. **B,** Inferior surface.

The *frontal lobe* is located in the anterior fossa and extends from the anterior portion of each hemisphere to the central sulcus (fissure of Rolando) posteriorly. The inferior border is the lateral cerebral fissure (fissure of Sylvius). The frontal lobe controls psychic and higher intellectual functions. It also contains higher-level centers for autonomic functioning, such as cardiovascular responses and gastrointestinal activity. Broca's area, which assists in the formation of words, is also located in the frontal lobe.

The *parietal lobe* is located in the middle fossa in the area between the central sulcus (fissure of Rolando) and the parieto-occipital fissure. The major functions of the parietal lobe are position sense, touch, and motor movement.

The *occipital lobe* is a pyramidal structure in the middle fossa, behind the parietooccipital fissure and just above the cerebellum. The occipital lobe contains the primary vision centers (primary vision cortex).

The *temporal lobe* also is located in the middle fossa. Primary functions of the temporal lobe are memory storage and hearing. Wernicke's area, the auditory association area, is found in the temporal lobe.

The *rhinencephalon (limbic lobe)* is anatomically part of the temporal lobe but has different functions. It consists of cortical and subcortical structures that form the border of the lateral ventricles of each cerebral hemisphere. The functions of the rhinencephalon involve self-preservation, visceral activities, instincts, feeling states, and moods.

The *basal ganglia* are gray nuclei located deep within the white matter of each cerebral hemisphere. They consist of the paired anatomic structures of the lenticular nucleus, caudate nucleus, amygdaloid body, and claustrum. The lenticular and caudate nuclei together are called the corpus striatum. Functions include motor control of fine body movements, particularly in the hands and lower extremities.

The *internal capsule,* located in the thalamic-hypothalamic area, is a massive bundle of white matter. It consists of afferent and efferent fiber tracts that transmit impulses from the cerebrum to the brainstem and spinal cord.

The *oval diencephalon* forms the rostral (toward the head) end of the brainstem and consists of gray matter. The diencephalon contains pathways for visceral, sensory, somatic, and motor impulses and consists of the epithalamus, thalamus, hypothalamus, and subthalamus. The epithalamus, located in the most dorsal aspect of the diencephalon, is made of the pineal body, habenula, habenular commissure, posterior commissure, and striae medullares. The pineal body is the most important structure of the epithalamus and is composed primarily of neuroglia cells. It plays a role in growth and sexual development. The thalamus consists of two connected oval masses of gray matter in the dorsal portion of the diencephalon. Each half of the thalamus is located deep within the corresponding cerebral hemisphere. The thalamus functions as a relay and integration station for cerebral, cerebellar, and brainstem activity. The hypothalamus lies inferior to the thalamus, forming the floor and portions of the walls of the third ventricle. Functions of the hypothalamus include mediating most endocrine and autonomic functions (i.e., blood pressure regulation) and emotional responses such as panic, fear, rage, blushing, and depression.

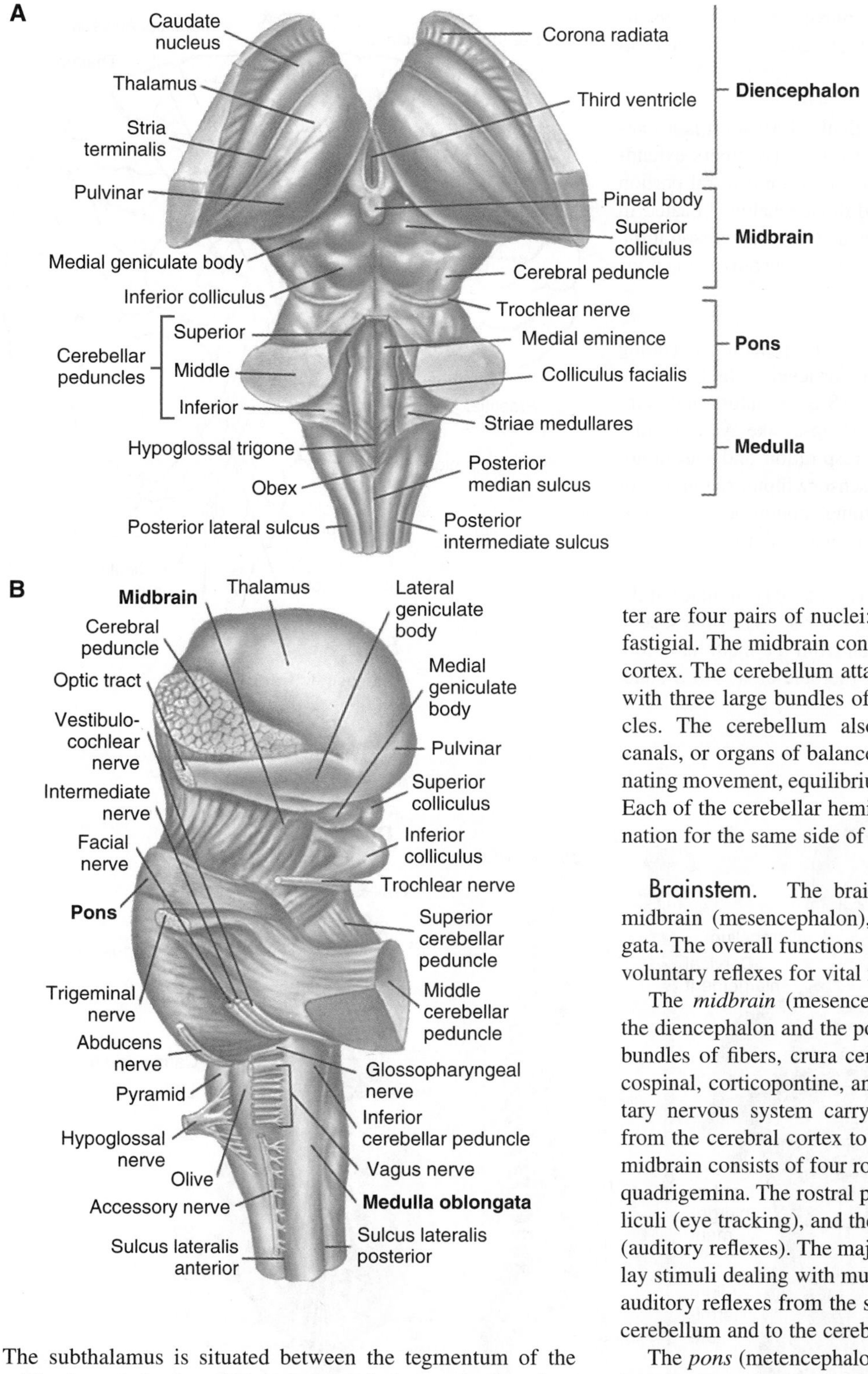

FIG. 5-12
Brainstem. **A,** Posterior view. **B,** Lateral view.

The subthalamus is situated between the tegmentum of the midbrain and the dorsal aspect of the thalamus. Its functions are part of the extrapyramidal system of the autonomic nervous system.

Cerebellum. The cerebellum (FIG. 5-11) is approximately one fifth the size of the cerebrum and consists of two lateral hemispheres and a medial portion, the vermis. It is separated from the cerebrum by the tentorium cerebelli. The cerebellum has an outer cortex of gray matter and an internal medulla of white matter. Embedded deep within the white matter are four pairs of nuclei: dentate, emboliform, globose, and fastigial. The midbrain connects the cerebellum to the cerebral cortex. The cerebellum attaches on each side of the brainstem with three large bundles of nerve fibers, the cerebellar peduncles. The cerebellum also connects with the semicircular canals, or organs of balance. It is involved primarily in coordinating movement, equilibrium, muscle tone, and position sense. Each of the cerebellar hemispheres controls movement coordination for the same side of the body (ipsilateral).

Brainstem. The brainstem (FIG. 5-12) consists of the midbrain (mesencephalon), the pons, and the medulla oblongata. The overall functions of the brainstem are to maintain involuntary reflexes for vital functioning of the body.

The *midbrain* (mesencephalon) forms a junction between the diencephalon and the pons. The lower surface contains two bundles of fibers, crura cerebri, which are made of the corticospinal, corticopontine, and corticobulbar tracts of the voluntary nervous system carrying descending motor fiber tracts from the cerebral cortex to the pons. The upper surface of the midbrain consists of four rounded elevations called the corpora quadrigemina. The rostral pair of elevations is the superior colliculi (eye tracking), and the caudal pair is the inferior colliculi (auditory reflexes). The major function of the midbrain is to relay stimuli dealing with muscle movement, visual reflexes, and auditory reflexes from the spinal cord, medulla oblongata, and cerebellum and to the cerebrum.

The *pons* (metencephalon; see FIG. 5-12) connects the midbrain to the medulla oblongata and relays impulses to the brain centers and to the lower spinal centers of the nervous system. Sensory and motor nuclei of the trigeminal (cranial V), abducens (cranial VI), facial (cranial VII), and acoustic (cranial VIII) nerves originate in the pons. The corticobulbar and corticospinal tracts make up the white matter of the pons.

The *medulla oblongata* (myelencephalon; see FIG. 5-12) contains the reflex centers for controlling involuntary functions such as breathing, sneezing, swallowing, coughing, salivation, vomiting, and vasoconstriction. The medulla also provides points of origin for the glossopharyngeal (cranial IX), vagus (cranial X), spinal accessory (cranial XI), and hypoglossal (cranial XII) nerves.

Reticular Formation. The reticular formation is a scattered, interconnected complex of sensory nerve fibers extending from the upper spinal cord through the midventral portion of the medulla, pons, midbrain, and diencephalon. Located in the reticular formation are centers that regulate respiration, blood pressure, heart rate (medulla), and vegetative functions (FIG. 5-13).

Reticular Activating System. The reticular activating system (RAS) extends from the superior level of the brainstem to the cerebral cortex. Most of the RAS is excitatory and is involved in maintaining attention, the sleep-awake cycle, regulation of visceral functions such as respiration and vasomotor tone, consciousness, perception of sensory input, regulation of temperature, emotional states, learning, conditioned reflexes, and regulation of skeletal muscle tone and activity.

Spinal Cord. The spinal cord (FIG. 5-14) originates at the foramen magnum and ends at the superior border of the second lumbar vertebrae. It is a continuation from the medulla oblongata. The cord tapers in the lower thoracic area into a cone-

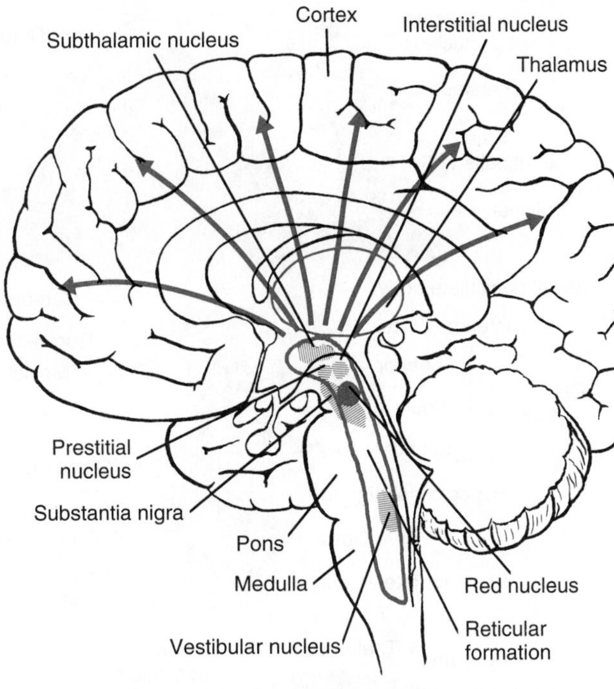

FIG. 5-13
Reticular activating system.

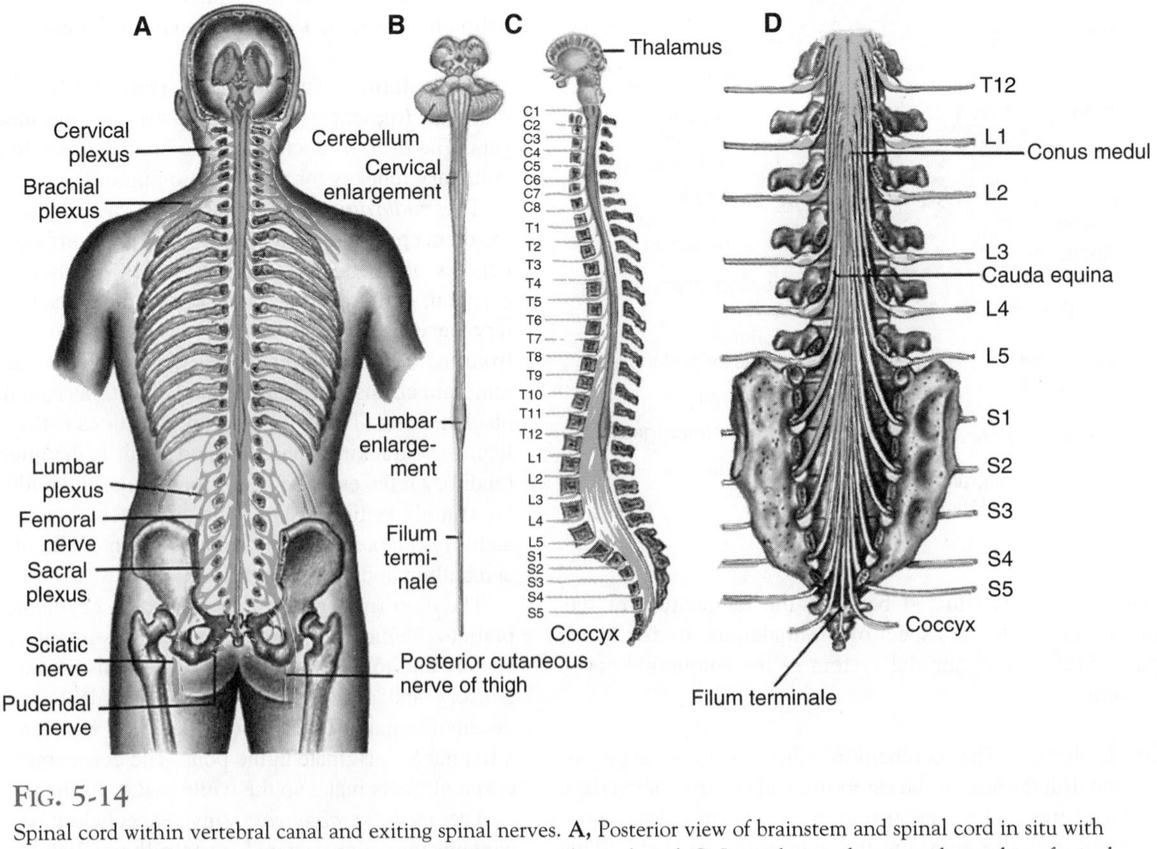

FIG. 5-14
Spinal cord within vertebral canal and exiting spinal nerves. **A,** Posterior view of brainstem and spinal cord in situ with spinal nerves and plexuses. **B,** Anterior view of brainstem and spinal cord. **C,** Lateral view showing relationship of spinal cord to vertebrae. **D,** Enlargement of caudal area showing termination of spinal cord (conus medullaris) and group of nerve fibers constituting the cauda equina. (From Rudy.[11])

shaped structure called the conus medullaris. Extending inferiorly from the *conus medullaris* is a thin prolongation, the *filum terminale,* that anchors the spinal cord to the coccyx. The spinal cord consists of 31 segments, each giving rise to a pair of spinal nerves.

Microscopically, the spinal cord consists of gray (unmyelinated) and white (myelinated) matter. The *gray matter* integrates the cord reflexes and is concentrated into an internal core. When this internal core is viewed in cross section, it resembles a butterfly (FIG. 5-15). The paired gray matter projections forming the front "wings" of the butterfly are the anterior, or ventral, horns. The pair of projections forming the back "wings" is called the posterior, or dorsal horns. The ventral horn consists of multipolar neuron structures (e.g., cell bodies, dendrites) that together form the motor efferent neurons of the ventral roots and spinal nerves. The dorsal horn contains cell bodies and dendrites of sensory (afferent) neurons and sensory receptors from the periphery.

The gray matter also contains internuncial (association) neurons. The internuncial neurons transmit impulses from one lateral half of the cord to the other, from the dorsal portions to the ventral portions, and to other levels of the CNS.

Surrounding the gray matter of the spinal cord is the *white matter,* comprising long ascending and descending tracts that serve as pathways between the spinal cord and brain for afferent and efferent impulses. The white matter is grouped into anatomic and functional bundles called fasciculi.

The spinal cord is divided into lateral halves by the *anterior fissure* and the *posterior sulcus.* Each lateral half is connected to the other half by commissures of gray and white matter. Each lateral half of the spinal cord is divided into three sections that run the length of the spinal cord: dorsal, lateral, and ventral. Within each of these divisions are distinct fiber tracts: ascending fibers, which bring sensory information to the CNS; descending fibers, which carry impulses from the brain to motor neurons of the brainstem and the spinal cord; and internuncial (association) neurons, which form short ascending and descending tracts that travel between spinal segments. These short tracts are called intersegmental tracts or pathways.

The neurons in the *ascending* pathways transmit sensory information from peripheral receptors to the spinal cord and brain. The sensory chain consists of a three-neuron pathway. The first-order neuron's cell body originates in the dorsal root ganglion and conducts impulses from peripheral receptors to the spinal cord. The second-order neuron's cell body is found at various levels of the gray matter of the spinal cord and brainstem. These neurons conduct impulses, in the white matter, to the thalamus. The third-order neuron's cell body lies in the thalamus and conducts impulses from the thalamus to the cerebral cortex. Ascending pathways include the lateral spinothalamic, ventral spinothalamic, and fasciculi gracilis and cuneatus.

The pathways are organized according to body surface areas and cross in the brain so that sensory information enters the cerebral cortex from the opposite side of the body. This crossing over is usually done by the second-order neuron.

The descending pathways are made of two principal types of neurons: the upper motor neurons and lower motor neurons. The upper motor neuron has its cell body in the cerebral motor areas or subcortical areas (i.e., brainstem) of the CNS. It transmits impulses from the brain to motor neurons in the anterior (ventral) horn of the spinal cord and to motor neurons in the cranial nerves. The lower motor neuron begins in the CNS and terminates in the peripheral nervous system. The lower motor neurons consist of motor nuclei of the cranial nerves and the motor cells in the anterior horn of the spinal cord. The two major subdivisions of the descending pathways originate from the cerebral cortex and are called the pyramidal and extrapyramidal tracts.

The *pyramidal tracts* (corticospinal tracts) originate from the large pyramid-shaped motor neurons in the cerebral cortex of the parietal lobe. They descend through the diencephalon, midbrain, pons, medulla, and white matter of the spinal cord to the motor cells in the anterior horns of the gray matter. In the medulla the pyramidal tracts form the medullary pyramids

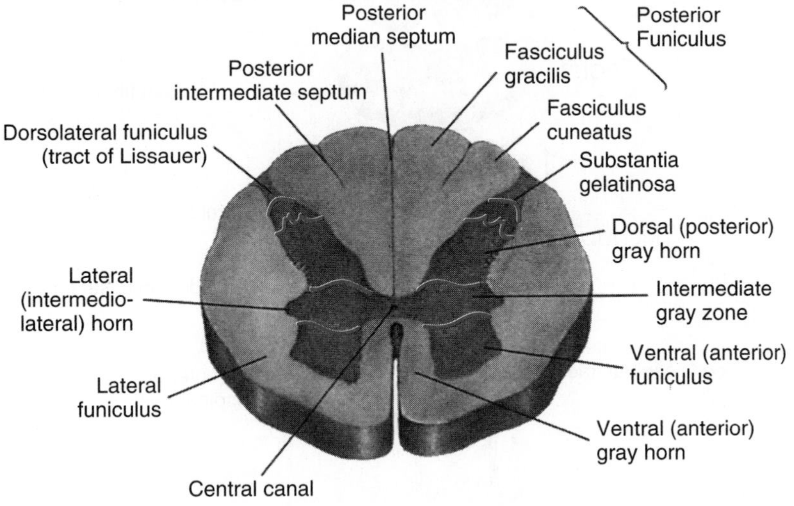

FIG. 5-15
Cross section of spinal cord illustrating subdivisions of white and gray matter. (From Rudy.[11])

where the majority of fibers decussate (cross over) to the other side and form the larger of the two corticospinal tracts, the *lateral corticospinal tract.* Fibers that do not decussate at the medulla form the *ventral corticospinal* tract, which descends (on the same side of origin) in the spinal cord in the anterior white matter to the cervical and upper thoracic regions. Many fibers of the ventral corticospinal tract decussate at respective levels of the anterior white commissure before synapsing with the lower motor neurons. The pyramidal tracts conduct voluntary impulses and reflex muscle contractions (FIG. 5-16).

The *extrapyramidal tracts* (FIG. 5-17) originate in the brainstem, basal ganglia, and cerebellum. These pathways are motor systems that coordinate muscular activity. The medial reticulospinal tract originates in the reticular formation of the brainstem and descends uncrossed. It stimulates flexor responses and inhibits extensor responses. The lateral reticulospinal tract also originates from the brainstem and is primarily uncrossed. The lateral tract stimulates extensor responses and inhibits flexor responses to maintain posture. Table 5-1 summarizes the principal ascending and descending tracts of the spinal cord and their respective functions.

The extrapyramidal system is a functional unit, not an anatomic one, and depends on an intact pyramidal system. This system consists of extrapyramidal areas of the cerebral cortex, the corpus striatum, thalamic nuclei connected to the corpus striatum, the subthalamus, and the rubral and reticular systems. The extrapyramidal system coordinates associated movements and changes in posture and integrates functions of the autonomic nervous system. The system has fibers that originate from the cerebral cortex and project to the basal ganglia. The basal ganglia of the extrapyramidal system act to coordinate movement.

Reflexes

The reflex arc (FIG. 5-18, p. 230) is the basic functional unit that maintains body integrity by automatically conducting impulses from sensory receptors (afferent) to efferent neurons. In the reflex arc or loop a sensory nerve ending is stimulated and then conveys the impulse via sensory (afferent) neurons to gray matter nuclei in the spinal cord. In the gray matter the afferent neuron may synapse directly with lower motor neurons, or it may synapse with one or more internuncial (association) neurons, which transfer the impulse to the lower motor neuron. The lower motor neurons (efferent) carry the impulse via the ventral roots of the spinal cord to the neuroeffector junction. The effector organ then responds to stimulation (e.g., by muscle contraction or glandular secretion). An example of a simple reflex involving only two neurons and one synapse is the knee-jerk (patellar) reflex. When the knee is tapped, afferent receptors are stimulated and send the impulse to the spinal

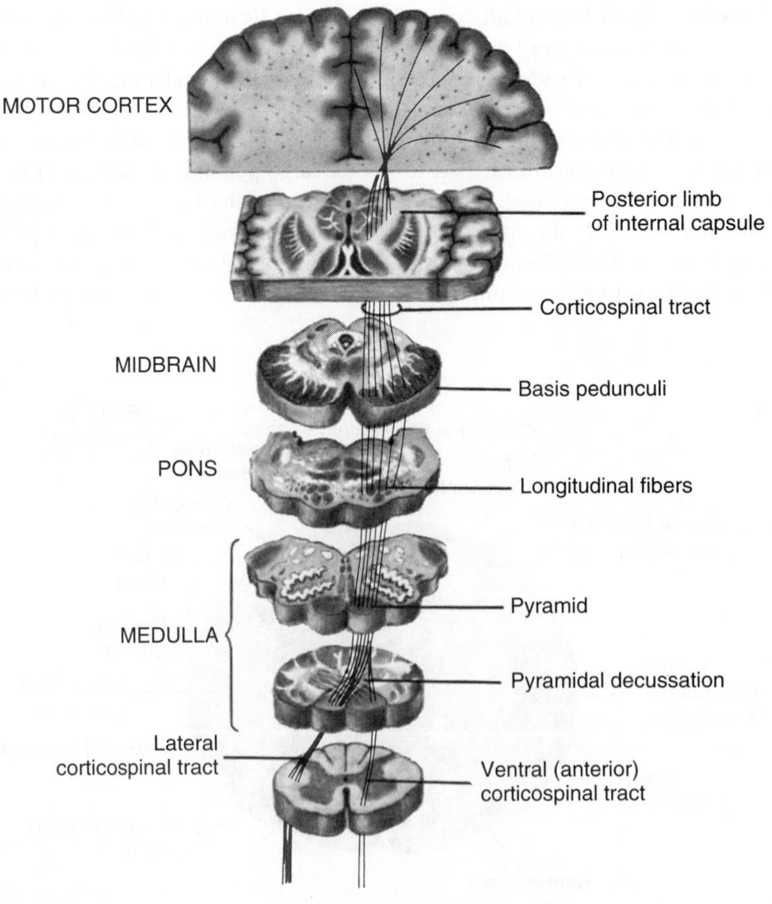

FIG. 5-16

Schematic drawing to show decussation of pyramids at level of medulla. (From Rudy.[11])

cord. In the spinal cord the impulse is directly relayed to the lower motor neuron. As a result, the quadriceps muscles contract and jerk the leg.

Unlike the knee-jerk reflex, which is the only monosynaptic reflex in the body, most reflex pathways involve numerous synaptic connections (polysynaptic). Reflex response time increases proportionately with the number of synapses. Some reflexes involve only one half of the body (e.g., flexor reflex) and are called ipsilateral reflexes. Other reflexes cross over, eliciting responses on the opposite side of the body (e.g., crossed extensor reflex). These are called contralateral reflexes. For example, when someone steps on a tack, there is a reflex flexion in one leg to move away from the tack, while in the opposite leg there is extension to maintain body balance.

Finally, both the brain and the spinal cord contain reflex centers that provide important data about level of functioning. Pupillary response, cardioregulatory mechanisms, and the medullary vasomotor mechanisms are all brain reflexes. Reflexes controlled predominantly by the spinal cord include emptying of the bowel and bladder, withdrawal from painful stimuli (known as a nociceptive reflex), increased blood flow to the skin, and stretch reflexes that maintain normal posture and position. Specific reflexes and responses elicited are discussed in the section on normal findings of the neurologic system.

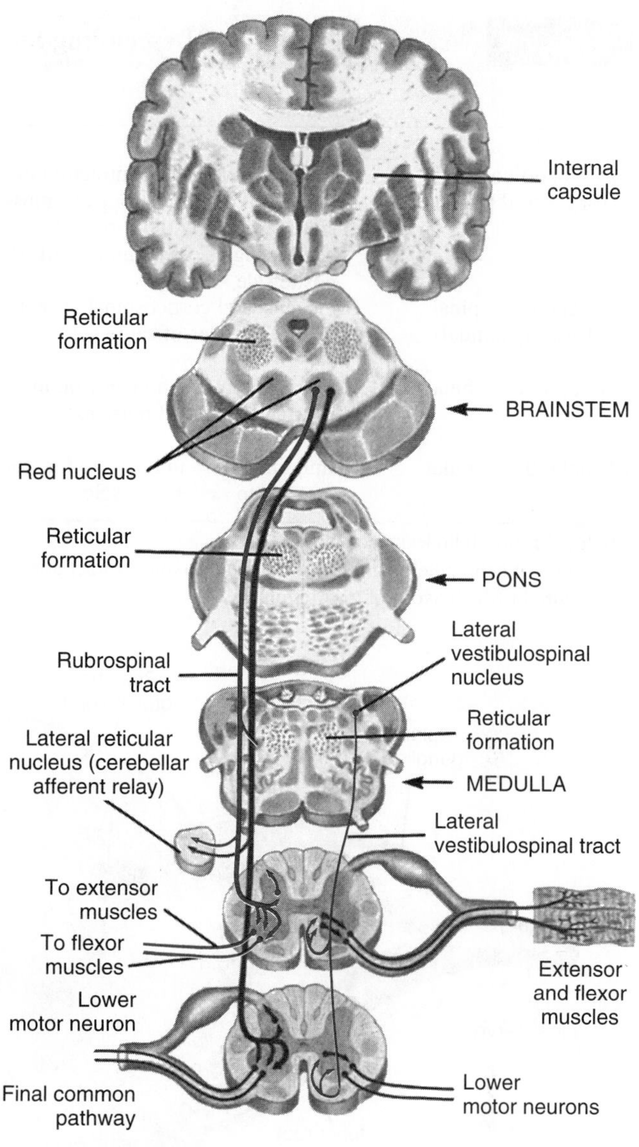

FIG. 5-17
Extrapyramidal descending tracts. Upper motor neurons originate below level of cortex and converge on lower motor neurons (final common pathway) along with upper motor neurons of pyramidal tracts. Rubrospinal tract originates in red area.

Table 5-1 Major Ascending and Descending Spinal Cord Tracts

Name	Function	Location	Origin*	Termination†
ASCENDING				
Lateral spinothalamic	Pain, temperature, and crude touch opposite side	Lateral white columns	Posterior gray column opposite side	Thalamus
Ventral spinothalamic	Crude touch, pain, and temperature	Anterior white columns	Posterior gray column opposite side	Thalamus
Fasciculi gracilis and cuneatus	Discriminating touch and pressure sensations, including vibration, stereognosis, and two-point discrimination; also conscious kinesthesia	Posterior white columns	Spinal ganglia same side	Medulla
Spinocerebellar	Unconscious kinesthesia	Lateral white columns	Posterior gray column	Cerebellum

Modified from Thibodeau and Patton.[15]
*Location of cell bodies of neurons from which axons of tract arise.
†Structure in which axons of tract terminate.

Continued

Table 5-1 Major Ascending and Descending Spinal Cord Tracts—cont'd

Name	Function	Location	Origin*	Termination†
DESCENDING				
Lateral corticospinal (or crossed pyramidal)	Voluntary movement, contraction of individual or small groups of muscles, particularly those moving hands, fingers, feet, and toes of opposite side	Lateral white columns	Motor areas of cerebral cortex (mainly areas 4 and 6) opposite side from tract location in cord	Intermediate or anterior gray columns
Ventral corticospinal (direct pyramidal)	Same as lateral corticospinal except mainly muscles of same side	Lateral white columns	Motor cortex but on same side as tract location in cord	Intermediate or anterior gray columns
Lateral reticulospinal	Mainly facilitatory influence on motor neurons to skeletal muscles	Lateral white columns	Reticular formation, midbrain, pons, and medulla	Intermediate or anterior gray columns
Medial reticulospinal	Mainly inhibitory influence on motor neurons to skeletal muscles	Anterior white columns	Reticular formation, medulla mainly	Intermediate or anterior gray columns

Modified from Thibodeau and Patton.[15]
*Location of cell bodies of neurons from which axons of tract arise.
†Structure in which axons of tract terminate.

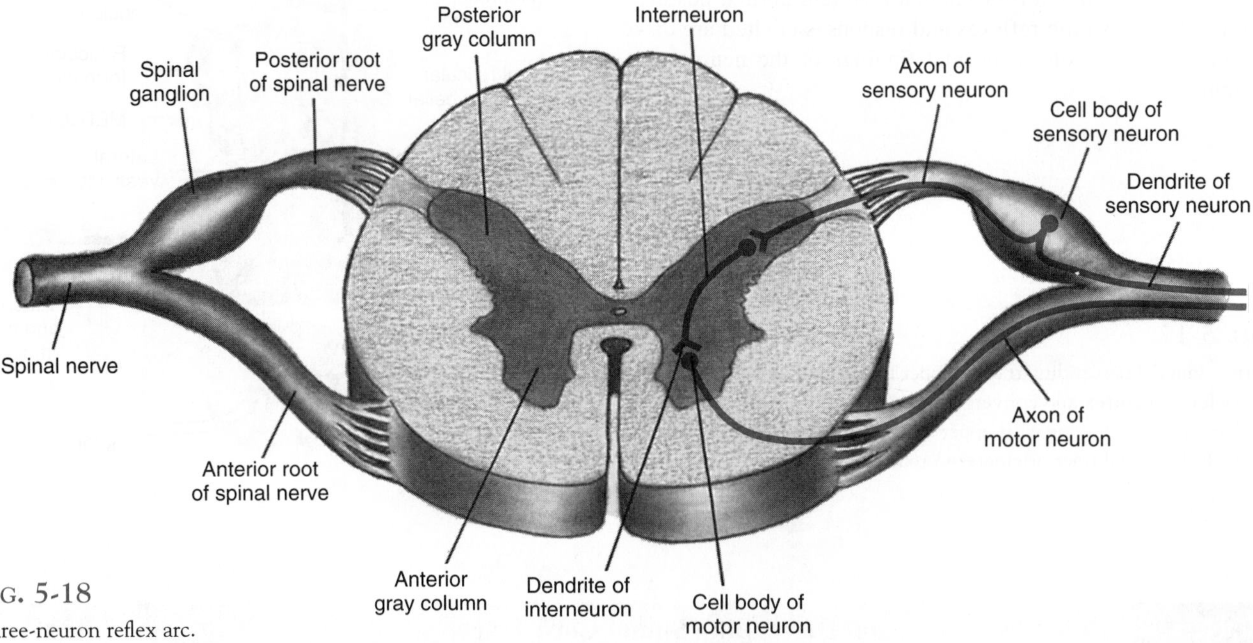

FIG. 5-18
Three-neuron reflex arc.

Peripheral Nervous System

Cranial Nerves.

The 12 pairs of cranial nerves form the peripheral nerves of the brain. Some have only motor fibers (five pairs), some have only sensory fibers (three pairs), and the rest (four pairs) have both sensory and motor fibers. The cranial nerves correspond to the spinal nerves serving common sensation, voluntary control of muscles, and autonomic functions in the head; in addition, they include the mechanism for the special senses of vision, hearing, smell, and taste.

Table 5-2 summarizes origin, functional class, and primary functions of the cranial nerves. Assessment of their functions is in the section on neurologic assessment.

Spinal Nerves.

The 31 pairs of spinal nerves arise from different segments of the spinal cord. Each pair of spinal nerves is formed by the union of anterior and posterior roots attached to the spinal cord. Each pair of spinal nerves and its corresponding part of the spinal cord constitute a spinal segment. Individual spinal segments in turn innervate specific body segments.

Some spinal nerves join at the anterior rami to form a complex network of nerve fibers called a *plexus.* The *cervical* and *brachial plexuses* provide peripheral nerves for innervation to the upper extremities. The lower extremities are innervated by peripheral nerves from the *lumbar* and *sacral plexuses.* Unlike the cervical and thoracic spinal nerves, the lumbar and sacral nerves do not exit from the intervertebral foramen at right angles. Instead, these nerves extend obliquely and inferiorly and form a large bundle of nerve fibers called the *cauda equina.*

Table 5-3, p. 233 summarizes the spinal nerves, corresponding plexuses, and peripheral innervation (see also Table 5-4, p. 234).

Table 5-2 Cranial Nerves

		Sensory Fibers†		Motor Fibers†		
Nerve*	Receptors	Cell Bodies	Termination	Cell Bodies	Termination	Functions‡
I Olfactory	*Nasal mucosa*	*Nasal mucosa*	Olfactory bulbs (new relay of neurons of olfactory cortex)			*Sense of smell*
II Optic	*Retina*	*Retina*	*Nucleus in thalamus (lateral geniculate body): Some fibers terminate in superior colliculus of midbrain*			*Vision*
III Oculomotor	*External eye muscles except superior oblique and lateral rectus*			**Midbrain (oculomotor nucleus and Edinger-Westphal nucleus)**	**External eye muscles except superior oblique and lateral rectus; fibers from Edinger-Westphal nucleus terminate in ciliary ganglion and then to ciliary and iris muscles**	**Eye movements, regulation of size of pupil, accommodation,** *proprioception (muscle sense)*
IV Trochlear	*Superior oblique*			**Midbrain**	**Superior oblique muscle of eye**	**Eye movements,** *proprioception*
V Trigeminal	*Skin and mucosa of head, teeth*	*Gasserian ganglion*	*Pons (sensory nucleus)*	**Pons (motor nucleus)**	**Muscles of mastication**	*Sensations of head and face,* **chewing movements,** *muscle sense*
VI Abducens	*Lateral rectus*					**Abduction of eye,** *proprioception*
VII Facial	*Taste buds of anterior two thirds of tongue*	*Geniculate ganglion*	*Medulla (nucleus solitarius)*	**Pons**	**Lateral rectus muscle of eye Superficial muscles of face and scalp**	**Facial expressions, secretion of saliva,** *taste*

From Thibodeau and Patton.[15]

*The first letters of the words in the following sentence are the first letters of the names of the cranial nerves. Many generations of anatomy students have used this sentence as an aid to memorizing these names. It is "On Old Olympus' Tiny Tops, A Finn and German Viewed Some Hops." (There are several slightly differing versions of this mnemonic.)

†Italics indicate sensory fibers and functions. Boldface type indicates motor fibers and functions.

‡An aid for remembering the general function of each cranial nerve is the following 12-word saying: "Some say marry money but my brothers say bad business marry money." Words beginning with "S" indicate sensory function. Words beginning with "M" indicate motor function. Words beginning with "B" indicate both sensory and motor functions. For example, the first, second, and eighth words in the saying start with "S," which indicates that the first, second, and eighth cranial nerves perform sensory functions.

Continued

Table 5-2 Cranial Nerves—cont'd

Nerve*	Receptors	Sensory Fibers† Cell Bodies	Sensory Fibers† Termination	Motor Fibers† Cell Bodies	Motor Fibers† Termination	Functions‡
VIII Acoustic						
1 Vestibular branch	*Semicircular canals and vestibule (utricle and saccule)*	*Vestibular ganglion*	*Pons and medulla (vestibular nuclei)*			*Balance or equilibrium sense*
2 Cochlear or auditory branch	*Organ of Corti in cochlear duct*	*Spiral ganglion*	*Pons and medulla (cochlear nuclei)*			*Hearing*
IX Glossopharyngeal	*Pharynx; taste buds and other receptors of posterior one third of tongue*	*Jugular and petrous ganglia*	*Medulla (nucleus solitarius)*	**Medulla (nucleus ambiguus)**	**Muscles of pharynx**	*Taste and other sensations of tongue,* **swallowing movements, secretion of saliva,** *aids in reflex control of blood pressure and respiration*
	Carotid sinus and carotid body	*Jugular and petrous ganglia*	*Medulla (respiratory and vasomotor centers)*	**Medulla at junction of pons (nucleus salivatorius)**	**Otic ganglion and then to parotid gland**	
X Vagus	*Pharynx, larynx, carotid body, and thoracic and abdominal viscera*	*Jugular and nodose ganglia*	*Medulla (nucleus solitarius), pons (nucleus of fifth cranial nerve)*	**Medulla (dorsal motor nucleus)**	**Ganglia of vagal plexus and then to muscles of pharynx, larynx, and thoracic and abdominal viscera**	*Sensations and* **movements** *of organs supplied; for example,* **slows heart, increases peristalsis, and contracts muscles for voice production**
XI Spinal accessory				**Medulla (dorsal motor nucleus of vagus and nucleus ambiguus)**	**Muscles of thoracic and abdominal viscera and pharynx and larynx**	**Shoulder movements, turning movements of head, movements of viscera, voice productions,** *proprioception?*
				Anterior gray column of first five or six cervical segments of spinal cord	**Trapezius and sternocleidomastoid muscle**	
XII Hypoglossal				**Medulla (hypoglossal nucleus)**	**Muscles of tongue**	**Tongue movements,** *proprioception?*

From Thibodeau and Patton.[15]

*The first letters of the words in the following sentence are the first letters of the names of the cranial nerves. Many generations of anatomy students have used this sentence as an aid to memorizing these names. It is "On Old Olympus' Tiny Tops, A Finn and German Viewed Some Hops." (There are several slightly differing versions of this mnemonic.)

†Italics indicate sensory fibers and functions. Boldface type indicates motor fibers and functions.

‡An aid for remembering the general function of each cranial nerve is the following 12-word saying: "Some say marry money but my brothers say bad business marry money." Words beginning with "S" indicate sensory function. Words beginning with "M" indicate motor function. Words beginning with "B" indicate both sensory and motor functions. For example, the first, second, and eighth words in the saying start with "S," which indicates that the first, second, and eighth cranial nerves perform sensory functions

Table 5-3 Spinal Nerves and Peripheral Branches

Spinal Nerves	Plexuses Formed From Anterior Rami	Spinal Nerve Branches From Plexuses	Parts Supplied
Cervical		Lesser occipital	Sensory to back of head, front of neck, and upper part of shoulder, motor to numerous neck muscles
1		Great auricular	
2	Cervical Plexus	Cutaneous nerve of neck	
3		Anterior supraclavicular	
4		Middle supraclavicular	
		Posterior supraclavicular	
		Branches to numerous neck muscles	
		Phrenic (branches from cervical nerves before formation of plexus; most of its fibers from fourth cervical nerve)	Diaphragm
		Suprascapular and dorsoscapular	Superficial muscles* of scapula
		Thoracic nerves, medial and lateral branches	Pectoralis major and minor
		Long thoracic nerve	Serratus anterior
Cervical		Thoracodorsal	Latissimus dorsi
5		Subscapular	Subscapular and teres major muscles
6	Brachial plexus	Axillary (circumflex)	Deltoid and teres minor muscles and skin over deltoid
7		Musculocutaneous	Muscles of front of arm (biceps brachii, coracobrachialis, and brachialis) and skin on outer side of forearm
8			
Thoracic (or dorsal)		Ulnar	Flexor carpi ulnaris and part of flexor digitorum profundus; some of muscles of hand; sensory to medial side of hand, little finger, and medial half of fourth finger
1			
2			
3		Median	Rest of muscles of front of forearm and hand; sensory to skin of palmar surface of thumb, index, and middle fingers
4			
5			
6		Radial	Triceps muscle and muscles of back of forearm; sensory to skin of back of forearm and hand
7	No plexus formed; branches run directly to intercostal muscles and skin of thorax		
8		Medial cutaneous	Sensory to inner surface of arm and forearm
9		Iliohypogastric (Sometimes fused)	Sensory to anterior abdominal wall
10		Ilioinguinal (Sometimes fused)	Sensory to anterior abdominal wall and external genitalia; motor to muscles of abdominal wall
11			
12		Genitofemoral	Sensory to skin of external genitalia and inguinal region
		Lateral cutaneous of thigh	Sensory to outer side of thigh
Lumbar		Femoral	Motor to quadriceps, sartorius, and iliacus muscles; sensory to front of thigh and medial side of lower leg (saphenous nerve)
1			
2			
3			
4		Obturator	Motor to adductor muscles of thigh
5			
Sacral	Lumbosacral plexus	Tibial† (medial popliteal)	Motor to muscles of calf of leg; sensory to skin of calf of leg and sole of foot
1			
2		Common peroneal (lateral popliteal)	Motor to evertors and dorsiflexors of foot; sensory to lateral surface of leg and dorsal surface of foot
3			
4		Nerves to hamstring muscles	Motor to muscles of back of thigh
5		Gluteal nerves, superior and inferior	Motor to buttock muscles and tensor fasciae latae
Coccygeal		Posterior cutaneous nerve	Sensory to skin of buttocks, posterior surface of thigh, and leg
1			
		Pudendal nerve	Motor to perineal muscles; sensory to skin of perineum

From Thibodeau and Patton.[15]

*Although nerves to muscles are considered motor, they do contain some sensory fibers that transmit proprioceptive impulses.

†Sensory fibers from the tibial and peroneal nerves unite to form the *medial cutaneous* (or sural) *nerve* that supplies the calf of the leg and the lateral surface of the foot. In the thigh the tibial and common peroneal nerves are usually enclosed in a single sheath to form the *sciatic nerve,* the largest nerve in the body with its width of approximately ¾ inch. About two thirds of the way down the posterior part of the thigh, it divides into its component parts. Branches of the sciatic nerve extend into the hamstring muscles.

Autonomic Nervous System

The autonomic nervous system is considered part of the peripheral nervous system. It regulates the body's internal environment in close conjunction with the endocrine system. It is responsible for the unconscious moment-to-moment functioning of all internal systems, including visceral organs (e.g., digestive, urogenital), involuntary muscle fibers (e.g., smooth muscle), and glandular functions (e.g., adrenal medulla, islets of Langerhans in the pancreas). The autonomic nervous system is activated by centers in the hypothalamus, brainstem, and spinal cord. It is characterized by a two-neuron chain consisting of a preganglionic neuron and a postganglionic neuron.

Preganglionic neurons have cell bodies in the CNS and efferent fibers that terminate in the autonomic ganglia. *Postganglionic neurons* have cell bodies outside the CNS in the autonomic ganglia and innervate the target, or effector, organ (e.g., cardiac muscle). The purpose of the postganglionic neuron is to relay impulses beyond the ganglia.

The autonomic nervous system has two major subdivisions (*sympathetic* and *parasympathetic*), and both consist of autonomic ganglia and nerves. Generally, each effector organ has both sympathetic and parasympathetic innervation. The subdivisions differ in the type of neurotransmitters released, distribution of nerve fibers, and effects on organs innervated, in that the subdivisions produce antagonistic physiologic responses.

The *sympathetic* (thoracolumbar) subdivision is activated during internal and external stress situations (the flight-or-fight phenomenon). During those stressful situations, sympathetic responses include increases in blood pressure and heart rate and vasoconstriction of peripheral blood vessels. The sympathetic division is also called adrenergic because the transmitter substance norepinephrine (noradrenalin) is secreted by its postganglionic nerve terminals.

The *preganglionic* fibers of the sympathetic system are located in the intermediolateral columns of the thoracic and first two lumbar segments in the spinal cord (i.e., T1 to T2); thus this system is sometimes called the thoracolumbar system. After leaving the spinal nerves, the small, myelinated, preganglionic, sympathetic fibers enter the sympathetic trunk via the white ramus. The sympathetic trunk is a chain of ganglions extending from the base of the skull to the coccyx on either side of the spinal cord.

Most axons of sympathetic neurons synapse in the sympathetic trunk or travel up and down the trunk before synapsing. Some axons do not synapse within the sympathetic trunk; instead they exit to synapse in collateral ganglia nearer to the organ of innervation. Acetylcholine is the neurotransmitter at all preganglionic nerve terminals of the sympathetic division. Norepinephrine is the neurotransmitter at all postganglionic nerve terminals of the sympathetic system. Because of the sympathetic chain ganglia, the nerve fibers of the sympathetic system generally have short and long postganglionic fibers. Fibers terminate on two receptor sites (α or β), which determine the effects of the neurotransmitters. β receptors are divided into β_1 and β_2 receptors because some drugs affects some, but not all, β receptors.

The *adrenal medulla* is a functional extension of the sympathetic nervous system. Its postganglionic neurons are specialized secretory cells. Epinephrine and norepinephrine are secreted by the adrenal medulla at the same time the sympathetic nerves are stimulating afferent organs and have almost the same effect as direct sympathetic stimulation. As a result, body tissues are stimulated simultaneously, directly by the sympathetic nerves and indirectly by the hormones of the adrenal medulla. After their release the hormones are rapidly metabolized, primarily by the liver. Approximately one half of the catecholamines are excreted in the urine as free or conjugated normetanephrine and metanephrine. Daily normal urinary output of the catecholamines equals approximately 6 mg of epinephrine and 30 mg of norepinephrine. Chapter 11 gives further detail on the adrenal medulla and the catecholamines.

The *parasympathetic* (craniosacral) subdivision of the autonomic nervous system consists of preganglionic fibers arising from cell bodies in cranial nerves III, VII, IX, and X, as well as sacral spinal nerves II through VII. This division is activated when an individual is at rest or relaxed, protecting and restoring the body's resources. It works slower than the sympathetic division, has a more discrete effect, and dominates control over the sympathetic subdivision during nonstressful conditions. Parasympathetic fibers in the cranial and sacral nerves form synaptic connections only with terminal ganglia located near the organs innervated. Therefore in the parasympathetic division, preganglionic fibers are long and postganglionic fibers are short. Both preganglionic and postganglionic fibers secrete the neurotransmitter acetylcholine; therefore the parasympathetic subdivision is called cholinergic.

The organs innervated and effects of stimulation by sympathetic and parasympathetic subdivisions are summarized in Tables 5-3 and 5-4.

Table 5-4 Cranial Nerves Contrasted With Spinal Nerves

	Cranial Nerves	Spinal Nerves
Origin	Base of brain	Spinal cord
Distribution	Mainly to head and neck	Skin, skeletal muscles, joints, blood vessels, sweat glands, and mucosa except of head and neck
Structure	Some composed of sensory fibers only; some of both motor axons and sensory dendrites; some motor fibers belong to somatic nervous system, some to autonomic	All of them composed of both sensory dendrites and motor axons; some of latter somatic, some autonomic
Function	Vision, hearing, sense of smell, sense of taste, eye movements	Sensations, movements, and sweat secretion

From Thibodeau and Patton.[15]

Vascular Supply to Brain and Spinal Cord

Maintaining adequate blood supply to the brain and spinal cord is vital for proper functioning of the nervous system. The blood removes metabolic waste products and supplies the cells with nutrients.

Brain. The blood supply to the brain comes principally from two pairs of arteries: the *internal carotid* and the vertebral arteries. The internal carotid arteries arise from the common carotid artery at the level of the thyroid cartilage. They supply approximately 80% of the blood to the brain. The internal carotid arteries then give rise to the anterior and middle cerebral arteries at about the level of the optic chiasm. The *anterior cerebral artery* supplies portions of the medial surfaces of the frontal and parietal lobes, nuclei of the basal ganglia, caudate putamen, and portions of the internal capsule and corpus callosum. The *middle cerebral artery* supplies lateral surfaces of the parietal, frontal, and temporal lobes. It is the major source of blood supply to the precentral (motor) and postcentral (sensory) gyri. The vertebral arteries arise from the right and left *subclavian arteries* and provide the remaining 20% of cerebral blood supply. The vertebral arteries join at the base of the brain and form the basilar artery. The *basilar artery* enters the skull at the foramen magnum and ascends to the midbrain. Branches of the vertebral and basilar arteries supply the brainstem and cerebellum. In the midbrain the basilar artery splits into the paired *posterior cerebral arteries,* which supply portions of the temporal and occipital lobes of each hemisphere, the vestibular organs, and the cochlear apparatus. FIG. 5-19 illustrates the vessels supplying the brain tissue.

At the base of the brain the cerebral arteries are connected, by their communicating branches, into an arterial circle called the *circle of Willis* (FIG. 5-20). More specifically, the posterior cerebral artery is connected to the middle cerebral artery by the

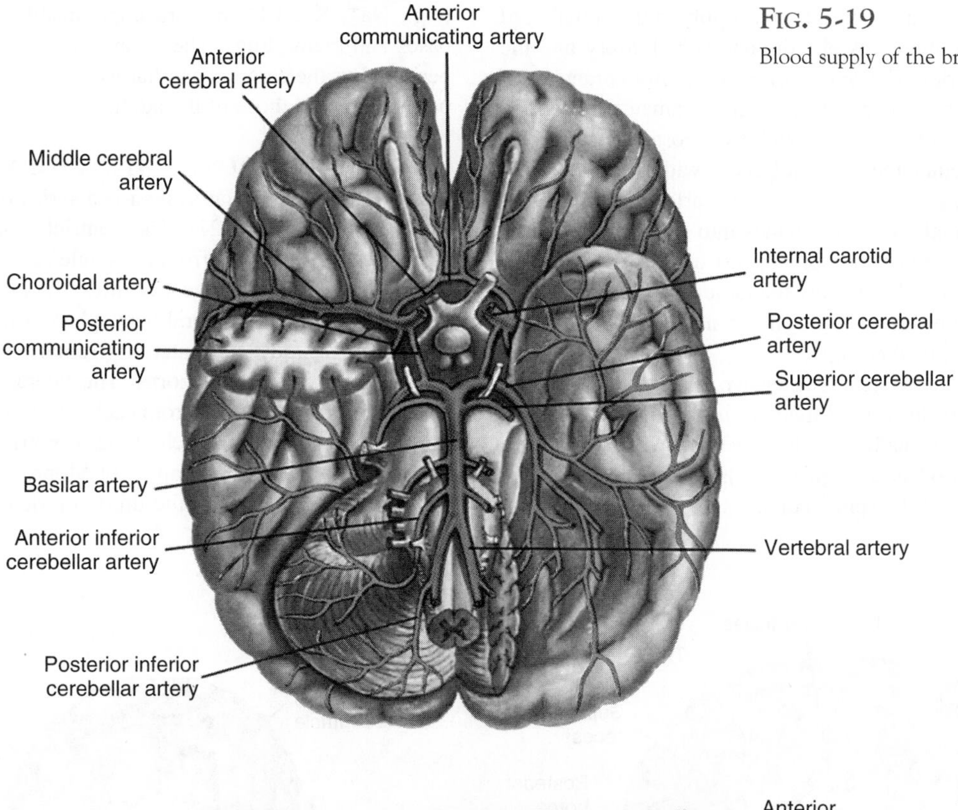

FIG. 5-19
Blood supply of the brain. (From Rudy.[11])

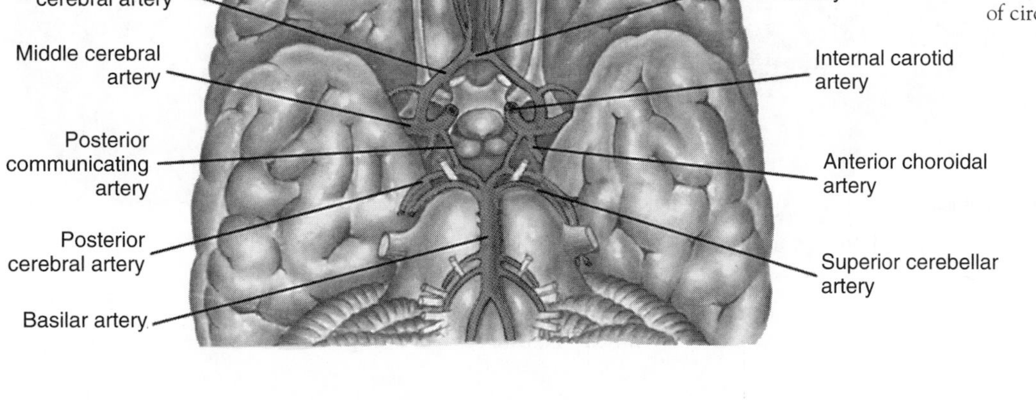

FIG. 5-20
Anatomic diagram of circle of Willis.

posterior communicating branches. The anterior cerebral arteries are connected by the anterior communicating branches. The purpose of the circle of Willis is to ensure circulation if one of the four main blood vessels is interrupted.

Branches of cerebral arteries extend throughout the brain. These branches are called end arteries because they have few branching connections. This lack of branching results in decreased potential for collateral circulation.

Dense networks of capillaries are found in the gray matter of the brain. These capillaries are surrounded by a protective membrane formed by the end-feet of *astrocyte cells.* The capillary blood enters the deep veins, which then empty into the superficial venous plexuses and dural sinuses (principally the superior longitudinal sinus). The venous blood is drained from these sinuses by the internal jugular veins, which return the blood to the general circulation (a small volume of blood drains via the *pterygoid* and ophthalmic venous sinuses).

The anterior, middle, and posterior meningeal arteries provide an abundant blood supply to the cranial meninges.

Spinal Cord. The arterial blood supply to the spinal cord comes from three main vessels: the one spinal artery and the two radicular arteries. The *spinal artery* arises from branches of the vertebral arteries at the level of the foramen magnum. It then divides into one anterior and two posterior branches. These branches enter the vertebral canal with the dorsal and ventral nerve roots. The *radicular artery* arises from the thoracic and abdominal aorta and divides into anterior and posterior branches that enter the spinal cord at the intervertebral foramina. At the spinal segments the radicular arteries connect with the spinal arteries to form an extensive vascular plexus around the entire spinal cord.

The spinal venous system is extensive, with many intradural veins exiting from the ventral median fissure. In addition, numerous extradural veins form a dense venous plexus in the pia mater. Venous blood is drained from the plexus by veins accompanying roots of the spinal nerves.

Brain Barriers. The neuronal tissues of the brain are extremely sensitive to any changes in the ionic concentration of their environment. Therefore the composition of the brain's internal environment must be delicately balanced to ensure normal functioning. The *blood-brain barrier* is a physiologic mechanism that helps maintain and protect this homeostatic balance by way of selective capillary permeability. Since substances from the blood enter the brain either through capillaries into the cerebrospinal fluid or through capillaries into the extracellular fluid, there are actually two barrier mechanisms. The blood-brain and blood-cerebrospinal barriers function together to protect the neuronal brain tissue. The complex of intermembranes that form these barriers is found in most regions of brain parenchyma, the choroid plexus, and the vasculature of the brain. Unlike most capillaries in the body, these capillaries are surrounded by astrocyte end-feet that form tight junctions of the endothelial cells. It is thought the tight junctions and glial end-feet affect capillary permeability. Both the blood-brain and blood-cerebrospinal barriers are permeable to oxygen, carbon dioxide, and water. They are slightly permeable to electrolytes (e.g., Na^+, K^+, Cl^-) but are impermeable to fixed acids and bases and many drugs. These barriers develop in the postnatal period; thus the cerebral capillaries of the newborn are far more permeable than those of the adult.

Cerebral Ventricular System

The cerebral ventricular system is a series of four ependymal-lined cavities (FIG. 5-21). The ventricles are interconnecting structures that originate from the single cavity of the embryonic neural tube. The two largest cavities, the lateral ventricles, are located within each cerebral hemisphere. Each lateral ventricle consists of a body and anterior (frontal), inferior (temporal), and posterior (occipital) horns. The lateral ventricles in each hemisphere are separated from each other by a thin layer called the septum pellucidum. Each of these ventricles communicates, via the interventricular foramen of Monro, with a central cavity. This central cavity is the third ventricle, which is a small

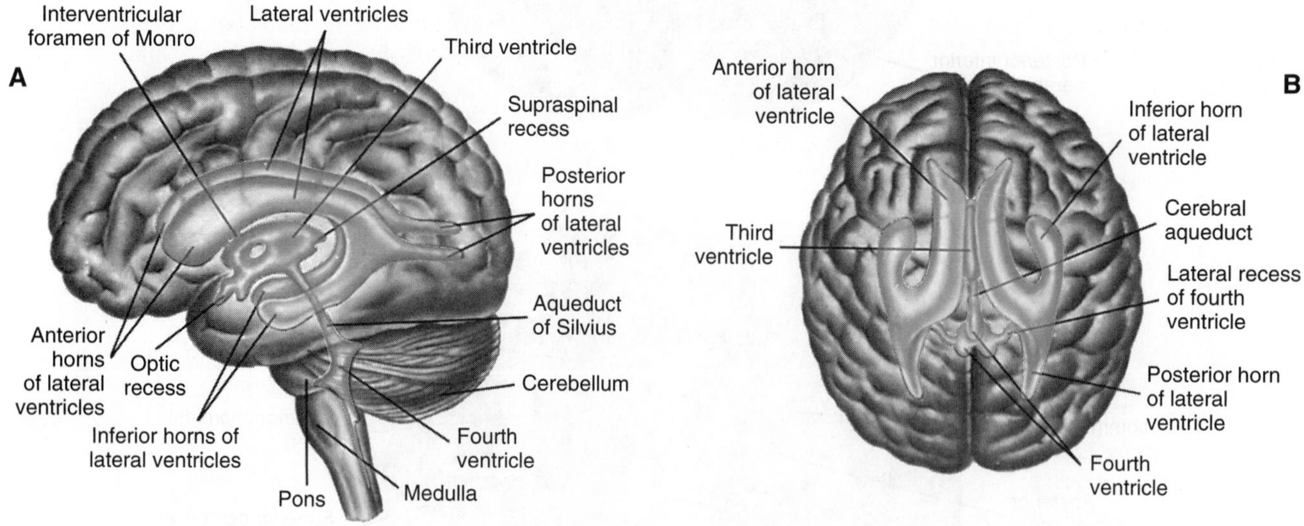

FIG. 5-21
Cerebral ventricles. **A,** Lateral view. **B,** Superior view.

cleft space between the thalamic structures of the diencephalon. In the midbrain the third ventricle communicates with the fourth ventricle via the aqueduct of Sylvius. The rhomboid fourth ventricle is located posterior to the pons and anterior to the cerebellum, extending down to the central canal of the upper cervical portion of the spinal cord. The fourth ventricle is connected by three foramina to the subarachnoid space.

Cerebrospinal Fluid

Parts of the lateral, third, and fourth ventricular structures are lined with dense networks of capillaries called the choroid plexus (tela choroidea). The choroid plexus secretes cerebrospinal fluid (CSF), which is a colorless, clear, and odorless fluid that contains glucose, electrolytes, oxygen, water, carbon dioxide, small amounts of protein, and a few leukocytes. The CSF removes metabolic wastes, provides nutrition, performs some mechanical function (i.e., shock absorber), and participates in maintaining normal intracranial pressure (ICP). In 24 hours the choroid plexuses secrete approximately 500 to 750 ml of CSF; however, only about 125 to 150 ml is present in the system at any one time.

From the choroid plexuses in the lateral ventricles, the CSF passes through the foramen of Monro to the third ventricle. From there, it slowly flows through the aqueduct of Sylvius to the fourth ventricle. The fluid then leaves the fourth ventricle through the single medial foramen of Magendie (located in the roof of the fourth ventricle) and the paired foramina of Luschka (located in the lateral portion of the fourth ventricle). After leaving the fourth ventricle the CSF enters the subarachnoid space, where it fills the spinal cisterns and slowly diffuses upward over the convexities of the brain. The fluid is slowly absorbed from the subarachnoid space by the arachnoid villi, which are clusterlike protrusions extending into the superior sagittal sinus. The CSF diffuses from the arachnoid villi into the intradural venous sinuses, where it is reabsorbed into the venous system.

Variations in Older Adults

Like other systems in the body, the neural structures undergo significant changes as a person ages. Understanding these anatomic and physiologic changes assists the practitioner to establish realistic normative behaviors for the elderly population.

Brain. The neuronal cells of the CNS (brain and spinal cord) of all adults are postmitotic and therefore do not regenerate once destroyed. Studies indicate that the aging process causes a loss of brain cells and that cells not destroyed may undergo significant structural changes. Brain cells decrease in number at a rate of about 1% a year after age 50 years. However, this rate of loss is not consistent throughout the brain, so that certain areas may lose cells at a faster (e.g., cortex) or slower (e.g., brainstem) rate than others. Other cells, such as the neurons of the prefrontal neocortex, undergo structural changes that result in a progressive decline in dendritic interconnections. In addition, neuronal cells of the elderly contain the age pigment *lipofuscin* in the storage granules, as well as senile plaques and neurofibrillary tangles.

Cerebral blood flow studies indicate there is a change with age in cerebral blood flow and oxygen utilization. Cerebral blood flow showed a decline from 79.3 ml/min/100 g of brain tissue at the mean age of 17 years to 46 ml/min/100 g at the mean age of 80 years, a net loss of 33.3 ml/min/100 g of brain. The rate of cerebral oxygen consumption declined from 3.6 ml/min/100 g of brain tissue at the mean age of 17 years to 2.7 ml/min/100 g at the mean age of 80 years.

Nerve conduction velocity of the individual over age 50 years also differs from that of younger adults. By age 80 to 90 years, conduction velocity equals abut 50 m/sec, whereas a young adult has a conduction velocity of approximately 60 m/sec. This loss of conduction velocity appears to be slightly greater in aging women. Nerve conduction velocity in the elderly is also affected by an increased synaptic delay and a change in neurotransmitters. Recent studies indicate that in the human brain, monoamine oxidase (MAO) and serotonin increase with age whereas norepinephrine decreases.

Vertebrae. The vertebral column may show advancing kyphosis in the thoracic region of the elderly patient. This degenerative change is the result of osteoporosis, vertebral collapse, or changes in vertebral cartilage. As the vertebral cartilage calcifies, there is decreased mobility of the vertebral column.

Spinal Cord. The basic reflex arc does not change with the aging process. The spinal cord may show changes in sensory conduction because of decreased vascularity of the white matter in the cord. Therefore diminished reflexes in the distal portion of the lower extremities (e.g., ankle) are not uncommon. Degenerative changes in the peripheral nerves are responsible for the loss of vibratory sense at the ankles. Reflexes of the upper extremities should be intact in the healthy elderly individual.

NORMAL FINDINGS*

"Normal" behaviors must be evaluated in terms of the patient's baseline pattern, as well as significant variables (e.g., anxiety) affecting the assessment process. One way to establish the patient's baseline is through a careful and thorough health history. Whenever the health history or the physical examination provides data indicating a deviation from normal, that symptom or complex of symptoms requires a comprehensive symptom analysis.

Normative behaviors of the geriatric patient may vary from source to source. Therefore it is recommended that the examiner cross-reference the assessment findings with the patient's previous patterns of behavior. The examiner also must carefully consider the effect on behavior of such variables as physical illness, displacement, examiner approach, change in self-image, and physiologic changes (i.e., diminished sense of hearing or vision).

General Cerebral Functions

Appearance and behavior: Age, height, weight; body proportionate in size in terms of body parts; clean; groomed; dressed appropriate to age, sex, peers, and background; ⭘ Length of trunk decreased in relation to extremities

Posture: Shoulders back and relaxed; arms rest at sides; feet rest on floor (if applicable); stands with narrow base;

*⭘ = Older adult.

○ may assume posture with slight semiflexion at principal joints; stands with narrow to medium base; may exhibit kyphosis in thoracic spine region with accompanying backward tilt of head

Gestures: Smooth; coordinated; deliberate

Movements: Coordinated; smooth; deliberate; able to change positions with smooth, even movements; ○ changes position with slow, even movements

Facial expression: Facial features symmetric; establishes eye contact; acknowledges examiner's presence; uses eye contact throughout interview

Attention: Able to complete thought processes (e.g., able to repeat series of numbers forward and backward); has continuity of ideas

Level of consciousness: Responds appropriately to visual, auditory, tactile, and painful stimuli; oriented to person, place, time; able to carry out simple and complex commands; opens eyes spontaneously; extraocular eye movement present; ○ may respond more slowly but still appropriately to visual, auditory stimuli; may demonstrate diminished response to tactile and painful stimuli; able to carry out simple and complex commands, with slower response time

A reliable guide to the quick determination of the level of neurologic status in an individual who may or may not be able to participate in more advanced testing is the Glasgow coma scale (GCS) (Table 5-5). This scale measures three faculties: Eye opening, best motor response, and best verbal response. Numbers are assigned to each of the responses in the three categories. The lowest possible score is 3; 15 is the highest. A GCS score of less than 7 indicates a coma state. Serial scores have value in trending patient status. To score, the patient's best response is elicited in each category and the points added.

Intellectual functions: Memory: immediate; able to repeat a series of numbers (e.g., 12, 9, 5, 1, 6); recent: able to repeat correct series of numbers after 5 minutes; remote: able to state correct birthplace; able to correctly state personal and vocational history; abstract reasoning: able to describe meaning of simple proverbs such as "A stitch in time saves nine," or "Rome wasn't built in a day"; insight: demonstrates consistent awareness of reality and perception of self; ○ may demonstrate increased resistance to "new" ideas

Specific Cerebral Functions

Sensory interpretation: Visual: recognizes objects; differentiates between size and shape; auditory: able to identify sound made by ringing bell; tactile: able to recognize familiar objects through use of touch (stereognosis); ○ longer response time

Cortical: Motor integration: able to carry out a skilled act such as protruding tongue, using a comb; comprehension: able to answer questions correctly throughout history, interview, and examination; judgment: able to discuss plans for future

Language and speech: Smooth, flowing; easily able to formulate words; varied inflections; pace, clarity, tone, volume, and vocabulary appropriate to age and educational level; demonstrates ability to read appropriate to educational level; able to write letters and numbers to dictation; ○ flow may be slightly decreased

Table 5-5 Glascow Coma Scale

Category	Response	Score (points)
Eye opening	Eyes open spontaneously	4
	Eyes open in response to voice	3
	Eyes open in response to pain	2
	No eye opening response	1
Best verbal	Oriented (e.g., to person, place, time)	5
	Confused, speaks but is disoriented	4
	Inappropriate, but comprehensible words	3
	Incomprehensible sounds but no words are spoken	2
	None	1
Best motor	Obeys command to move	6
	Localizes painful stimulus	5
	Withdraws from painful stimulus	4
	Flexion, abnormal decorticate posturing	3
	Extension, abnormal decerebrate posturing	2
	No movement or posturing	1
TOTAL POINTS POSSIBLE		**3-15**

! EMERGENCY ALERT

ALTERED LEVEL OF CONSCIOUSNESS

Changes in a person's level of consciousness (LOC) can be serious, must be assessed further, and are symptoms, not a diagnosis. LOC is an important vital sign because it reflects cerebral perfusion and function.

ASSESSMENT

- Determine patient's baseline status.
- Assess ability to verbalize.
- Assess ability to follow commands.
- Assess orientation to person, time, place, and situation.
- Assess response to pain, light pressure.
- Assess pupillary response.
- Use the Glasgow Coma Scale to score.

INTERVENTIONS

- Maintain airway, breathing, and circulation.
- Ensure patient safety.
- Interventions are directed as underlying cause is discovered.

Emotional status: Affect: appropriate to verbalization; body behaviors indicative of mild to moderate anxiety: mood: consistent with conversation; cooperates with examiner

Thought processes: Content: spontaneous, natural, logical, and free flowing; ○ thought patterns become more concrete; thought patterns increase in orderliness

Cranial Nerves

Olfactory (I): Able to identify aromatic, volatile, nonirritating substances (e.g., lemon, peppermint) with each nostril; ○ may demonstrate diminished sense of smell;

able to identify changes in aromatic substances with each nostril

Optic (II): See Chapter 8

Oculomotor, trochlear, abducens (III, IV, VI): Eyelids symmetric and not drooping; pupils equal in size, regular in outline, with prompt and equal reaction (direct and consensual) to light stimulus; conjugate gaze; smooth conjugate eye movements intact through six cardinal positions of gaze; prompt accommodation to distant and near objects; bilaterally, equal corneal light reflex; eyelids appear less elastic; eye movements intact with some limitation of upward gaze; eyes may be unable to converge

Trigeminal (VP): Sensory: bilateral blink when limbus of cornea touched with cotton wisp; symmetric tickling sensation when cotton wisp touched to anterior scalp, paranasal sinuses, and jaws; symmetric pressure and pain sensation when alternating blunt and sharp ends of a safety pin are touched to anterior scalp, paranasal sinuses, and jaws; symmetric warm and cold sensation felt when patient is tested for temperature over anterior scalp, paranasal sinuses, and jaws; motor: patient experiences bilaterally strong contractions of temporal and masseter muscles

Facial (VII): Sensory: able to correctly identify sweet, sour, salty, and bitter substances placed on anterior tongue; motor: symmetry of facial movements such as smiling, frowning, closing eyes, raising eyebrows, showing teeth, and puffing out cheeks

Acoustic (VIII)

Cochlear division: bilateral ability to hear whispered voice (from distance of 1 to 2 feet); able to hear watch ticking (from distance of 1 to 2 inches); Weber test: sound heard equally in both ears; Rinne test: sound heard twice as long by air conduction as by bone conduction

Vestibular division (tested only with history of vertigo): B-r-ny test: demonstrates a feeling of nausea, slow horizontal nystagmus toward side irrigated, with past pointing and falling; B-r-ny chair rotation: nystagmus, past pointing, and postural deviation in direction of chair movement; vertigo and sensation of continued movement in opposite direction of chair movement; electronystagmography: no displacement of corneal-retinal potential bilaterally

Glossopharyngeal and vagus (IX, X): Immediate contraction of pharyngeal muscles, with or without gagging, with lateral, upper, lower, and posterior stimulation; speech smooth, without hoarseness; able to identify tastes of sweet, salty, sour, and bitter on posterior third of tongue

Spinal accessory (XI): Able to turn head against resistance: sternocleidomastoid muscle bilaterally equal in strength and symmetry; able to shrug shoulders against resistance with bilaterally equal strength of upward movement

Hypoglossal (xii): Able to protrude tongue in midline; able to move tongue in and out of mouth rapidly; able to wiggle tongue from side to side (Table 5-6)

Proprioception; Cerebellar and Motor Function

Gait: Maintains upright posture of trunk; walks unaided with narrow base, weight shifts from one extremity to another, pelvis approximately at right angle to weight-bearing extremity; maintains balance; opposing arm swing; maintains upright posture of trunk (if no kyphosis); walks with narrow to medium base

Table 5-6 Mnemonic for Learning Cranial Nerves

#	Nerve	First Initial
I	Olfactory	On
II	Optic	Old
III	Oculomotor	Olympus'
IV	Trochlear	Towering
V	Trigeminal	Top
VI	Abducens	A
VII	Facial	Finn
VIII	Acoustic	And
IX	Glossopharyngeal	German
X	Vagus	Viewed
XI	Spinal Accessory	Some
XII	Hypoglossal	Hops

Romberg test: Slight swaying, but upright posture and narrow foot stance maintained

Tandem walk: Able to walk heel to toe in straight line

One-foot balance: Able to maintain position for at least 5 seconds; bilaterally equal response with eyes open and eyes closed

Hop in place: Able to maintain balance, hop on one foot, and stay in place: bilaterally equal response

Knee bends: Able to perform knee bends while maintaining balance

Upper extremity testing: Able to rapidly pronate and supinate hands with bilaterally equal timing, purposeful movement; able to touch nose repeatedly, alternating index fingers in rhythmic fashion (eyes open and eyes closed); able to rapidly and purposefully touch each finger to thumb; able to move index finger from nose to examiner's finger in coordinated fashion (each hand tested)

Lower extremity testing: Able to purposefully run heel down contralateral shin with bilaterally equal coordination

Muscle strength and tone: See Chapter 6

Sensory Functions

Primary: Light touch: able to perceive light or tickling sensation; able to identify location touched correctly; pain: able to perceive pain sensation as sharp or dull; able to identify area touched correctly; temperature: able to perceive sensation as hot or cold; vibration: able to perceive sensation of vibration

Discriminating sensation: Stereognosis: able to identify common object (e.g., key, pencil) by handling it; two-point discrimination: able to distinguish whether touched by one or two objects; palms, 8 to 12 mm; dorsum of hands, 20 to 30 mm; fingertips 2.8 to 5 mm; dorsa of fingers, 4 to 6 mm; chest and forearm, 40 mm; back, 40 to 70 mm; upper arms and thighs, 75 mm; shins, 30 to 40 mm; may evidence diminished values from normal adult findings; graphesthesia: can recognize traced letter or number on hand, back; double simultaneous sensation: able to distinguish if touched on one or two sides of body (at same level); may not be able to distinguish; kinesthetic: able to identify change in position of fingers as up or down

GRADING AND RECORDING OF DEEP TENDON REFLEXES

Deep tendon reflexes (DTRs) are graded according to the following scale:

0	Absent
1+	Present, but diminished
2+	Normal
3+	Increased, slightly hyperactive
4+	Brisk, hyperactice; clonus may also be present

Patient's reflex scores are recorded by entering the correct scores at the correct location on a stick figure.

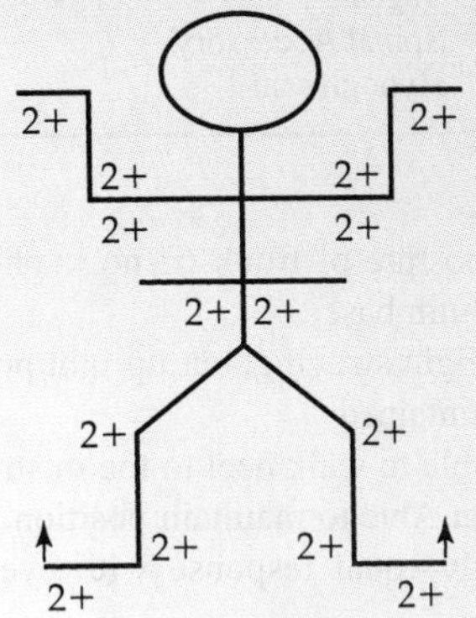

Reflexes

Superficial: Upper abdominal (T8, T9, T10): upward movement of umbilicus toward area of stimulus; older adult: may be diminished or absent; lower abdominal (T10, T11, T12): downward movement of umbilicus toward area of stimulation; ⭘ may be diminished or absent; cremasteric (T12, L1): elevation of ipsilateral testicle as cremaster muscle contracts (males only); gluteal (L4 to S3): contraction of anal sphincter

Deep tendon: Biceps (C5, C6): flexion of arm at elbow; triceps (C6, C7, C8): extension of arm at elbow and contraction of triceps muscles; finger flexion (C7 to T1): fingers flexed; brachioradialis (C5, C6): flexion at elbow and pronation of forearm; patellar (L2 to L4): extension of leg at knee and contraction of quadriceps; older adult: may be diminished; Achilles (1, S2): plantar flexion of foot at ankle; ⭘ may be absent; see box for grading and recording of deep tendon reflexes

Pathologic: Plantar (Babinski) (L4, L5, S1, S2): dorsal flexion of great toe with fanning of other toes; Chaddock (L4, L5, S1, S2): dorsal flexion of great toe with fanning of other toes; clonus: no movement of foot

CONDITIONS, DISEASES, AND DISORDERS

BRAIN ABSCESS

A brain abscess is a suppurative infection consisting of a collection of pus within the parenchyma of the brain and the meningeal structures covering the brain and spinal cord.

Brain abscess accounts for only 2% of intracranial lesions. Current mortality rates range from 5% to 15%, depending on the location of the abscess and the preexisting condition of the patient. Surgical intervention may reduce the mortality, but this depends on accessibility of the abscess and the general condition of the patient. Morbidity after a brain abscess presents continued difficulties. Individuals surviving brain abscesses may experience different types of neurologic deficits, including paralysis and seizures.

PATHOPHYSIOLOGY

Currently the most common cause of brain abscess in many of the larger health systems is toxoplasmosis occurring in conjunction with human immunodeficiency virus (HIV) infection. Brain abscess may also result from extension of extracranial infections, such as chronic middle ear, sinus, or mastoid infections. Penetrating head injuries, compound skull fractures, and osteomyelitis of the skull may lead to the formation of a brain abscess. Patients with right-to-left cardiac shunts are susceptible to the formation of brain abscesses because of polycythemia, which causes cerebral ischemia and necrosis.

Organisms commonly isolated as the cause of brain abscesses include streptococci, aerobic Enterobacteriaceae, and staphylococci. Anaerobic bacteria (i.e., *Bacteroides fragilis*) and aerobic Enterobacteriaceae (i.e., *Escherichia coli, Klebsiella*) are found in suppurative ear infections. Staphylococci frequently are associated with penetrating head injuries and endocarditis. In patients with impaired host resistance, disseminated fungal infections (e.g., candidiasis) may also result in brain abscesses. In the patient with acquried immunodeficiency syndrome (AIDS), brain abscess usually is caused by the protozoal organism *Toxoplasma gondii.*

After the initial implantation of bacteria, there is a localized inflammatory reaction (i.e., focal cerebritis or encephalitis) that is characterized by local edema, hyperemia, leukocyte infiltration, parenchymal softening, and petechial hemorrhage. Several days to weeks after bacterial invasion of the brain tissue, there is central liquefaction and necrosis of brain tissue that produce a cystic mass of pus. The cystic mass is encapsulated by a wall of granulated tissue from the migration of fibroblasts. Continued fibroblastic activity and gliosis result in the replacement of granulation tissue of the abscess wall by collagenous connective tissues. The encapsulation process usually is completed within about 3 weeks. A free, or nonencapsulated, abscess is associated with a higher mortality rate.

DIAGNOSTIC STUDIES AND FINDINGS

Roentgenograms (skull, sinuses, mastoid processes, chest): Helpful in locating associated suppurative processes

CT scan: Locates well-formed and encapsulated abscesses; visualizes ventricle size and midline displacement

Brain scan: Locates abscesses over 1 cm in size; sensitive in early cerebritis when local alteration in permeability of blood-brain barrier can be visualized

Magnetic resonance imaging (MRI) (with gadolinium contrast): Enhanced view of brain and brainstem; extent of mass; effect of cerebritis; associated venous thrombus

Electroencephalogram (EEG): Marked slowing at sites of abscess

Multidisciplinary Plan

Surgery

Aspiration or complete excision and evacuation of abscess (method depends on site and accessibility of lesion)
Stereotaxic biopsy (for lesions deep in the brain)
Craniotomy (done only when abscess is encapsulated)

Medications

Antiinfective agents: Course of therapy may be 6 wk
- Penicillin G, 20 million units IV q4h
- Metronidazole (Flagyl) (given in combination with penicillin)
  - Loading dose: 15 mg/kg IV over 1 h
  - Maintenance dose: 7.5 mg/kg IV over 1 h q6h
  - If staphylococcal infection is suspected, add Vancomycin, 7.5-15 mg/kg IV q12h

For abscesses associated with *Toxoplasma gondii:*
- Pyrimethamine (Fansidar), 25-50 mg PO
- Clindamycin (Cleocin), 900-1200 mg IV q6h (for patients allergic to sulfa drugs)

Anticonvulsants
- Phenytoin (Dilantin), 300 mg PO qd
- Phenobarbital (Luminal), 100-200 mg PO in divided doses
- Mannitol 20%, 1.5-2 g/kg IV infused over 30-60 min
- Dexamethasone (Decadron), 6-12 mg IV q6h

General Management

Serial-order computed tomography (CT) scans to monitor effectiveness of therapy
Support of vital functions (e.g., ventilator) if indicated
Physical therapy
Nutritional services: High caloric intake
Treatment of elevated ICP
Social services
Occupational therapy

NURSING CARE

Nursing Assessment

Pain related to increased cerebral pressure: Headache (70% of patients) that becomes increasingly severe
- Activation phase: Increased pulse; increased blood pressure; increased respiratory rate; dilated pupils; pallor; increased muscle tension; cold perspiration
- Rebound phase: Blood pressure lower than before pain experience; pulse rate slower than before pain experience
- Adaptation phase: Pain occurring frequently or for long duration; pulse rate and blood pressure not increased as much as in activation phase
- Stress reaction: Pain persisting for many days; increased production of 17-ketosteroids; increased production of eosinophils; increased susceptibility to other infections
- Vocalizations: Grunt, whimper, groan, sob, cry, gasp
- Facial expressions: Clenched teeth, eyes open wide or tightly shut lids, wrinkled forehead, biting lower lip
- Other: May withdraw socially; may not initiate conversation

Airway clearance: Patient's ability to handle secretions; audible breath sounds in all lobes
Breathing patterns: Monitor arterial blood gases per protocol: report changes in arterial oxygen pressure (Po_2) of 10 to 15 mm Hg, report changes in Pco_2 of 10 to 15 mm Hg; monitor pulse oximetry: change in respiratory rate or depth, change in breath sounds
Level of consciousness: Assessment of vital signs and neurologic status every 1 to 2 hours and as needed; note level of consciousness, orientation, and ability to understand: lethargy, irritability, confusion or coma
Meningeal irritability: Nuchal rigidity (25% of patients)
Seizure activity: Generalized or focal (30% of patients); monitor for effects and side effects of anticonvulsants; monitor for therapeutic serum levels of anticonvulsants
Fluid balance: Intake and output
Anxiety
- Appearance: Increased perspiration, clammy skin; fatigue; increased muscle tension (rigidity); skin blanches, pale; increased small motor activity (i.e., tremors, restlessness)
- Behavior: Decreased attention span; increased immobility; decreased ability to follow directions
- Other: Increased heart rate; rapid shifts in body temperature, blood pressure; urinary urgency; diarrhea; dry mouth; decreased appetite; pupillary dilation

Skin integrity: Assess skin turgor and pressure for areas of breakdown
Other: Selective aphasia (if temporal lobe involved); weakness of lower facial muscles; ataxia, nystagmus, incoordination of extremities, and occasionally intention tremors (cerebellar abscess); impaired two-point discrimination, altered position sense, astereognosis, visual inattention, and impaired opticokinetic nystagmus (parietal lobe abscess)
Findings related to specific location of brain abscess
- Temporal lobe
  - Dysphasia (sensory): Palsies of cranial nerves III and VI; disturbances in upper quadrant visual fields; contralateral facial paresis; localized headache
  - Frontal lobe: Frontal headache; focal or jacksonian seizure; lethargy, disorientation; contralateral paralysis/hemiparesis; dysphagia (motor)
  - Cerebellum: Nuchal rigidity (stiff neck); ipsilateral ataxia and limb paralysis; dystonia; occipital or postauricular headache; nystagmus; dysfunction of cranial nerves III, IV, V, and VI

Potential Complications

Seizures
- Preconvulsive (preictal) stage: Aura—flash of light, sense of loss or fear, weakness, dizziness, peculiar taste, smell, and sounds; cry or scream; fall to floor; loss of consciousness; tachypnea
- Convulsive stage: Tonic—rigid body, flexed jaws, clenched fists, extended legs, cyanosis, holding breath; clonic—urinary and/or fecal incontinence, jerking of facial muscles and extremities, biting tongue, frothing at mouth
- Postconvulsive (postictal) stage: Altered level of consciousness; headache; nausea and/or vomiting; malaise; muscle soreness; aspiration; breathing difficulty, choking, cyanosis, decreased breath sounds, tachycardia, tachypnea

Hypoxia: Confusion, restlessness, increased heart rate, early hypertension, late hypotension, cyanosis
Intracranial hypertension: Changing level of consciousness (see p. 238) for additional signs and symptoms of increased ICP; decreased pulse; increased systolic blood pressure; widened

pulse pressure; irregular and decreased respirations; pupillary changes (papilledema—late sign); seizures; worsening of focal neurologic signs

Patient Problems/Nursing Diagnoses & Interventions

NIC Respiratory Management

Ineffective airway clearance related to altered cerebrovascular status
Ineffective breathing pattern related to altered cerebrovascular status
Impaired gas exchange related to altered breathing pattern

- Maintain patent airway; avoid flexion of neck if patient is comatose.
- Keep emergency drugs and ventilator at bedside; intubation and assisted ventilation may be indicated *to maintain adequate respiratory function.*
- Suction as needed *to prevent obstruction.*
- Maintain nothing-by-mouth (NPO) status *to prevent risk of choking and aspiration.*
- Administer medications per protocol.
- Instruct/assist with coughing, deep breathing, and incentive spirometry.
- Regulate fluid intake *to optimize fluid balance.*

NIC Tissue Perfusion Management

Ineffective tissue perfusion related to high risk for intracranial hypertension
Risk for imbalanced fluid volume related to cerebral edema and use of osmotic diuretics

- Monitor ICP (if monitoring device is used) every 30 minutes to 1 hour for waveform changes or spikes *to evaluate for intracranial hypertension.* **Continuous flushing devices must not be used for measuring ICP.**
  Monitor cerebral perfusion pressure.
  Monitor insertion site for signs of infection.
  Space care activities *to minimize elevations in intracranial pressure.*
  Minimize environmental stimuli.
- Maintain head of bed at 20- to 30-degree elevation *to facilitate cerebral venous drainage.*
- Maintain body alignment.
- Maintain fluid restrictions as ordered.
- Measure intake and output. Report hourly output less than 30 ml *to identify potential hypotension or fluid overload.*

NIC Physical Comfort Promotion

Acute pain related to increased ICP

- Administer medications as indicated.
- Improve effectiveness of pain reduction medications by using them before pain becomes intense.

NIC Risk Management

Disturbed sensory perception (visual, tactile, and kinesthetic) related to altered cerebrovascular status
Risk for injury related to seizures or altered level of consciousness
Risk for infection related to hematogenous dissemination of pathogen

Preconvulsive care

- Have oral airway at bedside *to prevent airway obstruction.*
- Have suction equipment available at bedside.
- Administer oxygen per protocol.
- Identify auras if possible.

Convulsive care

- Maintain patent airway.
- Support and protect head; turn to side if possible *to protect airway.*
- Place pillows along side rails if patient is in bed *to prevent injury.*
- Provide privacy as necessary.
- Stay with patient; remain calm to provide reassurance.
- Note frequency, time, involved body parts, and length of seizure *to establish the type of seizure activity.*

Postconvulsive care

- Maintain patent airway.
- Suction as indicated.
- Administer oxygen per protocol.
- Reorient patient to environment *to minimize sensory-perceptual alteration.*
- Place patient in position of comfort; turn head to side.
- Administer oral hygiene as necessary for secretions and bleeding.
- Prepare for diagnostic tests if ordered: CT scan, skull series, arteriogram, electroencephalogram (EEG).

Injury prevention

- Keep side rails up at all times when patient is alone. Maintain fall precautions at all times *to prevent injury.*
- Maintain bed in low and locked position.
- Implement use of bed alarm, as appropriate, *to alert caretakers that patient is getting out of bed.*
- Ensure the patient's call light is within reach.
- Answer call light immediately.
- Reorient patient frequently to time, person, and place.
- Repeat explanations frequently and simply *to facilitate understanding.*
- Place articles within easy reach for the patient.
- Instruct patient to request assistance with movement, as appropriate.
- Maintain quiet environment, reducing external stimuli to minimum *to reduce sensory overload.*
- Maintain planned rest periods *to allow sufficient time for REM sleep.*

Infection protection

- Administer selected antiinfective therapy as prescribed.
- Evaluate white blood cell (WBC) count daily *to monitor effectiveness of drug therapy.*
- Maintain aseptic technique for all dressing changes.
- Maintain strict use of universal precautions *to prevent secondary infection.*
- Promote proper nutritional intake.
- Monitor for signs of meningitis: nuchal rigidity, headache, chills, and diaphoresis.

Patient Education/Continuum of Care Plan

1. Ensure the patient and family know and understand the following:

   a. Nature of a brain abscess, treatments, and procedures; explain as they occur
   b. Need to ambulate as tolerated
   c. Importance of maintaining planned rest periods
   d. Names of medications, dosages, frequency of administration, purposes, and toxic or side effects
   e. Need to avoid taking over-the-counter medications without consulting physician
   f. Possible residual effects such as headaches, sensory or motor deficits, seizures
2. Discuss with the patient and the family ways to recognize seizure activity and appropriate course of action:
   a. Sit or lie down.
   b. Avoid trying to stop seizure or restraining patient.
   c. Protect patient from injury.
   d. Observe and record body parts involved and duration of seizure activity.
3. Ensure that the patient and family understand importance of ongoing outpatient care (i.e., physician's visits and physical therapy).
4. Explain to the patient and family the importance of maintaining a well-balanced diet.

EVALUATION/PATIENT OUTCOMES

Respiratory Management: Patent airway is maintained. Chest excursion is symmetric. Breath sounds are normal, or there is no increase in adventitious sounds. Arterial blood gas values are within normal ranges or consistent with patient's baseline. Vital signs are within normal ranges or consistent with patient's baseline. Hemoglobin levels are 14 to 18 g/dl (male) and 12 to 16 g/dl (female). Intake and output are stable. Resonance of all lobes is evident on percussion. Skin color is without cyanosis. There are no subjective or objective findings of shortness of breath, air hunger, or dyspnea on exertion.

Tissue Perfusion Management: There is no change in level of consciousness. There is no evidence of neurologic deficits or intracranial hypertension. There is no seizure activity. Pattern of electrolytes is stable. Intake and output are stable.

Physical Comfort Promotion: Patient openly verbalizes feelings of discomfort when they occur. Patient is able to use measures to decrease discomfort. Patient verbalizes a decrease in subjective feelings of discomfort. There is a decrease in objective findings of pain.

Risk Management: Patient maintains optimal level of mobility. Patient remains free of injury. Skin integrity is maintained. Nutritional status is adequate. Patient demonstrates minimal self-care deficits. Patient remains free of seizures. Safety measures appropriate to level of physiologic status are used. Skin is free of bruises, burns, abrasions, redness, etc. Patient is free of nosocomial infections. Patient is afebrile, and WBC count is 5000 to 10,000/mm^3. Patient's vital signs are stable.

HYDROCEPHALUS

Hydrocephalus is characterized by an abnormal accumulation of CSF within the cranial vault with subsequent dilation of the cerebral ventricles.

Hydrocephalus has an incidence of 4 per 1000 births through age 3 months but it can occur at any age. In infants it is considered a primary disease, whereas in later life it occurs as a complication of other diseases.

Hydrocephalus has several known causes, which can be categorized as congenital or acquired. Congenital abnormalities obstruct the flow of CSF; 70% of these obstructions result from stenosis of the aqueduct of Sylvius. Other anomalies causing or associated with hydrocephalus are the Arnold-Chiari malformation, Dandy-Walker syndrome, and spina bifida cystica.[8] Flow and absorption of CSF also can be affected by fibrosis of the meninges and obstruction of the aqueduct and basal cisterns caused by inflammatory lesions.

Causative mechanisms of hydrocephalus are (1) excessive secretion of CSF as a result of a choroid plexus papilloma, (2) obstruction of CSF flow in the ventricles or subarachnoid space, (3) obstruction by pacchionian granulations, and (4) hemodynamic production. Common sites for obstruction of CSF are the third ventricle, the fourth ventricle, the foramina of Monro, and the aqueduct of Sylvius. Each site may be obstructed by a mass within or outside the lumen. Pacchionian granulations caused by inflammatory processes and fibrosis can occlude the arachnoid villi, preventing the escape of CSF from the subarachnoid space and resulting in hydrocephalus.

Although most causes of hydrocephalus are associated with intraventricular hypertension, there are two types in which intraventricular pressure is not elevated. Hydrocephalus ex vacuo results in ventricular dilation to fill spaces caused by a decreasing neural mass (e.g., Alzheimer's disease and stroke). Normal pressure hydrocephalus is characterized by dilated ventricles, normal neural tissue mass, and normal ICP. The etiology and pathology of normal pressure hydrocephalus remain to be elucidated.

Communicating Versus Noncommunicating Hydrocephalus

A communicating or extraventricular hydrocephalus occurs when the obstruction is outside the ventricular system; therefore flow between the ventricles is not blocked. Excessive CSF accumulates in the ventricles because the fluid is not adequately absorbed from the cerebral subarachnoid space. Noncommunicating, or intraventricular, hydrocephalus results in an accumulation of CSF from a block of the normal flow at some point in the ventricular system. The cerebral ventricles proximal to the blockage then dilate.

PATHOPHYSIOLOGY

When there is an obstruction in the ventricular system or in the subarachnoid space, the cerebral ventricles dilate, causing the ventricular surface to stretch, disrupting its ependymal lining. The underlying white matter atrophies and may be reduced to a thin ribbon. There is selective preservation of the gray matter, even when the ventricles have attained enormous size. The dilation process may be an insidious or acute process and may be selective, depending on the site of blockage. The acute process may cause a medical emergency. In the infant and young child the cranial sutures split and widen to accommodate the increasing cranial mass. If the anterior fontanel is not closed, it bulges and feels tense to palpation. Aqueductal stenosis, a sex-linked familial disease, causes a marked dilation of the lateral and third ventricles. This dilation gives the head a characteristic dominant frontal brow appearance. The Dandy-Walker syndrome occurs when there is an obstruction of the exit foramina of the fourth ventricle. Consequently, the fourth ventricle dilates, with the posterior fossae becoming prominent and bulging below the tentorium. This type of hydrocephalus gives the patient generalized symmetric enlargement of the cerebrum, and the face appears disproportionately small.

In the older individual the cranial sutures have closed; therefore the space is fixed and limits expansion of the brain mass. As a result, the older person usually exhibits the signs and symptoms of increased ICP before the cerebral ventricles become greatly enlarged.

Defects of CSF absorption and circulation in hydrocephalus are not complete. Formation of CSF exceeds the capacity of the normal ventricular system every 6 to 8 hours, and a total lack of reabsorption is incompatible with life. Ventricular dilation causes a disruption of the normal ependymal lining of the walls of the cavities, permitting increased absorption. If the collateral route is adequate to prevent progressive ventricular dilation, a state of compensation may exist.

Diagnostic Studies and Findings

Angiography: Detection of vessel abnormalities caused by stretching; vascular lesions

CT scan/MRI: Detection of variations in tissue density; presence of cysts or masses; visualization of the ventricular system

Lumbar puncture: Diagnosis of communicating hydrocephalus; lumbar puncture on a patient with increased ICP must be done with caution because of the risk of brain herniation

Ventriculography: Visualization of ventricular system configuration; shows ventricular dilation with hydrocephalus

Multidisciplinary Plan

Surgery

Correction of CSF obstruction such as resection of cyst, neoplasm, or hematoma

Ventricular bypass into normal intracranial channel (i.e., Torkildsen procedure where CSF is shunted from lateral to cisterna magna) in noncommunicating hydrocephalus

Ventricular bypass into extracranial compartment (i.e., ventriculoperitoneal or ventriculoatrial shunt)

Reduction of CSF production as in third or fourth ventriculostomy or endoscopic choroid plexus extirpation (plexectomy or electric coagulation)

Medications

Acetazolamide (Diamox), 8-30 mg/kg in divided doses IV

Dexamethasone (Decadron), 6-20 mg q6h IV

General Management

ICP monitoring

Cardiac monitoring

Respiratory management
- Monitor pulse oximetry
- Assess arterial blood gases as ordered:
  - Report decrease of P_{O_2} of 10 to 15 mm Hg.
  - Report increase of P_{CO_2} greater than 10 to 15 mm Hg.

Physical therapy

Speech/occupational therapy

Dietary consultation

NURSING CARE

Nursing Assessment

Head circumference (pediatrics): Severely enlarged head; bulging fontanels after pulsation; fixed downward gaze of eyes with visible sclera above (sunset gaze); visible, distended scalp veins; radiation of light throughout accumulated CSF with transillumination

Vomiting: More frequent in older patient; likely to occur in morning (frequency may increase with increased ICP)

Seizures: History of previous seizure activity; monitor for effects and side effects of anticonvulsants; monitor serum for therapeutic levels of anticonvulsants; focal or general tonic-clonic seizures; may assume opisthotonic position

Behavioral changes: Feeds poorly (pediatrics); lethargy; irritability when stimulated; apathy, inattentiveness

Muscle tone: Alteration of muscle tone in extremities

Later assessment findings: Physical and/or mental development lag; prominence of forehead; scalp shiny, with scalp veins prominent; optic atrophy, strabismus, nystagmus, exposed sclera

Potential Complications

Intracranial hypertension: Change in level of consciousness, restlessness, lethargy; decreased pulse; increased systolic blood pressure; widened pulse pressure; irregular and decreased respirations; pupillary changes (late sign); seizures; worsening of focal neurologic signs

Patient Problems/Nursing Diagnoses & Interventions

NIC Respiratory Management

Ineffective airway clearance related to impaired cough reflex and decreased level of consciousness

Ineffective breathing pattern related to impaired respiratory mechanics

Impaired gas exchange related to altered breathing patterns

- Maintain patent airway.
- Have intubation and assisted ventilation equipment at bedside.
- Suction as needed.
  - Use universal precautions, as appropriate.
  - Hyperoxygenate with 100% oxygen before suctioning *to prevent suction-induced hypoxia.*
  - Auscultate breath sounds before and after suctioning *to determine effectiveness of secretion removal.*
- Position for maximum lung expansion; elevate head of bed slightly (10 to 20 degrees).

- Limit fluid intake per protocol; include titrating according to intracranial pressure.
- Measure and record intake and output; report hourly output less than 30 ml *to detect hypervolemia.*

NIC Neurologic Management

Ineffective cerebral tissue perfusion related to enlarged ventricular system

Decreased intracranial adaptive capacity related to intracranial hypertension

- Monitor values and waveforms of ICP line, if appropriate **(continuous flushing devices are not used for ICP measurement).**
  - Maintain patency and sterility of system.
  - Note effects of nursing care on ICP.
  - Correlate neurologic status with ICP values, and notify physician if inconsistent.
  - Space nursing care *to prevent intracranial hypertension.*
- Assist with drainage of CSF from system, if indicated, *to prevent or control intracranial hypertension.*
- Intervene to prevent increased ICP.
  - Administer medications, treatments, and intravenous fluids per protocol.
  - Maintain elevation of head of bed per protocol *to maximize cerebral venous drainage.*
  - Accurately record intake and output
- Intervene to monitor or prevent seizures. Institute seizure precautions to minimize potential for injury to the patient.
  - Keep airway at bedside.
  - Maintain bed height at lowest level *to prevent falls.*
  - Keep side rails up at all times.
  - Have oxygen and suction equipment at bedside.
  - Place emergency medications at bedside.
  - Administer anticonvulsants per protocol.
- Provide preoperative nursing care for patient who will have shunt implantation.
  - Suction or aspirate mucus as needed *to prevent airway obstruction.*
  - Administer medications (i.e., antibiotics and anticonvulsants).
  - Turn every 2 hours and provide skin care every 2 hours *to protect skin integrity.*
  - Insert nasogastric tube *to decompress abdomen.*
- Provide postoperative nursing care after shunt implantation.
  - Position patient and pump shunt per protocol *to maintain maximum effectiveness.*
  - Compress valve specified number of times at regular intervals.
  - Accurately measure intake and output and record on flow sheet.
  - Administer parenteral fluids per protocol.
  - Administer feedings per protocol *to provide adequate nutrition.*
  - Monitor for complications, such as dehydration, infection, or fluid overload.

NIC Risk Management

Disturbed sensory perception (visual, auditory, tactile, and kinesthetic) related to altered sensory integration

Risk for injury related to altered level of consciousness or seizures

Preconvulsive care

- Have oral airway and suction equipment at bedside.
- Administer oxygen per protocol.
- Identify auras, if possible.

Convulsive care

- Support and protect head, turn to side *to protect airway.*
- Prevent injury, place pillows along side rails if indicated.
- Provide privacy and stay with patient *to provide safety and reassurance.*
- Establish the type of seizure activity and note frequency and time involved.

Postconvulsive care

- Maintain patent airway; suction as indicated.
- Administer oxygen per protocol.
- Place in position of comfort, turn head to side *to maintain patent airway.*

Injury prevention

- Have side rails up at all times when patient is alone *to prevent injury or fall.*
- Maintain fall precautions at all times.
- Judiciously use soft restraints; monitor patient's response.
- Implement use of bed alarm *to alert caregivers that patient is getting out of bed.*
- Frequently reorient patient to time, person, and place.
- Reintroduce yourself each time you reorient patient.
- Have family bring in familiar objects *to promote sense of security.*
- Allow family to stay with patient.
- Maintain planned rest periods *to allow sufficient time for REM sleep.*
- Use day and night lighting appropriately *to promote normal sleep-wake cycle.*

NIC Skin/Wound Management

Risk for impaired skin integrity related to physical immobilization

- See general intervention strategies, p. 255.
- Prevent pressure sores and contractures:
  - Keep scalp dry and clean.
  - Reposition every 2 hours; turn head frequently. (Maintain neck in neutral alignment *to facilitate cerebral venous drainage and prevent increased ICP.)*
- Rotate head and body together *to prevent strain on neck.*
- Provide passive ROM exercise, especially of lower extremities, every 4 hours and as needed *to prevent contractures.*

Patient Education/Continuum of Care Plan

1. Make certain the patient and family know and understand the following:
   a. Nature of hydrocephalus, treatments, and procedures; explain as they occur
   b. Care of shunt devices if indicated
   c. Need to ambulate as tolerated

   d. Importance of maintaining planned rest periods
   e. Names of medications, dosages, frequency of administration, purposes, and toxic or side effects
   f. Need to avoid taking over-the-counter medications without consulting physician
   g. Possible residual effects such as headaches, sensory or motor deficits, seizures
2. Discuss with the patient and the family ways to recognize seizure activity and the appropriate course of action:
   a. Assist patient to sit or lie down.
   b. Avoid trying to stop seizure or restraining patient.
   c. Protect patient from injury.
   d. Observe and record body parts involved and duration of seizure activity.
3. Ensure that the patient and family understand the importance of ongoing outpatient care (i.e., physician's visits and physical therapy).
4. Explain to the patient and family the importance of maintaining a well-balanced diet.

EVALUATION/PATIENT OUTCOMES

Respiratory Management: Patent airway is maintained. Chest excursion is symmetric. Breath sounds are normal, or there is no increase in adventitious sounds. Arterial blood gas values are within normal ranges or consistent with patient's baseline. Vital signs are within normal ranges or consistent with patient's baseline. Hemoglobin levels are 14 to 18 g/dl (male) and 12 to 16 g/dl (female). Intake and output are stable. There are no signs of respiratory distress. Resonance of all lobes is evident on percussion. Skin color is without cyanosis.

Neurologic Management: There is no change in level of consciousness. There is no evidence of neurologic deficits. Pattern of electrolytes is stable. There is no seizure activity.

Risk Management: Optimum level of orientation is maintained. The patient remains free of injury. Skin integrity is maintained. Nutritional status is adequate. Self-care deficits are minimal. Patient remains free of seizure activity.

Skin/Wound Management: Skin is intact. Nutritional status is adequate. Electrolyte balance is maintained. Patient remains free of pressure sores and contractures.

CRANIAL AND PERIPHERAL NERVE DISORDERS

BELL'S PALSY

Bell's palsy (facial paralysis) is the paralysis of the facial nerve (cranial nerve VII), resulting in a sudden loss of ability to move the muscles of expression of the face (FIG. 5-22).

Any or all of the three branches of the facial nerve may be affected. The disorder can be unilateral or bilateral, transient or permanent. Generally, the disorder appears static for about 10 days to 2 weeks, at which time muscle tone begins to reappear. Voluntary movement of the muscles may appear within 3 or 4 weeks. However, some individuals manifest no recovery for almost 6 months, and maximum recovery (which may not be complete) may occur in approximately a year. More than 80% of the patients with Bell's palsy recover without residual neurologic deficits.[10]

PATHOPHYSIOLOGY

Bell's palsy develops as a result of a viral infection produced by reactivation of the herpes simplex virus. After a primary infection the virus becomes latent in the cranial and spinal sensory ganglia. When a state of immunosuppression exists, the virus is reactivated within the ganglion cells and produces local damage that is characterized by hypoesthesia of the head, face, neck, and pharynx. The virus then travels up and down to the axons, where

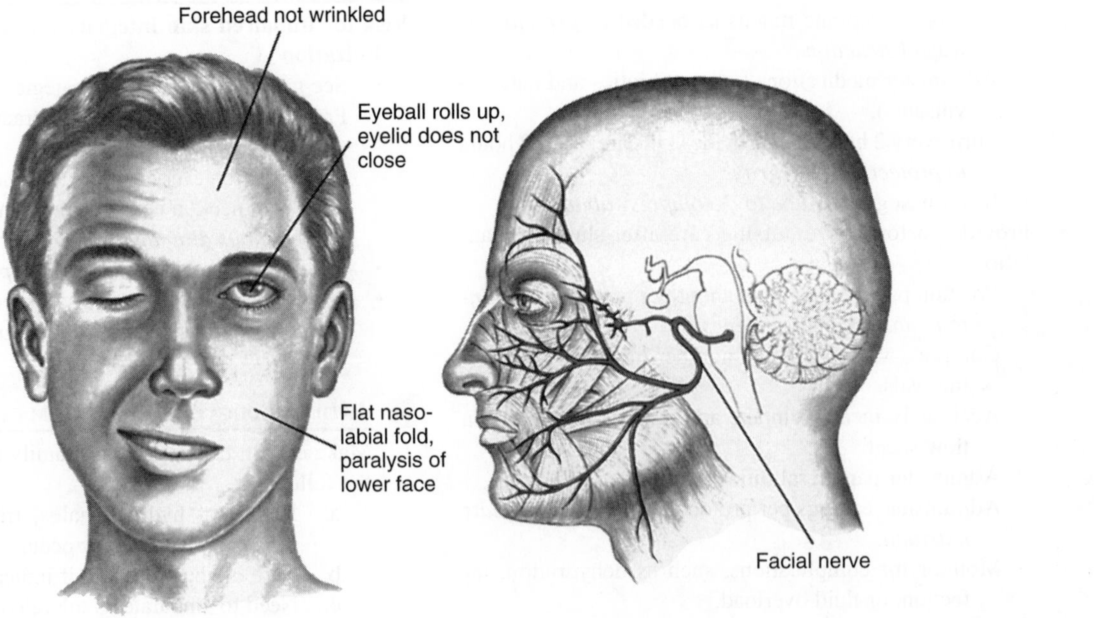

FIG. 5-22 Bell's palsy. (From Chipps, Clanin, and Campbell.[1a])

it induces an inflammatory response with antibody and lymphocytic infiltration. The end result is segmental demyelination that manifests as nerve paralysis. When the infection is resolved, remyelination follows and innervation to muscles is restored.

The disorder can occur at any age but most frequently occurs in individuals between ages 20 and 60 years. The incidence of Bell's palsy increases with age. It is twice as common in women between age 10 and 19 years, but is 1.5 times more common in men after age 40 years. The diagnosis of Bell's palsy is made by the characteristic presenting symptoms and the patient's history.

Multidisciplinary Plan

Medications

Prednisone (Deltasone), 60-80 mg/day PO for 5 days; dosage is tapered over next 5 days
Acyclovir (Zovirax), 200 mg PO, five times per day for 10 days
Analgesics as required

General Management

Surface electromyography feedback
Warm, moist heat
Massage
Facial sling to prevent muscle stretching and to facilitate eating (by improving lip alignment)
Visual facial exercises (i.e., wrinkling brow, forcing eyes closed, puffing out cheeks in a mirror) for 5 minutes three or four times daily, as muscle tone returns
Swallowing precautions
Nutritional consultation

NURSING CARE

Nursing Assessment

Pain: Usually begins behind the ear; may or may not be accompanied by herpetic vesicles in the external ear
Paralysis: Drawing sensation on affected side, followed by complete paralysis of affected side (ipsilateral) of face; all muscles powerless and flaccid (i.e., cannot smile, wrinkle forehead, or close eye; drooling of saliva; constant eye tearing)
Taste: Loss of taste sensation over anterior two thirds of tongue on affected side
Eating and drinking difficulties: May see anorexia and weight loss; impaired ability to chew and swallow increases potential for choking and aspiration

Potential Complications

Drying keratitis: Pain, photophobia, blepharospasm

Patient Problems/Nursing Diagnoses & Interventions

NIC Physical Comfort Promotion

Acute or chronic pain related to cranial nerve VII irritation
Chronic pain related to chronic irritation of cranial nerve VII

- Administer pain medications per protocol.
- Provide gentle massage, as needed, *to relieve pain and promote relaxation.*
- Provide warm moist heat per protocol.
- Provide for electrical stimulation per protocol *to relieve severe pain.*
- Apply facial sling as needed *to prevent muscle stretching and facilitate eating.*
- Provide eye care every 1 to 2 hours and as needed *to prevent corneas from drying and suffering injury.*
- Apply moist eye pads as indicated *to prevent injury and to minimize eye strain;* tape eye closed during sleep *to prevent keratitis*
- Teach patient to perform facial exercises three or four times daily for 5 minutes *to promote muscle tone:* wrinkling brow, grimacing, whistling, puffing out cheeks, and forcing eyes closed.
- Provide patient with sunglasses as needed *to prevent eye strain.*

NIC Nutrition Support

Imbalanced nutrition, less than body requirements, related to inability to ingest food

- Offer patient frequent, small feedings *to maintain adequate caloric intake.*
- Maintain soft diet as indicated *to minimize choking.*
- Avoid hot fluids and foods *to prevent burns to insensitive areas.*
- Provide patient with privacy at mealtimes *to minimize anxiety and embarrassment.*
- Provide patient with adequate time for eating meals.
- Teach patient to take foods on unaffected side *to minimize discomfort.*
- Apply facial sling *to improve lip alignment.*
- Teach patient to chew food on unaffected side.
- Provide meticulous mouth care before and after meals.
- Provide dietary supplements as indicated *to maintain adequate caloric intake.*

Patient Education/Continuum of Care Plan

1. Discuss with the patient the possible causes, involvement, symptoms, treatments, and usual course of Bell's palsy (explain procedures as they occur).
2. Discuss signs of complications and progression of the disorder.
3. Explain special techniques such as the use of facial slings, massage, dietary adjustments, and exercise program to minimize discomfort.
4. Stress importance of continued eye care.
5. Explain safety measures for minimizing trauma to insensitive areas.
6. Explain names of medications, dosage, frequency of administration, purpose, and toxic or side effects of the medication.
7. Stress importance of ongoing outpatient care: physician's visits, physical therapy and exercise program, and support groups.

Evaluation/Patient Outcomes

Physical Comfort Promotion: Patient is able to use measures such as facial sling and warm massage as needed. Patient openly expresses feelings of discomfort when they occur. Patient or caregiver instills eyedrops appropriately. Eye is taped shut during sleep. Patient is able to perform facial exercises as indicated.

Nutrition Support: Weight pattern is stable: normal for height, age, sex, and previous baseline. Intake and output balanced and stable. Diet is appropriate to age. Skin turgor is good. There is fluid and electrolyte balance. Dietary supplements are used as appropriate.

Guillain-Barré Syndrome

Guillain-Barré syndrome (acute inflammatory demyelinating polyradiculoneuropathy) is an immune-mediated syndrome characterized by widespread inflammation or demyelination of ascending or descending nerves in the peripheral nervous system that results in impaired nerve impulse conduction between the nodes of Ranvier (Fig. 5-23).

Guillain-Barré syndrome has an incidence of 1 to 2 cases per 100,000 persons in the United States. Eighty-five percent of individuals affected by Guillain-Barré syndrome have complete functional recovery. The recovery period usually extends over several weeks, but it may last months or even years. The remaining 15% of affected individuals experience some degree of permanent neurologic deficit.

Pathophysiology

The pathogenesis of Guillain-Barré syndrome is thought to be related to the sensitization of peripheral nerve myelin and is characterized by infiltration of mononuclear cells at all levels of the peripheral nervous system. Approximately two thirds of the individuals affected have had an acute nonspecific infection 10 to 14 days before the onset of Guillain-Barré symptoms, suggesting that sensitized lymphocytes may produce demyelination. The syndrome may also occur in association with such diseases as infectious mononucleosis, HIV infections, lymphoma, leukemia, Epstein-Barr virus, and viral hepatitis. The syndrome occurs in both sexes and can affect persons of any age.

Morphologic alterations that characterize Guillain-Barré syndrome include (1) widespread monocytic inflammatory infiltrate around blood vessels throughout the cranial and spinal nerves, including nerve roots, ganglia, and distal nerves; (2) segmental demyelination of peripheral nerves; and (3) in severe cases, axon destruction with resultant axonal reaction and wallerian degeneration. Anterior horn cells and neurons in dorsal root ganglia occasionally show central chromatolysis. If the axon loss is severe, denervation group atrophy can be seen in distal muscles.

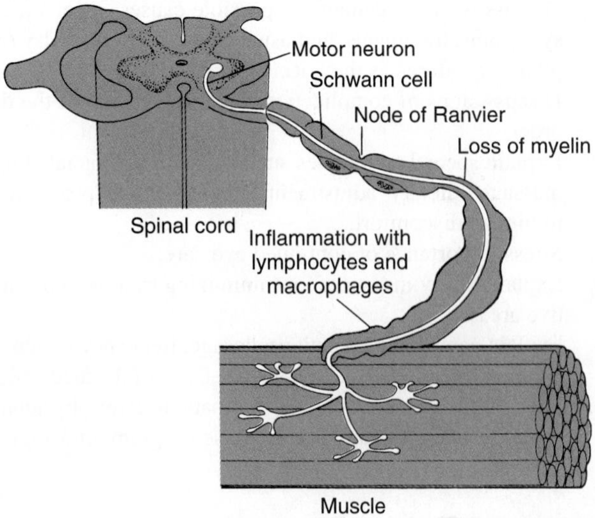

Fig. 5-23

Demyelination of nerve segments in Guillain-Barré syndrome. (From Chipps, Clanin, and Campbell.[1a])

Diagnostic Studies and Findings

CSF sampling: Albuminocytologic dissociation: Decreased protein initially (15 to 45 mg), then increases as high as 600 mg; followed by return to normal; CSF is normal in pressure and acellular (or contains a few lymphocytes)

Electromyography (EMG): Reduced amplitudes of muscle action potentials, slowed conduction velocity, or conduction block in motor nerves; fibrillations and positive sharp waves (more common in late stages)

Pulmonary function tests (PFT): Below normal for patient's height and weight

Multidisciplinary Plan

Surgery

Tracheotomy (see Chapter 4) indicated if respiratory failure occurs

Medications

Corticosteroids: Given in conjunction with plasmapheresis
  Prednisone (Deltasone), 5-80 mg/day in divided doses
Intravenous immune globulin (IVIg), 0.4 g/kg/day for 5 consecutive days
Antiinfective agents
Prophylactic antibiotics
Anticoagulants (heparin): Low-dose for prevention of deep venous thrombosis (DVT)/pulmonary embolus

General Management

Cardiac monitoring
Hemodynamic monitoring
Mechanical ventilation/respiratory support
Intubation or tracheostomy
Plasmapheresis (plasma exchange): Given in conjunction with or in place of immune globulin
Chest physiotherapy
Arterial blood gas monitoring
Nutritional maintenance (e.g., total parenteral nutrition [TPN] or nasogastric feedings)
Nutritional consultation
Special eye care

Bowel/bladder management
Physical therapy
Psychosocial counseling

NURSING CARE

Nursing Assessment

Autonomic function: Hypertension; sinus tachycardia or bradycardia; postural hypotension; chest and abdominal tightness; profuse diaphoresis; urinary incontinence, constipation; paroxysmal facial flushing; heart block

Cranial nerve function: Cranial nerve VII most commonly involved; abnormal testing response elicited; dysphagia; dysarthria

Motor function: Patient's ability to provide self-care varies; weakness after paresthesia; most common type of weakness is ascending (i.e., lower to upper limbs to trunk); equal involvement of proximal and distal muscles; atrophy possible

Reflex status: Deep tendon reflexes absent or diminished

Sensory function: Usually less severe than motor involvement; superficial or deep sensory involvement: usually stocking-glove distribution

Level of consciousness: Usually not affected; patient's anxiety level must be monitored closely

Respiratory status
- Airway patency
- Assess breath sounds
- Monitor pulse oximetery
- Monitor arterial blood gases:
  - Report decease in Po_2 of 10 to 15 mm Hg
  - Report increase in Pco_2 greater than 10 to 15 mm Hg
- Respiratory muscle paralysis

Potential Complications

Respiratory failure
- Hypoxia: Restlessness, confusion, cyanosis, tachycardia, hypotension, impaired motor function
- Hypercapnia: Dizziness, confusion, headache, unconsciousness, hypertension, diaphoresis, flushed face
- Air hunger, shortness of breath, tachypnea, use of accessory muscles, flared nostrils

Sepsis: Hyperventilation, decreased $Paco_2$; respiratory alkalosis (early); respiratory acidosis (late); decreased pulse pressure, tachycardia, hypotension; decreased urinary output; cool, clammy skin; increased WBC count; organ system dysfunction

Syndrome of inappropriate antidiuretic hormone (SIADH): Serum hypoosmolality and hyponatremia; urine hyperosmolarity and hypernatremia; decreased urinary volume; disorientation, anxiety, anorexia, nausea, vomiting, muscle weakness, seizures

Patient Problems/Nursing Diagnoses & Interventions

NIC Respiratory Management

Ineffective airway clearance related to weakened cough reflex

Ineffective breathing pattern related to neuromuscular paralysis

Impaired gas exchange related to ineffective breathing pattern

Risk for aspiration related to use of enteral feedings

- Suction as needed *to prevent airway obstruction.*
  - Maintain use of universal precautions.
  - Hyperoxygenate with 100% oxygen before suctioning.
  - Auscultate breath sounds before and after suctioning *to determine effectiveness of secretion removal.*
  - Intubation, tracheostomy, and mechanical ventilation may be indicated *to maintain airway patency and effective breathing.*
- Monitor mechanical ventilation, if used.
  - Ensure that tidal volume, rate, mode, and oxygen concentration are set as ordered.
  - Ensure that ventilator alarms are on and functional.
  - Check all ventilator connections regularly.
- Assist and teach patient to cough, deep breathe, use incentive spirometry every 2 hours *to improve respiratory functioning.*
- Administer medications per protocol. Maintain adequate fluid and nutritional intake.

Enteral feeding care
- Confirm initial enteral tube placement by physician verification of chest X-ray.
- Confirm feeding tube placement before, during, and after each tube feeding.
- Keep suctioning equipment available.
- Tape nasogastric tube securely per protocol.
- Avoid tube feeding implementation if residuals are high.
- Hold tube feedings if bowel sounds are absent and if diarrhea/constipation or nausea/vomiting are present.
- Maintain optimal patient positioning.
  - Elevate head of bed 30 to 40 degrees.
  - Position on right side, if possible, *to facilitate drainage through pylorus.*
- Discontinue continuous feeding 30 to 40 minutes before activity/procedure that requires lowering the patient's head.
- Put food coloring into enteral feeding.
- Check pulmonary secretions *to determine presence of enteral feeding in lungs.*

NIC Immobility Management

Impaired physical mobility related to neuromuscular impairment

Risk for disuse syndrome related to muscle paralysis and prolonged immobility

- Provide ROM exercises every 2 hours and as needed.
- Monitor nutritional intake *to ensure adequate caloric resources for activity.*
- Assist with care activities as indicated; encourage patient participation to tolerance.
- Maintain rest periods between care activities.
- Maintain bowel program.

NIC Self-Care Facilitation

Feeding, bathing/hygiene, dressing/grooming, and toileting self-care deficits related to impaired neurologic and mobility status

- Avoid giving oral feedings *to minimize risk of aspiration;* administer intravenous or nasogastric feedings per protocol.
- Administer oral hygiene every 2 hours and as needed.
- Provide daily hygiene care *to promote cleanliness and self-esteem.*
- Provide eye care every 2 hours *to prevent injury.*
  - Cleanse eyes and remove crust.
  - Apply eye shields or tape eyes closed *to protect cornea.*
  - Administer artificial tears or eyedrops per protocol *to provide lubrication.*
- Maintain bowel function with regular evacuation *to prevent constipation.*

NIC Psychologic Comfort Promotion

Anxiety related to altered sensory and motor functions

- Deal realistically and honestly with patient's anxiety about the disorder, the discomfort, and the change in self-image
- Explain potential treatments for the disorder.
  - State simply and monitor patient's reactions.
  - Repeat explanations, as indicated.
- Teach basic relaxation techniques. Reinforce teaching, as indicated.
- Teach the essential aspects of care, as indicated by the patient's condition.
- Assist the patient to participate in making decisions about care, as indicated by patient's condition.
- Alert staff to possible emotional changes; expect mood swings.

Patient Education/Continuum of Care Plan

1. Encourage open verbalization regarding fears of permanent disability, loss of function, and dying, as well as changes in body image.
2. Stress importance of avoiding individuals who have upper respiratory infections.
3. Emphasize importance of maintaining planned rest periods.
4. Stress need for independence and socialization.
   a. Encourage self-care.
   b. Encourage patient to eat meals with family.
5. Explain each medication, dosage, frequency of administration, purpose, and toxic or side effects.
6. Stress need to check with physician before taking any over-the-counter medication.
7. Emphasize need to exercise to tolerance level and avoid fatigue.
8. Stress need for high-caloric, high-protein diet; progress from soft to solid as tolerated.
9. Emphasize need to arrange utensils and food so they are easily managed by the patient.
10. Discuss need to maintain fluid intake at 2000 ml daily, unless contraindicated.
11. Stress need to avoid constipation.
    a. Drink fluids.
    b. Use stool softeners (as approved by physician).
    c. Eat foods and fruits high in roughage.
12. Emphasize need for diversional activities (e.g., watching television, reading, listening to radio).
13. Stress importance of ongoing outpatient care: physician's visits, physical therapy, and occupational therapy.
14. Ensure the patient or family demonstrates the following: speech exercises, active and/or passive ROM exercises with massage to all extremities, and exercises that increase strength and mobility of fingers (e.g., squeeze toys, balls, clay).
15. Discuss importance of warm baths to alleviate pain and stiffness.

Evaluation/Patient Outcomes

Respiratory Management: Airway remains patent. Chest excursion is symmetric. Vesicular, bronchial, and bronchovesicular breath sounds are normal with no adventitious sounds. Arterial blood gas values are within normal ranges or consistent with patient's baseline. Vital signs are within normal limits or consistent with patient's baseline. Hemoglobin levels are 14 to 18 g/dl (male) and 12 to 16 g/dl (female). Intake and output are stable. There are no signs of respiratory distress (i.e., nasal flaring, increased pulse rate, air hunger). All lobes are resonant on percussion. Skin color is not cyanotic. Patient reports no subjective or objective findings of choking or coughing. Pattern of residuals remains within acceptable range. Tube placement is verified. Pulmonary secretions show no evidence of enteral feedings. Patient experiences no nausea/vomiting and no diarrhea or constipation.

Immobility Management: Skin integrity is maintained. Contractures and deformities do not form. Level of mobility is appropriate to physiologic status. Intake and output pattern is stable. Nutritional status is adequate. There are no signs or symptoms of thrombophlebitis. There are no signs or symptoms of local infection.

Self-Care Facilitation: Outcome criteria stated for impaired physical mobility are met. Level of self-care is appropriate to physiologic status. Diet is high in calories and protein. Physical and occupational therapy is given as indicated.

Psychologic Comfort Promotion: Patient demonstrates a low level of anxiety. Patient openly verbalizes concerns and feelings of grief, loss, and discomfort. Patient openly verbalizes feelings, supported by health-care professionals and significant others. Patient verbalizes essential aspects of care. Patient is able to demonstrate relaxation techniques when feelings of anxiety begin.

Trigeminal Neuralgia

Trigeminal neuralgia, or tic douloureux, is a neurologic condition that affects the sensory distribution of the trigeminal facial nerve (cranial nerve V) and is characterized by flashing, stablike paroxysms of pain radiating along the course of a branch of cranial nerve V from the angle of the jaw (Fig. 5-24).[7]

Terminal neuralgia is caused by degeneration of or pressure on the nerve. Any of the three branches of the nerve may be affected. Attacks of lancinating pain, caused by trigeminal neuralgia, often cause the person to wince with facial contractions, thus the term *tic douloureux.*

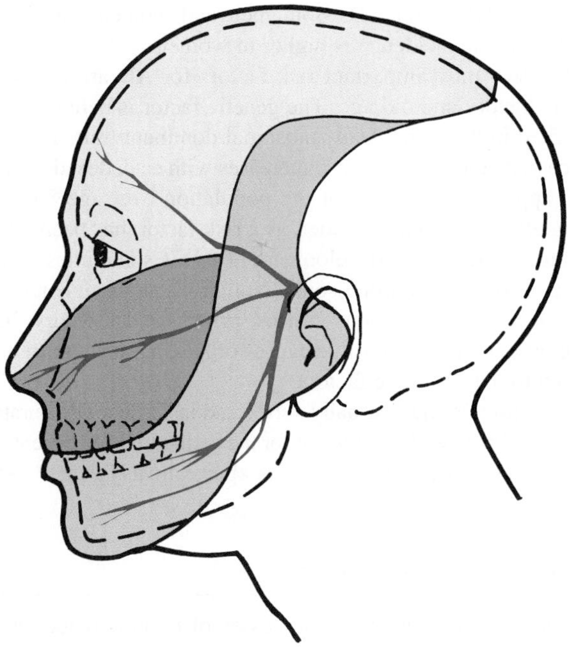

FIG. 5-24
Pathway of trigeminal nerve and facial areas innervated by each of the three main divisions of this nerve. (From Phipps, Sands, and Marek.[10])

PATHOPHYSIOLOGY

The etiology of trigeminal neuralgia is unknown. The term *neuralgia* is used because there is no demonstrable structural lesion along the course of the nerve. A similar syndrome can occur in cases of multiple sclerosis, gasserian ganglion tumor, cerebellopontine tumor, or brainstem infarction. The idiopathic form of trigeminal neuralgia affects 15,000 individuals in middle adult to late adulthood each year. There is a slightly higher incidence in women.

Although any of the trigeminal nerve's three branches can be affected, the second (maxillary) and third (mandibular) divisions are most commonly involved. Neuralgia of the first division (ophthalmic) results in pain over the forehead and around the eyes. Neuralgia of the second division results in pain in the nose, cheek, and upper lip, and when it occurs in the third division, it causes pain in the lower lip and on the side of the tongue. Episodes of the pain recur over weeks or months, although there may be spontaneous remissions. Triggering stimuli may include any mechanical activity such as smiling, talking, or touching the face. Frequently the pain occurs spontaneously either from environmental stimuli or without an apparent trigger.

The diagnosis of trigeminal neuralgia is based on the characteristic history and clinical presentation of the disorder.

MULTIDISCIPLINARY PLAN

Surgery

Microvascular decompression procedure for selective cutting of fibers within the trigeminal nerve
Glycerol injection of gasserian ganglion
Stereotactically controlled thermocoagulation of trigeminal nerve roots using radiofrequency generator
Posterior fossa craniotomy

Medications

Carbamazepine (Tegretol), 600-1200 mg/day PO
Phenytoin (Dilantin), 300-400 mg/day PO (mechanism of action in relieving pain is unknown)
Valproic acid (Depakene), 800-1200 mg/day PO
Clonazepam (Klonopin), 2-6 mg/day PO
Butorphanol (Stadol) nasal spray, 1 spray insufflated on side of pain every 3-4 h
Proparacaine (5%) eyedrops
Analgesics

General Management

Semisolid, fluid diet; nutritional consultation
Psychosocial counseling
Social services
Home health consult

NURSING CARE

NURSING ASSESSMENT

Pain: Severe, shooting pain, starting at a particular point with a repetitive tic and increasing in severity to where it shoots violently and with explosive force through the face on the affected side; discover what precipitates pain
Apprehension prevention: Protects face from any stimulation
Imbalanced nutrition: Food must be proper temperature and consistency

POTENTIAL COMPLICATIONS

Chronic pain: Verbal report or observed evidence of discomfort experienced for more than 6 months; guarding, protective movements; change in appetite; fatigue; physical or social withdrawal; shortened attention span; altered perception of time

PATIENT PROBLEMS/NURSING DIAGNOSES & INTERVENTIONS

NIC PHYSICAL COMFORT PROMOTION

Acute or chronic pain related to pressure on trigeminal nerve

- Promote rest and relaxation *to increase coping skills.*
- Modify anxiety associated with the pain experience.
- Administer medications per protocol.
- Improve effectiveness of pain relief measures by using them before the pain becomes intense
- Remain with the patient *to minimize anxiety.*
- Provide other sensory input *to serve as diversional therapy.*

NIC NUTRITION SUPPORT

Imbalanced nutrition: less than body requirements, related to inability to ingest food as a result of pain

- Offer small, frequent feedings *to encourage adequate intake.*

- Complete nursing care before feeding times.
- Allow ample time for feeding.
- Encourage a high-protein, semisolid diet.
- Accurately measure and record intake on a flow sheet *to establish if intake is adequate.*
- Administer parenteral fluids per protocol.
- Administer tube feedings per protocol.

NIC PSYCHOLOGIC COMFORT PROMOTION

Anxiety related to pain and threat to self-concept

- See general strategies on pp. 250-251.

PATIENT EDUCATION/CONTINUUM OF CARE PLAN

1. Ensure patient's understanding of involvement, symptoms, treatments, and usual course of trigeminal neuralgia (explain procedures as they occur).
2. Discuss signs of complications and progression of the disorder.
3. Discuss measures for minimizing stimulation of affected areas and trigger zones.
4. Discuss name of medications, dosage, frequency of administration, purpose, and toxic or side effects of the medication.
5. Stress the importance of ongoing outpatient care and physician's visits.
6. Refer patient to support groups.
7. Ensure family members' understanding of possible dietary alterations.

EVALUATION/PATIENT OUTCOMES

Physical Comfort Promotion: Patient openly expresses feelings of discomfort when they occur. Patient is able to use measures to decrease discomfort such as decreasing stimuli to affected areas and judicious use of analgesics.

Nutrition Support: Patient demonstrates adequate nutritional status. Weight pattern is stable. Intake and output pattern is stable. Skin turgor is good. There is fluid and electrolyte balance. Dietary supplements are taken as appropriate.

Psychologic Comfort Promotion: Patient demonstrates low level of anxiety. Patient openly verbalizes concerns and feelings of grief, loss, and discomfort.

DEGENERATIVE DISORDERS

ALZHEIMER'S DISEASE

Alzheimer's disease (AD, senile disease complex) is a chronic neurologic disorder characterized by progressive and selective degeneration of neurons in the cerebral cortex and certain subcortical structures, as well as a clinical syndrome of behavioral disturbances, memory loss, and difficulty with thought processes.

AD is the fourth leading cause of death among elderly persons in the United States.[6] The most common forms of the disorder are late-onset familial Alzheimer dementia (FAD) and nonhereditary late-onset AD. Both men and women may be affected, but the incidence is higher in women.

The two most important risk factors for AD are a positive family history and old age. The genetic factor is believed to be inherited in the form of an autosomal dominant trait. The incidence of Alzheimer's disease increases with each decade of life, with approximately 47% of the population over age 85 years being affected. Female gender, as a risk factor, has been attributed to the belief that development of AD is sometimes related to a gene on the X chromosome. Numerous environmental factors, including aluminum, viruses, prions, and mercury, have been investigated as possible causes of AD, but none have been proven to the causative factors.

The onset of AD is usually subtle and insidious. The duration and rate of progression vary, but for the well-cared-for patient, the average survival rate from onset is approximately 8 to 9 years.

PATHOPHYSIOLOGY

The basic pathophysiologic processes of brain damage occurring with AD are not known. Early-onset FAD includes at least three gene defects on chromosomes 14, 19, and 21 and possibly another gene that has not yet been mapped. Late-onset FAD is linked to a defect on chromosome 19. Cellular changes and injury associated with aging, such as decreased oxygen and glucose transport, mitochrondial defects, and loss of the blood-brain barrier may contribute to the development of AD.

Gross examination of the brain demonstrates varying degrees of cortical atrophy with widening of the cerebral sulci, particularly in the temporal, frontal, and parietal lobes. At the cellular level the major abnormalities are neurofibrillary tangles, senile plaques, and amyloid angiography. Neurofibrillary tangles (NFTs) are composed of paired helical filaments in the cytoplasm of neurons that displace or encircle the cell nucleus. Nerve processes in the cortex become twisted and distorted because of the accumulation of filaments that form the tangles. Terminal axons and clusters of nerve cells degenerate and coalece around a central amyloid core, forming patches or flat areas of senile (neuritic) plaques. These plaques disrupt nerve-impulse transmission. The greater the number of neurofibrillary tangles and senile plaques, the more dysfunction is present.[8] Amyloid angiography develops as a result of the accumulation of amyloid peptide in the cerebral arteries.

DIAGNOSTIC STUDIES AND FINDINGS

CT scan (serial): Cerebral ventricular and subarachnoid space enlargement because of diffuse brain atrophy (later stages)

MRI: Same as CT scan

EEG: Diffuse slowing of brain waves and diminished voltage (advanced stages)

Comprehensive history: Identification of symptoms listed in the assessment section for this disorder; family history of similar disorders; careful attention to medication history

Psychometric and behavioral rating scales: Mini Mental State (MMS); Mental Status Questionnaire (MSQ); Alzheimer's Disease Assessment Scale (ADAS); Wechsler Memory Test, Revised

Multidisciplinary Plan

Medications

Cognition

Tetrahydroaminoacridine (tacrine), 80-160 mg/day PO (NOTE: Must check alanine aminotransferase [ALT] level every other week until highest stable dose for 6 weeks, then check every 3 months.).

Donepezil (Aricept), 5 mg PO qd for 1 month, then 10 mg PO qd

Agitation/psychosis

Haloperidol (Haldol), 0.5-2 mg/day PO (NOTE: Haloperidol has reported risk of inducing dyskinesia tarda.[6])

Thioridazine (Mellaril), 10-25 mg PO tid

Olanzapine (Zyprexa), 5-10 mg PO qd

Risperidone (Risperdal), 0.5-2 mg PO qd or bid

Sedative/hypnotics

Zolpidem (Ambien), 5-10 mg PO hs prn

Chloral hydrate, 500-1000 mg PO prn (up to 2/day or 10/week)

Trazodone (Desyrel), 50 mg PO hs may increase gradually to 50 mg PO bid or tid

Antianxiety agents: NOTE: May produce side effects of sedation, confusion, increased muscle tone, and adventitious movements.

Lorazepam (Ativan), 0.5 to 1 mg/day PO in divided doses

Alprazolam (Xanax), 0.25-1 mg/day PO in divided doses

Buspirone (Buspar), 5-10 mg PO tid for up to several weeks

Depression

Fluoxetine (Prozac), 20-40 mg PO qAM

Paroxetine (Paxil), 20-40 mg PO qAM

Sertraline (Zoloft) 50-100 mg PO qd

Anticonvulsants

Phenytoin (Dilantin), 300 mg PO in single or divided doses

Carbamazepine (Tegretol), 200 mg PO bid on day 1; increase by 200 mg/day or less at weekly intervals until best response is attained

Laxatives/stool softeners

Ducosate sodium (Colace)

General Management

Nutritional support: Soft or liquid diet

Social services consultation

Physical therapy

Psychologic counseling and support

Community referrals

Occupational therapy

Home nursing services

Extended care facility referrals

NURSING CARE

Nursing Assessment

The literature has described three stages of AD.[4a]

Initial Stage (2 to 4 Years)

Level of consciousness is a factor to document.

Absentmindedness

Lack of spontaneity

Time and spatial disorientation

Loss of memory and emotional control

Changes in affect

Depression

Diminished ability to concentrate

Perceptual alterations

Neglectfulness in appearance

Careless actions

Judgment mistakes

Delusions (transitory) of persecution

Muscle twitching

Epileptiform seizures

Ability to provide self-care is a factor

Patient has potential for injury

Patient' level of mobility is a factor

Middle Stage (2 to 12 Years)

Assess and document level of consciousness.

Nocturnal restlessness

Apraxia (impaired ability to perform purposeful activity)

Alexia (inability to comprehend written words)

Astereognosis (inability to identify objects by touch)

Auditory agnosia (total or partial inability to recognize familiar objects by the sense of sound)

Agraphia (inability to write)

Hypertonia

Increased aphasia

Hyperorality

Complete disorientation

Unsteady gait

Progressive memory loss

Increase in socially unacceptable behaviors

Decreased ability to comprehend

Preservation phenomenon (i.e., repetitive actions such as chewing, tapping)

Ability to provide self-care is a factor

Patient's skin condition may become red when cleaned

Patient's potential for injury is a factor

Patient's level of mobility is a factor

Terminal Stage (Up to 1 Year)

Level of consciousness is documented

Seizures (rare)

Marked weight loss; emaciation

Decreased appetite

Bulimia

Apraxia

Visual agnosia

Incontinence (bowels and/or bladder)

Hyperorality

Paraphasia

Hypermetamorphosis

Increased irritability

Feelings of helplessness

Bedridden

Unresponsive or comatose

Anxiety

Appearance

Increased perspiration, clammy skin

Fatigue

Increased muscle tension (rigidity)
Skin blanches: Pale
Increased small motor activity (i.e., tremors, restlessness)
Behavior
Decreased attention span
Increased immobility
Decreased ability to follow directions
Other
Increased rate or depth of respirations
Increased heart rate
Rapid shifts in body temperature, blood pressure
Urinary urgency
Diarrhea
Dry mouth
Decreased appetite
Pupillary dilation
Altered elimination
Patients demonstrate varying voiding patterns.
Urine is checked for sediment, concentration, and color.
Altered sleep patterns.
Current sleep patterns can be compared with normal sleep patterns.
Various factors may cause sleep pattern to be interrupted.
Patient's daytime habits and activities should be noted.

Potential Complications

Aspiration: Breathing difficulty, choking, cyanosis, decreased breath sounds, tachycardia, tachypnea
Seizures: Generalized or focal
Preconvulsive (preictal) stage: Aura: flash of light, sense of loss, fear or weakness, dizziness, peculiar taste, smell, sounds; cry or scream; fall to floor; loss of consciousness; tachypnea
Convulsive stage: Tonic: rigid body, flexed jaws, clenched fists, extended legs, cyanosis, holding breath; clonic: urinary and/or fecal incontinence, jerking of facial muscles and extremities, biting tongue, frothing at mouth
Postconvulsive (postictal) stage: Altered level of consciousness; headache; nausea and/or vomiting; malaise; muscle soreness; breathing difficulties/aspiration

Patient Problems Nursing Diagnoses & Interventions

NIC Risk Management

Disturbed sensory/perception alterations related to dementia and cognitive impairment
Risk for injury related to falls or seizures

- Keep side rails up at all times when patient is alone *to minimize risk for falls and injury.*
- Maintain fall precautions at all times *to prevent accidental injury.*
- Maintain quiet environment, reducing external stimuli to a minimum.
- Reorient patient frequently to time, place, and person.
- Introduce yourself each time you reorient patient.
- Repeat explanations frequently and simply *to facilitate understanding; speak slowly in a calm voice.*
- Have family bring in familiar objects *to provide memory aids.*
- Maintain planned rest periods *to allow sufficient time for REM sleep.*
- Use day and night lighting appropriately *to promote normal sleep-wake cycle.*
- Stimulate senses of touch, taste, position.
- Have visitors or staff wear name tags.
- Document observation of patient's memory skills.
- Call patient by preferred name *to aid in self-recognition.*
- Maintain consistent caregivers.
- Maintain a simple and consistent schedule of care activities.
- Post large calendar *to aid in time and date orientation.*
- Institute safety measures *to prevent falls and protect during seizures;* implement fall precautions as appropriate.
- Maintain bed in low position at all times unless side rails are up or when nurse is with the patient.
- Provide the patient with a call light within easy reach; maintain items within easy reach for the patient.
- Maintain side rails in up position at bedtime, after sedation, when patient is confused, and as needed.
- Pad side rails if patient is overactive.

Preconvulsive precautions

- Have oral airway at bedside *to prevent obstruction.*
- Support and protect head; turn to side if possible *to prevent aspiration.*
- Prevent injury.
  - Ease to floor if in chair.
  - Place pillows along side rails if in bed.
  - Remove surrounding furniture.
  - Loosen constrictive clothing.
- Provide privacy as necessary *to protect patient's dignity.* Stay with patient; remain calm.
- Note frequency, time, involved body parts, and length of seizure *to determine type of seizure.*

Postconvulsive care

- Maintain patent airway.
- Suction as indicated.
- Administer oxygen per protocol *to minimize cerebral hypoxia.*
- Reorient patient to environment *to minimize perceptual alteration.*
- Place patient in position of comfort; turn head to side *to prevent aspiration.*
- Administer oral hygiene as necessary for secretions and bleeding.

NIC Respiratory Management

Risk for aspiration related to enteric feeding via nasoenteric tube

- Confirm initial tube placement with physician confirmation of chest x-ray.
- Confirm feeding tube placement after insertion, every 4 hours, and as needed; confirm tube placement before and after each intermittent tube feeding.
- Tape nasogastric tube securely per protocol.
- Aspirate stomach contents to determine gastric pH.

NIC Self-Care Facilitation

Feeding, bathing/hygiene, dressing/grooming, and toileting self-care deficits related to dementia and progressive neuromuscular impairment

Disturbed sleep pattern related to sensory alterations

- Encourage independent performance of daily activities to level of ability; assist with daily hygiene as indicated.
- Provide adaptive devices for personal hygiene, dressing, grooming, toileting, and eating; establish and maintain consistent care routines
- Assist with feeding, as indicated; use intravenous or nasogastric feedings per protocol.
- Maintain regular bowel and bladder routines *to promote regularity.*
- Administer oral hygiene every 2 hours and as needed *to remove secretions and promote comfort.*
- Administer eye care every 2 to 4 hours if indicated *to prevent dryness and injury.*

Sleep promotion

- Assist patient/family to eliminate stressful factors/situations before bedtime.
- Encourage patient to express concerns when unable to sleep.
- Adjust medication regimen *to support sleep/wake cycle.*
- Evaluate daytime habits and activities:
  - Assist in planning daytime activities.
  - Discourage daytime napping if it negatively affects nighttime sleep patterns.
- Provide comfortable environment *to promote rest or sleep.*
- Teach patient simple relaxation techniques *to promote rest or sleep.*
- Decrease fluid intake before bedtime.
- Discourage intake of food or caffeine at bedtime.
- Assist patient to maintain a normal day-night pattern *to facilitate sleeping at night.*
- Provide sedation per protocol if necessary. Evaluate effectiveness and side effects of sedatives.

NIC Nutrition Support

Imbalanced nutrition: less than body requirements, related to sensory and neuromuscular impairment

- Offer small, frequent feedings *to encourage adequate intake.*
- Complete nursing care before feeding times.
- Allow ample time for feeding.
- Encourage a high-protein, low-calcium diet.
- Accurately measure and record intake on a flow sheet *to establish adequate intake.*
- Administer parenteral fluids per protocol.
- Administer tube feedings per protocol.
- Elevate head to prevent aspiration

NIC Immobility Management

Impaired physical mobility related to perceptual-cognitive impairment

Risk for disuse syndrome related to prolonged immobility and altered cognition

- Document patient's baseline level of mobility.
  - Change position slowly *to prevent orthostatic hypotension.*
  - Position in proper body alignment.
- Use firm mattress or bed board *to support back and spine.*
- Apply antiembolus stockings to lower extremities *to promote venous return.*
- Administer anticoagulation therapy per protocol *to prevent embolus formation.*
- Observe for signs of thrombophlebitis.
- Provide passive ROM exercises *to maintain joint mobility.*

NIC Skin/Wound Management

Risk for impaired skin integrity related to altered mobility and sensation

- Prevent pressure sores and contractures.
  - Keep skin dry and clean.
  - Reposition every 2 hours; massage pressure areas after turning *to stimulate circulation.*
  - Provide passive ROM exercises every 4 hours and as needed *to prevent contractures.*
    - Perform ROM exercises gently, slowly, and rhythmically.
    - Repeat each ROM exercise three times every 4 hours
    - Use footboard or Spence boots *to prevent foot drop.*
- Maintain high-protein, low-calcium diet *to prevent muscle wasting.*

NIC Elimination Management

Impaired urinary elimination related to sensory and neuromuscular impairment

- Perform intermittent catheterization per protocol.
- Monitor intake and output. Maintain fluid intake at 2000 ml/day unless contraindicated.
- Acidify urine with foods such as orange juice and cranberry juice *to minimize potential for infection.*
- Administer urinary tract germicides (e.g., methenamine mandalate [Mandelamine]) as ordered.

NIC Coping Assistance

Chronic confusion related to organic or cognitive impairment

Impaired thought processes related to progressive dementia

Powerlessness related to sensory and neuromuscular impairment

Impaired adjustment related to impaired cognition

- Evaluate previous interests.
- Ensure optimal sensory input (e.g., eyeglasses, hearing aid) is available.
- Evaluate stimulation threshold *to prevent overstimulation.*
- Provide for structured repetitive group activities.
- Provide rest periods between activities *to minimize fatigue.*
- Monitor for changes in physical, functional, and psychologic status.

- Maintain calm, reassuring demeanor when interacting with patient *to promote sense of trust.*
- Encourage patient to participate in care as tolerated *to minimize feelings of powerlessness.*
- Provide positive feedback for tasks/activities that are mastered.
- Assist patient to reestablish as much physiologic control as condition allows.
  - Share information about physiologic functioning with the patient.
  - Focus on functions that remain intact.
- Assist patient to reestablish some means of psychologic control.
  - Encourage patient to express feelings as long as possible.
  - Encourage patient to participate in care as long as able to do so.
  - Encourage patient to become an active decision maker about care and immediate environment as able.
- Encourage patient to express feelings and fears regarding disease and disabilities.
- Assist patient to examine own responses to the threatening situation.
- Avoid judgment, criticism, or belittling of feelings and ideas.
- Encourage focus on remaining strengths and intact roles.
- Support patient's spiritual beliefs.
- Assist patient to develop problem-solving skills regarding disappointments and dissatisfactions.
- Assist patient to develop a stress management plan with simple relaxation exercises, self-monitoring activities, and use of imagery.

Social isolation related to altered mental status

- See Functional Health Pattern VII in Chapter 23.

NIC LIFE SPAN CARE

Caregiver role strain related to severity of patient's illness

Impaired family processes related to situational transition and/or crisis

Anticipatory grieving related to potential for loss of loved one

- Obtain assistance with meeting of caregiver role.
- Assist caregiver to identify/utilize caregiving resources such as family members, friends, or community agencies.
- Assist caregiver to develop plan of care with paced direct-care activities.
- Assist caregiver to develop support systems with alternate caregivers/friends.
- Assist caregiver to identify and address personal healthcare needs.
- Assist family to identify and understand what is occurring as specifically as possible *to focus on the situational factors.*
- Assist family to redefine situation in favorable terms.
- Support family in efforts to clarify family interactions.
- Assist family to express ideas assertively *to resolve the problem or situation.*
- Assist family in exploring alternatives for problem solution.
- Provide family with information about dynamics that enhance family's problem-solving skills.
- Assist family in identification of consequences of proposed options for resolutions of the problem.
- Support family members in efforts to implement problem resolution.
- Assist family in evaluating effectiveness of problem solving.
- Encourage patient and family to identify and describe their perceptions of potential loss.
  - Provide family with ongoing information regarding patient's progress, care, and prognosis.
  - Encourage family to express need for information and desires in caring for the patient.
  - Facilitate family participation in patient's care as appropriate *to decrease feelings of isolation and loss.*
  - Arrange flexible visiting hours *to promote family interactions.*
  - Assist patient and family to share feelings, concerns, and fears with each other.
  - Assist family members to maintain own self-care needs *to promote and maintain physical health.*
  - Evaluate need for referral to resources such as the social services department.
- During period of mourning before patient's death:
  - Promote expression of what family expects when death occurs.
  - Discuss indicators of impending death as appropriate.
  - Provide comfort measures for the patient.
  - Encourage family to maintain verbal communication and touch with patient even though patient may not respond.
  - Provide privacy to protect patient and family dignity.

PATIENT EDUCATION/CONTINUUM OF CARE PLAN

1. Discuss each medication's dosage, time of administration, purpose, and side effects.
2. Reinforce physician's explanation of medical management.
3. Emphasize need to avoid taking over-the-counter medications without notifying the physician.
4. Emphasize need for adequate nutritional status.
   a. Give diet as tolerated.
   b. Offer small, frequent feedings.
   c. Instruct to chew thoroughly and eat slowly and in small pieces.
5. Emphasize need for activity and exercise to tolerance.
   a. Plan activities of daily living.
   b. Maintain rest periods as planned.
   c. Do active and passive ROM exercises.
   d. Get at least 8 hours of sleep at night, if possible.
6. Encourage independent activities, as possible.
   a. Alert patient to limitations.
   b. Avoid overprotection.
   c. Stress need for supportive devices, as indicated.
7. Emphasize importance of ongoing outpatient care.
8. Give outpatient, home nursing care, or extended care facility referral, as appropriate.
9. Emphasize safety measures: side rails, ramps, shower chairs, walkers, and canes.

Evaluation/Patient Outcomes

Risk Management: Patient demonstrates minimal complications of sensory/perceptual alterations. Level of orientation is optimum. Patient is free of injury. Self-care deficits are minimum. Safety measures are appropriate to physiologic status. Skin integrity is maintained. Skin is free of bruises, burns, abrasions, and redness. Environment is safe. Patient is free of nosocomial infections. Airway is patent. Vital signs are stable.

Respiratory Management: Patient reports/demonstrates no signs of choking. Breath sounds are normal. Nasoenteric tube placement is verified.

Self-Care Facilitation: Patient demonstrates minimal self-care deficits. Outcome criteria listed for impaired physical mobility are met. Level of self-care activities is appropriate to physiologic status. Patient participates in physical and occupational therapy.

Actual and potential causes of disturbances for inadequate sleep are identified. Management plan to correct or minimize causes of inadequate sleep is developed. Patient verbalizes feelings of being rested or refreshed.

Nutrition Support: Patient demonstrates adequate nutritional status. Weight pattern is stable. Intake and output pattern is stable. Diet is appropriate to physiologic status. Skin turgor is good. Fluid and electrolyte balance is maintained. Patient takes dietary supplements as appropriate.

Immobility Management: Patient demonstrates an optimum level of mobility. Skin integrity is maintained. Patient remains free of contractures and deformities. Level of mobility is appropriate to physiologic status. Intake and output pattern is stable. Nutritional status is adequate. Patient is free of thrombophlebitis. Patient is free of local infection. Patient participates in an ongoing physical therapy program.

Skin/Wound Management: Patient demonstrates skin integrity. Skin is intact. Nutritional status is adequate. Electrolyte balance is maintained. Patient is free of pressure sores and contractures.

Elimination Management: Patient demonstrates minimum complications from alterations in urinary elimination patterns. Intake and output pattern is stable. Urine is clear, yellow to amber in color, and without sediment. Skin in perineal area is clean and dry. Urine is acidic (pH 6.0). Patient is free of urinary tract infections. Patient is free of bladder distention. Patient or family can describe symptoms of urinary tract infections that require medical intervention.

Coping Assistance: Patient demonstrates minimal confusion/thought process alterations. Available sensory aids (e.g., eyeglasses, hearing aid) are used appropriately. Patient is able to participate in structured repetitive group activities. Rest periods between activities are maintained. Patient is able to participate in care to tolerance.

Patient demonstrates minimal feelings of powerlessness. Optimum level of physiologic control, as possible for current health status, is maintained. Optimum level of psychologic control, as possible, is maintained. Patient participates, as possible, in decision making about care. Patient participates, as possible, in self-care.

Patient demonstrates social participation. Patient states importance of interpersonal relationships. Patient relates to self and others. Patient participates, as possible, in unit and group activities. Patient participates, as possible, in family activities.

Life Span Care: Caregiver demonstrates minimal role strain. Caregiver appropriately uses available resources. Caregiver develops adequate support systems. Caregiver addresses personal needs.

Patient's family demonstrates intact family processes. Family demonstrates role congruence. Family demonstrates clear communication. Family demonstrates constructive interactions. Family achieves resolution to the problem situation. Family learns and uses new approaches to problem solving.

Patient and family demonstrate constructive anticipatory grief work. Patient and family demonstrate ability to discuss thoughts and feelings about impending loss. Patient and family verbalize needs for information. Patient and family demonstrate appropriate use of available resources. Patient's family demonstrates ability to meet ongoing self-care needs. Patient (as appropriate) and family participate in mutual decision making regarding anticipated loss. Patient and family demonstrate constructive interactional patterns.

Patient demonstrates effective coping mechanisms. Patient is able to express fears and concerns. Patient participates in care as able.

Amyotrophic Lateral Sclerosis

Amyotrophic lateral sclerosis (ALS; Lou Gehrig's disease) is a relentlessly degenerative, fatal disease of the upper and lower motor neurons of the cortex, brainstem, and spinal cord. It is characterized by atrophy of the muscles of the hands, forearms, and legs that eventually spreads to involve most of the body.[3]

ALS is the most common variant of motor neuron disease (MND). Possible causes of the disorder include exposure to heavy metals, lymphoma, viral infections, gammopathy, and hexosaminidase A deficiency. ALS has also occurred in association with the HIV virus. Other hypotheses of causation include autoimmune destruction and motor neuron death by excitotoxic neurotransmitters.

ALS usually occurs between ages 40 and 70 years, but it also may occur in the very aged. The disorder has an annual incidence of 0.4 to 1.76 per 100,000 population, and the incidence increases with each decade of life. The majority (95%) of cases are sporadic, but 5% are familial, resulting from some type of inherited autosomal dominant gene. Men have a higher incidence, and the disease is more common among whites than blacks. The disorder usually is fatal within 2 to 3 years after diagnosis, with death primarily caused by respiratory failure. However, a small number of the patients may survive for up to 10 years.

Pathophysiology

ALS is characterized by deterioration of the anterior horn cells. Atrophy of the cortex, particularly of the precentral gyrus, may be grossly apparent in the cerebrum. Other pathologic changes include reduced numbers and size of the Betz cells of the motor cortex. In the brainstem there is a loss of the motor neurons except for those serving the extraocular muscles. In the spinal cord there is a loss of large motor neurons and degeneration of the corticospinal tract.[2] The surviving motor neurons are atrophic and show pyknotic nuclei. The loss of the anterior horn cells results in denervation of the muscle fibers.

Diagnostic Studies and Findings

Serum: Creatinine phosphokinase (CPK) slightly elevated when there is rapidly progressive muscle weakness and atrophy
CSF sampling: Protein normal or slightly elevated with normal IgG concentration and normal cell count
Myelography: Normal or shrunken spinal cord
MRI: Some atrophy of motor cortices and degeneration of motor tracts in the spinal cord and brainstem
Muscle biopsy: Abnormalities and changes of denervation
Electromyography: Widespread fibrillations and fasciculations indicating muscle wasting and denervation

Multidisciplinary Plan

No specific treatment for amyotrophic lateral sclerosis has been established. Therapy is primarily supportive in nature.

Surgery

Cricopharyngeal myotomy to alleviate dysphagia
Cervical esophagostomy
Transtympanic neurectomy to control neural supply to parotid glands (to decrease salivation)
Tracheostomy
Gastrostomy or jejunostomy tube placement

Medications

Riluzole (Rilutek), 50 mg PO q12h
Antianxiety agents (also used for muscle relaxant effect)
- Diazepam (Valium), 5 mg PO bid to tid
- Lorazepam (Ativan), 1 mg PO bid

Muscle relaxants (for spasticity): Baclofen (Lioresal), 5 mg PO tid; up to 15-25 mg PO tid (therapy initiated at low dosage and increased gradually until optimum results are achieved)

General Management

Cardiac monitoring
Mechanical ventilation (respiratory support)
Long-term assisted ventilation
Splints to support weakened muscles/limbs
Physical therapy to maintain muscle strength
Psychosocial counseling and support
Nutritional support: Soft or liquid diet
Occupational therapy to assist with performance of activities of daily living (ADLs)
Community referrals
Social service referral
Available resources: American Lateral Sclerosis Association (*www.alsa.org*)

NURSING CARE

Nursing Assessment

Symptoms of ALS vary, depending on which motor neuron cells are affected. The rate of progression of the disorder is "stuttered," with periods of stability followed by intervals of more rapid deterioration.

Muscle functioning
- Respiratory muscle paralysis
- Monitor pulse oximetry
- Monitor arterial blood gases
  - Report decrease in $Pa{O_2}$ of 10 to 15 mm Hg
  - Report increase in $Pa{CO_2}$ of 10 to 15 mm Hg
- Loss of swallow and choking reflex; increased risk of aspiration
- Assess ability to handle secretions and swallow
- Fasciculation of muscles; may be accompanied by weakness
- Upper extremity (usually unilateral) atrophy evident in palms and both sides of thumbs
- Loss of dexterity for fine hand movements
- Lower extremities (usually affected late): Spasticity and progressive weakness until flaccidity and atrophy occur

Sensory function: Not usually affected
Bulbar palsy: Fasciculations and atrophy of the tongue, dysphagia, dysphonia, dysarthria, excessive drooling (sialorrhea), choking
Reflexes: Progressive decrease, increase in pathologic reflexes
Mental faculties: Not affected
Altered communication: Weakened muscles of speech; patient's ability to communicate may be altered
Fear: Subjective statements of feeling fearful about health status and future lifestyle
Imbalanced nutrition: Dysphagia; determine need for enteral feedings; monitor recorded intake for nutritional content and calories; monitor laboratory values relevant to fluid deficit; monitor vital signs for dehydration

Potential Complications

Respiratory failure: Air hunger, shortness of breath, tachypnea, use of accessory muscles, flared nostrils; hypoxia: restlessness, confusion, cyanosis, tachycardia, hypotension, impaired motor function; hypercapnia: dizziness, headache, unconsciousness, hypertension, diaphoresis, flushed face
Aspiration: Subjective/objective sensation of choking/gagging; loud, sonorous respiration; air hunger; change in breath sounds; nausea/vomiting; change in level of consciousness

Patient Problems/Nursing Diagnoses & Interventions

NIC Respiratory Management

Ineffective airway clearance related to high risk for obstruction
Ineffective breathing pattern related to neuromuscular impairment

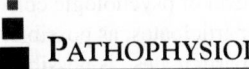

Impaired gas exchange related to ineffective breathing pattern
Risk for aspiration related to enteral feeding via nasogastric tube

- Maintain patent airway; avoid flexion of the neck if patient is comatose.
- Suction as needed *to prevent obstruction and manage secretions;* maintain equipment at bedside.
    - Hyperoxygenate with 100% oxygen with mechanical ventilator or manual resuscitation bag before and after suctioning *to prevent suction-induced hypoxia.*
    - Limit suctioning time to 15 seconds or less.
    - Monitor oxygen saturation ($Sa{O_2}$) before, during, and after suctioning.
    - Maintain universal precautions.
- Assist ventilation per protocol.
- Keep emergency drugs at the bedside.
- Remain with patient during meals *to monitor for choking and possible aspiration.*
- Confirm initial enteral tube placement by physician examination of chest x-ray.
- Confirm tube placement at least q8h; before and after each intermittent feeding
- Tape nasogastric tube in place securely.
- Elevate head of bed 30 to 40 degrees *to reduce risk of aspiration.*
- Keep suction equipment available *to maintain patent airway.*
- Hold feedings if residuals are greater than 150 ml, or more than 110% to 120% of hourly rate.
- Provide more frequent feedings in smaller amounts.
- Discontinue continuous feedings 30 to 45 minutes before activity/procedure that requires lowering the patient's head.
- Hold tube feedings if bowel sounds are absent and if diarrhea/constipation or nausea/vomiting are present.
- Add blue food coloring to tube feeding *to detect aspiration or fistula.*

NIC SELF-CARE FACILITATION

Feeding, bathing/hygiene, dressing/grooming and toileting self-care deficits related to neuromuscular impairment

- See general intervention strategies on pp. 249-250.

NIC IMMOBILITY MANAGEMENT

Impaired physical mobility related to progressive muscle weakness
Risk for disuse syndrome related to progressive muscle impairment

- Administer skeletal muscle relaxants *to reduce spasticity.*
    - Turn and reposition patient every 2 hours and as needed *to reduce potential for spasticity that occurs as a result of spinal cord involvement.*
    - Perform passive ROM exercises *to maintain muscle strength.*
- Use braces (hand splint, ankle-foot braces) *to maintain function.* Collaborate with physical therapy *to maintain maximal mobility and motor function.*
- Schedule activities and nursing care *to allow rest periods.*
- Teach family turning, positioning, and transfer techniques.
    - Maintain bowel program.
    - Provide nutritional foods and fluids *to maximize muscle strength.*
    - Consult nutritional services, as appropriate.

NIC NUTRITION SUPPORT

Imbalanced nutrition: less than body requirements, related to impaired ability to ingest food
Deficient fluid volume related to impaired ability to drink fluids

- Have suction equipment at bedside at all times *to prevent aspiration.*
- Administer anticholinergic drugs *to reduce oral secretions.*
- Have patient eat and drink in an upright position with neck flexed.
- Apply soft cervical collar if patient is unable to hold head upright.
- Maintain soft or liquid diet as indicated *to prevent aspiration.*
- Offer patient frequent, small feedings *to promote adequate nutrition and fluid intake.*
- Avoid mucus-producing foods such as milk *to control secretion production.*
- Institute intravenous, nasogastric, or gastric feedings per protocol *to provide adequate fluids and nutrition.*
    - Provide free water and tube feedings, as appropriate.
    - Weigh daily; maintain intake and output records *to ensure adequate intake.*
- Provide frequent mouth care.

NIC COMMUNICATION ENHANCEMENT

Impaired verbal communication related to neuromuscular impairment

- Develop a means of communication with patient.
    - When patient is restricted to eye or eyelid movement, develop a code with the patient.
    - Reinforce the techniques established.
    - Provide verbal prompts/reminders.
    - Use picture board, if appropriate.
    - Listen attentively.
- Assist patient and family to identify other outlets for communication.
- Continue to use sense of touch and nonverbal forms of communication.

PATIENT EDUCATION/CONTINUUM OF CARE PLAN

1. Encourage open verbalization of feelings and fears about loss of function, changes in body image, and dying.
2. Emphasize importance of maintaining planned rest periods.
3. Stress need for independence and socialization.
    a. Encourage self-care to tolerance.
    b. Encourage family to eat meals together for as long as possible.
4. Emphasize need to exercise to tolerance levels.
    a. Tell the patient to avoid fatigue.
    b. Teach the patient and family active exercises and ROM exercises.

5. Discuss name of each medication, dosage, frequency of administration, purpose, and toxic and side effects.
6. Stress need to check with physician before taking any over-the-counter medications.
7. Emphasize need to maintain fluid intake at 200 ml daily, unless contraindicated.
8. Discuss proper techniques for turning, positioning, and transfer.
9. Stress importance of ongoing outpatient care:
   a. Physician's visits
   b. Physical therapy
   c. Occupational therapy
   d. Home nursing care, if indicated
   e. ALS Foundation referral
10. Ensure that the patient and family can demonstrate application of hand splints and ankle-foot braces.

Evaluation/Patient Outcomes

Respiratory Management: Airway remains patent. Chest excursion is symmetric. Vesicular, bronchial, and bronchovesicular breath sounds are normal. Arterial blood gas values are within normal limits or consistent with patient's baseline. Vital signs are within normal limits or consistent with patient's baseline. Hemoglobin levels are 14 to 18 g/dl (male) or 12 to 16 g/dl (female). Intake and output are stable. There are no signs of respiratory distress. Skin tone is appropriate to racial background. Patient demonstrates/reports no episodes of choking. Nasoenteral tube placement is verified. Residuals are within acceptable range. No nausea, vomiting, diarrhea, or constipation is seen.

Self-Care Facilitation: Outcome criteria listed for impaired physical mobility are met. Level of self-care is appropriate to physiologic status. Patient participates in physical and occupational therapy.

Immobility Management: Skin integrity is maintained. Patient remains free of contractures or deformities. Patient demonstrates a level of mobility appropriate to physiologic status. Intake and output are stable. Nutritional status is adequate. There are no signs or symptoms of local infection.

Nutrition Support: Weight pattern is stable. Intake and output pattern is stable. Diet is appropriate to physiologic status. Skin turgor is good. There is fluid and electrolyte balance. Dietary supplements are taken, as appropriate.

Communication Enhancement: Patient verbalizes feelings as long as physically able to do so. Patient develops alternative methods of communication.

Multiple Sclerosis

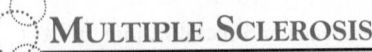

Multiple sclerosis (MS), or disseminated sclerosis, is a chronic disorder characterized by inflammation, demyelination, and gliosis (scarring) of brain, optic nerves, and spinal cord.

MS is the most prevalent of the human demyelinating diseases, with an incidence of 1.5 to 11 per 100,000 persons. Worldwide prevalence varies according to geography, with incidence increasing in temperate zones. Women are affected twice as often as men. In the United States the disease is twice as common in Caucasians as in African-Americans. The onset of symptoms most commonly occurs between ages 20 and 50 years. Incidence of the disease is rare in childhood, and the onset of symptoms rapidly decreases in old age. The severity, duration, and prognosis of MS vary. The diagnosis of this disorder is based on the presence of multiple lesions in the CNS and dissemination over time.

The cause of MS is unknown, but the most common hypothesis is that it is an autoimmune disease related in some way to a viral infection. Individuals with MS have elevated (i.e., up to twofold) serum and CSF titers of antibodies to many viruses, including herpes simplex type I, parainfluenza, rubella, mumps, measles, and Epstein-Barr virus.

Pathophysiology

The neuropathologic changes in MS include multifocal plaques of demyelination distributed randomly within the white matter of the brainstem, spinal cord, optic nerve, and cerebrum. The active changes include three essentially concurrent processes: breakdown of myelin structure, lysis of oligodendrocytes, and activation of astroglial processes.[2] Within the cerebrum there is a predilection of plaques in the periventricular areas, particularly around the third and fourth ventricles. A mild lymphocytic meningitis mainly in deep sulcal recesses may accompany the parenchymal changes. The external surface of the brain appears normal. Brain weight may be diminished, and the ventricles may be enlarged. The most characteristic feature of the chronic lesions is a proliferation of astrocytic processes, which transform the lesion into a glial scar. As lesions age, the lipid products of myelin breakdown are phagocytosed.

During the demyelination process (termed *primary demyelination*) the myelin sheath and the myelin sheath cells are destroyed. The demyelination process leads to four significant central disturbances: a decrease in nerve conduction velocity, nerve conduction block (frequency related), differential rate of transmission of impulses, and complete failure of impulse transmission. These disturbances account for the variety of clinical signs and symptoms. Symptom remission occurs when demyelinated areas are healed by sclerotic tissue. However, when the nerve fiber degenerates, symptoms become permanent. The clinical course of multiple sclerosis is classified as follows[3]:

1. Relapsing-remitting: Discrete motor, sensory, visual, or cerebellar attacks that begin over a 1- to 2-week period, and resolve in 4 to 8 weeks, with or without treatment with corticosteroids. Patient returns to preattack baseline.
2. Relapsing-remitting progressive (transitional): Patient experiences acute attack but does not return to preattack baseline and develops progressive disability.
3. Progressive: Patient experiences progressive worsening of disabilities with no periods of stability.
4. Stable MS: Patient has had no clinical disease activity and reports no subjective worsening in condition over the previous 12 months.

DIAGNOSTIC STUDIES AND FINDINGS

CSF sampling: Mononuclear cell pleocytosis, elevation in the level of total immunoglobulin G (Ig), and presence of oligoclonal Ig; elevated total protein
CT scan: Hypodense areas in white matter; may show ventricular enlargement and cerebral atrophy (with long-term disease)
MRI scan (serial): Disseminated lesions predominately in periventricular white matter, corpus callosum, cerebellar punduncles, brainstem, and spinal cord
Visual evoked potentials (VEP): Increased latency

MULTIDISCIPLINARY PLAN

Surgery

Contralateral thalamotomy
Rhizotomy
Nerve root blocks
Tenotomy
Myotomy

Medications

Methotrexate (Rheumatrex), 7.5 mg PO q wk
Azathioprine (Imuran), 2-3 mg/kg PO qd
2-Chloradeoxyadenosine (Cladribine), 0.1 mg/kg qd times 1 wk every month for 4 mo
Immunotherapy
Interferon beta-1b (Betaseron), 1 ml, SC, qod
Interferon beta-1a (Avonex), 30 μg IM weekly
Glatiramer acetate (Copaxone), 20 mg SC qd
ACTH: Aqueous ACTH, 80 U/500 ml D_5W IV over 6-8 h for 3 days, followed by ACTH gel, 40 U, IM bid for 7 days, followed by tapering of 35 U, IM bid for 3 days; 30 U bid IM for 3 days; 50 U IM qd for 3 days; 40 U IM qd for 3 days; 30 U IM qd for 3 days; 20 U IM qd for 3 days; 20 U IM qod for 3 doses
Corticosteroids: Methylprednisolone (Solu-Medrol), 1000 mg IV for 5 days with or without oral taper (given for acute attacks)
Muscle relaxants
Dantrolene sodium (Dantrium), initial dose of 25 mg PO qid; maintenance dose up to 400 mg/day
Tizanidine hydrochloride (Zanaflex), initial dose of 4 mg PO q8h, then increase dose in 2- to 4-mg steps to optimum effect
Baclofen (Lioresal), 15-25 mg PO tid (institute slowly to avoid sedation and weakness)
Baclofen, 200-800 μg/day via implanted intrathecal infusion pump
Pain (neuralgia and dyesthesias)/depression
Phenytoin (Dilantin), 300 mg/day PO
Carbamazepine (Tegretol), 100-1200 mg/day PO in divided doses
Amitriptyline hydrochloride (Elavil), 50-200 mg/day PO
Anticholenergics
Oxybutyrin (Ditropan), 5 mg PO bid or tid
Propantheline (Pro-Banthine), 7.5-30 mg PO tid
Hyoscyamine (Levsin), 0.125-0.25 mg PO q4h
Plasmapheresis

General Management

Braces
Splints
Wheelchair, walker, cane
Nutritional consultation
Physiotherapy
Occupational therapy
Home nursing services
Extended care facility referrals
Hydrotherapy
Speech therapy
Social services
Home health consultation
Resources available: National Multiple Sclerosis Society *(www.nmss.org)*

NURSING CARE

NURSING ASSESSMENT

Sensory symptoms: Numbness and tingling of involved extremity or face; loss of joint sensation and proprioception (generally accompanies extremity edema); loss of sense of position, shape, texture, and vibration (50% of patients)
Ocular symptoms: Optic neuritis (pain with eye movement, visual clouding, decrease in visual field); internuclear ophthalmoplegia (INO): delay of adduction of one eye with nystagmus of the abducting eye on lateral gaze
Diplopia: Marcus-Gunn phenomenon (failure to maintain pupillary constriction when light is shined into eye); swinging-flashlight sign (dilation of affected pupil when light is moved from intact eye to eye with defect)
Motor symptoms: Weakness in lower extremities (initially); decline in motor function after hot bath or shower (Uhthoff's phenomenon); incoordination; intentional tremors of upper extremities and ataxia of lower extremities; motor weakness and ability to carry out ADL varies; staggering gait and spastic weakness of speech muscles; facial palsy
Vestibular/Auditory functions: Vertigo
Mental/Behavioral symptoms: Anxiety, irritability, inattentiveness, emotional lability, mild depression, poor judgment; LATER: memory deficits, depression, confusion, disorientation, impaired communication patterns, dementia
Other: Hyperactive reflexes; positive Babinski's sign; ankle clonus (50%); impotence; loss or impairment of sphincter control; loss of abdominal reflexes (80%); Lhermitte's phenomenon: flexion of neck results in tingling and parenthesias into legs; Charcot triad (intentional tremors, nystagmus, and staccato speech) with brainstem involvement; urine and fecal incontinence; loss of swallow and gag reflex
Nutritional status changes: determine need for enteral feedings; monitor laboratory values relevant to fluid deficit; monitor vital signs for dehydration

POTENTIAL COMPLICATIONS

Aspiration: Coughing and/or gagging sensation; loud, sonorous respirations; air hunger; increase in adventitious breath sounds; nausea and/or vomiting; change in level of consciousness
Respiratory failure: Hypoxia: restlessness, confusion, cyanosis, tachycardia, hypotension, impaired motor function;

hypercapnia: dizziness, headache, unconsciousness, hypertension, diaphoresis, flushed face; air hunger, shortness of breath, tachypnea, use of accessory muscles, flared nostrils

Seizures: Pain or paresthesias in the face or a limb, followed by painful tonic contraction, lasting 1 to 2 minutes and occurring several times per day

Chronic pain: Verbal report or observed evidence of discomfort experienced for more than 6 months; guarding, protective movements; change in weight, appetite; fatigue; facial mask (of pain); physical and social withdrawal; hopelessness, helplessness; shortened attention span; altered perception of time; impaired thought processes; altered ability to participate in previous activities

Patient Problems/Nursing Diagnoses & Interventions

NIC Respiratory Management

Ineffective airway clearance related to decreased energy and fatigue

Ineffective breathing pattern related to musculoskeletal impairment

- Maintain patent airway and avoid flexion of the neck if patient is immobile.
- Suction as needed *to prevent obstruction.*
  - Hyperoxygenate with 100% oxygen before and after suctioning *to prevent suction-induced hypoxia.*
  - Limit suctioning time to 15 seconds or less.
- Maintain NPO status *to prevent risk of choking or aspiration.*
- Monitor for any increase in adventitious breath sounds *to detect possible aspiration.*
- Assist ventilation as indicated.
- Keep emergency drugs at bedside.

Risk for aspiration related to enteral tube feedings

- Confirm initial enteral tube placement by physician examination of chest x-ray.
- Confirm tube placement every 8 hours and as needed, before and after each intermittent feeding.
- Keep suction equipment at bedside *to maintain patent airway.*
- Tape enteral tube securely in place.
- Provide small frequent feedings.
- Hold tube feedings if residuals are greater than 150 ml or more than 110% to 120% of hourly rate.
- Elevate head of bed 30 to 40 degrees *to reduce risk of aspiration.*
- Discontinue feedings 30 to 45 minutes before any activity/procedure that involves lowering the patient's head.

NIC Self-Care Facilitation

Bathing/hygiene, dressing/grooming, feeding, and toileting self-care deficits related to neuromuscular weakness

- Assist with daily hygiene care, as indicated.
- Assist with feeding, as indicated:
  - Use of hand braces
  - Use of IV or nasogastric feedings, as ordered
- Administer oral hygiene every 2 hours and as needed.
- Administer eye care every 2 to 4 hours.
- Perform intermittent catheterization as per protocol *to maintain adequate bladder elimination and prevent infection.*
- Maintain bowel function with regular evacuation.

NIC Nutrition Support

Imbalanced nutrition: less than body requirements, related to decreased strength and ability to ingest food

- See general intervention strategies on p. 247.

NIC Elimination Management

Impaired urinary elimination related to neuromuscular impairment

- See general intervention strategies on p. 255.

Patient Education/Continuum of Care Plan

1. Discuss nature of multiple sclerosis and treatment modalities (explain procedures as they occur).
2. Stress importance of routines for activities of daily living.
3. Emphasize importance of avoiding fatigue, overwork, and emotional stress.
4. Stress importance of regular exercise and planned rest periods.
5. Emphasize importance of diversional activities.
6. Stress importance of speech therapy, physical therapy, and occupational therapy.
7. Encourage verbalization about feelings.
8. Emphasize need for socialization with significant others.
9. Stress need for independence and self-care to level of tolerance.
   a. Support the patient when ambulating.
   b. Help the patient to walk with a wide base.
10. Discuss symptoms of disease progression and flu or cold to report to the physician.
11. Emphasize need to avoid persons with upper respiratory infections.
12. Stress need to avoid extremes of hot and cold.
13. Discuss the name of medication, dosage, frequency of administration, purpose, and toxic or side effects.
14. Emphasize importance of avoiding over-the-counter medication.
15. Stress importance of ongoing outpatient care.
   a. Physician's visits
   b. Physical therapy
   c. Speech therapy
   d. Occupational therapy
   e. Home nursing services
   f. MS Society referral
16. Ensure that the patient and family demonstrate the following:
   a. Active and/or passive ROM exercises
   b. Proper techniques of ambulation
   c. Proper techniques for turning, positioning, and transfer
   d. Application of hand splints and braces
   e. Methods for maintaining patient safety

17. Ensure the patient understands factors that exacerbate symptoms of multiple sclerosis.
    a. Overexertion
    b. Hot baths
    c. Fever
    d. Emotional stress
    e. Cold
    f. High humidity
    g. Pregnancy

Evaluation/Patient Outcomes

Respiratory Management: Airway is patent. Chest excursion is symmetric. Breath sounds are normal, or there is no increase in adventitious sounds. Arterial blood gas values are within normal ranges or consistent with patient's baseline. Hemoglobin levels are 14 to 18 g/dl (male) or 12 to 16 g/dl (female). Intake and output are stable. There are no signs of respiratory distress. All lobes are resonant on percussion. Skin color is not cyanotic.

No report/observation of coughing or choking sensation. Abdomen soft with normal bowel sounds. Tube placement is verified with each tube feeding. Pattern of residuals is within acceptable range. No signs of nausea, vomiting, diarrhea, or constipation are present.

Self-Care Facilitation: Level of orientation is optimum. Patient remains free of injury. Skin integrity is maintained. Nutritional status is adequate. Self-care deficits are minimal. Participation in care is appropriate to physiologic status.

Nutrition Support: Weight pattern is stable. Intake/output pattern is stable. Diet is appropriate. Good skin turgor is noted. Fluid and electrolyte balance is maintained.

Elimination Management: Intake and output patterns are stable. Urine is clear, yellow to amber in color, and without sediment. Skin in perineal area is clean and dry. Urine is acidic (pH 6.0). Patient remains free of urinary tract infections. Patient remains free of bladder distention. Patient can describe symptoms of urinary tract infections that require medical intervention. Patient remains free of constipation. Patient maintain regular bowel pattern.

Parkinson's Disease

Parkinson's disease (paralysis agitans) is a chronic, slowly progressive degeneration of the brain's dopamine neuronal systems. It is characterized by the clinical syndrome of masklike facies, trunk-forward flexion, muscle weakness and rigidity, shuffling gait, resting tremors, finger pill-rolling, and bradykinesia (Fig. 5-25).

The progressive, degenerative course of Parkinson's disease varies from individual to individual. Approximately 30% of persons with Parkinson's disease experience dementia.

The possible causes of Parkinson's disease include known genetic, viral, vascular, and toxic factors and many unknown factors. Parkinson's disease occurs in all ethnic groups; however, the incidence in African-Americans is one fourth that in Caucasians. A slightly larger proportion of men are affected. The disease has an incidence of about 1 to 2 per 1000 of the general population. The disorder is uncommon in individuals under age 40 years, with the mean age of onset at 60 years. The prevalence of Parkinson's disease increases with age. Familial cases are rare.

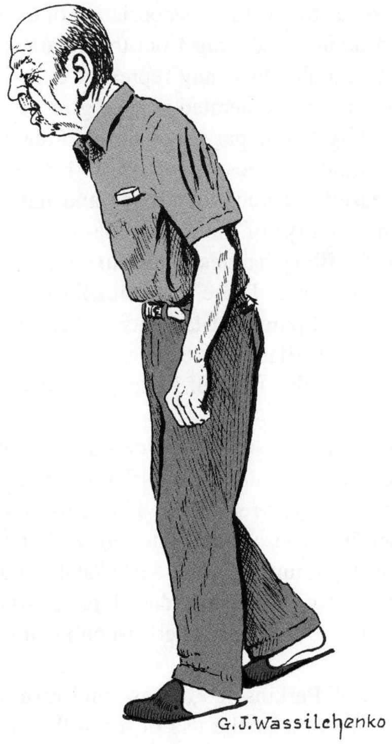

Fig. 5-25
Posture and shuffling gait associated with Parkinson's disease. (From Rudy.[11])

Recent advances in the treatment of Parkinson's disease include the transplantation of fetal midbrain dopaminergic (nigral) cells into the putamen of individuals with the disorder. Fetal nigral transplantation remains experimental, and any long-term benefits are unknown. The transplantation of autologous adrenal medullary tissue into patients with Parkinson's disease has produced mixed results and remains investigational

Pathophysiology

Parkinson's disease can be divided into three major types of pathophysiologic mechanisms: parkinsonism-dementia complex, Lewy body Parkinson's disease, and neurofibrillary tangle Parkinson's disease. Parkinsonism-dementia complex is unique to certain Pacific islands and is often associated with ALS. The pathologic characteristics of this complex include neurofibrillary tangles found throughout the neuraxis, atrophy of the thalamus and temporal and frontal lobes, and granulovascular degeneration in structures such as the hippocampus.

Lewy body Parkinson's disease involves the degeneration of the pigmented neurons of the substantia nigra and locus ceruleus. Other melanin-bearing neurons of the brainstem and spinal cord also degenerate, such as the dorsal motor nucleus of the vagal nerve and paravertebral ganglia. The surviving melanin-bearing cells contain structures known as Lewy bodies, which are cytoplasmic inclusions consisting of a central core of filamentous proteins. Radiating from the central core is a less dense array of tubules that may represent excess axoplasmic transport material or degenerated storage granules.

Neurofibrillary tangle parkinsonism demonstrates the following pathologic changes: atrophy of the cerebral cortex with an increased subarachnoid space and narrow gyri, depigmentation (usually) of the substantia nigra, and the presence of neurofibrillary tangles in the surviving neuronal cells of the substantia nigra. These neurofibrillary tangles consist of helically twisted pairs of filaments and result from proliferation of the neurofilaments. Studies suggest a possible relationship between this form of Parkinson's disease and viral encephalitis.

Iatrogenic parkinsonism, which closely resembles Parkinson's disease, may be induced by different drugs, such as the major tranquilizers or, rarely, methyldopa, α-methyl-paratyrosine, and reserpine. These agents interfere with the synthesis or the storage of dopamine or block the striatal dopamine receptors. The effects of chemical-induced parkinsonism are reversible within 1 to 2 weeks after discontinuation of the offending agent.

Progression of Parkinson's disease and resultant disabilities may be evaluated by the use of the following classification system:

Stage I	Unilateral involvement
Stage II	Bilateral involvement
Stage II	Mild to moderate impairment; impaired postural reflexes
Stage IV	Marked impairment; fully developed, severe disease
Stage V	Confined to bed or wheelchair

Diagnostic Studies and Findings

Serum examination: Mild microcytic anemia
Chest roentgenograms: Slight scoliosis
CT scan, skull films: Normal results (CT scan may show cerebral atrophy, with history of chronic dementia)
EEG: Normal results or shows minimum slowing and/or disorganization; with marked dementia and bradykinesia, may show moderate to marked slowing and diffuse disorganization
Swallowing studies: Abnormal pattern: delayed relaxation of cricopharyngeal muscles
Gastrointestinal studies: Hypomotility; delayed emptying of stomach; varying degrees of large bowel distention (frank megacolon in patients with severe constipation)

Multidisciplinary Plan

Surgery

Unilateral posteroventral pallidotomy
Stereotactic thalamotomy: Produces small lesion in ventrolateral nucleus of thalamus to alleviate contralateral tremor and rigidity
Gastrostomy or jejunostomy tube placement

Medications

Anticholinergic agents
Benztropine (Cogentin), 0.5-2 mg PO tid
Biperiden (Akineton), 1-3 mg PO qid
Procyclidine (Kemadrin), 2.5-10 mg PO tid
Trihexyphenidyl (Artane), 2-5 mg PO tid

Antiparkinsonism agents
Selegiline hydrochloride (Eldepryl), 5-10 mg/day PO in divided doses (use is controversial)
Carbidopa-Levodopa (Sinemet), 25-250 mg PO daily in divided doses
Amantadine (Symmetrel), 100-300 mg PO bid

Dopamine antagonists
Bromocriptine mesylate (Parlodel), 1.25 mg/day for 1 wk and 2.5 mg/day the next week; dose increased by 2.5 mg increments every week, depending on response and tolerance
Usual maintenance dose: 2.5-10 mg PO tid
Pergolide (Permax), 0.05 mg qd times 2 days; dose then increased by 0.1-0.15 mg/day every 3 days for 12 days, and by 0.25 mg PO every 3 days thereafter
Usual maintenance dose: 1 mg PO tid

Antidepressant agents:
Amitriptyline (Elavil), 75-150 mg/day PO

Insomnia agents
Diphenhydramine (Benadryl), 10-50 mg PO hs prn
Chloral hydrate, 1000 mg PO h prn
Trazodone (Desyrel), 50-150 mg, PO qd in divided doses

General Management

Heat massage
Walkers, canes, wheelchairs
Physical therapy
Bowel and bladder program
Nutritional program
Social services
Occupational therapy
Extended care facility referral
Speech therapy
Resources available: Parkinson's Disease Resource Center *(http//members.aol.com./healwell/parkinsons.htm)*

NURSING CARE

Nursing Assessment

Initial symptoms: Weakness, tendency to tremble (usually in one hand); slowness or awkwardness of affected limb; some loss of facial expression; deliberate quality of speech; tendency to maintain arm flexed at elbow; may progress to other side of the body after 1 to 2 years
Autonomic dysfunction: Increased secretion of sebum resulting in scaly erythematous eruptions of skin (particularly by ears and eyebrows and in scalp and nasolabial folds); intermittent, profuse diaphoresis; gastric retention; urgency or hesitancy in micturition; urinary retention; monitor intake and output; orthostatic hypotension; dysphagia
Equilibrium: Festination (leaning of the trunk farther and farther with each step)
Propulsion (forward stepping with leaning of trunk)
Retropulsion (backward stepping with leaning of trunk)
Lateropulsion (sidewise stepping with leaning of trunk)

Face: Masklike facies; decreased eye blinking

Gradual dementia: Monitor neurologic status on an ongoing basis

Initial: Forgetfulness, minor confusional episodes, depression

Later: Irritability, paranoia and visual hallucinations, frank delirium, social isolation

Hands: Fingers extended, with metacarpophalangeal joints flexed approximately 30 degrees

Handwriting: Letters becoming progressively smaller (micrographia), tremulous writing

Nutrition: Impaired deglutition; drooling; weight loss: determine need for enteral feedings; monitor laboratory values for fluid volume deficit and electrolyte imbalances; monitor vital signs for dehydration

Failure of cricopharyngeal muscles to relax/choking: Bowel dysfunction/constipation

Posture and rigidity: Shuffling gait without arm swing (see FIG. 5-25); akinesia (most evident in spinal musculature): cogwheel rigidity; bradykinesia; hypertonicity; stooped body posture; impaired mobility; self-care deficits

Speech: Involuntary repetition of sentences; decreased amplitude; soft, rapid monotone

Toes: Toe flexion with dorsiflexion of proximal phalanges; great toe may assume continuous dorsiflexion position

Tremors: Lips, jaws, tongue, facial muscles, axial muscles, and limb muscles; usually resting tremors (most apparent when affected area is at rest): paralysis agitans; "pill-rolling" motion of the hand

POTENTIAL COMPLICATIONS

Aspiration: Subjective/objective reports/signs of choking; air hunger; loud sonorous respirations; change in breath sounds

A change in level of consciousness

Nausea/vomiting

PATIENT PROBLEMS/NURSING DIAGNOSES & INTERVENTIONS

NIC RESPIRATORY MANAGEMENT

Risk for aspiration related to impaired swallowing

- Maintain patent airway.
- Maintain swallowing precautions.
- Maintain suction equipment nearby; suction as needed *to prevent obstruction.*
- Assist ventilation as indicated.
- Help patient select foods that are easy to swallow.
  - Remain with patient during meals.
  - Teach family members Heimlech maneuver.
- Give oral medications (crushed) in gelatin or custard.
- Provide frequent mouth care.

Acute or chronic confusion, chronic, related to organic or cognitive impairment

- Maintain hazard-free environment.
- Allow patient to maintain rituals that minimize anxiety.
- Ensure optimal sensory input (i.e., eyeglasses, hearing aid) is available.
- Provide adequate surveillance/supervision.
- Minimize stimulation *to prevent overstimulation.*
- Provide for structured repetitive group activities.
- Provide adequate rest and proper nutrition.
- Maintain calm, reassuring demeanor when interacting with patient *to promote sense of trust.*
- Provide positive feedback for tasks/activities that are mastered.

NIC IMMOBILITY MANAGEMENT

Impaired physical mobility related to decreased neuromuscular functioning

- Administer medications in a timely fashion *to avoid symptom aggravation.*
- Collaborate with physical therapist *to maintain maximal mobility and motor strength.*
- Institute gait-retraining program if indicated *to maintain balance and to improve walking.*
- Apply splints and braces as indicated.
- Encourage patient to dress daily *to promote self-esteem.*
- Avoid shoes with laces or snaps.
- Avoid clothes with buttons; use zippers.
- Place head of bed or chair on blocks *to facilitate getting up.*
- Provide raised toilet seat and side rails *to facilitate sitting and standing.*
- Encourage outdoor ambulation (avoid extremes of hot and cold).

NIC SELF-CARE FACILITATION

Bathing/hygiene, dressing/grooming, and toileting self-care deficits related to impaired neuromuscular function

- Assist with daily hygiene care, as indicated.
- Perform intermittent urinary catheterization per protocol *to maintain adequate bladder elimination and to prevent infection.*
- Administer skin care every 2 to 4 hours and as needed *to remove skin oil and perspiration.*
- Perform ROM exercises *to prevent stiffness, muscle wasting, and contractures.*
- Assist with feeding, as indicated.
  - Use of hand braces
  - Use of IV or nasogastric feedings, as ordered
- Administer oral hygiene every 2 hours and as needed *to control drooling.*
- Administer eye care every 2 to 4 hours *to remove crustations.*
  - Maintain regular bowel evacuation program.

NIC NUTRITION SUPPORT

Imbalanced nutrition: less than body requirements, related to impaired neuromuscular function

Risk for fluid volume deficit related to inability to drink sufficient fluids

- Promote oral intake of fluids as appropriate.
- Offer small, frequent feedings *to minimize risks of dysphagia and aspiration.*
- Encourage a high-bulk, high-roughage diet. Provide supplements as needed. Control protein intake *to minimize blocking of effects of L-dopa.*

- Complete nursing care before mealtimes.
- Apply braces to minimize tremors.
- Allow ample time for eating and keep food warm.
  Place utensils within easy reach.
  Cut foods for patient.
  Use blender for thick foods.
- Use bib or straw as indicated.
- Weigh daily; monitor intake for calories and nutrition.

NIC Elimination Management

Constipation related to neuromuscular impairment
Impaired urinary elimination related to neuromuscular impairment

- Administer urinary tract germicides as ordered.
- Maintain regular bowel evacuation with stool softeners, rectal suppositories, mild cathartics, and natural laxatives such as prune juice.
- Provide high-residue diet *to promote gastrointestinal motility.*
- Monitor intake and output. Maintain fluid intake at 2000 ml/day unless contraindicated.
- Perform intermittent catheterization per protocol.
- Monitor urine for sediment, concentration, color, and odor.
- Acidify urine with foods such as orange juice and cranberry juice *to minimize potential for infection.*
- Maintain activity level to tolerance.

NIC Communication Enhancement

Impaired verbal communication related to neuromuscular status

- Evaluate patient's ability to communicate and develop means of communication with the patient, such as pad and pencil, Magic Slate, call light.
- Teach patient to speak in a slow, unhurried manner. Provide electronic amplifiers as needed *to augment decreased amplitude of speech.*
- Obtain referral for speech therapy.
  Provide verbal prompts/reminders.
  Use picture board, if appropriate.
  Listen attentively.
- Assist patient and family to identify other outlets for communication.
- Continue to use sense of touch and other nonverbal forms of communication.

NIC Behavior Therapy

Social isolation related to alterations in mental status

- See Functional Health Pattern VII in Chapter 23.

NIC Life Span Care

Caregiver role strain related to severity of patient's illness

- Assist caregiver to identify/use caregiving resources such as family members, friends, and community agencies.
- Assist caregiver to develop plan of care with paced direct-care activities.
- Assist caregiver to develop support systems with alternate caregivers/friends.
- Assist caregiver to identify and address personal health care needs.

Patient Education/Continuum of Care Plan

1. Discuss causes, symptoms, and treatment modalities for Parkinson's disease (explain procedures as they occur).
2. Stress importance of verbalization about loss of self-esteem, sexuality, and body functions.
3. Emphasize importance of verbalization about feelings.
4. Encourage social participation.
5. Emphasize capabilities.
6. Encourage independence and self-care; avoid overprotection.
7. Stress need for daily exercise program.
8. Emphasize need for high-calorie, low protein, soft diet; instruct the patient to eat slowly and take small bites.
9. Stress need for diversional activities.
10. Discuss safety measures to prevent injury.
11. Emphasize need for speech therapy.
12. Stress need for frequent skin care and oral hygiene.
13. Emphasize need for bowel and bladder programs.
14. Discuss name of medication, dosage, frequency of administration, purpose, and toxic or side effects.
15. Ensure that the patient understands he or she must take medications with food to reduce gastric irritation and nausea.
16. Stress importance of ongoing outpatient care.
    a. Physician's visits
    b. Physical therapy
    c. Home nursing care
    d. Parkinson's Disease Information Center; Parkinson's Foundation

Evaluation/Patient Outcomes

Respiratory Management: There are no subjective or objective findings of shortness of breath, air hunger, coughing, or choking. Tube placement is verified with each feeding. Abdomen is soft with normal bowel sounds. There is no nausea, vomiting, diarrhea, or constipation. Tube feeding residuals are within acceptable range. Available sensory aids are used appropriately. Patient is able to participate in structured repetitive group activities.

Immobility Management: Patient demonstrates optimum level of mobility. Skin integrity is maintained. There are no contractures or deformities. Patient's level of mobility is appropriate to physiologic status. Intake and output pattern is stable. Nutritional status is adequate. There is no thrombophlebitis. There is no local infection. Patient participates in an ongoing physical therapy program.

Self-Care Facilitation: Patient demonstrates minimum self-care deficits. Outcome criteria listed for impaired physical mobility are met. Level of self-care activities is appropriate to physiologic status. Patient participates in physical and self-care activities to tolerance.

Nutrition Support: Patient demonstrates adequate nutritional status. Weight pattern is stable. Intake and output pattern is stable. Diet is appropriate to physiologic status. Skin turgor is good. Fluid and electrolyte balance is maintained. Patient takes dietary supplements, as appropriate.

Elimination Management: Patient demonstrates minimum complications from alterations in urinary elimination patterns. Urine is clear, yellow to amber in color, and without sediment. Skin in perineal area is clean and dry. Urine is acidic (pH 6.0). Patient is free of urinary tract infections. Patient is free of bladder distention. Patient can describe symptoms of urinary tract infections that require medical intervention. Fluid intake is adequate (2000 ml/day unless contraindicated). Intake and output patterns are stable. Patient remains free of fecal impaction. Patient demonstrates a regular bowel evacuation pattern.

Communication Enhancement: Patient verbalizes feelings for as long as physically able to do so. Patient develops alternative methods of communication.

Behavior Therapy: Patient demonstrates social participation. Patient states importance of interpersonal relationships. Patient relates to self and others. Patient participates, as possible, in unit and group activities. Patient participates, as possible, in family activities.

Life Span Care: Caregiver demonstrates minimal role strain. Caregiver appropriately uses available resources. Caregiver develops adequate support systems. Caregiver addresses personal needs.

Myasthenia Gravis

Myasthenia gravis is a neuromuscular disease involving lower motor neurons and muscle fibers that is characterized by abnormal fatigue and motor weakness of skeletal muscles that increases with effort and improves with rest. Voluntary muscles most commonly affected in myasthenia gravis include the oculomotor, facial, laryngeal, pharyngeal, limb, and respiratory muscles.

Muscle involvement may be focal (i.e., only extraocular muscles), regional (i.e., ocular and bulbar muscles), or generalized. The underlying problem is a defect in the number of acetycholine receptors (AChRs) at the postsynaptic muscle membrane.[3]

The cause of the deficiency of AChRs is unknown, although considerable data suggest that it is a systemic autoimmune disease. Myasthenia gravis is not a hereditary condition, but 15% of infants born to myasthenic mothers manifest transitory symptoms lasting from 7 to 14 days after birth. The incidence of myasthenia gravis is estimated at between 43 to 84 per million of the population. Myasthenia gravis affects all age groups, but there are two characteristic ages of onset: women between ages 20 and 30 years and men between ages 60 and 70 years. The course of myasthenia gravis is variable and is characterized by exacerbations and remissions.

Pathophysiology

Regardless of the cause of myasthenia gravis, the basic physiologic defect is that nerve impulses do not pass onto the skeletal muscle at the neuromuscular junction. This defect is characterized by the presence of AChR-ab and a reduction in the number of AChRs on the postsynaptic folds of the neuromuscular junction.[3] Although acetylcholine is released in normal amounts, there is insufficient depolarization of the postsynaptic membrane to initiate muscle excitation. The end result is extreme muscle weakness and fatigability. Myoid cells in the thymus, which have AChRs on their surface, may provide the source of autoantigen, which then triggers an autoimmune response in the gland itself. Involved skeletal muscles usually do not atrophy, and there is no loss of sensation.

Diagnostic Studies and Findings

Chest roentgenogram, CT scan of chest: May indicate presence of thymoma

Edrophonium (Tensilon) test: Intravenous injection of 1 mg of edrophonium chloride (Tensilon); if no symptoms (i.e., nausea, diarrhea, salivation, fasciculations, and syncope) occur within 1 minute, another 3 mg is injected. Many patients with myasthenia gravis will demonstrate improved muscle tone within 30 to 60 seconds of giving the initial 4 mg, and the test can be stopped at this point. If after 1 minute there is no improvement, another 3 mg is given; if there is still no response 1 minute later, the final 3 mg is injected. The test is positive when there is clear-cut improvement in muscle tone. (NOTE: Intravenous atropine, 0.4 mg, should be readily available in the event of sudden cardiorespiratory depression.)

Electromyogram (EMG): Muscle fiber contraction with rapid (i.e., greater than 10% to 15%) reduction in amplitude of evoked responses (NOTE: Anticholinesterase medications should be stopped 6 to 24 hours before testing.)

Anti-AChR radioimmunoassay (antibody detectable in 80% of individuals with myasthenia gravis): Four-panel test:

1. AChR-binding antibody test
2. AChR-modulating antibody test
3. AChR-blocking antibody test
4. Striational antibody test

CSF analysis: CSF protein levels elevate as disease progresses

IgA deficiency screening

Multidisciplinary Plan

Surgery

Tracheotomy (see Chapter 4)

Thymectomy
- Suprasternal approach
- Transsternal approach

Medications

Cholinesterase inhibitors (CEIs)
- Neostigmine bromide (Prostigmin), 7.5-45 mg PO q3-4h
- Pyridostigmine bromide (Mestinon), individualized size and frequency of dosage (average dose: 30-60 mg PO q4-6h)
- Ambenonium chloride (Mytelase), 2.5-5 mg PO q4-6h

Immunosuppressive drug therapy (used when symptoms are uncontrolled on CEIs)
Prednisone, 60-80 mg PO qod (dose gradually reduced at a rate of 10 mg every 1-2 mo)
Azathioprine (Imuran), 2-3 mg/kg/day PO
Cyclophosphamide (Cytoxan), 3-5 mg/kg/day PO (used for severe refractory myasthenia gravis)
Cyclosporine (Sandimmune), 3-5 mg/kg/day PO in two divided doses
High-dose intravenous immunoglobulin (IVIg), 0.4 g/kg/day IV over 5 consecutive days
Plasma exchange (plasmapheresis): Removes ACh receptor antibodies and results in rapid clinical improvement

General Management

Mechanical ventilation, if indicated
Bronchoscopy
Physical therapy
Occupational therapy
Social services
Swallow precautions
Resources available: Myasthenia Gravis Foundation of America *(www.myasthenia.org)*

NURSING CARE

NURSING ASSESSMENT

Eye muscles (usually affected first): Ocular palsy, ptosis (unilateral or bilateral); diplopia
Facial muscles: Masklike expression and mobility (weakness) of face; weak voice that may fade to a whisper; dysphagia; choking; aspiration, impaired swallowing; drooling; nasal speech
Neck muscles: Head bobbing up and down
Respiratory muscles: Breathlessness; respiratory weakness; reduced vital capacity
Other muscles: Stress incontinence; anal sphincter weakness
Other findings: Imbalanced nutrition (ability to chew and swallow is a factor); monitor intake for nutritional content and calories; monitor laboratory values for fluid deficit; monitor vital signs for dehydration
Reflexes: Normal or brisk

POTENTIAL COMPLICATIONS

Myasthenia gravis crisis: NOTE: Myasthenic crisis is a medical emergency characterized by respiratory failure and severe oropharyngeal weakness leading to aspiration. There may be respiratory distress; respiratory arrest; cyanosis; hypertension and tachycardia; diaphoresis; weak cough; dysphagia; weakness; improves with edrophonium
Cholinergic crisis: Respiratory distress; vertigo; blurred vision; sweating; lacrimation; salivation; anorexia; dysarthria; dysphagia; abdominal cramps; diarrhea; nausea and vomiting; muscular spasms or cramps; generalized muscle weakness; dyspnea and wheezing; bradycardia; hypotension; worse with edrophonium
Respiratory failure: Air hunger, shortness of breath, tachypnea, anxiety, use of accessory muscles, flared nostrils; hypoxia: confusion, restlessness, cyanosis, tachycardia, hypotension, impaired motor function; hypercapnia: dizziness, confusion, headache, unconsciousness, hypertension, diaphoresis, flushed face
Aspiration: Subjective/objective report/observation of choking; air hunger; loud sonorous respirations; change in breath sounds; change in level of consciousness; nausea/vomiting

PATIENT PROBLEMS/NURSING DIAGNOSES & INTERVENTIONS

NIC RESPIRATORY MANAGEMENT

Ineffective airway clearance related to impaired/weak cough reflex
Ineffective breathing pattern related to impaired neuromuscular function
Impaired gas exchange related to ineffective breathing pattern
Risk for aspiration related to enteral feedings

- Maintain patent airway, and avoid flexion of the neck if patient is comatose; monitor effectiveness of gag reflex.
- Suction as needed *to prevent obstruction.*
  - Hyperoxygenate with 100% oxygen before and after suctioning *to minimize suction-induced hypoxia.*
  - Limit suction time to 15 seconds or less *to minimize airway trauma and hypoxemia.*
  - Monitor Sao_2 before, during, and after suctioning *to detect any arrhythmias.*
- Assist ventilation as indicated.
- Keep emergency drugs and suction equipment at the bedside.
- Teach family members Heimlich maneuver. If patient has thymectomy, monitor for signs of pneumothorax, restlessness, tachycardia; maintain patency of chest tubes.
- Administer enteral feedings as ordered.
  - Confirm initial placement by physician evaluation of chest x-ray.
  - Confirm tube placement at least every 8 hours as necessary, and before and after each intermittent tube feeding.
  - Tape nasogastric tube securely in place.
  - Administer small, frequent feedings.
  - Hold tube feedings if residuals are greater than 150 ml, or more than 110% to 120% hourly rate.
  - Discontinue tube feedings 30 to 45 minutes before activity/procedure that requires patient's head to be lowered.
  - Elevate head of bed 30 to 40 degrees during administration of tube feeding.

NIC IMMOBILITY MANAGEMENT

Impaired physical mobility related to neuromuscular impairment

- See general intervention strategies on p. 249.

NIC SELF-CARE FACILITATION

Feeding, bathing/hygiene, dressing/grooming, and toileting self-care deficits related to neuromuscular impairment

- See general intervention strategies on pp. 249-250.

NIC NUTRITION SUPPORT

Imbalanced nutrition: less than body requirements, related to impaired swallowing

Risk for deficient fluid volume related to impaired swallowing

- Administer medications 30 minutes before eating *to maximize muscle strength needed for chewing and swallowing of food.*
- Maintain swallow precautions.
- Allow ample time for eating. Stay with patient.
- Encourage a high-protein, high-bulk, high-roughage diet.
- Give fluids, as appropriate.
- Accurately measure and record intake on a flow sheet.
- Administer parenteral fluids per protocol *to ensure adequate fluid intake.*
- Administer enteral feedings as ordered.
- Report any significant changes in the patient's weight.
- Obtain nutritional services consultation.

NIC COMMUNICATION ENHANCEMENT

Impaired verbal communication related to neuromuscular impairment

- Develop means of communication with patient: pad and pencil, Magic Slate, call light.
  Reinforce established techniques.
  Provide verbal prompts/reminders.
  Use picture board, if appropriate.
  Listen attentively.
- Teach patient to speak in a slow, unhurried manner *to avoid voice strain.*
- Obtain referral for speech therapy. Reinforce technique established.
- Assist patient and family to identify other outlets for communication.
- Continue to use sense of touch and other nonverbal forms of communication.

PATIENT EDUCATION/CONTINUUM OF CARE PLAN

1. Discuss names of medications, dosage, time of administration, purpose, and side effects. For anticholinesterase medications:
   a. Stress importance of dosage.
   b. Instruct patient to take at scheduled times.
   c. Instruct patient not to skip doses.
   d. Instruct patient to avoid taking with fruit, tomato juice, coffee, or other medications.
   e. Instruct patient to take medications with food to minimize gastric irritation and nausea.
   f. Inform patient of toxic side effects (i.e., diarrhea, abdominal cramping, muscular weakness).
2. Stress need to avoid taking over-the-counter medications without notifying the physician.
3. Discuss symptoms of progression or recurrence to report to physician.
4. Emphasize need to wear medical alert tag.
5. Stress importance of avoiding individuals with upper respiratory infection.
6. Discuss symptoms of upper respiratory infection to report to physician (i.e., chills, cough, low-grade temperature).
7. Stress need to avoid alcohol, tobacco, and prolonged exposure to heat or cold.
8. Emphasize need for adequate nutritional status.
   a. Give diet as tolerated.
   b. Arrange food and utensils so they can be managed by patient.
   c. Instruct to chew thoroughly, and eat slowly and in small pieces.
9. Stress need for activity and exercise to tolerance.
   a. Plan activities of daily living.
   b. Maintain rest periods as planned.
   c. Do active and passive ROM exercises.
   d. Get at least 8 hours of sleep at night.
10. Emphasize need for diversional activities.
11. Stress importance of avoiding physical and emotional stress.
12. Emphasize need for speech therapy.
13. Stress importance of avoiding constipation.
14. Emphasize importance of ongoing outpatient care.
15. Give available agencies for reference (e.g., Myasthenia Gravis Foundation).
16. Give outpatient or home nursing care referrals.

EVALUATION/PATIENT OUTCOMES

Respiratory Management: Airway is patent. Chest excursion is symmetric. Breath sounds are normal, or there is no increase in adventitious sounds. Arterial blood gas values are within normal ranges or consistent with patient's baseline. Vital signs are within normal ranges or consistent with patient's baseline. Hemoglobin levels are 14 to 18 g/dl (male) or 12 to 16 g/dl (female). Intake and output are stable. Cough is effective. There are no signs of respiratory distress. There are no subjective or objective findings of shortness of breath, air hunger, or dyspnea on exertion. All lobes are resonant on percussion. Skin is not cyanotic. No objective/subjective findings of nausea, vomiting, coughing, or choking. Abdomen is soft with normal bowel sounds. Tube feeding placement is verified. Pattern of tube feeding residuals is within acceptable range.

Immobility Management: Skin integrity is maintained. Patient is free of contractures and deformities. Level of mobility is appropriate to physiologic status. Intake and output pattern is stable. Nutritional status is adequate. Patient remains free of thrombophlebitis. Patient remains free of local infection.

Self-Care Facilitation: Outcome criteria stated for impaired physical mobility are met. Level of self-care is appropriate to physiologic status. Patient participates in physical and occupational therapy as physically able to do so.

Nutrition Support: Intake and output pattern is stable. Weight pattern is stable. Diet is appropriate to physiologic status. Dietary intake is high in calories and protein. Patient takes dietary supplements, as appropriate. Skin turgor is good. Fluid and electrolyte balance is maintained.

Communication Enhancement: Patient verbalizes feelings for as long as physically able to do so. Patient develops alternative methods of communication.

TUMORS

INTRACRANIAL TUMORS

Intracranial tumors (brain tumors) include both benign space-occupying (primary) and malignant (metastatic) lesions. The incidence of intracranial tumors in the United States is about 25,000 annually. Intracranial tumors can occur in any structural area of the brain and in all age groups. Growth rates range from the rapid growth of glioblastomas to the almost imperceptible changes of some meningiomas (FIG. 5-26).

Brain tumors are named according to the tissues from which they arise. Primary brain tumors include oligodendrogliomas, ependymomas, astrocytomas and glioblastomas, medulloblastomas, and meningiomas. Secondary or metastatic tumors include metastatic carcinoma or sarcoma. (See Chapter 18 for a discussion of malignant brain tumors.)

Gliomas

Oligodendrogliomas evolve slowly and may be detected on a routine skull roentgenogram because of intracranial calcification. The most common sites for oligodendrogliomas are the frontal and temporal lobes, but they are also found in the brainstem, cerebellum, and spinal cord. This type of tumor makes up only 5% of all intracranial tumors. There is a high incidence of this tumor among young adults who have a childhood history of temporal lobe epilepsy.

Ependymomas (grades I to IV) are fairly rare in the general adult population and make up only 6% of all intracranial tumors. They are more commonly found in young children and adolescents and account for 20% of brain tumors in this age group. Ependymomas form in the ependymal cells and astrocytes that line the walls of the cerebral ventricular system and most commonly affect the fourth ventricle.

Astrocytomas form in astrocyte cells at any level of the CNS. In the adult they are usually lateral and supratentorial, whereas astrocytes in children are in or near the midline. Cerebellar astrocytomas, which constitute 30% of all pediatric brain tumors, are usually located just lateral to the midline in the cerebellar hemisphere. Simple surgical excision provides a long survival rate. Brainstem astrocytomas primarily affect school-age children, who have a high mortality rate because of destruction of the local cranial nerve nuclei and the long tracts.

Cerebral astrocytomas are classified by grade (Table 5-7). Cerebral astrocytomas are common between ages 30 and 50 years, making up 30% of the brain tumors for this age group. These tumors have a growth rate proportional to their grade. For example, grades I and II grow slowly, whereas grades III and IV grow rapidly.[8]

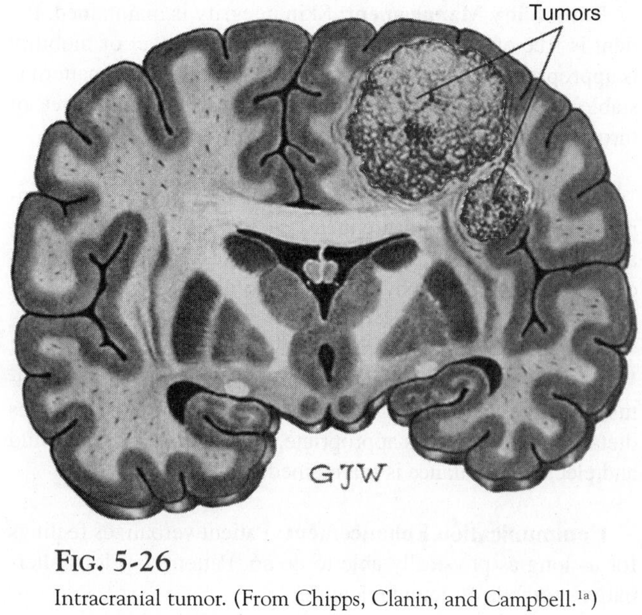

FIG. 5-26
Intracranial tumor. (From Chipps, Clanin, and Campbell.[1a])

Neuronal Cell Tumor

Medulloblastomas constitute 30% of brain tumors in children and 4% of brain tumors found in adults. Medulloblastomas are found in the posterior cerebellar vermis and roof of the fourth ventricle. The tumor eventually obstructs the flow of CSF from the aqueduct, resulting in hydrocephalus and cerebellar signs. Without irradiation the tumor is fatal; with irradiation there is a 30% survival rate.

Meningiomas are adult tumors arising from the cells of vessels, pia-arachnoid, and surrounding fibroblasts. Meningiomas make up 15% of all adult tumors of the CNS and its coverings. These tumors are found in the parasagittal falx of the frontal lobe, sylvian fissure region, olfactory groove wing of the sphenoid bone, superior surface of the cerebellum, and cerebellopontine angle. They occur more frequently in women and are found in approximately 40% to 50% of patients with von Recklinghausen's disease (neurofibromatosis). The symptoms of a meningioma are manifested as the tumor indents a local area of the brain and raises the ICP.

PATHOPHYSIOLOGY

An *oligodendroglioma* can be seen microscopically as small round cells with spherical nuclei. Many of these tumors have an astrocytic component; therefore recurrence of the tumor may have astrocytic characteristics.

An *ependymoma* has several variants. The myxopapillary ependymoma is a special variant occurring in adolescents. It develops in the fifth ventricle (ventriculus terminalis), formed by the caudal opening of the central canal of the spinal cord.

Table 5-7 Grades of Astrocytoma

Grade	Growth Rate	Prognosis
Astrocytoma		
Grade I	Slow	Good; 15-20 yr after surgery
Grade II	Slow	Good; 10-15 yr after surgery
Glioblastoma		
Grade III	Rapid, invasive	Poor; less than 2 yr without therapy
Grade IV (glioblastoma multiforme)	Rapid, invasive	Very poor; 6-9 mo without surgery

Generally symptoms of increased ICP are manifested when the ependymoma fills the fourth ventricle, blocking the flow of CSF.

An *astrocytoma* of low grade (I or II) is gelatinous and frequently indistinguishable from cerebral gliosis. This type of tumor is slow growing and infiltrative. Astrocytomas commonly arise in the white matter. Their cellularity is almost normal. Astrocytomas of grades III and IV are rapidly growing tumors characterized by a high degree of macroscopic necrosis. An astrocytoma of this grade is not confined to white matter and may grow into areas of the subarachnoid space and brainstem. These tumors are very cellular, pleomorphic, and necrotic and demonstrate marked endothelial proliferation.

A *medulloblastoma* arises in the caudal cerebellar vermis and is markedly cellular. The cells in the tumor have little cytoplasm and are undifferentiated. When medulloblastomas occur beyond the first decade of life, they arise more rostrally and laterally in the cerebellar hemispheres.

A *meningioma* may have one of several cell types, each with a different prognosis, depending on the cellular variety. The tumor cells are commonly uniform and may form characteristic whorls. Frequent locations for these tumors include the ethmoid regions, parasagittal region, sphenoid ridge, and dorsal roots of the spinal cord.

Regardless of the pathologic type of intracranial tumor, signs and symptoms reflect progressive neurologic deficits caused by focal disturbances and increased ICP. Focal disturbances are caused by increasing compression of brain tissue and the infiltration or direct invasion of brain parenchyma, resulting in destruction of neural tissue.[8] Cerebral blood supply may also be altered by the tumor's compression of blood vessels, resulting in necrotic cerebral tissue or seizures. Approximately 30% of adults with intracranial tumors develop focal or generalized seizure activity. Increased ICP may result from regional edema, alterations in CSF circulation, and increased tissue within the skull. Hydrocephalus results from disruption in the circulation of CSF from the cerebral ventricles to the subarachnoid spaces (FIG. 5-27).

The size and location of the specific tumor can cause shifts of brain tissue with associated brain herniation syndromes. If left untreated, herniation can lead to infarction and hemorrhage in the upper pons and the midbrain, resulting in pontomedullary decompensation.

DIAGNOSTIC STUDIES AND FINDINGS

Skull roentgenograms: Erosion of posterior clinoid process or presence of intracranial calcifications
Chest roentgenograms: Detection of primary lung tumor or metastatic disease
CT scan (with or without contrast): Identification of vascular tumors; shifts in midline structures; changes in cerebral ventricular sizes
MRI with gadolinium enhancement: Same as CT scan
EEG: Marked focal slowing (with rapidly developing tumors); rhythmic, periodic, and high-voltage slowing (with increased ICP)
Ophthalmoscopic examination: Papilledema (late sign of increased ICP)
Brain scan: Increased uptake of isotope in the tumor
Cerebral angiography: Cerebral vascularity; blood vessel deviations
Stereotaxic biopsy: Identifies histologic cell type

MULTIDISCIPLINARY PLAN

Surgery

ICP monitoring
Tumor excision or debulking; craniotomy (supratentorial; infratentorial)
Image-directed surgery
Shunting procedure to treat secondary complications of hydrocephalus
Ommaya reservoir for intraventricular chemotherapy

Medications

Corticosteroids: Dexamethasone (Decadron), 4 mg q6h PO
Anticonvulsants: Phenytoin (Dilantin), 100 mg PO tid
Phenobarbital (Luminal), 60-200 mg/day in single or divided dose PO
Gabapentin (Neurontin), 900-1800 mg/day in divided doses PO (Initial dose is usually titrated up over 3 days.)
Chemotherapeutic agents
Lomustine (CCNU), 100 mg/m^2 PO q6-8 wk
Carmustine (BCNU), 200 mg/m^2 (single dose or divided doses of 100 mg/m^2) IV q6 wk
Procarbazine (Matulane), 100-150 mg/m^2 PO for 10 days
Vincristine (Oncovin), 1-2 mg/m^2 IV q wk
Analgesic/antipyretics: Acetaminophen, gr X PO q4h prn
Histamine blocker: Famotidine (Pepcid), 20 mg PO bid

Radiation Therapy

Proton beam
Stereotactic radiosurgery with gamma knife or linear accelerator
Interstitial brachytherapy

General Management

Mechanical ventilation, if indicated
Controlled hyperventilation (for management of intracranial hypertension)
Cardiac monitoring
Nutritional consultation
Physical therapy
Speech therapy
Occupational therapy
Social services
Resources available: American Brain Tumor Association *(www.abta.org)*

NURSING CARE

NURSING ASSESSMENT

Neurologic disturbance: Gradually increasing weakness; subtle sensory loss; adult-onset seizures not always relieved by medications: monitor for effects and side effects of anticonvulsants, monitor for therapeutic serum levels of anticonvulsants

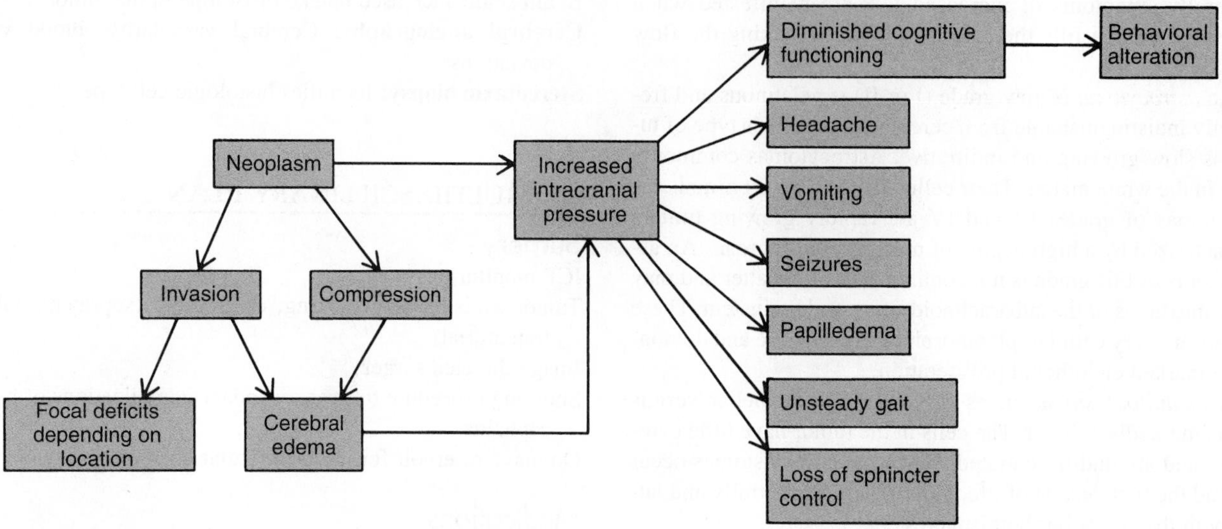

FIG. 5-27
Origin of clinical manifestations associated with an intracranial neoplasm. (From McCance and Huether.[18])

Mentation: Patient's level of consciousness must be carefully monitored (see Table 5-5); personality changes (e.g., loss of emotional restraints); depression; memory deficits; judgment deficits; self-care deficits; lethargy; obtundation; stupor; coma

Pain: Headaches with steady, persistent, or intractable dull pain; changes in character of headaches; stress-induced headaches

POTENTIAL COMPLICATIONS

Increased ICP: Generalized effects of increased ICP summarized in FIG. 5-27: restlessness, lethargy; changes in level of consciousness; changes in vital signs; pupillary changes (i.e., mydriasis); impaired pupillary reflex; papilledema (70% to 75% of patients); vomiting (may be projectile); Fluctuations in temperature—temperature must be taken every 20 minutes and prn

Brain herniation: Change in level of consciousness; change in response to painful stimuli; change in pupil size or shape; widening pulse pressure; change in respiratory pattern; bradycardia

Seizures: Seizure history; potential for injury; initial symptom in 15% of patients

Preconvulsive (preictal stage): Aura: flash of light, sense of loss, fear, weakness, dizziness, peculiar taste, smell, and sounds; cry or scream; fall to floor; loss of consciousness; tachypnea

Convulsive stage: Tonic: rigid body, fixed jaws, clenched fists, extended legs, cyanosis, holding breath; clonic: urinary and/or fecal incontinence, jerking of facial muscles and extremities, biting tongue, frothing at mouth

Postconvulsive (postictal stage): Altered level of consciousness; headache; nausea or vomiting; malaise; muscle soreness; aspiration: breathing difficulty, choking, cyanosis, decreased breath sounds, tachycardia, tachypnea

PATIENT PROBLEMS/NURSING DIAGNOSES & INTERVENTIONS

NIC TISSUE PERFUSION MANAGEMENT

Impaired cerebral tissue perfusion related to cerebral edema and cerebral hyoxia

Decreased intracranial adaptive capacity elated to cerebral edema

- Intervene to monitor waveforms of ICP line and to prevent increased ICP. **(Continuous flushing systems must not be used for ICP measurement.)**
- Maintain patency and sterility of the system.
- Assist with drainage of CSF from the system *to lower intracranial hypertension.*
- Evaluate effects of treatments of ICP.
- Administer corticosteroids *to control cerebral edema.*
- Administer anticonvulsants as ordered.
- Provide adequate ventilation and oxygenation; controlled ventilation may be indicated.
- Plan nursing care to minimize elevation in ICP.
- Institute seizure precautions: airway at bedside, bed height at lowest level, side rails up at all times, oxygen and suction equipment at bedside, emergency medications at bedside.
- Maintain normothermia.
- Elevate head of bed 30 to 45 degrees *to facilitate cerebral venous drainage.*
- Avoid flexion of hip, isometric exercises, Valsalva's maneuver, hypoxemia, and hypercapnia.
- Accurately record intake and output *to monitor for imbalance.*

NIC RESPIRATORY MANAGEMENT

Ineffective airway clearance related to high risk for tracheobronchial obstruction

Ineffective breathing pattern related to potential ineffective airway clearance

Risk for aspiration related to use of enteral feedings

- See general intervention strategies listed on p. 249.
- Confirm feeding tube placement after insertion, every 4 hours and as needed.
- Confirm initial enteral tube placement by physician examination of chest x-ray.
- Confirm tube placement before and after each intermittent tube feeding.
- Tape nasogastric tube securely per protocol.
- Hold feedings if residuals are greater than 150 ml or more than 110% to 120% hourly rate.
- Hold feedings if nausea/vomiting or diarrhea/constipation present.
- Maintain proper patient positioning.
- Elevate head of bed 30 to 40 degrees.
- Turn patient to right side *to facilitate stomach drainage through pylorus.*
- Discontinue continuous feedings 30 to 40 minutes before activity/procedure that requires lowering the patient's head.
- Hold tube feedings if abdominal distention, diarrhea/constipation, nausea/vomiting are present.
- Check pulmonary-tracheal secretions every 4 hours and as needed *to detect presence of enteric feeding.*

Risk for injury related to seizure activity

- Protect patient safety before, during, and after seizure activity.

Preconvulsive care

- Have oral airway at bedside.
- Support and protect head; turn to side if possible.

Injury prevention

- Ease patient to floor if in chair.
- Place pillows along side rails if in bed.
- Remove surrounding furniture.
- Loosen constrictive clothing.
- Provide privacy as necessary.
- Stay with patient; remain calm.
- Note frequency, time, involved body parts, and length of seizure.

Postconvulsive care

- Maintain patent airway.
- Suction as indicated *to prevent airway obstruction.*
- Administer oxygen per protocol *to minimize cerebral hypoxia.*
- Reorient patient to environment.
- Place patient in position of comfort; turn head to side.

NIC Risk Management

Disturbed sensory perception related to neurologic impairment

Chronic confusion related to organic or cognitive impairment

- Maintain bed in low position at all times unless side rails are up or when nurse is with the patient.
- Provide the patient with a call light within easy reach.
- Maintain frequently used items within patient's reach.
- Maintain side rails in up position.
- Maintain quiet environment *to reduce external stimuli to a minimum.*
- Reorient patient frequently to time, place, and person. Introduce yourself each time you reorient patient.
- Repeat explanations frequently and simply.
- Assist patient in judgments, perceptions, and reorientation as needed.
- Plan care with frequent rest periods.
- Use day and night lighting appropriately *to promote nocturnal wake-sleep pattern.*
- Identify and remove potential dangers in environment.
- Provide consistent physical environment and daily routine.
- Provide appropriate level of surveillance/supervision.
- Ensure optimal sensory input (i.e., eyeglasses, hearing aid) is available.
- Evaluate stimulation threshold *to prevent overstimulation.*
- Provide for structured repetitive group activities.
- Provide for adequate rest periods between activities and proper nutrition.
- Maintain calm, reassuring demeanor when interacting with patient *to promote sense of trust.*
- Encourage patient to participate in care as tolerated *to minimize feelings of powerlessness.*
- Provide positive feedback for tasks/activities that are mastered.

NIC Thermoregulation

Ineffective thermoregulation related to cerebral edema or increased ICP

- Administer steroids per protocol *to reduce cerebral edema.*
- Administer antipyretic agents per protocol.
- Adjust patient temperature as indicated, using cooling blanket, heat mattress, or warm blankets.
- Administer IV fluids at room temperature *to promote adequate fluid intake and prevent chilling.*
- Adjust environmental temperature as indicated.

NIC Physical Comfort Promotion

Acute or chronic pain related to increased tumor mass; nausea or vomiting

- Administer analgesics as ordered.
- Monitor effects of analgesics on level of consciousness and ICP.
- Administer antiemetics per protocol.
- Offer frequent mouth care.

NIC Self-Care Facilitation

Bathing/hygiene, dressing/grooming, and feeding self-care deficits related to perceptual cognitive impairment

- Assist with daily hygiene care as indicated.
- Assist with feeding as indicated. Use intravenous or nasogastric feedings per protocol.
- Administer eye care every 2 to 4 hours if indicated *to prevent crustation and infection.*
- Maintain bowel function with regular evacuation.

NIC IMMOBILITY MANAGEMENT

Impaired physical mobility related to perceptual cognitive impairment

- See general intervention strategies listed on p. 249.

NIC SKIN/WOUND MANAGEMENT

Risk for impaired skin integrity related to impaired physical mobility

- See general intervention strategies listed on p. 255.

PATIENT EDUCATION/CONTINUUM OF CARE PLAN

1. Involve the family in care, as possible; teach essential aspects of care.
2. Reinforce the physician's explanation of medical management.
3. Stress importance of ongoing outpatient care and follow-up visits.
4. Encourage independent activities, as possible.
   a. Alert the patient to limitations.
   b. Avoid overprotection.
   c. Stress need for supportive devices as indicated.
5. Stress need for a regular exercise program. Teach ROM exercises to family.
6. Stress importance of diet as ordered.
   a. Offer supplemental feedings.
   b. Offer small portions, and instruct the patient to chew slowly.
7. Stress importance of safety measures: side rails, ramps, shower chairs, and walkers and canes.
8. Discuss each name of medication, dosage, time of administration, and toxic or side effects.
9. Ensure the patient understands the need to avoid over-the-counter medications without first consulting physician.
10. Encourage socialization with friends and family.
11. Stress importance of verbalization of feelings about anxiety, fear, and body image changes.
12. Discuss with the patient and family about seizures: safety measures and whom to contact.

EVALUATION/PATIENT OUTCOMES

Tissue Perfusion Management: Level of consciousness is unchanged. Neurologic functioning is stable, and there is no evidence of additional neurologic deficits. Pattern of electrolytes is stable. There are no signs of increased ICP. There is no seizure activity.

Respiratory Management: Airway is patent. Breath sounds are normal. Chest excursion is bilateral and symmetric. Rate and depth of respirations are normal. Cough is effective. There are no subjective or objective findings of shortness of breath, air hunger, choking, or dyspnea on exertion. Breath sounds are normal, or there is no increase in adventitious sounds. Arterial blood gas values are within normal ranges or consistent with patient's baseline. Vital signs are within normal ranges or consistent with patient's baseline. Hemoglobin levels are 14 to 18 g/dl (male) or 12 to 16 g/dl (female). Intake and output are stable. All lobes are resonant on percussion. Skin color is not cyanotic. Enteric tube placement is verified. No symptoms of choking, nausea, or vomiting.

Risk Management: Safety measures are appropriate to physiologic status. Skin is free of bruises, burns, abrasions, and redness. Environment is safe. Patient is free of nosocomial infections. Patient remains free of traumatic injury. Patient experiences minimal fatigue. Patient demonstrates minimal confusion and is able to participate in structured activities.

Thermoregulation: Vital signs are within normal range for patient. Serum electrolytes and fluid balance are within normal limits. Patient's body temperature is maintained between 35.8° and 37.3° C (96.4° and 99.2° F). Patient remains free of symptoms of hypothermia or hyperthermia, including flushing or cyanosis, irritability, and seizures.

Physical Comfort Promotion: Patient experiences no or minimal pain. No reports/observations of nausea or vomiting are made. Level of consciousness is not affected by analgesic agent.

Self-Care Facilitation: Outcome criteria for impaired physical mobility are met. Level of self-care consistent with physiologic functioning. Patient participates in physical and occupational therapy.

Immobility Management: Patient demonstrates an optimum level of mobility. Skin integrity is maintained. Patient remains free of contractures and deformities. Level of mobility is appropriate to physiologic status. Intake and output pattern is stable. Nutritional status is adequate. Patient is free of thrombophlebitis. Patient is free of local infection. Patient participates in an ongoing physical therapy program. Patient is able to participate in structured repetitive group activities. Rest periods between activities are maintained. Patient is able to participate in care.

Skin/Wound Management: Skin integrity is maintained. Nutritional status is adequate. Electrolyte balance is maintained. Patient is free of pressure sores and contractures.

SPINAL TUMORS

Spinal tumors, although less common than intracranial tumors, are similar in pathologic types. They can arise from spinal nerve roots, the meninges, parenchyma of the cord, vertebral column, or the spinal vascular network (FIG. 5-28).

Spinal tumors frequently affect young and middle-age adults and usually involve the thoracic (50%), cervical (30%), and lumbosacral (20%) areas. The tumors are rare in children and elderly persons. Spinal tumors are classified according to their location; those occurring within the spinal cord tissue are called intramedullary, and those outside the spinal cord are called extramedullary. Extramedullary tumors are categorized further as intradural, extradural, or extravertebral. Spinal lesions constitute approximately 1% of all tumors in the general populaton. Men and women are affected about equally, except that meningiomas affect women more frequently. Approximately 85% of intraspinal tumors are benign.

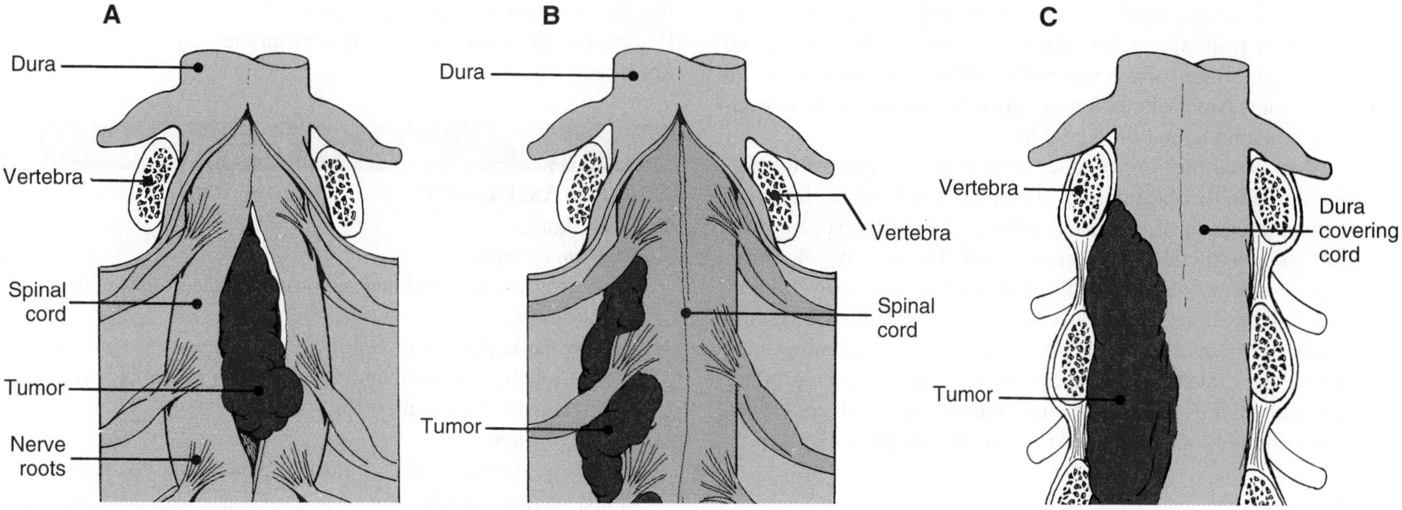

FIG. 5-28
Spinal cord tumors. **A,** Intramedullary tumor. **B,** Intradural-extramedullary tumor. **C,** Extradural-extramedullary tumor.

PATHOPHYSIOLOGY

Intramedullary tumors within the tissue of the spinal cord arise primarily from astrocyte or ependymal cells. Expanding intramedullary lesions may compress the spinal cord and nerve roots and destroy the parenchyma. Extramedullary tumors can be inside or outside the dural sac and produce spinal cord and spinal nerve root compression. Lesions outside the dural sac are called extradural and include herniated vertebral disks, acute and chronic infectious processes, metastatic lesions, meningiomas (5% to 10%), schwannomas (25% to 30%), and epidural hemorrhages. Tumors located within the dural sac but outside the spinal cord and nerve roots are called extramedullary intradural tumors; they include several types of glial tumors (e.g., ependymoma), most meningiomas and schwannomas, hemorrhages, and embryonic or congenital lesions. Extramedullary extravertebral tumors are commonly associated with bony destruction of vertebrae.

Schwannomas are the spinal tumors most commonly arising from the nerve sheath and can be found in all portions of the spinal cord. These tumors appear as a firm, encapsulated, rounded mass that contains many small cysts. Schwannomas consist of interlacing bands of cells with parallel intracellular fibrils and elongated nuclei that are usually arranged in parallel rows. There are also a number of star-shaped cells resembling astrocytes loosely arranged in the microscopic structure. Small foci of degeneration with cysts are common. First, the schwannoma compresses at the spinal nerve root in the foramen of the canal, producing localized nerve root symptoms. As the lesion progresses, it further compresses other nerve roots and the spinal cord, producing neurologic findings of cord compression. Symptoms are usually asymmetric. Extradural schwannomas are often hourglass or dumbbell in shape, with a portion in the spinal canal attached by a narrow band of tumor through the foramen to a part outside the spinal canal. This type of tumor can compress cervical, mediastinal, or abdominal tissue.

Meningiomas constitute approximately 22% of all primary spinal tumors. Most meningiomas are extramedullary. Eighty percent of meningiomas affect women, usually in the fourth, fifth, or sixth decade of life. These tumors can appear anywhere in the spinal canal but are most common in the region of the nerve roots, particularly in the thoracic region (two thirds of meningiomas occur in this region). They appear as small, rounded, nodular masses that frequently attach to the insertion of the denticulate ligament and extend dorsally or ventrally. Meningiomas consist of groups of elongated cells with round or oval nuclei. There is a tendency toward the formation of whorls, and calcification frequently is present in the center of the whorls. Symptoms are initially produced by traction or irritation of the nerve roots (i.e., radicular pain) and progress to long motor tract signs (i.e., spasticity) as a result of compression. Meningiomas can undergo malignant changes.

Ependymomas make up approximately 13% of all spinal cord tumors. They arise from the internal lining of the CNS and are usually intramedullary. Ependymomas are found throughout the spinal cord but commonly are located caudally in the conus medullaris and the filum terminale (cauda equina ependymoma). They are more common in men, generally appearing in the fourth or fifth decade of life. These tumors occur as loculated masses in the spinal canal, frequently with fusiform swelling. Microscopically, an ependymoma appears as a crowded mass of polygonal-type cells. In the filum it appears as a central core of connective tissue and blood vessels surrounded by a single layer of ependymal cells. Ependymomas may extend to 10 vertebral spaces in length and produce symptoms resulting from cord compression.

Astrocytomas and oligodendrogliomas are similar clinically. The oligodendroglioma is a rare type of spinal cord tumor. Astrocytomas are less common than ependymomas, generally intramedullary, and more common in men. Astrocytomas appear as elongated, fusiform swellings of the spinal cord. (See Table 5-7 for grading of astrocytomas.) Symptoms result from compression of the long tracts of the spinal cord.

The pathologic processes occurring with any spinal tumors can result from spinal cord destruction and infiltration, spinal cord displacement and compression, spinal nerve root irritation and compression, disruption in spinal blood supply, or disruption of cerebrospinal fluid circulation.[2]

Most benign lesions produce neurologic symptoms by compression and displacement of the spinal cord and by irritation and compression of the spinal nerve roots rather than by invasion and destruction of the spinal cord. The severity of neurologic symptoms depends on the degree of compression and how rapidly it develops. With slower-growing tumors the spinal cord can accommodate the mass by compressing itself into a slender, ribbonlike tissue. Such a slow-growing tumor may produce minimum deficits. Fast-growing tumors can produce sudden cord compression, edema, and severe neurologic deficits.

Diagnostic Studies and Findings

Roentgenograms: Determine presence of vertebral column lesions and bony destruction
Myelography (with contrast): Identifies size, boundaries, and level of tumor (with incomplete blockage of subarachnoid space)
CSF sampling (serial): Froin's syndrome (xanthochromatic CSF with large amounts of protein, rapid coagulation, and absence or decreased number of cells, immediate clotting)
Electromyogram (EMG): Assistive in differential diagnosis
Queckenstedt test: Positive
CT scan: Lesion location identified
Spinal angiograms: Differentiates vascular lesions from tumors
Positron emission tomography (PET): Lesion location identified

Multidisciplinary Plan

Surgery
Tumor excision
Laminectomy
Tracheotomy, if indicated
Spinal fusion

Other Treatments
Chemotherapy: Systemic chemotherapy, intrathecal chemotherapy
Radiation therapy

Medications
Corticosteroids (to control cord edema): Dexamethasone (Decadron), 10-40 mg IV qid

General Management
Mechanical ventilation, if indicated
CT scans (serial)
Soft cervical collar, if indicated, to alleviate discomfort
Spinal prostheses
Physiotherapy
Nutritional consultation
Psychosocial counseling and support
Extended care facility referral, if appropriate
Social services

NURSING CARE

Nursing Assessment

General Signs

Sensory impairment
- Slow, progressive numbness or tingling, and coldness in an extremity
- Hyperesthesia at level of lesion
- Loss of touch, vibration, and position sense (later signs)
- Skin integrity has potential for breakdown

Motor impairment
- Weakness, spasticity, and clumsiness; spreading contralaterally or ipsilaterally
- Self-care deficit
- Hyperactive reflexes
- Hypotonia and ataxia (cerebellar signs)
- Spasticity
- Positive Babinski's reflex
- Paresis
- Assess patient's mobility level

Pain
- Intermittent nerve root (radicular) pain, aggravated by straining, movement, and coughing
- Persistent back pain
- Monitor vital signs
- Observe for nonverbal cues of discomfort

Sphincter disturbances
- Urinary urgency
- Difficulty in initiating urination
- Retention and overflow incontinence
- Decreased sphincter control (later sign)

Other
- Brown-Séquard syndrome
- Contralateral loss of temperature and pain
- Ipsilateral motor loss
- Ipsilateral loss of vibration, touch, and position sense
- Potential for injury exists

Cervical Tumors

C4 and above
- Sensory: Vertigo
- Motor
  - Quadriparesis
  - Atrophy of sternocleidomastoid muscles
  - Dysphagia
- Dysarthria
- Tongue deviation
- Respiratory insufficiency
- Respiratory failure
  - Monitor vital signs frequently
  - Monitor Sa_{O_2}
- Monitor arterial blood gases
  - Report decrease in P_{O_2} of 10 to 15 mm Hg to prevent hypoxemia.
  - Report increase in P_{CO_2} greater than 10 to 15 mm Hg to prevent hypercapnia.

Other
Occipital headaches
Nuchal rigidity
Downbeat nystagmus
Papilledema (late sign of increased ICP)
C4 and below
Sensory
Paresthesia
Horner's syndrome (ipsilateral pupillary constriction, ptosis, and anhidrosis)
Motor
Weakness
Muscle fasciculations
Muscle atrophy
Other: Shoulder and arm pain

Thoracic Tumors
Sensory: Hyperesthesia band immediately above level of lesion
Motor
Spastic paresis of lower extremities
Positive Babinski's sign
Lower motor neuron deficits
Other: Sphincter impairment

Lumbar Tumors
Sensory: Localized loss in legs and saddle area
Motor
Footdrop
Diminished or absent patellar and Achilles reflexes
Other
Severe low back pain with radiation down legs
Perineal and bladder discomfort
Decreased libido
Impotence
Bladder disturbances
Bowel dysfunction

POTENTIAL COMPLICATIONS

Respiratory failure: Air hunger, shortness of breath, tachypnea, use of accessory muscles, flared nostrils; hypoxia: restlessness, confusion, cyanosis, tachycardia, hypotension, impaired motor function; hypercapnia: dizziness, confusion, headache, unconsciousness, hypertension, diaphoresis, flushed face

Chronic pain: Verbal report or observed evidence of discomfort experienced for more than 6 months; guarding, protective movements; change in appetite; fatigue; physical or social withdrawal; shortened attention span; altered perception of time

PATIENT PROBLEMS/NURSING DIAGNOSES & INTERVENTIONS

NIC RESPIRATORY MANAGEMENT

Ineffective airway clearance related to weakened cough reflex
Ineffective breathing pattern related to impaired respiratory muscle function.
- Suction as needed *to prevent airway obstruction and secretion stasis.*
  Hyperoxygenate lungs with 100% oxygen via mechanical ventilator or manual resuscitation bag for 1 minute before and 1 minute after suctioning, unless contraindicated, *to minimize hypoxia during suctioning.*
  Limit suction time to 15 seconds or less.
  Monitor Sa_{O_2} before, during, and after suctioning *to detect suction-induced hypoxia.*
- Monitor mechanical ventilation, if used.
  Ensure that tidal volume, rate, mode, and oxygen concentration are set as ordered.
  Ensure that ventilator alarms are on and functional.
  Check ventilator connections regularly.

NIC RISK MANAGEMENT

Disturbed sensory perceptions (kinesthetic, tactile) related to motor/sensory changes
- See general intervention strategies on p. 245.

Risk for injury related to impaired muscle strength
- Maintain bed in low position at all times unless side rails are up or nurse is with patient *to prevent patient falls.*
- Provide patient with a call light within easy reach.
- Maintain side rails in up position at bedtime, after sedation, when patient is confused, and as needed.
- Maintain bed, carts, and wheelchairs in locked position when transferring patient *to minimize risk of falling.*

NIC PHYSICAL COMFORT PROMOTION

Acute pain related to spinal cord compression
- Provide analgesic agents, as ordered.
  Use pain control measures before pain becomes severe.
  Medicate before activity *to increase participation.*
  Administer antiemetic medications as needed *to prevent nausea.*
- Modify anxiety associated with the pain experience.
- Provide other sensory input *to minimize focus on painful stimuli.*
- For patients receiving radiation or chemotherapy, explain procedure or medication before implementing.

NIC IMMOBILITY MANAGEMENT

Impaired physical mobility related to muscle weakness or spasticity, paralysis, pain
Risk for disuse syndrome related to paralysis
- Administer anticoagulation therapy per protocol.
- Apply antiembolus stockings to lower extremities *to promote venous return.*
- Obtain physical therapy referral.
- Document the following interventions:
  Use firm mattress or bed board *to support back and spine.*
  Use footboard or Spence boots *to prevent footdrop*
  Administer ROM every 4 hours and as needed.
  Reposition every 2 hours; use support devices *to maintain proper alignment/position.*
  Encourage self-care activities to tolerance.
  Maintain planned rest periods *to avoid fatigue.*

NIC Self-Care Facilitation

Feeding, bathing/hygiene, dressing/grooming, and toileting self-care deficits related to altered motor/sensory changes

- Encourage patient to perform normal activities to level of ability.
  - Assist with daily hygiene care as indicated.
  - Provide desired personal articles (e.g., soap, toothbrush, deodorant)
  - Use consistent pattern for ADL as means *to establish routine.*
  - Assist with feeding, as indicated; use intravenous or nasogastric feedings per protocol.
  - Administer oral hygiene every 2 hours and as needed.
  - Administer eye care every 2 to 4 hours if indicated.
- Perform intermittent urinary catheterization in accordance with protocol.
- Maintain bowel function with regular evacuation *to prevent constipation.*

NIC Skin/Wound Management

Risk for impaired skin integrity related to musculoskeletal impairment and prolonged immobility

- Administer skin care every 2 hours *to prevent breakdown and decubitus ulcers.*
- Turn patient every 2 hours and as needed, unless contraindicated:
  - Change position slowly.
  - Position in proper body alignment.
  - Massage pressure points every 2 hours *to stimulate circulation;* give gentle back rubs every shift and as needed.
  - Keep skin dry and clean.
  - Provide passive ROM exercises every 4 hours and as needed *to maintain joint mobility.*
- Maintain high-protein, low-calcium diet.

NIC Elimination Management

Risk for constipation or incontinence or altered urinary elimination because of sensory-motor impairment

- Use rectal suppositories, as needed.
- Initiate bowel training program, as appropriate.
- Ensure adequate fluid intake.
- Maintain regular toileting intervals.

Patient Education/Continuum of Care Plan

1. Involve family in care, as possible; teach essential aspects of care.
2. Reinforce physician's explanation of medical management.
3. Stress importance of ongoing outpatient care and follow-up visits.
4. Encourage independent activities, as possible.
   a. Be alert to limitations.
   b. Avoid overprotection.
   c. Stress need for supportive devices as indicated.
5. Stress need for regular exercise program; teach ROM exercises to family.
6. Stress importance of diet as ordered.
   a. Offer supplemental feedings.
   b. Give small portions, and instruct patient to chew slowly.
7. Stress importance of safety measures.
   a. Side rails
   b. Ramps
   c. Shower chairs
   d. Removal of scatter rugs
   e. Walker, canes
8. Discuss name of medication, dosage, time of administration, and toxic or side effects.
9. Stress need to avoid over-the-counter medication without first consulting physician.
10. Encourage socialization with friends and family.
11. Stress importance of verbalization of feelings about anxiety, fear, and body image changes.
12. Ensure patient and family understand about seizures (i.e., safety measures and whom to contact).

Evaluation/Patient Outcomes

Respiratory Management: Patient demonstrates an effective breathing pattern. Airway is patent. Chest excursion is symmetric. Breath sounds are normal, or there is no increase in adventitious sounds. Arterial blood gas values are within normal ranges or consistent with patient's baseline values. Vital signs are within normal ranges or consistent with patient's baseline values. Hemoglobin levels are 14 to 18 g/dl (male) and 12 to 16 g/dl (female). Intake and output are stable. There are no signs of respiratory distress. All lobes are resonant on percussion. Skin color is not cyanotic.

Risk Management: Level of orientation is optimum. Patient remains free of injury. Patient demonstrates skin integrity. Nutritional status is adequate. Self-care deficits are minimum. Social participation is appropriate to physiologic status. Safety measures are appropriate to level of physiologic status. Skin integrity is maintained. Skin is free of bruises, burns, abrasions, and redness. Environment is safe. Patient is free of nosocomial infections.

Physical Comfort Promotion: No objective/subjective observations/reports of discomfort. Vital signs are stable. No nausea or vomiting is observed or reported.

Immobility Management: Patient demonstrates an optimum level of mobility. Patient exhibits skin integrity. Patient is free of contractures and deformities. Level of mobility is appropriate to physiologic status. Nutritional status is adequate. Intake and output pattern is stable. Patient is free of thrombophlebitis. Patient is free of local infection. Patient participates in an ongoing physical therapy program.

Self-Care Facilitation: Patient demonstrates minimum self-care deficits. Outcome criteria listed for impaired physical mobility are met. Level of self-care activities is appropriate to physiologic status. Patient participates in physical and occupational therapy.

Skin/Wound Management: Patient demonstrates skin integrity. Skin is intact. Nutritional status is adequate. Electrolyte balance is maintained. Patient is free of pressure sores and contractures.

Elimination Management: Normal pattern of urinary output is maintained. No urinary or bowel incontinence is observed. Regular bowel evacuation is maintained.

VASCULAR DISORDERS

ANEURYSM

An intracranial aneurysm (cerebral aneurysm) is a localized dilation that develops secondary to a weakness of the arterial wall.

Cerebral aneurysm is the fourth most frequent cerebrovascular disorder, with an incidence of 10 cases per 100,000 in the general population. The peak incidence is in the 40- to 65-year-old age group, and women are affected slightly more often than men (ratio of 3:2). Cerebral aneurysms rarely occur in children and adolescents. Saccular aneurysms are associated with an increased incidence of congenital polycystic disease of the kidney and coarctation of the aorta. Hypertension is found more frequently in persons who have aneurysms than in the average population; however, aneurysms also occur in normotensive individuals.

Ruptured cerebral aneurysm is the most common cause of nontraumatic subarachnoid hemorrhage. At least 28% of individuals with ruptured cerebral aneurysm die immediately. Of individuals who survive the initial hemorrhage but are not treated, approximately 50% experience rebleeding within a year. Approximately one third of individuals who survive ruptured cerebral aneurysms demonstrate some residual paralysis, headaches, and mental changes, or epilepsy. Aneurysmal rupture often is associated with physical exertion (e.g., sports or coitus), severe emotional excitement, and a sudden rise in blood pressure, but it can also occur during sleep.

PATHOPHYSIOLOGY

No single mechanism has been identified in the pathogenesis of intracranial aneurysm. Possible causes are congenital structural defects in the media and elastica of the vessel well, incomplete involution of embryonic vessels, and secondary factors such as arterial hypertension, atherosclerotic changes, hemodynamic disturbances, and polycystic disease. Intracranial aneurysms also may result from the shearing forces produced during craniocerebral trauma. These shearing forces may weaken the arterial wall, which expands or dilates with each arterial pulsation until bleeding or symptoms occur.

Aneurysms are generally classified according to their predominant characteristics into (1) saccular or berry, (2) fusiform or atherosclerotic, and (3) mycotic (FIG. 5-29). Saccular aneurysms are the fourth most common cerebrovascular disorder. They appear as small, thin-walled "berries" protruding from arteries of the circle of Willis, or its major branches,

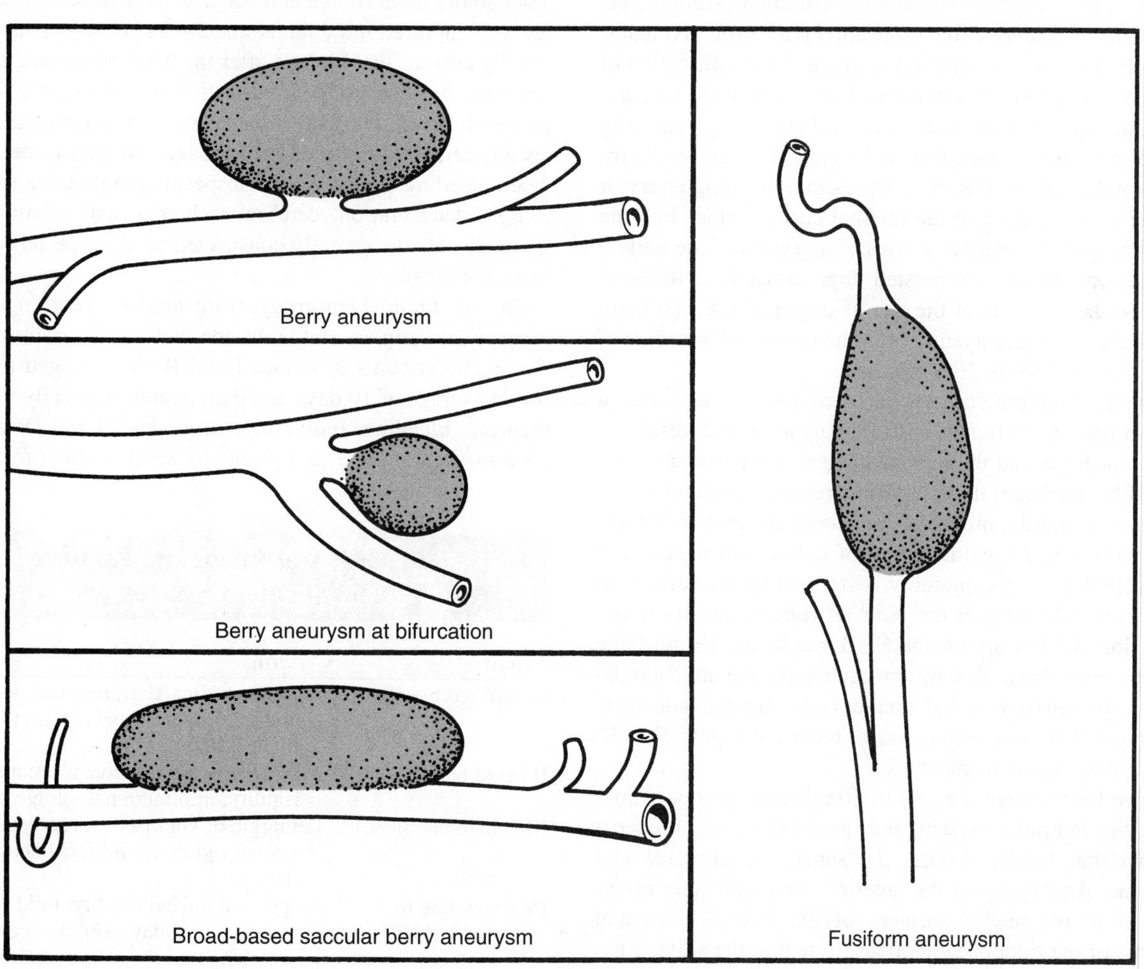

FIG. 5-29
Types of aneurysms. (From McCance and Huether.[8])

primarily at points of bifurcations and branchings. Because of the local weakness in the vessel, the intima bulges outward and the sac slowly enlarges until finally the wall ruptures and floods the subarachnoid space with blood under high pressure.

Fusiform (ectatic) aneurysms are spindle-shaped dilations of the entire circumference of an artery for several centimeters. They are characterized by degenerative changes in the elastic fibers and deposits of cholesterol in the intima and by fibrous replacement of smooth muscle.[2] These aneurysms most commonly occur along the trunk of the basilar artery. They infrequently rupture and generally produce symptoms by compression of adjacent cerebral tissue or cranial nerves. When rupture does occur, the atherosclerotic or fusiform aneurysm is often fatal.

Mycotic aneurysms are rare and can result when a septic embolus from acute or subacute bacterial endocarditis or other infectious process causes arterial necrosis that may lead to thrombosis or aneurysm formation. Mycotic aneurysms usually arise in a characteristic location along the distal branches of the middle and anterior cerebral arteries. They tend to be multiple.

The majority of ruptured aneurysms are saccular, or berry, aneurysms. Saccular aneurysms characteristically occur at specific locations in the intracranial circulation. Approximately 90% to 95% of berry aneurysms are found in the anterior portion of the circle of Willis, and the rest are situated in the vertebral or basilar arteries. Within the circle of Willis there are four main sites of rupture: The anterior communicating artery; the origin of the posterior communicating artery, the first major bifurcation of the middle cerebral artery, and the bifurcation of the internal carotid artery into the middle and anterior cerebral arteries. Aneurysms of the internal carotid artery are frequently large and may be situated either in the angle formed by the internal carotid artery and the posterior communicating artery or at the site of bifurcation of the internal carotid artery into the anterior and middle cerebral arteries. Aneurysms of the middle cerebral artery usually are located approximately 2 to 3 cm from the vessel's origin, at the site of origin of the first main branches. Multiple aneurysms, often bilateral and symmetric, may be found in 15% to 20% of cases.

Aneurysmal rupture occurs when the pulse pressure tears a very small hole in the fundus of the aneurysm, which results in direct hemorrhage into the leptomeningeal compartment (subarachnoid hemorrhage) under arterial pressure. Such a hemorrhage spreads rapidly, producing localized changes in the underlying cortex and focal irritation of the cranial nerves and arteries. The bleeding commonly is stopped by the formation of a fibrin-platelet plug at the point of rupture and by tissue compression. Within approximately 3 weeks the hemorrhage undergoes resorption. Resorption occurs by the arachnoidal villi after the leukocytes and macrophages have begun their scavenging.[2] There is a serious risk of recurrent rupture 7 to 10 days after the original hemorrhage.

Massive hemorrhage (i.e., 30 to 50 ml) may produce rapid filling of the ventricular system and vasal cisterns or produce a hematoma that locally distorts the subarachnoid space and brain tissue. Aneurysms of the anterior communicating artery lying next to the medial surfaces of the frontal lobes and aneurysms of the middle cerebral artery within the sylvian fissure next to the frontal and temporal lobes are particularly prone to rupture into the parenchyma of the brain. Aneurysms of the anterior communicating artery may rupture into the frontal lobes. Aneurysms of the basilar artery may rupture into the midbrain or diencephalon. Secondary rupture into the cerebral ventricles can occur because these intracerebral hemorrhages commonly extend through the brain tissue. Aneurysmal rupture may include bleeding in nearby cranial nerves. The most commonly affected cranial nerve is the oculomotor, or cranial nerve III, because of rupture of an aneurysm at the origin of the posterior communicating artery from the internal carotid artery. The optic nerve frequently is involved with ophthalmic artery aneurysms. Carotid aneurysms in the cavernous sinus involve cranial nerves III, IV, and VI, which act on the muscles and the first division of the trigeminal nerve. Increased ICP results in distortions that can produce unilateral or bilateral sixth nerve palsies. Most of the cranial nerve palsies that develop result from hemorrhage in the nerve and not from compression of the nerve by the aneurysm.

Increased ICP is frequently a sequela of acute subarachnoid hemorrhage and occurs because of several mechanisms. First, an expanding hematoma acts as a rapidly enlarging space-occupying lesion that compresses or displaces adjacent brain tissue. Second, blood in the basal cistern may impede or interrupt the flow of CSF. Last, if the pacchionian granulations become distended with blood, the spinal fluid resorption is impeded. The increased ICP may retard subsequent hemorrhage.

Cerebral vasospasms are a frequent complication of subarachnoidal hemorrhage and occur in 35% to 40% of individuals with ruptured intracranial aneurysms. Cerebral vasospasms usually appear 3 to 14 days after the hemorrhage and are characterized by measurable constriction or reactive narrowing of the cerebral arteries. The vasospasms are most evident in arteries adjacent to the site of hemorrhage and tend to be lessened when bleeding is minimal. Vasospasms can produce focal neurologic deterioration, cerebral ischemia, and infarction. Angiography shows severely constricted cerebral vessels and confirms the diagnosis.

Subarachnoid hemorrhages are graded according to their severity and clinical status. In one method for grading hemorrhages, individuals in grades I and II are managed medically for an average of 10 days and then treated surgically to prevent recurrent bleeding. Individuals in grades III and IV are managed medically for 3 to 4 weeks to stabilize them for surgery.

Table 5-8 Cerebral Aneurysm Rupture Classification System

Grade	Criteria
I (minimal bleed)	Asymptomatic: Alert, minimal headache and minimum nuchal rigidity; no neurologic deficits
II (mild bleed)	Mild to severe headache; alert; nuchal rigidity; minimum neurologic deficits
III (moderate bleed)	Lethargic or confused; severe headache; nuchal rigidity; mild focal neurologic deficits
IV (moderate to severe bleed)	Stuporous; nuchal rigidity; mild to severe hemiparesis; may exhibit decerebrate posturing
V (severe bleed)	Comatose; decerebrate posturing

Individuals in grade V are not surgical candidates unless they have life-threatening complications. The complete cerebral aneurysm classification system is listed in Table 5-8.

DIAGNOSTIC STUDIES AND FINDINGS

Lumbar puncture: NOTE: Contraindicated in presence of suspected increased intracranial pressure; elevated protein content (80 to 130 g/dl); increased WBC count; slightly decreased glucose; bloody CSF with deep xanthochromia (hemolyzed red blood cells) after centrifugation

CT scan (serial): Demonstration of blood in the subarachnoid space, within the brain or ventricular system (within 48 hours of initial bleeding); displaced cerebral midline structures; localized blood clots; baseline evaluation of ventricles (for later determination of hydrocephalus)

MRI or MR angiography (MRA): Same as CT scan, but with lower index of accuracy

Cerebral angiogram: Diagnostic tool of choice. Identification of local or general vasospasm; outlining of cerebral vasculature, characteristics of the aneurysm

Skull roentgenograms: May reveal calcified wall of aneurysm and areas of bone erosion

Brain scan: May indicate the presence of local diminution of flow

ECG: Shortened P-R interval; increased, peaked, or inverted T waves, increased U waves

Serum tests: Electrolyte imbalances; changes in bleeding parameters (i.e., prothrombin time, partial thromboplastin time, and platelet count); leukocytosis, normal sedimentation rate

Regional cerebral blood flow (rCBF): Mean flow values for both hemispheres and determination of status of cerebral vasospasm

MULTIDISCIPLINARY PLAN

Surgery

Tracheostomy or endotracheal intubation
ICP monitoring
Cerebral ventriculostomy to treat increased ICP and hydrocephalus
Ventriculoatrial shunting (hydrocephalus)
Clipping of aneurysm
Wrapping of aneurysmal sac
Endovascular obliteration
Vascular bypass
Evacuation of intracerebral clot

Medications

Anticonvulsants
- Phenytoin (Dilantin), 100 mg PO or IV tid or qid (do not exceed 50 mg/min IV to prevent hypotension and cardiac arrhythmias)
- Phenobarbital, 50-100 mg PO in two or three divided doses

Antihypertensive agents (used with caution)
- Nitroprusside (Nitropress), average 3 μg/kg/min IV
- Propranolol (Inderal), 40 mg PO bid

Calcium channel blockers (to reduce incidence of stroke from vasospasm)
- Nimodipine (Nimotop), 60 mg PO q4h for 21 days

Corticosteroids: Dexamethasone (Decadron), 6-10 mg IV q6h
Antibiotics (for mycotic aneurysm)
Analgesic/antipyretics: Acetaminophen (Tylenol), gr X PO or rectal suppository q4h prn
Narcotic analgesics: Acetaminophen with codeine, 30 mg PO or IV q4-6h prn
Stool softeners: Docusate sodium (Colace), 100 mg PO or nasogastric bid

General Management

Ventilatory support
Hypothermia blanket
ECG; cardiac monitoring
Arterial blood pressure monitoring
Elevation of head of bed
Serial arterial blood gases
Subarachnoid precautions
Strict intake and output
Volume expansion (treatment of cerebral vasospasms)
Intermittent catheterization
Seizure precautions
Antiembolus stockings; sequential compression devices (SCDs)
Hemodynamic monitoring
Complete bed rest
Soft, high-fiber diet
Physical therapy consult
Occupational therapy consult
Social services consult
Home health referral
Nutritional consultation

NURSING CARE

NURSING ASSESSMENT

Before rupture, aneurysms are usually asymptomatic.
Assessment findings depend on the location of the hemorrhage.

Level of consciousness: Varies from brief loss of consciousness to persistent coma; level of consciousness checked every 15 to 30 minutes; frequent monitoring of neurologic status

Meningeal irritation: Nuchal rigidity; positive Kernig's sign; positive Brudzinski's sign; fever; irritability; restlessness; later stages: Seizures and blurred vision

Visual disturbances: Blurred vision; double vision; visual field defects; unilateral blindness

Cranial nerve involvement: Ptosis and dilation of pupil; inability to move eye upward or inward; papilledema (late sign of intracranial hypertension); photophobia;

Autonomic function: Diaphoresis; chills; heart rate changes; changes in blood pressure; slight temperature elevation (37.8° to 38.9° C; 100° to 102° F); altered respiratory rhythm

Motor function: Onset and worsening of hemiparesis; aphasia; dysphagia; hemiplegia; unilateral or bilateral transient paresis of lower extremities; ability to communicate varies

Pain: Sudden onset of a violent headache usually beginning as localized frontally or temporally and then generalizing to involve entire head

Other: Dizziness, nausea, and vomiting frequent; cranial bruits may sometimes be auscultated on affected side; Babinski's sign

Potential Complications

Increased ICP/acute communicating hydrocephalus: Restlessness and lethargy; changes in level of consciousness; changes in vital signs (e.g., Cushing response with increased systolic blood pressure, wide pulse pressure, and decreased pulse rate); pupillary changes (i.e., mydriasis); impaired pupillary reflex; papilledema (late symptom); vomiting; fluctuations in temperature; seizures; worsening of focal neurologic signs; changes in respiratory patterns

Seizure activity

Preconvulsive (preictal stage): Aura: flash of light, sense of loss, fear, weakness, dizziness, peculiar taste, smell, sounds; cry or scream; fall to floor; loss of consciousness; tachypnea

Convulsive state: Tonic: rigid body, fixed jaws, clenched fists, extended legs, cyanosis, holding breath; clonic: urinary and/or fecal incontinence, jerking of facial muscles and extremities, biting tongue, frothing at the mouth

Postconvulsive (postictal) stage: Altered level of consciousness; headache; nausea or vomiting; malaise; muscle soreness; aspiration: breathing difficulty, choking, cyanosis, decreased breath sounds, tachycardia, tachypnea

Cerebral vasospasms: Highest incidence 3 to 14 days after initial hemorrhage; impaired level of consciousness; fluctuating hemiparesis; aphasia; cranial nerve deficits

Rebleeding: Highest incidence 2 weeks after initial hemorrhage; new headache; cranial nerve deficits; hemiparesis, hemiplegia, cognitive deterioration, aphasia; increased ICP; stiff neck, nausea/vomiting; pain in neck or back; photophobia (result of meningeal irritation)

Diabetes insipidus: Polyuria (hourly output greater than 200 ml); low specific gravity of urine (1.001 to 1.005); polydipsia; high serum osmolality

Patient Problems/Nursing Diagnoses & Interventions

NIC Respiratory Management

Ineffective airway clearance related to impaired cough reflex

Ineffective breathing pattern related to neuromuscular dysfunction

- See general intervention strategies on pp. 244 and 249.

NIC Tissue Perfusion Management

Ineffective tissue perfusion related to increased ICP secondary to subarachnoid hemorrhage

Impaired adaptive capacity related to intracranial hypertension, intracranial hemorrhage

- Monitor closely for signs of increased ICP (greater than 15 mm Hg for 5 minutes or longer); report any changes to physician.
- Maintain patency and sterility of ICP monitoring device, if used

  Use surgical asepsis for all dressing changes.

  Monitor ICP responses to care and treatments.

  NOTE: **Continuous flushing devices must not be used for measuring ICP.**
- Administer medications per protocol: anticonvulsants, steroids, antibiotics, and analgesics.
- Administer calcium channel blocking agents per protocol *to treat cerebral vasospasms.*

Bradycardia

- Regulate mechanical ventilation to maintain $Paco_2$ 25 to 30 mm Hg *to reduce cerebral vasodilation.*
- Institute subarachnoid precautions, if appropriate:

  Provide private room with controlled lighting (e.g., dim artificial lighting).

  Maintain complete bed rest *to keep physical activity and exertion to a minimum.*

  Provide all nursing care for the patient.

  Limit visitors to immediate family members *to prevent overstimulation.*

  Have patient wear elastic stockings or sequential compression devices *to prevent venous stasis.*

  Maintain dietary restrictions (no stimulants such as coffee, tea, or soda).

  Administer stool softeners *to prevent straining during bowel movement.*

  Instruct patient on need to avoid coughing and sneezing *to prevent sudden increases in ICP.*

  Instruct patient not to watch television, listen to radio, or read.
- Elevate head of bed 30 to 40 degrees, unless contraindicated, *to facilitate venous return.* Maintain head and neck in neutral position.
- Avoid hip flexion.
- Maintain strict intake and output (1500 to 1800 ml for 24 hours) *to maintain fluid balance.*

NIC Risk Management

Disturbed sensory/perception (kinesthetic, tactile) related to altered sensory perception

- See general intervention strategies on p. 245.

Risk for injury related to seizures, altered consciousness

- Maintain bed in low position at all times unless side rails are up or nurse is with patient.
- Provide patient with a call light within easy reach.
- Maintain side rails in up position at bedtime, after sedation, when patient is confused, and as needed *to prevent falls.*
- Maintain bed and carts in locked position when transferring patient *to prevent falls.*
- Prevent injury before and during seizures.

Preconvulsive care

- Maintain seizure precautions.
- Have oral airway at bedside *to maintain patent airway.*
- Have suction equipment available at bedside *to prevent aspiration.*
- Pad side rails, if indicated.
- Administer oxygen per protocol *to prevent cerebral hypoxia.*
- Identify auras if possible.

Convulsive care
- Maintain patent airway.
- Support and protect head; turn to side if possible *to maintain airway.*
- Prevent injury:
  Ease patient to floor if patient is in chair.
  Place pillows along side rails if patient is in bed.
  Loosen constrictive clothing.
- Provide privacy as necessary; stay with patient.
- Note frequency, time, involved body parts, and length of seizure *to provide accurate description of seizure activity.*

Postconvulsive care
- Maintain patent airway.
- Suction as indicated *to maintain open airway.*
- Administer oxygen per protocol *to prevent hypoxia.*
- Reorient patient to environment *to minimize sensory-perceptual alteration.*
- Place patient in position of comfort and turn head to side.
- Administer oral hygiene as necessary *to remove secretions and bleeding.*

NIC Immobility Management

Impaired physical mobility related to prolonged bed rest
- See general intervention strategies listed on p. 277.
- Encourage mobility to tolerance, unless contraindicated by subarachnoid hemorrhage precautions.
- Encourage self-care activities to tolerance unless contraindicated by subarachnoid hemorrhage precautions.

NIC Skin/Wound Management

Risk for impaired skin integrity related to sensory and perceptual alterations
- See general intervention strategies listed on p. 255.

NIC Communication Enhancement

Impaired verbal communication related to altered sensory and neuromuscular function
- Develop a means of communication with the patient: pencil, Magic Slate, or call light within easy reach.
- Reinforce the techniques established.
- Assist patient and family to identify other outlets for communication.
- Continue to use sense of touch and nonverbal forms of communication.

Patient Education/Continuum of Care Plan

1. Involve family in patient care, as possible; teach essential aspects of care.
2. Reinforce physician's explanation of medical management.
3. Stress importance of ongoing outpatient care and follow-up visits.
4. Stress need for regular exercise program.
   a. Teach ROM exercises to family.
   b. Instruct patient or family to perform ROM exercises to all body joints every 2 to 4 hours.
5. Encourage independent activities, as possible.
   a. Be alert to limitations.
   b. Avoid overprotection.
   c. Instruct regarding need for supportive devices as indicated (wheelchairs, braces, walker, canes, overhead trapeze).
6. Stress importance of diet as ordered.
   a. Offer supplemental feedings.
   b. Offer small portions, and instruct patient to chew slowly.
   c. Arrange food and utensils within easy reach.
   d. Avoid foods such as soft breads, mashed potatoes, semicooked vegetables, and large pieces of meat that can cause choking.
7. Stress importance of safety measures.
   a. Side rails
   b. Ramps
   c. Shower chains
   d. Removal of scatter rugs
   e. Walker, canes, flat shoes
8. Discuss each name of medication, dosage, time of administration, and toxic or side effects.
9. Ensure that patient understands need to avoid over-the-counter medications without first consulting physician.
10. Encourage socialization with friends and family.
11. Stress importance of communication.
    a. Speak slowly and distinctly.
    b. Use one-word commands and short sentences. Repeat as needed.
    c. Use gestures and touch when giving directions. Maintain eye contact.
    d. Implement speech exercises twice a day.
12. Stress importance of verbalization of feelings about anxiety, fear, and body image changes.
13. Discuss with patient and family about seizures (i.e., safety measures and whom to contact).

Evaluation/Patient Outcomes

Respiratory Management: Patient demonstrates a patent airway. Breath sounds are normal, or there is no increase in adventitious sounds. Chest excursion is bilateral and symmetric. Rate and depth of respirations are normal. Cough is effective. There are no subjective or objective findings of shortness of breath, air hunger, or dyspnea on exertion. Arterial blood gas values are within normal ranges or consistent with patient's baseline. Vital signs are within normal ranges or consistent with patient's baseline. Hemoglobin levels are 14 to 18 g/dl (male) and 12 to 16 g/dl (female). Intake and output are stable. Skin color is not cyanotic.

Tissue Perfusion Management: Patient maintains adequate cerebral tissue perfusion. Level of consciousness is unchanged. There is no evidence of neurologic deficits. Pattern of electrolytes is stable. There is no seizure activity.

Risk Management: Patient demonstrates minimum complications of sensory/perceptual alterations. Level of orientation is optimum. Environment is safe. Patient remains free of injury. Skin integrity is maintained. Skin is free of bruises, burns, abrasions, and redness. Patient is free of nosocomial infections. Nutritional status is adequate. Self-care deficits are minimum.

Immobility Management: Patient demonstrates optimum level of mobility. Skin integrity is maintained. Patient remains free of contractures and deformities. Level of mobility is appropriate to physiologic status. Nutritional status is adequate. Intake and output pattern is stable. Patient remains free of thrombophlebitis. Patient remains free of local infection. Patient participates in an ongoing physical therapy program.

Skin/Wound Management: Patient demonstrates skin integrity. Skin is intact. Nutritional status is adequate. Electrolyte balance is maintained. Patient remains free of pressure sores and contractures.

Communication Enhancement: Patient demonstrates minimum impaired verbal communication. Patient verbalizes feelings for as long as is physically able to do so. Patient develops alternative methods of communication.

STROKE

In stroke, or cerebrovascular accident (CVA), the cerebral vessels are occluded by an embolus or cerebrovascular hemorrhage, resulting in ischemia of the area of the brain normally perfused by the damaged vessels.[8]

The sequelae of a stroke depend on the extent and location of the ischemia (FIG. 5-30). Death rates from stroke decreased by 32% from 1980 to 1990. However, stroke remains the third leading cause of death in the United States and the second most common cause of neurologic disability after Alzheimer's disease. Persons ages 25 to 64 years are affected, but incidence increases rapidly from age 35 years upward. The greatest increase in frequency occurs between ages 75 and 85 years.

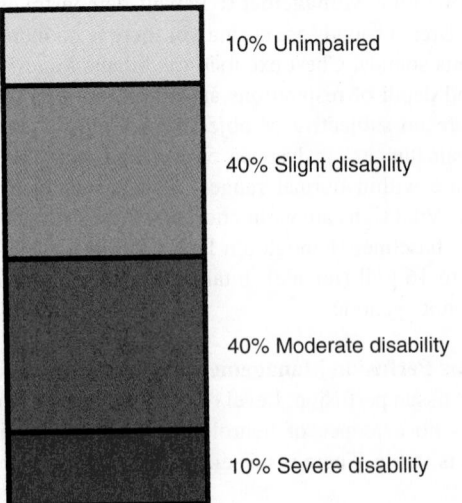

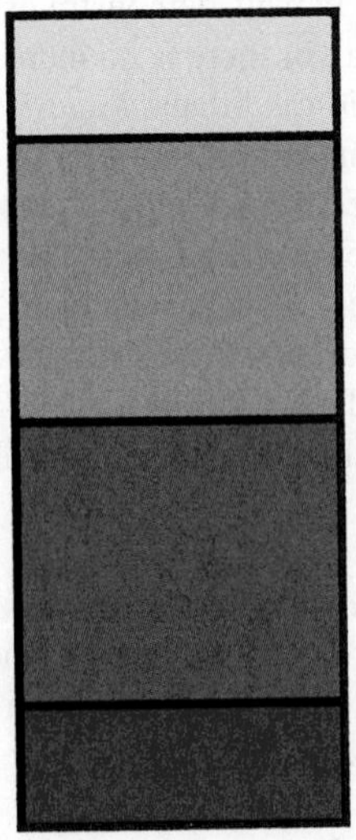

FIG. 5-30
Degree of disability in survivors of stroke. (From Chipps, Clanin, and Campbell.[1a])

Certain risk factors may predispose an individual to a stroke; hypertension is the major risk factor. Risk factors showing some familial tendencies include diabetes mellitus, hypertension, cardiac disease, subclavian steal syndrome, and high serum cholesterol level. Obesity, sedentary lifestyle, cigarette smoking, stress, and high serum levels of cholesterol, lipoprotein, and triglycerides make the individual a high-risk candidate for stroke. In women the use of oral contraceptives and cigarette smoking increase the risk of stroke. Combinations of risk factors put the individual at a greater risk.[8]

PATHOPHYSIOLOGY

The pathologic mechanisms of stroke are classified as hemorrhagic, thrombotic, and embolic. Hemorrhage may be subarachnoid from rupture of the subarachnoid artery or intraparenchymal from rupture of an intraparenchymal artery. Embolic occlusion stems from tumors, valvular cardiac diseases, and, most commonly, plaques released from cerebral vessels that produce infarction. Thrombotic arterial occlusion produces various ischemic or hypoxic insults.

Cerebral Hemorrhage

Hypertensive cerebral hemorrhage usually occurs in relation to some mild exertion, and it occurs in individuals who have experienced significant increases in systolic-diastolic pressures for several years. Some researchers theorize that microaneurysms, known as Charcot-Bouchard aneurysms, in small arteries or arteriolar necrosis may precipitate the bleeding.

Resolution of the hemorrhage occurs via resorption and begins when macrophages and reactive fibrillary astrocytes appear. After the tissue has been cleared of blood by the macrophages, there is a cavity surrounded by dense fibrillary gliosis and hemosiderin-laden macrophages.

! EMERGENCY ALERT

CEREBROVASCULAR ACCIDENT

Cerebrovascular accident (CVA) is a cerebral infarct that results from a decrease in cerebral blood flow, cerebral embolus, and commonly cerebral thrombosis. Patients at risk are those with hypertension, diabetes, cardiac disease, hyperlipidemia, polycythemia, family history, smoking, and use of oral contraceptives.

ASSESSMENT

- HA, progressive or sudden neurologic deficits
- Decreased carotid pulse or carotid bruit
- Hypertension
- Signs of cerebral ischemia: Hypotension, shock, arrest

INTERVENTIONS

Maintain airway, breathing, circulation.

- Closely monitor vital signs.
- Administer anticoagulant therapy if indicated.
- Obtain IV access.
- *If patient is hypertensive,* reduce blood pressure slowly to minimize risk of hemorrhage or extension of the infarct.
- Administer diuretics and/or corticosteroids as ordered to reduce cerebral edema.

Cerebral Infarction

Cerebral infarction occurs when a local area of brain tissue is deprived of blood supply because of vascular occlusion. The pathogenesis of cerebral infarcts includes abrupt vessel occlusion (i.e., embolus), gradual vessel occlusion (i.e., atheroma), and vessels that are stenosed but not completely occluded.

Common causes of vascular occlusions are cerebral thrombi and cerebral emboli. Thrombi usually occur in larger vessels (e.g., internal carotid arteries) and are associated with localized damage to the vessel wall at the point of occlusion. Atherosclerosis and hypotension are important underlying processes, but other types of vascular injury (e.g., arteritis) can initiate thrombosis. Emboli usually affect smaller vessels and are commonly found at points of narrowed vessel lumen and bifurcation. The sources of cerebral emboli vary, but the most common is a mural thrombus in the left atrium or ventricle. Septic emboli may originate from bacterial endocarditis. Cerebral infarcts from embolic occlusions frequently are hemorrhagic, whereas thrombotic infarcts are bland or ischemic. Emboli occur most frequently in the middle cerebral artery.

A cerebral infarction may be ischemic or hemorrhagic. Ischemic infarctions usually are not demonstrable on gross examination for 6 to 12 hours. The initial change of the affected area is a slight discoloration and softening, with the gray matter taking on a muddy color and the white matter losing its normal fine-grained appearance. After 48 to 72 hours, infarction, necrosis, circumlesional swelling, and disintegration of the affected area are evident. Eventually there is liquefaction and formation of a cyst surrounded by a firm glial tissue.

Hemorrhagic infarctions usually occur in the cerebral cortex and result from a reflow of blood into the infarcted area. This reperfusion is caused by a fragmentation or lysis of the embolus or a reduction of vascular compression and reestablishment of blood flow.

Hemorrhagic infarcts therefore are ischemic in origin.

Diagnostic Studies and Findings

CF scan (without contrast): Infarct: Appears initially (first 24 hours) as area of decreased density surrounded by area of intermediate density; shifts in midline structures and ventricular system; older infarct (NOTE: Contrast-enhancing agents have a small risk of neurotoxicity and may normalize density of small hypodense infarct.)

MRA: Visualization of occluded vessels, clots

Pulsed transcranial Doppler (PTCD): Direction and velocity of blood flow in intracranial blood vessels

EEG: May show focal slowing around area of lesion

Brain scan: Diminished perfusion; detection of infarction, encapsulated hemorrhage, hematoma, and arteriovenous malformations

Digital subtraction arteriography: Shows occlusion or narrowing of large vessels

Duplex ultrasound: Outlines with ultrasound the flow of blood through large neck vessels

Skull roentgenogram: Pineal body position; intracranial calcifications

Multidisciplinary Plan

Surgery

Carotid endarterectomy

Anastomosis of superior temporal artery and middle cerebral artery (STA-MCA anastomosis)

Intralumenal stent placement

ICP monitoring: **Contraindicated in patients with coagulopathy or on anticoagulation therapy**

Endotracheal intubation or tracheostomy

Evacuation of intracerebral clot or hematoma

Medications

Antiplatelet agents
- Aspirin, 75-1300 mg PO qd
- Indomethacin (Indocin), 25-50 mg PO bid or tid
- Dipyridamole (Persantine), 150-400 mg/day PO
- Ticlopidine (Ticlid), 250 mg PO bid

Anticoagulants: Heparin to partial thromboplastin time (PTT) of 1.5-2 times control for 3-5 days, then warfarin (Coumadin) to prothrombin time (PT) of 1.3-1.7 times control or international ratio 2-3.

Thrombolytics (treatment of ischemic stroke): Recombinant tissue plasminogen activator (t-PA), 0.9 mg/kg to maximum of 90 mg IV 10% given as a bolus over 1 min, and the remainder over 1 h (NOTE: Patient **must** meet eligibility criteria for t-PA administration.)

Calcium channel blockers: Nimodipine (Nimotop), 30 mg PO q6h for 4 wk

Diuretic: Furosemide (Lasix), 40-80 mg IV 30-60 min before each dose of diazoxide

Corticosteroids
- Prednisone
- Dexamethasone (Decadron), 10 mg initially, then 4 mg q4-6h IV or IM

Anticonvulsants: Phenytoin (Dilantin), 100-600 mg/d orally or IV

Narcotic analgesic: Codeine, 30-60 mg q3-4h

Analgesic/antipyretics: Acetaminophen, gr X q4h PO or rectal suppository

General Management

Mechanical ventilation

Coagulation studies (i.e., PT, PTT, INR): Bleeding precautions

Hypothermia blanket

ECG and cardiac monitoring

Subarachnoid precautions

Strict intake and output
- Volume expansion (intravenous saline)
- Anticoagulation therapy
  - Monitor serum coagulation studies
  - Check stool and urine for occult blood
- Electrolyte and blood sugar monitoring

Bed rest

Elevation of head of bed

Nasogastric tube

Foley or indwelling catheter

Elastic stockings; sequential compression devices

Serial arterial blood gases

Seizure precautions

Hemodynamic monitoring
Nutritional consultation
Physical therapy
Social services
Home health referral
Resources available: American Stroke Association *(www.americanheart.org/catalog/stroke)*

NURSING CARE

Nursing Assessment

See Assessment Considerations table.

Potential Complications

Cerebral reperfusion injury: Intracranial hypertension; cerebral edema; neurologic deficits; symptoms of CVA
Cerebral vasospasms: Drowsiness, change in level of consciousness; fluctuating hemiparesis; aphasia; cranial nerve deficits

Patient Problems/Nursing Diagnoses & Interventions

NIC Tissue Perfusion Management

Ineffective tissue perfusion related to hemorrhage and/or increased ICP

Decreased intracranial adaptive capacity related to intracranial hypertension

- Intervene to monitor waveforms of ICP and to prevent increased ICP. **Continuous flushing devices should not be use to monitor ICP.**
  Maintain patency and sterility of ICP monitoring device.
  Use surgical asepsis for all dressing changes.
  Monitor ICP responses to care and treatments.
  Correlate neurologic status with ICP values; notify physician if inconsistent.
  Assist with drainage of CSF from the system *to decrease intracranial hypertension.*
- Institute subarachnoid precautions, if appropriate.
  Provide private room with controlled lighting (i.e., dim artificial lighting).
  Maintain complete bed rest *to keep physical activity and exertion to a minimum.*
  Provide all nursing care for the patient.
  Limit visitors to immediate family members only *to prevent overstimulation.*
  Have patient wear elastic stockings at all times *to prevent venous stasis.*
  Maintain dietary restrictions (no stimulants).
  Administer stool softeners *to prevent straining during bowel movement.*
  Instruct patient on need to avoid coughing and sneezing *to prevent sudden increases in ICP.*
  Instruct patient not to watch television, listen to radio, or read.
  Maintain bleeding precautions for patients receiving fibrinolytic or anticoagulant agents.
- Administer medications per protocol: Anticonvulsants, steroids, antibiotics, antifibrinolytics, analgesics, and agents/fluids *to control vasospasms.*
  Implement seizure precautions.
- Maintain normothermia per protocol *to minimize cerebral metabolic demands.*
  Administer antacids per protocol *to decrease or prevent gastric irritation.*
  Accurately record intake and output *to monitor for imbalances.*

Assessment Considerations

The following table summarizes assessment findings and diagnostic studies in seven types of strokes.

	Intracerebral Hemorrhage	Subarachnoid Hemorrhage	Subdural Hemorrhage
Onset	Rapid; minutes to 1-2 hours	Sudden; varied progression	Insidious; occasionally acute
Duration	Permanent if lesion is large; small lesions are potentially reversible	Variable, complete clearing may occur in days or weeks	Hours to months
Relation to activity	Usually occurs during activity	Most commonly related to head trauma	Usually related to head trauma
Contributing or associated factors	Hypertensive cardiovascular disease; coagulation defects	Intracerebral arterial aneurysm; trauma; vascular malformations	Chronic alcoholism
Sensorium	Coma common	Coma common	Generally clouded
Nuchal (neck) rigidity	Frequently present	Present	Rare
Location of cerebral deficit	Focal; arterial syndrome not common	Diffuse aneurysm may give focal sign before and after	Frontal lobe signs; ipsilateral pupil may dilate
Convulsions	Common	Common	Infrequent
CSF	Bloody unless hemorrhage entirely intracerebral	Grossly bloody; increased pressure	Normal to slightly elevated protein
Skull roentgenograms	Pineal shift, edema, hemorrhage, or hematoma	Normal or calcified aneurysm	Frequent contralateral shift of pineal gland

NIC Risk Management

Disturbed sensory perception (visual, auditory, kinesthetic, gustatory, tactile, olfactory) related to cerebral hemorrhage and/or increased ICP

- See general interventions listed on p. 273.

Risk for injury related to seizures

- Maintain bed in low position at all times unless side rails are up or nurse is with patient.
- Provide patient with a call light within easy reach.
- Maintain side rails in up position at bedtime, after sedation, when patient is confused, and as needed.
- Maintain wheelchairs and stretchers in locked position when transferring patient *to prevent falls.*

Preconvulsive care

- Maintain seizure precautions.
  - Have oral airway at bedside *to provide for adequate oxygenation.*
  - Have suction equipment available at bedside *to prevent aspiration.*
  - Administer oxygen per protocol *to prevent cerebral hypoxia.*
  - Establish means of communication; identify auras if possible.

Convulsive care

- Maintain patent airway.
- Support and protect head; turn to side if possible *to prevent aspiration.*
- Prevent injury.
  - Ease patient to floor if in chair.
  - Place pillows along side rails if patient is in bed.
  - Loosen constrictive clothing.
- Provide privacy as necessary. Stay with patient.
- Note frequency, time, involved body parts, and length of seizure.

Postconvulsive care

- Maintain patent airway.
- Suction as needed.
- Administer oxygen per protocol.
- Reorient patient to environment *to minimize sensory-perceptual alteration.*
- Place patient in position of comfort, and turn head to side.
- Administer oral hygiene as necessary *to remove secretions and bleeding.*

Risk for aspiration related to enteric feeding via nasoenteric tube

- Confirm feeding tube placement after insertion every 4 hours and as needed.
  - Confirm tube placement before and after each intermittent tube feeding.
  - Confirm initial enteral tube placement by physician examination of chest x-ray.
- Tape nasogastric tube securely per protocol.
- Aspirate stomach contents *to determine gastric pH.*
- Assess patient for abdominal distention, nausea/vomiting, and diarrhea/constipation.
  - Hold tube feedings if bowel sounds are absent and if diarrhea/constipation or nausea/vomiting is present.
- Maintain proper patient positioning.
  - Elevate head of bed 30 to 40 degrees.
  - Turn patient to right side *to facilitate stomach drainage through pylorus.*
- Discontinue continuous feedings 30 to 40 minutes before activity/procedure that requires lowering the patient's head.
- Check pulmonary-tracheal secretions every 4 hours and as needed *to detect presence of enteral feeding.*

Extradural Hemorrhage	Focal Cerebral Ischemia	Cerebral Thrombosis	Cerebral Embolism
Rapid; minutes to hours	Rapid; seconds to minutes	Minutes to hours	Sudden
Initially fluctuating; then steadily progressive	Seconds to minutes	Permanent if lesion is large; potentially reversible if lesion is small	Rapid improvement may occur depending on collateral flow
Almost always related to head trauma	Occurs during activity if related to decreased cardiac output	Usually occurs at rest	Unrelated to activity
Any condition that predisposes to trauma	Peripheral and coronary atherosclerosis; hypertension	Peripheral and coronary atherosclerosis; hypertension	Atrial fibrillation; aortic and mitral valve disease; myocardial infarct; atherosclerotic plaque
Rapidly advancing coma	Usually conscious	Usually conscious	Usually conscious
Rare	Absent	Absent	Absent
Temporal lobe signs; ipsilateral pupil may dilate; high intracranial pressure	Focal; or arterial syndrome	Focal; or arterial syndrome	Focal; or arterial syndrome
Common	Rare	Rare	Rare
Increased pressure; color and cells usually normal	Usually normal	Usually normal	Usually normal
Frequently fracture across middle meningeal artery groove	May show calcification of intracranial arteries	Possible arterial calcification and pineal shift from edema	Usually normal

SIGNS AND SYMPTOMS FOR STROKE

Restlessness and lethargy
Changes in level of consciousness
Changes in vital signs (increased systolic blood pressure; widened pulse pressure, decreased pulse rate)
Pupillary changes (i.e., mydriasis)
Improved pupillary reflexes
Papilledema (late sign)
Nausea and vomiting (may be projectile)
Other
Feelings of powerlessness
Improved mobility: Skin condition and pressure points should be checked every 20 min, as well as phonation, respiration, and articulation-resonance (PRA)
Impaired communication: Assess ability to communicate

NIC Immobility Management

Impaired physical mobility related to altered sensory and neuromuscular status

- Apply elastic stockings *to prevent thrombus and embolus formation.*
  Monitor for signs of thrombophlebitis and deep vein thrombosis, including redness, tenderness, localized swelling, warmth, and upward red streaking on an extremity.
- Administer anticoagulation therapy per protocol.
- Encourage self-care activities to tolerance unless contraindicated by subarachnoid hemorrhage precautions.
- Plan all activities and maintain planned rest periods *to avoid fatigue.*
- Obtain physical therapy referral.
- Turn, reposition, and provide skin care every 2 hours *to prevent skin breakdown.*
- Perform active or passive ROM exercises every 2 to 4 hours *to prevent contractures.*
- Assist patient out of bed to chair two or three times daily unless contraindicated *to promote mobility.*

NIC Self-Care Facilitation

Feeding, bathing/hygiene, dressing/grooming, and toileting self-care deficits related to neurologic impairment

- Assist with daily hygiene care as indicated.
- Assist with feeding if indicated; use intravenous or nasogastric feedings as ordered.
- Administer oral hygiene every 2 hours and as needed *to keep mucous membranes moist.*
- Administer eye care every 2 to 4 hours if indicated.
- Insert indwelling urinary catheter or perform intermittent urinary catheterizations per protocol.
- Maintain bowel function with regular evacuation.

NIC Skin/Wound Management

Risk for impaired skin integrity related to prolonged immobility

- See general intervention strategies on p. 278.

NIC Coping Assistance

Powerlessness related to neurologic impairment

- Assist patient to reestablish some means of psychologic control.
  Encourage patient to express feelings.
  Encourage patient and family to participate in care.
  Encourage patient to become an active decision maker about care and immediate environment.
- Share knowledge of physiologic functioning with patient and family.

NIC Cognitive Therapy

Chronic confusion related to organic or cognitive impairment

- Ensure optimal sensory input (i.e., eyeglasses, hearing aid) is available.
- Evaluate stimulation threshold *to prevent overstimulation.*
- Provide for structured repetitive group activities.
- Provide rest periods between activities *to minimize fatigue.*
- Maintain calm, reassuring demeanor when interacting with patient *to promote sense of trust.*
- Encourage patient to participate in care as tolerated *to minimize feelings of powerlessness.*
- Provide positive feedback for tasks/activities that are mastered.

Patient Education/Continuum of Care Plan

1. Involve the family in care, as possible. Teach essential aspects of care.
2. Reinforce the physician's explanation of medical management.
3. Stress importance of ongoing outpatient care and follow-up visits.
4. Stress need for regular exercise program.
   a. Teach ROM exercises to family.
   b. Perform ROM exercises to all body joints every 2 to 4 hours.
5. Encourage independent activities, as possible.
   a. Be alert to limitations.
   b. Avoid overprotection.
   c. Emphasize need for supportive devices as indicated (wheelchair, braces, walker, canes, overhead trapeze).
6. Stress importance of diet as ordered.
   a. Offer supplemental findings.
   b. Offer small portions, and instruct patient to chew slowly.
   c. Arrange food and utensils within easy reach.
   d. Avoid foods such as soft breads, mashed potatoes, semicooked vegetables, and large pieces of meat that can cause choking.
7. Stress importance of safety measures: side rails; ramps; shower chains; removal of scatter rugs; and walker, canes, and flat shoes.
8. Discuss name of each medication, dosage, time of administration, and toxic or side effects.
9. Stress need to avoid over-the-counter medications without first consulting physician.

10. Encourage socialization with friends and family.
11. Stress importance of communication.
    a. Speak slowly and distinctly.
    b. Use one-word commands and short sentences. Repeat as needed.
    c. Use gestures and touch when giving directions. Maintain eye contact.
    d. Implement speech exercises twice a day.
12. Stress importance of verbalization of feelings about anxiety, fear, and body image changes.
13. Ensure the patient and family understand about seizures (i.e., safety measures and whom to contact).

Evaluation/Patient Outcomes

Tissue Perfusion Management: Patient maintains adequate cerebral tissue perfusion. Level of consciousness is maintained or improved. There are no signs of increased ICP. Vital signs are stable. There is no evidence of neurologic deficits. Electrolyte pattern is stable. There is no seizure activity. Patient is normothermic. Arterial blood gas values are within normal limits or consistent with patient's baseline. Intake and output are stable.

Risk Management: Patient demonstrates minimal complications of sensory/perceptual alterations. Optimum level of orientation is maintained. Patient remains free of injury. Patient demonstrates skin integrity. Nutritional status is adequate. Self-care deficits are minimum. Social participation is appropriate to physiologic status. Patient remains free of injury. Safety measures are appropriate to physiologic status. Skin integrity is maintained. Skin is free of bruises, burns, abrasions, and redness. Environment is safe. Patient is free of nosocomial infections. Patient remains free of aspiration. Airway is patent. Vital signs are stable. Patient reports/demonstrates no signs of choking. Breath sounds are normal. Nasoenteric tube placement is verified.

Immobility Management: Patient demonstrates an optimum level of mobility. Skin integrity is maintained. Patient remains free of contractures and deformities. Level of mobility is appropriate to physiologic status. Intake and output pattern is stable. Nutritional status is adequate. Patient remains free of thrombophlebitis. Patient remains free of local infections. Patient participates in an ongoing physical therapy program. Patient demonstrates minimum self-care deficits. Outcome criteria listed for impaired physical mobility are met. Level of self-care activities is appropriate to physiologic status. Patient participates in physical and occupational therapy.

Self-Care Facilitation: Patient demonstrates optimal self-care activities. Level of self-care is appropriate to physiologic status. Patient participates in self-care to optimal level.

Skin/Wound Management: Patient demonstrates skin integrity. Skin is intact. Nutritional status is adequate. Electrolyte balance is maintained. Patient remains free of pressure sores and contractures.

Coping Assistance: Patient demonstrates minimum feelings of powerlessness. Optimum level of physiologic control, as possible for current health status, is maintained. Optimum level of psychologic control, as possible, is maintained. Patient participates, as possible, in decision making about care. Patient participates, as possible, in self-care.

Cognitive Therapy: Patient demonstrates minimal confusion. Available sensory aids (i.e., eyeglasses, hearing aid) are used appropriately. Patient is able to participate in structured repetitive group activities. Rest periods between activities are maintained. Patient is able to participate in care to tolerance.

TRAUMA

Craniocerebral Trauma

Craniocerebral trauma is physical injury to the brain or structures within the cranium.

Each year, there are more than 2 million head injuries in the United States. Approximately 120,000 of these injuries are classified as severe head trauma, which is defined by a score of 8 or less on the Glasgow Coma Scale (GCS). For individuals who survive head injury, 70,000 to 90,000 will experience serious functional losses for the rest of their lives.

General effects of moderate to severe head injuries include cerebral edema, sensorimotor deficits, and increased ICP. After the initial brain injury, secondary damage can result from brain herniation, cerebral ischemia, and hypoxemia. Leading causes of craniocerebral trauma include falls, industrial accidents, vehicular accidents, assaults, sport accidents (e.g., football, boxing, diving), and intrauterine and birth injuries.[6]

Pathophysiology

Craniocerebral injuries can result from primary or secondary trauma to the head. Primary trauma occurs when traumatic forces directly impact the head, setting into action the mechanisms of injury. The mechanisms of primary trauma that produce actual brain deformation include acceleration-deceleration with cavitation, as well as rotation of the skull and its cranial contents. These forces can occur simultaneously or in succession and damage the brain by compression, shearing, or tension. Acceleration injuries result when the head is struck by a moving object and set in motion. The slower-moving brain tissue is damaged by sudden contact with the edges of the dural membrane or the bony prominences of the skull. As a result of acceleration forces, there may be bruising or contusion of the undersurfaces of the occipital lobes, the brainstem, the superior surface of the cerebellum at the edge of the tentorium, or the tips of the frontal and temporal lobes.

Deceleration occurs when the moving head strikes a solid, immovable object (as when the head hits a windshield). There is rapid deceleration of the skull, but the brain decelerates more slowly (20 msec), and the brain tissue may travel 2 to 3 cm in that time period.

Acceleration-deceleration movements from lateral flexion, hyperflexion, hyperextension, and turning movements during the injury cause the cerebrum to rotate about the brainstem and produce shearing, straining, and distortion of neural tissue.

Microscopically, the stretching or tension causes fracture of axons in the longitudinal bundles of the cerebrum and the long axons in the brainstem. This rotational mechanism is a major cause of contrecoup lesions and may account for most of the contusions to the brain tissue. Areas most frequently injured during rotation are the frontal and temporal lobes.

Primary trauma to the head may be followed by secondary injury that increases the morbidity and mortality of head-injured patients. Secondary trauma to the head may result when tension strains and shearing forces are transmitted to the cranium by extreme torsion and stretching of the neck, as in a hard fall on the buttocks. Other factors such as sustained intracranial hypertension, sustained cerebral edema, hypercapnia, hypoxemia, systemic hypotension, infections, and respiratory trauma and its complications may contribute to secondary injury to the brain.

Head injuries can be classified as open or closed. Open head injuries result from skull fractures or penetrating wounds (FIG. 5-31). The velocity, mass, shape, and direction of impact are the major determinants of brain injury. With an open head injury there is some type of skull fracture, such as linear, comminuted, depressed, or perforated.

A linear fracture is a simple break in bone continuity that produces an inbending of the bone at the point of impact and an outbending of the skull in the surrounding area. A comminuted skull fracture occurs when two or more communicating breaks divide the bone into two or more fragments. Depressed fractures result when the bone is forced below the line of normal contour as a result of impact with a moving object. Compound fractures may be linear, comminuted, or depressed.

Another, serious type of skull fracture is the basal fracture, which can be linear, comminuted, or depressed. Structures most commonly damaged with this type of fracture include the internal carotid artery and cranial nerves I, II, VII, and VIII. Basal skull fractures usually traverse the paranasal sinuses (frontal, maxillary, or ethmoid). The fragility of the bones and the close adherence of the dura account for the frequency of this type of fracture and the subsequent leakage of CSF through the dural tear.

With open head injuries there can be high- or low-velocity impacts. The higher the velocity of impact, the greater is the explosive effect within the cranium. For example, in high-velocity impacts, as with gunshot wounds, there is laceration at the entry site, cerebral edema, hemorrhage into the destroyed area, and remote contusions (secondary to tissue displacement).[6] Lower-velocity impacts usually result in distortion and linear fractures of the skull.

A closed, blunt head injury can produce the pathologic signs of cerebral concussion, contusion, or laceration. A concussion is a transient neurologic dysfunction of paralysis and is the least serious type of brain injury. With a concussion there may be immediate and transitory disturbances in equilibrium, consciousness, and vision. Contusions result in bruising of brain tissue, usually accompanied by hemorrhages of surface vessels. Lacerations are the actual tearing of the cortical surface. Contusions and lacerations result in microscopic hemorrhages around blood vessels with destruction of surrounding brain tissue.

A contusion or laceration directly beneath the site of impact is a coup lesion; those occurring opposite the site of impact are contrecoup lesions (FIG. 5-32). The two major factors that determine the distribution of coup and contrecoup lesions are the ability of CSF to act as a shock absorber and shifts of the intracranial contents. With a coup lesion the impact causes greater displacement of the skull than the brain. At the site of impact the CSF is squeezed out from between the brain and skull, and the skull hits the brain at the point of impact. Contrecoup lesions occur because of dissipation of the CSF between the trailing edge of the brain and the trailing surface of the skull and because of a compensatory increase in the volume of CSF between the leading edge of the brain and the leading surface of the skull. The coup or contrecoup lesion may be accompanied by cavitation, which is the release of dissolved gases from CSF, blood, or brain tissue. The release of these gases produces microscopic bubbles that extensively disrupt

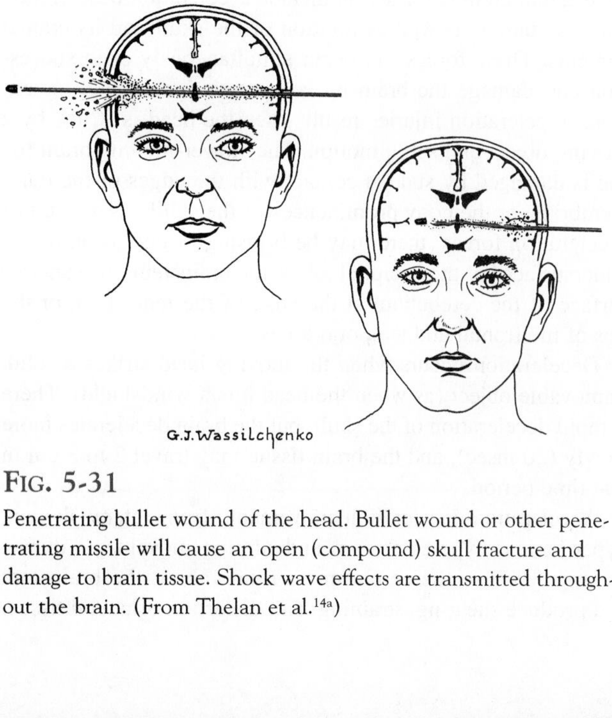

FIG. 5-31
Penetrating bullet wound of the head. Bullet wound or other penetrating missile will cause an open (compound) skull fracture and damage to brain tissue. Shock wave effects are transmitted throughout the brain. (From Thelan et al.[14a])

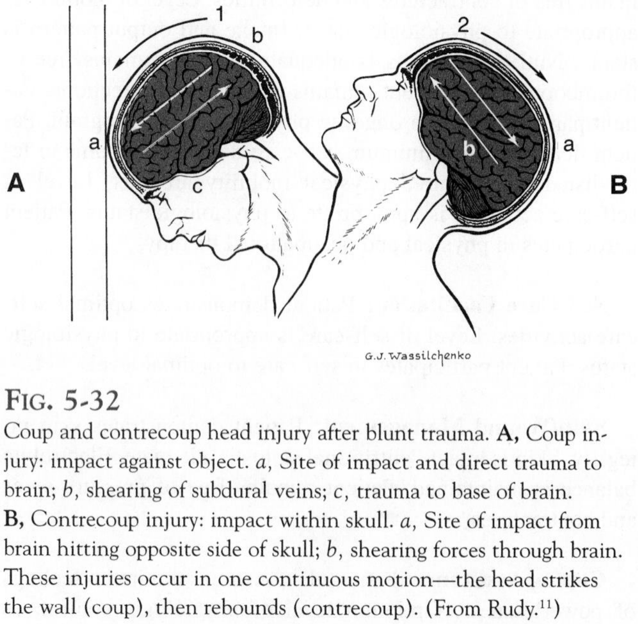

FIG. 5-32
Coup and contrecoup head injury after blunt trauma. **A,** Coup injury: impact against object. *a,* Site of impact and direct trauma to brain; *b,* shearing of subdural veins; *c,* trauma to base of brain. **B,** Contrecoup injury: impact within skull. *a,* Site of impact from brain hitting opposite side of skull; *b,* shearing forces through brain. These injuries occur in one continuous motion—the head strikes the wall (coup), then rebounds (contrecoup). (From Rudy.[11])

neural tissue, primarily in cerebrospinal pathways and near blood vessels.

Secondary responses to craniocerebral trauma may include the formation of an epidural, subdural, or intracerebral hematoma, a subarachnoid hemorrhage, cerebral edema, and brain herniation (FIG. 5-33). An epidural hematoma usually occurs when there is a linear fracture of one of the skull's membranous bones, such as the temporal area near the meningeal artery and vein. After rupture the arterial blood forms a convex mass that indents the brain. If the hemorrhage continues, the hematoma may break periosteal attachments and the dural collagen.

A subdural hematoma may result from cerebral hemorrhage in the temporal, frontal, or midline region or in any region where there is a laceration of brain tissue or its parenchymal vessels. Because the subdural hematoma is venous, symptoms appear much later than with the arterial epidural hematoma and therefore can be classified as acute, subacute, or chronic. Acute subdural hematomas usually manifest symptoms within 24 to 48 hours after severe trauma. Symptoms of subacute subdural hematoma may develop anywhere from 48 hours to 2 weeks after severe head injury. Chronic subdural hematomas develop weeks, months, and possibly years after an apparently minor head injury. The chronic type of subdural hematoma is most common for individuals in the 60- to 70-year age group because atrophy of the brain permits more room for expansion.

An intracerebral hematoma is a collection of blood within the actual brain tissue that usually occurs in the temporal or frontal region. Extensive removal of the hematoma and surrounding necrotic brain tissue generally is necessary to prevent further brain injury.

Subarachnoid hemorrhage is a frequent complication of head trauma. The pathologic processes of subarachnoid hemorrhage are presented in the discussion of vascular lesions.

Cerebral edema after craniocerebral trauma can occur locally around the injury and throughout the brain. Cerebral edema that develops after a traumatic head injury is not a single clinical or pathologic entity but exists in three forms: vasogenic, cytotoxic, and ischemic. Vasogenic edema results from an increase in capillary permeability, which then permits transudation of plasma out of the cerebral vessels and into the compliant brain tissue. Cytotoxic edema occurs with impairment or failure of the cation pump, allowing infiltration of water and sodium into the intracellular space. Ischemic edema encompasses both previous types. Mechanisms of ischemic cerebral edema are initiated by the infiltration of water and sodium into the intracellular space (cytotoxic edema). This intracellular edema then affects the tight junction of the endothelial cell, with resultant infiltration of plasma across the damaged capillaries into the extracellular space (vasogenic edema).

The mechanisms of traumatic cerebral edema are significant factors affecting both an individual's physiologic responses and survival after a severe head injury. If untreated or uncontrolled, cerebral edema produces a cycle of intracranial hypertension, reduced cerebral perfusion, and increased cerebral hypoxia. These mechanisms then produce more cerebral edema, and results are often fatal.[2]

The peak of cerebral edema is usually around 72 hours after the traumatic injury. Responses to the cerebral edema include increased ICP and the cerebral herniation syndromes.

Brain herniation is a secondary complication that can develop as a result of a primary head injury. The main types of brain herniation syndromes are uncal, transtentorial, and cerebellar. Uncal (lateral transtentorial) herniation involves displacement of the medial portion of the temporal lobe across the tentorium into the posterior fossa, compressing the midbrain and brainstem. Transtentorial (central) herniation involves downward displacement of the cerebral ventricles through the diencephalon against the midbrain. Cerebellar herniation results when the cerebellar tonsils move downward through the foramen magnum and compress the medulla.

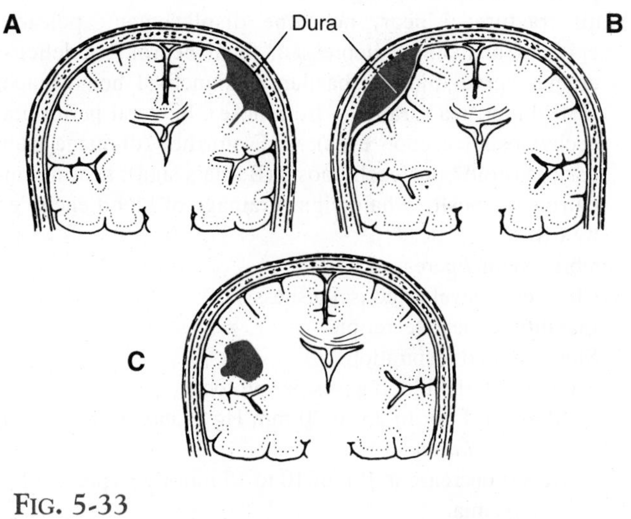

FIG. 5-33
Different types of hematomas. **A,** Subdural. **B,** Epidural. **C,** Intracerebral. (From Thelan et al.[14a])

DIAGNOSTIC STUDIES AND FINDINGS

Skull roentgenograms: Detection of skull fractures (simple, compound, depressed, or comminuted); visualization of bone fragments

Cervical roentgenogram: To confirm or rule out cervical spinal injury (assume neck injury until proven negative)

Chest roentgenogram: Indicates presence of aspiration, chest injuries, and atelectasis; indicates placement of endotracheal tube

CT scan (serial): May indicate subdural hematoma, intracerebral hematoma, or shift and distortion of cerebral ventricles

Pulsed transcranial Doppler (PTCD): Flow velocities of cerebral vessels

MRI: Detection of small extraaxial fluid collections and parenchymal injuries.

CSF sampling: May be contraindicated with increased ICP; normal in cerebral edema and brain concussion; increased pressure and blood with laceration and contusion

Cerebral angiography: May indicate intracerebral or subdural hematoma by showing avascular areas with displacement of surrounding vessels

EEG (done serially): Appearance or development of pathologic waves; determination of brain death

Serum osmolarity: Hyperosmolar state (i.e., diabetes insipidus); hypoosmolar state (syndrome of inappropriate secretion of antidiuretic hormone [SIADH])

Serum electrolytes: Natriuresis; hypernatremia and hyponatremia; elevated plasma cortisol; increased serum lactic dehydrogenase
Urine osmolarity: Dilute urine or concentrated urine
Arterial blood gases: Hypoxemia; hypercapnia

MULTIDISCIPLINARY PLAN

Surgery

Suturing of head and scalp lacerations
Debridement of wounds
Ventricular catheter, subarachnoid bolt, and epidural sensor
Ventriculostomy
Cranioplasty
Shunting procedures for hydrocephalus
Craniectomy
Craniotomy
Tracheostomy
Skull trephine (burr holes); twist-drill ventriulography

Medications

Diuretics
- Mannitol 20% (osmotic diuretic), 0.25-1.0 mg kg IV q3-4h (used with caution)
- Furosemide (Lasix) (loop diuretic), 0.5-1.0 mg/kg IV q6-8h

Anticonvulsants
- Phenytoin sodium (Dilantin), 18 mg/kg; then maintenance dose of 5 mg/kg/day
- Phenobarbital sodium, 1-3 mg/kg IV (continuous infusion)
- Carbamazepine (Tegretol), 200 mg bid initially; gradually increased up to 800-1200 mg/day in divided doses

Sedative/hypnotics
- Lorazepam (Ativan), 0.5 to 2 mg/h IV
- Midazolam (Versed), 1-2 mg/h IV (continuous)
- Propofol (Diprivan), 100-150 μg/kg/min IV (continuous)
- Fentanyl (Sublimaze), 2-20 μg/kg IV

Neuromuscular blockade: Pancuronium (Pavulon) 1-4 mg IV q4h
Histamine antagonist: Ranitidine (Zantac), 50 mg IV q6h
Cimetidine (Tagamet), 300 mg IV q6h
Analgesic/antipyretic: Acetaminophen, 325-650 mg PO or rectal suppository q4h prn
Antacids
- Maalox, 30 ml PO or nasogastric (NG) q2h
- Artificial tears prn
- Stool softeners
- Colace, 100 mg PO or NG tid

Antibiotics: Broad-spectrum agents used to prevent (controversial) or control infection

General Management

Controlled mechanical ventilation
Hyperventilation to control intracranial hypertension
Cervical collars
Central venous pressure line
Arterial pressure line
ICP monitoring; **contraindicated in patients with coagulopathy**
Hypothermia-hyperthermia balance
Incentive spirometry
Cardiac monitoring
Salem sump, nasogastric tube
Swan-Ganz catheterization
GCS
Endotracheal intubation
Physical nerve stimulation (used with neuromuscular blockade agents)
Nutritional support (i.e., enteral feedings, intravenous hyperalimentation)
Physical therapy program
Warm or cold compresses for periorbital edema and ecchymosis
Indwelling urinary catheter
Speech therapy, if indicated
Psychosocial counseling
Seizure precautions
Nutritional consultation
Social services consultation
Home health referral

NURSING CARE

NURSING ASSESSMENT

Cranial nerve palsies: bilateral anosmia; agnosia (less common); paralysis of ocular movements: diplopia, nystagmus; partial or complete blindness; vertigo; deafness; numbness, paresthesias, or neuralgia of areas supplied by trigeminal nerve; strabismus
Level of consciousness: Mental changes; irritability; anxiety; restlessness; confusion; delirium; stupor; coma
Pain: Headache
Motor function: Concussion; transitory extensor spasms; contusion; weakness; paresis; paralysis; decorticate (flexor) posturing: upper extremity flexion, lower extremity extension; decerebrate (extension) posturing: extension and internal rotation of upper extremities, extension of lower extremities; areflexia
Meningeal irritability: Nuchal rigidity; positive Kernig's sign; positive Brudzinski's sign
Skull fracture: Linear; no bone displacement; possible epidural hematoma; depressed; focal neurologic deficits; cranial nerve injuries; basilar; conjunctival hemorrhage; CSF rhinorrhea (drainage from nose); bilateral periorbital ecchymosis (raccoon eyes); CSF otorrhea (drainage from ear); mastoid bone ecchymosis (Battle's sign); hearing impairments; positive halo sign (drainage of blood encircled by CSF)
Cerebral edema/increased ICP
- Changes in level of consciousness
- Inability to clear secretions
- Slow, labored respirations
- Monitor arterial blood gases per protocol
  - Maintain Pco_2 to 25 to 30 mm Hg *to minimize cerebral vasodilation*
  - Report decrease in Po_2 of 10 to 15 mm Hg to prevent hypoxemia.
  - Report increase in Pco_2 greater than 10 to 15 mm Hg to prevent hypercapnia.

Reflexes: Pupils dilated; loss of cutaneous and tendon reflexes (concussion); Babinski's reflex positive (with increased ICP)
Vital signs: Decreased blood pressure; pulse slow (associated with intracranial hypertension) or rapid and feeble (associated with hemorrhage); respirations shallow or temporary cessation (concussion)
Hyperventilation: Cheyne-Stokes, apneustic, ataxic, or cluster respirations (depending on level of function); hyperthermia associated with hypothalamic injury; widening pulse pressure with hypertension and bradycardia (Cushing's syndrome) associated with intracranial hypertension and cerebral ischemia
Other: Dehydration; polyuria; shock
Late signs of cerebral edema/increased ICP
Bradycardia
Anorexia
Pupillary dysfunction
Papilledema (late sign)
Changes in motor function (e.g., posturing)
Nausea and vomiting (may be projectile)
Positive Babinski's sign (usually contralateral to lesion)
Visual abnormalities (e.g., diplopia, visual blurring, decreased visual acuity)
Monoparesis or hemiparesis (usually contralateral)
Seizures

Potential Complications

Posttraumatic seizure disorder: Clonic-tonic seizures
Hemorrhage: Epidural hematoma; transient loss of consciousness; increasing ICP (rapid development); ipsilateral dilated pupil; subdural hematoma; increasing lethargy; headache; seizures; minimal dilation of unilateral pupil; intracerebral hematoma; sensory and motor deficits
Brain herniation
Uncal: Decreased level of consciousness with almost simultaneous rapid motor function changes (decerebrate or decorticate posturing) and rapid changes in pupillary equality; respiratory acidosis or alkalosis; loss of oculocephalic reflex
Transtentorial: Decreased level of consciousness; nuchal rigidity; headache; unilateral or bilateral pupil dilation; elevated blood pressure; bradycardia; Cheyne-Stokes respiration; cardiac arrhythmias; decerebrate or decorticate posturing
Cerebellar: Pupils constricted and nonreactive: decreased level of consciousness, apnea or ataxic respirations
SIADH: Serum hypoosmolality and hyponatremia; urine hyperosmolality and hypernatremia; decreased urinary volume; generalized weight gain; disorientation, anxiety, anorexia, nausea, vomiting, muscle weakness, seizures.
Diabetes/Insipidus: polyuria (hourly output greater than 200 ml); low specific gravity of urine (1.001 to 1.005); polydipsia; high serum osmolality
Posttraumatic amnesia: Loss of day-to-day memory after the injury
Retrograde amnesia: Loss of memory regarding events immediately preceding the injury
Punch-drunk encephalopathy: Memory impairment, dysarthria, ataxias, tremors, parkinsonian manifestations
Postconcussion syndrome: Headache, insomnia, nervousness, fatigability, giddiness

Patient Problem/Nursing Diagnoses & Interventions

NIC Respiratory Management

Ineffective airway clearance related to impaired cough reflex
Ineffective breathing pattern related to neuromuscular impairment and/or increased ICP
Impaired gas exchange related to ineffective breathing pattern
Risk for aspiration related to enteric feeding via nasoenteric tube

- Maintain patent airway; avoid flexion of the neck until cervical films rule out neck injury. Intubation/tracheostomy and mechanical ventilation may be indicated.
- Suction as needed *to remove secretions and blood.* Hyperoxygenate lungs with 100% oxygen for 1 minute before and 1 minute after suctioning, unless contraindicated; limit suctioning to less than 15 seconds *to prevent suction-induced hypoxemia.*
- Monitor mechanical ventilator, if used. Controlled ventilation may be indicated.
  Ensure that tidal volume, rate, mode, and oxygen concentration are set as ordered.
  Ensure that ventilator alarms are on and functional. Check ventilator connections regularly.
- Keep emergency drugs and ventilator at bedside.
- Maintain NPO status, if indicated, *to prevent risk of choking or aspiration.*
- Maintain neck in neutral position *to promote optimal cerebral venous drainage.*
- Confirm feeding tube placement after insertion every 4 hours and as needed.
  Confirm tube placement before and after each intermittent tube feeding.
  Confirm initial enteral tube placement by physician examination of chest x-ray.
- Tape nasogastric tube securely per protocol.
- Aspirate stomach contents *to determine gastric pH.* Hold tube feedings if bowel sounds are absent and if diarrhea/constipation or nausea/vomiting are present.

NIC Tissue Perfusion Management

Ineffective tissue perfusion related to primary injury or increased ICP
Decreased intracranial adaptive capacity related to cerebral edema

- Intervene to monitor values and waveforms of ICP line and prevent intracranial hypertension. **Continuous flushing systems must not be used for measuring ICP.**
- Maintain patency and sterility of the system.
- Monitor effects of treatments on ICP.
- Space out nursing care activities.
- Correlate neurologic status with ICP values; notify physician if inconsistent.

- Assist with drainage of CSF from the system *to control intracranial hypertension.*
- Administer diuretics, hyperosmotics, and corticosteroids as directed.
- Intervene to monitor or prevent seizures. Maintain seizure precautions.
- Administer anticonvulsant agents per protocol.
  - Monitor effects and side effects.
  - Monitor for therapeutic serum levels of anticonvulsants.
- Prevent initiation of Valsalva's maneuver *to avoid increase in intrathoracic pressure.*
- Maintain elevation of head of bed per protocol *to facilitate cerebral venous drainage.*
- Test urine pH every two hours *to detect onset of diabetes insipidus.*
- Accurately record intake and output. Maintain slight state of dehydration.
- Post fluid restriction chart that clearly indicates amount of fluid permitted for a 24-hour period and how restriction is allocated for each work shift.
- Test urine pH and osmolarity every 2 hours *to detect onset of diabetes insipidus or SIADH.*

NIC RISK MANAGEMENT

Risk for injury related to seizures

Disturbed sensory/perception (visual, auditory, gustatory, kinesthetic, tactile, olfactory) related to altered cerebrovascular status

- Maintain bed in low position at all times unless side rails are up or nurse is with patient.
- Provide patient with a call light within easy reach. Maintain care items within easy reach of patient.
- Maintain side rails in up position at bedtime, after sedation, when patient is confused, and as needed.
- Maintain wheelchairs and stretchers in locked position when transferring patient.

Preconvulsive care

- Maintain seizure precautions.
- Have oral airway at bedside *to provide for adequate oxygenation.*
- Have suction equipment available at bedside *to prevent aspiration.*
- Pad side rails if indicated *to prevent injury.*
- Administer oxygen per protocol *to prevent cerebral hypoxia.*
- Establish means of communication; identify auras if possible.

Convulsive care

- Maintain patent airway.
- Support and protect head; turn to side if possible.
- Prevent injury.
  - Ease patient to floor if in chair.
  - Place pillows along side rails if patient is in bed.
  - Remove surrounding furniture.
  - Loosen constrictive clothing.
- Provide privacy as necessary; stay with patient.
- Note frequency, time, involved body parts, and length of seizure.

Postconvulsive care

- Maintain patent airway.
- Suction as needed, as indicated.
- Administer oxygen per protocol *to prevent hypoxia.*
- Reorient the patient to environment.
- Provide emotional support.
- Place patient in position of comfort; turn head to side.
- Administer oral hygiene as necessary for secretions and bleeding.
- Keep side rails up at all times when patient is alone *to prevent falls.*
- Maintain patient safety at all times; implement fall precautions as indicated.
- Avoid sedative agents, if possible.
- Maintain quiet environment, reducing external stimuli to a minimum.
- Reorient patient frequently to time, place, and person. Introduce yourself each time you reorient the patient.
- Repeat explanations frequently and simply.
- Have family bring in familiar objects *to minimize depersonalization.*
- Maintain planned rest periods, allowing sufficient time for REM sleep.
- Use day and night lighting appropriately *to promote natural sleep-wake cycle.*
- Address patient by preferred name.

NIC IMMOBILITY MANAGEMENT

Impaired physical mobility related to neuromuscular or musculoskeletal impairment

- Apply antiembolus stockings or sequential compression devices to lower extremities *to promote venous return.*
- Administer anticoagulation therapy per protocol *to prevent thrombus or embolus formation.*
- Monitor for signs of thrombophlebitis and deep vein thrombosis, including redness, tenderness, localized swelling, warmth, and upward red streaking on an extremity.
- Administer skin care every 1 to 2 hours.
- Turn patient every 2 hours and as needed, unless contraindicated.
- Change position slowly *to prevent orthostatic hypotension.*
- Position in proper body alignment; may need to use log-roll technique when turning.
- Massage pressure points every 2 hours *to stimulate circulation;* give gentle back rubs every shift and as needed.
- Obtain physical therapy referral.
- Use firm mattress or bed board *to support back and spine.*
- Use footboard or Spence boots *to prevent footdrop.* Instruct patient not to push against footboard *to prevent Valsalva's maneuver.*
- Encourage mobility to tolerance or per protocol.
- Avoid isometric exercises.
- Encourage self-care activities to tolerance.
- Plan all activities to avoid fatigue; maintain planned rest periods.

NIC SELF-CARE FACILITATION

Feeding, bathing/hygiene, dressing/grooming, and toileting self-care deficits related to neurologic disorder

- Assist with daily hygiene care as indicated.
- Assist with feeding as indicated.
- Use intravenous or nasogastric feedings per protocol.
- Administer oral hygiene every 2 hours and as needed.
- Administer eye care every 2 to 4 hours if indicated *to prevent drying of corneas.*
- Maintain bowel function with regular evacuation.

NIC SKIN/WOUND MANAGEMENT

Risk for impaired skin integrity related to prolonged immobility

- See general intervention strategies on p. 278.

NIC COMMUNICATION ENHANCEMENT

Impaired verbal communication related to neurologic impairment

- Develop a means of communication with the patient: pencil, Magic Slate, or call light within easy reach.
- Reinforce the techniques established.
- Assist patient and family to identify other outlets for communication.
- Continue to use sense of touch and nonverbal forms of communication.
- Maintain neutral body alignment with head of bed elevated at 30 degrees, unless contraindicated *to facilitate cerebral venous drainage.*

NIC COPING ASSISTANCE

Chronic confusion related to organic or cognitive impairment

- Evaluate previous interests.
- Ensure optimal sensory input (i.e., eyeglasses, hearing aid) is available.
- Provide for structured repetitive group activities.
- Provide rest periods between activities *to minimize fatigue.*
- Maintain calm, reassuring demeanor when interacting with patient *to promote sense of trust.*
- Encourage patient to participate in care as tolerated *to minimize feelings of powerlessness.*
- Provide positive feedback for tasks/activities that are mastered.

PATIENT EDUCATION/CONTINUUM OF CARE PLAN

1. Involve family in care, as possible; teach essential aspects of care.
2. Reinforce physician's explanation of medical management.
3. Stress importance of ongoing outpatient care and follow-up visits.
4. Encourage independent activities, as possible.
   a. Alert to limitations
   b. Avoid overprotection.
   c. Stress need for supportive devices as indicated.
5. Emphasize need for regular exercise program. Teach ROM exercises to family.
6. Stress importance of diet as ordered.
   a. Offer supplemental feedings.
   b. Offer small portions; instruct patient to chew slowly.
7. Stress importance of safety measures: side rails; ramps; shower chairs; walker, canes.
8. Instruct patient regarding name of medication, dosage, time of administration, and toxic or side effects.
9. Stress need to avoid over-the-counter medications without first consulting physician.
10. Encourage socialization with friends and family.
11. Emphasize importance of verbalization of feelings about anxiety, fear, and body image changes.
12. Ensure that patient and family understand about seizures (i.e., safety measures and whom to contact).

EVALUATION/PATIENT OUTCOMES

Respiratory Management: Breath sounds are normal. Chest excursion is bilateral and symmetric. Rate and depth of respirations are normal. Cough is effective. There are no subjective or objective findings of shortness of breath, air hunger, or dyspnea on exertion. Arterial blood gas values are within normal ranges or consistent with patient's baseline. Vital signs are within normal ranges or consistent with patient's baseline. Hemoglobin levels are 14 to 18 g/dl (male) or 12 to 16 g/dl (female). Intake and output are stable. All lobes are resonant on percussion. Skin color is not cyanotic. There are no signs or symptoms of choking. Tube feeding residuals are within acceptable range.

Tissue Perfusion Management: Level of consciousness is unchanged. There is no evidence of neurologic deficits. Electrolyte pattern is stable. There is no seizure activity. Vital signs are stable. No signs of increased ICP are present. Patient is normothermic. Arterial blood gas values are within normal limits or consistent with patient's baseline. Intake and output are stable.

Risk Management: Optimum level of orientation is maintained. Patient remains free of injury. Patient demonstrates skin integrity. Nutritional status is adequate. Self-care deficits are minimum. Safety measures are appropriate to level of physiologic status. Skin integrity is maintained. Skin is free of bruises, burns, abrasions, and redness. Environment is safe. Patient is free of nosocomial infections.

Immobility Management: Patient exhibits skin integrity. Patient remains free of contractures and deformities. Level of mobility is appropriate to physiologic status. Intake and output pattern is stable. Nutritional status is adequate. Patient remains free of thrombophlebitis. Patient remains free of local infection. Patient participates in an ongoing physical therapy program.

Self-Care Facilitation: Outcome criteria listed for impaired physical mobility are met. Level of self-care activities is appropriate to physiologic status. Patient participates in physical and occupational therapy.

Skin/Wound Management: Skin is intact. Nutritional status is adequate. Electrolyte balance is maintained. Patient remains free of pressure sores and contractures.

Communication Enhancement: Patient demonstrates minimum impaired verbal communication. Patient verbalizes feelings for as long as is physically able to do so. Patient develops alternate methods of communication.

Coping Assistance: Patient demonstrates minimal confusion. Available sensory aids (i.e., eyeglasses, hearing aid) are used appropriately. Patient is able to participate in structured repetitive group activities. Rest periods between activities are maintained. Patient is able to participate in care to tolerance.

Spinal Cord Trauma

Spinal cord trauma is physical injury to the spinal cord caused by violent or disruptive action.

Each year in the United States, there are 8000 to 10,000 new cases of spinal cord injury (SCI). Approximately one third of the individuals who experience an SCI die before reaching an acute care facility. About 60% of individuals sustaining an SCI are between ages 16 and 30 years, and most (85% to 90%) are male. Causes of spinal cord trauma include assaults (e.g., bullet wounds), falls, sport injuries (e.g., diving accidents), industrial accidents, birth injuries, degenerative changes (e.g., vertebral disk deterioration), and vehicular accidents. Presently, there are more than 200,000 individuals in the United States who are severely disabled as a result of spinal cord trauma.

> **! EMERGENCY ALERT**
>
> **NEUROGENIC (SPINAL) SHOCK**
>
> Neurogenic shock is a form of vasogenic or distributive shock that results when the vascular system dilates. In neurogenic shock this generally occurs when there is disruption of the spinal cord leading to loss of sympathetic tone and resultant dilation of the arterioles and venules.
>
> ASSESSMENT
> - Decreased blood pressure
> - Rapid, shallow respirations
> - Slowed pulse rate
> - Paraplegia, quadriplegia, or priapism
> - Diaphoresis above the level of the cord injury
> - Loss of vasomotor tone and ability to control heat
> - Warm and dry skin
>
> INTERVENTIONS
> - Maintain airway, breathing, and circulation.
> - Protect cervical spine from displacement or injury.
> - Obtain IV access and administer fluids (avoid overload).
> - Administer vasoconstricting medications as ordered.
> - Monitor vital signs.
> - Monitor urinary output.

The most common sites of injury are the lower cervical region (C4-7 and T1) and the thoracolumbar junction (T12, L1, and L2). Trauma to the spinal cord includes concussion, contusion, laceration, hemorrhage, transection (partial or complete), or impairment in the spinal vascular supply.

Pathophysiology

The spine and spinal cord can be injured by direct or indirect forces. Direct injuries such as falls on the head or buttocks can cause spinal cord lesions from fractured vertebrae or direct compression of the cord by depressed bone fragments. Indirect injuries (the major type of SCIs) can occur when excessive forces accelerate the cranium in relation to the trunk (i.e., whiplash injury) or when the trunk is suddenly decelerated in regard to the lumbar spine. Whether the forces are direct or indirect, the subsequent fractures of vertebrae seriously injure the neural elements of the spinal cord.

Vertebral Injuries

The primary mechanisms of vertebral injury, occurring alone or in combination, include hyperextension, hyperflexion, vertical compression trauma, and rotation.

Hyperextension injuries (FIG. 5-34) (commonly termed *whiplash*) occur frequently in the cervical region, and damage results from the forces of acceleration-deceleration and the sudden reduction in the anteroposterior diameter of the spinal canal. Since the spinal canal is full of neural tissue in the cervical area, injury can produce profound disability. With a hyperextension injury the cord can be compressed between the body of one vertebra and the leading edge of the laminal arch of adjacent vertebrae, causing complete or partial transection. In addition, the ligamentum flavum may be torn or bulge inward, and intervertebral discs may tear. Severe hyperextension injuries can produce complete transverse fracture of the vertebral body. With the compression and shearing forces of a hyperextension injury, gray matter of the cord is destroyed and microcirculation at and around the level of the injury is disrupted.

Hyperflexion injury (FIG. 5-35) results in an overstretching, compression, and deformation of the spinal cord from a sudden and excessive force that propels the neck forward or an exaggerated lateral movement of the neck to one side or another. Hyperflexion injuries can occur with wedge or compression fractures of the vertebral body with or without dislocation, fracture of the pedicle with or without dislocation of intraspinal ligaments, or fracture of the vertebral body and rupture of the intervertebral discs.

Vertical compression (FIG. 5-36) trauma primarily occurs around the area of the thoracolumbar junction (T12 to L2) and results from a force applied along an axis from the top of the cranium through the vertebral bodies. With compression injuries the vertebral body bursts, compressing the spinal cord and damaging nerve roots with bony fragments.

Rotation (FIG. 5-37) can involve all portions of the vertebral body, including pedicles, ligaments, and the articulation. Fracture of the pedicles or locked facets of the vertebrae can rupture ligaments and shear spinal cord tissue.

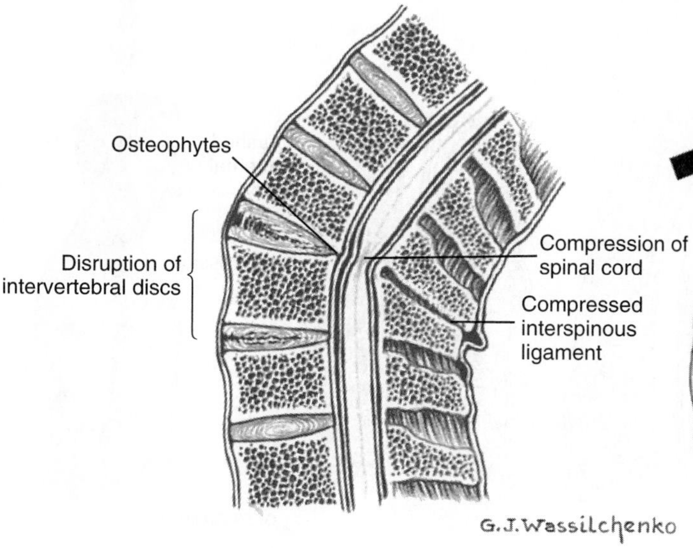

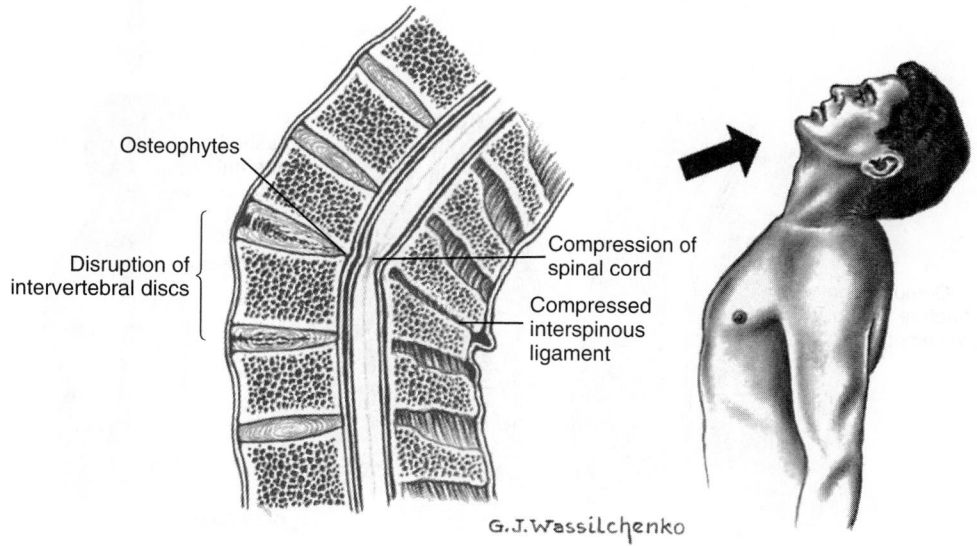

Fig. 5-34
Hyperextension injuries of the spine. (From Rudy.[11])

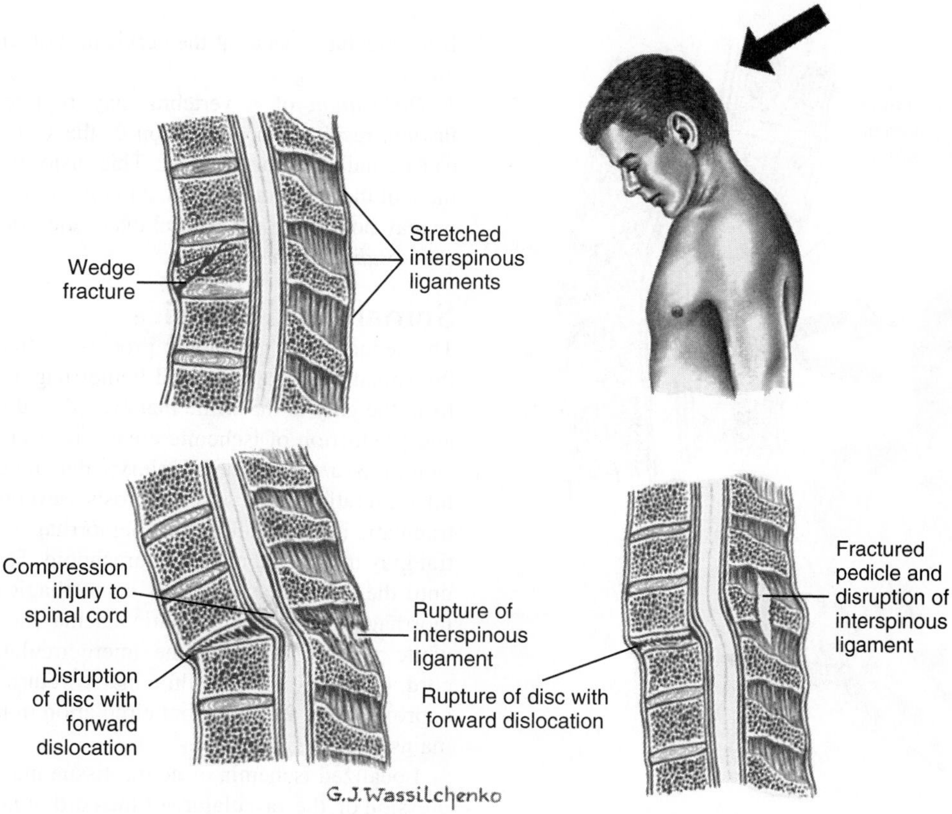

FIG. 5-35
Hyperflexion injury of the spine. (From Rudy.[11])

Vertebral injuries can be classified as simple fractures, compressed or wedged fractures, comminuted fractures, and vertebral dislocation. A simple fracture is a single break usually affecting transverse or spinous processes. Vertebral alignment usually remains intact, and compression of the spinal cord is not usually present.

Compressed, or wedged, vertebral fractures occur when the vertebral body is compressed anteriorly. Spinal cord

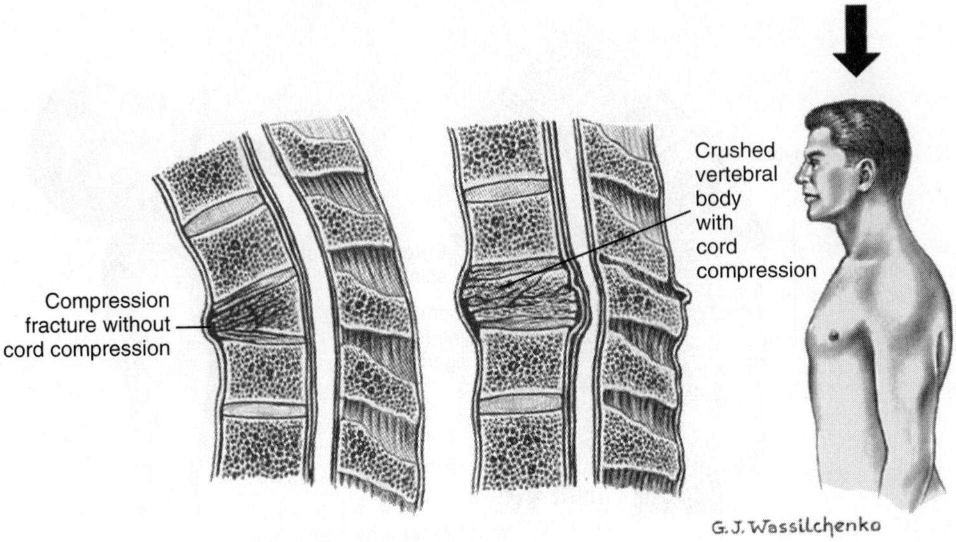

FIG. 5-36
Vertical compression injuries of the spine. (From Rudy.[11])

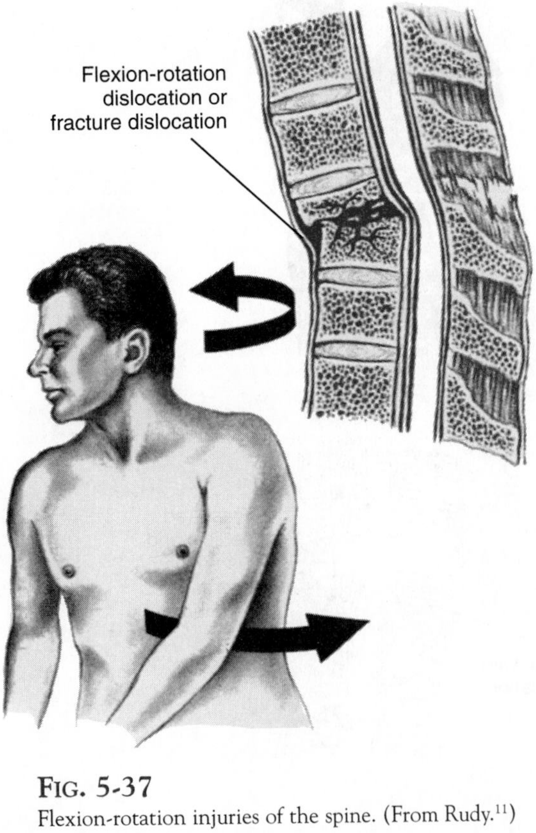

FIG. 5-37
Flexion-rotation injuries of the spine. (From Rudy.[11])

compression may or may not be present with a wedged fracture.

Comminuted, or burst, fractures can cause serious injury to the spinal cord. The vertebral body shatters into multiple fragments, and these fragments may penetrate the spinal cord. Burst fractures occur at the cervical, thoracic, and lumbar regions.

Dislocation of a vertebra may rupture the ligamentum flavum, resulting in dislocation of the vertebral facets, which can be unilateral or bilateral. This dislocation disrupts alignment of the vertebral column, and injury to the spinal cord may or may not be present. Partial dislocation of the spinal cord is called *subluxation.*

Spinal Cord Injuries

The sequence of pathologic processes after impact injury to the spinal cord are localized hemorrhaging, which advances from the gray to the white matter; reduced vascular perfusion and production of ischemic areas and decreased oxygen tension in tissue at the site of injury; edema; cellular and subcellular alterations; and tissue necrosis. Several minutes after the traumatic injury, microscopic hemorrhages appear in the central gray matter and in the pia-arachnoid. They increase in size until the entire gray matter is hemorrhagic and necrotic. Hemorrhaging and peritraumatic edema then progress to the white matter, impairing the microcirculation to the spinal cord. Circulation in the white matter returns to normal within approximately 24 hours, but circulation in the gray matter remains altered.

Localized ischemia of neural tissue may result from compression on the vasculature of the cord or nerve roots by bony fragments or herniated discs. If the flow of blood from the vertebral artery to the anterior spinal artery or to the branches of the radicular arteries is impaired, severe cord ischemia results. Hemorrhage, other than with contusion and edema, usually does not produce significant neural impairment. Although subarachnoid bleeding is usual, it is of little clinical significance.

In the third to fourth week after the injury, the traumatized section of the cord is gradually replaced with connective scar tissue or glial fibers. Injured segments of the spinal cord are replaced with acellular collagenous tissue, which connects the meninges to the cord and central canal. Scarring in the injured area consists mainly of thickened meninges and connective tissue.

Spinal Shock

Spinal shock at the area of transection occurs after complete severing of the spinal cord. It causes a complete loss of sensory, motor, autonomic, and reflex functioning below the level of the lesion.

Autonomic Hyperreflexia

Autonomic hyperreflexia may occur after spinal shock has been resolved and reflex activity has returned. The syndrome is associated with a massive uncompensated cardiovascular response to stimulation of the sympathetic division of the autonomic nervous system.[2] Individuals most likely to be affected with autonomic hyperreflexia have lesions at the level of T6 or above.

Cord Syndromes

Trauma to the spinal cord results in several syndromes that develop from the specific area of cord damaged and vary in severity depending on the amount of cord compression or transection.

The *anterior cord* syndrome occurs after an acute flexion injury to the cervical area and is rare in its pure form. Clinical manifestations are caused by anterior compression of the spinal cord, which injures the lateral corticospinal and spinothalamic tracts.

The *posterior cord* syndrome, although rare, is associated with cervical hyperextension trauma.

Central cord syndrome results primarily from hyperextension injuries. Neurologic deficits are caused by central hemorrhage in the cord, which affects lower motor neurons and decussating tracts, but spares the lateral corticospinal tracts.

The *Brown-Séquard syndrome* results from rotation-flexion injuries where subluxation or dislocation of the fracture occurs. This type of injury is seen most often with blunt trauma.

The *herniated disc syndrome* is one of the most common spinal cord syndromes. The severity of symptoms depends on quantity of herniated disc tissue, number of involved discs, amount of nerve root compression, and amount of spinal canal narrowing. Herniated discs most frequently (90%) affect the lower lumbar and lumbosacral regions.

Diagnostic Studies and Findings

Roentgenograms (anterior-posterior and especially lateral): Vertebral fractures in the cervicothoracic junction, thoracic spine, and thoracolumbar regions (**NOTE: Assume presence of a cervical fracture until it is ruled out by x-ray.)**

CT scan: Spinal cord edema

MRI: Spinal cord edema and compression

Spinal puncture: Establishes presence or absence of spinal block

Myelography: Establishes presence of spinal block

Multidisciplinary Plan

Surgery

Decompression laminectomy
Harrington rods
Endotracheal intubation (nasal) (NOTE: Cricothyrotomy and tracheostomy should be avoided, if possible, because these procedures put pressure on vertebral column.)
Gardner-Well tongs
Spinal fusion for stabilization
Wound debridement; suturing of lacerations
Myotomies, tenotomies, neurectomies, rhizotomies, and muscle transplants (treatment for spasticity)
Gastrostomy or jejunostomy tube placement

Medications

Corticosteroid protocol (must be started within 8 h of injury): Methyprednisolone (loading dose), 30 mg/kg IV over 30 min, then IV methylprednisolone, 5.4 mg/kg/h IV for 23 h

Antianxiety agents
- Lorazepam (Ativan), 0.5-1 mg, PO, q4-6h
- Diazepam (Valium), 2-10 mg tid or qid PO

Muscle relaxants
- Baclofen (Lioresal), 15-80 mg/day PO in divided doses
- Dantrolene sodium (Dantrium), 25 mg tid to 100 mg qid
- Clonazepam (Klonopin), 0.1-0.5 mg/day PO or transdermal patch
- Tizanidine (Zanaflex), 4 mg PO hs—increase slowly to maximum dose of 36 mg/day in three divided doses

Anticoagulants (prophylactic for deep vein thrombosis and pulmonary embolism): Heparin, 5000 U SC q12h

Agent for heterotopic ossification (HO): Etidronate disodium (Didronel), 20 mg/kg/day for 2 wk; then 10 mg/kg/day for 10 wk

Laxatives: Glycerin or bisacodyl (Dulcolax), as rectal suppository

Histamine blocker: Famotidine (Pepcid), 20 mg q6h PO

Antihypertensives (autonomic dysreflexia)
- Nifedipine (Procardia), 10 mg bitten and swallowed; may repeat in 15 min, if needed
- Hydralazine (Apresoline), 5 mg IV q5-10 min, up to maximum of 20 mg

Antacids: Magnesium hydroxide and aluminum hydroxide (Maalox TC), 20 ml PO q4h

General Management

Halo vest or brace with skeletal traction
Splints and braces
Phrenic nerve pacemakers
Functional electrical stimulation
Meticulous chest physiotherapy and pulmonary toilet
Mechanical ventilation
Cardiac monitoring
Rotating of flotation beds
Bed board and firm mattress
Indwelling and intermittent urinary catheterization
Intake and output recording
Cervical collar (soft or rigid)
Serial measurement of arterial blood gases

Urine sugar and acetone; guaiac
Antiembolus stockings or sequential compression devices
Nasogastric tube
Physical therapy
Foley catheter; intermittent catheterization
Occupational therapy
Social services
Dietary consultation
Urodynamic testing
Sexual counseling
Psychosocial counseling for individual and family

NURSING CARE

NURSING ASSESSMENT

Anterior cord syndrome: Weakness and loss of pain and temperature sensation below level of injury

Posterior cord syndrome: Power and gross sensation preserved; loss of vibratory and fine touch sensation and proprioception

Central cord syndrome: Sensation variably altered; spasticity below level of injury; disproportionate loss of motor power in upper extremities (termed *upside-down tetraplegia*)

Herniated disk syndrome

- Lumbar: Pain in lower back with radiation down back of one leg; restricted spinal mobility; walking painful; back appears straight with loss of lumbar curve; spastic paravertebral muscles; impaired sensation of affected leg and foot; less active ipsilateral ankle jerk may be present; pain aggravated by jugular compression
- Cervical: Stiffness of neck; pain radiating down arm to fingers

Pain: Hyperesthesia immediately above level of lesion; intense tingling and burning pain below level of lesion (in paraplegia)

Spasticity: Partial or complete loss of voluntary control; exaggerated deep tendon reflexes

Sexual function irregularities: Varies from normal function to complete impotence; menstrual irregularities for short time after injury

POTENTIAL COMPLICATIONS

Spinal shock: Complete neurologic assessment every 15 to 30 minutes until stable: flaccid paralysis below level of lesion; loss of proprioception, pain, temperature, touch, and pressure below level of lesion; loss of all spinal reflexes below level of lesion: paralytic ileus, loss of bladder and bowel tone; loss of vasomotor tone; loss of visceral and somatic sensations below level of lesion; loss of ability to perspire below level of lesion; bradycardia; hypotension; loss of temperature control: poikilothermia, loss of ability to perspire or shiver below level of lesion

Autonomic hyperreflexia: Complete neurologic assessment every 15 to 30 minutes until stable; paroxysmal hypertension; pounding headache; diaphoresis below level of lesion; flushing above level of lesion; cutis anserina below level of lesion; nasal congestion; nausea; bradycardia

MUSCLE FUNCTION ACCORDING TO LEVEL OF SPINAL CORD INJURY

C4 and above	Loss of all muscle function, including respiratory (usually fatal)
C5	Quadriplegia with poor respiratory functioning
C6-C8	Quadriplegia with sparing of some arm and hand muscles
T1-T3	Quadriplegia with loss of muscle function below nipple line
T4-T10	Paraplegia with some chest and trunk muscles intact
T11-L2	Paraplegia with muscles intact through upper thigh
L3-S1	Paraplegia with muscles of chest, trunk, thigh, and most of leg intact; loss of voluntary bowel and bladder control
S2-S4	Loss of voluntary bowel and bladder control

PATIENT PROBLEMS/NURSING DIAGNOSES & INTERVENTIONS

NIC RESPIRATORY MANAGEMENT

Ineffective airway clearance related to impaired cough reflex
Impaired breathing related to respiratory muscle weakness or paralysis
Impaired gas exchange related to ineffective breathing

- Maintain patient airway and avoid flexion of the neck.
- Suction as needed *to remove secretions and prevent aspiration.*
  - Hyperoxygenate lungs with 100% oxygen for 1 minute before and 1 minute after suctioning, unless contraindicated, *to prevent hypoxemia.*
- Assist ventilation as indicated. Keep Ambu-bag at bedside.
- Monitor mechanical ventilator, if used.
  - Ensure tidal volume, rate, mode, and oxygen concentration are set as ordered.
  - Ensure ventilator alarms are on and function *to prevent accidental disconnection.*
- Maintain nothing by mouth status to prevent aspiration.

NIC TISSUE PERFUSION MANAGEMENT

Altered spinal tissue perfusion related to spinal tissue edema and hypoxia

- Ensure immobilization of vertebral column.
  - Maintain skeletal traction.
  - Maintain cervical skeletal traction.

Halo traction

- Assess traction pins to ensure they are tight and secure.
- Assess fiberglass cast jacket for proper fit (should be able to insert index finger between cast and skin).
- Assess cast edges for roughness and crumbling or petal rough edges.
  - Provide routine cast care.
  - Provide pin site skin care: clean site with hydrogen peroxide and then apply povidone-iodine solution *to prevent infection.*

Cover with sterile dressing.

- Administer medications as ordered.
- Maintain parenteral fluids per protocol.

NIC Risk Management

Disturbed sensory perception (visual, auditory, kinesthetic, gustatory, tactile, olfactory) related to neuromuscular dysfunction

- See general intervention strategies on p. 294.

Risk for injury related to tissue hypoxia and/or integrative dysfunction

- Maintain bed in low position at all times unless side rails are up or nurse is with patient.
- Provide patient with a call light within easy reach.
- Maintain side rails in up position at bedtime, after sedation, and as needed.
- Maintain stretchers in locked position when transferring patient.
- Pad side rails if patient is overactive.

NIC Immobility Management

Impaired physical mobility related to instability of spine or paralysis

Risk for disuse syndrome related to muscle paralysis and prolonged immobility

- Apply antiembolus stockings or sequential compression devices to lower extremities.
- Administer anticoagulation therapy per protocol.
- Administer skin care every 2 hours.
  - Turn patient every 2 hours and as needed, unless contraindicated, *to prevent respiratory complications.*
  - Change position slowly *to prevent orthostatic hypotension.*
  - Position in straight body alignment; use log-roll technique when turning.
- Keep skin dry; give perineal care as needed.
- Perform active or passive ROM exercises every 2 to 4 hours *to promote circulation and improve muscle tone.*
- Obtain physical therapy referral.
- Use heel and elbow guards as needed *to prevent skin irritation and breakdown.*
- Use firm mattress.
- Use footboard or Spence boots *to prevent footdrop.*
- Encourage mobility to tolerance or per protocol.
- Encourage self-care activities to tolerance.
- Plan all activities *to avoid fatigue.*

NIC Self-Care Facilitation

Feeding, bathing/hygiene, dressing/grooming, and toileting self-care deficits related to neuromuscular impairment

- See general intervention strategies listed on p. 295.

NIC Elimination Management

Bowel incontinence related to neuromuscular impairment

- Maintain fluid intake of 2000 ml/day, unless contraindicated.
- Provide patient with diet that is high in roughage, protein, and bulk.
- Keep patient's skin clean and dry.
- Check patient for impaction every 1 to 2 days.
- Institute a regular bowel evacuation program.
  - Begin bowel retraining program *to prevent constipation.*
  - Instruct patient to take 8 to 10 ounces of prune juice 12 hours before time set for defecating; insert glycerin suppository high in rectum 15 to 20 minutes before set time, then place patient on bedpan, toilet, or commode.
  - Insert lubricated glycerin suppository 2 hours before set time, and position patient in sitting position or transfer to bedpan or commode at set time.
  - Instruct patient to drink 4 to 8 ounces prune juice each night.
  - Instruct patient to drink a warm drink (water, coffee, milk) 30 minutes before set time.
  - Insert laxative suppository for 2 to 4 days, then glycerin suppository for 2 to 4 days; note length of time between insertion and defecation; place patient on bedside commode at appropriate time; if no bowel movement, give small tap water enema.[6]

Impaired urinary elimination related to neuromuscular and/or sensory motor impairment

- Check for bladder distention every 2 to 4 hours.
- Perform intermittent catheterization per protocol.
- Perform catheter care every shift.
  - Maintain closed system.
  - Tape catheter to thigh *to prevent pulling and tension (female).*
  - Tape catheter to lower abdomen *to prevent pulling and tension (male).*
- Monitor intake and output. Maintain fluid intake of 2000 ml daily unless contraindicated.
- Acidify urine with foods such as cranberry juice.
- Administer urinary tract germicides (e.g., methenamine [Mandelamine]) as ordered.
- Begin bladder retraining program.
  - Upper motor neuron bladder
    - Administer fluids between 7 AM and 7 PM.
    - Remove urinary catheter at 7 AM.
    - Force fluids (i.e., 240 ml) every hour.
    - After approximately 3 to 4 hours, trigger areas (i.e., digital stimulation of rectum) until stimulated and attempt to void is made; if patient is able to void, residual urine is immediately checked.
      - Residual urine of less than 100 ml is needed to continue with training.
      - Residual urine of greater than 100 ml requires catheter reinsertion. Bladder retraining is then resumed another day.
  - Lower motor neuron bladder
    - Administer fluids between 7 am and 7 pm.
    - Remove urinary catheter at 7 am.
    - Force fluids (i.e., 240 ml) every hour.
    - After approximately 3 to 4 hours, patient attempts to void by Valsalva's maneuver, Credé's maneuver of bladder, or contraction of abdominal muscles (suprapubic stimulation).
    - If patient is able to void, residual urine is immediately checked.

Residual urine of less than 50 to 75 ml is needed to continue with training.
Residual urine of greater than 75 ml requires catheter reinsertion. Retraining is then resumed on another day.

NIC SKIN/WOUND MANAGEMENT

Risk for impaired skin integrity related to prolonged immobility
- See general intervention strategies listed on p. 278.

NIC COPING ASSISTANCE

Disturbed body image related to change in body functioning
- Provide a safe, comfortable environment.
- Carefully explain what you are doing and why you are doing it.
- Listen to the feelings the patient expresses (e.g., feelings of grief and loss).
- Answer questions simply and honestly.
- Correct misinformation.
- Protect the patient's privacy.
- Provide gentle physical care in a caring environment.
- Assist the patient to become involved in self-care.
- Assist the patient to become involved in unit activities.

NIC PSYCHOLOGIC COMFORT PROMOTION

Anxiety related to threat to self-concept
- See general intervention strategies on p. 250.

NIC LIFE SPAN CARE

Caregiver role strain related to severity of patient's illness
- Obtain assistance with meeting of caregiver role. Assist caregiver to identify/utilize caregiving resources such as family members, friends, and community agencies.
- Assist caregiver to develop plan of care with paced direct-care activities.
- Assist caregiver to develop support systems with alternate caregivers/friends.
- Assist caregiver to identify and address personal health care needs.

PATIENT EDUCATION/CONTINUUM OF CARE PLAN

1. Discuss name of each medication, dosage, time of administration, purpose, and side effects.
2. Avoid over-the-counter medications without first checking with physician.
3. Discuss muscle-building exercises: rubber balls, clay, trapezes, pulleys, squeeze toys, and sit-ups.
4. Stress importance of bladder retraining.
   a. Avoid food low in calcium.
   b. Force fluids to 2000 ml/day unless contraindicated.
   c. Maintain an acidic urine by drinking cranberry juice and taking ascorbic acid if ordered.
   d. Avoid alcoholic beverages, coffee, and tea.
   e. Maintain mobility as tolerated.
   f. Stress that rehabilitation may be a long process.
   g. Instruct regarding signs of full bladder.
   h. Avoid use of penile clamp to control incontinence.
   i. Avoid persons with infections, especially upper respiratory infections.
   j. Instruct regarding care of indwelling catheter.
   k. List symptoms to report to physician: urinary tract infection, kidney stone, upper respiratory infection, or skin lesions.
5. Ensure that the patient or family demonstrates:
   a. Bladder exercises every 2 to 4 hours:
      (1) Tighten rectum or vaginal vault.
      (2) Hold contraction for 5 seconds; then relax.
      (3) Continue tightening and relaxing for 5-minute period.
   b. Credé's maneuver for manual bladder stimlation:
      (1) Apply manual pressure over suprapubic region.
      (2) Contract abdominal muscles.
   c. Palpation of bladder distention
   d. Intake and output measurement
   e. Recording of time and amount of fluid intake
   f. Recording of time and amount of urine voided
   g. Testing of urine for pH
   h. Application of condom catheter if necessary
   i. Self-catheterization
6. Discuss importance of bowel retraining program.
   a. Encourage patient participation in developing program.
   b. Evaluate previous bowel habits.
   c. Establish regular bowel habits: (1) time of day that will be convenient for patient once discharged (e.g., after breakfast) and (2) development of program to have bowel evacuation at same time of day or every 3 days.
   d. Discuss exercises that will help to develop abdominal muscles and tone: pushing up, bearing down, and contracting abdominal muscles.
   e. Ensure privacy.
   f. Provide bedside commode rather than bedpan when possible: encourage sitting position rather than lying position.
   g. Keep equipment easily available at bedside.
   h. Ensure that the patient recognizes signals that may indicate full bowel: goose pimples, perspiration, rising of hair on arms or legs, and sense of fullness.
   i. Assist the patient to develop exercise or signals that may help to stimulate urge to defecate: (1) pressure on inner thigh, (2) stroking anus, (3) digital rectal stimulation, (4) drinking coffee, and (5) massaging abdomen downward or side to side.
   j. Discuss ways to respond to signals of defecation promptly.
   k. Discuss importance of establishing well-balanced diet that includes bulk and roughage.
   l. Discuss foods to avoid: bananas, beans, and cabbage.

m. Assist the patient to recognize impaction: (1) no formed stool for 3 days, (2) semiliquid stools, and (3) restlessness and increased feeling of discomfort.
n. Discuss treatment for impaction: (1) laxative suppository, (2) tap water or oil retention enema, or (3) manual clearing of bowel followed by enema.
o. Stress importance of reporting symptoms of autonomic hyperreflexia to physician immediately.
p. Discuss possibility of accidental incontinence once program has been established.
q. Instruct the patient to relate incontinence to change in diet or daily routine.

7. Stress importance of ongoing outpatient care such as physician's visits and physical therapy.
8. Refer to Spinal Cord Injury Foundation.

Evaluation/Patient Outcomes

Respiratory Management: Airway is patent. Breath sounds are normal. Chest excursion is bilateral and symmetric. Rate and depth of respirations are normal. Cough is effective. There are no subjective or objective findings of shortness of breath, air hunger, or dyspnea on exertion. Arterial blood gas values are within normal ranges or consistent with patient's baseline. Vital signs are within normal ranges or consistent with patient's baseline. Hemoglobin levels are 4 to 18 g/dl (male) or 12 to 16 g/dl (female). Intake and output are stable. Skin color is not cyanotic.

Tissue Perfusion Management: Neurologic and vital signs are stable. Spinal column is immobilized via appropriate method. Straight body alignment is maintained. Intake and output are adequate.

Risk Management: Level of orientation is optimum. Patient remains free of injury. Nutritional status is adequate. Self-care deficits are minimum. Social participation is appropriate to physiologic status. Safety measures are appropriate to level of physiologic status. Skin integrity is maintained. Skin is free of bruises, burns, abrasions, and redness. Environment is safe. Patient is free of nosocomial infections.

Immobility Management: Skin integrity is maintained. Patient remains free of contractures and deformities. Level of mobility is appropriate to physiologic status. Intake and output pattern is stable. Nutritional status is adequate. Patient remains free of thrombophlebitis. Patient remains free of local infection. Patient participates in an ongoing physical therapy program.

Self-Care Facilitation: Outcome criteria listed for impaired physical mobility are met. Level of self-care activities is appropriate to physiologic status. Patient participates in physical and occupational therapy.

Elimination Management: Skin in perineal area is clean and dry. Dietary intake is adequate. Fluid intake is adequate (2000 ml/day unless contraindicated). Intake and output pattern is stable. Urinary output is stable. Urine is clear, yellow, and odorless. Urine residuals are less than 100 ml when bladder training is implemented. Patient remains free of fecal impaction. Patient demonstrates a regular bowel evacuation pattern.

Skin/Wound Management: Skin is intact. Nutritional status is adequate. Electrolyte balance is maintained. Patient remains free of pressure sores and contractures.

Coping Assistance: Patient demonstrates intact self-concept. Patient openly verbalizes feelings of grief and loss. Patient verbalizes positive feelings about self. Patient acknowledges actual change in self-image. Patient focuses on present and future appearance and function. Patient verbalizes feelings of hopefulness, helpfulness, and powerfulness.

Psychologic Comfort Promotion: Patient demonstrates a low level of anxiety. Patient openly verbalizes concerns and feelings of grief, loss, and discomfort. Patient openly verbalizes feelings supported by health-care professionals and family. Patient verbalizes essential aspects of care. Patient identifies methods to effectively deal with anxious feelings.

Life Span Care: Caregiver demonstrates minimal role strain. Caregiver appropriately uses available resources. Caregiver develops adequate support systems. Caregiver addresses personal needs.

Headache

Headache, or cephalalgia, is any ache or pain in the head that results from the stimulation of pain-sensitive structures in the cranium or the extracranial tissues in the head and neck.

Headaches range in severity from a benign and transient discomfort to a severe, incapacitating pain. They may be the symptom of some potentially destructive pathologic process such as cerebral hypoxia, head trauma, inflamed meninges,

> **! EMERGENCY ALERT**
>
> **HEADACHE**
>
> Headache is an extremely common complaint. Causes may include acidosis, hypoglycemia, dehydration, *glycemia,* toxicologic factors, infections both local and systemic, trauma, and toothaches. Each is treated accordingly.
>
> **Assessment**
>
> - Nausea, vomiting, family history
> - Use PQRST assessment
> - Pain: Mild, throbbing, stabbing, unilateral, localized, photophobia, buzzing sounds, euphoria, intense yawning, depression
> - Weight gain, generalized edema
> - Visual field changes
> - Miscellaneous paraesthesia
>
> **Interventions**
>
> - Assess stability of vital signs.
> - Rule out injury and try to determine underlying cause of headache.
> - Place patient in darkened room (decreased light may relieve visual disturbances).
> - Administer medications and obtain laboratory work as indicated.

cerebral hemorrhage, or expanding cranial mass. Therefore headaches, and particularly recurring headaches, require thorough investigation, including a complete history and neurologic examination.

In 1988 the International Headache Society published a classification system to distinguish between different types of headaches. Headaches such as migraine, cluster, and tension are designated as *primary headaches.* Headaches associated with another medical diagnosis (e.g., headache accompanying head trauma) are termed *secondary headaches.*

PATHOPHYSIOLOGY

Primary Headaches

Migraine Headaches. Migraine headache generally begins in childhood, adolescence, or early adult life. It is frequently familial. Young women appear most susceptible, particularly just before or during the menstrual period. Migraine is characterized by a paroxysmal, throbbing, unilateral head pain that frequently is accompanied by autonomic symptoms such as nausea and vomiting. Attacks generally decrease in frequency and intensity with advancing are.

The exact pathogenesis of migraine is unknown. The initial physiologic change is that of vasospasm in the intracranial and extracranial arteries and their branches on one side of the head. From 10 to 30 minutes later, dilation of the same vessels occurs. The constriction of the arteries is responsible for the symptoms of the aura (if experienced), while vessel dilation produces the headache part of the syndrome.

Agents and circumstances thought to precipitate migraine attacks include emotional stress and tension, menstruation, too much or too little sleep, and dietary agents such as tyramine, nitrate, and glutamate. However, none of these affect all individuals or consistently produce attacks in the same individual. There is no evidence to support allergy or autonomic disorders as being responsible for migraine attacks.

According to the International Headache Society there are seven subtypes of migraine headaches, including migraine without aura (common migraine); migraine with aura (classic migraine); ophthalmoplegic migraine; retinal migraine; childhood periodic syndromes; complications of migraine (i.e., status migrainous, migrainous infarct); and migrainous disorder.

Cluster Headaches. Cluster headaches are four times more common in men, with a mean age of onset of 25 years. They are characterized by a distinct episode of excruciating pain, usually unilateral, that lasts from 10 minutes to less than 2 hours and is accompanied by ipsilateral lacrimation, nasal stuffiness, and drainage. Usually the same side of the head is involved in the cluster of attacks. There is no prodrome and usually only slight nausea. The attack may occur at any time (generally they are nocturnal), and multiple attacks are common.

Headaches may occur in an episodic or chronic pattern. The episodic pattern of cluster headaches is characterized by recurring headaches for several weeks to months, followed by months to years during which no headaches occur. The exact mechanism of cluster headaches is unknown. Increased histamine with resultant vasodilation has been implicated.

Tension Headaches

Muscle Contraction Headaches. Muscle contraction headaches are the most common type of head pain. Research studies indicate a preponderance of muscle contraction headaches in women and a higher incidence in adults from age 20 to 40 years. This headache is usually bilateral and may be diffuse or confined to the frontal, temporal, parietal, or occipital area. The onset of an attack is more gradual than with a migraine, and duration is highly variable, but it may last for several days up to several months or years.

Muscle contraction headaches are frequently accompanied by contraction of skeletal muscles of the face, jaw, and neck. Concurrent arterial vasodilation may contribute further to the discomfort. There are no structural changes in the involved muscle groups.

Secondary Headaches

Traumatic Headaches. The posttraumatic, or postconcussion, headache, which consists of a dull, generalized pain, may develop after head injury and may be coupled with other symptoms such as lack of concentration, giddiness, or dizziness. Symptoms are much the same whether the head injury is mild or severe. Traumatic headaches usually are nonfocal, appearing for at least part of every day and persisting over days, weeks, or months. The headache is made worse by coughing and straining, both of which raise the pressure in the intracranial and extracranial venous systems. Posttraumatic headaches are thought to be caused by vascular dilation, muscle contraction, or direct injury to the scalp.

Traction-Inflammatory Headaches

Traction Headaches. Traction headaches may result from increased ICP, cerebral hemorrhage, decreased ICP (e.g., lumbar puncture), and inflammatory processes (e.g., encephalitis, meningitis). The discomfort produced with traction headaches occurs because of referred pain when the pain-sensitive structures (e.g., cranial nerves, arteries) are stretched or displaced by a mass lesion.

Temporal Arteritis. Temporal arteritis, also called cranial arteritis or giant cell arteritis, generally affects individuals over age 60 years. This headache usually is located in the temporal area and may be accompanied by visual loss, which is caused by ophthalmic artery involvement.

Temporal arteritis is thought to result from an autoimmune mechanism and is included in the group of collagen-vascular diseases. The temporal arteries may be palpated as firm, tender cords or may be seen as tortuous, enlarged vessels.

DIAGNOSTIC STUDIES AND FINDINGS

Cervical and skull roentgenograms: Detection of abnormalities at base of brain
CT scan (contrast enhanced): Possible intracranial lesions

MRI: Same as CT scan
Diagnostic lumbar puncture (suspicion of meningitis or subarachnoid hemorrhage)
Cerebral angiography: Detection of vascular abnormalities
Neurologic history and examination: Identification of precipitating influences; effects on ADLs; neurologic deficits

MULTIDISCIPLINARY PLAN

Medications

Analgesic/antiinflammatory agents

Ergots

Ergotamine tartrate (Wigraine), 1-6 mg/attack or 10 mg/wk PO
Dihydroergotamine (DHE), up to 3 mg/24 h or 6 mg/wk PO

Narcotic analgesics

Codeine, 30-60 mg PO q4h prn
Meperidine (Demerol), 50-75 mg IM q4-6h prn

Calcium channel antagonists

Verapamil (Calan) 240-640 mg PO

β-Adrenergic blocking agents

Propranolol (Inderal), 80-320 mg PO
Atenolol (Tenormin), 50-200 mg PO
Timolol (Blocadren), 10-60 mg PO qd
Nadolol (Corgard), 40-240 mg/qd PO

Nonsteroidal antiinflammatory drugs (NSAIDs)

Naproxen (Naprosyn), 1000 mg/day in divided doses PO
Ibuprofen (Ibuprin), 400-800 mg/day in divided doses PO

Tricyclic antidepressants

Amitriptyline (Elavil), 25-100 mg PO qid
Amitriptyline (Elavil), 10-100 mg at bedtime (hs)
Methysergide (Sansert), 4-8 mg PO with meals (not for long-term use)

Other

Sumatriptan (Imitrex), 100 mg PO or 6 mg SC taken at onset of attack; NOTE: Cannot be taken within 24 h of last dose of DHE or Wigraine
Isometheptene (Midrin), 2 tablets at onset, then qh until relief PO (do not exceed 5 tablets/24 h)
Nasal butorphanol (Stadol), 1-2 mg

General Management

Application of heat or cold to affected areas
Short-term use (i.e., 10 to 15 minutes) of 100% oxygen (cluster headache)
Dietary counseling to eliminate food items that may provoke headaches
Psychologic counseling for behavioral modification, stress management, and biofeedback

NURSING CARE

NURSING ASSESSMENT

See Assessment Considerations table.

POTENTIAL COMPLICATIONS

Chronic pain

PATIENT PROBLEMS/NURSING DIAGNOSES & INTERVENTIONS

NIC PHYSICAL COMFORT PROMOTION

Acute and chronic pain related to severe headache

- Administer medication per protocol. Dosages of ergot drugs greater than 10 mg per week can lead to ergotism and cumulative effects.
- Improve effectiveness of pain relief measures by using them before the pain becomes intense. Have patient lie in quiet, dark room after taking the medication.
- Document degree of pain and effect of medication administered.
- Promote rest and relaxation.
- Decrease noxious stimuli.
- Modify anxiety associated with the pain experience.
- Provide other sensory input *to reduce focus on noxious stimuli.*
- Teach patient about his or her discomfort.
- Use other professionals, as appropriate.
- Apply cold compresses or dry heat to head.

NIC PSYCHOLOGIC COMFORT PROMOTION

Anxiety related to discomfort

See general intervention strategies listed on p. 250.

PATIENT EDUCATION/CONTINUUM OF CARE PLAN

1. Reinforce physician's explanation of medical management.
2. Instruct regarding name of medication, dosage, time of administration, and toxic or side effects.
3. Instruct regarding proper use of ergot drugs.
   a. Take medication at earliest symptom of a headache.
4. Stress need to avoid over-the-counter medications without first consulting physician.
5. Emphasize need for regular exercise program.
6. Instruct regarding possible food causes of headaches.

EVALUATION/PATIENT OUTCOMES

Physical Comfort Promotion: Patient openly verbalizes feelings of discomfort when they occur. Patient can use measures to decrease discomfort. Patient verbally validates a decrease in subjective feelings of discomfort. Objective findings of pain are decreased.

Psychologic Comfort Promotion: Patient experiences minimal feelings of anxiety. Patient is able to express feelings of anxiety and ways to minimize those feelings.

SEIZURE DISORDER

Seizures (convulsions, epilepsy) are paroxysmal episodes in which there are excessive, abnormal, and hypersynchronous discharges from a group of neurons in the CNS.[2]

Although used interchangeably, the term *seizure* is not synonymous with epilepsy. Epilepsy denotes a group of clinical disorders characterized by the repeated occurrence of any of the various forms of seizures. Approximately 2 million people in the

Assessment Considerations

Classic migraine	Throbbing, high-intensity; unilateral discomfort in temporal area, upper cranium, or lower hemicranium (rare)	Usually unilateral in temporal area, but may occur in any area of the head	Hours	Hours to days	Prodrome/aura; visual disturbances; sensory symptoms; mild paresis; nausea, vomiting, or anxiety
Common migraine	Throbbing, intense pain; progresses to generalized nonthrobbing head pain	Usually frontal or temporal region	Gradual	Hours to days	Prodrome; photophobia; nausea; irritability; vomiting; anxiety
Cluster	Sudden, intense, and unilateral pain	Orbitotemporal area; may begin in area of nostril and spread to adjacent eye and sometimes forehead	Sudden	Hours; occurs in clusters	No prodrome; anxiety; lacrimation; rhinorrhea; nasal congestion; flushing of face; Horner's sign with ptosis and pupillary constriction
Muscle contraction	Aching, tightness, or pressure	Suboccipital, occipital, frontal areas	Gradual	Hours to days	Muscle tension; anxiety
Posttraumatic headaches	Dull, generalized pain	Varies	Gradual	Varies	Intensified by physical exertion; anxiety; personality changes; insomnia; lack of concentration; nausea, vomiting; dizziness; fatigue; unsteadiness
Traction headaches	Deep, dull, steady ache usually worse in morning and aggravated by coughing or straining	Varies	Varies	Varies	Varies
Temporal arteritis	Variable intensity; unilateral or bilateral tenderness of painful area	Temporal, occipital, fronto-occipital regions; may be accompanied by tenderness of painful areas	Gradual	Weeks	Visual loss

From Hickey.[6]

United States are affected with epilepsy, the greatest number among children under age 2 years and persons over age 65 years.

PATHOPHYSIOLOGY

Seizure disorders may result from pathologic processes, endogenous or exogenous poisons, metabolic disturbances, or fever, or may be idiopathic. Pathologic processes include formation abnormalities (e.g., vascular anomalies), space-occupying lesions (e.g., brain abscess, tumors, hematomas), craniocerebral trauma, acute cerebral edema (e.g., secondary to acute renal failure), infection (e.g., encephalitis), degenerative changes (e.g., leukodystrophies), vascular lesions (e.g., embolus, cerebrovascular accidents, and hemorrhages), and neuronal injury (e.g., anoxia from deficient oxygen).

Toxic endogenous substances (e.g., uremia) or exogenous substances such as certain mediations (e.g., phenothiazines), lead ingestion, and alcohol intoxication or sudden withdrawal may precipitate seizure activity. Metabolic disturbances (e.g., electrolyte imbalances) that cause an interference with crucial substances such as oxygen, glucose, or calcium being delivered to cerebral tissues can result in seizures. Individuals with decreased neuronal thresholds may experience a seizure secondary to a febrile state. Finally, *idiopathic* seizures may occur without any identifiable cause. The basis of idiopathic seizure disorders may be a biochemical imbalance.

These causative agents are either genetic or acquired factors. Genetically, epilepsy is rarely a predictable, inherited entity. The only well-defined inherited seizure pattern is that of the classic 2.5- to 3-second spike-and-wave pattern on the electroencephalogram (EEG).[14] Therefore, although inheritance may be a risk in developing seizures, environmental risk factors (e.g., trauma) play a significant role. Acquired factors include pathologic processes (e.g., infection), trauma that produces epileptogenic lesions, toxic substances, metabolic disturbances, and febrile states.

In 1981 the International League Against Epilepsy published a modified version of the International Classification of Epileptic Seizures that remains a useful clinical guide. This classification includes the following:

1. Partial or focal seizures (seizures that begin locally)
2. Generalized seizures (seizures that are without local onset and are bilateral and symmetric)
3. Special epileptic syndromes.

Partial seizures are subdivided into partial-simple (without loss of consciousness) and partial-complex (with impaired consciousness) types. Generalized seizures include tonic, clonic, or

! EMERGENCY ALERT

SEIZURE

Seizures are classified as partial, generalized, and unclassified and are a symptom rather than a diagnosis. Seizures are characterized as an abnormal period of electrical activity in the brain.

ASSESSMENT

- Patient may report an aura.
- Can be localized and then progress (partial).
- Sudden loss of consciousness with contractions of large muscle groups, apnea, dilated/unresponsive pupils, biting the tongue, incontinence of bladder/bowel, hyperventilation, sweating, rapid pulse, excessive salivation.
- Frequently a postictal phase follows a seizure where muscles relax, consciousness is depressed, and respirations are deep; confusion, disorientation, and headache may follow; the patient may be fatigued and sleep for several hours.

INTERVENTIONS

- Ensure patent airway.
- Position patient on side if possible.
- Protect the patient's body from injury.
- Treat underlying cause.
- Administer high-flow oxygen by mask (10 L), if possible.
- Obtain IV access; administer medications to suppress seizures if required.

absence (petit mal), tonic-clonic (grand mal), and atonic seizures.

Partial Seizures

Partial seizures start with a localized activation of neurons (the *epileptogenic focus*) and generally do not involve the whole brain or significantly impair consciousness or memory. Simple-partial seizures cause symptoms of which the individual is aware, including motor, sensory, autonomic, or psychic symptoms, depending on which cortical area is affected. Simple motor seizures may start with clonic (jerking) or tonic (stiffening) movement of a single muscle group and may be self-limiting. If the simple motor seizure spreads to involve contiguous areas of the motor cortex, clonic movements progress in an orderly fashion (the jacksonian march). Simple sensory seizures are uncommon but, when present, they originate from hyperexcitable neurons in the postcentral gyrus. Symptoms of a partial sensory seizure include various degrees of numbness and paresthesias. Autonomic seizures result from hyperexcitable neurons of the frontal, temporal, mesial, orbital, or insular cortices. These seizures may begin with disturbances in gastric motility, which may progress to nausea and vomiting, tenesmus, or sudden bowel evacuation. Partial seizures with only autonomic symptoms are rare.

Partial seizures with complex symptoms generally produce some type of transitory loss of consciousness. This type of seizure may include cognitive, affective, psychosensory, or psychomotor symptoms. Events that trigger the seizure occur within the structures of the temporal lobe. Partial-complex seizures begin with various types of auras such as sensory illusions, déjà vu, or unusual smells. The individual may recognize these auras, or the memory of them may be lost in postictal amnesia. In partial-complex seizures, EEG abnormalities are localized in temporal or frontotemporal areas, including rhinencephalic structures. Partial-complex seizures are characterized by purposeful behavior that is inappropriate for the time and place. Automatisms such as lip smacking, walking aimlessly, or picking at one's clothing are common. The individual with this type of seizure usually cannot remember the seizure, but consciousness is not lost totally.

Generalized Seizures

Generalized seizures begin locally but almost immediately result in bilateral involvement of the corticoreticular and reticulocortical systems of the diencephalon. Generalized seizures are usually absence seizures (petit mal) or tonic-clonic (grand-mal) in nature. Absence seizures usually affect children after age 4 years and before puberty, and although rare, they can occur in adults up to age 70 years. Absence seizures consist of a sudden cessation of conscious activity without convulsive motor activity or loss of postural control. These absence attacks usually last for seconds or minutes. The brief lapses of consciousness may be accompanied by minor motor manifestations (e.g., eyelid flickering and isolated myoclonic jerks). After an absence seizure the individual quickly regains consciousness or awareness and usually experiences no postictal confusion.

Tonic-clonic seizures are one of the most common epileptic paroxysms and may be generalized seizures or the result of secondary generalization of partial seizures. Tonic-clonic seizures usually occur without warning and follow a common pattern: (1) tonic phase; forceful contraction of axial and appendicular muscles, loss of postural control, epileptic cry, cyanosis; usually lasts 2 or 3 minutes; (2) clonic phase, characterized by gradual transition from tonic contractions to intermittent bilateral brisk clonic movements; this phase represents recurring inhibition phases interrupting the initial tonic phase; and (3) postictal phase; amnesia of seizure and possibly even retrograde amnesia.

Generalized seizures also can result from secondary generalization of focal cortical discharges and are identical to primary generalized seizures. These facts make it difficult to distinguish secondary generalized seizures from primarily generalized tonic-clonic seizures. With secondary generalized seizures, however, there are usually diffuse cerebral pathologic findings.

Generalized seizures such as myoclonic seizures, tonic seizures, infantile spasms, and atonic seizures usually occur during childhood and generally are associated with some type of genetic, perinatal, or metabolic brain disease.

The microscopic changes leading to pathologic processes occurring during the different types of seizure activities are essentially the same. The major alteration in the physiologic state is a hypersynchronous discharge in a localized area of the brain. This localized area of hypersynchronized discharge is called the epileptogenic focus, producing a large, sharp EEG waveform known as the spike discharge.

Metabolic changes occurring within the cerebrum during the epileptic discharges include release of unusually large amounts of neuropeptides and neurotransmitters during the seizure, increased cerebral blood flow to primary involved areas, increased extracellular concentrations of potassium and decreased extracellular concentrations of calcium, changes in oxidative metabolism and local pH, and increased utilization of glucose.

Termination of seizure activity appears to be related to the large and lasting hyperpolarization of the neuronal cell membrane. This hyperpolarization is possibly generated by an electrogenic sodium pump. As the hyperpolarization is sustained, the neuronal cells cease firing, and the surface potentials of the brain are suppressed.

DIAGNOSTIC STUDIES AND FINDINGS

History and neurologic examination: Pattern of onset and characteristics of seizure activity; precipitating factors

Blood studies: Fasting glucose; serum calcium; electrolytes; complete blood count; erythrocyte sedimentation rate, renal function, liver function

CT scan: Structural changes

MRI: Structural changes

Positron emission tomography (PET): Altered brain metabolism

Single photon emission computed tomography (SPECT): Alterations in cerebral blood flow

Skull roentgenogram: Evidence of fractures; shift of calcified pineal gland; bony erosion; separated sutures

Echoencephalogram: Possible midline shifts of brain structures

Lumbar puncture: Not routinely done except when encephalitis or meningitis is suspected.

Cerebral angiography: Possible vascular abnormalities; evaluation of a subdural hematoma

EEG: Grand mal: high, fast voltage spiked in all leads; petit mal: 3/sec, rounded spike wave complexes in all leads; psychomotor (temporal lobe): square-topped 4- to 6-second spike wave complexes over involved lobe; delta waves: usually associated with destroyed brain tissue; theta waves: not always abnormal

Toxicology screen

MULTIDISCIPLINARY PLAN

Surgery

Focal cortical resection

Medications

Antiepileptic drugs (AED) (used alone or in combination)

- Phenytoin (Dilantin), 100 mg PO or IV tid or qid
  - Generalized tonic-clonic
  - Simple and complex partial
  - Status epilepticus, 15-20 mg/kg IV with 10 mg IV diazepam
- Valproate (Divalproex), 1000-3000 mg PO qd
  - Generalized tonic-clonic
  - Absence
  - Myoclonic
- Carbamazepine (Tegretol), 800-1600 mg PO qd
  - Generalized tonic-clonic
  - Simple and complex partial
- Gabapentin (Neurontin), 900-3600 mg/day PO
  - Simple and complex partial
  - Secondary generalized
- Phenobarbital (Luminal), 90-150 mg PO qd
  - Status epilepticus
- Ethosuximide (Zarontin), 750-1250 mg PO qd
  - Absence

General Management

Emergency equipment at bedside

Blood antiplystic drug (AED) concentrations

Seizure precautions

NURSING CARE

NURSING ASSESSMENT

Simple-Partial Seizures

Motor signs: Involuntary recurrent contractions of muscles (e.g., face, hand, arm, finger) of one body part; may be confined to one body area or spread to contiguous ipsilateral body parts (spread of activity such as left thumb to left hand to left arm to left side of face is known as jacksonian march)

Behavoral manifestations

- Sensory: Auditory or visual hallucinations; paresthesias; vertigo
- Autonomic and psychic: Sensation of déjà vu; complex hallucinations; illusions; unwarranted feelings of anger or fear; pupillary dilation; sweating

Level of consciousness: No loss of consciousness

Complex-Partial Seizures

Onset: May consist of variety of auras (e.g., sensory hallucinations, déjà vu, unusual smells)

Motor activity

- Compulsive patting or rubbing of body parts, lip smacking, walking aimlessly, swallowing, picking at clothing (termed automatisms)
- Unconscious performance of highly skilled acts

Level of consciousness

- Episodic loss of conscious contact with environment
- Postictal amnesia
  - Amnestic for seizure events
  - May be amnestic of auras

Generalized Seizures

Absence

- Transient loss of consciousness for few seconds to minutes; may be accompanied by flickering eyelids or intermittent jerking movements of hands

Tonic-clonic: See findings listed on p. 307

Myoclonic

- Sudden brief contraction of muscle groups producing rapid jerky movements in one or more extremities or entire body
- May be accompanied by violent fall without loss of consciousness

Tonic

Sudden assumption of an abnormal dystonic posture for a few seconds to minutes
Consciousness usually retained
Head and eyes may deviate toward one side

Potential Complications

Injury secondary to falling during seizure; injury secondary to body trashing during seizure; aspiration of oral secretions during seizure; airway impairment resulting from improper positioning during seizure

Patient Problems/Nursing Diagnoses & Interventions

NIC Respiratory Management

Ineffective airway clearance related to obstruction with secretions
Ineffective breathing pattern related to obstructed airway
Impaired gas exchange related to ineffective breathing

- See general intervention strategies listed on p. 242.

NIC Risk Management

Disturbed sensory/perception (visual, auditory, kinesthetic, gustatory, tactile, olfactory) related to change in level of consciousness

- See general intervention strategies listed on p. 242.

Risk for injury related to seizures

Preconvulsive care

- Maintain seizure precautions.
  - Have oral airway at bedside.
  - Have suction equipment available at bedside to prevent aspiration.
  - Pad side rails, if indicated.
  - Administer oxygen per protocol *to prevent cerebral hypoxia.*
  - Establish means of communication. Identify auras if possible.

Convulsive care

- Maintain patent airway.
- Support and protect head; turn to side if possible *to maintain airway.*
- Prevent injury.
  - Ease patient to floor if in chair.
  - Place pillows along side rails if patient is in bed.
  - Loosen constrictive clothing.
- Provide privacy as necessary; stay with patient.
- Note frequency, time, involved body parts, and length of seizure *to provide accurate description of seizure activity.*

Postconvulsive care

- Maintain patent airway.
- Suction as indicated.
- Administer oxygen per protocol *to prevent hypoxia.*
- Reorient patient to environment *to minimize sensory-perceptual alterations.*
- Place patient in position of comfort, and turn head to side.
- Administer oral hygiene as necessary *to remove secretions and bleeding.*

Patient Education/Continuum of Care Plan

1. Discuss with patient the nature of the seizure disorder and need to adopt positive attitude.
2. Stress importance of verbalizing feelings of shame, humiliation, anxiety, and fears regarding seizure disorder. Assist in clarifying common fears regarding seizure disorder. Assist in clarifying common fears and myths about epilepsy (e.g., not a form of insanity).
3. Emphasize need to avoid overprotection.
4. Stress need to continue with normal work and recreation routines. Assure patient that activity may inhibit seizure activity.
5. Emphasize need to avoid excessive stress or emotional excitement.
6. Discuss importance of wearing a medical alert band or carrying a medical alert card at all times.
7. Stress importance of well-balanced diet and avoidance of excessive use of stimulants such as alcohol.
8. Emphasize importance of identifying aura and course of action to take.
9. Discuss name of medication, action, side effects, dosage, and frequency of administration.
10. Stress need to avoid taking over-the-counter medications without first consulting physician.
11. Emphasize importance of ongoing outpatient care.

Evaluation/Patient Outcomes

Respiratory Management: Airway is patent. Breath sounds are normal. Chest excursion is bilateral and symmetric. Rate and depth of respirations are normal. Cough is effective. There are no subjective or objective findings of shortness of breath, air hunger, or dyspnea on exertion. Arterial blood gas values are within normal ranges or consistent with patient's baseline. Vital signs are within normal ranges or consistent with patient's baseline. Hemoglobin levels are 14 to 18 g/dl (male) or 12 to 16 g/dl (female). Intake and output are stable. There are no signs of respiratory distress. All lobes are resonant on percussion.

Risk Management: Safety measures are appropriate to physiologic status. Skin integrity is maintained. Skin is free of bruises, burns, abrasions, and redness. Environment is safe. Patient is free of nosocomial infections.

Collaborative Interventions and Related Nursing Care

Chordotomy

Description and Rationale

A chordotomy is a surgical procedure in which the lateral spinothalamic tract of the spinal cord is divided to relieve pain. The lesion is created on the contralateral side, approximately two to three spinal segments above the desired level of anesthesia, which then severs the pain pathways. If the pain is midline, the lesions must be made bilaterally. The preferred surgical technique is the percutaneous chordotomy.

The procedure consists of stereotactic insertion of a spinal lumbar puncture needle laterally between C1 and C2 (at the cervical level). A wire electrode then is inserted into the anterior quadrant, and a lesion is made by use of a radio frequency generator at a designated site to destroy ascending pain fibers. The percutaneous chordotomy may be repeated if pain recurs or the level of anesthesia falls. The other method for performing a chordotomy consists of a surgical thoracic resection approach. After exposure of the spinal cord the dendate ligament is divided at the level selected for the chordotomy. After a chordotomy the patient may experience an interruption in respiratory reflex pathways, causing periods of apnea or respiratory arrest, temporary paralysis, permanent loss of temperature sensation, and loss of bowel and bladder control.

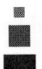

MULTIDISCIPLINARY PLAN

Surgery

Laminectomy (open chordotomy)

Medications

Local anesthesia (percutaneous chordotomy)
General anesthesia
Regional anesthetic blocks (preoperatively)

General Management

Radiofrequency generator (percutaneous chordotomy)
Mechanical ventilator, if indicated (i.e., high cervical chordotomy)
Pulmonary function testing (preoperatively and postoperatively)
Cardiac monitoring
Counseling and support regarding coping effectively with diffuse pain
Occupational therapy
Physical therapy

NURSING CARE

NURSING ASSESSMENT

Pain; discomfort at puncture or incision site

POTENTIAL COMPLICATIONS

Paralysis: Leg weakness, temporary paralysis
Bowel/Bladder control: Temporary (i.e., several weeks) urine retention, incontinence
Respiratory function: Periods of apnea, respiratory arrest (with cervical chordotomy)
Sensation: Permanent loss of temperature sensation below level of interruption, paresthesias, decreased position sense

PATIENT PROBLEMS/NURSING DIAGNOSES & INTERVENTIONS

NIC RESPIRATORY MANAGEMENT

Ineffective breathing pattern related to interrupted respiratory reflex pathway

- Maintain patent airway; intubation and mechanical ventilation may be indicated. Suction as needed. Hyperoxygenate lungs with 100% oxygen for 1 minute before and 1 minute after suctioning, unless contraindicated, *to prevent hypoxemia.*
- Maintain aseptic technique during suctioning *to prevent infection.*
- Monitor mechanical ventilator, if used.
  - Ensure that tidal volume, rate, mode, and oxygen concentration are set as ordered.
  - Ensure that ventilator alarms are on and functional.

NIC TISSUE PERFUSION MANAGEMENT

Ineffective tissue perfusion related to high risk for spinal cord edema

- Administer medications as ordered (e.g., steroids) *to control cord edema).*
  - Administer antacids per protocol *to decrease gastric irritation.*
- Maintain parenteral fluids as ordered.
- Measure intake and output every hour. Immediately report urine output of less than 30 ml per hour.

NIC IMMOBILITY MANAGEMENT

Impaired physical mobility related to surgical procedure

- Apply antiembolus stocking to lower extremities *to prevent thrombus and embolus.*
- Administer prophylactic anticoagulation therapy as ordered.
- Administer skin care every 2 hours:
  - Turn patient every 2 hours and as needed unless contraindicated.
  - Change position slowly.
  - Position in straight body alignment.
  - Use log-roll technique when turning.
  - Keep skin dry; give perineal care as needed.
- Perform active or passive ROM exercises every 2 to 4 hours.
- Encourage mobility to tolerance or as ordered.
- Encourage self-care activities to tolerance.
- Plan all activities to avoid fatigue.
- Maintain planned rest periods.
- Obtain physical therapy referral.

PATIENT EDUCATION/CONTINUUM OF CARE PLAN

1. Stress need to continue with physical and occupational therapy as ordered.
2. Discuss methods of avoiding injury (e.g., burns) to lower trunk and legs.
3. Discuss methods and routine for inspecting lower portion of the body and feet for infection and breaks in the skin.
4. Discuss care of surgical incision (with thoracic approach chordotomy).
5. Emphasize importance of ongoing outpatient care by physician.

EVALUATION/PATIENT OUTCOMES

Respiratory Management: Airway is patent. Chest excursion is symmetric. Breath sounds are normal or there is no increase in adventitious sounds. Arterial blood gas values are within normal ranges or consistent with patient's baseline. Vital signs are within normal ranges or consistent with patient's baseline. Hemoglobin levels are 14 to 18 g/dl (male) or 12 to 16 g/dl (female). Intake and output are stable. There are no signs of respiratory distress. All lobes are resonant on percussion. Skin color is not cyanotic.

Tissue Perfusion Management: There is no evidence of further neurologic deficits. Pattern of electrolytes is stable. There is no seizure activity. Vital signs are stable.

Immobility Management: Skin integrity is maintained. Patient remains free of contractures and deformities. Level of mobility is appropriate to physiologic status. Intake and output pattern is stable. Nutritional status is adequate. Patient remains free of thrombophlebitis. Patient remains free of local infection. Patient participates in an ongoing physical therapy program.

CRANIOTOMY

Description and Rationale

A craniotomy is a surgical procedure in which an opening is made into the cranium for removal of a tumor, control of bleeding, or relief of ICP. A flap is created by leaving the bone attached to the muscle so that the tissue can be turned down. Next the dura is incised in the opposite direction so its base is near the midline. After the surgery's purpose is accomplished, closure is done in layers (i.e., dura, muscles, fascial, galea, and scalp). Craniotomies can be classified into two major categories: supratentorial and subtentorial.

Supratentorial craniotomy refers to a surgical procedure performed on the brain structures located above the tentorium for removal of space-occupying lesions in the frontal, temporal, parietal, and occipital lobes. The incision usually is made behind the hairline. Subtentorial craniotomy is performed to relieve the discomfort of trigeminal neuralgia and for tumor removal from the cerebellum or cerebellar-pontine angle. The incision usually is made slightly above the nape of the neck.

Complications after a craniotomy can include any or all of the following: increased ICP, seizures, meningitis, respiratory distress, cardiac arrhythmias, wound infection, diabetes insipidus, thrombophlebitis, visual disturbances, personality changes, bowel or bladder dysfunction, periocular edema, motor and sensory disturbances, headache, and postoperative hydrocephalus.

If part of the cranium is removed without replacement (i.e., to provide decompression from cerebral edema), the procedure is termed a *craniectomy.* Cranioplasty is the surgical repair of a cranial defect to reestablish the integrity and normal contour of the skull. The area of cranial defect is repaired using substitute bone materials (i.e., tantalum, vitallium, or plastic).

MULTIDISCIPLINARY PLAN

Surgery

Intracranial pressure monitoring

Medications

Corticosteroids: Dexamethasone (Decadron), 20-40 mg/day PO (dosage gradually tapered)
Anticonvulsants: Phenytoin (Dilantin), 100 mg PO tid
Stool softener: Docusate sodium (Colace), 100 mg PO bid or tid
Histamine-blocking agents: Cimetidine (Tagamet), 300 mg PO qid
Antacids: Magnesium hydroxide (Maalox), 30 ml PO or NG qid
Antiinfective agents: Organism specific

General Management

Mechanical ventilation, if indicated
Cardiac monitoring
Nutritional consultation
Physical therapy

NURSING CARE

NURSING ASSESSMENT

Focal neurologic disturbance: Gradually increasing weakness; subtle sensory loss; adult-onset seizures not always relieved by medications
Mentation: Personality changes; insidious decrease in mentation; depression; memory deficits; judgment deficits
Pain: Headaches with steady, persistent, or intractable dull pain; changes in character of headaches; stress-induced headaches
Other: Periocular edema; thrombophlebitis

POTENTIAL COMPLICATIONS

Increased ICP: Restlessness, lethargy; changes in level of consciousness; changes in vital signs (i.e., Cushing response with increased systolic blood pressure, wide pulse pressure, and decreased pulse rate); pupillary changes (e.g., mydriasis); impaired pupillary reflex; papilledema (late sign); vomiting; fluctuations in temperature; seizures; worsening of focal neurologic signs; changes in respiratory patterns; impaired swallow/gag reflex

Seizure activity
- Preconvulsive (preictal) stage: Aura: flash of light, sense of loss, fear, weakness, dizziness, peculiar taste, smell, and sounds; cry or scream; fall to floor; loss of consciousness; tachypnea
- Convulsive stage: Tonic: rigid body, fixed jaws, clenched fists, extended legs, cyanosis, holding breath; clonic: urinary or fecal incontinence, jerking of facial muscles and extremities, biting tongue, frothing at mouth
- Postconvulsive (postictal) stage: Altered level of consciousness; headache; nausea and/or vomiting; malaise; muscle soreness; aspiration; breathing difficulty; choking; cyanosis; decreased breath sounds; tachycardia; tachypnea; pneumonia

Diabetes insipidus: Marked polyuria; marked polydipsia; anorexia; weight loss; dehydration; dry skin; poor turgor; headache; general weakness; irritability; apathy; laboratory studies: urinary specific gravity of 1.001 to 1.005, electrolyte imbalance, increased plasma osmolality

Patient Problems/Nursing Diagnoses & Interventions

NIC Respiratory Management

Ineffective airway clearance related to impaired cough reflex

Ineffective breathing pattern related to high risk for increased ICP

- See general intervention strategies on p. 242.

NIC Tissue Perfusion Management

Ineffective tissue perfusion related to increased ICP

- Intervene to prevent increased ICP.
  - Administer hyperosmotics, diuretics, and corticosteroids as ordered.
  - Administer supplemental oxygen *to prevent hypoxia and hypercapnia.*
  - Regulate mechanical ventilation to maintain $Paco_2$ 25 to 30 mm Hg *to reduce cerebral vasodilation.*
- Monitor values and waveforms of ICP line for increased pressure readings.
  - Maintain patency and sterility of system.
  - Maintain normothermia to reduce cerebral metabolic demands.
- Intervene to monitor and prevent seizures.
  - Obtain patient's seizure history.
  - Institute seizure precautions.
    - Padded tongue blade and airway at bedside
    - Bed height at lowest level
    - Side rails up at all times and padded *to prevent injury*
    - Oxygen and suction equipment at bedside *to prevent hypoxia and aspiration*
    - Emergency medications at bedside
  - Administer anticonvulsants as ordered.
- Maintain head elevation at 30 to 45 degrees if supratentorial approach used *to promote cerebral venous return.*
- Keep head of bed flat with infratentorial approach *to prevent pressure on brainstem;* avoid neck flexion *to prevent stress on suture line.*
- Check head dressing every hour and as needed. Report any new or increased drainage. Measure and mark all drainage.
- Change head dressing as needed *to prevent infection.*
- Provide wound care every shift and as needed when head dressing is removed.

NIC Risk Management

Disturbed sensory/perceptions related to altered neurologic status

Risk for injury related to seizures

- Keep side rails up at all times when patient is alone.
- Maintain patient safety at all times.
- Maintain quiet environment, reducing external stimuli to a minimum.
- Reorient patient frequently to time, place, and person.
- Introduce yourself each time you reorient the patient.
- Repeat explanations frequently and simply.
- Set realistic goals.
- Have family bring in familiar objects.
- Maintain planned rest periods, allowing sufficient time for REM sleep.
- Use day and night lighting appropriately.
- Stimulate senses of touch, taste, and position.

Preconvulsive care

- Maintain seizure precautions.
  - Have oral airway at bedside *to provide for adequate oxygenation.*
  - Have suction equipment available at bedside *to prevent aspiration.*
  - Pad side rails if indicated.
  - Administer oxygen per protocol *to prevent cerebral hypoxia.*

Convulsive care

- Maintain patent airway.
- Support and protect head; turn to side if possible.
- Prevent injury.
  - Ease patient to floor if in chair.
  - Place pillows along side rails if patient is in bed.
  - Remove surrounding furniture.
  - Loosen constrictive clothing.
- Provide privacy as necessary to protect patient's dignity.
- Note frequency, time, involved body parts, and length of seizure.

Postconvulsive care

- Maintain patent airway.
- Suction as needed *to prevent aspiration.*
- Administer oxygen as ordered *to prevent hypoxia.*
- Reorient patient to environment *to minimize sensory-perceptual alteration.*
- Place patient in position of comfort; turn head to side.
- Administer oral hygiene as necessary for secretions and bleeding.

NIC Immobility Management

Impaired physical mobility related to postoperative recovery

- See general intervention strategies listed on p. 1500.

NIC Self-Care Facilitation

Self-care deficit related to altered level of consciousness

- Assist with feeding as indicated; use IV or nasogastric feedings as ordered.
- Administer oral hygiene every 2 hours and as needed.
- Assist with daily hygiene care as indicated *to promote self-esteem.*
- Administer eye care every 2 to 4 hours if indicated.
- Perform intermittent urinary catheterization as ordered.

NIC Physical Comfort Promotion

Acute or chronic pain related to craniotomy incision

- Improve effectiveness of pain relief measures by using them before the pain becomes intense.
- Provide pain medications per protocol.

NIC COPING ASSISTANCE

Disturbed body image and personal identity and situational low self-esteem related to neurologic changes/deficits

- See general intervention strategies listed on p. 302.

PATIENT EDUCATION/CONTINUUM OF CARE PLAN

1. Involve family in care, as possible; teach essential aspects of care.
2. Reinforce physician's explanation of medical management.
3. Emphasize the importance of ongoing outpatient care and follow-up visits.
4. Encourage independent activities, as possible.
    a. Alert the patient to limitations.
    b. Avoid overprotection.
    c. Stress need for supportive devices as indicated.
5. Explain the need for regular exercise program and need for ROM exercises to family.
6. Discuss the importance of diet as ordered.
    a. Offer supplemental feedings.
    b. Offer small portions; instruct the patient to chew slowly.
7. Discuss the importance of safety measures: side rails, ramps, shower chairs, removal of scatter rugs, walker, and canes.
8. Explain name of medication, dosage, time of administration, and toxic or side effects.
9. Explain need to avoid over-the-counter medications without first consulting physician.
10. Encourage socialization with friends and family.
11. Explain the importance of verbalization of feelings about anxiety, fear, and body image changes.
12. Instruct the patient and family about seizures (i.e., safety measures and whom to contact).

EVALUATION/PATIENT OUTCOMES

Respiratory Management: Airway is patent. Breath sounds are normal. Chest excursion is bilateral and symmetric. Rate and depth of respirations are normal. Cough is effective. There are no subjective or objective findings of shortness of breath, air hunger, or dyspnea on exertion. Arterial blood gas values are within normal ranges or consistent with patient's baseline. Vital signs are within normal ranges or consistent with patient's baseline. Hemoglobin levels are 14 to 18 g/dl (male) or 12 to 16 g/dl (female). Intake and output are stable. There are no signs of respiratory distress. All lobes are resonant on percussion. Skin color is not cyanotic.

Tissue Perfusion Management: Level of consciousness is unchanged. There is no evidence of neurologic deficits. Pattern of electrolytes is stable. There is no seizure activity.

Risk Management: Patient experiences minimum complications of sensory/perceptual alterations. Patient maintains an optimum level of orientation. Patient remains free of injury. Skin integrity is maintained. Nutritional status is adequate. Self-care deficits are minimal. Social participation is appropriate to physiologic status.

Patient remains free of traumatic injury. Safety measures are appropriate to level of physiologic status. Skin integrity is maintained. Skin is free of bruises, burns, abrasions, and redness. Environment is safe. Patient is free of nosocomial infections.

Immobility Management: Patient's level of mobility is optimum. Skin integrity is maintained. Patient remains free of contractures and deformities. Level of mobility is appropriate to physiologic status. Intake and output pattern is stable. Nutritional status is adequate. Patient remains free of thrombophlebitis. Patient remains free of local infection. Patient participates in an ongoing physical therapy program.

Self-Care Facilitation: Self-care deficits are minimized. Criteria listed for impaired physical mobility are met. Level of self-care activities is appropriate to physiologic status. Patient participates in physical and occupational therapy.

Physical Comfort Promotion: Alterations in comfort are minimized. Patient openly verbalizes feelings of discomfort when they occur. Patient can use measures to decrease discomfort. Patient verbally validates a decrease in subjective feelings of discomfort. There is a decrease in objective findings of pain.

Coping Assistance: Patient maintains intact self-concepts. Patient openly verbalizes feelings of grief and loss. Patient verbalizes positive feelings about self. Patient acknowledges actual change in self-image. Patient focuses on present and future appearance and function. Patient verbalizes feelings of hopefulness, helpfulness, and powerfulness.

INTRACRANIAL PRESSURE MONITORING

Description and Rationale

ICP monitoring devices now make it possible to reliably measure the parameters of intracranial dynamics, such as volume-pressure relationships, pressure waves, and cerebral perfusion pressures. Indications for ICP monitoring include any of the following: head trauma; cerebral hemorrhage; massive brain lesions; encephalitis; congenital hydrocephalus; hydrocephalus resulting in an alteration of CSF production or absorption; and symptoms of increased ICP such as change in level of consciousness, headache, vomiting, or deterioration in respiratory status and motor function. ICP can be measured continuously via three basic monitoring systems: the ventricular catheter, the subarachnoid bolt, and the epidural sensor (FIG. 5-38).

The *ventricular* catheter consists of a cannula that is implanted, via burr holes, into the anterior horn of the lateral ventricle of the nondominant cerebral hemisphere. The catheter then is connected by pressure-resistant, fluid-filled tubing to a transducer and recording instrument. (**NOTE: Continuous flushing devices are not used for ICP measurement.**) The transducer is positioned so the dome is at the level of the foramen of Monro. The external anatomic landmarks for this position are the tragus of the ear or the edge of the brow. An error

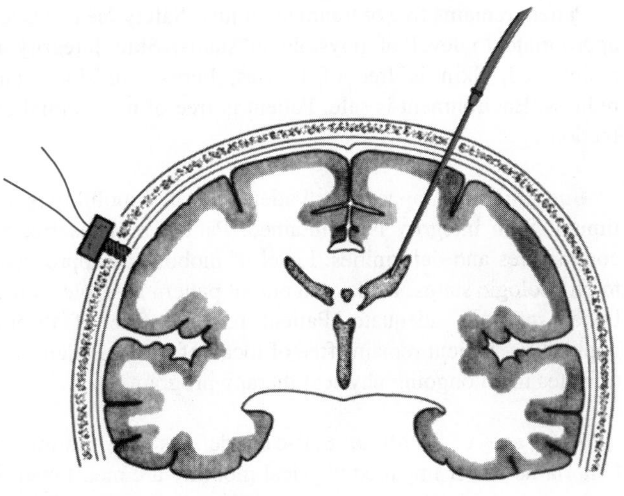

FIG. 5-38
Subarachnoid screw monitoring *(left)* and intraventricular *(right)* devices for measuring ICP. Both require attachment to transducer using a stopcock or pressure tubing. (From ENS.[2a])

of approximately 2 torr exists for each inch of discrepancy between the level of the transducer and the pressure source.

Advantages of the ventricular catheter include accurate measurement of ICP; instillation of a contrast medium; evaluation of pressure/volume responses; and ability to drain large amounts of CSF, if needed.

Disadvantages of the ventricular catheter are that catheter placement may be difficult if the lateral ventricle is displaced, swollen, or collapsed; the catheter is the most invasive type of monitoring and can provide another route for infection; excessive CSF drainage can occur if the stopcock is not positioned properly; brain tissue or blood may occlude the catheter; false pressure readings may occur if the ventricle collapses and compresses the catheter; and frequent recalibration of the transducer and monitor is necessary for accurate readings.

The *subarachnoid bolt* method of ICP measurement began in the early 1970s. The device consists of a metal screw with a sensor tip that is inserted through a twist drill hole into the subdural or subarachnoid space. Although the cerebrum is not penetrated, the ICP is measured directly from the CSF. The bolt is connected to a transducer and recording device via pressure-resistant, fluid-filled tubing. Here, as with the intraventricular catheter, continuous flushing devices are contraindicated. Indications for use of the subarachnoid bolt are to provide a means to measure and monitor ICP and to provide access for sampling of the CSF.

Advantages of the bolt are that ICP is measured directly and accurately from CSF; it provides access for CSF sampling and drainage; it provides access for volume-pressure responses; and it can be placed quickly without penetrating the cerebrum.

Disadvantages of the bolt are that it may become occluded with tissue or blood; the infection rate is comparable to that of the ventricular catheter; it requires a closed skull; and frequent recalibration of the transducer and monitor is necessary for accurate readings.

The epidural sensor consists of placement of a fiber-optic sensor, radio transmitter, or tiny balloon with radioisotopes in the epidural space through a burr hole in the skull. The sensor cable then plugs directly into the monitor.

! EMERGENCY ALERT

INCREASED INTRACRANIAL PRESSURE

Increased ICP reflects three volumes in the cranial vault: brain, CSF, and blood. Normal ICP is 10-15 mm Hg. ICP is controlled by autoregulatory mechanisms that may fail after injury. This failure leads to cerebral vasodilation, increased blood volume, and cerebral engorgement as well as edema.

ASSESSMENT

- Cerebral ischemia, evidence of hypoxia
- Headache, nausea, vomiting
- Amnesia, altered level of consciousness
- Altered speech, drowsiness, agitation
- Dilated, nonreactive pupil
- Unresponsive to verbal, painful stimuli
- Abnormal posturing
- Increased blood pressure and decreased pulse
- Altered respiratory pattern
- Herniation of the brain may occur

INTERVENTIONS

- Maintain airway, breathing, circulation.
- Administer high-flow oxygen by mask (10-15 L).
- Obtain IV access.
- Position patient's head to decrease ICP (usually low Fowler's); local guidelines may vary.
- Hyperventilate patient to maintain $Pa{CO_2}$ (26-30 mm Hg); local guidelines may vary.
- Administer mannitol, anticonvulsant, antipyretic as ordered.
- Do not occlude CSF leak from nose, ears, etc.
- Obtain CT scan, MRI.
- If patient has been injured and if there is drainage from nose or ears, test drainage with dextrose stick to determine whether fluid is CSF.

Advantages of the sensor are that it is less invasive, it can be easily placed, and it cannot become occluded. The major disadvantage of the sensor is its questionable reliability. Other disadvantages are that the system cannot be recalibrated if the sensor is affected by pressure or heat, CSF sampling and drainage are not possible, and volume/pressure responses cannot be evaluated.

The *fiber-optic transducer-tipped catheter* is a relatively new device for monitoring ICP. This catheter can be placed intraventricularly, intraparenchymally, in the subarachnoid space, or in the subdural space. Advantages of the fiber-optic transducer-tipped catheter are that it may be placed in three different areas of the cerebrum, is capable of monitoring intraparenchymal pressure, provides for CSF drainage with a ventricular system, and requires no adjustment of the transducer with head movement. Disadvantages of the fiber-optic catheter are that it is relatively fragile, cannot be recalibrated or reset to zero after placement, and requires a separate monitoring system.

Pressure Waves

ICP's dynamic state is reflected by the pressure waves produced. These waveforms are most commonly known as A waves, B waves, and C waves (FIG. 5-39).

A waves (or plateau waves), which occur at variable intervals, are spontaneous, rapid increases in pressure between 50 and 200 torr. Plateau waves usually occur in patients with mod-

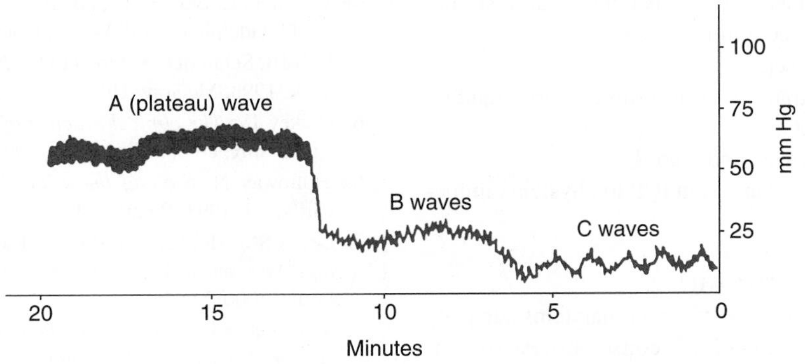

FIG. 5-39
ICP waves. Composite drawing of A (plateau) waves, B waves, and C waves. (From Lewis.[7])

erate ICP elevations and last 5 to 20 minutes, falling spontaneously. Factors that can trigger plateau waves include REM sleep, emotional stimuli, isometric muscle contractions, the rebound phase of the Valsalva's maneuver, hypercapnia, hypoxemia, sustained coughing and sneezing, arousal from sleep, and certain positions such as neck flexion or extreme hip flexion. A waves are known to cause cerebral ischemia and brain damage and can produce paroxysmal or transient symptoms of change in level of consciousness, headache, nausea and vomiting, altered motor function, abnormal pupillary reactions, changes in vital signs (i.e., increased blood pressure, widened pulse pressure, and decreased pulse rate), and respiratory patterns (i.e., ataxic breathing and central neurogenic hyperventilation).[1] Because of the ischemia and previously stated symptoms, A-waves are the most clinically significant ICP waveforms and require immediate intervention to prevent further brain injury.

B waves appear as sharp, rhythmic, sawtooth waves that occur every half minute to 2 minutes and have pressures up to 50 torr. B waves correlate to changes in respiration, such as Cheyne-Stokes respirations. B waves can also occur in patients with normal ICP.

C waves are small, rapid, rhythmic waves that occur at a rate of approximately 4 to 8 per minute and increase pressures up to 20 torr. C waves are also called Traube-Herring-Mayer waves. These waveforms correspond to normal changes in the systemic arterial pressure and are not clinically significant.

MULTIDISCIPLINARY PLAN

Surgery
ICP monitoring
Tumor excision
Shunting procedure

Medications
Corticosteroid agents: Dexamethasone (Decadron), 20-40 mg/day PO
Anticonvulsant agents: Phenytoin (Dilantin), 100 mg PO tid
Laxative agents: Docusate sodium (Colace), 100 mg PO bid or tid
Antiemetic agents: Cimetidine (Tagamet), 300 mg PO tid
Antacids: Magnesium hydroxide (Maalox), 30 ml PO qid
Antiinfective agents: Organism specific

General Management
Radiation therapy
Mechanical ventilation, if indicated
Cardiac monitoring
Arterial blood pressure monitoring
Nutritional consultation
Physical therapy

NURSING CARE

NURSING ASSESSMENT
See specific disorder for specific physical assessment findings.

POTENTIAL COMPLICATIONS
Loss of ICP waveform: Transducer may be incorrectly connected; monitoring device could be occluded; air may be between pressure source and transducer diaphragm
Low ICP: Cerebral ventricles may have collapsed; transducer may have been incorrectly zeroed and calibrated
High ICP: Excessive activity; body posture with neck or extreme hip flexion; use of positive end-expiratory pressure (PEEP); hyperthermia; respiratory distress; fluid and electrolyte imbalances; infection; blood pressure changes
False high ICP: Transducer too low or incorrectly balanced; system incorrectly calibrated; air in system
False low ICP: Transducer too high; air in system

PATIENT PROBLEMS/NURSING DIAGNOSES & INTERVENTIONS

NIC TISSUE PERFUSION MANAGEMENT

Ineffective tissue perfusion related to altered cerebrovascular dynamics
- Maintain sterility of the ICP monitoring equipment.
  Maintain strict sterile technique *to prevent infection.*
  Change equipment (i.e., tubing) daily or as ordered.
- Maintain patency of ICP monitoring device.
  Keep all stopcock ports capped to keep system closed to air.
  Never flush the system.
  Observe for CSF leaks and blood in the tubing.
- Obtain accurate pressure measurements.
  Place patient in baseline position.

Obtain measurements when patient is at rest, not when moving, coughing, sneezing, etc.
Level the transducer.
Recalibrate the transducer according to the manfacturer's instructions.
Obtain measurements and record.
Report significant changes in ICP to physician immediately.

EVALUATION/PATIENT OUTCOMES

Tissue Perfusion Management: Patient maintains adequate cerebral tissue perfusion. Level of consciousness is unchanged. There is no evidence of neurologic deficits. Pattern of electrolytes is stable. There is no seizure activity. Vital signs are stable.

REFERENCES

1. Bennett JC, Plum F, eds.: *Cecil textbook of medicine,* Philadelphia, 1996, WB Saunders.
1a. Chipps E, Clanin N, Campbell V: *Neurologic disorders,* St. Louis, 1992, Mosby.
2. Cotran RS, Kumar V, Robbins SL: *Robbins pathologic basis of disease,* ed. 6, Philadelphia, 1999, WB Saunders.
2a. ENS: *Sheehy's emergency nursing principles and practice,* ed 4, St. Louis, 1997, Mosby.
3. Fauci AS et al: *Harrison's principles of internal medicine,* ed 14, New York, 1998, McGraw-Hill.
4. Genvik A, Senior Editor: *Textbook of critical care,* ed 4, Philadelphia, 2000, WB Saunders.
4a. Goldman L, Bennett JC, editors: *Cecil's textbook of medicine,* ed 21, Philadelphia, 2000, WB Saunders.
5. Hall JB, Schmidt GA, Wood LDH: *Principles of critical care,* New York, 1998, McGraw-Hill.
6. Hickey JV: *The clinical practice of neurological and neurosurgical nursing,* ed 2, Philadelphia, 1997, Lippincott.
6a. Holloway N: *Nursing the critically ill adult,* ed 4, Englewood Cliffs, NJ, 1993, Prentice Hall.
7. Lewis SM, Heitkemper MM, Dirksen SR: *Medical-surgical nursing: Assessment and management of clinical problems,* ed 5, St. Louis, 2000, Mosby.
8. McCance KL, Heuther SE: *Pathophysiology: the biologic basis for disease in adults and children,* ed 3, St. Louis, 1998, Mosby.
9. McCloskey JC, Bulechek GM, editors: In *Nursing interventions classification (NIC),* ed 3, St. Louis, 2001, Mosby.
10. Phipps WJ, Sands JK, Marek JF: *Medical-surgical nursing: concepts and clinical practice,* ed 5, St. Louis, 1999, Mosby.
11. Rudy EB: *Advanced neurological and neurosurgical nursing,* St. Louis, 1984, Mosby.
11a. Schottelius BA, Schottellius DD: *Textbook of physiology,* ed 18, St. Louis, 1978, Mosby.
12. Simon RP, Aminoff MJ, Greenberg DA: *Clinical neurology,* ed 4, Stamford, Conn., 1999, Appleton & Lange.
13. Spratto GR, Woods AL: *PDR nurse's drug handbook,* Montvale, NJ, 2000, Delmar Publishers & Medical Economics.
14. Stein JH, Editor-in-chief. *Internal medicine,* ed 5, St. Louis, 1998, Mosby.
14a. Thelan LA et al: *Critical care nursing: diagnosis and management,* ed 3, St. Louis, 1998, Mosby.
15. Thibodeau GA, Patton KT: *Anatomy and physiology,* ed 4, St. Louis, 1999, Mosby.

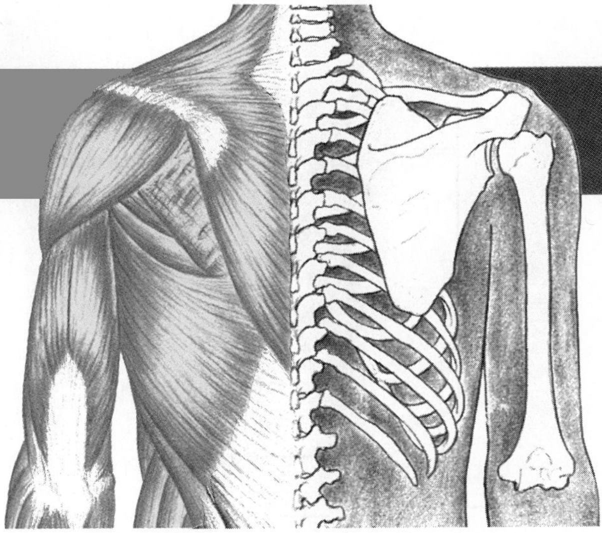

6 Musculoskeletal System

Leona A. Mourad

OVERVIEW

The tissues of the musculoskeletal system are the framework for the rest of the body and provide the means for easy, comfortable movement. Because of their many important structures and functions, they greatly affect the body's general health when they are inflamed, injured, or anomalous. Musculoskeletal anomalies and birth injuries affect newborns and lead to disability in growth, development, and productivity throughout life. Injuries from sports or physical fitness activities are major factors in the health of young to middle-age adults. Trauma, primarily from automobile accidents, is the number one cause of death among people age 16 to 24 years. Inflammatory, rheumatic, and degenerative diseases of the musculoskeletal tissues are significant causes of death among young adults and account for a large portion of the illness and disability of middle-age and elderly adults. Billions of dollars are spent yearly for care and treatment of people of all ages with musculoskeletal conditions. The economic cost is a major health-care problem.

ANATOMY, PHYSIOLOGY, AND RELATED PATHOPHYSIOLOGY

Skeleton

According to Wolff's law, which states that bones are shaped according to their function, the 206 bones of the skeleton are shaped according to their specific functions. Thus they may be long (arm or leg), short (wrist or ankle), flat (sternum or scapula), irregular (vertebrae), or rounded (patella). The skull, face and auditory ossicles, vertebrae, ribs, sternum, and hyoid bone make up the axial skeleton; the appendicular skeleton consists of the bones in the upper and lower extremities, shoulders, and pelvis (FIG. 6-1).

Bones support the body, enabling it to stand erect; protect internal organs and other soft tissues; assist movement by leverage and in coordination with muscles; make blood cells within the red bone marrow; and provide for storage of minerals, particularly calcium and phosphorus.

Structure of Bone Tissue. Long bones of the extremities and thorax consist of a long shaft, the diaphysis, and two ends, the epiphyses. The epiphyses are covered with cartilage and are separated from the shaft by the growth plate and nutrient arteries of the metaphysis (FIG. 6-2). The outer surface (cortex) of a bone is hard, dense tissue called compact bone. The ends of long bones, the flat bones, and the ridges or crests of the ilium and tibia contain cancellous bone, which is soft and spongy and has cavities containing the red bone marrow for hematopoiesis. Red bone marrow depletions are replaced by fat cells of the yellow bone marrow, which is found in the shafts of long bones.

The periosteum is the tough outer membrane that covers each bone and provides protection and nutrition. Blood vessels in the inner layer of the periosteum bring nutrients and remove wastes. The periosteal blood vessels communicate with vessels in the central canal of the haversian system, which is the microscopic unit of compact bone.

The haversian system contains layers or plates of compact bone cells called lamellae. These lamellae surround the haversian canal, which contains two blood vessels and a nerve. The lamellae are aligned parallel to the shaft of the bone and encompass the lacunae, which are small cavities filled with bone cells and tissue fluids. The lacunae are connected to the blood vessels in the haversian canal by smaller canals, the canaliculi (FIG. 6-3). The haversian canal provides nutrients to osteocytes for bone building and removes wastes and debris from bone growth and resorption. *Osteocytes,* mature bone cells that develop from osteoblasts, are found in and surrounded by bone matrix. *Osteoblasts* are spindle-shaped cells derived from uncommitted cells located in the periosteum and in the inner regions of bones, the endosteum.[49a] Osteoblasts remain dormant until needed for new bone growth, after which they mature into osteocytes. A third type of cell, the *osteoclast,* is needed for shaping and remodeling bone. Osteoclasts are the cells primarily responsible for resorbing unneeded or necrotic bone cells.

Bones are in a constant process of resorption counterbalanced by new bone formation. The skeleton replaces itself approximately every 3 months, so bones do not become excessively thick or heavy from new bone formation, nor do they

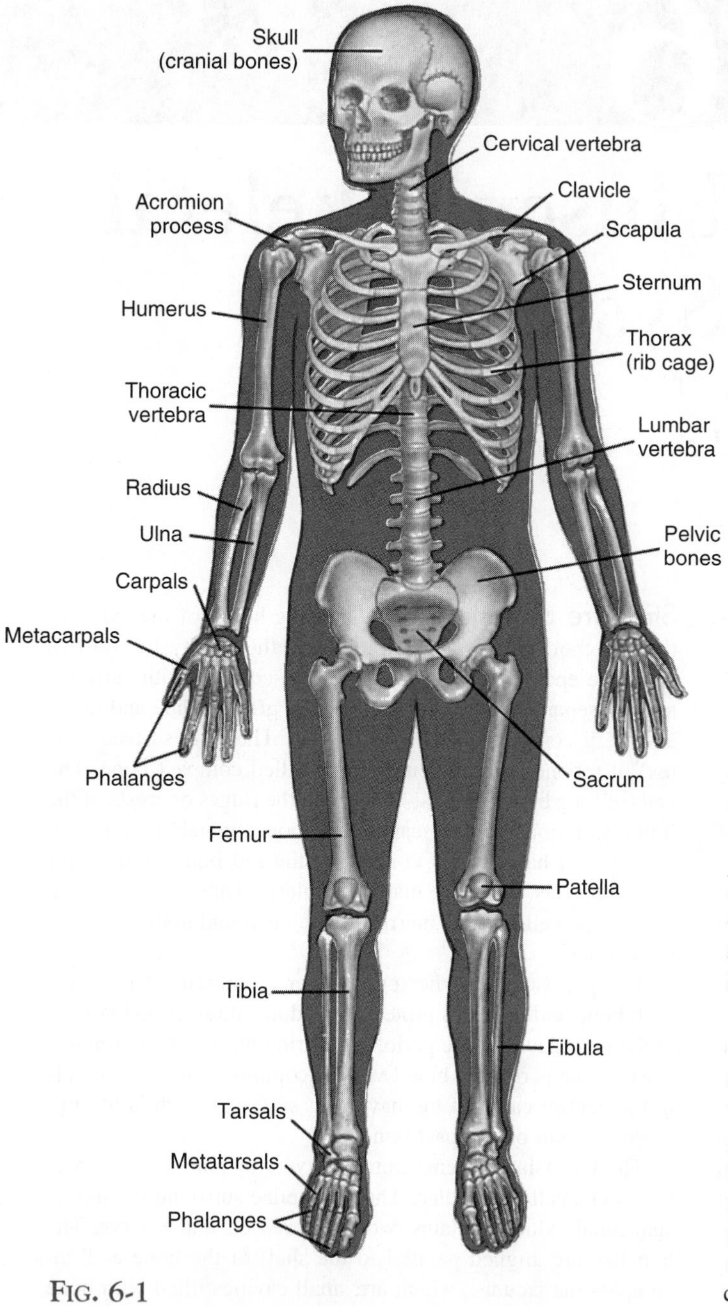

FIG. 6-1

Bones that make up axial and appendicular skeletons (see text for content).

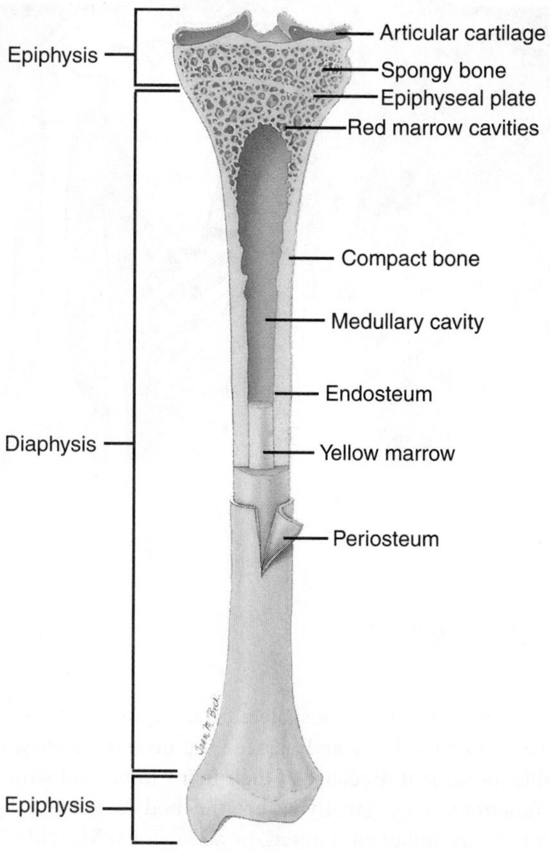

FIG. 6-2

Cross section of bone. Longitudinal section of long bone (tibia) showing cancellous and compact bones. (From Thibodeau and Patton.[57a])

become thinner or weaker from bone resorption. Bone formation and resorption processes are related to calcium and phosphate levels and metabolism in the body.

Approximately 99% of the calcium in the body is contained in bones; the remaining 1% circulates in the blood plasma and interstitial fluid. Extracellular calcium and phosphate concentrations are regulated by secretions of parathyroid hormone from the parathyroid glands, by absorption in the intestinal tract, and by retention or excretion by the kidneys so that relatively stable concentrations are maintained. Low calcium levels stimulate parathyroid hormone production, which stimulates osteoclasts to break down bone structure. The breakdown of bone frees calcium phosphate crystals to be available to increase serum calcium concentrations. The gastrointestinal ion transport system absorbs calcium and moves the ion from the gut lumen to the blood. Resorption of calcium increases in the renal tubules to raise serum calcium levels, which concurrently reduces the resorption of phosphate. Through these processes, calcium levels remain relatively constant in healthy people, and bone remains strong with relatively stable calcium concentration through bone formation and resorption.

Bone strength, formation, and resorption are also affected by the amount and metabolism of vitamin D, which facilitates the absorption of calcium and phosphorus from the intestine. A deficiency of either vitamin D or sunshine (needed to activate sterol precursors to vitamin D in the skin) will cause changes in bones, known as rickets in children and osteomalacia in adults.

The skeleton begins to develop from mesenchymal cells in the first prenatal month and is completely formed by the third month. Bones form through intramembranous and endochondral formation. In both processes the first stage involves formation of cancellous or spongy bone tissue, which later becomes compact bone through deposition of bone matrix. The bone matrix then becomes calcified. The bones of the skull and other flat bones are formed through intramembranous pathways, and all long bones are formed from endochondral tissues within a preformed cartilage framework. After birth, secondary centers for ossification develop in the epiphyseal regions of the bones. The

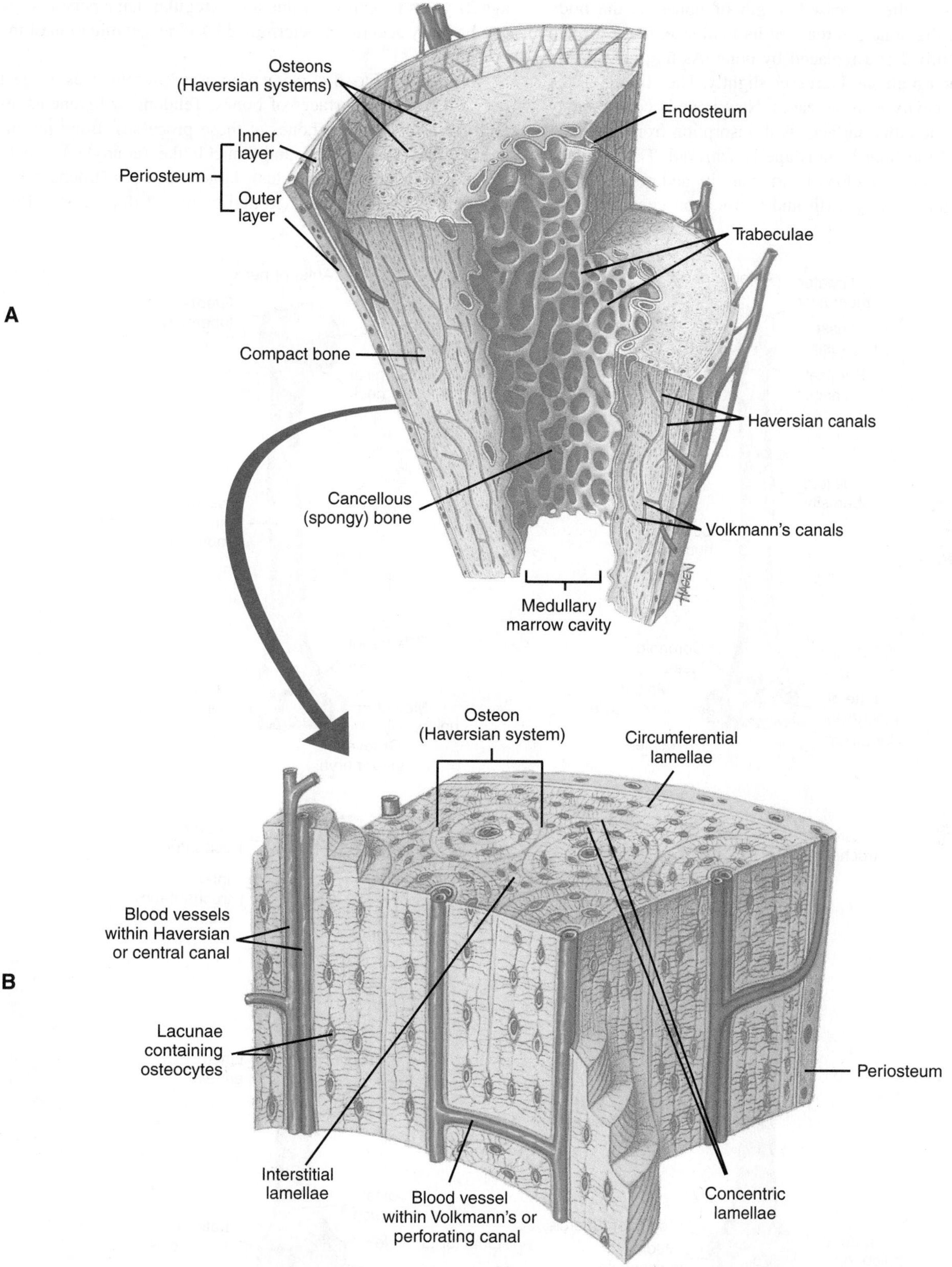

FIG. 6-3

Structure of compact and cancellous bone. **A,** Longitudinal section of a long bone showing both cancellous and compact bone. **B,** Magnified view of compact bones. (From Thibodeau and Patton.[57a])

cartilage that remains in this region becomes the epiphyseal plate. The growth or proliferation of the cartilage cells in this region results in the increased length of bones as the body grows. When the bone has reached its final size, these growth zones are resorbed and replaced by bone. As the bone grows longer, its outer diameter increases slightly. The volume in the bone marrow cavity also increases. New bone is continuously deposited on the outer surfaces with resorption from the inner surfaces, until the final bone shape is achieved. The shape of each bone maximizes its load-bearing ability and minimizes its mass or weight. Bone growth and ossification generally continue longitudinally until age 15 years in girls and age 16 years in boys. Bone maturation and shaping, however, continue until age 21 years in both sexes and are so regular that a person's age can be fairly accurately determined by x-ray examination of the bones.

As shown in FIG. 6-4, many processes (prominences) project outward from the surfaces of bones. Tendons or ligaments attach themselves to the bones at these processes. Bony prominences may be rounded and knucklelike (condyles); small, rounded projections (tubercles); large processes (trochanters); or narrow ridges or crests (frontal bone and iliac crests). Pro-

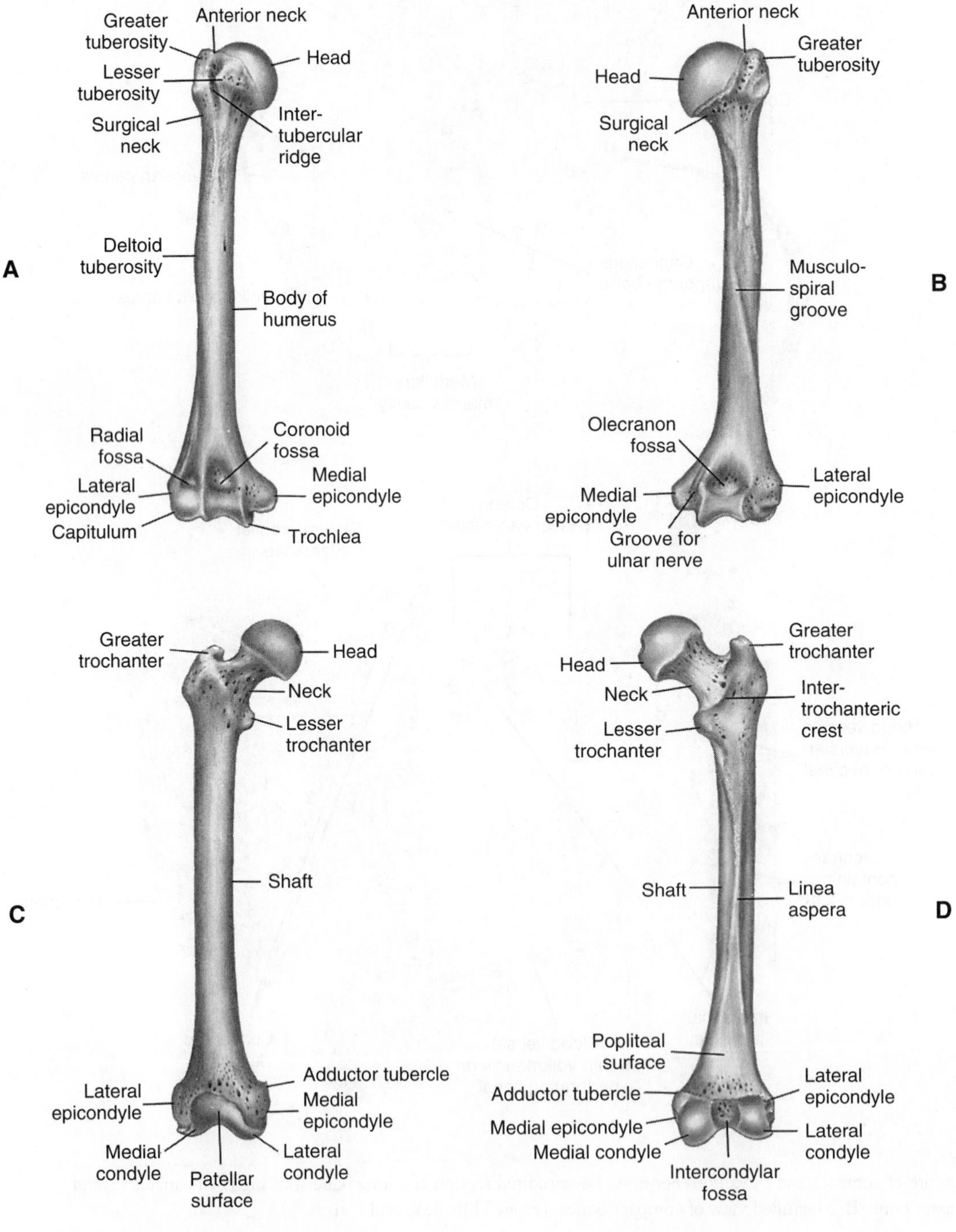

FIG. 6-4

A, Anterior and, **B,** posterior of right humerus. **C,** Anterior and, **D,** posterior views of right femur.

jections may be transverse (transverse processes of vertebrae and ear), or they may project posteriorly (posterior spinous processes) or anteriorly (nasal cartilages). Bones may contain alveoli (sockets), fossae (depressions), fissures (narrow slits), foraminae (openings for nerves, muscles, and blood vessels), sinuses (cavities), and sulci (grooves); some are shown (groove, fossa) on the A and B surfaces of the humerus in Fig. 6-4.

Muscles

Structure of Skeletal Muscles. Skeletal muscles make up 40% to 45% of the body's weight and 50% of a child's body weight. Generally, muscles are 75% water, 20% protein, and 5% organic and inorganic compounds. Approximately 30% of all protein stores available for energy and metabolism is contained in the body's muscles (Fig. 6-5). Through their contractions, they move the whole body or just parts of it. They cover the skeletal bones and help produce the contours of the body. Muscles are attached at each end to a bone, ligament, tendon, or fascia. One end of the muscle, the more fixed end, is referred to as the origin; the more movable end is the muscle insertion. Muscles of the skeletal system are voluntary muscles controlled by the will; in contrast, visceral muscles move involuntarily.

Muscles of the skeletal system (striated muscles) are generally long, slender bundles containing dark cross-markings or lines called striations. Each muscle is made up of fibers enclosed in a sarcolemma and bound together in bundles (fasciculi) by a connective tissue sheath (perimysium). The fasciculi are further bound together by a stronger sheath (epimysium). These bundles of bound fibers make up the muscle belly, the fleshy part of the muscle. The epimysium extends beyond the belly of the muscle to form a tendon (Fig. 6-6). The muscles of the limbs are bound together by a layer of connective tissue called fascia, a tough, silvery-appearing covering, which also covers individual muscle groups.

Skeletal muscles vary in length, width, and diameter and are red or white. Red muscle gets its color from the pigment myoglobin. Being closely related to hemoglobin, myoglobin acts as a temporary oxygen store for the muscle. White muscle fibers contain less myoglobin. White muscles react rapidly when stimulated, whereas red muscles carry out slower, sustained movements.

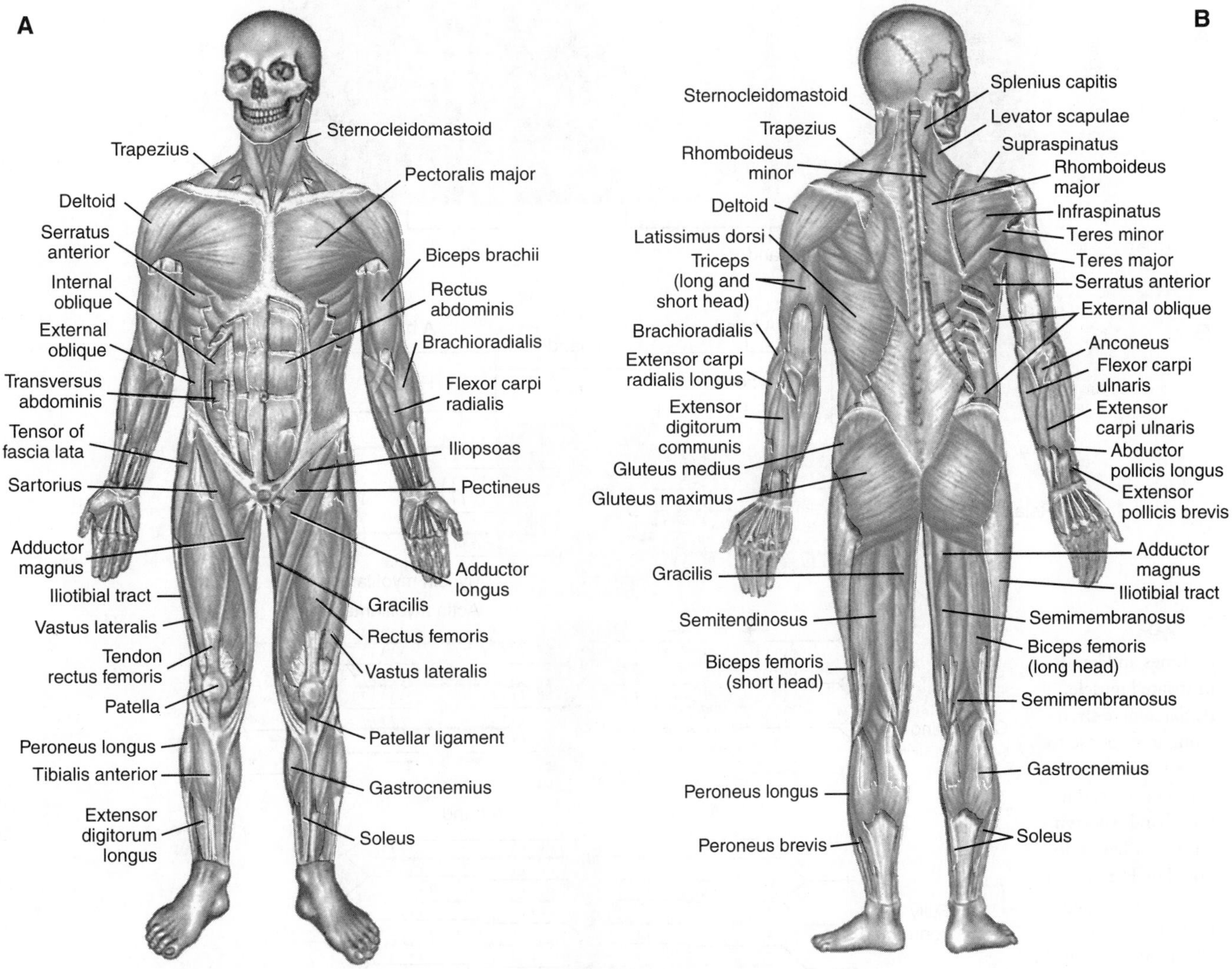

Fig. 6-5
Muscles of body. **A,** Anterior view. **B,** Posterior view.

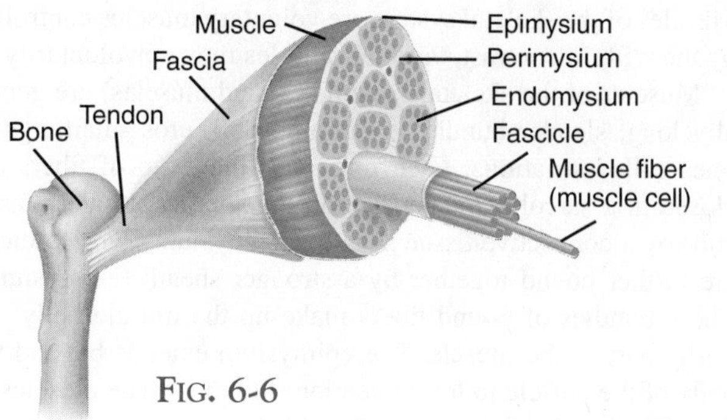

FIG. 6-6

Cross section of skeletal muscle showing muscle fibers and their covering. (From Thibodeau and Patton.[57a])

The striations of skeletal muscles result from bands of muscle fibers made up of cylindric cytoplasmic elements called myofibrils. Myofibrils form the longitudinal striation of the muscle; transverse striations form the banding patterns in the myofibrils. Each myofibril consists of smaller myofilaments, which form a regular repeating pattern along the length of the fibril. One unit of this repeating pattern is called a sarcomere. The sarcomere is the functional unit of the contractile system in muscles.

Each sarcomere contains two types of myofilaments: thick and thin. The thick myofilaments are found in the central region of the sarcomere, where their orderly, parallel arrangement results in the dark bands, called A bands, that are seen in striated muscles. The thick filaments contain the protein myosin. The

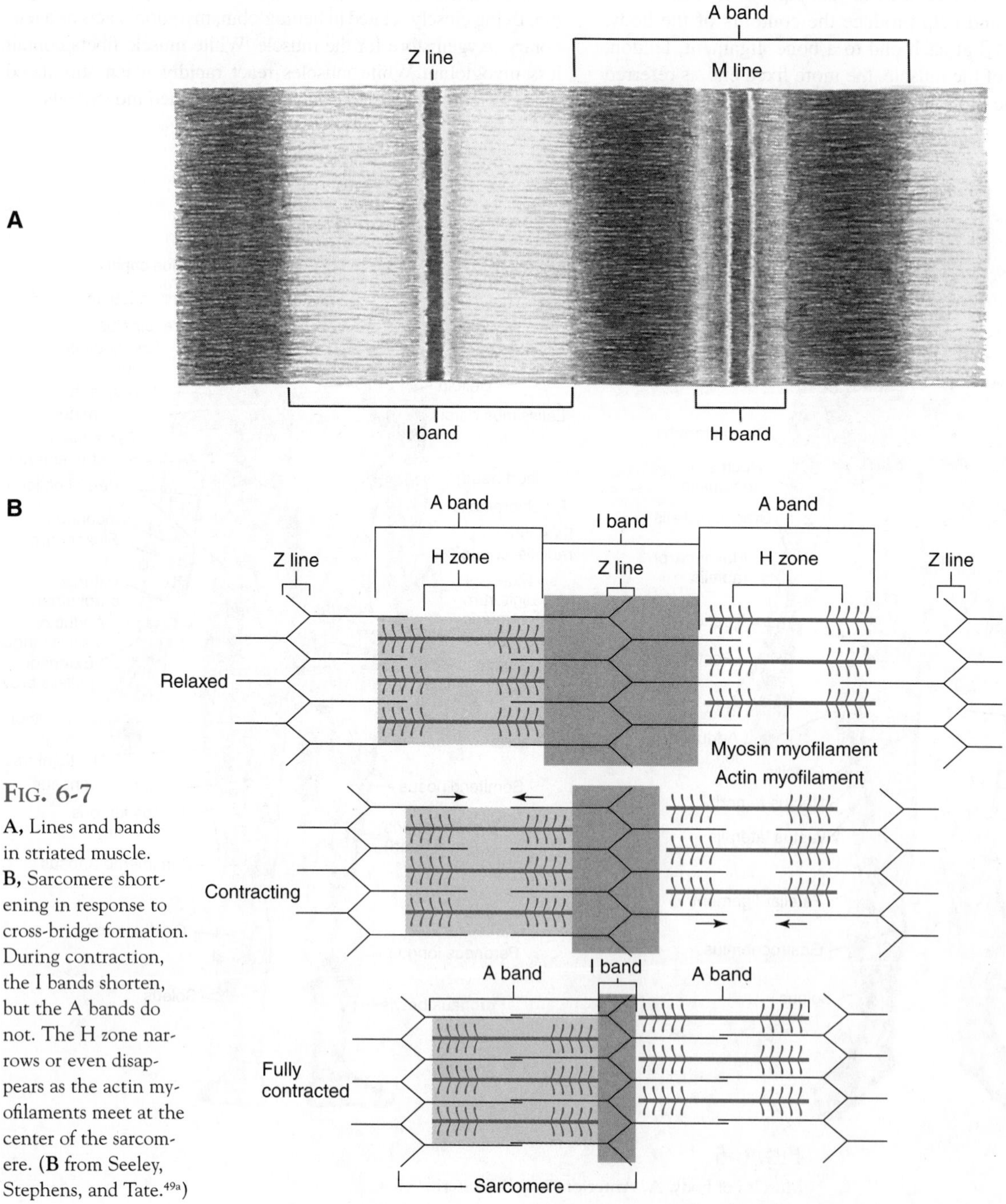

FIG. 6-7

A, Lines and bands in striated muscle. **B,** Sarcomere shortening in response to cross-bridge formation. During contraction, the I bands shorten, but the A bands do not. The H zone narrows or even disappears as the actin myofilaments meet at the center of the sarcomere. (**B** from Seeley, Stephens, and Tate.[49a])

thin myofilaments contain the protein actin and are attached at either end of the sarcomere to a structure known as the Z line. Two successive Z lines define the limits of one sarcomere. The Z lines contain short elements that interconnect the thin filaments from two adjoining sarcomeres to provide an anchoring point for the thin filaments. The thin elements extend from the Z lines toward the center of the sarcomere, where they overlap with the thick filaments (FIG. 6-7).

Two other bands, the I band and the H zone, change during contraction in relation to the positions of the thick and thin filaments in the sarcomere. The I band is between the ends of the A bands in two adjoining sarcomeres. Because it contains only thin filaments, it usually appears as a light band separating the dark A bands. The H zone is a thin, lighter band in the center of the A band that corresponds to the space between the ends of the thin filaments. Only thick filaments are found in the H zone.

Muscle Contraction. Muscles move the body through tightening and shortening of their fibers (contraction) brought about through the motor unit. Each motor unit has 100 to 200 muscle fibers innervated by a single motor nerve axon that stimulates the motor unit and sends the contraction through the muscle body. The muscle responds either entirely or not at all to the stimulus. The strength of the muscle contraction is determined by the number of motor units contracting and by the number of times per second each motor unit is stimulated.

The type of peripheral nerve influences muscle fibers in the motor units for fast or slow contractions. White or fast-twitch motor fibers (type II) have fast conduction velocities, relying on short-term anaerobic glycolytic reactions for rapid energy transfer and muscle contraction. Slow-twitch (type I) fibers, called red muscle, use aerobic oxidative metabolism and are slower responders. Postural muscles have more type I fibers, with the high resistance to fatigue necessary to maintain a position or positions for extended periods. Ocular muscles contain more type II fibers and respond rapidly to needed visual changes (Table 6-1).

During muscle contraction the thick (myosin) and thin (actin) filaments slide past each other, but the lengths of the individual thick and thin filaments do not change. As the thin filaments move past the thick filaments, the width of the H zone between the ends of the thin filaments becomes smaller and shorter. These changes in the banding pattern during contraction led to the sliding-filament theory of muscle contraction, that is, that muscle shortening results from the relative movement of the thick and thin filaments past each other.

Sliding of the filaments is produced by the myosin cross-bridges, which swivel in an arc around their fixed positions on the surface of the thick filament. The cross-bridges undergo many repeated cycles of movement during a contraction. The myosin bridges detach themselves from actin, rebind to new actin sites, and repeat these cycles of movements, brought about by the binding of a molecule to adenosine triphosphate (ATP) to myosin. The process of binding ATP appears to break the linkage between actin and myosin. The reaction returns the bridge to its initial state so it can repeat the cycle of bridge movement.

Muscle contraction results from a series of interactions at the myoneural junction in the muscle tissue. The stimulus travels along the motor nerve to the motor end plate (myoneural junction) of the muscle fiber. Acetylcholine is produced at this synapse (junction) and released. It causes the muscle to contract by depolarizing the sarcolemma. Depolarization permits interstitial calcium ions to enter the muscle membrane to aid the contraction. The wave of depolarization travels through the muscle fiber until it is deactivated by the enzyme acetylcholinesterase (FIG. 6-8). The fiber is then ready for reactivation. The positive calcium ions catalyze an energy-releasing reaction to cause the actin to slide along the myosin, which results in contraction and shortening of the muscle.

Table 6-1 Characteristics of Muscle Fibers

Characteristic	Type I (Red)	Type II (White)
Anatomic location	Deep axial portion of surface muscle	Surface portion of surface muscle
Contraction speed	Slow	Fast
Motor neuron type	Type I, small alpha	Type II, large alpha
Firing frequency	Low, long duration	Rapid, short duration
Resistance to fatigue	High	Low
Myoglobin	High	Low
Capillary supply	Profuse	Intermediate to sparse
Metabolism	Oxidative	Glycolysis
Mitochondria	Many	Few
Enzymes	Lactate dehydrogenase, types 1-3	Lactate dehydrogenase, types 4 and 5
Creatine kinase	Cardiac type	Fast, skeletal
Example (most muscles are mixed)	Greater proportion of slow-contracting fibers in soleus	Greater proportion of fast-contracting fibers in laryngeal and ocular muscles
Mitochondria	Many	Few
Glycogen content	Low	High
Intensity of contraction	Low	High
Aerobic metabolic capacity	High	Low
Fiber diameter	Small	Large
Myosin–adenosine triphosphatase (ATPase) activity	Low	High

From Mourad.[38]

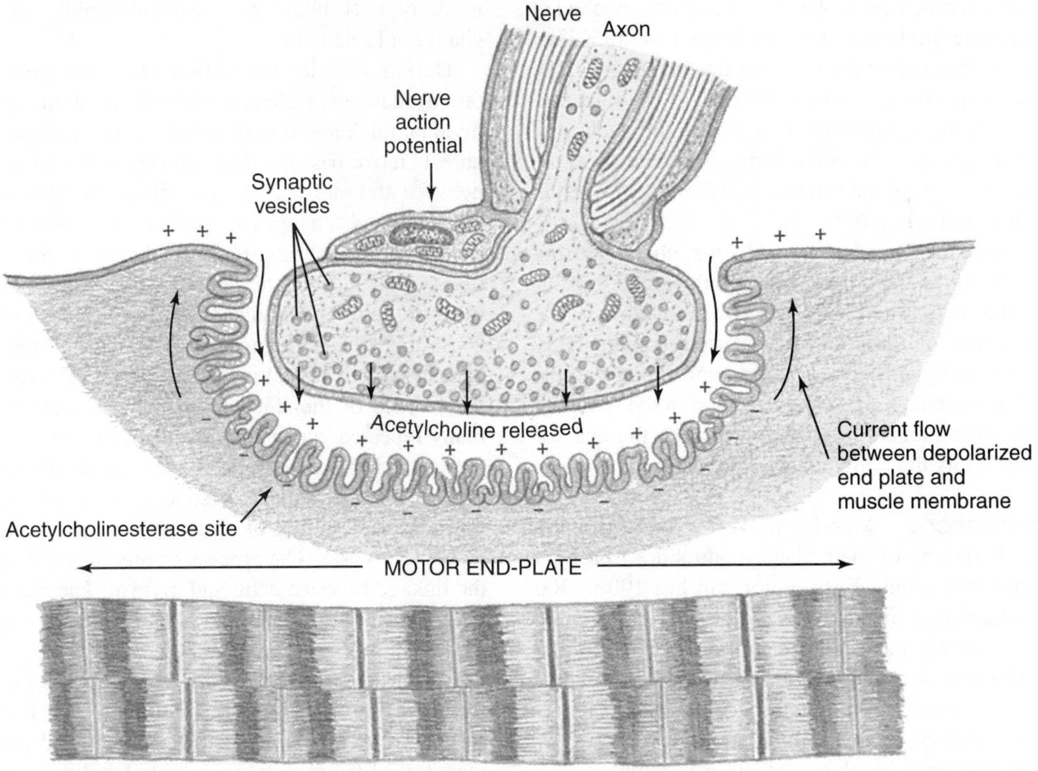

FIG. 6-8
Motor end plate and myoneural junction involved in muscle contraction (see text for content).

The energy for muscle contraction comes from the hydrolysis of ATP into ADP + phosphate + energy. Additional energy sources are phosphocreatine, a protein-energy source found only in muscle tissues, and oxygen, which aids contraction by oxidizing the lactic acid that results from the anaerobic hydrolysis of the high-energy ATP bonds.

Muscle spasm is an involuntary contraction of one muscle or a group of muscles caused by repetitive activation of entire motor units from the repetitive firing of a motor nerve. Tetanus is a sustained contraction caused by a repetitive series of stimuli conducted along the sarcolemmal membrane.

Muscles also have the ability to relax. A relaxing factor called relaxin acts by rendering ATP inactive until the next stimulus reaches a particular fiber, thereby keeping the muscle relaxed.

Muscle Twitch.

A muscle twitch occurs when a minimal stimulus is attained. All muscle fibers associated with the stimulated nerve contract and then relax.

An isotonic twitch causes the muscle to change length when constant tension is applied throughout its contraction. An isometric twitch is one in which the muscle remains or retains a constant length even with a sudden increase in muscle tension.

Muscle Tone.

Tone in muscles provides resistance to passive elongation or stretch and ensures a rapid reaction to an external stimulus. It results from a continuous flow of stimuli from the spinal cord to each motor unit. Muscle tone can be increased or decreased depending on the activity within the nervous system. Tone is increased in anxiety states and decreased during restful periods.

Ligaments

Ligaments hold bones to bones. They may encircle a joint to add strength and stability, as they do around the hip joint (FIG. 6-9), or they may hold obliquely or parallel to the ends of bones across the joint, as they do in and around the knee joint (FIG. 6-10). Ligaments are relatively long bands. They are made up of tough bands of collagen fibers arranged in parallel bundles of fibers to add strength. Type I collagen produces these large, densely packed fibers (see p. 328 for discussion of collagen structure and types). Type I collagen gives ligaments great tensile strength with limited extensibility. When ligaments are taut, they provide the greatest stability to the specific joint. Ligaments allow movement in some directions while restricting movement in other directions. Ligaments differ from tendons by their lower percentage of collagen fibers, which are also less compact, and not necessarily parallel, and ligaments are usually flatter than tendons.

Tendons

Tendons hold muscles to bones (FIG. 6-11, *A* and *B*). They form at the ends of muscles into strong, nonelastic cords of collagen, which gives them great strength. The cells of tendons are arranged in coarse, parallel bundles bound together into fascicles to provide high tensile strength while allowing them to transmit forces from contractile muscle to bone or cartilage and still remain undamaged. Tendons vary in length from 1 inch to

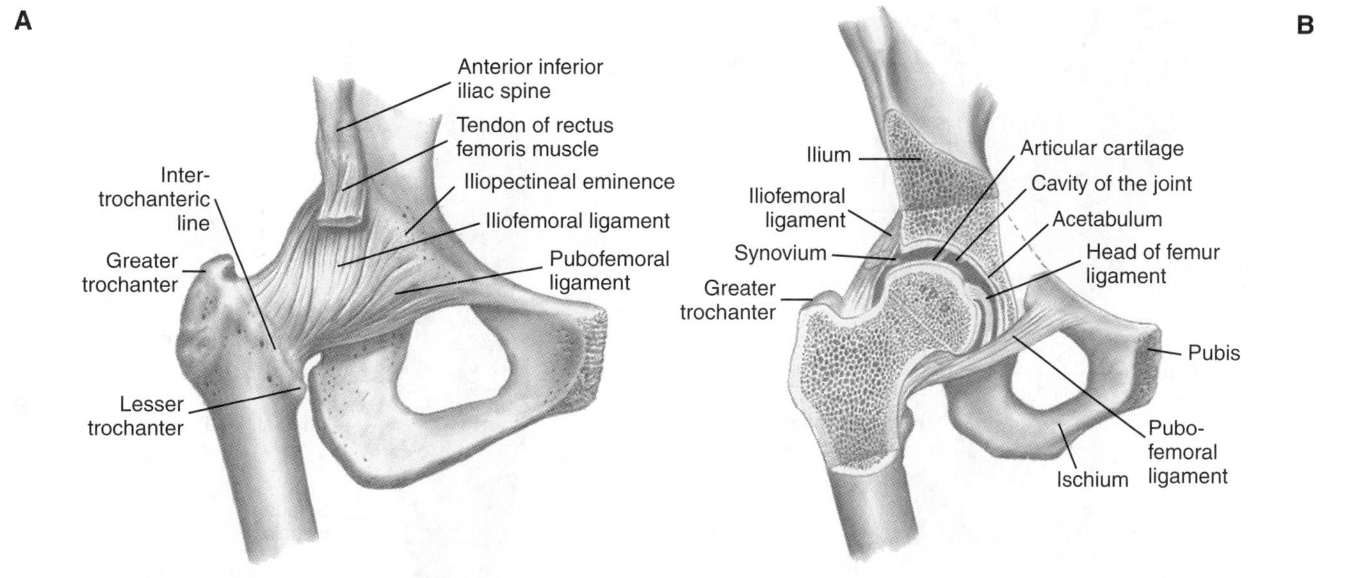

FIG. 6-9
A, Ligaments surrounding hip joint. **B,** Ligaments holding structures in hip joint.

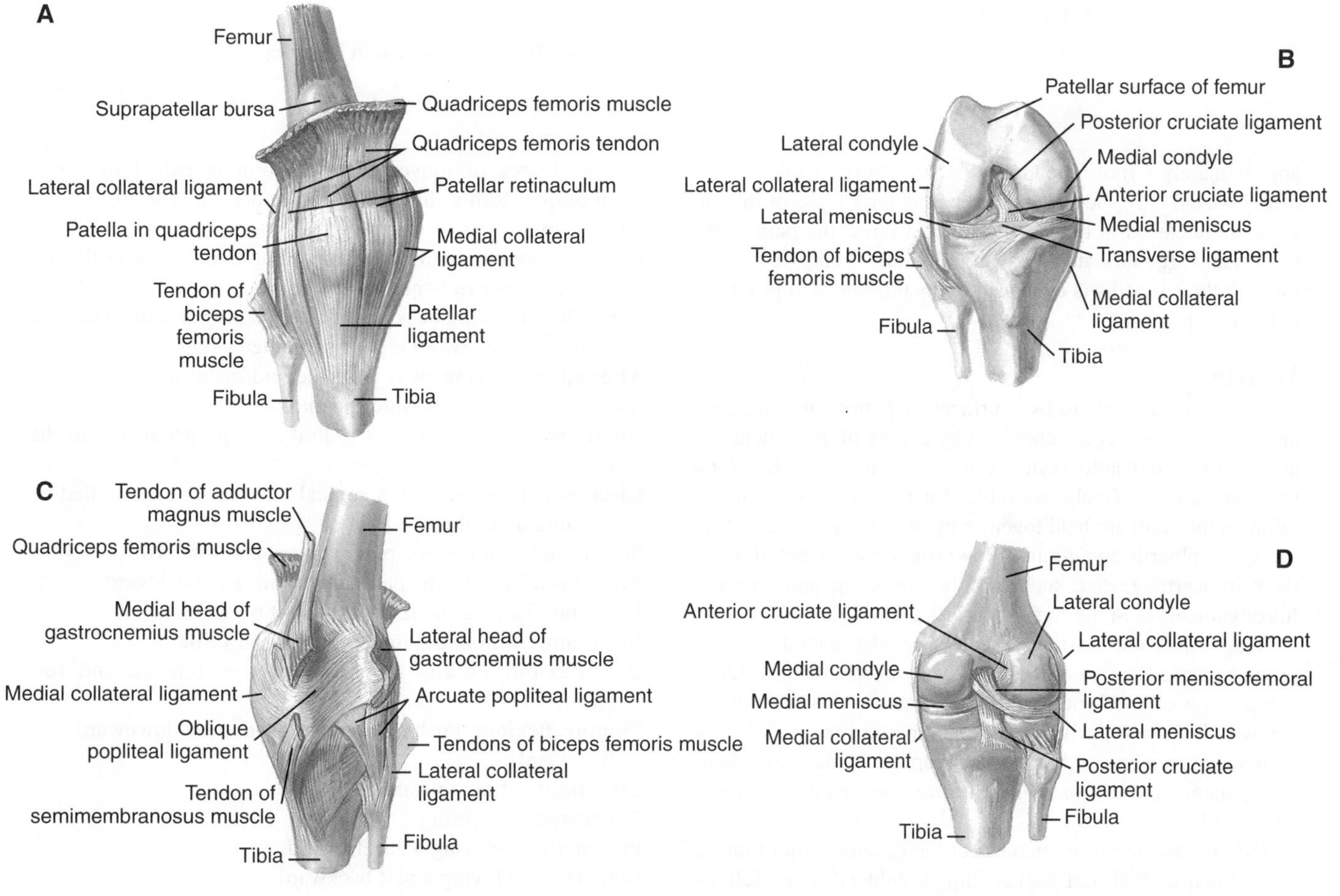

FIG. 6-10
Ligaments of knee joint. **A,** Anterior superficial view. **B,** Anterior deep view. **C,** Posterior superficial view. **D,** Posterior deep view.[49a]

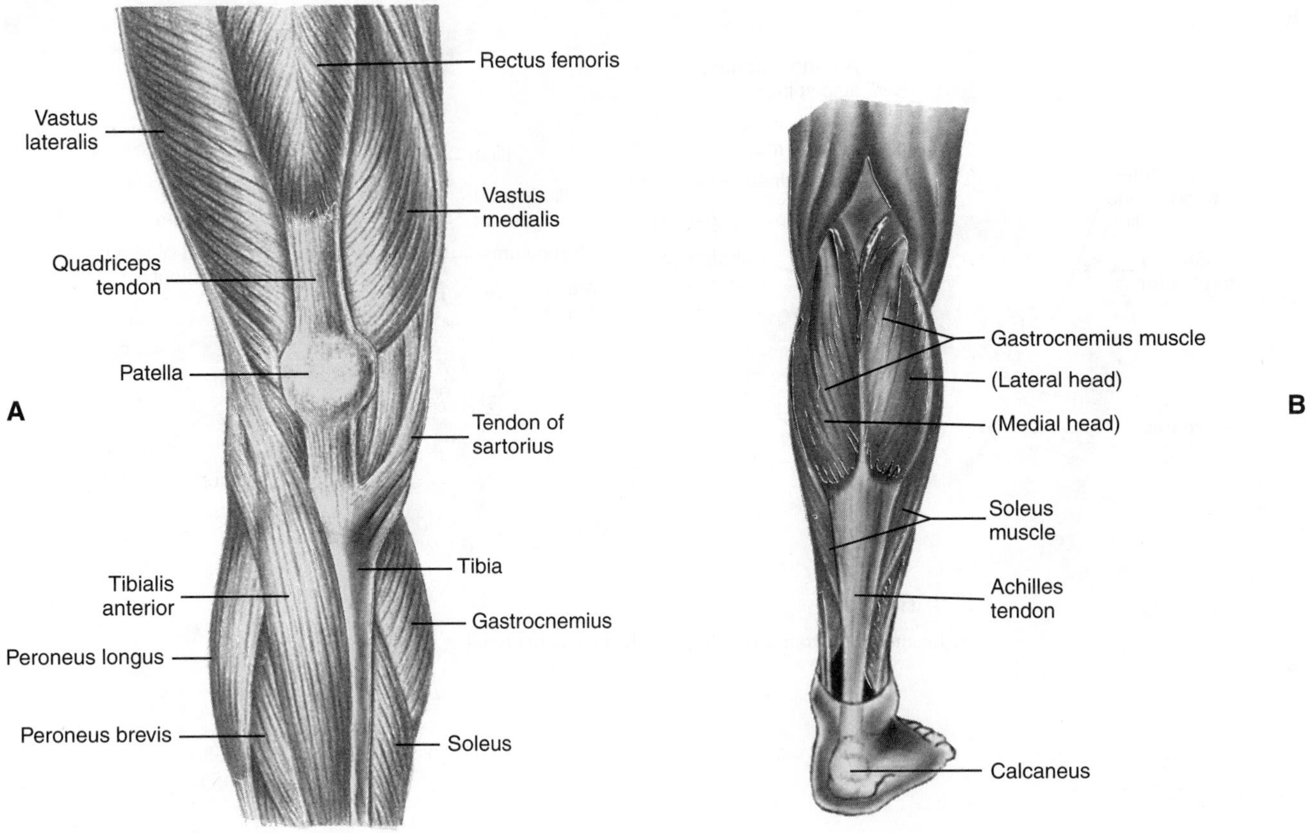

FIG. 6-11
A, Tendons and muscles around knee joint (anterior view). **B,** Achilles tendon in lower leg.

approximately 1 foot. The longest is the Achilles tendon of the heel (FIG. 6-11, *B*). Some tendons, particularly those of the fingers, are enclosed in tendon sheaths that direct the path of the tendon and are lubricated by synovial fluid. Gliding of tendons through their sheaths is enhanced by hyaluronic acid produced in the lining cells.

Joints

Joints are formed where two surfaces of bones come together and articulate. Joints are classified by degree of movement and are either immovable (synarthrotic), slightly movable (amphiarthrotic), or freely movable (diarthrotic). Synarthrotic joints in the skull are held together by fibrous tissues called sutures. Amphiarthrotic joints allow slight movement through their fibrocartilage disc, such as in the symphysis pubis, or by a fibroligament, as in the radioulnar articulation.

Most joints are diarthrotic. They are also called synovial joints because they are lined with synovial membranes. Other components of diarthrodial joints are bones, articular cartilage, synovial fluid, nerves, lymphatics, and blood vessels. All these components are encased in the joint capsule, which is made up of ligaments and tendons encircling or surrounding the joints (FIG. 6-12).

Diarthrodial joints are named for their major form of movement, such as ball and socket (hip, shoulder), hinge (elbow, knee), pivot (atlas, axis), condyloid (wrist), saddle (first metacarpal, trapezium), and gliding (intervertebral).

The degree of movement of a joint is called its range of motion. Joints have one or more of the following movements:

Flexion: Bending forward or shortening that decreases the angle between two bones.
Extension: Bending backward or lengthening that increases the angle between two bones or straightens the joint.
Abduction: Moving away from the midline of the body.
Adduction: Moving toward the midline.
Rotation: Moving around a central axis, perpendicular to the axis.
Circumduction: Making a conical movement, exemplified by winding up to throw a ball.
Supination: Turning the palm upward and forward.
Pronation: Turning the palm downward and backward.
Eversion: Turning the sole of the foot outward.
Inversion: Turning the sole of the foot inward.
Dorsiflexion: Pulling the foot and toes upward and forward.
Plantar flexion: Pushing the foot and toes downward and backward.
Elevation: Lifting upward.
Depression: Lowering.
Protraction: Moving a part forward.
Retraction: Moving a part backward.
Apposition: Moving the thumb toward the little finger to touch together.

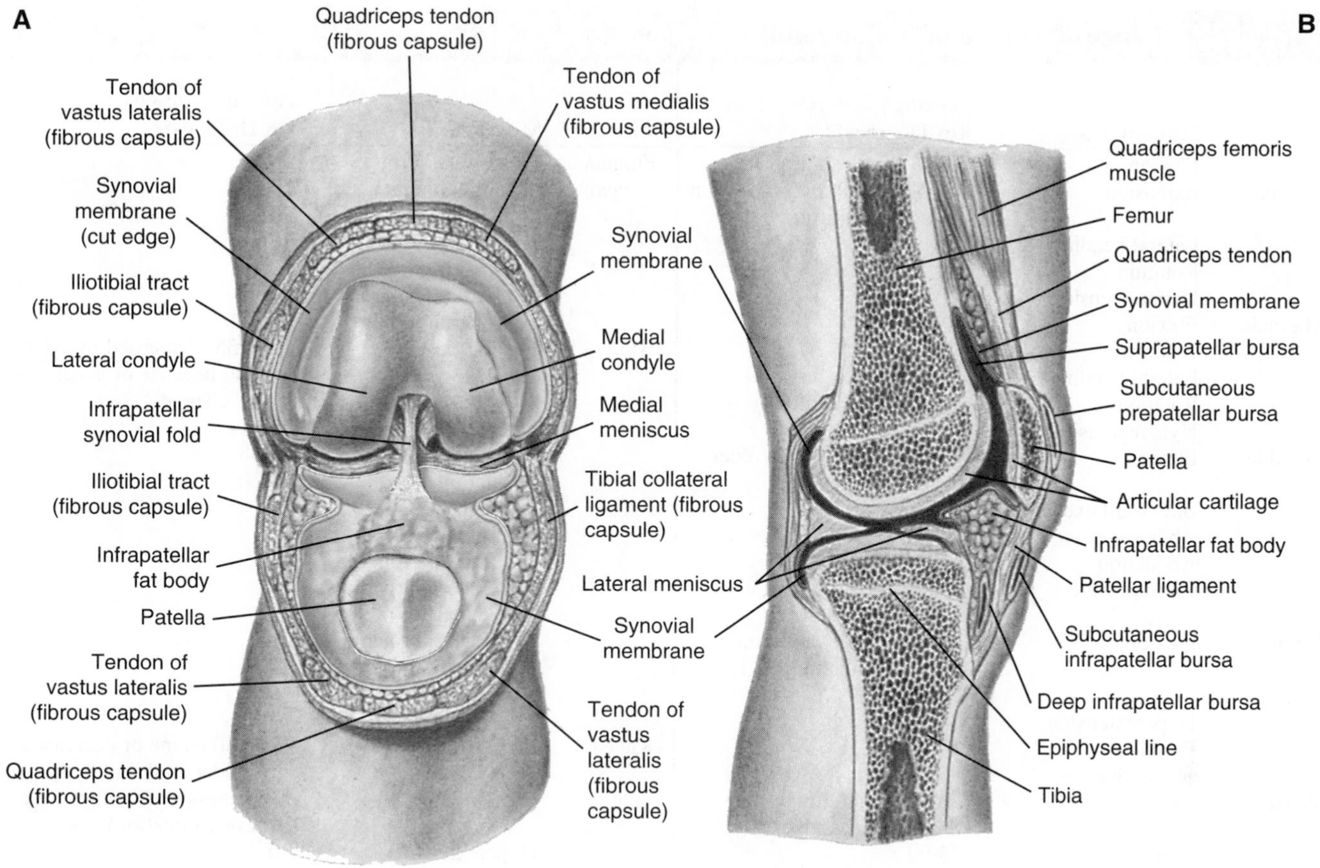

FIG. 6-12

Knee joint (synovial joint). **A,** Frontal view. **B,** Lateral view.

When joints cannot or do not maintain their usual range of motion (ROM), they affect all musculoskeletal tissues and other body tissues. Table 6-2 gives the ROM of major joints.

Synovium

The synovium is a membrane that loosely lines the inner surfaces of the joint (see FIG. 6-12). It forms from cells within the inner layer of the joint capsule. The membrane has many folds that contain the blood vessels and lymphatic vessels. The membrane is made up of cells derived primarily from type I collagen molecules, although the blood vessels are derived from type III collagen (see p. 328).

The folds of the synovial membrane are filled with fluid, called synovial fluid, that bathes the articular cartilage to facilitate articulation and to provide nutrients, phagocytes, and other immunologic functions within the joints. Synovial fluid is a protein-rich filtrate of blood containing hyaluronate, a glycoaminoglycan and lubricating glycoprotein that makes the joint fluid very slippery, facilitating smooth movement within the joint.

Cartilage

Cartilage is a smooth, white or yellow, resilient supporting tissue made up of elastic fibers containing the protein chondrin. There are three types of cartilage:

Hyaline: Bluish white, elastic cartilage covering the ends of bones, synovial joints, the ends of the ribs, the nasal septum, and the walls of the trachea; made up of type II collagen molecules with some type I cells.

Fibrous: White fibers that are particularly resistant to tension and are found in the symphysis pubis and the knee; made up of type I collagen molecules.

Yellow: Elastic yellow fibers found in the epiglottis and the pinna (outer ear); made up of type I collagen molecules.

Hyaline cartilage provides a smooth, low-friction surface for the articulating bones in a joint. It also absorbs weight and distributes it to reduce the forces of weight bearing. Cartilage is elastic and moldable to prevent or lessen injury to the bones and other tissues in a joint (see FIG. 6-10).

Cartilage contains no intrinsic blood vessels. It receives its nutrition from the synovial fluids forced into its porous cellular network by the movements and weight bearing of the joints. Therefore, when a particular joint ceases to bear weight or develops limitations of its usual ROM, articular cartilage atrophies until joint motion and weight bearing are resumed.

Joint cartilage is composed of 65% to 80% water, approximately 2% cartilage cells (chondrocytes), from 10% to 36% collagen as the intercellular matrix, and 5% to 10% protein polysaccharides. The collagen fibers in the cartilage are a highly organized system, making them resistant to physical, metabolic, or chemical breakdown. About 90% of the joint collagen is made up of type II fibers (see Table 6-3 for types of collagen in musculoskeletal tissues).

Table 6-2 Range of Motion of Major Joints

Joint	Movements	Average Ranges (in Degrees)*
Cervical spine	Flexion	35-45 (older adult 35)
	Extension	35 (older adult may have pain and some stiffness)
	Lateral bending	45
	Rotation	45
	Hyperextension	45
Thoracic and lumbar spine	Flexion	80-90
	Extension	30
	Lateral bending	28-35
	Rotation	35-38 (older adult 30)
	Hyperextension	30
Shoulder	Flexion	90 (some stiffness in older adult)
	Backward extension	44-55
	Abduction	90
	Adduction	45-50
	Circumduction	360 (older adult may have crepitation)
Elbow	Flexion	145-160 (older adult may only be able to flex 135 degrees)
	Hyperextension	0
Forearm	Pronation	70-90
	Supination	85-90
Wrist	Extension	70 (older adult may have soreness or stiffness)
	Flexion	73-90
	Ulnar deviation	33-55
	Radial deviation	19
Thumb	Abduction	58
Fingers	Flexion	Decreased (in older adult may be caused by Heberden's or Bouchard's nodes)
	Distal joint	80
Fingers, *cont'd*	Flexion, *cont'd*	
	Middle joint	100
	Proximal joint	90
	Extension	
	Distal joint	0
	Middle joint	0
	Proximal joint	45
Hip	Flexion	120-135 (decreased in older adult because of degenerative changes)
	Extension	28
	Abduction	45-48
	Adduction	20-30
	Rotation	
	In flexion	
	Internal rotation	45
	External rotation	45
	In extension	
	Internal rotation	35
	External rotation	48
	Abduction in 90-degree flexion	45-60
Knee	Flexion	120-130 (same or decreased in older adult but with soreness and stiffness; may have crepitation)
	Hyperextension	10
Ankle	Flexion	48-50
	Extension	18-20
Forefoot	Inversion	30-33 (same or decreased in older adult because of hallux valgus or degenerative changes)
	Eversion	18-20
	Dorsiflexion	20
	Plantar flexion	45-50

*Zero degrees is the extended position; movement is measured by degrees in the specific directions in which the joint moves.

Table 6-3 Types of Collagen in Musculoskeletal Tissues

Type of Collagen*	Distribution in Musculoskeletal Tissues
I	Bone, tendon, ligament, intervertebral disk
II	Cartilage, intervertebral disk
III	Skin, blood vessels
IV	Basement cell membrane
V	Codistributed with type I
VI	Widespread distribution
IX	Codistributed with type II
X	Cartilage growth plate; hypertropic cartilage
XI	Cartilage with type II
XII	Codistributed with type I
XIII	Endothelial cells
XIV	Codistributed with type I

*To date, 14 different types of collagen have been identified.
Modified from McCance and Huether[34]

Bursa

A bursa is an enclosed fluid-filled sac situated between muscles or tendons and bony prominences. Bursae are lined with synovium and are filled with synovial fluid. They serve to cushion, separate, and lubricate the tissues where they are located (see FIG. 6-13). Adventitious bursae may form secondary to pressure or friction over a prominent part. Just such a bursa forms with a bunion in hallux valgus deformity in the foot (see p. 352).

Collagen

The protein collagen is the principal supporting structural element in connective tissues and bone matrix. Collagen makes up over one third of the total body protein in fully developed adults. Collagen fibers are approximately 90% type I fibers, which are synthesized and secreted by osteoblasts. Collagen molecules assemble into *alpha* chains, which combine in threes to form a fibril. The fibrils form a staggered pattern, overlapping contiguous fibrils by approximately one fourth their length. This staggered, overlapping pattern creates gaps, called hole zones, into which crystals are deposited. Then the

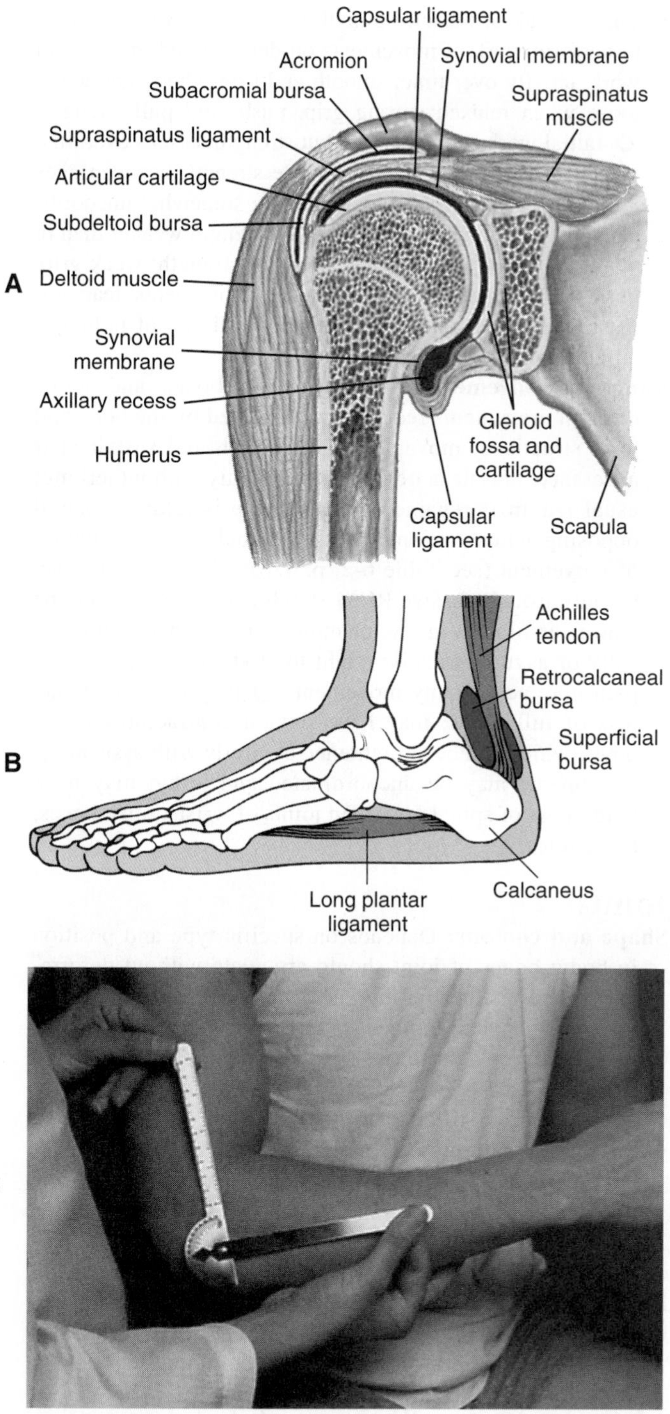

FIG. 6-13

A, Bursae of shoulder joint. **B,** Bursae of the heel. **C,** Goniometer for joint measurements.

fibrils link together and twist to form ropelike fibers. Collagen fibers form a framework that gives bone its tensile strength and enables it to bear weight. Collagen is found in nearly all tissues, and, to date, 14 different types of collagen have been identified (see Table 6-3). Articular cartilage contains types II and IX collagen, which is thought to be the "glue" that holds together the type II collagen scaffold of the articular cartilage. Type IX collagen also helps to maintain the structural integrity of cartilage and resists tensile forces on the joint cartilage.

Collagen also plays an active role in developmental processes, cell attachment, chemotaxis, and the binding of antigen-antibody complexes, making collagen more than an inert structural protein.

NORMAL FINDINGS* MUSCULOSKELETAL EXAMINATION

The orthopedic examination should take into account both the history and the physical examination of the patient. The history should include any past and present musculoskeletal, rheumatic, and orthopedic problems; patterns of local and systemic signs and symptoms; review of all body systems; social, marital, employment (occupational), and psychologic state; habits or hobbies; and living locale and home situation. Assessment should include the effects of any musculoskeletal conditions on the patient's lifestyle, employment, family, and activities of daily living (ADLs). Past medical and family histories are elicited and recorded. The patient's age, sex, general appearance, and any deformities or assistive devices are noted. Presence of a brace, cast, belt, or other wrapping is noted. Skin color and texture are observed and noted. The patient's height and weight are checked, as are temperature and vital signs. Presence of glasses or hearing aids is noted.

The physical examination includes an overall general inspection; observance of gait, posture, and movements while walking, sitting, and standing; and assessment of bilateral symmetry, strength, size, and shape of musculoskeletal tissues, muscular development, generalized or localized edema, ROM of each joint, deep tendon reflexes, and condition of skin and hair distribution, of body, and of fingers and toes (with presence or complaints of Raynaud phenomenon). Note lesions, rash (color and site), pain at rest or with movement in one or more joints, hair growth and distribution, evidence of bruises or hemorrhage, bone or joint deformity, congenital defects or deformities, condition of blood vessels, peripheral pulses, color of tissues, lymph nodes, leg length equality, and "point" tenderness (patient can point to area of greatest tenderness). Note patient's indications of pain by observing frequent shifts in position, wincing, grimacing, sighing, or even crying from pain; facial appearance as sad or frowning; complaints of "pinches," spasms, numbness, tingling, inability to stand straight without pain; need to support self on or with furniture while rising or sitting; pressing palm or fist over specific part or area of body; inability to find a comfortable position, and such.

The following equipment is needed: goniometer to measure ROM (see FIG. 6-13, *C*), percussion hammer, paper clip and needle (for dull and sharp sensory determinations), cotton, sphygmomanometer, thermometer, tourniquet, tape measure, and stethoscope.

The following principles should be kept in mind in performing an orthopedic examination:

- Normal tissues are examined before injured, inflamed, or otherwise involved ones.
- Local signs and symptoms are assessed along with systemic findings.
- Bilateral local and systemic observations are made and compared.

*✪ = Older adult.
✪ = An elderly adult, a person age 85 years and above.[56]

PERIPHERAL NEUROVASCULAR ASSESSMENT*

Vascular assessment	Neurologic assessment
Color	Sensation
Temperature	Motor function
Capillary refill	Pain: Increased pain on passive
Peripheral pulses	movement is a hallmark of
Edema	compartment syndrome (see
	p. 408 for content)

*All parameters must be assessed each time checks are done to determine current status.

- Palpation is gently performed while observing facial or other reactions to note tenderness or sensitivity within the tissues.
- Movements are assessed within norms for ROM of all joints from head to foot.

Physical examination is one part of the orthopedic examination, along with the history and the radiologic, serologic, surgical biopsy or exploratory procedure, and consultative examinations. Special assessment techniques may also be done to aid in diagnosis (see p. 331).

Skeleton

Posture: Stands upright; head perpendicular to shoulders and pelvis; shoulders and pelvis aligned; convex curve to thoracic spine; concave curve to lumbar spine; arms hang freely from shoulders; legs straight with feet aligned with toes pointing straight ahead; ○ stance less upright, with head and neck more forward; thoracic curvature more pronounced; lumbar curvature less pronounced; shoulders may be hunched or rolled forward; angle of head of femur into acetabulum changes, leading to varus planting or placement of thighs, legs, and feet; height is decreased; may have kyphotic thoracic curve; may have less lordotic curve; ✪ frail; functional disabilities in walking, maintaining balance, and pain-free mobility often caused by osteoporosis and decreased muscle mass. It has been noted that adults between ages 20 and 70 years often lose up to 2 inches of their height.

Gait: Smooth, coordinated, easy, and rhythmic with push off and swing through; arms move freely at sides; easy acceleration and deceleration; can stand still without swaying or tilt; ○ gait slow to initiate and stop; gait may be shuffling at times, with less knee and ankle lifts; more stiffness of hips, knees, and back; steps may be shorter and more rapid but cover less overall distance, may limp; ✪ slow gait, may need to hold onto furniture or another person to maintain balance; shuffles when stepping; less bending at knees; may have varus planting of feet if female.

Muscles

Shape and contour: "Full-bellied"; firm and supple; muscle mass in overall conformity with body build; tapered at either end of muscle mass; ○ shape and contour decrease, with less belly and mass common; ✪ smaller muscle mass with somewhat flaccid "belly" of muscle.

Strength: Peak of muscle strength is age 25 to 30 years; able to perform work of movements on demand and to maintain work activity over time; smooth and firm when contracted; loose when relaxed; strong grip, push, and pull strength; ○ initial work energy strong, but strength lessens over time (gradual 10% yearly loss in muscle strength between ages 30 and 60 years); movements may be somewhat uncoordinated and jerky; grip, push, and pull strength weaker than in young adults; ✪ poor muscle mass or strength; weak grip, push, and pull strength; uncoordinated movements; fears going to unfamiliar places because of possibility of falling in unfamiliar surroundings.

Range of movements: Able to move bones and joints through movements required or permitted by the bone and joint structures; movements are smooth and sustained if necessary; muscle action begins smoothly without jerking; usual length is regained when muscle is relaxed; paired opposing actions are smooth; there should be no limitation of movement (see Table 6-2, p. 328); ○ all muscles can be put through passive ROM slowly; active ROM may be slower or limited in one or more joints, either symmetrically or asymmetrically; slight to moderate tenderness or pain may accompany movement; ✪ may have moderate loss of full ROM; may have flexion contractures of elbows, which can be straightened carefully with assistance; movements may be uncoordinated and jerky; may have tenderness of spinal areas and joints of wrists, hips, knees, and ankles.

Joints

Shape and contour: Depends on specific type and position in body; bones of joint should articulate without deformity on one another in alignment; joint is firm and strong; ○ joints appear larger than surrounding tissues; contour may be irregular in one or more joints; bones may glide over one another with slightly audible click, crepitus, or sound; joint is stiffer than in younger adult; ✪ joints are misshapen and irregular; are large, do not glide easily; may have pain on weight bearing in back and hips or knees; may have limp.

Temperature: Warmth around joint should be same as surrounding tissues; may have some redness (erythema).

Swelling/edema: None; ○ may have slight edema of fingers, feet, or lower legs; ✪ may have edema under lower eyelids and edema of fingers, feet, and lower portion of legs

Ligaments, Cartilage, and Tendons

Shape and contour: Taut, elastic, and firm; permit weight bearing; ○ taut but may be tighter and less elastic; may limit bone and joint contour.

Movements: Easily moves through ROM and holds joints and muscles according to place or function; movements of joints can be sustained without deformity or curvature; weight bearing is pain free; ○ less ease and range of movements; joints are stiffer; may have some joint laxity and weakness; weight bearing may cause some soreness or pain; ✪ jerky, uncoordinated movements; movements are slower and with some soreness and pain; joints are stiff, weaker, and with some mild to moderate laxity.

CONDITIONS, DISEASES, AND DISORDERS

INFLAMMATORY CONDITIONS

Inflammatory conditions are those that result in local or systemic responses to noxious stimuli (temperature extremes, chemicals, microorganisms, and others). These conditions can affect cells locally, resulting in cellular and tissue alterations while attempting to initiate, maintain, and resolve the inflammatory reaction. Initial reactions are referred to as acute, which are rapid and short lived; reactions that are longer lasting or prolonged are referred to as chronic inflammatory conditions. Inflammatory conditions of musculoskeletal tissues include both acute and chronic types.

Inflammatory conditions can affect one or more muscles, tendons, ligaments, bones, and structures in and around the joints. Because of the interaction of the structures, diagnosis and treatment of specific tissue inflammations may be difficult. Overlapping therapy may be needed to ensure relief of the condition. Treatment methods for many specific musculoskeletal inflammatory conditions are often identical. Also, inflammatory or degenerative effects in one musculoskeletal tissue may have long-term effects on contiguous tissues. Therefore inflammatory conditions must be considered serious alterations even if only one small area of localized inflammation is noted.

ANKYLOSING SPONDYLITIS

Ankylosing spondylitis (AS) is a chronic inflammatory disease characterized by low back pain initially, with progressive stiffening and eventual fusion (ankylosis) of the vertebrae and sacroiliac joints. These fusions result in deformities of the vertebral column, joints, and adjacent tissues, which together progressively inhibit mobility.

AS is approximately three times more common in men than in women. Men also experience more severe disease than women. Ankylosing spondylitis appears to affect persons between the ages of 20 and 40 years with a peak around age 20 years. The prevalence of AS in the United States is approximately 1% in Caucasians, 3% to 4% in African-Americans, and 18% to 50% in Native Americans.[18] Many persons with AS remain undiagnosed or misdiagnosed. There is a marked hereditary factor, histocompatibility antigen HLA-B27, associated with AS. It is inherited as a mendelian-dominant trait.

Special Assessment Techniques*

Examination or Test	Site	Normal Findings	Abnormal Findings
Joint range of movements	Any or all joints	Specific range of motion (ROM) as per Table 6-2; no soreness or pain; no edema or elevated temperature in or around joints	Limitation of range of movements in one or more spheres; pain, soreness, muscle weakness, edema, elevated temperature in or around joint or joints; deformity, lump or mass around joint
Straight leg raising (Lasègue)	Legs (one at a time)	No pain or soreness in back, buttocks when leg is raised while fully extended at knee; patient lies on back	Pain, soreness, or radiation of pain from low back to buttocks; may spread down leg to toes
McMurray	Knee	No excessive or palpable pop or click in knee noted when ankle is grasped to turn knee medially and laterally, and while moving knee backward and forward from full flexion to extension	Click or pop felt or heard; pain or local tenderness is positive for meniscal damage to tears
Fabere-Patrick	Knee and hip	Knee can be flexed and brought to almost horizontal position to body with heel resting on opposite knee	Knee cannot be brought to horizontal position; limitation may be in hip, knee, or back (usually hip disease prevents knee rotation to horizontal position)
Drawer: Anterior and posterior	Knee	Knee has slight forward or backward movement while flexed on tibia and fibula	Knee has more movement forward or backward (direction indicates tear of either anterior or posterior cruciate ligament).
Trendelenburg	Pelvis and gluteus muscles	With weight on one leg, pelvis on opposite side will be slightly elevated (observed posteriorly)	With weight on one leg, pelvis will drop (because of weakness or pain in hip joint or its muscles) on opposite side
Thomas	Hip, knee, and lumbar spine	With patient on back, hip and knee are flexed to abdomen without flexion simultaneously occurring in lumbar spine	When patient flexes knee and hip to abdomen, lumbar spine will flex if there is a pathologic condition of the hip, and opposite leg will rise from table

*These tests are examples of those most commonly done. The reader is referred to Seidel HM et al: *Mosby's guide to physical examination,* ed 3, 1995, Mosby, or to Wilson SF, Giddens J: *Health assessment for nursing practice,* ed 2, 2001, Mosby, for additional special assessments.

Continued

Special Assessment Techniques—cont'd

Examination or Test	Site	Normal Findings	Abnormal Findings
Phalen	Wrists	No tingling of fingers with wrists maximally flexed against each other and held for 1 minute	Tingling felt in the thumb, the index finger, and the middle and lateral half of the ring finger
Tinel	Carpal tunnel of wrist or tarsal tunnel at ankle	No tingling into thumb, index, and middle fingers when median nerve is tapped at the wrist or posterior tibial nerve is tapped at medial malleolus	Tingling felt as above for Phalen test of wrist; tingling in toes for entrapped posterior tibial nerve
Brudzinski	Back and neck	With patient lying on back, no pain is felt in neck or back when head is passively flexed to chest	Pain in back and neck felt with passive flexion of head; knees and hips involuntarily flex to relieve pain (sign of meningeal irritation)
Kernig	Back and leg	No back or leg pain felt when leg is extended (patient lies on back with hip and knee flexed)	Pain is felt in lower back, neck, or head when leg is extended from flexed position (sign of meningeal irritation)

*These tests are examples of those most commonly done. The reader is referred to Seidel HM et al: *Mosby's guide to physical examination,* ed 3, 1995, Mosby, or to Wilson SF, Giddens J: *Health assessment for nursing practice,* ed 2, 2001, Mosby, for additional special assessments.

PATHOPHYSIOLOGY

Ankylosing spondylitis frequently begins with the complaint of low back pain, which is caused by the chief pathologic condition of inflammation of the *enthesis,* the place in which ligaments and tendons insert into bones of the vertebrae. The end results of the inflammatory changes are scarring (fibrosis), ossification, and fusion of the affected joints, primarily those of the lower vertebral column and the sacroiliac joints. Eventually all of the vertebral joints become fused and fibrotic and lose flexibility as the inflammation moves up the vertebral column. The vertebrae lose their normal contour and appear square on radiographs, displaying the characteristic "bamboo spine" appearance diagnostic of AS. Achilles tendinitis may also be noted in AS.

Extraskeletal manifestations of AS occur in up to 25% to 30% of persons at some time during the course of their disease. The most common extraskeletal manifestation is acute anterior uveitis, noted by acute pain, increased lacrimation, photophobia, and blurred vision.[24a] In addition, there may be edema around the eye and the iris, which appears discolored compared to the contralateral side.

Rarely occurring conditions associated with AS include ascending aortitis, aortic valve incompetence, cardiac conduction abnormalities, myocardial dysfunction, and pericarditis.[24a] Incidence of cardiovascular conditions varies from 4% to 10% after 30 or more years of AS. Another late extraskeletal manifestation of AS is pleuropulmonary involvement, with progressive fibrosis of the upper lobes of the lungs, which can develop cysts over time.

Some patients with AS develop "silent" (asymptomatic) mucosal inflammatory lesions in the terminal ileum and colon detected on radiologic studies. These lesions may have some role in the pathogenesis of AS.[24a]

DIAGNOSTIC STUDIES AND FINDINGS

Physical examination of back and all musculoskeletal tissues: Local and systemic limitations: initial complaint of low back pain with morning stiffness; has difficulty turning, extending, or twisting back; may have Reiter's syndrome (see p. 334), consisting of conjunctivitis with uveitis, urethritis and arthritis (occurs in 30% of patients); may have progressive kyphosis of cervical, thoracic, and lumbar spine with eventual loss of ability to look forward or upward (FIG. 6-14); sacroiliac and hip abnormalities and pain and stiffness may cause severe disability and limitations in mobility; kyphosis may limit chest expansion and pleural functions, leading to pleuritic pain and lessened chest movements and tenderness over the entire thorax; pain over the iliac crests and ischial tuberosities may make lying and sitting painful, disrupting sleep cycles and social interactions; walking causes tender areas in heels with cautious placement of the feet or even a limp noted; rest of affected areas makes symptoms worse; fatigue and weight loss occur frequently; aortic insufficiency may be noted by heart block resulting from Stokes-Adam's attacks, requiring a follow-up pacemaker; may have pacemaker in place because of arrhythmias and/or syncope

Roentgenograms: Reveal the inflammatory, fibrotic, and fused vertebral joints, with "squared" vertebrae and "bamboo spine" configuration; sacroilitis is usually noted; colonoscopic studies may show inflammatory lesions in terminal ileum

Serologic examination: Positive serum analysis for presence of histocompatibility antigen B-27, present in 80% to 90% of Caucasian patients with AS, but in only 8% of general population; HLA-B27 present in only 50% of African-Americans with AS[18]; rheumatoid factor is negative in most patients; erythrocyte sedimentation rate is elevated throughout the disease, at 10 to 15 mm/h in both males and females (normal is 0 to 9 mm/h in males and 0 to 20 mm/h in females); alkaline phosphatase levels are frequently elevated; hypochromic anemia may be present; serum IgA is frequently elevated; generally, serologic studies are not strongly relied on for the diagnosis of AS; its diagnosis is based mainly on the patient history, physical examination, and radiologic findings

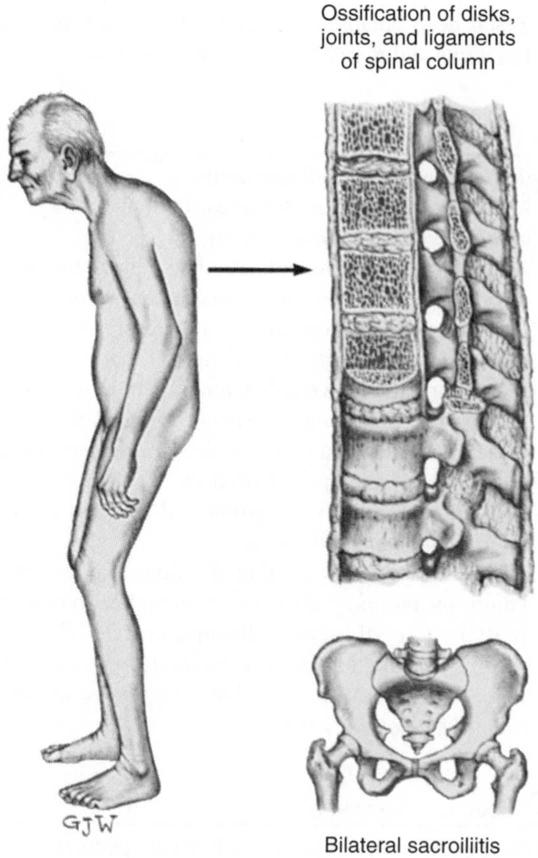

FIG. 6-14

Characteristic posture and site of ankylosing spondylitis. (From Mourad.[39])

MULTIDISCIPLINARY PLAN

Surgery

Total hip replacement to correct fixed fusion of hip
Cervical spinal fusion to prevent osteoporotic fracture
Osteotomy of thoracic or lumbar vertebrae and to allow patient to see straight ahead

Medications

Analgesic-antipyretic agents: Salicylate analgesics (aspirin), 600 mg q4h (with buffering)
Nonsteroidal antiinflammatory drugs (NSAIDs)*
- Ibuprofen, 400-600 mg tid or qid
- Indomethacin (Indocin), 25-50 mg tid; may be increased to a maximum of 200 mg/day
- Naproxen (Naprosyn), 500 mg at bedtime; 250 mg bid: dosage may be increased to 1.5 g daily for symptom relief from acute exacerbations
- †Celecoxib (Celebrex), 100 mg bid
- †Rofecoxib (Vioxx), 12.5 mg once daily; may increase to total of 25 mg total daily

Antibacterial agents: Sulfasalazine; in individualized doses, if inflammatory bowel disease is present

General Management

If smoker patient should stop smoking
Occupational therapy for identification and learning of modifications in ADLs, employment, and changes in lifestyle necessary because of rigidity and curvature of spinal column: focus on ergonomic work stations and furniture for optimal spinal positioning while standing, sitting, lying down, and walking
Consultation with a rheumatology clinical nurse specialist for assistance with overall patient management
Education related to role of patient to become an active participant in care in the early stages before permanent rigidity and deformity have developed
Assessment of daily activities, lifestyle patterns, visual difficulties resulting from spinal rigidity; use of aids such as elastic laces or stocking aids to facilitate grooming, hygiene, and other daily activities
Provide continuous reinforcement of purposes of treatments and patient's role in self-care to achieve short- and long-term goals; patient's own efforts are the key to long-term success in managing AS
Education related to avoidance of trauma to prevent vertebral fracture in neck or lumbar areas
Weight monitoring with weight reduction and stabilization as needed
Physical therapy for exercises of the entire back, specific joint and muscle exercises, and deep-breathing exercises or other respiratory exercises
Physical therapy using pulsed short-wave therapy, application of local heat or cold, local ultrasound or transcutaneous nerve stimulation, teaching optimal posture positions, chest expansion, and breathing techniques
Exercises to maintain mobility, including swimming and aqua therapy; walking (rest is not beneficial in AS); if able, playing sports, such as volleyball or cross-country skiing (helps counteract kyphosis and decreases stiffness)
Use of nonpharmacologic pain management techniques, including use of music, audio and/or video tapes, imagery, and other such techniques
Apply heat to spinal column to lessen pain and inflammation
Local injection of corticosteroid to lessen enthesopathy as needed
A firm mattress and bed with only a small pillow or no pillow for good sleep posture
Lying prone 15 to 30 minutes once or twice daily to lessen tendency to kyphosis
Occasionally, use of a neck or back brace or other orthosis
Occasionally, use of cervical or pelvic belt traction for short periods
Consultations with social service and community nursing personnel to plan for long-term care and follow-up
Driver mirrors on both sides of car to increase safety while driving; car should have air bags for safety in event of accident

NURSING CARE

NURSING ASSESSMENT

Back, hips, legs, and feet: Pain: may alternate side to side, usually is worse on rising in morning; stiffness along entire

---

*A variety of NSAIDs may be used at different times for individual patients. See table on p. 337 for additional NSAIDs.
†New cyclooxygenase-2 (COX-2) inhibiting agents.

vertebral column, hips, and shoulders; limitation of movements: check ROM of all joints (see Table 6-2, p. 328); radiation to buttocks, down one or both legs; posture; gait; use of cane or furniture for balance; note caution in placing of feet when moving or walking

Cervical or thoracic areas: Loss of normal curves, kyphosis, fixed flexion of cervical vertebrae—ability or inability to look forward or upward (see FIG. 6-14); loss of full inhalation or exhalation, respiratory limitations or excursions

Systemic responses: Polyarthritis: asymmetric and affecting the large joints of the lower limbs; malaise, fatigue, weight loss, vague chest pains; Reiter's syndrome may be present (Table 6-4); uveitis is commonly spread throughout spinal column as disease progresses and to sacroiliac, hips, knees, neck, and shoulder joints; cannot hold head upright because of inflammatory changes

Psychosocial concerns: Self-concept and body image concerns from limitations of social interactions and loss of mobility and independence; sleep deprivation; position in bed—supine or prone (should sleep in supine position to lessen kyphotic changes)

POTENTIAL COMPLICATIONS

Fracture of cervical and/or lumbar vertebrae; decreased respiratory reserve; pneumonia; fusion of hips and vertebrae from inflammatory changes; risk for fall and injury

PATIENT PROBLEMS/NURSING DIAGNOSES & INTERVENTIONS

NIC IMMOBILITY MANAGEMENT

Impaired physical mobility related to spinal inflammatory condition

- Observe while walking, sitting, or lying *for signs of relief or progressive impairment, and site of pain or soreness.*
- Assist with ROM exercises *to maintain joint mobility.*
- Encourage performance of prescribed exercises (swimming and walking) *to maintain mobility.*
- Massage back as needed *to relieve tense or tired muscles.*
- Assist patient to positions of comfort; keep bed flat *to maintain extension of the spine.*
- Assist with immersion in Hubbard tank or spa *to lessen muscle spasms and strengthen extensor muscles.*
- Teach deep-breathing exercises to maintain respiratory functions and *to aid peripheral oxygenation.*

NIC PHYSICAL COMFORT PROMOTION

Chronic pain related to inflammation

- Monitor patient for the presence, amount, and severity of pain *to determine current status.*
- Administer analgesic and antiinflammatory medications as prescribed *to relieve pain and inflammation.*
- Observe patient's movements for increasing ease and frequency *to note effects of medications.*
- Listen for patient's verbalization of pain relief or continuing pain *to determine if changes are needed.*
- Observe all involved points *to note abatement or continuation of inflammation, if possible.*
- Encourage proper use of pillow and mattress *to prevent additional trauma and pain.*
- Observe for side effects of medications (e.g., gastric irritation or burning; changes in complete blood count [CBC] and erythrocyte sedimentation rate [ESR]; diarrhea or constipation) *to note reactions to medications.*
- Place soft pillow in chair for sitting *to ease soreness around ischial tuberosities.*

NIC COPING ASSISTANCE

Disturbed body image and ineffective role performance related to severe kyphosis and rigidity of spine

- Monitor for implicit and expressed concerns.
- Encourage socialization with family and friends *to help maintain usual roles.*
- Encourage team recreational activities and games, or sports such as volleyball or cross-country skiing, *to maintain patient's inclusion in activities, and counteract effects of inflammation.*
- Encourage compliance with treatment regimen *to prevent severe deformity and effects on body image.*
- Encourage patient to continue seeing physician for continuity of care and for current or recent developments in treatment of ankylosing spondylitis *to aid in maintaining long-term health status.*
- Stress need to remain active and mobile *because rest is detrimental in AS and may accelerate joint fusion.*

Table 6-4 Syndromes Associated With Arthritic Diseases

Syndrome	Patterns	Associated Diseases
Reiter	Triad of conjunctivitis, urethritis, and arthritis; oral, genital, and mucocutaneous lesions (stomatitis, ulcerations, papules)	Ankylosing spondylitis; rheumatoid arthritis
Behcet	Triad of iritis, oral lesions, and genital lesions; cutaneous lesions; phlebitis; colitis; polyarthritis	Polyarthritis of unknown etiology
Sjogren	Patterns of dryness (sicca) of conjunctivae and salivary glands; arthritis, swelling of parotid gland; Raynaud phenomenon in some patients	Connective tissue diseases such as systemic lupus erythematosus (SLE), progressive systemic sclerosis (PSS), polymyositis
Stevens-Johnson (variant of erythema multiforme)	Stomatitis with ulcerations of oral mucosa; high fever; genital ulcerations; erythematous skin eruptions; arthritis	Erythema multiforme; erythema nodosum; rheumatic fever; rheumatoid arthritis and juvenile rheumatoid arthritis; ulcerative colitis

- Apply heat to spinal column *to lessen pain and inflammation.*

NIC SELF-CARE FACILITATION

Disturbed sleep pattern related to results of inflammatory changes, joint fusion, kyphotic changes, or others

- Observe for disruptions in sleep cycles, when possible, *to determine effects on sleep and rest.*
- Place foam corrugated pad over mattress *to lessen pressure on sore or tender areas.*
- Discuss need to "leave stresses or concerns at bedroom door" *to encourage longer, restorative sleep periods.*
- Encourage use of firm mattress on bed with only a small pillow under head *to lessen progression of kyphotic curvature or increase of cervical flexion contracture.*
- Instruct to lie prone 15 to 30 minutes one to two times daily *to lessen pressure over ischial tuberosities and skin tissues.*
- Stress need to stop use of tobacco or smoking, if a smoker, *to increase circulation to all body tissues.* Nicotine decreases circulation to vertebral and other areas.
- Assist to positions of comfort with bed flat *to maintain extension of spine.*
- Discuss with physician possible need for short-term use of cervical collar, back belt, or other orthosis *to lessen strain on inflamed tissues.*
- Consult with respiratory therapist for exercises to enhance deep breathing and pulmonary functions that *should increase oxygenation to all tissues.*
- Encourage coughing to clear secretions from respiratory passages *to aid restful sleep.*
- Gently massage back areas *to relieve tense or tired muscles.*
- Teach use of imagery and relaxation techniques *to aid rest and sleep.*

NIC PATIENT EDUCATION

Deficient knowledge related to lack of information about disease process

- Reiterate, if or as needed, physician's explanations of patient's diagnosis, treatments, and prognosis *to assure patient's and significant others' understanding.*
- Clarify that active exercises are necessary for regaining or maintaining strength and mobility *because rest is contraindicated in AS.*
- Explain need to use care and caution in all daily activities and movements *to prevent injury or fall related to inflammatory changes, spinal rigidity, and painful or limited movements of joints and muscles.*
- Consult with dietitian for foods *to prevent the possibility of osteoporosis* and teach about high calcium foods.
- Explain need for driver and passenger side mirrors on car *to increase safety while driving;* car should also have air bag(s) *for prevention of injury in the event of an accident.*
- Discuss need to lie prone *to lessen kyphotic changes.*
- Reiterate relaxation techniques *to increase self-care and confidence.*
- Encourage to seek medical care for increases in vertebral rigidity, kyphosis, or other changes *to determine causes of changes or necessity of treatment change.*
- Discuss ways to lessen development of osteoporosis, including activity, nutrition, exercises, and weight bearing, *to lessen possibility of fracture.*
- Observe patient for weakness or loss of motor functions *to note possible signs of paraplegia related to kyphosis.*

PATIENT EDUCATION/CONTINUUM OF CARE PLAN

1. Reiterate explanations of inflammatory processes and rationale for medical care to ensure that patient and family understand.
2. Discuss rationale for exercise as opposed to rest of affected tissues, since rest is detrimental in AS.
3. Explain action and side effects of antiinflammatory medications. The patient should understand and be alert to the many side effects of ordered medications. List names, dosages, and common side effects for patient safety.
4. Demonstrate deep-breathing, ROM, and joint mobility exercises to encourage patient to comply.
5. Include family members in evaluation, practice, and performance of ADLs as necessary for home care continuity.
6. Explain benefits of aqua therapy (especially swimming and water aerobics) to maintain mobility.
7. Refer patient and family to community health club, nursing organization, and support groups for continuing care after discharge, such as the Arthritis and Rheumatism Council, National Spondylitis Society of America, and Arthritis Foundation.

EVALUATION/PATIENT OUTCOMES

Immobility Management: Patient retains adequate vertebral mobility and satisfactory curvature. Patient's inflammation abated without ankylosis or severe curvature.

Physical Comfort Promotion: Patient experiences pain relief with medications. Patient continues own ADLs and usual employment activities, interactions, and recreation.

Coping Assistance: Patient maintains independence, recreational/sports activities, social interactions, and ADLs. Patient states pain is tolerable with analgesic medication and other treatments. Patient does not experience vertebral fracture. Patient appears to accept change in appearance. Patient does not require surgical intervention for joint repair or respositioning. Patient copes satisfactorily with limitations of disease and required vigilance and care.

Self-Care Facilitation: Patient has a consistent, restful sleep pattern.

Patient Education: Patient verbalizes understanding of condition and need for ongoing care.

FIBROMYALGIA

Fibromyalgia is a chronic syndrome of musculoskeletal tissues characterized by its core symptom of chronic widespread pain.[3]

The condition is often misdiagnosed because of the vagueness of the symptoms that bring the person to the physician.

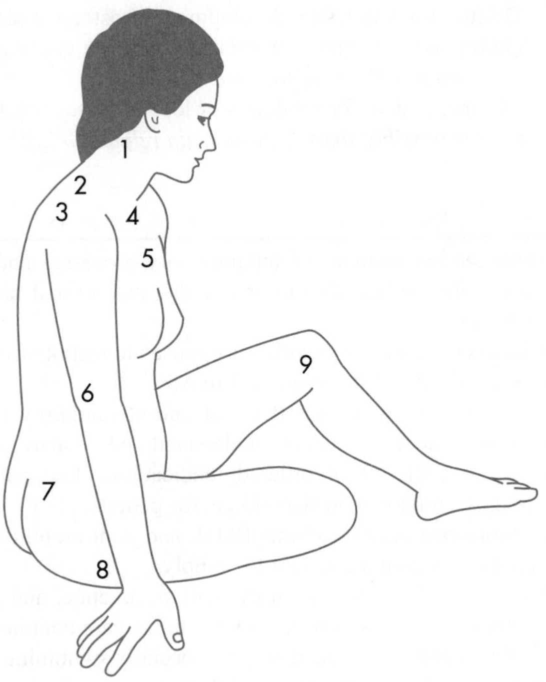

FIG. 6-15

Tender points. The nine paired tender points recommended by the 1990 American College of Rheumatology Criteria Committee for establishing a diagnosis of fibromyalgia are as follows: (1) insertion of nuchal muscles into occiput; (2) upper border of trapezius—midportion; (3) muscle attachments to upper medial border of scapula; (4) anterior aspects of the C5, C7 intertransverse spaces; (5) second rib space about 3 cm lateral to the sternal border; (6) muscle attachments to lateral epicondyle—about 2 cm below bony prominence; (7) upper outer quadrant of gluteal muscles; (8) muscle attachments just posterior to greater trochanter; and (9) medial fat pad of knee proximal to joint line. A total of 11 or more tender points in conjunction with a history of widespread pain is characteristic of the fibromyalgia syndrome.

Fibromyalgia occurs much more commonly in women than in men, increasing progressively from ages 18 to 70 years, with a 23% prevalence in the seventh decade,[3] contrary to the widespread belief that fibromyalgia is predominantly a disorder of young and middle-age women; however, the peak age of all patients is 30 to 50 years.[15]

PATHOPHYSIOLOGY

The major pathologic symptom is the diffuse pain and tender points on the skin. Some of the tender points are exquisitely tender on palpation and are localized to common sites (FIG. 6-15), and the tender points or areas are paired on both sides of the body. The soreness is thought to arise from muscle fibers in the affected muscle mass. The number of tender points varies from 9 to 18 or more; however, the American College of Rheumatology Criteria Committee recommended in 1990 that the nine symmetric tender points shown in FIG. 6-15 be present for the diagnosis of fibromyalgia.[3]

The source of the pain appears to arise from nociceptors in the muscle, leading to unremitting pain. Some characteristic situations causing the painful muscles include increased pain after exertion, although not severe for approximately 24 hours; decreased pain after epidural blocks; or injections in "trigger points," with less regional pain after injections, and focal areas of increased electromyographic (EMG) activity on needling of tender point areas.[3] Biopsy specimens of trigger points have shown some quantitative changes compared with nonaffected persons but no qualitative changes. Bennett[3] has hypothesized that, because of the delayed onset of pain after unaccustomed exertion, the focal "microlesions" may result from postexertional muscle microtrauma. Increased sarcolemmal levels of calcium are the postulated mechanism of postexertional muscle microtrauma.[3] Patients with the diagnosis of fibromyalgia have other complaints, along with the multiple tender points, including sleep disturbances, specifically awakening often and being a "light sleeper." Sleep apnea is particularly common in male fibromyalgia patients.[3] Fatigue is another common complaint, with more than a majority of women having pain and profound fatigue for more than 90% of their time awake.[33] Headaches, restless leg syndrome, excess response to cold, and periods of depression are common. Memory loss is also common in fibromyalgia.

DIAGNOSTIC STUDIES AND FINDINGS

History: Complaints of multiple tender points in symmetric sites over body; sleep disturbances; extreme fatigue when awake; headaches; restless legs at night; depression; memory loss; numbness and tingling in the extremities present in more than 75% of patients.[15]

Physical examination: Palpation gives evidence of multiple tender points (see FIG. 6-15), most commonly in the neck, shoulders, occipital area of head, and others as shown; muscles may appear slightly swollen; the patient may appear tired, anxious, and/or depressed; neurologic examination is usually normal

Serologic examination (to rule out other rheumatic diseases, which at times coexist with fibromyalgia): Rheumatoid factor negative; erythrocyte sedimentation rate normal (0-20 mm/h in men and 0-25 mm/h in women); thyroid hormone within normal limits

Sleep laboratory studies: May indicate sleep apnea more commonly in male patients; rapid eye movement (REM) sleep reduced by about 50%[3,15] (may appear to sleep all night yet wake up feeling exhausted)

MULTIDISCIPLINARY PLAN

Surgery

No specific procedure performed

Medications

NSAIDs
- Ibuprofen (Motrin), 400 mg PO q4h
- See table on p. 337 for additional NSAIDS

Narcotic analgesics (used infrequently): Oxycodone (Percodan), 30-60 mg PO q4-6h (for short-term treatment of headaches)

Nonsteroidal Antiinflammatory Agents

Generic Name	Trade Name	Adult Dosage Ranges
Acetylsalicylic acid	Aspirin	600-1000 mg 3-4 times daily
Ibuprofen	Motrin, Advil, Nuprin	300-400 mg 3-4 times daily
Naproxen	Naprosyn	250-375 mg bid
Tolmentin	Tolectin	200-400 mg 3-4 times daily
Sulindac	Clinoril	150-200 mg bid
Piroxicam	Feldene	20 mg daily
Diclofenac	Voltaren	25-75 mg bid
Oxaprozin	Daypro	600-1200 mg daily
Choline magnesium trisalicylate	Trilisate	500-100 mg tid or 1500 mg bid
Indomethacin	Indocin	25-50 mg 3-4 times daily
Celecoxib	Celebrex	100 mg bid
Rofecoxib	Vioxx	12.5 mg daily
Ketorolac	Toradol	15-30 mg IM or IV q4h
Fenoprofen	Nalfon	1200-3200 mg daily
Acetaminophen	Tylenol (and others)	600-1000 mg 3-4 times daily
Ketoprofen	Orudis	25-75 mg 3-4 times daily
Mefenamic acid	Ponstel	250 mg 4 times daily
Meclofenamate	Meclomen	50-100 mg 3-4 times daily

Antidepessant agents (may be used to enhance sleep patterns if patient not depressed)
- Amtriptyline (Elavil), 25-50 mg at bedtime
- Cyclobenzaprine, 20-40 mg in divided doses
- Fluoxetine (Prozac), 10-20 mg, initial dose daily

Antiparkinsonism agents (for restless legs[3])
- Carbidopa (Sinemet), 10-100 mg at suppertime
- Clonazepam (Klonopin), 0.5-1 mg at bedtime

General Management

Massage back, neck, or shoulders as desired
Use heat via ultrasound for tender points
Group therapy to assist with problem solving
Ongoing education about fibromyalgia
Passive stretching exercises by physical therapist
Active exercises, including stretching, gentle strengthening, and aerobic conditioning guided by physical therapist; regular aerobic exercises a minimum of 30 minutes, three times weekly
Aqua therapy program
Continuous positive airway pressure (CPAP) machine used for sleep apnea during naps or nighttime sleep, pressure prescribed by physician

NURSING CARE

Nursing Assessment

Muscle processes: Tender points: sites (see Fig. 6-15); edema; heat; joint ROM; color; pain: degree, duration

Systemic responses: Fatigue: when, severity; sleep disturbances; "restless legs" syndrome; headache: type, frequency; depression; anxiety

Psychosocial concerns Severe fatigue during awake hours; effects on self, family, employment; lack of correct diagnosis for long period of time; associated rheumatic disease

Potential Complications

Hypoxia (from sleep apnea) without use of CPAP therapy; Severe depression

Patient Problems/Nursing Diagnoses & Interventions

NIC Activity and Exercise Management

Activity intolerance related to profound fatigue

- Determine status of or degree of fatigue, when occurs, and such *to learn extent of condition.*
- Clarify activities that cause fatigue *to gauge pattern.*
- Discuss effects of rest on fatigue: Help? Make worse?
- Consult with occupational therapist for home, family situation, or employment evaluation as contributing to fatigue.
- Consult with physical therapist for program of exercises according to physician's prescription; should include stretching, strengthening, and conditioning exercises for greatest benefits.
- Massage neck, shoulders, and back *to ease fatigued or tender areas.*
- Discuss benefits of aqua therapy to lessen effects of gravity on tissues *to enhance anticipation of beneficial effects:* generally must do aerobic exercises a minimum of 30 minutes, 3 times weekly to maintain effects

NIC Physical Comfort Promotion

Acute or chronic pain related to tender or trigger points over body

- Monitor areas indicated as tender or trigger points by patient: locate sites, estimate extent of pain/tenderness on scale of 0 to 10 (or other suitable scale) *to determine condition.*
- Apply heat by hot compresses to tender points *to ease soreness.*
- Clarify effects of heat as beneficial or unsatisfactory with patient *to evaluate effects of treatment.*
- Discuss use of antiinflammatory medications and mutually decide to hold or administer prescribed medications *to enhance patient's decision-making process.*
- If medication administered, evaluate its effects to relieve soreness of muscles *to determine if changes needed.*
- Clarify concerns or appearance of depressed persons, feelings, or statements of sadness regarding condition *to have current information pertinent to care.*
- Clarify patient's statements of feeling anxious or concerned over uncertainty of prognosis.
- Consult with mental health practitioner for techniques to assist patient with feelings *to provide support.*
- Encourage diversionary activities such as walking, reading, imagery, and relaxation techniques *to lessen attention to body signals,* if feasible.
- Use consultant's suggestions to help patient become more self-sufficient and to assume responsibility for

ongoing management of symptoms *to enhance overall outcomes.*

NIC SELF-CARE FACILITATION

Disturbed sleep pattern related to sleep apnea and restless legs syndrome

- Monitor sleep patterns if present when asleep *to note signs of sleep apnea:* periods of loud snoring and apnea up to 25 to 30 seconds, followed by gasping, gurgling, or thrashing about to catch breath; repeated with each respiratory cycle.
- Observe leg movements to note restless legs: one or both legs move frequently; movements are jerky, jumpy, and uncoordinated; legs are seldom quiet or still.
- Note if patient wakes frequently and quickly, rouses with minor noise in room, or stays awake for indefinite periods during sleep time.
- Teach good sleep hygiene techniques: Get up if waken and have difficulty returning to sleep; divert attention from daily worries or stresses; drink some warm milk; maintain cool bedroom temperatures and use loose coverings; read a book, if desirable; listen to audiotapes with or without soft music.
- If apnea undiagnosed, discuss data with physician for diagnostic study in sleep laboratory, if available.
- Have patient ready for sleep laboratory study at appointed time, if it is to be done from current setting.
- If prescribed, administer medication (see above) for restless legs; note effects *to learn if therapeutic.*
- Have CPAP machine, if used, checked by respiratory therapist for proper pressure setting, filter condition, and water level in machine *for safety of care.*
- Record sleep patterns when CPAP machine used during sleep cycles: patient sleeping longer periods; no snoring, gasping, or apnea noted; legs quieter; movements somewhat more coordinated; no hypoxia noted if oximeter in use (oxygen levels between 95% and 100%).

PATIENT EDUCATION/CONTINUUM OF CARE PLAN

1. Reiterate physician's explanations about diagnosis of fibromyalgia.
2. Discuss treatment plan as beneficial over the future.
3. Stress continued consultation with sleep management physicians for follow-up care, as needed, for sleep apnea.
4. Stress need to continue prescribed exercise regimen for maintaining muscle functions and strength.
5. Reiterate benefits of aqua therapy.
6. Discuss use of medications; list them, along with dosages and side effects when used for pain, depression, anxiety, or mood treatment.
7. Assure patient/family of continued contact after discharge.

EVALUATION/PATIENT OUTCOMES

Activity and Exercise Management: Patient continues to have fatigue over long periods, but attempts to do own ADLs, home activities, and employment activities when able. Patient uses techniques and utensils to ease work and home energy expenditure. Patient seeks guidance to help manage exercises and aqua therapy programs for greatest benefits. Patient is positive participant in exercise regimen.

Physical Comfort Promotion: Patient uses antiinflammatory medications sparingly and infrequently; pain is still present but diverts self to lessen focus. Patient has a more positive attitude toward future. Depression is lessened and sleep is improved with prescribed medication and no change needed.

Self-Care Facilitation: Patient uses CPAP machine continuously during naps or nighttime sleep; no hypoxia is noticed, no snoring, and legs less restless with prescribed medication.

BURSITIS

Bursitis is the inflammation of a bursa.

A bursa is an enclosed fluid-filled sac situated between muscles or tendons and bony prominences. When a bursa becomes inflamed, the inflammation may spread to contiguous structures or may be confined to the bursal fluid and sac.

One or more bursae can become inflamed, but the most common sites are the subdeltoid and subacromial bursae of the shoulder (see FIG. 6-13, *A,* p. 329), the olecranon (elbow) bursa, the greater trochanteric bursa lateral to the hip, the anserine bursa in the medial aspect of the upper tibia, and the Achilles bursa of the heel. One common but often overlooked site of bursitis is the obturator internus bursa, which inserts into the greater trochanter.

Bursitis is more common in athletes and persons who do repetitive motions. It can cause significant morbidity and may also be associated with low back pain.

PATHOPHYSIOLOGY

Bursitis usually results from constant friction between the skin and the musculoskeletal tissues around the affected joint. Bursitis from friction would be sterile or aseptic without pathogenic organisms. Rarely, bursitis results from a foreign body or microorganism invasion. The area around the bursa becomes exquisitely tender. Motion is either partially or greatly limited by the swollen, enlarged sac, which causes pressure and pain when the tissues are moved. The area may be reddened, hot, and edematous with only point tenderness (the patient can point to the spot or area of greatest tenderness) or with soreness radiating to the tendons at the site. Tendinitis may also occur, further limiting motion and prolonging recovery. Calcium may be deposited in the bursal sacs in long-standing or recurring bursitis.

DIAGNOSTIC STUDIES AND FINDINGS

History: Repetitive motions for throwing; running or bicycling long distances; overuse; low back pain

Physical examination: Localized inflammation in bursal area; point tenderness; limitation of motion of one or more bursae and involved joints; movements elicit complaints of pain; may be pain-free at rest

Roentgenograms: May or may not show calcified deposits

Multidisciplinary Plan

Surgery

Open removal of the calcified deposits
Aspiration of fluid within the sac (infrequently) for persistent edema and pressure
Removal of the bursal sac (rarely needed)

Medications

Analgesic-antipyretic agents: Salicylates (aspirin), 500-1000 mg q4h
NSAIDs
- Ibuprofen, 400-600 mg qid or tid
- Celecoxib (Celebrex), 100 mg bid or rofecoxib (Vioxx), 12.5 mg qd
- See table on p. 337 for additional NSAIDs

Antibiotic agents: If the bursa is infected, antibiotics specific for the offending organism after culture
Others: Injections of steroid into the sac to relieve the inflammation; dosage is individualized

General Management

Avoidance of activities (e.g., bicycling, walking long distances, or kneeling) that cause pressure
Avoidance of constant friction movements (e.g., throwing or hitting a ball) that may cause an inflammatory reaction
Avoidance of repetitive motions that affect bursa and joint
Moist heat applications every 4 hours to inflamed area
ROM exercises to help regain or maintain motion
Wrapping with elastic bandages, if bursa is accessible, to reduce edema

NURSING CARE

Nursing Assessment

Inflammatory process: Area around joint; degree of inflammation; heat; redness; swelling; tenderness and pain with use, aching around joint; limitation of movement: initiation, duration; point tenderness; onset of pain, increased with which specific activities; treatments, if any, used to date
Systemic response: Similar responses in one or more joints or bursae; fever and malaise if pathogen is involved
Psychosocial concerns: Limitation of use of muscles and joints, possibly curtailing income, livelihood, or other activities

Potential Complications

Prolonged painful episodes in affected tissues; potential for bursal infection; limited use of affected muscles/joint tissues; calcification of affected bursa

Patient Problems/Nursing Diagnoses & Interventions

NIC Immobility Management

Impaired physical mobility (limitation of motion) related to inflammation of bursa
- Observe amount of edema, pain, and redness related to limiting or increasing motion *to note progression or regression*
- Teach to apply warm compresses every 4 hours as prescribed *to aid resolution or easing of inflammation.*
- Encourage stretching exercises to maintain ROM as prescribed *to maintain functions.*
- Caution against continuing activities that may cause recurrence *to lessen chance of chronicity.*
- Remove bandages, observe site, and rewrap bandages (if used) *to prevent loosening or tightening of bandages.*

NIC Physical Comfort Promotion

Acute pain related to inflammation of bursa
- Listen to complaint of pain; have patient describe amount of pain on scale of 1 to 10, or other suitable scale *to note extent and severity.*
- Gently palpate area of pain *to determine exact site.*
- Handle inflamed tissues gently when moving joint *to prevent additional trauma.*
- Administer medications as prescribed *to relieve pain and inflammation.*
- Note continuation or relief of pain, tenderness, or inflammation *to note efficacy of medications.*
- Observe for side effects of medications *to note presence or need for other medications.*
- Discourage activities that increase pain or discomfort until inflammation has subsided *to lessen chance of recurrence.*

Patient Education/Continuum of Care Plan

1. Discuss ROM exercises to lessen possibility of bursal inflammation.
2. Give the patient a written list of names, dosages, and side effects of medications and instruct the patient to report to physician as needed.
3. Alert the patient to the possibility that pain may increase temporarily after injection of steroid (1 to 24 hours) to be followed by noticeable pain relief and increasing ROM.
4. Instruct patient that applying ice or Cryopac will lessen pain after injection.
5. Caution the patient to avoid activities that could cause exacerbation until inflammation is resolved (1 to 2 weeks in some instances).

Evaluation/Patient Outcomes

Immobility Management: Patient regains ROM of affected joint. Patient can engage in usual activities with affected joint and contiguous tissues.

Physical Comfort Promotion: Patient no longer needs medication to relieve pain. Patient feels no pain with ROM actions or when using joint for usual activities. Patient is avoiding use of affected joint and tissues for prolonged distances or activities.

Epicondylitis and Tendinitis (Tenosynovitis)

Epicondylitis is an inflammation of the tendons of the medical or lateral epicondyles of the radius, ulna, or other bones. Tendinitis (tenosynovitis) is an inflammation of the tendons and their sheaths.

Epicondylitis and tendinitis may occur together and, with some variations, the local sites of inflammation are next to one another, which makes proper diagnosis more challenging.

Lateral epicondylitis, commonly called tennis elbow, is caused by repetitive twisting and swinging movements of the elbow that accompany, among other activities, swinging a tennis racket or using a hammer or other tools. Inflammation affects the tendons that originate in the medial or lateral epicondyles of the radius or ulna. The tendons and their sheaths may both become inflamed (tendinitis and tenosynovitis, respectively). Medial epicondylitis is called golfer's elbow and is primarily related to repetitive swings of the elbow, such as those made by the golfer, although other activities may cause medial epicondylitis.

Tenosynovitis affects joints other than the elbow, with the shoulder and knee joints frequently affected in baseball pitchers, football players, soccer players, and other athletes. Tenosynovitis also frequently affects tendons of the fingers of one or both hands and often the Achilles tendon.

Tenosynovitis is a common condition. It may be caused by infection, diabetes, or gout and can accompany pregnancy, especially during the third trimester. It may be unilateral or bilateral.

Some tendon injuries result from overuse injuries causing multiple microtrauma, disrupting the internal structure of the tendon and degeneration of the cells and matrix, which fail to mature into normal tendon, resulting in tendinosis, rather than tendinitis. Tendinosis is a degenerative rather than inflammatory process.[26]

PATHOPHYSIOLOGY

Repetitive trauma damages and tears the fibers of the common extensor tendon of the involved joint. Extravasation of tissue fluids sets up inflammatory reactions, and healing produces scar tissue and adhesions that limit the ROM of the joint. The joint can then become inflamed by repetitive trauma to the scarred, inelastic fibers. The inflammation can spread to the tendon sheath, with fibrosis binding the sheath to the tendon and thus further limiting joint movements. Classic symptoms of epicondylitis include tenderness (frequently point tenderness), pain, and edema. Pronation or supination of the hand when the elbow is in 45 degrees of flexion causes severe medial and epicondylar pain if the inflamed joint is the elbow. In the hand, pain is increased on passive extension of the affected digit or digits.

Tendinitis is characterized by the presence of an increased number of lymphocytes or neutrophils (sign of inflammation, whereas tendinosis is characterized by the presence of dense populations of fibroblasts, vascular hyperplasia, and disorganized collagen, signs of degenerative processes.[26] It is not clear why tendinosis is painful, given the absence of acute inflammatory cells, nor is it known why the collagen fails to mature.[26]

Tendons involved in locomotion (such as the Achilles tendon) and ballistic performance (such as the rotator cuff tendons) are most likely to suffer overuse injuries. Other tendons likely to be injured because of their vulnerable anatomic positions are the patellar tendon at the knee and the adductor tendons of the hip. Tennis elbow, or lateral epicondylitis, is a prime example of an overuse injury. It more correctly should be termed a tendinosis because it is a degenerative rather than an inflammatory condition.[26] Golfer's elbow, or *medial* epicondylitis, is also associated with overuse. Its symptoms are pain and tenderness poorly localized to the medical epicondyle of the humerus, which becomes worse with resisted wrist flexion.

DIAGNOSTIC STUDIES AND FINDINGS

History: Flexion, rotation, and repetitive ROM actions from occupational or sports activities resulting in localized joint pain, tenderness, and limitation of motion in involved joint, such as elbow, shoulder, knee, or heel

Physical examination: Point tenderness and increased pain with flexion or supination and pronation of hand, arm, or foot; edema and tenderness radiating along the affected tendon and its sheath; weak grasp or loss of strength of affected joint; decreased ROM of affected joint

MULTIDISCIPLINARY PLAN

Surgery

Removal of calcium deposits from the inflammatory processes occasionally required

Removal of a degenerated (scarred and bound-down) tendon sheath for chronic, persistent synovitis or a shoulder, elbow, or heel because of calcium deposits from repeated trauma

Incision of infected tissues, if indicated by severity of condition and release of scar tissue (repair bypasses the area of tendinosis)

Medications

Corticosteroids
- Oral in individualized doses (rarely used)
- Injected into the inflamed area to relieve pain if not sufficiently relieved by analgesic medications, may need to be repeated at intervals for complete pain relief; dosage and type individualized

Analgesic-antipyretic/antiinflammatory agents
- Ibuprofen, 400-800 mg tid or bid
- Salicylates (aspirin), 600 mg q4h for mild conditions
- Celicoxib (Celebrex), 100 mg bid or rofecoxib (Vioxx), 12.5 mg daily
- See table on p. 337 for additional NSAIDs

General Management

Cold or moist head applications to area every 4 hours

Rest to the part or parts for varying periods of time

Occasionally, splint or other orthosis applied to the forearm and elbow, sling for shoulder; knee immobilizer (rarely used); crutches for Achilles tendinitis (if danger of rupture of tendon)

ROM exercises per physical therapist plus low impact, low velocity exercises to increase strength, flexibility, and endurance through resistance exercises and stretching protocols

NURSING CARE

Nursing Assessment

Inflammatory process: Localized or point tenderness (can point to site of pain) in shoulder, elbow, wrist, hand, knee, or heel, and pain radiating to arm, forearm, leg, or heel and foot; assess amount, degree, duration, and type of pain (using pain scale appropriate to patient), activities or treatments that increase or decrease pain; tenderness with movement or use; edema in shoulder, elbow, knee, or heel; edema in one or more fingers, local area of knee, or heel; presence and use of sling, elastic wrap, or crutches

ROM: Pain increased with supination and pronation of hand or flexion and extension of fingers or foot; pain with throwing motions of shoulder; pain with lateral movements of knee; pain with walking or pressure on heel

Systemic response: Elevated temperature if infection present (rare).

Psychosocial concerns: Concern for ability to earn a living if in an occupation requiring full elbow, hand, shoulder, knee, or foot ROM or other joint movements

Potential Complications

Prolonged painful episodes of affected tissues; marked limitation or use of affected tissues; scarring of involved tissues; loss of income from professional activities; tear or avulsion of inflamed tendon(s); calcification of affected tendon(s)

Patient Problems/Nursing Diagnoses & Interventions

NIC Immobility Management

Impaired physical mobility related to limitation of joint functions and pain

- Observe amount of edema, pain, and redness related to limiting or increasing motion *to note progression of inflammation;* note complaint of numbness, if indicated (occurs with some frequency).
- Caution against continuing activities that may cause recurrence until relief of symptoms has occurred.
- Apply prescribed cold or warm compresses every 4 hours as ordered *to relieve inflammation* (whirlpool may be used, alternating with cryotherapy or ice).
- Encourage exercises *to maintain ROM as prescribed;* exercise under guidance of physical therapist.

NIC Physical Comfort Promotion

Acute pain related to inflammation of tendons and their sheaths

- Handle inflamed tissues gently *to avoid additional pain.*
- Observe activities that increase or decrease pain episodes *to determine extent of inflammation* or injury.
- Administer medications as prescribed *to relieve pain.*
- Note continuation or relief of pain, tenderness, or inflammation *to assess effect of medications.*
- Observe for side effects of medications *to note problem that may need treatment.*
- Apply splint, sling, or joint immobilizer as ordered, if used.
- Administer prescribed antibiotic *to resolve infection if present.*

NIC Coping Assistance

Ineffective role performance related to presence and severity of condition

- Encourage patient to comply with treatment regimen and to continue medical care to note recovery.
- Encourage expression of concerns; seek guidance to resolve concerns about employment and recurrence of condition.
- Discuss preventive techniques, therapies, or other strategies to ease concerns.
- Refer to community agencies for assistance with financial or other concerns.

Patient Education/Continuum of Care Plan

1. Explain inflammatory processes and effects of repetitive trauma to lessen painful episodes and inflammation.
2. Provide written list of medications, dosages, and side effects of medications; clarify to ensure understanding.
3. Alert the patient to the possibility that pain may increase temporarily after injection of steroid (1 to 24 hours), to be followed by noticeable pain relief and increasing ROM.
4. Caution to avoid activities that could cause exacerbation until inflammation is resolved (1 to 2 weeks).
5. Discuss the effects of application of heat or cold with patient and family.

Evaluation/Patient Outcomes

Immobility Management: Patient regains joint mobility without limitation. Patient can put joint through normal ROM without limitation, hesitation, or loss of strength.

Physical Comfort Promotion: Patient experiences relief of pain. Patient has no pain on usual ROM activities and has stopped use of oral steroid and analgesics.

Coping Assistance: Patient returns to employment as before. No restrictions necessary on employment activities. Patient expresses awareness of possible causes of recurrence of conditions.

Rheumatoid Arthritis

Rheumatoid arthritis (RA) is a chronic systemic autoimmune disease characterized by inflammation of the connective tissues throughout the body, but primarily in the joints.

RA affects 7 million persons in the United States, occurring 4.1 to 2:1 in females over males. It affects about 1% to 2% of the population worldwide and affects about 5% of the population age 70 years and older.

This severely disabling chronic disease is one of the major rheumatic diseases. Although the disease is a systemic disorder, this discussion concerns the local effects on the tissues in and around the joints. The disease appears to be decreasing in its incidence and severity, although 65% to 70% of patients have severe, progressive disease processes.[20]

Table 6-5 The Stages of RA

Stage	Pathologic Process	Symptoms	Physical Signs	Radiographic Changes
1	Presentation of antigen to T cells	Probably none	—	—
2	T cell and B cell activation	Malaise, mild joint stiffness and swelling	Swelling of small joints of hands or wrists, or pain in hands, wrists, knees, and feet	None
3	Accumulation of neutrophils in synovial fluid; synovial cell proliferation without polarization or invasion of cartilage	Joint pain and swelling, morning stiffness, malaise, and weakness	Warm, swollen joints, excess synovial fluid, soft tissue proliferation within joints, pain and limitation of motion, rheumatoid nodules	Magnetic resonance imaging (MRI) reveals proliferative pannus; radiographic evidence of periarticular osteopenia
4	Polarization of synovitis—invasive pannus; activation of chondrocytes; initiation of enzyme (proteinase) degradation of cartilage	Same as stage 3	Same as stage 3, but more pronounced swelling	Early erosions and narrowing of joint spaces
5	Erosion of subchondral bone; invasion of cartilage by pannus; stretched ligaments around joints	Same as stage 3, plus loss of function and early deformity (e.g., ulnar deviation at metacarpophalangeal [MCP] joints)	Same as stage 3, plus instability of joints, flexion contractions, decreased ROM, extraarticular complications	Progression of stages 3 and 4; subluxation

Modified from Pope.[42]

RA is an autoimmune phenomenon, along with evidence of a genetic predisposition, especially related to HLA-DR4, HLA-DR, HLA-DP, and HLA-DQ areas of the major histocompatibility complex,[12] although recent authors[50] believe that the HLA genes, immune response genes, immunoglobulin genes, and T cell receptor (TCR) genes may have an impact later in the chain of pathologic events. Synovial tissue injury, which may result from an infection, is considered characteristic of stage 1 of RA (Table 6-5). Individuals with RA do not follow just one pattern of response to the tissue infection, but each person with RA has his or her own pattern, which complicates the overall symptomatology and treatment regimens, as shown later.[50]

Most patients develop RA between ages 25 and 55 years, but the mean age at onset appears to be increasing, with a simultaneous deadline in the age-specific incidence in younger individuals.[13] Younger person's disease is called juvenile RA or Stills disease, with symptoms developing between ages 8 and 15 years. RA has increased probability of going into remission during pregnancy with almost equal high probability of postpartal relapse.[2]

PATHOPHYSIOLOGY

The disease begins in the synovial membrane within the joint, usually in one of the smaller joints of the wrist, fingers, or hand, and bilateral symmetric joint involvement is characteristic of RA. The synovial membrane becomes inflamed from the autoimmune antigen-antibody effects, and the membrane becomes swollen, irritated, and painful. There is an abundance of activated T cells in joints affected by RA, whereas virtually no T cells are present in normal joints. These T cells are antigen specific, and T cells are the crucial regulators in the immune system and determine when, where, or whether specific immune responses occur. There are also abundant macrophages and monocytes present in affected joints, which produce cytokines that affect immune responses and inflammatory reactions. These cytokines include interleukins 1 through 8, tissue necrosis factor, transforming growth factor alpha and beta, granulocyte-macrophage colony-stimulating factors, and platelet-derived growth factors alpha and beta.[12] Some of these cytokines cause cartilage destruction and amplify the inflammatory focus, causing overgrowth of the synovial membrane and leading to decreased blood flow to the synovium, with less oxygen and nutrients to the synovial cells. With less blood supply, yet increased metabolic needs because of synovial cell hypertrophy and hyperplasia, hypoxia and metabolic acidosis occur, both being detrimental to the inflamed cells and synovial membrane. Acidosis causes release of hydrolytic enzymes from synovial cells, initiating erosion of the cartilage in the joint and inflaming the surrounding ligaments and tendons.[64] Thus RA affects all the soft tissues in and around the diseased joint(s). Eventually, with continued inflammation, the synovial tissues develop fibrosis and overgrowth of granulation tissue called pannus, extending from the synovium over the joint cartilage, destroying the cartilage cells, and leading to immobilization of the affected joint or joints. Ligaments and tendons become scarred and shortened, contributing to joint deformities, subluxations (partial dislocations), and contractures. Loss of cartilage leads to pain and grating of bones with weight bearing and movements. Bone spurs, bone cysts, erosions, fissures, and osteophytes (outgrowths of bone) develop, further limiting joint mobility and use. The entire joint(s) and the joint structures remain inflamed, edematous, and painful. Additionally, collections of fibroblasts in collagen tissues near joints enlarge into rheumatoid modules, a classic feature of RA.

Characteristically, RA affects smaller joints symmetrically before involving the larger weight-bearing joints. Bouchards nodes are the classic enlargements of the proximal phalangeal and metacarpophalangeal (MCP) joints. The foot and ankle areas ultimately become involved in more than 95% of patients with RA.[47a]

Eventually the local disease in the joints involves major organ systems in the remainder of the body, including the heart, kidneys, lungs, skin, eyes, and hematologic tissues.

Diagnostic Studies and Findings

History: Monoarticular or polyarticular inflammation, with a slow, insidious onset (about 8% to 15% have an acute onset[20])

Physical examination: Criteria for the diagnosis of RA have been established by the American Rheumatism Association (ARA); presence of four or more of the following is needed for the diagnosis[20]: morning stiffness on arising; pain and tenderness in at least one joint; swelling in at least one and possibly two joints; symmetric joint swelling bilaterally; fatigue, malaise, and weight loss; paresthesias of hands or feet; Raynaud phenomenon of fingers and toes; development of subcutaneous nodules; involvement of major organs such as heart and kidney; pericarditis; valvular lesions; vasculitis; pneumonitis; fibrosis; tenosynovitis; ankylosis of joints; joint contractures; presence of Bouchard nodes, Felty syndrome (splenomegaly and leukopenia); deformities of joints; ulnar drift of wrists; sicca syndrome and scleritis of eyes

Serologic examination: Rheumatoid factor (autoantibody directed against antigenic determinants on a fragment of immunoglobulin G [IgG] generally associated with RA): Positive in 70% or higher in patients with RA[58]

- Erythrocyte sedimentation rate (ESR): Elevated (moderate to severe elevation [to 15 mm/h in males and 25 mm/h in females]); normal 0-9 mm/h in males and 0-20 mm/h in females
- C-reactive protein: Present during acute phases
- Red cell count: Anemia, primarily hypochromic (normocytic is common)
- White cell count: Elevated over all cell types
- Serum complement: Decreased
- Antinuclear antibody: May be positive
- Creatinine levels may be elevated related to disease activity or side effects of some medications used as treatments (cyclosporine)

Synovial fluid aspiration and analysis: may reveal immune complexes and IgG rheumatoid factors; elevated white cell counts

Synovial membrane biopsy: Positive for pannus formation and inflammatory changes

Roentgenograms: Rarefaction of bones, plus erosions of involved bone, as disease progresses; subluxation (partial dislocation) of bones from joints; MRI shows proliferative pannus; and may show osteopenia around the affected joints; narrowing of joint spaces; erosions of subchondral bone

NOTE: Laboratory studies are not "diagnostic" of RA but are used in conjunction with careful evaluation of the history, physical findings, laboratory tests, and radiographic changes.

Multidisciplinary Plan

Surgery

Synovectomy of inflamed synovial membranes to relieve pain and maintain muscle and joint balance

Repair of ruptured or fibrotic tendon sheaths to prevent deformity and subluxations

Total joint replacement to increase mobility

Arthrodesis (fusion of a joint): May be done to decrease deformity and joint instability; spinal fusion may be required to treat subluxation

Osteotomy to change weight-bearing surfaces and relieve pain

Arthroplasty to correct deformities

Medications

Analgesic/antipyretic agents: Aspirin, divided doses up to 6 g/day

NSAIDs (one or more may be prescribed during course of patient's RA)

- Ibuprofen (Motrin), 1200-3200 mg/day
- Fenoprofen (Nalfon), 1200-3200 mg/day
- Tolmentin (Tolectin), initially 400 mg tid to reach optimum daily dose of 600-1800 mg/day
- Naproxen (Naprosyn), 750-1500 mg/day
- Diclofenac (Voltaren), 75-150 mg/day
- Piroxicam (Feldene), 20 mg/day
- Celecoxib (Celebrex), 100 mg bid
- Rofecoxib (Vioxx), 12.5 mg qd or bid

See table on p. 337 for additional NSAIDs.

Antirheumatic agents

- Gold thiomaleate (Myochrysine), 20-50 mg/wk IM, or auranofin (Ridaura), 3-6 mg/day PO, to decrease inflammation
- Penicillamine (Cuprimine, Depen), 125-250 mg/day increased to 500-750 mg/day; may be used as a substitute for patients sensitive to gold
- Sulfasalazine, 500 mg/day initially; may be increased weekly

Immunosuppressive agents

- Azathioprine (Imuran), 305 mg/kg/day initially, then 1-2 mg/kg/day maintenance dose
- Cyclosporine, 2-3 mg/kg/day

Antimalarial agents: Hydroxychloroquine, 400 mg/d PO

Antineoplastic agents

- Methotrexate (Rheumatrex), 7.5 mg PO or IM weekly; may increase 2.5 mg/wk
- Cyclophosphamide; dosage is individualized; may start at 50 mg/day

Corticosteroids

- Primarily prednisone (Deltasone, others) or prednisolone (Delta-Cortef, others) in titrated doses of 2-10 mg/day (usually 7.5 mg/day) used before or after other medications for antiinflammatory effects
- Hydrocortisone (Cortef, other), 100 mg injected into the joint to reduce inflammation

General Management

Immersion in paraffin "glove" (rarely used currently)

Immersion in whirlpool or spa; aqua therapy for joint exercises

MULTIPLE TREATMENTS* IN MANAGEMENT OF RHEUMATOID ARTHRITIS

Education for patient and family
Heat/cold applications
Therapeutic exercises
Rest
Salicylates at therapeutic doses
Occupational and physical therapies
Orthotic devices
Gold salts, antimalarial drugs, D-penicillamine
NSAIDs and analgesic drugs
Glucocorticoids in low or high doses
Intraarticular glucocorticoids
Reconstructive surgery
Immunosuppressive drugs, such as azathioprine
Cytotoxic drugs, such as methotrexate

*Treatments generally include each of the above modalities during the course of the disease process.

Application of splints to inflamed joints to maintain proper position (used during rest periods mainly)
Moist, warm applications to joints
Applications of cold alternating with heat
ROM exercises to maintain motion
Prescribed rest periods in morning and afternoon
Well-balanced diet; avoidance of obesity because of increased joint stress
Instruction and practice in home maintenance technique
Instructions about the disease to ease patient's fears and increase compliance with treatment regimen
Ocular examination every 6 months if taking hydroxychloroquine
See box above

POTENTIAL COMPLICATIONS

Avascular necrosis of bones in one or more joints because of intraarticular steroids or high doses of oral steroids; cerebral vascular accident (CVA); myocardial infarction; vasculitis; pleuritis and/or pulmonary nodules, plus pneumoconiosis (Caplan syndrome); pericarditis plus valvular deformities; splenomegaly; renal infarctions

NURSING CARE

NURSING ASSESSMENT

Local inflammatory processes in or around joint: Symmetric joint involvement bilaterally, edema, boggy joint, skin of joints may have bluish hue; hyperkeratosis; ulceration; pain and tenderness in and around joint, amount, severity; heat in and around joint; redness; limitation of motion, stiffness lasting 1 hour or longer after arising; deformity, numbness of fingers or toes, atrophy of surrounding muscles; flexion contractures; ulnar drift, boutonniere and swan-neck deformities of one or more joints; rheumatoid nodules

Systemic processes: Malaise, degree of fatigue, muscle weakness; pale color of skin, anemia; fever; multiple joint involvement; subcutaneous rheumatoid nodules (may be multiple throughout body); weight loss, anorexia, nausea, food likes or dislikes; color of fingers or toes (redness, whiteness, blueness), changes at times; pulmonary, cardiac, and renal changes (see Potential Complications at left)

Psychosocial concerns: Lack of thorough understanding of RA; concern about disease; concerns with self-concept, body image disturbances, loss of mobility because of chronicity, deformity; concern about ability to care for and maintain home/employment; multiple treatments without cure in near future; interference with roles or role performance; sleep disruption; severity of disease may shorten life expectancy

Economic concerns: Major costs for treatments over extended periods; possible loss of employment because of nature of disease and joint involvement; lack of insurance coverage

BIOLOGIC AGENTS IN THE TREATMENT OF RHEUMATOID ARTHRITIS

Antibodies
  Immunoglobulin preparations
  Monoclonal antibodies (various preparations)
Cytokines and cytokine inhibitors
  Interleukin-1 and its inhibitors
  Interleukin-2 and its inhibitors
  Interferon gamma
Peptides such as V_β-17
Collagen II
Immunotoxins
Photopheresis
T cell vaccination

Data from Strand and Keystone.[55]

PATIENT PROBLEMS/NURSING DIAGNOSES & INTERVENTIONS

NIC COPING ASSISTANCE

Ineffective coping related to depression of chronic illness of RA

Anxiety related to recently identified diagnosis without a current cure

Disturbed body image and altered role performance related to deformities and chronic disease

- Observe for signs of mild, moderate, or severe depression; *mild:* sadness; dejected appearance; needs extra effort to concentrate or do usual activities; *moderate:* inability to experience joy; feelings of powerlessness; lack of energy; pessimistic; sleep disturbances; slowed speech and thought processes; *severe:* despair, hopelessness, emptiness; limited ability to respond to teaching, stimuli, or do life-sustaining activities; anorexia; constipation; decreased libido.
- Ascertain from patients if having suicidal ideations *to provide safe care.*
- Ascertain ability to do self-care (grooming, hygiene, nutrition, and elimination) *to determine present status of depression.*
- Observe interactions with health professionals, family members, friends: Does patient initiate or wait to be addressed?

- Discuss perceptions of RA as a chronic condition and outlook on treatments *to find areas of concern that should be addressed.*
- Encourage to express expectations of self, family members, health-care members *to determine feelings of being wanted, appreciated, or tolerated; anger; or other feelings.*
- Ascertain ability or desire to participate in goal setting *to determine self-esteem, passivity, or positive outlook.*
- Monitor energy level and sleep patterns *to determine depth of depression or need for protective measures.*
- Assist with self-care activities and make decisions for patient until energy levels and self-esteem increase *to aid recovery efforts.*
- Provide care for physical symptoms, such as anorexia, constipation, or insomnia, *to demonstrate acceptance of concerns or condition.*
- Prepare patient for diagnostic tests to determine personality traits or as part of patient interview or history *to provide data for physician's evaluation.* (Tests include Symptom Checklist 90R, Center for Epidemiologic Studies—Depression Scale, Beck Depression Inventory, and Arthritis Impact Measurement Scale, or others as needed).
- Assist patient to identify people to turn to for assistance *to help patient feel more hopeful and positive.*
- If prescribed, administer antidepressant medication *to aid efforts to overcome depression.*
- When energy level rises, have patient do simple to complex care as condition permits *to strengthen self-esteem and sense of accomplishment.*
- Assist to set goals for self and others *to help develop realistic expectations for self and others.*
- Seek guidance from health-care team members to help deal with patient's depression *for safe and effective care and environment.*
- Monitor level of anxiety *to determine optional nursing measures required.*
- Clarify physician's explanations, as needed, *because anxiety may preclude patient's and family's clear understanding of diagnosis and proposed regimen of care.*
- Review specifics of regimen, as needed, *to aid understanding and patient's and family's full participation.*
- Review characteristics of patient's "stage" of RA (see Table 6-5, p. 342); correlate symptoms with relief to be achieved by treatment regimen *to lessen anxiety.*
- Discuss patient's daily roles and responsibilities to determine optimal times for specific care (e.g., time of day for aqua therapy if employed during day or evening hours) *to facilitate achieving treatment goals.*
- Remind patient and family of health team members' availability *to clarify regimen as needed.*
- Answer questions as honestly as able *to establish trust and ease concerns when possible.*
- Encourage active participation in usual roles as able *to maintain self-concept.*
- Allow to ventilate feelings about deformities and limitation of movements *to determine needs.*
- Offer support and encouragement *to help maintain a positive attitude about the disease and its treatment.*

PRINCIPLES OF JOINT PROTECTION IN PATIENTS WITH ARTHRITIS

Do:
- Use the strongest and largest joints available for a specific task
- Carry objects close to the body
- Spread the weight of objects over many joints
- Use both hands to slide objects
- Organize work areas to reach most frequently used equipment easily
- Use assistive devices as needed and available

Avoid:
- Sitting or standing in given position for long periods
- Using force in the direction of flexion and ulnar deviation of wrist, hands, and fingers
- Laterally deviating pressures on hands or wrists
- Pressures against the volar surface or undersurface of the fingers
- Activities requiring a tight grasp to manipulate
- Constant pressure or force against the pad of the thumb

Modified from Stucki and Sangha.[55a]

- Encourage family members to maintain open communication *to help maintain usual roles.*
- Confer with health team members to discuss clinical care plan *to provide continuity of care and to build trust relationships with patient and family.*

NIC IMMOBILITY MANAGEMENT

Impaired physical mobility related to joint and systemic involvement

- Check degree and amount of joint movements or limitations *to learn patient's condition.*
- Assist with treatment regimen (e.g., medications, heat, cold, or paraffin) *to maintain joint mobility.*
- Provide ROM exercises as able *to prevent stiffening of joints.*
- Provide splint and walking aid such as cane *to lessen joint stress.*
- Turn and reposition every 2 to 4 hours *to prevent joint deformity.*
- Maintain joints in functional (extended) positions *to prevent joint contractures.*

NIC LIFE SPAN CARE

Impaired home maintenance management related to joint and muscle weakness

- Secure physical therapy consultation.
- Secure occupational therapy consultation to teach modifications in home environment *to lessen joint and systemic stress.*
- *Consult community health nurses* for home evaluation and continuity of care.
- Encourage practice with and use of implements and utensils *to gain skill and independence.*
- Encourage self-care, modify utensils, and provide learning experience *to gain skills.*

- Clarify safety measures for home/employment area *to lessen possibility of injury.*

NIC Physical Comfort Promotion

Acute pain related to inflammatory process and joint deformities

- Administer medications as prescribed *to relieve pain and inflammation.*
- Discuss relief of pain, length of relief, or other evidence of medications' efficacy *to determine if change is needed.*
- Encourage patient to be active during periods of pain relief *to maintain usual roles.*
- Encourage patient to express thoughts and feelings about pain, disease, and loss of independence *to ease concerns.*
- Provide quiet periods *for medications to be effective over time.*
- Encourage diversionary activities *to decrease focus on pain.*
- Encourage to participate actively and positively in each type of treatment *to increase comfort and sense of control.*
- Provide list of common side effects of medications *for safety and to relieve concern.*

NIC Drug Management

Risk for injury related to medications, their side effects, and treatments with hot and cold applications.

- Provide a written list of common side effects of medications, along with expected action of the medications, *to increase patient's comfort and knowledge.*
- Discuss measures to lessen side effects of medications, such as enteric coatings, taking with food or sufficient fluids, or use of antacids or gastric reflux–controlling medications.
- Discuss responsibility to report occurrence of side effects to physician or nurses *for safe care.*
- Discuss techniques, expected actions, and purposes of aqua therapy or hot and cold applications; provide written list of actions of each therapy *to increase patient's understanding, safety, and compliance.*
- Remind patient to report untoward responses, such as increased pain, stiffness, or blisters, *to prevent injury to susceptible tissues* (see Emergency Alert box).

NIC Nutrition Support

Imbalanced nutrition: less than body requirements, related to inadequate intake of iron, anorexia, and depression

- Observe intake for types and amounts of foods; appetite; presence of nausea, vomiting, or lack of interest in eating.
- Discuss food likes and dislikes *to determine if changes are needed.*
- Weigh daily before breakfast *to note weight losses or gains.*
- Provide oral hygiene before meals *to enhance taste for foods.*
- Encourage eating of four to six smaller meals daily instead of three large ones *to conserve energy; eating smaller meals is less fatiguing.*
- Discuss and assist selections from menu and iron-containing foods *to increase iron intake to lessen anemia.*
- Clarify that iron absorption is increased by intake of orange juice, and provide when taking medication *to lessen anemia.*
- Provide food or milk when administering NSAIDs *to reduce or prevent gastric irritation.*
- Provide snack at bedtime *to aid intake and lessen effects of gastric secretions on empty stomach.*
- Use health-care team members for guidance to deal with patient's depression *to provide safe and effective care and environment.*

NIC Activity and Exercise Management

Activity intolerance related to anemia and disease state

- Observe levels of energy, tiredness, and fatigue; elicit patient's statements when possible.
- Provide rest periods in morning and afternoon *to help maintain strength and lessen fatigue.*
- Provide 8 to 10 hours for uninterrupted nighttime sleep if possible *to help maintain strength.*
- Alternate activities with rest periods *to prevent fatigue.*
- Provide trapeze, assistive devices, and side rails as needed to help conserve energy and muscle and joint functions.
- Seek consultation with physical and occupational therapists for exercises and other aids *to maintain or increase strength.*
- Monitor laboratory data such as hematocrit and hemoglobin *to note current anemia* (levels of hematocrit <30% and hemoglobin <12 g are indicative of anemia); monitor ESR as sign of disease activity and inflammation status (normal ESR for males, 0 to 20 mm/h; for females, 0 to 25 mm/h).

NIC Self-Care Facilitation

Disturbed sleep pattern related to pain and joint or muscle disease

- Observe sleep patterns over time, noting snoring or periods of apnea if present (may be signs of sleep apnea).
- Prepare for rest with massage and straightening of bed linens *to aid relaxation.*
- Position with small pillow under head and lower back *to prevent flexion contractures;* mattress should be firm.
- Administer medications *to relieve pain and inflammation.*
- Maintain a quiet environment *to promote and maintain sleep periods.*
- Avoid caffeine-containing foods *to promote restful sleep.*
- Monitor, and possibly change, hours of administration of medications, such as diuretics and steroids, that could interfere with sleep *to promote sleep.*

NIC Patient Education

Deficient knowledge related to disease and progression

- Determine through discussion present understanding of RA.

EMERGENCY ALERT

CAUTIONS WHEN ADMINISTERING MEDICATIONS TO TREAT RHEUMATOID ARTHRITIS

Side effects of one or more medications used to treat RA must be observed for by health team members as they interact with patients and family members. Major side effects for the various categories of medications are listed here.

Assessment

Category	Major Side Effects*
• Nonsteroidal analgesic/antiinflammatory drugs (NSAIDs)	Potential for GI bleeding Interference with antihypertensives Interference with platelet function/can lead to bleeding Increase in creatinine levels/azotemia
• Oral corticosteroids	Risk of osteoporosis (dose related) Risk of osteonecrosis, often affecting head of femur Increased risk of infection (may mask infection) May increase risk of peptic ulceration and/or GI bleeding May precipitate or exacerbate hyperglycemia or development of diabetes May lead to myopathy and/or weakening of collagen fibers May precipitate adrenal insufficiency if withdrawn too rapidly May lead to increased sodium retention and excretion of potassium May increase blood glucose levels
• Disease-modifying antirheumatic drugs (DMARDs):	
Sulfasalazine	Do not administer if patient allergic to sulfa drugs; skin rash may develop Lowers platelet and total WBC counts; may also lead to anemia Affects liver function tests, increasing normal results to upper limits
Hydroxychloroquine	Retinopathy, blurred vision, halos around lights; do not administer if patient has known retinopathy or other serious ophthalmic condition May cause irritability and nervousness Hemolytic anemia (rare) Alopecia
Methotrexate	Leukopenia; thrombocytopenia; anemia; bleeding Oral and GI ulcerations Increased toxicity if renal function impaired
Methotrexate—cont'd	Skin rash Development of opportunistic infections Increases liver function tests Pulmonary changes: Shortness of breath, cough, chest pain, abnormal chest x-ray Severe GI effects of nausea and vomiting
Azathioprine	Increased liver function tests Increased risk of infection such as herpes zoster Skin rash Decreased WBC and platelet counts Severe GI upsets of nausea and vomiting
Cyclosporine	Marked decrease in glomerular filtration rates; may lead to decreased renal function Gingival hypertrophy Hirsutism of face, arms, trunk Gout Tremors, paresthesias Hypertension Hyperglycemia Rise of opportunistic infections
Cyclophosphamide	Hemorrhagic cystitis Leukopenia; thrombocytopenia Anemia Risk of bladder cancer Alopecia Severe GI upsets of severe vomiting, nausea Increased risk of infections
D-Penicillamine	Skin rash with pruritus Leukopenia; thrombocytopenia Proteinuria Bronchiolitis Rarely: Development of myasthenia gravis Mouth ulcers
• Gold therapy: Auranofin; gold sodium aurothiomalate; aurothioglucose	Decreased WBC and platelet counts Skin rash with marked pruritus Oral ulcers Persistent diarrhea Proteinuria

Interventions

- Evaluate patient's side effects carefully; may need to hold medication until consultation with medical personnel.
- Secure prescription for medication to alleviate side effects, such as an antiemetic, antacid, analgesic (aspirin, if not contraindicated) for headache, antidiarrheal, antipruritic, or other medication as needed.
- Monitor laboratory data closely to note responses to specific medications.
- Offer mouthwashes and secure prescription for soothing oral medication to ease oral ulcerations.
- Observe urine for hematuria; monitor output closely.
- Offer cool damp cloths to ease pruritus or apply emollients as needed.
- Monitor liver function test results.
- Use medical asepsis to help prevent nosocomial infections.
- Monitor vital signs closely to note early changes.
- Monitor patient's ROM of joints to note response to medications.
- Encourage participation as able in aqua therapy or other prescribed therapies for condition.
- Record and report to health team members patient's responses to treatment regimen; initiate changes as prescribed.

*Many medications have common side effects, including anorexia, nausea or vomiting, headache, diarrhea, or constipation. Those side effects will not be listed but must be observed for in daily care.

- Clarify inflammatory process *to increase understanding of condition.*
- Reiterate physician's explanations of the different treatments and their purposes *to increase understanding and compliance.*
- Provide a quiet environment *to aid teaching/learning process.*

Patient Education/Continuum of Care Plan

1. Reiterate explanations of chronicity and controllability of RA and its symptoms to aid compliance.
2. Reiterate necessity for patient compliance with multiple treatment regimen for maximum benefits.
3. Discuss with patient and family members each medication and common side effects to be noted or reported to the physician; provide written lists.
4. Encourage patient to participate actively and fully in each aspect of the disease, its treatments, and alternatives for long-term care.
5. Explain the necessity for cooperative family relationships in the patient's care and treatments to maintain self-worth and role relationships.
6. Teach foods needed for a balanced diet or others needed to regain positive nutritional status.
7. Explain community resources to deal with future depressive episodes, if they occur.
8. Refer to community agencies for long-term association related to RA.

Evaluation/Patient Outcomes

Coping Assistance: Patient experiences only mild anxiety; anxiety is relieved by repeated explanations and visits over time. Patient regains positive outlook. Depression is treated with appropriate medications; patient has set realistic goals. Patient has a positive body image and has returned to usual roles; verbalizes acceptance of RA and its possible progression over time; has slowly regained roles in family hierarchy and usual behaviors.

Immobility Management: Patient has satisfactory physical mobility; can walk several miles daily with assistive aid; can walk up and down stairs, using the railing for support; uses aqua therapy daily. Patient moves slowly and deliberately with use of cane or other assistive device; can walk recreationally up to 2 miles several times a week. Patient demonstrates proper use of assistive devices. Medications and massage ease backache.

Life Span Care: Patient can maintain activities at home; has learned to use modified utensils to maximize muscle strengths; can use home appliances by self.

Physical Comfort Promotion: Patient has adequate pain relief; experiences long, pain-free periods when complying with analgesic antiinflammatory medication regimen.

Drug Management: Patient has manageable side effects from medications; experiences no injury from hot/cold applications.

Nutrition Support: Patient has intake of iron-containing foods and proteins to overcome anemia; has normal hematocrit (over 33%) and hemoglobin (over 12 g); has increased appetite and eats four to six small meals per day; has not lost weight and is maintaining satisfactory weight for size, age, and sex.

Activity and Exercise Management: Patient has a satisfactory tolerance of daily activities; can maintain ADLs with mild restrictions on lifting because of limited strength and joint deformities.

Self-Care Facilitation: Patient has long periods of sleep; achieves 7 to 8 hours of restful sleep at night; can return to sleep after changing position.

Patient Education: Patient can explain symptoms of RA, verbalizes changes resulting from inflammation and purposes of multiple treatments necessary.

Osteomyelitis

Osteomyelitis is an infection of the bone and its marrow.

Osteomyelitis concerns those who have a fractured bone and/or an open wound. It may start by direct invasion into bone tissues from the open wound or fractured bone (referred to as exogenous spread), or it may spread from an infected throat or bacterial pneumonia or other infection to a distant site in the host bone, referred to as endogenous or hematogenous spread. Approximately 56% of open tibial fractures develop osteomyelitis.[24] Long-standing or inadequately treated osteomyelitis can be destructive of many tissues and may be life threatening.

Some of the major organisms causing osteomyelitis are *Staphylococcus aureus, Streptococcus pneumoniae, Escherichia coli, Pseudomonas aeruginosa,* and *Haemophilus influenzae.* Children usually develop osteomyelitis as a result of hematogenous spread from "strep" throat. Adolescents and adults develop it from direct invasion after trauma and surgical procedures. Sickle cell disease also predisposes the person to osteomyelitis after a "sickling" episode in which ischemia may lead to necrosis of bone. Some persons with pulmonary tuberculosis also develop osteomyelitis of joints or vertebrae. Persons with open pressure sores may develop osteomyelitis in underlying bones.

In addition, osteomyelitis may be caused by viruses, fungi, or parasites, although osteomyelitis caused by these organisms occurs less frequently than that caused by bacteria. Bacteria that cause infection can colonize the host tissue and produce damage as they adhere to the host tissue. Also, bacterial adherence requires some form of damage to the bone, either mechanical or chemical, or the insertion of a foreign body to reliably establish infection.[60]

Pathophysiology

The longer and larger the bone, the more susceptible it is to osteomyelitis, which involves the interaction between host and pathogen in a specific environment. Entry into the host is accomplished as the pathogen breaches the barriers of skin or mucus membranes or through the blood. The pathogen must colonize and reproduce in the host tissue. Hematogenous seeding is thought to be one method of developing osteomyelitis after an open fracture; however, the incidence of osteomyelitis is much higher in open fractures when bacteria enter the wound directly from the environment. The bacteria colonize and cause more tissue damage as they set up an acute inflammatory response at the site of adherence to the injured bone and the surrounding soft tissues. Traumatized soft tissue and bone expose potential binding sites such as collagen, which have receptors that accept *S. aureus* organisms. *S. aureus* is the most common cause of posttraumatic osteomyelitis.[60] The established colonies grow in the area, leading to edema, blood vessel engorgement, multiple white cell invasion, and tissue responses. The bacteria adhere to the bone and soft tissue by producing biofilm, which forms strong bonds with the glycoproteins in the tissues. Biofilm may be a key factor contributing to the difficulty in eradicating bacteria from bone. Biofilm protects bacteria from the action of antibiotics, inhibits phagocytosis, impedes the ingress of antibodies, and impairs T and B lymphocyte functions.[60]

In hematogenous osteomyelitis the pathogenic organisms travel to a site within the metaphysis of the bone. The metaphysis provides a warm, secluded area where the organisms can grow and multiply. The result of either the direct invasion or hematogenous routes is the inflammatory response, which, through phagocytosis, attempts to contain the spread of bacteria. Cytokines initiate or amplify the inflammatory response. Cytokines can mediate and help regulate the body's immune responses, but trauma impairs the body's ability to overcome the pathogens as the inflammatory processes continue. Ultimately, purulent material accumulates from dead cell bodies, extravasated fluids, and toxins, causing more swelling and pain. As more purulent matter is produced, the enlarging mass blocks blood flow in the bone, producing an area of infarction and causing the bone to become necrotic. The body's response to the mass and necrotic tissue brings polymorphonuclear macrophages to the site to combat and ingest the pathogens. Purulent matter continues to be produced, and the enlarging mass spreads out of the confined area, through the cortex of the bone, into contiguous tissues, and into the bone marrow. Pain ensues as the mass presses against the rigid walls of the infected bone. The exudate matter flows through the least resistant pathways to the skin surface through a sinus tract. The infected bone attempts to keep the infection localized by forming new bone trabeculae called involucrum, and the necrotic or dead bone tissue is called sequestrum. The infection spreads into the bone marrow, along fascial planes in the affected areas, and to the skin through the sinus tract. The weakened, infected bone may fracture, and the patient may be hesitant to move, may have pain or soreness, and may experience edema or increased warmth in the area as the osteoclasts attempt to destroy or resorb small, dead, sequestered bone. Large sequestra must be surgically removed because they are a source for continued infection (Fig. 6-16). Osteomyelitis may spread to a joint, leading to septic arthritis, or to the vertebra, especially if the osteomyelitis is caused by tuberculosis organisms.

Occasionally a Brodie's abscess may develop in an area of osteomyelitis if the pathogenic organisms are insufficient in number or virulence to lead to a full-scale infection. Macrophages enclose the area, and a cold abscess (Brodie's) forms, surrounded by fibrous (scar) tissue and a ring of dense bone. The pathogens inside the abscess remain alive and virulent, and they may flare up and cause a reinfection, or they may all die. The resultant cavity will eventually fill with serum or blood.

Osteomyelitis may become subacute or chronic, related to incomplete resolution of the initial infection, which occurs in 15% to 30% of patients. Children and adolescents may also develop chronic recurrent multifocal osteomyelitis with multiple sites of bone involvement.

Diagnostic Studies and Findings

History: Antecedent infection or open trauma in the previous 3 to 4 weeks; history of pulmonary tuberculosis; sickle cell disease; dental, urinary, or respiratory infection

Physical examination: Area of tenderness, edema, warmth, redness, and possibly mass or drainage around an open fracture site or near the ends of a long bone; increased pain with movement or weight; spiking fevers in the 39° to 40° C (103° to 104° F) range intermittently noted, chills, and diaphoresis; headache and nausea; fracture of involved bone; presence of open pressure sore or puncture wound of foot or other bone and tissue; symptoms may be vague in subacute or chronic osteomyelitis

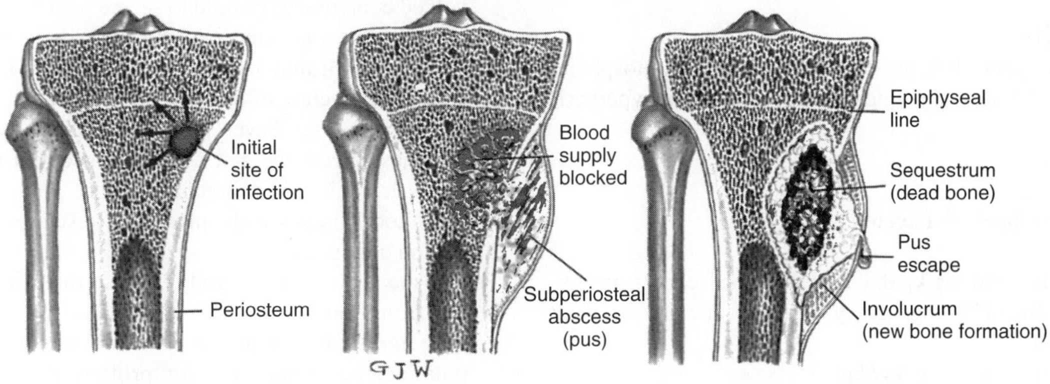

Fig. 6-16

Development of osteomyelitis infection with involucrum and sequestrum. (From Mourad.[39])

Aspiration of mass: May aspirate purulent material
Culture of mass or drainage: Infecting pathogenic organisms: bacteria or fungi; an increasing number of joint replacement patients have fungal infections resulting from overgrowth or superinfection after the use of antibiotics
WBC count: Elevated with increased levels of polymorphonuclear neutrophils (PMNs) indicative of bacterial infection
ESR: Increased (normal rate in males, 0 to 20 mm/h; females, 0 to 25 mm/h)
X-rays: Initially may not reveal the destructive processes but will later show rarefaction of the involved bone with evidence of formation of sequestrum and involucrum; chest x-ray may reveal lesions of tuberculosis, if present
CT scan: May show spread along fascial planes into surrounding tissues
Serum cultures: Pathogenic organism, most commonly *S. aureus,* in about 55% of cases of osteomyelitis
MRI: May show soft tissue mass or sinus tract, bone marrow changes, or vertebral osteomyelitis
Bone scan: May show "hot" area of inflammation or "cold" area that may be associated with Brodie's abscess

MULTIDISCIPLINARY PLAN

Surgery

Aspiration of abscess for culture purposes only
After "sterilization" of abscess, sequestrum is removed and replaced by bone grafts
Saucerization is performed: involved bone is scraped to remove all necrotic cells, after which bone regenerates; if the defect is pronounced, bone grafts or metallic fixation may be applied (the latter never used in infected areas or if uncertainty exists about the possibility of lingering pathogens)
External fixation devices such as Hoffman or Ilizarov apparatus (pp. 414-417) may be used to hold bones weakened from the initial infection, from saucerization during treatments, or from fracture
Amputation of limb (done less frequently now because of improved treatment modalities)
Removal of implants until infection is cleared
Reaming of intramedullary canal for long-term chronic osteomyelitis[39]

Oxygen Therapy

Hyperbaric oxygen therapy: 100% oxygen at 2 atmospheres pressure for 2 hours six times a week, given in hyperbaric chamber

Medications

Antibiotic/antibacterial agents

Children

Oxacillin, 150 mg/kg/day for staphylococcal organisms
Cefazolin, 100 mg/kg/day if child allergic to penicillin
Clindamycin, 25 mg/kg/day
Vancomycin, 40 mgk/kg/day if allergic to both penicillin and cephalosporin
Antibiotics given for 5-10 days IV, followed by PO administration for up to 6 weeks

Adolescents and adults

IV antibiotic therapy for 4-12 weeks, depending on causative organism
Antibiotics impregnated in bone and cemented into beads for placement at site of infection
Cefazolin or moxalactam, 6 g
Cefotaxime, 10 g
Tobramycin, 9.6 g
Vancomycin, 5 g
Ticarcillin, 12 g
Ciprofloxacin, PO or IV for 4-6 weeks, individualized dose (IV 2 weeks, then PO for 4 weeks or longer)

For fungal osteomyelitis: Fluconazole or itraconazole, individualized dose

Analgesic/antipyretic agents

Acetaminophen, 325-500 mg q4h prn
Aspirin, 500-650 mg 1-2 tabs q4h prn (only for adolescents age 18 years or over to avoid Reye's syndrome)

Narcotic analgesic agents

Oxycodone (Percodan), 15-60 mg q4h prn
Morphine, 10-15 mg q4h PO or IM for severe pain
Hydrocodone/APAP (Vicodin) 30-60 mg q4-6h

General Management

Splints to decrease joint pain
Bed rest to conserve energy while acutely ill
Sling for the arm, if site of infection is in arm
Cast to prevent a fracture of weakened bones; should have "windows" for dressing changes, if needed
Frequent dressing changes of draining area
Frequent checks of external fixation apparatus, if in use
Ambulation to maintain muscle and joint strength after initial bed rest
Ilizarov fixator to prevent pathologic fracture of weakened bone, if extremity involved
As condition permits, child may be taken to playroom

NURSING CARE

NURSING ASSESSMENT

Inflammatory processes of infected area: Redness, increased warmth at site, edema, tenderness on use or palpation of involved bone/tissues or mild to severe pain or sharp pain with bone fracture; affected part may not be used or have decreased ROM; may have palpable mass or sinus tract, may have open fracture of bone
Systemic response: Fever and chills, diaphoresis; malaise; weakness; headache and nausea; concurrent or past infection; back pain if vertebrae involved
Spread: Local tissues with sinus tract; distant sites, where infection continues
Psychosocial concerns: Body image disturbance, disability from long-term disease processes and compliance with medication regimen, concern about possible amputation, economic cost for prolonged treatments, lack of insurance coverage, concern about nonhealing of fracture

Potential Complications

Development of chronic osteomyelitis, metastasis to additional sites, delayed healing of fracture, allergic response to one or more antibiotics, amputation

Patient Problem/Nursing Diagnoses & Interventions

NIC Immobility Management

Impaired physical mobility related to bone involvement

- Observe effects on mobility and joint use.
- Encourage ROM of unaffected joints *to decrease tiredness and prevent weakening.*
- Encourage self-care *to maintain muscle strength.*
- Encourage hobby and diversionary activities *to maintain motion and strength in all uninvolved joints.*
- Use walker or crutches *to aid ambulation if necessary and to increase socialization.*

NIC Thermoregulation

Ineffective thermoregulation related to infection in bone and soft tissue

- Monitor temperature and other vital signs as prescribed or indicated.
- Administer prescribed antipyretic medication *to reduce hyperpyrexia if present.* Antipyretics will mask fevers.
- Monitor for diaphoresis and patient's response of drop in fever; change clothing and bed linens as needed *to maintain skin integrity.*
- Monitor for additional signs of pyrexia: flushed skin, headache, malaise, sleepiness, or restlessness *to determine patient's reaction to fever and infection.*
- Maintain room temperature; keep consistently in normal temperature range (70° to 74° F [21° to 23.3° C]) *to aid patient's comfort.*
- Provide light bed covers only *to lessen possible elevation of temperature* from excess covers.
- Provide adequate fluid replacement *to prevent dehydration.*
- Record and report temperature elevations as necessary.

NIC Physical Comfort Promotion

Acute pain related to presence of abscess in bone and soft tissue

- Determine amount, site, severity, and duration of pain.
- Maintain limited activity *to lessen stress on involved tissues.*
- Administer analgesics as prescribed *to relieve pain.*
- Handle affected limb gently *to lessen pressure and pain.*
- Use sling when appropriate for arm infections.
- Administer IV antibiotics as prescribed *to clear infection and thereby lessen pain.* Monitor patient's responses to therapy.
- Use care when initiating IV therapy and during therapy *to preserve venous integrity for long-term need* (therapy may be via a central venous catheter).
- Use care to maintain asepsis of all equipment *to prevent nosocomial infection.*
- Encourage activities to divert attention from condition (e.g., with children, take to playroom, outside).

NIC Risk Management

Risk of infection or spread related to pathogens and site of osteomyelitis

- Observe site of infection: observe for local changes (sinus tract with purulent drainage; palpate contiguous tissues and joints for signs of inflammation or infection).
- Listen to complaints of pain in back or joints distant to initial site of osteomyelitis *to determine if infection has spread,* especially if infection is caused by tubercle bacilli.
- Monitor body temperature *to determine if infection if systemic.*
- Monitor initial infection site for increase in drainage and hesitancy to use part *to determine if infection is abating or increasing.*
- Monitor IV site *for signs of inflammation or infection.*
- Monitor serum hematologic study or culture results *to determine if patient's defenses are responding to the infectious process;* check complete blood count, including hematocrit and hemoglobin, blood or wound culture results, and antibiotic sensitivity data.
- Use universal precautions *to prevent spread of infection to others.*
- Wash hands before and after patient contacts *to prevent spread of nosocomial infection to others.*

NIC Tissue Perfusion Management

Ineffective tissue perfusion related to surgery or oxygen therapy

- Perform neurovascular checks *to determine tissue perfusion in affected areas.*
- Note skin color and condition of wound after each treatment in hyperbaric chamber.
- Monitor patient's response to being in enclosed chamber for hyperbaric therapy (may become claustrophobic) *for greatest patient benefits.*
- Remove jewelry, watch, synthetic clothing, and perfume before hyperbaric therapy *for patient safety and to prevent possible combustion.*

NIC Skin/Wound Management

Impaired skin integrity related to incision and surgery

- Observe skin surfaces *for wound closure and condition.*
- Loosen splint if used *for care and to check skin condition.*
- Change dressings as needed *to remove drainage and to lessen odor and skin maceration.*
- Reposition patient every 2 hours *to maintain healthy skin tissues.*
- Massage skin areas *to increase tissue perfusion.*
- Assist to be out of bed and to ambulate as condition indicates.

NIC Coping Assistance

Disturbed body image related to pathology
Anxiety related to economic costs of prolonged treatment

- Discuss concerns related to condition or treatments.
- Explain rationale for long-term therapy *to clear disease.*
- Check equipment (splint, Hoffman or Ilizarov apparatus, etc.) for proper functioning, as well as patient's responses, *to monitor effects of treatments.*
- If amputation is required, do preoperative preparation, encouraging patient to talk about concerns over loss of body part. After amputation, do necessary care to promote wound healing and prevent complications (see p. 390).
- Encourage patient and family interaction *to maintain relationships and usual roles.*
- Discuss patient's and family's verbalized concerns about cost of treatments, hospitalization, lack of insurance, or extent of insurance reimbursement.
- Observe for signs of anxiety, such as sighing, crying, wringing hands, restlessness, apprehension, irritability, ability to listen, and ability to understand explanations.
- Provide privacy to discuss concerns *to learn extent of problems.*
- Maintain a safe and quiet atmosphere.
- If a child patient, take child to playroom for supervision while discussing concerns with parents *to lessen child's anxiety.*
- Teach or explain to patient and family self-care activities *to help ease anxiety.*
- Seek consultation with social service personnel for explanation of financial or home care needs *to lessen anxiety or seek solutions.*
- Discuss option of home care with patient and family *to provide a sense of control of future care or needs.*
- Discuss home care needs with community health nurse *to determine feasibility of home treatment plan or regimen.*
- Secure home care equipment, if needed, and teach patient and family how to use and maintain *for safe care.*
- Discuss community resources available for family's use, such as Meals on Wheels and Home IV Therapy Team, *to ease anxiety about home care.*

Patient Education/Continuum of Care Plan

1. Reiterate the need for prompt medical attention for local or systemic infections to prevent the recurrence or the spread of infection; discuss how osteomyelitis occurs.
2. Discuss the rationale, purposes, and expected outcomes for long-term antibiotic therapy to increase the patient's understanding and compliance.
3. Discuss home care for long-term IV antibiotic treatments and other home care needs as necessary.
4. List the side effects of long-term antibiotic therapy, and clarify with patient and family.
5. Discuss purposes for continuing ROM exercises to maintain strength and mobility.
6. Use pictures to clarify characteristics of the hyperbaric oxygen chamber and the external fixator.
7. Discuss community resources available for care or financial aid.

Evaluation/Patient Outcomes

Immobility Management: Patient has satisfactory mobility; walks about easily without aid; has no muscle or joint soreness.

Thermoregulation: Patient's temperatures are within normal ranges. Wound drainage has ceased.

Physical Comfort Promotion: Patient has experienced relief of pain; takes no analgesic for pain; states that no longer has pain in wound site.

Risk Management: Patient has no evidence of continuing infection; has no wound drainage and wound is healing well. Vital signs and laboratory data are within normal ranges.

Tissue Perfusion Management: Patient has satisfactory tissue integrity; has well-healed, 3-inch scar on right lateral surface of thigh; has no tenderness, numbness, or unusual skin color at site; neurovascular checks are all in normal limits.

Skin/Wound Management: Patient has regained skin integrity. Patient's scar edges are approximated with scar remaining slightly pink; has no skin lesions or pressure areas.

Coping Assistance: Patient has a positive body image; is outward looking, in high spirits, eager for new experiences, and seems to have no fear of recurrent disease. Anxiety has markedly lessened. Patient is restless no longer, with no crying noted; responses to questions are pertinent to discussion. Family's financial concerns have been addressed by appropriate personnel. Patient and family are looking forward to continued treatments at home.

DEGENERATIVE CONDITIONS

As people age, they experience some musculoskeletal conditions resulting from degeneration. Even though such conditions may begin in a specific tissue, such as the cartilage or bone, they affect not only that tissue but also other musculoskeletal tissues because of their anatomic and physiologic interrelationships. Therefore these conditions have local and systemic effects, as do the conditions previously discussed. Degenerative conditions are usually noninflammatory.

Age-related changes in the feet are listed in Table 6-6, leading to many musculoskeletal effects throughout the body.

Hallux Valgus

Hallux valgus is deviation of the great toe toward the other toes.

In hallux (great toe) valgus the great toe deviates toward the other toes either from congenital abnormality or from tendon and ligament degeneration caused by increasing weight and weight-bearing activities. The forefoot becomes splayed (spread out), allowing the first metatarsal bone to deviate into a more varus position (Fig. 6-17).[47a]

Usually hallux valgus is bilateral, with one side more prominent and symptomatic than the other. It is most commonly

Table 6-6 Age-Related Changes in Feet

Tissue	Common Changes
Skin	Dryness; atrophy; hyperkeratosis (marked thickening, especially skin of heels and balls of feet); cracking, scaling; corns, calluses; ulcerations
Bones	Osteoporosis with diffuse osteopenia
Toenails	Onychauxis (thickened and discolored nails) Onychocryptosis (ingrown nails) Onychomycosis (fungal infections of nails) Corns on top of or between toes
Ligaments and tendons	Tendinitis; rupture of tendon (Achilles); claw or hammer toes; overlapping toes; weakened ligaments; bursitis retrocalcaneal (above heel); tendinitis of tibialis posterior tendon; flattening of arch; splaying of toes and metatarsal bones, mid-foot pronation
Joints	Hallux valgus; hallux rigidus; joint instability
Nerves and circulation	Acrocyanosis (blue color) of feet; cold feet; ulcerations; hair loss; smooth skin; inelastic skin; edema; nail dystrophy; limb or foot ischemia leading to gangrene; paresthesia; numbness

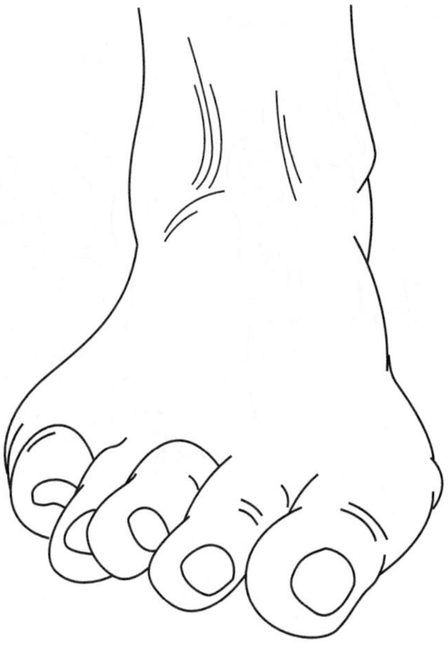

FIG. 6-17
Hallux valgus and bunion deformity. Note hammertoe (third toe) and nearly covered fourth toe.

noted in women during the sixth decade, with a strong familial tendency. Adolescents also may have hallux valgus (hallux refers to the great toe, and valgus refers to lateral deviation away from the midline).

The etiology of hallux valgus remains controversial related to its basis in wearing constrictive footwear or having a genetic basis. Its genetic role was first addressed in the 1920s, but studies have continued to yield conflicting information about genetic influence. It is possible that juvenile hallux valgus is transmitted as an autosomal dominant trait, but it is also possible that it may be passed as an X-linked dominant trait or as a polygenic trait, and studies are presently ongoing to determine whether constrictive footwear merely aggravates hallux valgus and if a significant hereditary predisposition is the major causative factor in its development.

PATHOPHYSIOLOGY

Hallux valgus is most obvious from the increasing prominence and deformity of the first metatarsal bone, with this bone's shaft deviated medially away from the second metatarsal. The head of the first metatarsal bone develops a protective bursa (bunion) wherever it rubs against a shoe. As the valgus deformity of the proximal phalanx of the great toe increases, the second toe is crowded and may also become deformed.

DIAGNOSTIC STUDIES AND FINDINGS

History: Familial occurrence, primarily in mother, rarer in father; may be ballet dancer or wear high-heeled shoes during most waking hours

Physical examination: Valgus deformity of great toe, with or without bursa development (bunion), hammertoe, corns, calluses, often bilateral; great toe and second toe may be over or under each other; forefront splays bilaterally; arch of foot weakened (may show "flat" foot); tailor's bunion may be present at the outer base of the small toe

Roentgenogram: Deformities described above

MULTIDISCIPLINARY PLAN

Surgery

Usually as outpatient procedure

Osteotomy to realign bones, such as Mitchell osteotomy or other osteotomy

Arthroplasty: Keller operation; Stone procedure (FIG. 6-18)

Arthrodesis of first metatarsal joint of great toe

Bunionectomy

Medications

NSAIDs
- Ibuprofen, 400-600 mg tid or qid
- Naproxen, 250-500 mg bid or tid
- Celecoxib (Celebrex), 100 mg bid
- Rofecoxib (Vioxx), 12.5 mg daily
- See table on p. 337 for additional NSAIDs

Analgesic/antipyretic agents
- Aspirin, 600-1000 mg qid
- Acetaminophen, 600-1000 mg qid
- Codeine phosphate, 30-60 mg PO q4h (rarely needed or used because of side effects)

General Management

Tape pad under metatarsal heads to change weight-bearing pressure

Change shoe style to wider, open-toed shoe with soft upper portions, cushioned sole

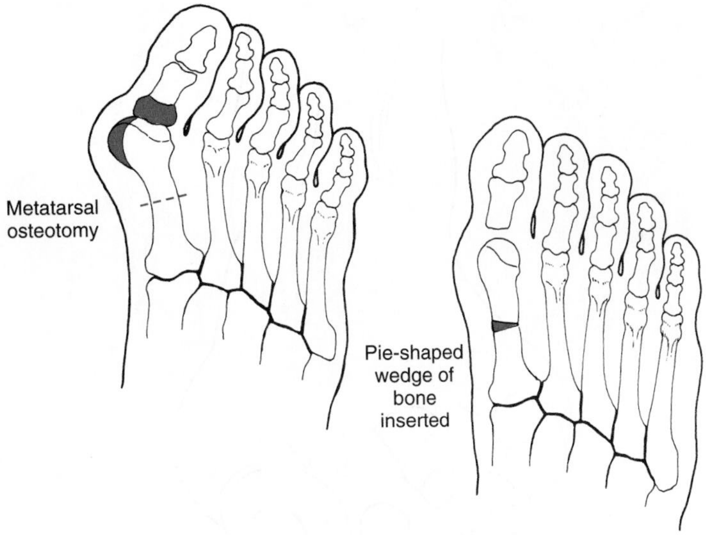

FIG. 6-18

One type of operative repair.

Wear low-heeled shoes
Foot exercises to lessen splayfoot
Application of ice compress to site of bunion
Form-fitting insole in shoe to cushion foot
Use of toe pad over corn or bunion
Custom-molded shoes occasionally necessary

NURSING CARE

NURSING ASSESSMENT

Signs of degeneration: Valgus (away from midline) deformity of great toe and varus deformity of first metatarsal bone, splaying of metatarsal bones; presence of bunion on great toe; corn development from pressure on other toes, may have corns between toes; deformity or crowding of second toe; hammertoe possible in other toes; callus possible under metatarsal heads of other toes; possible presence of tailor's bunion at base of small toe; toenails: thickened, discolored; may have ingrown toenails, fungal infections; pain may be marked with use; amount, duration, types, and sites of pain

Other accompanying signs: Presence of inflamed bursa, producing tenderness and often exquisite pain in and around joint (metatarsophalangeal joint of great toe); condition usually bilateral, although one side may have more deformities; hallux rigidus: painful hallux valgus with marked movement limitations; skin may be dry, itching, loss of patches of skin if vigorous scratching; hyperkeratosis of heel with marked thickening; cracks in heel areas[47a]

Psychosocial concerns: Concern with body image from deformity, pain, and effects on mobility; concern with need to change shoe styles and sizes; concern with need to correct deformities; concern with need to change career (possible, if ballet dancer) or employment

POTENTIAL COMPLICATIONS

Recurrence: osteoarthritis

PATIENT PROBLEMS/NURSING DIAGNOSES & INTERVENTIONS

NIC IMMOBILITY MANAGEMENT

Impaired physical mobility related to deformity of one or more toes and feet

- Discuss effects of deformities on mobility and use.
- Encourage use of padding in shoes *to change weight-bearing sites.*
- Encourage usual activities when pain free *to increase mobility.*
- Encourage consulting with physician to remove bursa or bunion if necessary *to relieve condition and increase mobility.*
- Encourage consultation with physician or podiatrist for need to change shoe styles or sizes *to decrease progression of foot abnormalities.*

NIC PHYSICAL COMFORT PROMOTION

Chronic pain related to bunion, inflammation, and deformity

- Determine severity, type, and sites of pain in foot or toes.
- Administer ordered medication *to ease discomfort.*
- Teach side effects of medications *to increase understanding.*
- Apply ice compress to inflamed bursa *to lessen edema and pain.*
- Encourage temporary cessation of weight bearing when pain is acute *to increase comfort or lessen discomfort.*
- Encourage wearing of shoes with wider box and soft tops *to increase comfort and lessen pressure on tender areas.*
- Discuss need to wear lower-heeled (rather than high-heeled) shoes *to decrease progression of deformities.*

NIC COPING ASSISTANCE

Disturbed body image related to perception of deformities

- Discuss concerns about presence of hallux valgus *to determine effects on body image.*
- Encourage wearing of well-fitted footwear *to lessen progression.*
- Encourage consulting with physician for probable surgical removal *to aid in regaining positive feelings.*
- Encourage exercises *to lessen progressive deformity.*
- Consult physician for placement or use of orthoses in shoes *to lessen effects of deformities before and after surgical correction, if performed.*

PATIENT EDUCATION/CONTINUUM OF CARE PLAN

1. Clarify bunion as accompanying hallux valgus.
2. Instruct about preventive measures with proper footwear, use of orthoses, and exercises.
3. Explain surgical options previously discussed with physician, as necessary, for clarity.
4. Provide list of medication side effects and instruct to notify physician if any occur.
5. Teach care of the feet to prevent infection or deal with age-related changes.

6. If surgical correction done, instruct on home care, use of ambulatory aid, if prescribed, and analgesic use as prescribed.

Evaluation/Patient Outcomes

Immobility Management: Patient again walks without deformity of toe joint, uses orthotic devices as needed, and wears well-fitted shoes. Patient applies ice during acute inflammation and rests the joint. Patient undergoes surgical correction if necessary to relieve deformity and regain painless mobility.

Physical Comfort Promotion: Patient's pain and inflammation are relieved. Surgical procedure removes bunion and corrects toe alignment, thereby relieving pain. Orthoses ease discomfort of splayfoot. Side effects of medications are few and manageable.

Coping Assistance: Patient has positive body image. Better-looking feet have a positive effect on patient's body image; states principles and practices for proper foot care: keep skin of feet clean and dry; dry between toes after cleansing; apply moisturizing lotion to prevent drying or cracking; check feet daily to note early signs of inflammation or pressure; wear properly fitted shoes with low heels; alternate shoes to permit shoes to dry between wearing. Patient can continue present employment after corrective measures.

Osteoarthritis

Osteoarthritis (OA) is a condition characterized by degenerative changes initially in the cartilage covering the ends of bones, primarily in the major weight-bearing joints: hip and knee and, later, other joints throughout the body.

It is the most common of all joint diseases.[52]

The development of OA involves a process of dynamic changes taking place initially in the macromolecules of joint cartilage. These changes factor into the degradation, synthesis, structure, and interaction of its macromolecules, leading to changes in the functional properties and failure of the joint cartilage. The cartilage cannot fully repair itself after injury, causing it to wear down or erode more easily. Thus OA results from altered cartilage physiology.[32]

OA is classified as type I (primary) or type II (secondary). A genetic cause has been determined for primary OA, located on chromosome 12, associated with specific alleles of the gene COL 2A1.[53] Linkage of this gene with the development of OA has been demonstrated in several families, and the gene COL 2A1 is linked with type II collagen, the most common collagen in joint cartilage.[52] It has also been seen that mutations in genes other than COL 2A1 have been responsible for some cases of primary OA.[23] Also, the role of other extracellular matrix proteins must be investigated as to their linkage to type I OA. The genetic basis for type II OA has not yet been determined. Type II is secondary to trauma or other conditions.

OA is considered a disease of older persons, with more than 50 million people in the United States affected, and will continue to be a very significant disease entity as increasing numbers of persons are older, elderly, and even centenarians. At least 70% of persons over age 65 years show radiographic evidence of OA, with the knee joint being affected most often. Increasing age is the major risk factor for the development of OA.[32] Obesity is also a major factor, since being only 10 pounds overweight increases the load at the hip by 30 pounds.[44] Studies have also shown that 76% to 79% of persons with OA of the hip have evidence of previously unrecognized childhood hip disease.[44]

Pathophysiology

Osteoarthritis is characterized by loss of articular cartilage and by successive destruction of the musculoskeletal tissues of the

HEALTHY PEOPLE 2010

Health Status—Arthritis, Osteoporosis, and Chronic Back Conditions

Goal: Prevent illness and disability related to arthritis and other rheumatic conditions, osteoporosis, and chronic back conditions.

Arthritis and Other Rheumatic Conditions

- (Developmental) Increase the mean number of days without severe pain among adults who have chronic joint symptoms.
- Reduce the proportion of adults with chronic joint symptoms who experience a limitation in activity because of arthritis.
- Reduce the proportion of all adults with chronic joint symptoms who have difficulty performing two or more personal care activities, thereby preserving independence.
- (Developmental) Increase the proportion of adults age 18 years and older with arthritis who seek help in coping if they experience personal and emotional problems.
- Increase the employment rate among adults with arthritis in the working-age population.
- (Developmental) Eliminate racial disparities in the rate of total knee replacements.
- (Developmental) Increase the proportion of adults who have seen a health-care provider for their chronic joint symptoms.
- (Developmental) Increase the proportion of persons with arthritis who have had effective, evidence-based arthritis education as an integral part of the management of their condition.

Osteoporosis

- Reduce the overall number of cases of osteoporosis.
- Reduce the proportion of adults who are hospitalized for vertebral fractures associated with osteoporosis.

Chronic Back Conditions

- Reduce activity limitation resulting from chronic back conditions.

Modified from U.S. Department of Health and Human Services: *Healthy people 2010* (conference edition, in two volumes), Washington, DC, January 2000.

NOTE: *Developmental* indicates that criteria for measurement and strategies to improve health have not as yet been specified.

affected joint. Enzymes in the cartilage matrix initiate the cartilage destruction. These enzymes are markedly elevated in OA, and these enzymes, particularly stromelysin and metalloproteinase, cause breakdown of the collagen fibers in the cartilage.[25] Collagen breakdown destroys the fibrils that give joint cartilage its tensile strength and exposes the cartilage cells (chondrocytes) to mechanical stress and continued enzyme attack, with resultant changes in the normal, whitish, smooth hyaline cartilage in the joint. The cartilage shows an increase in its water content and a decrease in the amount of proteoglycan (complex protein-carbohydrate molecules). The cartilage begins to look irregular, becomes softer, and is pitted. It undergoes fibrillation, and cartilage flakes (detritus) are shed into the joint. This shedding rubs away the cartilage, primarily from sites where the maximum load is greatest. Repeated wear and erosion continue to thin the cartilage.

Although the cartilage is not rubbed away or thinned in nonstress areas, it is unhealthy from undernourishment. Cartilage is nourished during compression by synovial fluid and transudates from subchondral vessels. This pumping action does not occur in nonstress areas, so there is undernourishment. The subchondral vessels hypertrophy and invade the cartilage, which calcifies and later ossifies, forming osteophytes. The hyperemia spreads into the bone beneath the stress area, but pressure in this area prevents the vessels from penetrating into the cartilage. The cartilage continues to be rubbed away, exposing the underlying bone. Stress (fatigue) fractures occur in the subchondral trabeculae, and cysts and osteophytes develop where pressure is greatest. Bone ends become reshaped and remodeled as OA progresses.

During cartilage erosion, detritus is deposited on the synovial lining, which then hypertrophies. Flakes of cartilage also penetrate into the subsynovial layer, where they induce fibrosis that extends into the joint capsule. The ligaments and tendons of the capsule become thickened, inelastic, and stiff. The fibrous tissue shrinks as it matures, thereby limiting joint movement and causing deformity (FIG. 6-19). Thus all the joint tissues—cartilage, bone, synovium, ligaments, tendons, muscles, and skin—are eventually involved in OA, and the diseased cartilage and other tissues cannot carry out their normal weight-bearing loads.

Restriction of movement resulting from fibrosis is the main feature of OA. Symptoms appear early in joints such as the hip, where full extensions and stability are required for walking. Because the hip joint capsule is well supplied with pain fibers, slight restriction is noted by pain with attempts at full extension. Thus major weight-bearing joints show earlier symptoms. Weight bearing continues as an aggravation in OA. Sometimes no cartilage remains as bone ends are exposed, causing osteophytes to form in greater numbers.

Besides the hip and knee, the carpometacarpal joint at the base of the thumb, the vertebrae and sacroiliac joints, and the distal joints of the fingers are also affected by OA.

Limitation of movements and pain are the major symptoms. Pain frequently occurs during and after a night's rest. Usually there are no systemic signs, just the local signs confined to the joints and their contiguous tissues.

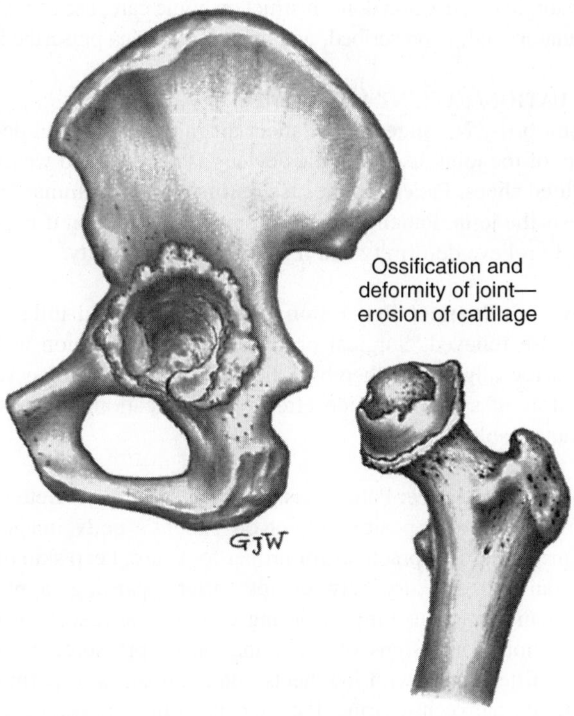

FIG. 6-19
Osteoarthritis of hip joint. Note erosion of cartilage from head of femur and osteophytes around acetabulum. (From Mourad.[39])

DIAGNOSTIC STUDIES AND FINDINGS

History: Patient has complaints of stiffness and limitation of movement of one or more weight-bearing joints, usually the hip or knee; states has pain radiating down thigh to knee and has pain at night when adjusting position in bed and on arising; pain limits mobility and activities and, if used, joint pain may lead to limping while walking; may complain of pain down sciatic nerve distribution down leg and into sacroiliac joints

Physical examination: Enlarged edematous joint with some stiffness and deformity; usually one joint has most pronounced signs, although more than one can be involved; if hip is involved, patient may hold it flexed, adducted, and externally rotated; joint may be tender but rarely feels hot; movements of joint limited; crepitus common; Heberden's nodes may be present in distal interphalangeal joints of fingers, and Bouchard's nodes occur in the proximal interphalangeal joints; gait analysis is done to determine weight-bearing patterns and stability; limp may be noted; varus deformity may be noted if one or both knees affected; obesity may be present; may have hallux valgus (see FIG. 6-17, p. 353)

ESR: Usually normal; may be slightly elevated in generalized polyarticular OA

Roentgenogram/MRI: Shows decreased or diminished joint space; necrotic or sclerotic bone; osteophytes and lipping in some joints; subchondral bone cysts; loss of joint cartilage; various deformity of peripheral joints, especially knees; valgus deformity of great toe

Arthroscopy: Can reveal cartilage damage long before any bone changes become evident[52]

Multidisciplinary Plan

Surgery

Percutaneous diskectomy, if indicated
Arthroscopic debridement of joint
Arthroplasty to repair the joint if only one surface of joint involved
Total joint replacement to replace diseased tissues if both surfaces involved
Osteotomy to change weight-bearing surfaces
Arthrodesis to limit joint movements (done to abolish pain)
Spinal fusion to maintain posture and eliminate pain
Muscle release if flexion contracture present

Medications

Analgesic-antipyretic agents: Aspirin (enteric-coated), 600-1000 mg 3-4 times daily

NSAIDs (one or more may be used at various times for treatment)
- Ibuprofen (Motrin), 300-400 mg 3-4 times daily
- Naproxen (Naprosyn), 250-375 mg bid
- Tometin (Tolectin), 200-400 mg 3-4 times daily
- Indomethacin (Indocin), 25-50 mg 3-4 times daily
- Sulindac (Clinoril), 150-200 mg bid
- Piroxicam (Feldene), 20 mg/day
- Diclofenac (Voltaren), 25-75 mg bid
- Oxaprozin (Daypro), 600-1200 mg/day
- Choline magnesium trisalicylate (Trilisate), 500-1000 mg tid or 1500 mg bid
- Celecoxib (Celebrex), 100 mg bid
- Rofecoxib (Vioxx), 12.5 mg/day
- See table on p. 337 for additional NSAIDs

Intraarticular agents
- Betamethasone, 3 mg/ml, 0.25-2.0 ml, based on joint size—small, medium, or large
- Dexamethasone, 8 mg/ml, 0.5-2.0 ml
- Hydrocortisone acetate, 25-50 mg/ml, 0.2-2.0 ml
- Prednisolone tebutate, 20 mg/ml, 0.4-2.0 ml
- Triamcinoline acetonide, 10-40 mg/ml, 9.25-1.0 ml

General Management

Moist heat applications with diathermy, ultrasound, and radiant heat
Exercises in aqua therapy to loosen stiff joints and ease soreness
Rest and modified weight-bearing activities beneficial
Canes, crutches, or walkers to aid walking, decrease joint stress, and increase stability; use of a cane in the contralateral hand decreases load on the hip by 50%[3a]
Soft collar and cervical traction to lessen pain in neck areas
Back brace or support to lessen pain and maintain posture
Elastic bandage to wrist or knee for support; orthosis for knee (brace)
Massage around painful joints
Wearing sturdy, low-heeled shoes
Weight reduction, if overweight

NURSING CARE

Nursing Assessment

Local (joint) signs of degeneration: Limitation of full extension; pain on arising and on weight bearing in joint; gait may be antalgic (pain avoiding); pain disturbing sleep as disease progresses; joint stiffness and deformity from fibrosis, shrinkage, and muscle imbalance; limp; joint feels unstable, may give way; pain radiating to soft tissues around joint; Heberden's nodes on distal phalangeal joints and Bouchard's nodes on proximal phalangeal joints
Systemic signs: None
Psychosocial concerns: Body image changes; pain; limitation of movement or weight bearing; difficulty managing home and meal preparation; loss of socialization/isolation; economic costs of medications, prolonged medical care, and procedures, and lack of insurance coverage for expenses

Potential Complications

Herniation of joint capsule, most commonly behind knee (Baker's cyst); locking of affected joint caused by loose bodies (cartilage and bone fragments) in joint(s); spinal stenosis from osteophytes; spondylolisthesis

Patient Problems/Nursing Diagnoses & Interventions

NIC Immobility Management

Impaired physical mobility related to joint pathology
- Check ROM, mobility limitations, and gait *to determine present condition.*
- Encourage and assist with ambulation as needed *to maintain joint functions and mobility.*
- Assist with ADLs as needed *to aid in completing activities.*
- Use ambulatory aid as prescribed *to facilitate walking with less discomfort and more stability.*
- Assist with ambulation after pain is relieved with heat or medication *to increase distances and muscle strength.*
- Encourage exercises in water to increase joint movement without increasing joint stress (immersion in water removes most of effects of gravity on joints).

NIC Physical Comfort Promotion

Chronic pain related to joint pathology and pressure on contiguous tissues
- Monitor amount, site, duration, time of day, and severity of pain.
- Administer prescribed analgesic or antiinflammatory medications *to lessen pain and aid relaxation.*
- Observe for effects and side effects of medications for pain relief *to note efficacy or untoward reactions.*

- Use heat and diathermy as prescribed *to relieve pain.*
- Discuss and demonstrate strategies to relieve pain such as imagery, relaxation techniques, and diversion *to increase patient's sense of control over pain episodes.*
- Stress proper posture when walking, standing, or sitting *to aid in proper muscle use.*
- Encourage weight loss, if overweight, *to decrease joint stress.*
- Apply traction or collar if necessary and prescribed *to lessen muscle pain; use knee brace as prescribed.*
- Encourage use of assistive devices *to aid activities in home or place of employment.*

NIC Coping Assistance

Disturbed body image and ineffective role performance related to progressive degenerative condition

- Determine effects of condition on self, ADLs, and usual daily regimen *to evaluate current condition.*
- Encourage to do usual activities and ADLs *for self-esteem and to maintain fitness and strength.*
- Encourage patient to comply with plan of medical care *to lessen joint deformity and decrease pain.*
- Encourage planned rest *to maintain strength.*
- Discuss weight reduction strategies if person is overweight.
- If surgery is contemplated, review and clarify options discussed by physician with patient *to lessen anxiety.*

NOTE: Nursing care after surgical treatments for OA begins on p. 397.

Patient Education/Continuum of Care Plan

1. Clarify understanding of degenerative nature of this disease and effects on mobility.
2. List side effects of medications; clarify with patient.
3. Caution about effects of heat on less sensitive tissues.
4. Discuss benefits of exercises in water (aqua therapy).
5. Discuss weight loss if overweight.

Evaluation/Patient Outcomes

Immobility Management: Patient walks with minimum limitation of motion. Patient maintains self-care, ADLs, and employment for as long as desired without experiencing uncontrollable pain or joint movement limitations or deformity.

Physical Comfort Promotion: Patient has relief of severe pain; takes medications as prescribed without nausea, vomiting, GI burning, bleeding, pain, or hematologic changes. Pain is relieved with medications, and joint mobility is enhanced. Patient uses imagery and relaxation techniques periodically.

Coping Assistance: Patient is gradually regaining normal range of weight. Patient returns to social interactions, has positive body image. Patient returns to usual family, social, and employment roles. Patient engages in exercises in water alone and in groups.

Muscular Dystrophy

The muscular dystrophies consist of a group of X-linked recessively inherited diseases of childhood characterized by progressive weakness and atrophy of symmetric groups of skeletal muscles. The prototype of all muscular dystrophies is Duchenne's muscular dystrophy.

The study of muscle pathology began in the early 1830s with a paper presented on the subject of progressive muscular atrophy with fatty transformation. However, the most rapid strides toward understanding the bases of many muscle pathologic conditions have been made since 1978 with the discovery of the structure of the gene and with the analysis of the human genome, which is still ongoing. Since 1978 the protein product of the muscular dystrophy gene, dystrophin, has been localized to the sarcolemma membrane of muscles. Much research has since been done attempting to devise new treatments for a great many hereditary human diseases.

One group of muscular diseases encompasses the muscular dystrophy diseases listed in Table 6-7; with their sexual and genetic transmission, rates of occurrence of children affected, symptoms, diagnostic studies, and usual treatments. The muscular dystrophy diseases cause degeneration of skeletal muscle fibers by progressive, symmetric weakness and wasting of these muscle groups leading to increasing disability and deformity. Presently most children with the major muscular dystrophies rarely live beyond age 20 to 25 years.[64a]

Not only are the skeletal muscles affected in the muscular dystrophies, but also other organs, joints, and bones are involved. Cardiac involvement, smooth muscles, and at times moderate mental retardation may affect some children. Many variations or mutations are now being diagnosed because of DNA and genetic research and studies of the human genome.

Pathophysiology

The muscular dystrophies listed in Table 6-7 appear to be X-linked recessive genetic diseases. They are associated with progressive muscle degeneration of predominantly male children. Duchenne's muscular dystrophy is the most severe form of muscular dystrophy; it affects 1:3000 boys in early childhood.[1] Mutations of the gene lead to a premature termination of dystrophin, a protein vital to normal muscle function, which is localized to the sarcolemmal membrane covering muscle fibers. Dystrophin is a large protein consisting of domains referred to as A through D. The A and C domains have homology (similarity) with alpha-actinin, the B domain has homology to spectrin, and the D domain has recently been shown to be homologous to a chromosome 6–encoded dystrophin-like protein.[1] The D domain is essential in the association of dystrophin with the sarcolemma. No dystrophin has been detected in muscle biopsies of patients with Duchenne's muscular dystrophy, whereas in a milder form (Becker's muscular dystrophy) the dystrophin is of abnormal size or quantity. During fetal development, COOH-truncated dystrophin is initially present in the myotubes of fetuses with Duchenne's muscular dystrophy, with the same location as in a normal fetus. It is

Table 6-7 Classifications of Muscular Dystrophy

Type	Sex Affected	Prevalence (Rate of Occurrence)	Symptoms	Diagnostic Studies	Usual Treatments
Duchenne's muscular dystrophy (major)	Males only, X-linked, recessive	1:33,000 births	Progressive muscle wasting and weakness leading to difficulty running, stair climbing, rising from the floor without use of the upper extremities for "climbing up the legs" support (positive Gower's sign); may have hypertrophy of calf muscles from fatty degeneration; loss of ability to walk; may develop scoliosis and joint contractures; many have cardiac sinus tachycardia and right ventricular hypertrophy; eventually develop dysrhythmias and heart failure; may have poor gastric motility; moderate mental retardation may be noted; pulmonary failure; waddling gait	Creatine phosphokinase elevated often up to 50 to 100 times normal (normal: cord blood, 70-380 U/L; 5-8 h, 24-1175 U/L; 24-33 h, 130-1200 U/L; 72-100 h, 87-725 U/L); electrocardiogram may show units of decreased amplitude and short duration; muscle biopsy shows dystrophic degeneration and fibrosis, with some regeneration but no dystrophin; dystrophin immunotesting; DNA mutation analysis by polymerase chain reaction and Southern blot analysis—help determine correct diagnosis; dystrophin RNA testing can detect some DNA mutations; electromyogram shows lack of contractility	Physical therapies; education of patient/family related to use of orthotic devices, braces, wheelchair, exercises, and use of parallel bars; myoblast cell therapy (recent development) with myoblasts injected into muscles of boys with Duchenne's—unknown yet if muscle functions will be restored; prednisone therapy has some short-term benefit to slow progression of muscle weakness; pulmonary breathing exercises; spinal fusion with metallic implants, such as Harrington, Luque, or Cotrel-Dubousset (CD) rods (less use of CD rods)
Becker's muscular dystrophy (milder form of Duchenne's)	Males; X-linked; female carriers	1:30,000 live births	Develops later in childhood than Duchenne's; has longer course and less severe involvement; can usually walk fast and longer in teen years; less muscle degeneration and fewer respiratory problems	Same as for Duchenne's; DNA analysis differentiates Duchenne's from Becker's; there is some dystrophin in muscle fibers on biopsy	Release of contracted muscles of hips, knees, ankles, and feet and tenotomy of tendons; electromyogram shows lack of contractility (same as for Duchenne's but later in course of disease)
Variant of Becker's muscular dystrophy: myalgia without weakness	Males only; female carriers	None noted yet	Milder symptoms than Becker's; less skeletal muscle weakness	Same as above	Individualized according to patient's symptoms; physical therapy, education as above
Emery-Dreifuss muscular dystrophy	Males only, X-linked recessive; female carriers; rarer autosomal dominant form has also been described		Muscle weakness in first few years of life; awkward gait; tendency to toewalk; by the middle of the second decade may see fixed equinus ankle deformities, flexion contracture of the elbows, extension contracture of the neck, tightness of the lumbar paravertebral muscles, and cardiac abnormalities (bradycardia; later complete heart block); patient is able to walk up to ages 50 to 60 years	Electromyogram shows muscle myopathy; muscle biopsy shows muscle myopathy; creatine phosphokinase: only mild to moderate elevations	Heel-cord lengthening for equinus contracture; transfer of posterior tibial tendon; release of elbow contractures; medications for cardiac involvement and use of a pacemaker if indicated
Facioscapulohumeral muscular dystrophy	X-linked, autosomal dominant; both sexes		Slowly progressive weakness of face as patient cannot close the eyes, whistle, purse the lips, or drink through a straw; weakness of shoulder girdle and shoulder muscle; begins in late childhood or early	Similar to above	Operative stabilization of shoulders to eliminate winging of scapulae; arthrodesis of scapula to ribs with metallic plate and screws; other treatments for individual patient needs

Data from Aminoff[1] and Scully.[49]

Continued

Table 6-7 Classifications of Muscular Dystrophy—cont'd

Type	Sex Affected	Prevalence (Rate of Occurrence)	Symptoms	Diagnostic Studies	Usual Treatments
			adulthood; scapular winging; limited abduction of arms; weakness in dorsiflexion of foot; foot drop; weakness of muscles of forearms, thighs, and pelvis; scoliosis is rarer than in other muscular dystrophies; affected person can usually live a full life		
Infantile facioscapulohumeral muscular dystrophy (variant of adult form)	Autosomal recessive		More severe than adult form; infant develops facial diplegia in early months of life; sensorineural hearing loss, often by age 5 years; scapular winging; lumbar lordosis; foot drop; loss of ability to walk by second decade of life; severe weakness of gluteus maximus muscles		Use of ankle-foot orthosis; heel-cord lengthening; use of spinal orthosis; scapulopexy; use of hearing aid; use of wheelchair; spinal arthrodesis
Limb-girdle muscular dystrophy	Autosomal recessive; autosomal dominant in some families		Shoulder and hip weakness; weak distal muscles of the limbs	Creatine phosphokinase levels may be 10 times higher than normal; electromyogram (EMG) shows myopathy; muscle biopsy shows myopathy	Similar to that for Becker's
Congenital muscular dystrophy (Fukuyama-type congenital muscular dystrophy is prevalent in Japanese infants)	Males and females; autosomal recessive		Affected babies are weak at birth; have severe joint stiffness; variable course—some have rapid degeneration and do not survive beyond first year, whereas others live full life expectancy; muscle/joint contractures; Japanese infants have central nervous system involvement	Creatine phosphokinase levels elevated; dystrophin gene or protein has no abnormalities; EMG abnormal; muscle biopsy shows perimysial and endomysial fibrosis	Passive ROM exercises; use of splints; osteotomy rarely done; use of various orthoses
Myototonic dystrophy	Males and females; autosomal dominant		Delayed muscle relaxation (delayed release of hand grip); frontal baldness in affected males; glaucoma in both sexes; normal muscle motor strength	Serum creatine phosphokinase levels normal; EMG shows "dive bomber pattern"—diagnostic of this condition	Treatments are individualized
Congenital myotonic dystrophy			Severe hypotonia; facial diplegia; long, narrow face; problems feeding, respiratory problems; club foot common; many have moderate to severe mental retardation; walking onset delayed	Radiologic studies of feet and lungs, prenatal gene study may show presence of this condition	Use of serial manipulation of feet; cast immobilization; ankle-foot orthosis; possible use of Lofstrand crutches for foot problems; use of foot-leg brace; spinal fusion for scoliosis if develops in adolescence

thought that the COOH-terminal domain of dystrophin is involved in the integration in the plasma membrane and that this domain is missing in the dystrophin of fetuses with Duchenne's muscular dystrophy mutations; it is a plausible proposal that dystrophin is degraded when no integration in the sarcolemma of the muscle cell can take place.[1] Without dystrophin, muscles suffer complete loss of function, resulting in progressive muscle wasting and leading to early death. Dystrophin deficiency probably leads to instability of the plasma membrane of skeletal muscle fibers, with two immediate consequences: leakage of cellular contents out of the cell and influx of extracellular material into the cell.[49] The extremely high muscle creatine kinase (CK) found in dystrophin-deficit species from birth is evidence of the efflux of cytoplasm from muscle fibers. However, the unregulated influx of extracellular material into the myofiber, especially calcium ions, usually leads to cell death. Biochemical and physiologic differences between specific muscle fibers and muscle groups may explain the different degrees of muscle cell death noted.

Diagnostic Studies and Findings

History: Parents note progressive muscle weakness and wasting; the child has delayed sitting, standing, or walking, seems clumsy, and falls easily and often; may not be able to whistle, purse lips, or close eyes

Physical examination: Marked wasting and muscle weakness progressing to increasing disability, deformity, and eventually death; loss of strength; atrophy of muscle mass; delayed motor development; difficulty in running, climbing, and riding tricycle; abnormal gait; enlarged calves (hypertrophy of muscle with fatty infiltration); positive Gowers' sign; process of rising from sitting or squatting position by using hands to "walk up" thighs until upright (Fig. 6-20); mild mental retardation; decreased deep tendon reflexes

Roentgenograms: Contractures of hips, knees, and ankles; lordosis of lumbar spine; scoliosis; may have megacolon or volvulus of bowel

Muscle biopsy: Reveals lack of dystrophin degeneration of muscle fibers; fatty infiltration of muscle fibers

Blood serum studies: Greatly elevated creatine phosphokinase (CPK) levels (diagnostic of Duchenne's muscular dystrophy), with lesser elevations in the other forms of muscular dystrophy; serum glutamic-oxaloacetic transaminase (SGOT) levels are sharply elevated

Electromyogram (EMG) studies: Reveal decreased amplitude and duration of motor unit potentials[1]

Multidisciplinary Plan

Surgery

Release of contractures

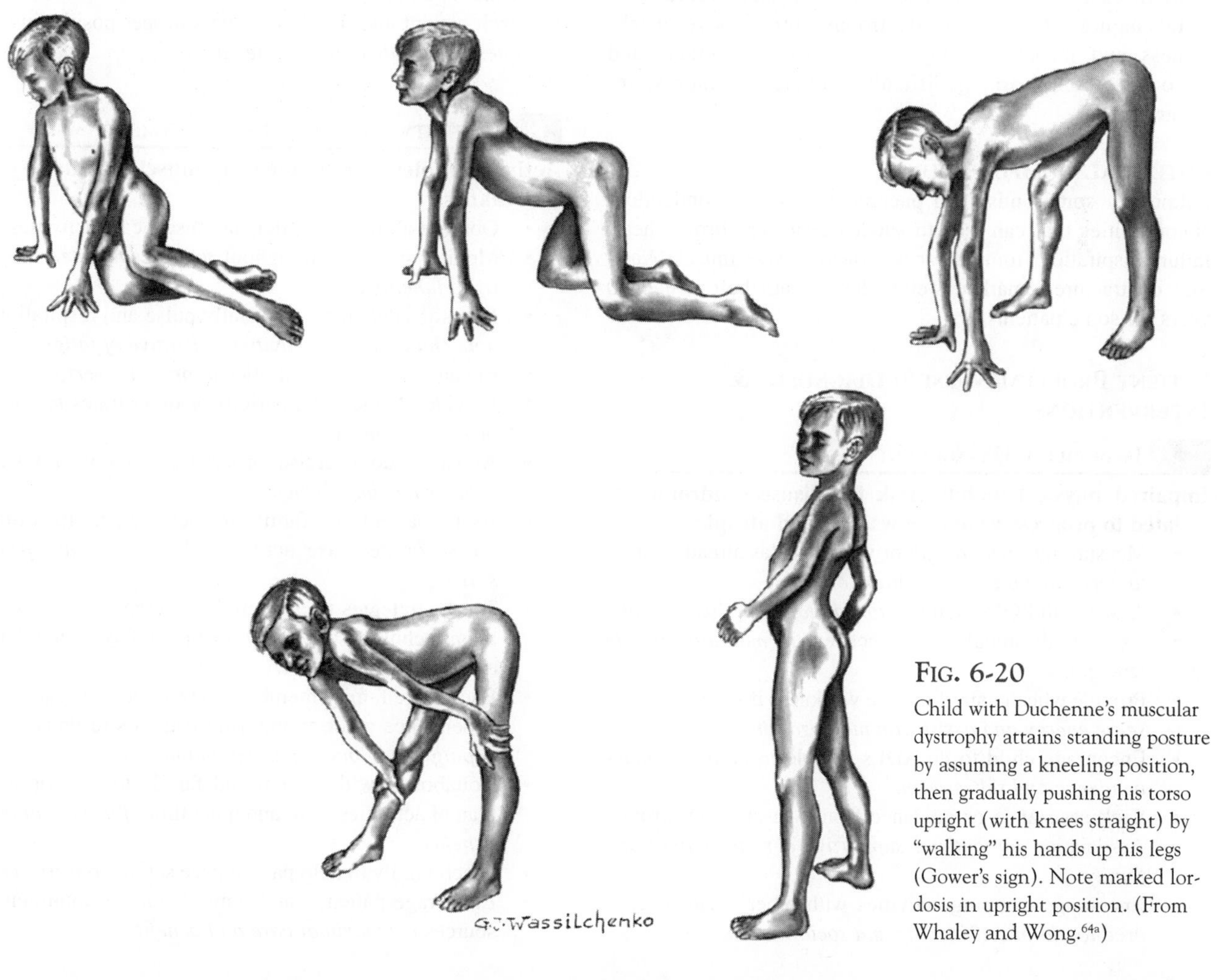

Fig. 6-20

Child with Duchenne's muscular dystrophy attains standing posture by assuming a kneeling position, then gradually pushing his torso upright (with knees straight) by "walking" his hands up his legs (Gower's sign). Note marked lordosis in upright position. (From Whaley and Wong.[64a])

General Management

Gentle ROM exercises to maintain functions
Assistance with ADLs
Use of brace to affected joints to prevent contractures
Consultation with Muscular Dystrophy Association for guidance and support as needed
Use of wheelchair for movement from place to place
Home teaching for educational progress
Specialized nursing assistants as muscular weakness progresses for home care
Nutritional guidance as needed
Genetic counseling

NURSING CARE

NURSING ASSESSMENT

Whole body assessment: Muscle strength, grip, pull and push strength; deep tendon reflexes charted; presence of contractures; muscle atrophy; age-related motor development; gait may be "waddling" as a result of pelvic muscle weakness; posture: lordosis, scoliosis; enlarged calves from fatty deposits; age-related mental development

Systemic processes: Pulmonary functions compromised, breath sounds, cardiac size and heart sounds, systemic infections, obesity or weight loss

Psychosocial concerns: Parental guilt related to transmittal of disease, self-concept and independence, eventual fatal nature of muscular dystrophy, progressive weakness and muscle atrophy, loss of social contacts and socialization, learning difficulties related to mental retardation

POTENTIAL COMPLICATIONS

Pulmonary compromise and pneumonia; cardiac conduction; abnormalities that can lead to sudden death or chronic heart failure; aspiration from bulbar weakness; severe muscle wasting; contractures; marked weight loss; death before age 30 years for some patients

PATIENT PROBLEM/NURSING DIAGNOSES & INTERVENTIONS

NIC IMMOBILITY MANAGEMENT

Impaired physical mobility/risk for disuse syndrome related to progressive muscle wasting and atrophy

- Measure muscle strength or weakness (as already listed) *to determine present condition.*
- Assist with ROM exercises *to maintain functions as able.*
- Assist with ambulation, if needed, *to maintain muscle strength.*
- Provide wheelchair, if muscle weakness if severe, *to conserve energy and assist with mobilization.*
- Encourage child to do ADLs as able *to maintain independence and self-esteem.*
- Seek assistance or guidance from Muscular Dystrophy Association *for optimal supportive care to patient and family.*
- Encourage camping activities with other disabled children *to aid in self-identity and socialization.*

NIC SKIN/WOUND MANAGEMENT

Risk for impaired skin integrity related to pressure on bony prominences from wheelchair or brace use

- Observe all skin surfaces and bony prominences carefully *to note condition.*
- Assist to bathe and carefully dry all skin surfaces *to prevent skin abrasion or maceration.*
- Teach patient and family to do "minishifts" *to relieve pressure on bony prominences and skin surfaces.*
- Apply lotion to skin tissues *to help keep skin surfaces supple and moisturized.*
- Encourage fluid intake *to maintain skin hydration.*
- Monitor patient for bowel or bladder incontinence, diarrhea, and excess perspiration *to prevent skin maceration or breakdown.*
- Encourage changing from wheelchair to bed or couch *to change pressure areas to prevent breakdown.*
- Use elbow and heel pads, pillows, or blankets *to relieve pressure on bony prominences and skin surfaces.*
- Turn or reposition patient every 2 hours *to promote circulation.*
- Lift patient gently and carefully *to avoid breaking skin surfaces with fingernails or fingers.*
- Have patient help lift self to prevent dragging body *to prevent shear forces that could break skin.*
- Keep head of bed in low-Fowler's position (about 30-degree elevation) *to prevent skin shearing forces and prevent ischemia of bony prominences.*
- Teach patient and family members proper positioning principles *to provide optimal safe care.*

NIC ACTIVITY AND EXERCISE MANAGEMENT

Activity intolerance related to muscle pathology and weakness

- Observe ability to participate in self-care activities.
- Monitor strength throughout activities *to determine ability to function.*
- Monitor vital signs, especially pulse and respirations, *to note changes with activities indicative of fatigue.*
- Encourage to pace activities *to prevent overtiring.*
- Provide planned rest periods or quiet times *to conserve or restore energy.*
- Assist to do exercise programs when well rested *to achieve maximal benefits.*
- Assist patient and family to identify activities that increase or decrease activity tolerance *to aid problem solving.*
- Teach strategies to aid activity tolerance, such as relaxation techniques, imagery, or biofeedback (age dependent), *to increase activity tolerance.*
- Encourage family members to promote self-care and independence while monitoring patient's responses *to aid coping behaviors of patient and family.*
- Collaborate with patient and family to develop a daily plan of activities, rest, and quiet times *for optimal patient benefits.*
- Teach family to help patient pace self *to conserve energy.*
- Encourage patient's and family's use of community resources *for maximal care and benefits.*

NIC Life Span Care

Readiness for enhanced family coping related to ultimate death of child with muscular dystrophy

- Assist patient and family to identify changes in family situation and dynamics because of illness and its eventual outcome *to determine effects and possible options for change.*
- Assist patient and family to adapt to muscular dystrophy and to continue living rather than dealing with dying *to foster adjustment to muscular dystrophy.*
- Offer support and guidance to help family deal with the stress of an ill child on individual members and the family as a whole *to determine requirements for resources if needed.*
- Assist family's problem-solving efforts by clarifying or providing information, discussing alternatives, summarizing current and future needs, and discussing family and individual roles *to help maintain day-to-day coping behaviors.*
- Help family members and patient plan and implement home maintenance or changes (e.g., ramps, wheelchair access, van for transporting) *to promote family and patient independence and comfort.*
- Encourage use of Muscular Dystrophy Association support groups *to aid adjustments to changing family situation.*
- Teach family strategies to access community resources *to maximize growth.*
- Encourage patient's participation in Special Olympics or other group activities for maintenance of self-esteem and achievement *to aid acceptance and adaptation to own circumstances.*

NIC Respiratory Management

Impaired gas exchange related to weak pulmonary muscles and kyphoscoliosis

- Observe use of accessory respiratory muscles, dyspnea, production of sputum, ability to cough; listen to breath sounds.
- Monitor vital signs frequently *to detect early signs of infection.*
- Encourage deep-breathing exercises *to promote maximal oxygenation.*
- Reposition patient from side to side with head lower than body *to promote postural drainage* if able.
- Encourage use of incentive spirometry *to promote pulmonary functions.*
- If necessary, and patient is congested and unable to cough, suction as needed *to maintain clear respiratory passages.*
- Use aseptic techniques for suctioning *to avoid introducing infective organisms.*
- Teach patient and family members positioning, postural drainage, and suctioning, if necessary, *to lessen their anxiety and increase comfort.*

NIC Tissue Perfusion Management

Risk for decreased cardiac output related to cardiac muscle decompensation

- Check vital signs, heart sounds, and pulse for rate or dysrhythmias to determine present condition.
- Administer prescribed medications, if any, *to strengthen cardiac functions.*
- Observe for edema throughout body *to determine peripheral circulatory status or decompensation.*
- Monitor patient's color and mental alertness *to determine peripheral circulation and oxygenation.*
- Monitor ECG, if on monitoring, for changes in rhythms *to determine need for additional medications or other treatments.*
- If on IV therapy, monitor type of solution and medication infusion, rate, and effects on patient *to determine if changes are needed.*

Patient Education/Continuum of Care Plan

1. Reiterate explanations of muscular dystrophy and specific status of patient's condition, treatment regimen, and prognosis, if pertinent.
2. Clarify need for exercise programs, use of ambulatory aid as needed, and positions required for safety and to maintain muscular and skin integrity as well as cardiac and pulmonary functions.
3. Emphasize patient's participation in self-care, sports, or other activities for living life to fullest possible.
4. Encourage use of Muscular Dystrophy Association services and support groups for long-term benefits.
5. Refer family to community nursing services for follow-up care.

Evaluation/Patient Outcomes

Immobility Management: Patient uses wheelchair or walker to move about when able. Patient does some self-care when strength is present—washes face by self. Patient and family use community muscular dystrophy resources. Patient no longer goes on camping trips.

Skin/Wound Management: Patient's skin tissues remain intact; uses padding in wheelchair. Patient mini-shifts frequently and lies on chaise lounge to alter pressure on skin. Patient has normal fluid intake to hydrate skin. Family members use proper litfing and positioning techniques to avoid skin trauma.

Activity and Exercise Management: Patient participates in planned daily activities and education as strength and energy permit. Patient assists in exercise program when able. Patient uses relaxation techniques to conserve energy, takes rest and nap breaks appropriately, and paces self as able. Patient uses physical therapist to assist with strengthening exercises.

Life Span Care: Patient and family continue positive coping behaviors with realistic outlook related to patient's prognosis. Family encourages patient to participate in age-appropriate activities with use of community resources. Muscular Dystrophy Association offers guidance and educational assistance as requested by family. Patient observes rather than participates in Special Olympics activities because of limited energy reserves.

Respiratory Management: Patient does deep breathing exercises satisfactorily. Breath sounds remain clear. Cough is nonproductive.

Tissue Perfusion Management: Vital signs are within norms for age. Patient takes prescribed medications at appropriate times. Patient has mild peripheral edema of feet and legs. Color remains pale because of mild anemia.

BONE DEFICIENCY DISEASE

OSTEOPOROSIS

Osteoporosis is a systemic condition of overall reduction in bone mass or density in which bone resorption has outstripped bone formation, thereby upsetting the normal balance.

The bone that remains is biochemically normal, but there is not enough of it to maintain skeletal integrity and mechanical support.[39] Osteoporosis is classified as type I—primary, consisting of juvenile and postmenopausal osteoporosis—and type II—secondary, consisting of cases caused by endocrine abnormalities; estrogen and testosterone deficiency; medications such as corticosteroids, heparin, anticonvulsants, and methotrexate; and chronic diseases of the lungs or kidneys. The disease may be generalized throughout the body or only in a region or localized area.

Osteoporosis is most common in older, postmenopausal women, probably because of endocrine involution and inactivity. Younger people may develop osteoporosis after severe injuries, with paralysis and long periods of immobility. People with rheumatoid arthritis, endocrine abnormalities, and chronic pulmonary or renal disease may also develop osteoporosis. Men can develop osteoporosis but do so less frequently than women (ratio is 1:4). It has been estimated that 33% of postmenopausal women have osteoporosis, and risk of an osteoporotic fracture is one in three women and one in six men.[39]

One goal in the care of persons with osteoporosis is to prevent fractures, with their resultant morbidity and mortality. Ninety percent of the men and women who suffer a hip fracture are over age 70 years; there is a 20% mortality in this group.[56] Annual expenditure on short-term care after an osteoporotic hip fracture exceeds $8 million. There are 1.5 million osteoporotic fractures annually, including 250,000 hip, 250,000 wrist, and 55,000 vertebral fractures.[29] About 20% of patients with hip fractures will die within the first 4 to 6 months, and 50% will be unable to walk independently, requiring long-term nursing home care.[29]

PATHOPHYSIOLOGY

Osteoporosis develops when the bone remodeling cycle—process of bone formation or resorption—is disrupted for whatever reason or cause. More bone is lost or resorbed than is formed. The loss may be fast or slow, being relatively fast in the first 3 to 5 years after menopause, then slowing with less loss over the remaining lifetime of the person. The normal remodeling cycle usually takes about 4 months; however, in a person with osteoporosis, the cycle may take up to 2 years to complete a cycle. The rate of resorption is increased, while the rate of new bone formation is delayed, resulting in a disrupted cycle and a decrease in total bone mass. Some hormones or drugs may cause an imbalance in the rate of resorption and the rate of new bone formation, also leading to either a speedup in resorption or a slowdown in formation, thereby weakening the remaining bone. Age-related losses are greater in women than in men because men have greater overall bone mass than women, so their losses are not as critical as losses for women.

The vertebral column's overall mass is diminished, leading to increasing kyphosis and loss of height. Backache is common, and there may be radiation to the buttocks or down the legs.

Risk factors for osteoporosis include a family history of osteoporotic fracture; small stature; fair, pale skin; thinness (being overweight or obese is protective); early menopause, late menarche, exercise-induced amenorrhea, or oophorectomy; sedentary lifestyle; smoking; alcohol intake (may both increase and decrease bone density); rheumatoid arthritis treated with corticosteroids (osteoporotic fractures develop in an estimated 30% to 50% of glucocorticoid-treated patients[29]; paralytic conditions; Caucasian rather than African-American; and women more than men. Also, hyperparathyroidism and insufficient intake of calcium or excess intake of proteins may lead to the development of osteoporosis.

DIAGNOSTIC STUDIES AND FINDINGS

History: Prolonged immobility; menopause; decreased activity; oophorectomy; chronic disease; smoker; excessive alcohol intake; bed rest; lack of weight bearing (see risk factors already listed)

Physical examination: Increased kyphosis; backache or neck ache with radiation to legs and arms; fractures; small frame; decreased height; fair, thin

Roentgenograms: Soft vertebral bodies that are indented by the disks and become biconcave; vertebrae possibly wedged from fractures; thoracic vertebral curvature increased; absorptiometry studies: single-photon, dual-photon, dual-energy x-ray, and quantitative computed tomography; each will show specific peripheral bone or cortical bone mass results according to its purpose

Blood serum study: Low levels of alkaline phosphatase (alkaline phosphatase increases bone formation); high levels of serum total hydroxyproline (increases bone resorption); high levels of serum osteocalcin may indicate a high rate of bone loss,[29] low serum calcium levels

MULTIDISCIPLINARY PLAN

Medications

See Table 6-8 for list of new drug treatments.

Etidronate (Didronel), 400 mg daily for 2 weeks only every 3 months with 1500 mg calcium daily during etidronate-free periods; etidronate has been shown to be an effective, safe, nonhormonal treatment to prevent early menopausal bone loss[22]

Estrogens for postmenopausal women who have undergone hysterectomy; because of increased risk of endometrial cancer and cardiovascular complications, use of estrogens for

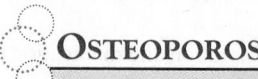

Table 6-8 New Drugs as Treatments for Osteoporosis

Class	Dose	Benefits	Side Effects/Risks
BIPHOSPHONATES			
Alendronate (Fosamax)	Prevention: 5 mg/day Treatment: 10 mg daily on an empty stomach	Reduces bone loss in postmenopausal women; increases bone density at spine and hip; reduces risk of spinal or hip fractures; slows loss of height; impairs function of osteoclasts	Abdominal or musculoskeletal pain; nausea; heartburn; esophageal irritation (minimized) if person remains upright for at least 30 minutes after taking.
Pamidronate (Aredia)	30 mg IV every 3 months	Increases lumbar density; decreases femoral neck fractures	Ototoxicity rare but can occur; similar effects as alendronate
Risedronate (Actonel)	25 mg/day with glass of water 30 minutes before eating	Increases bone mass; aids in glucocortoid-induced osteoporosis	Gastrointestinal irritation (less if person remains upright for 30 minutes after taking)
Clodronate*	200 mg IV every month	Decrease in loss of spinal density; decrease in vertebral fracture	Unknown at present
Tiludronate (Skelid)	100 mg/day	Prevents postmenopausal bone loss; decreases activity of osteoclasts in paraplegia and immobilization; preserves bone mass and a parallel increase in biomechanical bone strength	Stomach upset; heartburn; intestinal cramping
SELECTIVE ESTROGEN RECEPTOR MODULATORS (SERMS)			
Raloxifene (Evista)	60 mg/day PO	Prevents bone loss at spine, hip, and whole body; may protect against heart disease; does not increase risks of breast cancer	Hot flashes; deep vein thrombosis
HORMONE			
Calcitonin (Miacalcin)	Nasal spray: 200 U daily; parenteral: 100 U, SC or IM 3 times weekly	Slows bone loss in postmenopausal women; increases spinal bone density; relieves pain associated with bone fracture; reduces risk of hip or spinal fracture	Injection may cause allergic reaction; flushing of face, hand; urinary frequency; nausea; skin rash; nasal spray may cause runny nose and itching of nasal mucosa
OTHER			
Sodium fluoride, sustained release	Individualized, may be given with calcium citrate	Decreased spinal and hip fracture rates; increased femoral neck bone density; increased cancellous and trabecular bone quality	Gastrointestinal irritation; lower extremity pain

From Licata AA,[30] National Osteoporosis Foundation, 1998, Washington, DC.

osteoporosis is controversial; however, estrogen-progestin combinations are now advocated as estrogen 0.625 mg/day; progesterone may be added to the estrogen (estrogen taken for 25 days/mo, combined with progesterone for days 16-25, then both stopped for rest of month), or 50-100 μg/day of transdermal estradiol; addition of progesterone may not protect against breast cancer risk, although to date there is no increase in breast cancer related to these medications

Testosterone in individual doses for men

Nutritional Supplements

Calcitonin, subcutaneously, individualized dosage

Calcium carbonate, 1 g/day

Vitamin D, 50,000 IU once or twice per week

General Management

Application of back corset or neck support to prevent stress fractures

Ambulation and maintaining active weight-bearing exercises to hold calcium in bones

Passive exercises if unable to do active exercises

Deep breathing exercises to maintain pulmonary healthy tissues

NURSING CARE

NURSING ASSESSMENT

Skeletal tissues: Degree of strength in muscles and joints, ROM of joints; presence of increased kyphosis; loss of height over time; fracture of hip, compression fractures of vertebrae, or fracture of radius

Other tissues: Fair skin, thin; backache; neck pain; pain radiating to legs and arms; effects of pain on mobility

Psychosocial concerns: Self-concept: disturbances in self-esteem and body image; alteration in physical mobility, possibility of fractures; pain in neck, back, or hips; fear of falling; fear of fracture

POTENTIAL COMPLICATIONS

Fracture of vertebra, hip, wrist, or other bone; increased kyphosis; respiratory compromise; fat embolism after surgical repair of fracture; shock or hemorrhage

Patient Problems/Nursing Diagnoses & Interventions

NIC Immobility Management

The use of splinting and a wheelchair may be required by some patients with severe osteoporosis.

Impaired physical mobility related to decreased bone mass

- Perform ROM exercises actively and passively if necessary *to maintain muscle and joint strength.*
- Use sling or ambulatory aid (cane or crutch) if needed *to lessen stress on bones.*
- Apply back corset or neck collar *to lessen pain and increase mobility* (use is controversial because such aids limit muscle movements).
- Encourage active exercises in water *to maintain ROM of joints* (water immersion markedly decreases effects of gravity on bones and joints).
- Encourage weight-bearing exercises *to stimulate bone mineralization*

NIC Physical Comfort Promotion

Acute or chronic pain

- Observe limitations of movement because of acute pain in thoracic, lumbosacral, and hip areas *to determine sites and amount of pain.*
- Assist with moving if needed *to lessen acute symptoms.*
- Gently massage tender and painful areas *to ease soreness and pain.*
- Administer medications as prescribed for pain; monitor responses or modifications of pain *to determine if changes are needed.*
- Administer medications to counteract osteoporosis as prescribed (see Table 6-8) *to slow or stop continuation of condition.*
- Discuss intake of calcium *to improve concentration in serum and bones.*

NIC Coping Assistance

Risk for situational low self-esteem and ineffective role performance related to kyphosis and associated pain

- Observe ability to carry out self-care, ADLs, and usual roles.
- Explain or clarify the processes accompanying menopause as normal and natural *to ease concerns.*
- Encourage usual ADLs and other activities *to maintain bone mass.*
- Encourage fashion consultation for clothing to lessen evidence of increased kyphosis *to increase self-esteem.*
- Consult with physical and occupational therapists for techniques to improve performance *to maintain usual self-care and roles.*

NIC Respiratory Management

Impaired gas exchange related to kyphosis

- Check respiratory rates, depth, and breath sounds *to evaluate effects of kyphosis.*
- Encourage attempts to maintain upright posture *to aid ventilation.*
- Check vital capacity to determine if level is satisfactory.
- Encourage deep-breathing exercises *to aid gas exchanges.*
- Encourage shoulder-strengthening exercises *to enhance breathing.*
- Suggest lying on back *to lessen furthering of kyphosis* (may not be able to lie completely on back).

NIC Risk Management

Risk for injury related to fall or fracture of radius, hip, or vertebra

- Observe ability to move easily and freely or limitations on movements.
- Observe gait and placement of feet when walking, especially in postmenopausal women, to determine risk of a hip fracture. (With aging the normal 150-degree angle of fit of the femur into the acetabulum shortens to 135 degrees, resulting in a more varus placing of each foot when walking. Varus placement puts a strain on the neck of the femur, which in the case of a minor twist in the presence of osteoporosis can easily lead to a fractured femoral neck.)
- Caution to walk carefully and to observe surfaces ahead to lessen possibility of a slip, ankle twist, or fall *to prevent possible fracture.*
- Encourage gentle extension hip exercises in pool (with water above waist level to negate effects of gravity) *to increase hip ROM to help maintain 150-degree angle of hip and femur.*
- Instruct to remove loose rugs or carpeting and long cords from walking areas *to lessen danger of tripping or falling.*
- Clarify effects of shadows or wearing bifocal glasses as influencing depth perception when walking on uneven surfaces *to lessen risk of falling.*
- Encourage wearing of well-repaired shoes and, in rain and in icy conditions, wearing proper footwear *to prevent slipping and falling.*

Patient Education/Continuum of Care Plan

1. Discuss perception of osteoporosis as "thin" bones; bone mass is decreased, but bones are not thinner; there is just less bone mass in body.
2. List advantages of active weight-bearing exercises and activity to maintain bone mass and calcium in bones.
3. Clarify effects of increased calcium intake and reiterate need for serial examinations of serum calcium levels.
4. Encourage patient to read current research data and treatment modalities and discuss with physician.
5. Encourage compliance with taking prescribed medications correctly to increase bone mass.
6. Encourage use of community resources and facilities to lessen effects of osteoporosis on self and family.
7. Contact National Osteoporosis Foundation for current information for family or patient use as needed.

Evaluation/Patient Outcomes

Immobility Management and Physical Comfort Promotion: Patient maintains pain-free ambulation and joint mobility. Patient's disease is controlled by medication, calcium intake, or activity. Patient has no continued major loss of bone density on x-ray studies.

Coping Assistance: Patient has positive self-esteem and has maintained roles; is outward looking; participates in usual roles and responsibilities; wears clothing to disguise kyphosis.

Respiratory Management: Patient has satisfactory gas exchange. Patient has normal color, respiratory rates, and depth; vital capacity is in low normal range.

Risk Management: Patient does not experience a fractured radius, vertebra, or hip. Patient exercises in water four or more times weekly.

TRAUMA

Musculoskeletal injury or trauma is a major factor in the care of persons in all age groups. Injuries become more common as persons grow and age. By the year 2040, more than 20% of the people in the United States will be over age 65 years.[59] Persons in this age group suffer more injuries, with morbidity and mortality three times higher than their representative numbers.[59] Many of the 6.2 million persons with fractures of the hip or other musculoskeletal fractures in the United States have difficulty healing because of poor nutritional status, decreased cardiopulmonary reserves, and an increased propensity for extensive bleeding after their fractures. More services from health-care providers are required to prevent infections, pulmonary problems, or thrombus formations and to assist these injured persons to regain their health and mobility, when possible. National competitive and regulatory pressures are dramatically changing health-care programs[57] and will continue to have marked impact on the care of all persons experiencing trauma and injuries. Musculoskeletal conditions and trauma rank second only to respiratory conditions as reasons for hospitalization among the older population. Even though some injuries are not fatal or life threatening, there is no assurance that there will be no future pain, disability, or periods of decreased mobility that will further tax health-care facilities, personnel, or community resources.

Less serious injuries comprise bruises or contusions of the skin; strain (stretch) of tendon or ligament fibers; and sprains (tearing) of some, many, or all tendons, ligaments, or even bones in and around a joint. These three conditions (contusion, strain, or sprain) have similar initial signs, require similar assessments, and have similar treatments.

CONTUSIONS, STRAINS, AND SPRAINS

A contusion is a bruise without an external break in the skin.

A strain is a "pull" in a muscle, ligament, or tendon caused by excessive stretch.

A sprain is a tear in a muscle, ligament, or tendon; it may be mild to severe.

PATHOPHYSIOLOGY

Contusions are bruises from sudden external pressure that tears the subcutaneous circulatory veins and capillaries. Bleeding occurs in the injured subcutaneous tissues and is noted by bluish discoloration of the injured tissues, with edema or swelling accompanying the vessel or tissue injury. Depending on the extent or severity of the contusion, the edema and discoloration begin to abate in 48 to 72 hours. A "charley horse" is a contusion of a muscle.

A *strain* is caused by an undue force applied to muscles, ligaments, or tendons. It stretches the fibers, causing a temporary weakness, numbness, and some bleeding if the veins or capillaries within the injured tissues are excessively stretched. The weakness may last 24 to 72 hours, but the numbness usually disappears within hours. Bleeding may continue for 30 minutes or longer unless pressure or cold is applied to stop it. A strained muscle, ligament, or tendon can regain its full function after conservative treatments, which are discussed later. Muscles that are frequently strained are the hamstring and pectineus (hamstring and groin pull, respectively).

A *sprain* is a partial or full tearing off or away (avulsion) of one or more ligaments or tendons or portions of the bone in and around a joint. Sprains are caused by undue force, twisting, or pull exerted during sports or work activities. Most sprains occur in the ankles, wrists, fingers, and toes. Other joints can be sprained if undue force, pressure, or pull is applied without relief.

Sprains are classified as first degree (some tearing of fibers with some bleeding); second degree (moderate tearing and more extensive bleeding or hemorrhage); and third degree (full tearing or avulsion of the tendon or ligament from its bony attachment, with or without some bone attached, accompanied by marked hemorrhage, pain, edema, and loss of function).

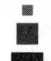

DIAGNOSTIC STUDIES AND FINDINGS

History: Pressure applied to area, usually unanticipated; undue force; pull without relief (if strain or sprain); pain with use; mechanism of injury; surface where injury occurred

Physical examination: Skin, circulatory, and musculoskeletal signs as described on pp. 327-330.

MULTIDISCIPLINARY PLAN

See Multidisciplinary Plan table.

NURSING CARE

NURSING ASSESSMENT

See Assessment Considerations table.

POTENTIAL COMPLICATIONS

Posttraumatic arthritis of joint; avascular necrosis of bone with avulsion injury, meniscal degeneration

PATIENT PROBLEMS/NURSING DIAGNOSES & INTERVENTIONS

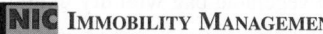

NIC IMMOBILITY MANAGEMENT

Impaired physical mobility related to specific injury

- Observe injured area *to determine condition.*
- Handle injured tissues gently *to avoid further trauma.*

Multidisciplinary Plan

	Contusion	Strain	Sprain
SURGERY			
Open reduction and repair of torn or avulsed tissues	None	None	May be needed for full joint function; ligament or tendon may be reattached or may need to be removed and replaced if severely damaged; avulsed fragment may require screw for reattachment to bone
MEDICATIONS			
Analgesics	None	Aspirin, 300-600 mg qid prn; acetaminophen, 300-600 mg qid prn	Aspirin, 300-1000 mg q4h to relieve pain and inflammation; NSAIDs in individualized doses
Narcotics	None	None	Codeine, 30-60 mg po q4-6h for severe pain
GENERAL MANAGEMENT*			
Cold application	Ice application for 24 h	Ice application for 24 h	Ice application for 24 h or longer
External wrap	None	Elastic wrap or sling	Elastic wrap or soft cast; sling for upper extremity
Elevation	None	Elevate if extremity	Elevate if extremity
Exercises (ROM)	Gentle exercises after 48 h	Gentle exercises and use as able after 48 h	No exercises while severe edema and bleeding present; gentle exercises may be begun after 3-5 days, depending on tissue injured and severity of sprain
Weight bearing	Full use	As able; full use	Cessation of weight bearing with crutch use for 7 days or longer, depending on tissues involved

*Part of treatment of musculoskeletal injuries referred to as RICE:

R = Rest for injured part. May be temporary nonuse or more prolonged non–weight bearing, depending on injury.

I = Ice. Applications of ice lessen bleeding and edema. Ice is needed for 24-72 h or longer, depending on the injury.

C = Compression. Elastic bandages or at times a circular cast may be used for compression. Compression is to be of the *venous* vessels; therefore the wrapping should be applied only snugly enough that it does not compromise the *arterial* flow. Application of the bandages or cast should be from distal to proximal on the limb to aid venous constriction and venous return.

E = Elevation. The injured part is elevated to heart level to aid venous return and thereby lessen edema. Elevation of the part too high (or above the patient's central venous pressure) should be avoided because too high elevation could impede arterial flow and increase rather than decrease edema. Normal central venous pressure (CVP) ranges from 6-13 cm H_2O pressure. Elevation should not exceed 5 inches above the heart level (2.5 cm = 1 inch; 5 inches = 12.5 cm), assuming the patient has the highest CVP. Accurate elevation can be achieved if the patient has a CVP line in place. If not, elevation to heart level is safest.

Assessment Considerations

	Contusion	Strain	Sprain
Specific tissue or tissues	Skin and subcutaneous tissue	Tendon, ligament, bone, and entire joint	Same as with strain
Local processes	Bluish discoloration and edema; skin openings; pain; soreness	Weakness, numbness, bleeding noted by discoloration; assess for skin opening; joint mobility, stability, or laxness; pain; edema; ability to bear weight or use joint normally	Same as with strain only more pronounced: more edema, bleeding, and discoloration; inability to use joint, muscles, or tendons normally; cannot bear weight; pain more severe and constant
Systemic processes	Other bruises or contusions possibly present	Distant joints possibly sore from initial injury; generalized muscle soreness	Same as with strain
Psychosocial concerns	Minor discomfort; no major concerns	Temporary (24-72 h) impairment of mobility	Mobility impaired for varying periods (10 days to 3 or more weeks); may develop posttraumatic arthritis later if severe sprain

- Provide support under affected joints *to prevent lever actions of muscles.*
- Apply ice or bag of frozen vegetables to site *to decrease edema and bleeding.*
- Cover ice bag or frozen vegetable bag with dry cloth *to prevent tissue damage.*
- Elevate injured part or parts to heart level *to decrease edema and increase venous return.*
- Assist with ROM exercises when allowed; perform as able *to increase mobility.*
- Use sling for upper extremity injury *to lessen pain and increase comfort.*
- Perform neurovascular checks (see p. 331) as prescribed *to determine condition and to note possible complications.*
- Assist with crutch walking, as needed; measure crutches for proper length *to provide safety.*

- Caution patient not to rest axillae on crutches *to prevent nerve damage.*
- Administer analgesics and NSAIDs *to lessen pain and aid in relief of inflammation.*
- Assist with personal hygiene as needed *to maintain healthy tissues.*
- Assess concerns with immobility *to lessen anxiety.*

NIC Coping Assistance

Ineffective role performance related to injury

- Assure patient that full function should be regained after treatment *to ease concerns.*
- Encourage resumption of ADLs and usual activities as able *to enhance self-concept.*
- Caution about possibility of reinjury if self-care and preventive measures are not learned or practiced.
- Discuss concerns related to employment or future sports activities *to elicit thoughts or fears, if present.*

Patient Education/Continuum of Care Plan

1. Be sure the patient knows the nature and extent of injury.
2. Demonstrate the use of crutches, if necessary.
3. Discuss the effects of cold, then hot applications if the patient has future trauma.
4. Consult physicians or trainers to teach the patient preventive measures in sports or exercise activities.
5. Clarify with the patient or family the use of medications, dressing changes, and need for limited mobility, if necessary.
6. List and explain the signs and symptoms that require physician's attention.

Evaluation/Patient Outcomes

Immobility Management: Patient recovers ROM of affected joints and tissues without limitations and experiences no pain, tenderness, limitation of motion, edema, or loss of function of tissues. Patient needs no long-term analgesic medication.

Coping Assistance: Patient regains social interactions and returns to usual family, social, and employment roles.

Dislocation

A dislocation is a displacement of a part, usually a bone, from its normal anatomic position within a joint.

Dislocations may be complete or partial (called subluxations). They usually result from a blow, force, or pull strong enough to cause the bone to be forced or pulled from the joint. For some people, repeated dislocations are common because of repetitive or chronic trauma to a joint, which weakens ligaments, tendons, or muscles. Some joints, such as the shoulder, elbow, fingers, and knee, are more commonly dislocated than others.

Subluxations are partial dislocations and are more common in people with long-standing rheumatoid arthritis because fibrosis shortens the tendons, forcing the bones to sublux; this is referred to as a swan-neck or boutonniere deformity, common in some arthritic conditions.

Pathophysiology

The major signs of dislocation are deformity and inability to use the part or joint normally. Tendons or ligaments can become interposed, making reduction and replacement of the dislocated part into the joint difficult or impossible without open surgical reduction. Reduction and replacement within the joint space without surgery are more commonly impossible in cases of subluxations associated with rheumatoid arthritis because of the shortening of the tendon from inflammatory changes. Trapping of nerves or blood vessels between dislocated bones is a surgical emergency.

Diagnostic Studies and Findings

History: Repetitive trauma, such as throwing or hitting a ball; presence of rheumatoid arthritis; acute injury during work, recreational activity, or auto accident

Physical examination: Head or other part of bone out of the normal anatomic position; tendon shortening; deformity; inability to use joint normally; tenderness; possible edema and bleeding into joint tissues

Roentgenogram: Dislocated parts noted; position of parts not in normal anatomic sites

Multidisciplinary Plan

Surgery

Open reduction of the dislocated bone or bones, if not able to reduce dislocation manually or if nerve is trapped

Tendon debridement or transplant for swan-neck and boutonniere deformities to prevent recurrence

General Management

Manual closed reduction of the dislocated bone into the joint

Application of a sling for the upper extremity to lessen stress on shoulder joint

Elastic wrap of lower extremity joint

Ice applications for 24 hours, then warm applications to joint

Active exercises under physical therapist's direction as prescribed by physician

Application of skin traction, especially Buck extension, for a short period of time if hip dislocated with acetabular damage

NURSING CARE

Nursing Assessment

Joint and bones of joint: Palpation of dislocated part out of usual position; deformity; inability to use joint normally; tenderness, soreness, or pain; bleeding into joint

Psychosocial concerns: Self-concept if repeated dislocations, disturbances of role expectations, impaired mobility and ROM

Potential Complications

Nerve entrapment, avascular necrosis if blood vessel inflow is disrupted, posttraumatic arthritis, permanent deformity

Patient Problems/Nursing Diagnoses & Interventions

NIC Immobility Management

Impaired physical mobility related to dislocation

- Observe effects of dislocation on patient's mobility and ROM of affected joint.
- Apply sling or elastic wrap *to maintain reduction.*
- Perform ROM to all unaffected joints *to maintain strength.*
- Assist with ambulation four or more times daily *to maintain strength,* depending on which joint is involved.

NIC Coping Assistance

Ineffective role performance related to injury or condition

- Clarify any statements of limitations.
- Assure that full ROM should be regained after reduction and healing *to lessen concerns.*
- Assist with hygiene and ADLs as needed *to lessen patient stress.*
- Provide postoperative care as needed *to aid recovery.*

NIC Risk Management

Risk for injury related to shortening, laxity, or weakness of joint ligaments, tendons, or muscles

- Check previously dislocated joints for stability, laxness, or weakness of joint tissues.
- Discuss current activities related to affected joints regarding possible recurrence (Is person doing same activities as previously? Is person using a protective device to prevent recurrence? Is person doing strengthening exercises?) *to determine risk of recurrence.*
- Consult with physical therapist for exercises to strengthen joint tissues *to lessen risk of recurrence.*
- Encourage patient to comply with prescribed medical plan and exercises *to lessen risk of recurrence.*

Patient Education/Continuum of Care Plan

1. Clarify how repetitive trauma weakens joint supports and predisposes to repeated dislocations.
2. Explain that prompt treatment lessens long-term effects of repetitive dislocations.
3. Encourage continued compliance with prescribed therapy to lessen risk of recurrence.

Evaluation/Patient Outcomes

Immobility Management: Patient has normal ROM of affected joint and no limitation of mobility. Patient performs ROM exercises without pain, limitation, or recurrence of dislocation.

Coping Assistance: Patient returns to usual roles and activities and does own ADLs unassisted. Patient has returned to employment or sports activities as before dislocation. Patient has no discomfort with use and has experienced no recurrence of dislocation.

Risk Management: Patient has no recurrence of dislocation. Tissues around joint slowly regain strength and function. Patient does strengthening exercises to prevent recurrence.

Fractures

A fracture is a discontinuity or break in a bone.

Fractured bones cause major trauma to musculoskeletal tissues. Not only is the most vital part (bone) unable to perform its normal functions, but all the surrounding tissues also are unable to function normally. The cumulative effects may or may not be in direct relationship to the severity of the injury because of the interrelationship of these tissues.

The type of fracture is usually related to the source or force of the blow (see box on pp. 371-373). Only minor force may be needed for a greenstick fracture of one bone cortex, whereas more powerful forces cause comminuted fractures with associated soft tissue trauma.

Anyone is susceptible to fractures; however, younger children and elderly people may suffer fractures from minor forces. Young and middle-age adults have stronger musculoskeletal tissues; therefore greater force is required to fracture a bone, and there is more associated soft tissue trauma.

Each year there are 6.2 million fractures in the United States,[59] and more than 150,000 persons die from trauma and fractures. An additional 33 million or more persons are treated at hospitals. Trauma costs Americans over $200 billion annually, and these costs will probably increase as the population ages. By the year 2040, more than 20% of Americans will be over age 65 years. These older persons suffer injuries (often fatal) at three times the rate of their representative numbers.[10,11]

Pathophysiology

Bones are held relatively firmly in their normal anatomic positions by their shape, bony projections and processes, and the strong ligaments and tendons that hold them in their joints. Muscles surrounding the bones along their shafts also provide protection. However, either direct or indirect forces against the bone that are superior to the strength of the bone, muscles, tendons, or ligaments cause the tissues to "give in." Bones break when they cannot continue to resist the strength, duration, or repetitive nature of the applied forces.

Aging also affects bones, making them more subject to a fracture. Cortical bone in the human femur, for example, becomes less stiff, less strong, and more brittle with aging. Age-related fractures are an enormous problem in the United States, especially related to the vertebrae, proximal femur, and distal radius, which are frequent sites of fractures. Aging causes trabecular loss, less bone mass, and changes in the "architecture" of the bones. Bone mineral density is decreased, more so in females than in males, leading to fracture risk. Osteoporotic changes in bones, especially in the lumbar spine, have shown a decrease in trabecular bone density of approximately 50% from ages 20 to 80 years and older.[29]

A fractured bone can no longer maintain its normal length unless the two fragments forcibly contact each other at the time of the fracture. Usually there will be shortening of the tissues around the fractured bone because of muscle contraction and spasms as the muscles respond to the stimulus of trauma. As the muscles contract and shorten, they move the distal fragment upward (cephalad). The distal fragment is less stable and more movable than the proximal fragment, which is held more firmly

TYPES AND CAUSES OF FRACTURES

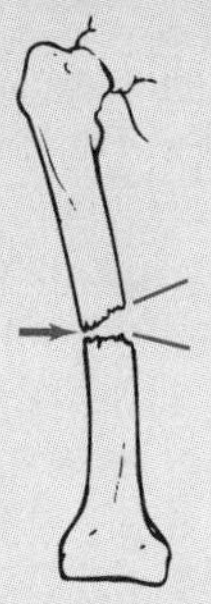

Angulated

Angulated: Fracture with fragments at angles to each other. *Cause:* Direct or lateral force, causing break and loss of anatomic positions

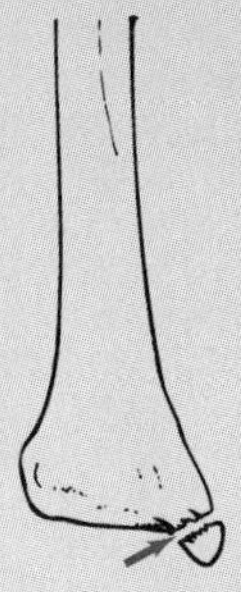

Avulsed

Avulsed: Fracture that pulls bone and other tissues from usual attachments. *Cause:* Direct energy or force, with resisted extension of bone and joint

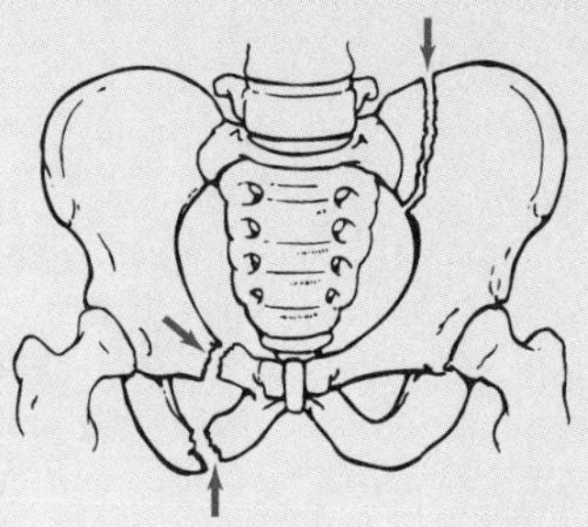

Bucket-handle

Bucket-handle: Double vertical fractures of pelvis on same side, resulting in pelvic dislocation. *Cause:* Direct blow or anterior compression force, with or without sacral torsion

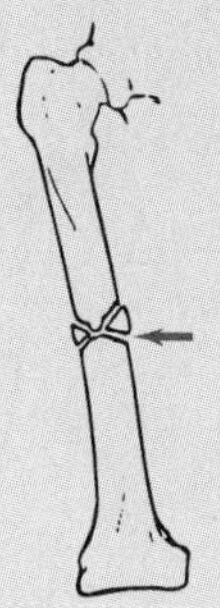

Butterfly

Butterfly: Butterfly-shaped piece of fractured bone, usually accompanying comminuted fracture. *Cause:* Direct, indirect, or rotational force to bone

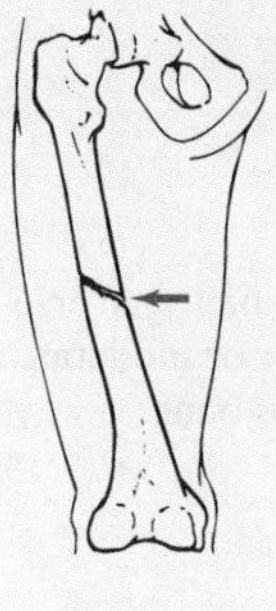

Closed

Closed: Skin intact over fracture. *Cause:* Minor force or energy

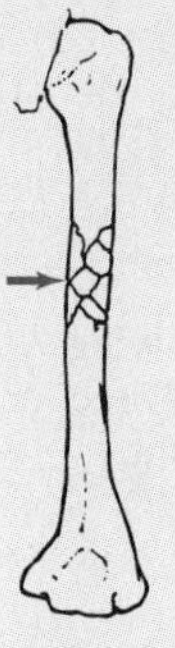

Comminuted

Comminuted: Fracture with more than two pieces; may have significant associated soft tissue trauma. *Cause:* Direct crushing injury or force to tissues and bone

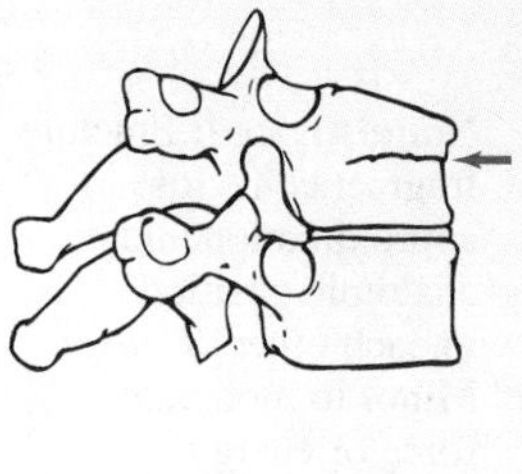

Compression

Compression: Fracture is squeezed or wedged together at one side. *Cause:* Compressive, axial energy or force applied directly from above fracture site

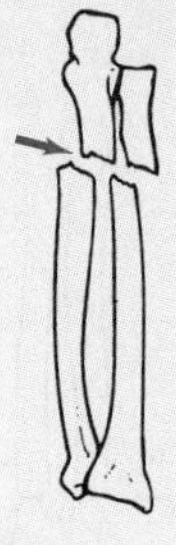

Displaced

Displaced: Fracture with one, both, or all fragments out of normal alignment. *Cause:* Direct energy or force to site

From Mourad.[38]

Continued

TYPES AND CAUSES OF FRACTURES—cont'd

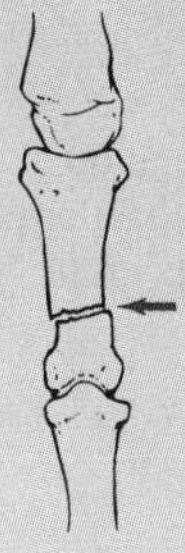

Extraaraticular

Extraarticular: Fracture near but outside a joint. *Cause:* Direct energy above or below a joint

Greenstick

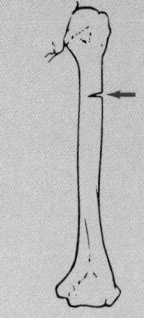

Greenstick: Break in only one cortex of bone. *Cause:* Minor direct or indirect energy

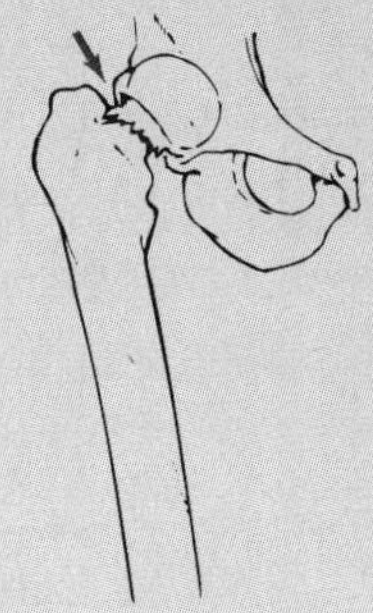

Impacted

Impacted: Fracture with one end wedged into opposite end or inside fractured fragment. *Cause:* Compressive axial energy or force directly to distal fragment

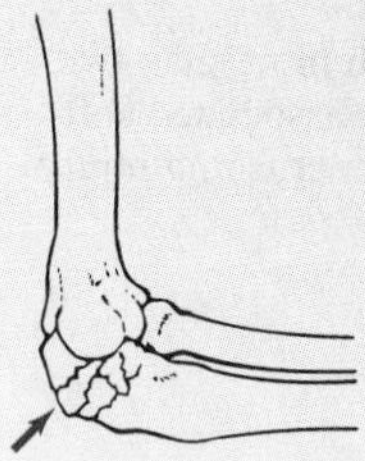

Intraarticular

Intraarticular: Fracture involving bones inside a joint. *Cause:* Direct or indirect energy or force to joint

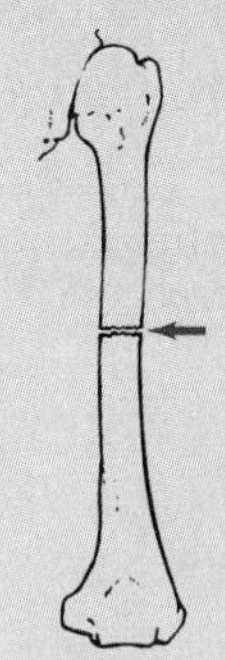

Linear

Linear: As a line, so can be transverse or oblique. *Cause:* Minor or moderate energy or force directly to bone

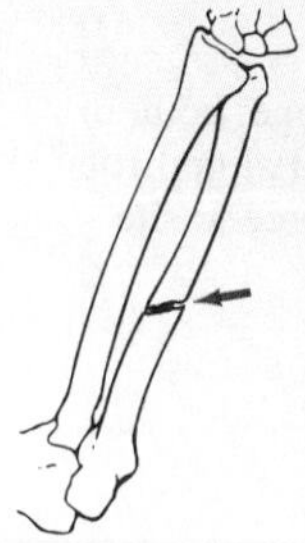

Nightstick

Nightstick: Fracture of ulna caused by blow to forearm elevated in defensive position. *Cause:* Direct force or blow to forearm

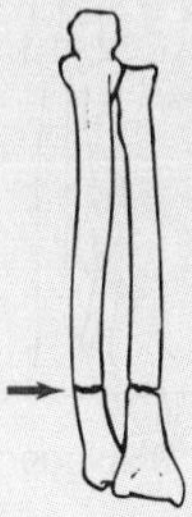

Nonangulated

Nonangulated: Fracture with fragments in anatomic relationship to each other. *Cause:* Minor force or energy

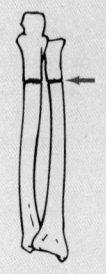

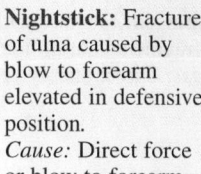

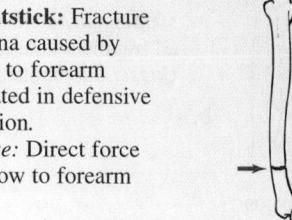

Nondisplaced

Nondisplaced: Fracture fragments in close approximation and anatomic position to each other. *Cause:* Minor to moderate force or energy

TYPES AND CAUSES OF FRACTURES—cont'd

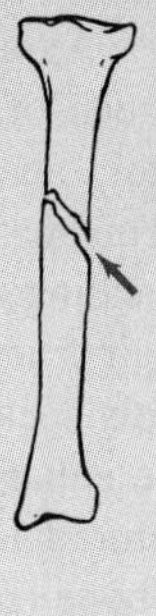

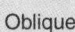

Oblique: Fracture at oblique angle across both cortices. *Cause:* Direct or indirect energy, with angulation and some compression

Oblique

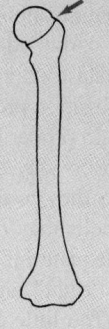

Occult: Fracture that is hidden or not readily discernible. *Cause:* Minor force or energy

Occult

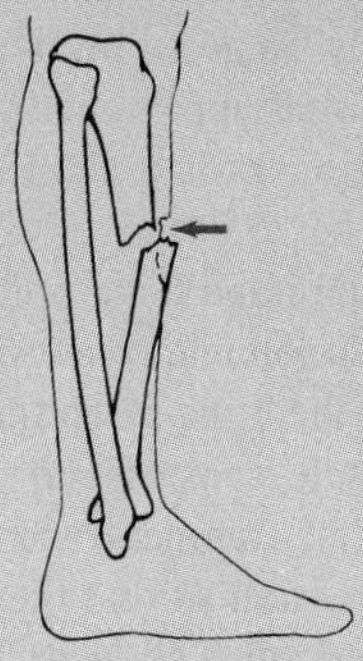

Open: Skin broken over fracture; possible soft tissue trauma. *Cause:* Moderate to severe energy that is continuous and exceeds tissue tolerances

Open

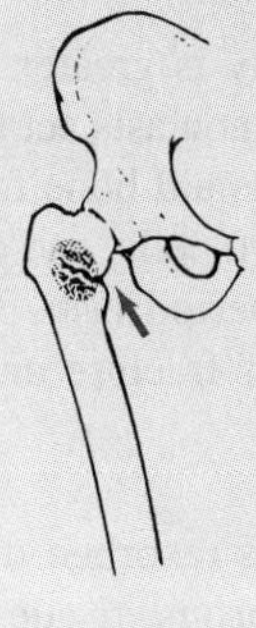

Pathologic: Transverse, oblique, or spiral fracture of bone weakened by tumor pressure or presence. *Cause:* Minor energy or force, which may be direct or indirect

Pathologic

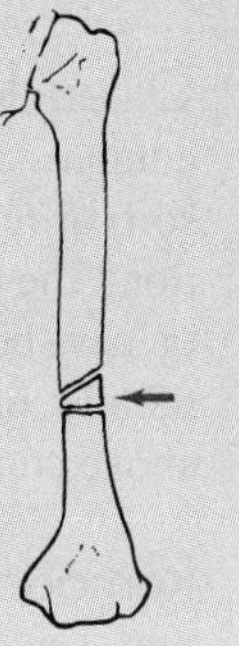

Segmented: Fracture with two or more pieces or segments. *Cause:* Direct or indirect moderate to severe force

Segmented

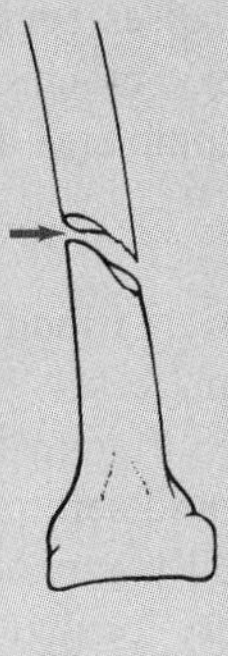

Spiral: Fracture that curves around cortices and may become displaced by twist. *Cause:* Direct or indirect twisting energy or force with distal part held or unable to move

Spiral

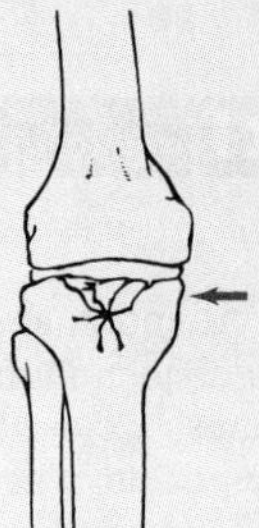

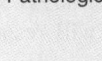

Stellate: Central fracture point from which fissures radiate. *Cause:* Direct blow or force of moderate energy

Stellate

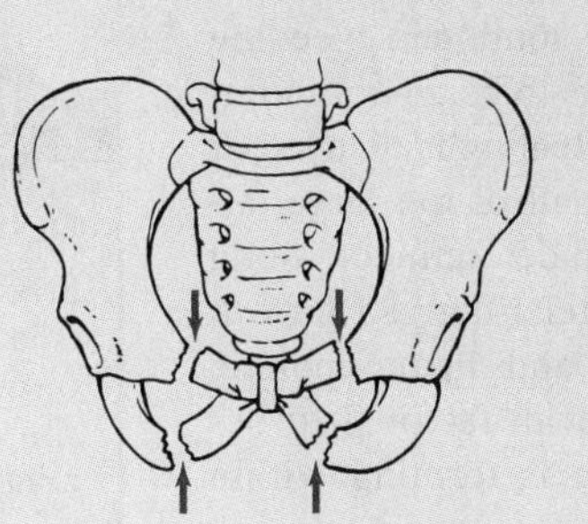

Straddle: Bilateral fractures of pelvic and pubic rami. *Cause:* Fall that causes or results in straddling of hard object

Straddle

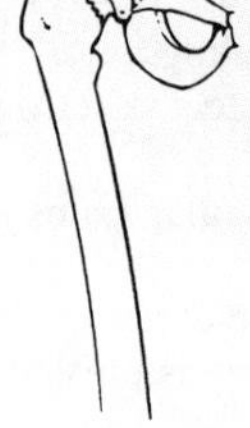

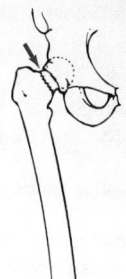

Stress: Crack in one cortex of bone. *Cause:* Repetitive direct energy or force, as from jogging, running, or striking a lever, or from osteoporosis

Stress

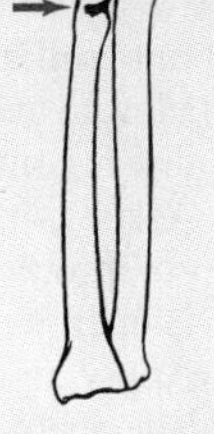

Torus: Fracture of one cortex of shafts of radius and ulna (one cortex of each bone), shown as wrinkle or buckle. *Cause:* Direct blow to forearm or indirect compressive force, as from fall

Torus

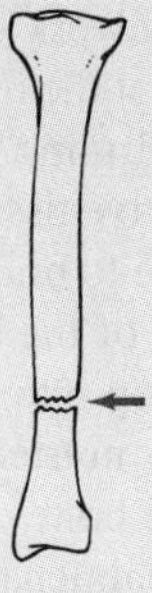

Transverse: Horizontal break through bone. *Cause:* Direct or indirect energy toward bone

Transverse

from the muscles' originations (the origins of muscles are less movable than their insertions). The shortening of the muscles and the displacement of the distal fragment result in deformity, overriding, and displacement, characteristic signs of a fracture. The deformity can generally be noted on physical examination as a deviation from the normal appearance of the tissues. Displacement of the distal fragment is a significant sign because the distal fragment must be replaced in continuity with the proximal fragment for healing and bone union. The amount of displacement and the angulation and rotation of the distal fragment are caused by loss of the bone's continuity and the severity or strength of the muscle spasms and contraction. Force must be applied to the distal fragment and to the muscles to overcome the muscle contraction so that the two or more fracture fragments can again become aligned. Terms used to describe the position of the distal fragment include varus or valgus displacement, rotation, and medial, lateral, anterior, or posterior displacement.

When a bone is fractured, many or all of the following processes occur. These processes begin immediately with the injury and continue for weeks, months, and in some situations even years before they are completed and bone union has been achieved.

Hematoma Formation. Blood and blood cells move into the injured tissues from vessels broken or bruised at the time of injury and from the inflammatory response to release of histamine, bradykinins, and serotonin into the injury site. White blood cells, especially monocytes, phagocytize debris to keep the area of injury localized and prevent spread to contiguous tissues. Bleeding into the tissues causes a hematoma to form. Blood cells, especially thrombocytes, begin to work with fibroblasts to form a fibrin (clot) meshwork within the hematoma. Usually the hematoma is well formed in 24 to 48 hours, and frank or continued bleeding slows or ceases completely. There appears to be an optimum-size hematoma to facilitate bone union. Healing is delayed or prevented by hematomas that are too small or too large, although the exact favorable size is still undetermined. Along with fibroblasts, platelets also make platelet-derived growth factor, macrophages, T lymphocytes, and hematopoietic growth factors such as transforming growth factor-β to begin new bone formation, and new bone is forming within 24 hours.[39]

Consolidation, Angiogenesis, and Cartilage Formation. During this period of fracture healing, a fascinating phenomenon occurs because osteoblasts (bone-forming cells) move into the fibrin meshwork to make new *bone,* not scar tissue. No other tissue except the liver regenerates itself as itself. The osteoblasts help in firming the fracture site, intertwining it with collagen connective tissue fibers to form strong cartilage and then with new bone to bridge the gap between the fractured ends—all as attempts of the bone cortex to reestablish itself. Capillary buds develop into new blood vessels (angiogenesis), which bring more nutrients and calcium molecules into the area to form soft bone callus. A tissue oxygen gradient is necessary for the maintenance of angiogenesis in the injury area. This bone-forming period lasts 3 to 6 weeks or longer.

Callus Formation. This is probably the most vital period for bone healing for two reasons: (1) Enough nutrients must be present to provide a continuous supply to support bone formation to its completion. Oxygen is a major nutrient, as is alkaline phosphatase, along with sufficient amounts of vitamins A, B, C, and D, carbohydrates, proteins, minerals, and water. Alkaline phosphatase may be a key enzyme that governs much of the mineralization process. Insulin, a potent growth factor, must be present in proper amounts for healing at this stage. This may be one reason why diabetics have impaired fracture healing; not only do they have circulatory disturbances, but their fracture callus cells may respond ineffectively to other signals because of inadequate insulin. (2) Callus formation must be enhanced by the "right" amount of compression of the fractured fragments. Too little compression may result in pseudobone (false bone), and too much compression may decrease oxygen supply and tension, resulting in bone-end absorption and creating too large a gap for the collagen fibers to bridge. This decreases or prevents formation of strong callus.

Osteoclast Activity. Osteoclast activity is greater when compressive forces are too great, because osteoclasts act to absorb or resorb bone cells, whereas osteoblasts aid bone formation. The balance is disrupted between the two cells, and callus or new bone formation is decreased. This period lasts 3 to 6 months or longer, depending on the type of fracture and the above conditions.

Remodeling. If present, excess bone is resorbed during this period. The collagen fibers and fibrous tissues are aligned to form trabeculae along the lines of stress according to Wolff's law, which states that bone will respond to

> **! EMERGENCY ALERT**
>
> **DISLOCATIONS AND FRACTURES**
>
> Fractures and dislocations occur frequently. Attention to circulatory and neurovascular status is essential to minimize further damage. One classification of fractures is closed or simple and open or compound. Dislocations occur when a joint exceeds its ROM and joint tissues are disrupted (usually a bone).
>
> **ASSESSMENT**
>
> - Assess vital signs; rule out life-threatening injury.
> - Assess for swelling, discoloration, abrasions, contusions, or obvious deformity.
> - Assess neurovascular status (the five *P*s and others; see box on p. 330), and reassess frequently.
>
> **INTERVENTIONS**
>
> - Immobilize limb; note and observe for swelling.
> - Elevate and apply cold pack as possible (protect skin from direct contact with ice).
> - Assist with traction application if neurovascular status is compromised.
> - If open wound is present, apply a dry sterile dressing.
> - Apply a pressure dressing if profuse bleeding is present.
> - Manage pain.
> - Keep person warm to help prevent shock.

stress by becoming thicker and stronger and that the structure of a bone depends on its function. Osteoclasts resorb the excess callus or poorly aligned trabeculae until they are firm and strong. Remodeling may continue for up to 2 years after injury.

Bone Healing. Bone healing, then, depends on several *local* factors, including the severity of the injury, nutrient supply, amount of bone bridge or gap, degree of immobilization, infection or necrosis of bone cells, and type of bone fractured. Cancellous bone fractures heal more quickly than fractures of compact bone because of the presence of blood and blood cells in greater quantities than in compact bone. *Systemic* factors influencing bone healing include the patient's age (children heal more quickly), concomitant diseases such as diabetes, hormonal balances (growth hormones aid healing, and excess corticosteroids delay healing), and stress, immobility, or movement at the fracture site. Application of electric current aids bone healing and has become a valuable adjunct in recent years for delayed fracture healing.

Bone Union. Fractures of bones may not heal well or form bone union in the usual amount of time, or they may not even unite. There may be *delayed* union, in which bone union does not occur for 9 months or longer after a fracture; there may be *malunion,* in which the bones unite in a less than optimal position; and there may be *nonunion,* in which no fracture healing has occurred. Open fractures (fractures in which the skin has been torn or disrupted) must be carefully cleaned, definitively treated, and closed as soon as feasible to prevent possible infection and to promote proper healing.

Diagnostic Studies and Findings

History: Sudden, unexpected trauma; chronic, repetitive forces rather than sudden force usually cause stress fractures

Physical examination: Local deformity; edema or a mass; distal tissues held at abnormal angles or positions; limitation of use of part; crepitation; pain or tenderness at or around the site; subjective signs of numbness, tingling, weakness, or inability to use part normally; distal tissues cooler than proximal; peripheral pulses should be palpable; skin over injury site open or intact

Roentgenograms: Complete break in bone continuity or in one cortex; rarely, may fail to reveal fracture initially; repeat in 10 days for certainty because bone resorption at fracture site makes diagnosis easier

Multidisciplinary Plan

Emergency Care

Application of splint to hold fractured bones to prevent additional injury
Nonuse or non–weight bearing
Application of cryotherapy
Initiation of IV therapy to prevent shock, if possible
Transport to medical facility

Surgery

Open reduction with internal fixation (ORIF) of the fracture fragments with pins, nails, screws, staples, plates, intramedullary nails, or wire
Arthroplasty and replacement of injured or crushed bone with prosthesis
Total joint replacement for crush injuries
Amputation for severe crush injuries if circulation/nerve cannot be restored
Microvascular surgery (see box, p. 391)
Application of external apparatus such as the Hoffman, Ilizarov, Ace-Fischer, or other device

Medical Care

Closed reduction with cast
Application of skin or skeletal traction (depends on type of bone or fracture severity; traction used less now because of extended hospitalization and costs)
Use of bone "glue" to aid fracture "setting" and healing

Medications

Narcotic analgesic agents
- Meperidine (Demerol), 50-100 mg q3h IM for acute pain
- Morphine, 5-20 mg q4h subcutaneously, or hydromorphone (Dilaudid), 2-4 mg q4h subcutaneously; for acute pain (may use patient-controlled analgesic [PCA] pump for IV self-medication

Analgesic/antipyretic agents
- Aspirin, 600-1000 mg q4h between narcotic administration times; aspirin also has anticoagulant effects to prevent deep vein thrombosis
- Acetaminophen (Tylenol), 600-1000 mg q4h between narcotic administration times

Antiinflammatory agents
- Ibuprofen (Motrin), 400-800 mg q4h PO
- Piroxicam (Feldene), 20 mg daily PO
- Ketorolac (Toradol), 15-30 mg IM or IV q4h
- Celecoxib (Celebrex), 100 mg bid PO
- Rofecoxib (Vioxx), 12.5 mg daily PO, up to 25 mg/day
- See table on p. 337 for additional NSAIDs

Anticoagulants: Heparin in individualized doses IV (after bleeding ceased), then enoxaparin (Lovenox), 30 mg subcutaneously bid, then coumadin (Warfarin), individualized doses PO

Tranquilizers: Hydroxyzine (Vistaril), 25-50 mg IM, with narcotic as a narcotic potentiator (used less presently)

Muscle relaxants
- Cyclobenzaprine (Flexeril), 10-20 mg PO tid
- Methocarbamol (Robaxin), 500-750 mg PO q4-6h; metaxalone (Skelaxin), 400-800 mg tid or qid

Antiinfective agents: Specific to the invading organisms (noted by culture) if the skin is open; after surgery, antibiotics:
- Cefoxitin (Mefoxin), 1 g q8h IV for 3 days
- Cefoperazone (Cefobid), 2-4 g q2h IV for 48-72 h (or longer)
- Vancomycin (Vancocin), 1 g q12h or 400 mg q6h IV

General Management

Restrict to bed rest, if necessary, because of severity of injuries

Ensure patient does not bear weight on affected bone and joints; have patient use cane, crutches, or walker to avoid bearing weight on injured extremity initially
Well-balanced diet high in vitamins, proteins, carbohydrates, and minerals
Force fluid intake
Concurrent treatment of systemic disease of present
Begin physical therapy exercises early in postoperative period
Use of cryotherapy to decrease bleeding and edema for 48 to 72 hours postoperatively
Continue prescription of antiinflammatory/analgesic medications over time

NURSING CARE

NURSING ASSESSMENT

Fracture site and surrounding tissues: Edema; color changes in tissues at fracture site and distal to site; deformity; temperature of affected tissues: colder or hotter than normal; paresthesia with numbness and tingling; pain, acute and unremitting; limitation of movement or inability to use part; skin closed or open; crepitation (movement of parts normally not movable, causing noise, crackling, or rubbing together of fractured ends); bruising, blisters on skin at fracture site (related to loss of proper circulation); bleeding or hematoma (noted by mass) or frank bleeding; presence or absence of pulses distal to injury; capillary refill; petechial rash over upper chest, eyelids
Systemic concerns: Pallor; confusion or disorientation; dyspnea; shock: may be neurologic, cardiogenic, toxic, hemorrhagic; changes in blood pressure and other vital signs; sweating or perspiring; fear and anxiety; concomitant diseases or injuries to other organs or tissues
Psychosocial concerns: Self-concept, separation from significant other, family, or friends; disturbances in body image and impairment of physical mobility; alteration in comfort, severe pain; inability to carry out usual roles and responsibilities; economic costs of treatments, hospitalization, and long-term recovery; lack of insurance coverage

POTENTIAL COMPLICATIONS

Pulmonary embolism; fat embolism syndrome; osteomyelitis; nonunion; malunion; delayed union; amputation; compartment syndrome

PATIENT PROBLEMS/NURSING DIAGNOSES & INTERVENTIONS

NIC IMMOBILITY MANAGEMENT

Impaired physical mobility related to fractured bone and soft tissue trauma

- Observe area around fractured bone. Look for open areas of skin.
- Gently handle injured tissues by supporting joint above and below site *to prevent additional injury and lessen pain.*
- Apply cold pack to site *to lessen edema formation and bleeding.*
- Elevate extremity as prescribed; support with pillows *to aid venous return.*
- Restrict patient to bed rest, if prescribed, *to put body and part at rest.*
- Explain purposes for rest and not bearing weight on injured extremity *to ease patient's concerns.*
- Perform neurovascular checks at minimum of every 8 hours *to note condition of affected tissues.*
- Check integrity of the cast, function of traction or wrapping every 1 to 2 hours initially, then every 4 hours *to note condition or proper functions.*
- Explain position required for maximum healing *to aid compliance.*
- Assist to proper position; change position every 2 hours, if can be repositioned, or help to position self correctly *to ease tired muscles.*
- Teach patient the "post position" for lifting self (patient plants [posts] unaffected foot flat on bed with knee bent at right angle; lifts body using trapeze while pushing down with foot and leg). Help by lifting patient's buttocks if needed *to encourage independence and self-care.*
- Teach exercises to maintain strength and facilitate resolution of inflammation; have quadriceps, buttocks, and triceps setting exercises done every 4 hours when allowed *to retain or maintain muscle strength.*

NIC PHYSICAL COMFORT PROMOTION

Acute pain related to pressure on nerve endings

- Ask about amount, type, severity, site, and duration of pain.
- Help patient assume a position of comfort if possible *to lessen pain or discomfort.*
- Monitor patient's use of narcotic in PCA or administer prescribed narcotic analgesics: every 3 hours for meperidine (action is lost after 3 hours) or every 4 hours for opiate narcotics. Administer narcotics "around the clock" for 3 to 5 days or longer as prescribed *to maintain adequate blood levels to relieve pain.* Periods between narcotics may be increased with use of muscle relaxants for acute muscle spasms *to lessen dependence on narcotics and to decrease muscle spasms.*
- Administer nonnarcotic analgesics or NSAIDs as prescribed every 4 hours between narcotic administrations to enhance pain relief. Antiinflammatory medications *aid resolution of inflammation.*
- Change position every 2 hours *to lessen muscle fatigue, when possible.*
- Massage back and buttocks *to decrease pressure and fatigue and to increase circulation in those areas.*
- Administer muscle relaxant or sedatives as prescribed *to aid reduction of muscle spasms and lessen pain episodes.*

NIC COPING ASSISTANCE

Disturbed body image and ineffective role performance related to temporary loss of independence

- Discuss self-concept and dependency concerns *to determine appropriate care.*
- Maintain privacy while helping perform ADLs and hygienic care *to aid personal cleanliness and self-esteem.*
- Offer oral hygiene and back care frequently *to maintain healthy tissues.*

- Explain that proper positioning and non–weight bearing are required *to facilitate bone healing.*
- Encourage to express feelings about enforced immobility and displacement from familiar surroundings *to foster comfort and lessen undue concerns.*
- Arrange for physical therapy and occupational therapy consultations *to maintain muscle strength and self-esteem and to prepare for self-care after discharge.*
- Encourage family members to interact with patient *to maintain customary roles and esteem.*
- Help patient comply with high-nutrient diet *to lessen weight loss (a patient in skeletal traction may lose weight quickly) and to maintain positive body image.*

NIC PATIENT EDUCATION

Deficient knowledge related to shock (from severity of injury) and to unfamiliar terms or treatments

- Clarify understanding of condition, if feasible; if in shock or unconscious, do assessment when condition has improved.
- Clarify misconceptions or lack of understanding; may use pictures or patient's x-rays *to provide needed explanations.*
- Show videotape, if available, or similar-age or same-sex patient with same type of injury or treatment *to clarify a specific regimen or action.*
- Ask about understanding by having patient draw picture *to ascertain level or degree of understanding.*
- Continue teaching as needed at current time or later period *if patient appears tired or uncomfortable.*
- Provide a quiet, calm atmosphere *for optimal learning.*
- Seek questions from patient and family *to determine if additional teaching is needed.*

NIC TISSUE PERFUSION MANAGEMENT

Ineffective tissue perfusion related to impaired circulation from trauma

- Monitor condition of affected tissues.
- Perform all parts of neurovascular checks every hour initially. Check color; temperature; peripheral pulses; edema; presence, amount, and type of pain; motor functions (patient should be able to move parts proximal to injury); sensory functions (complaints of numbness, tingling, or pins and needles indicate sensory compromise); and capillary refill (compress nail of middle finger or toe, release; nail should pink up in 2 to 4 seconds for normal capillary refill; 4 to 6 seconds is abnormal and should be reported); compare the injured area with the same tissues on the opposite side of the body. Another critical finding, along with prolonged capillary refill, is increased pain on passive movement of the fingers or toes or pain not relieved by narcotic administration, which could signify that the patient may be developing compartment syndrome. Increased anoxia caused by the stretching of the muscle with the passive movement causes the increased pain (see FIG. 6-32, p. 409). Report abnormal findings to physician.
- Elevate limb to heart level *to increase venous return, thereby lessening edema.*
- Loosen circumferential dressings, if present, or bivalve cast *to increase arterial circulation to tissues.*

NIC SKIN/WOUND MANAGEMENT

Risk for impaired skin integrity related to immobility, presence of a cast, or traction equipment

- Observe skin surfaces for signs of pressure, such as redness, blistering, soreness, or open lesion.
- Reposition patient every 2 hours if possible *to relieve pressure.*
- Turn to side if permitted *to distribute pressure to other areas and to relieve tired or sore muscles.*
- Massage around bony prominences *to increase circulation.*
- Use foam or lamb's wool bed pads *to distribute pressure.*
- Encourage to eat adequately from a high-protein, high-carbohydrate, high-vitamin diet *to maintain healthy cellular tissues and to aid fracture healing.*
- Be sure patient gets at least 3000 ml of fluid daily *to maintain skin turgor and renal functions.*
- Teach how to move self in bed *to lessen friction and shearing forces and maintain healthy skin surfaces.*
- Use turning sheet, if allowed, to turn side to side *to relieve pressure on skin and bony prominences.*

PATIENT EDUCATION/CONTINUUM OF CARE PLAN

1. Reiterate reasons for rest and not bearing weight on injured limb (anxiety may prevent the patient from hearing or understanding initial explanations).
2. Explain reasons for weight loss and how it can lessen through exercise and diet.
3. Explain measures for dealing with acute pain and changes in using medications as pain decreases.
4. Show pictures of bone healing processes to elicit the patient's cooperation and understanding.
5. Explain turning and moving techniques to prevent skin breakdown.
6. List purposes and techniques for neurovascular checks.
7. Encourage patient to notify physician if concerned about healing processes or prolonged pain.
8. Discuss signs and symptoms to report to physician and signs and symptoms that require medical attention.
9. Coordinate teaching with physical or occupational therapists for self-care at home.
10. Provide needed aids (walker, crutches) or equipment (bed pad, abduction pillow) before discharge for self-care at home.
11. Teach significant other or family member care patient is unable to do for self, such as dressing changes, care of cast, or other required care.

EVALUATION/PATIENT OUTCOMES

Immobility Management: Patient resumes walking and bearing full weight on limb without limitation or discomfort in usual time frame after healing—may be 6 weeks to 2 months or longer. Patient feels no discomfort or pain when walking or bearing weight on limb or using part normally.

Physical Comfort Promotion: Pain is relieved as bone union occurs in anatomic position; can use part without pain.

No deformity is present. Patient is using no analgesics for pain after 2 to 3 months.

Coping Assistance: Patient resumes social interactions and roles. Patient returns to family, social, and employment roles after 3 months or later, according to bone fractured and treatment.

Patient Education: Patient is able to explain type of injury, purposes, and results of treatments.

Tissue Perfusion Management: Patient has normal tissue perfusion. Patient has normal color, temperature, capillary refill, motor and sensory functions, and no edema of healed tissues after 6 to 9 months.

Skin/Wound Management: Patient has healthy skin turgor without developing pressure areas. Patient has pink, well-nourished skin with good turgor. Patient is regaining lost weight over 3 months or longer.

CURVATURES OF THE SPINAL COLUMN

The spine develops its characteristic curves during fetal growth (FIG. 6-21). Both prenatally and postnatally the curves may become abnormal because of defective bone, muscle, nerve, or other growth factors. The abnormal curves are called kyphosis (excessive curvature of thoracic spine), scoliosis (lateral or rotary curvature of thoracic spine), and lordosis (excessive curvature of lumbar spine) (FIG. 6-22).

KYPHOSIS

Kyphosis is excessive curvature of the thoracic vertebrae.

The various types of kyphosis, related to their causes, include congenital, developmental, metabolic, infective, inflammatory, neuromuscular, tumor, skeletal dysplasia, posttraumatic, and iatrogenic. Idiopathic kyphosis has no apparent cause.

It is important to identify a cause for the patient's kyphosis, if possible, because congenital kyphosis has a virtual guarantee of progression. It is also important to determine if the curve is smooth and gradual or sharp and angular because the latter curves are often associated with neurologic risk.

A progression of curve of 5 to 10 degrees per year is estimated for type I (failure of formation of the anterior bodies) congenital kyphosis, with an estimated incidence of neurologic problems of 25% to 30% related to cord compromise at the gibbus (hump) of the kyphosis. Type II congenital kyphosis also progresses in curve deformity at a slightly slower rate, but still about 5 degrees per year. Type II is a failure of anterior vertebral segmentation. Type III is a condition of mixed anomalies and has no specific curve progression rates.

Kyphosis occurs in various age groups. When it occurs in young children, it is usually congenital. It may become apparent in the adolescent years, when it is referred to as juvenile kyphosis, or Scheuermann's disease. Occasionally kyphosis may develop to compensate for lumbar lordosis, and kyphosis may also be associated with scoliosis. Kyphosis is also a classic symptom of ankylosing spondylitis. When kyphosis occurs in postmenopausal women, it is called senile kyphosis.

PATHOPHYSIOLOGY

Because the thoracic vertebrae have a physiologic posterior curve normally, the curvature becomes pathologic only when it becomes excessive or exaggerated. In young children the abnormal curvature may be the only pathologic sign until the curve progresses. As children become adolescents, the curvature may become pronounced, especially with Scheuermann's disease, which produces irregular epiphyseal plate growth and ossification. Scheuermann's disease is often confused with type II congenital kyphosis; however, the progressive ossification and fusion of Scheuermann's disease by the end of skeletal growth clarifies the difference.

In older people with kyphosis, some degenerative changes usually occur in the intervertebral cartilages. These changes lead to the excessive curvature. In postmenopausal women, kyphosis is commonly associated with osteoporosis and degeneration in the annulus fibrosus rings between the vertebrae.

Kyphotic curves may occur mainly in the thoracic vertebra or lower in the thoracolumbar vertebrae, primarily in congenital kyphosis, where the progressive curve growth compromises the spinal cord, leading to motor and sensory changes in the lower body and extremities if the curve progression is left untreated.

DIAGNOSTIC STUDIES AND FINDINGS

Physical examination: Excessive thoracic spinal curvature, rounded shoulders; occasional low back pain (40% of adolescents with Scheuermann's disease have back pain, as do many children with congenital kyphosis); easy fatigability; exaggerated lumbar lordosis to compensate for the kyphosis; respiratory deficit

Roentgenograms: Marked curvature of thoracic spine; geriatric patients: possible osteoporosis with vertebral wedging; wedging and narrowing of anterior portions of thoracic vertebral bodies (T6-T10); lateral tomograms may show spinal deformities not clear on plain x-ray; MRI or myelograms may show sites of neurologic pressures

Histocompatibility testing: Serum HLA-B27 antigen present in young adults with ankylosing spondylitis

MULTIDISCIPLINARY PLAN

Surgery

Halo traction; osteotomy

Spinal fusion for severe kyphosis, especially if signs of neurologic deficit begin

Spinal instrumentation (see p. 426)

Medications

Older adults may have hormonal treatment or mineral administration for treatment of osteoporosis, if present

Younger adults with ankylosing spondylitis receive several drugs (pp. 331-332) for treatment of their disease processes

General Management

Milwaukee brace or other brace for adolescents

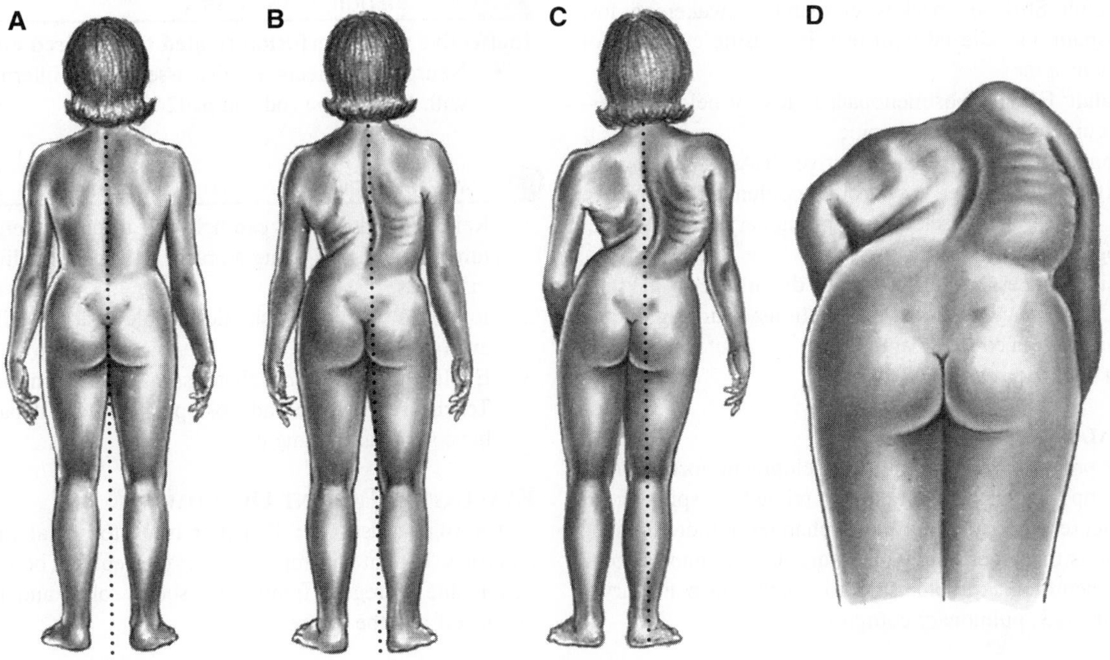

FIG. 6-21
Normal spinal alignment and abnormal spinal curvatures associated with scoliosis. **A,** Normal; **B,** mild; **C,** severe; **D,** rotation and curvature of scoliosis.

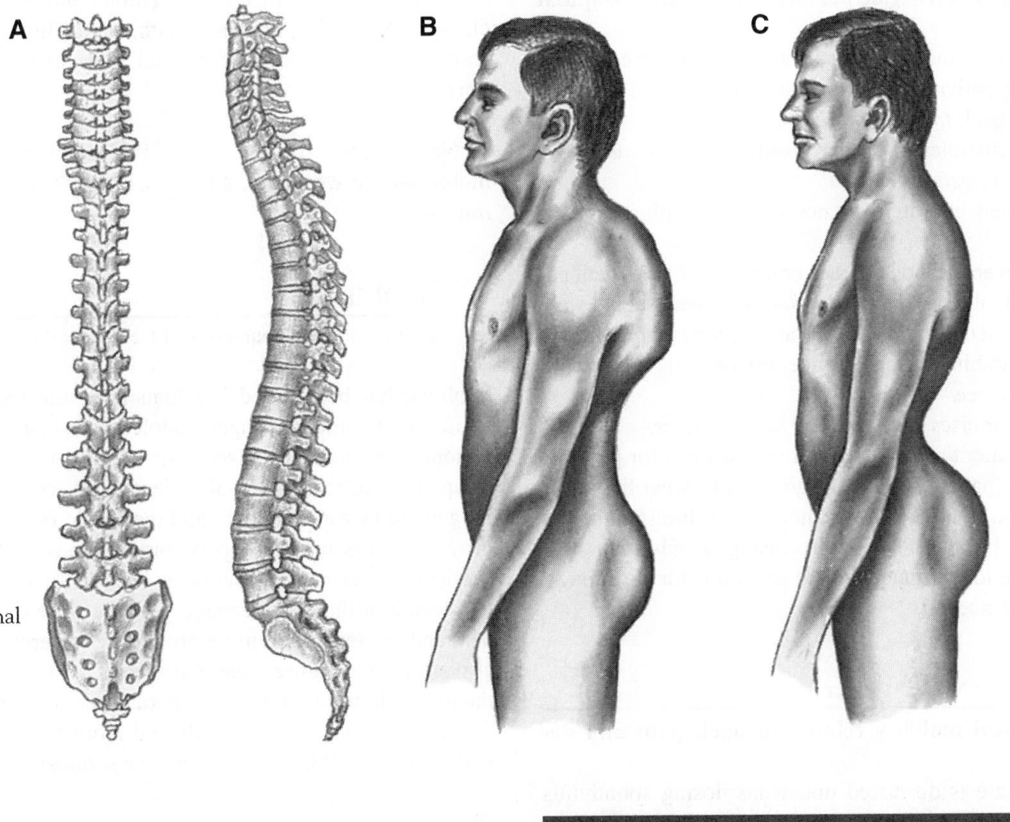

FIG. 6-22
A, Normal spinal alignment and curvatures.
B, Kyphosis.
C, Lordosis.

Back corset for older adults
Orthotic devices (plastic or canvas/metal splint) for adolescents
Teaching patient to stand up as straight as possible
Exercise program to strengthen muscles and ligaments
Deep-breathing exercises for any respiratory compromise

NURSING CARE

NURSING ASSESSMENT

Thoracic spine

Adolescent: Rounded shoulders, backache, excessive curvature of thoracic spine, lumbar lordosis increased

Young adult: Stiff, sore back when rising on awakening; low back pain not relieved with rest; increasing curvature of thoracic spine
Older adult: Female, postmenopausal, loss of height, excessive curvature of thoracic spine

Systemic processes: Young adult: positive HLA-B27 histocompatibility antigen, Reiter's syndrome (conjunctivitis, uveitis, genital lesions, low back pain), pulmonary compromise, neurologic compromise

Psychosocial concerns: Self-concept; disturbances in self-esteem, body image, and role expectations; neurologic: possible paralysis, need to use ambulatory aid (crutches, wheelchair) if severe disease

Potential Complications

Continuing progression of curvature development, formation of gibbus (hump), pain and dysfunction related to spinal cord compromise, respiratory compromise, changes in motor or sensory functions in tissues below curvature area; kyphosis complications: neurologic problems, cord compromise at curve, possible paralysis, pulmonary compromise

Patient Education/Nursing Diagnoses & Interventions

NIC Coping Assistance

Ineffective coping, chronic low self-esteem, disturbed body image, and ineffective role performance related to spinal deformity

- Observe back and spine for excessive thoracic curvature by having patient bend over, turn side to side, and face front and back *to note condition.*
- Discuss principles of proper posture *to aid in maintaining upright posture.*
- Explain that condition is not life threatening *to ease concern.*
- Assist with application of brace or orthosis, if used, until patient can do it alone *to aid compliance.* Patient should wear cotton T-shirt under orthosis or brace *to protect skin surfaces.*
- Discuss clothing to make brace less obvious *to increase self-confidence.*
- Discuss exercises *to strengthen back muscles.*
- Discuss patient's life goals and review need for possible alteration (patient should set goals as to what he or she desires and is able to do without many limitations; see p. 331 for limitations with ankylosing spondylitis).
- Encourage to continue medical checkups for early interventions if needed.

NIC Immobility Management

Impaired physical mobility related to back pain and deformity

- Nursing care is discussed under ankylosing spondylitis on p. 331.

NIC Respiratory Management

Impaired gas exchange related to pulmonary compromise

- Nursing interventions are discussed under care of a person in a cast on p. 412.

NIC Neurologic Management

Ineffective tissue perfusion related to impaired circulation

- Neurologic effects are discussed under internal fixation with Harrington rods on p. 426.

Patient Education/Continuum of Care Plan

1. Reiterate that patient can help self through exercises, posture changes, and using a brace, orthosis, or splint, in most instances.
2. Reiterate that patient should be able to achieve life's goals even with kyphosis.
3. Explain clothing types that lessen curvature noticeability.
4. Teach preoperative and postoperative care if patient is to have surgical treatment.

Evaluation/Patient Outcomes

Coping Assistance: Patient returns to social interactions and roles. Patient has improved self-concept and body image, is better able to regain family and social roles, and is positive about self and the future.

Immobility Management: Patient's posture has improved and curvature is lessened after treatment and mobility is increased. Patient stands straighter with less curvature or rotation. Hips and shoulders are more normally aligned.

Respiratory Management: Patient has adequate gas exchange. Patient has normal breath sounds in all lobes and has respiratory excursions of normal rates and depth. Color is normal.

Neurologic Management: Patient has not developed motor/muscle weakness, and muscle strength is maintained or improved.

Scoliosis

Scoliosis is lateral curvature of the vertebral column.

Scoliosis has been noted in infants (infantile scoliosis), young children (juvenile), teenagers (adolescent), and adults. For most patients the cause of the scoliosis is unknown; thus it is called idiopathic scoliosis (15% of patients with scoliosis).[36] A familial genetic factor, hormonal and metabolic factors, and skeletal growth factors may also play parts in causing some cases of scoliosis. Most cases of scoliosis become more prominent and noticeable in the early teenage years because of uneven shoulders and hip levels and more pronounced laterality and rotatory curvatures. Curvatures may vary from 20 degrees (considered the lowest limit of clinically important scoliosis) to curves of 60 degrees or more. Girls are affected more than boys. Approximately 1.5 per 1000 population have scoliosis.

Pathophysiology

The curvatures of scoliosis have more than one dimension because they occur in the vertically stacked vertebrae. Three curve planes are involved: concave curvature on the anterior vertebral bodies, convex posterior curves, and lateral rotation of the thoracic spine on bending or flexing forward. Lordosis is present in the thoracic vertebral curve. As the person with scoliosis bends forward, the thoracic lordosis causes lateral flexion of the affected thoracic vertebrae. The lateral curvature is thus secondary to the thoracic lordosis. Also, the larger the lordosis, the greater is the rotation and lateral curvature on flexion. The risk of curve progression is greatest for children with larger curves who are in the adolescent growth spurt.[34a]

Curves can also stop growing and restart during adult years. Muscles, ligaments, and other soft tissues become shortened on the concave side of the curve and can influence the "growth" of the curve, or compression of one side of the vertebral bodies. Usually curves greater than 20 degrees require treatment. Curves of 60 degrees affect pulmonary functions.

Scoliotic curves are referred to as thoracic (the most common thoracolumbar) and lumbar. Curves may be double, with a right thoracic curve and left lumbar curve, left thoracic curve and right lumbar curve, or variations of these. Interestingly, true wry neck (torticollis) is scoliosis of the cervical spine.

DIAGNOSTIC STUDIES AND FINDINGS

History: Asymmetry of shoulders or hips; uneven hemlines, pant length, or waistline; forward bending in school screening may show lateral curvature

Physical examination: Lateral deviation with or without rotation of vertebrae; curvature may become more pronounced when patient bends forward; rotation may also be more noticeable when patient bends forward; when hands of examiner are placed on patient's hips, one hand is higher than other when patient is standing upright; examination of leg length reveals one leg is shorter, and when patient sits, the curvature disappears, rib angles may protrude, and one hip may stick out; asymmetric shoulder levels; prominence of one shoulder, parents may be unaware of curvature until it is significant; deep tendon reflexes may be abnormal; absent abdominal reflexes

Roentgenograms: Curvature and angle of curvature, plus rotation; special x-ray studies can detect lordosis, concave curves, and convex curves; X-rays show skeletal maturity by evaluating ossification of the iliac apophysis (anterior iliac spine), classified as Risser 1 through 4—ranges from 25% to 100% ossification; Risser 5—fusion of the apophysis, cessation of skeletal growth has occurred

Bone scan: Bone scans, MRI, CT, tomogram, or myelogram may be done if patient has back pain or abnormal neurologic findings on physical examination

Pulmonary consultation: Arterial blood gas levels

MULTIDISCIPLINARY PLAN

Surgery

Straightening of curve with Harrington or Luque rods, Wisconsin segmental system, Texas Scottish Rite Hospital system, Isola spine implant system, the Moduloc posterior spinal system, or Cotrel-Dubousset instrumentation (CDI) for internal fixation with bone grafts to fuse spine; may be anterior, posterior, or both

Dwyer procedure: Staples and screws fixed to the vertebral bodies; a cable is inserted through the screw heads; tightening the cable closes the vertebral areas and straightens the curve

Anterior diskectomy with interbody fusion

Pedicle screw fixation is investigational under Food and Drug Administration (FDA) regulations

General Management

Use of Milwaukee, Boston, or similar brace or orthotic device

Application of Cotrel's traction or halo-femoral traction

Regimen of exercises to strengthen back muscles

Electrical stimulation to paraspinous muscles—no longer used because does not alter the natural history of curve progression[34a]

NURSING CARE

NURSING ASSESSMENT

Entire spinal column: Spinal column will curve away from the midline in thoracic and lumbar areas; one shoulder or hip will be a different height than the other, legs of unequal length; spine will rotate laterally when patient bends over; use scoliometer to measure angle of trunk rotation; may have upper and lower (sacral) curves; arm-to-body space will be different on one side

Systemic concerns: Patient may have muscle weakness throughout body; cardiac or respiratory signs such as pulse rate or rhythm changes, dyspnea, or shortness of breath may be noted in more severe scoliosis of thoracic area; vital capacity may be decreased

Psychosocial concerns: Self-concept; alteration of body image and role expectations; impaired physical mobility; impaired gas exchange

POTENTIAL COMPLICATIONS

Marked progression of curve, respiratory compromise

PATIENT PROBLEMS/NURSING DIAGNOSES & INTERVENTIONS

NIC COPING ASSISTANCE

Disturbed body image and ineffective role performance related to spinal deformity

- Observe degree or severity of curvature; assist with measuring degrees of curve or curves.
- Discuss patient's feelings of inadequacy because of deformity *to aid in ventilation of feelings.*
- Discuss clothing to make curve or brace less noticeable *to ease concerns.*
- Discuss need to continue wearing brace *to prevent increase in rotation or lateralization.* Orthosis or brace is worn for 23 hours per day in most instances.
- Discuss adjustments to clothing hemlines *to negate effects of scoliosis.*
- Encourage usual peer relationships and activities *to aid psychosocial development.*

NIC SKIN/WOUND MANAGEMENT

Risk for impaired skin integrity related to presence and use of brace or other orthotic devices

- Check all skin tissues for condition, presence of skin irritation, color changes, or open areas.

- Clarify necessity to wear proper clothing such as cotton T-shirt under brace or orthosis *to maintain skin integrity.*
- Encourage proper skin cleansing and use of lotions *to maintain intact and healthy skin tissues.*
- Monitor fit of brace or orthosis *to detect early signs of improper fit or pressure areas.*
- Encourage child or parents to check with orthotist if signs of skin pressure develop *to prevent progression of skin irritation.*

NIC Immobility Management

Impaired physical mobility related to deformity or treatment

- Discuss purposes of bed rest and Cotrel's or halo-femoral traction before surgical correction.
- Change patient's position every 2 to 3 hours *to maintain tissue integrity.*
- Discuss need to limit activities to maintain traction or brace use *to increase compliance.*
- If surgery is performed, discuss need for bed rest *to permit healing.* (See p. 429 for nursing care for spinal fusion.)
- Encourage patient to maintain peer visits and interactions while movement is restricted *to foster personal growth and esteem.*
- Arrange for tutoring *to help patient keep up with schoolwork* if needed.
- Arrange for occupational therapy and physical therapy consultations *to maintain muscle strength, keep spirits up, and gain skill in equipment use.*
- Provide well-balanced diet *to promote healing after surgery and to lessen risk of infection.*

NIC Respiratory Management

Impaired gas exchange related to pulmonary compromise

- Nursing care is discussed under fracture/cast care, p. 411

Patient Education/Continuum of Care Plan

1. Clarify usual progression of lateralization without treatment.
2. Encourage continuity of medical care to monitor status of scoliosis and postoperative progress and healing.
3. Reiterate need to wear brace as prescribed to prevent progression of scoliosis before surgical correction.
4. After surgery, explain bone healing processes and cautions to permit healing to proceed.
5. Teach pulmonary and breathing exercises to improve pulmonary functions postoperatively.
6. Encourage communication and use of National Scoliosis Foundation or Scoliosis Association materials and services.
7. Encourage continuance of school-age children's screening for early detection of spinal abnormalities.

Evaluation/Patient Outcomes

Coping Assistance: Patient returns to social interactions and roles, has improved self-concept and body image, is better able to regain family and social roles, and is positive about self and future.

Skin/Wound Management: Patient uses brace or orthosis as prescribed. Skin tissues develop no redness or chafing. Patient wears proper underclothing under device.

Immobility Management: Posture and mobility have improved and curvature is lessened after treatment. Patient stands straighter with less curvature and rotation, hips and shoulders are more normally aligned, and mobility is improved.

Respiratory Management: Patient has satisfactory gas exchange. Patient has clear breath sounds and normal respiratory rates. No cough is noted. Patient's color is normal. Vital capacity has decreased minimally.

Lordosis

Lordosis is a normal curvature of the lumbar spine.

Lordosis may become exaggerated during pregnancy or in cases of large abdominal tumors or obesity, when overcorrection may be necessary to maintain balance when upright. Structural changes do not occur, and the condition is relieved with delivery, removal of the tumor, or weight loss.

Hyperlordosis, or "swayback," is fairly common in young children, especially girls, before puberty. The cause is thought to be rapid skeletal growth without appropriate stretching of the posterior soft tissues, such as the lumbar fascia and paraspinal muscles.

Permanent hyperlordosis, although very rare, can occur from degenerative conditions (e.g., osteoporosis) of the lumbosacral disks or vertebral bodies. Treatments for hyperlordosis include use of a brace or lumbar belt, spinal fusion, or osteotomy.

PERIPHERAL NERVE INJURIES

During a difficult delivery the baby may be injured around the neck and shoulder because of the force required for delivery through a tight pelvis and vagina. The injuries may be traction injuries to the nerves of the brachial plexus, but as a result, such injuries produce musculoskeletal injury from weakness and atrophy. Table 6-9 presents several injuries that can occur at birth or develop later in life from trauma. Nerve damage at any time of life causes significant musculoskeletal defects.

Without stimuli, muscles become weakened and flaccid and eventually shrink and atrophy. As muscles atrophy, they pull the tendons, ligaments, bones, and skin with them. Because the flexor muscles are generally stronger than the extensors, flexion contractures usually result. Adduction is frequently more noted than abduction, although either may be present. Rotation and pronation of the muscles and joints are also common. Changes may also accompany the motor losses.

Carpal and Tarsal Tunnel Syndromes

Carpal tunnel syndrome is a cluster of symptoms affecting the functions of the wrist, hand, and fingers.

Tarsal tunnel syndrome is a group of symptoms caused by pressure on the posterior tibial nerve in the medial side of the ankle.

Both syndromes have similar concerns but carpal tunnel syndrome will be discussed first.

Table 6-9 Musculoskeletal Effects of Nerve Injuries

Nerve	Site of Injury	Cause of Injury	Effects of Injury
Brachial plexus	Cervical roots of C5-7	Traction to arm or shoulder during delivery; gunshot wound; avulsion of nerves from excess traction accidentally applied; injury to cervical vertebrae	Erb's palsy: Affected arm, forearm, and hand internally rotated and pronated. Injury may cause temporary weakness and palsy; if severe, it will cause permanent paralysis with contracture of lower forearm, wrist, and fingers; sensory loss to outer arm
Brachial, axillary, and musculocutaneous	Cervical roots of C8 and T1	Breech delivery with arm above head; gunshot wound	Klumpke's palsy: Intrinsic muscles of hand and flexor muscles of fingers are paralyzed; some sensory loss may be present in ulnar forearm and hand; permanent effects: a claw hand develops in a flaccid, weak limb
Radial	Shoulder or elbow	Leaning on crutches in axillae; elbow: fracture; other: cutting of nerve, pressure of cast at wrist	Radial weakness from leaning on crutches with axillary pressure is fully reversible; elbow lesions; may have paralysis of wrist extensor and supinator muscles; eventually may need tendon transplants to wrist and fingers
Ulnar	Shoulder to elbow and to forearm	Open wounds (cut); fracture of medial epicondyle or lateral condyle; osteoarthritic or rheumatoid arthritis changes	Ring and little fingers may be temporarily or permanently held in hyperextended positions while rest of the hand is clawed; sensation is lost over ring and little fingers; there is muscle wasting of intrinsic muscles of hand
Median	Wrist under transverse carpal ligament	Trauma; pregnancy; rheumatoid arthritis; postmenopausal state; overuse (carpal tunnel syndrome)	Wasting of palmar thenar prominence (base of thumb); edema of hand; heavy, "clumsy" hand; sensory loss over radial 3½ fingers; if median nerve is severed without repair, paralysis of middle finger or index finger causes it to point ahead while other fingers are held in flexion; muscle wasting of hand (see below for carpal tunnel syndrome)
Peroneal	Neck of fibula	Pressure of splint; traction with leg in external rotation	Patient cannot dorsiflex or evert foot and toes; outer side of leg is wasted; foot drop is present; sensation is lost over front and outer half of leg and dorsum of foot and toes
Posterior tibial	On, by, or below medial malleolus	Overuse; injury from sprain of ankle, fracture of fibula or tibia; rheumatoid arthritis, diabetes mellitus, pregnancy (third trimester)	Patient may develop atrophy of the abductor hallucis (cannot abduct great toe), loss of sensory functions over heel, sole, and lateral plantar areas of foot; motor weakness of foot and lower leg

Carpal Tunnel Syndrome

Carpal tunnel syndrome results from compression of the median nerve in the tendon sheath under the transverse ligament on the ventral surface of the wrist (Fig. 6-23). Because the tissues in this part of the wrist normally fit closely together, any swelling usually brings on the compressive symptoms. The syndrome usually develops after trauma with subsequent inflammation, fibrosis, and scarring of the tendon sheath. However, no previous trauma may be noted.

Certain repetitive movements involving wrist twisting, turning, or pounding, such as those experienced when using a computer for many hours daily or when using a jackhammer, may cause the syndrome. Carpal tunnel syndrome has become one of the three most common industrial or work-related conditions and is related to the increased computer usage in all industries and government.

Curiously, pregnant women may develop carpal tunnel syndrome during their last trimester. The reasons for this have not yet been determined, although fluid retention, hypoxia from decreased circulation, and edema may be contributing factors.

More women than men develop carpal tunnel syndrome. Menopausal women and people with rheumatoid arthritis also show a higher incidence of the condition. It is seen bilaterally in nearly half of those affected.

Pathophysiology

Carpal tunnel syndrome develops secondary to repetitive motions of the wrist area, secondary to trauma, ganglion or neuroma, or tenosynovitis. Pain is one of the first symptoms of carpal tunnel syndrome. It often occurs at night, waking the patient with burning, tingling, and numbness. The fingers feel swollen, and the hand feels heavy. The patient usually hangs the arm over the bed or gets up and walks around to relieve the pain. The fingers may have paresthesias, including the thumb and the second, third, and radial side of the fourth fingers.

During the day the patient has few symptoms except when doing things that require turning the wrist, such as word processing and construction work. The hand is weaker and feels clumsy, and sometimes pain radiates up the arm. The thenar muscles develop atrophic changes with noticeable loss of muscle mass. Either one hand or both hands may be involved. Factors that correlate with carpal tunnel syndrome caused by repetitive motion include the following:

- Age 50 years or older
- Symptoms that have occurred for more than 10 months
- Constant tingling and burning sensation in fingers or hand
- Trigger finger (one finger locks, indicating that a broader area of inflammation is present)
- Positive Phalen test (see Fig. 6-24, *A*)

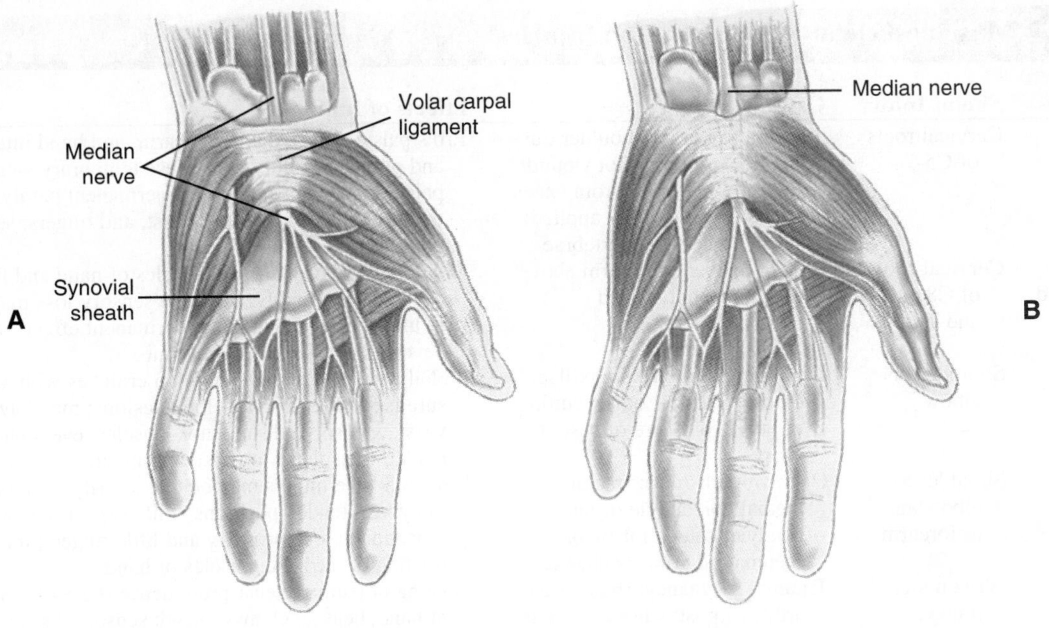

FIG. 6-23
A, Wrist structures affected in carpal tunnel syndrome. **B,** Decompression of median nerve.

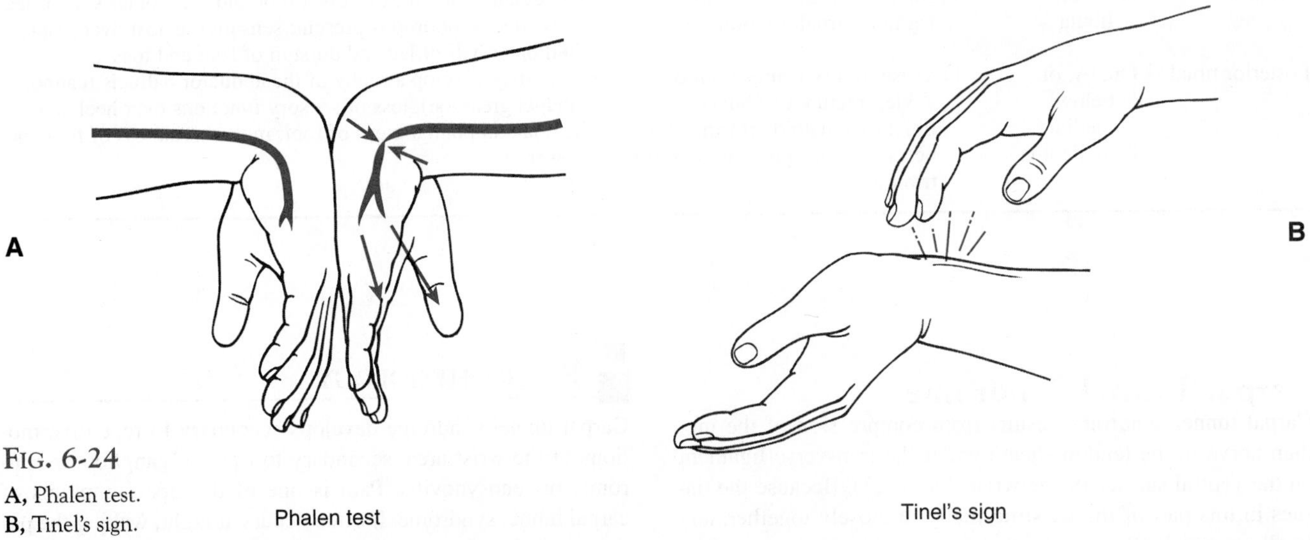

FIG. 6-24
A, Phalen test.
B, Tinel's sign.

A condition similar to carpal tunnel syndrome can occur in one or more other peripheral nerves, including the radial and ulnar tunnels in the upper extremity. Tarsal tunnel syndrome, which is similar to carpal tunnel syndrome, may occur in the lower extremity and foot. Radial nerve weakness can temporarily occur from improper use of crutches. This clears when the person stops resting on the axillary supports of the crutches. Ulnar nerve injuries frequently accompany elbow trauma. When severe, such upper extremity nerve injuries can cause clawing of and loss of sensation in the ring and little fingers.

DIAGNOSTIC STUDIES AND FINDINGS

History: History of repetitive activities of wrist(s); sensory changes: paresthesia and numbness of thumbs, index fingers, and ring fingers, pain waking patient at night; motor changes, with clumsiness, heaviness of hand, and edema; thenar muscle atrophy; pain, possibly radiating up arm; correlation with pregnancy, rheumatoid arthritis, postmenopausal state, diabetes, thyroid dysfunction; similar symptoms in lower extremity with tarsal tunnel syndrome (see later)

Physical examination: Deficits in sensory mapping along median nerve innervation pathways; positive Tinel's sign (FIG. 6-24, *B*): increased tingling with gentle tap over tendon sheath on ventral surface of central wrist; edema of fingers noted; thenar surfaces of palm thinner than normal (wasting); holding wrists against each other in forced palmar flexion for 1 minute can elicit sensory changes of numbness and tingling, which is a positive Phalen test (FIG. 6-24, *A*), one indication of carpal tunnel syndrome

Electromyogram: Weakened muscle response to stimulation

MRI: Shows compression and flattening of the median nerve; increased signal intensity within the median nerve; abrupt changes in diameter of the median nerve

Handheld electroneurometer: Used if EMG services not available; predicts motor latency of median nerve that is diagnostic of carpal tunnel syndrome

MULTIDISCIPLINARY PLAN

Surgery

Release of carpal ligament and tendon to relieve compression (see FIG. 6-23, *B*); surgery may be done endoscopically

Medications

Injection of hydrocortisone (dosage varies) into tendon sheath to relieve inflammation

Antiinflammatory agents

- Ibuprofen, 400-600 mg bid
- Celecoxib (Celebrex), 100 mg bid
- See table on p. 337 for additional NSAIDs

General Management

Use of a cock-up splint to relieve pressure and to lessen wrist flexion

Elevation to relieve edema

ROM exercises to lessen sense of clumsiness

Restriction of twisting and turning activities of wrist

Continuation of usual medical care for systemic illness (rheumatoid arthritis) if present

NURSING CARE

NURSING ASSESSMENT

Wrist, hand, and fingers (both extremities) and both ankles and feet: Inability to use hands and fingers through normal ROM; inability to walk or use pressure on heel and sole of foot—compare with opposite foot; movements limited; presence or absence of edema, numbness, tingling, pain; assessment of time when pain is present, severity, and activities that increase or decrease pain; assessment of palmar thenar (base of thumb) surfaces for atrophy, may have slight atrophy of foot muscles; assessment of distribution of paresthesia (if present) into fingers or up arm, and/or assessment of numbness of heel, sole, and toes

Systemic concerns: Rheumatoid arthritis, postmenopausal state, pregnancy in last trimester, diabetes, thyroid dysfunction, overuse

Psychosocial concerns: Self-concept, disturbance in body image, role performance; impaired physical mobility

POTENTIAL COMPLICATIONS

Return of carpal tunnel syndrome, lingering numbness, tarsal tunnel syndrome (see p. 386)

PATIENT PROBLEMS/NURSING DIAGNOSES & INTERVENTIONS

NIC PERFUSION MANAGEMENT

Ineffective tissue perfusion related to compression and edema of nerve

- Check circulatory status of limb by neurovascular checks (p. 330).
- Apply ice bag or cryotherapy or similar apparatus to wrist area *to decrease edema.*
- Report increasing numbness to physician *for patient's safety.*
- Apply splint *to prevent flexion of wrist;* flexion increases numbness and tingling in presence of syndrome.
- Compare both wrists and hands *to note if symptoms are bilateral.*

NIC IMMOBILITY MANAGEMENT

Impaired physical mobility related to pain, edema, and motor changes

- Clarify effects of condition on wrist and hand ROM *to determine severity of condition.*
- Explain inflammatory processes to correlate need to limit activities of wrist and hand *to ease concerns or anxiety.*
- Assist with and teach proper splint application and need to wear at night *to prevent flexion of wrist;* assist with hygienic care if necessary *to increase independence and compliance.*
- Elevate hand and wrist or foot if edema present *to aid venous return.*
- Assist with ROM exercises if ordered *to maintain functions.*
- Continue care for concomitant illnesses *to relieve symptoms.*
- Observe and assess site for relief of symptoms after injection of hydrocortisone, if used, or after surgical release *to note effects of treatment.*
- Encourage continuing follow-up medical care until recovery is complete *to aid resolution of condition.*

NIC PHYSICAL COMFORT PROMOTION

Acute pain related to edema and compression of nerve

- Ask about amount, type, and severity of pain.
- Administer pain medication as prescribed; monitor and report patient's response *to note efficacy.*
- Apply ice bags *to decrease edema and pain.*
- Do preoperative preparation and teaching *to ease anxiety and promote safe care.*
- Monitor relief of numbness, tingling, and pain after surgical procedure *to determine effect of ligament release.*

PATIENT EDUCATION/CONTINUUM OF CARE PLAN

1. Reiterate explanations of inflammatory processes as bases for symptoms.
2. Discuss activities to lessen stress on inflamed tissues.
3. Reassure about relief of symptoms after surgical release or injection of steroid that follows reduction of edema and healing of involved tissues.
4. If patient is pregnant, discuss probable relief of symptoms after delivery.
5. If condition is employment related, discuss possible need for changing to alternate job activities or seek changes in equipment to prevent recurrence.

Evaluation/Patient Outcomes

Tissue Perfusion Management: Patient regains adequate tissue perfusion. Patient has no numbness, tingling, or edema after treatments.

Immobility Management: Patient regains joint ROM and muscle strength over time. Patient performs self-care and regains strength after incision heals. Thenar pad gradually regains muscle mass.

Physical Comfort Promotion: Patient experiences pain-free wrist and hand functions. Patient has no pain, edema, numbness, or tingling when using wrist and hand. Heel and foot are pain free without numbness.

Tarsal Tunnel Syndrome

Tarsal tunnel syndrome (TTS) is a condition analogous to carpal tunnel syndrome, but involving the posterior tibial nerve in the foot rather than the median nerve in the wrist. It is believed to be more common than previously thought because it may be misdiagnosed initially. TTS may accompany rheumatoid arthritis and diabetes mellitus. It may also have no known cause. It is also diagnosed in runners and aerobic dancers.

TTS involves compression of the posterior tibial nerve and its branches (see Fig. 6-25) where the nerve crosses through the fibro-osseous tunnel below the medial malleolus—the tarsal tunnel.[27] Along with the posterior tibial nerve, other structures in this tunnel are the posterior tibial artery and vein and the tendons of the posterior tibialis, flexor degitorum longus, and flexor hallucis longus muscles. The nerve divides into branches that innervate various parts of the foot sole and heel areas with both sensory and motor functions.

Pathophysiology

The nerve and its branches are very susceptible to injury because of the many structures within the tarsal tunnel. Compression leads to inflammation of the tendon sheaths, causing local ischemia, pain, swelling or edema, and tenosynovitis, tightening and inflammation of one or more of the tendon sheaths in the tarsal tunnel. Inflammatory changes and pressure may lead to permanent destruction of the nerve and its branches. The person with TTS may have sharp, shooting pains in the heel, sole, or plantar and lateral surfaces of the foot, with aching and cramping at times. Pain may even radiate up the lower leg areas. Activities, such as walking, running, and jumping, make the pain more intense and lead to restricting use of the affected foot. There may be numbness with flexion of the foot and paresthesias into the heel, foot, and toes, along with "burning" sensations. Pain may be worse and awaken the patient at night in untreated TTSs.[27]

Diagnostic Studies and Findings

History: History of engaging in sports activities such as basketball, soccer, volleyball, or aerobics; history of recent fracture of tibia and/or fibula or severe, third-degree sprain of ankle; history of rheumatoid arthritis or diabetes mellitus; is a runner and jogger

Physical examination: Positive Tinel's sign over distribution of posterior tibial nerve (see Fig. 6-24, *B*); sensory losses over heel, plantar, and lateral surfaces of the foot and toes; motor weakness of ankle flexion, plantar flexion, and up and down movements of toes; may have ankle, foot, and/or toe edema, with weak ability to abduct great toe against examiner's pressure

Nerve conduction studies: May indicate slowed responses or motor latency

Electromyogram: May indicate slower action potentials

MRI: May show inflammation in tendon sheaths with tendon sheath effusion

Multidisciplinary Plan

Conservative Treatment

Rest of leg and foot
Immobilization in a splint, cast, or ankle brace

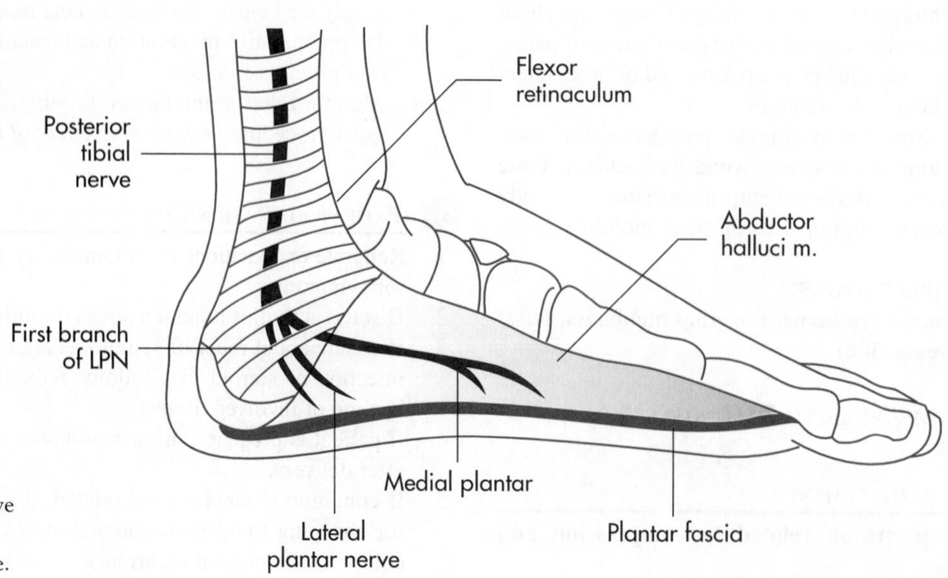

Fig. 6-25
Posterior tibial nerve with its branches, medial side of ankle.

Application of alternating ice/heat compresses as prescribed
Physical therapy with foot/ankle exercises
Use of orthosis in shoe and crutches for ambulation
Injection of steroid into tarsal tunnel
Stop activities that aggravate the condition
Intake of NSAID as prescribed
Phenytoin (Dilantin), 100 mg tid or Elavil (amitriptyline), 25-50 mg daily for neuritic pain or depression

Surgery

Decompression of the tarsal tunnel and all branches of the posterior tibial nerve

Medications

Narcotic analgesic agents
- Ketorolac (Toradol), 10 mg IV or PO q4h as needed
- Hydrocodone/APAP (Vicodin), 60 mg, PO q4-6h as needed

Antiinflammatory agents
- Ibuprofen (Motrin), 400-600 mg q4-6h as needed
- Celecoxib (Celebrex), 100 mg bid
- Rofecoxib (Vioxx), 12.5 mg daily

General Management

Bed rest with operative leg elevated after decompression
Use crutches for ambulation with non–weight bearing initially
Wound care with dressing changes and suture removal in approximately 2 weeks
Physical therapy and aqua therapy exercises with heel stretching

NURSING CARE

Nursing Assessment

NOTE: The nursing diagnoses and interventions are very similar for TTS and carpal tunnel syndrome (see pp. 382-387); thus they will not be repeated. The reader need only substitute lower leg, ankle, and foot for wrist, hand, and fingers in most instances. Also, mobility aids are necessary for TTS until healing has progressed. Patient education, continuity of care, and evaluation goals are also too similar to repeat.

Potential Complications

Recurrence of TTS, calcaneal neuroma, tibial neuritis

Sciatic Nerve Injury

Sciatic nerve injury is a pathologic condition usually caused by external trauma to the nerve.

Injury to the sciatic nerve may be primary, from a gunshot wound, stabbing, fall, or other cause, or it may result from pressure caused by rupture of an intervertebral nucleus pulposus. The pathologic nucleus pulposus exerts pressure on the spinal nerves as they exit the spinal cord and traverse the sciatic nerve. The intervertebral disks that rupture most often (95%) are at the L5-S1 and L4-L5 interspaces. Cervical intervertebral disks rupture less frequently, although they can become painful from degenerative changes and may lead to spinal stenosis from osteophyte formation.

The following discussion focuses on pathologic findings in the sciatic nerve resulting from herniation (rupture) of one or more lumbar intervertebral nuclei pulposi.

Low back pain, with or without sciatica, is a symptom complex reported in nearly 60% to 80% of persons in the general population with a cost of over $24 billion per year. The medical treatment of low back pain is one of the leading compensable costs injuries in the workplace. The following discussion focuses on degenerative disk disease in the lower back as the cause of low back pain.

Pathophysiology

The nucleus pulposus is a semigelatinous mass inside the cartilaginous annulus (disk) between the bodies of each vertebra. It plays a key role in the structural stability of the spine by providing load absorption and distribution while anchoring the vertebral bodies to one another through a wide range of motions. When the cartilage of the annulus cracks or degenerates, it allows the nucleus pulposus to rupture through the cracks. A ruptured disk is a twofold process of degeneration of the annulus with herniation of the nucleus pulposus material. It appears that the intervertebral disk undergoes dramatic age-related changes.

Rupture of the annulus is generally caused by degenerative changes in the cartilaginous structures of the annulus. As the disk (annulus) ages, it loses elasticity, partly from changes and increases in proteoglycans in its collagen fibers and partly from decreases in its fluid content. These changes weaken the disk, making it unable to tolerate even usual body weight. The disk flattens or bulges, and additional pressure from lifting, straining, increased weight, or a sudden twist, turn, or sharp bending of the back may cause the annulus to bulge backward or tear. The nucleus pulposus can then extrude through the crack. The mass can extrude anteriorly toward the cord, laterally toward the lamina and facets, or posteriorly toward the posterior spinous processes (FIG. 6-26). The extruded mass presses on the dura mater, nerve roots, or both, causing pain in the back that radiates to the sciatic nerve. The presence of the extruded mass plus the pressure causes edema to develop, which also increases pain. At times, if the entire nucleus mass has not extruded, it may move back inside the disk when the edema subsides. If the mass stays extruded, it can adhere to the nerve roots or their dural sheaths, adding to the scarring and pain. Eventually the prolapsed material can also disturb the functioning of the facets or the vertebrae, leading to further degeneration of these joints, through the formation of osteophytes and hypertrophy of the facet joints.[19]

The incident that causes the acute rupture can be as trivial as a sneeze or cough while the person is bent forward. Usually the rupture is caused by lifting something while the body is not in optimum lift position, lifting an unexpectedly heavy load, or lifting a load that shifts suddenly. Excessive pressure is referred from tensed abdominal and back muscles to the annulus and then to the nucleus, which ruptures through the weakened, cracked annulus. Signs of sciatic nerve pressure follow the rupture. Approximately one third or more of patients who have a first episode of back pain still have significant problems years later.

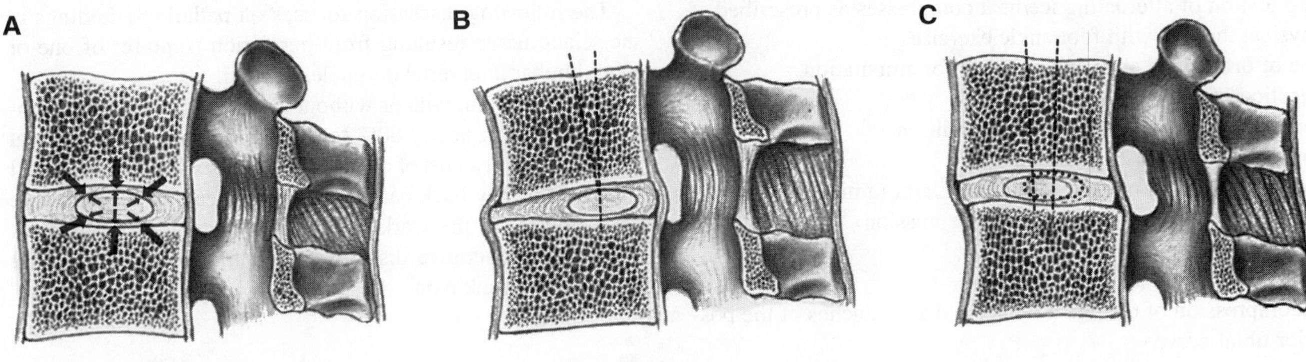

FIG. 6-26
Mechanisms that can cause degeneration of the annulus leading to herniation of the nucleus pulposus. **A,** Axial pressure. **B,** Lateral pressure. **C,** Posterior pressure.

Recent studies of degenerative disk disease found this condition to have a heritable incidence in twins studied. Researchers[40] found disk height and bulge as well as formation of osteophytes to be heritable in 79% of twins with "severe disease." The gene or genes have not been discovered to date.[46]

DIAGNOSTIC STUDIES AND FINDINGS

History: Sudden acute pain in low back, with or without radiation to hips or down one or both legs

Physical examination: Loss of normal lordotic curve; "list" or tilt to side; tense, tight back muscles; tenderness in low back that may radiate to buttocks; ROM movements limited in forward flexion, in lateral flexion, and sometimes in extension; pain radiating down (usually) one leg to foot and toes; straight leg raising limited by pain; pain increased with foot dorsiflexion; sensations impaired on outer thigh, calf, and foot; paresthesia with numbness and tingling; knee and ankle reflexes possibly diminished or absent (knee reflex rarely lost)

Roentgenograms of back: Tilt; diminished disk space (not necessarily diagnostic)

Myelogram: Location of rupture revealed by impaired dye flow

CT scan: Ruptured disk or spinal stenosis

MRI: Ruptured disk shows clearly and reveals where pressure is on nerves or other tissues; also identifies changes in facet joints

Discogram: Should differentiate between disk infection and rupture

MULTIDISCIPLINARY PLAN

Surgery

Arthroscopic diskectomy
Percutaneous diskectomy
Microdiskectomy
Nuclear diskectomy
Hemilaminectomy with removal of extruded nucleus and degenerated annulus
Spinal fusion, if more than one disk is involved and patient does heavy lifting
Lumbar arthrodesis to relieve pain
Fenestration to open nerve root exit sites

Chemonucleolysis

Done less frequently now and tends to be concentrated in a few centers

Medications

Analgesic/antipyretic agents
- Aspirin (ASA), 600-1000 mg q4h
- Acetaminophen (Tylenol), 600-1000 mg q4h

Antianxiety agents
- Diazepam (Valium), 2-10 mg PO q4-6h

Narcotic analgesic agents
- Oxycodone (Percodan), 30-60 mg q4h for severe pain uncontrolled by aspirin
- Meperidine (Demerol), 50-150 mg IM q3h

Muscle relaxants
- Cyclobenzaprine (Flexeril), 10-20 mg PO tid
- Methocarbamol (Robaxin), 500-750 mg PO q4-6h
- Metaxalone (Skelaxin), 400-800 mg tid or qid

NSAIDs
- Naproxen (Naprosyn), 250-500 mg bid
- Diclofenac (Voltaren), 25-75 mg bid
- Choline magnesium trisalicylate (Trilisate), 750-1000 mg q4h
- Ibuprofen (Motrin), 400-60 mg bid or tid
- Ketorolac (Toradol), 10 mg q4-6h
- Celecoxib (Celebrex), 100 mg bid
- Rofecoxib (Vioxx), 12.5 mg daily

General Management

NOTE: Many patients are outpatients for these care and management techniques. Application of skin traction (pelvic belt) (no study to date indicates any positive influence on low back pain with traction)
Williams' position in bed (head of bed and knee gatch each elevated 45 degrees to relax lumbosacral muscles)
Diathermy to low back three or four times daily; ice massage; hydrotherapy
Application of canvas back support or metal back brace
Physical therapy with specific exercises to strengthen back and abdominal muscles

Bed rest on firm mattress during acute rupture for 1 to 3 days only because there is up to a 3% loss of muscle strength per day during bed rest
Cessation of lifting and stooping
Back massage after diathermy
Use of transcutaneous electrical nerve stimulation (TENS)
Avoidance or cessation of smoking (nicotine decreases circulation in intervertebral disks)
Maintenance of normal weight (some patients overeat and gain weight with chronic low back pain syndromes)

NURSING CARE

Nursing Assessment

Vertebral column, lumbar back, and sciatic nerve dermatomes (areas on the skin surface innervated by spinal nerve roots): Degree of lumbar lordotic curve; ROM of back (forward, backward, lateral to each side) slightly less than normal: "list" or tilt to either side, tenderness or painful areas; pain in back or buttocks, radiating down posterior thighs and legs to feet and toes; may be only unilateral; assessment of muscles for spasm, tenseness, tightness, or weakness; leg-raising assessments—may be diminished or less than 90 degrees; sensory functions around thigh, leg, and foot (bilaterally)—check sharp and dull sensitivity; strength or absence of knee and ankle reflexes; bowel or bladder function changes; may have constipation and bladder retention
Systemic concerns: Concomitant systemic diseases: rheumatoid arthritis, ankylosing spondylitis, osteoarthritis, osteoporosis
Psychosocial concerns: Body image disturbance and altered role performance; impaired physical mobility; acute pain in lower back with radiation; failure of conservative care, necessitating surgery; economic costs for prolonged disability, long-term care, and possible loss of employment; lack of insurance coverage (if not injured on the job)

Potential Complications

Permanent numbness of foot, heel, lower leg; development of degenerative joint disease (osteoarthritis); failed back surgery; spinal stenosis

Patient Problems/Nursing Diagnoses & Interventions

NIC Immobility Management

Impaired physical mobility related to back and leg pain and muscle spasms

- Observe ability to move and limitations of movements.
- Explain purposes of hospitalization, temporary bed rest, and traction *to increase compliance.*
- Explain use of firm mattress and bed position (Williams' position) *to relax spasm of back muscles.*
- Prepare patient for physical therapy, diathermy, and massage; assist with hygienic care to have patient ready and to lessen strain on back *to aid compliance and lessen anxiety.*
- Help apply back support, brace, or belt; teach self-application *to increase independence.*
- Place in skin traction belt; observe responses; remove traction while sleeping *to lessen muscle spasms and muscle strain.*
- Monitor relief of pain or numbness *to determine efficacy of treatments.*

NIC Coping Assistance

Disturbed body image and ineffective role performance related to condition

- Ask about condition's effects on usual roles and self-concept.
- Encourage to discuss usual roles and temporary adjustments needed with family members *to ease patient's concerns.*
- Seek assistance from social services *for continuity of care after discharge.*
- Encourage to ventilate stresses or other concerns *to aid relaxation.*

NIC Physical Comfort Promotion

Acute pain in back and legs related to condition

- Determine amount, sites, and severity of pain by discussion with patient.
- Keep patient on bed rest *to relieve inflammation with acute low back pain,* if prescribed—usually not longer than 48 to 72 hours because it decreases muscle strength.
- Administer analgesics around the clock as prescribed *to maintain an adequate blood level for first 2 to 3 days.*
- Administer NSAIDs as prescribed *to block effects of prostaglandins to relieve pain.*
- Administer muscle relaxants as ordered *to relieve spasms.*
- Assess effect of Williams' position *in relieving spasms and pain.*
- Offer back massage *to relax muscles and relieve inflammation.*
- Clarify relief of pressure signs on sciatic nerve by determining relief of paresthesia, numbness, and so forth *to note resolution of symptoms.*
- Perform "laminectomy checks" *to note progression or regression of symptoms:* check sites and amount of numbness, tingling, motor functions, leg strength, temperature of extremities, sites and amount of pain, sites of radiation of pain, color, and temperature of affected tissues.
- Report continued presence of pain, paresthesia, and muscle spasms to physician.
- Teach muscle relaxation techniques *to aid relaxation of tense muscles.*
- Use dietary measures, high fluid intake, and medication *to prevent constipation (straining increases pain).*
- Encourage weight loss through diet, if overweight, *to lessen strain on weak muscles of back and abdomen.*

Patient Education/Continuum of Care Plan

1. Discuss purposes of bed positions to relieve pain and inflammation.
2. Demonstrate proper lifting postures, when feasible.

3. Demonstrate exercises to strengthen muscles.
4. Encourage maintenance of normal weight for size, sex, and age.
5. Provide pamphlet and explain use of proper body mechanics.
6. Encourage to seek medical care if symptoms continue.
7. Stress cessation of smoking.

EVALUATION/PATIENT OUTCOMES

Immobility Management: Patient regains physical mobility with treatments; resumes walking with less back pain. Patient returns to work while continuing treatments. Back muscle spasms are no longer present.

Coping Assistance: Patient resumes many social interactions and roles; returns to family, social, and employment roles and activities. Patient takes rest periods periodically.

Physical Comfort Promotion: Patient's back pain and muscle spasms are mostly relieved. Patient uses back for ADLs without pain, numbness, radiation to legs, or muscle spasms and has no limitations in ROM. Patient needs only nonnarcotic analgesics for comfort.

COLLABORATIVE INTERVENTIONS AND RELATED NURSING CARE

AMPUTATION

Description and Rationale

Amputation is the removal of all or part of a specific tissue or organ. Musculoskeletal tissues are frequently amputated because of crush injuries, severe sepsis, malignant tumors, or gangrene resulting from loss of arterial or venous circulatory integrity. Less frequently a limb may be amputated because of intractable pain from paralysis or because of multiple recurrent flare-ups of osteomyelitis that threaten not only the limb but also the individual's life.

The following terms refer to amputations involving the extremities:

Forequarter: Removal of entire arm, forearm, and hand; extremity disarticulated at shoulder joint.

Arm: Amputation above elbow or along forearm.

Hemipelvectomy: Removal of thigh at hip joint, leg, and foot; also referred to as hindquarter amputation or hip disarticulation.

Thigh: Amputation above the knee (above-knee amputation, AKA).

Lower Leg: Amputation below the knee (below-knee amputation, BKA).

Foot: Amputation of toes and foot at metatarsal joints (Syme's amputation).

Finger or toe: Amputation of part or all of one or more fingers or toes.

The three types of amputations are *provisional,* which is done when primary healing is unlikely; *definitive end bearing,* which is done when weight will be borne through the end of the stump; and *definitive non–end bearing,* which is done when weight will not be borne at the end of the stump. When weight will be borne through the end of the stump, the incision is not made at the end but is cut through or near a joint; if weight will not be borne at the end of the stump, the incision can be terminal (at the end of the stump). Also, the incision may be cut perpendicularly to the bone through all the tissues, called a guillotine incision, with little or no incisional closure and only loosely applied dressings. The guillotine incision is used in grossly infected tissues. The more frequently used incision is closed and snugly dressed after the tissues are amputated; it is commonly done in noninfected tissues.

During the surgical procedure, bleeding is controlled through application of a tourniquet unless there is arterial insufficiency. Skin flaps are made, usually of equal length for upper limb or above-knee amputations and with a longer posterior flap for below-knee amputations. The muscles are divided distal to the intended site of bone resection, and later opposing muscle groups are sutured over the bone end to each other and to the periosteum to provide better muscle control and circulation. Nerves are divided proximal to the bone end. After the bone is cut, all vessels and bleeders are ligated carefully and the skin flaps are sutured closed (unless tissues are infected), drains are inserted, and the stump is firmly dressed.

Contraindications and Cautions

1. If the amputation is to be done to remove a malignant tumor, metastasis to distant sites is usually a contraindication.
2. Lack of arterial circulation requires that the amputation be proximal to the gangrenous or necrotic tissues.
3. Enough tissues must be left on and over the stump for fitting of a prosthesis when possible.

Preprocedural Nursing Care

1. Meticulous skin cleansing with antiseptic solutions removes transient and some resident bacteria.

EMERGENCY ALERT

UNINTENTIONAL TRAUMATIC AMPUTATION

Unintentional traumatic amputation occurs when a limb or digit is partially or totally severed from the body.

ASSESSMENT

- Assess presence of and amount of bleeding or hemorrhage at site(s) of amputation.
- Assess condition and reactions to injury: level of consciousness, awareness of traumatic event, confusion or disorientation, fainting, color of skin, and shock.
- Assess respirations for rate, depth, and regularity.

INTERVENTIONS

- Establish or maintain airway, breathing, and circulation.
- Control bleeding, support limb in functional position.
- Administer high-flow oxygen by mask (10 to 15 L).
- Obtain IV access.
- Locate amputated part(s); wrap in gauze saturated with normal saline or lactated Ringer's solution.
- Maintain amputated part(s) at 40° C; *do not* place directly on ice.
- Keep limb in anatomically correct position.
- Transport to medical facility.

2. Determine presence of peripheral pulses as distally as possible; for crush injuries, may need Doppler for most accurate assessment.
3. Compare edema, color, temperature, skin condition, and pain (when present) with tissues on the opposite side of the body. Edema may be pronounced in venous obstruction.
4. Observe the skin for open or draining areas.
5. Check vital signs for evidence of systemic infection and to monitor the patient's general condition.
6. With crush injuries, observe the patient for hemorrhage, possible shock, and renal functions.
7. If the patient is a child or older adult, determine factors related to age and developmental or educational level that could affect recovery and self-care after the amputation.
8. A rehabilitated person with a similar amputation may visit the patient preoperatively when possible or when requested by the patient.
9. Monitor control of chronic diseases, such as diabetes or peripheral vascular diseases, related to preoperative and postoperative care.
10. Begin discussion of phantom limb pain before surgery to enhance positive patient outcomes and to reduce anxiety and fear. Include family or significant others in discussion, if appropriate.

MULTIDISCIPLINARY PLAN

Surgery

Wound suction continuously postoperatively
Change of dressings as needed

Medications

Antiinfective agents
- Cephalothin sodium (Keflin), 500-1000 mg IV q4-6h for 48-72 h (or longer, if prescribed)
- Cefazolin (Ancef), 250-1000 mg q4-6h IV for 3-5 days
- Vancomycin (Vancocin), 500-1000 mg q6-8h for 24 h

Narcotic analgesic agents
- Meperidine (Demerol), 50-100 mg IM q3h for pain (may use PCA IV)
- Morphine 1.5-2 mg q10min with 20-30 min lockout per PCA pump

IV fluid replacement with 5% dextrose in 0.45 normal saline solution, 2000-3000 ml for 24 h

MICROVASCULAR REPAIR AND REPLANTATION

Although not thoroughly discussed here, major advances in the care of patients with severe musculoskeletal trauma have been made with the development of microvascular surgical techniques. These include replantation of completely amputated body parts and revascularization of crush, avulsion, and other soft tissue injuries.

Before replantation or microsurgical repair, data are gathered and evaluated to determine whether functional return is possible, particularly if the injuries involve an upper extremity. Functional return is more likely when the injury is to a finger or fingers or low on the forearm because of the shorter distances for nerve regeneration. Repair or replantation should be performed as soon as possible after the injury because ischemic tissues must be reperfused within 12 hours for function to be regained. Necrosis of tissues may preclude functional return if tissues are ischemic longer than 24 hours.

Surgical repair or replantation is done under a microscope and usually follows a pattern of stabilization of fractured bones followed by repair of arteries for restoration of blood flow. With circulation restored, nerves, veins, tendons, and ligaments are repaired, and skin closure, which may necessitate placement of a skin graft, is done. Nerves may not be repaired during the initial surgery but may be repaired 2 to 3 weeks later because the injuries or scarring from inflammatory processes and healing may delay or preclude nerve regeneration.

Postoperatively, nursing observations and care are critical for the success of the repair or replantation. Tissue pressure monitoring may be required in crush injuries to detect rising interstitial pressures, which may signal the development of compartment syndrome (see box, p. 408). The digits are monitored closely for evidence of capillary refill and arterial flow through the use of Doppler detectors, arteriography, and plethysmography. Tissue temperatures are checked with thermometers, and edema, skin color, and turgor are closely assessed. Bleeding is carefully monitored, especially if anticoagulants are being administered. The external fixator or splint is checked for proper position and function. Dressings are changed as required to aid healing, and antibiotics are administered to prevent infection.

Leeches *(Hirudo medicinalis)* may be used in the early postoperative period to decrease venous congestion and edema by promoting bleeding. At times each leech will ingest 5 to 10 times its own weight in secretions and fluid. Leeches are used carefully and are closely monitored. They loosen their hold after 10 to 30 minutes of feeding. Each leech is placed individually in a congested area. The leech is placed on a bleeding puncture wound made by a sterile needle. The leech quickly attaches to the site. Its bite is painless because the leech secretes a natural anesthetic to lessen pain. Once the leech has become attached to the site, it is covered and confined with a sterile clear specimen cup taped over the area. The leech will loosen its hold or attachment when it is full (some leeches can ingest up to 50 ml). As the leech loosens its hold, it is removed and put in alcohol or saline solution to destroy it. Leeches may be needed for 3 to 5 days or until the congestion is markedly lessened.

A complication of the use of leeches is a bacterial infection that responds to cephalosporin or aminoglycoside therapy.

The patient, relatives, visitors, and all health-care personnel in contact with the patient are not permitted to smoke because the nicotine in the tobacco could lead to vasospasm, vasoconstriction, and ischemia, which could threaten the tissue perfusion and healing processes.

Initial outcomes after repair or replantation vary with the extent of trauma, the adequacy of tissue repairs, the degree of inflammatory responses, scarring, and absence of complications of arterial and venous occlusion and infection. Long-term success depends greatly on physical therapies and psychosocial rehabilitation.

General Management

Stump elevated for 24 hours, then kept flat and extended (elevation depends on presence or amount of edema in stump)
Adduction exercises of amputated extremity, 10 times per hour after 24 hours
For lower extremity amputation, turning to prone position four times daily to extend hip and knee
Thigh (hamstring) tightening exercises in prone position begun after 24 hours (10 times q4h)
Up with crutches three times daily on first postoperative day
Physical therapy consultation for exercise regimen, to assist with ambulation, and for shoulder or elbow exercises, if upper extremity amputation
Occupational therapy consultation for rehabilitation care
Regular diet as desired
Stump wrapping after sutures are removed
Orthotic technician (prosthetist) to measure for prosthesis
Stump check every hour for first 24 hours to note color, drainage, edema, bleeding, sutures (wound), and pulses proximal to incision site; measure amount of drainage in suction system, if used
Tourniquet always present at bedside
Up in chair after recovery from anesthesia
Pulmonary deep breathing and coughing every 4 hours
Analysis of gait problems and progress by gait laboratory personnel

NOTE: Some patients may return from surgery with a prosthesis already in place, held to the stump with plaster (an immediate postsurgical fitting). It is usually left in place up to 10 days, after which it is removed, the sutures are removed, and a new cast is applied. This fitting lessens edema and pain, although the rigidity of the plaster delays the shaping of the stump into a conical shape. However, the immediate postsurgical prosthesis does permit earlier ambulation and discharge, particularly in younger patients.

NURSING CARE

NURSING ASSESSMENT

Site of amputation (stump): Drainage or bleeding scant and serosanguineous; edema slight; dressing intact without constriction; pain may be sharp and acute in incisional area; if drain is present, drainage may be scant to moderate, although still serosanguineous; drainage in a suction setup, such as a Hemovac or Jackson-Pratt, may be moderate and serosanguineous; tourniquet should be at bedside in the event of arterial bleeding
Entire extremity: Extremity should remain extended to prevent contracture; ROM of muscles and joints may be slightly limited by pain, stiffness, or edema; only incisional area may have edema or erythema unless infection develops
Psychosocial concerns: Concern with alteration in body image and appearance; presence of phantom pain—feeling as if fingers or hand, toes, foot, arm, or leg is still present, pinched, or painful; may have burning, crushing sensations, cramping, or spasmodic sensation; alteration in mobility and ability to maintain livelihood and income

POTENTIAL COMPLICATIONS

Hemorrhage, wound infection, or dehiscence; development of contractures; persistence of phantom pain; development of neuromas; excessive scar formation; inability to use prosthesis for ADLs and mobility; development of limp

PATIENT PROBLEMS/NURSING DIAGNOSES & INTERVENTIONS

NIC COPING ASSISTANCE

Disturbed body image related to loss of limb

- Discuss effects of amputation on body image.
- Allow and encourage patient to express feelings of mutilation, grief, anger, and loss, as well as avoidance of looking at stump, *to aid adaptation processes.*
- Encourage patient to help with dressing changes and wrapping of stump as able. Teach family member wrapping techniques if necessary *to increase competence and independence.*
- Encourage family members to walk with patient *to maintain strength and social contacts.*
- Encourage grooming and wearing of personal clothing *to maintain individuality and personality.*
- Encourage activities for self-care and ambulation *to maintain positive outlook and maximum strength.*
- Arrange for consultation with gait laboratory *for assistance with gait management to increase self-esteem in use of prosthesis.*
- Encourage or arrange for social services consultation *for economic and employment aid.*
- Arrange for follow-up care referral *to aid rehabilitation.*

NIC IMMOBILITY MANAGEMENT

Impaired physical mobility related to loss of limb

- Determine ability to use remaining limbs.
- Turn and position on side, back, and abdomen (after 24 h) *to maintain muscle and joint ROM.*
- Teach adduction and extension exercises and help patient perform them every 4 hours *to prevent abduction and flexion contractures.*
- Assist with sitting in chair and ambulation with aid as able *to maintain muscle strength.*
- Prepare for physical therapy, transportation for exercises, and stump wrapping if appropriate.
- Encourage family members to learn wrapping (FIG. 6-27).
- Encourage family members to walk with patient during initial ambulation periods, accompanied by health professionals, *to increase independence.*
- Teach purposes of prone and extension positions *to prevent contractures.*
- Assist prosthetist with prosthesis measurements and fitting as needed *to aid rehabilitation.*
- Contact personnel in gait laboratory, per physician's prescription, for gait analysis *to increase patient's mobility and confidence.* Gait analysis helps determine the optimal type of prosthetic foot for amputee.

NIC PHYSICAL COMFORT PROMOTION

Acute pain (nerve trauma after surgery) related to surgical transection

- Determine type, amount, and severity of pain. Clarify site of pain (i.e., in the stump, missing body part or where in body. See p. 390 for definitions)

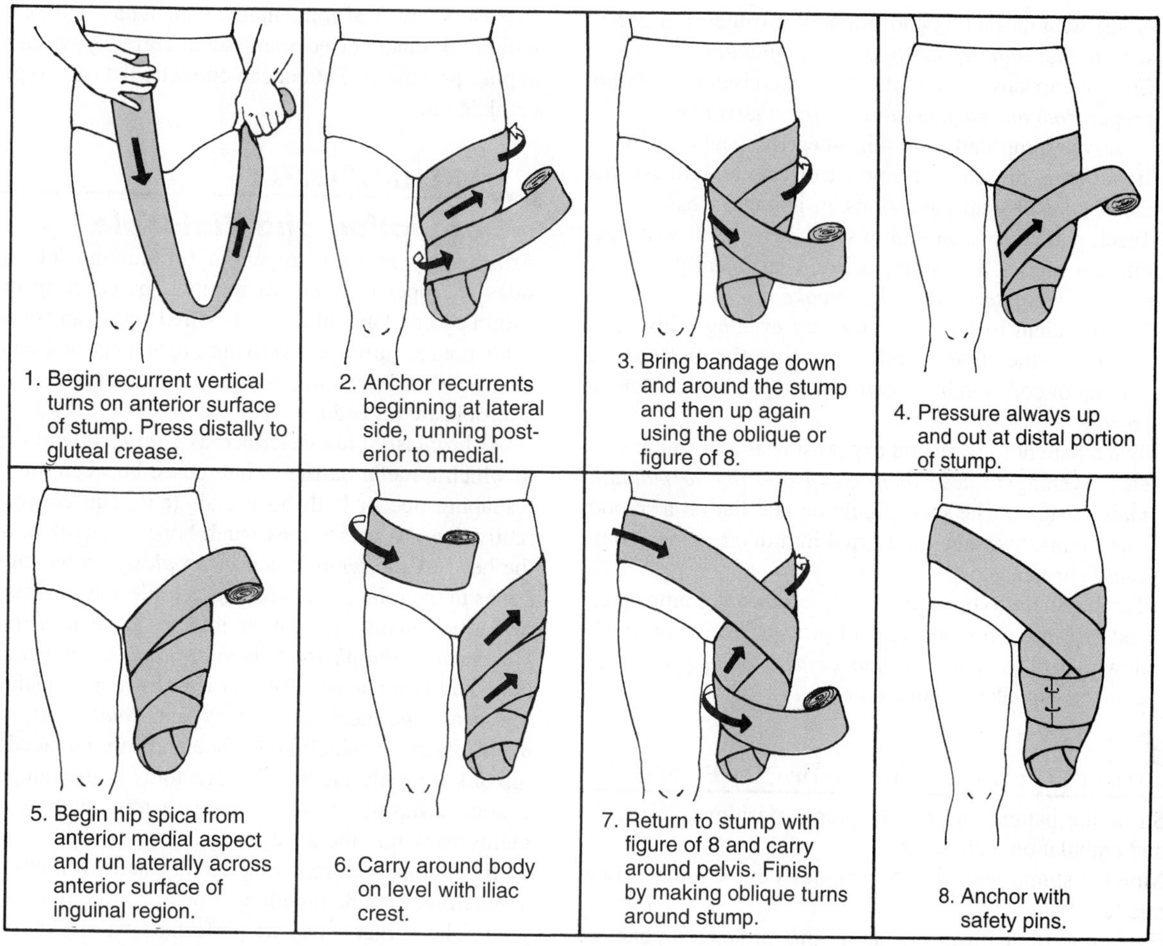
1. Begin recurrent vertical turns on anterior surface of stump. Press distally to gluteal crease.
2. Anchor recurrents beginning at lateral side, running posterior to medial.
3. Bring bandage down and around the stump and then up again using the oblique or figure of 8.
4. Pressure always up and out at distal portion of stump.
5. Begin hip spica from anterior medial aspect and run laterally across anterior surface of inguinal region.
6. Carry around body on level with iliac crest.
7. Return to stump with figure of 8 and carry around pelvis. Finish by making oblique turns around stump.
8. Anchor with safety pins.

FIG. 6-27

One method of wrapping to help shape stump after above-knee amputation.

- Administer narcotics as ordered every 3 hours for first 24 to 48 hours until surgical trauma is lessened; then administered as needed *to aid pain relief* (may have PCA).
- Explain causes for phantom pain sensations and techniques to overcome them *to ease concerns.* Phantom limb pain is defined as painful sensations perceived as in the missing body part; residual limb pain is perceived as emanating from the residual portion of the limb (the stump).[51a]
- Teach patient other pain-relieving techniques, including use of diversionary measures such as listening to music, listening to radio, watching television or videotapes, using relaxation techniques, and guided imagery, *to lessen need for narcotic usage and divert attention.*
- Massage back and other bony prominences *to ease soreness or pain.*
- Administer antibiotics as ordered to prevent infection, thereby *lessening pain and scarring.*

NIC SKIN/WOUND MANAGEMENT

Impaired skin integrity related to healing wound on stump and pressure of prosthesis

- Observe wound for signs of healing: amount of redness, edema; condition of sutures or skin clips, if present, approximation of wound edges, pain, functions, sensory deficits.
- Reinforce or change wound dressings using strict aseptic techniques *to hasten wound healing and to prevent wound infection.*
- Monitor cast, if present, for tightness or loosening, edema above edges, and other signs of integrity of the cast *to determine the viability of the cast and need for changes.*
- Monitor the pressure in the Jobst air splint, if in use. Pressure is usually inflated to 20 mm Hg for 22 hours per day *to control edema and aid shaping the stump.*
- Wrap stump when prescribed with proper techniques *to aid molding and shaping of stump and control edema.*
- Demonstrate proper wrapping techniques to patient and family members *to increase self-reliance and self-care.*
- Teach patient and family that elastic wraps must be removed and reapplied *to maintain their snugness and effectiveness.*
- Assist with removal of (or remove, if unit policy) sutures or skin clips, as prescribed, *to permit wound maturation and reduce inflammation.*
- Teach stump skin care; clean incisional area with prescribed solution or soap and water *to decrease resident bacteria to reduce possibility of infection.*

- Assist with measuring and fitting of prosthesis, if necessary, *to facilitate regaining physical mobility.*
- Continue extension and adduction exercises *to maintain proper limb muscle functions for prosthesis use.*
- Observe stump daily for skin integrity: healing of incisional area, presence or amount of edema, redness, hot areas, conical shape, abrasions, or irritated areas.
- Teach patient to wear stump sock, if required with specific prosthesis, over stump and to change daily, or more often if damp, *to prevent skin breakdown.*
- Teach patient to wash stump every evening with warm water, dry the stump carefully and gently, and apply a coating of cornstarch or powder *to help maintain skin integrity.*
- Teach patient to wash and dry prosthesis and stump sock each evening *to keep them clean and dry to maintain their integrity.* The sock should be laid flat on a smooth surface after washing, not dried in a dryer, which could cause shrinkage.
- Teach patient to do careful daily checks of stump, sock, and prosthesis for any signs of pressure, wear, or breakdown *to prevent any wound or skin breakdown.* Skin damage can take months to heal.

Patient Education/Continuum of Care Plan

1. Show the patient and family proper positions, exercises, and ambulation techniques.
2. Monitor stump-wrapping techniques done by the patient and family.
3. Explain to the patient and family that prolonged phantom pain experiences are unusual and should receive medical attention, if persistent.
4. Discuss skin care with the patient and family to prevent stump irritation or breakdown.
5. List signs of a wound infection, and discuss these with the patient and family.
6. Provide information about gait analysis to the patient and family.
7. Explain community resources available for financial, rehabilitative, or home care, as needed.
8. Discuss daily care principles of stump, sock, and prosthesis.

Evaluation/Patient Outcomes

Coping Assistance: Alteration in body image and self-concept is achieved. Patient has positive outlook about condition and can resume personal and employment roles after convalescence.

Immobility Management: Patient has regained mobility after wound healing. Patient's scar has healed well on stump. Stump fits into prosthesis well. Patient walks with slight limp only. Patient uses upper extremity prosthesis satisfactorily and continues care with occupational and physical therapists. Patient uses gait analysis personnel and techniques to increase ambulation skills.

Physical Comfort Promotion: Patient experiences pain relief over time. Patient needs no analgesics. Patient has no phantom pain.

Skin/Wound Management: Patient has well-healing stump without drainage or edema. Patient correctly wraps stump and applies prosthesis. Patient can correctly list care to prevent skin breakdown.

Arthroplasty

Description and Rationale

Arthroplasty refers to repair or refashioning of one or both sides of upper or lower extremities, parts, or specific tissues within a joint. Parts of a joint repaired during an arthroplasty include bones, cartilage, synovium, ligaments, and tendons. Bursae are outside a joint, but they may be removed during an arthroplastic procedure.

Arthroplasties are described as *interpositional arthroplasty,* in which a metal barrier is interposed between the bones after reshaping one or both bone ends (e.g., cup arthroplasty, currently done to preserve as much bone as possible, particularly the head of the femur); *gap arthroplasty,* in which one of the bones in the joint is excised (e.g., Girdlestone arthroplasty, now performed mainly to remove infected bones); *partial joint replacement arthroplasty,* or *hemiarthroplasty,* in which one joint bone end is replaced with a prosthesis (e.g., prosthesis replacing head and neck of femur); and *total joint replacement arthroplasty,* in which both bone ends are replaced (e.g., total hip or knee replacement). Synovectomy is an example of an excisional arthroplasty, as is a meniscectomy with removal of the meniscus within the knee joint.

Refashioning or repairing a joint usually follows trauma, degeneration, or inflammation of one or more tissues within the joint. The surgery may be performed within hours of a traumatic injury, such as a hip fracture or meniscus tear, or it may be done after years of inflammation in a joint, such as occurs with rheumatoid arthritis or after degenerative erosions accompanying osteoarthritis.

An arthroplasty, therefore, is usually performed to relieve restrictive movements of a joint, to relieve pain, to remove loose or torn tissues (ligaments, cartilage, or calcium deposits), to reshape one or both bone ends to make a joint perform more smoothly, or to remove overgrown, hypertrophied tissue (synovium) or atrophic, avascular tissue (avascular head of femur).

Contraindications and Cautions

The age of a specific patient may be a contraindication to a particular arthroplasty. Arthroplasties are performed infrequently in children because they may damage the growth epiphyses and the immature cartilage and bones. Surgical repair of childhood conditions such as Legg-Perthes disease is undertaken only after more conservative medical treatments fail to resolve the condition. Adolescents with large, unsightly bunions may have an arthroplasty to correct them, but often surgical correction is required again in later years. Older adults with rheumatoid arthritis or degenerative osteoarthritis may have their surgical procedures delayed to correct a concurrent endocrine, cardiac, or respiratory condition, as also will those patients having arthroplastic surgery after trauma. Elderly persons often require arthroplastic procedures as treatment for rheumatoid arthritis and osteoarthritis. They require careful monitoring, at times, for concomitant medical conditions.

Bunionectomy: Keller or Mayo Arthroplasty

Description and Rationale

Keller arthroplasty is one of the most commonly performed corrective procedures for hallux valgus and bunions. It involves excision of the proximal part of the proximal phalanx plus trimming of the prominent portion of the metatarsal head. The Mayo procedure involves excision of the first metatarsal head and trimming of the prominent portion of the proximal phalanx. Both procedures are examples of gap arthroplasty; the gap is usually filled with a Silastic implant. The bunion (enlarged bursa and knob of bone) is also removed during the arthroplasty. A plaster toe cap or splint is then applied to some patients.

Contraindications and Cautions

1. Hallux valgus in an adolescent is primarily unsightly and deforming; surgical correction may be delayed until the patient is older because osteotomy is a radical procedure at this age.
2. Surgery may be delayed or avoided in some patients through careful attention to wearing properly fitted footwear. Padding may protect the bunion to lessen pain. Exercise and use of a metatarsal arch support may lessen splayfoot, delaying the need for surgical intervention.
3. Surgery may not be entirely successful or satisfactory. Bunions can recur, and surgery may weaken the foot slightly.

Multidisciplinary Plan

Surgery

Arthroplasty or osteotomy
Bunionectomy

Medications

Narcotic analgesic agents
- Meperidine (Demerol), 75-100 mg IM q3h for 24-48 h for severe pain (may have PCA pump with smaller doses—see box on p. 403)
- Morphine, 1-2 mg q10min with 10-15 min lockout per PCA pump (if elderly person)
- Codeine (codeine sulfate or phosphate), 30-60 mg
- Oxycodone (Percodan), 5-10 mg PO

Analgesic/antipyretic agents
- Aspirin, 600-1000 mg PO q4h for minor pain
- Acetaminophen, 500-1000 mg q4h rectally until can take PO

NSAIDs
- Ibuprofen (Motrin), 400-600 mg q4-6h
- Ketorolac (Toradol), 10 mg PO q4-6h
- See table on p. 337 for additional NSAIDs

General Management

Up with crutches when edema lessens, usually in 1 day (depends on whether surgery is bilateral)
Check cast or splint for tightness, intactness, and drainage
Wear wooden shoe in place of splint
Assess wound for edema, pain, and drainage
Elevate foot (feet) on pillows
Elevate foot of bed
Keep patient on bed rest for 12 to 24 hours and then up in chair without weight bearing, if prescribed
Apply ice bags to operative site continuously
Assess motor and sensory functions in toes and feet postoperatively

NURSING CARE

Nursing Assessment

Before Surgery

Area of great toe (bilateral): Presence of deformity, swelling over first metatarsal head (bursa), pain and throbbing in bunion area, limitation of movement of joint with or without pain, presence of hallux valgus deviation (see Fig. 6-17, p. 353), hammertoe, crowding of second toe, splayfoot, calluses or corns
Foot: Varus or valgus deviation of one or both feet usually noted
Shoes: Condition; type; evidence of wear, sites of wear; softness; data indicative of footwear contributing to hallux condition
Systemic: Evidence of gout—tophi, elevated serum uric acid levels, pattern of acute pain in great toe joint and other joints

After Surgery

Great toe or toes and incisional site: Assessment of plaster cast, splint, or wooden shoe for intactness: visible portions of toes: color, edema, pain, pulses proximal or distal to incision (if able to locate in toe), drainage, bleeding; dressing: tightness; amount of sensation and motion in operative area (splint, shoe, or dressing may limit movement)
Psychosocial concerns: Alteration in body image, comfort, and mobility; possibility of recurrence or lack of wound healing

Potential Complications

Excessive scarring or recurrence of bursa, weakening of foot joint or joints of or near one or more toes

Patient Problems/Nursing Diagnoses & Interventions

NIC Physical Comfort Promotion

Acute pain related to corrective procedures
- Determine amount, type, and severity of pain; discuss using pain scale.
- Put bed cradle on bed to cover feet without pressure of linens *to aid comfort.*
- Keep foot of bed and feet elevated *to lessen edema.*
- Administer narcotics as prescribed *for acute pain relief.*
- Administer analgesics or antiinflammatory medications as prescribed *to continue pain relief.*
- Apply ice bags *to lessen bleeding and edema.*
- Assist with position changes and skin care; do back massage as needed *to relieve tired muscles.*
- Instruct patient about analgesic and antiinflammatory effects of medications and ice *to increase compliance and use.*

NIC Immobility Management

Impaired physical mobility related to foot surgery
- Observe limitations on mobility.

- Help patient up in chair when prescribed *to increase mobility.*
- Assist with use of crutches when up *to aid mobility efforts.*
- Encourage activities as strength, cast, splint, or wooden shoe permit *to maintain mobility.*
- Encourage return to social activities despite cast, splint, or crutches *to lessen isolation.*
- Help with fitting of soft shoes if or when cast is removed (to lessen pressure or rubbing on tender tissues) *to prevent additional injury.* Often, open, laced shoes are used after bunion surgery.

NIC Tissue Perfusion Management

Ineffective tissue perfusion related to surgery or cast

- Perform neurovascular check (see p. 330).
- Remainder of nursing care is discussed on p. 411.

Patient Education/Continuum of Care Plan

1. Explain wound healing and signs of wound dehiscence to report to physician.
2. Discuss principles and examples of proper footwear.
3. Explain that friction and pressure of snug footwear can precipitate recurrence.
4. Discuss bone and wound healing for long-term follow-up.
5. Provide list of signs or symptoms of infection

Evaluation/Patient Outcomes

Physical Comfort Promotion: Patient is relieved of acute pain. Patient can walk easily without pain. Deformity has been removed. ROM in normal scar formation is not excessive. Pain in and around joint is gone.

Immobility Management: Patient has satisfactory physical mobility. Patient returns to usual activities with unassisted,

TOTAL HIP REPLACEMENT

Sir John Charnley of England first reported his experiences with low-friction arthroplasty in the hip joint in 1961. Since that time, total hip replacement has become one of the most frequently performed orthopedic surgical procedures. Over 300,000 total hip replacements are done yearly in the United States, and over 1 million are done worldwide. Also 100,000 total knee replacements/revisions or more are done yearly. Revisions are often required about 10 years after placement because of loosening of one or both prostheses in the joint. Approximately three fourths of the revisions are done because of loosening; others are done because of deep infection (about 5%), implant fracture (5%), or other individual reasons, such as marked pain or discomfort or the need to replace a particular prosthesis (some last longer than others).

Currently, prostheses are being developed with new instruments and techniques for inserting them (FIG. 6-28). Prostheses now have matching parts that fit snugly into each other, allowing

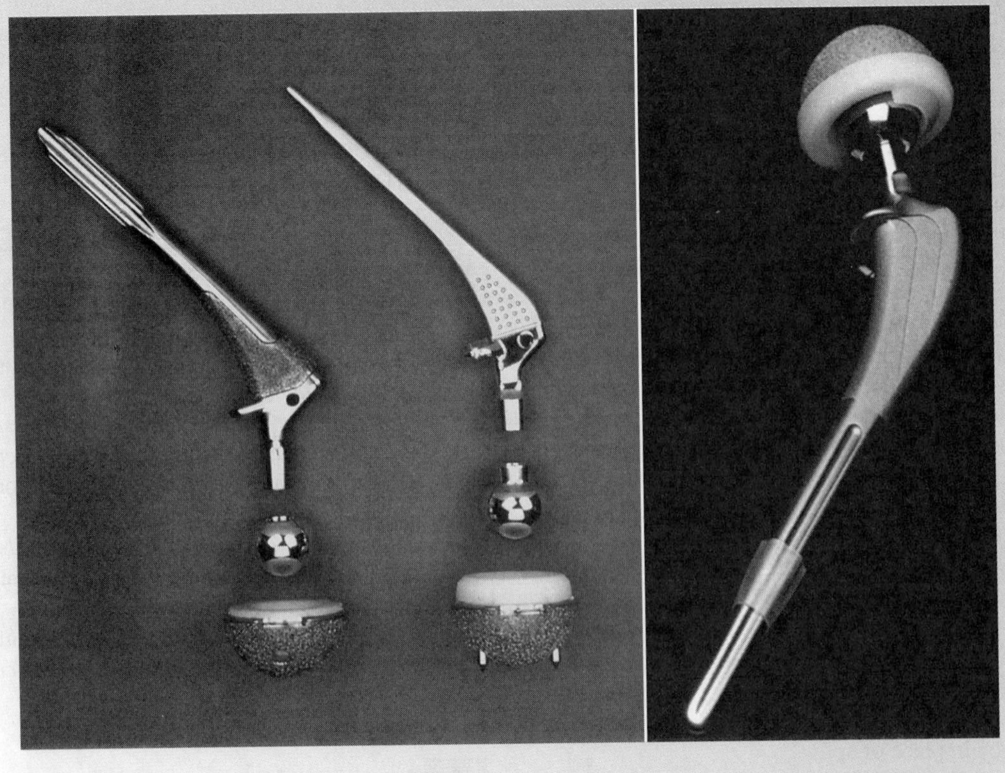

FIG. 6-28

Several types of total hip replacement prostheses. (**A** courtesy Zimmer, Warsaw, Ind.; **B** courtesy Biomet, Warsaw, Ind.)

pain-free mobility. Footwear is comfortable. Patient feels better about body image.

Tissue Perfusion Management: Patient has normal peripheral perfusion. Neurovascular checks are within normal limits with minimal edema of toes; operative wound is well approximated with minimal edema of suture line; no drainage is present.

Total Joint Replacement Arthroplasty

Description and Rationale

Work done since the late 1950s and early 1960s has made it possible to repair and replace bone surfaces on both sides of many joints. Work with total replacement of hip joints has led to the ability to totally replace many joints, including ankles, knees, shoulders, elbows, wrists, and joints of the fingers and toes. Not all prosthetic materials or arthroplastic procedures work entirely satisfactorily in the joints with more and varied movements, such as the elbow, wrist, knee, and ankle. To date, more successful replacements have been achieved in the ball-and-socket joints, the hip and shoulder. Research and design changes continue to perfect the prostheses and the techniques for all total arthroplastic procedures.

Replacement of both joint surfaces is required primarily in inflammatory or degenerative conditions within the joint, such as those accompanying rheumatoid arthritis or osteoarthritis from deterioration of the synovium or cartilage (Fig. 6-30). As one or more of the normal joint tissues deteriorate or degenerate, the bone ends are exposed, causing pain and limitation of joint movements. Joint stiffness and muscle atrophy follow, further increasing pain and limiting movement and mobility, both locally in the involved joint and systemically as other joints become involved. Exposed bone surfaces will lead to bone growth that may eventually adhere to the opposing bone ends, causing bony ankylosis and loss of joint movements. Therefore replacement of the deteriorated or degenerated tissues and bones restores movement and relives pain.[9]

Total joint replacements involve removal of some or all of the synovium, cartilage, and bone on both sides of the joint. One of the joint bone surfaces is then replaced with a metallic prosthesis while the other surface is replaced with a ceramic or plastic, silicone-lined prosthesis. This metallic-plastic approximation is necessary to prevent metal-to-metal wear, friction, and possible electrolytic reactions from the interactions and intermingling of joint fluids. Individual physicians prefer specific

TOTAL HIP REPLACEMENT—cont'd

only one part (not two, three, or more) to be replaced as needed; they also have a porous coating to be press fit into the bone shaft or socket. The porous coating blends with the bone through bio-ingrowth of bone cells. Another substance, hydroxyapatite, is now being applied to prostheses, bonding the replacement directly to bone without intervening fibrous tissue. This substance may strengthen the bone-prosthesis bonding. At present, methylmethacrylate polymer (a substance that helps glue the prostheses in place) is used in less than 50% of total hip replacements because it was found to contribute to loosening, as well as joint infection.[4]

Ball-and-socket joints (hip and shoulder joints) succeed better when replaced than do joints that are more complex and have more functions, such as the knee, wrist, elbow, or ankle (Fig. 6-29).

Total hip replacement requires special operative tables and instruments and careful, extensive physician-patient contact with consultation before and after surgery. When successful, as are the great majority of joint replacements, this surgery provides the patient with relief from pain, increased mobility, and a freedom not available with more conservative procedures.

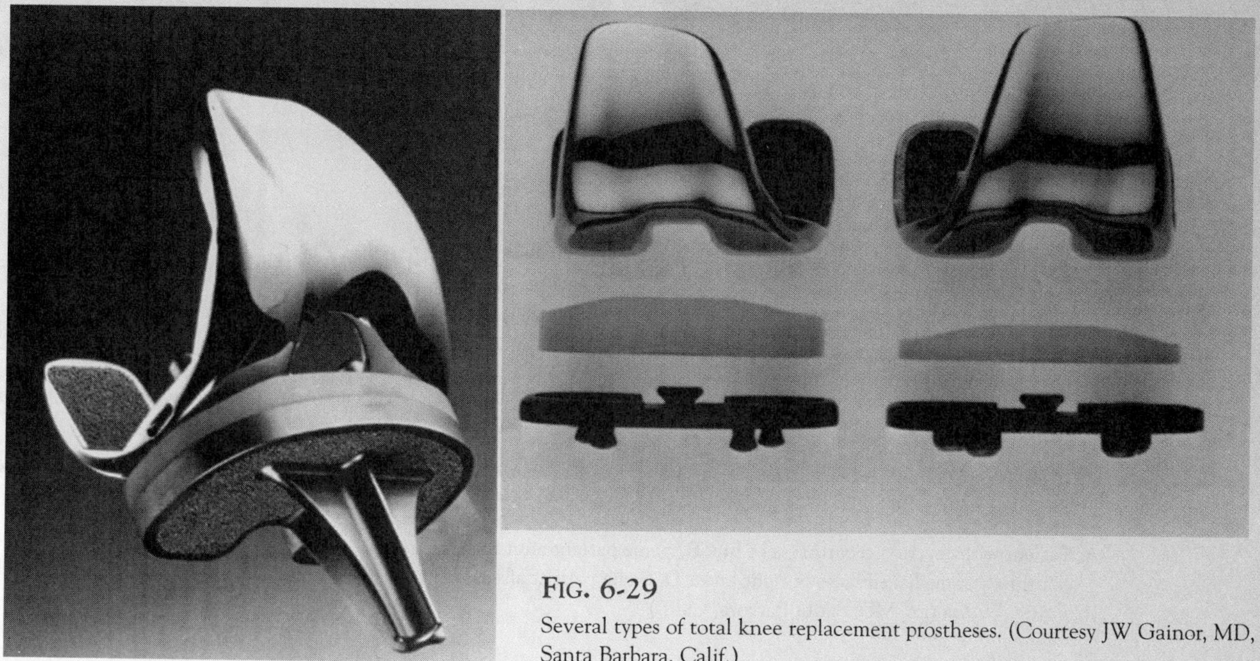

Fig. 6-29

Several types of total knee replacement prostheses. (Courtesy JW Gainor, MD, Santa Barbara, Calif.)

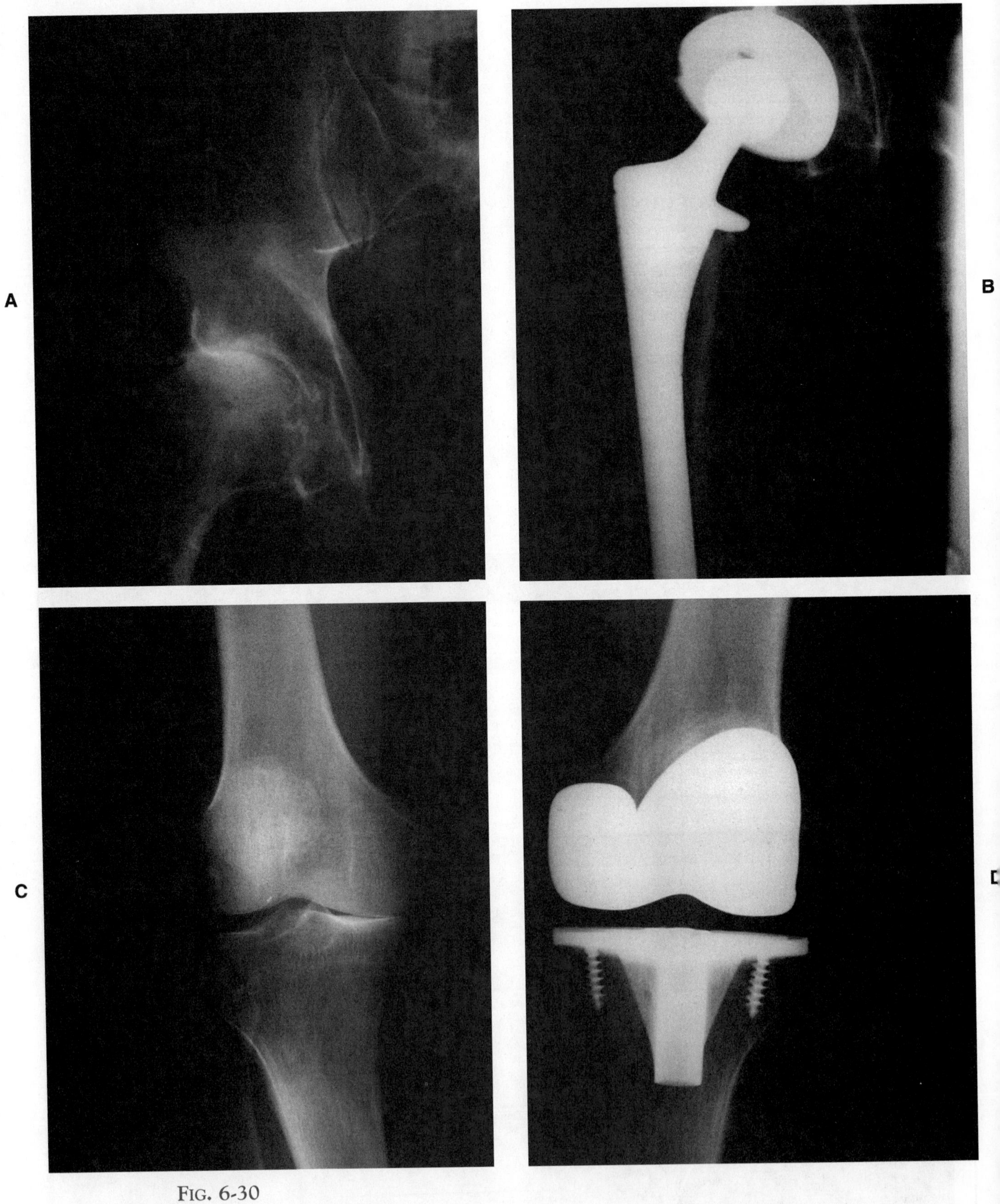

FIG. 6-30

A, Patient with severe osteoarthritis of hip. **B,** Same patient after total hip replacement. **C,** Patient with osteoarthritis of medial surfaces of right knee. **D,** Same patient after total knee replacement. (Courtesy JW Gainor, MD, Santa Barbara, Calif.)

combinations of prostheses for particular joints according to the patient's condition. Also, the timing for total joint replacement varies with the physician and patient because this procedure is usually elective except in situations of trauma.

Currently each prosthetic replacement on both sides of the joint may be secured with or without methyl methacrylate, a pliable polymer that hardens to hold the prostheses more firmly. Through research and development, ceramic and metallic components have been designed that are self-adhering and immovable and do not require methacrylate adherence.[9] These self-adhering replacements currently are being used in many centers. They have become more widespread as the technique for their insertion and the differences in postoperative recovery and rehabilitation have been accepted. Patients may take longer to start walking and use crutches or other aids for a longer time with the adhering replacements because the bone particles used as the natural interfacing material must granulate and ossify for solid adherence to the prosthetic replacements. Obviously, using the patient's own bone for the interface with the prosthesis is desirable because methyl methacrylate sets up an inflammatory response that may eventually lead to loosening or instability within the joint (see boxes on specific joint replacements).

The most important goal in replacement of any joint, after pain relief, is restoration of function so the patient can use the operative limb or limbs effectively and carry out the activities desired or required of the specific joint or joints.

Contraindications and Cautions

1. Joint infection with or without an associated systemic infection is the major deterrent to total replacement. Infection loosens components, prevents healing, and may eventually lead to osteomyelitis.
2. Active flare-up of a chronic rheumatic or other inflammatory disease is another deterrent. Flare-ups of such disorders as rheumatoid arthritis, ulcerative colitis, or systemic lupus preclude surgery until the condition is controlled or becomes quiescent.
3. Respiratory diseases and limitations from chronic conditions may preclude surgery. Methyl methacrylate is excreted through the lungs; this may set up a pneumonitis that could severely limit respiratory reserves.
4. Chronic renal conditions or mild renal failure may also preclude replacement because prolonged hypotension could lead to acute renal shutdown.
5. Bleeding or clotting disorders would usually preclude surgery unless special care is taken to prevent hemorrhage, such as use of fresh frozen plasma for hemophiliacs.
6. Insertion of the femoral component into the femoral shaft during total hip replacement causes pressure changes in the venous system, which can lead to thrombophlebitis and pulmonary or fat embolization.
7. Limb length inequality can occur from inadequate muscle strength or improper operative fit. If limbs are unequal in length preoperatively, the inequality can possibly be corrected with the surgical procedure.
8. Porous-coated prostheses used for noncemented total joint replacements must be "press fit" for bio-ingrowth to occur.

Preprocedural Nursing Care

1. Preadmission patient data are gathered, usually by phone or in the physician's office.
2. Preoperative teaching is begun by the nurse/assistant in the physician's office or in group teaching sessions, if feasible. Written materials are provided to the patient for continued self-study.

TOTAL SHOULDER ARTHROPLASTY

Total shoulder arthroplasty (TSA) can be dated to 1973. It was preceded by more than 20 years of shoulder surgical approaches and development of improved prostheses.

TSA is performed as treatment to relieve intractable pain associated with arthritic conditions, osteonecrosis of the humeral head, fracture of the humeral head or neck, rotator cuff arthropathy, neoplasms, and chronic shoulder pain and instability problems. Because the shoulder joint is similar to a ball-and-socket joint, the TSA arthroplasty has achieved successful outcomes. However, because the shoulder lacks a true bony socket, it relies heavily on the support and integrity of its soft tissues for stability through its extensive ROM (the shoulder is capable of a wider ROM than any other joint in the body). It can perform flexion/extension, abduction/adduction, and internal rotation/external rotation.[6] (See Table 6-2 on p. 328 for shoulder ROM compared with other joints.)

TSA is a technically challenging surgery because of all the structures articulating with the humerus and glenoid cavity, including the tendons and muscles of the rotator cuff, the deltoid muscle, the subacromial and subscapsular bursae, the acromion process of the scapula, and the multiple nerve plexus around the joint.

The designs of the humeral prosthesis and the glenoid component are vital to the successful outcome of TSA. The humeral prosthesis is now a two-piece modular unit that permits the best fitting of the distal humeral shaft portion, coupled with the best fit of available proximal stem portion, thus producing a custom-fit prosthesis. The glenoid component is vital for the ultimate success of TSA because the weight of the extremity when in 90 degrees of abduction causes a force against the glenoid that may represent many times the weight of the extremity, which can lead to loosening of the glenoid component. This component may be all plastic, metal-backed plastic, all metal, smooth-fit cemented, porous-coated cementless with screw fixation, or pegged, there being no consensus as to the best glenoid component among the varieties.

TSA involves removal of the head of the humerus, preparing the humeral shaft for the distal and proximal humeral components, and smoothing the glenoid for placement of the glenoid component, which may be cemented or held in place with screws.

Complications include infection, dislocation or subluxation, intraoperative fracture, nerve weakness, loosening, impingement, pulmonary embolus, and pneumonia.

The ultimate success of TSA includes a planned rehabilitative coordinated recovery protocol involving exercises to restore ROM and strengthen muscles. The patient must actively participate in the program for the time required. To achieve the relief of preoperative pain, patients usually are highly motivated and compliant.

Preoperative preparations and postoperative care are similar to those for other joint arthroplasties, discussed on p. 397.

3. Blood serum studies and chest x-ray, electrocardiogram, and x-ray of operative joints are done, either in the family physician's or the orthopedic surgeon's office. Leg length measurements are also done, and a thorough physical examination is completed.
4. Physical therapy teaching may be begun 2 to 10 days before hospital admission for surgery.
5. Respiratory care is begun preoperatively, including deep-breathing and coughing exercises and use of respiratory aids such as Triflow or Voludyne apparatus for incentive spirometry.
6. Patient is made NPO at midnight the day of surgery.
7. All operative permits and informed consent must be understood and signed before surgery.
8. Preanesthesia visit with anesthesiologist is usually done as part of preoperative admission and laboratory periods before the day of surgery.
9. Patient or family may have donated blood for use during surgery as needed.
10. Patient is admitted to hospital on morning of surgery, and all preparations are completed expeditiously.
11. Antibiotics are begun intravenously preoperatively to establish a therapeutic blood level.
12. Many patients go to surgery in their hospital bed rather than on a gurney to minimize trauma after hip replacement.

TOTAL ELBOW REPLACEMENT

Total elbow replacement (TER) is done primarily to relieve the severe pain of and repair the destruction of the elbow joint secondary to rheumatoid arthritis.

TER involves resurfacing and use of either nonconstrained or semiconstrained implants. The resurfacing components provide resurfacing areas for the bones making up the joint. The semiconstrained implants are either hinged or of a snap-fit design. The most successful replacements are those with the fewest constraints and those that most closely resemble the anatomic elbow. In addition, there must be sufficient metaphyseal bone stock and intact collateral ligaments for stability. TER is done to reestablish the alignment of the humerus with the ulnar components to treat elbow instability.[43]

TER consists of removal of the diseased trochlea of the intra-articular humerus and ulna with replacement by the capitellocondylar nonconstrained resurfacing implant, which is made of metal with a long humeral stem, and replacement of the diseased ulnar surfaces with a metal-stemmed polyethylene ulnar "tray." Each prosthetic component is cemented in place with the use of methyl methacrylate. After the incision is closed and a drain inserted, the operative arm is placed in a protective sling or splint secured with elastic bandages. The elbow and splint are placed in approximately 90 degrees of flexion.

Postoperative physical therapy, occupational therapy, administration of intravenous antibiotics, neurovascular checks, pain management, and wound care are all vital to the successful outcome of TER.

Complications of TER are similar to those seen with other total joint arthroplasties, including wound or joint infection, dislocation of prostheses, deep vein thrombosis or pulmonary embolism, joint instability, and loosening of prostheses. TER continues to have a rather disappointingly high rate of complications.[43]

TOTAL ANKLE REPLACEMENT

Total ankle replacement (TAR) has been available to orthopedic surgeons since the early 1970s. It is indicated as treatment for the severe pain and disability of older patients with rheumatoid arthritis and less frequently for older patients with posttraumatic arthritis of the ankle. TAR is indicated after there have been less than satisfactory results with nonoperative management, including use of antiinflammatory medications, analgesics, and supportive devices. Younger patients may have an ankle arthrodesis, considered the "gold standard" for younger patients with posttraumatic arthritis who place a high physical demand on their ankle joints.

TAR involves preparation of the patient as for other surgical procedures, meticulous skin cleansing, and administration of an intravenous prophylactic antibiotic after the induction of anesthesia. Anesthesia may be given as general anesthesia or regional anesthesia via a spinal-subarachnoid block.

Preparation of the dome of the talus is done for the prosthesis, along with subperiosteal dissection of the distal tibia. Osteophytes are removed, as is some synovial tissue. The medial malleolus is resected, and trial spacers are inserted to assess the sufficiency of the preparations. The tibial prosthesis is placed, after removal of the trial components, and held with the use of polymethyl methacrylate cement. The talar component is inserted and held in place with a small amount of cement. The ankle joint is reduced and held in dorsiflexion compression until the cement is fully polymerized. The types of prostheses used include two types of porous-coated prostheses, currently used with cement. Tibial components may be multiaxial, allowing unrestricted movement about any of the three major axes, or a single-axis joint prosthesis that allows flexion or extension only, with various degrees of constraint to internal-external rotation and abduction-adduction. After the components are inserted, the tourniquet is released, and hemostasis is done. Sutures are placed, and a small drain may be inserted. The wound is covered with a bulky, soft compressive dressing, and a plaster splint is placed. The operative leg and ankle are kept elevated for up to 3 days. A short-leg walking cast is applied and worn for 2 to 3 weeks to permit soft tissue healing. After cast removal, ROM exercises are done by the patient, and ambulation progresses as tolerated. Exercise protocols follow the physician's prescription under physical therapy guidance.

Complications include infection, incomplete pain relief, reoperation to remove excess (impinging) bone, and loosening of one or both components. Positive outcomes vary with the purpose of doing the TAR related to patient's condition and whether or not there has been previous ankle surgery. Pain is usually relieved with TAR.

MULTIDISCIPLINARY PLAN

Medications

Antiinfective agents (may vary per physician and patient sensitivity)
- Cefamandole (Mandol), 1000 mg q8h IM or IV
- Cefazolin (Ancef), 1000 mg q6-8h for 24 h
- Ciprofloxacin (Cipro), 500 mg q12h
- Cephalexin (Keflex), 250-500 mg q6h PO when IV antibiotics are discontinued

Narcotic analgesic agents (may be administered per PCA):
- Morphine, 1.5-2 mg q10min with 20-30 min lockout

NSAIDs
- Ibuprofen (Motrin), 400-800 mg tid or qid
- Ketorolac (Toradol), 10-20 mg tid or qid
- See table on p. 337 for additional NSAIDs

Antianxiety agents: Hydroxyzine (Vistaril), 25-50 mg IM q6h (may not be used for elderly patients—see Emergency Alert box, p. 403)

Anticoagulants
- Low-molecular-weight heparin enoxaparin (Lovenox), 30 mg q12h subcutaneously for 7-10 days postoperatively
- Warfarin (Coumadin), 5 mg/day beginning after heparin has been discontinued

Sedative-hypnotic agents: Flurazepam (Dalmane), 15-30 mg at bedtime

Cathartic or laxative agents: Bisacodyl (Dulcolax), 1-2 tablets PO or rectal suppository prn

Analgesic/antipyretic agents
- Acetaminophen (Tylenol), 600-1000 mg q4h prn for elevated temperature or as analgesic

If rheumatic or inflammatory disease is present, antirheumatic or antiinflammatory medications are begun postoperatively as soon as the patient can tolerate oral intake

General Management

Empty and record suction drainage every 4 hours, if prescribed; otherwise, empty as needed (some physicians have discontinued use of drainage systems).

Give oxygen at 2 to 3 L per nasal cannula for 12 to 24 hours, then as needed.

Perform respiratory therapy with IPPB every 4 hours, and instruct patient in use of incentive spirometer every 2 to 4 hours.

Help patient do deep breathing and coughing every 2 to 3 hours; encourage family members to remind patient to do breathing exercises.

Record intake and output every 8 hours.

Maintain bed rest for 8 to 16 hours (varies with specific joint replaced, the security of the replacement prostheses, and physician's choice).

Change dressing after 24 to 48 hours; may reinforce dressing as necessary.

Give nothing by mouth for 12 to 24 hours, then clear liquids and advance to regular diet as tolerated.

Perform neurovascular checks every hour for 24 hours, then every 2 hours for 24 hours, and then every 4 hours (see box on p. 330 for checks).

Check vital signs every hour, initially, then every 2 to 4 hours.

Maintain position of operative area with sling, splint, abduction pillow, immobilizer, brace, or elastic wrappings (varies with specific joint replaced); after a total knee replacement, a continuous passive motion (CPM) machine may be present and in use.

Patient should be up but bearing no weight on operative limb after bed rest order expires (may be after 12 to 24 hours, depending on joint replaced and whether cemented or noncemented replacement was done); some physicians permit touch-down weight bearing after total hip replacement.

Begin physical therapy exercises on first or second postoperative day; exercises and schedule vary with joint replaced; exercises are either active or passive to all joints, excluding the operated joint, and include quadriceps setting, straight leg raising, flexion and extension, or other individually prescribed exercises for the particular joint replaced; total shoulder replacement therapy is begun later in the postoperative period.

Patient should be up with walker or crutches two to three times daily; ambulation should increase as patient is able, with up to 25 pounds weight on operative limb, gradually increasing to full weight bearing with crutches (time frame varies with type of prostheses used, cemented or uncemented replacement, and physician's choice).

Patient should sit in chair for 10 to 15 minutes only (after hip replacement), two or three times daily for first week; then may sit in chair 20 to 30 minutes four times daily.

Patient should wear antiembolism hose or have an athrombic (pneumatic compression) pump system in use for operative extremity or both extremities.

Encourage fluid intake and high-fiber foods (if tolerated) to prevent constipation; administer rectal suppository if needed to empty rectum; indwelling bladder catheter is in place for 12 to 24 hours, then removed.

Patient should use toilet riser for toilet (prevents hyperflexion of hip after total replacement—may lead to dislocation of prosthesis).

Patient should wear a sling and swathe after total shoulder replacement for 7 to 10 days per physician's prescription.

Monitor suction-reinfusion drainage system for possible reinfusion or for homologous transfusion of blood (some postoperative suction-reinfusion drainage systems are neither physiologically beneficial nor cost-effective.

NURSING CARE

NURSING ASSESSMENT

Joint and incisional area: Presence, amount, and type of drainage; edema; color of tissues and capillary refill of fingers or toes; presence, type, and tightness of dressings or bandages; presence of peripheral pulses; pain in incision or distal to operative site; presence of immobilizing device, splint, or pillow to maintain proper position of prostheses within joint; leg in abducted position after total hip replacement; sling and swathe, knee immobilizer, or passive movement machine in place

Respiratory status: Excursion with respirations; dyspnea, shallow respirations; orthopnea; pain in chest or lung areas; cough, sputum expectoration—note color; decreased breath sounds; color of nail beds: pink, pale or bluish

Urinary status: Presence of indwelling catheter in urinary bladder, later removed; intake and output

Vascular and cardiac functions: Hypertension, peripheral vascular disease, cardiac irregularities, congestive heart condition; varicose veins

Psychosocial concerns: Concern with body image; acute pain; regaining mobility and weight bearing; risk of death with surgery

Potential Complications

Pneumonitis; pneumonia; wound infection (superficial or deep); limb inequality or limp; urinary tract infection after catheter use; dislocation of prostheses; thrombophlebitis or deep vein thrombosis (it is estimated that deep vein thrombosis occurs after total hip replacement in over 50% of patients; it occurs in 40% to 84% of patients after total knee replacement; pulmonary embolism—fatal in 0.5% to 2% after total hip replacement[47] and 1% to 3% after knee arthroplasty[9]; fat embolism—occurs in 0.5% to 0.8% after total joint replacement[37,41]

Patient Problems/Nursing Diagnoses & Interventions

NIC Immobility Management

Impaired physical mobility related to surgical and soft tissue trauma

- Check ROM of unaffected joints
- Maintain bed rest as prescribed *to promote recovery.*
- Begin ambulation with ambulatory aid and weight-bearing restrictions as prescribed *to aid early rehabilitation and to prevent complications.* Start slowly with rest periods, and increase gradually.
- Assist with gluteal and quadriceps setting exercises *to maintain muscle strength.*
- Monitor use of walker or crutches to ascertain proper use and amount of weight bearing.
- Encourage performance of active and passive ROM exercises, isometric exercises, and other specific exercises *to aid muscle strength and decrease immobility.*
- Encourage use of trapeze to assist with lifting, turning, and positioning *to increase independence.*
- Assist to be up in chair twice daily with increases to four times daily.
- Secure physical therapist's assistance with being up and ambulating.
- Encourage participation after discharge in activities such as swimming, stationary bike riding, and calisthenics *to increase physical and cardiovascular fitness.*
- Stress compliance with prescribed rehabilitation program for full recovery.

NIC Skin/Wound Management

Impaired skin integrity related to incision through tissues to joint structures

- Monitor condition of all skin surfaces.
- Reinforce and then change dressing with strict aseptic technique: note wound edge approximation, redness, edema, hematoma, or unusual tenderness of wound *as signs of possible wound infection.* Infection after total hip arthroplasty varies from 0.1% to 1%[44]; after total knee arthroplasty infection varies from 1% to 4%, although it may approach 15% with metal-hinged prostheses.[66]
- Listen to patient's complaints of deep, dull, aching pain in hip operative areas *as a sign of possible joint infection;* report complaints to surgeon.
- Maintain serum levels of IV antibiotics as prescribed *to lessen possibility of infection.*
- Measure and empty drainage (may reinfuse) in suction setup as prescribed.
- Monitor vital signs, note elevations, and report *as possible signs of wound infection.*

NIC Tissue Perfusion Management

Ineffective tissue perfusion related to surgery and immobility

Risk for injury related to development of deep vein thrombosis

- Check circulatory condition of operative limb; compare with nonoperative limb for color, edema, temperature (operative limb may feel cooler).
- Apply ice to operative site for 24 hours *to lessen edema and bleeding.*
- Do circulation checks and record findings; note presence or absence of pain, swelling, redness, or heat in calf and positive Homans' sign *as signs of developing thrombophlebitis.* Homans' sign is a nonspecific sign.
- Check drainage in suction apparatus and record. Report unusual amounts *as signs of hemorrhage.*
- Remove antiembolism hose twice daily; check color, presence of pulses, and skin condition; replace hose after 15 to 30 minutes off *to aid circulation and venous return.*
- Check vital signs; note presence of hypotension and elevated pulse or temperature; record and report *as signs of infection or sepsis.*
- Maintain prescribed flexion, extension, or abduction of operative tissues according to specific joint replaced *to aid recovery and increase mobility.*
- Maintain IV therapy as prescribed *to aid circulation and tissue perfusion and means for antibiotic administration.*
- Administer low-molecular-weight heparin or coumadin as prescribed *to prevent thrombophlebitis.*
- Check antithrombotic hose and external compressive system functioning for normal or abnormal status; correct as needed *to maintain a safe environment.*
- Elevate legs as prescribed *to increase venous return and lessen stasis.*
- Keep patient well hydrated *to decrease blood viscosity to lessen stasis.*
- Encourage deep breathing *to promote venous return through vena cava.*
- Maintain antiembolism hose or pneumatic compression device *to promote venous return and prevent stasis.*
- Administer low-molecular-weight heparin, 30 mg every 12 hours, *to lessen possibility of deep vein thrombosis.* Orthopedic surgery patients are at high risk of developing deep venous thrombosis and pulmonary embolism. The incidence of deep vein thrombosis increases with age.[44]

- Monitor bleeding and clotting times while patient is receiving heparin (therapeutic range of partial thromboplastin time is up to 1.5 times normal—normal is 30 seconds). Prothrombin times are done with warfarin administration; therapeutic ranges are 1.3 to 1.5 times the patient's control.[37]
- Monitor stools, urine, and emesis for blood and skin areas for bruising or ecchymosis while patient is receiving heparin or warfarin.
- Use external pneumatic compression devices as prescribed *to lessen possibility of deep vein thrombosis.*
- Continue anticoagulation with warfarin (Coumadin) as prescribed after heparin discontinued *to continue to prevent deep vein thrombosis.*
- Advise of agents that interact with warfarin anticoagulation such as cefamandole, cimetidine, phenytoin, and trimethoprim.[37]

NIC PHYSICAL COMFORT PROMOTION

Acute pain related to tissue trauma

- Monitor amount, type, site, and severity of pain.
- Monitor narcotic use via PCA to determine if change is needed *to increase comfort.*
- Turn, raise, or adjust position *to prevent pressure and lessen fatigue.*
- Administer prescribed antiinflammatory medications *to enhance pain relief.*
- Administer medications for concomitant disease as prescribed *to relieve symptoms and pain.*
- Administer sedative at bedtime if prescribed *to provide for restful sleep.*
- Assess bowel and bladder output; may need laxative, suppository, or enema *to aid elimination and relieve pain (straining increases pain).*
- Convalescent care: Encourage self-care and return to ADLs as able *to aid recovery.*
- Stress alternatives to medication for restful sleep (activity to become tired, reading, warm milk, snack, or massage) *to lessen dependence on medications, if pertinent.*

NIC RISK MANAGEMENT

Risk for injury related to dislocation of prostheses

- Assess postoperatively for required position *to maintain prostheses inside joint* (abduction of operative limb after hip replacement).
- Reiterate preoperative instructions *to prevent dislocation:* avoid adduction of legs and do not cross ankles; keep head to bed below 90 degrees *to prevent unsafe hip flexion;* keep operative leg abducted by using abduction pillow or two to three pillows placed between legs; use the knee immobilizer, if prescribed, *to prevent knee flexion, which could cause hip flexion;* keep leg abducted when turned to side.
- Teach the "post" position *to prevent dislocation:* patient bends knee of nonoperated leg and firmly plants (posts) foot on mattress, then grasps trapeze, stiffens back and pelvis, and lifts body from bed by pushing on posted foot and leg while pulling up. Assist with lifting as needed.

! EMERGENCY ALERT*

PRINCIPLES FOR MANAGING POSTOPERATIVE PAIN IN OLDER/ELDERLY PATIENTS AFTER ORTHOPEDIC PROCEDURES

ASSESSMENT

- Assess for general condition and tolerance of operative procedure (most are older or elderly patients who have total joint replacements).
- Assess for complaints of pain; degree, site, severity, and frequency—use appropriate pain scale.
- Assess for relief of pain from anesthetic or administration of analgesic for pain.
- Assess patient's position in bed and operative site for deformity or signs of dislocation, which could contribute to the patient's pain.
- Assess circular dressings for tightness, which may cause pain if too tight.

INTERVENTIONS

- Review postoperative pain management with previous teaching used for individual patient.
- Reiterate explanations postoperatively to reorient patient recovering from anesthesia.
- Use IV or intraspinal, not IM, analgesia to control severe pain quickly.
- Initiate opioid therapy with 25% to 50% lower dose than recommended for adults.
- Titrate doses upward slowly (with 25% increases), since elders experience higher peak effects and longer duration of action.
- Combine opiate medications with in-between administration of NSAID medications for sustained pain relief.
- Use around-the-clock (ATC) dosing for all routes, but evaluate the intervals; may need to be longer than in younger persons.
- Cautiously use NSAIDs for pain control between opioid doses by limiting daily dose of, for example, ketorolac (Toradol) to 60 mg/day if patient has impaired renal function, serum creatinine level is moderately elevated, or patient weighs less than 50 kg (and not over 3 to 5 days in use).
- Substitute acetaminophen if NSAIDs are contraindicated.
- Monitor sedation levels carefully to prevent opioid-induced respiratory depression; if prescribed, administer naloxone titrated in small doses.
- Use oral route for medications as early as possible and evaluate before discharge to ascertain safe and effective dosages.
- Postoperative pain may be more severe and last longer in elderly patients than in younger patients; may need to consider use of oral morphine or hydromorphone rather than opioid-acetaminophen combinations.
- Be aware that pain perception does not decrease with age.

*Content modified from Pasero and McCaffery.[40]

- Listen to patient's complaints of increased pain in operative area and observe position of the limb; if it is held in external or internal rotation, could indicate dislocation of hip prostheses.
- Use toilet riser to elevate seat *to prevent hyperflexion of hip, which could dislocate prosthesis.*
- Maintain patient on bed rest for 1 day, then help patient up in a chair; use caution to avoid adduction of the operative limb and to avoid 90-degree flexion of the hip.

TOTAL KNEE ARTHROPLASTY

Total knee arthroplasty (TKA) is a more difficult procedure than total hip arthroplasty because of the multiple functions of the knee, including flexion, extension, and rotation, in the course of weight bearing. No single prosthetic design type for the femoral, patellar, or tibial components has been entirely satisfactory because of the knee joint's complexity, and the prostheses have undergone revisions and are continuing to be redesigned. When a primary knee implant is well aligned, balanced, and firmly fixed, it can withstand 20 years or more of wear in some patients, and 90% to 95% of all primary knee replacements still perform well up to 15 years postoperatively. However, revisions of TKA are being done in up to 20% of patients because of aseptic loosening or osteolysis.[8] Because of these concerns, TKA is usually done for patients over age 60 years.[66]

TKA is done to relieve the constant pain associated with osteoarthritis, rheumatoid arthritis, traumatic arthritis, or chondromalacia. Lingering pain may not entirely disappear, occasionally remaining up to 1 year after TKA. However, the operation corrects deformity, restores function, and usually provides pain relief.[9]

TKA involves preparing the femoral condyles for the femoral prosthesis; preparing the tibial surface for the prosthesis while attempting to preserve as much bone stock as possible and creating a level surface in the bone; and preparing the patella for the patellar component. Diligence must be taken to carefully align the femur and tibia in as anatomically correct a position as possible to prevent undue wear or loosening of either prosthesis.[48] It is also vital to prevent shearing of the patellar component by recessing it to help maintain joint stability.

Prostheses presently being used include a cobalt-chrome femoral prosthesis, usually noncemented, with a cemented or noncemented polyethylene tibial prosthesis, with additional fixation using screws, stems, or pegs.[66] The patellar component is usually a metal-backed polyethylene prosthesis. Bioingrowth occurs on the porous-coated prostheses in the majority of patients.

Meticulous preoperative preparation and postoperative care must be done to prevent complications after TKA. Included are superficial wound and deep, periprosthetic infections; deep vein thromboses; pulmonary emboli; acute compartment syndrome; osteolysis, especially in the tibial plateau; aseptic loosening; patellar maltracking; patellar fracture; reflex sympathetic dystrophy; and hemorrhage or blood loss.[21]

Rehabilitative exercises must be performed by the patient to restore stability and improve motion, under the guidance of physical therapists, over a long (6 months to 1 year) period of time. If exercises are not done, the joint will have less than optimal results because of weak quadriceps and hamstring muscles.

See nursing interventions after total hip arthroplasty because they are similar to those for TKA.

PATIENT EDUCATION/CONTINUUM OF CARE PLAN

1. Stress that rehabilitation of muscles and joint tissues, locally and systemically, will require daily practice over time.
2. Discuss compliance with the medication regimen for chronic disease, if present.
3. Discuss the fact that joint ROM and mobility should be regained after recovery and rehabilitation are accomplished.
4. Stress the use of antiembolism hose as prescribed to prevent deep vein thrombosis.
5. Caution patient to notify physician if chest, calf, or pelvic pain develops after discharge.
6. Avoid sources of infection (e.g., use prophylactic antibiotics before dental or genitourinary procedures).
7. Teach signs indicating dislocation of the prosthesis and to notify physician if one or more signs occur.
8. Provide list of medications that interact with warfarin.

EVALUATION/PATIENT OUTCOMES

Immobility Management: Patient has regained physical mobility. Patient walks with ambulatory aid as required until healing occurs. Patient walks daily without pain or soreness of operative joint.

Skin/Wound Management: Patient has regained skin integrity. Patient's incision heals well without excess scarring or keloid. Scar is maturing normally (beginning to contract).

Tissue Perfusion Management: Patient has regained peripheral tissue integrity. Patient does not develop any neurologic deficit. Patient performs ROM and ankle exercises as required. Patient's color and temperature of extremities are within normal ranges.

Patient developed no wound or joint infection. Patient's incision heals well with no drainage. There are no fluctuant masses, no temperature elevations, and no joint pain or soreness.

Patient developed no thrombophlebitis. Patient has no vein problems during postoperative period. Patient is taking warfarin 3 months postoperatively.

Physical Comfort Promotion: Patient has minimal pain. Patient no longer needs narcotic or nonnarcotic analgesics but continues to take NSAID two or three times daily for muscle and joint soreness. Patient states is doing well with pain control.

Risk Management: Patient has experienced no displacement of prostheses. X-rays show excellent position of prostheses. Patient has no joint deformity.

ARTHROSCOPY

Description and Rationale

With the advent and development of the arthroscope, many advances and changes have occurred in the operative examination and treatment of pathologic joint conditions. Although the knee joint is still a major focus, nearly all joints can be examined with the arthroscope. The multiple benefits of early arthroscopic treatment with specialized techniques and instruments in the hands of a skilled practitioner include lessened inflammation, degeneration, and posttraumatic arthritis. With the advent of same-day surgical settings, patients experience decreased hospital stays and can usually return to their daily activities much sooner with full use of the involved joint after arthroscopic examination and repair.[65]

Arthroscopy is most frequently done for the diagnosis and treatment of knee injuries, primarily torn or damaged menisci.

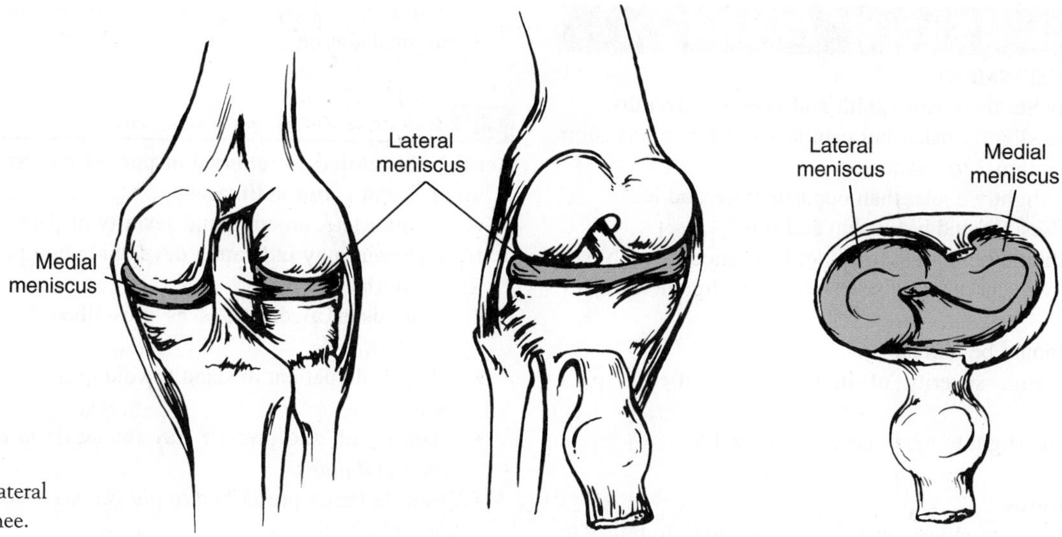

FIG. 6-31
Medial and lateral menisci of knee.

The menisci, C-shaped rings of cartilage covering the ends of the tibia within the knee joint, are subject to degeneration, tears, and wear (FIG. 6-31). Cartilage has no intrinsic blood supply, and if torn, worn, or degenerated, it rarely heals without developing unsatisfactory fibrocartilage. Trauma to the meniscus is greatest among athletes, who suffer tears from external forces, such as a tackle, or from internal forces when a load exceeds the compressibility and resilience of the cartilage; this may occur in a single incident or over time from repeated stressors. The meniscal tear may cause slight, partial, or complete avulsion from adjoining bone tissues.

The discussion that follows focuses on the knee because it is the joint most commonly examined and treated arthroscopically, although arthroscopy is also commonly done in the shoulder, ankle, elbow, and hip. In the hip, arthroscopy is the most useful procedure for diagnosing and treating loose bodies, torn labra, foreign bodies, and synovial pathology of the hip joint, since hip pain may be, and often is, referred to the knee.

Loose or torn pieces of meniscus 1 inch or slightly larger in size can be removed arthroscopically. One or more small incisions may be required for full visualization of the joint. Incisions or "ports" for arthroscopic procedures are on the mediolateral or posterolateral surfaces of the knee joint superior to the patella. The exact incidence of knee arthroscopic procedures is difficult to determine; however, it is a very common procedure.

Contraindications and Cautions

1. Arthoscopy requires skilled practitioners, as well as more specialized techniques and equipment than extensive arthrotomy procedures.
2. Using more than one port for visualization of the joint may lead to infection.
3. Small pieces of torn or loose cartilage may be missed if hidden under other joint tissues.
4. Hemorrhage must be prevented to lessen posttraumatic arthritis.
5. Scar formation may predispose to future tears in ligaments or cartilage.
6. Postoperative physical therapy and individualized exercise programs must be prescribed and performed to maintain or regain the muscles' and joints' mobility, stability, and strength.
7. Many arthroscopic procedures are same-day surgeries; the patient must be stable for discharge.

MULTIDISCIPLINARY PLAN

Medications

Finish IV fluids, as prescribed, then discontinue
Narcotic analgesic agents
  Ketorolac (Toradol), 30 mg IV or IM q4h while hospitalized
  Oxycodone (Percodan), 30-60 mg q4h prn
Antiinfective agent
Cefazolin (Ancef), 1000 mg IV preoperatively and q8h × 3 doses postoperatively
Antiinflammatory agents
  Ibuprofen, 600-800 mg q4h
  See table on p. 337 for additional NSAIDs

General Management

Bed rest until patient is fully alert; then can be up with crutches four times daily, depending on operative findings, and joint examined or treated
Check vital signs every 2 hours for 6 hours, then every 4 hours as needed
Do neurovascular checks every hour for 24 hours
Apply ice bags to knee continuously; keep leg elevated, if knee joint operated
Change dressing as needed
Advance to regular diet as tolerated
Physical therapy consultation for knee exercises
Knee immobilizer to operative knee as prescribed
Perform discharge preparation and teaching if to be discharged same day
Continuous passive motion machine, degrees of motion, and times prescribed for postoperative treatment after ligament repairs.

NURSING CARE

Nursing Assessment

Neurovascular Status of Knee Joint and Lower Extremity

Color: May be slightly paler, but capillary refill and perfusion should be within 2 to 4 seconds

Temperature: Slightly cooler than opposite knee and leg

Peripheral pulses: Should be present and full

Movement: Should be normal in ankle; knee should be able to be flexed with moderate discomfort, if no ligament repair done

Sensations: Should be normal

Pain: Varies with severity of injuries and patient's pain threshold

Edema: May be slight to moderate around patella

Physical Concerns

Concern with regaining knee mobility and strength to return to usual ADLs and activities without impairment

Potential Complications

Hemorrhage: Bleeding into the joint is associated with an anterior cruciate ligament tear[17]; thrombus formation (deep vein thrombosis) or arterial occlusion; posttraumatic degeneration and arthritis; infection; weak ligaments with possibility of tear or retear; compartment syndrome (see pp. 408-409).

Patient Problems/Nursing Diagnoses & Interventions

NIC Tissue Perfusion Management

Ineffective tissue perfusion related to use of tourniquet during arthroscopy

- Monitor neurovascular status as prescribed *to determine current status;* report abnormal data to physician.
- Apply ice bags to knee continuously *to lessen bleeding and edema.*
- Encourage patient to report severity of pain *to help determine if amount is normal or if a complication (arterial occlusion) is developing.*
- Determine amount of active and passive movement (increased pain on passive movement is one indication of compartment syndrome).

NIC Immobility Management

Impaired physical mobility related to knee arthroscopy

- Observe effects of surgery on mobility.
- Assist to positions of comfort; assist to ambulate as prescribed *to maintain strength.*
- Monitor drainage and change dressing as needed (drainage should be scant, serosanguineous) *to note condition of wound and healing.*
- Assist with physical therapy exercises as needed *to regain joint functions, if still in surgical setting.*
- Teach walking up and down stairs with crutches *to regain joint motion.*
- Assist with straight leg raising exercises as needed *to increase muscle strength.* Ability to lift leg while keeping it straight is frequently one criterion for discharge from surgical setting.

NIC Physical Comfort Promotion

Acute pain related to removal of part of meniscus or to ligament repair and arthroscopy

- Monitor site, amount, and severity of pain carefully; severe pain may indicate a developing complication, such as arterial occlusion.
- Administer medications as prescribed for pain *to aid comfort.*
- Help male patient to stand to void (easier while standing if male).
- Assist with and prepare tray for meals *to aid intake of food and fluids.*
- Elevate leg as prescribed *to aid venous return and to decrease edema.*
- Apply ice bags *to lessen edema and thereby decrease pain.*
- Apply knee immobilizer *to prevent flexion;* may have long, layered dressing on operative leg that prevents knee flexion.
- Monitor use of continuous passive motion machine, if and when in use.

Patient Education/Continuum of Care Plan

1. Discuss physical therapy exercises needed to gradually increase strength and mobility.
2. List for the patient the signs or symptoms that would require return to see physician, such as increased pain, redness around arthroscopy portals, drainage from portals, swelling of knee, pain in calf or lower abdomen (may indicate proximal vein thrombus), redness and heat in calf, or elevated body temperature.
3. Discuss with the patient appropriate use of pain medications and adequate diet to promote healing.

Evaluation/Patient Outcomes

Tissue Perfusion Management: Patient regains normal peripheral perfusion. Patient has pink color to skin. Patient has capillary refill in 2 to 4 seconds. Color is the same in both legs. Patient has no numbness or swelling.

Immobility Management: Patient regains joint motion. Patient has full ROM without pain or limitation, has returned to usual activities, and does not have degenerative changes at this time.

Physical Comfort Promotion: Patient has relief of pain. Patient needs only an occasional analgesic for pain.

Meniscectomy/Meniscal Repair

Description and Rationale

Traditional meniscectomy for the removal of larger portions of damaged or degenerated cartilage from the knee joint is still required at times, although the incidence of this more extensive procedure continues to lessen as arthroscopic techniques and skilled practitioners have become more available. The techniques and equipment have been in use in the United States only since 1974, but the knowledge and understanding gained in the past 25 years are revolutionizing the thinking and surgical treatment of meniscal lesions. Open meniscectomy is still required for some patients, however, and some nursing care differs from that of closed arthroscopy.

Meniscal repair is now the major treatment for meniscal injuries because the importance of meniscal preservation has been recognized, influenced, and aided by the use of arthroscopy.

Meniscal tears suitable for repair include those located no more than 3 mm from the meniscosynovial junction; those in which there is minimal damage to the body of the meniscus; and those in which the length of the tear is such that it subluxes into the joint and is obviously unstable.

A meniscal tear should be suspected in a patient with a history of intermittent locking, joint effusions, pain, a positive McMurray's test (see p. 331), and an unstable knee. Meniscal repairs involve a short hospital stay but extensive postoperative rehabilitation.

Diagnostic studies needed to determine the repairability of a torn meniscus include a double contrast arthrogram and MRI. The patient's age must be considered because vascular penetration has been shown to be greater in skeletally immature individuals. Acute tears also yield slightly improved results compared with the repair of chronic tears. The reparable meniscus is finally determined through arthroscopy.

Tears not suitable for arthroscopic repair include those greater than 5 mm from the meniscosynovial junction and tears in which the displaceable portion of the meniscus is grossly deformed or torn.

Meniscal repair is preferred to partial meniscectomy because it offers the chance to restore the normal anatomy and function of the knee (see FIG. 6-31).

Contraindications and Cautions

1. Small pieces of torn or loose cartilage may be missed if hidden under other joint tissues during arthroscopy; however, newer positioning techniques help locate the torn meniscal pieces.
2. Hemorrhage must be prevented to lessen posttraumatic arthritis.
3. Scar formation may predispose to future tears of ligament or cartilage (menisci).
4. Postoperative physical therapy and individualized programs of exercises must be prescribed and performed to maintain or regain the joint's mobility, stability, and strength.
5. Degenerative arthritis is a common long-term complication.[17]

MULTIDISCIPLINARY PLAN

Medications

Narcotic analgesic agents
- Meperidine (Demerol), 75-100 mg IM q3h for severe pain or use of PCA protocol according to age
- Morphine, 1.5-2 mg q10min with 20-30 mg lockout with PCA pump

Analgesic-antipyretic/antiinflammatory agents
- Aspirin, 600-1000 mg PO q4h prn
- Ibuprofen, 400-800 mg q4h
- Acetaminophen, 650 mg q4h
- See table on p. 337 for additional NSAIDs

Antiinfective agents
- Cefazolin sodium (Ancef) or cephalothin sodium (Keflin) (or other cephalosporin), 500-1000 mg q6-8h for 3 doses
- Cephalexin (Keflex), 250-500 mg q6h PO, after IV antibiotic is discontinued, if necessary to prevent infection

General Management

NOTE: Many patients are outpatients for these care and management techniques.

Crutch walking with minimal weight bearing; varies with specific procedure but may begin as early as 6 to 8 hours postoperatively; continue for 3 to 6 weeks, if necessary

Knee immobilizer splint applied between exercise periods, prescribed for 4 to 6 weeks after meniscal repair

Use of hinged knee brace for 2 weeks postoperatively, locked in extension; followed by ROM from 20 to 80 degrees, then free motion is permitted after 4 weeks

Maintain postoperative dressing and immobilization as prescribed (varies with specific procedure; for meniscectomy, 24 hours and then up with crutches four times as tolerated)

Check peripheral pulses every 2 hours with neurovascular checks (should feel posterior tibial and dorsalis pedis)

Elevate operative leg and foot of bed

Apply ice or cold packs to incisional area

On first postoperative day, begin straight leg raising exercises if prescribed; may not begin until second to third postoperative day with anterior cruciate ligament repair

Begin active and passive ROM knee exercises in physical therapy on first postoperative day (varies with procedure and patient need, but specific program will be prescribed)

Do quadriceps setting exercises, 10 repetitions per set, every hour (see Table 6-10)

Table 6-10 Techniques For Muscle Setting Exercises

Muscle	Technique
Quadriceps setting	Ask patient to straighten leg and thigh; then ask patient to lower knee joint to bed while contracting quadriceps muscle. Have patient hold contraction for 4-6 sec, then relax muscle and knee joint. Repeat exercise 10-15 times q3-4h. Patella should move proximally when quadriceps contracts.
Gluteal setting	Have patient either flat in bed or in low-Fowler's position; ask patient to tighten (squeeze) buttocks (gluteal muscles) and hold for 5 sec; relax buttocks muscles, and repeat tightening (setting) 10-15 times q3-4h.
Triceps setting (in preparation for crutch walking)	Have patient extend forearm and hold elbow straight, with fingers spread apart on bed; then have patient press hands into mattress while trying to lift shoulders (tenses triceps muscles). Head of bed can be in low-Fowler's position to aid in doing this exercise. Repeat exercise 10-15 times q3-4h.

EMERGENCY ALERT

COMPARTMENT SYNDROME

Compartment syndrome occurs after soft tissue or musculoskeletal injury or surgery in which the amount of swelling, accumulation of fluid, or hematoma constricts circulation, perfusion, and oxygenation to the area. Each compartment contains at least one muscle, nerve, artery, and vein.

Assessment

- Assess capillary refill (normal refill is 2 to 4 sec).
- Assess for pulses above and below the site of trauma.
- Assess neurovascular status (the five P's): pallor, pulselessness, paralysis, paresthesia, pain.
- Assess for presence of infection, condition of affected tissues.
- Increased pain is common; pain is increased when limb is moved passively by health team member (stretch increases ischemia, causing increased pain): **increasing pain on passive movement is a hallmark of compartment syndrome.**
- Assess color of limb; compare with opposite limb.

Interventions

- Elevate limb and reposition frequently.
- Apply cold packs to area (protect skin from direct contact with ice).
- Perform frequent neurovascular assessments (once every hour).
- Monitor interstitial pressures as prescribed.
- Manage pain.
- Obtain IV access.
- Prepare for surgical incision and fasciotomy, if indicated.

NURSING CARE

Nursing Assessment

Knee joint and incisional area: Presence, amount, and type of drainage (usually is scant, serosanguineous); skin color is paler than nonoperated knee but should not be bluish, which could indicate an arterial clot; edema and pain (increasing edema and pain are untoward signs of excessive bleeding); ability or inability to move leg with knee extended; complaint of increasing amounts of pain; may signify compartment syndrome (see box above).

Psychosocial concerns: Alteration in or concerns with body image and return to usual activities and sports (if an athlete); limitation of mobility over time; development of arthritis

Potential Complications

Development of hematoma or thrombus in or distal to knee or calf; instability of knee joint, knee stiffness; recurrence of pain with or without degeneration or reinjury of tissues of knee joint (patellofemoral pain); reflex sympathetic dystrophy; compartment syndrome also possible (ischemia of muscles leading to necrosis of tissues); reinjury of same or injury of opposite knee

Patient Problems/Nursing Diagnoses & Interventions

NIC Immobility Management

Impaired physical mobility related to surgery and meniscal repair

- Monitor ROM of unaffected joints.
- Maintain bed rest as prescribed *to aid recovery.*
- Begin straight leg raising exercises as prescribed *to regain strength.*
- Encourage performing quadriceps setting exercises every 2 hours when prescribed *to maintain strength.*
- Encourage setting of gluteus muscles every 2 hours when prescribed *to maintain functions.*
- Help patient up in a chair with minimal weight bearing initially; then progress to helping patient walk with crutches as needed. Monitor patient's response *to note progress.*
- Emphasize necessity to continue exercise program at home and in rehabilitation setting *to aid full recovery.*
- Apply continuous passive motion machine (used when meniscal repair is combined with anterior cruciate ligament reconstruction).[9] The machine is kept at full extension and 30 degrees of flexion of knee.[9]
- Teach patient how to put on knee immobilizer, splint, or brace if required *to aid independence and self-care.*
- Assist with ADLs as required *to increase independence.*
- Encourage weight lifting of operative leg as prescribed *to regain full function* (usually done in rehabilitation center).

NIC Tissue Perfusion Management

Ineffective tissue perfusion related to surgery and use of tourniquet

- Monitor color and temperature of operative limb *to determine circulatory adequacy.*
- Perform neurovascular checks every 2 hours, including check of color, edema, temperature, pain, sensory or motor changes, ability to use or lift leg, peripheral pulses, extension of inflammation to contiguous tissues above or below knee, and comparison of operative leg characteristics with nonoperated leg *to note current status.*
- Report changes in findings; may require removal of constricting dressings or additional surgery if pulses are absent *to aid perfusion and relieve pressure.*
- Elevate leg and foot of bed *to increase venous return.*
- Note patient's complaint of increased pain on passive movement *as one sign of compartment syndrome* (see box above).
- Apply ice to site *to decrease edema.*
- Continue checks every 4 to 6 hours *to note changes early.*

NIC Skin/Wound Management

Impaired skin integrity related to surgical incision

- Check condition of wound or incision.
- Change dressings of wound as needed *to aid healing.*

- Observe drainage characteristics and amount; report findings to physician if drainage cloudy or odorous—may be signs of infection.
- Obtain culture of cloudy or odorous drainage *to determine type or presence of infective organisms.*

NIC PHYSICAL COMFORT PROMOTION

Acute pain related to surgical procedure

- Clarify presence, amount, type, and severity of pain *to determine present status.*
- Administer narcotics as prescribed every 3 hours, or encourage patient's use of PCA medication. Increase time between administration of narcotics or analgesics as acute pain abates *to lessen need.*
- Administer aspirin or ibuprofen between narcotics (enhances pain relief and relief of inflammation). Encourage use of aspirin as antiinflammatory drug if prescribed (patients are usually discharged with either aspirin or acetaminophen "prescription" to buy over the counter) *to substitute for narcotics.*
- Encourage position changes *to lessen pressure and fatigue.*
- Report continuing severe pain, change in peripheral pulses, or increasing edema as signs *indicative of ischemia, thrombus formation, or developing compartment syndrome** (FIG. 6-32).

PATIENT EDUCATION/CONTINUUM OF CARE PLAN

1. Clarify recovery program and exercises to aid recovery.
2. Clarify rationale for each part of neurovascular check to gather thorough information about tissues.
3. Reiterate the need for continuing the exercise and walking programs prescribed for long-term recovery.
4. Encourage return to social contacts to regain mobility and comfort even though having only partial weight bearing initially.

---

*A compartment contains one or more muscles, along with at least one artery, vein, and nerve held enclosed in a covering of inflexible fascia. The interstitial pressure rises with edema and bleeding into injured muscles. The pressure rises because the fascia does not allow the muscle to swell with the edema and bleeding. Unless the fascia is opened, the muscle will die in 6 to 12 hours from ischemia because the elevated venous and interstitial pressure or slow arterial inflow of blood delays removal of wastes.

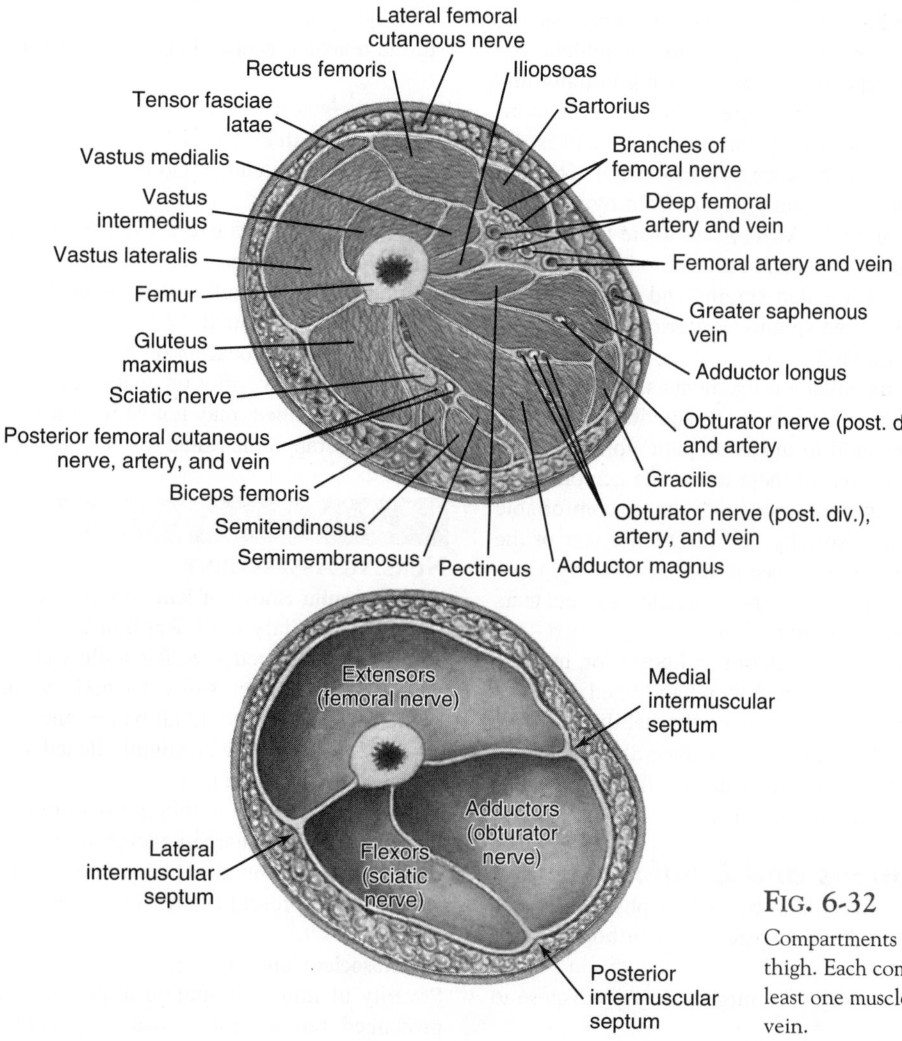

FIG. 6-32 Compartments and cross section of the thigh. Each compartment contains at least one muscle, nerve, artery, and vein.

5. Stress need to refrain from sports activities that could retraumatize unhealed tissues until physician permits resumption.
6. Encourage compliance with low-impact, in-line sports activities such as swimming, rowing machine, or level-surface jogging *to aid full recovery.*

Evaluation/Patient Outcomes

Immobility Management: ROM of knee joint is regained. Patient has 90 to 125 degrees of flexion and full extension of knee with minimal pain over time.

Tissue Perfusion Management: Patient has normal peripheral tissue integrity. Patient returns to sports activities or usual ADLs with protective knee covering, if required. Patient has normal color, normal temperature of legs, and no swelling.

Physical Comfort Promotion: Patient has pain easily controlled with nonnarcotic analgesics, with only intermittent use after several weeks. Patient is continuing rehabilitation exercise program as prescribed.

Arthroscopic Ligament Repair

Description and Rationale

Ligaments in and around joints, particularly of the knee, shoulder, fingers, and ankles, are often injured or torn in athletic activities or are torn from repetitive stresses causing initially microscopic tears and eventually complete tears of one or more ligaments in a joint. The most frequently torn ligament is the anterior cruciate ligament in the knee (see Fig. 6-10). The tear can be partial or complete. It usually occurs from hyperextension or abnormal rotation of the knee. A complete tear creates laxity in the knee and must be repaired to restore joint stability. Tears in ligaments are also called sprains and referred to as first-, second-, or third-degree sprains. Posterior cruciate ligaments can also be torn inside the knee.

The medial and lateral collateral ligaments surrounding the knee joint are also torn frequently in sports activities. Swelling, tenderness, and at times mild to moderate pain along the ligament pathways are indications of these tears. The person is unable to continue to play after the injury and is more comfortable keeping the affected knee partially flexed. Often a tear of the medial collateral ligament of the knee is accompanied by a medial meniscal injury. One half of anterior cruciate ligament tears are accompanied by meniscal injury.[17]

Cruciate ligament tears, both anterior and posterior, must be repaired carefully for the knee to be fully rehabilitated. With the development of the arthroscope, the overall rehabilitative time and process decreases. Athletes, however, face a long, intense process of exercises to restore strength and stability to the knee. Often rehabilitation takes 1 year or longer.

Contraindications and Cautions

1. Arthroscopic repairs are done by skilled physicians, frequently by sports medicine physicians or orthopedic surgeons.
2. Multiple ports for arthroscopic surgery may predispose to infection.
3. Younger patients or children whose growth plates are still open may be treated more conservatively with braces and rehabilitative exercises.
4. If the young child or athlete's knee remains unstable, surgery may need to be considered despite the risk of growth arrest.
5. Surgery may be done within 1 or 2 days after injury to the athlete or may be delayed until some of the bleeding and edema have subsided.
6. The injured athlete will be placed on crutches to preclude additional injury related to the knee instability.
7. The knee and anterior cruciate ligament have a direct relationship to the foot and hip for walking, during which a stable knee is required.

Multidisciplinary Plan

Medications

Antiinflammatory agents
- Ibuprofen, 400-800 mg tid or qid
- Ketorolac (Toradol), 10-30 mg IV or PO q4h
- See table on p. 337 for additional NSAIDs

Antiinfective agent: Cefazolin (Ancef), 1000 mg IV before surgery and q8h × 3 IV postoperatively

Narcotic analgesic agents: Oxycodone (Percodan), 30-60 mg PO q4h prn

Muscle relaxant: Metaxalone (Skelaxin), 10-20 mg q4-6h

General Management

Ambulation with crutches
Elevation of affected leg and knee
Ice to knee
Neurovascular checks every 1 to 2 hours as prescribed
Dressing changes as needed
Elastic bandages or bulky dressing postoperatively
Regular diet as tolerated
Up without weight bearing or as prescribed with crutches
Continuous passive motion machine, degrees of motion and times prescribed, may not be used for all patients
Physical therapy rehabilitative exercises as prescribed

NURSING CARE

Nursing Assessment

Neurovascular Status of Knee Joint and Lower Extremity

Color and capillary refill: Refill in 2 to 4 seconds is normal
Temperature: Injured knee/leg slightly cooler than opposite leg
Discoloration or contusions around knee joint
Peripheral pulses: Should all be present and full
Movement: Knee may be slightly flexed, but can be moved; extension will cause pain
Sensation: Should be within normal limits
Edema: May have marked edema around knee
Pain: Varies with number and site of ligament tear or sprain
Hemarthrosis present if anterior cruciate ligament tear[17]

Psychosocial Concerns

Severity of injury; limitation after injury and surgical repair; prolonged rehabilitation needed; possible end of career or sports activities; reinjury possible; postinjury joint instability, disability, or arthritis

POTENTIAL COMPLICATIONS
Hemorrhage or hematoma; thrombus formation or deep vein thrombosis; infection; posttraumatic degeneration and arthritis; possible repeat tear; compartment syndrome; loss of livelihood, financial problems

PATIENT PROBLEMS/NURSING DIAGNOSES & INTERVENTIONS
See pp. 410-411.

FIXATION FOR IMMOBILIZATION OF BONES (EXTERNAL)

CASTS

Description and Rationale

Casts are hard structures of plaster, fiberglass, or plastic materials used to immobilize musculoskeletal tissues after injuries. Although plaster (gypsum) is still the most frequently used material for casts, newer fiberglass, soft plastic, and cast-tape casts are being used more often. Each of the particular materials requires specific application techniques and has advantages and disadvantages, such as being heavy, cumbersome, or expensive or requiring special drying procedures and care to prevent skin breakdown. The use of a particular material is determined by the patient's injury, the length of time needed for immobilization, and the physician's preference (FIGS. 6-33 and 6-34).

Preparation for encasement in a cast varies from simply explaining its application and purpose to complete physical preparation, including an enema, bath, and skin cleansing with antiseptic solutions. Explanations and care should be geared to the patient's level of comprehension and need to prevent undue fear or anxiety. Handling the patient gently, especially the parts to be encased in a cast, alleviates tension and facilitates application without additional trauma.

Depending on the type of cast and the materials used, all supplies should be assembled and assistance for positioning and holding arranged in advance. Privacy is required when the skin is exposed, and breast and genital areas should be covered for the patient's ease of mind. Padding may be used over bony prominences before the cast is applied.

Once a cast is applied, drying times vary with the material used, the amount of plaster used, the areas of the body put into the cast, and the weather conditions. Plaster casts dry more slowly in damp, high-humidity conditions and can take 2 or 3 days to dry thoroughly. While drying, the areas in a cast must remain uncovered for drying to proceed from inside out. Drying is also facilitated by using fans (except with open wounds) and lamps with low-wattage bulbs.

During the drying periods, care must be taken to avoid making finger indentations in the cast, which would be reflected inward and cause a pressure area on the skin under the indented area. Pressure is also eased by turning the patient every 2 hours while the cast is drying to prevent molding and deformation. Propping or elevating with pillows helps maintain proper positioning. The pillows used should not have a plastic or rubber covering because the heat given off by the cast material will be trapped by the rubber or plastic and reflected back to the tissues in the cast, causing injury to the skin. Plastic and rubber also delay drying of plaster.

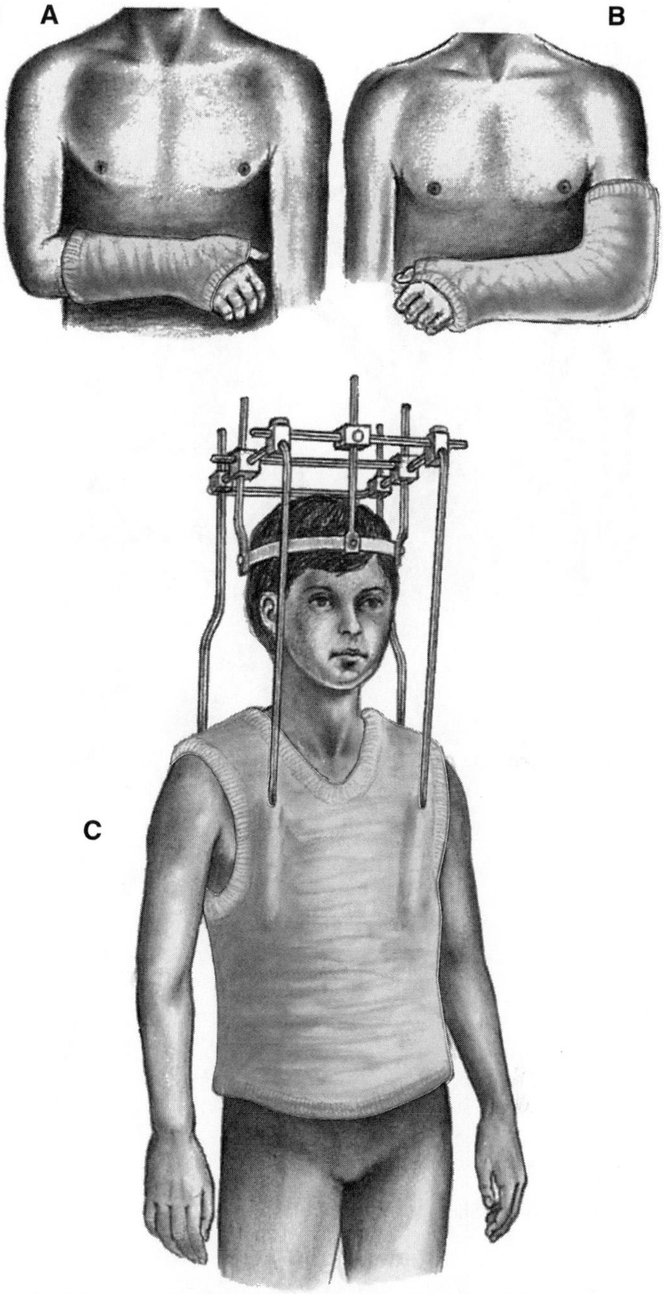

FIG. 6-33
Examples of casts for upper extremity and cervical spine injuries. **A,** Short arm cast. **B,** Long arm cast. **C,** Body jacket with halo apparatus attached; apparatus may be used with a brace, not cast.

Contraindications and Cautions

1. Open fractures may not be treated with casts initially because of the need to observe the injury site over an extended period. If in a cast, a window may be cut for dressing changes or to observe the open area more easily.
2. Plaster casts must be kept dry to prevent disintegration and weakening of the cast.

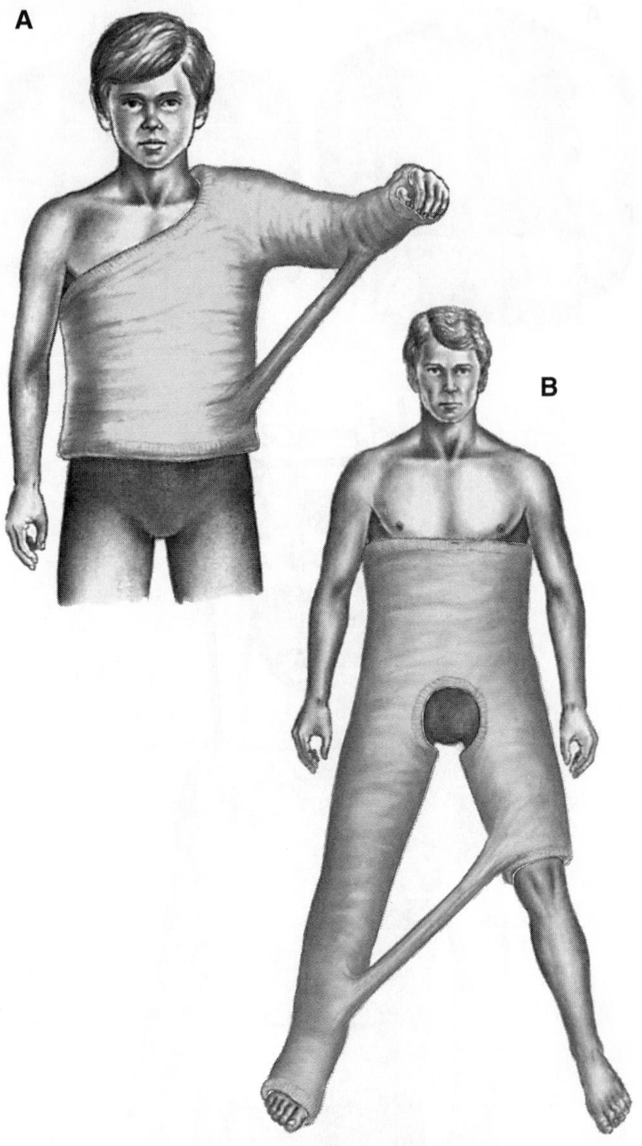

FIG. 6-34
Spica casts. **A,** Shoulder spica. **B,** One and one-half leg hip spica.

3. Fiberglass, plastic, and cast-tape casts can become wet without weakening; however, the skin under the cast must be dried if it becomes very wet to prevent maceration under the cast; drying is done with a hair dryer on low setting only to prevent a burn inside the cast.
4. Abdominal distention should be treated before placing a patient in a spica cast because the distention may increase, causing respiratory or circulatory compromise. A circular abdominal window may be cut out of the cast to lessen pressure over tissues.

Preprocedural Nursing Care

1. The skin areas to be encased must be clean, dry, and free of open lesions or blisters that occur with some fractures.
2. X-rays are taken to ascertain the extent of trauma.
3. All equipment and supplies must be assembled before the procedure is begun for ease and safety of application without unnecessary delay.
4. Sufficient skilled personnel should be present to assist with the application; two or three people may be needed to assist the physician with a spica or body cast.
5. A sedative, narcotic, or anesthetic may be given before cast application to ease pain and calm the patient.

MULTIDISCIPLINARY PLAN

Medications

Narcotic analgesic agents
- Meperidine (Demerol), 25-100 mg IM q3h (exact dosage varies with age and trauma), if pain severe
- Morphine, 10-15 mg IM once before application of spica cast if pain is severe (dosage varies with age)

Analgesic/antipyretic agents
- Aspirin, 300-600 mg PO or rectally (if NPO) for moderate pain q4h prn (not used for persons under age 18 years because of association with Reye's syndrome)
- Acetaminophen, 325-600 mg q4h up to 1000 mg q4h, age-dependent dose

Sedative-hypnotic, nonbarbiturate agents: Flurazepam (Dalmane), 30 mg PO hs prn

NSAIDs
- Ibuprofen, 400-600 mg q4-6h
- Ketorolac (Toradol), 10-30 mg IV or IM q4h
- See table on p. 337 for additional NSAIDs

General Management

Ice bags prescribed to a specific site—place carefully to avoid causing indentation of a damp plaster cast

Bed rest until cast is dry, if plaster cast is large, or to abdomen and lower extremities

Elevation of cast (extremity) on pillows

Neurovascular checks every hour for 24 hours, then every 2 hours for 24 hours, and then every 4 hours

For open reduction: Recording and reporting amount of drainage or bleeding

Forcing fluids to maintain hydration

Begin regular diet as prescribed

Seek consultation with physical therapist for exercises to maintain muscle strength, for use of crutches, if needed, and for assistance with ambulation

Apply sling for cast to upper arm for comfort and safety

NURSING CARE

NURSING ASSESSMENT

Cast and contiguous tissues: Extent of cast and type of materials used; neurovascular condition of tissues around cast; position of tissues in cast (e.g., in flexed or extended position) or functional position of fingers in forearm cast; condition of cast (damp or dry); temperature of cast and tissues around cast; ice bags: ice melted or still frozen and properly placed, cover dry; reaction of patient to being in a cast; compare with tissues from opposite side to detect changes

POTENTIAL COMPLICATIONS

Cast syndrome; refracture; development of pressure areas; delayed or nonunion

! EMERGENCY ALERT

TROUBLESHOOTING SPLINTS AND CASTS

The goal is to prevent circulatory compromise or extension of the injury.

ASSESSMENT

- Assess neurovascular status (see p. 330 for check areas).
- Assess for new injury, pressure areas, or open lesions.
- Inspect for signs of infection at suture lines, surgical sites, and open skin.
- Assess stability of surgical hardware if present.

INTERVENTIONS

- Obtain order, if needed, to loosen or bivalve cast or splint while maintaining anatomic position; assess for restored color, circulation, sensation, and lessened pain.
- Obtain order for radiographs to assess for new injury or to ensure corrective measures were effective.
- Pad pressure points and areas adequately.
- Reposition limb frequently (q2h, minimum).
- Maintain elevation of affected area to lessen edema.

PATIENT PROBLEMS/NURSING DIAGNOSES & INTERVENTIONS

NIC IMMOBILITY MANAGEMENT

Impaired physical mobility related to presence of the cast

- Check ROM of unaffected muscles.
- Teach isometric exercises as feasible, such as quadriceps and gluteus setting exercises. If fracture is below knee, quadriceps setting exercises of affected leg are vital *to retain muscle strength and prevent atrophy of thigh and leg muscles.*
- Assist with ambulation as needed *to increase mobility.*
- Teach techniques for walking with crutches *for safety.*
- Apply sling to upper extremity *to hold cast snugly and lessen edema formation.*
- Teach patient to allow cast to lie in sling with shoulder loose *to prevent shoulder pain or "freeze" of muscles of joint, for upper extremity cast.*
- Assist physical therapist with rehabilitation program.

NIC PHYSICAL COMFORT PROMOTION

Acute pain related to cast or trauma

- Determine presence, site, and degree and duration of pain.
- Stress that return of pain after pain-free period should be reported to physician (may indicate loss of reduction or other complication).
- Administer narcotic or analgesic as necessary and prescribed *to relieve pain.*
- Note increase in pain, numbness, or tingling and decrease or absence of pulses as indicative of compartment syndrome or that cast may be too tight; report promptly to physician because cast may need to be cut (bivalved) *for safe care.*
- Stress need to elevate extremity if edema recurs after discharge *to relieve edema by increasing venous return.*
- With body cast, note signs of increasing anxiety, dyspnea, nausea or vomiting, or eructation or complaints of abdominal distention; may be caused by "cast syndrome" from excessive aerophagia (air swallowing) or from kinking of the superior mesenteric artery, leading to gastric or intestinal distention and ileus; cast may need to be bivalved, and a nasogastric tube may be inserted *to relieve ileus and vascular compromise.* If no abdominal window is present, one may be cut in cast.
- Consult occupational therapist and physical therapist for activities *to relieve boredom and maintain muscle strength.*

NIC TISSUE PERFUSION MANAGEMENT

Ineffective tissue perfusion related to fracture, soft tissue trauma, and cast with a potential of causing neurovascular dysfunction

- Check status of injured leg or arm and compare with opposite extremity: skin color, edema, temperature, presence of contusions or other lesions; cast: type and dryness; complaints of soreness or pressure from cast *to determine if changes are needed.*
- Perform neurovascular checks as prescribed: Check color, temperature, edema, peripheral pulses and capillary refill, motor and sensory functions, and pain (type, amount, and site) *to determine current neurovascular status.*
- Elevate casted tissues *to increase venous return, thereby decreasing edema.*
- Change patient's position every 2 hours *to lessen pressure on sensitive tissues and relieve muscle tension.*
- Monitor patient's complaint of increasing severity of pain and increasing pain on passive movement *as one sign of developing compartment syndrome.* Report to physician, if present.
- Monitor interstitial tissue (compartment) pressures as prescribed *to detect rising venous pressures as a sign of developing compartment syndrome.*
- Perform capillary refill of toes or fingers to detect prolonged refill as a sign of decreased arterial inflow and developing ischemia *as a sign of compartment syndrome.*
- Release constricting dressings or bivalved cast to relieve compressive forces *to reduce interstitial pressures.*
- Prepare patient for surgical fasciotomy, if physician determines its necessity, from unrelieved increased interstitial pressures *to prevent permanent loss of muscle/nerve functions.*

After Removal of Cast

NIC IMMOBILITY MANAGEMENT

Impaired physical mobility related to edema and muscle weakness from being in cast for period of time

- Check for presence of edema and amount of muscle function after cast removed.
- Explain that affected tissues may develop edema and tenderness with reuse *to ease concern.*
- Explain to patient that he or she must elevate extremity for 24 hours and when sitting thereafter *to lessen edema.*

- Caution patient to resume usual activities slowly *to lessen edema and soreness.*
- Explain that soreness and pain are common after cast removal *to ease concern;* explain that patient should take nonnarcotic analgesic to ease soreness for 24 to 48 hours
- Explain to continue ROM exercises as usual *to regain or maintain strength.*
- Explain that muscle atrophy and an accumulation of dead skin cells are common after cast removal *to prepare patient for appearance of tissues.*

PATIENT EDUCATION/CONTINUUM OF CARE PLAN

1. Explain techniques to keep cast clean and dry.
2. Explain not to put anything inside cast.
3. Explain use of hair dryer on cool setting to ease itching under cast.
4. Explain need for well-balanced meals and adequate fluids.
5. Explain proper crutch and walking techniques, including not to lean on axillary supports and to bear weight on hand grips.
6. Explain skin care after cast removal: gently cleanse skin with cold-water wash containing enzymes; allow to soak into skin for 20 to 30 minutes, then flush with clear water; dry carefully and apply a lubricating lotion to prevent cracking or drying of the skin. Caution not to scrub skin tissues because this could cause skin openings and sores.
7. Explain that the patient should report persistent pain, weakness, and edema to the physician (usually all symptoms are relieved in 3 or 4 days after cast removal, although muscle weakness may persist longer); at times special exercises may be prescribed.
8. Teach signs and symptoms of compartment syndrome (see pp. 408-409).

EVALUATION/PATIENT OUTCOMES

Immobility Management: Patient regains mobility and ROM. Patient uses muscles and joints normally, without limitation or edema, and has minimum initial postremoval discomfort.

Physical Comfort Promotion: Patient is relieved of pain. Patient needs only occasional analgesic for muscle soreness. Acute pain is gone; only occasional sore joint pain is noted. X-rays show fracture union.

Tissue Perfusion Management: Patient regains usual peripheral vascular perfusion. Patient has no numbness or edema of extremity or digits. Color returns to normal 1 to 2 days after cast removal. Patient has not developed compartment syndrome.

EXTERNAL FIXATION DEVICES

Description and Rationale

Several types of externally applied fixation devices are currently used for immobilization of bones, including the Roger Anderson, Ilizarov, Monticelli-Spinelli, Hoffman, and Ace-Fischer apparatuses. The Hoffman apparatus consists of pins placed at right angles to the long axis of a bone and held by the clamps and screws of the device. The Ilizarov or Ace-Fischer devices have pins, rods, and rings placed in oblique and vertical angles to the long axis of the bone and then attached to the retaining devices. The use of one or the other device depends on the patient's condition and physician choice, as with any medical treatment (FIG. 6-35).

Externally applied fixation is used in many sites and for many conditions. Sites where such fixation may be applied include bones of the face, jaw, upper and lower arm or leg, pelvis, ribs, and fingers or toes. Pins used vary in number, length, and thickness according to the bones or area to be treated. The major reasons for use of these devices are that they allow increased use of contiguous joints while maintaining local immobility, permit the patient's discharge to home, hold unstable fractures or reductions and weakened muscles while allowing ambulation, and hold bones with tissue or bone infection (pins are above and below the infected areas). They are also currently used for nonunions, leg-lengthening procedures, traumatic injuries that have a lot of soft tissue damage that precludes use of a cast, and bone transport for limb salvage. A portion of bone is moved to a new site to fill a void, and new bone forms behind the transported segment through distraction osteogenesis with the external fixator in place.[31] Dr. Ilizarov developed and perfected the operative techniques of distraction osteogenesis and built the external fixator that bears his name to immobilize the operative tissues for the time required to lengthen limbs.[31]

Contraindications and Cautions

1. Severely comminuted bone fractures may be a contraindication because the multiple pins needed may cause more fractures or weakening. Comminution with good alignment may be an indication for use, as it is for the Ilizarov or Monticelli-Spinelli fixators.
2. Severe or *spreading* osteomyelitis may be another contraindication because the multiple sites can be sources for progressive infection; localized osteomyelitis may allow use of an external fixator to help hold the weakened bones to prevent fracture.
3. Overuse or excessive muscular movements may cause loosening or pin movements.
4. The multiple pin entrance and exit sites can be sources of skin and bone infection.
5. After removal of the pins, bones can be refractured because of the multiple tracts through the bones; patients must be cautioned to increase activities slowly to prevent reinjury.
6. Self-care techniques must be learned by the patient and family.
7. Limb-length discrepancy of less than 2 cm requires no specific treatment, other than use of orthotic devices.[45] The current indication for lengthening is a limb length inequality exceeding 5 to 6 cm.[54]

MULTIDISCIPLINARY PLAN

Surgery

Pin care according to institution policy: Some physicians do not prescribe pin care; there is no one method in current use[35]

Turning of nuts, as required, every 6 hours for some fixators

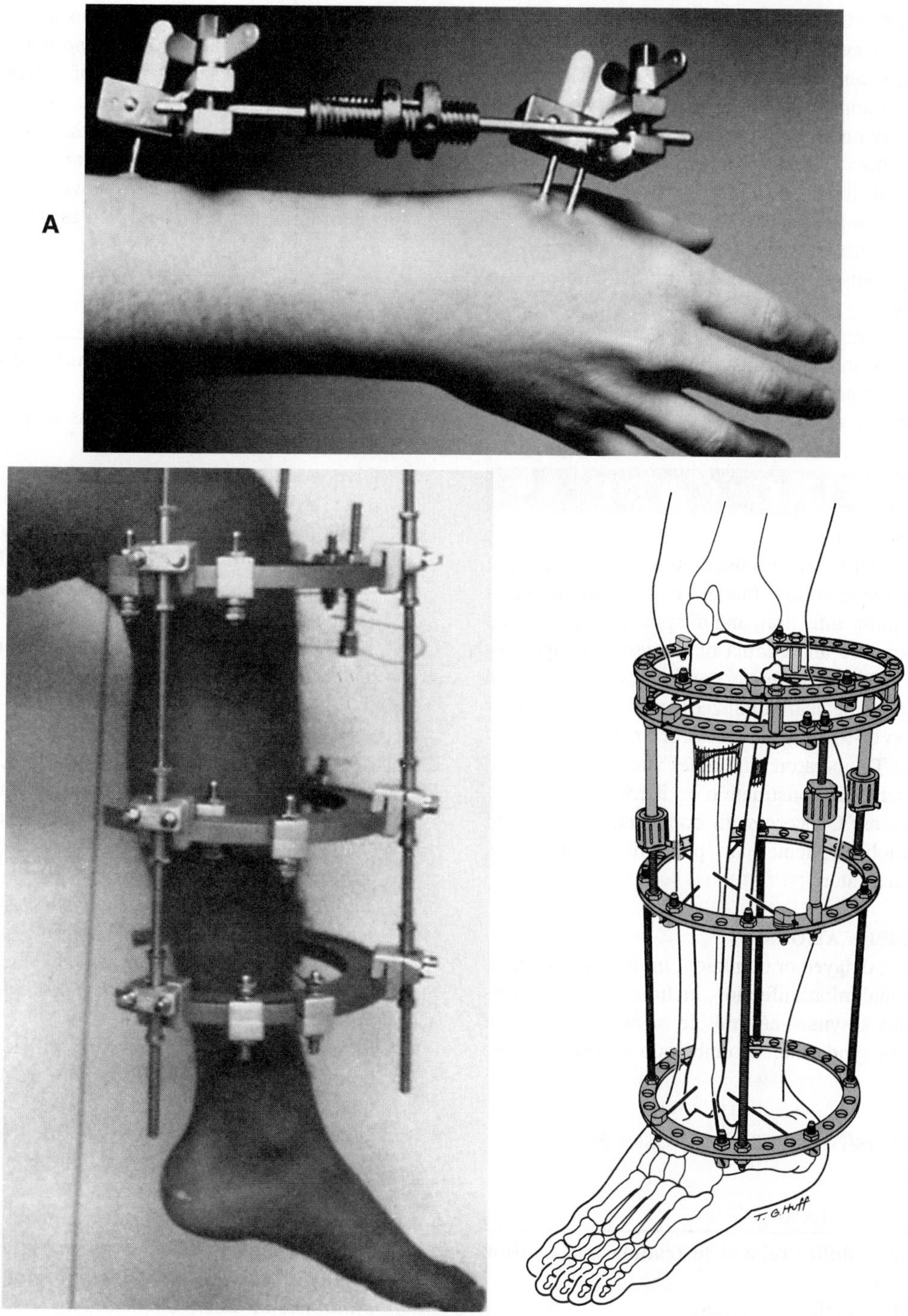

FIG. 6-35
External fixation apparatuses. **A,** Hoffman. **B,** Monticelli-Spinelli circular fixator. **C,** Ilizarov apparatus for lower leg.

Medications

Narcotic analgesic agents

Meperidine (Demerol), 50-100 mg IM q3h (dosage varies with age and trauma); may use PCA with age-appropriate dosage

Morphine, 1.5-2 mg q10min with 20-30 min lockout

Antiinfective agents

Cefamandole (Mandol) or cefazolin (Ancef), 250-1000 mg IV q6h for 7 days

Vancomycin (Vancocin), 1 g q8 or 12h IV

Cephalexin (Keflex), 500 mg q6h PO after IV antibiotic is discontinued

Analgesic/antipyretic agents

Aspirin, 600 mg PO q4h for moderate pain or temperature above 38.3° C (101° F) (aspirin should not be given to persons younger than age 18 years because of its association with Reye's syndrome)

Acetaminophen, 325-650 mg PO q4h prn for moderate pain or temperature above 38.3° C (101° F)

General Management

Neurovascular checks every hour for 24 hours, then every 2 hours for 24 hours, and then every 4 hours
Ice bags to site continuously, if able to be placed at site
Elevation of extremity on pillows
Up with sling (if upper extremity) or with crutches and no weight bearing (if lower extremity; after recovery from anesthetic); may also use wheelchair
ROM of unaffected joints and muscles
Turning (tightening) nuts as prescribed every 6 hours for limb lengthening only
Begin regular diet as prescribed
Inspect pin sites every shift for signs of inflammation or infection; do pin site care per institution policy or physician's prescription (see box, p. 417).

NURSING CARE

NURSING ASSESSMENT

Site of injury and external apparatus: Assessment of each pin entrance and exit site: color—marked redness and purulent drainage may signify infection, and the pins may need to be removed; temperature and edema of tissues; drainage; peripheral pulses; ability to move contiguous muscles and joints (unless to be held immobilized); pain, numbness, or tingling; position of fixator; intactness of fixator parts
Systemic concerns: Temperature and other vital signs, nausea, headache or other pain, constipation or diarrhea
Psychosocial concerns: Concern with body image, degree of mobility or immobility, acute pain, possibility of infection, length of time in fixator

POTENTIAL COMPLICATIONS

Infection; refracture; delayed or nonunion; limb length discrepancy; nonunion or malunion; infection, including osteomyelitis and rarely toxic shock syndrome; muscle or nerve damage or injury; compartment syndrome; fat embolism syndrome; deep vein thrombosis

PATIENT PROBLEMS/NURSING DIAGNOSES & INTERVENTIONS

NIC IMMOBILITY MANAGEMENT

Impaired physical mobility related to trauma and fixation device

- Check ROM of unaffected tissues.
- Maintain bed rest until recovered from anesthesia *to aid recovery and for safety.*
- Ambulate as prescribed with sling or crutches *to enhance mobility; may use wheelchair.*
- Turn and alter bed position as need *to prevent development of pressure areas.*
- Seek assistance of physical therapist for strengthening exercises to unaffected tissues.

NIC COPING ASSISTANCE

Disturbed body image related to limb length discrepancy and need for external apparatus

- Determine implicit or expressed concerns.
- Clarify purposes of multiple pins and external device *to increase understanding and compliance.*
- Stress positive aspects of use of external devices *to increase self-concept and body image.*
- Discuss having equal limb lengths after treatments *to aid development of positive body image.*
- Reiterate that pins can be removed in physician's office when union has been achieved as determined by x-rays *to ease concern.*

NIC SKIN/WOUND MANAGEMENT

Impaired skin integrity related to multiple pins, skin openings, and trauma

- Observe all skin areas for signs of pressure or inflammation.
- Give wound care as needed and pin site care (see box, p. 417).
- Teach patient and family members how and when (usually q6h) to turn nuts, if to be done, for limb lengthening *to increase skill and confidence in ability to do self-care.*
- Teach recording screw adjustments when completed q6h.

NIC PHYSICAL COMFORT PROMOTION

Pain related to trauma or fixation apparatus

- Check site and amount of pain (may initially be acute, sharp pain at pin insertion sites on skin) *to determine current status.*
- Administer narcotics and analgesics as needed and prescribed *to relieve pain or discomfort.*
- Stress that recurrence of pain at site is a sign to be reported to physician—*may indicate a developing problem.*
- Stress that acute pain episodes will lessen in 24 to 48 hours and that most pain will be relieved in approximately 7 to 10 days *to ease concern.*
- Note localization of pain to one site (may be sign of infection or inflammation); continue hourly neurovascular checks *to note early changes.*
- Note change in sensation or numbness and tingling as signs of neurovascular pressure; report increases in either sign *because these may signify beginning compartment syndrome, or other complication.*
- Apply ice bags as prescribed *to lessen edema and pain.*

PATIENT EDUCATION/CONTINUUM OF CARE PLAN

1. Explain to the patient and family pin care techniques to continue at home as needed; provide instructions in writing to avoid confusion or forgetting.
2. Stress the need to increase movements and weight bearing slowly to lessen tenderness and to permit the muscles to regain strength.
3. Discuss and list expected effects and side effects of medications and what to report to physician.
4. Reiterate treatment goals and stress need for compliance with regimen.

RECOMMENDATIONS FOR PIN-SITE SKIN CARE

Cleansing solution	Normal saline solution
Ointments	Use of ointments is not recommended
Sterile versus clean technique	Use sterile technique during hospitalization and clean technique after discharge
Dressings	Loosely apply gauze dressings to pin sites
Frequency of care	Conduct pin-site skin care q8h in the presence of drainage, or daily if no drainage present

From McKenzie LL: In search of a standard for pin site care, *Orthop Nurs* 18(2):73, 1999.

5. Stress 24-hour availability of health team personnel to ease concerns.

EVALUATION/PATIENT OUTCOMES

Immobility Management: Patient regains mobility and ROM. Patient uses muscles and joints normally, without limitation or edema, and with minimum initial postremoval pain and discomfort.

Coping Assistance: Patient has a positive body image. Patient has equal leg lengths. Patient has become more outgoing and sociable.

Skin/Wound Management: Wound sites remain free of infection. No drainage, redness, or erythema is noted at pin sites. No fracture has occurred. Skin openings are closing without signs of infection.

Physical Comfort Promotion: Patient is relieved of pain. Patient has only occasional pain or muscle soreness.

TRACTION

Description and Rationale

Traction is the application of force to the skin, muscles, and bones to aid in reduction of fractures, hold the reduced bones in alignment for healing, relieve muscle spasms and pain, and exert sufficient pull on muscles and bones to relieve pressure on peripheral spinal nerves. Traction can be applied to the skin and thus indirectly to the bones and muscles, or it can be applied directly to the bones through skeletal pins inserted through the skin and bones, with the pins then being attached to ropes, pulleys, and weights. The particular type of skin or skeletal traction applied is determined by the physician with regard to the patient's injury or condition, the purpose of the traction, the age of the patient, the weight of the patient, the condition of the skin tissues to be placed in traction, and the length of time the patient will need to be kept in traction. Table 6-11 summarizes the various types of skin and skeletal traction and the specific points pertinent to each type of traction (FIGS. 6-36 and 6-37).

Because time is required to overcome muscle spasms, bone overriding, angulation, and shortening, patients may be in traction for as short a time as 24 to 48 hours or as long as 4 to 6 weeks or more. Generally, patients in skeletal traction must remain hospitalized for the entire time because of the specialized care and equipment required (except for patients being treated

Table 6-11 Traction Types and Considerations for Care

Type	Patient's Age	Amount of Weight	Purposes and Principles	Considerations for Care
Buck's extension (one or both legs) (see FIG. 6-36, *A*)	Any age; most commonly used in adults	5-7 lb/leg	Applied preoperatively for hip fractures; for "pulling" contracted muscles; for relieving muscle spasms of legs or back; patient usually lies in recumbent position; may be turned to either side if no fracture is present; if there is a fracture, patient is turned to unaffected side; pillows to back and between legs	Skin of older patients is more "friable" and subject to loosening because of less subcutaneous fat; patient's complaints of burning under tape, moleskin, or traction boot should be assessed; traction may be removed for skin care even in presence of fracture; check heels for pressure areas
Russell's (one or both legs) (see FIG. 6-36, *B*)	Children 5 years or older to older adults	2-5 lb/leg	Applied for "pulling" contracted muscles; preoperatively for hip fractures; uses principle that "for every force in one direction, there is an equal force in the opposite direction" for the pulley placement and amount of weight used because weight pull is doubled	Patient is positioned on back for most effective pull; knee sling can be loosened for skin care and checking pulses in popliteal area

Continued

Table 6-11 Traction Types and Considerations for Care—cont'd

Type	Patient's Age	Amount of Weight	Purposes and Principles	Considerations for Care
Pelvic belt or girdle (abdomen and pelvis are enclosed) (see FIG. 6-36, *C*)	Adults or older adolescents	20-35 lb	Relieve muscle spasms and pain associated with "disk" conditions; pull is from iliac crests to relieve spasm	Patient may be positioned in Williams' position, which permits 45 degrees of flexion of the knees and hips to relax the lumbosacral muscles; orders usually state to be "in traction 2 h, out 2h" and out of traction at night; traction straps should not put pressure over sciatic nerves
Pelvic sling (under pelvis and buttocks like a hammock); is not traction per se but suspension	Adults	20-35 lb	For holding fractured pelvic bones; buttocks must be slightly off bed	Patients are comfortable in the sling even with extensive pelvic bruising; they may become dependent on being in the sling, and gradual "weaning" may be required; the sling should be kept clean and dry, and the patient can be removed from the sling for care and toileting, if institutional policies permit
Cervical head halter (under chin, around face, head, and back of head)	Adults	5-15 lb	For relieving muscle spasms caused by degenerative or arthritic conditions in or of the cervical vertebrae; halter should be applied so pull comes from occipital area, not through chin portion	Patients may be in low- or high-Fowler's position depending on the purpose of the traction; halter is usually incorrectly positioned if the patient complains of pain of chin, teeth, or temporomandibular joint; the side straps usually should be adjusted to relieve these complaints; patients should be removed from the traction for sleeping; patients may also use this type of traction at home for cervical arthritic conditions
Cotrel's (cervical head halter to head and pelvic belt to pelvis)	Adolescents	5-7 lb to head halter and 10-20 lb to pelvic belt	For stretching muscles preoperatively for scoliosis; principle is to pull muscles and joints apart	Patient is put in this traction to relax muscles and curvature; should be in traction except for sleeping; rarely, patient may be placed in Cotrel's postoperatively, too, although less frequently because of newer operative techniques such as Harrington or Luque rods or Cotrel-Dubousset instrumentation
Dunlop's (lower humerus and forearm)	Children to adults	5-7 lb to humerus; 3-5 lb to forearm	For realigning fractures of the humerus; body is used for countertraction by slightly elevating side of bed of arm in traction; forearm is merely held at right angles to the humerus for comfort, by using Buck's extension to the forearm	Dunlop's can be totally skin traction by Buck's extension to the humerus or can be skeletal with a Steinmann pin inserted through the distal humerus; use of either depends on the patient's injury; traction to the *forearm* should be removed daily for skin care, pulse checks, and ROM exercises because the forearm traction is merely a means to keep the forearm vertically at a right angle to the humerus; patients must have assistance during ADL because they are held flat on their backs; they can turn enough for back care only
Cervical via skull tongs (skull bones bilaterally)	Any age (most commonly young adults)	20-30 lb (depends on weight of patient)	To realign fractures of cervical vertebrae and to relieve pressure on cervical nerves; patient must be on a special bed or frame such as a CircOlectric bed or Stryker frame to facilitate care; traction weights must never be "lifted"; traction must be continuous	Patients with this traction may be severely injured, having either upper or lower spinal cord injury or complete transection, making them develop quadriplegia or paraplegia; neurovascular checks are required hourly to assess progression or relief of symptoms; patients also may develop paralytic ileus (therefore are given nothing by mouth), may have a nasogastric tube inserted to suction, and have an indwelling urinary catheter; pin care is done according to institutional policies and physician's preference

Type	Patient's Age	Amount of Weight	Purposes and Principles	Considerations for Care
Balanced suspension to femur (Steinmann pin or Kirschner wire inserted through upper tibia; thigh and leg are suspended in a splint and leg attachment) (see FIG. 6-37)	Any age from 3 yr	20-35 lb	For realignment of fractures of the femur; to overcome muscle spasms associated with fractures of the femur; suspension of the thigh and leg is "balanced" by countertraction attached to the top of the thigh splint with weights equal to those of suspension (usually 7-8 lb)	Patients in this traction should be recumbent for best effects; they can turn approximately 30 degrees to either side briefly for back care or can lift themselves using the trapeze and by using the uninjured leg and foot; neurovascular checks are vital to assess circulatory status and to prevent compartment syndrome (see box, p. 408)

A

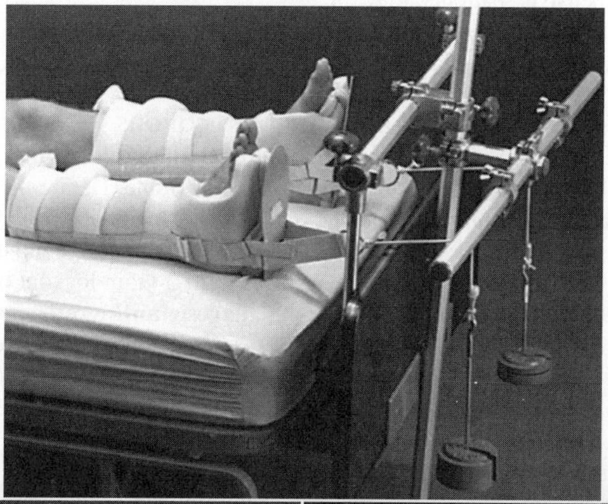

B

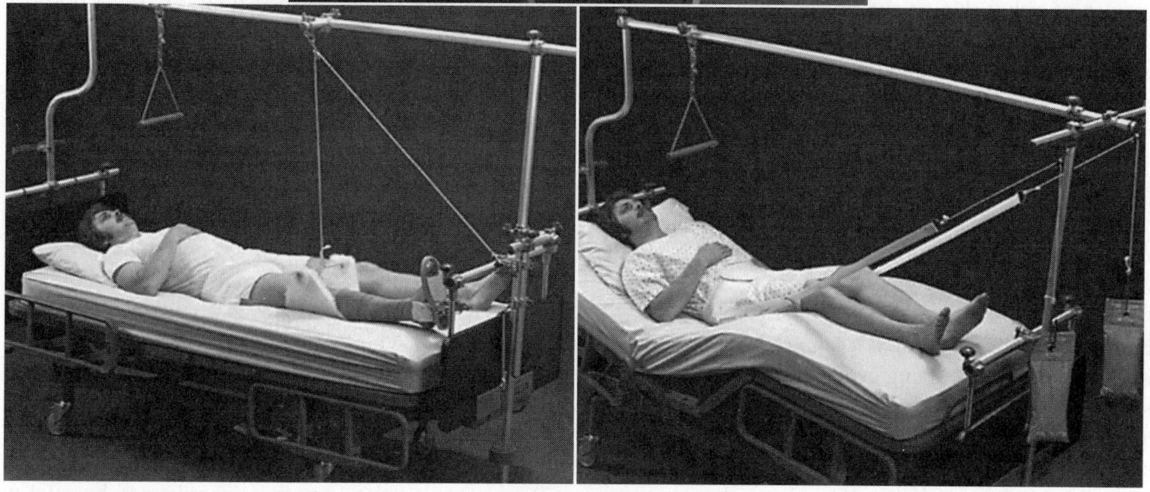

C

FIG. 6-36

Types of skin traction. **A,** Buck's extension. **B,** Russell's traction. **C,** Pelvic belt (patient in Williams' position; see Table 6-11 for explanation).

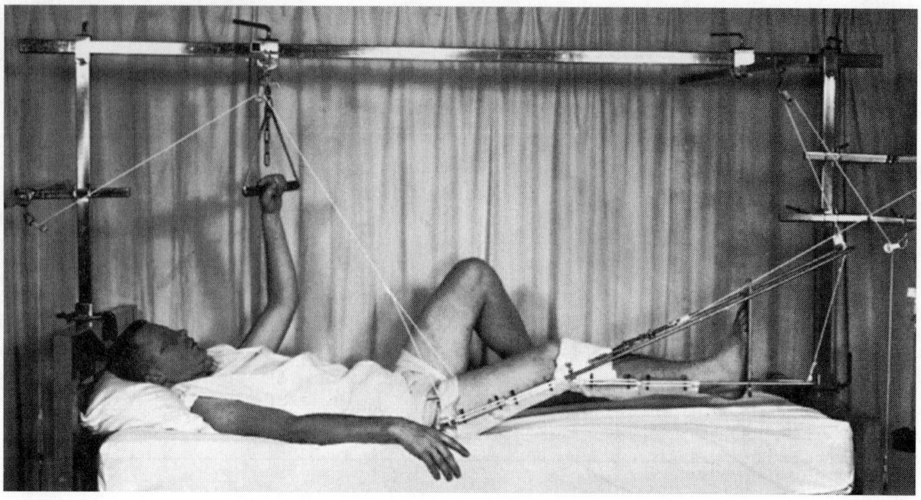

FIG. 6-37
Balanced suspension skeletal traction to the femur.

with home cervical traction with a head halter or in rare instances in other types of traction). Because hospitalization in traction is both extensive and expensive, patients may be placed in traction for periods only to achieve relief of muscle spasms and to correct fracture overriding or angulation; once alignment is regained, the patient may be taken to surgery to have internal metallic fixation. Therefore, although traction is still frequently required for specific treatment of an individual patient's injuries, the traction may be removed sooner than in the past because metallic implants are used to maintain the reduction.

Contraindications and Cautions

1. Age is a restriction for the application of one or more types of skin or skeletal traction (see Table 6-11). Because of lack of muscle mass or strength, a newborn baby or an elderly adult may not benefit from traction.
2. Open draining wounds or lesions are also contraindications to the use of either skin or skeletal traction because such wounds predispose to infection.
3. The amount of weight applied must be determined by the physician, who will consider the amount of muscle spasm, the degree of overriding and angulation, and the specific purposes of the treatment. The weight may be increased or decreased as x-rays indicate the need for weight changes.
4. Buck traction with a foam boot should not be applied over or under a pneumatic compression device that covers the calf.[5]

Preprocedural Nursing Care

1. Reiterate or clarify upcoming events for patient's traction.
2. Assess local and systemic physical condition for indications or contraindications to placement in traction (e.g., open lesions or blisters, deep calf pain, or diabetes).
3. Assist with hygienic self-care for clean, dry skin surfaces.
4. Assist with positioning for x-rays.
5. Administer preprocedural medication if prescribed.
6. Assemble all equipment for application of specific traction.
7. Assist with application of specific traction.

MULTIDISCIPLINARY PLAN

Medications

Opioid analgesic agents

Meperidine (Demerol), 50-100 mg IM q3h for 72 h (may use PCA with age-specific dosages)
Morphine, 10-15 mg IM q4h, or 1.5-2 mg q10min with 20-30 min lockout per PCA pump (rarely needed)

Analgesic-antipyretic agents

Aspirin, 600-1000 mg q4h prn for moderate pain
Acetaminophen, 325-650 mg q4h for moderate pain
Celecoxib (Celebrex), 100 mg bid
Rofecoxib (Vioxx), 12.5 m daily
See table on p. 337 for additional NSAIDs

Tranquilizers: Diazepam (Valium), 2-10 mg PO q4-6h

Muscle relaxants

Baclofen (Lioresal), 40-80 mg/day
Cyclobenzaprine (Flexeril), 10-20 mg PO tid
Metaxalone (Skelaxin), 400-800 mg tid or qid

General Management

Application of skin or skeletal traction (see Table 6-11)
Diathermy to back (lumbar area) twice daily
Bed rest; specific position or positions (see Table 6-11)
Neurovascular checks qh for 24 hours, then every 2 hours, and then every 4 hours
Monitoring of tissue pressure if prescribed
Ice bags to affected tissues (site always indicated for application)
Diet: High protein, high vitamin, low fat; force fluids
Physical therapy for ROM and isometric exercises
Pin care for skeletal traction according to hospital policies or physician's preference (see box, p. 417; nursing research has demonstrated no differences in outcomes related to use of various methods for pin/site care[35])

NURSING CARE

NURSING ASSESSMENT

Area of Body in Traction*

Type of traction; area of body involved; tissues: color, edema, signs of pressure around traction, pain—sensations for sharp, dull perception, motor functions of extensor longus muscle that extends great toe—compare strength of extension with opposite great toe; weakness may indicate pressure on peroneal nerve, one indication of developing anterior compartment syndrome[5]; amount of weight; direction of pull; weights hanging freely in holder and off the bed, not over patient

Systemic Concerns

Patient: Pressure areas over bony prominences, muscle strength or weakness, weight loss, position in bed

Traction (entire traction setup) and principles of maintaining traction:

Ropes: Riding freely in pulleys, no frayed ends, knots intact; *never reuse rope* as it may fray and break

Pulleys: Moving freely

Weights: Hanging freely in holder; correct prescribed amount

Knots: Intact; no rope fraying

Pins: Straight, unbending; not moving in tissues

Slings: Under or around appropriate tissues

Belts: Intact; under appropriate tissues; clean and dry; padded properly; each part of setup (see Table 6-11)

Complications of immobility: Weight loss

Development of osteoporosis

Possible pulmonary infections

Pressure areas or sores

Development of compartment syndrome

Psychosocial Concerns

Concern with changes in body image, immobility and loss of livelihood, acute pain, bone healing over time

POTENTIAL COMPLICATIONS

Nonunion, malunion, embolic phenomena, pin necrosis, skin lesions or pressure areas, compartment syndrome

PATIENT PROBLEMS/NURSING DIAGNOSES & INTERVENTIONS

NIC PHYSICAL COMFORT PROMOTION

Acute pain related to trauma and traction

- Clarify pain experiences *to determine extent, etiology, and patient's reactions.*
- Help patient alter position within traction limitations *to relieve muscle and joint stiffness or soreness.*
- Administer narcotic analgesics as prescribed *to relieve acute pain* and nonnarcotic analgesic (aspirin or acetaminophen) *to relieve inflammation.*
- Review patient's entire pain experiences: local pain at site of injury and *systemic* spread (e.g., chest pain, dyspnea, calf pain, headache, confusion); *may be indications of pulmonary, circulatory, neurologic, or other complications.*
- Monitor for evidence of fat embolism with symptoms of mental confusion, dyspnea, chest pain, and vital sign changes. A petechial rash may also develop over upper chest and neck with fat emboli, which are more common with long-bone fractures.
- Perform Homans' procedure to determine possible cause of calf pain; could indicate thrombophlebitis if positive Homans' sign; may also have redness, swelling, increased warmth in calf. A positive Homans' sign does not always signify thrombophlebitis.
- Determine degree of muscle spasms at injury site; clarify causes of and measure *to relieve spasms through traction and muscle-relaxant medications.*
- Compare both legs *for similarities or differences in symptoms.*
- Monitor entire traction setup for proper functioning *to decrease friction, which decreases effectiveness of traction.*
- Observe all bony prominences for signs of pressure or irritation on skin and nerves.
- Clarify use of ice bags and apply ice bags *to help relieve muscle spasms, bleeding, and edema.*
- Assist with ROM exercises *to maintain strength in unaffected muscles.*
- Monitor effects of diathermy *in relieving pain and muscle spasms* if pertinent to injury.
- Perform pin care if needed *to remove secretions and to lessen possibility of infection.* Follow institutional policies or physician's preference for pin care (see box, p. 417).

NIC COPING ASSISTANCE

Disturbed body image related to weight loss and weakness

- Clarify effects of injury on body image and self-concept.
- Explain purposes of traction repeatedly because patient's anxiety and pain may preclude hearing or full understanding during initial explanations *to lessen concerns.*
- Explain reasons for bed rest, weakness, and anorexia. Encourage patient to eat more as appetite returns *to help regain weight and to aid in tissue and bone healing.* Some patients lose from 10 to 20 pounds in skeletal traction because of decreased muscle activity over time.
- Explain purposes of position changes *to maintain healthy tissues.*
- Observe appetite and intake and output *to note current status and to encourage intake.*
- Provide 3000 ml fluid intake *to maintain hydration and to perfuse kidneys properly to prevent renal complications.*

NIC IMMOBILITY MANAGEMENT

Impaired physical mobility related to traction, hospitalization, and loss of livelihood

- Monitor effects of injury and traction on mobility.

*See Table 6-11, p. 417 for specific tissues.

- Clarify use of traction as one part of treatment regimen for patient's specific injury *to increase understanding and compliance.*
- Encourage patient and family communications with physician for "timetable" for overall treatment *to aid compliance.*
- Seek consultations (per physician's prescription) for occupational therapy and physical therapy *to assist patient's recovery and adjustment to treatment regimen and hospitalization.*
- Seek consultation with social service personnel to help patient and family plan and prepare for possible economic needs *to regain livelihood* (may lose employment while hospitalized).
- Encourage patient's self-care activities *to maintain mobility within traction limits.*
- If surgical repair follows traction use, assist to ambulate *to regain mobility.*

PATIENT EDUCATION/CONTINUUM OF CARE PLAN

1. Ensure that patient and family can apply traction correctly if it is to be used in the home.
2. Explain to patient and family the use of muscle relaxants and pain medications if prescribed for use at home.
3. Ensure that patient and family recognize when to contact physician if symptoms recur.
4. Explain that patient should maintain intake of well-balanced diet to regain weight and strength.

EVALUATION/PATIENT OUTCOMES

Physical Comfort Promotion: Patient has minimal pain experiences. Patient has moderate soreness of operative site after surgical repair, relieved with narcotic, analgesic, and muscle relaxant occasionally. No other pains are noted.

Coping Assistance: Patient has a positive body image. Patient has positive outlook toward full recovery in 3 to 6 months. Patient regains some weight (5 pounds) and some muscle strength, and feels positive and sure of full recovery.

Immobility Management: Patient regains more physical mobility and ROM. Patient tolerates traction well and undergoes insertion of intramedullary rod to fractured femur. Patient walks with crutches and cane for next 10 days and longer. Patient performs ROM for unaffected muscles.

FIXATION FOR IMMOBILIZATION OF BONES (INTERNAL)

Description and Rationale

Surgical implantation of metallic pins, nails, screws, plates, and other devices for immobilizing or repairing traumatized or damaged bones and joints is major orthopedic treatment. With the development in the early 1930s of nonreactive metal alloys, surgical repair has provided greatly decreased hospitalization periods, a more rapid return to home and social and employment opportunities, and a more rapid regaining of mobility. Surgical repair requires the concurrent administration of antibiotics to prevent infection, the major hazard and deterrent to use of more orthopedic surgical and metallic implants for a wider range of injuries. However, in most instances the advantages of internal metallic fixation far exceed the disadvantages.

Fractures of bones may be surgically immobilized by screws attached to a compression plate; nails or pins, as in a hip nailing; a rod or nail placed within the intramedullary canal (intramedullary rod) or parallel to the bones (Harrington rods, Cotrel-Dubousset instrumentation, or Luque rods); screws or staples to hold fracture fragments together; or natural bone grafts to fill in gaps in bones or to fuse two bone surfaces together, as in a spinal fusion.

This section will focus on several procedures representative of internal fixation procedures: hip nailing or pinning, spinal fusion by Harrington or Luque rods or Cotrel-Dubousset instrumentation, spinal fusion by natural bone grafts, and internal fixation with compression plate and screws.

INTERNAL FIXATION WITH HIP NAILS OR PINS

Description and Rationale

The patient's specific injury, general physical and mental condition, and the physician's choice from the many available metallic nails and pins determine which type will be used for the particular patient. The injury may be a fairly stable fracture that requires only a single nail, such as a compression nail or screw or a sliding compression nail. Unstable fractures may require multiple pins, such as Knowles pins, or use of a nail with a side plate.

The type of internal fixation used is also determined by the particular fracture type and site. Hip fractures are referred to as intracapsular or extracapsular. Intracapsular fractures are those of the femoral head or neck that are contained within the hip capsule (FIG. 6-38). Intracapsular fractures may disrupt the blood supply of the head of the femur, with subsequent development of avascular necrosis of the head of the femur. Therefore fractures of the head or proximal femoral neck may be treated with insertion of a femoral prosthesis (hemiarthroplasty). Subcapital or distal neck fractures may heal without avascular necrosis; thus these latter fractures may be nailed or pinned (FIG. 6-39).

Extracapsular fractures are those around or through the trochanters and are referred to as intertrochanteric or subtrochanteric fractures. These fractures heal well with the use of compression screws or nails because the blood supply to the fracture site comes from the surrounding vessels outside the capsule. Side plates attached to the nails help maintain a stable reduction while healing progresses (see FIG. 6-39, *A*).

Finally, the patient's physical and mental condition may also help determine which type of internal fixation is performed. The weak or confused patient would benefit from a compression interlocking nail, which can withstand some weight bearing; a single nail with or without a side plate would be appropriate for a stable fracture in a mentally clear patient who could be cautioned and expected to walk with only minimum or touchdown weight bearing initially. Thus the specific internal fixation and repair require careful evaluation and assessment by the surgeon and other health professionals for the patient's greatest benefit.

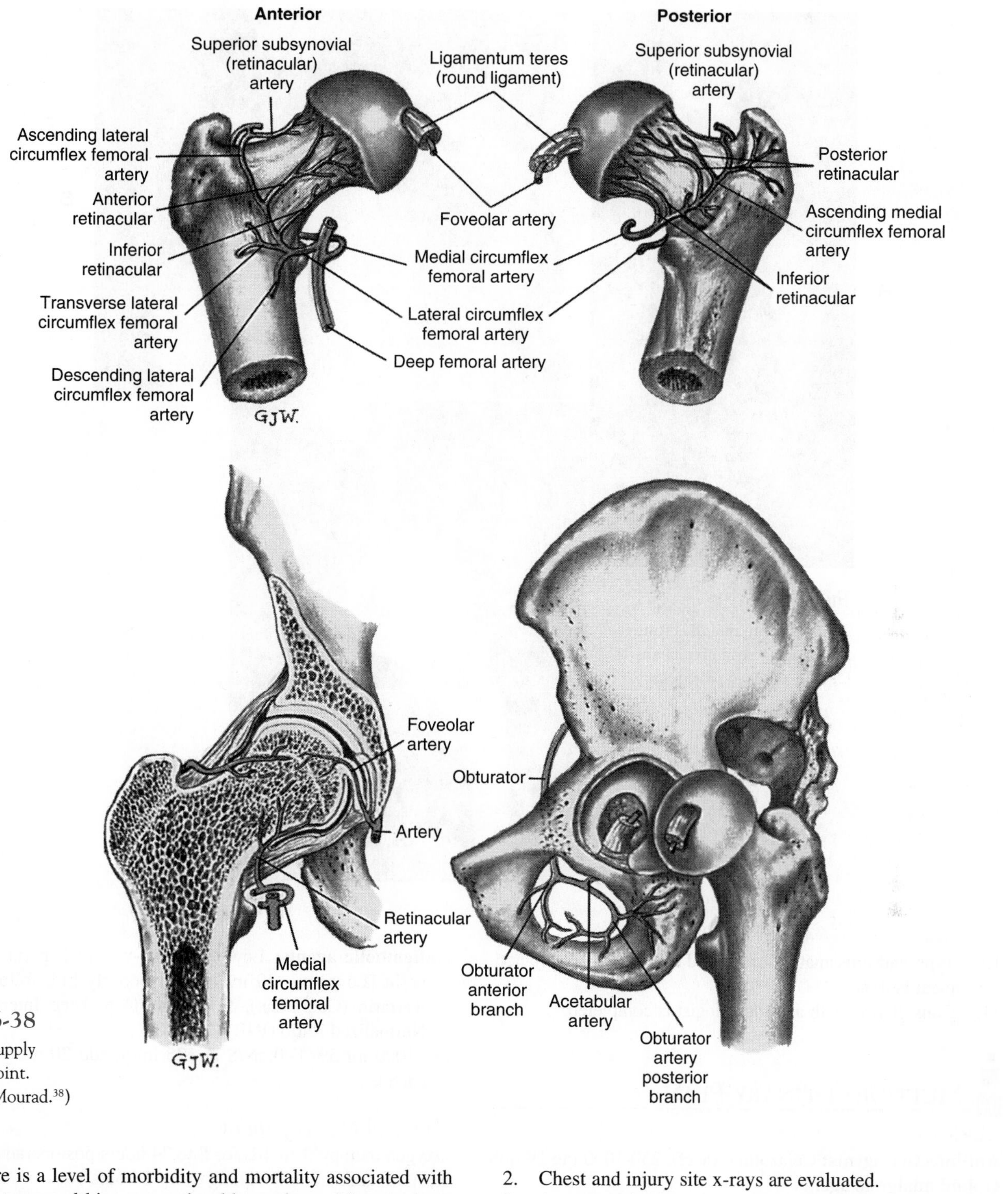

FIG. 6-38 Blood supply to hip joint. (From Mourad.[38])

There is a level of morbidity and mortality associated with hip fractures and hip surgery in older patients. Many patients never regain ambulatory status after surgery and require long-term care. The mortality rate of postoperative hip surgery patients who experience pulmonary embolism approaches 50,000 per year, secondary to thromboembolic disease. Without anticoagulation, as many as 75% of patients will show deep vein thrombosis, with a mortality rate of 2%.[37]

Preprocedural Nursing Care

1. The patient may be placed in traction, usually Buck's extension or Russell's traction, while preparations for surgery are completed.
2. Chest and injury site x-rays are evaluated.
3. An enema is given, if needed, and an indwelling catheter may be inserted.
4. An electrocardiogram is done to determine cardiovascular status.
5. Complete consultation for medical clearance is done before surgery if the patient is older or elderly.
6. Serologic studies are done for chemistry analysis; urinalysis is done.
7. Preoperative medication is administered.
8. Intravenous therapy is initiated for fluid intake.
9. Skin cleansing is done to decrease organisms in the operative site in the prep room.

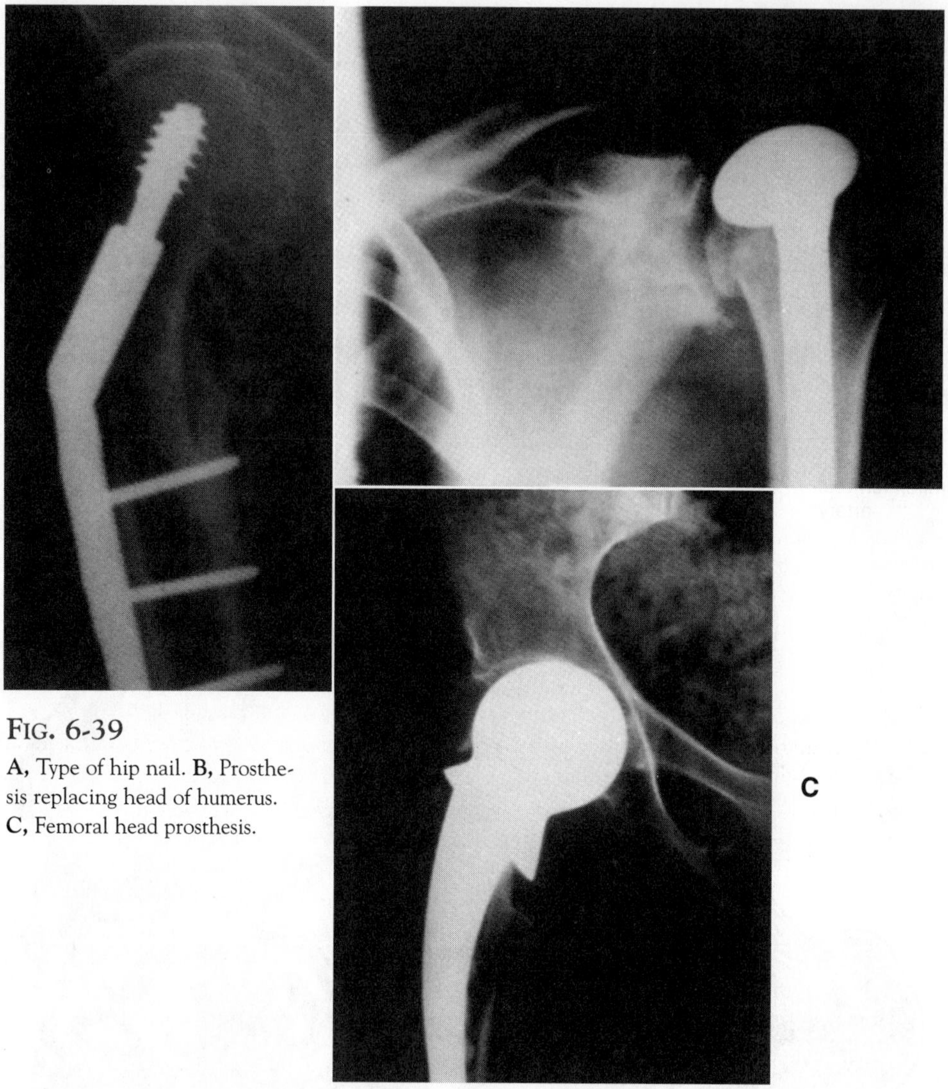

FIG. 6-39
A, Type of hip nail. **B,** Prosthesis replacing head of humerus. **C,** Femoral head prosthesis.

10. Type and crossmatch for packed red blood cell replacement is done.
11. Consultation with anesthesiologist is completed.

MULTIDISCIPLINARY PLAN

Medications

Antiinfective agents: Cefazolin (Ancef), 250-1000 mg IV q6h

Opioid analgesic agents

Meperidine (Demerol), 50-100 mg q3h for 24 h, then q3h prn (may have PCA administration in smaller dosages); may not be used for elderly patients because it may cause delirium[40]

Morphine, 1-2 mg q10min with 20 min lockout per PCA pump

Analgesic-antipyretic agents: Aspirin, 600 mg q4h for temperature elevation above 38.3° C (101° F) and for moderate pain

NSAIDs

Ibuprofen, 400-600 mg q4-6h

Ketorolac (Toradol), 10 mg PO q4h or 10 mg IV q4h (for elderly patients)

See table on p. 337 for additional NSAIDs.

Antiembolic agents: Low-molecular-weight heparin (enoxaparin [Lovenox], 30 mg subcutaneously bid, followed by warfarin (Coumadin), 5-10 mg PO to keep International Normalized Ratio (INR) (2.0-3.0)[57]

IV: 1000 ml 5% D/0.2N/S at 125 ml/h; add 20 mEq KC1 to each liter

General Management

Oxygen therapy, 1 to 4 L for 8 to 24 hours postoperatively

Deep breathing and coughing every 2 hours

Respirex (or Triflow) 10 times every hour for incentive spirometry

Pulmonary IPPB every 4 hours

Bed rest with operative leg in neutral position

Turning to nonoperated side and back every 2 hours

Change of dressing as needed; reinforce as needed

Record input and output; record wound drainage separately

Vital signs every 15 minutes for four times, every 30 minutes for four times, every hour for four times, then every 4 hours

Up in chair three times on first postoperative day with no or touch-down weight bearing on operated leg

Up with walker on second postoperative day; weight bearing on operated leg must be specifically prescribed
Clear liquids after nausea has subsided; advance to regular diet as tolerated
Complete blood count, electrolytes, and CO_2 measurements in morning and daily for 4 days
Physical therapy to help with walking and ROM exercises
Perform neurovascular checks as prescribed
Apply antithrombotic hose or pneumatic compression hose to prevent deep vein thrombosis

NURSING CARE

Nursing Assessment

Hip and upper thigh incisional and wound area: Assessment: dressing—type, drainage—type, amount, wound suction equipment, if present—may not be used, drainage in container or on dressing; presence of edema at wound site; position of thigh and leg; complaints of pain in operative area or calf; color of tissues; antiembolism hose presence
Systemic concerns: Respiratory and circulatory status; vital signs: temperature elevation; mental state and recovery from anesthesia; muscle strength or weakness; urinary output, catheter-drainage setup, and voiding after catheter removal; intravenous fluid type, amount, and rate
Psychosocial concerns: Concern with body image; immobility; confusion; acute pain; postoperative lack of ambulation; fear of falling; economic cost of hospitalization, rehabilitation, and long-term care; limited or partial insurance coverage only

Potential Complications

Deep vein thrombosis, pulmonary embolism, dislocation of prosthesis, loss of reduction or dislocation, thrombophlebitis, pneumonia, cardiac arrhythmias, wound infection, compartment syndrome

Patient Problems/Nursing Diagnoses & Interventions

NIC Coping Assistance

Disturbed body image related to trauma

- Discuss concerns, if patient can verbalize them.
- Maintain bed rest; clarify need for bed rest *to aid compliance.*
- Help with ADLs as needed *to help patient regain positive feelings.*
- Massage back *to aid comfort and circulation.*
- Encourage use of lipstick and personal makeup *to enhance self-concept and appreciate regaining health.*
- Discuss recovery processes and future outlook for full ambulation *to aid becoming more outward looking.*
- Discuss home situation, family/friend supports *to encourage planning for post-discharge care.*

NIC Immobility Management

Impaired physical mobility related to modification in weight bearing

- Determine ability to understand instructions and limitations; check visual and hearing acuity for safety.
- Assist to dangle at bedside on first postoperative day, then to pivot to chair with no weight on operative leg, or touchdown weight if prescribed.
- Stress that operative foot should be placed on floor but weight should be borne on nonoperated leg (refer to limb as either left or right leg so patient has a clear understanding) *to maintain safety in care.*
- Turn every 2 hours; prop with pillows between legs or back *to maintain position.*
- Assist with ROM, quadriceps, and gluteal setting exercises *to maintain muscle strength.*
- Help physical therapist walk patient with walker and limited weight to operative limb *for comfort and safety.*
- Encourage patient and family members to walk together *for patient's safety.* Instruct family about weight-bearing techniques *for clarity and safety.*
- Discuss transfer to rehabilitation unit for convalescent care to continue recovery.

NIC Physical Comfort Promotion

Acute pain related to trauma and surgery

- Observe wound for evidence of resolution of surgical trauma and inflammation.
- Listen to patient's complaints of pain; clarify site, type, and amount of pain.
- Administer analgesics judiciously because of patient's age (see box, p. 403). Dosage should be sufficient to relieve pain without causing confusion (may need to vary dosage within ordered ranges) *for safety in care.*
- Turn or reposition patient and massage back *to increase comfort.*
- If patient complains of calf pain, perform Homans' test *to help determine possibility of thrombophlebitis, which could lead to pulmonary embolism.*
- Observe for chest pain, dyspnea, and changes in vital signs, *which could indicate pulmonary embolism, atelectasis, or pneumonia.*
- Observe autologous blood transfusion equipment for amount and type of reinfusion, if needed and prescribed; note and investigate any complaint of soreness or pain at needle site as signs of infiltration.
- When pain is lessened, assist with meal and food selections *to aid in healing, resolution of inflammation, and enhancement of bone calcification.*
- Force fluids *that aid digestion and bowel and bladder elimination,* which could be decreased from narcotic administration.

Patient Education/Continuum of Care Plan

1. Clarify need for weight-bearing restrictions for bone union to proceed.
2. Clarify signs to report to the physician: increased soreness or pain at operative site, fever, decreased urine output or burning with urination.
3. Reiterate techniques for use of walker or crutches.
4. Teach patient and family necessity to continue eating a well-balanced diet and drinking plenty of fluids for healing, circulation, and elimination.

5. Explain transfer procedures to rehabilitation unit for continued recovery care.

EVALUATION/PATIENT OUTCOMES

Coping Assistance: Patient has positive body image. Patient has positive outward-looking demeanor. Patient appreciates ability to get around with aid.

Immobility Management: Patient regains some mobility. Patient walks with progressive weight bearing as healing occurs, with minimum discomfort and satisfactory ROM.

Physical Comfort Promotion: Patient is free of pain. Patient has no pain in fracture site. Muscle and joint strength is regained. Patient has lessened fear of falling. Patient is progressing in rehabilitation efforts for discharge to home.

INTERNAL FIXATION WITH HARRINGTON OR OTHER RODS TO VERTEBRAL COLUMN

Description and Rationale

Harrington rods are long metallic implants attached posteriorly to the vertebral column after corrective repair and fusion as treatment for scoliosis or vertebral burst fractures. The rod or rods (they may be used bilaterally) hold the vertebrae in the corrected alignment to permit the bones to heal and fuse the vertebrae solidly. The rods may remain in the site for extended periods or may be removed (rarely done) after x-rays indicate there is sound, solid fusion. In the early postoperative period some patients may wear a fitted brace to help the rods maintain spiral immobility if the curvature was marked preoperatively and multiple bone grafts were implanted during surgery. The brace is worn during waking hours and removed for sleep.

Luque rods are another kind of metallic implant used for corrective spinal surgery. Luque rods are used on both sides of the vertebral column with multiple attachments to each spinal segment to add corrective forces throughout the preoperative deformity. In addition, Luque rods are contoured to aid in correcting the deformation. Luque rods can also be combined with an L-shaped segment in a new technique for spiral instrumentation referred to as spinopelvic transiliac fixation (STIF), which provides a more stable construct.

Cotrel-Dubousset rods are a third type of internal fixation rod used to straighten and fuse the vertebrae. The patient's specific condition and the physician's preference determine which rods will be used (FIG. 6-40).

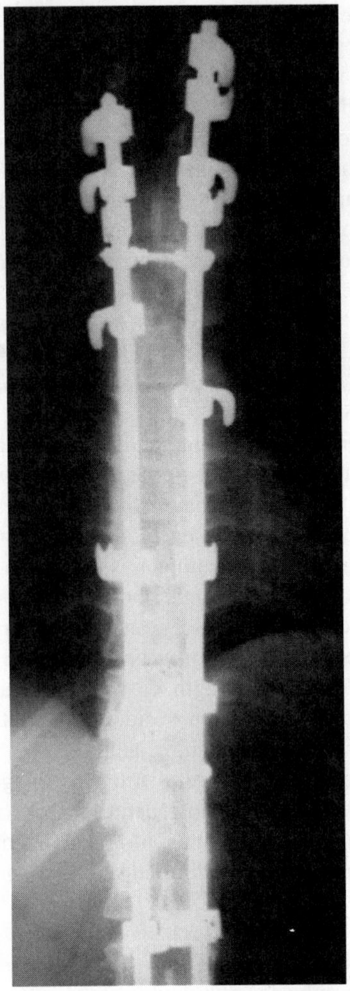

FIG. 6-40
Cotrel-Dubousset rods used to treat scoliosis. (From Mourad.[38])

Contraindications and Cautions

1. Harrington and other rods are foreign bodies, as are all metallic implants; thus they may cause a severe inflammatory reaction and infection, which may necessitate their removal.
2. Open surgery may predispose to local wound infection or lead to meningeal infections.
3. One or more bone grafts may be needed to maintain correction of the curvature or fracture; parts of or whole grafts may not unite firmly, which may require prolonged wearing of a brace, encasement in a plaster cast, or even reoperation.
4. The spinal attachments holding the rods may loosen, allowing the rods to move. Major movement of either end of the attachments would necessitate reoperation.
5. Complete medical evaluation is done to determine the current status of chronic conditions, if present.

Preprocedural Nursing Care

1. The patient may be placed in Cotrel's or halo-femoral traction (see Table 6-11, p. 417) before surgery to stretch muscles contracted from scoliosis.
2. Meticulous skin cleansing is done to remove organisms to prevent infections.
3. X-rays determine respiratory and spinal conditions; respiratory therapy with IPPB and use of a respiratory apparatus, such as Respirex or Triflow, is done every 4 hours.
4. Serologic and urologic studies are done.
5. An enema is administered to clear the lower bowel.
6. An indwelling catheter is inserted into the urinary bladder.
7. A full-length bed pad or alternating pressure mattress is placed on mattress.

8. Autologous blood donations may have been made every 7 to 14 days and stored frozen before use at the time of surgery.
9. An anesthesia consultation is completed before operation.

MULTIDISCIPLINARY PLAN

Medications

Opioid analgesic agents
- Meperidine (Demerol), 50-100 mg IM q3h
- Morphine, 10-15 mg IM q4h or PCA with 1-2 mg (depending on patient's age) q10min with 20 min lockout

Analgesic/antipyretic agents
- Aspirin, 600 mg rectal suppository for moderate pain q4h prn or for temperature over 38.3° C (101° F) (aspirin should not be given to persons under age 18 years because of its association with Reye's syndrome)
- Acetaminophen, 325-650 mg q4h prn

Antiinfective agents: Cefazolin (Ancef) or cefamandole (Mandol), 250-500 mg q6 or 8 h IV

Intravenous 1000 ml 5% D/0.45N/S at 75 ml/h with 10 mEq KCl in every other liter

Muscle relaxants
- Cyclobenzaprine (Flexeril), 10-20 mg tid
- Diazepam, 10-15 mg q4-6h
- Metaxalone (Skelaxin), tab q12h

NSAIDs
- Ibuprofen, 400-800 mg tid or qid
- Celecoxib (Celebrex), 50-100 mg bid (age-dependent dose)
- Rofecoxib (Vioxx), 12.5 mg daily
- See table on p. 337 for additional NSAIDs

General Management

IPPB every 4 hours
Maintain patient flat in bed
Logroll patient every 2 hours
Help patient deep breathe and cough every 2 hours, use respiratory aid 10 times every hour
Do not change dressing; reinforce if needed
Do neurovascular checks every hour
Give clear liquids after patient has had nothing by mouth for 24 hours; advance to regular diet as tolerated
Force fluids after intravenous line is discontinued
Do ROM exercises to arms and legs every 4 hours
Keep cast uncovered until dry or keep brace on at all times (if prescribed and in place)
Consult physical therapist for ROM and isometric exercises
Begin ambulation with assistance as prescribed

NURSING CARE

NURSING ASSESSMENT

Vertebral column, incisional wound site: check alignment and position of back and entire patient; check wound: drainage (may have suction drainage), edema, dressing, presence of brace or plaster cast with open window in back portion; skin condition of formerly contracted tissues; respiratory excursions; depth, rate, and character of respirations; breath sounds in all lobes; site and amount of pain

Systemic concerns: Assessment of motor and sensory functions by neurovascular checks; catheter drainage; intravenous fluid infusion site, solution, and rate; presence of nausea or vomiting; abdominal distention or ileus

Psychosocial concerns: Self-concept and body image; immobility; acute pain; length of convalescence; cost of hospitalization and long-term care; employment possibilities and concerns

POTENTIAL COMPLICATIONS

Infection, loss of reduction or loosening of rods, nonunion, wound dehiscence, cast syndrome, shock, hemorrhage, meningitis, pneumonia, thrombophlebitis, urinary tract infection

PATIENT PROBLEMS/NURSING DIAGNOSES & INTERVENTIONS

NIC COPING ASSISTANCE

Disturbed body image related to deformity and dependence because of bed rest and surgery
- Clarify patient's concerns with self-concept and image.
- Stress patient's improved appearance after fusion *to aid positive self-concept.*
- Encourage self-care as able; help with placement and removal of supplies *to maintain an asthetic atmosphere.*
- Assist with bath or shower *to provide security and encourage self-care.*

NIC IMMOBILITY MANAGEMENT

Impaired physical mobility related to prolonged convalescence and muscle weakness and spasms
- Monitor ROM of unaffected tissues.
- Turn, with assistance of another health professional, by logrolling every 2 hours. (Teach family logrolling technique if possible, and use their assistance.) Do not let patient turn self; logrolling cannot be accomplished safely by self because patient would twist. Twisting could disrupt fibrin meshwork (see pp. 372-375 for bone healing), thereby delaying or preventing bone union and fusion. Brace will hold back sufficiently rigid after discharge so patient can safely turn or get up unassisted.
- Encourage deep breathing and leg exercises *to increase self-activities and independence and promote healing and circulation,* and help prevent thrombophlebitis.
- Perform neurovascular checks qh; that is, observe and compare in all four extremities: color, temperature, edema; ROM; grip, push, and pull strength; sharp and dull discrimination; presence and type of pain, radiation, numbness, and tingling *to note signs of pressure.*
- Massage exposed areas of shoulders, neck, back, and buttocks *to relieve tiredness and muscle spasms.*
- Assist with stretching exercises if needed *to relieve skin restrictions from preoperative curvature limitations.*
- Caution patient to avoid bending, twisting, stooping, or lifting more than 10 pounds until physician permits *to enhance healing processes.*

NIC Neurologic Management

Risk for altered neurologic function related to insertion of metallic implants and bone grafts

- Monitor muscle strength or weakness in muscle groups *to detect early signs of pressure or palsy.*
- Monitor urinary and bowel output *to detect early signs of paralysis or weakness.*
- Perform neurovascular checks to all extremities as prescribed *to determine current status;* compare with previous data *to note any deterioration;* report untoward changes to physician.
- Consult with physical therapist for exercises *to increase or maintain muscle functions.*
- Monitor temperature and all vital signs; *elevations could indicate meningeal inflammation or infection.*

NIC Respiratory Management

Impaired gas exchange related to operative procedure and anesthesia

- Check rate, quality, and depth of respirations, cough, sputum production and color of sputum, and skin tissues as signs of possible pulmonary infection if out of normal ranges.
- Encourage deep breathing and coughing *to enhance and clear respiratory efforts and excursions.*
- Have patient use Respirex or Triflow *to increase respiratory excursions and strengthen respiratory muscles.*
- If chest tube is present, splint the chest or incision area while assisting patient to cough *to enhance respiratory excursions and lessen pain during procedure.*
- Monitor breath sounds in all lobes *to detect signs of respiratory complications.*
- Encourage family members to assist patient with pulmonary exercises *to encourage their participation in care as able.*

NIC Physical Comfort Promotion

Acute pain related to surgical trauma and muscle stretching

- Listen to patient's complaints of pain; clarify site, type, duration, and amount of pain *to determine proper interventions.*
- Administer medication (dosage adjusted to age, for younger child or adolescent, and severity of pain) as ordered *to maintain therapeutic levels,* or monitor use of PCA medications. Carefully monitor children to determine amount of pain and pain medication dosage and administration *to help maintain pain relief.*
- Check wound as pain source; note signs of resolution of inflammation and surgical trauma. Report continued edema, redness, and increased drainage *as untoward signs.*
- Help patient increase amount and time of walking (when allowed) *to help resolve muscle soreness and weakness and to lessen soreness and pain in operative site.*
- Change dressings over incision (after initial dressing change by physician) as needed; note lessening of soreness and acute pain as healing proceeds *to note resolution of inflammation.*
- Check bowel sounds, abdominal distention, passage of flatus (ileus may be source of pain).
- Administer prescribed muscle relaxant medication *to relieve muscle spasms.*
- Encourage use of measures to divert focus on pain; use music, television, imagery, or relaxation techniques that are age appropriate.

Patient Education/Continuum of Care Plan

1. Demonstrate to the patient and family how to put on brace, when prescribed.
2. Clarify that muscle stiffness, weakness, and soreness may increase with increase in activities but will last for brief periods only.
3. Reiterate stages to bone healing for strong union; stress need for caution against sudden position changes and need to continue wearing the brace.
4. Stress that the patient must eat a well-balanced diet to regain muscle strength, promote healthy bone growth, and promote wound healing.
5. Explain that sudden or gradually increasing pain should be reported to physician.
6. Stress walking program to increase strength and endurance.
7. Discuss continued use of diversions to enhance continued recovery.
8. Emphasize use of continued physical therapy program to help full recovery.
9. Stress need to refrain from sexual activity until incisions are healed and patient has few aches or pains; patient should wear thoracolumbosacral orthosis during sexual activity until full healing of bone grafts (bone union has occurred by x-ray evidence).

Evaluation/Patient Outcomes

Coping Assistance: Self-concept is positive. Patient resumes social contacts after convalescent period. Patient wears brace without difficulty or embarrassment. Patient enjoys new "straightened" appearance.

Immobility Management: Patient regains independence, mobility, and spinal motion with limited flexion. Patient moves freely with minimal muscle weakness, discomfort, or pain and has learned to use muscles of lower extremities and hips to assist lumbar muscles (must kneel or bend from hips rather than from lumbar area).

Neurologic Management: Patient has not developed motor/muscle weakness but is slowly regaining normal muscle strength. Patient walks upright with less curve evident. Patient has normal bowel and bladder functions. Temperatures are within normal ranges.

Respiratory Management: Patient has clear breath sounds in all lobes; cough is nonproductive. Patient deep breathes easily.

Physical Comfort Promotion: Patient is relatively pain free. Patient takes only occasional nonnarcotic analgesic for muscle and bone pain.

Spinal Fusion With Bone Grafts

Description and Rationale

Spinal fusion with natural autogenous bone grafts is done as treatment of a herniated nucleus pulposis. Nursing care of patients after spinal fusion for treatment of a ruptured disk is similar to that discussed previously, with the addition of assessing relief of sensory pressure signs, numbness, and tingling as surgical wound healing progresses. Autogenous bone grafts usually provide solid union without the problems associated with metallic implants, such as foreign body reactions, loosening, or infections.

Nursing care for spinal fusion is the same as for internal fixation with Harrington rods (see pp.426-428.)

Hemilaminectomy (Laminectomy)

Description and Rationale

Hemilaminectomy is the partial removal of the lamina to gain access to the intervertebral space to remove a ruptured disk. It may also just be called a laminectomy. From 200,000 to 500,000 laminectomies are done yearly in the United States, although newer percutaneous techniques have somewhat lessened the incidence of laminectomies. The pathophysiology leading to disk degeneration and rupture is discussed on p. 387 (Figs. 6-41 and 6-42).

Indications of a need for a laminectomy include intolerable pain unrelieved by bed rest and recurring episodes of incapacitating pain. Laminectomy for definite disk herniation remains a

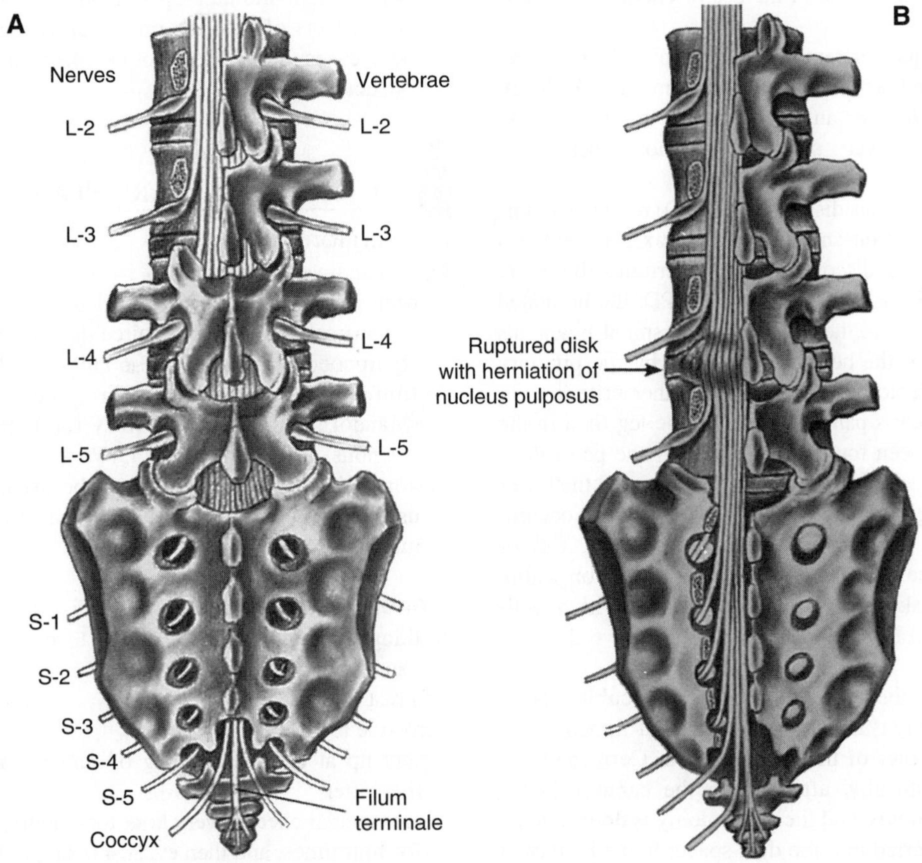

Fig. 6-41
A, Spinal nerves exiting from cord. **B,** Herniated nucleus pulposus; note pressure on nerve.

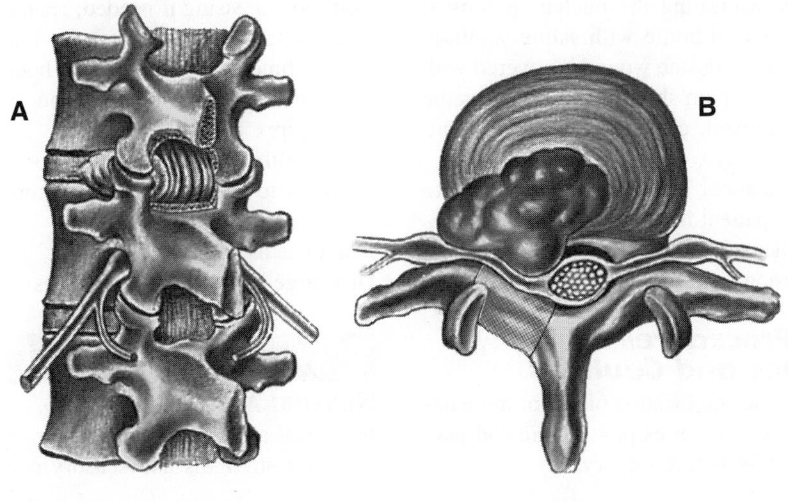

Fig. 6-42
Laminectomy for herniation of nucleus pulposus. **A,** Area of lamina removed during a laminectomy. **B,** Herniated nucleus pulposus.

highly successful procedure,[30a] and 96% of operative patients have improvement, especially if the disk herniation was a prolapse through the annulus.[30a] Success rates vary if the disk herniation is concealed in scar tissue after an inflammatory reaction. Only about 15% have complete and permanent relief after laminectomy with diskectomy.[30a]

Other treatments for herniated nucleus pulposus include injection of the disk space with chymopapain, referred to a chemonucleolysis. Previous success rates of about 75% for a good result (relief of pain) were similar to laminectomy with diskectomy. Only a few centers in the United States continue to do this procedure, since a complication of chymopapain is allergic reaction, with anaphylaxis the most severe form. Additionally, a small risk of transverse myelitis with irreversible paraplegia has led to a decline in the use of chemonucleolysis in this country.[30a]

The latest technique for removal of a herniated disk is referred to as automated percutaneous diskectomy. It was developed in the early 1980s as an alternative to the use of chymopapain. It is now a very safe and commonly performed procedure.

Automated percutaneous diskectomy (APD) requires a thorough physical examination and history, plain x-rays, either a CT scan or MRI, and discography to determine the exact pathology of the disk. As one criterion for APD, the herniated disk fragments must be contained within paraspinal ligaments to achieve removal of the herniated particles by the pituitary rongeur or the Nucleotome instrument. Another criterion for APD is that the patient's pain is greater in the leg than in the back because it has been found that the higher the percentage of leg pain, the more suitable the decompression, and the lower the percentage of leg pain, the poorer the results from decompression. Additional APD indications are that MRI, CT, or discographic evidence indicates only a single herniation within the annulus of the disk and failure to be benefited with a well-managed course of conservative treatment to relieve the pain and symptoms.

APD is done with the patient in the lateral decubitus position. A local anesthetic is injected, and diamond-tipped trocar is inserted into a corner of the affected disk. Correct site is confirmed fluoroscopically, after which the cannula is inserted against the annulus, and the annulotomy is done. An aspiration probe is inserted into the disk space; it can be turned 180 degrees in a reciprocal cutting action. Suction is applied through the inner cannula, aspirating the nucleus pulposus, which is then put in a collection bottle with saline solution. The equipment is removed and the stab wound is covered with a small adhesive dressing. Leg pain should be relieved as the herniated fragments are removed, confirmed by the patient, who is awake.

The success rate averages about 75%, varying from 49% to 85% in various groups. The patient is discharged the next day.

Complications include hematoma and disk space infection, nerve root injury, and occasional cauda equina injury.

Disk Removal Procedures Contraindications and Cautions

1. Determination of the cause and location of one or more degenerated or ruptured disks requires physiologic and psychologic diagnostic profiles before surgery.
2. Removal of a degenerated or ruptured disk may not relieve the patient's complaints of pain.
3. Patients for lumbar spine surgery are admitted the morning of surgery after extensive preadmission testing has been done.
4. Postoperative rehabilitation requires the patient's cooperation and performance of daily exercises to strengthen the spinal and abdominal muscles
5. The specific operative procedure varies with the site of disk rupture and the patient's and physician's preference. Percutaneous diskectomy and microdiskectomy are now being done almost exclusively because these are less invasive procedures for a single herniated disk than laminectomy.
6. The patient should stop smoking, if a smoker, because of the effects of nicotine on the disk; nicotine in the blood decreases blood flow to the disks and other vertebral structures.

Multidisciplinary Plan

Medications

Opioid analgesic agents
- Meperidine (Demerol), 50-100 mg q3-4h for pain before surgical removal of ruptured disk, if hospitalized
- Hydrocodone (Vicodin), 30-60 mg PO q4-6h if at home

Antiinfective agents: Cefazolin (Ancef) or cefamandole (Mandol), 250-500 mg q6-8h IV for 48 h

Intravenous, 1000 ml 5% D/0.45N/S at 75-100 ml/h

Postoperative PCA analgesia may be used, if needed (rarely used because pain is relieved by the surgical procedure for majority of patients).

General Management

Nothing by mouth until morning; then clear liquids and advance to regular diet

Bed rest until evening of surgery

Turn side to side every 2 hours

Patient up at bedside evening of surgery and up as tolerated thereafter

Neurovascular checks every hour for 4 hours, then every 2 hours for four times, and then every 4 hours, if still hospitalized

Male patient may stand to void if necessary

Reinforce dressing if needed; change dressing after 24 hours

Check vital signs every hour for 4 hours, then every 2 hours for four times, and then every 4 hours

Have patient deep breathe and cough every 2 hours; use Respirex 10 times each hour

Physical therapy consultation for exercise regimen and program, to be started after postoperative visit to physician's office

Ambulate as prescribed

Discharge as physician prescribes

NURSING CARE

Nursing Assessment

Incisional area of lumbar back or cervical area: Assessment of motor strengths and sensory condition of feet and legs or

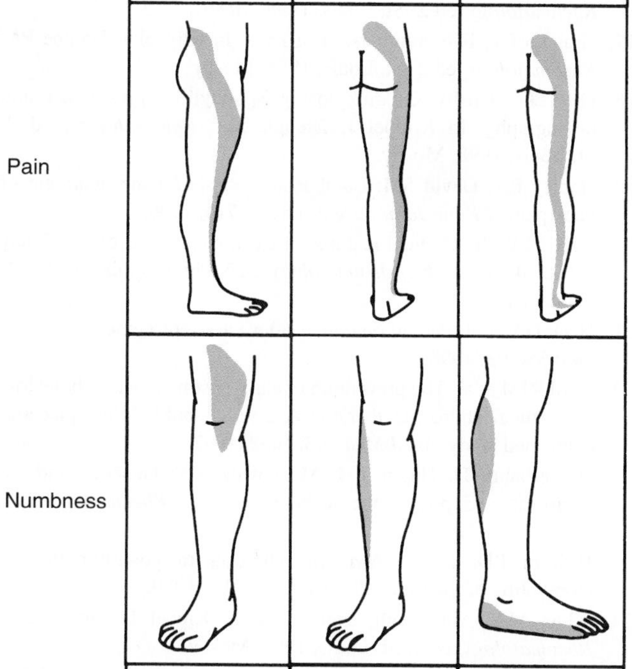

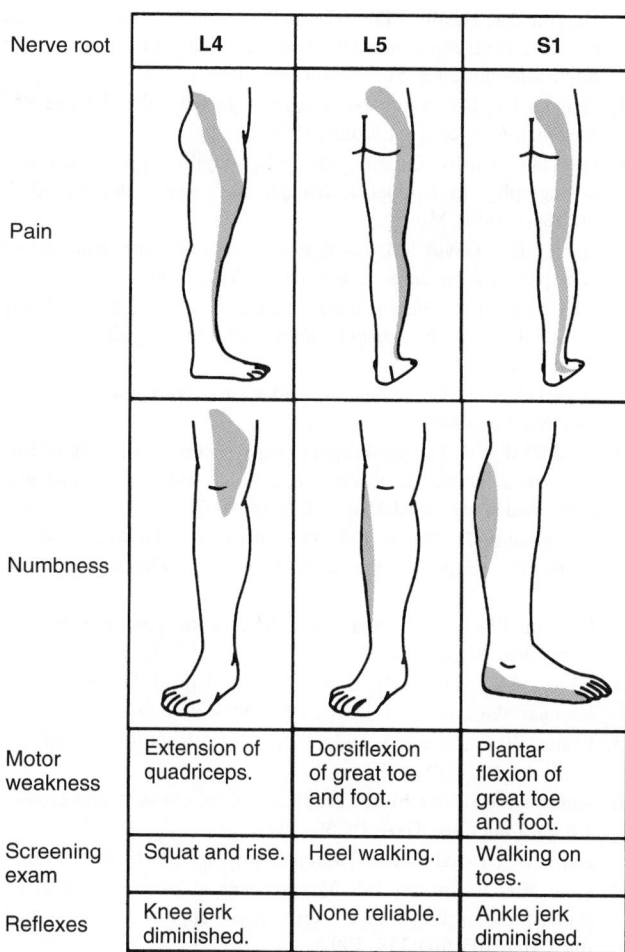

Nerve root	L4	L5	S1
Motor weakness	Extension of quadriceps.	Dorsiflexion of great toe and foot.	Plantar flexion of great toe and foot.
Screening exam	Squat and rise.	Heel walking.	Walking on toes.
Reflexes	Knee jerk diminished.	None reliable.	Ankle jerk diminished.

FIG. 6-43
Testing for lumbar nerve root compromise. The *colored areas* are assessed for changes as indicated in the content below each area.

arms and hands bilaterally (usually are within normal limits for push, pull strength; may have some remaining sensory changes such as lingering numbness or decreased sensitivity to sharp pinpricks) (FIG. 6-43); all peripheral pulses palpable; skin temperature of feet, legs, arms, and hands: may be slightly cool and pale; drainage on dressing scant to moderate amount and serosanguineous; pain mild to moderate in operative area with some radiation to shoulders and occipital area (if cervical) and to hips and buttocks (if lumbar); if cervical ruptured disk, may have soft surgical collar in place.

Systemic concerns: Headache, nausea, abdominal distention, urinary retention (may need to stand to void)

Psychosocial concerns: Acute pain, lingering chronic pain, limitation of neck or back muscle and joint mobility and strength, preoperative numbness remains postoperatively

POTENTIAL COMPLICATIONS

Hemorrhage, hematoma; motor and sensory weakness; continued pain; wound infection; disk infection

PATIENT PROBLEMS/NURSING DIAGNOSES & INTERVENTIONS

NIC PHYSICAL COMFORT PROMOTION

Chronic pain related to pressure on the nerve and surgical trauma

- Monitor degree, site, type, and amount of pain; medicate as necessary, according to physician's prescription, *to increase comfort.*
- Turn or adjust position *to relieve fatigue and discomfort.*
- Get patient up to change position and ease pain. Instruct on proper techniques to turn, sit up, and walk *to maintain safe care.*
- Increase up time as able *to increase activity.*
- Perform neurovascular checks. Report any decreases in motor or sensory functions.

NIC IMMOBILITY MANAGEMENT

Impaired physical mobility related to surgery

- Monitor ROM of unaffected tissues.
- Encourage physical therapy as ordered and prescribed *to increase muscle strength.*
- Note muscle spasms or limitation of movements when moving and doing wound care or hygienic care *to note current conditions or continuation of pain or soreness.*
- Teach patient how to logroll, if required or prescribed.

NIC SKIN/WOUND MANAGEMENT

Risk for impaired skin integrity related to wound infection

- Observe incisional area for relief of inflammation and evidence of wound healing (approximation of wound edges, no drainage, and later removal of sutures or staples).
- Refer patient to rehabilitation for work-hardening program, which is a program of graduated activities that simulate the individual's work tasks and the physical demands of the patient's job.
- Assess vital signs for fluctuations *that could indicate inflammation or infection.*
- Encourage fluid and food intake of regular diet *to aid wound healing.*
- Change wound dressing as needed; remove sutures or staples, if permitted when prescribed.

PATIENT EDUCATION/CONTINUUM OF CARE PLAN

1. Reiterate need to do exercises to regain muscle strength after surgery. Provide written list and pictures of exercises.
2. Clarify and stress normal motor and sensory functions as evidence of regaining full functions with relief of inflammation.
3. Explain lingering numbness as sign of former nerve pressure that may or may not completely abate.
4. Clarify physician's limitations in lifting and driving for 1 to 3 weeks or longer (individualized, based on specific condition). Stress follow-up visit to physician to determine recovery status.

5. Explain signs of fever, continued pain, and wound drainage as reportable to physician.

Evaluation/Patient Outcomes

Physical Comfort Promotion: Neck or back pain is relieved. Patient has some residual motor or sensory impairment with less pain, locally or systemically.

Immobility Management: Patient has satisfactory ROM without muscle spasms. Patient can move about more comfortably and easily and can do prescribed exercises satisfactorily. Patient returns to family, social, and, later, employment activities.

Skin/Wound Management: Patient has no wound or disk infection and wound and incision heal well. There is no drainage. Scar is contracting normally over time.

References

1. Aminoff MJ: *Electromyography in clinical practice: clinical and electrodiagnostic aspects of neuromuscular disease,* ed 4, London, 1999, Churchill Livingstone.

1a. Asher MA, Burton DC: A concept of idiopathic scoliosis deformities as imperfect torsion(s), *Clin Orthop* 364:11, 1999.

2. Barrett JH, et al: Does rheumatoid arthritis remit during pregnancy and relapse portpartum? Results from a nationwide study in the United Kingdom performed prospectively from late pregnancy, *Arthritis Rheum* 42(6):1219, 1999.

3. Bennett RM: The fibromyalgia syndrome. In Kelley WN, et al: *Textbook of rheumatology,* ed 5, Philadelphia, 1997, WB Saunders.

3a. Brandt KD: Management of osteoarthritis. In Kelley WN et al: *Textbook of rheumatology,* ed 5, Philadelphia, 1997, WB Saunders.

4. Brown EC, III, Lachiewicz PF: Precoated femoral component in total hip arthroplasty, *Clin Orthop* 364:153, 1999.

5. Byrne T: The setup and care of a patient in Buck's traction, *Orthop Nurs* 18(2):79, 1999.

6. Cofield RH: The shoulder. In Kelley WN et al: *Textbook of rheumatology,* ed 5, Philadelphia, 1997, WB Saunders.

7. Coughlin MJ: Hallux valgus: heredity or bad shoes? *Biomechanics* 2(8):31, 1995.

8. Duffy GP, Berry DJ, Rand JA: Cement versus cementless fixation in total knee arthroplasty, *Clin Orthop* 356:66, 1998.

9. Duffy GP, Trousdale RT, Stuart MJ: Total knee arthroplasty in patients 55 years old or younger, *Clin Orthop* 356:22, 1998.

10. Einhorn TA: The cell and molecular biology of fracture healing, *Clin Orthop* 355S:S7, 1998.

11. Einhorn TA, Lane JM: Editorial, *Clin Orthop* 355S:S3, 1998.

12. Firestein GS: Rheumatoid arthritis: Etiology and pathogenesis. In Kelley WN et al: *Textbook of rheumatology,* ed 5, Philadelphia, 1997, WB Saunders.

13. Gabriel SE, Crowson CS, O'Fallon WM: The epidemiology of rheumatoid arthritis in Rochester, Minnesota, 1955-1985, *Arthritis Rheum* 42(3):415, 1999.

14. Garr JL et al: Monitoring for compartmental syndrome using near-infrared spectroscopy: a noninvasive, continuous, transcutaneous monitoring technique, *J Trauma* 46(4):613, 1999.

15. Goldenberg DL: Fibromyalgia and related syndromes. In Klippel J, Dieppe PA: *Rheumatology,* ed 2, St. Louis, 1998, Mosby.

16. Gordon DA, Hastings DE: Rheumatoid arthritis: clinical features of early, progressive and late disease. In Klippel J, Dieppe PA: *Rheumatology,* ed 2, St. Louis, 1998, Mosby.

17. Graham GP, Fairclough JA: The knee. In Klippel J, Dieppe PA: *Rheumatology,* ed 2, St. Louis, 1998, Mosby.

18. Gran JT, Husby G: Ankylosing spondylitis: prevalence and demography. In Klippel J, Diepple RA: *Rheumatology,* ed 2, St. Louis, 1998, Mosby.

19. Hanley EN, David SM: Lumbar arthrodesis for the treatment of back pain. *J Bone Joint Surg Am* 81(5):716, 1999.

20. Harris ED, Jr: Clinical features of rheumatoid arthritis. In Kelley WN et al: *Textbook of rheumatology,* ed 5, Philadelphia, 1997, WB Saunders.

21. Heck DA et al: Patient outcomes after knee replacement, *Clin Orthop* 356:93, 1998.

22. Herd RJM et al: The prevention of early postmenopausal bone loss by cyclical etidronate therapy: A 2-year, double-blind, placebo-controlled study, *Am J Med* 103(2):92, 1997.

23. Holderbaum D, Haggi TM, Moskowitz RW: Genetics and osteoarthritis: Exposing the iceberg, *Arthritis Rheum* 42(3):397, 1999.

24. Holtom PD, Smith AM: Introduction to postraumatic osteomyelitis of the tibia, *Clin Orthop* 360:6, 1999.

24a. Khan MA: Ankylosing spondylitis. In Kippel J, Dieppe RA: *Rheumatology,* ed 2, St. Louis, 1998, Mosby.

25. Kraus VB: Pathogenesis and treatment of osteoarthritis, *Med Clin North Am* 81(1):85, 1997.

26. Kraushaar BS, Nirschl RP: Tendinosis of the elbow (tennis elbow), *J Bone Joint Surg* 81-A(2):259, 1999.

27. Kuper BC: Tarsal tunnel syndrome, *Orthop Nurs* 17(6):9, 1998.

28. Lane NE, Thompson JM: Management of osteoarthritis in the primary-care setting: an evidence-based approach to treatment, *Am J Med* 103(6A):25S, 1997.

29. Le Boff MS: Metabolic bone disease. In Kelley WN et al: *Textbook of rheumatology,* ed 5, Philadelphia, 1997, WB Saunders.

30. Licata AA: Biphosphonate therapy, *Am J Med Sci* 313(1):17, 1997.

30a. Lipson JJ: Low back pain. In Kelley WN et al: *Textbook of rheumatology,* ed 5, Philadelphia, 1997, WB Saunders.

31. Maciocchi AB: Historical review of the method according to Ilizarov, *Bull Hosp J Dis* 56(1):16, 1997.

32. Mankin HJ, Brandt KD: Pathogenesis of osteoarthritis. In Kelley WN et al: *Textbook of rheumatology,* ed 5, Philadelphia, 1997, WB Saunders.

33. McBeth J et al: The association between tender points, psychological distress, and adverse childhood experiences, *Arthritis Rheum* 42(7):1397, 1999.

34. McCance KL, Huether S: *Pathophysiology,* ed 3, St. Louis, 1998, Mosby.

34a. McCullough FL: Alterations of musculoskeletal functions in children. In McCance KL, Huether SE: *Pathophysiology,* ed 3, St. Louis, 1998, Mosby.

35. McKenzie LL: In search of a standard for pin site care, *Orthop Nurs* 18(2):73, 1999.

36. Monney G, Kaelin AJ: Short posterior fusion for patients with thoracolumbar idiopathic scoliosis, *Clin Orthop* 364:32, 1999.

37. Morris BA, Colwell CW, Hardwick ME: The use of low molecular weight heparins in the prevention of venous thromboembolic disease, *Orthop Nurs* 17(6):23, 1998.

38. Mourad LA: *Orthopedic disorders,* St. Louis, 1991, Mosby.

39. Mourad LA: Alterations in musculoskeletal function. In McCance KL, Huether SE: *Pathophysiology,* ed 3, St. Louis, 1998, Mosby.

40. Pasero CL, McCaffery M: Managing postoperative pain in the elderly, *Am J Nurs* 96(10):39, 1996.

41. Pitto RP, Koessler M, Draenert K: Prophylaxis of fat and bone marrow embolism in cemented total hip arthroplasty, *Clin Orthop* 355:23, 1998.
42. Pope RM: Rheumatoid arthritis: pathogenesis and early recognition, *Am J Med* 100(Suppl 2A):2A, 1996.
43. Ramsey ML, Adams RA, Morrey BF: Instability of the elbow treated with semiconstrained total elbow arthroplasty, *J Bone Joint Surg Am* 81(1):38, 1999.
44. Ranawat CS et al: The hip. In Kelley WN et al: *Textbook of rheumatology,* ed 5, Philadelphia, 1997, WB Saunders.
45. Rose R et al: Pediatric leg length discrepancy: causes and treatments, *Orthop Nurs* 18(2):21, 1999.
46. Sambrook PN, MacGregor AJ, Spector TD: Genetic influences on cervical and lumbar disc degeneration, *Arthritis Rheum* 42(2):366, 1999.
47. Sarmiento A, Goswami ADK: Thromboembolic prophylaxis with the use of aspirin, exercise, and graded elastic stockings or intermittent compression devices in patients managed with total hip arthroplasty, *J Bone Joint Surg Am* 81(3):339, 1999.
47a. Scardina RJ, Wood BT: Ankle and foot pain. In Kelley WN et al: *Textbook of rheumatology,* ed 5, Philadelphia, 1997, WB Saunders.
48. Schmalzreid TP, Callaghan JJ: Wear in total hip and knee replacements, *J Bone Joint Surg Am* 81(1):115, 1999.
49. Scully RE: Becker's muscular dystrophy involving skeletal muscle and myocardium, *N Engl J Med* 337(2):182, 1998.
49a. Seeley RR, Stephens TD, Tate P: *Anatomy and physiology,* ed 3, St. Louis, 1995, Mosby.
50. Seldin MF et al: The genetics revolution and the assault on rheumatoid arthritis, *Arthritis Rheum* 42(6):1071, 1999.
51. Sledge CB: Reconstructive surgery for rheumatic disease. In Kelley WN et al: *Textbook of rheumatology,* ed 5, Philadelphia, 1997, WB Saunders.
51a. Smith DG: Phantom limb, residual limb, and back pain after lower extremity amputation, *Clin Orthop* 361:29, 1999.
52. Solomon L: Clinical features of osteoarthritis. In Kelley WN et al: *Textbook of rheumatology,* ed 5, Philadelphia, 1997, WB Saunders.
53. Spector TD, Cicuttini IM: The genetics of osteoarthritis. In Klippel J, Dieppe PA: *Rheumatology,* ed 2, Philadelphia, 1997, WB Saunders.
54. Stanitski D: Limb length inequality: assessment and treatment options, *J Am Acad Orthop Surg* 7(3):143, 1999.
55. Strand V, Keystone EC: Biologic agents in the treatment of rheumatoid arthritis. In Kelley WN et al: *Textbook of rheumatology,* ed 5, Philadelphia, 1997, WB Saunders.
55a. Stucki G, Sangha O: Principles of rehabilitation. In Klippel J, Dieppe PA: *Rheumatology,* ed 2, St. Louis, 1998, Mosby.
56. Swezey RL: Preventing osteoporotic fractures: the role of exercise, posture, and safety, *J Musculoskeletal Med* 14(4):9, 1997.
57. Theis LM: Cost containment and quality: coexisting in total joint care, *Orthop Nurs* 17(6):70, 1998.
57a. Thibodeau GA, Patton KI: *Anatomy and physiology,* ed 3, St. Louis, 1996, Mosby.
58. Tighe H, Carson DA: Rheumatoid factors. In Kelley WN et al: *Textbook of rheumatology,* ed 5, Philadelphia, 1997, WB Saunders.
59. Tornetta P, III et al: Morbidity and mortality in elderly trauma patients, *J Trauma* 46(4):702, 1999.
60. Tsukayama DT: Pathophysiology of posttraumatic osteomyetitis, *Clin Orthop* 360:22, 1999.
61. van der Linden S: Ankylosing spondylitis. In Kelley WN et al: *Textbook of rheumatology,* ed 5, Philadelphia, 1997, WB Saunders.
62. Xenos JS et al: The porous-coated anatomic total hip prosthesis, inserted without cement, *J Bone Joint Surg Am* 81(1):74, 1999.
63. Walsh DA, Sledge CB, Blake DR: Structure and function of joints connective tissue, and muscle. In Kelley WN et al: *Textbook of rheumatology,* ed 5, Philadelphia, 1997, WB Saunders.
64. Weyand CM, Goronzy JJ: Pathogenesis of rheumatoid arthritis, *Med Clin North Am* 81(1):29, 1997.
64a. Whaley LF, Wong DL: *Nursing care of infants and children,* ed 5, St. Louis, 1995, Mosby.
65. Whipple T, Duval MJ: Arthroscopy and synovectomy. In Kelley WN et al: *Textbook of rheumatology,* ed 5, Philadelphia, 1997, WB Saunders.
65a. Wilson SF, Giddens J: *Health assessment for nursing practice,* ed 2, St. Louis, 2001, Mosby.
66. Windsor RE, Insall JN: The knee. In Kelley WN et al: *Textbook of rheumatology,* ed 5, Philadelphia, 1997, WB Saunders.
67. Wolfe F: The prognosis of rheumatoid arthritis: assessment of disease activity and disease severity in the clinics, *Am J Med* 103(6A):12S, 1997.

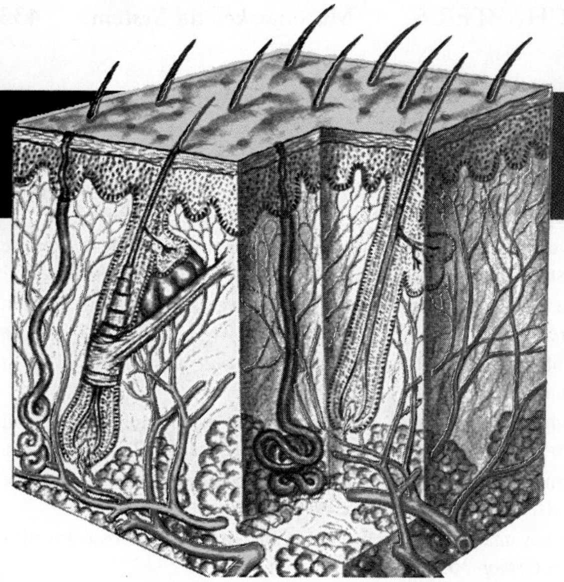

7 Integumentary System

Joyce E. Dains

Overview

The integument, or skin, is the largest organ of the body. It is a protective barrier between the internal structures of the body and the external environment. Tough, resilient, and virtually impermeable, it is also affected by changes within the body. The condition of the skin can indicate a great deal about a person's health and how the environment affects that person.

Skin disorders and diseases are common; approximately 3% of all annual office visits are made to dermatologists. An estimated 2% of the U.S. population experiences an acute skin condition, but the true extent of skin disorders is difficult to determine because many persons with skin problems treat themselves rather than seek medical care. The economic cost of skin diseases is substantial.

Anatomy, Physiology, and Related Pathophysiology

Structure

The skin comprises two principal layers: an outer layer, the epidermis, and an underlying connective tissue layer, the dermis. Beneath the dermis is the hypodermis (subcutaneous tissue), which technically is not part of the skin. The hypodermis is composed of loose connective tissue and fat cells that provide a layer of insulation. Specialized structures of the epidermis include glands, hair, and nails.

The anatomy of the skin varies from one part of the body to another, so the diagram of the skin in Fig. 7-1 shows only the main parts and their approximate relationships. The pathologic conditions that arise in skin disorders occur in one or more of the various layers. The variation in anatomy often accounts for the distribution of skin diseases.

Epidermis. The epidermis is composed of stratified squamous epithelium. Two cell types, keratinocytes and melanocytes, make up most of the epidermal cells. The epidermis is composed of two major sublayers: the stratum corneum, which protects the body against harmful environmental substances and restricts water loss, and the cellular stratum, where keratin cells are synthesized. The basement membrane lies beneath the cellular stratum and connects the epidermis to the dermis. The epidermis has no blood or lymph channels and depends on the underlying dermis for its nutrition.

The stratum corneum is the outer horny layer of closely packed dead squamous cells that contain the waterproofing protein keratin and form the protective barrier of the skin. The variation in skin thickness (0.5 mm in the eyelids to 4 mm in the palms and soles) is caused mostly by differences in the thickness of the stratum corneum.

The cellular stratum is composed of three or four layers; from the most superficial to the deepest they can be identified as follows:

Stratum lucidum: This is a thin translucent layer of protein-filled cells found only in the thicker skin of the palms and in the soles.

Stratum granulosum: This granular layer is composed of cells containing granules of keratohyaline, an intermediate in keratin formation.

Stratum spinosum: This is the prickle cell layer, where cells begin to flatten and precursors of keratin appear.

Stratum germinativum: This is the basal cell layer, where mitotic activity occurs to replace the cells in the upper epidermal layer. The basal layer also contains the melanocytes, which synthesize the melanin that gives the skin its color.

The keratinocytes in the basal layer evolve into cells of the stratum corneum as they mature (keratinize) and make their way to the surface, where they are eventually desquamated. The transit time of basal layer cells to the final stage of desquamation is approximately 28 days.

Appendages. The epidermis invaginates into the dermis and forms eccrine sweat glands, apocrine sweat glands, sebaceous glands, hair, and nails.

The *eccrine sweat glands* are small, convoluted secretory coils that extend from the dermis and open directly on the skin's surface. Only humans have eccrine glands. They are dis-

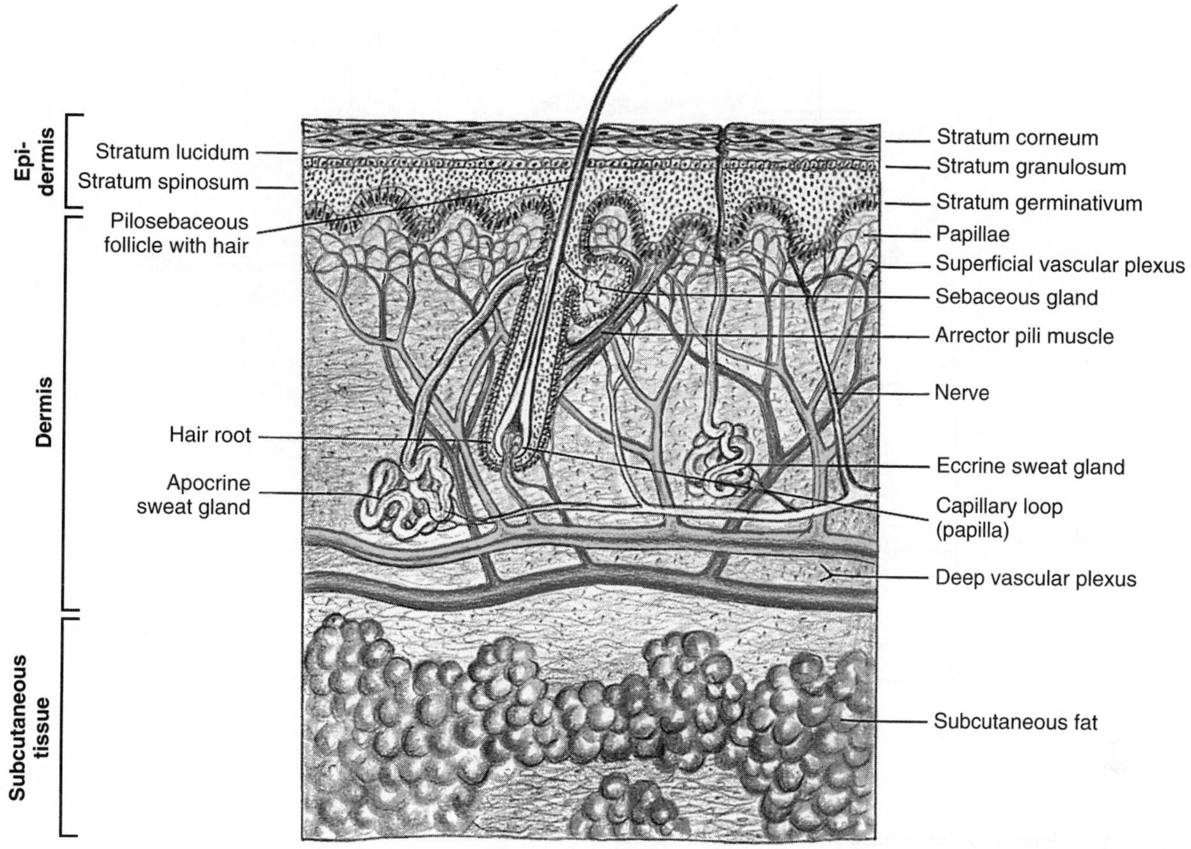

FIG. 7-1
Structures of skin.

tributed throughout the body except for the lip margins, eardrums, nail beds, inner surface of the prepuce, and glans penis. The main function of the sweat glands is regulation of body temperature through water secretion. The eccrine sweat glands are innervated by sympathetic cholinergic nerve fibers, and heat is the primary stimulus for their secretion. Muscle exertion and emotional stress also stimulate the secretion of water, chlorides and other electrolytes, and waste products such as lactate and urea.

The apocrine sweat glands are special structures found only in the axilla, nipple and areola, anogenital area, eyelids, and external ear. They do not develop fully until puberty. These glands are much larger and located deeper than the eccrine glands. The apocrine glands are adrenergic and secrete a white fluid containing water, salt, protein, carbohydrate, and other substances in response to emotional stimulation. Secretions from these glands are initially odorless, but bacteria on the skin decompose the organic components of sweat and cause distinctive body odors.

The *sebaceous glands* occur everywhere on the body except the palms and soles. Sebaceous glands secrete sebum, a lipid-rich substance that helps keep the skin and hair from drying out. These glands are stimulated by sex hormones, primarily testosterone, and their action varies according to hormonal levels throughout life.

Hair is formed by epidermal cells that invaginate into the underlying dermal layers. Hair consists of keratin that is synthesized by cells in the papilla at the base of the hair shaft. The papilla provides nourishment for mitosis, which causes the hair to grow. The hair shaft projects above the skin surface and at an acute angle with the hair root. Hair goes through cyclic changes: growth (anagen), atrophy (catagen), and rest (telogen), after which the hair is shed. Normal hair loss is not noticeable because neighboring follicles have differently timed cycles. Hair grows on most of the body except for the palms, soles, and parts of the genitalia. Men and women have about the same number of hair follicles, which are stimulated to differential growth by hormones. Melanocytes in the hair shaft give the hair its color. Hair follicle muscles, called arrectores pilorum, are immediately beneath the sebaceous glands. When innervated by adrenergic fibers, they elevate the hair to a more vertical position and indent the surrounding skin, producing "goose bumps."

The *nails* (FIG. 7-2) are epidermal cells converted to hard plates of keratin. The nail root lies beneath the skin; the nail body (plate) is the visible part lying on the nail bed. The nail bed is highly vascular, giving the transparent nail body a pink color. The white crescent-shaped area extending beyond the proximal nail fold (lunula) marks the end of the matrix. This is the site of mitosis and nail growth. The stratum corneum of the skin covering the nail root is the cuticle, or eponychium, which pushes up and over the lower part of the nail body. The paronychium is the soft tissue surrounding the nail border.

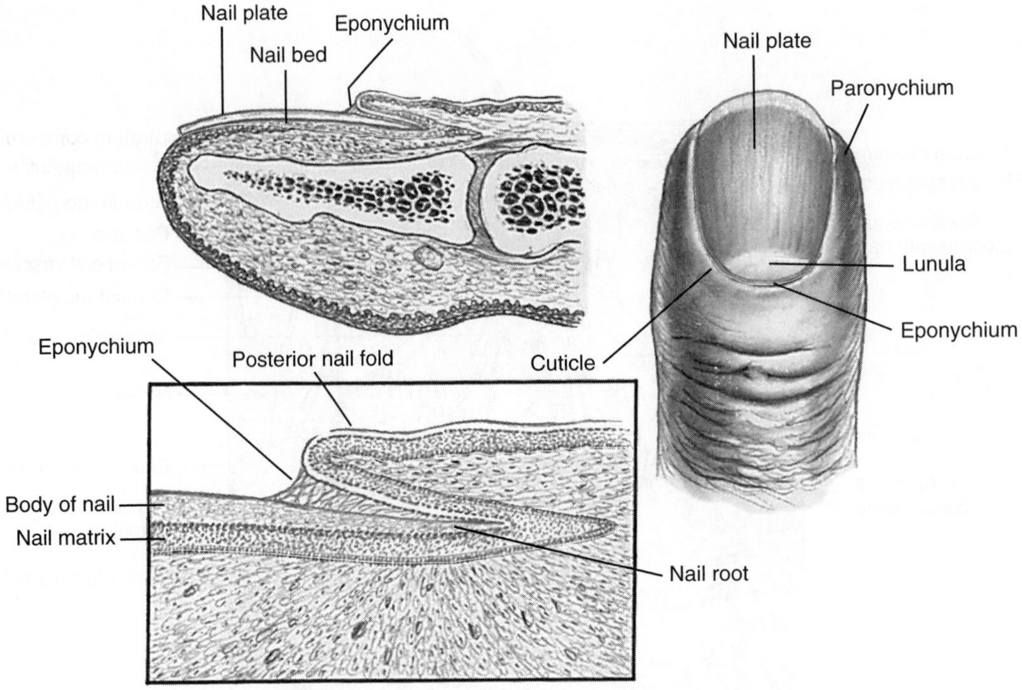

FIG. 7-2
Structures of nail.

Dermis. The dermis is the connective tissue layer of the skin that supports the epidermis and separates it from the cutaneous adipose tissue. The dermis is highly vascular and provides nutrition for the epidermis. The vascular structure also controls body temperature and blood pressure. The appendages of the epidermis are located in the dermis.

The dermis is composed of two parts: the papillary layer and the reticular layer. The papillary layer contains blood vessels and some nerve elements that respond to stimuli applied to the skin. This layer is folded into ridges, or papillae, extending into the upper epidermal layer. Folding produces ridges on the surface of the skin—notably on the palms of the hands. The papillae also nourish living epidermal cells and maintain a strong attachment between the dermis and epidermis.

The *reticular layer* contains elastin fibers for resilience, collagen fibers for strength, and reticulin fibers for stability. This connective tissue portion also contains blood vessels, lymphatics, nerves, matrix, and various cells. Collagen forms the greatest part of the dermis.

The skin is actually the body's major sensory organ. The sensory fibers in the dermis form a complex network to provide the sensations of pain, touch, and temperature. The dermis also contains autonomic motor nerves that innervate blood vessels, glands, and the arrectores pilorum muscles.

Hypodermis (Subcutaneous Tissue). The dermis is connected to underlying organs by a layer of subcutaneous tissue that is composed of loose connective tissue filled with fatty cells. This layer of adipose tissue provides heat, insulation, shock absorption, and a reserve of calories. Sensory and autonomic motor nerve fibers are located in the subcutaneous tissue.

Function

The skin serves several functions that are integral to the functioning of the entire body.

Protection. An intact stratum corneum creates a physical barrier against invasion by bacteria and foreign substances and minor physical trauma. Glandular secretions wash microorganisms from the pores, and colonies of nonpathogenic bacteria on the skin retard the growth of pathogens. Hairs in the nose, ears, anogenital areas, eyebrows, and eyelid act as barriers against the entry of foreign materials. Sebaceous gland secretions, along with the skin, prevent absorption of water during immersion. The skin reduces potential damage to deoxyribonucleic acid (DNA) from ultraviolet radiation through thickening of the stratum corneum that disperses radiation and through melanin production that forms a protective cap over the nucleus of the cell.

Retardation of Body Fluid Loss. The skin acts as a barrier to minimize loss of internal contents and to prevent the internal fluid environment from leaking out.

Excretion. The skin acts as a minor organ of excretion. Some urea and lactic acid are lost through the skin, along with sweat and sodium chloride.

Regulation of Body Temperature. The skin controls body temperature by four processes: radiation of heat energy from the body surface; conduction of heat from the skin to other objects or the air; convection or removal of heat by air currents; and evaporation of perspiration stimulated by the sympathetic nervous system when the body is overheated.

Blood vessels of the skin help control body temperature by dilating in warm environments to promote heat loss through radiation and by constricting in cold environments to help conserve heat. If the skin is directly exposed to temperatures below 15° C (59° F), blood vessels begin to constrict to prevent the tissues from freezing.

Blood Pressure Regulation. During strenuous exercise, anxiety, or hemorrhage, constriction of skin blood vessels through sympathetic stimulation reduces blood flow to the skin, promotes increased venous return, increases cardiac output, and thereby increases blood pressure.

Tissue Repair. The skin maintains itself and repairs its own wounds through exaggeration of the normal process of replacement of desquamated stratum corneum and formation of scar tissue.

Vitamin D Production. The skin provides an area for irradiation of vitamin D precursors. Through catalytic action, ultraviolet light converts the precursor found in the skin to vitamin D_3, which is reabsorbed into blood vessels. Vitamin D is necessary in the metabolism of calcium and phosphorus.

Sensory Perception. Free nerve endings and special receptors in the skin function alone or together to detect environmental stimuli, including pain, touch, heat, cold, pressure, vibration, tickle, itch, wetness, oiliness, and stickiness.

Expression. Feelings such as anxiety, fear, and anger may be visible on the skin through sweating, pallor, or flushing. Because of its visibility, skin is also closely connected with an individual's body image.

NORMAL FINDINGS*

Skin

Tone: Deep to light brown in blacks; whitish pink to ruddy with olive or yellow overtones in whites; ○ skin of whites tends to look paler and more opaque

Uniformity: Sun-darkened areas; areas of lighter pigmentation in dark-skinned people (palms, lips, nail beds); labile pigmented areas associated with use of hormones or pregnancy; callused areas appear yellow; crinkled skin areas darker (knees and elbows); dark-skinned (Mediterranean origin) people may have lips with bluish hue; vascular flush areas (cheeks, neck, upper chest, or genital area) may appear red, especially with excitement or anxiety; skin color masked through use of cosmetics or tanning agents; ○ more freckles; uneven tanning; pigment deposits; hypopigmented patches

Moisture: Minimum perspiration or oiliness felt; dampness in skin folds; increased perspiration associated with warm environment or activity; wet palms, scalp, forehead, and axilla associated with anxiety; ○ increased dryness, especially of extremities; decreased perspiration

Surface temperature: Cool to warm

Texture: Smooth, even, soft; some roughness on exposed areas (elbows and soles of feet); ○ flaking and scaling associated with dry skin, especially on lower extremities

Thickness: Wide body variation; increased thickness in areas of pressure or rubbing (hands and feet); ○ thinner skin, especially over dorsal surface of hands and feet, forearms, lower legs, and bony prominences

Turgor: Skin moves easily when lifted and returns to place immediately when released; ○ general loss of elasticity; skin moves when lifted but does not return to place immediately when released; skin appears lax; increased wrinkle pattern more marked in sun-exposed areas, in fair skin, and in expressive areas of face; pendulous parts sag or droop (under chin, earlobes, breasts, and scrotum)

Hygiene: Clean, free of odor

Alterations: Striae (stretch marks) usually silver or pinkish; freckles (prominent in sun-exposed areas); some birthmarks; ○ nevi often become lighter or disappear; seborrheic keratosis (pigmented, raised, warty, slightly greasy lesions most often found on trunk or face); senile (actinic) keratosis on exposed surfaces, first seen as small reddened areas and then as raised, rough, yellow to brown lesions; senile sebaceous adenomas (yellowish flattened papules with central depressions); cherry adenomas (tiny, bright, ruby red, round; may become brown with age)

Nails

Configuration: Nail edges smooth and rounded; nail base angle 160 degrees; nail surface flat or slightly curved; ○ toenails may be thickened and distorted.

Consistency: Smooth, hard surface; uniform thickness; ○ fingernails may be more brittle or peel

Color: Variations of pink; pigment deposits in nail beds of dark-skinned individuals; ○ toenails may lose translucence and luster and become yellow

Adherence to nail bed: Nail base feels firm when palpated

Hair

Surface characteristics: Scalp smooth; hair shiny; vellus hair short, fine, inconspicuous, and unpigmented; terminal hair coarser, thicker, more conspicuous, and usually pigmented; ○ sebaceous hyperplasia may extend into scalp

Distribution and configuration: "Normal" varies with individual; hair present on scalp, lower face, nares, ears, axillae, anterior chest around nipples, arms, legs, back, buttocks; female public configuration forms inverted triangle; hairline may extend up linea alba; male pubic configuration is upright triangle with hair extending up linea alba to umbilicus; ○ increased facial hair (especially in women), bristly quality; men may have coarse hair in ears, nose, and eyebrows; decreased scalp hair; symmetric balding in men (most often frontal or occipital); decreased pubic and axillary hair

Texture: Scalp hair may be fine or coarse; fine vellus hair over body; coarse terminal hair in pubic and axillary areas; ○ facial hair coarse; body hair fine

Color: Wide variation from pale to black; color may be masked or changed with rinses or dyes; older adults: graying; whitening; hairs that do not lose pigment often become darker

Quantity: "Normal" varies with individuals; gradual symmetric balding of scalp hair in some men; ○ general decrease of body and scalp hair

*○ = Older adult.

Common Abnormal Findings: Descriptions and Characteristics of Skin Lesions

Primary Skin Lesions

Primary skin lesions occur as initial spontaneous manifestations of an underlying pathologic process.

Lesion

Macule: Flat; nonpalpable; circumscribed; less than 1 cm in diameter; brown, red, purple, white, or tan in color
Examples: Freckles; flat moles; rubella; rubeola; drug eruptions

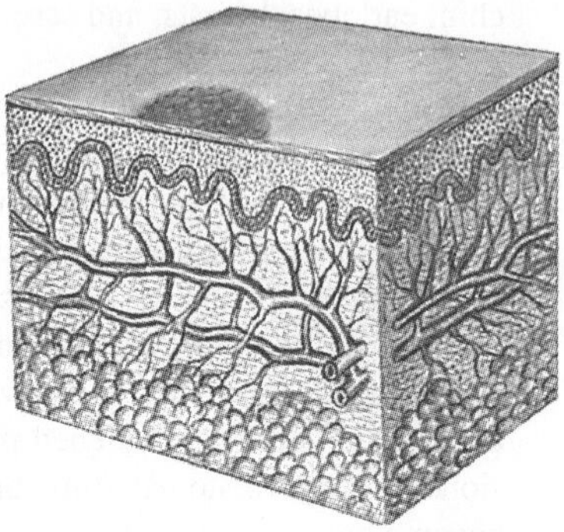

Patch: Flat; nonpalpable; irregular in shape; macule greater than 1 cm in diameter
Examples: Vitiligo; port-wine stain

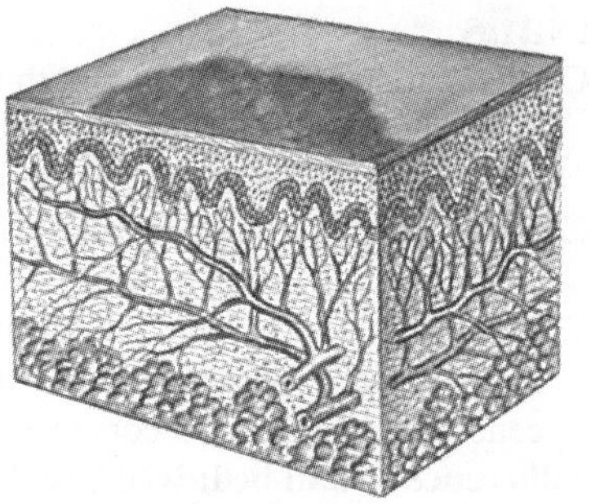

Papule: Elevated; palpable firm; circumscribed; less than 1 cm in diameter; brown, red, pink, tan, or bluish red in color
Examples: Warts; drug-related eruptions; pigmented nevi

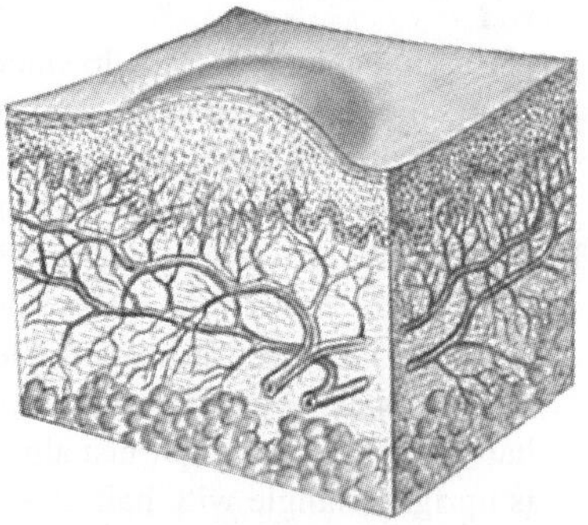

Plaque: Elevated; flat-topped; firm; rough; superficial papule greater than 1 cm in diameter, may be coalesced papules
Examples: Psoriasis; seborrheic and actinic keratoses; eczema

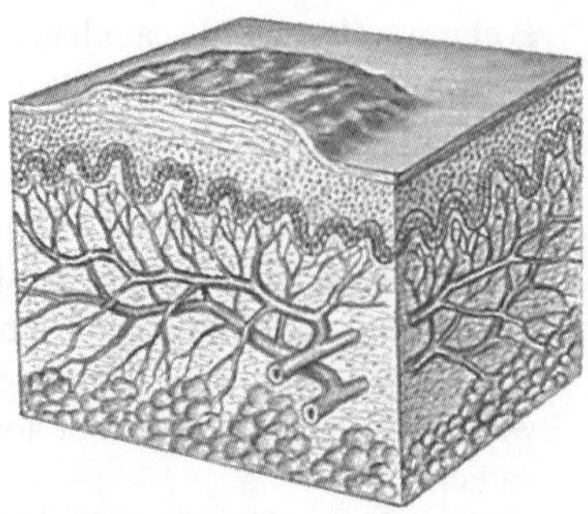

Wheal: Elevated, irregular-shaped area of cutaneous edema; solid, transient, changing; variable diameter; pale pink in color
Examples: Urticaria; insect bites

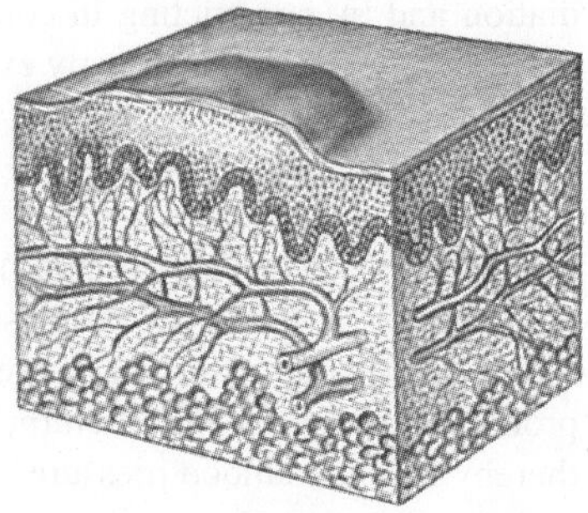

Nodule: Elevated; firm; circumscribed; palpable; deeper in dermis than papule; 1 to 2 cm in diameter
Examples: Erythema nodosum; lipomas

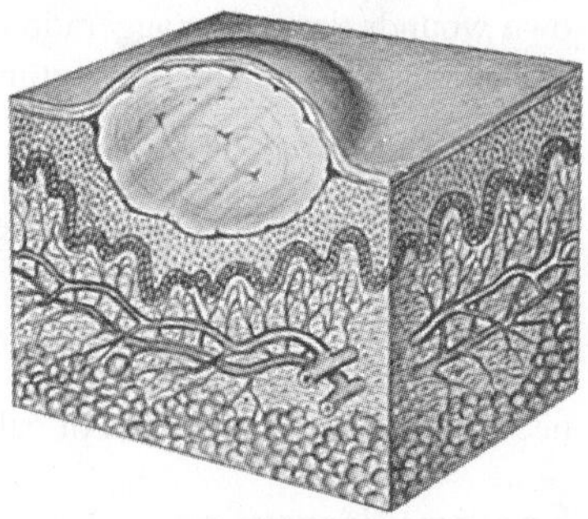

Tumor: Elevated; solid; may or may not be clearly demarcated; greater than 2 cm in diameter; may or may not vary from skin color
Examples: Neoplasms

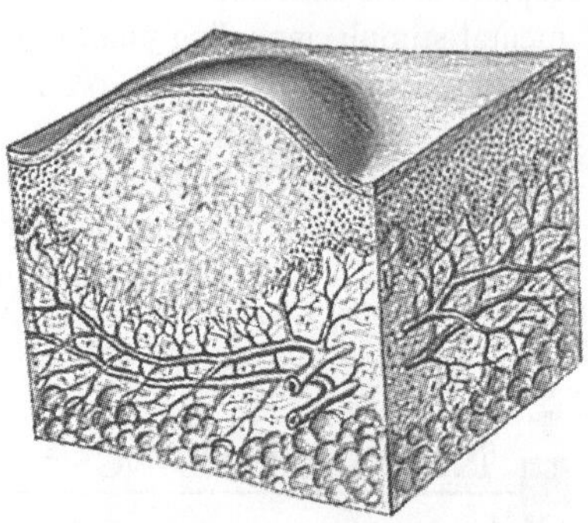

Vesicle: Elevated; circumscribed; superficial; filled with serous fluid; less than 1 cm in diameter
Examples: Blister; varicella

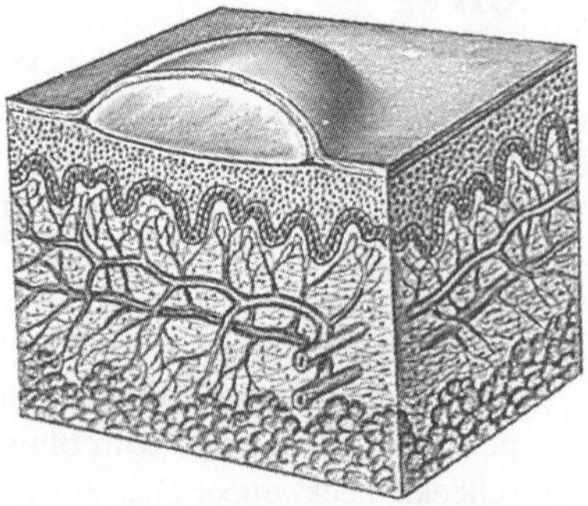

Bulla: Vesicle greater than 1 cm in diameter
Examples: Blister; pemphigus vulgaris

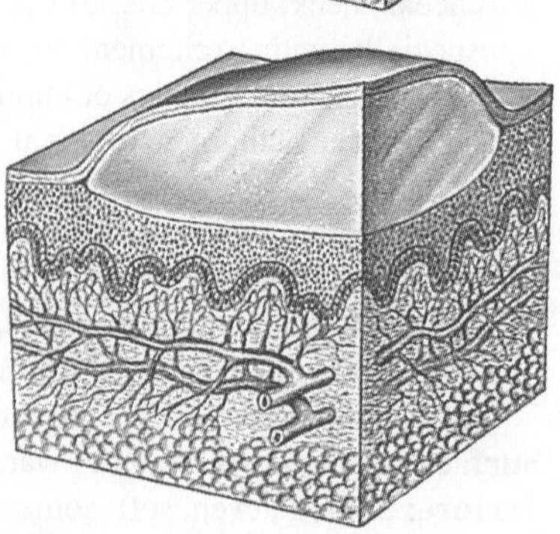

Pustule: Elevated; superficial; similar to vesicle but filled with purulent fluid
Examples: Impetigo; acne; variola; herpes zoster

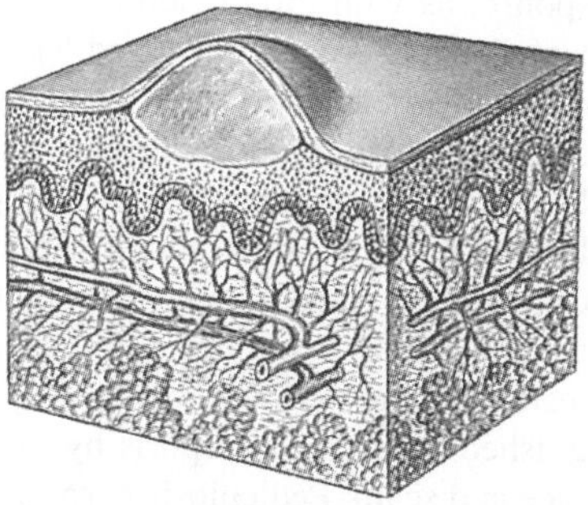

Cyst: Elevated; circumscribed; palpable; encapsulated; filled with liquid or semisolid material
Example: Sebaceous cyst

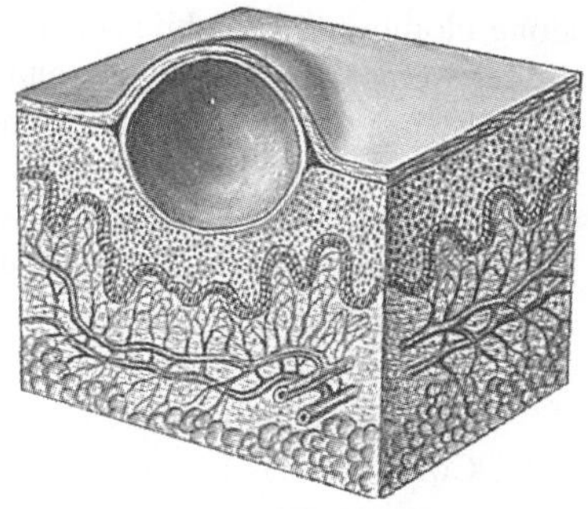

Telangiectasia: Fine, irregular red line produced by dilation of capillary
Example: Telangiectasia in rosacea

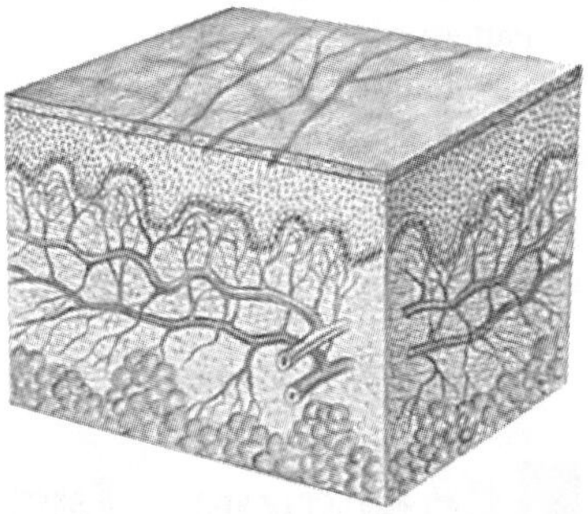

Secondary Skin Lesions

Secondary lesions are a result of later evolution of a primary lesion or are induced by external trauma to the primary lesion.

Lesion

Scale: Heaped-up keratinized cells; flaky exfoliation; irregular; thick or thin; dry or oily; varied size; silver, white, or tan in color
Examples: Psoriasis; exfoliative dermatitis

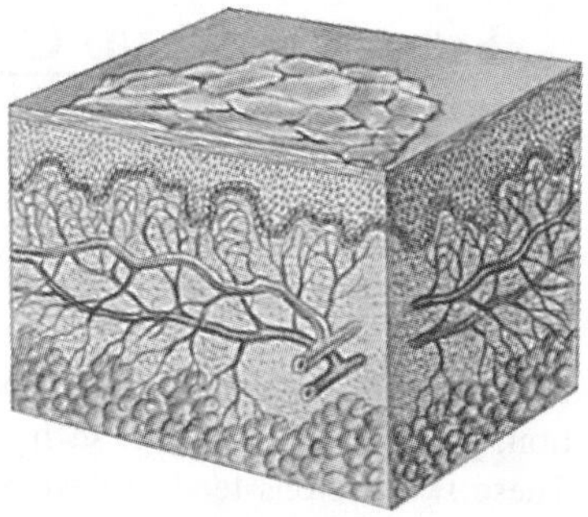

Crust: Dried serum, blood, or purulent exudate; size varies; brown, red, black, tan, or straw in color
Examples: Scab on abrasion; eczema; impetigo

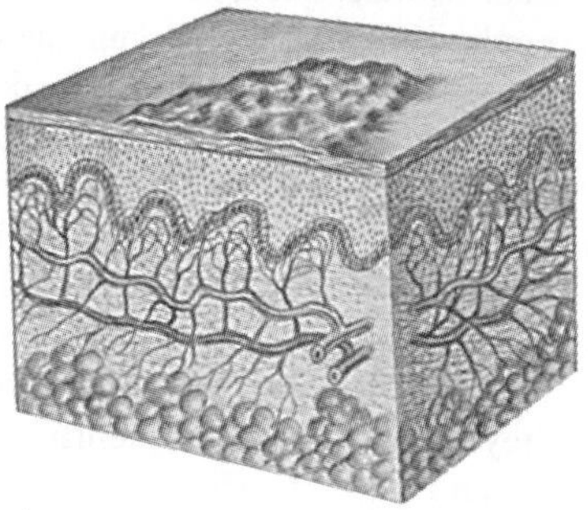

Lichenification: Rough, thickened epidermis; accentuated skin markings due to rubbing or irritation; often involves flexor aspect of extremity
Example: Chronic dermatitis

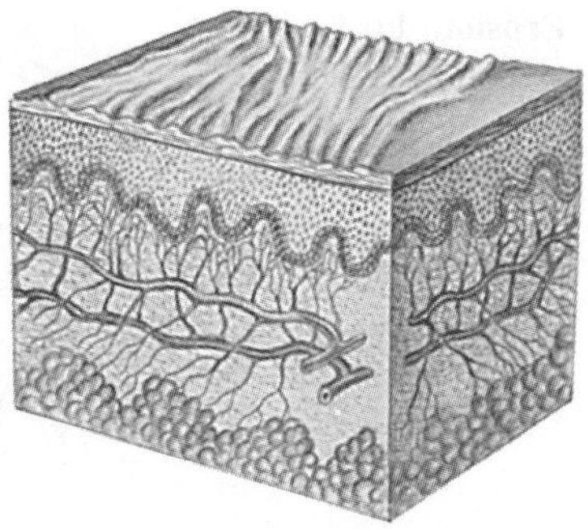

Scar: Thin to thick fibrous tissue replacing injured dermis; irregular; pink, red, or white in color; may be atrophic or hypertrophic
Examples: Healed wound or surgical incision

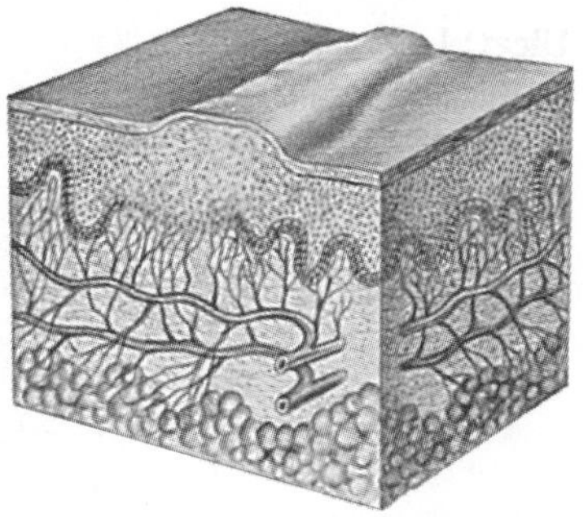

Keloid: Irregularly shaped, elevated, progressively enlarging scar; grows beyond boundaries of wound; caused by excessive collagen formation during healing
Examples: Keloid from ear piercing or burn scar

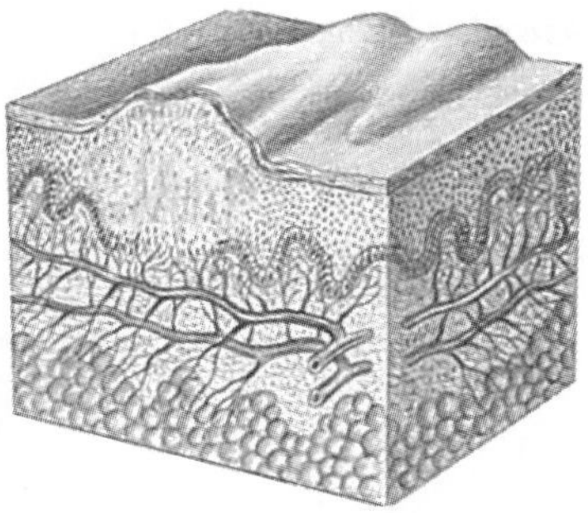

Excoriation: Loss of epidermis; linear or hollowed-out crusted area; dermis exposed
Examples: Abrasion; scratch

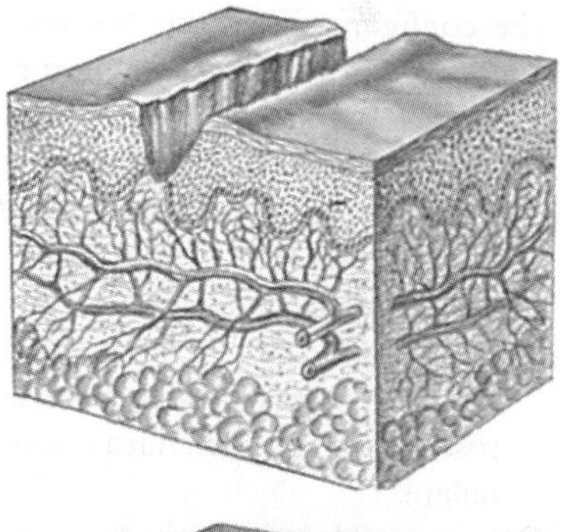

Fissure: Linear crack or break from epidermis to dermis; small; deep; red
Examples: Athlete's foot; cheilosis

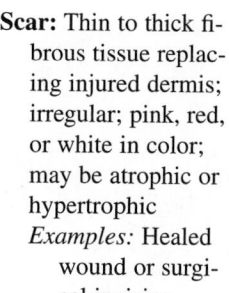

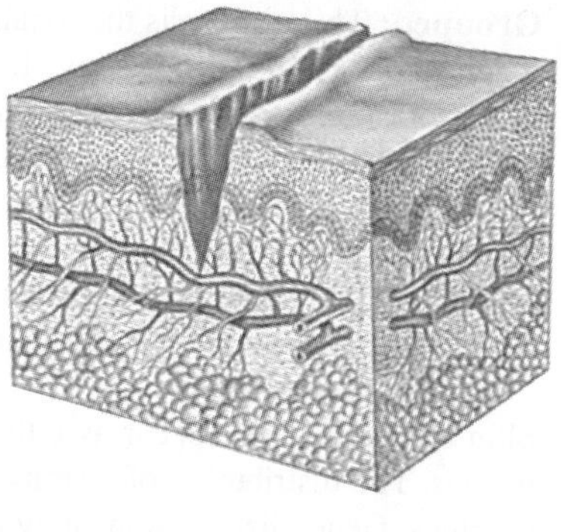

Erosion: Loss of all or part of epidermis; depressed; moist; glistening; follows rupture of vesicle or bulla; larger than fissure
Examples: Varicella; variola after rupture

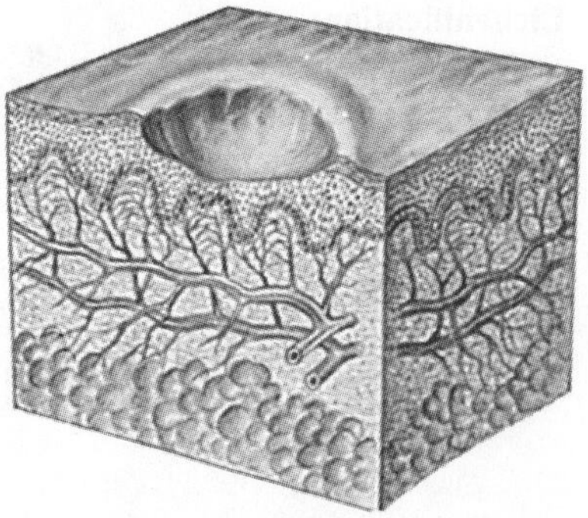

Ulcer: Loss of epidermis and dermis; concave; varies in size; exudative; red or reddish blue
Examples: Decubiti; stasis ulcers

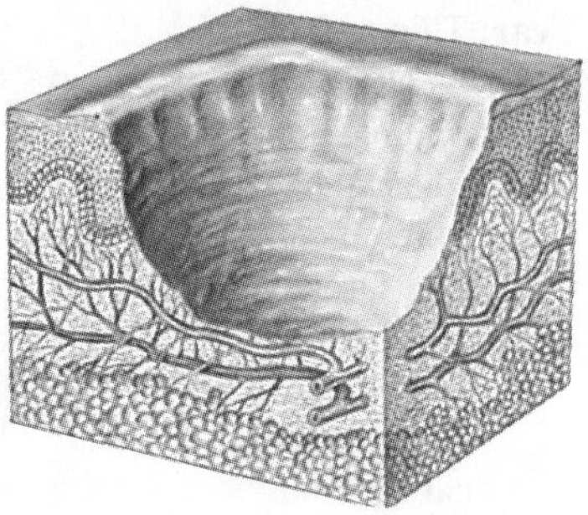

Atrophy: Thinning of skin surface and loss of skin markings; skin translucent and paperlike
Examples: Striae; aged skin

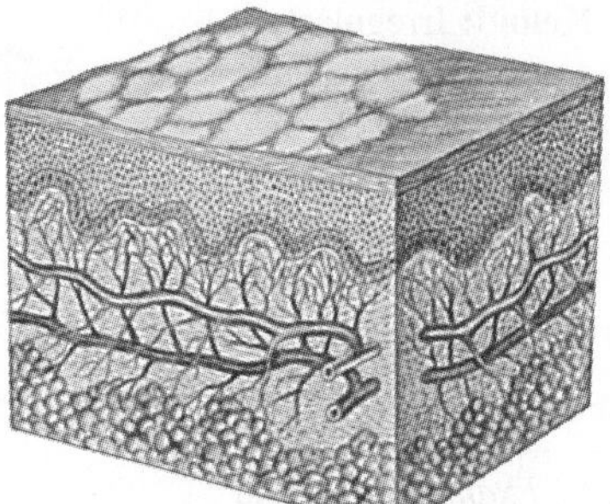

Attributes of Lesions

The configuration of skin lesions often has diagnostic value. These patterns can sometimes be explained by their pathogenesis. There are three common patterns of arrangement:

Annular: The formation of rings indicates extension of the lesion from the initial location to the periphery with clearing in the center. The skin may revert to normal appearance or may be scarred. Annular configuration can also result from an allergic process in which the central area becomes refractory. Annular patterns are commonly seen in pityriasis rosea, tinea corporis, tinea cruris, urticaria, and erythema annulare.

Grouped: This pattern is the localization of numerous small primary lesions in one area. It may be from mechanical factors (as in insect bites) or from a predisposition of a particular body area to a specific lesion, as in herpes simplex.

Linear: This arrangement may be caused by external factors such as trauma or may occur in contact dermatitis. It may also be determined by developmental origins of the lesions, as in herpes zoster.

Skin disorders may appear as either generalized or localized lesions. The distribution of lesions may also provide diagnostic clues. Generalized lesions may indicate an underlying systemic disorder, as in erythema multiforme; an allergic response, as with drug reactions; or a genetic disorder, as with lamellar ichthyosis. Localized lesions occur frequently as the result of a primary irritant or allergic eczematous dermatitis. Many disorders produce lesions in specific regions of the body. For example, erythema nodosum produces nodules that are limited to the legs and thighs. Acne vulgaris produces lesions on the face, chest, back, and shoulders. Candidal infections usually manifest in intertriginous areas. Tinea cruris produces lesions in the perineal region. Pityriasis rosea may be distinguished from tinea corporis by the absence of lesions on the face and scalp. Pediculosis corporis is characterized by lesions along clothing lines, while scabies lesions are found in interdigital webs along the fingers and on the wrist and penis. In contrast, lesions from flea bites are limited to the ankles and lower legs.

In assessing skin lesions, the following characteristics should be considered and described:

- Characteristics of the lesion
  - Size
  - Shape or configuration
  - Color
  - Consistency
  - Elevation or depression
- Pattern of arrangement
  - Annular
  - Grouped
  - Linear
- Location and distribution
  - Generalized or localized
  - Region of the body
  - Discrete or confluent

Conditions, Diseases, and Disorders

BACTERIAL CONDITIONS

Furuncles and Carbuncles

A furuncle is an acute localized staphylococcal infection that is initially limited to a hair follicle but spreads rapidly to the surrounding dermis and subcutaneous tissue. A carbuncle is a group of furuncles combined as one larger lesion and involving adjoining hair follicles.

Furuncles and carbuncles usually occur in areas exposed to friction, pressure, or plugging, such as sweat glands in the axilla. These skin lesions tend to develop in people who are debilitated, malnourished, fatigued, or obese. They also develop in people who have altered immune mechanisms, diabetes mellitus, severe acne, or seborrheic dermatitis. Poor personal hygiene is another predisposing factor.

Furuncles occur most frequently on the neck, breasts, face, and buttocks. The condition may be recurrent and troublesome (furunculosis) and often occurs in healthy young adults.

Carbuncles develop more slowly than single furuncles. They occur most frequently on the nape of the neck in men.

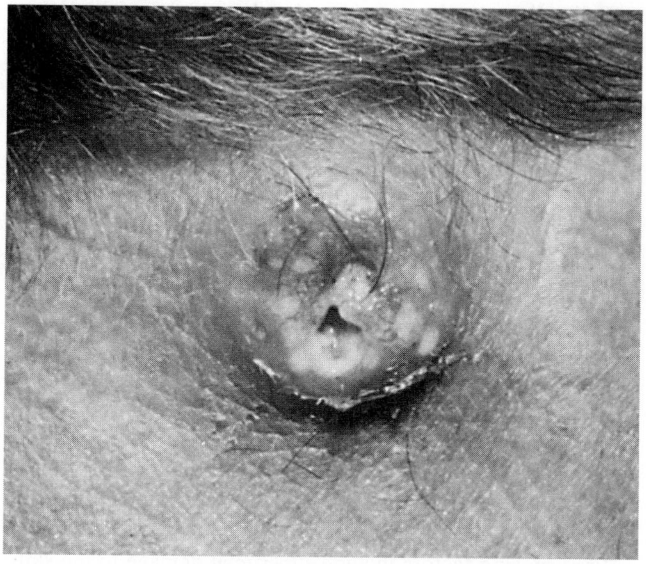

FIG. 7-3

Furuncle. (Courtesy Jaime A. Tschen, MD, Department of Dermatology, Baylor College of Medicine, Houston, Tex.)

PATHOPHYSIOLOGY

A furuncle develops as a small perifollicular abscess that ordinarily destroys the hair and follicle during its early stages. A carbuncle involves more than one pilosebaceous unit and may involve many.

The invading organism is usually *Staphylococcus aureus,* which is found anywhere on the body. It usually gains entry after trauma causes a break in the skin. The organism produces an acute inflammatory process around the hair follicle. The initial nodule becomes a pustule that is 5 to 20 mm in diameter at the base of the hair follicle. The surrounding skin becomes red, hot, and tender. Local edema occurs in 3 to 5 days. The center of the lesion fills with yellow pus and forms a core that may rupture spontaneously or require surgical incision (FIG. 7-3). The initial drainage is purulent and progresses to a serosanguineous discharge. Healing occurs gradually, usually with residual scarring.

The infection is usually walled off by local defense mechanisms. However, if the inflammatory process spreads to the deeper structures of the dermis and subcutaneous tissue (cellulitis), the bacteria may reach the dermal vascular plexus and cause septicemia. This complication is more likely to occur in people with altered immune status and in infants, whose defense mechanisms are less efficient.

DIAGNOSTIC STUDIES AND FINDINGS

Physical examination: Characteristic lesion

Culture of lesion discharge: Presence of infecting organism *(S. aureus)*

MULTIDISCIPLINARY PLAN

Surgery

Incision to promote drainage after lesion has become localized and filled with pus

Medications

Antiinfective agents

Systemic antibiotics

- Amoxicillin plus clavulanate potassium (Augmentin), 500-875 mg PO bid
- Clarithromycin (Biaxin), 250-500 PO bid
- Cephalexin (Keflex), 250-500 PO qid
- Ciprofloxacin (Cipro), 500 mg PO bid for methicillin-resistant *Staphylococcus aureus (MRSA)*
- Dicloxacillin (Dycill, Dynapen, Pathocil), 250-500 mg PO q6h
- Rifamycin (rifampin), 600 mg PO qd for recurrent furunculosis
- Trimethoprim-sulfamethoxazole (Bactrim DS), 1 tablet PO bid for MRSA
- Mupirocin (Bactroban) 2% topical, applied intranasally tid to eliminate nasal carriage of *S. aureus*

Topical antibiotics: Once the lesions begin to drain, bacitracin or Neosporin applied locally tid or qid

Analgesic agents: If lesions are extensive or pain is severe

General Management

Warm, moist compresses to promote suppuration; nutritional therapy for underlying malnourishment, obesity, or debilitation; appropriate therapies for underlying disease

NURSING CARE

NURSING ASSESSMENT

Inflammatory process: Tenderness; pain; swelling; redness around infected follicle; drainage and signs of systemic infection

Systemic response to infection: Malaise; fever; regional lymphadenopathy; increased white blood cell count; increased eosinophils; decreased neutrophils; increased lymphocytes; increased erythrocyte sedimentation rate

Spread of infection: Personal hygiene; family hygiene

Psychosocial concerns: Concern with body image

POTENTIAL COMPLICATIONS

Scarring; antibiotic-resistant infection

PATIENT PROBLEMS/NURSING DIAGNOSES & INTERVENTIONS

NIC SKIN/WOUND MANAGEMENT

Impaired skin integrity related to inflammatory process

Risk for impaired skin integrity related to exudates

Risk for infection related to inadequate primary or secondary defenses

- Use meticulous hand washing *to prevent spread of infection.*
- Apply hot, moist compresses *to promote suppuration.*
- Change sterile dressing frequently after spontaneous drainage or surgical incision; properly dispose of contaminated articles *to prevent spread of infection.*

- Teach importance of not picking or squeezing lesions *to decrease the spread of infection and the risk of scarring.*
- Instruct patient in correct use of antibiotic therapies.
- When drainage begins, eliminate compresses *to prevent skin maceration and infection.*
- Teach meticulous hand washing and proper hygiene practices *to prevent autoinoculation.*
- Teach the importance of not picking or squeezing lesions *to decrease the risk of scarring.*
- Instruct patient to bathe daily with bacteriostatic soap and to avoid using oily preparations *to reduce the risk of recurrence.*
- Address predisposing factors such as altered nutritional status and obesity; patient should modify intake of fats and sugars.

NIC PHYSICAL COMFORT PROMOTION

Acute pain related to etiologic factors

- Apply warm, moist compresses.
- Instruct patient in use of analgesics.

PATIENT EDUCATION/CONTINUUM OF CARE PLAN

1. Discuss with the patient or family members to make sure that:
   a. The patient bathes daily with a bacteriostatic soap.
   b. The patient uses towels, linens, and clothing separate from the rest of the family.
   c. The patient's clothing, linen, and towels are changed and washed daily.
   d. A clean washcloth is used each time lesions are cleaned or soaked; lesions should be washed gently, not scrubbed.
2. Ensure that the patient and family know how to apply warm compresses and to change dressings using aseptic technique.
3. Ensure that the patient and family understand the need to maintain the correct regimen of antibiotic therapy.

EVALUATION/PATIENT OUTCOMES

Skin/Wound Management: Therapeutic effect is achieved. Existing lesions heal. Skin is intact and free of infection. Scarring is minimal. Hygiene measures to prevent spread or recurrence are instituted. Lesions do not recur. Infection does not spread to family members.

Physical Comfort Promotion: Pain is alleviated

FOLLICULITIS

Folliculitis is a superficial or deep bacterial infection and irritation of the hair follicle usually caused by *S. aureus.*

The bacterial infection can be limited to the hair follicle, resulting in its destruction, or the process can extend deeper to involve all of the hair follicle and the surrounding dermis.

Newborns have multiple lesions of the forehead, face, and neck. In adults the lesions are found in hairy areas such as the thigh, face, scalp, groin, or axilla.

Folliculitis may become chronic when the hair follicles are deep in the skin, as in the bearded area. Stiff hairs in the bearded area may emerge from the follicle, curve, and reenter the skin, producing a chronic low-grade irritation without significant infection (pseudofolliculitis). Pseudofolliculitis occurs most often in black men.

PATHOPHYSIOLOGY

Folliculitis is a variable condition, with lesions ranging from minute, white-topped pustules in newborns to large, yellow, tender, pus-containing lesions in adults.

The primary lesion is a small pustule 1 to 2 mm in diameter located over the pilosebaceous orifice. It is sometimes perforated by a hair. The pustule may be surrounded by inflammation or nodular lesions. A crust develops after the pustule ruptures.

Predisposing factors include superficial damage to the skin; exposure to certain chemicals, solvents, and greases; and the presence of staphylococci. Other bacteria can also cause folliculitis, especially after antibiotic therapy. Gram-negative folliculitis occurs in patients who receive long-term tetracycline or erythromycin therapy for acne.

DIAGNOSTIC STUDIES AND FINDINGS

Physical examination: Characteristic lesions
Culture of lesions: Presence of infecting organism: gram-positive *S. aureus* or gram-negative organisms

MULTIDISCIPLINARY PLAN

Medications

Antiinfective agents

Systemic antibiotics

Cephalexin (Keflex), 250-500 mg PO q6h
Ciprofloxacin (Cipro), 500 mg PO bid for *Pseudomonas*
Dicloxacillin (Dycill, Dynapen, Pathocil), 125-250 mg PO q6h
Erythromycin (E-Mycin, Ery-Tab, ERYC, others), 250 mg PO q6h for 10 days
Penicillin V (Pen-Vee K, V-Cillin K), 125-500 mg PO q6h for 10 days
Rifampin (Rifadin, Rimactane), 600 mg/day PO for recalcitrant condition

Topical antibiotics: Mupirocin 2% (Bactroban); apply topically to affected area bid

NURSING CARE

NURSING ASSESSMENT

Inflammatory process: Tenderness; pain; swelling or redness around infected follicle; presence of precipitating factors such as exposure to oils, greases, and solvents

POTENTIAL COMPLICATIONS

Spread of infection

Patient Problems/Nursing Diagnoses & Interventions

NIC Skin/Wound Management

Impaired skin integrity related to inflammatory process
Risk for impaired skin integrity related to exudates, chemical substance, or mechanical factors
- Use meticulous hand washing *to avoid spread of infection.*
- Apply hot, moist compresses *to promote suppuration.*
- Prevent maceration of skin *to avoid delay in healing.*
- Instruct patient *to use antibacterial soap.*
- Instruct patient in correct use of antibiotic therapies.
- Teach meticulous hand washing and proper hygiene practices *to avoid autoinoculation.*
- Help patient identify and eliminate precipitating factors such as skin maceration and exposure to oils, greases, and solvents *to prevent occurrence of new lesions.*
- Encourage men with chronic folliculitis or pseudofolliculitis in bearded area to grow a beard *to prevent occurrence of new lesions.*

Patient Education/Continuum of Care Plan

Discuss with the patient or family members to make sure that:
1. The patient bathes daily with a bacteriostatic soap.
2. The patient uses towels, linens, and clothing separate from the rest of the family.
3. The patient's clothing, linen, and towels are changed and washed daily.

Evaluation/Patient Outcomes

Skin/Wound Management: Lesions heal. Skin is intact and free of infection. Hygienic measures to prevent spread of recurrence are instituted. Lesions do not spread; no new lesions develop. Lesions do not spread to family members. Precipitating factors are avoided. No new lesions develop.

Impetigo and Ecthyma

Impetigo (impetigo contagiosa) is a superficial vesiculopustular infection. Ecthyma is an ulcerative form of impetigo.

Impetigo and ecthyma occur primarily in infants, children, and the elderly. They are highly contagious among newborns in nurseries and young children and less contagious in older people.

The arms, legs, and face are more susceptible to impetigo and ecthyma than unexposed areas, although lesions may occur anywhere. Impetigo occurs most commonly on the face. It usually appears first around the nose and mouth. Ecthyma occurs most often on the legs, the posterior aspect of the thighs, and the buttocks.

Impetigo occurs most frequently during the late summer and early fall. Biting insects, mosquitoes, and flies appear to be the most frequent transmitters. Predisposing factors include poor hygiene, anemia, and malnutrition. The infection spreads easily among family members and from one child to another in a classroom or playgroup.

Pathophysiology

Impetigo is produced by coagulase-positive staphylococci and β-hemolytic streptococci. The bacteria may be found alone or in combination. Staphylococci are usually seen in very early lesions, but streptococci predominate in chronic lesions.

The infectious process is located beneath the corneum. The initial lesion is a small erythematous macule that changes into a vesicle or bulla with a thin roof. In streptococcal impetigo the vesicle becomes pustular in a matter of hours. A characteristic thick, honey-colored crust forms when the vesicle ruptures. In staphylococcal impetigo the thin-walled bulla breaks and a thin, clear crust forms from the exudate. Both forms usually produce pruritus, burning, and regional lymphadenopathy. Autoinoculation from scratching may cause satellite lesions to form. Because the process is superficial, healing can occur spontaneously in the center of the lesion. This results in the formation of annular or circinate patterns.

A serious complication that develops in 2% to 5% of patients is acute glomerulonephritis from a nephritogenic strain of β-hemolytic streptococci. Impetigo in adults may have a more serious prognosis than impetigo occurring during childhood.

Ecthyma is a deeper infection than impetigo. It often develops in neglected superficial abrasions or from the scratching of insect bites. The inflammatory process is deeper and involves both the dermis and epidermis, so scarring results.

Ecthyma is characterized by localized thick, adherent, crusted plaques with underlying ulceration and purulent exudate. The early lesions may appear as a vesicle or pustule surrounded by an area of erythema. Itching is common; an autoinoculation from scratching can transmit ecthyma to other parts of the body.

Diagnostic Studies and Findings

Physical examination: Characteristic lesion
Gram's stain: Identification of infecting organism (gram-positive or gram-negative)
Culture: Identification of infecting organism (coagulase-positive staphylococci; β-hemolytic sreptococci)

Multidisciplinary Plan

Medications

Antiinfective agents

Systemic antibiotics

Cephalexin (Keflex), 250-500 mg PO q6h
Clarithromycin (Biaxin), 250 mg PO bid
Dicloxacillin (Dynapen) if initial treatment fails, 250-500 mg PO q6h
Erythromycin, E-Mycin, Ery-Tab, ERYC, others), 250-500 mg PO q6h for 10-14 days
Oxacillin (Bactocil), 250-500 mg PO qid
Penicillin V (Pen-Vee K, V-Cillin K), 125-500 mg PO q6-8h for 10-14 days
Penicillin G benzathine (Bicillin, Permapen), 1.2 million U IM as single injection
Trimethoprim-sulfamethoxazole (Bactrim DS), 1 PO bid for MRSA

Topical antibiotics
Mupirocin 2%, bacitracin, or Neosporin, applied locally tid or qid
Antihistamines for itching

General Management

Crust removal through soap-and-water washing and cool, moist compresses; nutritional therapy for underlying malnourishment or debilitation; appropriate therapies for underlying disease

NURSING CARE

Nursing Assessment

Lesion: Vesicle, bulla, exudate, or ulceration; satellite lesions; itching
Spread of infection: Personal hygiene, particularly fingernails; family hygiene; contact with others; presence of lesions in other family members
Psychosocial concerns: Concern that others may react to highly contagious disease; concern with body image

Potential Complications

Acute glomerulonephritis (impetigo), scarring (ecthyma)

Patient Problems/Nursing Diagnoses & Interventions

NIC Skin/Wound Management

Impaired skin integrity related to infectious process
Risk for impaired skin integrity related to exudates and mechanical factors
Risk for infection related to inadequate primary defenses and environmental exposure

- Use meticulous hand washing *to prevent spread of infection.*
- Remove crusts: clean lesion with bactericidal soap and water; apply compresses of Burow's solution and cool water *to soften crust;* gently scrub crust; dispose of contaminated articles *to prevent spread of infection.*
- Apply topical antibiotics to area of lesion for 2 days after lesion disappears.
- Cut patient's fingernails short *to minimize damage to lesion and to prevent autoinoculation from scratching.*
- Cut patient's fingernails short *to prevent autoinoculation and new skin breaks.*
- Teach patient and family meticulous hand washing *to prevent autoinoculation and spread to family members.*
- Have patient and family bathe daily with bactericidal soap *to reduce recurrences and prevent spread to family members.*
- Check family members for lesions *for early detection and treatment.*
- Address predisposing factors such as insect control and nutrition.

NIC Coping Assistance

Disturbed body image related to cognitive-perceptual factors

- Recognize importance of body image in growth and development.
- Encourage patient to express feelings about body appearance and fear of reaction or rejection by others *to begin process of realistic self-evaluation.*

Patient Education/Continuum of Care Plan

1. Ensure that the patient or family members understand that:
   a. The patient and all family members must bathe daily with bacteriostatic soap.
   b. The patient or any family member with lesions must use towels, linens, and clothing separate from the rest of the family.
   c. The patient's clothing, linen, and towels must be changed and washed daily.
   d. A clean washcloth must be used each time lesions are cleaned or soaked.
2. Ensure that the patient and family know how to remove the crust from the lesions: apply cool compresses of water and Burow's solution to soften the crust, and then scrub the crust gently.
3. Instruct parents to check other family members, particularly other children, for lesions, and have infected family members treated.
4. Ensure that the patient and family understand the need to maintain the correct regimen of antibiotic therapy even though the skin lesions have healed.

Evaluation/Patient Outcomes

Skin/Wound Management: Lesions resolve. Skin is intact and free of infection. Hygienic measures are instituted. Lesions do not spread to other areas of the body; lesions do not recur. Measures to prevent spread of infection are instituted. Infected family members are treated. Infection does not spread to noninfected family members. Complications do not occur.

Coping Assistance: Patient evaluates self-concept in realistic manner. Patient engages in usual activities and relationships.

Cellulitis and Erysipelas

Cellulitis is a diffuse, acute streptococcal or staphylococcal infection of the skin and subcutaneous tissue. Erysipelas is a rarer form of streptococcal cellulitis.

Cellulitis occurs most frequently in the lower extremities, usually from bacterial invasion through a wound in the skin or an open lesion. The infection may also spread through the lymphatic system from an existing infection site, but often there is no predisposing condition or site of entry.

Erysipelas occurs on the face (bilaterally), ears, arms, and legs. Recurrences in the same area are not uncommon.

Pathophysiology

Cellulitis is most commonly caused by group A β-hemolytic *Streptococcus* or *Staphylococcus aureus.* Diffuse spread of the infection occurs because enzymes produced by the organism break down cellular components that would otherwise localize the inflammatory process. Areas of skin trauma,

! EMERGENCY ALERT

CELLULITIS

Cellulitis is an infectious process in which devitalized tissue or a dirty wound becomes infected with growth of often anaerobic bacteria.

ASSESSMENT

- There is an erythemous area and an open wound.
- Exudate and foul smell may be present.
- Pain is usually minimal.
- Patient appears healthy otherwise.

INTERVENTIONS

- Obtain intravenous (IV) access.
- Administer antibiotics as ordered.
- Physician may consider incision and drainage or fasciotomy.
- Physician may consider hyperbaric oxygen treatments if gas formation is present.

ulceration, or lymphedema are especially susceptible to developing cellulitis.

The area of infection is diffuse and involves all layers of the skin and subcutaneous tissue, with ill-defined borders. The skin is red, hot, indurated, and tender. Sometimes pitting is evident with pressure. Irregular lymphangitic streaks (seen as red streaks) may extend from the periphery, and regional lymphadenopathy may be present. The skin frequently has an infiltrated surface resembling the skin of an orange (peau d'orange). Breakdown of the infected area can occur with purulent discharge. Local abscesses form occasionally and require surgical incision.

Erysipelas occurs at the dermal level of the skin. It is caused specifically by group A β-hemolytic streptococci. The inflammatory process is acute, with sudden onset. The area of infection is characterized by an erythematous, hot, and tender raised plaque with well-defined, sharply demarcated margins. Burning and pain, which may be severe, are common at the lesion site. Vesicles and bullae may develop and rupture, occasionally with necrosis of the involved skin. There is a great deal of exfoliation of the overlying skin as erysipelas heals.

Both cellulitis and erysipelas may be accompanied by systemic symptoms.

DIAGNOSTIC STUDIES AND FINDINGS

Physical examination: Characteristic lesion

Culture of lesion: For infecting organisms (group A β-hemolytic *Streptococcus* or *Staphylococcus aureus*); organism difficult to isolate unless drainage is present

Blood culture: For infecting organism: only occasionally positive

MULTIDISCIPLINARY PLAN

Surgery

Incision and drainage of localized abscesses; debridement of devitalized structures

Medications

Antiinfective agents

Systemic antibiotics

Should be continued for 1 week after infection has cleared; may need to be prolonged for several weeks for erysipelas

Ampicillin (Unasyn), 1.5-3 g IV q6h

Cefazolin (Kefzol, Ancef), 1.0 g IV q6-8h

Ceftriaxone (Rocephin), 1-2 g IM or IV q24h

Cephalexin (Keflex), 500 mg PO qid

Ciprofloxacin (Cipro), 500-750 mg PO bid for MRSA

Dicloxacillin (Dynapen, Pathocil), 500 mg PO q6h

Erythromycin (E-Mycin, Ery-Tab, ERYC, others), 250-500 mg PO q6h for 10-14 days

Minocycline (Minocin), 100 mg PO bid

Analgesic agents

Aspirin (ASA) or acetaminophen (Tylenol), alone or combined with codeine

General Management

Immobilization and elevation of affected limb to reduce edema; hospitalization for patients with severe infections or systemic symptoms; cool compresses for discomfort alternated with warm compresses or soaks to increase circulation; appropriate therapies for underlying disease

NURSING CARE

NURSING ASSESSMENT

Inflammatory process: Cellulitis: tenderness, pain; redness; heat; swelling; lymphangitic streaks; peau d'orange skin; purulent discharge; abscesses; erysipelas: tenderness, pain; redness; heat; swelling; raised plaque; vesicles; bullae; purulent exudate

Systemic response to infection: Regional lymphadenopathy; fever; chills; tachycardia; headache; hypotension; malaise; increased white blood cell count; decreased neutrophils; increased eosinophils; increased lymphocytes; increased erythrocyte sedimentation rate

POTENTIAL COMPLICATIONS

Systemic infection

PATIENT PROBLEMS/NURSING DIAGNOSES & INTERVENTIONS

NIC SKIN/WOUND MANAGEMENT

Impaired skin integrity related to the inflammatory process

- Elevate and immobilize affected area for 2 to 3 days *to decrease edema and increase circulation for healing.*
- Use meticulous hand washing *to prevent spread of infection.*
- Use sterile dressing changes for ulcers and open or draining lesions *to prevent spread of infection.*
- Instruct patient in correct use of antibiotic therapies *to obtain maximum benefit.*

NIC PHYSICAL COMFORT PROMOTION

Acute pain related to biologic factors

- Assess for discomfort.

- Elevate and immobilize affected area *to promote lymphatic drainage.*
- Apply cool wet compresses alternated with warm compresses or soaks.
- Instruct patient in use of analgesics.

NIC Immobility Management

Impaired physical mobility related to pain and discomfort

- Elevate affected area *to decrease edema and pain.*
- Explain need to maintain elevation and immobility for at least 2 to 3 days.
- Discuss with patient options to maximize elevation and immobility depending on patient's situation and severity of infection: bed rest, sling, crutches, or leg propped above heart level.

Patient Education/Continuum of Care Plan

1. Explain the need to elevate and immobilize the affected area for at least 2 to 3 days or until redness and edema decrease.
2. Demonstrate how to wash an open or draining wound gently with clean washcloth, soap, and water and to change dressings using aseptic technique.
3. Demonstrate how to apply a cool compress for discomfort, alternating with a warm compress or warm soak to increase circulation.

Evaluation/Patient Outcomes

Skin/Wound Management: Infection resolves. Lesions heal. Skin is intact and free of infection. Systemic infection does not occur or is quickly resolved. Laboratory values are normal; temperature is normal.

Physical Comfort Promotion: Pain is relieved. Symptoms of pain, burning, and discomfort are alleviated.

Immobility Management: Mobility is regained. Patient engages in usual activities.

Acne Vulgaris

Acne vulgaris is an inflammatory disease of the pilosebaceous follicles characterized by comedones, pustules, papules, or nodular lesions.

Acne occurs during puberty, although lesions may occur as early as age 8 years and continue through the twenties and thirties. The peak incidence appears to be around age 14 years for girls and 16 years for boys. Acne occurs more frequently in boys but tends to be more severe and prolonged in girls. Almost all adolescents experience some degree of acne, and about 80% have substantial lesions that range from superficial noninflammatory comedones to cysts and scars. Only a small percentage of these people seek medical attention; most treat themselves with over-the-counter preparations that may be ineffective.

Acne lesions occur most frequently on the face, neck, upper back, and chest. The precise cause of acne is unknown. Androgenic activity with an overproduction of sebum, follicular keratinization, bacterial proliferation, and the development of inflammation are the primary pathogenic factors.[23] The course and severity of the disease seem to be genetically determined. Dietary factors have little or no influence on the development of the disease, although certain foods may aggravate the condition in some patients. Predisposing factors include the use of cosmetics, steroids, oral contraceptives, and certain drugs (iodides, bromides, phenytoin, phenobarbital, trimetadione, isoniazid, ethionamide, rifampin, and lithium); exposure to heavy oils, greases, and tars; friction or occlusion from clothing such as sweatbands, shoulder straps, and football shoulder pads; emotional stress; hyperalimentation; or an unfavorable climate. Acne seems to improve during the summer and worsen in the fall and winter. This is probably because exposure to sunlight lessens the severity of acne during the summer months. However, a hot, humid climate can produce severe acne in some people.

The clinical presentation of acne can range from a mild noninflammatory form to severe inflammatory cystic acne. In the mildest forms only comedones may be present. Moderate involvement also produces some papules or pustules. The most severe forms manifest inflammatory papules, pustules, cysts, abscesses, and scarring.

Pathophysiology

The sebaceous gland increases in size and produces more sebum because of androgenic activity. This is accompanied by abnormal keratinization of the middle third of the hair follicle, which results in obstruction of the pilosebaceous unit. This blockage prevents the normal flow of sebum to the skin surface, causing retention of cells, lipids, fatty acids, hair, and focal masses of *Corynebacterium acnes (Proprionibacterium acnes).* Comedones then form either as open comedones (blackheads) or closed comedones (whiteheads). Open comedones have a raised opening that allows the contents to escape to the skin surface. The black appearance is caused by melanin granules or oxidation of the keratinous material. Closed comedones have a skin covering that prevents extrusion of the contents and promotes further retention of keratin and sebum. The open or closed comedones can remain free of inflammation, despite the presence of bacteria. As the contents of the structure continue to accumulate, the enlarging comedone becomes visible. This process may take weeks, months, or a year. If the wall of the upper third of the hair follicle becomes disrupted, its contents are discharged onto the epidermis and a pustule develops.

An enlarged follicle can eventually rupture and discharge its contents into the surrounding dermis. The result is the development of the inflammatory papule, nodule, or cyst. There is usually a combination of acute inflammation and foreign body reaction induced by keratin and hair in the dermis. Rupture of the follicle can occur spontaneously because of the inflammatory effects of the bacteria or can be caused by trauma such as squeezing the comedone. The deeper the lesions, the more severe is the potential for and degree of scarring.

The regeneration of the ruptured follicular wall is accomplished by proliferating keratinizing epidermis, but cystic structures with surrounding fibrosis can form in the process. These can develop into deep cystic processes with interconnecting channels, gross inflammation, and abscess formation. Chronic, recurring lesions produce distinctive acne scars.

DIAGNOSTIC STUDIES AND FINDINGS

Physical examination: Characteristic lesions and scarring

MULTIDISCIPLINARY PLAN

Management usually includes a combination of modalities that depends on the severity and type of lesions.

Surgery

Surgical removal of fibrotic cysts that have not responded to intralesional injections or liquid nitrogen therapy; excision should not be performed on actively inflamed acne cysts

Intralesional injections of corticosteroids (triamcinolone [Aristocort, Kenalog]) into cysts, 2.5 to 5 mg/ml of injectable steroid in saline or lidocaine, 0.1 to 0.3 ml in each cyst

Medications

Vitamins

Oral retinoids (for severe acne)

Isotretinoin (Accutane, 1-2 mg/kg/day PO in two divided doses for 20 weeks; initial dose individualized for patient's weight and severity of disease, with dosage adjusted after 2 weeks according to response of disease; second course may be initiated for persistent acne after 2 months without therapy

Topical: Vitamin A acid (retinoic acid) (Retin-A) gel or cream, 0.01%-0.1%, applied nightly 30 min after washing face and 1 h before bedtime

Antiinfective agents

Systemic antibiotics (for moderate acne)

Tetracycline, 250-500 mg PO qid for 4 weeks, then decreased to lowest maintenance dose that gives good response; ibuprofen (Motrin), 2.4 g/day will enhance the effect of 1 g of tetracylcine daily

Minocycline (Minocin), 100 mg/day PO in divided doses when no response to tetracycline

Erythromycin (EES, E-Mycin, Ery-Tab, ERYC, others), 250-500 mg PO in two divided doses

Trimethoprim-sulfamethoxazole (Bactrim DS), 1 tablet PO qd

Doxycycline (Vibramycin, Monodox), 50-200 mg PO qd

Topical antibiotics (for mild acne)

Clindamycin, 1%, apply tid or qid to lesions

Erythromycin, 2%, apply tid or qid to lesions

Tetracycline, apply tid or qid to lesions

Sodium sulfacetamide 10% and sulfur 5% tid to lesions

Keratolytic agents

Salicylic acid gel, apply nightly to affected areas

Benzoyl peroxide, 2.5%-10%, 3-4 h/day for 4 days, then overnight if tolerated; patient establishes own level of tolerance for strength and time

Hormones

Ethinyl estradiol, 0.035-0.05 mg PO in cyclic monthly routine

Spironolactone (Aldactone), 50-200 mg PO in divided doses with meals; for antiandrogenic effect

Prednisone, 5.0-7.5 mg PO qd, PM administration

General Management

Cryotherapy: Liquid nitrogen applied with cotton-tipped applicator or fine spray onto cysts

Expression of comedones by means of Schamberg or other extractor

Ultraviolet light in increasing doses at least once a week

Well-balanced diet to eliminate foods known to aggravate condition; foods will be specific to each individual

NURSING CARE

NURSING ASSESSMENT

Lesion: Presence of comedones (open or closed), pustules, papules, nodules, cysts, pitting scars on face, neck, shoulders, upper back, or chest; seasonal or monthly pattern and history of past inflammatory lesions; evidence of picking or squeezing lesions

Inflammatory process: Tenderness; pain; swelling; redness; and infected follicle

Psychosocial concerns: Concern with body image and social relationships; patient's perception of his or her appearance

POTENTIAL COMPLICATIONS

Secondary infection; scarring

PATIENT PROBLEMS/NURSING DIAGNOSES & INTERVENTIONS

NIC SKIN/WOUND MANAGEMENT

Impaired skin integrity related to inflammatory process

Risk for infection related to mechanical factors and internal factors

- Encourage patient to seek medical attention when acne develops.
- Stress importance of adhering to therapeutic regimen; assist in setting up overall schedule for managing regimen on daily basis.
- Plan schedule for facial hygiene: clean skin with acne soap or mild soap once or twice a day, keep skin clean and dry, and avoid abrasive soaps.
- Give written instructions for use of peeling agents such as benzoyl peroxide or retinoic acid. Alternating the creams can give better results. Never apply the two together.
- Discourage squeezing, picking, and rubbing of lesions to prevent infection.
- Teach patient how to use comedone extractor. Set up criteria for which comedones can be removed. Establish limited schedule for removal *to prevent further tissue damage.*
- Apply hot packs to cystic lesions *to promote circulation and suppuration.*
- Encourage frequent shampooing and hairstyle that keeps hair off face.
- Analyze diet and help patient identify foods that cause flare-ups.

- Help patient deal with stress; help patient label feelings, identify alternative courses of action, and set reachable goals.
- Identify and eliminate predisposing factors.
- Dispel myths that sexual activity or abstinence causes or affects acne.
- Instruct patient in correct use of antibiotic therapies.

NIC COPING ASSISTANCE

Situational low self-esteem; disturbed body image related to cognitive perceptual factors

- Recognize importance of body image in growth and development.
- Teach importance of not picking or squeezing lesions *to decrease risk of scarring.*
- Encourage patient to express feelings about body, body appearance, or fear of reaction or rejection by others *to begin process of realistic self-evaluation.*
- Encourage patient to develop interests and other attributes *to support positive self-image, feelings of self-worth, and self-confidence.*
- Help patient evaluate facial scarring in realistic perspective *so it does not become focal point of existence.*
- Advise patient of availability of tinted acne lotions that can mask lesions and scars.
- Arrange for individual or group therapy if patient is unable to adjust to appearance.

PATIENT EDUCATION/CONTINUUM OF CARE PLAN

1. Discuss and provide written instructions regarding the following:
   a. Side effects of systemic antibiotics and oral retinoids (isotretinoin should not be given to women of childbearing potential because fetal abnormalities have been reported with use of this drug).
   b. Need for and schedule of follow-up laboratory work for long-term antibiotic therapy or with oral retinoids.
   c. Untoward effects of topical preparations:
      (1) For increased redness and peeling, reduce time and strength of preparation until symptoms subside, then increase slowly.
      (2) Photosensitizing properties of retinoic acid: use only at bedtime; do not go out into sunlight with it on; use sunscreen with SPF of 15.
   d. Safe use of ultraviolet lamp: Eyes covered, timed exposure with backup timer, and measured distance.
2. Discuss good hygiene practices to prevent secondary infection.
3. Discuss with the patient how to maintain a well-balanced diet and get adequate rest.
4. Encourage the patient to go out into the sunlight unless contraindicated.
5. Discuss with the patient and family that successful therapy requires the patient's full cooperation and patience and that therapy is long-term and results may not be immediate.
6. Discuss with the patient the importance of continuing local lesion care even after the lesions have resolved.

EVALUATION/PATIENT OUTCOMES

Skin/Wound Management: Disease condition improves. Patient has fewer comedones, pustules, papules, nodules, or cysts. Acne lesions improve. Lesions heal with as little scarring as possible. There is no secondary infection. Inflammatory process recedes. There is no pain, tenderness, swelling, or redness around affected follicle. Side effects or untoward effects of medications are recognized and treated quickly. Patient seeks medical attention for untoward or side effects.

Coping Assistance: Patient has realistic self-concept. Acne disorder is not used as excuse for unsuccessful interpersonal relationships. Patient has realistic perception of his or her appearance.

ROSACEA

Rosacea is a chronic inflammatory disorder involving the central area of the face, which is characterized by erythema, telangiectasia, papules, and pustules.

Rosacea tends to occur in people who blush easily and sunburn easily. It appears most often in white women in their forties and fifties. When it occurs in men, it is usually more severe and is often associated with rhinophyma. Rhinophyma is characterized by thickened red skin on the nose that can be disfiguring.

The cause of rosacea is unknown, although alcohol, coffee, spicy foods, stress, and sun exposure may precipitate or exacerbate it in some people. Physical activity, infection, endocrine abnormalities, use of tobacco, and extreme heat or cold—anything that produces flushing—can also aggravate rosacea. The use of fluorinated steroid creams can also cause rosacea.

PATHOPHYSIOLOGY

The main pathologic processes of rosacea are instability of the superficial blood vessels, which results in persistent erythema and telangiectasia; overgrowth of normal bacteria, which results in pustules; and a granulomatous inflammation, which results in popular localization.

Rosacea develops gradually, beginning with periodic flushing across the forehead, nose, chin, and cheeks. The redness is intermittent at first but later becomes permanent. Telangiectasia develops along with pustules and papules. The inflammatory process causing the papules is granulomatous, differentiating it from the papules of acne. The pustules of roacea appear similar to those of acne but do not have the characteristic comedones of acne. Rhinophyma is seen in advanced cases, where there is marked hyperplasia of the sebaceous glands of the nose. Rhinophyma develops on the lower half of the nose and produces red, thickened, bulbous skin with dilated follicles.

Rosacea is sometimes associated with ocular symptoms of keratitis, corneal vascularization and blepharitis, and uveitis. Rosacea usually spreads slowly and does not subside without treatment.

Diagnostic Studies and Findings

Physical examination: Characteristic vascular flushing and acneiform lesions without comedones of acne vulgaris; rhinophyma

Multidisciplinary Plan

See Chapter 8 for treatment of eye symptoms.

Surgery

Excision of excess tissue in rhinophyma

Medications

Antiinfective agents

Systemic antibiotics

Tetracylcine, 250-500 mg PO qid initially for 1- to 2-week periods to prevent pustules; decrease doses as symptoms subside

Metronidazole (Flagyl), 200 mg PO bid

Erythromycin, 250 mg PO q6h

Topical antibiotics

Topical erythromycin 2% or clindamycin 2% alternated with hydrocortisone cream

Topical metronidazole gel 0.75% or cream 1%

Corticosteroids (topical preparations)

Sulfur 20% in hydrocortisone cream 1% applied bid

Hydrocortisone cream 1% applied bid

Isotretinoin (Accutane), 0.5 mg/kg/day for 20 weeks

Spironolactone, 50 mg/day for 4 weeks for antiandrogenic effect

Oral isotretinoin (Accutane), 1-2 mg/kg body weight/day

General Management

Prevention: Avoidance of hot food, drinks, and activities that precipitate or aggravate condition; electrolysis for large dilated blood vessels; cryotherapy for rhinophyma; carbon dioxide laser therapy for rhinophyma

NURSING CARE

Nursing Assessment

Inflammatory process: Erythema, telangiectasia, papules, and pustules across forehead, nose, chin, and cheeks; rhinophyma

Extension of inflammation: Ocular symptoms of keratitis, conjunctivitis, uveitis, and vascular dilation

Precipitating factors: Erythema in response to sunlight, hot beverages, spicy foods, vegetables, vinegar, alcohol, physical activity, and stress

Psychosocial concerns: Concern with body image; patient's perception of his or her appearance

Potential Complications

Rhinophyma; extension of inflammation to eye

Patient Problems/Nursing Diagnoses & Interventions

NIC Skin/Wound Management

Impaired skin integrity related to inflammatory process

Risk for impaired skin integrity related to environmental or internal factors

- Instruct patient not to squeeze or pick pustules *to prevent infection.*
- Instruct patient to keep skin clean and oil free but *to avoid excessive dryness and irritation to prevent aggravation of condition.*
- Instruct patient to shampoo hair often *to avoid oiliness.*
- Instruct patient in correct use of antibiotic and medication therapies *to maximize therapeutic benefit.*
- Help patient identify factors that cause exacerbations, and work with patient *to eliminate them.*

NIC Coping Assistance

Disturbed body image related to cognitive-perceptual factors; situational low self-esteem

- Encourage patient to express feelings about body, body appearance, and fear of reaction or rejection by others *to begin process of realistic self-evaluation.*
- Help patient evaluate his or her appearance in a realistic manner.

Patient Education/Continuum of Care Plan

1. Discuss with the patient the need to eliminate factors leading to facial hyperemia: consuming hot beverages, spicy foods, or alcohol; exposure to external irritants; and extremes of environmental heat or cold.
2. Discuss with the patient the need to avoid excessive sun exposure.
3. Teach the patient about the effects of long-term antibiotic therapy and to report untoward reactions.

Evaluation/Patient Outcomes

Skin/Wound Management: Pustular lesions resolve. Skin is intact with no papules or pustules. Exacerbations are not triggered by avoidable factors. Patients avoids factors leading to facial hyperemia.

Side effects or untoward reactions from long-term antibiotic therapy are recognized and treated. Patient seeks medical attention for untoward or side effects.

Coping Assistance: Patient evaluates appearance in a realistic manner. Patient engages in usual activities and relationships.

BENIGN SKIN CHANGES

Corns and Calluses

A corn (clavus) is a painful circumscribed area of hyperkeratosis caused by external pressure. A callus is a superficial area of hyperkeratosis that forms at the site of repeated pressure or friction.

A corn is a flat or slightly elevated circumscribed lesion with a smooth hard surface. "Soft" corns are caused by the pressure of a bony prominence. They appear as whitish thickenings usually between the fourth and fifth toes. "Hard" corns have a sharply defined conical appearance. They appear most frequently over bony prominences, such as the interphalangeal joints of the toes at the site of pressure from footwear. Hard corns are usually painful. The pain may be dull and constant or sharp when pressure is applied, similar to the sensation of stepping on a pebble.

Calluses are not well demarcated and may be large. They are elevated, with a normal pattern of skin ridges running over the surface. Calluses usually occur on the weight-bearing areas of the feet, overlying bony prominences. Calluses may form over plantar warts and must be differentiated from them. They are also common on the palmar surface of the hands, particularly in people who work with their hands. Calluses are usually not tender, but pressure may produce dull pain.

PATHOPHYSIOLOGY

A corn contains a localized pinpoint accumulation of keratin that forms an elongated hard plug in the horny layer of the epidermis with thinning of the underlying epidermis. The plug presses downward on the dermal structures.

In callus formation the epidermis reacts to repeated friction with an increased mitotic rate that results in hyperkeratosis and thickening of the stratum corneum. The severity of a corn or callus depends on the degree and duration of the trauma that caused it to form.

DIAGNOSTIC STUDIES AND FINDINGS

Physical examination: Characteristic lesion consistent with history of chronic pressure or friction

MULTIDISCIPLINARY PLAN

Surgery

Excision of superficial cornified layer of corn

Medications

Keratolytics: 40% salicylic acid plaster or ointment

Corticosteroids: Injection of triamcinolone (Kenalog, Aristocort), 10 mg/ml at base of corn to relieve pain

General Management

Orthopedic correction of weight-bearing mechanics through use of bars and support devices; corn pads to redistribute weight and relieve pressure

NURSING CARE

NURSING ASSESSMENT

Lesion: Thickened skin, may be tender to touch

Pain: Location, duration, and intensity

POTENTIAL COMPLICATIONS

Secondary infection from improper home interventions such as cutting or paring

PATIENT PROBLEMS/NURSING DIAGNOSES & INTERVENTIONS

NIC SKIN/WOUND MANAGEMENT

Impaired skin integrity related to mechanical factors

- Teach patient how to apply keratolytic substance and to avoid normal skin *to prevent tissue damage.*
- Demonstrate proper application of corn pads.

NIC PHYSICAL COMFORT PROMOTION

Acute pain related to physical factors

- Teach patient use of corn pads *to relieve pressure.*

PATIENT EDUCATION/CONTINUUM OF CARE PLAN

1. Explain the importance of not paring away existing corns and calluses.
2. Discuss with the patient the use of keratolytic plaster: apply sticky side to skin, making sure plaster is large enough to cover affected area; cover the plaster with adhesive tape and leave in place for designated period of time (overnight to 7 days); after the plaster is removed, soak the area in warm water and rub the soft macerated skin with a rough towel or pumice stone; reapply the plaster and repeat the process until all hyperkeratotic skin is removed.
3. Teach patient that most corns and calluses on feet are caused by tight, ill-fitting shoes and that new lesions can be avoided by wearing shoes that fit properly.
4. Show patient potential areas of pressure and how shoes should fit.

EVALUATION/PATIENT OUTCOMES

Skin/Wound Management: Source of pressure is relieved. Shoes fit properly. Orthopedic correction is used. Corn pads redistribute weight. Thickened areas disappear. Existing lesions resolve. New lesions do not form.

Physical Comfort Promotion: Symptoms of pain are alleviated.

SEBACEOUS, EPIDERMAL, AND DERMOID CYSTS

Sebaceous, epidermal, and dermoid cysts are slow-growing, benign, cystic, intradermal, or subcutaneous tumors.

Cysts are classified into three basic types depending on their histopathology: epidermal cysts, pilar or trichilemmal cysts (sebaceous cysts), and dermoid cysts.

Epidermal cysts are usually found on the face, scalp, neck, and back. Epidermal cysts include milia, acne cysts, and traumatic inclusion cysts. Only a few lesions are usually present unless the patient has had severe acne, in which case multiple lesions may be seen.

Pilar or trichilemmal cysts (wens) occur most frequently on the scalp but may also occur elsewhere. These cysts are usually referred to as sebaceous cysts. However, this is a misnomer. True sebaceous cysts are seen only in steatocystoma multiplex, a relatively rare inherited condition.

Dermoid cysts are usually found at birth. They are located deep in the subcutaneous tissue and may adhere to the periosteum.

Cystic lesions vary in size from 1 mm to several centimeters. Most cysts are less than 3 cm in diameter but they can enlarge to the size of an orange. On palpation the mass is firm, movable, round, globular, and nontender unless infected.

PATHOPHYSIOLOGY

The wall of the epidermal cyst is composed of keratinizing epidermis. The cyst contains keratin in laminated layers. The wall of the pilar cyst is made up of epidermal cells from the central part of the hair follicle. The contents of the pilar cyst are homogeneous rather than in laminated layers. The walls of the dermoid cyst are composed of keratinizing epidermis containing hair follicles, sebaceous glands, and sweat glands.

Cyst formation may occur after inflammation, trauma, or rupture of closed comedones. A person may also have a genetic predisposition to cyst formation. The contents of the cyst result from the obstructed hair follicle, with the exact nature depending on the level of the obstruction. The contents are soft and yellow-white and have a rancid odor.

DIAGNOSTIC STUDIES AND FINDINGS

Physical examination: Characteristic lesion

MULTIDISCIPLINARY PLAN

Surgery

Excision of cyst, including wall, to prevent recurrence incision and drainage of infected cysts

Medications

Corticosteroids: Triamcinolone (Aristocort, Kenalog) by intralesional injection

NURSING CARE

NURSING ASSESSMENT

Lesion: Size; location; number; presence of tenderness, inflammation, or infection; on palpation, firm, movable, round, globular, and nontender

POTENTIAL COMPLICATIONS

Infection

PATIENT PROBLEMS/NURSING DIAGNOSES & INTERVENTIONS

NIC SKIN/WOUND MANAGEMENT

Risk for impaired skin integrity related to mechanical factors

- Teach importance of not picking or squeezing lesions *because this may lead to infection of cyst.*

PATIENT EDUCATION/CONTINUUM OF CARE PLAN

Demonstrate and discuss with the patient dressing changes and suture care after excision of the cyst.

EVALUATION/PATIENT OUTCOMES

Skin/Wound Management: Nonexcised lesions do not become infected. There is no redness, swelling, tenderness, pus, or fever; scarring is minimal. Excised lesions heal. Skin is intact and smooth.

CUTANEOUS TAG

Cutaneous tags (acrochordon) are common, small, flesh-colored or pigmented pedunculated lesions.

Acrochordons are found most often in middle-aged and elderly people. The number increases with pregnancy and menopause. The lesions occur most frequently around the neck, upper chest, axilla, and groin and with seborrheic keratoses. They may occur singularly or in the hundreds. Although the lesion is benign, it may cause concern because of cosmetic embarrassment or because of irritation by clothing.

PATHOPHYSIOLOGY

The cutaneous tag consists of an outpouched core of loose connective tissue and dilated capillaries covered by normal epidermis. The papilloma is pedunculated and varies in size from 1 to 2 mm in diameter to considerably larger, soft, baglike, fibrous lesions.

DIAGNOSTIC STUDIES AND FINDINGS

Physical examination: Characteristic lesion

MULTIDISCIPLINARY PLAN

Surgery

Removal with scalpel or scissors, with electrocoagulation of central vessel if needed

General Management

Removal through electrodesiccation or cryotherapy

NURSING CARE

NURSING ASSESSMENT

Lesion: Location; number; size; presence of irritation, tenderness, and inflammation

POTENTIAL COMPLICATIONS

Irritation, inflammation from friction

PATIENT PROBLEMS/NURSING DIAGNOSES & INTERVENTIONS

NIC SKIN/WOUND MANAGEMENT

Risk for impaired skin integrity related to mechanical factors

- Evaluate with patient the potential for irritation of tags through friction from clothing or rubbing against other body parts.

Patient Education/Continuum of Care Plan

1. Discuss with the patient the benign nature of the lesions.
2. Explain to the patient that lesions can be removed relatively easily for cosmetic purposes or if tags become irritated.

Evaluation/Patient Outcomes

Skin/Wound Management: Patient seeks treatment for lesions that are irritated or inflamed. Lesions are removed if they become irritated or if patient is embarrassed.

Keloid

A keloid is an overgrowth of fibroelastic tissue that occurs spontaneously or at the site of dermal trauma.

The factors that trigger keloid formation are unknown. There appears to be a genetic predisposition and a regional susceptibility because keloids commonly occur on the sternum, chest, upper back, and earlobes and where an injury crosses normal flexion creases. Keloids occur predominantly in children or young adults, particularly in dark-skinned persons (Fig. 7-4).

Pathophysiology

In susceptible people keloids form after any skin trauma, or they may arise spontaneously. Keloids are an abnormal progressive deposition of collagen that exceeds the requirements for wound repair. This may be the result of immune activity. The lesions are soft and pink in the early stages and then become firm and white. Keloids are raised, smooth, or ridged; extend beyond the edges of the initial wound; and may continue to grow for many months or years to form large irregular lesions. Keloid scars are frequently tender and pruritic.

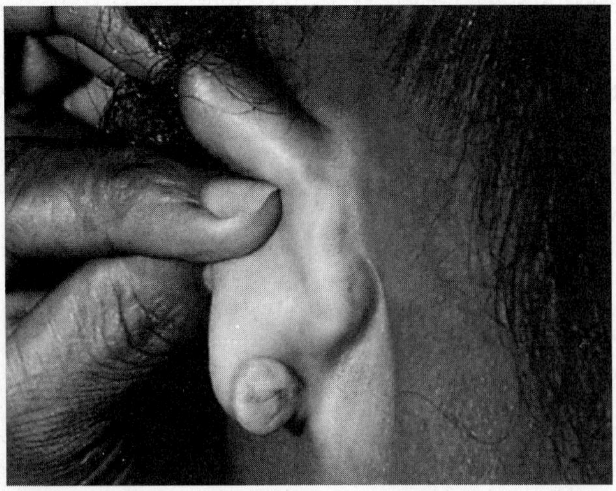

Fig. 7-4

Keloid. (Courtesy Stephen B. Tucker, MD, Department of Dermatology, University of Texas Health Science Center at Houston, Tex.)

Diagnostic Studies and Findings

Physical examination: Characteristic lesion; clinical differentiation from hypertrophic scar not possible in first 3 months of lesion, but thereafter any continued increase in size and sensitivity of firm, indurated scar is indicative of keloid formation

Multidisciplinary Plan

Keloids may become worse as the result of treatment; therefore the need for intervention must first be carefully assessed. Small keloids are often best left untreated. Many keloids gradually soften and flatten out over a period of years, even without treatment

Surgery

Surgical or carbon dioxide laser excision combined with radiation therapy or intralesional injection of steroids for large keloids; surgical excision alone will result in the formation of new and larger keloids

Medications

Corticosteroids: Triamcinolone (Aristocort, Kenalog), 24-40 mg/ml by intralesional injection; may require repeated injections at monthly intervals until keloid remains flattened and asymptomatic

Topical retinoic acid, 0.05% applied bid for 3 months

General Management

Solid carbon dioxide or liquid nitrogen applied topically at 2-week intervals

NURSING CARE

Nursing Assessment

Lesion: Size, location, color, tenderness, pruritus

Psychosocial concerns: Concern about body image, perception of his or her appearance

Potential Complications

Worsening secondary to treatment

Patient Problems/Nursing Diagnoses & Interventions

NIC Skin/Wound Management

Impaired skin integrity related to mechanical factors

- Discuss nature of keloid formation and help patient find skilled practitioners for therapeutic intervention.
- Inform patient that optimum time for treatment is within first few months of scar formation, while lesions are still vascular and growing, and that older keloids may be resistant to treatment.
- Instruct patient not to scratch keloid that itches *to avoid skin trauma that could cause further keloid formation.*

- Discuss safety habits *to avoid injury that leads to keloid formation* such as protective clothing and proper equipment.

NIC COPING ASSISTANCE

Disturbed body image related to cognitive-perceptual factors; situational low self-esteem

- Help patient express feelings about body, body appearance, and fear of reaction or rejection by others *to assist in process of realistic self-evaluation.*

PATIENT EDUCATION/CONTINUUM OF CARE PLAN

1. Discuss with the patient the nature of keloid behavior and the need to evaluate therapeutic intervention carefully with practitioners familiar with and skilled in treating keloids.
2. Explain to the patient that many keloids gradually soften and flatten out over a period of years, even without treatment.

EVALUATION/PATIENT OUTCOMES

Skin/Wound Management: Patient is knowledgeable about keloid therapies and risks. Patient seeks intervention early and from practitioners familiar with and skilled in keloid treatment. Patient avoids surgical excision of keloids. Patient takes measures to prevent injury that would result in keloid formation. Patient uses safety measures, such as protective clothing and use of proper equipment, to avoid injury. Patient refrains from scratching or irritating scar tissue.

Coping Assistance: Patient evaluates appearance in a realistic manner. Patient engages in usual activities and relationships.

SEBORRHEIC KERATOSES

Seborrheic keratoses are common, benign, superficial, epithelial, pigmented tumors.

The cause of seborrheic keratoses is unknown. They occur most frequently after age 40 years. They most commonly occur on the back, central chest, face, and scalp. In African-Americans the lesions tend to be more numerous and smaller and occur earlier. The lesions are inherited as a dominant trait.

Seborrheic keratoses vary in color from yellow to brownish black. They are elevated plaques with sharply circumscribed borders and appear to be stuck on the skin. The size of the lesion varies from a few millimeters to several centimeters. They almost always occur in multiples rather than singly. These lesions do not become malignant, but a sudden increase in the number and degree of itching of the lesions can occur in association with an internal malignancy.

PATHOPHYSIOLOGY

Immature keratinocytes accumulate, causing the formation of seborrheic keratoses. Keratinization eventually occurs, causing the lesions to become warty, dry, and fissured. The surface of the lesions often appears greasy, with pits filled with keratotic material. These represent invaginations of the epidermis. There is also a papular variant of the lesion that has a smooth surface. Epidermal thickening is associated with an increase of dermal papillae and the formation of the verrucous surface. The lesions grow slowly and are round or oval.

Seborrheic keratoses are usually asymptomatic unless they become irritated. They may itch occasionally. Irritation of the lesions by physical or chemical trauma results in tenderness, itching, erythema, and an increase in the size of the lesion.

DIAGNOSTIC STUDIES AND FINDINGS

Physical examination: Characteristic lesion
Biopsy: Done if squamous cell carcinoma is suspected

MULTIDISCIPLINARY PLAN

In most instances, small, asymptomatic seborrheic keratoses require no treatment. Treatment is instituted for lesions that itch, are irritated, or are cosmetically embarrassing.

Surgery

Shave ablation or curettage using local anesthesia

General Management

Liquid nitrogen cryotherapy at 2- to 3-week intervals; carbon dioxide pencil applied with light to moderate pressure for 12 to 20 seconds

NURSING CARE

NURSING ASSESSMENT

Lesion: Location, size, number, appearance, color, surface characteristics, borders, pruritus, changes in characteristics
Irritation of lesion: Erythema, tenderness, increased pruritus
Psychosocial concerns: Concern with body image, perception of his or her appearance

POTENTIAL COMPLICATIONS

Irritation, inflammation

PATIENT PROBLEMS/NURSING DIAGNOSES & INTERVENTIONS

NIC SKIN/WOUND MANAGEMENT

Risk for impaired skin integrity related to mechanical factors

- Reassure patient that this lesion has no potential for malignancy.
- Have patient identify lesions that itch, are irritated, or are cosmetically embarrassing *for potential treatment.*
- Evaluate with patient lesions that are likely to become irritated from clothing or rubbing against other body parts *to identify for potential treatment.*

NIC COPING ASSISTANCE

Disturbed body image related to cognitive-perceptual factors; situational low self-esteem

- Encourage patient to express feelings about body, body appearance, or fear of reaction or rejection by others *to assist in process of realistic self-evaluation.*
- Inform patient that bothersome lesions can be removed, usually with minimal or no scarring.

PATIENT EDUCATION/CONTINUUM OF CARE PLAN

1. Explain to the patient that the lesion has no potential for malignancy.
2. Discuss with the patient the availability of medical therapy for lesions that become irritated or bothersome or that are cosmetically embarrassing.

EVALUATION/PATIENT OUTCOMES

Skin/Wound Management: Treated lesions heal. Skin is intact with minimum scarring and is free of infection. Patient evaluates lesions realistically. Patient seeks treatment for lesions that itch, are irritated, or are cosmetically embarrassing.

Coping Assistance: Patient evaluates appearance realistically. Patient engages in usual activities and relationships.

ERYTHEMA MULTIFORME

Erythema multiforme is an acute inflammatory eruption characterized by symmetric erythematous, edematous, or bullous lesions precipitated by numerous factors.

The cause and pathogenesis of erythema multiforme are unknown. The mechanism of response seems to be an allergic hypersensitivity.

The disease is associated with herpes simplex, bacterial and other infections, endocrine changes, and internal malignancies. Almost any drug can cause erythema multiforme; penicillin, sulfonamides, salicylates, and barbiturates are the most commonly implicated drugs. Bacterial and viral infections are often implicated in children and young adults, but associations with drugs and malignancy are more common in adults. Attacks sometimes last for 2 to 4 weeks and recur in the fall.

PATHOPHYSIOLOGY

In mild cases of erythema multiforme, eruption occurs only in cutaneous lesions of erythematous macules, papules, and plaques located predominantly in the distal portion of the extremities and face and symmetrically distributed. The classic lesion (target or iris lesion) is a dark, urticarial plaque with elevated circular borders and a depressed inner ring (FIG. 7-5). After a few days the central area of erythema develops a dusky purplish discoloration that can become bullous.

In more severe cases fever, coryza, malaise, and athralgia may also occur. In these cases the lesions are predominantly vesiculobullous and involve mucous membranes as well as skin. In children and young adults a severe and sometimes fatal form of erythema multiforme known as Stevens-Johnson syndrome can develop. In this syndrome mucous membrane lesions are present and may or may not be accompanied by cutaneous lesions. Vesicles and ulcerations develop in the mucous membrane of the lips, mouth, nasal passages, eyes, and genitalia. Conjunctival and corneal lesions are present in 90% of the cases.

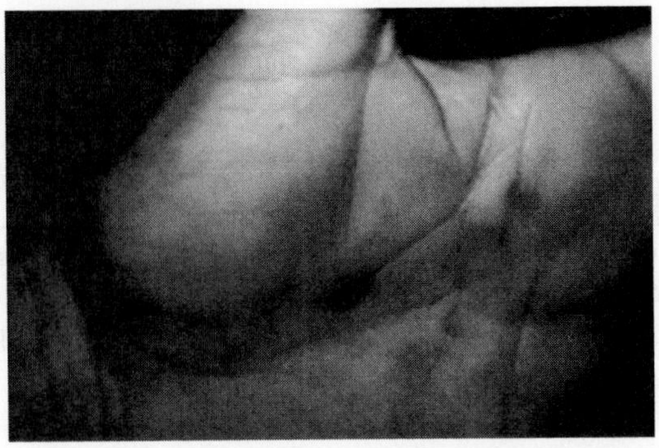

FIG. 7-5
Erythema multiforme (target lesion). (Courtesy Stephen B. Tucker, MD, Department of Dermatology, University of Texas Health Science Center at Houston, Tex.)

Genitourinary lesions in erythema multiforme can compromise bladder function, and the inflammatory process can involve the kidneys with consequent hematuria and renal tubular necrosis. Mucous membrane ulceration can extend into the pharynx, esophagus, larynx, trachea, and bronchi.

The variety of histologic changes in erythema multiforme depends on the site of involvement and the degree of the inflammatory process. The blood vessels are dilated and are surrounded by lymphohistiocytic infiltrate with substantial edema of the papillary dermis. Edema of the upper dermis leads to the formation of bullae that are subepidermal without acantholysis. Epidermal necrosis occurs primarily in the center of the lesion, the site of the dusky iris (target) lesion.

DIAGNOSTIC STUDIES AND FINDINGS

Physical examination: Characteristic lesion, particularly iris or target lesion; lesions fixed and do not fade or change location; absence of itching

Complete blood count: Increased white blood cell count, increased erythrocyte sedimentation rate

Urinalysis: Red blood cells and albumin in urine if genitourinary lesions are present

Antistreptolysin titer: Elevated if disease occurs after streptococcal infection

MULTIDISCIPLINARY PLAN

Mild erythema multiforme clears spontaneously and may require no treatment other than elimination of the precipitating factor. For treatment of eye symptoms, see Chapter 8.

Medications

Antiinfective agents

Systemic antibiotics for underlying infection or control of secondary infection; specific drug and dosage depend on infection and its severity and age of patient

Corticosteroids

Systemic glucocorticoids: Prednisone, 60-80 mg PO qd in divided doses, then decreased; controversial[21,23]

Topical corticosteroids

Betamethasone (Diprolene) 0.05% bid

Clobetasol propionate (Temovate) 0.05% bid

Antiviral agents for underlying viral infection

Local anesthetic agents: Viscous lidocaine (Xylocaine) swish for mouth lesions

Analgesics: Aspirin (ASA), 600 mg PO q4-6h

General Management

Wet dressings to debride crusted lesions; bed rest, hospitalization for severe cases; bland diet for mouth lesions; intravenous fluids for hydration in severe cases

NURSING CARE

Nursing Assessment

Lesion: Erythematous macules, papules, vesicles, or bullae at distal aspect of extremities and face; target or iris lesion; vesicles or ulcerations of mucous membranes; discomfort from mucous membrane lesions

Systemic involvement: Fever; coryza; arthralgia; malaise; chest pain; vomiting; diarrhea; hematuria; albuminuria; increased erythrocyte sedimentation rate; increased white blood cell count; radiologic changes in lungs

Nutritional status: Inability to eat because of mouth ulcerations

Psychosocial concerns: Body image

Potential Complications

Systemic involvement; Stevens-Johnson syndrome; secondary infection

Patient Problems/Nursing Diagnoses & Interventions

NIC Skin/Wound Management

Impaired skin integrity related to mechanical factors

Altered oral mucous membrane related to pathologic condition

- In collaboration with physician, apply wet dressings to debride lesions.
- Scrub crusted lesions gently with antibacterial soap *to promote healing and prevent infection.*
- Teach meticulous hand washing and good hygiene *to prevent secondary infection.*
- Provide soft, bland diet *to prevent tissue damage.*
- Avoid astringent or acidic liquids *to promote comfort.*
- Provide mouth care with alkaline or saline mouthwash *to promote comfort and prevent infection.*

NIC Physical Comfort Promotion

Acute pain related to physical factors

- Apply cool compresses or soaks.
- Encourage bed rest.
- Instruct patient in use of analgesics.
- Instruct patient in use of viscous lidocaine mouth swish *to promote comfort.*

NIC Nutrition Support

Imbalanced nutrition: less than body requirements, related to inability to ingest food

- Provide soft, bland diet *to promote comfort while eating.*
- In collaboration with physician, offer viscous lidocaine mouth swish 15 minutes before eating *to promote comfort.*

NIC Coping Assistance

Disturbed body image related to cognitive-perceptual factors

- Help patient express feelings about body, body appearance, or fear of reaction or rejection by others *to assist in process of realistic self-evaluation*

Patient Education/Continuum of Care Plan

1. Demonstrate to the patient and family the application of cool compresses or soaks using aseptic technique.
2. Discuss with the patient and family the need for follow-up urinalysis to detect the presence of renal tubular necrosis.
3. Discuss with the patient and family signs and symptoms of secondary infection and to seek medical attention if they occur.
4. Help the patient identify potential precipitating factors and to eliminate those factors when possible.

Evaluation/Patient Outcomes

Skin/Wound Management: Existing lesions heal. Ulcerations and erosions reepithelialize. Skin and mucous membrane heal. Secondary infection is avoided. There is no swelling, redness, or pus in healing lesions. Systemic involvement resolves. There are no red blood cells or protein in urine. White blood cell count is 5000 to 10,000/mm^3. Erythrocyte sedimentation rate is normal (depends on method). Complications are recognized early. Patient has follow-up urinalysis. Patient seeks medical attention for vision changes.

Physical Comfort Promotion: Discomfort is alleviated.

Nutrition Support: Nutritional status is adequate. Weight is maintained.

Coping Assistance: Patient evaluates appearance in a realistic manner. Patient engages in usual activities and relationships.

ERYTHEMA NODOSUM

Erythema nodosum is an acute inflammatory nodular eruption that involves primarily the lower extremities and is precipitated by various factors.

Erythema nodosum is found equally in boys and girls but is more common in adults, particularly young women. It occurs more commonly from January to June.

There are many precipitating factors, including various infections, drugs, diseases, and pregnancy. Erythema nodosum frequently follows an infection of the upper respiratory tract, especially from streptococci. In adults, streptococcal infections and sarcoidosis are the most common causes. An underlying systemic cause is identifiable is more than 50% of cases. The remainder of the cases occur in apparently healthy young adults.

The prodromal symptoms may be fever, chills, malaise, and arthralgia, which occur a few days or several weeks before the onset of the eruption. Some of the prodromal symptoms may be from the underlying condition.

Pathophysiology

Erythema nodosum is a vascular reaction pattern, most likely a hypersensitivity response involving both cellular and humoral mechanisms (see Chapter 16). The eruption is sudden with discrete, erythematous, hot, and very tender nodules on the shins, knees, ankles, thighs, buttocks, and sometimes lower arms. The nodules are bright red initially but change to a purplish color and finally become a flat brown pigmentation that slowly fades completely. The total evolution of lesions takes 3 to 4 weeks.

The nodules vary in size from 6 to 8 mm and are usually bilaterally symmetric. There may be only a few lesions or many appearing in crops. New crops may occur periodically. Edema of the ankles and general aching of the legs are common and are aggravated by ambulation.

Cellular changes are probably caused by the immunologic processes. Deep dermal inflammation extends down into subcutaneous tissue. Small blood vessels experience mild vasculitis and inflammatory infiltrate with partial obstruction of blood flow.

Diagnostic Studies and Findings

Physical examination: Characteristic lesion; history consistent with possible precipitating factors

Complete blood count: Increased erythrocyte sedimentation rate; platelet estimate

Biopsy: Deep excision biopsy, including subcutaneous tissue; shows histologic changes described previously

Diagnostic studies to isolate underlying disorders: Antistreptolysin titer; throat culture; tuberculosis test; rheumatoid factor; antinuclear factor

Multidisciplinary Plan

Management of the disease is aimed at identifying and treating the precipitating factor or underlying disorder.

Medications

Analgesics: Aspirin (ASA), 600 mg PO q4-6h

Antiinfective agents: Systemic antibiotics for underlying infection; may require long-term therapy; specific antibiotic depends on the underlying infection

Corticosteroids

Prednisone, 40-60 mg PO qd tapered over 7-10 days

Intralesional injection of triamcinolone (Aristocort, Kenalog), 5 mg/ml

Potassium iodide, 360-900 mg PO qd for 3-4 weeks

Nonsteroidal antiinflammatory drugs (NSAIDs)

General Management

Bed rest with legs elevated to reduce pain and swelling; cool compresses applied to nodules; support stockings or elastic bandages

NURSING CARE

Nursing Assessment

Lesions: Red, hot, tender nodules (initially) on anterior aspect of lower extremities; discomfort

Systemic involvement: Fever, chills, malaise, arthralgia, ankle edema, aching legs

Underlying disorder: Complete blood count, urinalysis, antistreptolysin titer, tuberculosis test, rheumatoid factor, throat culture, antinuclear factor

Psychosocial concerns: Body image

Potential Complications

Infection

Patient Problems/Nursing Diagnoses & Interventions

NIC Physical Comfort Promotion

Acute pain related to biologic factors

- Encourage bed rest and elevation of legs *to alleviate aching.*
- Have patient use support hose and elastic bandages *to prevent venous pooling.*
- Apply cool compresses.

Patient Education/Continuum of Care Plan

1. Help the patient identify potential precipitating factors and eliminate them when possible (such as with drugs).
2. Explain the effects of long-term antibiotic therapy if indicated.
3. Discuss with the patient the management of symptoms: elevation of legs, rest, use of support hose or elastic bandages, and application of cool compresses.

Evaluation/Patient Outcomes

Physical Comfort Promotion: Nodules resolve. Underlying condition is identified and treated. Symptoms of underlying disorder improve and resolve. Precipitating factors are eliminated when possible. Condition does not recur. Discomfort is alleviated.

INFESTATIONS AND PARASITIC DISORDERS

PEDICULOSIS

Pediculosis is an infestation by lice of the head (pediculosis capitis), the body (pediculosis corporis), or the genital area (pediculosis pubis).

Pediculosis is a highly pruritic and often secondarily infected disorder that results from two species of lice: *Pediculus humanus,* which affects the head and body, and *Phthirus pubis,* which infects the pubic area, the lower abdomen, and sometimes the eyebrows, eyelashes, and scalp.

Pediculosis capitis occurs most frequently in schoolchildren and is easily transmitted by personal contact and by objects such as combs and hats. Itching and excoriation are present. The posterior aspect of the scalp commonly shows the most involvement. The posterior occipital nodes may be enlarged and tender.

Pediculosis corporis is characterized by pruritus and parallel linear excoriations that are frequently secondarily infected. The infesting lice live in the seams of clothing and move onto the skin to feed frequently. Lesions are most common on the shoulders, buttocks, and abdomen. Infestation is associated with unhygienic living conditions.

Pediculosis pubis is transmitted by close personal contact, usually through sexual contact. Infestation is usually in the pubic hair but may occur in the chest or axillary hair, eyebrows, or eyelashes. A sign of infestation is the presence of reddish brown specks on undergarments as a result of the excreta of lice.

PATHOPHYSIOLOGY

In pediculosis capitis, injection of saliva from the lice during feeding produces severe pruritus. Scratching causes excoriation, and secondary infection is common. Each day the female louse lays 7 to 10 eggs that hatch in 8 days. The eggs (nits) are cemented to the hair shaft and cannot be dislodged.

In pediculosis corporis the primary lesion is an urticarial papule, which is often obscured by secondary excoriation and infection. With prolonged infestation the skin becomes dry, scaly, and hyperpigmented.

Pediculosis pubis is manifested primarily by itching. The lice ova are commonly attached to the skin at the base of the hair follicle. Discrete, small, 1- to 3-cm, gray-blue macules can be seen on the trunk, thighs, and axillae. These lesions result from a reaction of the lice's saliva with bilirubin, converting it to biliverdin. Excoriation and secondary infection are uncommon.

DIAGNOSTIC STUDIES AND FINDINGS

Physical examination: Presence of lice or eggs; presence of nonspecific lesion with characteristic distribution
Wood's light: Fluorescence of adult louse
Microscopic examination: Examination of hair shaft for eggs

MULTIDISCIPLINARY PLAN

Medications

Antiinfective agents

Synthetic pyrethrin (RID) liquid applied to dry hair, scalp, and any other infested area; left on 10 min then rinsed with warm water, soap, and shampoo; dead lice and eggs removed with nit comb; treatment repeated in 7 to 10 days; must not exceed two consecutive applications within 24 h

Permethrin (Nix) 1% creme rinse for head lice; applied to towel-dried hair; left on 10 min and rinsed out

Lindane (Kwell) shampoo, cream, or lotion, applied qd for 2 days; application repeated in 10 days; used with caution with young children because of neurotoxicity

Ophthalmic preparation of yellow mercury oxide qd for infested eyelashes

Colinergic agents

Physostigmine (Eserine) 0.25% ophthalmic ointment qd for infested eyelashes

General Management

Combing to remove lice and nits from hair shaft; rinsing with white vinegar diluted with equal amounts of water followed by washing to remove residual nits from hair; lice removed from eyelashes with forceps; body lice eliminated from clothing and bedding by thorough hot washing, hot ironing, boiling, and steaming; personal articles sealed in a plastic bag for 10 days

NURSING CARE

NURSING ASSESSMENT

Infestation: Presence of lice, eggs, and lesions; location and distribution of lesions

Local response to infestation: Pruritus, excoriation, secondary infection

Psychosocial concerns: Concern that others may react to transmissible infestation; low self-esteem: assess for defining characteristics

POTENTIAL COMPLICATIONS

Allergy to antiinfective agents, neurotoxicity from lindane, secondary infection from scratching, resistant organisms

PATIENT PROBLEMS/NURSING DIAGNOSES & INTERVENTIONS

NIC SKIN/WOUND MANAGEMENT

Impaired skin integrity related to mechanical factors

- Instruct patient in use of antiinfective agents *to kill parasite.*
- Instruct patient to comb hair with fine-toothed comb *to remove eggs after preparation is used.*
- Instruct patient to remove lice from eyelashes with cotton-tipped applicator.

- Instruct patient in good hygiene, meticulous hand washing, and need for short fingernails t*o avoid secondary infection.*

NIC Risk Management

Risk for infection related to close personal contact
- Teach patient how to decontaminate sources of infestation.
- Treat all family members and sexual partners.
- Advise patient that recurrence is common.
- Teach patient importance of not borrowing personal items such as combs.

NIC Coping Assistance

Situational low self-esteem related to negative self-appraisal
- Encourage patient to express feelings about the infestation, embarrassment, or fear of rejection by others *to begin the process of realistic self-evaluation.*
- Assure patient and family that infestation can be treated successfully.

Patient Education/Continuum of Care Plan

1. See under Patient Problems/Nursing Diagnoses & Interventions.
2. Explain to the patient that prolonged use of lindane may result in dermatitis.
3. Advise that all household members and sexual partners be treated.

Evaluation/Patient Outcomes

Skin/Wound Management: Infestation is cleared in patient and affected family members and partners. Pruritus subsides. No new areas of itching or excoriation develop. There are no lice or eggs on examination. Lesions heal. Excoriations resolve. Skin is intact. Secondary infection is resolved or avoided. Lesions heal without redness, swelling, or pus.

Risk Management: Infestation does not spread to unaffected family members or intimate contacts. Associates of patient do not develop symptoms. Hair and skin are free of lice or eggs. All family members and sexual partners receive treatment.

Coping Assistance: Patient evaluates self realistically. Patient verbalizes positive feelings about self.

Scabies

Scabies is a transmissible parasitic infestation characterized by burrows, pruritus, and excoriations with secondary infection.

Scabies is caused by the *Sarcoptes scabiei* mite. The infestation and lesions occur most commonly on the finger webs, the flexor surfaces of the wrist, and the elbows and axillary folds, along the belt line, and on the lower buttocks. The areolae in women and the genitalia in men are particularly susceptible. Lesions do not extend to the face in adults but may do so in infants.

Scabies is transmitted readily by personal contact. It characteristically spreads to other family members, to intimate contacts, and between schoolchildren. It is not transmitted by clothing, bedding, or inanimate objects. Infestation can occur from cats, dogs, and other small animals, but the animal scabies mite does not burrow, only feeds.

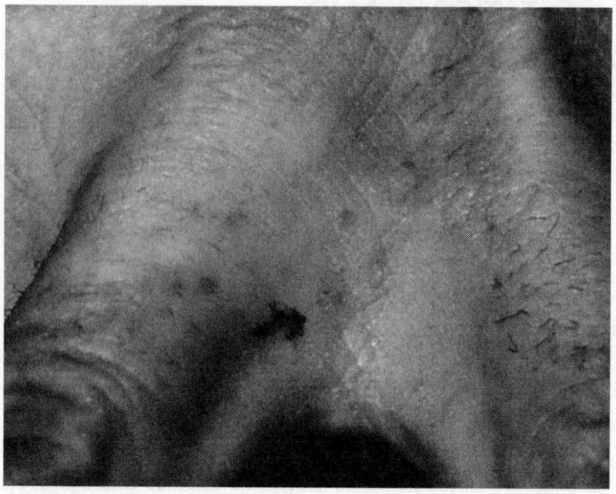

Fig. 7-6
Scabies burrow. (Courtesy Stephen B. Tucker, MD, Department of Dermatology, University of Texas Health Science Center at Houston, Tex.)

Pathophysiology

The impregnated female mite burrows into the stratum corneum and forms a small tunnel that is seen as a fine, wavy, dark line. The burrow is a few millimeters to 1 cm long with a minute papule at the open end. The mite extends the burrow daily and deposits eggs and feces in it (Fig. 7-6).

The lesions are at first asymptomatic. After several weeks the person becomes sensitized to the mite and itching becomes noticeable. The itching is intense and more severe at night. The itching intensifies over a period of several weeks. The burrows and papules are often obscured by secondary excoriation, bacterial infection, crusting, and lichenification. A fine rash is present that consists of papules of various sizes.

Diagnostic Studies and Findings

Physical examination: Burrows; nonspecific excoriations; papules with characteristic distribution; intense itching that worsens at night; burrow ink test (BIT): blue or black felt-tipped pen is applied to suspected lesions and partially removed with alcohol pad; ink is retained in the burrows
Scrapings: Taken from burrow and placed in oil; presence of mite on microscopic examination

Multidisciplinary Plan

Medications

Antiinfective agents
Permethrin cream 5% (Elimite) applied to entire body and left on 18-24 h and then washed off; lacks systemic toxicity

Benzyl benzoate topical emulsion 20%-25% applied to entire cutaneous surface from neck down; left on 12-24 h and then washed off; procedure repeated after 2 days; third treatment may be necessary in 2 weeks

Lindane (Kwell) 1% cream or lotion applied according to above instructions; not used for young children because of neurotoxicity; not recommended during pregnancy

Sulfur ointment 5%-10% applied nightly for 3 nights, with previous applications washed off before new application; washed off thoroughly 24 h after final application; used for infants

Crotamiton (Eurax) 10% applied with benzyl benzoate; less irritating than benzyl benzoate; repeat nightly for 3-5 nights

Corticosteroids

Fluorinated corticosteroid ointment 1% applied topically bid, tid, or qid for persistent itching

General Management

Clothing and linens washed and dried on hot cycles; personal articles sealed in a plastic bag for 10 days

NURSING CARE

NURSING ASSESSMENT

Lesion: Linear gray-brown burrows a few millimeters in length; excoriation; secondary infection; crusting; papules; vesicles; lichenification

Local response to infestation: Intense itching out of proportion to visible signs; itching worse at night

Psychosocial concerns: Concern that others may react to transmissible infestation; assess for defining characteristics: low self-esteem

POTENTIAL COMPLICATIONS

Secondary infection from scratching, neurotoxicity from lindane

PATIENT PROBLEMS/NURSING DIAGNOSES & INTERVENTIONS

NIC SKIN/WOUND MANAGEMENT

Impaired skin integrity related to mechanical factors

- Isolate patient until treatment is completed *to prevent transmission.*
- Instruct patient in meticulous hand washing and good hygiene *to avoid secondary infection.*
- Have patient's fingernails cut short *to avoid excoriation from scratching.*
- Instruct patient in use of treatment lotion; all skin surfaces except face must be covered.

NIC RISK MANAGEMENT

Risk for infection related to close personal contact

- Have all family members and sexual partners treated.
- Have patient notify sexual contacts.
- Instruct patient and family in modes of infestation and transmission.

NIC COPING ASSISTANCE

Situational low self-esteem related to negative self-appraisal

- Prepare patient and family for potential reaction of others to transmissible infestation.
- Encourage patient to express feelings about the infestation, embarrassment, or fear of rejection by others *to begin the process of realistic self-evaluation.*
- Assure patient and family that infestation can be treated successfully.

PATIENT EDUCATION/CONTINUUM OF CARE PLAN

1. Explain to the patient and family that treatment irritates the skin and does not quickly reduce the pruritus; discomfort may persist for a few weeks.
2. Demonstrate the use of cool soaks and compresses to reduce itching after treatment is complete.
3. Stress the importance of the correct use of treatment lotion to avoid neurotoxicity and undue irritation.
4. Advise that all family members and sexual partners be treated.

EVALUATION/PATIENT OUTCOMES

Skin/Wound Management: Infestation is cleared in patient and affected family members and partners. No new papules, burrows, or areas of itching develop. Lesions heal. Excoriations resolve. Skin is intact. Secondary infection is resolved or avoided. Lesions heal without redness, swelling, crusts, or pus.

Risk Management: Infestation does not spread to seemingly unaffected family members or sexual partners. Exposed persons do not develop symptoms of infestation, or they seek treatment if symptoms develop.

Coping Assistance: Patient evaluates self realistically. Patient verbalizes positive feelings about self.

ARACHNID AND HYMENOPTERA BITES

Arachnids are ticks, spiders, and scorpions; hymenoptera are bees, wasps, yellow jackets, and ants. Their bites cause toxic and allergic reactions as a result of the injection of a venom or toxin.

Tick Bites. Tick bites are common in woods and fields throughout the United States. The tick attaches itself to a passing animal or person and after biting remains attached to the skin for several days or longer. Ticks transmit Rocky Mountain spotted fever, Q fever, relapsing fever, and Lyme disease. (See Chapter 15.) The tick bite is initially painless but begins to itch after several days. Infiltration and erythema develop around the bite with formation of firm, discrete, intensely pruritic nodules that may be present for several months or longer.

Systemic symptoms attributed to a toxin include fever, malaise, headache, and abdominal pain. Several species of ticks inject a salivary neurotoxin that causes paralysis. Paresthesia and pain in the lower extremities, weakness, and incoordination develop. The condition may progress to respiratory failure and death from bulbar involvement. Symptoms clear dramatically once the tick is removed.

Spider Bites.

The most important spider bites are caused by the black widow and brown recluse spiders. The black widow is common throughout the United States and southern Canada. It lives in old lumber, unused sheds, and outdoor toilets and may be found in attics, drawers, and closets. Only the female bites and only in self-defense. The female is recognized by her coal black coloring with an hourglass-shaped red or orange marking on the underside of the abdomen.

The black widow bite results from the injection of a neurotoxic venom through a clawlike appendage. The bite, which may go unnoticed, is felt as a pinprick followed by a dull numbing pain. Local necrosis may cause a small ulcer at the site. Within 10 to 60 minutes muscle spasms occur locally and then spread to include all extremities and the trunk. Excruciating pain is felt in waves. The attack subsides after several hours.

Systemic symptoms may include restlessness, vertigo, sweating, chills, pallor, hyperactive reflexes, hypertension, tachycardia, thready pulse, nausea and vomiting, headache, eyelid edema, urticaria, pruritus, and fever. Ascending paralysis, severe hypotension, circulatory collapse, convulsions, and death may result. Mortality is less than 1%.

The brown recluse spider is common in the south-central United States and is usually found in dark areas such as drawers and closets. It commonly bites people when they are asleep. The spider is small and light to dark brown, with a light violin-shaped mark on its head. The female is more dangerous than the male. Most bites occur between April and October.

Brown recluse venom is coagulotoxic. Pain and local symptoms develop 2 to 8 hours after the bite. Localized vasconstriction causes ischemic necrosis at the site. The area is red with blisters and blebs surrounded by ischemia. After several days the center becomes dark and hard. After 2 weeks it becomes depressed, demarcated, and necrotic, and a large open ulcer forms. The ulcer may take several weeks to heal and may require grafting.

Systemic symptoms include fever, chills, malaise, weakness, arthralgia, nausea, vomiting, petechiae, hemolysis, and thrombocytopenia.

Scorpion Bites.

Scorpions are found throughout the United States but are most common in the southern United States and Mexico. The two deadly species are found in the southwest United States.

Scorpions are nocturnal and photophobic. They sting by means of a hooked caudal stinger that discharges venom. Most stings occur during the warmer months. Nonlethal bites cause local swelling, tenderness, pain, a sharp burning sensation, skin discoloration, paresthesia, regional lymphadenopathy, and, rarely, anaphylaxis. Lethal bites are neurotoxic and result in pain, hyperesthesia followed by hypoesthesia, drowsiness, itching of the nose, mouth, and throat, slurred speech, incontinence, vomiting, and convulsions. Symptoms last 24 to 48 hours. Death may follow cardiovascular or respiratory failure. Mortality is less than 1%.

Bee, Wasp, Hornet, Yellow Jacket, and Ant Stings.

All female Hymenoptera have an egg-laying organ (stinger) that can be used for defense or offense. The venom of bees, hornets, wasps, and yellow jackets contains four to six distinct chemical compounds, each of which can produce an allergic reaction. The venoms of all stinging Hymenoptera are closely related and therefore cross-sensitizing.

Local reactions include swelling, pain, erythema, urticaria, and pruritus. Generalized allergic reactions include nausea, vomiting, diarrhea, urticaria, pruritus, and anaphylaxis, with shortness of breath, tightness in the chest, difficulty swallowing, anxiety, convulsions, or unconsciousness. Delayed reaction (serum sickness) occurs 1 to 4 weeks after the sting and is characterized by fever, malaise, lymphadenopathy, rash, urticaria, and arthralgia.

PATHOPHYSIOLOGY

The local or systemic response to injection of a venom occurs as a result of direct action of the venom on susceptible cells, IgE-mediated humoral immune response (type I), and immune complex humoral response (type III).

The arthropod or Hymenoptera venom is toxic to all humans. The biologically active venom works directly on susceptible cells (such as nerve cells and blood cells). The protein component of the venom may contain enzymes that cause cell lysis, histamine release, anticoagulation, or interference with neuromuscular transmission.

The IgE-mediated immune response occurs in people who are sensitive to the protein component of the venom, which acts as an antigen. These individuals have come in contact with the allergen in the past and have become sensitized rather than immunized. Sensitization triggers the synthesis of specific antiallergenic IgE antibodies. On subsequent contact with the allergen the person responds with a type I immune reaction.

IgE immunoglobulins are bound to mast cells and basophils. Mast cells are found in all body tissues, close to blood vessels, and in abundance in the skin. Basophils circulate as leukocytes in the blood. Both mast cells and basophils contain potent pharmacologically active substances such as histamine, bradykinin, serotonin, and other vasoactive amines. The venom (antigen) becomes bound to the IgE on the surface of the cell, creating degranulation of the cell that releases the active agents. These mediators cause increased vascular permeability and smooth muscle contraction. Histamine seems to be the most important agent. Its release causes peripheral vasodilation, increased permeability of capillaries with subsequent loss of plasma from the circulation, smooth muscle constriction (as in the bronchi), and increased mucous gland secretion. If the agents remain confined to the area of the bite, the tissue reaction remains localized (local anaphylaxis) with tissue swelling, wheal formation, and itching. If the mediators are released systemically, systemic anaphylaxis (anaphylactic shock) may result. The widespread response to histamine release causes profound bronchoconstriction and vasodilation with subsequent circulatory collapse. The severity of the reaction depends on the amount of the sensitizing dose, the amount and distribution of the IgE antibodies, and the dose of toxin that causes the reaction.

A type III (immune complex) reaction, or serum sickness, can develop 1 to 3 weeks after the antigen is injected. The antigen initiates an immune response, and antibodies are formed. The response is mediated by IgG or IgM and complement. The immune complexes are deposited in joints, blood vessels, kidneys, and the heart. Platelet aggregation is caused by the collection of immune complexes and complement along blood vessel walls. Anaphylatoxins are released during activation of the complement system, causing a severe inflammatory response.

Diagnostic Studies and Findings

Physical examination: Puncture wound with characteristic symptoms
Complete blood count: Eosiniphilia in type I reaction
Direct immunofluorescence: Presence of antigen, immunoglobulin, or complement in type III reaction

Multidisciplinary Plan

Surgery

Skin grafting: Split-thickness graft to close necrotic ulcers

Medications

For anaphylaxis

Bronchodilators

Epinephrine (Adrenalin), 1:1000 for allergic reactions, 0.3-0.5 ml subcutaneously or IM for mild or severe reactions repeated q5-20 min as needed; 0.1-0.2 ml subcutaneously injected into site to decrease absorption of antigen; 0.25-0.5 ml IV in 10 ml saline solution repeated in 5-10 min for severe anaphylaxis with cardiovascular involvement

Epinephrine 1:200 aqueous suspension, 0.3 ml subcutaneously; long-acting for severe reactions without cardiovascular involvement after edema has subsided

Aminophylline (Aminodur, Lixaminol, Phyllocontin, Somopyllin) for bronchospasm, 6 mg/kg IV over 10-20 min followed by 0.5 mg/kg/h IV

Antihistamines: Diphenhydramine (Benadryl), 50-100 mg IV

Adrenergic agents

Isoproterenol (Isuprel, Drafylin, Nophyl, Triphylline), 1 mg diluted in 500 ml D_5W infused at rate of 0.5-1 ml/min for myocardial insufficiency

Vasoconstrictors for prolonged hypotension

Norepinephrine (Levophed, levarterenol), 8-12 mg/min IV of 4 mg/ml dilution, titrated

Metaraminol (Aramine), 15-100 mg/500 ml D_5W IV, titrated, for adults; 0.4 mg/kg IV for children

Corticosteroids: Hydrocortisone, 100 mg IV for prolonged symptoms

Oral antihistamines: Diphenhydramine (Benadryl), 25-50 mg PO qid for mild reaction

For toxins

Antivenin: 1 ampule IV in 10-50 ml saline solution for black widow and scorpion bites

Anticonvulsant muscle relaxants

Calcium gluconate 10%, 10 ml IV slowly q4h

Methocarbamol (Forbaxin, Robaxin, others), 300 mg/min IV to total of 3 g/day

Orphenadrine (Flexon, Flexoject, Norflex, others), 60 mg IV q12h

For convulsions from scorpion bites: phenobarbital, 30-60 mg/min IV up to 600 mg

Corticosteroids: Dexamethasone (Decadron, Hexadrol), 4 mg IM q6h for brown recluse spider bites during acute phase, then in decremental doses

Antihistamines: Diphenhydramine (Benadryl), 25-50 mg PO qid

Antiinfective agents: Bacitracin or Neosporin applied tid or qid as topical antibiotic for brown recluse spider bite

Immunologic agents: Tetanus prophylaxis as indicated with tetanus toxoid, 0.5 ml IM

Intravenous infusion with D_5W or lactated Ringer's solution

General Management

Scraping to remove stinger if present; do not squeeze or pinch because retained venom sacs discharge residual venom
Application of meat tenderizer paste (containing proteolytic enzyme) to sting site
Hospitalization for observation or ventilator support
Prevention (see Patient Education/Continuum of Care Plan)

NURSING CARE

Nursing Assessment

Local response: Presence or absence of stinger; pain, itching; edema; blister; ulcerations; tissue necrosis. Discomfort
Systemic response: Anxiety, feeling of doom, fever, malaise
Respiratory response: Respiratory distress, tightness in chest, shortness of breath, wheezing, dyspnea
Cardiovascular response: Tachycardia, bradycardia, hypotension, imperceptible pulse, pallor
Musculoskeletal response: Cramping, pain, rigidity, weakness
Gastrointestinal response: Nausea, vomiting, diarrhea, cramping, constipation
Skin: Flushing, diffuse erythema, urticaria, pruritus
Delayed response: From 1 to 4 weeks after sting, fever, malaise, lymphadenopathy, arthralgia, rash, urticaria
Psychosocial concerns: Concern about body image as a result of disfigurement, depending on severity of tissue damage; fear of insects, spiders, bees, and scorpions

Potential Complications

Allergic reaction (local or generalized), secondary infection, serum sickness, tissue necrosis from spider bites, death

Patient Problems/Nursing Diagnoses & Interventions

NIC Respiratory Management

Ineffective breathing pattern related to tracheobronchial obstruction

- Maintain airway.
- In collaboration with physician, perform oropharyngeal suctioning as needed *to clear secretions.*
- Provide oxygen by cannula or mask.
- Position for ease of respiration.
- Administer drugs as indicated *for control of symptoms.*

NIC Tissue Perfusion Management

Decreased cardiac output related to mechanical factors; deficient fluid volume related to failure of regulatory mechanisms

- Monitor vital signs *to detect circulatory compromise.*
- Initiate intravenous line in collaboration with physician *to provide vascular access for fluids and medications.*
- Administer drugs as indicated *to control symptoms.*

NIC Skin/Wound Management

Impaired skin integrity related to chemical substance

- Apply meat tenderizer paste *to neutralize venom.*
- Apply ice packs to decrease pain and swelling and *to limit venom absorption.*
- Keep patient quiet *to limit venom circulation.*
- Remove stinger by scraping *to prevent further discharge of retained venom by squeezing.*
- Remove tick; do not pull because head and mouth may remain embedded; apply heat to body and tick will back out, or cover with oil, *which blocks its breathing and causes it to withdraw.*
- Clean bite with antiseptic *to prevent infection.*
- Clean brown recluse bite with 1:20 Burow's solution *to prevent infection.*

NIC Physical Comfort Promotion

Acute pain related to biologic factors

- Apply ice packs to area *to reduce swelling.*
- Apply meat tenderizer *to neutralize venom.*

NIC Coping Assistance

Fear (of arachnids and Hymenoptera) related to environmental stimuli

Disturbed body image related to cognitive-perceptual factors

- Encourage patient to express fears.
- Help patient develop preventive measures (see under Patient Education).
- Encourage patient to express feelings about body, body appearance, or fear of reaction or rejection by others *to begin process of realistic self-evaluation.*
- Reassure patient with disfiguring ulcer that skin grafting can improve appearance.

Patient Education/Continuum of Care Plan

1. Explain to patients who are sensitive to stings the need to carry an emergency kit that has an antihistamine and epinephrine.
2. Teach the patient, a family member, or a friend how to inject epinephrine.
3. Explain to patients who are sensitive to stings to wear or carry medical alert information and identification.
4. Refer the patient to an allergist for desensitization.
5. Explain to the patient how to remove ticks and stingers.
6. Discuss with the patient and family preventive measures such as wearing protective clothing when outdoors, spraying areas of spider infestation with creosote every 2 months, inspecting clothing before putting it on in infested areas, not wearing bright colors or scents that attract bees when outdoors, and inspecting pets and people for ticks after a visit to a tick-infested area.
7. Instruct patient/family in correct procedure of removing stinger or tick.
8. Encourage the patient and family to keep the site of the bite clean by washing two or three times daily with warm soapy water or water with hydrogen peroxide; apply antibiotic ointment as needed.
9. Demonstrate how to change the dressing if needed.
10. Assist patient in process of skin grafting if needed for resolution of spider bite wound.

Evaluation/Patient Outcomes

Respiratory Management: Respirations are regular and easy.

Tissue Perfusion Management: Systemic response is avoided or resolved. Cardiovascular, neurologic, musculoskeletal, or gastrointestinal symptoms are avoided or resolved. Pulse rate is 60 to 100 beats/min and regular. Blood pressure is within patient's usual limits. Reflexes, sensation, and motion are intact. Patient has urinary continence and bowel function.

Skin/Wound Management: Local toxic reaction is minimized. Stinger or tick is removed correctly, and treatment is initiated immediately. Areas of ulceration and necrosis are limited. There is no malaise, fever, lymphadenopathy, arthralgia, rash, or urticaria after delayed response. Lesions heal. Areas of necrosis, ulceration, and blistering reepithelialize. Skin is intact and free of infection.

Physical Comfort Promotion: Pain is alleviated.

Coping Assistance: Psychosocial concerns are addressed. Patient expresses feelings about body appearance. Patient with disfiguring ulcer has opportunity to seek surgical interventions. Patient expresses fears about arachnids and hymenoptera. Patient discusses preventive measures.

Lesions Caused by Beetles and Caterpillars

Toxic reactions to beetles and caterpillars occur from contact with the toxin on the skin.

Blister beetles produce local irritation and blistering if they are crushed while on the skin surface. Damage to the beetle causes release of a toxic substance in the insect's body fluids.

More than 50 species of caterpillars possess spines that contain a venom capable of producing dermatitis on human skin. These caterpillars are widely distributed throughout the United States and Canada. Contact with the venom occurs from direct contact with the insect or its nest or from wind-blown hairs. Papular lesions or urticaria may develop at the site or elsewhere on the body. The venom produces a stinging sensation followed by swelling and erythema. Symptoms can occur systemically, depending on the species and the amount of venom the person receives. Painful and persistent nodules are formed if the toxin comes in contact with the conjunctiva.

PATHOPHYSIOLOGY

The venom produces a direct toxic response to human tissue. The caterpillar's venom is biologically active and causes histamine release, anticoagulation, fibrinolysis, and plasminogen activity. The toxins are capable of producing impaired cellular activity or cellular destruction.

DIAGNOSTIC STUDIES AND FINDINGS

Physical examination: Lesion consistent with history of beetle or caterpillar contact

MULTIDISCIPLINARY PLAN

Medications

Corticosteroids

Topical corticosteroid for skin inflammation; hydrocortisone 1% applied tid

Ophthalmic corticosteroid and analgesic for eye injury; Cortisporin ophthalmic solution, 1-2 drops qid

NURSING CARE

NURSING ASSESSMENT

Local reaction: Pain, swelling, blister, papule, urticaria, necrosis

Systemic reaction: Widespread papular lesions, urticaria

POTENTIAL COMPLICATIONS

Systemic symptoms, secondary infection

PATIENT PROBLEMS/NURSING DIAGNOSES & INTERVENTIONS

NIC SKIN/WOUND MANAGEMENT

Impaired skin integrity related to chemical factors

- Flush skin with copious amounts of water and scrub gently with soap and water *to remove toxin.*
- Irrigate eye with copious amounts of normal saline solution *to remove toxin.*

PATIENT EDUCATION/CONTINUUM OF CARE PLAN

1. Instruct the patient to avoid crushing beetles.
2. Teach the patient how to flush the skin and eye.
3. Teach the patient to keep the site clean by washing two or three times a day with soap and water.
4. Show the patient how to use eyedrops.

EVALUATION/PATIENT OUTCOMES

Skin/Wound Management: Lesions heal. Urticaria, blisters, or papules resolve. Necrotic areas reepithelialize. Pain is alleviated. Skin is intact and free of infection. Eye symptoms or visual disturbances resolve.

LESIONS CAUSED BY FLEAS, FLIES, AND MOSQUITOES

Toxic reactions to fleas, flies, and mosquitoes occur as a result of saliva that is injected during feeding.

Fleas. Any of the human or domestic animal fleas will attack humans. Adult fleas are attracted to moving objects and leap to attack them. Thus flea bites are often found on the ankles or lower legs. The bites are characteristically found in groups of three on the ankles, legs, or waist. The flea penetrates the skin, feeds, and then crawls to a higher location until stopped by constrictive clothing.

A flea bite usually results in a small wheal with a hemorrhagic puncture at the center. In susceptible persons the flea bite produces larger wheals, urticaria, intensely pruritic papules, bullae, and small necrotic ulcers. Flea bites are usually harmless but can produce a severe reaction in sensitive persons.

Flies. There are innumerable biting flies in the United States. Most common are the blackflies, houseflies, deer flies, gadflies, and dog or stable flies. Most flies feed during the day or at dusk and attack in swarms on exposed parts of the body, such as the face, neck, and arms. Fly-transmitted tularemia occurs in the central and western United States.

Fly bites are painful and pruritic for several days. Urticaria may occur as a result of a protein in the fly's saliva.

Mosquitoes. Mosquitoes are important because they transmit viral encephalitis, dengue fever, yellow fever, malaria, and filariasis. Lesions are produced on the skin when the mosquito feeds and deposits droplets of saliva. These lesions commonly occur on exposed areas of the hands, arms, face, and legs.

Mosquitoes are attracted by lights, dark clothing, and the presence of warm-blooded creatures. In most species the female mosquito is the bloodsucking biter.

The usual mosquito bite produces transient local irritation and pruritic erythematous papules. Large numbers of bites can produce intense pruritus. Urticaria and serum sickness can develop in sensitive people.

PATHOPHYSIOLOGY

For an explanation of toxic reactions and antigen-antibody reactions, see p. 460.

DIAGNOSTIC STUDIES AND FINDINGS

Physical examination: Puncture wound with characteristic symptoms

MULTIDISCIPLINARY PLAN

For treatment of systemic reactions see p. 461

Medications

Corticosteroids: Glucocorticoid ointment (e.g., hydrocortisone 1%) with 0.5% menthol and 0.5% phenol applied topically to lesion q1-2h

Antiinfective agents

Topical antibiotic agents: Bacitracin or Neosporin applied qd or bid

General Management

Prevention (see Patient Education)

NURSING CARE

NURSING ASSESSMENT

Local response: Puncture wound with any of the following: pain, pruritus, wheal, urticaria, erythematous papule, bullae, or small necrotic ulcer; secondary infection; pain, swelling, tenderness, exudate

Systemic response: See p. 461.

Serum sickness: Fever, malaise, lymphadenopathy, arthralgia, rash, urticaria

POTENTIAL COMPLICATIONS

Secondary infection; serum sickness; viral encephalitis (mosquito transmission); dengue fever, yellow fever, malaria, and filariasis (mosquito transmission)

PATIENT PROBLEMS/NURSING DIAGNOSES & INTERVENTIONS

NIC SKIN/WOUND MANAGEMENT

Impaired skin integrity related to chemical and mechanical factors

- Apply ice to puncture wound *to decrease pain and swelling.*
- Instruct patient to trim fingernails *to decrease damage and prevent secondary infection from scratching.*
- Instruct patient in good hygiene and hand washing *to prevent secondary infection.*
- Instruct patient in personal and prophylactic environmental control (see under Patient Education).

PATIENT EDUCATION/CONTINUUM OF CARE PLAN

1. Discuss with the patient how to keep the lesion clean by washing two or three times a day with soap and water.
2. Teach the patient how to change the dressing for infected lesions.
3. Explain to the patient the correct use of appropriate insect repellents:
   a. For flies: Repellent should contain at least 20% N,N-diethyltoluamide (DEET); reapply every 1 to 2 hours or after swimming.
   b. For mosquitoes: Repellent should contain at least 20% N,N-diethyl-m-toluamide, or dimethyl phthalate; reapply every 1 to 2 hours or after swimming. Use caution in employing DEET around young children or persons allergic to it.
4. Instruct in use of appropriate protective clothing.
5. Explain to the patient the control of fleas in the environment and on animals.
   a. Environment: Apply insect growth regulator [methoprene (Precor)] as spray or fogger plus an insecticide such as pyrethrin, lindane 1%, or malathion 1%; use according to the instructions on the container; vacuum the house 1 to 2 times/week.
   b. Animals: Use topical application or oral agent of product such as fipronil (Frontline, TopSpot), imdoclopid (Advantage), or selmectin (Revoluation); use according to instructions.
6. Instruct patient/family in infected areas to observe for signs and symptoms of viral encephalitis (headache, fever, disorientation) and to seek care immediately.
7. Instruct international travelers to obtain appropriate chemoprophylaxis for mosquito-transmitted disease and to observe appropriate preventive measures.

EVALUATION/PATIENT OUTCOMES

Skin/Wound Management: Lesions heal. Puncture wound resolves. Pain disappears. Skin is intact and free of infection. Systemic responses resolve. There is no fever, malaise, lymphadenopathy, arthralgia, rash, or urticaria. Cardiovascular, neurologic, gastrointestinal, and musculoskeletal symptoms are also resolved. Patient takes precautionary measures and uses environmental control. No new lesions occur.

DERMATITIS

ECZEMATOUS DERMATITIS (ECZEMA)

Eczematous dermatitis is a superficial inflammation of the skin characterized by vesicles, redness, edema, oozing, crusting, scaling, and itching.

Eczematous dermatitis is a reaction pattern of the skin. Several forms of dermatitis occur, including primary contact dermatitis, allergic contact dermatitis, atopic dermatitis, diaper dermatitis, and seborrheic dermatitis. The common feature of the various forms is the breakdown of the epidermis, usually as a result of intracellular vesiculation. Eczematous dermatitis is the model for understanding the other forms of dermatitis. The treatments are similar, and the nursing care is virtually the same. Individual differences are identified in the following discussion when appropriate.

PATHOPHYSIOLOGY

Eczematous dermatitis can be classified as acute, subacute, or chronic. The skin responds to a wide variety of noxious stimuli with a limited number of changes, including vasodilation, edema of the upper dermis, inflammatory cell infiltration of the upper dermis and epidermis, and breakdown of epidermal cells. Vesicles or bullae form when fluid accumulates between epidermal cells (spongiosis) or when there are changes within the cell itself.

The result of this inflammatory process is a skin surface that is erythematous (from vasodilation), edematous, exudative, or eroded (from vesicle formation), and crusted or scabbed (from infection or an accumulation of serous exudate). Thickening and scaling occur from attempted or exaggerated repair effort (hyperkeratosis or parakeratosis).

Table 7-1 summarizes the clinical features and changes occurring in eczematous dermatitis. Acute dermatitis becomes subacute as it heals, as a result of either treatment or natural repair processes. Subacute eczematous dermatitis can resolve or become chronic if exposure to noxious stimuli persists. Acute, subacute, and chronic eczematous dermatitis may occur simultaneously.

DIAGNOSTIC STUDIES AND FINDINGS

See discussion of contact dermatitis, atopic dermatitis, and seborrheic dermatitis.

Physical examination: Characteristic eruption; history congruent with specific forms of eczematous dermatitis

MULTIDISCIPLINARY PLAN

Table 7-2 summarizes the specific treatment measures for the different classes of eczematous dermatitis.

Medications

Antipruritic agents

Antihistamines

Cyproheptadine (cyproheptadine, Periactin), 12-16 mg/d PO in divided doses

Trimeprazine (Temaril), 2.5 mg PO qid

Hydroxyzine (Atarax, Vistaril), 25-100 mg PO tid or qid

Corticosteroids

Systemic: Prednisone, 40-80 mg PO in divided doses; dosage depends on severity of condition

Topical ointment:

Hydrocortisone (Cort-Dome, others) 1% tid or qid for mild eczema

Betamethasone valerate (Valisone) 0.1% tid or qid for mild eczema

Triamcinolone 0.1% (Aristocort A, Kenalog) bid or tid for moderate eczema

Fluticasone propionate 0.05% (Cutivate) qd or bid for moderate eczema

Fluocinolone acetonide 0.025% (Synalar) bid to qid for moderate eczema

Fluocinonide 0.05% (Lidex) bid to qid for severe eczema; avoid prolonged use

Antiinfective agents

Systemic: For secondary infection; specific drug and dosage depend on infecting organism and severity of condition

Topical antibacterials

Bacitracin or Neosporin applied tid or qid

Mupirocin 2% (Bactroban) applied tid

Topical antifungals: Nystatin (Mycostatin, Nilstat, others), miconazole (Monistat-Derm), or clotrimazole (Lotrimin, Mycelex), applied bid

Keratolytics

Salicylic acid, 3%-5% added to topical corticosteroid

Urea, 10%-20% added to topical corticosteroids

General Management

Wet Burow's dressings, saline solution, and plain water dressings; occlusive dressings; oil-in-water compresses; hydration

See pp. 500-502

NURSING CARE

NURSING ASSESSMENT

Local responses

Eruption: Clinical features as described in Table 7-1; discomfort

Secondary infection: Purulent drainage, fever, tenderness, regional lymphadenopathy

Psychosocial concerns: Concern with body image; inability to sleep because of pruritus; perception of personal appearance

Table 7-1 Clinical Features and Changes in Eczematous Dermatitis

	Acute	Subacute	Chronic
Clinical features	Erythema; exudate; weeping vesicles; crusts; pruritus	Less erythema; involuting vesicles; excoriation; some scaling; pruritus	Dryness; scaling; lichenification; pruritus
Microscopic changes	Vasodilation; edema; inflammatory infiltrates; spongiotic vesicles	Less vasodilation, inflammatory infiltrates, and vesiculation; parakeratosis; hyperkeratosis; acanthosis	Hyperkeratosis; no frank vesicles; acanthosis

Table 7-2 Summary of Treatments for Eczematous Dermatitis

	Acute	Subacute	Chronic
Chemotherapeutic	Antihistamines; systemic corticosteroids; topical corticosteroids (water miscible); topical antibacterials; topical antifungals	Topical corticosteroids in emollient base	Keratolytic agents; tars; topical corticosteroids
Supportive	Wet dressings (Burow's solution, saline solution, or tap water)	Oil-in-water compresses; emollient creams	Oil soaks or compresses; occlusive dressings; hydration

POTENTIAL COMPLICATIONS

Secondary infection

PATIENT PROBLEMS/NURSING DIAGNOSES & INTERVENTIONS

NIC SKIN/WOUND MANAGEMENT

Impaired skin integrity related to mechanical factors

- Instruct patient in hand washing and good hygiene *to prevent secondary infection.*
- Instruct patient to cut fingernails short *to decrease trauma and secondary infection.*
- Apply dressings, wet, oil, or occlusive, as indicated (see p. 500).
- Scrub crusted lesions gently with antibacterial soap *to debride.*
- Establish realistic therapeutic regimen with patient *to alleviate patient's frustration.*
- Instruct patient in use of medications.

NIC PHYSICAL COMFORT PROMOTION

Patient problem: Pruritus related to inflammatory process*

- Apply cool compresses for wet skin or oil compresses *for dry skin to soothe itching and discomfort.*
- Instruct patient in use of antipruritics *to relieve itching.*

NIC COPING ASSISTANCE

Disturbed body image related to cognitive-perceptual factors

- Encourage patient to express feelings about body, body appearance, or fear of reaction or rejection by others *to begin process of realistic self-evaluation.*
- Encourage development of other interests *so skin condition does not become focal point of patient's existence.*

PATIENT EDUCATION/CONTINUUM OF CARE PLAN

1. Demonstrate the application of compresses, soaks, and scrubs using aseptic technique.
2. Discuss the use and side effects of medications.
3. Explain to the patient and family that successful therapy requires patience, that therapy may be long term, and that results may not be immediate.
4. Discuss the signs and symptoms of secondary infection and the necessity of seeking medical treatment if they occur.

EVALUATION/PATIENT OUTCOMES

Skin/Wound Management: Eruption improves. Erythema, exudate, crusts, dryness, scaling, and pruritus are decreased. Excoriated areas reepithelialize. Secondary infection is avoided. Lesions heal without purulent exudate. Temperature is normal.

Physical Comfort Promotion: Pruritus is alleviated. There are fewer areas of excoriation. Patient is able to sleep.

Coping Assistance: Patient evaluates his or her appearance in a realistic manner. Patient engages in usual activities and relationships.

*Not a NANDA diagnosis.

CONTACT DERMATITIS

Contact dermatitis is an acute or chronic inflammation of the skin caused by external factors (primary irritant dermatitis) or specific sensitizers (allergic contact dermatitis).

Contact dermatitis is a form of eczematous dermatitis (see p. 464). Primary irritant dermatitis is caused by irritation from various chemical and biologic substances, including acids, alkalies, solvents, detergents, oils, salts, secretions, and excretions. Chronic hand dermatitis ("housewife's eczema") and industrial dermatoses are common primary irritant dermatoses. The degree of irritation depends on the physical and chemical characteristics of the substance and the degree and time of exposure. The amount of inflammation varies from person to person and depends on factors such as race, degree and pH of perspiration, type of skin, preexisting disease, and family history. People with little skin pigmentation are more susceptible to the effects of irritants.

Allergic contact dermatitis is a manifestation of delayed hypersensitivity. The allergen is an environmental substance to which the person has become sensitized. Genetically predisposed people and those who have had a previous episode of allergic contact dermatitis are more likely to experience episodes of the disorder. The most common causes of allergic contact dermatitis are chemicals that have a high sensitizing index, including certain plants (tulips and chrysanthemums), plant oils (poison ivy, oak, and sumac), nickel, chrome, rubber, and paraphenylenediamine (an ingredient in many dyes).

The severity of the reaction depends on how long and frequent the contact is. Because allergic contact dermatitis is enhanced by friction and pressure, the addition of these factors to simple exposure produces a more severe reaction.

PATHOPHYSIOLOGY

The irritating substances of primary irritant dermatitis cause damage to the stratum corneum, alter its elasticity, and change the physical features of the skin's lipid film. This impairs the barrier function of the skin and allows absorption of the irritating substance and the subsequent changes of eczematous dermatitis. The basic features of primary irritant dermatitis are the same as those of eczematous dermatitis (see pp. 464-466). The condition can be acute, subacute, or chronic. Primary irritant dermatitis is frequently complicated by secondary bacterial infection.

Allergic contact dermatitis is a cell-mediated, type IV immune response (see Chapter 16). The sensitizing chemical (hapten) enters the epidermis through the stratum corneum and combines with epidermal proteins to form a new molecule (hapten-protein or hapten-carrier complex) that has antigenic potential. This molecule enters the local cutaneous lymphoid tissue, where specific committed lymphocytes are developed and selectively directed against the antigen. Subsequent exposure to the hapten results in release of the committed lymphocytes around the capillary endothelial cells with the development of inflammation and eczematous dermatitis.

Diagnostic Studies and Findings

Physical examination: Characteristic history of contact with irritating or sensitizing substance; detailed history essential

Patch test: Usually positive to allergen in allergic contact dermatitis; should not be performed if patient has active acute dermatitis

Multidisciplinary Plan

Management is directed toward identification and elimination of the precipitating factor.

Medications

Antipruritic agents

Antihistamines

Cyproheptadine (Periactin), 12-16 mg/day PO in divided doses

Trimeprazine (Temaril), 2.5 mg PO qid

Hydroxyzine (Atarax, Vistaril), 25-100 mg PO tid or qid

Corticosteroids

Systemic: Prednisone, 40-80 mg PO in divided doses; dosage depends on severity of condition; tapered over 2-3 weeks

Topical

Hydrocortisone (Cort-Dome, others), 1% tid or qid

Betamethasone diproprionate 0.05% (Diprolene) qd or bid

Antiinfective agents

Systemic (for secondary infection): Specific drug and dosage depend on infecting organism and severity of condition

Topical antibacterials: Bacitracin or Neosporin applied tid or qid

General Management

Tepid tub baths with Aveeno, 1 cup to ½ tub, bid-tid for acute, severe conditions with marked edema and bullae

NURSING CARE

Nursing Assessment

Eruption: Erythema; exudate, vesicles; crusts; scaling; dryness; lichenification; pruritus; location and distribution of eruption; history of eruption; site of initial eruption; history of contact with irritating or sensitizing substances; pattern of flare-ups

Secondary infection: Purulent drainage, fever, tenderness, regional lymphadenopathy

Psychosocial concerns: Concern with body image, inability to sleep

Potential Complications

Secondary infection

Patient Problems/Nursing Diagnoses & Interventions

NIC Skin/Wound Management

Impaired skin integrity related to mechanical factors

- Instruct patient in hand washing and good hygiene *to prevent secondary infection.*
- Instruct patient to cut fingernails short *to decrease trauma and secondary infection.*
- Apply dressings, wet, oil, or occlusive, as indicated (see p. 500).
- Scrub crusted lesions gently with antibacterial soap *to debride.*
- Establish realistic therapeutic regimen with patient *to alleviate patient's frustration.*
- Instruct patient in use of medications.

NIC Physical Comfort Promotion

Patient problem: Pruritus related to inflammatory process*

- Apply cool compresses for wet skin or oil compresses for dry skin *to soothe itching and discomfort.*
- Instruct patient in use of antipruritics *to relieve itching.*

NIC Coping Assistance

Disturbed body image related to cognitive-perceptual factors

- Encourage patient to express feelings about body, body appearance, or fear of reaction or rejection by others *to begin process of realistic self-evaluation.*
- Encourage development of other interests *so skin condition does not become focal point of patient's existence.*

Patient Education/Continuum of Care Plan

1. Discuss with the patient how to eliminate or avoid the precipitating factors.
2. Instruct patient in use of blocking agents (e.g., Ivy Block) for prevention of plant oil contact dermatitis.
3. Instruct patient in use of protective clothing to prevent irritant dermatitis.

Evaluation/Patient Outcomes

Skin/Wound Management: Lesions heal. Precipitating factor is identified and avoided. There are no recurrent episodes of dermatitis.

Physical Comfort Promotion: Pruritus is alleviated. There are fewer areas of excoriation. Patient is able to sleep.

Coping Assistance: Patient evaluates his or her appearance in a realistic manner. Patient engages in usual activities and relationships.

Atopic Dermatitis

Atopic dermatitis is a chronic, superficial, pruritic, inflammatory response of the skin that is often associated with other atopic diseases (asthma, hay fever, and allergic rhinitis).

*Not a NANDA diagnosis.

Atopy refers to a type I immunologic response that is hereditary (see Chapter 16). Patients with atopic dermatitis usually have high serum levels of IgE. Patients with atopic dermatitis experience vasomotor changes, great susceptibility to environmental irritants, and susceptibility to bacterial and viral infections. Atopic dermatitis is associated with ichthyosis and xerosis and with numerous abnormalities of humoral and cell-mediated immunity.

Patients with atopic dermatitis have dry, highly sensitive skin with a lowered threshold to pruritus, so that a minor stimulus causes exaggerated itching. Scratching leads to epidermal breakdown and damage to nerve endings, which in turn increase the itch sensation. This itch-scratch cycle is characteristic of atopic dermatitis.

Atopic dermatitis can begin at any time. There are usually three phases: an infantile phase (age 3 or 4 months to 2 years), the childhood phase (age 4 to 10 or 12 years), and the adolescent and young adult phase. The condition gradually improves. This section addresses only the adolescent and young adult phase.

Pathophysiology

The disease is the result of a type I immunologic response. The findings are the same as those of eczematous dermatitis and may be acute, subacute, or chronic (see discussion of eczematous dermatitis).

There is a great tendency toward vasoconstriction of superficial blood vessels, decreased response to cooling and warmth, increased sweat production in flexor areas, and a blanch phenomenon on stroking (white dermographia). Cold and low humidity are poorly tolerated. Heat and high humidity are also poorly tolerated; vasodilation increases the inflammatory response, thereby aggravating the dermatitis and causing increased itching. Psychologic and emotional factors do not play a causative role but do modify symptoms. Food allergies may exacerbate the skin disease in some patients, and a good history is extremely important.

Diagnostic Studies and Findings

Physical examination: Characteristic eruption with typical distribution; personal or family history of allergies
Immunofluorescence: Serum IgE may be elevated

Multidisciplinary Plan

Atopic dermatitis presents the whole range of the eczematous process from acute to chronic, and treatment must be directed accordingly. The focus of therapy is to interrupt the itch-scratch cycle.

Medications

Corticosteroids
Topical steroids with menthol or camphor 0.25%-0.5% applied bid or tid
Systemic: Prednisone (Deltasone, Orasone, others), 60-80 mg/day as single morning dose for 1-2 weeks only
Keratolytics: Coal tar 3% (Zetar) applied topically at bedtime
Antihistamines
Hydroxyzine (Atarax, Vistaril), 25-100 mg PO tid or qid
Diphenhydramine (Benadryl), 25-50 mg PO tid or qid
Tripelennamine (pyribenzamine, PBZ), 10 mg PO bid or tid
Third-generation multifunction antihistamines (cetrizine [Zyrtec], fexofenadine [Allegra], loratadine [Claritin])
Antiinfective agents: Systemic antibiotics for secondary infection; drug and dosage dependent on causative organism and severity of infection

General Management

Burow's dressings and saline compresses (see p. 500); oatmeal and oil baths (see p. 500); occlusive dressings (see p. 500); allergy diet (controversial); house humidified; light, cotton clothing; UVA-UVB phototherapy; PUVA therapy (see Psoriasis)

NURSING CARE

Nursing Assessment

Eruption: Lichenification, excoriation, subacute papular eruptions, generalized erythema, pruritus
Location: Face, neck, upper chest, flexor surfaces, wrists, feet, upper back, generalized
Special disease manifestations: Chronic hand eczema, nummular eczema (coin-shaped eczematous plaques)
Secondary infection: Purulent drainage, fever, tenderness, regional lymphadenopathy
Psychosocial concerns: Concern with body image, inability to sleep because of pruritus, exacerbations caused by stress

Potential Complications

Secondary infection

Patient Problems/Nursing Diagnoses & Interventions

NIC Skin/Wound Management

Impaired skin integrity related to mechanical factors
- Instruct patient in hand washing and good hygiene *to prevent secondary infection*
- Instruct patient to cut fingernails short *to decrease trauma and secondary infection.*
- Apply dressings, wet, oil, or occlusive, as indicated (see p. 500).
- Scrub crusted lesions gently with antibacterial soap *to debride.*
- Establish realistic therapeutic regimen with patient *to alleviate patient's frustration.*
- Instruct patient in use of medications.

NIC Physical Comfort Promotion

Patient problem: Pruritus related to inflammatory process*
- Apply cool compresses for wet skin or oil compresses for dry skin *to soothe itching and discomfort.*
- Instruct patient in use of antipruritics *to relieve itching.*

*Not a NANDA diagnosis.

NIC COPING ASSISTANCE

Disturbed body image related to cognitive-perceptual factors

- Encourage patient to express feelings about body, body appearance, or fear of reaction or rejection by others *to begin process of realistic self-evaluation.*
- Encourage development of other interests *so skin condition does not become focal point of patient's existence.*

PATIENT EDUCATION/CONTINUUM OF CARE PLAN

1. Discuss with the patient and family that the patient should avoid the following:
   a. Heat, high humidity, and rapid changes of temperature
   b. Sweating
   c. Excessive bathing
   d. Strong soaps and detergents that can irritate skin
   e. Emotional stress
   f. Wools, coarse synthetic fabrics, and tight-fitting clothing
   g. Primary irritants
2. Discuss with the patient and family that the patient should:
   a. Keep skin well lubricated
   b. Wear light, loose, cotton clothing that "breathes"
   c. Bathe in lukewarm, not hot, water
3. Discuss with the patient and family the signs and symptoms of secondary infection and the need to seek medical attention if they occur.
4. Explain to the patient and family that therapy requires patience and results may not be immediate.
5. Teach the adolescent or young adult to manage the skin condition as soon as possible.

EVALUATION/PATIENT OUTCOMES

Skin/Wound Management: Known causative agents are avoided. Eruption subsides. Exacerbations are limited. Excoriations heal. Secondary infection is avoided. Eruption is free from tenderness and purulent exudate. There is no fever or lymphadenopathy.

Physical Comfort Promotion: Pruritus is relieved. Scratching decreases. Patient is able to sleep.

Coping Assistance: Patient assesses appearance in realistic manner. Patient engages in usual relationships and activities when possible.

SEBORRHEIC DERMATITIS

Seborrheic dermatitis is a chronic, recurrent, erythematous scaling eruption that is localized in areas where sebaceous glands are concentrated.

In infants, seborrheic dermatitis may develop on the scalp, back, and intertriginous and diaper areas. The scalp lesions are scaling, adherent, thick, yellow, and crusted. Lesions elsewhere are erythematous, scaling, and fissured.

After puberty lesions tend to occur in the scalp, eyebrows, eyelids, nasolabial areas, postauricular areas, and presternal and intertriginous areas (FIG. 7-7). Lesions may be mild or severe and vary from dry, greasy scales to erythema, excoriation, and crusting. Secondary bacterial or fungal infection may occur. Genetic factors seem to affect the incidence and severity of the disease. The disorder is worse during the winter months.

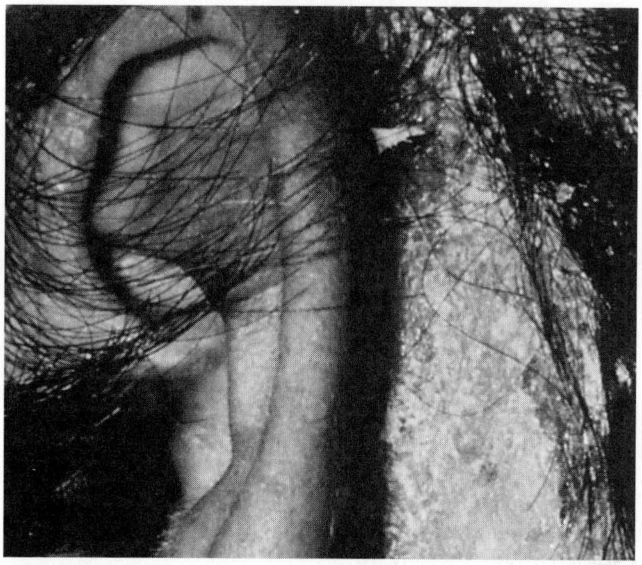

FIG. 7-7
Seborrheic dermatitis. (Courtesy Stephen B. Tucker, MD, Department of Dermatology, University of Texas Health Science Center at Houston, Tex.)

PATHOPHYSIOLOGY

The cause of seborrheic dermatitis is unknown. Histologic changes include vasodilation and discharge of inflammatory cells into the epidermis from the capillary loops. Epidermal inflammation and eczema may be present. Scales are produced as a result of an increased mitotic rate and an accumulation of corneocytes. Despite the name, the composition, production, and flow of sebum are normal.

DIAGNOSTIC STUDIES AND FINDINGS

Physical examination: Characteristic lesions and distribution

MULTIDISCIPLINARY PLAN

Medications

Corticosteroids

Topical

Fluocinolone (Synalar), 0.01% bid
Fluocinonide (Lidex), 0.05% bid
Hydrocortisone (Hytone), 2.5% bid
Betamethasone (Valisone), 0.05% bid in hairy areas

Antiseborrheic shampoos

Coal tar (Denorex, 9%; DHS tar 0.5%; others), 2-3 times/week in the first week, then once weekly as needed; leave on for 5 min before rinsing

Ketaconazole shampoo 2% (Nizoral), use every 3-4 days for up to 8 weeks; leave on 5 min before rinsing
Selenium sulfide (Selsun Blue 1%; others), 2-3 times/week; leave on 2-3 min before rinsing
Pyrithione zinc (Danex 1%; DHS Zinc 2%; others), 2 times/week
Combinations (Sebulex, 2% sulfur, 6% salicylic acid; others) 2 times/week

Antifective agents
Topical antibiotics for secondary infection
Neomycin 0.1% bid or tid
Chloramphenicol (Chloromycetin cream) 0.1% bid to tid

Keratolytics
Salicylic acid 1%-3% topically bid
Precipitated sulfur 1%-5% topically bid
Tar cream 4% topically bid

General Management

Oils: Castor, mineral, and olive, rubbed into scalp lesions and left overnight; frequent shampooing; Burow's solution for weeping lesions

NURSING CARE

NURSING ASSESSMENT

Eruption: Erythema, scaling, fissures, inflammation, pruritus
Secondary infection: Purulent discharge, fever, tenderness, increased inflammation, regional lymphadenopathy
Psychosocial concerns: Concern about body image

POTENTIAL COMPLICATIONS

Secondary infection

PATIENT PROBLEMS/NURSING DIAGNOSES & INTERVENTIONS

NIC SKIN/WOUND MANAGEMENT

Impaired skin integrity related to pathologic process and mechanical factors

- Instruct patient in use of medications and topical preparations.
- Instruct patient to shampoo daily *to alleviate scaling and crusting.*
- Instruct patient not to scratch or rub lesions *because that will prolong course of disease.*

NIC COPING ASSISTANCE

Disturbed body image related to cognitive-perceptual factors

- Encourage patient to express feelings about body, body appearance, or fear of reaction or rejection by others *to begin process of realistic self-evaluation.*
- Assure patient that treatment can be successful.

PATIENT EDUCATION/CONTINUUM OF CARE PLAN

1. Explain to the patient the use of medications and preparations.
2. Explain the care regimen to the patient.
3. Discuss with the patient the signs and symptoms of secondary infection and how to seek medical care if these occur.
4. Explain to the patient to avoid external irritants, excessive heat, and excessive perspiration.

EVALUATION/PATIENT OUTCOMES

Skin/Wound Management: Eruption resolves. Erythema and inflammation disappear. Scaling decreases. Fissures heal. Pruritus is relieved. Skin is intact. Secondary infection is resolved or prevented. There is no purulent discharge, fever, or lymphadenopathy.

Coping Assistance: Patient evaluates his or her appearance in a realistic manner. Patient engages in usual activities and relationships.

HERPES ZOSTER

Herpes zoster is an acute cutaneous vesicular eruption caused by the varicella-zoster virus.

Herpes zoster, also known as shingles, occurs as a result of reactivation of a dormant varicella virus. Reactivation can occur at any time. Older adults and human immunodeficiency virus (HIV)–positive individuals are more likely to develop the condition because of their diminishing immunologic functioning.

The eruption is generally limited to the skin of a single dermatome, although one or two adjacent dermatomes may be involved. Pain, itching, and burning along the dermatome precede the eruption by 4 to 5 days. The pain is often mistaken for pleurisy, myocardial infarction, or appendicitis, and diagnosis may be difficult until the characteristic eruption occurs. The eruption begins with erythematous plaques of various size that involve all or part of a dermatome. Purulent, fluid-filled vesicles arise in clusters from the erythematous base. Successive crops continue to appear for 7 days. The vesicles either involute or rupture and then heal in 10 to 14 days, frequently with residual scarring.

Postherpetic neuralgia, the most common complication, is a dermatomal pain syndrome that persists beyond the time of complete cutaneous healing. Pain can persist in a dermatome for months or years after the lesions have disappeared. Most cases resolve in a few months. The pain is often severe, intractable, and exhausting. The incidence of postherpetic neuralgia increases with the age of the patient.

PATHOPHYSIOLOGY

Herpes zoster occurs as a result of reactivation of the varicella virus that entered the cutaneous nerves during an earlier episode of acute infection with the virus. The virus remains dormant in the sensory root ganglia for the lifetime of the patient and can be reactivated at any time. Reactivation can be triggered by local trauma, acute illness, a compromised immunologic state, fatigue, emotional upsets, or chronic debilitation. Once reactivated, the virus travels down the sensory nerve and infects the skin of the affected ganglion.

Diagnostic Studies and Findings

Physical examination: Characteristic lesion: clusters of painful, itching vesicles along a single dermatome
Cytologic smear: Direct identification of multinucleated cells
Culture: Vesicular fluid to determine presence of virus

Multidisciplinary Plan

Medications

Analgesic agents
ASA (Aspirin), 300 mg PO q4h for mild pain
Acetaminophen (Tylenol, Datril), 250 mg PO q4h for mild pain
NSAIDs for mild pain
Codeine PO in dosages sufficient for more severe pain relief during eruptive phase or for postherpetic neuralgia
Tranquilizers: Chlorpromazine (Thorazine), 25 mg PO qid for severe postherpetic neuralgia
Antiviral agents
Acyclovir (Zovirax), 800 mg PO q4h for 7-10 days during eruptive phase
Acyclovir sodium (Zovirax), 10 mg/kg IV q8h; for immunocompromised patients
Famciclovir (Famvir), 500 mg PO tid for 7 days
Valacyclovir (Valtrex), 1000 mg PO tid for 7 days
Systemic steroids
During eruptive phase for prevention of postherpetic neuralgia; use is controversial[21,23]
Prednisone, 20 mg PO tid for 7 days, followed by 20 mg PO bid for 7 days, followed by 20 mg each morning for 7 days
For postherpetic neuralgia
Capsaicin cream (Zostrix), 0.075%, applied topically
Amitryptyline (Elavil), 75-100 mg PO qd, with perphenazine (Trilafon), 4 mg PO tid-qid, or fluphenazine hydrochloride (Permitil), 1 mg PO tid-qid, or thioridazine (Mellaril), 25 mg PO qid; may be necessary to continue medication for months
Chlorprothixene (Taractan), 25-50 mg PO q6h for 4-10 days
Carbamazepine (Tegretol), 600-800 mg PO qd, with nortriptyline (Pamelor), 500-100 mg PO qd
Intralesional injection of triamcinolone (Aristocort, Kenalog), 0.2 mg/ml daily
Lidocaine 5% or EMLA cream for topical anesthesia

General Management

Cryosurgery (for postherpetic neuralgia): Affected area sprayed with refrigent (Freon, Frigiderm) until blanching occurs, repeated every 2 weeks for three to six treatments; if relief occurs, it is rapid and limited to specific area treated; produces relief in about 50% of affected patients; transcutaneous electric nerve stimulation (TENS) treatments (for postherpetic neuralgia)

Burow's solution tid for symptomatic relief (see table on p. 500).

NURSING CARE

Nursing Assessment

Lesions (eruptive phase): Location and characteristics, crusting, scarring with healing
Secondary infection (eruptive phase): Erythema, swelling, purulent drainage from lesions
Discomfort (eruptive phase): Pain, burning, itching of lesions; intensity
Discomfort (postherpetic phase): Intensity and location, interference with activity

Potential Complications

Postherpetic neuralgia

Patient Problems/Nursing Diagnoses & Interventions

NIC Skin/Wound Management

Impaired skin integrity related to pathologic process and mechanical factors
- Assess for lesion characteristics and location.
- Apply wet compresses with Burow's solution for 20 minutes three times a day *to macerate vesicles, remove serum and crust, and suppress bacterial growth.*
- Assess for secondary infection from scratching.
- Trim fingernails short *to prevent secondary infection.*

NIC Physical Comfort Promotion

Acute pain related to biologic factors
- Assess for pain, itching, and burning during eruptive phase.
- Assess for pain during postherpetic phase.
- As physician directs, provide analgesic medications.
- Provide empathy, understanding, and emotional support for patient with persistent pain.
- Investigate alternate means of pain management with patient and physician (e.g., biofeedback, transcutaneous nerve stimulation).

Patient Education/Continuum of Care Plan

1. Discuss with the patient the course of the disease process.
2. Discuss the correct use of analgesics.
3. Demonstrate the application of wet compresses with Burow's solution (p. 500).

Evaluation/Patient Outcomes

Skin/Wound Management: Eruption improves. Lesions resolve; secondary infection does not occur. Pruritus is alleviated. Areas of excoriation resolve or do not occur.

Physical Comfort Promotion: Pain is relieved. Patient is able to resume usual activities without fear of triggering paroxysms of pain. Patient successfully manages intractable pain. Patient engages in usual activities and maintains interpersonal relationships; patient is not withdrawn or suicidal.

ICHTHYOSIS

Ichthyosis is a common inherited keratinization disorder that is characterized by varying degrees of dryness, scaling, and exfoliation.

Several genetic keratinization abnormalities result in dry, scaly skin. The most common condition is ichthyosis vulgaris, an autosomal dominant inherited disease that occurs in 1 in 1000 people. The other forms of ichthyosis are rarer.

PATHOPHYSIOLOGY

In ichthyosis vulgaris the mitotic rate is decreased and the stratum corneum fails to desquamate normally. The granular layer is reduced or absent, and sweat and sebaceous glands may be reduced. The follicular orifices are hyperkeratotic and are often plugged with keratin. The ability of the stratum corneum to retain water is decreased. Aggravation during the winter months and improvement during the summer are common. The other forms of ichthyosis show similar pathologic changes.

Table 7-3 summarizes the clinical, pathologic, and genetic features of the four patterns of inherited ichthyosis (FIG. 7-8).

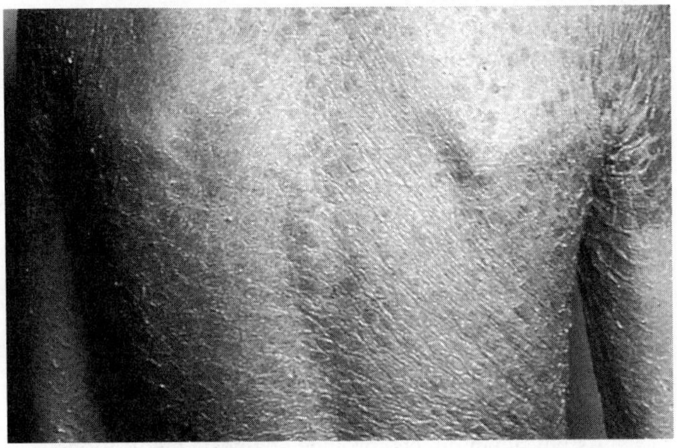

FIG. 7-8

Lamellar ichthyosis. (Courtesy Stephen B. Tucker, MD, Department of Dermatology, University of Texas Health Science Center at Houston, Tex.)

DIAGNOSTIC STUDIES AND FINDINGS

Physical examination: Characteristic lesion

MULTIDISCIPLINARY PLAN

Medications

Emollients: Apply to moist skin bid after bathing
- Propylene glycol 40%-50%
  - Propylene glycol 60%, ethanol 2%, and salicylic acid 6% in gel base under occlusive dressing for 1-4 days and then every third night
- Ammonium lactate 12% (LacHydrin) bid, rubbed in
- Hydrophilic petrolatum
- Water-miscible bath oil

Keratolytics: Apply after bathing to moist skin for 3-7 times/week
- Salicylic acid 5% in emollient base
- Urea 10% in water-miscible base
- Sodium chloride 10% and salicylic acid 5%

Vitamins
- Tretinoin (Retin-A) 0.1% (vitamin A, retinoic acid), applied topically for lamellar ichthyosis
- Oral synthetic retinoids: Etretinate (Tegison), 0.3-0.5 mg/kg/day; up to 0.75 mg/kg/day as tolerated for lamellar ichthyosis

Table 7-3 Summary of Ichthyosis Disorders

Disorder	Inheritance Pattern	Age of Onset	Prognosis	Histopathology	Type of Scale	Distribution
Vulgaris	Dominant	Childhood (1-4 years)	Improves during adult years	Increased mitotic rate; retained stratum corneum; decreased granular layer; plugged follicular orifices	Fine, small, thin, light	Back and extensor surfaces; flexures spared; increased markings on palms and soles
Male, sex linked	Recessive X-linked	Birth	Persistent	As above; increased plugging	Large, brown	Neck and trunk; total extremities; flexures spared; normal markings
Lamellar nonbullous	Recessive	Birth	Persistent	Increased mitotic rate; granular layer present; acanthosis; hyperkeratosis; plugged follicular orifices	Large, coarse, yellow, raised corners	Generalized; thick palms and soles
Bullous epidermolytic hyperkeratoses	Dominant	Birth	Persistent; severe forms may cause death in early infancy from secondary infection	As above; vacuolation of epidermal cells	Thick, gray-brown, coarse, warty, vesicular, and bullous lesions	Patchy or generalized; flexures affected

NURSING CARE

Nursing Assessment

Lesions: Type of scale and distribution as in Table 7-3; severity
Secondary infection: Redness, tenderness, swelling, exudate, odor
Comfort and mobility: Discomfort from dry, cracked skin; limitation on mobility
Psychosocial concerns: Concern about body image; patient's perception of appearance

Potential Complications

Secondary infection

Patient Problems/Nursing Diagnoses & Interventions

NIC Skin/Wound Management

Impaired skin integrity related to biologic and mechanical factors

- Assess for distribution and severity of lesions.
- Instruct patient and parent in use of topical preparations.
- Stress importance of good hygiene *to prevent secondary infection.*

NIC Physical Comfort Promotion

Chronic pain related to physical factors
Impaired physical mobility related to pain and discomfort

- Instruct patient in use of emollients *to decrease dryness.*
- Instruct patient not to use soap or to use it sparingly while bathing *to prevent drying and cracking of skin.*
- Instruct patient to maintain humidity in living environment *to prevent drying and cracking of skin.*

NIC Coping Assistance

Disturbed body image related to cognitive-perceptual factors

- Assess patient's or parent's perception of patient's appearance.
- Encourage patient to express feelings abut body, body appearance, and fear of reaction or rejection by others *to begin process of realistic self-evaluation.*
- Encourage patient to develop interests and other attributes *to support positive self-image, feelings of self-worth, and self-confidence.*
- Help patient evaluate appearance in a realistic manner *so it does not become focal point of existence.*
- Inform parents that condition may improve as child matures.

Patient Education/Continuum of Care Plan

1. Instruct the patient and family in the use of emollients and keratolytics.
2. Instruct the patient in the signs and symptoms of secondary infection and to seek medical care if they occur.
3. Inform the patient and family that successful therapy requires the patient's full cooperation and patience, that therapy is long term, and that results may not be immediate.

Evaluation/Patient Outcomes

Skin/Wound Management: Secondary infection is avoided. There is no redness, tenderness, swelling, or purulent exudate.

Physical Comfort Promotion: Discomfort is relieved. Dryness decreases. Cracks and fissures improve. Limitations on mobility lessen.

Coping Assistance: Patient makes successful adaptations in self-concept. Patient develops interests and participates in activities compatible with degree of mobility. Patient engages in satisfying relationships. Patient does not use disorder as excuse for unsuccessful relationships.

LICHEN PLANUS

Lichen planus is a chronic pruritic inflammatory eruption of the skin and mucous membrane. It is characterized by small angular papules that may combine to form larger plaques.

Lichen planus occurs most frequently in adults. The onset may be gradual or abrupt. The average duration of the disease is 15 to 24 months, but it may persist or recur for years. Healing is followed by residual pigmentation that eventually fades.

Pathophysiology

The cause of lichen planus is unknown. However, certain drugs and chemicals used in developing color photographs can cause an eruption.

Inflammation occurs primarily at the dermal level with lymphocytic infiltrate. There are hyperkeratosis and prominence of the granular layer. Vacuolation, degeneration, and inflammatory changes occur in the basal layer. Fibrin and IgM are deposited in the papillary dermis.

Cutaneous lesions are pruritic, flat-topped, reddish violet, angular papules that are 0.5 to 5 mm in diameter. The papules have a sheen on cross-lighting. Whitish gray lines (Wickham's striae) are seen on the skin. The individual papules can combine to form larger plaques, becoming more scaly and verrucous. The lesions are usually symmetrically distributed and occur most commonly on the flexor surfaces of the wrist, forearm, and ankles and on the abdomen and sacrum. The face, palms, and soles are rarely affected. Eruption can occur at the site of minor trauma (Kobner's phenomenon).

Lesions of the buccal mucosa are present in 50% to 60% of cases. These gray lacy lesions may ulcerate and be painful. Malignant degeneration occurs in about 1 in 100 cases.

Clinical variants of lichen planus include annular, bullous, hypertrophic, and atrophic lesions. Nails can be involved, with pitting, thinning, and increased longitudinal ridging. In severe cases the nail may be shed completely.

Diagnostic Studies and Findings

Physical examination: Characteristic lesion
Biopsy: Characteristic histologic findings
Immunofluorescence: IgG deposits in papillary dermis

MULTIDISCIPLINARY PLAN

Medications

Corticosteroids

Topical

Hydrocortisone (Cort-Dome, others) 0.1% or triamcinolone (Aristocort, Kenalog, others) 0.1% in occlusive dressing at bedtime; must be maintained until all signs of lesions disappear

Triamcinolone 0.1% in dental paste (Kenalog in Orabase), applied q3-5h for mouth lesions

Intralesional injection: Triamcinolone (Aristocort, Kenalog), 5 mg/ml (see p. 502)

Systemic corticosteroids: For very severe or generalized lesions

Prednisone, 40-60 mg/day PO tapered over 2-8 weeks

Clobetasol propionate (Temovate) 0.025% ointment in adhesive paste to yield a 0.25% concentration for oral lesions; under investigation

Vitamins: Tretinoin (Retin-A) 0.1% applied with cotton-tipped applicator at night followed by triamcinolone 0.1% tid

Local anesthetics: Viscous lidocaine (Xylocaine), mouth swish before meals

Antihistamines

Cyproheptadine (Periactin), 4 mg PO tid

Hydroxyzine (Atarax, Vistaril), 25-100 mg PO tid or qid

Diphenhydramine (Benadryl), 25-50 mg PO q6h

General Management

Withdrawal of all current medications and replacement with substitutes

NURSING CARE

NURSING ASSESSMENT

Lesion: Angular papules; bullous, hypertrophic, and atrophic lesions; coalesced plaques; mucosal plaques, or ulceration; distribution of lesions

Discomfort: Pruritus, pain from buccal ulceration

Nutrition: Inability to eat because of buccal ulceration

Psychosocial concerns: Concern with body image

POTENTIAL COMPLICATIONS

Malignant degeneration of oral lesions

PATIENT PROBLEMS/NURSING DIAGNOSES & INTERVENTIONS

NIC SKIN/WOUND MANAGEMENT

Impaired skin integrity related to inflammatory process

Altered oral mucous membrane related to pathologic condition

- Assess for location and characteristics of lesions.
- Instruct patient in good hygiene and need for short fingernails *to prevent secondary infection.*
- Apply cool compresses *to relieve itching.*
- Obstruct patient in use of occlusive dressing (see table on p. 500) *to promote healing.*
- Instruct patient in use of viscous lidocaine (Xylocaine): 15 min before eating, swish in mouth *to promote comfort.*
- Instruct patient to avoid astringent and acidic fluids *to avoid tissue trauma.*
- Provide mouth care with alkaline or saline mouthwash *to promote comfort and prevent infection.*

NIC PHYSICAL COMFORT PROMOTION

Acute pain related to physical factors

- Assess for discomfort.
- Provide soft diet *to prevent mechanical irritation.*
- Provide bland foods *to prevent mechanical irritation.*

PATIENT EDUCATION/CONTINUUM OF CARE PLAN

1. Discuss with the patient the treatment regimen, medications, and dressings.
2. Discuss with the patient the side effects of medications.
3. Teach the patient the signs and symptoms of secondary infection and to seek medical treatment if they occur.
4. Discuss the long-term nature of the disorder and the fact that treatment requires persistence and patience.
5. Discuss with the patient the avoidance of precipitating drugs and chemicals.

EVALUATION/PATIENT OUTCOMES

Skin/Wound Management: Eruption improves. Papules, bullae, and plaques resolve. Ulcerations reepithelialize. Pruritus resolves. Secondary infection does not occur.

Physical Comfort Promotion: Discomfort from buccal lesions is alleviated. Patient is able to eat and does not lose weight. Pruritus is alleviated. Areas of excoriation resolve or do not recur.

PIGMENTED DISORDERS

PIGMENTED NEVI, BLUE NEVI, AND MONGOLIAN SPOTS

Pigmented nevi, blue nevi, and mongolian spots are benign skin lesions that are caused by an accumulation of pigment in the dermis.

Pigmented nevi occur in various forms that vary in size and degree of pigmentation. Nevi are present on most persons and may occur anywhere on the body. They may be flat, slightly raised, dome shaped, smooth, rough, or hairy. Their color ranges from tan, gray, and shades of brown to black.

The blue nevus usually occurs as a single nodular lesion on the dorsal surface of the hands, face, or buttocks. The nevus is present at birth and remains unchanged through life.

Mongolian spots have a dusky blue color and blend into the surrounding normal skin. The spots occur primarily in Asian and dark-skinned infants, usually in the lumbosacral area. The spots vary in diameter from 1 cm to several centimeters. They cause no symptoms and usually disappear during childhood.

Table 7-4 Features and Occurrence of Various Types of Pigmented Nevi

Type	Features	Occurrence	Comments
Halo nevus	Sharp, oval, or circular; depigmented halo around mole; may undergo many morphologic changes; usually disappears and halo repigments (may take years)	Usually on back in young adult	Usually benign; biopsy indicated because same process can occur around melanoma
Intradermal nevus	Dome shaped; raised; flesh to black color; may be pedunculated or hair bearing	Cells limited to dermis	No indication for removal other than cosmetic
Junction nevus	Flat or slightly elevated; dark brown	Nevus cells lining dermoepidermal junction	Should be removed if exposed to repeated trauma
Compound nevus	Slightly elevated brownish papule, indistinct border	Nevus cells in dermis and lining dermoepidermal junction	Should be removed if exposed to repeated trauma
Hairy nevus	May be present at birth; may cover large area; hair growth occurring after several years		Should be removed if changes occur

PATHOPHYSIOLOGY

The lesions occur as the result of nevus cells that migrate to the dermis during embryonic development. The nevus cells have the same origin as melanocytes and are closely associated with them. The nevus cells contain melanin pigment, which give the lesions their color. The blue color of the blue nevus and the mongolian spots is caused by the concentration of melanin and its depth below the epidermis.

Table 7-4 summarizes the features of the various types of pigmented nevi.

DIAGNOSTIC STUDIES AND FINDINGS

Physical examination: Characteristic lesion
Biopsy: Shows histologic configuration

MULTIDISCIPLINARY PLAN

Most nevi do not require any treatment. Surgical removal may be indicated for cosmetic purposes or if changes occur in the nevus (see box at right). Mongolian spots require no treatment.

Surgery

Shave ablation with electrodessication of base for intradermal nevus; excisional or punch biopsy removal of junction nevus; excision of hairy nevus with full-thickness skin grafting (see p. 503)

Laser Therapy[22,56,57]

Argon laser treatment for some pigmented lesions; pulsed tunable dye laser for some pigmented lesions; Q-switch ruby Candela laser for some pigmented lesions

MALIGNANT CHANGES IN NEVI

Some changes in preexisting nevi may indicate malignancy. Moles that exhibit any of the following changes or irregularities should receive medical evaluation:

A Asymmetry of one half compared to the other
B Borders irregular
C Color blue-black or variegated, with red, white, blue, pink, gray
D Diameter 0.6 mm or greater
E Elevation from change in thickness
F Fading of the borders, with notches or streams of pigmentation
G Growing
H Halo formation (depigmented area) around the nevus

NURSING CARE

NURSING ASSESSMENT

Lesion: Location, size, color, shape
Lesion changes: Enlargement, darkening, crusting, bleeding, inflammation, ulceration, appearance of satellite lesions
Psychosocial concerns: Concern about body image

POTENTIAL COMPLICATIONS

Irritation; malignant changes

PATIENT PROBLEMS/NURSING DIAGNOSES & INTERVENTIONS

NIC SKIN/WOUND MANAGEMENT

Risk for impaired skin integrity
- Inform patient of options for treatment.
- Instruct patient to watch for changes that signal dysplastic changes in nevi (see box) and to seek treatment.

NIC COPING ASSISTANCE

Disturbed body image related to cognitive-perceptual factors
- Encourage patient to express feelings about body, body image, or fear of reaction or rejection by others *to begin process of realistic self-evaluation.*

Patient Education/Continuum of Care Plan

1. Discuss with the patient the benign nature of the lesions.
2. Explain to the patient about changes that might indicate malignancy, and encourage the patient to seek medical attention if they occur.

Evaluation/Patient Outcomes

Skin/Wound Management: Patient seeks treatment for changes in lesions. Patient seeks medical attention if color or size of nevus changes, if it bleeds, or if it is exposed to repeated trauma.

Coping Assistance: Patient evaluates appearance in realistic manner. Patient seeks removal if lesion is cosmetically embarrassing.

Chloasma

Chloasma is a diffuse, mottled brown pigmentation that appears over areas of the face and forehead.

Pathophysiology

Chloasma is a blotchy brown pigmentation that involves the forehead, malar prominences, and preauricular area. The distribution is usually symmetric. Chloasma occurs primarily in women during and after childbearing years. Increased activity of melanocytes and the increase in melanin deposits in the basal cells of the epidermis can occur with pregnancy or from the use of anovulatory hormones. Exposure to sunlight exaggerates the pigmentation. It fades somewhat after childbirth or after the hormones are discontinued. Rarely, chloasma occurs idiopathically in dark-skinned men.

Diagnostic Studies and Findings

Physical examination: Characteristic pigmentation and distribution; in women, history congruent with pregnancy or anovulatory hormones

Multidisciplinary Plan

Medications

Topical depigmenting agents

Hydroquinone (Eldopaque, Eldoquin) 2%-4% applied sparingly bid

Compound of retinoic acid 0.1%, hydroquinone 5%, and dexamethasone 0.1% applied sparingly bid

Sunscreen: With or without para-aminobenzoic acid (PABA 5%) applied every 3 h after swimming for prevention

Topical preparations

Azelaic acid 20% (Azelex) bid

Glycolic acid 35%-70% weekly

Tretinoin (Retin-A) 0.05%-0.1% at bedtime

Laser Therapy[52]

Argon laser treatment; Q-switch ruby laser treatments

General Management

Discontinuation of anovulatory hormones

Nursing Care

Nursing Assessment

Pigmentation: Severity and extent of pigmentation, questioning to determine if woman is pregnant or taking anovulatory hormones

Psychosocial concerns: Concern about body image; assess patient's self-perception

Potential Complications

None

Patient Problems/Nursing Diagnoses & Interventions

NIC Skin/Wound Management

Risk for impaired skin integrity

- Instruct patient in treatment options.
- Inform patient of contributing causes.

NIC Coping Assistance

Disturbed body image related to cognitive-perceptual factors

- Encourage patient to express feelings about body, body image, or fear of reaction or rejection by others *to begin process of realistic self-evaluation.*
- Inform patient that pigmentation fades in time.
- Instruct patient in use of medications.

Patient Education/Continuum of Care Plan

1. Discuss with the patient the need to avoid sun exposure, which will worsen the condition.
2. Explain to the patient the need to use sunscreens.
3. Discuss with the patient the side effects of depigmenting agents.

Evaluation/Patient Outcomes

Skin/Wound Management: Existing pigmentation fades. Blotchy brown areas become less noticeable. Patient avoids sunlight and use of anovulatory hormones. New areas of pigmentation do not occur.

Coping Assistance: Patient evaluates appearance in realistic manner. Patient seeks treatment for areas that are cosmetically embarrassing. Patient engages in usual activities and relationships.

Depigmentation: Albinism and Vitiligo

Albinism and vitiligo are depigmentation that results from a congenital or acquired decrease in melanin production.

Albinism is a rare inherited disease that may be complete or partial. Partial albinism is autosomal dominant. The affected areas are usually linear and unilateral. The same area may be affected in more than one family member. A small area on the scalp with a streak of white hair is frequently seen.

Complete or universal albinism is autosomal recessive or irregularly dominant. There is no pigmentation in the skin, hair, and eyes. (Some pigmentation may occur with increasing age.) The skin is pale, the hair white, and the iris pink or red. Nystagmus and errors of refraction are common. Skin cancer and premature actinic keratosis are common.

Vitiligo is localized areas of depigmentation that are caused by the disappearance of previously active melanocytes. Vitiligo is fairly common, occurring in 1% of the world's population. It is a familial trait and can occur at any age. It has been associated with autoimmune and endocrine disorders. The depigmentation can also result from exposure to phenols, thiols, and quinones. Initial lesions frequently develop in areas exposed to the sun. The process may remain stable for years and involve only small areas, or it may progress to affect more extensive areas or the entire skin surface and hair. The eyes do not lose their pigment.

The lesions are completely depigmented and have well-demarcated borders that may be hyperpigmented. Vitiligo usually develops symmetrically and may follow trauma to the area. The hands, axillae, perineum, and periorbital areas are usually involved. The surface of the depigmented skin is normal except for the absence of pigmentation. There is no scaling. Some spontaneous repigmentation occurs in about 10% of patients, but complete repigmentation is rare.

Vitiligo is associated with thyroid dysfunction, diabetes mellitus, Addison's disease, and pernicious anemia.

PATHOPHYSIOLOGY

In partial albinism, melanocytes are not present in the depigmented area because they failed to migrate to the skin during embryonic development. In complete albinism, melanocytes are present in the dermis, but they are unable to synthesize pigment because of a block in the formation of melanin from its precursor.

The cause of vitiligo is unknown. It is considered an autoimmune process that causes destruction of preexisting melanocytes. The melanocytes are abnormal and in various stages of cell death at the periphery of the lesions. Repigmentation is thought to result from the migration of melanocytes from residual areas of melanocytic activity within hair follicles.

DIAGNOSTIC STUDIES AND FINDINGS

Physical examination: Distinctive lesions with characteristic configuration and distribution

MULTIDISCIPLINARY PLAN

There is no treatment for albinism other than protection from sun exposure and actinic damage. The treatment for vitiligo is protracted and has mixed results.

Medications

Photosensitizers

Psoralen therapy with 8-methoxypsoralen or methoxsalen (Oxsoralen) or trioxsalen (Trisoralen) to repigment; psoralen, 40-50 mg PO 2 h before sun exposure; sun exposure time initially 20 min, then gradually increased

Psoralen, 40-50 mg PO with long-wave ultraviolet light (PUVA), exposure time gradually increased (see p. 504)

Sunscreens

Sunblock (Umbrelle, Total Block) or sunscreen, with or without PABA to prevent sunburn; apply typically q3h and after swimming

Skin dyes: contain dihydroxyacetone to stain stratum corneum; applied topically several times a week

Corticosteroids: Oral glucocorticoids or topical glucocorticoids used in occlusive dressings to repigment

Depigmenting agents: For surrounding area in extensive vitiligo; 20% monobenzyl ether or hydroquinone

NURSING CARE

NURSING ASSESSMENT

Lesions: Location and distribution, extent of involvement

Psychosocial concerns: Concern about body image; patient's perception of his or her appearance

POTENTIAL COMPLICATIONS

Actinic damage from sun exposure

PATIENT PROBLEMS/NURSING DIAGNOSES & INTERVENTIONS

NIC SKIN/WOUND MANAGEMENT

Risk for impaired skin integrity related to radiation

- Instruct patient to protect skin exposure to sun through use of protective clothing and hats.
- Instruct patient to use PABA as sunscreen *to protect skin from actinic damage.*

NIC COPING ASSISTANCE

Disturbed body image related to cognitive-perceptual factors
Situational low self-esteem

- Encourage patient to express feelings about body, body image, or fear of reaction or rejection by others *to begin process of realistic self-evaluation.*
- Encourage development of interests and other attributes *to support positive self-image and feelings of worth and self-confidence*
- Help patient evaluate appearance in realistic way *so it does not become focal point of patient's existence.*
- Advise patient of cosmetic products (Covermark) available for use on small areas.
- Facilitate initiation of counseling if patient is unable to adjust to appearance.

PATIENT EDUCATION/CONTINUUM OF CARE PLAN

1. Discuss with the patient the need to protect against exposure to the sun to prevent premature actinic damage.

2. Discuss with the patient the use and side effects of medication and preparations.
3. Explain to the patient that treatment for vitiligo is protracted and results vary.

Evaluation/Patient Outcomes

Skin/Wound Management: Actinic damage is avoided. Epidermis is not dry or fissured. There are no actinic keratoses. Skin remains smooth and elastic.

Coping Assistance: Patient evaluates appearance in realistic manner. Disorder is not used as excuse for unsuccessful interpersonal relationships. Patient develops interests and relationships so appearance is not focal point of existence.

PITYRIASIS ROSEA

Pityriasis rosea is a self-limiting inflammation of unknown etiology.

The disease peaks in spring and fall. It is less likely to occur on tanned skin, and sunlight apparently hastens the course. Onset is sudden, with occurrence of a herald patch followed 1 to 3 weeks later by a generalized eruption. New lesions continue to appear for about a week after onset of the generalized eruption. A gradual involution follows. Total duration is 4 to 12 weeks with rare recurrence. The disease is not infectious or contagious.

Pathophysiology

The cause of pityriasis rosea is unknown. Pathogenesis may be related to a cell-mediated immunity. The primary (herald) patch is a single oval or round plaque with fine superficial scaling. The remainder of the lesions are smaller but similar in configuration to the primary lesions. The lesions develop in the trunk and extremities. The palms and soles are not involved, and facial involvement is rare. The lesions are characteristically distributed in parallel alignment following the direction of the ribs in a Christmas tree–like pattern. An inverse pattern can occur, with concentration of the lesions on the extremities and few lesions on the trunk. The lesions are usually pale, erythematous, and macular with the fine scaling, but they may be papular or vesicular. Pruritus may be present.

Microscopic examination reveals nonspecific inflammation of the dermis, perivascular infiltrates, and localized epidermal changes with spongiosis and focal parakeratosis.

Diagnostic Studies and Findings

Physical examination: Characteristic lesion with distinct distribution and congruent history

VDRL or rapid plasma reagin (RPR) test: Done to rule out secondary syphilis

Multidisciplinary Plan

Treatment is usually unnecessary.

Medications

Antipruritic effects
- Antipruritic agents
  - Menthol 0.25% in cream base applied topically bid or tid
- Antihistamines
  - Cyproheptadine (Cyproheptadine, Periactin), 4 mg PO tid
  - Hydroxyzine (Atarax, Orgatrax, Vistaril), 25-100 mg PO tid or qid

Corticosteroids
- Prednisone, 10 mg PO qid for severe pruritus until itching subsides, tapered over 2 weeks
- Topical triamcinolone 0.1% (Arestocort), applied qd to bid

General Management

Exposure to short-wave ultraviolet light (UVB)—five consecutive daily doses to level of erythema to decrease pruritus and extent of eruption

NURSING CARE

Nursing Assessment

Lesion: Pale, erythematous macules with fine scaling or papules and vesicles; herald patch larger than new lesions; characteristic distribution

Psychosocial concerns: Concern with body image

Potential Complications

Secondary infection from scratching

Patient Problems/Nursing Diagnoses & Interventions

NIC Skin/Wound Management

Impaired skin integrity related to inflammatory process and mechanical factors
- Assess for lesions and pruritus.
- Lubricate skin with emollient and water-miscible bath oil *to alleviate dryness and scaling.*
- Stress importance of good hygiene *to avoid secondary infection.*
- Have patient cut fingernails short *to avoid tissue trauma from scratching.*

NIC Coping Assistance

Disturbed body image related to cognitive-perceptual factors
- Reassure patient that lesions will clear in 4 to 12 weeks.
- Encourage patient to express feelings about body, body appearance, or fear of reaction or rejection by others *to begin process of realistic self-evaluation.*

Patient Education/Continuum of Care Plan

1. Explain to the patient that the disease is self-limiting and will resolve.
2. Explain to the patient that exposure to sunlight may hasten the course of the disease.
3. Teach the patient the signs and symptoms of secondary infection and to seek medical attention if they occur.

4. Discuss with the patient the use and side effects of medications.

EVALUATION/PATIENT OUTCOMES

Skin/Wound Management: Lesions resolve. Macules, papules, vesicles, and scaling disappear. Pruritus is relieved. Skin is intact. Secondary infection is resolved or avoided. There is no tenderness, swelling, purulent discharge, or fever.

Coping Assistance: Patient evaluates appearance in realistic manner. Patient engages in usual activities and relationships.

PSORIASIS

Psoriasis is a chronic and recurrent disease of keratin synthesis that is characterized by dry, well-circumscribed, silvery, scaling papules and plaques.

Psoriasis occurs in 3% to 5% of the population. Onset is usually between ages 10 and 40 years. A family history of psoriasis is common.

The onset of the disease is slow, and the course is characterized by periods of inactivity and exacerbation. Emotional stress may cause exacerbations. Spontaneous remission may occur. Psoriasis characteristically involves the back, buttocks, and extensor surfaces of the extremities, particularly the knees and elbows, and the scalp. The nails, axillae, umbilicus, eyebrows, and anogenital areas may be affected. Generalized eruptions can occur. Approximately 5% of people with psoriasis have associated arthritis. Lesions may develop at sites of recent epidermal injury.

The characteristic lesions of psoriasis are raised, erythematous, sharply demarcated papules covered with overlapping, silvery or shiny scales. The papules may combine as large plaques. When the scales are removed, a deep red base, covered with a thin membrane that bleeds, is revealed.

PATHOPHYSIOLOGY

The basic defect in psoriasis is in the control of the growth of epidermal cells. This defect may be genetic, biochemical, or immunologic. The three main components of the psoriatic process are increased mitotic rate that results in rapid cellular turnover and shortened transit time of the epidermal cell from the basal layer to the epidermis (4 to 7 days versus the normal 28 days); faulty keratinization of the horny layer, which desquamates readily and affords little protection to the underlying skin; and dilation of upper dermal vessels and intermittent discharge of polymorphonuclear leukocytes into the dermis.

The three processes occur in different degrees that result in varying forms of psoriasis with differing clinical features. If the increased mitotic rate predominates, the result is a thick silvery scale because of the separation of corneocytes and the presence of air between them. If vasodilation predominates, the result is diffusely red, hot, slightly scaling skin.

The forms of psoriasis and their clinical features are summarized in Table 7-5.

DIAGNOSTIC STUDIES AND FINDINGS

Physical examination: Characteristic lesions

MULTIDISCIPLINARY PLAN

Medications

Corticosteroids

- Topical nonfluorinated corticosteroids for lesions on face and intertriginous areas: hydrocortisone (Cort-Dome, others) 2%-3% applied sparingly bid
- Topical corticosteroids for lesions on scalp, body, and extremities
  - Fluocinolone (Fluonid, Synalar) 0.025%-0.01% applied sparingly bid, tid, or qid
  - Betamethasone (Valisone) 0.05%-0.1% applied sparingly bid, tid, or qid
  - Triamcinolone (Aristocort, Kenalog) 0.05%-0.1% applied sparingly bid, tid, or qid
  - Mometasone furoate (Elocon) 0.1% applied once daily
- High-potency topical steroids
  - Clobetasol propionate (Temovate) 0.05% applied sparingly bid or tid
  - Betamethasone dipropionate (Diprolene) 0.05% applied sparingly bid or tid
- Topical corticosteroids in conjunction with tar preparations or in occlusive therapy (see p. 500)
- Intralesional injections of corticosteroids: Triamcinolone (Kenalog), 10 mg/ml

Table 7-5 Clinical Features and Distribution of the Various Forms of Psoriasis

Clinical Pattern	Clinical Features	Distribution
Localized plaques	Erythematous plaques with silver scales; nails pitted, thickened, discolored, and crumbling beneath free edge	Extensor aspect of extremities; elbows; knees, scalp; nails
Generalized plaques	As discussed above	Disseminated
Guttate	Tiny plaques (0.5-2 cm); sudden onset usually after streptococcal infection; may progress to other types; may itch	Disseminated
Pustular	Pustular lesions covered by thin scale	Palms and soles only or generalized
Erythrodermic exfoliative	More inflammatory; skin red and hot; deep erythema with massive shedding of scales; usually follows overly aggressive therapy; can cause temperature and fluid imbalances	Generalized

Systemic corticosteroids: Individualized treatment regimen; use is controversial[1]

Topical vitamin D_3 preparations: Calcipotriene 0.005% (Dovonex) applied qd to bid and rubbed in; use for at least 6 weeks, do not use on face

Keratolytics

Coal tar preparations (Alphosyl, PsoriGel, Balnetar), added to bath oil or shampoo or applied sparingly to lesions

Dianthrol compounds: Anthralin (Drithocreme 0.1%-0.5%, Anthra-Derm 1%) apply to chronic plaque for 15-60 min then shower off

Phenol-saline mixture (P & S liquid), massaged into scalp and left for 3-4 h for scalp lesions, followed by tar shampoo

Photosensitizing agents

Psoralen (Trisoralen, Oxsoralen), 0.6 mg/kg 2-4 h before exposure to ultraviolet light; used as photoactivator in combination with long-wave ultraviolet light therapy (see p. 504)

Oral retinoids

Etretinate (Tegison), 1 mg/kg/day PO up to maximum of 75 mg/day; for severe recalcitrant forms; used especially in combination therapy

Acetritin (etretin): For severe recalcitrant forms; used especially in combination therapy

Antineoplastic agents: Used for antimetabolite effect in recalcitrant cases

Methotrexate, 5-7.5 mg in a single weekly PO, IM, or IV dose, increased by a 2.5-5 mg increment each week up to 30 mg/week, then tapered after clearing; or 2.5 mg q12h in 3 doses in a 24-h period, increased by 2.5 mg each week up to 30 mg/week, then tapered after clearing; for severe recalcitrant disease

Cyclosporine, 3 mg/kg/day as initial dose, altered according to clinical state; dose not to exceed 5 mg/kg/day; for severe disease

Antiinfective agents: Penicillin (Pen-Vee K, V-Cillin K, others), 250 mg PO qid for 10 days for underlying streptococcal infection in guttate psoriasis

General Management

See pp. 503-504 for steroid therapy

Exposure to short-wave ultraviolet light (UVB): One to three times weekly with increasing UVB exposure; kept below level that would cause erythema

Goeckerman therapy: UVB therapy in combination with coal tar applications that are photosensitizing; coal tar ointment applied and left on for several hours and then washed off; UVB therapy then administered in doses to account for photosensitization; tar finally reapplied

Long-wave ultraviolet light (UVA) in combination with psoralen as a photosensitizer (PUVA therapy): Psoralen administered in initial dose of 0.6 mg/kg; UVA irradiation delivered 2 to 4 hours after psoralen administration; dosage and exposure determined by individual response; special equipment and careful monitoring required, so therapy is usually provided in special treatment centers; treatment usually reserved for chronic, severe, refractory psoriasis

Combination therapies

PUVA-UVB: PUVA plus UVB

Methotrexate-PUVA: Methotrexate plus PUVA

Methotrexate-UVB: Methotrexate plus UVB

RePUVA: Etretinate plus PUVA

Acitretin-UVB: Etretin plus UVB

Topical, soak, or both PUVA: Topical Oxsolaren plus PUVA

X-ray therapy and Grenz-ray therapy: Used to provide temporary clearing of stubborn plaques; of limited value as therapeutic tools in psoriasis therapy

Occlusive dressings with topical corticosteroids or tar preparations or both (see p. 500)

Day care treatment centers for psoriasis: Patients with severe psoriasis can undergo treatment regimens that are intensive or that require special equipment and supervision

NURSING CARE

Nursing Assessment

Lesions: Characteristics and distribution as in Table 7-5

Psoriatic arthritis: Pain, tenderness, stiffness in small distal joints (early), larger joints involved later

Environment: Presence of mechanical injury that can exacerbate lesions; stress factors

Potential Complications

Scarring; psoriatic arthritis

Patient Problems/Nursing Diagnoses & Interventions

NIC Skin/Wound Management

Impaired skin integrity related to the pathologic process and mechanical factors

- Assess for lesion characteristics, distribution, and severity.
- Explain disease process regarding exacerbations and remissions.
- Stress importance of adhering to therapeutic regimen; help patient set up overall schedule for managing regimen on daily basis *to maximize therapeutic value.*
- Give written instructions for use of topical preparations, tar baths, and shampoos.
- Instruct patient in application of occlusive dressings.
- Instruct patient to scrub scales gently during daily bath with soft brush and to apply medications after removing scales *to maximize absorption and therapeutic value.*
- Instruct patient not to apply keratolytics and tar to unaffected area *because they may precipitate new lesions.*
- Explore stress factors affecting patient and alternatives for dealing with stress *to help prevent exacerbations.*

NIC Coping Assistance

Disturbed body image related to cognitive-perceptual factors

Impaired social isolation related to alterations in physical appearance

Powerlessness related to illness-related regimen

- Recognize importance of body image in growth and development.
- Assess patient's perception of his or her appearance.
- Encourage patient to express feelings about body, body appearance, or fear of reaction or rejection by others to begin process of realistic self-evaluation.

- Encourage patient to develop interests and other attributes *to support positive self-image, feelings of worth, and self-confidence.*
- Facilitate initiation of individual or group therapy if patient is unable to adjust to appearance.
- Involve family members in treatment regimen.
- Stress that psoriasis is not communicable.
- Refer patient for counseling if patient is socially disabled by disease.
- Assess for presence of defining characteristics.
- Observe for signs of depression and apathy.
- Involve patient in decision making *to increase sense of power and control.*
- Encourage patient to express dissatisfaction and frustration.

PATIENT EDUCATION/CONTINUUM OF CARE PLAN

1. Discuss with the patient the treatment regimen and the use of medications.
2. Discuss with the patient the side effects of medications.
3. Explain to the patient that anthralin (Dithranol) stains skin, sheets, and clothing. Skin discoloration resolves in a few weeks as the stratum corneum is shed.
4. Evaluate the patient's ability to carry out home care and reteach procedures as necessary.
5. Discuss with the patient the need for good hygiene to avoid secondary infection.

EVALUATION/PATIENT OUTCOMES

Skin/Wound Management: Lesions improve. Scaling, pustules, erythema, and size of plaques decrease.

Exacerbating factors are avoided. Patient takes precautions against skin trauma. Patient avoids or tries alternative strategies for reducing stress factors.

Untoward effects from therapies are minimized. Patient seeks medical attention for untoward or side effects from medications or therapies.

Coping Assistance: Patient copes with disorder in an effective manner. Patient engages in satisfying relationships. Patient seeks counseling when feeling overwhelmed by disease. Patient does not use disorder as excuse for failures in life or in relationships. Patient participates actively in treatment regimen.

PRURITUS

Pruritus is a localized or generalized itching sensation that elicits the desire to scratch.

Pruritus may occur as a primary disorder or may be a symptom of a systemic disorder. Pruritus may result from inflammations caused by various factors, including irritation, infection, infestations, and allergic reactions. It may result from systemic disease, malignancy, and altered physiologic states.

Three areas of the body are most frequently affected by pruritus: the anus (pruritus ani), vulva (pruritus vulvae), and ear (otitis externa). These are body orifices that have an abundance of sensory nerve endings.

Pruritus ani occurs primarily in men. It is caused by many factors and is associated with various diseases. Perianal erythema and scratches or gross excoriation are evident. Lichenification or fissures occur in long-term cases. The entire gluteal fold may be involved. Aggravating factors include contact dermatitis, anatomic abnormalities, infection, and systemic disorders. Aggravating factors include contact dermatitis, anatomic abnormalities, infection, and systemic disorders. Common irritating factors include feces, toilet tissue, tight clothing, sweating, and long periods of sitting. The itching is often associated with tension, irritability, and depression.

Pruritus vulvae is caused by many factors and is associated with various diseases. Pruritus vulvae begins with intermittent episodes that can develop into unremitting pruritus. Erythema develops in the labia majora, with lichenification in long-standing disease. The perianal region may also be affected. Tight clothing, heat, perspiration, motion, sitting, and lying down aggravate the condition.

Otitis externa occurs in the external ear, usually as a result of trauma, moisture in the ear, and bacterial colonization. The distal third of the external canal and the meatal skin develop a scaling erythema that becomes moist and oozing as the condition worsens. Itching is the main complaint. Otitis externa is aggravated by heat, humidity, moisture, and overzealous cleansing (see Chapter 9).

Generalized pruritus can signify a systemic disorder. Diabetes mellitus, thyroid disorders, HIV infection, drug reactions, biliary obstruction, renal disease, malignancy, and pregnancy are common causes of generalized pruritus.

PATHOPHYSIOLOGY

The exact mechanism of pruritus is undetermined. The itch sensation seems to arise from nerve endings just below the epidermis and in the dermis. Itching may be a result of repetitive, low-frequency stimulation of C fibers that are similar to but distinct from those that transmit pain.

Persistent scratching may produce erythema, urticarial papules, excoriation, and fissures. Prolonged scratching and rubbing may produce lichenification and pigmentation. Many factors, including personality, determine whether itching will be ignored, rubbed, or scratched and excoriated.

DIAGNOSTIC STUDIES AND FINDINGS

Physical examination and history: To determine underlying cause or systemic disorder

Laboratory studies with generalized pruritus: To determine possible systemic cause: complete blood count, blood urea nitrogen, serum bilirubin, serum iron, blood glucose, sulfobromphthalein retention, stool for occult blood, and parasites

Biopsy: To determine histopathologic changes

MULTIDISCIPLINARY PLAN

Treatment is aimed at the specific underlying cause (see specific diseases for treatments) and at eliminating aggravating factors (see Patient Education/Continuum of Care Plan, p. 482).

Medications

Topical preparation: Combination of menthol 0.5%, phenol 0.5%, and betamethasone 0.1% applied sparingly tid

Antiinfective agents: Topical antibiotics if pruritus has bacterial etiology; gentamicin (Garamycin) or polymycin, applied tid

Antihistamines: Used for antipruritic effect
- Hydroxyzine (Atarax, Vistaril), 25 mg PO at bedtime or q6h for localized itching
- Cyproheptadine (Periactin), 4 mg PO tid
- Cetirizine (Zyrtec), 10 mg PO qd
- Fexofenadine (Allegra), 60 mg PO bid
- Loratadine (Claritin), 10 mg PO bid

Psychotherapeutic agents: Used for antipruritic effect
- Chlorpromazine (Thorazine), 10-25 mg PO q6-8h for severe generalized itching

General Management

Sitz baths; Burow's compresses; emollients for dry skin; UVB phototherapy in suberythemogenic doses

NURSING CARE

Nursing Assessment

Pruritus: Severity, localization, diurnal or seasonal patterns, distribution

Lesion: Erythema, scaling, excoriation, fissures

Environment: Aggravating factors; stress, tension; depression; irritability

Potential Complications

Secondary infection from scratching

Patient Problems/Nursing Diagnoses & Interventions

NIC Skin/Wound Management

Impaired skin integrity related to mechanical factors

- Instruct patient in good hygiene *to prevent secondary infection.*
- Instruct patient to cut fingernails short *to avoid tissue damage from scratching.*

NIC Physical Comfort Promotion

Acute pain related to biologic and physical factors

- Help patient identify and eliminate potentially aggravating factors (see under Patient Education/Continuum of Care Plan).
- Help patient identify stress factors and alternative approaches to dealing with stress *to avoid aggravating the condition.*
- Apply cool compresses and Burow's compresses *to alleviate itching.*
- Offer sitz baths *to alleviate itching.*
- Apply emollients *to prevent dry skin.*
- Instruct patient in use of medications.

Patient Education/Continuum of Care Plan

1. Explain to the patient the need to avoid aggravating factors.
   a. Heat and humidity
   b. Rubbing and friction from clothing
   c. Tight clothing
   d. Wool and rough fabrics
   e. Fabrics that do not allow ventilation
   f. Excessive perspiration
   g. External irritants (such as soap)
   h. Dry skin
   i. Temperature changes
2. Discuss with the patient the use and side effects of medications.
3. Discuss with the patient the use of compresses (see p. 500).
4. Discuss with the patient the signs and symptoms of secondary infection.

Evaluation/Patient Outcomes

Skin/Wound Management: Aggravating factors are avoided. Pruritus decreases. Exacerbations do not occur.

Underlying disease is identified and treated. Erythema, scaling, excoriation, and fissures resolve. Pruritus is alleviated.

Secondary infection is resolved or avoided. There is no tenderness, swelling, or purulent exudate in resolving lesions.

Physical Comfort Promotion: Discomfort is alleviated. Scratching and excoriations decrease. Patient is able to sleep.

TINEA (DERMATOPHYTOSIS)

Tinea is a group of superficial fungal infections.

Dermatophytes (ringworm fungi) cause various superficial fungal infections through invasion of the stratum corneum, nails, or hair. The disorders are usually classified according to the anatomic location because treatment of most superficial fungal disorders is the same and the clinical appearance of the eruption is not always related to the species of fungus. The disorder varies from mild inflammation to acute vesicular infection. Remissions and exacerbations may occur. Itching is usually present. The condition is transmissible from other persons or from animals.

Pathophysiology

The local response to fungal invasion is inflammation, scaling, erythema, and pruritus. A cell-mediated immunologic response may develop, with the production of further erythema, spongiosis, vesicles, and oozing. Table 7-6 summarizes the features of tinea.

Diagnostic Studies and Findings

Physical examination: Characteristic lesion and distribution

Potassium hydroxide (KOH) scraping: Presence of branching mycelia or spores

Fungal culture: Infecting organism

Wood's light: Affected hairs fluoresce

Table 7-6 Summary of Tinea

Type	Distribution	Occurrence	Clinical Features
Tinea corporis	Nonhairy parts of body; face; neck; extremities	More common in hot and humid climates; more common in rural than in urban settings; occurs in both adults and children	Pruritus; papulosquamous annular lesions with raised borders; lesions expand peripherally with central clearing
Tinea cruris	Groin; inner thigh; scrotum or labia not involved	More common in adult men; tends to recur; flare-ups common in summer; aggravated by tight clothes, perspiration, and physical activity	Pruritus; hypopigmented; well-demarcated lesions; dryness and scaling; pustules present at margins; central clearing sometimes present; secondary bacterial or candidal infection and maceration common
Tinea capitis	Scalp	More common in children; contagious	Lesions vary: small gray scaly patches with short broken hairs; mild erythematous papules; raised, boggy, inflamed nodules dotted with perifollicular abscesses; thick, yellow, suppurative lesions; lesions may be small, coalesced, or cover entire scalp; hairless patches
Tinea pedis	Feet; begins in third and fourth interdigital spaces and spreads to involve plantar surface; may involve nails	Rare in children; not transmitted by simple exposure	Lesions vary: maceration, scaling, fissuring of interdigital space; vesicular scaling, erythema of plantar surface; chronic, noninflamed, diffuse scaling; nails brittle, discolored; pruritus
Tinea unguium	Toenails and (less commonly) fingernails		Nails thickened, lusterless, and discolored; subungual debris; nail plate crumbling or absent

MULTIDISCIPLINARY PLAN

Medications

Antiinfective agents

Griseofulvin microsize (Grifulvin V), 50 mg PO qd or ultramicrosize (Gris-PEG), 330-750 mg qd for tinea capitis and severe cases of other tineas; continue therapy for 2 weeks after last sign of clinical activity

Ketaconazole (Nizoral), 200-400 mg/day PO for 6-8 weeks

Itraconazole (Sporanox), 100 mg/day PO for 15 days for tinea corporis and tinea cruris; 100 mg PO for 30 days for tinea pedis; 200 mg/day PO for 12 weeks or 200 mg bid for 1 week, then off for 3 weeks, then repeat for 1 week for onychomycosis

Terbinafine, 250 mg PO bid for 2-6 weeks; under investigation

Topical antifungals rubbed in bid for 3 weeks

- Tolnaftate 1% (Aftate, Tinactin)
- Miconazole 2% (Monistat-Derm)
- Clotrimazole 1% (Lotrimin, Mycelex)
- Econazole 1% (Spectazole)
- Cyclopiroxolamine 1% (Loprox)
- Ketoconazole cream 2% (Nizoral), qd
- Naftifine cream 1% qd, gel 1% (Naftin) bid
- Terbinafine cream 1% (Lamisil)

Keratolytic agents: For noninflammatory scaling

Salicylic acid 3% and benzene acid 6% in ointment or alcohol

General Management

Preventative measures (see Patient Education/Continuum of Care Plan)

1. Avoid aggravating factors: tight clothing, moist skin, excess humidity
2. Dry thoroughly after bathing.
3. Wear nonocclusive footwear, cotton socks, and cotton underclothing.
4. Launder towels and clothes in hot water.

NURSING CARE

NURSING ASSESSMENT

Lesion: For description and distribution, see Table 7-6

Secondary infection (bacterial or candidal): Itching, exudate, inflammation, odor, tenderness, maceration

Environment: Aggravating factors, hygiene, contacts

POTENTIAL COMPLICATIONS

Secondary infection, reinfection

PATIENT PROBLEMS/NURSING DIAGNOSES & INTERVENTIONS

NIC SKIN/WOUND MANAGEMENT

Impaired skin integrity related to infectious process and mechanical factors

- Assess for lesion characteristics and distribution
- Decrease moisture in affected areas.
- Stress importance of good hygiene and hand washing *to prevent secondary infection.*
- Have patient's fingernails cut short *to avoid tissue trauma from scratching.*
- For tinea capitis, remove scales with shampoo and gently scrub before medication is applied *to maximize absorption of medication.*
- Instruct patient in use of medications and preparations *to avoid recurrence.*

NIC Risk Management

Risk for infection related to transmissibility

- Inform patient that contacts should be screened and referred for treatment if symptoms appear *to avoid reinfection.*
- Instruct patient that pets should be checked and treated for fungal infection *to avoid reinfection.*
- Instruct patient and family to protect themselves and others by not sharing towels or personal articles and by wearing protective footwear in public showers.

NIC Physical Comfort Promotion

Acute pain related to biologic and physical factors

- Assess for discomfort and itching.
- Instruct patient not to wear tight clothing *to avoid aggravating the condition.*
- Instruct patient to wear cotton next to skin *to avoid aggravating the condition.*
- Instruct patient to stay in areas of decreased humidity *to avoid aggravating the condition.*
- Instruct patient in use of medications and preparations as prescribed.

Patient Education/Continuum of Care Plan

1. Teach the patient and family about the transmission, recurrence, and reinfection of the disease.
2. Discuss with the patient the necessity of avoiding aggravating factors: tight clothing, moist skin, and excessive humidity.
3. Teach the patient to thoroughly dry intertriginous and interdigital areas after bathing; to wear nonocclusive footwear; to wear cotton socks; to change clothes and towels frequently; and to launder them in hot water.
4. Stress the importance of following the therapeutic regimen to avoid recurrence of reinfection.
5. Discuss with the patient and family the side effects of medications.
6. Discuss with the patient and family the signs and symptoms of secondary infection and the necessity of seeking medical attention if they occur.

Evaluation/Patient Outcomes

Skin/Wound Management: Eruption clears up. Papules, scaling, pustules, erythema, vesicles, and pruritus resolve. Nails resume smooth texture.

Risk Management: Secondary infection is avoided or resolved. There is no tenderness, swelling, or purulent exudate. Spread of infection is contained. Contacts are notified and treated if symptoms appear. Personal articles and items are not shared. Aggravating environmental factors are avoided. Eruption clears. Exacerbations do not recur.

Physical Comfort Promotion: Discomfort is alleviated. Patient stops scratching

URTICARIA

Urticaria is a reaction pattern characterized by hives or wheals.

Urticaria is a common disorder that can occur at any age. It can be acute, chronic, or physical. Most cases are acute, lasting from hours to a few weeks. This condition is self-limited, and most people do not seek medical treatment. Patients who have a history of hives lasting 6 weeks or longer are considered to have chronic urticaria. The course of chronic urticaria is unpredictable and may last for months or years, followed by spontaneous resolution. The physical urticarias include dermographia, pressure urticaria, and cholinergic urticaria. Hives are elicited by physical stimuli to the skin; the attacks are brief and transient.

Drugs, foods, and environmental antigens are common causes of acute and chronic urticaria. Emotional stress should also be considered in the evaluation of chronic urticaria.

Pathophysiology

A hive or a wheal is a nonpitting edematous plaque that results from localized capillary vasodilation followed by transudation of protein-rich fluid into the surrounding tissue. The hive may be erythematous or white with irregular borders that extend or recede during the evolution of the hive. The hive resolves when the fluid is reabsorbed.

Histamine is the primary chemical mediator of urticaria. Histamine induces vascular changes resulting in vasodilation and pruritus. It also causes endothelial cell contraction, which allows vascular fluid to leak between the cells through the vessel wall. A variety of immunologic, nonimmunologic, physical, and chemical stimuli may cause release of histamine from the mast cells. Other factors that contribute to vascular dilation include alcohol ingestion, emotional stress, endocrine factors, exercise, fever, and heat.

Diagnostic Studies and Findings

Physical examination: Characteristic lesion, location, pattern, and history; inducement of hive by physical stimuli to determine physical urticaria

Sinus and dental radiographic examination: For chronic urticaria; a percentage of these patients exhibit sinusitis

Change of environment: For chronic urticaria; separation from the home and work environment for a 1- to 2-week trial period

Food challenge: For chronic urticaria, foods containing salicylate, azo dyes, and benzoic acid preservative; to elicit hive development

Biopsy: For chronic urticaria; to rule out urticarial vasculitis

Laboratory tests: For specific suspected causes in internal diseases such as hyperthyroidism, systemic lupus erythematosus, and carcinomas; there are no routine laboratory studies for acute urticaria

Multidisciplinary Plan

Treatment is aimed at identifying and eliminating known causes or aggravating factors.

Medications

For symptom control

- Epinephrine 1:1000, 0.2-1 ml subcutaneously or IM for severe urticaria and laryngeal edema

Antihistamines

- Hydroxyzine (Atarax, Vistaril), 10 mg q4h, then increase dosage as required to 25-100 mg q4h
- Cyproheptadine (Periactin), 4 mg qid
- Cetirizine (Zyrtec), 10 mg PO qd
- Fexofenadine (Allegra), 60 mg PO bid
- Loratadine (Claritin), 10 mg PO tid
- Cromolyn sodium (Intal) oral nebulizer, 20 mg tid for refractory chronic urticaria

Antidepressant: For antihistamine effect

- Doxepin (Sinequan) 10-25 mg PO tid

NURSING CARE

Nursing Assessment

Lesion: Edematous plaques of 1 to 3 mm; erythematous or white, either uniform or varied; approximately round or oval with borders that extend and recede; new hives appear as old ones resolve; duration varies from hours to weeks; generalized distribution with inhalants, ingestions, and internal disease; localized distribution with contact urticaria

Pruritus: Intensity and interference with activities

Secondary infection: Erythema, excoriation, purulent exudate from scratching

Patient Problems/Nursing Diagnoses & Interventions

NIC Skin/Wound Management

Impaired skin integrity related to mechanical factors

- Assess for lesion characteristics and distribution
- Assess for excoriation and secondary infection from scratching.
- Trim fingernails short *to prevent secondary infection.*
- Apply cool compresses to localized lesions or use cool baths for generalized eruption *to soothe pruritus.*

Patient Education/Continuum of Care Plan

1. Discuss with the patient the possible causes of condition and help identify and eliminate precipitating or aggravating factors: foods, drugs, emotional stress, exercise, heat, pressure or physical stimuli, other vasodilating factors.
2. Discuss with the patient a diet free of salicylates, azo dyes, and benzoic acid preservatives if indicated.
3. Discuss with the patient the use of antihistamines.
4. Discuss with the patient the chronic nature of urticaria, that evaluation may be lengthy and unrewarding, and that in most cases the disorder resolves spontaneously.

Evaluation/Patient Outcomes

Skin/Wound Management: Eruption improves. Hives resolve and do not recur. Pruritus is alleviated. Areas of excoriation resolve or do not occur. Patient stops scratching.

VASCULAR DISORDERS OF CUTANEOUS BLOOD VESSELS

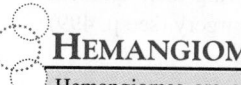

Hemangioma

Hemangiomas are congenital vascular lesions of the skin and subcutaneous tissue.

Pathophysiology

The three common types of hemangiomas are nevus flammeus, capillary hemangiomas, and cavernous hemangioma.

Nevus flammeus (port-wine stain) is a flat purple-red lesion that is present at birth and is caused by a mass of mature, dilated, congested capillaries in the dermis. The color depends on whether the superficial, middle, or deep dermal vessels are involved. The lesion does not disappear or fade over time, does not enlarge, and may develop a thickened nodular surface.

The occipital area of the scalp is the most common site of occurrence. The lesion may occur elsewhere and is frequently seen on the face. The lesions are usually unilateral and tend to follow the course of a cutaneous nerve.

Capillary hemangioma (strawberry mark) is a common, raised, bright red lesion that usually appears in the third to fifth week of life. It consists of a proliferation of endothelial cells arranged in strawberry-like lobules. It may occur anywhere on the body. It may enlarge for the first several months but rarely enlarges after the first year. It involutes spontaneously and is usually completely regressed by 3 to 5 years of age. Involution begins with an area of fibrosis in the center. The lesion may leave a brownish pigmentation or scarring and wrinkling of the skin as it involutes. No treatment is required unless the lesion is massively disfiguring or is near the eye or a body orifice where it might interfere with body functioning.

Cavernous hemangioma is a large vascular pool lined with mature epithelial cells that are located in the subcutaneous tissue of the dermis. It is deeper than the other types of hemangiomas and may contain many arteriovenous shunts and vascular formations.

The lesion, which is present at birth, is reddish blue and round and may be elevated and compressible. It can occur on any part of the body. Most lesions eventually involute at least partially.

Diagnostic Studies and Findings

Physical examination: Characteristic lesion and congruent history

Multidisciplinary Plan

Laser Therapy

Nevus flammeus: Argon laser, pulsed-dye laser, candela laser, CW dye laser, copper vapor laser

Capillary hemangioma: Argon laser, pulsed-dye laser

Cavernous hemangioma: Argon laser, ND-YAG laser

Surgery

Used for capillary or cavernous hemangiomas only if lesion does not involute; may leave more scarring than spontaneous resolution; excision with grafting; cryosurgery (see p. 499)

Medications

Capillary or cavernous hemangiomas

Corticosteroids; efficacy questionable1

- Prednisone, 10 mg PO bid or tid with decremental doses until lesion resolves
- Intralesional injection of triamcinolone (Kenalog, Aristocort); may cause scar formation

NURSING CARE

NURSING ASSESSMENT

Lesion history: Present or absent at birth; rate of growth or involution

Lesion: Size, color, texture, elevation, location, secondary trauma or bleeding

PATIENT PROBLEMS/NURSING DIAGNOSES & INTERVENTIONS

NIC SKIN/WOUND MANAGEMENT

Risk for impaired skin integrity related to mechanical factors

- Assess lesion for characteristics.
- Instruct patient in ways to protect lesions from scratching (cut nails short) and trauma *to avoid tissue damage and bleeding and secondary infection.*
- Stress importance of good hygiene *to avoid secondary infection.*
- Advise patient that it is better to wait for involution of capillary and cavernous hemangiomas *to avoid complications and scarring through early treatment.*

NIC COPING ASSISTANCE

Disturbed body image related to cognitive-perceptual factors

- Assess for defining characteristics.
- Advise patient of excellent prognosis for involution of capillary and cavernous hemangiomas, but warn that lesion may grow before it involutes.
- Use accurate measurements or photographs *to show progress of involution.*
- Assess patient's self-perception or parents' perception of child's appearance.
- Encourage patient to express feelings about body, body image, and fear of reaction or rejection by others *to begin process of realistic self-evaluation.*
- Help patient or parent evaluate appearance in realistic manner *so lesion does not become focal point of existence.*

PATIENT EDUCATION/CONTINUUM OF CARE PLAN

1. Discuss with the patient and family the likelihood of involution.
2. Discuss with the patient and family the hazards of unnecessary treatment.

EVALUATION/PATIENT OUTCOMES

Skin/Wound Management: Secondary trauma and infection are minimized. Lesion remains intact and free of bleeding, crusting, excoriation, and purulent exudate. Unnecessary scarring is avoided. Family waits for spontaneous involution in capillary and cavernous hemangiomas before seeking treatment.

Coping Assistance: Patient and parents evaluate appearance in realistic manner. Patient develops interest and attributes and engages in activities so hemangioma is not focal point of existence. Lesion is not used as excuse for unsuccessful interpersonal relationships.

TELANGIECTASIA AND HEREDITARY HEMORRHAGIC TELANGIECTASIA

Telangiectasia is a network of dilated superficial dermal capillaries and venules.

PATHOPHYSIOLOGY

Essential telangiectasia is a disorder that is characterized by a network of small dilated veins on the thighs and calves of adult women. The condition is localized and often symmetric. The vessels involved are the superficial venous plexuses. The condition affects the appearance only, not the health, of the person.

Telangiectasia is also a component of certain systemic diseases, such as lupus erythematosus and scleroderma, and certain hereditary disorders. Hereditary hemorrhagic telangiectasia (Rendu-Osler-Weber disease) is a rare, autosomal dominant, inherited disorder. Telangiectatic lesions of the skin, mucous membranes, and internal organs are present in this disease. Lesions occur most commonly after puberty and increase throughout adult life. The small, red to violet lesions consist of thin, dilated vessels that blanch with pressure and tend to bleed spontaneously or with minor trauma. Bleeding may also occur from lesions in the mouth, pharynx, and gastrointestinal and genitourinary tracts. Anemia may result from continued oozing. Bleeding tends to become more severe with age. Systemic problems may arise from associated pulmonary arteriovenous fistulas and cerebrovascular malformations.

DIAGNOSTIC STUDIES AND FINDINGS

Physical examination: Characteristic lesions

Complete blood count: Iron deficiency anemia

MULTIDISCIPLINARY PLAN

For treatment of anemia see Chapter 17. For treatment of underlying systemic disorders see the specific diseases.

Medications

For Rendu-Osler-Weber disease

Estrogens: Cyclic therapy to decrease bleeding tendency

Corticosteroids: Nasal spray to control bleeding
Hematinic agents: Iron PO for loss through repeated bleeding

General Management

For localized lesions: Electrolysis—free hydrogen via electric current to obliterate vessels
Blood transfusion for acute hemorrhage

Laser Therapy[3,29,46]

Argon: Pulsed dye laser

NURSING CARE

NURSING ASSESSMENT

Lesion: Number, location, and bleeding tendency; symptoms of anemia (see Chapter 17)

PATIENT PROBLEMS/NURSING DIAGNOSES & INTERVENTIONS

NIC SKIN/WOUND MANAGEMENT

Impaired skin integrity related to pathologic process and mechanical factors

Impaired oral mucous membrane related to pathologic condition and trauma

- Assess lesions for characteristics.
- Instruct patient to avoid trauma to lesions; wear protective clothing and cut fingernails short.
- Instruct patient to eat soft foods to avoid mechanical trauma.
- Instruct patient to use soft toothbrush to avoid mechanical trauma.

NIC COPING ASSISTANCE

Disturbed body image related to cognitive-perceptual factors

- Assess for defining characteristics.
- Encourage patient to express feelings about body, body image, or fear of reaction or rejection by others *to begin process of realistic self-evaluation.*
- Advise patient of availability of covering makeup (Covermark).

PATIENT EDUCATION/CONTINUUM OF CARE PLAN

1. Discuss with the patient protective measures to avoid trauma that may cause bleeding (see under Patient Problems/Nursing Diagnoses & Interventions).
2. Discuss with the patient the use and side effects of medications.
3. Discuss with the patient the advisability of seeking medical attention if unable to stop a bleeding episode.

EVALUATION/PATIENT OUTCOMES

Skin/Wound Management: Trauma is minimized. Bleeding episodes are less frequent.

Coping Assistance: Patient assesses self-concept in realistic manner. Patient engages in activities compatible with limitations of disorder. Patient engages in interpersonal relationships. Patient employs protective measures and seeks medical attention as needed.

VASCULITIS

Vasculitis is a range of cutaneous lesions associated with inflammation of the wall of blood vessels of the skin and subcutaneous tissue.

Vasculitis is a general term for a large number of disorders that cause skin lesions as a result of inflammation of the walls of cutaneous blood vessels. The diseases range in severity from mild to fatal. The cutaneous lesions appear as erythematous papules and plaques, nodules, urticaria, purpuric or hemorrhagic papules and vesicles, and pustular and necrotic lesions.

Lesions, which tend to develop in crops, occur most commonly on the legs, thighs, and buttocks. Some lesions begin as erythematous papules or plaques and progress to ulcerations that heal slowly. In severe ulcerative forms, lesions are progressive and involve other body organs. There is currently no universal or satisfactory classification system for the vasculitis disorders.

PATHOPHYSIOLOGY

Vasculitis involves intravascular and extravascular changes. The sequence of events occurs as a result of damage to the vessel that is precipitated by numerous factors and modified by the body's response to noxious stimuli.

The inflammatory process of the vessel includes increased permeability; epithelial shedding; increased deposition of fibrin, platelets, and leukocytes; changes in endothelial cells during repair; and thrombosis. The cutaneous changes that occur as a result of the inflammation processes depend on the degree of inflammation and the size of the involved vessel.

The pathogenesis of vasculitis can be summarized as follows:

Intravascular component
- Deposition of circulating antigen-antibody complexes with chemotaxis of leukocytes and release of mediators of inflammation
- Direct toxic effect of circulating chemicals, drugs, and bacterial antigens
- Bacterial emboli and reaction to products of bacterial breakdown

Vascular wall component
- Endothelial proliferation in reparative attempt
- Infiltration by lymphocytes and polymorphonuclear leukocytes
- Fibrinoid necrosis and scarring from fibrin deposits
- Granulomatous infiltrates

Extravascular component
- Leakage of red blood cells and fibrin into surrounding tissue
- Deposition of inflammatory infiltrates
- Thrombosis of small vessels with secondary tissue; ischemia
- Increased fibrosis
- Venous stasis

Diagnostic Studies and Findings

Physical examination: Lesions and history as described under Nursing Assessment

Biopsy of blood vessel: Immunofluorescence shows cellular changes as already described; will determine type and severity of vasculitis

Further studies to determine systemic involvement and underlying conditions: Complete blood count; antinuclear factor, serum protein, and rheumatoid factor; serum fibrinolytic activity; VDRL test or rapid plasma reagin test; culture and antistreptolysin titer; urinalysis for red blood cells and casts; serum complement and cryoglobulin; x-rays of chest, sinuses, and teeth; x-ray of gastrointestinal tract if symptoms indicate

Multidisciplinary Plan

Specific treatment is aimed at the particular clinical condition or underlying disease process.

Medications

Antihypertensive agents: If needed to minimize small vessel damage

Antiinfective agents: Agent-specific to clear infection

Corticosteroids: Systemic glucocorticoids for deep, tender nodular lesions

Antiinflammatory agents: Aspirin, potassium iodide, indomethacin (Indocin), ibuprofen (Motrin), celecoxib (Celebrex), rofecoxib (Vioxx)

NURSING CARE

Nursing Assessment

Lesion: Erythematous papules, plaques, or nodules; persistent urticaria; purpuric papules and vesicles; pustules; necrotic lesions

Surrounding tissue: Abnormal vascular patterns; abnormal reactions to cold

History: Precipitating factors; infection; food and drug allergies or sensitivity

General medical problems: Diabetes mellitus; arthritis; cardiovascular diseases; respiratory diseases; connective tissue diseases

Patient Problems/Nursing Diagnoses & Interventions

Nursing interventions other than those listed depend on the symptoms produced by the particular clinical condition and disorder.

NIC Skin/Wound Management

Impaired skin integrity related to inflammatory process and altered circulation

- Assess lesions for characteristics.
- Instruct patient in good hygiene and hand washing *to prevent secondary infection.*
- Apply dressings on open or draining lesions.
- Encourage elevation of affected part *to promote lymphatic drainage.*
- Initiate range of motion exercises *to maintain blood flow.*
- Protect affected area from cold *to prevent vasoconstriction.*

NIC Physical Comfort Promotion

Acute or chronic pain related to physical factors

- Assess for defining characteristics.
- Encourage patient to rest affected area.
- Apply cool compresses to hot, nodular lesions.

Patient Education/Continuum of Care Plan

1. Teach the patient how to change dressings, if indicated, using aseptic technique.
2. Teach the patient how to use cool compresses as needed.
3. Discuss with the patient the use of medications and their side effects.
4. Discuss with the patient the signs and symptoms of secondary infection and the need to seek medical attention if they occur.

Evaluation/Patient Outcomes

Skin/Wound Management: Clinical disorder is identified and treated. Inflammatory response is not exacerbated or does not recur. Cutaneous lesions improve. Erythema and lesions resolve. Necrotic areas reepithelialize. Skin is intact. Secondary infection is resolved or avoided. There is no swelling, purulent exudate, fever, or lymphadenopathy.

Physical Comfort Promotion: Discomfort is alleviated.

BURNS (THERMAL, CHEMICAL, AND ELECTRICAL)

Thermal burns are caused by exposure to flames, hot liquids, and radiation. Chemical burns are caused by contact, ingestion, inhalation, or injection of acids, alkalies, or vesicants. True electrical burns occur when electrical current passes through the body to the ground. Electrical current can also cause secondary flash or flame burns.

More than 2 million people in the United States are burned each year. Although most of these burn injuries are minor, approximately 3% to 5% are life threatening. Burn injury is the second-leading cause of death among young children and is the fourth overall cause of accidental death for people of all ages.

Pathophysiology

Thermal and chemical injury disrupts the normal protective barrier function of the skin, causing a wide range of sequelae. In electrical injury, heat is generated as the electricity passes through tissues. The thermal energy released is the cause of the injury.

The extent and depth of the burn injury determine the extent and severity of burn sequelae. Injury to the stratum corneum results in evaporative heat and water loss as a result of the loss or disruption of the lipid-water barrier of that layer. Injury to the stratum germinativum results in delayed or absent reepithelization and healing. Injury to the deeper structures results in scarring and tissue damage that may require skin grafting.

Vascular changes are caused by direct cellular damage or inflammatory processes. During the first few hours after the burn, vasoactive substances are released from the injured cells and vasoconstriction occurs. Vasodilation then occurs as a result of kinin release. During this period, histamine causes increased capillary permeability, which allows plasma to leak into the burn area.

There are three zones of associated tissue damage:

Zone of coagulation: This is the area of greatest destruction, where coagulation and irreversible cellular death occur. The area remains white because all viable tissue has been destroyed. Leukocytosis is inhibited or totally blocked. The zone can extend deeply into the tissue structures, causing full-thickness skin destruction.

Zones of stasis: This area surrounds the zone of coagulation and involves the vasculative dermis. Shortly after the burn, leukocytes and platelets aggregate in underlying capillaries, causing thrombosis. This, combined with the vasoconstriction, causes decreased circulation and transient ischemia to the area. With appropriate protection and treatment, circulation to the area can be restored and the tissue saved. However, the tissue in this area is very fragile, and any further trauma because of rough handling or infection can convert this zone to one resembling the zone of coagulation.

Zone of hyperemia: This area, which is the least affected, forms the border of the burn wound. Vascular integrity is maintained with no cellular death. The area is bright red and blanches with pressure. The inflammatory processes are present.

In electrical injury, vessel wall changes occur that are characterized by cellular disintegration of the media of the arteries and arterioles and by severe arterial spasm.

Vascular changes and tissue loss cause fluid shifts. The first of these shifts, the hypovolemic stage, occurs during the first 24 to 48 hours. It is characterized by a rapid shift of fluid and protein from the vascular compartment into the interstitial spaces, causing blisters, edema, and fluid escape. Deep in the wound, sodium is translocated into skeletal muscle and other tissues and pulls water with it, which results in hyponatremia and hyperkalemia. This fluid shift, along with evaporative fluid loss from the surface of the wound, causes an abrupt decrease in the circulating blood volume resulting in hypovolemic shock. In turn, hypovolemic shock causes decreased cardiac stroke volume, decreased blood pressure, increased peripheral resistance, decreased tissue perfusion, and circulatory collapse. Anuria, renal failure, and death result if treatment is delayed or inadequate.

Uninjured cells may become dehydrated as a result of this fluid shift. Hypoproteinemia develops from continued loss of protein as a result of increased capillary permeability. Nitrogen is lost through renal catabolism, and a negative nitrogen balance develops. Metabolic acidosis can occur as a result of decreased tissue perfusion, anaerobic metabolism, and retained acid end products.

Within 18 hours after the burn injury, the sodium and water shunting reverse. Within 48 to 72 hours of the burn, a second fluid shift occurs in the opposite direction that causes fluid to return to the vascular compartment. In this phase the rapidly increasing blood volume causes diuresis and hemodilution that may result in dehydration, hyponatremia, and hypokalemia. Metabolic acidosis may occur because of bicarbonate loss in the urine and the catabolic state. Protein continues to be lost through the burn wound. Hypovitaminosis and weight loss also occur.

The evaporative fluid loss that occurs after the burn may be five to 19 times the normal loss. Associated with this fluid loss are tremendous heat loss and hypermetabolism that cause enormous caloric expenditure and hypothermia.

Erythrocyte hemolysis and a decrease in red blood cell mass occur as a result of direct damage and a decreased half-life of damaged red cells. Platelet function and half-life are also diminished. Hemoconcentration occurs as a result of fluid loss from the vascular system, which causes hematocrit values to rise.

Patients who have been injured in a fire also have carbon monoxide poisoning from inhaling the gas that results from incomplete burning of some materials. Poisoning occurs because carbon monoxide has 200 times the affinity of oxygen to combine with hemoglobin.

DIAGNOSTIC STUDIES AND FINDINGS

Physical examination: Determination of extent of injury using rule of nines (FIG. 7-9); Lund and Browder charts (FIG. 7-10); determination of degree of injury (Tables 7-7 and 7-8).

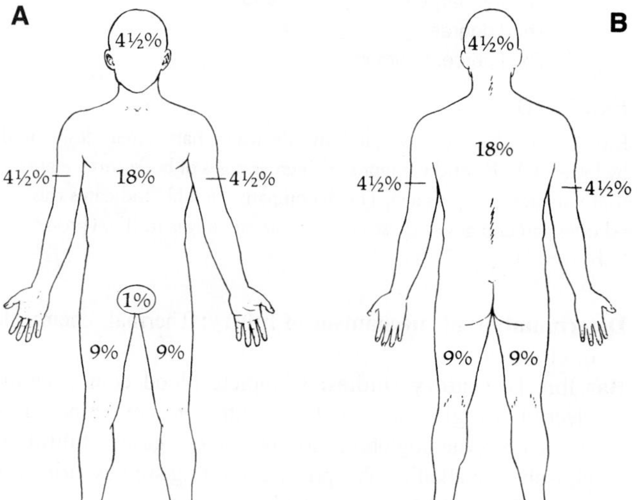

FIG. 7-9

Estimation of adult burn injury: rule of nines. **A,** Anterior view. **B,** Posterior view. (From Rosen and Barkin.[59])

Table 7-7 Assessment of Burn Injury

Degree	Depth	Characteristics
Superficial (first degree)	Epidermis only; revitalization of epidermis and dilation of intradermal vessels	Pain; erythema; blanching with pressure; normal texture
Partial-thickness (second degree)	Destruction of epidermis and part of dermis	Erythema; blisters; pain; blanching with pressure; firm texture
Full-thickness (third and fourth degree)	Destruction of all layers of skin extending into subcutaneous tissue, muscle, nerves, and bone	Dryness; pale, white, brown, or red color; charring; no capillary refill; no pain; firm and leathery texture

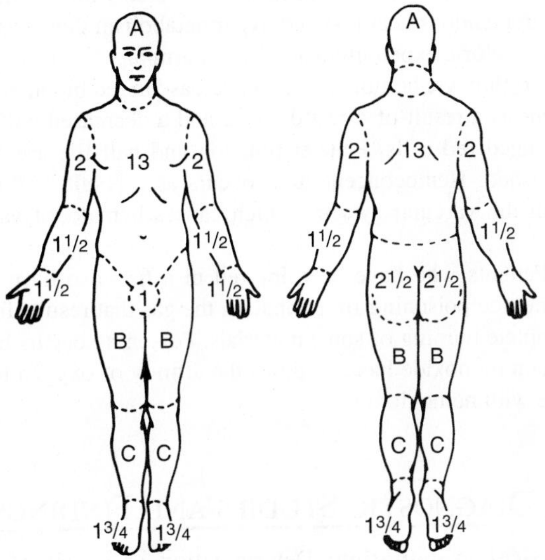

Relative percentages of areas affected by growth (age in years)

	0	1	5	10	15	Adult
A: half of head	9 1/2	8 1/2	6 1/2	5 1/2	4 1/2	3 1/2
B: half of thigh	2 3/4	3 1/4	4	4 1/4	4 1/2	4 3/4
C: half of leg	2 1/2	2 1/2	2 3/4	3	3 1/4	3 1/2

Second degree __________ and
Third degree __________ =
Total percent burned ___

FIG. 7-10

Estimation of burn injury: Lund and Browder chart. Areas designated by letters (A, B, and C) represent percentages of body surface area that vary according to age. The accompanying table indicates the relative percentages of these areas at various stages in life. (From Sabiston.[61])

Determination of mechanism of injury: Thermal, chemical, or electrical

Baseline laboratory studies: Complete blood count; serum electrolytes; glucose; blood urea nitrogen; creatinine; arterial carboxyhemoglobin; arterial blood gases; bilirubin; phosphorus; alkaline phosphatase; clotting studies; urine for myoglobin and hemoglobin levels

Fiberoptic bronchoscopy: Inspection of major and proximal airways to determine upper airway injury

Xenon lung scan: Determination of small airway and parenchymal burns; bolus of xenon is injected; as xenon gas is expired from lungs, injured areas trap gas and show high density levels.

Table 7-8 American Burn Association Classification of Burn Injury

Class	Description
Major	Full-thickness burns over 10% or more of body surface area (BSA) Partial-thickness burns over 25% of BSA All burns on face, hands, eyes, ears, feet, or perineum All inhalation and electrical burns All burns complicated by trauma All burns in poor-risk patients
Moderate	Full-thickness burns over 2%-10% of BSA Partial-thickness burns over 15%-25% of BSA
Minor	Full-thickness burns over less than 2% of BSA Partial-thickness burns over less than 15% of BSA

MULTIDISCIPLINARY PLAN

Short-Term Care of Major Burns

Surgery

Escharotomy: May be needed for circumferentially burned extremities or chest

Fasciotomy: May be needed for electrical injuries

Medications

Narcotic analgesics: Meperidine (Demerol) for pain, 20-25 mg IV

Immunologic agents: Tetanus immunization

Diphtheria tetanus (DT)
- 0.5 ml IM for immunized patients
- 0.5 ml IM plus 250 U tetanus immune globulin (Hypertet) for nonimmunized patients

General Management

Airway maintenance; intubation if needed

Humidification with 10% oxygen for inhalation injuries

Emergency treatment of musculoskeletal injuries or hemorrhage

Fluid replacement
- Parkland (Baxter formula): 2 to 4 ml lactated Ringer's solution/kg/% of BS burned/24 hours; give half of total amount in first 8 hours and half during next 16 hours
- Brooke formula (after first 24 hours): Colloids (plasma, plasmanate, or dextran), 0.5 ml/kg/% of BSA burned plus 2000 ml of dextrose in water
- Electrical and inhalation injuries require more fluids

Urethral catheterization

Table 7-9 Comparison of Topical Burn Agents

Agent	Advantages	Disadvantages
Mafenide acetate (Sulfamylon)	Penetrates rapidly; not inactivated by pus or body fluids; softens wound, allowing better mobility; more effective in established infection	Painful; sulfa sensitivities; acidosis with renal or pulmonary impairment; antibacterial activity lasts 4-6 h
Silver sulfadiazine (Silvadene)	Penetrates slowly; not inactivated by pus or body fluids; minimum systemic absorption; painless; antibacterial activity lasts up to 48 h	Sulfa sensitivities; not as effective in established infection
Silver nitrate	Wet dressings retain heat, moisture, and reduce evaporation; no sensitivities	Painful; staining

! EMERGENCY ALERT

THERMAL INJURY: BURNS

Burn injury occurs from human contact with flame, hot liquids and objects, chemicals, electricity, and radiation. The surface burn is a low priority during initial contact with the patient; maintaining airway, breathing, and circulation is the top priority.

Assessment

- Assess airway and respiratory status for burns and inhalation injury; prepare for emergency intubation.
- Obtain history of events, time of incident, duration, and nature of chemicals if known.
- Assess physical area of injuries and burns.
- Assess circulatory status of affected extremities.

Interventions

- Maintain airway, breathing, and circulation.
- Stop burn process by removing clothing.
- Administer high-flow humidified oxygen (10-15 L) by mask.
- Obtain IV access and administer fluids.
- Maintain temperature by covering burns with dry sterile dressings and ensuring warm room temperature.
- Elevate affected extremities.
- Manage pain.
- Physician may consider escharotomies for compromised circulation.
- Prevent infection by using aseptic technique.
- If chemical burn: Thoroughly rinse off chemical.
- If electrical burn: be alert that as electricity passes through the body, muscle damage, including to the heart, may have occurred.
- If tar burn: Cool tar, remove with oil-based product such as antibiotic ointment or De-Solv-It solvent.

Nasogastric tube insertion

Wound cleansing with povidone-iodine (Betadine), saline solution, or hydrogen peroxide

Central venous line insertion

Swan-Ganz catheter to monitor pulmonary arterial and capillary wedge pressures

Long-Term Care of Major Burns

Surgery

Skin grafts (see p. 503)

Split-thickness: Autograft from unburned area; postage stamp or strip application

Mesh graft: Split-thickness graft meshed with special instrument to cover large areas; held in place by dressing or sutures

Homograft: Skin from deceased person; used as temporary cover for about 10 days; may survive 4 to 5 weeks

Heterograft: Pigskin or synthetic substitute; acts as biologic dressing

Autologous cultured human epithelium: Epidermal cells from unburned area cultured into sheets in flask; cultured sheets then attached to petrolatum gauze squares and sutured in place in wound; petrolatum gauze removed 7 to 10 days later

Amputation of limb severely injured from electrical injury

Medications

Antiinfective agents

Topical (Table 7-9)

Mafenide acetate 10% (Sulfamylon); sterile application of amounts sufficient to just cover wound; wound left open to air; reapplied bid after washing off previous application and debriding wound

Silver sulfadiazine 1% (Silvadene) cream applied tid or qid; left open or covered with mesh gauze dressing; washed off before application, but no wound debridement done

Silver nitrate solution 0.5%; saturated thick gauze pads replaced q12-24h

Parenteral: Aqueous penicillin G for prophylaxis against gram-positive organisms; 1.2-2 million U IV in divided doses

Narcotic agents

Codeine, meperidine (Demerol), methadone (Dolophine); dosage determined on individual basis

General Management

Wound debridement (see p. 499)

Hydrotherapy (see p. 500) once or twice daily for 20 to 30 minutes for dressing removal and debridement

Dressings, wet or dry (see p. 500 for wet dressings)

Dry dressing: Single layer of nonadherent fine mesh gauze held in place by coarse gauze wrap

Nutrition

2 to 4 g protein/kg/day

3500 to 5000 calories daily

Vitamin and iron replacement

Total parenteral nutrition (hyperalimentation) if needed

Physiotherapy

Care of Minor Burns

Medications

Immunologic agents: Tetanus immunization, 0.5 ml IM for immunized patients

Diphtheria tetanus: 0.5 ml IM plus 250 U tetanus immune globulin (Hyper-Tet) for nonimmunized patients

Antiinfective agents

Topical (applied with sterile tongue blade to completely cover wound with ⅛-inch thickness)

Mafenide acetate (Sulfamylon) 5%

Silver sulfadiazine (Silvadene) 1%

Povidone-iodine (Betadine)

Polymyxin B, Bacitracin, Neosporin

Nystatin combined with Silvadene

Narcotic agents

Codeine, 30-60 mg PO or subcutaneously q4-6h

Morphine, 8-10 mg subcutaneously

Meperidine (Demerol), 50-100 mg PO q4-6h

Analgesic/antipyretic agent: Aspirin, 650 mg PO q4-6h

General Management

Wound cleansed with one-half strength Betadine solution

Wound debridement (see p. 499)

Dressing: Innermost layer of nonadherent, porous, fine mesh gauze (fine enough to prevent epithelialization into gauze); second layer of bulky, fluffed coarse mesh gauze to absorb exudate; outer layer of semielastic coarse mesh to apply even pressure and hold dressing in place; change once or twice daily

Polyurethane dressing (Epi-Lock), left on for 1 week

Hydrocolloid dressings (DuoDerm), left on for several days

Dimac with silver sulfadiazine (Sildimac), dressing left on for several days

NURSING CARE

Nursing Assessment

Wound: Degree and extent of injury; see Tables 7-7 and 7-8; mechanism of injury (thermal, chemical, or mechanical)

First fluid shift and hypovolemic shock: Vital signs: Decreased blood pressure, increased pulse, urinary output (desirable: 50 ml/h); monitoring of central venous pressure; potassium levels increased

Second fluid shift: Hyperpnea; blood pH less than 7.35; CO_2 combining power less than 21 mEq/L; $Paco_2$ less than 40 mm Hg

Airway: Pulmonary edema (see Chapter 4); singed nasal hair; soot in mouth or nose; darkened septum; rales, cough, or cyanosis; dyspnea or stridor

Carbon monoxide poisoning: Vomiting, chest pain, tachycardia, confusion, agitation, decreased coordination

Neurologic response: Changes in level of consciousness

Cardiovascular response: Vital signs, dysrhythmias, fluid shifts, cyanosis, capillary refill, pulses

Musculoskeletal response: Fractures, decreased mobility, deformities, exposed bone or muscle

Hypermetabolism and heat loss: Body temperature, weight loss

Hemopoietic response: Increased hematocrit, hemoglobinuria

Gastrointestinal response: Mouth injuries, nausea and vomiting, blood in gastric contents, bowel sounds, paralytic ileus, stress ulcer, constipation

Renal response: Renal failure resulting from hypovolemic shock; oliguria; anuria; desirable output 50 ml/h for adults, 1 ml/kg/h for children; myoglobinuria; hemoglobinuria; diuresis (second phase)

Nutrition: Nutritional status and weight loss

Pain: Presence or absence, location, intensity, severity

Psychosocial concerns: Body image

Infection: Inflammation, exudate, odor

Potential Complications

Systemic complications and organ failure, hypothermia, hypovolemic shock, infection, scarring, contractures, death

Patient Problems/Nursing Diagnoses & Interventions

NIC Skin/Wound Management

Impaired skin integrity related to hyperthermia

- Handle wounds gently *to avoid converting zone of stasis to zone of coagulation.*
- Provide hydrotherapy *to debride burn.*
- Provide wound care to graft donor site *to promote healing.*
- Use bed cradles to prevent pressure *to injured tissue.*
- Assess for signs and symptoms of first and second fluid shifts.

NIC Risk Management

Risk for infection related to impaired skin integrity

- Implement isolation precautions *to prevent infection.*
- Use sterile technique in wound care: Debridement, topical preparations, and dressing changes *to prevent infection.*
- Use sterile linen *to prevent infection.*

NIC Electrolyte and Acid/Base Management

Deficient fluid volume related to active loss

- Observe patency of urinary catheter.
- Monitor intake and output.
- Replace fluids *to achieve output of 50 ml/h.*
- Monitor vital signs.
- Monitor urine specific gravity.
- Monitor central venous pressure.

NIC Tissue Perfusion Management

Ineffective tissue perfusion (renal, cardiopulmonary, gastrointestinal, and peripheral) related to hypovolemia

- Maintain adequate fluid replacement *to maintain circulating volume.*
- Maintain optimum mobility *to promote circulation.*
- Provide adequate nutrition *to promote tissue healing.*

NIC Immobility Management

Impaired physical mobility related to musculoskeletal impairments

Risk for disuse syndrome related to immobilization

- Provide active and passive range-of-motion exercises *to prevent muscle wasting and contractures.*
- Use CircOlectric bed per physician order.

- Refer patient for physiotherapy *to establish therapeutic regimen of motion and exercise.*
- Apply splints *to prevent contractures.*
- Have patient participate in water exercises *to maintain limb mobility.*

NIC Nutrition Support

Imbalanced nutrition: less than body requirements, related to hypermetabolism

- Monitor protein intake: 2 to 4 g/kg/day.
- Monitor caloric intake: 3500 to 5000 calories daily *to meet necessary requirements and promote healing.*
- Monitor vitamin replacement.
- In collaboration with physician, institute total parenteral nutrition *to replace or supplement oral intake.*
- Provide high-protein powdered milk preparations.
- Encourage self-feeding.
- Offer favorite foods *to stimulate appetite.*
- Avoid performing painful procedures near mealtime.
- Offer snacks.

NIC Elimination Management

Constipation related to immobilization, ineffective tissue perfusion or medications

- Assess for defining characteristics.
- Give nothing by mouth until bowel sounds return.
- Provide bulk foods *to promote peristalsis.*
- Provide fruit juices *to promote peristalsis.*
- Administer stool softeners to aid elimination.

NIC Thermoregulation

Hypothermia related to fluid loss

- Keep patient warm through control of environmental temperature *to prevent heat loss.*
- Maintain adequate caloric intake (see under Nutrition) *to provide energy and heat replacement.*

NIC Physical Comfort Promotion

Acute or chronic pain related to chemical or physical agents

- Administer analgesics as ordered.
- Position patient for comfort.
- Provide or refer patient for hydrotherapy.
- Instruct in relaxation techniques.
- Refer patient for biofeedback training.

NIC Coping Assistance

Disturbed body image related to cognitive-perceptual factors; situational low self-esteem

Anticipatory grieving related to potential loss of physiosocial and psychosocial well-being

Powerlessness related to illness-related regimen

- Assess for defining characteristics.
- Encourage patient to express feelings about body, body appearance, or fear of reaction or rejection by others *to begin process of realistic self-evaluation.*
- Spend time with patient *to reassure patient that appearance is not repulsive.*
- Prepare visitors for patient's appearance *to reduce overt negative reactions.*
- Encourage self-esteem by continued interest in patient and attentiveness to patient's needs.
- Assess for defining characteristics.
- Encourage patient to express distress, anger, sorrow, guilt, and fear *to assist patient in movement through stages of grieving.*
- Observe for signs of depression or apathy.
- Involve patient in decision making *to increase sense of control.*
- Encourage patient to express dissatisfaction and frustration.
- Accept patient's feelings of anger.

Patient Education/Continuum of Care Plan

1. Demonstrate to the patient the care of minor burns.
   a. Cleanse wound with one-half strength Betadine using sterile gauze; rub gently to remove existing topical agent.
   b. Apply topical agent thickly enough to cover wound with ⅛ inch of agent to provide healing and prevent bandage from adhering.
   c. Apply nonadherent fine mesh gauze (fine enough not to be epithelialized), then fluffed bulky coarse gauze to trap exudate; hold in place with semielastic net to exert even pressure.
2. Discuss with the patient the care of healed burns.
   a. Wash skin gently, rinse well, dry thoroughly, and apply cream.
   b. Avoid exposure to sunlight, harsh detergents, fabric softeners, and irritation by rubbing of clothing.
3. Discuss with the patient the importance of watching for signs of infection and the need to seek early treatment to avoid further complications.
4. Explain to the patient that increased calories and protein may be required until healing is complete.
5. Advise the patient of available support groups and community resources to assist in the resumption of usual activities and relationships.

Evaluation/Patient Outcomes

Skin/Wound Management: Burn area heals. Reepithelialization occurs. Skin is intact and free of infection. Home care is satisfactory. Healing remains uninterrupted. Scar tissue remains soft and pliable.

Risk Management: New tissue is free of irritation or infection.

Electrolyte and Acid/Base Management: State of homeostasis exists. Normal blood values include the following: pH of 7.35 to 7.45; $PaCO_2$ of 40 to 43; CO_2 combining power of 21 to 28 mEq/L; sodium 136 to 145 mEq/L; potassium 3.5 to 5 mEq/L; chloride 100 to 106 mEq/L. Nitrogen is in balance. Fluids are in balance.

Tissue Perfusion: Complications are recognized, and treatment is sought. Patient seeks medical attention for infection, weight loss, contracture, or changes in scar tissue.

Immobility Management: Patient is free of contractures. Patient has full extremity flexion and extension.

Nutrition Support: Nutrition is adequate. Patient eats diet high in protein, calories, minerals, and vitamins. Patient does not lose weight. Wounds heal.

Elimination Management: Patient has usual elimination pattern.

Thermoregulation: Patient maintains appropriate temperature.

Physical Comfort Promotion: Patient remains as comfortable as possible. Pain from interventions is minimized.

Coping Assistance: Patient resocializes and evaluates appearance in realistic manner. Patient returns or plans to return to former activities if possible. Patient develops interests and activities compatible with degree of limitation. Patient engages in satisfactory interpersonal relationships.

COLD INJURY (FROSTBITE)

Frostbite is a localized cold injury caused by exposure to freezing temperatures.

Several predisposing factors are associated with the occurrence of frostbite. People who are not acclimated to the cold and those from warmer climates have more vasospasm and less heat production in their extremities when exposed to cold temperatures; thus their risk of cold injury is increased. A racial predisposition of blacks to cold injury has been noted. Fatigue, hunger, young or old age, circulatory disorders, fear, use of alcohol, and hypoxia increase the risk of cold injury. Factors that promote heat loss such as contact with metal, wet skin, and high wind velocity contribute to the occurrence and severity of frostbite injuries.

PATHOPHYSIOLOGY

Cellular injury in frostbite is caused by direct freezing of cells at the time of injury or by inadequate tissue perfusion resulting from vascular spasm and occlusion of small vessels in the injured area.

With direct freezing of cells (crystallization), ice crystals form in extracellular fluids and osmotically draw intracellular fluid, thereby causing cell dehydration. Vascular changes include vasoconstriction, decreased capillary perfusion, and increased viscosity of the blood with sludging and thrombus formation.

After thawing, vascular stasis occurs in the injured area as a result of obstruction in the vascular bed. Edema occurs in the injured area and peaks 2 to 3 days after thawing. Thrombi, interstitial hemorrhaging, and leukocyte infiltration are present. Tissue necrosis occurs and becomes more prominent as the edema resolves. It may take 60 to 90 days before the necrotic tissue becomes fully evident.

The extent of the injury is determined by the amount and rate of heat loss from the skin. Frostbite is classified as superficial or deep. Superficial injury involves the skin and subcutaneous tissue. The injured area is white, waxy, soft, and anesthetic. Capillary refill is absent. On thawing the area becomes flushed, edematous, and painful and then may turn mottled or purplish. Large blisters may develop within 24 hours and resolve in about 10 days, leaving a hard, dark eschar. After 3 to 4 weeks the eschar separates, leaving sensitive new epithelium. Throbbing and burning pain lasts for several weeks. The area is sensitive to heat and cold for months, and the frostbitten part may perspire excessively.

Deep frostbite injures the skin, subcutaneous tissue, muscle, tendon, and neurovascular structures. The injured part is hard and solid and remains cold, mottled, and blue or gray after thawing. Blisters may be absent or may form after several weeks at the point where viable and nonviable tissue meet. Edema occurs in the entire limb and may take months to resolve. When the blisters dry, blacken, and slough off, a line of demarcation remains where the viable tissue separates and retracts from the dead tissue.

DIAGNOSTIC STUDIES AND FINDINGS

Physical examination: Characteristic findings with congruent history

MULTIDISCIPLINARY PLAN

Surgery

Escharotomy; sympathectomy for severe vasospasm and pain; debridement after retraction of viable tissue (13 weeks to 4 months after injury); amputation of nonviable extremity after retraction of viable tissue and medical intervention, may be several months after injury

Medications

Immunologic agents: Tetanus immunization, 0.5 ml IM for immunized patients

Diphtheria tetanus: 0.5 ml IM plus 250 U tetanus immune globulin (Hypertet) for nonimmunized patients

Plasma expanders: Low-molecular-weight dextran 40, 20 ml/kg IV q24h to decrease sludging; this therapy is controversial[59]

Antiinfective agents: Tetracycline or ampicillin (Amcill, Omnipen, others) for prophylaxis, 250 mg PO q6h

Narcotic agents: Morphine, up to 15 mg IM q3h

Analgesic-antipyretic agents: Aspirin, 650 PO q3h

Fibrinolytic agents, antiprostaglandins, thromboxane inhibitors, calmodulin antagonists: experimental therapies[59]

General Management

Rapid rewarming by immersion for 20 minutes in water at 38° to 41° C (100° to 106° F); protective isolation of patient or extremity; whirlpool baths three times a day at 32° to 37° C (90° to 98° F)

NURSING CARE

NURSING ASSESSMENT

Injured area: Color of skin; resilience of tissue; extent of limb involvement; duration of contact with cold; superficial in-

! EMERGENCY ALERT

THERMAL INJURY: COLD

Frostbite is irreversible, but minimizing the damage is of top priority. Frostbite occurs when ice crystals form in the intracellular space; they then enlarge and compress cells. This results in rupture that ultimately leads to microvascular occlusion. Hypothermia may also be present. Frostbite is classified as superficial or deep.

ASSESSMENT

Superficial

- Assess for tingling, numbness, burning sensation, and whitish color, usually on tips of toes.
- Assess circumstances, duration of exposure, temperature, wind chill, and other risk factors (e.g., homeless, peripheral vascular disease).

Deep

- White to waxy appearance.
- Burning pain followed by warmth, then numbness.
- Edema, blistering 1-7 days after injury.
- Black or gray mottling.

INTERVENTIONS

Superficial

- Handle skin extremely gently; do not rub.
- Apply warm soaks and elevate injured area.
- Avoid friction and weight on affected parts.
- Manage pain

Deep

- Handle skin extremely gently; *do not rub.*
- Obtain IV access.
- Manage pain (thawing tissue is extremely painful).
- Prevent body heat loss by keeping patient covered and ensuring warm room temperature.
- Assess neurovascular status frequently.
- Once at health-care facility, immerse injured part in warm water: 38°-41° C (100°-106° F).

jury: white, waxy, soft, no capillary refill; deep injury: hard, solid, mottled, blue or gray

Healing process: Pain, edema, color, blister formation, eschar formation, line of demarcation between viable and nonviable tissue

Infection: Pus, odor, redness, heat, fever

Other: Impaired mobility

Psychosocial concerns: Patient's perception of self and appearance, powerlessness and loss

POTENTIAL COMPLICATIONS

Vasospasm, pain, hyperesthesia, increased perspiration; loss of body part

PATIENT PROBLEMS/NURSING DIAGNOSES & INTERVENTIONS

NIC TISSUE PERFUSION

Ineffective tissue perfusion related to interruption of arterial or venous flow

- In collaboration with physician, initiate rapid rewarming in water at 38° to 41° (100° to 106° F) until the skin becomes soft and pliable and develops color.
- Completely immerse affected area in water, avoiding contact of skin with container.
- Instruct patient not to smoke *to avoid vasoconstriction.*

NIC SKIN/WOUND MANAGEMENT

Impaired skin integrity related to hypothermia

- Use sterile sheets *to prevent infection.*
- Isolate patient or extremity if necessary *to prevent infection.*
- Use bed cradle *to prevent mechanical trauma to injured tissue.*
- Keep blisters intact *to avoid introducing pathogens.*
- Keep extremity exposed to air *to prevent maceration.*
- Avoid debridement *to prevent further tissue injury.*

NIC IMMOBILITY MANAGEMENT

Impaired physical mobility related to pain and tissue damage

- Elevate extremities periodically *to promote venous return and prevent stasis.*
- Initiate range-of-motion exercises *to promote circulation and prevent contractures.*

NIC PHYSICAL COMFORT PROMOTION

Acute and chronic pain related to physical factors

- Keep sheets off extremity *to avoid pressure.*
- Administer analgesics as ordered.
- Instruct patient in relaxation techniques.
- Refer patient for biofeedback training.

NIC COPING ASSISTANCE

Disturbed body image related to cognitive-perceptual factors

Anticipatory grieving related to risk for loss of physiosocial or psychosocial well-being

Powerlessness related to illness-related regimen

- Encourage patient to express feelings about body, body appearance, or fear of reaction or rejection by others *to begin process of realistic self-evaluation.*
- Encourage patient to express distress, anger, sorrow, guilt, and fear about potential loss of extremity part or function *to assist in movement through stages of grieving.*
- Observe for signs of depression and apathy.
- Inform patient that healing process is long-term, slow, and uncertain; provide accurate information about healing.
- Encourage patient to express dissatisfaction and frustration.
- Involve patient in decision making *to increase sense of control.*
- Accept patient's feelings of anger.

PATIENT EDUCATION/CONTINUUM OF CARE PLAN

1. Discuss with the patient the need to protect the extremity from temperature extremes and rapid changes in temperature because the tissue is sensitive to temperature changes and refreezing will cause tissue loss.

2. Discuss with the patient the need to avoid tight, constrictive clothing or pressure to an area that might decrease circulation.
3. Demonstrate to the patient the application of dry, sterile dressing to small, open areas.
4. Explain to the patient the need to avoid smoking to reduce vasoconstriction.
5. Discuss with the patient preventive measures to avoid future episodes of reinjury of the frostbitten part: protective, multilayered, warm, nonconstrictive clothing; avoidance of fatigue, hunger, and use of alcohol when exposed to the cold.

EVALUATION/PATIENT OUTCOMES

Tissue Perfusion: Maximum tissue is preserved. Initial rapid thawing with no refreezing of tissue occurs. Tissue is free of infection. Healing is allowed to occur without premature surgical intervention.

Skin/Wound Management: Patient prevents further injury to area. Patient avoids tight, constrictive clothing or pressure to area. Patient does not smoke. Joints are functional. Patient has full extension and flexion of joints.

Patient prevents further episodes of cold injury. Patient wears protective clothing and avoids hunger, fatigue, and use of alcohol when exposed to cold.

Immobility Management: Pain is alleviated. Patient verbalizes relief of pain.

Physical Comfort Promotion: Patient remains as comfortable as possible. Pain from interventions is minimized.

Coping Assistance: Patient evaluates self in realistic manner. Patient resumes former activities if possible. Patient develops interests and activities compatible with degree of limitation. Patient engages in satisfactory interpersonal relationships.

DISEASES OF THE NAILS

FUNGAL INFECTIONS

See Tinea, p. 482.

PARONYCHIA

Paronychia is an acute or chronic inflammation of the proximal nail fold.

Erythema, induration, and swelling of the nail folds and consequent pain and tenderness are the primary features of paronychia. Staphylococci, streptococci, and sometimes *Candida* are the organisms usually responsible for the infection. One or more fingers or toes may be involved. Paronychia may be acute or chronic. Acute paronychia usually results from minor trauma or a hangnail. Chronic paronychia occurs in people whose hands are exposed to chronic irritation and moisture.

PATHOPHYSIOLOGY

In acute paronychia, organisms enter through a break in the epidermis. The infection may follow the nail margin or extend beneath the nail and suppurate. Purulent exudate may drain from beneath the nail fold. The eponychium remains attached to the nail plate. This separation creates a space in which foreign material and inflammatory exudate accumulate. Such an environment is conducive to bacterial and yeast growth. Chronic paronychia usually leads to nail ridging, distortion, and discoloration.

DIAGNOSTIC STUDIES AND FINDINGS

Physical examination: Characteristic lesion
Culture: Growth of infecting organism

MULTIDISCIPLINARY PLAN

Surgery

Incision and drainage of purulent pocket

Medications

Antiinfective agents

- Systemic antibiotics; depending on infecting organism
- Anticandidal solutions or lotions applied topically tid: clotrimazole (Lotrimin, Mycelex), miconazole (Monistat-Derm)
- Naftifine (Naftin), terbinafine (Lamasil), ciclopirox (Loprox)
- Thymol 4% in chloroform solution, 1 drop tid to affected area

NURSING CARE

NURSING ASSESSMENT

Inflammatory and infectious processes: Erythema; swelling; heat; tenderness; pain; purulent exudate; nails ridged, distorted, and discolored

Environmental factors: Constant moisture and trauma to hands or feet; history of previous infections

POTENTIAL COMPLICATIONS

Nail ridging, distortion, discoloration

PATIENT PROBLEMS/NURSING DIAGNOSES & INTERVENTIONS

NIC SKIN/WOUND MANAGEMENT

Impaired skin integrity related to inflammatory and infectious processes

Risk for impaired skin integrity related to mechanical factors

- Apply hot soaks *to promote suppuration and drainage.*
- Instruct patient in proper hand washing *to reduce existing pathogens.*
- Instruct patient to scrupulously dry hands and feet, especially around nails, and to use hot air drying rather than towel when possible *to prevent a wet environment that predisposes to infection.*

- Instruct patient to protect hands and feet from moisture by wearing cotton socks and rubber gloves with cotton liners when hands are in water.
- Discuss with patient role of environmental factors such as moisture and trauma, and explore ways to eliminate them.

NIC PHYSICAL COMFORT PROMOTION

Acute pain related to physical factors

- Offer hot soaks *to decrease swelling.*
- Elevate affected limb *to prevent throbbing.*

PATIENT EDUCATION/CONTINUUM OF CARE PLAN

1. Discuss with the patient prevention strategies regarding hand washing, drying, protection from moisture, and trauma (see under Patient Problems/Nursing Diagnoses & Interventions).
2. Discuss with the patient the use of medications and their side effects.
3. Demonstrate to the patient aseptic dressing changes if needed for draining lesions or after incision and drainage.

EVALUATION/PATIENT OUTCOMES

Skin/Wound Management: Inflammation subsides, and infection resolves. There is no erythema, swelling, heat, tenderness, pain, or purulent exudate. Chronic moisture and trauma are avoided. Paronychia does not recur.

Physical Comfort Promotion: Pain is relieved.

DISEASES OF THE HAIR

ALOPECIA

Alopecia is a partial or complete loss of hair.

Alopecia may occur as a result of genetic factors, the aging process, or local or systemic disease. Alopecia can be scarring or nonscarring and localized, patterned, or diffuse. The biologic dysfunctions of hair have little clinical importance, but the psychologic and social importance is substantial (FIG. 7-11).

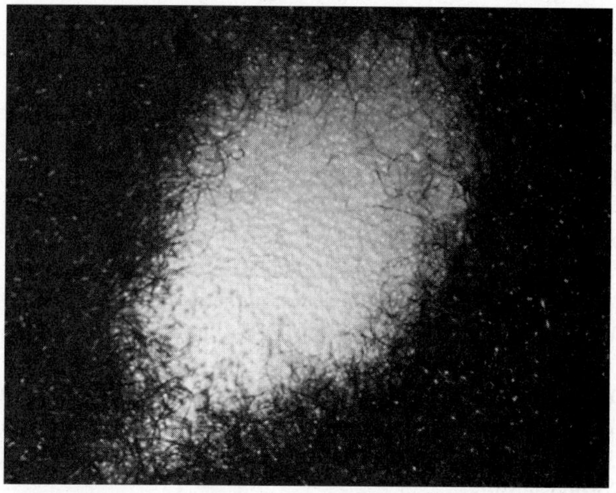

FIG. 7-11

Alopecia areata. (Courtesy Stephen B. Tucker, MD, Department of Dermatology, University of Texas Health Science Center at Houston, Tex.)

Table 7-10 Clinical Features and Pathology of Various Forms of Alopecia

Disease	Type	Features	Pathology
Areata	Nonscarring; localized or general	Occurs on any part of body; associated with family incidence; skin soft, smooth, not inflamed; one or several patches of loss; loss sudden; regrowth may occur with fine, light hair; hair pigments eventually	Inflammatory infiltrate around hair bulb; retraction in anagen hair; abnormal keratinization; loss of melanin and melanocytes; increased number of hair follicles in telogen phase
Androgenetic	Nonscarring; patterned	Occurs on scalp; in men frontal and temporal loss; thinning over vertex in women; mild, severe, or complete loss; familial trait	Androgens cause hair follicles to become smaller in size; terminal hair no longer formed; most hair follicles eventually disappear
Mechanical and chemical	Nonscarring; localized	Acute or chronic; attributable to hair-dressing procedures or habitual hair pulling; skin may show trauma from tight braids or curlers	Trauma to hair shaft; localized breakage of hair
Telogen effluvium	Nonscarring; diffuse	Occurs 6-16 weeks after precipitating episode; hair loss seen on shampooing or brushing; occurs as diffuse thinning; common precipitating factors are pregnancy, hormone therapy, stress, surgery, fever, and illness	Increased percentage of hairs in resting phase and subsequently in normal process of shedding
Drug related	Nonscarring; diffuse	Caused by antimitotic drugs (anagen hair loss) or by oral contraceptives, anticoagulants, propranolol (telogen hair loss); usually temporary	Antimitotic drugs cause decreased mitosis and decreased number of anagen hairs; hair shaft constricted; cause increase in percentage of hairs in telogen phase and subsequently in normal process of shedding
Scarring	Scarring	Due to systemic diseases such as lupus erythematosus, scleroderma, lichen planus, folliculitis decalvans; regrowth does not occur	Follicle destroyed by infection or scarring

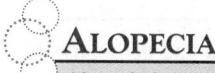

PATHOPHYSIOLOGY

Table 7-10 summarizes the clinical features and pathophysiology of the various types of hair loss.

DIAGNOSTIC STUDIES AND FINDINGS

Physical examination: Hair loss distribution, characteristics, and history
Biopsy: Reveals hair phase and structural damage
Damage: Infecting bacteria or fungus

MULTIDISCIPLINARY PLAN

Surgery

Hair transplant for androgenetic hair loss

Medications

Finasteride (Propecia), 1 mg/kg/day; use with males only
Topical minoxidil 2%-3% for androgenetic alopecia
Topical minoxidil 2% plus Retin-A for androgenetic alopecia; under investigation
Topical minoxidil 5% plus 0.5% anthralin for alopecia areata
Topical sensitizers: Dinitrochlorobenzene (DNCB); for many months
Corticosteroids
- Intralesional injection of 1-2 ml of triamcinolone (Kenalog), 10 mg/ml
- Topical glucocorticoids under occlusive dressing (see pp. 500)
  - Betamethasone (Valisone) 0.1%
  - Fluocinolone (Fluonid, Synalar, Flurosyn, Synemol) 0.025%

Chemotherapeutic agents: Cyclosporine, 6 mg/kg/day PO

General Management

Prolonged phototherapy (PUVA) (see p. 504)

NURSING CARE

NURSING ASSESSMENT

Lesion: As described in Table 7-10; location; distribution; scarring
Precipitating factors: Trauma, drugs, family history, systemic diseases
Psychosocial concerns: Concern about body image, patient's self-perception

POTENTIAL COMPLICATIONS

Untoward effects from treatments

PATIENT PROBLEMS/NURSING DIAGNOSES & INTERVENTIONS

NIC SKIN/WOUND MANAGEMENT

Impaired skin integrity related to hair loss
- Inform patient about treatment options.

NIC COPING ASSISTANCE

Disturbed body image related to cognitive-perceptual factors; situational low self-esteem
- Encourage patient to express feelings about body, body appearance, or fear of reaction or rejection by others *to begin process of realistic self-evaluation.*
- Advise patient that regrowth will occur in certain temporary conditions.
- Discuss use of wigs and hairpieces.

PATIENT EDUCATION/CONTINUUM OF CARE PLAN

1. Advise the patient that commercial preparations will not restore hair or encourage hair growth.
2. Discuss with the patient the cause and course of the disease.
3. Discuss with the patient the use of glucocorticoids under an occlusive dressing when indicated (see p. 500).

EVALUATION/PATIENT OUTCOMES

Skin/Wound Management: Underlying cause of hair loss is diagnosed and treated. There is no new hair loss. Hair regrowth occurs in some conditions.

Coping Assessment: Patient evaluates appearance in realistic manner. Patient does not use commercial hair restorative preparation. Patient uses wigs or hairpieces. Patient engages in satisfactory interpersonal relationships.

HYPERTRICHOSIS AND HIRSUTISM

Hypertrichosis refers to nonspecific hair growth of all types. Hirsutism is excessive hair growth induced by androgens in women.

PATHOPHYSIOLOGY

Hypertrichosis occurs as a result of increased activity of the hair follicle with the production of a coarse terminal hair. Localized hypertrichosis can be the result of persistent trauma that causes chronic hyperemia and inflammation of the dermis. Hypertrichosis can also be caused by systemic disorders, including severe infection, gross malnutrition, and gluten enteropathy.

Hirsutism occurs as a result of increased androgen activity and simulates the male pattern of hair distribution, with increased coarse terminal hair on the face, areolae, midline of the abdomen, and extremities. Hirsutism may be familial. Onset usually occurs slowly with no other symptoms of virilization. It may occur after menarche. Sudden onset of hirsutism may be from increased androgen production from adrenal, ovarian, or pituitary sources or by certain drugs such as systemic steroids, androgens, testosterone, progesterone, norethindrone, and phenytoin.

DIAGNOSTIC STUDIES AND FINDINGS

Physical examination: Distribution of hair with congruent history
Screening for adrenal, ovarian, and pituitary disorders

Multidisciplinary Plan

For treatment of adrenal, ovarian, or pituitary disorders, see the specific diseases. Generally, tumors are removed surgically; glucocorticoids are used for adrenal hyperplasia.

General Management

Electrolysis: Hair follicle destroyed by passage of galvanic electric current

Diathermy: Tissue destroyed through electrocoagulation; not recommended because it may cause scarring

Depilatories (wax or chemical): Chemicals can be irritating

Shaving

Bleaching with hydrogen peroxide and ammonia to depigment hair

NURSING CARE

Nursing Assessment

History: Onset, menstrual history, family history of hirsutism

Hair characteristics: Description of hair type, distribution, and pattern

Systemic features: Signs of virilization, size of ovaries and clitoris, uterine development

Psychosocial concerns: Concern abut body image, patient's self-perception

Potential Complications

From underlying disorder

Patient Problems/Nursing Diagnoses & Interventions

NIC Skin/Wound Management

Impaired skin integrity related to nonspecific or excessive hair growth

- Discuss treatment options with patient.

NIC Coping Assistance

Disturbed body image related to cognitive-perceptual factors; situational low self-esteem

- Encourage patient to express feelings about body, body image, and fear of reaction or rejection by others *to begin process of realistic self-evaluation.*
- Advise patient of treatments available for hair removal or bleaching.

Patient Education/Continuum of Care Plan

1. Discuss with the patient the advantages and disadvantages of the methods to remove or bleach the hair.
2. Discuss with the patient the cause and course of the disorder.

Evaluation/Patient Outcomes

Skin/Wound Management: Underlying or systemic disorders are diagnosed and treated. Hair growth diminishes or ceases. Patient chooses acceptable method for removing or bleaching hair. Patient is satisfied with method and appearance.

Coping Assistance: Patient evaluates appearance in realistic manner. Patient engages in usual activities and relationships.

Collaborative Interventions and Related Nursing Care

See table on p. 500.

Cryosurgery

In cryosurgery, tissue is frozen to remove hyperkerolytic growths (such as warts) or to cause involution of cysts.

Contraindications and Cautions

1. Overfreezing can cause scarring and hyperpigmentation.
2. Application of liquid nitrogen can be painful and is not well tolerated by children.

Procedural Guidelines

1. Liquid nitrogen is applied with a cotton-tipped applicator and is held in place for 10 to 20 seconds.
2. Carbon dioxide is applied via CO_2 pencil, which is held in place with moderate pressure for 20 to 30 seconds; or with CO_2 spray for 5 to 20 seconds depending on size of lesion.

Nursing Interventions

1. Inform patient before treatment of possibility of scarring or hyperpigmentation, and help patient evaluate the benefit/risk trade-off.
2. Instruct patient in the procedure.
3. Observe for blister formation immediately with CO_2 or in 5 to 10 hours with liquid nitrogen.
4. Instruct patient to prevent infection by keeping area clean and dry, not puncturing blister, and not picking at scab.
5. Instruct patient to observe for signs of infection and to seek medical attention if they occur.

Debridement

In debridement, dead tissue or eschar is removed to facilitate healing or in preparation for skin grafting.

Procedural Guidelines

Surgery

Surgical excision: Large areas removed down to fascia

Tangential excision: Layers of eschar removed with dermatome or scalpel to point of capillary bleeding; edge of tissue picked up with forceps and necrotic tissue cut with scissors; margin of 0.5 cm left to avoid cutting viable tissue; debridement limited to area of 10 cm; bleeding controlled by direct pressure; topical agent applied

Medications

Proteolytic enzymes applied with saline solution to erode and consume eschar

Mechanical

Removal through mechanical action in dressing changes, hydrotherapy, and showers

Common Therapeutic Interventions and Topical Preparations and Medications

Common Therapeutic Interventions	Therapeutic Effect	Nursing Care/Patient Education
Balneotherapy	Treat large areas of body or widely disseminated lesions	Fill tub full (20-25 gallons) at room temperature. Keep water from cooling. Bathe for 20-30 min. Use safety mat because medications make tub slippery. Keep room warm. Remove loose skin and crusts after bath. Apply medications while skin is still moist. Blot dry. Have patient dress in light, loose clothing.
Tap water	Antipruritic cooling; antiinflammatory	
Colloid, oatmeal, 1 cup	Antipruritic; nondrying	
Colloid, cornstarch, 2 cups	Antipruritic; drying	
Tar, commercial preparations, 2 teaspoons	Antipruritic; nondrying	
Carbonis detergens liquor, 1 ounce	Antipruritic; nondrying	
Oil (e.g., Alpha Keri, Domol, Lubath, Jeri-Bath)	Lubrication	
Burn hydrotherapy May add prescribed amounts sodium chloride, potassium chloride, calcium hypochlorite, or detergent	Facilitate dressing change and debridement	Immerse in water at temperature of 100° F (37.8° C) for 20-30 min. Stay with patient. Administer pain medications. Plug catheter. Shave and debride as needed. Use aseptic technique.
Occlusive dressings	Increased absorption and penetration of topical preparations; produces moisture retention, skin maceration, and decreased evaporation to increase effect of topical preparations	Apply airtight plastic film over medicated skin. Remove for 12 of 24 h to prevent complications. Watch for complications: bacterial and candidal infections, sweat retention, folliculitis, and side effects of medications.
Shampoos		Lather sufficiently. Gently work into scalp. Avoid contact with eyes.
Selenium sulfide	Antiseborrheic	
Betadine	Antibacterial	
Zinc pyrithione 2%	Antiseborrheic	
Carbonis detergens liquor, 5 %	Antiseborrheic Antipruritic	
Triethanolamine sulfate 40%	Bland (can add medications)	
Wet dressings and compresses	Cool and dry acute inflammation through evaporation	Soak compress to point of dripping. Keep at room temperature. Remoisten every few minutes. Apply for 15-30 min every 2 to 3 h. Do not rub or blot. Do not treat more than one third of the body at one time. Keep patient warm and covered. Advise patient that potassium permanganate stains skin, clothing, and tub. Instruct patient to use soft towels or cotton sheeting for home care to avoid irritating skin. Instruct patient to use clean towel or sheet each time compress is used, to keep them separate from rest of family linens, and to launder between each use.
Tap water or normal saline solution	Antipruritic; antiinflammatory through evaporation	
Aluminum acetate (Burow's solution)	Antipruritic; antiinflammatory used in acute, oozing dermatoses	
Potassium permanganate 1:10,000 solution; 5 grains/3 quarts water	As above; also antibacterial As above; also antifungal and antibacterial	
Dry burn dressing		Cleanse wound with one-half strength Betadine using sterile gauze; rub gently to remove existing topical agent. Apply topical agent thick enough to cover wound with ⅛ inch of agent to provide healing and prevent bandage from adhering. Apply layers of dressing: fine gauze, bulky coarse gauze; semielastic mesh. Change dressing one or two times daily.
Nonadherent, porous, fine mesh gauze	First layer; nonadherent; fine enough to prevent epithelialization into gauze	
Bulky, fluffed, coarse, mesh gauze	Second layer; absorbs exudate	
Semielastic coarse mesh	Outer layer; applies even pressure; holds dressing in place	
TOPICAL PREPARATIONS		
Creams and ointments Petrolatum, mineral oil, lanolin, Eurin, Qualatum, Unibase, Dermabase	Lubrication; protection; vehicle for medications; decrease water loss; ointments greasy with oil base; creams lighter and water washable	Rub into skin by hand. Cover ointments with light dressing to protect clothing. Apply frequently. Wash off before reapplication.
Gels Contain propylene glycol and carboxymethylene	Like creams and ointments; clear and nongreasy; may be used on hairy areas	Apply with fingers. Avoid rubbing because gels are thixotropic agents (become thinner with rubbing). Apply frequently.
Lotions	Liquid vehicles for medications; lubrication; cooling through evaporation	Apply with cotton gauze. Lotions are usually not washed off between applications.
With 0.5% menthol and 0.25% phenol	Antipruritic; drying	
Pastes	Stiff vehicle of powder and ointment; porous and less occlusive than ointments; protective	Apply with tongue depressor. Wash off between applications. Scrub gently if paste is difficult to remove.

Common Therapeutic Interventions	Therapeutic Effect	Nursing Care/Patient Education
Powders Talc, zinc oxide, cornstarch	Absorbent; hygroscopic (take up water); reduce friction	Apply with shaker. Avoid accumulation in intertriginous areas.
TOPICAL MEDICATIONS		
Antiseptic agents Chlorhexidine, povidone iodine, hexachlorophene	Treat carriers of pathogens; reduce overall skin bacterial count	Observe for sensitivities. Do not use hexachlorophene for infants and children.
Antibacterial agents	Like antiseptic agents	Observe for sensitivities. Cover with light dressing to protect clothing. Apply two to four times a day. Wash off before reapplication. With sulfamylon, debride wound before reapplication.
Neomycin	For gram-negative and gram-positive organisms	
Bacitracin	For gram-negative organisms and *Pseudomonas*	
Silver sulfadiazine (Silvadene)	For burns; for gram-negative and gram-positive organisms and yeast	
Sulfamylon	For burns; bacteriostatic only; for gram-negative and gram-positive organisms	
Precipitated sulfur 3%	Antiseborrheic	Observe for irritation.
Salicylic acid 3%-5%; urea 10%-20%	Keratolytic; increases absorption of other medications	Observe for irritation.
Corticosteroids Hydrocortisone 1%; fluocinolone 0.01%; triamcinolone 0.025%-0.1%; betamethasone	Decrease inflammation through vasoconstriction and direct action on leukocytes; decrease prostaglandin synthesis; decrease mitotic rate of epidermal cells	Apply sparingly to skin or apply in occlusive dressing. When used for prolonged periods, especially under occlusive dressings, watch for thinning of skin, striae formation, telangiectasia, and follicular hyperkeratosis.

Nursing Interventions

1. Describe procedure to patient.
2. Administer analgesics 20 minutes before debridement.
3. After procedure, assess area for exudate, color, sensation, bleeding, and size of area debrided.
4. Assess patient's response: pain, stress, or fear.

BLUNT DISSECTION

Blunt dissection is an office surgical procedure for removal of epidermal tumors, using a blunt dissector. Normal tissue is not disturbed, and scarring does not usually occur.

Procedural Guidelines

1. Before procedure, patient is given systemic analgesics if lesions are such that postoperative pain is anticipated, as with large plantar or periungual warts.
2. Local anesthesia with lidocaine is provided via needle injection or jet injector.
3. Plane of dissection is established by inserting tip of blunt-tipped scissors between lesion and normal skin and cutting skin circumferentially.
4. Blunt dissector is then inserted into the opened plane, which is separated from normal underlying tissue with short firm strokes.
5. After lesion is removed, dissector is drawn back and forth over the exposed surface of the bed to remove tissue fragments.

Nursing Interventions

1. Instruct patient in the procedure.
2. After procedure, cover wound with Band-Aid. Advise patient to change it daily for 3 to 4 days and thereafter to leave wound exposed to air.
3. Advise patient that moderate to intense pain may occur for 30 minutes to 2 hours after blunt dissection of periungual and plantar warts.

ELECTRODESICCATION AND CURETTAGE

In electrodesiccation an electric current is used to remove superficial lesions. In curettage a dermal curette with round or oval sharp surfaces is used to remove superficial lesions. The procedures may be used together or separately.

Contraindications and Cautions

1. High-frequency current can deactivate a pacemaker. Special precautions are required in patients with indwelling cardiac pacemakers.
2. Electrodes should be changed after each use or sterile disposable needle electrodes used to prevent the transmission of viral-associated infections.

Procedural Guidelines

Fulguration

1. Surface to be treated is cleaned so it is dry and free of blood.

2. Pointed electrode is held slightly away from tissue surface, and unit is activated.
3. A sparking occurs, resulting in tissue dehydration and charring of immediate surrounding area.

Desiccation

1. Pointed electrode is placed in contact with the skin surface or inserted slightly in the tissue, and unit is activated.
2. Resulting tissue char is produced by fulguration.

Electrocoagulation

1. Bipolar setting is used.
2. Active electrode is placed in contact with the tissue, and unit is activated.
3. Tissue necrosis is more extensive than with fulguration or desiccation.

Curettage

1. Area is anesthetized with lidocaine via needle injection or jet injector.
2. Skin around lesion is supported with fingers of the hand not holding the instrument.
3. With several smooth strokes, curette is drawn through the tissue.

Nursing Interventions

1. Instruct patient in procedure.
2. Clean surrounding skin with antibacterial agent.
3. If oozing occurs after procedure, cover with sterile gauze.
4. Leave area exposed to air or covered with light dressing.
5. Encourage daily washing with soap and water.

Intralesional Injections

Intralesional injections are injections of a corticosteroid into a lesion. The antiinflammatory action helps clear lesions and reduce the size of cysts.

Contraindications and Cautions

Injection into subcutaneous tissue can result in transient or permanent atrophy and local tissue depression.

Procedural Guidelines

Aqueous suspension (usually triamcinolone, 5 to 10 mg/2 ml) is injected intracutaneously into the lesion or cyst with a fine-gauge needle. The more superficial the injection, the better is the result.

Nursing Interventions

1. Inform patient before treatment of possibility of atrophy, and help patient evaluate benefit/risk trade-off.
2. Instruct patient to observe for side effects of treatment: bleeding, hemorrhaging, pigmentation, and atrophy; adrenal suppression may occur with multiple injections.
3. Instruct patient to observe for desired effects: cyst decreases in size, and lesion clears.
4. Instruct patient to keep area clean to avoid secondary infection.

Laser Therapy

Laser (light amplification by stimulated emission of radiation) therapy is used to treat certain vascular, pigmented, and other lesions of the skin. The most commonly used laser systems are the pulsed-dye laser, argon laser, and carbon dioxide laser.

Procedural Guidelines

Pulsed-Dye Laser

1. Anesthesia is seldom required. Topical or local anesthesia may be used, especially in children.
2. Most patients feel the laser pulse as a snapping sensation against their skin.
3. A gray-blue bruise is produced that resolves in 7 to 14 days, or the bruise may take up to 3 months to resolve in darker-skinned patients.
4. Wound care is usually not necessary.

Argon Laser

1. Local or general anesthesia is usually administered.
2. The potential for scarring is higher than with the pulsed-dye laser.
3. Testing is usually performed with both the argon and the pulsed-dye laser to select the most effective treatment.
4. A superficial burn wound is created that requires dressing changes for 1 week or for several weeks.

Carbon Dioxide Laser

1. The laser beam can be focused to bloodlessly excise lesions, or it can be defocused to vaporize tissue.
2. Local anesthesia is usually used.
3. Evaporation of tissue during excision and vaporization produces steam that requires removal by smoke evacuation equipment.
4. Postoperative pain is minimal.
5. Excision produces an incision that may require closure with sutures, staples, or other wound-closure materials. Wound healing may be delayed; therefore sutures or staples are commonly left in place longer than with a comparable scalpel wound.
6. Vaporization produces minimal thermal damage to surrounding tissue that will turn it brown; it will remain brown until it is healed.

Nursing Interventions

1. Assist in discussing all treatment options with the patient. Discuss with the patient that patch testing may be used to assist in determination of efficacy or to select the most effective system of treatment. Such testing may delay actual therapy.
2. Assist in discussing potential adverse outcomes with the patient: hypertrophic scarring, hypopigmentation, hyperpigmentation, incomplete removal of the lesion, and infection.
3. Prepare the patient for any draping or safety equipment that may be used during the procedure, such as patient eye protectors and wet draping, depending on the laser and on the area being treated.
4. Assist in ensuring appropriate safety precautions:
   a. Limited access to the surgical area
   b. Internally controlled door locks
   c. Proper testing of equipment before each use

d. Eye protection designed for the specific laser being used
e. Removal of reflective jewelry and surgical instruments
f. Wet draping if required

5. Cleanse the area to be treated. Remove all makeup or skin lotions, and dry the area.
6. Provide assistance and support to the patient to remain stationary during the procedure.
7. Discuss postprocedure care with the patient, depending on the laser system used. Discuss with the patient the need to:
   a. Avoid trauma to the area.
   b. Pat dry the skin after bathing, rather than rubbing it.
   c. Avoid sunlight to the area, and use a sunscreen with an SPF of 15 or higher; this precaution may need to be observed for several months.

SKIN GRAFT

In a skin graft a section of skin tissue that is separated from its blood supply is transferred to a recipient site to provide tissue for epithelization.

Split-thickness graft: Composed of epidermis and superficial layers of dermis.
Full-thickness graft: Composed of epidermis and all layers of dermis.
Homograft (allograft): Skin from a deceased person that is used as temporary cover for about 10 days and may survive for 4 to 5 weeks.
Heterograft (xenograft): Pigskin or synthetic substitute that acts as biologic dressing.
Autograft: Skin from another part of the patient's own body.
Mesh graft: Slit-thickness graft meshed with a special instrument to cover large areas and held in place by a dressing or sutures.
Autologous cultured human epithelium: Unburned epidermal cells cultured into sheets in a flask. The cultured sheets are then attached to petrolatum gauze squares and sutured in place in the wound. The petrolatum gauze is removed 7 to 10 days later.

Procedural Guidelines

1. Donor site is prepared by surgical scrub. Recipient site is debrided and cleansed.
2. Split- or full-thickness graft is taken from the donor site with a dermatome. Graft is cut as "postage stamps" or strips or is meshed and placed on recipient sites.
3. Graft is held in place by a pressure dressing or sutures.
4. Donor site is covered with nonadherent gauze held in place by a gauze dressing.

Nursing Interventions

Donor Site

1. Remove outer dressing in 24 hours.
2. Inspect site daily.
3. Assess for bleeding, pain, and infection.
4. Leave nonadherent gauze in place until it separates spontaneously.
5. If infection occurs, treat it with medicated wet dressing.

Recipient (Graft) Site

1. Inspect site daily.
2. Assess for edema, hematoma formation, fluid collection, infection, and viability of graft tissue.
3. Immobilize affected part to avoid disrupting graft.
4. Elevate grafted extremity for 7 to 10 days.
5. Protect graft from scratching by patient.
6. If infection occurs, treat it with a medicated wet dressing.
7. Heterograft acts as a biologic dressing; expect it to slough off in 10 days to 5 weeks.

Healing Phase

1. Inform patient about changing hues of graft scar tissue: pale, then pink, then red, then fading to resemble surrounding skin; a full-thickness graft may remain deeply red for several months.
2. Anticipate skin scaling with a full-thickness graft.
3. Lubricate donor site with lanolin or cocoa butter to keep the tissue soft and pliable.
4. Apply mineral oil or lanolin to graft site after second or third week to remove superficial crusts, moisten graft, and stimulate circulation.
5. Instruct patient who will be at home to avoid overexposure of graft site to the sun because site is sensitive to the sun and can burn easily.
6. Encourage patient to express feelings about body, body appearance, or fear of reaction or rejection by others.

SYSTEMIC STEROID THERAPY

In systemic steroid therapy, parenteral or oral glucocorticoids are used for their antiinflammatory action.

Contraindications and Cautions

1. Hypertension and diabetes mellitus can be exacerbated.
2. Concurrent infections can be masked.
3. Therapy is used with caution in patients who are predisposed to peptic ulceration, thrombophlebitis, adrenal suppression, and mood swings.

Procedural Guidelines

Dose and duration of treatment depend on the severity of the disease and the patient's response. The patient should receive a dose sufficient to produce a therapeutic response and then be maintained with a minimum effective dose; the dose should be tapered slowly after the lesions have cleared.

Approximate equivalent doses of various steroids are as follows:

Betamethasone, 0.5 mg	Methylprednisolone, 4 mg
Dexamethasone, 0.75 mg	Prednisolone, 5 mg
Fludrocortisone, 2 mg	Prednisone, 5 mg
Hydrocortisone, 20 mg	Triamcinolone, 4 mg

Nursing Interventions

1. Inform patient about side effects to watch for and to seek medical attention if they occur: euphoria, gastrointestinal pain or bleeding, bruising, thrombophlebitis, hypertension, moonface, cushingoid features, acne, hirsutism, osteoporosis, and mood swings.

2. Instruct patient to take medication with milk or antacids to decrease gastric irritation.
3. Instruct patient to increase protein intake to combat osteoporosis.

TOPICAL STEROID THERAPY

Topical steroids are used therapeutically for their antiinflammatory, immunosuppressant, and antimitotic effects on the skin.

Contraindications and Cautions

For use of superpotent topical steroids:

1. All local side effects from less potent topical steroids may be accentuated with superpotent steroids.
2. Systemic side effects may include suppression of the hypothalamic-pituitary-adrenal axis or development of Cushing's syndrome.
3. Superpotent topical steroids should not be used in children because of their increased ratio of skin surface to body weight.
4. Superpotent topical steroids should not be used in occlusive dressings because enhanced absorption could lead to atrophy and bacterial infection.
5. Superpotent topical steroids should not be used for longer than 2 weeks in flexor areas because these areas are sites of natural occlusion.
6. Prolonged usage of superpotent topical steroids should be avoided in the elderly because they have thinner skin and the drug clears more slowly.
7. Superpotent topical steroids should not be used on the face, eyelids, scrotum, or mucous membranes because of the enhanced degree of penetration in these areas.

Procedural Guidelines

Topical steroids in general are used alone, though they are often used under occlusive dressings. Topical steroids can be classified in terms of their relative potency. The superpotent steroids (i.e., betamethasone dipropylene, clobetasol propionate, and diflorasone diacetate) produce a highly effective and enhanced therapeutic effect; however, they require special guidelines for use.

1. Proper potency is selected. The lowest-potency preparations are used for dermatoses that are mild and chronic and involve the face, intertriginous regions, and genitalia. Medium- and high-potency preparations are used for dermatoses that are more severe and recalcitrant to treatment.
2. The proper vehicle is selected. Ointments are occlusive and are best used for chronic inflammation characterized by dryness, scaling, and lichenification. Lotions, creams, and gels are nonocclusive and are used for acute and subacute inflammations that are oozing or vesiculated. Lotions and gels are best used on hairy areas such as the scalp.
3. Frequency of application is determined. The stratum corneum acts as a reservoir and continues to release topical steroid into the skin after the initial application. Application one to two times is usually sufficient. Some chronic dermatoses become less responsive after prolonged or more frequent use of topical steroids.

Nursing Interventions

1. Instruct patient in proper application of the preparation. Application right after bathing improves penetration of the preparation into skin. The product should be spread as thinly as possible until it disappears. It is not necessary to leave a visible layer.
2. Inform patient of potential topical side effects: Atrophy and striae formation, acne, enhanced fungal infection, retarded wound healing, and contact dermatitis. Glaucoma or cataracts can occur with application to the eyelids.
3. Inform patient of potential risk of systemic absorption and side effects with extensive and chronic use of potent topical steroids.

ULTRAVIOLET LIGHT THERAPY

Short-wave ultraviolet light (UVB) is used for the treatment of psoriasis and acne. In Goeckerman therapy, ultraviolet light therapy is used in combination with coal tar applications that are photosensitizing; it is used for the treatment of psoriasis. In PUVA therapy, long-wave ultraviolet light (UVA) is used in combination with psoralen, which is a photosensitizer (PUVA); it is used for treating psoriasis.

Procedural Guidelines

Short-Wave Ultraviolet Light

1. Patient is exposed one to three times per week.
2. Exposure time is increased to keep skin just below erythema level.

Goeckerman Therapy

1. Coal tar ointment is applied, left on for several hours, and then washed off.
2. UVB therapy is given in doses to account for photosensitization.
3. Skin is kept just below erythema level.
4. Coal tar ointment is reapplied after UVB exposure.

PUVA Therapy

1. Psoralen is administered in an initial dose of 0.6 mg/kg.
2. UVA irradiation is delivered 2 to 4 hours after psoralen administration.
3. Dosage and exposure are determined by individual response.
4. Therapy is usually provided in specific treatment centers because specialized equipment, careful calibration, and close monitoring are required.

Contraindications and Cautions

PUVA Therapy

Long-term effects of PUVA therapy remain controversial, and treatment is usually reserved for chronic, severe, refractory psoriasis.

Nursing Interventions

1. Instruct patient in the procedure.
2. Assist patient in setting up a schedule to maintain therapeutic regimen.
3. Instruct patient who is using short-wave ultraviolet light therapy at home to:

   a. Use a lamp with an automatic timer to shut off.
   b. Use a backup timer.
   c. Measure the distance from the lamp carefully and maintain correct distance.
   d. Increase exposure time slowly and keep skin below erythema level.
   e. Wear an occlusive protective eye covering.
4. Advise patient who is using concomitant photosensitizing agents to avoid lengthy exposure to sunlight.
5. Advise patient who is receiving PUVA therapy of undetermined long-term effects, and assist patient in evaluating risk/benefit trade-off.

REFERENCES

1. Arndt K: *Manual of dermatologic therapeutics,* ed 5, Boston, 1995, Little, Brown.
2. Barone E et al: *Skin disorders, the Academy collection quick reference guides for family physicians,* ed 1, Philadelphia, 2000, Lippincott Williams & Wilkins.
3. Bergler W et al: Argon plasma coagulation for the treatment of hereditary hemorrhagic telangiectasia, *Laryngoscope* 109(1):15, 1999.
4. Berman B, Flores F: Comparison of a silicone gel-filled cushion and silicon gel sheeting for the treatment of hypertrophic or keloid scars, *Dermatol Surg* 25(6):484, 1999.
5. Bevier DE: Insect and arachnid hypersensitivity, *Vet Clin North Am Small Anim Pract* 29(6):1385, 1999.
6. Boguniewicz M: Advances in the understanding and treatment of atopic dermatitis, *Curr Opin Pediatr* 9(6):577, 1997.
7. Brehler R et al: Recent developments in the treatment of atopic eczema, *J Am Acad Dermatol* 36(6 Pt 1):983, 1997.
8. Bright RD: Methotrexate in the treatment of psoriasis, *Cutis* 64(5):332, 1999.
9. Caceres-Rios H et al: Comparison of terbinafine and griseofulvin in the treatment of tinea capitis, *J Am Acad Dermatol* 42(1 Pt 1): 80, 2000.
10. Chen J et al: A comparison among four regimens of itraconazole treatment in onychomycosis, *Mycoses* 42(1-2):93, 1999.
11. Correale CE et al: Atopic dermatitis: a review of diagnosis and treatment, *Am Fam Physician* 60(4):1191, 1999.
12. Cribier B et al: Treatment of lichen planus: an evidence-based medicine analysis of efficacy, *Arch Dermatol* 134(12):1521, 1998.
13. Downs AM et al: Head lice: prevalence in schoolchildren and insecticide resistance, *Parasitol Today* 15(1):1, 1999.
14. Droogan J: Treatment and prevention of head lice and scabies, *Nurs Times* 95(29):44, 1999.
15. Dubertret L: Strategy for treatment of psoriasis: systemic treatments, *J Dermatol* 25(12):788, 1998.
16. Elewski BE: Treatment of tinea capitis: beyond griseofulvin, *J Am Acad Dermatol* 40(6 Pt 2):S27, 1999.
17. Federman DG, Froelich CW: Topical psoriasis therapy, *Am Fam Physician* 59(4):957, 1999.
18. Feldman SR et al: New topical treatments change the pattern of treatment of psoriasis: dermatologists remain the primary providers of this care, *Int J Dermatol* 39(1):41, 2000.
19. Fernandez-Obregon AC: Azithromycin for the treatment of acne, *Int J Dermatol* 39(1):45, 2000.
20. Fish RM: Electric injury, part I: treatment priorities, subtle diagnostic factors, and burns, *J Emerg Med* 17(6):977, 1999.
21. Fitzpatrick T et al: *Color-atlas and synopsis of clinical dermatology,* ed 3, New York, 1997, McGraw-Hill.
22. Goldberg DJ: Laser treatment of pigmented lesions, *Dermatol Clin* 15(3):397, 1997.
23. Goldstein B, Goldstein A: *Practical dermatology,* ed 2, St. Louis, 1997, Mosby.
24. Gollnick H, Schramm M: Topical drug treatment in acne, *Dermatology* 196(1):119, 1998.
25. Goolsby MJ: The elusive itch. assessment, diagnosis and management of pruritis, *Adv Nurse Pract* 6(11):61, 1998.
26. Greenwald D et al: An algorithm for early aggressive treatment of frostbite with limb salvage directed by triple-phase scanning, *Plast Reconstr Surg* 102(4):1069, 1998.
27. Gross WL: New concepts in treatment protocols for severe systemic vasculitis, *Curr Opin Rheumatol* 11(1):41, 1999.
28. Habif T: *Clinical dermatology: a color guide to diagnosis and therapy,* ed 3, St. Louis, 1996, Mosby.
29. Harries PG et al: Treatment of hereditary haemorrhagic telangiectasia by the pulsed dye laser, *J Laryngol Otol* 111(11):1038, 1997.
30. Harris DR: The art of treating psoriasis: practical suggestions for improved treatment, *Cutis* 64(5):335, 1999.
31. Hartley AH: Pityriasis rosea, *Pediatr Rev* 20(8):266, 1999.
32. Janniger C, Schwartz R: Seborrheic dermatitis, *Am Fam Physician* 52(1):149, 1995.
33. Johnson RW: Herpes zoster and postherpetic neuralgia: optimal treatment, *Drugs Aging* 10(2):80, 1997.
34. Kakourou T et al: Corticosteroid treatment of erythema multiforme major (Stevens-Johnson syndrome) in children, *Eur J Pediatr* 156(2):90, 1997.
35. Kanzenbach TL, Dexter WW: Cold injuries: protecting your patients from the dangers of hypothermia and frostbite, *Postgrad Med* 105(1):72, 1999.
36. Kim M et al: *Pocket guide to nursing diagnoses,* ed 7, St. Louis, 1997, Mosby.
37. Kullavanijaya P et al: Treatment of psoriasis vulgaris with topical vitamin D analogue (calcipotriol): open multicenter study, *J Med Assoc Thai* 82(10):974, 1999.
38. Kumar SA, Martin BL: Urticaria and angioedema: diagnostic and treatment considerations, *J Am Osteopath Assoc* 99(3 Suppl):S1, 1999.
39. Lange DS et al: Ketoconazole 2% shampoo in the treatment of tinea versicolor: a multicenter, randomized, double-blind, placebo-controlled trial, *J Am Acad Dermatol* 39(6):944, 1998.
40. Layton A: Know how treatment for childhood eczema, *Nurs Times* 94(41):30, 1998.
41. Lim JT: Treatment of melasma using kojic acid in a gel containing hydroquinone and glycolic acid, *Dermatol Surg* 25(4):282, 1999.
42. Linden KG, Weinstein GD: Psoriasis: current perspectives with an emphasis on treatment, *Am J Med* 107(6):595, 1999.
43. Lookingbill D, Jr, Marks JM: *Principles of dermatology,* ed 2, Philadelphia, 1993, WB Saunders.
44. Lord RW, Jr: Treatments for atopic eczema, *J Fam Pract* 48(9):663, 1999.
45. Martin BG: Contact dermatitis: evaluation and treatment, *J Am Osteopath Assoc* 99(3 Suppl):S11, 1999.
46. McCoy SE: Copper bromide laser treatment of facial telangiectasia: results of patients treated over five years, *Lasers Surg Med* 21(4):329, 1997.
47. Milles CL et al: Onychomycosis: Diagnosis and systemic treatment, *Nurse Pract* 23(12):40, 1998.

48. Moghetti P et al: Comparison of spironolactone, flutamide, and finasteride efficacy in the treatment of hirsutism: a randomized, double blind, placebo-controlled trial, *J Clin Endocrinol Metab* 85(1):89, 2000.
49. Monroe EW: Loratadine in the treatment of urticaria, *Clin Ther* 19(2):232, 1997.
50. Noble SL et al: Diagnosis and management of common tinea infections, *Am Fam Physician* 58(1):163, 1998.
51. Nolting SK et al: Continuous itraconazole treatment for onychomycosis and dermatomycosis: an overview of safety, *Eur J Dermatol* 9(7):540, 1999.
52. Nouri K et al: Combination treatment of melasma with pulsed CO_2 laser followed by Q-switched alexandrite laser: a pilot study, *Dermatol Surg* 25(6):494, 1999.
53. O'Dell ML: Skin and wound infections: an overview, *Am Fam Physician* 57(10):2424, 1998.
54. Orfanos CE: Treatment of psoriasis with retinoids: present status, *Cutis* 64(5):347, 1999.
55. Parsons L: Office management of minor burns, *Prim Care* 1(1):40, 1997.
56. Raulin C et al: Treatment of a nonresponding port-wine stain with a new pulsed light source (PhotoDerm VL), *Lasers Surg Med* 21(2):203, 1997.
57. Raulin C et al: Q-switched ruby laser treatment of tattoos and benign pigmented skin lesions: a critical review, *Ann Plast Surg* 41(5):555, 1998.
58. Reamy BV: Frostbite: Review and current concepts, *J Am Board Fam Pract* 11(1):34, 1998.
59. Rosen P, Barkin R, editors: *Emergency medicine concepts and clinical practice,* ed 4, St. Louis, 1998, Mosby.
60. Rushton DH: Androgenetic alopecia in men: the scale of the problem and prospects for treatment, *Int J Clin Pract* 53(1):50, 1999.
61. Sabiston D, Jr, editor: *Textbook of surgery: the biological basis of modern surgical practice,* ed 11, Philadelphia, 1977, WB Saunders.
62. Saurat JH: Retinoids and psoriasis: novel issues in retinoid pharmacology and implications for psoriasis treatment, *J Am Acad Dermatol* 41(3 Pt 2):S2, 1999.
63. Sawaya ME: Novel agents for the treatment of alopecia, *Semin Cutan Med Surg* 17(4):276, 1998.
64. Scow DT et al: Medical treatments for balding in men, *Am Fam Physician* 59(8):2189, 1999.
65. Seidel H et al: *Mosby's guide to physical examination,* ed 4, St. Louis, 1999, Mosby.
66. Sharma PK et al: Erythromycin in pityriasis rosea: a double-blind, placebo-controlled clinical trial, *J Am Acad Dermatol* 42(2):241, 2000.
67. Soltz-Szots J et al: A randomized controlled trial of acyclovir versus netivudine for treatment of herpes zoster, International Zoster Study Group, *J Antimicrob Chemother* 41(5):549, 1998.
68. Sommer S et al: Ruby laser treatment for hirsutism: clinical response and patient tolerance, *Br J Dermatol* 138(6):1009, 1998.
69. Stary A, Sarnow E: Fluconazole in the treatment of tinea corporis and tinea cruris, *Dermatology* 196(2):237, 1998.
70. Tharp MD: Chronic urticaria: pathophysiology and treatment approaches, *J Allergy Clin Immunol* 98(6 Pt 3):S325, 1996.
71. The American Academy of Dermatology, Committee on Guidelines of Care: Guidelines of care for acne vulgaris, *J Am Acad Dermatol* 22:676, 1990.
72. The American Academy of Dermatology, Committee on Guidelines of Care: Guidelines of care for contact dermatitis, *J Am Acad Dermatol* 32:109, 1995.
73. Thissen M, Westerhof W: Laser treatment for further depigmentation in vitiligo, *Int J Dermatol* 36(5):386, 1997.
74. Toubi E et al: Low-dose cyclosporin A in the treatment of severe chronic idiopathic urticaria, *Allergy* 52(3):312, 1997.
75. Toyoda M, Morohashi M: An overview of topical antibiotics for acne treatment, *Dermatology* 196(1):130, 1998.
76. Treseler KM: *Clinical laboratory and diagnostic tests,* ed 3, Norwalk, 1995, Appleton & Lange.
77. Tristani-Firouzi P, Krueger GG: Efficacy and safety of treatment modalities for psoriasis, *Cutis* 61(2 Suppl):11, 1998.
78. Van Laborde S, Scher RK: Developments in the treatment of nail psoriasis, melanonychia striata, and onychomycosis: a review of the literature, *Dermatol Clin* 18(1):37, 2000.
79. Wahn U et al: Atopic eczema: how to tackle the most common atopic symptom, *Pediatr Allergy Immunol* 10:10, 1999.
80. Wood MJ et al: Treatment of acute herpes zoster: effect of early treatment, *J Infect Dis* 178(Suppl 1):S81, 1998.
81. Young E et al: *Geriatric dermatology,* Philadelphia, 1993, Lea & Febiger.

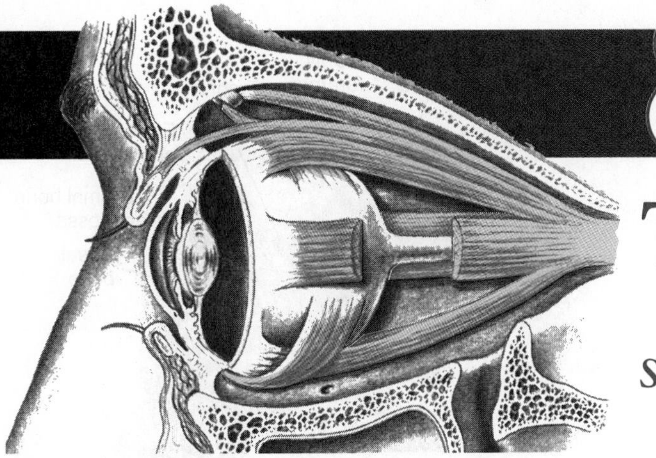

8 The Eye

Sarah C. Smith

Overview

Preserving vision and preventing blindness are important to everyone. A recent poll found that Americans fear blindness more than any other disorder except cancer.[8] The American Academy of Ophthalmology's Committee on Eye Care for the American People reports that "approximately 1,000,000 Americans are legally blind, more than 11.4 million are visually impaired because of chronic or permanent defects, 80 million have a disease in one or both eyes, and additional millions need eyeglasses or contact lenses to see clearly."[8] Eye care has become the focus of more attention in recent years because expanding knowledge and technology have increased the opportunity for early diagnosis and successful treatment of eye disorders. Technologic advances include microsurgical techniques, laser surgery, contact lens refinement, development of intraocular lenses, and corneal replacement. Screening programs offered by schools and community agencies have enhanced public awareness of eye disorders and preventive eye care. This greater awareness of the need for periodic eye examinations, of specific measures for preventing eye injuries, and of the early signs or symptoms of eye disorders has contributed to the prevention of visual impairment. Major eye disorders include cataract, corneal impairments and injuries, glaucoma, retinal diseases, strabismus, and amblyopia. All these impairments can cause blindness, but most of them are partially or fully treatable if diagnosed early. Nurses can contribute significantly to the prevention of visual impairment by becoming knowledgeable about the cause and prevention of eye disorders and by urging patients to follow through with self-care and health promotion measures. For example, the American Academy of Ophthalmology's Committee on Eye Care for the American People has made the recommendations in the box on p. 508.

Anatomy, Physiology, and Related Pathophysiology

External Structures

Orbit and Its Contents

The human eye is approximately 24 mm in diameter. It rests within a fatty cushion in a bony orbit of the skull. The orbit comprises six bones forming a cavity that converges into two major posterior openings, the optic foramen and the superior orbital fissure (Fig. 8-1). Through these openings run blood vessels and nerves that connect the eyeball to the brain and the body's blood supply. The ophthalmic artery, the optic nerve, and sympathetic nerves from the carotid plexus enter the orbit through the optic foramen. The oculomotor nerve (cranial nerve [CN] III), trochlear nerve (CN IV), abducent nerve (CN VI), and ophthalmic branch of the trigeminal nerve (CN V) pass through the superior orbital fissure.[36]

The orbit contains the eyeball, which is cradled in the anterior portion; six oculomotor muscles, which surround and insert into the eyeball; a muscle for elevating the eyelid; and fat, ligaments, and connective tissue in the posterior section that cushion and support the eyeball and the extrinsic muscles. The anterior orbital walls are relatively thick and provide good protection for the eye. The orbit contains a fibrous sheet that encircles the optic foramen and is the origin for the extrinsic muscles, which stretch forward to encircle and insert into the anterior and medial aspects of the eyeball (Fig. 8-2). The orbital contents are supported and separated from the bone by a periosteal lining and fascial tissue that form the eye socket in which the eyeball rests.

Eyelid. The exposed part of the eye is protected by a lid that serves as a shield from external injury and exposure to excessive light. As the upper lid blinks, it distributes tears over the surface of the eye to keep it moist. When the lids are open, they form the palpebral fissure (the elliptic opening). As a result, the upper lid covers part of the iris (Fig. 8-3). The lids meet at the medial (inner) canthus and fold over a small elevation, called the lacrimal caruncle. This caruncle contains large sebaceous glands. The inner canthus is sometimes obscured by a vertical skin fold (epicanthus) in Asian people and young children. The central portion of the upper and lower lid is thickened with a firm connective tissue (tarsal plate) that protects the eye and maintains the shape of the lid. The eyelids are lined with a thin, transparent mucous membrane (palpebral conjunctiva) that continues as an outer cover for the sclera of the eyeball (bulbar conjunctiva) (see Fig. 8-2). The conjunctiva contains blood vessels, nerves, hair follicles, and sebaceous glands (meibomian glands). The meibomian glands are found along the margin of the lids. Their secretions prevent rapid evaporation and

GUIDELINES FOR EYE EXAMINATIONS FOR ADULTS AND THE ELDERLY

All adults with decrease in visual acuity for distant or near objects should have an ophthalmologic eye examination or refractive eye examination.

All adults should have an eye examination by a family physician, internist, or other health care professional as a component of regular health care.

Adults with risk factors such as a family history of glaucoma, cataract, retinal detachment, or significant degenerative eye disease should have an ophthalmologic eye examination early in adult life and at medically appropriate intervals thereafter.

Adults with diabetes mellitus should have an ophthalmologic eye examination at the time of diagnosis and at medically appropriate intervals thereafter.

Adults with systemic disease and/or medical treatment known to be associated with increased risk of eye disease should have an ophthalmologic eye examination at the time of diagnosis and/or treatment onset.

All adults 65 or more years of age should have an ophthalmologic eye examination at least every 2 years.

Adults should participate in vision screening programs conducted by eye care and health care professionals, industry representatives, or volunteer organizations annually or every 2 years.

From Comprehensive adult eye examination.[8]

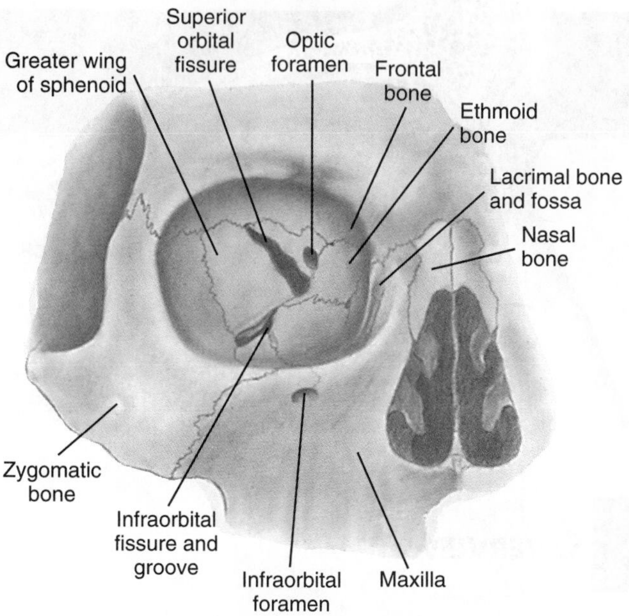

FIG. 8-1
Right bony orbit.

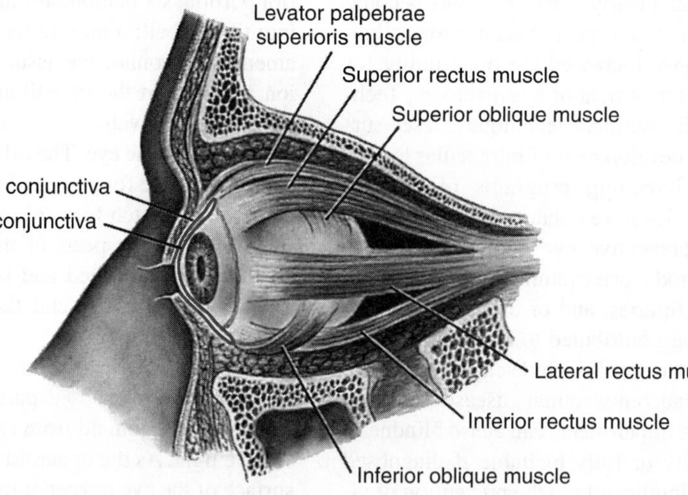

FIG. 8-2
Diagrammatic section of orbit.

overflow of tears and create an airtight seal when the eyelids are closed.

Lid movement is supplied from the superior division of the oculomotor nerve (CN III), which activates the superior palpebral levator muscle for upper lid elevation and the retractor muscle for lower lid retraction. The facial nerve (CN VII) activates the orbicularis oculi muscle, an oval sheet of fibers that surrounds the palpebral fissure, for lid closure. Superior and inferior palpebral smooth muscles and a central portion of the orbicularis oculi muscle respond to sympathetic innervation for involuntary blinking. The upper lid receives its sensory innervation from the ophthalmic division of the trigeminal nerve (CN V), and the lower lid is innervated by the maxillary branch of the trigeminal nerve.

The eyelids are the only portion of the eye that has a lymphatic system. The medial portions of the upper and lower lids drain into the submaxillary nodes, and the lateral aspects drain into the preauricular nodes.[36]

Lacrimal Apparatus. The lacrimal system secretes and drains a fluid that moistens and lubricates the anterior surface of the eye. Tears are produced in the lacrimal gland, which is located in the anterior lateral fossa of the orbit. Smaller accessory glands scattered throughout the palpebral conjunctiva also secrete fluid. Lacrimal fluid is normally clear and does not overflow unless reflex or mental-emotional stimuli produce excessive tearing or unless there is a blockage in the normal drainage channels. Sebaceous gland secretion and a thin mucin

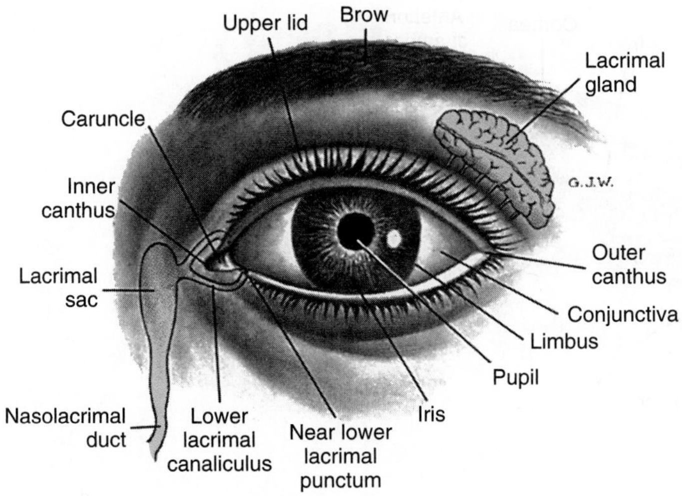

FIG. 8-3

Visible surface of eye.

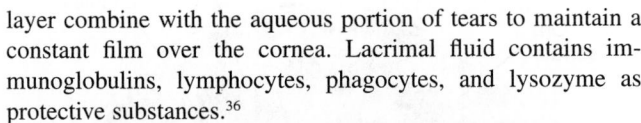

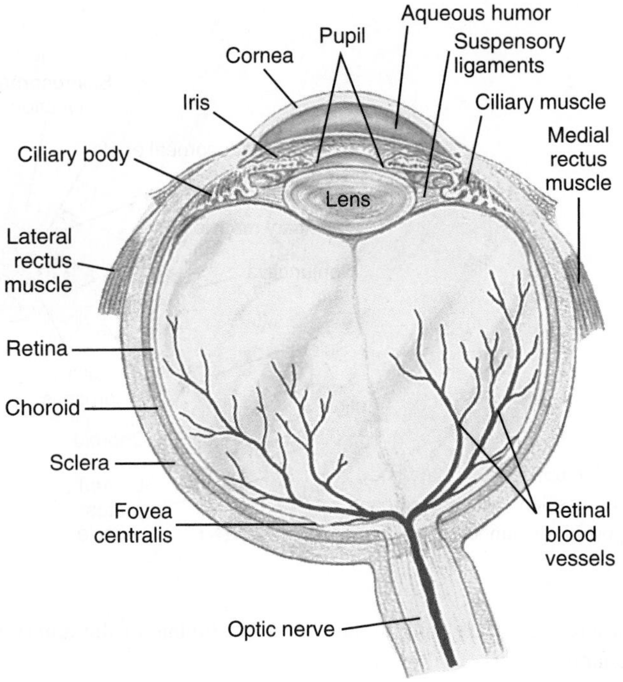

FIG. 8-4

Cross section of eye.

layer combine with the aqueous portion of tears to maintain a constant film over the cornea. Lacrimal fluid contains immunoglobulins, lymphocytes, phagocytes, and lysozyme as protective substances.[36]

Lid blinking helps distribute tears over the eye and draws the tears inward to the puncta, which are small openings in the margins of the upper and lower lids at the inner canthus (see FIG. 8-3). The puncta empty into the lacrimal canaliculi, which join to form the common canaliculus. Tears empty next into the lacrimal sac (see FIG. 8-3). The adjacent lacrimal duct empties into the nasal cavity in the inferior nasal meatus.

Eyeball

Layers of the Eye

Outer Layer: Cornea and Sclera. The eyeball is surrounded by the sclera, the "white" of the eye. It is a tough fibrous layer that covers the posterior five sixths of the eye.

The cornea covers the anterior one sixth of the eye. It is transparent, avascular, and richly innervated with sensory nerves (trigeminal [CN V]). The anterior surface of the cornea is convex, and irregularities of the curvature cause astigmatism. Because the cornea is avascular, it depends on the atmosphere, tears, and aqueous humor for oxygenation and nourishment. The cornea has five layers: the superficial epithelial layer, which is continuous with the bulbar conjunctiva; Bowman's membrane; stroma, which constitutes 90% of corneal thickness; Descemet's membrane; and an endothelial layer.[47]

The epithelial layer is a regenerative multilayered barrier. If its cells are injured, uninjured cells migrate to the traumatized area and form a new barrier one cell thick within an hour of the injury.[36] Total repair of the corneal epithelium takes approximately 48 to 72 hours in a normal, healthy person. Because of its dependence on exposure to tears, corneal epithelium is subject to edema if deprived of oxygen. (The implications for contact lenses are discussed later.) The stroma is faced anteriorly with a collagenous membrane (Bowman's membrane) that resists infection and trauma. If Bowman's membrane is destroyed, it re-forms with scarring and irregular cell formation that contribute to astigmatism. The endothelial layer pumps fluid from the other corneal layers into the aqueous humor. A relatively diminished fluid volume is necessary for corneal transparency. If the endothelium is destroyed, it does not regenerate, and the remaining corneal layers become edematous.

The sclera and cornea merge at a junction called the limbus (see FIG. 8-3). The corneoscleral limbus has a rich vascular supply that encircles and nourishes the outer edges of the cornea. At the limbus, corneal cells are mixed with conjunctival and scleral layers. Bowman's membrane ends abruptly at this junction. The posterior inner surface of the limbus adjoins the trabecular meshwork and the canal of Schlemm, which drain aqueous fluid from the anterior chamber.[47]

The sclera is the outer layer that surrounds most of the eye. It is adjacent to the second layer, the uveal tract, which includes the choroid layer, the ciliary body, and the iris (FIG. 8-4). The sclera has three layers. The outermost is the episclera, which merges with fascial tissue at the limbus; it is vascular and dense, and the minute vessels can be seen through the conjunctiva. The middle layer, the scleral stroma, is composed of tough collagenous fibers that create the white appearance of the sclera. The innermost layer, the lamina fusca, contains melanocytes that may contribute to a yellow-brown scleral hue in dark-skinned people. The lamina fusca contains collagenous fibers that filter into the choroid layer for adherence. The oculomotor muscles attach to the sclera at various points near the midsection of the eyeball (see FIG. 8-2). The sclera also has numerous openings through which nerves and blood vessels pass. The two major openings are the posterior foramen, which admits the optic nerve into the eye, and the anterior foramen,

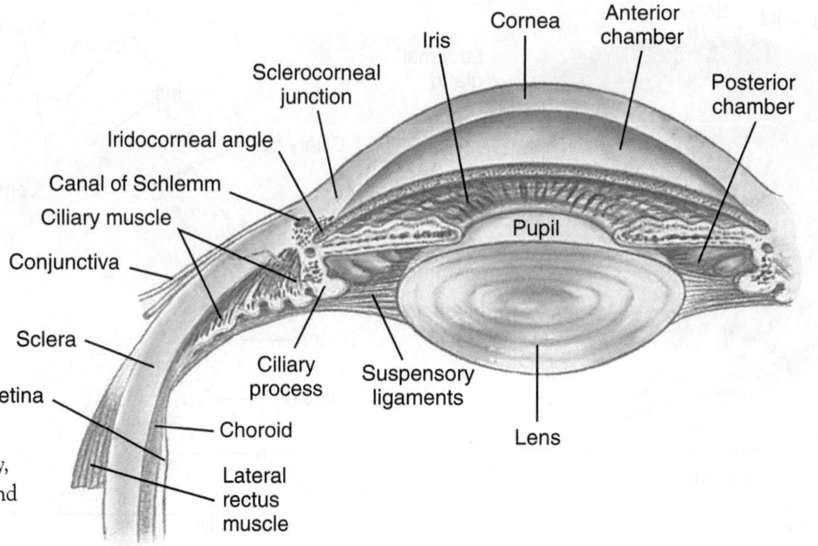

FIG. 8-5
Close-up view of ciliary body, zonules, lens, and anterior and posterior chambers.

where the ciliary muscle adjoins at the limbus in the anterior chamber.

Middle Layer: Choroid, Ciliary Body, and Iris.

The middle layer of the eyeball (the uveal tract) comprises the choroid, a vascular layer; the ciliary body, which contains smooth muscles attached to the lens and an epithelial portion for secreting aqueous humor; and the iris, which surrounds the pupil (see FIG. 8-4).

The choroid adheres to the sclera at the entrance point of the optic nerve and extends anteriorly to the ciliary body. It has five layers. The outer layer, the suprachoroid, contains melanocytes, smooth muscle fibers, and ciliary arteries that nourish a portion of the choroid. The three middle layers contain veins and arterioles that feed into the ciliary body, the iris, and the outer portion of the retina. The inner layer of the choroid is called Bruch's membrane. It is multilayered and collagenous and contains cells from the adjacent retinal and choroid layers.

The ciliary body has both a muscular and a secretory function. The ciliary muscles expand from the choroid and extend anteriorly and medially toward the lens (FIG. 8-5). The body forms a ring of smooth ciliary muscle that surrounds the lens and parallels the overlying sclera. There are three groups of ciliary muscles. Muscles in the outer division are longitudinal and parallel and adjacent to the sclera. Contraction of these fibers opens the canal of Schlemm, a thin-walled vessel that encircles the eye and drains aqueous fluid from the anterior chamber. The canal of Schlemm is located at the inner aspect of the sclerocorneal junction (limbus) (see FIG. 8-5). A series of delicate ligaments (zonular fibers) attaches the ciliary muscles to the equator of the lens (see FIG. 8-5). The tension of the zonular fibers suspends the lens and stabilizes its position. The zonular tension relaxes with ciliary circular muscle contraction to increase the convexity of the lens for accommodation.[36]

The ciliary body ends in ciliary processes behind the peripheral portion of the iris. The processes are lined with nonpigmented epithelium that secretes aqueous humor. The retina joins the inner lining of the ciliary epithelium (the pars plana) at a serrated structure called the ora serrata, which corresponds in shape to the ciliary processes (FIG. 8-6).

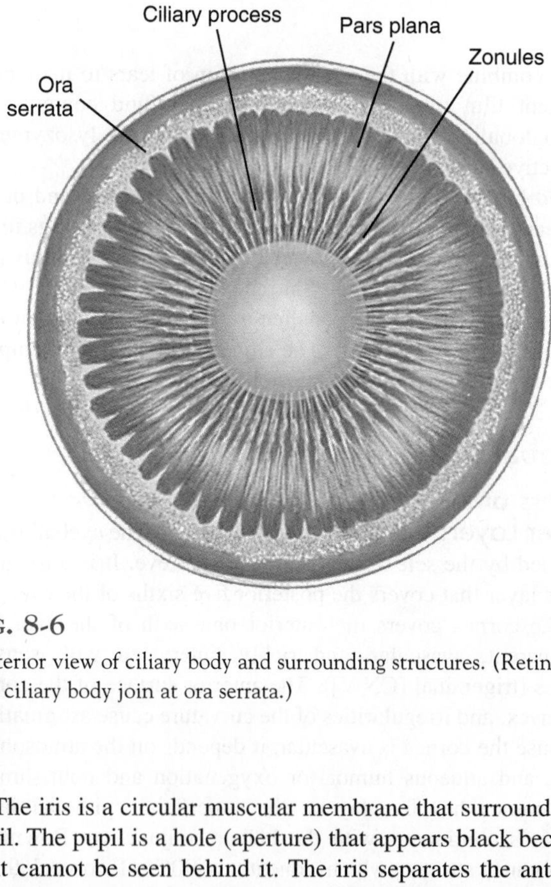

FIG. 8-6
Posterior view of ciliary body and surrounding structures. (Retina and ciliary body join at ora serrata.)

The iris is a circular muscular membrane that surrounds the pupil. The pupil is a hole (aperture) that appears black because light cannot be seen behind it. The iris separates the anterior and posterior eye chamber and rests in front of the lens (see FIG. 8-5). The amount of melanin in the iris determines the color of the eyes; the more melanin, the darker the iris. The iris sphincter surrounds the pupil, and its contraction decreases pupil size. The pigmented epithelial layer contains the dilator pupillae muscle, which dilates the pupil when contracted. Pupillary response is described in more detail in the discussion of the nervous system of the eye.

Inner Layer: Retina.

The retina is an extension of the central nervous system. This inner layer of the eye begins pos-

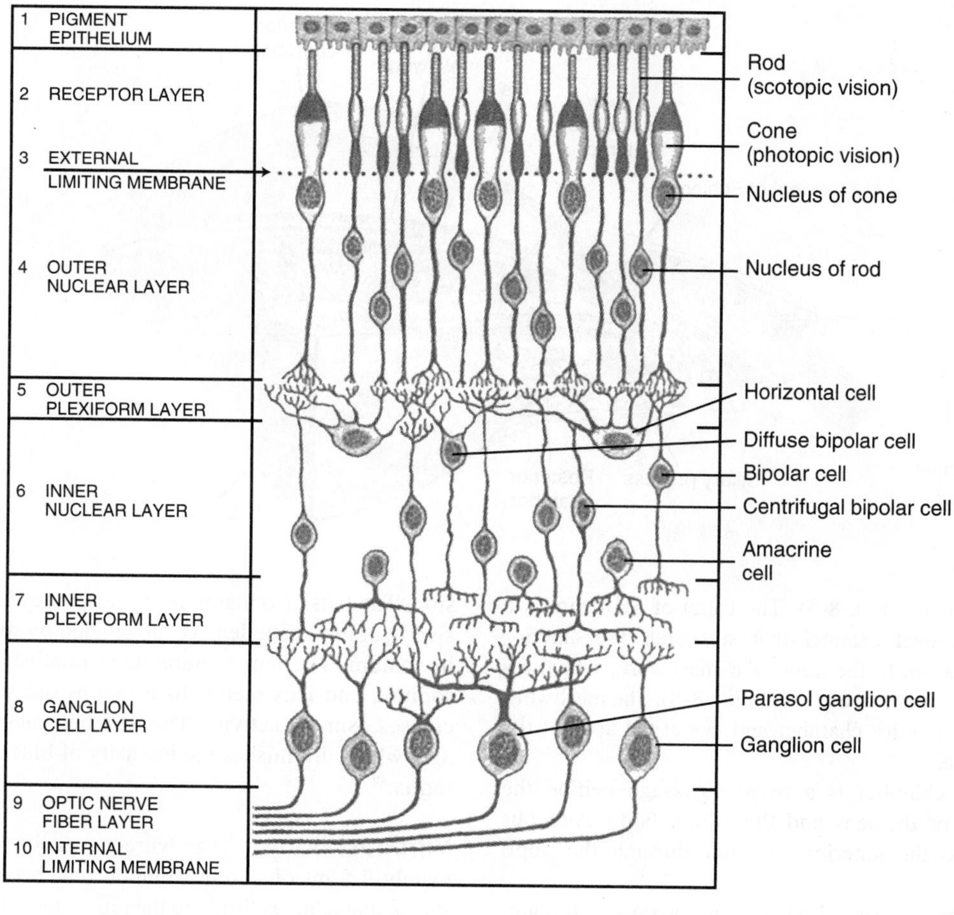

FIG. 8-7
Layers of retina.

teriorly at the optic nerve, coats the inside of the sphere, and ends at the ora serrata, where it joins the ciliary body (see FIGS. 8-4 and 8-6). The retina is normally transparent. It has 10 layers and contains rods and cones (photoreceptor cells), which are connecting cells that synapse with ganglion cells in a peripheral layer. Optic nerve fibers (axons) pass into the optic nerve (FIG. 8-7). The pigmented epithelium (adjacent to the choroid surface) contains enzymes and protein binding sites for vitamin A. These protein sites are necessary for the photochemical visual process. The rods and cones are elongated cells that respond to light and convert it into electrical energy. They pass through the next four layers. Both types of cells contain light-sensitive pigments that undergo chemical changes necessary for neural transmission of light. Rods are light sensitive in low levels of light (scotopic vision). Cones perceive images and color in higher levels of light (photopic vision). Rods and cones are so named because of their microscopic appearance; rods are more cylindric and generally more elongated. Rods and cones connect with each other in the plexiform layer and synapse with a variety of cells that ultimately reach the ganglion cells. The ganglion cells transmit electrical discharges through their axons to the midbrain.

Rods and cones are scattered throughout the retinal surface. If the retina were laid out on a flat surface, its center would be the fovea centralis. The fovea is a small depression that contains no rods but is densely packed with cones. Each cone synapses with more than one foveal photoreceptor and ganglion cell but with fewer of these cells than elsewhere in the retina. Visual acuity is sharpest in this area if enough light is available for photopic vision. The fovea is surrounded by the macula lutea, a pigmented area about 4.5 mm in diameter. Rods are densely packed in the periphery of this region (approximately 150,000 rods/mm^2) and become less dense as they extend toward the periphery. Cones average about 4500/mm^2 and also become sparse in the periphery.[36] The optic disc (the head of the optic nerve) perforates the retina about 3 mm toward the nose from the fovea. The disc is approximately 1.5 mm in diameter and contains no rods or cones. This results in a small blind spot for each eye located about 15 degrees laterally from the center of vision. The viewer is not aware of this because the other eye compensates for the loss. The periphery of the retina contains primarily rods. When viewed through the ophthalmoscope, the fovea appears as a small pinpoint of light surrounded by a yellow-brown pigmented area (the macula). The head of the optic nerve appears as a pink or cream-colored circle with a white depression in the center. This depression is where the central retinal artery and central vein bifurcate, emerge, and feed into smaller branches throughout the retinal surface.

Chambers, Fluids, and Inner Structures of the Eye

Aqueous Fluid and Intraocular Pressure. The eye contains three chambers: the anterior, the posterior, and the vitreous body. The anterior chamber rests between the cornea (in front) and the iris (behind). It is filled with aqueous humor, which flows from the posterior chamber and empties at the

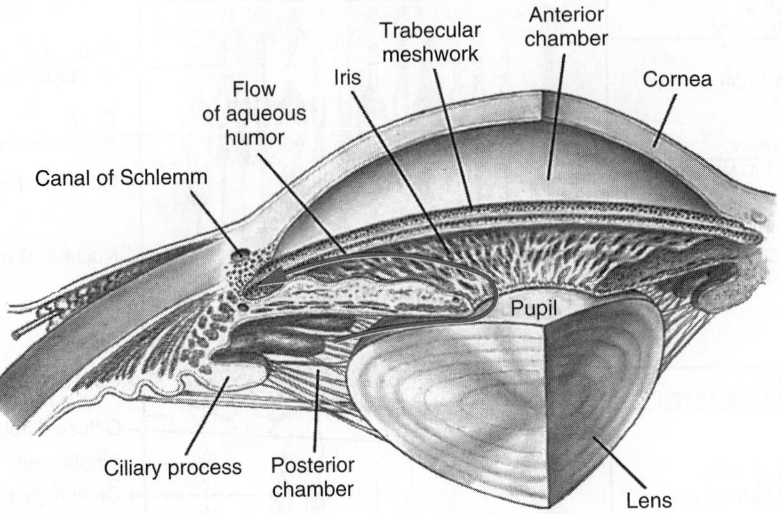

FIG. 8-8
Close view of trabecular meshwork and flow of aqueous humor.

canal of Schlemm (see FIG. 8-5). The canal of Schlemm is a highly permeable oval channel that surrounds the anterior chamber. It is adjacent to the trabecular meshwork, which filters the fluid before it enters the canal (FIG. 8-8). The meshwork also encircles the anterior chamber and lies at the apex of the irido-corneal angle.

The posterior chamber is a narrow passage behind the iris and in front of the lens and the ciliary body. Aqueous humor flows into the anterior chamber through the pupil (see FIG. 8-8).

Aqueous humor is secreted by the ciliary processes. It maintains intraocular pressure (normally within a range of 10 to 22 mm Hg), contributes to metabolism of the lens, and nourishes the cornea. Intraocular pressure is maintained by the rate of fluid secretion and the resistance to outflow by the trabecular meshwork. Eyeball pressure must exceed atmospheric pressure to maintain the shape of the sphere. Intraocular pressure fluctuates 1 to 2 mm Hg with each heartbeat. Pressure fluctuations are based on the pressure within the episcleral veins, which connect to the canal of Schlemm, and the osmotic pressure of the blood. Normal pressure changes (up to 5 mm Hg) are usually quickly compensated for by trabecular meshwork distention, which lowers outflow resistance.[36] Valsalva's maneuver (bearing down to complete a bowel movement) increases venous pressure and so greatly increases intraocular pressure, which quickly returns to normal when the maneuver ends. Drinking large quantities of water or receiving saline intravenous fluids causes a slight increase in intraocular pressure.

Lens. The lens separates the posterior chamber from the vitreous body. It is biconvex and transparent and is held in position by suspensory ligaments attached to the ciliary body. The lens comprises a capsule that encases it, a cortex (the peripheral portion), and a central core. It is transparent because most of its cells do not have a nucleus. Newly formed cells, with nuclei, originate at the periphery and "move toward the center, where mature fibers have lost their nuclei. New fibers are formed throughout the life span of the lens and continue to migrate to the center core and become compressed. Therefore an older lens is larger, denser, less elastic, and less able to contract to accommodate for near vision. The lens also maintains transparency by avoiding excessive hydration. The lens is surrounded by media that are high in sodium. The lens membrane is relatively impermeable to sodium, and lens metabolism pumps out sodium, which decreases osmotic activity. The lens becomes yellow in middle age, which diminishes the intensity of blue-toned light on the retina.[47]

Vitreous Body. The vitreous cavity contains approximately 4.5 ml of vitreous humor, which is a gelatinous substance that adheres firmly to the retina, the ciliary epithelium (at the base of the lens), and the margin of the optic nerve. If the vitreous humor diminishes in volume or degenerates, retinal tears may occur because of traction on the retina.

Image Formation

Light Reception and Refraction. The receptors of the eye are sensitive to only a small portion of the light spectrum. Light in wavelengths less than 400 nm or greater than 700 nm is not absorbed by rods and cones and therefore is not seen.

To reach the retina, light must pass through the clear media of the cornea, aqueous fluid, the lens, and the vitreous body. Light rays are emitted in all directions from any source. These light rays pass through the optic system, which focuses them at a specific point to achieve image accuracy.

A ray of light that passes from one clear medium into another is affected by the density of the medium. The density of the cornea slows the light ray, and the curvature of the cornea bends it. This process is known as refraction. The surface of the cornea is curved so light rays hit the surface at different angles but are bent to redirect them to the lens. The lens further bends and directs them to a single point on the retina (FIG. 8-9, *A*). When a person focuses on an object, the light waves from that object are directed to the fovea centralis for image identification and clarity (called focal vision). Light waves also enter the eye from a wide visual field (approximately 170-degree arc for each eye) that surrounds the object of focus (FIG. 8-9, *B*). These peripheral sources focus on the outer areas of the retina (ambient vision) and help with spatial sense.[36]

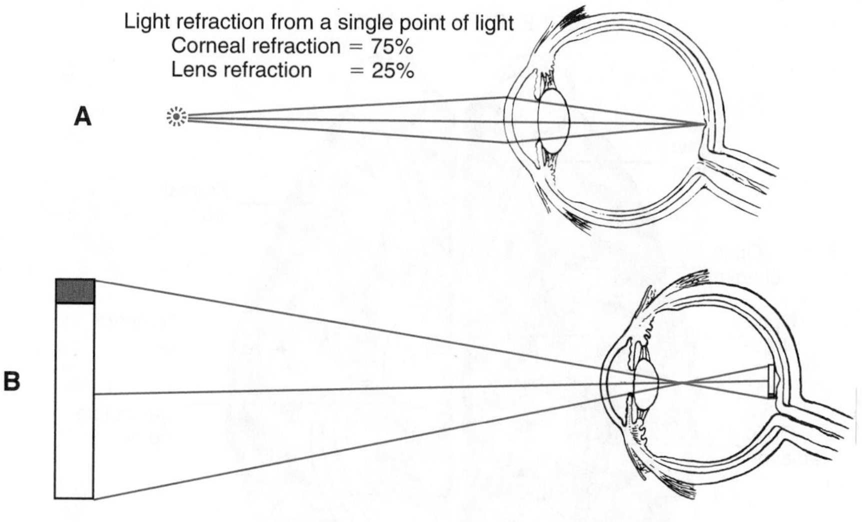

FIG. 8-9
A, Light refraction from single point of light. **B,** Light refraction from object with more than one point of light.

The anterior surface of the cornea is the primary refractive area of the eye. The more a surface bends light rays, the greater the refractive power. The shift in the direction of light when it moves through the corneal surface is greater than the second shift at the lens surface.

Accommodation. Accommodation is the process by which the lens alters its shape for visual clarity when the eye is viewing an object at close range. In other words, the lens surface increases its refractive power by becoming thicker and more convex to accommodate near objects. The lens is constantly adjusting to stimuli at different distances. Ciliary branches of the oculomotor nerve respond to brain signals for this automatic response.

Binocular Vision and Vergence. Normal eyes are aligned in their orbits so that they can direct light rays to the fovea centralis of each eye. The visual axis is an imaginary line drawn from each fovea centralis to a fixation point. When a three-dimensional object is focused on the back of both eyes, there is a slight difference in the horizontal placement of the two images. This slight difference sets up two images in the brain, which permits the binocular viewer (using both eyes) to experience the visual sensation of depth (stereopsis).

Vergence is a visual reflex of simultaneous eye movements. When distant objects are viewed, the visual axes of the eyes become more parallel and the eyes are rotated outward (divergence). As the object draws nearer, the medial rectus muscles contract and pull the eyes inward (convergence).[47] This reflex is necessary to prevent diplopia (double vision). If a person holds a finger about 10 inches in front of his or her nose and focuses on the finger, he or she sees one finger. If the person suddenly shifts his or her focus to a distant object, the person sees two fingers because the parallel visual axes do not meet at the finger.

Image Interpretation

Visual Pathway. We are able to see because refracted light rays stimulate retinal photoreceptors and are changed into electrical energy. This energy is transmitted to different cerebral cortical areas for interpretation. Light rays constantly stimulate photoreceptors. Rods and cones contain specific pigments (opsins) that combine with a form of vitamin A to absorb light and convert it to an electrical potential. The optic nerve forms the optic disc and exits the eyeball at the posterior region. The choroid and all the retinal layers except the nerve fiber layer end at the edge of the disc.

The optic nerve contains more than 1 million fibers (axons of ganglion cells) that control vision, eye movement, and pupillary reflexes. As the optic nerve exits the sphere, it is encased in dura mater, an arachnoid sheath, and pia mater. It forms an S-shaped curve that allows it to stretch when the eye is moved. The optic nerve also contains the central retinal artery and vein, which bifurcate and branch into the eyeball near the head of the nerve (the disc). The central artery and vein exit the optic nerve about 12 mm behind the eyeball.[36]

The optic nerves from each eye pass through the optic foramen and meet at the optic chiasm, which lies above and in front of the pituitary gland. Optic tracts emerge from the chiasm and encircle the hypothalamus. They terminate in the lateral geniculate bodies in the temporal lobes (FIG. 8-10). Cells in the lateral geniculate bodies send fibers (optic radiation) to the occipital lobe of each cerebral hemisphere. The visual cortex in the posterior aspect of the occipital lobe receives most of the visual fibers representing central vision (stimuli from the fovea centralis and surrounding macula). Adjacent occipital lobe areas receive fibers representing the more peripheral portions of the retina. Reversed images are righted when perceived in the cortex.

Objects in the visual field stimulate the opposite side of the retina. When nerve fibers pass into the optic nerve, the nasal (closest to the nose) and temporal (closest to the side of the face) fibers are separate within the sheath. Temporal fibers pass on the temporal side of the nerve, nasal fibers are on the nasal side, and central (foveal) fibers are in the center of the nerve. When the nerves merge at the chiasm, nasal fibers cross (decussate) to the opposite optic tract. Temporal fibers do not cross but continue in the optic tract on the same side as the nerve that conveys them to the chiasm (FIG. 8-11). Therefore the pathway of vision for an object seen on a person's right side would be through nasal receptors in the right eye and then through the

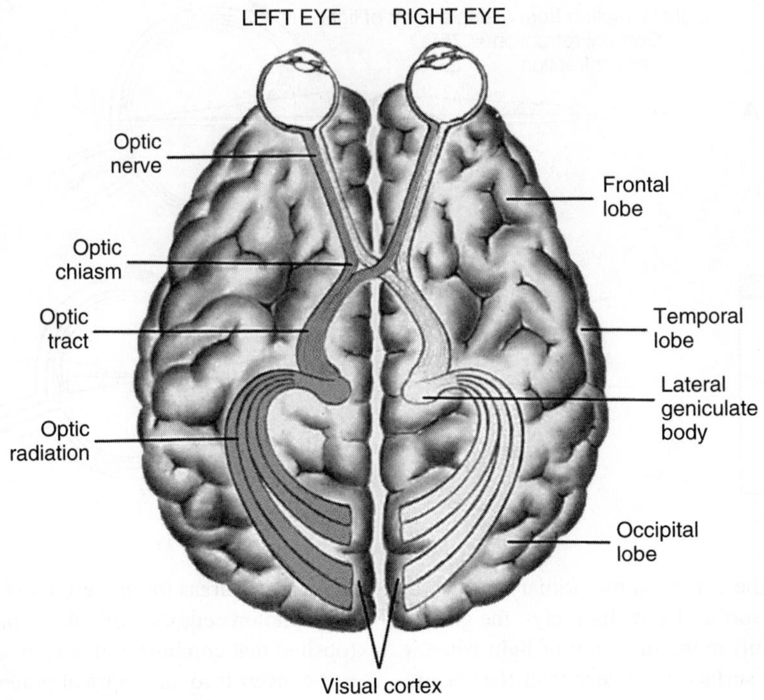

FIG. 8-10
Visual pathway.

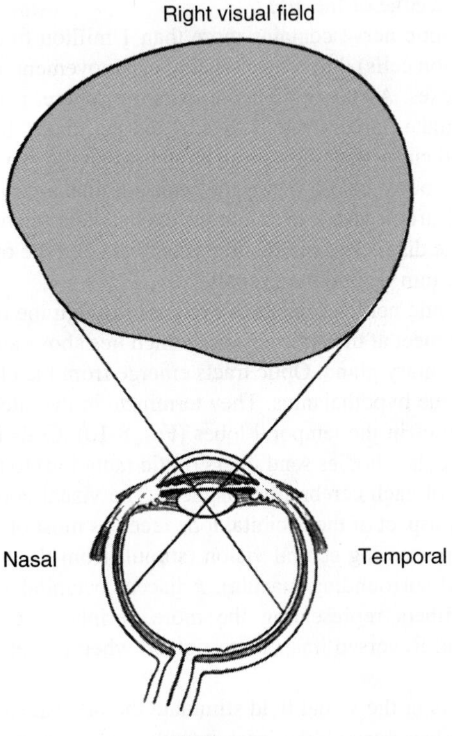

FIG. 8-11
Image placement on retina.

nasal side of the optic nerve to the chiasm, where it would cross to the left optic tract and proceed to the left cerebral occipital lobe. Visual field defects can often be traced to disorders in specific anatomic locations because of the arrangement of nerve fibers. A left or right optic nerve lesion would cause a corresponding defect in the left or right eye. Chiasm lesions can cause a variety of defects depending on the location of the lesion. A common defect is bitemporal hemianopia, which results from a pituitary tumor. A left optic tract lesion would result in a bilateral right visual field deficit. These defects are depicted in FIG. 8-12.

Light and Dark Adaptation. The concentration of pigment in the photoreceptor cells of the retina determines the sensitivity of these cells to light. Photoreceptive pigments are constantly being used and replaced through chemical changes in the retina. When the eyes are exposed to bright light, the pigments become bleached and the sensitivity of the photoreceptors diminishes. Bright light causes discomfort for several minutes until breakdown of the photopigments produces a gradual rise of the visual threshold. Together with pupillary constriction, decreased rod and cone sensitivity to light protects the retinal cells in bright light. This is called light adaptation.[47]

Exposure to darkness tends to increase photopigment regeneration to increase sensitivity to light. Rhodopsin, the photopigment in rods, is particularly sensitive to dim light and enables a person to visualize dim forms and shapes in near darkness. Rhodopsin does not absorb color wavelengths, so color is not perceived in dim light.

Color Perception. Light waves do not contain color. Color is perceived according to the wavelength (frequency) of a light ray. Colors are determined by hue (the standard recognition of a particular shade) and saturation (the intensity of a color). A less intense color contains larger amounts of white and appears relatively pale. Any object that reflects all visible light rays evokes a sensation of white. The absence of light rays is perceived as black.

The retina contains three types of cones, and each has a different photopigment that absorbs light waves of different frequencies. Each type of cone responds to a primary color: red,

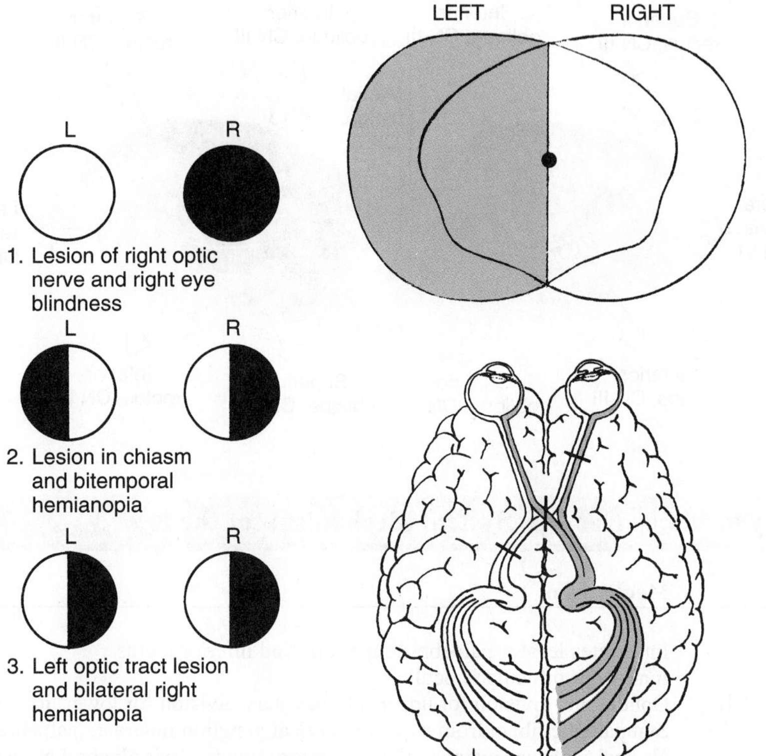

FIG. 8-12
Visual pathway defects.

green, or blue. If all of the cones are equally stimulated, white is perceived. Rods do not perceive color.

Eye Movement

The movement of each eye is controlled by six muscles. Four of these (the recti) originate behind the eyeball, move forward around the sphere, and insert into the sclera about 7 mm behind the limbus (FIG. 8-13, *A*). The superior oblique muscle begins at the posterior orbit, passes forward to the anterior orbital rim, loops through the trochlea (a fibrocartilaginous structure) to return to the eyeball, and inserts into the sclera under the belly of the superior rectus muscle (FIG. 8-13, *B*). The sixth muscle, the inferior oblique, originates at the nasal side of the orbit and passes under the eyeball to attach at its lateral surface (see FIG. 8-13, *B*). The oculomotor nerve (CN III) supplies the medial, inferior, and superior rectus muscles and the inferior oblique muscle. The trochlear nerve (CN IV) supplies the superior oblique muscle, and the abducens nerve (CN VI) supplies the lateral rectus muscle (FIG. 8-14).

Contraction of an eye muscle turns the eye toward that muscle. All six muscles are constantly coordinating stretch and contraction functions to permit full and continuous eye movement.

Both eyes must move together to maintain a clear focus. When a person looks to the right, the right lateral rectus muscle and the left medial rectus muscle contract. The innervation stimulus to both muscles is equal, so the speed and destination of the two eyeball movements are equal. Muscles that produce equal movement of each eye in the same direction are called yoke muscles. Eye movements that are simultaneous, equal, and coordinated are called conjugate eye movements.

The fibers within the extraocular muscles are highly differentiated. Eye muscles are capable of slow graded contractions

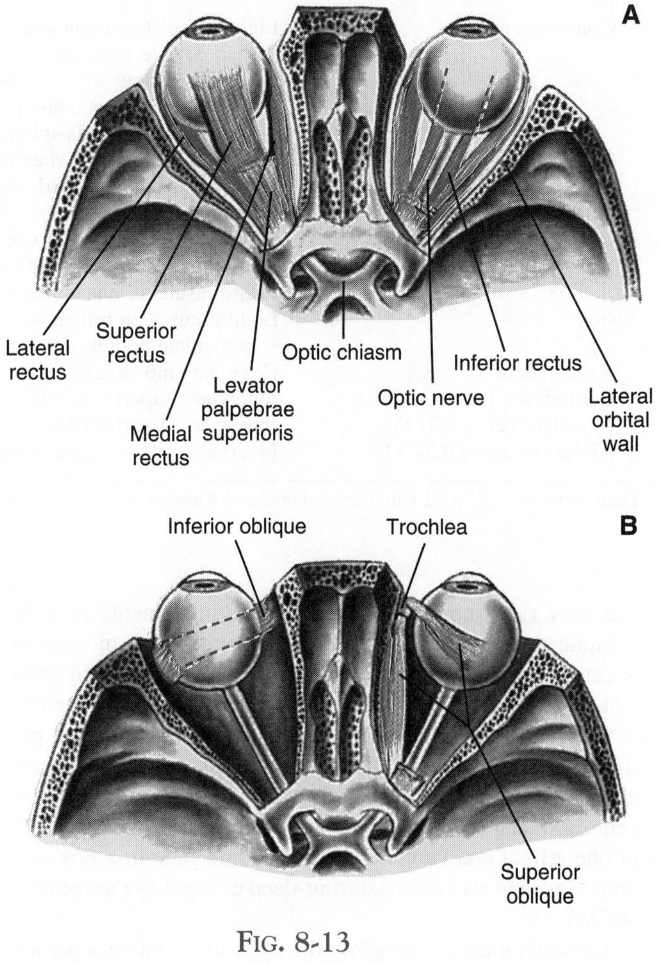

FIG. 8-13
Extraocular muscles.

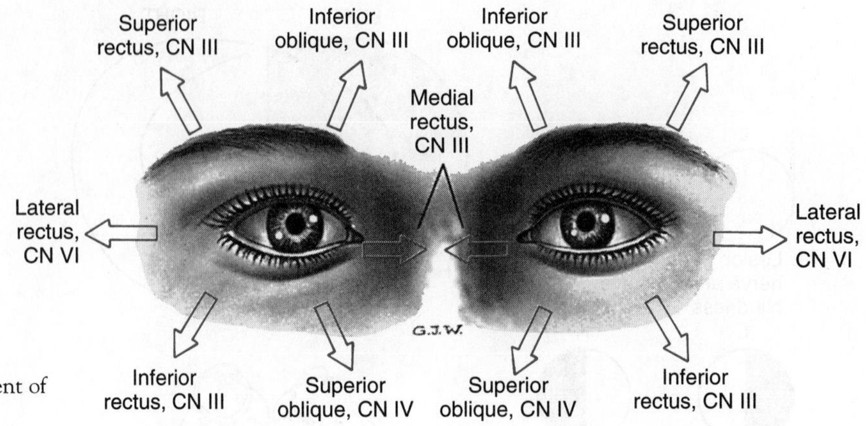

FIG. 8-14
Innervation of movement of extraocular muscles.

Table 8-1 Summary of Major Nervous System Mechanisms of the Eye

Function	Mechanism
Lid movement	
Oculomotor (CN III)	Innervates levator palpebrae superioris and inferior rectus
Facial (CN VII)	Innervates orbicularis oculi
Sensation (trigeminal [CN V])	Ophthalmic division for upper lid; maxillary division for lower lid
Reflex response	Sympathetic fibers from superior cervical ganglion innervate palpebral muscles
Tears	Normal moisture maintained by secretory function of palpebral accessory glands; excess tears mediated through stimulation of facial nerve (CN VII) and trigeminal nerve (CN V)
Corneal sensation	Trigeminal nerve (CN V)
Pupil	
Constriction	Light stimulates retina and afferent fibers that pass through optic nerve (CN II) and chiasm and then deviate from tract to area of midbrain (superior colliculus); axons leave this area and connect to nucleus of oculomotor nerve (CN III), which sends efferent fibers to ciliary ganglion (between optic chiasm and posterior orbit); parasympathetic fibers leave ciliary ganglion and enter eye to stimulate iris sphincter
Consensual response	Both pupils constrict when only one is stimulated; oculomotor nucleus responds to afferent fibers from one eye and sends signals through its fibers and parasympathetic fibers to both iris muscles
Dilation	Reduction of parasympathetic tonic flow to iris sphincters in dim light; sympathetic stimulation of fibers from carotid plexus occurs with startle or pleasure responses
Lens accommodation	Oculomotor nerve (CN III) mediates parasympathetic stimulation for ciliary muscle contraction and resultant lens convexity
Vision	Light focuses on retinal receptors; axons pass into optic nerve (CN II), chiasm, optic tracts, lateral geniculate bodies, and optic radiation to occipital lobe and visual cortex
Eye movement	Conjugate movements occur because nuclei of CN III, IV, and VI connect in fiber tract in midbrain
Oculomotor nerve (CN III)	Innervates superior rectus, medial rectus, inferior rectus, and inferior oblique muscles
Trochlear nerve (CN IV)	Innervates superior oblique muscle
Abducens nerve (CN VI)	Innervates lateral rectus muscle

Data from Newell[36] and Vaughan, Asbury, and Riordan-Eva.[47]

and very rapid contractions. Rapid eye movements may be voluntary or involuntary. One type of rapid reflex movement is called saccade. Saccadic movements are small rapid jerks that alternate with steady fixation (particularly when the eye is focusing on a near object). Saccadic movements bring peripheral retinal images to the fovea centralis for clarity. These movements also sweep images over retinal receptors to prevent light adaptation. If a person continued to focus an image in one retinal area, color and detail would fade in a few seconds. Saccade also occurs during sleep as rapid eye movement (REM).

Certain reflexes also allow the eyes to maintain a steady gaze of fixation despite head movements. If the head turns to the right, the eyes can shift an equal rotation to the left. Upward head movement causes downward rotation of the eyes.

In summary, eye movements can be classified as tracking (slow, smooth, coordinated rotations for maintaining the image of an object on the fovea centralis); vergence (slow, smooth movements that rotate the eyes inward or outward to track an object as being near or far); saccadic movements (rapid reflexes that alternate with fixation to keep the image clear and steady); and compensatory movements (reflexes that coordinate head movement with object fixation and steady gaze). Table 8-1 summarizes the major nervous system mechanisms of the eye.

NORMAL FINDINGS*

Eyelids: Blink response to light or corneal touch; frequent involuntary bilateral blinks (average 15 to 20 per minute); lid margins rest over inferior and superior borders of cornea

Eyeball: Anterior-posterior diameter 22 to 27 mm; whites: eyeball does not protrude beyond supraorbital bridge of frontal bone; blacks: eyeball may protrude slightly beyond ridge

Lacrimal function: Eyeball surface moist; excess tears in response to emotion or noxious atmospheric stimuli; puncta nontender and without discharge on palpation; ○ over 50 years: diminished reflex response for excess tearing

Conjunctivae: Palpebral: pink with uniform small vessels showing no discharge; bulbar: clear, tiny, red vessels may be visible; ○ bulbar: may lack luster of young adult

Sclera: White; slight overall yellowish cast or black dots (pigmentation) in dark-skinned individuals

Cornea: Transparent, smooth surface; convex curvature; ○ arcus sinilis (gray ring of lipid deposit around limbus)

Iris: Rounded; consistent, bilateral coloration; ○ bilateral irregularity of pigment density (color may appear paler)

Pupil: Equal; round; reacts to light and accommodation; consensual response; ○ often miotic with slower dilation reaction to dark

Anterior chamber: Clear; approximately 3.3 mm between cornea and iris; ○ becomes slightly shallower with aging

Lens: Clear, biconvex refractile body, enclosed in a capsule; becomes yellowish with age ○ when opaque deposits are numerous enough to cause vision deficit that interferes with normal activities of daily living (ADLs), a significant cataract exists and may ethically be surgically removed

Internal eye: Full, round, bilateral red reflex

- **Retina:** Uniform pink and granular texture (surface uniformly more pigmented in blacks); choroid layer may be visible showing linear light orange vessels; ○ may appear slightly paler or yellowish
- **Vessels:** Central vein and artery emerge on nasal side of physiologic cup within disc, and each immediately breaks into two branches; arteries light red and 25% narrower than dark red veins; narrow band of light may appear at center of arteries; vessel caliber regular and uniformly decreases as vessel branches toward periphery; venous pulsations more prominent in young adults; ○ arteries slightly narrower; arterial light reflex may be widened; arterial caliber may be slightly irregular
- **Disc, cup:** Whitish, cream, or pink; vertically oval or round with distinct border (nasal side may be slightly less demarcated, and temporal border may appear as grayish crescent); approximately 1.5 mm diameter (magnified 15 times through ophthalmoscope); cup is small, white or pale depression in center of disc and occupies approximately half of disc diameter; ○ disc may appear slightly smaller and more opaque
- **Macula, fovea:** Macula is darker area two disc diameters temporally from disc; fovea is pinpoint bright light in center of macula

Visual acuity

- **Distant vision:** 20/20 (able to read designated-size letter on standardized chart at 20-foot distance); ○ 20/20 to 20/30
- **Near vision:** Able to read newsprint at 14 inches; ○ presbyopic owing to loss of lens refractive power (average person over 60 years cannot focus more closely than 3 feet without corrective lenses)
- **Peripheral vision:** Temporal vision 90 degrees from central visual axis; upward: 50 degrees; nasalward: 60 degrees; downward: 70 degrees; ○ may be slightly diminished but usually not measurable with confrontation testing

Eye movement, coordination, and interpretation: Both eyes demonstrate coordinated, parallel movements in six cardinal fields of gaze; physiologic nystagmus (mild rhythmic twitching if eye held in extreme gaze); eyes converge and diverge in smooth coordinated fashion as person focuses on near and far objects; tracking, saccadic, and compensatory movements enable person to perceive objects clearly in depth and accurately in terms of distance and surrounding space

Color perception: Able to identify all colors accurately when tested with series of pictures or cards that present multicolored field for color differentiation; ○ brightness of colors may be dimmed; yellow overcast to hues owing to aging lens

*○ = Older adult.

HEALTHY PEOPLE 2010

HEALTH STATUS–VISION

Goal: Improve the visual health of the nation through prevention, early detection, treatment, and rehabilitation.

VISION

- (Developmental) Increase the proportion of persons who have a dilated eye examination at appropriate intervals.
- (Developmental) Increase the proportion of preschool children age 5 years and under who receive vision screening.
- (Developmental) Reduce uncorrected visual impairment due to refractive errors.
- (Developmental) Reduce blindness and visual impairment in children and adolescents age 17 years and under.
- (Developmental) Reduce visual impairment due to diabetic retinopathy. Potential data source: National Health Interview Survey (NHIS), CDC, NCHS.
- (Developmental) Reduce visual impairment caused by glaucoma.
- (Developmental) Reduce visual impairment caused by cataract.
- (Developmental) Reduce occupational eye injury.
- (Developmental) Increase the use of appropriate personal protective eyewear in recreational activities and hazardous situations around the home.
- (Developmental) Increase the use of vision rehabilitation services and adaptive devices by people with visual impairments.

Modified from U.S. Department of Health and Human Services: *Healthy people 2010* (conference edition, in two volumes), Washington, DC, January 2000.

NOTE: *Developmental* indicates that criteria for measurement and strategies to improve health have not as yet been specified.

CONDITIONS, DISEASES, AND DISORDERS

DISORDERS OF THE EYELID

Lid disorders are extremely common and varied. Because the lids are responsible for tear maintenance and dispersion, structure and position defects can result in excess tears or drying of the eyeball surface. Deformities and movement abnormalities interfere with the lid's vital protective function and with vision. Structure and movement malfunctions alter facial expression and appearance and create cosmetic concerns. Many pain receptors are near the lid margin, and stretching and inflammation of the tissue result in acute discomfort. Because the palpebral conjunctiva is adjacent to the lid margin, disorders in this area can produce acute and diffuse redness of the eye.

Two types of lid disorders will be discussed: those involving position, structure, and movement and those involving inflammatory disorders. Most disorders of lid structure and function require surgical intervention if localized nerve or muscle malfunction is diagnosed as the causative factor. Inflammatory disorders can affect the glands in the eyelids, the eyelid margins, and the meibomian glands. The skin of the eyelids may also be involved in a variety of inflammations because of the skin's looseness, its exposed position, and the secondary involvement of the eye. Contact dermatitis is common in the eye area because of use of cosmetics and frequent rubbing of the eyes.[36]

ENTROPION

Entropion is an abnormal inward turning of the margin of the eyelid.

PATHOPHYSIOLOGY

The lower lid is most commonly involved. Involution of the lid can be caused by atrophy of the lower lid retractor muscle (atonia), spasms of the orbicularis oculi muscle, or scarring and deformity of the tarsal plate resulting from trauma or chemical or inflammatory assaults. Atonia is relatively common in the elderly and can occur in varying degrees of severity. If the lashes are turned inward, corneal and conjunctival inflammation may occur. Spastic entropion results from chronic or acute irritation of the horizontal muscle. Corneal inflammation, conjunctivitis, and ocular surgery are common causes of spasm. Congenital entropion occurs with a deformity of the tarsal plate.[36]

MULTIDISCIPLINARY PLAN

Surgery

Orbicularis procedure: Small section of orbicularis oculi muscle is resected to tighten remaining muscle farthest from lid margin, which results in peripheral lid eversion

Tarsal resection: Wedge of tarsal plate is removed, which prevents lid margin from rotating inward

Mucosal graft: Scarred, atrophied conjunctiva may be replaced with section of mucous membrane from mouth[36]

General Management

For entropion (spasm from irritation), remove irritation (e.g., eye dressing) to reduce or relieve spasms; stabilize lower lid with pressure patch or tape lower lid to cheek for temporary relief

NURSING CARE

NURSING ASSESSMENT

Eyelid(s) and Lashes

Misdirected eyelashes may result in corneal rubbing, irritation, or exposure and/or epiphora (tear spillage)

Cornea and Conjunctiva

Possible corneal and/or conjunctival infection secondary to irritation from eyelashes

Possible exposure problems, including dryness, abrasion(s), and chronic erosion syndrome secondary to the malpositioned eyelid(s)

Possible discomfort ranging from feelings of dryness to irritation, to constant foreign body sensation, to stinging and/or constant pain

Various levels of visual dysfunction ranging from mild blur to significant loss of visual acuity, depth perception, contrast, and/or color discrimination

Possible anxiety secondary to vision loss, anticipation of surgical intervention, and/or pain

PATIENT PROBLEMS/NURSING DIAGNOSES & INTERVENTIONS

NIC SKIN/WOUND MANAGEMENT

Risk for impaired tissue integrity related to surgical intervention and possible eyelid malposition

Before surgery

- Evaluate cornea/conjunctiva for signs of inflammation and/or abrasion, including redness, dull-looking or opaque areas, and/or infiltrates.
- Stabilize eyelid position by taping lid to cheek if entropic or by patching lid closed *to protect exposed cornea/conjunctiva if cause is ectropic, ptotic, lagged or diminished rate of blinking.*
- Apply artificial moisturizers as ordered/desired by patient.

After surgery

- Apply antibiotic ointment as ordered *to prevent infection.*

NIC PHYSICAL COMFORT PROMOTION

Acute pain related to exposure secondary to eyelid(s) malposition and/or surgical intervention

- Monitor and document patient's level of discomfort.
- Administer analgesia as ordered.
- Report pain unrelieved by ordered analgesia.

NIC PSYCHOLOGIC COMFORT PROMOTION

Anxiety related to fear of vision loss and/or potential disfigurement

- Evaluate patient's level of anxiety and/or body image disturbance.

- Listen to patient's concerns.
- Provide supportive counseling and explanations about disorder, surgical procedure, and expected outcomes.

NIC Risk Management

Risk for infection: eyelid(s), cornea, and/or conjunctiva secondary to surgical repair and suture site(s)

Disturbed sensory perception (visual) related to disorder and/or postsurgical patching

- Warn patient that depth perception is reduced when one eye is patched, necessitating extra care in activities (e.g., maneuvering stairs and sidewalk curbs and when pouring liquids from one container to another).
- Warn patient that peripheral vision on affected side is reduced, necessitating exaggerated head turning *to compensate for field reduction.*
- Inform patient that proceeding slowly and cautiously will often increase safety in environment *by enabling identification of problematic activity in time to take appropriate counteraction.*

Patient Education/Continuum of Care Plan

1. Ensure patient understanding of surgical site care, including cleaning with mild soap and water, and observe a return demonstration of the application of antibacterial/antiinflammatory ointment(s) to suture line(s).
2. Teach patient to remove crust(s) by soaking with a warm, wet washcloth and not to pick at or remove crusts with fingers, etc.
3. Encourage patient to perform ADLs independently as much as possible.
4. Reinforce need for adequate nutritional intake to promote healing.
5. Encourage reduced activity for first 24 to 72 hours and then to resume activity as tolerated.
6. Encourage use of localized ice packs to reduce swelling and increase comfort.

Evaluation/Patient Outcomes

Skin/Wound Management: Cornea and conjunctiva are healthy, transparent, smooth, glossy, and moist. Visual symptoms are improved. Patient is able to care for nonsurgically treated eyelid(s). Surgically repaired eyelid(s) maintain adequate anatomic positioning and movement. Epiphora is improved. Patient administers prescribed ocular medications properly and sucessfully. Patient is able to monitor condition of eye/eyelid(s) and report adverse signs appropriately.

Physical Comfort Promotion: Pain is minimized and/or absent. Patient understands and complies with follow-up regimen.

Psychologic Comfort Promotion: Patient reports decreased feelings of anxiety and has less or no negative body image perception.

Risk Management: There is no burning, itching, redness, or evidence of infection of cornea, conjunctiva, and/or eyelid(s).

Ectropion

Ectropion is an abnormal outward turning of the margin of the eyelid.

Pathophysiology

Ectropion occurs in two main forms, atonic and cicatricial. Only the lower eyelid is involved in the atonic type, which is the more common. Older adults are frequently subject to the atonic type from the bulbar conjunctiva owing to relaxation of the orbicularis oculi muscle. This condition can occur in all degrees of severity and may cause corneal drying, irritation, and conjunctivitis. Paralysis of the orbicularis oculi muscle (CN VII) also results in atonic ectropion. Cicatricial ectropion can affect either the upper or lower eyelid and follows burns, lacerations, and infections of the eyelid skin.

Multidisciplinary Plan

Surgery

Ectropion repair: Wedge of skin, muscle, and tarsal plate removed to tighten lower lid(s)[13]

Skin grafting: Replacement of scar tissue that relieves constriction of inferior part of lower lid

General Management

Monitoring of exposed conjunctiva for infection and drying; lubricating ointment as needed

Ptosis

Ptosis is a drooping of the upper eyelid.

Pathophysiology

Ptosis can be bilateral or unilateral, constant or intermittent, and congenital or acquired. Congenital deformity usually involves malfunction of the levator muscle and is often accompanied by limited eye movement associated with superior rectus muscle failure. Acquired ptosis is mechanical, neurogenic, or myogenic in origin. Mechanical factors usually stem from abnormal weight of the eyelid imposed by such conditions as chronic edema, tumor, or excess tissue. Malfunction of the oculomotor nerve (CN III) interferes with lid elevation, eye movement, and pupillary constriction. Carotid aneurysms and diabetic neuropathy are common causes of CN III degeneration. Interruption of the sympathetic innervation of the smooth muscle that maintains lid tone and dilates the pupil causes ptosis. Horner's syndrome (a miotic pupil and drooping lid) occurs with sympathetic pathway lesions such as goiter, cervical lymph node enlargement, or apical bronchogenic carcinoma.[36] Unilateral ptosis is frequently the first sign of myasthenia gravis, which is characterized by fatigability of striated muscles. Bilateral involvement with progressive diminished eye movement may ensue. Aging eyes lose muscle tone of the lid elevator and the smooth muscle within the lid, and a general mild lid sag may occur.[36]

MULTIDISCIPLINARY PLAN

Surgery

Resection of levator palpebrae superioris muscle: If functioning, muscle is reattached to tarsus at shorter length to increase muscle strength and lid-raising capacity

Upper eyelid suspension: When levator muscle is not functioning, supportive band of material is threaded within lid and attached to frontalis muscle to provide sling effect; lid movement is not affected, but cosmetic effect is improved.[36]

General Management

Glasses with "crutch" can be worn to suspend inoperable lid; treatment of systemic disorders (such as treatment of myasthenia gravis or removal of sympathetic pathway lesion) may relieve lid drooping[36]

LAGOPHTHALMOS

Lagophthalmos is inadequate closure of the eyelids. Lagophthalmos may result from facial nerve (CN VII) weakness or enlargement or protrusion of the eyeball.[36]

MULTIDISCIPLINARY PLAN

Surgery

Immediate surgical closure of lids may be necessary to prevent corneal drying and trauma; upper and lower eyelid adhesions can be temporarily or permanently created

General Management

When only small portion of central cornea is exposed:

Lubricating ointment instilled at bedtime for protection during sleep

Soft contact lens worn or artificial tears administered several times a day

Sustained-release tear insert in each eye once a day[36]

BLINKING DISORDERS

Blinking disorders may occur as excessive blinking or a diminished rate of blinking.

PATHOPHYSIOLOGY

Blinking is both a voluntary and an involuntary action. The rate of involuntary blinking varies among individuals, but blinking occurs frequently enough to spread tears over the surface of the eye. Reflex blinking increases in response to conjunctival or corneal irritation or pain in the eye. Chronic irritation may result in a continuous clonic response that is sustained until the stimulus is removed. Rapid blinking also accompanies anxiety and may become a prolonged pattern with chronic stress. Spasms of the orbicularis oculi muscle (blepharospasm) sometimes occur in elderly people. These spasms are involuntary, tonic, spasmodic, usually bilateral contractions. They range from an annoying tic to a dangerous level during which the person cannot see. They are also unattractive. Causes include irritation of the eyes, facial nerve lesions, fatigue, and anxiety. Absence or diminution of blinking may accompany parkinsonism or hyperthyroidism.

MULTIDISCIPLINARY PLAN

Blinking disorders may be relieved when the cause (systemic origin, anxiety, or local irritation) is treated or removed. When a systemic origin cannot be determined, rapid bilateral blinking is labeled as essential blepharospasm. In many cases, botulinum toxin is injected, in minute doses, every few months, to paralyze the obicularis oculi muscle and decrease the frequency and intensity of the spasms.[13,37]

NURSING CARE

NURSING ASSESSMENT

Blinking disorder

Rapid bilateral blinking: Multiple anxiety behaviors

Tics: Anxiety; statements of stress

Cornea and conjunctiva: Diminished blinking: Conjunctival drying and irritation or corneal drying; keratitis

Psychosocial concerns: Anxiety

PATIENT PROBLEMS/NURSING DIAGNOSES & INTERVENTIONS[24]

NIC SKIN/WOUND MANAGEMENT

Impaired tissue integrity of cornea and conjunctiva related to inadequate tear dispersion

- Assess eye for symptoms of dryness.
- Administer artificial tears, sustained-release tear insert, or lubricating ointment as ordered *to improve lubrication.*
- Be certain lid is closed when applying dressing *to prevent injury to cornea.*

NIC PSYCHOLOGIC COMFORT PROMOTION

Anxiety related to fear about disorder

- Assess patient's level of anxiety and stressors.
- Listen to patient's concerns.
- Provide supportive counseling.

PATIENT EDUCATION/CONTINUUM OF CARE PLAN

1. Educate patient about disorder.
2. Discuss alternative care plans, rationale, and consequences.
3. Ensure that patient can administer eyedrops, lubricant, or tear insert if ordered; discuss with patient the need to wash hands before and after procedure.
4. Caution patient not to rub or pick at eyes.
5. Encourage patient to avoid noxious odors or fumes such as cigarette smoke.
6. Suggest that patient use a humidifier in home if atmosphere is dry.
7. Show patient how to monitor eye for signs and symptoms of dryness or irritation.

EVALUATION/PATIENT OUTCOMES

Skin/Wound Management: Cornea and conjunctiva are healthy. Cornea is transparent, smooth, glossy, and moist.

Palpebral conjunctiva is homogeneous pink color, and bulbar conjunctiva is clear. There is no burning, itching, or evidence of infection. Lid movement is normal. Open and closure movement of lid is not excessive. Vision is not obscured. Source of nervous mannerisms or local irritant has been removed.

Psychologic Comfort Promotion: Anxiety is decreased. Patient is able to discuss and cope with the disorder.

BLEPHARITIS

Blepharitis is an inflammation of the eyelid margins.

PATHOPHYSIOLOGY

Blepharitis is a chronic condition that can be caused by organisms (chiefly *Staphylococcus*), associated with seborrheic dermatitis, or aggravated by allergies. Often the causative factors are inseparable. Other conditions commonly associated with chronic blepharitis are diabetes, gout, anemia, and rosacea.[36] Infections of the nose and mouth can be transferred to the eyes and lids by frequent eye rubbing. Staphylococcal lesions usually ulcerate and often involve the conjunctiva and meibomian glands. Chalazions and hordeola (styes) may develop and recur. Seborrheic blepharitis is frequently accompanied by dermatitis of the scalp, eyebrows, and external ears. Some people first have this chronic condition in childhood and continue to have intermittent exacerbations throughout life.

MULTIDISCIPLINARY PLAN

Medications[30,36,47]

Antiinfective agents: Ointment applied locally qd or bid, usually at bedtime if infection is present

Sulfacetamide sodium (Sulamyd, others), 10%-30% solution or 10% ointment

Bacitracin (Baciguent), 500 U/1 g ointment

Neomycin sulfate (Myciguent), 0.5% ointment

General Management

Eyelid Hygiene

Drape warm washcloth over both eyes for 10 minutes; warm the cloth every 2 minutes

Wash face with warm soap and water

Mix one part "no-tears" baby shampoo with two parts water in a clean container

Wrap your finger in a washcloth

Rub eyelids (along lashes) with wet, warm washcloth dipped in baby shampoo and water mixture

Rinse face with warm water and dry

Do above three to four times a day for 4 to 6 weeks; thereafter only once daily

NURSING CARE

NURSING ASSESSMENT

Eyelids and lashes: Red lid margins; flaking and scaling around lashes; localized discomfort; loss of lashes; ingrown lashes; thickening and eversion of lid margins; tear spillage; in ulcerative staphylococcal blepharitis, pus, multiple lesions and crusting at lid margins, development of ulcers, lids glued shut by dried drainage

Cornea and conjunctiva: Light sensitivity; possible chronic conjunctivitis; possible corneal inflammation[36]

PATIENT PROBLEMS/NURSING DIAGNOSES & INTERVENTIONS[24]

NIC SKIN/WOUND MANAGEMENT

Impaired tissue integrity; risk for impaired tissue integrity related to lesions or ulcerations

Risk for infection of eye tissue related to organism transfer from nose or mouth

- Assess lids and conjunctivae for crusting or inflammation.
- Perform eyelid hygiene as appropriate *to minimize skin injury.*
- Assess patient's self-care and hygiene habits (e.g., hand washing, avoidance of rubbing eyes).
- Instruct patient in self-care *to prevent reinfection.*
- Demonstrate and instruct patient in self-administration of ointment *to prevent injury and contamination.*

PATIENT EDUCATION/CONTINUUM OF CARE PLAN

1. Ensure that patient can perform eyelid hygiene regimen, and apply antibiotic ointment if ordered.
2. Discuss with patient hygiene practices related to self-care of eye, such as washing hands before and after self-care and avoiding fumes, smoke, and other external irritants.
3. If patient uses eye makeup, encourage patient to avoid use during acute phase of lid infection because makeup is a common allergen and also may become contaminated with the causative organisms.

EVALUATION/PATIENT OUTCOMES

Skin/Wound Management: Eyelids are normal. Lid margins are smooth and without scaling. Conjunctiva is normal. Palpebral conjunctiva is homogeneous pink color, and bulbar conjunctiva is clear. There is no excessive tearing or evidence of infection.

CHALAZION

Chalazion is a granulomatous inflammation of a meibomian gland.

PATHOPHYSIOLOGY

A chalazion forms on the conjunctival aspect of the upper or lower eyelid because glands in both are affected. It begins as a nontender swelling and may take several weeks to develop. It does not appear inflamed unless a secondary infection occurs. If large enough, the nodule can compress the eyeball and cause an astigmatism, resulting in blurred vision. A large nodule also produces discomfort as the upper lid closes, causing pressure on the cornea. Some chalazia disappear in a few months without ever causing symptoms. Chronic chalazia tend to subside partially and reactivate periodically.[36,47]

MULTIDISCIPLINARY PLAN

Medical Treatment

Hot-packing chalazia several times daily often causes them to open and drain; however, unless antibiotic eyedrops are prescribed to destroy the bacteria, they recur chronically

Surgery

Localized excision of chronic chalazion with patient under local anesthesia; antibiotic eyedrops administered three to four times a day before and after surgery

Medications

Antiinfective agents: Ointment applied locally 4 times a day postoperatively

Sulfacetamide sodium (Sulamyd, others), 10%-30% solution or 10% ointment
Bacitracin (Baciguent), 500 U/1 g ointment
Neomycin sulfate (Myciguent), 0.5% ointment

NURSING CARE

NURSING ASSESSMENT

Eyelids: Small, nontender, noninflamed lump on outer lid; lid eversion reveals nodule that points toward conjunctiva; secondary infection produces redness, pain, and suppuration; sensitivity to light

See Hordeolum (below) for nursing care.

HORDEOLUM

A hordeolum (sty) is an acute infection of an eyelash follicle or the glands of Moll or Zeis (sebaceous glands).

PATHOPHYSIOLOGY

The offending organism is usually *Staphylococcus.* The lesion becomes a pustule that eventually points and may rupture. Multiple pustules may occur along adjacent lash follicles because of reinfection.[36,47]

MULTIDISCIPLINARY PLAN

Medications

Antiinfective agents: Ointment applied locally 2-4 times a day

Sulfacetamide sodium (Sulamyd, others), 10%-30% solution or 10% ointment
Bacitracin (Baciguent), 500 U/1 g ointment
Neomycin sulfate (Myciguent), 0.5% ointment

General Management

Warm compresses with clean cloth for 10 to 20 minutes two or three times a day; local incision of pustule if rupture is not spontaneous

NURSING CARE

NURSING ASSESSMENT

Eyelids: Initial tenderness with localized redness and swelling that forms pustule at lid margin; may be multiple pustules; generalized lid edema; pain that increases as pustule enlarges and ceases with rupture

PATIENT PROBLEMS/NURSING DIAGNOSES & INTERVENTIONS

NIC RISK MANAGEMENT

Risk for infection related to secondary contamination or surgical alteration in skin integrity

- Evaluate patient's hygiene practices (e.g., hand washing before touching eye) *to prevent spread of infection.*
- Assess the patient for *Staphylococcus* infections or lesions elsewhere on the body *to monitor potential for or presence of systemic staphylococcal infection.*

NIC SKIN/WOUND MANAGEMENT

Impaired tissue integrity; risk for impaired tissue integrity related to presence of pustule/inflamed chalazion lump

- Apply warm compresses with clean cloth for 10 to 20 minutes two or three times a day *to expedite healing.*

PATIENT EDUCATION/CONTINUUM OF CARE PLAN

1. Demonstrate to patient the application of warm compresses and antibiotic ointment if ordered.
2. Discuss with patient hygiene practices related to self-care of eye, such as washing hands before and after self-care and avoiding fumes and smoke.
3. If patient uses eye makeup, encourage patient to avoid use during acute phase of lid infection because makeup is a common allergen and also may become contaminated with the causative organism.

EVALUATION/PATIENT OUTCOMES

Risk Management: Eyelids are normal. Lid margins are smooth, without lesions. There is no evidence of infection.

Skin/Wound Management: Conjunctiva is normal. Palpebral conjunctiva is homogeneous pink color, and bulbar conjunctiva is clear. There is no excessive tearing.

LACRIMAL APPARATUS DISORDERS

Patients with lacrimal disorders usually complain of "dry eyes," excessive tearing, or pain and swelling of the lacrimal duct. Inadequate tearing can result in drying and severe damage to the cornea. Excessive tearing can be caused by overproduction of tears by the lacrimal gland or a faulty drainage system that results in tear spillage. Tear accumulation can interfere with vision and irritate the eyeball. Inflammation of the lacrimal sac and adjacent canaliculi can be associated with conjunctivitis, nasal disease, or drainage obstruction.

Dry Eye Syndrome

Dry eye syndrome is a condition in which tear production is inadequate. The signs and symptoms may occur in any age group; however, they are most common in women 50 to 60 years old.

Pathophysiology[36,47]

Dry eye syndrome occurs for three primary reasons: lacrimal gland malfunction, mucin deficiency, and mechanical abnormalities that interfere with the spread or maintenance of tears over the eyeball surface. Lacrimal gland malfunctions can be congenital or acquired. The most common congenital disorders are lacrimal gland aplasia, ectodermal dysplasia, and trigeminal nerve (CN V) malfunction, which disrupts sensory stimulation to the upper lid. Acquired disorders that affect lacrimal gland function can be systemic, infectious, or related to trauma. Common systemic disorders that may be associated with diminished tear production are rheumatoid arthritis (Sjögren's syndrome), leukemia, lymphoma, sarcoidosis, and systemic sclerosis. Facial nerve (CN VII) palsy inhibits tearing. Mumps and some forms of conjunctivitis may obstruct tear flow. Chemical burns and irradiation may reduce lacrimal gland function. Some medications such as antihistamines, atropine, and beta-blockers decrease tear production. Even if the lacrimal gland is not functioning, accessory glands in the palpebral conjunctiva may secrete sufficient tears to prevent severe corneal damage.

A layer of mucin, produced by goblet cells in the lid, maintains a homogeneous tear spread over the eyeball surface. The absence of mucin causes the tear film to break up, leaving "dry holes" over the cornea. Mucin deficiency is commonly associated with some forms of chronic conjunctivitis, vitamin A deficiency, and medications such as antihistamines and beta-blockers.

Mechanical defects that contribute to dry eyes include abnormalities of eyelid structure and function, protrusion of the eyeball (proptosis), and use or misuse of contact lenses.[36,47]

The symptom most commonly associated with inadequate tearing is keratoconjunctivitis sicca (KCS). The person experiences burning, itching, and a foreign body sensation in the eyes. The cornea and conjunctiva may show inflammation, erosion, or keratinization. Untreated or severe KCS can result in blindness.

Diagnostic Studies and Findings[36,47]

Rose Bengal staining: Drop of 1% or 2% solution placed in conjunctival sac; 2% solution demonstrates loss of corneal and conjunctiva epithelium in keratoconjunctivitis sicca; 1% solution valuable in demonstrating conjunctival and corneal epithelial cell loss and degeneration; patients with deficiency of aqueous portion of tears have punctate staining of lower two thirds of cornea and bright red staining of bulbar conjunctiva in area corresponding to palpable aperture

Schirmer's test: Topical anesthetic administered to eyeball; strip of filter paper, 3.5 × 0.05 cm, placed in temporal aspect of conjunctival cul-de-sac of lower lid for 5 minutes; 10- to 15-mm length of paper wetted with tears considered normal; more than 25 mm moistened paper indicates excessive tearing.

Multidisciplinary Plan[13,36]

A correlation does not always exist between the failure of tear production and inflammatory or degenerative changes on the surface of the eye. The mechanisms that connect tear and mucin production to ocular surface maintenance are not fully understood. Depending on the cause and severity of the condition, the examiner may select from or combine the following therapeutic approaches:

Restoration or stimulation of tears
- Estrogen replacement therapy has been associated with relief of dry eye symptoms in some postmenopausal women[11,47]
- Elimination of systemic medications that have created the problem
- Treatment and resolution of eyelid or conjunctival inflammation
- Alteration in contact lens prescription or patient's self-care methods

Preservation of existing tears
- Surgically induced punctal occlusion
- Eyelid repair (ectropion) or lid closure repair
- Wearing of airtight goggles to prevent tear evaporation

Tear replacement

Maintenance and treatment of ocular surface
- Antibiotic ointments
- Lubricating ointments
- Some studies have reported success with the use of topical vitamin A preparations in the maintenance of healthy conjunctival tissue[13]

Surgery

Occlusion of puncta to conserve tears; surgical repair of lid position or movement abnormalities

Medications

Antiinfective Agents

Ointment applied locally for existing inflammation
- Polysporin Ophthalmic Ointment (polymyxin, 10,000 U; bacitracin, 500 U), 2-4 times a day

Tear Substitutes

There are literally dozens of tear substitutes available, but there is no scientific way to determine which type of tear is best for each patient. There are some basic differences in tear substitutes that the nurse should know about both as a clinician and as a patient educator.

Tears are either thin (watery), thick (like honey), or so thick they are an ointment. In addition, either they contain a preservative to increase their shelf life and the length of time they can be used without fear of microbial growth or they contain no preservative because some people are sensitive to the preservatives in artificial tear preparations.

If the preparation contains a preservative, the container will have a screw cap. Containers of nonpreserved tears hold only 4 to 6 drops. They should be used or thrown away within 24 hours because they contain nothing to hamper bacterial growth.

Thin tears do not blur vision when used; however, they also do not remain in contact with the ocular surface very long, necessitating frequent use. Thick tears and ointments soothe the ocular surface for much longer but cause various amounts of visual blurring. Therefore the contact lens wearer who needs tear replacement during the workday will need to use a thin, watery tear substitute. The elderly patient in long-term care who no longer has useful vision in an eye that needs lubrication to increase comfort will be better served by a thick tear or a lubricant ointment.[3]

General Management

Humidifier in environment; airtight goggles or eye shield

NURSING CARE

NURSING ASSESSMENT

Dry eyes: Burning; itching; foreign body sensation; sensitivity to light; blurred vision; lack of tears; loss of glossy appearance of cornea; tear film interspersed with mucus strands

PATIENT PROBLEMS/NURSING DIAGNOSES & INTERVENTIONS1[3,24,47]

NIC SKIN/WOUND MANAGEMENT

Risk for impaired tissue integrity of cornea and conjunctiva related to lack of tears

- Evaluate eye for signs and symptoms of irritation (itching, burning, and loss of glossy appearance of eyeball surface).
- Administer artificial tears, sustained-release tear insert, or lubricating ointments as ordered *to prevent tissue damage to ocular surface.*

NIC PHYSICAL COMFORT PROMOTION

Acute pain related to localized inflammation

- Monitor and document patient's degree of discomfort.
- Provide analgesics as ordered *to promote patient's comfort.*

PATIENT EDUCATION/CONTINUUM OF CARE PLAN

1. Demonstrate to patient how to administer eyedrops, lubricant, or a tear insert; stress importance of washing hands before and after procedure.
2. Ensure that patient knows to avoid rubbing or picking at eyes.
3. Encourage patient to avoid noxious odors or fumes and to use a humidifier in home if atmosphere is dry.
4. Demonstrate to patient how to monitor eye for signs and symptoms of dryness or irritation.

EVALUATION/PATIENT OUTCOMES

Skin/Wound Management: Cornea and conjunctiva are healthy. Cornea is transparent, smooth, glossy, and moist. Palpebral conjunctiva is homogeneous pink color, and bulbar conjunctiva is clear. There is no burning, itching, or evidence of infection. Visual alteration is improved. Patient experiences no sensitivity to light; blurred vision improves.

Physical Comfort Promotion: Patient experiences minimal or no discomfort.

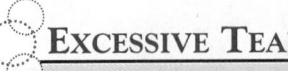

EXCESSIVE TEARS

Excessive tears can occur from overproduction or inadequate drainage of tears.

PATHOPHYSIOLOGY[36,47]

Tear spillage most commonly occurs because the drainage system is faulty (epiphora). The puncta can be occluded because of congenital absence of an opening or because of infection in the lacrimal sac. Lid abnormalities, such as ectropion, cause abnormal alignment of the lacrimal tear pool and the puncta. An accumulation of tears in the inner canthus is an irritant that stimulates more tear production. Obstructions may also occur in the lacrimal duct or the meatus in the nasal cavity.

Lacrimation (excessive tear production) occurs most commonly with reflex stimulation of the lacrimal gland. Corneal injury, eye pain, noxious odors, eyestrain, bright light, and allergies are examples of sensory stimuli affecting the trigeminal nerve (CN V). Glaucoma often stimulates tear production because of trigeminal irritation. Facial nerve (CN VII) irritation during vomiting or laughter also stimulates tear production. Abnormal regeneration of the facial nerve following Bell's palsy causes "crocodile tears," a phenomenon of excess tearing that occurs during eating. Parasympathetic stimulants (cholinergic drugs) and some endocrine disorders (such as hyperthyroidism) can also increase tearing.

DIAGNOSTIC STUDIES AND FINDINGS

Dye disappearance: Cul-de-sac of lower lid flooded with 2% fluorescein solution; fluorescein normally disappears from cul-de-sac in 1 minute

Computed tomography: Computed tomography (CT), with or without contrast, shows normal versus abnormal lacrimal passages

MULTIDISCIPLINARY PLAN

Surgery

Repair of lid structure abnormalities to enhance punctal access to tear pool

Probing of obstructed punctum

Construction of tube connecting conjunctival cul-de-sac to nasal cavity

Dacryocystorhinostomy (DCR): Creation of a new pathway for tear drainage, bypassing the nasolacrimal duct by making an opening in the nasal bone

General Management

Related to removal of cause of lacrimation

NURSING CARE

NURSING ASSESSMENT

Eyes: Tear spillage; blurred vision; puncta red and swollen; puncta may exude purulent material on mild compression over lacrimal sac; conjunctivitis (reddened conjunctiva)

Patient Problems/Nursing Diagnoses & Interventions

NIC Skin/Wound Management

Risk for impaired tissue integrity related to infection secondary to contamination

- Assess eye for amount of lacrimation or increased symptoms of irritation or infection.
- Encourage patient to maintain hygiene *to prevent infection.*

Patient Education/Continuum of Care Plan

Discuss with patient hygiene practices related to self-care of eyes, such as washing hands before and after self-care and keeping hands away from eyes.

Evaluation/Patient Outcomes

Skin/Wound Management: Lacrimal drainage system is patent. There is no excess tearing. Inner canthus of eye is homogeneous pink color. When eye is compressed at medial infraorbital rim, punctum does not exude any material. Underlying endocrine cause, if any, is corrected. Amount of tears produced is not excessive.

Dacryocystitis

Dacryocystitis is an inflammation of the lacrimal sac.

Pathophysiology

Dacryocystitis can be acute or chronic and is caused by blockage of tear drainage from the punctum or lacrimal sac.

Normal newborns often do not have patent nasolacrimal ducts. The duct usually opens about the third week of life. If the duct fails to open, tearing occurs and eventually purulent material exudes from the punctum. The condition often corrects itself by 3 to 6 months of age. Lacrimal probing may be performed if spontaneous patency does not occur. Surgical construction of a duct is rarely needed, but if necessary it is performed when the child reaches 3 or 4 years of age.[47]

Chronic dacryocystitis most often occurs in middle-age adults. Spontaneous punctum obstruction is followed by bacterial infection with a mucopurulent discharge. The nasolacrimal duct can also be obstructed by injury or nasal lesions, causing an inflammatory response.

Acute dacryocystitis has a rapid onset, with marked swelling and tenderness of surrounding tissue.[47]

Multidisciplinary Plan[36,47]

Surgery

Incision and drainage of abscess

Dacryocystorhinostomy for construction of passage between lacrimal sac and nasal cavity

Medications

Antiinfective agents: Systemic antibiotics for acute, severe infection; instillation of antibiotic or sulfonamide eyedrops 4-5 times a day until infection subsides

General Management

Daily massage of lacrimal sac to rid it of purulent material (often assists spontaneous opening of nasolacrimal duct system in newborns)

Warm compresses over affected eye during acute phase

Lacrimal probing with graduated sizes of probe while patient is under local anesthesia

NURSING CARE

Nursing Assessment

Lacrimal inflammation: Tear spillage; purulent material exuding from punctum on compression; punctum swollen, and surrounding tissue may be reddened; localized pain

Patient Problems/Nursing Diagnoses & Interventions

NIC Skin/Wound Management

Risk for impaired tissue integrity related to infection secondary to obstruction of tear drainage

- Assess punctum and surrounding tissue for inflammation.
- Apply warm compresses over affected eye for 10 to 20 minutes three to four times a day.
- Lightly massage lacrimal sac at medial infraorbital rim *to rid sac of accumulated purulent material.*
- Administer antibiotic or sulfonamide eyedrops or ointment as ordered.
- Wash hands thoroughly before and after care of affected eye *to prevent spread of infection.*

Patient Education/Continuum of Care Plan

Discuss with patient hygiene practices related to self-care of eyes, such as washing hands before and after self-care and keeping hands away from eyes.

Evaluation/Patient Outcomes

Skin/Wound Management: Cornea and conjunctiva are healthy. Cornea is transparent, smooth, glossy, and moist. Palpebral conjunctiva is homogeneous pink color. Bulbar conjunctiva is clear. There is no burning, itching, or evidence of infection. Lacrimal drainage system is patent. There is no excess tearing. Inner canthus of eye is homogeneous pink color. Punctum does not exude any material when eye is compressed at medial infraorbital rim.

CONJUNCTIVAL DISORDERS

The bulbar conjunctiva is a protective coating for the scleral portion of the eyeball. It can be affected by many injuries or infections from the environment. It adjoins the palpebral conjunctiva in the lid cul-de-sac and is susceptible to infection because it is close to the eyelid. The conjunctiva also responds to internal infections or diseases such as measles, diabetes mellitus, or riboflavin deficiency. This outer layer contains blood vessels that dilate rapidly and pain receptors that register mild to moderate discomfort in response to inflammation. The conjunctiva is adjacent to the cornea and can be an avenue for spreading infection to this vital area.

CONJUNCTIVITIS

Conjunctivitis is an inflammation or infection of the conjunctiva.

Conjunctival tissue can become inflamed by dust, smog, tobacco smoke, noxious fumes, wind, sun, and airborne allergens. Conjunctivitis is common and easily spread, particularly in crowded environments such as schools and nursing homes.

PATHOPHYSIOLOGY[36,47]

Conjunctivitis varies in severity. Vascular dilation and engorgement can be a response to external irritants such as smog, hair sprays, or noxious fumes. The person may experience lacrimation and a foreign body sensation, but no discharge or progressive infectious process appears. Generalized hyperemia and burning are initial responses to insufficient tearing, and a secondary infection can follow rapidly. Allergic responses may be seasonal and include vascular injection, moderate tearing, and severe itching.

Viral conjunctivitis is characterized by generalized hyperemia, profuse tearing, and little exudate. Preauricular nodes are commonly associated with viral infections. Some adenoviruses invade the upper respiratory or gastrointestinal systems, causing fever and acute systemic signs along with the conjunctivitis. Viral infections may be mild and self-limited or may quickly invade the cornea and surrounding tissue and cause severe ocular surface and periorbital pain. Type I herpes simplex conjunctivitis has been diagnosed more often in recent years with fluorescent antibody staining of corneal scrapings. Herpes conjunctivitis often invades the cornea with inflammation, erosion, and ulceration. Usually only one eye is involved initially, but both may be affected eventually. Recurrent eye lesions that may cause scarring and diminished vision can be brought on by stress, immunosuppression, menstruation, fever, or exposure to ultraviolet light.

Bacterial conjunctivitis, the most common type, is frequently called pinkeye. Almost any bacterium can be involved, but *Pneumococcus, Staphylococcus,* and *Streptococcus* organisms are common. The infection usually begins in one eye and is transferred to the other eye through contamination. The onset is acute, with a mucopurulent exudate, tearing, generalized hyperemia, and moderate discomfort. This form of conjunctivitis is highly contagious.

Some organisms rapidly invade the cornea and the conjunctiva and lead to corneal ulceration and perforation. Two of the most virulent organisms are *Neisseria gonorrhoeae* and *Chlamydia trachomatis.* Ophthalmia neonatorum, a conjunctivitis that occurs in newborns, is commonly transmitted from the mother with acute gonorrheal urethritis during birth. Ophthalmia neonatorum occurs within the first 10 days of life and is characterized by a rapid progression of signs from mild inflammation to marked redness, swelling, and purulent exudate. Corneal involvement is common and severe. *C. trachomatis* organisms can also be transmitted during a newborn's passage through the vagina. The early symptoms are similar to those of gonococcal conjunctivitis, but the incubation period is slightly longer (5 to 14 days). *Chlamydia* organisms do not respond to silver nitrate, which has been traditionally administered prophylactically to newborns. Since 1980 erythromycin has been more commonly used because it is effective against both *N. gonorrhoeae* and *Chlamydia.* Both gonococcal and chlamydial organisms (which are transmitted venereally) can invade adult conjunctivae and cause severe, acute, purulent infection.

The conjunctival infections that have been described are generally acute and can be successfully treated. Some persons have a chronic recurrent conjunctivitis characterized by periodic eye discomfort, redness, and discharge. Repeated inflammatory episodes can cause thickening of the conjunctiva and lid margins. The causes are numerous, but the most common are contact allergens (e.g., cosmetics or chlorine), airborne allergens, excessive meibomian gland secretions, and chronic blepharitis. Trachoma (a chronic *C. trachomatis* conjunctivitis) has been described as the leading cause of blindness in the world. It is prevalent in warm climates where living conditions are crowded and hygienic practices are poor. Insects may transmit the disease. In some cases the disease heals spontaneously, but in other cases it leads to conjunctival or corneal scarring and loss of vision if left untreated.

DIAGNOSTIC STUDIES AND FINDINGS[36,47]

Microscopic examination of stained conjunctival scrapings: Numerous polymorphonuclear neutrophils in bacterial infections; monocytes in viral infections or trachoma; eosinophils and basophils in allergies

Culture of exudate or conjunctival scrapings: Organism identification

MULTIDISCIPLINARY PLAN[13,36,47]

Medications

Antiallergic agents: Most cell stabilizers (e.g., Alamast, Alocril, Alomode Crolom, Opticrom) and decongestants (e.g., Albalon, Clear Eyes, Naphon-A, Visine-A)

Nonsteroidal antiinflammatory drugs (NSAIDs): Ketorolac tromethamine (Acular)

Antiinfective agents: Medication varies with causative organism
- Sulfacetamide sodium (Sulamyd, Bleph 10), 10%-30% solution or 10% ointment for 3-7 days
- Erythromycin (Ilotycin), topical 0.5% ointment for 3-7 days

Antiviral agents
- Trifluridine (Viroptic), 1% solution, 1 drop q2h during waking hours during epithelial healing, then 1 drop q4h for 7 days
- For gonococcal or chlamydial conjunctivitis or severe purulent conjunctivitis
  - Tetracycline (Achromycin, Oxytetracycline), 250-500 mg PO qid for 21 days
  - Erythromycin (E-Mycin, others), 250 mg qid for 21 days

Prophylactic dose within first hour of life for newborns
- Erythromycin ophthalmic ointment 0.5%, ¼-inch strip in each eye
- Tetracycline ophthalmic ointment 1%, ¼-inch strip in each eye

General Management

Saline irrigation for purulent discharge; warm compresses for discomfort and inflammation, 10 to 15 minutes two to three times a day; cold compresses for allergic itching, 10 to 15 minutes two or three times a day; eyelid hygiene regimen for softening, loosening, and removing crusts on eyelids[36]

NURSING CARE

NURSING ASSESSMENT

Allergic and general irritant responses: Lacrimation; generalized hyperemia; gritty, sandy sensation; severe itching (with allergies)

Viral inflammation: Lacrimation, minimum mucopurulent discharge; generalized hyperemia; possible preauricular nodes; some lid swelling; moderate discomfort; possible photophobia

Bacterial inflammation: Purulent discharge; lid swelling; generalized hyperemia; moderate discomfort; possible photophobia; complaints of blurred vision (owing to excess exudate over eye surface); blurring may disappear with blinking

Severe (corneal) involvement: Moderate discomfort that becomes severe

PATIENT PROBLEMS/NURSING DIAGNOSES & INTERVENTIONS[24]

NIC SKIN/WOUND MANAGEMENT

Risk for impaired tissue integrity related to infection secondary to organism contamination

Risk for impaired tissue integrity related to excessive irritation

- Assess patient's eyes for presence of mucopurulent discharge *to confirm presence of bacterial, possible gonococcal, or chlamydial infection.*
- Isolate patient from others (in institutional setting) and use precautions *to prevent spread of infection.*
- Administer prescribed topical ointments or systemic antibiotics.
- Administer saline irrigations for excessive discharge *to prevent crusting and expedite healing.*
- Cleanse lids and lashes with mild shampoo and water mixture and clean, wet washcloth *to remove crusts.*

NIC PHYSICAL COMFORT PROMOTION

Acute pain related to localized inflammation

- Apply warm compresses to eyes *to increase comfort.*
- Administer analgesics as ordered.

PATIENT EDUCATION/CONTINUUM OF CARE PLAN

1. Demonstrate to patient how to perform saline irrigation of eye.
2. Demonstrate to patient how to apply warm compresses with clean cloth or cold compresses (ice should not be applied directly to eyelids).
3. Instruct patient to wash hands thoroughly before and after treating each eye.
4. Encourage patient to keep hands away from face.
5. Encourage patient to avoid crowded environments when possible.
6. Discuss with family members the need to avoid touching their faces and to wash hands thoroughly when contact has occurred.
7. Encourage patient to avoid noxious fumes and smoke.
8. Discuss with patient the importance of not wearing contact lenses during suppuration period.

EVALUATION/PATIENT OUTCOMES

Skin/Wound Management: Conjunctiva and cornea are healthy. Palpebral conjunctiva is homogenous pink color. Bulbar conjunctiva is clear and glossy. Cornea is clear and glossy.

Physical Comfort Promotion: There is no eye discomfort, lacrimation, or discharge.

SUBCONJUNCTIVAL HEMORRHAGE

Subconjunctival hemorrhage is a common phenomenon caused by the rupture of a blood vessel. It appears suddenly as a well-defined bright red area on the surface of the eyeball and gradually disappears in 2 to 3 weeks.

A large hemorrhage may be darker in color and expand for the first few days. The patient feels no discomfort but is usually alarmed. The ruptured vessel is usually the result of localized increased pressure (following severe coughing, vomiting, or sneezing) or minor trauma. Often a cause cannot be found, and no treatment exists. In rare instances blood dyscrasias, hypertension, or viral conjunctivitis is associated with this hemorrhage.[36,47]

CONJUNCTIVAL DISCOLORATION AND GROWTHS

Conjunctival discoloration is different from the normal yellowish pigmentation that occurs with increased melanin deposits in darker-skinned people.

The conjunctiva is subject to a large variety of growths, tumors, and discoloration. Bilirubin is absorbed in the conjunctiva with jaundice and gives the underlying sclera a yellow coloring.

Two of the most common benign growths are pterygium and pinguecula. A pterygium is a triangular growth of connective tissue that usually advances from the nasal side of the conjunctiva and encroaches on the cornea. It occurs more commonly among people who are frequently exposed to the sun and wind. It is not surgically removed unless it creates a cosmetic concern or threatens to involve the central cornea. A pinguecula is common in older adults and appears as a yellow nodule on either side of the cornea at the limbus. It usually involves both eyes. It may be periodically inflamed but does not invade the cornea and is usually not treated unless the patient is concerned about its appearance.

DISORDERS OF THE CORNEA AND SCLERA

The cornea is the main exterior protector of vision. Visual clarity depends on uniformity, smoothness, and transparency throughout the corneal layers. The avascular central cornea depends on its periphery (the limbus) for nourishment and on its epithelial (outer layer) and endothelial (inner layer) activity for hydration stability. Because the cornea is exposed to the external environment, it is more vulnerable to trauma and infection. Injury to the outer epithelial layer exposes Bowman's membrane and the substantia propria (stromal layer) to infection. If untreated infection perforates the cornea, the eye may be lost. The epithelial layer regenerates rapidly without scarring, but the deeper layers form opacities that may cause astigmatism or mild to severe visual loss. Corneal transplant and implications for nursing are covered in the last section of this chapter (p. 564).

The sclera surrounds the eyeball and is adjacent to the uveal tract (including the choroid layer). It opens posteriorly to admit the optic nerve and other nerves and vessels into the eye. Scleral inflammation and disease are often associated with systemic connective tissue disorders.

KERATITIS

Keratitis is an inflammation of the cornea.

PATHOPHYSIOLOGY[36,47]

The cornea can be injured by exposure (drying), ischemia, nutritional deficiency, microbe invasion, anesthesia (sensory interruption), and trauma. Keratitis (corneal inflammation) may be superficial (epithelial), invade the stroma (subepithelial) or eventually break through the inner layer (Descemet's membrane) to the endothelium. Most organisms require a break in the epithelium before they can enter the cornea. The epithelium can be damaged by hypersensitivity to conjunctival inflammation, corneal drying, mechanical injury, or chemical irritants. Because the epithelium is richly innervated, superficial inflammation causes moderate to severe pain. Epithelial erosions may appear in the form of tiny pits or small or coarse lesions scattered over the surface. Central ulcers (or craters) may invade deeply into the underlying layers. Some of the medical treatments prescribed for therapy or relief of discomfort may facilitate bacterial invasion. People whose immune systems have been suppressed are more vulnerable to infection; the misuse of local corticosteroid therapy increases the tissue destruction activity of collagenase, which is produced when epithelial cells are injured. Immunosuppression also makes a person more vulnerable to invasion by fungi, which easily penetrate Descemet's membrane. Fluorescein solution, which is used to stain and detect epithelial damage, is easily contaminated and can inoculate the epithelium with organisms. Patients should never be given local anesthetics for use at home because they can further abrade the cornea without knowing it. Besides inhibiting the protective corneal reflex, anesthesia of the eye interrupts epithelial regeneration.

Almost any bacterium can invade the cornea. *Pneumococcus, Staphylococcus, Streptococcus,* and *Pseudomonas* organisms are the most common. Fungal infections have become much more common since the introduction of topical corticosteroids and antibiotics. Chronic debilitating disease increases vulnerability to fungal infections. Viral infections, most commonly caused by herpes simplex, are also prevalent.

Herpes zoster can also invade the eye through inflammatory lesions of areas served by the trigeminal nerve. The lesions, in the form of scattered erosions or plaques, may be superficial or embedded in the deeper corneal layers. Residual corneal stromal infiltrates and scarring may ensue. The acute phase of herpes zoster keratitis resolves in 4 to 6 days. Treatment is primarily aimed at relieving the symptoms. Topical and systemic steroids and some newly approved antiviral topical medications speed recovery.

Pneumococcus and *Pseudomonas* organisms tend to spread rapidly and form ulcers that penetrate deep into the stroma. Herpes keratitis can be recurrent; it is triggered by stress, exposure to ultraviolet light (sunlight), or by other illness. It is relatively asymptomatic because it attacks the trigeminal nerve (CN V) and diminishes pain. Corneal ulceration and optic atrophy develop rapidly in neonates contaminated with herpes virus at birth. Adults with recurrent herpes keratitis may heal with or without scarring. Herpes virus is also activated with the use of topical steroids. Some virus forms are highly contagious and cause outbreaks, especially in schools, institutions, and eye clinics. Chronic disabling illness increases an individual's vulnerability to corneal damage, as do certain diseases, such as diabetes mellitus, leukemia, chronic alcoholism, severe vitamin A deficiency, and autoimmune diseases.

Recent reports have created concern about the increasing incidence of *Acanthamoeba* keratitis. *Acanthamoeba* is commonly found in fresh water, soil, and airborne dust. The organisms have been recovered from the nose and throat of seemingly healthy individuals, suggesting that they can be inhaled, as well as acquired through contaminated water. The amoebae are resistant to freezing, to most antimicrobial agents, and to levels of chlorine used to disinfect swimming pools, public drinking water, and hot tubs. Most people who have this infestation are contact lens wearers who use distilled or tap water to clean or rinse their lenses. The organism is devastating because it is resistant to most antimicrobials, it is often misdiagnosed as herpes simplex keratitis and treated without success, and it tends to cause recurrent epithelial breakdown. A large percentage of patients with this disorder have had to undergo a corneal transplant to regain useful vision.[13]

The severity of corneal destruction depends on the virulence of the organism, the degree of corneal destruction, the accuracy and promptness of therapy, and the immunocompetence of the host.

DIAGNOSTIC STUDIES AND FINDINGS[36,47]

Fluorescein stain (2%): Sterile paper strips most commonly used; breaks in epithelium are stained green

Ulcer scrapings for microscopic viewing (Gram's or Giemsa stain): Organism identification

Ulcer scrapings for culture: Organism identification

MULTIDISCIPLINARY PLAN[36]

Surgery

Corneal transplantation; enucleation (or evisceration)

Medications

Mode, frequency, and duration of therapy depend on identified organism and degree of corneal penetration[13,36,47]

Antiinfective agents
Topical
Erythromycin, 5 mg/g
Tobramycin
Penicillin G, 10,000-20,000 U/ml
Bacitracin, 10,000 U/ml
Sulfacetamide sodium, 10% solution
Amphotericin B, 1.5-3 mg/ml
Idoxuridine, 0.1% solution or 0.5% ointment
Subconjunctival injections of antibiotics for acute, severe central ulcerations
Systemic antibiotics (intravenous [IV] or by mouth [PO]) for acute severe central ulcerations, if sclera is involved, or if perforation threatens
Antiviral agent: Trifluridine (TFT, Viroptic), 1% solution, 1 drop q2h during waking hours during epithelial healing, then 1 drop q4h for 7 days
Mydriatic-cycloplegic agent: Atropine, 1% solution bid or tid for painful inflammation of iris and inflammatory constriction of pupil
Mucolytic agent: Acetylcysteine, 10% to 20% solution for inhibiting collagenase
Analgesics: For severe pain
Acetaminophen (Tylenol), 650 mg PO q4h prn
Acetaminophen (Tylenol 650 mg) with codeine (30 mg), 1-2 tablets PO q4h prn
Codeine, 30-60 mg PO q4h prn
Antiamoeba agents
Brolene
Polyhexamethylene biguanide (PHMB), 0.02%
Chlorhexidine, 0.02%
Clotrimazole, 1% drops
Ketoconazole, 200 mg bid PO
Itraconazole, 200 mg bid PO

General Management

Supportive therapy according to severity of condition
Hospitalization for extensive central ulcer (over 2 to 3 mm in diameter or penetrating deep into stroma)
Pressure dressings (often over both eyes) for discomfort
Loose epithelium mechanically removed with applicator and local anesthetics for viral keratitis.
Ice compresses for 10 to 15 minutes two or three times a day for discomfort and inflammation
Therapeutic soft contact lenses for recurrent corneal erosion or other chronic keratopathy

NURSING CARE

Nursing Assessment

Corneal epithelium: Moderate to severe pain; blurred vision; halos seen around lights; lacrimation; generalized hyperemia; fluorescein stains green on corneal surface; possible photophobia; possible purulent exudate, especially with accompanying conjunctivitis
Scarring: Opacity or irregular light reflection may be visible on corneal surface; diminished vision if opacity in visual axis
Edema: Cornea appears dull and uneven; visual loss (blurring)
Ulceration: Ulcers vary in appearance and size; whitish gray opacity with overhanging margins; fungous ulcer may be white, fluffy, and elevated; severe pain with epithelial damage or iritis; lacrimation and possible purulent discharge; generalized hyperemia

Patient Problems/Nursing Diagnoses & Interventions

NIC Risk Management

Risk for infection related to epithelial erosion
- Monitor for purulent exudate. If purulent exudate is present, isolate patient (in institutional setting) and practice precautions *to prevent spread of infection.*
- Administer topical and systemic medications as ordered for infection.

NIC Skin/Wound Management

Impaired tissue integrity related to epithelial erosion
- Instill mydriatic-cycloplegic topical solutions as ordered *to prevent inflammatory constriction of pupil and iritis.*

NIC Physical Comfort Promotion

Acute pain related to localized inflammation
- Administer topical anesthetic if ordered.
- Apply pressure bandage to eye; be certain eye is closed before covering (one or both eyes may be covered) *to prevent further damage to ocular surface.*
- Apply warm compresses for 10 to 15 minutes two or three times a day *to relieve discomfort.*
- Provide systemic analgesic as ordered *to promote comfort.*

NIC Self-Care Facilitation

Disturbed sensory perception (visual) related to use of bilateral eye patches or decreased vision
- Encourage patient to perform self-care with personal hygiene *to promote independence.*
- Provide patient's privacy, and assure patient that privacy is provided.
- Help patient with walking *to avoid injury.*
  - Walk slowly and slightly ahead of patient: patient's hand should rest on your arm at the elbow.
  - If possible, allow patient to trace progress by running dorsal aspect of his or her free hand along a wall.
  - Describe surroundings as you proceed.
  - Allow patient to feel chair, toilet, or bed before turning to sit.

Patient Education/Continuum of Care Plan

1. Explain to patient the self-care of corneal abrasion.
2. Demonstrate to patient how to instill eyedrops or ointments as ordered.
3. Demonstrate to patient the application of warm or cold compresses.
4. Discuss with patient the need to wear dark glasses if cycloplegic drug is ordered.
5. Discuss with patient the need to wash hands before and after treating each eye.

6. Encourage patient to keep hands away from face and eyes except when treating condition.
7. Explain to patient not to use soiled handkerchief or tissue on eyes.
8. Encourage patient to avoid noxious fumes and smoke.
9. Discuss with patient how to monitor eye for increased pain or change in discharge.
10. Explain visual changes (increased blurring) or visual blockage.

EVALUATION/PATIENT OUTCOMES

Risk Management: There is no evidence of infection.

Skin/Wound Management: Cornea is healthy. Cornea is clear and glossy. There is no eye discomfort, lacrimation, or discharge. Visual alteration is improved.

Physical Comfort Promotion: The patient does not experience discomfort.

Self-Care Facilitation: Patient is able to perform ADLs and return to precondition level of functioning.

CORNEAL INJURIES

Corneal injuries are injuries to the surface epithelium or deeper layers of the eye in the form of contusions, abrasions, perforations, lacerations, burns, or damage from chemical irritants.

PATHOPHYSIOLOGY[36,47]

Contusions result from blows that do not penetrate the corneal surface. Frequently the protective lid suffers the most damage, with edema and bruising. A subconjunctival hemorrhage may result, which looks alarming but usually heals spontaneously over 2 to 3 weeks without residual effects. The anterior chamber should be examined for repository blood, which gravitates to the lower segment and is absorbed within a few days, leaving no aftereffects. If the entire chamber is filled with blood, normal intraocular pressure is threatened and surgical evacuation through an incision at the corneal margin may be required. Severe blows may dislocate the lens, which causes visual distortion and possible ciliary spasms that are extremely painful. Surgical intervention with lens removal may be necessary. Retinal hemorrhages may occur; they are usually self-limited and without complications unless the macula is the site of bleeding. A large retinal hemorrhage might invade the vitreous, permanently obscuring vision, and increase the risk of a retinal tear.

Corneal abrasion is the disruption of cells and the loss of the superficial epithelium. This outer surface is easily separated from the underlying layers and can be injured or destroyed by exposure (lack of moisture), chemical irritants that dissolve in the protective tear film, and scrapes from foreign bodies. Drying of the surface occurs with structural or functional alterations of the eyelids, which normally blink and spread tears to maintain moisture. Some studies have shown that eye surface irritation is a risk with individuals who work with computer visual display terminals (VDTs) for prolonged periods. There is some evidence that the rate of blinking is reduced during the intense staring at the VDTs, and heated or air-conditioned offices with low humidity contribute to drying and irritation of the eye surface. Contact lenses, eyelashes, dust and dirt particles, fingernails, and crusted matter from purulent eye drainage are among the most common offenders for scraping the corneal surface.

The epithelium heals quickly (within 24 to 48 hours) and leaves no scarring or residual damage. However, severe pain occurs with even minor abrasions because of the numerous pain receptors in the epithelium. Lacrimation and photophobia accompany the pain. Short-acting anesthetic drops may be administered to provide immediate relief and ease the eye examination, but the drops are not given after the examination because the anesthetic slows epithelial repair. The extent of the abrasion can be viewed with fluorescein dye. Foreign bodies are often spotted during examination of the surface. If no foreign bodies are found, the upper eyelid may need to be everted and examined. Even with removal of the foreign body and rapid healing, the eye surface must be monitored (and is often treated) for possible secondary infection because epithelial breaks invite a variety of bacteria that cannot normally invade an intact epithelium.

Lacerations and perforations are serious emergencies because of invasion and disruption of the underlying stroma, endothelium, lens, and vitreous. The eye should be patched or shielded (if a foreign body is protruding) until surgery is performed. The iris may fall forward to close a corneal wound and may need to be partially excised before the wound is closed. Lens perforations usually result in cataract formation, which may result in a need to remove the lens. After surgical repair the eye is treated for potential massive infection and monitored for uveitis (see p. 533), vitreous clouding, scarring, and changes in vision. Mydriatic-cycloplegic agents may be given

! EMERGENCY ALERT

TRAUMA TO THE EYE

Reasons vary greatly, but over half of eye injuries are occupational incidents, and 90% of ocular trauma is preventable.

ASSESSMENT

- Obtain thorough history; sensation of foreign body.
- Assess area; obtain visual acuity if possible.
- Assess for tearing.
- Look for hemorrhage, hyphema, foreign body, impaled object, and eviscerated eye tissue or vitreous humor.
- Assess for facial fractures, head injury.

INTERVENTIONS

- Do not instill anesthetic drops before eye is examined or without an order from the physician.
- If patient is in severe pain, patch both eyes.
- Check to see if patient is wearing contact lenses.
- Prevent drying by instilling ointment or artificial tears.
- Lightly apply ice pack for ecchymosis or abrasions.
- Decrease intraocular pressure by keeping patient's head still and head of bed elevated.
- Prepare for an ophthalmology consultation.
- If an impaled object is in the eye, stabilize the object and patch both eyes. Do not attempt to remove the object.

to maintain pupil dilation and thus prevent adhesions from forming on the underlying lens.

Many perforations occur in industrial settings, where flying metal flakes or particles are produced by high-speed drilling, riveting, and grinding. Workers are encouraged to wear protective goggles to prevent such injuries. The Occupational Safety and Health Administration (OSHA) mandates the use of protective eyewear or goggles whenever there is even minimal risk. Foreign bodies with iron or rusted particles may leave a deposit in the form of a rust ring. This deposit can be surgically removed after the epithelium has healed if it is superficially deposited. Deeply dispersed iron particles may interfere with an individual's vision in the future. Some foreign bodies, such as glass, are inert and can remain embedded in the eye tissue for years without harmful effects.

Chemical irritants, depending on the substance, can burn and destroy the underlying corneal layers. Regardless of the substance, the eye should be irrigated with copious amounts of water or sterile saline. Alkaline substances (such as ammonia, lime and cement dust, and sodium hydroxide) penetrate the tissues rapidly and continue to burn into the cornea unless they are removed. Acids coagulate the protein and often result in relatively superficial reversible damage. Local anesthetic drops may be used initially to provide comfort and ease irrigation and examination, but they are not used more than twice because they obstruct the healing process of the epithelium.

Ultraviolet burns (or irritation) can occur with sun exposure and are a risk for welders who are not protected from welding flashes. Epithelial irritation, swelling, and possible desquamation may occur. Desquamation is usually repaired without visual loss or changes.

EMERGENCY ALERT

CHEMICAL BURNS TO THE EYE

Chemical burns are caused by acids, alkaline substances, or irritants such as Mace. Acid burns are usually superficial, whereas alkaline burns are progressive and represent an extreme emergency. An alkali chemical can penetrate the cornea in as little as 15 seconds.

ASSESSMENT

- Attempt to measure visual acuity.
- Determine the chemical.
- If burn is from an alkaline source, there may be tissue destruction, which may be seen as white spots on the eye.
- The damage from an alkaline burn may not be evident until 3 to 4 days after the injury.

INTERVENTION

- Regardless of the chemical, irrigate the eye immediately with copious amounts of normal saline or tap water. Continue to irrigate until the pH of the eye returns to 7.0, which is normal. The irrigation may take as long as 30 minutes. Do not be afraid to irrigate too much.

Acid

- Irrigate as directed above.
- Apply topical applications of antibiotics and cycloplegic agents as ordered.

Alkaline

- Irrigate as directed above.
- Apply topical applications of antibiotics, steroids, and cycloplegic agents as ordered.

DIAGNOSTIC STUDIES AND FINDINGS

Fluorescein stain (2%): To identify corneal surface disruption
Slit lamp examination: To view the eye surface, anterior chamber, deeper layers of the cornea, and anterior eye
Indirect ophthalmoscopy: To view vitreous and retina

MULTIDISCIPLINARY PLAN

Surgery

Removal of foreign objects; removal of damaged or prolapsed eye tissue; repair of wounds

Medications[13]

Mode, frequency, and duration of therapy depend on degree of corneal penetration and potential for secondary infection.

Topical anesthetic agents: Administered once or twice for pain relief during examination or removal of foreign body
- Proparacaine (Alcaine, Ophthetic), 0.5% solution, 1-2 drops in injured eye; onset within 2 min; duration, 20 min
- Tetracaine, 0.5% solution or ointment, 1-2 drops in injured eye; onset within 1 min; duration, 20 min

Antiinfective agents: Type and duration of medication depend on extent of injury

Topical
- Erythromycin (Ilotycin), 1% ointment applied qd or bid in conjunctival cul-de-sac
- Combination of bacitracin 400 U, polymyxin B 5000 U, and neomycin 0.25% (Neosporin) ointment, applied tid or qid in conjunctival sac
- Tetracycline (Achromycin), 1% suspension or ointment, 1-2 drops bid or qid

EMERGENCY ALERT

CORNEAL ABRASION

Corneal abrasion is common; it usually occurs when a foreign body scratches the corneal epithelium.

ASSESSMENT

- Tearing and eyelid spasms
- Pain
- Diagnosed by using fluorescein staining and observing the abrasion with a blue light

INTERVENTION

- Test visual acuity.
- Apply topical anesthesia if indicated and in collaboration with a physician.
- Patch eye for 24 hours after examination.
- Instruct patient to avoid blinking eyelid as much as possible.
- Instruct patient to avoid driving while patch is in place.

Mydriatic-cycloplegic agents: May be given to prevent inflammatory pupillary constriction, uveitis

Scopolamine hydrobromide (Isopto Hyoscine), 0.25% solution, 1-2 drops in injured eye; duration, 48-72 h

Systemic antibiotic agents: May be prescribed for severe invasive trauma

Systemic analgesic agents: May be prescribed for severe invasive trauma

General Management

Protective eye patch or shield applied until patient is examined

Eye irrigation: Normal saline is commonly used

Bilateral pressure dressing often prescribed for 24 to 72 hours to promote rest, reduce discomfort, and aid corneal reepithelialization

Tinted glasses to reduce discomfort of photophobia

NURSING CARE

NURSING ASSESSMENT

Corneal epithelium: Moderate to severe pain; blurred vision; lacrimation; photophobia; generalized redness; fluorescein stains green on disrupted corneal surface; presence of foreign body

Surrounding conjunctivae: Generalized redness, bleeding, excoriation, presence of foreign body; evert upper lid to inspect for foreign body if discomfort persists and foreign body is not present on eye surface

Anterior chamber: May be partially or completely filled with blood

Surrounding eye tissue: A portion of the iris may prolapse through open corneal wound

PATIENT PROBLEMS/NURSING DIAGNOSES & INTERVENTIONS

NIC PHYSICAL COMFORT PROMOTION

Acute pain related to corneal injury

- Evaluate and document patient's level of discomfort. If discomfort is severe, delay visual testing or other assessment until topical or systemic anesthetic or analgesic has been ordered and has taken effect.
- Administer medications as ordered immediately *to relieve discomfort.*
- After treatment, apply pressure bandage to eye *to relieve discomfort* (be certain eye is closed before applying bandage).
- Apply a warm compress for 10 to 15 minutes as ordered *to relieve discomfort and inflammation.*
- Administer cycloplegic medication as ordered *to prevent pain from inflammatory pupil constriction and iritis.*
- Ensure safety and comfort of hospitalized patient.

NIC SKIN/WOUND MANAGEMENT

Impaired tissue integrity related to corneal surface disruption
Risk for infection related to corneal surface disruption

- Apply bandage or shield to eye until patient can be examined.
- Warn patient not to touch eye for duration of topical anesthetic *to avoid self-injury.*
- Administer topical and systemic medications as ordered *to prevent infection.*

NIC PSYCHOLOGICAL COMFORT PROMOTION

Fear related to discomfort and uncertainty about present and future visual loss

- Relieve discomfort as quickly as possible.
- Assess patient for signs of fear.
- Provide comfort and realistic reassurance.
- Keep patient informed about all procedures as they occur *to alleviate as much uncertainty as possible.*

NIC SELF-CARE FACILITATION

Disturbed sensory perception (visual) related to use of eye patch or decreased vision in one or both eyes

- Warn patient that depth perception will be lost and 50% of peripheral vision will be lost on affected side.
- Caution patient to bring hand forward slowly to touch objects (especially containers of hot liquid and containers receiving poured liquids) *to ensure safety.*
- Explain that patient should turn head fully to affected side to view objects or obstacles.
- Teach patient to use up and down head movements to judge stair dimensions and oncoming objects *to promote safety.*
- Teach patient to proceed slowly with all movement *to prevent injury.*

  NOTE: Patients with ocular trauma only are usually not hospitalized. However, patients with multiple injuries including ocular trauma will need interventions for sensory alterations as described here.
- Evaluate patient for level of fear or disorientation related to sudden loss of vision.
- Review events since injury and present situation with patient *to reorient patient and to maximize patient's capacity to deal with present circumstances.*
- Raise side rails *to ensure safety.*
- Address patient by name and identify yourself *to reduce anxiety.*
- Complement voice stimulation with touch *to notify patient of your proximity.*
- Orient patient to equipment (such as call light) and personal belongings at bedside by directing patient's hand.
- Encourage patient to perform self-care with personal hygiene *to maximize independence.*
- Ensure patient's privacy, and assure patient that privacy is provided.
- Provide patient with television set or radio *to encourage mental and memory stimulation.*
- Provide patient with a clock that can be felt, and remind patient of date.
- Continue to assess patient for evidence of sensory deprivation signs (e.g., withdrawal, anxiety, depression).
- Balance privacy and quiet with stimulation events.
- Help patient with meals *to promote the needed caloric intake.*

  Read menu selections.
  Guide hand to utensils and food on tray.
  Describe food on tray in clock terms.

Help with cutting meals, removing lids from containers, buttering bread, and so on.

- Help with walking *to promote safety.*
  Walk slowly and slightly ahead of patient; patient's hand should rest on your arm at elbow *to maximize patient's capacity to maintain balance and assurance of attending support.*
  If possible, allow patient to trace progress by running dorsal aspect of his or her free hand along a wall.
  Warn of steps, turns, and narrow passageways in advance.
  Allow patient to feel chair, toilet, or bed before turning to sit.

Patient Education/Continuum of Care Plan

1. Demonstrate to patient how to apply eyedrops or ointment as ordered.
2. Demonstrate to patient how to apply warm or cold compresses as ordered.
3. Tell patient to wash hands well before treating eye(s).
4. Discuss with patient the need to wear dark glasses if a cycloplegic drug is ordered.
5. Encourage patient to keep hands away from face and eyes except when treating condition.
6. Instruct patient not to use soiled handkerchief or tissue on eyes.
7. Encourage patient to avoid noxious fumes and smoke.
8. Discuss with patient how to monitor eye for increased pain and for blood or discharge from eye or on dressing.
9. Interpret any temporary or permanent visual alterations patient might experience (e.g., blurring with corneal healing, swelling, blurring with ointment over eye surface, blurring and photophobia with pupil dilation).
10. Review with patient the need for eye protection at work (e.g., protective goggles) or at other times (e.g., care of contact lenses—see p. 562.)

Evaluation/Patient Outcomes

Physical Comfort Promotion: Patient does not experience pain.

Skin/Wound Management: Cornea is healthy. Cornea is clear and glossy. There is no discomfort, visual loss, distortion, or evidence of infection.

Psychologic Comfort Promotion: Patient does not exhibit anxiety or fear.

Self-Care Facilitation: Visual alteration is improved. Patient is able to perform ADLs and has returned to preinjury level of function.

Scleritis[15]

Scleritis is an inflammation of the sclera.

Scleral inflammations are uncommon. The sclera has a poor blood supply and a low metabolism that does not encourage infection. Deep-seated aching and tenderness to touch without loss of vision are early indicators of the disease. An ocular muscle may contract and turn the eye if the inflammation is near its insertion. Because of the proximity of the sclera to the uveal tract, secondary choroiditis or retinal detachment may occur.

The episclera (located anteriorly) is more vascular than the rest of the sclera, and infections in this area may be worse. Infection is usually unilateral, has a sudden onset, and is accompanied by marked generalized hyperemia and pain. The cause is not always apparent, and the inflammation often subsides spontaneously.

Chronic or recurrent scleritis may result in scleral thinning with a localized outward bulging of the choroid layer. Perforation may occur.

DISORDERS OF THE UVEAL TRACT AND PUPIL

The uveal tract comprises the iris, ciliary body, and choroid layer. The iris surrounds the pupil and controls its size; the ciliary body secretes aqueous humor and controls accommodation; and the vascular choroid nourishes the anterior uveal tract and part of the retina. The location and extent of uveal lesions determine the variety and severity of signs, symptoms, and visual alterations. Deep corneal inflammation often spreads to the iris and results in a painful contraction of the iris and ciliary body. Iris abnormalities or inflammation can alter the shape of the pupil, disrupt the pupillary light reflex, or form adhesions to the cornea or lens to cause glaucoma. Ciliary body lesions can interfere with accommodation or cause anterior chamber or vitreous clouding with exudates, which diminishes visual acuity. Choroidal inflammation can spread to the sensory retinal layer and destroy central or peripheral vision. Retinal detachment may occur because of vitreous pull on the retina.

Uveitis[44,51]

Uveitis is an inflammation or infection of the uveal tract.

Uveitis is the most common uveal condition. Organisms can be identified if the inflammation is peripheral enough to give the examiner access to infected tissue for staining or culture. Often the cause is unknown, and the inflammation is treated on the basis of the presumed cause. Some inflammatory processes are associated with endogenous causes or chronic conditions that can be diagnosed and treated systemically. Acute inflammations vary in severity and may subside without residual alterations. The uveal tract is also subject to congenital or developmental lesions that may or may not affect vision.

Pathophysiology[36,47]

Inflammation of the uveal tract can be acute or chronic, can be mild or severe, and can involve primarily the anterior tract (iris, ciliary body, and anterior choroid), the posterior choroid, or the entire eye. The most common form of uveitis is acute anterior inflammation. The onset is sudden, and the symptoms of pain and visual loss appear abruptly and are sometimes severe. The arteries of the anterior ciliary body become engorged and dilated, creating a purplish discoloration around the limbus (circumcorneal flush). The iris and the ciliary body release an exudate that increases protein and inflammatory cells in the anterior chamber. The protein causes clouding of the chamber (aqueous flare), and the cells form in clumps that adhere to the posterior cornea (keratic precipitates). Keratic precipitates, a diagnostic determinant, can be viewed with a slit lamp and occasionally with the ophthalmoscope if the deposits are large enough. A massive production of cells forms pus in the anterior chamber (hypopyon). The ciliary body also releases exudate into the vitreous to cause clouding and cell production. The iris is usually constricted (miotic pupil) and does not respond to light. The constriction is painful, and pain intensity increases with light stimulation. If the pain is severe, it is difficult to open the lid for examination. If the iris remains constricted, it quickly forms adhesions to the underlying lens (posterior synechiae) that may obstruct aqueous flow and cause a pupillary block glaucoma. With anterior inflammation the iris, ciliary body, and anterior choroid are usually all involved because of a common blood supply.

Posterior uveitis is usually confined to the posterior choroid and quickly spreads to the sensory retina. The vitreous becomes clouded with cells and exudate that can be viewed with an ophthalmoscope. Chorioretinal lesions can also be seen as irregular gray-white areas on the retinal surface. Vision impairment is the chief symptom of posterior choroiditis. Often there is no pain, redness, or photophobia. The degree of visual impairment depends on the extent of vitreous clouding and the location of retinal sensory layer inflammation. If the macula is involved, central vision is severely impaired. Retinal inflammations often leave scars that permanently impair the patient's vision.

Acute uveitis results from external infection, trauma (laceration, puncture, or contusion) or chemical burns. Herpes simplex, herpes zoster, and fungal infections are common causes of iritis. There are many endogenous sources. Rubella, rubeola, or mumps may cause a mild, transient uveitis. A hypermature cataract may release exudate into the anterior chamber and cause severe inflammation. Systemic diseases such as rheumatoid arthritis, regional enteritis, ankylosing spondylitis, and collagen disorders may contribute to uveitis. Many uveitis exacerbations are idiopathic and treated symptomatically. Acute uveitis can recur, particularly if the cause is endogenous and chronic.

Chronic uveitis is usually a continuous and progressive inflammation that involves cell production in the anterior and posterior chambers, frequent posterior synechia formation, retinal involvement, minimum exterior inflammatory signs or pain, and residual scarring of inflammatory sites. Some organisms invade and remain in the uveal tract. Tuberculosis, herpes zoster, and some forms of fungi are common causes of chronic inflammation. Systemic diseases such as sarcoidosis, rheumatoid arthritis (Still's disease), and histoplasmosis may be implicated. Some of the chronic syndromes are caused by local eye degenerative reactions. Chronic infections resulting from the degenerative changes in blind eyes may force a decision to perform enucleation for relief. Pars planitis is a chronic inflammation of the posterior choroid that involves vitreous opacities with a chief complaint of "floaters," retinal inflammation, and scarring. The cause is unknown, and the disease extends over 5 to 10 years.

In severe infections the entire inner eyeball may become inflamed (panophthalmitis). Pyogenic bacteria may penetrate to the uvea with trauma, through rupture of a corneal ulcer, or through endogeneous sources such as septicemia, meningitis, or bacterial endocarditis. *Staphylococcus aureus, Pseudomonas,* and *Proteus* are commonly involved organisms. Suppurative panophthalmitis is acute and severe. Severe pain, visual loss, and necrosis of the sclera may be followed by rupture of the globe. Sometimes the infection does not invade the sclera but remains confined to the inner eyeball (endophthalmitis). In this case the onset and course are less severe and the infection is more responsive to treatment.

Diagnostic Studies and Findings[36,47]

Staining and culture of scraping: Performed if uveitis is associated with peripheral inflammation or ulceration; organism is identified through culture and Gram's stain

Slit lamp (binocular microscope) examination: Focuses on thin sections of cornea, anterior chamber, lens, or anterior vitreous; presence and extent of inflammatory cells or pus in anterior chamber and anterior vitreous can be viewed

Gonioscopy: Corneal contact lens (goniolens) is placed over anesthetized cornea to permit viewing of anterior chamber angles with microscopic lens; cellular debris and adhesions are seen in anterior chamber; angles can be viewed

Ophthalmoscopy: Vitreous opacities and chorioretinal lesions can be viewed

Diagnostic studies to rule out or identify systemic disease

Multidisciplinary Plan[36,47]

Acute uveitis is often treated symptomatically because the cause cannot be identified.

Surgery

Enucleation for ruptured globe or marked eye degeneration[22]; lens extraction for lens-induced uveitis

Medications

Mydriatic-cycloplegic agents: Duration of administration depends on severity of infection

Atropine sulfate, 1% solution bid or tid to maintain full pupillary dilation

Corticosteroids: Topical (often the choice with anterior uveitis)

Instilled as frequently as q1-2h initially for severe inflammation, or bid or tid, to reduce inflammation and prevent iritic adhesions; patient response must be carefully supervised because herpes simplex and fungal organisms increase in activity and growth with steroid therapy; immunosuppression may increase host susceptibility to secondary infection; because open-angle glaucoma is a common complication of topical steroid treatment, ocular tension must be carefully monitored.

Dexamethasone alcoholic suspension (Maxidex), 0.1% suspension, 1-2 drops 4-6 times a day

Fluorometholone suspension (FML Liquifilm), 0.1%, 1-2 drops 4-6 times a day

Corticosteroids: Subconjunctival injections (sometimes administered along with topical medication; administration and dosage determined by physician)

Dexamethasone sodium phosphate (Decadron Phosphate), 4 mg/ml
Hydrocortisone acetate (Hydrocortone Acetate, Cortef Acetate), 25 mg/ml or 50 mg/ml

Topical antiinfective agents: Type and duration of medication depend on severity of infection
Erythromycin (Ilotycin), 1% ointment applied qd or bid in conjunctival sac
Combination of bacitracin 400 U, polymyxin B 5000 U, and neomycin 0.25% (Neosporin) ointment, applied tid or qid in conjunctival sac
Tetracycline (Achromycin), 1% suspension or ointment, 1-2 drops bid or qid

Systemic medications
Analgesics
Acetaminophen (Tylenol), 650 mg PO q4h as needed (prn)
Acetaminophen (Tylenol), 650 mg with codeine (30 mg), PO q4h prn
Corticosteroids
For posterior uveitis and inflammations that do not respond to local treatment

NURSING CARE

NURSING ASSESSMENT

Anterior uveitis: Moderate pain; severe pain if associated with keratitis; intense photophobia; no visual change; possible blurred vision if eye chambers clouded with exudate, or possible blurred distant vision with ciliary spasm; circumcorneal flush (purplish coloration); pupillary constriction

Posterior uveitis: Minimum or no pain; blurred vision from vitreous opacities or sensory retina inflammation (may be central [macular] or peripheral, depending on extent and location of inflammation); ophthalmoscopy may reveal vitreous opacities as black dots

PATIENT PROBLEMS/NURSING DIAGNOSES & INTERVENTIONS

NIC PHYSICIAN COMFORT PROMOTION

Acute pain related to acute anterior iridocyclitis

- Administer cycloplegics as ordered *to reduce painful pupillary constriction.*
- Apply warm and cold compresses for 10 to 15 minutes two or three times a day as ordered.
- Administer systemic analgesics as ordered *to promote comfort.*
- Instruct patient to wear dark glasses or avoid light *to reduce photophobic discomfort.*

NIC SKIN/WOUND MANAGEMENT

Impaired tissue integrity related to adhesions and increased intraocular pressure, secondary to iridocyclitis

Risk for infection related to penetration of bacteria to the uvea

- Administer cycloplegics as ordered *to prevent adhesions from iris to lens.*
- Monitor patient for signs of increased intraocular pressure, increased haziness of vision (corneal edema), extreme pain, nausea, vomiting, or onset of conjunctival injection.
- Administer topical and systemic medications (steroids, antiinfective agents) as ordered *to prevent infection.*

PATIENT EDUCATION/CONTINUUM OF CARE PLAN

1. Demonstrate to patient how to apply eyedrops and ointments.
2. Demonstrate to patient how to apply warm and cold compresses.
3. Encourage patient to wear dark glasses.
4. Discuss with patient how to monitor eye for increased pain, visual changes (increased blurring), and inflammatory signs.
5. Review with patient that vision will be blurred because pupil will be dilated.

EVALUATION/PATIENT OUTCOMES

Physical Comfort Promotion: Patient does not experience pain.

Skin/Wound Management: Uveal tissue is healthy. Cornea is clear and glossy. There is no photophobia, eye discomfort, inflammation (corneal, circumcorneal, or conjunctival), or discharge. Vision is restored. There is no blurring at close or distant range.

UVEAL TRACT DEFORMITIES[38,44,47]

Uveal tract deformities range from minor defects to severe impediments to visual functioning.

A coloboma is a localized absence of uveal tissue. An absence of a portion of the iris may cause a pupil shape defect (see p. 537) with no visual defects. If the choroidal coloboma is large, the overlying retina is deprived of blood supply in that area, which affects sensory vision. Aniridia is absence or diminishment of the iris. The pupil appears greatly enlarged, and no iris is showing. Photophobia and severe reduction of visual acuity follow. Aniridia may be inherited or associated with other chromosomal disorders such as mental retardation, Wilms' tumor, and urogenital abnormalities. The iris can atrophy over a period of years, leaving a misshapen pupil or holes (looking like additional pupils) over the visible surface of the iris. The presence of holes can cause diplopia. Atrophy can follow severe eye inflammation or trauma or occur as a primary disease. Choroid atrophy can be a benign disorder or result in marked retinal degeneration. Some forms of choroid atrophy cause progressive night blindness and diminished visual acuity.

The size of the pupil is controlled by dilator and constrictor muscles in the iris. There are no disorders of the pupil, but its size, response to light (accommodation), uniformity of shape, and symmetric responses with the corresponding eye are indicators of iris, eye, or systemic disorders.[36,47] Table 8-2 gives a summary of pupil abnormalities.

Table 8-2 Pupil Abnormalities

Abnormality	Contributing Factors	Appearance
BILATERAL		
Miosis (pupillary constriction; usually less than 2 mm in diameter)	Iridocyclitis; miotic eyedrops (such as pilocarpine given for glaucoma)	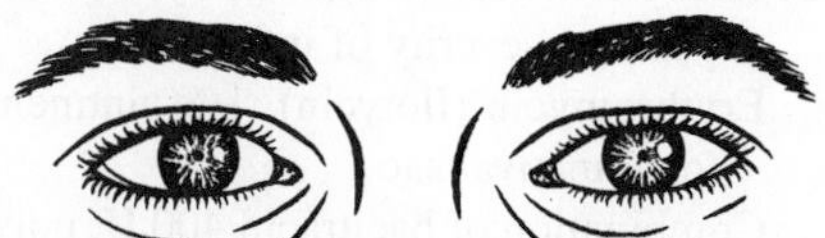
Mydriasis (pupillary dilation; usually more than 6 mm in diameter)	Iridocyclitis; mydriatic or cycloplegic drops (such as atropine); midbrain (reflex arc) lesions or hypoxia; oculomotor (CN III) damage; acute-angle glaucoma (slight dilation)	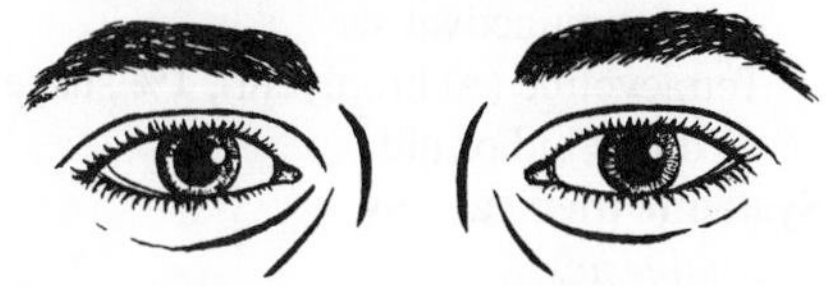
Failure to respond (constrict) with increased light stimulus	Iridocyclitis; corneal or lens opacity (light does not reach retina); retinal degeneration; optic nerve (CN II) destruction; midbrain synapses involving afferent pupillary fibers or oculomotor nerve (CN III) (consensual response is also lost); impairment of efferent fibers (parasympathetic) that innervate sphincter pupillae muscle	
Argyll Robertson pupil	Bilateral, miotic, irregular-shaped pupils that fail to constrict with light but retain constriction with convergence; pupils may or may not be equal in size; commonly caused by neurosyphilis or lesions in midbrain where afferent pupillary fibers synapse	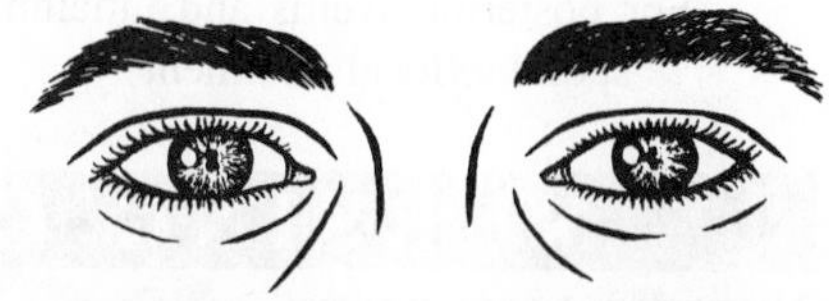
Oval pupil	Sometimes occurs with head injury or intracranial hemorrhage; transitional stage between normal pupil and dilated, fixed pupil with increased intracranial pressure (ICP); in most instances returns to normal when ICP is returned to normal	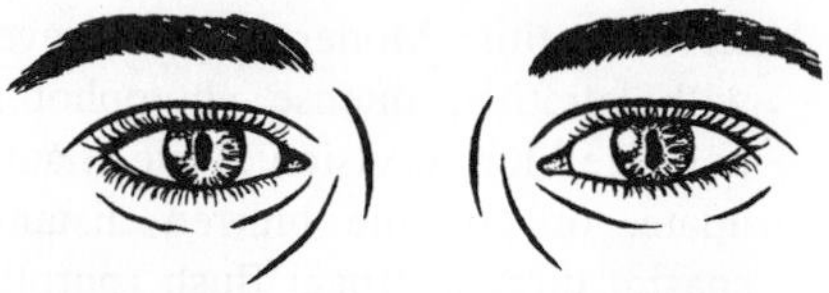
UNILATERAL		
Anisocoria (unequal size of pupils)	Congenital (approximately 20% of normal people have minor or noticeable differences in pupil size, but reflexes are normal) or caused by local eye medications (constrictors or dilators), amblyopia, or unilateral sympathetic or parasympathetic pupillary pathway destruction (NOTE: Examiner should test whether pupils react equally to light; if response is unequal, examiner should note whether larger or smaller pupil reacts more slowly [or not at all] because either pupil could be abnormal size)	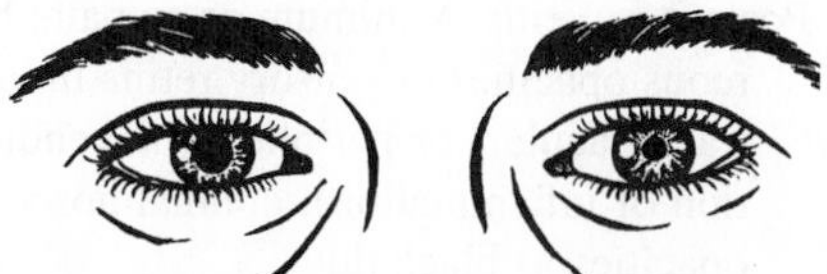
Iritis constrictive response	Acute uveitis is frequently unilateral; constriction of pupil accompanied by pain and circumcorneal flush (redness)	Normal eye Affected eye 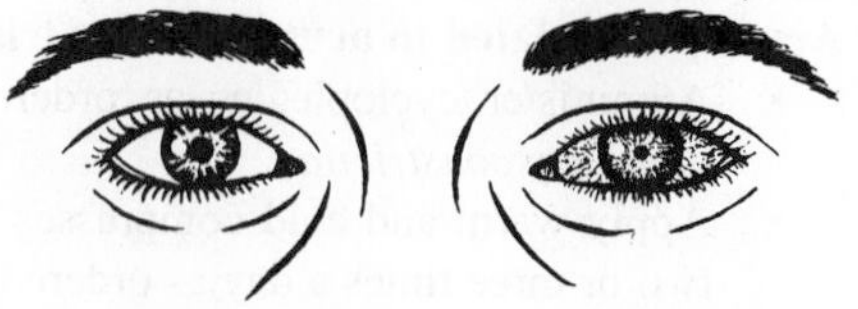
Oculomotor nerve (CN III) damage	Pupil dilated and fixed; eye deviated laterally and downward; ptosis	Normal eye Affected eye 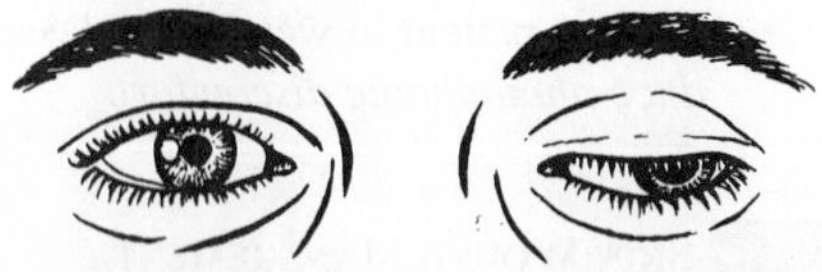
Horner's syndrome	Miotic pupil; ptosis; interruption of sympathetic nerve supply to dilator pupillae muscle; may be caused by goiter, cervical lymph enlargement, apical bronchogenic carcinoma, or surgical injury to neck	Normal eye Affected eye 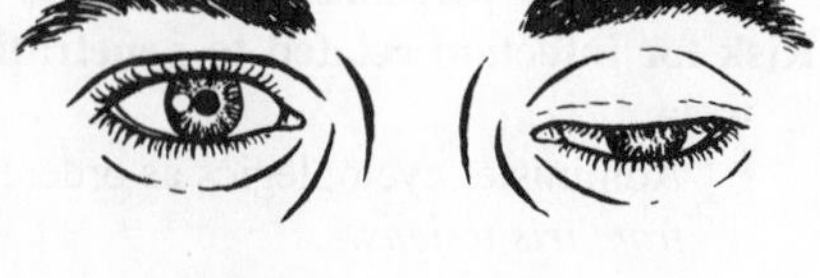

Abnormality	Contributing Factors	Appearance
Adie's pupil (tonic pupil)	Affected pupil dilated and reacts slowly or fails to react to light; response to convergence normal; caused by impairment of postganglionic parasympathetic innervation to sphincter pupillae muscle or ciliary malfunction; often accompanied by diminished tendon reflexes (as with diabetic neuropathy or alcoholism)	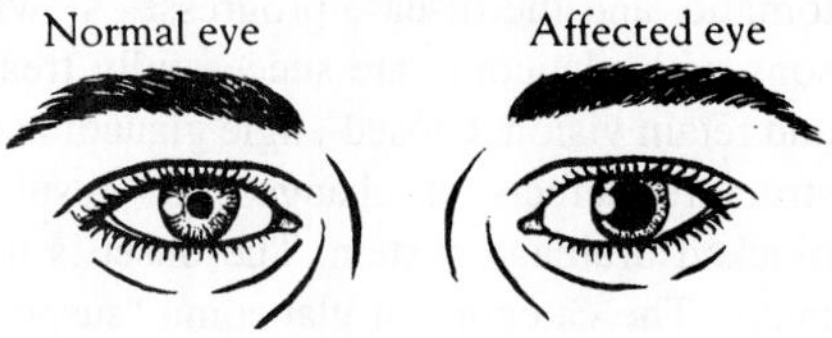
OTHER IRREGULARITIES		
Iridectomy	Sector iridectomy	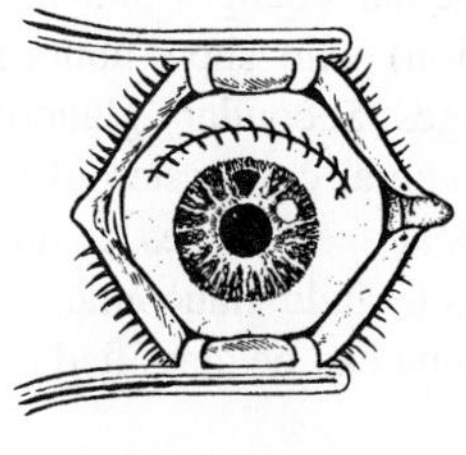
	Peripheral iridectomy Surgical excision of portion of iris usually done in superior area so upper lid will cover additional exposure	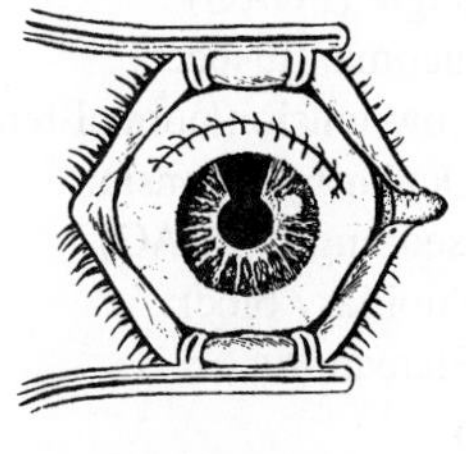
Coloboma (localized absence of portion of iris)	Congenital absence of area of iris; remaining iris shows normal light response	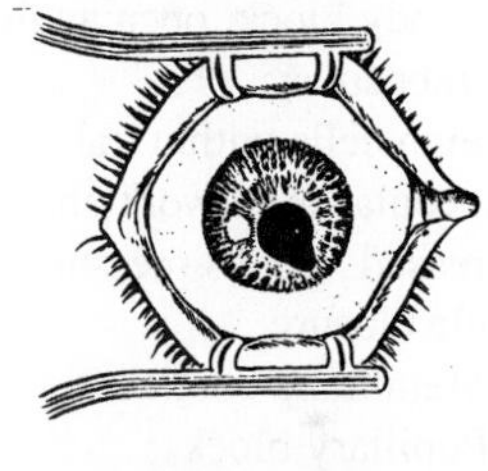
Iridodialysis (circumferential tearing of iris from scleral spur)	Blunt trauma; more than one "pupil" in eye can cause diplopia	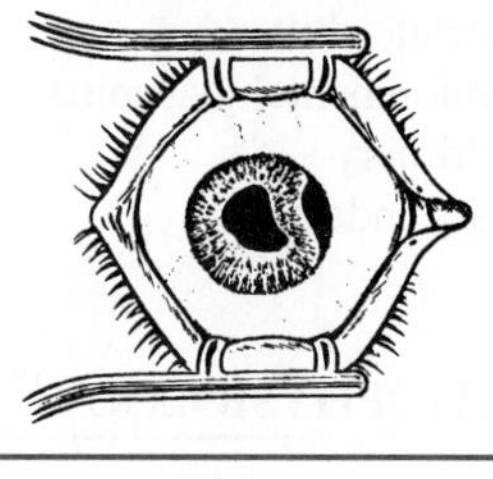

GLAUCOMA

Glaucoma incorporates a variety of diseases that exhibit all or at least one of the following abnormalities: increase in intraocular pressure, degeneration of the optic nerve (disc), and visual field losses that may lead to total loss of vision.

The prevalence of glaucoma is difficult to determine because of the different screening methods and criteria for diagnosis among physicians and regions of the world. An estimated 1.5% of persons over 40 years of age have glaucoma, and approximately 100,00 persons in the United States are blind as a result of this disease.[10]

Glaucoma is detected in a variety of ways. Simple tonometry testing reveals intraocular pressure (IOP) that exceeds the normal range of 10 to 22 mm Hg. Only 5% to 10% of persons with IOP over 21 mm Hg have visual defects or optic nerve changes. A variety of variables (discussed later) determine whether an unaffected person with a high IOP will only be monitored or will be treated for glaucoma. When screening methods include ophthalmoscopy or perimetry testing for visual field defects, some patients with a normal IOP exhibit optic nerve degeneration or visual field losses. Approximately one third of the visual defect population have a normal IOP when first examined.[17] Tonometry alone is not an adequate screening method for detecting glaucoma, and higher incidences are reported when persons are more thoroughly examined.

Glaucoma occurs because aqueous fluid cannot be drained adequately from the anterior chamber to maintain a normal IOP. Excessive pressure results in optic nerve degeneration.

Primary glaucomas (from an unknown cause) include open-angle, closed-angle, and glaucoma "suspect" disorders. Open-angle glaucoma is the more common and generally affects adults over 40 years of age. The onset is insidious and asymptomatic, and the disease progresses slowly. Many elderly persons with glaucoma are successfully treated with medications and retain vision. Closed-angle glaucoma occurs because of eye structure defects or changes and results in a mechanically blocked drainage system. The onset is usually acute and dramatic. The category of glaucoma "suspect" disorders includes individuals with an elevated IOP (above 24 mm Hg) who exhibit no ocular changes and persons with normal IOP levels (low tension) who show abnormal optic disc and peripheral field changes. Secondary glaucomas can be caused by inflammation, trauma, corticosteroid administration, systemic disorders, or local eye changes. In addition, a number of congenital syndromes include glaucoma.

Glaucoma can be classified as follows[36]:

Primary
- Open-angle (POAG)
  - Glaucoma "suspect"
    - Low-tension/normal-tension
    - Ocular hypertension
  - Closed-angle (PCAG)
    - Pupillary block
    - Plateau iris

Secondary
- Ciliary body block, open angle
  - Pretrabecular
  - Foreign cells within trabecular meshwork
  - Trabecular meshwork abnormality
  - Increased venous pressure
  - Angle closure
    - Membrane contracture
    - Pupillary block
    - Angle shift
  - Developmental glaucoma
    - Primary
    - Secondary

PATHOPHYSIOLOGY[17,23,31,36,47]

Open-Angle Glaucoma

Approximately 90% of cases of primary glaucoma are of the open-angle type. The incidence of this disease increases with age. Population studies have shown that less than 1% of persons under 65 years of age have glaucoma and that approximately 3% of the population over 75 years of age have this disorder. Other risk factors for open-angle glaucoma have been identified. Nonwhites have a much higher incidence and frequently exhibit an earlier onset and a more rapid eye degeneration. Hypertension has been linked to glaucoma, as have the hypotensive episodes associated with treatment for hypertension. Approximately 20% to 25% of patients with elevated IOP have a family history of this disease. Persons with myopia and diabetes are reported to have a higher incidence of glaucoma.

Increased IOP occurs because of degenerative changes of unknown cause in the trabecular meshwork and the canal of Schlemm. Excess fluid cannot be emptied from the anterior chamber.

Intraocular pressure is not static but normally varies 2 to 5 mm Hg with increased heart rate, activity, or excitement. One high reading does not constitute a basis for diagnosis. Some persons exhibit visual field defects and optic nerve changes with normal or near-normal IOP, whereas others are able to tolerate elevated IOP without eye damage. Elevated IOP without ocular damage is called ocular hypertension. Some physicians believe that this elevation is a precursor of glaucoma, but others think that a mildly elevated IOP (20 to 24 mm Hg) is a normal state. The risk for eye damage increases with age, a family history of glaucoma, diabetes, and systemic vascular disorders.

Early open-angle glaucoma may be difficult to diagnose because it is asymptomatic. Even persons with visual field defects do not usually perceive them until they become extensive. There is no pain or blurred vision, and the outer eye does not appear inflamed or abnormal to the examiner. Tonometry usually shows an elevated IOP. Schiøtz's tonometer is less accurate in higher pressure ranges and consistently shows lower pressures than applanation or noncontact tonometers. Direct ophthalmoscopy may reveal the earliest finding if the examiner is sufficiently skilled. The physiologic cup (a depression in the center of the disc) may be larger in one eye than the other. As the disease progresses, the cup widens and extends toward the disc temporal margin. The temporal vessels appear to drop (or bend) abruptly into the cup. The large vessels become displaced and crowded toward the nasal side of the disc. The temporal disc border atrophies and loses its pink coloration to appear a flat white. The cup widens and deepens (excavation) as the surrounding optic nerve margin diminishes and atrophies.

Visual field testing often shows the most tangible alterations. Visual field testing by confrontation does not measure early or limited defects. The Goldmann perimeter measures both central and peripheral losses. Characteristic defects (blind areas or scotomas) appear and enlarge as the disease progresses. Nerve fiber bundles originating from the optic nerve cease to function as the nerve head atrophies. The nasal visual field is often first affected, and eventually the periphery is diminished. The person may retain only a small portion of central vision with acuity of the unaffected area.

Many older adults are treated successfully with medication. Parasympathomimetic agents (miotic eyedrops) increase the outflow of fluid by enlarging the area around the trabecular meshwork. Beta-blockers (eyedrops) and oral and/or topical carbonic anhydrase inhibitors decrease aqueous production. These drugs are given in various combinations. Miotic drops disturb vision because of pupillary constriction and may cause ciliary spasms. Beta-blockers must be administered cautiously to asthmatic patients. Epinephrine drops are sometimes prescribed to increase outflow, but their use should be evaluated carefully because of potential systemic effects (tachycardia) and occasional local effects (macular edema). Diuretics deplete potassium and may cause thirst and drinking of large amounts of fluids, which could increase pressure. Patients receiving medication need careful and continuous supervision.

If IOP cannot be controlled through medication, laser trabeculoplasty (creating openings in the trabecular meshwork with laser beams), laser iridotomy, or surgery may be performed. Surgery usually involves the creation of an opening between the anterior chamber and the subconjunctival space. Many physicians prefer laser therapy because it is less damaging to the eye (see p. 566). Success rates for laser and surgical therapies are variable. The openings or filter systems may not remain patent. Invasive therapy for open-angle glaucoma is a last resort for eyes that do not respond to chemotherapeutic regimens.

Normal Tension Glaucoma

Angle-closure

Angle-closure glaucoma occurs because mechanical blockage of the anterior chamber angle results in accumulation of aqueous fluid and increased IOP. Most persons with angle-closure glaucoma have shallow anterior chambers (less than 3-mm depth between the iris and the posterior corneal surface), which is often a familial trait. These persons do not exhibit IOP elevations unless the angle is closed and obscures the trabecular meshwork, which ordinarily drains fluid from the anterior chamber. The shallow chamber is often accompanied by narrowed anterior angles (FIG. 8-15). Narrow angles are more vulnerable to other physiologic events that cause further crowding of the angles.

Angle closure occurs because of pupillary dilation or forward displacement of the iris. In some instances pupillary dilation (physiologic or induced) causes the iris to crowd into the anterior angle, resulting in obstruction. Forward displacement of the iris occurs with enlargement of the lens, which normally thickens with aging. The iris can also be pushed forward with physiologic pupillary block. In a shallow anterior chamber the iris may press against the lens and obstruct aqueous flow from the posterior chamber to the anterior chamber. As fluid accumulates posteriorly, it bulges forward against the iris. A bulging iris can be viewed by an examiner with a penlight aimed obliquely at the cornea. The bulge casts a shadow on the opposite side of the light source (FIG. 8-16).

Acute angle closure causes a dramatic response. A sudden onset of blurred vision, severe ocular pain, and halos seen around lights is followed by a progression of symptoms as the pressure increases. Ciliary injection (a purplish red coloration around the limbus), profuse lacrimation, a mildly dilated, nonreactive pupil (5 to 6 mm in diameter), and nausea and vomiting may occur. Corneal edema causes the cornea to appear hazy. An acute episode constitutes a medical emergency. If the pressure is not relieved within several hours, permanent eye damage occurs.

Emergency medical treatment consists of oral or intravenous administration of carbonic anhydrase inhibitors to suppress aqueous humor secretion, miotic eyedrops to pull the iris away from the inner angle, osmotic agent to reduce pressure, and systemic analgesics to reduce pain. Surgical treatment (usually laser iridotomy) follows as soon as ocular pressure is stabilized.[2] Although usually only one eye is affected at a time, surgery is eventually performed on the other eye as a preventive measure. When narrow angles are apparent on ocular examination, prophylactic laser iridotomies are often performed today, dramatically reducing the number of acute attacks. Regular ophthalmic care is key to this diagnosis and preventive therapy.

Secondary Glaucomas

Trabecular meshwork obstruction or closed-angle glaucoma can occur because of eye deformities, inflammation, or trauma (surgical or accidental). Corticosteroid therapy increases IOP; this may be transient or may cause permanent eye damage.

A displaced, enlarged, hypermature, or ruptured lens can result in a crowding of the angle, an associated trabecular meshwork obstruction, or uveitis. Uveitis may cause a pupillary block with ciliary spasms or posterior synechiae (adhesions of the iris to the lens), which ultimately obstructs angle drainage. Trabeculitis with resultant scarring and damage may follow iridocyclitis when inflammatory cells and fibrous material are deposited in the anterior angles. Eye contusions elevate IOP, usually temporarily. If hemorrhage or edema of the iris or ciliary body ensues, the IOP increase is sustained and the angle flow may be compromised. If the anterior eye is traumatized through

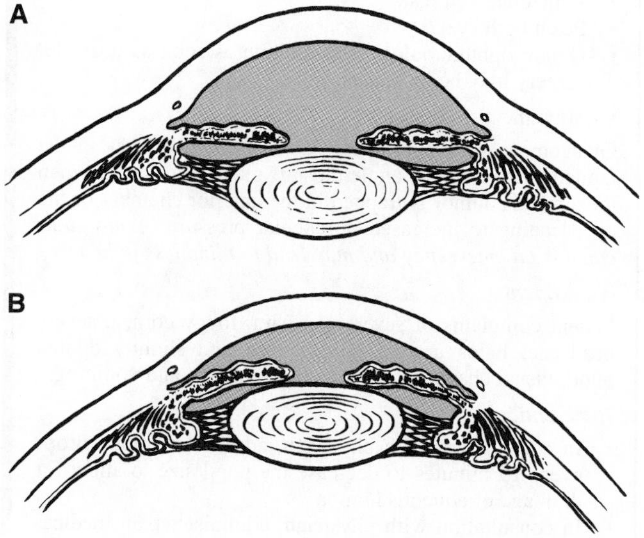

FIG. 8-15

A, Normal anterior chamber. **B,** Shallow anterior chamber. Shallow chamber shows forward displacement of iris and narrow anterior angle.

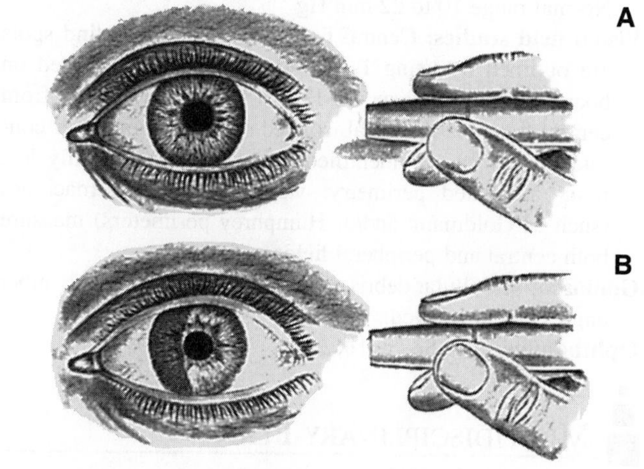

FIG. 8-16

A, Normal anterior chamber: iris is flat. **B,** Shallow anterior chamber: iris is bulging, and crescent shadow appears on far side. (From Seidel et al.[39])

surgery or laceration, the iris root may re-form or adhere to the ciliary body to obstruct the anterior angle.

Congenital Glaucoma[50]

Primary congenital glaucoma is a hereditary disease. It occurs when the structures of the anterior chamber angle do not fully develop at about the fifth month of fetal life. A thin remnant of iris tissue inserts into the trabecular meshwork and partially or fully covers it. The IOP increases, and corneal and optic nerve destruction ensues. Boys are affected more often than girls, and the disease is most commonly diagnosed at birth or within the first 2 years of life. The disease is most often bilateral. The earlier the symptoms, the less favorable the prognosis because earlier onset indicates a greater anatomic abnormality. Other systemic congenital defects may accompany primary congenital glaucoma. Early symptoms are excessive tearing and photophobia. A hazy cornea eventually becomes opaque because of edema and stretching with breaks in Descemet's membrane, which allows fluid into the cornea. The eye enlarges because the tissue is elastic, and the diameter of the cornea increases. Optic nerve deterioration occurs rapidly, resulting in total loss of vision. If the symptoms are diagnosed early, goniotomy (cutting away the tissue covering the meshwork) is performed. In some instances the goniotomy must be repeated a number of time to ensure adequate drainage. Approximately 80% of these surgeries are successful.

Secondary congenital glaucomas are associated with a variety of systemic and eye disorders. Aniridia, the absence of an iris, may be associated with other anterior eye deformities to cause glaucoma. A dystrophic cornea or a congenital cataract may be associated with glaucoma. Neurofibromatosis and Sturge-Weber syndrome (hemangioma of the face) are two of the more common systemic disorders that accompany congenital glaucoma. Usually filtering or trabeculoplasty procedures are performed with varying success, depending on the severity of the anatomic abnormality.

Diagnostic Studies and Findings

Tonometry (Schiøtz's, applanation, or contact methods): Normal range 10 to 22 mm Hg

Visual field studies: Central field tangent screen: blind spots are outlined by using 1- to 3-mm white target placed on board; normal blind spot is 13 to 18 degrees temporal from central fixation; abnormal isolated spots (scotomas) or confluent areas can be identified; nasal areas are usually lost first; automated perimetry: various automated machines (such as Goldmann and/or Humphrey perimeters) measure both central and peripheral fields

Gonioscopy: Cellular debris and adhesions in anterior chamber angles can be viewed

Ophthalmoscopy: See p. 1363.

Multidisciplinary Plan

Open-Angle Glaucoma[41]

Surgery

Surgery performed if medications do not control pressure

Laser trabeculoplasty: Almost always done on outpatient basis; 100 to 120 laser impacts aimed evenly spaced around anterior portion of trabecular meshwork through a goniolens; resultant scarring thought to increase tension within meshwork to maintain openings; success rate not fully determined

External trabeculectomy: Favored over other filter device procedures because it does not disrupt anterior chamber and adhesions do not form between iris and posterior canal; portion of meshwork is removed through scleral flap incision; flap is replaced over surgical site to keep anterior chamber intact; procedure performed in hospital with patient under general anesthesia; usually discharged the same day

! EMERGENCY ALERT

SUDDEN VISUAL CHANGES

Sudden changes in vision may be suggestive of an acute eye emergency, which may lead to blindness.

Central Retinal Artery Occlusion

Assessment

- Produces sudden blindness; prognosis is poor.

Interventions

- Interventions are directed at returning the blood supply to the retina and dilation of the artery.
- Possible interventions include amyl nitrate inhalation, sublingual nitroglycerin, and alternating administration of carbon dioxide and oxygen.

Retinal Detachment

Assessment

- Once detached, the retina is unable to perceive light because the blood and oxygen supply to the retina is compromised.
- Patient may report flashes of light, veil in visual field, or dark spots or particles in the visual field.

Interventions

- Immediate bed rest.
- Patch both eyes.
- Obtain ophthalmology consultation as soon as possible; surgery may be indicated.

Glaucoma

Glaucoma causes 1 of every 10 cases of blindness in the United States. Acute angle-closure glaucoma occurs when the aqueous humor is trapped in the anterior chamber of the eye, leading to increased intraocular pressure. *Acute glaucoma is an emergency and may lead to blindness in hours.*

Assessment

Patient complains of severe eye pain, foggy cornea, severe headache, halos around lights, fixed and slightly dilated pupil, visual changes, and sometimes nausea and vomiting.

Interventions

- In consultation with physician, administer miotic drops every 15 minutes to decrease the pupil size to allow for drainage of aqueous humor.
- In consultation with physician, administer pain medications and medications that will lower intraocular pressure (Diamox is generally used).
- Surgical and/or laser intervention may be necessary.

Glaucoma: Practical Therapeutic Approach

The goal of glaucoma therapy is the preservation of good visual function for the lifetime of the patient. Treatment is individualized to each patient with the aim of using as few medications as possible to maintain a predetermined target pressure that results in stable visual fields and optic nerve health.

There are numerous antiglaucomatous agents available, and they are changing rapidly. The commonly accepted treatment algorithm follows.

Topical agents are the first line of therapy and include nonselective beta-blockers such as timolol maleate and selective beta-blockers such as brimonidine, latanoprost, and topical carbonic anhydrase inhibitors such as dorzolamide. When

Only when all combinations of treatment options fail and damage to the optic nerve and visual receptor cells continue to cause vision loss is a treatment destructive of the ciliary body structure that produces aqueous humor employed.[43]

Angle-Closure Glaucoma

Surgery

Laser iridotomy: Lens placed over anesthetized cornea; argon laser aimed at iris for approximately 50 deliveries to penetrate iris and create openings for aqueous flow; laser sessions repeated several times if necessary; ultimately both eyes usually treated

Peripheral iridectomy: Incision of 3 to 4 mm made at limbus or parallel to limbus over cornea; iris prolapses through limbus, or forceps is inserted into anterior chamber to pull portion of iris outward so small wedge or piece of iris can be excised; remaining iris is massaged back into chamber, and pupil is constricted to assure surgeon that it is intact and round surrounding excised wedge; incision is then closed; pupil is dilated postoperatively, and steroid eye medication is given for few days so inflamed iris will not form adhesions; iridectomy opens channel between anterior and posterior chambers and creates opening in anterior angle for aqueous flow

Medications

In acute attacks, medications given to lower and control IOP so surgery can be performed

Hyperosmotic agents

Glycerin (glycerol, Osmoglyn), 50% solution, 1.5 g/kg body weight PO; duration, 4-6h

Mannitol (Osmitrol), 20% solution, 2 g/kg body weight, IV

Carbonic anhydrase inhibitors: Acetazolamide (Diamox), 250 mg PO bid or qid, or 500 mg followed by 250 mg IV q4h; should be given immediately to abort acute attack

Narcotic analgesic agents: Meperidine (Demerol), 100 mg intramuscularly (IM) q4-6h prn

Miotic agents: Pilocarpine hydrochloride (Isopto Carpine, Pilocar) 0.25%-8% solution, 1-2 drops q4-6h

See Common Glaucoma Medications table.

Congenital Glaucoma

Surgery

Goniotomy: Knife inserted near limbus to penetrate anterior chamber and reach area of trabecular meshwork in anterior angle; special goniolens used to scrutinize angle while knife tears away tissue covering meshwork; procedure may be repeated a number of times to ensure patency of drainage system

Tonometry

IOP usually elevated (more than 24 mm Hg) but may be within normal limits (under 22 mm Hg)

Visual fields (perimetry)

Typical central blind spots (scotomas) identifiable; superior/nasal vision usually lost before peripheral vision

Angle-Closure Glaucoma

Excessive lacrimation; acute, severe ocular pain (usually bilateral); blurred vision; halos seen around lights; pupil in mild dilation (5 to 6 mm diameter); corneoscleral flush (purplish red coloration at limbus); cornea may appear hazy; possible nausea and vomiting

Tonometry

IOP usually sharply elevated (may be over 50 mm Hg)

Congenital Glaucoma

Excessive lacrimation; photophobia; hazy opaque cornea; affected eye enlarged (both eyes may be affected); affected cornea enlarged in diameter

Tonometry

IOP usually elevated, but elastic eye tissue may stretch and give false low reading

PATIENT PROBLEMS/NURSING DIAGNOSES & INTERVENTIONS[31,45,48]

Open-Angle Glaucoma

NIC SKIN/WOUND MANAGEMENT

Risk for impaired tissue integrity related to deficient knowledge of therapeutic regimen or noncompliance with regimen secondary to undesirable side effects of medications

- Monitor patient's needs and response to medications *to see if negative responses are occurring* (physician

Common Glaucoma Medications

Type/Class	Medication	Trade Name	Action	Side Effects
Beta-blocker, nonselective	Timolol Maleate	Timoptic	Aqueous suppressant	Bronchospasm, bradycardia, depression, impotence
	Timolol Hemihydrate	Betimol		
	Levobunolol	Betagan	Aqueous suppressant	Bronchospasm, bradycardia, depression, impotence
	Carteolol	Ocupress	Aqueous suppressant	Bronchospasm, bradycardia, depression, impotence
	Metipranolol	Optipranolol	Aqueous suppressant	Bronchospasm, bradycardia, depression, impotence
Beta-blocker, selective	Betaxolol	Betoptic	Aqueous suppressant	Same as above, but bronchospasm less likely
Alpha and beta agonist	Epinephrine		Increases outflow	Stinging, allergic conjunctivitis, adrenochrome deposits
Alpha agonist	Apraclonidine HCl	Iopidine	Aqueous suppressant	Allergic conjunctivitis, tachyphylaxis
Alpha-2 agonist	Brimonidine	Alphagan	Aqueous suppressant	Dry eye, dry mouth, drowsiness
Carbonic anhydrase inhibitors	Topical Dorzolamide	Trusopt	Aqueous suppressant	None identified
	Dorzolamide	Diamox	Aqueous suppressant	Paresthesias of extremities, malaise, depression, nausea, vomiting, diarrhea, kidney stones, decreased serum K^+, blood dyscrasias, aplastic anemia
	Methazolamide	Neptazane	Aqueous suppressant	Same as above but less frequent
	Dichlorphen-amide	Daranide	Aqueous suppressant	Same as above but less frequent
Prostaglandin	Latanoprost	Xalatan	Increases uveoscleral outflow	Iris color change, longer eyelashes
Parasympatho-mimetics	Pilocarpine	Pilo-car Sopto-carpine	Increases aqueous outflow	Headache, browache, decreased night vision, fluctuating vision, burning
	Carbachol	Iosopto-carbachol		
Combinations	Trusopt and Timolol	Cosopt	Aqueous suppressant	See individual medications

may be able to change medication if side effects are severe).

- Evaluate patient's knowledge about disease and its insidious progress unless treated *to anticipate noncompliance.*
- Be certain patient can read medication labels.
- Explain that number of medications and number of administrations can be confusing, inconvenient, and easy to forget. Enlist patient's assistance and understanding in devising medication schedule that patient can meet *to reduce noncompliance.*
- Discuss with patient that medications do not relieve any symptoms and may cause unpleasant side effects.
- Ensure that patient is aware of possible side effects.
  - Miotics—blurred vision for 1 to 2 hours after administration, diarrhea
  - Timolol—fatigue, weakness, depression
  - Diamox—numbness, tingling of extremities and lips, decreased appetite or nausea, impotence
  - (See table above.)
- Instruct patient with new prescription that frequent checkups by physician are needed *to detect side effects and other symptoms such as increased IOP, sudden blurred vision, and inflammation of eyes.*
- Teach patient about possible side effects (see table above).
- Demonstrate correct method for administration and storage of eyedrops. Have patient repeat demonstration *to ensure proper technique.*

NIC SELF-CARE FACILITATION

Disturbed sensory perception (visual) related to symptoms of disease or side effects of medication

Risk for injury related to diminished peripheral vision

- Review patient's family and support system for assistance in dealing with visual loss.
- Evaluate patient's feelings about visual loss or changes.
- Review patient's lifestyle, and suggest adjustments to blurred vision associated with miotics.
- Offer support for feelings of loss and helplessness.
- Inform patient that diminished peripheral vision is a great safety hazard and that peripheral vision may be markedly reduced with advanced glaucoma.
- Explain that patient must learn to turn head to visualize either side *to ensure safety.*
- Ask patient to reduce clutter in home (such as electrical cords, loose rugs, and items on floor) *to prevent falls.*
- Inform patient that home should be well lighted (especially stairways) and that night-light in bathroom is helpful.
- Warn patient that seeing at night, at dusk, or in dim lighting will be difficult *because miotic pupils do not dilate to admit more light to retina in subdued lighting or darkness.*

Surgical and/or Laser Procedures for Glaucoma

NIC PATIENT EDUCATION

Deficient knowledge related to lack of information about the procedure

- Describe procedure carefully to patient and family members, including discussion of equipment, length of procedure, nature of procedure, and postoperative events.

- Educate patient about administering eye medications and necessity for maintaining prescribed therapy because iris may become inflamed postoperatively and IOP may be increased.
  - Glaucoma medications—resumed until inflammatory process subsides and then discontinued or adjusted
  - Topical steroid drops—often prescribed for approximately 1 week after surgery; reduce inflammation but may raise IOP
- Inform patient that IOP may rise postoperatively and must be carefully monitored.
- Educate patient about necessity for keeping appointments for monitoring IOP.
- Educate patient about self-monitoring for symptoms (especially sudden onset).
  - Excessive lacrimation
  - Photophobia
  - Severe ocular pain
- Advise patient that vision will be blurred for first day or two after procedure but should then be stable or improve.

NIC PHYSICAL COMFORT PROMOTION

Acute pain related to surgical procedure

- Administer systemic analgesics as ordered for headache that may occur a day or two after procedure.
- Apply eye patch or wear sunglasses for a few hours postoperatively *to avoid discomfort associated with light exposure.*

PATIENT EDUCATION/CONTINUUM OF CARE PLAN

Specific knowledge needs are described under Patient Problems/ Nursing Diagnoses & Interventions because glaucoma is commonly managed on an outpatient basis.

1. Review with patient that glaucoma is not curable but can be controlled.
2. Explain to patient that medications *must* be taken regularly and at the prescribed intervals.
3. Encourage patient to visit physician regularly as prescribed.
4. Ensure that patient understands need to monitor himself or herself for side effects[29] and report any to physician because therapy may be changed according to patient's response to medications (either undesirable side effects or ineffective therapy).
5. Explain to patient to watch for sudden changes, including severe eye pain, inflamed eye, excessive lacrimation, marked photophobia, and visual field losses (inability to use peripheral vision), which may be noted because of bumping into obstacles from the side or at patient's feet.
6. Remind patient of any existing limited vision and related safety concerns.
7. Review with patient factors that may increase IOP, such as constrictive clothing around neck or torso, constipation (straining), heavy exertion or lifting, and sneezing or coughing (upper respiratory infection).
8. Explain that family members should be examined regularly because glaucoma and shallow anterior chambers are often familial.

EVALUATION/PATIENT OUTCOMES

Skin/Wound Management: IOP is under control, and visual fields remain stable over time, indicating that eye damage is not present or not increasing. Eye examination shows normal findings. Eyeball surface is moist without excessive tearing. Conjunctiva is clear without injection. Cornea is clear, and no redness appears at limbus. Pupil may be constricted because of medication. Red reflex is full and round. Retinal surface is pink, granular, and uniform in color and consistency. Optic disc is pinkish white and translucent with physiologic cup that occupies no more than half of disc diameter. Both optic cups are same size. Central vessels emerge evenly from optic disc and are not crowded toward nasal side.

Self-Care Facilitation: Patient can perform ADLs and returns to usual level of function.

Patient Education: Patient verbalizes understanding of therapeutic regimen and importance of medication administrations as ordered.

DISORDERS OF THE LENS[18,36,47]

The lens is a 4-mm (sagittal diameter) by 9-mm (equatorial diameter) transparent structure between the anterior chamber and the vitreous body. Its transparency and biconvex shape enable it to focus light rays on the retina through refraction. The lens is suspended by fibers (zonules) that attach to the ciliary muscles, and it is stabilized behind the iris. The elasticity of the lens enables it to increase its spheric shape in response to ciliary contraction for near vision (accommodation). Loss of elasticity with aging results in diminished refractive power for near vision (presbyopia).

Diseases of the lens result in either opacity or dislocation of the lens. Because the lens contains no pain fibers or blood vessels, usually the only symptom is blurred vision without discomfort.

LENS DISLOCATION[36,47]

The lens can be dislocated by trauma (a blow to the eye), systemic congenital disorders, or deformities of the lens itself.

In most instances the lens loses the full support of the zonular fibers and is either partially dislocated or fully detached and floating in the vitreous. Iritis and glaucoma are common complications of a lens in the vitreous. The detached lens may be surgically removed to prevent further eye damage, although complications may ensue because of disruption and loss of vitreous. Partially dislocated lenses are often successfully treated with glasses to correct blurred vision.

CATARACT[20,21,28,36]

Cataract is an opacity of the lens.

The prevalence of the disease is difficult to determine because in some studies cataracts are defined as lens changes, whereas in others the disease is reported when vision is altered or the lens must be surgically removed. A summary of available cation and lens suction have all contributed to an improved prognosis and rapid recovery from surgery. In the past, patients had to wait for the cataract to become "ripe" (develop marked edema and liquefaction) before surgery was possible. Newer techniques permit the decision to be made jointly by the patient and physician on the basis of visual impairment and the patient's need for visual clarity. Extended-wear soft contact lenses and surgically implanted lenses allow monophakic persons (those with one lens removed) to enjoy binocular vision. Over 95% of surgically treated cataract patients can now look forward to restored useful vision.

a temporary improvement and is followed by increased opacities that ultimately reduce vision. Opacities may develop very slowly and form different configurations. An early symptom may be glare (especially at night) because the opacities reflect light rays inefficiently. In some instances central opacities split light rays and cause a monocular diplopia. This symptom disappears as the opacity increases. Vision may improve in dim light (or with pupil dilation) because the person has more pupil available to see around the opacity. Some patients are able to "see" the dark spots, which remain fixed in the visual field, unlike floaters (debris in the vitreous), which move around.

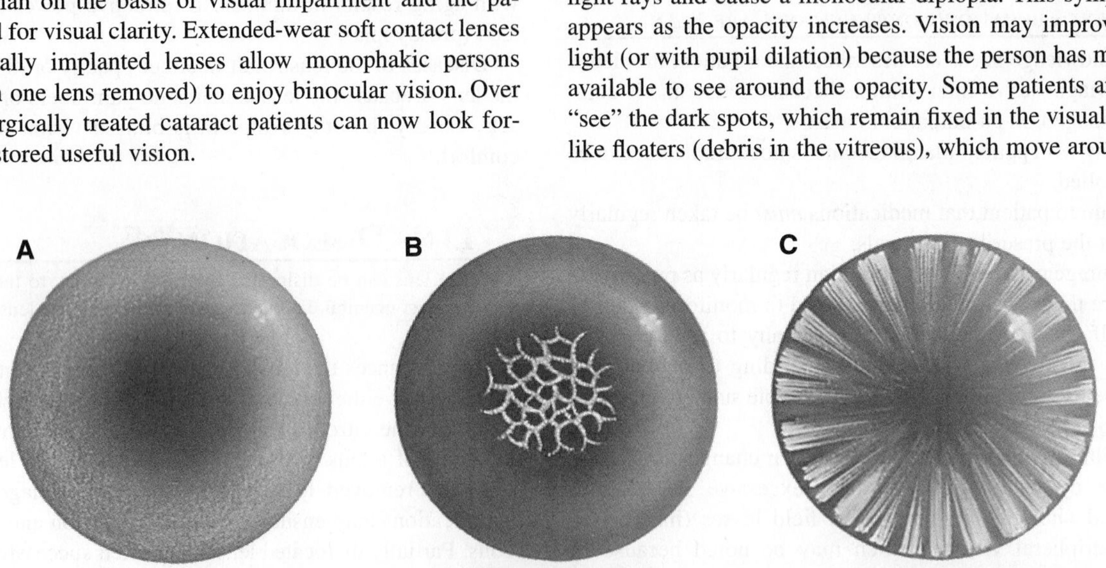

FIG. 8-17

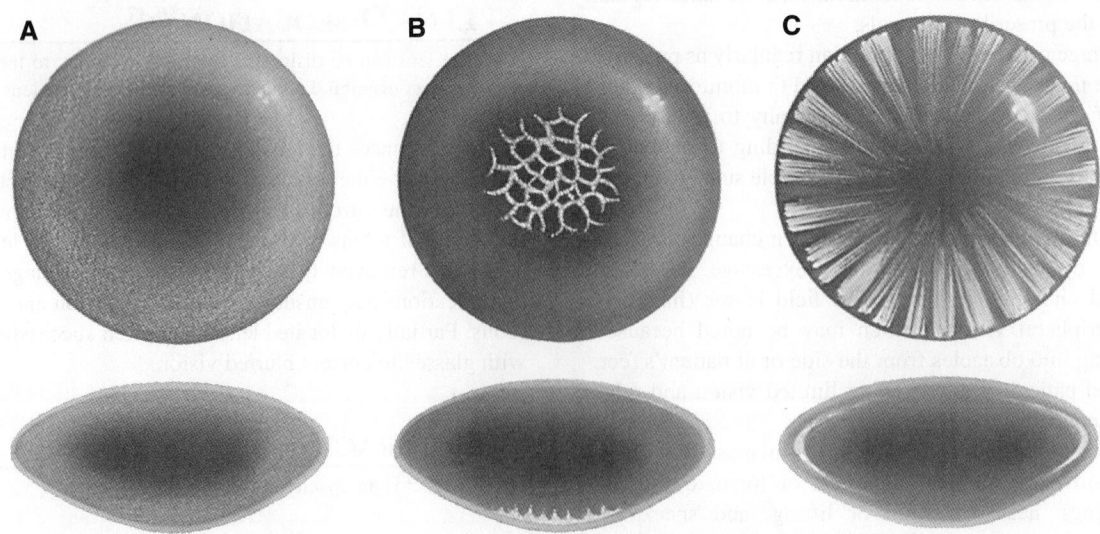

Appearance of various types of aging cataracts. **A,** Nuclear sclerosis. ***B*,** Nuclear sclerosis and posterior subcapsular cataract. **C,** Nuclear sclerosis and anterior and posterior cortical cataracts. (From Newell.[36])

If the cataract is not removed, it may eventually cause the entire lens to be opaque. This can be seen with gross observation as a whitish discoloration of the entire pupil. Less advanced opacities may be seen through the ophthalmoscope as dark spots, patches, or networks of lines that disrupt the red reflex.

Decision for removal of the lens is usually based on the patient's need to see. Vision is evaluated by examining both eyes. If one eye enables the patient to maintain adequate vision, the failing eye may not be surgically treated. In some instances the lens swells and encroaches on the anterior chamber angle to cause glaucoma. Hypermature cataracts may release toxic products that cause a secondary uveitis or glaucoma or both. Surgical intervention is sometimes undertaken to prevent eye damage regardless of visual acuity.

Risk factors other than age have been identified as possible sources of cataract formation. Women over 65 years of age are reported to have a higher rate of cataract formation than men. Some studies have shown that people living in warm, sunny climates have a significantly higher incidence of cataracts. The correlation between cataract formation and ultraviolet light exposure is under further investigation. The lens is susceptible to heat because its avascular tissue does not transfer heat efficiently.

High-dose radiation has been proved to cause cataracts. Survivors of atomic bomb explosions have exhibited a high prevalence of this disease. Study findings of the effects of exposure to low doses of radiation over a prolonged period are not conclusive. Some concern has been raised about computed tomography scans of the skull as a direct source of radiation to the eyes.

Some drugs are reported to be associated with early cataract formation. Corticosteroids, phenothiazines, and some cancer chemotherapy agents are commonly used medications cited in clinical and animal studies.

Diabetes is associated with an earlier onset of cataracts. Young adults with poorly controlled diabetes may rarely exhibit fulminating bilateral cataracts. Sorbitol, a by-product of excessive glucose, is known to accumulate in and damage the lens. Hypertensive patients also have a higher incidence of cataracts.

Blunt trauma (contusion) to the eye may result in opacification of the lens that occurs several months after the injury. If the trauma is invasive, localized opacification occurs as a response to rupture of the lens capsule.

Congenital cataracts may be associated with multiple systemic disorders or other eye deformities, or they may occur in the absence of other signs or symptoms. Maternal rubella in the first trimester often results in infant cataracts that may be accompanied by other signs of deformity. Down syndrome is commonly associated with cataracts, which usually do not progress sufficiently to impair vision. Infants with identifiable cataracts should be examined and monitored for other physical abnormalities, developmental delay, impaired hearing, and mental retardation.[53]

Most infants and children with cataracts do not exhibit enough opacification to interfere with normal vision. If a newborn has dense opacities, surgery is often performed shortly after birth to prevent permanent sensory loss from disuse of the eye. Foveal stimulation must occur in both eyes in the first 4 months of life to allow normal visual development. Long-wearing contact lenses may be prescribed for monophakic infants if the parents are able to manage the care involved. Children with slowly progressive cataracts have a better prognosis for normal binocular vision if surgery can be delayed until 10 to 12 years of age.

Congenital cataracts can be detected at birth if severe opacification is present. Marked density can be seen with gross observation. The newborn normally manifests a full round red reflex when examined with an ophthalmoscope. Lens opacities interrupt the red reflex and require further examination with a gonioscope. In some instances the parent may notice that the infant is not responding visually at home. The family of the affected child should be examined for cataracts.

Diagnostic Studies and Findings

Cataracts are identified through ophthalmoscopy or slit lamp examination. Visual acuity is measured periodically to assess visual function in both the impaired eye and the less impaired eye.

Multidisciplinary Plan[33,35,36,47]

Surgery

Surgical Removal of the Lens. Indications for surgical intervention include diminished visual acuity (by definition of the patient's lifestyle needs), hypermature cataracts that threaten to cause eye damage (glaucoma, uveitis), and the necessity to treat or view the structure behind the lens.

Two procedures are used for extraction: intracapsular and extracapsular. Intracapsular extraction is removal of the entire lens, including its surrounding capsule. An 18- to 20-mm incision is made at the superior limbus arc, and the entire lens is extracted through the incision. A peripheral iridectomy may be performed at the same time. The lens is extracted by forceps or a cryoprobe (which has a low-temperature tip that freezes and adheres to the lens surface so that it can be easily extracted). Chymotrypsin, a proteolytic enzyme, is sometimes briefly instilled in the anterior chamber to dissolve resistant zonular fibers in younger patients. Total lens extraction has traditionally been performed on elderly patients. This procedure is no longer common in the Western Hemisphere.

Extracapsular extraction is removal of the anterior portion of the capsule and the lens, leaving the posterior capsule intact. This is the standard in the United States and most of the Western Hemisphere. A 2- to 3-mm incision at the limbus provides access to the anterior capsule, which is mechanically disrupted so the lens nucleus can be removed. The remaining lens cortex is irrigated and suctioned out, leaving the posterior capsule in place. Leaving the capsule in place avoids disruption and loss of vitreous. This method is favored by some surgeons to accommodate placement of a lens implant. The posterior capsule often becomes opaque and has to be opened with the use of a laser. This creates a clear pathway for light to reach the retina, and visual acuity returns to its previous level.[5]

With younger adults, ultrasonic fragmentation (phacoemulsification) is used to disintegrate the lens so it can be aspirated. A rapidly vibrating needle powered by ultrasonic energy breaks ambulatory within an hour. An eye patch may be applied to the operative eye for a brief period or longer if the physician prefers. A metal eye shield is applied to the eye at night for several weeks to prevent accidental rubbing or injury. The postoperative phase requires patient precautions to avoid increased intraocular pressure.

Lens Implantation. Lens implantation offers many advantages over the use of eyeglasses and is particularly useful for patients with good vision in the unoperated eye. Binocular vision is rapidly restored, with improved depth perception and good distant visual acuity. The lens implant provides accurate distant vision, and glasses are prescribed to correct near vision difficulties. Recently Food and Drug Administration (FDA) approval was granted for a multifocal intraocular lens (IOL) (i.e., one that corrects for both distance and near vision). The technology for this lens, however, is very new, and it is not often prescribed currently.

A variety of materials are used for today's intraocular lenses. All have been proven to be nontoxic to the intraocular contents (FIG. 8-18).

Some patients are not good candidates for implantation because of potential postoperative complications. Patients with severe myopia, a history of chronic iritis, retinal detachment, diabetic retinopathy and glaucoma, congenital cataracts, or complications during surgery may not be advised to receive an implant. The rate of surgical complications is reported to be less than 1%, including corneal edema, secondary glaucoma, iritis, hemorrhage, retinal detachment, and lens displacement.

Medications[36,47]

A wide variety of medications are ordered before and after surgery according to the surgeon's preference, the patient's condition, and the nature of the procedure.

infants must have corrective lenses to permit development of vision in the first 6 months of life.

Eyeglasses are still prescribed for patients who cannot tolerate contact or implanted lenses. Adjusting to eyeglasses is difficult because image magnification of approximately 30% is still present and peripheral vision and depth perception are obscured. Binocular vision is not possible with a unilateral cataract removal unless contact lenses are prescribed. Corrective lenses are usually bifocal, and the prescription may have to be changed several times over a period of months until the most effective visual correction is attained.

Contact lenses are usually the prescription of choice for adults and infants if the wearer can tolerate them. Increased depth perception, less image magnification (approximately 7%), and binocular vision are attained. Many elderly patients who cannot remove and insert lenses visit a physician weekly and later monthly or quarterly for removal and cleansing of extended-wear lenses and examination of the eyes. Parents of infants receiving contact lenses must be capable of removing, inserting, and cleansing the lenses and monitoring the eyes for complications. For further discussion of contact lens care and precautions see p. 562. A permanent corrective lens can usually be prescribed within 4 to 6 weeks after surgery.

A protective patch is worn postoperatively for 24 to 72 hours. Dark glasses are worn to relieve photophobic discomfort, if the patient's pupil(s) are dilated, and a protective eye shield is worn at night to prevent injury to the eye during sleep.

NURSING CARE

NURSING ASSESSMENT

Cataract: Glare at night and in bright light; blurred vision; peripheral vision may diminish before central vision; near vision may improve temporarily (with nuclear cataract); monocular diplopia if central opacity splits visual axis

Advanced cataract: Pupil cloudy and white on gross examination; minimal to no visual perception

Aphakia with implanted lens correction (pseudophakia): Treatment most often performed today; full binocular vision restored; minimum magnification; peripheral vision intact; improved near and far visual acuity; reading glasses are needed because unlike the human lens, the lens implant can only focus vision at either distance or near (reading); most patients receive implants designed for distant viewing; occasionally, a lens is implanted that corrects to near viewing (e.g., if the patient's occupation is performed with mostly near vision, such as accounting)

Aphakia with contact lens correction: Seven percent to 10% magnification of images; peripheral vision intact; monocular aphakic patient able to experience binocular vision (improved depth perception); improved near and far visual acuity; reading glasses may be needed

Psychosocial concerns: Fears regarding blindness, pain, and surgical procedure

PATIENT PROBLEMS/NURSING DIAGNOSES & INTERVENTIONS

NIC SELF-CARE FACILITATION

Disturbed sensory perception (visual) related to unilateral eye patch

Before surgery

- Help in measuring visual acuity of unoperated eye preoperatively.
- Have patient's glasses available for immediate use postoperatively.
- Warn patient that depth perception will be lost and 50% of peripheral vision will be lost on affected side.

After surgery

- Help patient with activities of daily living.
- Caution patient to bring hand forward slowly to touch objects (especially containers of hot liquids and containers receiving poured liquids).
- Teach patient to turn head fully toward affected side to view objects or obstacles *to avoid falls.*
- Tell patient to use up and down head movements to judge stairs and oncoming objects and to go slowly.

NIC PHYSICAL COMFORT PROMOTION

Acute pain related to surgery

- Assess patient for postoperative discomfort (which is usually mild) and itching and administer analgesics as ordered *to prevent patient from inadvertently rubbing eye.*

PATIENT EDUCATION/CONTINUUM OF CARE PLAN

1. Discuss with patient the need to avoid heavy lifting, straining with elimination, and strenuous exercise for 6 weeks because increased intraocular pressure should be avoided until eye is healed.
2. Alert patient to wear an eye shield at night for 2 to 6 weeks to avoid injury to eye.
3. Inform patient that dark glasses may be worn during the day to avoid pupil constriction and glare associated with mydriatic medication. Eye is sensitive to light after surgery, and tearing or squinting may occur in bright natural or artificial light.
4. Review with patient the correct procedures for instilling eyedrops and ointments and applying eye shield (without touching or applying pressure on eyeball) to avoid self-inflicted injury.
5. Discuss with patient and family that patient's lifestyle must be altered to deal with continued diminished vision in one or both eyes because final prescription eyeglasses or contact lenses take 4 to 8 weeks to attain.
6. Explain to patient receiving eyeglasses that images will be magnified 30%, peripheral vision will be obscured and distorted, and the lenses will probably be bifocal or trifocal. Therefore lifestyle changes and safety concerns will need to be assessed; for example, patient must learn to judge distances when descending stairs or viewing oncoming objects and must turn head from side to side to see peripheral environment. Several recent studies have shown an association between loss of peripheral vision and driving performance. A few states require some form of visual field testing before awarding or renewing a driver's license, but most do not. The visual acuity testing that is ordinarily performed does not usually pick up peripheral loss. Patients with peripheral loss will need to be evaluated and counseled about their driving potential. Losing the ability to drive is a huge alteration for most people. Follow-up in the form of support is necessary to ensure compliance with driving ban, continued access to community, and maintenance of patient's well-being in the face of this loss of independence.
7. Explain to patient receiving contact lenses that images will be magnified 7% to 10%, peripheral vision will be intact, and reading glasses may also be prescribed. Therefore patient must learn to care for, insert, and remove lenses (see p. 562) or arrange to visit a physician routinely for removal, cleansing, and reinsertion of extended-wear lenses.
8. Review with patient that it will be necessary to adjust to mild magnification when performing daily activities.
9. Alert patient and family to signs and symptoms of complications to watch for and report: sudden onset of eye pain, redness and watering of eyes; photophobia, and sudden onset of visual changes.

EVALUATION/PATIENT OUTCOMES

Self-Care Facilitation: Patient with cataracts has adjusted to visual changes. Lifestyle needs are not hampered by diminished vision. Patient is able to participate in activities requiring near and far vision. Patient understands cause of visual changes and recognizes that further changes will ensue. Patient expresses feeling of self-control in terms of participating in future decisions about cataract surgery. Patient is not endangering himself or herself with activities requiring more vision than patient has, such as driving, venturing into the community without assistance, home maintenance, self-care activities (self-administering medication), or working at a job.

Patient with cataract removal has adjusted to visual correction with contact lenses. Patient can demonstrate insertion, eases vary in severity from total blindness at birth or a slowly deteriorating condition to minor defects that are unnoticed by the person. The cause and cure for many of these diseases are unknown. Photocoagulation can sometimes arrest the pathologic process, but treatment is difficult if the lesion is in the macular area because photocoagulation causes scarring and further vision reduction. Alterations in the configuration of the retina can cause traction, hole formation, and tearing that are surgically treatable.

RETINAL VASCULAR OCCLUSION

Occlusion of the retinal artery or vein can cause loss of vision.

PATHOPHYSIOLOGY

Retinal arterial occlusion causes a sudden, unilateral, painless loss of vision. The severity of vision diminishment ranges from total loss with an occluded central artery to a visual field defect that corresponds to blockage of a branch. Emboli associated with atherosclerosis, valvular heart disease, and blood hyperviscosity are among the most common causes. Emboli sometimes form in elderly patients with carotid plaques. Retinal arterial spasms cause transient vision losses that often progress to a permanent loss. Treatment for occlusion must be swift (within 2 hours) to restore vision. Massage of the eyeball (intermittent moderate pressure on the globe) may dislodge an embolus and send it to a more peripheral branch. Evaluation and treatment of the systemic disorder that led to the retinal artery occlusion follow emergency treatment.

Retinal vein occlusion results in a more gradual loss of vision, occurring over several hours in contrast to the abrupt loss

(crowding, shunts, obliteration); vessel leakage; microaneurysms; neovascularization

MULTIDISCIPLINARY PLAN[13,16,36,47]

Retinal Artery Occlusion

Surgery

Anterior chamber paracentesis: With patient under local anesthesia, needle is inserted through limbus into anterior chamber; 1 or 2 drops of aqueous fluid are removed to cause sudden lowering of intraocular pressure, which might dislodge embolus

Medications

Anticoagulant agents: May be prescribed in early phases of occlusion

- Heparin, IV loading dose of 5000-10,000 U followed by 5000-10,000 U q4-6h for adult

General Management

Intermittent massage of eyeball: Physician applies moderate pressure to globe for 5 seconds, releases pressure for another 5 seconds, and then repeats maneuver in attempt to dislodge embolus to more peripheral branch

Oxygenation: 95% oxygen for 10 minutes each hour over period of hours

Evaluation and treatment of systemic cardiovascular dysfunction

Retinal Vein Occlusion

Recovery may be spontaneous, and no curative therapy exists. Therapy is given to prevent further retinopathy in the affected eye and occlusive responses to the other eye.

Surgery

Photocoagulation (see pp. 566-567) to burn small or new vessels

Medications

Anticoagulant agents

Heparin, for adult, IV loading dose of 5000-10,000 U followed by 5000-10,000 U q4-6h, followed by bishydroxycoumarin (dicumarol), 25-150 mg/day as maintenance dose

Acetylsalicylic acid (aspirin), for adult, 200 mg every third day; may be given for antithrombotic effect as preventive measure for remaining eye

Corticosteroids: Prednisone (Deltasone, others), 30 mg PO qd in divided doses for retinal edema

General Management

Monitoring of eye for increased intraocular pressure

NURSING CARE

NURSING ASSESSMENT

Central retinal artery occlusion: Monocular event; sudden (within seconds), painless loss of vision; fovea cherry red in contrast to surrounding whiteness; no pupil constriction response; consensual response present

Central retinal vein occlusion: Usually monocular event; gradual (within hours), painless loss of vision; retinal veins dilated and tortuous; neovascularization; cotton wool patches; visible hemorrhages

Psychosocial concerns: Anxiety

PATIENT PROBLEMS/NURSING DIAGNOSES & INTERVENTIONS

NIC SELF-CARE FACILITATION

Disturbed sensory perception (visual) related to sudden unilateral loss

- Offer support and comfort.
- Keep patient informed of status, progress, and events during emergency care *to decrease anxiety.*

NIC PSYCHOLOGIC COMFORT PROMOTION

Anxiety related to threat of further visual loss

- Inform patient of related systemic disease and its effect on present and future visual dysfunction *to reduce anxiety.*
- Be realistic in describing health status assessment and prognosis to patient.
- Offer continuing support and comfort to patient and family.

NIC TISSUE PERFUSION MANAGEMENT

Risk for injury related to altered clotting factors

- Monitor patient for spontaneous bleeding, such as hematuria, tarry stools, bleeding gums, or bruising, *to determine response to anticoagulant therapy.*
- Observe patient for allergic responses (pruritus, rash, or wheals).
- If medication is continued at home, educate patient concerning dosage, frequency, signs of bleeding, necessity for keeping appointments with physician, drug interactions, and necessity for keeping laboratory appointments for prothrombin time monitoring.

PATIENT EDUCATION/CONTINUUM OF CARE PLAN

1. Review with patient the systemic disease that contributes to vascular problem.
2. Explain degree of visual loss (usually unilateral) and its effect on patient's lifestyle.

EVALUATION/PATIENT OUTCOMES

Outcomes vary from a fully restored healthy retina with fully functional vision to total loss of central vision, peripheral vision, or both, with marked retinal destruction. Expected outcomes include the following: vision returns to or approaches previous acuity, and appearance of retina returns to normal or shows improvement.

Self-Care Facilitation: Patient has adjusted to partial or complete loss of vision. Patient is fully informed about present visual status and prognosis. Patient is able to draw on effective support system to supplement self-care. Patient is aware of safety measures to use at home or in community related to visual changes or loss.

Psychologic Comfort Promotion: Patient's anxiety has been minimized.

Tissue Perfusion Management: Patient experiences no bleeding. There is no hematuria, bruising, tarry stools, or bleeding gums from anticoagulant therapy.

DIABETIC RETINOPATHY[6,27,32,36,47]

Diabetic retinopathy is a vascular disorder that occurs in patients with diabetes.

Diabetic retinopathy is one of the leading causes of blindness in the Western world. The prevalence of retinal pathologic findings is directly related to the length of time that diabetes has been present. Newell[36] states that 7% of diabetics who have had the disease less than 10 years have retinopathy, as do 26% of those with diabetes of 10 to 14 years' duration and 63% of those with diabetes for 15 years or more. These figures are estimates because the onset of type 2 diabetes is not easily determined. The incidence of retinopathy is increasing as diabetics receive better treatment and live longer. Retinopathy is also related to the degree of control of diabetes in early years of the disease.

PATHOPHYSIOLOGY[36,47]

Diabetic retinopathy exists in all degrees of severity, and the loss of visual acuity depends on the location of the lesion rather than its extent. An early lesion in the central retina (macular area) can obliterate central vision. Multiple scattered lesions throughout the periphery may not affect visual acuity. Clinicians divide

Eventually the vessels and surrounding tissue become fibrous and the vitreous contracts and fully detaches.

The course of retinopathy varies greatly. The pathologic changes may take many years to develop, and the patient may or may not lose functional vision.

Photocoagulation of the vascular abnormalities frequently slows the progress of microaneurysm formation and neovascularization. However, photocoagulation cannot be used in the macular area. Control of diabetes after retinopathy has begun is less effective in reducing retinal damage than careful control at the onset of diabetes.

Diagnostic Studies and Findings

Indirect ophthalmoscopy: Venous dilation and tortuosity; arterial narrowing or obliteration; opacities, hemorrhage; microaneurysms; neovascularization

Slit lamp examination (biomicroscopy): Magnification of lesions

Fluorescein angiography: Vessel leakage; microaneurysms; neovascularization

Multidisciplinary Plan

Surgery

Photocoagulation (see pp. 566-567) to destroy neovascularization sites, prevent retinal edema, and seal small leaking vessels

Vitrectomy: If portion of vitreous is clouded with blood or fibrous membrane, opacities can be removed with fine probe passed through anterior scleral incision; fiberoptic light attached to probe permits direct viewing of vitreous and retina with microscope and special contact lens; cannulated probe cuts and removes vitreous fragments; removed vitreous is replaced with a basic salt solution; simultaneous infusion and aspiration maintain intraocular pressure during surgery; after surgery, gas (sulfur hexafluoride or perfluorocarbon) mixed with air may be introduced into the eye to support the retinal layer in proper position until adequate scar formation creates permanent adhesion of the detached area; silicone oil may also be used as a vitreous replacement; air-gas mixtures are absorbed and replaced by aqueous humor; silicone oil remains in the eye permanently

Medications

Vitrectomy

Cycloplegic agents: Prescribed before and for 4-6 weeks after surgery
- Atropine sulfate (Atropisol, Isopto Atropine), 1% solution bid or tid

Topical antiinfective/steroid agents: To prevent inflammation and secondary infection
- Combination of dexamethasone, alcohol 0.1%, neomycin 3.5 mg, polymyxin B, 6000 U (Maxitrol), suspension or ointment, 1-2 drops qid for 4 weeks

Systemic analgesic agents
- Acetaminophen (Tylenol), 650 mg PO q4h prn
- Acetaminophen (Tylenol) with codeine (30 mg) PO q4h prn

General Management

Vitrectomy

Pressure patch to operative eye immediately after surgery

Ice packs to operative eye as ordered to reduce inflammation and discomfort

PERIOPERATIVE CARE FOR PATIENTS WITH MONOCULAR VISION AND POSTOPERATIVE EYE PATCH

Before Surgery

- Be sure patient's glasses are available for immediate use postoperatively.
- Warn patient that depth perception will be lost and 50% of peripheral vision will be lost on affected side.
- Notify patient that no reading will be permitted while operative eye is patched *to prevent eye movement;* however, watching television may be permitted.

resting on a table (to permit air in eye to float against retina); this positioning is not necessary if oil is injected into the eye

Dark glasses worn postoperatively to reduce discomfort from photophobia

Assessment and careful control of diabetes; some think this is more effective in preventing or delaying retinopathy during first 5 years of disease, although this is controversial

The Diabetes Complications Control Trial (DCCT), a national, multicenter randomized clinical trial, proved that tight glucose control reduces the incidence and severity of diabetic retinopathy, heart and kidney disease by 50%.[10,25]

NURSING CARE

Nursing Assessment

Background Retinopathy

General factors: Visual loss may be total, partial, or absent; may not correspond to number or severity of lesions seen; possible complaints of glare; absence of pain; visible retinal changes

Hard yellow exudates: Yellow, waxy, confluent deposits that surround microaneurysm area

Cotton wool patches: Fluffy, white, soft deposits scattered over retinal surface

Subretinal hemorrhages: Small, round, red spots, less circumscribed and usually larger than microaneurysms

Preretinal hemorrhages: Larger, blotchy, red spots

Dilated retinal veins: Enlarged and tortuous; may appear "beaded" (irregular in caliber)

Proliferative Retinopathy

Neovascularization: Minute network of fine vessels (often at arteriovenous crossing)

Retinal opacification: Increased clouding or whitening of area surrounding neovascularization

Vitreous hemorrhage: Large, red blotches (may obscure much of retina); patient may "see" vitreous hemorrhage as red shower over eyes or multiple floaters, or vision may suddenly be obscured; lesions described in background retinopathy may also be present

Patient Problems/Nursing Diagnoses & Interventions[24, 47]

NIC Coping Assistance

Risk for ineffective coping related to situational crisis of vi-

NIC Self-Care Facilitation

Ineffective health maintenance related to diminished vision

- Help patient to adapt self-care practices to visual handicaps.
- Review activities that require close vision and color differentiation (e.g., urine testing, reading medication labels [use large print], and administering insulin injections).
- Help patient identify resources available in community for other assistance as needed.
- Ensure that small personal items are within easy reach.

NIC Psychologic Comfort Promotion

Anxiety related to hospitalization and uncertainty about outcome of vitrectomy

- Evaluate patient for present visual acuity, other physical problems, frailty, knowledge about condition, and available support system.
- Offer support and comfort.
- Orient patient to room and surroundings.
- Describe procedure and warn patient that eye will be patched after surgery and will be swollen and bruised for a period of time.
- Inform patient that outcome for functional vision depends on condition of retina.
- Patient should be able to learn his or her visual status from physician (to the extent that physician can offer prognosis).
- Inform patient that decision for using general or local anesthetic will be made by physician.

NIC Physical Comfort Promotion

Acute pain related to postoperative status and restricted positioning

- Monitor patient's ocular-orbital-muscle discomfort, and administer analgesic-muscle relaxant as ordered.

- Offer frequent (every 2 to 4 hours) neck and back rubs *to relieve discomfort and muscle tension occurring from prolonged positioning restriction.*
- Provide skin care for knees and elbows; suggest sheepskin if at risk for skin breakdown—may purchase from local medical supply house.
- Limit time in elbow-flexed position and with head resting on forearms *to prevent ulnar and radial nerve compression, respectively.*

NIC COMMUNICATION ENHANCEMENT: VISUAL DEFICIT

Disturbed sensory perception (visual) related to binocular patches

- Evaluate patient for restlessness, anxiety, depression, or disorientation.
- Keep side rails up at all times *to ensure safety.*
- Identify yourself when entering room; touch patient as you approach, and identify yourself and what you are doing *to maintain patient orientation.*
- Put note at door instructing all who enter to identify themselves and explain reason for being there (e.g., cleaning staff).
- Help with feeding and hygienic measures as needed. (Patient may have entered hospital with severely diminished vision and may have some self-care skills.)
- Place call bell and all personal articles within reach; have patient locate them with hand.
- Maintain patient's independence as much as possible.
- Describe events and nursing activities as they occur.
- Visit patient frequently and offer back rubs, deep breathing, range-of-motion exercises, and conversation *to provide stimulation.*

PATIENT EDUCATION/CONTINUUM OF CARE PLAN

1. Maintain patient's awareness of diabetic state and self-care needs.
2. Reinforce with patient the need for regular visual examinations.
3. Ensure that patient knows to monitor visual responses and changes at home and to report any sudden changes to physician.
   a. Sudden loss of vision (usually unilateral; loss may be within seconds or persist over a day or two)
   b. Increase in floaters or persistent floaters
   c. Flashes of light
   d. Sharp pain in or around eyes
4. Ensure that patient is aware of any changes in visual status, especially changes in peripheral vision (as evidenced by running into large objects, "blind" spots on either side of central vision, or changes in ability to differentiate colors).
5. Review with patient that visual changes may be very gradual (over many years). Give patient realistic reassurance to help him or her continue an independent lifestyle to fullest extent and develop ways to adapt to diminishing vision.
6. If patient has had a vitrectomy:
   a. Cycloplegic, antibiotic, and antiinflammatory eyedrops will be continued at home. Review the procedure for administering eyedrops, and emphasize the importance of maintaining the prescribed dosage. Tell the patient to wash hands before administering drops.
   b. Tell the patient to avoid constipation (straining), sneezing, coughing, heavy lifting (more than 5 pounds), rapid or jarring head movements, and heavy exercise the first week or two at home.
   c. Watching television or reading is acceptable.
   d. Have patient make an appointment with physician for a week after discharge.
   e. Visual function should be restored to the extent that retina is intact. Tell patient to review visual prognosis with physician.
7. If gas or air bubble was injected intraoperatively, caution patient to secure advice from ophthalmologist regarding air travel while bubble is present.

EVALUATION/PATIENT OUTCOMES

Outcomes vary from a healthy retina with fully functional vision to total loss of central vision, peripheral vision, or both, with marked retinal destruction. Generally the condition of retina is optimal for patient. Changes in retinal appearance are slowed or stopped.

Coping Assistance: Patient is able to draw on effective support system to supplement self-care.

Self-Care Facilitation: Patient has adjusted to partial or complete loss of vision. Patient is fully informed about present visual status and prognosis.

Psychologic Comfort Promotion: Patient's anxiety has been minimized.

Physical Comfort Promotion: Pain has decreased or been eliminated. Patient experiences no pain or discomfort in eye area or in other areas because of restricted positioning.

Communication Enhancement: Patient has learned and accepted alternative methods for living with diminished vision.

RETINAL DEGENERATION[36,47]

Degenerative changes in the retina cause a partial or complete loss of vision.

PATHOPHYSIOLOGY

Retinal degeneration may occur because of genetic defects, inflammation, vascular insufficiency, or aging. In many instances the cause of the disorder is unknown; the defect is often familial. Some defects occur at birth, with total blindness, whereas others develop insidiously and lead to severe visual loss. Some degenerative changes only minimally affect vision or are considered harmless. The extent, spread, and location of the deterioration and ensuing lesions determine the effect on visual acuity. Lesions that encroach on the macula often diminish vision dramatically.

Age-related macular degeneration (ARMD) occurs because layers of the choroid thicken and the capillaries of the choroid are sclerosed and deprive the fovea centralis of nourishment. It is divided into two forms: dry (atrophic) and exudative (wet). The onset of the dry form is slow, involving both eyes, but deterioration may progress faster in one eye than the other. Near and central vision diminishes over a period of years, but most of the peripheral vision remains intact.[1]

The wet form of ARMD comes on acutely, over a period of days or weeks. It involves serous detachment of the pigment epithelium, followed by neovascularization, hemorrhaging, and eventually scarring of the overlying retina. Photocoagulation destroys the neovascular network and may prevent further visual loss if the macula is not destroyed in the process. Elderly adults (9 out of 10) with macular degeneration experience the dry form with gradual (bilateral) loss of central vision and are eventually classified as legally blind.[14] One out of 10 develops the wet form.

Diagnostic Studies and Findings

Indirect ophthalmoscopy: Opacities; hemorrhage; microaneurysms; neovascularization; retinal pallor, detachment, breaks, and folds.

Slit lamp examination (biomicroscopy): Magnification of lesions

Fluorescein angiography: Retinal vessel irregularities, neovascularization, vessel leakage, and detached pigment epithelium

Multidisciplinary Plan

Surgery

Photocoagulation (see pp. 566-567) used when degenerative site is not over macula to destroy neovascularization sites, prevent retinal edema, and seal small leaking vessels

NURSING CARE

Nursing Assessment

Age-related macular degeneration: Bilateral event (pathologic progress usually not the same in both eyes); gradual diminishment of vision over months or years

Psychosocial concerns: Ability to carry out ADLs with level of independent functioning

Patient Problems/Nursing Diagnoses & Interventions[24,29]

NIC Self-Care Facilitation

Disturbed sensory perception (visual) related to gradual bilateral loss

- Assess visual acuity and review ADLs that are affected or diminished because of loss.
- Devise strategies for carrying out activities of daily living.
- Refer patients with 20/40 or worse vision to a low vision center to access specialized magnifying devices and other daily living aids for the visually impaired. (For a national listing contact the Light House, New York City.)
- Assess patient's support system at home, and encourage full use of it.
- Give realistic encouragement for maintenance of independent functioning.
- See pp.1516-1530.

Patient Education/Continuum of Care Plan

Education depends on the extent of visual changes (usually bilateral) and whether the prognosis indicates that further changes will occur.

1. Inform patient or family that patient should have regular visual examinations.
2. Provide full information to patient or family about visual status and prognosis (realistic reassurance about a gradual loss may help patient maintain an independent lifestyle).

Evaluation/Patient Outcomes

Outcomes vary from mild to severe loss of vision.

Self-Care Facilitation: Patient has adjusted to loss of vision. Patient is fully informed about present visual status and prognosis. Patient is able to draw on effective support system to supplement self-care. Patient is aware of safety measures to use.

Retinal Holes, Tears, and Detachment

Retinal holes and tears are breaks in the continuity of the retina. Detachment is a separation of the sensory layers of the retina from the pigmented epithelium.

Pathophysiology[26,36,47]

The retina is a smooth, unbroken, multilayered surface that attaches to the hyaloid membrane of the vitreous on its inner aspect. The posterior retinal lining (pigmented epithelium) attaches to Bruch's membrane of the choroid layer on its outer aspect. Breaks in the continuity of the retina can occur in the form of small holes caused by degeneration or tearing (tears are U shaped, with flaps over the holes).

Degenerative holes usually occur in the retinal periphery and are the result of retinal thinning that often parallels the ora serrata. Multiple holes form a row of latticework that is fluid filled and covered by vitreous that adheres to either side of the series of holes. Latticework degeneration occurs in about 8% of the population in all age groups and contributes to about 30% of hole-formation retinal separations. The holes are often missed during general ophthalmoscopic inspection and can be seen only with scleral depression and an indirect ophthalmoscope. Many of these patients are asymptomatic, and retinal detachment does not occur. They are carefully monitored for further degeneration or tearing throughout their lifetimes.

Retinal tears occur most often because of vitreous traction. The vitreous degenerates with age and falls forward, resulting in fluid-filled cavities and collagenous areas that tug on the inner lining of the retina. The vitreous also contracts with fibrous separation gives the sensation that a curtain is being pulled over the eyes. A slow separation may offer no symptoms until the macular area is invaded or the person closes the unaffected eye and notes decreased vision in the affected eye.

Examination with an indirect ophthalmoscope shows the detached portion of the retina as a gray bulge, ripple, or fold in contrast to the pink attached retina.

that eventually hold implant in place; rectus muscles tied with sutures so eyeball can be rotated to expose equator; detached area may be treated with diathermy before implant is put in place; encircling rod or strap often used if multiple retinal holes exist; implant sutured in place, and subretinal fluid drained from site of detachment; air, other gases such as sulfur hexafluoride and perfluorocarbon, or liquids such as silicone oil may be injected into vitreous to flatten detached retina against choroid surface; air or liquid is absorbed and eventually replaced with vitreous fluid

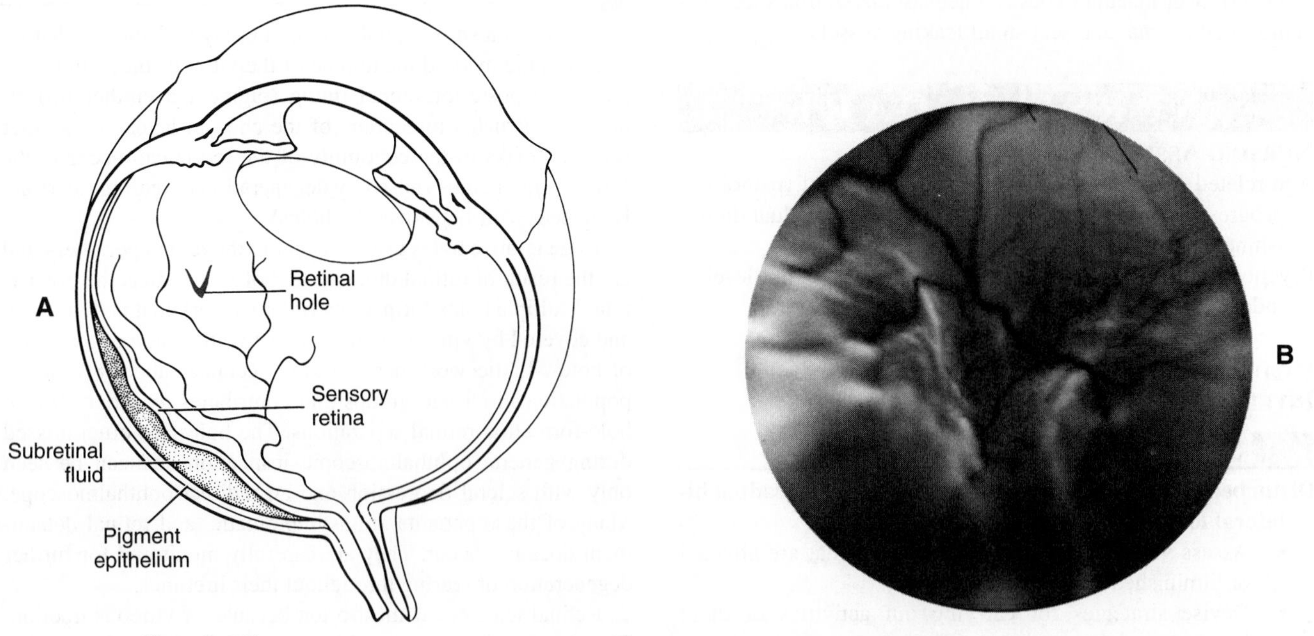

FIG. 8-19

A, Retinal detachment with horseshoe-shaped hole in superior temporal quadrant. **B,** Ophthalmoscopic appearance of a retinal detachment. (From Newell.[36])

Medications

Adrenergic-mydriatic agents: Phenylephrine (Neo-Synephrine), 2.5%-10%, 1-2 drops instilled for preoperative pupil dilation

Mydriatic-cycloplegic agents: Cyclopentolate (Cyclogyl), 1 drop of 1% solution or 2 drops of 0.5% solution preoperatively and postoperatively; frequency and duration of postoperative dosage vary with degree of inflammation

Antiinfective agents: Postoperative eyedrops to prevent uveitis complications

Gentamicin sulfate (Garamycin), 3 mg/ml topical solution, 1-2 drops qid

Neomycin sulfate and prednisolone sodium phosphate, neomycin 3.5 mg/ml, and prednisolone 5 mg/ml; frequency and duration of prescription vary according to physician's order, usually 1 drop tid or qid for 4-6 weeks

General Management

Postoperative monocular or binocular eye patches (according to physician's preference) to rest eyes for day or two (usually bilateral patches because operated eye may move when unoperated eye moves)

If air is injected into vitreous cavity, head positioned so air bubble will rise and remain flush against detached retinal segment; physician specifies optimum head position and duration for positioning (usually 4 to 8 days); usual position is face down or angled to unoperated side; pillows or rubber or plastic ring used to support head; pillows under abdomen for support

Dark glasses to reduce discomfort from photophobia

NURSING CARE

NURSING ASSESSMENT

Visual symptoms reported by patient: Flashing lights (unilateral, may be repeated over a period of days, months, or years); shower of floaters (black dots within visual field); sensation of curtain folding over eyes

Appearance of retina: Vessels over detached portion dark red in color; holes or breaks within detached area cherry red, in contrast to the grayish area

PATIENT PROBLEMS/NURSING DIAGNOSES & INTERVENTIONS

NIC PSYCHOLOGIC COMFORT PROMOTION

Anxiety related to sudden loss of unilateral vision

- Offer comfort, support, and realistic reassurance (about 90% of retinal detachment repairs are successful).

NIC SKIN/WOUND MANAGEMENT

Risk for impaired tissue integrity or tissue injury related to preoperative status: detached retina

- Supervise limited activities or bed rest as ordered.
- Maintain eye patch and/or shield as ordered.
- Keep room dark.
- Keep patient supine.
- Keep side rails up if patient is bedfast.
- Assist with walking and avoid jarring, bumps, or fall *to prevent further detachment.*
- Administer drops as ordered.
- Position patient as ordered. (If gas or air has been injected into vitreous, head position may need to be maintained for several days to several weeks.)
- Keep patient's head parallel to floor when patient is out of bed for brief periods.
- Check dressing for excessive bleeding.
- Report sudden severe pain or pain that is unrelieved by ordered analgesics.
- Assess and document marked swelling and serous drainage, which is present for first 42 to 48 hours.
- Initiate deep-breathing exercises 4 times a day, if indicated, *to prevent respiratory infection.*
- Administer cycloplegic, mydriatic, antibiotic, and antiinflammatory eyedrops as ordered.
- Assess patient for nausea, coughing, excessive restlessness, and disorientation t*o avoid impairing tissue integrity.*
- Avoid excessive restlessness, jarring or bumping head, sneezing, coughing, or vomiting *to avoid tissue injury.*

NIC PHYSICAL COMFORT PROMOTION

Acute pain related to postoperative status

- Monitor patient's pain (which is usually moderate), and administer analgesics according to physician's orders.

PATIENT EDUCATION/CONTINUUM OF CARE PLAN

1. Inform patient that cycloplegic and antibiotic eyedrops will be continued at home. Review the procedure for administering eyedrops, and emphasize the importance of maintaining the prescribed dosage and washing the hands thoroughly before administration.
2. Tell patient to avoid constipation (straining), sneezing, jarring head movements, and heavy exercise for the first 4 to 6 weeks at home.
3. Inform patient that television watching/reading is permitted. Patient should rest eyes when he or she feels tired or strained.
4. Work may be resumed after first week depending upon occupation. Physician will discuss.
5. Discuss with patient the need to be aware of visual changes or sensation and to report sudden loss of vision, severe pain in eyeball, a heavy shower of floaters, or flashing lights to physician. (Usually some floaters are seen for a period of weeks postoperatively, but they should be reported.)
6. Have patient schedule appointment with physician a week after hospital discharge.
7. With patient and physician, review and ensure that patient understands visual status, including possibility of recurrence of detachment in affected eye, ultimate visual acuity and macular damage, and potential for retinal detachment or holes in other eye.

EVALUATION/PATIENT OUTCOMES

Outcomes vary from a fully restored healthy retina with fully functional vision to total loss of central vision, peripheral vision, or both, with marked retinal destruction.

States and does not reflect the universal visual status and complementary needs for visual assistance that people present to the health professions.

The World Health Organization and a variety of experts have attempted to define and standardize categories of visual impairment to serve as guidelines for research and reporting. Table 8-3 is adapted from the International Classification of Diseases, published by the World Health Organization in 1977.

PATHOPHYSIOLOGY[11,12,34,39]

The categories of impairment are helpful to health professionals but still do not incorporate the vast array of visual alterations that must be assessed, managed, or prevented. Regard-

Table 8-3 Categories of Visual Impairment

Category	Visual Acuity (With Optimum Correction)	Visual Field Radius
LOW VISION STATUS		
1	20/70	Not defined
2	20/70 to 20/200	Not defined
BLINDNESS STATUS		
3	Able to count fingers at 3 m; 20/200 to 20/400	Radius reduced to 5-10 degrees regardless of visual acuity status
4	Able to count fingers at 1 m; 20/400 to 20/1200 (5/300)	Radius reduced to 5-10 degrees regardless of visual acuity status
5	No light perception	

cidence of diabetic retinopathy by 50%. However, as more diabetic individuals survive early and middle adulthood because of better care, the number of visually handicapped people is likely to increase. At present about 413,000 people in this country have visual impairments, and 192,500 are legally blind because of retinal diseases. Further research is in progress in the areas of diabetic care, laser therapy, and other forms of retinal therapy. Genetic counseling and research are expected to reduce the incidence of some disorders. Early detection and careful monitoring of a number of systemic diseases, especially diabetes and cardiovascular disorders, will eliminate or slow visual complications. In addition, rehabilitative services for the visually handicapped continue to improve the quality of life for these individuals.

Cataract, another disease associated with aging, is usually treatable with surgery (removal of the lens), and vision is usually restored so the individual can function at least as well as before the surgery. The surgical procedure has become more available and simpler because patients no longer have to wait for surgery until they are severely handicapped and they do not have to endure long recovery periods. The incidence of cataract is increasing because Americans are living longer. One study reported that 18% of the group between the ages of 65 and 74 years showed a decrease in vision to 20/30 or less, and 46% of those between 75 and 85 years of age showed the same effect; in both sets the effect was related to cataract. Yet even with improved and simplified treatment, about 71,500 people in this country are legally blind because of cataract.

Glaucoma is still a leading cause of blindness in this country, but it is becoming less so because detection and early care have enabled people to control intraocular pressure and prevent optic nerve deterioration. Vision screening, compliance with prescribed care, and familial screening and counseling are major issues with this disorder.

Blindness from ambylopia can be prevented with comprehensive eye examination of infants and acuity screening and follow-up with preschool children.[12,34]

The World Health Organization estimates that 10 million people throughout the world are totally blind and that millions more have incapacitating impairments. The leading worldwide causes of blindness are trachoma, leprosy, onchocerciasis, and xerophthalmia. Trachoma, a form of chronic keratoconjunctivitis caused by *C. trachomatis,* currently affects about 400 million people. It exists primarily in rural areas of the Middle East, Africa, and Asia, where poverty, crowding, flies, lack of sanitation, and malnutrition dominate. It can be cured with sulfonamides and tetracyclines, but if it is not treated, recurrent scarring leads to total blindness. In the United States, the disease exists among Indians in the Southwest and in some rural areas. Leprosy (Hansen's disease) affects about 15 million people throughout the world. Chronic eyelid inflammation, keratoconjunctivitis, and iritis result in granuloma formation and eventual blindness. The disease is treated systemically, and topical rifampin is used with severe corneal involvement. Because international reporting systems are vague, the estimates of the percentage of eye involvement from the systemic disease range from 6% to 90%. The disease is uncommon in the United States. Onchocerciasis (river blindness) is transmitted by black fly bites. Infected larvae are deposited in clear running streams in Central Africa, Mexico, and Central and South America. Microfilariae from the adult female enter the eyes and cause corneal opacification, inflammation and atrophy of the iris, and eventual destruction of the eyes. Treatment is not very effective, and attempts are being made to rid areas of the fly with insecticides. It is estimated that this disease affects about 40 million people. Xerophthalmia (dry eye) is caused by protein, calorie, and vitamin A deficiency. If the cornea is not protected with moisture, it softens, becomes vulnerable to fungal and bacterial invasion, or becomes necrotic. Eventually retinal deterioration and destruction of the optic nerve result in blindness. In countries where malnutrition is common (India, Somalia), infants with this disorder frequently die of infection or pneumonia before reaching adulthood. Supplemental vitamin A (along with antiinfective agents) can reverse early eye complications and prevent blindness.

Besides the most common causes of blindness, other disorders contribute greatly to visual impairment. Corneal diseases and infestations are not the major contributors to blindness that they are in other parts of the world because Americans have better access to a higher quality of care. However, herpes simplex virus is being reported and treated increasingly in the United States. The treatments are partially successful, and new antiviral agents are being explored, but the disease tends to recur or reactivate and threatens the corneal structure. Some corneal problems have occurred because of use or misuse of contact lenses (see p. 560). The cornea is also vulnerable to damage from exposure to toxic agents (in vapor, spray, dust, or liquid form) such as ammonia, butanol, lime and cement dust, some forms of detergents and pesticides, and other concentrated liquid alkalies or acids. People must be educated and counseled about early symptoms of eye irritation or inflammation and measures to protect the eyes.

Safety regulations need to be explored and put into practice to assist the public with eye protection. Protective goggles should be worn in some work settings and while traveling in vehicles in the open air. Some sports activities require eye protection. The scrutiny of children's toys and the laws that some states have passed regulating the sale of BB guns have helped reduce eye injuries.

Many other varieties of eye diseases threaten visual functioning. Most are treatable if detected early and followed by skilled therapy. The American Academy of Ophthalmology's Committee on Eye Care states, "Despite the fact that an increasing number of people seek out and utilize eye care services, approximately a third of all new blindness is potentially avoidable if only Americans had access to or could take full advantage of existing and available technology."[8]

NURSING CARE

Nursing Assessment

Signs and symptoms for further evaluation or referral: Blurred vision (uncorrectable with lenses; uncorrectable by wiping film from eyes); double vision; sudden loss of vision; alternating dimming and clearing of vision; red eye; traumatized eye; eye pain; loss of side vision; halos (colored rays or circles around lights); crossed, turned, or wandering eye; twitching or shaking eye; flashes or streaks of light; floaters (dots, streaks, or strands, especially in showers or large numbers, or a floater that does not go away); a sense of pressure or "pulling" within the eye; discharge, crusting, or excessive tearing; swelling of any part of the eye; bulging of one or both eyes; difference in size of eyes or pupils

Emotional reactions: Fear; immobilization (physical and emotional); anxiety; disorientation; altered self-esteem; and altered body image

Chronic visual impairment: Possible unsafe living conditions; possible isolation; possible nutritional deficit (related to self-care); possible general ineffective coping (with activities of daily living; earning income; maintaining support system; intellectual stimulation; or recreational activities)

Patient Problems/Nursing Diagnoses & Interventions

NIC Risk Management

Risk for injury related to sudden onset of alteration in eye or vision

Risk for infection related to alteration in eye integrity

- Apply pressure patch or shield (with trauma) *to protect from further injury.*
- Refer patient to physician *to secure medical diagnosis, care, and prognosis.*
- Provide wheelchair, put up side rails, or assist with walking by offering arm for patient's hand *to ensure safety while transporting patient.*
- Administer topical and systemic antiinfectives as ordered.

NIC Physical Comfort Promotion

Acute pain related to traumatic eye injury

- Administer topical analgesic as soon as ordered.
- Apply eye patch after treatment as ordered *to alleviate discomfort from photophobia.*

arrangement *to avoid or reduce disorientation.*

- Arrange for placement of personal belongings in advance, and review plan with patient.
- Warn patient that side rails will be raised *for safety.*

After surgery (most patients are admitted after surgery)

- Assess patient's level of anxiety and disorientation.
- Reorient patient to equipment (such as call light) and personal belongings at bedside by directing patient's hand.
- If necessary, review immediate past events and procedures with patient *to assist in reorientation.*
- Raise side rails *to ensure safety.*
- Address patient from doorway and identify yourself.
- Complement voice stimulation with touch *to notify patient of your proximity.*
- Help family members and other staff to use vocal and touch approach *to reduce patient's anxiety.*
- Encourage patient to perform self-care with personal hygiene.
- Ensure patient's privacy, and assure patient that privacy is being provided.
- Provide patient with television set or radio *to encourage mental and memory stimulation.*
- Provide patient with clock that can be felt and remind patient of date.
- Help patient with meals. Read menu selections *to encourage patient to eat.*
    - Guide hands to utensils and food on tray.
    - Describe food on tray in clock terms.
    - Help with cutting meats, removing lids from containers, buttering bread, and so on.
- Assist with walking *to prevent injury.*
    - Walk slowly and slightly ahead of patient; patient's hand should rest on your arm at elbow.

procedures taking place *to alleviate as much uncertainty as possible.*

- Constantly reassure patient that he or she is being cared for: speak in a soothing voice, and use touch as a comfort.
- Avoid lengthy and complicated explanations *to avoid sensory overload.*
- Maintain a quiet atmosphere.

Decisional conflict related to deficient knowledge of cause of visual loss and ways to prevent further loss or maintain present vision

Impaired adjustment related to irreversible loss of vision

Situational low self-esteem related to irreversibly impaired vision

Readiness for enhanced family coping related to acceptance of patient's altered visual status

- Evaluate patient's knowledge about events and localized or systemic causes for visual alteration.
- Evaluate patient's level of knowledge about the treatment prescribed.
- Evaluate patient's capacity and motivation for further learning *to avoid patient education that is not usable* (because of anxiety, inability to take in too much or too complicated information at one time, or because patient cannot read directions or labels).
- Plan to extend elaborate teaching beyond hospital stay *to avoid sensory overload.*
- Evaluate patient's personal reactions to present level of visual functioning.
- Evaluate patient's reactions to anticipated discharge from hospital and functioning at home.
- Help patient identify specific fears in terms of self-care.
- Provide specific information about visual capacity and changes that will have to be made at home.

- Evaluate patient's feelings about himself or herself in the context of living and functioning with visual loss.
- Evaluate family's perception of patient's ability to function with impaired vision.
- Identify specific self-care capabilities in the hospital and encourage patient to exercise self-care *to help patient achieve a sense of independence.*
- Encourage patient to make as many decisions as possible about daily routines *to enhance competence.*
- Evaluate family's reaction to patient's altered visual status.
- Discuss family's changed perceptions with family members *to make them more aware of altered behavior toward patient.*
- Encourage family to help patient toward independent living as quickly as possible.
- Recognize that family dynamics will change over a long period of time and that continuing counseling should be available.

Patient Education/Continuum of Care Plan

1. Describe anatomy and function of normal eye.
2. Describe alterations in visual function that have occurred.
3. Clarify prognosis so that patient understands time frame and degree of recovery or degree of irreversible visual impairment.
4. While patient is in hospital or clinic teach and help him or her practice self-assistance skills to maximize independence.
   a. Exploring and mapping out furniture, steps, and doorways in room through guidance and touch
   b. Using another's arm to serve as a guide when walking
   c. Tracing wall (or rail) with free hand to orient to perimeters of room while walking
   d. Using a lightweight walking stick when walking alone to identify obstacles
   e. Exploring food, containers, liquids, and utensils with touch before eating
   f. Feeling chairs or toilet before turning to sit
   g. Obtaining assistance with selection of clothing before dressing and approval and support of appearance afterward
   h. Placing articles for grooming and hygiene near bed and arranging them so they can be retrieved whenever patient wishes
5. On discharge, review specific hazards in home with patient and family.
   a. Patient's room arrangement and living quarters should not be altered once patient is familiar with placement of furniture and furnishings.
   b. Patient should proceed slowly and with assistance in exploring living arrangements.
   c. Family must evaluate and maintain living quarters for a clutter-free environment (e.g., loose throw rugs, loose articles on floor or stairways, electric cords).
   d. Exploration of the outdoors must proceed carefully and with assistance (uneven ground, steps, loose gravel, and icy sidewalks are some additional hazards of outdoors).
   e. Exploration of community must proceed slowly and with assistance.
6. Discuss with patient and family that progress will be slow; they must allow for frustration and should seek additional support from community or health agencies.
7. Encourage family to explore future for increased independence when patient has made initial adjustments to impaired vision. State agency for the blind should be contacted immediately upon discharge; this agency can give early assistance and provide support for future concerns (e.g., computer-assisted reading, talking books, time and temperature devices, rehabilitation for future employment, acquisition of new skills).
8. In collaboration with physician, demonstrate to patient how to care for eye(s) at home.
   a. Administering drops or ointment as prescribed
   b. Keeping eye(s) free of infection by washing hands, not contaminating dropper, using clean tissues or cloth to wipe eyes, and gently wiping from inner to outer canthus
   c. Monitoring eye(s) for signs and symptoms of infection (pain, itching, redness, swelling, discharge)
   d. Monitoring eye(s) for signs and symptoms of the specific disorder

Evaluation/Patient Outcomes

Risk Management: No injury occurs after alteration in vision. No signs of injury are present during acute phase of visual impairment.

Infection is absent. No signs or symptoms of infection exist.

Physical Comfort Promotion: Pain is absent. Patient experiences no pain or discomfort from photophobia or pupillary constriction.

Self-Care Facilitation: Patient adjusts to visual impairment. Patient reports no signs or symptoms of infection or disease. Patient reports no accidents in home or community. Patient reports satisfaction with self-care abilities. Patient reports progress with (or mastery of) selected visual handicap aids. Patient reports ability to earn income or is seeking or getting employment training.

Coping Assistance: Patient reports interpersonal relationships are satisfactory. Patient reports resumption of old recreational or diversional skills or acquisition of new ones. Patient exhibits confidence in caring for self and in relating to others.

Collaborative Interventions and Related Nursing Care

Contact Lenses

Description and Rationale

Contact lenses are rounded plastic discs that are curved and shaped to fit over the cornea and beneath the eyelid. As methods for producing them improve, contact lenses are being used increasingly as a substitute for eyeglasses to correct refractive errors.

correction of marked corneal irregularities because their shape does not conform to the corneal surface as readily as soft lenses and they provide better peripheral vision. Hard lenses can be worn only for a limited time (10 to 14 hours) and are not worn during sleep. They eventually change the shape of the corneal surface and therefore cannot be worn alternately with eyeglasses.

Soft lenses are made of hydrophilic plastics that increase access of fluid to the cornea. They are usually larger in diameter and more easily tolerated than hard lenses and can be worn longer. They are regarded as a medical device and are regulated by the Food and Drug Administration. Soft lenses absorb medications, cleaning solutions, and chlorinated water from swimming pools and gradually release them into the tear film.[36] This can cause local irritation and systemic side effects. Soft lenses are removed every day for cleansing and are not worn during sleeping hours to allow the cornea to recover.

Extended-wear lenses are designed to provide continuous oxygen to the cornea. One type of lens is ultrathin and permits absorption of oxygen through it. The other type is thicker but has a higher concentration of water (70% to 80%), which continuously bathes the corneal surface. Extended-wear lenses can be worn for periods ranging from a few days to several months, depending on patient tolerance, self-care habits, and the patient's eye condition. The effects of extended wear and the development of new materials are the subjects of considerable research. In late 1993 the introduction of daily-wear disposable lenses began a movement to change the way people think about contact lenses. New materials enabled the creation of an ultrathin, highly oxygen permeable lens, which can be used for 24 hours and then disposed of for about the same cost as a standard set of contact lenses and the cleaning solutions needed to maintain them for 1 year.

for lens wearing and the appropriate type of lens. After the lenses are prescribed and fitted, the patient is closely followed for signs of complications. The major complications are corneal abrasion, corneal edema, infection, ulceration, tight lens syndrome, and giant papillary syndrome.

Corneal Abrasions

Corneal abrasions occur when hard lenses are left in too long (overwear syndrome) and drying of the corneal surface results in minute epithelial breaks. Abrasions also form if foreign bodies lie between the lens and the cornea or if the corneal surface is scraped during insertion or removal. A fluorescein stain can be used to identify epithelial breaks. The patient experiences severe pain and usually seeks care immediately. Epithelial abrasions can heal in 24 to 48 hours.

Medications

Antiinfective agents

- Sulfacetamide sodium (Sulamyd), bacitracin, Ilotysin, neomycin, ointment applied to affected eye before 24-h patching

Anesthetics

- Proparacaine (Ophthaine), 0.5% solution, 1-2 drops in each eye, gives relief for 10-15 min (used to facilitate examination; never sent with patient)
- Cycloplegic agents
- Cyclogyl, 0.5%-1% solution, 1-2 drops bid or tid for 24 h

General Management

Binocular tight patches for 24 hours (if patient has someone to care for him or her) or monocular patch on more painful eye and cycloplegic drops in open eye to reduce ciliary spasm and pain (see above for dosage); reexamination of patient in 24 hours

Corneal Edema

Corneal edema most commonly occurs with soft or extended-wear lenses because of a more gradual oxygen deprivation to the cornea. The epithelium becomes edematous, and vision becomes blurred. There is usually no pain, but slight redness of the eye may be evident.

General Management

Removal of contact lens reverses condition; lens prescription may have to be changed.

Corneal Ulceration and Infection

Corneal ulceration and infection occur if corneal abrasions or edema is not successfully treated. A secondary uveitis may ensue and require intensive emergency care to prevent loss of vision (see pp. 533-535 for pathophysiology and interventions). Infection also occurs if insertion, removal, and lens care are not managed hygienically by the patient.

Medications

Antiinfective agents
- Sulfacetamide sodium (Sulamyd), 10% or 30% solution, 1-2 drops several times a day for 3-7 days (varies with severity of infection)
- Fortified bacitracin, fortified gentamycin, or other antiinfective appropriate to the invading organism is prescribed

General Management

Cool compresses for discomfort and inflammation for 10 to 15 minutes two or three time a day

Culture and sensitivities laboratory test of corneal and conjunctival mucus and drainage

Tight Lens Syndrome

Tight lens syndrome occurs in soft lens wearers. The lens tends to change shape and become more curved and less mobile over the cornea. The change may take place within hours after the fitting or within several days (with extended-wear lenses). The wearer experiences decreased visual acuity and conjunctival congestion.

General Management

Removal of lens reverses process; wearer may have to be refitted with new prescription

Giant Papillary Syndrome

Giant papillary syndrome occurs after several months or years of lens wearing and manifests itself as a cobblestone-appearing inflammation of the inner lining of the upper lid. Redness, tearing, and discharge accompany the tissue inflammation. The cause is unknown, and the treatment is removal of the lens.[47]

NURSING CARE

Nursing Assessment[36,47]

Corneal abrasion (epithelial): Moderate to severe pain; blurred vision; halo seen around lights; generalized hyperemia; lacrimation; fluorescein stains (green) on corneal surface; patient unable to open eyes (because of pain)

Corneal edema: Blurred vision; absence of pain; dull appearance of cornea; slightly reddened conjunctiva

Corneal ulceration: Ulcers varying in appearance and size; severe pain associated with epithelial damage; iritis; lacrimation and possible purulent discharge; generalized hyperemia

Localized infection: Purulent discharge; generalized hyperemia; moderate discomfort; possible photophobia; crusting around lids; eyes may be "stuck together" in morning (or on awakening); complaints of blurred vision (because of excessive exudate over eye surface, which disappears with blinking)

Tight lens syndrome: Eye discomfort; decreased visual acuity (onset may be sudden [within hours] or more gradual); patient unable to remove lens; conjunctival congestion with some redness

Giant papillary syndrome: Slow onset over months or years; lacrimation; conjunctival redness; discharge may be present

Patient Problems/Nursing Diagnoses & Interventions

NIC Skin/Wound Management

Risk for impaired tissue integrity and injury related to epithelial damage to cornea with potential for stroma injury

- Assist with identification of epithelial breaks with fluorescein stain as ordered.
- Instill medications as ordered, such as topical antibiotics and cycloplegic drops.

NIC Physical Comfort Promotion

Acute pain related to corneal epithelial damage

- Apply pressure bandage to eye(s) as ordered, being certain that covered eye is closed *to reduce blinking and eye movement.*
- Apply topical anesthetic as ordered *to reduce pain.*
- Apply cool compress as ordered for 10 to 15 minutes *to reduce inflammation or discomfort.*
- Administer systemic analgesic as ordered and document response.
- Discourage patient from reading *to reduce eye movement.*

NIC Self-Care Facilitation

Disturbed sensory perception (visual) related to total loss of vision with binocular patches

Disturbed sensory perception (visual) related to blurred vision with corneal edema or tight lens

- Raise side rails *to ensure safety.*
- Address patient by name from doorway, and identify yourself and reason for presence.
- Complement voice stimulation with a touch *to notify patient of your proximity.*
- Orient patient to bedside equipment (such as call light, bed control, and side rails) and personal belongings at bedside by directing his or her hand over objects.
- Encourage patient to perform self-care with personal hygiene *to maximize independence.* Provide support and supervision.

to be certain that they can be performed safely by patient or with assistance from someone else.

Patient Education/Continuum of Care Plan

1. Caution patient to wash hands and dry well before inserting and removing lenses.
2. Explain to patient that eyelashes and face should be thoroughly cleansed before lenses are inserted.
3. Inform patient that instructions for care and follow-up should be carried out meticulously.
4. Explain care of hard contact lenses.
   a. Encourage patient to monitor himself or herself for sudden onset of pain, excessive eye redness, sudden decrease in vision, mucus discharge, or foreign body sensation. Tell patient to remove lenses and report to physician.
   b. Inform patient that adjustment to new lenses may take 2 to 3 weeks and that mild photophobia, tearing, and lid edema may occur.
   c. Inform patient that hard lenses are not recommended for wearing alternately with glasses or on a part-time basis after initial adjustment and that wearing time will increase to 10 to 14 hours after adjustment period.
   d. Inform patient that hard lenses should not be worn when engaging in contact sports.
   e. Tell patient that lenses must be removed at night or before sleeping.
   f. Explain that lenses must be cleaned after each removal according to manufacturer's directions and stored in their case.
   g. Explain that lens is wetted with an approved wetting solution before being placed over cornea.

   d. Tell patient that soft lenses can be alternated with glasses.
   e. Caution patient not to wear soft lenses while swimming, applying eye medications, or using hair or body sprays because soft lenses absorb chemicals easily.
   f. Explain that soft lenses are usually removed at night and that wearing time will increase to 12 to 14 hours after adjustment time.
   g. Tell patient that lenses must be cleaned after each removal according to manufacturer's instructions and stored in a specified solution. Soft lenses should not be permitted to dry out.
   h. Explain that storage solution must be changed as directed.
   i. Inform patient that soft lenses are fragile and can be damaged by exposure to makeup, creams, or mascara or nicked by fingernails.
   j. Tell patient that lenses should be checked daily for scratches, tears, loose debris, or clouding. Tell patient to report to physician if unable to wash lenses clear.
   k. Explain that lens must be wetted with approved wetting solution before being placed in eye.
   l. Review insertion and removal procedure with patient, and have patient demonstrate it to ensure competence.
   m. Inform patient of importance of consistently applying one lens before the other to avoid mixing lenses. If vision is blurred immediately after application, lenses may be reversed.
   n. Stress the need to keep appointment with physician because eyes and lenses should be checked regularly.

Evaluation/Patient Outcomes

Skin/Wound Management: Cornea is healthy. Cornea is clear and glossy without eye discomfort, redness, or discharge.

Physical Comfort Promotion: Patient does not experience pain.

Self-Care Facilitation: Contact lenses are successfully worn. Visual acuity is 20/20 for right eye (OD), left eye (OS), and both eyes (OU). Near vision is clear at 14 inches.

Patient is aware of high risk for injury with lenses. Patient can verbalize the need to care for lenses properly; no signs or symptoms of infection, corneal damage, or lack of proper fit are present.

ENUCLEATION

Description and Rationale

Enucleation, or surgical removal of the eyeball, is performed when other treatment of the eyeball is insufficient to prevent pain, disfigurement, or spread of malignant disease.

Indications include severe infections, malignancies such as melanoma and retinoblastoma, large and infiltrating tumors, extensive trauma to the eye, blindness when severe eye pain is also present, and end-stage glaucoma, when the patient is blind with no light perception and has increased intraocular pressure. Enucleation may also be performed as a prophylactic measure when sympathetic ophthalmia is likely to occur. Sympathetic ophthalmia is a rare granulomatous inflammation that usually develops within 3 months of an injury to one eye and involves the entire area. The injured eye is called the exciting eye, and the other eye (the sympathizing eye) can also become inflamed with uveitis unless the exciting eye is enucleated before the inflammation spreads.

Enucleation can be performed with the patient under local or general anesthesia. During surgery a 360-degree peritomy is performed at the limbus, opening the conjunctiva and allowing Tenon's fascia to be separated between the rectus muscles. The rectus muscles are separated, hooked, and cut with scissors near their insertion into the sclera. The inferior oblique muscle and superior oblique tendons are hooked and cut, the medial rectus muscle is clamped, and enucleation scissors are placed between the sclera and Tenon's capsule. The optic nerve is then cut as far behind the globe as possible, and the eye is removed. After adequate hemostasis is obtained at the socket, the muscles may be sutured to each other around a plastic or Teflon sphere to build up the eye and provide a more acceptable cosmetic appearance.

After the enucleation a "conformer" is placed in the socket until postoperative edema subsides and an artificial eye can be placed, usually 10 to 14 days after enucleation.

Two relevant surgical procedures are evisceration and exenteration. In evisceration the entire contents of the eyeball and sometimes the cornea are removed but the sclera remains. This procedure may be used when panophthalmitis, an inflammation of the entire inner eye including the sclera, is present. Exenteration is a more radical procedure in which the eyelids, eyeball, and orbital contents are removed, usually in cases of malignancies of the lacrimal gland, extension of eyelid malignancies in the orbit, malignant melanoma of the conjunctiva, or melanoma or retinoblastoma that has invaded the orbit.

Contraindications and Cautions

Panophthalmitis is a contraindication to enucleation because the risk of postoperative meningitis is increased after removal of an actively infected eyeball.

Multidisciplinary Plan

Surgery

Removal of the eyeball as described previously

Medications

Narcotic-analgesic agents

Meperidine (Demerol), 50-75 mg IM q4-6h prn for severe pain

Acetaminophen with codeine (Tylenol with Codeine), 30-60 mg PO q4-6h prn for less severe pain

General Management

Firm pressure dressing applied to operative site for 24 to 48 hours; activity progression without restrictions as tolerated; progressive diet as tolerated

NURSING CARE

Nursing Assessment

Eye socket: Pain at enucleation site; headache on side of enucleation; no fever or bleeding

Patient Problems/Nursing Diagnoses & Interventions

NIC Physical Comfort Promotion

Acute pain related to surgical intervention

- Administer pain medications as ordered by physician and document response.
- Notify physician if pain or headache persists *because this may indicate infection.*
- Notify physician if temperature is elevated *because this may indicate infection.*

NIC Skin/Wound Management

Risk for impaired tissue integrity and injury related to postoperative bleeding

- Evaluate dressing at operative site frequently for signs of oozing or frank bleeding.
- Document absence of blood or amount if present.
- Maintain firm pressure dressing at operative site until removal is ordered by physician.
- Monitor and document patient's vital signs according to protocol, and report any change in pulse and blood pressure.

NIC Self-Care Facilitation

Disturbed sensory perception (visual) related to enucleation procedure

- Help patient walk as tolerated *to avoid injury.*
- Ensure that patient's call light and personal belongings are close by on unaffected side.

4. Educate patient regarding signs and symptoms of infection, abscess, and meningitis.
5. Discuss limited field of vision and need to exaggerate head movement to achieve a full visual field, for example, when driving. Discuss changes in depth perception.

Evaluation/Patient Outcomes

Physical Comfort Promotion: Patient does not experience pain.

Skin/Wound Management: There is no infection. Patient and family demonstrate ability to care for eye socket and artificial eye after discharge from hospital. Patient verbalizes knowledge of signs and symptoms of possible infection: pain, headache, drainage, and elevated temperature.

Self-Care Facilitation: Patient is fitted with and wears artificial eye, if appropriate, after discharge from hospital, to improve appearance. Patient verbalizes understanding of need for eye removal.

Coping Assistance: Body image is adequate. Patient expresses concerns and frustrations regarding disease process and body image.

Keratoplasty[36,40,47]

Description and Rationale

Keratoplasty, or corneal transplant, is the excision of corneal tissue and its replacement by a cornea from a human donor.[36]

This procedure may be performed to replace a corneal opacity, which is a lack of corneal transparency resulting from injury or inflammation, or to correct a variety of corneal abnor-

people who have died as a result of injury or acute disease or from patients whose eyes have been surgically removed for some reason but whose corneas are normal. Ideally the donor is between 25 and 35 years of age. Corneas should not be used from patients who were ill for a long time before death or who had such diseases as leukemia, sepsis, hepatitis, human immunodeficiency virus (HIV) positivity, or certain tumors of the eye.

If it is known when a patient dies that the eyes are to be donated, the lids should be closed and covered with small ice bags. Nothing should touch the corneas themselves. The donor eyes should be enucleated within an hour after death, but up to 5 hours is acceptable if ice bags have been placed on the eyes at death. Ideally corneas are transplanted into the recipient immediately after removal, but many eye banks can now safely store corneas for longer periods. Whole eyes can be stored from 24 to 48 hours if refrigerated; corneal tissue can be kept longer if removed with a 3-mm rim of scleral tissue attached. Corneas must not be folded during storage, because this damages the endothelium. They must be stored at a temperature of 4° C (39° F) in a modified tissue culture medium.[36]

Transplantation is usually performed with the patient under topical and retrobulbar anesthesia. The surgeon removes the cornea from the donor's eye with a trephine and then removes the impaired areas from the recipient eye using another trephine the same size or slightly larger. The donor cornea, called the donor button, is sutured into place with continuous or interrupted sutures to align and graft and ensure a watertight wound (Fig. 8-20).

Contraindications and Cautions

Light perception and projection must be normal before surgery will be considered.

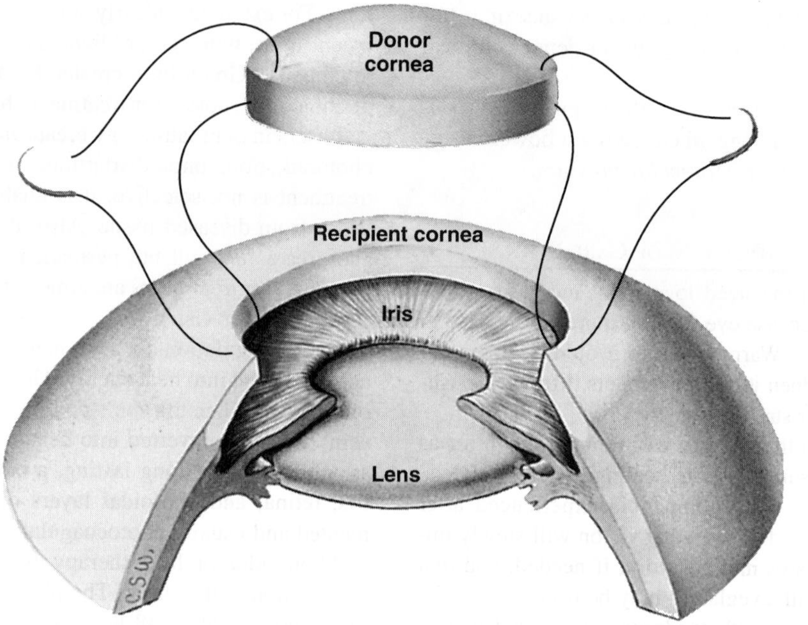

FIG. 8-20

The excised portion of the cornea is being replaced with a clear donor cornea in a partial penetrating keratoplasty. (From Newell.[36])

There is the possibility that some corneal dystrophy will occur in the transplanted cornea.

Corneal graft rejection may occur. This starts 3 weeks or more after keratoplasty and is limited to the donor cornea, because there are no blood vessels or lymphatics to sensitize the recipient. The inflammatory process begins at the graft margin and spreads to involve the entire graft.

MULTIDISCIPLINARY PLAN

Surgery

Lamellar or penetrating keratoplasty as described previously

Medications

Narcotic analgesic agents: Meperidine (Demerol), 50-100 mg IM q4h for pain

Antiemetic agents: Prochlorperazine (Compazine), 25 mg by rectum bid or 5-10 mg IM q4-6h for nausea

Corticosteroids: Pred-Forte eyedrops, 1 drop qid

Laxatives: Docusate sodium (Colace), 240 mg to prevent straining during bowel movement

General Management

Unilateral eye patch for 24 hours; activity and diet progress as tolerated

NURSING CARE

NURSING ASSESSMENT

Cornea: Wound edema; inflammation; photophobia; decreased vision; clouding caused by vascularization as result of graft rejection

PATIENT PROBLEMS/NURSING DIAGNOSES & INTERVENTIONS

NIC RISK MANAGEMENT

Disturbed sensory perception (visual) related to unilateral eye patch

- Ensure that eye patch remains securely in place for at least 24 hours.
- Help patient with walking postoperatively *because patient may be unsteady and must be prevented from falling and injuring eye.*
- If patient stays in the hospital overnight, ensure that call light is in place, side rails are up, and items at bedside are in familiar place for patient *to ensure safety.*
- Administer eyedrops, as ordered by physician.

NIC PHYSICAL COMFORT PROMOTION

Acute pain related to surgical intervention

- Administer pain medication as ordered, particularly on first postoperative night if patient remains in the hospital, *to decrease discomfort and promote rest and healing of eye.*

NIC SKIN/WOUND MANAGEMENT

Risk for impaired tissue integrity and injury related to potential increase in IOP causing displacement of graft

- Institute measures designed to prevent increases in intraocular pressure that might push healing graft forward.
- Administer antiemetics as ordered *to prevent vomiting.*
- Encourage patient not to cough but to breathe deeply often *to increase lung expansion.*

so treatment can begin promptly.

EVALUATION/PATIENT OUTCOMES

Risk Management: Patient does not fall or sustain injury as a result of visual impairment.

Physical Comfort Promotion: No pain is experienced after graft heals.

Skin/Wound Management: Corneal graft heals adequately. Wound edema and inflammation dissipate. Photophobia decreases. Vision improves slowly. No evidence of graft rejection occurs. No injury is caused to the graft from increase in intraocular pressure.

LASER THERAPY[5,13,47]

Description and Rationale

Laser is the application of a light wavelength to tissue for therapeutic purposes.

The word "laser" is an acronym for *l*ight *a*mplification by *s*timulated *e*mission of *r*adiation. Experimentation with the effect of light on the retina began in the 1800s after the invention of the ophthalmoscope, when ophthalmologists began noticing solar burns in patients' eyes after solar eclipses. Early investigators used the effects of the sun or the carbon arc to produce a lesion in the retina. Since that time, research with laser therapy has refined and broadened its use, and lasers are now the treatment of choice for a wide variety of ophthalmic disorders.

Ophthalmic lasers differ by the type of energy they create and the color(s) they are able to emit. Interestingly, over time and with research, we have come to use specific colors in the light spectrum to treat specific ophthalmic diseases and condi-

Photodisruption is the term used to describe the effect of the neodymium:yttrium-aluminum-garnet (Nd:YAG) laser. This white laser light is aimed at the target tissue extremely precisely. When the light strikes the tissue, small explosions occur on the surface that eventually disrupt the tissue and create a hole or opening. This technique is most commonly performed on patients who have had cataract surgery. At the time of primary extracapsular cataract surgery the posterior lens capsule is left intact. This provides support for the vitreous jelly and retina and is proven to lower the incidence of retinal detachments in postcataract patients. However, approximately 6 months to 2 years after surgery this capsule, which is clear at the time of surgery, becomes cloudy or opaque to light, and patients note a loss in visual acuity. The Nd:YAG laser is used to "blast" an opening in the center of this capsule, recreating a clear pathway for light. This usually results in a sudden and dramatic improvement in visual acuity. It is one example where laser treatment does result in visual improvement rather than a stabilization of vision and prevention of further loss.

Photovaporization therapy is the use of carbon dioxide laser radiation to vaporize malignant intraocular and extraocular tumors in a precise manner. When repeated surface impacts are made with the carbon dioxide laser, carbon dioxide radiation is highly absorbed by ocular tissue, with almost complete absorption and conversion to heat within a tissue depth of 100 μm.[5]

Laser therapy provides a nonsurgical approach to many ophthalmic disorders and can usually be performed on an outpatient basis. The goal of most ophthalmic laser therapy is to stabilize vision and to prevent further visual loss. It offers hope to patients with diabetic retinopathy and glaucoma.

Two types of laser treatments are performed for the treatment of diabetic retinopathy. Panretinal photocoagulation (PRP) treatment is the application of several thousand laser spots or burns to the peripheral areas of retina. The laser burns create scars, destroying the retinal tissue where it is applied. The macular area is spared to maintain central vision. Theoretically, abnormal blood vessels, which occur in diabetic retinopathy and threaten vision by hemorrhaging or causing traction retinal detachments, regress after laser therapy because they are perceived by the body as no longer needed. The goal of the treatment is to sacrifice some areas of retinal tissue to spare and protect central vision.

Focal laser treatment is performed for diabetic persons whose blood vessels are leaking fluid and plasma into the retina, creating edema and blurring central vision. A localized application of laser spots is aimed directly at the leaky blood vessels to seal them closed, preventing additional leakage. In approximately 2 months the remaining fluid is absorbed and the macular area dries out. Vision usually does not improve after focal laser therapy; however, if diabetic-related edema is identified early, when vision is minimally affected, good stabilization is usually accomplished, as well as no further vision loss.

Photocoagulation has also become useful in the treatment of glaucoma to control intraocular pressure. A procedure called laser trabeculoplasty can control pressure successfully in about 85% of cases, especially in eyes with wide angles and slight pigmentation of the trabecular meshwork.

Laser therapy is also useful in treating chronic primary closed-angle glaucoma. The aim of therapy is to prevent the pressure in the posterior chamber from exceeding that of the anterior chamber by creating an opening that eliminates the accumulation of aqueous humor in the posterior chamber. The surgeon performs a laser iridotomy in which a localized area of the midperipheral iris is caused to bulge forward by means of mild laser burns. The central portion of this area is then perforated by laser burns of much higher energy. Many applications of the beam may be necessary.[5]

Contraindications and Cautions

Before photocoagulation therapy each segment of the eye must be closely examined for factors that would diminish the effectiveness of therapy.

NURSING CARE

Nursing Assessment

Vision: Constriction of peripheral fields; temporary decrease in central vision; slight decrease in night vision; headache from bright laser light; pain unrelieved by acetaminophen

Patient Problems/Nursing Diagnoses & Interventions

NIC Coping Assistance

Anxiety related to lack of information about laser procedure

- Explain purpose of laser therapy.
- Assure patient that procedure causes little pain and that topical anesthetic (eyedrops) will be administered *to alleviate anxiety related to fear of pain.*
- Describe procedure to patient and family. Explain that patient will be awake and sitting up in a chair and may have special contact lens placed on eye.
- Describe bright lights caused by laser beam that patient will see during procedure.
- Explain that procedure may take 15 to 40 minutes.
- Tell patient that family member or friend should accompany patient and drive home *because patient's eye will be dilated and vision may be temporarily blurred.*

NIC Physical Comfort Promotion

Acute pain related to laser treatment

- Explain to patient that headache may develop after treatment because of bright laser light. Suggest acetaminophen *to relieve discomfort.* Warn patient not to use aspirin for 24 hours after the procedure *because of its anticoagulant effect.*

Patient Education/Continuum of Care Plan

1. Emphasize importance of not increasing venous pressure in head, neck, and eyes, particularly with Valsalva's maneuver. Instruct patient to keep head up and to move slowly and not to bend over or make sudden movements.
2. Caution patient not to lift anything heavier than 5 pounds and not to strain for any reason, as when having bowel movement, for 24 hours after procedure. Encourage patient to take a stool softener to avoid constipation.
3. Explain that spots may be seen before eyes for 24 to 48 hours after treatment. Inform patient that eye may be bloodshot, vision may be somewhat blurred temporarily, and night vision may be temporarily decreased.
4. Advise patient to avoid coughing and sneezing and not to blow nose vigorously. (However, sneezes should not be stifled because this raises pressure in eyes.)
5. Teach patient not to rub eyes.
6. Instruct patient to avoid medications that contain epinephrine, such as nose drops or sprays, because these may raise blood pressure.
7. Instruct patient to use nonaspirin pain relievers for 24 hours after laser surgery to avoid bleeding and to reduce antiinflammatory response. (Laser creates scarring by heat and inflammation.)

Evaluation/Patient Outcomes

Coping Assistance: Patient does not experience anxiety during procedure. Blurred vision decreases after about 3 weeks, and normal or improved vision returns.

Physical Comfort Promotion: Pain is relieved with acetaminophen; pain is absent.

Refractive Surgery

Regardless of the procedure used, the goal of refractive surgery is to reshape the cornea to permit the light rays to more accurately fall exactly on the macula of the retina so that static visual acuity is at or very near 20/20 without any optical aid. The techniques fall into several categories; however, the most commonly performed and currently "popular" modes are photorefractive keratectomy (PRK) and laser in situ keratomileusis, or LASIK. Both of these techniques utilize an excimer laser to idated various refractive procedures, refractive surgery has been accepted by many surgeons who were previously skeptical. The first approved procedure for refractive therapy was radial keratotomy (RK). In RK 8 to 16 partial-thickness incisions were made in the cornea excluding the pupillary zone. The resultant flattening reduced myopia. Although this procedure is still an approved technique, few ophthalmologists today continue to utilize it because laser intervention has replaced reshaping the cornea with a knife blade. The technology in this arena of eye care is very dynamic and will continue to be so for a long time to come. Both the procedures and the equipment used to perform them are in a constant state of change. As quickly as one procedure is approved, another one enters the clinical trials phase. Our responsibilities to patients who desire refractive surgery center around informed consent and an unequivocal understanding of the risks versus benefits of this "high-tech" and highly desired procedure. Refractive procedures are primarily aimed at reducing either myopia (nearsightedness) or astigmatism (irregular curvature of the cornea). A small percentage of refractive procedures reduce hyperopia (farsightedness).

Patients who already have presbyopia requiring a bifocal or reading lens for near vision may opt to undercorrect one eye. By doing this they become somewhat monocular, using one eye for distance visual acuity and the other for clear vision up close.

The most recent innovations in this fast-paced arena are an implantable but removable ring of plastic in the cornea and the implantation of an intraocular lens in a patient who is highly myopic but does not yet need cataract surgery. Both of these procedures received FDA approval in late 1999. However, the permissible criteria under which either of these procedures may be performed are quite stringent at this point. Intacs, the im-

Louis, 1992, Mosby.

12. Flynn JT: 17th Annual Frank Costenbader lecture, amblyopia revisited, *J Pediatr Ophthalmol Strabismus* 28(4):183, 1991.
13. Fraunfelder FT, Roy FN, editors: *Current ocular therapy,* Philadelphia, 1995, WB Saunders.
14. Freund KB, Yannuzzi LA, Sorenson JA: Age-related macular degeneration and choroidal neovascularization, *Am J Ophthalmol* 115(6):786, 1993.
15. Friedlander MH: The eye in immunologic disease, *J Fla Med Assoc* 81(4):252, 1994.
16. Groer MW, Shekleton ME: *Basic pathophysiology: a holistic approach,* ed 3, St. Louis, 1989, Mosby.
17. Grosskreutz C, Netland PA: Low tension glaucoma, *Int Ophthalmol Clin* 34(3):173, 1994.
18. Hart W Jr, editor: *Adler's physiology of the eye,* ed 9, St. Louis, 1992, Mosby.
19. Helveston EM: *Surgical management of strabismus: an atlas of strabismus surgery,* ed 4, St. Louis, 1993, Mosby.
20. Hockwin O: Cataract classification, *Doc Ophthalmol* 88(3-4):264, 1994-1995.
21. Hurst MA, Douthwaite WA: Assessing vision behind cataract: a review of methods, *Optom Vis Sci* 70(11):903, 1993.
22. Jaffe NS: *Atlas of ophthalmic surgery,* ed 2, St. Louis, 1995, Mosby.
23. Jay JL: Primary open angle glaucoma, *Practitioner* 236(1511):199, 1992.
24. Kim MJ, McFarland GK, McLane AM: *Pocket guide to nursing diagnoses,* ed 7, St. Louis, 1997, Mosby.
25. Kohner EM: The effect of diabetic control on diabetic retinopathy, *Eye* 7(pt 2):309, 1993.
26. Lewis H, Ryan SJ, editor: *Medical and surgical retina: advances, controversies, and management,* St. Louis, 1994, Mosby.
27. MacCuish AC: Early detection and screening for diabetic retinopathy, *Eye* 7(pt 2):254, 1993.

28. MacInnis B: Update in cataract and refractive surgery, *Can J Ophthalmol* 30(1):1, 1995.
29. Mattingly WB: Advanced low vision optics, *Ophthalmic Nurs Technol* 13(4):161, 1994.
30. Mauger TF, Craig EL: *Mosby's ocular drug handbook,* St. Louis, 1996, Mosby.
31. Migdal C: What is the appropriate treatment for patients with primary open-angle glaucoma: medicine, laser or primary surgery, *Ophthalmic Surg* 26(2):108, 1995.
32. Murphy RP: Management of diabetic retinopathy, *Am Fam Physician* 51(4):785, 1995.
33. Murray S: Cataract surgery: new techniques, better results, *Practitioner* 239(1549):272, 1995.
34. Navon SE, McKeown CA: Amblyopia, *Int Ophthalmol Clin* 32(1):35, 1992.
35. Nelson LB, Wagner RS: Pediatric cataract surgery, *Int Ophthalmol Clin* 34(2):165, 1994.
36. Newell FW: *Ophthalmology: principles and concepts,* ed 8, St. Louis, 1996, Mosby.
37. Osako M, Keltner JL: Botulinum A toxin (oculinum) in ophthalmology, *J Am Optom Assoc* 65(9):621, 1994.
38. Salasche SJ et al: The retinoblastoma gene and its significance, *Ann Med* 26(3):177, 1994.
39. Seidel HM et al: *Mosby's guide to physical examination,* ed 4, St. Louis, 1999, Mosby.
40. Serdarevic ON: Refractive corneal transplantation: control of astigmatism and ametropia during penetrating keratoplasty, *Int Ophthalmol Clin* 34(4):13, 1994.
41. Serle JB: Pharmacologic advances in the treatment of glaucoma, *Drugs Aging* 5(3):156, 1994.
42. Smith SC: Diabetic retinopathy, *Nurs Clin North Am* 27(3):745, 1992.
43. Stamper RL et al: *Practical therapeutic approaches in Becker-Shaffer's diagnosis and therapy of the glaucomas,* ed 7, St. Louis, Mosby, 1999.
44. Swanson MW: Ocular metastatic disease, *Optom Clin* 3(3):79, 1993.
45. Thompson JM, Wilson SF: *Health assessment for nursing practice,* St. Louis, 1996, Mosby.
46. Tusa RJ, Newman SA, editors: *Neurophthalmological disorders: diagnostic work-up and management,* New York, 1995, Marcel Dekker.
47. Vaughn D, Asbury T, Riordan-Eva P: *General ophthalmology,* ed 14, Norwalk, Conn, 1995, Appleton & Lange.
48. Vernon S: How to screen for glaucoma, *Practitioner* 239(1549):257, 1995.
49. vonNoorden GK: *Binocular vision and ocular motility: theory and management of strabismus,* ed 5, St. Louis, 1996, Mosby.
50. Wagner RS: Glaucoma in children, *Pediatr Clin North Am* 40(4):855, 1993.
51. Weiter JJ, Roh S: Viral infections of the choroid and retina, *Infect Dis Clin North Am* 6(4):875, 1992.
52. Wright KW: *Pediatric ophthalmology and strabismus,* St. Louis, 1995, Mosby.
53. Wong DL: *Whaley and Wong's nursing care of infants and children,* ed 5, St. Louis, 1995, Mosby.

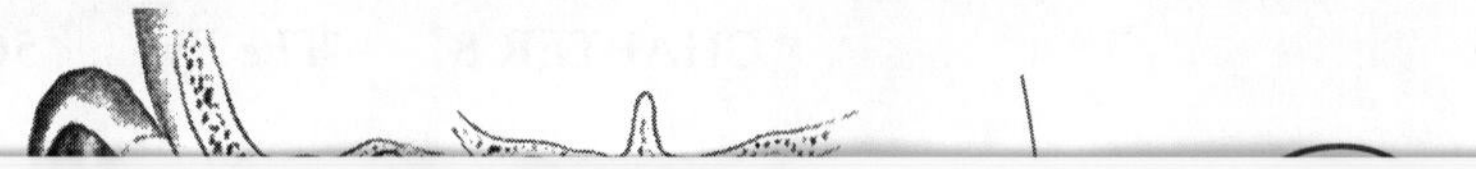

with disorders affecting these areas must be highly sensitive and skilled in assessing the symptoms of disorders that may have a great impact on a patient's life or self-perception.

Ear, nose, and throat disorders can cause painful, incapacitating illnesses and major disruptions in communication, appearance, eating, swallowing, and breathing. Neoplastic disorders of the ear, nose, and throat may be fatal.

Because many ENT disorders are treated on an outpatient basis, patient and family education is a focus of this chapter.

The development of antibiotics and new surgical techniques has greatly reduced the impact of many ENT diseases. Hearing loss was once a common occurrence after severe or repeated ear infections, but now infection-related hearing loss has been nearly eliminated in the United States. Other diseases that once were life threatening are now considered minor if treated early. Surgical techniques such as microsurgery, stapedectomy, cochlear implant, and tympanoplasty have greatly improved the management of the patient with a hearing loss.

Anatomy, Physiology, and Related Pathophysiology

Ear

The ears are responsible for both hearing and equilibrium. The ear is divided into three anatomic sections: The external ear, the middle ear, and the inner ear (Fig. 9-1).

External Ear. The function of the external ear is to receive sound waves and direct them to the tympanic membrane. The external ear includes the outer projection (known as the auricle or pinna) and the ear canal, called the external auditory meatus or the external auditory canal. The auricle is attached to the

gus nerve, the auriculotemporal nerve, and the fifth, seventh, and tenth cranial nerves.

The external auditory meatus or ear canal has a slight downward curve; it ends at the tympanic membrane. The outer half is cartilaginous, and the inner half is bony except in infants, in whom ossification has not yet occurred. The skin that lines the cartilaginous portion of the canal is thick and contains fine hairs, large sebaceous glands, and ceruminous glands. Cerumen (earwax), the combined secretion of the sebaceous and ceruminous glands, may accumulate, obstructing sound transmission. The epithelium that lines the bony half of the external canal is very thin and does not contain hair or glands. In adults the external canal is approximately 24 mm long, and the bony portion is slightly longer than the cartilaginous portion (Fig. 9-3).

The temporomandibular joint is anterior to the ear canal. Diseases of this joint can cause referred pain to the ear.

Tympanic Membrane. The tympanic membrane, which separates the external ear from the middle ear, is composed of three layers: the outer squamous layer, the inner cuboidal layer, and a middle layer of fibrous collagen tissue. New cells of the tympanic membrane are produced in the periphery and migrate toward the center of the drum. The drum is somewhat conical and slightly inclined; the concavity of the drumhead (umbo) and its position in relation to the ear canal vary and may be greatly altered during disease.

The fibers of the tympanic membrane condense into an incomplete, dense, fibrous ring called the annulus, which fits into the tympanic sulcus. The annulus contains a superior break, the notch of Rivinus, between the anterior and posterior malleolar ligaments. The portion of the tympanic membrane closing this area is the pars flaccida, so named because it does not contain a fibrous collagen layer.

HEALTHY PEOPLE 2010

HEALTH STATUS—HEARING

Goal: Improve the visual and hearing health of the nation through prevention, early detection, treatment, and rehabilitation.

AUDIOLOGY

- Increase the proportion of newborns who are screened for hearing loss by age 1 month, have audiologic evaluation by age 3 months, and are enrolled in appropriate intervention services by age 6 months.
- Reduce otitis media in children and adolescents.
- (Developmental) Increase access by persons who have hearing impairments to hearing rehabilitation services and adaptive devices, including hearing aids, cochlear implants, or tactile or other assistive or augmentative devices.
- (Developmental) Increase the proportion of persons who have had a hearing examination on schedule.
- (Developmental) Increase the number of persons who are referred by their primary care physician for hearing evaluation and treatment.
- (Developmental) Increase the use of appropriate ear protection devices, equipment, and practices.
- (Developmental) Reduce noise-induced hearing loss in children and adolescents under age 17 years.
- (Developmental) Reduce adult hearing loss in the noise-exposed public.

U.S. Department of Health and Human Services: *Healthy people 2010* (conference edition, in two volumes), Washington, DC, January 2000.

NOTE: *Developmental* indicates that criteria for measurement and strategies to improve health have not as yet been specified.

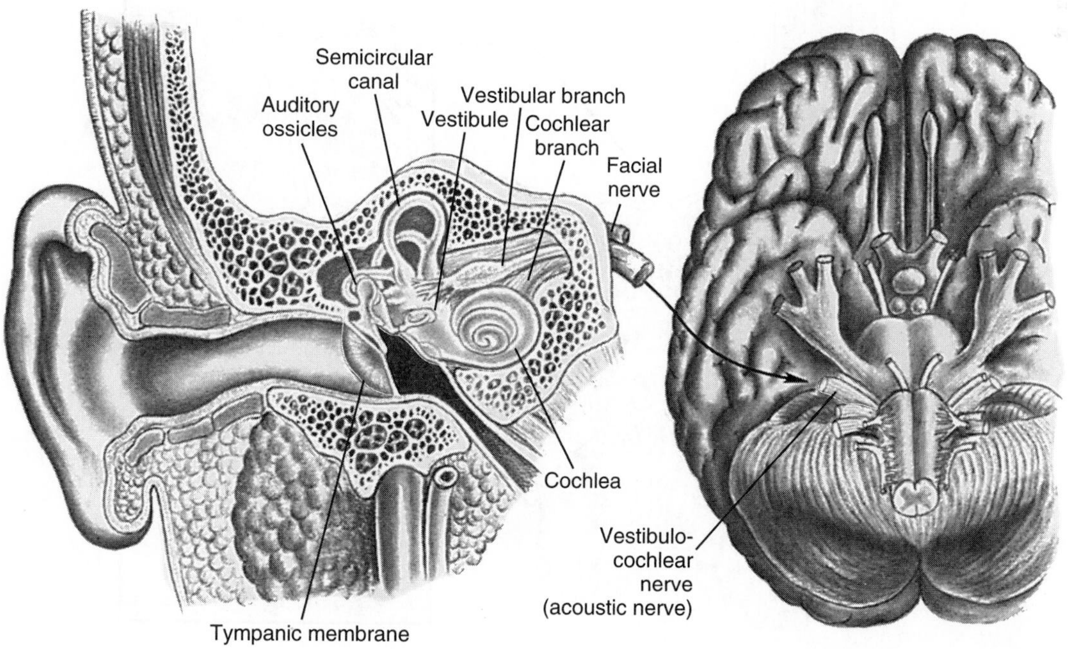

FIG. 9-1

Relationship of external, middle, and inner ear.

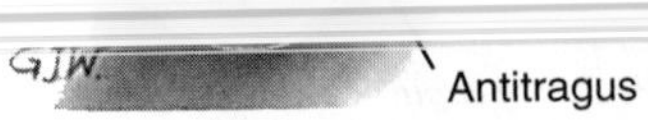

FIG. 9-2

Anatomic structures of the external ear. (From Seidel et al.[21])

more audible.

The middle ear communicates directly with the nasopharynx by the eustachian tube. This tube, which leads downward and medially to the nasopharynx, carries air into the middle ear to

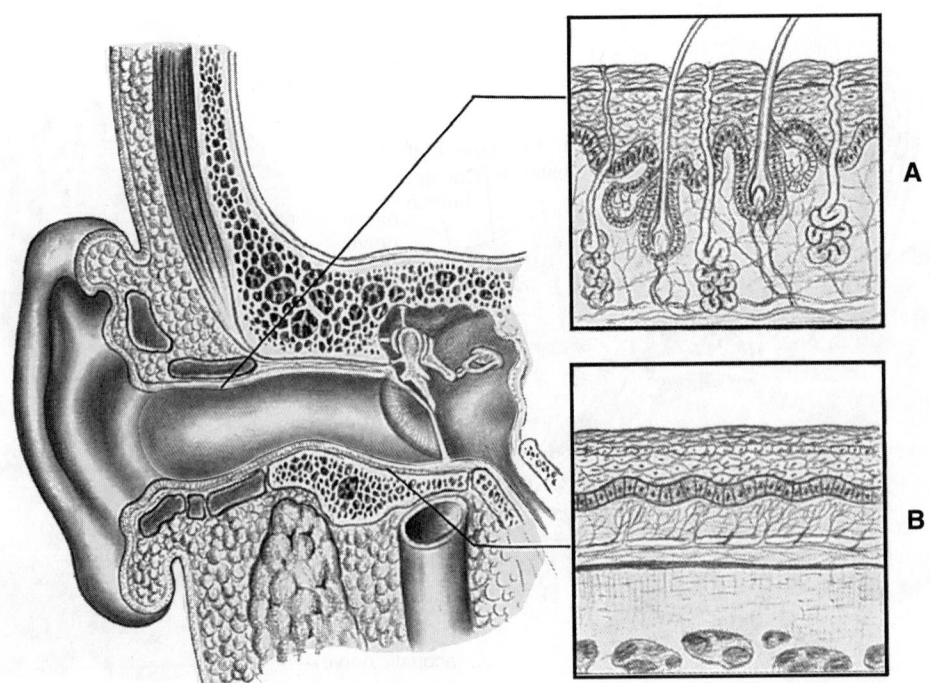

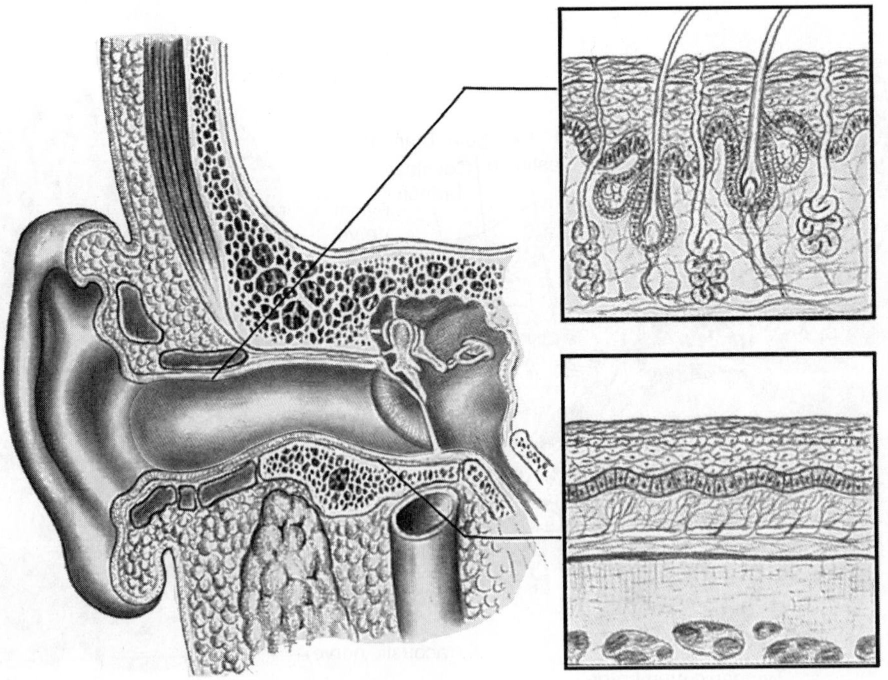

FIG. 9-3

External auditory canal. **A,** Cartilaginous ear canal showing hair follicles, sebaceous glands, and ceruminous glands. **B,** Bony ear canal with thin epithelial lining, containing no hair or glands.

equalize pressure on both sides of the tympanic membrane. The mucosal lining of the middle ear is continuous with that of the nasopharynx by way of the eustachian tube. Normally the eustachian tube is passively closed; it opens by action of the tensor and levator muscles of the palate, usually, although not always, during swallowing, yawning, or sneezing to equalize middle ear pressure with atmospheric pressure. The eustachian tube can serve as a direct route for infection to reach the middle ear from the upper respiratory tract.

A third structure of the middle ear is the collection of mastoid air cells. These are air-filled spaces in a portion of the temporal bone in the skull. They communicate posteriorly with the middle ear. They are present at birth but are small and filled with diploic bone and loose osseous tissue between the two tables of cranial bones. Between the ages of 2 and 6 years the diploic bone is gradually replaced by air cells that bud off from the mastoid antrum, which is the first and largest air cell and connects directly to the middle ear.

Inner Ear. The end organs for hearing and equilibrium are housed in the inner ear. The inner ear, or labyrinth, is composed of two portions, one inside the other (FIG. 9-6). The bony

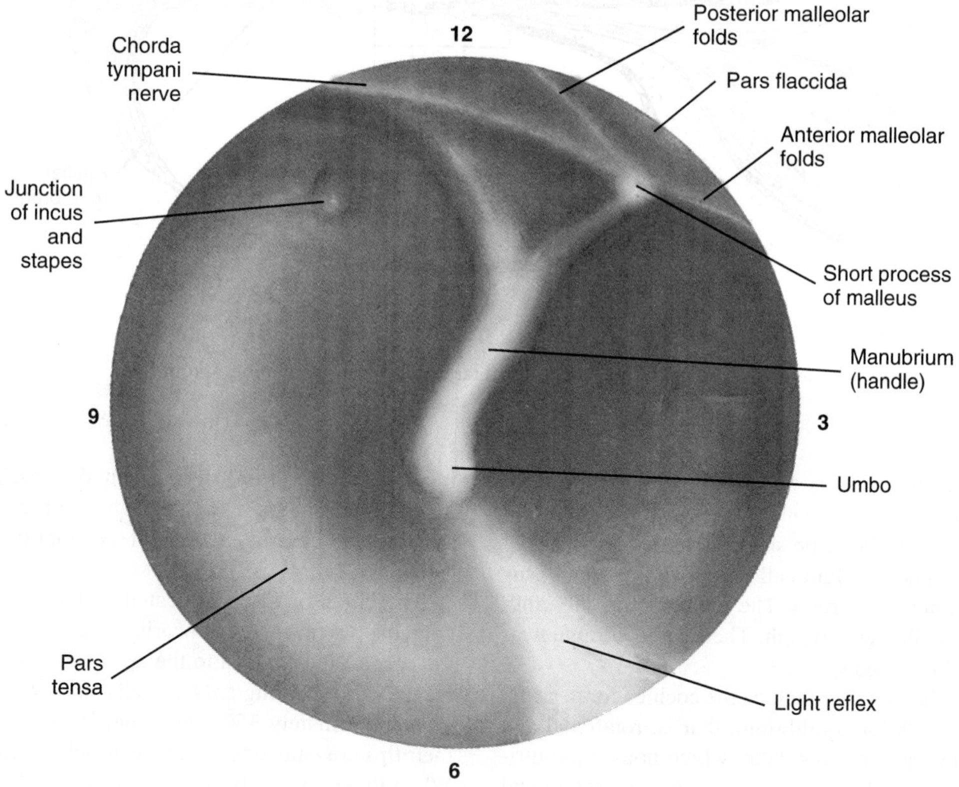

FIG. 9-4
Normal tympanic membrane. (From Wong.[24])

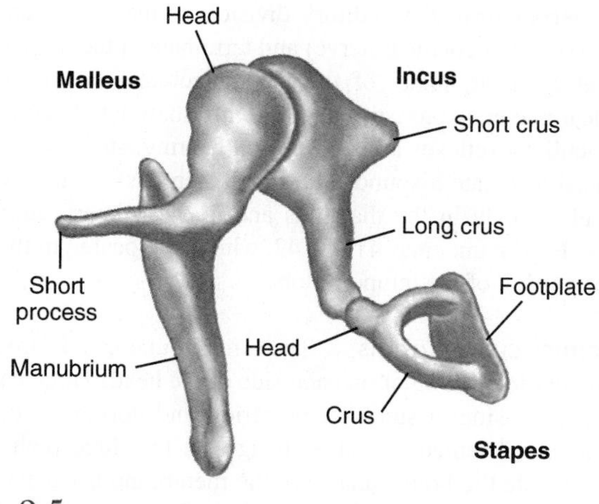

FIG. 9-5
Ossicles of right middle ear.

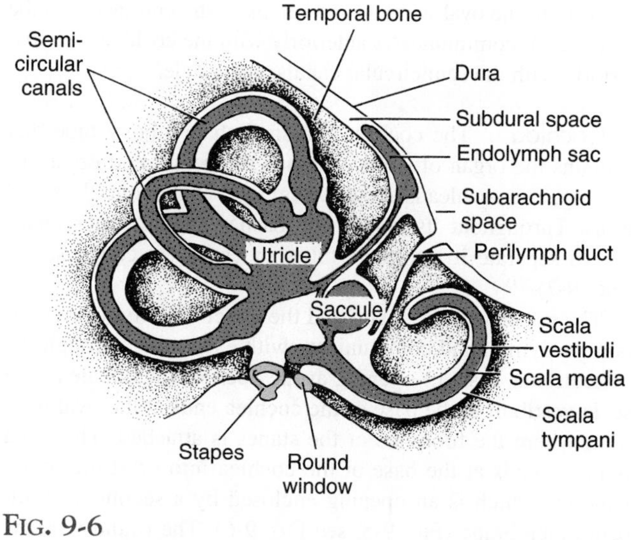

FIG. 9-6
Bony labyrinth and membranous inner labyrinth. (From Sigler and Schuring.[22])

labyrinth is a series of channels within the petrous portion of the temporal bone. Lining the bony labyrinth is the membranous labyrinth, which is the same shape as the bony channels. Inside the bony channels is fluid called perilymph, which surrounds the membranous labyrinth. The membranous labyrinth is filled with fluid called endolymph. There is no communication between the fluid-filled spaces.[2,23]

Components of the inner ear include the cochlea for hearing, the semicircular canals for equilibrium, that is, rotational and angular acceleration, and the vestibule, which houses the utricle and saccule responsible for sensing changes in gravity and linear and angular acceleration. The vestibule is a space that opens onto the oval window and serves as the entrance into the inner ear. It communicates anteriorly with the cochlea and posteriorly with the semicircular canals and utricle.

Cochlea. The cochlea is a snail-shaped bony tube that contains the organ of Corti, which is the neural end organ for hearing. The cochlea is about 3.5 cm long with about $2^1/_2$ spiral turns. Throughout its length, the basilar and Reissner membranes separate it into three tubes or chambers called scalae (FIG. 9-7).[2,23]

The upper scala vestibuli and the lower scala tympani contain perilymph and communicate with each other through the helicotrema, a small opening at the apex of the cochlea. The scala vestibuli at the base of the cochlea ends at the oval window, where the footplate of the stapes is attached. The scala tympani ends at the base of the cochlea into or at the round window, which is an opening enclosed by a secondary tympanic membrane (FIG. 9-8, see FIG. 9-6). The round window bulges outward to dissipate the pressure waves that are set up in the inner ear fluid during sound transmission. The scala media, or the middle cochlear chamber, contains endolymph and does not communicate with the other two scalae (see FIGS. 9-6 and 9-8).[2,23]

The organ of Corti is located on the basilar membrane and contains the receptors of hearing (FIG. 9-9, *A*). It extends from the base of the cochlea to the apex and has a spiral shape. The receptors for hearing are hair cells arranged in two rows. There are approximately 3500 inner and 20,000 outer hair cells, and their tips are embedded in the tectorial membrane (FIG. 9-9, *B*). When these hair cells are bent or distorted by pressure waves, sound is changed (transduced) into electromechanical impulses. These impulses are carried by the afferent neuron to the spiral ganglion in the bony core of the cochlea. The axons of these nerves form the auditory division of the eighth cranial nerve (vestibulocochlear nerve) and terminate in the dorsal and ventral cochlear nuclei of the medulla oblongata. From the cochlear nuclei, axons carry auditory information to the inferior canaliculi for reflexes associated with hearing, such as turning the head to locate a sound. The fibers then pass to the medial geniculate body in the thalamus and to the primary auditory cortex, Brodmann areas 41 and 42, which are located in the superior portion of the temporal lobe.

Semicircular Canals. The semicircular canals are perpendicular to each other on each side of the head. Three canals are on each side: a superior, posterior, and horizontal canal; they are so oriented to sense changes in the three planes of space. Inside the bony canals are the membranous canals suspended in the perilymph. Near the end of each canal is an enlargement called the ampulla, which houses the crista am-

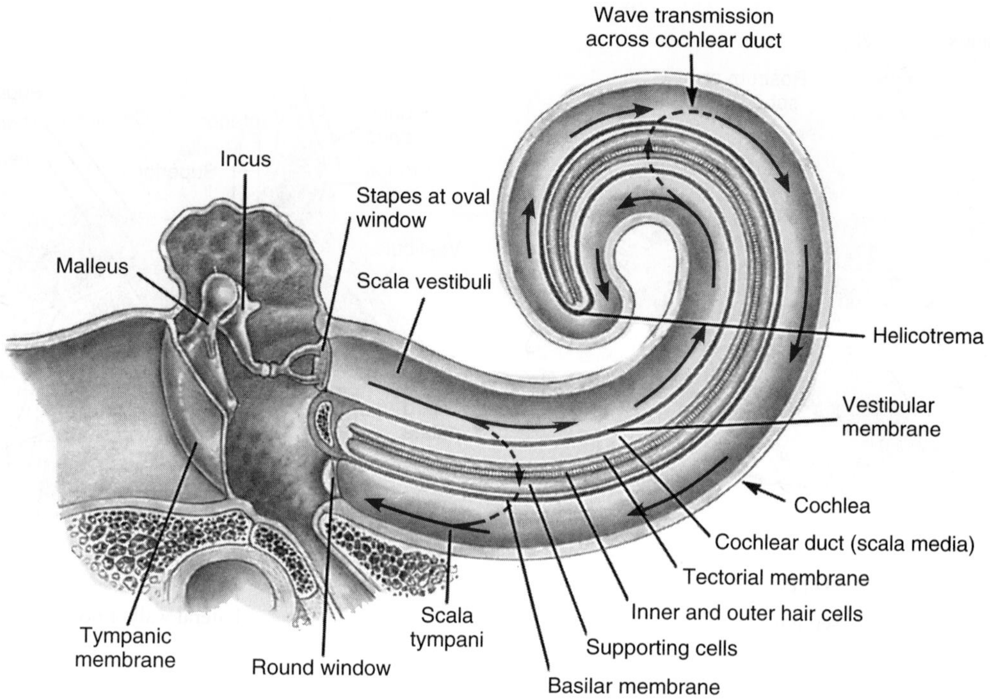

FIG. 9-8

Middle ear, showing relationship of ossicles and cochlea. Communication between scala vestibuli and scala tympania is shown. Arrows indicate displacement of liquid inside bony cochlea and round window from movement of stapedial footplate and displacement of oval window.

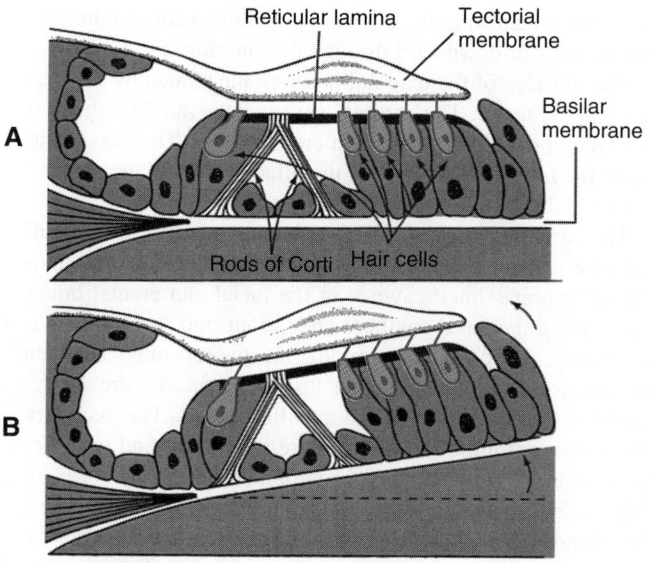

FIG. 9-9

A, Organ of Corti on basilar membrane. **B,** Hair cells embedded in tectorial membrane. (From Berne and Levy.[6])

pullaris, or the vestibular receptors. The hair cells of the crista ampullaris are stimulated with rotation. The pattern of stimulation varies with the direction and plane of rotation. Nerve fiber tracts compose the vestibular portion of the vestibulocochlear nerve, or cranial nerve VIII, to the vestibular nuclei and terminate in the four vestibular nuclei at the level of the pons and medulla in the brainstem. Tracts that descend from the vestibular nuclei into the spinal cord are responsible for head-righting reflexes and changes with muscle tone associated with rotation. Ascending fibers from the vestibular nuclei are concerned with eye movements, that is, nystagmus associated with rotation.

Utricle and Saccule. Housed within the vestibule are the utricle and saccule, which are responsible for sensing changes in gravity and forward and backward movement. Hair cells in the macula of the utricle and saccule are stimulated by head tilting and by jumping or falling, respectively. Both macular structures are sensitive to forward and backward movement. Fibers from the utricle and saccule compose portions of the vestibular division of cranial nerve VIII, which is the vestibulocochlear nerve. The vestibular division is important for the control of posture and the maintenance of balance. The cochlear division is responsible for hearing.

Nose

The nose is composed of bone in the upper third segment and cartilage in the lower two thirds. The midline point where the nose joins the forehead is called the nasion. The bridge of the nose is called the dorsum, and the base, which includes the nares (nostrils), is the point where the nose joins the upper lip.[22] The two nares are separated by the columella and allow air to enter and pass posteriorly to the nasopharynx. The nose is divided in the midline by the septum, which is composed of both prevents the roof from collapsing. The anterior cartilaginous portion melds into the medial margins of the lateral cartilage and holds them in place.[22]

The nasal cavity is an irregularly shaped space that extends from the bony palate, which separates the nose and mouth cavities, upward to the frontal, ethmoid, and sphenoid bones of the cranial cavity. The walls of the nasal cavity are made of bone covered with mucous membrane.

The vestibule of the nostril is lined with skin containing vibrissae, or nasal hairs, and some sebaceous and sweat glands. The nose is lined with respiratory mucosa, except for the skin in the vestibule and the olfactory epithelium. Mucus secreted by the mucosa is carried back to the nasopharynx by the cilia of the mucosa. The nasal mucosa is extremely vascular, which makes it appear redder than the oral mucosa.

The lateral wall of the nose has three and occasionally four nasal turbinates or conchae: the inferior, middle, superior, and supreme (FIG. 9-11). The supreme turbinate, if present, is quite small and cannot be seen during examination. The inferior turbinate is a separate bone, but the other three are part of the ethmoid bone. The turbinates greatly increase the surface area of the mucous membrane over which air travels as it passes through the nasal passages and into the nasopharynx. The nasolacrimal duct communicates indirectly with the lacrimal gland and opens onto the lateral surface of the inferior meatus of the nose. Tears drain continuously into the nose. If any part of the system becomes blocked or if tears are formed at an unusual rate, the fluid runs out onto the face.

The blood supply to the nose comes from the external and internal carotid arteries. The external carotid artery supplies blood primarily through one of its terminal divisions, the internal maxillary artery. This artery and its terminal branch, the sphenopalatine artery, supply blood to most of the posterior

system. The ethmoidal artery supplies blood to the anterosuperior part of the septum and the lateral wall of the nose. The external nose receives blood mainly from the same arteries as the internal nose, but venous drainage is partly through the angular vein, which leads into the inferior ophthalmic vein and the cavernous sinus or downward through the anterior facial vein.

The muscles of the external nose are innervated by the seventh cranial nerve. The external skin is innervated by the first and second divisions of the fifth cranial nerve. The nerve supply to the internal nose is from the olfactory nerve and the first and second divisions of the fifth cranial nerve.

The paranasal sinuses, which lighten the weight of the skull and give resonance and timbre to the voice, are air-filled, mucous membrane–lined cavities in the facial and cranial bones surrounding the nasal cavities. They drain into the nasal cavities through the ostia of the middle meatus (openings between the inferior and middle turbinates). The sinuses are in the frontal, sphenoid, ethmoid, and maxillary bones. The maxillary sinuses (or antrum of Highmore) are the largest and most accessible of the sinuses. They are within the maxillary bones on either side of the nose. The frontal sinuses are above the eyes, the ethmoid sinuses are between the eyes and nose, and the sphenoid sinuses lie at the rear of the nasal cavity. The sphenoid sinuses, which are the most deeply placed of the sinuses, are directly below the sella turcica, from which pituitary tumors can erode downward to fill them. Only the maxillary and ethmoid sinuses are present at birth; the frontal sinuses form during the second year of life, and the sphenoid sinuses form during the third year.

The normal physiologic functions of the paranasal sinuses are unknown. It has been proposed that they did not develop for any specific biologic reason but were formed incidentally to the forward and downward growth of the face during transition from infancy to adulthood.

Functions of the Nose. The major functions of the nose are air conditioning and olfaction; air conditioning refers to temperature and humidity control and to filtering of particles and bacteria in inspired air before it reaches the trachea, bronchi, and lungs. Inspired air reaches the nasopharynx in about ¼ second; during this short period, the temperature of the air reaches 36.11° to 36.67° C and the humidity becomes a constant 75% to 80%.[20]

Serum and mucus cover the surface of the nasal mucosa and can provide large amounts of water to be absorbed by cold, dry air. As much as 1 L of moisture can evaporate from the nose during 24 hours of normal breathing; the submucosal glands replenish this moisture as the water evaporates. The turbinates are covered with erectile tissue that can rapidly fill with blood, which allows greater control of temperature and humidification. The nose, sinuses, pharynx, trachea, bronchi, and bronchioles are covered by a continuous mucous blanket to which airborne particles cling on contact. The blanket contains lysozyme, an enzyme that causes most bacteria to disintegrate on contact. Cilia carry the mucous blanket with its trapped particulate matter back toward the nasopharynx where it is swallowed. Residual bacteria are then destroyed by hydrochloric acid and gastric juices.

The olfactory sense organs are located in the olfactory membrane that covers the roof of the nose and is reflected medially downward over the superior turbinate. The olfactory receptors are hair cells or chemoreceptors that are stimulated when air is inspired through the nose.

Pharynx

The pharynx, from the Greek word for throat, is the muscular tube that is behind the oral cavity and extends downward from the base of the skull to the larynx. The pharynx is a somewhat conical chamber. It conducts air between the nasal cavities and larynx and conducts food from the mouth to the esophagus.

The pharynx is divided into three sections: nasopharynx, oropharynx, and laryngopharynx. The nasopharynx is above the margin of the soft palate posterior to the nose; the oropharynx is the area behind the mouth that is visible when the tongue is depressed with a tongue blade; and the laryngopharynx is dorsal to the larynx (Fig. 9-12).

The nasopharynx lies behind the nasal cavities and communicates with them through the posterior nasal apertures. The nasopharynx also communicates with the middle ear through the eustachian tube about 1 cm behind the posterior end of the inferior turbinate. Near these openings are patches of lymphoid tissue called the pharyngeal tonsils, which lie in the mucous membrane at the junction of the posterior wall and roof. (Hypertrophied pharyngeal tonsils are adenoids.) The nasopharyngeal space opens inferiorly into the oropharynx so the floor is formed by the dorsal part of the soft palate, which is its only movable boundary. At birth the mucosal lining of the nasopharyngeal cavity is columnar ciliated epithelium, but this changes to patchy squamous epithelium between the ages of 10 and 80 years. Squamous epithelium covers about 80% of the posterior wall, and surface mucosa becomes stratified squamous epithelium after about age 10 years. Glands secreting mucus and serous fluid are scattered throughout the mucous membrane.

The oropharynx communicates with the nasopharynx above and the laryngopharynx below to the level of the epiglottis. The oropharynx contains the palatine tonsils, which with the pharyngeal and lingual tonsils (on the dorsum of the tongue) comprise Waldeyer's ring. This ring is a protective barrier of lymphoid tissue between the mouth and throat and the respiratory and digestive tracts. This lymphoid tissue is considered important in the development of immune bodies. If stimulated by bacterial infection, immune bodies promote the production of additional immune factors that provide future protection from bacterial infection.

The laryngopharynx boundaries are the superior constrictor muscle and vertebrae posteriorly, the larynx and pyriform fossa below, and hyoid bone, base of the tongue, and constrictor muscle above. The upper end of the epiglottis projects into the laryngopharynx.

The oropharynx and laryngopharynx are spaces surrounded by muscles that provide support to the surrounding tissue and a passageway through which air, food, and fluids can be ingested. Swallowing is accomplished by the action of the constrictor muscles in the pharynx and by the suprahyoid and infrahyoid muscles. Action of these muscles and their nerves is also responsible for the gag reflex, which protects the air and food passages from the entrance of any unwanted material. Two cranial nerves are responsible for the gag reflex: the glossopharyngeal nerve (cranial nerve IX) and the vagus nerve (cranial nerve X). The glossopharyngeal nerve has sensory and motor divisions. The sensory division supplies sensation to the pharynx, and the motor division innervates the posterior wall of the pharynx. The vagus nerve innervates all of the thoracic and abdominal viscera and conveys impulses from the walls of the intestines, the heart, and the lungs.

Tonsils. The tonsils are small masses of primarily lymphoid tissue. They are covered by mucous membrane and contain small openings that deliver phagocytes to the mouth and pharynx.

In the past, removal of the tonsils and adenoids was commonplace, but it is now known that the lymphoid tissue of the pharynx plays an important role in the immune system of the body, and they are not removed as routinely (Table 9-1).

The lymphoid tissues of Waldeyer's ring drain into the lymph nodes of the neck. The adenoids in the nasopharynx drain into the posterior cervical lymph glands, and the palatine and lingual tonsils drain into the anterior cervical lymph nodes.

Larynx

The larynx has several functions: (1) it is the air passageway between the pharynx and the lungs; (2) it prevents food and fluid from entering the lungs; and (3) it is involved in sound production or phonation.

The larynx is a roughly tubular structure with an irregular shape. It is somewhat wider at the top where it is attached to the pharynx and narrower below where it attaches to the trachea. The larynx is composed of cartilages, ligaments, and muscles that prevent the walls from collapsing on inspiration (Fig. 9-13). Three of the cartilages are paired and three are unpaired, for a total of nine cartilages (Table 9-2).

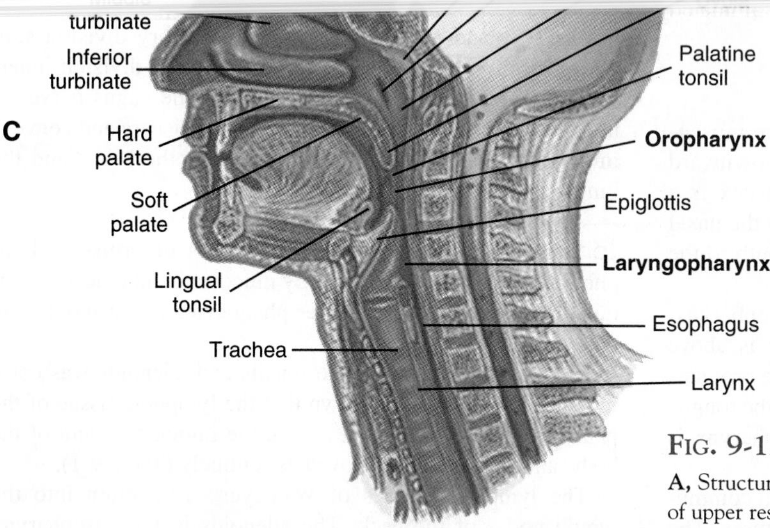

pharynx:

Two posterior nares (into the nasopharynx)
Two eustachian tubes (into the nasopharynx)
The fauces (into the oropharynx)
The larynx (into the laryngopharynx)
The esophagus (into the laryngopharynx)

FIG. 9-12

A, Structures of pharynx: Uvula, epiglottis, and tonsils. **B,** Structures of upper respiratory tract. **C,** Hypopharynx (posterior view).

Table 9-1 Types of Tonsils

Structure	Description
Pharyngeal tonsil or adenoid	Mass of lymphoid tissue in nasopharynx; extends from its roof almost to free end of soft palate; present in all infants and children; starts to regress just before puberty; normally absent in adults
Lateral pharyngeal bands	Extend down lateral wall of pharynx from adenoids; located behind posterior tonsillar pillar; gradually become thinner until they disappear below level of faucial tonsil
Faucial (palatine) tonsil	Located laterally at junction of oropharynx and oral cavity; composed of large lymphoid follicles; contains numerous crypts lined with squamous epithelium; supplied by tonsillar and palatine arteries, which come from external carotid artery
Lingual tonsils	Two masses of lymphoid tissue located on dorsum of tongue; extend from circumvallate papillae of tongue to epiglottis

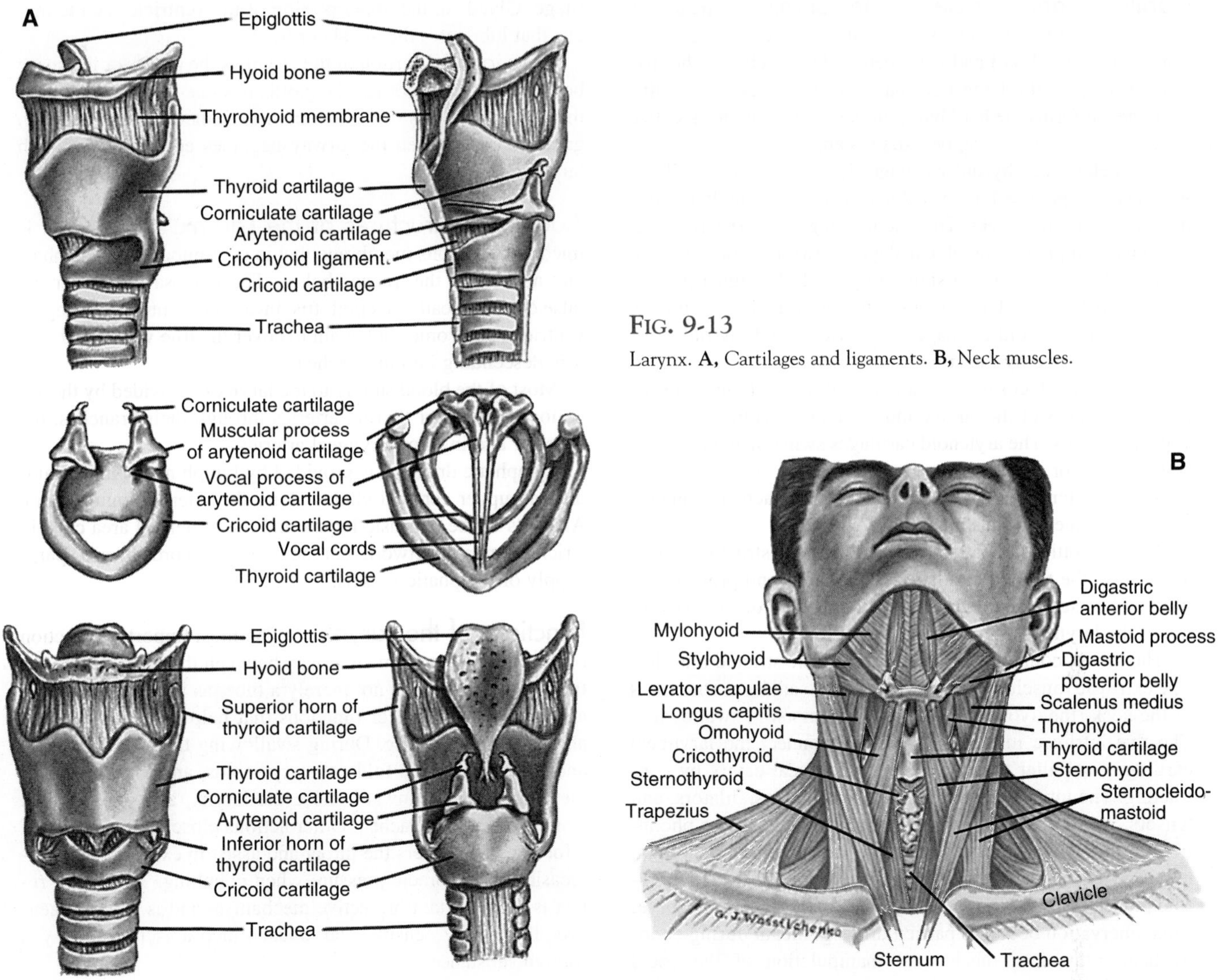

FIG. 9-13

Larynx. **A,** Cartilages and ligaments. **B,** Neck muscles.

Table 9-2 Cartilages and Muscles of the Larynx

Structure	Description
UNPAIRED CARTILAGES	
Thyroid	Largest cartilage of larynx; forms anterior midline shield called laryngeal prominence or Adam's apple
Cricoid	Only complete cartilaginous ring in respiratory tract; located just below thyroid cartilage
Epiglottis	Leaf shaped; projects upward at base of tongue and guards opening of larynx
PAIRED CARTILAGES	
Arytenoid, corniculate, and cuneiform	Serve as attachment for vocal ligaments; movement of cartilages controls tension of vocal ligaments
INTRINSIC MUSCLES	
Thyroarytenoideus	Tilts arytenoid cartilages toward thyroid; results in shortening and relaxation of vocal cords
Arytenoideus	Approximates arytenoid cartilages and closes glottis
Cricothyroideus	Lifts anterior section of cricoid cartilage; results in increased tension on vocal cords
POSTERIOR	
Cricoarytenoideus	Produces lateral rotation of arytenoid cartilages; results in separation of vocal cords and opening of glottis
LATERAL	
Cricoarytenoideus	Produces medial rotation of arytenoid cartilages; results in approximation

of the neck (the hyoid and sternum) and assist in swallowing. The five intrinsic muscles (Table 9-2) connect the laryngeal cartilages and alter the shape of the laryngeal cavity by contracting. The intrinsic muscles act as constrictors, dilators, and tensors, so they are important in sound production or phonation. A branch of the vagus nerve, the recurrent laryngeal nerve, supplies the intrinsic muscles except for the cricothyroid muscle, which is supplied by the superior laryngeal nerve. This innervation becomes particularly significant during endotracheal intubation; mechanical manipulation of the vocal cords and musculature may result in bradycardia from vagal stimulation.

Internal Structures of the Larynx. The internal structures are protected by the thyroid cartilage in front and include the vestibule, the false vocal cords, the true vocal cords, the laryngeal ventricle, and the glottis.

The inlet to the larynx lies in the anterior wall of the pharynx and is bordered by the epiglottis and arytenoid cartilages. From the inlet the larynx expands into a wide vestibule that ends at the level of the true vocal folds.

Inside the larynx are two pairs of shelflike folds that project inward from the lateral walls of the larynx. The superior folds, or false vocal cords, are attached to the cartilage anteriorly and the arytenoid cartilage posteriorly. They do not produce sound. Just under the false vocal cords are the true vocal cords. The true vocal cords are joined anteriorly where they attach to the inner surface of the thyroid cartilage. This is a fixed point at which the cords are held immobile, but they attach posteriorly to the movable arytenoid cartilages, which allow them to adduct and abduct.

The laryngeal ventricle, a fold of mucous membrane between the true and false cords, extends up under the thyroid car-

an organ with sphincter functions that help prevent aspiration and assist in coughing. During swallowing the larynx elevates and the aryepiglottic folds, the arytenoids, and the tubercle of the epiglottis fold inward, close the larynx, and prevent food from entering the trachea. Other actions close the glottis when a foreign body enters the throat and assist in expelling it by increasing intrathoracic pressure when coughing. The cough reflex is an important protective mechanism and is set off whenever the highly sensitive laryngeal mucosa is touched by a foreign substance.

Phonation, or the formation of speech sounds, is also an important function of the larynx. Although phonation is not its only purpose, the larynx is sometimes called the "voice box." During phonation, tracheal air pressure increases and decreases; as the edges of the vocal cords firm and relax, the larynx moves up and down so the air columns above and below are lengthened and shortened. The larynx creates sounds (humming or buzzing) as a result of vocal cord vibration. Words are formed when the vibrating column of air comes up from the larynx to the tongue, lips, palate, and teeth (FIG. 9-14). Movements of the mouth (articulation) actually form the words.

NORMAL FINDINGS*

Ear

External ear: Height and size equal; skin clean; no evidence of injury or trauma; ○ earlobes may appear pendulous

*○ = Older adult.

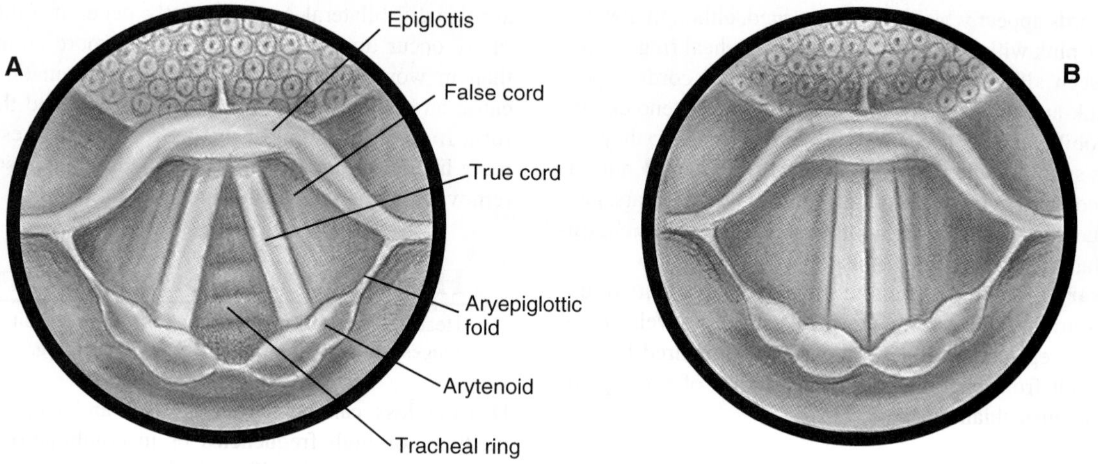

FIG. 9-14
Larynx. **A,** In quiet respiration. **B,** In phonation.

Auricle: Moves freely without causing pain; ⭘ may be more prominent

Tympanic membrane: Drumhead slightly conical, quite shiny, and pearl gray in color; oblique position when viewed with otoscope; cerumen color varying from black to brown to creamy pink; cerumen waxy or flaky; depending on translucency, should be possible to visualize the following in normal drumhead: malleus, anterior and posterior malleolar folds, annulus (whiter and denser than rest of drumhead), long process of incus (frequently seen posterior to manubrium of malleus), occasionally chorda tympani nerve seen crossing transversely behind drumhead at about level of short process of malleus; ⭘ some landmarks may appear more pronounced because of atrophied or sclerotic tympanic changes; cerumen may appear very dry as fewer sebaceous glands are active

Eustachian tube: Eardrum moves with Valsalva's maneuver if tube is patent

Vestibulocochlear nerve (cranial nerve VIII): Patient able to hear whisper from distance of 2 feet; tuning fork placed in middle of head heard equally well in both ears; ⭘ presbycusis (hearing loss from senile degenerative changes) may be present

Nose

Nares: Oval and symmetric

Mucosa: Nose lined with respiratory mucosa that is deep pink and glistening; ⭘ may be somewhat drier

Septum: Septum usually not straight but deviates from midline; posterior two thirds bony, anterior one third cartilaginous; ⭘ usually deviates

Turbinates: Turbinates deep pink and similar in color to rest of nasal mucosa; firm consistency

Sinuses: No tenderness, swelling, or purulent secretions from sinus ostia

Olfactory nerve (cranial nerve I): Patient able to identify odor of substances such as lemon or coffee; ⭘ sense of smell may be somewhat depressed

Pharynx

Oropharynx: Soft palate pink, showing fine vessels under mucosa; hard palate white, more irregular, showing rugae running transversely; ducts of mucous glands may be seen in back of hard palate; uvula may vary greatly in size and may be bifid or "split"; tonsils same color as rest of oral mucosa, with crypts of whitish epithelium showing; small irregular red or pink spots of lymphoid tissue commonly seen in mucosa of posterior pharyngeal wall; gag reflex induced by touching posterior wall of pharynx

Nasopharynx: Superior, middle, and inferior turbinates can be seen and may vary in size and appearance; orifice of eustachian tube seen, usually pale, yellowish, and small; orifice normally closed but opens during yawning and swallowing; adenoids seen growing from roof and posterior wall if not surgically removed, usually small after puberty

Hypopharynx: Circumvallate papillae in inverted V found on posterior tongue, may vary greatly in size; lingual tonsils on either side of tongue, may vary in size; small white spots that are debris in tonsillar crypts frequently seen; valleculae seen as cup-shaped spaces between tongue and epiglottis, may have large veins; epiglottis varies in size, shape, and color, free edge thin and slightly curved

Larynx

External (by visual examination): Thyroid cartilage (Adam's apple) protrudes, more obvious in men; laryngeal crepitation should occur when thyroid cartilage is grasped between thumb and forefinger and is moved from side to side; cricoid cartilage can be seen in thin persons with head extended and can be easily palpated; hyoid bone palpable above thyroid cartilage; cricoid cartilage drawn upward when patient says high-pitched E-E-E as normal cricothyroid muscle contracts; ⭘ thyroid cartilage may be very noticeable

Internal (by indirect laryngoscopy): Cords move only slightly during normal respiration; phonation causes adduction of cords, which should approximate perfectly; true

Nonmalignant tumors may develop on the external ear or anywhere in the ear canal. They rarely become malignant, but they may occlude the ear canal and cause retention of cerumen and a conductive hearing loss. The prognosis is excellent with proper diagnosis and treatment.

PATHOPHYSIOLOGY

Keloids are large overgrowths of hypertrophied scar tissue that result from surgery or trauma. They are much more common in blacks than in whites. In the ear keloids commonly form as a result of ear piercing; however, other trauma to the auricle can also cause them. Keloids may also appear with no history of trauma. The treatment is excision, followed by repeated injections of a long-lasting steroid. Recently, carbon dioxide laser resection of the keloid has been performed, allowing the wound bed to heal by secondary intention with good results.

Nodules may form along the superior rim of the auricle and become indurated or painful. The cause is unknown. Treatment is excision or injection of a long-lasting steroid such as methylprednisolone or triamcinolone (Kenalog).

Sebaceous cysts are sebaceous glands that become obstructed with sebum, a soft, cheesy material. These cysts may occur in the meatus of the canal or just behind the earlobe. They are normally painless, but can enlarge quickly and become painful if infected. Acute sebaceous cysts are incised and drained, and hot, moist compresses are applied.

Exostoses are small, hard, bony lumps covered with normal epithelium. They arise from the osseous ear canal near the tympanic membrane and are attached to the posterior wall. The bases of these exostoses are close to the facial nerve. Exostoses

function, depending on the severity.

Many individuals in industrialized societies are exposed to high levels of noise. Noise exposure is the major cause of acquiring hearing loss in the United States; it is ranked as one of the country's major health problems by the National Institute of Occupational Safety and Health. Permanent threshold shifts can also result from exposure to a number of ototoxic agents—ototoxic compounds, such as aspirin, are the most commonly used drugs in industrialized societies.

PATHOPHYSIOLOGY

The six types of hearing loss are sensorineural, conductive, mixed, congenital, simulated, and central.

Sensorineural Hearing Loss. Sensorineural hearing loss is the result of disease within the cochlea, the cochlear nerve, or the brain. It usually results from trauma, an infectious process, a degenerative process such as presbycusis, a senile degenerative change in the hair cells in the organ of Corti, a congenital abnormality, or exposure to ototoxic substances such as certain drugs.

Exposure to high-level noise appears to damage the cochlea in a temporary and in a permanent manner. Extremely high level exposures, such as impulse noise, may cause direct mechanical damage of the hair cells and supporting cells in the organ of Corti and the lateral wall of the cochlea.

Ototoxic drugs (aminoglycoside antibiotics and cisplatin) clearly increase damage caused by concurrent exposure to noise; ototoxic drugs also cause permanent damage when administered alone. The initial site of damage appears to be the hair cells.

HEARING AND BALANCE DISORDERS IN THE ELDERLY

Presbycusis is hearing loss in the elderly patient. Changes in the inner ear result in a predominantly high-frequency sensorineural hearing loss. The hearing loss may be associated with tinnitus (ringing in the ears). Although presbycusis cannot be cured, some patients may benefit from the use of a hearing aid. Consultation with an audiologist will allow the patient to experiment with various techniques to enhance hearing and communication.

Presbyvertigo (presbyastasis) is the vestibular disorder associated with aging. When a balance disorder occurs in this group of patients, it is usually associated with a decrease in visual acuity and altered proprioception. The three systems are necessary to maintain balance; therefore the elderly may have more difficulty ambulating, resulting in falls and injury. As with presbycusis, presbyvertigo cannot be cured but the symptoms can be controlled. Consultation with a physical therapist can provide the patient with vestibular (balance) exercises to help accommodate to the vertigo. In addition, the use of a cane or walker can be attempted to compensate for the loss of stability.

This may also be called perceptive or nerve-type hearing loss. Patients with sensorineural hearing losses are often unable to use hearing aids satisfactorily.

Conductive Hearing Loss. Conductive hearing loss is also called transmission hearing loss. It occurs in disorders of the external or middle ear such as otitis media, otosclerosis, or a perforated eardrum. These patients have a normal inner ear, but sound waves are prevented from reaching the inner ear normally. If sound is amplified, these patients may be able to hear very well, and therefore a hearing aid can be beneficial. With the exception of otosclerosis in which the drumhead usually appears normal, disorders that cause conductive hearing loss also cause changes in the normal appearance of the drumhead, such as thickening or retraction.

Mixed Hearing Loss. Some patients have both conductive and sensorineural hearing losses.

Congenital Hearing Loss. Congenital hearing loss is present from birth or early infancy. "Neonatal" causes may be anoxia, trauma during delivery, or Rh incompatibility. Other causes may be maternal exposure to syphilis or rubella during pregnancy or the use of ototoxic drugs during pregnancy. Infants with serum bilirubin levels greater than 20 mg/dl may also incur hearing losses from the toxic effect of high bilirubin levels on the brain.

Simulated Hearing Loss. Simulated hearing loss is also called functional, psychogenic, or nonorganic hearing loss. It means that an apparent hearing loss is not the result of an organic cause and may represent malingering or a functional disorder.

Central Hearing Loss. Central loss is caused by damage to the brain's auditory pathways, as in a cerebrovascular accident.

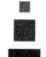

Diagnostic Studies and Findings

Weber's test: The tip of the handle of a vibrating tuning fork is placed on the patient's forehead or front teeth. The patient is asked if the sound is heard in the head, right ear, or left ear. Sound is heard in the head or equally in both ears if the patient has normal hearing. Lateralization of sound to the deaf ear occurs in conductive hearing loss; lateralization of sound to the better ear occurs in sensorineural hearing loss.

Rinne test: A vibrating tuning fork is alternately placed against the mastoid bone (to determine bone conduction) or in front of the ear (for air conduction). Bone conduction is heard longer than or equal to air conduction in conductive hearing loss; air conduction is heard longer but not twice as long as bone conduction in sensorineural hearing loss.

Schwabach's test: Schwabach's test compares the hearing of the examiner with the patient. The vibrating tuning fork is placed on the mastoid bone of both the examiner and patient. The patient hears longer than the examiner in conductive hearing loss; the examiner hears longer than the patient in sensorineural hearing loss.

Audiometric tests: Speech and impedance audiometry, tympanometry, and electrocochleography are used to differentiate between types of hearing loss and to identify the degree of hearing impairment.[2]

Multidisciplinary Plan

Surgery

Depending on the type of hearing impairment, a variety of surgical interventions may be appropriate

Stapedectomy: See p. 624

Cochlear implant: Provides auditory sensation to patients with severe bilateral hearing loss who have not had any successful hearing with a hearing aid; complex procedure in which inferior aspect of the basal scala tympani is exposed; bone is removed from inferior margins of scala tympani for distance of approximately 4 to 5 mm from round window; surgeon then negotiates the tip of the Silastic-sheathed multielectrode around the first turn of the basal cochlea in the bony groove in the posterior canal wall, which is then covered with cortical bone and temporalis fascia; device electrically stimulates remaining, intact, and excitable auditory neurons in profoundly deaf individuals; electronic "heart" of device is small processor that can be carried on belt and can receive sound through microphone and electronically break signal into four channels; a tiny transmitter, which is mounted behind ear, sends signal to receiver implanted under skin; from internal receiver, fine wire leads to electrode, which is implanted against auditory nerves in cochlea.

Environmental and speech sounds are picked up by a microphone and sent to a sound processing unit that filters the stimuli. The auditory stimuli are changed into an electrical pattern that goes to the external transmitter.

recommended

NURSING CARE

NURSING ASSESSMENT

Stares blankly or has strained facial expression; speaks loudly; asks to have things repeated; gives irrelevant answers to questions; may not participate in conversations; withdraws; may hear much better when watching speaker's face; inattentive; daydreams; scholastic performance below apparent ability (if school age); delayed speech and language development (if small child); may complain of sound distortion; intolerant of loud noise

POTENTIAL COMPLICATIONS

Safety

PATIENT PROBLEMS/NURSING DIAGNOSES & INTERVENTIONS

NIC COMMUNICATION ENHANCEMENT

Disturbed sensory perception (auditory) related to hearing impairment

- Assess patient's degree of hearing impairment and concomitant ability to communicate with others.
- Ensure that other health-care providers are aware of patient's hearing impairment; place a note in computer, on door, and at intercom at nursing station.
- When conversing, speak slowly and distinctly and face patient directly *so patient can see your face.* Do not shout or overexaggerate words.
- Ensure that patient has heard and understood everything said.

PATIENT EDUCATION/CONTINUUM OF CARE PLAN

1. Demonstrate for the patient the proper use and maintenance of hearing aid, if prescribed (see below).
2. Ensure that the patient and family are aware of any postoperative instructions, if appropriate.
3. Encourage the patient to ask people to speak more slowly or clearly or to repeat statements so the patient does not feel left out of conversations.
4. Encourage referral for aural rehabilitation, if indicated.

Care of a hearing aid

1. Turn the hearing aid off when not in use.
2. Open the battery compartment at night to avoid accidental drainage of the battery.
3. Keep an extra battery available at all times.
4. Wash the earmold frequently (daily if necessary) with mild soap and warm water, using a pipe cleaner to cleanse the cannula.
5. Dry the earmold completely before reconnecting it to the receiver.
6. Do not wear the hearing aid if an ear infection is present.

What to do if hearing aid fails to work

1. Check the on-off switch.
2. Inspect the earmold for cleanliness.
3. Examine the battery for correct insertion.
4. Examine the cord plug for correct insertion.
5. Examine the cord for breaks.
6. Replace the battery, cord, or both, if necessary. The life of batteries varies according to the amount of use and the power requirements of the aid. Batteries last from 2 to 14 days.

7. Check the position of the earmold in the ear. If the hearing aid "whistles," the earmold is probably not inserted properly into the ear canal, or the person needs to have a new earmold made.

EVALUATION/PATIENT OUTCOMES

Communication Enhancement: Patient recovers uneventfully (if surgery performed). Hearing level is improved to normal. Patient verbalizes ear regimen and any symptoms to be re- [illegible]

[illegible] tient has learned to use strategies, such as lip reading or sign language.

EXTERNAL OTITIS

External otitis is a general term used to describe inflammatory diseases of the auricle and the external auditory canal. [illegible]

a combination of the two. It is [illegible] sometimes called swimmer's ear. External otitis varies in severity; occasionally no infection is present, and it may result from either contact or seborrheic dermatitis. Either bacteria or fungi may produce infectious external otitis. Bacterial causes are usually attributed to *Pseudomonas, Proteus, Streptococcus,* or *Staphylococcus.* Fungi are usually *Aspergillus* and *Candida.* Predisposing factors include allergies that may increase the likelihood of external otitis; irritants such as hair sprays, hair dyes, or dust that cause the person to scratch the ear canal, resulting in excoriation; cleaning or scratching the ear canal with a foreign object, such as a cotton swab, bobby pin, or finger, which causes irritation and possible introduction of infectious organisms; continual use of earphones, earplugs, hearing aid, or earmuffs, which trap moisture in the ear, thereby creating a medium for infection; and swimming in contaminated water, which is absorbed by the wax in the ear, macerates the skin of the canal, and allows the introduction of organisms.

PATHOPHYSIOLOGY

Acute external otitis is frequently caused by *Pseudomonas,* which can be cultured from the auditory canal. The infection begins in the external auditory canal, usually after minor trauma, and may spread to involve the cartilage and perichondrium. If left untreated, the infection can progress to involve the brain and cranial nerves.

Acute external otitis can range from mild to severe. Pain is moderate to severe and is aggravated by traction on the auricle or pressure on the tragus. The patient may have a low-grade fever and a sticky, yellow discharge from the ear canal. There may be a loss of hearing or the feeling of a blocked ear if the ear canal is swollen or obstructed with debris.

The external auditory canal is swollen or entirely closed, and the tragus and external meatus are also swollen. The epithelium of the canal is usually soggy and pale. Desquamated epithelium and wax are often present in the canal. However, the canal may be reddened rather than pale, or the epithelium may be dry instead of wet. Patients may also have lymphadenopathy anterior to the tragus, behind the ear, or in the upper neck. If the auricle is involved, the skin is crusted and oozing. Pustules may be present, and the ear may be swollen and tender. If the infection did not originate on the face or scalp, it may spread to these areas. The eardrum frequently cannot be seen well in acute external otitis because of [illegible]

[illegible] usual complaint. There is no pain even with manipulation of the auricle or tragus. The epithelium is thickened and red, and the canal and drumhead are insensitive to pressure from cotton applicators. A discharge is usually present.

[illegible] external otitis, is caused by *Pseudomonas* and occasionally by [illegible]

[illegible] ish with *Aspergillus niger*) forms in the ear canal. Removal reveals a hyperemic, edematous epithelium that may be denuded. Fungal infections may be asymptomatic because frequently the growth is found only on wax or other debris in the ear and has not invaded the tissue.

Furunculosis is a localized type of external otitis in the outer half of the ear canal. Glands and hair follicles in this area may become infected and form boils or furuncles. The onset of a furuncle may be acute; the patient may notice a feeling of fullness in the ear, loss of hearing, adenopathy, and swelling behind the ear. The area is reddened. It may be very swollen and may obstruct the entire canal. Pain is intense; even a small furuncle causes severe pain until it is surgically drained or breaks spontaneously. Movement of the auricle and tragus causes pain, as does chewing if the furuncle is on the canal floor or anterior wall.

DIAGNOSTIC STUDIES AND FINDINGS

Culture of drainage: Identification of causative organisms

MULTIDISCIPLINARY PLAN

Surgery

Surgery not performed unless furuncle needs incision and drainage

Medications

Narcotic analgesics such as codeine, 30 mg PO q4h

Corticosteroids: A wick is inserted into the ear canal; hydrocortisone and acetic acid otic solution may be used to reduce swelling and to allow penetration of antibiotics

Antiinfective agents: Antibiotic or antifungal ear drops may be prescribed, which usually contain 0.5% neomycin or 10,000

U/ml of polymyxin; if ear canal is swollen, a wick may be inserted to allow drops to reach ear canal; systemic antibiotics: may be prescribed if infection is severe; specific drug depends on causative organism

General Management

Careful cleaning of ear canal to remove debris and impacted cerumen

Heat therapy to external ear for pain relief

For malignant external otitis: hyperbaric O_2 therapy may be used to reverse tissue hypoxia and augment the action of aminoglycoside antibiotics (for advanced or recurrent cases)[3]

NURSING CARE

Nursing Assessment

Infection of External Ear

Acute: Moderate to severe pain in the ear, which is exacerbated by chewing and manipulation of the auricle or tragus; headache; fever; feeling of fullness or blockage in ear; foul-smelling, yellow, sticky discharge from ear (black if from fungal infection); hearing normal or decreased; tinnitus; localized swelling; erythema; lymphadenopathy

Chronic: Chief complaint itching rather than pain; discharge usually present

Patient Problems/Nursing Diagnoses & Interventions

NIC Skin/Wound Management

Impaired skin integrity related to involvement of skin by infectious process

- Assess ear canal and auricle for swelling, crusting, scabs, pustules, and drainage.
- Keep ear canal clean: Cleanse gently with cotton swab soaked with Burow's solution (as ordered) and also apply directly to auricle. Dry gently and completely.
- Administer antibiotics as ordered.
- Instill medicated ear drops as ordered.
- Observe and record amount of aural drainage.

NIC Physical Comfort Promotion

Acute pain related to ear infection

- Assess need for pain medication and in collaboration with physician, provide medication as required *for pain relief;* evaluate and document effectiveness.
- Monitor vital signs, especially temperature.
- If chewing is painful, arrange for soft or full-liquid diet.

NIC Communication Enhancement

Disturbed sensory perception (auditory) related to obstruction of ear canal from edema or debris

- Assess degree of hearing impairment.
- If patient's hearing is diminished, be sure that alternate method of communication is used.
- Speak slowly and clearly and stand directly in front of patient when speaking.

Patient Education/Continuum of Care Plan

1. Discuss with the patient and family the necessity of completing the prescribed course of medication, whether antibiotics or ear drops, to avoid inadequate treatment or possible recurrence.
2. Demonstrate to the patient and family the proper way to instill ear drops (Box 9-1).

INSTRUCTIONS FOR USING EAR WASH AND DROPS — Box 9-1

The patient will need a 2- or 3-ounce ear syringe and a prescription for ear wash and drops. The patient should have a family member or another caregiver perform the ear washing according to the following instructions:

1. Wash hands before and after the earwashing procedure.
2. Fill the ear syringe with the solution.
3. The solution must be at body temperature. If the solution is too warm or too cool, the patient will feel dizzy. Warm the solution by placing the syringe in a pan of hot water. Do *not* warm the solution on the stove or in the microwave.
4. Have the patient lie down with the ear to be washed facing up. Pull up and out on the external ear. Place the tip of the ear syringe into the ear canal. Do not be afraid to push it down into the ear. However, a return flow of solution should be noted. If not, the syringe is in too far. Pull the syringe out slightly.
5. Pump the warmed solution from the syringe back and forth into the ear by squeezing and releasing the bulb of the syringe. Do this very vigorously and repeatedly. The ear wash must be forced back and forth, in and out of the ear canal.
6. Have the patient lean over the side of the sink or basin and let the solution run out of the ear.
7. Pull the ear up, back, and out to straighten the ear canal.
8. Put 3 to 5 warmed drops into the ear.
9. If the solution burns too much at first, it may need to be diluted. Mix 2 ounces of water with 2 ounces of the solution. Later, decrease the amount of water used with each irrigation.
10. Use the solution and drops twice a day for 2 weeks and then until the ear stops running or becomes dry. If it is uncertain whether the ear is dry, check it by putting a cotton swab down into the ear canal. If the cotton swab comes out dry, stop using the solution and drops. If the cotton swab is wet or there is an odor from the ear, continue using the solution and drops for 4 days.
11. Do not use the solution and drops as long as the ear remains dry and is not running, and as long as there is no odor. Should the ear start to run after being dry for a period of time, start using the ear solution and drops until the ear is once again dry.

Instruct the patient to prevent any water from getting into the ear. Instruct the patient to refrain from swimming. Whenever there is a chance that water may get into the ear, such as when the patient showers or washes the hair, the patient should put cotton in the ear. First, place a dry piece of cotton in the ear, then a second piece of cotton that has been saturated with petroleum jelly.

Instruct the patient to call the physician if there are questions.

3. If Burow's soaks are done, give instructions in the proper method.
4. Instruct patient and family about factors contributing to development of external otitis and encourage patient to keep foreign objects such as bobby pins out of ears.
5. Encourage patient to use earplugs when swimming and to minimize amount of water that gets into ears when showering and shampooing.

EVALUATION/PATIENT OUTCOMES

lymphadenopathy. Patient and family verbalize increased knowledge of disease and its treatment.

Physical Comfort: No pain is present in the ear.

Communication Enhancement: Hearing is within normal

PERICHONDRITIS

Perichondritis is an inflammation of the auricular cartilage.

Perichondritis may follow a skin infection or trauma, which causes exposure of the cartilage to bacteria.

PATHOPHYSIOLOGY

Perichondritis may be initiated by trauma, insect bites, or incision of superficial infections of the pinna, which causes pus to accumulate between the cartilage and the perichondrium. The causative organism is usually a gram-negative rod, frequently *Pseudomonas.* Perichondritis can cause a loss of blood supply to the cartilage, resulting in breakdown and necrosis of the cartilage. The pinna appears enlarged, inflamed, and shiny. Pain is usually severe, and localized fluctuant areas may be present on the auricle. Perichondritis must be treated early and aggressively to prevent a lengthy, destructive course.

DIAGNOSTIC STUDIES AND FINDINGS

Culture of purulent material: Identification of causative organism

MULTIDISCIPLINARY PLAN

Surgery

Incision and drainage of any purulent material; removal of any necrotic cartilage

Medications

Antiinfective agents: Systemic parenteral antibiotic therapy, depending on cultured organisms; local irrigations with antibiotic solutions

Narcotic analgesics or analgesic/antipyretic agents: Analgesia for pain relief; aspirin or acetaminophen (Tylenol), 650 mg, with codeine, 30 mg PO q4h

General Management

Small polyethylene tube inserted into area beneath nonpressure dressing to facilitate irrigation; local heat applications for relief

NURSING ASSESSMENT

the cartilage; fluctuant areas on auricle; severe pain; may have fever or lymphadenopathy; history of trauma, insect bite, or incision of superficial infection on pinna

POTENTIAL COMPLICATIONS

Recurrent infection; deformity of ear

PATIENT PROBLEMS/NURSING DIAGNOSES & INTERVENTIONS

lage

- Assess need for pain medication and provide analgesic medications for pain relief as ordered. Evaluate and document effectiveness.

NIC COMMUNICATION ENHANCEMENT

Disturbed sensory perception (auditory) related to obstruction of ear canal or use of ototoxic drugs

- Assess patient's hearing ability before and during treatment with ototoxic drugs.

NIC SKIN/WOUND MANAGEMENT

Impaired skin integrity related to inflammation of and altered circulation to auricular cartilage

- Assess auricular cartilage for inflammation, swelling, and presence of pus.
- Perform wound care of affected area if incision and drainage have been done.
- Apply local heat for comfort as ordered.
- Administer antibiotics as ordered.
- Perform irrigations as ordered with room-temperature antibiotic solution.
- Be aware that irrigating solution contains potentially ototoxic drugs.
- Monitor vital signs, especially temperature.

PATIENT EDUCATION/CONTINUUM OF CARE PLAN

1. Discuss with the patient and family the necessity of completing the prescribed course of antibiotics to avoid recurrence or complications.
2. If wound care is being done, be sure that the patient and family know the procedures to change the dressing and aseptic techniques to avoid wound contamination.

EVALUATION/PATIENT OUTCOMES

Physical Comfort Promotion: Patient is free of pain. Patient can tolerate pain or is comfortable with analgesia prescribed.

Communication Enhancement: No hearing impairment exists. Patient's hearing remains at pretreatment level.

Skin/Wound Management: Inflammation of auricular cartilage is absent. There is no drainage from affected ear. Temperature is within normal limits for patient. There are no fluctuant areas on auricle. Patient and family demonstrate ability to change dressing properly using aseptic technique. Patient and family verbalize and demonstrate knowledge of treatment. Patient and family verbalize understanding of necessity of completing prescribed course of antibiotics to prevent recurrence of infection.

OTITIS MEDIA

Otitis media is an inflammation of the middle ear and can be classified as acute and suppurative or subacute (otitis media with effusion).

Acute Otitis Media

Acute otitis media is very common in young children and is usually the result of a bacterial or viral infection of the upper respiratory tract. Organisms travel from the nasopharynx to the middle ear by way of the eustachian tube. Infants and children have shorter, straighter eustachian tubes than do adults; this easier access to the middle ear is probably the reason otitis media is common in children. Another contributing factor is that children have not developed immunities to the organisms that cause the infection. Children also have a large mass of adenoid tissue that usually disappears during adolescence. If this lymphoid tissue is swollen, it can obstruct the opening of the eustachian tube and contribute to the development of otitis media by preventing equalization of the atmospheric pressure in the ear, thereby causing a vacuum and effusion of the middle ear.

Most episodes of recurrent acute otitis media occur between 6 and 36 months of age and in the winter and early spring.

Although the prognosis for acute otitis media is good, successful treatment requires patients to follow medical regimens and to keep scheduled appointments with caregivers for proper follow-up.

Epidemiologic studies have shown that up to 80% of all children who have not yet attained school age have episodes of eustachian tube dysfunction and secretory otitis media of varying duration. In addition to causing reduced hearing and various eardrum changes, secretory otitis media predisposes to acute middle ear infection and perhaps even chronic otitis media and cholesteatoma later in life.

Otitis Media With Effusion (Subacute)

Otitis media with effusion results from incomplete resolution or inadequate treatment of acute otitis media. The most recent evidence indicates that bacteria or bacterial products are trapped in the middle ear as a result of poor eustachian tube function. This situation causes a high negative pressure in the middle ear and produces transudation of fluid from the blood vessels in the membranes of the middle ear. Another factor may be failure to clear the bacteria and bacterial products by dysfunctional phagocytes or inadequate host-immune response to eradicate bacteria. These trapped bacteria in the middle ear initiate a host response that causes tissue injury leading to otitis media with effusion. Otitis media with effusion can also be caused by allergies that produce edema in the lumen of the eustachian tube or by barotrauma that results from external pressure markedly exceeding lowered pressure of the middle ear, as during diving or the descent of an airplane. It is common in children.

Patients feel a fullness in their ears but have no pain or fever. A conductive hearing loss may occur, especially in chronic otitis media with effusion. Otoscopic examination reveals mild retraction of the tympanic membrane with a clear transudate from the blood vessels. The tympanic membrane is immobile and amber colored, and a fluid level or air bubbles may be seen through the tympanic membrane. The meniscus of the fluid may appear as a thin black hair or line across the tympanic membrane. If blood is present, as with barotrauma, the fluid may appear blue-black.

Treatment consists of inflation of the eustachian tube, a Valsalva's maneuver (in which the patient inspires, holds the breath, and bears down as though having a bowel movement) several times a day, myringotomy to drain fluid from the middle ear, or decongestant therapy to improve eustachian tube function.

Chronic otitis media with effusion that results from inadequate treatment of acute otitis media or from overgrowth of the lymphoid tissue in the nasopharynx caused by sinonasal infections or allergies poses a serious threat to the patient's hearing. There are few symptoms; a fluctuating hearing loss or a feeling of heaviness on one side of the head is most common. Treatment is directed at the underlying cause and the removal of fluid by myringotomy. A small tube is frequently inserted during myringotomy to equalize pressure on both sides of the eardrum and is left in place for 8 to 9 months, when it is usually falls out by itself. If the condition does not resolve, the tube may be replaced. Patients should be instructed not to swim while a tube is in place.

Not to be overlooked as a cause of chronic otitis media with effusion in adults is carcinoma of the nasopharynx; if the effusion is unilateral, a thorough workup must be done to rule out carcinoma.

Chronic otitis media caused by repeated attacks of acute otitis media, and acute mastoiditis may result in a permanent perforation of the tympanic membrane. Chronic changes such as thickening and scarring of the mucosa eventually occur in the middle ear, and the ossicles may be destroyed. These permanent tympanic perforations result in a conductive hearing loss. If the ossicles are involved, the hearing loss may be greater.

There are two types of perforations: central and marginal. In central perforations the margin of the eardrum is not involved; in marginal perforations the annulus or margin of the drum is destroyed. Central perforations are more benign than marginal ones and less likely to result in cholesteatomas. Cholesteatomas occur when the marginal perforation of the eardrum allows squamous epithelium of the external auditory canal to grow into the middle ear, which then becomes lined with squamous epithelium. As the epithelium grows, it desquamates and the debris collects inside the middle ear. Cholesteatomas enlarge slowly, expand into the mastoid antrum, and destroy adjacent structures.

The most common symptom of chronic otitis media is a constant, painless, serous discharge from the ear, which varies from foul smelling to nearly odorless. The discharge becomes much worse when the patient has an infection of the upper respiratory tract, and it occasionally causes slight discomfort in the ear.

Treatment consists of thoroughly cleaning the ear and in-

(See p. 630.)

Pathophysiology

The usual pathogens of acute otitis media are gram-positive

as a barrier to infection is lost. Edema decreases the size of the lumen, and inflammation causes hyperemia of the mucosal lining of the middle ear, which results in increased oxygen absorption. This leads to decreased aeration, development of a partial vacuum, retraction of the tympanic membrane, and serous exudation. This stage is common in viral infections of the upper respiratory tract, but the infection does not progress if the middle ear is reaerated. However, if bacterial superinfection is present, the exudate becomes purulent and causes bulging of the tympanic membrane as the pus collects behind it. This is called purulent otitis media.

Diagnostic Studies and Findings

Culture of purulent drainage: Identification of causative organisms

Multidisciplinary Plan

Surgery

Myringotomy: To drain pus and fluid from middle ear (see p. 623)

Medications

Antiinfective agents

Amoxicillin (Amoxil, Wymox), 500 mg PO tid for 10 days

Sulfamethoxazole with trimethoprim (Septra or Bactrim), 1 tab PO bid for 10 days (if allergic to penicillin)

Penicillin G or V, 250-500 mg PO q6h for 10 days for patients older than 8 years

Ampicillin (Ampicin, others), 50-100 mg/kg/day for 10 days for children under 8 years because of frequency of *H. influenzae* infections in this age group

If patient is allergic to penicillin, erythromycin (E-Mycin, others), 250 mg PO q6h for adults and older children; combination of erythromycin and sulfisoxazole for children younger than 8 years

Analgesic-antipyretic or narcotic analgesics: Codeine, 30 mg PO q4h (for severe pain); sedatives sometimes given to small children

Antihistamines: Chlorpheniramine (Chlor-Trimeton), 4 mg PO q4-6h for 7-10 days for adults; 0.35 mg/kg qid for

General Management

A new therapy involves teaching children a method of autoinflation using a special tube designed to improve middle ear ventilation and thereby reduce the need for inserting ventilation tubes.

Infectious process: Fever that may be as high as 40° C (104° F); chills; malaise, weakness and dizziness; nausea and vomiting; tympanic membrane appears red, inflamed, and bulging; if it is perforated, pulsating purulent material can be seen coming through drum after ear is cleaned of pus and debris

Potential Complications

Hearing loss, perforation of tympanic membrane, mastoiditis, cholesteatoma

Patient Problems/Nursing Diagnoses & Interventions

NIC Skin/Wound Management

Impaired skin integrity related to skin contamination by purulent material

- Assess patient's ear canal for purulent drainage.
- If patient has had myringotomy, keep ear clean and dry.
- Place sterile cotton in outer ear *to absorb drainage and prevent possible contamination of outer ear (external otitis.)*
- Monitor vital signs, especially temperature, and report any changes.
- Instruct patient/family to avoid introduction of water in ear canals, which can produce an environment for bacterial growth.

NIC Physical Comfort Promotion

Acute pain related to buildup of pus behind tympanic membrane

- Determine need for pain medication and provide analgesia as ordered; evaluate and document effectiveness.
- Administer sedatives, if ordered, to young children as needed, *to assist with relaxation and sleep.*

- Instruct parents in appropriate dosages of medication to give child at home.
- Encourage bed rest if patient is weak, complains of malaise, or has nausea and vomiting.

NIC Communication Enhancement

Disturbed sensory perception (auditory) related to fluid in middle ear

- Assess patient for symptoms of hearing deficit.
- If patient is child, ask parents if they have noticed any signs of hearing loss: inattentiveness, blank stares, lack of response to questions, or pulling at affected ear. (Ear pain is frequently so severe that hearing loss is not noticed.)
- Administer antibiotics as ordered and instruct patients and family about appropriate dosages.
- Instruct patient or family to monitor level of hearing (it should return to normal with appropriate antibiotic therapy).

Patient Education/Continuum of Care Plan

1. Discuss with the patient and family the necessity for completing the entire course of antibiotics to prevent a recurrence or complications.
2. Explain to the parents the need to feed children in an upright position and not lying down to prevent reflux of nasopharyngeal flora through the eustachian tube into the middle ear.
3. Explain to the patient the need to avoid blowing the nose forcefully, which can force contaminated material into the eustachian tube.
4. If the patient has had a myringotomy, demonstrate to the patient and family how to change the cotton in the outer ear at least twice a day.
5. Instruct patient/parents to avoid the introduction of water in ear by using earplugs or inserting a cotton ball coated with petroleum jelly into ear canal when showering or shampooing hair.

Evaluation/Patient Outcomes

Skin/Wound Management: Skin integrity is maintained. There is no purulent drainage from tympanic membrane. Tympanic membrane appears normal with no bulging, redness, retraction, or inflammation.

Physical Comfort Promotion: Patient's comfort level is increased. Pain is decreased. Patient can sleep through the night and experiences no nausea or vomiting. Patient is afebrile. Activity level is normal.

Communication Enhancement: Hearing is intact. Patient's hearing is at preinfection level, or the family knows to monitor carefully for return of hearing.

Patient and family have increased knowledge of treatment. Patient and family verbalize understanding of necessity for completing prescribed course of antibiotics and the need to seek medical intervention if symptoms persist or recur.

Mastoiditis

Mastoiditis is an inflammation of the air cells of the mastoid cavity.

Usually of bacterial origin, mastoiditis is the result of the extension of a middle ear infection. It was quite common before the discovery of antibiotics but is now found only in patients with inadequately or untreated otitis media.

Pathophysiology

Mastoiditis occurs when infection progresses into the bony portion of the mastoid antrum and cells. This can cause bony necrosis of the mastoid process and breakdown of its bony structure.

With mastoiditis, large amounts of thick purulent material usually fill the external auditory canal, which indicates perforation of the tympanic membrane. The soft tissue that is next to the eardrum may be ruptured and sagging. X-ray examinations of the mastoid are needed to determine the extent of involvement. Findings vary from clouding of the air cells and some decalcification of the bony walls to complete coalescence of the air cells. If early decalcification is present, intense antibiotic therapy and myringotomy can usually cure mastoiditis; if it has progressed to further destruction, simple mastoidectomy is necessary. Chronic infection can also lead to the development of a cholesteatoma.

Diagnostic Studies and Findings

Mastoid x-ray examinations: May show cloudy air cells and decalcification of cell walls; cholesteatoma

Audiometric testing: To show and document amount of hearing loss and middle ear impedance

Multidisciplinary Plan

Surgery

Mastoidectomy if necessary; involves removing involved bone and cleansing area; can be performed through postaural or endaural incision

Myringotomy to drain fluid and pus from middle ear (see p. 623)

Medications

Antiinfective agents
- Penicillin G procaine suspension 600,000-1,200,000 U IM
- Penicillin G aqueous, 1.5 million U q4-6h for severe infections
- Other agents specific to organism

Analgesics: Acetaminophen, 650 mg with/without codeine 30 mg q-4h prn

NURSING CARE

Nursing Assessment

Ear: Thick purulent discharge from ear; dull aching behind ear; low-grade fever; auricle may be pushed out from head by edema; erythema; hearing loss; presence of cholesteatoma

Potential Complications

Subperiosteal abscess, meningitis, facial paralysis, brain abscess, sigmoid sinus thrombosis

Patient Problems/Nursing Diagnoses & Interventions

NIC Physical Comfort Promotion

Acute pain related to perforation of tympanum and necrosis of mastoid process

[illegible]

NIC Skin/Wound Management

Impaired skin integrity related to bony necrosis of mastoid process

- Administer antibiotics as ordered.
- [illegible]

[illegible]

- Assess incision for separation, abscess, erythema, tenderness after mastoidectomy.
- Avoid introduction of water into ear canal.

NIC Communication Enhancement

Disturbed sensory perception (auditory) related to rupture of tympanic membrane or ear surgery

- Assess patient's hearing before and after mastoidectomy and myringotomy.
- If patient experiences hearing loss, speak slowly and clearly when talking with patient.
- Ensure that family and other staff members are aware of hearing loss and use appropriate methods of communication.
- Assist patient with standing and ambulation initially *because patient may experience some vertigo.* Administer antivertiginous medications, as ordered.

Patient Education/Continuum of Care Plan

1. Discuss with the patient and family the necessity of completing the prescribed course of antibiotics to prevent recurrence or complication.
2. Demonstrate dressing change technique to patient and family, if necessary.
3. Discuss possible hearing loss with the patient and family and refer to medical or community resources as appropriate.
4. Reassure patient that cracking and popping noises are normal if mastoid surgery performed.
5. Inform the patient that ear discomfort is normal. Increased ear pain should be reported to the physician.
6. Instruct the patient to avoid the introduction of water into the ear. Demonstrate the procedure of inserting a cotton ball coated with petroleum jelly into the ear canal when showering or shampooing the hair.
7. Advise the patient to consult with physician regarding specific instructions on flying.

Evaluation/Patient Outcomes

Skin/Wound Management: Skin integrity is intact. There is no drainage in external canal. If mastoidectomy was performed, wound is well healed. Patient and family verbalize knowledge of treatment of mastoiditis. Patient and family ver- [illegible]

Physical Comfort Promotion: Patient's comfort is increased. There is no pain in ear. Patient's temperature is within normal limits. Activity level is normal for patient.

Communication Enhancement: Hearing is maintained. Patient's hearing is assessed and, if diminished, the patient is referred to appropriate medical and community resources.

[illegible]

Labyrinthitis is quite rare, and it is usually classified into four types: paralabyrinthitis, serous, purulent, and viral. Because the membranous labyrinth is protected by bone, it is difficult for microorganisms to enter the area unless the bony labyrinth is eroded, as it is with cholesteatoma formation in chronic otitis media. However, organisms can gain entry through the oval and round windows during acute otitis media or through the cochlear aqueduct or internal auditory canal during meningitis. Symptoms are usually severe vertigo and nystagmus followed by total sensorineural hearing loss on the affected side.

Paralabyrinthitis causes the least serious symptoms of the four types of labyrinthitis. A fistula between the bony and membranous labyrinths is caused by erosion of the bone from granulation or cholesteatoma formation, but no inflammation or infection exists. There is no spontaneous nystagmus, and vertigo may be present only because the membranous labyrinth is exposed when exogenous stimulation occurs. A diagnosis is usually made when alternating positive and negative pressures are applied to the external meatus: applying positive pressure may induce nystagmus toward the affected ear, and negative pressure has the opposite effect. Nystagmus is not always produced, however, and the presence of vertigo usually assists in making the diagnosis. Treatment consists of surgically exteriorizing the fistula.

In *serous labyrinthitis* the membranous labyrinth is inflamed and direct labyrinthine stimulation occurs, probably by a direct effect on the nerve endings. This stimulation produces nystagmus on the affected side. Nystagmus may also result from the caloric effect caused by the hyperemia. The patient experiences severe vertigo and nausea and vomiting, characteristically lies quietly with the affected side down, and looks up in an attempt to decrease the nystagmus. The patient may experience some deafness. Any type of movement may worsen the vertigo, and an attempt to stand results in a fall. Heavy sedation, bed rest, and systemic antibiotics in high doses are indicated. If the patient's hearing returns, the labyrinthitis was serous rather than purulent.

Purulent labyrinthitis causes destruction of the labyrinth and cochlea, resulting in permanent deafness in the affected ear. Symptoms and treatment are the same as for serous labyrinthitis; massive doses of antibiotics are administered to prevent the spread of infection and pus and resultant meningitis. Drugs such as ampicillin are usually prescribed because penicillin does not easily cross into the labyrinth. Patients may require intravenous hydration and administration of antivertigo drugs such as meclizine.

Viral labyrinthitis is a common condition that can affect both hearing and balance. It may occur after an infection of the upper respiratory tract; as a sequelae of mumps, measles, rubella, or encephalitis; or following herpes infections of cranial nerves VII or VIII.

Nursing care is aimed at preventing falls. Bed rails are kept up, and the patient is instructed to lie quietly and not to get out of bed without assistance. Antiemetic and antivertigo medications are administered for patient comfort. Antibiotics are given if ordered. The patient's intake and output are monitored for symptoms of dehydration, and IV fluids are given if ordered.

If not hospitalized, the patient should stay in bed at home and request assistance from a family member before getting up during acute episodes. Vestibular suppressants (buclizine, meclizine) may be prescribed to decrease the severity of vertigo. Labyrinthine (vestibular) exercises may also be suggested to assist the patient in compensating for the dizziness. See Patient Education/Continuum of Care Plan for exercises to strengthen the balance system.

If the symptoms persist for a prolonged period, vestibular nerve resection or labyrinthectomy may be performed.

Patient Education/Continuum of Care Plan

Review balance exercises with patient.

Balance exercises can decrease dizziness. Although the exercises are accomplished by turning the head and neck, the exercises are performed to help the brain compensate for the injury to the balance system.

The balance exercises are done while the patient is sitting with feet on the floor for stability. The balance exercises may make the patient dizzy. If dizziness occurs, have the patient wait for the dizziness to subside, but then continue with the exercises.

The head is turned quickly in six different directions. A "sequence" consists of quickly jerking the head right, left, up, down, tilt right, and tilt left. The distance that the head is turned is unimportant. An inch in each direction is sufficient as long as the head is stopped suddenly. After each position, the head should be returned to the midline before beginning the next position. The entire sequence should be repeated 10 times, twice per day. The diagrams illustrate how these balance system exercises should be done (Box 9-2). Over a period of months, these will help the balance system to compensate.

Any physical activity or movement that causes dizziness should be repeated several times. For example, if turning quickly to the right or looking up causes dizziness, these maneuvers should be repeated often. Instead of avoiding certain situations or positions that cause dizziness, repeat them. These repetitions will hasten the recovery process. Although avoiding dizziness is more comfortable for most patients, the only way for the patient to regain complete balance function is to use the balance system. The goal of these exercises is to improve compensation over a period of several months.

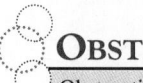

QUICK TURNS **Box 9-2**

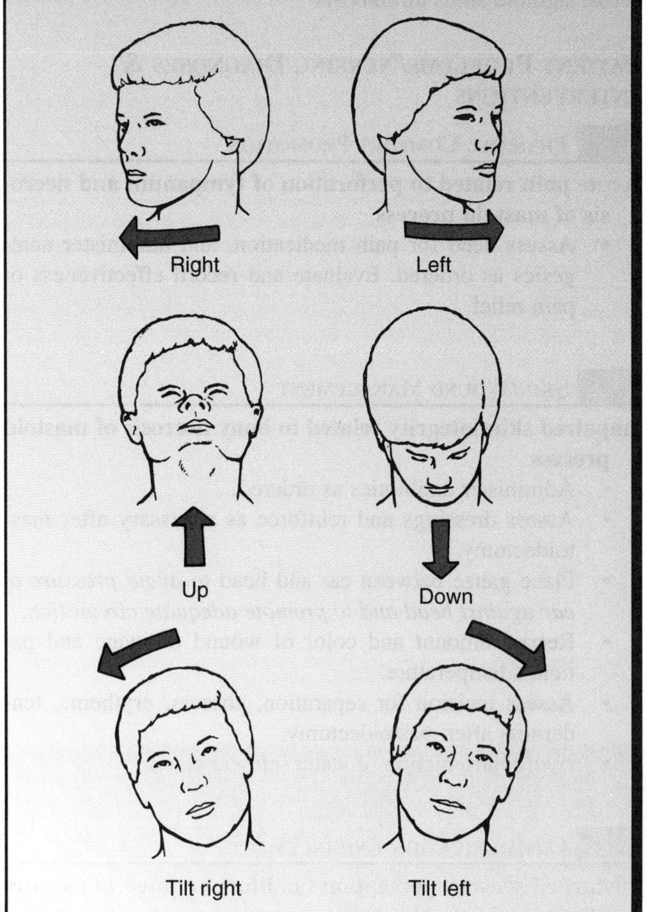

Obstruction

Obstruction of the ear canal is usually caused by excessive secretion or impaction of cerumen or by foreign bodies, including insects.

Young children put various objects, such as beads, pebbles, beans, and small toys, into their ears. An obstruction of the ear canal can lead to infection and to conductive hearing loss if auditory function is disrupted.

Pathophysiology

Cerumen is normally produced in small amounts and dries in the ear, where it is forced out during chewing and talking. Some people have overactive glands that produce excessive amounts

> **! EMERGENCY ALERT**
>
> **FOREIGN BODY REMOVAL: EAR, NOSE**
>
> **ASSESSMENT**
>
> - Patient complains of a foreign body (FB) in the ear or nose.
>
> ***Ear***
>
> - There may be evidence of purulent drainage or odor from the ear. This is most commonly seen in children.
>
> [illegible]
>
> further injury.
>
> ***Nose***
>
> - Administer nasal decongestants and topical anesthetic drops.
> - Place patient in a head-down Trendelenberg position.
> - Remove the foreign body with alligator or ring forceps.
> - If necessary, restrain patient and manage pain to prevent further injury.

of cerumen that can completely occlude the ear canal and others have narrow or tortuous ear canals that can become impacted with cerumen.

Insects occasionally fly into the ear, which causes an unpleasant sensation as they beat their wings.

Foreign objects, which children frequently put into their ears, may not cause symptoms or may cause intense pain if deep in the canal. Physicians occasionally find foreign objects in children's ears during a routine examination.

DIAGNOSTIC STUDIES AND FINDINGS

Otoscopic examination: Visualization of obstructing object

MULTIDISCIPLINARY PLAN

Surgery

Surgical removal of foreign object under anesthesia may be necessary if patient, who is often a child, is unable to remain still during removal

Medications

Carbamide peroxide 6.5% (Debrox drops), 5-10 gtts in ear canal to soften cerumen

General Management

Removal of cerumen by irrigation or with cerumen spoon

If insect is cause of obstruction, it is smothered with drops of oily substance and removed with forceps

Other foreign objects removed with forceps if possible (see Emergency Alert box)

[illegible]

- Assess degree of hearing impairment or tinnitus.
- Instill eardrops or perform irrigation if ordered. Use solution at room temperature *to avoid stimulating a caloric response.*
- Warn patient and family not to put foreign objects in ears.

PATIENT EDUCATION/CONTINUUM OF CARE PLAN

1. For patients who produce excessive cerumen, suggest a method for preventing impaction or obstruction: Once a week put 1 or 2 drops of an oily substance in the ears at night. In the morning put 1 or 2 drops of hydrogen peroxide in the ears and clean gently with a soft cotton wick.
2. Discourage use of foreign objects in ear (e.g., cotton-tipped applicator, hair pins).

EVALUATION/PATIENT OUTCOMES

Communication Enhancement: Sensory/perceptual integrity is restored. Obstruction, if present, is removed. There is no feeling of occlusion or tinnitus in the ear. Hearing is normal for the patient.

OTOSCLEROSIS

> Otosclerosis is a disease of the bone in the bony labyrinth (cochlear otospongiosis) or the otic capsule, in which normal bone is replaced by the formation of highly vascular, "spongy" otosclerotic bone.

Otosclerosis most commonly (85%) occurs at the oval window and eventually causes a conductive hearing loss. Most patients have the disease in both ears, although not to the same degree. It is unilateral in about 10% to 15% of patients.[13]

Otosclerosis is present to some degree in about 10% of whites. It is not found as frequently in Asians and blacks but is reported as common in southern India. About half of patients with otosclerosis have a family history of the disease. Women are apparently affected more often than men, and although the etiology is unclear, pregnancy frequently triggers a rapid onset of this condition. It is usually noticed first in the late teens or early twenties.[13]

PATHOPHYSIOLOGY

The precise pathophysiologic process that causes otospongiotic and otosclerotic disease is still unclear. It is not thought to have any relationship to previous ear infections. During the process, however, normal bone in the otic capsule is gradually replaced by otosclerotic bone that is highly vascular and described as spongy. Although it is controversial, one theory postulates that the destructive process causes the release of proteolytic enzymes, which destroy the capsular bone, freeing other destructive enzymes. As these enzymes enter the labyrinthine fluid, they may affect the neural elements of the inner ear, causing vestibular and cochlear functional impairment. The second stage of this process is the body's natural reaction to heal the involved area by calcification. The calcification causes local expansion of the bone and leads to progressive fixation of the stapes with physical intrusion into labyrinthine spaces and virtual immobilization of the footplate in the oval window.[13] This produces a conductive hearing loss because sound pressure vibrations can no longer be transmitted to the fluid media. Patients may also experience a sensorineural hearing loss if the cochlea is involved. This is referred to as a mixed hearing loss.

In otosclerosis the eardrum usually appears normal, although a pink blush called Schwartz's sign can occasionally be seen through the eardrum. This indicates a high degree of vascularity in active otosclerotic bone.

DIAGNOSTIC STUDIES AND FINDINGS

Rinne test: Bone conduction lasts longer than air conduction in affected ear (negative Rinne)
Weber's test: Tone lateralizes to poorer ear
Audiometric tests: Hearing loss ranges from 60 dB in early stages to total loss in later stages; sound lateralizes more to affected ear; on examination with otoscope, tympanic membrane appears normal

MULTIDISCIPLINARY PLAN

Surgery

Stapedectomy: See p, 624.
Stapedotomy: Minimal (0.4 mm) opening of oval window; ribbon-shaped, platinum Teflon prosthesis is crimped to long process of the incus through opening into footplate before rather than after disrupting the incudostapedial joint and breaking off the stapes arch; this causes less trauma to inner ear, prevents migration of prosthesis, and produces better hearing results[22]

Medications

Antiinfective agents: Amoxicillin, 250 mg po tid for 10 days (after surgery)
Vestibular suppressants may be ordered to control postoperative vertigo

General Management

Air conduction hearing aid if stapedectomy is not indicated

NURSING CARE

NURSING ASSESSMENT

Auditory function: Slowly progressive conductive hearing loss; low- to medium-pitched tinnitus

POTENTIAL COMPLICATIONS

Total unilateral hearing loss

PATIENT PROBLEMS/NURSING DIAGNOSES & INTERVENTIONS

NIC IMMOBILITY MANAGEMENT

Risk for activity intolerance related to bed rest and vertigo after stapedectomy

- Assess patient for pain, nausea, or dizziness.
- Encourage activity level within physician's protocol. (Most patients can be up the day of surgery, others require bed rest for at least a day.)
- Instruct the patient to lie flat with head turned to side and operated ear facing upward *to maintain position of inserted prosthesis.*
- Explain to the patient that vertigo, pain, nausea, and vomiting may occur.
- Administer analgesic, vestibular suppressant, or antiemetic medication as needed.
- Use precautions to prevent falls from dizziness.
- *Convalescent care:* Assist patient to begin ambulation gradually *to minimize vertigo.*

PATIENT EDUCATION/CONTINUUM OF CARE PLAN

1. Encourage the patient not to cough, sneeze, or blow the nose for at least 1 week to prevent increased pressure by way of the eustachian tube, which may dislodge the prosthesis and graft over the oval window. Instruct the patient to cough or sneeze with the mouth open, if coughing or sneezing cannot be avoided. Nose should be blown gently if necessary.
2. Encourage the patient to avoid loud noises, although no evidence exists that any damage is caused.
3. Explain that a decrease in hearing may occur after surgery because of packing, edema, or increased fluid in the middle ear.
4. Encourage the patient to discuss with the physician when flying will be permitted because pressure changes may cause injury to the prosthesis and graft. This varies greatly from physician to physician and can range from 2 to 3 days after surgery to 1 to 2 months after surgery.
5. Caution the patient to avoid the introduction of water into the ear. Demonstrate technique of placing cotton ball

coated with petroleum jelly into ear canal when showering or shampooing hair.

Evaluation/Patient Outcomes

Immobility Management: Patient activity level returns to normal. Patient experiences no vertigo or pain. Hearing is improved to normal (remember that patient may experience decrease in hearing after surgery until packing is removed and blood in middle ear is reabsorbed). Patient and family verbalize understanding of treatment. Patient verbalizes understanding of importance of completing medication regimen and knowledge of convalescent care.

Acoustic Neuroma

Neuromas are benign lesions that arise from the neurilemma or Schwann cell sheath in the covering of the axon of a neuron.

Acoustic neuromas actually arise from the vestibular portion rather than from the cochlear portion of the eighth cranial nerve; the origin is only occasionally found to be the acoustic nerve. Thus these tumors are also called vestibular schwannomas, tumors of the eighth cranial nerve, or cerebellopontine angle tumors. Because most of these neuromas arise within the internal auditory meatus, early effects may be from pressure on the meatus, the cochlear division of the eighth cranial nerve, and the vestibular nerve. Initially patients have tinnitus, unilateral hearing loss, and nystagmus.[3] Although these tumors can affect people at any age, most patients are age 40 to 50 years, with women affected slightly more frequently (60%) than men. Acoustic neuromas comprise approximately 8% to 10% of all intracranial tumors.[8]

During the past 20 years, advances in diagnosis and techniques for removal of these tumors, such as the use of lasers and microsurgery, have greatly reduced morbidity and mortality.

Pathophysiology

The neuroma is a well-defined, fleshy, lobulated mass that is soft and cystic in some areas. It has a variegated appearance that may be caused by areas of old hemorrhage, although the tumor itself is quite avascular. Small, white, patchy areas of calcification may also be present.

The tumor usually arises in the internal auditory meatus. It is called an intracanalicular tumor if it lies entirely within the auditory canal and is considered an ear tumor. As the tumor increases in size, it grows into the cerebellopontine angle and may begin to erode the wall of the internal meatus above and below. After the tumor grows out of the bony canal, it can expand medially, anterosuperiorly, and posteroinferiorly. As it grows medially, the tumor encroaches on the brainstem in the region of the pons. As the tumor enlarges, it may come in contact with the anterior inferior cerebellar artery, which is responsible for the blood supply to the side of the pons and medulla. Continued enlargement medially compresses and distorts the pons and aqueduct, producing brainstem signs and causing an obstructing hydrocephalus.[3]

As the tumor expands anterosuperiorly, it displaces the facial nerve and stretches it over the surface of the tumor. Although it may adhere to the facial nerve, the tumor can usually be separated from the nerve at surgery because the tumor does not normally wrap itself around the nerve. As the tumor extends farther, it may involve the trigeminal nerve, lifting it up from below and causing facial numbness, pain, and decreased corneal sensation.

If the tumor extends inferiorly and posteriorly, it may compress the middle cerebellar peduncle and the cerebellum. It also stretches the ninth, tenth, and eleventh cranial nerves as it approaches the foramen magnum.

Most acoustic neuromas grow within the subarachnoid space. They are usually considered slow growing, although this can vary from patient to patient. Tumors seem to grow more rapidly in young adults and more slowly in the elderly.

Substantial cochlear and labyrinthine changes occur with these space-occupying lesions of the internal meatus (Fig. 9-15), causing abnormalities of the cochlear and eighth cranial nerves. There may be chemical alterations, such as high concentrations of protein in the perilymph, and the sense organs themselves may be destroyed, although the hair cells of the organ of Corti often remain quite normal.

Von Recklinghausen's disease, or neurofibromatosis, can also cause acoustic neuromas that are usually bilateral and expand within the nerve rather than against the nerve, such as in isolated neuromas.[3]

Diagnostic Studies and Findings

Audiometry, electrocochleography (ECOG), and auditory brainstem response (ABR): Performed to evaluate degree of hearing loss and to differentiate between conductive and sensorineural hearing losses

Cerebral arteriography: Used less frequently in recent years but may be performed to diagnose aneurysms, to outline size and location of tumors, and to determine location and deviation of major vessels (see p. 1393, for description)

Computed tomography (CT) and magnetic resonance imaging (MRI) scan: Can indicate presence of tumor, pinpoint location, and show evidence of enlarged ventricles (see p. 1390, for description)

Lumbar puncture: Cerebrospinal fluid examined for increased protein; should not be performed if increased intracranial pressure is suspected to prevent herniation of cerebellar tonsils through foramen magnum or uncal herniation through tentorial notch (see p. 1373 for description)

Multidisciplinary Plan

Surgery

Historically, surgery has been the treatment of choice because acoustic neuromas do not respond well to chemotherapy or radiation; the objective is to remove the tumor completely while saving the facial nerve and acoustic nerve; suboccipital or transpetrosal approach can be used for tumor of any size; for suboccipital approach, small portion of hair at base of neck is

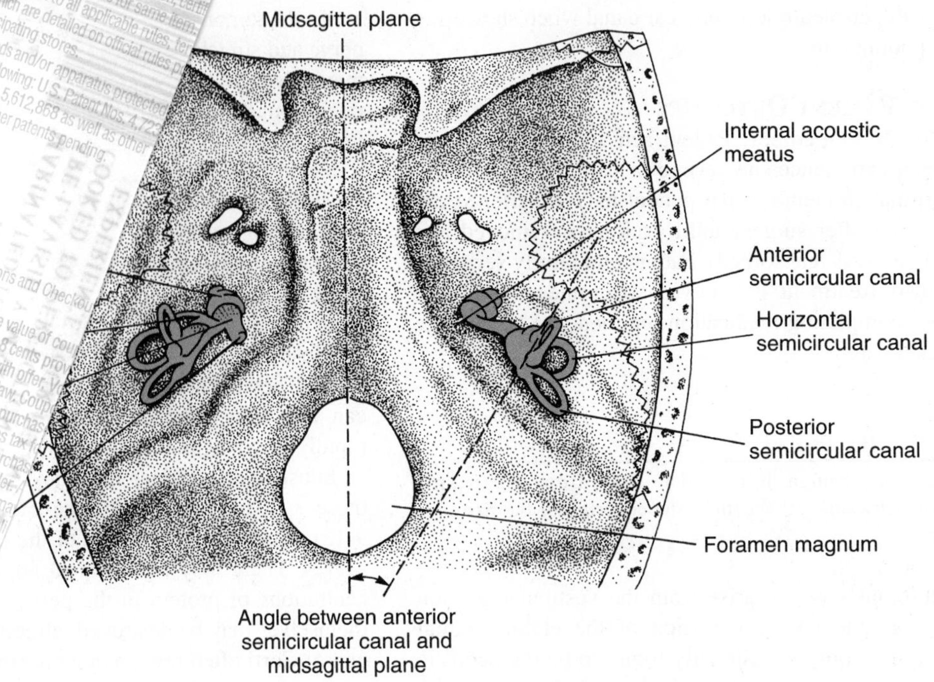

… surgeons prefer translabyrinthine approach, … appropriate for the patient with a tumor 1.5 to 4 cm in size and no usable hearing; one institution reports that all acoustic neuromas, regardless of size, can be removed with this approach, although there may be technical problems with very large tumors; translabyrinthine approach associated with lower mortality, better facial nerve function, less postoperative ataxia, and much less postoperative hydrocephalus than with suboccipital approach but greater loss of hearing

If tumor is large and adheres to facial nerve, total removal of tumor may necessitate sacrifice of facial nerve; if possible, reconstruction of the facial nerve is performed at the time of surgery and should result in return of nerve function

Ventriculostomy: Sometimes performed during surgery so intracranial pressure can be monitored after surgery

Fractionated stereotactic radiosurgery has recently been used for treatment of acoustic neuroma; as with other forms of radiation, effects may not be immediate; the radiation may continue to work on the tumor, decreasing its size over several weeks or even months; fractionation is dividing the radiation dosage, allowing a higher dosage to be delivered to the tumor while minimizing effects on the normal surrounding tissue; radiation is administered by way of a gamma knife when a small amount of tissue is to be treated or with a linear accelerator-based system for larger lesions[17]; stereotactic radiosurgery is used most often for patients who refuse or are otherwise unable to undergo conventional microsurgery; procedure is done on an outpatient basis and allows patient to return to normal activities with a few days of recovery[1]

Medications

Corticosteroids: Dexamethasone (Decadron), 4-6 mg IV q4h to decrease cerebral edema

Antihypertensives: Propranolol (Inderal), 160 mg PO over 24 h before operation for prophylaxis, then nitroprusside (Nitropress) during operation and after operation as needed

Osmotic diuretics to decrease cerebral edema

General Management

Cardiac, hemodynamic, and intracranial pressure monitoring; intubation with mechanical ventilation during and immediately after surgery; oxygen administered by face mask after extubation

Nothing by mouth and intravenous feedings until patient is able to eat; tube feedings necessary in some patients until gag reflex or ability to chew returns

Physical therapy and possibly speech therapy after surgery

NURSING CARE

NURSING ASSESSMENT

Symptoms depend on size and location of tumor.

Auditory function: Sensorineural hearing loss, usually unilateral and slowly progressive; tinnitus; dizziness and transient unsteadiness; true vertigo (sense of rotation, nausea, or vomiting) in some patients; otalgia (ache within ear or mastoid); tension or neck pain on same side as otalgia; occasional facial numbness; occasional tic douloureux (trigeminal neuralgia)

Visual function: Decreased tear production; eyes feel dry and gritty; nystagmus, with eye movement slower and coarser toward side of tumor; with large tumors, diplopia, ataxia, headaches, loss of vision

Gustatory function: Diminished sense of taste on anterior two thirds of tongue; difficult chewing and/or swallowing

Motor function: Poor coordination and gait disturbances; patient leans toward affected side; impairment of fine movements

Potential Complications

Hearing loss, cerebral edema, cerebrospinal fluid leak, facial nerve paralysis, infection, meningitis

Patient Problems/Nursing Diagnoses & Interventions

NIC Tissue Perfusion Management

Ineffective cerebral tissue perfusion related to surgical procedures

Ineffective tissue perfusion related to rebound hypertension

- Establish neurologic baseline and assess neurologic status and vital signs every 15 minutes until stable, then hourly, then every 4 hours. Notify physician of any changes.
- Monitor and record amount of and describe ventricular drainage.
- Assess for signs of increasing intracranial pressure: Widening pulse pressures, decreased level of consciousness, papilledema, seizures, hyperactive deep tendon reflexes, complaints of headache, vomiting.
- Avoid or limit any activity that may increase intracranial pressure.
- Administer osmotic diuretics or dexamethasone as ordered *to decrease cerebral edema.*
- Observe for symptoms of hydrocephalus from edema or bleeding into ventricles, which is possible after surgery.
- Assess for presence of cerebrospinal fluid leak.
- Observe cardiac monitor *to detect any dysrhythmias* resulting from cerebral edema or vagal stimulation during surgery.
- Keep head of bed elevated 45 degrees *to promote venous drainage and minimize cerebral edema.*
- Assess for seizure activity.
- Assess patient's blood pressure frequently; be alert for hypertension, which could be significant after surgery.
- Monitor antihypertensive medication per protocol.

NIC Electrolyte and Acid-Base Management

Risk for deficient fluid volume related to dehydration necessary to decrease congestion in vasculature and to minimize effects of postoperative swelling

- Assess skin turgor, mucous membranes, and lung sounds *to monitor fluid status.*
- Maintain and record intravenous infusions at ordered rate. Titrate to maintain serum osmolarity between 300 and 310 mOsm/L.
- Permit nothing by mouth initially.
- Maintain strict intake and output records.
- Monitor electrolyte levels because patients are given diuretics *to decrease brain bulk during surgery.*
- Perform care of Foley catheter *to prevent urinary tract infection;* patient will have catheter until able to void normally.
- Provide frequent mouth care; patient may suck on lollipops.

NIC Physical Comfort Promotion

Acute pain related to surgical procedure

- Assess for pain and give medication as needed *to minimize pain, nausea, and vomiting.* Evaluate and document effectiveness.

NIC Skin/Wound Management

Impaired skin integrity related to surgical incision

- Assess dressing for drainage and bleeding and reinforce or change as needed.
- Remove dressing 3 to 5 days after surgery. Observe for redness, inflammation, drainage, or edema near operative site. Edema may be from accumulation of subgaleal fluid because dura was entered; fluid should be reabsorbed in few days. Position patient comfortably and change position frequently until patient is mobile *to prevent skin breakdown.*
- Provide adequate support to head and back when positioning *because neck muscles may be weak.*

NIC Respiratory Management

Ineffective breathing pattern related to decreased gag reflex, mechanical ventilation

- Assess patient's arterial blood gases and chest expansion for adequate ventilation.
- Maintain ventilator settings and suction airway as needed (patient may be mechanically ventilated for 1 or 2 days after surgery).
- Observe patient after extubation for return of gag reflex and ability to cough effectively.
- Provide oxygen by face mask as ordered after extubation.
- Continue suctioning or physical therapy of the chest as needed.

NIC Nutrition Support

Imbalanced nutrition: less than body requirements, related to NPO status; decreased gag reflex; discomfort from surgery

Disturbed sensory perception (gustatory) related to surgical procedure

- Administer antacids *to decrease gastric acidity and prevent stress ulcers.*
- Maintain nothing by mouth until gag reflex returns.
- Assess for gag reflex; symmetry and movement of tongue, soft palate, and pharynx.
- Evaluate patient's ability to swallow without evidence of aspiration or collection of food in mouth *to promote swallowing.*
- Provide tube feedings, as ordered, until patient is able to swallow *to avoid aspiration.*
- Begin offering patient soft or pureed foods when gag reflex has returned, feeding on unaffected side if patient experiences difficulty or facial weakness or numbness.
- Evaluate need for dietary consultation.
- Inspect oral cavity and provide oral care after meals.

- Consult with dietitian and/or swallowing therapist to determine food consistencies best tolerated and techniques to improve swallowing.

NIC Communication Enhancement

Disturbed sensory perception (visual, auditory) related to surgical procedure

Visual

- Assess cornea for excessive dryness.
- Provide artificial tears/lubricants to patient's eyes as needed (hourly) *to maintain lubrication because of loss of corneal reflex and decreased ability to close eye.*
- Place moisture chamber (clear plastic occlusive eye shield) over affected eye *to collect moisture and protect the cornea.*
- Tape eye closed and apply patch, if indicated. Check frequently *to ensure eyelid closure under patch.*
- Adapt patient's environment to accommodate for visual changes.

Auditory

- Assess for hearing loss.
- Indicate **patient with hearing loss** on chart, room intercommunication system.
- Speak slowly and distinctly with adequate lighting on your face. Face the patient directly and do not shout or overexaggerate words.
- Place items such as the telephone and call light on unaffected side.

NIC Coping Assistance

Disturbed body image related to facial weakness/ paralysis

- Encourage patient to discuss feelings and concerns.
- Discuss patient's perception of body.
- Evaluate coping mechanisms used in the past.
- Encourage participation in self-care activities.
- Facilitate social interactions with family, other patients, staff.
- Assist patient to identify realistic goals and ways to achieve these goals.
- Provide information on support groups.

The Acoustic Neuroma Association, PO Box 12402, Atlanta, GA 30355; 404-237-2704; E-mail: ANAUSA@aol.com.

Patient Education/Continuum of Care Plan

1. Explain to the patient and family signs and symptoms of wound infection.
2. Discuss with the patient and family signs and symptoms of hydrocephalus or increased intracranial pressure, which in rare cases occurs several weeks after surgery (onset of new motor weakness, stiff neck, fever, visual disturbance, seizures, drainage from incision or ear).
3. Ensure that the patient and family understand the need for continued physical therapy rehabilitation and possible speech therapy.
4. Explain to the patient and family the need for maintenance of nutrition, especially if a chewing or swallowing deficit remains. If the patient is discharged but will continue tube feedings, instruct the patient or a family member in performing the procedure safely.
5. Ensure that the patient and family understand that deficits may take several months to resolve or may not resolve at all; assess family's coping mechanisms and the possible need for assistance in dealing with these deficits.
6. Instruct patient to avoid crowds, persons with upper respiratory infections.
7. Provide instruction on eye care/protection, if facial weakness present.
8. Provide written information on support group (The Acoustic Neuroma Association).

Evaluation/Patient Outcomes

Tissue Perfusion Management: Adequate cerebral tissue perfusion is maintained. Neurologic signs are stable. Ventricular drainage is minimal or absent. Intracranial pressure remains normal; patient experiences no seizures, vomiting, decreased level of consciousness, or cerebrospinal fluid leak. Cardiac status is stable. Peripheral tissue perfusion remains normal. Patient's blood pressure is normal.

Electrolyte and Acid-Base Management: Patient's fluid volume status is normal. Patient experiences no dehydration. Electrolyte levels remain within normal limits for patient. Patient voids with no problems when Foley catheter is removed.

Physical Comfort Promotion: Comfort level is maintained. Patient experiences minimal pain at operative site. Nausea and vomiting are absent. Headaches are absent. Hearing, dizziness, and tinnitus have improved or are stable.

Skin/Wound Management: Skin integrity is maintained. Operative site heals normally, with no inflammation or drainage. Patient experiences no skin breakdown caused by bed rest or decreased activity. Preoperative gait and coordination difficulties have improved.

Corneal tissue is protected and maintained. Corneal lubrication is maintained, and patient experiences no dryness or loss of corneal reflex.

Respiratory Management: Breathing pattern improves. Arterial blood gases are normal; patient is weaned from ventilator soon after surgery. Gag reflex returns to normal. Patient experiences no need for suctioning.

Nutrition Support: Nutritional status is maintained. Patient receives adequate nutrition while NPO; when gag reflex returns, patient is able to maintain normal caloric intake by mouth. Dietary consult is provided if appropriate. Patient can swallow normally. Gag reflex returns to normal soon after extubation.

Communication Enhancement: Patient's visual and auditory alterations have been managed and communication is clear.

Coping Assistance: Body image change is accepted. Patient discusses feelings, uses appropriate coping strategies, interacts with family and friends, and sets realistic goals.

MÉNIÈRE'S DISEASE

Ménière's disease, also called *idiopathic endolymphatic hydrops,* is a labyrinthine dysfunction associated with dilation of the membranous labyrinth with a resultant abnormal fluid balance of the inner ear.

Ménière's disease has three typical symptoms: severe vertigo, tinnitus, and a sensorineural hearing loss, which is usually fluctuating, progressive, and initially of low tones. Although never fatal, Ménière's disease is nonetheless quite incapacitating during attacks, which occur periodically between intervals of remission. As hearing decreases, the attacks become less frequent, and they may stop altogether when the patient's hearing loss is almost total. The acute attacks usually last for several hours, but between attacks the patient may have no symptoms except for tinnitus and a gradually progressive hearing loss. In severe or untreated cases, however, the patient may have daily attacks, although with periods of complete relief from vertigo between attacks.

Adults between ages 30 and 60 years are usually affected. Although it can occur at any age, Ménière's disease is rare in children (it has been seen in a 6-year-old). It is distributed equally by sex; the condition is more often unilateral than bilateral, although the likelihood of bilaterality increases as patients grow older.[4]

PATHOPHYSIOLOGY

The most widely accepted theories regarding the cause of Ménière's disease are (1) an overproduction of endolymph from some disturbance in the formation of fluid in the inner ear and (2) a decreased absorption of endolymph from a disturbance in the sac, which leads to an accumulation of endolymph.

Many other theories have been postulated, but few have been widely accepted. Endolymphatic hydrops, however, is thought to cause degeneration of the neural end organ of the labyrinth and cochlea. Some researchers believe that fluid disturbances are caused by sodium retention, allergies, or vascular spasm. Small vesicles may form in the walls of the endolymphatic system, and the sudden rupture of these vesicles may cause acute attacks of vertigo. The cause of the formation of these vesicles is unclear.

The principal cause appears to be failure of the resorption mechanisms of the endolymphatic sac, resulting in slow accumulation of endolymph with distention and rupture of the membranous labyrinth. Potassium-rich neurotoxic endolymph may then enter the perilymphatic space, causing temporary paralysis of sensory and neural structures. As the disease progresses, there are permanent morphologic changes in sensory and neural structures and persistent losses in auditory and vestibular function.

These patients have hypocellular mastoid processes and deficiencies of the vestibular aqueduct. Trautmann's triangle is often small or distorted, primarily because of the anatomy of the lateral sinus, which is displaced anteriorly and more medially in most patients.

A fundamental problem seems to be malabsorption in the duct or sac. All forms of Ménière's disease develop after some inciting cause that may have occurred years earlier. Known or inciting factors include infection, trauma, otosclerosis, and syphilis, although the disease may be idiopathic. The syndrome is probably related to developmental abnormalities of the endolymphatic duct or sac, hypodevelopment of Trautmann's triangle, anterior displacement of the lateral sinus, and sometimes vascular anomalies, especially in venous drainage. Thus the quality of the endolymph is affected.

Characteristically, in advanced Ménière's disease, endolymphatic hydrops is seen in the scala media and saccule. It fills the vestibule and scala vestibuli in many cases. Because of the displacement of perilymph in advanced disease, the radial fluid flow decreases and longitudinal blood flow becomes dominant. Less often, the utricle or cochlear duct extends to occupy the vestibule. Stagnation of outflow can occur, and such distention can interfere with traveling waves and alter cochlear function.

DIAGNOSTIC STUDIES AND FINDINGS

Audiology: Tuning fork test shows sensorineural deficit; Rinne test may be false positive if severe unilateral hearing loss is present; pure tone test shows sensorineural hearing loss involving low tones

Electrocochleography: Used frequently to aid in differential diagnosis of auditory diseases

Electronystagmography (ENG): Measurement and graphic recording of electrical potentials of eye movements during spontaneous, positional, and caloric evoked nystagmus; normal to decreased vestibular response on affected side

Caloric tests: 5 ml ice water instilled into each ear with patient's head elevated 30 degrees to cause acute attack with nausea, vomiting, vertigo, and nystagmus; response is occasionally hypoactive in involved ear and sometimes in both ears

X-ray examinations of petrous bones: Internal auditory meatus examined carefully; patients with Ménière's disease usually have shorter, straighter vestibular aqueducts than do patients without Ménière's disease

MULTIDISCIPLINARY PLAN

Goals are preservation of hearing and control of vertigo.

Surgery

There is recent increased interest in surgical therapies because medical therapy has failed to halt hearing losses; if medical therapy has failed, two surgical procedures may be performed.

Decompression of endolymphatic sac: Done by inserting Teflon endolymphatic subarachnoid shunt or by incision in sac; kept patent by muscle flap or Teflon sheet; has some benefit in about one half to two thirds of patients[4]

Destruction of end organ and neural connections by labyrinthectomy or vestibular neurectomy; labyrinthectomy performed only as last resort when vertigo is persistent and little or no hearing is left because cochlear function is destroyed; vertigo disappears in almost every case, but tinnitus may remain; vestibular neurectomy may be regarded as operation of choice; middle cranial fossa approach is used; 90% of patients have relief from vertigo, some with improvements in hearing[13]

Medications

Vasodilators

Histamine (Diphosphate), 2.75 mg given in 200-500 ml of 5% glucose drip over 1 h (in remission); based on theory that labyrinthine ischemia is cause of disease; most have not been found to be effective, but β-histamine may improve vertigo, hearing, and tinnitus

Papaverine hydrochloride (Pavabid), 150 mg PO bid

Nicotinic acid (Niacin), 50-200 mg/day PO

Vestibular suppressants

Prochlorperazine (Compazine), 10 mg PO q6h

Droperidol (Inapsine), 25-50 mg/day IV

Haloperidol (Haldol), 5 mg IV q8h

Diazepam (Valium), 2.5-5 mg PO q6h

Lorazepam (Ativan), 0.5-1 mg PO q4-6h prn

Diuretics (used as vestibular suppressant): Hydrochlorothiazide (HydroDiuril), 25-200 mg/day

Cholinergic blocking agents

Atropine, 0.01 mg/kg to maximum of 0.04 mg/kg subcutaneously or IM

Scopolamine (Transderm Scop), 0.5 mg patch every 3 days

Adrenergic agents: Epinephrine, 0.2-0.5 mg IV may be administered to stop an attack; sedatives and antiemetics such as meclizine (Antivert), 25 mg PO qid, and prochlorperazine (Compazine), 10 mg PO q6h, may be used

General Management

Bed rest maintained during acute attack; low sodium diet (2 g) may be used to control symptoms; restriction of salt and water intake; avoidance of tobacco, alcohol, caffeine, and high triglycerides

NURSING CARE

NURSING ASSESSMENT

During Acute Attack

Balance: Sudden onset of acute vertigo (sensation of movement)

Auditory function: Tinnitus described by patient as a persistent background hum; decreased hearing

Visual function: Nystagmus

General: Nausea and vomiting; sweating; abdominal pain; diarrhea; and bradycardia

Between Attacks

Auditory function: Gradually progressive sensorineural hearing loss; tinnitus; loudness intolerance; some patients describe a fullness, pressure, or dull ache in ear; normal tympanic membranes

POTENTIAL COMPLICATIONS

Complete hearing loss, decreased quality of life

PATIENT PROBLEMS/NURSING DIAGNOSES & INTERVENTIONS

NIC RISK MANAGEMENT

Risk for trauma related to fall during vertigo attacks

- Assess patient for vertigo, nystagmus, nausea, and vomiting.
- Keep side rails of bed up *to prevent a fall.*
- Encourage patient to lie quietly and *not* to get up without assistance during attack.
- Instruct patient to avoid sudden head movements or position changes, since *attacks may begin without warning.*
- Administer antiemetics, antivertiginous medications, and/or vestibular sedatives *to help prevent vomiting and promote rest.*

NIC COMMUNICATION ENHANCEMENT

Disturbed sensory perception (auditory) related to degeneration of neural end organs of hearing

- See section on hearing loss, p. 582.

PATIENT EDUCATION/CONTINUUM OF CARE PLAN

1. Discuss with the patient theories about the etiology of the disease and acute attacks.
2. Ensure that the patient is aware that hearing loss may be progressive unless treatment is successful.
3. Explain to the patient ways to minimize tinnitus.
4. Explain to the patient that the attacks will last a few hours and will stop on their own, but that treatment is available to diminish or stop them if necessary.
5. Ensure that the patient understands the danger of trying to walk unassisted during an attack of vertigo.
6. Assist patient and family to identify hazards in home environment. Recommend adaptations.
7. Discuss with the patient and family dietary or medical regimen, if used, or about surgical interventions, if used.
8. Reinforce vestibular/balance exercise, if ordered.

EVALUATION/PATIENT OUTCOMES

Risk Management: Patient safety is maintained. Patient verbalizes understanding that attacks will eventually stop of their own accord. Patient verbalizes understanding that sudden movements and hazardous tasks should be avoided because of sudden onset of vertigo. Patient expresses knowledge of side effects of medical regimen if ordered or of surgical intervention if used.

Communication Enhancement: Auditory function is monitored. Patient understands possibility of hearing loss.

TINNITUS

Tinnitus is the perception of sound in the absence of an acoustic stimulus.

Tinnitus is usually described as a ringing in the ears, although it may also be perceived by the patient as roaring, sizzling, whistling, or humming. Although usually a subjective experience, tinnitus occasionally can be heard as a blowing sound or bruit by the examiner.

The intensity of tinnitus varies greatly from patient to patient. It is often slight and is noticed by the patient only at night when other sounds are minimal. At other times it can be loud and continuous. Tinnitus can be unilateral or bilateral, intermittent or continuous, and may be accompanied by a hearing loss.

Although the mechanism that produces tinnitus is not thoroughly understood, it can be a symptom of nearly all ear disorders. In many cases it is the first or only symptom of disease, and any patient complaining of tinnitus must have a thorough examination to determine the cause. It is estimated that more than 50 million Americans have tinnitus.[5]

PATHOPHYSIOLOGY

The exact mechanism that causes tinnitus is unknown. However, it is known that tinnitus can be caused by a disturbance anywhere in the ear, as well as in the acoustic nerve, brainstem, or cortex (FIG. 9-16). Two disorders with tinnitus as a major symptom, Ménière's disease and acoustic neuroma, are discussed separately in this section.

External ear causes include obstruction of the canal by foreign bodies or cerumen; patients usually describe the sound as low pitched, muffled, and intermittent. These patients may perceive their own voices as having a hollow sound.

Most middle ear disorders can also cause tinnitus. Otosclerosis is usually accompanied by tinnitus, which is described by patients as a ringing or whistling. It is constant, and some patients experience more than one sound. Infectious or inflammatory processes usually produce tinnitus, which is described as pulsating. This type of tinnitus usually ends when the infection is cleared.

Acoustic trauma caused by very loud noises frequently produces high-pitched tinnitus and may be associated with a temporary hearing loss. These symptoms should warn the patient that the ears should be protected before exposure to loud noises or a permanent hearing loss may result. The pitch of tinnitus in these patients is usually near the frequency where their hearing loss is the greatest.

Tinnitus is commonly caused by certain drugs. Quinine, salicylates, some diuretics, aminoglycoside antibiotics, and cisplatin frequently cause tinnitus and can also cause a hearing loss. These drugs damage the cochlea and the eighth cranial nerve; the tinnitus is usually high pitched and may or may not continue after the drug is stopped.

Other causes of tinnitus include anemia and hypotension. This tinnitus usually resolves when the underlying condition is

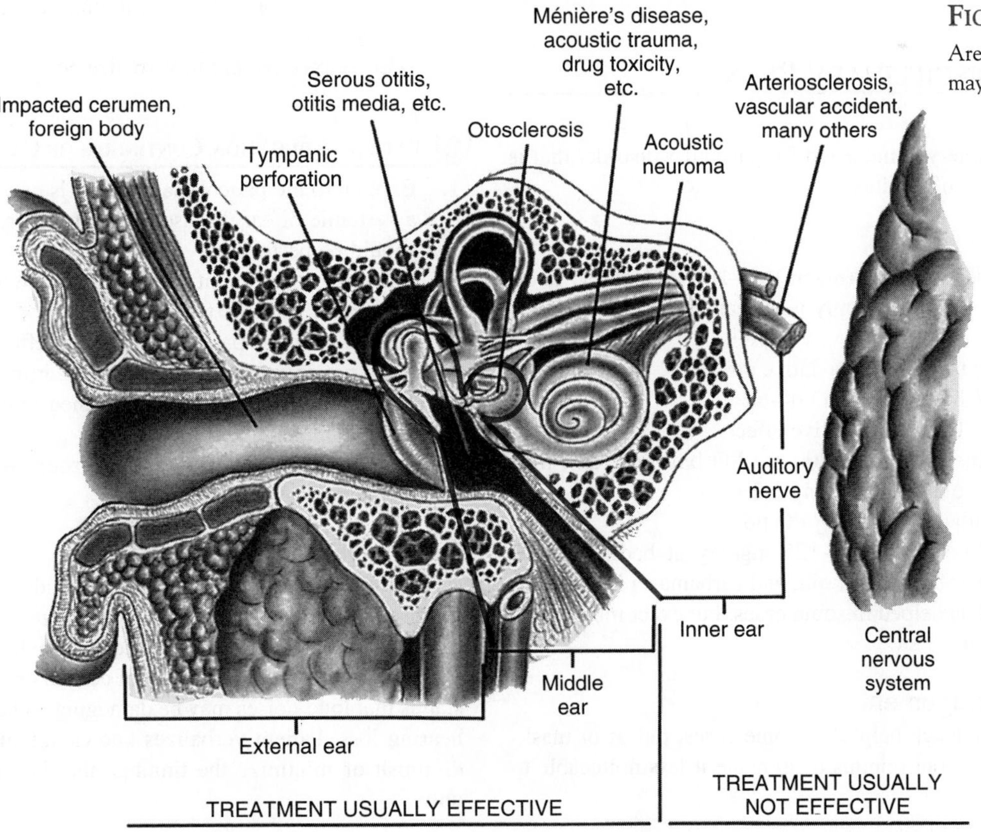

FIG. 9-16 Areas where tinnitus may occur.

corrected. Cardiovascular diseases, such as arteriosclerosis and hypertension, may also produce a tinnitus that may fluctuate with the patient's blood pressure.

Audible or objective tinnitus can be heard by another person. Possible causes include vascular abnormalities, an abnormally patent eustachian tube, repetitive muscular contractions, or defects in the structure of the inner ear. Tinnitus that sounds like a rushing noise caused by the patient's pulse is called pulsatile tinnitus. The examiner can hear objective tinnitus by using a stethoscope.

DIAGNOSTIC STUDIES AND FINDINGS

Audiology: Presence or absence of concurrent hearing loss; any diagnostic study may be performed to rule out the presence of systemic or ear diseases known to produce tinnitus; pitch—the patient manipulates the frequency of tone until the pitch is equal to the most prominent pitch of the tinnitus; loudness—can be evaluated by adjusting the level of pure tone until it has the same loudness as tinnitus; if a profound hearing loss is present, the measurement may be only a few decibels sensation level, whereas in regions of normal hearing, the measurement may be 40 dB sensation level; pure tone masking—measures the minimum level of a pure tone required to mask the tinnitus as a function of the masker frequency.

Auditory brainstem response (ABR): Also known as the *brainstem auditory evoked response (BAER);* used to detect electrical activity in the cochlea and auditory brain pathways; will indicate normal vs. abnormal cochlear activity

MULTIDISCIPLINARY PLAN

Surgery

None, unless surgery is indicated for particular disorder that is found to be cause of tinnitus

Medications

Vasodilators: Nicotinic acid (niacin), 50-200 mg/day PO to dilate blood vessels that supply inner ear; its efficacy is questionable

Antianxiety agents: Used for sedative effect
- Diazepam (Valium), 5 mg PO q4-6h

Anticonvulsants: Used for sedative effect
- Carbamazepine (Tegretol), 200 mg PO bid for 1 day, then maintenance dose of 800 mg-1.2 g qd
- Phenytoin (Dilantin), 100 mg PO tid
- Primidone (Mysoline), 100-125 mg/day at bedtime for 3 days, then 250 mg tid or qid, and carbamazepine in combination; has helped in some cases, but exact mechanism is unknown

General Management

Hypnosis, biofeedback helpful in some cases; radios or masking units to drown out tinnitus or to make it less noticeable to the patient

NURSING CARE

NURSING ASSESSMENT

Auditory function: Patient describes sound in one or both ears as ringing, sizzling, whistling, roaring, humming, or hissing; may be intermittent or continuous; may be high pitched; history of acoustic trauma, that is, exposure to loud noise; history of ototoxic drugs; hearing may be normal to decreased; may be associated with vertigo

POTENTIAL COMPLICATIONS

Inability to adapt

PATIENT PROBLEMS/NURSING DIAGNOSES & INTERVENTIONS

NIC COMMUNICATION ENHANCEMENT

Disturbed sensory perception (auditory) related to tinnitus; hearing impairment
- Assess patient for hearing impairment and degree of tinnitus.
- Encourage use of background noise, that is, radios or masking units, *to present a more pleasant noise.*
- Ensure that the use of any ototoxic substances is discontinued, if possible.
- Assist with any procedures necessary for diagnosis or treatment.

NIC COPING ASSISTANCE

Anxiety related to constant tinnitus
- Assess successful coping mechanisms used in past.
- Provide information about tinnitus, its causes, and its treatment.
- Encourage patient to verbalize concerns.

PATIENT EDUCATION/CONTINUUM OF CARE PLAN

1. Explain to the patient that tinnitus is usually a symptom of a systemic or ear disease and that a thorough examination should be performed.
2. Encourage the patient to avoid exposure to loud noises that may cause acoustic trauma.
3. Discuss with the patient the ototoxic effects of some drugs. If the patient must take an ototoxic drug, be sure that periodic audiologic testing is performed to detect any hearing loss.
4. Refer to counseling or support group (American Tinnitus Association, www.ata.org).

EVALUATION/PATIENT OUTCOMES

Communication Enhancement: Auditory symptoms are improved or managed. Patient verbalizes understanding of cause of tinnitus if known. Patient verbalizes understanding that tinnitus can be a side effect of certain drugs. Patient understands that loud noises may be damaging and cause tinnitus and hearing loss. Patient verbalizes knowledge of various ways to diminish or minimize the tinnitus, that is, radios or masking units.

Coping Assistance: Patient successfully uses coping skills, and anxiety is diminished or relieved.

NOSE DISORDERS

EPISTAXIS

Epistaxis is bleeding from the nose caused by irritation, trauma, coagulation disorders, hypertension, chronic infection, or tumor.

Epistaxis is thought to have occurred at least once in over 10% of the normal population. It is either a primary disorder or secondary to another condition such as hemophilia or leukemia, and many cases are idiopathic.

In children, who are twice as likely to have epistaxis as adults, the bleeding is usually mild and tends to originate from the anterior nasal septum. In older adults bleeding is more likely to originate from the posterior septum, so that the bleeding point is more difficult to locate, and the bleeding may be profuse. Epistaxis is equally common in men and in women and occurs more frequently in winter, probably because of the dryness of the air.

Although epistaxis is a frightening experience for the patient, it generally looks and feels worse than it actually is. The blood is usually bright red and the patient may swallow some of it, which is an unpleasant sensation. Although adults can lose up to 1 L per hour during severe bleeding, the mortality is extremely low. When the patient bleeds enough to show signs of shock, the nosebleed usually stops because of low blood pressure. Some deaths are thought to have been caused by coronary ischemia from blood loss.[12]

PATHOPHYSIOLOGY

The most common cause of epistaxis is trauma to the nasal mucosa from damage by a foreign object, picking crusts from the nasal septum, or dryness of the nasal mucosa. Nosebleeds are fairly common in patients with coagulation defects such as hemophilia, leukemia, and purpura. Infection, tumors, and some drugs and toxins may cause nosebleeds; in many instances, however, the cause is not identified or is considered idiopathic.

There may be some relationship between menstruation and epistaxis. It may be that in some women with premenstrual syndrome the nasal mucosa becomes congested at the time of menstruation, setting the stage for epistaxis.[12]

The incidence of epistaxis is no higher in hypertensive patients than in normotensive patients. However, hypertensive patients may bleed more profusely, partly because of the direct effect of the increased pressure and also because the small nasal arteries and arterioles of hypertensive patients tend to have much of their muscular walls replaced by fibrous tissue and are incapable of contracting adequately to attain hemostasis.[12]

Children experience frequent nosebleeds from the anteroinferior part of the septum known as Little's area or Kiesselbach's plexus (FIG. 9-17). The etiology is not clear, but the area is richly vascular, and children have hyperemic and congested upper respiratory tracts. Children also pick and rub their noses in the area where the mucosa is stretched over cartilage and bone.

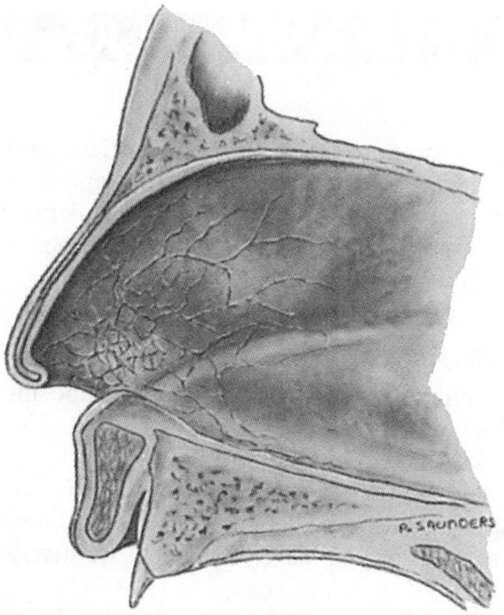

FIG. 9-17
Kiesselbach's plexus. (From DeWeese and Saunders.[10])

Digital trauma or intractable nose picking is another cause of anterior nosebleeds. Constant nose picking can cause septal ulceration or even a perforation, which leads to epistaxis.

A hereditary disease that is an unusual cause of epistaxis is Rendu-Osler-Weber disease or hemorrhagic hereditary telangiectasia. This disease is gene dominant and may be passed from either parent to a child of either sex. Epistaxis is usually the initial symptom, but telangiectasis is commonly found in other mucous membranes or anywhere on the external surface of the body. Bleeding usually occurs from the nose and gastrointestinal tract because mucosa in those areas is very fragile, whereas other areas have protective layers of squamous epithelium.

Most nosebleeds in the anterior part of the nose originate from Kiesselbach's plexus, the highly vascular network in the anterior nasal septum. It is also anatomically closer to the rapid inspiratory airflow, which may dry the normal mucus flow, especially in cold, dry weather. Because the vessels are fairly small and easily accessible, these nosebleeds are the easiest to treat. If bleeding is from the posterior part of the nose, the exact source of bleeding is more difficult to locate because it is sometimes impossible to see and bleeding is more profuse. (See Emergency Alert box.) Usually just one source on one side of the nose bleeds, although bleeding frequently originates from both sides in patients with blood dyscrasias.

DIAGNOSTIC STUDIES AND FINDINGS

Hematocrit, hemoglobin, platelets, prothrombin time, partial thromboplastin time, reticulocyte count, and differential: Done to rule out coagulation defect; results usually normal; bleeding from other parts of body likely in patients with hematologic disorders

Rhinoscopy and nasopharyngoscopy: To detect and localize site of bleeding

EMERGENCY ALERT

EPISTAXIS

Epistaxis is common. It may be minor or major and may actually become so severe that it is life threatening. Patients at risk for bleeding and those taking anticoagulants are more prone to nosebleeds. Epistaxis is most commonly seen in children and individuals age 50 years and older.

ASSESSMENT/INTERVENTION

Anterior Bleeding

The most common spot for bleeding is from the anterior and posterior septum.

- Assess the location of the bleeding.
- Pinch the nose firmly and hold for at least 10 minutes. It is best if you pinch the patient's nose instead of asking the patient to do so. This way, you can ensure steady and firm pressure.
- If bleeding continues beyond the pinching 10-minute period, prepare the patient for additional treatment.
- With the patient in a high-Fowler position's, slightly hyperflex the head and suction the clots in the nasal passage.
- Observe the canal for continued bleeding. If present, and in conjunction with physician, apply vasoconstricting agent such as 10% cocaine solution.
- If bleeding continues, the nose may need to be cauterized with silver nitrate or anterior nasal packing inserted.

Posterior Epistaxis

Posterior bleeding is more difficult to manage. It usually results from a chronic condition such as hypertension, atherosclerotic heart disease, or blood dyscrasia. The bleeding usually originates from the sphenopalatine artery, anterior ethmoid artery, or nasopalatine artery.

- Assess that the bleeding is posterior.
- Place the patient in a high-Fowler's position.
- In conjunction with a physician, anesthetize the posterior nasal passage with 10% cocaine solution.
- Pack the bleeding site with packing materials such as an epistaxis catheter, Foley catheter tip, and/or tampon.
- Monitor vital signs and estimate blood loss. If necessary, provide fluid volume replacement.
- Instruct patient to (1) tilt head forward if bleeding occurs; (2) not to blow nose; and (3) apply steady pressure to nose for at least 5 minutes if bleeding recurs.

MULTIDISCIPLINARY PLAN

Surgery

Endoscopic cautery: Chemical or electrical cauterization of bleeding vessels using nasal endoscope to visualize bleeding

Arterial ligation of ethmoid, maxillary, or carotid artery if proper packing fails to control nosebleed

Septal dermoplasty for Rendu-Osler-Weber disease: Skin graft is placed in nose to cover anterior parts of septum and floor and walls of nose anteriorly to provide protective covering over fragile mucosa; combined with laser therapy gains control of epistaxis for several years

Medications

Fibrinolytics: Vitamin K (AquaMEPHYTON), 10 mg PO or IM; useful in some cases of epistaxis, but packing remains therapy of choice

Antiinfective agents: Antibiotic prophylaxis because packing obstructs drainage of paranasal sinuses and may precipitate a sinus infection

General Management

Nosebleed from anterior part of nose

Easiest to treat; source of bleeding located, and clots and fresh blood aspirated with suction; cotton ball saturated with 1:1000 epinephrine inserted into bleeding nostril, and strong pressure applied to compress cotton ball against septum for several minutes; after cotton ball is removed, cauterization performed by means of silver nitrate or electric cautery; packing unnecessary if bleeding is controlled with cauterization; pressure alone may control bleeding; if bleeding is not controlled, the nose may be packed with gauze strips saturated with antibiotic ointment

Epistaxis from posterior part of nose

Postnasal packing: With patient sitting to prevent aspiration of blood, bleeding site located by advancing strong suction tip until nose fills with blood when suction tip has passed; large postnasal pack introduced through mouth by attaching it to catheter that is inserted into nostril and out mouth (FIG. 9-18); catheter pulled through nose, lodging pack in posterior part of nose and providing compression to bleeding site; packing remains in place for 5 days; if both choanae occluded because of large size of pack, patient must be checked daily for ear or eustachian tube symptoms; patient will have some difficulty swallowing

Posterior nasal pack: A silicone balloon is used to occlude the posterior choana; this configuration provides a good fit, using several milliliters of fluid without placing painful pressure on the soft palate that is often associated with Foley catheters; a suction channel is opened when the stylette, which allows accurate placement along the floor of the nose or around a septal deviation, is removed; to control epistaxis, an anterior pack may be placed easily because the parallel suction and inflation channels have a narrow diameter; discomfort is minimal, and patient may often be treated in an outpatient setting

NURSING CARE

NURSING ASSESSMENT

Nasal bleeding: Bright red blood comes from the nares; patient may also swallow or expectorate blood; history of trauma, such as nose picking or direct injury; hypertension; long-term use of anticoagulants, chemotherapy, or intranasal cocaine; nasal dryness; hereditary hemorrhagic telangiectasia; blood dyscrasia; tumors

General examination: Examination of patient's body for bruises or petechiae that may indicate underlying hematologic disorder

PATIENT PROBLEMS/NURSING DIAGNOSES & INTERVENTIONS

NIC TISSUE PERFUSION MANAGEMENT

Risk for deficient fluid volume related to nasal bleeding

Ineffective cerebral and cardiopulmonary tissue perfusion related to large-volume blood loss

- Practice universal precautions.

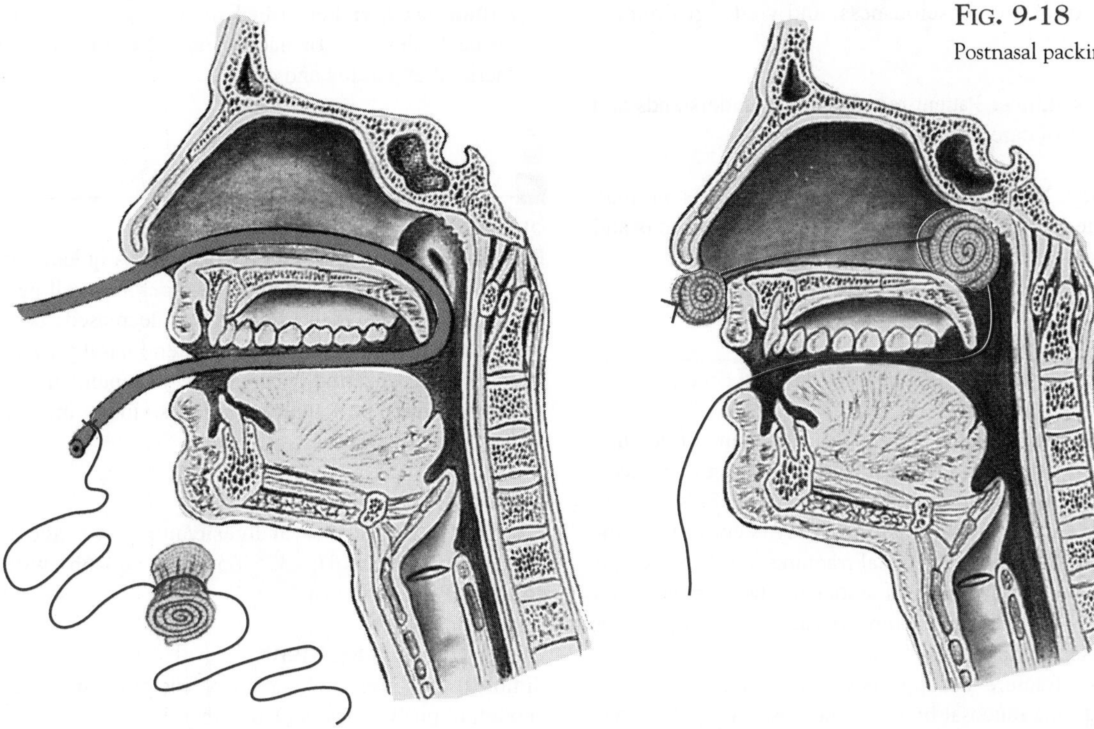

FIG. 9-18
Postnasal packing for epistaxis.

- Maintain patient in sitting position *to prevent aspiration of blood.*
- Initiate first aid measures such as pinching anterior nasal ala(e) for 10 to 15 minutes; apply ice compresses *to promote vasoconstriction.*
- Assess patient's vital signs and level of consciousness.
- Record color and amount of blood loss.
- Encourage patient to minimize activity.
- Encourage patient not to swallow blood *to prevent nausea and vomiting.*
- Monitor fluid, electrolyte, and hemodynamic values.
- Assess blood pressure, pulse, and level of consciousness.
- Administer intravenous fluids or blood products as ordered.

NIC Coping Assistance

Fear related to loss of blood

- Prepare patient for all procedures.
- Assess patient's emotional state.
- Reassure patient.

NIC Respiratory Management

Risk for aspiration related to inability to clear secretions; gagging

- Assess patient's ability to expectorate and clear secretions.
- Elevate head of bed or have patient sit with head tipped forward *to prevent aspiration of blood.*
- Pinch patient's nostrils together for 5 to 10 minutes *to compress soft portion of nostril against septum.*
- Apply ice or cold compress to nose *to help stop bleeding.*
- Notify patient's physician if bleeding cannot be stopped.
- Assist with packing if necessary.
- If nasal packing is in place, encourage fluids and provide frequent oral hygiene *to decrease mucosal dryness because patient will be breathing through mouth.*
- Have patient breathe through mouth.
- Have basin nearby for patient *to expectorate blood.*
- Inspect oropharynx for presence of blood.

Patient Education/Continuum of Care Plan

1. Explain to the patient the inherent dangers in nose picking or of inserting foreign objects into the nose.
2. Encourage the patient and family to seek medical assistance immediately if nasal infection or epistaxis occurs.
3. If epistaxis is from dryness of mucous membranes, discuss with the patient benefits of using a humidifier or vaporizer to provide additional humidity in the home especially during the winter months.
4. Encourage patient to sneeze with mouth open and avoid vigorous nose blowing.
5. Instruct patient in first aid measures if nasal bleeding recurs.
    a. Pinch nostrils tightly for 10 to 15 minutes.
    b. Apply ice compresses.
    c. Instill nasal decongestant spray to provide vasoconstriction, per physician's order.

Evaluation/Patient Outcomes

Tissue Perfusion Management: Epistaxis is well controlled and patient's fear is minimized. Bleeding is absent. Patient's hematocrit value and hemoglobin level are normal. Mucous membranes are healed if bleeding is from picking or ulceration. Patient verbalizes understanding of cause of epistaxis, if known, and ways to prevent bleeding in the future. Tissue perfusion remains adequate. Patient experiences no loss of consciousness, and vital signs remain stable.

Coping Assistance: Patient remains calm; understands and engages in plan of care.

Respiratory Management: Breathing pattern is normal. Patient experiences no aspiration of blood during epistaxis and is able to clear secretions.

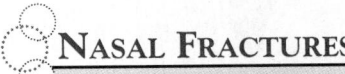

NASAL FRACTURES

A nasal fracture is a traumatic injury to the nasal bones.

Nasal fractures occur quite commonly and more often than fractures of the other facial bones. Common causes are accidents, sports injuries, and assaults. In children, falls are the most common cause of nasal fractures. They occur more commonly in men. However, when nasal fractures are diagnosed, it is essential to rule out fractures of associated facial bones such as zygomatic or mandibular fractures because facial injuries or trauma may also damage these bones.

Even a nasal fracture that appears simple usually has associated damage to the mucosal lining of the nose. If a patient has suffered a facial trauma that causes epistaxis, damage to the bone-cartilage structures of the nose is likely.

PATHOPHYSIOLOGY

A nasal fracture occasionally occurs in the birth canal during delivery. These are usually "greenstick" fractures, and the baby's nose inclines slightly to one side. The nose can be grasped at the tip and pulled toward the midline to realign it in these cases.

Nasal fractures can be classified as unilateral, bilateral, or complex. A unilateral fracture may produce little or no displacement and may appear on an x-ray examination as a simple crack. Bilateral fractures, which are the most common, may be caused by a swinging punch or blow that pushes both nasal bones to one side or by a frontal blow that depresses the nasal bones and gives a flattened look to the nose. The entire nose may be deviated, and the nose may have a C or S deformity.

Complex fractures are usually caused by powerful frontal blows. Such blows may shatter the nasal pyramid and frequently the frontal bones as well, causing a marked depression of the nasal and facial bones.

The usual findings are epistaxis, a noticeable facial deformity, and a history of trauma. Edema occurs quickly at the injury site and depending on the severity may include periorbital swelling. Ecchymosis is common, the nose is exquisitely tender, and nasal obstruction occurs. Complex fractures of the nose and face may result in diplopia or subscleral hemorrhage.

DIAGNOSTIC STUDIES AND FINDINGS

X-ray examination of face and nose: Shows fractures and depressed area of facial and nasal bones; done to complement clinical, visual evaluation

Ophthalmoscopy: Performed to rule out eye injury such as corneal abrasion or laceration, also to check status of lacrimal apparatus and orbit

MULTIDISCIPLINARY PLAN

Surgery

Reduction and fixation of the fractures as quickly as possible after injury (within first hour or two before swelling begins, or after 3 or 4 days when swelling has decreased) because fragments tend to stabilize quickly; bilateral nasal packing or nasal splints usually inserted during surgery to maintain stability and position of nasal structure; wiring or splinting may be required for complex fractures

Medications

Narcotic analgesics or analgesic/antipyretic agents: Acetaminophen (Tylenol), 325-650 mg q4-6h with/without codeine, PO q4-6h prn

General Management

Simple thumb pressure on convex side of the nose occasionally enough to push bones back together

NURSING CARE

NURSING ASSESSMENT

Facial swelling: Deformity; ecchymosis; epistaxis; pain; history of trauma to face and nose; possible accompanying lacerations; possible bony crepitus; if leak of cerebrospinal fluid is present, clear fluid dripping from nose and/or ears

Respiratory status: Difficulty in breathing through the nose; mouth breathing

POTENTIAL COMPLICATIONS

Hematoma; infection; altered sense of smell

PATIENT PROBLEMS/NURSING DIAGNOSES & INTERVENTIONS

NIC PHYSICAL COMFORT PROMOTION

Acute pain related to facial trauma

- Assess need for pain medication and provide adequate analgesia for pain relief; evaluate and document effectiveness.

NIC RESPIRATORY MANAGEMENT

Ineffective breathing pattern related to nasal obstruction and swelling

- Assess for shortness of breath, dyspnea from nasal obstruction, or difficulty in swallowing.
- Apply ice to face and nose *to minimize swelling and bleeding without pressure to nose.*
- Monitor amount and color of epistaxis and record.
- Keep head of bed elevated, even when sleeping, *to prevent aspiration of blood or secretions and minimize edema.*

- Prevent patient from swallowing blood or aspirating; encourage patient to breathe through mouth.
- Have basin nearby for patient *to expectorate blood.*
- Provide frequent oral hygiene and encourage intake of oral fluids.
- Monitor vital signs and level of consciousness.

NIC NEUROLOGIC MANAGEMENT

Disturbed sensory perception (visual) related to periorbital edema

- Assess for eye swelling; apply ice *to minimize edema.*
- Observe for scleral hemorrhage and periorbital edema.
- If eyes are not completely closed, assess patient's ability to see.

PATIENT EDUCATION/CONTINUUM OF CARE PLAN

1. Ensure that the patient knows to keep head elevated, even while sleeping.
2. Explain to the patient the timing of pain medication for maximum effectiveness.
3. Encourage the patient to seek medical assistance immediately if there is a decrease in vision, level of consciousness, or ability to breathe.

EVALUATION /PATIENT OUTCOMES

Physical Comfort Promotion: Comfort is maintained. Pain is minimized or managed effectively with oral pain medications.

Respiratory Management: There is no facial deformity. There is no nasal obstruction; patient can breathe normally through nose.

Neurologic Management: Vision remains normal for patient. Sclera is clear without redness or swelling.

NASAL POLYPS

Polyps are benign growths that appear as soft, pale gray, nontender masses and gradually form from recurrent localized swelling of the sinuses or nasal mucosa (FIG. 9-19).

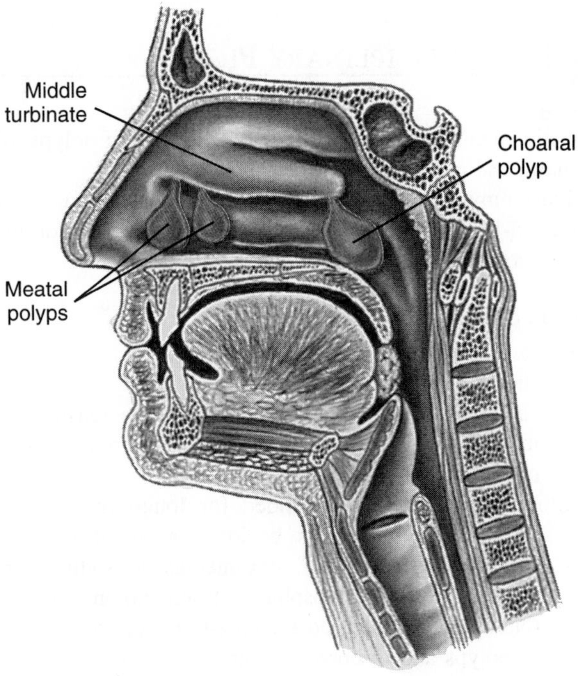

FIG. 9-19
Nasal polyps.

Polyps may become quite large. They are usually bilateral, occur in multiples, and may cause actual distention and enlargement of the bony structures of the nose. Even after surgical removal, some nasal polyps recur. Although rare in children, polyps are occasionally found in children with cystic fibrosis and allergies and in those with Puetz-Jeghers syndrome. The symptoms of this syndrome include pigmented spots on the skin, especially around the mouth, and polyposis of the gastrointestinal tract.

Many patients with polyps have anosmia or hyposmia.

PATHOPHYSIOLOGY

The etiology of nasal polyps is not clear. They are often pedunculated and suspended in the nasal cavity by stalks of varying lengths. The polyps and stalks usually originate in the paranasal sinuses, particularly the ethmoid sinuses, and pass into the middle meatus of the nose through the ostia connecting them to the nasal cavities. They are often called pseudotumors. Their pathogenesis is thought to be the result of focal mucosal edema that causes a polypoid swelling. Because of the polyp's weight, the swelling tends to enlarge and eventually becomes suspended on a stalk.

Polyps are usually found in the middle meatus near the openings of the sinuses and occasionally on the roof of the nose. They are never found on the septum or in the lower meatus; the reason for this is not known.

Nasal polyps are often found in patients with allergy, cystic fibrosis, asthma, disorders of ciliary motility, chronic rhinitis, and chronic sinusitis. The exact relationship is unknown but may be related to an inflammatory response causing hypertrophy of the mucosa, edema, and thinning of the mucous membranes. Polyps may be exacerbated by allergic symptoms but are not caused by allergies.[14]

An interesting phenomenon that occurs in some patients with asthma and nasal polyposis is an intolerance to aspirin, indomethacin, and some coal tar dyes. This intolerance is severe and can cause respiratory arrest if these substances are ingested. This is thought to be related to the inhibitory action of these substances on prostaglandin synthesis.

DIAGNOSTIC STUDIES AND FINDINGS

CT-scan of sinuses: Opaque areas in affected sinuses
Immunologic assessment: Performed if allergy is considered a causative factor

MULTIDISCIPLINARY PLAN

Surgery

Functional endoscopic sinus surgery: Removal of polyps using nasal endoscope is the surgery of choice

Polypectomy: Each polyp avulsed with wire snare

Caldwell-Luc procedure: May be performed if polyps originate in maxillary sinus

Medications

Corticosteroids

Predisone (Deltasone), high dose for 5 days

Methylprednisolone (Medrol Dosepack), decreasing doses may be used for severe nasal obstruction to decrease size of polyps

Steroids are not recommended for long-term use; local steroid sprays such as beclomethazone diproprionate (Beconase, Vancenase), dexamethasone sodium phosphate (Decadron Phosphate), triamcinolone acetonide (Nasacort) can be used for long-term control of the size of polyps and to prevent recurrence by reducing the inflammatory response[19]

Antihistamines

Aztemizole (Hismanal), 10 mg PO qd

Loratadine (Claritin), 10 mg PO qd

Decongestants

Pseudoephedrine hydrochloride (Sudafed), 30 mg PO q4-6h

Phenylpropanoline hydrochloride (Entex, Ornade), 1 capsule PO bid

Pseudoephedrine hydrochloride with guaifenesin (Deconsal II, Guaifed), 1 PO bid

Antiinfective agents: Organism-specific antibiotics to treat infection

NURSING CARE

NURSING ASSESSMENT

Nasal Obstruction: Feeling of fullness in face or nose; nasal obstruction; difficulty breathing through nose; nasal discharge; anosmia; symptoms of allergic rhinitis, such as sneezing, watery eyes, eczema and asthma

PATIENT PROBLEMS/NURSING DIAGNOSES & INTERVENTIONS

NIC RESPIRATORY MANAGEMENT

Ineffective airway clearance related to swelling of the nasal mucosa and nasal obstruction

- Assess patient's ability to clear secretions.
- Assess amount of swelling.
- Increase humidification.
- After surgical intervention, elevate head of bed, and apply ice compresses to nose *to minimize swelling and bleeding.*
- Change nasal drip pad as indicated and record amount and consistency of drainage.
- Encourage patient not to swallow blood or secretions but to expectorate into basin *to prevent nausea.*
- Monitor patient's vital signs.
- Instruct patient not to blow nose *to prevent tissue trauma and bleeding.*
- Convalescent care: Observe for bleeding.
- If bleeding occurs, instruct patient to notify physician, elevate head of bed, check vital signs, compress outside of nose against septum, and apply ice compresses to nose.
- If bleeding persists, packing may be necessary.

NIC NEUROLOGIC MANAGEMENT

Disturbed sensory perception (olfactory) related to anosmia, presence of nasal edema

- Assess patient's ability to smell.
- Assure patient that sense of smell should return postoperatively after swelling has decreased.
- Instruct patient to make appropriate adaptations to environment.

PATIENT EDUCATION/CONTINUUM OF CARE PLAN

1. Ensure that the patient knows how to reach the physician immediately if bleeding begins after surgical removal of polyps.
2. Encourage the patient with allergies to avoid known allergens if possible and to take antihistamines early to minimize allergic reactions. May be referred for immunologic evaluation if local treatment ineffective.
3. Explain to the patient the need to use decongestant nose drops and sprays cautiously because of the rebound effect on the mucous membranes.
4. Instruct patient to make appropriate changes in environment.
   a. Install smoke detectors.
   b. Check appearance of food for spoilage.
   c. Check gas lines for leaks.

EVALUATION/PATIENT OUTCOMES

Respiratory Management: Normal airway clearance is maintained. Bleeding, nasal obstruction, shortness of breath, or nausea is not present after surgery. Patient's knowledge of polyps is increased. Patient verbalizes understanding of possible causes and ways to prevent recurrence of nasal polyps. Patient seeks early treatment for sinusitis or minimizes severity of allergies by taking antihistamines and receiving immunologic evaluation and treatment.

Neurologic Management: Olfactory sense is maintained. Patient verbalizes understanding that sense of smell will return after swelling decreases.

SEPTAL DEVIATION AND PERFORATION

A deviated septum is a shift of the septum from the midline, which is common in many adults. It is either S or C shaped.

Although the septum is usually straight at birth, it may shift from one side to another as a result of trauma or injury.

A septal perforation is a hole in the nasal septum between the nostrils, which is usually in the anterior or cartilaginous septum but may occasionally occur in the bony septum. A small perforation, which can be caused by infections, nasal crusting, or nose picking, is often asymptomatic, although a slight whistle may be heard as the patient breathes. Larger perforations may produce rhinitis, nasal crusting, or epistaxis.

PATHOPHYSIOLOGY

The nasal septum is usually straight. The septum is occasionally bent during birth, and the infant may have a twisted-appearing nose. This can usually be corrected when first noticed by placing light pressure on the convex side of the nose. There is no need for packing or a splint. Minor degrees of deviation go unrecognized in the newborn period.

With aging, the septum has a tendency to become deviated or to form a hump. There is frequently no history of injury to account for the deviation. As a result, few adults have a totally straight septum. Trauma during childhood may also contribute to septal deviation in the adult.

Although frequently no symptoms are associated with a deviated septum, some patients have moderate to severe degrees of nasal obstruction. Other, less well-defined symptoms include headaches, which occur in some patients who have a septal spur impinging on the inferior turbinate; epistaxis; and symptoms of sinusitis, which are rare but may be influenced by a deviated septum that obstructs a sinus opening.

Septal perforations may be small or large. They may be asymptomatic or may cause annoying symptoms, such as crusting, a watery discharge, or a whistling noise as the patient breathes. Small perforations are usually caused by repeated irritation of the nose such as picking it; they may also be caused by septal surgery. Less frequent causes are repeated cauterizations because of epistaxis, abuse of intranasal cocaine, and chronic nasal infections. Once quite common, perforations resulting from syphilis and tuberculosis are now rare. Approximately 25% to 30% of perforations are of unknown etiology. Ninety percent of perforations are in the anterior cartilaginous portions of the nose, less than 10% are in posterior or superior bony portions. The margins of many are lined by smooth, shiny, flat mucosa; others have elevated edges of granulation tissue and crusted edges. These latter types should be fully evaluated for the presence of serious underlying disease.

DIAGNOSTIC STUDIES AND FINDINGS

Facial x-ray examination; examination with nasal speculum or endoscope: Show a shift of the septum or septal perforation

MULTIDISCIPLINARY PLAN

Surgery

For deviation

Submucous resection: May be performed to reposition septum and relieve nasal obstruction

Rhinoplasty: May be done to correct nasal structure deformity and enhance external appearance of nose

Septoplasty to replace septum in midline: May be done to relieve nasal obstruction

For perforation: Surgical closure: possible but not always successful; a Silastic "button" prosthesis may be inserted to close perforation

Medications

Analgesic/antipyretic agents: Acetaminophen (Tylenol), 650 mg PO q4-6h to relieve headache if present (for deviation)

Antihistamines
- Aztemizole (Hismanal), 10 mg PO qd
- Loratadine (Claritin), 10 mg PO qd

Decongestants
- Pseudoephedrine hydrochloride (Sudafed), 30 mg PO q4-6h
- Phenylpropanolamine hydrochloride (Entex, Ornade), 1 PO bid
- Pseudoephedrine hydrochloride with guaifenesin (Deconsal II, Guaifed), 1 capsule PO bid

Antiinfective agents: Antibiotic ointment topically applied to prevent infection; bacitracin (Baciquent), 500 U/g in petrolatum base

General Management

Local application of lanolin or petrolatum twice a day to prevent crusting (for perforation)

Irrigate nose with normal saline solution or a dilute solution of sodium bicarbonate two or three times a day to keep the nasal mucosa hydrated (for perforation) (Box 9-3)

Packing to control bleeding if present (for deviation)

POTENTIAL COMPLICATIONS

Complications related to surgery

INSTRUCTIONS FOR NASAL IRRIGATIONS — Box 9-3

NASAL IRRIGATIONS

USING A SYRINGE

1. Purchase an "ear syringe" (small rubber bulb syringe) from the drugstore.
2. Purchase normal saline solution or prepare by mixing 1 teaspoon salt per 1 quart water (boiled). Store solution in a clean bottle.
3. Squeeze bulb of syringe to withdraw solution from storage container.
4. Leaning over a sink, insert tip of syringe about 1½ to 2 inches into nostril.
5. Gently squeeze bulb to irrigate nose.
6. Blow nose gently after first irrigation.
7. Repeat the irrigation with second syringeful.

NOTE: The normal saline solution also can be placed in a nasal spray bottle for moisturizing the nasal mucosa.

USING A WATER PIK

1. Mix solution as above.
2. Set irrigator to lowest pressure setting.
3. Insert irrigator tip into nose or oral cavity.
4. Leaning over a sink, irrigate nose or sinus through oral cavity defect. Keep your mouth open as some solution will come out through the mouth.
5. Repeat the irrigation.

NURSING CARE

NURSING ASSESSMENT

Nasal Obstruction

Irregularities or deformity of external nose; obstruction to nasal breathing; feeling of facial fullness, headaches, epistaxis; crusting of nasal mucosa; whistle sound when breathing (perforation); or sinusitis

PATIENT PROBLEMS/NURSING DIAGNOSES & INTERVENTIONS

NIC RESPIRATORY MANAGEMENT

Ineffective breathing pattern related to septal deformity causing obstruction

- Assess and record respiratory status.
- Postoperative care includes explanation to patient that facial and periorbital edema may be present and that nasal packing or nasal splints may be used.
- Instruct patient to breathe through mouth during this time.

NIC SKIN/WOUND MANAGEMENT

Impaired skin integrity related to surgery on septum
Risk for injury related to bleeding or tissue trauma

- Keep head of bed slightly elevated *to prevent edema and promote drainage.*
- Use ice compresses on face *to decrease edema, pain, and bleeding.*
- Use cool mist vaporizer *to assist in liquefying secretions.*
- Point out that patient may experience difficulty swallowing if nasal packing used.
- Change drip pad as necessary, recording color, consistency, and amount of drainage.
- Provide meticulous mouth care *because the patient is breathing through mouth.*
- Assess and report presence of excessive bleeding, swallowing, or purulent drainage.
- Caution patient against attempting to blow nose, *which may cause bruising, edema, and bleeding.*
- Caution patient not to smoke and to limit physical activity for several days *to prevent increase in intranasal pressure and irritation or trauma to tissues, which may cause bleeding.*

PATIENT EDUCATION/CONTINUUM OF CARE PLAN

1. To prevent tissue trauma, encourage the patient not to smoke or blow the nose.
2. Encourage the patient to avoid strenuous activity and exercise for several days.
3. Instruct patient in techniques for supplemental humidification.
   a. Vaporizer or humidifier
   b. Normal saline nasal spray
   c. Normal saline irrigations (see Box 9-3)
   d. Apply ointment to nose

EVALUATION/PATIENT OUTCOMES

Respiratory Management: Nasal obstruction is lessened. The patient breathes comfortably. No epistaxis or headache is present.

Skin/Wound Management: Skin integrity is maintained. Septum heals well, with no evidence of infection. Injury does not occur to nasal tissue. Patient verbalizes understanding of the need not to blow the nose, smoke, or participate in excess physical activity for several days.

SINUSITIS

Sinusitis is an inflammatory process caused by bacterial, viral, fungal, or allergic conditions that change the mucosa of a sinus.

Sinusitis is frequently blamed for such symptoms as headaches or nasal problems and accounts for about 25 million visits to a health care facility.[16] Sinusitis can be acute or chronic.

The changes in the sinus mucosa caused by sinusitis produce definite signs and symptoms, most of which can be assessed during a physical examination or on an x-ray examination.

An attack of sinusitis may follow a common cold (0.5% of the time) because nasal edema results in blockage of the sinus ostia, resulting in retained secretions in the sinuses; excessive or forceful nose blowing may also force infected material into the sinuses. Because the sinuses drain secretions through their normal routes into the meatus, any condition that obstructs these openings and forces the secretions to remain in the sinuses may cause infection. These conditions may include the presence of nasal polyps, a deviated nasal septum, or nasal edema resulting from an allergic disorder.

The maxillary sinus (antrum) is the one most frequently affected with acute sinusitis, although the entire group of sinuses may be involved. These are maxillary, frontal, ethmoid, and sphenoid sinuses, all of which drain into the middle meatus of the nose.

The prognosis for sinusitis is usually good with identification and adequate treatment, but some complications may result from sinusitis if the infection spreads. These complications include septicemia, periorbital abscesses, brain abscesses, and osteomyelitis.

Regardless of the type of sinusitis, patients should avoid cold, damp conditions and maintain a constant room temperature and humidity. Smoking may aggravate sinusitis because smoke irritates the mucous membranes and inhibits the normal self-cleansing ciliary action.

PATHOPHYSIOLOGY

Acute suppurative sinusitis may follow a common cold, swimming, or diving when infected water may be forced into the nose and sinuses, resulting in a bacterial infection, or following dental manipulation.

Bacteria that are commonly responsible include gram-positive cocci, such as *Streptococcus, Staphylococcus moraxella catarrhalis,* and *Haemophilus influenzae.* Other organisms are less commonly responsible.

Swimming and diving may cause an acute onset of sinusitis; otherwise the symptoms occur gradually as the involved sinus becomes more inflamed. The nasal mucosa appears red and swollen, and purulent discharge is obvious in the middle meatus. The discharge increases, may be blood tinged in the first 24 to 48 hours, and may cause an inflamed, sore throat from the postnasal discharge. As fluid fills the sinuses, they become opaque to transillumination and an actual fluid level may be seen on x-ray examinations of the sinus.

Pain varies from low-grade to intense as the oxygen in the sinus is absorbed into the blood vessels. This creates negative pressure in the sinus and allows it to be filled with exudate, which produces a painful positive pressure. Tenderness is also present over the involved sinus.

Most cases of acute sinusitis are cured with conservative treatment, including antibiotics, decongestants, and mucoevacuants. Purulent secretions may be present for 3 to 4 days and then slowly resolve over the next 10 days to 2 weeks. In a few cases, however, a purulent nasal discharge persists, and the patient may continue to complain of nasal congestion and vague discomfort over the sinuses or face. This is classified as subacute sinusitis. These patients may have persistent pus in the nose for more than 3 weeks after the acute infection. Because antibiotic therapy will be needed, a culture of the exudate should be obtained and x-ray examinations may be done to determine if more than one sinus is involved.

Frontal sinusitis can cause severe intracranial complications because these sinuses are in close physical relationship with the orbits and are separated from them by thin bony walls. Infection spreads easily from these sinuses to the orbits either through dehiscences in the bones or through infected thrombophlebitic veins. Spread of the infection is made easier by the rich plexus of valveless veins passing between the frontal and ethmoid sinuses and the orbits. Fungal sinusitis may occur both in healthy persons and in persons who are compromised by immunosuppression, debilitation, diabetes, or malignancies being treated with cytotoxic drugs. Depending on the particular fungus and the health of the affected person, fungal sinusitis may be fatal. It is being increasingly recognized in otherwise healthy individuals and should be suspected as well in immunocompetent individuals who have nasal polyposis and sinusitis refractory to standard medical management.

The most common infecting fungal agent is *Aspergillus.* Patients usually have a unilateral infection of the maxillary sinus after a long-standing sinus infection. Similar infections may be caused by *Alternaria, Petriellidum,* or *Paecilomyces,* all commonly found soil organisms.[15]

Patients with persistent subacute sinus infections may have an allergy; recognition of this obviously aids in treatment.

If sinus infections are neglected or a patient has repeated attacks, the mucosal lining of the sinus may become permanently damaged. This is known as chronic suppurative sinusitis. Often the only symptom is continued purulent nasal discharge. If the patient seems unable to overcome the infection, the physician must look for systemic conditions that may lower resistance to infection, such as anemia, malnutrition, or hypometabolism.

Allergic sinusitis occurs only in conjunction with allergic rhinitis. The symptoms are the same, and the sinus mucosa undergoes the same changes as the nasal mucosa. Patients with allergic rhinitis probably also have allergic sinusitis; polyps, which are common with allergic rhinitis, also occur with regularity in the mucosal lining of the sinuses.

Purulent sinusitis superimposed on allergic rhinitis and sinusitis is called hyperplastic sinusitis. The lining of the mucosa

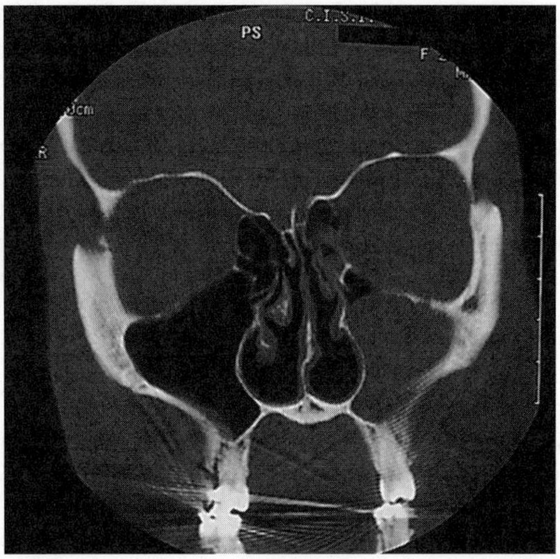

FIG. 9-20
CT scan showing ethmoid and maxillary sinusitis. (From Sigler and Schuring.[22])

and submucosa becomes chronically thickened, and nasal polyps tend to form and recur even after surgical removal. These polyps may block the natural openings to the meatus and obstruct drainage of purulent material. Tissue swelling remains severe, and the nasal tissue does not respond to the usual decongestant solutions. The nose feels plugged most of the time, and a frontal headache is common.

Diagnostic Studies and Findings

Transillumination: Examiner shines bright light in patient's mouth with lips closed around bulb; involved sinus appears dark, whereas normal sinus transilluminates; has limited use but may be used as a screening tool.

Sinus x-ray examinations: Involved sinuses appear clouded or actual fluid level may be seen (FIG. 9-20); screening sinus CT—best diagnostic method to evaluate significant sinonasal inflammatory disorder

Culture of sinus discharge: To identify causative organism

Sinus endoscopy: To evaluate drainage, edema, obstruction of sinus ostia

Multidisciplinary Plan

Surgery

Most now can be performed through sinus endoscopy (functional endoscopic sinus surgery) to open sinus ostia and drain sinuses.

Acute maxillary sinusitis: Creation of nasal window to open sinus and allow pus and secretions to drain through nose

Chronic maxillary sinusitis: Caldwell-Luc procedure (radical antrum operation) through incision under lip to remove diseased mucosa and periosteum

Chronic ethmoid sinusitis: Ethmoidectomy to remove infected tissue through incision into ethmoid sinus

Chronic frontal sinusitis: Creation of osteoplastic flap involves incision across skull and behind hairline to drain sinuses
Frontoethmoidectomy allows removal of infected frontal sinus tissue through external ethmoidectomy approach
Sphenoid sinusitis: External sphenoethmoidectomy performed through incision that begins under eyebrow and extends along side of nose, allowing removal of infected sinus tissue
Fungal sinusitis: Aggressive comprehensive surgical debridement of diseased tissue

Medications

Antiinfective agents
Penicillin G or V, 250-500 mg PO q6h for 10 days
Erythromycin (E-Mycin), 250-500 mg PO q6h for 10 days
Clarithromycin (Biaxin), 500 mg PO bid for 10-14 days
Amoxicillin (Amoxil), 500 mg PO tid for 10 days
Amoxicillin-clavulanate (Augmentin), 500 mg PO q6h for 10-14 days
Sulfamethoxazole (Bactrim, Septra), 1 tab PO bid or qid
Cefaclor (Ceclor) 250 mg PO tid
Cephalexin (Keflex), 500 mg PO qid
Ampicillin, 500 mg PO q6h (for chronic sinusitis)
Loracarbef (Lorabid), 400 mg PO bid for 10-14 days
Amphotericin (Fungizone), 1 mg in 250 D5W over 2-4 h, or 0.25 mg/kg daily by slow infusion over 6 h; increase gradually as patient's tolerance develops, to a maximum of 1 mg/kg/day; dosage must not exceed 1.5/mg/kg/day; premedicate patient with acetaminophen (Tylenol) and diphenhydramine (Benadryl) as a prophylactic measure to avoid some of the unpleasant side effects

Narcotic analgesic agents: Used to relieve headache from acute sinusitis
Codeine, 30-60 mg PO q4-6h
Meperidine (Demerol), 50 mg PO q4-6h

Antihistamines: Used to decrease secretions and congestion in patients with allergic component
Iodinated glycerol, 2 tablets qid, with liquid
Azatadine (Optimine), 1 or 2 mg PO q12h

Decongestants
Pseudoephedrine (Sudafed), 30 mg PO q4-6h prn
Phenylpropanolamine HCl (Entex) PO bid for 10-14 days

Vasoconstrictors
Nose drops or nasal spray containing vasoconstrictor to keep the nose open; Afrin or Neo-Synephrine (1 spray in each nostril q12h) is commonly prescribed for 3-5 days only

Mucolytic agents: Used to thin secretions

General Management

Drainage of involved sinus if usual therapy fails
Antral puncture (puncture of medial wall of maxillary sinus) to provide means of irrigation (may also be done to collect specimen for diagnosis)
Steam inhalation to encourage drainage and promote vasoconstriction
Hot, wet packs applied locally for relief of pain and congestion at least four times a day

Potential Complications

Periorbital abscess, brain abscess, septicemia, osteomyelitis

NURSING CARE

Nursing Assessment

Acute sinusitis: Malaise, anorexia; nasal congestion; purulent nasal discharge; cough; sore throat; fever, usually low grade; pain over sinus areas that worsens as patient bends over; pressure over involved areas and upper teeth; orbital or facial edema; constant, severe headaches; loss of vocal resonance, hyposmia; halitosis
Subacute sinusitis: Stuffy nose; vague intermittent discomfort in involved areas; fatigue; pus in nose more than 3 weeks after acute infection; nonproductive cough
Chronic sinusitis: Persistent purulent nasal discharge; occasional slight headache (from nasal edema or allergic rhinitis and not necessarily from sinuses) that is worse in the morning and relieved slightly during the day; postnasal drip; halitosis
Allergic sinusitis: Nasal stuffiness; symptoms of allergic rhinitis; watery eyes, eczema, and asthma; itching and burning of nose and eyes; sneezing; frontal headache; thin nasal discharge

Potential Complications

Postoperative hemorrhage

Patient Problems/Nursing Diagnoses & Interventions

NIC Physical Comfort Promotion

Acute pain related to edema of nasal tissue and infection
- Assess and document level of comfort.
- Encourage bed rest with head of bed slightly elevated *to promote drainage of secretions.*
- In collaboration with physician, give decongestants and antihistamines as needed for relief. Assess and document effectiveness.
- Administer antibiotics as ordered.
- Medicate with analgesics as needed and evaluate effectiveness. Avoid use of aspirin and NSAIDs.
- Encourage steam inhalation *to liquefy secretions and promote drainage.*
- Apply warm, moist compresses locally at least four times a day *for pain relief and promotion of drainage.*
- Monitor vital signs, especially temperature.
- Watch for and report increase in headaches, blurred vision, periorbital edema, chills, or vomiting.

Disturbed sleep pattern related to pain and edema
- Assess patient's comfort and relaxation level at bedtime.
- Give analgesic medications per physician's orders before patient goes to bed *to minimize headaches.* Administer antihistamines, decongestants, or nose drops at bedtime *to clear nasal passages.*
- Make sure that patient understands importance of using nose drops as prescribed *to prevent rebound effect on mucous membranes if drops are used for a long time.*

Disturbed sensory perception (olfactory) related to nasal congestion
- Assess patient's ability to smell.

- Administer antihistamines, decongestants, and nose drops or spray in collaboration with physician *to relieve nasal congestion.*
- Reassure patient that condition is temporary.

NIC Respiratory Management

Risk for ineffective breathing pattern related to the presence of nasal packing

- Assess and document patient's respiratory status frequently.
- Inform patient before surgery that nasal packing may be in place, that breathing through the mouth will be necessary, and that nose blowing cannot be performed postoperatively *to prevent tissue trauma and bleeding.*

NIC Skin/Wound Management

Impaired skin integrity related to surgical intervention

- Assess surgical site every 1 to 2 hours.
- Place patient in semi-Fowler's position *to minimize edema and promote drainage.*
- Use iced compresses *to minimize swelling and bleeding for first 24 hours.*
- Apply cool or warm vapor inhalations as ordered.
- Provide meticulous mouth care *because patient will be breathing through mouth and may have copious bloody secretions.*
- Change dressing or nasal drip pad and record amount and color of drainage. (There will normally be small amounts of bright red blood with some clots.)
- Inform patient that some numbness of upper lip and teeth may be present after Caldwell-Luc procedure and that ecchymosis and some swelling of operative area are not uncommon for about a week after sinus surgery.
- Instruct patient not to brush teeth in the surgical area during this time *to prevent tissue trauma, if Caldwell-Luc procedure performed.*
- Assess patient for bleeding after surgery.
- Monitor vital signs and watch for frequent swallowing, which may indicate hemorrhaging and swallowing of blood.

Patient Education/Continuum of Care Plan

1. Encourage the patient not to smoke after surgery to minimize irritation of the mucous membranes.
2. Discuss with the patient the need to watch for bleeding after surgery and to notify the physician immediately if it occurs.
3. Explain to the patient the early signs and symptoms of sinusitis so prompt treatment can be obtained.
4. Caution patient about overuse of nasal decongestant sprays (longer than 3 to 5 days), which can cause rebound edema (rhinitis medicamentosa).

Evaluation/Patient Outcomes

Physical Comfort Promotion: Pain and sensory alterations are improved. There is no headache, nasal congestion, or purulent discharge. Patient is able to sleep comfortably. Patient verbalizes an understanding of ways to enhance relaxation and the ability to sleep by using relaxation techniques, analgesics, decongestants, and antihistamines.

Respiratory Management: Normal breathing pattern is maintained. Patient verbalizes an understanding of the need for postoperative mouth breathing, being unable to blow the nose. Patient's breathing returns to normal when edema subsides.

Skin/Wound Management: There is no blood loss after surgery. Patient's vital signs remain stable; no hemorrhage occurs. Tissue integrity is maintained. There is no excessive bleeding or postoperative infection; the wound is completely healed. Patient returns to preoperative level of activity.

THROAT DISORDERS

Abscesses

Throat abscesses are infections in the fascial spaces.

The most common throat abscesses are peritonsillar (quinsy), retropharyngeal, and pharyngomaxillary (lateral pharyngeal space). These abscesses may form after tonsillitis or an infection of the upper respiratory tract. A peritonsillar abscess forms in the space between the tonsil and the fascia that covers the superior constrictor muscle; a retropharyngeal abscess forms between the posterior pharyngeal wall and the prevertebral fascia; and a pharyngomaxillary abscess forms in the deep space between the fascia of the parotid gland, the internal pterygoid muscle, and the superior constrictor muscle (Fig. 9-21).

Pathophysiology

A peritonsillar abscess usually forms after a patient has had tonsillitis and appears to improve. Peritonsillar abscesses are usually caused by group A β-hemolytic streptococci, *Staphylococcus aureus,* or occasionally anaerobic organisms. They are rare in children but fairly common in young adults.

Retropharyngeal abscesses historically were found almost exclusively in infants and children less than 6 years old because the lymph nodes in the retropharyngeal space usually atrophy by young adulthood. Adult cases have been reported with increasing frequency in the medical literature, possibly because of underlying systemic pathologic conditions, or anaerobes and multiple organisms involved with deep neck infections.[15] These are usually found as complications of infections that have spread from the pharynx, sinuses, adenoids, or ears to the retropharyngeal lymph nodes.

Pott's disease, or tuberculosis of the cervical spine, can also cause a "cold" retropharyngeal abscess that may appear at any age.

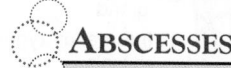

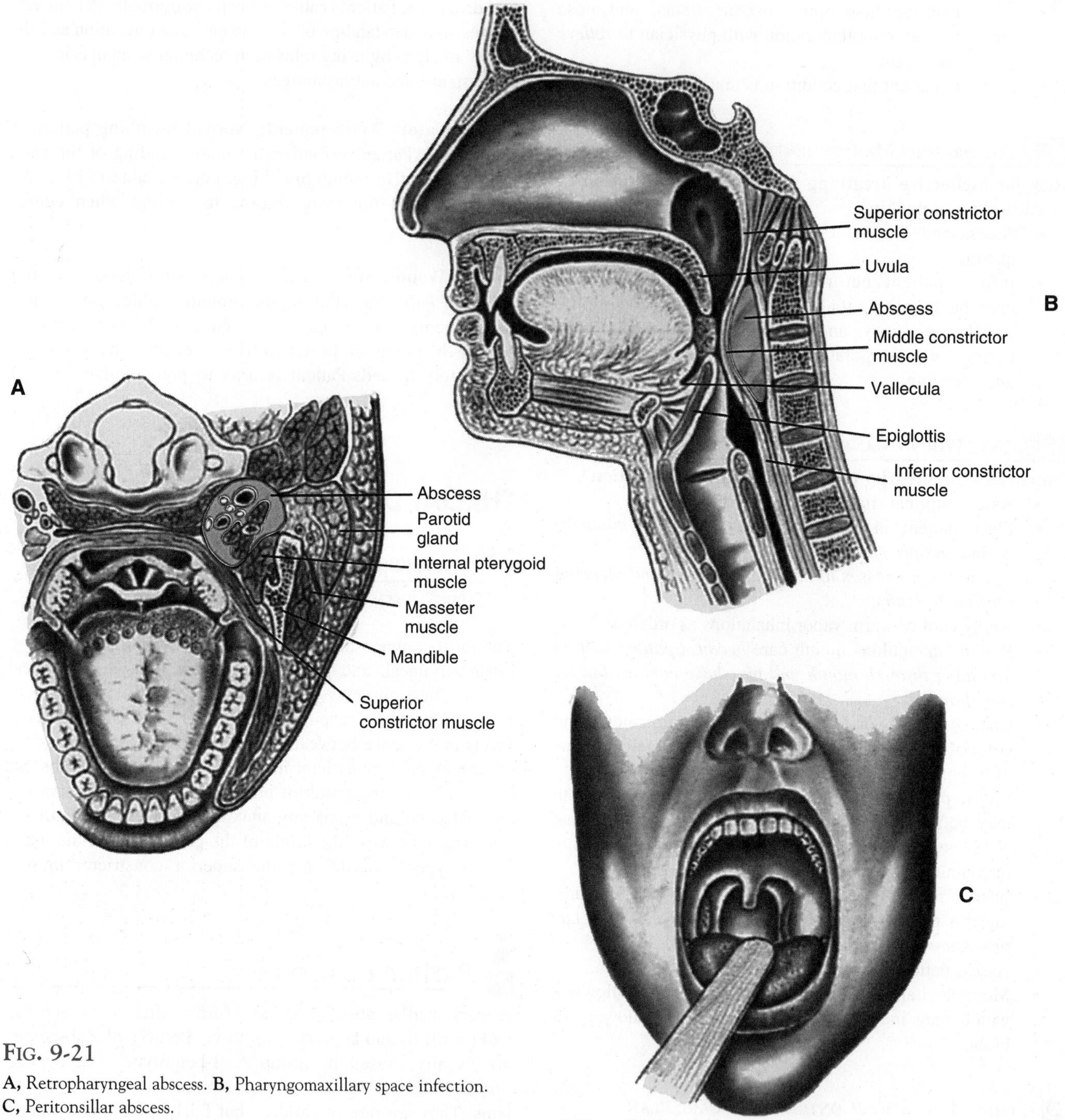

FIG. 9-21

A, Retropharyngeal abscess. **B,** Pharyngomaxillary space infection. **C,** Peritonsillar abscess.

Pharyngomaxillary abscesses are less common than peritonsillar abscesses but more common than retropharyngeal abscesses. Pharyngomaxillary abscesses usually result from the spread of an adjacent infection from the pharynx, tonsils, teeth, parotid gland, or lymph nodes.

Diagnostic Studies and Findings

CT or MRI scan: Mass shows in posterior pharynx with retropharyngeal abscesses
Culture of abscess: To identify causative organism
Visual examination: Tonsil appears pushed toward midline forward and downward; uvula may rest against tonsil or palate in peritonsillar abscess

Multidisciplinary Plan

Surgery

Guided needle aspiration with CT
Incision and drainage of abscess with or without local anesthetic, if needed
External drainage of pharyngomaxillary space abscess

Tonsillectomy during acute episode or about 1 month after peritonsillar abscess has healed to prevent recurrence

Medications

Antiinfective agents

- Clindamycin (Cleocin), 300 mg IV, IM, or PO q6h for 10-14 days
- Ampicillin-sulbactam (Unasyn), 1.5-3 g IM, IV q6h for 7-10 days
- Amoxicillin-clavulanate (Augmentin), 500 mg PO q8h for 10-14 days

POTENTIAL COMPLICATIONS

Septic thrombosis of internal jugular vein (most common complication of pharyngomaxillary abscess); recurrent infection or spread into pharyngomaxillary space with peritonsillar abscess; rupture of abscess with aspiration; airway obstruction

NURSING CARE

NURSING ASSESSMENT

Peritonsillar area: Severe sore throat; difficulty in swallowing; trismus; drooling; muffled voice; "hot-potato" voice; thick secretions; fever, chills, nausea, and malaise; displacement of uvula to unaffected side

Retropharyngeal area: Stridor and nasal obstruction; muffled cry; child lies with head extended; fever; posterior pharyngeal wall soft, red, and bulging

Pharyngomaxillary area: Fullness behind jaw; trismus

PATIENT PROBLEMS/NURSING DIAGNOSES & INTERVENTIONS

NIC PHYSICAL COMFORT PROMOTION

Acute pain related to swelling from abscess

- Assess and record amount of pain experienced and need for pain medication.
- Administer analgesic and antipyretic agents as ordered and document effectiveness.

NIC RESPIRATORY MANAGEMENT

Ineffective breathing pattern related to pressure on airway from abscess

Risk for aspiration related to spontaneous rupture of abscess

- Observe airway until edema subsides.
- Assess for dyspnea, restlessness, stridor, and cyanosis.
- Before abscess is drained, assess patient closely for signs of spontaneous rupture of abscess and possible aspiration of pus. (When abscesses are drained, it is not unusual for pus to pour out.)
- Avoid use of oral thermometer and gargles, which could precipitate spontaneous rupture of abscess.
- Keep patient upright with oral suction available *to prevent aspiration of pus.*
- After incision and drainage or evacuation of abscess administer antibiotics as ordered.
- Monitor and document vital signs, skin color, and presence of bleeding.

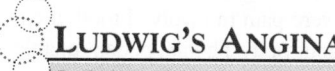

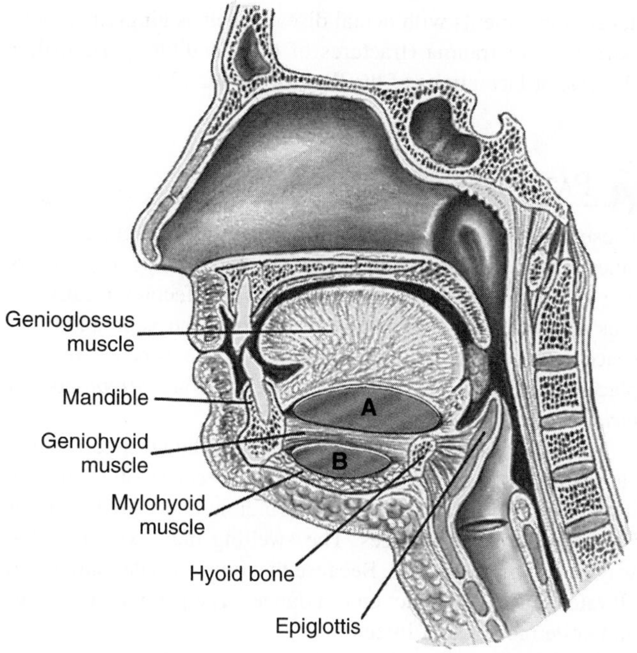

FIG. 9-22

Ludwig's angina. *A* and *B* indicate spaces in which infection may start.

- Ensure adequate fluid intake; intravenous therapy will probably be ordered.

PATIENT EDUCATION/CONTINUUM OF CARE PLAN

1. Explain to the patient or family the necessity of continuing antibiotic therapy for the entire prescribed course to prevent recurrence or complications.
2. Review signs of abscess with patient and family. Encourage patient to seek medical attention if symptoms recur.
3. Discuss with the patient that peritonsillar abscesses are likely to recur and if tonsillectomy has not been performed during acute episode, about a month after the abscess has healed, a tonsillectomy will be performed to prevent recurrence.

EVALUATION/PATIENT OUTCOMES

Physical Comfort Promotion: Patient's comfort is improved. There is no pain in throat. Temperature is within normal limits for patient. Trismus and drooling are absent. Incised area is healing well.

Respiratory Management: Normal breathing pattern is maintained. Patient's airway is maintained. There is no stridor, dyspnea, or aspiration. Vital signs and fluid intake remain at normal levels.

LUDWIG'S ANGINA

Ludwig's angina is a virulent, rapidly spreading cellulitis of the floor of the mouth that occurs in the submental, sublingual, and submaxillary spaces (FIG. 9-22).

Ludwig's angina is actually not an abscess, although it resembles one, and there is no lymphatic involvement. Most cases develop in patients with dental disease such as gingivitis, tooth extraction, or trauma (fractures of the mandible, peritonsillar abscess, or lacerations of the floor of the mouth).[7]

PATHOPHYSIOLOGY

These patient's lower molars oddly have the roots closer to the inner than to the outer side of the jaw, and the tips of the roots may extend below the mylohyoid line. The infection usually begins around a tooth root that drains into the submandibular space rather than into the sublingual space because of root placement. The usual causative organisms are *Streptococcus viridans* and *Escherichia coli.*

The infection spreads rapidly to the sublingual space, which causes the floor of the mouth to become very swollen. It may involve all the tissues under the mandible and usually one or both submandibular spaces. The swelling may extend all the way down to the clavicle. Because the tongue is edematous and elevated, airway obstruction is a danger. The patient has a fever and systemic signs of infection.

Pus is seldom found if an incision and drainage are performed, although they must occasionally be done to drain fluid and relieve the pressure on the swollen tissues.

Tracheotomy must often be performed because the patient's airway is greatly compromised from both swelling and excessive secretions.

DIAGNOSTIC STUDIES AND FINDINGS

Identification of causative organism: Culture of exudate; visual examination

CT scan: Indicates presence of and pinpoints location of cellulitis

MULTIDISCIPLINARY PLAN

Surgery

Incision and drainage to relieve pressure; tracheotomy if airway is impaired

Medications

Antiinfective agents

- Penicillin G aqueous, 1-2 million U q4h IV
- Cefotaxime (Claforan), 1-2 g q6-8h IM or IV (given if patient is allergic to penicillin)

NURSING CARE

NURSING ASSESSMENT

Infectious process in mouth: Severe pain in involved tooth area; trismus (difficulty opening mouth); dysphonia; patient unable to eat; excessive secretions and drooling; swelling of the floor of the mouth causing the tongue to be pushed up and back

Respiratory function: Dyspnea and stridor

POTENTIAL COMPLICATION

Airway obstruction

PATIENT PROBLEMS/NURSING DIAGNOSES & INTERVENTIONS

NIC RESPIRATORY MANAGEMENT

Ineffective airway clearance related to swelling, airway obstruction

- Maintain emergency airway equipment in case it is needed.
- Assess patient for signs of airway obstruction.
- Perform usual tracheostomy care and frequent suctioning; assist patient in suctioning secretions.
- Encourage patient to expectorate secretions, if possible.
- Observe vital signs and symptoms of dyspnea and stridor.
- Elevate head of bed.
- Administer antibiotics, antipyretics, and steroids as ordered.

NIC PHYSICAL COMFORT PROMOTION

Acute pain related to swelling in the floor of the mouth

Fear related to inability to open mouth, pain, and airway obstruction

- Assess level of pain experienced and need for medication.
- Provide adequate analgesia for pain relief; assess and document effectiveness.
- Perform wound care gently but thoroughly if incision and drainage were performed.
- Assure patient that he or she is closely monitored.
- Explain all procedures, progress, and areas of concern.
- Explain tracheostomy procedure and suctioning, and assure patient it will assist with breathing.

NIC NUTRITION SUPPORT

Imbalanced nutrition: less than body requirements, related to trismus, pain, and swelling in the floor of the mouth

- Maintain NPO status until patient is able to swallow.
- Assess and document patient's fluid and nutrition status.
- Ensure adequate fluid intake *to prevent dehydration.*
- Monitor intravenous line closely.
- When patient can take food and fluids orally, have nutritionist visit patient to plan diet *to provide needed caloric intake.*

NIC PATIENT EDUCATION

Deficient knowledge related to lack of information about Ludwig's angina

- Inform patient of cause of Ludwig's angina.
- Encourage good oral hygiene and dental care.

PATIENT EDUCATION/CONTINUUM OF CARE PLAN

1. Stress the importance of good dental hygiene to prevent recurrence of Ludwig's angina or other oral or dental problems.
2. Ensure that patient and family can perform wound care if tracheotomy is performed.
3. Discuss with patient and family the nutritional needs after discharge.

4. Discuss the need for the patient to complete course of antibiotics.

Evaluation/Patient Outcomes

Respiratory Management: Airway clearance is adequate. Airway is patent without respiratory difficulty. Tracheostomy stoma is healing well. There is no swelling in the floor of the mouth. Tongue is not elevated or edematous.

Physical Comfort Promotion: Comfort is increased. Pain is diminished to absent. Temperature is within normal limits. Wound is healing normally if incision and drainage are performed. Fear is resolved.

Nutrition Support: Patient's nutritional status is adequate. Patient eats with no difficulty and understands the need to maintain adequate caloric and fluid intake.

Patient Education: Patient's knowledge base is increased. Patient verbalizes understanding of importance of prophylactic dental care and early treatment of any oral inflammation.

Laryngitis

Laryngitis, or inflammation of the larynx, is a common disorder that may be either acute or chronic.

Acute laryngitis may be found as part of a viral or bacterial infection of the upper respiratory tract, or it may be an isolated infection limited to the vocal cords. Trauma such as voice abuse or gastroesophageal reflux may also cause acute laryngitis.

Chronic laryngitis implies inflammatory changes in the laryngeal mucosa. It can be progressive and may lead to a serious voice disability.

Pathophysiology

Acute laryngitis is often found in combination with viral or bacterial infections of the upper respiratory tract. Viral infections are the most common, but organisms such as β-hemolytic streptococci and *Streptococcus pneumoniae* are also causative agents. Laryngitis may occur with colds, bronchitis, pneumonia, or influenza.

Noninfectious causes include excessive use of the voice, such as in public speakers or singers; chronic reflux of gastric acid; inhalation of toxic or irritating fumes; or aspiration of caustic chemicals.

Chronic laryngitis can be caused by frequent attacks of acute laryngitis, chronic abuse of the voice, and smoking. Chronic tonsillitis and adenoiditis, allergies, or hypermetabolic states may occasionally cause chronic laryngitis.

Diagnostic Studies and Findings

Laryngoscopy, direct or indirect: Shows abnormalities in true cords, reddened mucosa, and secretions on vocal cords; acute: hoarseness to aphonia; nonproductive cough; rough, scratchy throat; edema, stridor, and dyspnea in severe cases; fever or malaise; chronic: progressive hoarseness, if present, is worse in morning because of dried secretions in larynx; voice improves during day and deteriorates again toward evening with voice use; usually no throat pain; nonproductive cough

Multidisciplinary Plan

Surgery

None unless tracheotomy is required because of severe laryngeal edema

Medications

Antiinfective agents: Penicillin G, 250 mg PO q6h for 10-12 days

Analgesic/antipyretic agents: Acetaminophen (Tylenol), 650 mg PO q4-6h prn

Analgesic agents: Throat lozenges (Chloraseptic or Cepacol) if necessary for throat pain

Antitussive agents: Guaifenesin (Robitussin), 100-400 mg q4h to relieve cough

General Management

Voice rest; steam inhalation; speech therapy for chronic laryngitis

Potential Complications

Abnormal voice, airway obstruction

NURSING CARE

Nursing Assessment

General: Hoarseness; rough, scratchy throat; fever, malaise; cough

Patient Problems/Nursing Diagnoses & Interventions

NIC Physical Comfort Promotion

Acute pain related to sore throat, laryngeal edema

- Assess level of pain experienced.
- Administer analgesics, throat lozenges, or antitussives *for comfort.*
- Administer antibiotics as ordered.
- Provide for inhalation of warm steam *for symptomatic relief.*
- Enforce that patient does not smoke.

NIC Communication Enhancement

Impaired verbal communication related to poor voice quality, hoarseness

- Assess patient's understanding of need for voice rest.
- Encourage complete voice rest or minimal use of voice. Encourage patient not to whisper *as more force is needed to approximate vocal cords.*
- Provide Magic Slate or paper and pencil *to facilitate communication.* Provide communication board, if patient is illiterate.

- Anticipate patient's needs as much as possible *to eliminate need for patient to talk.*
- Encourage family and friends to assist patient by asking questions patient can answer by nodding.
- If patient is hospitalized, mark on intercom that patient cannot respond and notify patient that someone will come to room when light is turned on.

PATIENT EDUCATION/CONTINUUM OF CARE PLAN

Ensure that the patient understands possible sequelae of constant voice abuse and smoking and encourage improvement of these habits.

EVALUATION/PATIENT OUTCOMES

Physical Comfort Promotion: Comfort is improved. There is no hoarseness and voice is normal for patient. Raw, tickling feeling in throat is gone. Cough and throat pain are absent. Temperature is within normal limits for patient. There is no inflammation or swelling in laryngeal mucosa or vocal cords.

Communication Enhancement: Patient's understanding of laryngitis is increased. Patient verbalizes understanding of causes of laryngitis and preventive measures: no smoking, no voice abuse, early treatment of colds, and recognition of symptoms of bronchitis.

PHARYNGITIS

Pharyngitis is an acute or chronic inflammation of the pharynx, including the pharyngeal walls, tonsils, uvula, and palate.

PATHOPHYSIOLOGY

Pharyngitis is the most common of the throat disorders. It frequently precedes or accompanies the common cold and is characterized by a mild sore throat, difficulty and pain in swallowing, and a low-grade fever. In more than 50% of cases pharyngitis is viral in origin.[15] The bacterial cause is usually *Streptococcus,* especially in children. Unless complicated by other bacteria, pharyngitis usually resolves in 4 to 6 days. It is communicable for 2 to 3 days after the initial symptoms appear. Fungal pharyngitis is usually seen in immunocompromised patients and may result from prolonged use of antibiotics.

If follicular pharyngitis develops, usually from infection by β-hemolytic streptococci, the mucous membrane becomes severely inflamed and studded with white or yellow follicles. If these follicles are present, most are on the tonsils; if the tonsils have been removed, the follicles appear on the lymphoid areas in the posterior pharynx and also on the lingual tonsils and in the nasopharynx.

In approximately 10% of cases, pharyngitis is a result of infection with adenovirus. Primary infections occur during childhood; summer epidemics may result from waterborne vectors. In winter the mode of transmission is mainly respiratory. This can cause a severe and rapidly infectious, diffuse respiratory infection known as acute febrile respiratory disease, often accompanied by primary atypical pneumonia.[15] Infectious mononucleosis, caused by the Epstein-Barr virus, may also cause pharyngitis.

DIAGNOSTIC STUDIES AND FINDINGS

Throat culture: Taken to determine causative organism
Heterophil agglutination antibody (monospot): To rule out mononucleosis
WBC count

MULTIDISCIPLINARY PLAN

Medications

Antiinfective agents
Erythromycin, 250-500 mg q6h
Azithromycin, 500 mg PO × 1 time, then 250 mg qd for 4 days
Clarithromycin, 250-500 mg q12h for 10 days
Penicillin G or V, 250 mg PO q6h for 10 days (if pharyngitis has bacterial cause)

For fungal pharyngitis
Fluconazole (Diflucan), 100-200 mg PO qd for 1-5 days
Nystatin (Mycostatin), 100,000 U/ml; 400,000-600,000 U PO (swish and swallow) qid for 10-14 days
Clortrimazole (Mycelex troche), 10 mg (dissolve in mouth) qid for 14 days

Analgesic/antipyretic agents
Acetylsalicylic acid (aspirin), 300-600 mg PO q4-6h
Acetaminophen, 650 mg q4h prn

General Management

Bed rest; humidification; warm saline throat irrigations; adequate fluid intake: if throat is so painful and swollen that adequate fluids cannot be taken orally, the patient is often hospitalized for intravenous fluid intake for 24 to 72 hours or until inflammation subsides

NURSING CARE

NURSING ASSESSMENT

Infectious Process in Throat
Sore throat, with slight difficulty swallowing, including saliva; mild fever; headaches, malaise, and joint pain; earache; cervical lymphadenopathy; pharynx reddened and inflamed; blisters or follicles on tonsils or lymphoid areas
Patients with mononucleosis may have enlargement of the spleen in addition to local symptoms

POTENTIAL COMPLICATIONS

Retropharyngeal abscess, parapharyngeal abscess, peritonsillar abscess

PATIENT PROBLEMS/NURSING DIAGNOSES & INTERVENTIONS

NIC PHYSICAL COMFORT PROMOTION

Acute pain related to infectious process in throat
- Assess level of pain experienced.
- Administer antiinfective agents and analgesics as ordered.

- Assess and document effectiveness.
- Provide warm saline throat irrigations for comfort.
- Encourage bed rest.

NIC TISSUE PERFUSION MANAGEMENT

Risk for deficient fluid volume related to pain and an inability to drink fluids normally

- Assess patient's fluid intake, skin turgor, and urine output.
- Encourage a fluid intake of at least 2500 ml/day.
- Monitor intake and output; observe for signs of dehydration (dry skin, cracked lips, and decreased urine output).
- If intravenous fluid is ordered, maintain adequate flow rate.
- Assist patient with frequent oral hygiene; patient may be mouth breathing, which adds to discomfort.
- Monitor patient's temperature and report abnormalities.

NIC PATIENT EDUCATION

Deficient knowledge related to lack of information about pharyngitis

- Teach the patient the early signs of infection.
- Provide information to patient and family about transmission of pharyngitis.
- Reinforce information provided about treatment of pharyngitis.
- Encourage patient to complete medications prescribed.

PATIENT EDUCATION/CONTINUUM OF CARE PLAN

1. Instruct the patient and family about the necessity of completing the prescribed course of antiinfective agents to prevent complications or recurrence of infection.
2. Inform the patient and family of possible irritants (smoking and lack of humidity) and ways to prevent inflammation.
3. Instruct patient/caregiver about fluid requirements and signs of dehydration.

EVALUATION/PATIENT OUTCOMES

Physical Comfort Promotion: Pharyngitis is resolved. Sore throat is gone. Patient is afebrile. Activity level is normal for patient. There is no swelling or infection in throat. Cervical lymphadenopathy is absent.

Tissue Perfusion Management: Patient maintains adequate hydration. Fluid and nutritional status are adequate for patient's needs. Skin turgor is normal.

Patient Education: Patient verbalizes knowledge of treatment. Patient verbalizes understanding of necessity of completing prescribed course of antiinfective agents.

TONSILLITIS

Tonsillitis is an inflammation of the palatine tonsil(s).

Tonsillitis may be acute or chronic. It usually remains localized in the tonsillar tissue and is considered mildly contagious. It is characterized by a sore throat, but the patient may experience referred pain to the ears.

Tonsillitis is usually an airborne bacterial infection. It can occur at any age but is most frequently found in children between the ages of 5 and 10 years. If uncomplicated, it usually resolves after 5 to 7 days. Treatment makes the patient more comfortable and may prevent serious complications such as arthritis, glomerulonephritis, or chronic tonsillitis. A less common cause of tonsillitis is viral infection.

Several years ago the role of the tonsils and adenoids in the immune system was not as well known as it is today, and surgical removal of the tonsils and adenoids was common. However, these procedures are performed less today because the importance of this lymphoid tissue to the body's immune system has been established.

PATHOPHYSIOLOGY

Tonsillitis begins as a sore throat accompanied by fever, chills, headache, myalgia, joint pain, and anorexia. The patient may also have enlarged and tender anterior cervical lymph nodes. The tonsils appear enlarged, reddened, and inflamed with pus or exudate projecting from between the pillars of the fauces or in the crypts. Some of the exudate can be pulled away from the tonsil, which causes bleeding. The white blood cell count is frequently increased.

A throat culture should be obtained to identify the infecting organism. *Streptococcus* (β-hemolytic streptococci group A) is the most common organism. If this is the cause, the tonsils appear studded with yellow follicles. Other causative agents are *Pneumococcus* and gram-negative organisms (*Proteus, Pseudomonas,* or coliforms) and viruses.

DIAGNOSTIC STUDIES AND FINDINGS

Throat culture: Identification of causative organism

MULTIDISCIPLINARY PLAN

Surgery

Tonsillectomy, if indicated, after acute infection has subsided

Medications

Analgesic/antipyretic agents: Acetaminophen (Tylenol), 650 mg PO q4-6h for adults with /without codeine

Antiinfective agents

- Penicillin V (Pen-V), 250-500 mg PO q6h
- Penicillin G (Bicillin), 600,000-1,200,000 U IM
- Dicloxacillin, 250-500 mg PO q6h
- Cephalexin, 250-500 mg PO q12h

NURSING CARE

NURSING ASSESSMENT

Infectious Process in Throat

Moderate to severe sore throat; pain referred to ears; anterior cervical lymphadenopathy; fever and chills; headache; muscle and joint pain; anorexia; increased secretions from throat; enlarged, reddened, inflamed tonsils; pus or exudate on tonsils; halitosis; edematous or inflamed uvula; elevated white blood count

Potential Complications

Peritonsillar abscess, glomerulonephritis

Patient Problems/Nursing Diagnoses & Interventions

NIC Physical Comfort Promotion

Acute pain related to severe sore throat

- Assess level of pain experienced and need for pain medication.
- Provide adequate analgesia *for relief of throat pain;* assess and document effectiveness.
- Administer antibiotics as ordered.
- Perform throat irrigations; provide warm saline gargles or ice collar *as comfort measure.*
- Maintain bed rest during acute phase and emphasize importance of rest while convalescing.

NIC Nutrition Support

Imbalanced nutrition: less than body requirements, related to difficulty in swallowing food

Risk for deficient fluid volume related to difficulty in swallowing fluids

- Assess patient's nutritional status and ability to eat.
- Ensure that patient has adequate intake of soft, nourishing foods.
- Encourage patient to eat foods that are minimally irritating to throat and provide adequate caloric intake, that is, soups and milkshakes.
- Assess skin turgor, intake and urine output, and ability to swallow fluids.
- Encourage increased fluid intake, keeping in mind that children can become dehydrated very quickly. Note that the child may like ice cream, sherbet, or flavored drinks; avoid citrus juices *because they may irritate throat.*
- If patient is hospitalized, monitor intravenous intake *to ensure adequate intake of fluid.*

Patient Education/Continuum of Care Plan

1. Stress to the patient and family the importance of completing the prescribed course of antibiotics to prevent complications or recurrence.
2. Ensure that patient and family understand which foods and fluids maintain adequate nutrition and hydration without irritating throat.
3. Instruct patient and family about signs of dehydration.

Evaluation/Patient Outcomes

Physical Comfort Promotion: Comfort is improved. Patient is afebrile. Tonsils are normal in size and free of pus and exudate. There is no pain in throat. Lymph nodes are not enlarged, although this might persist after other symptoms have disappeared. White blood count is within normal limits. Patient and family verbalize understanding of necessity of completing the required course of medication.

Nutrition Support: Nutrition and hydration are adequately maintained. Patient is able to eat and drink to maintain nutritional and hydration status within normal limits.

Vocal Cord Paralysis

Vocal cord paralysis is the loss of nerve and motor supply to the vocal cords resulting in fixation and abnormal position of one or both cords.

Paralysis of the vocal cords is the result of either disease or injury to the superior laryngeal nerve or the recurrent laryngeal nerve, which is the branch of the vagus nerve that provides the entire motor supply to the larynx.

Vocal cord paralysis may be unilateral or bilateral. The quality of the voice depends on whether one or both cords are affected, as well as the position and tenseness of the affected cord. Paralysis of the vocal cords may also be described as complete versus incomplete or abductor versus adductor. Lesions of the central nervous system, such as multiple sclerosis, syringomyelia, brain tumors, and vascular accidents can produce paralysis of the vocal cords.

Pathophysiology

The left recurrent laryngeal nerve, which follows a longer path, is paralyzed in more than 70% of cases, in contrast to about 15% for the right recurrent laryngeal nerve. Men are affected about 10 times more commonly than women, and the most common age is during the seventies. The most common cause of injury to the nerve is thyroid surgery, with other causes following surgery such as anterior cervical fusion or carotid endarterectomy. Cancer of the larynx and lung can also result in vocal cord paralysis or fixation of the vocal cord.

Peripheral causes are also common. These include stretching of the nerve, as occurs with aortic aneurysms and mitral stenosis. Stretching causes enlargement of the left auricle and also stretches the left recurrent laryngeal nerve. The nerve can be infiltrated or stretched by lung or bronchial tumors. Thyroid carcinomas may cause paralysis, and tumors of the vocal cords eventually cause fixation of one or both cords as the tumor invades the muscle or nerve.

Some cases of vocal cord paralysis are unexplained and are called idiopathic. These cases may be from viral infections that remain undiagnosed. In many of these cases the function of the vocal cord recovers spontaneously. The high incidence of infections of the upper respiratory tract suggests a viral cause in many cases.

The most common form of paralysis is unilateral; one cord is paralyzed, and the other remains normal. If the affected cord is paralyzed in the midline, the normal cord can usually approximate it and the patient may have a normal voice. However, if the paralyzed cord is abducted, the normal cord cannot meet it and the patient has a husky, "breathy" voice and may be at risk for aspiration.

PRESBYLARYNGEUS: SPEECH DISORDER IN THE ELDERLY

Presbylaryngeus is dysphonia of the elderly. The patient's vocal cords undergo a loss of muscle tone resulting in bowing of the vocal cords. This bowing prevents the normal approximation of the cords, causing a breathy, weak voice. Consultation with a speech therapist may provide the patient with strengthening exercises to improve the voice.

Dyspnea is not associated with unilateral cord paralysis because the laryngeal airway is adequate; the good cord abducts enough for the airway. However, bilateral cord paralysis affects the airway more seriously. The cords are usually paralyzed in the adducted position. The cords may be within 2 to 3 mm of the midline, and the patient suffers both stridor and dyspnea on exertion. Anything causing even minimal vocal cord edema may precipitate respiratory distress.

Diagnostic Studies and Findings

Laryngoscopy: Shows paralyzed condition of vocal cord(s)
Bronchoscopy and esophagoscopy: Done as part of malignancy workup
Videostroboscopy: Records vocal cord movement
Electromyography: Determines vocal cord innervation
Skull x-ray examinations, CT scan to visualize the course of the recurrent laryngeal nerve from the skull base to the chest, thyroid scan, upper gastrointestinal series, and complete neurologic examination: Performed to rule out other causes of vocal cord paralysis

Multidisciplinary Plan

Surgery

For unilateral paralysis

Injection of measured amounts of silicone or Teflon into paralyzed cord under direct laryngoscopy; enlarges or swells cord and brings it closer to midline so normal cord can better approximate it; strengthens voice and prevents aspiration

Thyroplasty: Involves an external incision in the neck with insertion of a stent to move the paralyzed cord toward the midline

For bilateral paralysis

Tracheotomy may be needed because of inadequate airway

Alternative therapy is arytenoidectomy in which one arytenoid cartilage is removed and glottis is opened posteriorly

King procedure is another alternative in which suture is passed around arytenoid cartilage and through adjacent cricoid cartilage; arytenoid is rotated and fixed laterally; improves airway patency but may adversely affect quality of voice; many patients decide to conserve their voices and keep tracheotomy tube

Medialization laryngoplasty: Generally performed under local anesthesia with little discomfort to the patient; involves creation of a window into the larynx, centered over the thyroid ala; a Silastic implant (1×0.5 cm) is placed after the cartilage is pushed inward[14a, 17a]

NURSING CARE

Nursing Assessment

Voice: Vocal weakness; hoarse, breathy quality
Respiratory function: Stridor and dyspnea on exertion if paralysis is bilateral; aspiration on swallowing, coughing

Potential Complication

Airway distress

Patient Problems/Nursing Diagnoses & Interventions

NIC Respiratory Management

Ineffective breathing pattern related to excessive secretions

- Assess patient closely for excessive secretions and need for suctioning.
- Increase humidification.
- Elevate head of bed.
- Minimize patient's activity.
- Instruct patient to avoid upper respiratory infection.
- Provide usual postoperative care after tracheotomy is performed.
- After assessing patient's readiness, teach patient to care for tracheotomy tube: suctioning, cleaning, and changing tube.

Risk for aspiration related to paresis or paralysis

- Evaluate swallowing ability and cough.
- Provide foods with thick consistency; avoid liquids.
- Consult with speech/swallowing therapy for assistance with determining food consistency and swallowing techniques.
- Auscultate lungs for signs of aspiration pneumonia.

NIC Communication Enhancement

Impaired verbal communication related to poor voice quality and to surgical procedure

- Assess and document quality of patient's voice before and after operation.
- Ensure that patient understands surgical procedure.
- Indicate to patient that voice will be improved but may not be completely normal.

Patient Education/Continuum of Care Plan

1. Instruct patient to avoid smoking, smoke-filled environment.
2. Encourage follow-up with rehabilitation team members (speech therapist, gastroenterologist).
3. Encourage patient to avoid crowds, upper respiratory infections, strenuous exercise.
4. If a tracheotomy has been performed:
   a. Remind the patient that speaking can be accomplished normally by using a tracheotomy plug or by occluding the lumen of the tracheotomy with a finger.

b. Advise the patient to wear a medical alert bracelet indicating that a tracheotomy is present.
c. Ensure that the patient and family can care safely for the tracheotomy tube at home; evaluate the need for community resource assistance to provide care.

EVALUATION/PATIENT OUTCOMES

Respiratory Management: Breathing pattern improves. Patient demonstrates ability to suction, clean, and humidify tracheotomy tube. No signs of aspiration or aspiration-related complications.

Communication Enhancement: Communication has improved. Voice maintains good quality. Secretions have diminished, and patient requires minimal suctioning.

VOCAL CORD POLYPS AND NODULES

Polyps are edematous masses of mucous membrane that attach to the vocal cords by either broad or narrow bases.

Polyps usually develop on the vocal cords from chronic abuse of the voice, allergies, or chronic inhalation of irritants, which frequently starts during an acute infection of the upper respiratory tract. Most have a broad base, so there is permanent interference with voice production; however, some polyps are pedunculated, hang under the vocal cord, and cause only intermittent symptoms. Polyps are usually unilateral and may appear anywhere on the vocal cord. They are common in adults who smoke, have allergies, or live in very dry climates. Polyps are far more common in men and rarely found in children. Because the vocal cords are inhibited from approximation, painless hoarseness is the only symptom.

Polyps are gelatinous and telangiectatic, but mainly transitional types of polyps can be seen. Examination may show a change in the permeability of blood vessels, allowing extravasation of fluid, fibrin, or erythrocytes. After this, reactive processes develop and labryinthine vascular spaces form. This process is similar to the formation of a thrombus. The polyps develop at the site of maximum muscular and aerodynamic forces exerted during phonation and are considered a sequela of phonotrauma.

Vocal cord nodules, also called singer's, teacher's, or screamer's nodules, are caused by chronic voice abuse, such as singing, screaming, or constantly speaking outside the natural voice range. Nodules occur at any age and usually in girls and women, although they are sometimes found in young boys who scream and shout excessively.

The nodules are benign growths that first appear red and raised above the vocal cord surface. They later change into small white lumps that touch when the cords approximate. Because they are raised, the cords are kept apart and produce a characteristic hoarse, breathy voice (FIG. 9-23). The patient may complain of a foreign body sensation in the throat.

Conservative treatment of nodules and complete voice rest often cause even large nodules to disappear. After voice rest, speech therapy may be indicated to prevent recurrence of the nodules and restore a normal voice. In contrast, polyps usually require surgical removal; they do not disappear with voice rest. Direct laryngoscopy is performed, and the polyps are removed by laser or surgical excision. If a patient has bilateral polyps, the excision should be done in two stages because doing both sides at the same time may cause a laryngeal web to form between the two raw surfaces.

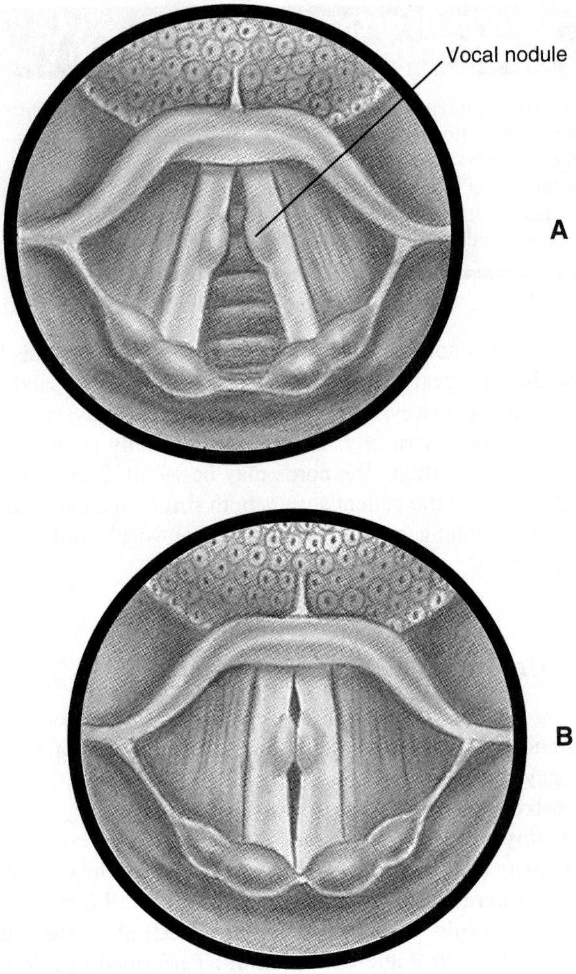

FIG. 9-23
Vocal cord nodules. **A,** During respiration. **B,** During phonation.

PATIENT PROBLEMS/NURSING DIAGNOSES & INTERVENTIONS

NIC COMMUNICATION ENHANCEMENT

Impaired verbal communication related to prescribed voice rest

- Assess patient's understanding of need for voice rest.
- Ensure that patient does not speak or whisper during period of voice rest; provide patient with Magic Slate or paper and pencil *to encourage nonverbal written communication.*
- Remind visitors and staff members that patient is not to speak; attempt to anticipate patient's needs so patient will not have to speak.
- Use humidifier in room *to provide adequate moisture in air and decrease throat irritation.*

- Encourage patient to avoid smoking *to minimize exposure to irritants.*

PATIENT EDUCATION/CONTINUUM OF CARE PLAN

1. Refer the patient to a speech therapist after discharge to prevent recurrence of nodules or polyps.
2. Discourage the patient from smoking because exposure to irritants such as smoke predisposes patients to changes in membrane lining the larynx.
3. Discuss with the patient the importance of adequate humidification in the home to prevent throat irritation.

EVALUATION/PATIENT OUTCOMES

Communication Enhancement: Patient's communication has improved. There are no nodules or polyps on vocal cords. Patient is able to speak in a normal voice. Patient verbalizes understanding of stresses on voice and how to minimize these: no smoking, avoidance of allergens, and no excessive shouting or screaming.

COLLABORATIVE INTERVENTIONS AND RELATED NURSING CARE

MYRINGOTOMY

Description and Rationale

Myringotomy is an incision in the tympanic membrane, usually to drain fluid from the middle ear. A local or general anesthetic may be used, although the procedure is relatively painless. A curved incision is made in the posteroinferior portion of the drumhead with a very sharp myringotomy knife. The physician wears a head mirror and uses an aural speculum, or microscope, to visualize the drumhead to avoid injuring the ossicles.

After the drumhead is incised, suction may be used to remove fluid. Cotton is then placed in the ear to absorb the drainage, which may continue for several days.

A myringotomy incision heals quickly with only minimal scarring and does not disrupt hearing.

A ventilating tube may be inserted after a myringotomy to assist in equalizing pressure. The ventilating tube normally remains in place for 6 to 9 months. The tube usually falls out of the tympanic membrane as the membrane regenerates. Myringotomy can be performed with or without the use of ventilating tubes.

Contraindications and Cautions

When making the incision, the physician must carefully avoid injuring the ossicles and cutting too deep. A deep incision may cut the mucous membrane covering the promontory, causing bleeding and pain. If it is cut, however, the injury is not serious. The drumhead can be easily visualized posteriorly and inferiorly, which is where the incision should be made to avoid injury to the medial wall of the middle ear and the ossicles.

There are no apparent contraindications to myringotomy if the disease process requires its performance. Most third-party payers require precertification and evidence of alternative therapy before approving a myringotomy.

MULTIDISCIPLINARY PLAN

Surgery

Incision of eardrum with sharp myringotomy knife for evacuation of fluid; possible insertion of ventilating tubes.

Medications

Antiinfective agents
- Amoxicillin, 250-500 mg PO q6h
- Gentamicin otic drops indicated only if patient has mucoid effusions because risk is significantly higher for developing postoperative otorrhea

Analgesic agents: Acetaminophen (Tylenol), 650 mg with codeine 30 mg q4-6h prn

General Management

Cotton in ear to absorb drainage

NURSING CARE

NURSING ASSESSMENT

Tympanic membrane: Drainage from eardrum; bleeding and pain at incision site; no impairment of hearing

POTENTIAL COMPLICATIONS

Hearing loss, injury to ossicles, persistent otorrhea

PATIENT PROBLEMS/NURSING DIAGNOSES & INTERVENTIONS

NIC PHYSICAL COMFORT PROMOTION

Acute pain related to surgical incision
- Assess degree of discomfort.
- Provide analgesia as needed *for pain relief;* assess and document effectiveness.
- Administer antibiotics and eardrops as ordered.
- If patient is child, instruct parents in treatment regimen and proper instillation technique for eardrops.

NIC SKIN/WOUND MANAGEMENT

Impaired tissue integrity related to surgical incision
- Assess amount of drainage from ear.
- Change cotton as needed.
- Teach technique to patient or to parent.
- Because drainage is usually infected, wash hands well after handling drainage and teach patient or parents to do same *to prevent contamination.*
- Keep external ear dry and clean.
- Assess for and report symptoms such as headache, nausea, fever, or increased ear pain.

PATIENT EDUCATION/CONTINUUM OF CARE PLAN

1. Explain to patient and family the necessity for completing prescribed course of antibiotics to prevent recurrence or complications.
2. Discuss with patient or family the need to monitor for hearing loss or increased ear pain. Myringotomies

occasionally must be performed again for reaccumulation of fluid.

3. Ensure that patient and family understand how to assess amount of drainage and how to change cotton in the ear.
4. Explain to patient and family that no water should enter the ear. Ear plugs or cotton balls coated with petroleum jelly may be used.

EVALUATION/PATIENT OUTCOMES

Physical Comfort Promotion: Comfort is improved. Patient experiences no pain at myringotomy site. Patient is afebrile.

Skin/Wound Management: Tissue integrity is maintained. Myringotomy incision is healed well with no evidence of pus or fluid behind eardrum. There is no drainage from eardrum. Patient does not experience hearing loss.

STAPEDECTOMY AND STAPEDOTOMY

Description and Rationale

Stapedectomy is the removal of the footplate and the stapes and replacement with a prosthesis that allows the reestablishment of normal sound pathways. The prostheses are made of various materials, depending on the physician's preference.

Stapedotomy is the removal of the stapes with placement of a hole in the footplate. A prosthesis is inserted into the hole to improve hearing.[18]

Attempts to reverse hearing losses that result from otosclerosis have been made for almost 100 years. Stapedectomy is the result of refinement of these various attempts and is now the operation of choice in many patients with hearing losses from otosclerosis.

If patients are appropriately selected for the procedure and the surgeon has the necessary skills, 90% of patients experience an improvement in the level of hearing and in many instances hearing is almost normal.

Patients who may benefit from stapedectomy include those with a negative Rinne test of at least 572 Hz with a vibrating tuning fork and an air-bone gap of at least 20 dB for speech frequencies. Patients with otosclerosis and accompanying tinnitus may experience relief from tinnitus after stapedectomy.

Because the "worst" ear is the one operated on, patients selected for this surgery must have one ear functioning at a fairly adequate level. The operative ear must have a mobile malleus and a normally situated tympanic membrane.

Contraindications and Cautions

Active external otitis or otitis media must be well healed before stapedectomy will be considered
Severe vertigo from Ménière's disease
Occupation that requires frequent or large changes in barometric pressure, that is, divers, pilots, and those who work at heights
"Dead" or nonfunctioning ear on one side, unless patient has reached stage at which hearing aid can no longer be satisfactorily used
Patients younger than age 25 years because otosclerosis may still be in an active stage
Older patients assessed carefully for general health status and adequate sensorineural reserve and for evidence of vestibular damage; caution exercised in patients with any vestibular damage and poor sensorineural reserve because results may not be satisfactory
Perforation of tympanic membrane

MULTIDISCIPLINARY PLAN

Surgery

With patient under local anesthesia and sedation, surgeon turns eardrum back on itself like omelette; microscope used to magnify bones of middle ear; stapes and footplate removed by means of various picks and sometimes electric drill; when footplate is removed, open oval window sealed with fascial graft from temporal muscle and prosthesis connected to incus to restore normal sound conduction; several types of prostheses used; one end attached to the incus and other to graft or plug in oval window; external ear canal packed to ensure healing of tympanum; packing left in place 5 to 7 days

Medications

Analgesic agents
- Meperidine (Demerol); 50-100 mg IM q4h prn
- Ketorolac (Toradol), 30-60 mg IM q6h prn

Antiemetic agents
- Prochlorperazine (Compazine), 10-25 mg q4-6h prn
- Meclizine (Antivert) for antivertigo effect, 25 mg PO $^1/_2$ h ac and hs

Sedative agents
- Sedation before surgery
- Phenobarbital, 60-100 mg PO or Midazolam HCl (Versed), 2.5-5 mg IM before surgery

Antiinfective agents
- Amoxicillin, 250 mg PO tid for 10 days

General Management

Bed rest for 24 hours (may vary with physician) with operative side facing upward to maintain position of prosthesis and graft

NURSING CARE

NURSING ASSESSMENT

Infectious process: Fever or other symptoms of infection; pain in operated ear
Auditory function: Hearing ability; vertigo
Gustatory function: Ability to taste with anterior tongue
Reparative granuloma: Occurs in about 1% of stapedectomies; cause is unknown, but it may be related to contamination of the implant or trauma to the tissue; can be recognized if the flap and tympanic membrane still appear reddened and inflamed and there has been no hearing improvement 1 week after surgery; granulomas can fill much of middle ear and must be completely removed along with prosthesis; different type of prosthesis must then be inserted

Patient Problems/Nursing Diagnoses & Interventions

NIC Immobility Management

Impaired physical mobility related to decreased activity and vertigo

- Assess patient's understanding of need for decreased activity and immobility.
- Enforce bed rest if ordered; patient should lie flat with operative side up *to maintain position of prosthesis and graft.*
- Assist patient with ambulation because *vertigo may be present.*
- Begin movement and ambulation gradually and provide medication for pain or dizziness as needed.
- Instruct patient to avoid normal activity for 1 week and strenuous activity for 2 to 3 weeks.

NIC Communication Enhancement

Disturbed sensory perception (auditory) related to ear packing postoperatively

- Assess patient's hearing levels before and after operation.
- Improvement in hearing may not be noticeable immediately because of packing in ear and bleeding. Make sure that patient is aware of this fact *to avoid disappointment immediately after surgery.*
- Speak distinctly, facing patient.
- Alert patient to cracking and popping sounds during healing.

NIC Skin/Wound Management

Risk for impaired skin integrity related to surgical intervention, draining, and possible bleeding

- Assess for excessive bleeding, drainage, fever, and ear pain and report any symptoms immediately.
- Instruct patient to cough and sneeze with mouth open to prevent dislodgment of prosthesis.
- Inform patient that after packing is removed, a piece of cotton may be placed in ear for few days *to provide protection.*
- Instruct patient in appropriate technique of changing cotton and tell patient to do it once or twice a day.
- Instruct patient to avoid the introduction of any water in the ear.

NIC Physical Comfort Promotion

Acute pain related to surgical procedure

- Assess patient's degree of pain and report excessive ear pain immediately.
- Administer pain medication and antiemetics as needed; assess and document effectiveness.
- Encourage patient to move gradually, avoiding sudden movement *to minimize pain at operative site and vertigo*

Patient Education/Continuum of Care Plan

1. Encourage the patient to sneeze or blow the nose with the mouth open for at least 1 week to prevent dislodgment of the prosthesis and graft.
2. Ensure that the patient is aware of the necessity for careful ear care both immediately before surgery and on an ongoing basis.
3. Explain to the patient that the ear must not become wet (as by shampooing) while deep external packing remains in place. Instruct patient to insert cotton coated with petroleum jelly into ear canal.
4. Explain to the patient that smoking is contraindicated after stapedectomy.
5. Instruct patient to confer with surgeon about instructions for flying and exercise.
6. Encourage patient to wear noise protective devices when around loud noises.

Evaluation/Patient Outcomes

Immobility Management: Patient mobility is normal. Activity level is normal for patient; no weakness or vertigo is present.

Communication Enhancement: Hearing improves after surgery. Hearing is improved to normal.

Skin/Wound Management: Tissue integrity is maintained. There is no pain or excessive drainage from operated ear. Patient verbalizes understanding of ear care regimen and symptoms to report to physician.

Physical Comfort Promotion: Comfort is improved. Patient experiences no pain and is afebrile.

Tonsillectomy

Description and Rationale

Tonsillectomy is the surgical removal of the tonsils and sometimes the adenoids (adenoidectomy). The rationale for this procedure is usually the removal of chronically infected tissue. A general anesthetic is used; the most common method for removal of the tonsils is dissection and snare because it can be used for all sizes of tonsils whether they are in shallow or deep fossae. Although it has disadvantages, the guillotine method is chosen by some physicians. Injury to the tonsillar pillar is more common with this method, and it is not suitable for deeply recessed tonsils. It may also not reach the base of the tonsils and will leave a tonsil tag. Adenoids are removed with an adenotome; a curette may also be used to remove adenoid tissue. Laser excision of the tonsils can also be performed.

Contraindications and Cautions

Presence of any acute infection, especially tonsillitis
Active tuberculosis
Presence of hematologic disorders, such as hemophilia, leukemia, or aplastic anemia

Multidisciplinary Plan

Surgery

Tonsil and adenoidal tissue removed

Medications

Narcotic analgesic agents: Acetaminophen (Tylenol), 650 mg with codeine, PO q4-6h prn (avoid aspirin because of possibility of bleeding)

Antibiotic agents: May be prescribed by some physicians

General Management

Intravenous fluids until nausea has subsided and patient is drinking well; soft or liquid diet; minimize activity

NURSING CARE

NURSING ASSESSMENT

Postoperative status: Vital signs stable; no fever; pulse and blood pressure normal for patient; skin warm and dry; level of consciousness appropriate for recovery from anesthesia; no bleeding at operative site; if adenoidectomy is done, there may be some serosanguineous nasopharyngeal drainage trickling down back of throat

POTENTIAL COMPLICATIONS

Bleeding from failure to secure bleeding points during surgery; airway obstruction from blood or secretions; aspiration of blood or secretions

PATIENT PROBLEMS/NURSING DIAGNOSES & INTERVENTIONS

NIC PHYSICAL COMFORT PROMOTION

Acute pain related to surgical intervention

- Assess patient's degree of pain.
- Provide adequate pain relief; assess and document effectiveness.
- Ensure adequate fluid intake.
- Monitor intravenous intake at prescribed rate until discontinued and then provide soothing fluids *to prevent dehydration.*
- Instruct patient to avoid citrus juice, *which would cause irritation in the throat.*
- Offer ice chips or popsicles *to encourage fluids and provide comfort.*
- Monitor vital signs, level of consciousness, and presence of bleeding and report any change immediately.
- Provide ice collar for comfort, if ordered.

NIC RESPIRATORY MANAGEMENT

Risk for aspiration related to postoperative bleeding

- Maintain patent airway; keep patient on bed rest lying on side as much as possible until awake and alert *to prevent aspiration.*
- Observe for vomiting of dark brown fluid because of "swallowed" blood during surgery.
- Watch for frequent swallowing, which may indicate bleeding; check frequently with flashlight *to see if blood is trickling down back of throat.*

PATIENT EDUCATION/CONTINUUM OF CARE PLAN

1. Explain to patient the need to avoid clearing the throat, to watch for bleeding, and to call the physician immediately if any symptoms occur. They may occur about 5 to 10 days after surgery when the scab sloughs from the operative area.
2. Because tonsillectomy is routinely performed as outpatient surgery, give patient a preprinted list of instructions for postoperative care at home (see box below).

EVALUATION/PATIENT OUTCOMES

Physical Comfort Promotion: Comfort is improved. There is no bleeding from operative site. Patient is afebrile and takes fluids and food well. Activity level is normal for patient. Patient verbalizes understanding of necessity of watching for late postoperative bleeding and calling physician immediately. Patient verbalizes knowledge of when to return to physician for postoperative visit.

Respiratory Management: Airway remains patent. Patient experiences no bleeding; no aspiration occurs.

POSTOPERATIVE INSTRUCTIONS FOR TONSILLECTOMY AND ADENOIDECTOMY

1. For the first 7 to 10 days after surgery there may be pain and soreness in the throat and ears.
2. Small amounts of bleeding occur during this period. If bleeding persists, call the physician immediately.
3. If signs and symptoms of infection occur, such as purulent exudate or increase in pain or fever, call the physician immediately.
4. Keep the fluid intake high for the first few days after surgery, which will help keep the temperature down.
5. The diet should consist of soft bland foods, gelatin, cooked cereals, ice cream, soft-boiled eggs, custard, broth, mashed potatoes, and noncitrus juices for about 1 week. Apple and grape juice are the best liquids. Carbonated beverages may be taken if the patient tolerates them. Well-ground meat should be added as soon as tolerated.
6. Activity should not cause overexertion for the next 7-10 days. If tolerated, the patient may go outside after the second day. Persons with acute infections should be kept away. Bathing may be carried out in the usual manner.
7. Acetaminophen (Tylenol) (if patient is not allergic) may be taken by mouth, 650 mg q4h for pain, especially ½ h before meals. If the patient is given medications to take home from the hospital, they may be substituted for Tylenol.
8. The patient should not gargle but only gently rinse mouth.
9. Avoid throat clearing.
10. Do not smoke.
11. If you have any questions or concerns, call your physician to discuss these areas.

Courtesy Ruth Weddle, RN, and Eden Rivera, RN, University of California, San Francisco Medical Center.

TRACHEOTOMY

Description and Rationale

A tracheotomy is an incision into the trachea to form a temporary or permanent opening, which is called a tracheostomy. The incision is made through the second, third, or fourth tracheal ring, and a tube is inserted through the opening to allow the passage of air and the removal of tracheobronchial secretions.

Except in the cases of head, neck, and face trauma, a tracheotomy is rarely performed as an emergency procedure. If immediate airway control is needed and the patient is hospitalized, endotracheal intubation is usually performed; a tracheotomy is performed as an elective procedure if an artificial airway is necessary longer than an endotracheal tube should be left in place.

Aside from tracheotomy performed to reduce anatomic dead space (by approximately 150 cc) in patients with chronic pulmonary disease or to aid in mechanical ventilation of an unconscious patient, most tracheotomies are performed on patients in two categories. Patients in the first group have an obstruction at or above (see Emergency Alert box) the level of the larynx, such as foreign body obstruction, carcinoma of the head and neck, severe infection (such as Ludwig's angina), trauma to the tongue or mandible, or stenosis from prolonged intubation. Patients in the second group have no actual obstruction but are unable to raise their own secretions and are in danger of anoxia if secretions accumulate and are not removed from the chest. These patients include those with paralysis of the chest muscles and diaphragm (as in Guillain-Barré syndrome), patients who are unconscious or semiconscious with head injuries, and patients with fractured ribs or other chest injuries causing severe pain that inhibits them from coughing.

Tracheotomy is an excellent way to provide access to the trachea when a patient needs frequent suctioning. Other indications include patients with smoke inhalation or severe burns around the head and neck, patients who are at risk of edema from surgery in the head and neck, and patients with central obstructive sleep apnea.

Contraindications and Cautions

Caution is exercised in infants because of extremely small size of their tracheas and small size of tube that must be used.

MULTIDISCIPLINARY PLAN

Surgery

Incision in midline of neck from lower border of thyroid cartilage to slightly above suprasternal notch; soft tissue and muscle layers divided and isthmus of thyroid exposed and divided between clamps or retracted upward, which exposes rings of trachea; vertical or transverse incision made, usually between third and fourth rings, secretions thoroughly suctioned, and tracheostomy tube of correct size for patient inserted; the anterior portion of the tracheal ring may be removed to create a window (FIG. 9-24); complete hemostasis ensured after procedure; if procedure is elective, endotracheal tube left in place and tracheotomy performed over tube; endotracheal tube can be removed after airway is secured; traction structures may be inserted above and below the window or opening (stoma) for reopening the stoma in case of accidental decannulation

Medications

Drugs prescribed depending on reason for tracheotomy, that is, infection or laryngeal edema

> **EMERGENCY ALERT**
>
> **FOREIGN BODY IN THROAT**
>
> Foreign bodies in the throat may penetrate or obstruct the airway, or the object may be aspirated into the lungs. Fish and chicken bones are commonly found foreign bodies.
>
> **ASSESSMENT**
>
> - History of foreign body.
> - The patient may appear fearful and anxious.
> - Assess for difficult breathing, noisy respirations, coughing, and/or choking.
> - The patient may complain of pain or sharpness in the throat.
>
> **INTERVENTION**
>
> - If the patient is coughing, do not perform the Heimlich maneuver. This may actually suck the foreign body deeper into the airway.
> - If the patient is not able to cough and evidence of complete airway obstruction exists, attempt to clear the airway with a finger sweep.
> - Proceed with the Heimlich maneuver: four abdominal thrusts, and repeat if necessary.
> - Attempt to clear airway with suction, and prepare for an emergency tracheotomy.

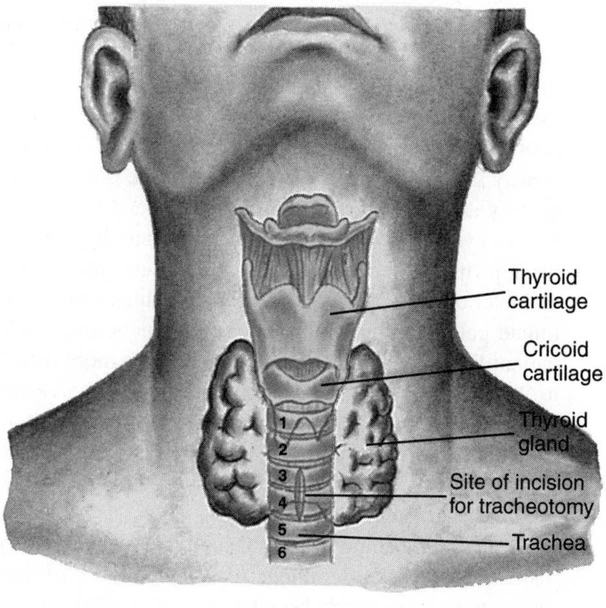

FIG. 9-24
Correct area of trachea for incision and insertion of tracheotomy tube.

General Management

Tracheobronchial suctioning; humidification of inspired air

NURSING CARE

NURSING ASSESSMENT

Respiratory function: Respiratory rate; amount and color of tracheal secretions; need for and frequency of suctioning; anxiety level; arterial blood gases; presence of bleeding at tracheostomy site (should be minimal); no excessive coughing after suctioning; adequate humidification provided to tracheostomy (mucus is thin and without thick plugs); breath sounds audible in all lobes after suctioning; tracheostomy ties securely fastened

Pneumomediastinum: No dyspnea, crepitus, or edema of face and neck

Pneumothorax: No cough, anxiety, sharp chest pain, or tachycardia

Cardiac tamponade: No increase in central venous pressure, narrowed pulse pressure, paradoxic pulse, decreased pressure, dyspnea, or decreased level of consciousness

POTENTIAL COMPLICATIONS

Bleeding, subcutaneous emphysema, mucous plug with airway obstruction, accidental decannulation, tracheal stenosis, pneumothorax

PATIENT PROBLEMS/NURSING DIAGNOSES & INTERVENTIONS

NIC RESPIRATORY MANAGEMENT

Ineffective airway clearance; risk for aspiration; impaired gas exchange related to obstruction or excessive secretions

- Assess for and report any symptoms suggesting obstruction, pneumomediastinum, pneumothorax, cardiac tamponade, hemorrhage, or subcutaneous emphysema.
- Assess rate, rhythm, depth of respirations; auscultate lung fields; monitor ABGs and pulse oximetry.
- Encourage coughing and deep breathing.
- Elevate head of bed.
- Suction airway as often as necessary *to maintain patent airway and remove secretions.* This can be done as frequently as every 5 to 10 minutes immediately after surgery to every 3 to 4 hours after tracheostomy has been in place awhile. Use catheter that is no greater than ½ the diameter of tracheostomy tube. Preoxygenate and hyperinflate patient using Ambu bag before suctioning. Give patient five sigh breaths. Do not suction for more than 5 to 10 seconds *because suctioning decreases alveolar oxygen pressure by 30 mm Hg.* Keep bypass port open on catheter while inserting it *to minimize oxygen removal.* Gentle twisting motion of catheter should be used when removing catheter.
- Stop suctioning immediately if any signs of respiratory distress occur *because mucus blockage may be present and patient may quickly become hypoxic.* Postoxygenate patient after suctioning by giving five sigh breaths, with Ambu bag to reopen small airways. Maintain adequate humidification *to keep secretions loose and minimize difficulty in secretion removal.* (Sputum is 95% water and mucous membranes dry out easily without proper hydration.)
- Clean inner cannula (if present) of tracheostomy tube every 4 to 8 hours as necessary or discard disposable inner cannula.
- If appropriate, ensure that patient receives chest physiotherapy, depending on condition and reason for tracheostomy.
- Document suctioning, patient response, result of chest assessment, and all treatments.
- If patient is receiving ventilation assistance or intermittent positive pressure breathing treatments or is at risk for aspiration, a cuffed tracheostomy tube is used. The cuff pressure should be maintained at a level that just occludes trachea. Pressure should be less than 20 cm H_2O.[9]
- Observe for any frank bleeding from tracheostomy or pulsation of cannula. *(Innominate artery is in close proximity, and tracheostomy tube may erode through the artery wall.)*
- Ensure that tracheostomy ties are secured at all times *to prevent tube from falling out or becoming dislocated.*
- When tracheotomy has just been performed, change ties with assistance *so tracheostomy tube is held in place while ties are replaced.* Institutional policy may vary regarding whether nurses may change tracheostomy ties within first 48 hours after surgery. Two nurses should be present during tracheostomy tie changes.
- Avoid using aerosol sprays, talcum powder, or tissue or gauze containing cotton *to prevent patient from inhaling foreign particles.*
- Use precut tracheostomy gauze or unlined gauze opened full length and folded into U shape under neck plate of outer cannula. Replace when soiled.

NIC COMMUNICATION ENHANCEMENT

Impaired verbal communication related to the inability to talk

- Assess patient's understanding of inability to communicate verbally.
- Evaluate patient's ability to read and write.
- Provide patient with Magic Slate or pen and paper *to facilitate communication.*
- Use word cards with commonly used phrases or flash cards/picture communication board, if patient is illiterate.
- Instruct patient to occlude tracheostomy opening with finger or plug *to allow verbal communication,* only if tube is uncuffed.
- Consult with physician and speech therapist to use alternative speech devices (electrolarynx, speech valve, fenestrated tracheostomy tube).
- Observe patient for nonverbal cues.

NIC SKIN/WOUND MANAGEMENT

Impaired skin integrity related to stoma incision, to decreased activity, or to immobility

- Assess stoma during every shift and note any bleeding, purulent drainage, and condition of surrounding tissue.

- Check skin under tracheostomy dressing and note areas of breakdown.
- Wear gloves to change dressing when soiled or at least every shift.
- Clean wound thoroughly with hydrogen peroxide and water or normal saline solution when changing dressing.
- Clean inner cannula of tracheostomy tube during every shift or as necessary.
- Ensure that sterile technique is maintained while suctioning.
- Make sure that patient is turned at least hourly if condition warrants and that areas of breakdown are noted and treatment begun promptly.
- Change tracheostomy ties, as needed.

NIC Nutrition Support

Imbalanced nutrition: less than body requirements, related to the inability to eat or drink normally, to discomfort, and to anorexia

- Assess closely for signs of dehydration and malnutrition and report immediately.
- Monitor intravenous or tube feedings as necessary and document appropriately.
- Weigh patient daily.
- Assess patient's ability to swallow.
- If patient is eating, has a cuffed tracheostomy tube, and is prone to aspiration, inflate cuff while patient eats and deflate after meals.
- Instruct patient to assume sitting position for meals and for 1 hour afterward.
- Consult nutritionist and swallowing therapist to determine food consistency and adequate calories.
- Provide high-calorie snacks and supplements if needed.
- Provide attractive, clean environment at meals and meticulous mouth care before meals *because patient may experience loss of taste because of decreased sense of smell.*
- Weigh patient daily and maintain accurate record of intake and output.
- If patient is receiving tube feedings, ensure that they are of sufficient caloric value *to maintain weight and promote wound healing.*
- Monitor patient's hydration and nutritional status.
- Follow established guidelines for tube feedings; that is, check for placement in stomach and residual before next tube feeding.
- Replace residual, and hold feeding if greater than 100 ml.
- Feed patient with head of bed elevated *to prevent aspiration.*
- Assess patient's bowel activity.

NIC Coping Assistance

Anxiety related to presence of tracheostomy, the inability to speak, and concern about breathing pattern

- Assess patient's level of anxiety and carefully explain suctioning procedure to patient.
- Provide assurance that patient will be closely observed for respiratory distress or need for suctioning and that call light will be answered promptly.

Disturbed body image related to presence of tracheostomy

- Encourage patient to discuss feelings and concerns.
- Identify, with patient, successful coping strategies used in the past.
- Assess patient's readiness to perform self-care procedures.
- Remain with patient during self-care to provide needed support.
- Demonstrate techniques/coverings to camouflage tracheostomy.
- Provide privacy for patient and significant other to discuss possible societal reactions, sexual concerns.
- Encourage participation in support/self-help organizations.

NIC Patient Education

Deficient knowledge related to the need for information about continued tracheostomy care

Convalescent care

- If patient will be discharged with tracheostomy, ensure that patient and family have been instructed in and understand management of tracheostomy at home, including suctioning, cleaning, wound care, humidification, changing tracheostomy ties, and tube feeding if necessary. Discuss changes in activities of daily living, such as no water in stoma; tracheostomy tube protection; sexual activity.
- Ensure that family and patient know where to purchase supplies and when to return to see physician.
- Arrange for home health services and equipment, as ordered.
- Provide patient and caregivers with resources and emergency instructions (cardiopulmonary resuscitation, medic alert bracelet).

To prepare patient for tracheostomy tube removal

- Assess patient's ability to breathe and cough effectively, gag reflex, and swallowing reflexes.
- Report any symptoms of distress to physician immediately.
- "Plug" tracheostomy tube intermittently and increase length of time for occlusion as patient tolerates.
- Remove tracheostomy tube or assist physician with removal of tube when patient tolerates occlusion well.
- Apply Steri-Strips or tape *to approximate wound edges.*
- Apply occlusive dressing over Steri-Strips.
- Stress need for patient to splint stoma site with finger when coughing or speaking.
- Check and cleanse wound site daily.
- Observe for signs of infection; opening should heal within a few days.
- Make referral to home health nurse.

Patient Education/Continuum of Care Plan

See deficient knowledge above.

1. Inform the patient that there will be frequent suctioning, a loss of speech, and decreased ability to smell and that he or she will not be breathing through the nose or mouth while the tracheostomy is present.

2. Refer the patient to a speech therapist, if appropriate, to learn alternative method of speech.
3. Reinforce need for supplemental humidification (normal saline instillation, humidifier, moist bib).

Evaluation/Patient Outcomes

Respiratory Management: If short-term tracheostomy is used, respiratory status is within normal limits. Patient has no excess secretions, and tracheostomy stoma is healed without signs of infection. Patient does not experience dyspnea or shortness of breath.

Communication Enhancement: Verbal communication is improved. Patient can enhance speech by occluding tracheostomy tube with finger or plug, uses alternative devices as indicated.

Skin/Wound Management: Skin integrity is maintained. Stoma is healed. No drainage or bleeding is present.

Nutrition Support: Nutritional status is maintained. Weight and caloric intake are normal for patient. Patient eats regularly; patient and family demonstrate the ability to administer tube feedings as necessary.

Coping Assistance: Patient and family anxiety is decreased. Patient and family demonstrate an understanding of and are at ease in caring for the tracheostomy tube and in the suctioning procedure. Patient/family adjusts to changes in body image. Patient and significant other able to provide care, able to socialize with others.

Patient Education: If long-term tracheostomy is needed, patient and family demonstrate ability to care for all aspects of tracheostomy at home. Patient and family demonstrate suctioning and cleaning techniques, wound care, changing ties, and methods for humidification. Home health nurse assists patient and family if necessary.

Tympanoplasty

Description and Rationale

Tympanoplasty is a reconstructive or reparative procedure of the tympanic membrane that is usually performed to correct conductive hearing loss, to close a perforation of the tympanic membrane, to prevent recurrent infections, and to provide adequate aeration of the middle ear.[18] The procedure involves rebuilding the structures of the middle ear or replacing them with prostheses and closing the perforation. Tympanoplasty may also be indicated in patients with ossicular problems such as dislocation of the incus from trauma, congenital middle ear problems, or tympanosclerosis, in which the malleus is fused to the incus. In these cases metal or plastic prostheses, autogenous material, or cadaveric ossicles are commonly used.[3,18]

The principle rationale for tympanoplasty is to improve hearing in patients with conductive hearing loss but intact nerve function or cochlear reserve. The greatest improvement is seen in patients with bilateral disease and a large difference between air and bone measurements. In chronic otitis media the tympanic membrane, malleus, and incus are frequently damaged or destroyed. If this occurs, sound waves can enter the oval and round window with equal intensity and cancel each other, because the tympanic membrane is not there to protect the round window from sound pressure. Chronic otitis media also disrupts the tympanic membrane–stapes footplate ratio or the tympanic membrane–footplate ratio, thereby negating the transformer action of the middle ear.

Tympanoplasty, of which there are five types described here, improves hearing by reestablishing two important middle ear functions: restoring the tympanic membrane–stapes footplate ratio and creating sound protection for the round window.

Contraindications and Cautions

Presence of infection; procedure to clear infection must be performed before tympanoplasty

Patients with poor nerve function as determined by bone conduction tests

Hearing loss from otosclerosis or serous otitis media rather than chronic suppurative otitis media

Multidisciplinary Plan

Surgery

See Fig. 9-25

Postaural or endaural approach: With operating microscope at high magnification, surgeon performs one of five types of tympanoplasty, using either temporal fascia or tissue from nearby vein as graft; tympanic membranes from human cadavers sometimes used as graft, although this technique is still being evaluated. Teflon or stainless steel wires also used occasionally

Type I (myringoplasty): Performed for closure of perforation; epithelium removed from edge of perforation and graft of autogenous tissue, usually fascia or vein placed under tympanic membrane; tympanic membrane–footplate ratio and round window sound protection restored

Type II: Performed when malleus is eroded; perforation closed with graft against incus or what remains of malleus; enough ossicular chain must remain to create new tympanic membrane–footplate ratio

Type III: Also restores both areal ratio and sound protection of round window by means of autogenous graft; performed when tympanic membrane and ossicular chain are destroyed but normal stapes remains; graft is placed in contact with stapes.

Type IV: Tympanic membrane–footplate ratio cannot be restored, but round window sound protection is provided; only footplate remains intact, and air pocket is placed between round window and graft to provide sound protection

Type V: Only round window sound protection provided; footplate is fixed and fenestration into inner ear must be performed; replaced by stapes surgery

Medications

Narcotic analgesic agents

Meperidine (Demerol), 50 mg IM q4h prn

Acetaminophen (Tylenol), 650 mg with codeine q4-6h prn

Antiinfective agents

Antiemetics (for antivertigo effect): Meclizine (Antivert), 25 mg PO 1/2 h ac and hs

NURSING CARE

Nursing Assessment

Middle ear function: Bleeding; amount, color, and consistency of drainage; temperature elevation; dizziness when getting out of bed or with sudden movement; nausea; vertigo

Potential Complications

Graft failure, facial nerve injury, vertigo

Patient Problems/Nursing Diagnoses & Interventions

NIC Skin/Wound Management

Risk for impaired tissue integrity related to a fall or a disruption of graft

- Assess, record, and report unusual bleeding or drainage from operative site.
- Encourage patient to maintain bed rest until first morning after surgery.
- Keep patient from lying on operative side *to prevent pressure on graft.*
- Elevate head of bed 40 degrees.
- Assist with ambulation when patient is allowed to get up.
- Administer antivertiginous medications, as ordered.

NIC Communication Enhancement

Disturbed sensory perception (auditory) related to postoperative edema

- Assess patient's hearing ability before and after operation.
- Reassure patient that hearing improvement, if expected, will not be noticed until edema and drainage at operative site have decreased.

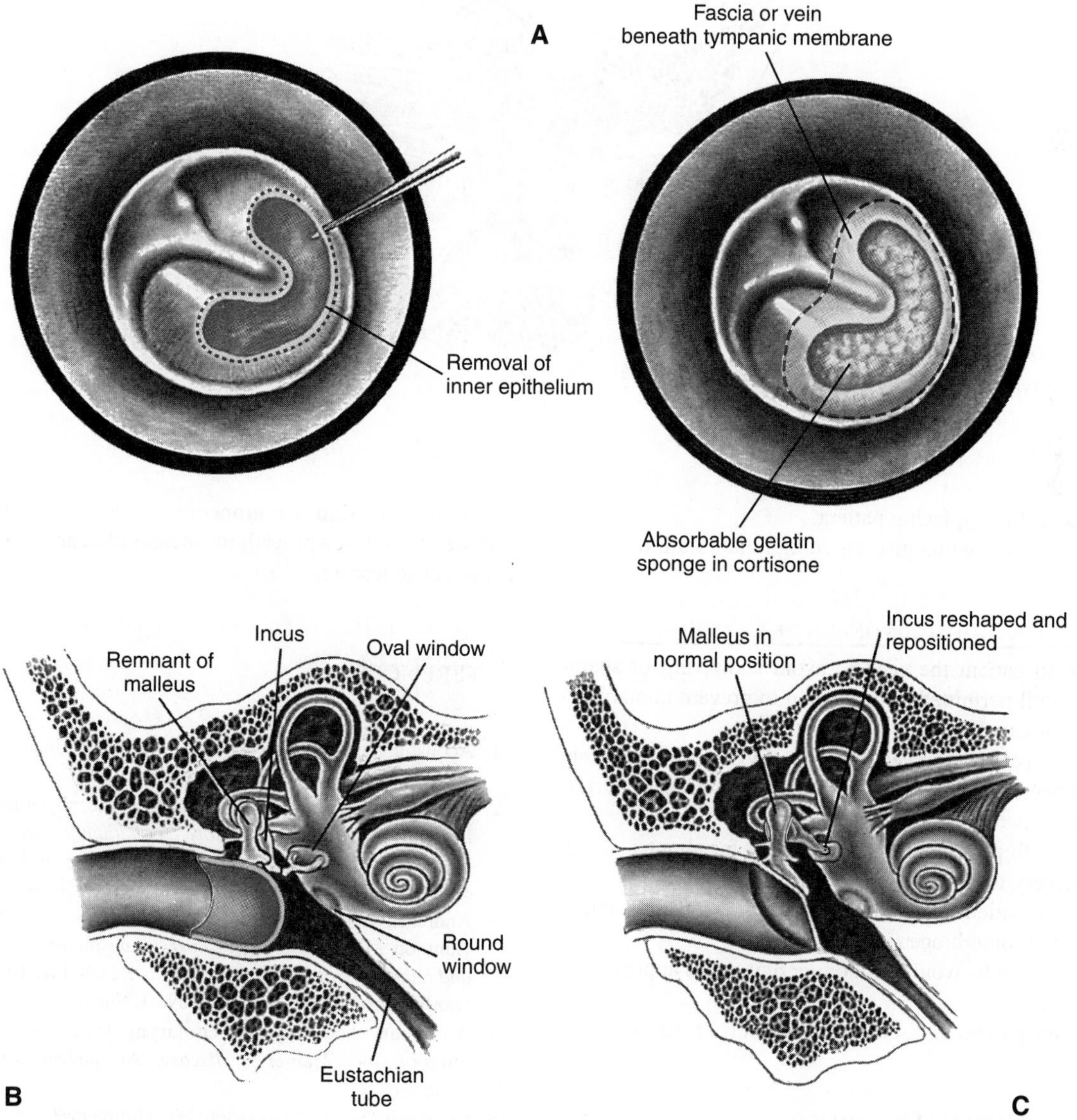

FIG. 9-25
Various types of tympanoplasty. **A,** Type 1 (myringoplasty). **B,** Type 2. **C,** Variation of type 2.

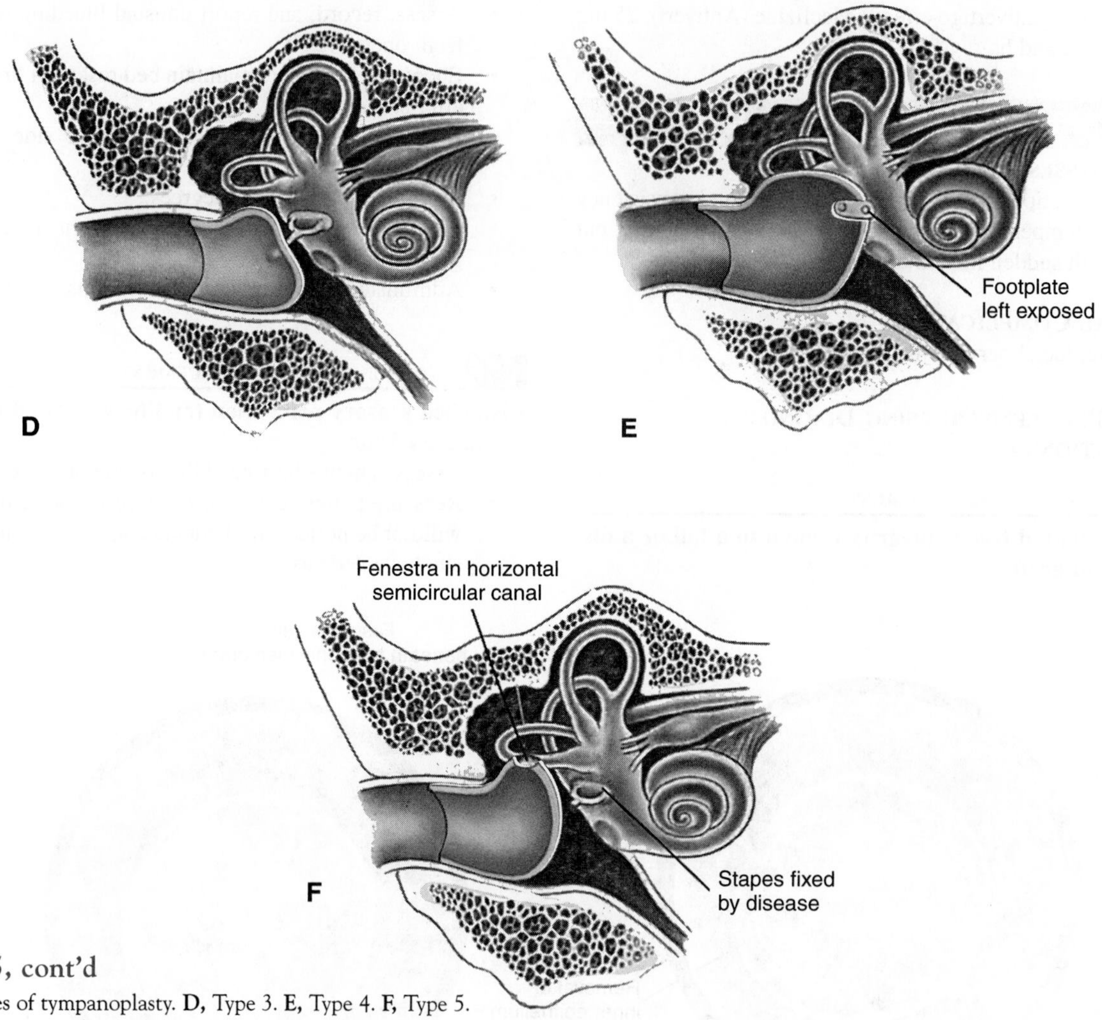

FIG. 9-25, cont'd
Various types of tympanoplasty. **D,** Type 3. **E,** Type 4. **F,** Type 5.

- Speak distinctly, facing patient.
- Consult with audiologist regarding rehabilitation.

PATIENT EDUCATION/CONTINUUM OF CARE PLAN

1. Explain to patient the need to avoid showering or shampooing until permitted by physician to prevent contamination of ear canal.
2. Explain to patient the need to notify physician immediately if evidence of fever, bleeding, increased drainage, or dizziness exists.
3. Discuss with patient the use of Antivert for about 1 month after surgery to minimize dizziness.
4. Encourage patient to avoid blowing nose with force and to sneeze with mouth open.
5. Inform patient to avoid strenuous activity until approved by physician.
6. Encourage patient to discuss with physician restrictions for flying.

EVALUATION/PATIENT OUTCOMES

Skin/Wound Management: Graft heals well. There is no fever, excessive drainage, or dizziness.

Communication Enhancement: Hearing is improved if this was reason for procedure. Increased hearing is verified by audiometric testing.

REFERENCES

1. Acoustic Neuroma Association: Treatment choices for acoustic neuromas, *http://anausa.org/treat.htm, 1999.*
2. Andreson HG et al: Normal anatomy and physiology. In Harris LL, Huntoon MB, editors: *Core curriculum for otorhinolaryngology and head-neck nursing,* New Smyrna Beach, Fla, 1998, Society of Otorhinolaryngology and Head-Neck Nurses.
3. Andresen HG et al: Auditory conditions and care. In Harris LL, Huntoon MB, editors: *Core curriculum for otorhinolaryngology and head-neck nursing,* New Smyrna Beach, Fla, 1998, Society of Otorhinolaryngology and Head-Neck Nurses.
4. American Academy of Otolaryngology—Head and Neck Surgery, Inc: *Meniere's disease,* Alexandria, Va, 1995, The Academy.
5. American Tinnitus Association: What is tinnitus? *http://www.ata.org/WHAT.HTM, 1999.*
6. Berne RM, Levy M: *Physiology,* ed 3, St. Louis, 1992, Mosby.

7. Byrne MN, Lee KJ, Neck spaces and fascial planes. In Lee KJ, editor: *Essential otolaryngology: head and neck surgery,* ed 6, Norwalk, Conn, 1995, Appleton & Lange.
8. Clayton H et al: Acoustic neuroma standard of care, *ORL—Head Neck Nurs* 13(1):15, 1995.
9. Cyr MH, Hickey MM, Higgins TS: Tracheal, esophageal conditions and care. In Harris LL, Huntoon MB, editors: *Core curriculum for otorhinolaryngology and head-neck nursing,* New Smyrna Beach, Fla, 1998, Society of Otorhinolaryngology and Head-Neck Nurses.
10. DeWeese DD, Saunders WH: *Textbook of otolaryngology—head and neck surgery,* ed 7, St. Louis, 1988, Mosby.
11. el-Kashlan HK et al: Direct electrical stimulation of the cochlear nucleus: surface vs. penetrating stimulation, *Otolaryngol Head Neck Surg* 105:533, 1991.
12. Feldman BA, Feldman DE: The nose and sinuses. In Lee KJ, editor: *Essential otolaryngology: head and neck surgery,* ed 6, Norwalk, Conn, 1995, Appleton & Lange.
13. Graham MD, Lee KJ, Goldsmith MM: Noninfectious disorders of the ear. In Lee KJ, editor: *Essential otolaryngology: head and neck surgery,* ed 6, Norwalk, Conn, 1995, Appleton & Lange.
14. Higgin ST et al: Nasal cavity, paranasal sinuses, nasopharynx conditions and care. In Harris LL, Huntoon MB, editors: *Core curriculum for ortorhinolaryngology and head-neck nursing,* New Smyrna Beach, Fla, 1998, Society of Otorhinolaryngology and Head-Neck Nurses.
14a. Isshiki N: Laryngeal framework surgery. In Myers EN et al: *Advances in otolaryngology—head and neck surgery.* St. Louis, 1991, Mosby.
15. Johnson JT, Yu VL: *Infectious diseases and antimicrobial therapy of the ears, nose, and throat,* Philadelphia, 1996, WB Saunders.
16. Kennedy DW: *Sinus disease: guide to first-line management,* Darien, Conn, 1995, Health Communications.
17. Lederman G et al: Fractionated stereotactic radiosurgery for acoustic neuroma, Acoustic Neuroma, *http://www.interstat.net/siuh/radonocology/acoustic.html, 1999.*
17a. Lee KJ: *Essential otolaryngology: head and neck surgery,* ed 6, Norwalk, Conn, 1995, Appleton & Lange.
18. Luckmann J, editor: *Saunders manual of nursing care,* Philadelphia, 1997, WB Saunders.
19. Mabry CS, Mabry RL: Making the diagnosis of allergy, *ORL—Head Neck Nurs* 14(1):13, 1996.
20. Proetz AW: *Essays on the applied physiology of the nose,* ed 2, St. Louis, 1953, Mosby.
21. Siedel HM et al: *Mosby's guide to physical examination,* ed 2, St. Louis, 1991, Mosby.
22. Sigler BA, Schuring LT: *Ear, nose, & throat disorders,* St. Louis, 1993, Mosby.
23. Thibodeau GA, Patton KT: *Anatomy & physiology,* St. Louis, 1999, Mosby.
24. Wong DL: *Nursing care of infants and children,* ed 5, St. Louis, 1995, Mosby.

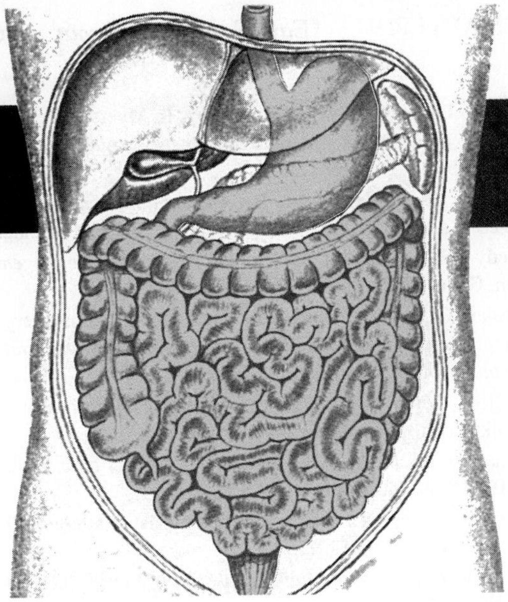

10 Gastrointestinal System

Mary G. Hirsch

OVERVIEW

Disorders or inflammation of any organs in the gastrointestinal system are commonly called digestive diseases. Examples of digestive diseases are reflux esophagitis, peptic ulcer disease, ulcerative colitis, pancreatitis, and cancer. The diagnosis, treatment, and management vary with each digestive disease.

More Americans are hospitalized with disorders of the digestive system than any other group of disorders. The National Institute of Diabetes and Digestive and Kidney Diseases reports that more than 40 million people are chronically ill with digestive diseases. This results in 158 million restricted activity days and 22 million work-loss days. In 1985, the direct health care costs associated with digestive diseases were more than $40 billion, or at least 10% of all U.S. health-care costs. Approximately 191,000 people die each year from digestive diseases.[13] Thus this group of diseases may have devastating long-term personal, social, and economic effects. There are more than 25 lay organizations and 18 professional associations involved in digestive disease programs and education. This reflects the national concern with the management of digestive diseases.

The importance of digestive diseases and their implications for health care have often been minimized. The group of diseases involving the gastrointestinal tract may vary from mild to severe. The chronicity of the diseases and the symptoms can affect the person's ability to maintain a desired lifestyle. Psychosocial stressors often intensify the symptoms.

The National Digestive Disease Advisory Report[32] showed that research involving the gastrointestinal tract is also relevant to the study of acquired immunodeficiency syndrome (AIDS). The immune dysfunction damages the gastrointestinal tract, and this damage contributes to the malnutrition and wasting syndrome observed in AIDS. The latest research on neuropeptides found in the intestine indicates that these substances may modulate immune function. This finding may have significance for future research.[32]

ANATOMY, PHYSIOLOGY, AND RELATED PATHOPHYSIOLOGY

The gastrointestinal tract is a series of connected organs and accessory organs whose overall purpose is to break down food products that can be used by the body as a source of energy. Three key processes are associated with the gastrointestinal tract: digestion, absorption, and metabolism. Digestion is the mechanical and chemical breakdown of food into amino acids, glucose, and fatty acids that can be used by the body for cellular functions. Absorption is the passage of the digested food products (essential nutrients) from the lumen of the gastrointestinal tract into the blood and lymphatic system. Metabolism is the use of the basic food product by the cell. Digestion and absorption can be affected by age-associated physiologic changes, infections, inflammatory diseases, surgery, or other alterations of the gastrointestinal tract. To adequately assess the effects of digestive diseases, the nurse must have a basic understanding of the alimentary, or gastrointestinal, system.

The gastrointestinal system consists of the mouth, pharynx, esophagus, stomach, and small and large intestines. Accessory organs include the liver, gallbladder, and pancreas. The accessory organs in the mouth are the teeth and salivary glands (FIG. 10-1).

The gastrointestinal system produces both exocrine and endocrine secretions. Exocrine secretions prepare food for absorption by diluting it to the osmolality of plasma (isotonic), altering the pH for hydrolysis, and hydrolyzing complex foods. The exocrine secretions also protect the mucosa from physical and chemical irritants. Endocrine secretions are important in the control and coordination of secretory and motor activities involved in the digestion and absorption of food. The types and functions of the secretions are discussed as they appear in the gastrointestinal tract.

Indigenous bacteria, or microflora, are present throughout the gastrointestinal tract. The flora's most important function is to protect the host from pathogens; however, in certain pathologic conditions, otherwise normal flora may have unfavorable effects on the host. Normal flora of the intestinal organs are discussed as they appear in the gastrointestinal tract.

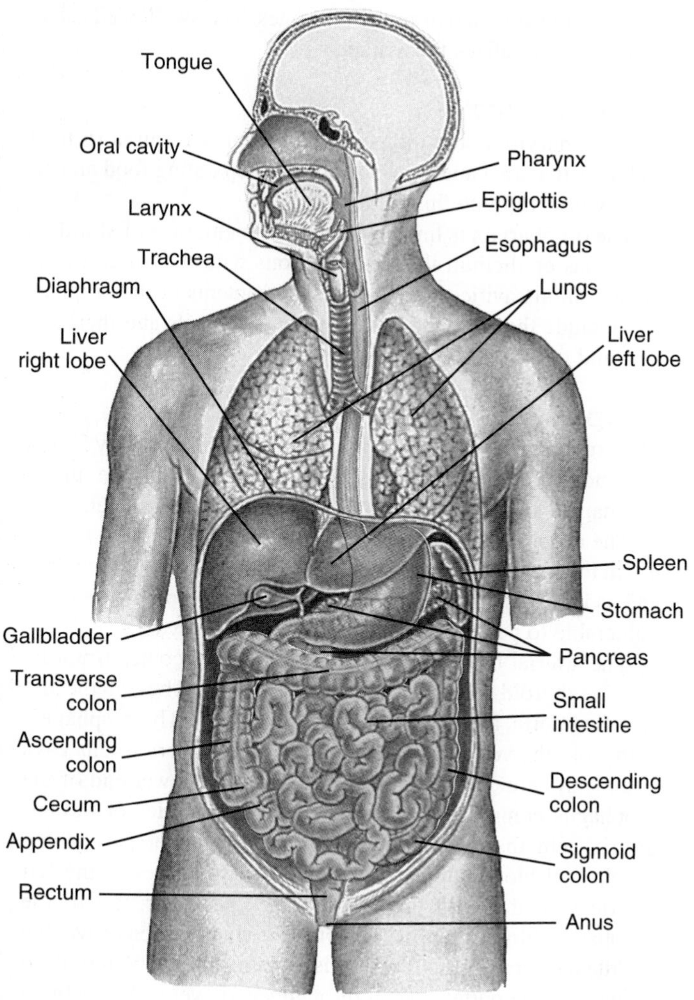

FIG. 10-1
Anatomy of gastrointestinal system.

Mouth

The mouth, also called the buccal cavity or oral cavity, is the beginning of the gastrointestinal tract. Mechanical and chemical digestion begins in the mouth. The teeth and tongue aid in mechanical breakdown, and the secretions of the salivary glands begin basic starch digestion and lubricate food to aid in swallowing.

The vestibule is the region between the lips, cheeks, teeth, and gums. The region posterior to the teeth and gums is the mouth cavity proper. Saliva from the salivary glands is received by the mouth cavity proper and aids in digestion.

The lips keep food and saliva in the mouth during chewing (mastication). The lips are covered externally by skin and internally by mucous membrane. The bulk of the lips is composed of orbicularis oris, a sphincterlike muscle.

The internal cheeks are composed of muscle, fat, areolar tissue, nerves, vessels, and buccal glands covered by an inner mucous membrane. The gums, or gingivae, are dense fibrous tissue covered by a smooth mucous membrane.

The roof of the mouth is formed by the hard and soft palates. The hard palate is formed by two palatine bones and parts of the superior maxillary bone. The midline of the hard palate is called the palatine raphe. The mucous membrane of the hard palate is thick, pale, and corrugated anterior to and to either side of the palatine raphe. The posterior mucous membrane is thin, smooth, and a deeper pink. Attached to the posterior portion of the hard palate is the soft palate. The soft palate forms the partition between the mouth and the nasopharynx. In a relaxed position the anterior surface of the soft palate is concave and continuous with the roof of the mouth, whereas the posterior surface is convex and continuous with the nasal cavities. The uvula is the conical fingerlike projection of the posterior border of the soft palate. During swallowing the soft palate moves upward, closing off the nasopharynx and preventing foods and fluids from entering the pharynx.

The tongue is a muscular organ anchored to the hyoid bone and the mandible and covered with a mucous membrane. The frenum, or frenulum, is a fold of mucous membrane under the tongue that attaches the tongue to the floor of the mouth. Mucous membrane also attaches the tongue to the epiglottis, soft palate, and pharynx. The tip of the tongue is the apex.

The tongue contains mucous and serous glands. The mucous glands are behind the apex and secrete mucin. The serous glands, also called Ebner's glands, are found in the back of the tongue. Ebner's glands assist in the distribution of substances to be tasted over the tongue.

The muscles of the tongue are divided into lateral halves by a median fibrous septum. The two groups of muscles can be identified by their role in the tongue's functions. The muscles that assist the tongue in protrusion, retraction, elevation, and depression during mastication are the genioglossus, hyoglossus, chondroglossus, styloglossus, and palatoglossus. The muscles that are responsible for altering the shape of the tongue (shortened, curved, narrowed) include the longitudinalis superior, longitudinalis inferior, transversus, and verticalis. These movements are important in the enunciation of different letters and words.

The four types of papillae that contain taste buds are located on the anterior two thirds of the dorsum of the tongue. They are fungiforme papillae, filiforme papillae, foliate papillae, and circumvallate papillae. Taste buds are concentrated in the circumvallate and fungiform papillae. Adults have up to 10,000 taste buds.[18] As a person ages, the taste buds begin to degenerate and perception of taste becomes less acute.

The four primary sensations of taste are sweet, sour, salty, and bitter. Taste buds detecting a primary taste tend to be localized in certain areas of the tongue. Sweet taste is primarily on the anterior surface and the tip of the tongue; sour taste on the two lateral sides; bitter taste on the papillae vallatae; and salty taste over the entire tongue. Taste buds respond in varying degrees to all four taste sensations. A taste bud may be very sensitive to one or two tastes but respond moderately to the other taste sensations.

The sense of smell also affects the sense of taste. Odors from food stimulate the olfactory system. When the sense of smell is decreased, the degree of taste is often reported as diminished. Taste preference is used by animals and humans to regulate diet.

Adults have 32 teeth, and children have 20. Teeth serve as an accessory to digestion by cutting and mixing food. Mixing the food with saliva begins some chemical digestion and lubricates the food for swallowing.

Chewing involves the stimulation of jaw muscles. Much of the chewing process is innervated by the motor branch of the fifth cranial nerve. Because digestive enzymes work only on the surface of food particles, chewing increases the surface area exposed to the enzymes. Chewing food also increases the ease with which food is swallowed and affects the ease of emptying of food from the stomach into the small intestine.

The composition of bacteria varies from place to place in the mouth, but bacteria adhere most efficiently to the tooth surfaces, the buccal mucosa, and the surfaces of the tongue and pharynx. Normal oral flora is similar to that found in the distal colon. Good dental hygiene removes most detrimental oral flora, although poor dental hygiene contributes greatly to the development of oral disease. Oral bacteria is killed as it enters the stomach and therefore has little significance for the remainder of the gastrointestinal tract.

Salivary Glands

The salivary glands are the parotid, submaxillary, and sublingual glands. Some small salivary glands are found in the lips, buccal mucosa, and palate. These are exocrine glands that secrete a mixture of serous and mucous fluid into the oral cavity.

The parotid gland is anterior to the external ear and wraps around the mandible. The parotid glands are the largest of the salivary glands. The parotid gland produces ptyalin (salivary amylase), which begins the chemical breakdown of starches. The action of ptyalin in the mouth breaks down only 5% to 10% of ingested starches. The action of the enzyme continues in the stomach for 30 minutes to several hours, until the pH falls, rendering the enzyme inactive.

The submaxillary gland is smaller. It is located in the submandibular fossa. The submaxillary gland produces a mixture of mucous and serous secretions.

The sublingual glands are located beneath the floor of the mouth. The sublingual glands produce primarily mucous secretions. The primary purpose of the sublingual gland secretions is lubrication.

Approximately 1000 to 1500 ml of saliva is produced by the salivary glands in 24 hours. The parotid and submaxillary glands account for almost 90% of the total production of saliva. The pH of the saliva is maintained between 6.0 and 7.0 by a complex autonomic mechanism that controls salivary secretion of sodium, potassium, chloride, and bicarbonate ions. The superior and inferior salivatory nuclei are located in the brainstem and may be stimulated by taste and tactile sensations from the tongue and mouth. Pleasant taste stimuli result in more salivation than unpleasant tastes, and smooth-textured foods stimulate more saliva production than rough-textured foods. Less salivation may result in less lubrication of food and more difficulty in swallowing. More saliva is produced when a person is eating a food he or she likes than when eating a disliked food. Thus salivation may be divided into three phases: psychic, gustatory, and gastrointestinal. The psychic phase occurs when the mouth is preparing itself to receive food. It is stimulated by thoughts or smells of pleasant foods. The gustatory phase occurs while one is chewing or swallowing food. The saliva is stimulated to aid in mastication and lubricate the food for swallowing. The gastrointestinal phase occurs when one has eaten irritating foods. The salivation is a response to reflexes originating in the stomach or upper intestines. The swallowed saliva dilutes or neutralizes the irritant.

Oropharynx

The oropharynx is the midpoint of the upper respiratory tract and digestive tract and is responsible for separating food and air as they pass through this area.

The oropharynx is lined by a mucous membrane of stratified squamous epithelium that is continuous with the lining of the mouth, nasal cavities, and larynx. The contents of the oropharynx include the soft palate, the uvula, the tonsils and their pillars, and the base of the tongue.

Esophagus

The esophagus is a hollow muscular tube approximately 25 cm (10 inches) long. It is closed at both ends by the upper esophageal sphincter and the lower esophageal sphincter.

The esophagus narrows slightly at three points: near its origin in the region of the cricoid cartilage, at the arch of the aorta, and as it passes through the diaphragm. The esophagus is more vulnerable to perforation and trauma in these areas.

The arterial blood supply of the esophagus comes from the inferior thyroid artery in the neck, from branches of the descending aorta, and from the left gastric artery. The esophageal veins join the vena azygos, which joins the superior vena cava and the systemic circulation. The veins at the lower end of the esophagus communicate freely with the tributaries of the left gastric vein that join the portal vein. The upper part of the esophageal blood supply drains into the tributaries of the left gastric vein that join the portal vein. The upper part of the esophageal blood supply drains into the superior vena cava; the middle part drains into the azygos system; and the bottom third drains into the portal system through gastric veins. When there is increased pressure in the portal system, there is increased pressure in the esophageal veins, leading to the development of esophageal varices.

The wall of the esophagus has all the characteristics of the gastrointestinal tract except for the serosa. Absence of serosa becomes important when esophageal surgery (i.e., anastomosis) has been performed because an increased chance for leakage may be present postoperatively. The esophageal lumen is lined with stratified squamous mucosa that is continuous with the oral cavity and pharynx. At the lower end of the esophagus the luminal lining changes to a simple columnar (transitional) epithelium that merges with the gastric mucosa in the cardiac portion of the stomach. The esophageal mucosa functions as a barrier to noxious luminal contents. The mucosa is repeatedly exposed to potentially damaging intraluminal materials, including oral intake and hypertonic gastric contents associated with gastroesophageal reflux. However, esophageal injury does not occur in most individuals. The esophageal mucosa maintains its protective function even when normal protective mechanisms, such as the lower esophageal sphincter, esophageal peristalsis, and salivary bicarbonate, fail.[17]

The submucosa layer underlying the squamous epithelium contains the blood vessels, nerves, mucous cells, and connective tissues. The mucous cells secrete mucus to further lubricate the food and protect the wall of the esophagus. The secretions are amphoteric, neutralizing both acid and base.

The muscle layer is composed of an internal circular and outer longitudinal layer. It differs from the remainder of the alimentary tract in several ways. First, the longitudinal layer is thicker than the inner circular layer. Second, the upper third of the esophagus is striated muscle. This portion of the esophagus receives its innervation from lower motor neurons and is dependent on cholinergic mechanisms. The middle third of the esophagus is mixed muscle tissue, and the lower third is primarily smooth muscle. The innervation of the smooth muscle found in the lower two thirds of the esophagus is from preganglionic fibers of the autonomic nervous system.

Swallowing

Deglutition (swallowing) can be divided into several phases. In the voluntary phase the tongue moves upward and backward, forcing a bolus of food into the pharynx. During the voluntary stage of swallowing, the bolus of food stimulates swallowing receptors around the pharynx. A series of involuntary events follows.

The esophageal phase of swallowing moves the bolus from the pharynx to the stomach by peristalsis. There are three types of esophageal peristalsis: primary, secondary, and tertiary. Primary peristalsis is a continuation of the movement begun in the pharynx. If a person is upright, downward gravity also affects the travel time through the esophagus. If primary peristalsis fails to move all the food that has entered the esophagus into the stomach, secondary peristalsis is stimulated from the distention of the esophagus by the retained bolus. The only difference is that primary peristalsis is initiated in the pharynx and secondary peristalsis is initiated in the esophagus at the level of the aortic arch.

Tertiary contractions may occur in some individuals, particularly after middle age. These are nonperistaltic contractions and do not assist in transport of food through the esophagus. The autonomic mechanisms of swallowing are usually preserved as an individual ages.[21]

Approximately 1 to 3 cm above the junction of the esophagus and stomach lies the lower esophageal sphincter. It has a higher resting pressure than the body of the esophagus or the stomach. Under normal circumstances this area relaxes with primary or secondary peristalsis. The purpose of this high-pressure area is to prevent reflux of acid gastric contents into the esophagus. Certain factors increase or decrease this high-pressure zone[54]:

- Increase high-pressure zone
  - Gastrin
  - Cholinergic agents
    - Methacholine (Mecholyl)
    - Bethanechol (Urecholine)
  - Prostaglandin F_2
  - Alpha-adrenergic agonists
  - Protein meal
  - Serotonin
  - Bombesin
- Decrease high-pressure zone
  - Secretin
  - Cholecystokinin
  - Glucagon
  - Gastric inhibitory polypeptide
  - Vasoactive intestine peptide
  - Prostaglandins E, E_2, A_2
  - Isoproterenol
  - Dopamine

Peritoneal Cavity

The abdomen is the largest cavity in the human body. It contains the stomach, small intestine, kidneys, adrenal glands, uterus in women, liver, colon, gallbladder, pancreas, and major vessels.

The structures in the cavity are protected and covered by peritoneum, which is made up of serous membrane composed of mesothelium and a thin layer of irregular connective tissue. The parietal peritoneum is the tissue that lines the abdominal wall. The mesentery is a double fold of parietal peritoneum that is fan shaped and encircles the jejunum and ileum, attaching them to the posterior abdominal wall. The blood vessels and nerves of the small intestine pass though the mesentery. The greater omentum is an apron-shaped double fold of peritoneum that hangs loosely over the intestines. The greater omentum is attached to the upper border of the duodenum, the lower edge of the stomach, and the transverse colon.

A small amount of serous fluid separates the space between the parietal and visceral peritoneum. The fluid provides lubrication between the organs and the abdominal wall.

Stomach

The function of the stomach is to alter the consistency and the composition of ingested foods. The ingested foods are liquified, increasing the surface area of food particles to facilitate the digestive process. The food particles mixed with gastric secretions create a solution called chyme. The chyme is then released in a regulated manner into the duodenum for further digestion and absorption.

The stomach connects to the esophagus 3 cm below the diaphragm. The stomach lies obliquely beneath the cardiac sphincter of the esophagus, above the pyloric sphincter next to the small intestine, and under the left lobe of the liver and diaphragm. The size, shape, and position of the stomach vary depending on body size, posture, degree of gastric retention, degree of gastric muscle development, and effects of pressures from adjacent organs. Its normal capacity is 1 to 2 L. The stomach functions as a reservoir where mechanical and chemical breakdown of food continues.

The stomach is divided into the cardia, fundus, body, antrum, and pylorus (FIG. 10-2). The cardia is the proximal portion of the stomach. The fundus is the uppermost portion of the stomach. The antrum is the peristaltic portion of the stomach and is distal to the body. The pylorus is the portion just before the duodenum.

The wall of the stomach is composed of four layers (from the innermost lining layer out): the mucosa, the submucosa, the muscle layer, and the serosa. The mucosa layer is separated from the submucosa by the muscularis mucosae and is composed of gastric epithelium. The mucosa is arranged in longitudinal folds called rugae found most predominantly in the fundus and body regions of the stomach. The rugae are invaginated with gastric pits, or openings to gastric glands, which are responsible for gastric acid secretion (FIG. 10-3). The rugae are low and flat in the lesser curvature and are sometimes absent in the antrum.

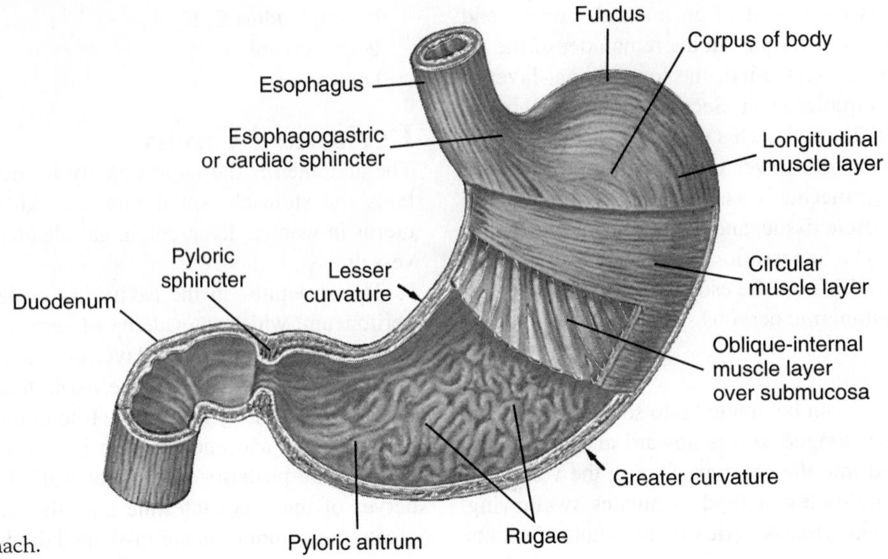

FIG. 10-2
Gross anatomy of stomach.

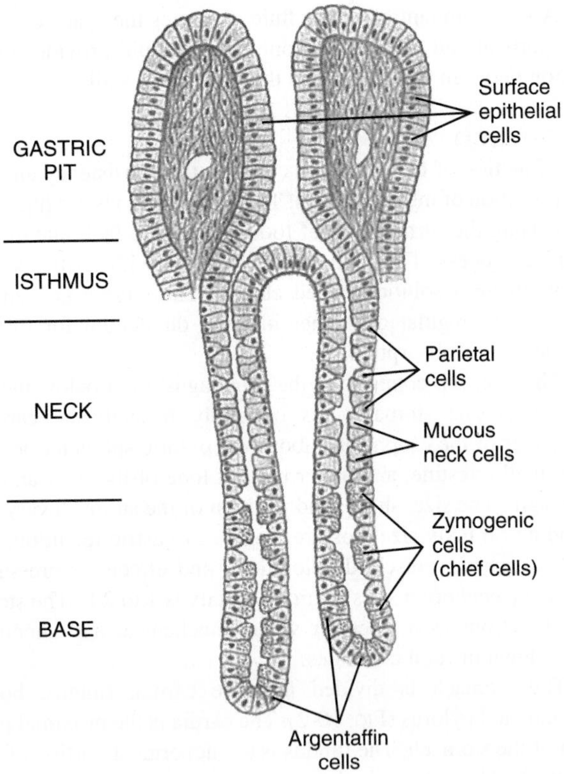

FIG. 10-3
Human gastric mucosa. Diagram of tubular gland from fundic area of stomach.

There are three distinct areas of cells within the stomach: the cardia, the oxyntic, and the antral, or pyloric. The mucosa of the cardia is columnar epithelium that secretes mucus. This zone or area has also been referred to as the transitional or junctional mucosa.

The glands of the fundus and body are straight, closely packed, and tubular. These glands contain neck cells, parietal (oxyntic) cells, chief (zymogenic) cells, and argentaffin cells. Mucous neck cells are most numerous and play a role in mucosal cell renewal. Parietal cells are located at the upper portion of the gland. Parietal cells produce hydrochloric acid (HCl) and intrinsic factor. Chief cells are most abundant in the deeper portion of the gland and secrete pepsinogen (type I). Argentaffin cells are in the deeper portion of the gland and produce serotonin.

The fundus and body are often referred to as the acid-pepsin secreting area. The pepsinogen is activated in a pH less than 5.0. The optimum level of pH is 1.8 to 3.5. The hydrochloric acid provides the acidity necessary for the pepsinogen to convert to its active form, pepsin.

The antrum mucosa is thinner than the oxyntic, and the gastric pits are deeper. The glands are tubular and coiled. Gastrin-producing G cells are located in the mucosa adjacent to the tubular glands. The tubular glands secrete mucus and pepsinogen II.

The submucosa is composed of loose areolar and elastic tissue. It contains vascular and lymphatic channels and an intrinsic nerve plexus, Meissner's plexus. The muscle layer is thick and is composed of three separate strata of smooth muscle. The outer, longitudinal layer extends downward from the esophagus along the greater and lesser curvatures to the pyloric sphincter. The middle circular muscle forms a uniform layer over the entire stomach. There is a second nerve plexus found between the two muscle layers, Auerbach's plexus. The inner oblique muscle is continuous with the circular muscle of the esophagus and is thickest in the fundus region. It extends to the pyloric sphincter. The outermost layer is the serosa and is an extension of the peritoneum.

The blood supply to the stomach is from large branches of the celiac artery. There may be variation in the branching pattern of the celiac axis. In approximately one fourth of all people, the left hepatic artery arises in part or totally from the left gastric artery. It is therefore critical that the surgeon first assess the pattern of arterial blood flow before relevant operative procedures.[7] Arterial branches passing through the muscle layer form an extensive plexus of blood vessels in the submucosa.

These vessels then enter the mucosa and subdivide to form a capillary network in the lamina propria surrounding the gastric glands and pits. Blood can be shunted from one area of the stomach to another or from one layer of the stomach to another by submucosa anastomoses and numerous submucosa arteriovenous communications. Mucosal ischemia can be caused by a redistribution of blood flow from vasoconstrictor activity of the sympathetic nervous system and by vasoconstrictor drugs. Venous blood from the right and left gastric veins of the stomach empties directly into the portal vein.

The vagus and splanchnic nerves innervate the stomach. Branches of the left and right vagus nerves join to form the anterior esophageal plexus, and branches of the right vagus form the posterior esophageal plexus. At the distal esophagus they join to form the anterior and posterior vagal trunk. The anterior trunk provides the anterior gastric and hepatic divisions. The anterior gastric division goes along the lesser curvature to the pyloric sphincter with branches to the anterosuperior wall of the stomach. The hepatic division supplies the gallbladder, biliary tree, and proximal duodenum.

The posterior trunk of the vagus nerve divides into the posterior gastric and celiac divisions. The posterior gastric division goes along the lesser curvature with branches to the posteroinferior wall of the stomach. The celiac division descends with the left gastric artery through the celiac plexus to the superior mesenteric plexus, supplying the small intestine and ascending and transverse colon to the splenic flexure.

The splanchnic nerves contain sensory fibers and postganglionic sympathetic fibers (whose transmitters are catecholamines). The vagi contain sensory fibers, preganglionic parasympathetic fibers, and postganglionic (sympathetic) fibers.[18] These fibers synapse with the ganglion cells of the myenteric (Auerbach's) plexus and the submucosal (Meissner's) plexus. The postganglionic fibers end in the gastric glands and muscle fibers, stimulating gastric secretion and muscle contraction.

The reservoir function of the stomach is the capacity of the stomach to accommodate a meal. A vagal-mediated reflex relaxes the body of the stomach so that it accepts the ingested meal with minimal increase in intragastric pressure. Once swallowing is completed, the gastric wall tension increases and intragastric pressure is proportional to the volume ingested. This also helps to modulate gastric emptying. If the normal vagal reflex activity is inhibited or if the capacity of the stomach is reduced, the reservoir function is altered. People with significantly compromised reservoir functions need to eat frequent, smaller meals to avoid or minimize symptoms such as early satiety, postprandial epigastric pain, and nausea and vomiting.

Gastric secretions include mucus, pepsinogen, hydrochloric acid, intrinsic factor, and the hormone gastrin. Gastric mucus is composed of proteins, glycoproteins, mucopolysaccharides, and blood group substances. The principal component is glycoprotein. Gastric mucus is a thin layer of mucus adherent to the cell surface. The gastric mucosal barrier helps separate acid in the lumen from bicarbonate on the epithelial cell surface. The mucosal barrier prevents diffusion of hydrogen ions from lumen to mucosa and diffusion of sodium ions from mucosa to lumen.

The surface mucous cells are stimulated by vagus nerve and acetylcholine in response to chemicals (e.g., ethanol) and physical contact and friction from roughage in the diet. They protect the mucosa with an alkaline layer of lubricant.

Pepsinogen is secreted by the chief cells of glands in the body and fundus with a small amount secreted by neck cells and by Brunner's glands in the duodenum. Pepsinogen is converted to active pepsin at a pH less than 6.0. The optimum pH of pepsin is 1.8 to 3.5 with no activity greater than a pH of 5.0. Pepsinogen is stimulated by both vagal stimulation and a local reflex activity. Pepsinogen secretion is increased by the presence of gastrin, calcium, histamine, and secretin. Pepsin is responsible for initiating protein digestion, particularly collagen, a major protein component of meat.

Hydrochloric acid is secreted by the parietal cells. Endogenous stimuli for hydrochloric acid production are acetylcholine, gastrin, and histamine. Histamine, secreted by mast cells in the stomach, plays a critical role in regulating gastric acid secretion through the activation of the parietal H_2 receptor.

The production of intrinsic factor by the parietal cells is a critical function of the stomach. Intrinsic factor is a mucoprotein that binds with vitamin B_{12}. This bond is essential for the absorption of vitamin B_{12} at specific receptor cells in the terminal ileum. The stimuli that increase secretion of intrinsic factor are the same as those stimulating hydrochloric acid production. The failure to secrete intrinsic factor is associated with achlorhydria and the absence of parietal cells. The condition results in vitamin B_{12} deficiency and subsequent pernicious anemia.

The hormone gastrin is secreted by the antral G cells and is the primary mediator of gastric acid secretion. Gastrin is also secreted by cells in the duodenum, pancreatic islets, and jejunum. Vagal stimulation, gastric distention, and the presence of amino acids, peptides, and calcium ions stimulate the secretion of antral gastrin. Antral gastrin then circulates in the blood system with the parietal cells as the target organ. When the gastric pH is less than 1.5, gastrin release is inhibited. Duodenal gastrin is secreted in response to distention and protein.

Gastric secretion has been divided into three phases (cephalic, gastric, and intestinal) that occur almost simultaneously. The cephalic phase includes the sight, smell, taste, thought, and chewing of food, as well as conditional reflexes and intracellular hypoglycemia. The vagus nerve releases acetylcholine by postganglionic fibers in the gastric mucosa, causing the secretion of hydrochloric acid, intrinsic factor, and pepsinogen. The gastric phase constitutes the major physiologic stimulus for gastric secretion and is activated by the presence of food in the stomach. The intestinal phase serves mainly to inhibit gastric secretions. Duodenal gastrin that is released in response to protein digestion products and distention functions in the same way as antral gastrin (FIG. 10-4).

Inhibition of gastric secretions in the intestinal phase is related to the actions of cholecystokinin (CCK), secretin, gastric inhibitory polypeptide (GIP), vasoactive intestinal peptide (VIP), glucagon, and prostaglandins (FIG. 10-5). CCK is stimulated by L-amino acids and fatty acids in the duodenum. When CCK and gastrin are both present, a competitive inhibition of gastrin occurs because both have the same active terminal tetrapeptide. Thus the secretory function of gastrin is inhibited. Hydrogen ions in the duodenum stimulate the release of secretin. Secretin inhibits acid output and blocks the secretory effects of gastrin and histamine. Secretin stimulates pepsinogen

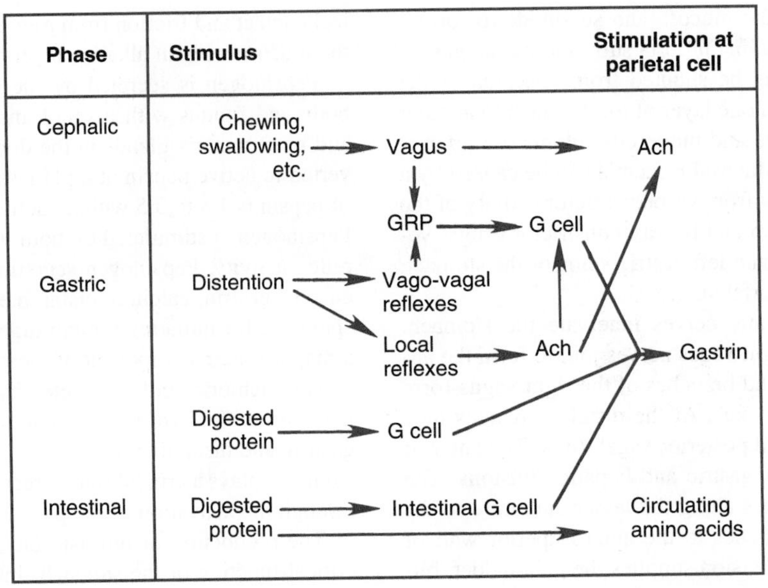

FIG. 10-4
Mechanisms for stimulation of acid secretion. (From Johnson.[25])

Region	Stimulus	Mediator	Inhibit gastrin release	Inhibit acid secretion
Antrum	Acid (pH <3.0)	Somatostatin	+	
Duodenum	Acid	Secretin	+	+
		Nervous reflex		+
	Hyperosmotic solutions	Unidentified enterogastrone		+
Duodenum and jejunum	Fatty acids	GIP	+	+
		Unidentified enterogastrone		+

FIG. 10-5
Mechanisms for inhibition of acid secretion. (From Johnson.[25])

output. Both CCK and secretin stimulate pancreatic secretion of bicarbonate.

GIP is found throughout the intestinal tract, although it is concentrated in the duodenum. GIP has a wide range of functions, including inhibition of food-stimulated release of gastrin, gastric acid secretion, and pepsinogen secretions. VIP and glucagon inhibit gastric secretion and stimulate intestinal electrolyte secretion.

Prostaglandins are a group of cyclic fatty acid compounds that act to inhibit parietal cells, effecting a prostaglandin-mediated negative feedback loop that regulates gastric acid secretion.

Enterogastrone is a general term often used to designate hormones released from duodenal mucosa in response to glucose, long-chain fatty acids, and triglycerides that inhibit gastric acid secretions.[7] There are still unanswered questions regarding gastric inhibition. Future research should answer many of the uncertainties in the understanding of hormonal inhibition of gastric secretion.

Gastric motility can be divided into tonic, mixing, and peristaltic contractions. Gastric tone controls luminal volume and maintains a relatively constant pressure despite changes in volume. The fundus and body serve as a receptacle and the antrum as a pump. Circular muscle contractions in the body of the stomach mix the food with the gastric secretions. Contractions in the antrum are stronger and produce considerable mixing motions and propulsion of gastric contents into the duodenum in a controlled fashion.

Antral peristaltic contractions force the chyme into the pyloric canal and then into the duodenum. The pyloric sphincter is a high-pressure zone that relaxes with antral peristalsis and contracts in response to acids, fats, amino acids, and nonisotonic solutions in the duodenum. Gastric distention stimulates stretch receptors, which results in increased gastric peristalsis and increased gastric emptying. The stimulus for rapid gastric emptying is gastric distention.

There are three receptors in the duodenum that release substances inhibiting gastric emptying: osmoreceptors, acid-

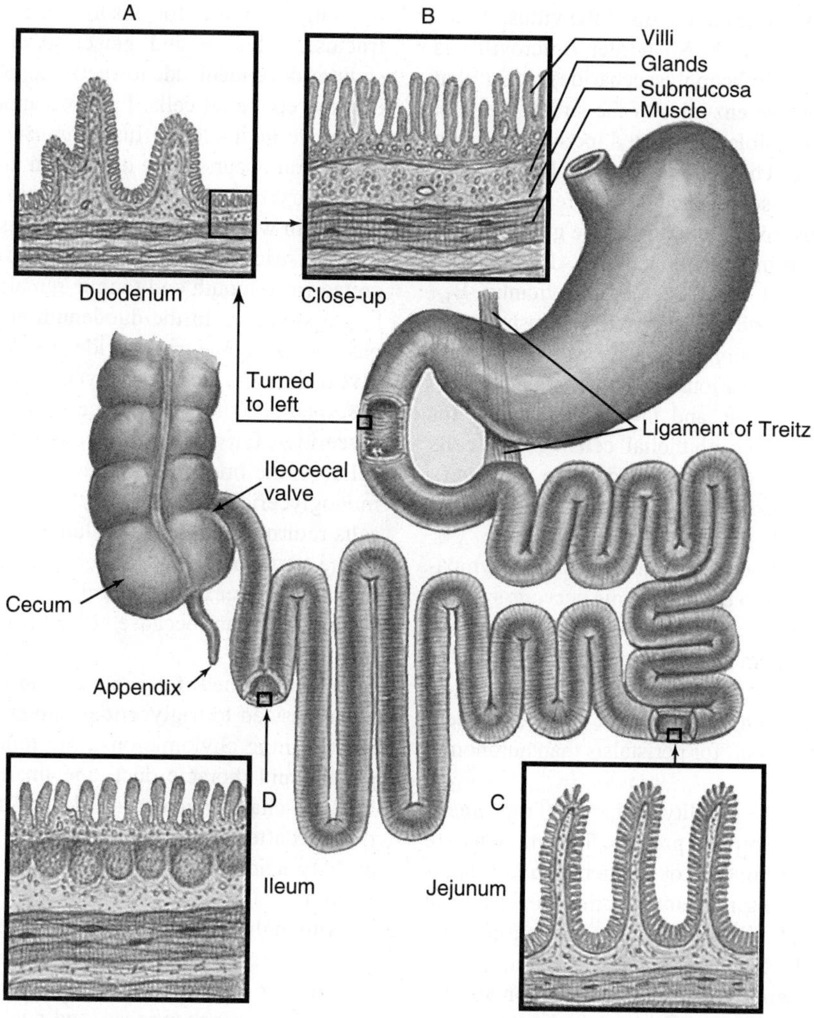

FIG. 10-6
Clinical anatomy of small intestine.

sensitive receptors, and fat-sensitive receptors. Feedback control by the small intestine is one of the most important regulators of gastric emptying. Duodenal perfusion of nutrients such as amino acids can almost abolish gastric emptying of solids and, to a lesser extent, can delay the intestinal delivery of liquids.[54]

Gastric emptying can be impaired by drugs, diseases, and surgery. Incomplete emptying may result in early satiety, postprandial epigastric pain, and vomiting. Rapid gastric emptying may occur with duodenal ulcers and after surgery for peptic ulcers. Prokinetic oral medications may be effective in increasing gastric emptying time.

The microflora of the stomach are comparatively sparse. Only relatively acid-resistant organisms survive any length of time. *Lactobacillus, Candida, Streptococcus, Neisseria, Staphylococcus,* and *Peptostreptococcus* are the genera best represented. *Helicobacter pylori* may colonize the stomach, it is not clear whether this organism should be considered part of the indigenous flora or a pathogen.

Small Intestine

In the small intestine, ingested food is mixed, digested, and absorbed. The small intestine is divided into three segments: duodenum, jejunum, and ileum. The first portion is the duodenum; at 20 to 30 cm (8 to 12 inches) long, it is the shortest segment. The ligament of Treitz is the dividing point between the duodenum and jejunum, although histologic changes cannot be demonstrated. The jejunum is 2.5 m (8 feet) long, and the ileum is 3.5 m (11⅓ feet) long. The jejunum and ileum have no specific anatomic division (FIG. 10-6). The common bile duct and main pancreatic duct empty into the duodenum at the ampulla of Vater.

The wall of the small intestine is divided into four layers: mucosa (innermost layer), submucosa, muscularis externa, and serosa (outer layer). As in other segments of the gastrointestinal tract, the mucosa is separated from the submucosa by the muscularis mucosae. The submucosa contains the connective tissue, lymphatics, blood vessels, and nerves. Meissner's plexus is in the submucosa. The muscularis externa consists of an inner circular layer and an outer longitudinal layer. Auerbach's (myenteric) plexus lies between the two muscle layers.

The duodenum contains Brunner's glands in the submucosa, which secrete an alkaline fluid containing pepsinogen. The hormones secreted in the duodenum include gastrin, CCK, secretin, GIP, VIP, and enterogastrone.

The jejunum and ileum have a greatly increased mucosa and submucosa surface area for absorption. Three characteristic features of this portion of the small intestine are a large series of circular folds of mucosa and submucosa; minute, fingerlike projections of the mucosa called villi; and microvilli, or brush border. Mucosal crypts at the base of the villi extend into the wall of the small intestine to the muscularis mucosae. Epithelial cells migrate from the crypts to extrude from the tip of the villi. As an epithelial cell migrates to the tip of the villus, its absorptive capacity increases. The brush border (microvilli) is covered with a glycocalyx (mucopolysaccharide) cover that contains many of the digestive enzymes of the small intestine. Hosoda et al[21] describe a possible age-related increase in brush border membrane enzymes. This may indicate higher turnover of small intestinal cells with senescence or may reveal an age-related reduction in the absorptive function of the gut that leads to a compensatory increase in enzyme activity. Also found in the microvillus-calyceal area are receptors for vitamin B_{12}. The surface epithelial cells and the microvillus brush border constitute the digestion-absorption unit. Several enzymes are found in this unit, including various hydrolases, peptidases, transport proteins, adenylcyclase, and the "active pump" for sodium.[7] In addition to surface epithelial cells, goblet cells (mucin secreting), crypt cells (fluid and electrolyte secreting), and enteroendocrine cells (hormonal) are found in the small intestine.

The small intestine has both sympathetic and parasympathetic stimulation. In addition to the autonomic nervous system, the enteric nervous system also regulates small bowel activities. The autonomic nervous system stimulation can be interrupted with vagotomy and sympathectomy without significant alteration in intestinal motility. An intact enteric nervous system may therefore be more important for peristalsis than autonomic innervation.

The primary function of the motility of the small intestine is to facilitate the digestive-absorptive process. Two motions are found in the small intestine: mixing, or segmental, and propulsive, or peristaltic. The mixing movements bring the chyme in contact with pancreatic and biliary secretions. The musculature constricts at the rate of 11 to 12 contractions per minute, resulting in segmentation resembling links. Segmentation also increases the contact of the chyme with the intestinal villi and microvilli, enhancing absorption. Peristalsis propels chyme forward. The myenteric plexus supplies the sympathetic and parasympathetic stimulation for segmentation and peristalsis.

The terms *digestion* and *absorption* emphasize two phases of a single continuing process. The digestion of dietary lipids, carbohydrates, and proteins is initiated in the lumen of the duodenum and proximal jejunum and is completed at the glycocalyx and microvilli plasma membrane of enterocytes (jejunal absorptive cells). Most absorption occurs in the jejunum. Vitamin B_{12} is absorbed in the terminal ileum, and bile salts are reabsorbed by active transport in the terminal ileum. Otherwise, minimum absorption occurs in the ileum unless the jejunum is nonfunctioning or diseased. The processes of absorption in the small intestine are passive absorption and active transport. Passive absorption resembles diffusion of a substance through a membrane, and the rate of movement depends on a higher concentration in the lumen than in the bloodstream. Active transport is more rapid, more complex, more efficient, and requires energy.

Carbohydrate absorption requires conversion of starches to monosaccharides. Starch digestion by pancreatic amylase yields oligosaccharides and disaccharides. Disaccharides are further hydrolyzed by brush border enzymes. Active absorption of sugars occurs primarily in the brush border and at the apex of the epithelial cell. Brush border enzymes include lactase, sucrase, maltase, isomaltase, and trehalase. The sugars that are normally available for absorption are glucose, galactose, and fructose. Glucose and galactose are transported through a sodium-dependent adenosinetriphosphatase (ATPase) process into the epithelial cells. Fructose appears to be absorbed by a nonactive facilitated diffusion transport process. Carbohydrate absorption occurs in the duodenum and jejunum.[54]

Dietary fat consists of long-chain triglycerides that are insoluble in water. In the stomach, fat is shaken into a fine emulsion. Gastric pepsin strips fat of its protein wrapper. Lipase secreted from mouth and tongue remains active in digesting fats in the stomach. In the duodenum and jejunum, pancreatic lipase breaks down triglycerides to diglycerides, then to monoglycerides, and finally to glycerol and fatty acids. Glycerol is absorbed into the epithelial cell and capillaries directly. Monoglycerides, fatty acids, and conjugated bile salts form the micelle. At the brush border the micelle breaks up, allowing the monoglyceride and free fatty acid to enter the cells. The bile salts return to the intestinal lumen, where they are reabsorbed in the terminal ileum. Resorbed bile salts are cycled through the liver and reexcreted in bile. Bicarbonate from the pancreas is also important because efficient lipolysis occurs in an alkaline pH.

The absorbed fatty acids and beta-monoglycerides are resynthesized to triglycerides, are enclosed in a protein covering (forming chylomicrons), are transported through the lymphatics and thoracic duct, and finally reach the blood. Some medium-chain triglycerides do not depend on micelle formation and after hydrolysis can be absorbed by the epithelial cell as fatty acids and transported directly into the portal venous system.

Although gastric pepsin begins protein digestion, it is not essential for protein digestion. Pancreatic proteases include trypsinogen, chymotrypsinogen, procarboxypeptidases A and B, leucine aminopeptidase, and nucleases. The hormone CCK is the primary stimulator of the pancreatic acinar cells. CCK is released in the duodenum and jejunum in the presence of amino acids and fatty acids. The presence of hydrogen ions, or a low pH, stimulates the release of the hormone secretin. Secretin stimulates the bicarbonate and fluid responses of the pancreas. The activation of the pancreatic enzyme trypsinogen depends on the intestinal secretion of the enzyme enterokinase. Thus pancreatic functioning depends on the presence and functioning of a normal proximal small bowel.

The intraluminal protein digestion by-products are peptides of two to six amino acids. The brush border and intracellular enzymes further break down these products to free amino acids, dipeptides, and some tripeptides that can enter the epithelial cell. In the cell the small peptides are hydrolyzed into free amino acids, which are absorbed into the capillary, where further protein breakdown occurs.

Vitamin B_{12} binds with intrinsic factor (gastric secretion) to protect it from gastric digestion and bacterial digestion in the small bowel. The intrinsic factor also is essential for attachment of vitamin B_{12} to receptors of the glycocalyx membrane of the ileal absorptive cell. Calcium, magnesium, and pH greater than 5.6 are also necessary for the attachment of vitamin B_{12} and the transport through the cell. The vitamin B_{12} is then transported in the portal blood bound to a carrier (transcobalamin). Pancreatic insufficiency may be associated with a vitamin B_{12} deficiency because R binders found in saliva, gastric secretions, bile, and intestinal secretions can bind with vitamin B_{12} instead of intrinsic factor. Pancreatic proteases degrade the R binders, making it possible for vitamin B_{12} to bind with the intrinsic factor. Intestinal microflora are capable of synthesizing vitamin B_{12}. When oral vitamin B_{12} is reduced, the use of antibiotics may alter intraluminal flora, resulting in vitamin B_{12} deficiency. The body stores of vitamin B_{12} may be adequate for years. Thus clinical signs of vitamin B_{12} deficiency are unusual.

Calcium absorption is highest in the upper small intestine where the pH is lowest. Its absorption and transport are enhanced by vitamin D. Calcium is transported against a concentration gradient. Passive absorption occurs when intraluminal concentrations are greater than 6 mmol/L. Calcium absorption is decreased by phosphate ingestion, anticonvulsant drugs, alcohol, and steroids.

Dietary folate is composed of multiple glutamyl units, and the linkage is broken by the jejunal brush border enzymes to monoglutamate. Absorption occurs primarily in the proximal small bowel by a saturable, carrier-mediated process that is maximal at a luminal pH between 5.5 and 6.0. Folate enters the portal circulation and functions as a cofactor in many enzyme systems.

Iron absorption depends on the physiologic demands of the body. When iron stores are low or when red blood cells are being rapidly formed, iron absorption is increased. Iron absorption occurs primarily in the duodenum and proximal jejunum against a concentration gradient. Iron is absorbed in the ferrous form, bound to globulin (transferrin), then released into the portal circulation or stored within cells as apoferritin.

One of the major functions of the small intestine is fluid and electrolyte shifts from gastrointestinal lumen to blood and from blood to lumen. In a 24-hour period, approximately 9 L of fluid enters the lumen of the small intestine. Approximately 7.5 to 8.2 L is endogenous secretions (saliva, gastric, intestinal, pancreatic, and bile). Another 1 to 1.5 L is exogenous. Most of the fluid is reabsorbed, and only 500 to 1000 ml passes through the ileocecal valve into the colon. The duodenum and jejunum are primarily responsible for the large amounts of absorption of fluids, electrolytes, and nutrients because of large pores that allow rapid flow of solutes and water in both directions. Isosmolarity in the lumen is rapidly attained and maintained throughout the small intestine. Several factors help prevent osmotic disequilibrium, including the relative impermeability of gastric mucosa, the regulation of gastric emptying, the fact that nutrients are largely macromolecules with low osmotic activity, and rapid absorption of products of macromolecule digestion or breakdown. Fat is high in most diets, but because its osmotic potential is low, it does not impede osmotic equilibrium. Maintaining osmolarity requires rapid flow of salt and water through the intestinal membrane. The direction of the flow is determined by hydrostatic and osmotic forces.

Sodium absorption is a major function of the small intestine. Sodium absorption plays a part in regulating cellular absorption of electrolytes and water. The brush border contains a carrier that binds sodium and glucose. When intraluminal glucose is present, sodium is actively reabsorbed by the shared carrier. Sodium is also absorbed from the lumen by a sodium-hydrogen exchange mechanism. A sodium pump at the basolateral border of epithelial absorbing cells transports sodium from intracellular to intercellular spaces by means of sodium-potassium ATPase activity. The decrease of intracellular sodium concentration enhances the sodium-glucose carrier mechanism.

In the ileum a chloride-bicarbonate exchange mechanism is present. The bicarbonate concentration in the ileum is much higher than in the jejunum. Potassium is absorbed based on sodium-potassium ATPase and hydrostatic and osmotic forces.

Water transport is passive and depends on osmotic and hydrostatic pressures. Increased solute concentration in the intercellular space (e.g., from sodium pump activity) provides osmotic forces for water absorption. As water flows through the pores, it brings small solutes with it. This is referred to as solvent drag. Hydrostatic forces from the serosa layer will restrict passive water and solute absorption. Water from the interstitial fluid will enter the lumen when solutes accumulate in the lumen. The flow continues until osmotic equilibrium is reached.

The secretory function of the intestinal epithelium appears to be the result of electrogenic activity. If the secretory function is greater than the absorption function, significant fluid and electrolyte loss can occur. This is frequently seen in diseases of abnormal states (malabsorption syndromes).

Immunologic function of the small bowel is regulated through Peyer's patches, lymphoid cells, and nonorganized cells in the lamina propria. Peyer's patches are found in the submucosa and contain small lymphocytes from the mesenteric nodes. IgA is the prominent immunoglobulin found in the small bowel, but IgM, IgG, IgD, and IgE are also present. The IgA found in the small bowel differs from serum IgA. An infant is born without secretory or serum IgA. The secretory IgA appears first and reaches adult levels sooner. The secretory IgA has antiviral and antibacterial activities. The immune system of the small bowel is complex. Clinically important immune responses to invasive intracellular organisms and to tumors include responses of T cells, B cells, M cells, plasma cells, phagocytic cells, and mast cells present in the submucosa, lymphoid, and lamina propria tissues.

Hormonal function of the small intestine is of great interest. The small intestine may be the body's largest and most diffuse endocrine organ. To be classified a hormone, a substance should be released in response to physiologic stimulation into the circulation in amounts sufficient to account for the target organ response, its action should be replicated by intravenous administration of the putative peptide, and blocking the substance's activity abolishes the target organ response. Secretin, gastrin, CCK, enteroglucagon, and GIP meet the criteria for an intestinal hormone. A large number of other small- and moderate-sized peptides are also found in the gastrointestinal tract that may meet these criteria. These include vasoactive intestinal peptide, motilin, pancreatic polypeptides, somatostatin, neurotensin, substance P, and glucagon-related gut peptides. The actions of the hormones are complex, and many have more than one action. The activity may be as a paracrine agent, a neuroendocrine or neurotransmitter substance, or an exocrine agent. Table 10-1 summarizes several small intestinal hormones and their activities.[7]

The numbers and types of bacteria found in the small intestine depend on the flow rate of the intestinal contents and are highest when stasis occurs, such as in a bowel obstruction. Streptococci, lactobacilli, yeasts, staphylococci, clostridia, bacteroides, and coliforms may be present, particularly in the distal ileum.

Table 10-1 Gastrointestinal Hormones and Their Actions

Hormone	Location	Primary Action	Secondary Action
Gastrin	Antrum, duodenum, proximal jejunum	Stimulates gastric acid secretion	Trophic effect on gastrointestinal mucosa
Cholecystokinin	Throughout small intestine, but primarily found in jejunum	Stimulates contraction of gallbladder Stimulates secretion of pancreatic enzymes	Motility of stomach and small intestine
Secretin	Throughout gastrointestinal tract, except colon; primary sites are duodenum and jejunum	Stimulates pancreatic bicarbonate secretions	Numerous interactions with other gastrointestinal hormones
Gastric inhibitory peptide	Small intestine, primarily jejunum	Increases release of insulin from pancreas	Decreases gastric acid secretion Increases intestinal secretion
Enteroglucagon	Primarily lower ileum and colon	Inhibits motility	May be trophic for mucosa
Vasoactive intestinal peptide	Esophagus to rectum	Increases intestinal and pancreatic secretions	Decreases gastric acid secretion Increases insulin secretion Causes peripheral vasodilation

Large Intestine (Colon) and Rectum

The colon is approximately 150 cm ($4^1/_2$ to 5 feet) long. The terminal ileum joins the colon at the ileocecal valve. The appendix arises from the cecum medially, about 2 cm below the junction of the ileum and cecum. The cecum is continuous with the ascending colon, which goes from the cecum to the undersurface of the right lobe of the liver. The colon bends to the left, forming the hepatic flexure. The colon then extends to the left, becoming the transverse colon. The transverse colon has a mesentery and therefore a wide range of movement. The cecum, ascending colon, and proximal half of the transverse colon are derived from the midgut. The innervation and vascular supply are shared with the small intestine.

The transverse colon continues to the left and slightly upward, forming the splenic flexure. The splenic flexure is slightly higher than the hepatic flexure and is in front of and above the left kidney. As the colon turns downward, it becomes the descending colon. The sigmoid colon begins at the point where the descending colon crosses the iliac artery at the rim of the pelvis. The mesentery of the sigmoid colon attaches it to the posterior (retroperitoneal) wall of the pelvis. Near the midsacrum, the sigmoid colon becomes the rectum. The rectum descends in front of the sacrum and coccyx. The rectum becomes the anal canal approximately 2 cm anterior to the tip of the coccyx. The upper portion of the rectum is in the peritoneal cavity, but the distal 12 to 15 cm has no peritoneal covering. This area lies behind the bladder in the male with the seminal vesicles on either side. In the female the distal 12 to 15 cm is posterior to the uterus. The rectal ampulla is the lowest part of the rectum and is anterior to the posterior aspect of the prostate in the male. In the female the rectal ampulla is attached to the posterior wall of the vagina.

The wall of the colon is divided into the same four layers as the small intestine: mucosa, submucosa, muscularis externa, and serosa. There are no villi in the large intestine. The simple columnar epithelial surface is flat and is broken into polygonal units by clefts. Goblet cell openings occur on the epithelial surface. In the center of polygonal units are crypts of Lieberkühn. These crypts are lined with goblet cells and extend into the muscularis mucosae. At the bottom of the crypts are proliferating undifferentiated epithelial cells and occasionally argentaffin cells. Cell renewal begins in the crypts. The cells then migrate upward to the surface and extrude into the lumen. The renewal time is approximately $3^1/_2$ to 4 days.

The mucosa, submucosa, and circular muscular layer form semilunar folds (plicae semilunares) dividing the haustra (sacculations). The semilunar folds are crescent shaped and extend one third of the way around the wall of the intestine. The longitudinal muscle layer is incomplete in the large colon. It is called teniae coli and is the noticeable band in the colon wall. Fatty tags (appendices epiploicae) project from the serosa coat of the colon; this is another difference between the large and small intestines.

The musculature of the rectum is a continuation of the colonic muscular layers. The outer longitudinal layer spreads from the teniae of the sigmoid colon to form a continuous even coat. The superficial fibers insert into the perianal body and merge with the levator ani muscles of the pelvic floor. The deep fibers insert into the perianal skin. The circular muscle forms the internal sphincter surrounding the anal canal. The pectinate line marks the boundary between the anal canal and rectum. At this anorectal junction, the lining layer changes from columnar to squamous epithelial cells. The external sphincter is striated muscle and lies outside the internal sphincter. The external sphincter encircles the terminal portion of the anal canal.

The mesenteric attachments of the colon permit considerable mobility of the ileocecal junction and sigmoid colon. Two potential problems are a volvulus, or twisting of the bowel on itself, and intussusception. The hepatic and splenic flexures, descending colon, and rectum are relatively fixed.

The major blood vessels of the large colon and rectum are the superior and inferior mesenteric arteries as previously stated. The superior rectal artery is a branch of the inferior mesenteric and branches as low as the proximal anal canal. The middle and inferior rectal arteries are branches of the internal iliac artery and supply the anal canal and subcutaneous perianal area. The superior hemorrhoidal vein empties into the inferior mesenteric vein, which drains into the portal system. The inferior hemorrhoidal veins drain into pudendal veins and the systemic venous system. Because of the venous relationship with

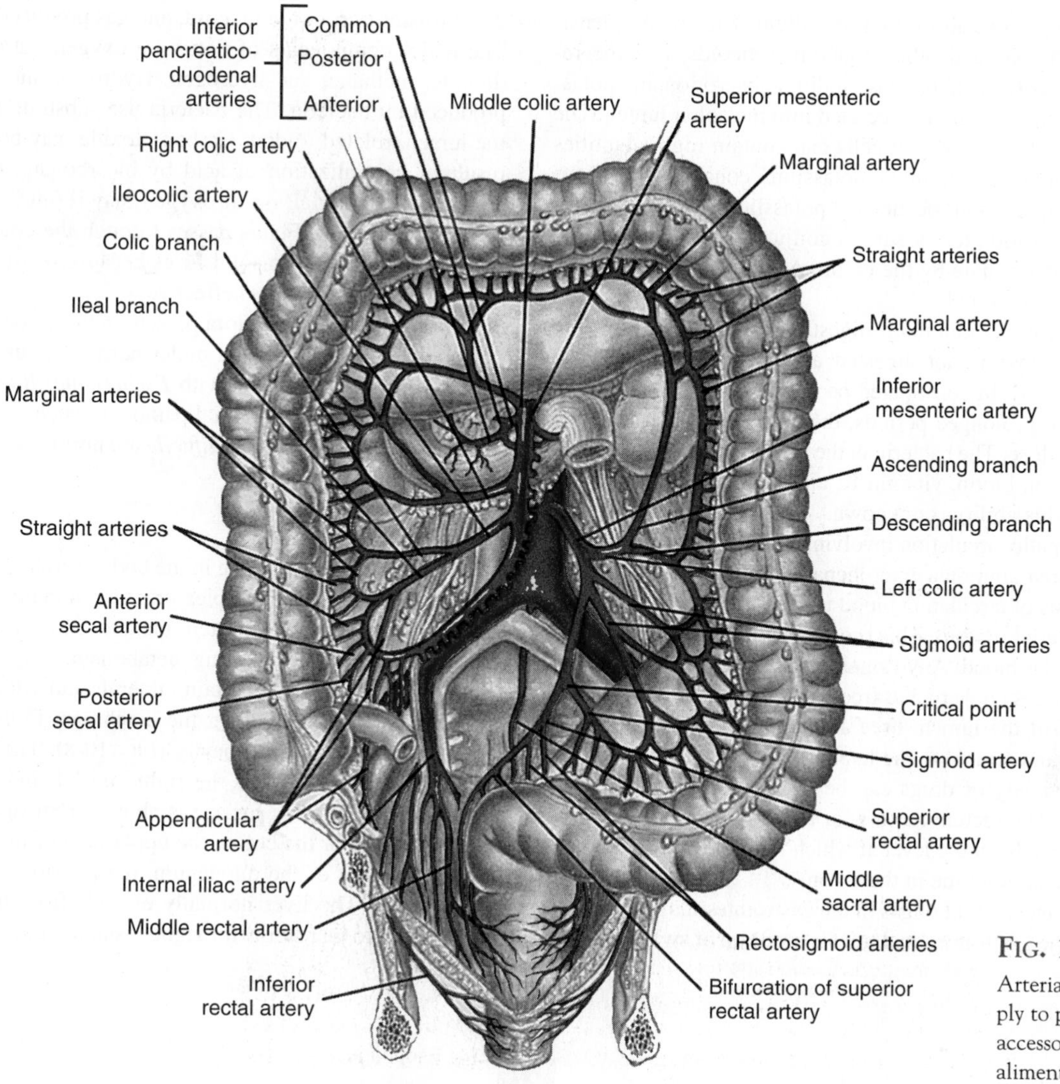

FIG. 10-7
Arterial blood supply to primary and accessory organs of alimentary canal.

the portal system, portal hypertension can lead to congestion and enlargement of the hemorrhoidal system and hemorrhoids (FIG. 10-7).

Nervous innervation includes external sympathetic and parasympathetic fibers and submucosal and myenteric nerve plexuses. Sympathetic innervation is from segments T2 to L2. These form the mesenteric hypogastric nerves. The parasympathetic fibers to the right colon are through the vagus nerve. The left colon parasympathetic fibers are from the second to fourth sacral segments by way of the pelvic nerves.

The integrated functions of the colon, rectum, and internal and external sphincters require both sensory and motor innervation. The sensory pathways for the anal canal and perianal skin go through the somatic nerves to S2, S3, and S4. Proprioceptive spindles are found in the striated muscle of the external sphincter. Autonomic sensory innervation for the rectum passes through the same segments (S2, S3, and S4) but through parasympathetic pathways. The pudendal nerve and coccygeal plexus originating in S2 to S5 form the motor fibers for the external sphincter. The hypogastric nerve provides excitatory motor stimuli of the parasympathetic fibers. The rectal sympathetic fibers are from L2 through L4, and the parasympathetic fibers are from S2 through S4.

The normal functions of the colon include controlling transit of waste, absorption, and limited secretion. Defecation is the mechanism for eliminating metabolic waste and dietary residue. Colonic motor activity includes segmentation (mixing) and peristaltic movement. Segmentation occurs by alternate formation and relaxation of haustral folds. Peristalsis is a forward movement over longer segments of bowel. Colonic activities increase after a meal. There is an increase in ileal activity resulting in a slow filling of the cecum and ascending colon. The fluid contents of the right colon are moved back and forth (segmentation) over the absorptive epithelium. The proximal colon retains the contents longer than the distal colon.

Gradually the sigmoid colon fills, and the stool periodically passes into the rectum. Distention of the rectum causes an urge to defecate. Defecation can be a simple emptying of the rectal area, or it may stimulate mass propulsion and empty the distal half of the colon. Defecation in a continent person includes voluntary relaxation of external sphincters, relaxation of internal sphincters, increase in intraabdominal pressure, tensing of the pelvic floor, and colon contraction.

Most absorption of fluid and electrolytes occurs in the right colon. The mechanism for water absorption is passive flow in response to an osmotic gradient. The osmotic gradient is produced by active absorption of sodium. The colon is sensitive to aldosterone and other mineralocorticoids, and the response of the colon is to increase sodium absorption and potassium secretion. Potassium is secreted into the colon lumen. The mucus secreted by the goblet cells can contain high quantities of potassium. If the luminal potassium concentration goes above 15 mEq/L, a shift occurs and potassium is absorbed. Absorption of chloride ion occurs in conjunction with secretion of sodium bicarbonate by the colon. As chloride is absorbed, bicarbonate is secreted.

The colon has a minimum digestive or synthetic function. Ingested cellulose is not digested and passes into the colon largely unaltered. In constipated people, when feces remain in the lumen for prolonged periods, the colon can digest and absorb the cellulose. The bacteria in the colon can synthesize folic acid, riboflavin, biotin, vitamin K, and nicotinic acid. The importance of this ability is unknown.

Enterohepatic circulation involving the colon has been identified. The urea-ammonia enterohepatic circulation is related to the hydrolysis of circulating blood urea in the colonic epithelial wall by bacterial ureases. This produces ammonia, which is absorbed into the blood. Any remaining ammonium ion that enters the lumen is converted to free ammonium as a result of the alkaline pH of the lumen. Free ammonium readily penetrates the mucosa and returns to the liver.

A wide variety of drugs can be administered by enema or suppository. The rectum has a poor absorptive capacity, so absorption depends on the level at which the preparation is in the colon and retention time in the colon.

The average amount of gas in the gastrointestinal tract is 100 ml. Gas in the gastrointestinal tract is made up of swallowed air, gas diffusing across the mucosa, and gas produced by bacteria. The major components of flatus are oxygen, nitrogen, carbon dioxide, methane, and hydrogen. Hydrogen and methane are produced by bacteria. The bacteria use substrate found within the lumen, related to diet. Carbon dioxide may be formed as a result of neutralization of acid by bicarbonate, or it may be swallowed. Bacterial use of oxygen may result in low concentrations of oxygen. Flatus passes through the colon more rapidly than liquid or semisolid feces because resistance to flatus flow by haustration is less effective.

Most of the intestinal flora present in the colon is anaerobic, with little invasive potential under normal circumstances. The colon is heavily populated with *Escherichia, Bacteroides,* and *Eubacterium* genera. Potential pathogens such as *Staphylococcus aureus* and *Clostridium difficile* are normally present in low numbers.

Liver

The liver is the largest organ in the body, weighing 1.4 to 1.8 kg (3 to 4 pounds). It is a complex organ with many functions, including bile production, protein metabolism, carbohydrate metabolism, fat metabolism, drug metabolism, coagulation, detoxification, and storage of certain minerals and vitamins.

The liver is located under the diaphragm in the upper right portion of the abdominal cavity (FIG. 10-8). The superior surface of the liver is under the right and left halves of the diaphragm. The inferior surface is above (from right to left) the hepatic flexure of the colon, the upper pole of the right kidney, the first portion of the duodenum, the inferior vena cava, and the stomach. The liver normally extends from the fifth intercostal space to just below the right costal margin. The right lobe

FIG. 10-8
Liver, gallbladder, and pancreas.

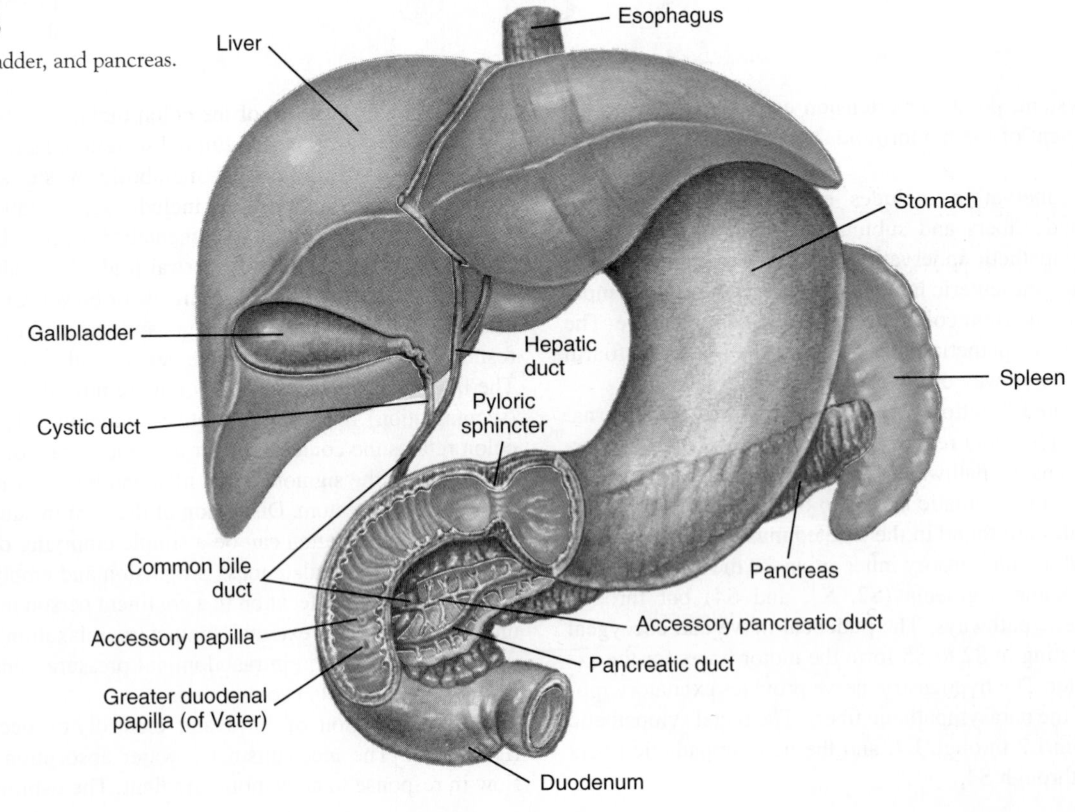

is normally palpable on inspiration 1 to 2 cm below the right costal margin. The left lobe is rarely palpable in the epigastric region of a healthy person.

The liver is divided into two lobes, with the right six times larger than the left in an adult and three times larger in an infant. The falciform ligament separates the lobes. The right lobe is further subdivided into quadrate and caudate lobes. Riedel's lobe is a common accessory lobe on the right that is lateral to the gallbladder. This is a functional and anatomic division of the liver created by the falciform ligament. The division is determined largely by the liver's vascular supply.

The liver has a dual blood supply: the portal vein and the hepatic artery. The portal vein brings nutrients from the gastrointestinal system, and the hepatic artery provides the arterial circulation. The origin of the hepatic artery varies. In approximately 55% of individuals the hepatic artery originates from the celiac artery. The remainder have hepatic arteries arising from the left gastric or splenic artery. Off the hepatic artery is the gastroduodenal artery; then the hepatic artery enters the porta hepatis, divides into the right and left hepatic arteries, and enters the corresponding lobes of the liver. A middle hepatic artery originates from one branch and supplies the quadrate lobe. The possible variations in blood flow play an important role in surgical interventions in the gastrointestinal tract. Blood flow to the liver can be disturbed if the origin of the hepatic artery is not carefully noted. In 25% of individuals the left hepatic artery originates from the left gastric artery and this may be the only left hepatic artery present. Occasionally the right hepatic artery arises from the superior mesenteric artery. Another deviation is for the entire hepatic artery to arise from the superior mesenteric artery. In reading arteriograms, it is helpful to know of possible alternative patterns of blood flow. Arteriography can be useful before abdominal surgery. Also, for effective intraarterial chemotherapy, a knowledge of possible anomalies of the hepatic arteries is necessary. The right, middle, and left hepatic arteries supply different areas and do not anastomose with each other to any significant degree.

Within the liver, branches of the hepatic artery, the portal vein, and bile ducts in the portal tract, described as the portal triad, accompany each other and empty into sinusoids. The portal vein is formed by the superior mesenteric vein at its junction with the splenic vein. The inferior mesenteric vein also empties into this system. The portal vein has several tributaries, of which the left gastric or coronary vein is the most important. The left gastric vein anastomoses with the esophageal veins, which empty into the vena cava.

The branches of the hepatic artery and portal vein are next to each other within the substance of the liver, with the portal vein emptying into the sinusoids. Approximately 1500 ml of blood passes through the liver every minute. Seventy percent of the blood flow is from the portal vein, which is derived primarily from the inferior and superior mesenteric veins, with one third or less coming from the splenic vein. The remaining 30% of the blood flow is from the hepatic artery.

Sinusoidal outflow is into central veins that flow into the hepatic veins. The three hepatic veins (right, middle, and left) enter the inferior vena cava separately. Normal portal pressure is 8 to 10 mm Hg. Arteriolar resistance, pressure in the aorta, and pressure in the inferior vena cava are important determinants of hepatic blood flow. Exercise, standing, or assuming an erect position reduces hepatic blood flow.

In the liver a superficial subcapsular lymphatic network communicates with the gallbladder and a deep lymphatic network that runs in the portal triad with branches of the portal vein, hepatic artery, and bile ducts. The lymphatic drainage is primarily to the nodes at the hilum of the liver and eventually into the thoracic ducts.

The innervation of the liver is sympathetic (paravertebral ganglia, T7 to T10) and parasympathetic (vagus). Although neuronal stimulation affects hepatic blood flow and biliary tree pressures, there are no known direct effects on parenchymal cell function.

The stroma is the connective tissue of the liver. It includes Glisson's capsule, which covers the liver and the connective tissue around the vascular and biliary branches. A reticular framework extends into the lobules and lies between the liver plates and sinusoidal lining cells.

The liver is composed of a complex circulatory system involving the hepatic artery, portal vein, sinusoids, central vein, and hepatic vein. The biliary system includes the bile canaliculi, ductules (or cholangioles), hepatic duct, and common duct.

Several cell types are present in the liver. The parenchymal cell, or hepatocyte, is the most important. The chemical actions that occur in the liver take place in the parenchymal cells. Kupffer's (reticuloendothelial) cells line the sinusoids.

The flow of bile is in the opposite direction of the flow of blood through the liver. The bile canaliculi carry the bile from the central vein area to the portal triads. The bile canaliculi are small, intercellular channels between parenchymal cells. The canaliculi join the bile ductules, which are lined by columnar epithelium. The ductules join together to form the bile ducts, which form part of the portal triad with the hepatic artery and portal vein. The bile ducts go toward the hilum of the liver and join, forming the right and left hepatic ducts. The common hepatic duct joins the cystic duct from the gallbladder to form the common bile duct.

The common bile duct is joined by the pancreatic duct, and the two combined ducts form the ampulla of Vater on the duodenal mucosa. Oddi's sphincter at the opening regulates the one-way flow of bile and pancreatic secretions into the duodenum.

Heme, a source of bile pigments, is an end product of the breakdown of hemoglobin and accounts for about 80% of the bilirubin produced daily in adults. Hemoglobin is broken down into globin, iron, and protoporphyrin heme. The metabolic process for the conversion of protoporphyrin heme to bilirubin is not well understood. The bilirubin is taken up by the parenchymal cells (hepatocytes) by active transport. This is unconjugated bilirubin, a lipid-soluble pigment that cannot be excreted by the liver unless it is conjugated, increasing its water solubility. Within the parenchymal cell the bilirubin is conjugated. The enzyme located on the endoplasmic reticulum, glucuronyl transferase, stimulates this process.

Conjugated bilirubin is not absorbed from the intestine or gallbladder. In the colon, bacteria hydrolyze conjugated bilirubin to urobilinogen. Urobilinogen is found in feces, bile, and urine. It is partially absorbed and reexcreted by the liver and kidneys. Most urobilinogen is found in the feces.

In the kidneys, urobilinogen is secreted by the proximal tubules and partially reabsorbed. The amount of reabsorption is increased in acid urine. Urine urobilinogen is influenced by the amount of hemolysis of red cells: an increase in hemolysis increases urine urobilinogen. In the presence of decreased bowel motility and stagnation of the small bowel contents, small bowel bacterial colonization and hence bacterial activity are increased. This increases the formation of urobilinogen from bilirubin. Absorption in the small bowel is more efficient, and the absorbed urobilinogen is excreted by the kidney, increasing urine urobilinogen. Hepatocellular disease or transhepatic shunting of portal blood increases the amount of urobilinogen in the systemic circulation, increasing excretion by the renal system. In the presence of biliary tract obstruction, less bilirubin enters the intestines, decreasing both fecal and urine urobilinogen.

The formation of bile is a major function of the liver. Hepatic bile contains approximately 97% water, cholesterol, bile salts, phospholipids, mucin, conjugated bilirubin, electrolytes (sodium, potassium, chloride, and bicarbonate), calcium, and many enzymes. The liver secretes approximately 700 ml of bile per day. Although bile is secreted continuously, a meal augments the rate of secretion. The volume of bile produced by the liver is determined by the amount of bile salts synthesized. Conjugated bile salts are secreted by the hepatocytes, and this provides an osmotic pressure for the movement of water into bile. The volume of bile increases as it flows through the biliary tree because of active secretion of an electrolyte solution high in bicarbonate by the biliary epithelium.

Secretion of bile is increased by vagal stimulation and by the action of secretin, cholecystokinin-pancreozymin, vasoactive intestinal peptide, gastrin, and glucagon. Vagal stimulation and cholecystokinin-pancreozymin cause relaxation of Oddi's sphincter. Exogenous agents that increase hepatic bile secretion and contraction of the gallbladder include bile salts, acetylsalicylic acid, pilocarpine, acetylcholine, choline, histamine, and insulin.

Bile is composed of bile acid, phospholipids, cholesterol, and bile pigments. Bile salts are necessary for micellular solubilization of dietary lipids and to maintain biliary cholesterol in solution. They are synthesized in the liver from cholesterol, are conjugated with glycine and taurine, and then form salts with sodium and potassium. Most bile salts are reabsorbed in the terminal ileum by an active transport process. New bile acids account for 10% of the total amount each day, replacing the amount lost in the feces.

The formation of bile is only one function of the liver. Protein, carbohydrate, and lipid metabolism are additional functions. The liver is the source of albumin, which is 50% to 60% of the total plasma protein. For protein synthesis the liver uses dietary amino acids, amino acids formed by endogenous protein catabolism, and amino acids formed during carbohydrate and fat metabolism. Deamination of amino acids in the liver releases nitrogen, which is converted to urea. The liver also converts ammonia formed in other parts of the body to urea. Other functions related to protein metabolism include uric acid formation from nucleoprotein, creatine formation from glycine, and synthesis of methionine and arginine. Other proteins of importance to coagulation include haptoglobin, C-reactive protein, several glycoproteins, transferrin, serum enzymes, and ceruloplasmin.

Albumin has two major functions. First, it helps maintain the plasma colloid osmotic pressure because of its small molecular size and high charge. About one third of the body's albumin (4.5 to 5 g/kg) is intravascular, and the rest is extravascular. Second, albumin plays a role in active transport.

Carbohydrate metabolism involves the liver's ability to store glycogen within the hepatocyte. The liver converts glucose, fructose, and galactose to glycogen. If a diet is low in carbohydrates, or in the presence of prolonged fasting, the liver can convert protein and fat to glycogen. This is referred to as gluconeogenesis. Glucose not stored as glycogen or aminated to amino acids is converted to fatty acids, carbon dioxide, and water.

A normal blood glucose level depends on the liver's ability to remove glucose from the blood, store glucose as glycogen, break glycogen into glucose, and release glucose into the blood. Glycogenolysis (breaking glycogen to glucose) is increased by a decreased blood glucose, exercise, glucagon, and epinephrine. In a fasting state, glucose stores can be significantly depleted in approximately 12 hours. In hepatocellular disease, glycogen stores may be reduced, resulting in hypoglycemia. This may also occur during stress and exercise.

Dietary lipid enters the liver in the form of chylomicrons. Triglycerides are hydrolyzed to glycerol and fatty acids. The liver also takes up fatty acids mobilized from fat depots and synthesizes fatty acids from carbohydrates and amino acids. The fatty acids are used in oxidation for energy production, resynthesis of triglycerides, formation of cholesterol esters, and conversion to phospholipids. Hepatic triglyceride accumulation, or fatty liver, may be the result of an excess of fatty acids, reduced lipid oxidation, or decreased lipoprotein formation.

Cholesterol is synthesized in the liver from acetate. Other sources of cholesterol are the kidneys, adrenal glands, and small bowel mucosa. The liver removes cholesterol from the blood and excretes cholesterol into bile, forming a bile acid. Cholesterol may also combine with fatty acids to form cholesterol esters. Serum cholesterol is kept in solution by phospholipids.

The liver plays a major role in coagulation in that it is the site of production of coagulation factors I, II, VI, VII, VIII, IX, and X. Vitamin K is required for the synthesis of factors II, VII, IX, and X. Natural vitamin K is lipid soluble. There are synthetic forms of vitamin K that are water soluble. Vitamin K is stored in the liver. Oral anticoagulants such as coumarin interfere with the action of vitamin K within the parenchymal cell. The liver also removes active clotting factors from the circulation, contributing to coagulation homeostasis.

Plasminogen (profibrinolysin), the inactive form of plasmin (fibrinolysin), is believed to be synthesized by the liver. Plasmin is a proteolytic enzyme that dissolves fibrin, the plasma protein responsible for the semisolid character of a blood clot. Plasminogen levels may be decreased in hepatocellular disease. Antiplasmin, a proteinase inhibitor found in plasma and serum, is also formed in the liver.

Clotting abnormalities may accompany almost any type of liver disease. The severity of acquired clotting problems associated with hepatic disease depends on the extent of hepatocellular damage. Vitamin K deficiency is uncommon because vitamin K is found in food and is synthesized by colonic bacteria. Vitamin K deficiency may be seen in chronically ill people with limited oral intake who are taking broad-spectrum antibiotics.

Chronic alcohol abusers may be vitamin K depleted because of their diets and liver disease. Also, patients on long-term total parenteral nutrition may develop clotting abnormalities if their diet is not supplemented with vitamin K. Malabsorption of vitamin K may result from problems that cause a decrease in lipid absorption, for example, biliary obstruction. Coagulation problems seen in hepatocellular damage are usually caused by increased use of clotting factors, decreased production of clotting factors, production of abnormal clotting factors, or platelet abnormalities.

The liver also plays a role in detoxification of many materials, particularly drugs. Most drugs undergo significant metabolism during their first pass through the liver, resulting in a significant drop in their systemic availability. Basically, the liver process involves making the substance water soluble for excretion in bile or urine. Enzymes from the smooth endoplasmic reticulum oxidize, reduce, hydrolyze, and conjugate foreign compounds. The enzymes have a low substrate specificity and readily detoxify substances. The processes that determine whether a compound is excreted in the urine or the bile are multiple and not always understood. Substances that are highly polar and those with molecular weights greater than 200 are excreted in the bile. Substances with smaller molecular weights are excreted in the urine.

The effectiveness of lipid-soluble drugs may be altered by their conversion in the liver to a water-soluble state. Some drugs, such as phenylbutazone, become more potent after conversion in the liver to oxyphenbutazone. However, oxidation of barbiturates decreases their effect and may produce a toxic byproduct. Some drugs require metabolic transformation in the liver for production of a therapeutic action. In a patient with liver disease it is important to know the effects of a drug. Certain medications should be avoided, and others should be given in reduced dosages.

Gallbladder

The gallbladder (see FIG. 10-8) is a pear-shaped sac 6 to 8 cm (3 to 4 inches) long and attached to the inferior surface of the liver. It is joined to the biliary tree by the cystic duct at the point where the hepatic duct becomes the common bile duct.

The mucosa of the gallbladder is columnar epithelium overlying a lamina propria. The mucosa is in multiple, irregular folds that increase its absorptive area. The fibromuscular layer forms the framework of the sac. It is a mixture of longitudinal smooth muscle fiber and dense fibrous tissue. The fibromuscular layer is covered by a subserous adventitia. The serous layer is continuous with the serosa of the liver.

The gallbladder is supplied by the superior and inferior cystic artery, which branches off the hepatic artery. The venous system consists of capillary plexuses that drain into superficial veins on the gallbladder surface. These superficial veins empty directly into the liver. The gallbladder also has an extensive lymphatic system that connects with the lymphatic channels draining the liver. This system then combines with the lymphatic vessels of the cystic duct and proximal sections of the extrahepatic ductal system and drains into the nodes at the porta hepatis.

Innervation of the gallbladder and biliary tree is from the sympathetic and parasympathetic systems. Parasympathetic stimulation causes contraction of the gallbladder. Sympathetic stimulation is inhibitory. Preganglionic sympathetic fibers are from the seventh or tenth thoracic segment, and postganglionic fibers are from the celiac ganglia.

The hepatic division of the vagal nerve supplies parasympathetic preganglionic fibers that synapse with postganglionic fibers in the gallbladder wall. Afferent fibers travel with the splanchnic nerves and the right phrenic nerve. Right referred shoulder pain in gallbladder disease is related to this shared course with the right phrenic nerve.

The function of the gallbladder is to concentrate and store bile. The organ stores 30 to 50 ml of bile. In the presence of CCK the gallbladder contracts, forcing bile through the cystic duct into the common bile duct and hence the duodenum (see the discussion of bile under Liver).

Pancreas

The pancreas (see FIG. 10-8) is an important accessory organ of digestion. It is located transversely across the posterior wall of the abdomen. It is about 20 cm (10 inches) long and weighs 60 to 160 g. The pancreas can be divided into the head, the body, and the tail. The common bile duct passes through the head of the pancreas. The terminal portion of the pancreas is the pancreatic tail.

The pancreas resembles the salivary glands histologically. The difference between the two is the presence of islets of Langerhans within the pancreas. The pancreas has both exocrine and endocrine functions. Acinar cells secrete the exocrine products (bicarbonate and pancreatic enzymes) and the endocrine secretions of insulin, glucagon, and gastrin are from the alpha, beta, and delta cells of islets of Langerhans.

The blood supply of the pancreas is from the superior and inferior pancreaticoduodenal arteries and from branches of the splenic artery. The venous flow from the body and tail of the pancreas is through the splenic vein, and the head empties directly into the portal vein. The lymphatic system drains through the pancreaticoduodenal nodes to the celiac nodes.

The innervation of the pancreas is sympathetic and parasympathetic. The sympathetic fibers follow the arterial blood vessels and play a part in regulating blood flow to the pancreas. The parasympathetic fibers terminate at the acinar cells, the islet cells, and the smooth muscle cells and regulate pancreatic secretion.

The pancreas is divided into lobules; each lobule empties into a branch of the main pancreatic duct that joins the common bile duct at the ampulla of Vater before entering the duodenum. Each individual lobule is a group of acini formed from acinar cells and drained by a ductule that forms intralobular ducts that empty into the pancreatic duct. Dark zymogenic granules that are the precursors of pancreatic enzymes form the acinar cells. With the enzymes stored and secreted in an inactive form, and with the presence of inhibitors of proteolytic enzymes in the pancreatic juice, the pancreas protects itself from autodigestion.

The exocrine secretion of the pancreas is approximately 1 to 2 L per day. The secretions are aqueous and clear, rich in bicarbonate, digestive enzymes, and electrolytes. The enzymes formed in the acinar cells are secreted into the ducts. Water and electrolytes are secreted by the ductular epithelium. The major pancreatic exocrine function is digestion and absorption in the small intestines. The bicarbonate, calcium, and magnesium in the pancreatic secretions are necessary for creating an optimum environment for enzyme activity. Interference with the exocrine function may lead to severe malabsorption of the dietary fats, fat-soluble vitamins, protein, and carbohydrates in starch form.

The four major enzyme groups secreted by the pancreas are amylolytic, lipolytic, proteolytic, and nucleolytic. Of these, the proteolytic enzymes (trypsinogen, chymotrypsinogen, procarboxypeptidase, and pro aminopeptidase) account for most enzymes in the juice.

The hormones involved in the regulation of pancreatic exocrine secretions are gastrin, secretin, and CCK. Gastrin is released by the antral mucosa in response to the presence of food in the stomach, distention, a decrease in hydrogen ion concentration, and vagal stimulation. In the duodenum, gastrin release is stimulated by distention and the presence of protein. Cholecystokinin is secreted by the duodenal and proximal jejunal mucosa by the presence of L-amino acids, long-chain fatty acids, and hydrogen ions. The response of the pancreas to gastrin and cholecystokinin is the secretion of enzyme-rich fluid. There is a minimum increase in volume in bicarbonate output, and chloride concentration decreases slightly. Calcium and magnesium secretions parallel enzyme output. Secretin is released from duodenal and proximal jejunal mucosa in response to hydrogen ion. Secretin stimulates large volumes of pancreatic secretions, which are high in bicarbonate, with little increase in enzyme output. The concentration of cations (sodium and potassium) remains relatively constant. Anion concentration varies with the flow rate. As bicarbonate concentration increases, chloride concentration decreases. Secretin does interact with gastrin and cholecystokinin to augment the secretory response.

Vagal stimulation augments the hormonal stimulation of the exocrine secretions. The sight, smell, and taste of food stimulate the vagus. Also, gastric distention stimulates the vagus nerve. Vagal stimulation of the pancreas results in the secretion of pancreatic enzymes with a minimum increase in bicarbonate concentration or volume.

Any disease process that obstructs the duct system or destroys the acinar cells reduces the secretion of enzymes and bicarbonate and progresses to malabsorption and damage of the duodenal mucosa from unneutralized hydrochloric acid. In the presence of pancreatic disease, secretory functions can be decreased by limiting or eliminating food ingestion, minimizing vagal stimulation with anticholinergics, and reducing acids by nasogastric suctioning and use of histamine$_2$ (H_2) blockers or antacids. A pancreas that is not secreting properly may be partially compensated for by an increase in fat and protein in the diet, use of medium-chain triglycerides, or administration of pancreatic enzyme extracts.

The islets are spheric cells that are outgrowths from the walls of the pancreatic duct during embryonic life. The hormones released from the islets directly enter the circulation.

The endocrine functions are the secretion of glucagon (alpha cells), insulin (beta cells), and gastrin (delta cells). Glucagon causes glycogenolysis in the liver. A blood glucose level less than 60 to 80 mg/dl stimulates the alpha cells to release glucagon, causing the breakdown of glycogen to glucose in the liver. A normal blood glucose level "turns off" the alpha cells.

The beta cells of the islets of Langerhans secrete insulin, which increases glucose use. It carries glucose by active transport through the cellular membrane. An increased blood glucose level, usually after a meal, stimulates the beta cells to release insulin. The insulin carries the glucose across the cell membrane, reducing the blood level to normal.

NORMAL FINDINGS*†

Mouth

Temporomandibular joint: Mobility: smooth jaw excursion; 3.5 to 4.5 cm; tenderness: absent on palpation; crepitus: absent; referred pain: absent on closing jaw

Occlusion: Top back teeth rest directly on lower teeth; upper incisors slightly override lowers; ⭘ may change because of missing teeth; marked overclosure may be associated with edentulous patient; individuals who stoop and thrust head forward tend to habitually protrude lower jaw

Lips: Color: pink; symmetry: vertical and lateral symmetry at rest and on movement; moisture: smooth and moist; surface characteristics: slight vertical linear markings: ⭘ decreased saliva production may contribute to drier lips and difficulty swallowing foods; vertical markings increased; "purse-string" appearance associated with edentulism or overclosure of jaws

Inner lips and buccal membrane: Color: pale coral, pink; increased pigmentation, general or localized, in darker-skinned individuals; parotid duct: pinpoint red marking; may be slightly elevated; surface characteristics: where teeth meet, occlusion line may appear on adjacent mucosa; clear saliva over surface ⭘ surface characteristics: mucosa becomes thinner and less vascular; may appear shinier than in younger adults; Fordyce's granules common

Gums: Color: pink, coral; surface characteristics: slightly stippled, clearly defined, tight margin at tooth; patchy brown pigmentation in darker-skinned individuals; hypertrophy may appear during puberty or pregnancy; if inflammation (gingivitis) appears, refer to dentist; ⭘ color: may be slightly paler; surface characteristics: stippling may be decreased

Teeth: Number: 32 (adult); upper and lower third molars may be absent; color: white, yellowish, or grayish hues; form: smooth edges; surface characteristics: smooth; dental restorations; movement: none or slight movement: ⭘ color: may appear more yellowish or slightly darker; form and surface characteristics: teeth may appear elongated as more root surface or neck of tooth is exposed with resorption of supporting bone

Tongue: Symmetry and movement: forward thrust smooth and symmetric; tongue appears symmetric; color: pink; surface characteristics: dorsal and lateral is moist and glistening, with papillae; elongated vallate papillae; fissures: smooth, even tissue; ventral surface: pink and smooth with large veins: ⭘ papillae may appear slightly smoother and shinier; epithelium is thin and loosely attached; veins may be varicosed

Floor of mouth: Frenulum is centered; submaxillary duct opening can be found; color: pale, coral pink

Hard and soft palate: Color: hard palate: pale; soft palate: pink; surface characteristics: hard palate; immovable, irreg-

---

*Modified from Thompson and Wilson.[47]

† ⭘ = Older adult.

ular transverse rugae, midline exostosis (torus palatinus) may be present; soft palate: movable, symmetric elevation, smooth

Mouth odor: Absent or sweet

Oropharynx

Landmarks: Anterior and posterior pillars symmetric; uvula midline; tonsils; color: posterior wall pink; surface characteristics: smooth; tonsils may be cryptic; slight vascularity on posterior wall

Abdomen

Inspection: On inspection the following are normal findings: skin color: may be pale in comparison to body parts that are more exposed; surface characteristics: smooth, soft, silver-white striae; scars: configuration, location, and length; venous network: faint, fine network; umbilicus: centrally located; usually shrunken, but may protrude slightly; should be smooth and noninflamed; contour: flat, rounded, or concave (scaphoid); symmetry: evenly rounded with maximum height of convexity at umbilicus; surface motion: peristalsis usually not visible but may be visible in thin people; movement with respirations: smooth and even; female primarily exhibits costal movements whereas males evidence primarily abdominal movements; contour remains smooth and symmetric when patient takes a deep breath and holds it; rectus abdominis muscles are prominent; on tightening muscle, midline bulge may appear: ◯ contour: geriatric patients may have an increase in fat deposits over abdominal area even though subcutaneous fat over extremities is decreased

Auscultation: Bowel sounds: usually 5 to 34 per minute; irregular; gurgles, clicks, and quality vary greatly; all four quadrants; absence of vascular sounds; absence of friction rub

Percussion

Four abdominal quadrants: Tone: general distribution of tympany depending on amount of air and solid material in bowel, suprapubic dullness over distended bladder

Liver percussion: Lower border: usually at costal margin or slightly below; upper border: begins in fifth to seventh intercostal space; midclavicular liver span: 6 to 2 cm ($2^{1}/_{2}$ to $4^{1}/_{2}$ inches); liver span usually greater in men than women; liver span greater in taller individuals; right midaxillary liver: liver dullness; may be heard in fifth to seventh intercostal space; midsternal liver span: 4 to 8 cm ($1^{1}/_{2}$ to 3 inches); liver descent with deep inspiration: lower border should move inferiorly to 2 to 3 cm ($^{3}/_{4}$ to 1 inch); ◯ lower border: in elderly patient with distended lungs, liver border is 1 to 2 cm ($^{1}/_{2}$ to $^{3}/_{4}$ inch) into abdominal cavity; upper border: with distended lung may descend 1 to 2 cm ($^{1}/_{2}$ to $^{3}/_{4}$ inch); deep inspiration may be difficult for elderly individual

Spleen percussion:* Left posterior midaxillary line: small area of splenic dullness at sixth to tenth rib, or tone may be tympanic (colonic); left intercostal space in anterior axillary line: tympanic; left lower rib cage: gastric "bubble"; tympanic; varies in size

*If an enlarged spleen is suspected, it may be advisable to perform palpation before percussion.

Palpation:

Four abdominal quadrants

Light and moderate palpation: Tenderness: none; muscle tone: abdomen relaxed; muscular resistance may be seen in anxious patients; surface characteristics: smooth, consistent tension opposed to localized area of rigidity (increased tension); masses: none ◯ muscle tone: often more lax

Deep palpation: Tenderness: often present in midline near xiphoid process over cecum, over sigmoid colon; masses: aorta often palpable at epigastrium and pulsates in forward direction; can palpate borders of rectus abdominis muscles; feces may be palpated in ascending or descending colon; sacral promontory may be palpable; umbilicus: check for bulges, nodes, and umbilicus ring; normal findings include umbilicus ring with no irregularities or bulges; umbilicus may be inverted or slightly everted ◯ muscle tone: often more lax

Liver: Liver border and contour: liver often not palpable; liver may "bump" against fingers on inspiration, especially in thin people; liver border surface: smooth; tenderness: none ◯ liver commonly palpated 1 to 2 cm ($^{1}/_{2}$ to $^{3}/_{4}$ inch) below costal margin in patients with distended lungs, emphysema, and lowered diaphragm

Spleen: Spleen not normally palpable

Kidney: Occasionally lower pole of kidney may be palpable in thin individuals; right kidney most often palpable; contour: smooth, firm; tenderness: none

Inguinal nodes: Note presence of nodes: small, mobile; none tender; nodes often present; contour: smooth or nonpalpable; consistency: soft or nonpalpable

Assessment for abdominal fluid: None should be found; techniques for assessment include flank bulging and fluid shift

Rectal-Anal Region

Perianal area: Skin and surface characteristics: smooth, clear; no tenderness in coccygeal area; anus: surface characteristics include increased pigmentation, coarse skin

Rectal examination: Sphincter muscle: tightens evenly around finger with minimal discomfort for patient; anal muscular ring: smooth, even pressure on finger; rectal wall: continuous, smooth surface (examination should cause minimal discomfort for patient); stool: brown, soft

Common Abnormal Findings*†

Mouth

Temporomandibular joint: Mobility: limited excursion; tenderness: present on palpation; crepitus: present ◯ joint may dislocate when mouth opened wide associated with loss of elasticity of joint ligaments

Occlusion: Protrusion of upper incisors; protrusion of lower incisors

Lips: Color: pale, cyanotic, reddened; swelling ◯ dry, flaking, cracked; inflamed fissures at corners

*Modified from Thompson and Wilson.[47]

† ◯ = Older adult.

Inner lips and buccal membrane: Color: pale, cyanotic, reddened, local deposits of brown pigmentation; surface characteristics: ulcers, white patches, swelling, excessively dry mouth, excessive salivation

Gums: Color: reddened, pale; surface characteristics: swelling, bleeding with slight pressure, enlarged crevice between teeth and gums ○ lesions, redness, uneven ridges, spurs, white patches or tenderness of edentulous gums; enlarged crevices between teeth and gums

Teeth: Missing teeth; color: darkened, stained; form: irregular notching; surface characteristics: caries, much tooth neck exposed with receding gums; movement: marked movement (generalized or localized) ○ loose or broken teeth; deterioration of old dental restorations; dentin surface abraded; occlusal surfaces markedly worn

Tongue: Symmetry and movement: unilateral atrophy, lateral movement, fasciculation; color: red; surface characteristics: papillae absent, lesions ○ tongue lies limp on floor of mouth; very smooth tongue associated with vitamin deficiency

Floor of mouth: Color: pallor, redness; frenulum: lesions, lumps

Hard and soft palate: Color: hard palate: reddened; soft palate: pallor, redness; surface characteristics: patches, lesions, petechiae

Mouth odor: Fetid, musty, or acetonic

Oropharynx

Landmarks: Pulled laterally; hypertrophied (adult); color: reddened; surface characteristics: lesions, plaques, increased vascularity, swelling, exudate, grayish membrane

Abdomen

Inspection: Color: jaundice, redness, lesions, bruises, discoloration, cyanosis (localized at umbilicus or generalized); surface characteristics: rashes, lesions, glistening taut appearance, pink, red or purple striae; venous network: prominent venous pattern, engorgement of veins around umbilicus; umbilicus: displaced, visible hernia; contour: distended, concave; symmetry: distention, visible masses or bulges; surface motion: visible, marked pulsation; on deep breathing or tightening muscle: bulges or masses appear

Auscultation: Absence of sound established after listening 5 minutes; high-pitched, tinkling noises; bruits, venous hum, friction rub

Percussion

Tone: Marked dullness in local area

Liver percussion: Upper border lowered; lower border exceeds 2 to 3 cm below costal margin; dullness extending above fifth intercostal space; midclavicular liver span exceeds 12 cm; midsternal liver span exceeds 8 cm; liver does not move with inspiration or movement less than 2 cm

Spleen percussion: Dullness extends above sixth rib or covers large area; tympany changes to dullness on inspiration

Palpation

Light and moderate palpation: Tenderness; involuntary resistance; superficial masses; localized areas of rigidity or increased tension

Deep palpation: Local or generalized tenderness; masses that descend on inspiration, are pulsatile, laterally mobile, or fixed; umbilical ring may be incomplete or soft in center ○ aortic pulsations directed laterally

Liver: Liver border and contour: irregular surface or edge; tenderness

Spleen: Palpated as a firm mass

Inguinal nodes: Enlarged, hard, tender

Rectal-Anal Region

Perianal area: Skin and surface characteristics: lumps, rash, inflammation, scars, pilonidal dimpling, tuft of hair at pilonidal area, tender; anus: inflammation, lesions, scars, skin tags, fissures, lumps, swelling, excoriation, hemorrhoids, mucosal bulging

Rectal examination: Sphincter muscle: hypotonic or hypertonic sphincter, tenderness, nodules, irregularities; stool: presence of blood, pus; black or tarry stool; pale, yellow, light tan, or gray stool

CONDITIONS, DISEASES, AND DISORDERS

ORAL CAVITY DISORDERS

Oral cavity disorders may result in localized inflammation or infection, pain, and difficulty eating. The diagnostic studies, multidisciplinary plan, and nursing care will therefore be related to all oral cavity disorders at the end of this section.

GLOSSITIS

Glossitis is a chronic or acute inflammation of the tongue.

Glossitis is manifested as a reddened, inflamed, smooth, and sore tongue, and it usually has one of several causes:

1. Ulcerations, from stomatitis, lichen planus, or carcinomas of the tongue, can cause glossitis.
2. Anemia (usually iron deficiency or pernicious anemia) is one of the most common causes of glossitis. Other vitamin B group deficiencies can also produce glossitis (vitamin B_6, vitamin B_{12}, folate).
3. Sometimes a patient's tongue appears normal, but the patient complains of soreness. In these cases anemia must be ruled out, but depression and other psychogenic causes or factors have been known to cause a painful tongue.
4. Chemical irritants, drug reactions, amyloidosis, microbial infections (candidiasis), vesiculoerosive diseases, and systemic infections may cause glossitis. Median rhomboid glossitis, believed to stem from erythematous candidiasis on the dorsum of the tongue, is a common oral manifestation of patients infected with human immunodeficiency virus (HIV).[28]
5. Geographic tongue, which may be genetic in origin, is manifest as irregular, smooth, red areas with sharply defined borders that heal and then reappear in a few days. Examination reveals thinning of the epithelium in the middle of the lesion with mild hyperplasia and hyperkeratosis around the edges. Some chronic inflammatory cells can be found in the underlying tissue. Most patients are asympto-

matic, but some complain of soreness and hypersensitivity to certain foods.

A variation in geographic tongue is hairy tongue, in which the filiform papillae become elongated and stained, resembling hair. The papillae can vary in length and color; the cause is unknown, but usually only adults are affected. Some drugs, including antibiotics, corticosteroids, and methyldopa, can also cause these papillae.[43]

Treatment for glossitis consists of correcting the underlying cause, if known. Pain relief (both analgesics and viscous lidocaine), meticulous mouth care, and, if necessary, a bland diet may aid patient comfort.

LEUKOPLAKIA

Leukoplakia is persistent white patches in the oral mucosa that cannot be removed by simply rubbing the surface. The term "leukoplakia" is a clinical description and not a diagnosis of a pathologic condition. Diagnosis must be made by exclusion.

Increased keratin production is known to cause the whitish appearance, but its development can be the result of many factors. A small percentage of nondysplastic leukoplakias (about 5%) undergo malignant change and become squamous cell carcinomas. Biopsies should be done on all leukoplakias to determine the probable cause.[9]

PATHOPHYSIOLOGY

The causes of leukoplakia vary. Friction from cheek biting or prolonged denture wearing can cause lesions that are initially pale and translucent and later become white and thick with a rough surface. Smoking, usually pipe smoking, may cause a lesion that is probably formed from both chemical components of the smoke and irritation from the heat.

An uncommon cause is white spongy nevus, a familial disorder characterized by large, soft thickening of the superficial epithelial layers. The entire inner surface of the mouth can be affected by the thick, white plaque. Although untreatable, this is a benign condition.

Patients who have chronic candidal infections in their mouths have plaque formed from epithelial overgrowth. This is another uncommon cause and is treated with local or systemic antifungal agents.

A type of leukoplakia called hairy leukoplakia (named for its characteristic hairy or corrugated appearance) has a high association with HIV infection. It is not known to be premalignant but is a predictor of poor prognosis.[40] Hairy leukoplakia usually occurs on the side of the tongue and is caused by the Epstein-Barr virus.[43]

Most commonly, leukoplakias are of unknown etiology. In these patients the degree of hyperkeratosis ranges from simple to severe. Treatment of choice may be local excision of the leukoplakia.

Recently laser excision of oral soft tissue lesions with the CO_2 or neodymium:yttrium-aluminum-garnet (Nd:YAG) laser has been used with good results and offers comparative advantages over traditional scalpel excision.[42] However, recurrence is common, so many physicians simply choose to see the patient frequently to observe for any changes in the appearance of the leukoplakia; if changes do occur, they perform periodic biopsies to assess for malignancy.

There are three types of leukoplakia: simplex, verrucous, and erosive, depending on its degree and likelihood of malignant transformation. Leukoplakia simplex, which is the smooth and nonindurated type, rarely results in malignant change, whereas verrucous and erosive leukoplakia more commonly become malignant.

PERIODONTAL DISEASE

The term *periodontal disease* refers to diseases of the supporting tissues of the teeth that are usually inflammatory.

The characteristic feature of chronic periodontitis is the destruction of these supporting tissues; almost every case begins with gingivitis, which, if not treated properly, progresses to irreversible chronic periodontitis and loosening, and loss of teeth.

There is now a clear association between smoking and periodontal diseases, independent of oral hygiene, age, or any other risk factor.[14]

Acute Gingivitis

Acute ulceromembranous gingivitis is usually seen in young adults who have neglected oral hygiene.

Although the exact cause is unclear, plaque bacteria are thought to be implicated in this infection that may also require lowered host resistance. The inflammation starts at the tips of the interdental papillae and progresses quickly to involve the gingival membranes and periodontal tissues. Crater-shaped ulcers with erythematous, edematous edges are characteristic, with a thick yellowish or grayish material over the surface of the ulcer. Bleeding occurs if this material is removed.

The infection remains localized; although the mouth is very sore and the gums bleed, the patient experiences no fever, malaise, or lymphadenopathy.

Acute gingivitis also is seen frequently in patients who are HIV positive, and infection can be progressive and aggressive.

Treatment is with antibiotics for the specific organism and oral hygiene measures to reduce the acute oral infection. The patient and family must be given explicit instructions in the performance of meticulous oral hygiene. Excellent lifelong plaque control will decrease or eliminate gingival inflammation in most patients.[24]

Plaque control may be achieved by mechanical or chemical methods. Mechanical plaque removal may be aided by new manual and electric toothbrushes and interproximal cleaning tools. Chemical supragingival plaque control with safe and effective agents such as chlorhexidine are available.

The antiplaque properties of chlorhexidine are currently unsurpassed by other agents and have much greater and more prolonged effects than other agents[12]; however, it may cause tooth staining and alter taste sensation. Research is ongoing into improved chemical antiplaque agents.

Chronic Gingivitis

Almost everyone has a degree of chronic gingivitis. It is probably caused by the accumulation of plaque around the neck of the tooth, which if not removed adequately by oral care, involves the epithelium and progresses to the periodontal tissues. Gingivitis can develop in 2 days if plaque is allowed to accumulate, and there is a correlation between the amount of plaque and the severity of the gingivitis.

Although the exact relationship between gingivitis and the destruction of the supporting tissues is not clearly understood, it is probable that the bacteria present in the plaque begin an inflammatory response that is assisted by interactions between antibodies, complement, neutrophils, lymphocytes, and macrophages. Immunologic responses have also been implicated.

As plaque begins to collect at the neck of the teeth, inflammatory changes occur in the gingiva. The epithelium becomes hyperplastic, blood vessels dilate, and some extend almost to the surface, causing the gums to appear darker than normal, even purplish, as a result of congestion. These inflammatory cells spread so that the gingiva appears edematous, soft, and slightly glazed. The gums bleed easily, and there is usually a collection of calculus, or calcified plaque, above the gingival margins.

Chronic gingivitis, if it has not progressed further than the gingiva, will subside if meticulous oral hygiene is begun and followed strictly. Part of the treatment must be aimed at teaching the patient and family about oral hygiene and the progression of the disease if these instructions are not followed.

Periodontitis

Acute periodontitis is quite uncommon and usually does not last long. It can be caused by trauma, most often from biting on a hard object, which may produce some minor damage that heals quickly; a periodontal abscess, which is a complication of periodontal disease; or progression from ulceromembranous gingivitis if untreated.

Premature, progressive periodontitis is common in HIV-infected patients and is thought to be caused by an overgrowth of microorganisms.

Chronic periodontitis is very common and is the main reason for loss of teeth in adults. Up to 70% of adults have at least mild periodontitis, whereas less than 15% are affected by severe disease and tooth attachment loss.[24] Untreated infection of the gingiva leads to progressive inflammation and destruction of the supporting structures of the teeth.

The four main features of chronic periodontitis are destruction of periodontal membrane fibers, resorption of alveolar bone, migration of the epithelial attachment along the root toward the apex, and formation of pockets around the teeth.[24]

The pocket formation is characteristic of periodontitis; these pockets form a closed space where bacteria (and possibly anaerobic bacteria) grow. The infected material cannot drain, and these bacteria irritate the tissues.

Clinical symptoms include bleeding from the gums, a bad taste in the mouth, and foul-smelling breath; later there is gum recession and loosening of the teeth. The gingiva appears purplish and swollen, and plaque and calculus are evident.

The best treatment is prevention; regular and thorough toothbrushing and removal of plaque would make any further treatment or surgery unnecessary. However, surgery is necessary when the disease has been neglected, pockets have formed, and the gingiva cannot be restored to normal without surgical intervention.

> **! EMERGENCY ALERT**
>
> **DENTAL AVULSION**
>
> Avulsion of the teeth usually occurs as a result of injury. It may be possible to replant the tooth if medical attention is obtained immediately after the injury.
>
> **INTERVENTIONS**
>
> - Ensure that the patient's airway is patent and is not obstructed with teeth/tooth.
> - Place the tooth/teeth immediately into a normal saline solution.
> - Control bleeding at the site with pressure using a gauze sponge.
> - Obtain dental consultation as soon as possible. Time is important for the successful replantation of the tooth/teeth.

Patients who are considered for surgery must realize that they will have to expend some effort to maintain their teeth during the postoperative period. The rationale for surgery includes debridement and removal of plaque and calculus and restoring soft tissue and bone to its normal contour and state of health.

Several surgical procedures may be carried out, depending on the severity of the periodontal disease. A local anesthetic is used in most cases, and patients rarely require hospitalization. Patient education remains a vital part of the overall treatment because, if a patient is unaware of or fails to comply with meticulous oral hygiene measures, the disease will undoubtedly recur or progress. When the disease has reached the point where surgery would not be useful, the teeth must be extracted and the patient will have to wear dentures.

SALIVARY GLAND DISORDERS

Disorders or inflammation can occur in the parotid, sublingual, or submaxillary glands.

Salivary gland disorders can be classified into several categories: inflammation, as in mumps and acute and chronic sialadenitis; obstruction, as in calculi; and degenerative diseases and neoplasms, which are not discussed here. Dry mouth (xerostomia), which may be caused by damaged salivary glands, is an unpleasant problem and can be the result of local or systemic causes and chronic anxiety states.

PATHOPHYSIOLOGY

Inflammation of the salivary glands is most commonly caused by mumps. Mumps is discussed further in Chapter 15. Of the salivary glands, the parotid gland is most commonly affected by an inflammatory process.

Less common infections are acute ascending parotitis and chronic sialadenitis. Acute parotitis is most frequently seen in postoperative patients who have poor oral hygiene and who are dehydrated. Usually, the patients have prolonged nasogastric intubation and are elderly, debilitated, and malnourished. Infection is caused by ascending bacteria from the oral cavity (staphylococcal or gram-negative) and can lead to abscesses. If not treated, the infection may occlude the trachea, causing acute respiratory failure. Parotitis begins with pain or tenderness in the angle of the jaw.

This disorder can be prevented by proper hydration, good oral hygiene, and care taken during surgery to avoid trauma to the duct orifices. Treatment of acute parotitis includes rehydration, the discontinuation of all medications that may decrease salivary flow, parotid massage, broad-spectrum antibiotic therapy, oral hygiene, and hard candies to suck to stimulate salivary flow. Response to therapy should be observed within 48 to 72 hours after initiating treatment. Despite antibiotic therapy, the mortality rate of acute suppurative parotitis approaches 25%.[38]

Chronic sialadenitis is usually caused by chronic duct obstruction, which may be due to mucus plugs or other causes. It is usually unilateral, and the patient experiences painful swelling of the gland accompanied by an inflamed duct and purulent discharge from the orifice. Treatment is usually conservative, but occasionally removal of the obstruction or excision of the gland is necessary.

Obstructions of the salivary glands are usually caused by calculi, although mucoceles and cysts may also form, and these must be excised. Calculi formation is quite common, and most (80%) of them form in the parotid gland or Stensen's duct; the rest are in the sublingual and minor salivary glands. Although salivary calculi occur at any age, they are uncommon in children. Men are affected twice as often as women. Diagnosis is based on recurrent, painful enlargement of the gland and is confirmed by physical examination, palpation, and imaging techniques.

Calculi are composed mainly of calcium and phosphate and tend to form more frequently in the submandibular gland because its saliva has a high pH and is viscous because of a high mucin content. This gland also may be irritated by the teeth during chewing, and it is larger in diameter and longer than the parotid duct.

Pain and swelling may occur suddenly during eating and subside within a short time. Symptoms may not occur with every meal, and sometimes the patient is asymptomatic until the stone enlarges, moves along the duct, and can be felt in the mouth. Usually no inflammation is present, but occasionally a gland or duct becomes infected, indicated by increased swelling and tenderness over the gland and purulent discharge from the orifice. Pain and fever accompany this infection. Treatment is the same as for acute parotitis.

Xerostomia, or dry mouth, can result from a variety of transient and chronic causes. Fear and acute anxiety are the most common causes of transient dry mouth. Chronic conditions can be caused by mouth breathing; heavy smoking; some drugs such as antihistamines, antidepressants, and sympathomimetics; chronic anxiety states; and treatment with radiation to the head and neck, which causes irreversible damage to the salivary glands. With xerostomia, the lubrication, mastication, and digestion of food may become difficult. This may lead to depression, poor nutrition, and weight loss. The rate of opportunistic infection increases with xerostomia; the most common of these infections is candidiasis.

STOMATITIS

Stomatitis is ulceration in the mouth that may be on the gums or the oral mucosa.

Stomatitis may be a single lesion, as from a local injury, or widespread, caused by systemic factors. Stomatitis is mainly inflammatory, and there are several types: viral, bacterial, noninfective, and drug related. It may result from excessive smoking, spicy foods, poor nutrition, poor oral hygiene, or allergic responses. All types of stomatitis are usually quite painful and therefore may inhibit food ingestion; this can be a major problem in an already debilitated patient.

PATHOPHYSIOLOGY

Herpetic stomatitis is the most common form of viral stomatitis; after an initial infection, usually in infancy or childhood, it begins with vesicle formation. After the rupture of the vesicles and the shedding of the cells, an ulcer is visible. These ulcers are usually scattered over the mucous membranes and are circular and about 3 to 4 mm in diameter. The gingivae are swollen and inflamed, and the local lymph nodes are usually swollen. The patient may have an elevated temperature, increased salivation, and severe mouth pain. These lesions usually clear in 7 to 10 days.

After the primary infection, many people are subject to recurrent infections. These are not usually within the mouth but affect the skin around the lips at the mucocutaneous junctions. These infections, known as herpes labialis, are caused by the herpes simplex virus and are discussed further in Chapter 15.

Angular stomatitis, which is the result of iron deficiency anemia, causes inflammatory changes at the angles of the mouth that vary from reddening to ulcerated, crusting fissures. More common in elderly patients with full dentures, it can cause deep folds at the corners of the mouth, where infection can spread if not treated, making the condition much more extensive. Lack of vitamins such as niacin and riboflavin can cause cellular weakening because cell growth, oxidation, and metabolism are impaired.

Denture stomatitis is caused by occlusion of the mucous membranes by a tight-fitting denture for a long time. This creates a closed environment in which organisms can grow. Although the patient may be asymptomatic, there is normally a reddened, erythematous area corresponding to the area covered by the denture. These patients should leave their dentures out, at least at night, to allow the mucous membranes to heal.

Aphthous stomatitis (canker sores) is one of the more common diseases affecting the mucous membranes. The underlying cause of these small, yellowish, very painful ulcers is unclear, although several factors have been implicated (virus, allergy, gastrointestinal disease, psychosomatic causes). Women are affected slightly more often than men. The disease is most troublesome in adolescence or early adult life and often clears up by early middle age. The first sign of aphthous stomatitis is usually a pricking feeling in the mucous membrane, followed soon after by eruption of painful ulcers that may appear alone or in groups. They resemble craters with red, raised margins, and they usually heal in a week or so without scarring. These lesions do not vesiculate like herpetic lesions.

Thrush, or oral candidiasis, is one of the most common types of stomatitis. This mycotic stomatitis is characterized by white plaques on the oral mucous membrane, gums, and tongue. It is frequently seen in patients who are malnourished, diabetic, immunosuppressed, or taking antibiotics that destroy the normal oral flora.

Although *Candida* is part of the normal mouth flora, some weakening of the body's resistance can permit an increase in its growth (usually *Candida albicans* or *Candida tropicalis*). Fungal spores lodge between the epithelial cells and cause a gradual separation of the layers, spreading the infection to the surface of the mucous membrane and the rest of the mouth. White patchy growths appear in several areas of the mucous membrane and spread, so a continuous membrane forms. Oral candidiasis occurs in over 60% of patients with HIV infection and AIDS.[43]

One of the more distressing types of stomatitis appears as a result of drug treatment. It is frequently seen in patients who have been taking systemic antibiotics for long periods and who have bacterial overgrowth in the mucous membranes or in patients receiving chemotherapy for cancer treatment, and it may be quite debilitating because the patient may already have a lowered resistance to infection. In a severely leukopenic patient, necrotizing ulceration of the mucous membranes, gums, and throat may occur, which can in turn cause septicemia. Usually, these ulcers appear on the mucous membranes in any number and are very painful. They may cause increased salivation and prevent the patient from eating normally.

Diagnostic Studies and Findings

X-ray examination of lateral and oblique views of jaw and upper neck: May demonstrate large stones

X-ray examination using dental film to project through floor of mouth from below: May demonstrate small stones

Sialograpy: May demonstrate partial or complete filling defects in the ductal system with retention of dye on evacuation films; not advisable in acute stage of inflammation

Ultrasonography: May demonstrate suppuration within the gland or presence of sialoliths

Microbiologic studies: Culture and sensitivity of oral ulcerations, plaque bacteria, or purulent matter expressed from periodontal pockets/abscesses

Multidisciplinary Plan

Surgery

Surgical removal of sialoliths if stone cannot be removed by manual manipulation

Laser excision of oral lesions with CO_2 or ND:YAG laser

Medications

Anesthetic agents: Topical anesthetics (viscous lidocaine [Xylocaine]) as needed

Vitamins: Vitamin replacement if condition caused by underlying deficiency

Glucocorticoid ointment: Kenalog in Orabase (aphthous ulcers)

Antiinfective agents

Topical

Nystatin (Mycostatin) oral suspension or lozenges for *Candida* q6h PO

Clotrimazole vaginal tablets for *Candida* q6h PO

Systemic

Oral or intravenous antibiotics as indicated by culture, sensitivity

Narcotic analgesic agents

Acetominophen (Tylenol) with codeine, 30-60 mg PO q4-6h as needed

Meperidine (Demerol), 50-75 mg IM q4-6h as needed for acute pain relief

General Management

Many sialoliths can be removed by manipulation of duct

Mild mouthwashes for comfort

Synthetic saliva for comfort

Meticulous oral hygiene to include plaque removal

Dietary

Well-balanced diet; bland if necessary; high in protein, calories, and needed vitamins

Nutritional consultation if necessary

NURSING CARE

Nursing Assessment

Nutritional status: Anorexia, weight loss; dehydration; history of poor dietary habits: poor oral intake or decrease in oral intake associated with discomfort when eating; debilitated physical appearance; presence of dentures in angular and denture stomatitis; vitamin deficiency; sensitivity to spicy foods

Infection: Fever, malaise; lymphadenopathy with parotitis, primary herpetic stomatitis; recent or recurrent chemotherapeutic or antibiotic regimen; history of HIV or other immunocompromised state

Oral examination: Reddened, inflamed, smooth tongue; dry oral membranes; localized swelling; purulent discharge from orifice of duct: signs of infection in open or excised duct, if stone has been surgically removed; palpation of stone in gland or duct; increased or decreased salivation; halitosis; painful, ulcerated areas on oral mucous membranes that may appear yellowish with reddened, raised areas; white coating on the tongue

Laboratory values: Serum B_{12}, folate levels decreased with anemia; white blood cell (WBC) count normal or slightly elevated in presence of acute inflammation or infection

Potential Complications

Anorexia, dehydration, tooth loss, malignant changes in oral lesions

Patient Problems/Nursing Diagnoses & Interventions

NIC Nutrition Support

Imbalanced nutrition: less than body requirements, related to disruption of oral mucous membrane secondary to infection, ulcerations, or inflammation

Imbalanced nutrition: less than body requirements, related to oral pain when eating

- Ensure adequate hydration.
- Provide mouthwashes, avoiding those with alcohol *because they may be irritating.*
- Assist with and instruct patient about thorough but gentle mouth care.
- Keep lips lubricated *to prevent further drying and further irritation.*
- Offer ice chips *for numbing effect.*
- Provide hard, sour candies for patient to suck *to stimulate salivary flow.*
- Change texture of food to soft or pureed if necessary; avoid extremes of temperature in food.
- Provide dietary consultation to offer a palatable, nourishing diet that is high in protein, calories, and vitamins.
- Instruct patient to avoid spicy foods, alcohol, and citrus juices if they are irritating. A bland diet may be more tolerable.

NIC Physical Comfort Promotion

Acute pain related to inflammation, ulcerations

- Provide analgesics for pain relief as prescribed, especially before meals, and assess and document effectiveness.
- Topical anesthetic agents such as viscous lidocaine (Xylocaine) may help to *relieve minor discomfort.*
- Apply warm, moist packs to affected area *to decrease swelling and discomfort.*
- Advise frequent gargles, mouth irrigation, and synthetic saliva (with xerostomia) *to improve comfort.*

NIC Risk Management

Risk for infection related to presence of plaque bacteria

- Monitor oral temperature bid.
- Administer oral or intravenous antibiotics as ordered *to prevent or treat infection.*
- Administer topical antiinfective agents as ordered. Freezing nystatin may make it more tolerable for the patient.

Patient Education/Continuum of Care Plan

1. Explain to patient the importance of continued meticulous mouth care. Instruct patient in effective plaque removal techniques.
2. Discuss with patient and family the need for maintenance of a proper diet.
3. If stomatitis is herpetic, inform patient of its infective nature and instruct in isolation and hand-washing techniques.
4. Ensure patient's understanding of prescribed medications, including application, dosage, and side effects.
5. Ensure that patient knows ways to prevent or minimize dry mouth.

Evaluation/Patient Outcomes

Nutrition Support: Adequate nutrition maintained. Patient's weight and hydration are maintained at normal levels.

Physical Comfort Promotion: Oral pain is manageable. Patient is able to eat with relative comfort. There is no localized pain. Oral mucous membrane is healing. Absence of halitosis.

Risk Management: Inflammation/infection is resolved. Patient is afebrile. There is no localized swelling. Patient verbalizes understanding of oral hygiene measures to prevent recurrence.

ESOPHAGEAL DISORDERS

Achalasia

Achalasia is a disorder of esophageal motility in which there is degeneration of parasympathetic innervation to the lower esophageal sphincter (LES). It is characterized by failure of the lower esophageal sphincter to relax, by dilation of the esophagus, and by loss of esophageal peristalsis. Most patients with achalasia have progressive dysphagia, first with solid then with liquid foods. Other classic symptoms include chest pain, hiccups, regurgitation, and weight loss.[3]

Achalasia is more common in adults, but it may also be seen in children and infants. The incidence of achalasia is 1 in 100,000 population per year.[15] In a geriatric patient, achalasia may be related to cancer of the lower end of the esophagus. Also, an increased risk (2% to 7%) of esophageal cancer exists for patients with long-standing achalasia that was never treated or was minimally treated.[52]

The cause is unknown.

No therapy can reverse or even halt the degeneration of neurons that occurs in primary achalasia. The treatment is functional and aimed at decreasing resting pressure in the lower esophageal sphincter so that the sphincter does not pose a substantial barrier to the passage of ingested material.[1]

Pathophysiology

There are three pathophysiologic changes in achalasia: elevated resting lower esophageal sphincter pressure, residual pressure after swallowing because of poor relaxation of the lower esophageal sphincter, and loss of peristalsis in the body of the esophagus.

The esophageal sphincter pressure is elevated to approximately 50 mm Hg (twice normal level). This high pressure does not relax with swallowing. In a normal situation the lower esophageal sphincter pressure drops to the level of the stomach pressure. In achalasia the pressure drops but not enough to permit unrestricted passage of food into the stomach.

Motility disturbances in the body of the esophagus mean that the peristalsis is weak and ineffectual in pushing a bolus of food through the closed sphincter. Aperistalsis may be located throughout the length of the esophagus. The esophagus may empty only when the hydrostatic pressure of its contents is great enough to overcome the pressure resistance in the lower esophageal sphincter. Because esophageal emptying depends on gravity in this case, emptying is improved if the person is sitting rather than lying down.

In the early stages the body of the esophagus is dilated symmetrically. In later stages the esophagus dilates considerably, lengthens, and curves. The body of the esophagus may bend and rest on the diaphragm. A dilated esophagus in achalasia may hold 1 to 2 L of fluid.

DIAGNOSTIC STUDIES AND FINDINGS

Barium swallow with fluoroscopy: Absent peristalsis in esophageal body; dilated esophagus; conically narrowed LES ("beaklike" tapering); retained food in the esophagus; identification of esophageal lesions that may pose threat to endoscopy

Manometry: Pressure readings: elevated resting lower esophageal sphincter pressure (50 mm Hg or greater) and residual pressure after swallowing; intraesophageal resting pressure greater than intragastric pressures; absence of primary peristalsis in esophageal body

Endoscopy (to rule out cancer and other conditions that mimic achalasia): Dilation, atony of esophageal body; puckered and closed lower sphincter that does not open during the procedure

MULTIDISCIPLINARY PLAN

NOTE: Therapy chosen depends on availability of local experts in either medical or surgical area.

Forceful pneumatic dilation of esophagus is primary treatment and is done to decrease ability of sphincter to react to stretch

Surgery

May be required when dilation cannot be done or is unsuccessful; surgical treatment is a distal esophagomyotomy (Heller's esophagomyotomy) in which the muscle fibers enclosing the esophagus are divided, allowing mucosa to pouch out through divisions in muscle layers; when this surgery includes the cardiac end of the stomach, it is referred to as a cardiomyotomy; the most common complication after Heller's esophagomyotomy is gastroesophageal reflux; an antireflux operation (loose fundoplication) is frequently performed at the same time as myotomy

Medications

All have a direct relaxant effect on the smooth muscle fibers of LES. Not proven to be of substantial value in changing the clinical symptomatology of patients with achalasia; however, may be used in patients with significant concomitant disease where dilation or surgery is considered too risky

Nitrates: Sublingual isosorbide dinitrate (Isordil), 5 to 10 mg before meals

Oral isosorbide dinitrate (Isordil), 10 mg

Often must be discontinued because of undesirable side effects; patients may become refractory after initial good response[1]

Calcium channel blockers: Verapamil (Isoptin) or nifedipine (Procardia XL capsules PO); dosage varies in clinical studies; give close to mealtimes for optimal effect

Botulinum toxin (BoTox): Injection into the LES is a recent treatment approach. A potent inhibitor of acetylcholine release, BoTox may poison the excitatory neurons responsible for the LES tone, therapeutically decreasing LES pressure. BoTox is very expensive, and though initial response rates are high and morbidity is low, symptom relapse often occurs.[1,3]

General Management

Carcinoma after treatment remains a possibility, and diagnosis may be more difficult because of lack of early symptoms; a tumor in the dilated esophagus may be large before obstructive symptoms develop; pain and dysphagia associated with carcinomas may be assumed to be part of the primary diagnosis of achalasia

Pulmonary problems may still develop after dilation from reflux at night, and patient instruction should include refraining from oral intake 1 to 2 hours before bedtime

Nutritional Consultation

To help patient select and plan diet that is easily swallowed

Gradual symptoms and adaptation techniques of patients include fullness after meals; swallowing water or bicarbonate of soda after a meal; and using a modified Valsalva's maneuver after a meal

NURSING CARE

NURSING ASSESSMENT

Nutritional status: Dysphagia; vomiting; weight loss

Respiratory status: History of hoarseness, night cough, chronic laryngitis, and bronchitis from aspiration of retained food and fluids; chest discomfort and spasms, nocturnal coughing spells; signs of pulmonary problems, especially in the morning after patient awakens

POTENTIAL COMPLICATIONS

Aspiration, weight loss

NURSING DIAGNOSES/PATIENT PROBLEMS & INTERVENTIONS

NIC RESPIRATORY MANAGEMENT

Risk for aspiration related to esophageal regurgitation with food accumulation

- Elevate head of bed while patient sleeps *to avoid regurgitation or aspiration.*
- Instruct patient to eat evening meal in early evening *to allow food time to pass into stomach before going to sleep.*

NIC NUTRITION SUPPORT

Imbalanced nutrition: less than body requirements, related to difficulty swallowing

- Provide diet that avoids alcohol, spicy foods, or foods at temperature extremes *because these items may be irritating to the esophagus.* A soft diet encourages more rapid esophageal emptying.
- Instruct patient to eat slowly, chew food thoroughly, and arch the back while swallowing *to facilitate swallowing.*

- Instruct patient to eat sitting upright and to remain sitting after completion of meal *because emptying of esophagus is improved if patient is sitting.*
- Administer medications as ordered *to relieve discomfort,* thus promoting appetite.

Patient Education/Continuum of Care Plan

1. Explain to patient the importance of not eating for at least 2 hours before bedtime to decrease symptoms and to prevent aspiration.
2. Discuss with patient the need to try using more than one pillow to elevate head and shoulders slightly or to raise head of bed.
3. Instruct patient to prepare liquid foods to maintain nutritional status, if solid foods cause dysphagia.
4. Discuss with patient the signs and symptoms of pneumonia or other pulmonary problems related to aspiration of food.
5. Discuss with patient the relationship between achalasia and a slightly higher incidence of esophageal cancer. If patient's symptoms change, he or she should be encouraged to see a physician.
6. Explain to patient the procedure for care before and after dilation, with explanation of surgical treatment, if necessary.

Evaluation/Patient Outcomes

Respiratory Management: Airway is clear. There is no evidence of aspiration or other pulmonary problem.

Nutrition Support: Nutrition is adequate. Patient maintains stable weight.

Esophageal Diverticulum

An esophageal diverticulum is a hollow outpouching of one or more layers of the esophageal wall.

The symptoms associated with esophageal diverticulum depend on where the diverticulum is located. Esophageal diverticuli occur in three main areas. The most common, Zenker's diverticulum, develops through the space at the junction of the hypopharynx and the esophagus. A Zenker's diverticulum is three times more common in men than in women and usually occurs in patients who are 70 years of age or older. It is rare in children.[49]

A second type of diverticulum, midesophageal diverticulum, occurs at the midpoint of the esophagus and is caused by esophageal dysmotility. The third type, epiphrenic diverticulum, occurs immediately above the lower esophageal sphincter. Midesophageal and epiphrenic diverticula are associated with several manometric abnormalities. They are usually asymptomatic.[49]

Pathophysiology

The only diverticula of clinical consequence are those that retain food or fluid. Most patients present with progressive upper esophageal dysphagia. Zenker's diverticulum is related to a developmental weakness of the muscular coat of the posterior portion of the pharynx. A small hernia of the esophageal wall is pushed out with swallowing and forms a diverticulum. Zenker's diverticulum can enlarge and obstruct the esophagus.

Bronchitis and bronchiectasis can result from nocturnal regurgitation and aspiration associated with both Zenker's and epiphrenic diverticulum.

Diagnostic Studies and Findings

Barium swallow: Herniation of esophageal wall; patient should be rotated during procedure so barium does not miss small diverticula; also shows unusual complication of esophagotracheal fistula

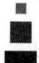

Multidisciplinary Plan

Surgery

Epiphrenic diverticulum: Dilation, myotomy

Zenker's diverticulum: Diverticulectomy with myotomy or diverticulopexy with myotomy; endoscopic treatment with electrocautery, diathermy, CO_2 laser therapy, endoscopic stapling

General Management

Careful assessment of patient so that other esophageal diseases are not overlooked in managing esophageal diverticulum

NURSING CARE

Nursing Assessment

Nutritional status: Regurgitation of undigested food eaten hours earlier; dysphagia, late symptom, indicates obstruction of esophagus; intermittent vomiting; noisy deglutition; bad taste in mouth (sour, metallic); halitosis

Respiratory status: Choking, aspiration with pulmonary symptoms

Potential Complications

Aspiration, pneumonia, dysphagia, weight loss

Nursing Diagnoses/Patient Problems & Interventions

NIC Respiratory Management

Risk for aspiration related to esophageal regurgitation with food accumulation

- Elevate head of bed while patient sleeps *to avoid regurgitation or aspiration;* aspiration at night may lead to chronic pulmonary disease
- Instruct patient to eat evening meal in early evening *to allow food time to pass into stomach before going to sleep.*

NIC Nutrition Support

Imbalanced nutrition: less than body requirements, related to difficulty in eating

- Obtain daily weights, measure intake and output (I&O).

- Instruct patient to eat slowly, chew food thoroughly, and arch the back while swallowing *to facilitate swallowing.*
- Instruct patient to eat sitting upright and to remain sitting after completion of meal *because emptying of esophagus is improved if patient is sitting.*

Patient Education/Continuum of Care Plan

1. Ensure that patient understands relationship between potential pulmonary problems (aspiration) and lying down after eating.
2. Nutritionist will review with patient which foods to avoid, will demonstrate menu planning, and will discuss follow-up procedures.

Evaluation/Patient Outcomes

Respiratory Management: Aspiration is prevented. Patient's breath sounds are heard over all lung fields. No evidence of any other pulmonary problem exists.

Nutrition Support: Nutritional status is adequate. Patient maintains stable weight.

Hiatal Hernia

Hiatal hernia refers to the presence in the chest, above the diaphragm, of part of the stomach that has passed through the normal esophageal hiatus.

Hiatal hernia is very common, occurring in up to 60% of the elderly Western population.[7] A hiatal hernia is clinically significant when it is accompanied by a reflux of acid.

Pathophysiology

Muscle weakness is a primary factor in hiatal hernia development. Loss of muscle tone in middle age or after a long illness weakens the muscles around the diaphragmatic opening, predisposing the person to hiatal hernia. Increased intraabdominal pressure helps to push the upper portion of the stomach through the large opening of the diaphragm.

Intraabdominal pressure may be increased by the effort needed to evacuate firm stools associated with low-residue diets or constipation. Hiatal hernia is uncommon in countries where the diet is high in fiber. Obesity, pregnancy, and ascites are associated with hiatal hernia, as are the use of girdles and tight-fitting belts and clothes. Esophagitis may lead to secondary shortening of the esophagus and spasm, which may pull part of the stomach upward, creating a small hiatal hernia. Esophageal carcinomas may also pull upward on the stomach. This may cause confusion in diagnosing the primary cause. Hiatal hernia is also seen with kyphoscoliosis.

Hiatal hernia may develop after surgical treatment for achalasia. After partial gastrectomy, hiatal hernia may be found because of the straightening and opening of the gastroesophageal junction angle and the elimination of the sphincter.

Paraesophageal and sliding hiatal hernia are two types of hiatal hernia. Paraesophageal hernias involve the herniation of the cardia of the stomach up into the chest, with the gastroesophageal junction remaining below the diaphragm. Acid reflux is not present in this type. Less than 10% of all hiatal hernias are paraesophageal. Complications associated with paraesophageal hernias are incarceration, hemorrhage, obstruction, and strangulation. These disorders are treated operatively.[19]

The sliding hiatal hernia is the most common type of esophageal hernia. In these patients the cardioesophageal junction and a portion of the fundus of the stomach are above the diaphragm. This condition creates a weakened LES, allowing reflux of acid into the esophagus. Patients with reflux symptoms typically respond well to acid suppression, but those with persistent or refractory symptoms may require surgery.[7]

If a portion of the stomach is fixed above the diaphragm, congestion of the gastric mucosa may lead to gastritis and ulcerations in the herniated portion of the stomach. The size of the hiatal hernia does not affect the development of esophagitis or the severity of the symptoms.

Diagnostic Studies and Findings

Esophagography (barium swallow): Outpouching, depending on patient's position when the test is performed

Fiberoptic esophagoscopy with biopsy: Assessment of degree of esophagitis and to rule out carcinoma; retroflexion of scope allows identification of sliding hiatal hernia

Multidisciplinary Plan

Surgery

Conservative medical management usually successful; surgery is indicated in the following situations:

Persistent or recurrent symptoms not responding to medical treatment

Complete mechanical incompetence of the sphincter (less than 6 mm Hg)

Strictures

Strangulation or incarceration (paraesophageal hiatal hernia)

Type of Procedure

Nissen fundoplication: The fundus of the stomach is wrapped around the lower 3 to 4 cm of esophagus, creating an area of higher pressure; procedure may be done laparoscopically

Belsey fundoplication: The fundus is wrapped around 270 degrees of the lower esophagus, and the operation is performed through a left thoracotomy

Medications

Antacids: 1 ounce taken 1 and 3 h after eating and at bedtime

H_2 receptor blockers: Ranitidine (Zantac), 300 mg at dinnertime or bid. If no symptomatic response after 2 weeks, increase dose or begin treatment with proton pump inhibitors.

Proton pump inhibitors

Omeprazole, 20 mg qd

Lansoprazole, 15 mg qd

Gastrointestinal stimulants: Metoclopramide (Reglan), 10 to 20 mg/day; will increase the rate of gastric and esophageal emptying by stimulating the smooth muscles of the intestine; monitor for signs of acute agitation with metoclopramide

Cisapride (Propulsid), 10 to 20 mg qid before meals and at bedtime; improves esophageal peristalsis, increases LES tone, and promotes gastric emptying

General Management

Instruct patient to use 4- to 10-inch bed blocks to raise the head of the bed so that he or she lies on an incline; pillows are not effective

Avoid eating foods that are irritating

Avoid wearing tight belt, corset, or girdle, which increases intraabdominal pressure

Avoid eating 1 to 2 hours before bedtime; avoid lying down after eating

Walk around after eating

Weight reduction

Take medications with an ample amount of water; always take medications in an upright position

NURSING CARE

NURSING ASSESSMENT

Pain

Reflux esophagitis: Symptoms include heartburn or pain; the condition is worsened by lying down or stooping over; pain is relieved by sitting up or by antacids

Epigastric pain

Pattern of discomfort in relation to food ingestion

Nutritional status: History of foods that irritate or worsen symptoms; dysphagia

Gastrointestinal status: Gaseous eructations, water brash (mouth filling with fluid from esophagus), regurgitation; sudden onset of vomiting, pain, and complete dysphagia indicates incarceration of paraesophageal hiatal hernia

Respiratory status: Chronic lung disease after nocturnal regurgitation and aspiration; may include hoarseness, chronic laryngitis, bronchospasm

POTENTIAL COMPLICATIONS

Incarceration, hemorrhage, obstruction, strangulation, aspiration

PATIENT PROBLEMS/NURSING DIAGNOSES & INTERVENTIONS

NIC NUTRITION SUPPORT

Imbalanced nutrition: less than body requirements, related to postprandial pain and dysphagia

- Provide small meals; avoid gastric distention.
- Provide a bland diet, avoiding foods that are irritating. Chocolate is associated with relaxation of esophageal sphincter and is contraindicated.
- Have patient avoid eating 1 to 2 hours before bedtime *to reduce heartburn of reflux esophagitis.*
- Have patient sip a half glass of water after a meal *to cleanse the esophagus.*
- Consult with nutritionist for meal planning, as well as weight reduction for those who are obese.

NIC PHYSICAL COMFORT PROMOTION

Chronic pain related to gastroesophageal reflux

- Provide 4-inch blocks to elevate head of bed (and help patient find out where they can be purchased for home use); *this will maintain patient in an inclined plane, reducing abdominal pressure.*
- Provide antacids at bedside for frequent use during acute phase. Administer antacids to patients with poor memory or who are confused.
- Explain relationship between food and pain patient is experiencing; that is, that pain is related to reflux of gastric contents.
- Administer H_2 blockers and gastrointestinal stimulants as ordered.

PATIENT EDUCATION/CONTINUUM OF CARE PLAN

1. Discuss with patient the relationship between hiatal hernia, reflux esophagitis, and treatment plan.
2. Provide instructions on use of prescribed medications. If patient has other medical problems and is taking other medications, check with pharmacist before choosing antacid to be used.
3. Provide information on use of 4- to 10-inch blocks under head of bed; patient may also need help to prevent sliding out of bed.
4. Other substances that reduce pressure in lower esophageal sphincter and should be avoided include chocolate, peppermint, nicotine, anticholinergics, calcium channel blockers, nitrates, diazepam, beta-adrenergic agonists (Isuprel; Alupent), dietary fat, caffeine, and alcohol.

EVALUATION/PATIENT OUTCOMES

Nutrition Support: Nutrition is maximized. Patient takes in small, frequent, low-fat, high-protein meals, avoiding irritating substances. Patient's weight remains stable.

Physical Comfort Promotion: Pain is minimized. Patient understands medication regimen and importance of raising head of bed; patient reports a decrease in pain associated with eating and sleeping.

ESOPHAGEAL VARICES

Esophageal varices are dilated blood vessels in the esophagus caused by portal hypertension.

Portal hypertension results in the enlargement of collateral blood vessels and the predisposition to ascites. Normally blood flows from the higher pressures of the portal system through the liver sinusoids and then through the hepatic vein to the lower pressure of the vena cava and the systemic venous system. As long as this normal flow is uninterrupted, the potential collateral circulation between the portal and systemic circulations remains closed. Potential collateral circulation exists at the cardioesophageal junction, in the lower rectum, and around the umbilicus. When the normal hemodynamics are disturbed by portal hypertension, the flow of blood that normally goes from the coronary veins into the splenic vein is reversed.[53] This forces open the collaterals between the esophagus and the gastric veins, leading to esophageal varices. Internal hemorrhoids and dilated veins around the umbilicus also occur.

Portal hypertension is the result of blockage or increased resistance to the inflow of blood into the liver or decreased outflow of blood from the portal system into the vena cava. Causes of portal hypertension include congenital obstruction of the portal vein, thrombosis of the splenic vein from acute pancreatitis, liver parenchymal disease, occlusion of the hepatic vein, and cirrhosis.

Thirty percent of patients with compensated liver disease and 60% of those with decompensated liver disease will have varices. Thirty percent of these will go on to bleed. Once varices occur, they tend to progressively increase in size. Risk of bleeding has been shown to be related to the size of the varices and the severity of underlying liver disease.[30]

PATHOPHYSIOLOGY

The veins from the small segment of the abdominal esophagus and the fundus and cardia of the stomach drain into the left coronary vein. These two venous systems are connected by small veins that lie in the esophageal submucosal plexus and normally remain closed. When these veins become dilated, they quickly become tortuous and variceal because of poor support in the esophageal submucosa. In portal hypertension the pressure of the portal system is transmitted through these collateral vessels, which dilate and then produce large esophageal varices. The focus of care is on the management of massive gastrointestinal hemorrhages that occur in these patients. Priorities of treatment include correction of hypovolemia, achievement of hemostasis at the bleeding site, and prevention of pulmonary aspiration. The long-term goal is to prevent recurrent hemorrhage.

DIAGNOSTIC STUDIES AND FINDINGS

Endoscopy: Tortuous protrusions into lower end of esophagus; may show large amount of blood and possibly source of bleeding; excludes other causes of upper gastrointestinal (GI) tract blood loss

MULTIDISCIPLINARY PLAN

Surgery

Surgery is recommended if patient has bled once because 60% to 90% run a risk of further bleeding

Endoscopy with surgical ligation during acute bleeding episode; does not correct underlying pathologic condition

Shunt procedures: High morbidity caused by anatomic variations created from shunting procedure; hepatic encephalopathy common

- Portacaval shunt: Portal vein or one of its tributaries is connected to the inferior vena cava, and portal vein blood flow bypasses diseased liver; complication: hepatic encephalopathy
- Mesocaval shunt: Unites high-pressure superior mesenteric vein of patient with portal hypertension to low-pressure inferior vena cava, directly or with a synthetic graft
- Distal splenorenal shunt: Uses spleen to conduct blood from high pressure of esophageal and gastric varices to low-pressure renal vein; lower incidence of hepatic encephalopathy
- Transjugular intrahepatic portosystemic shunt (TIPS): Catheter-directed percutaneous shunt using stainless steel balloon expandable wire mesh stent to connect portal vein to hepatic vein to decompress portal system; minimizes hepatic encephalopathy; no general anesthesia required
- Liver transplantation for intractable esophageal bleeding

Medications

Focus is on management of the massive gastrointestinal hemorrhages that occur

Vasoconstrictors: Terlipressin or vasopressin (Pitressin) to reduce portal and mesenteric blood flow, given intravenously or during endoscopy or angiography; side effects include abdominal cramps, diarrhea, hyponatremia, peripheral vasoconstriction, hypertension, decreased cardiac output, angina, dysrhythmias, and infarction of bowel

Vasodilators: Nitroglycerin patch, 10 mg replaced after 24 h, concurrent administration with vasoconstrictors may help to minimize their undesirable side effects

Octreotide or somatostatin: Intravenous infusion for 5 days to reduce splanchnic blood flow and hepatic blood flow with little systemic effect

Coagulants: Vitamin K, intramuscularly (IM); fresh frozen plasma; platelets

Propranolol (beta-blocker), 20-80 mg bid; lowers portal pressure; decreases splanchnic blood flow

General Management

Nothing by mouth (NPO)

Sclerotherapy of varices may be done by a transhepatic approach or through an endoscope; involves injecting varices with agents that irritate them, causing thrombosis; complications include perforation of esophagus, aspiration pneumonia, pleural effusions, increased ascites, and ulceration of esophagus; takes several sessions to obliterate esophageal varices; repeated sclerotherapy results in the development of supportive scar tissue around the vessel

Esophageal tamponade to control bleeding

- Minnesota (quadruple lumen) tube: Improvement over Sengstaken-Blakemore tube; additional lumen for esophageal aspiration
- Sengstaken-Blakemore tube (triple lumen): Gastric aspiration with two balloons (esophageal and gastric); need additional nasogastric tube to empty esophagus if patient is not alert

Complications of esophageal tamponade include rupture or erosion of esophagus, occlusion of airway by balloon, and aspiration of secretions

Blood transfusions: Volume replacement: keep Hct about 30% (overtransfusion can contribute to portal hypertension and potentiate variceal rupture)

Removal of ascitic fluid (paracentesis)

NURSING CARE

NURSING ASSESSMENT

Fluid volume

Signs and symptoms of hypovolemic shock: Postural pulse and blood pressure changes; cool, clammy skin; increased respiratory rate; change in mental status; decreased urine output; hemoglobin and hematocrit levels decreased over 24 hours

Blood transfusion reaction

Gastrointestinal status: Complications associated with esophageal tamponade: rupture or erosion of esophagus; occlusion of airway by balloon; aspiration of secretions; massive hematemesis; melena; amount of blood loss; history of liver disease

Mental status: See Nursing Assessment under Hepatic Coma on p. 718

POTENTIAL COMPLICATIONS

Esophageal rupture, hypovolemic shock, hepatic coma

PATIENT PROBLEMS/NURSING DIAGNOSES & INTERVENTIONS

NIC TISSUE PERFUSION MANAGEMENT

Ineffective cerebral, cardiopulmonary, gastrointestinal, and peripheral tissue perfusion related to variceal hemorrhage

- Start intravenous (IV) line with large-bore catheter and administer IV fluids as ordered by physicians *to begin fluid replacements and to facilitate possible blood transfusions.*
- Assist with insertion of Swan-Ganz or central venous pressure (CVP) catheter and perform ongoing hemodynamic monitoring.
- Perform gastric lavage with room temperature saline or water as ordered by physician. If patient vomiting or at high risk for aspiration, notify physician. Endotracheal intubation may offer best airway protection from aspiration of blood or gastric contents.
- Assist with esophageal tamponade *to control bleeding* if ordered, and monitor patient closely after insertion of the tube.
- Monitor esophageal balloon pressure: prevent pressure from exceeding 45 mm Hg. Limit inflation time to 24 to 36 hours.
- If patient has diarrhea, assist with gentle cleansing and application of moisture barrier ointment to soothe and protect perianal skin.

NIC RISK MANAGEMENT

Acute confusion related to biochemical abnormalities associated with shunting of portal blood into systemic circulation

- If confusion or disorientation occurs, frequently reorient patient to time, date, and place.
- If patient is disoriented or combative, ensure patient's safety by placing side rails up or restraining patient if necessary.
- Stay with patient or enlist assistance from family members *to keep patient from harming himself or herself.*
- Continue to administer lactulose or neomycin as ordered by physician. These agents help eliminate blood from patient's gut; if untreated, hepatic encephalopathy could occur from by-products of protein metabolism produced by bacterial action in gut.
- Provide usual care necessary for comatose patient if hepatic coma should occur.

PATIENT EDUCATION/CONTINUUM OF CARE PLAN

1. Prepare patient for all diagnostic procedures, treatments, or surgery so patient will understand what will happen and what to expect.
2. Review with patient the effects of high-protein diets and alcohol consumption in preventing future complications. Include nutritionist.
3. Discuss with patient the relationship of esophageal varices to primary diagnosis that resulted in portal hypertension.
4. Instruct patient to avoid alcohol, salicylates, and other medications that may irritate gastric or esophageal mucosa.
5. Instruct patient to avoid activities that increase intraabdominal pressure, including heavy lifting, straining to stool, vomiting, and ingestion of large meals.
6. Instruct patient in early detection of bleeding, including weakness, dizziness, dark stool, "coffee ground" emesis.
7. Assist patient with location of community resources that offer rehabilitation from alcohol abuse, if applicable.

EVALUATION SUPPORT/PATIENT OUTCOMES

Tissue Perfusion Management: There is no gastrointestinal bleeding. Hematocrit and hemoglobin are normal for patient. Vomiting and diarrhea are not present. Vital signs are stable. Skin turgor is normal for patient.

Risk Management: Mental status is normal for patient. Patient is alert and oriented to time, date, and place.

STOMACH DISORDERS

GASTRITIS

Gastritis is inflammation of the mucosa of the stomach.

Gastritis has been classified in several different ways, including acute or chronic and erosive or nonerosive. For the purposes of this chapter gastritis will be discussed as two separate but related entities: acute and chronic gastritis. The similarities are histologic; the clinical manifestations and morbidity are discussed separately.

Infections of *Helicobacter pylori* are responsible for most cases of chronic gastritis.[7] Multiple other factors also contribute to the development of or are directly responsible for clinical gastritis; definitive diagnosis must be verified by endoscopic gastric biopsy.[7]

Acute gastritis is predominantly an erosive process. It is responsible for 10% to 30% of upper gastrointestinal bleeding.[52]

Acute damage to the gastric mucosa may be caused by a wide range of substances, including alcohol, cortisone, aspirin, nonsteroidal antiinflammatory drugs (NSAIDs), and shock associated with trauma, surgery, sepsis, burns, or hypothermia.[7]

Chronic gastritis, also classified as erosive and nonerosive, implies a duration of at least 6 months. Chronic erosive gastritis is rare, and the symptoms, if present, are anorexia, nausea, and a vague upper abdominal discomfort.

The more common, chronic nonerosive gastritis increases in frequency with age and is seen more often in women than in men. The incidence increases given chronic alcoholism and postgastrectomy. By 50 or 60 years of age, 50% or more of the population can be shown to have *H. pylori* gastritis.[54] Other possible causes include gastric stasis, duodenal regurgitation, repeated mucosal injury, immunologic factors, endocrine disturbances, radiation treatment, ulcerative colitis, genetics, diet, environment, and debility.[16] Gastric ulcer, gastric cancer, and pernicious anemia are associated.

PATHOPHYSIOLOGY

Acute gastritis is a brief inflammatory process affecting the stomach mucosa. It involves erosion of the mucosa. The mucosa is spotted with submucosal hemorrhages that resemble ecchymoses and may be round or linear. There may also be shallow erosions that appear as brown spots or red petechiae or small breaks in the mucosa. The hemorrhagic erosions usually involve only the glandular layer, are extremely shallow, and are found anywhere in the stomach. Acute gastritis is more common in gastric ulcer than in duodenal ulcer. The difference between gastritis erosion and gastric ulcer is that in erosion the muscularis mucosae is uninvolved and healing leaves no scar.

Erosion and hemorrhage are caused by a back-diffusion of hydrogen ions and mucosal ischemia. The disruption of the gastric mucosal barrier allows the back-diffusion of the hydrogen ion, which stimulates the release of vasoactive substances, increased capillary permeability, and inflammation (FIG. 10-9).

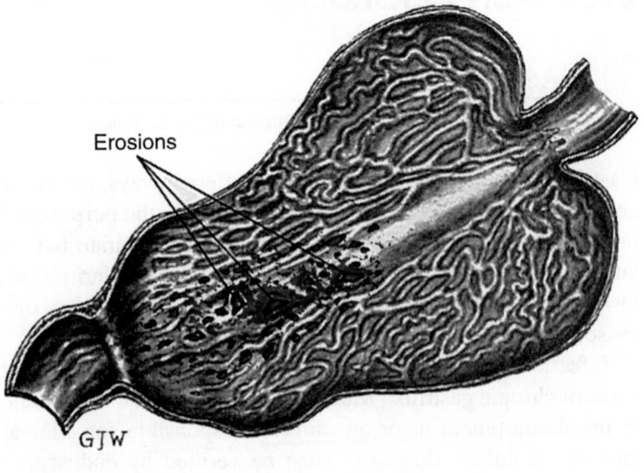

FIG. 10-9

Erosive gastritis (disruption of "tight cellular junctions" with back-diffusion of H^+). (From Doughty.[10])

Steroids appear to potentiate the action of other factors in acute gastritis. Nonsteroidal antiinflammatory agents probably affect gastric mucosa because they work by inhibiting prostaglandin synthesis. Prostaglandins have a cytoprotective function on the gastric mucosa. Apparently, patients taking both nonsteroidal antiinflammatory agents and aspirin are at a greater risk for bleeding from acute erosive gastritis. In these cases, the patient must be observed, medications adjusted, and the patient treated for erosion as indicated.

If the irritating agent or stimulus is removed, a spontaneous remission often results.

Chronic gastritis is often referred to as a nonerosive, nonspecific gastritis that is further differentiated by the histologic appearance of the gastric mucosa into superficial gastritis, atrophic gastritis, or gastric atrophy.

Superficial gastritis is characterized by an inflammatory infiltration of the lamina propria. Lymphocytes, plasma cells, and eosinophils are found in the outer one third of the mucosa. The gastric cells are not involved.

Atrophic gastritis shows a loss of fundic glands, parietal cells, and chief cells. The muscularis mucosae is split and thickened, and marked inflammation is present.

Gastric atrophy refers to marked or total gland loss with minimum inflammation. The mucosa is thinned.

Two additional features, intestinal metaplasia and pseudopyloric metaplasia, may be seen in the three types of chronic gastritis. Intestinal metaplasia is the replacement of normal gastric cells by cells identical to those of the normal small intestine. Intestinal metaplasia is greater in more severe degrees of gastric atrophy. The surface of the normal stomach is columnar, whereas the small intestine has a prominent brush border and may contain goblet and Paneth's cells. When intestinal metaplasia occurs, the stomach acquires the appearance and absorptive capacity of the small intestine. Cancer is much more likely to develop in intestinalized gastric mucosa in comparison with the rare instances of carcinoma of the intestinal epithelium in the small intestine.

In pseudopyloric metaplasia the normal fundic glands are replaced by clear-staining mucous glands that cannot be distinguished from mucous glands in the antral gland or cardial gland mucosa. The replacement may be partial or total. Diagnosis of pseudopyloric metaplasia is made by biopsy. It is imperative that the location of the biopsy be carefully stated on pathology slips so that the pathologist does not mistake normal antral gland mucosa for pseudopyloric metaplasia or vice versa.

Chronic gastritis has also been divided into type A and type B. Type A gastritis involves the fundus. There are circulating parietal cell antibodies and high serum gastrin levels. The destruction of parietal cells by the inflammatory process results in a marked reduction in acid secretion and impaired intrinsic factor production or binding. There is decreased binding of intrinsic factor with dietary vitamin B_{12} in the stomach, impairing vitamin B_{12} absorption and eventually resulting in pernicious anemia. Pernicious anemia is generally associated with type A gastritis.[7] The relationship of the parietal cell antibodies and intrinsic factor lends support for the hypothesis that type A gastritis has an autoimmune background.

Type B gastritis involves the fundus and the antrum. Type B gastritis increases with age and is probably caused by *H. pylori* infection. This infection can be eradicated with several therapy regimens. Type B has less reduction of acid secretions, normal gastrin levels, and only rare impairment of vitamin B_{12} absorption. As the mucosa of the stomach changes with atrophy, the acid secretion is reduced, resulting in achlorhydria or hypochlorhydria.

Atrophic gastritis and gastric atrophy are associated with an increase in gastric malignancies. There is a high rate of cell death and increased cell turnover in atrophic gastritis. Mucosal nuclear activity is increased during the premalignant state. The highest mitotic rates are found in areas of intestinal metaplasia.

Diagnostic Studies and Findings

Acute Gastritis

Endoscopy: Erosions, superficial ulcerations, and diffuse oozing of blood when procedure is done during acute phase; best performed within 24 hours of admission or lesions will begin to heal

Angiographic visualization: If bleeding has not stopped, used to detect and treat lesions with infusion of vasopressin

Double-contrast barium study: Superficial gastric erosions; cannot be used to detect bleeding lesions

Enzyme-linked immunosorbent assays (ELISAs): For detection of serum antibodies to *H. pylori*

Urea breath test: For detection of enzyme produced by *H. pylori,* patient drinks carbon-labeled urea solution; in an infected patient, labeled carbon dioxide can be detected in expired air; fasting usually required; 30-minute delay between preurea and posturea breath sampling[46]

Chronic Gastritis

Serum gastrin: Elevated in type A

Serum parietal cell antibodies: Presence in type A, high association with pernicious anemia

Intrinsic factor antibodies: Presence in type A

Antibodies to gastrin-producing cells: Presence in type B

Gastric secretory testing (pentagastrin): Requires intubation; superficial gastritis: normal or slightly decreased acid secretion; atrophic gastritis: hypochlorhydric; gastric atrophy: achlorhydric

Serum pepsinogen I levels: Elevated in superficial gastritis; low level in atrophic gastritis reflects absence of chief cells

Schilling test: Assessment of vitamin B_{12} absorption by measuring urinary excretion of an oral dose of radiolabeled vitamin B_{12}

Barium swallow with double contrast: Appearance of a "bald fundus" and thinning of gastric rugae

Endoscopy with biopsy and cytology: Biopsy necessary to obtain a definitive diagnosis; cytologic examination of multiple biopsy sites through the stomach is used to rule out gastric carcinomas

ELISAs: For detection of serum antibodies to *H. pylori*

Urea breath test: For detection of enzyme produced by *H. pylori,* patient drinks carbon-labeled urea solution; in an infected patient, labeled carbon dioxide can be detected in expired air; fasting usually required; 30-minute delay between preurea and posturea breath sampling[46]

Multidisciplinary Plan

Acute Gastritis

Surgery

Partial gastrectomy, pyloroplasty, or vagotomy (truncal, selective, or highly selective) may be indicated for managing patients with major bleeding from erosive gastritis

Medications

Histamine receptor antagonists
- Ranitidine (Zantac), 100 mg PO qid
- Cimetidine (Tagamet), 300 mg PO qid

Antacids
- Antacids recommended to help maintain alkaline pH
- Antacids (30 ml q2h) have been shown to be 80% to 90% effective in keeping pH above 4.0

Fluid volume replacement
- Intravenous fluid replacement during a bleeding episode to maintain volume
- Blood replacement may be required when gastrointestinal hemorrhage is associated with acute gastritis

Pituitary hormone
- Vasopressin (Pitressin) per angiography or IV, 20 U in 100 ml 5% dextrose in water (D_5W) over 10 min; may be used in severe cases and may be repeated q3-4h if bleeding recurs; may lose efficacy after repeated doses

General Management

Room temperature water or saline lavage used in patient with gastrointestinal bleeding

Laser therapy with direct coagulation of bleeding spots through an endoscopic approach may be used

Removal of causative agents (alcohol, aspirin, nonsteroidal antiinflammatory agents)

Withholding of food and fluids until vomiting and inflammation subside; then bland diet of medium temperature in acute gastritis without bleeding will assist healing process

Nutritional Consultation

To help patients identify foods that exacerbate symptoms and select diet that minimizes symptoms

Chronic Gastritis

Symptomatic treatment only

Medications

Antacids to reduce or alleviate symptoms

Vitamins
- Vitamin C (ascorbic acid) to facilitate iron absorption in the patient with achlorhydria
- Vitamin B_{12} injections (cyanocobalamin), 1 mg/ml (1000 μg) if pernicious anemia diagnosed

Multiple **antibacterial regimens** identified/investigated to eradicate *H. pylori;* none achieve cure rate greater than 85%; these include:*

---

*Not all medication protocols are Food and Drug Administration (FDA)–approved for gastritis/peptic ulcer disease.

Combination proton pump inhibitor or ranitidine bismuth citrate with two antibiotics, including clarithromycin, amoxycillin, and metronidazole or tinidazole

Combination of a proton pump inhibitor or H_2 receptor antagonist with bismuth subcitrate or tripotassium dicitrato bismuthate, metronidazole, and tetracycline.[29]

General Management

Endoscopy with any change in symptoms to assess formation of gastric polyps and gastric carcinomas in patients diagnosed with atrophic gastritis and gastric atrophy

Routine Schilling tests or serum vitamin B_{12} levels to evaluate intrinsic factor deficiency

Nutritional Consultation

To help patients identify foods that exacerbate symptoms and select diet that minimizes symptoms

NURSING CARE

NURSING ASSESSMENT

Acute Gastritis

General status: Malaise; hypovolemic shock

Pain

Asymptomatic; or vague complaints of postprandial distress after a large meal; or vague dyspepsia, particularly relieved by food

Epigastric discomfort or fullness, cramping

Pattern of discomfort in relation to food or drug ingestion

History of ethyl alcohol (ETOH) or aspirin (ASA) intake

Gastrointestinal status: Early signs of gastrointestinal bleeding; nausea, vomiting, eructation; hematemesis, melena; hemorrhage

Abdominal examination: Abdominal tenderness

Nutritional status: Anorexia, early satiety; weight loss

Chronic Gastritis

General status: Often asymptomatic

Gastrointestinal status: Dyspepsia, epigastric fullness after eating, diarrhea, flatulence, steatorrhea, bleeding

Pain: No relief with antacids

Nutritional status: Intolerance of fatty or spicy foods; anorexia, weight loss

Oral examination: Cheilosis, glossitis, stomatitis (associated with pernicious anemia)

Extremities: Numbness and tingling

POTENTIAL COMPLICATIONS

Hypovolemic shock, hemorrhage, weight loss

PATIENT PROBLEMS/NURSING DIAGNOSES & INTERVENTIONS

NIC TISSUE PERFUSION MANAGEMENT

Deficient fluid volume related to active upper gastrointestinal bleeding

- Permit nothing by mouth; keep patient quiet if hemorrhage is considered a possibility.
- Maintain intravenous fluids and blood as ordered and observe for transfusion reactions.
- Prepare patient for endoscopy as a diagnostic or treatment procedure.

NIC NUTRITION SUPPORT

Imbalanced nutrition: less than body requirements, related to postprandial distress

- Identify foods or fluids that irritate or exacerbate, and avoid these.
- Monitor intake and output.
- Record nausea and vomiting.
- Administer antiemetics as ordered.
- Provide frequent small feedings (approximately six per day) a day if acute gastritis *to relieve postprandial distress associated with large meals.*

PATIENT EDUCATION/CONTINUUM OF CARE PLAN

Acute gastritis

1. Assist patient in identifying agents that irritate the gastric mucosa, including aspirin, aspirin-containing compounds, over-the-counter agents, alcohol, and prescription drugs, such as indomethacin, phenylbutazone, reserpine, nicotine, ibuprofen, sulindac, and naproxen.
2. Discuss with patient the alternatives to irritating substances.
3. Provide patient with information related to cause-and-effect relationship of above agents and gastritis.
4. Discuss patient's diet, as well as amounts of food eaten, and use of antacids with patient, to demonstrate their relationship to pain management.

Chronic gastritis

Following regimen for eradication of *H. pylori,* discuss with patient the importance of medical follow-up if he or she notes a change in his or her symptoms.

EVALUATION SUPPORT/PATIENT OUTCOMES

Tissue Perfusion Management: Volume status is within normal limits. Bleeding has stopped (hematemesis and melena are absent). Blood pressure and pulse are within normal limits for patient. Patient is taking oral fluids.

Nutrition Support: Nutrition is adequate. Patient has an appetite, and weight is stable. Serum vitamin B_{12} level is within normal limits. Schilling test is normal (8% to 40% of original oral dose of radioactive vitamin B_{12} appears in a 24-hour urine specimen).

GASTRIC ULCERS

A gastric ulcer is a well-defined break in the gastric mucosa that penetrates the muscularis mucosae.

A gastric ulcer (FIG. 10-10) must be differentiated from a duodenal ulcer and from gastric erosion. Often gastric ulcers are included with duodenal ulcers and discussed under the classification of peptic ulcer disease. However, the incidence and pathophysiology of gastric and duodenal ulcers are not the same. *H. pylori* is the etiologic factor in most patients with gastric and duodenal ulcers, with NSAID use the other major

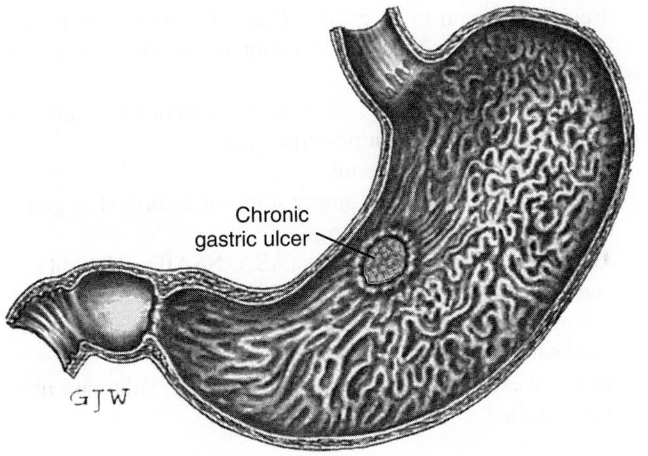

FIG. 10-10
Gastric peptic ulcer. (From Doughty.[10])

cause. Other associated risks (smoking, alcohol use, and socioeconomic status) are negligible when compared to the primary causes.[7] About 5% of patients with symptomatic or asymptomatic *H. pylori* develop gastric ulcers. Patients with *H. pylori* infection are three times more likely to develop gastric ulcers than are noninfected persons.[7]

NSAIDs are believed to increase the rate of ulcer complications by fourfold in the elderly. Among chronic NSAID users, the prevalence of ulcer is 15% to 30% and correlates with the dose and potency of the drug.[7] Because of the widespread therapeutic use of NSAIDs, major research investigations are currently focused on the development of new NSAIDs that are devoid of or have reduced gastroduodenal toxicity. The most promising of these are nitric oxide–releasing NSAIDs.[20] Research has also concentrated on coprescribed cytoprotective drugs such as misoprostol (Cytotec) and omeprazole (Prilosec).

Fewer than 5% of gastric ulcers are deemed idiopathic today, although this number may be higher in the elderly.[7]

PATHOPHYSIOLOGY

Gastric ulcers are generally found at the junction of the fundus with the pyloric mucosa. Ulcers in the antrum are usually smaller than those in the proximal part of the stomach. Gastritis is more common in patients with gastric ulcers and is often seen around the ulceration. The relationship of gastritis and gastric ulcer can be stated as follows: it appears that a gastric ulcer is more than a localized lesion and that gastritis contributes to the hyposecretion of gastric acid and to the susceptibility of the mucosa to ulcerate.

Patients with gastric ulcers have normal to below normal gastric acid secretion. If gastritis is also present, this will contribute to the hyposecretion of acid. An exception to the decreased acid production occurs when the gastric ulcer is close to the pylorus or is associated with a duodenal ulcer, in which case hypersecretion of acid occurs.

Gastric ulcer develops when aggressive factors overwhelm protective mechanisms, such as occurs with an overabundance of acid or pepsin (rare) or with a loss of normal defenses (common). *H. pylori* and NSAID use both reduce protective factors.[7]

The mechanism by which *H. pylori* infection produces gastric ulcers is under investigation. A possible mechanism is that the bacteria's spiral shape and flagella allow it to penetrate the mucous layer, where it delivers soluble phospholipases and proteases that may harm the mucosal layer and underlying cells. Ammonia generated by *H. pylori* urease damages the gastric mucosa. *H. pylori* also releases chemotactic proteins, which begins an inflammatory response that may further contribute to mucosal injury.[7]

Agents that are barrier breakers (e.g., aspirin, alcohol, and NSAIDs) disrupt the intercellular barriers regulating paracellular transport, and acid flows back into the mucosa. Detergents, such as bile salts, and toxic agents can destroy the lipid plasma membrane. When the mucosal barrier is damaged, acid diffuses back from the stomach into the mucosa. Histamine is released, stimulating more acid production, vasodilation, and increased capillary permeability. Bleeding may develop. Protein loss may occur, and an increased sodium content may be found in the stomach.

Bile is generally prevented from contact with the gastric mucosa by a competent pyloric sphincter. In gastric ulcer disease the pyloric sphincter does not respond normally to secretin or cholecystokinin; thus bile is allowed to reflux into the stomach.

The four layers of a peptic ulcer include the superficial layer, which lines the ulcer with a white fibrinous coat composed of leukocytes and erythrocytes; a second layer of fibrinoid necrosis; a third layer of inflammatory granulation tissue containing blood vessels; and the fourth layer, a dense scar of fibrous tissue lacking elastic tissue. The dense scar forms the base of the ulcer and extends beyond the margins of the mucosal defect. In a rapidly developing ulceration, massive bleeding may develop in asymptomatic patients when the vessel wall erodes. When the ulceration develops at a slower rate, inflammatory responses, thrombosis, and endarteritis occur and inhibit massive bleeding, and the patient experiences symptoms of peptic ulcer disease.

DIAGNOSTIC STUDIES AND FINDINGS

Endoscopy and biopsy: Primary diagnostic tool; allows differentiation between benign and malignant lesions; endoscopy combined with optimal biopsy and brush cytology is 96% to 99% accurate in detecting malignancy; need for serial examinations is assessed on an individual basis[7]

Double-contrast barium study (upper GI): Detection of a gastric ulcer; when present, radiologist must determine whether lesion is a gastric ulcer or a gastric carcinoma

Gastric cytologic findings: Abnormal findings would indicate gastric carcinoma

ELISAs: For detection of serum antibodies to *H. pylori*

Urea breath test: For detection of enzyme produced by *H. pylori,* patient drinks carbon-labeled urea solution; in an infected patient, labeled carbon dioxide can be detected in expired air; fasting usually required; 30-minute delay between preurea and posturea breath sampling[46]

MULTIDISCIPLINARY PLAN

Surgery

Medical management usually successful; surgery is indicated in the following situations: recurrent gastric ulcer, persistent bleeding or hemorrhage, perforation, penetration, obstruction, intractability

Types of procedures: Partial gastrectomy; parietal cell vagotomy and excision of ulcer; vagotomy and pyloroplasty; parietal cell vagotomy

Medications

Histamine receptor antagonists

- Cimetidine (Tagamet), 300 mg PO qid, 400 mg PO bid, 800 mg PO at bedtime
- Ranitidine (Zantac), 150 mg PO bid, 300 mg PO after dinner
- Famotidine (Pepcid), 40 mg PO after dinner
- Nizatidine (Axid), 300 mg PO qd, 150 PO bid

Proton pump inhibitor: Omeprazole (Prilosec), 20-40 mg/day

Multiple **antibacterial regimens** identified/investigated to eradicate *H. pylori:* none achieve cure rate greater than 85%; these include*:

- Combination of a proton pump inhibitor or ranitidine bismuth citrate with two antibiotics, including clarithromycin, amoxycillin, and metronidazole or tinidazole
- Combination of a proton pump inhibitor or H_2 receptor antagonist with bismuth subcitrate or tripotassium dicitrato bismuthate, metronidazole, and tetracycline[29]

Buffers: Antacids, 500-1000 mmol/day, 1 and 3 h after eating and at bedtime

Cytoprotective: Sucralfate, 1 g qid on an empty stomach

General Management

Esophagogastroduodenoscopy (EGD) to manage bleeding

Room temperature water or saline lavage if massive hemorrhage

Arteriography with intraarterial vasopressin if intractable bleeding

Avoid spicy foods, coffee (both decaffeinated and caffeinated), tea, 80 proof alcohol, smoking, known ulcerogenic substances (ASA, steroids, NSAIDs); discontinue NSAIDs if possible

Rest

Nutritional Consultation

To help patient identify foods that irritate gastric mucosa and develop dietary plan that minimizes symptoms

NURSING CARE

NURSING ASSESSMENT

General status: Fatigue

Pain: No symptoms to vague symptoms and atypical symptoms

- Heartburn, dyspepsia
- Relation of pain to ingestion of food (pain in gastric ulcer usually occurs closer to ingestion of food than in duodenal ulcer)
- Location of pain in left midepigastric area or pain radiating to the back (ulcer on posterior wall)
- Relief of pain with antacids
- Epigastric distress on an empty stomach described as gnawing, burning, hunger pangs
- Use of ulcerogenic substances (ASA, NSAIDs, alcohol)
- Sudden onset of severe, diffuse abdominal pain

Gastrointestinal status: Anorexia; vomiting, fullness, distention

Nutritional status: Weight loss common

Abdominal examination: Epigastric tenderness, voluntary muscle guarding

POTENTIAL COMPLICATIONS

Hemorrhage, perforation, obstruction (see signs and symptoms in Duodenal Ulcer, p. 671)

PATIENT PROBLEMS/NURSING DIAGNOSES & INTERVENTIONS

NIC TISSUE PERFUSION MANAGEMENT

Ineffective renal, cerebral, cardiopulmonary, gastrointestinal, and peripheral tissue perfusion related to blood loss

- Monitor vital signs, central venous pressure, Swan-Ganz catheter pressure, laboratory values, urinary output, and early signs of hypovolemic shock.
- Maintain intravenous fluids and blood replacements as ordered *to replace fluid volume loss.*
- Prepare patient for endoscopic procedures: permit nothing by mouth, explain procedure, and administer preprocedural medications as ordered.
- Institute room temperature lavage if ordered *for gastrointestinal bleeding not controlled by endoscopy.*

NIC NUTRITION SUPPORT

Imbalanced nutrition: less than body requirements, related to abdominal pain after eating

- Monitor intake and output.
- Record complaints of fullness, nausea, and vomiting *because these symptoms may indicate delayed gastric emptying.*
- Consult with nutritionist.

NIC PHYSICAL COMFORT PROMOTION

Acute or chronic pain related to presence of gastric ulcer

- Provide antacids as needed *because pain is often relieved by small amounts of antacids.*

PATIENT EDUCATION/CONTINUUM OF CARE PLAN

1. Discuss with patient the relationship of causative agents to development of gastric ulcers, recurrence rate (approximately 40%), and repeat of endoscopy.
2. Provide written information on medication regimen, and ensure that patient can identify drugs and when each is to

---

*Not all medication protocols are FDA–approved for gastritis/peptic ulcer disease.

be taken, which require empty stomach or should be taken after a meal, and so forth.

3. Discuss with patient diet management during acute phase: avoid spices, avoid alcohol, avoid any type of coffee or tea, avoid citrus acid juices, avoid binges and overdistention.
4. Ensure that patient understands that milk ingestion is not encouraged because of increased gastric acid secretion.
5. Give patient a list of over-the-counter remedies that contain salicylates.
6. Discuss importance of continued treatment, even in the absence of overt symptoms.

Evaluation Support/Patient Outcomes

Tissue Perfusion Management: Volume status is normal. Bleeding has stopped (hematemesis and melena are absent). Blood pressure and pulse are within normal limits for the patient. Patient is taking oral fluids.

Nutrition Support: Nutrition is adequate. Patient tolerates recommended diet. Patient has an appetite. Patient's protein and calorie intake is adequate.

Physical Comfort Promotion: Pain is relieved. Patient is able to identify irritating substances in diet and to avoid them. Patient understands medication regimen and how medications are used to alleviate symptoms.

INTESTINAL DISORDERS

Duodenal Ulcers

A duodenal ulcer is a chronic circumscribed break in the duodenal mucosa extending through the muscularis mucosae that leaves a residual scar with healing. The duodenal ulcer is the most common form of peptic ulcer disease.

The incidence of duodenal ulcers has been decreasing since the 1950s. Currently, there are about 200,000 to 400,000 new cases a year. Men and women are equally likely to develop duodenal ulcers. Risk factors include *H. pylori* infections, use of NSAIDs, and cigarette smoking. Genetic and environmental factors have also been implicated in the development of duodenal ulcer disease.[7]

More efficient diagnostic techniques and treatment may also have a role in the decline of duodenal ulcers. The duodenal ulcer (Fig. 10-11) can be differentiated from dyspepsia, duodenitis, and gastric ulcer. Medical treatment with H_2 receptor antagonists has been successfully used, and patients often undergo diagnostic techniques and treatment as outpatients. Surgery is used only to manage complications of duodenal ulcers such as perforation.

H. pylori infection, NSAID use, and hypersecretory states appear to account for nearly all duodenal ulcers.[7]

Pathophysiology

The duodenal ulcer usually is less than 3 mm in diameter and is located 0.5 to 2 cm from the pylorus. Duodenal ulcers occur on both the anterior and posterior walls. The ulcers on the anterior wall appear to have a greater incidence of perforation. Posterior wall ulcers tend to be larger.

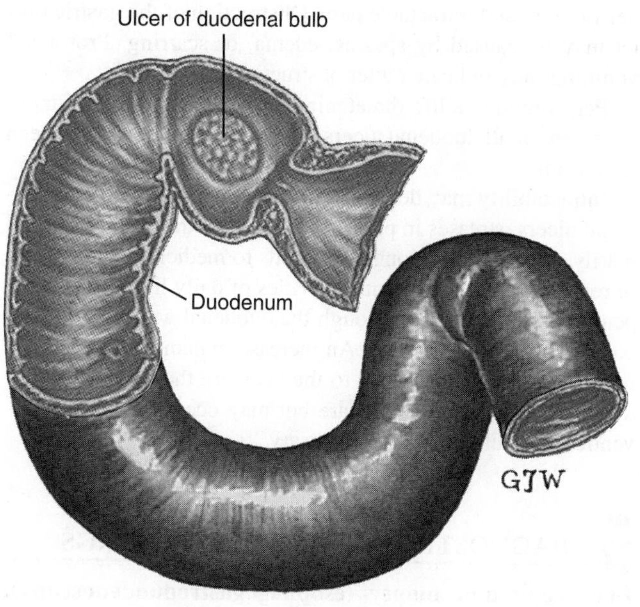

Fig. 10-11
Duodenal peptic ulcer. (From Doughty.[10])

Patients with duodenal ulcers secrete more gastric acid than normal in basal states and in response to stimuli. The increased acid production may be the result of an increased capacity to secrete hydrochloric acid because of increased parietal cell mass, or heightened vagal activity increasing the response to stimuli to overproduce acid, or a decreased ability to stop or "turn off" gastric secretions.

The nervous system phase of gastric secretions includes impulses from the cortex (limbic system and hypothalamus) to the vagal nerve. Vagal stimulation acts directly on the parietal cells and indirectly on the antral G cells to release gastrin. Pepsin and hydrochloric acid secretions are stimulated. The stimuli to the nervous system may include food in the mouth (tactile), thoughts and anticipation of food, or the sight of food.

Gastric activity also affects the regulation of secretions. The person with a duodenal ulcer secretes larger amounts of gastric juices and may be unable to stop the release of gastrin in response to normal hormonal stimuli. The concentration of acid in the duodenum is higher than normal. Hypersecretion of acid, in and of itself, does not result in a duodenal ulcer but has been shown to be a factor in its development.

The more rapid the development of the ulcer, the more likely that blood vessels in the ulcer will show inflammatory changes, medial hypertrophy, or endarteritis. Blood vessels adjacent to the ulcer will have arteriosclerotic changes. The blood vessels 5 cm away from the ulcer will appear normal. In rapidly developing ulcers, bleeding is more common and may be massive because the blood vessel wall may erode in an asymptomatic patient. In instances where the duodenal ulcer develops slowly, thrombosis, endarteritis, and inflammatory changes result in an avascular, scarred area that heals slowly.

In addition to upper gastrointestinal bleeding, other complications of duodenal ulcer disease include gastric outlet obstruction, perforation, and intractable pain. Obstruction of the gastric outlet may be caused by spasms, edema, or scarring. Protracted vomiting may indicate outlet obstruction.

Perforation is a life-threatening event. Perforation occurs in 2% to 5% of all duodenal ulcers. The overall incidence has been decreasing.

Intractability may develop from other complications of duodenal ulcers, stresses in patients' lives, and other disorders. Primarily, the patient no longer responds to medical management, or recurrences interfere with activities of daily living. Posterior penetration of the ulcer through the duodenal wall and into the pancreas will alter the pain. An increase in pain, loss of antacid relief, and radiation of pain to the back are the primary symptoms. Acute pancreatitis is rare but may occur. Surgical intervention may ultimately be necessary.

Diagnostic Studies and Findings

Endoscopy and biopsy (esophagogastroduodenoscopy): Presence of an ulcer; degree of healing; differential diagnosis

Double-contast barium studies (upper GI): Presence of a crater, scar, or deformity in duodenum; delayed gastric emptying of barium (gastric outlet obstruction); not as effective in detection of small ulcers

ELISAs: For detection of serum antibodies to *H. pylori*

Urea breath test: For detection of enzyme produced by *H. pylori,* patient drinks carbon-labeled urea solution; in an infected patient, labeled carbon dioxide can be detected in expired air; fasting usually required; 30-minute delay between preurea and posturea breath sampling[46]

Multidisciplinary Plan

Surgery

Medical management usually successful; surgery is indicated usually for complications: Bleeding, perforation, penetration, obstruction, and intractability

Types of procedures: Removal of a portion of gastrin-producing portion of stomach (antrectomy or partial gastrectomy) with attachment of duodenum to stomach (Billroth I) or attachment of stomach to jejunum (Billroth II) and vagotomy

Complications of surgical procedures: Alkaline reflux gastritis; afferent loop syndrome; bezoar formation; malnutrition

Medications

Histamine receptor antagonists: Do not take within 2 h of antacids
- Cimetidine (Tagamet), 800 mg PO at bedtime
- Ranitidine (Zantac), 300 mg PO at bedtime
- Famotidine (Pepcid), 40 mg PO at bedtime
- Nizatidine (Axid), 300 mg PO at bedtime

Antacids: Aluminum-magnesium regimen, PO: provide 120-414 mEq buffering capacity per day (amount required varies based on commercial antacid used; Table 10-2)

Proton pump inhibitor
- Omeprazole (Prilosec), 20 mg/day for 4-8 weeks
- Lansoprazole 30 mg/day

Table 10-2 Relative Potency of Liquid Antacids

Antacid	Potency*
Concentrated Aluminum and Magnesium Hydroxides	
Delcid	100
Maalox	75
Mylanta II	75
Gelusil II	60
Regular Aluminum and Magnesium Hydroxides	
Maalox	45
Mylanta	40
Gelusil	40
Riopan	40
Aluminum Hydroxide	
Alternagel	40
Amphojel	20

Modified from Sleisenger and Fordtram.[44]
*Millimoles of neutralizing capacity per 15 ml.

Multiple **antibacterial regimens** identified/investigated to eradicate *H. pylori:* None achieve cure rate greater than 85%; these include*:
- Combination of a proton pump inhibitor or ranitidine bismuth citrate with two antibiotics, including clarithromycin or amoxycillin and metronidazole or tinidazole
- Combination of a proton pump inhibitor or H_2 receptor antagonist with bismuth subcitrate or tripotassium dicitrato bismuthate, metronidazole, and tetracycline.[29]

Cytoprotective agents: Sucralfate (Carafate), 1 g qid on empty stomach for 4-8 weeks; avoid other medications 30 min before and after dose

Prostaglandin E_1 analog: Mucosal protective effect; antisecretory properties
- Misoprostol (Cytotec), 200-400 μg bid to qid; take before eating and at bedtime to decrease adverse effects; used prophylactically to prevent duodenal ulcer in patients taking NSAIDs

General Management

Esophagogastroduodenoscopy (EGD) to manage bleeding

Room temperature water or saline lavage, if massive hemorrhage

Arteriography with intraarterial vasopressin for intractable bleeding

Avoid smoking, known ulcerogenic substances (ASA, steroids, NSAIDs) when possible

Rest

Nutritional Consultation

To assist patient in identification of foods and eating patterns that contribute to increased gastric acid secretion and subsequent mucosal irritation, and to develop diet that minimizes gastric acid secretion and ulcer symptoms

*Not all medication protocols are FDA–approved for gastritis/peptic ulcer disease.

NURSING CARE

NURSING ASSESSMENT

Pain: No symptoms to vague symptoms and atypical symptoms
- Heartburn, dyspepsia
- Relation of pain to ingestion of food (pain in duodenal ulcer); usually occurs 2 to 3 hours after eating, and there is pain; at night
- Chronic or periodic symptoms
- Relief of pain with antacids
- Well-localized epigastric pain occurring when stomach is empty, relieved by food, vomiting, or antacids
- Use of ulcerogenic substances (ASA, NSAIDs, alcohol)

Gastrointestinal status: Constipation (may be related to diet and drugs); diarrhea (may be present from antacid therapy)

Nutritional status: Weight gain (patient may eat more frequently in attempt to alleviate symptoms)

Abdominal examination: Epigastric tenderness, voluntary muscle guarding

POTENTIAL COMPLICATIONS

Bleeding, perforation, penetration, pyloric outlet obstruction

PATIENT PROBLEMS/NURSING DIAGNOSES & INTERVENTIONS

NIC TISSUE PERFUSION MANAGEMENT

Ineffective renal, cerebral, cardiopulmonary, gastrointestinal, and peripheral tissue perfusion related to blood loss

- Monitor vital signs, central venous pressure, Swan-Ganz catheter pressure, laboratory values, urinary output, and early signs of hypovolemic shock.
- Maintain intravenous fluids and blood replacements as ordered *to replace fluid volume loss.*
- Prepare patient for endoscopic procedures: permit nothing by mouth, explain procedure, administer preprocedural medications as ordered.
- Institute room temperature lavage if ordered for gastrointestinal bleeding not controlled by endoscopy.

NIC PHYSICAL COMFORT PROMOTION

Acute pain related to presence of duodenal ulcer

- Provide antacids at the bedside *to relieve well-localized epigastric pain.*

PATIENT EDUCATION/CONTINUUM OF CARE PLAN

1. Provide instructions (verbal and written) on medication regimen; ensure that patient can identify drugs and understand when each is to be taken, which medicines require an empty stomach or should be taken after a meal, and so forth.
2. Provide information on relationship of duodenal ulcers and aspirin-containing compounds, milk, various antacids, and NSAIDs.
3. Give patient a list of over-the-counter remedies that contain salicylates.
4. Discuss the importance of continuing treatment, even in the absence of overt symptoms.
5. Ingestion of alcohol and H_2 blockers (except famotidine) may result in increased absorption of oral alcohol, higher blood levels, and greater susceptibility to alcohol toxicity.

EVALUATION SUPPORT/PATIENT OUTCOMES

Tissue Perfusion Management: Volume status is normal. Bleeding has stopped. Hematemesis and melena are absent. Blood pressure and pulse are within normal limits for patient. Patient is taking oral fluids.

Physical Comfort Promotion: Pain is relieved. Patient is able to identify irritating substances in the diet and avoids them. Patient will tolerate recommended diet.

APPENDICITIS

Appendicitis is the inflammation of the vermiform appendix; it may be classified as simple, gangrenous, or perforated. Simple appendicitis involves an inflamed and intact appendix, whereas in gangrenous appendicitis the appendix may have focal or extensive necrosis with microscopic perforations. Gross disruption of the appendix wall occurs in perforated appendicitis.

Acute appendicitis is the most common cause of acute abdomen in the United States and is one of the most common indications for emergency abdominal surgery. The rate of appendicitis is approximately 7%,[7] and the disorder is more common in adolescents and young adults. The diagnosis is difficult to determine in very young and elderly individuals. A very young child is often unable to describe the symptoms that are key clues to the diagnosis. In an elderly person the symptoms are vague and may cause the person to delay seeking medical assistance, and then the physician may not consider appendicitis as a possibility. The abdominal tenderness in the elderly may be mild, making diagnosis more difficult. Perforation rates range from 11% to 32% and are probably related to delay in patient consultation.[6]

PATHOPHYSIOLOGY

Appendicitis can be compared to a closed-loop obstruction in which obstruction occurs first and inflammation and infection second. In acute appendicitis (FIG. 10-12) the long narrow tube of the appendix is obstructed, hypoxia develops, the mucosa ulcerates, and bacteria invade the wall. The lumen of the appendix may be obstructed by a kinking of the appendix (this is uncommon), edema of the lymphoid tissue, or a fecalith. The lymphoid hyperplasia or edema may develop in response to a viral or bacterial infection. A fecalith is a formed, hard mass of feces. Fecaliths are associated with diets deficient in fiber. After the lumen becomes obstructed, the mucosa continues to secrete fluid until the intraluminal pressure exceeds the venous pressure. Hypoxia develops because blood flow is impeded. The mucosal wall ulcerates, and bacterial invasion occurs. The infection results in more edema, which further impedes blood flow. Gangrene and perforation occur in 24 to 36 hours. Perforation of the appendix creates serious complications, including periappendiceal abscess, pelvic abscess, or peritonitis.

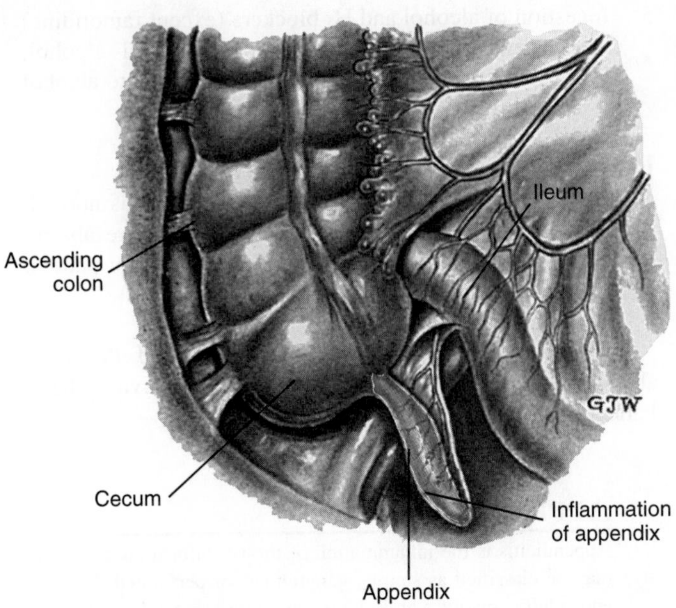

FIG. 10-12
Appendicitis (acute). (From Doughty.[10])

Atypical appendicitis refers to situations in which the symptoms do not follow the classic presentation of appendicitis. The position of the appendix (retrocecal, pelvic, retroileal, preileal, subcecal), the age of the patient, and pregnancy may affect the symptoms of appendicitis, making diagnosis more difficult.

Diagnostic Studies and Findings

White blood cells: Elevated, with shift to the left; 10,000 to 16,000/mm^4; 75% neutrophils; 10% have normal differential cell counts; WBC counts greater than 20,000 frequently are associated with perforation or other septic complications.
Urinalysis: Small number of erythrocytes and leukocytes; excludes urinary tract infection and renal stones
Ultrasound: May be helpful in patients in whom the clinical features of appendicitis are ambiguous; dilated appendiceal lumen and a thickened wall
Computed tomography (CT) scan (indicated if mass): Identifies abscesses and appendicoliths
Pregnancy test: To rule out ectopic pregnancy
Nuclear medicine: Radionuclide studies with technetium 99m–labeled substances are being evaluated for predictive value in diagnosing appendicitis

Multidisciplinary Plan

Surgery
Appendectomy; may be done laparoscopically

Medications
Antiinfective agents: Broad-spectrum antibiotic therapy as prophylaxis before surgery or for a period postoperatively (to prevent wound infection or pelvic abscess)

NURSING CARE

Nursing Assessment
Pain: Pain in epigastrium or periumbilical area that is colicky, peaks in 4 hours, and subsides (see Emergency Alert box); pain reappears in right lower quadrant, is progressively severe, and is exacerbated by movement
Gastrointestinal status
- May vomit once or twice: anorexia present
- Constipation and failure to pass flatus
- Abdominal examination
  - Patient can point to localized pain at McBurney's point (midway between iliac crest and umbilicus)
  - Coughing or moving abdominal wall up and out will reproduce or exacerbate pain
  - Rebound tenderness; muscle rigidity (palpate abdomen with *one* finger)
  - Pain on palpation or percussion can be localized to a spot

General status: Anxiety level; low-grade fever, does not usually exceed 39° C (102° F)
Atypical appendicitis
- Retrocecal or retroileal
  - Pain less intense (no discomfort with walking or coughing) and poorly localized
  - Urinary frequency (irritation of ureter)
- Pelvic
  - Very severe, constant pain
  - Localized pain on left
  - Urge to urinate and defecate
  - Tenderness on rectal examination
  - Absence of muscle rigidity and abdominal tenderness
- In elderly persons
  - Symptoms vague; pain minimal
  - Pain
- In pregnancy
  - Late in gestation, diagnosis more difficult because of displacement of cecum by uterus

Potential Complications
Perforation, peritonitis

Patient Problems/Nursing Diagnoses & Interventions

NIC Physical Comfort Promotion

Acute pain related to appendiceal inflammation
- Help patient reduce pain by having him or her lie still and avoid sudden movements, such as coughing.
- Administer analgesics as ordered after diagnosis has been established.

Patient Education/Continuum of Care Plan
1. Wound or incisional care instructions should be provided.
2. A pattern of increasing activities (e.g., walking, driving) should be provided as recommended by physician.

Evaluation Support/Patient Outcomes
Physical Comfort Promotion: Comfort level is achieved. Reduction or absence of guarding, protective behavior. Uses

EMERGENCY ALERT

ACUTE ABDOMINAL PAIN

Acute onset of abdominal pain needs immediate evaluation.

ASSESSMENT

- Determine *PQRST*
  - P = Precipitating factors
  - Q = Quality
  - R = Radiation
  - S = Severity
  - T = Time of onset
- Assess associated symptoms such as nausea, vomiting, diarrhea, constipation, fever, chills, urinary tract symptoms (frequency, burning, pain), gynecologic symptoms (pain, discharge, missed menses), gastrointestinal upset.
- Conduct a thorough physical assessment of the abdomen, including inspection, auscultation, palpation, and percussion.
- Determine laboratory tests to be obtained specific to symptoms.
- Determine radiologic studies to be obtained specific to symptoms.

INTERVENTIONS

- Obtain IV access as indicated by vital signs and hydration.
- Obtain results of relevant laboratory and radiologic studies.
- If indicated, keep client NPO until possible surgical evaluation is completed.
- Surgical intervention may be indicated for the following problems:
  - Appendicitis
  - Bowel obstruction
  - Cholecystitis
  - Diverticulitis
  - Massive GI bleeding
  - Pancreatitis
  - Peritonitis
  - Perforation of viscus
  - Ruptured ectopic pregnancy
  - Ruptured intraabdominal aneurysm
  - Urethral stone

pain control strategies appropriately. Verbalizes increased control over pain.

DIVERTICULAR DISEASE

Diverticulosis is the presence of diverticula, pouchlike herniations through the muscular wall of the intestine. They may occur anywhere throughout the gut but are most common in the sigmoid colon. Diverticulitis is the most frequent complication of diverticular disease and the result of inflammation or perforation of one or more diverticula.

Diverticular disease is common in developed Westernized countries. It is probably secondary to a diet that is low in fiber. African, Asian, and Third World countries have low rates of diverticular disease; however, when a Western diet is adopted by blacks in Africa, diverticular disease develops.[7]

The incidence of diverticular disease increases with age. One third of North Americans can expect to develop colonic diverticula by age 50; two thirds by age 80. Most diverticula are

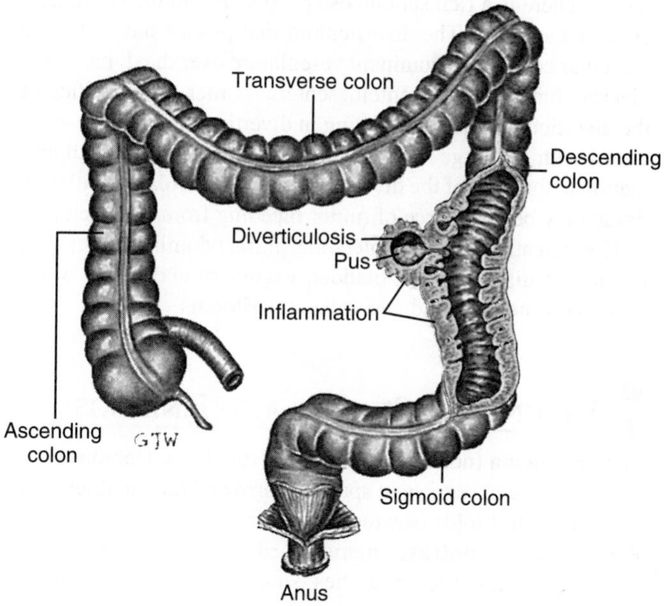

FIG. 10-13

Diverticulosis (diverticulitis). (From Doughty.[10])

in the sigmoid colon.[52] (FIG. 10-13). Bleeding from diverticular disease is one of the most common causes of lower gastrointestinal hemorrhage and tends to be from diverticula located on the right side of the colon.[7]

PATHOPHYSIOLOGY

The development of diverticula is related to the pressures generated in the bowel lumen. Normal intraluminal pressure is less than 10 mm Hg in the sigmoid colon. The normal pressure can be increased significantly when the bowel is divided into segments by the muscular contraction rings. The muscular activities in the localized segments can exert enough pressure to increase intracolonic pressure to 90 mm Hg, and this high pressure may push out diverticula through "weak spots" where blood vessels enter the colon wall.[7]

Symptoms of diverticular disease that are considered complications are caused by the associated motility disorder and not by the presence of the diverticula. Intraluminal pressures in diverticular disease are excessive in response to food ingestion, morphine, and parasympathomimetic agents. These pressures are virtually identical to intraluminal pressures recorded in patients with irritable bowel syndrome.

Constipation has been associated with diverticular disease. More pressure is required to move hard, dry fecal material through the lumen. Moist, soft stools and multiple bowel movements each day are associated with high-fiber diets. The decrease in segmentation and intracolonic pressures with high-fiber diets may lessen the symptoms of diverticulosis and impede progression of the disease.

The blood flow to the large colon runs from the mesentery around the bowel and divides into branches that go subserosally. These vessels enter the circular muscle obliquely from the mesenteric side of the bowel between the mesenteric and lateral teniae. There is a rich submucosa plexus around the circumference of the colon. The diverticulum that pushes out under the muscular coat has a prominent vasculature over the dome of the diverticulum and at the antemesenteric border of the orifice of the diverticulum. Major bleeding in diverticular disease is associated with the large vessel over the dome. Localized inflammation at the base of the diverticulum with vascular granulation tissue may be the source of minor bleeding from diverticula.

Complications include bleeding, intraabdominal abscesses, fistulas (to distant bowel, bladder, vagina, or abdominal wall), bowel obstructions, and generalized peritonitis.

DIAGNOSTIC STUDIES AND FINDINGS

Barium enema (not used in acute diverticulitis): Demonstrates diverticulum, segmental spasms, narrowed lumen, thickened interhaustral folds (sawtooth appearance)

Water-soluble contrast enema (used in acute diverticulitis): Demonstrates abscess cavities, sinus tracts, fistula, intramural abscesses, extrinsic compression; if CT unavailable

Plain abdominal films: Free abdominal air (perforation); ileus (localized inflammation); small bowel obstruction; normal in uncomplicated diverticular disease

CT scan (with IV and oral contrast): Effacement of pericolic fat, abscess, fistulas (diverticulitis); confirms diagnosis

Ultrasonography: May demonstrate extracolonic fluid collections

Sigmoidoscopy or colonoscopy: Orifices of the diverticula may be visible (high risk of perforation if instrument enters a diverticulum); excludes other diseases that may mimic diverticulitis

MULTIDISCIPLINARY PLAN

Surgery

Surgery reserved for management of complications or for recurrent attacks; hemorrhage, obstruction, perforation, and fistula

Primary resection with anastomosis (if bowel not edematous or if there is no gross infection present)

Primary resection with temporary colostomy (two-stage procedure) if bowel is edematous or in presence of gross infection

Medications

Diverticulosis

- Bran, 10 to 25 g/day in divided doses: Must slowly increase to develop tolerance; will help relieve abdominal pain; lowers intraluminal pressure
- Laxatives: Hydrophilic colloid laxatives rather than bran in acute phases may be better tolerated; slowly decrease amount as bran and fiber in diet increase

Diverticulitis

- Intravenous fluid therapy
- Narcotic analgesic: Meperidine (Demerol) for analgesia (dose calculated for patient)
- Antibiotic therapy
  - Gentamicin (Garamycin), 5 mg/kg/day, *and* clindamycin, 300 mg q6h IV, or metronidazole, 500 mg q8h IV
  - Cefoxitin (Mefoxin), 4-6 g/day parenterally in divided doses
  - All antiinfective agents continued for 7-10 days; not all listed would be used; agents chosen should cover the major colon pathogens: anaerobes, gram-negative bacilli, and gram-positive coliforms

General Management

Nasogastric tube inserted if nausea, vomiting, and abdominal distention are severe

Radiographic studies and ultrasonography used to evaluate the response to therapy (e.g., resolution of abscess)

Carcinoma: Difficult to detect in bowel with narrowed areas and partial obstruction; use colonoscopy procedures to distinguish between acute diverticular disease and carcinoma after an acute episode

Bleeding: Angiographic injection of vasopressin, 0.5 to 1 ml/min

High-fiber diet for managing diverticulosis

Give nothing to eat initially in acute diverticulitis; slowly resume diet; when inflammation has resolved and bowel functioning returns to normal, resume high-fiber diet

For acute diverticulitis, bed rest

Nutritional Consultation

To advise patient in choices for selecting a high-fiber diet

NURSING CARE

NURSING ASSESSMENT

General status: Sepsis

Pain

- Diverticulosis: Ranges from no pain to intermittent cramping, left lower abdominal pain
- Diverticulitis: Pain more intense; may be severe pain; in the elderly it is often difficult to assess pain

Abdominal examination

- Diverticulosis: Tenderness in left lower colon, palpable colon, distention; sometimes there are no symptoms
- Diverticulitis: Palpable colon, tenderness in the left lower quadrant, distended and tympanic abdomen, decreased bowel sounds; may hear increased bowel sounds with abdominal distention if obstruction is present

Gastrointestinal status: Constipation or alternating constipation and diarrhea; blood in stools

Urinary status: Dysuria; frequency (associated with bladder involvement); passage of gas or stool through urethra (colovesicular fistula)

POTENTIAL COMPLICATIONS

Lower GI bleeding, abscess, fistula, bowel obstruction, peritonitis

PATIENT PROBLEMS/NURSING DIAGNOSES & INTERVENTIONS

NIC TISSUE PERFUSION MANAGEMENT

Ineffective renal, cerebral, cardiopulmonary, gastrointestinal, and peripheral tissue perfusion related to sepsis and bleeding

- Maintain intravenous fluids, monitor vital signs, intake and output if complications occur *to prevent intravascular fluid imbalance.*

NIC Elimination Management

Constipation related to diverticular disease, low-fiber diet

- In acute phase, provide low-fiber diet *to allow bowel inflammation to resolve.*
- In diverticulosis, initiate bran therapy or hydrophilic colloid laxative, increase oral fluid intake, and increase patient's activity level with instructions on slowly increasing the amount of fiber: *to reduce constipation and dry stools.*
- Instruct patients with diverticular disease to avoid nuts and popcorn.

Patient Education/Continuum of Care Plan

1. Dietary instructions on high-fiber diet should be provided. Teach patient ways to make bran more palatable (e.g., muffins, use on cereals).
2. Discharge instructions should include relationship of diet to diverticular disease, assessment of bowel movements to evaluate dietary intake of bran and fluids, and signs of complications of acute diverticular disease.
3. Instruct patient in bowel training, that is, to set aside a time daily without anxiety or interruption to have a bowel movement.
4. See p. 732 for colostomy care instructions.

Evaluation/Patient Outcomes

Tissue Perfusion Management: There is no gastrointestinal bleeding. Hematocrit and hemoglobin levels are normal for patient. Patient's vital signs are stable. Stool for occult blood negative.

Elimination Management: Patient experiences regular bowel movements. Patient reports that stools are soft, brown, and regular in caliber. Patient verbalizes knowledge of need for high-fiber diet.

Herniation (External)

A hernia is a protrusion of an organ (usually bowel) through an abnormal opening in the muscle wall. Hernias may be congenital (failure of certain structures to close after birth) or acquired when muscle weakens (associated with obesity, surgery, or illness or from increased abdominal pressure as a result of straining or ascites).

Hernias can occur in any age group. Lifting heavy objects is commonly associated with hernia formation. Approximately 75% of hernias occur in the groin (indirect inguinal, direct inguinal, or femoral). Kinds of hernias include reducible, irreducible, incarcerated, and strangulated. Reducible hernias may be returned to their proper position. They return spontaneously, or they are returned manually. An irreducible hernia (incarcerated) cannot be returned to the abdomen. It is trapped by the narrow neck of the opening or defect. An incarcerated hernia that becomes gangrenous because the contents are constricted is called a strangulated hernia.

Pathophysiology

External hernias include inguinal, femoral, umbilical, and incisional hernias. The inguinal hernia is the most common. It is a weakness in the abdominal wall where the spermatic cord (men) or the round ligament (women) emerges. In an indirect inguinal hernia the herniation protrudes through the inguinal ring and follows the round ligament or spermatic cord. A direct inguinal hernia goes through the posterior inguinal wall. Inguinal hernias are more common in men.

A femoral hernia, or protrusion through the femoral ring into the femoral canal, is seen as a bulge below the inguinal ligament. It occurs more frequently in women. Femoral hernias strangulate easily.

The umbilical hernia is caused by a gradual yielding of the scar tissue closing the umbilical ring. Predisposing factors include (1) multiple pregnancies with prolonged labor, (2) ascites, (3) obesity, and (4) large intraabdominal tumors.[52] Ventral and incisional hernias are associated with muscle weakness from abdominal incisions. Hernias after surgery are more common in obese persons, the elderly, those with wound infections, and those with general debility.

Multidisciplinary Plan

Surgery

Herniorrhaphy (surgical repair of hernia) or hernioplasty (reinforcement of weakened area with wire, fascia, or mesh) may be done laparoscopically

Temporary colostomy (for complications of intestinal obstruction or strangulation of hernia)

General Management

Binder or truss (to reduce hernia and to prevent protrusion; danger: strangulation if not reduced properly)

NURSING CARE

Nursing Assessment

Abdominal examination

Examine patient supine and sitting

Can often see hernia "bulge" or protrude as person changes position or coughs (many patients have a history of being able to reduce their own hernias before seeking repair)

Palpate weakened muscle area

Pain of increasing severity, fever, tachycardia, and abdominal rigidity are signs of strangulation

Potential Complications

Incarceration, strangulation

Patient Problems/Nursing Diagnoses & Interventions

NIC Skin/Wound Management

Impaired skin integrity related to hernia repair

- Prevent or manage any increased abdominal pressure (coughing, straining at stool, hiccups) that could impair healing at the hernia site.
- Optimize nutrition for adequate wound healing.
- Apply scrotal support for inguinal hernia repairs.

Patient Education/Continuum of Care Plan

1. Inform patient of the need to lose weight if patient is obese.
2. Patient should avoid heavy lifting for 6 to 8 weeks, unless otherwise specified by the physician. Give patient a limit of weight not to carry or lift.
3. If patient will use a binder at home, provide correct instructions for application. Teach patient to observe for skin irritation.
4. Teach patient to splint incision with hands or pillow to provide incisional support if it is necessary to cough or sneeze.
5. Instruct patient to increase fiber and fluids postoperatively to prevent constipation. If the patient is discharged home on codeine, he or she may need a bulk laxative.
6. See pp. 730 to 732 for management of temporary colostomy and interventions related to care and adaptation.

Evaluation/Patient Outcomes

Skin/Wound Management: No injury is present. Patient verbalizes understanding of preventing increased abdominal pressure. Incision is healing without signs of infection.

Intestinal Obstruction

An intestinal obstruction occurs when the contents of the intestines fail to propel forward through the lumen. Intestinal obstructions may be mechanical or functional.

Mechanical obstructions are caused by a blockage of the bowel lumen by adhesion, hernia, volvulus, tumor, inflammation (as in Crohn's disease), impacted feces, or intussusception. Functional obstructions, also referred to as ileus, occur when there is a loss of propulsive peristalsis associated with abdominal surgery, hypokalemia, intestinal distention, peritonitis, severe traumas, spinal fractures, ureteral distention, or the effects of some narcotic drugs and diphenoxylate (Lomotil).

Intestinal obstructions are more common in persons who have undergone abdominal surgery or who have had congenital abnormalities of the bowel. An intestinal obstruction, if untreated, can progress to a life-threatening disorder. The severity and types of symptoms vary according to the cause and location of the intestinal obstruction. Ninety percent of intestinal obstructions are the result of adhesions or incarcerated hernias.

Mechanical obstructions can be caused by factors that block the lumen of the bowel wall, in which case they are referred to as obturation obstructions. This category includes intussusception, large gallstones, feces, bezoars, and ingested foreign objects. Intrinsic factors that may progress to mechanical obstructions include stenosis, strictures associated with chronic inflammation or neoplasms, iatrogenic strictures after intestinal surgery or radiation therapy, and mesenteric vascular occlusion. Extrinsic factors that may lead to mechanical obstructions of the intestine are the most common cause of intestinal obstructions and include adhesions, hernias, neoplasms, abscesses, and volvulus.

A volvulus is a twisting of the bowel on itself. The two most common sites for the development of a volvulus are the cecum and the sigmoid colon. A cecal volvulus may occur any time from adolescence but is most common in the fifth decade of life. Sigmoid volvulus is more common in the elderly and has been associated with chronic constipation. A volvulus usually develops in an area where an underlying abnormality exists.

Mechanical obstructions may be simple obstructions in the small bowel or colon or strangulation obstructions. The location of a mechanical obstruction is important in determining the sequelae. Simple mechanical obstructions may resolve medically, whereas strangulation obstructions require surgical intervention.

The paralytic ileus or functional obstruction is a state of inhibited motility in the gastrointestinal tract that is temporary and reversible.

Pathophysiology

An accumulation of fluid and gas proximal to an obstruction occurs in a simple mechanical obstruction of the small bowel. Initially, the pooled fluids include ingested foods and digestive enzymes. Intestinal gas, in obstruction, is primarily made up of swallowed air that has high concentrations of nitrogen and is not absorbed by the intestinal mucosa. The distention of the bowel by the trapped fluids and gases causes the small bowel to secrete water and electrolytes into the obstructed lumen.

The distention impedes venous return and inhibits the absorptive quality of the mucosa. The bowel wall becomes edematous. The bowel continues to secrete water, sodium, and potassium into the obstructed segment. As the obstruction continues, the intestinal distention is self-perpetuating. Distention increases the intestinal secretions of water and electrolytes into the lumen. As fluid and gas pour into the intestine, motility is further compromised and the distention enlarges proximally. Successive loops of proximal bowel distend, fill with fluid, and stop absorbing. Transudation of water through the wall of the obstructed segment may develop, leading to the development of peritoneal fluid. Distention may lead to pressure necrosis of the bowel wall.

Bacteria are not usually found in the small intestine, but during intestinal obstruction an abnormal bacterial flora that rapidly proliferates is found in the intestinal lumen. The bacteria produce hydrogen or methane gases that contribute to the gaseous distention. Also, the small bowel contents become feculent during obstructions as a result of the bacterial proliferation.

The site and duration of intestinal obstruction affect the symptoms and potential metabolic effects. Obstructions in the upper jejunal area usually result in vomiting and little abdominal distention. Dehydration and electrolyte depletion occur.

In distal small bowel obstruction or ileal obstructions, constipation is an early symptom. Vomiting, which is not a prominent symptom, is less effective in reducing intestinal decompression. Reflex vomiting may result from intestinal distention. In distal small bowel obstruction, large quantities of fluid and electrolytes may become trapped in the intestinal lumen, resulting in nausea and passage of gas. The patient has classic signs and symptoms of circulatory shock (severe hypovolemia). Before the development of shock, dehydration and metabolic acidosis accompanied by oliguria, azotemia, and hemoconcentration occur. Early circulatory changes may be detected by tachycardia, low central venous pressure, and hypotension. Hypovolemic shock develops if the obstruction is not treated.

The intestinal distention can impair breathing because abdominal distention causes elevation of the diaphragm. The increased intraabdominal pressure caused by the intestinal distention may impede venous return from the legs.

Death of the bowel wall (bowel necrosis) complicates intestinal obstructions. Shock can quickly develop when long loops of bowel are affected. Short-segment involvement progresses quickly to perforation and peritonitis.

Impaired circulation to the bowel wall during obstructions is referred to as a strangulation obstruction. The circulation may be impeded by a closed-loop obstruction that causes occlusion of the lumen at two points along the length of the bowel segment. Volvulus is an example of a closed-loop obstruction. The closed-loop obstruction progresses to strangulation more rapidly than a simple mechanical blockage of the lumen. The circulation to the bowel may also be impaired by a sustained increase in intraluminal pressure, as with intestinal distention.

When the circulation is impaired, the venous outflow is impaired and the mural veins become engorged. The bowel wall becomes ischemic. An arterial spasm follows, and the bowel responds to anoxia with increased peristalsis. Within 15 minutes, blood escapes from the engorged veins and infiltrates the submucosa and mucosa, resulting in a hemorrhagic infarction of the tissues. Venous thrombosis occurs, further compromising circulation. The necrosis develops from the mucosa outward. Small intravascular thrombi extend the area of necrosis. The lymph channels dilate and may carry bacteria from the lumen into the serosa. Initially the fluid accumulating resembles plasma, and it gradually becomes bloody and contains bacteria and toxins.

Strangulation results in loss of blood and plasma from the affected segment. Shock occurs quickly if the patient has been dehydrated before strangulation developed. Gangrene may develop and progress to peritonitis. Perforation of the strangulated segment may occur, releasing a toxin that may be absorbed from the peritoneal cavity, producing systemic effects. Bacterial infection and toxemia are generally thought to be responsible for the shock that can quickly develop in strangulation obstructions.

In colonic obstructions the colon may become massively distended by gas. Fluid and electrolyte losses are not as significant as in small bowel obstructions and occur when the obstruction is prolonged. When the ileocecal valve is competent, there is little if any small bowel distention. However, a competent ileocecal valve may resist backward decompression enough to produce a closed-loop obstruction. If this develops, cecal distention may be significant and may progress to perforation of the cecum.

The most common cause of colon obstruction is cancer, and perforation during obstructive episodes is adjacent to the tumor. As in small bowel obstructions, the patient must be carefully observed for signs and symptoms of strangulation obstruction.

Diagnostic Studies and Findings

Serial abdominal x-rays—plain films: Abnormally large amounts of gas in the bowel; films taken with patient standing or sitting, supine, and on left side; gas- and fluid-filled loops of bowel; gas does not progress downward in serial examinations; cecal volvulus: marked distention of cecum; sigmoid volvulus: large dilated loop, from right to left side of abdomen; two fluid levels can be visualized

Barium enema*: Barium will clear entire colon or stop at site of obstruction; cecal volvulus: conical narrowing at the twist; sigmoid volvulus: narrowing at the twist

Serum electrolytes: Demonstrates electrolyte losses

White blood cell count: Sudden rise greater than 10,000/mm^3 indicates strangulation

Serum amylase: Normal value rules out acute pancreatitis; concentration as a result of fluid losses

Arterial blood gas: Acid-base deficits

Multidisciplinary Plan

Surgery

Used when cause of obstruction is thought to be adhesions, necrosis, tumor, or unresolved inflammatory lesions (e.g., strictures found in Crohn's disease)

Surgical resection of mechanical obstruction after patient's fluid and electrolytes are stabilized; strangulation obstructions are a surgical emergency; in colonic obstructions, surgery is almost always required

Cecal volvulus: Untwisting bowel; if viable, the cecum and ascending colon are anchored in place; if gangrene is present, bowel resection of involved parts

Sigmoid volvulus: Elective resection of twisted segment; if later viability is questioned, operate without decompression

Obstructing lesions of the right colon: Either a one-stage ileotransverse colostomy or two-stage procedure, with diverting ileostomy in a fragile patient

Obstructing lesions of the left colon

- Temporary end colostomy, with resection and later colostomy take-down
- Intraoperative colonic lavage, with primary anastomosis
- Primary intestinal anastomosis using resection, with intraluminal bypass tube

Cecostomy: In patients with high surgical risk

Transverse colostomy: Requires three operations; the first is a decompressing colostomy; the second surgical procedure is resection and anastomosis; the third surgical stage is closure of colostomy

Medications

Antibiotics if strangulation is present or peritonitis is suspected

*Meglumine diatrizoate (Gastrografin) used if perforation is suspected.

Prophylactic perioperative antibiotics (for anaerobes and gram-negative organisms) in unprepared bowel; surgery to prevent wound infection and sepsis

General Management

Fluid and electrolyte replacement critical

Nasogastric (for upper or jejunal obstruction) or intestinal suctioning (for distal obstructions); Cantor or Miller-Abbott tubes (used rarely) when obstruction is caused by infection or inflammation and can resolve with medical therapy (intravenous fluids and electrolytes, administration of blood or plasma)

Colonoscopy may assist with reduction of volvulus by releasing trapped gas and fluid (surgery may still be advised after reduction of volvulus if mucosal viability is in doubt)

NURSING CARE

Nursing Assessment

General Status

Loss of skin turgor and dry mucous membranes: dehydration

Fever (high fever with strangulation of small bowel; peritonitis)

Anxiety level

Tachycardia and hypotension (may indicate dehydration or peritonitis)

Metabolic acidosis

Hypovolemic shock

Pain

Crampy abdominal pain; onset clearly recalled

Severe continuous ache (strangulation)

Increased severity and diffuseness of pain, rebound tenderness, guarding (perforation, peritonitis)

Gastrointestinal Status

Vomiting

Proximal jejunal obstructions: profuse vomiting unassociated with abdominal distention

Distal small bowel obstruction: feculent odor (secondary to bacterial proliferation in obstructions)

Colonic obstructions: vomiting after prolonged obstructions; usually secondary to pain; may contain fecal material

Obstipation

Obstipation and failure to pass gas are signs of a complete obstruction after the bowel distal to the obstruction has been evacuated

Constipation

Blood in stools (may indicate strangulation, cancer, intussusception, or infarction of obstructing lesions)

History of previous surgeries, inflammatory bowel disease, diverticulitis, or symptoms of malignancy

Abdominal Examination

Observe and palpate carefully for presence of hernias

Note amount of abdominal distention; girth measurements may be beneficial in observing the progress of an obstruction

Mechanical obstruction: peristalsis is high-pitched, tinkling sound with rushes

Visible peristalsis: seen moving toward obstruction and reversing

Paralytic ileus: absence of bowel sounds or low infrequent sounds

Auscultate abdomen for full 5 minutes before palpating

Localized tenderness, constant pain, guarding, and rebound tenderness are signs of strangulation obstructions

Sigmoid loop volvulus may be palpable

Potential Complications

Hypovolemic shock, perforation, peritonitis

Patient Problems/Nursing Diagnoses & Interventions

NIC Tissue Perfusion Management

Deficient fluid volume related to vomiting, third spacing of fluids

- Administer intravenous fluids and electrolytes, blood, and plasma *to replace and maintain fluid volume.*
- Monitor vital signs, central venous pressure, blood pressure, urinary output, and nasogastric aspirations every hour.
- Measure abdominal girth every 4 to 8 hours *to assess distention.*
- Notify physician of changes in patient's status *because they generally indicate a decline in patient's stabilization for surgical intervention.*

NIC Physical Comfort Promotion

Acute pain related to intestinal distention, ischemia, or obstruction

- Help patient assume a comfortable position (one that places minimum stress on the abdominal muscles); limit sudden movement and abdominal examination.
- Provide analgesics as prescribed.

NIC Coping Assistance

Anxiety related to fear of the unknown and impending surgery

- Provide emotional support for patient and family *because the pain is acute and frightening and surgery is often imminent.*
- Reassure patient and explain to patient and family all the tests and procedures. Provide preoperative teaching.

Patient Education/Continuum of Care Plan

1. Do primary postoperative teaching if resection and anastomosis of small bowel obstruction were performed. This includes showering, activity progression, driving, and returning to work.
2. Colonic obstructions are often treated with a temporary diverting colostomy, and patient requires instruction in colostomy care and plans for continued surgical intervention, and education about primary cause of obstruction (see pp. 730-732).

Evaluation/Patient Outcomes

Tissue Perfusion Management: Fluid balance is maintained. Patient returns to normal hydration levels as assessed by skin turgor, color, and mucous membrane, blood pressure and pulse, and urinary output.

Physical Comfort Promotion: Comfort level is achieved. Patient shows reduction or absence of guarding or protective behavior. Patient uses pain control strategies appropriately. Patient verbalizes increased control over pain.

Coping Assistance: Anxiety is reduced. Patient shows absence or reduction of defining characteristics indicating presence of anxiety.

INTESTINAL ISCHEMIA

Intestinal ischemia may develop when the mesenteric vascular supply is insufficient. Acute and chronic occlusion of blood flow to the splanchnic bed, thrombosis or embolus of the superior mesenteric artery, strangulation obstructions, chronic vascular insufficiency, anoxia, hypotension, or other low-flow states may lead to intestinal ischemia.

Intestinal ischemia has in the past been difficult to diagnose. The symptoms initially do not correspond with physical examination and laboratory findings. As the ischemia progresses, the severity of the patient's condition becomes apparent, and perforation and peritonitis may have already occurred. Advances in angiography have assisted the physician in diagnosing intestinal ischemias. Awareness of intestinal ischemias is increasing, and angiography is being used to rule out acute occlusion of vessels when patients are seen with sudden onset of severe abdominal pain. Poor perfusion of the intestine is known to result in ischemia, and the syndromes of poor perfusion are gaining more attention. The frequency of thrombosis or embolus as the cause of mesenteric ischemia has been reported to be as high as 50%.[7]

Advances in vascular surgery and advances in nutritional and fluid replacement after intestinal resections have allowed a more aggressive approach in the treatment of intestinal ischemias. Knowledge of predisposing factors may improve the likelihood of clinical awareness and suspicion leading to earlier diagnosis and more favorable outcomes. These include cardiac dysrhythmias, myocardial infarction, peripheral vascular disease, embolic disease, hypotension, and postoperative status.[33]

PATHOPHYSIOLOGY

The blood flow to the intestines may be affected by a variety of factors.[26] The following factors increase splanchnic blood flow:

- Presence of food
- Digestive hormones: gastrin, secretin, and cholecystokinin
- Metabolite-produced muscle activity
- Beta-stimulating sympathomimetic amines

The following factors decrease splanchnic blood flow:

- Physical activities
- Abdominal distention (marked intraluminal pressure)
- Alpha-stimulating sympathomimetic amines
- Cardiac glycosides (digitalis)

The response to the alteration in blood flow depends on the degree of obstruction of blood flow, the rapidity of onset, the duration of the process, and the efficiency of the collateral circulation. Disease processes may affect both large and small vessels. This section reviews the normal pattern of blood flow to the intestines; the cause of alteration of blood flow, including a variety of diseases that affect blood distribution to the bowel; and the pathophysiology of events.

The intestine receives its blood supply from the celiac, the superior mesenteric, and the inferior mesenteric arteries. These three major vessels arise from the abdominal aorta and subdivide into a complex collateral circulation. The celiac artery divides into the splenic, left gastric, and hepatic arteries to supply the stomach, proximal duodenum, liver, pancreas, and spleen. The hepatic artery divides into the gastroduodenal artery, which divides to form the superior pancreaticoduodenal and right gastroepiploic arteries. The celiac axis is interconnected with the superior mesenteric artery through pancreaticoduodenal arcades. Ischemic necrosis of the stomach is uncommon because of this rich collateral network.

The superior mesenteric artery divides into the ileocolic, middle colic, and right colic arteries. The terminal ileum, cecum, and proximal ascending colon are supplied by the ileocolic artery. The ascending colon and hepatic flexure are supplied by the right colic artery. The middle colic vessel supplies the proximal portion of the transverse colon.

In addition to the above branches, the superior mesenteric artery divides into smaller arteries that supply the jejunum and ileum. The superior mesenteric artery connects with the celiac axis through the pancreaticoduodenal artery. In this way the small intestine receives its blood flow.

The vessels originating from the superior mesenteric artery ultimately enter the wall of the intestine as end arteries. Few anastomotic connections are found in the bowel wall. Vasculitis may result in the selective occlusion of the distal vessels and may lead to segmental infarction and small bowel ischemia and necrosis.

The superior mesenteric artery is susceptible to atherosclerotic changes and is a common site for thrombosis and embolus. The inverted Y shape of the superior mesenteric artery as it leaves the aorta provides a channel for emboli. Thromboses and emboli tend to occlude the superior mesenteric artery within 2 cm of its origin off the aorta.

The inferior mesenteric artery supplies blood to the distal transverse colon, the descending and sigmoid colon, and proximal portions of the rectum. The distal transverse colon and the splenic flexure appear to be more vulnerable to ischemia. A "watershed" area refers to branches of the inferior mesenteric artery anastomosing with the superior artery branches in the rectosigmoid area. The branches involved are the inferior mesenteric and the hypogastric.

Acute vascular occlusion may be the result of thrombosis or embolus to the superior mesenteric artery. The development of emboli is associated with atrial fibrillation in patients with subacute bacterial endocarditis and cardiac valve disease, mural thrombosis of myocardial infarct, and post-intracardiac surgery. Thrombosis of mesenteric vessels is associated with polycythemia, sickle cell trait, intraabdominal sepsis, pancreatic disorders, and blood dyscrasias. It may also occur after bowel surgery, other major surgery, or abdominal trauma, when there may be a decrease in blood flow to the mesentery. Infarction of the bowel results in a sudden onset of severe abdominal pain, distention, fluid loss, and shock.

Chronic intestinal angina is an obstructive vascular disease involving atherosclerotic changes in two of the three major vessels. An increase in mesenteric blood flow is required to supply oxygen for the metabolic processes of digestion, absorption, and increased peristalsis. Abdominal pain occurs when the superior mesenteric artery supply is less than the demand of the smooth muscle activity in the intestine. The patient may fear eating and begin losing weight. Between meals, the patient is free of pain. Diagnosis may be delayed because many physicians first test the patient for cancer because weight loss and pain in older persons are associated with malignancies. Intestinal ischemia may progress to frank infarction of the intestine.

Nonocclusive intestinal ischemia accounts for up to 50% of the cases.[33] Patients with recent myocardial infarctions, severe congestive cardiac failure, shock, anoxia, or hypotension may have a nonocclusive intestinal ischemia develop. An episode of inadequate cardiac output and poor tissue perfusion results in shunting of blood away from the gut to vital organs. The use of alpha-adrenergic vasoconstrictors in patients in shock adds to the effect of the increased secretions of endogenous catecholamines, further reducing mesenteric blood flow. Other drugs that may negatively influence intestinal circulation include vasopressin, propranolol, estrogens, and ergot derivatives.

The mucosa layer is the most sensitive to oxygen deprivation because it has the highest energy requirement as a result of its high metabolic activity and rapid cell turnover. The mucosa undergoes hemorrhagic necrosis. As the anoxia continues, the necrosis becomes transmural (involving all layers of the bowel wall).

The patient who has nonocclusive intestinal ischemia develop may have evidence of some degree of occlusive or atherosclerotic changes in smaller splanchnic vessels.

Digitalis has been associated with the development of poor perfusion syndromes. Digoxin constricts splanchnic vessels. In patients with early intestinal infarction, considerations should be made regarding discontinuation of digoxin therapy.[7]

Vasculitis has been associated with mesenteric infarction in approximately 3% of reported cases. However, the vasculitis associated with systemic disorders may be seen as intestinal angina or frank infarction. The systemic disorders include polyarteritis nodosa, lupus erythematosus, dermatomyositis, rheumatoid vasculitis, scleroderma, anaphylactoid purpura, and Degos' disease. Table 10-3 examines the bowel involvement that occurs as a result of systemic vasculitis.

Certain surgical procedures such as coarctation of the aorta, excision of abdominal aneurysms, and iliac or femoral grafts are associated with mesenteric vascular insufficiency.

The oxygenation of the bowel depends on patency of the major arterial vessels, arteriolar resistance, adequacy of perfusion pressure, arterial oxygen saturation, and oxygen need.

Table 10-3 Systemic Disorders Affecting Splanchnic Perfusion

Disorder	Definition	Gastrointestinal Implications
Polyarteritis nodosa	A progressive, polymorphic disease of connective tissue characterized by numerous large, palpable or visible nodules in clusters along segments of medium-sized arteries	Segmental ischemia with ulceration, hemorrhage, or perforation to massive infarction of bowel; may also have hepatic artery thrombosis; nodules obstruct lumen of vessels
Lupus erythematosus	A chronic inflammatory collagen disease affecting many systems; includes severe vasculitis, renal involvement, and lesions of skin and nervous system.	Segmental lesions of ischemia progressing to necrosis and perforation; involvement of submucosa and muscularis leads to protein-losing enteropathy; abdominal pain may be caused by serositis or acute pancreatitis; ulcerative colitis and Crohn's disease have been associated with lupus erythematosus; diagnosis of gastrointestinal involvement difficult to evaluate
Dermatomyositis	A disease of the connective tissue characterized by pruritic or eczematous inflammation of skin and tenderness and weakness of muscles	Vasculitis associated with ischemia of bowel; increased incidence of gastrointestinal cancers with this disorder
Rheumatoid vasculitis	A collagen disease that affects the connective tissue by inflammation and fibrinoid degeneration	Vasculitis associated with intestinal ischemia; occurs with abdominal pain
Scleroderma	A relatively rare autoimmune disease affecting blood vessels and connective tissue; most common in middle-age women	Bowel symptoms arise from fibrosis of the intestinal wall and loss of muscle; focal areas of vasculitis may lead to ischemia
Anaphylactoid purpura (Henoch-Schönlein syndrome)	A self-limited hypersensitive vasculitis that occurs primarily in young children; palpable purpuric skin lesions appear on lower abdomen, buttocks, and legs; arthritis and abdominal pain are also seen; occasionally seen in adults, whose prognosis is not as favorable as in children	Colicky abdominal pain; surgery demonstrates submucosal and subserosal hemorrhages; may have upper or lower gastrointestinal bleeding; segmental ischemic bowel episodes may occur but do not generally progress to gross infarction or perforation
Degos' disease (malignant atrophic papulosis)	A rare syndrome of progressive occlusive vascular disease affecting small- and medium-size arteries; primarily involves the skin (malignant atrophic papulosis) and intestine; skin lesions usually precede gastrointestinal symptoms; primarily affects young men	Lesions (identical to skin lesion) are found in mucosa and serosa of bowel; weight loss and diarrhea develop; progresses to intestinal infarction and perforation

Acute or chronic changes of any or all of the above affect the blood flow to the bowel.

The events of intestinal ischemia include structural changes in the cells within 5 minutes of the occlusion of the superior mesenteric artery. The epithelium becomes detached from the basement membrane at the villus tips, and subepithelial blebs form. Within 30 to 60 minutes, the villi are denuded of epithelium. The mucosa undergoes necrosis and ulceration with an inflammatory cell infiltration. A secondary bacterial invasion occurs. In acute ischemic necrosis, massive submucosa edema and bleeding into the mucous membrane develop because of an increase in capillary permeability followed by loss of capillary integrity.

The submucosal edema and hemorrhage are seen as the "thumbprint" pattern in radiographic studies. The exudation of protein-rich fluid, and later blood, found in the intestinal lumen is the result of the loss of epithelial and vascular integrity. Fluid loss and hypovolemia further compromise blood flow to the intestine.

The development of peritonitis indicates the involvement of the muscle and serosa layer and that the perforation is imminent or has occurred. If the ischemic episode is self-limited and does not progress to perforation and resection, the acute inflammatory response resolves spontaneously with stricture formation.

In chronic or gradual reduction of blood flow, the anoxia damages the mucosa initially. The necrosis may be limited to the mucosa, in which event the mucosa will slough with regeneration occurring in 4 to 5 days. The villi may recover, but their shape and functioning abilities are affected and a temporary malabsorption develops that is seen clinically as enterocolitis. As the anoxia continues, the necrosis progresses. A microscopic examination of the bowel may reveal a coagulative necrosis of the inner two thirds of the wall with muscle and serosa uninvolved. A scar may form.

The bowel totally deprived of its blood supply ultimately becomes black and necrotic. The bowel perforates, with leakage of intestinal contents. Bacterial invasion of the necrotic bowel produces gas cysts, massive sepsis, and shock. Repair cannot take place when this degree of injury has occurred, and bowel death usually results. If surgery is performed, it is usually a massive bowel resection resulting often in short bowel syndrome.

Diagnostic Studies and Findings

Plain films of the abdomen (kidney, ureter, and bladder [KUB]): Dilated loops of bowel with air-fluid levels; complete absence of small bowel air; generalized distention (later sign); thickening of bowel wall with "thumbprinting" pattern with edema and fluid (ischemic colitis); string or ring of gas outside lumen of bowel (marked necrosis); gas in portal vein (evidence of leak of bacteria from infarcted bowel); blunt plicae

Angiograpy: Abnormal vascular tree (intestinal angina); demonstrates site of arterial blockage or spasm; absence or severe flow impairment of two of the three vessels supplying the bowel (chronic mesenteric ischemia); angiographic studies generally indicated only in patients with disorders predisposing to embolization but may be used when other tests are negative and patient is symptomatic; also used preoperatively to map vessels that are narrowed or occluded

CT scan: Small bowel distended with fluid and air; wall thickened; may show immediate cause of ischemia or infarction; engorgement of mesenteric veins

Hematocrit: In presence of necrosis, hemoconcentration (decreased fluid volume)

White blood cell count: Leukocytosis (20,000/mm^3 and higher)

Amylase and lipase: Elevated (from leakage into peritoneum or from back-pressure resulting from development of intestinal obstruction)

Multidisciplinary Plan

Surgery

Chronic: Balloon angioplasty (intestinal angina) to improve blood flow; bypass graft, embolectomy, endarterectomy, and reimplantation procedures have been used effectively

Acute: Resection of infarcted bowel, temporary colostomy or ileostomy, and subsequent reanastomosis (colonic ischemia)

Medications

Acute ischemia

- Antiinfective agents: Broad-spectrum antibiotics given to reduce bacterial flora of bowel and treat sepsis
- Vasodilators: Intraarterial infusion of vasodilators (papaverine, telazoline, Urotensin II), for up to 5 days; stop digitalis unless absolutely necessary
- Anticoagulation with heparin followed by bishydroxycoumarin (dicumarol): Used in patients with mesenteric venous occlusion that tends to recur; dosages adjusted based on patient's coagulation time; not recommended for first 48 h after operation because of concern for hemorrhage

General Management

Correction of predisposing factors

Patients with abdominal pain but no evidence of peritonitis or systemic toxicity should be treated conservatively

Acute ischemia

- Intraoperative fluorescein angiography (may be used during surgery to determine viability of bowel and evaluate mesenteric vessels)
- Intravenous fluid replacements, volume expanders
- Nasogastric or intestinal suctioning preoperatively for treatment of ileus
- Total parenteral nutrition (TPN) postoperatively

NURSING CARE

Nursing Assessment

This section is divided into assessments of chronic ischemia of the bowel (i.e., intestinal angina) and acute episodes of ischemia. The acute episodes are similar in progression of symptoms, and therefore not all causes are outlined. Acute occlusive ischemia is used as the example. Exceptions are noted. The assessment of abdominal pain is an example of an area where differences do exist in the acute episodes.

Pain

Intestinal angina: Severe crampy or colicky pain around umbilicus; radiates to back; lasts 2 to 4 hours; no pain between meals

Acute occlusive ischemia: Severe colicky pain in the periumbilical area; as ischemia progresses, pain becomes more severe and poorly localized

Ischemic colitis: Lower abdominal pain of abrupt onset

Mesenteric venous thrombosis: Gradual progression of abdominal pain until it resembles acute occlusive ischemia

Degree of pain out of proportion to findings on abdominal examination

Gastrointestinal Status

History: Recurring pain after meals; sudden onset in patient with atrial fibrillation, prosthetic heart valves, bacterial endocarditis

Intestinal angina: Nausea and vomiting; abdominal bloating; malabsorption with steatorrhea and diarrhea

Acute occlusive ischemia: Copious vomiting and hematemesis indicate necrosis adjacent to ligament of Treitz; gross rectal bleeding

Enterocolitis symptoms: Malabsorption; diarrhea, may be hemorrhagic (seen regardless of cause of ischemia, results from sloughing of mucosa and bacteremia)

Maroon or red blood from rectum

Abdominal Examination

Absence of significant abdominal findings initially; hyperperistalsis, with no tenderness or resistance

After necrosis occurs: Classic signs of peritonitis with rebound tenderness, rigidity, abdominal distention, and ileus

General Status

Mental confusion (elderly in particular); fever; fluid and electrolyte loss, metabolic acidosis, hypovolemic shock

Nutritional Status

Intestinal angina: Weight loss; fear of eating because of chronic malabsorption syndrome; malnutrition

Cardiovascular Status

Shock; hypotension; anoxia; severe congestive heart failure; recent myocardial infarction or some cause that results in shunting of blood away from the gut to "vital" organs; tachycardia

Potential Complications

Hypovolemic shock, perforation, peritonitis

Patient Problems/Nursing Diagnoses & Interventions

NIC Tissue Perfusion Management

Deficient fluid volume related to acute ischemic event

- Replace intravenous fluids and electrolytes, blood, and plasma as ordered.
- Monitor vital signs, central venous pressure, blood pressure, urinary output, diarrhea, and nasogastric aspirations every hour.
- Measure abdominal girth every 8 hours *to assess distention.*
- Notify physician of changes in patient's status, *because they generally indicate a decline in patient's stabilization for surgical intervention*

NIC Physical Comfort Promotion

Acute pain related to acute ischemia

- Help patient assume a comfortable position; limit sudden movement and abdominal examination
- Provide analgesics as prescribed.

NIC Elimination Management

Diarrhea related to colitis caused by ischemia

- Document episodes of steatorrhea and diarrhea (intestinal angina); gross rectal bleeding (acute occlusive ischemia); and hemorrhagic diarrhea (enterocolitis), *which are diagnostic assessments of ischemia of the intestine.*
- Assist patient with cleansing of perianal area. Apply moisture barrier ointment after cleansing *to protect perianal skin.*

NIC Nutrition Support

Imbalanced nutrition: less than body requirements, related to chronic intestinal pain after eating or after resection for acute ischemia

- Provide enteral nutrition as tolerated.
- Initiate and monitor TPN as ordered after operation for significant small bowel resections.
- Nutritionist to see patient for both ongoing assessment and recommendations.

Patient Education/Continuum of Care Plan

Chronic ischemia

1. Help patient understand relationship of eating and pain in intestinal angina.
2. After surgery for venous thrombosis, patient may need instruction regarding anticoagulant therapy.

Acute ischemia

1. In colonic ischemia a temporary colostomy may be performed. If so, patient requires colostomy teaching and plans for surgical closure at a later date.
2. Patient who has had a massive bowel resection may be on home total parenteral nutrition. In these cases patient and family require extensive discharge preparation (i.e., central line care; management of total parenteral nutrition).
3. Help patient deal with increase in diarrhea, especially for first 6 months postoperatively, caused by rapid transit time or varying degrees of malabsorption.

Evaluation/Patient Outcomes

Tissue Perfusion Management: Fluid balance is maintained. Patient returns to normal hydration levels as assessed by skin turgor, color, moist mucous membranes, blood pressure, pulse, and urinary output. Serum electrolytes, hematocrit, and WBC count are within normal limits.

Physical Comfort Promotion: Comfort level is achieved. Reduction in or absence of guarding or protective behavior. Patient uses pain control strategies appropriately. Patient verbalizes increased control over pain.

Elimination Management: Diarrhea is manageable. Patient's perianal skin is intact. Patient understands the use of diet to decrease bowel transit time.

Nutrition Support: Nutritional status is normal. Patient maintains normal body weight. Nutritional status is maintained through home TPN (major resection of small bowel).

IRRITABLE BOWEL SYNDROME

Irritable bowel syndrome (IBS), or functional bowel syndrome, is a disorder of the large bowel that results in altered bowel habits, abdominal pain, and absence of structural or biochemical abnormalities. It is the most common gastrointestinal disorder seen in primary care and gastroenterology practice.

The patient may have diarrhea or constipation or both. Abdominal pain and distention are common.

It is important to recognize the mislabeling of IBS in the past. Nervous colon, spastic colon, and mucous colitis are incorrect terms. Nervous colon recognizes only one aspect of the possible cause of IBS. Spasticity is one sign or response of the colon to the altered motor activity. Inflammation is not present, making "colitis" a misnomer. IBS does not progress or predispose individuals to inflammatory bowel disease or cancer.

The incidence of IBS is considered high, but accurate data on the prevalence are not available. IBS does not lead to death and therefore does not appear on death certificates. Rarely does IBS require hospitalization. IBS is a leading cause of absenteeism from work. Many people with IBS do not seek medical attention because they have mild symptoms, making it more difficult to estimate the prevalence.

PATHOPHYSIOLOGY

IBS is a functional disorder of gastrointestinal motility. The abdominal pain and altered bowel pattern are caused by altered motility of the small and large intestines that may be affected by stress and certain foods. Visceral hypersensitivity has been noted in this patient population.[7]

Two patterns of IBS are identified: painful IBS with diarrhea, constipation, or both and IBS with painless diarrhea. The two types of IBS may be differentiated on observations of motility recordings.

Segmental contractions are the predominant form of normal motor activity in the colon, consisting of 90% of recorded motor activity. Segmental contractions slow the forward progress of stool, promoting mixing, absorption, and dehydration. Segmental contractions appear as haustral markings on barium studies. Increasing segmental contractions produce constipation, whereas decreasing segmentation results in diarrhea.

Although motility studies demonstrate abnormalities throughout the alimentary tract in patients with IBS, no one abnormality clearly separates IBS from organic gastrointestinal disease or even from normal bowel function.[54] Some of the more common (but not pathognomonic) abnormalities are described below. In general, a diagnosis of IBS is based on recognition of characteristic symptom patterns, probability, and exclusion of organic gastrointestinal disease.

A pattern of hypermotility with high-amplitude pressure waves is common in patients with painful IBS. Motility in the pain-free diarrheal-predominant IBS is normal or lower than normal.

Motility of the bowel may be affected by a variety of factors. For example, sleep lowers the motor activity in the colon. This may account for the infrequency of nocturnal symptoms. The presence of nocturnal symptoms usually indicates an organic etiology rather than the functional cause of IBS.

Anxiety, depression, fear, and hostility have been identified in IBS, as well as in other gastrointestinal disorders. Stress and emotions alone do not cause IBS but are related to the clinical course. Stress can be related to the onset of symptoms. Diarrhea can readily be associated with stressful situations such as test taking or job interviews. Constipation is not apparent for several days, and it may be more difficult to pinpoint the source of anxiety or generalized depression.

Meals, or the ingestion of food and caffeine, will stimulate colonic hypermotility in irritable bowel syndrome. The postprandial symptoms are related to this effect. Normally, a meal will lengthen segmental contractions, allowing for additional mixing and absorption, and the effect of the meal slows after approximately 50 minutes. In IBS the meal stimulation of segmental contractions may be blunted and the effect continues postprandially, gradually becoming stronger.

The gastroileocolic response to food ingestion moves intestinal contents forward, emptying material in the distal colon and creating distention. Colon distention may induce exaggerated spastic contractions in IBS. Patients with alternating diarrhea and constipation or diarrhea-predominant IBS often have a bowel movement after every meal. For some this may be the only symptom of IBS.

Neurohumoral agents, such as cholinergic, anticholinergic, adrenergic, and adrenergic-blocking substances, produce hyperactivity of the colon in both normal bowels and in irritable bowel syndrome. In IBS, response to neurohumoral agents is more pronounced and occurs during both symptomatic and asymptomatic periods.

Anticholinergic agents affect colonic activity induced by meals. Anticholinergics suppress an early neurogenic myoelectric and motor reflex component of the gastrocolic reflex in normal subjects. In IBS the myoelectric and motor reflex is not suppressed, but anticholinergics inhibit the second, delayed component of gastrocolic reflex, which is hormonally mediated.

The gastrointestinal hormones that affect motility include cholecystokinin, gastrin, glucagon, and vasoactive intestinal peptide. Cholecystokinin is associated with abdominal pain and colonic hypermotility when given through infusion. Because cholecystokinin is released after a meal, this may account for the postprandial pain in IBS. Also, the delayed hormonally meditated phase of the gastrocolic reflex depends on the fatty content of the meal. This indicates a relationship with cholecystokinin that produces colonic contractions.

New therapies being studied for the treatment of IBS include serotonin antagonists, which may inhibit excitation of extrinsic sensory nerves without interfering with intrinsic enteric reflexes, and somatostatin analog, which reduces visceral sensation, inhibits tonic response, and increases phasic response to a meal.[8]

Diagnostic Studies and Findings

No specific radiographic, endoscopic, or biochemical abnormalities are associated with the diagnosis of IBS. A detailed history using established symptom criteria can often exclude most organic diseases that can cause symptoms consistent with IBS. The extent of the diagnostic evaluation required to exclude organic disease is guided by the patient's symptoms and history.[7] Diagnosis is made by the exclusion of organic diseases with similar symptoms, as follows:

Sigmoidoscopy: Spastic contractions may prevent passage of the instrument beyond 10 to 12 cm; reproduction of symptoms with air insufflation; mucosa free of ulcers, bleeding, friability, and masses; do not use enemas or cathartics before sigmoidoscopy (may produce edema, obscuring the normal colon appearance); to rule out colon cancer, polyps, colitis, diverticulosis, and hemorrhoids

Manometric studies: May be used to evaluate electric response to colon; balloons are placed in rectosigmoidal colon (cephalad balloon) and rectum (caudad balloon), and 20 mm of air is instilled into the cephalad balloon every 20 minutes; balloon mimics presence of stool in the area; a graph recording is made of the bowel response to the stimulus; response in a normal bowel is a brief contraction in the rectosigmoid colon and rectum, with a rapid return to the prestimulus state; in patient with IBS, the distention may produce a diffuse spastic contraction in the rectosigmoid colon and rectum

Biopsy: To rule out other disorders; not helpful in diagnosing IBS

Stool test for guaiac: To rule out inflammatory bowel diseases and malignancy

Stool stains: To rule out motile amebic trophozoites, leukocytes, and mucus

Stool cultures: To rule out ova and parasites, specifically *Giardia*

Complete blood count (CBC): To rule out anemia and inflammation

Differential blood cell count (eosinophilia): To rule out parasitosis, cytosis (suggests tuberculosis), and vacuolated cells (suggest inflammation)

Three-day trial on lactose-free diet, lactose tolerance test, or breath hydrogen test: To rule out lactose insufficiency in patients with distention and bloating or diarrhea

Double-contrast barium enema: Exaggerated haustral contractions or absence of haustrations; narrow lumen with pellet stones; lumen easily dilated; rule out colon cancer, polyps, diverticulosis

Cholecystogram or ultrasonography of gallbladder: To rule out gallbladder disease in presence of dyspepsia

Small bowel series: To rule out obstruction of bowel, if diarrhea and symptoms suggest obstruction

Colonoscopy: To rule out inflammatory bowel disease, polyps, diverticulosis, or colon cancer when clinically justified as in change in symptoms in patient with long-standing IBS; uncontrollable exacerbation of IBS

Thyroid function: To rule out hyperthyroidism or hypothyroidism if constipation predominates

Multidisciplinary Plan

Surgery

Rare

Medications

Bulk-forming laxatives: Psyllium preparations (Metamucil, Konsyl, Mitrolan) taken at mealtimes; in obese patients before meals and in thin patients after meals (hydrophilic properties bind water, preventing excessive dehydration of stool and excess liquidity); may improve symptoms

Antidiarrheal agents
- Loperamide (Imodium), 2 mg q6-8h (preferred, does not cross blood-brain barrier)
- Diphenoxylate (Lomotil), 2.5 to 5 mg q4-6h
- Dependency on antidiarrheals can develop; slow withdrawal of medicines as coping abilities are developed is recommended; may improve symptoms

Antispasmodic agents
- *Anticholinergics*
  - Dicyclomine (Bentyl), 20 mg 30-45 min before meals
  - Propantheline (Pro-Banthine), 15 mg 30-45 min before meals
  - Hyoscyamine (Levsin), 1-2 tablets q4h as needed, *not* before meals
- *Calcium channel blockers:* Currently under investigation for treatment of IBS based on smooth muscle relaxant properties and inhibitory effects on gastrocolonic response

General Management

Patient should be placed on high-fiber (12 to 16 g/day as 2 tablespoons of bran qid; gradually reduced), low-lactose, no-caffeine diet before trying drug therapy

Low-fat diet (to reduce stimulation of cholecystokinin)

NURSING CARE

Nursing Assessment

General status: Tense, anxious patient who may be unaware of features of tenseness; no evidence of weight loss

Pain: Lower abdominal pain: often precipitated by meals; often relieved by defecation

Gastrointestinal status: Alternating diarrhea and constipation, diarrhea, or constipation
- Constipation
  - Episodic initially, becomes continuous, increasingly intractable to laxatives and later to enemas
  - Stools: Hard and narrow
  - Objectively defined as passage of fewer than three stools per week; sometimes patient will have diarrhea following a week of constipation
  - Subjectively defined as difficult or painful evacuation

Diarrhea
- Defined as loose, mushy, or watery stools
- Urgency and tenseness in the morning or after meals, followed by evacuation
- Initial movement may be of normal consistency and is rapidly followed by a softer, unformed stool and then by increasingly loose stools
- Postprandial diarrhea correlates with quantity rather than type of food
- Patients with diarrhea-only type of IBS more likely to have explosive, watery stools

Abdominal examination: Palpable, tender sigmoid colon

Potential Complications
Diarrhea, constipation, anxiety

Patient Problems/Nursing Diagnoses & Interventions

NIC Elimination Management
Constipation related to gastrointestinal motility disorder and stress

Diarrhea related to gastrointestinal motility disorder and stress
- Administer bulk laxatives as ordered.
- Administer antidiarrheal medications as ordered.
- Help patient identify irritating or troublesome foods *because diet may affect motility in IBS.*

NIC Coping Assistance
Ineffective coping related to stress
- Help patient recognize role of emotions, stress, and diet in symptoms of IBS.
- Help patient and family understand that symptoms are based on functional motility problems and that psychosocial stress accentuates rather than causes symptoms.
- Help patient identify sources of stress and counterbalancing relaxation techniques.
- Encourage patient to keep a diary of events and symptoms.
- Psychotherapy may be helpful for patients who do not show improvement on medications.

Patient Education/Continuum of Care Plan
1. Provide information on irritable bowel syndrome. Patient education material is available through National Digestive Disease Education Information Clearinghouse, NIH, 1555 Wilson Blvd., Suite 600, Rosslyn, VA 22209-2461.
2. Instruct patient in necessary diet alterations. Inform patient that often it is possible to manage with diet and stress reduction without using any medications.
3. Provide written instructions for medications prescribed for the management of IBS by physician. Ensure that patient knows names, amounts, and rationales for treatment plan.

Evaluation/Patient Outcomes
Elimination Management: Bowel functioning is normal. Diarrhea and constipation are relieved, and recurrences are managed through medical regimen and stress reduction.

Coping Assistance: Psychosocial stress is reduced. Patient can identify sources of stress and uses effective coping mechanisms. Combination of counseling, relaxation techniques, modification of diet (avoiding irritating foods), and medications is effective in relieving symptoms. Symptoms are managed so that lifestyle does not center around bowel elimination.

Lactose Intolerance

Lactose intolerance results from a deficiency of the enzyme lactase. Lactase (found in the brush border of the intestinal villi) is necessary for the digestion or breakdown of the disaccharide lactose (found in milk and milk products). Lactose intolerance is a common cause of diarrhea, crampy abdominal pain, gas, and bloating.

Lactase deficiency may have a genetic basis and certainly is expressed more in some population groups than in others. In the United States, the prevalence of lactose maldigestion has been estimated at about 25% of the population, with extensive occurrence in Mexican-Americans, Native Americans, African-Americans, and Asian-Americans.[23]

Primary disaccharidase deficiency is a congenital, hereditary absence of the lactase enzyme. The symptoms may be present from birth or may become apparent in middle life. By the age of 10 to 20 years, most persons with genetic tendencies for lactase deficiency have the same low level of lactase as adults. Primary lactase insufficiency is associated with a normal bowel mucosa and epithelial cells.

Secondary disaccharidase deficiency occurs when injury or disease damages the brush border of the intestinal mucosa. The secondary lactase deficiency is usually temporary. Diseases or disorders associated with secondary lactase insufficiency include gastroenteritis, ulcerative colitis, Crohn's disease, operative procedures (partial gastrectomy, small bowel resection), and cholera.

Lactose maldigestion does not mean that one is allergic to milk, dairy foods, or dairy products. A milk allergy is an allergy related to proteins in milk, not lactose. Dairy products provide key nutrients such as calcium, vitamins A and D, riboflavin, and phosphorus. Research suggests that people with medically confirmed lactose maldigestion can include the recommended number of servings of milk and other dairy foods in their diets without experiencing gastrointestinal discomfort.[23]

Pathophysiology

The basis of the symptoms found in lactose intolerance is an excessive amount of sugar in the bowel lumen. Disaccharides form a large part of the dietary carbohydrate, and the three predominant forms are maltose (glucose and glucose), lactose (glucose and galactose), and sucrose (glucose and fructose). The disaccharides are not digested by enzymes in the lumen of the bowel but are taken into the brush border of the intestinal mucosal cell. The disaccharide is split by enzymes in the brush border into the simple sugars (glucose, galactose, and fructose), which can be further absorbed and metabolized. The enzymes of the brush border are lactase, sucrase, and a series of four enzymes that are called maltase.

The lactose absorption begins in the duodenum, and lactase activity is highest in the jejunum and nearly absent in the ileum. The process of lactose digestion is slower, normally, than sucrose and maltose. The blood sugar level after a meal of lactose will show little increase.

Lactase is present in the microvillus membrane of the columnar epithelial cells. Many intestinal bacteria also contain lactases. The two forms of lactase differ in their actions. Gut lactase splits the disaccharide, lactose, into glucose and galactose. Bacterial lactase results in the formation of hydrogen gas, carbon dioxide, and short-chain organic acids.

The diarrhea associated with lactose intolerance is caused by the osmotic effect of the lactose in the small bowel. The osmotic load of the lactose increases fluid secretion into the small bowel. The organic acids and fermentation products of the bacterial lactase in the colon impede colonic absorption. The pH of the stools in children may drop to 5.5 in response to the presence of organic acids.

The bloating and gaseous symptoms are the end products of bacterial lactase breaking down lactose.

DIAGNOSTIC STUDIES AND FINDINGS

Dietary trial: 3 weeks on a lactose-free diet: Absence of gastrointestinal symptoms

Lactose tolerance test: Positive for lactose intolerance: blood sugar rise less than or equal to 20 mg/dl after lactose load of 50 g/m^2 in children or 50 g in adults; accompanied by characteristic symptoms

Hydrogen breath test: A rise of more than 20 parts per million after administration of oral lactose is consistent with lactose intolerance (NOTE: Oral antibiotics can suppress bacteria that produce hydrogen; smoking increases breath hydrogen concentrations; small percentage of individuals do not normally produce hydrogen gas)

Stool pH: Drop from the normal pH of 7.0 or 8.0 to 5.5 (more common in children)

MULTIDISCIPLINARY PLAN

Medications

Commercial lactase enzyme preparation can be used in milk for patients with limited tolerance to milk

General Management

Lactose-controlled diet (is tolerated well by most individuals; lactose added until symptoms appear and then decreased until asymptomatic)

Calcium supplements (particularly in postmenopausal women)

Nutritional Consultation

For nutritional prescription, lactose and diet intake, focusing on calcium

NURSING CARE

NURSING ASSESSMENT

Gastrointestinal status: Excessive gas and flatus; abdominal gurgling and pain; persistent to profuse diarrhea; may vary from mild to extreme

Nutritional status: Relationship between foods and onset of abdominal symptoms; history as to dietary sources of calcium, milk intolerance

POTENTIAL COMPLICATIONS

Diarrhea

PATIENT PROBLEMS/NURSING DIAGNOSES & INTERVENTIONS

NIC ELIMINATION MANAGEMENT

Diarrhea related to osmotic effect of unhydrolyzed sugars in the colon

- Record amount, frequency, and consistency of bowel movements.
- Administer commercial lactase enzyme preparations as ordered.

NIC NUTRITION SUPPORT

Imbalanced nutrition: less than body requirements, related to inability to eat calcium-rich (Ca^{++}) foods; related to undiagnosed lactose intolerance with weight loss

- Provide calcium supplements as ordered.
- Refer mothers of infants with diarrhea and failure to thrive to physician *for evaluation of lactase deficiency versus other malabsorption syndromes.*
- Ensure patient's understanding of lactose-controlled diet and potential to add lactose-containing foods as tolerated.

PATIENT EDUCATION/CONTINUUM OF CARE PLAN

1. Provide oral and written instructions on lactose-controlled diets.
2. Patients should be taught to read all packaged food labels for lactose content and to select foods per nutrition prescription.

EVALUATION/PATIENT OUTCOMES

Elimination Management: Bowel elimination is normal. There are no symptoms with lactose-controlled diet.

Nutrition Support: Nutritional status is good. Calcium level is normal; there are no signs of bone disease.

CELIAC SPRUE

Celiac sprue is a malabsorption disease that can occur at any age. The mucosa of the small intestine is damaged by gluten-containing grains (wheat, barley, rye, and oats).

Celiac sprue (FIG. 10-14) may cause severe malabsorption from the small bowel, resulting in marked malnutrition, debilitation, dehydration, and complications of nutrient and vitamin deficiencies. Other associated disorders include depression, thyroid disease, peptic ulcer disease, and diabetes mellitus.

Only 50% of patients have gastrointestinal symptoms when initially examined. Other complaints include dermatitis herpetiformis, anemia, tetany, osteopenia, muscle atrophy, fatigue, and weight loss.[7]

The onset of celiac sprue symptoms occurs at three peak periods. The first peak occurs when the infant's diet is changed

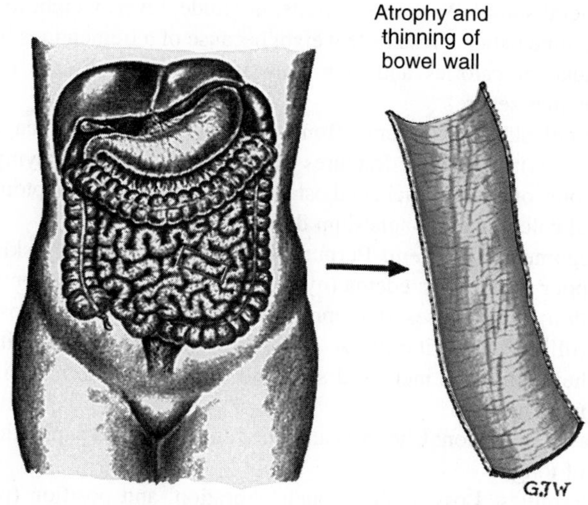

FIG. 10-14
Celiac sprue (primary malabsorption). (From Doughty.[10])

to include cereals. There is a period during late childhood when the disease becomes asymptomatic; however, in the third and fourth decades the second onset of symptoms occurs. The third peak occurs after the age of 60.[7] Unequivocal evidence of celiac sprue in childhood indicates a need to remain on a gluten-free diet indefinitely to avoid recurrent disease during adult life.

PATHOPHYSIOLOGY

In celiac sprue the interaction of the water-soluble protein moiety (gluten) with the mucosa of the small bowel changes the absorptive surface structures of the mucosa. Ingestion of gluten-containing foods subsequently causes bloating, malaise, abdominal cramps, and diarrhea within a few hours. The fecal fat excretion increases. The intestinal absorptive cells are damaged. The dying absorptive cells are sloughed from the mucosal surface more rapidly than normal. The number of proliferating cells increases, and the crypts become hyperplastic to compensate for the excessive loss of absorptive cells. The mucosal layer of the small bowel appears flat, the villi are absent, and the intestinal crypts are markedly elongated and open onto a flat, absorptive surface. These structural changes decrease the amount of epithelial surface available for digestion and absorption. Many of the mucosal enzymes necessary for digestion and absorption are altered in the damaged mucosal cells. Thus the absorptive cells are reduced in number and functionally compromised. The crypt cells are increased in number, which accounts for the elongation of the crypts.

Celiac sprue may involve varying lengths of small intestine. The amount of involved bowel does correlate with the severity of the clinical symptoms. The proximal bowel is always involved and is usually more severely involved than the distal bowel. In mild cases of celiac sprue, some villous structure will remain even in the proximal bowel.

Treatment with a gluten-free diet results in significant improvements in the intestinal mucosa. The absorptive cells improve in days. The mucosa of the distal small intestine improves more rapidly than the proximal bowel, which is more severely involved. It may take months or years to reach its full recovery. Complete reversion to normal is uncommon. This may be in part related to inadvertent gluten ingestion.

The cause of gluten damage to the intestinal mucosa is not known. Four possible mechanisms are an immune response to dietary gluten, a genetic disorder, a metabolic disorder, and a viral disorder. Circulating antibodies to gluten fractions have been found in patients with celiac sprue. However, there does not appear to be a correlation between the presence of the circulating antibodies and the severity of the disease. Researchers have also found that immunoglobulins synthesized by celiac sprue mucosa have antigluten specificity. Other data link celiac disease to a rare virus, human adenovirus 12. This virus may be responsible for initiating the immune system's reaction to gluten, thus causing the disease. Although evidence implicates the immune response theory, it is inconclusive at this time.

Genetic factors do play a role in celiac sprue. Celiac sprue occurs in 5% to 15% of first-degree relatives with celiac sprue.[7]

Antigens have been detected on the surface of B lymphocytes that are identified from antisera of celiac sprue patients. These antigens are present in most patients with celiac sprue and in all the parents of celiac sprue patients. This suggests a recessive inheritance.[37] It may be that the cause is a combined genetic and immune response.

Several factors contribute to the diarrhea in celiac sprue. The stool volume and osmotic load entering the colon are increased by the malabsorption in the small bowel. Water and electrolytes are secreted into the upper small bowel lumen rather than being absorbed. Cholecystokinin and secretin release is impaired in celiac sprue, decreasing pancreatic and biliary secretions and compromising digestion. Thus the digestion and absorption of nutrients, fluids, and electrolytes is impaired in the small bowel, resulting in higher stool volume and the osmotic load. The diarrhea is aggravated by the presence of dietary fats and bile salts. The excessive dietary fat is broken down by the colon bacteria into hydroxy fatty acids, which are potent, irritating cathartics. If the terminal ileum is involved, conjugated bile salts are absorbed and enter the colon. Bile salts have a direct cathartic action in the colon.

Esophageal cancer and intestinal lymphomas have been associated with celiac sprue. Patients who have been responding well to a gluten-free diet and who suddenly have gastrointestinal systems develop (weight loss, malabsorption, abdominal pain, bleeding) should undergo diagnostic studies to rule out carcinoma. Before the diagnostic workup, it is necessary to ask the patient about adherence to the gluten-free diet. Any amount of gluten can damage the mucosa and create symptoms.

Refractory sprue is another complication. In refractory sprue, patients initially respond to a strict gluten-free diet and then relapse despite maintaining the diet. Some of these patients respond to corticosteroids. If patients do not respond, malabsorption becomes progressive and may lead to death. Since the advent of home total parenteral nutrition, however, death is less common.

Mucosal ulceration and intestinal strictures can develop in celiac sprue. The ulcers may perforate, with ensuing peritonitis. Intestinal strictures may lead to intestinal obstructions.

DIAGNOSTIC STUDIES AND FINDINGS

Jejunal biopsy (serial sections): Most valuable diagnostic procedure; flat mucosal surface; shortened or absent villi; elongated intestinal crypts; villous atrophy with crypt hyperplasia.

Quantitative stool for fat, 72- to 96-hour collection: Normal results: 2 to 7 g of fat per 24 hours while ingesting 100 g/day; not specific for malabsorption

Hemoglobin, hematocrit, folic acid, and vitamin B_{12} levels: Anemia common in celiac sprue; anemia may be related to folic acid or vitamin B_{12} deficiencies

IgG antigliadin, IgA antigliadin, and IgA antiendomysial antibodies: If all detected, positive predictive value for celiac sprue is 99%; expensive; poorly standardized among laboratories

Barium contrast studies: barium swallow: Dilation of small intestine; marked coarsening of mucosal pattern or complete obliteration of mucosal folds; fragmentation of barium; delayed transit time of barium

Gluten challenge: After response to gluten-free diet, rechallenge bowel to establish diagnosis unequivocally

MULTIDISCIPLINARY PLAN

The only treatment is a permanent gluten-free diet.

Medications

Used to manage effects of malnutrition and malabsorption

Hematinic agent

Anemia: Iron

Vitamins

Anemia: Folic acid, vitamin B_{12}

Multivitamins daily to replace vitamins A, C, and E; thiamine; riboflavin; niacin; and pyridoxine

Electrolyte and nutritional replacements

Dehydration: Intravenous fluid with potassium chloride added

Calcium: Tetany, 1-2 g IV calcium gluconate

Magnesium: Tetany, 0.5 g magnesium sulfate in dilute solution IV, *or*

100 mEq magnesium chloride PO

Osteomalacia: Calcium gluconate or calcium lactate, 6-8 g/day and oral vitamin D

Nutritional Consultation

Nutritional assessment to instruct patient regarding gluten-free diet

NURSING CARE

NURSING ASSESSMENT

Gastrointestinal status

Diarrhea: Watery, bulky, semiformed, light tan or grayish, greasy-appearing, rancid odor; frequency, volume, consistency of stools

Constipation: Large quantities of "puttylike" stool

Abdominal examination: Excessive amounts of malodorous flatus; protuberant and tympanic; "doughy" consistency; ascites (hypoproteinemia)

General status: Weakness, fatigue, lassitude, fever; weight loss (some patients lose little weight because of a tremendous intake of calories and enormous appetite until disease becomes severe)

Musculoskeletal system: Bone pain (low back, rib cage, pelvis); pathologic fractures (uncommon); signs and symptoms of osteomalacia and osteoporosis; signs and symptoms of calcium and magnesium depletion

Integumentary system: Purpura; clubbing of nails; dry skin; poor skin turgor; edema (hypoproteinemia); skin pigmentation; ecchymoses (hypoprothrombinemia); hyperkeratosis follicularis (vitamin A deficiency); pallor; dermatitis herpetiformis; increased skin and mucous membrane pigmentation

Oral examination: Cheilosis and glossitis; decreased papillation of tongue

Extremities: Loss of light touch, vibration, and position (peripheral neuropathy)

Psychosocial concerns: Coping with diagnosis; compliance with diet; relationship support

POTENTIAL COMPLICATIONS

Marked malnutrition, dehydration, cancer, refractory sprue

PATIENT PROBLEMS/NURSING DIAGNOSES & INTERVENTIONS

NIC NUTRITION SUPPORT

Imbalanced nutrition: less than body requirements, related to malabsorption

- Weigh patient daily.
- Provide dietary supplements as ordered; in severe malabsorption, TPN may be used during initial stabilization period.
- Check dietary trays for foods containing gluten.
- Support patient and family as they learn the implications of a gluten-free diet.
- Evaluate patient's comprehension of dietary patient education.
- Evaluate, in outpatient setting, patient's dietary intake and nutritional status (weight gain and stabilization); a diary may be helpful.

NIC ELIMINATION MANAGEMENT

Diarrhea related to gluten sensitivity

- Ensure patient's understanding of relationship between diarrhea and gluten-containing foods.
- Replace intravenous fluids and electrolytes, vitamins, and minerals as ordered.

NIC COPING ASSISTANCE

Anxiety related to strict nutritional restrictions and increased chances of cancer

- Discuss with patient the implications of diet restrictions on social functioning, allowing patient to verbalize his or her concerns.
- Enlist help of family members or significant others in assisting patient to follow recommended diet.

- Provide patient with specific information regarding increased risk of cancer.

Patient Education/Continuum of Care Plan

1. Provide written and oral instructions on a gluten-free diet (no wheat or wheat products).
2. Encourage patient to buy a cookbook on gluten-free cooking.
3. Instruct patient to read packaged food labels carefully. Wheat flour is often used as an extender in processed foods and is in many brands of ice cream, salad dressings, canned foods, instant coffee, catsup, mustard, and candy bars.
4. Provide consultation with a nutritionist to teach patient about presence of gluten in many foods.
5. Ensure that patient understands increased risk of cancer and understands importance of reporting any changes in symptoms to health care provider.

Evaluation/Patient Outcomes

Nutrition Support: Nutrition is adequate. Patient tolerates recommended diet. Patient has an appetite. Patient is able to plan menus around dietary restrictions. Patient achieves and maintains usual weight.

Elimination Management: Gastrointestinal function is normal. Bowel elimination is normal with no steatorrhea.

Coping Assistance: Anxiety is reduced or decreased. Absence or reduction of defining characteristics indicating presence of anxiety.

Short Bowel Syndrome

Short bowel syndrome refers to the severe diarrhea and significant malabsorption symptoms that develop after small bowel resections. The severity of short bowel syndrome is influenced by the amount of bowel resected and the portion of small bowel resected. Symptoms are related to diarrhea (fluid and electrolyte losses) and malnutrition (mineral, vitamin, fat, carbohydrate, and protein deficiencies).

Catastrophic malabsorption may develop from massive resections of the small bowel. The total length of resected bowel and the bowel lost must be considered in establishing the prognosis and treatment. As much as 50% of the small bowel may be resected and tolerated well, *if* the duodenum, proximal jejunum, distal half of the ileum, and ileocecal sphincter are spared. Severe diarrhea and malabsorption may result if the distal two thirds of the ileum and ilocecal valve are removed.[7] The advent of TPN has improved the survival rate of people who have lost significant amounts of small bowel. Small intestine transplants and operative procedures to expand intestinal surface area for improved function of the intestinal remnant are currently being studied.[48]

Short bowel syndrome may develop after major resection of the small intestine for mesenteric thrombosis, volvulus of the small intestine, and strangulated internal or external hernias. Less common causes include Crohn's disease, trauma, and radiation enteropathy. Jejunal bypass procedures for obesity are no longer recommended because of the severe malabsorption associated with the surgery.

Pathophysiology

The loss of small bowel affects the body's ability to absorb nutrients and vitamins. The pathophysiologic response to resections of small bowel varies, depending on the length and the segments involved. Long-term parenteral nutrient supplements are likely if less than 50 cm of residual jejunum remains.[54]

The pathophysiologic response to resections of small bowel varies depending on the length and segments involved. The ileocecal valve plays an important role in reducing contamination of residual small bowel by colonic flora. The valve also controls transit time of the contents. When short bowel syndrome occurs, absorption of water, electrolytes, fat, protein, carbohydrates, vitamins, and trace elements is reduced. Fluid loss is greatest in the first few days after surgery. Fluid loss is also higher when all or part of the colon has also been resected.

The small bowel absorbs nutrients and vitamins in different segments. Resections of small portions of the midintestine do not generally create clinical problems. However, smaller resections involving proximal or distal segments result in more significant clinical symptoms. The duodenum is responsible for iron, folate, and calcium absorption. Resection or bypass of the duodenum may result in anemia. The distal or terminal ileum is responsible for bile salt and vitamin B_{12} absorption. Reduction or absence of the active absorptive sites for bile salts will disrupt the enterohepatic circulation of bile salts.

Two forms of diarrhea may develop: cholerheic or steatorrheic. Cholerheic diarrhea is a watery diarrhea that is common if less than 100 cm of distal ileum is resected.[54] In cholerheic diarrhea the hepatic synthesis of bile salts partially compensates for the bile salts not being absorbed in the ileum. Fat digestion remains normal. The bile salts in the colon impair fluid and electrolyte absorption and stimulate further secretions of fluid into the colon. Steatorrheic diarrhea occurs when more than 100 cm of distal ileum is removed. Bile salt loss cannot be compensated by hepatic synthesis, and fat digestion is impaired (this can be resolved by using an agent such as cholestyramine). Undigested fat in the colon also impairs fluid and electrolyte absorption and stimulates colonic secretions. Steatorrheic diarrhea contains water, electrolytes, bile salts, and undigested fats. After ileal resections, gallstones have been reported to be two to three times higher than in the general population. This has been related to the depletion of the bile salt pool.[34]

Interestingly, the small bowel undergoes an adaptive process after bowel resections. The remaining villi enlarge and lengthen, increasing the absorptive surface area. The epithelial hyperplasia is associated with accelerated cell renewal and migration. It appears that exposure to nutrients (oral feedings), exposure to bile and pancreatic enzymes, and response to trophic gut peptides influence the adaptative process. Cholecystokinin and secretin support the adaptative process. The presence of oral feedings is necessary for adaptation to occur, but the oral intake should be gradually started and advanced. Clinically, the patient tends to improve in absorptive ability with time.

Gastric hypersecretion occurs in approximately half of the patients who have massive small bowel resections, and the mucosa distal to the stomach can be injured by high gastric output.[51] This can impair intestinal absorption by damaging the mucosa. This is often a temporary effect and decreases to normal levels.

Diagnostic Studies and Findings

Double-contrast barium films: Estimation of amount of small bowel remaining; increase in caliber of remaining segment several weeks after surgery (adaptation)
Laboratory studies: Folate, iron, vitamin B_{12}, vitamin A, calcium, magnesium, potassium, mean corpuscular volume (MCV), mean corpuscular hemoglobin concentration (MCHC), mean corpuscular hemoglobin (MCH), sodium, carotene, cholesterol, zinc: Reduced
Prothrombin time: Lengthened
Quantitative stool test for fat: Steatorrhea normal: 2 to 7 g of fat per day on diet of 100 g of fat per day
Culture of intestinal fluid: Bacterial overgrowth
D-Lactate levels (serum): Elevated

Multidisciplinary Plan

Medications

Parenteral replacement of fluid loss
Antidiarrheal agents: Liquid form may be absorbed better than tablets or capsules
- Diphenoxylate (Lomotil), 2.5-5 mg q4h PO
- Loperamide (Imodium), 2 mg q6h PO
- Somatostatin, 50 μg subcutaneously q6h bid to tid (may be added to parenteral nutrition fluids)

Antiinfective agents: Broad-spectrum antibiotic therapy if bacterial overgrowth suspected
Histamine receptor antagonist
- Cimetidine (Tagamet), 300 mg IV q6h then qid with meals and at bedtime (for gastric hypersecretion)
- Omeprazole (Prilosec), 60 mg qd

Bile salt binders: Ileal resections with cholerheic diarrhea: Cholestyramine, 8-12 mg/day
Vitamins
- Cyanocobalamin (vitamin B_{12}), 1000 μg IM monthly (if extensive ileal resection)
- Folate, 1 mg PO daily
- Other vitamin and mineral supplements as needed (may be added to TPN)

General Management

Intravenous fluids and replacement of K^+, Mg^{++}, Ca^{++}
TPN for nutrition, especially immediately postoperatively
Gradual oral feedings: Elemental diet initially; followed by polymeric supplements; add milk carefully (a low-lactose diet may be preferred)
High caloric intake; six meals per day
Home TPN
Protection of perianal skin from diarrhea

Nutritional Consultation

To advise on preparation of TPN; to advise on progression to enteral feedings; to instruct patient regarding dietary selections/avoidance at home (if applicable)

NURSING CARE

Nursing Assessment

General status: Purpura; generalized bleeding; poor skin turgor; severe weight loss; fatigue; lassitude; weakness
Nutritional status: Weight; diarrhea (cholerheic or steatorrheic); monitor for signs and symptoms of nutritional deficiencies

Potential Complications

Severe diarrhea, malabsorption

Patient Problems/Nursing Diagnoses & Interventions

NIC Nutrition Support

Imbalanced nutrition: less than body requirements, related to decreased intestinal absorptive area
- Help patient design a nutritional plan to meet lifestyle and caloric needs.
- Provide nutritional replacements as ordered *to prevent complications of malabsorption.*
- Provide total parenteral nutrition as ordered.
- Observe catheter site (Broviac, Hickman, central line).
- Change dressing per protocol.
- Observe for signs of infection (fever or redness at insertion site).
- Monitor vital signs, intake and output, urine for sugar and acetone, and daily weights while receiving parenteral nutrition.
- Record description of stools, including frequency, characteristics, and odor.

NIC Tissue Perfusion Management

Deficient fluid volume related to increased fluid losses from diarrhea
- Provide fluid replacement as ordered.
- Measure and record stool volume and urinary output.

NIC Elimination Management

Diarrhea related to decreased intestinal absorptive area
- Provide antidiarrheal agents as ordered.
- Record accurate description of stools and frequency.
- Provide fluid replacements as ordered.
- Assist patient with cleansing of perianal area and apply moisture barrier ointment as needed *to prevent skin breakdown.*

NIC Coping Assistance

Ineffective coping related to need for lifestyle change
- Provide opportunities for patient to verbalize concerns and feelings regarding the possibility of home

TPN for an undetermined time after major bowel resection.

- Consider having the patient meet other home TPN patients *for support and inspiration.*
- Discuss with the family and significant others their fears and concerns related to the new diagnosis and assist them in providing support for the patient.

Patient Education/Continuum of Care Plan

1. Provide information, oral and written, on dietary restrictions, dietary supplements, and medications regarding nutritional effects of malabsorption.
2. Discuss with patient the possibility of home TPN if necessary. Provide home care referral to evaluate and assist patient and family.
3. Provide patient with information about signs and symptoms of key electrolyte, fluid, and nutritional losses and complications from increased acidity and oxalate stones.
4. Instruct patient to notify physician immediately if gastroenteritis develops because patient can become seriously dehydrated quickly.

Evaluation/Patient Outcomes

Nutrition Support: Nutritional status is normal. Patient gains weight. Degree of diarrhea is minimized. Dietary plans provide adequate nutrition for absorptive capacity of the bowel. Nutritionist remains involved with dietary planning.

Tissue Perfusion Management: Fluid status is adequate. Patient has moist mucous membranes. Patient has balanced intake and output. Patient's blood pressure and pulse rate are within normal limits. Patient's urine specific gravity and osmolality are within normal limits.

Elimination Management: Diarrhea is controlled. Patient's fluid status and electrolytes are within normal limits.

Coping Assistance: Patient is coping with the situation or recognizes resources. Patient performs activities of daily living. Patient appropriately uses others for support. Patient has clear, realistic goals regarding situation.

Peritonitis

Peritonitis is the inflammation of the peritoneum. The inflammatory response may be localized or generalized.

The cause of peritonitis is contamination of the peritoneal cavity by bacteria or chemicals. Peritonitis is also classified as primary and secondary. Primary peritonitis is an acute (Fig. 10-15) or subacute bacterial infection of the peritoneum not associated with any underlying bowel disorder. It is often seen in children with underlying nephrotic syndromes and urinary tract infections. Cirrhosis with ascites is most commonly associated with primary peritonitis. Secondary peritonitis is the result of contamination of the peritoneum from perforation of the gastrointestinal tract (peptic ulcer, diverticulum, or appendix), gangrene of the bowel, salpingitis, traumatic injuries, and surgical contaminants. Peritonitis is a common complication of many diseases and can progress to perforation or rupture of the organs of digestion. In secondary peritonitis the inflammation is a result of bacterial and chemical irritation.

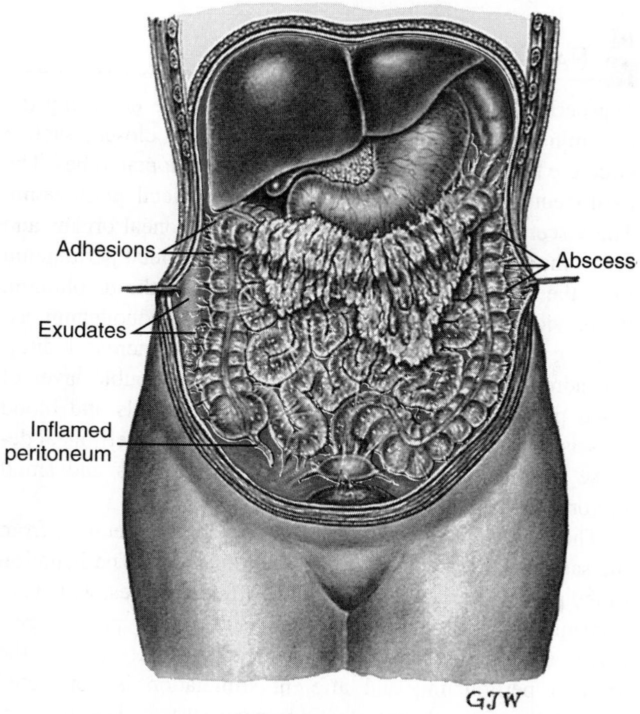

Fig. 10-15
Peritonitis (acute). (From Doughty.[10])

Secondary (generalized) peritonitis is a serious complication of an acutely ill patient. The overall mortality of generalized peritonitis is 40% with the use of antibiotics and intensive support systems.[52] Three factors that negatively affect the prognosis are age, type of contamination, and tissue perfusion. An older patient is at a higher risk for a poor prognosis or poor response to treatment. Fecal contamination is the most serious. Poor tissue perfusion indicates a poor prognosis. Poor tissue perfusion is associated with hypotension, acidosis, hypokalemia, or respiratory difficulties. Perforated peptic ulcer, ruptured appendix, trauma, ischemic bowel disease, intestinal obstruction, pancreatitis, and perforated colon are common causes of a generalized peritonitis.

Primary peritonitis may be divided into idiopathic (or spontaneous) and tuberculous peritonitis. Spontaneous bacterial peritonitis is associated with 2% of all abdominal emergencies and 13% of diffuse peritoneal sepsis in children.[44]

Tuberculous peritonitis is caused by a reactivation of latent tuberculosis in the peritoneum. The patient may not have active pulmonary, intestinal, or genital tuberculosis. Peritonitis from fungi and parasites is uncommon. *C. albicans* may cause severe peritonitis, but it requires a contamination of the peritoneum, usually from an occult gastrointestinal perforation.

Complications of peritonitis include abscess formation in the pelvis, the subphrenic space, and the abdomen.

PATHOPHYSIOLOGY

The peritoneum is a semipermeable membrane enclosing the abdominal viscera and mesentery. It forms a closed, saclike structure that is opened in the female at the fallopian tubes. The peritoneum is divided into visceral and parietal peritoneum. The visceral peritoneum covers the intraperitoneal organs and forms the mesenteries of these organs. The parietal peritoneum lines the abdominal wall, the undersurface of the diaphragm, the pelvic floor, and the retroperitoneal viscera (duodenum, ascending and descending colon, portions of the pancreas, kidney, and adrenals). The omentum is formed by a double layer of fused peritoneum and enclosed lymphatic vessels and blood vessels. The omentum plays a primary role in the peritoneal defense mechanism against impending perforations and small perforations.

The nervous innervation of the parietal peritoneum is from the same nerves that supply the abdominal wall. The irritation of the parietal peritoneum stimulates afferent nerves, which are transmitted through the intercostal nerves. The pain is perceived as somatic pain. No pain receptors are identified in the visceral peritoneum, and afferent stimulation is conducted through the visceral sympathetic nervous system. The different responses or symptoms of irritation are related to the nerve pathways. The symptoms of parietal peritonitis include a sharp, localized pain, whereas the pain in visceral peritonitis is poorly characterized and poorly localized.

The diaphragmatic peritoneum is innervated in the central portion from phrenic nerves and in the peripheral portion by branches of the intercostal nerves. Symptoms vary depending on the location of the pathologic process. Phrenic nerve stimulation would result in referred pain to either shoulder. Intercostal nerve stimulation may cause pain in the thoracic or the abdominal wall, as occurs in cholecystitis.

The peritoneal defense mechanism is the body's attempt to localize or wall off any contamination of the peritoneal cavity and prevent diffuse peritonitis. The first response is vascular dilation and increased capillary permeability. Large numbers of polymorphonuclear leukocytes pour into the area and through phagocytosis remove bacteria and foreign matter. Fibroblastic exudate is deposited and plasters the adjacent bowel, mesentery, and omentum to the inflamed area, forming a watertight seal. Thus the inflammation is enclosed as an abscess. Peritoneal injuries heal without fibrous adhesions unless infection, ischemia, or foreign bodies are associated with the peritonitis.

The body's response to secondary (acute bacterial) peritonitis includes removal of the bacteria through diaphragmatic lymphatics; phagocytosis and destruction of bacteria by opsonins, polymorphonuclear leukocytes, and macrophages; and localization by the omentum and fibroblastic exudate. Vascular dilation, hyperemia, and a fluid shift occur. The vascular dilation and hyperemia lead to an increase in polymorphonuclear leukocytes and macrophages. The absorption capacity of the peritoneum increases, facilitating the absorption of bacteria and toxins. A fluid shift occurs from the extracellular fluid compartment into the free peritoneal space, into the loose connective tissue (as edema), and into the lumen of the atonic gastrointestinal tract. The translocation of water, electrolytes, and protein into this third-space compartment depletes the circulating fluid volume. The rate of fluid shift is proportional to the degree of peritoneal involvement and the success of the body's peritoneal defense mechanism.

Early diagnosis and treatment are necessary to prevent severe shock from the loss of fluid into the peritoneal space. The principal complications of untreated peritonitis are septicemia, shock, ileus, and major organ failure including respiratory, renal, hepatic, and cardiac systems. The patient has symptoms of an acute condition in the abdomen, and it is necessary to rule out other causes of the symptoms.

DIAGNOSTIC STUDIES AND FINDINGS

Laboratory studies: WBC count: increased leukocytes; red blood cell (RBC) count: hemoconcentration; metabolic acidosis; respiratory alkalosis; electrolytes: vary

Plain films of the abdomen (KUB): Intestinal distention (small and large); gas and fluid collections in both the large and small bowel; free air (perforations); bowel walls may appear thickened

Peritoneal aspiration: Identification of organisms (primary peritonitis); appearance of aspirate (cloudy, blood-tinged, etc.); amylase, protein measurement, cytologic examination

MULTIDISCIPLINARY PLAN

Surgery

Operative procedure determined by primary cause

Objectives of surgery are to close perforation, to prevent septicemia, and to prevent abscess formation (or to drain abscess)

Medications

Aggressive volumes of electrolytes and colloid solutions to correct hypovolemia

Analgesics to control pain

Antibiotic therapy to cover multiple bacterial flora contaminating the peritoneal cavity; usually includes aminoglycoside (aerobic gram negative), clindamycin or metronidazole (anaerobes), ampicillin (enterococci), and cephalosporins (broad spectrum); beta-lactam antibiotics (carbapenems), a new class of broad-spectrum antibiotics, are being evaluated in the treatment of bacterial peritonitis

General Management

NPO

Nasogastric suctioning

Hourly vital signs, urinary output measurement, central venous pressure (CVP)

Monitoring: CBC, electrolytes, creatinine, arterial pH, Po_2, Pco_2, blood clotting profiles, liver and renal function tests

CVP or Swan-Ganz catheter for pulmonary capillary wedge and pulmonary artery pressure determinations

Oxygen (increased metabolic demand and respirations decreased because of pain and abdominal distention)

Respiratory assist devices or endotracheal intubation

Cultures: Blood, urine, sputum, peritoneal fluid

Nutritional supplements: TPN, providing 3000 to 4000 calories per day (to avoid major catabolic losses)

NURSING CARE

NURSING ASSESSMENT

Abdominal examination: Abdominal pain; diffuse tenderness and rigidity; often rebound; diminished or absent bowel sounds; abdominal distention

Respiratory status: Shallow and rapid; limited intercostal respirations; pain associated with deep respirations and coughing

Cardiovascular status: Rapid, weak, thready pulse; decreased blood pressure; hypovolemic shock

Urinary status: Decreased urinary output

General status: Fever; lying quietly in bed with knees flexed; guards abdomen against sudden movements or physical examination

Gastrointestinal status: Vomiting; nausea; anorexia

POTENTIAL COMPLICATIONS

Septicemia, shock, major organ failure

PATIENT PROBLEMS/NURSING DIAGNOSES & INTERVENTIONS

NIC TISSUE PERFUSION MANAGEMENT

Deficient fluid volume related to fluid shifts associated with inflamed peritoneum

- Replace intravenous fluids and electrolytes, blood, and plasma as ordered.
- Monitor vital signs, central venous pressure, urinary output, and nasogastric aspirations every hour.
- Notify physician of changes in patient's status *because they generally indicate a decline in patient's stabilization for surgical intervention.*

NIC PHYSICAL COMFORT PROMOTION

Acute pain related to irritation of parietal peritoneum

- Help patient assume a comfortable position (one that places minimum stress on the abdominal muscles); limit sudden movement and abdominal examination.
- Provide analgesics as prescribed. (Some surgeons will not order analgesics because they may mask signs and symptoms.)

NIC COPING ASSISTANCE

Anxiety related to pain, fear of death, and fear of the unknown

- Reassure patient and family, providing a calming influence.
- Explain all tests, procedures, and upcoming surgery.
- Use comfort measures.
- Encourage patient to ventilate feelings.

PATIENT EDUCATION/CONTINUUM OF CARE PLAN

1. Patient manages any wounds, abscesses, or incisions that have not closed or continue to drain before and after discharge from the hospital.
2. Patient identifies purpose of discharge medications and appropriate method of administration, including times, route, and length of course of medications.

EVALUATION/PATIENT OUTCOMES

Tissue Perfusion Management: Adequate fluid volume is maintained. Patient has moist mucous membranes. Patient has a balanced intake and output. Patient's urine output and specific gravity are within normal limits. Vital signs are stable.

Physical Comfort Promotion: Pain is tolerable. Patient understands that staff is doing all they can for the pain. Pain resolves with resolution of peritonitis.

Coping Assistance: Anxiety has decreased. Patient and family verbalize concerns and understanding of tests and procedures.

POLYPS

The term *polyp* refers to a discrete tissue mass that is elevated above the mucosal surface. A polyp may be described according to histologic examination, presence or absence of a stalk, and whether it is one of multiple similar protrusions in the gastrointestinal tract.

The histologic examination of a polyp determines the tissue from which the polyp developed and the descriptive name. For example, adenoma develops from epithelium, myoma from smooth muscle, and hemangioma from blood vessels. The most common type of colonic polyp is an adenoma. Pedunculated polyps are attached to the mucosa by a stalk, whereas sessile polyps rest on a broad base of mucosa. Although polyps may occur throughout the gastrointestinal tract, the predominant site is in the distal 25 cm of the colon. Colonic polyps may be classified as neoplastic or nonneoplastic. Neoplastic polyps include adenomas and carcinomas. Categories of nonneoplastic polyps include mucosal polyps, hyperplastic polyps, pseudopolyps of inflammatory bowel disease, and juvenile polyps. Syndromes that involve multiple gastrointestinal polyps include familial polyposis, Gardner's syndrome, Turcot's syndrome, Peutz-Jeghers syndrome, and juvenile polyps.

The frequency of colonic adenomas, although varying widely among populations, tends to be highest in North America and Europe. Autopsy surveys in the United States indicate that 50% of the population have at least one adenomatous colonic polyp. When age is considered as a variable, it is noted that two thirds of those 65 years of age and older have colonic adenomas. Adenomas in the colon and rectum are more likely to become malignant. The diagnosis and removal of polyps play an important role in preventing colon and rectal cancers.

Familial polyposis, an inherited autosomal dominant trait, is characterized by progressive development of hundreds of polyps (adenomas) throughout the colon. Familial polyposis is a precancerous condition. The development of colon cancer in familial polyposis is inevitable without surgical intervention. The polyps begin to develop after puberty, and the patient may remain asymptomatic for several years. The presence of multiple cancers at the time of diagnosis is high. Family assessments and genetic counseling are important in reducing the rates of early death from colon cancer by identifying family members who have the gene for familial polyposis.

Gardner's syndrome is a variant of familial polyposis and consists of gastrointestinal polyposis, osteomas of the skull, mandible, and long bones, and soft tissue tumors. Gardner's syndrome is inherited as an autosomal dominant trait. The gastrointestinal polyps appear in the small and large intestine and are precancerous.

Turcot's syndrome describes the combination of familial polyposis and malignant central nervous system (CNS) tumors. The CNS tumors include glioblastomas and medulloblastomas.

Peutz-Jeghers syndrome involves mucocutaneous pigmentation of the mouth, lips, hands, and feet and multiple polyps in the small and large intestines. The polyps are hamartomas; that is, they develop from glandular epithelium supported by smooth muscle. The pigmentation generally fades after puberty with the exception of those found in the mouth.

Juvenile polyps are distinctive hamartomas found in the rectums of children. The polyps do not tend to be precancerous lesions but are removed because of the associated problems of bleeding, obstructions, and intussusception.

PATHOPHYSIOLOGY

Colonic polyps or adenomas are composed of immature epithelial cells that continue to proliferate. Normally, the lower third of the colonic crypt is the site of cell division. As the cells move upward toward the lumen of the colon, they differentiate into colonic epithelium that secretes mucus. When the normal processes of cell proliferation and differentiation are altered, cells migrate to the surface, where they continue to synthesize DNA and divide. The surface epithelium of undifferentiated cells accumulates and leads to the formation of a polyp. The same steps are found in familial polyposis, where normal-appearing mucosa is found to be mature and differentiated epithelium and polyps are composed of proliferative cells.

Adenomatous polyps may develop as tubular adenomas, villous adenomas, or tubulovillous adenomas. Tubular adenoma is used to describe polyps that consist of densely packed colonic cells with loss of goblet cell mucin, branching of glands, and varying degrees of nuclear atypia. Tubular adenomas are more common and usually smaller. Villous adenomas contain a proliferation of villi. Villous adenomas are larger than tubular adenomas. The polyps that contain villi and tubular epithelium are referred to as tubulovillous adenomas. The involvement of the villi is associated with a higher incidence of cancer.

The relationship between polyps and cancer has been developed through longitudinal observations. Dysplasia, in varying degrees, is found during histologic examination of polyps after biopsy. Evidence supporting the relationship between polyps and colon carcinomas is based on three major findings: location of clusters of cancers within adenomatous polyps, findings in patients with multiple polyposis, and epidemiologic studies. Although small, isolated colon carcinomas are rare, small groups of cancers are found within adenomatous polyps. The development of carcinomas in patients with colonic polyps is usually 10 to 15 years after the appearance of benign adenomas. Data supporting the time span are based on patients with familial polyposis. However, residual adenomatous tissue may be found surrounding malignant tissue in patients with early colon cancer lesions at diagnosis and surgery. The same population groups tend to have high rates of colon cancer and colonic adenomas, further supporting the relationship.

When a polyp is removed, cytologic and histologic studies are performed to carefully assess the patient for further medical or surgical intervention. Polyps may be associated with mild to severe degrees of dysplasia. When the polyp contains foci in which the nuclei are large and irregular, cells are crowded, polarity is lost, and cribiform glands are present, the cytologic appearance is malignant. The interpretation of the finding is then made by examining the entire polyp. If the foci do not extend into the muscularis mucosae, the polyp contains carcinoma in situ. If there is extension into the muscularis mucosae and submucosa (and thus lymphatic and blood supply), the polyp is considered invasive carcinoma.

The development of polyps in familial polyposis is through the alteration of the normal cell proliferation and differentiation as previously described. In familial polyposis, young people develop hundreds to thousands of colonic polyps. Cancer, in one or more polyps, generally develops before 40 years of age.

Studies of skin fibroblasts of patients with familial polyposis and Gardner's syndrome have demonstrated abnormal growth characteristics in culture. The cells have normal contact inhibition; they grow in multilayered, crisscrossed patterns and have decreased serum requirements for growth. The study of skin fibroblasts in patients to detect the familial polyposis trait may be a diagnostic tool for the future.[44]

In Gardner's syndrome precancerous polyps may be found throughout the gastrointestinal tract. Duodenal polyps are more common than jejunal or ileal polyps. Multiple polyps may also be found in the stomach. Extracolonic manifestations include osteomas of the mandible, skull, and long bones (e.g., epidermoid cysts, fibromas, lipomas, and desmoid tumors), dental abnormalities (e.g., impacted teeth, mandibular cysts), and soft tissue tumors (e.g., carcinoma of the thyroid and adrenal glands).

DIAGNOSTIC STUDIES AND FINDINGS

Proctosigmoidoscopy: Visualization of bowel lumen demonstrates presence of polyps (flexible fiberoptic sigmoidoscopy is better tolerated, but only 30 cm in length)

Colonoscopy: Visualization and polypectomy; biopsy (total excision of polyp is the accepted method of providing an accurate histologic diagnosis)

Radiography studies: Osteomas found in Gardner's syndrome

MULTIDISCIPLINARY PLAN

Surgery

Colonic adenomas: Require colon resection with wide margins for invasive carcinoma, sessile polyps, cancer in situ, cancer at margin of resection by polypectomy, and undifferentiated cancer in any polyp

Inherited multiple polyposis syndromes: Require prophylactic proctocolectomy with end ileostomy, continent ileostomy, or ileoanal reservoir

General Management

Colonic adenomas: Colonic polypectomy by colonoscopy for benign polyp, pedunculated polyp, and carcinoma in situ when confined to head of polyp

Juvenile polyps: Colonoscopy with polypectomy

Routine or periodic proctosigmoidoscopy or colonoscopy in patients at risk for developing familial polyposis or Gardner's syndrome; screening should begin at 10 to 12 years of age if symptoms have not already led to a diagnosis.[54]

Genetic counseling and screening

NURSING CARE

Nursing Assessment

Gastrointestinal status: Hematochezia (blood per rectum), occult and overt; diarrhea in villous adenoma; constipation or a change in the caliber of stools

Abdominal examination: Crampy, lower abdominal pain (caused by intermittent intussusception in Peutz-Jeghers syndrome)

History: Family history of deaths from colon cancer or known relatives with familial disease

Integumentary system: Macular lesions (brown to greenish black) around the mouth, nose, lips, buccal mucosa, hands, feet, and occasionally in the perianal and genital regions (Peutz-Jeghers syndrome)

Psychosocial concerns: Assess individual's ability to cope in relation to the presence of familial disease that may require surgery

Potential Complications

Cancer

Patient Problems/Nursing Diagnoses & Interventions

NIC Coping Assistance

Ineffective coping related to situational crisis of treatment

- Provide opportunities for patient to verbalize concerns and feelings regarding the possibility of surgery.
- Consider having patient meet other patients of same age and with same disease for support.
- Discuss with family and significant others their fears and concerns related to new diagnosis; assist them in providing support for patient.
- Assess patient who is to undergo surgery for familial polyposis regarding verbal responses to the actual change in structure of his or her body function; physical changes anticipated with surgery; and age, sex, and developmental level.
- Assist patient by providing information on rationale of total colectomy for familial polyposis and available surgical procedures, including conventional ileostomy, continent ileostomy, and anal sphincter–saving surgeries.
- Refer patient to enterostomal therapy (ET) nurse and ostomy organization for support.

Patient Education/Continuum of Care Plan

Close follow-up should be planned because of recurrence rates.

Evaluation will require barium enema, proctosigmoidoscopy, or colonoscopy. The pattern should be as follows:

Benign colonic adenoma: Every 2 to 3 years
Carcinoma confined to polyp: In 6 months, then yearly
Multiple polyps and family history of cancer: Yearly
Asymptomatic familial polyposis: Every 6 months
Familial polyposis, following surgery when rectal segment is left: Every 6 months

See pp. 730-736 for instructions on ostomy care or care of the patient with an ileoanal reservoir, if appropriate

Evaluation/Patient Outcomes

Coping Assistance: Patient is coping with situation or recognizes resources. Patient performs activities of daily living. Patient appropriately uses others for support. Patient has clear, realistic goals regarding the situation.

Pseudomembranous Colitis (Antibiotic-Associated Colitis)

Pseudomembranous enterocolitis is an inflammation and necrosis of the bowel that primarily affects the mucosa and occasionally the submucosa. Pseudomembranous exudative plaques are found attached to the mucosal surface of the small bowel (enteritis), colon (colitis), or both (enterocolitis).

C. difficile has been identified as the enteric pathogen responsible for pseudomembranous colitis after antibiotic therapy. Although many antimicrobial agents have been implicated in pseudomembranous colitis, the most common agents include clindamycin, lincomycin, cephalosporins, ampicillin, penicillin, metronidazole, and amoxicillin. Antimicrobial therapy is by far the most common risk factor, although there are others, including surgery of the colon, stomach, or pelvic region complicated by shock during or after the surgery; spinal fractures; intestinal obstructions; Crohn's disease; uremia, leukemia, colonic carcinoma, and heavy metal poisoning.

If untreated, pseudomembranous colitis leads to severe dehydration, electrolyte imbalance, toxic megacolon, and colonic perforation.

Pathophysiology

Antibiotic-induced pseudomembranous colitis develops when the normal bowel flora is altered by antibiotic therapy. The *C. difficile* organisms multiply, producing two toxins. The toxins damage the membranes of the epithelial cells, leading to cell necrosis. Poor vascular perfusion to the mucosa may also progress to necrosis of the mucosal layer of the gut. Antibiotic-induced pseudomembranous enterocolitis tends to be primarily a disease of the colon, whereas studies of pseudomembranous enterocolitis not associated with antibiotics have demonstrated lesions in the small bowel as well.

The pseudomembrane is composed of fibrin, mucin, sloughed epithelial cells, and leukocytes. The mildest form of pseudomembranous enterocolitis consists of focal necrosis. A characteristic "summit" lesion develops from a collection of fibrin and polymorphonuclear cells. As the disease progresses, the appearance changes to a "volcanic" lesion that includes glandular cell disruption and the typical pseudomembrane of elevated yellow-white plaques. As the necrosis worsens, there is an extensive involvement of the lamina propria and a thick overlaying of the pseudomembrane. If the pseudomembranes slough, the bowel is left with large denuded areas.

Pseudomembranous colitis can progress to a life-threatening illness. The symptoms may not develop for 4 to 7 weeks after the antibiotic therapy has been discontinued. Patients generally have severe diarrhea, abdominal tenderness, fever, and leukocytosis. As the bowel wall necrosis continues, the patient begins to lose fluids, electrolytes, and albumin. Toxic megacolon may develop. The colon may perforate, leading to the sequelae of peritonitis and sepsis.

Early diagnosis is important in initiating oral treatment and preventing the disorder from becoming fulminant or intractable to medical management. The medical management consists of antimicrobials that are effective against *C. difficile.* In patients with a less severe disease, an anion exchange resin (cholestyramine) has been used to bind the toxins produced by *C. difficile.* Cholestyramine should not be used in combination with antimicrobials because the resin will bind the antimicrobial and reduce the drug levels in the colon.

Diagnostic Studies and Findings

Colonoscopy and sigmoidoscopy: Yellowish white plaques; erythema; friable mucosa; ulcerations; hemorrhage; endoscopic procedures only when rapid diagnosis is needed and test results are delayed, or patient has ileus and a stool sample is not available, or when other colonic diseases are included in the differential diagnosis.

Stool analysis: *C. difficile* toxin assay; stool culture for *C. difficile*

Laboratory studies: Leukocytosis (10,000 to 20,000/mm^3 or higher)

Multidisciplinary Plan

Surgery

For Perforation or Toxic Dilation

Severely ill patients with fulminant or intractable symptoms may require colectomy or diverting ileostomy (rare)

Medications

Metronidazole, 250 mg PO qid or 500 mg PO tid
Vancomycin, 125 mg PO qid
Cholestyramine, 4 g q6h for 5 days PO (mild cases only; not with concomitant antimicrobial therapy)
Antimotility agents contraindicated

General Management

Intravenous fluids; total parenteral nutrition; bowel rest; discontinue inciting antibiotic; no antidiarrheal drugs

NURSING CARE

Nursing Assessment

General status: Fever; history: recent exposure to antibiotic agent (within last 2 months)

Gastrointestinal status: Diarrhea consisting of watery stools containing mucus, severity varies up to 30 loose stools per day, may begin during antibiotic therapy or after drug is discontinued, stool may occasionally be bloody; abdominal cramps; vomiting

Integumentary system: Assess perianal area for irritation from diarrhea

Abdominal examination: Abdominal pain and tenderness on palpation; decreased bowel sounds

Cardiovascular status: Signs of acute dehydration

Potential Complications

Severe diarrhea, toxic megacolon, perforation, peritonitis, sepsis

Patient Problems/Nursing Diagnoses & Interventions

NIC Elimination Management

Diarrhea related to effect of *C. difficile* toxin on bowel mucosa

- Report to physician if patient is experiencing loose, watery, frequent diarrheal stools.
- Observe patient for signs and symptoms of fluid loss, electrolyte imbalance, abdominal pain or tenderness, and fever.
- Document number, description, amount, and frequency of bowel movements.
- Follow standard body substance isolation: *C. difficile* toxin is often spread among patients and among patients and staff. Spores can also be found on inanimate objects.
- Replace fluid losses as ordered with isotonic solution.
- Measure I&O accurately.

NIC Perfusion Management

Ineffective renal, cerebral, cardiopulmonary, gastrointestinal, and peripheral tissue perfusion related to massive fluid shifts and losses

- Record blood pressure, pulse, temperature, and respirations, reporting any signs of shock.
- Maintain patient's intravenous fluids as ordered.

NIC Skin/Wound Management

Risk for impaired skin integrity related to massive diarrhea

- Cleanse skin carefully after each bowel movement; warm sitz baths will help cleanse skin and soothe irritated perianal skin.
- Apply barrier ointments to perianal area as long as patient has diarrhea.

Patient Education/Continuum of Care Plan

1. Patients will be given oral medications, and it is important that patient understand rationale for agent and importance of compliance with prescribed protocol.
2. If surgery is required for fulminating disease, patient and family will require instructions in management of diverting or permanent ileostomy. The surgery is rarely necessary.

3. Ensure that patient understands he or she must notify his or her health provider if diarrhea recurs. Symptoms of a relapse (diarrhea; with or without fever, cramps) occur 3 to 10 days after treatment is discontinued.

Evaluation/Patient Outcomes

Elimination Management: Bowel functions normally. Patient has no diarrhea, nor does diarrhea recur after discontinuation of treatment.

Tissue Perfusion Management: Fluid balance is maintained. Patient returns to normal hydration levels as assessed by skin turgor, mucous membranes, color, blood pressure, and pulse. Serum electrolytes, hematocrit, and WBC count are within normal limits.

Skin/Wound Management: Skin integrity is maintained. Patient has no signs of perianal irritation or breakdown.

Crohn's Disease

Crohn's disease, a chronic inflammatory disorder of the gastrointestinal tract, may occur in any part of the gastrointestinal tract from the mouth to the anus, but the most common sites are the terminal ileum and colon.

Crohn's disease, granulomatous colitis, regional enteritis, transmural colitis, and transmural ileitis all refer to the same disease process. Crohn's disease is segmental in nature, and normal mucosa will be found between diseased segments (skip lesions). Crohn's disease and ulcerative colitis are often called inflammatory bowel diseases (IBDs), and differential diagnosis between the two diseases is important in planning treatment. A chronic disorder, Crohn's disease frequently recurs after surgical resection of diseased segments.

The prevalence of Crohn's disease is 7 to 10 cases per 100,000 population in Northern countries.[2] Crohn's disease is reported with increasing frequency throughout the world, but it is hard to determine if the increase is in actual numbers of cases or whether it is related to an increased awareness of Crohn's disease and improved diagnostic techniques. Crohn's disease is more common among Jews than non-Jews and among whites than nonwhites. The age at onset of the disease is the early teens and early twenties, with a range of 15 to 30 years of age.[2] A positive family history for inflammatory bowel disease may be found in patients.[2] The frequency among siblings is higher than with more distant relatives, yet no genetic markers have been found to support a genetic basis.

Crohn's disease is described by the anatomic location of the disease. Crohn's disease may be limited to the small bowel, involve both small bowel and colon (ileocolitis), be limited to the colon, or be present in the stomach or duodenum. A small group of patients may have Crohn's disease that is limited to the anorectal region. Most patients have Crohn's disease involving both the small bowel and the colon.

The cause of Crohn's disease is unknown. Research funded through the Crohn's and Colitis Foundation of America and other digestive disease groups is directed toward discovery of the cause and cure for this chronic illness.

Pathophysiology

Although the cause of Crohn's disease is unknown, the foundation for its occurrence is probably at the primary genetic level, and the expression of genetic susceptibility is triggered by environmental factors.[35] It has been hypothesized that an exogenous agent penetrates the intestinal epithelium, creating a cytopathic immune response in a susceptible individual. Factors that have been examined as possible causes include infectious agents (bacteria and viruses), altered host susceptibility, immune-mediated intestinal damage, psychologic factors, and dietary and environmental factors.

The role of infectious agents has been studied to identify a specific myobacteria or virus responsible for Crohn's disease. Recent studies have explored the possibility of cell wall–defective variants of enteric bacteria, whereas other research suggests a viruslike agent. So far, studies have failed to document a specific cause in Crohn's disease.

Altered host susceptibility has been considered in the cause of Crohn's disease. Although a specific infectious agent has not been identified, some researchers suggest that an impaired immune or inflammatory response to an infectious agent might progress to Crohn's disease. Impairment of various manifestations of cell-mediated immunity has been found in a substantial portion of patients with Crohn's disease, but this may be due to drug therapy or to malnutrition. Genetic transmission of specific histocompatibility antigens has also been explored, without conclusive findings.

Immune mechanisms have been implicated in the cause of Crohn's disease because of the recurrent inflammatory process, presence of granulomatous lesions, systemic manifestations, and the positive response to corticosteroids and other immunosuppressives. Studies have examined the following as possible immune causes: hypersensitivity reaction in the intestines, "autoimmune" antibody–mediated damage to intestinal epithelium, tissue deposition of antigen-antibody complexes, lymphocyte-mediated cytotoxicity, and impairment of cellular immune mechanisms.[35]

Dietary and environmental factors have also been questioned in the cause of Crohn's disease. Chemical food additives, such as carrageenan, reduced dietary fibers, smoking, oral contraceptives, and increased refined sugars have been studied. No evidence firmly links dietary or environmental factors to Crohn's disease at this time.

In Crohn's disease the inflammatory process extends through the layers of the bowel wall, hence the term *transmural.* Microscopically the following are found in the intestines: transmural inflammation, submucosal infiltration, submucosal thickening and fibrosis, ulceration through the mucosa, fissures, and focal granulomas. As the disease progresses, the bowel wall thickens and the lumen narrows. Stenosis is common. The mucosa show skip lesions, with normal bowel between diseased segments. The mesentery thickens and may extend over the serosal surface toward the antimesenteric border of the bowel. The intestinal segment may become fixed as the mesentery becomes fibrotic and contracts. The mesenteric nodes are enlarged and firm and may come together to form an irregular mass. The lymphatic vessels dilate and may be visible in the involved mesentery and serosal layer of the bowel.

The mucosal layer in advanced Crohn's disease consists of deep mucosal ulcerations and nodular submucosal thickening, producing a cobblestone appearance to the surface layer. The ulcers usually extend into the submucosa, and two or more ulcers may coalesce to form deep longitudinal ulcers traversing long segments. These ulcers are often referred to as *rake* ulcers. As the disease progresses, the mucosa becomes denuded.

The inflammation of the serosa and mesentery leads to a characteristic tendency in Crohn's disease for involved loops of bowel to adhere to one another. Fissures extend through the entire wall of the bowel and erode into adjacent loops of bowel or bladder, forming a fistula. It is not unusual for a fistula tract to develop to the skin (enterocutaneous), the umbilicus, or the perineum. When the rectum is diseased, ulcers arising in the rectal crypts may end in the perirectal fat and form abscesses. Rectal abscesses may erode into the anal sphincter and the supporting muscles. Abscesses can occur anywhere in the peritoneum, retroperitoneal area, or pelvis.

The severity of the malabsorption depends on the severity of the Crohn's disease, the amount of gut involved, and the treatment regimen. Crohn's disease in the jejunum and ileum decreases the capacity of the small bowel mucosa to absorb multiple nutrients, including carbohydrates, amino acids, folate, water-soluble vitamins, fats, and fat-soluble vitamins. Disease in the terminal ileum may lead to vitamin B_{12} (cobalamin) malabsorption and bile salt reabsorption, resulting in increased diarrhea because of increased osmolality of bile salts in the colon and decreased fat absorption. Lactase deficiency may develop with small bowel disease. The presence of ulcerations in extensive disease may result in protein loss. Iron deficiency anemia may develop from a chronic, slow blood loss and decrease in iron absorption. Bleeding in Crohn's disease is often mild, and the stool color may not change. The characteristic changes of the lymphatic system in Crohn's disease contribute to an impaired fat absorption.

The strictures and internal fistulas common in Crohn's disease may lead to stasis of intestinal contents in the bypassed segment, which results in bacterial overgrowth in the lumen; bacterial overgrowth impairs absorption of carbohydrates, fats, and vitamin B_{12} and alters bile salt metabolism, affecting fat absorption.

Therapy may also affect nutrition. Some patients impose dietary restrictions on themselves or limit their oral food intake. Patients should be tested for lactose intolerance before a lactose-free diet is imposed. Surgical resection of diseased segments of small bowel and colon may also affect nutrition. Resection or bypass of an intestinal segment may decrease the absorptive surface area. Resection of the terminal ileum may lead to vitamin B_{12} and bile salt malabsorption. The distal ileum is the site for reabsorption of conjugated bile salts, and the loss of ileum results in loss of bile salts through the colon, thereby decreasing the total bile salt pool and decreasing biliary secretion of bile salts, resulting in fat malabsorption. Unabsorbed bile salts stimulate the colon mucosal secretion and reduce the net absorption of water and electrolytes in the colon, and the patient experiences increased diarrhea.

Surgeries that result in enteroenterostomies (bowel anastomosis to bowel), surgical blind loops, and loss of ileocecal valve create conditions in which bacterial overgrowth frequently occurs. The effect of overgrowth of enteric microorganisms was discussed previously.

Folate deficiency is common in patients with Crohn's disease. Decreased dietary intake and decreased absorption affect folate levels. In addition, sulfasalazine (which is frequently used in treating Crohn's disease) impairs the absorption of folate. Patients with Crohn's disease may also have an increased requirement for folate because of increased catabolism and chronic blood loss.

Patients with Crohn's disease frequently have increased caloric and protein requirements because of the catabolic effects of the chronic inflammation and superimposed infection. This further depletes the patient's nutritional status. The consequences of the impaired absorption and nutritional deficiencies are more serious in children than in adults. Growth retardation and delayed sexual maturation occur in 20% to 30% of young patients. The use of corticosteroids over a prolonged period also contributes to growth retardation.

Complications of Crohn's disease are either intestinal (e.g., small bowel obstructions, abscesses, cancer, perforation, or fistula formation) or systemic. Obstructions are usually the result of inflammation and edema in a strictured or narrowed segment of bowel. The typical obstruction tends to progress slowly to a complete obstruction. Sudden complete obstruction may occur if the bowel becomes kinked by adhesions.

Fistula formation is very common in Crohn's disease and is a characteristic that often distinguishes Crohn's disease from ulcerative colitis. Perianal and perirectal fistulas and fissures can be extremely severe and may cause more problems for the patient than other clinical symptoms. Enterocutaneous fistulas can also cause severe management problems for the patient. A fistula between the bowel and bladder is infrequent, but when it occurs, it leads to chronic urinary infections and if untreated may progress to irreversible renal damage. Free perforation is rare in Crohn's disease because of the more frequent fistula and abscess formation.

Systemic manifestations include arthritis, iritis, erythema nodosum, ankylosing spondylitis, pyoderma gangrenosum, aphthous mouth ulcers, and occasionally liver disease. Arthritis is the most common systemic manifestation. Arthritic symptoms may be present several years before bowel symptoms appear. Children with arthritic symptoms should have tests done to rule out inflammatory bowel disease. The arthritis may be migratory arthritis involving large joints, sacroilitis, or ankylosing spondylitis. In Crohn's disease the arthritis does not seem to reflect the degree of intestinal disease. (However, in ulcerative colitis, arthritis tends to be more severe, and the patient experiences exacerbations or remissions depending on the intestinal state.)

Erythema nodosum and pyoderma gangrenosum are inflammatory disorders of the skin that may occur with Crohn's disease. Pyoderma gangrenosum is the more severe disorder and may be found during a recurrence of active Crohn's disease in a patient after a surgical resection. The lesion may develop before the bowel symptoms.

Although liver disease is unusual in patients with Crohn's disease, mild abnormalities of liver function may be observed in hospitalized patients. Sclerosing cholangitis occurs more frequently in patients with Crohn's disease than in the general population. Renal disorders may also be a complication of

> **! EMERGENCY ALERT**
>
> **GASTROINTESTINAL BLEEDING**
>
> The upper and lower gastrointestinal (GI) tract may experience hemorrhage and may produce significant pain. Upper GI bleeding is most commonly caused by peptic ulcers that erode through a vessel. Ruptured esophageal varices produce upper GI bleeding and are often associated with chronic hepatic disease; one third of these individuals die. Lower GI bleeding from the large bowel and rectum is typically caused by ulcerative colitis, cancers, ulcers, hemorrhoids, diverticulitis, or polyps.
>
> ASSESSMENT
>
> - History: Determine history, including alcohol use, previous bleeding or ulcers, history of pain or gastric upset.
> - Assess hemodynamic stability, including vital signs, skin color and moisture, and other signs that may indicate hypovolemia or shock.
> - Presence of hematemesis (vomiting of blood), black tarry stools, or bright red stools.
> - Presence of epigastric tenderness, jaundice, enlarged spleen, or enlarged liver.
>
> INTERVENTIONS
>
> - Keep client NPO until source of bleeding is determined.
> - Obtain IV access and maintain fluid hydration as indicated by signs of hypovolemia.
> - Obtain laboratory specimens as indicated, including hemoglobin, hematocrit, and possible specimens for type and crossmatching of blood.
> - Prepare for possible endoscopy to determine source of bleeding.

Crohn's disease. The infections related to enterovesical fistulas may lead to urinary tract infections. The ureters may also be affected by the bowel and mesenteric inflammation, leading to obstruction and hydronephrosis. Oxalate stones and hyperoxaluria have been associated with steatorrhea in patients with Crohn's disease.

Cancer of the colon occurs three times more often in patients with Crohn's disease than in the general population. This is less frequently than colon cancer is found in patients with ulcerative colitis.

Crohn's disease may vary from a mild to severely debilitating disease. An individual may experience one acute episode and be asymptomatic for years. Medical management is the primary form of therapy; however, most patients will require surgery at some time to manage intestinal complications of the long-term effects of the disease. The recurrence of Crohn's disease after surgical resection is about 20% overall.[5]

DIAGNOSTIC STUDIES AND FINDINGS

Stool cultures: Negative (used to rule out infections)
Stool guaiac: Positive (shows blood loss)
Laboratory studies: Serum albumin: low (protein loss through lesions and increase in protein catabolism); liver function: abnormal (pericholangitis or fatty liver); serum cobalamin: low (ileal disease); serum folic acid: low (malabsorption); hemoglobin, hematocrit: anemia; leukocytes (marked elevation may suggest presence of abscess or other suppurative condition)
Platelets: Greater than 300,000/ml^3 (may occur with active disease)
Lactose tolerance test: To rule out lactase deficiency
Sigmoidoscopy: Rectum: rectal mucosa may be free of disease; perianal or perirectal fissures, fistulas, or abscesses may be found; distal colon: aphthous ulcers or erosions; deep longitudinal fissures with intervening edematous mucosa
Colonoscopy: Skip lesions; cobblestone mucosa; patchy erythema, edema, and granularity
Biopsy: Aids in differentiation of pseudopolyposis, ulcerative colitis, adenomatous polyp, and cancer; discontinuous crypt distortion and inflammation; presence of epithelioid granulomas
Double-contrast barium studies: Upper small bowel, barium enemas; asymmetric disease, skip lesions, pseudodiverticula, linear ulcerations, transverse fissures, cobblestone mucosa, strictures, fistulas (NOTE: Routine preparation of colon should be omitted because it may initiate an exacerbation of the disease; prepare patient with a clear liquid diet for 2 to 3 days)
CT scan: Prominent wall thickening, occasional stricture formation; increased pericolic fat in areas of disease activity, adenopathy, skip lesions, and perianal sinus tracts

MULTIDISCIPLINARY PLAN

Surgery

Strictureplasty: A conservative approach for high-risk patients with chronic bowel obstruction
Surgical resection of diseased segments of bowel (operative therapy reserved for complications of Crohn's disease or unequivocal failure to respond to medical management)
Total colectomy with ileostomy (when disease is limited to the colon and is not responsive to medical management or cancer is found)
Subtotal colectomy with temporary ileostomy or with ileorectal anastomosis (when the rectum is not involved)

Medications

5-ASA formulations: May inhibit inflammatory or immune-mediated injuries
- *Sulfasalazine (Azulfidine):* Acute phase: 3 to 4 g/day in divided doses tid; maintenance: 1 to 2 g/day tid
- *Mesalamine*
  - Asacol, 2-4 g/day PO
  - Pentasa, 2-4 g/day PO
  - Dipentum, 500 mg bid PO

Prednisone: Acute phase: 50-80 mg/day (intravenously in severely ill patient); maintenance 5-15 mg/day PO
Antibiotics
- Metronidazole (Flagyl), 20 mg/kg/day in divided doses
- Ciprofloxacin being studied

Immunomodulatory agents
- "Third-line" drugs: These have significant side effects, and their use is somewhat controversial
- 6-Mercaptopurine (6-MP): Acute phase: 1.5 mg/kg/day PO (has a steroid-sparing effect and may be more useful in patients with fistulas and perianal disease)
- Azathioprine, 50 mg/day initial dose; may be gradually increased if tolerated

Cyclosporine A, 8-10 mg/kg/day; still being studied
Methotrexate, 8-10 mg/kg/day; still being studied

Anti–tumor necrosis factor-α (TNF)[41]
Infliximab: Monoclonal antibody works against the key cytokine relevant to intestinal inflammation; single-dose IV infusion; still in clinical trials

Antidiarrheal agents: Loperamide, diphenoxylate, codeine; if diarrhea related to bile salt malabsorption: cholestyramine, aluminum hydroxide; metamucil may be used for watery stools in the chronic phase

Vitamin B_{12} supplementation: Every month if terminal ileum disease is present

Calcium supplement

General Management

Acute phase: Intravenous fluids, nothing by mouth, bed rest or limited activity

Complication of small bowel obstruction: Nasogastric suctioning

Stenosis or narrowing of lumen: Avoid high-fiber foods containing cellulose or those foods that are not readily digested

Nutritional support: Vitamin replacement, folic acid, iron, TPN, enteral alimentation; lactose restrictions (if indicated); some institutions use peripheral amino acids, fat for 1 to 5 days, with bowel rest and then start food or TPN

Nutritional Consultation

To assist patient in identification of foods that exacerbate symptoms; to assist in planning for enteral/parenteral supplementation

NURSING CARE

Nursing Assessment

Gastrointestinal status
- Initially, diarrhea, abdominal cramping, and fever; as disease progresses, must observe patient for signs of complications: bloody diarrhea or steatorrhea
  - Diarrhea: When disease confined to ileum, five or six loose bowel movements per day; when colon involved, urgency and incontinence frequent
  - Abdominal cramping: Mild to severe, lower quadrant, intermittent periumbilical colic experienced during bowel movements
  - Gastrointestinal complications
    - Fistulas
      - Stool in urine
      - Passing gas via vagina
      - Fecal drainage through skin (enterocutaneous)
    - Small bowel obstructions
    - Toxic megacolon
    - Cancer
    - Free perforations (rare)
    - Hemorrhage (infrequent)

Nutritional status: Anorexia, nausea, dietary intolerance, weight loss

Perianal examination: Presence of fissures, fistulas, or abscesses; irritation from diarrhea or fistula drainage

Extracolonic manifestations: Arthritis; inflammation of eye, skin, or mucous membrane in form of iritis, pyoderma gangrenosum, erythema nodosum, or aphthous ulcers of mouth and tongue

General status: Low-grade fever; low energy level

Psychosocial emotional status; interactions with significant others and health care providers; effect on social activities and work; involvement with local support organizations; seeks psychiatric help; influence on sexuality and sexual activity

Knowledge level: Disease process, complications, manifestations, usual tests and procedures, local support organizations

Musculoskeletal system: Joint pains, back pain

Potential Complications

Severe malabsorption, small bowel obstruction, abscess, fistula, cancer, perforation, systemic manifestations

Patient Problems/Nursing Diagnoses & Interventions

NIC Elimination Management

Diarrhea related to intestinal inflammatory process
- Protect the perianal skin with barrier ointments.
- Provide for privacy and odor control.
- Check stools for occult blood.
- Provide antidiarrheal medications as ordered.
- Replace losses as needed (fluids, electrolytes, and blood products).

NIC Nutrition Support

Imbalanced nutrition: less than body requirements, related to decreased intake, nausea, abdominal pain and cramping, food intolerance, and diarrhea
- Monitor weight, serum albumin (or prealbumin if available), folate, hemoglobin, magnesium, iron, and vitamin B_{12}.
- Obtain nutritional consultation.
- Provide nutritional supplements, enteral or parenteral formulas as ordered.
- Assist the patient in identifying irritating foods if the disease is new to him or her.

NIC Coping Assistance

Risk for compromised family coping related to the nature of the disease symptoms and the chronicity of the disease and the effect on sexuality
- Provide sensitive, caring approach to patient and his or her family.
- Help patient and family support one another as they manage effects of chronic illness in their lives; refer as needed for support.
- Provide opportunities for patient and family to express their feelings regarding the illness and to identify their perceptions for a successful outcome (including changes in sexuality patterns).

NIC Physical Comfort Promotion

Acute pain related to intestinal inflammation
- Monitor change in intensity of pain, effectiveness of narcotics, relation of pain to stress, passage of bowel movements, and eating.

- Provide for adjunctive treatments that help manage pain (relaxation, music, massage, diversion).
- Provide analgesics as ordered.

NIC SKIN/WOUND MANAGEMENT

Risk for impaired skin integrity related to diarrhea, incontinence, and perianal disease

- Protect perianal skin in patients with frequent bowel movements.
  - Use gentle cleansing solutions, such as Periwash or Tucks.
  - Do not use toilet paper; have patient use squirt bottle to rinse perineum after bowel movements instead of wiping.
  - Apply barrier cream to protect skin.
  - If area is denuded, use sitz baths or cleanse with cotton balls soaked in mineral oil.
  - Use Anusol suppositories or Nupercainal ointment.
- Provide interventions or treatment for perianal fissures as ordered; treatment includes sitz baths and keeping the perianal area cleansed after bowel movements.

PATIENT EDUCATION/CONTINUUM OF CARE PLAN

1. Discuss with patient the usual treatments, procedures, and natural history of the disease.
2. Teach patient the importance of optimal nutrition in cooperation with nutritionist.
3. Explain to patient the schedules of medications. Ensure that patient understands how prednisone affects adrenal glands and how he or she must not abruptly stop taking the medication.
4. Provide patient with information on drug toxicities. For example, sulfasalazine is associated with rashes, and patients may be desensitized with small doses.
5. Inform patient of Crohn's and Colitis Foundation of America as a source of support and information.
6. Provide specific instructions for procedures and allow return demonstrations: TPN or central line care.

EVALUATION/PATIENT OUTCOMES

Elimination Management: Number and consistency of stools are within normal limits. Patient has a decrease in episodes of fecal incontinence. Patient has fewer episodes of diarrhea and incontinence.

Nutrition Support: Nutrition is adequate. Patient's weight is in positive nitrogen balance. Patient has an appetite. Patient's protein and caloric intake is adequate.

Coping Assistance: Patient and family are able to cope with chronic illness or an acute exacerbation. Patient and family are able to verbalize factors that create anxiety and stress. Patient and family are aware of resources available to them for further supportive care. Patient and family are able to verbalize mechanisms that help them deal with stressors.

Physical Comfort Promotion: Comfort level is achieved. Patient is able to perform activities of daily living (ADLs). Patient has stopped using all injectable narcotics by discharge. Patient is able to use alternate methods for relief of pain.

Skin/Wound Management: Skin integrity is maintained. No evidence of irritation from diarrhea or perianal fistula drainage.

ULCERATIVE COLITIS

Ulcerative colitis is a chronic mucosal inflammatory disease limited to the colon and rectum.

The disease generally starts in the rectum and progresses uninterrupted through the colon. The mucosa and submucosa layers of the colon and rectum are affected by ulcerative colitis. It is often difficult to differentiate the symptoms of ulcerative colitis from Crohn's disease of the large colon. The distinction between the two diseases is important in planning treatment and long-term prognosis. Ulcerative colitis is cured by total proctocolectomy. The incidence of cancer associated with long-standing ulcerative colitis is four times greater than in Crohn's disease. Ulcerative colitis is characterized by bloody, frequent, watery diarrhea. Patients report as many as 20 to 30 diarrheal stools per day. Remissions and exacerbations of the disease are common.

The annual incidence of ulcerative colitis has been relatively stable, with 6 to 12 cases per 100,000 persons per year in Northern countries.[2] The incidence of ulcerative colitis is more common among Jewish than non-Jewish populations and among whites than nonwhites. The disease is seen with highest frequency between the ages of 15 and 25 years.

There is a higher frequency of additional cases of ulcerative colitis in families than in control populations. It is not uncommon to have family members with ulcerative colitis and Crohn's disease. A small percentage of patients may demonstrate features of both ulcerative colitis and Crohn's disease.

As with Crohn's disease, research continues to focus on discovery of the cause. Surgery is no longer considered a "last resort," and newer surgical techniques have improved the outlook for patients. Continent ileostomies and ileoanal reservoir procedures have eliminated the need for conventional ileostomies in selected patient populations.

PATHOPHYSIOLOGY

The cause of ulcerative colitis is unknown. Proposed causes include infectious agents, genetic factors, immunologic mechanisms, environmental, and psychosomatic determinants. No specific bacterium or virus has been found to be the exogenous agent producing the inflammatory reaction seen in ulcerative colitis. The genetic hypothesis is suggested because of the familial tendency for the disease, the higher incidence in Jews, and the low incidence among nonwhites.

An immunologic contribution has been suggested for ulcerative colitis because of the presence of extraintestinal manifestations and the presence of antibodies to colonic epithelial cells and of cytotoxic T cells. Like Crohn's disease, the foundation for the occurrence of ulcerative colitis is probably at the primary genetic level, and the expression of genetic susceptibility is triggered by environmental factors.[35]

Environmental factors may have a role in the pathogenesis of ulcerative colitis because of the increased incidence of the disorder in industrialized nations. An increased incidence of ulcerative colitis occurs in nonsmokers or in heavy smokers who quit. Environmental factors (infectious, noninfectious antigens, or toxins) may trigger a sequence of events in which altered immunologic responses result in inflammatory bowel disease. Studies investigating dietary factors as causative agents have not provided definitive answers.

Stress and tension may influence the symptoms of ulcerative colitis and have been known to cause exacerbations.

Ulcerative colitis is an inflammatory disease confined primarily to the mucosa and to a lesser degree to the adjacent submucosa. The primary lesion appears to be crypt abscess formation in the crypts of Lieberkühn. Polymorphonuclear cells accumulate near the tip of the crypt, and degenerative changes occur in the crypt epithelial cells. As the crypt abscess progresses, frank necrosis of the crypt epithelium occurs and the polymorphonuclear infiltrate extends through the colonic epithelium. A more chronic inflammatory infiltrate composed of mast cells, lymphocytes, plasma cells, and eosinophils develops. Vascular engorgement appears in the submucosa. The microabscesses in the crypts are not visible to an unaided eye. However, as the microabscesses coalesce by lateral enlargement, they produce shallow ulcerations of the mucosa extending down to the lamina propria. In some areas the extensions of the abscesses undermine the mucosa on three sides, producing an area of ulceration adjacent to a hanging fragment of mucosa, which is referred to as a pseudopolyp during radiographic or endoscopic procedures.

The body attempts to heal itself even as the destruction of the mucosa is occurring. Highly vascular granulation tissue may develop in ulcerated, denuded areas. Collagen is deposited in the lamina propria. Fibrosis is minimal. In long-standing disease the muscularis mucosae may hypertrophy. The hypertrophy and spasms of the muscularis mucosae may result in shortening and narrowing of the colon, loss of haustral markings, and apparent stricture formation. All of these are reversible in ulcerative colitis because they are not caused by fibrosis.

The two most prominent symptoms of ulcerative colitis are hematochezia and diarrhea. (See Emergency Alert box on p. 699.) The bleeding is the result of the mucosal changes: ulceration, vascular engorgement, and highly vascular, friable granulation tissue. As the mucosa is destroyed or damaged, it loses its ability to absorb sodium and water, resulting in watery diarrhea. The absence of involvement of the muscularis and serosa layers accounts for the lack of localized abdominal pain, fistula formation, and well-defined peritoneal signs observed frequently in Crohn's disease.

Complications of ulcerative colitis include perforation, toxic megacolon, adenocarcinoma of the colon, massive hemorrhage, and extracolonic manifestations. Perforation of the colon may develop if the disease process extends through the muscle and serosa layers of the colon. Toxic megacolon is a severe and serious complication of ulcerative colitis. Toxic megacolon is associated with fulminant disease, in which the circular and longitudinal muscles have been destroyed. Damage to the myenteric ganglia in the wall of the colon produces a loss of contractibility, and peristalsis ceases with marked dilation of the colon developing. The transmural inflammation may lead to necrosis and perforation. Narcotics, anticholinergics, and hypokalemia may precipitate toxic megacolon because they produce atony of the smooth muscles of the colon.

Cancer of the colon and rectum occurs at a much higher rate in patients with ulcerative colitis than in the general population. Two factors appear to be related to the incidence of adenocarcinoma of the colon and rectum. First, the duration of the disease process has been related to the cancers. Ulcerative colitis of 10 years' duration increases the risk, and the risk continues to increase thereafter. Second, the extent of colonic involvement influences the risk of colorectal cancers. The more universal (affecting the entire colon and rectum) ulcerative colitis is, the higher the incidence of cancer. Patients with the disease limited to the rectum have no greater risk of colon cancer than persons of the same age and sex without ulcerative colitis. The cancerous lesions tend to be flat and infiltrative in nature and are multicentric. Early diagnosis is important. In patients with ulcerative colitis of 10 years' duration or longer, frequent colonoscopy with biopsy is recommended (at least yearly). Even with close follow-up, colon cancer may be detected too late for curative therapy.

The question often arises of whether to perform a prophylactic colectomy after a duration of 10 years. Colectomy does cure ulcerative colitis and also prevents colon cancer. Of course, the person will have some type of diversional procedure (conventional ileostomy, continent ileostomy, ileorectal pouch). One question concerning length of duration is the actual beginning of the disease. Patients may have the ulcerative colitis for a year or two before diagnosis. The decision to have surgery is a serious one with which patients are faced. By the time a patient with long-standing disease is admitted for surgery, he or she has dealt with a variety of emotions and may be "ready" for surgery. Other patients prefer to wait until it is essential that surgery be done. Although it is impossible to generalize and recommend surgical interventions for all patients, the nurse does play an important role in educating patients to the risk of cancer, the long-term effects of the disease, its treatments, and the need for consistent follow-up, even when the patient is asymptomatic.

A medical emergency for a person with ulcerative colitis is a massive hemorrhage, which occurs in approximately 4% of patients.[2] Patients with ulcerative colitis are often severely ill, with high temperatures, tachycardia, and fluid depletion. Massive fluid replacements are required to replace the circulating volume and maintain blood pressure. The hemorrhage usually subsides spontaneously. Surgical intervention (total proctocolectomy) is rarely necessary.

The mortality of an acute initial episode of ulcerative colitis is approximately 5%. The prognosis is negatively affected by total colonic involvement, age at onset older than 60 years, and presence of toxic megacolon.

Extracolonic manifestations can also be serious complications of ulcerative colitis. Arthritis, uveitis, and skin disorders reflect the disease process and will have remissions and exacerbations with the disease. The arthritis of ulcerative colitis involves the larger joints and is migratory. The joint is frequently swollen, erythematous, and tender. Steroids also cause osteonecrosis, and patients should have bone scans or magnetic resonance imaging (MRI) if they complain of bone pain while receiving long-term steroids.

Uveitis (iritis) is the most common eye lesion seen accompanying ulcerative colitis. The patient may experience blurred vision, eye pain, and photophobia. An acute attack of iritis may be followed by atrophy of the iris, anterior and posterior synechiae, and old pigment deposits on the lens.

The extracolonic skin disorders consist of erythema nodosum and pyoderma gangrenosum. Erythema nodosum consists of raised, tender, erythematous swellings of 2 to 3 cm on the arms and legs. The condition often develops during an exacerbation of the colitis and is frequently found when arthritis is associated with the exacerbation of the primary disease. Occasionally arthritis and erythema nodosum appear just before the first overt bowel symptoms of ulcerative colitis. Pyoderma gangrenosum is less frequent than erythema nodosum and is usually associated with severe ulcerative colitis. Pyoderma gangrenosum first appears as a pinpoint lesion, a boil, or an infected hair follicle. The lesion collects purulent drainage that contains few polymorphonuclear cells and no bacteria. The lesion may drain spontaneously. There is a characteristic purple border around the lesion. As the lesion becomes gangrenous, progressive necrosis of the dermis occurs and the area is deeply ulcerated. Healing of the lesions requires control of the ulcerative colitis through corticosteroids or surgical removal of the colon and rectum.

Liver diseases have also been associated with ulcerative colitis. The pathogenesis is not understood, and the incidence of liver disease is approximately 7%. Liver disease may range from minor abnormalities in one or more liver function tests to more serious changes in liver structure and function. Diseases of the liver associated with ulcerative colitis include fatty infiltrations, pericholangitis, chronic active hepatitis, postnecrotic cirrhosis, amyloidosis, and sclerosing cholangitis. The question remains as to the degree of improvement in liver diseases after colectomy.

Renal stone formation is associated with ulcerative colitis and is probably related to dehydration, inactivity of the patient, and changes in the composition of the urine.

Ulcerative colitis may range from mild to severe. The degree of involvement of the colon influences the severity. For many patients, ulcerative colitis will remain in remission for years after an acute phase of the illness. The treatment and the nursing interventions will be influenced by the degree of involvement and the severity of the colitis.

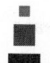

Diagnostic Studies and Findings

Stool cultures: Negative

Laboratory studies: Hemoglobin, hematocrit: anemia; liver function: abnormal; serum albumin: low; erythrocyte sedimentation rate (ESR): elevated; white blood cell count (acute episode): elevated

Sigmoidoscopy: Submucosal inflammation and edema; subepithelial infiltration and edema; microscopic mucosal erosions; crypt abscesses; granular appearance; friable (bleeds easily)

Rectal biopsy: Inflammatory changes in the mucosa; helps to differentiate between ulcerative colitis and Crohn's colitis

Colonoscopy: Superficial mucosal changes in early disease: hyperemia, mucosal friability, fine granular pattern, shallow ulcerations; late disease: coarse, granular appearance; deep mucosal ulcerations; pseudopolyps; shortening of colon; loss of haustrations (NOTE: Colonoscopy should be avoided in acute situations because of danger of perforation.)

X-ray examination: Plain film of abdomen: shortening of colon; loss of haustrations; irregular mucosa caused by pseudopolyps, ulcerations, and mucosa tags; midtransverse colon dilated with air in toxic megacolon; thickened bowel wall

Double-contrast barium enemas: Evaluates disease above the sigmoidoscopy level (preferred over colonoscopy); early disease: study may appear normal, or there may be a reticulated pattern denoting the denudation of the mucosa; late disease: ulceration of mucosa; shortening of the bowel; pseudopolyps (NOTE: Under no circumstances should a patient with ulcerative colitis be prepared with irritant cathartics; such treatment may worsen the disease; barium enemas should be avoided in acute situations because of danger of perforation.)

Multidisciplinary Plan

Surgery

Emergency operations (fulminant disease, hemorrhage, perforation, toxic megacolon)
- Total abdominal colectomy (subtotal colectomy) with end ileostomy and distal mucous fistula or Hartmann's pouch

Elective operations (intractability, dysplasia, or cancer)
- Mucosal proctectomy with ileoanal anastomosis performed in one or two stages; if the operation is done in one stage, there is no diverting ileostomy; stage I: subtotal colectomy, rectal mucosal stripping, creation of ileal reservoir, anastomosis of reservoir to upper anal canal after pulling it down through the rectal muscle tube, formation of diverting ileostomy; stage II: takedown of the diverting ileostomy and reestablishing bowel continuity
- Continent ileostomy: Total proctocolectomy with the creation of an ileal reservoir with an intussuscepted ileal segment or nipple valve formation creating continence
- Total proctocolectomy with permanent ileostomy

Medications

Choice depends on location and severity of disease; if the disease is confined to the rectum or left colon, suppositories or enemas may be all that are needed

Corticosteroids
- In mild disease (ulcerative proctitis), acute phase: Hydrocortisone retention enemas, 100 mg in 60 ml nightly, should retain for 20 min
- In mild disease, remission: Hydrocortisone retention enemas several times per week, slowly tapering down and discontinuing
- In moderate disease, acute phase: Prednisone, 40-60 mg/day PO
- In moderate disease, remission: Taper off prednisone slowly

In severe disease, acute phase: Prednisolone, 100 mg IV over 24 h (need intravenous potassium to prevent steroid-induced hypokalemia) q10-14d followed by prednisolone, 60-100 mg/day PO (If patient does not respond, surgery may be indicated)

5-ASA derivatives: Need weeks to months for response

Rectal preparations

Rowasa enema, 4 g/60 ml buffered suspension suppository 0.5 g/kg

Oral preparations

Sulfasalazine (Azulfidine): Acute phase, 3-4 g tid PO; maintenance 4-6 g/day

Pentasa, 2-4 g/day

Asacol, 2-4 g/day

Dipentum, 500 mg bid

Topical corticoids: Decreased systemic effects, decreased systemic absorption—clinical trials only

Budesonide, 2 mg/dl enema (100 times more potent than topical hydrocortisone)

Tixocortol pivalate, 250 mg nightly enema

Immunosuppressives

6-Mercaptopurine (6-MP), 50 mg/day to 1.5 mg/kg/day

Azathioprine, 50 mg/day initially; dosage may be increased if well tolerated

Cyclosporine (clinical trials only), 8-10 mg/kg/day PO

Methotrexate (clinical trials only), 8-10 mg/kg/day PO

Antidiarrheal agents:

Loperamide (Imodium), 4 mg/day and 2 mg after each unformed stool up to a maximum of 16 mg/day

Diphenoxylate hydrochloride (Lomotil), 5 mg qid (codeine and Lomotil used with caution because opiates and atropine in Lomotil can precipitate toxic megacolon)

Metamucil, 1 teaspoon qid (used to add bulk to watery stools; avoid in the very ill patient)

Folate supplementation

General Management

Acute phase: Intravenous fluids, limited activity or bed rest, TPN (for severe dehydration and cachexia); blood replacement usually required; nasogastric tube if dilated colon; no opiates or anticholinergics if risk of toxic megacolon

Nutrition: No general restrictions; patients should avoid foods that they identify as irritating; usually a low-fiber diet advanced as tolerated with one food added at a time; milk can be a problem for some patients; need extra calories and protein

NURSING CARE

Nursing Assessment

General status: Low energy level, fever

Pain: Location and nature of pain

Use pain scale for rating both intensity of pain and ability to tolerate pain

Nutritional status: Anorexia, nausea, dietary intolerances, weight loss

Abdominal examination: Localized areas of tenderness, bowel sounds

Gastrointestinal system

Diarrhea: Amount and frequency; presence of blood or mucus; relation to eating, stress, activity; tenesmus; incontinence

Hemorrhoids

Integumentary system: Pyoderma gangrenosum, erythema nodosum; perianal skin for fissures, fistulas, abscesses, irritation

Psychosocial concerns: Emotional status; interactions with significant others; interactions with health care providers; impact on social activities and work; involvement with local support organizations or psychiatric help; impact on sexuality and sexual activity

Knowledge level: Disease process, complications, manifestations, usual tests and procedures, local support organizations

Musculoskeletal system: Joint pains, back pain

Potential Complications

Toxic megacolon: severe abdominal distention; increasing abdominal pain; fever; tachycardia; sharp decrease in number of stools and in gas; rectal bleeding; hypoactive or absent bowel sounds

Patient Problems/Nursing Diagnoses & Interventions

NIC Elimination Management

Diarrhea related to intestinal inflammatory process

- Protect patient's perianal skin with barrier ointments.
- Provide privacy and odor control for patient.
- Check patient's stools for occult blood.
- Provide patient with antidiarrheal medications as ordered.
- Replace patient's losses as needed (fluids, electrolytes, and blood products).

NIC Nutrition Support

Imbalanced nutrition: less than body requirements, related to decreased intake, nausea, abdominal pain and cramping, food intolerance, and diarrhea

- Monitor patient's weight, serum albumin (or prealbumin, if available), folate, hemoglobin, magnesium, iron, and vitamin B_{12}
- Request a consultation with the nutritionist for the patient.
- Provide the patient with nutritional supplements, enteral, or parenteral formulas as ordered.
- Assist the patient to identify irritating foods if the disease is new to him or her.

NIC Coping Assistance

Risk for compromised family coping related to nature of disease symptoms and the chronicity of the disease, and the effect on sexuality

- Provide sensitive, caring approach for patient and family.
- Help patient and family support each other as they manage the effects of chronic illness in their lives. Refer patient for support as needed.
- Provide opportunities for patient and family to express their feelings regarding the illness and to identify their

perceptions for a successful outcome (including changes in sexuality patterns).

NIC Physical Comfort Promotion

Acute pain related to intestinal inflammation

- Monitor changes in patient for intensity of pain, effectiveness of narcotics, relation of pain to stress, passage of bowel movements, and eating.
- Provide for adjunctive treatments for patient that help manage pain (relaxation, music, massage, diversion).
- Provide analgesics as ordered.

NIC Skin/Wound Management

Risk for impaired skin integrity related to diarrhea, incontinence, and perianal disease

- Protect perianal skin in patients who have frequent bowel movements.
  - Use gentle cleansing solutions (Periwash, Tucks) on patient.
  - Do not use toilet paper; have patient use squirt bottle to cleanse perineal area after bowel movements instead of wiping.
  - Apply barrier cream to protect patient's skin.
  - If area is denuded, have patient use sitz baths or cleanse with cotton balls soaked in mineral oil.
  - Have patient use Anusol suppositories or Nupercainal ointment.
- Provide interventions or treatment for patient's perianal fissures as ordered: sitz baths; keep area cleansed after bowel movements.

Patient Education/Continuum of Care Plan

1. Discuss with patient the usual treatments, procedures, and natural history of the disease.
2. Teach patient the importance of optimal nutrition, using nutritionist.
3. Explain schedules of medications. Ensure that patient understands how prednisone affects adrenal glands and explain that patient must not abruptly stop taking the medication.
4. Provide patient with information about drug toxicities. For example, sulfasalazine is associated with rashes, and patients may be desensitized by taking small doses.
5. Inform patient of Crohn's and Colitis Foundation of America as a source of support and information.
6. Provide patient with specific instructions for procedures and allow return demonstrations: TPN, central line care.

Evaluation/Patient Outcomes

Elimination Management: Number and consistency of stools are within normal limits. Patient has a decrease in episodes of fecal incontinence and in the number of stools. Patient has fewer episodes of diarrhea and incontinence. Patient knows which foods to avoid.

Nutrition Support: Nutrition is adequate. Patient is in positive nitrogen balance. Patient has an appetite. Patient's protein and caloric intake is adequate.

Coping Assistance: Patient and family are able to cope with chronic illness or an acute exacerbation. Patient and family are able to verbalize factors that create anxiety and stress. Patient and family are aware of resources available to them for further supportive care. Patient and family are able to verbalize mechanisms that help them deal with stressors.

Physical Comfort Promotion: Comfort level is achieved. Patient is able to perform ADLs. Patient has stopped using all injectable narcotics by discharge. Patient is able to use alternate methods for relief of pain.

Skin/Wound Management: Skin integrity maintained. Patient's perianal skin is intact.

Benign Tumors

The term *tumor* is used to refer to neoplasm, a new growth of tissue characterized by uncontrolled proliferation of cells. A tumor may be malignant or benign.

The benign tumors of the small and large intestines include colonic adenomas (polyps), villous or papillary adenomas, lipomas, leiomyomas, and lymphoid hyperplasia. Polyps have been discussed on p. 693. A villous adenoma is a rare tumor found most often in the rectosigmoid area; it may be benign or contain foci of carcinoma. Lipomas are smooth, round tumors found in the submucosal layer of the colon. Leiomyomas are found in the small intestine and are submucosal or subserosal growths that protrude intraluminally, extraluminally, or in both directions. Malignant tumors of the colorectal area are covered in Chapter 18.

Benign tumors in the intestines occur equally in men and women. The benign tumors are most often discovered between the ages of 50 and 80. Symptomatic benign tumors are commonly diagnosed between the ages of 30 and 60. Most benign tumors in the small and large intestines are asymptomatic and may be discovered during routine examinations or surgery. Symptoms, when present, are generally related to the size of the tumor. A benign tumor may block the lumen, resulting in obstruction or intussusception. If the mucosa covering a tumor is irritated and becomes ulcerated, the patient may have signs of intestinal bleeding.

The cause of isolated benign tumors of the small intestine is unknown. Benign tumors in the small bowel include adenomas, leiomyomas, lipomas, hamartomas (associated with Peutz-Jeghers syndrome), and neurogenic tumors. Pseudotumors may also be found in the small intestine, and surgical excision is required for histologic studies and differential diagnosis.

The most common benign tumor of the colon is the polyp (or colonic adenoma). Neurofibromas, leiomyomas, and lipomas are found, but the incidence is low. Histologic examination of the tissue is required to determine the type of tumor.

PATHOPHYSIOLOGY

Adenomas in the intestines may be tubular, villous, or tubulovillous. Adenomas in the small intestine are generally found near the ileum. Villous adenomas are rare in the small intestine and when they occur are found in the duodenum. The villous adenoma is most often found in the rectosigmoid areas. It tends to recur, to secrete large amounts of mucus, and to act as a site for development of cancer.

The primary symptoms of villous adenomas in the rectosigmoid area include increased colonic motility, diarrhea, and electrolyte loss. A villous adenoma higher in the gastrointestinal tract does not seem to precipitate the electrolyte loss, probably because of the reabsorption capacity of the colon distal to the adenoma. Villous adenomas consist of branching papillary fronds lined with goblet cells. The villous adenoma secretes large amounts of mucus. If the villous adenoma is large, the amount of fluid lost through mucous secretions can be significant. Sodium and potassium are lost in the mucus diarrhea. The fluid and electrolyte imbalance may divert attention away from the presence of a villous adenoma as other conditions and causes are considered during diagnosis.

Lipomas may occur anywhere in the small and large intestines, but they are more common in the colon. Lipomas tend to be single lesions averaging 4 cm in diameter. Most lipomas are found incidentally during surgery. Symptoms are associated with intussusception, obstruction, or bleeding. Lipomas in the colon may be detected during water enemas when the returns contain fat. An enlargement of the ileocecal valve may be caused by lipomatosis or by a tumor in the cecum. Lipomatosis is more common, and differential diagnosis can be made by colonoscopy.

Leiomyomas in the small intestine are found in the jejunum and tend to produce more symptoms than other benign tumors of the small intestine. Ulceration of the mucosa is common, and patients' initial complaint is bleeding. Obstruction and intussusception are rare.

Lymphoid hyperplasia of the colon is found more often in children than in adults. An enlarged lymphoid follicle may occur in the rectum. No intervention is required. When lymphoid hyperplasia appears in multiple numbers throughout the rectum and colon, it can be confused with familial polyposis. Differential diagnosis is important because treatment is not indicated in lymphoid hyperplasia and total colectomy is used to treat familial polyposis.

DIAGNOSTIC STUDIES AND FINDINGS

Small bowel: Barium studies; prograde enteroclysis or retrograde infusion through ileocecal valve: small isolated tumors, multiple small tumors; exploratory laparotomy: biopsy and removal of tumor for histologic studies

Colon: Sigmoidoscopy, colonoscopy: visualization, biopsy, and removal of tumor; double-contrast barium enema: villous adenoma; reticulated appearance; presence of tumors in colon and rectum

MULTIDISCIPLINARY PLAN

Surgery

Laparotomy may be used for diagnosis and removal of tumors in small bowel when patient is symptomatic

Villous adenoma

- Above peritoneal reflection: Resection of bowel containing villous adenoma
- Below peritoneal reflection: Local excision
- With evidence of frank invasive carcinoma: Abdominoperineal resection

NURSING CARE

NURSING ASSESSMENT

Abdominal examination: Signs of intestinal obstruction: abdominal pain, distention, nausea and vomiting, absence of peristalsis, absence of bowel movements; large bowel or distal small bowel obstructions: fecal odor to emesis

Gastrointestinal status: Occult, blood-tinged, or black tarry stools

POTENTIAL COMPLICATIONS

Blockage, intussusception, cancer

PATIENT PROBLEMS/NURSING DIAGNOSES & INTERVENTIONS

NIC ELIMINATION MANAGEMENT

Constipation related to partial obstruction of bowel lumen

- Determine whether patient has regular bowel habits and whether bowel pattern has changed.
- Observe stool for shape, consistency, color, quantity, and odor.
- Note and report any signs of blood-tinged stools.
- Check stool for occult blood, an early sign of a bowel tumor.

PATIENT EDUCATION/CONTINUUM OF CARE PLAN

1. Provide patient with information about type of tumor and any impact regarding long-term care (e.g., after removal of villous adenoma, regular follow-up required if a focus of carcinoma is present).
2. Provide routine postoperative information on activity, diet, driving, and returning to work associated with any abdominal surgery.

EVALUATION/PATIENT OUTCOMES

Elimination Management: Bowel functions normally. Bowel elimination is adequate.

ANAL AND RECTAL DISORDERS

ANORECTAL ABSCESS

An anorectal abscess is a localized infection with pus found in the tissue spaces adjacent to and in the anorectal area.

Anorectal abscesses are classified according to location (FIG. 10-16):

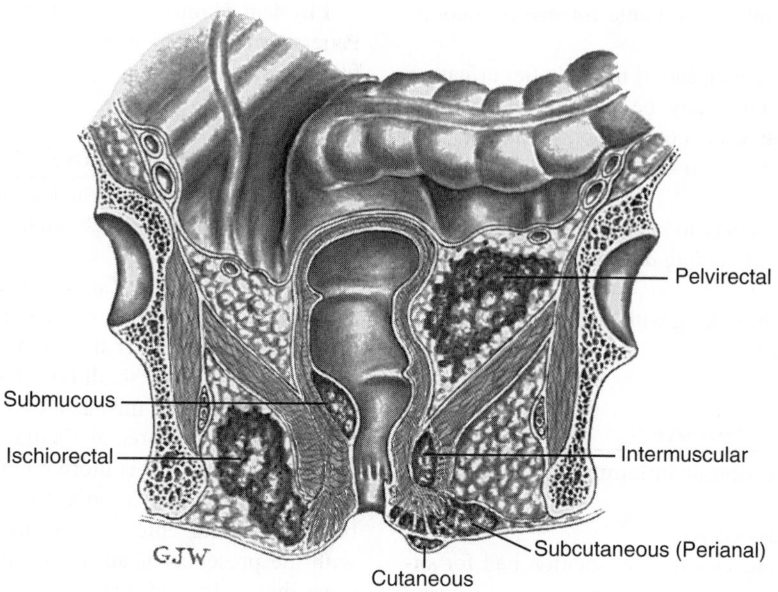

FIG. 10-16
Anorectal abscesses. (From Doughty.[10])

Perianal: Beneath perianal skin
Ischiorectal: Ischiorectal fossa
Intersphincteric: Between internal and external sphincters
Pelvirectal or supralevator: Above the levators ani and below the pelvic peritoneum

Anorectal abscesses are more common in men. Certain diseases and conditions increase the likelihood of anorectal abscesses developing. Anorectal abscesses are common in patients with Crohn's disease and in homosexual men who engage in traumatic anal intercourse. Hematologic and immune-deficient conditions have also been associated with anorectal abscesses.

PATHOPHYSIOLOGY

Anorectal abscesses develop from infections beginning in an anal crypt and moving along anal ducts through the internal sphincter before spreading in different directions. An infection may also develop in anal fissures, prolapsed internal hemorrhoids, traumatic injuries, and superficial skin lesions that progress to form anorectal abscesses. Extension of the abscess formation is the most common complication. An abscess may eventually progress to an anorectal fistula.

DIAGNOSTIC STUDIES AND FINDINGS

Anoscopy (proctoscopy): Visualization of lesions above the pectinate line

MULTIDISCIPLINARY PLAN

Surgery

Prompt surgical drainage of abscess, with or without excision of fistula tracts associated with anorectal abscesses

Medications

Antibiotic therapy based on causative organisms
Stool softeners: Docusate (Colace), 50-200 mg/day; dose based on individual's response

General Management

Sitz baths

NURSING CARE

NURSING ASSESSMENT

General status: Fever, malaise
Pain: Throbbing, constant pain exacerbated by sitting or walking (superficial abscess); pain decreases if abscess drains spontaneously; pain with defecation
Gastrointestinal status: Change in bowel habits (purulent discharge, increased odor); time of last bowel movement; use of laxatives or stool softeners, anal intercourse, anal dilators (e.g., vibrators or other instruments)
Perianal examination: Assess for signs of a tender, erythematous and indurated area that displaces the anus (superficial abscess), erythema, purulent drainage

POTENTIAL COMPLICATIONS

Anorectal fistula

PATIENT PROBLEMS/NURSING DIAGNOSES & INTERVENTIONS

NIC SKIN/WOUND MANAGEMENT

Impaired tissue integrity related to presence of infection or surgical wound
- Keep perianal area clean.
- Provide sitz baths, *for comfort and for cleansing purposes.*
- Apply dressing over wound; change frequently, noting color and amount of drainage; dressing may be held in

place with mesh "panties" available for use in incontinence management.
- Keep surgical wound clean; care is needed after urination and defecation; packing may be used to ensure that wound heals from the inside out; after bowel and bladder elimination, it is necessary to check dressing and replace if soiled.
- Shave perianal area weekly to keep hair from the wound *(hair will delay wound healing and is often the cause of infection or irritation).*
- Irrigate wound before packing with normal saline or irrigation solution as ordered.

NIC PHYSICAL COMFORT PROMOTION

Acute pain related to infection or inflammation in sensitive area
- Provide analgesics as ordered.
- Provide a thick pillow, cushion, or flotation pad for sitting (avoid air rings and rubber donuts *because they tend to spread the buttocks apart).*

PATIENT EDUCATION/CONTINUUM OF CARE PLAN

Demonstrate to patient how to irrigate wound (Water Pik or shower massager may be used) and to reinsert dressing. Family member may need to assist patient. Patient should comprehend necessity of keeping wound clean and free of fecal soiling.

EVALUATION/PATIENT OUTCOMES

Skin/Wound Management: Wound heals without complication. Skin integrity is maintained.

Physical Comfort Promotion: Comfort level is achieved. Patient verbalizes increased comfort and is able to have pain-free bowel movements.

ANORECTAL FISTULA

An anorectal fistula is a hollow, fibrous tunnel or tract with two openings lined by granulation tissue.

The internal opening of an anorectal fistula is inside the anal canal or rectum and leads to the secondary, or external, opening (FIG. 10-17). The external opening is in the perianal skin. Fistulas from the colon, small bowel, or urethra may exit through the perineum and be mistaken for anorectal fistulas.

Although an anorectal fistula may occur without predisposing conditions, it is more common to find anorectal fistulas associated with Crohn's disease in the large or the small bowel (regional enteritis). Anorectal fistulas are associated with the presence of an anorectal abscess. An anorectal abscess that is drained may reduce the discomfort and pain, but a fistulous tract may remain through which the abscess continues to drain.

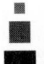

PATHOPHYSIOLOGY

The primary, or internal, opening of an anorectal fistula is usually at a crypt near the pectinate line. Infection in the crypt progresses to form an abscess that drains (spontaneously or with surgical drainage), and the tract is preserved as the abscess heals. Anorectal fistulas are associated with traumatic injury, fissures, Crohn's disease, chlamydial infections, tuberculosis, cancer, and radiation therapy. Once the tract is fibrosed, it will

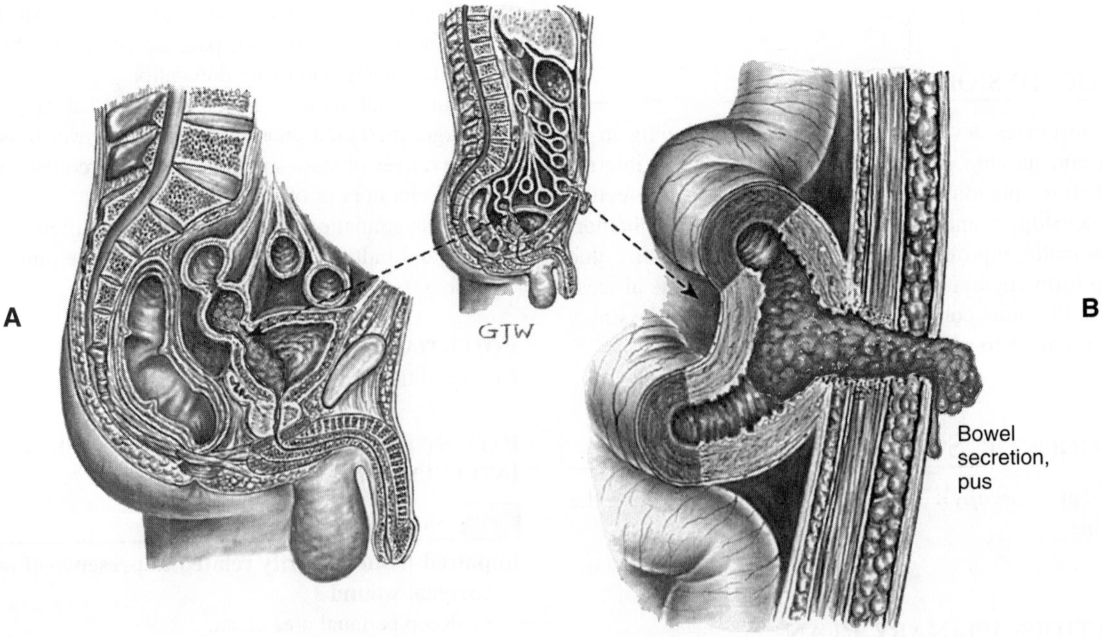

FIG. 10-17
Fistulas. **A,** Internal fistula with escape of bowel into the bladder and urethra. **B,** Enterocutaneous fistula into the abdominal wall. (From Doughty.[10])

not close on its own and surgical intervention is indicated. Stool, pus, mucus, blood, and flatus may drain through the fistula. Patients may have single or multiple anorectal fistulas. The skin opening may seal over temporarily, but it will reopen spontaneously and drain.

After treatment, recurrent fistulas in the anorectal area are associated with inadequate exposure of the tract, with primary openings not being identified, and with failure of the tract to heal from the inside out. When a patient has Crohn's disease, recurrent anorectal fistulas are associated with exacerbation of the inflammatory bowel disease.

Diagnostic Studies and Findings

Digital rectal examination: Palpate tract direction internally
Anoscopy (proctoscopy): May reveal the primary opening in a crypt
Sigmoidoscopy: Used to rule out other sources of fistula formation in patients with symptoms suggesting inflammatory bowel disease
Fistulography: Used if the tract is of questionable origin; rules out colonic, small bowel, and urethral fistulas

Multidisciplinary Plan

Surgery

Fistulotomy or fistulectomy may be indicated depending on location and depth of the fistula tract

Medications

Antibiotics per sensitive organism
Stool softener: Docusate (Colace), 50-200 mg/day; dose based on individual's response
Metronidazole (Flagyl), 20 mg/kg/day in divided doses (for perianal disease associated with inflammatory bowel disease)

General Management

Sitz baths as needed and after defecation

NURSING CARE

Nursing Assessment

Perianal examination: Raised, red papules; drainage of pus, blood, mucus, or stool through the open skin lesions; pruritus; inundated, "cordlike" pattern may be palpated from cutaneous opening toward anus
Pain: Complaints of pain and discomfort, complaints are greater when lesions are sealed and not draining
Gastrointestinal status: Change in bowel habits (purulent discharge, increased odor); time of last bowel movement; use of laxatives or stool softeners; anal intercourse; anal dilators (e.g., vibrators or other instruments); history of anorectal abscesses or inflammatory bowel disease

Potential Complications

Perianal irritation

Patient Problems/Nursing Diagnoses & Interventions

NIC Skin/Wound Management

Risk for impaired skin integrity related to presence of infection or surgical incision
- Estimate amount of drainage; note color, odor, and consistency of drainage.
- Keep perianal area clean after bowel movements with sitz baths and irrigation of site.
- Replace dressings as soiled and assess appearance of wound, signs of healings, and early signs of postoperative infection.
- Irrigate wound before packing or dressing.
- Shave perianal area regularly *to prevent hair from irritating or infecting wound as granulation tissue develops after surgery.*

NIC Physical Comfort Promotion

Acute pain related to perianal inflammation
- Provide pain medication as needed.
- Provide a thick foam cushion or pillow for patient to use in sitting (avoid air rings and rubber donuts *because they tend to spread the buttocks apart).*
- Provide sitz baths or warm compresses as needed.

Patient Education/Continuum of Care Plan

1. Instruct patient how to irrigate wound with Water Pik or shower massager, to shave perianal area, and to redress wound.
2. Show patient how to use a mirror to inspect area and look for redness or firm reddened areas of increased itching and tenderness.
3. Mesh panties can be used to hold dressings in place, or sanitary pads or belts may be used in the underwear. Jockey shorts will be more effective than boxer shorts for managing dressings.
4. A family member's help may be needed.
5. Sitz baths can be used for cleansing and for comfort. (Sitz bath does not replace irrigation procedure.)

Evaluation/Patient Outcomes

Skin/Wound Management: Skin integrity maintained. Perianal skin free of irritation.

Physical Comfort Promotion: Comfort level is achieved. Patient verbalizes increased comfort and is able to have pain-free bowel movements.

Anal Fissure

An anal fissure is a small tear in the lining of the anus. The tear resembles a slitlike crack and may extend from the anal verge to the pectinate line.

Fissures are most common in young and middle-age adults. The posterior midline is the most common site, but occasional anal fissures will be found in the anterior wall. Fissures in other positions on the anal wall are usually associated with Crohn's disease or ulcerative colitis.

Pathophysiology

Anal fissures are usually caused by trauma from passing large, hard stools. Acute fissures are tears that may become chronic when the patient has an elevated resting anal pressure and contraction of the internal anal sphincter after rectal distention. Defecation stimulates spasms of the internal anal sphincter, which causes the edges of the sphincter to adhere, trapping any drainage. Edema and fibrosis of adjacent tissue develop and progress to hypertrophied anal papillae and a tag of skin at the anal verge.

Loss of elasticity of the anal canal may predispose a person to anorectal fissures. Laxative abuse, scarring from anal surgery, and chronic diarrheal diseases may lead to a loss of elasticity, as will frequent anal intercourse.

Diagnostic Studies and Findings

Digital rectal examination: Use topical anesthesia before digital examination to decrease pain from the procedure; induration; tenderness; sphincter spasm; hypertrophied anal papillae

Anoscopy (proctoscopy): Visualization of the anorectal fissure: a superficial tear that bleeds easily and has a reddish base

Multidisciplinary Plan

Surgery

Lateral subcutaneous sphincterotomy (internal sphincter is divided up to the pectinate line, hypertrophied papillae and anal tag are excised, and fissure is left to heal); for chronic anal fissures

Medications

Bulk agents
- Psyllium (Metamucil or Effersyllium), 1 teaspoon (7 g) 1-3 times per day

Emollient suppositories

Analgesic ointments
- Dibucaine (Nupercaine) prn topically

Tucks or witch hazel pads to cleanse

1% hydrocortisone cream topically to fissure

Chronic Anal Fissures (Experimental Treatments)

0.2% topical nitroglycerine ointment to decrease mean resting sphincter pressure

Botulinum toxin (BoTox), 2.5-5 U injected into external sphincter to decrease mean resting sphincter pressure

General Management

Sitz bath; warm compresses

NURSING CARE

Nursing Assessment

Pain: Complaints of pain and discomfort during evacuation; described as tearing or burning; associated with slight bleeding; evacuation stimulates spasms that result in prolonged, gnawing discomfort for extended periods

Gastrointestinal status: Change in bowel habits (constipation, bright red blood after bowel movements); pruritus; time of last bowel movement; history or use of laxatives or stool softeners, anal intercourse, anal dilators (e.g., vibrators or other instruments), enema abuse, or inflammatory bowel disease; obtain dietary history

Perianal examination: Rectal tag of skin, rectal discharge

Potential Complications

Anal pain, constipation

Patient Problems/Nursing Diagnoses & Interventions

NIC Elimination Management

Constipation related to avoidance of painful defecation
- After surgery, record consistency of stool and effectiveness of stool softeners.
- Keep the postoperative site clean and free of stool by using sitz baths and careful cleansing after surgery.
- Administer bulk laxatives as ordered.

NIC Physical Comfort Promotion

Acute pain related to inflammation of anal area
- Provide warm compresses, sitz baths, and analgesic ointments for pain and discomfort.
- Patients often postpone or delay having bowel movements because of the pain.
- Premedicate before bowel movement and/or have sitz bath ready.

Patient Education/Continuum of Care Plan

Provide patient with information on natural methods of relieving or preventing constipation (i.e., diet high in bulk and fiber, increased fluid intake, avoidance of harsh laxatives and constipating medications such as codeine).

Evaluation/Patient Outcomes

Elimination Management: Gastrointestinal function is normal. Patient has no constipation or hard, formed stools.

Physical Comfort Promotion: Comfort level is achieved. Patient verbalizes increased comfort and has no pain with evacuation or delayed pain.

Hemorrhoids

Hemorrhoids are masses of vascular tissue found in the anal canal.[22]

Internal hemorrhoids are found above the pectinate line, arise from the superior hemorrhoidal venous plexus, and are covered with mucosa. External hemorrhoids are found below the pectinate line, arise from the inferior hemorrhoidal venous plexus, and are covered by anoderm and perianal skin. Patients may have a combination of internal and external hemorrhoids.

Internal hemorrhoids may also be classified according to the degree of involvement:

First-degree: Project slightly into the anal canal
Second-degree: Prolapse with defecation and reduce spontaneously
Third-degree: Prolapse with defecation and reduce manually
Fourth-degree: Irreducible

One commonly accepted cause is that hemorrhoids are varicose veins. The basis of the varicose vein theory of hemorrhoids is that increased pressure in the veins results in congestion. Certain occupations, the erect positions of humans, structural absence of valves in the veins, and increased abdominal pressure from straining at defecation, constipation, and pregnancy have been associated with the development of hemorrhoids. Another related cause is increased maximal resting anal pressure, which has been the most consistently reported physiologic abnormality associated with hemorrhoids.[22]

Pathophysiology

An internal hemorrhoid is a prolapse of normal vascular mounds or a prolapse of normal anal canal lining. The prolapse may be caused by spasms of the internal sphincter that require straining or increased pressure to push the stool through the internal sphincter which results in the hemorrhoid.

The complications associated with internal hemorrhoids include bleeding, prolapse, and thrombosis. Because the hemorrhoid is composed of spongy vascular tissue, bleeding tends to be an oozing of bright red blood. The blood may appear as a bright spot on toilet paper or on the surface of the stool. Blood may drip from the anus for a few minutes after the stool has been expelled. Iron deficiency anemia may develop if blood loss continues over a period of time.

Prolapse of hemorrhoids is first perceived as a mass of tissue that protrudes from the anus after a bowel movement. Initially, it slips back into the anal canal spontaneously. As the condition continues, the hemorrhoid will later need to be manually replaced and may become irreducible. A mucous discharge is associated with irreducible hemorrhoids because of the mucosal covering of the internal hemorrhoid. Protection of undergarments will be required. Pain is associated with prolapsed and inflamed hemorrhoids but is not a general symptom of internal hemorrhoids. Patients whose initial complaint is pain should be assessed for other anorectal conditions (fissure, abscess) and colorectal diseases.

Thrombosis of prolapsed hemorrhoids can create severe pain. This is also referred to as strangulated hemorrhoids. Ulceration and secondary infections can develop. One or all hemorrhoids may be affected.

A thrombosis of an external hemorrhoid is a blood clot within a hemorrhoidal vein. The pectinate line is visible and separate from the mass or lump that forms. Thrombosis of external hemorrhoids has been associated with heavy lifting, straining at defecation, and childbirth. The patient has a painful lump that appears suddenly at the anus. Pain may be constant and is increased with sitting and defecation. It usually disappears in a week. The thrombosed external hemorrhoid should not be confused with prolapsed, thrombosed internal hemorrhoids. If the skin covering the clot becomes ulcerated, bleeding may be noted.

Diagnostic Studies and Findings

Digital rectal examination. Tone of internal sphincter: usually increased in young men with hemorrhoids; may be low in older patients and women with hemorrhoids; palpation of third-degree internal hemorrhoids

Anoscopy: Visualization of hemorrhoids as instrument is removed

Sigmoidoscopy and barium enema: To rule out carcinoma and inflammatory disease; particularly important in patients 40 years old and older who complain of abdominal symptoms, altered bowel habits, or a family history of colon cancer

Multidisciplinary Plan

Surgery

Injection of sclerosing solutions (5% morrhuate sodium or ethanolamine in vegetable oil) submucosally around hemorrhoid; complications: sloughing of overlying mucosa, prostatic or rectal infection, reaction to injected material

Rubber band ligation: Placement of rubber band over base of hemorrhoid causes necrosis and sloughing of hemorrhoid in 7 days; complications: rarely, rectal infection

Photocoagulation: Application of infrared light or lasers to coagulate hemorrhoids

Electrocoagulation: Application of low voltage to destroy hemorrhoidal tissue

Hemorrhoidectomy: Surgical excision of the hemorrhoidal masses; complication: anal stenosis

Excision under local anesthesia of thrombosed external hemorrhoid if seen in a day or two of onset

Medications

Anesthetic ointments and suppositories
Dibucaine (Nupercaine) prn
Stool softeners, bulk laxatives
Analgesics
Topical hydrocortisone ointments

General Management

High-fiber diet, adequate hydration, and exercise to minimize constipation and straining; warm sitz baths; compresses

Nutritional Consultation

To educate patient regarding high-fiber dietary selections

NURSING CARE

Nursing Assessment

Perianal skin examination: External hemorrhoids visible in subcutaneous skin at anus; if hemorrhoids are thrombosed, tender, bluish spheric mass at anal verge; prolapsed internal hemorrhoids: moist, red mucosa covering upper portion; presence of mucoid discharge or staining of undergarments

Pain: Size and type of hemorrhoid determine amount of pain: internal hemorrhoids may have no symptoms; thrombosis of prolapsed hemorrhoids causes severe pain; pain related to bowel movements

Gastrointestinal status: Change in bowel habits (constipation, bright red blood after bowel movements); pruritus; last bowel movement; history of use of laxatives or stool softeners, straining at the toilet, enema abuse; obtain dietary history

Potential Complications

Bleeding, prolapse, thrombosis

Patient Problems/Nursing Diagnoses & Interventions

NIC Physical Comfort Promotion

Acute pain related to inflammation and increased pressure

- Use thick foam pillows or pads under buttock; avoid air or rubber donuts *because they spread the buttocks apart.*
- Promote the use of sitz baths *for comfort and for cleansing* after bowel movements.
- Assess patient during sitz bath for hypotension resulting from vasodilation of pelvic blood vessels.
- Provide oral and topical analgesics as ordered.
- Use ice packs as ordered *to reduce congestion and edema.*
- Use warm compresses *to promote circulation* (also soothing).

NIC Elimination Management

Constipation related to poor dietary habits and fear of defecation

- Instruct patient to defecate promptly with the urge, to avoid sitting on toilet for prolonged periods, and to avoid straining.
- Provide adequate fluids *to maintain hydration.*
- Encourage patient to exercise (mild at first).
- Give patient medication before first bowel movement.
- Encourage patient to have a bowel movement after surgery even though patient may be afraid of increased pain *(prevents formation of strictures and preserves lumen size of anus).*
- Administer laxatives as ordered.
- Educate patient regarding a high-fiber diet.

Patient Education/Continuum of Care Plan

1. Management and prevention of constipation with diet, fluids, and physical activities should be discussed with patient.
2. Patient needs to respond to urge to defecate, to avoid straining, and to keep stool soft and moist.

Evaluation/Patient Outcomes

Physical Comfort Promotion: Comfort level is achieved. Patient verbalizes increased comfort and has no pain with evacuation. Patient has no delayed pain.

Elimination Management: Gastrointestinal function is normal. Patient has no constipation or hard, formed stools. Patient eats a high-fiber diet with good hydration.

Pilonidal Disease

Pilonidal disease occurs in the midline of the upper portion of the gluteal fold. A sinus channel develops that is lined with epithelium and hair.

The sinus channel may appear as a hairy dimple that is asymptomatic unless it becomes infected or inflamed. A cyst or abscess may develop. Pilonidal disease affects men more than women, probably because of the increased amount of hair.

Pathophysiology

The trapping of hair beneath the skin and the enlargement of hair follicles probably causes infection and irritation.

Diagnostic Studies and Findings

Refer to diagnostic studies on anorectal fistulas.

Multidisciplinary Plan

Surgery

Incision and drainage under local anesthesia; removal of hair and granulation tissue; wound may be closed or left open and packed

Medications

Antibiotic therapy to treat the infection per organism

NURSING CARE

Nursing Assessment

Pain: Tenderness, erythema, and induration in sacral region

Perianal examination: Hairy dimple in gluteal fold; open draining lesion in sacral region with hair protruding from sinus opening

Potential Complications

Infection, abscess formation

Patient Problems/Nursing Diagnoses & Interventions

NIC Physical Comfort Promotion

Acute pain related to surgical drainage of cyst or abscess

- Apply hot moist compresses when an abscess is present.
- Assist patient with sitz bath.
- Position patient on abdomen or side.

Patient Education/Continuum of Care Plan

1. Prepare patient or family member to change dressing as needed, to keep wound free of fecal and urinary contamination, and to cleanse wound as needed.
2. Avoid direct trauma.

3. Shave skin regularly or apply a depilatory regularly to prevent hair growth.

EVALUATION/PATIENT OUTCOMES

Physical Comfort Promotion: Comfort level is achieved. Patient uses pain control strategies appropriately. Patient verbalizes increased control over pain.

LIVER DISORDERS

CIRRHOSIS

Cirrhosis is a chronic degenerative disease of the liver in which diffuse destruction and regeneration of hepatic parenchymal cells have occurred.

In cirrhosis the lobes are covered with fibrotic tissue, and the lobules are infiltrated with fat (FIG. 10-18). The diffuse increase in connective tissue results in disorganization of the lobular and vascular structure of the liver, affecting the many functions of the liver and its blood flow. Cirrhosis is characterized by nodular regeneration, which is an attempt by the liver to heal itself by fibrosis or scar tissue. Cirrhosis is the end result of pathologic changes associated with liver disease.

A variety of conditions may progress or lead to cirrhosis of the liver and range from genetic disorders to alcohol abuse. The genetic disorders include galactosemia, $alpha_1$ antitrypsin deficiency, and Wilson's disease. Biliary atresia, a congenital malformation of bile ducts, may progress to cirrhosis. Chemical agents that may be toxic to the liver include acetaminophen, thorazine, ether, amitriptyline (Elavil), and various household cleansers (carbon tetrachloride). Infectious causes, such as viral hepatitis, syphilis, and schistosomiasis, may progress to cirrhosis. Alcoholic cirrhosis is the most common and accounts for approximately 80% of the liver disease in urban areas.

Cirrhosis develops in approximately 10% to 20% of alcoholics. Of interest to clinicians and researchers is why all individuals who abuse alcohol do not develop cirrhosis. Alcohol ingestion in a susceptible host in the presence of an unknown factor may lead to cirrhosis of the liver.

PATHOPHYSIOLOGY

The pathophysiology of cirrhosis will vary according to the initial cause (e.g., viral hepatitis, biliary obstruction, or alcohol abuse). The symptoms and results of cirrhosis are the same. For this reason and because of the high incidence of alcohol abuse–related cirrhosis, the pathophysiology of the alcohol-induced cirrhotic changes will be described. Alcoholic cirrhosis is also referred to as portal cirrhosis, Laënnec's cirrhosis, and micronodular cirrhosis.

Several steps occur before the liver becomes cirrhotic. Initially, subcellular changes develop and may progress to a fatty liver. (Fatty livers are not limited to alcoholic cirrhosis.) The fatty liver is a reversible stage if alcohol intake is eliminated. The fatty liver can be recognized by its increased size and the marked degree of fatty infiltration seen microscopically. The fatty liver in the presence of continued alcohol ingestion may progress to alcoholic hepatitis. It is the continuing use of alcohol that causes development of cirrhosis versus the progression from fatty liver to hepatitis to cirrhosis. These may not be related. The patient could have cirrhosis, and acute hepatitis could develop because of a drinking bout if the patient has cirrhotic changes. In alcoholic hepatitis the fatty infiltration is combined with liver cell necrosis, leukocytic inflammation, and fibrosis. As the disease progresses, the inflammatory changes decrease and fibrotic changes increase. Continued alcohol ingestion leads to chronic changes (i.e., alcoholic cirrhosis).

The microscopic changes in cirrhosis consist of degeneration and death of hepatocytes, proliferation of connective tissue, and regeneration of hepatocytes. The connective tissue spreads from the portal tracts and from the central veins throughout the liver, changing the normal lobular architecture. The extension of fibrous cords throughout the liver alters the

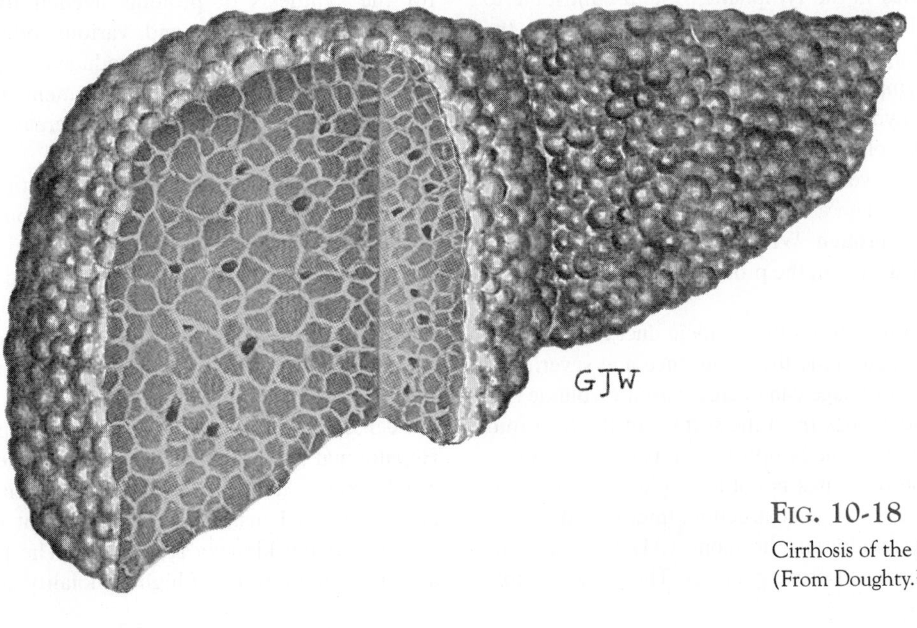

FIG. 10-18
Cirrhosis of the liver (septal cirrhosis). (From Doughty.[10])

relationship between the hepatic veins and the portal veins. Scar tissue and nodular regeneration of hepatocytes may compress small branches of the portal vein. The compression of the vessels leads to an increased alteration in the vascular system. The veins become engorged and dilated, and portal hypertension develops. The nodular regeneration of the hepatic cells produces postsinusoidal obstruction, which causes the portal system to become congested and contributes to portal hypertension.

The overall effects of the structural and vascular changes are seen in the resulting dysfunction of the liver and the changes in the portal circulation. The liver is a very complex organ and plays a major role in metabolism; detoxification; blood-forming functions; storage of iron, copper, and various vitamins; and formation of bile. As the liver functions are altered, various clinical manifestations develop, including bleeding disorders (decreased clotting factors), muscle wasting (decreased protein metabolism), hepatic coma (detoxification of ammonia), jaundice (inability to conjugate bilirubin), and peripheral edema (low serum albumin and an increase in hydrostatic pressure). The changes in the portal circulation result in portal hypertension, one of whose clinical manifestations is esophageal varices. Ascites and mesenteric congestion are other clinical manifestations.

Ascites in chronic liver disease has been associated with portal hypertension, low serum albumin, and abnormalities in the lymphatic system. The transudation of fluid between capillaries and tissue spaces is determined by the equilibrium of hydrostatic and osmotic forces in the two compartments. In the normal situation the hydrostatic pressure is higher at the arterial end of the capillary and promotes the passage of protein-free fluid into the pericapillary space. The hydrostatic pressure is lower than the osmotic pressure and the extravascular tissue pressure at the venous end of the capillary, and reabsorption of the fluid occurs.[45] The patient with advanced cirrhosis and portal hypertension has an increased intravascular hydrostatic pressure (portal hypertension) and decreased vascular osmotic pressure (low serum albumin). The combination of the changes in hydrostatic pressure and osmotic pressure leads to the loss of fluid into the peritoneal cavity, an extravascular space.[45] Abnormalities in the lymphatic system contribute to ascites formation. In cirrhosis with portal hypertension, the thoracic duct is enlarged and lymph flow is significantly increased. The high lymph flow may decompress the hepatic or splanchnic vessels. Lymph from the liver is generally high in protein. When the lymph flow is greater than the thoracic duct can manage, a hepatic venous outflow obstruction develops, with resultant ascites. The ascitic fluid in a venous outflow obstruction is high in protein. When the obstruction is an extrahepatic venous obstruction, the protein concentration is low in the fluid.[7]

The communication between the thoracic duct and the subclavian vein helps to determine the occurrence and severity of ascites. Thoracic duct drainage can decrease ascitic volume and portal pressure. Fluid exudes from the surface of the liver into the peritoneal cavity when the lymph system is unable to manage it. The formation of ascites is not a simple reaction to increased hepatic venous outflow obstruction. Interrelated factors include aldosterone, antidiuretic hormone (ADH), renin, angiotensin, vasopressins, and prostaglandins. The pathophysiology of ascitic fluid formation in cirrhosis has not been successfully described to include all the interrelated factors.[7]

There are three types of jaundice: obstructive, hemolytic, and hepatocellular. Obstructive jaundice develops in association with obstruction of the biliary ductal system. There is marked elevation of alkaline phosphatase, mild elevation of serum glutamic-oxaloacetic transaminase (SGOT) and lactate dehydrogenase (LDH), and significant bile in the urine. Hemolytic jaundice is associated with an increased load of bilirubin from hemolysis that a diseased liver is unable to manage. Large amounts of urobilinogen may be found in the urine. Anemia is generally associated with hemolytic jaundice. Hepatocellular jaundice develops because of a failure of the liver cells to metabolize bilirubin. In acute hepatocellular failure, the LDH and SGOT are markedly increased and urine contains both bile and urobilinogen. In chronic cirrhosis or hepatocellular failure, there may be no elevation of enzymes and the jaundice may not correlate with the severity of the liver disease. Its presence usually indicates acute disease, and in the patient with chronic cirrhosis the presence of jaundice indicates a poor prognosis. Severe hepatic parenchymal necrosis may develop in the absence of jaundice.[45] Hemolysis is common in cirrhosis and may contribute to jaundice. Biliary obstruction may also occur in cirrhosis.

Hepatic encephalopathy encompasses several stages of mental deterioration culminating in coma. The pathophysiology and treatment are presented on pp. 717-718. Bleeding esophageal varices are a major complication associated with portal hypertension and are discussed on p. 661.

The healthy liver plays a role in the metabolism of estrogens. In cirrhosis, hyperestrogenism develops, which includes an increase in sex hormone–binding globulin and other hormone-binding proteins and an increase in the secretion of prolactin.[45] Clinically, the male patient shows signs of feminization, including gynecomastia, spider angiomas, palmar erythema, and testicular atrophy. The distribution of body hair changes, with less chest hair and axillary hair being noted. In women testosterone may accumulate with some masculinization.

Hematologic disorders associated with cirrhosis include impaired coagulation and anemia. The liver is responsible for the synthesis of proteins needed for coagulation: fibrinogen, prothrombin, and various other clotting factors. The liver uses vitamin K to produce prothrombin. Vitamin K absorption depends on bile. Treatment of cirrhosis by wiping out intestinal bacteria will decrease the production of vitamin K.

Anemia in cirrhosis may be microcytic, hypochromic anemia resulting from gastrointestinal blood loss and iron deficiency; macrocytic anemia from folic acid deficiency, leukopenia, or thrombocytopenia; or hemolytic anemia. Hemolysis may be indicated by reticulocytosis, hyperbilirubinemia, or increased levels of serum LDH. Splenomegaly may be associated with leukopenia, thrombocytopenia, and hemolytic anemia.

A major complication of cirrhosis is hepatorenal syndrome. Hepatorenal syndrome occurs when a patient with decompensated cirrhosis has developed functional renal failure. The usual causes of renal insufficiency are present in hepatorenal syndrome, but the kidneys are normal. The patient has oliguria, azotemia, and a urine of high osmolality and low sodium content. Oliguria and azotemia will persist in hepatorenal syndrome even if blood volume and cardiac output are normal. Hepatorenal syndrome carries a very high mortality rate and does not respond well to medical management.

Hypotension in liver failure is common and may lead to oliguria, azotemia, hyponatremia, and changes in potassium levels. Clinically, the patient may have a high cardiac output and a low total peripheral resistance. Changes in the liver circulatory system may be responsible for this development, and treatment focuses on improving liver function. In addition, oliguria may be associated with a depletion of circulatory blood volume (decreased cardiac output) and decreased renal perfusion. Treatment requires volume expanders.

The patient with cirrhosis has a complex, interrelated group of clinical manifestations. The symptoms observed in cirrhosis can be correlated with a particular dysfunction in the liver or its vascular system. The nurse must be able to identify potential life-threatening complications of advanced liver failure.

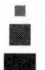

Diagnostic Studies and Findings

Serum bilirubin: Elevated in jaundice
SGOT, Serum glutamate pyruvate transaminase (SGPT), LDH: Elevated (SGOT may be higher if alcoholic cirrhosis)
Serum albumin: Decreased (tissue edema)
Prothrombin time: Prolonged
Complete blood count: Anemia, leukopenia, thrombocytopenia
Blood glucose: Hypoglycemia (from impaired gluconeogenesis)
Serum ammonia: Elevated (sign of impending hepatic coma)
Urinalysis: Sodium and potassium levels; urine dark, bile colored; presence of urobilinogen
Endoscopic retrograde cholangiopancreatography (ERCP): May show common bile duct obstruction
Esophagoscopy: Presence of esophageal varices
Percutaneous liver biopsy: Histologic changes found in cirrhosis of liver: fatty infiltration; degeneration and regeneration of hepatocytes; increase in connective tissue
Ultrasonography: Evaluates patency of splenic and portal veins; differentiates biliary obstruction from nonobstructive, parenchymal jaundice; documents presence of occult ascites; assesses liver size
Liver scans: Decreased uptake in liver (caused by intrahepatic shunts that bypass liver cells); cold spots of cirrhosis can be differentiated from hepatocellular carcinoma by gallium scans
Barium contrast esophagography: Documents esophageal varices
Angiography: Detects sites of upper gastrointestinal bleeding
Percutaneous transhepatic portography (angiographic study): Visualization of portal venous system
Paracentesis: Clear, straw-colored fluid; decreased total protein

Multidisciplinary Plan

Surgery

Refer to discussions of esophageal varices, hepatic coma, liver transplant

Ascites: Peritoneovenous shunt: LeVeen valve, ascites drainage system implanted in abdominal wall and connected to peritoneal cavity and to venous system

Medications

Diuretics: Used to promote fluid loss; recommended weight loss 1-1$^1/_2$ pounds/day
- Spironolactone (Aldactone, potassium-sparing diuretic), 100 mg/day (higher dosage may be used initially or given in combination with other diuretics)
- Hydrochlorothiazide (Esidrix) or furosemide (Lasix); dosage varies; given with spironolactone

Digestants: Pancreatin (Panteric), 1 or 2 tablets PO with meals; each tablet contains 2400 mg; use in presence of steatorrhea; promotes fat digestion

Vitamins
- Menadiol sodium diphosphate (Synkayvite; vitamin K), 5-15 mg IM, subcutaneously, or IV; repeat dosage in 12 h if no improvement or give 10 mg for 3 days
- Vitamin C (decreased vitamin C associated with gastrointestinal bleeding)
- Folic acid, 1 mg/day PO (for anemia)

Cathartics and laxatives
- Stool softeners: To reduce straining and thereby reduce chance of bleeding from hemorrhoids; docusate (Colace), 50-200 mg/day
- Lactulose (Cephulac), 30 ml 3-4 times/day PO, 300 ml in 700 ml normal saline (NS) or sorbitol per rectum as retention enema for 30-60 min (to decrease serum ammonia levels)

General Management

Paracentesis: Indicated for diagnostic purposes, relief of abdominal pain, relief of dyspnea or orthopnea, reduction of intraabdominal pressure; complications: perforation of abdominal viscera, hemorrhage, infection, shock, hyponatremia syndromes
Oxygen and incentive spirometer if respiratory complications develop
Intravenous fluids
Fresh whole blood during acute bleeding episodes
Abstinence from alcohol
Adequate rest
Albumin replacement: Considered on individual basis
Vitamin supplements, including thiamine, iron, and vitamins K and C
Fresh frozen plasma or platelets
Diet: High in protein (70 to 90 g), high in carbohydrates, approximately 3000 calories
Diet: With impending liver failure, restrict protein and fluids

Nutritional Consultation

To counsel patients regarding sodium restrictions, salt substitutes, high- or low-protein dietary selections, fluid restrictions

Psychologic Consultation

May be advised to counsel patient, family members regarding alcoholism; refer patient and family members to Alcoholics Anonymous and affiliated family organizations

NURSING CARE

Nursing Assessment

General status: Fatigability; fever; weakness; signs of bleeding

Gastrointestinal status: History of hepatitis or previous liver disease, drug use, toxic substance ingestion, alcohol use; nausea, vomiting, hematemesis; change in bowel habits; hemorrhoids; glossitis, cheilosis

Psychosocial concerns: Ability to give up alcohol ingestion (if alcoholic cirrhosis); assess coping level and support

Mental status: Changes in thinking and mental function resulting from increased serum ammonia levels; may progress to hepatic coma (serum ammonia levels do not always correlate with mental functions; that is, some patients with very high levels have minimum mental function alteration, whereas others with low levels may progress to coma)

Nutritional status: Recent changes in weight (loss or gain); anorexia

Integument: Jaundice, spider angiomas, spider telangiectasis, palmar erythema, purpuric lesions, loss of chest hair

Urinary status: Changes in urine output, oliguria; color of urine: dark yellow, amber, mahogany

Respiratory status: Shortness of breath, decreased lung expansion; congestion

Extremities: Nail changes (transverse pale bands); signs of tissue wasting (legs); asterixis, tremors

Sexual functioning: Impotence, loss of libido, sterility, amenorrhea

Abdominal examination: Ascites; abdominal pain; splenomegaly; hepatomegaly; caput medusae: dilated veins around the umbilicus secondary to portal hypertension

Potential Complications

Impaired coagulation, hepatic encephalopathy, hepatorenal syndrome

Patient Problems/Nursing Diagnoses & Interventions

(See also Hepatic Coma, Esophageal Varices)

NIC Tissue Perfusion Management

Risk for impaired tissue integrity related to altered clotting factors

Deficient fluid volume related to use of diuretics and third spacing of fluids (ascites and edema)

- Help patient minimize trauma (e.g., forceful nose blowing, harsh toothbrush, safety razors).
- Provide stool softener and remind patient not to strain during bowel movements.
- Use small-gauge needles for injections and apply pressure after injections.
- Record any indications of small bleeding sites.
- Monitor platelet count and prothrombin time.
- Maintain accurate intake and output records, reporting abnormalities.
- Record daily weights.
- Measure abdominal girth daily *to monitor ascites.*
- Monitor serum and urine electrolytes.
- Provide diuretics as ordered.
- Restrict fluid intake if ordered.
- Perform frequent mouth care.
- Administer IV fluids and colloids as ordered.

NIC Nutrition Support

Imbalanced nutrition: less than body requirements, related to poor nutritional intake and anorexia

- Provide small frequent feedings high in calories, carbohydrates, and fats; low in proteins and low in sodium.
- Provide salt substitutes if ordered.

NIC Respiratory Management

Ineffective breathing pattern related to ascites

- Place patient in semi-Fowler's or high-Fowler's position *to increase lung expansion compromised by ascites.*
- Turn frequently from side to side.
- Monitor blood gases.
- Monitor vital signs.
- Assist patient with ADLs if patient is short of breath.

NIC Risk Management

Acute confusion and disturbed thought processes related to increased serum ammonia levels

- Observe for early signs of mental changes: lethargy, confusion, drowsiness, and irritability.
- Avoid use of sedatives or tranquilizers.
- Refer to section on hepatic coma.

NIC Coping Assistance

Compromised family coping related to chronic irreversible illness, progressive debility, and changes in sexuality

- Provide sensitive, caring approach to patient and family.
- Assess patient's and family's coping patterns and use of support groups or psychiatric services.
- Provide opportunities for patient and family to express fears and concerns regarding the illness.

Patient Education/Continuum of Care Plan

1. Stress importance of avoiding alcohol, and provide information on alcoholic cirrhosis.
2. Help patient identify community resources available for alcohol rehabilitation.
3. Provide patient with information on altered drug effects with cirrhosis, and caution to use only physician-prescribed or physician-approved medications.
4. Have nutritionist ensure that patient and family understand written dietary instructions. Stress role of nutrition in recovery. Include any restrictions required, specifically sodium or protein.
5. Instructions should include need for rest and diversional activities to prevent boredom.
6. Provide and ensure that patient understands written instructions of signs and symptoms that warrant seeing a physician: increased abdominal girth, rapid weight gain or loss, edema, fever, blood in urine or stool, bleeding that does not cease with pressure in a short time (nosebleeds,

cuts, gums), gross upper gastrointestinal bleeding, or tarry stools.
7. Instruct family in all of the above plus signs of mental changes: confusion, untidiness, night wandering, personality changes, irritability, and sleeplessness.

EVALUATION/PATIENT OUTCOMES

Tissue Perfusion Management: Patient's risk of bleeding diminishes. Platelet count, bleeding times are normal. Patient verbalizes common signs of abnormal bleeding times and how to minimize trauma during these times.

Fluid volume is maintained. Serum electrolytes (sodium, potassium, and magnesium) are normal. Fluid weight loss is 1-1½ pounds per day. Abdominal girth decreases. Peripheral edema is reduced. Vital signs are stable. Urinary output is adequate.

Nutrition Support: Nutrition is adequate: Patient does not experience anorexia, nausea and vomiting, indigestion, or muscle wasting. Calorie and protein intake is sufficient for healing. Patient does not drink alcohol.

Respiratory Management: Breathing pattern is normal. Patient does not experience atelectasis or pneumonia. Ascites decreases or disappears; therefore lung expansion improves.

Risk Management: Thought processes are normal. Thought processes are not altered. Patient is not confused and is oriented. Serum ammonia levels are controlled.

Coping Assistance: Patient and family are able to cope with chronic illness or an acute exacerbation. Patient and family are able to verbalize factors that create anxiety and stress. Patient and family are aware of resources available to them for further supportive care. Patient and family are able to verbalize mechanisms that help them deal with stressors.

HEPATIC COMA

In acute and chronic liver diseases, a series of neuropsychiatric manifestations may develop that range from hepatic encephalopathy to precoma to hepatic coma. Hepatic coma is the end stage of the neuropsychiatric manifestations.

The pathophysiology of hepatic coma has become better understood and has been related to the presence of two factors: the shunting of blood around the liver so that substances toxic to the brain are no longer completely metabolized or cleared by the liver, and hepatic insufficiency. The syndrome is currently referred to as portal-systemic encephalopathy (PSE). PSE is characterized by recurrent changes in consciousness, impaired intellectual function, neuromuscular abnormalities, metabolic slowing of electroencephalogram, and elevated serum ammonia levels.[45]

Most patients who have hepatic coma (or PSE) develop cirrhosis. However, PSE may develop in fulminant liver failure, deficiency of urea cycle enzyme, and Reye's syndrome. PSE occurs in patients with cirrhosis who have portal hypertension or portal-systemic shunting. Hepatic coma also develops in half of those patients who have portacaval shunts.

Several clinical situations have been associated with the initiation of PSE and include azotemia; medications such as sedatives, tranquilizers, and analgesics; gastrointestinal bleeding; high dietary protein; sepsis; hypokalemia; hypovolemia; paracentesis; and hypokalemic alkalosis. The cause is iatrogenic in approximately half of the cases of hepatic coma.

PATHOPHYSIOLOGY

Most episodes of PSE are caused by ammonia intoxication. Ammonia is a by-product of nitrogen metabolism. Nitrogen is a by-product of amino acid digestion. The bacteria in the colon break down nitrogen to ammonia. The ammonia is absorbed and carried through the portal veins to the liver, where it is converted to glutamine, a nontoxic form. Glutamine is later synthesized by the liver into urea, which is excreted.

The colon, when in a fasting state, is a continuous source of ammonia. When the portal vein flow bypasses the liver, such as with a portal-systemic anastomosis, the systemic blood ammonia levels increase to toxic levels.

The following equation refers to the ammonia and ammonia hydroxide balance:

$$NH_4OH \leftrightarrows NH_4^+ + OH^-$$

Only ammonia hydroxide can cross the cell membrane and thus create toxic effects. The pH of the extracellular and intracellular compartments affects this equation. Abnormalities of acid-base balance, primarily alkalosis associated with hypokalemia, result in an increase in ammonia hydroxide and passage of the substance into the cells. Hypokalemia in alcoholic cirrhosis may be related to vomiting, diarrhea, diuretics, and secondary aldosteronism.

Ammonia is also released during muscle activities from the muscles of the extremities. Under normal resting conditions, a small quantity of ammonia uptake occurs. This uptake may increase when arterial levels of ammonia are increased.[45]

PSE may be initiated by conditions that increase nitrogen levels. Endogenous factors include azotemia, blood in the gastrointestinal tract, and constipation. Azotemia affects the kidney's ability to excrete nitrogen. Blood is a source of more ammonia than dietary protein, and the ammonia is liberated from the blood in the colon. Constipation may exaggerate other factors. In constipation the waste products remain in the colon for longer periods, providing more opportunity for colonic bacteria to convert nitrogenous products to ammonia.

Exogenous factors that contribute to the nitrogenous cause of PSE include dietary protein, ammonia salts, urea, cation exchange resins, amino acids, and diuretics. In addition to these factors potassium depletion is associated with nitrogenous PSE.

Several noncirrhotic clinical conditions in which ammonia levels are associated with PSE include hereditary deficiencies of urea cycle enzymes and Reye's syndrome.

The blood ammonia levels do not always correlate well with the clinical manifestations of PSE. Venous blood levels do not reflect what is delivered to the tissues. Arterial ammonia blood levels are recommended, and because individuals respond differently to various levels of ammonia, serial studies of ammonia levels would provide a better indication of the relationship of increasing symptoms to blood levels. Blood ammonia levels are also affected by potassium levels and food ingestion. Hypokalemia results in more tissue uptake of ammonia with a resultant low serum ammonia level. Serum levels of ammonia increase after meals and vary according to the amount of protein consumed. Fasting and serial arterial ammonia levels are more likely to correlate with the clinical symptoms of PSE.

Diagnostic Studies and Findings

Ammonia blood levels (fasting): Elevated
Serum electrolytes: Hypokalemia; alkalosis
Blood glucose: Hyperglycemia: iatrogenic hyperglycemia may cause coma; in cirrhosis there is little glycogen stored, so patients are usually hypoglycemic
Electroencephalogram (EEG): Paroxysms of bilateral, synchronous, symmetric slow waves at a rate of $1^1/_2$ to 3/sec. Four grades of EEG: grade 0: normal; grade 1: mild impairment; grade 2: moderate impairment; grade 3: severe impairment; grade 4: coma; rule out other causes of coma such as subdural hematomas and nonnitrogenous causes of PSE

Multidisciplinary Plan

Medications

Antiinfective agents: Nonabsorbable
To decrease bacterial action in colon
Neomycin sulfate, 0.5-1 g PO q6h for 7 days
Broad-spectrum antibiotics: Ampicillin
Ammonia detoxicants: Lactulose (Cephulac), 300 ml syrup diluted with 700 ml NS or sorbital by enema (retain 20-30 min), or 30-45 ml tid or qid PO

General Management

Removal of blood from gastrointestinal tract: Cathartics
Gastric lavage with room temperature saline or water
Cleansing enemas with dilute acetic acid or neomycin
Discontinuation of any precipitating substance: Dietary proteins, sedatives, diuretic therapy, analgesics
Intravenous glucose: Minimizes protein breakdown
Oxygen: Respiratory or metabolic alkalosis
Correction of any electrolyte imbalances
Parenteral or enteral nutrition

NURSING CARE

Nursing Assessment

(See also Cirrhosis)

Mental Status

Appearance and behavior
Level of consciousness: Drowsiness, hypersomnia, insomnia, or inversion of sleep pattern; slow responses; lethargy; minimum disorientation, somnolence, confusion, semistupor, stupor, coma
Posture and motor behavior: Metabolic tremor, muscular incoordination, impaired handwriting, asterixis (liver flap), hypoactive or hyperactive reflexes, ataxia, slowed movements of depression, nystagmus
Speech and language: Slurred speech
Mood: Unusual mood, thoughts of hopelessness; exaggeration of normal behavior; euphoria or depression; garrulousness; irritability; decreased inhibitions; overt changes in personality; anxiety or apathy; inappropriate behavior; bizarre behavior; paranoia or anger to rage
Thought processes, thought content, and perceptions: Shortened attention span, amnesia for past events
Cognitive functions: Loss of orientation to time, place, and person; grossly impaired computations to inability to compute
Integumentary system: Perianal erythema or erosions (diarrhea)

Potential Complications

Cirrhosis, fulminant liver failure

Patient Problems/Nursing Diagnoses & Interventions

NIC Risk Management

Acute confusion and disturbed thought processes related to impaired liver clearance
Risk for injury related to changes in mentation

- Document changes in mental status (may have patient do simple math, serial handwriting).
- Monitor arterial ammonia and potassium levels.
- Provide sedatives, tranquilizers, and analgesics as ordered with caution; note any delayed or prolonged reactions; avoid use if possible.
- Protect patient from injury as personality behaviors become more overt and inappropriate and as neuromuscular activities alter.
- Reorient patient frequently.
- Ensure side rails up on bed at all times.
- Ensure that call-light device is within patient's reach or attached to patient's bedclothes.
- Assist patient with ambulation.
- Toilet patient frequently.
- Identify personality and behavior changes and relate them to progression of disease and help family and staff understand and learn about disease progression.
- Document treatment ordered by physician as it is implemented (e.g., retention or cleansing enemas, gastric lavage, medications).

NIC Skin/Wound Management

Risk for impaired skin integrity related to incontinent diarrhea

- Begin protective perianal skin care before beginning lactulose or neomycin orally or rectally. Diarrhea stools will be more acidic. Cleanse skin with gentle, nondetergent solutions such as commercial perineal cleansers.
- If skin already eroded, cleanse perianal area with aluminum subacetate (Domboro) solution and cotton balls. Dust eroded areas with stoma powder and cover with barrier ointment.
- Pat the skin dry or use a hair dryer on cool or warm; avoid hot settings.
- Use a barrier ointment, skin sealant, or fecal collector.

- Document signs of fungal infection—red, itchy rash with papules, pustules, or white curdy exudate—and obtain order for antifungal powder or cream.
- Repeat procedures with each bowel movement.

PATIENT EDUCATION/CONTINUUM OF CARE PLAN

1. Provide family with and ensure understanding of written signs of changes in mental functions that are related to early PSE: confusion, untidiness, night wandering, and personality changes. They should notify physician if symptoms occur.
2. Have nutritionist ensure that patient and family understand dietary instructions for reduced protein intake.

EVALUATION/PATIENT OUTCOMES

Risk Management: Thought processes are not impaired. Thought processes, personality, behavior, consciousness, and neuromuscular activities are not altered. Patient is oriented and not confused. Blood ammonia levels are normal. Patient remains injury-free.

Skin/Wound Management: Skin integrity is maintained. There are no signs of irritation or erosion.

GALLBLADDER DISORDERS

CHOLECYSTITIS WITH CHOLELITHIASIS (GALLSTONES)

Cholecystitis refers to the acute or chronic inflammation of the gallbladder.

Acute cholecystitis is associated with gallstones (cholelithiasis) in 95% of cases (FIG. 10-19).[7] Less than 5% of cases of acute cholecystitis are acalculous or unrelated to stone formation. Chronic cholecystitis refers to repeated attacks of acute cholecystitis and an abnormal-looking gallbladder. Pain often follows a meal in chronic cholecystitis. Chronic cholecystitis predisposes to acute cholecystitis (FIG. 10-20), common duct stones, and adenocarcinoma of the gallbladder.

Acute cholecystitis is common and accounts for one fourth of all gallbladder surgeries. Although it may occur in all ages, it is more common in middle age.

The overall death rate is about 5%, occurring almost entirely in patients over 60 years or in those with diabetes.

Cholesterol gallstones are most common in developed countries. Several mechanisms are being studied to explain cholesterol stone formation.

PATHOPHYSIOLOGY

Acute cholecystitis consists of acute inflammation of the wall of the gallbladder. In calculous cholecystitis an obstruction of the cystic duct by a stone or from edema resulting from the passage of a stone is the underlying problem. The cystic duct is obstructed. The gallbladder distends, and the wall becomes edematous, compressing the capillaries and lymphatics and resulting in ischemia and inflammation. The inflamed mucosa allows bile salt to be reabsorbed, further damaging the mucosa. If the inflammation continues, the wall will become friable and necrosis may develop. Perforation of the gallbladder may occur. The perforation may be small and localized, forming an abscess, or there may be free perforation, causing generalized peritonitis. In severe acute cholecystitis, inflammation spreads to the serosal layer of the gallbladder and may progress to form inflammatory adhesions to adjacent structures. Bacteria may be found in the bile and is associated with secondary infections.

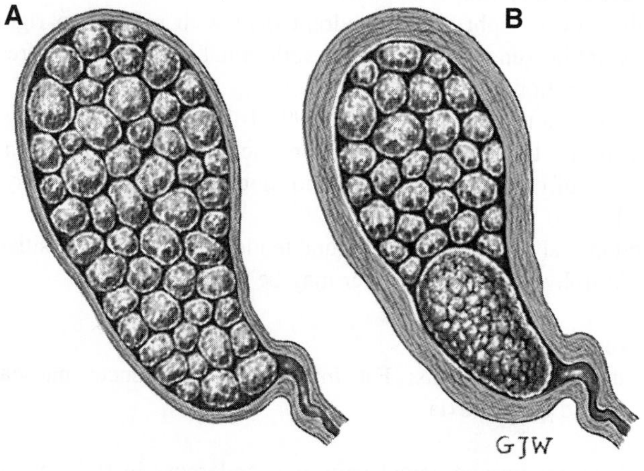

FIG. 10-19
Cholelithiasis. **A,** Multiple-faced stones. **B,** Large and numerous small stones in chronic cholecystitis. (From Doughty.[10])

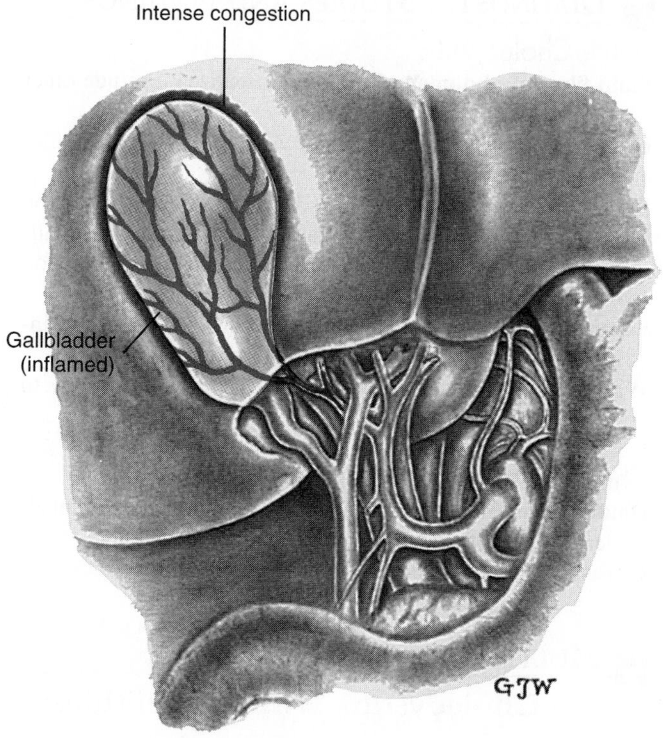

FIG. 10-20
Cholecystitis (acute). (From Doughty.[10])

The gallbladder heals after the acute attack with scarring and decreased absorptive capacity. The mucosa of the gallbladder in a patient with chronic cholecystitis is also ulcerated and scarred. Chronic cholecystitis may develop from repeated intermittent episodes of cystic duct obstruction resulting in chronic inflammation. The gallbladder is contracted, white in color, and thick walled. The bile is turbid and filled with debris.

Acute cholecystitis in the absence of stones has been associated with sudden starvation and immobility. These are changes that affect the regular filling and emptying of the gallbladder. A patient hospitalized for cardiovascular disease, burns, traumas, or biliary surgery may have acalculous acute cholecystitis develop. The patient on TPN may also have cholecystitis develop as a result of gallbladder distention and biliary stasis.

The primary symptom associated with acute cholecystitis is pain. The pain of acute cholecystitis has been described as colicky. However, this is not a true colic pain that waxes and wanes. The pain of acute cholecystitis is abrupt in onset, reaches a peak intensity quickly, and remains at that level for 2 to 4 hours. Initially the pain may be poorly localized, but as it becomes more severe, it localizes in the right upper quadrant epigastric region. The pain radiates around the midtorso to the right scapular area. Guarding and rigidity represent peritoneal involvement. Tenderness may be elicited at the tip of the ninth costal margin during inspiration (Murphy's sign). Jaundice may be found in acute cholecystitis. The jaundice may be related to edema of the ducts or to direct involvement of the liver by inflammation because stones are not always found in patients with jaundice.

Diagnostic Studies and Findings

Acute Cholecystitis

Plain films of abdomen: Gallstones visualized; exclude other causes of pain

Ultrasonograpy: Gallstones; thickening of wall; ductal dilation

Biliary scintigraphy: Scans 15 to 30 minutes after IV injection of radionuclide show the ducts but not the obstructed gallbladder; recommend repeat scan 90 minutes after injection to rule out late filling of gallbladder

Serum amylase: Elevated may indicate concomitant acute pancreatitis; usually indicates common duct stone

White blood cell count: Leukocyte count of 12,000 to 15,000/mm^3 with left shift

Chronic Cholecystitis

Double-dose oral cholecystogram: Nonfunctioning gallbladder; patency of cystic duct

Ultrasonograpy: Presence of gallstones; ductal dilation

Multidisciplinary Plan

Acute Cholecystitis With Cholelithiasis

Surgery

Laparoscopic cholecystectomy: The gallbladder and the stones can be removed laparoscopically; this will often replace open cholecystectomy because more surgeons are learning the laparoscopic technique, and hospital stays are shorter

Cholecystectomy with operative cholangiography and exploration of common bile duct

Percutaneous cholecystotomy: In critically ill patients: a tube is inserted into the gallbladder to drain the abscess; when the patient recovers from acute attack, cholecystectomy can be performed

Medications

Narcotic analgesic agents: For acute pain, meperidine (Demerol), 100 mg, and atropine, 0.6 mg IM

Antiinfective agents

Average severity

Ampicillin, 4 g/day IV

Cefazolin, 2-4 g/day IV

Severe disease

Penicillin, 20 mU/day IV

Clindamycin and aminoglycosides

General Management

Intravenous fluids to correct dehydration

Nasogastric tube; nothing by mouth

Chronic Cholecystitis

Surgery

Cholecystectomy with exploration of common bile duct

Medical Management

Stone dissolution: Ursodeoxycholic acid orally for stones smaller than 5 mm and devoid of calcium

Extracorporeal shock wave lithotripsy used in conjunction with dissolution for stones that are initially larger than 5 mm

General Management

Avoidance of offending foods

NURSING CARE

Nursing Assessment

Acute Cholecystitis With Cholelithiasis

Pain: Severe right upper quadrant pain with referral to right scapula; sudden, generalized abdominal pain indicates free perforation

General status: Fever 37°-39° C (99°-102° F)

Gastrointestinal status: Anorexia, nausea, vomiting; mild jaundice of the skin; dry mouth and mucous membranes (dehydration)

Abdominal examination: Rebound tenderness, rigidity; positive Murphy's sign; gallbladder may be palpable

Chronic Cholecystitis

Gastrointestinal status: Fat intolerance; flatulence; nausea, vomiting; anorexia

Pain

Nonspecific abdominal pain and tenderness in right hypochondrium; episodic abdominal pain; dyspepsia; biliary colic; steady pain that begins abruptly and subsides gradually; pain lasts from a few minutes to several hours

Potential Complications
Perforation

Patient Problems/Nursing Diagnoses & Interventions

NIC Physical Comfort Promotion

Acute pain related to biliary colic (obstruction of cystic duct)
- Provide pain medication as ordered and record patient's response.
- Allow patient to assume position that is least painful.
- Allow patient to express feelings and fears.

NIC Tissue Perfusion Management

Risk for deficient fluid volume related to emesis and NPO status
- Maintain careful intake and output records, including emesis and nasogastric aspiration.
- Monitor serum electrolytes.
- Provide intravenous fluids as ordered.
- Maintain frequent oral hygiene.

Patient Education/Continuum of Care Plan

1. During acute phase, patient will need explanation of all procedures and may require pain medication before moving. Patient should be made aware that nurse recognizes severity of pain during acute cholecystitis.
2. After or during resolution of acute phase, patient will need information about cholecystectomy to make an informed decision regarding surgery.
3. Patients electing medical management will need information on chronic cholecystitis; signs and symptoms of recurrence; signs of potential complications (recurrent attacks, jaundice, obstruction of common bile duct, cholangitis, pancreatitis, internal biliary fistula, carcinoma); and low-fat diets.

Evaluation/Patient Outcomes

Physical Comfort Promotion: Comfort level is achieved. Patient verbalizes increased control over pain. Patient uses pain-control strategies appropriately.

Tissue Perfusion Management: Adequate hydration is maintained. Intake and output equal; vital signs stable; mucous membranes moist; serum electrolytes within normal limits.

PANCREATIC DISORDERS

Pancreatitis

Pancreatitis is an inflammation of the pancreas that may be acute or chronic

Acute pancreatitis (Fig. 10-21) involves a diffuse inflammation caused by premature activation of pancreatic enzymes into active, potent proteolytic enzymes. Acute pancreatitis is a process of autodigestion. The two types of acute pancreatitis are interstitial or edematous pancreatitis and hemorrhagic or necrotizing pancreatitis. The two forms may be a continuum of the same process. Interstitial pancreatitis is milder and characterized by interstitial edema, with exudation into the surrounding retroperitoneal structures. As the disease progresses, frank necrosis develops with disruption and thrombotic occlusion of blood vessels. Bleeding, ischemic necrosis, and fat necrosis are found throughout the pancreas.

Most cases of acute pancreatitis are caused by biliary tract disease or heavy alcohol intake; yet many other causes of acute pancreatitis exist, including postoperative states (pancreas, stomach, biliary tract), infections (mumps, hepatitis, coxsackie B), drugs (thiazides, steroids, azathioprine, pentamidine), and vasculitis. More conditions are being recognized all the time. The incidence varies with location and is higher in urban populations. Complications include abscess, pseudocyst formation, hemorrhage, ascites, and local effects on contiguous organs (portal vein

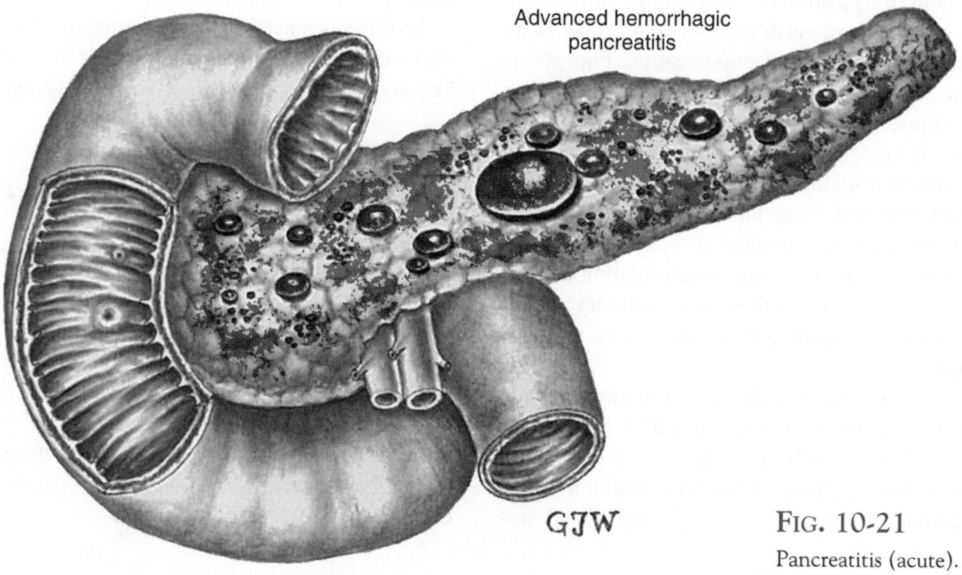

Fig. 10-21
Pancreatitis (acute). (From Doughty.[10])

thrombosis, bowel necrosis, intraperitoneal bleeding, and obstruction of the common duct). Systemic effects include pleural effusions, atelectasis, acute renal failure, gastritis, disseminated intravascular coagulation (DIC), hypotension, hypoglycemia, and hyperglycemia. Mortality of acute necrotizing pancreatitis ranges from 10% to 80% (if infected).[7]

Chronic pancreatitis is characterized by progressive functional damage to the pancreas even if the initiating cause is removed. The primary causative factor is chronic excessive alcohol ingestion. Clinical features include pain, malabsorption, diabetes mellitus, and intraductal calcifications. Complications consist of loss of exocrine and endocrine function, pseudocysts, biliary and duodenal obstruction, malnutrition, and drug addiction.

A pseudocyst occurs when an accumulation of tissue debris, blood, fat droplets, and pancreatic juice develops within confluent areas of necrosis. A pseudocyst may arise within or adjacent to the pancreas. Pancreatic ascites develops when the accumulation of active pancreatic enzymes and leukocytes irritates the peritoneal surfaces and fluid accumulates in the peritoneal cavity. The same process of irritation through the diaphragmatic lymphatics leads to pleural effusion. Abscesses result from secondary infection of necrotic tissue and fluid collection.

PATHOPHYSIOLOGY

Acute Pancreatitis

Acute pancreatitis is a process of autodigestion, but the agent that prematurely triggers the activation of the enzymes is unknown. Several theories have been proposed, including the theory involving the obstruction of the pancreatic ducts, reflux of bile, reflux of duodenal contents, and the toxic effect of alcohol. Unfortunately, none of the proposed theories has proven to be the cause.

The process of enzyme activation regardless of the cause is the basis of the disease process. Trypsinogen may undergo spontaneous activation to trypsin in the presence of an alkaline pH. Trypsin is inactivated by a specific trypsin inhibitor found in the pancreatic secretions and in the pancreatic tissue. However, the small amount of trypsin may activate other proteolytic enzymes. Phospholipase A and elastase have been proposed as the primary enzymes responsible for autodigestion. Phospholipase A, in the presence of bile, results in severe pancreatic parenchymal and adipose tissue necrosis. Elastase dissolves the elastic fibers of blood vessels and is implicated in the hemorrhage associated with necrotizing pancreatitis.

Many substances released from the injured pancreas will have systemic effects. Two low–molecular weight vasoactive peptides (kinins) are released and result in vasodilation and increase in vascular permeability, resulting in circulatory shock. Severe pulmonary edema and pain are also associated with the vasoactive peptides.

Hypocalcemia develops when a decreased binding of calcium to serum protein occurs as a result of a drop of albumin levels. In addition, a decrease in ionized serum calcium occurs in acute pancreatitis. Damage to the islet cells results in mild, transient hyperglycemia from release of glucagon and decreased release of insulin. The glucose levels are too high for the insulin production to control.

Patients with acute pancreatitis are at risk for developing adult respiratory distress syndrome (ARDS). Arterial hypoxia occurs when intrapulmonary right-to-left shunting develops. Pulmonary edema from disruption of the alveolar-capillary membrane is a serious complication. In addition, renal function may be altered during acute pancreatitis. Hypovolemia and shock are not always the causative factors in altered renal function. The blood flow may be reduced and the vascular resistance increased in the kidney in the absence of hypovolemia.

Another major potential complication of acute pancreatitis is DIC, which involves the development of microthrombi and consumption of clotting factors. Mild DIC may play a role in the development of early hypoxia and renal impairment.

Chronic Pancreatitis

Chronic pancreatitis generally develops from an insidious sclerosing process in the pancreas; however, it may develop from repeated bouts of acute inflammation and necrosis. The histologic changes in the pancreas include irregularly distributed fibrosis, reduced number and size of acini and islet cells, and obstruction of the pancreatic ductal system.

The clinical signs of chronic pancreatitis include pain and functional impairment of the pancreas. The pain may be intermittent or chronic and affects the productivity of the patient and his or her activities of daily living. Nausea and vomiting often accompany the pain. The pain is described as steady, boring, dull, or sharp and radiates from the epigastrium to the back. The pain may be lessened by leaning forward from a sitting position. Eating or lying down may increase the pain.

Malabsorption and weight loss develop during the course of the chronic illness. Patients may limit food intake because of the pain. Secretions of pancreatic enzymes decrease in chronic pancreatitis, and fat and protein are poorly digested. Steatorrhea and azotorrhea are observed. Carbohydrate malabsorption is clinically not seen because salivary amylase is unimpaired. Pancreatic amylase is highly efficient and in fact would have to be reduced by 97% before carbohydrate malabsorption would develop.[44]

Insulin response to glucose is impaired in chronic pancreatitis. Overt diabetes mellitus will occur in most of these patients. The ability of the pancreas to release glucagon is also affected.

DIAGNOSTIC STUDIES AND FINDINGS

Acute Pancreatitis

Amylase: Greater than 500 U/dl; highest levels 2 to 12 hours after onset, drop to normal (60 to 180 U/dl) within 48 to 72 hours

Lipase: Elevated; may remain elevated for 5 to 10 days

WBC count: Greater than 12,000/mm^3 with suppurative complications

Glucose: Greater than 180 mg/dl with no prior history of hyperglycemia

CT scan: Pancreatic enlargement

Chronic Pancreatitis

Amylase and lipase: Usually normal; increased in presence of pseudocysts and pancreatic ascites
Alkaline phosphate: Increased five times normal for 4 weeks; indicates common bile duct stenosis
Glucose: Elevated
Urine: Glycosuria (diabetes mellitus)
CT scan: Calcifications
ERCP: Ductal stones and irregularity with dilation and stenoses; rule out carcinoma and pseudocyst
Plain films of abdomen: Sentinel loop sign: isolated dilation of a segment of bowel; colon cutoff sign: gas distending the right colon that abruptly stops in the mid or left transverse colon; demonstration of pancreatic calculi
Upper gastrointestinal series: Widened duodenal loop, swollen ampulla of Vater
CT scan with IV contrast media: Necrosis, abscess, phlegmon (complications)

MULTIDISCIPLINARY PLAN

Acute Pancreatitis

Surgery

Debridement of dead peripancreatic tissue in necrotizing pancreatitis
Surgical drainage of pancreatic pseudocyst may be indicated if it does not resolve spontaneously
Surgical drainage of pancreatic abscesses may be indicated
Laparotomy for common duct obstruction

Medications

Narcotic analgesic agents: Meperidine (Demerol), 75-125 mg IM q4h or prn (hold analgesics until initial laboratory samples are drawn because many will cause elevations in serum amylase and lipase)
Antacids: Aluminum-magnesium preparation, 30-40 ml (clamp nasogastric tube for 15 min after dosage)
H_2 receptor antagonists: Cimetidine or ranitidine, 300 mg IV qid if any evidence of upper gastrointestinal bleeding
Antiinfective agents: Cephalothin (Keflin), 2 g q6h IV or with peritoneal lavage
  For abscess, chloramphenicol (Chloromycetin), 0.5 g q6h IV, and penicillin G, 5-10 million U/day IV, *or* cefoxitin, 1 g q6h IV (used before cultures are known)
Adrenergic agents: For hypotension, dopamine (Intropin), 2-5 μg/kg/min, diluted in solution and titrated as needed or isoproteronol (Isuprel) may be used

General Management

Endoscopic sphincterotomy for biliary pancreatitis
Continuous hemodynamic and arterial blood gas monitoring; Swan-Ganz or CVP catheter
Nasogastric suctioning
Peritoneal lavage for persistent hypotension (removes pancreatic exudate, which contains large amounts of vasoactive kinins)
ARDS: Endotracheal intubation and controlled ventilation with positive end-expiratory pressure (PEEP)
Restoration and maintenance of intravascular volume including human serum albumin, low–molecular weight dextran 40
Correction of electrolyte imbalances: Hypocalcemia, hypomagnesemia, hyperglycemia, hyperkalemia, and metabolic acidosis
Nutritional support with TPN or feeding jejunostomy
Discontinue offending drugs associated with pancreatitis

Chronic Pancreatitis

Surgery

Not primary treatment but may be used to treat intractable pain and complications (e.g., pseudocysts or abscesses)
Drainage procedures
  Longitudinal pancreaticojejunostomy (modified Puestow procedure)
  Sphincteroplasty plus extraction of pancreatic calculi
Resection
  Subtotal or total pancreatectomy
  Pancreaticoduodenostomy (Whipple procedure)
To preserve islet cell function
  Islet cell autotransplantation by infusion of islet cell preparations into portal system
  Segments of pancreas autotransplanted
  Insertion of closed-loop insulin infusion system

Medications

Analgesics: Acetaminophen or narcotics prn for pain
Pancreatic enzyme supplements: Use one of the following (dosage chosen should administer 25,000 to 40,000 U of lipase per meal):
  Pancreatin (Viokase), 6 tablets with each meal
  Pancrelipase (Cotazym), 5 capsules with each meal
  Pancrelipase (Pancrease), enteric-coated, 2-3 capsules with each meal
Antacids and absorbents: Sodium bicarbonate or aluminum hydroxide antacids may be used with pancreatic enzyme supplements to improve results
H_2 receptor antagonists: Cimetidine, 300 mg PO 30 min before meals (may be used to improve effects of pancreatic enzyme supplements)
Medium-chain triglycerides (MCT) supplements (temporary)
Insulin therapy: Does vary with individual (remember that glucagon deficiency is present and patient may have hypoglycemic reactions easily)

General Management

Enteral nutritional support or TPN as indicated by nutritional status and weight loss
Discontinue alcohol intake

NURSING CARE

NURSING ASSESSMENT

Acute Pancreatitis

General status: Fever of 38° C (100°-101° F)
Abdominal examination
  Grey Turner's sign: Bluish brown discoloration of flanks

Cullen's sign: Bluish brown discoloration in periumbilicus area
Absent bowel sounds with intestinal ileus
Palpation: Localized epigastric tenderness intensifies with deep palpation
Soft abdomen: Retroperitoneal location of pancreas means that signs of peritoneal irritation, rigidity, and rebound tenderness will not be present initially
Mild abdominal swelling and mild ascites
Abdominal mass with pseudocyst

Integumentary system
Subcutaneous fat necrosis occurring as tender, red subcutaneous nodules
Jaundice in some patients; hyperbilirubinemia of 3 mg/dl
Spontaneous drainage of pancreatic abscess through an abnormal tract to skin or after surgical drainage of an abscess (pancreatic cutaneous fistula)

Respiratory status: Pleuritic pain; pleural rub; decreased breath sounds; increased respiratory rate

Cardiovascular status: Tachycardia, hypovolemia, and hypotension may progress to circulatory shock and coma

Pain: Steady, dull, boring, severe pain in epigastrium or left upper quadrant: poorly localized; reaches peak intensity within 15 minutes to 1 hour; radiates to lower thoracic vertebral area; worsens in supine position; partially relieved by leaning forward; sometimes patient has referred shoulder pain from irritation of diaphragm

Nutritional status: Weight loss, if related to alcohol intake may show signs of chronic malnutrition from alcoholism

Chronic Pancreatitis

Pain: Intermittent or chronic pain; boring, dull, or sharp pain that is steady; epigastric, right or left subcostal region, periumbilical region, or lower abdomen; radiates to patient's back; patient observed sitting up and leaning forward to relieve pain

Nutritional status: Weight loss, steatorrhea, voluminous diarrhea, nausea, and vomiting (associated with pain and with complications)

Endocrine system: Signs and symptoms of diabetes mellitus; reactive hypoglycemia to insulin therapy

Potential Complications

DIC, ARDS, diabetes mellitus

Patient Problems/Nursing Diagnoses & Interventions

NIC Tissue Perfusion Management

Risk for deficient fluid volume related to fluid exudation in acute pancreatitis

- Document intake and output, central venous pressure, Swan-Ganz catheter pressure, daily weights.
- Document vital signs and blood pressure every 4 hours, more often if indicated.
- Monitor laboratory values, particularly hematocrit and hemoglobin, which will decrease after volume is restored.
- Provide fluid volume replacement as ordered; intravenous fluids, dextran, fluid expanders.

NIC Respiratory Management

Ineffective breathing pattern related to pulmonary complications of acute pancreatitis

- Document breath sounds, cough, sputum, fluid accumulation, elevated diaphragm, shallow breathing *because patients are candidates for ARDS.*
- Monitor arterial blood gas levels.

NIC Skin/Wound Management

Risk for impaired skin integrity related to presence of pancreatic fistula

- Monitor output of any fistula.
- Provide skin protection for a pancreatic fistula with a clean pouch with skin barrier or with barrier ointments and dressings.

NIC Physical Comfort Promotion

Acute or chronic pain related to acute or chronic inflammatory process

- Allow patient to assume a comfortable position; usually sitting up and leaning forward will help relieve pain.
- Provide analgesics as ordered *because pain may be severe and steady; analgesics before procedures alleviate or minimize discomfort.*

NIC Nutrition Support

Imbalanced nutrition: less than body requirements, related to pain and malabsorption

- Give patient nothing by mouth during acute pancreatitis episodes *to eliminate unnecessary secretion of pancreatic enzymes.*
- Measure and record nasogastric output.
- Provide frequent mouth care.
- Monitor blood and urine glucose levels *because damage to islet cells may result in mild transient hyperglycemia.*
- Assess stools for diarrhea and steatorrhea, a sign of malabsorption of fats.
- Provide insulin as ordered for endocrine dysfunction in chronic pancreatitis (note possibility of reactive hypoglycemia to insulin therapy).
- Provide medium chain triglycerides (MCTs) orally if tolerated as supplement *to relieve steatorrhea, increase calorie absorption.*
- When eating, provide small, frequent, low-fat meals that are high in protein and carbohydrates.
- Avoid coffee, spicy foods, and alcohol.
- Administer pancreatic enzyme supplements before meals as ordered

Patient Education/Continuum of Care Plan

1. Assist patient in understanding cause or causal relationships of pancreatitis with alcohol use or gallstones.
2. Plan an appropriate rehabilitation program if alcohol abuse is related to disease process.
3. Provide written dietary instructions.
4. Provide written medication instructions.

5. Provide patient with information about diabetes mellitus: signs, symptoms, and insulin therapy.
6. Discuss with patient ways to avoid another attack (abstain from alcohol; quit smoking; follow prescribed diet).

EVALUATION/PATIENT OUTCOMES

Tissue Perfusion Management: Fluid status is stable. Patient's hydration and electrolyte balance are adequate.

Respiratory Management: Respiratory function is normal. Patient shows no signs of respiratory distress. Patient's arterial blood gas levels are within normal range.

Skin/Wound Management: Skin integrity is maintained. Perifistular skin is effectively protected from enzymatic drainage.

Physical Comfort Promotion: Comfort level is achieved. Patient shows reduction or absence of guarding or protective behavior. Patient uses pain control strategies appropriately. Patient verbalizes increased control over pain.

Nutrition Support: Nutritional status is stable. Patient's nutrition is adequate. Patient's weight is stable. Patient does not experience steatorrhea or diarrhea. Patient's serum glucose is stabilized. Patient does not experience anorexia, nausea, or vomiting.

COLLABORATIVE INTERVENTIONS AND RELATED NURSING CARE

ABDOMINAL SURGERIES FOR SELECTED DISEASES OF GASTROINTESTINAL TRACT

Description and Rationale

Abdominal surgeries involve an incision into the abdomen with the patient under general anesthesia. A variety of abdominal surgeries may be required under the broad scope of gastrointestinal diseases. Commonalities exist in the preoperative and postoperative patient care assessment and interventions that will be covered in this section. Examples of abdominal surgeries in which a portion of the gastrointestinal tract is surgically removed include appendectomy (appendix), cholecystectomy (gallbladder), colectomy (colon); and gastrectomy (stomach). An intestinal resection may be referred to as an ileotransverse colostomy (ileum is reanastomosed to transverse colon with removal or bypass of the ascending colon: in this case there is no externalization of the bowel even though the term "colostomy" is used).

Laparoscopic surgical techniques are being used increasingly for abdominal surgeries. Laparoscopic cholecystectomies are now done routinely, and techniques are being developed for antireflux procedures, appendectomy, hernia repair, colectomy, vagotomy, and hysterectomy. Although laparoscopic surgeries may require increased intraoperative time, they often result in decreased hospitalization time, less discomfort and pain postoperatively, smaller scars, lower costs, and less time away from work and usual activities.

Surgery is indicated in many gastrointestinal diseases when medical management is ineffective or when complications develop. Surgery may be palliative, as in the case of Crohn's disease, or curative, as with ulcerative colitis and familial polyposis.

Contraindications and Cautions

1. Patients with signs and symptoms of an acute condition in the abdomen or an emergency situation will need to be quickly stabilized with fluid and electrolyte replacements.
2. The surgical intervention in an emergency may be considered a first stage, diverting the problem, with a required second operation for definitive treatment.
3. For patients with permanent colostomies, ileostomies, continent ileostomies, and ileoanal reservoirs, recommend medical alert card stating: "No rectal temperatures, no rectal enemas, no rectal suppositories: the rectum has been removed." Provide definition of above procedures.

Preprocedural Nursing Care

1. Thorough bowel preparation is required for many abdominal surgeries, including oral cathartics, antibiotics, and enemas. The trend is toward eliminating the preoperative day and having the patient perform bowel preparation at home. Caution must be used not to deplete weakened or elderly patients with multiple tap water enemas.
2. Drains such as Penrose, silicone dual sump, Shiley sump, and tubes, such as nasogastric tubes, T tubes, gastrostomy tubes, and Foley catheters are often used after surgery, and patients should be prepared for their presence.
3. All postoperative general management interventions should be explained preoperatively.

MULTIDISCIPLINARY PLAN

Medications

Bowel preparation: For elective large intestinal surgery; nonabsorbable antiinfective agent (done preoperatively)
  Neomycin, 1 g at 2 PM, 6 PM, and 11 PM
  Erythromycin (base), 1 g at 2 PM, 6 PM, and 11 PM
Postoperatively, broad-spectrum antibiotic prophylaxis for 24-36 h
Narcotic analgesic agents given by intramuscular, subcutaneous injections q3-4h; by patient-controlled IV analgesia (PCA); by epidural catheter

General Management

Pulmonary care: Incentive spirometry, splinting, and coughing
Gastrointestinal decompression: Nasogastric tube, gastrostomy tube
Early and progressive ambulation
Embolus prevention: Thromboembolic disease support hose (TEDs) and pneumatic compression stockings
Pain management: Subcutaneous and intramuscular injections; PCA; continuous epidural narcotics; transcutaneous electrical nerve stimulation (TENS)
Intravenous fluids with electrolytes (particularly potassium)
Nutrition: Enteral or intravenous feedings as supplement or maintenance

Respiratory Therapy
May be used to assist patient with pulmonary toilet

Physical Therapy
May be used to assist patient with progressive ambulation or mobility exercises

Nutritional Consultation
May be necessary to assist patient with postoperative dietary selections for well-balanced diet if surgery necessitates significant dietary changes; may be used to recommend formulations for enteral or parenteral therapy

NURSING CARE

Nursing Assessment

General Status
Low-grade fever first 24 to 48 hours common
Fever of 38° C (100° F) or fever that does not subside may indicate pulmonary complications, wound infection, urinary infection, or thrombophlebitis
Fever of 38.3° C (101° F) occurring suddenly and accompanied by chills, weakness, fatigue, rapid respiration, tachycardia, and sudden drop in blood pressure indicates septic shock

Gastrointestinal Status
Gas pains, passage of gas, bowel movement, hunger and appetite, constipation, diarrhea, nausea, vomiting

Pain
Assess intensity of pain using pain scale; note location, type, duration, intensity, pattern of pain occurrence, narcotic usage patterns, effectiveness of narcotics, and what makes the pain better or worse

Determine previous narcotic use or history of substance abuse (to plan for higher postoperative dosages)

Nutritional Status
Usual weight, percent change on admission, change in dietary habits
Assess patient for nutritional deficiencies; see nutritional assessment chart

Psychosocial Concerns
Assess emotional reaction to surgery and consequences
Assess level of support and coping mechanisms
Assess health information needs

Ability for Self-Care
Determine usual activities and restrictions
Determine perception of responsibilities after surgery

Urinary Status
Dehydration: Urinary output less than 30 ml/h; urine specific gravity
Voiding problems after indwelling catheter removal, or secondary to temporary nerve damage after rectal manipulation

Abdominal Examination
Observations: Distention (note shape and contour); presence of drains or tubes; staples, sutures, Steri-strips, dressing (dry or with drainage); incision (dry, draining, erythematous, indurated); presence of skin color changes (e.g., mottling, erythema, ecchymosis, rash)
Auscultation: Presence or absence of bowel sounds; character (frequency and pitch) of bowel sounds
Palpation: Soft, firm, location and intensity of pain, rigidity, rebound tenderness, and ascites
Percussion: Dull, tympany (distinguish air from fluid from solid mass)

Integumentary System
Assess nares for pressure from nasogastric tubes
Assess incision for erythema, induration, drainage, wound edge separation, and bleeding
Assess wound healing by secondary intention: presence or absence of granulation tissue, necrotic tissue, exudate, odor, and evidence of contraction
Identify impairments to wound healing: steroids, malnutrition, obesity, sepsis, and so forth
Assess patient's risk for developing pressure ulcers
Assess for skin breakdown from excess drainage, shearing tape, and pressure

Mental Status
Evaluation of effects of narcotics, anesthesia, and fatigue
Encephalopathy after surgery on patients with cirrhosis

Respiratory Status
Decreased respiratory stimulus from respiratory depressants such as narcotics and anesthesia
Shallow breathing and inadequate coughing as a result of abdominal pain

Oral Examination
Hydration, presence of thrush, and cleanliness

Cardiovascular Status
Shock and circulatory failure associated with hemorrhage, sepsis, fluid, and electrolyte imbalance
Thrombophlebitis, pulmonary emboli: Assess calves for tenderness, warmth, or cords, Homans' sign

Fluids and Electrolytes
Nausea, vomiting, diarrhea, and nasogastric and intestinal suctioning may affect fluid and electrolyte balance

Potential Complications
Pneumonia, wound infection, urinary tract infection, thrombophlebitis

Patient Problems/Nursing Diagnoses & Interventions

NIC Tissue Perfusion Management

Risk for ineffective renal, cardiopulmonary, gastrointestinal, and peripheral tissue perfusion related to postoperative fluid shifts and complications
Risk for deficient fluid volume related to postoperative fluid shifts

- Monitor intake and output, including all drainage from nasogastric, gastric, intestinal, and T tubes, as

well as wound drainage or fistula output and urinary output.
- Monitor patient's vital signs and central venous pressure or Swan-Ganz catheter for changes in cardiac output and tissue perfusion.
- Weigh patient daily.
- Monitor color, consistency, amount, and odor of any drainage; test drainage (i.e., nasogastric aspirate, stool, urine, fistula) for blood or pH if indicated.
- Provide fluid replacement as ordered.
- Encourage patient to do leg exercises, and measure and apply elastic hose *to facilitate venous circulation.* Provide pneumatic compression stockings, if indicated.

NIC Respiratory Management

Ineffective breathing pattern related to narcotic use and abdominal pain
- Auscultate lungs every 2 to 4 hours.
- Encourage patient to turn, deep breathe, and cough every 2 hours.
- Encourage use of incentive spirometer *to promote maximal inspiratory maneuvers.*
- Provide pain medications and splint abdomen with pillow *to decrease abdominal pain associated with deep breathing and coughing.*
- Assist patient with early and progressive ambulation.
- Peripheral pulse oximetry may provide useful information regarding oxygen saturation levels.
- Administer O_2 prn or as ordered.

NIC Physical Comfort Promotion

Acute pain related to surgical incision and manipulation, and gas
- Discuss with patient the importance of pain relief postoperatively *to prevent complications.*
- Provide analgesics as ordered for pain, keeping physician informed of patient's level of comfort and response to medication.
- Premedicate patient before ambulation, dressing changes, or other painful procedures.
- Assist patient in proper positioning.
- Use adjunctive pain-relieving strategies (massage, heat or cool pads, relaxation techniques, and music). Document the effectiveness on the care plan.
- Reassure patient and family that usual postoperative patient does not become addicted to narcotics.
- Evaluate patient for side effects of narcotics, and discuss with patient respiratory depression, itching, nausea, and hallucinations.
- Be supportive of patient while he or she is having pain; at the same time, evaluate nature and location of pain.
- Gradually discontinue intravenous and intramuscular injections, and ease the patient on to oral analgesia when patient is eating or able to tolerate it.

NIC Skin/Wound Management

Risk for infection related to preoperative contamination

Risk for impaired skin integrity related to tissue ischemia; excessive wound drainage
- Assess wound during postoperative period for redness, pain, edema, unusual drainage, odor, and separation of the suture line.
- Observe wound dressing frequently for signs of bleeding.
- Protect nares when nasogastric tube is to be left in place several days.
- Keep primary dressing intact for 48 hours. Reinforce if saturated.
- After 48 hours, change wound dressings frequently if output is high *to protect skin from moisture maceration.*
- Evaluate patient with wound drainage for a wound pouching system *to contain the drainage, protect the skin, allow for accurate measurement, and decrease cost of dressing changes* (see box, p. 728).
- Ensure that all tubes and drains are well secured *to prevent accidental removal.* Provide skin protection if there is leakage around a tube (see box, p.729).
- Apply a pectin-based (Stomahesive, Hollihesive) wafer to the skin and tape to the wafer rather than applying tape on the skin. Montgomery straps can be applied on top of the pectin-based wafer. Keep in mind that drainage from the gastrointestinal tract continues to contain very irritating digestive enzymes (bile, gastric, pancreatic, intestinal).

NIC Elimination Management

Constipation related to altered bowel motility postoperatively

Diarrhea related to altered bowel motility postoperatively

Impaired urinary elimination related to use of catheters or local trauma
- Observe and record intake and urinary output.
- Observe color, consistency, frequency, and amount of stools.
- Provide privacy and promote relaxation when patient needs to void or defecate.
- Palpate bladder for distention if patient has not voided for 6 to 8 hours or patient is voiding small amounts frequently (overflow voiding). Catheterize patient if ordered.
- Evaluate bowel pattern change after gastrointestinal surgery (e.g., diarrhea related to bile in colon after cholecystectomy or small bowel resection; constipation related to narcotic use).
- Administer stool softeners/laxatives/antidiarrheal agents as ordered.

NIC Nutrition Support

Imbalanced nutrition: less than body requirements, related to disease process, postoperative ileus, nausea, and vomiting
- Weigh patient every day, and record the findings.
- Document percentage of oral intake. Do calorie counts as needed.
- Obtain nutritional consultation if indicated.
- Monitor laboratory values that reflect nutritional status—albumin, prealbumin.

CONTAINMENT OF WOUND DRAINAGE AND FISTULA OUTPUT

Pouch Method

1. Premedicate patient if procedure will be painful.
2. Gather supplies:
   a. Ostomy or wound pouch (with skin barrier attached) that will accommodate wound. The pouch should be designed to attach to a bedside bag.
   b. Scissors, plastic film, marker.
   c. Skin barrier paste (e.g., Premium or StomaHesive).
3. Make a pattern of the wound or fistula using a piece of plastic film. Carefully label the patient's left side, right side, head and feet; pouch side and skin side.
4. Trace the pattern onto the skin barrier on the back of the pouch. Be sure to match up the patient's right side, left side, head, and so forth, so that the pouch will not be positioned backwards or upside down.
5. Cut the opening in the barrier following the pattern.
6. Cleanse the patient's skin with warm water, and pat dry. Fill in any folds or creases with paste.
7. Remove the paper backing from the back of the pouch, and apply a thin coat of paste around the cut opening.
8. Center the cut opening over the wound, pressing firmly at the wound edges. Cover any exposed skin with paste through the access cap or through the end of the pouch.
9. Close the spout, or apply a clamp. If the drainage is liquid, attach the spout to a bedside drainage bag.
10. Check the system each shift for signs of leakage; change when necessary.
11. If pouching system leaks consistently and you are unable to achieve an adequate seal, an enterostomal therapist consultation may be required to assess the need for a different pouching system.

Suction and Transparent Dressing Method

1. Premedicate the patient if the procedure will be painful.
2. Gather supplies:
   a. Skin barrier, if the skin is intact; hydrocolloid wafer, if the skin has open ulcers or eroded areas near the wound
   b. Paste
   c. Powder (Premium or StomaHesive)—used if there are eroded, weeping areas near the wound
   d. Transparent dressing or polyurethane film in the size that corresponds to the wound size
   e. Catheters—soft, large lumen with hand-cut side holes; need 1 to 3 catheters, depending on the size of the wound and whether the wound is being irrigated
   f. Connectors for catheters
   g. Scissors, pattern, black marker, normal saline, if using flush and irrigation, razor, and washcloth
3. Turn off the wound irrigation before changing the pouch, if using irrigation.
4. Gently remove the old skin barrier/hydrocolloid and transparent film. Use a warm washcloth as needed.
5. Clean surrounding skin gently, and remove all accumulated pastes and so forth. To remove residual soft paste, use a dry facial tissue in a gentle, pinching and rolling motion. Shave any hair that will come into contact with the paste or barrier to make removal easier.

NIC Self-Care Facilitation

Bathing/hygiene self-care deficit related to postoperative pain and immobility

- Assist patient with activities of daily living after surgery.
- Encourage patient to participate in self-care as tolerated.
- Encourage patient to assume primary responsibility for care as tolerated as nasogastric tube and IV lines are removed.
- Provide or assist patient with regular mouth care *to prevent problems associated with nasogastric tubes, limited oral intake for several days, and mouth breathing.*

NIC Coping Assistance

Anxiety related to change in body image, fear of the future, unfamiliar environment, feelings of lack of control, and separation from home and work roles

- Provide information related to patient's fears and concerns *so that he or she can gain understanding.*
- Set aside time to listen actively, allowing patient to sort out vague or anxious feelings. Help patient to verbalize and understand the feelings he or she is having.
- Provide for continuity in staffing or assign a primary nurse, if possible.
- Introduce patient to other patients who are in similar situations and can provide mutual support.
- Make a referral to a local support organization (United Ostomy Association, American Cancer Society, Crohn's and Colitis Foundation of America).
- Provide patient with quiet time alone or with significant others *to allow him or her uninterrupted time to sort through emotions.*
- Refer patient for psychologic follow-up in the hospital or after discharge, if indicated.
- Talk with family and significant others *to help them understand patient's situation better and to assist them in supporting patient.*

Patient Education/Continuum of Care Plan

1. Ensure that patient understands that routine care follows major abdominal surgery: ambulate at regular times, rest frequently, and slowly increase activities as tolerated; report any signs of redness, pain, or drainage from incision; avoid heavy lifting for 6 to 8 weeks, and splint abdomen when coughing or sneezing. Ensure that patient understands that pain may accompany these activities and that pain medications are available and should be taken as necessary and as prescribed.
2. Explain medications and medication schedule to patient.
3. Discuss with patient the importance of regular follow-up care.
4. Review with patient information related to primary diagnosis, type of surgery, and expected outcomes.
5. Review with patient written instructions for any at-home care: wound, T tube, gastrostomy tube, and so on.
6. Arrange for home health nurses for the patient if needed.

CONTAINMENT OF WOUND DRAINAGE AND FISTULA OUTPUT—cont'd

6. Let dry thoroughly.
7. Make a pattern of the wound opening using a black marker and clear piece of plastic, or use the existing pattern. If using an existing pattern, make certain it is still a good fit.
8. Trace the edges of the wound and any surrounding drains, ostomies, and so forth. Transfer pattern to the skin barrier or hydrocolloid (it may have to be in two separate pieces). When in doubt where the skin edge lies, make the pattern slightly larger than the wound to avoid having the skin barrier on the wound surface.
   a. Make sure you mark which is up and which is down or which is right and which is left; this will ensure that the pieces will not be upside down or backwards.
9. Place a bead of paste at the edge of the skin near the wound; place the cut barrier on the surrounding skin. Cover any exposed skin at the wound edge with the paste. Apply the paste with a slightly damp gloved finger. The paste seals the area between the skin barrier and the wound.
10. Now that the periwound skin is completely protected, squeeze a bead of paste about an inch away from the wound on the top of the skin barrier. This is the seal for the transparent dressing. If this bead of paste is too close to the edge, it will be sucked onto the wound when suction is applied.
11. If using irrigation, you will need two catheters. One at the top for the NS and the other at the bottom for suction of drainage. The dependent catheter can have side holes cut into it for better suction. Lay catheters in the wound, with one in the superior portion of the wound and one in the most inferior portion of the wound. Lay them on top of the paste just applied. Apply another bead of paste over the top of each catheter. Make sure the tips of the catheters are not lying in paste, or they will clog.
   a. You can bevel the tips of the catheters and lay them bevel down in the wound. If the suction is too high or the wound tissue friable, the tip should be placed on top of the skin barrier at the most dependent part.
12. Lay a piece of transparent dressing over the entire wound. If it is not big enough, lay it over the bottom of the wound first (this is where it is most likely to leak). *DO NOT remove the paper backing of the larger sizes before application because it becomes more difficult to apply the dressing.* Remove the paper backing after laying it over the wound. If there are still exposed areas on the superior aspect, cover them with an additional piece of transparent dressing. DATE the system!
13. Connect the lower catheter to suction (as low suction as possible to do the job); connect the upper catheter to the irrigant—usually NS.
14. Change the dressing on a regular schedule to prevent skin irritation. These systems can be patched by recaulking with the paste and applying more transparent dressing if the skin is still protected. The dressing can last as long as a week.
15. If pouching system leaks consistently and you are unable to achieve an adequate seal, an enterostomal therapist consultation may be required to assess the need for a different pouching system.

7. Provide patient with unit phone number and physician's phone number in case questions or problems should arise after patient's discharge.

EVALUATION/PATIENT OUTCOMES

Tissue Perfusion Management: Fluid status is normal. Vital signs at baseline, adequate intake and output reflect adequate circulation and tissue perfusion, no thrombophlebitis.

Respiratory Management: Pulmonary status at baseline. Breathing and oxygenation normal for patient; patient demonstrates splinting and use of pain medications to assist with proper breathing techniques.

Physical Comfort Promotion: Comfort level is achieved. Patient has reduction or absence of guarding or protective behavior. Patient uses pain control strategies appropriately. Patient verbalizes increased control over pain.

Skin/Wound Management: Surgical incision is healing. Absence of erythema or drainage, and wound is well approximated. Patient demonstrates wound care, if applicable. There is no evidence of infection.

Elimination Management: Bowel and bladder are functioning normally. Patient is experiencing minimal or no diarrhea or constipation. Patient's abdomen is not distended; patient is without nausea or vomiting. Patient voids large amounts

GASTROSTOMY TUBE CARE

A variety of tube retention devices are manufactured and may be available at your institution. If not, the following steps may be taken to secure the tube and protect the skin around the tube from drainage:

1. Use a pectin-based wafer (skin barrier) around the tube. Cut a small opening in the wafer ⅛ inch larger than the skin exit site.
2. Cleanse the skin with warm water and pat dry.
3. Apply the wafer, and seal to the skin.
4. Apply a thin coat of paste (Stomahesive) to any exposed skin around the tube.
5. Anchor the tube to the wafer with use of a baby bottle nipple. Cut open the end of the nipple. Cut the end of the nipple large enough to accommodate the tube. Cut up through the side of the nipple (base to top), open the nipple, and wrap around the tube. Then tape the base of the nipple to the pectin-based wafer.
6. Tape the tube to the top of the nipple.
7. Remove the nipple daily and assess the exit site. If needed, gently cleanse around the tube exit site and dry, reapply paste, and replace nipple. If the skin barrier has drainage leaking under the seal, remove and replace. The wafer should be changed weekly otherwise.

spontaneously and is able to completely empty the bladder. Patient shows no signs of urinary tract infection.

Nutrition Support: Nutrition is adequate. Patient tolerates recommended diet by time of discharge. Weight is stable.

Self-Care Facilitation: Patient returns to activities of daily living. Patient is able progressively to do the things he or she was doing before surgery

Coping Assistance: Anxiety is reduced. Patient gains understanding of anxious feelings and is able to verbalize fears and concerns to the staff or significant others.

DIVERSIONS: COLOSTOMY AND ILEOSTOMY

Description and Rationale

A colostomy is a diversion involving the colon in which a segment of diseased or injured colon is bypassed or removed and an end or loop of colon is brought through a small opening in the abdominal wall and matured, forming a stoma. The anatomic location in the colon is an important description and influences the care. Ascending, transverse, and sigmoid colostomies may be performed. Transverse colostomies are most often loop ostomy stomas and are temporary. A loop means that the intact bowel has been brought through the abdominal wall, a rod placed under the bowel, the incision closed, and a cautery used to open the top wall of the bowel (the lower wall remains intact). The proximal opening will drain the stool while the distal opening may drain mucus and leads to the rectum. The patient may have bowel movements from the rectum that consist of stool remaining in the bowel before surgery, or the patient may continue to pass mucus. The stool is semiformed, odorous, and unpredictable.

The sigmoid colostomy is the most common permanent stoma and is indicated for cancer of the rectum. The stool from the sigmoid colostomy is similar to normal bowel movements. Generally, stool is evacuated once or twice a day. A regular pattern before surgery is used to predict the possibility of regulation of the sigmoid colostomy with diet or with colostomy irrigations.

For patients with a sigmoid colostomy a device that plugs the stoma is available.

The removal of the entire colon and rectum (total proctocolectomy) results in the ileum being brought through the abdominal wall, forming an ileostomy stoma. The stool from the ileostomy is liquid to semiformed and contains residual digestive enzymes. The drainage from the ascending colostomy is similar, and the nursing interventions are the same for both. Fluid and electrolyte imbalance is a potential problem with an ileostomy and may result in significant problems.

Contraindications and Cautions

1. Only a sigmoid colostomy should be irrigated (see box on p. 733) to obtain regular bowel eliminations. The decision to do so is left up to the patient.
2. An ileostomy lavage for a food blockage refers to the insertion of 30 to 50 ml of normal saline through a small catheter using an Asepto syringe. *This is not a colostomy irrigation and should not be performed by patients.*
3. Laxatives should *never* be given to a patient with an ileostomy. The result can be severe fluid and electrolyte imbalance.

Preprocedural Nursing Care

1. Consultation with an ET nurse is arranged.
2. A preoperative visit by a United Ostomy Association (UOA) trained visitor (rehabilitated person with an ostomy) is recommended.
3. Stoma site selection is marked by the ET nurse for the surgeon.

NURSING CARE

NURSING ASSESSMENT

Gastrointestinal status: Abdominal distention, nausea and vomiting, absence of stool; food blockage (ileostomy)

Perianal examination

- Perineum: Perineal incision: redness, tenderness, drainage
- Stoma: Color (necrosis); perfusion (moisture and color); protrusion (flush, retracted, prolapsed)
- Peristomal skin: Erythema; erosion; rash; parastomal hernia

Sexual functioning: Wide resections in perineal care for cancer of rectum may damage nerves responsible for erection, ejaculation, and orgasm in men; no impairment or one or a combination of all functions may be affected. (NOTE: Physiologic effects on women have been poorly studied.)

Self-concept and body image

- Adjustment and integration of ostomy require time and support from family and health care providers
- Complications: Prolonged use of defense behaviors, noninvolvement in physical care, social isolation

POTENTIAL COMPLICATIONS

Fluid/electrolyte imbalance, dehydration, blockage

PATIENT PROBLEMS/NURSING DIAGNOSES & INTERVENTIONS

NIC TISSUE PERFUSION MANAGEMENT

Risk for deficient fluid volume related to postoperative diarrhea

- Observe patient with ileostomy for diarrhea: high-volume, watery, pouch emptied every 20 to 30 minutes.
- Monitor intake and output, vital signs, daily weights, and electrolytes.
- Replace fluids and electrolytes orally or intravenously as ordered.
- Administer antidiarrheal agents as ordered.

NIC COPING ASSISTANCE

Disturbed body image related to external abdominal stoma

Ineffective sexuality patterns related to external abdominal stoma

- Provide patient and family an opportunity to express their feelings regarding the ostomy preoperatively and postoperatively.

- Remind patient that an ostomy is an alternative pattern of elimination, that it will take time to adjust to, both physically and emotionally, and that people are available to help.
- Encourage patient to return to all presurgical activities as soon as possible.
- Recommend a trained ostomy visitor of same age and sex as patient and preferably one who has had same type of ostomy procedure.
- Allow patient to grieve for loss of a body part and loss of control of elimination.
- Be realistic and positive: negative reactions and facial expressions will be picked up by patient and will make adjustment harder; most people adapt successfully to ostomy surgery.
- Allow patient and significant other to discuss concerns and fears regarding sexual activities. Many patients fear rejection by spouse or by a significant other. In addition, many spouses and significant others worry about hurting patient.
- Remind patient that he or she must first be comfortable with self. Spouse or significant other is most often kind, gentle, and caring. Communication between partners is extremely important.
- Refer men who have had nerve damage and are unable to obtain an erection to a urologist for information on penile prosthesis or vacuum erection devices.
- Refer to family and sexual counselors as indicated by poor coping or maladaptation.

NIC Skin/Wound Management

Risk for impaired skin integrity related to improper pouch fit, allergic reaction, fungal infection, or folliculitis

Impaired skin integrity related to improper pouch fit, allergic reaction, fungal infection, or folliculitis

- Assess skin integrity with each pouch change.
- Protect peristomal skin with skin barriers: pectin-based wafers and paste, skin sealant wipes or sprays.
- Change pouching system whenever pouch first begins to leak (an early sign is odor); ***do not*** tape a leaking pouch seal and plan on changing it later.
- Treat erythematous, noneroded skin reactions that are secondary to ileostomy drainage, stool, glue, solvents, and soaps as follows:
  - Remove source of irritation (frequently it is a too-large pouch opening or a sensitivity to adhesive).
  - Cleanse skin with warm water and pat dry or use a hair dryer set on cool.
  - Cover all irritated skin with skin barrier; the opening in the skin barrier must be cut to exact size and shape of stoma.
  - Select a different pouch or adhesive if patient shows an allergic reaction to a particular pouch.
- Treat skin that is eroded or ulcerated as follows:
  - Use normal saline to cleanse skin (less painful).
  - Dust eroded area with stoma powder; dust off excess powder. Dab skin sealant wipe over powder to set powder.
  - If eroded areas are caused by diarrhea washing away barrier, use stoma paste around stoma or on the cut opening in skin barrier; advise patient ahead of time that it may burn for a few minutes.
  - Change pouch every 24 to 48 hours until erosion or ulceration heals, then resume usual pouching schedule.
- Avoid mechanical injury to skin by gentle removal of tape and skin barriers.
- Empty pouches rather than changing and discarding pouches that are full.
- Observe for monilial *(C. albicans)* reactions associated with antibiotics and changes in normal bowel flora. Skin appears bright red with weepy papulae, satellite lesions, and secondary crusting. Patients may complain of intense itching.
- Assess other sites for monilial infection: under arms, under breasts, around groin, and in mouth.
- Consult physician for order of nystatin (Mycostatin) powder. Rub into affected area and dust off excess. Dab skin sealant wipe over powder to set powder. Ointments will keep pouch from sealing.
- Prevent radiation dermatitis by not having any portion of pouch or pouch adhesive in the field of radiation. If pouch must be removed daily for treatments, use a karaya-only backed pouch that is belted in place.

NIC Elimination Management

Altered bowel elimination related to colostomy*

- Notify ET nurse to fit patient for pouching system.
- Select a system that is invisible under clothing, is odor-proof, and fits the body size.
- Suggest fabric pouch covers; other patients have recommended crotchless panties for women and binders for men to hold pouch in place.
- Provide consistent management of the ostomy, control odor, and prevent leaking, *giving patient a sense of control over stoma.*
- Evaluate output for color, consistency, frequency, and amount.
- Identify, report, and manage constipation.

Risk for intestinal injury related to blockage of ileostomy

- Perform an ileostomy lavage.
  - Remove pouch; stoma will become edematous.
  - Apply irrigation sleeve.
  - Have patient assume knee-chest position and massage abdomen under stoma; if blockage is removed, stop here and reapply pouching system; if not, continue.
  - Insert catheter gently into stoma to level of blockage (usually at fascia level).
  - Irrigate with 30 to 50 ml normal saline using Asepto syringe; allow to return.
  - Repeat instillation of 30 to 50 ml of saline.
  - Procedure may take 1 to 2 hours; may try knee-chest position between irrigations if patient is stable.
  - Assess for dehydration; fluid becomes trapped behind food blockage, which acts as an intestinal obstruction.

---

*Not a NANDA diagnosis.

Provide intravenous fluids as ordered.

NOTE: Ileostomy lavage is *not* taught to patients. However, patient should be taught to recognize early signs and symptoms and seek medical assistance.

Assist patient in returning to regular diet, avoiding only foods that give that person problems.

- Instruct patient to chew food carefully and eat slowly.

PATIENT EDUCATION/CONTINUUM OF CARE PLAN

1. Colostomy and ileostomy care involves the following:
   a. Stomal and skin assessment: stoma should be red and moist; skin should be free of irritation.
   b. Management of frequently encountered skin problems.
      (1) Usual causes include fungal infections, pouch opening cut too large, or an allergic reaction to barriers, paste, or tape. See interventions under Impaired Skin Integrity for management.
      (2) Remind patient that weeping skin may prevent pouch or skin barrier from adhering to skin for long periods. If skin is severely irritated and weeping, it may be necessary to change pouch more frequently to prevent leakage and further damage until the skin heals.
      (3) Remind patient that hair under barrier should be removed by electric razor or safety razor.
   c. Principles of changing a pouching system should be accompanied by several opportunities for practicing the procedure.
      (1) Instruct patient to assemble all equipment: tissues, toilet paper, wash cloths, towels, cut-to-fit stoma pouch; paste (if stool is liquid); pouch closure; tape or belt; and equipment for cleansing or disposing of used pouches.
      (2) A paper towel or template may be used to trace a pattern, which should hug the stoma but not ride up on it, and top should be labeled. Outer dimensions of the pattern (avoiding hip bones, pubic areas, ribs and folds at waist and navel) should be considered.
      (3) Instruct patient to trace pattern on paper side of pouch, to cut out hole using pattern, and to remove paper backing from pouch.
      (4) Empty and remove pouch being worn. Cleanse and dry skin.
      (5) Patient should note any changes in skin or stoma (color, size, ulcerations, irritations), center and apply skin barrier and pouch, close end, and tape edges (if necessary).
      (6) Instruct patient to check supplies and reorder as necessary.
   d. Dietary considerations should be discussed with patient. Use a nutritionist, if one is available.
      (1) Foods associated with odor are fish, eggs, asparagus, onions, garlic, and some spices.
      (2) Foods associated with diarrhea are green beans, broccoli, spinach, raw fruits, highly seasoned foods, and beer.
      (3) Foods used to manage diarrhea (low-residue diet) are strained bananas, peanut butter (without nuts), rice, and applesauce.
      (4) Foods used to manage constipation are high-fiber foods (bran, celery), increased raw fruits and vegetables, and increased fluid intake (water, fruit juices).
      (5) Foods associated with gas are brussels sprouts, cabbage, beans, peas, mushrooms, carbonated drinks, onions, cucumbers, and beer.
      (6) Patients are encouraged to eat all above foods in moderation, chewing well, and adding one new food at a time to evaluate tolerance.
   e. Provide patient with written instructions for follow-up, and initiate home care referral if indicated.
2. Ileostomy patient teaching should include the following:
   a. Instruct patient about symptoms of food blockage and what to do if it occurs.
      (1) Discharge changes from semisolid to a thin liquid; lumen is blocked by food, but water passes around it.
      (2) Total volume of output increases and functions almost constantly; water is drawn from bloodstream in attempt to rid bowel lumen of blockage, and intestines become hyperactive.
      (3) There is an objectionable odor; bacterial overgrowth occurs at blockage and causes fermentation of foodstuff.
      (4) Cramping occurs, usually followed by increase in watery output; this is caused by increased bowel activity to rid itself of blockage.
      (5) Abdomen is distended; blockage traps gas and liquids in bowel lumen.
      (6) Vomiting occurs; this is a further attempt of body to rid itself of blockage by traveling in direction of least resistance.
      (7) There is no ileostomy output because of complete blockage.
      (8) Instruct patient to get into a knee-chest position for a few minutes or take a hot shower to relax and then try the knee-chest position.
      (9) Many blockages relieve themselves; however, if the blockage persists more than 3 to 4 hours, contact physician.
   b. Foods associated with blockage include celery, Chinese foods, corn, nuts, coleslaw, dried fruits, coconut, wild rice, popcorn, whole vegetable skins, and fibrous vegetables. Do not eliminate from diet. Eat in moderate amounts and chew well.

EVALUATION/PATIENT OUTCOMES

Tissue Perfusion Management: Hydration is adequate. Fluid intake meets needs for increased output.

COLOSTOMY IRRIGATION

1. Explain procedure to the patient.
2. Collect equipment:
   a. Irrigation sleeve (either 2¼ or 2¾, depending on the size of the flange on the patient)
   b. Irrigation kit with cone or enema bag with Laird tip (do not use catheter for irrigations)
   c. Water-soluble jelly
   d. Disposable face cloths and toilet paper
   e. Disposable gloves
   f. Patient handout on colostomy irrigations to help the patient follow along
3. With the patient sitting on a chair facing the toilet (see note), remove pouch (leave skin barrier), and attach irrigation sleeve. Sleeve end will be in the toilet. (Have the patient wear something warm so that he or she does not get chilled.)
4. Fill the irrigation bag with lukewarm tap water. The extra water in the bag can be used to rinse the sleeve out. The first irrigation should only have 250 to 300 ml; gradually increase the amount. Never use more than 1500 ml.
5. Clear the tubing of air.
6. Hang the bag so it is about 18 inches above the stoma.
7. To determine the direction of the colon, insert a lubricated gloved finger into the stoma about 1 to 2 inches. Insert the cone in the direction of the colon. This only needs to be done with the first irrigation.
8. Lubricate the end of the cone with lubricant, and gently insert the cone into the colostomy. Do not force it. Hold the cone firmly in position.
9. Allow a little water to run into the intestine by releasing the clamp. If water leaks around the stoma, insert the cone in further.
10. The water must go in slowly. It should take at least 3 to 5 minutes (time it) for the water to enter the intestine. If the patient experiences cramping while the water is running in, clamp the tube and have the patient take several deep breaths. When the cramping subsides, allow more water to run in. *Do not* remove the cone until the irrigation is finished.
11. When all the water has run in, hold the cone in place 1 to 2 minutes to allow the fluid to remain in the colon to achieve good results. Gently remove the cone.
12. Clip or secure the top of the irrigating sleeve shut. NOTE: Expect returns of the first irrigation to be stool-colored water. As the patient's diet and the amount of water increases, the irrigation will be more successful: the patient will expel soft stools after irrigation.
13. Most of the water and stool will be eliminated in 5 to 10 minutes. After that time, lift the sleeve out of the toilet, rinse the sleeve clean, and clip the bottom of the sleeve to the top of the sleeve. Have the patient walk around, go back to bed, or sit in a chair, to stimulate a better return from the irrigation.
14. After 20 minutes in the bathroom, use the remaining water in the bag to flush the sleeve clean; remove the sleeve. Wipe the skin barrier clean, and attach a clean pouch and clip.
15. Wash the irrigation sleeve and bag with warm water, and store it in the bathroom. (NOTE: If the patient is not able to perform the procedure at the toilet because he or she has had an abdominal perineal resection or because he or she is debilitated, the procedure can be performed in bed. Protect the bed with disposable pads, and place the sleeve off the side of the bed. Keep the sleeve clamped and empty to prevent odors from escaping.)

Coping Assistance: Patient begins to incorporate ostomy into self-concept. Patient verbalizes feelings related to ostomy and external pouching system. Patient can care for ostomy. Patient resumes normal patterns of sexuality and sexual activity. Patient's and significant other's questions and concerns regarding sexuality and sexual changes have been discussed.

Skin/Wound Management: Peristomal skin is intact. Patient has no redness or eroded areas near stoma or under pouch.

Elimination Management: Patient understands to eat and chew slowly. There is no intestinal blockage, or ileostomy blockage has been effectively resolved with lavage.

Diversion: Continent Ileostomy

Description and Rationale

The continent ileostomy, or Kock pouch, was first described by Nils Kock in 1969.[27] Other surgeons have developed adaptations of Kock's procedure. The procedure involves the creation of an internal pouch constructed of ileum and of a nipple valve that maintains continency of stool and flatus. The patient has a stoma flush with the skin located in the lower right quadrant, which is intubated with a large-bore tube several times a day to evacuate the stool and flatus. Most patients who have this procedure have already had their rectums removed at a prior operation.

The continent ileostomy is an alternative for people who do not want to wear an external pouch. Some patients also believe a flush stoma rather than a protruding stoma is an advantage. Patients do not find the intubation or catheterization procedure bothersome once the pouch capacity increases.

The advantages of the continent ileostomy include the following:[31]

No appliance required
No noise or odor from stoma except during emptying
No skin irritation
Improved psychosocial adjustment

The continent ileostomy has a higher risk of complications than conventional ileostomies. Long-term problems are common and may be associated with loss of continency.

The disadvantages of the procedure are associated with the high percentage of nipple valve dysfunction and the reoperative rate. Even with the high rate of reoperation, many patients who have converted to a continent ileostomy state that it is a more satisfactory procedure.

The continent ileostomy is constructed from a long segment of terminal ileum after the colectomy has been performed. After the pouch is constructed, the nipple valve is constructed by one of several techniques. The pouch is then sutured closed and assessed for adequacy of the valve and the suture line by filling it with a saline solution and air. If no signs of leakage are noted from the valve or from the sutures, the pouch is inserted into the abdominal cavity and anchored. The end portion of the distal ileum is brought through the abdominal wall, and a flush stoma is constructed. A catheter is placed in the reservoir during surgery and remains in the pouch for 3 to 4 weeks.

Complications of continent ileostomies include the following:

Leakage of nipple valve
Valve prolapse
Skin stricture
Pouch perforation
"Pouchitis": local crampy pain, diarrhea that may be bloody, fever, valve leakage, intubation difficulty

Contraindications and Cautions

1. The diagnosis must be familial polyposis or ulcerative colitis. This procedure is *not* performed for Crohn's disease because of the risk of ulcerations in and subsequent failure of the pouch.
2. The patient needs medical alert cards because the continent ileostomy is an uncommon procedure.
3. Obesity is considered a contraindication.

Preprocedural Nursing Care

1. There should be a preoperative consultation with an ET nurse to answer the patient's questions about possible surgical options; conventional ileostomy, continent ileostomy, and ileoanal reservoir.
2. If possible, a rehabilitated patient with a continent ileostomy should visit preoperatively.

NURSING CARE

Nursing Assessment

Self-concept and body image: Presence of stoma and no external pouch more positive; if valve leaks, requires external pouch (p. 728)

Peristomal skin: Erythema, erosions from leakage, or excess mucus secretion

Potential Complications

Nipple valve dysfunction, pouch perforation, "pouchitis"

Patient Problems/Nursing Diagnoses & Interventions

NIC Coping Assistance

Disturbed body image related to presence of abdominal stoma

- Allow patient opportunity to explore feelings regarding surgery.
- Provide trained visitor for patient.
- Assist patient in getting used to intubating abdominal stoma.

NIC Skin/Wound Management

Risk for impaired skin integrity related to leakage or mucus on the peristomal skin

- Protect peristomal skin with skin sealant (Bard Protective Barrier, Hollister Skin Gel) from moisture in mucus.
- Cover stoma with small pad.
- Protect skin from ileostomy drainage if nipple valve leaks (p. 729).

Patient Education/Continuum of Care Plan

1. Intubation and irrigation of continent ileostomy involve the following procedures (procedures vary with surgeon). The goal is to gently increase pouch capacity without straining new suture lines.
   a. First 3 weeks (catheter in place)
      (1) Irrigate internal continent ileostomy pouch; insert 30 ml water and allow to drain out by gravity; irrigate every 3 hours during day and once at night.
      (2) Attach bedside bag or leg bag.
      (3) Clean bedside and leg bags with soapy water; allow to dry; have two bags and one alternate.
      (4) Eat a low-residue diet.
   b. Week 4
      (1) Catheter is removed in outpatient clinic, and patient is taught to intubate continent ileostomy.
      (2) Intubate and irrigate every 3 hours during day.
      (3) Intubate with catheter to straight drainage at night; irrigate once at night.
   c. Week 5
      (1) Intubate every 3 hours, and irrigate twice a day.
      (2) Connect to gravity drainage at night; irrigate once at night.
   d. Week 6
      (1) Intubate every 4 hours, and irrigate twice during day.
      (2) Intubate at night only if sign of fullness or uncomfortable.
   e. Week 7 and thereafter
      (1) Intubate pouch four times each day.
      (2) Irrigate pouch once each day until return is clear.
2. The following procedure is used for emptying and intubating the continent ileostomy:
   a. Patient sitting on commode inserts well-lubricated catheter into stoma and through nipple valve. Stool and flatus will drain through catheter directly into toilet. If stool is thick, water can be inserted through catheter to loosen stool. Catheter may need to be removed and flushed if lumen becomes blocked with undigested residue. Grape juice and prune juice are often ingested by patients to keep their stool "thin."
   b. Several types of catheters are available (Marlen, Atlantic). Patient should have at least two catheters and should know how to order additional ones. It is important to discard catheters when they become old. Hard, brittle catheters are more likely to damage valve or pouch.
3. Patient should be provided with written instructions on signs and symptoms of "pouchitis" and procedures if he or

she experiences difficulty intubating pouch or leakage of nipple valve develops.
4. Patient should be given instructions on low-residue diet and advancing to a regular diet.

EVALUATION/PATIENT OUTCOMES

Coping Assistance: Patient begins to incorporate change in body image into new self-image. Patient verbalizes positive feelings related to the ostomy and the necessity for intubation. Patient can care for the new continent ileostomy.

Skin/Wound Management: Peristomal skin is intact. Patient has no redness or eroded areas near the stoma.

DIVERSION: ILEOANAL RESERVOIR

Description and Rationale

The ileoanal reservoir is the procedure performed for patients with ulcerative colitis and familial polyposis that provides the most normal mechanism for maintaining continency and the most natural method of evacuation. Factors that are assessed when evaluating a patient for this procedure include normal anorectal sphincter mechanism, absence of perianal disease, good physical condition, motivation, and age. It is important that the patient understand that it is a one-, two-, or three-stage procedure and that close follow-up is important throughout. A temporary ileostomy requires that the patient learn stomal care. The patient must also be aware that diarrhea may be a problem for 6 months to 1 year after the closure of the ileostomy. During this time, incontinence may occur but is usually minimal and is more common at night.[11]

Four types of procedures may be done to preserve normal bowel elimination. Each involves removal of the rectal mucosa. The first step in constructing the ileoanal reservoir is the mucosal stripping of the rectal segment to form a muscular cuff through the mucosa and submucosa of the rectum for 2 to 3 cm above the dentate line. The rectal muscle layers and the anal sphincters are left intact while the primary disease is removed. During the abdominal colectomy, the rectosigmoid is removed with care to preserve the autonomic nerves on the posterior and lateral pelvic walls.

When no reservoir is constructed, diarrhea and incontinence are major problems. In 1978, Parks and Nicholls[36] added an ileoanal reservoir to the previously described rectal mucosectomy and ileorectal pull-through. The reservoir provided an important addition, a means by which the liquid effluent could be held until evacuation was appropriate. Thus the patient undergoing total colectomy also has rectal mucosectomy, construction of an ileal reservoir, ileoanal anastomosis, and a temporary ileostomy during the first stage of the procedure. During the second stage, the ileostomy is closed. The ileoanal reservoir may be constructed in three configurations. It is constructed from 30 to 50 cm of terminal ileum. In the S reservoir, three loops of ileum, approximately 12 to 15 cm in length, are aligned side by side. The reservoir is constructed by suturing the limbs and opening the segments, creating a pouch. A remaining 5 cm of ileum forms a spout that is sutured to the dentate line, completing the ileoanal portion of the procedure.

The J reservoir consists of two loops of ileum. The ileum is brought down to the rectal cuff, and one limb is looped upward, creating a J shape. The loops are anastomosed in a side-by-side fashion by use of a stapler. The portion where the ileum curves upward is sutured to the anus and opened.

In the isoperistaltic reservoir, a single lumen of 25 to 30 cm of ileum is brought down and through the rectal cuff. The distal end is sutured to the anus, and the proximal end is closed. An ileostomy is performed. In the second stage the ileostomy is taken down and a lateral side-to-side ileal anastomosis is performed to create the reservoir.

The operation is done occasionally in one stage, avoiding an ileostomy. The patient should be in excellent health, and no tension should be on the rectal reservoir anastomosis during the operation. The adjustment period after a one-stage procedure is often more difficult (more frequency and incontinence) because of the diarrhea seen immediately after colectomy.

If a patient is very ill and malnourished, he or she will initially have a colectomy with end ileostomy. The patient returns in approximately 6 months for the creation of the ileal reservoir; at that time the end ileostomy is converted to a loop ileostomy. The third operation, the ileostomy takedown, restores bowel continuity.

The diverting loop ileostomy protects the ileal reservoir during the healing period—usually 6 to 8 weeks. The management of these loop ileostomies can be challenging and may require a convex pouch.

Because it is the most common approach, the nursing care plan focuses on the patient undergoing this operation in two stages.

The advantages of the ileoanal reservoir include the following:

- Avoidance of a permanent abdominal stoma
- Avoidance of repeated stomal catheterizations
- Avoidance of body image alterations
- Decreased incidence of sexual dysfunction
- Provision of a near-normal pattern of defecation

The disadvantages of the procedure are as follows:

- Possible residual rectal mucosa
- Problems with differentiation of gas, fluids, and solids
- Tenesmus or fecal urgency
- Nocturnal incontinence
- Diarrhea
- Perianal skin denudation

Complications of the ileoanal reservoir include:

- Anal stenosis
- Ischemia of reservoir
- Rectal cuff abscess
- Nocturnal leakage
- Fecal incontinence
- "Pouchitis" (sudden onset of high-volume diarrhea, cramping, and bleeding)

Contraindications and Cautions

Crohn's disease or cancer of the rectum; obesity; short mesentery; decreased sphincter control

MULTIDISCIPLINARY PLAN

Medications

Bulk-forming agents: Psyllium (Metamucil), 1 teaspoon prn for diarrhea

Antidiarrheal agents: Loperamide (Imodium), up to 8 capsules PO per day for diarrhea
Dermatologic agents: Balneol cleansing agent; skin barrier ointments
Antifungal agents: Clotrimazole (Mycelex cream) 1%, prn for pruritus

General Management

Sitz bath; meticulous skin care after each stool

Nutritional Consultation

To advise patients regarding dietary management of diarrhea

NURSING CARE

NURSING ASSESSMENT

Perineum: Skin erosions from mucus, frequent bowel movements, incontinence, pruritus, and perianal pain
Fluids and electrolytes: Urine output is decreased; output is greater than input; sudden weight loss; hypotension

POTENTIAL COMPLICATIONS

Anal stenosis, abscess, reservoir ischemia, fecal incontinence, "pouchitis"

PATIENT PROBLEMS/NURSING DIAGNOSES & INTERVENTIONS

Stage 1: Ileostomy; Ileoanal Reservoir Constructed

NIC TISSUE PERFUSION MANAGEMENT

Deficient fluid volume related to postoperative diarrhea

- Monitor fecal output from ileostomy; 800 to 1200 ml/day is not uncommon.
- Replace fluid and electrolytes as ordered.
- Monitor daily weights.

NIC SKIN/WOUND MANAGEMENT

Impaired skin integrity related to incontinence of mucus

- Provide perianal skin care *because mucus contains residual enzymes, is copious, and is odorous.*
- Use skin sealants and moisture barrier creams before skin breaks down.
- Instruct patient in wearing absorbent pads at night.
- Protect peristomal skin and maintain pouch seal.

Stage 2: Ileostomy Closure; Ileoanal Reservoir Functioning

NIC SKIN/WOUND MANAGEMENT

Impaired skin integrity related to stool frequency or incontinence

- Avoid irritants such as nylon underwear, harsh or deodorant soaps, and fragrant toilet papers. Have patient flush perianal area after each stool; do not have patient wipe with toilet paper.
- Protect skin with barrier ointments containing petrolatum or zinc oxide *because of frequency of bowel movements and residual enzymes present in stool.*
- Provide sitz baths, Balneol cleansing agents, or Tucks pads *to help with perianal cleansing and to reduce pruritus.*

NIC ELIMINATION MANAGEMENT

Diarrhea; bowel incontinence related to postoperative reservoir adaptation

- Expect 10 to 20 bowel movements per day in early postoperative period; frequency slows to 6 to 12 per day as diet increases and averages 3 to 4 per day after 1 year.
- Instruct patient in high-fiber diet *to decrease number of stools.*
- Provide psyllium (Metamucil) or loperamide (Imodium), as ordered and as needed for diarrhea.

PATIENT EDUCATION/CONTINUUM OF CARE PLAN

The following list applies to stage 1.

1. Teach patient ileostomy management. Wearing time is decreased with loop ileostomies.
2. Perianal skin care is essential. Mucous drainage through anus is expected and may be irritating. Skin can be protected by use of skin barrier ointments. Minipads may be worn at night to absorb the drainage.
3. Approximately 6 to 8 weeks after surgery, a Gastrograffin x-ray film is taken to assess reservoir, ruling out anastomotic leaks and checking anatomic position of reservoir. Gastrograffin is water soluble and easier to evacuate from reservoir than barium would be.

The following list applies to stage 2.

1. For perianal skin care:
   a. Avoid nylon underwear, harsh or deodorant soaps, and fragrant toilet papers.
   b. Cleanse perianal skin with water and dry with hairdryer.
   c. Protect skin with barrier ointments.
   d. Manage pruritus with sitz baths. Balneol cleansing agents, or Mycelex cream.
2. Frequency of bowel movements will drop to 6 to 12 per day for first year and then decrease to 3 or 4 per day. Diarrhea associated with flu or viral infection will increase number and amount of bowel movements.

EVALUATION/PATIENT OUTCOMES

Tissue Perfusion Management: Patient maintains adequate fluid and electrolyte balance. Patient has balanced intake and output. Patient's vital signs are normal.

Skin/Wound Management: Perianal skin is normal. Patient's perianal skin is intact with no signs of irritation orpruritus.

Elimination Management: Bowel adapts to reservoir. Frequency of stooling decreases.

LIVER TRANSPLANTATION

Orthotopic liver transplantation (OLT) has been performed since the early 1960s. Improved survival rates in the last decade have made it a more common therapeutic option for patients with liver failure. One-year patient survival rates were 83% in 1995 compared with 77% in 1988.[7] These improved statistics are the result of better surgical techniques and immunosuppressive medications, including cyclosporine (CSA), improved preoperative and postoperative care, careful patient selection, and increased donor availability.[7] The procedure involves the removal of the recipient's liver (hepatectomy) and the transplantation of a donor liver. There are many more potential recipients than donors, especially in children.

Despite widespread publicity and availability of information about organ donation, many potential donors are lost. The Omnibus Budget Reconciliation Act of 1986 states that hospitals participating in Medicare programs must establish protocols to identify potential donors. Families of potential donors must be assured information about the options for donation of organs and tissue, as well as the right to refuse consent. The law also encourages discretion and sensitivity concerning the circumstances, views, and beliefs of the donor family. This law encourages organ and tissue donation when appropriate criteria are met.

A national organ sharing system was instituted in 1987. The system offers available livers first locally, then regionally, and then nationally until a suitable recipient is found. Improved techniques for preserving the liver graft allow for a day of safe storage,[7] thereby increasing the opportunity for a good match and making a more equitable distribution of donor livers.

Indications for liver transplantation vary somewhat from center to center, but the United Network for Organ Sharing (UNOS) indicates that the most common indications for liver transplantations include the following: (1) alcoholic cirrhosis, (2) hepatitis C, (3) cryptogenic cirrhosis, (4) hepatitis B, (5) autoimmune cirrhosis, (6) primary biliary cirrhosis, (7) primary sclerosing cholangitis, (8) fulminant hepatic failure, (9) malignancy, and (10) metabolic disorders.[50]

Once it has been determined that a patient is a candidate for liver transplantation the patient is listed by weight and blood type. Only in cases of absolute emergency are ABO-incompatible donors used because of a decreased survival rate. Orthotopic liver transplantation in pediatric patients has been limited because of the size match needed between donor and recipient. Some surgeons now reduce the size of the donor liver for pediatric patients.[39]

Complications of liver transplantation can be divided into surgical and nonsurgical. Surgical complications are most commonly biliary in origin (12% to 13%), including disruption of the anastomosis and strictures. Other surgical complications include hepatic artery thrombosis (3% to 10%) and portal vein thrombosis (1.8%)—the former being very serious in the postoperative period, often necessitating retransplant. Nonsurgical complications include renal dysfunction most often related to cyclosporine; infections, including bacterial, viral, and fungal (40% to 50%); and rejection of the donor liver (70% to 80%). Rejection is diagnosed by percutaneous liver biopsy (performed weekly after transplant). When two biopsies in a row are normal, the biopsies are done yearly.

Contraindications and Cautions

1. An extensive work-up and evaluation by the transplant team is required before transplantation. The work-up includes a complete history and physical examination of the patient to establish a primary diagnosis and prognosis; an evaluation of the patient's psyche, financial status, and family situation; a determination of portal vein patency with ultrasonography; chest x-ray examination; electrocardiogram, pulmonary function tests; and computed tomography scans of the abdomen to detect malignancies. Blood tests include ABO typing; HIV, hepatitis B and C, VDRL, and cytomegalovirus serologic screening; liver function tests; electrolyte, blood urea nitrogen, and creatinine panels; ammonia level; cholesterol and triglyceride levels; alpha-fetoprotein levels; and urinalysis.
2. Percutaneous transhepatic cholangiography with brushings may be used to rule out cholangiocarcinoma in patients with sclerosing cholangitis.
3. Patients and families should be provided with ongoing support and evaluations as they make the decision to undergo this major procedure. An evaluation of the educational needs is also made to provide the patient and family with the information needed to manage these life changes. Most transplant teams have nurse coordinators and social workers who monitor patients and families during evaluation and transplantation, as well as postoperatively.
4. Absolute contraindications may include (depending on the center) active infection or sepsis, extrahepatic malignancy, advanced cardiopulmonary or cerebrovascular disease, positive HIV test, and active alcohol or drug abuse. Relative contraindications include renal failure, age older than 60, positive test for hepatitis B surface antigen (HBsAg), hepatobiliary malignancy, previous portocaval shunt surgery, and portal vein thrombosis.

Preprocedural Nursing Care

1. Liver transplant patients usually are extremely ill and require expert nursing care to manage the primary diagnosis and any existing complications.
2. Inform the patient and family about the specific procedure and the rationale for the diagnostic procedure.
3. Inform the patient and family about the general postoperative course and any drains and tubes that will be present after surgery. Encourage attendance at a transplant support group, if one is available.

Multidisciplinary Plan

Medications

Dosages and type vary by physician and center protocol
No one protocol or dosages will be referred to

Antibiotic agents
- Ampicillin or cephalosporin
- Trimethoprim and sulfamethoxazole (Bactrim), prophylaxis against *Pneumocystis carinii* pneumonia
- *Or* Pentamidine puff, if allergic to Bactrim

Antiviral agents
- Acyclovir, prevent herpes simplex virus (HSV) infections
- Ganciclovir (DHPG), treat cytomegalovirus (CMV) infections for 5-7 days

Antifungal agents: Clotrimazole (Mycelex) troche/nystatin, or oral fluconazole to prevent *Candida* infections

Immunosuppression: Maintenance to prevent rejection; dose based on blood level and renal function; CSA may be given IV initially, then PO; azathioprine (Imuran); prednisolone or prednisone, often given IV, then PO; tacrolimus (FK506)

Acute rejection: Often based on biopsy

Initial therapy: Corticosteroids given in large initial doses and gradually tapered; may be repeated if no improvement

Subsequent therapy: If no improvement with steroids:

Polyclonal preparations (e.g., Minnesota antilymphocyte globulin [MALG]), for 5-14 days IV; antithymocyte globulin (ATG) for 14 days IV

Orthoclonal preparations (e.g., Orthoclone OKT3), for 5-14 days IV

Patients with chronic or irreversible rejection may be candidates for retransplantation

General Management

Mechanical ventilation for 24 to 48 hours, then oxygen by mask or nasal prongs

If patient has been encephalopathic preoperatively, intracranial pressure monitoring may be done until patient is awake

T tube

Jackson-Pratt drains

Intravenous fluids

Nasogastric drainage

NURSING CARE

NURSING ASSESSMENT

Abdominal examination: Surgical incision for drainage (note character, color, amount); monitor for signs and symptoms of infection; abdominal girth measurements to monitor postoperative complications

Cardiovascular status: Shock and circulatory failure associated with hemorrhage, sepsis, and fluid and electrolyte imbalance

Metabolic functioning: Decreased urine output, increased serum creatinine level and urine electrolyte levels (early nephrotoxicity associated with cyclosporine use); lethargy, decreased response to stimuli, glycosuria, osmotic diuresis, changes in mental status (hypoglycemia)

Infection: Early signs of infection: fever, herpes-virus infections (oral, esophageal, or gastric), *Candida* or CMV, pulmonary infiltrate *(Pneumocystis),* wound or urinary tract systems

Rejection

Malaise, fever, graft tenderness, diminished graft function as evidenced by decreased bile output

Increased bilirubin and transaminase levels

Monitor to evaluate liver function and evidence of increased cerebral pressure because intracranial bleeding is a major complication. Cyclosporine may also affect mental status. Notify physician of any of the following: decreased intellectual function; altered state of consciousness; mild to moderate EEG abnormalities; altered behavior; asterixis; agitation; drowsiness; confusion

Psychosocial concerns: Emotional reaction to surgery and consequences; level of support and coping mechanisms; health information needs

POTENTIAL COMPLICATIONS

Biliary complications, hepatic artery or portal vein thrombosis, renal dysfunction, infection, organ rejection

PATIENT PROBLEMS/NURSING DIAGNOSIS & INTERVENTIONS

NIC TISSUE PERFUSION MANAGEMENT

Ineffective renal, cerebral, cardiopulmonary, gastrointestinal, and peripheral tissue perfusion related to major surgical procedure with multiple anastomoses in compromised patient

- Monitor vital signs every 15 minutes until patient is stable and then every hour. Monitor intake and output every hour (include all drainage tubes: nasogastric, Jackson-Pratt [J-P], Foley, T tube).
- Monitor and document any incisional drainage.
- Monitor hourly central venous pressure, pulmonary artery pressure, pulmonary capillary wedge pressure, and right arterial pressure *because hemodynamic instability is a potential problem in the early postoperative period.* Intraoperative blood loss may be extensive.
- Observe carefully for signs of transfusion reactions *because patients may receive multiple units of blood during and after surgery.* Fresh frozen plasma may also be ordered.
- Weigh patient daily.
- Monitor serum electrolytes, CBC, prothrombin time, partial thromboplastin time, platelets, blood urea nitrogen (BUN), creatinine, bilirubin (total/direct), SGOT, SGPT, alkaline phosphatase, albumin, and CSA levels.
- Monitor electrocardiogram (ECG) for signs of hyperkalemia (T-wave elevation and widening of QRS complex on ECG) and hypokalemia (U-wave on ECG, ectopic beats, leg cramps) consistent with cyclosporine use.
- Check blood glucose levels qid *because the transplanted liver may be unable to control glucose metabolism in the early postoperative period; also steroid-induced diabetes may develop.*
- Test urine for glucose and ketones.

NIC DRUG MANAGEMENT

Risk for infection related to immunosuppressive medications

Risk for injury: rejection of donor organ, related to patient's functioning immune system

- Monitor and educate patient regarding cyclosporine side effects: hypertension, hyperkalemia, decreased renal function, and gingival hyperplasia.
- Monitor serum cyclosporine level every day to maintain a level of 250 to 350 mg/dl. *Toxic levels may lead to tremulousness and nephrotoxicity.*
- Observe patient for side effects of Orthoclone OKT3 or other drugs used to treat rejection (MALG, ATG, prednisone): chills, fever, development of ARDS and anaphylaxis, rigors, hypotension, chest pain, nausea, vomiting, diarrhea, pulmonary edema (if patient is fluid overloaded, no Orthoclone OKT3 should be administered), joint pain, shortness of breath, and hypotension. If acute

respiratory symptoms occur, discontinuation of the drug is necessary.
- Patient is maintained on a low dose of immunosuppressive medications.

NIC Coping Assistance

Risk for ineffective coping and compromised family coping related to near-death experience before transplant, prolonged recuperation, mental status changes, medication regimen, rejection, or infection episodes
- Provide continuity of nursing care as able.
- Allow time for patient and family to verbalize fears and concerns.
- Refer patient to a psychiatrist or social worker *for further support.*
- If support group is available, encourage patient and family to participate.
- Encourage other transplant patients and their families to network and provide mutual informal support.
- Encourage family to take breaks from the hospital.

NIC Risk Management

Risk for disturbed thought processes related to medications, intracranial hemorrhage, and encephalopathy
- Monitor small changes in mental status closely. Inform the transplant team.
- If cause is known, reassure family about duration of changes and help them cope with changes.
- Minimize number of people in room at any one time if patient is confused or combative *to reduce environmental stimuli.*
- Reorient patient frequently.
- Continue to explain and reassure patient even though it may appear that he or she does not follow.

Patient Education/Continuum of Care Plan

Patient education can be done effectively on a day-to-day or a group basis.
1. Instruct patient on routine care after any major surgery; ambulate at regular times; rest frequently; increase activities slowly; keep incision dry; report any signs of redness, pain, or drainage; avoid heavy lifting; keep appointments for follow-up visits.
2. Provide written instructions on medication schedule and side effects.
3. Provide written instructions on signs and symptoms that should be reported to physician.
4. Provide written instructions on any procedures for at-home care. Make sure that patient has had an opportunity to practice procedures before discharge.
5. Provide written instructions on need for follow-up laboratory work and communication of laboratory values to transplant program.

Evaluation/Patient Outcomes

Tissue Perfusion Management: Patient maintains adequate fluid and electrolyte balance. Intake and output are balanced. Patient's vital signs are normal. Patient's blood sugar level is within normal limits.

Drug Management: Patient verbalizes knowledge of immunosuppressive drug regimen, including side effects. Patient verbalizes common signs and symptoms of infection and organ rejection.

Coping Assistance: Patient verbalizes feelings regarding new liver, serious illness, and prolonged recuperation. Patient identifies positive support system through family, friends, support groups.

Risk Management: Patient's mental status returns to baseline. Patient is oriented and not confused.

References

1. American Gastroenterologic Association: AGA technical review on treatment of patients with dysphagia caused by benign disorders of the distal esophagus, *Gastroenterology* 117:233, 1999.
2. Andres PG, Friedman LS: Epidemiology and the natural course of inflammatory bowel disease, *Gastroenterol Clin North Am* 28(2):255, 1999.
3. Andrews CN, Anvari M, Dobranowski J: Laparoscopic Heller's myotomy or botulinum toxin injection for management of esophageal achalasia: patient choice and treatment outcomes, *Surg Endosc* 13:742, 1999.
4. Barkin GJS, Rogers AL: *Difficult decisions in digestive diseases.* St. Louis, 1994, Mosby.
5. Becker JM: Surgical therapy for ulcerative colitis and Crohn's disease, *Gastroenterol Clin North Am* 28(2):371, 1999.
6. Bergeron E et al: Appendicitis is a place for clinical judgement, *Am J Surg* 177:460, 1999.
7. Brandt LJ: *Clinical practice of gastroenterology,* Philadelphia, 1999, Current Medicine.
8. Camilleri M: Review article: clinical evidence to support current therapies of irritable bowel syndrome, *Aliment Pharmacol Ther* 13(suppl. 2):48, 1999.
9. Crissman JD, Visscher DW, Sakr W: Premalignant lesions of the upper aerodigestive tract: pathologic classification, *J Cell Biochem Suppl* 17F:49, 1993.
10. Doughty DB: *Gastrointestinal disorders,* St. Louis, 1993, Mosby.
11. Dunne D: Common questions about ileoanal reservoirs, *Am J Nurs* 97(11):67, 1997.
12. Eley BM: Antibacterial agents in the control of supragingival plaque: a review, *Br Dent J* 186(6):286, 1999.
13. Everhart JE: Summary. In Everhart JE: *Digestive diseases in the United States: epidemiology and impact,* DHHS, PHS, NIH No. 94-1447, Washington, DC, 1994, U.S. Government Printing Office.
14. Fenesy KE: Periodontal disease: an overview for physicians, *Mt Sinai J Med,* 65(5&6):362, 1998.
15. Ferguson MK: Achalasia: current evaluation and therapy, *Ann Thorac Surg* 52:336, 1991.
16. Gitnick G: *Current gastroenterology,* St. Louis, 1994, Mosby.
17. Goldstein JL et al: The esophageal mucosal resistance: structure and function of a unique gastrointestinal epithelial barrier, *J Lab Clin Med* 123(5):653, 1994.
18. Guyton AC, Hall JE: *Human physiology and mechanisms of disease,* ed 6, Philadelphia, 1997, WB Saunders.

19. Hashemi M, Sillin LF, Peters JH: Current concepts in the management of paraesophageal hiatal hernia, *J Clin Gastroenterol* 29(1):8, 1999.
20. Hawkey CJ: Future treatments for arthritis: new NSAIDS, NON-SAIDS, or no NSAIDS? *Gastroenterology* 109(2):614, 1995.
21. Hosoda S et al: Age-related changes in the gastrointestinal tract, *Nutr Rev* 50(12):374, 1992.
22. Hussain JN: Hemorrhoids, *Gastroenterol Clin North Am* 28(2):35, 1999.
23. Inman-Felton AE: Overview of lactose maldigestion (lactase non-persistence), *J Am Diet Assoc* 99(4):481, 1999.
24. Jeffcoat MK: Prevention of periodontal diseases in adults: strategies for the future, *Prev Med* 23(5):704, 1994.
25. Johnson LR: *Gastrointestinal physiology,* St. Louis, 1997, Mosby.
26. Kinney MD et al: *AACN's clinical reference for critical care nursing,* New York, 1988, McGraw Hill.
27. Kock NG, Myrvold HE, Nilsson LO: Progress report on the continent ileostomy, *World J Surg* 4:143, 1980.
28. Kolokotronis A: Median rhomboid glossitis, *Oral Surg Oral Med Oral Pathol Oral Radiol Endod* 78(1):36, 1994.
29. Leheij RJF et al: Evaluation of treatment regimens to cure *Helicobacter pylori* infection: a meta-analysis, *Aliment Pharmacol Ther* 13:857, 1999.
30. McCormack G, McCormick PA: A practical guide to the management of oesophageal varices, *Drugs* 57(3):327, 1999.
31. Mullen P: Barnett continent intestinal reservoir: multicenter experience with an alternative to the Brooke ileostomy, *Dis Colon Rectum* 38:573, 1995.
32. National Institute of Arthritis, Diabetes, and Digestive and Kidney Diseases (NIADDK): *Second annual report,* DHHS, PHS, NIH Pub No. 83-2493, Washington, DC, U.S. Government Printing Office.
33. Newman TS et al: The changing face of mesenteric infarction, *Am Surg* 64(7):611, 1998.
34. Nightengale JMD: Management of patients with a short bowel, *Nutrition* 15(7,8):633, 1999.
35. Papadakis KA, Targan SR: Current theories on the causes of inflammatory bowel disease, *Gastroenterol Clin North Am* 28(2):283, 1999.
36. Parks AG, Nicholls RJ: Proctocolectomy without ileostomy for ulcerative colitis, *BMJ* 2:85, 1978.
37. Pena AS et al: Genetic bases of gluten-sensitive enteropathy, *Gastroenterology* 75:230, 1978.
38. Pou AM, Johnson JT, Weissman J: (1995). Management decisions in parotitis, *Compr Ther* 21(2):85, 1995.
39. Reyes J, Mazariegos GV: Pediatric transplantation, *Surg Clin North Am* 79(1):163, 1999.
40. Samet JH et al: Dermatologic manifestations in HIV-infected patients: a primary care perspective, *Mayo Clin Proc* 74:658, 1999.
41. Sands B: Novel therapies for inflammatory bowel disease, *Gastroenterol Clin North Am* 28(2):323, 1999.
42. Schoelch ML et al: Laser management of oral leukoplakias: a follow-up study of 70 patients, *Laryngoscope* 109:949, 1999.
43. Scully C: (1999). *Handbook of oral disease: diagnosis and management,* London, 1999, Martin Dunitz.
44. Sleisenger MH, Fordtran JS: *Gastrointestinal disease,* Philadelphia, 1993, WB Saunders.
45. Sorrell MF: *Schiff's diseases of the liver,* Philadelphia, 1999, JB Lipincott.
46. Stone MA: Non-invasive testing for *Helicobacter pylori, Postgrad Med J* 75:74, 1999.
47. Thompson JM, Wilson SF: *Health assessment for nursing practice,* St. Louis, 1996, Mosby.
48. Thompson JS, Langnas AN: Surgical approaches to improving intestinal function in the short-bowel syndrome, *Arch Surg* 134:706, 1999.
49. Tobin RW: Esophageal rings, webs, and diverticula, *J Clin Gastroenterol* 27(4):285, 1998.
50. UNOS: *The US Scientific Registry of Transplant Recipients and the Organ Procurement and Transplantation Network:* transplant data 1988-1995, 1996, U.S. Department of Health and Human Services, Health Resources and Services Administration.
51. Vanderhoof JA, Langnas AN: Short-bowel syndrome in children and adults, *Gastroenterology* 113:1767, 1997.
52. Way LW: *Current surgical diagnosis and treatment,* Norwalk, Conn, 1994, Appleton & Lange.
53. Wolf DC: The management of variceal bleeding: past, present and future, *Mt Sinai J Med* 66(1):1, 1999.
54. Yamada T et al: *Textbook of gastroenterology,* Philadelphia, 1999, JB Lipincott.

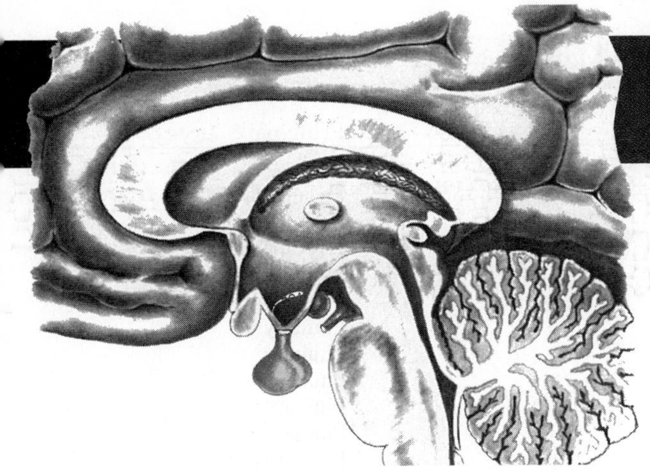

11 Endocrine-Metabolic System

Molly Solares
Rubi Agana-Defensor
Cynthia Song-Mayeda
Louise Dulaney Canada

OVERVIEW

Definitions

The *endocrine-metabolic system* is a widely diversified system of glands, hormones, intermediate metabolites, receptors, and cellular responses. *Endo* means internal. The *endocrine glands* secrete substances (hormones) directly into the bloodstream or lymphatic system. *Hormones* (derived from the Greek word meaning to "set in motion") are chemical messengers that are involved in both intracellular and extracellular communication. *Endocrinology* is the study of the endocrine glands and their functions. *Metabolism* is the action of the many diverse biochemical mechanisms that occur. The endocrine system controls or regulates growth, development and aging, energy metabolism, fluid and electrolyte balance, response to stress, and reproduction.

Endocrine glands include the following: hypothalamus, pituitary, thyroid, parathyroid glands, adrenal glands, gonads (ovaries and testes), and pancreas (islets of Langerhans of the pancreas). Other structures sometimes considered endocrine glands: pineal gland, thymus, gastrointestinal cells, and placenta (FIG. 11-1).

Hormones

There are three main types of hormones, depending on their chemical structure:

1. *Protein and polypeptide* are derived from amino acids and are water soluble. Some are from carbohydrate residues and are called glycoproteins.
2. *Steroid* hormones are derived from cholesterol and are fat soluble and can diffuse through membranes.
3. *Miscellaneous* hormones may be derived from either group but because they have overlapping functions, they can be considered as a separate group[36] (Table 11-1).

Action

The action of the hormones depends on how they are transported and able to enter their target cells. Some hormones become bound to plasma proteins, which act like a stored circulating form, allowing the hormone to be readily available at its target tissue when required.[36] Some hormones are present in a free (unbound) state. It is in this state that the hormone is biologically active both at its target tissue and at its own endocrine cells, where it may have a feedback-controlling influence on its own production. When target cells require free hormone for activity, more of the protein-bound hormone is released into the free state to allow its action by those target cells. A decrease in the free-hormone concentration in the blood stimulates the endocrine gland to secrete more hormone. Also, if the protein-binding capacity is increased, the amount of free hormone is taken up by the carrier protein, but the overall free-hormone level will be normal. An example of this is found in pregnancy or high estrogen states when the binding capacity is high, but the free hormone level is normal, so clinical abnormalities do not occur.

Usually, before hormones can exert an effect, they must also attach to receptors. The hormones become keys opening the receptor doors for subsequent cellular and system responses. Only one hormone acts as the key for each receptor, which are proteins at the plasma membrane or within the cell (FIG. 11-2).

Hormone Regulation

Hormones are regulated by feedback systems to maintain hormonal equilibrium. The endocrine gland receives constant rapid information from various sources, as well as the hormonal level, to regulate its hormone production, and it sends signals to reduce or increase its stimulation to return to the basal state.

Table 11-1 General Hormonal Classification into Three Main Groups[36]

Name and Common Abbreviation	Principal Source
PROTEIN AND POLYPEPTIDES	
Gonadotropin-releasing hormone (GnRH)	Hypothalamus
Thyrotropin-releasing hormone (TRH)	Hypothalamus
Corticotropin-releasing hormone (CRH)	Hypothalamus
Follicle-stimulating hormone (FSH)	Pituitary
Luteinizing hormone (LH)	Pituitary
Growth hormone (somatotropin) (GH)	Pituitary
Prolactin	Pituitary
Thyroid-stimulating hormone (thyrotropin) (TSH)	Pituitary
Adrenocorticotropic hormone (corticotropin) (ACTH)	Pituitary
Vasopressin (VP)	Pituitary
Oxytocin	Pituitary
Calcitonin (CT)	Thyroid
Parathyroid hormone (PTH)	Parathyroid glands
Insulin	Pancreas (islets)
Glucagons	Pancreas (islets)
Gastrin	Stomach
Secretin	Small intestine
Cholecystokinin/pancreozymin	Small intestine
Atrial natriuretic peptide (ANP)	Heart, brain
Somatomedins (IGF-I, IGF-II)	Liver
STEROID	
Aldosterone	Adrenal cortex
Cortisol	Adrenal cortex
17-β Estradiol	Gonads, placenta (adrenal cortex)
Progesterone	Gonads, placenta (adrenal cortex)
Testosterone	Gonads, (adrenal cortex)
1,25-Dihydroxyvitamin D_3 ($1,25[OH]_2)D_3$	Kidneys
MISCELLANEOUS	
Triiodothyronine (T_3)	Thyroid
Thyroxine (T_4)	Thyroid
Noradrenaline (Nadr)	Adrenal medulla
Adrenaline (Adr)	Adrenal medulla
Melatonin	Pineal gland

The pituitary or hypophysis, long considered to be the master endocrine organ, is subject to hypothalamic control via various stimulating and inhibiting hormones and substances as well as complex feedback systems. The release of these hormones is stimulated by chemical secretions from the hypothalamus called releasing factors or releasing hormones. The pituitary (stimulating) hormones stimulate the target organ to release its hormone, which circulates or feeds back to the pituitary gland, whose hormones, in turn, feed back to the hypothalamic hormones to regulate the pituitary hormones (FIG. 11-3). For instance, thyroid-stimulating hormone (TSH), which is released by the pituitary gland, stimulates the thyroid gland to produce thyroxine (T_4). The circulating blood levels of TSH are stimulated by hypothalamic thyroid-releasing hormone (TRH) and inhibited by increasing levels of circulating thyroid hormones so that the blood thyroid hormone levels are maintained within a narrow range. Damage to the thyroid gland reduces its ability to produce thyroid hormone levels, resulting in stimulation by the pituitary gland with increased TSH levels. Conversely, overgrowth of thyroid tissue results in overproduction of thyroxine, which feeds back to the pituitary gland, resulting in low TSH levels.

Hormone secretion is affected by time and outside influences. Some hormones are secreted minute by minute; some (estrogen, progesterone) are secreted in a monthly cycle; and some (cortisol) are secreted in a diurnal (circadian) rhythm in which a hormone fluctuates predictably. Some hormones are suppressed by certain substances (glucose levels suppress growth hormone), and some hormones are stimulated by other substances (growth hormone is stimulated by exercise). Therefore the interpretation of hormonal levels can be complex.

In the laboratory, some hormones are measured in units of weight, while some are measured in units of size. This varies between laboratories and countries. Conventional units are now being translated into international units, which are currently being accepted as the preferred medium for international communication. For example, testosterone levels are expressed as nanograms per milliliter (ng/ml) in the conventional method,

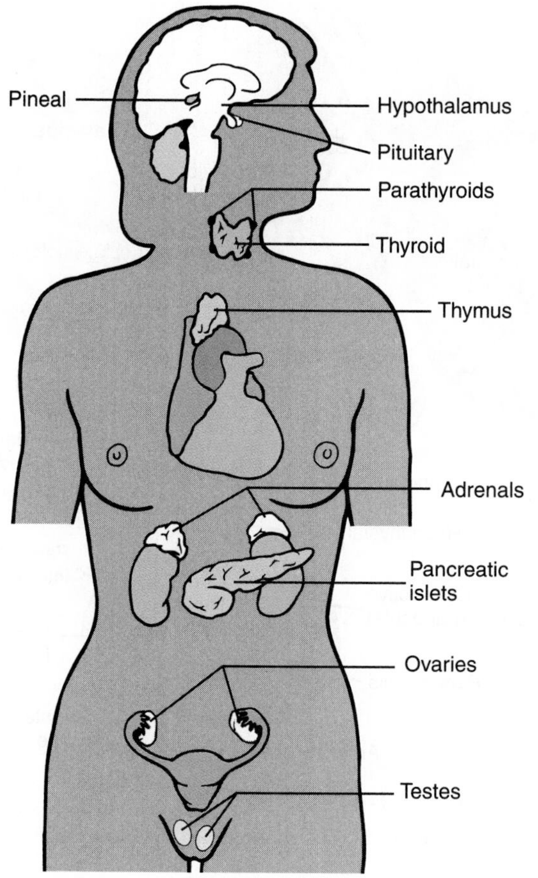

FIG. 11-1

Location of major endocrine glands. The parathyroid glands actually lie on the posterior surface of the thyroid. (From Haas.[26])

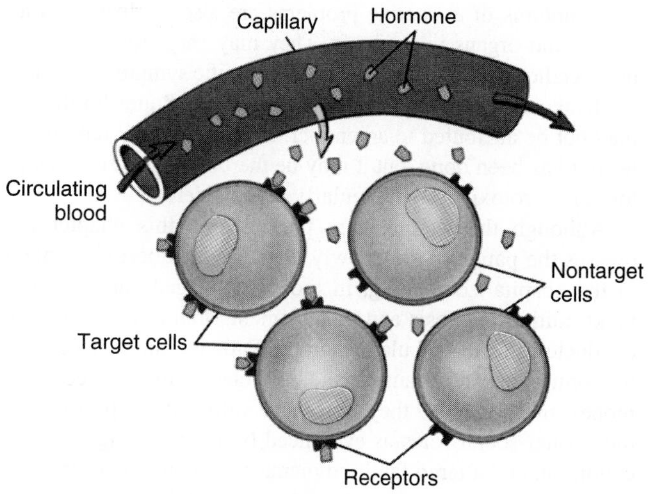

FIG. 11-2

The target cell concept. A hormone acts only on cells that have receptors specific to that hormone because the shape of the receptor determines which hormone can react with it. This is an example of the lock-and-key model of biochemical reactions. (From Haas.[26])

and nanomoles per liter (nmol/L) in the international method. The units of measurement are minute: nano is one billionth part of a whole. Blood glucose level is measured as milligrams per deciliter (mg/dl) at laboratories in the United States and as millimoles per liter (mmol/L) in Europe. One millimole is one eighteenth part of a milligram per deciliter.

Clinical problems in endocrinology were traditionally limited to whether there is a relative overproduction or underproduction of a hormone from a particular gland. Diseases are often referred to as primary or secondary. Primary disease is a failure or malfunction of the endocrine (target) gland, and secondary disease is failure or malfunction of the pituitary gland. Today, disruption of hormone transport, clearance, regulation, and binding also lead to clinical manifestations. The availability of diagnostic testing can also determine the clinical distinction between adequate hormone production in the basal state and the ability to increase hormonal production as required to meet physiologic needs in a stimulated, stressed, or maximal state.

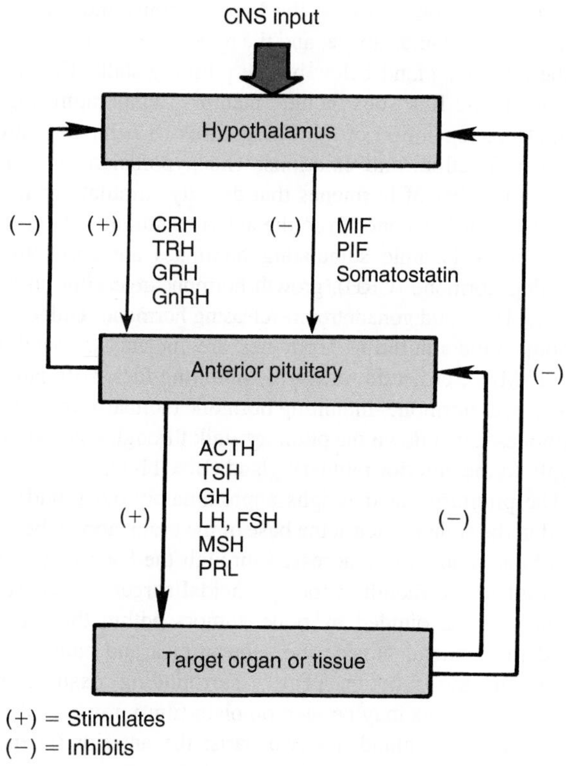

FIG. 11-3

Negative-feedback mechanism.

Symptoms of endocrine problems are also as diverse as all tissues and organs in the body. They may vary from a general nonspecific symptom like fatigue to a specific symptom like heat intolerance. Some symptoms such as atrial flutter/fibrillation may not be attributed to an endocrine problem until laboratory testing has been done, but it may be the only presenting symptom of thyrotoxicosis, particularly in the elderly.

Although the nursing care presented in this chapter addresses the patient with a newly diagnosed endocrine problem in the hospitalized setting, in today's managed care environment, initial diagnosis and management would most likely be conducted in the ambulatory arena. Patients might have very few symptoms, or because of the interrelationship between hormones and behavior, they may have difficulty in performing their usual social roles as evidenced by mood swings, altered cognition, and altered family dynamics. The nursing care ideas presented in this chapter will need minor modifications but can be equally applicable for ambulatory care. When a patient is hospitalized, it may be for surgical intervention or for an unrelated problem. In both cases the goal of nursing care would be maintenance of hormone-related therapies. The information in this chapter can be used to prevent a patient from getting out of endocrine physiologic balance.

Anatomy, Physiology, and Related Pathophysiology

Hypothalamus and Pituitary Gland

The hypothalamus is located at the ventral portion of the diencephalon, beneath the thalamus and subthalamus. There are neural connections between the hypothalamus and the limbic system and thalamus above, and the hypothalamus is connected to the pituitary gland below by the pituitary stalk (Fig. 11-4). Hypothalamic functions include memory, temperature regulation, sleep, regulation of food intake, sexual behavior, cardiovascular function, and emotions. The hypothalamus also secretes a number of hormones that directly stimulate or inhibit the release of hormones from the anterior pituitary gland.[33,34]

The hypothalamic stimulating hormones are corticotropin-releasing hormone (CRH), growth hormone–releasing hormone (GRH), TRH, and gonadotropin-releasing hormone (GnRH). The hypothalamic inhibiting hormones are melanocyte-inhibiting factor (MIF), prolactin releasing–inhibiting factor (dopamine), and growth hormone–inhibiting hormone (somatostatin). These hormones travel down the pituitary stalk through a portal blood supply to the anterior pituitary gland (Box 11-1).

The pituitary gland weighs approximately 0.6 g and is located in the sella turcica at the base of the brain, above the sphenoid bone, and can be accessed through the back of the nose and roof of the mouth in transphenoidal surgery. Because the pituitary is surrounded by bone, tumors within the pituitary gland may extend outside the sella turcica and cause disturbances in the function of the surrounding tissue. These anatomic changes may be seen on plain film x-rays.

The pituitary gland has two parts: the anterior (adenohypophysis) and the posterior (neurohypophysis).

The anterior pituitary releases luteinizing hormone (LH), follicle-stimulating hormone (FSH), growth hormone (GH), prolactin (PRL), adrenocorticotropic hormone (ACTH), TSH, and melanocyte-stimulating hormone (MSH). These hormones travel through the blood supply to specific glands called target organs (ACTH to the adrenal gland) as well as extraglandular cell-specific responses (Table 11-2).

The neurohypophysis secretes two hormones: vasopressin and oxytocin. Vasopressin is the primary regulator of water metabolism in human beings. Oxytocin is responsible for the milk letdown reflex and stimulates the contraction of uterine muscles. Neurogenic reflexes from the nipple travel through the spinal cord and midbrain to the hypothalamus. The neurohypophysis then releases oxytocin, which stimulates contractions of mammary myoepithelium; this results in the ejection of milk. Vasopressin and oxytocin are transported along the neurohypophyseal tract to the posterior lobe of the pituitary gland, where they are stored. Rapid release of these hormones occurs

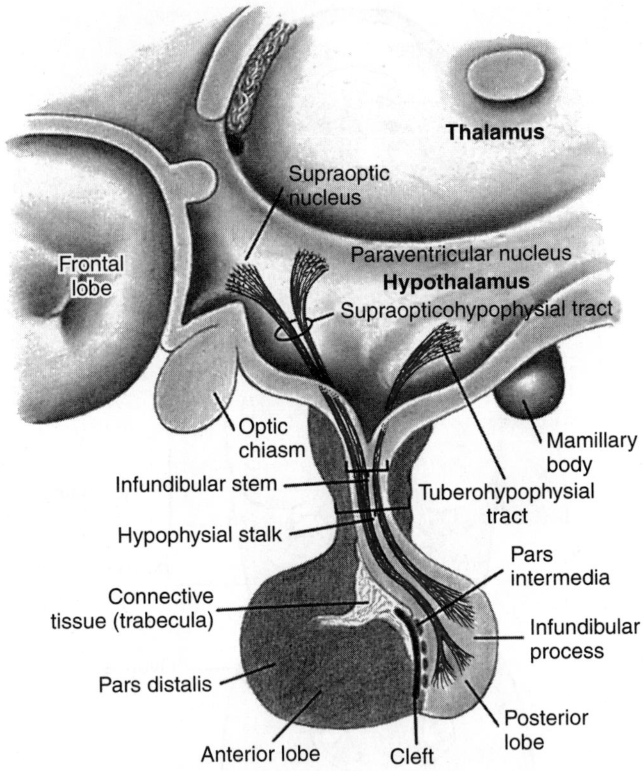

Fig. 11-4
Anatomy of the hypothalamus and pituitary.

HYPOTHALAMIC HORMONES — Box 11-1

Stimulating Hormones
Corticotropin-releasing hormone (CRH)
Growth hormone–releasing hormone (GRH)
Thyrotropin-releasing hormone (TRH)
Gonadotropin-releasing hormone (GnRH)

Inhibiting Hormones
Melanocyte-inhibiting factor (MIF)
Prolactin releasing–inhibiting factor (dopamine)
Growth hormone–inhibiting hormone (somatostatin)

Table 11-2 Major Endocrine Glands and Hormonal Function[26,33,37]

Gland/Hormone	Target Tissue	Functions
PITUITARY (ANTERIOR)		
Growth hormone (GH)	All body cells	Stimulates growth of body tissues and bones Decreases glucose uptake Promotes fat mobilization
Prolactin	Ovaries, breasts	Stimulates milk production, breast development Maintains corpus luteum and progesterone secretion during pregnancy
Thyroid-stimulating hormone (TSH)	Thyroid gland	Stimulates thyroid gland to synthesize and secrete thyroid hormones Promotes growth and development of thyroid gland
Adrenocorticotropic hormone (ACTH)	Adrenal cortex	Stimulates adrenal cortex to secrete glucocorticoids, mineralocorticoids, and androgens Promotes growth and development of adrenal cortex
Follicle-stimulating hormone (FSH)	Testes Ovaries	Stimulates development of seminiferous tubules and spermatogenesis Stimulates graafian follicles to mature and secrete estrogen
Luteinizing hormone (LH)	Testes Ovaries	Stimulates differentiation of Leydig cells to produce testosterone Produces ovulation Stimulates secretion of progesterone and estrogen
Melanocyte-stimulating hormone (MSH)	Skin	Promotion of skin pigmentation May stimulate adrenal cortex
PITUITARY (POSTERIOR)		
Oxytocin	Uterus, breasts	Stimulates uterine contractions Promotes lactation and uterine motility
Antidiuretic hormone (ADH, vasopressin)	Distal renal tubules, vascular smooth muscle	Promotes reabsorption of water, thus decreases urine excretion Triggers arteriolar constriction
THYROID		
Thyroxine (T_4) Triiodothyronine (T_3)	All body tissues	Regulates metabolic rate, controls rate of growth of body cells, especially bones, teeth, and brain Stimulates protein, carbohydrate, and fat metabolism Accelerates oxygen consumption
Calcitonin (CT)	Bone	Promotes calcium reabsorption from bone, blood, and intestines Inhibits bone resorption Promotes excretion of phosphorus
PARATHYROID		
Parathyroid hormone (PTH)	Bone, intestine, kidney	Increases calcium levels Decreases phosphorus levels Increases resorption of bone
ADRENAL (CORTEX)		
Glucocorticoids (cortisol)	All body tissues	Promotes fat, protein, and carbohydrate metabolism Mobilizes body defenses during stress Suppresses inflammatory reaction
Mineralocorticoids (aldosterone)	Kidney	Regulates sodium and potassium balance
Androgens (testosterone, estrogen)	Sex organs	Influences development of bone, reproductive organs, secondary sex characteristics, and virilization
ADRENAL (MEDULLA)		
Epinephrine (adrenaline 80%) Norepinephrine (noradrenaline 20%)	Sympathetic effectors	Responds to stress Produces vasoconstriction of heart and smooth muscles Converts glycogen to glucose Activates sweat glands
PANCREAS (ISLETS OF LANGERHANS)		
Insulin (from beta cells)	Liver, fat cells	Promotes utilization and storage of carbohydrates, protein, and fat, thus decreases blood sugar levels
Glucagon (from alpha cells)	Liver	Promotes hepatic glucogenolysis and gluconeogenesis, thus increases blood sugar levels
Somatostatin (from delta cells)	Pancreas	Inhibits insulin and glucagon secretion

Continued

Table 11-2 Major Endocrine Glands and Hormonal Function—cont'd

Gland/Hormone	Target Tissue	Functions
OVARIES		
Estrogen	Reproductive system, breasts	Stimulates sex and reproductive functions Stimulates development of secondary sexual characteristics Promotes epiphyseal closure of bones
Progesterone	Reproductive system	Effects repair and maintenance of endometrial lining
Androgens	Reproductive system	Stimulates sex and reproductive functions Stimulates development of secondary sexual characteristics
TESTES		
Testosterone, dihydrotestosterone	Reproductive system	Stimulates sex and reproductive functions Stimulates development of secondary sexual characteristics Promotes epiphyseal closure of bones

in response to various stimuli. Oxytocin may be inhibited by emotional stress, pain, or fright. Its release is stimulated by a crying baby, sexual excitement, and orgasm. Although oxytocin may be used to induce labor and control obstetric hemorrhage, its physiologic role in initiating and maintaining normal labor is unclear. Patients with complete hypophysectomy (surgical removal of the whole pituitary gland) seem to progress through labor normally.

Vasopressin conserves water in the renal collecting duct; thus it is also known as antidiuretic hormone (ADH). ADH causes an increase in the permeability of the renal collecting ducts to water, thereby increasing water retention and decreasing urine output. The production of ADH in the hypothalamus and the release of ADH from the posterior pituitary gland are determined by plasma osmolality and extracellular fluid volume.

ADH secretion is stimulated by such factors as hemorrhage, a reduction in cardiac output, dehydration, and hypoalbuminemic states. The limbic system also plays a role in the stimulation of ADH during stress, trauma, heat, fear, and pain. Certain drugs also promote ADH secretion, such as morphine, nicotine, barbiturates, beta-adrenergic agents, general anesthetics, vincristine, cyclophosphamide (Cytoxan), carbamazepine, and chlorpropamide. Inhibition of ADH occurs during states of hypervolemia and hypo-osmolality. Total body immersion in water and a sensation of cold also inhibit ADH secretion. Pharmacologic agents inhibiting ADH include morphine antagonists, α-adrenergic agents, and ethyl alcohol[8] (Table 11-3).

Free water loss leads to concentration of the blood, which causes plasma osmolality to rise. When plasma osmolality reaches about 288 mOsm/kg, two things occur. First, the osmoreceptors in the hypothalamus are stimulated and promote synthesis of ADH in the hypothalamic nuclei and release of ADH from the posterior pituitary gland. Second, a perception of thirst occurs, leading to the ingestion of water. ADH causes the kidney to increase water reabsorption, resulting in antidiuresis. As plasma osmolality returns toward normal, stimulation of osmoreceptors is reduced and ADH secretion decreases. The sensation of thirst is reduced. Overhydration dilutes the blood, and plasma osmolality decreases. When it reaches about 282 mOsm/kg, the synthesis and release of ADH are inhibited. The kidneys decrease water reabsorption, and diuresis begins. Serum osmolality returns toward normal (FIG. 11-5).

Table 11-3 Factors Influencing Antidiuretic Hormone Secretion

Stimulated	Inhibited
Hypovolemia in hemorrhage, dehydration	Hypervolemia
Hypoalbuminemia	Hypo-osmolality
Stress	Cold
Trauma	Total body emersion
Heat	Drugs: Morphine antagonists, ethyl alcohol, alpha-adrenergic agents
Fear	
Pain	
Drugs: Morphine, nicotine, barbiturates, general anesthetics, chlorpropamide, beta-adrenergic agents	

Thyroid Gland

The thyroid gland is located in the neck, just below the cricoid cartilage (FIG. 11-6).

The normal thyroid gland weighs approximately 15 to 25 g. It is composed of two encapsulated lobes positioned on either side of the trachea and joined by the isthmus. The right lobe is larger and more vascular than the left. The recurrent laryngeal nerves run in the grooves beside the trachea and behind the lobes of the thyroid gland. The main function of the thyroid gland is to produce, store, and release the thyroid hormones, thyroxine (T_4), triiodothyronine (T_3), and calcitonin.

The major function of thyroxine is to regulate body metabolism. The major function of calcitonin is to inhibit osteoclast-mediated bone resorption.

Because of the effects of the thyroid gland on growth and development, neonatal screening for congenital abnormalities is now standard, and treatment for congenital hypothyroidism is started as soon after birth as possible.[1] Several countries and all U.S. states now have a newborn screening program.

Thyroid blood supply is greater than the kidney blood supply. This blood supply is furnished by two major pairs of arteries that account for the rich vascularity of the gland and for the increased risk of hemorrhage that may occur postoperatively. The presence of a palpable thrill or audible bruit over the gland or surrounding area is indicative of an increased blood flow.

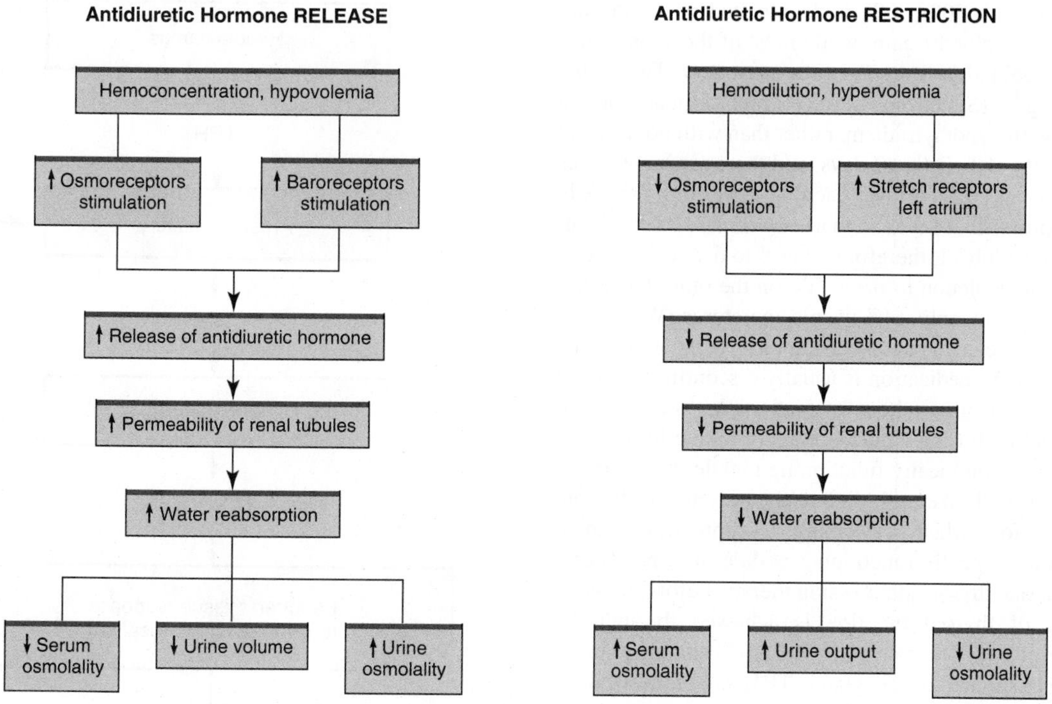

FIG. 11-5
Physiology of the release and restriction of antidiuretic hormone. (From Haas.[27])

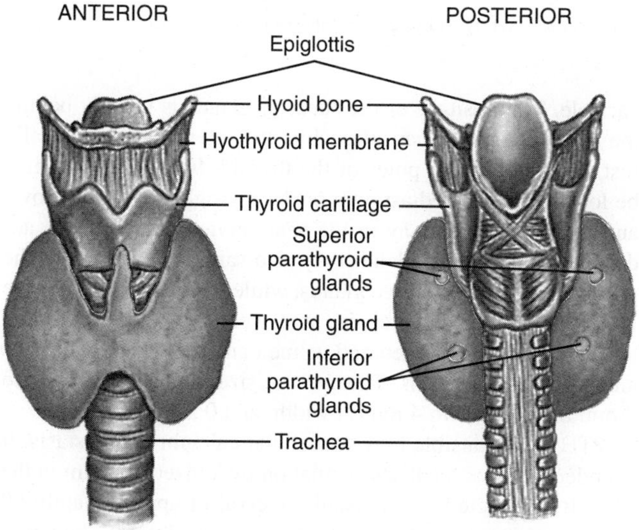

FIG. 11-6
Thyroid anatomy.

The thyroid is composed of follicular and parafollicular cells. The follicles are filled with proteinaceous colloid, which is the major constituent of total thyroid mass.

The function of the follicular cells is to secrete the two major thyroid hormones: thyroxine (T_4) and triiodothyronine (T_3). The parafollicular cells or C cells secrete a third hormone, calcitonin. Although calcitonin is a powerful inhibitor of bone resorption in pharmacologic doses, the physiologic role of calcitonin in humans is still unclear.[10]

The major component of thyroid hormones is iodine. Normal iodine balance depends on sufficient dietary intake. Seafoods and water are the major natural sources. Medications, diagnostic agents, dietary supplements (especially iodized salt), and the use of iodine by the food-processing industry and in the food given to animals have increased iodine ingestion in the more highly developed countries. Normal daily dietary intake of iodine varies widely throughout the world, primarily because of the varying iodine content of soil and water and cultural food preferences. The minimum recommended daily requirement for iodine is about 150 mg (50 to 75 mg is required for adults to prevent goiter or enlargement of the thyroid gland, caused by iodine deficiency).[8] However, dietary intake of iodine ranges from 300 to 1000 mg daily in the United States.

Iodine is rapidly absorbed from the gastrointestinal tract, primarily as iodide, the form in which it is carried in the blood, and is largely confined to the extracellular fluid (ECF) compartment. When absorbed in organic form, iodine is converted to iodide in the liver. Small quantities of iodine are lost in stool, in expired air, and through the skin. During lactation, more notable losses occur. Removal from the ECF pool occurs by excretion of iodine into the urine and by transport of iodine into the thyroid gland.[8]

Renal clearance of iodide is important because it determines the availability of iodide to the thyroid gland. The kidneys are considered passive participants in iodide metabolism and are not a part of the body's defense mechanism for the maintenance of thyroidal homeostasis.[8]

There is more T_4 produced intrathyroidally than T_3, with a total daily production rate of 80 to 100 mg. T_4 is converted to T_3 by the removal of one of the iodine atoms. This enzymatic reaction occurs in both the thyroid itself and in peripheral tissues. Only 10% to 30% of T_3 is deiodinated in the thyroid and secreted in the bloodstream, while most of the T_3 is generated by the deiodination from T_4 in the periphery. This is the reason for using T_4 (Synthroid, Levoxyl) replacement alone in most patients with hypothyroidism, rather than with both T_3 and T_4.[10] The half-life of T_4 is 6 to 7 days, and there are large stores in plasma allowing 10% turnover each day. (Missing one daily dose of thyroxine will not cause a marked decrease of drug concentration in the adult.) It therefore takes 4 to 6 weeks for total thyroid hormone depletion to occur. T_3, on the other hand, has a short half-life with only 14% in plasma stores. When performing a thyroid scan and uptake using radioactive iodine, any thyroid replacement medication is usually discontinued until it has been depleted from the body (4 to 6 weeks in the case of thyroxine) to allow for maximum uptake of iodine by the thyroid gland. An autonomically functioning nodule, which is not TSH dependent, will take up iodine in the presence of thyroid hormone. Therefore when performing a suppression scan to rule out an autonomically functioning nodule, it is not necessary to discontinue thyroid suppression therapy before the scan.

Regulation of thyroid function is achieved through the hypothalamic-pituitary-thyroid axis (FIG. 11-7) and an autoregulatory mechanism within the gland. TRH is synthesized by neurons in the hypothalamus and is transported to cells of the anterior pituitary gland that contain specific cell membrane receptors for TRH binding. TSH in the anterior pituitary gland is stimulated by the secretion of TRH. Most of the thyroid gland's metabolic processes are regulated by TSH. Although the primary action of TSH is the production and secretion of the thyroid hormones, it can also stimulate growth of the gland. The thyroid hormones, on the other hand, inhibit TSH secretion at the level of the anterior pituitary gland. Small alterations in serum T_4 and T_3 concentrations result in reciprocal changes in both TSH secretion and TSH response to exogenous TRH. Serum thyroid levels override the pituitary gland's response to TRH if the T_4 and T_3 levels are high.

Blockage or removal of TSH stimulation results in hypovascularity and atrophy of the thyroid gland. The reverse effects occur when stimulatory doses of TSH are produced. Secretion of TSH in serum is pulsatile and is subject to a circadian rhythm. TSH secretion is characterized by fluctuations at 15- to 20-minute intervals and by a nocturnal surge during sleep. If TSH secretion is completely destroyed (i.e., hypophysectomy or suppression), there is a decreased activity of the thyroid iodide transport mechanism and organic binding is inhibited. The reverse effect occurs with the administration of TSH.

Many factors influence thyroid hormone function. For example, TSH secretion is affected by somatostatin, dopamine, and the catecholamines. Other factors that influence thyroid hormone functioning include sex and sex hormones; pregnancy; the newborn state; age; glucocorticoids; environmental temperatures, especially exposure to extreme cold; alterations in nutritional states (i.e., starvation or overfeeding); and other nonthyroid illnesses, such as cirrhosis and chronic renal failure.

Parathyroid Gland

The two pairs of parathyroid glands arise from the brachial pouches and descend along with the thymus until the embryo is approximately 18 mm in size. Like the thyroid gland, the final location of any one of the parathyroid glands may be extremely

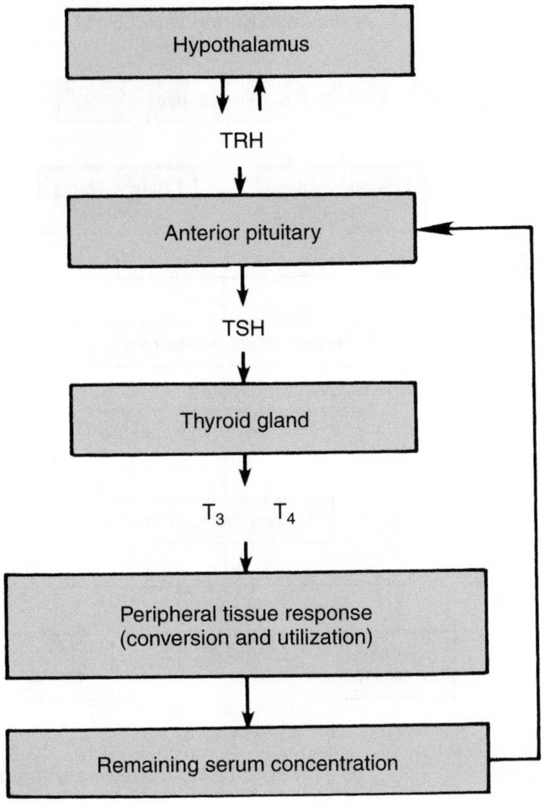

FIG. 11-7
Thyroid negative-feedback mechanism.

variable. The position of the superior glands is usually behind the superior thyroid capsule, while the inferior glands usually rest near the inferior poles of the thyroid. Inferior glands may be located in the mediastinum or the thyroglossal duct groove, and superior glands may reside near cervical vertebrae. In addition, the number of glands may also vary. Five percent of the population have only three glands, while 12% to 15% may have five or more glands. The size and weight of the parathyroid glands vary between men and women and between Caucasians and African-Americans. The average size of each gland is 2 to 7 mm in length, 2 to 4 mm in width, and 0.5 to 2 mm thick.

PTH is responsible for extracellular calcium homeostasis. It is under negative feedback regulation by ionized calcium in the ECF. It is secreted in a pulsatile interval of approximately 60 minutes with a peak circadian secretion at midnight. The target cells for PTH are specialized calcium transport cells in the skeleton, intestine, and kidneys.

There is constant remodeling of bone that takes place between osteoclast (bone-resorbing) and osteoblast (bone-building) cells. PTH increases osteoclastic activity while simultaneously inhibiting osteoblastic activity, yielding a net release of calcium from the skeleton into the ECF.

Calcium absorption from the intestine occurs as an active process and as passive diffusion. Passive diffusion relies on a concentration gradient and is responsible for the absorption of 10% to 15% of dietary calcium. Active transport occurs by a carrier mechanism regulated by 1,25-dihydroxyvitamin D (1,25 $[OH]_2D$). Although 1,25-dihydroxyvitamin D is synthesized in the kidneys as well as by skin cells, lack of vitamin D (high sun

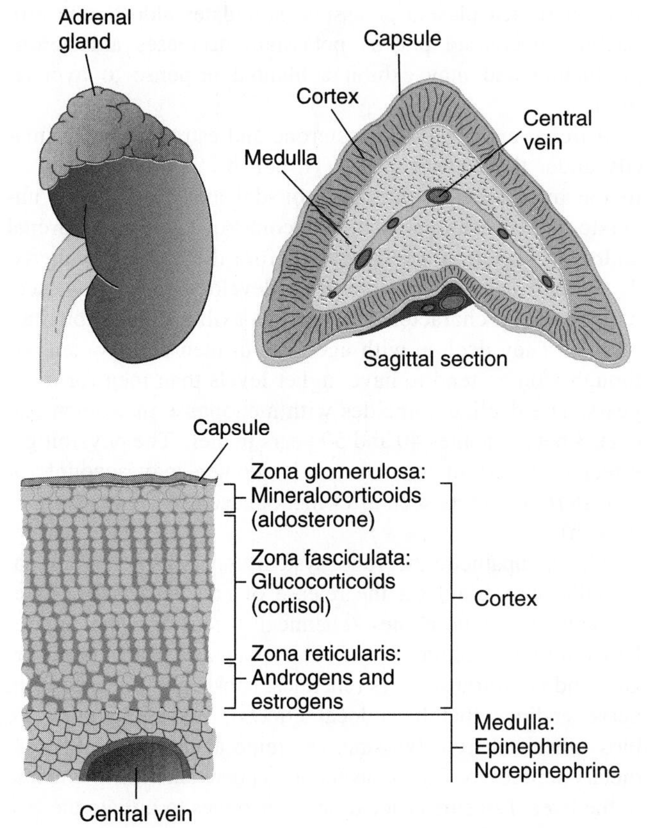

FIG. 11-8
Adrenal glands location, structure, and hormonal secretions. (From Matassarin-Jacobs.[37])

protection factor [SPF] sunblock, lack of exposure to sunlight, poor dietary intake of dairy products) affects the amount of calcium the intestine will reabsorb.

The kidney filters about 10 g of calcium per day with approximately 65% of the calcium reabsorbed by the proximal tubule.[11] PTH increases the reabsorption of calcium in both the proximal and distal segments of the nephron by increasing transport from lumen to plasma. Vitamin D–dependent calcium-binding protein in the distal tubule may also be modified by PTH. Along with renal calcium, PTH inhibits phosphate reabsorption from both proximal and distal sites and enhances 1,25-dihydroxyvitamin D in the proximal tubule. It also plays a role in the excretion or reabsorption of other ions and ion transporters.

Pathologic conditions arising within the parathyroid gland lead to alterations in skeletal, intestinal, and renal calcium homeostasis. Conversely, pathologic conditions arising in one of the three target areas lead to altered calcium balance and have secondary effects on the other two target areas and the parathyroid glands.

Adrenal Glands

The adrenal glands are located at the upper poles of the kidneys, on the posterior parietal wall on each side of the vertebral column and lateral to the eleventh thoracic and the first lumbar vertebrae. Each weighs approximately 4 to 6 g, is 2 to 3 cm wide, and is 4 to 6 cm long.

The cortex has three distinct zones containing specific cell types responsible for the production of glucocorticoids, mineralocorticoids, and androgens, which are essential for survival. Loss of glucocorticoids and mineralocorticoids leads to death (FIG. 11-8).

The precursor of all steroid biosynthesis in the adrenal gland is cholesterol. Cholesterol (FIG. 11-9), under the influence of two classes of enzymes (cytochrome P-450 and short-chain

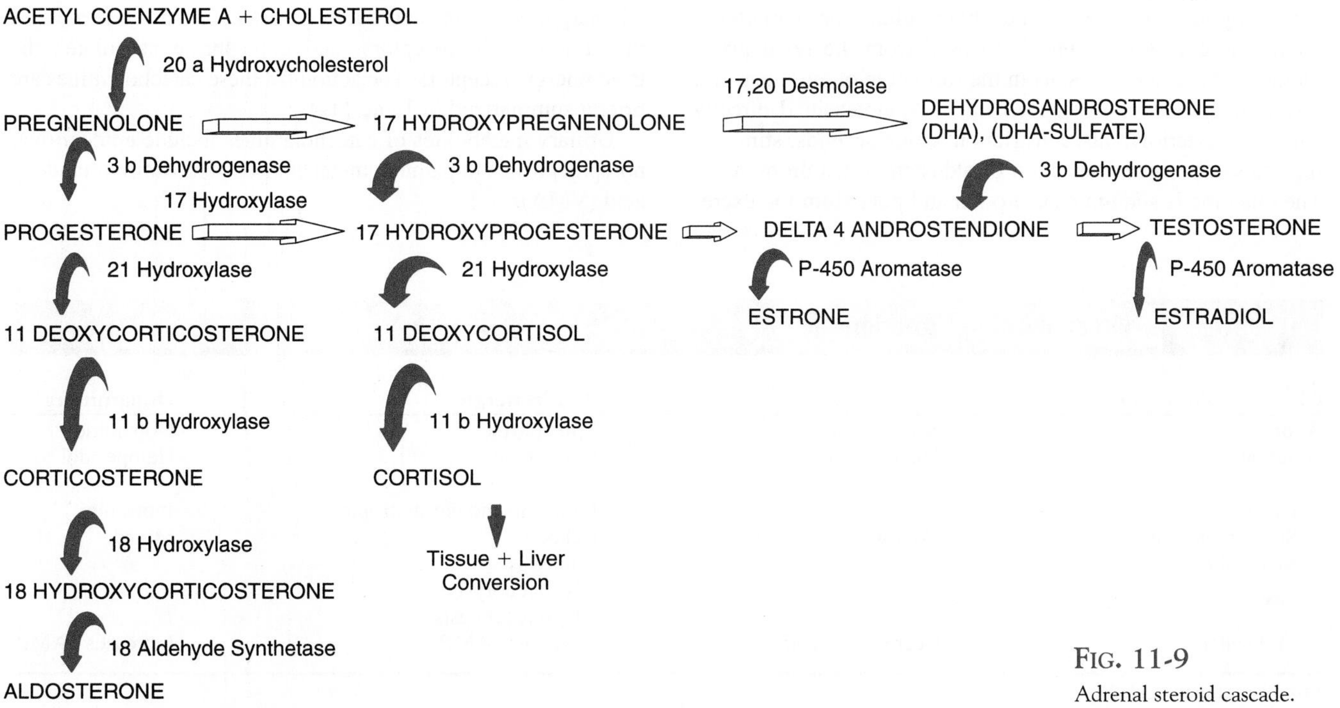

FIG. 11-9
Adrenal steroid cascade.

dehydrogenases), is converted into the primary hormones of cortisol (glucocorticoid), aldosterone (mineralocorticoid), testosterone, and estradiol (androgens). All of the final products as well as the intermediary hormones of the adrenal steroid cascade can be measured in the peripheral circulation.

Cortisol production and secretion are regulated by ACTH. The negative feedback effects of cortisol are exerted at both the level of the pituitary and the hypothalamus. Cortisol is secreted in a diurnal variation. The level is higher in the morning than in the evening. The rhythm is maintained in people who work night shift and maintain a conventional schedule on weekends. The rhythm changes gradually over 2 to 3 weeks when light/dark cycles are permanently changed or when time zones are crossed. Increased production during periods of stress results from increased central nervous system activity possibly mediated by vasopressin.

Cortisol has multiple effects throughout the body with important roles in carbohydrate, protein, and lipid metabolism. Cortisol increases glucose production by increasing hepatic gluconeogenesis. It stimulates glycolysis, proteolysis, and lipolysis to provide more substrate for gluconeogenesis and increases cellular resistance to insulin. Free fatty acid levels are increased through lipolysis and decreased glycerol production. A catabolic effect is exerted on protein metabolism in fat, skeletal muscle, bone, lymphoid tissue, and connective tissue. Glucocorticoids inhibit most immunologic and inflammatory responses. Other effects occur on connective tissues, calcium and bone metabolism, cardiac muscle, renal tubular excretion, growth and development, and central nervous system changes in mood.

Aldosterone is the most potent mineralocorticoid and accounts for 50% of plasma mineralocorticoid activity. The major function is to maintain intravascular volume by conserving sodium and eliminating potassium and hydrogen ions. Mineralocorticoids exert this effect in kidney, gut, salivary glands, sweat glands, vascular endothelium, and brain. The secretion of aldosterone is regulated by potassium ion concentration and the renin angiotensin system. When fluid-volume or intraarterial volume is decreased, renin is released from the renal juxtaglomerular cells. This results in the formation of angiotensin I, which then converts to angiotensin II. Angiotensin II directly stimulates arteriolar vasoconstriction within seconds, stimulating the synthesis and secretion of aldosterone within minutes. The outcome is sodium reabsorption and potassium ion excretion. Increased plasma potassium stimulates aldosterone production; decreased plasma potassium decreases aldosterone production and may exhibit a blunted response to hyponatremia.

Adrenal androgens, testosterone and estradiol, are primarily under the control of ACTH, but the linking mechanism to the hypothalamic-pituitary-gonadal axis is not well understood. Adrenarche is the outcome of increased adrenal androgen secretion a few years before the onset of puberty. These androgens play a role in the development of some secondary sexual characteristics such as axillary and pubic hair growth. They decline with age in both men and women, although women tend to have higher levels than men for more years. The decline coincides with menopause in women and occurs between ages 40 and 50 years in men. The physiologic effect is uncertain in men, but in women may account for testosterone effects seen after menopause (i.e., upper lip hair growth).

The sympathetic nervous system innervates the adrenal medulla and stimulates the release of catecholamines. Catecholamines are hormones (chemical substances that are released into the circulation and elicit a response from a target organ) and neurotransmitters (chemical substances released from nerve endings that have local effects). Catecholamines are biosynthesized from tyrosine, an amino acid that comes from dietary sources, or from conversion to phenylalanine to tyrosine in the liver. Tyrosine is acted on by enzymes to initiate the catecholamine pathway.

Norepinephrine and epinephrine are the main products of the pathway. Medullary catecholamine secretions are approximately 15% norepinephrine and 85% epinephrine. The medulla is the primary source of epinephrine production, whereas norepinephrine is secreted almost exclusively by the central nervous system. Epinephrine is five to ten times more potent than norepinephrine, although norepinephrine has a longer duration of action.

Norepinephrine and epinephrine are both alpha- and beta-adrenergic agonists, but norepinephrine primarily stimulates the α-adrenergic receptors, and epinephrine stimulates the β-adrenergic receptors. The actions of these catecholamines are briefly summarized in Table 11-4.

Urinary metabolites of catecholamines include epinephrine, norepinephrine, dopamine, metanephrine, and vanillylmandelic acid (VMA).

Table 11-4 Catecholamine Functions

Class and Function	α-Adrenergic	β-Adrenergic	Dopaminergic
Agonist	Norepinephrine	Epinephrine	Dopamine
Antagonist	Phentolamine	Propranolol	Haloperidol
Actions			
Heart		Inotropic and chronotropic	Inotropic
Smooth muscle	Contracts	Relaxes	Mixed
Metabolic		Lipolysis Glycogenolysis Gluconeogenesis	
Molecular	Decreases cAMP	Increases cAMP	Increases cAMP

From Korenman et al.[34]

Pancreas

The pancreas, both an endocrine and exocrine gland, lies behind the stomach to the left of the liver and is attached to the duodenum by ducts from the head and body section of the pancreas. It is through these ducts that the pancreatic digestive enzymes enter the small intestine (exocrine function).

The endocrine functions of the pancreas are carried out by the islets of Langerhans, which are a grouping of several hundred cells. The islets are scattered over the entire gland, and the cellular composition of each varies with the specific location within the pancreas. The islets contain at least four different types of cells. About 15% of islet cells are alpha cells that produce glucagon; 60% are beta cells that produce insulin; 10% are delta cells, producing somatostatin; and 15% are pancreatic polypeptide (PP) cells that produce pancreatic polypeptide.[23] Islets are organized with cells containing somatostatin, glucagon, and pancreatic polypeptide surrounding a core of insulin-producing cells. Biosynthesis of each of the islet cell hormones is similar. Prepropeptides give rise to propeptides that are packaged in secretory granules to provide bioactive hormone and a connecting or terminal peptide fragment.[18]

The islet cells have a large blood supply, and the pancreas is the most highly innervated of all endocrine glands. The central nervous system is linked to the islets through sympathetic and parasympathetic nerves of the autonomic nervous system. Stimulation of the sympathetic fibers increases the blood sugar level through stimulation of glucagon production and inhibition of insulin. Parasympathetic stimulation increases insulin secretion.

Glucagon is produced chiefly by the islet cells and plays an important role in maintaining blood glucose homeostasis. Glucagon production is stimulated by decreased blood glucose, fasting, and exercise. The primary target organ of this hormone is the liver, where it attaches to hepatic glucagon receptors. Glucagon acts to raise the blood glucose level by trapping amino acids in the liver and increasing gluconeogenesis, glycogenolysis, and ketogenesis. The fact that glucagon works in this manner to regulate glucose production is especially important in the fasting state. The secretion of glucagon and insulin are coordinated in a way that normally maintains the blood sugar level within a fairly narrow normal range. Glucagon and insulin have opposite actions, and the ratio, or relative concentration of both hormones, is important to blood glucose regulation.[23]

Insulin is synthesized in the endoplasmic reticulum of the beta cells under the direction of messenger RNA. After the terminal connecting C-peptide fragment is removed, the insulin molecule is folded and held together by disulfide bonds. Both insulin and C-peptide are secreted into the circulation along with small amounts of unchanged proinsulin. Since beta cell secretory granules contain equal amounts of C-peptide and insulin, C-peptide can be measured by radioimmunoassay to assess endogenous pancreatic beta cell function. Insulin is the primary hormone controlling the storage and metabolism of ingested nutrients. Glucose is the main stimulus for insulin secretion, with fat and protein being less potent stimuli for insulin secretion. Once secreted, insulin travels in the portal circulation to the liver and then through the general circulation. To be effective, insulin must bind to cell membrane receptors on target tissues (liver, fat, and muscle cells). Here it acts like a key to unlock the door to allow the entry of glucose into the cells. The metabolic effects of insulin include increased glucose transport into insulin-dependent cells and increased synthesis of protein, fat, and glycogen.[23] In the fasting state, decreased insulin levels and increased glucagon levels allow glucose production by the liver through the processes of glycogenolysis and gluconeogenesis to maintain the blood sugar level and an adequate glucose supply to cells for energy, since glucose is the main fuel for all cellular activity. In the fed state, glucagon levels drop and insulin levels rise to 30 to 100 mU/ml to prevent severe elevations in the blood sugar level by both suppressing liver production of glucose and stimulating glucose uptake by fat, muscle, and liver cells. An estimated 25% of glucose ingested is used by noninsulin-dependent cells (brain, eye, kidney, red blood cells) for energy.[23]

Although blood glucose regulation is primarily controlled by insulin and glucagon, three other counterregulatory hormones interact with glucagon to raise the blood glucose level. GH, secreted from the anterior pituitary gland, increases the blood sugar level by decreasing cellular glucose uptake; cortisol decreases cellular glucose uptake and increases gluconeogenesis; and catecholamines decrease cellular glucose uptake and increase glycogenolysis. The secretion of counterregulatory hormones is stimulated by hypoglycemia, exercise, and stress.[23]

Somatostatin is widely distributed in the central nervous system, stomach, intestines, and pancreatic islets. It acts as an inhibitor of insulin and glucagon secretion through direct action (paracrine effect). In addition, somatostatin acts to inhibit gastrointestinal hormones such as gastrin, secretin, and cholecystokinin, as well as pituitary hormones such as growth hormone and thyrotropin. Somatostatin secretion is stimulated by glucose, amino acids, and increased levels of extracellular calcium and potassium.[23]

PP secretion is increased with protein ingestion, fasting, exercise, and hyperglycemia. Increased PP levels have been noted in persons with diabetes mellitus and pancreatic endocrine tumors. The secretion of PP is thought to be under vagal control and does not influence carbohydrate metabolism. Its main action is to regulate gastrointestinal function such as exocrine pancreas secretion and gallbladder emptying.

Hormones produced by endocrine cells in the gastrointestinal tract include somatostatin, gastrin, secretin, cholecystokinin, motilin, neurotensin, enteroglucagon, peptide YY, and glucose-dependent insulinotropic peptide. These hormones mediate a variety of absorptive, secretory, digestive, motor, and tropic actions in the gastrointestinal tract and other organ systems that are essential to life.[23]

Gastrin is a peptide hormone that exists in three biologically active forms. It has various effects on the gastrointestinal tract, including (1) stimulation of gastric acid secretion; (2) stimulation of water and electrolyte secretion; (3) stimulation of digestive secretions from the stomach and pancreas; and (4) promotion of growth of the gastric mucosa. Excessive secretion of gastrin is responsible for a number of disease states that may include the occurrence of non–beta cell islet tumors (gastrinomas).[23]

Gonads

The testes are paired and oval in shape. Their size varies with age and degree of sexual maturity. Age-related testicular dimensions are found in Table 11-5.

Table 11-5 Assessment of Testicular Size

Method	Prepubertal	Pubertal	Adult
Orchidometer*	1-6	8-15	20-30†
Ruler measurement‡			
Length	1.6-2.9	3.1-4.0	4.1-5.5
Width	1.0-1.8	2.0-2.5	2.7-3.2

From Santen.[46]
*Measured in milliliters.
†2464SD ml; n544.
‡Measured in centimeters.

Clinically, testicular volume is measured with a Prader orchidometer in cubic centimeters. The testes are found within the scrotum and are maintained at a temperature approximately 2 degrees lower than the temperature of the abdomen.[46] Testes contain two functional areas: interstitial cells (Leydig cells) and seminiferous tubules (germinal and Sertoli cells).

Male gonadal hormone production in the testes is regulated by GnRH from the hypothalamus. Beginning at puberty, GnRH is secreted in a 24-hour pulsatile fashion. GnRH binds to receptors on anterior pituitary cells that subsequently produce and release LH and FSH. LH binds to Leydig cell receptors and stimulates androgen production, mainly in the form of testosterone. About 7 mg of testosterone is released each day (in a pulsatile manner) by adult testes into the peripheral circulation via the spermatic vein.[18,46]

Testosterone circulates attached to testosterone-binding globulin (TeBG) or albumin; 2% circulates unbound as free testosterone, the most biologically active form. The fractions of each are important in clinical evaluation.

Adrenal glands provide an additional source of testosterone in the amount of about 200 mg/day.[46] The hormonal effects of testosterone are direct in the testes (paracrine effect) and include the initiation of spermatogenesis. The peripheral effects of testosterone and a conversion product, dihydrotestosterone, are responsible for the masculinizing effects of androgens. The clinical actions of testosterone are summarized in Box 11-2.

After middle age, testosterone levels gradually decrease because of impaired hypothalamic control and Leydig cell attrition.

FSH binds to Sertoli cell receptors to stimulate the synthesis of proteins such as inhibin, transferrin, and androgen-binding protein (ABP). Inhibin is thought to provide negative feedback to inhibit FSH secretion at the pituitary gland level. ABP is thought to play a role in maintaining high testosterone levels in the seminiferous tubules and testes. FSH is also thought to be necessary for the completion of spermatogenesis and maintenance of normal sperm counts.[18,46]

Sperm are produced by germinal cells through the process of cell replication. FSH is thought to be required for initiating spermatogenesis; LH and testosterone maintain the process. Final maturation of spermatozoa occurs in the epididymus. During ejaculation, sperm are carried by fluid flow from the seminiferous tubules; through the rete testes, epididymus, and vas deferens; and finally into the urethra.[18]

The ovaries are paired, oval in shape, and situated on either side of the uterus, just posterior to the fallopian tubes. They are held in place by the mesovarium to the broad ligament that extends from the uterus to the pelvic cavity wall. Ovarian size and weight depend on normal development and degree of sexual maturity.

Each ovary consists of the cortex and the medulla. The cortex comprises maturing follicles that contain oocytes (eggs) and steroidogenic cells, called interstitial cells, that produce and secrete androgens. The loose connective tissue of the medulla contains nerves and blood vessels that course toward the cortex.

Female gonadal hormone production is regulated by GnRH secreted in pulsatile fashion from the hypothalamus. GnRH binds to receptors on anterior pituitary cells that in turn produce LH and FSH in pulsatile fashion every 60 to 90 minutes beginning at puberty.

CLINICAL ACTIONS OF TESTOSTERONE — **Box 11-2**

IN UTERO
External genitalia development
Wolffian duct development

PREPUBERTAL
Possible male behavioral effects

PUBERTAL
External genitalia
- Penis and scrotum increase in size and become pigmented
- Rugal folds appear in scrotal skin

Hair growth
- Mustache and beard develop; scalp line undergoes recession
- Pubic hair develops
- Axillary, body, extremity, and perianal hair appears

Linear growth
- Pubertal growth spurt
- Androgens interact with growth hormone to increase somatomedin C levels

Accessory sex organs
- Prostate and seminal vesicles enlarge and secretion begins

Voice
- The pitch is lowered because of enlargement of larynx and thickening of vocal cords

Psyche
- More aggressive attitudes are manifest
- Sexual potential develops

Muscle mass
- Muscle bulk increases
- Positive nitrogen balance is demonstrable

ADULT
Hair growth
- Androgenic patterns are maintained
- Male baldness may be initiated

Psyche
- Behavioral attitudes and sexual potency are maintained

Bone
- Bone loss and osteoporosis are prevented

Spermatogenesis
- Interaction with FSH to modulate Sertoli cell function and stimulate spermatogenesis

Hematopoiesis
- Erythropoietin-stimulated
- Direct marrow effect on erythropoiesis

Table 11-6 Summary of Hormonal Effects

Areas of Concern	Hormonal Influence
Normal growth	Thyroid Insulin Growth hormone Gonadotropins Sex steroids
Metabolic rate	Thyroid
Protein, carbohydrate, and fat metabolism	Thyroid Glucagon Insulin Gastrin, glucocorticoids
Cardiac contractility	Calcium, epinephrine
Blood pressure, pulse rate	Glucocorticoids, mineralocorticoids Epinephrine, norepinephrine
Muscle mass and contractility	Glucocorticoids Insulin Growth hormone Androgens
Skin turgor	Mineralocorticoids, glucocorticoids
Secondary sex characteristics	Gonadotropins Sex steroids
Lactation	Calcium Prolactin, oxytocin
Skin pigmentation	Melanocyte-stimulating hormone

From Santen.[46]

In response to LH and FSH secretion, females secrete three types of biologically active hormones in a process that depends on mixed-function oxidase enzymes. Steroidogenic cells convert cholesterol to pregnenolone, which is then converted enzymatically to progesterone, testosterone, and estrogen. FSH and LH control steroid metabolism enzymes and, thus, the conversion rates and amounts of active hormone. The principal actions of these ovarian hormones are (1) stimulation of growth of female reproductive organs (uterus, vagina, breasts) and (2) development of secondary sex characteristics.

Progesterone functions to (1) prepare the endometrium of the uterus for ovum implantation, (2) prepare the placenta, (3) prepare breasts for milk production, and (4) decrease uterine contractility. Estrogen affects the development and maturation of the breasts and genitalia. Androgens are responsible for the development of sexual hair. Table 11-6 summarizes the effects of these and other hormones.

Normal female reproductive function occurs when the hypothalamic-pituitary-ovarian axis is coordinated with uterine environment changes. LH and FSH levels follow a cyclic pattern of secretion each month beginning around puberty and continuing through the childbearing years until menopause, with the exception of pregnancy and lactation. FSH plays a key role in controlling the growth of the primary follicle to maturation; estrogen production regenerates the uterine lining each month. A surge in LH and fall in estrogen follows, causing the single follicle that reaches maturity to release an ovum into the peritoneal cavity (ovulation). The ovum is swept up into the fimbrae of the fallopian tube, where it can potentially be fertilized, and then implanted in the uterus. After ovulation the walls of the primary follicle form the corpus luteum and secrete progesterone. If implantation does not occur, the corpus luteum deteriorates into dense connective tissue called the corpus albicans. A subsequent fall in progesterone causes spasm of the spiral arterioles, the shedding of endometrium, menstruation, and the beginning of the next monthly cycle. (see FIG. 12-7, p. 645).

Nursing care in this chapter is based on the nursing process, which consists of assessment criteria, nursing diagnoses, interventions, education, and evaluation.[13,14,32,54,57]

CONDITIONS, DISEASES, AND DISORDERS

DISORDERS OF THE ADRENAL GLAND

ADRENAL INSUFFICIENCY

Adrenal insufficiency is caused by inadequate function of the adrenal cortex. There are two types: primary and secondary. Hypofunction of the adrenal cortex can originate from a disorder within the adrenal gland (primary adrenal insufficiency), or it may be due to hypofunction of the pituitary-hypothalamic unit (secondary adrenal insufficiency).

In primary adrenal insufficiency (Addison's disease), destruction of the adrenal cortex prevents adequate production of glucocorticoid (cortisol) and mineralocorticoid (aldosterone). In secondary adrenal insufficiency, hypothalamic-pituitary dysfunction prevents the adequate secretion of ACTH by the pituitary gland and leads to a relative cortisol deficiency.[8]

PATHOPHYSIOLOGY

Primary adrenal insufficiency can be insidious in onset; signs and symptoms appear after 90% of adrenocortical tissue has been destroyed.[59] Eighty percent of cases of Addison's disease are caused by autoimmune destruction of the adrenal glands. Other causes include infection (tuberculosis, fungus, human immunodeficiency virus [HIV], syphilis), hemorrhage, metastases, drugs, and congenital adrenal disease. Bilateral adrenal hemorrhage should be considered in patients receiving anticoagulation.

Primary adrenal insufficiency is the result of glucocorticoid and mineralocorticoid deficiency. Through negative feedback, low cortisol levels stimulate the pituitary gland to secrete increased amounts of ACTH. This compensatory overproduction of ACTH leads to the classic sign of primary adrenal insufficiency: hyperpigmentation. Hyperpigmentation is particularly obvious when examining scars, palmar surfaces, and skin creases. Other signs and symptoms include weakness and fatigue, anorexia, nausea, vomiting, diarrhea, weight loss, abdominal pain, muscle and joint pain, orthostatic hypotension, vitiligo, and changes in mentation.[18]

Secondary adrenal insufficiency occurs most commonly in patients recently withdrawn from exogenous glucocorticoid therapy. Recovery of a normal hypothalamic-pituitary-adrenal (HPA) axis can take months or years after this cessation of steroid administration. Other causes include pituitary tumors, hypophysectomy, pituitary radiation, postpartum pituitary necrosis, tumors of the third ventricle, and optic glioma.[18]

The clinical manifestations of secondary adrenal insufficiency are caused by glucocorticoid deficiency. Mineralocorticoid production is not impaired because its regulation by the renin-angiotensin system is independent of pituitary ACTH. Hypotension and shock are less common and less severe as a general rule.[59]

The central pathophysiologic alteration of adrenal insufficiency is cardiovascular: insufficient glucocorticoid reduces cardiac output, decreases vascular tone, and results in hypovolemia. This stimulates the release of vasopressin, causing water retention and hyponatremia. Cardiac contractility and output decrease, possibly leading to circulatory collapse. Reflex tachycardia results from a decrease in cardiac output. Free fatty acid mobilization is impaired, which reduces the free fatty acid levels. This in turn leads to increased utilization of glucose, resulting in hypoglycemia. Decreased cortisol increases ACTH and MSH production, causing hyperpigmentation, and there is a decrease in gastrointestinal enzymes. The loss of diurnal cortisol may cause a loss of vitality. Mineralocorticoid deficiency is reflected by hyperkalemia and hyponatremia.[8,18]

Adrenal crisis, or acute adrenal insufficiency, is characterized by an exacerbation of symptoms associated with adrenal insufficiency often precipitated by a major physiologic stress. It is usually associated with primary adrenal insufficiency, but can occur in secondary disease. Patients in adrenal crisis are usually dehydrated, hypovolemic, and hyponatremic. The hypotension resists volume repletion and requires glucocorticoid administration for rapid correction. Vomiting and diarrhea contribute to volume depletion. Other symptoms include nausea, anorexia, weakness, and fatigue. Mentation ranges from lethargy to coma. Hallmark signs include abdominal pain and fever. Fever can result from a precipitating infection or the glucocorticoid deficiency itself. Hyperpigmentation and weight loss can be seen in patients with chronic adrenal insufficiency. Adrenal crisis can be caused by inadequate glucocorticoid replacement or failure to compensate for major stressors such as surgery, trauma, or infection. The prophylactic use of exogenous steroids in trauma has greatly decreased the occurrence of adrenal crisis.[18]

Diagnostic Studies and Findings[8]

Imaging: Purified protein derivative (PPD) and/or chest x-ray: possible tuberculosis; abdominal computed tomographic (CT) scan: adrenal calcification or enlargement suggests infection, hemorrhage, or metastatic disease

Blood tests: Hyponatremia, hyperkalemia (in primary disease), azotemia (if severe), hypoglycemia

Endocrine tests: Plasma ACTH levels: increased in primary disease, decreased or normal in secondary disease; short ACTH stimulation test (Cortrosyn test): baseline cortisol level is drawn, then cortrosyn (ACTH) is administered; 30 minutes later, plasma cortisol level should rise; impaired response indicates adrenal insufficiency

Multidisciplinary Plan[18]

Medications

Hormone replacement

Glucocorticoid replacement: Hydrocortisone, 12-15 mg/m^2

Mineralocorticoid replacement: Fludrocortisone (Florinef), 0.05-0.1 mg/day

These medications are considered life-sustaining for the patient and cannot be discontinued. To avoid adrenal crisis, patients must be taught intramuscular self-injection of hydrocortisone (Solu-Cortef) to be administered when oral medication cannot be taken. A family member or significant other should be included in intramuscular injection instruction.

Special Considerations

Overtreatment with glucocorticoids can result in symptoms of hypercortisolism (Cushing's syndrome). Excess mineralocorticoids can result in fluid overload and hypertension. Evaluation of dosage adequacy can be done by monitoring clinical signs and symptoms and measuring 24-hour urinary free cortisol.[59]

NURSING CARE

Nursing Assessment

Circulation: Postural hypotension; dizziness, visual changes; serum electrolytes; hypopyrexia or hyperpyrexia*; shock*; vital signs, apical pulse—dysrhythmias; hydration status

Food and fluid needs: Salt craving, weight loss, nausea, vomiting, hyponatremia,* hyperkalemia,* skin turgor, dietary intake

Elimination: Diarrhea, oliguria, renal shutdown*

Mobility: Tires easily, muscle aches, muscle wasting, muscle weakness

Comfort and pain: Severe headache,* severe abdominal pain,* severe leg pain,* severe lower back pain*

Hygiene and skin care: Hyperpigmentation, decreased body hair, poor skin turgor

Sexuality: Amenorrhea, decreased libido

Potential Complications

Adrenal crisis from adrenal insufficiency, fainting, injuries from falls, shock, renal shutdown

Patient Problems/Nursing Diagnosis & Interventions

NIC Electrolyte and Acid-Base Management

Deficient fluid-volume and hypovolemia related to mineralocorticoid deficiency

- Provide aggressive fluid replacement in adrenal crisis.
- Administer glucocorticoid and mineralocorticoid as ordered.
- Administer medications to combat nausea, vomiting, and diarrhea *to maintain fluid and nutritional balance and to promote homeostasis.*
- Monitor patient's intake and output; be aware of the patient's high risk for renal shutdown in adrenal crisis.
- Monitor weight daily.
- Encourage high-sodium, low-potassium diet when tolerated.
- Instruct patient to change positions gradually (from lying to sitting or standing positions) *to avoid fainting from orthostatic hypotension.*

*Characteristic of adrenal crisis.

- Instruct patient to report early presyncopal signs (e.g., dizziness, light-headedness, and visual changes).
- Administer intravenous (IV) fluids rapidly as ordered to rehydrate patient, but use caution *to avoid cardiovascular overload.*
- Explain rationale for IV fluid therapy to patient.
- Note that shortened PR interval on electrocardiogram (ECG) can result from glucocorticoid deficiency.
- Hemodynamic monitoring may be indicated in adrenal crisis to monitor atrial filling pressure and peripheral vascular resistance.

NIC PHYSICAL COMFORT PROMOTION

Pain related to biochemical factors (metabolic imbalance)

- Monitor patient for development of pain (headache; abdominal, leg, or back pain); be aware that these signs may indicate adrenal crisis.
- Encourage the patient to report pain or discomfort.
- Provide hormonal replacement (hydrocortisone).
- Employ comfort measures for the patient as needed.

NIC ACTIVITY AND EXERCISE MANAGEMENT

Impaired physical mobility related to decreased strength and endurance (or musculoskeletal weakness)

- Provide rest periods for patient between nursing activities.
- Assist patient with task analysis of daily activities.
- Allow patient to increase strength and endurance at own pace; muscle weakness will improve as hormone replacement is achieved.

PATIENT EDUCATION/CONTINUUM OF CARE PLAN

1. Ensure that patient verbalizes the importance of taking medication and how to take it regularly and in emergency situations.
2. Discuss with patient the steps to follow when early symptoms of insufficiency are noted.
3. Discuss with patient the importance of regular medical follow-up and the wearing of medical identification.
4. Assist patient in identifying a support person/system.

EVALUATION/PATIENT OUTCOMES

Electrolyte and Acid-Base Management: Hydration and vital signs are normal. Patient's sodium and potassium blood levels are within normal limits. Patient's blood pressure is maintained within normal limits with no evidence of orthostatic hypotension. Patient makes no statements concerning syncope. Patient's peripheral pulses are adequate. Patient's output equals intake. Patient's urine output is greater than 40 ml/h. Patient's skin is intact, and turgor is normal. Electrolytes are within normal range. Weight is stable.

Physical Comfort Promotion: Pain is relieved (in adrenal crisis). Patient recognizes and reports onset of abdominal pain as a potential sign of acute adrenal crisis. Patient reports pain relief with cortisol replacement therapy.

Activity and Exercise Management: Activity pattern is improved. Patient is able to independently perform daily activities.

PRIMARY ALDOSTERONISM

Primary aldosteronism is the hypersecretion of aldosterone, resulting in renal wasting of potassium and reabsorption of sodium. This leads to hypertension, usually accompanied by hypokalemia.[59]

Primary aldosteronism is an uncommon disease accounting for about 2% of patients with hypertension. It must be distinguished from secondary aldosteronism, which is a normal adrenal response to hyperstimulation of the renin-angiotensin system (diuretic therapy, hepatic insufficiency, congestive heart failure, nephrotic syndrome, and licorice ingestion). Edema rarely occurs in primary aldosteronism, but can be seen in secondary aldosteronism.

PATHOPHYSIOLOGY[59]

Primary aldosteronism is a disorder of the adrenal cortex. It is most commonly caused by adrenal adenoma and idiopathic bilateral adrenal hyperplasia. In rare cases, adrenal carcinoma and dexamethasone-suppressible hyperaldosteronism can also cause primary hyperaldosteronism.

Primary aldosteronism is usually associated with asymptomatic hypertension and hypokalemia, but hypokalemia is not present in all cases. The diagnosis of primary aldosteronism should be suspected in all patients with spontaneous hypokalemia. Suppressed renin levels and aldosterone excess confirm the diagnosis. Excess aldosterone results in increased sodium reabsorption, increased total body sodium, water retention, and hypervolemia. Edema rarely occurs because of an "escape" mechanism wherein proximal tubular sodium reabsorption is inhibited by renal hemodynamic changes. Arterial hypertension results from volume expansion and increased vascular and sympathetic reactivity. The degree of hypertension ranges from mild to severe.

Aldosterone causes potassium depletion, both intracellular and extracellular, by increasing renal tubular excretion of potassium. The symptoms of muscle weakness, fatigue, and polyuria are related to the hypokalemia and thus are not seen in all cases. Hypokalemia can also cause altered electrical conductivity of the myocardium and diminished glucose tolerance.

Hydrogen ion secretion is increased, resulting in metabolic alkalosis. The alkalosis correlates with the degree of hypokalemia. The ability to concentrate urine diminishes, resulting in polyuria, and inappropriate excretion of potassium continues. Marked alkalosis is reflected by positive Chvostek's and Trousseau's signs.

Plasma renin activity is suppressed. Laboratory values reveal suppressed renin levels after the patient is exposed to conditions that cause elevated levels in normal patients. Simultaneous elevation of aldosterone secretion is also observed in these patients.

Diagnostic Studies and Findings[59]

Diagnosis of primary aldosteronism: Suggested by hypertension, hypokalemia, suppressed renin levels, and an elevated aldosterone level. Diuretics should be discontinued 2 to 4 weeks before diagnostic testing. The patient should eat a normal sodium diet.

Blood tests: Decreased potassium; decreased plasma renin activity (PRA); NOTE: If PRA is normal or elevated, secondary hyperaldosteronism is the probable cause of hypertension; increased plasma aldosterone concentration (PAC); increased PRA:PAC ratio

Urine tests: 24-hour collection: increased aldosterone

Imaging tests: CT scan used to define an adrenal mass; an adenoma is rarely too small to be seen on CT

Endocrine tests

Captopril test: 25-50 mg of captopril is administered orally to suppress renin activity; PRA and PAC are drawn 60 and 120 minutes later; the diagnosis of primary aldosteronism is reflected by the following results: decreased PRA, increased PAC, increased PAC:PRA ratio

Lying and standing renin and aldosterone levels: After confirming normal sodium diet, baseline renin and aldosterone levels are drawn after patient has been in a supine position for 30 minutes; normally, renin increases with ambulation; decreased PRA in primary aldosteronism; PRA remains low after ambulation; if resting and after ambulation levels are high, secondary aldosteronism is implied; increased PAC and an after-ambulation decrease suggest an aldosterone-producing adenoma

Normal saline infusion test: To test the response of aldosterone (PAC) to extracellular fluid volume expansion; testing should be performed in the afternoon because the circadian pattern of PAC is to decrease in the morning; patient must be supine for 30 minutes before the test; obtain baseline PAC level, administer 2 L of saline solution over 4 hours, obtain PAC level following infusion; if aldosterone (PAC) level is greater than 10 ng/dl and does not fall below 10 ng/dl, the test is positive for primary aldosteronism; a negative test suggests renin essential hypertension

Venous catheterization of adrenal glands with measurement of plasma cortisol and aldosterone: To distinguish between a unilateral and bilateral source of hyperaldosteronism

Multidisciplinary Plan[59]

Surgery

Unilateral adrenalectomy; to remove aldosterone-producing adenoma; preoperative spironolactone is administered for 2 weeks (200 to 400 mg/day)

Medications

Aldosterone receptor blockade with spironolactone (Aldactone), 200 to 400 mg/day

Antihypertensive therapy

General Management

Low sodium diet

NURSING CARE

Nursing Assessment

Circulation: Moderate to severe hypertension, vital signs, daily weights, hypokalemia, hypernatremia

Food and fluid needs: Polydipsia, intake and output, excessive ingestion of licorice (mimics mineralocorticoid activity), tobacco chewing (licorice-flavored tobacco)

Elimination: Polyuria, nocturia

Neurosensory concerns: Positive Chvostek's sign, Trousseau's sign

Mobility: Muscle weakness

Potential Complications

Severe hypertension

Patient Problems/Nursing Diagnoses & Interventions

NIC Electrolyte and Acid-Base Management

Fluid-volume excess/hypervolemia related to failure of regulatory mechanism—caused by sodium reabsorption due to overproduction of aldosterone

- Reinforce low-sodium diet *to decrease patient's fluid retention.*
- Monitor patient's serum electrolyte levels.
- Reassess Chvostek's and Trousseau's signs *to monitor patient for signs of alkalosis.*
- Monitor patient's respiratory status and quality of respirations *to monitor for early acidosis.*
- Administer spironolactone (Aldactone) to patient as ordered.

Patient Education/Continuum of Care Plan

1. Preoperative education to help patient and family prepare for unilateral adrenalectomy to remove aldosterone-producing adenoma (see discussion of adrenalectomy p. 804) and prepare for the postoperative care.
2. Preoperative preparation includes spironolactone therapy for 2 weeks. Medication teaching should include discussion of side effects. Women can expect menstrual disturbances; men can experience gynecomastia, impotence, and decreased libido.
3. Ensure that patient verbalizes importance of compliance with the regimen, knows importance of taking medication regularly, knows potential side effects to report, and knows symptoms associated with inadequate medication coverage.

Evaluation/Patient Outcomes

Electrolyte and Acid-Base Management: Excess fluid is decreased or absent. Patient's aldosterone level is not elevated but is within normal range. Patient's serum electrolyte levels are within normal limits. Patient's weight is within the normal range. Patient's vital signs are within the normal range; there is no evidence of dysrhythmias.

CUSHING'S SYNDROME (HYPERCORTISOLISM)[18,59]

Cushing's syndrome is caused by excess glucocorticoid secretion by the adrenal cortex or via the exogenous administration of glucocorticoids.

Cushing's syndrome is rare; its true incidence is not known. Sexual predominance relates to cause; Cushing's disease occurs four to six times more often in women, but ectopic ACTH syndrome occurs more frequently in men. Occurrence is usually during midlife.

The etiologies of Cushing's syndrome are divided into two groups: ACTH-dependent and ACTH-independent causes. In ACTH-dependent disease, adrenal activation is caused by excessive ACTH production, as in pituitary adenoma (80%), ectopic ACTH syndrome (20%), and, rarely, ectopic CRH secretion. In ACTH-independent disease, adrenal hyperactivity is independent of ACTH stimulation, for example, adrenal adenoma (40% to 50%), adrenal carcinoma (40% to 50%), and, less commonly, primary pigmented nodular adrenal disease (micronodular adrenal disease), McCune-Albright syndrome, and macronodular adrenal disease.

Seventy percent of all patients with Cushing's syndrome have Cushing's disease: hypersecretion of ACTH by a pituitary adenoma. Hypercortisolism can be caused by extrapituitary sources of ACTH, such as oat cell carcinoma of the lung. Cortisol production correlates directly with ACTH secretion. Hence, elevated ACTH levels result in adrenal hyperstimulation, hyperplasia, and hypercortisolism.

Diseases of the adrenal cortex, such as adrenal adenoma (benign) and adrenal carcinoma (malignant), can lead to hypercortisolism. When adrenal tissue becomes neoplastic, cortisol can be produced independently of ACTH stimulation. This overproduction of cortisol leads to low levels of ACTH because of the negative feedback effects of cortisol on the pituitary gland. Other conditions causing hypercortisolism include chronic alcoholism (alcoholic pseudo-Cushing's syndrome), depression, and the factitious administration of corticosteroid preparations.

The effects of glucocorticoid excess are reflected in changes in many tissue and organ systems. Early symptoms include weight gain, hypertension, and glucose intolerance. The majority of these clinical effects result from the direct antagonism of insulin by glucocorticoids. This leads to (1) impaired glucose tolerance and diabetes mellitus and (2) altered fat distribution. Normally, insulin inhibits the breakdown of fat (lipolysis), but glucocorticoid alters the pattern of the process leading to central obesity. In this state of impaired energy metabolism, cells are deprived of this major energy source. Hence, specialized functions such as the elaboration of skin and bone matrix are sacrificed. The effects of cortisol on gluconeogenesis result in hyperglycemia, polydipsia, polyuria, and polyphagia. Diabetes mellitus occurs in 10% to 15% of patients.

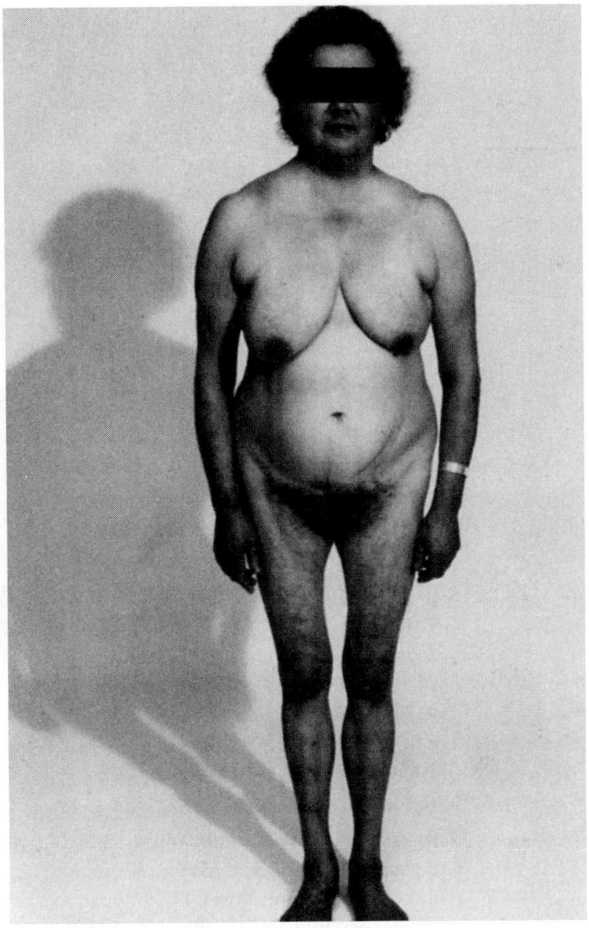

FIG. 11-10
Forty-six-year-old woman diagnosed with Cushing's disease. Note classic cushingoid habitus with prominent supraclavicular fat pads and muscle wasting in extremities. (Courtesy National Institutes of Child Health, Bethesda, Md.)

Weight gain is accompanied by a redistribution of fat, resulting in a protuberant abdomen, facial rounding (moon facies), supraclavicular fullness, dorsocervical fat pad (buffalo hump), and thinning of extremities (FIG. 11-10). Exophthalmos occurs in 6% of patients because of retroorbital fat accumulation. Weakness is associated with proximal muscle wasting, and patients can have difficulty rising from a squatting position and, in severe cases, getting up from a chair. Patients can experience a loss of height from severe osteoporosis. Loss of subcutaneous tissue produces thin, fragile skin (characteristically, "cigarette paper" thin). Facial plethora and erythema are common. Violaceous striae are the result of thin, fragile skin being pulled across a grossly enlarged abdomen. Striae can also be found on breasts, hips, shoulders, and upper thighs and are usually greater than 1 cm wide.

Wound healing is slowed, and immune function is suppressed. The normal sequelae of infection, fever, and pain can be masked by hypercortisolism.

Cardiovascular complications are a major cause of morbidity and mortality in patients with Cushing's syndrome. Hypertension is common and can be exacerbated by the excessive production of mineralocorticoid, which may contribute to dependent edema, possibly resulting in congestive heart failure. Vessel fragility and loss of connective tissue lead to bruising unrelated to trauma. Significant ecchymoses can occur with venipuncture. The use of pediatric-sized venipuncture needles for adults and neonatal venipuncture needles for pediatric patients may decrease bruising.

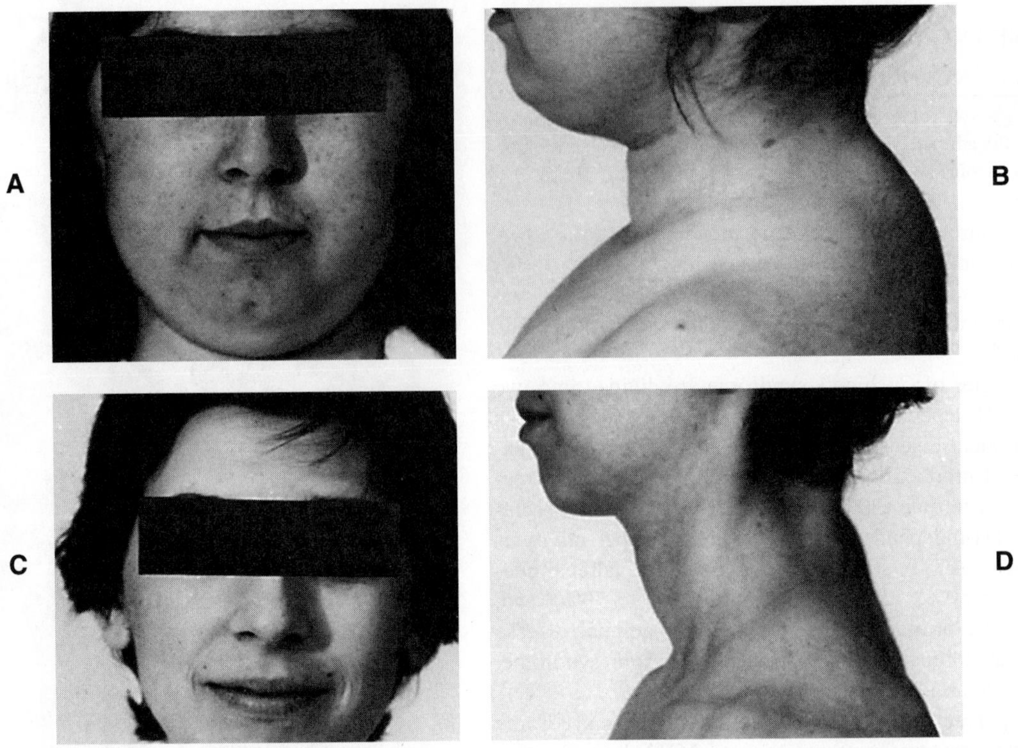

FIG. 11-11

Preoperative and postoperative appearance of 23-year-old woman with adrenal carcinoma. Note moon facies, buffalo hump, supraclavicular fat pads, and mild hirsutism. **A,** Preoperative adrenal carcinoma with moon facies and hirsutism. **B,** Preoperative adrenal carcinoma with buffalo hump. **C,** Postoperative adrenal carcinoma with loss of moon facies and hirsutism. **D,** Postoperative adrenal carcinoma with loss of buffalo hump. (Courtesy National Institutes of Child Health, Bethesda, Md.)

Androgen excess from adrenal hyperfunction can cause menstrual irregularities, hirsutism (in females) (FIG. 11-11), oily facial skin, acne, thinning scalp hair, and altered libido. Cortisol excess can lead to loss of bone density, back pain, compression fractures, and, rarely, long-bone fractures. Hypercalciuria and renal calculi accompany the bone disease. This also explains the presence of polydipsia and polyuria.

Emotional and cognitive changes from hypercortisolism can be severe. Effects include emotional lability, depression, impaired mentation and concentration, memory loss, irritability, anxiety, paranoia, and panic. Emotional and chemical depression may indicate the need for suicide precautions. Loss of the normal diurnal rhythm of cortisol has been associated with insomnia.

DIAGNOSTIC STUDIES AND FINDINGS

The diagnosis of hypercortisolism can be difficult. Examining old photographs can help assess the progression of physical changes associated with Cushing's syndrome: Truncal obesity with wasting of extremities; facial rounding and plethora; purplish red striae that are usually depressed below the skin surface of the abdomen, buttocks, and breasts; filling of supraclavicular areas and development of a "buffalo hump"; thinning of hair, especially at scalp line; and onset of hirsutism.[18] Cushing's syndrome in children is also manifested by short stature and obesity with a "falling off" of the growth curve.

Blood tests: Plasma cortisol: loss of diurnal rhythm (increased at night); plasma ACTH increased with ectopic syndromes; normal or slight increase with Cushing's disease; decreased with adrenal adenoma or carcinoma; potassium decreased; glucose increased; eosinophils decreased

Urine tests: 24-hour collection: 17-hydroxysteroids (17-OH) increased; urinary free cortisol 200 g/day (This is the single best test for identifying endogenous hypercortisolism and diagnosing Cushing's syndrome.)

Imaging: CT scan of sella to locate pituitary adenoma; CT scan of adrenal glands to locate adrenal adenoma, bilateral hyperplasia, macronodular hyperplasia; CT scan of chest to locate ectopic adenoma; magnetic resonance imaging (MRI) of pituitary gland to scan for adenoma

Endocrine tests

Dexamethasone suppression tests: Tests for negative feedback of the hypothalamic-pituitary-adrenal (HPA) axis by administering dexamethasone (synthetic cortisol); normal response: glucocorticoids directly inhibit ACTH secretion from the pituitary; false-positive results can occur with depression, alcoholism, and phenytoin, phenobarbital, or estrogen usage.

Overnight dexamethasone test: Oral administration of 1 mg of dexamethasone (10 μg/kg body weight in children) at 11 PM and with sample for cortisol drawn at 8 AM; normal response is ACTH secretion suppressing cortisol levels to less than 5 μg/100 ml.

Low-dose dexamethasone test, administration of 0.5 mg dexamethasone PO q6h for 48 hours; normal response is decreased ACTH, decreased urinary 17-OH (24-h urine); Cushing's disease: little or no effect; ACTH continues to be secreted despite attempts at negative feedback.

High-dose dexamethasone test: Administration of 2 mg dexamethasone PO every 6 hours for 48 hours; normal response is same as low-dose dexamethasone test; Cushing's disease: decreased urinary 17-OH by 50%.

Long dexamethasone suppression test: dexamethasone 0.5 mg every 6 hours for 2 days, followed by 2 mg every 6 hours for another 2 days; serum cortisol is measured at 8 AM on day 1, day 3 (after 2 days of low dose and before intake of high dose), and day 5 (after completion of 2 days of high dose); urine for free cortisol and creatinine is collected for 24 hours, three times: once before the start of the low dose, during the second day of the low dose, and during the second day of the high dose; in normal subjects the urinary 17-hydroxycorticosteroid levels on the second day of low-dose dexamethasone are usually less than 3 mg per 24 hours (1-2 mg/g creatinine), free cortisol is less than 5 μg/100 ml; higher values indicate Cushing's syndrome; suppression of the 17-hydroxycorticosteroids to less than 50% of the baseline level or normalization of the urine free cortisol on the second day of high-dose dexamethasone in a patient with abnormal values on the low dose indicates pituitary-dependent Cushing's syndrome (i.e., Cushing's disease); failure of suppression with the high-dose regimen suggests the presence of an adrenal adenoma or carcinoma or ectopic ACTH production; alternatives to standard dexamethasone suppression testing include the use of continuous intravenous infusion of dexamethasone (1 mg/h for 7 h), and an overnight high-dose (8-mg) dexamethasone test, but these have not been proven to be more reliable in diagnosing Cushing's disease.

Corticotropin releasing hormone (CRH) stimulation test: CRH administration, 1 mg/kg as an intravenous bolus, is the best way to separate ACTH-dependent from ACTH-independent disease; ACTH-dependent illness always responds to CRH with an ACTH level greater than 10 pg/ml.

Inferior petrosal sinus sampling (IPSS)[22]*:* Catheterization of the inferior petrosal sinuses (bilaterally) allows the measurement of ACTH secretion directly from the pituitary gland; ACTH levels from the petrosal sinuses ("central") and a peripheral venous site are compared; a pituitary adenoma is the likely cause of Cushing's syndrome if the ratio of central to peripheral ACTH is 2.0; if 1.0 mg/kg of ovine CRH is administered and the ratio is 3.0, the likelihood of pituitary adenoma is nearly 100%[22]; successful use of IPSS depends on local experience and expertise

MULTIDISCIPLINARY PLAN

Surgery

Pituitary adenomectomy, partial, or total hypophysectomy (see hypophysectomy section, p. 808)

Removal of microadenoma by transsphenoidal approach is treatment of choice; if tumor has not been located by imaging techniques, surgical exploration of the pituitary gland can lead to localization and removal of adenoma in 90% of patients; this treatment usually maintains normal pituitary function; if tumor is not identified, a partial or total hypophysectomy can be undertaken; lateralization during IPSS indicates which half of the gland contains the adenoma

Adrenalectomy

Treatment of choice only for non–ACTH-dependent hypercortisolism or Cushing's disease when pituitary surgery is unsuccessful (because it does not address the cause of ACTH hypersecretion, it blocks the adrenal response of cortisol overproduction); a complication that can develop is Nelson's syndrome; hypersecretion of ACTH continues, hyperpigmentation is evident, and the clinical manifestation of a pituitary tumor occurs; advantages include preservation of pituitary function; disadvantages include surgical risks and the need for lifelong glucocorticoid and mineralocorticoid replacement[18]

Ectopic tumor resection

Ectopic ACTH-producing tumors should be surgically resected when possible and may need to be followed with radiation or chemotherapy; if surgery is not possible, medications such as aminoglutethimide, metyrapone, and ketoconazole should be considered

Radiation

Pituitary irradiation is a treatment alternative when pituitary surgery is unsuccessful or not desired; therapeutic response, however, is slow; side effects include hypothalamic-pituitary dysfunction or panhypopituitarism; efficacy is related to dosage, and higher dosages increase the likelihood of side effects, including radiation necrosis of the brain

Medications

ACTH inhibitors

Cyproheptadine: Believed to exert an antiserotonin effect on hypothalamus; studies report successful treatment of symptoms in 60% of cases; symptoms usually recur when therapy is interrupted or discontinued; can be useful to treat metabolic imbalances while preparing for surgery, especially when impaired wound healing is anticipated from severe hypercortisolism[18]

Bromocryptine: A dopamine agonist commonly used to treat prolactinoma-secreting pituitary tumors; not usually effective in treating Cushing's disease

Sodium valproate: Suppresses ACTH secretion and lowers urinary free cortisol, 17-OH, and 17-KS levels; mechanism of action not known, but interference with ACTH response to CRH is suspected; not considered a standard treatment of Cushing's disease at this time

Adrenocortical inhibitors

Aminoglutethamide: An anticonvulsant that suppresses cortisol secretion by blocking conversion of cholesterol to 5-pregnenolone; particularly useful to treat cortisol-secreting adrenocortical carcinoma; not an effective treatment for Cushing's syndrome; side effects include nausea, vomiting, sedation, blurred vision, skin rash, headaches, and hypothyroidism

Metyrapone: Adrenal blockade decreases production of cortisol; side effects include hypertension and hypokalemic alkalosis, hirsutism, nausea, vomiting, dizziness
Ketaconazole: Inhibits adrenal and gonadal steroidogenesis; side effects include nausea, vomiting, abdominal pain, pruritus, and hepatoxicity
Trilostane: Decreases cortisol synthesis by blocking conversion of pregnenolone to progesterone; results in decreased production of cortisol and aldosterone
Mitotane: Inhibits biosynthesis of cortisol and chemically destroys adrenal cells secreting cortisol; can be combined with radiation therapy if surgery is not possible
RU-486 (mifepristone): A glucocorticoid antagonist effective in treating autonomous cortisol production, but as a receptor blockade, it can increase ACTH secretion, thus counteracting its antiglucocorticoid effect; it is well tolerated, but remains investigational

NURSING CARE

NURSING ASSESSMENT

Circulation: Mild to moderate hypertension; blood vessel fragility: plethora and easy bruising
Food and fluid needs: Moderate weight gain; fat distribution: truncal obesity, supraclavicular fat pads, buffalo hump, moon facies; hyperglycemia; increased appetite; daily weight
Elimination: Glycosuria, proteinuria, hypercalciuria, renal calculi
Neurologic concerns: Impaired memory, impaired concentration, impaired cognitive function, exophthalmos
Musculoskeletal concerns: Fatigue; muscle weakness: inability to rise from squat position; muscle wasting in extremities; activity intolerance; pathologic fractures; osteoporosis
Comfort and pain: Back pain, rib pain
Skin care: Blood vessel fragility: plethora and easy bruising; thin, translucent skin; hyperpigmentation; poor wound healing; hirsutism; abdominal striae; acne; thinning of scalp hair
Psychobehavioral concerns: Body image disturbance; irritability; emotional lability; anxiety, panic; paranoia; depression; insomnia (sleep pattern history); feelings of loss of control of body, powerlessness; current stressors of daily life; suicidal nature
Reproductive concerns: Amenorrhea, hirsutism (women), decreased libido, impotence

POTENTIAL COMPLICATIONS

Pressure ulcers, leg ulcers, severe obesity, severe depression, suicide

PATIENT PROBLEMS/NURSING DIAGNOSES & INTERVENTIONS

NIC NUTRITION SUPPORT

Imbalanced nutrition: more than body requirements, related to excessive intake greater than metabolic need (state of hypercortisolism causes increased hunger, increased propensity to gain weight, and central obesity)

- Relate changes in patient's appearance to onset of disease (compare old photographs with development of symptoms).
- Monitor patient's compliance to caloric restrictions.
- Encourage high-protein diet.
- Record patient's urine chemistry *to monitor metabolic balance.*

NIC ACTIVITY AND EXERCISE MANAGEMENT

Activity intolerance; generalized weakness related to muscle atrophy

- Identify patient's priorities for energy expenditures.
- Plan activity and rest periods with patient *to maximize energy and minimize fatigue.*
- Discuss limitations with patient.

NIC SKIN/WOUND MANAGEMENT

Impaired skin integrity related to altered metabolic and nutritional status

- Instruct patient concerning good skin hygiene.
  Wash and dry thoroughly.
  Use lotions as needed.
  Use antifungal cream as needed.
  Perform aseptic care to minor lacerations and abrasions.
- Provide adequate pressure to venipuncture sites *to prevent subcutaneous hematoma after using pediatric-size venipuncture needles.*
- Instruct patient to use caution during activities *to avoid minor bumps and trauma.*
- Keep patient's room clear of obstructions (e.g., excess furniture).
- Instruct patient in the use of protective clothing, especially shoes and socks, *to prevent trauma.*

NIC COPING ASSISTANCE

Risk for ineffective coping
Risk for violence: self-directed; related to depression (chemical) induced by hypercortisolism (see Chapter 19, pp. 1284-1287)
Disturbed body image related to biophysical changes (central obesity), moon facies, hirsuitism, facial plethora

- Assess degree of body image change since onset of disease *to determine what aspects of body image change are related to disease onset.*
- Discuss cushingoid features of the disorder with patient; give emotional support.
- Discuss palliative treatment for hirsutism (i.e., shaving or depilatories).
- Remind patient that symptoms are related to hypercortisolism and will resolve with treatment.
- Assess patient's emotional factors related to disorder.
- Reassess patient's current stressors as well as his or her effective and ineffective coping mechanisms.
- Give patient emotional support.
- Identify patient's sources of irritability and depression.
- Assist patient with problem solving *to minimize anxiety and frustration.*

- Collaborate with mental health nursing specialist or psychiatrist.
- Explain effect of hypercortisolism on cognitive function and memory.
- Assess presence of depression and suicidal ideation/intent.
- Establish supportive relationship *to demonstrate concern and caring.*
- Maintain close observation.
- Explain the relationship between depression and hypercortisolism, and that controlling disease state will also treat depression.

NIC Self-Care Facilitation

Disturbed sleep pattern related to elevated serum cortisol levels

- Assess current sleep patterns and identify patient's coping mechanisms.
- Discuss possible alternative measures that will help patient sleep better.

Patient Education/Continuum of Care Plan

1. Ensure that patient verbalizes the importance of taking medication and knows to report side or toxic effects.
2. Discuss with patient the importance of regular, lifelong medical follow-up.
3. Discuss with patient the importance of wearing or carrying medical alert information.
4. Discuss with family the relationship between depression and hypercortisolism and the need for observation before treatment.

Evaluation/Patient Outcomes

Nutrition Support: Nutrition is adequate. Weight is proportional to height and stature. Urine chemistry levels are within normal limits. Blood sugar level is within normal limits. Patient verbalizes use of appropriate dietary regimen.

Activity and Exercise Management: Activity tolerance increases. Patient maintains maximum activity levels for physical limitations. Patient verbalizes realistic plan for alternating activities and rest based on limitations. Patient participates in recreational activities.

Skin/Wound Management: Skin is intact. Patient shows no breaks, cracks, ulcers, or ecchymosis. There is no infection. Patient's wound healing is normal. Patient verbalizes a method for maintaining hygiene.

Coping Assistance: Patient's self-concept improves. Patient uses realistic self-care methods to enhance physical features. Patient is not preoccupied with negative aspects of physical appearance. Patient participates in age-related activities and groups. Patient maintains peer relationships. Patient expresses realistic expectations concerning physical abilities and appearance. Patient demonstrates increased problem-solving ability with assistance from others. Patient functions at maximum level of independence based on limitations.

Self-Care Facilitation: Patient's sleep patterns improve and patient verbalizes that he or she is sleeping better.

Pheochromocytoma

A pheochromocytoma is a tumor of the chromaffin cells of the adrenal medulla that produces excessive amounts of the catecholamines epinephrine and norepinephrine.

The incidence of pheochromocytoma is rare. Less than 0.5% of all patients with a recent diagnosis of hypertension have pheochromocytoma. The disorder is slightly more common in females, but has no age predominance. Tumors in children are usually associated with a familial tendency, are frequently bilateral, and are often malignant. Ninety percent of pheochromocytomas are sporadic; 10% are familial, inherited as an autosomal dominant trait. They are treatable when diagnosed, but if left untreated can be fatal. Pheochromocytomas are often linked with medullary carcinoma of the thyroid and multiple neoplasias (MEN II syndromes).[18]

Pathophysiology[8,59]

Ninety percent of pheochromocytomas are found in the adrenal medulla. The remainder are extraadrenal and are classified as paragangliomas; they usually are found in the abdomen. Most range in size from 3 to 5 cm. Multiple pheochromocytomas occur in approximately 20% of cases and often occur in patients possessing the inherited trait. Pheochromocytomas can occur in pregnancy and lead to increased morbidity and mortality for mother and fetus. Malignant pheochromocytomas are rare and occur in 5% of patients.

Pheochromocytomas can vary in clinical presentation from no symptoms to sudden heart attack, cerebral hemorrhage, or malignant hypertension. The hallmark sign is hypertension, occurring in 90% of patients. Hypertension is paroxysmal and characterized by a sudden and severe increase in blood pressure accompanied by a pounding headache, profuse sweating, palpitations, anxiety, pallor, nausea and possible vomiting, and abdominal or chest pain. Episodes can be spontaneous or induced by exercise, bending over, urination, defecation, abdominal pressure, or medications, but not usually by mental stress. Many patients are asymptomatic or experience only mild symptoms. A majority of pheochromocytomas are diagnosed during autopsy.

Pheochromocytomas produce excessive amounts of epinephrine and norepinephrine; however, norepinephrine is more prevalent and is responsible for most of the clinical manifestations. Norepinephrine, an alpha-adrenergic agonist, primarily causes the hypertensive effects of the disorder and is the principal hormone seen in extraadrenal tumors. Epinephrine, a beta-adrenergic agonist, is responsible for the hypertensive as well as the hypermetabolic and hyperglycemic effects of the disorder.

Overproduction of norepinephrine causes paroxysmal hypertension, the most outstanding clinical sign. Excess epinephrine production can also bring about hypertension and postural hypotension. Blood pressure measurements can range from 200 to 300/150 to 175 mm Hg. Patients may have widely fluctuating blood pressures with or without paroxysmal hypertensive episodes. Hypertensive episodes can be provoked by stimuli such as palpation of the tumor, emotional stress, or increased abdominal pressure (i.e., micturition). Extreme cases of hypertension may lead to cerebrovascular accidents that can be life threatening. Nephrosclerosis and retinopathy may accompany severe sustained hypertension. Myocarditis, dysrhythmias, and congestive heart failure are seen in patients who develop cardiomyopathies related to the direct effect of high levels of catecholamines on the myocardium.

Elevated levels of circulating epinephrine and norepinephrine can create a state of hypermetabolism similar to thyrotoxicosis. The patient can have tachycardia, tachyarrhythmias, weight loss, heat intolerance, tremors, and hyperreflexia. Sympathetic overstimulation can give rise to apprehension and emotional instability. Catecholamines suppress insulin secretion and stimulate the conversion of glycogen to glucose in the liver, resulting in hyperglycemia and glycosuria.

Diagnostic Studies and Findings

Pheochromocytoma must be distinguished from essential hypertension, anxiety or panic attacks (blood pressure does not significantly increase), drug-induced states (amphetamines, cocaine, PCP, LSD, cold preparations, and diet aids containing phenylpropanolamine [PPA]), myocardial infarction, or factitious administration of catecholamines.[8,18] The diagnosis can be made on the basis of a 24-hour urine collection.[59]

Urine tests: 24-hour collections (during hypertension) for free catecholamines or their metabolites, metanephrines and vanillylmandelic acid (VMA); refrigeration not necessary, but strong acid additive (20 ml 6N HCl) is required; the diagnosis of pheochromocytoma can be made on the basis of a 24-hour urine collection

Endocrine testing: Suppression tests—*clonidine:* obtain baseline catecholamine levels; administer oral clonidine (0.3 mg/70 kg body weight); repeat blood sampling after 3 hours; normal response (and patients with essential hypertension): decreased catecholamines (into normal range or by 50%); pheochromocytoma: increased or same

Provocative tests (rarely done, potentially hazardous): *Glucagon:* obtain baseline catecholamine levels; administer 1.0 mg IV bolus of glucagon; repeat blood sampling 2 minutes later; monitor blood pressure and heart rate every 60 seconds; phentolamine (5 mg IV bolus) must be on hand for treatment of severe hypertension; pheochromocytoma is indicated if catecholamine levels triple[18]

Imaging

Metaiodobenzylguanidine (MIBG) scan: Tumor uptake for localization of extraadrenal tumors; effective, but expensive

Adrenal CT scan: Tumor localization

MRI scan: Tumor localization

Ultrasonography: After localized, to determine attachment to nearby organs (liver or kidney)

Positron emission tomography (PET) scan: Localization of tumor

Multidisciplinary Plan

Surgery

Preoperative blockade with 7 to 10 days of phenoxybenzamine; dosage begins at 10 mg bid and increases to 0.5 to 1.0 mg/kg daily

Excision of pheochromocytoma

Medications[18]

Alpha-adrenergic blocking agents: Used to lower atrial pressure and to increase vascular volume

Phentolamine (Regitine), 0.5-5.0 mg IV and/or by continuous infusion at rate of 0.25 to 1.0 mg/min; short acting (carefully monitor blood pressure)

Phenoxybenzamine (Debenzyline), 10-60 mg/day PO; long acting

Prazosin (Minipress), 2.0-5.0 mg, 2 or 3 times a day

Beta-adrenergic blocking agents*: Propranolol (Inderal), 40 mg/day PO; used for tumors that secrete epinephrine, which causes tachycardia and dysrhythmias

Tyrosine inhibitors: Metyrosine (Demser), 250 mg orally q6-8h up to 4 g/day; interferes with catecholamine synthesis and decreases the amount of circulating catecholamines; useful before and during surgery; causes sedation and reversible extrapyramidal signs in elderly patients; can cause frightening dreams

NURSING CARE

Nursing Assessment

Circulation: Increased heart rate, palpitations, postural hypotension, sustained hypertension (one third of patients), paroxysmal hypertension (two thirds of patients), frequent vital sign checks

Food and fluid needs: Nausea, vomiting (possible)

Neurosensory concerns: Nervousness, flushing sensation

Comfort and pain: Headache (severe), abdominal or chest pain

Psychosocial concerns: Anxiety, sense of impending doom, coping skills

Hygiene and skin care: Profuse sweating (excessive and inappropriate), pallor

Potential Complications

Hypertensive crisis

Patient Problems/Nursing Diagnoses & Interventions

NIC Tissue Perfusion Management

Ineffective tissue perfusion (total body) related to hypervolemia from excess catecholamines

- Monitor patient's blood pressure and pulse (use same arm and position; routinely take measurements with patient lying and either sitting or standing).

*Beta-adrenergic blocking agents should be added only after *alpha* blockade has been achieved. Beta-adrenergic blockade alone may exacerbate hypertension.

- In hypertensive crisis:
  - Notify physician.
  - Have emergency cardiac drugs available (phentolamine, calcium channel blockers).
  - Monitor patient's neurologic status frequently.
  - Monitor patient's blood pressure and pulse electronically *to detect acute cardiovascular and neurologic changes.*
- Perform actions that minimize episode occurrence.
  - Do not palpate abdomen.
  - Assist patient to avoid constrictive clothing.
  - Elevate head of bed.
  - Restrict activity.
  - Do not allow smoking.
  - Eliminate patient's intake of beverages with caffeine.
  - Assist patient to avoid Valsalva's maneuver or straining at stools.
  - Monitor frequency of episodes.
  - Identify factor(s) that initiate an episode: coughing, micturition, any abdominal stimulation.

NIC Coping Assistance

Ineffective coping related to situational crisis

- Assess patient's coping skills (especially ability to tolerate episodic illness), support system, and adaptive skills that have been successful in the past.
- Collaborate with mental health nurse, specialist, or psychiatrist as necessary.
- Provide patient with opportunities to verbalize concerns and fears.
- Involve patient in plan of care *to decrease sources of feelings of powerlessness or loss of control.*

NIC Physical Comfort Promotion

Chronic pain related to sudden change in volume status

- Do not give patient pain medications; *may exacerbate episode.*
- Use supportive measures: dark room, cool cloth.
- Monitor patient's vital signs.
- Monitor duration of pain and relation to episodes.

Patient Education/Continuum of Care Plan

1. Ensure that patient verbalizes understanding of medication name, action, schedule, dose, and side effects.
2. Discuss with patient the importance of regular visits to physician and the need for lifelong follow-up.
3. Discuss with patient the need to carry or wear medical alert information.
4. Demonstrate to patient how to measure and record blood pressure at home.
5. Ensure that patient verbalizes understanding of episode stimulators and how to reduce or eliminate them.
6. Assist patient to identify support person(s).

Evaluation/Patient Outcomes

Tissue Perfusion Management: Tissue perfusion is normal. Blood pressure and pulse are within normal range, both lying and standing or sitting. There are no paresthesias, tremors, or palpitations.

Coping Assistance: Patient copes effectively. Patient identifies strengths and uses them in activities of daily living (ADLs). Patient verbalizes ability to manage stressful situations or decrease their frequency. Patient maintains relationships with family and contemporaries. Patient participates in independent self-care.

Physical Comfort Promotion: Pain tolerance is improved. Patient is able to tolerate pain without medications.

DISORDERS OF THE PITUITARY GLAND

Pituitary Tumors

Hypothalamic pituitary lesions have various manifestations, including pituitary hormone hypersecretion and hyposecretion, sellar enlargement, and visual loss. The approach to evaluation should be designed to ensure early diagnosis when the lesions are amenable to therapy.

Pituitary tumors are seldom malignant and seldom metastasize.[39] They are, however, the most common cause of pituitary hormone hypersecretion and hyposecretion syndromes in the adult.[38,50] Other problems they cause are related to their space-occupying effects and loss of function of the remaining gland.

Because the pituitary is a small endocrine gland (approximately 0.6 g) located adjacent to several vascular and neurologic structures, pathologic processes may have significant endocrinologic impact and/or mass effects, as briefly mentioned already. Although headaches and visual field defects are usually the first clinically evident symptoms, cranial nerve (III, IV, and VI) compression, bone erosions, and hormone hyposecretion are other signs commonly seen in patients harboring pituitary masses. Associated endocrinopathies vary according to the hormone produced by the adenoma.

Pituitary tumors represent at least 15% of operated intracranial tumors.[58] The true incidence of pituitary disease is probably higher, since studies using unselected adult autopsy material showed that pituitary tumors are incidentally identified in approximately 20% of men and women dying of different nonendocrine diseases.[12] Pituitary tumors are diagnosed more often in women, especially those of childbearing age, but autopsy results reveal an equal distribution between men and women. Prevalence increases with age, peak incidence being between ages 30 and 60 years. Rarely is the diagnosis made before puberty.[8] A hereditary predisposition exists for pituitary tumors; they can be part of the familial multiple endocrine neoplasia syndromes. Onset of disease can be slow and insidious, making diagnosis difficult.

The predominant focus to date has been on the major advances in both surgical and medical management of these patients, who often remain dependent on the exogenous administration of hormones to maintain equilibrium of their internal milieu. Yet many patients with pituitary disease experience problems with their day-to-day functioning that is more related to the impact that their pituitary disease has on their emotional, social, and family well-being. Many of these patients are devastated by the effects that their disease has on their mood, behavior, and interaction with family and society. Research efforts continue to improve our understanding of the hypothalamic–pituitary–target organ interaction.

PATHOPHYSIOLOGY

The origin of pituitary tumors is not fully understood. Two theories exist: some suspect that pituitary tumors result from hypothalamic dysfunction, while others believe tumors arise from an intrinsic pituitary defect. Almost all secreting pituitary tumors are monoclonal. Approximately 90% of pituitary tumors secrete one or more of the anterior pituitary hormones and can be classified functionally according to the hormone that is hypersecreted (Table 11-7). Most secreting tumors are prolactinomas (60%); GH-secreting (20%) and ACTH cell tumors (15%) comprise the rest of these tumors. Hypersecretion of TSH and the gonadotropins is unusual. One third of all pituitary tumors are nonfunctioning and yet usually large and do not produce a distinct hypersecretory syndrome.[38,50]

It has long been known that signs and symptoms of patients with pituitary tumor depend primarily on the size of the lesion and the state of endocrine function. In his landmark monograph, *The Pituitary Body and its Disorders,* published in 1912, Cushing formulated a provisional classification of these tumors into groups on the basis of the degree of neighborhood neurologic involvement and the presentation of endocrine glandular dysfunction. In essence, symptoms and signs are related to the compression of adjacent neural structures as the tumor expands from the confines of the pituitary fossa and/or endocrinopathy.[25]

Tumors are loosely classified by size: a microadenoma is less than 1 cm in diameter and has manifestations of hormonal excess without sellar enlargement or extension; a macroadenoma is greater than 1 cm in diameter and causes generalized sellar enlargement. Pituitary tumors that grow beyond the small, confined area of the sella turcica can impinge on or expand into surrounding structures and produce significant signs and symptoms. Macroadenomas by extracellular growth produce regional signs and symptoms in accordance with their particular direction of growth. Depending on location, macroadenomas arising from or adjacent to the pituitary gland may produce visual signs and/or symptoms, including optic atrophy, central visual loss, visual field defects, and nerve palsies. As diagnostic techniques have become more sophisticated, many tumors are diagnosed before visual symptoms appear. Nevertheless, ocular findings may still be the presenting or dominant sign of pituitary tumors.

Other structures that can be affected by large tumors include the bony sella turcica and the hypothalamus. Headache is not an uncommon symptom with relatively small pituitary tumors. However, with larger tumors the mechanism of headache is clearly the result of distention of surrounding, pain-sensitive structures.[25] Bailey[7] observed that in some patients, headaches that were present for some time suddenly ceased coincident with the development of visual difficulty. This train of events was attributed to rupture of the surrounding areas by the expanding tumor. Headaches seem to have no specific characteristics or localizing value, and although they are mostly supraorbital, they may be retroorbital, temporal, occipital, or even generalized in distribution.[25] Macroadenomas can further cause varying degrees of hypopituitarism (pituitary gland failure) as they impinge on normal pituitary tissue. Hypothalamic involvement can cause disturbances in temperature regulation, appetite, thirst, sleep, and behavior.

Aside from tumor size, the other factor that affects pathophysiology is the hormone secreted by the tumor and the varying degrees of clinical manifestations. Prolactin (PRL) hypersecretion is the most common pituitary hormone hypersecretion syndrome in both males and females. The primary physiologic actions of PRL are preparation of the breasts for lactation and stimulation of milk production postpartum. Hyperprolactinemic women and men present not only with galactorrhea but also with gonadal dysfunction, including amenorrhea, infertility, decreased libido, or impotence. Although the sex distribution of prolactinomas is approximately equal, microadenomas are much more common in females, presumably because of earlier recognition of the endocrine consequences of PRL excess.

Direct measurement of PRL can adequately diagnose this type of pituitary tumor. Dynamic testing is not indicated in the evaluation of PRL excess. However, it is recommended that multiple (at least three) measurements be drawn because of the pulsatile nature of PRL secretion. Because PRL may be increased by stress, inserting an intravenous catheter at least 30 minutes before sampling and encouraging bed rest and decreased stimulation can help avoid false-positive results caused by the stressors. The primary treatment for a prolactinoma is administration of a dopamine agonist such as bromocriptine. Bromocriptine directly inhibits PRL secretion by the tumor. Pergolide has been shown to reduce hypersecretion and shrink most PRL-secreting macroadenomas. With its dopaminergic properties, it is longer acting. Transphenoidal surgery may also be used, but a purely surgical cure for a prolactinoma is difficult to achieve. Radiotherapy can be used if all else fails.

GH is well-named because its primary function is the promotion of normal linear growth. In addition to its growth action on bone and soft tissues, GH affects protein, carbohydrate, and fat metabolism. GH-secreting tumors cause the syndrome called acromegaly in adults and gigantism in children and adolescence. The prevalence of acromegaly is five or six cases per 100,000 population, so even though it is the second most common disorder of pituitary overproduction, it is still relatively rare.[39] Acromegaly derives its name from the acral segments, which include the feet, hands, nose, chin, and forehead. Acral

Table 11-7 Incidence of Pituitary Tumors by Type

Type	Incidence
GH adenomas	17%
Prolactin PRL adenomas	30%
GH and PRL adenomas	10%
Corticotropin ACTH adenomas	14%
Gonadotropin GNRH adenomas	2%
Other (null cell, oncocytoma, unclassified)	25%

and soft tissue overgrowth is the hallmark of this disorder. This is usually accompanied by increased sweating, heat intolerance, oiliness of the skin, fatigue, and weight gain. Often a history of increased hand, feet, and heel pad thickness, with increased shoe, collar, shirt, hat, glove, and ring size, and a bulky handshake suggest the diagnosis. There is a generalized thickening of the skin, with increased oiliness and sweating. Acne, sebaceous cysts, and skin tags are not uncommon. These changes occur insidiously over many years, so patients and family often do not notice them. Skeleton overgrowth leads to mandibular enlargement with wide spacing of the teeth and frontal (skull) bossing. Linear growth does not occur because of prior fusion of the epiphysis of long bones.

These bony and soft tissue changes are accompanied by systemic manifestations, which include heat intolerance, fatigue, lethargy, and increased sleep requirement. Moderate weight gain usually occurs. Bone and cartilage overgrowth leads to arthralgias and, in long-standing cases, to degenerative arthritis of the spine, hips, and knees. Photophobia of unknown cause occurs in about half of cases and is most troublesome in bright sunlight and during night driving. Cardiovascular disease occurs in about a third of patients and consists of hypertension, coronary heart disease, cardiac enlargement, and cardiomyopathy with arrhythymias. Upper airway obstruction with sleep apnea occurs in about 60% of patients. Other endocrine and metabolic abnormalities are common, namely, glucose intolerance and hyperinsulinism caused by GH-induced resistance. Increased overall mortality, about threefold higher in men, has been reported as a result of cardiovascular and cerebrovascular disorders, malignancy, and respiratory disease.[38] Survival of these patients is reduced by an average of 10 years compared with the nonacromegalic population. Acromegaly increases the risk of malignancy and tissue polyps, most commonly colonic, gastric, and esophageal.

A random GH level is not an absolute criterion for the diagnosis or exclusion of acromegaly. This is because secretion remains episodic, with the number, duration, and amplitude of secretory episodes occurring randomly throughout a 24-hour period. An oral glucose tolerance test is the simplest and most specific dynamic test for acromegaly. Oral glucose load (50 to 100 g) normally suppresses GH levels to at least less than 1 μg/L within 1 to 2 hours, but acromegalic patients do not exhibit this suppression, and 20% of patients have a paradoxical rise.[38] This lack of response establishes the diagnosis. Serum IGF-I levels are elevated in virtually all patients with acromegaly and correlate better with the disease activity than single random GH measurements. Thus single elevated IGF-1 levels are highly specific for diagnosing acromegaly. Plain films show sellar enlargement in 90% of cases. Treatments for these patients include tumor resection. If surgery fails, medical management with the long-acting somatostatin analog octreotide should be initiated. This drug, administered subcutaneously in three daily injections, normalizes GH in half of acromegalic patients. Significant tumor shrinkage and normalization of IGF-1 occurs in up to 50% of patients. Sellar radiotherapy is selected only if medical therapy does not achieve biochemical remission. However, the slow rate of response and the high rate of late hypopituitarism are major disadvantages.

Pituitary ACTH hypersecretion causes the adrenal gland to secrete excess glucocorticoids (cortisol) and androgens (sex hormones). The resulting syndrome is called Cushing's disease. These patients typically are obese (with predominantly central fat distribution) and have hypertension, glucose intolerance or diabetes, and gonadal dysfunction (amenorrhea and impotence). The onset of these features is usually insidious, developing over months or years. Other common manifestations include purple abdominal striae, plethoric moon facies, signs of hyperandrogenism (hirsutism and acne), osteoporosis, and proximal muscle weakness. Psychologic disturbances, specifically, depression, can also be associated with Cushing's disease.

ACTH-secreting tumors are usually microadenomas and are much more common in women (female-to-male ratio 8:1), with a usual age range of 20 to 40 years.[39] The major challenge with diagnosing this syndrome is the differential diagnosis of ACTH-secreting pituitary tumor (Cushing's disease) from other causes of Cushing's syndrome, such as cortisol-secreting adrenal tumors and ectopic ACTH-secreting tumors. The diagnosis of Cushing's disease is established on biochemical documentation of endogenous hypercortisolism: serum and/or 24-hour urinary free cortisol, 1 mg overnight dexamethasone suppression test (cortisol levels fail to suppress), measurement of basal plasma ACTH levels, and inferior petrosal sinus sampling to detect a central to peripheral gradient of ACTH levels. Transphenoidal surgery is the procedure of choice in the management of ACTH-secreting pituitary tumors. Cases not controlled by surgery are referred for pituitary irradiation, which may cure up to 15% of patients after several years.[38,50] Irradiation may be combined with medical treatment to achieve early biochemical remission of hypercortisolism even before the effects of irradiation become established. Pharmocotherapeutic developments of effective cortisol-lowering agents, such as mitotane, ketoconazole, and aminoglutethimide, have significantly decreased the need for bilateral adrenalectomy, a procedure associated with morbidity, permanent hormone replacement, and subsequent risk for developing Nelson's syndrome. Nelson's syndrome is characterized by hyperpigmentation and is caused by excessive production of ACTH and MSH by a pituitary tumor. It is believed that this adenoma is the original cause of Cushing's disease and that it enlarges after adrenalectomy because of a lack of negative feedback, thereby increasing ACTH and MSH production.

Diagnostic Studies and Findings

Endocrine tests: Laboratory evaluations are critical. Tests can be performed under random or basal conditions. Assays of hormones in serum or urine can provide an indication of hormone levels at the time. Provocative challenge can demonstrate the inability to suppress or stimulate hormone secretion. In general, the diagnosis of pituitary hormone excess requires failure of suppression by peripheral hormones, whereas the diagnosis of hormone deficiency rests on an adequate rise during provocative testing.

Physical examination: Many manifestations of pituitary tumors frequently result from nonendocrine or unknown causes, which include tiredness, weakness, headache, anorexia, depression, and weight gain or loss, to name a few. Ophthalmologic examination includes visual acuity changes, such as blurring and diplopia, and visual field deficits. Neurologic examination for cranial nerve deficits associated with cranial nerves III, IV, and VI should also be assessed. These three cranial nerves are evaluated together because they control extraocular movements of the eyes. Testing cranial nerve V can be included by evaluating facial sensation, corneal reflex, and ability to chew food.

Imaging studies: Radiologic studies have gained increasing usage in the diagnosis and post test of pituitary adenoma. MRI scanning is the preferred method for localizing pituitary tumors. It has superseded the use of computed tomography (CT) scanning, since it allows better definition of normal structures and has better resolution in defining tumors.

MULTIDISCIPLINARY PLAN

Surgery

The past two decades have seen remarkable advances in the surgical management of pituitary adenomas with the development of refined transsphenoidal microsurgical techniques for resection of endocrine-active intrasellar microadenomas. Nevertheless, adenomas with major extrasellar extension still occur with significant frequency in contemporary neurosurgical practice, and most of these larger tumors are successfully treated by the transphenoidal route. Full appreciation of the variations in the neurological signs and symptoms seen with these larger pituitary tumors is essential for sound surgical planning in terms of probable direction of extrasellar growth and involvement of neighboring structures.

Medications

Hormone replacement therapy (thyroid, cortisone, estrogen, testosterone) following surgery and/or radiation is needed to treat any deficiencies. Dopamine agonists (Bromocriptine mesylate or Parlodel and cabergoline) should be the initial therapy for patients with prolactinomas whether microadenoma or macroadenoma; usual dosage is 2.5 to 10 mg/day for prolactinomas. These agonists are also useful for treating GH-secreting ademonas and require much higher doses, with the upper limit usually determined by patient tolerance. Common side effects include nausea and vomiting. As mentioned, octreotide (Sandostatin) is a somatostatin analog used to treat acromegaly. Subcutaneous injections of 50 to 150 ug are administered three times a day.

Radiation

Radiation therapy, formerly the initial treatment for pituitary tumors, has been replaced by microsurgical tumor removal and medications as preferred treatments of choice. However it is still used (1) following incomplete tumor resection, (2) for patients with persisting hypersecretion who have not responded to attempts to control their pituitary tumors with surgery or medications, (3) in conjunction with medication therapy, or (4) for patients who are not surgical candidates. Side effects may include panhypopituitarism and damage to optic chiasm or optic nerves and cranial nerves, resulting in visual deficits, cerebral ischemia, seizures, and development of malignancy.

NURSING CARE

NURSING ASSESSMENT

Macroadenomas

Sensory and vision concerns: Bitemporal hemianopsia, superior or bitemporal field defects, loss of red perception, decreased acuity, scotoma, papilledema, blindness

Neurologic concerns: Chronic headaches, intermittent or persistent, of moderate intensity and variably located; can be accompanied by nausea and vomiting; pain; fatigue; muscle weakness; possible neurologic changes, particularly those involving cranial nerves III, IV, V, VI (unequal pupil size, inappropriate reaction to light)

Endocrine concerns: Signs and symptoms of hypofunction (in regard to hormones other than those produced by the tumor)

Growth Hormone–Secreting Tumors (Acromegaly)

Musculoskeletal concerns: Coarse facial features (thick ears, nose); prognathism causing chewing difficulties; thick fingers and toes with concomitant increase in shoe or glove size; atrophied skeletal muscle; laryngeal hypertrophy causing voice to deepen; arthritis, arthralgia, backaches; osteoporosis; mobility difficulties related to pain, fatigue

Hygiene and skin care: Oily skin, acne, diaphoresis

Psychosocial concerns: Irritability, hostility, and other psychologic manifestations; body image disturbance; difficulty with social interactions, including sex partner and family (acting fearful, hostile, withdrawn); incongruity between self-concept and current self-image

Prolactin-Secreting Tumors

Gynecologic concerns: Galactorrhea involving one or both breasts, irregular menses, oligomenorrhea or amenorrhea, infertility

Androgenic concerns: Decreased libido, impotence, gynecomastia

Psychosocial concerns: Anxiety about fertility, sexual performance, and self-image

TSH-secreting tumors (see discussion of hyperthyroidism)

ACTH-secreting tumors (see discussion of Cushing's disease)

POTENTIAL COMPLICATIONS

Blindness, infertility

PATIENT PROBLEMS/NURSING DIAGNOSES & INTERVENTIONS

NIC PHYSICAL COMFORT PROMOTION

Pain related to physical factors of excess hormones or tumor compression

- Monitor type, location, intensity, and frequency of patient's pain. Inquire about successful and unsuccessful measures patient used in the past to control pain.
- Monitor use and schedule of medications and other physical comfort measures: heat, cold, light massage.
- Discuss with patient factors that precipitate pain and restructure the environment accordingly to decrease or eliminate these factors.

- Assist patient to use relaxation techniques; deep breathing, selective focusing.
- Discuss with patient realistic expectations about pain control.

NIC Coping Assistance

Disturbed body image related to biophysical changes
- See pp. 1534-1535.

Sexual dysfunction related to altered libido, menstrual pattern, or fertility
- Establish trusting relationship with patient and sex partner.
- Encourage patient to verbalize feelings with both healthcare provider and sex partner.
- Instruct patient and sex partner regarding relationship between disease process and sexual dysfunction.
- Provide patient and sex partner with information about various methods to obtain sexual gratification *to maximize skills of sexual expression.*

NIC Psychologic Comfort Promotion

Anxiety related to change in health status
- Reassess patient's coping behaviors, stresses, and adaptive skills.
- Discuss with patient and family the relationship of psychologic manifestations to the disease process *to increase family understanding and support.*
- Encourage family to avoid blaming patient for inappropriate behavior.
- See also pp. 1531-1533.

NIC Activity and Exercise Management

Activity intolerance related to generalized weakness
- Monitor patient's current activity levels and priorities for activity performance.
- Thoroughly evaluate patient's abilities and limitations at home and in the community.
- Discuss with patient alternate ways of performing limited activities.
- Help patient structure time to allow for rest periods throughout the day, especially after activities.
- Encourage patient to set realistic goals and prioritize activities *to maximize patient satisfaction.*

Patient Education/Continuum of Care Plan

1. Discuss with patient methods for modifying pain control program for use at home: structuring a supportive physical environment and appropriate self-administration of analgesics.
2. Discuss with patient community mental health resources (support groups, individual therapists, and so forth).
3. Discuss with patient methods for modifying activity program for use at home.
4. Ensure that patient verbalizes understanding of medication administration and need for follow-up examinations.

Evaluation/Patient Outcomes

Physical Comfort Promotion: Comfort is increased. Patient verbalizes a decreased frequency and amount of pain. Patient verbalizes pain-precipitating factors and means of decreasing or eliminating these factors. Patient demonstrates relaxation techniques. Patient follows a pain control program.

Coping Assistance: Body image improves. Patient verbalizes acceptance of body changes. Patient maintains relationships with others. Behavior is appropriate during interactions. Patient maintains physical appearance appropriate to age. Patient verbalizes and expresses feelings and concerns about differences between ideal self and realistic self.

Sexual functioning improves. Patient verbalizes feelings about sexual dysfunction. Patient expresses an understanding of the relationship between prolactinoma and sexual dysfunction or infertility. Patient verbalizes improvement in sexual functioning.

Psychologic Comfort Promotion: Anxiety is decreased. Patient can identify results of ineffective coping mechanisms. Patient used strengths in planning home care. Patient discusses alternate home care methods and makes positive choices.

Activity and Exercise Management: Activity tolerance improves. Patient identifies increased number of activities performed independently. Patient demonstrates active range-of-motion exercises and performs these three times daily. Patient demonstrates an ability to structure day, including all ADLs and appropriate rest periods.

Diabetes Insipidus

Hypofunction of the posterior pituitary gland creates the condition of diabetes insipidus from the lack of sufficient antidiuretic hormone (ADH) to control fluid balance. True primary disease is rare, but diabetes insipidus is a common secondary problem with a pituitary tumor or after surgery or trauma. Diabetes insipidus can be a transient or permanent disturbance of water metabolism that results in the excretion of a large volume of dilute urine. It may be hypothalamic, nephrogenic, or psychogenic.

Hypothalamic (or central) diabetes insipidus results from failure of the posterior pituitary to secrete adequate quantities of ADH. Nephrogenic diabetes insipidus results from renal insensitivity to ADH, from chronic renal disease, from drugs that inhibit ADH action, or from congenital (hereditary) defects in the ADH receptor pathway. Water conservation in the distal collecting tubules cannot occur because ADH is either not present or inactive. Psychogenic diabetes insipidus, commonly referred to as polydipsia, occurs when there is a large fluid intake that suppresses ADH secretion. Treatment for hypothalamic diabetes insipidus is the administration of potent vasopressin analogs, whereas nephrogenic etiologies are confined to genetic counseling. The treatment for psychogenic polydipsia (compulsive water drinking) is psychiatric in nature.

Pathophysiology

The maintenance of water homeostasis is a function of the posterior pituitary gland and the kidney. ADH, secreted by the gland, allows the body to produce concentrated urine. It does this by encouraging the kidneys to reabsorb water from the tubular filtrate. Without ADH the filtrate travels rapidly through the renal tubules and collecting ducts with little or no water absorption. Diabetes insipidus occurs with an insufficient amount of ADH or the ADH that is produced functions inadequately. Without sufficient ADH to stimulate water reabsorption from the renal tubules, large amounts of urine are excreted daily (polyuria). In the absence of ADH, an average adult produces 10 to 12 L of dilute urine daily, having a specific gravity of 1.001 or less and a urine osmolality of 100 mOsm/kg. The blood becomes concentrated and serum osmolarity increases. Osmolarity measures the relationship between the particles and water in the body. Other classic symptoms include polydipsia, weight loss, weakness, dizziness, dry mucous membranes, fever, palpitations, and tachycardia. Urinary loss becomes pronounced, creating the potential for severe fluid and electrolyte imbalance, dehydration, hypovolemia, and vascular collapse.

Diagnostic Studies and Findings

Diabetes insipidus should be suspected whenever the clinical presentation comprises unexplained thirst, high fluid intake, large urine volumes, and dilute urine (urine osmolality less than plasma osmolality). The initial challenge is distinguishing both types of diabetes insipidus from psychogenic polydipsia.

Evaluation of suspected diabetes insipidus begins with taking serum and urine samples simultaneously for osmolality and sodium. The diagnostic triad of diabetes is an increased serum sodium level (greater than 147 mEq/L), a decreased urine specific gravity (usually 1.001 or less), and increased serum osmolality (greater than 300 mOsm/L). In addition, the urine osmolality is decreased, meaning it is less concentrated than serum. The next step in the diagnosis is the water deprivation test. This examines the effect of water deprivation on urine osmolality under supervision. The patient should be weighed and denied access to water (usually for 8 to 10 hours before and during the test) and each voided urine sample is measured for specific gravity or osmolality or both. The test is continued until urine osmolalities stabilize (an hourly increase of less than 30 mOsm/kg for 3 successive hours), or 5% of body weight has been lost. Once the diagnosis of diabetes insipidus is established, ADH is administered to distinguish nephrogenic disease from the hypothalamic (central) form. An increase in urine osmolality of 15% or greater suggests hypothalamic diabetes insipidus; 15% or less suggests nephrogenic diabetes insipidus.[18]

Multidisciplinary Plan

Medications

The treatment and drug of choice is desmopressin (DDAVP; synthetic arginine, vasopressin), 5-40 μg/day in 1-3 divided doses; administer intranasally (high in nose, not inhaled into throat); onset 1 h; duration of effect 8-20 h; drug of choice for chronic treatment because of its long duration and infrequent side effects. The frequency of administration varies, depending on severity of the diabetes insipidus. This agent provides excellent control of polyuria and polydipsia. It is recommended that serum osmolality and sodium be monitored regularly. For patients who cannot tolerate intranasal therapy, desmopressin can be given subcutaneously in single doses of 1-2 μg once or twice daily.

Lypressin nasal solution (Diapid Nasal Spray; synthetic lysine), 1-2 sprays in one or both nostrils qid; onset 1 h; duration 3-8 h (shorter-acting); may be used alone or in conjunction with vasopressin tannate; if patient has nasal congestion, there will be decreased absorption of drug; can be administered subcutaneously, usually in doses of 5-10 units

Vasopressin (Aqueous Pitressin), 2-5 U 2-4 times daily IM, SC or IV; duration of drug 2-8 h; used in acute settings or initial emergency treatment; for close monitoring during transient episodes; too short acting for chronic use

NURSING CARE

Nursing Assessment

Circulation: Hypotension, tachycardia, dizziness

Food and fluid needs

- Thirst: Polydipsia, unquenchable thirst, preference for cold or iced water
- Hydration status: Dry mouth, poor skin turgor, dry skin, weight loss, daily weights, soft eyes, hypotension, urine output greater than PO intake, weakness

Elimination

- Urinary function: Polyuria (output greater than 2.5 L/24 h 2 days with ad lib fluid intake)[18]; frequency; nocturia; low specific gravity (1.001 to 1.005); urine output
- Bowel function: Constipation

Patient Problems/Nursing Diagnoses & Interventions

NIC Electrolyte and Acid-Base Management

Deficient fluid volume related to output greater than intake from loss of ADH

- Treat dehydration as ordered.
- Measure urine output. With diabetes insipidus, urine output is usually greater than 4 L/day and may exceed 10 L/day if severe. Rule of thumb: Patient voiding more than 200 ml/h of dilute urine indicates presence of diabetes insipidus.
- Specific gravity measurement is not necessary because urine excretion rates of this magnitude can occur only with dilute urine except in case of diabetes mellitus.
- Measure urine glucose level to exclude diabetes mellitus as cause of polyuria ("insipidus" means tasteless, "mellitus" means sweet).
- Measure plasma osmolality. If thirst mechanism is normal, plasma osmolality will be in high normal range. If thirst mechanism is abnormal, plasma osmolality will be above normal.

Patient Education/Continuum of Care Plan

1. Demonstrate to patient how to measure and record intake and output.

2. Demonstrate to patient how to administer vasopressin; discuss with patient side or toxic effects to report to physician and parameters for as-needed administration based on output volume and characteristics.
3. Demonstrate to patient how to check urine's specific gravity.
4. Discuss with patient the importance of wearing a medical alert bracelet to identify disorder.

EVALUATION/PATIENT OUTCOMES

Electrolyte and Acid-Base Management: Hydration is adequate. Adequate hydration is evidenced by moist mucous membranes, good skin turgor, firm eyes, normal vital signs, stable weight, and intake approximate to output. Urine output is less than 4 L/day. Plasma osmolality is normal (285 to 290 mOsm/L).

SYNDROME OF INAPPROPRIATE ANTIDIURESIS

Excess secretion of the posterior pituitary gland hormone ADH creates the syndrome of inappropriate ADH (SIADH). This leads to the retention of free water and loss of electrolytes, particularly sodium. Some of the most common causes of SIADH include CNS disorders, such as head trauma, brain tumor, cerebrovascular accident, and Guillian-Barré syndrome. Another common cause is malignant lung disease, particularly bronchogenic carcinoma. The continual hormone release is unrelated to the normal feedback mechanism of serum osmolality. Water is retained, extracellular fluid volume expands, and dilutional hyponatremia occurs.

PATHOPHYSIOLOGY

SIADH occurs when the posterior pituitary gland releases an excessive amount of ADH. When this happens, water that should be excreted into the urine is reabsorbed into the blood. This causes the blood volume to expand. Furthermore, water retention causes increased glomerular filtration along with a loss of electrolytes (particularly sodium) in the urine. Therefore no edema occurs because of the ongoing sodium excretion. The expanded plasma volume depresses aldosterone production, which further increases urine sodium loss. The resultant decreased osmolality in the blood causes water to move into the cells, possibly leading to cerebral swelling and overhydration.

Individuals with SIADH have increased urine output with an increased concentration of urine. The patient also has signs and symptoms of low sodium level, including fatigue, headache, decreased level of consciousness, nausea, vomiting, and possibly seizures and coma. These signs and symptoms generally develop slowly and only become pronounced with sodium deficits of less than 120 mEq/L.

DIAGNOSTIC STUDIES AND FINDINGS

Decreased plasma sodium level (less than 126 mEq/L)
Increased urine specific gravity (over 1.020)
Decreased serum osmolality (less than 285 mOsm/L)
Other findings: Increased urine sodium level (greater than 200 mEq/L) and increased urine osmolality (typically greater than 500 mOsm/L, but varies according to fluid intake)

MULTIDISCIPLINARY PLAN

Medications

Diuretics

Furosemide (Lasix), 40-80 mg/day in divided doses or 20-40 mg/day IV with salt supplementation; with severe hyponatremia, hypertonic saline solution in combination with diuretic therapy is used
Demeclocycline, 600-1200 mg daily to block antidiuretic action of vasopressin
Lithium carbonate: Has similar effect, but therapeutic doses are so close to toxic dose that this drug is rarely useful
Phenytoin: May occasionally suppress abnormal vasopressin secretion from the pituitary
Hypertonic saline infusion: Must be used with extreme caution to treat hyponatremia and should be reserved for emergency situations such as stupor or marked confusion

General Management

Focus on restoring plasma sodium level

Water intake restricted to no more than 500-1000 ml/day, depending on severity of sodium deficit; oral salt intake increased if patient is able to take oral nutrients; this allows blood volume to drop slightly, which triggers aldosterone release; increased aldosterone release leads to sodium conservation

NURSING CARE

NURSING ASSESSMENT

Fluids and electrolytes: Euvolemia, decreased volume of urine, increased specific gravity of urine, increased weight, abdominal and muscle cramping
Neurologic concerns: Early sign: change in level of consciousness, confusion; disorientation, uncooperativeness; hostility; increased deep tendon reflexes; drowsiness; lethargy; headache; increased seizure potential
Gastrointestinal concerns: Anorexia; nausea and vomiting; diarrhea (from water intoxication); constipation (from fluid restriction and hyponatremia motility)
Psychosocial concerns: Anxiety, frustration, irritability, uncooperativeness, hostility

POTENTIAL COMPLICATIONS

Severe hyponatremia, mental stupor, coma/death

PATIENT PROBLEMS/NURSING DIAGNOSES & INTERVENTIONS

NIC ELECTROLYTE AND ACID-BASE MANAGEMENT

Excess fluid volume related to decreased urine output

- Monitor for signs and symptons of water intoxication: increased irritability, change in sensorium, headache, and hyperreflexia.

- Maintain strict fluid limitations, especially free water intake and output, *to prevent water intoxication.*
- Monitor weight daily *to assess for fluid retention.*
- Monitor patient and visitor compliance with fluid restrictions; provide thorough explanations for restricting fluids.
- Monitor environment *to control patient's access to fluids.*

NIC COGNITIVE THERAPY

Disturbed thought processes related to fluid excess

- Check orientation to time, place, and person *to assess for confusion and level of consciousness.*
- Set limits as necessary *to maintain stable and safe environment.*
- Reduce confusing environmental stimuli.
- Explain rationale for disturbances in thought processes to family members.

PATIENT EDUCATION/CONTINUUM OF CARE PLAN

1. Discuss with patient and family the rationale for fluid restrictions.
2. Discuss with patient and family the importance of measuring intake and output (I&O); demonstrate to patient how to do I&O measurements.

EVALUATION/PATIENT OUTCOMES

Electrolyte and Acid-Base Management: Fluid volume is normal. Intake is approximately equal to output. Specific gravity is within normal limits. Vital signs are within normal limits. Weight of patient is stable.

Cognitive Therapy: Thought processes are normal. Patient is oriented to time, place, and person. There is no injury to self, others, or property. Statements are reality oriented. Patient performs ADLs, within physical limitations, independently.

DISORDERS OF THE THYROID GLAND

THYROTOXICOSIS/ HYPERTHYROIDISM[31]

Thyrotoxicosis is the term used to mean the clinical syndrome that results when circulating concentrations of thyroxine (T_4) or triiodothyronine (T_3) are increased. Hyperthyroidism is the term used to mean sustained increases in thyroid hormone biosynthesis and release from the thyroid gland.[10] The terms are not directly interchangeable, although many patients have both.

PATHOPHYSIOLOGY

There are many causes of thyrotoxicosis with and without hyperthyroidism. Table 11-8 presents an outline of possible disorders, their incidence, and underlying causes. Also included is whether the disorder is thyrotoxicosis alone (T) or thyrotoxicosis accompanied by hyperthyroidism (T&H).

Graves' Disease

Graves' disease is the most common cause of thyrotoxicosis with or without hyperthyroidism. It occurs from two to ten times more frequently in women than in men.[8] Graves' disease is an autoimmune disorder in which TSH receptor antibodies bind to the TSH receptors in the thyroid gland. These antibodies mimic pituitary TSH, causing an increase in thyroid hormone synthesis and release that is unresponsive to the normal negative feedback signals. The receptor antibodies are from two families of immunoglobulins called thyroid-stimulating immunoglobulins (TSIs) or thyroid binding–inhibiting immunoglobulins (TBIIs), both of which can be measured in serum. There is a genetic preponderance for the development of Graves' disease, although it is unknown what specifically triggers the production of the antibodies. The genetic linkage may be with other autoimmune thyroid disorders such as Hashimoto's thyroiditis, which is an underlying cause of hypothyroidism, or it may be with other systemic autoimmune disorders such as rheumatoid arthritis, pernicious anemia, or lupus. TSH stimulates growth as well as hormone synthesis, resulting in a diffusely enlarged thyroid gland (diffuse toxic goiter) with increased vascularity.

TSIs also have the ability to attach to TSH receptors outside of the thyroid gland and are the presumed causative agent for Graves' ophthalmopathy, which has been partially defined as T-lymphocyte infiltration and fibroblast proliferation of orbital connective tissue leading to edema and enlargement of eye muscles. Graves' ophthalmopathy can occur with or without hyperthyroidism. Infiltrative dermopathy, called pretibial myxedema, has also been described, but seems to occur less frequently than ophthalmopathy. The rarest complication is thyroid acropachy, which is a process of soft tissue swelling similar to localized myxedema, but is associated with clubbing of the digits and subperiosteal new bone formation.[10] These problems do not affect all patients with Graves' disease, although increased occurrence and severity of ophthalmopathy have been seen in people who smoke.

No treatment directly affects the presence or level of TSIs. They may increase and decrease over a person's lifetime. Treatment of Graves' disease is therefore directed to the target organ, the thyroid gland.

Clinical signs and symptoms of hyperthroidism may affect any body organ. The most common include tachycardia, heat intolerance, hyperkinesis, weight loss, tremor, fatigue, increased sweating, conjunctivitis or chemosis, anxiety, restlessness, and irritability. These symptoms may be absent in the older person, who may experience atrial flutter/fibrillation alone.

Laboratory tests usually show elevated levels of T_4 and T_3 with suppressed or undetectable levels of TSH.

There are three general treatments available for Graves' disease: antithyroid medication, radioactive iodine, and surgery. Antithyroid medication lowers thyroid hormone levels by blocking the synthesis of new thyroid hormone by the thyroid gland. It is usually combined with a beta-blocker to aid in adrenergic-related symptom relief. If the patient has a small gland and is willing to have frequent blood tests and take medication for 12 to 18 months, then there is approximately 50% chance of remission of the Graves' disease. Re-

Table 11-8 Varieties of Thyrotoxicosis (T) and Hyperthyroidism (H)

Disorder	Incidence	Cause
Graves' disease often referred to as toxic diffuse goiter)	More common in women during third and fourth decades of life; estimated to occur in 0.4% of U.S. population	An autoimmune disorder resulting from thyroid-stimulating immunoglobulins (T&H)
Subacute thyroiditis (granulomatous, giant cell)	Uncommon; more frequent in women; increased incidence during fourth and fifth decades; tendency for seasonal and geographic aggregations; mild hyperthyroidism in about 50% of cases	Probable viral infection of gland results in: Destruction of follicular epithelium; Loss of follicular integrity; Release of large quantities of preformed hormones and abnormal iodinated materials (T)
Painless thyroiditis/postpartum thyroiditis	Increasing in general population; occurs in 7% of pregnant women	Painless thyroiditis is a type of chronic autoimmune thyroiditis (T)
Toxic multinodular goiter	Unknown; more frequent in women in the sixth or seventh decade; usually a long history of gradually increasing thyroid enlargement	Hyperfunctioning autonomous thyroid tissue (T&H)
Toxic nodule (solitary autonomous nodule)	Female/male ratio: 3:1 to 6:1; U.S. incidence: 5% of hyperthyroid patients; adults: all ages, especially in younger age group in 30s and 40s; occasionally seen in children	Adenoma functions autonomously; with continued growth, the adenoma assumes a greater share of glandular function and ultimately results in atrophy and complete suppression of the remainder of the gland; adenoma may infarct, resulting in a change from hyperfunctioning to hypofunctioning nodule with relief from hyperthyroidism (T&H)
Exogenous hyperthyroidism, iatrogenic	Clinically has elevated hormone levels and symptoms; subclinical has suppressed TSH, normal T_4 and T_3, no symptoms	L-Thyroxine; L-Triiodothyronine (T)
Factitious (thyrotoxicosis factitia)	More common in women with background of underlying psychiatric disease, paramedical personnel with access to thyroid hormone, or patients for whom thyroid medications have been prescribed in the past	Chronic ingestion of excessive quantities of thyroid hormone (T)
Iodide-induced hyperthyroidism	Iodide-deficient populations (usually in patients with underlying thyroid disorders) or in multinodular goiter)	Administration of supplemental iodine to individuals with endemic, iodine-deficiency goiters; hyperthyroidism may be induced in patients with nonendemic goiter when large quantities of iodine are administered in the form of expectorants, x-ray contrast media, medications containing iodine, or any other form (T&H)
Ectopic hyperthyroidism	Very rare, usually mild, no exophthalmos	Dermoid tumor or teratoma of ovary that contains a hyperfunctioning thyroid adenoma (T)
Pituitary thyrotropin (TSH)	Rare tumor, usually large and seen on CT scan	Excessive TSH secretion from a pituitary tumor or inappropriate TSH secretion caused by pituitary resistance to thyroid hormone (T&H)
Trophoblastic tumor	Hyperthyroidism occurs in 10%-20% of patients	Tumors of trophoblastic origin: hydatidiform mole, choriocarcinoma or embryonal carcinoma of the testis with very high levels of chorionic gonadotropin, lower ratios of T_3/T_4 than Graves' disease

T, Thyrotoxicosis; *T&H,* thyrotoxicosis and hyperthyroidism.

currence could occur within the first year after treatment or at any time afterward. Long-term use of these agents is more frequently recommended in Europe or Japan than in the United States.[51]

A common goal of therapy is destruction or ablation of the thyroid gland so that the thyrotoxicosis cannot return. Although radioactive iodine is the usual treatment of choice in the United States, surgery of total or partial removal of the thyroid gland may be recommended in special circumstances.[51] The usual outcome of both total ablation or total thyroidectomy is hypothyroidism, so that the patient will require lifelong thyroid hormone replacement therapy. In the instance of partial ablation or partial thyroid removal, thyrotoxicosis could recur.

Toxic Nodule/Multinodular Goiter

A nodule is a lump in the thyroid gland; these lumps may be singular (solitary) or multiple (multinodular). Some of these nodules are considered nonfunctional (do not make thyroid hormone, cold on scintigraphy) or functional (make thyroid hormone; warm, hot on scintigraphy). A functional nodule that makes a continuous uninterrupted amount of thyroid hormone and is unresponsive to normal negative feedback signals is called autonomous. Cold nodules can be malignant, although most are benign. Malignancy can be diagnosed by *a fine needle aspiration,* an office procedure that is highly accurate. The patient is seated upright, and the neck is in an extended position, a needle is inserted into the nodule and fluid extracted into a syringe and analyzed in the laboratory. On removal of the needle, local pressure, with or without a cold pack, is applied to prevent bleeding, especially if the fluid obtained is bloody.

The symptoms can vary in intensity but are without the eye or skin complications of Graves' disease. Radioactive iodine is usually used for the treatment of hot nodules; however it is also used for cold nodules, which are nonmalignant. Surgery of total thyroidectomy is the treatment of choice for malignant nodules. Radioactive iodine ablation of thyroid remnants may be performed after surgery.

Antithyroid drugs are used to lower thyroid hormone levels before surgery.

Thyroiditis

Thyroiditis is inflammation of the thyroid gland that can occur at any time. It can occur postpartum when it is also an autoimmune disorder. The antibodies involved (antimicrosomal, antithyroglobulin) are associated with lymphocytic infiltration of the thyroid gland, which may interfere with thyroid hormone synthesis or release. Pregnancy decreases immunologic responsiveness to all types of antibodies, whereas parturition is a trigger for increased immunologic responsiveness. The chance of postpartum thyroiditis occurring increases with each subsequent pregnancy. Graves' disease may also occur in the first 6 to 9 months postpartum.

Subacute thyroiditis is a spontaneously resolving inflammation of the thyroid gland thought to be of viral origin. Like postpartum thyroiditis, it can have a hyperthyroid phase followed by a hypothyroid phase before the gland recovers with a return to normal thyroid hormone synthesis and release. Each phase may last 2 to 10 weeks. Unlike postpartum thyroiditis, antibodies are negative and the patient may experience fever or pain in the thyroid area that may radiate to the neck or jaw. Because the hyperthyroid phase is usually of short duration, beta-blockers, along with aspirin, provide symptomatic relief, although some patients may require corticosteroid therapy.

Subclinical Hyperthyroidism

Subclinical hyperthyroidism is defined as normal T_4 and T_3 levels with a suppressed or undetectable TSH level. It usually occurs as a result of exogenous thyroid hormone therapy. This may be purposeful as a goal of suppressive therapy for thyroid cancer, nontoxic multinodular goiter, or a solitary cold nodule. It may also occur inadvertently as a result of overzealous thyroid hormone replacement therapy. Hyperthyroidism is known to increase osteoclast activity of bone with a loss of bone mineral mass. The occurrence of fractures in postmenopausal women with hyperthyroidism, while no different in location, tend to occur about 10 years earlier than in postmenopausal women with other types of thyroid disorders. It has been postulated that subclinical hyperthyroidism may also decrease bone mass, increasing the risk of osteoporosis. Subclinical hyperthyroidism has recently been shown to be an independent risk factor for atrial fibrillation. A threefold higher risk was found in patients age 60 years or older.[47] This may put the patient at a higher risk for embolic events that may result from the atrial fibrillation.

Thyroid Storm

Thyroid storm may be life-threatening and is the usual reason a patient is admitted to a hospital for hyperthyroidism or thyrotoxicosis (see Emergency Alert Box). It is a very severe form of hyperthyroidism. Its most common cause is Graves' disease, although it has occurred in people with toxic multinodular goiters. Thyroid storm may occur if the patient has delayed seeking medical treatment, has not been compliant with antithyroid drug therapy, has not been responsive to antithyroid drug therapy, or has an additional insult of trauma or stress.

Diagnostic Studies and Findings

Laboratory findings: Serum T_4 increased; serum T_3 increased; serum free T_4 and T_3 increased; thyroid radioiodine uptake and scan, increased uptake in most patients with hyperthyroidism except patients with subacute thyroiditis, painless thyroiditis, and exogenous hyperthyroidism; TSH (third generation) sup-

! EMERGENCY ALERT

THYROID STORM

Thyroid storm is a complex hypermetabolic decompensation with symptoms and signs such as high fever, agitation, tachycardia, tachyarrhythmias, congestive heart failure, and often a psychotic component. Hyperthyroidism is generally categorized into three types: overproducing thyroid gland, thyrotoxicosis with an increased amount of hormone in circulation, and drug-induced hyperthyroidism (i.e., iodine, lithium). Thyroid storm does not occur at a specific hormone level threshold, but its onset appears to be precipitated by factors such as surgery, hospitalization, trauma, stress, cerebral vascular accident (CVA), diabetic ketoacidosis (DKA), congestive heart failure (CHF), or infection.

ASSESSMENT

- Obtain history to rule out hyperthyroidism.
- Assess body temperature (often fever of 100°-105° F).
- Assess cardiovascular status (often heart rate of 200 beats/min): Increased systolic blood pressure, premature ventricular contractions (PVCs), CHF.
- Assess CNS, gastrointestinal, or cardiovascular system dysfunction.
- Assess neurosensory system for presence of fine tremors, restlessness, anxiety, labile mood, manic behavior, or psychosis.
- Determine presence of diarrhea, nausea, vomiting, abdominal cramps, or jaundice.

INTERVENTIONS

- Aggressive intervention is important.
- Obtain IV access and provide fluid resuscitation.
- Administer high-flow oxygen (10-15 L/min) by mask.
- Reduce thyroid levels as rapidly as possible; possible therapies may include methimazole (Tapazole), Lugol's solution, propranolol, dexamethasone, occasionally peritoneal dialysis; plasmapheresis or charcoal hemodialysis may be indicated.
- Provide supportive care and fever control.

pressed and does not respond to TRH; TSI present in Graves' disease

MULTIDISCIPLINARY PLAN

Surgery

Thyroidectomy (toxic multinodular goiter or toxic nodule, occasionally in Graves' disease)

Medications

Thiomides

Propylthiouracil (PTU), 50-800 mg/day in 3-4 doses PO for adults; initially 300-600 mg/day; inhibits thyroid hormone synthesis but not release; inhibits extrathyroidal conversion of T_4 to T_3; used to lower thyroid hormone levels; agranulocytosis may occur in 1.4% of patients during first 2 months of therapy; skin rashes occur in roughly 3% of patients

Methimazole (Tapazole) (MMI), 5-80 mg/day PO in 2-3 doses for adults; initially 30-60 mg/day in either a single daily dose or 3-4 doses inhibits thyroid hormone synthesis but not release; similar to PTU; does not inhibit T_4 to T_3 conversion

Oral cholecystographic agents (Ipodate): Adults: Oral, 1.5-3 g; rapidly inhibits extrathyroidal T_3 production; may be useful for short-term therapy for the occasional patient in whom antithyroid drug treatment or ^{131}I is contraindicated

Beta-adrenergic blockers

Atenolol, 50 mg PO daily

Propranolol (Inderal), 20-80 mg/day PO in divided doses for adults; 5 mg or less IV at 1 mg/min or more slowly for adults; controls symptoms of hyperthyroidism but does not lower T_3 and T_4 levels; controls palpitations, tremor, sweating, proximal muscle weakness, and cardiac symptoms of hyperthyroidism by competitively blocking beta-adrenergic receptors; bronchospasm may occur in asthmatics

Iodides

Potassium or sodium iodide (strong iodine solution, SSKI, Lugol's solution), 0.1-0.3 ml PO tid for adults (SSKI 5-10 drops several times a day); IV 250-500 mg/day for adults in thyrotoxic crisis; produces short-term inhibition of thyroid hormone secretion; used as presurgical medication to reduce size of thyroid gland after thiomide therapy; used with thiomide and propranolol for hyperthyroid crisis

Radioactive iodine (^{131}I NaI)

Adults, up to 29.9 mCi as a single dose

Dose calculated from uptake and gland size; smaller doses are used for diagnostic purposes; concentrated in the thyroid and release radiation, which destroys thyroid tissue; used to destroy thyroid tissue without surgery for control of hyperthyroidism; hypothyroidism ultimately develops in most patients

General Management

Treatment of Graves' disease ophthalmopathy (often no cure)
- Palliative treatment
  - Corticosteroids
  - Surgical orbital decompression
  - Surgical correction of muscle imbalance
  - Radiation of orbit
  - 0.5% methylcellulose eyedrops for eye irritation and pain

Treatment of Graves' disease dermopathy (often no cure)
- Palliative treatment for extensive bulbous or ulcerated lesions
  - 0.2% fluocinolone or other corticosteroid cream

NURSING CARE

NURSING ASSESSMENT

Skin and appendages: Warm and moist, smooth velvety texture, erythema; increased body temperature (37.8° C or greater may indicate thyroid storm); increased sweating; hyperhidrosis; alopecia; hyperpigmentation; onycholysis; acropachy; pretibial myxedema; urticaria; pruritus; vitiligo

Eyes: Lid retraction and lag; proptosis; conjunctival irritation, lacrimation, chemosis; characteristic bright-eyed, frightened, or startled look (exophthalmos)

Cardiovascular concerns: Increased systolic blood pressure, wide pulse pressure; tachycardia, palpitations; presence of dysrhythmias; shortness of breath

Gastrointestinal concerns: Weight loss or modest weight gain (especially if large food intake; seen in younger patients); polyphagia, increased food intake; hyperdefecation or diarrhea; tremor of tongue; increased thirst

Musculoskeletal concerns: Generalized muscular wasting and weakness; hyperactive deep tendon reflexes; noticeable tremor

Nervous system concerns: Fatigue; restlessness, irritability; insomnia; heat intolerance

Mental and emotional concerns: Decreased ability to concentrate, memory loss, easily distracted; emotionally labile, irritable; manic behavior; family members report changes in performance; anxiety/depression

POTENTIAL COMPLICATIONS

Severe tachycardia, congestive heart failure, psychosis

PATIENT PROBLEMS/NURSING DIAGNOSES & INTERVENTIONS

NIC TISSUE PERFUSION MANAGEMENT

Decreased cardiac output related to alteration in rate

- Monitor patient's pulse, blood pressure, color, and temperature *to evaluate cardiovascular status and effectiveness of treatment.*
- Monitor intake and output *to detect fluid overload and impending heart failure.*

NIC ACTIVITY AND EXERCISE MANAGEMENT

Fatigue related to increased energy requirements

Activity intolerance related to imbalance between oxygen and demand

- Help patient identify work and home demands.
- Formulate with patient options for decreasing demands (delegating home tasks, reduction in work hours).

- Help patient plan a schedule that includes rest.
- Monitor patient's ability to perform ADLs.
- Provide rest periods for patient between all activities.
- Reassess need for assisting patient after discharge.

NIC THERMOREGULATION

Hyperthermia related to increased metabolic rate
- Regulate environmental temperature; place patient in cool and quiet room.
- Have patient wear light clothing.
- Provide light bed linens (sheet only).

NIC COGNITIVE THERAPY

Disturbed thought processes related to physiologic changes and sleep deprivation
- Avoid discrepancies in timing, activities, and methods of performing procedures.
- Provide physically and emotionally safe environment for patient.
- Explain procedures slowly and carefully *to facilitate patient concentration.*
- Repeat instructions to patient and limit number of instructions. Provide written instructions.
- Limit number of caregivers *to facilitate routines and decrease distractions.*
- Decrease external stimuli *to minimize distractions and increase the hyperactive patient's ability to concentrate.*

NIC RISK MANAGEMENT

Risk for injury (ocular damage, cornea and conjunctiva) related to inadequate tearing
- Monitor patient's eyes for symptoms of dryness.
- Give patient artificial tears frequently.
- Reassess patient's need for lubricated eye patch or gel.

PATIENT EDUCATION/CONTINUUM OF CARE PLAN

1. Patient verbalizes understanding of medication, name, dosage, action, frequency, and importance of taking medications on schedule.
2. Discuss with patient on outpatient follow-up visits whether plan needs modification after implementation.
3. Discuss with patient the importance of planned rest and avoidance of excessive exercise.
4. Discuss with patient and family the possibility that patient may have emotional outbursts and may need support.
5. Discuss with patient the importance of follow-up evaluations.
6. Give patient list of signs and symptoms of hypothyroidism.
7. Recommend patient and family read "Your Thyroid: A Home Reference."[60]

EVALUATION/PATIENT OUTCOMES

Tissue Perfusion Management: Cardiovascular function is normal. Dysrhythmias are absent or less frequent. Patient's skin remains warm and dry.

Activity and Exercise Management: Fatigue is managed. Patient establishes a plan of rest and activity that enables fulfillment of role and energy demands. Activity tolerance is improved. Patient is able to perform most ADLs independently.

Thermoregulation: Comfort is increased. Patient identifies and uses several techniques to control heat intolerance.

Cognitive Therapy: Thought processes are normal. Patient demonstrates increased problem-solving ability and judgment.

Risk Management: Eyes have adequate protection. Patient is able to self-administer artificial tears or lubricant.

HYPOTHYROIDISM

Hypothyroidism is the clinical and biochemical syndrome that results from deficient thyroid hormone production and is ameliorated by administration of exogenous thyroid hormone.

Hypothyroidism is a common disorder affecting both sexes from birth through old age. Overt hypothyroidism is a combination of low thyroxine (T_4) and low triiodothyronine (T_3) with increased TSH levels accompanied by easily identified physical signs and symptoms. Subclinical hypothyroidism denotes biochemical abnormalities without the presence of clinical signs or symptoms. Persons with subclinical hypothyroidism may have normal T_4 and T_3 levels, with either a slightly elevated TSH level or a normal TSH level that rises to higher levels only at the time of provocative testing.

Hypothyroidism occurs more often in women than in men, with the incidence increasing with age. The reported frequencies vary widely, depending on the population studied. Overt hypothyroidism may occur in from 1 to 2 per 1000 persons to as high as 18 per 1000 elderly persons. In persons seeking medical care, 5 to 20 per 1000 have had overt hypothyroidism. Subclinical hypothyroidism has reportedly been found in 20 to 120 per 1000 persons in the community.[8]

The many varieties of hypothyroidism are listed in Table 11-9. If the cause of the hypothyroidism is within the thyroid gland, it is called primary hypothyroidism. If the cause lies within the pituitary gland, it may be termed *secondary hypothyroidism,* while loss of TRH from the hypothalamus may be called *tertiary hypothyroidism.* These last two are also known as *central hypothyroidism.*

PATHOPHYSIOLOGY

Hashimoto's Thyroiditis

Hashimoto's thyroiditis, also known as chronic lymphocytic thyroiditis or autoimmune thyroiditis, is the most common cause of hypothyroidism in the United States, while iodine deficiency is the leading cause of hypothyroidism worldwide. Hashimoto's thyroiditis is characterized by the presence of circulating antimicrosomal antibodies (antiperoxidase autoantibodies) and/or antithyroglobulin antibodies, which are often at very high levels. These antibodies lead to infiltration of the thyroid gland with lymphocytes, designated killer or K lymphocytes, and plasma cells causing follicular destruction, fibrosis,

Table 11-9 Varieties of Hypothyroidism

Variety	Incidence	Cause
Chronic autoimmune thyroiditis: Hashimoto's thyroiditis	Most common cause of spontaneously occurring hypothyroidism in both children and adults More common in older women Strong hereditary risk factor (thyroid autoantibodies are found in up to 50% of siblings of patients) Patients and their relatives have a higher incidence of other associated autoimmune disorders	Autoimmune disorder; probably results from both cell- and antibody-mediated thyroid injury Characterized by antimicrosomal and antithyroglobulin antibodies in serum, often in very high titer; more prevalent in HLA-DR3 and DR5 haplotypes
Transient autoimmune thyroiditis	Most often occurs in postpartum period; rare in other populations Usually appears 3-6 months after delivery Recurrences after subsequent pregnancies are common	Autoimmune disorder; characterized by development of modest thyroid enlargement, hypothyroidism, and high titers of antithyroid microsomal antibodies may progress to permanent hypothyroidism
Hypothyroidism after radioiodine therapy and external neck radiation therapy	Common occurrence within a year after radioiodine therapy with ^{131}I for hyperthyroidism (thereafter it occurs at a rate of 0.5%-2% per year)	^{131}I therapy; external neck radiation therapy using doses of 2500 rad or more[51]
Postoperative hypothyroidism	After total thyroidectomy: Takes 3-4 weeks After subtotal thyroidectomy: Less predictable, ranges from 2%-75% in first few years after surgery After thyroidectomy for hyperthyroid Graves' disease: 25%-75% occurrence in first year	Surgery with loss of thyroid tissue or damage to it
Transient hypothyroidism from subacute painful thyroiditis	Several weeks or months after hypothyroidism	Part of recovery from initial viral insult
Thyroid dysgenesis (sporadic nongoitrous cretinism)	Most common cause of hypothyroidism in newborn; occurs in 1 of every 4000-5000 births)	Developmental defects of thyroid gland; cause unknown
Hypothyroidism caused by iodine deficiency	Most common cause of hypothyroidism in many parts of world	Iodine deficiency resulting in decreased production of thyroid hormones; important contributing factors are dietary goitrogens, genetic factors, and water pollution
Hypothyroidism caused by drugs and iodide excess	Exact prevalence unknown	Ingestion of compound with antithyroid potency Drugs: Thiocyanate, perchlorate, rifampin nitroprusside, sulfonamides, sulfonylureas, iodides, lithium, paraaminosalicylic acid Antithyroid drugs: PTU, MMI Goitrin plants: rutabaga, white turnips, soybeans, cabbage, peanuts
Hypothyroidism caused by hereditary defects in thyroid hormone biosynthesis	Rare	Defects caused by defective iodide transport Defective iodide organification caused by inadequate or defective thyroid peroxidase, thyroglobulin formation, or peroxide Defective or insufficient thyroglobulin biosynthesis and formation of abnormal iodoproteins Defective dehalogenation of iodotyrosines
Thyroid hormone resistance	Rare; also in some patients with pseudohypoparathyroidism	Autosomal recessive defects with point mutations of T_3 receptor
Hypothyroidism as a result of thyroid injury from other causes	Incidence unknown Occurs occasionally in patients with hemochromatosis, amyloidosis, sarcoidosis, scleroderma, cystinosis, and frequently in those with fibrous invasive thyroiditis (Riedel's thyroiditis)	Thyroid tissue damage
Pituitary hypothyroidism	Unknown, but common after pituitary surgery or radiation	Deficiency of TSH caused by destruction of pituitary tissue: Functioning or nonfunctioning pituitary macroadenomas, surgery, pituitary radiation, postpartum pituitary necrosis (Sheehan's syndrome), pituitary cysts, craniopharyngioma, carotid aneurysm, trauma, hemochromatosis, and infiltrative diseases such as metastatic tumor, tuberculosis, histiocytosis

Continued

Table 11-9 Varieties of Hypothyroidism—cont'd

Variety	Incidence	Cause
Hypothalamic hypothyroidism	Rare; occurs predominantly in children[51]	TRH deficiency caused by cranial irradiation; traumatic, infiltrative, and neoplastic diseases of hypothalamus; pituitary lesions that interrupt hypothalamic-pituitary portal circulation[51]
Spontaneous hypothyroidism after Graves' disease	Generally occurs after remission of Graves' disease; not associated with antithyroid drugs	May result from concomitant chronic autoimmune thyroiditis that frequently occurs with Graves' disease or may be an increase in thyroid-binding immunoglobulins (TBIs) with a concomitant decrease in TSIs

and colloid depletion. It is unknown when in a person's life these antibodies might become active, although iodine ingestion has been suggested as a trigger.[8] There is a genetic predisposition for this type of hypothyroidism. Patients with HLA-DR5 antigen exhibit an increased incidence of goitrous hypothyroidism. The effects of these antibodies against the thyroid gland is an extended process that may take many years. This is why more hypothyroidism is seen in older women than in younger women. In addition, environmental factors such as iodide or viral exposures may modify an already genetically predisposed gland to begin developing thyroiditis and hypothyroidism. Like autoimmune hyperthyroidism, autoimmune hypothyroidism may be associated with other organ-specific systemic autoimmune disorders such as idiopathic adrenal insufficiency, pernicious anemia, lupus, or rheumatoid arthritis.

An intermediary step in the development of hypothyroidism may be the formation of a goiter or nodules. As the thyroid gland begins to fail from destruction of individual follicles, feedback signals are sent to the pituitary gland, which increases its TSH output. TSH acts as a growth stimulator to increase the number of functional follicles. This may be adequate for a time until the antibodies cause more destruction.

When thyrotoxicosis occurs coincidentally with Hashimoto's thyroiditis, it is called hashitoxicosis. The patient's symptoms in this situation would be identical to those of any patient with thyrotoxicosis. These patients, however, have a greater chance of remission of their hyperthyroidism and are more prone to spontaneous hypothyroidism after treatment.

The clinical manifestations of hypothyroidism range from mild, with few signs or symptoms, to severe, culminating in life-threatening myxedema coma. The clinical manifestations depend on the degree and duration of thyroid hormone deficiency. Most of the signs or symptoms are a result of slowing of normal physical and mental activity and edema. The edema or myxedema is from increased interstitial glycosaminoglycan deposition, which is a highly hydrophilic substance. Although slight weight gain or an inability to lose weight while dieting may occur, morbid obesity does not occur from hypothyroidism. The skin, hair, nail, and voice changes are obvious in younger patients, but may be mistaken for normal aging in the older individual.

The treatment for hypothyroidism is levothyroxine. This is a synthetic preparation of only thyroxine. The T_4 is converted (deiodinated) to T_3 at peripheral cells. Therefore one medication is able to provide replacement of the two major thyroid hormones. The goal of treatment is called replacement therapy. This means that enough T_4 is prescribed to maintain the TSH level in a normal range without either the T_4 or T_3 levels being too high or too low. Levothyroxine has a long half-life; therefore if a patient is unable to take medication by mouth because of another illness or surgery, it may be withheld for up to 7 days. After 7 days, however, intravenous levothyroxine should be substituted for the oral preparation. The specific brand of levothyroxine is also important, since generic preparations do not always have the same bioavailability as the branded preparations, which can result in changing thyroid hormonal levels.

Nongoitrous Chronic Autoimmune Thyroiditis

Nongoitrous chronic autoimmune thyroiditis was previously called idiopathic hypothyroidism, primary myxedema, or primary thyroid atrophy. This form of hypothyroidism differs from Hashimoto's thyroiditis in that goiter does not develop. Pathologically, there is thyroid follicle atrophy, lymphocytic infiltration, and atrophy of the entire gland. Genetically, patients with HLA-DR3 tend to exhibit this form of hypothyroidism, which has the same clinical presentation, diagnostic test, and treatment as Hashimoto's thyroiditis.

Myxedema Coma

Myxedema coma is a life-threatening emergency. Long-standing, severe hypothyroidism compromises the patient's ability to withstand the trauma of an intercurrent illness. It occurs most often in the winter in older individuals. It may be precipitated by cold exposure, infection, cardiovascular or respiratory disease, or inappropriate use of narcotic and analgesic agents.[23] Clinically, nearly all these patients have hypothermia and hypoventilation with a metabolic acidosis. Survival of the patient depends on vigorous treatment of the precipitating nonthyroidal illness. Since patients may also have idiopathic adrenal insufficiency, they should be treated simultaneously with glucocorticoids. This is the primary reason a patient with previously undiagnosed hypothyroidism would be admitted to a hospital.

Diagnostic Studies and Findings

TRH stimulation tests: Primary hypothyroidism: TSH increases above normal basal level; pituitary hypothyroidism:

subnormal TSH response or no response to TRH; hypothalamic hypothyroidism: normal TSH, but retarded response to TRH

Radioactive iodine uptake (RAIU): Below normal uptake

Serum T_4: Decreased

Serum free T_4 and T_3: Decreased

Serum TSH: Elevated (primary hypothyroidism, chronic autoimmune thyroiditis, after subtotal thyroidectomy, ^{131}I therapy), normal or undetectable (pituitary or hypothalamic hypothyroidism, nonthyroidal illnesses)

MULTIDISCIPLINARY PLAN

Medications

Synthetic thyroid hormones: Levothyroxine sodium (Levothroid; Synthroid), dose depends on degree of hypothyroidism, age, and body weight of patient; may vary from 0.025 mg (25 μg) to 0.2 mg (200 μg) per day; each of these preparations is available in equivalent intravenous doses

TSH (Thytropar): Rarely used as a diagnostic agent to differentiate primary from central hypothyroidism; comes as a lyophilized powder containing 10 IU of bovine pituitary and is given IM or SQ

Protirelin (TRH) (Relefact TRH; Thypinone), 400-500 mg IV for adults; synthetic preparation of natural hypothalamic tripeptide hormone; diagnostic agent to differentiate pituitary-induced hypothyroidism from other types of hypothyroidism; may transiently produce nausea, facial flushing, hypertension, and urge to micturate

General Management

Thyroid hormone replacement; control of environment; high-protein, high-fiber, low-calorie diet

NURSING CARE

NURSING ASSESSMENT

Skin and appendages: Cool, pale, dry, coarse; yellowish tint; rough, scaly skin; puffy, masklike face; periorbital edema; brittle nails; hypothermia; myxedema

Cardiovascular concerns: Bradycardia, mild hypertension to decreased blood pressure; decreased exercise tolerance, vital signs, intake and output; weigh daily

Gastrointestinal concerns: Modest weight gain; constipation, fecal impaction; abdominal distention, myxedema ileus; nausea; enlarged tongue

Musculoskeletal concerns: Nonspecific fatigue, weakness; slow muscle movement, muscle cramps; delayed relaxation of deep tendon reflexes; aches and stiffness of joints; carpal tunnel syndrome

Nervous system concerns: General slowing of all intellectual functions, including speech; decreased hearing; lethargy and somnolence; impaired memory, inattentiveness; loss of initiative; harshness of voice; sensitivity to narcotics, sedatives; cerebellar ataxia

Mental and emotional concerns: Mental orientation to person, place, and time; paranoia; depression; agitation; apathy

POTENTIAL COMPLICATIONS

Congestive heart failure, depression

PATIENT PROBLEMS/NURSING DIAGNOSES & INTERVENTIONS

NIC TISSUE PERFUSION MANAGEMENT

Decreased cardiac output related to alteration in rate (myxedema, coma only)

- Observe level of consciousness and orientation.
- Monitor for potentiating effects of drugs (e.g., use lower doses of sedatives, narcotics.) *to identify cardiovascular depression caused by drug accumulation, resulting from lowered metabolic rate.*

NIC COGNITIVE THERAPY

Disturbed thought processes related to physiologic changes (myxedema, coma only)

- Provide tolerable activity schedule *to conserve energy.*
- Provide physically and emotionally safe environment.
- Explain procedures slowly and carefully *to support decreased concentration.*
- Assist family in accepting patient's dullness and slowness.
- Time nursing activities to patient's response level *to prevent further disorientation.*
- Explain procedures slowly and simply, reinforcing them repeatedly, *to support the patient with lethargy, impaired memory, and inattentiveness.*
- Schedule nursing activities around patient's activity cycles.

NIC THERMOREGULATION

Hypothermia related to decreased metabolic rate (myxedema coma)

- Use non–alcohol-containing, warmed lotions *to protect the patient's skin.*
- Use warmed blankets; however, do not increase the weight of the patient's clothing by using too many.
- Give patient warmed intravenous solutions slowly if ordered.

NIC ACTIVITY AND EXERCISE MANAGEMENT

Activity intolerance related to generalized weakness

- Reassess patient's ability to perform ADLs.
- Help patient take measures to conserve body temperature (warm blankets, robes, socks, bed jacket) *to prevent further hypothermia.*
- Provide safe environment *to protect patient with hypoactive reflexes, lethargy, or impaired memory.*
- Provide scheduled, uninterrupted rest.

NIC ELIMINATION MANAGEMENT

Constipation related to neuromuscular impairment

- Reassess patient's frequency, color, consistency, and amount of stool.
- Monitor effectiveness of anticonstipation aids.
- Provide high-protein, high-fiber, low-calorie diet in smaller, frequent meals.

- Encourage patient to increase fluid intake; record patient's I&O *to monitor dehydration.*
- Establish daily routine bowel training program.
- Avoid use of enemas *to prevent fluid retention in a patient with myxedema.*

Patient Education/Continuum of Care Plan

1. Give patient a list of signs and symptoms of hypothyroidism and hyperthyroidism and encourage patient to report occurrence of either to physician.
2. Discuss with patient that thyroid hormones are essential for life and treatment is therefore lifelong.
3. Discuss with patient medication administration: name, dosage, frequency of taking, and side effects.
4. Discuss with patient the importance of adequate rest alternated with increased periods of exercise.
5. Discuss with patient the importance of and necessity for follow-up evaluations.
6. Recommend patient and family read "Your Thyroid: A Home Reference."[60]

Evaluation/Patient Outcome

Tissue Perfusion Management: Cardiovascular function is normal. Patient demonstrates normal sinus rhythm. Skin remains warm and dry. Patient remains alert and fully oriented.

Cognitive Therapy: Thought processes are normal. Patient is oriented to person, place, and time. Patient validates thought processes with staff. Statements are reality oriented. Patient is interested in work, environment, friends, and family.

Thermoregulation: Normothermia exists. Temperature is normal; skin is intact, warm, and dry.

Activity and Exercise Management: Activity tolerance is improved. Patient is able to perform most activities independently.

Elimination Management: Constipation is absent or decreased. Bowel movements are regular and of normal consistency, color, and quantity. Patient verbalizes adherence to prescribed diet and fluid intake. Patient identifies high-fiber foods to use in diet plan. Nutrition is adequate. Patient verbalizes adherence to dietary plan.

Thyroid Cancer

Thyroid cancers are malignancies arising from cells normally found in the thyroid gland.

The incidence of thyroid cancer is about 17,000 new cases annually in the United States, with an estimated 1000 deaths per year. Papillary cancer accounts for about 80% of cases, with 5% to 10% from follicular cancer, 10% from medullary cancer, and 2% from anaplastic cancer. External radiation to the head or neck and environmental radiation exposure (nuclear reactors) increase the risk of thyroid cancer. An additional type of malignancy is thyroid lymphoma. Once thought to be rare, it now constitutes close to 8% of all thyroid malignancies.

All thyroid disorders, including thyroid cancer, are more common in women than in men, with a mean age at diagnosis of 40 years. Twenty percent of newly diagnosed cases occur in people less than age 30 years. Thyroid cancer can occur at any age, with an increased incidence occurring 15 to 20 years after radiation exposure and a prevalence of lymphoma after age 50 years (see box below). Papillary cancer (85%) is most often associated with radiation exposure.[8]

Pathophysiology

Thyroid tumors may be classified as epithelial (papillary, follicular, medullary, anaplastic) or nonepithelial (lymphoma). Some patients may have a mixed papillary-follicular pattern.

Epithelial Tumors

Papillary and follicular tumors specifically arise from the follicular cells of the thyroid gland and tend to be slow growing. These tumors usually appear as hypofunctioning nodules within the thyroid gland, alone, as a dominant nodule within a multinodular gland, or as a hypofunctioning nodule in a Graves' thyrotoxic gland. Cancer is occasionally found within a hyperfunctioning nodule, or it may occur with an extrathyroidal mass. Papillary cancer is usually nonencapsulated and may extend beyond the thyroid gland. Recurrence and metastasis are usually to local lymph nodes within the cervical region; less commonly these occur in the lung and bone.

Follicular cancers are usually encapsulated. Invasion of tumor through the capsule or local blood vessels or evidence of extrathyroidal involvement differentiates follicular cancer from the benign follicular adenoma. Distant metastasis is common; lung, lymph node, and bone are the common sites. This cancer may manifest as a lung or bone mass before any thyroidal abnormalities are found.

Medullary thyroid cancer arises from the calcitonin-secreting parafollicular or C-cells. It may occur in isolation (sporadic) or as part of Sipple's syndrome (multiple endocrine neoplasia [MEN type II]). If MEN is suspected, the patient is also evaluated for the simultaneous presence of pheochromocytoma and hyperparathyroidism. Medullary thyroid cancer may also have both local and distant metastases.

Anaplastic thyroid carcinoma is rarely discovered as a primary diagnosis. These are infiltrative tumors that grow rapidly,

RISK FACTORS FOR THYROID CANCER

1. Nodule greater than 3 cm
2. Solitary solid rather than cystic nodule
3. Female sex
4. Age less than 20 or greater than 70 years
5. Extrathyroidal masses at initial presentation
6. Rapidly growing mass
7. Growing nodule within a multinodular gland during thyroid hormone–suppressive therapy
8. Known family history of medullary cancer or multiple endocrine neoplasia

invade the trachea and major blood vessels, and metastasize to distant areas (bone, liver) rapidly.

Prognosis of cancer survival varies with the type, the extent of involvement at the time of diagnosis, and the presence of distant metastases. Papillary cancer generally shows the best survival, even with lymph node involvement. Follicular cancer tends to be more aggressive in affecting vital organs; however, if it is discovered early, life expectancy may not be decreased. Medullary cancer has a mortality of 35% in 10 years. Anaplastic cancer is resistant to all known therapy, and death usually occurs within months. Either papillary or follicular cancer may change aggressively and become anaplastic-like.

Nonepithelial Tumors

The last type of cancer is a non-Hodgkin's lymphoma that occurs as a nodule or mass, usually within a multinodular gland that may have an autoimmune lymphocytic component (Hashimoto's thyroiditis). These masses grow rapidly; they may or may not have extrathyroidal metastases. Patients with Hashimoto's thyroiditis are treated with standard lymphoma therapy—unlike other patients with thyroid cancers.

The goal of therapy for papillary and follicular tumors is first and foremost surgical removal of the thyroid gland. The procedure recommended would be a total or near-total thyroidectomy (see thyroidectomy). If local metastasis is identified at the time of surgery, a more extensive procedure may be required, including a modified radical neck dissection. Depending on the size of the cancer, and the presence of metastasis at presentation, the patient may or may not receive radioactive iodine to chemically kill any remaining thyroid tissue or microscopic cells (see radioactive iodine therapy). If the patient is to receive ^{131}I, an assessment of the amount of remaining tissue must be performed. This is done by a nuclear medicine ^{131}I uptake and whole body scan. Preparation for this procedure involves purposefully making the patient hypothyroid with a greatly elevated TSH. This process usually takes 4 to 6 weeks. Currently, Thyrogen (a DNA-recombinant TSH) may be used to increase TSH without making the patient hypothyroid as a result of withdrawal from thyroid hormone. If the patient receives ^{131}I that is 30 mCi, then, according to Nuclear Regulatory Commission guidelines, the patient must be placed in radiation isolation. The final step in treatment is lifelong thyroid hormone therapy. Unlike the patient with hypothyroidism, however, the goal in these patients is suppressive therapy. This means that enough levothyroxine is prescribed to lower the TSH to extremely low levels, sometimes called undetectable levels. This is to reduce any growth-stimulating or thyroid hormone production potential of any microscopic tumor cells that might remain. This amount of T_4 therapy may render the patient subclinically hyperthyroid, with all of the possible consequences to bone mass or cardiac abnormalities as endogenous subclinical hyperthyroidism (see thyrotoxicosis/hyperthyroidism).

The goal of therapy for medullary thyroid cancer is also a total or near-total thyroidectomy as a first step. ^{131}I is not indicated in this type of cancer because uptake of iodine by medullary tumor cells is negligible. External beam radiation may be used particularly in an attempt to reduce tumor mass when metastasis is present.

Diagnostic Studies and Findings

Fine needle aspiration: An outpatient cytologic procedure to obtain cells from the thyroidal or extrathyroidal mass and determine cell type (see p. 1385 for details)

Thyroid hormone levels: Serum TSH, serum T_4, possibly serum T_3 to exclude hyperthyroidism or hypothyroidism

Serum antibodies: Antimicrosomal, antithyroglobulin; may be positive in Hashimoto's thyroiditis and suspected lymphoma

Serum calcitonin: Elevated in medullary thyroid cancer

Calcium/pentagastrin stimulation test: A provocative test to further assess whether the patient may have medullary thyroid cancer; usually performed when baseline calcitonin level is in the normal range; elevated stimulated calcitonin levels may represent early medullary thyroid cancer

Serum thyroglobulin: Used as a tumor marker after total thyroidectomy; elevated levels indicate persistence or recurrence of papillary or follicular tumors; may also be elevated if normal thyroid tissue remains after treatment

Technetium scan: Used to identify whether presenting thyroidal mass is hypofunctioning (cold) or hyperfunctioning (warm, hot)

Thyroid ^{131}I uptake and scan: Used after total thyroidectomy to help determine amount of remaining tissue and amount of radioactive iodine to give the patient for papillary, follicular, or anaplastic tumors; also used to determine if there is new recurrence or metastasis of papillary or follicular tumors beginning 6 months after initial therapy; how often this procedure is done varies with type of tumor and patient's initial presentation

Multidisciplinary Plan

Surgery

Total thyroidectomy as first therapeutic step

Recurrence or metastasis may require additional surgical intervention; modified radical neck surgery

For all types except lymphoma

^{131}I ablation: Used primarily for epithelial tumors; dose varies depending on patient presentation; may not be given if tumor ≤ 2 cm. If dose is <30 mCi, give as an outpatient; if dose is ≥ 30 mCi, hospitalization and radiation isolation are required

Recurrence/metastasis: 150 to 400 mCi

Maximum cumulative dose: 1000 mCi before bone marrow dysfunction occurs

External beam radiation: Primarily used for recurrence of medullary and occasionally anaplastic tumor

Medications

Thyroid hormone to replace body requirement and to suppress possible cellular growth; long-term exposure to supraphysiologic doses of thyroid hormone may increase risk of osteoporosis

Chemotherapy

Adriamycin may be used in anaplastic tumors

NURSING CARE

Nursing Assessment

Psychosocial concerns: Anxiety

NOTE: All other assessment applies to posttreatment (see thyroidectomy, hypothyroidism, radioactive iodine)

Patient Problems/Nursing diagnoses & Interventions

NIC Psychologic Comfort Promotion

Anxiety related to change in health status

- Encourage patient to discuss feelings about diagnosis and planned therapies.
- Explore coping mechanisms with patient.
- Help patient identify a coping mechanism that will decrease anxiety.

Patient Education/Continuum of Care Plan

1. Discuss with patient before and after thyroidectomy care.
2. If necessary, discuss with patient the need to become hypothyroid (by end of 6 weeks postoperatively) in preparation for first ^{131}I treatment, including signs, symptoms, and ways to cope with symptoms.
3. Ensure that patient understands low-iodine diet in preparation for ^{131}I treatment and institution rules for radiation isolation.
4. Ensure that patient understands thyroid hormone suppressive therapy and need for periodic reevaluation for the rest of their life.
5. Discuss with patient the need to stop thyroid medication, start low-iodine diet, and become hypothyroid in preparation for ^{131}I neck and chest or whole body nuclear medicine scan, within first 6 months postoperatively.

Evaluation/Patient Outcomes

Psychologic Comfort Promotion: Anxiety is decreased. Patient demonstrates one coping mechanism that decreases anxiety. Patient is able to discuss diagnosis.

DISORDERS OF THE PANCREAS

Diabetes Mellitus: Types 1 and 2

Diabetes mellitus is a heterogeneous group of disorders caused by a relative or absolute lack of insulin that affects carbohydrate, protein, and fat metabolism.

In 1998 the National Center for Health Statistics estimated that 10.5 million people were diagnosed with diabetes mellitus.[29] Approximately 90% of these individuals had type 2 diabetes.[3,29] Approximately 10% of the other individuals had type 1 diabetes.[2,29]

Specific types of diabetes mellitus[2,3] are as follows:

1. Type 1 (previously known as insulin-dependent diabetes mellitus [IDDM], juvenile-onset diabetes mellitus); see Table 11-10.
2. Type 2 (previously known as non–insulin-dependent diabetes mellitus [NIDDM], mature-onset diabetes mellitus); see Table 11-10.
3. Impaired glucose tolerance
4. Gestational diabetes mellitus
5. Secondary diabetes mellitus
   a. Genetic defect of beta cell functioning
      (1) Mature-onset diabetes in the young (MODY)
      (2) Mitochondrial DNA
      (3) Others
   b. Genetic defect in insulin action
      (1) Type A insulin resistance
      (2) Leprechaunism

Table 11-10 Clinical, Genetic, and Immunologic Characteristics of Diabetes

	Type 1 Diabetes (Previously Known as IDDM or Juvenile-Onset Diabetes Mellitus)	Type 2 Diabetes (Previously Known as NIDDM or Mature-Onset Diabetes Mellitus)
Age of onset	Usually <30 years	Usually >40 years
Ketosis	Common	Rare
Body weight	Nonobesity	Obesity
Prevalence	0.5%	4%-5%
Genetics	HLA-associated; 25%-35% concordance rate in twins	Non-HLA associated; 95%-100% concordance rate in twins
Circulating islet cell antibodies	65%-85%	<10%
Treatment with insulin	Required	Not required, but insulin may be used to maximize glycemic control
Complications	Associated with poor glycemic control Diabetes Complications and Control Trial showed that poor glycemic control could accelerate or cause the development of microvascular complications[20]	Associated with poor glycemic, blood pressure, and lipid control United Kingdom Prospective Diabetes Study (UKPDS) demonstrates that optimizing glycemic control can cause a 15% decrease in major complications[56] Inference from the UKPDS are that optimization of blood pressure and lipid control also may ameliorate the development of major complications

(3) Rabson-Mendenhall syndrome
(4) Lipo-atrophic diabetes
(5) Others

c. Diseases of the exocrine pancreas
(1) Pancreatitis
(2) Trauma/pancreatectomy
(3) Neoplasia
(4) Cystic fibrosis
(5) Hemochromatosis
(6) Fibrocalculous pancreatopathy
(7) Others

d. Endocrinopathies
(1) Acromegaly
(2) Cushing's disease
(3) Glucagonoma
(4) Pheochromocytoma
(5) Hypothyroidism
(6) Somatostatinoma
(7) Aldosteronoma
(8) Others

e. Drug or chemical induced
(1) Vacor
(2) Pentamadine
(3) Nicotinic acid
(4) Glucocorticoids
(5) Thyroid hormone
(6) Diazoxide
(7) Beta-adrenergic agonists
(8) Thiazides
(9) Dilantin
(10) Interferon-alpha

PATHOPHYSIOLOGY

Type 1 diabetes mellitus is a condition of absolute insulin deficiency. Genetic predisposition for type 1 diabetes mellitus is conferred by a certain histocompatibility antigen, human leukocyte antigen (HLA) coded on chromosome 6.[9] Environmental factors can have a role in the development of insulin-dependent diabetes in the genetically susceptible individual. Virus (coxsackie, mumps, and rubella) can either cause direct destruction of the beta cell or induce an immunologic reaction to the beta cells of the pancreas.[9]

Autoimmunity plays a definitive role in type 1 diabetes mellitus. Autoantibodies directed against beta cells and insulin are present in type 1 diabetes mellitus and include islet cell antibodies (ICA), insulin autoantibodies (IAA), and anti–glutamic acid decarboxylase (anti-GAD). Several are present before the development of frank hyperglycemia. Why autoimmune destruction of the beta cells occurs, how it is activated, and whether or not the process of autoimmune beta cell destruction can be interrupted continues to be under worldwide clinical investigation.[41]

Once 80% to 90% of the beta cells are destroyed, metabolic compensation and the ability to maintain blood glucose levels within normal limits deteriorate steadily.[2] Symptoms are the direct result of the lack of insulin and subsequent deterioration of body processes and metabolism associated with requiring insulin.

HEALTHY PEOPLE 2010

HEALTH STATUS—DIABETES

Goal: Through prevention programs, reduce the disease and economic burden of diabetes and improve the quality of life for all persons who have or are at risk for diabetes.

DIABETES

- Increase the proportion of persons with diabetes who receive formal diabetes education.
- Prevent diabetes.
- Reduce the overall rate of diabetes that is clinically diagnosed.
- Increase the proportion of adults with diabetes whose condition has been diagnosed.
- Reduce the diabetes death rate.
- Reduce diabetes-related deaths among persons with diabetes.
- Reduce deaths from cardiovascular disease in persons with diabetes.
- (Developmental) Decrease the proportion of pregnant women with gestational diabetes.
- (Developmental) Reduce the frequency of foot ulcers in persons with diabetes.
- Reduce the rate of lower extremity amputations in persons with diabetes.
- (Developmental) Increase the proportion of persons with diabetes who obtain an annual urinary microalbumin measurement.
- Increase the proportion of adults with diabetes who have a glycosylated hemoglobin measurement at least once a year.
- Increase the proportion of adults with diabetes who have an annual dilated eye examination.
- Increase the proportion of adults with diabetes who have at least an annual foot examination.
- Increase the proportion of persons with diabetes who have at least an annual dental examination.
- Increase the proportion of adults with diabetes who take aspirin at least 15 times per month.

Modified from U.S. Department of Health and Human Services: *Healthy people 2010* (conference edition, in two volumes), Washington, DC, January 2000.
NOTE: *Developmental* indicates that criteria for measurement and strategies to improve health have not as yet been specified.

Insulin deficiency disrupts normal metabolism and results in hyperglycemia. In the absence of insulin, glucose uptake by the liver, muscle, and fat cells is inhibited; glucose production is promoted. Lack of the restraining effects by insulin on the liver processes of glycogenolysis and gluconeogenesis causes the liver to overproduce glucose. Synthesis of protein, fat, and glycogen is impaired. Muscle and fat are catabolized, freeing up more substrate for the liver to use in out-of-control gluconeogenesis. Although blood glucose levels are elevated, glucose is not available to cells as an energy source. If not corrected, lipolysis occurs to provide cells with needed energy. However, by-products of lipolysis, called ketones, are overproduced, excreted in the urine, and build up in the blood. Symptoms of hyperglycemia, including polydipsia, polyuria, polyphagia, fatigue, weight loss, and blurred vision, can occur whenever type 1 diabetes is poorly controlled.[41]

Type 2 diabetes mellitus comprises a group of disorders characterized by relative insulin deficiency, high hepatic glucose output, and insulin resistance. Individuals with type 2 diabetes mellitus have the following common features: usually are over age 30 years at the time of diagnosis, have a family history of type 2 diabetes mellitus, and are overweight or obese. Genetics, environment, and lifestyle factors play a role in the development of type 2 diabetes mellitus. Although type 2 diabetes mellitus is familial, a specific genetic marker has yet to be identified. The prevalence increases with age. African-Americans, Mexican-Americans, and Native Americans are at an increased risk for developing type 2 diabetes mellitus.[23,41]

Insulin resistance is a basic defect that occurs at the target cell. Beta cell defects and cell receptor defects are present in individuals with type 2 diabetes mellitus. Beta cell defects may include impaired insulin secretion because of the toxic effect of elevated glucose levels on the beta cell or diminished insulin response to usual stimuli. Low normal or elevated insulin levels may be present. At the target cell, malfunctioning of insulin receptors on target tissues and/or intracellular postreceptor processes can be present. The ability to identify exactly what defect(s) are present in any one individual with type 2 diabetes mellitus is still to be investigated.

The relative insulin deficiency of type 2 diabetes mellitus also results in hyperglycemia. However, because some insulin is produced, hyperglycemia is insidious and can be present for years before diagnosis. Symptoms of hyperglycemia can include polydipsia, polyuria, polyphagia, fatigue, and slowed wound healing. Often these signs and symptoms are attributed to a preexisting condition or the aging process.

Causes associated with the development of long-term complications of diabetes are hyperglycemia, hyperlipidemia, and hypertension. Long-term complications of diabetes include the following:

1. Macrovascular disease (coronary, cerebrovascular, and peripheral disease)
2. Microvascular disease (retinopathy and nephropathy)
3. Peripheral neuropathy (upper and lower extremities)
4. Mononeuropathy
5. Diabetic amyotrophy
6. Neuropathic cachexia
7. Autonomic neuropathy (gastroparesis, diabetic diarrhea, neurogenic bladder, sexual dysfunction in men and women, impaired cardiovascular reflexes)

Optimizing blood glucose control in individuals with type 1 diabetes mellitus reduces the risk for the development and progression of retinopathy, nephropathy, and neuropathy by approximately 60%.[20] The United Kingdom Prospective Diabetes Study[56] is demonstrating that aggressive glycemic, blood pressure, and lipid control for persons with type 2 diabetes mellitus is necessary to reduce the risk of developing microvascular and macrovascular complications. Consequently, diabetes management goals for persons with types 1 and 2 diabetes mellitus should include specific parameters identifying excellent glycemic, blood pressure, and lipid control.[16]

Table 11-11 Peptide and Insulin levels in Types 1 and 2 Diabetes

	Type 1 Diabetes (Previously Known as IDDM or Juvenile-Onset Diabetes Mellitus)	Type 2 Diabetes (Previously Known as NIDDM or Mature-Onset Diabetes Mellitus)
C-peptide, plasma	Low to absent	Low, normal, high
Insulin, plasma	Low to absent	Low, normal, high

Routine assessment for types 1 and 2 diabetes are as follows:

1. Blood pressure (every visit)
2. Weight (every visit)
3. Foot examinations (every visit)
4. Retinal examinations (every year)
5. Hemoglobin A1c (every 3 months)
6. Lipids (on initial visit and then yearly for adults)
7. Timed urine collection for microalbumin or protein

Diagnostic Studies and Findings

Diagnostic Criteria for Diabetes Mellitus[5]

1. Polyuria and polydipsia with a random plasma glucose level greater than or equal to 200 mg/dl

or

2. Two-hour plasma glucose level that is greater than or equal to 200 mg/dl

or

3. Fasting plasma glucose level greater than or equal to 126 mg/dl

The newest American Diabetes Association recommendation, a fasting plasma glucose level greater than or equal to 126 mg/dl, is known as impaired fasting glucose tolerance.[4,5] C-peptide and insulin levels differ between types 1 and 2 diabetes (see Table 11-11).

Multidisciplinary Plan

Standards of care for persons with diabetes are outlined in detail by the American Diabetes Association[2,3] and include the following:

1. Regular medical evaluation and follow-up
2. Medical nutrition therapy (refer to dietitian)
3. Exercise prescription
4. Education/behavior change (diabetes educator, dietitian, exercise specialist)
5. Psychosocial coping and support (diabetes educator, mental health professional)
6. Medications: Glycemic goals (Table 11-12), human insulins (Table 11-13) and oral hypoglycemia agents (Table 11-14)

Table 11-12 Glycemic Goals for People With Diabetes Mellitus*[5]

	Normal	Goal
Preprandial glucose (mg/dl)	<110	80-120
Bedtime glucose (mg/dl)	<120	100-140
Hemoglobin A1c (HPLC)	<6.0	<7.0

*Patients with severe cardiac arterial disease and/or who are being treated with beta-blocking agents may be managed with different glycemic goals (generally higher).

Table 11-13 Human Insulins

	Onset (h)	Peak (h)	Duration (h)
Lispro	<0.25	0.5-1.5	3-4
Regular	0.5-1.0	2-3	3-6
NPH	2-4	6-10	10-16
Lente	3-4	6-12	10-16
Ultralente	6-12	10-16	18-24

Modified from American Diabetes Association.[2]

Table 11-14 Oral Hypoglycemia Agents

Name	Description of Action
Sulfonylureas (Diabinese, Glucotrol, glyburide, Amaryl, repaglinide)	Increase hepatic levels of endogenous insulin and meet meal-related insulin requirements
Biguanides (metiformin)	Improves insulin sensitivity at the liver and reduces hepatic glucose production
Thiazelodiones (Rosiglitazone [Avandia], pioglitazone)	Improve insulin action in peripheral tissues and enhance glucose uptake
Alpha-glucosidase inhibitors (miglitol, acarbose)	Decrease postprandial glucose absorption by delaying carbohydrate metabolism

Modified from American Diabetes Association.[3]

NURSING CARE

NURSING ASSESSMENT

Circulation: Cold extremities; loss of hair on toes; skin shiny, thin, and atrophic; orthostatic hypotension; painful calves when walking; numbness and tingling of lower extremities; weak pedal pulse

Food and fluid needs: Hunger, thirst, nausea; weight loss or obesity; I&O, weigh daily

Elimination: Polyuria, nocturia

Neurosensory concerns: Decreased sensation to pain and temperature in feet; blurred vision; headaches, cataracts, halos around lights

Hygiene and skin care: Infection; rubeosis, dermopathy; foot ulcers

Psychosocial concerns: Verbalization of inability to cope; noncompliance with treatment plan; verbalization of change in lifestyle; negative feeling about body

Sexuality: Impotence, vaginal discharge/infection

Teaching and learning: Lack of exposure to diabetes if newly diagnosed; lack of recall; misinformation; inadequate demonstration of skills required (urine and/or blood testing, injection technique); lack of interest; unfamiliarity with survival level

POTENTIAL COMPLICATIONS

Leg ulcers (poor tissue healing), diabetic retinopathy

PATIENT PROBLEMS/NURSING DIAGNOSES & INTERVENTIONS

NIC ELECTROLYTE AND ACID-BASE MANAGEMENT

Deficient fluid volume related to failure of regulatory mechanisms

- Encourage patient to drink noncaloric fluids for hyperglycemia *to replace fluid loss resulting from polyuria.*
- Discuss causative factors with patient and family.
- Monitor indicators of patient's fluid balance (I&O, daily weights, signs of dehydration) during episodes of hyperglycemia.

NIC NUTRITION SUPPORT

Imbalanced nutrition: less than body requirements, related to inadequate intake of nutrients in diet (type 1)

- Reassess patient for factors that may influence diet preferences.
- Arrange a dietary consultation for patient.
- Reinforce the patient's meal plan as ordered.
- Encourage patient to verbalize feelings about weight, body size, and eating behavior.
- Monitor patient's laboratory and self-monitored blood glucose (SMBG) data *to monitor blood glucose control.*
- Discuss causative factors with patient and family.
- Monitor patient's compliance with all aspects of the diabetes treatment regimen.

Imbalanced nutrition: more than body requirements, related to long-established eating habits (type 2)

- Reassess for psychosocial concerns that may be related to overeating.
- Arrange a dietary consultation.
- Reinforce the meal plan as ordered.
- Suggest support group such as Weight Watchers *to provide group and peer support.*
- Allow patient to verbalize feelings regarding weight.
- Positively reinforce patient's effort at weight loss.
- Discuss causative factors with patient and family.
- Help patient develop a pattern of rewards other than food for weight loss.
- Teach patient the use of a food diary *for self-monitoring.*
- Suggest techniques to change patient's eating behaviors.
- Monitor patient's laboratory and SMBG data *to monitor blood glucose control and lipids.*
- Help patient to identify, select, and participate in energy-expending activities three times a week.
- Explore techniques to change eating behaviors.

NIC Skin/Wound Management

Risk for impaired skin integrity related to internal factors (altered metabolic state, altered circulation, altered sensation)

- Initiate health instruction for patient related to risks and referral to health-care professional, as needed.
- Minimize hazardous environmental factors.
- Provide assistive devices as needed.
- Discuss causative factors with patient and family.
- Keep patient's skin clean and dry.
- Monitor patient closely for signs and symptoms of infection.
- Observe patient performing daily foot care.
- Encourage measures to maximize patient's local circulation.

NIC Coping Assistance

Ineffective coping related to multiple life changes

- Offer patient support and positive reinforcement.
- Assess personal strengths and weaknesses, current stressors, and stress management skills.
- Emphasize that daily management can become as routine as personal hygiene.
- Encourage self-care to patient's maximum ability.
- Encourage participation in diabetic support groups through local American Diabetes Association (ADA) and Juvenile Diabetes Foundation (JDF).
- Teach problem-solving skills.

Ineffective sexuality pattern related to disordered metabolic function

- Encourage patient and partner to discuss sexual concerns.
- Acknowledge patient's feelings related to discussion of sexual concerns.
- Explore patient's knowledge regarding sexuality.
- Discuss causative factors with patient and partner.
- Offer patient some suggestions regarding alternative sexual expression.
- Provide patient with referrals to appropriate health-care professionals.

NIC Risk Management

Disturbed sensory perception (visual, kinesthetic, tactile) related to altered sensory perception

- Discuss causative factors with patient and family.
- Discuss patient's feelings about limitations.
- Assist patient to identify and to use assistive devices *to minimize injury.*
- Minimize hazardous environmental factors.
- Assist and support patient as needed *to reduce chance of injury.*
- Discuss injury prevention with patient and family.

NIC Behavior Therapy

Noncompliance related to inadequate knowledge, motivation, conflict in values, complexity of regimen

- Encourage and support patient's individual efforts.
- Give patient positive reinforcement for self-care efforts.
- Explore patient's feelings related to compliance.
- Provide patient with specific detailed instruction.
- Correct patient's misconceptions.
- Assist patient to use strategies to facilitate his or her behavior change.
- Use collaborative goal setting with patient.
- Assist patient in setting personal goals consistent with goals of treatment regimen.

Patient Education/Continuum of Care Plan

1. Demonstrate to patient how to administer insulin or oral hypoglycemics; teach patient to report side effects or toxic effects.
2. Demonstrate to patient the method for monitoring blood sugar level: SMBG (and urine ketone testing for type I with high blood glucose level).
3. Ensure that patient verbalizes understanding of prescribed diet and regular, routine exercise and activity needed to maintain blood sugar control.
4. Ensure that patient verbalizes early signs or symptoms and treatment of hypoglycemia and hyperglycemia.
5. Discuss with patient sick day management.
6. Discuss with patient personal hygiene, stressing specifics related to dental, foot, and skin care.
7. Discuss with patient the methods of care to prevent complications.
8. Discuss with patient the importance of regular medical care.
9. Discuss available community resources.

Evaluation/Patient Outcomes

Electrolyte and Acid-Base Management: Fluid balance is maintained. No signs of dehydration are present. Patient initiates fluid replacement during periods of hyperglycemia. Patient verbalizes causes of dehydration.

Nutrition Support: Intake of nutrients is adequate. Patient's blood sugar control is within individual target values. Patient ingests recommended types and amounts of nutrients. Patient describes causative factors. Patient's weight is within range for height and age (IDDM). Patient's glycosylated hemoglobin is within individual recommended range. Patient's weight gradually reduces no more than 1 to 2 pounds per week (NIDDM). Patient participates in support group. Patient uses strategies to facilitate behavior change.

Skin/Wound Management: Skin is intact. Patient performs daily foot, skin, and dental care correctly. Patient uses measures to minimize risk. Patient accepts referrals. Patient describes causative factors and rationale for measures to minimize risk. Patient has no infection present.

Coping Assistance: Patient copes effectively. Patient uses appropriate coping strategies. Patient accepts support. Patient shows increased independence in self-care.

Patient attains satisfying level of sexual functioning compatible with functional capability. Patient and partner verbalize concerns about sex. Patient and partner identify alternative expressions of sexuality. There is open communication about sexual concerns. Patient accepts referrals as appropriate. Patient resumes sexual activity.

Risk Management: Patient remains free of personal injury. Patient seeks assistance as needed. Patient uses assistive devices as needed. Patient verbalizes understanding of risk for injury with sensory/perceptual changes. Patient verbalizes cause of potential for injury. Patient recognizes environmental hazards and avoids them.

Behavior Therapy: Compliance is increased. Patient demonstrates accurate knowledge and skills for self-care. Patient demonstrates behaviors consistent with goals of treatment regimen. Patient accepts support. Patient identifies and uses strategies to facilitate behavior change. Patient sets personal goals that are consistent with goals of the treatment regimen.

Diabetic Ketoacidosis and Hyperglycemic Hyperosmolar Nonketotic Coma

Diabetic ketoacidosis (DKA) is a condition of severe metabolic disturbance caused by an absolute or relative insulin deficiency. Severe hyperglycemia, ketosis, and metabolic acidosis characterize DKA. DKA is considered to be a medical emergency. Individuals who develop DKA tend to have type 1 diabetes mellitus. DKA can occur in lean individuals with type 2 diabetes mellitus.[6]

Hyperglycemic hyperosmolar nonketotic syndrome (HHNS) is a condition of severe metabolic disturbance characterized by severe hyperglycemia, hyperosmolarity, and dehydration.

DKA occurs in 2% to 5% of patients and is always caused by insulin deficiency, which can be absolute, as when patients omit taking insulin or are newly diagnosed. Insulin deficiency can also be relative where there is an insufficient amount of circulating insulin to meet basal insulin requirements or antagonism by stress counterregulatory hormones.

Currently HHNS accounts for approximately 1 in 1000 hospital admissions.[6] Individuals tend to be elderly with type 2 diabetes mellitus.

Pathophysiology

Normally, insulin and counterregulatory hormones maintain metabolic homeostasis. Insulin has anabolic and anticatabolic actions. Growth hormone is also anabolic. Other counterregulatory hormones are catabolic.

An absolute or relative lack of insulin relative to basal insulin requirements can cause DKA. Insulin deficiency is absolute at presentation of newly diagnosed patients with type 1 diabetes mellitus. Counterregulatory hormone levels rise as a result of increased stress on the body.

Insulin deficiency can be relative if a major stress such as illness, trauma, or pregnancy increases counterregulatory hormone levels. Counterregulatory hormones antagonize or decrease the effects of insulin. The individual in DKA becomes more catabolic and begins to do the following[6]:

1. Increase glucose production by glycogenolysis and gluconeogenesis (catecholamines, glucagon)
2. Decrease glucose utilization by antagonizing the effects of insulin (catecholamines, glucagon, growth hormone)
3. Induce ketogenesis with an accumulation of organic acids, beta-hydroxybutyrate, and acetoacetic acid.

The events of DKA are summarized in Fig. 11-12.

In the absence of adequate insulin, peripheral fat, muscle, and liver cells cannot utilize glucose. Breakdown of fat and protein is accelerated, freeing up more substrate (fatty acids and amino acids) for use in gluconeogenesis and overproduction of glucose by the liver.

Excessive amounts of fatty acids are used by the liver (under the control of glucagon) to overproduce ketoacids (ketone bodies, beta-hydroxybuytyrate, and acetoacetic acids). Acetone, responsible for the characteristic fruity breath in DKA, is formed from acetoacetic acid. The ketone bodies are produced faster than they can be metabolized or excreted. Acetoacetic acid and beta-hydroxybutyric acid cannot be metabolized in the absence of insulin; therefore their levels also increase in the plasma. These strong organic acids dissociate at body pH and provide 1 mEq of hydrogen (H^+) cation and a ketoacid anion. Metabolic acidosis occurs when the body's buffer system and respiratory compensatory mechanisms cannot maintain normal pH.

Hyperglycemia results in glycosuria with a large osmotic water and electrolyte loss through the kidneys. Although glomerular filtration is increased initially, the development of hypovolemia is associated with decreased glomerular filtration and worsening of hyperglycemia. In addition, the organic acids are excreted through the kidneys as anions, significantly decreasing potassium and sodium in the body. The acidotic state creates a shift in electrolytes; extracellular H^+ is exchanged for intracellular potassium (K^+). Therefore serum K^+ may be elevated as H^+ moves intracellularly. Hypovolemia may seem to increase the degree of hyperkalemia, but eventually the loss of K^+ through the kidneys seriously depletes body K^+ levels. Once therapy is started for DKA, K^+ levels can fall rapidly. This is related to the direct action of insulin on K^+ uptake by cells, altered blood pH, decreased serum glucose level, or increased renal excretion. Many factors contribute to the changes in the level of consciousness in DKA patients, such as decreased oxygenation of tissues, increased H^+ levels, hyperosmolarity, and increased acetoacetic acid levels.

Many patients with DKA experience an abnormality of plasma serum enzymes, including serum amylase, creatine phosphokinase (CPK), transaminase (AST or SGOT and ALT or SGPT), and lysosomal enzymes.[39] The alkaline phosphatase level is often increased. Normal or elevated electrolyte levels should not be misinterpreted as adequate. Depletion of body stores and severe deficiency often are present with rehydration and insulin therapy. K^+ deficit is the most important, and recognition and intervention are essential. The diagnosis of DKA is made on the first clinical impression, with confirmation by bedside testing (blood glucose and urine ketone levels; laboratory values must be obtained before therapy is initiated). See FIG. 11-12.

In HHNS, seen in 1 of every 1000 hospital admissions,[6] severe hyperglycemic hyperosmolarity has been observed in association with intravenous therapy with large amounts of glucose solutions; dialysis of hyperosmolar dialysate; acromegaly; drugs such as the thiazide diuretics or phenytoin, cimetidine; and after the ingestion of large amounts of sugary beverages or high-protein gastric tube feedings.[44] Additional

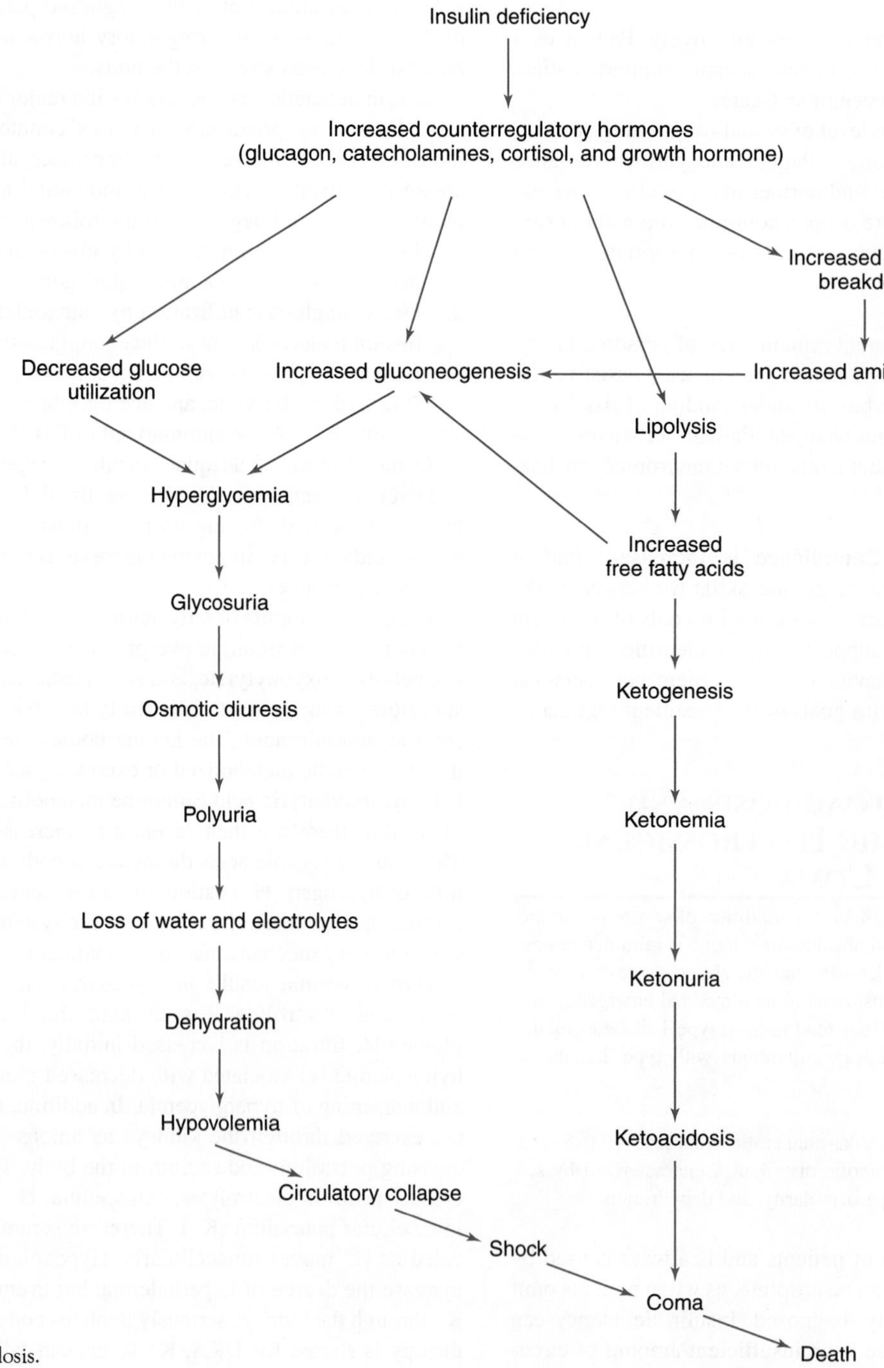

FIG. 11-12
Diabetic ketoacidosis.

precipitating factors for HHNS include acute pancreatitis, inadequate or limited access to fluids, impaired thirst, social isolation, massive fluid losses, or illness/infection.[18,38] About 80% of patients with HHNS have impaired renal function, a significant predisposing condition that contributes to the development of HHNS.[44] Most individuals who experience HHNS are elderly, infirm, institutionalized, or mentally impaired, with mild or previously undiagnosed diabetes. The mortality for HHNS is higher than for DKA.

HHNS is similar to DKA except that insulin deficiency is not as profound and develops over a longer period of time (Table 11-15). In HHNS, ketosis is suppressed, perhaps by more available endogenous insulin and by the serum hyperosmolarity.[6]

Decreased insulin leads to disrupted carbohydrate, fat, and protein metabolism (FIG. 11-13). Blood glucose level rises in response to decreased glucose use by the cells, increased glucose production by the liver because of insulin deficiency, and increased counterregulatory hormone effects. Osmotic water and electrolyte loss begin in response to glycosuria. Extracellular volume depletion is more pronounced in the elderly because of their decreased ability to concentrate urine, responsiveness to ADH, and conservation of body water. There is less total body water available to buffer losses. Hypovolemia and severe dehydration develop quickly, with concomitant mentation changes. Electrolyte losses include sodium, potassium, chloride, phosphate, magnesium, and calcium. Amino acid uptake and protein synthesis are halted. Breakdown of protein furnishes the liver with more substrate for gluconeogenesis. Increased lipolysis does not occur.[44]

The most significant factor differentiating HHNS from DKA is serum level of the free fatty acids, which is lower in HHNS than in DKA. This may be the most plausible explanation for the lack of ketosis in HHNS. Serum concentrations of the counterregulatory hormones differ significantly from those in DKA: serum glucagon levels are higher, and GH and cortisol levels are lowered in HHNS. The elevated glucagon levels appear to be primarily responsible for the elevations in blood glucose level, a direct result of stimulation of liver gluconeogenesis by glucagon.

Eighty percent of patients with HHNS have renal impairment related either to primary (kidney) or secondary (volume depletion) disease. This plays a significant role in elevating blood glucose levels in HHNS. The kidneys are unable to rid the body of excess glucose or maintain water balance. Inability to replace body water results in hyperosmolality and dehydration. Increased solutes increase osmotic pressure. The effective serum osmolarity (E_{osm}) is calculated as follows[44]:

$$E_{osm} = 2(N+K \text{ [in mEq]}) = \text{Glucose (mg/dl)}/18$$

When this value exceeds 350 mOsm/L, severe hyperosmolarity is present.[44] The hyperosmolarity of HNNS is a direct result of excessive blood glucose level and increasing sodium concentration in dehydration.

Insulin output continues to prevent ketosis. The steady loss of sodium, potassium, and water with hyperglycemia and glycosuria exacerbates the hyperosmolar state and ultimately results in hypovolemia, hypotension, hemoconcentration, and increased blood viscosity. It can contribute to

! EMERGENCY ALERT

DIABETIC KETOACIDOSIS (DKA)

This metabolic disturbance generally occurs in those with type I diabetes mellitus. DKA is always caused by insulin deficiency.

ASSESSMENT

- Determine compliance with taking insulin as ordered.
- Determine if insulin delivery system is working properly or insulin is drawn up correctly.
- Identify storage and handling of insulin. (Insulin can never be frozen or exposed to high temperatures. To maintain maximum insulin potency, insulin should not be exposed to temperature exceeding 86° F [21° C].)

INTERVENTIONS

- Obtain IV access and, in collaboration with the physician, provide fluid resuscitation using normal saline solution (can be as much as 1 L/h).
- In collaboration with physician, administer insulin therapy by IV infusion.
- Monitor electrolyte and arterial blood gas levels and, in collaboration with physician, correct imbalances.
- Provide periodic and careful monitoring of vital signs, urine output, mental status, and pulmonary status.

Table 11-15 DKA and HHNS: Comparison of Some Salient Features

Feature	DKA	HHNS
Age of patients	Usually <40 years	Usually >60 years
Duration of symptoms	Usually <2 days	Usually >5 days
Glucose level	Usually <600 mg/dl (<33.3 mmol/L)	Usually >800 mg/dl (>44.4 mmol/L)
Sodium concentration	More likely to be normal or low	More likely to be normal or high
Potassium concentration	High, normal, or low	High, normal, or low
Bicarbonate concentration	Low	Normal
Ketone bodies	At least 41 in 1:1 dilution	<2+ in 1:1 dilution
pH	Low	Normal
Serum osmolality	Usually <350 mOsm/kg (<350 mmol/kg)	Usually >350 mOsm/kg (>350 mmol/kg)
Cerebral edema	Often subclinical; occasionally clinical	Subclinical has not been evaluated; rarely clinical
Prognosis	3%-10% mortality	10%-20% mortality
Subsequent course	Insulin therapy required in virtually all cases	Insulin therapy not required in many cases

Modified with permission from Davidson[17]; from Peragallo-Dittko, Godley, and Meyer.[41]

the development of vascular occlusion, the most important complication of HHNS.[44] Most of the abnormal and confusing abnormalities resolve after treatment. It is suggested that the neurologic examination be repeated 48 hours after homeostasis has been restored by fluid and insulin replacement therapy.

Like DKA, clinical assessment and analysis as well as bedside testing (capillary blood glucose and urine ketones) are needed to make the diagnosis of HHNS. Initial laboratory values are obtained before treatment is initiated. Enormous fluid losses (up to 20 L) and deficits in sodium and potassium can be present. Other abnormal blood work findings can be present, such as elevations in hematocrit, triglycerides, cholesterol, liver function test, and various serum enzyme values.[44]

DIAGNOSTIC STUDIES AND FINDINGS

See Diagnostic Studies and Findings table on p. 789.

MULTIDISCIPLINARY PLAN

The goals of treatment are to accomplish the following:

1. Replace fluid and electrolyte losses.

FIG. 11-13

Pathogenesis of hyperosmolar nonacidotic uncontrolled diabetes.

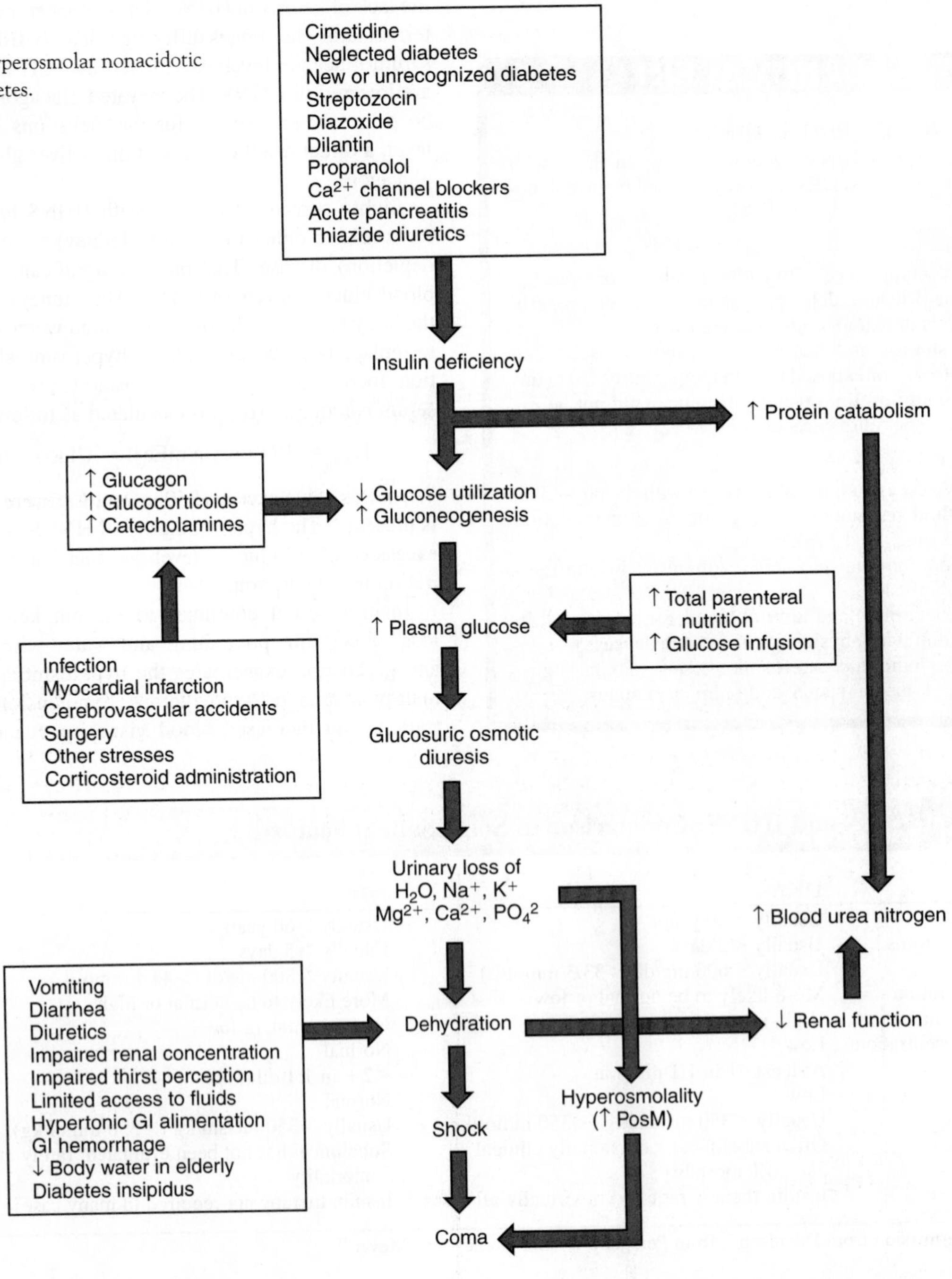

2. Provide insulin to normalize nutrient metabolism.
3. Correct acidosis (DKA).

Medications[2]

Fluid replacement depends on the hydration, blood pressure, age, weight, renal status, and cardiovascular status of the patient. Generally, fluid replacement is provided as follows:

Hour 1: 0.9% normal saline solution at 15-20 ml/kg.

Hour 2: Continue normal saline solution at 15-20 ml/kg. (If patient is hypernatremic, 0.5% normal saline solution is used.)

Hour 3: Reduce intravenous fluid rate for adults to 7.5 ml/kg/h. Switch to 0.5% normal saline solution.

Hour 4: Adjust intravenous fluid rate to meet the patient's clinical need. When blood glucose levels reach 250 mg/dl, add 5% dextrose.

U-100 regular insulin can be given IM or IV. Low-dose continuous infusion by IV is the preferred route of administration for insulin only if an IV pump is available to regulate the infusion.

Sodium, potassium, and phosphate are added to the IV fluid.

Continuous monitoring is required. Use of a flow sheet to follow essential laboratory data and patient assessment data is recommended. Monitoring should include but not be limited to electrolytes, blood glucose, serum/urine ketones, fluid balance, and level of consciousness.

Patients are kept NPO. If the patient is comatose, a nasogastric tube may be placed to prevent vomiting and possible aspiration of gastric contents.

When the patient is stabilized, an in-depth assessment must be performed to identify possible causes for the DKA or HHNS. Patients should be referred to a mental health-care professional for an assessment and intervention if psychologic or psychosocial barriers are suspected. All patients and their families/significant others require education on the causes, prevention, and principles of treatment of DKA and HHNS.

NURSING CARE

NURSING ASSESSMENT

See Assessment Considerations table below.

Diagnostic Studies and Findings

Study	(DKA)	HHNS
Blood glucose	High (>250 mg/dl)	Over 800 mg/dl
Plasma ketones	Strongly positive	Not present (or only in small amounts)
Serum sodium	Low, normal, or high	Normal or high
Serum potassium	Low, normal, or high	Low, normal, or high
Serum bicarbonate	4-15 mEq	Greater than 16 mEq
Blood pH	6.8-7.3	Normal
Serum osmolarity	Less than 350 mOsm/L	Greater than 350 mOsm/L

Assessment Considerations

Areas of Concern	DKA	HHNS
Circulation	Hypotension/orthostatic hypotension Tachycardia Weak, thready pulse ECG changes: Elevated or inverted P wave, prolonged QT interval Decreased neck vein filling	Tachycardia Rapid, thready pulse Cool extremities Normal to low blood pressure Orthostatic hypotension Shock Decreased neck vein filling
Gastrointestinal status	Nausea and vomiting Abdominal bloating Abdominal tenderness	Mild nausea and vomiting (if present)
Nutritional status	Weight loss	Weight loss
Fluid status	Polydipsia Weight loss Polyuria Nocturia Vomiting Hyperthermia/hypothermia Dry mucous membranes Sunken eyeballs Hot, dry, flushed skin Poor skin turgor	Polydipsia Weight loss Polyuria Hyperthermia Dry mucous membranes Sunken eyeballs

Continued

Assessment Considerations—cont'd

Areas of Concern	DKA	HHNS
Neurosensory status	Weakness Level of consciousness: Alert, drowsy Lethargy, coma Hyporeflexia	Diminished level of consciousness Visual changes Increased or decreased reflexes Positive Babinski's sign Various abnormal neurologic findings (aphasia, hemisensory defects, seizures, hemiparesis)
Pulmonary status	Hyperpnea (Kussmaul's respirations) Acetone breath	
Mobility	Decreased muscle tone Muscle wasting Muscle weakness	Muscle weakness
Psychosocial status	Frightened Crying Restless Unable to care for self because of high levels of anxiety or decreased consciousness	Inability to care for self because of change in level of consciousness

Patient Problems/Nursing Diagnoses & Interventions

NIC Electrolyte and Acid-Base Management

Deficient fluid volume related to failure of regulatory mechanism

- Reassess skin turgor to determine fluid balance.
- Reassess pulse, temperature, and blood pressure every 30 to 60 minutes.
- Monitor I&O every hour and urine specific gravity as ordered to assess changes in fluid balance.
- Administer intravenous fluids, insulin, potassium, and other electrolytes as ordered.
- Report signs and symptoms of circulatory collapse immediately.
- Start and maintain patent peripheral IV line.
- Provide mouth care every hour to maximize comfort.
- Monitor for circulatory overload during fluid replacement.
- Continue to monitor and report worsening of fluid volume deficit or electrolyte imbalance signs and symptoms.
- Record patient data on flow sheet.

NIC Nutrition Support

Imbalanced nutrition: less than body requirements, related to inadequate intake of nutrients in diet

- Monitor patient's laboratory data *to assess fluid and electrolyte balance.*
- Encourage patient to ingest small amounts of ice chips frequently and sip clear, cool fluids as tolerated.
- Encourage patient to maintain good oral hygiene.
- Discuss causes of nausea, vomiting, and thirst with patient.
- Treat underlying problem with intravenous fluids, insulin, potassium, and other electrolytes as ordered.
- Monitor patient's blood glucose and urine ketone levels as ordered.
- Review patient's diet prescription with dietitian before discharge.

NIC Coping Assistance

Ineffective coping related to situational crisis

- Explain all procedures to the patient and family.
- Encourage the patient's participation in self-care to maximum ability as soon as able.
- See p. 1583.
- Discuss causes of situational stress with the patient.
- Assist patient to identify and use appropriate coping strategies.
- Provide support and positive reinforcement.

NIC Risk Management

Risk for injury related to sensory dysfunction

- Assist and support patient as needed *to reduce chance of injury.*
- Provide assistive devices as needed.
- Minimize hazardous environmental factors.
- Discuss causative factors and prevention of injury with patient and family.
- Assess mental status frequently.

Patient Education/Continuum of Care Plan

Ensure patient verbalizes understanding of the essential skills and concepts of diabetes mellitus patient education (p. 784), especially sick day rules.

Evaluation/Patient Outcomes

Electrolyte and Acid-Base Management: Fluid balance is achieved. Patient's blood pressure is within normal limits. Patient's pulse is within normal limits. Shock is not present. Patient's circulation to peripheral tissues is adequate. Patient has no dehydration. Patient's output equals intake. Patient's skin turgor is normal. Patient's electrolyte levels are within normal limits.

Nutrition Support: Intake of nutrients is adequate. Patient's blood pH is normal, and blood sugar level is within normal limits. Patient is conscious and alert. Patient's respiratory rate and character are normal. Patient's electrolyte levels are within normal limits. Patient's ECG is at baseline. Patient has no ketonuria. Patient's weight is stable. Patient has ingested the recommended amounts and types of nutrients. Patient describes causative factors and rationale for treatment. Patient's fluid and electrolyte balance is normal. Patient has no nausea, vomiting, or thirst.

Coping Assistance: Patient copes effectively. Patient verbalizes concerns and fears. Patient's behavior is calm and appropriate. Patient discusses potential causes of condition. Patient verbalizes methods to prevent recurrence. Patient uses appropriate coping strategies. Patient accepts support. Patient shows increased independence in self-care.

Risk Management: Patient remains free of personal injury. Patient seeks assistance as needed. Patient uses assistive devices as needed. Patient verbalizes cause of potential for injury. Patient recognizes environmental hazards and avoids them.

HYPOGLYCEMIA

Hypoglycemia includes conditions of excess serum insulin, which causes a reduction in blood glucose level and produces symptoms of hypoglycemia. These symptoms are generally relieved when normal blood glucose levels are restored. (See Emergency Alert box on p. 792.) The presence of hypoglycemia, once proven, should be viewed as a marker of an underlying disorder and the etiology determined.[23]

Hypoglycemia is classified as follows:

Fasting
- Insulin-producing islet cell tumors (insulinomas)
- Islet cell hyperplasia (nesidioblastosis)
- Extrapancreatic tumors
- Hepatic disease
- Gluconeogenic substrate defects
- Insulin autoimmune syndromes

Reactive
- Reactive hypoglycemia
- Alimentary hypoglycemia
- Early diabetes mellitus

Induced
- Exogenous insulin or sulfonylurea use by persons with known diabetes
- Factitious use of insulin or sulfonylureas by patients without diabetes mellitus
- Drug/alcohol-induced

The following discussion will be limited to conditions that are endocrine in nature with hyperinsulinemia as a causative factor: Insulinoma, islet hyperplasia, reactive hypoglycemia, and induced hypoglycemia. Of all types of hypoglycemia, fasting hypoglycemia is the most serious.

The true prevalence of each entity is uncertain. Insulinomas are uncommon, with episodic hypoglycemia occurring in the fasting state. Episodes become more frequent and severe in nature. Insulinomas are the most common islet cell tumors. They arise from pancreatic beta cells and produce insulin. Tumors vary in size, but no relationship exists between the size of the tumor and the severity of symptoms. Most insulinomas are benign, and 90% occur in individuals over age 30 years.[23] Insulinomas can occur with other endocrine abnormalities, such as in type I multiple endocrine neoplasia (MEN-I), which is associated with adenomas of the pituitary and parathyroid tissue and with the occurrence of Zollinger-Ellison syndrome. Nesidioblastosis is a rare disease causing persistent hypoglycemia. This condition was formerly believed to affect only newborns and infants; however, it has recently been reported in adolescents and adults. Nesidioblastosis results from diffuse proliferation of beta cells and inappropriate insulin release.

Reactive hypoglycemia is somewhat poorly defined and controversial. Hypoglycemia occurs as a result of excessive or delayed insulin secretion. Early diabetes mellitus and alimentary hypoglycemia are conditions sometimes associated with reactive patterns of hypoglycemia. True reactive hypoglycemia is rare, occurring primarily in individuals who consume high amounts of refined carbohydrate calories. It is well documented that ingestion of large amounts of simple sugars often causes a transient drop in the blood glucose level. When meals contain a balance of complex carbohydrate, protein, and fat, the same degree of carbohydrate reactivity is not present.

Drug-induced hypoglycemia is commonly associated with diabetic persons who use blood glucose–lowering medication. Not only can the agent lower blood glucose levels, but it also can interact with other agents in an additive or synergistic way to produce hypoglycemia. Common causes of hypoglycemia in persons with known diabetes who use blood glucose–lowering medications include the following:

1. Error in dosage
2. Poor comprehension of medication information
3. Increased activity/exercise
4. Lack of sufficient food intake
5. Decreased insulin requirements

In these cases, hypoglycemia occurs as a complication of medical therapy; however, factitious use of these same medications by patients without diabetes mellitus is the result of a deliberate attempt to create the illusion of a hypoglycemic disorder. Hypoglycemia induced by factitious use of insulin was first described in 1947. C-peptide is useful in differentiating endogenous from exogenous hyperinsulinemia. The possibility of insulin self-injection in the patient without diabetes mellitus (surreptitious insulin use) should be considered in all cases of fasting hypoglycemia, particularly in instances involving health professionals or persons who have contact with those who have diabetes. These persons can be ingenious in concealing their use of insulin and often display no psychologic disturbance. Sulfonylurea abuse has also been reported as a cause of factitious hypoglycemia, together with surreptitious insulinomas.[44] Many other drugs have been reported to cause hypoglycemia, including pentamidine, quinine, and disopyramide.

PATHOPHYSIOLOGY

Insulin is responsible for maintaining normal blood glucose levels in conjunction with counterregulatory hormones (epinephrine, glucagon, cortisol, and growth hormones) that oppose

! EMERGENCY ALERT

HYPOGLYCEMIA

Hypoglycemia is defined as dangerously low glucose levels that are classified as either fasting or reactive. It results from an underproduction of glucose, oversupply of insulin, or some drug interactions.

ASSESSMENT

- Determine history of diabetes and management.
- Assess for the following:
  - Sweating
  - Tachycardia
  - Restlessness
  - Tremors
  - Headache
  - Appearance of drunkenness
  - Visual changes
  - Confusion
  - Personality changes
  - Seizures
  - Coma
  - Nightmares/vivid dreaming
- Test capillary blood glucose level (capillary blood glucose <60 mg/dl is too low).

INTERVENTIONS

If the patient is conscious, go to step 1.

1. Test capillary blood glucose level.
2. Administer 15 g of a fast-acting carbohydrate.
3. Wait 5 min.
   a. If signs and symptoms worsen before the 5 min ends, retreat. Go to step 2.
   b. If signs and symptoms improve, test the patient's blood glucose level.
      1. If the capillary blood glucose level is less than 60 mg/dl, go to step 2.
      2. If the capillary blood glucose level is greater that 60 mg/dl, go to step 4.
4. Consider when the next meal is scheduled.
   a. If the next meal/snack is <30 min away, feed the patient his or her usual meal or snack.
   b. If the next meal/snack is >30 min away, eat ½ bread exchange and ½ meat exchange.
   c. If it is at night, eat 1 bread and 1 meat exchange.

If the patient is unconscious and you have intravenous access, administer 1 ampule of dextrose 50%.

If the patient is unconscious and you have lost intravenous access:

1. Administer 1 unit of glucagon intramuscularly. (Glucagon can take as long as 20 min to raise the patient's blood glucose level.)
2. Establish intravenous access.
3. Monitor the patient's blood glucose level.
4. Feed the patient once he or she is able to swallow.
5. Notify the physician.

insulin action in the fasting and fed state. In hyperinsulinemia, excess insulin levels disrupt this balance by increasing glucose use and inhibiting hepatic glucose production. Negative feedback control over insulin secretion is lost; insulin secretion is not suppressed as plasma glucose levels decrease, and glucose utilization is increased. Disrupting this balance results in decreased serum glucose level. The clinical severity of hypoglycemia is not well correlated with specific blood glucose levels. The early symptoms of low blood glucose levels are associated with inhibition of glucose receptors in the ventromedial hypothalamic nucleus. This stimulates the sympathetic fibers of the autonomic nervous system to release epinephrine to restore blood glucose levels to normal. A decrease in blood glucose levels leads to an increased secretion of all four counterregulatory hormones. Glucagon plays the primary counterregulatory role by increasing hepatic glucose production. Catecholamines exert a major influence in counterregulation and are responsible for the appearance of early or adrenergic symptoms of hypoglycemia. These symptoms include sweating, palpitations, tachycardia, tremors, pallor, hunger, and nervousness. This adrenergic response serves as an early warning mechanism that precedes changes in cortical function occurring as a result of inadequate glucose to brain cells.

The brain depends completely on glucose as an energy source and, therefore, is extremely sensitive to hypoglycemia. Neuroglycopenic symptoms follow as a result of an inadequate supply of glucose to maintain normal function; they include headache, fatigue, irritability, visual disturbances, decreased attentiveness, amnesia, confusion, prosthesis, paralysis, seizures, and loss of consciousness. These symptoms can be most severe and occur at a higher blood level in elderly than in young individuals.[44] Some irreversible brain damage can occur as the result of frequent or prolonged hypoglycemia, including a decrease in intellectual function, impaired nerve function, and personality changes.

Insulin-producing islet cell tumors (insulinomas; islet cell hyperplasia nesidioblastosis) and induced forms of hypoglycemia produce absolute elevations in plasma insulin levels that are not responsive to changes in blood glucose levels. Hypoglycemia results from the following:

1. Elevated glucose uptake by insulin-dependent tissues
2. Inhibition of hepatic glucose production; exercise intensifies hypoglycemic symptoms because of additional glucose uptake by muscle cells

In contrast with fasting hypoglycemia, neuroglycopenic symptoms are not observed postprandially or in reactive patterns of hypoglycemia. In these cases, hypoglycemia is brief, mild, and accompanied by adrenergic and nonspecific symptoms. Alimentary hypoglycemia is thought to be mediated by rapid gastric emptying, rapid early glucose absorption with excessive hyperglycemia and hyperinsulinemia, and/or vagal interruption. Increased gut hormone secretion may also play a causative role.[23] Reactive hypoglycemia resolves spontaneously with counterregulation and does not require intervention with carbohydrate feeding.

Hypoglycemia is episodic; symptoms may recur, lasting for a few minutes to a few hours. If food ingestion does not occur to return blood glucose levels to normal, blood glucose continues to decline, leading to loss of consciousness, seizures, or death.[22] In most cases, symptoms of hypoglycemia are reversible within minutes after euglycemia is restored.

DIAGNOSTIC STUDIES AND FINDINGS[17,18]

Insulinomas: Blood glucose (low fasting or when symptomatic); plasma insulin (inappropirately elevated fasting or when symptomatic); plasma proinsulin and C-peptide (elevated fasting or when symptomatic); 72 hours supervised fast (elevated insulin, low blood glucose level; most are symptomatic within 24 hours); tumor localization by CT scan, ultrasound, percutaneous transhepatic portal venous sampling, and/or selective arteriography

Nesidioblastosis: Blood sugar (low fasting or when symptomatic); plasma insulin (inappropriately elevated fasting or when symptomatic); plasma proinsulin and C-peptide (elevated fasting or when symptomatic)

Exogenous insulin or sulfonylureas by patients with diabetes mellitus: Plasma glucose (low when symptomatic)

Factitious insulin use: Blood glucose (low when symptomatic); plasma insulin and C-peptide (low levels); plasma proinsulin and C-peptide (low levels); plasma insulin antibodies (may be present with use of nonhuman source insulin)

MULTIDISCIPLINARY PLAN

Surgery

Subtotal pancreatectomy (for nesidioblastosis); insulinoma resection

Medications

Insulinoma and nesidioblastosis
- Diazoxide (Proglycem), 150-600 mg/day
- Phenytoin (Dilantin), 300-600 mg/day
- Propranolol (Inderal), 80 mg/day

Malignant insulinoma
- Antineoplastic agents: Streptozocin, 5-fluorouracil, asparaginase, mithramycin, or adriamycin
- Somatostatin analog (octreotide), 200-675 μg/day

Unconscious hypoglycemia (all types)
- Glucagon, 1 mg SC, IM, or IV
- 50% dextrose, 25 g IV over 1-3 min

General Management

Diet

Insulinoma and nesidioblastosis
- Increase number of feedings per day, may need to ingest food every 2 to 4 hours through day and night
- During symptomatic episodes: rapidly absorbable forms of simple carbohydrates
- Continuous intravenous administration of glucose by infusion for severe refractory hypoglycemia

Exogenous insulin and sulfonylurea use by patients with diabetes mellitus
- Medical nutrition therapy (individualized)
- During symptomatic episodes: 10 to 15 g of simple carbohydrate for mild (adrenergic symptoms) reaction; 20 to 30 g of simple carbohydrate for moderate (adrenergic and neuroglycopenic symptoms) reaction
- May need to follow with mixed snack (complex carbohydrate and protein) if next meal is more than 1 hour after initial treatment

Reactive
- Carbohydrate restriction, especially with simple sugars
- Decrease meal size
- Increase meal frequency
- Dietitian referral

Factitious insulin and sulfonylurea use
- Before diagnosis, same as insulinoma and nesidioblastosis

Psychiatric Consultation

Factitious insulin and sulfonylurea use

NURSING CARE

NURSING ASSESSMENT

Circulation: Tachycardia, palpitations, vital signs

Food and fluid needs: Relief of symptoms with food intake: hunger, weight gain

Neurosensory concerns: Tremor, headache, mental dullness, confusion, amnesia, seizures, unconsciousness, paralysis, paresthesias, dizziness, irritability, visual disturbance

Psychosocial concerns: Change in role performance; resents enforced dependence; unable to stay alone: related to episodes of loss of consciousness; past history of destructive behavior

POTENTIAL COMPLICATIONS

Crisis hypoglycemia, coma, death

PATIENT PROBLEMS/NURSING DIAGNOSES & INTERVENTIONS

NIC NUTRITION SUPPORT

Imbalanced nutrition: more than body requirements, related to excess intake for metabolic needs
- Assess for symptoms that patient normally experiences with hypoglycemia and ask whether or not patient is awakened by symptoms at night.
- Assess patient for symptoms of low blood sugar level, and check blood glucose level by fingerstick using bedside blood glucose monitoring (BBGM): fasting, before and 2 hours after meals, at bedtime, and at 3 to 5 AM.
- Provide patient with 3 AM snack if needed *to prevent nocturnal hypoglycemia.*
- Arrange a dietary consultation.
- Identify symptoms of hypoglycemia experienced by patient.
- Provide prompt intervention for episodes of hypoglycemia.
- Monitor patient's blood sugar level frequently (q2-4h) including during the night.
- Discuss cause of weight gain.
- Discuss with patient the importance of frequent meals and monitoring *for prevention and early detection of hypoglycemia.*
- After successful treatment of underlying cause, assist patient to set realistic goals related to weight management.

NIC COPING ASSISTANCE

Ineffective coping related to situational crisis
- Assess patient's personal strengths and weaknesses and coping skills.
- Remove potentially dangerous articles from patient's room (factitious use of insulin or sulfonylureas).

- Encourage patient toward maximum independence.
- Assist patient to communicate with others.
- Discuss need for restrictions and precautions related to potential loss of consciousness *to maintain patient's safety and prevent injury.*
- Give information about disease to enhance feeling of control.
- Encourage patient to consult with psychiatrist.
- Offer support to patient.
- Discuss cause of situational stress with patient.
- Assist patient to identify and use appropriate coping strategies.
- See p. 1583.

NIC Risk Management

Risk for injury related to sensory dysfunction

- Provide patient with consistent daily meal plan, including 3 AM snack.
- Limit patient's physical activity or mobility during episodes of hypoglycemia.
- Minimize hazardous environmental factors.
- Discuss causative factors with patient and family.

Patient Education/Continuum of Care Plan

1. Explain to patient the signs and symptoms of hypoglycemia and importance of early recognition and prompt treatment.
2. Discuss with patient a 24-hour diet plan and the importance of adhering to it.
3. Provide patient with information regarding amounts and types of foods/fluids to treat hypoglycemia.

Evaluation/Patient Outcomes

Nutrition Support: Intake of nutrients is adequate. Patient has no hypoglycemia, or hypoglycemia is detected early and managed adequately. Patient experiences no seizures or loss of consciousness. Patient ingests the recommended types and amounts of nutrients at desired times. Patient describes causative factors and rationale for treatment. Patient's weight gain is minimized until the problem is resolved.

Coping Assistance: Patient copes effectively. Anxiety is decreased. Family verbalizes adapting to changes imposed by hypoglycemia. Patient accepts support from health professionals. Patient establishes and follows plan to minimize symptoms and maximize functioning. Maximum independence is maintained. Patient shows no self-destructive behavior. Patient complies with the precautions and restrictions imposed.

Risk Management: Patient remains free of personal injury. Patient identifies and avoids factors that increase potential for injury. Patient uses preventive measures. Patient verbalizes cause of potential for injury. Patient complies with diet and monitoring prescription, as well as activity restrictions during episodes of hypoglycemia. Patient shows no seizures or loss of consciousness.

Zollinger-Ellison Syndrome (Gastrinoma)

Zollinger-Ellison syndrome (ZES) is characterized by gastric acid hypersecretion and recurrent peptic ulcer disease. It is caused by excessive gastrin secretion from non–beta cell islet cell tumors, or gastrinomas, with accompanying diarrhea.

Although ZES is uncommon, it is not rare. Approximately 20% to 25% of pancreatic endocrine tumors are gastrinomas.[19] The tumors primarily arise from the pancreas and rarely may be found in the duodenum, stomach, spleen, ovary, and lymph nodes.

Gastrinomas vary in size and location, and approximately two thirds are malignant, 50% having metastasis at the time of diagnosis. Usual sites of metastasis are lymph nodes, liver, spleen, bone, skin, and peritoneum. Multiple endocrine neoplasia type I (MEN) is present in 25% to 30% of patients with ZES.

Before the development of potent antisecretory drug therapy, the mortality from ZES was high, not always from metastases of the malignant tumor, but often from the extreme effects of hypergastrinemia and complications of ulcers: hemorrhage, perforation or fistula formation leading to obstruction. Total gastrectomy was the only relatively successful treatment for ZES. The development of histamine H-receptor blocking agents and benzimidazole inhibitors of gastric acid secretion represented a major breakthrough in the management of ZES.

Pathophysiology

ZES is characterized by recurrent and severe peptic ulcer disease. Gastrin has various effects on the gastrointestinal tract. The major effect is the stimulation of gastric acid secretion from parietal cells, possibly through stimulation of a histamine or cyclic AMP–mediated process. The secretion of gastrin by tumor tissue (gastrinomas) is not responsive to the normal inhibitory stimuli of low gastric pH and secretin; secretin paradoxically stimulates gastrin release. The continuous high serum gastrin levels found in ZES produce a state of constant gastric acid hypersecretion that exceeds the duodenum's capacity to neutralize acid. This accounts for the upper gastrointestinal ulcerations found in sites as far distal to the stomach as the jejunum. Gastrin is also known to cause moderate stimulation of pepsin release from gastric chief cells. In the presence of low pH in the proximal and distal duodenum and jejunum, pepsin contributes to the development of mucosal erosion and ulceration at points as distal as the jejunum.[19] Gastrin also directly decreases salt and water absorption in the intestine, resulting in the presence of large amounts of fluid in both stomach and duodenum even in the fasting state. Marked hyperplasia of parietal cells and mucosal cell proliferation with hypertrophy of the pyloric gastric mucosa are the direct result of high serum gastrin levels, ultimately causing the development of prominent rugal folds in the stomach.[43] The increased number of parietal cells in ZES is significant in the development of hyperacidity because a close relationship exists between the number of parietal cells and the amount of gastric acid secreted.[19,53]

The other increasingly recognized feature of ZES is diarrhea and/or steatorrhea. The diarrhea and steatorrhea of ZES is caused by a number of factors, as follows:

1. Large amounts of hydrochloric acid irritate the gastrointestinal mucosa and increase peristalsis.
2. Gastrin increases intestinal motility.
3. Pancreatic lipase is inactivated in the presence of low intestinal pH and fat breakdown, and absorption is not accomplished.
4. Precipitation and inactivation of bile salts in the acid environment of the small intestine also prevent fat absorption.
5. The direct effect of gastrin stimulates gastric, pancreatic, liver, and intestinal secretion of water and electrolytes.
6. The malabsorption of various substances is caused by inactivation of intestinal enzymes in the presence of acidity.

Diarrhea and steatorrhea are accompanied by severe losses of potassium and magnesium in patients with ZES.

Gastrin also stimulates intrinsic factor secretion. In ZES, malabsorption of vitamin B_{12} is thought to result from the low intestinal pH, which may interfere with the action of intrinsic factor in facilitating the absorption of vitamin B_{12}. This condition is not corrected by the administration of intrinsic factor; only monthly vitamin B_{12} injections can ameliorate it.

Diagnostic Studies and Findings

Fasting elevated serum gastrin level: Level of 500 pg/ml diagnostic of ZES after exclusion of other disorders with hypergastrinemia[21]

Provocative testing: Gastric acid output test, basal acid concentration >15 mEq/h in previously unoperated patient and >5 mEq/h in previously operated patients; ratio of basal/maximal acid output (BAO/MAO) is 0.6 or greater[19]

Secretin test: Serum gastrin level rises by at least >200 pg/ml over baseline within 10 minutes of secretin injection[21]

Radiologic findings: Irregular thick gastric mucosal folds with ulcers at usual and unusual sites; pancreatic islet cell tumor demonstrated by angiography.

Tumor localization: Abdominal CT scan; abdominal ultrasound; selective mesenteric arteriography; transhepatic portal vein blood sampling

Multidisciplinary Plan

Surgery

Total gastrectomy (see Chapter 10); partial pancreatectomy (tumor excision)

Medications

Omeprazole, 20-60 mg/day (superior to histamine H_2 receptor antagonists because of its inhibition of gastric acid production)

Histamine H_2 receptor antagonists
- Cimetidine, 300-600 mg q6h
- Ranitidine, 150 mg qid or qid and hs
- Famotidine, 20-160 mg q6h

Benzimidazoles

Streptozocin, 5-FU, doxorubicin (see cancer section) for treatment of metastatic gastrinomas

Miscellaneous
- Octreotide (Sandostatin), inhibits gastric release, gastric acid secretion, diarrhea) long-acting, 220-675 μg/day

NURSING CARE

Nursing Assessment

Circulation: Decreased blood pressure; tachycardia; cold clammy skin; vital signs

Food and fluid needs: Burning, pain in epigastric region between meals; coffee-ground or frank blood emesis; thirst; decreased appetite; weight loss; weigh daily; intake and output; dry mouth

Elimination: Increased frequency of stools; foul-smelling, foamy stools; abdominal cramping/pain

Comfort and pain: Severe upper abdominal pain, may be referred to top of shoulders; abdomen rigid and tender

Psychosocial concerns: Feelings of helplessness, decreased participation in outside-the-home activities because of diarrhea, embarrassment

Potential Complications

Severe electrolyte imbalance, hyponatremia, hypokalemia, excessive vomiting and diarrhea, renal shutdown

Patient Problems/Nursing Diagnoses & Interventions

NIC Electrolyte and Acid-Base Management

Risk for deficient fluid volume related to excessive loss through normal routes
- Monitor fluid balance *to identify dehydration early.*
- Measure daily fluid loss in stools and drainage *to prevent undetected loss.*
- Replace fluids with water, tea, carbonated beverages, gelatin, popsicles, and broth.
- Have a dietary consultation to include foods high in potassium and magnesium *to replace losses in diarrhea.*
- Discuss causes of fluid loss with patient and family.
- Treat underlying cause as ordered.

NIC Elimination Management

Diarrhea related to inflammation, irritation, and malabsorption
- Monitor fluid losses in diarrhea by daily measurement.
- Check with physician about medication for perianal irritation from frequent stools.
- Replace lost fluid and electrolytes *to prevent fluid and electrolyte imbalance.*
- Observe patient for signs and symptoms of dehydration, decreased potassium, and magnesium.
- Discuss causative factors with patient and family.
- Treat underlying cause as ordered.

NIC Coping Assistance

Ineffective coping related to situational crisis
- Assess patient's and family's coping skills, support systems, and adaptive skills successful in the past.
- Encourage open communication between patient and family members.
- Assist patient in identifying strengths and positive coping skills *to cope with current stressors.*

- Offer suggestions as to how patient can cope with problem areas and function away from home.
- Discuss causes of situational stress.
- Offer support and positive reinforcement.
- Assist with problem solving.

NIC PHYSICAL COMFORT PROMOTION

Acute pain related to injuring agent
- Discuss causes of pain with patient and family.
- Assist patient to use pain control measures.
- Treat underlying cause as ordered.
- Monitor pain and effectiveness of comfort measures.

PATIENT EDUCATION/CONTINUUM OF CARE PLAN

1. Discuss with patient the importance of fluid and electrolyte replacement for diarrhea to prevent dehydration and changes in electrolyte balance.
2. Ensure patient understands the need for strict medication compliance to maintain status of healed ulcers and avoid pain.
3. Ensure patient understands the dose, schedule, action, and side effects of medication ordered to ensure safe and effective use of medication.

EVALUATION/PATIENT OUTCOMES

Electrolyte and Acid-Base Management: Fluid balance is achieved. Patient has no hemorrhage. Patient shows no changes in blood pressure or pulse. Patient verbalizes understanding of and complies with fluid and electrolyte (potassium, magnesium) replacement with diarrhea. Patient is not dehydrated.

Elimination Management: Normal bowel elimination pattern. Patient has a more normal pattern of bowel elimination. Patient describes causative factors and rationale for interventions. Patient shows no perineal irritation.

Coping Assistance: Patient copes effectively. Patient uses appropriate coping strategies. Patient accepts support. Open communication exists between patient and family. Patient uses suggestions to increase independence and ability to function away from home.

Physical Comfort Promotion: Pain is resolved. Patient uses suggested comfort measures. Patient describes causative factors. Patient verbalizes increased comfort

DISORDERS OF THE PARATHYROID GLANDS

PRIMARY HYPERPARATHYROIDISM (HPT)

Primary hyperparathyroidism (HPT) is caused by the excessive secretion of parathyroid hormone (PTH) from one or more of the four parathyroid glands.

Primary hyperparathyroidism is part of the differential diagnosis of hypercalcemia. It is the most common cause of hypercalcemia among nonhospitalized patients; malignancy accounts for the most common cause of hypercalcemia among hospitalized patients. The box below lists many of the causes of hypercalcemia. Only primary hyperparathyroidism is discussed in this section.

HPT may be triggered by a benign adenoma isolated to a single gland (80% of all HPT), more than one adenoma in a patient (1% to 2%), hyperplasia of all four glands (15%), or parathyroid carcinoma (1% of all HPT). The incidence of HPT increased greatly in the early 1970s when multichannel screening tests were first used. Today the incidence has stabilized at about 1:1000 and approximates the prevalence. It can occur at all ages but is unusual in children and peaks between ages 50 and 60 years. It is more frequent in women than in men, with a 3:2 ratio. A history of radiation to the neck may be a predisposing factor.[23]

Parathyroid hyperplasia occurs most frequently in conjunction with the multiple endocrine neoplasia (MEN) syndromes types I and IIA. MEN I is an autosomal dominant disorder with

CAUSES OF HYPERCALCEMIA

PARATHYROID GLAND
Idiopathic
Associated with MEN types 1 or 2a
Familial

MALIGNANCIES
Osteolytic hypercalcemia
Humoral hypercalcemia of malignancy
1,25-Dihydroxyvitamin D–mediated hypercalcemia
Hematologic malignancies

OTHER ENDOCRINE DISORDERS
Thyrotoxicosis
Pheochromocytoma
Addisonian crisis
VIPoma syndrome
Acromegaly
Familial hypocalciuric hypercalcemia (FHH)

MEDICATIONS
Vitamin D and A intoxication
Lithium
Thiazide diuretics
Estrogen/antiestrogens, androgens
Theophylline
Milk alkali syndrome (excess calcium drugs)
Parenteral nutrition

GRANULOMATOUS DISORDERS
Sarcoidosis
Tuberculosis
Histoplasmosis
Coccidioidomycosis
Candidiasis

MISCELLANEOUS
Dehydration
Renal failure
Advanced chronic liver disease
Immobilization
Serum protein disorders
Hypophosphatemia
Paget's disease

a high degree of penetrance. These patients usually have tumors of the pituitary, parathyroid, and endocrine pancreas. MEN IIA is also autosomal dominant and involves medullary thyroid carcinoma, HPT, and pheochromocytoma.

PATHOPHYSIOLOGY

Parathyroid hormone is usually regulated by the ionized calcium level. As ionized calcium decreases, it stimulates the release of PTH. Conversely, as ionized calcium increases, it suppresses the release of PTH. In primary hyperparathyroidism, PTH continues to be secreted in the presence of an elevated ionized calcium. It has been theorized that either the parathyroid cells have developed an altered set point so that they can only respond to a higher than normal ionized calcium or the parathyroid cells have increased in number without an altered set point.[23] The altered set point means that the gland still has the ability to be suppressed, such as by increasing dietary calcium intake. Both of these mechanisms may be operational in an adenoma, while hyperplasia is more closely linked to an increased number of parathyroid cells without alteration of the set point. In about 4% of adenomas, there is also evidence of a rearrangement involving the PTH gene and the parathyroid adenoma gene (PRAD1). PRAD1 is a monoclonal oncogene that may supplant PTH in the adenoma, leading to both growth of the cells and the altered set point. This rearrangement seems to be limited to the adenomatous gland and has not been found in the remaining normal parathyroid glands. In fact, the uninvolved glands become suppressed by the adenomatous gland, which means they are hormonally inactive. Hyperplasia, on the other hand, appears to be a polyclonal process. In parathyroid carcinoma, there seems to be true autonomy of one of the glands, which means that the gland no longer responds to any feedback mechanism and continues to secrete PTH unabated.

Primary hyperparathyroidism at present is recognized most frequently as an asymptomatic disease. The diagnosis is arrived at as a result of an elevated serum calcium level obtained on routine laboratory examination. If symptoms do occur, they have traditionally been described in relation to the primary target organs for PTH of bones and kidney. The patient may be predisposed to nephrolithiasis or to osteopenia, although it is rare for the patient to have both. The osteopenia may be seen as osteitis fibrous cystica on x-rays or as a decreased bone mineral density. Since HPT tends to occur in older postmenopausal women who may already have osteopenia, the onset of HPT may lead to osteoporosis. The gastrointestinal tract is the other major target organ. Peptic ulcer disease and acute pancreatitis have both been associated with HPT.

A number of other systemic effects accompany hypercalcemia. Intracellular to extracellular calcium balance in neurotransmission seems to be altered, leading to atrophy of type II muscle fibers and causing a proximal muscle weakness. Fatigue may be the nonspecific complaint voiced by the patient.

The area of greatest controversy today involves what has been termed the "psychic moans" of HPT. Distinct psychiatric manifestations of HPT have long included clinical depression, lethargy, stupor, and coma. The question remains whether, in mild HPT, the patients are truly asymptomatic, or there are more subtle psychologic alterations that increase the difficulty of completing ADLs and social responsibilities. Cognitive deficits have been described that include memory impairment and concentration difficulties. As in muscle cells, it has been postulated that the elevated PTH and calcium affect cerebral vascular adenyl cyclase and nerve conduction velocity. In addition to cognitive deficits, the following have also been described: Obsessive-compulsive behavior, psychoticism, anxiety, and paranoia.

The treatment for HPT varies from a wait-and-watch plan to surgical intervention. Some patients may have mild elevations in calcium and PTH levels that can remain unchanged over 5 or more years. These patients must be aware of symptoms of increasing calcium and be willing to have regular laboratory and physical reevaluations. Surgical intervention for an adenoma involves removal of the adenoma. The national consensus[15] criteria for surgery include (1) serum calcium level above 12 mg/dl, (2) 400 mg calcium/g creatinine in the urine, (3) worsening creatinine clearance, (4) nephrolithiasis, and (5) substantially reduced bone mass (osteoporosis). After surgery the patient is usually left with three healthy parathyroid glands that provide normal calcium/phosphorus metabolism. The surgical intervention for the patient with hyperplasia, however, involves removal of 3.5 to 3.75 glands. It is hoped that the remaining piece of a gland will eventually become hyperplastic and again provide normal calcium metabolism. If this does not occur and some of the removed tissue was cryopreserved, then minced pieces of parathyroid tissue might be implanted into a forearm muscle.

DIAGNOSTIC STUDIES AND FINDINGS

Total serum calcium: Greater than 11 mg/dl
Ionized calcium: Increased (varies by assay method)
Parathyroid hormone (PTH): Increased (>65 ng/ml)
Intact PTH better than C-terminal or N-terminal assay for differentiating primary hyperparathyroidism from renal disease and the hypercalcemia of malignancy
24-hour urine calcium: Normal to high
Creatinine clearance: Normal to high

MULTIDISCIPLINARY PLAN

Mild hyperparathyroidism: Wait and watch; may persist for months to years
Moderate/severe hyperparathyroidism: Parathyroidectomy
General: Increased hydration 2 to 3 L/day
Possible low-calcium diet
Psychologic/psychiatric evaluation

NURSING CARE

NURSING ASSESSMENT

No symptoms
Renal concerns: Polyuria, nephrolithiasis
Gastrointestinal concerns: Ulcer-type pain, constipation
Musculoskeletal concerns: Demineralization, pain, activity intolerance
Psychosocial concerns: Depression, paranoia, mood swings, anxiety, obsessive-compulsive behavior
Neuromuscular concerns: Weakness, fatigue

Potential Complications

Renal calculi, severe hypercalcemia, cardiac arrthymias

Patient Problems/Nursing Diagnoses & Interventions

NIC Activity and Exercise Management

Fatigue related to altered metabolic balance
Activity intolerance related to generalized weakness

- Help patient plan a daily schedule that includes pacing leisure activities, rest, and exercise.
- Help patient identify excessive demands of role obligations.
- Encourage patient to keep a diary of the degree of fatigue, precipitating factors, and specific symptoms that are perceived as fatigue.
- Observe patient for steadiness of gait.
- Assist patient with ambulation when necessary.
- Help patient identify environmental hazards at home and suggest alterations as necessary *to prevent injury.*

NIC Elimination Management

Constipation related to musculoskeletal impairment and less than adequate intake

- Encourage patient to ingest fluids to 3000 ml/day.
- Administer stool softeners to patient as ordered.
- Encourage patient to ingest a high-fiber diet.
- Avoid giving the patient enemas or laxatives.

NIC Coping Assistance

Ineffective coping related to personal identity vulnerability

- Help patient identify precipitating factors of stress.
- Help patient identify coping skills and adaptive behaviors used successfully in the past.
- Maintain a calm approach if the patient becomes agitated or irritable.
- Let patient know that the hormonal alteration reduces his or her ability to control his or her responses and that this is acceptable.

Patient Education/Continuum of Care Plan

1. Discuss with patient the need to keep follow-up appointments and have calcium levels rechecked.
2. Demonstrate to patient how to monitor and maintain adequate fluid intake.
3. Discuss with patient symptoms of kidney stones.
4. Discuss with patient the importance of proper body alignment and mechanics and the need to gradually increase activity tolerance.
5. Ensure that patient understands the importance of changing home environment to prevent accidents.
6. Discuss with patient the need for tolerance by family of patient's mood swings, irritability, or decreased decision-making ability until therapy is completed.

Evaluation/Patient Outcomes

Activity and Exercise Management: Comfort and activity level are increased. Patient's optimum level of mobility is maintained with little or no pain. Patient follows plan for using alternative pain-relieving methods. Patient uses pain medications infrequently. Patient verbalizes increased feelings of well-being. Patient participates in desired activities.

Elimination Management: Patient maintains good elimination pattern without constipation. Hydration is adequate. Patient's intake is at least 2 L/day.

Coping Assistance: Coping is improved. Patient can identify one stimulus to decreased coping. Patient uses one coping technique successfully.

Hypoparathyroidism

In hypoparathyroidism the parathyroid glands secrete an inadequate amount of parathyroid hormone (PTH) to maintain normal levels of serum calcium.

Hypoparathyroidism is manifested by hypocalcemia. This condition may occur at any age and is usually the result of damage to the parathyroid glands during parathyroid or thyroid surgery or purposeful removal of the parathyroid glands. It may also be from autoimmune destruction of the glands, either idiopathic or as part of a polyglandular autoimmune syndrome.

Pathophysiology

Although hypoparathyroidism is usually the result of damage to the parathyroid glands during surgical procedures, the disease may also be idiopathic. Idiopathic hypoparathyroidism is a rare autoimmune disorder that may occur before age 15 years. It is sometimes one of several endocrine disorders included in a polyendocrine syndrome, including hypoparathyroidism, Addison's disease, and moniliasis (HAM). Hypoparathyroidism has been acquired, in a few rare cases, after treatment with ^{131}I therapy. It has also been associated with metastases of malignant tumors to the parathyroid glands.[23]

The signs and symptoms of hypoparathyroidism are associated with hypocalcemia resulting from the decreased level of PTH. Neuromuscular irritability is the most common and recognizable feature of hypocalcemia, causing symptoms that range from mild parethesias to tetany and hypocalcemic seizures. These symptoms are caused by a decrease in resting ability and increased excitability of nerve and muscle membranes.

Bone resorption decreases in hypoparathyroidism, causing a decrease in osteoclastic activity. Bones remain normal or slightly denser in adults. New growth is suppressed and may cause dwarfism in children. Calcification of the basal ganglion, another clinical manifestation of hypoparathyroidism, results in a Parkinson-like syndrome with bizarre posturing and dystonic choreoathetoid movements. Other characteristics of the disease include dental abnormalities caused by decreased calcium levels, cataracts resulting from calcification of the lens, and hypotension caused by decreased cardiac contractility. Pseudohypoparathyroidism is a separate disease entity that is a familial disorder characterized by an atypical phenotype, chemical hypoparathyroidism, and increased circulating PTH levels.[23]

DIAGNOSTIC STUDIES AND FINDINGS

Serum calcium: Less than 8 mg/dl
Serum intact PTH: Less than 50 ng/ml

MULTIDISCIPLINARY PLAN

Medications

Calcium salts: Requirement 1500-2000 mg elemental calcium/day
- Calcium carbonate, 400 mg elemental calcium/1000 mg tablet
- Calcium citrate, 210 mg elemental calcium/1000 mg tablet
- Calcium lactate, 130 mg elemental calcium/1000 mg tablet
- Calcium gluconate, 90 mg elemental calcium/10 ml IV push in 3-5 min
- Calcium glubionate, 115 mg elemental calcium/5 ml syrup

Vitamin D
- Ergocalciferol, vitamin D_2, 50,000-100,000 U; 1.25-2.75 mg/day
- Dihydrotachysterol, 125-250 mg/day
- 25,Hydroxyvitamin D_3, cholecalciferol, 50-250 mg/day
- 1,25 Dihydroxyvitamin D_3, calcitriol, 0.5-1.0 mg/day

NURSING CARE

NURSING ASSESSMENT

Central nervous system concerns
- Personality disturbances: Lassitude, depression, irritability, cognitive deficits
- Increased neuromuscular excitability: Paresthesias, tetany, positive Chvostek's and Trousseau's signs
- Headache

Cardiovascular concerns: Decreased contractility, decreased output
Nutritional status: Dietary calcium intake, supplemental calcium intake
Skin: Dry, coarse, flaky
Eyes: Cataracts

POTENTIAL COMPLICATIONS

Severe hypocalcemia, tetany, seizures, coma/death

PATIENT PROBLEMS/NURSING DIAGNOSES & INTERVENTIONS

NIC NUTRITION SUPPORT

Imbalanced nutrition: less than body requirements, related to altered metabolism
- Identify food preferences that are high in calcium.
- Make high-calcium snacks available to patient at all times.
- Have the dietitian discuss dietary calcium supplements with the patient.
- Give calcium replacement medications on time *to enhance dietary intake of calcium.*
- Monitor Chvostek's and Trousseau's signs *to identify early loss of calcium.*

NIC COPING ASSISTANCE

Ineffective coping related to personal vulnerability
- Assess patient's current coping skills, support systems, and history of adaptive behaviors that worked in the past.
- Maintain a calm approach if the patient is agitated or irritable.
- Observe for precipitating factors causing stress; intervene when possible *to decrease stressors.*
- Observe for changes in mood and thought processes *to identify psychologic changes that may require medical interventions.*

NIC TISSUE PERFUSION MANAGEMENT

Decreased cardiac output related to alteration in conduction
- Assess vital signs, mental status, and urine output *for symptoms of hypoperfusion.*
- Check rhythm strip for QT interval changes and abnormal T wave and P wave changes *to identify hypocalcemia that is interfering with normal electrical activity of the myocardium.*

PATIENT EDUCATION/CONTINUUM OF CARE PLAN

1. Ensure that the patient verbalizes an understanding of calcium and vitamin D supplements and the reasons for the treatment.
2. Give the patient a list of the early signs and symptoms of hypocalcemia and its treatment.
3. Suggest patient wear medical alert bracelet.

EVALUATION/PATIENT OUTCOMES

Nutrition Support: Nutrition is adequate. Patient routinely consumes high-calcium foods without difficulty. Chvostek's and Trousseau's signs are negative.

Coping Assistance: Patient copes effectively. Patient expresses feelings and uses effective coping mechanisms for problems surrounding illness. Patient is able to identify factors leading to increased stress and possible solutions to prevent these situations. Patient's affect is appropriate to the situation.

Tissue Perfusion Management: Cardiac output is normal. Cardiac rate and rhythm are normal.

METABOLIC DISORDERS

DYSLIPIDEMIA (HYPERLIPIDEMIA)

Dyslipidemia is a condition of abnormal metabolism of plasma lipids that is manifested as abnormally high levels of lipids in the blood.

Hyperlipidemias are a group of disorders of lipid metabolism. They vary in cause, severity, response to treatment, and prognosis. Hyperlipidemias occur in all ages and races and in both sexes. *Primary hyperlipidemias* are often hereditary disorders caused by deficiencies of certain mechanisms involved in lipid metabolism. *Secondary hyperlipidemias* occur in relation to other conditions or disorders. The majority of hyperlipidemias seen in Western society are related to other conditions, the most common being diet. The American diet often includes foods that are high in cholesterol, total fat, saturated fat, and excess calories. Total fat and saturated fat have the most potent effect on cholesterol levels. Other common causes of secondary hyperlipidemia include the following:

1. Diabetes mellitus
2. Hypothyroidism
3. Renal disease, bile duct obstruction
4. Excessive alcohol intake
5. Drugs

Various medications such as beta-adrenergic blockers[30,35,42] retinoids, thiazide diuretics,[45] glucocorticoids,[28] and estrogen therapy[30] can cause blood lipid levels to increase significantly.

The most significant hyperlipidemias are those associated with atherosclerosis, narrowing of the blood vessels. Narrowing of the blood vessels results in diminished oxygen and nutrients to the affected organs. Restricted blood flow to the heart can cause cardiac ischemia and myocardial infarction. Restricted blood flow to the brain can cause transischemic attacks to the brain and stroke. Restricted blood flow to the lower extremities can cause intermittent claudication. Heart disease is responsible for 35% of all deaths in the United States.[59]

Compelling evidence[59] supports the Cholesterol-Diet-Heart Hypothesis, which states that:

1. Increased plasma cholesterol concentrations increase the risk of heart disease
2. Diets high in fat (especially saturated) and cholesterol result in increased levels of plasma cholesterol
3. Lowering plasma cholesterol levels results in a decreased risk of heart disease

Consequently, treatment of hyperlipidemias are targeted at:

1. Decreasing dietary intake of fat and overall caloric intake
2. Increasing exercise
3. The use of pharmacotherapeutic agents

Lipid Metabolism

Lipids have three major functions as follows:

1. Store nutrients (triglycerides)
2. Form the precursors for adrenal/gonadal steroids and bile acids (cholesterol)
3. Transport complex lipids throughout the body (lipoproteins)

Cholesterol comes from three sources. Cholesterol is absorbed from the gut, produced by the liver, and released by aging cells. Cholesterol is used to manufacture cell membranes, form precursors of adrenal/gonadal steroids, and form bile acids.

Triglycerides are composed of fatty acids and glycerol. Triglycerides are absorbed from the gut and produced by the liver.

Fatty acid components of triglycerides are used by the cells for energy or stored in adipose tissue. Excessive caloric intake and obesity encourage increased triglyceride synthesis by the liver and decreased removal from peripheral tissues. Phospholipids are synthesized mainly in the liver and intestines but are made by most body tissues. Phospholipids form cell membranes and lipoproteins.[23]

Lipids are important components of body tissue. Lipids are not water soluble and are unable to reach body tissues passively. Lipids must be transported to body tissues by lipoproteins. Lipoproteins contain an inner core of cholesterol and triglyceride, covered by a thin membrane of phospholipids, cholesterol, and protein. These membrane proteins are called apoproteins.

Apoproteins are made in the liver and intestines. Eleven apoproteins have been described, and genes responsible for their synthesis have been mapped. Apoproteins function to do the following:

1. Bind and transport lipids in the bloodstream
2. Inhibit lipid metabolism
3. Be enzyme cofactors

The major classes and functions of lipoproteins are shown in Table 11-16.

Lipoprotein (a) contains apoprotein (a). Apoprotein (a) is homologous to plasminogen and may contribute to atherogenesis by mechanisms related to thrombosis.[48] Remnants of lipoproteins containing apoprotein (b) may also be atherogenic.[59]

After a meal, fat and cholesterol are absorbed from the gut. Ingested fat is transported in the blood as chylomicrons (containing triglycerides) and carried to the tissues. Apoprotein C-II, located in the tissues, activates an enzyme in the capillary endothelium. The enzyme lipoprotein lipase removes fatty acids from the triglycerides. These fatty acids are either used by muscle tissue for energy or stored as fat in the adipocytes. A chylomicron remnant containing apoprotein E is left over from this process and is transported to the liver. Apoprotein E interacts with hepatocyte's surface receptors to facilitate the uptake of remnant particles from the plasma.

Cholesterol is synthesized by the liver at a rate regulated by the enzyme HMG CoA reductase enzyme. HMG CoA reductase is an enzyme that assists in the production of mevalonic acid. Mevalonic acid is converted to cholesterol. Cholesterol from dietary sources also adds to the body's cholesterol pool. About 40% of dietary cholesterol is absorbed by the intestines. A number of factors encourage cholesterol synthesis by the liver: Excessive caloric intake, excessive saturated fat in the diet, and high total dietary fat content.[23] Cholesterol-rich LDL is carried in the plasma to provide cholesterol to be used by cells for membrane synthesis, hormone production, bile acid synthesis, and production of vitamin D.

The liver is critical in the regulation of LDL levels. LDL receptors on the liver cells recognize the apoprotein B component of LDL. Apoprotein B binds LDL to these receptors. Apoprotein (b)–bound LDL is degraded by the liver to release cholesterol. Excess LDL is also removed by circulating macrophages, or scavenger white blood cells. Despite these regulatory mechanisms, excess LDL may accumulate, depositing cholesterol into arterial walls to form atheromatous plaques.

Table 11-16 Major Classes and Functions of Lipoproteins

Class of Lipoprotein	Source	Clearance	Function
Chylomicrons*	Gastrointestinal tract (The primary component of chylomicrons is triglycerides.)	Cleared from blood by lipoprotein lipase action Fragments cleared by liver cell receptors	Transport dietary fat from the intestines
Very-low-density lipoprotein (VLDL)*	Liver (produced from triglyceride, fatty aids, and carbohydrate)	Converted to intermediate density lipoproteins (IDL) and then to low-density lipoproteins (LDL)	Primary transporters for endogenous triglycerides from plasma to peripheral tissue
Low-density lipoprotein (LDL)*	Formed from the breakdown of VLDLs (contains 45% cholesterol by weight)	Removed from the blood by receptor binding with internalization into cells	Major carrier of cholesterol to nerve tissues, cell membranes, and other cholesterol-using cells
High-density lipoprotein (HDL)†	Produced by the liver and intestines Peripheral catabolism of chylomicrons and VLDLs	Removed by the liver	Carries cholesteryl ester Involved in the reverse transport of free cholesterol from peripheral tissues

*VLDL, LDL, and chylomicrons are considered to be atherogenic.
†One subfraction of HDL is associated with protection against premature atherosclerosis.

PATHOPHYSIOLOGY

Hyperlipidemias can be classified based on the plasma lipoprotein pattern produced by the phenotypic expression of identified genotypes. Of important note is that the clinical utility of this classification may be lost because individuals can manifest different phenotypes at different times.[24] Also, family members may share a genotype but have a different phenotypic expression of their hyperlipidemia.

Five basic plasma lipoprotein patterns for primary hyperlipidemia are shown in Table 11-17.

Common features of these plasma lipoprotein patterns are shown in Table 11-18.

Other primary disorders of the HDL metabolism are shown in Table 11-19.

Major Risk Factors for CHD

Major risk factors for the development of CHD include the following:

1. Age (male: greater than or equal to 45 years; female: greater than or equal to 55 years without hormone)
2. Family history of premature coronary heart disease (male parent or sibling less than age 55 years, female parent or sibling less than age 65 years)
3. Cigarette smoking
4. Hypertension
5. Diabetes mellitus
6. Low HDL cholesterol (less than 35 mg/dl)
7. High LDL cholesterol

Measurement of Plasma Lipids

Lipids level goals are shown in Table 11-20.

Recommendations[55] and treatment guidelines include the following:

1. With CHD (number of risk factors present is not relevant)
   - LDL ≥130 mg/dl
     - Treatment: Diet and drugs
   - LDL ≤130 mg/dl
     - Treatment: Diet and possibly drugs

Table 11-17 Primary Hyperlipidemia Classification

Lipoprotein Pattern	Laboratory Findings
I (lipoprotein lipase deficiency)	Lipoprotein: Elevated chylomicrons Plasma lipid: Elevated triglycerides
IIa (familial hypercholesterolemia)	Lipoprotein: Elevated LDL Plasma lipid: Elevated cholesterol
IIb (familial combined hyperlipidemia)	Lipoprotein: Elevated VLDL and LDL Plasma lipid: Elevated triglycerides and cholesterol
III (type III hyperlipoproteinemia)	Lipoprotein: Elevated remnant beta-VLDL Plasma lipid: Elevated triglycerides and cholesterol
IV (familial hypertriglyceridemia)	Lipoprotein: Elevated VLDL Plasma lipid: Elevated triglycerides
V (apo-CII deficiency)	Lipoprotein: Elevated chylomicrons and VLDL Plasma lipid: Elevated triglycerides, very low HDL

2. Without CHD (number of risk factors is relevant)
   - LDL ≥190 mg/dl
     - Number of risk factors present: 0 to 1
     - Treatment: Diet and drugs
   - LDL ≥190 mg/dl
     - Number of risk factors present: 2 or more
     - Treatment: Diet and drugs
   - LDL 160-189 mg/dl
     - Number of risk factors present: 0 to 1
     - Treatment: Diet
   - LDL 160-189 mg/dl
     - Number of risk factors present: 2 or more
     - Treatment: Diet and drugs
   - LDL 159 or less mg/dl
     - Number of risk factors present: Any
     - Treatment: Diet

Table 11-18 Lipoprotein Features

Lipoprotein Pattern	Occurrence	Pathophysiology	Clinical Features
I (lipoprotein lipase deficiency)	Rare	Lipoprotein lipase deficiency blocks clearance of triglyceride-rich lipoproteins from the plasma	Chronic features Eruptive xanthomas Lipemia retinalis Hepatomegaly Splenomegaly Acute features Recurrent abdominal pain or pancreatis Severe hypertriglyceridemia (>2000 mg/dl) Dyspnea Neurologic manifestation Overnight refrigeration of blood sample: Plasma Appearance Cream layer: Chylomicrons
IIa (familial hypercholesterolemia)	Common (1:300)	Deficiency of LDL receptors	Plasma cholesterol concentration is >300 mg/dl LDL is >250 mg/dl Tendon xanthomas (deposits on Achilles' tendons or extensor tendons of the hands) Premature arcus corneae (white ring around the eye) Xanthelasma (plaques on the skin) Premature CAD Overnight refrigeration of blood sample: Plasma Appearance Clear
IIb (familial combined hyperlipidemia)	Common (1:300)	Apoprotein (b) is elevated When the aproprotein (b) is degraded by hepatocytes, large amounts of cholesterol are liberated	Elevation of plasma cholesterol and triglycerides Increased susceptibility to CHD May be associated with syndrome X (insulin-resistant, increased plasma levels of LDL, elevated triglycerides, and low plasma HDL) (10) Overnight refrigeration of blood sample: Plasma Appearance Usually clear
III (type III hyperlipoproteinemia)	Uncommon	Accumulation of cholesterol-rich remnant particles in the plasma	Premature peripheral vascular disease and coronary artery disease Overnight refrigeration of blood sample: Plasma Appearance Turbid: Triglycerides
IV (familial hypertriglyceridemia)	Common (1:300)	Increased plasma concentrations of triglyceride-rich VLDL that cause elevations of plasma triglycerides but not plasma cholesterol	Plasma triglycerides 200-500 mg/dl Often associated with low plasma HDL Obesity and insulin resistance common Overnight refrigeration of blood sample: Plasma Appearance Turbid: Triglycerides
V (apo-CII deficiency)	Rare	Lack of apo-CII deficiency resulting in blocked clearance of triglycerides from the blood	Chronic features Plasma triglycerides 1000 mg/dl Acute features Recurrent abdominal pain or pancreatitis Severe hypertriglyceridemia Dyspnea Neurologic manifestation Overnight refrigeration of blood sample: cream layer: chylomicrons

Liver function tests are done to establish baseline function and to identify abnormalities necessitating discontinuation of medication.

Multidisciplinary Care Plan

Regular physical activity

Elimination or management of other risk factors: obesity/excess weight; cigarette smoking; hypertension; diabetes mellitus; alcohol abuse

Dietary Management[40]

For patients without CHD:

1. Complex carbohydrate: 50% of total caloric intake
2. Protein: 20% of total caloric intake
3. Saturated fat: <10% of total calories
4. Monounsaturated fat: 10% to 15% of total calories
5. Polyunsaturated fat: <10% of total calories
6. Cholesterol: <250 mg/dl

For patients with CHD:

1. Complex carbohydrate: 50% of total caloric intake

Table 11-19 Other Primary Disorders of HDL Metabolism

	Occurrence	Pathophysiology	Clinical Features
Tangier's disease	Rare	Associated with enhanced HDL catabolism where massive amounts of cholesteryl esters accumulate in macrophages of the reticuloendothelial system	1. Hypolipidemia (decreases in plasma HDL/LDL cholesterol levels) 2. Orange tonsils (result of cholesterol deposits) 3. Corneal opacities 4. Hepatosplenomegaly 5. Peripheral neuropathy 6. Premature CHD
Lecithin: Cholesterol acyltransferase deficiency	Very rare	Decreased esterification of cholesterol to cholesteryl esters on HDL particles, leading to accumulation of free cholesterol on lipoprotein particles and in peripheral tissues	1. Corneal opacities 2. Normochromic anemia 3. Renal failure 4. Premature CHD

From Wilson et al.[59]

Table 11-20 Lipids Level Recommendations

	Desirable	Borderline	High
Total cholesterol	Less than 200 mg/dl	200-239 mg/dl	240 mg/dl or more
HDL	As high as possible Range 29-67 mg/dl	—	—
LDL	Less than 130 (without CHD) Less than 100 (with CHD)	130-159 mg/dl	160 mg/dl or more
Triglycerides	Less than 200 mg/dl	200-399 mg/dl	400 or more mg/dl

Modified from Consensus Statement[16]; Expert Panel.[55]

Table 11-21 Antilipid Medications, Actions, and Side Effects

Class	Mechanism	Common Side Effects
Bile acid sequestrants (cholestipol, cholestyramine)	Decreases LDL (increases sterol production and LDL receptor-mediated removal of LDL)	Gastrointestinal symptoms Can increase triglycerides Can bind other drugs
Nicotinic acid (niacin)	Decreases VLDL/LDL (decreases VLDL production)	Flushing Hyperglycemia Abnormal liver enzymes Gout
Fibric acid derivitives (gemfibrozil, clofibrate)	Decreases VLDL/LDL (decreases VLDL production and enhances lipoprotein lipase action)	Gallstones Myopathy
HMG-CoA reductase inhibitors (lovastatin, pravastatin, simvastatin, fluvastatin, atorvastatin)	Decreases LDL (decreases cholesterol synthesis and increases LDL receptor-mediated removal of LDL)	Abnormal liver enzymes Myopathy
Probucol (probucol)	Decreases LDL/HDL (weak hypolipidemic agent; powerful antioxidant)	Diarrhea QT interval prolongation

Modified from Expert Panel.[55]

2. Protein: 20% of total caloric intake
3. Saturated fat: <7% of total calories
4. Monounsaturated fat: 10% to 15% of total calories
5. Polyunsaturated fat: <10% of total calories
6. Cholesterol: <200 mg/dl

Medications

Categories of medications[55] used to treat hyperlidemias and their common effects are listed in Table 11-21.

Special medication precautions are as follows:

1. Bile acid sequestrants can greatly reduce the absorption of other drugs administered, so medications should be taken 1 h before or 4-6 h after taking bile acid sequestrants. (Examples of drugs that may have interference of absorption include warfarin, levothyroxine, digoxin, and thiazide diuretics).
2. Sulfonylurea agents may antagonize the response to colestipol.
3. Oral contraceptives and rifampin may increase the effect of clofibrates.

4. Fibric acid derivatives may increase the anticoagulant effect of warfarin.

NURSING CARE

NURSING ASSESSMENT

Circulation: Signs and symptoms associated with coronary artery disease (CAD) (see Chapter 1)

Food and fluid needs: Gastrointestinal upset, nausea/vomiting, dyspepsia, excessive ETOH intake, obesity

Elimination: Constipation, diarrhea, flatulence

Psychosocial concerns: Noncompliance with diet, medications, exercise

POTENTIAL COMPLICATIONS

Severe electrolyte imbalances/crisis

PATIENT PROBLEMS/NURSING DIAGNOSES & INTERVENTIONS

NIC NUTRITION SUPPORT

Imbalanced nutrition: more than body requirements, related to excessive intake

- Reassess patient for psychosocial concerns that may be related to overeating.
- Arrange a dietary consultation.
- Encourage patient to choose foods that are low in fat, especially saturated fat and cholesterol, *to maintain nutritional balance and avoid elevating lipid levels.*
- Reinforce meal plan as needed.
- Suggest that patient join a support group such as Weight Watchers *to provide group and peer support.*

NIC PATIENT EDUCATION

Deficient knowledge related to lack of information

- Develop readiness for learning with patient.
- Provide information about disease, treatment, side effects, and reportable health changes.
- Include family in all instructions.

NIC BEHAVIOR THERAPY

Ineffective health maintenance related to ineffective coping

- Identify blocks to health maintenance.
- Support patient in organizing and using strengths *for health maintenance.*
- Collaborate with patient to determine and develop positive behaviors.

PATIENT EDUCATION/CONTINUUM OF CARE PLAN

1. Ensure that patient verbalizes understanding of dietary management of disease.
2. Discuss with patient the importance of achieving ideal body weight.
3. Discuss with patient the importance of engaging regularly in moderate physical exercise.
4. Discuss with patient the importance of eliminating other factors related to hyperlipidemia and coronary artery disease, such as cigarette smoking and hypertension.
5. Ensure that patient understands the name, action, dosage, schedule, side effects, and reportable health changes of ordered medications.
6. Ensure that patient understands the importance of regular reevaluations (follow-up medical care).

EVALUATION/PATIENT OUTCOMES

Nutrition Support: Nutrition is adequate. Patient verbalizes understanding of dietary restrictions. Patient complies with ordered diet.

Patient Education and Behavior Therapy: Patient is knowledgeable about disease cause, symptoms, and treatment. Patient and family verbalize understanding of disease, cause, symptoms, and treatment. Patient complies with medication regimen.

Health is maintained. Patient verbalizes one coping strategy and one positive health maintenance behavior. Patient demonstrates compliance with instructions and actions suggested by health team members.

COLLABORATIVE INTERVENTIONS AND RELATED NURSING CARE

ADRENALECTOMY

Description and Rationale

Adrenalectomy is the removal of one or both adrenal glands. Unilateral adrenalectomy can be indicated for pheochromocytoma, primary aldosteronism, and benign adrenal adenomas involving one gland. Treatment of adrenal carcinoma requires bilateral adrenalectomy. Bilateral adrenalectomy can be performed to treat Cushing's disease when other therapies have failed or when an ectopic ACTH-secreting tumor cannot be localized.[59]

Contraindications and Cautions

1. Bilateral adrenalectomy dictates lifelong glucocorticoid and mineralocorticoid replacement. (See discussion of adrenal insufficiency.)
2. Patients undergoing unilateral adrenalectomy are adrenally insufficient immediately after surgery and require glucocorticoid (but not usually mineralocorticoid) replacement for 6 months to 2 years or until the remaining adrenal gland recovers. Preoperative glucocorticoids are indicated.
3. Hyperglycemia should be controlled before surgery.
4. Patients undergoing adrenalectomy can have hypoaldosteronism or hyperkalemia after surgery.
5. Preoperative alpha blockade is essential for hypertension control in pheochromocytoma.

Preprocedural Nursing Care

Administration of preoperative steroids

Postoperative Nursing Care[18]

Administer supraphysiologic dosage of glucocorticoids (hydrocortisone, 300 mg) tapering over 3 to 4 days. Monitor blood and urine cortisol levels to assess potential onset of adrenal insufficiency. Later, administer replacement hormones.

Hydrocortisone, 12 to 15 mg/m² orally

Fludrocortisone (Florine), 100 mg/day orally (follow plasma renin activity levels)

NURSING CARE

NURSING ASSESSMENT

Skin: Poor wound healing, surgical incision

POTENTIAL COMPLICATIONS

Adrenal insufficiency, unresolved hypertension from primary aldosteronism or pheochromocytoma may require continued treatment with medication

PATIENT PROBLEMS/NURSING DIAGNOSES & INTERVENTIONS

NIC SKIN/WOUND MANAGEMENT

Impaired skin integrity related to surgical incision

- Monitor the patient's wound for edema, redness, warmth, induration, and drainage *to observe for signs of healing* or *infection.*

NIC RISK MANAGEMENT

Risk for infection

- Follow actions for adrenal insufficiency and for acute adrenal insufficiency when applicable.

PATIENT EDUCATION/CONTINUUM OF CARE PLAN

1. Teach patient wound care.
2. Give patient a list of early signs and symptoms of adrenal insufficiency. Inform patient to expect flulike symptoms during remission of hypercortisolism after surgery.
3. Demonstrate to patient how to use replacement steroids: dangers of glucocorticoid withdrawal, importance of compliance with medication administration, and need to double the dosage for nausea, diarrhea, and fever.
4. Instruct patient and family regarding emergency intramuscular injection of steroids during emesis, trauma, or severe stress. Medical follow-up should be pursued.
5. Discuss with patient the need to wear or carry medical alert information about the need for glucocorticoid replacement.

EVALUATION/PATIENT OUTCOMES

Skin/Wound Management: The patient's wound is healed. Patient's wound has closed without redness, edema, warmth, or drainage. Normal or subnormal plasma cortisol levels are present.

Risk Management: The patient is adrenally sufficient. Patient displays no symptoms of adrenal insufficiency.

CRISIS INTERVENTION FOR ADRENAL INSUFFICIENCY

Description and Rationale

The patient experiencing adrenal crisis must receive adrenocorticosteroids (glucocorticoids and mineralocorticoids).

The response to IV cortisol can be dramatic. Nelson[8] has reported blood pressure response from an unobtainable diastolic reading to one of over 80 mm Hg after the initial dose of cortisol was given. Therefore the patient must be treated with corticosteroids before other interventions, to enable the system to stabilize. The effects of corticosteroids on the electrolyte imbalance, hypovolemia, and blood pressure become apparent quickly. An IV infusion of 5% dextrose in saline solution should be part of the therapy because the patient is usually hypoglycemic as a result of the vomiting, diarrhea, and lack of food. Dehydration also compounds the problem. Response to therapy is encouraging; in fact, within 24 hours most patients are able to resume an oral course of corticosteroids.

Since most glucocorticoids (such as hydrocortisone) exert some mineralocorticoid effect, additional mineralocorticoid is not always necessary. Also, the sodium present in IV fluid can be sufficient to restore a normal level. However, if mineralocorticoid replacement is necessary, desoxycorticosterone pivalate can be given intramuscularly.[8]

Antibiotic therapy may also be necessary if the underlying cause of the adrenal crisis is infection.

Volume expanders may or may not be used, depending on how effective the steroid treatment and IV fluid are.

There is controversy in the literature regarding the use of vasopressors to treat hypovolemic shock. Response to initial glucocorticoid infusion and IV therapy should be evaluated before employing vasopressors.

Contraindications and Cautions

1. Complications associated with IV therapy
2. Severe hyperkalemia and hyponatremia may be present and require treatment

NURSING CARE

NURSING ASSESSMENT

Circulation: Hypotension, serum cortisol, hypopyrexia or hyperpyrexia,* shock*

Food and fluid needs: Vomiting, hyponatremia,* salt craving, hyperkalemia*

Elimination: Decreased urine output,* diarrhea

Neurosensory concerns: Confusion,* dizziness, coma,* visual changes, light-headedness

Mobility: Muscle weakness

Comfort and pain: Severe headache,* severe abdominal pain,* severe leg pain,* severe lower back pain*

Psychosocial concerns: Anxiety

Teaching and learning: Lack of knowledge about medications and crisis

POTENTIAL COMPLICATIONS

Severely low serum cortisol levels, coma/death

*Characteristics of adrenal crisis.

EMERGENCY ALERT

ADRENAL CRISIS

This metabolic disturbance is worsening of adrenal insufficiency and is exacerbated by major physiologic stress.

Signs and Symptoms

Vomiting and diarrhea
Pain
Hyponatremia
Lethargy
Dehydration
Fever
Hyperkalemia
Coma

Assessment

- Assess for worsening of shock, alertness, and coma level.
- Monitor vital signs, fluid balance, mental status, renal function, and cardiac function.

Interventions

- IV hormone replacement with hydrocortisone (Solu-Cortef)
- Rapid IV fluid replacement with normal saline solution followed by dextrose
- Monitor electrolytes, correct imbalances
- Investigative tests to determine cause

Patient Problems/Nursing Diagnoses & Interventions

NIC Risk Management

Risk for infection related to lack of primary defense

- Reassess patient's understanding of the risk of infection.
- Keep patient in an environment as free from stress as possible (low lighting, warm temperature, reduced noise level) *to minimize environmental stress.*
- Encourage frequent rest.
- Reinforce importance of medications, such as steroid replacement, to patient.

NIC Nutrition Support

Imbalanced nutrition: less than body requirements, related to inability to absorb nutrients

- Monitor the patient's intake of electrolytes, especially potassium and sodium.
- Encourage the patient to choose foods high in sodium and low in potassium.
- Take apical pulse *to detect cardiac dysrhythmias.*
- Employ means to combat nausea.
- Maintain intake and output records.

NIC Tissue Perfusion Management

Ineffective tissue perfusion related to hypovolemia

- Reassess for early presyncopal signs (dizziness, lightheadedness, visual changes).
- Have patient change positions (from lying to sitting to standing) slowly *to prevent orthostatic hypotension.*
- Take lying and standing blood pressures and pulses *to compare orthostatic values.*
- Administer IV fluids as ordered.
- Monitor intake and output.
- Monitor vital signs frequently (every 15 to 30 minutes).
- Explain rationale for IV therapy to patient.

NIC Immobility Management and Physical Comfort Promotion

Impaired physical mobility related to pain

- Give the patient cortisol replacement as ordered.
- Do not give the patient pain medications.
- Monitor degree and location of the patient's pain.
- Use only comfort measures: cool cloth; do not turn on lights (headache); reposition patient (back pain).
- Assist the patient with daily activities as needed.

NIC Coping Assistance

Anxiety related to threat of death

- Support the patient with comfort measures until the patient is alert enough for verbal communication.
- Identify whether the crisis is within the patient's ability to control: the patient purposely stops taking cortisone replacement versus other precipitating factors, such as an infection.
- Obtain psychiatric consult if the patient's intent is purposeful.

Patient Education/Continuum of Care Plan

1. Identify patient's readiness to learn.
2. Discuss with patient the steps to follow when early symptoms of adrenal insufficiency are noted.
3. Identify precipitating factors of adrenal crisis.
4. Discuss cause, signs, symptoms, and lifelong treatment with patient.
5. Discuss with patient the importance of regular medical follow-up and wearing medical identification.

Evaluation/Patient Outcomes

Risk Management: Patient is free of infection. Patient's temperature is within normal range. Patient has no signs or symptoms of infection. Serum cortisol and aldosterone levels are within normal range.

Nutrition Support: Electrolytes are within normal range. Patient's sodium and potassium blood levels are within normal limits.

Tissue Perfusion Management: Tissue perfusion is adequate. Patient's hydration is normal. Patient's intake equals output. Patient's electrolyte levels are normal. Patient's vital signs are normal.

Immobility Management and Physical Comfort Promotion: Patient is independently mobile. Patient is able to perform self-care without discomfort, although some weakness may be present.

Coping Assistance: Patient has decreased anxiety. Patient can verbalize precipitating factors for adrenal crisis and how these can be avoided. Patient agrees to continue counseling.

GONADOTROPIN REPLACEMENT THERAPY[23,59]

Description and Rationale

Approaches to treatment differ with individual clinical circumstances and preferences. Restoring gonadal function requires both gonadal steroid replacement and treatment of infertility for both men and women. In general, the lowest dose that produces the desired clinical effect is used.

Contraindications and Cautions

1. Human chorionic gonadotropin (HCG) is generally not given in the presence of the following conditions:
   a. Prostatic carcinoma
   b. Prior allergic reaction to HCG (rare)
   c. Pituitary hypertrophy or tumor
   d. Undiagnosed vaginal bleeding
   e. Uterine fibroids or cyst
   f. Pregnancy
   g. History of thrombophlebitis
2. Estrogen and progesterone are generally not given in the presence of the following conditions:
   a. Thromboembolic disorders
   b. Breast, reproductive, and genital cancers
   c. Pregnancy
   d. Abnormal genital bleeding
   e. Cardiac, renal, or hepatic disease
3. Testosterone is generally not given in the presence of the following conditions:
   a. Prostatic cancer, breast cancer
   b. Cardiac, renal, or hepatic disease
   c. Benign prostatic hypertrophy with obstruction
   d. Pregnancy, breast-feeding

MULTIDISCIPLINARY PLAN

Medications

In postmenopausal women without a uterus, estrogen can be taken alone and continuously

Estrogen replacement therapy can take one of the following forms:

Ethinyl estradiol, 5-20 mg/day

Conjugated estrogens (Premarin), 0.625-1.25 mg/day

Estradiol transdermal patch (Estraderm), 50-100 mg/day

In postmenopausal women with a uterus, estrogen can be taken cyclically or daily with progesterone

Estrogen is given 20-25 days per month and accompanied by:

Progesterone medication on the last 5-10 days each month:

Medroxyprogesterone (Provera), 5-10 mg/day or estrogen daily with 2-2.5 mg Provera daily

Androgens may be given in small amounts (specifically for decreased libido)

Testosterone enanthate, 50 mg q1-2months IM

Fluoxymesterone, 5-10 mg 1-2 times per week PO

Clomiphene citrate may be used to induce ovulation in women with hypothalamic gonadal deficiency; menotropins (Pergonal) and HCG or GnRH by intermittent infusion pump may be used to induce ovulation (restore fertility) in women with pituitary gonadal deficiency

In adult men

Androgen replacement therapy

Testosterone enanthate or cypionate, 200 mg IM q2weeks

Testosterone transdermal system (Testoderm), 4 mg/day, 6 mg/day

GnRH by intermittent infusion pump may be used to initiate spermatogenesis and restore fertility in men with hypothalamic gonadal deficiency

HCG alone or with menotropins (Pergonal) may be used in men with pituitary gonadal deficiency

NURSING CARE

NURSING ASSESSMENT

Musculoskeletal concerns: Bone density, strength/mass

Skin: Injection sites

Psychosocial concerns: Increase in libido, increase in self-esteem, increased confidence with both male and female peers, improved body image

Sexuality: Development/maintenance of secondary sex characteristics

POTENTIAL COMPLICATIONS

GH imbalances; if GH low, could have short stature; inadequate replacement could lead to decreased libido or poor development of secondary sexual characteristics

PATIENT PROBLEMS/NURSING DIAGNOSES & INTERVENTIONS

NIC COPING ASSISTANCE

Anxiety related to threat to self-concept

Sexual dysfunction related to lack of normal hormones

- Assess with the patient areas causing anxiety and usual coping mechanisms.
- Encourage open communication between patient and partner.
- Assist with problem solving.
- Explore alternative coping behaviors.
- Ask patient about any need for home health nurse visits for continued supervision of injections.
- Provide climate in which patient can openly discuss concerns and goals.
- Provide information and discuss length of time for improvement.
- Discuss expected changes in appearance, attitude, and behavior.
- Discuss possible need for contraception.
- Stress importance of medication compliance.

NIC PATIENT EDUCATION

Deficient knowledge related to self-administration of gonadotropins intramuscularly

- Demonstrate proper technique for preparation of medication, how to draw up medication in syringe, how to self-administer medication IM, and rotation of injection sites.

PATIENT EDUCATION/CONTINUUM OF CARE PLAN

1. Ensure that patient verbalizes name, dosage, action, side effects, and proper storage of medications.
2. Demonstrate to patient the procedure for intramuscular self-injection, including preparation and site rotation.
3. Discuss with patient the importance of follow-up medical care, including blood tests, Pap smears, mammograms, and prostate examinations.

EVALUATION/PATIENT OUTCOMES

Coping Assistance: Anxiety decreases. Patient discusses feelings about need for treatment. Patient continues open communication with partner regarding body changes. Patient complies with medical treatment program.

Patient Education: Patient complies with intramuscular injection of gonadotropins. Patient is able to prepare medication and perform self-injection without hesitance or difficulty. Partner demonstrates preparation of medication, injection, site rotation, and disposal of equipment.

HYPOPHYSECTOMY[59]

Description and Rationale

Surgical resection of a pituitary adenoma is the preferred treatment for tumors of the pituitary gland (Cushing's disease, prolactinomas, GH- and TSH-secreting adenomas). A hemihypophysectomy can be performed when an ACTH-secreting pituitary adenoma cannot be seen by MRI or CT scans, but inferior pertrosal sinus sampling (IPSS) indicates lateralization to one half of the gland (excessive ACTH levels from the left or right half of the pituitary gland). If the tumor cannot be localized, an adrenalectomy is usually preferred over a total hypophysectomy to preserve pituitary function. Total hypophysectomy is performed if multiple pituitary tumors exist, or if the tumor is very large despite conjunction with radiation therapy. Emergency hypophysectomy is occasionally required to treat pituitary apoplexy.

Surgical approach to the pituitary gland is by the transsphenoidal or transfrontal approach. The transsphenoidal route is preferred because it provides direct access to the contents of the sella turcica, is relatively safe, and avoids disruption of intracranial structures. It is a well-tolerated procedure that produces no visible scarring. The surgical goal is to remove as much tumor tissue as possible without impairing anterior pituitary function. Transsphenoidal adenomectomy or hypophysectomy is a microscopic surgery performed with the patient in a semi-sitting position. A gum-line incision is made, a nasal speculum is introduced, and the surgeon accesses the pituitary gland through the sphenoid sinus and floor of the sella turcica. Transfrontal craniotomy may be indicated if the tumor is inaccessible by the transphenoidal route because of its geometry or if carotid arteries obstruct access to the pituitary gland. After successful surgery, visual field deficits usually improve, and symptoms of hormone hypersecretion remit.[18]

Contraindications and Complications

Contraindications for transsphenoidal surgery include sphenoid or nasal infection or vascular anatomy that prevents access to the pituitary gland.

The incidence of postoperative complications increases with tumor size and difficulty of resection. Microadenoma resection rarely leads to permanent side effects. Cerebrospinal fluid (CSF) leakage, transient diabetes insipidus, or hypopituitarism occurs in up to 20% of patients. Permanent diabetes insipidus, cranial nerve damage, or visual deficits occur in up to 10% of cases. Meningitis is rare, and mortality occurs in 1% of cases.

Preprocedural Nursing Care

Provide explanations regarding diagnostic testing and procedures (MRI and CT scans, urine collection, blood work, and endocrine tests). Preoperative teaching specific to transsphenoidal hypophysectomy includes the following:

Presence of nasal packing postoperatively (2 or 3 days)
Mouth breathing while nasal packing is in place
Moustache dressing
Graft site on stomach or thigh (muscle plug removed for packing dura)
Expected decrease in sensation of smell and taste (few months)
Fluid restrictions possibly necessary
Possibly sent to intensive care unit (ICU), surgical ICU, or neurosurgical ICU (variable with institution)

NURSING CARE

NURSING ASSESSMENT

Neurologic concerns: Ophthamologic changes (PERRLA), postnasal drip (CSF rhinorrhea)
Fluid and electrolyte balance: Polydipsia, polyuria, decreased urine specific gravity, intake and output
Gum-line incision: Redness, swelling, drainage
Cardiovascular concerns: Blood pressure, heart rate stable; evidence of postsurgical hemorrhage
Graft site (stomach thigh): Redness, swelling, drainage
Respiratory concerns: Difficulty breathing because of mouth breathing, dry mouth

POTENTIAL COMPLICATIONS

CSF leak, permanent diabetes insipidus, severe hyponatremia

PATIENT PROBLEMS/NURSING DIAGNOSES & INTERVENTIONS

NIC SKIN/WOUND MANAGEMENT

Impaired oral mucous membrane related to mouth breathing and incision

- Reassess secretions from nasal drains; assess quality and quantity of drainage.
- Question the patient about postnasal drip.

- Perform frequent oral care with normal saline solution or half-strength H_2O_2 solution. Do not allow tooth brushing for 2 weeks, until sutures are healed.
- Apply petroleum jelly *to prevent the patient's lips from cracking as a result of mouth breathing.*
- Discuss with the patient the need to avoid sneezing, coughing, nose blowing, straining, and bending over *to protect muscle graft.*
- Monitor possible signs of infection of incision or graft sites

NIC ELECTROLYTE AND ACID-BASE MANAGEMENT

Risk for deficient fluid volume related to loss of regulatory mechanism (vasopressin) and leading to transient or permanent central diabetes insipidus

- Assess serum and urine osmolality and electrolytes.
- Check urine specific gravity *to identify early signs of diabetes insipidus.*
- Measure and record intake and output.
- Consider the need for vasopressin replacement therapy if serum sodium is 150 mmol/L and serum osmolality is 300 mOsm/kg (and greater than urine osmolality).
- See diabetes insipidus, p. 767.

PATIENT EDUCATION/CONTINUUM OF CARE PLAN

1. Provide instruction regarding hormone replacement therapy if indicated (glucocorticoids, thyroid hormone, LH, FSH, etc.).
2. Provide information regarding emergency medical alert identification if patient receives glucocorticoid replacement.
3. Provide instruction on emergency injection of hydrocortisone in the event of trauma, vomiting, or major stress.

EVALUATION/PATIENT OUTCOMES

Skin/Wound Management: Healing progresses normally. Patient shows no signs or symptoms of infection at operative sites (gum line, thigh). Signs and symptoms of meningitis (i.e., nuchal rigidity, fever, headache) do not develop. There is no evidence of CSF leak (rhinorrhea or postnasal leakage). No evidence of postoperative hemorrhage exists.

Electrolyte and Acid-Base Management: Fluid balance is normal. Patient's intake approximates output; weight is stable. Patient's urine output is less than 200 ml/h with a specific gravity of 1.005 to 1.015.

PARATHYROIDECTOMY

Description and Rationale

Surgical removal of hyperactive parathyroid tissue is the treatment of choice. Surgical techniques vary with different etiologies. When an adenoma is evident, surgical removal of the entire gland is necessary (there may be more than one adenoma present). Hyperplasia usually affects more than one gland; therefore three glands are removed completely, and three fourths of the remaining gland is removed, leaving enough tissue to maintain normal serum calcium levels. After parathyroidectomy, implantation of a portion of a gland may be performed (usually) in a muscle of the forearm. Sometimes a gland is frozen for implantation in the future.

Contraindications and Cautions

1. Contraindications for surgery
   a. Inability to locate the glands
   b. Underlying medical conditions such as renal failure or severe cardiac disorders
   c. Hypercalcemia from nonparathyroid etiology
2. Complications
   a. Hypocalcemia: Temporary (48 h) from "hungry bone syndrome" or permanent
   b. Edema
   c. Airway obstruction
   d. Paralysis of vocal cords

NURSING CARE

NURSING ASSESSMENT

Cardiovascular concerns: Dysrhythmias, bleeding
Respiratory concerns: Obstruction of airway, edema of incisional area
Neuromuscular concerns: Paresthesias, dysphagia, laryngeal spasm, positive Chvostek's and Trousseau's signs
Pain: Incision, shoulder, throat

POTENTIAL COMPLICATIONS

Aspiration, severe hypocalcemia

PATIENT PROBLEMS/NURSING DIAGNOSES & INTERVENTIONS

NIC RESPIRATORY MANAGEMENT

Risk for ineffective breathing pattern related to inflammatory process

- Keep a tracheostomy set at bedside.
- Elevate head of patient's bed 15 to 30 degrees.
- Monitor patient's vital signs and breathing pattern every 4 hours for first 48 hours.

NIC IMMOBILITY MANAGEMENT

Impaired physical mobility related to neuromuscular impairment

- Reassess patient for signs of pain during movement.
- Observe patient to assess steadiness on ambulation *to maintain patient safety.*
- Handle patient gently; allow patient to move slowly *to prevent injury.*

NIC PHYSICAL COMFORT PROMOTION

Pain related to physical factors

- Monitor type and degree of patient's pain.
- Administer pain medication to patient as needed.
- Provide ice chips to patient for pain from sore throat.
- Support patient's neck when the patient is turning or sitting *to protect the incision and to promote healing.*

- If pathologic fractures are apparent, splint ribs while the patient turns or coughs *to limit pain or additions to fractures.*

NIC NUTRITION SUPPORT

Imbalanced nutrition: less than body requirements, related to inability to absorb nutrients

- Reassess Chvostek's and Trousseau's signs *to identify symptoms of hypocalcemia.*
- Make high-calcium snacks available to patient at all times.
- Keep emergency calcium replacement medications available at bedside.
- Obtain a nutrition consultation for the patient.
- Monitor patient's serum electrolyte levels.

PATIENT EDUCATION/CONTINUUM OF CARE PLAN

1. Give patient a list of signs and symptoms of hypocalcemia (paresthesias, muscle cramps in extremities, and tingling in fingers and around the mouth) to report.
2. Demonstrate incisional care to patient.
3. Demonstrate body mechanics and importance of mobility (especially for patients with irreversible skeletal impairment).
4. Ensure patient verbalizes understanding of calcium replacement medications: actions, uses, side effects, and measures to use in case of emergencies.

EVALUATION/PATIENT OUTCOMES

Respiratory Management: Patient is able to breathe easily and adequately without mechanical or oxygen assistance. Oxygen saturation level maintained between 94% and 100% without oxygen therapy.

Immobility Management: Patient tolerates increased activity postoperatively without dizziness. Patient resumes independent ADLs.

Physical Comfort Promotion: Comfort level increases. Patient's incisional pain is minimal (can be tolerated without need for pain medication); sore throat is absent, and shoulder and posterior neck pain is minimal. Patient can perform a small neck and head circle movement.

Nutrition Support: Nutrition is adequate. Patient's electrolyte levels are in the normal range.

PARTIAL PANCREATECTOMY: INSULINOMA AND GASTRINOMA

Description and Rationale

Surgery is the treatment of choice for insulinoma and gastrinoma. Preoperative localization of the tumor by CT scan, venous sampling, or selective arteriography increases the chance of successful surgery; however, it is sometimes difficult. In the case of unsuccessful surgery or tumor metastasis, symptoms should be controlled by diet and medication. In nesidioblastosis an 80% pancreatectomy usually relieves the hyperinsulinemia. Usually no more than 85% of the pancreas is resected to prevent malabsorption problems.

Contraindications and Cautions

With gastrinoma, active bleeding ulcer

NURSING CARE

NURSING ASSESSMENT

Circulation: Decreased blood pressure, tachycardia, blood glucose checks, dehydration, vital signs, increasing abdominal girth

Food and fluid needs: Dry mouth, nausea, abdominal pain, intake and output, weigh daily

Comfort and pain: Describes incisional pain; splints, protects, or favors incisional area when moving; abdomen rigid and tender

Skin: Redness, swelling at incision; wound disruption; drainage from incision

POTENTIAL COMPLICATIONS

Severe hypoglycemia, postoperative pancreatitis, postoperative abdominal wound infection, coma/death

PATIENT PROBLEMS/NURSING DIAGNOSES & INTERVENTIONS

NIC TISSUE PERFUSION MANAGEMENT

Risk for deficient fluid volume related to loss of fluid through abnormal routes

- Observe patient for signs or symptoms of bleeding or shock.
- Check dressing and drainage tube every 1 to 4 hours postoperatively *to identify early signs of hemorrhage.*
- Discuss causative factors with patient and family.
- Monitor indicators of patient's fluid balance *to identify dehydration early.*
- Replace patient's fluids via intravenous line as ordered.

NIC NUTRITION SUPPORT

Imbalanced nutrition: less than body requirements, related to inability to ingest or digest nutrients

- Assess bowel sounds every shift postoperatively.
- Stop feeding if pain, vomiting, or nausea occurs.
- Monitor laboratory data *to assess patient's fluid and electrolyte status.*
- Encourage the patient to eat ice chips and to take sips of cool, clear fluids as tolerated.
- Teach the patient to maintain good oral hygiene.
- Discuss cause of gas pain or nausea with patient and family.
- Review the patient's diet prescription with dietitian before patient's discharge.

NIC PHYSICAL COMFORT PROMOTION

Acute pain related to surgical incision

- Monitor type, location, character, and duration of patient's pain.

- Evaluate effectiveness of pain medication.
- Report sudden increase in patient's incisional or abdominal pain.
- Discuss cause of pain with patient and family.
- Assist patient to use pain control measures.

NIC SKIN/WOUND MANAGEMENT

Impaired skin integrity related to external factors
- Monitor patient's incision site every shift for redness, swelling, and drainage.
- Report signs of wound infection or dehiscence immediately to physician.
- Perform prescribed dressing changes for the patient as ordered.
- Provide adequate nutrition for the patient as tolerated.

PATIENT EDUCATION/CONTINUUM OF CARE PLAN

1. Demonstrate proper wound care *to decrease the chance of infection.*
2. Discuss with patient the signs and symptoms and treatment of hypoglycemia (if surgery is unsuccessful) *to ensure correct management and no loss of consciousness (insulinoma only).*

EVALUATION/PATIENT OUTCOMES

Tissue Perfusion Management: Cardiac output is normal. Patient's vital signs are within normal limits.

Nutrition Support: Fluid balance is achieved. Patient's blood pressure is within normal limits. Pulse is within normal limits. Shock is not present. No signs of dehydration are present. Output equals intake.

Intake of nutrients is progressive. Patient ingests recommended amounts and types of nutrients. Patient describes causative factors. Patient's fluids and electrolytes are in balance. Patient has no nausea and no gas pain. Patient's bowel sounds return. Patient describes discharge diet planning.

Physical Comfort Promotion: Pain is relieved. Patient uses comfort measures and pain control measures. Patient describes causative factors. Patient verbalizes decreased pain.

Skin/Wound Management: Skin is intact. Wound healing is evident. Patient has no signs or symptoms of infection. Patient participates in prescribed dressing changes to promote wound healing.

RADIATION THERAPY FOR TREATMENT OF PITUITARY TUMORS

Description and Rationale[49]

Conventional radiation therapy administers 4500 to 5000 rad of high voltage cobalt-60 radiation to the region of the sella turcica. It is used as an alternative or adjunct to surgical excision of the tumor. Indications include tumors with suprasellar extension, presurgical removal or uncompleted surgical removal of the tumor, regrowth of a surgically treated tumor, or when surgery is contraindicated. Typically, radiation therapy reduces tumor size, but hormone levels do not always return completely to normal. The best results are seen in patients less than age 40 years. It can take 6 to 18 months to see the clinical results of radiation therapy.

Contraindications and Cautions[49]

1. Optimally, radiation therapy is not used with tumors large enough to mandate treatment faster than radiation therapy can provide (e.g., pressure on the optic nerve with ensuing partial blindness).
2. Often there is an initial acute inflammatory response with subsequent possible hydrocephalus and exacerbation of symptoms.
3. Destruction of normal tissue (pituitary, hypothalamus, or cranial nerves) and radiation necrosis of the brain is possible up to 20 years after therapy.
4. Pituitary tumors occasionally turn out to be radioresistant.
5. Hypopituitarism occurs in 30% to 50% of patients.

NURSING CARE

NURSING ASSESSMENT

Pain: Headache

Psychologic concerns: Level of anxiety initially and as therapy proceeds

Mobility: Decreased energy level

POTENTIAL COMPLICATIONS

Panhypopituitarism (loss of pituitary hormones, adrenal insufficiency), blindness, cerebrovascular accident, alopecia, burning of skin on the head

PATIENT PROBLEMS/NURSING DIAGNOSES & INTERVENTIONS

NIC PHYSICAL COMFORT PROMOTION

Pain related to injuring agent
- Encourage patient to report headache immediately.
- Provide analgesics and other supportive measures for headaches (quiet environment, cool compresses, etc.) *to minimize increased intracranial pressure.*

NIC COPING ASSISTANCE

Anxiety related to change in health status
- Assess patient frequently for psychosocial and physiologic manifestations of anxiety.
- Encourage the discussion of concerns and feelings regarding therapy, including the length of time needed to see the results of therapy, *to support realistic expectations.*

NIC ACTIVITY AND EXERCISE MANAGEMENT

Activity intolerance related to generalized weakness
- Monitor patient's activity tolerance and limitations; identify the patient's priorities regarding rest and activity.
- Help patient to structure each day to include frequent rest periods.

- Encourage patient to limit activities during the period of radiation therapy.

Patient Education/Continuum of Care Plan

1. Discuss importance of returning consistently for follow-up examinations.

Evaluation/Patient Outcomes

Physical Comfort Promotion: Pain is relieved. Patient reports no headache or worsening of headache if it is present at baseline.

Coping Assistance: Anxiety decreases. Patient verbalizes concerns regarding radiation therapy. Patient states general and specific facts about radiation therapy. Patient exhibits no observable signs of anxiety.

Activity and Exercise Management: Activity tolerance improves. Patient uses stress-reducing methods routinely. Patient structures each day to allow for rest periods and desired activities. Patient performs ADLs within limitations imposed by underlying disease state. Patient's statements about "feeling tired" are reduced.

Radioactive Iodine Therapy

Description and Rationale

The goal of radioactive iodine (RAI) therapy is to chemically destroy functioning thyroid tissue. This is called ablation therapy. ^{131}I is the isotope of choice in the treatment of thyrotoxicosis and thyroid cancer.

RAI is the preferred definitive therapy in the United States for Graves' disease. It is considered less costly and less traumatic than surgery and avoids surgery's complications. It may be used in the treatment of a toxic multinodular goiter when the patient is at risk from surgery. It may also be used to decrease the size of a large nontoxic substernal goiter with the goal of reducing the mass effect of the goiter around the trachea. The desired consequence of RAI therapy is complete thyroid gland destruction that renders the patient hypothyroid. This is usually achieved with a single dose, but in some patients with Graves' disease who have high TSIs and large glands, more than one dose may be required. It may take 3 to 6 months for ^{131}I to have its full destructive effect. Therefore, if a second dose is required, it would not be given until 6 months after the first dose.

Theoretically, in thyrotoxic patients ^{131}I may induce a sudden release of thyroid hormone from the gland into the bloodstream, causing thyroid storm. Patients are required to stop their antithyroid medication 3 to 5 days before treatment, since these drugs interfere with the uptake of the ^{131}I by the thyroid gland. They are then restarted on antithyroid medication 3 to 5 days after receiving treatment. On the other hand, stopping antithyroid drugs 3 to 5 days before RAI therapy has been found to increase thyroid hormone levels more than the RAI treatment itself.[11] Radioiodine is also given to patients without pretreatment with antithyroid drugs without any untoward effects. This last option is usually reserved for relatively young patients who have adequate beta blockade. The doses of ^{131}I for Graves' disease are relatively small, ranging from 6 to 15 mCi. Doses for toxic multinodular goiters tend to be higher, toward the outpatient limit of 30 mCi.

RAI use in the treatment of papillary and follicular thyroid cancer is quite variable. If the patient has a papillary tumor 2 cm or less without local or distant metastasis, 60% of physicians would recommend the patient receive ^{131}I after total thyroidectomy. The dose for this patient may range from 30 to 150 mCi. If the patient has a larger tumor or local or distant metastasis, almost 100% of physicians would recommend the patient receive ^{131}I and at a higher dose.[52]

When a patient with thyroid cancer has been on thyroid hormone suppression for 6 months or more, a ^{131}I whole body scan may be requested to assess whether the patient has developed new recurrence or to identify a metastasis previously unidentified. Scanning doses in thyroid cancer patients range from 1 to 10 mCi. Since levothyroxine has a very long half-life, the preparation for this study takes 4 to 6 weeks. The patient usually stops taking levothyroxine and is given pure T_3 (Cytomel) for 2 to 3 weeks. This medication has a short half-life and is usually prescribed at a dose of 25 mg three times per day. This allows the patient to stay relatively euthyroid while dissipating thyroxine stores. The patient then must stop the T_3 for the next 2 to 3 weeks. The goal is to have the patient become purposefully hypothyroid with a greatly elevated TSH. Because the TSH stimulates iodine uptake in thyroid tissue, when the scanning dose of ^{131}I is given, it should amplify any recurrent tissue. Another mechanism to enhance this effect is to have the patient follow a low iodine diet for the last 2 weeks before the test. Theoretically, this diet should enhance RAI uptake in both malignant and normal thyroid tissue, but this issue is still controversial. This diet is very difficult to follow because all water, except distilled water, has iodine added to it. Iodine is also in all processed flour and food products. As an alternative to this lengthy preparation, recombinant TSH (Thyrogen) is now available. The patient would be administered the drug by IM injection for a specified number of days, raising the TSH above the normal range just before the scan. The advantage to this newer investigational approach would allow the patient to continue taking thyroid hormone, eliminating the profound hypothyroidism and eliminating the need for the low iodine diet. If the results of the whole body scan indicate the presence of tissue, then the patient may require a second treatment dose of ^{131}I.

Contraindications and Cautions

1. ^{131}I crosses the placenta and can destroy the fetal thyroid. A pregnancy test should be performed on all women of childbearing age before treatment. Pregnancy is an absolute contraindication to its use.
2. Pregnant nursing personnel should be restricted from contact with patients receiving radiation therapy.
3. Complications (seldom) associated with RAI therapy include parotitis, radiation thyroiditis, exacerbations of hyperthyroidism, and thyroid crisis.
4. Antithyroid drugs may be given before radiation therapy. Drug therapy must be discontinued 3 to 7 days before the ^{131}I uptake is determined. Beta-adrenergic blocking agents may be continued.
5. Iodides, iodide-containing drugs, and contrast agents should not be given before therapy.

6. After therapy, saliva, perspiration, urine, feces, vomitus, wound drainage, and breast milk are radioactive.
7. Hyperthyroidism, increased swelling of the gland, pain, tenderness, and sore throat are signs of radiation thyroiditis. These signs may develop 1 to 2 weeks after therapy.

Preprocedural Nursing Care

1. Small doses of RAI are usually given on an outpatient basis. Special instructions are included in the section on patient education.
2. Large doses of radioiodine require hospitalization and radiation isolation.
    a. Private room at last 6 feet away from other patients or traffic flow
    b. Special protective measures for caregivers and visitors: Gowns, gloves, booties, dosimeter, radiation badges, and consultation by radiation safety branch of hospital
    c. Special precautions regarding visitors (no children or pregnant women)

NURSING CARE

NURSING ASSESSMENT

Thyroid gland concerns: Increased swelling, tenderness, and pain with pressure; difficulty swallowing
Respiratory concerns: Dyspnea, difficulty breathing
Psychosocial concerns: Social isolation, fear, anxiety

POTENTIAL COMPLICATIONS

Adverse effects on salivary glands

PATIENT PROBLEMS/NURSING DIAGNOSES & INTERVENTIONS

NIC COPING ASSISTANCE

Ineffective coping related to anxiety, fear, or social isolation

- Reassess patient's coping skills, support systems, and history of the adaptive skills that were successful.
- Listen attentively and provide an atmosphere of acceptance.
- Reduce situations that might startle or frighten patient.
- Avoid discrepancies in timing, activities, and methods of performing procedures.
- Anticipate and provide for patient's needs.
- Encourage expression and discussion of feelings.
- Help patient clarify source(s) of anxiety.
- Help patient identify strengths and resources.
- Encourage patient to learn and use diversional activities.
- Encourage use of telephone to communicate with family and friends.
- Keep patient informed of daily reductions in radioactivity.
- Remind patient that isolation is limited.

NIC PATIENT EDUCATION

Deficient knowledge related to lack of information about radiation isolation procedures

- Provide private room away from traffic flow; keep door closed.
- Explain rationale for isolation and visitor limitations.
- Explain purpose of gowns, gloves, booties, dosimeter, and radiation badges.
- Explain all procedures for handling secretions according to hospital radiation safety policies.
- Have patient handle own specimens if able.
- Explain rationale for rotation of nursing personnel assigned to patient.
- Instruct patient concerning signs and symptoms to report.
- Establish and practice procedures for communicating with nursing personnel.
- Check on patient approximately every 2 hours or more often as determined by his or her physical and emotional state to reduce social isolation.
- Establish patient's plan for diversional activities to reduce boredom of isolation.

NIC RESPIRATORY MANAGEMENT

Risk for ineffective breathing pattern or swallowing related to inflammation

- Provide respiratory support (oxygen, etc.) as needed.
- Monitor patient's ability to communicate verbally.
- Monitor patient's ability to eat and drink without difficulty.
- Notify physician if patient has difficulty with trying to swallow.
- Have patient suck on sour candy to increase salivary flow and reduce parotitis.
- Have patient drink 1.5 to 2 L of fluid per day.

PATIENT EDUCATION/CONTINUUM OF CARE PLAN

1. For an outpatient, discuss:
    a. The importance of a high fluid intake during the first 24 hours after dose
    b. The avoidance of contact with others (especially children) (Suggest sleeping alone for at least 2 nights after dose.)
    c. The avoidance of sharing eating utensils, kissing, and intercourse for at least 48 hours.
2. For an inpatient or outpatient, explain:
    a. Signs and symptoms of hypothyroidism and radiation thyroiditis
    b. Importance of follow-up care

EVALUATION/PATIENT OUTCOMES

Coping Assistance: Patient develops strategies for coping with anxiety, fear, or social isolation. Patient demonstrates ability to cope with restrictions imposed by isolation. Patient verbalizes fears and concerns regarding radiation isolation. Patient identifies source(s) of anxiety and fears. Patient verbalizes decrease in or absence of anxiety and fear. Patient uses strategies to reduce anxiety and fear. Patient verbalizes fears or concerns regarding radiation isolation. Patient verbalizes diversional activities to be used during isolation.

Patient Education: Patient understands radiation isolation procedure. Patient verbalizes rationale for isolation, visitor restriction, and special radiation precautions. Patient verbalizes procedures for nursing personnel entering and leaving isolation room. Patient verbalizes or demonstrates procedures for handling secretions. Patient verbalizes signs and symptoms to report. Patient verbalizes or demonstrates method(s) of communicating with nursing staff.

Respiratory Management: Patient denies dyspnea and is well hydrated.

THYROIDECTOMY

Description and Rationale

Partial, near-total (95%), or total thyroidectomy results in a decrease of thyroid hormones through permanent removal of thyroid tissue. Thyroidectomy may be used for patients with hyperthyroidism from a toxic adenoma or Graves' disease, large goiters, or nodules that suggest the presence of cancer.

Contraindications and Cautions

1. Patients may be euthyroid or mildly hyperthyroid at the time of surgery. Preoperative treatment is accomplished by antithyroid drugs for 1 to 2 months to bring the patient into a euthyroid state, and with iodine preparations for 7 to 10 days to reduce excessive vascularity of the gland.
2. Inadvertent removal or damage to the parathyroid glands may result in hypocalcemia and tetany.
3. Damage to the recurrent laryngeal nerves during surgery may result in aphonia or dysphonia because of vocal cord paralysis.
4. Permanent hypothyroidism after near-total or total thyroidectomy occurs in all patients.
5. Discharge occurs on second or third postoperative day.

NURSING CARE

NURSING ASSESSMENT

Respiratory concerns: Tachypnea; abnormal breath sounds; increased restlessness; complaints of tightness in throat, inability to swallow, inability to get air, pressure or fullness in neck, dressing too tight; change in level of orientation

Circulatory concerns: Variations in pulse and blood pressure readings; changes in skin condition: cool and clammy; increased swelling in tissue surrounding incision; decreased peripheral pulses; excessive bleeding on surgical dressing; hemorrhage

Electrolyte imbalance: Dysphagia: laryngeal spasms; headache; positive Chvostek's or Trousseau's sign; tetany: muscular twitching; personality changes; complaints of numbness and tingling of lips, fingers, and toes

Laryngeal nerve damage: Change in pitch and tone of voice; aphonia; hoarseness, weakness, "whispery" voice

Incision site: Redness, swelling, drainage, fever, pain, guarding behavior, distraction behavior (restlessness, moaning)

POTENTIAL COMPLICATIONS

Postoperative bleeding, airway obstruction, emergency tracheostomy

PATIENT PROBLEMS/NURSING DIAGNOSES & INTERVENTIONS

NIC TISSUE PERFUSION MANAGEMENT

Risk for decreased cardiac output related to hemorrhage

- Monitor pulse, blood pressure, color, and temperature.
- Monitor level of consciousness and orientation.
- Check dressing for evidence of excessive bleeding; watch for bleeding at the side of the neck and back of the head (immediately after operation, check every hour) *to identify signs of bleeding.*

NIC RESPIRATORY MANAGEMENT

Ineffective breathing pattern related to inflammation

- Monitor rate, depth, and character of respirations *to identify early signs of tracheal compression from edema.*
- Monitor level of consciousness.
- Monitor for apprehension, restlessness, and cyanosis.
- Keep suction equipment and tracheostomy set at bedside *to use in case of sudden tracheal compression.*

NIC NEUROLOGIC, ELECTROLYTE, AND ACID-BASE MANAGEMENT

Disturbed sensory perception (kinesthetic) related to chemical imbalance

- Monitor patient's calcium levels.
- Check reflexes every 2 hours; check vital signs every 4 hours.
- Check Chvostek's and Trousseau's signs every 2 hours.
- Observe for changes in personality.
- Have a 10% solution of calcium gluconate and equipment for IV administration at the bedside or readily available *to treat hypocalcemia.*

NIC PHYSICAL COMFORT PROMOTION

Pain related to physical factors

- Place patient in semi-Fowler's position *to promote ease in breathing.*
- Monitor edema surrounding incision.
- Observe body language for evidence of pain *to ensure comfort despite impaired communication.*
- Log-roll patient's head and chest *to prevent strain on sutures.*
- Teach patient to support the head and neck with a folded towel during mobility *to support surgical site.*

NIC COMMUNICATION ENHANCEMENT

Impaired verbal communication related to anatomic deficit

- Monitor pitch and tone of patient's voice every 1 to 2 hours postoperatively *to evaluate damage to recurrent laryngeal nerves (vocal cord paralysis).*
- Discourage talking *to prevent edema of vocal cords.*
- Monitor for edema of glottis and surgical incision.
- Establish alternate means of communication (i.e., pad and pencil).
- Reassure patient that hoarseness (from edema or pressure) will subside in a few days.

Patient Education/Continuum of Care Plan

1. Discuss with patient the name, action, dosage, schedule, route of administration, and side effects of thyroid hormone replacement if ordered.
2. Demonstrate to patient the care of the surgical incision.
3. Demonstrate to patient head and neck circle exercises.
4. Discuss with patient the need for follow-up medical care.

Evaluation/Patient outcomes

Tissue Perfusion Management: Cardiovascular function is normal. Patient's serum electrolyte levels, hemoglobin concentration, and hematocrit are normal. Patient's skin remains warm and dry. Patient's vital signs remain stable.

Respiratory Management: Respiratory function is normal. Patient demonstrates adequate respiratory depth and rate. Patient does not demonstrate cyanosis, dyspnea, or restlessness.

Neurologic, Electrolyte, and Acid-Base Management: Electrolyte balance is normal. Patient's serum calcium levels are normal. Chvostek's and Trousseau's signs are negative. Patient shows no signs of tetany.

Physical Comfort Promotion: Comfort increases. Patient verbalizes decreased pain or relief from pain. Signs of edema at surgical incision are decreased or absent. Patient demonstrates adequate support of head and neck during rest and mobility.

Communication Enhancement: Communication is normal or adequate. Pitch and voice tone of patient are normal. Patient shows no voice changes (i.e., hoarseness). Patient uses alternate means of communication to preserve voice.

References

1. American Academy of Pediatrics, Committee on Genetics: Newborn screening facts sheets, *Pediatrics* 98:473, 1996.
2. American Diabetes Association: *Medical management of type 1 diabetes,* ed 3, Alexandria, Va, 1998, The Association.
3. American Diabetes Association: *Medical management of type 2 diabetes,* ed 3, Alexandria, Va, 1998, The Association.
4. American Diabetes Association: Standards of medical care for patients with diabetes mellitus (Position Statement), *Diabetes Care* 21(suppl. 1):s23, 1998.
5. American Diabetes Association: Report of the Expert Committee on the Diagnosis and Classification of Diabetes Mellitus, *Diabetes Care* 20:1183, 1997.
6. American Diabetes Association: *Therapy for diabetes mellitus and related disorders,* ed 3, Alexandria, Va, 1998, The Association.
7. Bailey P: Intracranial tumors. In *Hypophyseal adenomas,* Springfield, Ill, 1983.
8. Becker KL et al: *Principles and practice of endocrinology and metabolism,* ed 3, Philadelphia, 2000, JB Lippincott.
9. Bennett PH: Epidemiology of diabetes mellitus. In Rifkin H, Porte D, editors: *Ellenberg and Rifkin's diabetes mellitus,* ed 4, New York, 1990, Elsevier.
10. Braverman EL, Utiger RD: *Werner and Ingbar's the thyroid,* ed 7, Philadelphia, 1996, Raven Press.
11. Burch HB et al: Discontinuing antithyroid drug therapy before ablation with radioiodine, *Ann Intern Med* 121:553, 1994.
12. Burrow GN et al: Microadenomas of the pituitary and abnormal sellar tomograms in an unselected autopsy series, *N Engl J Med* 304:156, 1981.
13. Carpentino LJ: *Nursing diagnosis: application to clinical practice,* ed 6, Philadelphia, 1995, JB Lippincott.
14. Collier IC, McCash KE, Bartram JM: *Writing nursing diagnoses—a critical thinking approach (with interactive case studies),* St. Louis, 1996, Mosby.
15. Consensus Development Conference Panel: Diagnosis and management of asymptomatic primary hyperparathyroidism: consensus development conference statement, *Ann Intern Med* 114:593, 1991.
16. Consensus Statement: Detection and management of lipid disorders in diabetes, *Diabetes Care* 116(Suppl 2):112, 1993.
17. Davidson JK: Diabetic ketoacidosis and the hyperglycemic hyperosmolar state. In Davidson J, editor: *Clinical diabetes mellitus: a problem-oriented approach,* ed 2, New York, 1991, Thieme Medical Publishers.
18. DeGroot LJ et al: *Endocrinology,* ed 3, Philadelphia, 1995, WB Saunders.
19. DelVallen J: Zollinger Ellison syndrome. In Yamada T, editor: *Textbook of gastroenterology,* ed 2, Philadelphia, 1995, JB Lippincott.
20. Diabetes Control and Complications Trial Research Group: The effect of intensive treatment of diabetes on the development and progression of long-term complications in insulin dependent diabetes mellitus, *N Engl J Med* 329:977, 1993.
21. Dons R: *Endocrine and metabolic testing manual,* ed 3, Boca Raton, 1998, CRC Press.
22. Doppman JL: The search for occult ectopic ACTH-producing tumors, *Endocrinologist* 2:41, 1993.
23. Felig P, Baxter JD, Frohman LA: *Endocrinology and metabolism,* ed 3, New York, 1995, McGraw-Hill.
24. Fredrickson DS: It's time to be practical, *Circulation* 51:209, 1975.
25. Goodrich I, Lee K: The pituitary: *Clinical aspects of normal and abnormal function,* Amsterdam, The Netherlands, 1993, Elsevier Publishers.
26. Haas LB: Nursing assessment endocrine system. In Lewis ML, Collier IC, Heitkemper MM, editors: *Medical-surgical nursing,* ed 4, St. Louis, 1996, Mosby.
27. Haas LB: Nursing role in management of the endocrine system. In Lewis ML, Collier IC, Heitkemper MM, editors: *Medical-surgical nursing,* ed 4, St. Louis, 1996, Mosby.
28. Haffner SM et al: Studies on the metabolic mechanism of reduced high density lipoproteins during anabolic steroid therapy, *Metabolism* 32:413, 1983.
29. Harris M: Diabetes in America: Epidemiology and scope of the problem, *Diabetes Care* 21(suppl. 3):23, 1998.
30. Henkin Y, Como JA, Oberman A: Secondary dyslipidemia: inadvertent effect of drugs in clinical practice, *JAMA* 267:961, 1992.
31. Kaplan MM, editor: Thyrotoxicosis. *Endocrinol Metab Clin North Am,* March 27(1):205, 1998.
32. Kim MJ, McFarland GK, McLane AM: *Pocket guide to nursing diagnosis,* ed 6, St. Louis, 1995, Mosby.
33. Kline N: The child with endocrine dysfunction. In Wong D et al, editors: *Whaley and Wong's nursing care of infants and children,* ed 6, St. Louis, 1999, Mosby.
34. Korenman et al: *Practical diagnosis and endocrine disease,* Boston, 1978, Houghton-Mifflin.
35. Lardinosis CD, Newman SL: The effects of hypertensive agents on serum lipids and lipoproteins, *Arch Intern Med* 1988.
36. Laycock JF, Wise PH: *Essential endocrinology,* ed 3, Oxford, 1996, Oxford University Press.

37. Matassarin-Jacobs E: Structure and function of the endocrine system. In Black JM, Matassarin-Jacobs E, editors: *Medical-surgical nursing,* ed 5, Philadelphia, 1997, WB Saunders.
38. Melmed S: Pathogenesis of pituitary tumors, *Endocrinol Metab Clin North Am* 28(1):1, 1999.
39. Niewoehner C: *Endocrine pathophysiology,* 1998, Madison, Conn, Fence Creek Publishing.
40. Nutrition Committee, American Heart Association: 1988 dietary guidelines for healthy American adults: a statement for physicians and health professionals, *Circulation* 77(3) 721A, 1988.
41. Peragallo-Dittko V, Godley K, Meyer J, editors: *A core curriculum for diabetes education,* ed 2, Chicago, 1993, American Association of Diabetes Educators and the AADE Education and Research Foundation.
42. Pollare T, Lithell H, Berne C: A comparison of the effect of hydrochlorothiazide and captopril on glucose and lipid metabolism in patients with hypertension, *N Engl J Med* 321:868, 1989.
43. Redfern J, O'Dorisio T: Gastrointestinal hormones and carcinoid syndrome. In Felig P, Baxter JD, Frohman LA, editors: *Endocrinology and metabolism,* ed 3, New York, 1995, McGraw-Hill.
44. Rifkin H, Porte D, editors: *Ellenberg and Rifkin's diabetes mellitus,* ed 4, New York, 1990, Elsevier.
45. Rohlfing JJ, Brunzell JD: The effects of diuretics and adrenergic-blocking agents on plasma lipids, *West J Med* 145:210, 1986.
46. Santen RJ: The testis. In Felig P, Baxter JD, Frohman LA, editors: *Endocrinology and metabolism,* ed 3, New York, 1995, McGraw-Hill.
47. Sawin CT et al: Low serum thyrotropin concentrations as a risk factor for atrial fibrillation in older persons, *N Engl J Med* 331:1249, 1994.
48. Scanu AM: Lipoprotein (a): a genetic risk factor for premature coronary heart disease, *JAMA* 267:3326, 1992.
49. Schteingart DE: Treating adrenal cancer, *Endocrinologist* 2:149, 1992.
50. Shimon I, Melmed S: Diagnosis and treatment of pituitary disease, *Psychother Psychosom* 67:119, 1998.
51. Solomon B et al: Current trends in the management of Graves' disease, *J Clin Endocrinol Metab* 70:1518, 1990.
52. Solomon BL, Wartofsky L, Burman KD: Current trends in the management of well differentiated papillary thyroid carcinoma, *J Clin Endocrinol Metab* 81:333, 1996.
53. Spiro H et al: *Clinical gastroenterology,* ed 4, New York, 1993, McGraw-Hill.
54. Taptich BJ, Iyer PW, Bernocchi-Losey D: *Nursing diagnoses and care planning,* ed 2, Philadelphia, 1994, WB Saunders.
55. The Expert Panel: Summary of the second report of the National Cholesterol Education Program (NCEP) Expert Panel on Detection, Evaluation, and Treatment of High Blood Cholesterol in Adults (Adult Treatment Panel II), *JAMA* 269:3015, 1993.
56. UK Prospective Diabetes Study (UKPDS) Group: Intensive blood glucose control with sulphonylureas or insulin compared with conventional treatment and risk of complications in patients with type 2 diabetes (UKDPS 33), *Lancet* 352:837, 1998.
57. Ulrich SP, Canale SW, Wendell SA: *Medical-surgical nursing care planning guides,* ed 4, Philadelphia, 1998, WB Saunders.
58. Weitzner M, Sonino N, Knutzen R: Introduction to pituitary disease, *Psychother Psychosom* 67:117, 1998.
59. Wilson JD et al: *Williams textbook of endocrinology,* ed 9, Philadelphia, 1998, WB Saunders.
60. Wood LC, Cooper DS, Ridgway EC: *Your thyroid: a home reference,* New York, 1995, Ballantine.

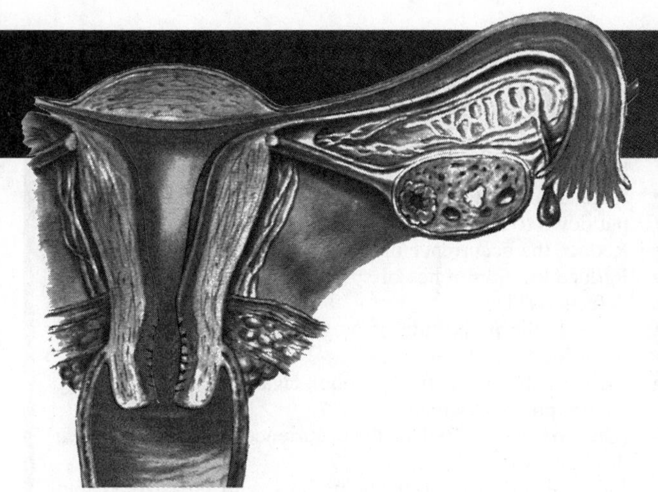

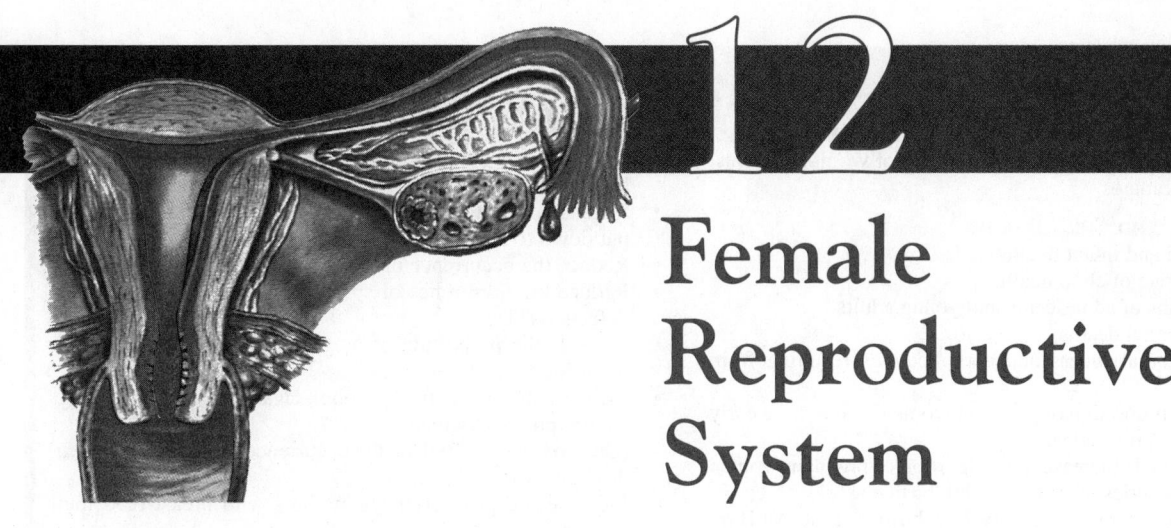

12 Female Reproductive System

Robert J. O'Malley
Susan M. Tucker

Overview

The major physiologic function of the reproductive system is the procreation of new life and perpetuation of the human species. This biologic process is primarily under endocrine control, but it is also influenced by neural and metabolic factors and human sexuality. Not merely a biologic phenomenon, human sexuality is the sum of physical, functional, and psychologic attributes that are expressed by a person's gender identity and sexual behavior. These factors interact when gynecologic and reproductive processes or conditions threaten, alter, or interfere with female sexual integrity.

The focus of this chapter is on the female organ system and includes those conditions for which patients are routinely hospitalized and those conditions that are commonly managed in the outpatient or ambulatory care setting. It was previously reported that data from 1988, 1989, and 1990 demonstrated that the five most frequent diagnoses for reproductive-age women were pelvic inflammatory disease, benign cysts of the ovaries, endometriosis, menstrual disorders, and uterine leiomyomas. Recent data from the National Hospital Discharge Survey (1997) demonstrate continued high incidence of these diagnoses. There were 212,000 admissions for uterine leiomyomas (109,000 reproductive age), 88,000 for endometriosis (66,000 reproductive age), 74,000 for pelvic inflammatory disease (PID) (61,000 reproductive age), 66,000 for ovarian cysts (51,000 reproductive age), and 11,000 for menstrual disorders.[26]

Pelvic inflammatory disease, benign cysts of the ovary, endometriosis, menstrual disorders, and uterine leiomyomas are discussed in this chapter, as well as other selected female organ dysfunctions. After a review of anatomy and physiology, the pathophysiology of each condition is presented, as well as diagnostic studies and findings, multidisciplinary plan of care, nursing assessment, diagnosis, intervention, evaluation, and patient education/continuum of care plan.

Anatomy, Physiology, and Related Pathophysiology

The female organ system consists of internal organs in the pelvic cavity and external organs in the perineum. The internal organs are the ovaries, fallopian tubes, uterus, and vagina. The external genitalia are the mons pubis, labia majora, clitoris, urethral opening, hymen, labia minora, and the vestibule of the vagina.

External Structures

The vulva includes all externally visible structures from the pubis to the perineum. These are the mons pubis, labia majora and minora, clitoris, vestibular glands, hymen, urethral opening, and perineum (Fig. 12-1).

Mons Pubis. The mons pubis or mons veneris is a cushionlike elevation of adipose tissue over the symphysis pubis. It is covered by pubic hair after puberty.

Labia Majora. The labia majora are two rounded folds of adipose tissue with overlying skin that extend from the mons pubis downward and backward, encircle the vestibule, and merge into the perineum. The outer surfaces are covered by hair, and the inner surfaces containing sebaceous follicles are smooth and moist. The labia majora are homologous with the male scrotum.

Labia Minora. The labia minora are two flat folds of skin medial to the labia majora. They are devoid of hair and fat and usually are in contact with each other. They come together

HEALTHY PEOPLE 2010

HEALTH STATUS—MATERNAL, INFANT, AND CHILD HEALTH

Goal: Improve the health and well-being of women, infants, children, and families.

FETAL, INFANT, AND CHILD DEATHS

- Reduce fetal and infant deaths.
- Reduce the rate of child death.
- Reduce deaths of adolescents and young adults.
- Reduce maternal deaths.
- Reduce maternal illness and complications resulting from pregnancy.
- Increase the proportion of pregnant women who receive early and adequate prenatal care.
- (Developmental) Increase the proportion of pregnant women who attend a series of prepared childbirth classes.
- Increase the proportion of very low–birth weight (VLBW) infants born at Level III hospitals or subspecialty perinatal centers.
- Reduce cesarean deliveries among low-risk (full-term, singleton, vertex presentation) women.

RISK FACTORS

Reduce low birth weight (LBW) and very low birth weight (VLBW).

- Reduce preterm births.
- (Developmental) Increase the proportion of mothers who achieve a recommended weight gain during their pregnancies.
- Increase the percentage of healthy full-term infants who are put down to sleep on their backs.
- Reduce the occurrence of developmental disabilities.
- Reduce the occurrence of spina bifida and other neural tube defects (NTDs).
- Increase the proportion of pregnancies begun with an optimum folic acid level.
- Increase abstinence from alcohol, cigarettes, and illicit drugs among pregnant women.
- (Developmental) Reduce the occurrence of fetal alcohol syndrome (FAS).
- Increase the proportion of mothers who breast-feed their babies.
- (Developmental) Reduce hospitalization for life-threatening sepsis among children age 4 years and younger with sickling hemoglobinopathies.
- (Developmental) Increase the proportion of children with special health-care needs who have access to a medical home.
- Increase the proportion of territories and states that have service systems for children with special health-care needs.

Modified from U.S. Department of Health and Human Services: *Healthy people 2010* (conference edition, in two volumes), Washington, DC, January 2000.

NOTE: *Developmental* indicates that criteria for measurement and strategies to improve health have not as yet been specified.

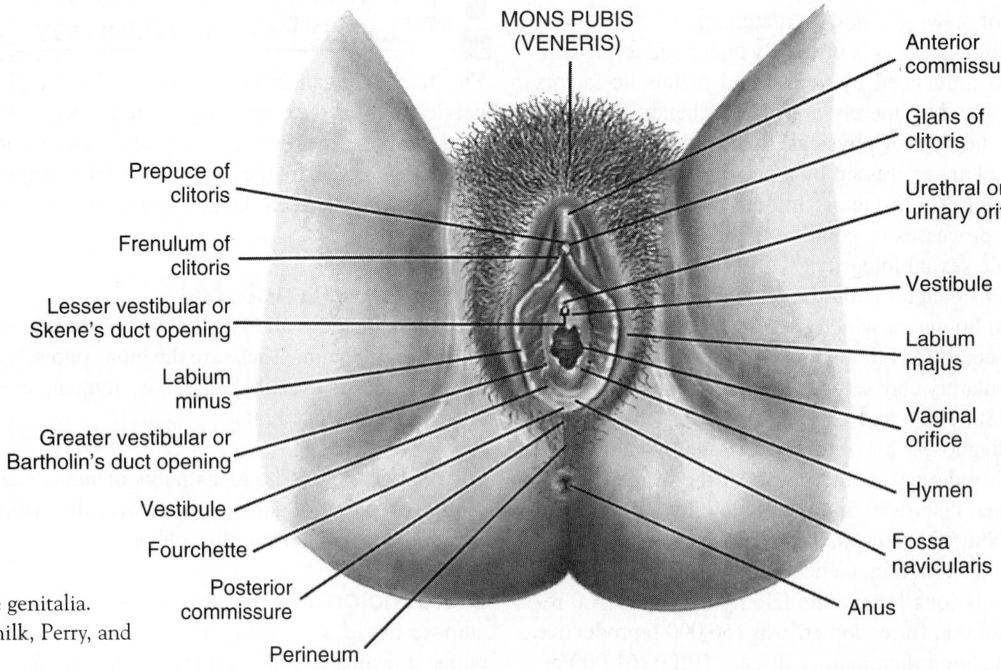

FIG. 12-1
External female genitalia. (From Lowdermilk, Perry, and Bobak.[22])

anteriorly at the frenulum of the clitoris and posteriorly at the frenulum of the labia.

Clitoris. The clitoris, situated at the anterior end of the labia minora, is a small, cylindric, erectile body consisting of a glans, a body (corpus), and two crura. It is partially covered by the anterior ends of the labia minora and is very sensitive to tactile stimulation. It consists of two corpora cavernosa enclosed in a dense fibrous membrane that is made up of smooth muscle and elastic fibers. It is connected to the ischiopubic rami by two crura. The clitoris, which corresponds to the male penis, rarely exceeds 2 cm in length even in a state of erection during sexual

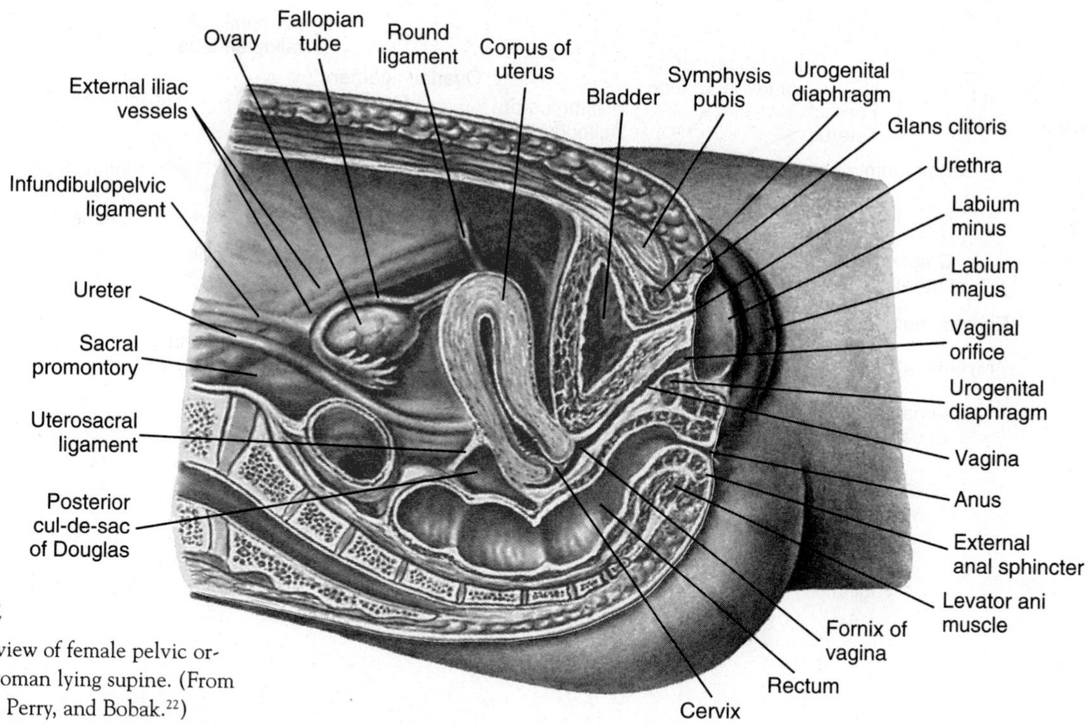

FIG. 12-2

Midsagittal view of female pelvic organs, with woman lying supine. (From Lowdermilk, Perry, and Bobak.[22])

arousal. The glans of the clitoris is covered by stratified epithelium that is richly supplied with free nerve endings within the fibers, terminating in small knoblike thickenings in or adjacent to the cells. Genital corpuscles, distributed in the glans and corpora, are considered the main mediators of erotic sensation.

Vestibule. The vestibule is the area between the labia minora. The hymen, vaginal orifice, urethral orifice, ducts of Bartholin's glands, and Skene's ducts are contained within the vestibule. The Bartholin's or greater vestibular glands secrete mucoid material during sexual excitement. They are on either side of the vaginal opening posteriorly under the constrictor muscle of the vagina.

Urethral Opening. The urethral opening, or urinary meatus, is in the midline of the vestibule posterior to the clitoris and anterior to the vaginal opening. The Skene's or paraurethral ducts open on the vestibule on either side of the urethra. Occasionally these openings are found on the posterior wall of the urethra just inside the meatus.

Hymen. The hymen is a fold of vascularized mucous membrane at the introitus of the vagina. It is not richly supplied with nerve fibers and has no glandular or muscular elements. The hymenal opening is usually very small in virgins who do not use tampons but is rarely imperforate, which would cause a retention of the menstrual discharge. During the first coitus or in certain other situations the hymen generally tears at several points. The edges of the tears soon cicatrize. Bleeding does not always occur when the hymen is ruptured.

Perineum. The perineum is a triangular area that is the inferior end of the trunk. It is situated dorsal to the pubic arch, superior to the tip of the coccyx, and lateral to the pubic and ischial rami. It supports and surrounds the distal portions of the urogenital and gastrointestinal tracts of the body. The central fibrous perineal body between the vagina and the anus divides the perineum into a posterior anal triangle and an anterior urogenital triangle.

Internal Structures

The internal organs include the ovaries, uterine (fallopian) tubes, uterus, and vagina (FIG. 12-2).

Ovaries. The ovaries are two oval structures in the upper part of the pelvic cavity, between the uterus medially and the uterine pelvic wall. They are suspended from the posterosuperior surface of the broad ligaments by the mesovarium. During the childbearing years each ovary is 2.5 to 5 cm in length, 1.5 to 3 cm in breadth, and 0.6 to 1.5 cm in thickness. After menopause the ovaries diminish markedly in size. In young women the ovary has a smooth, dull white surface through which glisten several small clear follicles. With advancing age the ovary becomes more corrugated, and in elderly women its exterior may appear convoluted. From the first states of development until after menopause, the ovary undergoes constant change. From birth to puberty an estimated 200,000 to 400,000 oocytes are present. It is evident that a few hundred ova suffice for reproduction because ordinarily only one ovum is cast off during a menstrual cycle. The glandular elements of the ovaries are described as interstitial, thecal, and luteal cells. The interstitial glandular elements are formed from cells of the theca interna of degenerating follicles. The thecal glandular cells are formed from the theca interna of ripening follicles. Luteal cells are derived from granulosa cells of ovulated follicles and from undifferentiated stroma surrounding them.

The ovarian cycle and its hormones are discussed in greater detail later in the chapter.

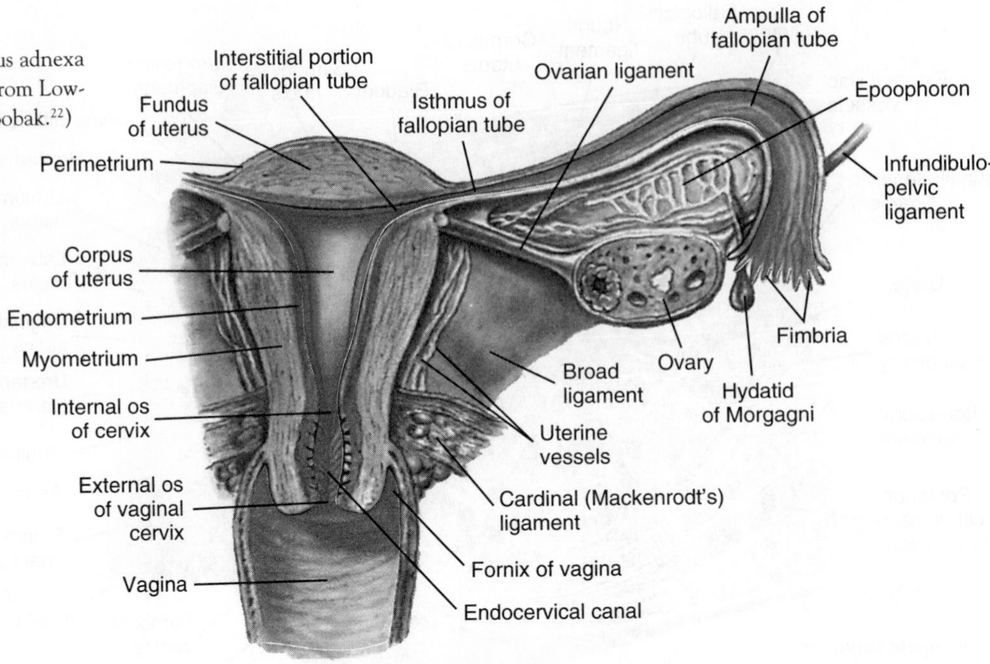

FIG. 12-3

Cross section of uterus adnexa and upper vagina. (From Lowdermilk, Perry, and Bobak.[22])

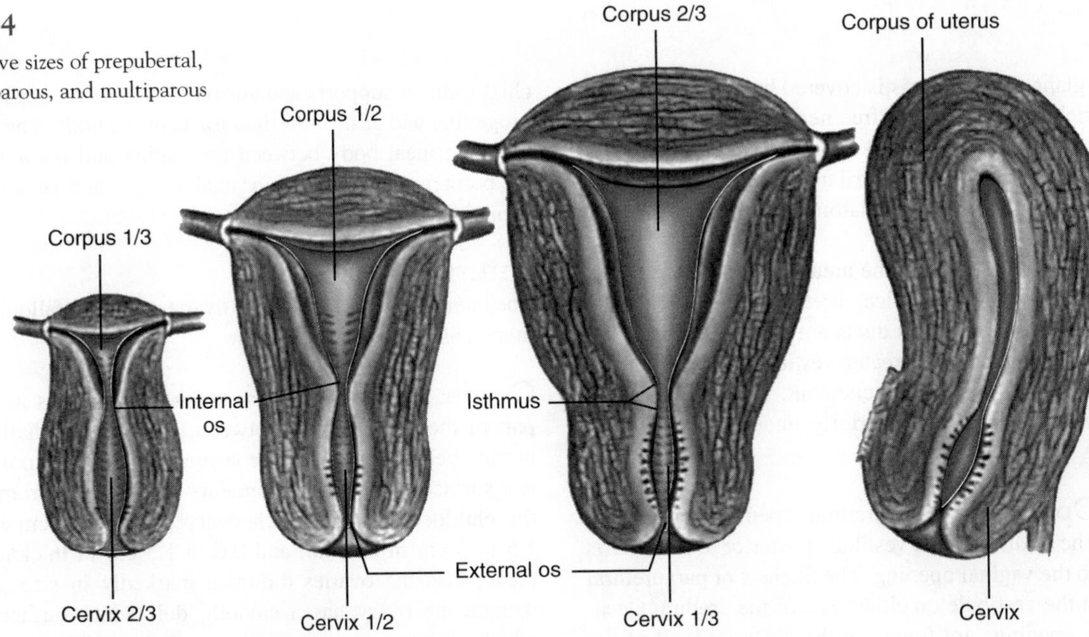

FIG. 12-4

Comparative sizes of prepubertal, adult nonparous, and multiparous uteruses.

Uterine (Fallopian) Tubes. The uterine (fallopian) tubes are two flexible, trumpet-shaped, muscular tubes that extend from the uterine cornua to the ovaries and provide the ova with access to the uterine cavity. They are approximately 10 cm in length in an adult and are suspended by a fold of the broad ligament called the mesosalpinx. The isthmus end of the tube opens into the uterine cavity. The ampulla is the dilated central part of the tube that is continuous with the infundibulum, the fimbriated funnel-shaped opening of the distal end of the tube. This fimbriated portion of the tube, which is adjacent to the ovary, draws the ovum into the tube, where fertilization may occur. The tubal musculature undergoes rhythmic contractions that transport the ovum into the uterus, and the lining cells produce secretions essential for the fertilized ovum.

Uterus. The uterus is a pear-shaped, thick-walled, muscular organ suspended in the anterior part of the pelvic cavity above and posterior to the bladder and in front of the rectum (FIG. 12-3). It consists of two major but unequal parts: an upper triangular portion, the body or corpus, and a lower cylindric or fusiform portion, the cervix. The isthmus divides these two portions. The uterine (fallopian) tubes emerge from the cornua of the uterus at the junction of the superior and lateral margins. The convex upper segment between the cornua is the fundus uteri. Before puberty the length of the uterus varies from 2.5 to 3.5 cm. In a mature nulliparous woman the uterus is 6 to 8 cm in length, as compared with 9 to 10 cm in a multiparous woman (FIG. 12-4). The uterus is covered with a layer of peritoneum from which arise the broad ligaments that extend from the lateral margins of the uterus to the pelvic walls and divide the pelvic cavity into anterior and posterior compartments. The base of the broad ligament, which is quite thick, is continuous with the connective tissue of the pelvic floor. The densest portion (cardinal ligament) surrounds the uterine blood vessels. The two round ligaments extend from each side of the uterus below and anterior to the uterine tubes. During pregnancy the round ligaments undergo considerable hypertrophy and increase in both length and diameter. The uterosacral ligaments extend from the sacrum around the rectum to the cervix of the uterus. They help support the uterus and maintain its position. The uterosacral and cardinal ligaments are the most important ligaments of the uterus; without them the uterus would tend to pass through the vagina, or prolapse.

The wall of the uterus comprises three layers: serosal, muscular, and mucosal. The serosal layer is formed by the peritoneum covering the uterus. The muscular portion, or myometrium, consists of bundles of smooth muscle that are united by connective tissue containing many elastic fibers. During pregnancy the thickness of the myometrium increases markedly. This occurs because of hypertrophy (enlargement of existing fibers) and addition of new fibers derived from transformation and division of mesenchymal cells. The innermost or mucosal layer that lines the uterine cavity in the nonpregnant state is the endometrium. It comprises surface epithelium, glands, and interglandular tissue. The uterine glands extend through the entire thickness of the endometrium to the myometrium and secrete a think alkaline fluid that keeps the uterine cavity moist.

Two types of arteries supply blood to the endometrium. The straight basal arteries extend to the basal layer of the endometrium from the radial and arcuate arteries in the myometrium. The coiled or spiral arteries, which are a continuation of the radial and basal arteries, supply the superficial layer of the endometrium. The coiled arteries play an important part in the mechanism of menstruation.

The cervix is the lower part of the uterus. The entrance of the uterus is the cervical os or opening, which changes in size and shape depending on pregnancy or previous deliveries. Hormonal changes influence mucus production by the endocervical glands.

Vagina. The vagina is a tubular canal 10 to 15 cm in length, directed backward and upward and extending from the vestibule to the uterus. It is located between the bladder anteriorly and the rectum posteriorly. It is the female organ of copulation, the birth canal, and the excretory duct of the uterus through which the menstrual flow escapes. In an adult the anterior wall of the vagina is approximately 8 cm long and the posterior wall is 9 to 10 cm long. The difference is due to the projection of the cervix into the anterior aspect of the superior end of the vagina. The anterior, posterior, and two lateral fornices are produced by the cervix projecting into the vagina. The fornices are of clinical importance because the internal pelvic organs can be easily palpated through the thin wall. The epithelium lining the vagina forms folds so that the vaginal walls are in contact with each other and kept moist by cervical secretions. The folds stretch with coitus and during the birth process.

Pelvis

The pelvis is composed of two innominate bones, the sacrum, and the coccyx. The innominate bones are formed by fusion of the ischium, ilium, and pubis and are joined to the sacrum and each other at the symphysis pubis. The pelvis has two parts: the shallow, upper, or false pelvis and the lower, smaller, or true pelvis. The false pelvis is bounded posteriorly by the lumbar vertebrae, laterally by the iliac fossa, and anteriorly by the abdominal wall. The true pelvis is bounded by the sacrum, the inner surface of the ischial bones, and the pubic bones. The shape and diameter of the true pelvis are important in obstetrics because it must accommodate the fetal head in a vaginal delivery.

Pelvic Inlet. The pelvic inlet is bounded posteriorly by the sacral promontory, laterally by the linea terminalis, and anteriorly by the horizontal rami of the pubic bones and symphysis pubis.

Breasts

The breasts, or mammary glands, are accessory organs of reproduction (FIG. 12-5). They consist of a glandular epithelium and a duct system embedded in interstitial tissue and fat. They lie anterior to the pectoralis major muscle and are separated from it by a layer of fat that is continuous with the fatty stroma of the gland itself. They extend from the anterior border of the axilla to the lateral edge of the sternum. Each gland consists of a comma-shaped mass of fat and collagenous tissue. The tail of Spence extends toward the axilla. The position of the breasts is maintained by suspensory (Cooper's) ligaments, which are condensations of connective tissue. They are easily stretched, especially if the breasts are large. Lymph drainage is mainly toward the axillary lymph nodes, with some drainage directed toward the substernal, diaphragmatic, and subclavicular nodes. Some women (as well as some men) have supernumerary nipples or breast tissue that developed during the early embryonic period along the longitudinal ridges extending from the axilla to the groin (FIG. 12-6).

The center of the fully developed breast in an adult woman is the nipple, which is elevated anterior to the breast. Bundles of smooth muscle fibers in the nipple have erectile properties. The areola that surrounds the nipple has a diameter of 1.5 to 2.5 cm. Small sebaceous glands located under the areola give it a rough appearance. Arranged radially under the areola are 15 to 20 lactiferous ducts. In a lactating woman these ducts drain milk from the lobes of glandular tissue embedded in the adipose tissue of the breast. The ducts enlarge slightly before reaching the nipple to form the short lactiferous sinuses in which the milk may be stored. From the sinuses the ducts extend toward the chest wall, uniting various lobules or acinar structures of the breast. Each lobule contains 10 to 100 alveoli or acini, and 20 to 40 lobules compose each of the 15 to 20 lobes that are distributed in each breast. The alveolus is lined by a single layer of milk-secreting epithelial cells, encased in a network of myoepithelial strands; it is surrounded by a dense capillary network.

Ovarian Cycle and Hormones

The purpose of the ovarian cycle is to provide an ovum for fertilization, whereas the purpose of the endometrial cycle is to furnish a suitable site for the fertilized ovum to implant and develop.

Follicle Development. Female primordial germa cells are derived from the germinal epithelium in the embryo. By

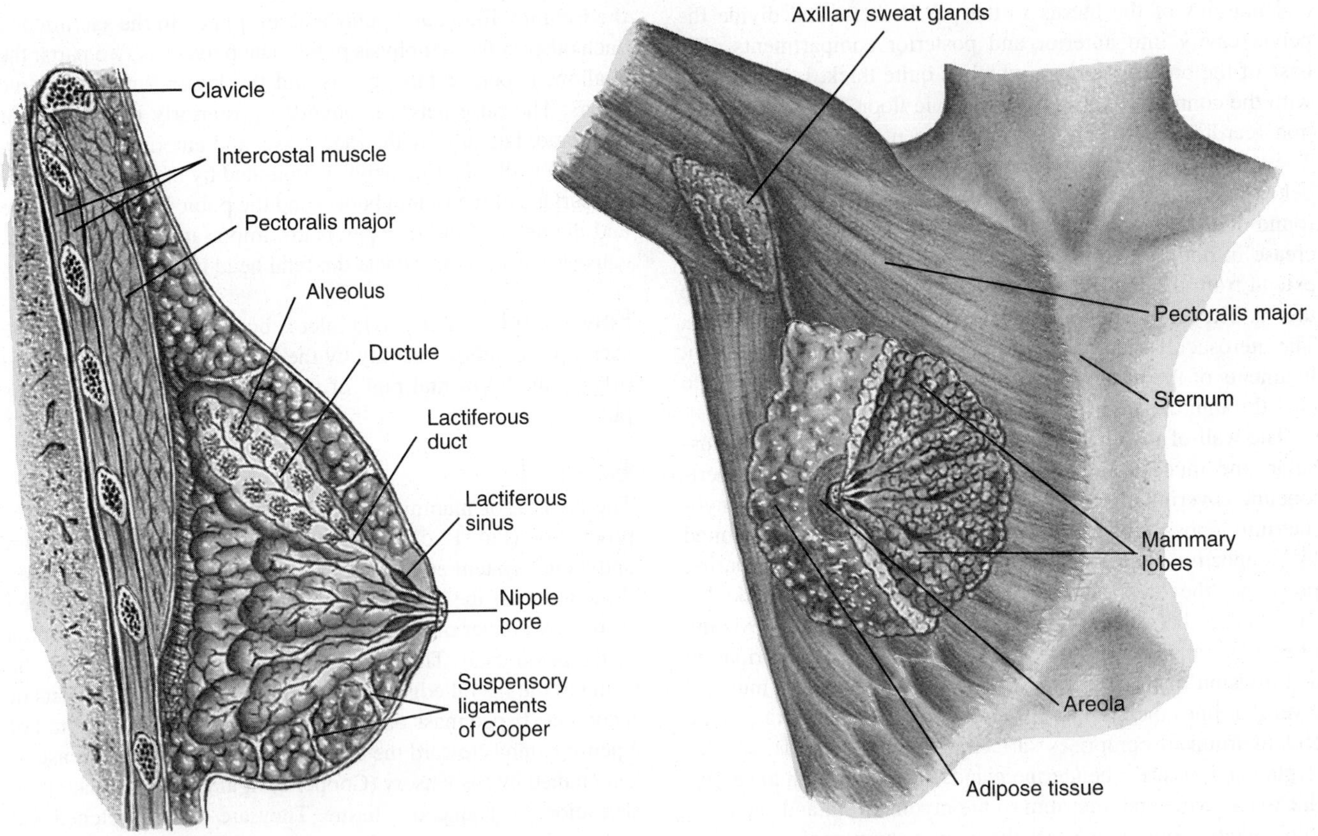

FIG. 12-5

Anatomy of breast.

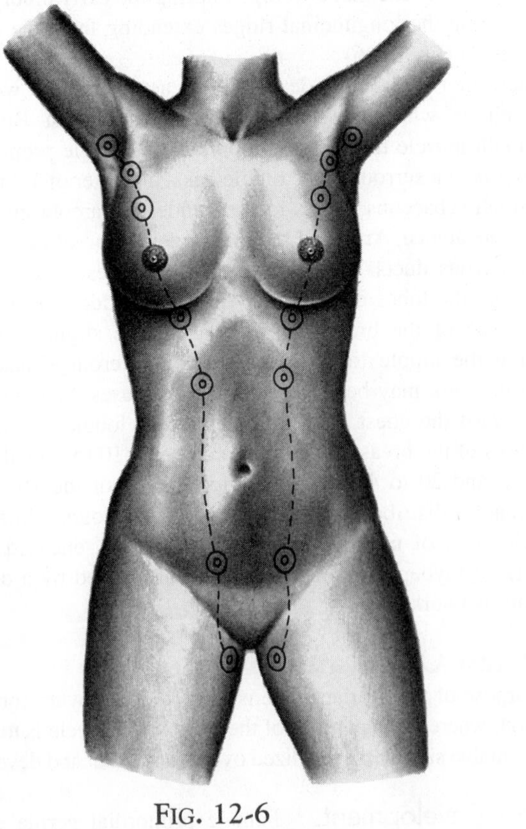

FIG. 12-6

Supernumerary nipples.

mitotic division these form primitive ova, or oogonia, until the fifth or sixth month of gestation. Between the second month of gestation and the sixth month of life some oogonia become primary oocytes through the prophase of meiosis. At birth some 2 million oocytes are in the ovary, decreasing through attrition to about 300,000 by the onset of puberty.

The first stage of follicle development occurs slowly during the childbearing years. The cells of the follicle divide, creating several layers of granulosa cells around the oocyte. Mucopolysaccarides secreted from the granulosa cells form a protective halo or zona pellucida around the oocyte. The primary oocyte, the surrounding layers of granulosa cells, and the outer basal lamina membrane make up the primary follicle.

The second stage of development occurs more rapidly, requiring 2 to 4 weeks for completion. During an ovarian cycle, approximately 6 to 12 primary follicles undergo growth and development but usually only one reaches maturity and ovulates. All others degenerate and become atretic follicles. The proliferating granulosa cells are separated into two parts. The cavity or antrum is filled with follicular fluid that presses the oocyte to one side. Several cells known as the cumulus oophorus surround the oocyte, forming a stalk that projects into the antrum. The follicle distends with fluid and moves outward to the surface of the ovary. The theca cells surrounding the antrum proliferate, and those nearest the basal lamina are transformed into cuboidal steroid-secreting cells called the theca interna. Spinal cells from the stroma form around this, composing the theca externa. At this point in development the entire complex is known as the graafian follicle.

The third and last stage of follicular development is complete within 48 hours. Before ovulation a single graafian follicle becomes dominant, and as the follicle ruptures, the oocyte is released into the fimbria. Because the initial meiotic division is complete at this time, this is called the secondary oocyte. Fertilization of this oocyte in the fallopian tube causes completion of the second meiotic division, resulting in a haploid ovum.

Ovulation. Ovulation is the actual discharge of the secondary oocyte from the graafian follicle. This usually occurs at the midpoint of both the ovarian and the menstrual cycle. The time from the first day of the menstrual period to ovulation is the follicular phase, or preovulatory period. The postovulatory period is the luteal phase.

Some women experience mittelschmerz, a lower abdominal discomfort at the time of ovulation. This is believed to be caused by peritoneal irritation from blood or follicular fluid that has escaped from the ruptured follicle. Another response to ovulation is an increase in basal body temperature caused by the thermogenic action of progesterone. Changes in the cervical mucus near the time of ovulation include decreases in viscosity and opacity, an increase in clarity, and an increase in sodium chloride content, which is demonstrated by arborization, or ferning, when mucus is allowed to dry on a glass slide. The signs and symptoms of ovulation are important both for women who wish to conceive during a particular cycle and for those who desire to avoid conception.

Corpus Luteum. A yellow glandular mass formed at the site of the ruptured follicle is called the corpus luteum. It secretes large amounts of progesterone and lesser amounts of estrogen. If fertilization occurs, the corpus luteum increases in size, remains enlarged for about 3 months until the placenta takes over secreting functions, and then degenerates. If fertilization does not occur, the corpus luteum degenerates and shrinks. The yellow or "luteal" tissue then changes to a white fibrous tissue known as the corpus albicans.

Estrogens. Estrogen is a generic term for substances capable of producing the typical changes of estrus. The common estrogens are estradiol, estrone, and estriol. They are secreted by the developing ovarian follicle and subsequently by the corpus luteum. Estrogens are secreted by the placenta during pregnancy.

Estrogens are responsible for the development of the female secondary sex characteristics, increased growth of the uterus at puberty, and repair of the endometrium after menstruation. They tend to increase uterine sensitivity to oxytocin and uterine motility. In this respect the actions of estrogens are opposite to those of progesterone. Estrogens also decrease resorption of calcium from bones, secondarily increasing bone matrix formation and slightly increasing sodium and water reabsorption by the renal tubules.

Progesterone. Progesterone is the principal hormone secreted by the corpus luteum. During pregnancy it is secreted by the placenta. Progesterone prepares the uterine endometrium for the reception and development of the fertilized ovum by converting a proliferative endometrium to the secretory stage. It also inhibits the contractility of smooth uterine muscle, which is the opposite action of estrogen. Progesterone is responsible for the development of acini and lobules in the breast during pregnancy. With estrogen, progesterone inhibits the action of prolactin. Removal of the placenta, a source of massive progesterone production, removes the inhibitory effect on prolactin, thereby permitting lactation. Progesterone is also called luteal or progestational hormone.

Androgens. Androgens are substances that produce masculine characteristics such as hair growth, lowering of the voice, muscularity, and, in the male, development of the genital system. The major androgen secreted by the female ovary is androstenedione, a biologically weak compound but one that can undergo peripheral conversion to testosterone. The adrenal gland also secretes androgens, androstenedione, and dehydroepiandrosterone (dehydroisoandrosterone). Dihydrotestosterone is formed in peripheral tissue by the action of an enzyme on testosterone. In addition, testosterone, which is secreted by the embryonic testicular Leydig's cells, is required in the male fetus for the differentiation of the genital tubercle, swellings, folds, and urogenital sinus into the penis, scrotum, penile urethra, and prostate. Testosterone stimulates fetal differentiation of the wolffian ducts into the epididymis, vas deferens, and seminal vesicles.

Pituitary Gonadotropic Hormones. The basophils of the anterior pituitary gland secrete follicle-stimulating hormone (FSH) and luteinizing hormone (LH). The acidophils secrete prolactin, which is also called lactogenic or luteotropic hormone (LTH).

Follicle-stimulating hormone stimulates ovarian follicle growth and maturation. The FSH level rises slightly before both ovulation and menstruation. This hormone is essential to the production of estrogen by the ovary. After menopause the level of FSH in the plasma and the amount excreted in the urine are increased.

Luteinizing hormone induces ovulation and stimulates formation of the corpus luteum and progesterone secretion.

Prolactin serves as a luteotropic hormone in helping to maintain the corpus luteum. This hormone stimulates the mammary glands to develop secretory alveoli and secrete milk.

Menstrual (Endometrial) Cycle

The menstrual cycle begins at puberty and continues until menopause some 40 years later (FIG. 12-7; Table 12-1). The day of onset of menstrual flow is considered to be the first day of the cycle. The cycle ends on the last day before the next onset of menstruation. The normal cycle can vary from 22 to 35 days but is generally 28 days.

The proliferative or follicular phase begins about the fifth day of the cycle and extends through ovulation. It is also known as the postmenstrual or estrogenic phase. During this phase the uterine endothelium thickens as estrogen secretion rises.

The secretory phase occurs after ovulation. It is also called the postovulatory, luteal, or progestational phase. During this phase the three endometrial zones become well defined. The basal zone is adjacent to the myometrium; the compact zone lies immediately below the endometrial surface; and the spongy zone lies between the compact and basal layers. The endometrium becomes extremely vascular and rich in glycogen,

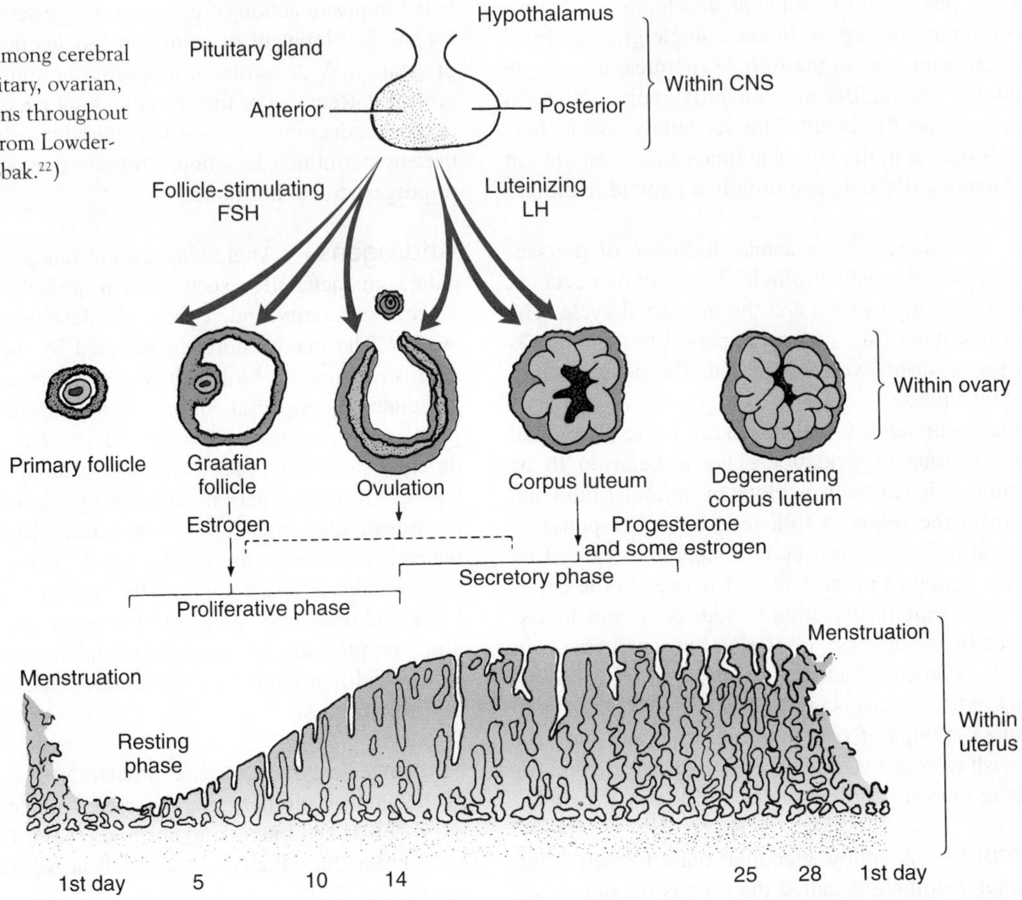

FIG. 12-7
Interrelationships among cerebral hypothalamic, pituitary, ovarian, and uterine functions throughout menstrual cycle. (From Lowdermilk, Perry, and Bobak.[22])

Table 12-1 Correlation of Ovarian and Endometrial Cycles (Ideal 28-Day Cycle)

	Menstrual (1-3 to 5 days)	Early Follicular (4 to 6-8 days)	Advanced Follicular (9 to 12-16 days)	Ovulation (12-16 days)	Early Luteal (15-19 days)	Advanced Luteal (20-25 days)	Premenstrual (26-32 days)
Ovary	Involution of corpus luteum	Growth and maturation of graafian follicle		Ovulation	Active corpus luteum		Involution of corpus luteum
Estrogen	Diminution	Progressive increase		High concentration	Secondary rise		Decreasing
Progesterone	Absent			Appearing	Rising		Decreasing
Endometrium	Menstrual desquamation and involution	Reorganization and proliferation	Further growth and watery secretion		Active secretion and glandular dilation	Accumulation of secretion and edema	Regressive
Pituitary secretion							
Follicle-stimulating hormone (FSH)	Fairly constant until just before ovulation			Moderate increase just before	Rapid decrease in previous levels		
Luteinizing hormone (LH)	Same as above			Marked increase just before	Same as above		

an ideal environment for implantation of the fertilized ovum. The uterine spiral arteries become more coiled and tortuous during this period, growing almost to the surface of the endometrium. If implantation of a fertilized ovum does not occur, the corpus luteum loses functional activity and degenerates. If fertilization and implantation occur, the secretion of human chorionic gonadotropin by the placenta maintains the corpus luteum. This promotes the continued secretion of progesterone and estrogen and prevents menstruation.

The premenstrual phase occurs 2 to 3 days before menstruation with infiltration of the stroma by polymorphonuclear or mononuclear leukocytes. The reticular framework of the stroma in the superficial zone disintegrates, resulting in a loss of tissue fluid and thinning of the endometrium. Some 4 to 24 hours before the onset of menstruation, a vasoconstriction in the arterioles and coiled arteries causes anoxia and shriveling of the compact and spongy zones. After a period of constriction the coiled arteries relax and bleeding occurs from them or their branches. This marks the onset of menstruation.

The menstrual phase lasts from the first to about the fifth day of the cycle. As the coiled arteries rupture, hematomas form that distend and eventually rupture the superficial endometrium. Fissures develop in adjacent layers and tissues, become fragmented, and detach. The entire functional layer of the endometrium is eventually sloughed, leaving only the deep basal layer intact. Bleeding stops when the coiled arteries return to a state of constriction.

Normal Findings*

External Genitalia

Surface characteristic: Homogeneous

Hair distribution: Variable in adults; usually inverse triangle with base over pubis; some hair may extend up midline toward umbilicus; ◆ pubic hair thinned, perhaps sparse, often gray

Inguinal and mons pubis skin surface: Smooth; clear

Labia and vestibule; labia majora, outer surface: Darker pigmentation; shriveled or full; gaping or closed; usually symmetric; skin surface smooth; may appear dry or moist; ◆ labial folds flattened or may disappear into surrounding skin; decrease in subcutaneous fat in folds that usually corresponds to degree of loss of subcutaneous fat elsewhere on body; skin appears smooth, often shiny, and paler than in younger adult

Labia majora, inner surface: Dark pink pigmentation; moist; usually symmetric; ◆ shiny; usually dry; paler than in young adult; fewer folds

Labia minora: Dark pink pigmentation; moist, usually symmetric

Vestibule surface: Dark pink pigmentation; moist, usually symmetric

Palpation of labia and vestibule: Soft, homogeneous consistency; nontender

Clitoris: Size: 2-cm length visible; 0.5-cm diameter; ◆ slightly smaller than in younger adult; surface: medial aspect covered by prepuce

Urethral meatus and surrounding tissue surface: Irregular opening or slit; may be close to or slightly within vaginal introitus; usually located midline; ◆ relaxed perineal musculature may result in meatus being situated more posteriorly; very near or within vaginal introitus; milking of urethral duct: nontender; no discharge

Vaginal introitus and surrounding tissue: Surface: thin vertical slit or large orifice with irregular edges (hymenal caruncles); moist tissue; ◆ may be smaller than in younger adult; multiparous client may manifest gaping introitus with vaginal walls rolling toward opening

Palpation of lateral and posterior introitus: Nontender; no discharge; ◆ opening may be very narrow and admit only one finger

Vaginal tone: Nullipara: squeezes tightly around examiner's index and middle fingers; unipara or multipara: squeezes firmly but with less tone than nullipara; no bulging or urinary incontinence when bearing down or pushing; ◆ may be relaxed; client has difficulty squeezing examiner's finger with voluntary vaginal constriction; vaginal wall may roll slightly outward; no incontinence

Perineum: Surface: smooth; midline or mediolateral episiotomy scar may be visible; palpation between index finger and thumb; nontender; nullipara: thick, smooth; unipara or multipara: thin, rigid, scarring; ◆ thin; rigid

Anal surface: Increased pigmentation and coarse skin

Internal Genitalia

Cervix

Color: Pink color evenly distributed; bluish in pregnancy; symmetric, circumscribed erythema surrounding os may indicate normal condition of exposed columnar epithelium, but inexperienced examiners should consider any reddened appearance a problem for consultation; ◆ paler than in younger woman; color evenly distributed

Position: Midline; cervix and os may be pointed in anterior or posterior direction; may project into vaginal tube 1 to 3 cm (resulting in 1- to 3-cm fornices surrounding cervix); ◆ cervix protrudes less into vaginal tube; may be flush against back of vaginal wall; surrounding fornices diminish or may disappear

Size: Usually 2.5-cm diameter; ◆ cervix decreases in size with age

Surface: Smooth; firm; occasional visible squamocolumnar junction (symmetric reddened circle around os); nabothian cysts (smooth, round, small, yellowish raised areas); ◆ smooth; may appear paler than in younger woman; occasional visible squamocolumnar junction (symmetric reddened circle around os)

Contour: Evenly rounded or slightly ovoid; ◆ nabothian cysts (smooth, round, yellowish, raised areas) common

Os: Nullipara: small, evenly round; unipara or multipara: slitlike, may be star shaped or irregular; ◆ often very narrow or stenosed; may be obliterated

Cervical discharge: Mucus plug may be present at os; odorless; creamy or clear; thin, thick, or stringy; discharge often heavier at midcycle or immediately before menstruation; ◆ Often scanty; if present, should be clear or slightly opaque and odorless

Vagina

Length: 10 to 15 cm; shortens with age

Color: Pink; ◆ paler than in younger women

*◆ = Older adult.

PERTINENT BACKGROUND INFORMATION

An additional consideration in assessment of the female organ system is a review of pertinent background information, including the following:

- Concurrent diseases or conditions
  - Menstruation
    - Age at onset
    - Length of cycles (duration)
    - Interval between cycles
    - Regularity of cycles
    - Duration, amount, and type of flow: Number of tampons or napkins used
    - Date of most recent douching
    - Date of last menstrual period (LMP)
    - Associated symptoms (such as dysmenorrhea, menorrhagia, metrorrhagia, abnormal pelvic or abdominal pain)
    - Premenstrual syndrome (PMS)
  - Obstetric history
    - Gravity, parity, abortions, number of living children
    - Complications of pregnancy and delivery or abortion
    - Contraceptive history: Method, duration, effectiveness, side effects
  - Infertility
    - Length of time attempting pregnancy
    - Knowledge of fertile period during menstrual cycle
    - Partner factors
    - Diagnostic evaluation studies to date
  - Menopause
    - When occurred
    - Related symptoms: Hot flushes, night sweats, dry vaginal mucosa
  - Gastrointestinal (GI) system
    - Constipation
    - Hemorrhoids
    - Vaginal protrusion on straining
  - Endocrine system
    - Hypothyroidism
    - Hyperthyroidism
    - Stein-Leventhal syndrome
    - Cushing's syndrome
  - Blood dyscrasias
  - Hypertension
  - Urinary system
    - Frequency
    - Nocturia
    - Urgency
    - Dysuria
    - Incontinence (stress, urgency)
- Previous surgery or illness
  - Gynecologic surgery
  - Other major surgery or illness (e.g., of abdomen or endocrine system)
  - Sexually transmitted diseases
  - Pelvic inflammatory disease
  - Vaginal infections
- Family history
  - Cancer
  - Sickle cell disease
  - Thyroid disorder
  - Diabetes
  - Other diseases
  - Death from gynecologic-related condition
  - Maternal diethylstilbestrol (DES) use
- Social history
  - Smoking, tobacco use, alcohol use
  - Illegal drug abuse or prescription drug abuse
  - Domestic/intimate partner abuse
- Sexual history
  - Age at first coitus
  - Frequency of coitus
  - Abnormal lesions or discharge in sex partner
  - Satisfaction and orgasmic response
  - Dyspareunia
  - Number of partners; lesions or discharge in sexual partner
- Medication history
  - Oral contraceptives
  - Estrogen therapy
  - Intrauterine contraceptive device (IUD)
  - Phenothiazines
  - Digitalis
  - Diuretics
  - Medical management medications

Data from Tucker et al[34] and Edge and Miller.[13]

Surface: Transverse rugae (diminish after vaginal deliveries); moist; smooth; ⭘ less moisture; smooth (rugae diminish with aging); shiny

Consistency: Smooth; homogeneous

Secretions: Minimum to moderate amount; thin; clear or cloudy; odorless; ⭘ May be absent or sparse; if present, should be clear or slightly opaque

Fornices: Pliable; smooth; ⭘ diminish and may disappear with aging; if palpable, should be pliable, smooth, and nontender

Uterus: Mobile; nontender; ⭘ diminishes greatly; often not palpable

Position: Fundus anteverted; palpable at level of pubis; ⭘ if palpated with internal hand, body of uterus should be smooth, firm, freely movable, and nontender

Contour of fundus: Rounded

Uterine wall: Firm consistency; smooth surface; pear shaped; 5.5 to 8 cm long

Ovaries: May not be palpable; slightly tender on palpation; firm; smooth; ovoid; mobile; diameter about 4 cm (size of walnut); ⭘ atrophy with age and rarely palpable in aged women; fallopian tube palpable

Breasts

Size: Varies; ⭘ decrease in adipose tissue

Symmetry: Bilaterally equal; slight asymmetry; breasts hang equally when woman is seated and leaning forward; breasts appear symmetric when woman is seated and pushing hands into hips or pushing palms together

Contour: Smooth; convex; even

Skin color: Even throughout

Skin texture: Smooth; elastic; movable; striae

⭘ = Older adult.

Venous patterns: Bilaterally similar
Moles, nevi: Long history of presence; nonchanging; nontender
Areolae
Size: Bilaterally equal
Shape: Round or oval
Surface characteristics: Smooth; bilaterally similar; Montgomery tubules
Nipples
Direction: Bilaterally equal in pointing direction
Size and shape: Bilaterally equal; long-standing inversion (unilateral or bilateral)
Color: Homogeneous
Surface characteristics: Smooth or may be slightly wrinkled; skin intact
Discharge: Absent
Suspensory ligaments: Equal bilateral pull when woman is seated with arms abducted over head; ⭘ relaxed; breasts may appear elongated or pendulous
Palpation of breasts
Tone: Bilaterally firm and equal; sagging of breast tissue may occur with aging or poor bra support
Tissue qualities: Smooth diffuse tissue bilaterally; nodular, bilateral granular consistency; premenstrual engorgement; elastic; nontender, firm mammary ridge along each breast at approximately 4 to 8 o'clock position; ⭘ decrease in granular tissue.
Lymph nodes: (including supraclavicular, infraclavicular, central and lateral axillary, pectoral, subscapular, scapular, brachial, intermediate, and internal mammary chains) Nonpalpable

CONDITIONS, DISEASES, AND DISORDERS

UTERINE AND OVARIAN DISORDERS

PELVIC INFLAMMATORY DISEASE

Pelvic inflammatory disease is an infectious process that may involve the fallopian tubes, ovaries, pelvic peritoneum, veins, or uterine connective tissue.

The incidence of PID is difficult to estimate because it is not a reportable disease and is not identified in a consistent manner; however, it is estimated that 1 million women are affected annually, with one third of them less than 19 years of age. It is not always treated, especially when symptoms are mild. It often occurs in sexually active women as the result of infection transmitted through sexual intercourse. It can also be associated with immunologic or renal disorders or through childbirth or abortion. In addition, frequent vaginal douching has been identified as a risk factor in predisposing women to PID.[31] It has been directly or indirectly linked to approximately one fifth of all of gynecologic problems. Specific risk factors include teenager (10 to 19), multiple sex partners, single status, previous diagnosis of PID, and sexual contact with urethritis or gonorrhea.

Pelvic inflammatory disease may be confined to one structure or involve the entire pelvis. Infections may be acute, subacute, recurrent, or chronic. Pelvic inflammatory disease in the fallopian tubes (the most common site) is referred to as salpingitis. Sequelae of PID include ectopic pregnancy, infertility, chronic pelvic pain, salpingitis, hydrosalpinx, and tubo-ovarian abscess.[25]

PATHOPHYSIOLOGY

Pelvic inflammatory disease begins in the vulva or accessory glands and spreads upward through the entire genital tract. One of the principal pathogens is *Chlamydia trachomatis,* but aerobic and anaerobic gram-negative bacilli and gram-positive cocci are also implicated as causative agents. Salpingitis resulting from tuberculosis has become rare. If PID follows childbirth or an abortion, anaerobic streptococci, staphylococci, coliform bacteria, or *Clostridium perfringens* are usually involved. Infections can also be caused by actinomycosis, schistosomiasis, leprosy, and oxyuriasis. Sarcoidosis and foreign bodies (such as radiographic contrast media) can cause inflammation.

The second principal pathogen is *Neisseria gonorrhoeae.* Gonococcal disease is characterized by an acute suppurative reaction with subsequent copious discharge of yellow pus. Hyperemia, edema, and tenseness occur in the involved structures, which are often bilaterally involved. The organisms spread over the mucosal surfaces, eventually involving the tubes and tubo-ovarian region. In an adult the vagina is resistant to the inflammation, but vulvovaginitis may develop in a child because of the more delicate mucosa. As the lumen of the fallopian tube fills with purulent exudate, some leaks out of the fimbriae. Over the course of days or weeks the fimbriae may seal or become adherent to the ovary, causing salpingo-oophoritis. The collection of pus in the sealed tube causes distention of the tube and is referred to as pyosalpinx. In this form the infection may persist for months. The demise of the organisms and sterilization of the infection occur eventually, owing to progressive anaerobiasis and increasing acidity. The pus then undergoes a slow proteolysis, and the exudate is transformed to a thin serous fluid in a condition known as hydrosalpinx.

Tubo-ovarian abscesses can occur when exudate collects where the tube is sealed against the ovary. This inflammatory process affects the most superficial layers of the ovary but spares the underlying ovarian tissue. Peritonitis resulting from spread of the exudate to the pelvic peritoneum is common. Infertility caused by mucosal destruction and tubal occlusion is a common sequela of salpingitis. Rupture of tubo-ovarian abscess and peritonitis can be life threatening.

DIAGNOSTIC STUDIES AND FINDINGS

Culture of purulent secretions: From cervix or posterior cul de sac during surgery; identification of organism and sensitivity to antibiotics
White blood cell count: Elevated, with increased differential
Erythrocyte sedimentation rate: Elevated

Laparoscopic examination: Visualization of pelvic inflammation; mild: erythema, edema, no obvious purulent exudate, tubes freely movable; moderate: gross, purulent material evident; marked erythema and edema; tubes not always freely movable; severe: pyosalpinx, severe inflammation, abscess

Gram's stain of secretions: Identification of gram-positive or gram-negative organisms

Ultrasonography: Visualization consistent with abscess or inflammation

Culdocentesis: White blood cells or nonclotting blood; purulent material

Urine or serum pregnancy test: Rule out pregnancy

MULTIDISCIPLINARY PLAN

Surgery

Hysterectomy with bilateral salpingo-oophorectomy: May be required for patients with abscesses, hydrosalpinx, and tubal obstruction if antibiotic therapy is unsuccessful

Laparotomy with incision and drainage of abscesses and lysis of adhesions

Colpotomy

Medications

Parenteral treatment[8,14]

Cefotetan, 2 g intravenously (IV) q12h, or cefoxitin, 2 g IV q6h plus doxycycline, 100 mg IV or by mouth (PO) q12h, or clindamycin, 900 mg IV q8h plus a loading dose of gentamicin, 2 mg/kg then 1.5 mg/kg q8h IV, or ofloxacin, 400 mg IV q12h plus metronidazole, 500 mg IV q8h, or ampicillin/sulbactam, 3 g IV q6h plus doxycycline, 100 mg IV or PO q12h, or ciprofloxacin, 200 mg IV q12h plus doxycycline, 100 mg IV or PO q12h plus metronidazole, 500 mg IV q8h

Parenteral treatment is given until evidence of clinical improvement; patient can be discharged with doxycycline, 100 mg PO bid to complete 14-day course

Oral treatment

Ofloxacin, 400 mg PO bid plus metronidazole, 500 mg PO bid for 14 days, or ceftriaxone, 250 mg IM times one plus doxycycline, 100 mg PO bid for 14 days, or trovafloxacin, 200 mg PO daily for 14 days

General Management

Pain management; bed rest in semi-Fowler's position; parenteral fluids; nasogastric suctioning if ileus is present; removal of intrauterine device (IUD); social services support; counseling and education (especially if sexually transmitted disease [STD] is precipitating factor)

NURSING CARE

NURSING ASSESSMENT

Subjective data: Abdominal and pelvic pain (aching, burning, cramping, and stabbing); low back pain; dyspareunia; menstrual irregularity; urinary discomfort (dysuria; frequency and urgency); constipation; malaise; nausea and vomiting; diarrhea; vaginal drainage (see Emergency Alert box)

> **! EMERGENCY ALERT**
>
> **ABDOMINAL PAIN—FEMALE**
>
> Commonly, women seek treatment for lower abdominal and pelvic pain. In the woman of childbearing age, a test for pregnancy is necessary to determine possibility of ectopic pregnancy.
>
> Ovarian cysts and PID are common causes of pelvic pain, although there are many others. Pelvic inflammatory disease is an infection that may involve the uterus, fallopian tubes, ovaries, and adjacent structures. It does not cause acute lower abdominal pain.
>
> **ASSESSMENT AND INTERVENTIONS**
>
> ***Ovarian Cyst***
>
> - Presentation is similar to ectopic pregnancy, although pregnancy test is negative.
> - Patient reports pain, often severe.
> - Vaginal or intraperitoneal bleeding may be present, and surgical intervention may be indicated.
> - Obtain IV access as indicated.
> - Obtain order for laboratory tests.
>
> ***Pelvic Inflammatory Disease***
>
> - Assess, for anorexia, fever, chills, nausea, and vomiting.
> - Evaluate pain without pelvic examination with purulent vaginal discharge.
> - Assess abdomen tenseness on palpation.
> - In collaboration with physician's orders, obtain complete blood count (CBC), sedimentation rate, smears to rule out pregnancy, and urinalysis.
> - Normal temperature, sedimentation rate, and white blood cell (WBC) count do not support PID as a diagnosis.
> - Provide antibiotic therapy as ordered.
> - Treat partner as indicated.
> - Provide emotional support and education.

Abdomen: Rebound tenderness; normal bowel sounds progressing to ileus in untreated persons

Cervix: Cervical motion tenderness; copious purulent discharge

Vulva: Pruritus; maceration

Temperature: Elevated above 100.4° F (38° C)

Fluid balance: Nausea; vomiting; dry skin; poor skin turgor

POTENTIAL COMPLICATIONS

Infertility, ectopic pregnancy, chronic pelvic pain, pyosalpinx/tubo-ovarian abscess, and recurrent pelvic inflammatory disease

PATIENT PROBLEMS/NURSING DIAGNOSES & INTERVENTIONS

NIC PHYSICAL COMFORT PROMOTION

Acute pain related to inflammation

- Maintain complete bed rest; semi-Fowler's position may be most desirable *to prevent pus from pelvis moving to upper abdominal area.*
- Explain cause of pain *to allay any undue anxiety.*
- Instruct patient to request analgesic before pain becomes severe *to avoid inconsistent control of pain.*

NIC SKIN/WOUND MANAGEMENT

Risk for impaired skin integrity related to drainage of purulent secretions on perineum

- Explain cause of vaginal discharge and pruritus if present.
- Assist and teach patient to perform perineal care every 3 to 4 hours or as needed *to maintain skin integrity.*
- Do not rub; blot skin dry *to prevent excoriation.*
- Prevent excessive warmth in room; lightweight covers over bed cradle may be indicated.

NIC TISSUE PERFUSION MANAGEMENT

Risk for deficient fluid volume related to fever

- Explain need to increase fluid intake during infectious processes.
- Encourage fluid intake of 3000 ml daily unless contraindicated.
- Monitor intake and output as indicated.

NIC PATIENT EDUCATION

Deficient knowledge regarding condition

- Explain importance of hand washing before and after contact with perineal area and of wiping from front to back after elimination *to prevent contamination of vaginal area with cross-contaminants from anal area.*
- Explain need to use perineal pads, which should be changed frequently according to amount of vaginal drainage. Instruct patient not to use tampons.
- Explain that a shower is preferable to a tub bath.
- Encourage patient to share concerns regarding sexual partner as probable source of infection *to promote health-seeking behaviors of partner.*
- Explain rationale for removal of IUD if this is ordered by physician.

PATIENT EDUCATION/CONTINUUM OF CARE PLAN

1. Explain need to avoid using tampons, having intercourse, or douching for at least 1 week after antibiotic therapy.
2. Explain methods to prevent venereal disease if condition is caused by gonorrhea or *Chlamydia.*
3. Explain importance of encouraging patient's sex partner to be examined and treated.
4. Explain alternative methods of conception control if condition is associated with an IUD.
5. Describe symptoms of recurrence that patient should report to physician.

EVALUATION/PATIENT OUTCOMES

Physical Comfort Promotion: Comfort is achieved and pain is controlled. Patient reports lower abdominal, low back, pelvic, or perineal pain is controlled.

Skin/Wound Management: Skin and mucous membrane color is good. There is no vaginal drainage or pruritus, inflammation, or maceration of vulva.

Tissue Perfusion Management: Hydration and body temperature are normal. There is no fever with temperature within normal limits. Patient is hydrated with balanced intake and output.

Patient Education: Patient understands home care and follow-up instructions. Patient understands that showers are permitted but not tub baths. Patient verbalizes methods to prevent sexually transmitted diseases. Patient understands necessity of avoiding douching, intercourse, or tampons for at least 1 week following completion of antibiotics. Patient wipes front to back after bowel movements. Patient understands medication schedule and signs or symptoms requiring contact with health care provider.

UTERINE BLEEDING: DYSFUNCTIONAL AND ABNORMAL

Dysfunctional uterine bleeding (DUB) occurs during the reproductive years and is associated with neuroendocrine factors.

Abnormal uterine bleeding can occur at any time and is associated with non–menstrual cycle factors, including tumors, inflammation, trauma, pregnancy, or exogenous hormone effects.

Abnormalities and variation in uterine bleeding are the most frequently encountered health care problems for women. Patients often think that abnormal uterine bleeding is life threatening or indicative of a major problem in reproductive or sexual functioning. Abnormal bleeding, varying from spotting to the passage of clots, may occur at any age and for a variety of reasons (see Emergency Alert box below).

DUB, which is always anovulatory and usually painless (whereas dysmenorrhea is associated with ovulatory cycles), can occur at any age from puberty through menopause. It generally occurs at the extremes of menstrual life, when disturbances in ovarian function are common. About 50% of dysfunctional bleeding occurs in premenopausal women (age 40 to 50), about 20% during the adolescent years, and about 30% during the reproductive period.

! EMERGENCY ALERT

VAGINAL BLEEDING/HEMORRHAGE

Commonly, women seek treatment for vaginal bleeding, which can occur for a variety of reasons. It is essential to rule out life-threatening illness or injury, search for a cause, and rule out normal menstruation and pregnancy.

ASSESSMENT

- Obtain history.
- Monitor vital signs. Determine the quantity and quality of vaginal bleeding and the duration and regularity.
- Determine pregnancy status.

INTERVENTIONS

- Direct interventions at stabilizing condition and managing the cause.
- Maintain airway, breathing, and circulation; oxygenization; and IV access as indicated.
- Obtain order for laboratory studies as relevant.
- Provide reassurance and support to the patient.

The following terms are often used to describe variations in uterine bleeding:

Dysfunctional uterine bleeding (DUB): Uterine bleeding during the reproductive period from neuroendocrinologic factors

Abnormal uterine bleeding: Can occur at any time during the life cycle and is generally associated with tumor, inflammation, pregnancy, trauma, or exogenous hormonal effects

Hypomenorrhea: Abnormally small amount of menstrual flow

Menorrhagia (hypermenorrhea): Increased amount (60 ml or more each period) or duration of menstrual bleeding

Metrorrhagia: Intermenstrual bleeding

Metrorrhea: Any pathologic uterine discharge

Oligomenorrhea: Infrequent menstruation

Polymenorrhea: Increased frequency of menstruation (not consistently associated with ovulation)

Postmenopausal bleeding: Bleeding from the reproductive tract occurring 1 year or more after menopause

Spotting: Small amounts of bloody vaginal discharge ranging from pink to dark brown

Medical therapy should be the first line of treatment for premenopausal women who are found to have no obvious cause for their abnormal uterine bleeding. For those who do not respond to treatment or who are unable to tolerate it, a conservative surgical solution is hysteroscopic resection of polyps or submucous fibroids. Hysteroscopic endometrial ablation may be used to treat women suffering from intractable menorrhagia. A hysterectomy is the final course of action if symptoms are not controlled or corrected.[18,33]

PATHOPHYSIOLOGY

The preceding terms used to describe abnormal bleeding do not indicate the cause of the abnormality or reason for bleeding. The following are the most common types of bleeding and their causes:

Midcycle spotting: Midcycle estradiol fluctuation associated with ovulation

Delayed menstruation with excessive bleeding: Anovulation or threatened abortion

Frequent bleeding: Chronic pelvic inflammatory disease, endometriosis, DUB, or anovulation

Profuse menstrual bleeding: Endometrial polyps, adenomyosis, DUB, submucous leiomyomas, or presence of intrauterine contraceptive device

Intermenstrual or irregular bleeding: Endometrial polyps, DUB, uterine or cervical cancer, or oral contraceptive use

Postmenopausal bleeding: Endometrial hyperplasia, estrogen therapy, or endometrial cancer

Other causes of bleeding include foreign bodies, lacerations, and systemic diseases such as leukemia, hypothyroidism, and blood dyscrasias. In addition, precocious puberty may warrant consideration as a cause, as may vaginal adenosis in young women with prenatal exposure to the synthetic estrogen diethylstibestrol (DES).

! EMERGENCY ALERT

ABORTION

In women of childbearing age, abortion is the leading cause of vaginal bleeding. Abortion occurs when the pregnancy ends before fetal viability, usually at 24 weeks, has been achieved. Abortions are classified as threatened, inevitable, incomplete, missed, septic, habitual, and therapeutic.

ASSESSMENT

- Determine signs of significant vaginal blood loss, shock.
- Determine pregnancy status, rule out ectopic pregnancy.
- Assess pain and cramping.

INTERVENTIONS

- Monitor vital signs closely.
- Obtain serum human chorionic gonadotropin (HCG) to verify pregnancy, HCG status.
- Obtain IV access, as needed.
- Assist physician during pelvic examination.
- Anticipate suction curettage.
- Administer medications as appropriate.
- Observe client for at least 2 hours after procedure.

Dysfunctional uterine bleeding is most common during the reproductive years and occurs as painless, irregular, heavy bleeding (menometrorrhagia), midcycle spotting, oligomenorrhea, or periods of amenorrhea. In most cases the cause is anovulation, but bleeding may reflect defects in the follicular or luteal phase of the ovulatory cycle.

With anovulation, the persistent unopposed estrogen stimulation may be endogenous from an ovarian tumor such as a granulosa cell tumor, polycystic ovaries (Stein-Leventhal syndrome), or abnormal metabolism of estrogen as in liver disease. Unopposed estrogen stimulation may cause endometrial hyperplasia; when the estrogen can no longer maintain the endometrium, sloughing and vaginal bleeding occur.

Follicular phase defects result from premature maturation of the ovarian follicle owing to pituitary hyperstimulation. The cycle is less than 22 days. Increased levels of FSH and slightly elevated estradiol levels result in a progressively shortened proliferative phase that can cause spotting in perimenopausal women. Oligomenorrhea most commonly occurs in young women and may result from a prolonged proliferative phase.

Luteal phase defects may result in profuse and prolonged bleeding caused by delayed involution of the corpus luteum. A corpus luteum cyst or persistent corpus luteum can cause a delay in menses, with premenstrual spotting.

The endometrium of women with menorrhagia has been found to have higher levels of prostaglandin E_2 and prostaglandin F_2 when compared with women with normal menses. Prostaglandin E_2 is associated with vasodilatory effects that contribute to bleeding.

DIAGNOSTIC STUDIES AND FINDINGS

Complete blood count: To determine the degree of anemia and to detect abnormal leukocyte production

Thyroid function tests: To assess thyroid function

Dilation and curettage with cervical or endometrial biopsy: To assess endometrium and identify carcinoma or polyps

Hysterography: To identify presence of endometrial polyps, submucous myomas, adenomyosis, endometrial carcinoma, and adnexal lesions

Hysteroscopy: To identify intrauterine abnormalities such as submucous myomas, endometrial polyps, and foreign bodies

Endovaginal ultrasonography: To differentiate endometrial polyps, hyperplasia, and carcinoma

Endocrine profile: To assess functioning of the adrenal glands, ovaries, and pituitary glands

Tests confirming luteinization: Endometrial biopsy to demonstrate secretory or menstrual endometrium; basal body temperatures: biphasic pattern is indicative of ovulation; examination of cervical mucus to determine presence of ferning; serum or urine progesterone levels to assess progesterone metabolites consistent with progestational phase of menstrual cycle

Measurement of blood loss: Weigh pads and tampons

MULTIDISCIPLINARY PLAN

The plan of medical care selected is contingent on the cause of the bleeding

Surgery

Dilation and curettage (see p. 853)

Hysteroscopic excision of polyps/myomas

Endometrial ablation: Done with a hysteroscopic resectoscope by applying a cauterizing current to the endometrium in women who are not candidates for hysterectomy, such as those with major medical diseases, severe heart disease, bleeding diatheses, and major respiratory difficulty

Abdominal or vaginal hysterectomy with partial or complete bilateral salpingo-oophorectomy (TAH/BSO) (see p. 853)

Medications

Oral contraceptive therapy

Progesterone or progestogen: Medroxyprogesterone (Provera, others), 2.5-10 mg/day PO or 100-400 mg/day intramuscularly (IM) (may be given if patient is anovulatory and infertility is not a concern)

Estrogens

Conjugated estrogens (Premarin), 0.625-3.75 mg/day followed by high doses of estrogen-progestin combinations (given for excessive anovulatory bleeding)

Clomiphene citrate can be used when excessive bleeding is caused by inadequate luteal phase or anovulation

Prostaglandin inhibitors: Meclofenamate sodium, 100 mg PO tid

Antigonadotropin: Danazol (Danocrine), 100-800 mg/day in divided doses

Gonadotropin-releasing hormone (Gn-RH) agonists: Nafarelin acetate (Synarel), 2 mg/ml nasal spray, 1 spray in nostril bid

Leuprolide acetate (Lupron), 3.75-7.5 mg IM once per month

Analgesics as indicated

General Management

Psychosocial services and counseling as indicated

NURSING CARE

NURSING ASSESSMENT

Variations depend on the cause of the bleeding.

Bleeding: Heavy menstrual flow; bleeding between periods; infrequent menstruation; increased frequency of menstruation; spotting

Pain: Menstrual cramps or pain with menses; low abdominal pain at midcycle*; uterine cramps at midcycle*

Vaginal secretions: Wet mucoid vaginal secretion at midcycle*

POTENTIAL COMPLICATIONS

Anemia; altered sexual function; psychosocial concerns

PATIENT PROBLEMS/NURSING DIAGNOSES & INTERVENTIONS

NIC TISSUE PERFUSION MANAGEMENT

Fatigue due to blood loss

- Explain importance of iron-rich foods to supplement iron.
- Explain methods of quantifying blood loss and reporting to health-care provider.

NIC PHYSICAL COMFORT PROMOTION

Pain related to uterine cramps

- Assist in and teach patient pain-relieving techniques *to promote self-sufficiency in managing pain.*

NIC COPING ASSISTANCE

Sexual dysfunction related to altered body function associated with uterine bleeding

Powerlessness related to illness-related regimen

- Explain importance of sharing concerns with sexual partner *to come to an understanding of preferences, concerns, and behavior related to uterine bleeding.*
- Assess meaning of dysfunction for patient *to explore self-concept issues.*
- Encourage patient to express her feelings *to increase understanding of individual coping style.*
- Consider nursing interventions associated with loss and grief if results of diagnostic studies confirm anovulatory cycle and infertility.

PATIENT EDUCATION/CONTINUUM OF CARE PLAN

1. Explain the importance of recording dates, type of flow, and number of pads or tampons used.
2. Explain the importance of ongoing care.
3. Explain medication schedule and purpose of each medication.

---

*Signs and symptoms suggestive of ovulation.

Evaluation/Patient Outcomes

Tissue Perfusion Management: Patient does not experience fatique. Patient quantifies and reports blood loss and understands need for iron-rich foods.

Physical Comfort Promotion: Comfort is achieved; there is no pain. Patient uses pain-relieving techniques or medication as ordered.

Coping Assistance: Patient demonstrates adaptive response related to self-concept. Patient asks appropriate questions. Patient shows signs of grief if she learns of undesired infertililty. Sexual adjustment is made. Patient indicates that she has discusssed concerns with partner.

Dysmenorrhea

Dysmenorrhea is menstruation that is painful enough to limit normal activity or cause a woman to seek medical treatment.

Dysmenorrhea is a common gynecologic complaint. It occurs in approximately 10% of high school–age girls, keeping them home from school for 1 or 2 days, and it also affects many college students and young women in the workforce. More than 50% of menstruating women have some degree of dysmenorrhea, with 5% to 20% of women being incapacitated. Dysmenorrhea is pain associated with menstruation during ovulatory cycles in the absence of organic disease. Secondary dysmenorrhea is due to an organic disease such as PID or endometriosis.

Pathophysiology

Primary dysmenorrhea usually develops 1 or 2 years after menarche, when ovulatory cycles are established. Increased amounts of prostaglandin are released from the endometrium under the influence of progesterone in the luteal phase of the cycle. Very little prostaglandin is produced during anovulatory cycles, which are almost never painful. Increased sensitivity of the myometrium and endometrium to prostaglandin F_2 can produce uterine contractions and ischemia, causing the cramping pain of dysmenorrhea.

Secondary dysmenorrhea is associated with pelvic disorders such as endometriosis, adenomyosis, or chronic pelvic inflammatory disease. It may appear after years of normal menstruation, and it is characterized by cramping. Dysmenorrhea caused by endometriosis is related to the number of endometrial implants.[27]

Diagnostic Studies and Findings

Pelvic examination: To rule out or confirm underlying disorders in secondary dysmenorrhea

Laparoscopy: To rule out or confirm underlying disorders in secondary dysmenorrhea

Dilation and curettage/hysteroscopy: To rule out or confirm underlying disorders in secondary dysmenorrhea

Hysterosalpingography: To rule out or confirm underlying disorders in secondary dysmenorrhea

Multidisciplinary Plan

Surgery

Laparoscopic CO_2 laser uterine nerve ablation (for treatment of drug-resistant primary dysmenorrhea)[12]

Laser ablation or fulguration of endometriosis

TAH/BSO: May be indicated for disorder associated with secondary dysmenorrhea

Presacral neurectomy (severance of nerve trunks in hypogastric plexus): Performed in *rare* cases when no underlying disorder can be found and there is no response to medications

Medications

Nonsteroidal antiinflammatory drugs

- Ibuprofen (Motrin), 400-600 mg PO q4-6h as prostaglandin synthetase inhibitor
- Naproxen sodium, 550 mg PO then 275 mg q4-8h

Oral contraceptives: May be ordered for hormonal effect to relieve pain by suppressing ovulation

General Management

Adequate exercise; balanced diet with increased consumption of complex carbohydrates, fruits, and vegetables, as well as a decreased consumption of salt, alcohol, sugar, and caffeine; adequate rest and sleep; attention to personal hygiene; no tobacco

NURSING CARE

Nursing Assessment

Pain: Colicky and cyclic pain, infrequently nagging and dull in low pelvis and often with radiation toward vulva, perineum, rectum, and down back of thighs; may be experienced 24 to 48 hours before menses or with start of menstruation; may be associated with symptoms of premenstrual tension, including nausea, vomiting, diarrhea, urinary frequency, chills, abdominal bloating, and breast tenderness

Psychoemotional status: Irritability, depression

Potential Complications

Loss of work; interference with activities of daily living (ADLs)

Patient Problems/Nursing Diagnoses & Interventions

NIC Physical Comfort Promotion

Pain related to uterine cramping

- Identify and help patient use pain-reduction methods, including relaxation techniques, heating pad, effleurage (abdominal massage), and orgasm (relieves cramps in some women).
- Evaluate patient's use of pain-control techniques and encourage use of those that reduce her pain.

NIC COPING ASSISTANCE

Disturbed body image related to negative feelings about menses

- Encourage patient to express feelings about any self-perceptions, as well as how she believes she is viewed by others.
- Explore patient's role and behaviors when dysmenorrhea is present *to identify effects on lifestyle.*
- Evaluate support system and coping strategies *to determine their effects on body image.*

PATIENT EDUCATION/CONTINUUM OF CARE PLAN

1. Explain the prescribed dosage and frequency of doses of prostaglandin antagonists or other medications.
2. Provide pain management information, including use of antiinflammatory and analgesic agents that should be taken every 4 to 6 hours instead of waiting for pain to peak before taking the next dose of medication.

EVALUATION/PATIENT OUTCOMES

Physical Comfort Promotion: Comfort is achieved. Patient uses pain-relieving techniques as ordered. Pain is gone. Patient initiates suggestions for coping with condition.

Coping Assistance: Body image is intact. Patient applies learned behaviors in dealing with stressful feelings. Patient verbalizes understanding of dysmenorrhea process and treatment.

ENDOMETRIOSIS

Endometriosis is an abnormal growth of endometrial tissue outside the uterine cavity.

Endometriosis is a benign disease, but it has certain characteristics of a malignancy, including the ability to grow, infiltrate, and spread. The ectopic tissue is responsive to hormonal variations of the menstrual cycle and is subject to menstrual-like bleeding.

Endometriosis is estimated to affect 1% to 5% of women of reproductive age. A familial incidence of endometriosis has been documented. A female patient who has an affected first-degree relative has an approximately tenfold increased risk for developing the disease. Cervical or vaginal atresia and müllerian fusion defects with obstructed outflow are commonly associated with pelvic endometriosis; this represents another genetic or at least congenital mechanism.[2] Characteristic lesions are found in at least 20% of patients undergoing gynecologic surgery. Endometriosis is a significant finding in only about one third of these patients. Symptoms severe enough to require treatment generally occur between the ages of 25 and 35 years. Endometriosis is rare in women over 50 years of age. The greatest incidence of the disease seems to be in women who tend to marry later and have fewer children. The fertility rate of patients with endometriosis is about 66%, compared with 88% for the general population. Endometriosis occurs in young women with congenital obstructions of the vagina or cervix that are associated with reflux menstruation.

Endometriosis is associated with infertility, pregnancy wastage, decreased fertilization, pain, and decreased pregnancy rates with in vitro fertilization. Recent studies suggest that endometriosis is associated with polyclonal B cell activation, which is a classic characteristic of autoimmune disease.

A rare but important complication of endometriosis that can mimic ovarian cancer is ascites. Most cases have been reported in nulliparous young black women who have massive ascites. It is important that this rare complication be considered in the presence of ascites with abdominal or pelvic masses and weight gain because this otherwise indicates the presence of malignant disease. Treatment is effected by ablation of ovarian function by surgery, radiotherapy, or suppression of endometriosis by endocrine therapy, which is the preferred treatment in very young women.

PATHOPHYSIOLOGY

Endometriosis has been identified in unusual sites in the body, but the majority of lesions are limited to the pelvis. The most common pelvic sites, in order of frequency, are the ovary, peritoneum of the cul-de-sac or pouch of Douglas, uterosacral ligaments, round ligament, oviduct, and peritoneal surface of the uterus (FIG. 12-8). Endometriosis of the cervix occurs infrequently but is associated with diagnostic and therapeutic traumatizing cervical procedures such as colposcopy. Isolated lesions in the appendix, bladder, ileum, cecum, cervix, or vagina are far less common. Endometriosis has been identified infrequently in laparotomy or episiotomy scars, in the umbilicus, and in distant sites (arms, legs, lungs, kidneys, and nose). There is a direct relationship between the number of endometrial implants and the severity of associated dysmenorrhea.[27]

Three major theories exist regarding the pathogenesis of endometriosis:

Transportation: Endometrium is regurgitated throughout the fallopian tubes during a normal menses. After the retrograde flow, endometrial fragments implant on the ovary, on peritoneal surfaces, and on other areas.

Metaplasia or formation in situ: Celomic epithelium differentiates to endometrial epithelium by inflammatory or hormonal influence and alteration.

Induction: This is a combination of transportation and metaplasia in which regurgitated endometrium liberates chemical-inducing substances that activate undifferentiated mesenchyme to form endometrial epithelium. This is believed to be the most likely pathogenesis of endometriosis.

The appearance of the lesions varies depending on the stage of the disease and its duration. The foci of endometrial tissue are under hormonal influence and bleed periodically. The foci appear as bluish red to yellow-brown nodules implanted on or lying beneath serosal surfaces. They may be microscopic or 1 to 2 cm in diameter. As individual lesions enlarge and coalesce, they can immobilize the affected structures and form adhesions. Endometriosis of the ovaries is characterized by endometriomas, cystic spaces 8 to 10 cm in size. Because they are filled with brown blood debris, they are also referred to as chocolate cysts.

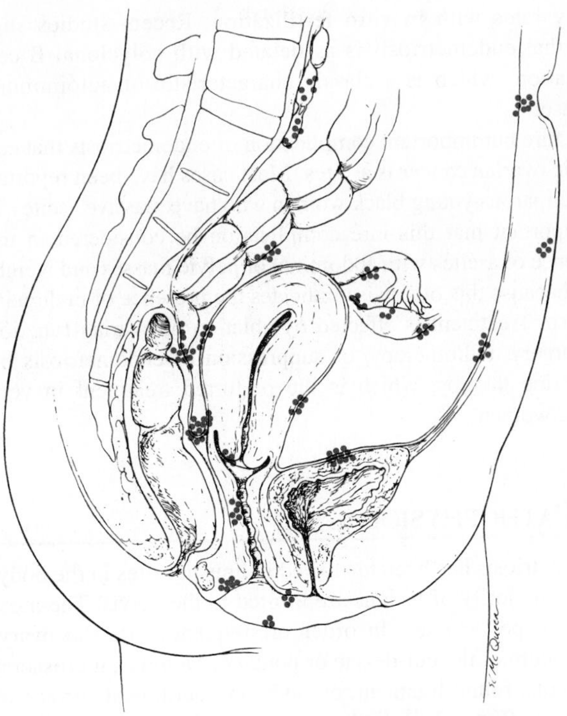

FIG. 12-8
Common sites of endometriosis. (From Herbst.[15])

DIAGNOSTIC STUDIES AND FINDINGS

Laparoscopy: To visualize foci and perform a biopsy of lesions (a conclusive diagnosis is based on surgical visualization)

Biopsy of lesions: To confirm histologic diagnosis by presence of glands, stroma, or hemosiderin pigment (an insoluble form of storage iron that indicates bleeding)

MULTIDISCIPLINARY PLAN

The treatment plan is directed toward producing maximum relief of symptoms and minimum interference with childbearing function in patients who desire children in the future.

Surgery

Laparoscopic removal of endometriotic implants, endometrioma capsules, and lysis of adnexal lesions surgically, using electrical or laser energy

Total abdominal hysterectomy and bilateral salpingo-oophorectomy

Resection or cautery destruction of visible lesions

Medications

Gn-RH agonists

Nafarelin acetate (Synarel), 2 mg/ml nasal spray, 1 spray in 1 nostril bid

Leuprolide acetate (Lupron), 3.75-7.5 mg IM once per month to once every 2 months

Leuprolide acetate for depot suspension (Lupron Depot), 11.25 mg q3 months

Progestins: Medroxyprogesterone acetate (Provera), 2.5-10 mg PO for 5 days every 2 months

Antigonadotropic agents: Danazol (Danocrine), 100-800 mg/day in divided doses for 6-9 months; produces hypoestrogenic state similar to menopause with eventually atrophy of endometrial lesions

Oral contraceptives

General Management

Psychosocial support services

NURSING CARE

NURSING ASSESSMENT

Pain: Pelvic pain with menstruation; vague aching, cramping, or bearing-down sensation in pelvis or lower back; dyspareunia; pain with defecation

Bimanual pelvic examination: Tender nodules along uterosacral ligaments; uterus may be immobile

Bleeding: Menses excessive, long, or both

Behavioral changes: Personality changes; depression

POTENTIAL COMPLICATIONS

Infertility; pregnancy wastage; pain; ascites

PATIENT PROBLEMS/NURSING DIAGNOSES & INTERVENTIONS

NIC PHYSICAL COMFORT PROMOTION

Pain related to chemical irritation of bleeding in pelvic cavity

- Assist with and explain pain-relieving techniques.
- Instruct patient to take analgesics as ordered.

NIC COPING ASSISTANCE

Disturbed body image related to altered biophysical function

Anticipatory grieving related to potential infertility

- Explore meaning of condition with patient *to establish plan of care.*
- Encourage patient to express feelings and to share these with her partner.
- Encourage verbalization of fears, concerns, and other emotions.
- Determine current sources of emotional support such as spouse, mother, or sister *because this can influence the extent of self-care management and coping behaviors.*
- Refer to nursing interventions for specific surgical procedure if done.

PATIENT EDUCATION/CONTINUUM OF CARE PLAN

1. Instruct the patient about the importance of ongoing patient care.
2. Provide information regarding goals of therapy and need to follow through.
3. Confirm patient's understanding of medication schedule and signs or symptoms to report to health-care provider.

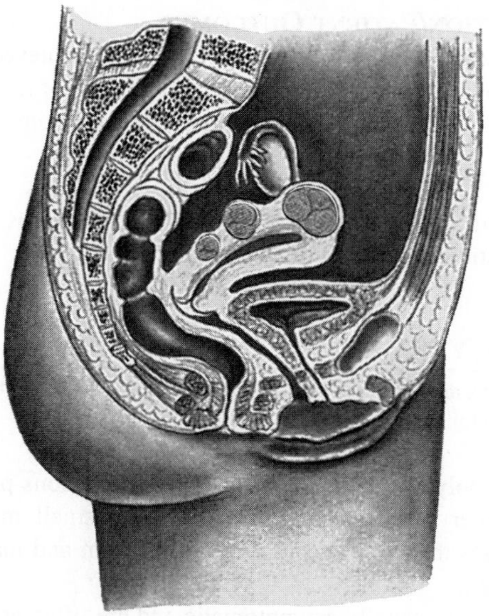

FIG. 12-9
Myomas of the uterus (fibroids). (From Seidel et al.[32])

EVALUATION/PATIENT OUTCOMES

Physical Comfort Promotion: Comfort is achieved. Intervention has relieved pain, ended abnormal bleeding, and preserved fertility if desired.

Coping Assistance: Body image is positive. Patient verbalizes increasing confidence in ability to cope with plan of care and verbalizes positive feelings about body.

Grief response is managed. Patient verbalizes fears and concerns and is able to cope in an adaptive manner with support of significant others.

LEIOMYOMAS

Uterine leiomyomas are well-circumscribed, nonencapsulated, benign tumors of the uterine musculature; they are also called myomas, fibromyomas, fibromas, or fibroids (FIG. 12-9).

Uterine leiomyomas are the most frequently occurring uterine neoplasm and can be found in at least 20% to 25% of all women of reproductive age. Leiomyomas are the most common indication for hysterectomy among the approximately 600,000 women who have this procedure each year in the United States. Almost one third of women undergoing a hysterectomy have a diagnosis of leiomyoma.[3] Most hysterectomies for uterine leiomyomas are performed for the relief of symptoms. Common complaints include abnormal uterine bleeding and pelvic pain or pressure. It has been determined that there is an increase in operative blood loss and postoperative morbidity, including urinary tract infections, vaginal cuff cellulitis, and febrile morbidity, when uterine weight exceeds 500 g. The use of Gn-RH agonists in the preoperative period to reduce the size of uterine leiomyoma is a preventive adjunct to surgical management. The benefits of a short course of Gn-RH agonists may also include the potential for conversion to a vaginal as opposed to an abdominal hysterectomy, reduction in preoperative bleeding accompanied by an increase in preoperative hematocrit, and decreased operative blood loss.[11,16]

PATHOPHYSIOLOGY

Leiomyomas are classified according to their location in the uterus as follows:

Intramural: Central portion of the uterine wall
Submucous: Beneath the endometrium protruding into the intrauterine cavity; may become pedunculated with growth, protruding into the cervix or vagina
Subserous: Beneath the peritoneal covering and projecting into the abdominal cavity; may become pedunculated with growth
Cervical: Within the musculature of the cervix
Intraligamentous: Lateral tumor growth between the leaves of the broad ligament
Wandering or parasitic: A subserous growth that has lost its connection to the uterus and receives blood from adjacent viscera, peritoneum, or omentum

Leiomyomas arise from smooth muscle within the myometrium, most commonly during the reproductive years. They increase in size during pregnancy, when estrogen production is high, and with the use of oral contraceptives. They generally regress after menopause. Symptoms occur in less than 50% of women who have fibroids.[17]

As the tumor enlarges, the blood supply may not increase as quickly as needed, resulting in degenerative changes. The most common type of degeneration is hyalinization, in which fibrous and muscle tissue is replaced by hyaline tissue that is smooth and soft and lacks the whorled fascicular pattern. Less commonly, cystic degeneration occurs, with the hyaline material breaking down further and undergoing liquefaction owing to a further decrease in blood supply. Calcification of the leiomyoma may occur. In a large tumor, areas of yellow-brown or red softening, referred to as red or carneous degeneration, may develop because of aseptic necrosis associated with hemorrhage into the tumor. Necrosis may also occur because of twisting or torsion of a pedunculated leiomyoma. Fertility may be impaired when leiomyomas occlude the endocervical canal, the tubal ostia, or the endometrial cavity.

DIAGNOSTIC STUDIES AND FINDINGS

Bimanual examination: Enlarged, bulky, or nodular uterus
Pregnancy test: To confirm or rule out pregnancy as a cause of symptoms
Dilation and curettage/hysteroscopy: To detect submucous leiomyomas
Hysterosalpingogram: To evaluate the endometrial cavity and fallopian tubes
Laparoscopy: To visualize subserous myomas
Ultrasonography: To distinguish adnexal inflammatory masses and endometriosis from pedunculated or subserous leiomyomas
Magnetic resonance imaging (MRI): Useful in differentiating subserasal fibroids from ovarian masses
Laboratory studies: Leukocytosis with degenerating tumor

MULTIDISCIPLINARY PLAN

Surgery

Hysteroscopic or laparoscopic myomectomy to preserve uterus for potential future childbearing in young women[36]

Total hysterectomy

Medications

Gn-RH agonists

Leuprolide acetate (Lupron), 3.75-7.5 mg IM once per month (to reduce size of myoma before surgery, which decreases operative blood loss and postoperative morbidity; or during short transition period before menopause in an effort to avoid surgery)[11]

General Management

Pelvic examinations at regular intervals to monitor status of leiomyoma

NURSING CARE

NURSING ASSESSMENT

Pain: Dull ache, soreness, or colicky pain; acute pain if torsion or twisting of pedunculated leiomyoma has occurred; bilateral pelvic discomfort if large tumor causes pressure on adjacent viscera; cramping pain if uterus attempts to expel submucous tumor; dysmenorrhea from intramural tumors; pelvic heaviness; feeling of bearing down; backache; dyspareunia

Elimination: Constipation from pressure on rectum; urinary frequency and urgency if leiomyoma causes pressure on bladder; nocturia, incontinence

Abdomen: Firm, irregular nodules palpated in lower abdomen; irregular abdominal contour; swelling

Bleeding: Profuse bleeding with flooding or clots; menses excessive, long, or both

Temperature: Elevated with degenerating tumor

POTENTIAL COMPLICATIONS

Anemia caused by gradual blood loss over time

PATIENT PROBLEMS/NURSING DIAGNOSES & INTERVENTIONS

NIC PHYSICAL COMFORT PROMOTION

Pain related to pressure of tumor on adjacent structures

- Assist and teach patient to use pain-relieving methods, including relaxation techniques and analgesics as ordered.

NIC COPING ASSISTANCE

Disturbed body image related to biophysical change

- Assess meaning of condition for patient.
- Encourage patient to express her feelings.

PATIENT EDUCATION/CONTINUUM OF CARE PLAN

Explain to patient the importance of obtaining follow-up care and regular examinations to check for unusual growth or complications.

EVALUATION/PATIENT OUTCOMES

Physical Comfort Promotion: Comfort is achieved. Patient is able to perform work activities and activities of daily living. Pain is controlled. Menses is normal if myomectomy was performed.

Coping Assistance: Patient's body image is positive with verbalization of feelings demonstrating same.

POLYPS

Polyps are benign neoplasms or protruding growths in the cervix or endometrium.

Cervical polyps are soft, red, pedunculated lesions protruding from the cervical os. Endometrial polyps are small, mostly sessile masses that project into the endometrium and may be pedunculated.

Polyps are usually asymptomatic and are often an incidental discovery during visual examination of the cervix, curettage, or hysterectomy. Because endometrial polyps may occur in association with leiomyomas and endometrial hyperplasia, specific symptoms are difficult to identify. The symptoms of cervical polyps are similar to those of chronic cervicitis with irregular bleeding. Polyps are the most common lesions of the cervix and occur most often during the reproductive years. Endometrial polyps can also occur at any age but are more common around the time of menopause. Polyps associated with the use of oral contraceptives tend to regress after the drug is discontinued.

PATHOPHYSIOLOGY

Cervical polyps most commonly arise from the lower end of the endocervix and vary from a few millimeters to 2 cm in diameter. The base of the pedicle is usually small. Polyps may develop as a result of inflammatory hyperplasia of endocervical mucosa owing to hyperestrinism, chronic inflammation, or vascular congestion. Microscopic examination shows a surface covered by columnar epithelium with areas of metaplasia and ulceration. The stroma is often congested with blood and infiltrated by inflammatory cells. The polyps may bleed after trauma from coitus or douching.

Endometrial polyps develop as single or multiple soft tumors composed of endometrium. Most arise from the fundus or cornua, and some may protrude through the cervix. They are usually paler and firmer than cervical polyps. Most frequently the polyp is made up of endometrium similar to that of the basalis and therefore does not show secretory changes. Polyps protruding into the cervix may become necrotic or inflamed, particularly if they are long.

DIAGNOSTIC STUDIES AND FINDINGS

Endometrial polyps are usually an incidental finding with curettage or hysterectomy, but it is possible to diagnose an endometrial polyp from a hysterosalpingogram or endovaginal sonography. Cervical polyps are diagnosed by inspection of the cervix.

Multidisciplinary Plan

Surgery

Curettage to remove endometrial polyps
Hysteroscopic resectoscope to remove polyps
Removal and cauterization of base of cervical polyps; can be performed in outpatient setting
Cryosurgery for cervical polyps (see discussion of cervical conization on p. 1388)

Uterine Prolapse

Uterine prolapse (pelvic relaxation, pudendal hernia) is an abnormal protrusion of the uterus through the pelvic floor and vaginal outlet (Fig. 12-10).

Approximately half of all parous women have some degree of vaginal or uterine prolapse. One or two women in 10 have symptoms severe enough to warrant surgical intervention. Most cases of pelvic relaxation are associated with cystocele and rectocele. A cystocele is a herniation of the bladder base into the vagina. Uterine prolapse is often seen in multiparous women during the postmenopausal period. Etiologically most cases appear to be the result of vaginal and chronic increases in intraabdominal pressure.[4]

Pathophysiology

Some authorities believe that probably all cases of vaginal or uterine prolapse are associated with some degree of endopelvic fascial weakness, neurologic impairment, and changes in the uterine axis secondary to childbirth. The aforementioned incidence of varying degrees of uterine prolapse presents a strong argument for this belief.

A more generally accepted belief is that the most common cause of uterine prolapse is childbirth trauma. Examples of

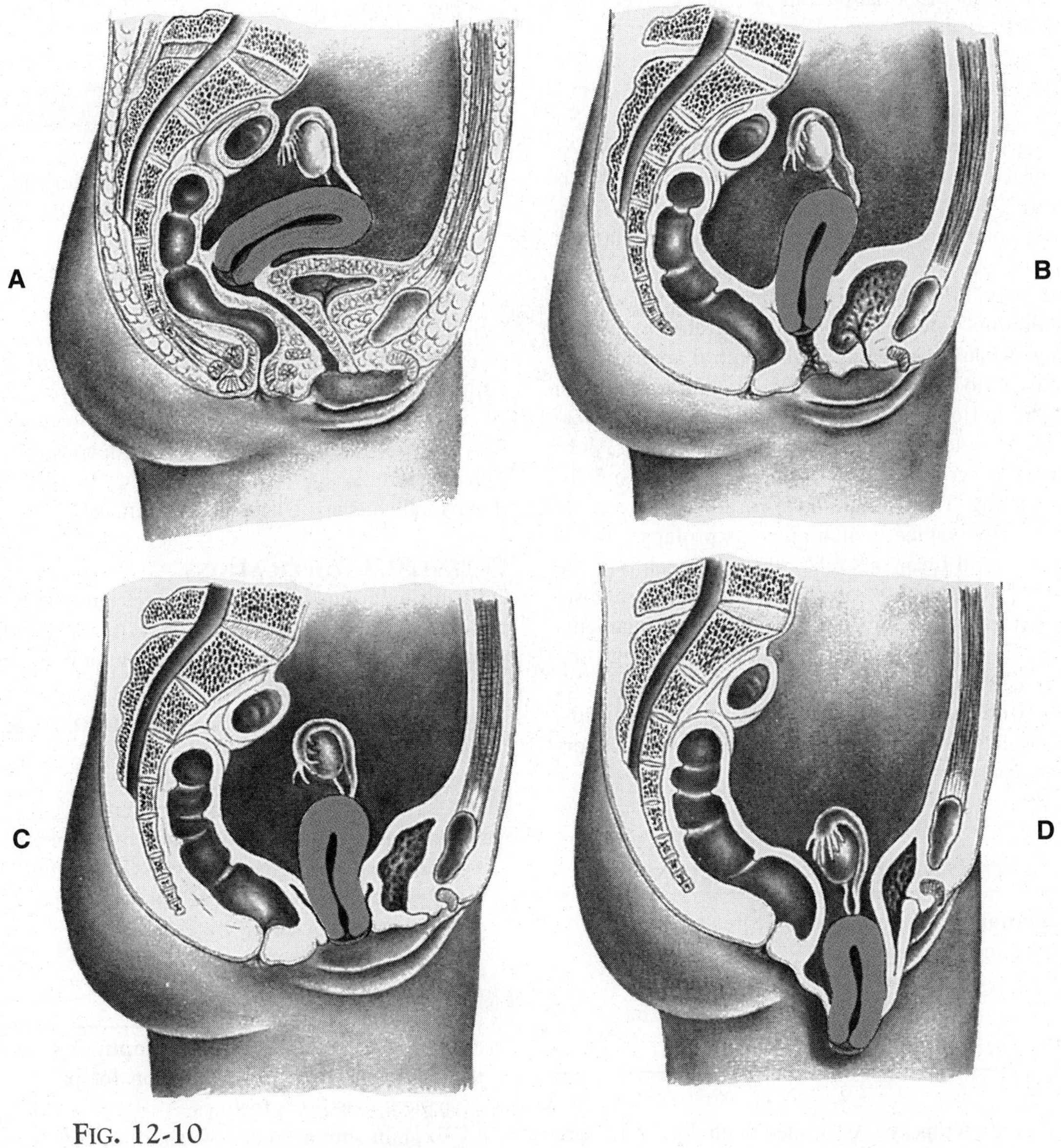

Fig. 12-10

Uterine prolapse. **A,** Normal uterus. **B,** First-degree prolapse of the uterus. **C,** Second-degree prolapse of the uterus. **D,** Complete prolapse of the uterus. (From Seidel et al.[32])

trauma are an episiotomy extension, laceration of the vagina or cervix, or improper episiotomy repair. Pelvic support tissues are damaged by the normal stretching, tearing, and pressure of a vaginal delivery. Other precipitating factors include these:

Pregnancy: Hormonal changes and the increased weight of the uterus during pregnancy contribute to softening or relaxation of uterine support structures.

Menopause: Decreased hormone levels after menopause contribute to atrophy of uterine support structures. If prolapse is present premenopausally, it will progressively worsen during this time.

Chronic pressure: Pelvic structures that are exposed to chronic abdominal pressure from asthma, chronic bronchitis, or obesity are weakened.

It appears that many factors contribute to progressive relaxation of uterine support structures, which eventually leads to varying degrees of uterine prolapse.

The amount of uterine descent into the vagina is measured in degrees:

A first-degree prolapse occurs when the cervix is between the ischial spines (normal placement is at the level of the ischial spines) and the vaginal opening.

A second-degree prolapse occurs when only the cervix, not the entire uterus, protrudes through the vaginal opening.

A third-degree prolapse occurs when the entire cervix and uterus extend beyond the vaginal opening. This is sometimes referred to as a procidentia. Some authorities use total procidentia as a fourth-degree classification.

Normally the pelvic floor supports the pelvic viscera and resists intraabdominal pressure from daily straining, lifting, and coughing. A narrow opening in the central anterior portion of the pelvic floor allows the urethra, vagina, and rectum to enter the pelvic floor, thus creating a weakened area. Certain members of the levator muscle group, puborectalis, pubococcygeal, and iliococcygeal, act as control mechanisms for this narrow opening. The uterus usually forms an acute angle with the axis of the vagina, which prevents prolapse. When the cardinal or sacral ligaments relax, the relationship of the uterus to the vagina is altered, which contributes to prolapse. When the levator muscles or cardinal and sacral ligaments weaken or are injured, the uterus can descend through the weakened area, which leads to uterine prolapse, cystocele, and rectocele. Both cystoceles and rectoceles can occur without uterine prolapse, depending on which pelvic support structures are weakened.

Diagnostic Studies and Findings

Pelvic examinations: To determine the degree of uterine prolapse, cystocele, and rectocele

Multidisciplinary Plan

Surgery

Retropubic cystourethropexy: Associated with long-term results in maintaining urinary continence

Transvaginal sacrospinous suspension of the vaginal vault for uterovaginal prolapse and vaginal vault prolapse

Vaginal hysterectomy: As indicated by symptoms associated with increased pelvic pressure

Anterior and posterior colporrhaphy: As indicated by symptoms

Colpocleisis (Le Fort's operation): Used for elderly, high-risk patients who are not sexually active

Medications

Hormones: Topical estrogen: Premarin vaginal cream inserted 2 times per week for 6 weeks; if effective, continued on a once-a-week basis; used to facilitate regeneration of support mechanism

General Management

Perineal exercise: Kegel exercises for relaxed vaginal outlet and minimum stress urinary incontinence

Pessaries: Devices worn in the vagina to support the uterus; once widely used, they are currently not the treatment of choice except for women who are poor surgical risks

Psychosocial services support

NURSING CARE

Nursing Assessment

Subjective data: A sense of heaviness or dragging in the low back or pelvis, a feeling of something falling out; bilateral groin pain, sacral backache

Vagina: Dyspareunia, excess vaginal mucus, spotting and bleeding in postmenopausal period

Cervix: Depending on degree of prolapse, may have constant irritation with tissue changes and cervical erosion

Urinary: Urinary frequency or urgency, urinary tract infection, stress urinary incontinence, nocturia; urine retention

Bowel: Hemorrhoids from straining with constipation

Constipation

Behavioral changes: Disturbed body image

Potential Complications

Difficulty with ambulation resulting from externally exposed portions of the uterus, bladder, or rectum. Possible excessive purulent discharge, decubitus ulceration, or bleeding.

Patient Problems/Nursing Diagnoses & Interventions

NIC Self-Care Facilitation

Deficient knowledge related to lack of information

- Teach patient perineal exercises *to improve pelvic tone.*
- If pessary is ordered, teach patient proper insertion and purpose of device.

NIC Coping Assistance

Disturbed body image related to biophysical change

- Assess meaning of dysfunction for patient. Encourage patient to express feelings.
- Explain importance of sharing concerns with sex partner

NIC PHYSICAL COMFORT PROMOTION

Pain related to pressure of protruding uterus

- Assess patient's degree of discomfort. Responses are varied and relate to gradual relaxation of pelvic floor over time. Often patients adjust to pressure changes.

PATIENT EDUCATION/CONTINUUM OF CARE PLAN

1. Explain Kegel's perineal exercises. Kegel exercises were designed to strengthen pubococcygeus muscle. (This is muscle that rims vagina.) To firm up pubococcygeus muscle, do this: When you urinate, try to stop in midstream. Then start again. Then stop again. When doing the exercise correctly, you will have sensation of "pulling up" into vagina with buttocks squeezed together. Pubococcygeus muscle, which controls starting and stopping, will be strengthened by this exercise. Muscles surrounding vagina and rectum should be squeezed off when doing this exercise, which will create a sensation of pulling everything up into vagina. Hold for 3 to 5 seconds, relax, and repeat 15 to 25 times in sequence each time the exercises are performed. These exercises should be performed at least four times daily. Once patient has learned to perform the exercises, she should perform them at times other than during urination.
2. Give written instructions to patient about need to change pessary every 2 to 3 months and to douche once or twice a week to prevent vaginitis from presence of pessary.
3. Explain importance of reporting any changes in vaginal secretions or elimination patterns to physician.

EVALUATION/PATIENT OUTCOMES

Self-Care Facilitation: Patient verbalizes proper technique for Kegal exercises and periodic accomplishment of same. Patient demonstrates proper use of pessary.

Coping Assistance: Patient demonstrates progress toward acceptance of altered body image and self-concept. Patient shows adaptive response to changes in self-concept and acceptance of treatment regimen.

Physical Comfort Promotion: Comfort is achieved. Discomfort is relieved, abnormal vaginal discharge is controlled, and skin integrity is maintained.

OVARIAN CYSTS

A cyst is a sac containing fluid or semisolid material. Ovarian cysts may develop at any time but are most common from puberty to menopause.

The ovary is a frequent location of a pelvic mass (FIG. 12-11). There are a variety of ovarian cysts, most being small and considered clinically unimportant. Only a few cysts require surgical removal. Most cyst enlargements disappear within a few months. However, malignancy must be considered when evaluating all pelvic masses.

Ovarian cysts are classified as follows.

Functional cysts: These are follicle and corpus luteum cysts that are normal transient physiologic structures.

Follicular cysts: These are common and appear on the ovary surface. They are usually asymptomatic and disappear spontaneously within 60 days.

Lutein cysts

Granulosa lutein cysts: These cysts are found within the corpora lutea. They are nonneoplastic enlargements of the ovary caused by an unexplained increase in fluid secretion by the corpus luteum after ovulation or during early pregnancy. They are 4 to 6 cm in diameter, raised, brown, and filled with tawny serous fluid. They may cause local pain and tenderness with either amenorrhea or delayed menses. Most cysts disappear within 2 months in nonpregnant women and gradually decrease in size during the third trimester of a pregnancy. A small percentage of cysts may rupture, requiring surgery.

Theca-lutein cysts: These cysts can vary in size from minute to several centimeters in diameter and are filled with straw-colored fluid. They appear in association with hydatidiform mole, choriocarcinoma, and gonadotropin therapy. Few abdominal symptoms are present, but the patient may feel a sense of pelvic aching or weight. Pregnancy signs and symptoms continue, especially hyperemesis and breast tenderness. A small percentage of cysts may rupture, requiring surgery, but most disappear spontaneously after removal of the causative factor.

Inflammatory cysts: Cysts of the fallopian tube and ovaries can form after an acute infection, such as gonorrhea. Pain is

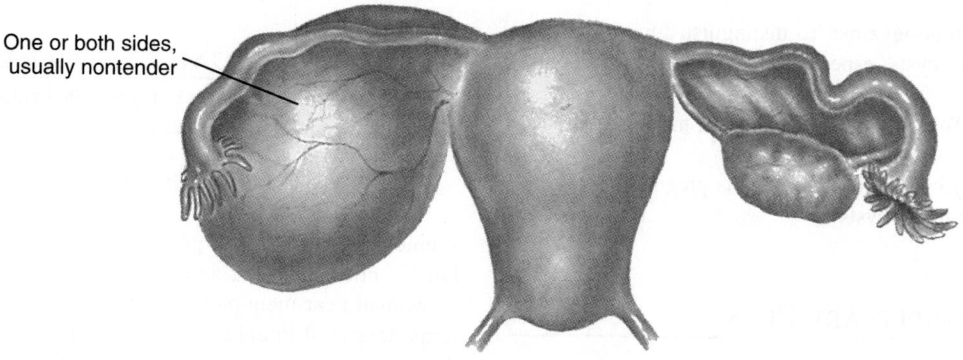

FIG. 12-11
Ovarian cyst. (From Seidel et al.[32])

persistent and severe in the pelvis and accompanied by hypermenorrhea. The white blood cell count is elevated, and a pregnancy test will be negative. Surgery is generally not required unless an ectopic pregnancy or acute appendicitis is suspected.

Endometrial cysts: Patients with endometriosis may have an endometrium implant on the ovary that will bleed with hormonal stimulation, thus forming a cyst through alternate oozing and healing. These cysts vary in size from microscopic to 10 to 12 cm in diameter. The cysts are filled with thick, chocolate-colored old blood. Large endometrial cysts should be surgically removed, leaving as much functioning ovary as possible. Endometrial cysts are sometimes referred to as chocolate cysts, although not all chocolate cysts are endometrial in origin.

Inclusion cysts: These cysts are most often microscopic in size and located just beneath the surface of the ovary. The cysts are filled with a minute amount of serous fluid and cause no discomfort. They occur after menopause or after an inflammatory state. No treatment is required.

Parovarian cysts: These cysts are located between the fallopian tube and ovary and are rarely larger than 4 cm in diameter. Found only in postpubertal females, these cysts are generally asymptomatic unless they grow in size to become palpable.

Dermoid cysts: These cysts are ovarian cysts composed primarily of skin and dermal appendages.

Follicular cysts: A follicular cyst is an ovarian follicle that fails to rupture.

Simple cysts: These cysts are fluid-filled sacs without solid or complex components.

The most important consideration in evaluating an ovarian cyst is the patient's age. Perimenopausal and postmenopausal women with palpable ovarian cysts stand a greater chance of having malignancy that is characterized by solid ovarian masses.

DIAGNOSTIC STUDIES AND FINDINGS

Pelvic and rectal examination: To determine location and size of ovarian cyst

Ultrasonography: To distinguish functional cysts from neoplastic cysts and to confirm findings of the pelvic examination

Laparoscopy: Used when the diagnosis of endometriosis is uncertain

Abdominal roentgenograms: To distinguish functional cysts from neoplastic cysts, especially when calcified structures are present

Barium enema: To determine if an adnexal mass is caused by a colonic disease; not done routinely

Pregnancy test: To determine if patient is pregnant, especially with suspected lutein cysts

MULTIDISCIPLINARY PLAN

Surgery

Laparoscopic cystectomy of ovarian dermoid cysts

Laparotomy to remove cysts, especially if they rupture, torse, and bleed, so as to control hemorrhage

Aspiration and tetracycline sclerotherapy for management of simple ovarian cysts[1]

General Management

Pelvic examinations at regular intervals to monitor reduction of cyst size; suppression of activity of functional cysts

NURSING CARE

NURSING ASSESSMENT

Pain: Dull ache, severe pain, local pain and tenderness depending on the type of cyst; severe pain if cyst ruptures

Abdomen: Some cysts are palpable, bilaterally or unilaterally, in the lower abdomen

Bleeding: Menses can be excessive when inflammatory cyst is present

POTENTIAL COMPLICATIONS

Differentiation between benign cyst and malignancy must be established.

PATIENT PROBLEMS/NURSING DIAGNOSES & INTERVENTIONS

NIC PHYSICAL COMFORT PROMOTION

Acute pain related to pressure of cyst on adjacent areas

- Assist with and teach patient to use pain-relieving methods, including relaxation techniques and analgesics as ordered.

PATIENT EDUCATION/CONTINUUM OF CARE PLAN

1. Provide information regarding type of cyst and expectations relative to menstrual cycle.
2. Explain the importance of obtaining follow-up care and regular examinations to check for any changes in size of cyst.

EVALUATION/PATIENT OUTCOMES

Physical Comfort Promotion: Comfort is achieved. There is no pain, and cyst had been reduced in size or was removed.

HORMONAL DISORDERS

PREMENSTRUAL SYNDROME

Premenstrual syndrome (PMS) may be defined as the cyclic recurrence, during the luteal phase of the menstrual cycle, of a combination of physical, psychologic, and behavioral changes sufficient to interfere with normal activities.[7]

Premenstrual syndrome generally occurs in women in their late twenties and older and increases in incidence and severity as women near menopause. The various behaviors and symptoms described in epidemiologic studies can be placed in the three major categories of edema, emotionality, and headache. The symptoms generally appear 7 to 10 days before menses and sharply decrease with the onset of menses. The cause of PMS remains obscure. The highest incidence occurs in the late twenties to early thirties. PMS is rarely encountered in adolescents.

Pathophysiology

The exact cause of premenstrual tension is unknown. Progesterone stimulates the production of aldosterone, which increases sodium retention and edema formation. Interestingly, no distinct differences in aldosterone levels have been shown between women with and those without premenstrual syndrome. The decrease in brain levels of monoamine oxidase that occurs as estrogen production falls before menses probably accounts for the feeling of depression. Fluctuation of monoamine oxidase and catecholamine levels in the brain may result in the frequently observed symptom of irritability. Studies have shown that carbohydrate metabolism and the adrenal production of corticosteroids change before menses. Serotonin levels are significantly lower during the last 10 days of the menstrual cycle in women with PMS. Decreased serotonin is known to be associated with depression in humans. The treatment of PMS must be individualized for each woman, and practices vary. For example, there is concern that even low doses of vitamin B_6 may result in potentially toxic effects. Premenstrual tension may be caused by a variety of factors.[5]

Diagnostic Studies and Findings

There are no specific tests for diagnosis of premenstrual syndrome. A personal log maintained by the woman can be helpful in diagnosis and efficacy of treatment.[5]

Multidisciplinary Plan

Medications

Hydrochlorothiazide, 50-100 mg/day PO, or spironolactone, 25-100 mg/day PO, during 7-10 days before cycle or 24-36 h before onset of expected symptoms
Mefenamic acid, 550 mg PO tid or qid from symptoms to menses
Naproxen sodium, 550 mg PO q12h during premenstrual period
Medroxyprogesterone (Provera), 10-20 mg/day PO during last half of cycle
Alprazolam (Xanax), 0.35 mg PO tid from cycle day 20 until second day of menstruation
Danazol, 200 mg PO qd from onset of symptoms, tapered dose until onset of menses
Gn-RH agonists
Nafarelin acetate (Synarel) nasal spray, 1 spray in one nostril bid
Leuprolide acetate (Lupron), 3.75-7.5 mg IM once per month
Antidepressants (serotonin uptake inhibitors), e.g., doxepin HCl, Elavil
Vitamins
  Vitamin B, 50 mg to 500 mg/day
  Vitamin E, 600 U/day

General Management

Limitation of intake of salt, refined sugars, caffeine, and animal fats; emotional and psychologic support; pain management; reflexology techniques of ear, hand, and foot to reduce somatic symptoms; exercise

NURSING CARE

Nursing Assessment

Hydration: Edema; weight gain; backache, breast tenderness, oliguria, palpitations; mastalgia
Gastrointestinal: Abdominal bloating; diarrhea or constipation; nausea; vomiting; food craving; compulsive eating
Affect and behavior: Irritability; anxiety; lability; fatigue; depression; crying; lethargy; agitation; insomnia; hypersomnia; difficulty in concentrating; decreased interest in usual activities; mood swings; confusion; forgetfulness; tension; increased libido
Neurologic: Headache; vertigo, fainting; migraine; paresthesias of head and feet
Respiratory: Increase in colds, asthma, or allergic rhinitis
Urinary: Cystitis; enuresis; urethritis
Ophthalmologic: Conjunctivitis; styes
Breasts: Tenderness; enlargement
Integument: Recurrence of herpes; acne; urticaria; boils; easy bruising

Patient Problems/Nursing Diagnoses & Interventions

NIC Coping Assistance

Anxiety related to cyclical change in health status
Ineffective coping related to inability to conserve adaptive energies

- Reassure patient that her symptoms are temporary.
- Assist patient in exploring her feelings about self-image, fears, and behaviors; clarify and correct any misconceptions.
- Help patient evaluate personal strengths and needs that affect health maintenance ability.
- Encourage participation in group therapy or sharing of feelings with family or significant other.
- Encourage patient to express her feelings and discuss or identify coping strategies *to manage mood swings.*
- Suggest that patient may wish to maintain a personal journal or diary to describe feelings, strengths, and needs on a daily basis. This should be reviewed on a regular basis *to identify any patterns or opportunities for changes in behavior or treatment regimen.*

Patient Education/Continuum of Care Plan

1. Involve patient in plan for care and information related to basis for plan.
2. Explain that fatigue exaggerates symptoms and that adequate rest and sleep are needed during premenstrual period.
3. Engage in some form of moderate exercise, such as brisk walking three to four times a week.
4. Encourage patient to avoid stressful activity during premenstrual period.
5. Give printed instructions to patient to avoid glucose fluctuation by taking small, frequent feedings of a high-protein,

complex carbohydrate diet and by decreasing sugar intake to less than 5 tablespoons daily.

6. Discuss with patient the need to reduce salt intake and to avoid foods with "hidden salts" such as soy sauce, salted crackers and bread, luncheon meats, dried meats, hot dogs, tomato juice, and cheeses. Discuss with patient the need to avoid dairy products and animal fats; the need to restrict caffeine by decreasing intake of coffee, tea, cola, and chocolate; and the need to restrict alcohol.
7. Discuss with patient the need to increase intake of leafy green vegetables, whole grain cereals, and complex carbohydrates.
8. Instruct patient to take medications as prescribed and explain reasons for taking specific medications. (For example, vitamin B_6 is taken to increase blood progesterone and promote diuresis, and vitamin E is taken to reduce breast tenderness.)
9. Suggest and offer printed educational materials.

Evaluation/Patient Outcomes

Coping Assistance: Comfort is achieved; there is little or no anxiety. Patient describes feeling of well-being and absence of bloating, weight gain, edema, mastalgia, irritability, anxiety, and other symptoms of PMS.

Patient uses strengths to cope and comply with plan of care. Patient recognizes personal strengths and needs that are directed toward elimination or reduction of symptoms.

Patient establishes appropriate coping with mood swings. Patient verbalizes about mood and advises others of her particular sensitivities. Patient develops a support system with significant others. Patient demonstrates increased interest in social and occupational activities.

Menopause and Climacteric

Menopause is the physiologic cessation of menses. The climacteric is the transitional period during which reproductive function diminishes and eventually ceases.

As the average life span has increased in the United States, so has the number of postmenopausal women. Of the 120 million women in the United States, 40 million are over 50 years of age. Postmenopausal women constitute one eighth to one sixth of the population. The average life span of women is 81 years, whereas that of men is only 72 years. As the ratio of men to women decreases with age, many women in the climacteric phase of life must cope with societal, as well as physical, changes.

The normal decrease in ovarian function begins during the fourth decade, and the majority of women cease to menstruate between the ages of 48 and 55. The average age at which menses disappears is 50 years, although some women cease to menstruate as early as 40 years and others continue until 55 years or older.

Induced or premature menopause is the cessation of ovarian function as a result of radiation, surgery, immunologic disease, or bacteriologic or viral agents. Although the signs and symptoms of natural and premature or artificial menopause are similar, the management may vary based on the patient's age.[19,20]

Physiology

A notable event of the climacteric phase of life is menopause, the complete cessation of menses. Before the actual menopause there are usually gradual changes, such as a decrease in the amount of menses, lengthening of the interval between menses, periodic amenorrhea, and finally slight spotting. These events are due to a progressive decline in the ovarian secretion of estrogen. When too little estrogen is secreted to cause endometrial growth, bleeding stops permanently. Irregular menses followed by amenorrhea for more than 1 year is indicative of menopause.

With menopause the estrogen fractions change and estrone becomes more available than estradiol. Peripheral conversion of androstenedione, a product of the adrenal glands, to estrone occurs principally in the fat. Some women produce enough estrone to cause endometrial growth and shedding or bleeding. Because obesity is a common factor in women with endometrial cancer, it has been hypothesized that production of estrone in the adipose tissue may contribute to the genesis of a tumor.

Changes in reproductive structures are related directly to decreased estrogen. Labial fat is reabsorbed; the labia majora become flattened, and the labia minora may disappear. The vaginal epithelium becomes thinner, the vagina smaller, and the fornices shallower. The myometrium thins, causing the uterus to decrease in size until it resembles that of a prepubertal girl.

Hot flushes, the most characteristic symptom of menopause, result in a slight increase in core body temperature and a higher increase in skin temperature. The sensation of heat is often accompanied by tachycardia, vertigo, palpitation, and a feeling of faintness.

The atrophic changes that result from estrogen deprivation may lead to dyspareunia owning to decreased precoital lubrication or constriction of the introitus or vagina.

Nervousness and other psychologic symptoms are not a direct result of estrogen deficiency. The patient's personality and response to aging are the keys to promoting adaptation to the climacteric.

Anthropometric studies, including weight, body mass index (BMI), waist-to-hip girth ratio, and body composition (particularly percentage of body fat and water), show a significant increase in body weight and fat mass in early postmenopausal women (44 to 54 years of age). A shift from gynecoid to android fat distribution is more likely to be observed in women who do not take hormone replacement therapy.[28]

Diagnostic Studies and Findings

Papanicolaou smear: Decrease in estrogen effect noted in vaginal mucosa

Blood chemistry: Estradiol less than 5 ng/dl; follicle-stimulating hormone greater than 40 mlU/ml

Multidisciplinary Plan

The use of hormonal therapy in the treatment of menopause is associated with a diminution of subjective complaints; a decrease in age-specific mortality for all categories of cause of death, including cardiovascular disease; and a decrease in osteoporosis.[9]

The decision to use hormone replacement therapy (HRT) should be made by the patient with full disclosure of the risks, side effects, and benefits by the physician. Cyclical bleeding, a common side effect associated with HRT, is unacceptable to most women who have looked forward to its absence, and this factor often contributes to the discontinuation of HRT in the long term. Although there is a correlation between estrogen and breast cancer, which is not ameliorated by the inclusion of oral progesterone agents, clinical studies do not demonstrate that the use of HRT is a significant risk factor for breast cancer.[20] Most practitioners believe that the overall benefits (relief of menopausal symptoms, and some protection from osteoporosis) outweigh any risks of HRT.[35]

Medications

Estrogens

Conjugated estrogen (Premarin), 0.3-2.5 mg/day PO, or ethinyl estradiol (Estinyl, others), 0.05-0.2 mg/day PO; initial doses should be lowest amount that will control symptoms; drug is taken for first 25 days of month or daily; withdrawal should be gradual over several months to prevent recurrence of hot flushes

Indications: Treatment of hot flushes and senile atrophic vaginitis; prevention of osteoporosis

Contraindications: Presence or history of breast or genital cancer (except cervical cancer in some cases); history of thromboembolism; fluid retention due to cardiac, renal, or hepatic disease, abnormal liver function

Cautions: Administration is closely monitored in women with uterine fibroids, endometriosis, hypertension, familial hyperlipidemia, gallbladder disease, or type 1 diabetes; annual endometrial biopsy needed for patient receiving long-term estrogen therapy

Transdermal estradiol (Estraderm), 0.05 mg transdermal patch changed twice weekly

Estrogen creams applied to vagina are more effective than oral estrogen in treatment of atrophic vaginitis

Progestins or progestogens

Medroxyprogesterone acetate (Provera), 2.5-10 mg/day PO for the first 25 days of the month or in last 10 days of estrogen cycle or daily

Indications: To prevent endometrial cancer, which may develop with unopposed estrogen stimulation

Cautions: May stimulate withdrawal bleeding; patients receiving long-term estrogen-only replacement therapy or those receiving progestogens on a quarterly basis should have annual endometrial biopsies

Bisphosphonates (as indicated for osteoporosis)

Fosamax, 10 mg PO qd, 30 min ac in morning

General Management

Psychosocial-educational support groups/classes

NURSING CARE

NURSING ASSESSMENT

Subjective data: Hot flushes; night sweats; diaphoresis; insomnia; headache; vertigo; syncope; numbness, tingling, or pain in joints; chilly sensation; lack of appetite or weight gain; constipation or diarrhea; nausea or vomiting; flatulence; fatigability; irritability; dyspareunia (resulting from vaginal atrophy); vaginal dryness, burning, and itching

Vulva: Decreasing labial fat; atrophy of muscle

Vagina: Decreased size with shallow fornices; dry appearance

Abdomen: Abdominal fat deposition

Cardiovascular: Tachycardia; palpitations

Breasts: Reduction in size

Body hair: Loss of pubic and axillary hair; increase in facial and lip hair

Behavioral changes: Anxiety; decreased tolerance level; body image change

POTENTIAL COMPLICATIONS

Without hormone replacement therapy, potential for increased risk of skeletal fractures with osteoporesis and coronary heart disease

PATIENT PROBLEMS/NURSING DIAGNOSES & INTERVENTIONS

NIC PATIENT EDUCATION

Deficient knowledge related to lack of information about self-care management

- Explain physiologic process of climacteric and menopause.
- Explain importance of keeping fit and eating well-balanced diet, getting adequate rest and sleep, avoiding stress and fatigue, and continuing contraception until health care provider indicates it is safe to stop.
- Inform patient about side effects of estrogen replacement therapy, need to report any vaginal bleeding occurring 6 months or more after last menstrual period, and availability of water-soluble lubricants if needed before coitus.

NIC COPING ASSISTANCE

Disturbed body image related to body change

Ineffective sexuality patterns related to knowledge deficit about alternative response to health-related topics

- Encourage patient to express concerns about femininity, sexuality, and aging.
- Reinforce correct information and provide factual information *to correct any misconceptions.*
- Encourage patient to express her concerns regarding sexuality.
- Encourage patient to discuss concerns with partner or significant other.
- Provide information for patient to access group or individual counseling and education.

EVALUATION/PATIENT OUTCOMES

Patient Education: Patient has acquired knowledge about climacteric. Patient expresses understanding of physiology and desired health behaviors. Patient relates understanding of prescribed medications including dose, route of administration, frequency, and side effects.

Coping Assistance: Patient demonstrates progress toward acceptance of altered body image, self-concept, and sexuality. Patient shows adaptive responses to changes in self-concept and movement toward acceptance of both physiologic and psychologic processes associated with climacteric.

FERTILITY CONTROL

Fertility can be controlled by natural, mechanical, chemical, hormonal, and surgical means.

Contraception has been identified by the World Heath Organization as one of the most important issues facing the world today. The birthrate in the United States is approximately 14.5 per 100,000 per year, reflecting a zero population growth; it is a phenomenon that is not occurring in many other countries. Continued population growth at current rates could have a negative impact on natural resources, food supply, and political stability, especially in Third World countries. The number of people the earth can sustain is unknown.

Fertility rates are higher among the poor and less educated, and the problem of teenage pregnancy remains unsolved. The goal of every pregnancy occurring as a result of an informed decision and resulting in a wanted child is far from being achieved.

Many factors affect the selection of a fertility control method, including the person's perception of the risk of pregnancy, knowledge of fertility control methods, and willingness and ability to use them; social pressures; the attitude of health-care providers; desires of the partner; and the cost and effectiveness of various methods. The methods most widely used in the United States in order of popularity are oral contraceptives, condoms, IUDs, rhythm, foam, diaphragm, and coitus interruptus. The method of fertility control varies according to the duration of the relationship or marriage. Young couples often use oral contraceptives until their first child is born and between pregnancies until their family is complete, and then select sterilization.

There has been an increase in those selecting sterilization in the last decade. Approximately equal numbers of men and women have undergone sterilization. Approximately 1 million Americans are sterilized annually.

Induced abortion, although not a contraceptive technique, is a method of preventing unwanted children. In January 1973 the U.S. Supreme Court declared all restrictive abortion laws by individual states unconstitutional. As a consequence, abortion in both the first and second trimesters is legal in all states, with the decision made by the woman. Since the Supreme Court decision, the numbers of illegal abortions and abortion-related deaths have fallen precipitously.

The health-care provider has a responsibility to provide information to women or couples choosing a method of contraception. The decision is a voluntary one based on explanation of the methods available, including their action, safety and effectiveness, expected effects, risks, and contraindications. The methods of fertility control can be divided into five major groups: natural or physiologic, mechanical, chemical, hormonal, and surgical.

Natural or Physiologic Methods

Rhythm. In the rhythm method, coitus is confined to phases in the menstrual cycle when conception is unlikely to occur. This can be determined by the calendar method, temperature method, or ovulation method. With the *calendar* method the fertile period is determined by recording the number of days of each menstrual cycle for a year, subtracting 18 days from the length of the shortest cycle to determine the beginning of the fertile period, and subtracting 11 days from the length of the longest cycle to determine the postovulatory safe period. The *temperature* method is based on abstinence from the end of the menses until 4 days after the rise in basal body temperature. The woman must take her temperature the first thing in the morning because the basal body temperature is the lowest temperature reached by the body during the waking hours. The *ovulation* method is based on the recognition of characteristic changes in cervical mucus. Initially after menstruation there is little mucus and the introitus is dry. The mucus becomes sticky

HEALTHY PEOPLE 2010

HEALTH STATUS—FAMILY PLANNING

FAMILY PLANNING

- Increase the proportion of pregnancies that are intended.
- Reduce the proportion of births occurring within 24 months of a previous birth.
- Increase the proportion of females at risk of unintended pregnancy (and their partners) who use contraception.
- Reduce the proportion of females experiencing pregnancy despite use of a reversible contraceptive method.
- (Developmental) Increase the proportion of health-care providers who provide emergency contraception.
- (Developmental) Increase male involvement in pregnancy prevention and family planning efforts.
- Reduce pregnancies among adolescent females.
- Increase the proportion of adolescents who have never engaged in sexual intercourse before age 15 years.
- Increase the proportion of adolescents who have never engaged in sexual intercourse.
- Increase the proportion of sexually active, unmarried adolescents ages 15 to 17 years who use contraception that both effectively prevents pregnancy and provides barrier protection against disease.
- Increase the proportion of young adults who have received formal instruction, before turning age 18 years, on reproductive health issues, including all of the following topics: birth-control methods, safer sex to prevent HIV, prevention of sexually transmitted diseases, and abstinence.
- Reduce the proportion of married couples whose ability to conceive or maintain a pregnancy is impaired.
- (Developmental) Increase the proportion of health insurance policies that cover contraceptive supplies and services.

Modified from U.S. Department of Health and Human Services: *Healthy people 2010* (conference edition, in two volumes), Washington, DC, January 2000.

NOTE: *Developmental* indicates that criteria for measurement and strategies to improve health have not as yet been specified.

and cloudy as estrogen stimulation increases, and as ovulation occurs, it becomes abundant, clear, and slippery and stretches without breaking: the spinnbarkeit phenomenon. Following ovulation and an increase in progesterone, the mucus becomes opaque and sticky again, with the woman experiencing a sensation of dryness. Coitus should be avoided from first recognition of the sticky mucus until after the watery discharge disappears.

Coitus Interruptus. Withdrawal of the penis from the vagina before ejaculation is probably the oldest and most frequently used fertility control method throughout the world. It is associated with a fairly high failure rate because live sperm may be present in the seminal fluid that leaks from the urethra during coitus.

Mechanical Methods

Condom. The condom or penile sheath must be applied over the erect penis, leaving space at the tip to contain the ejaculate. It must be removed before penile detumescence, with the rim held tightly to prevent leakage.

Diaphragm. The diaphragm is a latex dome-shaped cup that must be fitted to the patient to ensure that the cervix is covered. The woman must be instructed in its use and be able to demonstrate its application.

Cervical Cap. The cervical cap is smaller than the diaphragm and made of thick rubber or plastic. It may be applied some time before intercourse and left in place for at least 6 hours after intercourse. It is more difficult to apply than the diaphragm, and some women object to the odor when it is left in place for a long time.

Intrauterine Device. The IUD is a small plastic device connected to a string that protrudes into the vagina. IUDs are available in various sizes and shapes. A health-care provider inserts the device into the uterus, usually during menses when the cervix is partially open.

Chemical Methods

Spermicidal jellies, creams, suppositories, or aerosol foams are placed in the vagina immediately before intercourse and act as a chemical barrier to the sperm. They are often used in conjunction with another method such as a natural or a mechanical method. The spermicidal sponge inserted deep into the vagina at the cervical os blocks, absorbs, and kills sperms.

Hormonal Methods

The most popular form of hormonal contraception is the oral contraceptive ("the pill"). This is most commonly a combination of estrogen and progestin that inhibits ovulation and changes in the endometrium, cervical mucus, and probably tubal function. Oral contraceptives are extremely effective in preventing pregnancy but are known to affect every body system and may produce significant dangers with long-term use. Generally, the benefits and effectiveness outweigh the risk in healthy women below 30 years of age. See Table 12-2 for a summary of current agents.

Post-coital, or "morning after" contraceptive agents are commonly used in the United States. They are considered an emergency measure to be taken as soon as possible but no later than 72 hours after unprotected or condom-failure intercourse. These drugs should not be considered for routine use nor as a substitute for basic contraceptive methods. A kit called Preven is now available that includes a pregnancy test to ensure the absence of pregnancy before taking the pills.

Surgical Methods

Abortion. First-trimester abortion is done by dilation and curettage, aspiration of intrauterine contents through a suction device, or menstrual extraction. Second-trimester abortion is achieved by dilation and evacuation, intrauterine drug instillation, or hysterotomy.

Dilation and curettage is a painful procedure requiring general anesthesia; a sharp metal curette is inserted into the uterus to remove products of conception. When this surgical method of abortion fails because of uterine or cervical anomalies, methotrexate and misoprostol can be used to induce abortion in pregnancies up to 8 weeks of gestation. The methotrexate is administered by IM injection, and a misoprostol vaginal suppository is self-administered in 3 days.[24,30]

Vacuum aspiration can be done after a cervical block. The cervix is prepared by instillation of laminaria, an absorbent dried seaweed, into the cervix to expand the cervical canal. After the laminaria is removed, the aspiration curette is inserted and the products of conception are removed.

Menstrual extraction is the aspiration of endometrium and intrauterine contents through a polyethylene catheter that has been inserted into the uterus through the cervix. The procedure seldom requires cervical dilation and is performed not later than 8 weeks after the last menstrual period. Uterine injury and bleeding and continuation of pregnancy are the major risks associated with this procedure, which should not be considered a substitute for contraception.

The cervix must be more dilated for dilation and evacuation than for curettage. Dilation is usually effected with laminaria. The intrauterine contents are evacuated through a crushing instrument, followed by aspiration. The procedure is most frequently done in women who are 13 to 16 weeks pregnant.

Hypertonic saline solution is injected into the amniotic cavity to induce a second-trimester abortion. Complications are inadvertent infusion into the maternal bloodstream, producing salt intoxication; disseminated intravascular coagulation; and infection, especially if there is a long interval between instillation of the drug and uterine evacuation. Prostaglandin can be given by intramniotic or intravenous infusion or as a vaginal suppository. This method has virtually replaced use of hypertonic saline solution for abortion. Prostaglandins stimulate contractions of smooth uterine muscle and generally result in abortion within 24 hours. Side effects include nausea, vomiting, diarrhea, and abdominal cramping, which can be controlled with analgesics and antiemetics.

Hysterotomy is a surgical incision into the uterus for the removal of products of conception. It is associated with morbidity and is used only rarely for second trimester abortions.

Sterilization. Sterilization is the ultimate method of fertility control, rendering a person unable to reproduce. This is

Table 12-2 Summary of Methods of Conception Control

Method	Action	Safety-Effectiveness	Effects	Contraindications
ORAL CONTRACEPTIVE ("THE PILL")				
Combination pill: Each pill contains progestin and estrogen; schedule: one pill daily for 21 days, then discontinue for 7 days; placebo may be advised for last 7 days; pill cycle started and repeated on fifth day after onset of menstrual flow	Inhibits ovulation by suppression of pituitary gonadotropin Produces cervical mucus that is hostile to sperm Modifies tubal transport of ovum May have effect on endometrium to make implantation unlikely	Effective if taken accurately Failure results from failure to take pill regularly If woman forgets to take pill one day, she can "make up" by taking two pills next day Chances of pregnancy increased if pill is missed for even 1 day Highly acceptable to users; easy to take Linked with mortality caused by thromboembolus phenomena Does not alter fertility	Useful Relief of dysmenorrhea in 60% to 90% of cases Relief of premenstrual tension Regulation of menstrual cycles Relief of acne in 80% to 90% of cases Improved feeling of well-being Minor side effects (usually decrease after third cycle) Weight gain Breast tenderness Headaches Corneal edema Nausea Breakthrough bleeding Hypertension Major side effects Thromboembolus disorders Cerebrovascular accident (CVA), myocardial infarction (MI) May decrease lactation in breast-feeding women	Active thrombophlebitis Cerebrovascular or coronary artery disease Undiagnosed vaginal bleeding Breast or pelvic cancer Liver disease Use with caution if history of Epilepsy Multiple sclerosis Porphyria Otosclerosis Asthma Cardiovascular disease Renal disease Thyroid disease Diabetes Uterine fibroid tumors Smoker Age more than 35 years Deep vein thrombophlebitis
INTRAUTERINE CONTRACEPTIVE DEVICE (IUD OR IUCD)				
Small objects of various shapes made of plastic, nylon, or steel inserted into uterus; medicated with copper or a progestational agent Most have nylon string attached that protrudes from cervix into vagina; inserted using aseptic technique; follow-up visits in 1 month, then individualized Examples: ParaGard T 380A,	Unknown Copper may interfere with sperm transport Progestational agent causes progestin effects on cervical mucus and endometrial maturation	Easily inserted; highly effective: 97% to 99% Can be inserted anytime during cycle; presence of menstrual flow rules out early pregnancy Can be inserted immediately postpartum, but expulsion rate is higher Can be left in place indefinitely Effectiveness highly dependent on knowing IUD remains in place; women need to be taught to feel for string after each period Spontaneous expulsion occurs most often during menstruation (expulsion rates: 2% to 10%) Failure rate (pregnancy) 1.5% to 3% during first year of use; rate declines thereafter Does not alter fertility	Uterine cramping Heavy menstrual flow Irregular menses Vaginal discharge NOTE: Usually disappear in 2 to 3 months Problems Infection: Usually minor and occurs soon after insertion Perforation of uterus: Varies with types of device; highest rates in first 6 weeks postpartum; usually occurs at time of insertion	Current infection of reproductive tract Uterine fibroids Undiagnosed vaginal bleeding Nulligravida Multiple sexual partners History of salpingitis (PID) Known or suspected pregnancy Uterine abnormalities with distortion Immunosuppressive disorders Known or suspected uterine or cervical malignancy Genital actinomycosis Allergy to copper (copper-containing IUDs)

DIAPHRAGM (WITH SPERMICIDAL FOAM, CREAM, JELLY)				
Rubber dome attached to flexible metal ring; inserted into vagina to cover cervix; available in various sizes (requires careful fitting); self-inserted by user; surfaces and rim of diaphragm coated with spermicide before insertion; inserted no more than 2 h before intercourse and left in place at least 6 h after intercourse	Provides mechanical barrier to sperm Spermicidal preparation destroys large number of sperm	97% to 98% effective if fitted properly and used correctly Requires sustained motivation for repeated insertion and removal Refitting necessary after childbirth, surgery of cervix and vagina, or weight change of 10 pounds of more	None	Severe uterine prolapse History of reaction to product History of toxic shock
CERVICAL CAP				
A flexible natural rubber device available in various sizes (requires careful fitting); self-inserted by user; inserted before intercourse and left in place at least 6 h (but no more than 48 h) after intercourse	Provides mechanical barrier to sperm	82.6% to 93.6% effective if fitted properly and used correctly Requires 30-90 min education time to learn insertion procedure Requires sustained motivation for repeated insertion and removal	Potential for Papanicolaou test conversion from normal to abnormal at 3 months' follow-up (use of cervical cap is discontinued if this occurs) Cervicitis	Cervical dysplasia with abnormal Papanicolaou test History of toxic shock syndrome Concurrent vaginal or cervical infection History of reaction to product
CONDOM ("RUBBER," "SAFE," "PROPHYLACTIC")				
Thin, flexible plastic worn over penis; available without prescription; does not require medical supervision	Provides mechanical barrier to prevent sperm from entering vagina Prevents spread of venereal diseases	Effectiveness increased with use of diaphragm by woman Effectiveness decreased by tearing or slipping of condom during intercourse and by use of condoms without a reservoir end Failure rate 10% to 15%	None	None
NATURAL FAMILY PLANNING (OVULATION, SYMPTOTHERMAL, BILLINGS METHOD)				
Periodic abstinence from intercourse during fertile periods of menstrual cycle; days 12 to 16 before expected date of menstruation are possible ovulating days; because sperm can survive up to 48 h, days 11, 17, and 18 added to fertile period	Sexual abstinence around time of ovulation	Safe 65% to 85% effective Fertile period varies; precise time of ovulation not known Effectiveness increased with calculation of fertile period, high motivation to prevent pregnancy, determination of basal body temperature, and observation of mucous secretions' consistency	Frustration Lack of sexual gratification during period of abstinence	Irregular menstrual cycles Medical contraindications to pregnancy
CHEMICAL CONTRACEPTIVE (JELLIES, CREAMS, FOAMS, SUPPOSITORIES)				
Applied inside vagina by means of plunger-type applicator or aerosol spray	Contains spermicidal ingredients Partial barrier to entrance of sperm into cervix	Effectiveness increased when used with diaphragm or condom Easily available without prescription Effectiveness depends on dispersion of substance within vagina	None	History of reaction to product

Continued

Table 12-2 Summary of Methods of Conception Control—cont'd

Method	Action	Safety-Effectiveness	Effects	Contraindications
LEVONORGESTREL SUBDERMAL IMPLANT (NORPLANT)				
Six capsules of Silastic are implanted in the patient's arm; each capsule contains 36 mg of crystalline levonorgestrel	Inhibits ovulation by suppression of pituitary gonadotropin Produces thick cervical mucus that is hostile to sperm	Contraceptive failure rarely occurs Pregnancy rate 0.8/100 users over 5 years	Irregular bleeding, spotting, or amenorrhea may occur in the first year Headache	Hypertension History of thromboembolism, valvular heart disease; first 6 weeks postpartum; same as for oral contraceptives
INJECTABLE MEDROXYPROGESTERONE ACETATE (DEPO-PROVERA)				
Intramuscular injection of long-acting progestogen of 150 mg every 3 months	Inhibits ovulation	Efficacy similar to surgical sterilization	Amenorrhea may occur in women after 1 year of use Headache	Should be used by women only for long-term deferral of pregnancy; takes average of 22 weeks to ovulate after injection
EMERGENCY CONTRACEPTIVE PILL[6]				
Nordette, Levlen, Lo/Ovral, Triphasil, Tri-Levlen, and Ovral	Inhibits ovulation May affect endometrium to make implantation unlikely	Reduces risk of pregnancy by at least 75% if treatment initiated within 72 h of unprotected intercourse	Nausea Headache Breast tenderness	Reproductive cancers Cerebral hemorrhage
MEDICAL ABORTION				
Mifeprostone, 200 mg PO, is a synthetic steroid that must be followed 2 days later by misoprostol, 400 mg PO	Antiprogestational effects; contracts uterus	92% to 95% effective; remove IUD before use	Vaginal bleeding for 10 to 16 days	50 or more days since last menstrual period Presence of IUD Confirmed /expected ectopic pregnancy Chronic adrenal failure History of allergy to mifeprostone Hemorrhagic disorders
VAGINAL SPONGE				
Sponge is inserted adjacent to cervix and releases spermicide	Water activates sponge and facilitates insertion; spermicide is released for 24 h	At least 6 h should elapse after last intercourse before removal of sponge Sponge must be discarded after use and is not reusable	Irritation and allergic reactions in 2% to 3%; some increased risk of candidiasis; difficult removal reported in 6% of users	None
VAGINAL SHEATH (FEMALE CONDOM)				
Sheath is made of natural latex rubber with flexible rings at both ends; device is a combination of a diaphragm and condom; closed end of pouch is anchored around cervix, and open ring covers labia	Provides mechanical barrier to prevent sperm from entering vagina/cervix Spermicide jelly, foam, or cream should be added before intercourse	Effectiveness in excess of condom and diaphragm Failure rate of 15/100 (15%) May provide more protection than condoms against STDs	Relatively loose sheath provides heightened sensation for the man	None

EMERGENCY ALERT

SEXUAL ASSAULT

Sexual assault affects an estimated 80 per 100,000 women each year and is one of the four most violent and frequent crimes in the United States. Sexual assault can affect people of any age and of either sex.

Assessment and Interventions

- Recognize and acknowledge the victim.
- Place patient in quiet area or room; ideally do not leave victim alone; call sexual assault team or counselors if available in your community.
- Assess for life-threatening injury; record vital signs and obtain a *thorough* history, with details such as time, location, and use of weapons.
- Discuss forensic examination with patient and obtain consent. The forensic examination includes a battery of observations, specimen collecting, and historical information; the specific content varies from state to state, so be familiar with local requirements.
- Protect patient from pregnancy and STD by administering medications, as appropriate.
- Arrange follow-up care.

accomplished by vasectomy in men and tubal ligation or hysterectomy in women.

Vasectomy is a procedure for male sterilization involving the bilateral surgical removal of a portion of the vas deferens. It is most commonly performed on an outpatient basis with the patient under local anesthesia.

Tubal sterilization is the disruption of tubal patency to prevent the union of the ova and spermatozoa. It can be achieved through the vagina or by an abdominal approach through an incision or with laparoscopic visualization.

Laparoscope sterilization is often referred to as "Band-Aid" surgery because it can be performed in an ambulatory surgical center with general or occasionally local anesthesia. A pneumoperitoneum is produced with carbon dioxide, and the oviduct is ligated and most commonly electrocoagulated. In a vaginal tubal sterilization the peritoneal cavity is entered through the posterior vaginal fornix (culdotomy, colpotomy) and a ligation procedure or fimbriectomy is performed. The care of women undergoing tubal ligation is discussed on p. 855.

A summary of the common methods of conception control is provided in Table 12-2.

INFERTILITY

Infertility is the inability to conceive during a period of 1 year of unprotected intercourse. Primary infertility exists when there has been no prior conception. Secondary infertility follows at least one pregnancy.

Infertility affects 10% to 15% of couples in the United States. About 25% of women who do not use contraception and who have coitus regularly conceive within 4 months, more than 60% do so within 6 months, and about 80% within 1 year. The incidence of infertility shows a progression with advancing age of the woman. Fertility peaks between 20 and 25 years of age and decreases significantly after 40 years of age in women and 50 years of age in men.

It is estimated that male factors are responsible for about 30% of infertility problems. The cause of infertility is not identifiable in up to 15% of cases. Female factors are responsible for the remaining cases. Of these, around 20% to 30% are the result of disorders of the fallopian tubes, 10% to 15% lack of ovulation, and 50% cervical factors. It is believed that endometriosis is responsible for 30% to 40% of female infertility.

About 40% of those who seek medical attention for infertility eventually conceive. The identified cause of infertility cannot be corrected in 40% of the couples, and the cause of infertility in the remaining couples is never identified.

There are profound psychosocial effects of infertility on the couple. Nurses can play a crucial role in helping infertile couples cope by providing counseling and stimulating the adoption of strategies to manage the stress of infertility. Promotion of social support can also lead to a greater contentment over the course of time in infertile couples.[23]

PATHOPHYSIOLOGY

Normal fertility is dependent on many factors, including normal ovarian function, endocrine preparation of the uterus for implantation of the fertilized ovum, cervical mucus favorable for transport of sperm, normal anatomic structures, lack of obstruction to sperm and ovum, and normally functioning fallopian tubes. The male partner must have a sufficient number of motile and mature sperm that can be ejaculated without any anatomic or physiologic obstruction and that are capable of penetrating the egg.

The causes of infertility are as follows:

Female factors

Vaginal abnormalities: Rigid hymen or small hymenal orifice; psychogenic vaginismus; hyperacidity of vaginal secretions

Cervical abnormalities: Obstructive lesions such as polyps or congenital atresia; alterations in cervical mucus owing to bacteria or chemical agents; surgical destruction of endocervical glands

Uterine factors

Submucous myomas; structural malformations such as bicornuate or septate uterus; hypoplasia owing to endocrine disturbances; synechiae owing to endometritis; pelvic inflammatory disease

Uterine age greater than 40 years increases pregnancy losses in ovum donation patients after implantation is completed

Tubal and peritoneal abnormalities: Peritubal and periovarian adhesions following peritonitis; inflammatory damage owing to intrauterine devices, severe puerperal infections, and pelvic inflammatory disease; endometriosis

Ovarian abnormalities: Oligo-ovulation or anovulation owing to hypothalamic, pituitary, or ovarian deficits; hyperprolactinemia and galactorrhea associated with anovulation or luteal phase defects; faulty nutrition; metabolic dysfunction; luteal phase defects, which may be due to abnormal stimulation of the graafian follicle, hyperandrogen states, or increased prolactin levels; ovarian tumors (such as Stein-Leventhal syndrome)

Male factors

Sperm-related factors: Testicular hypoplasia; endocrine disorders such as hypopituitarism and hypothalamic disorders; cryptorchidism; varicocele; gonadal damage from trauma, surgery, or radiation; exposure of testicles to heat, including wearing of tight shorts; systemic infections, including mumps, tuberculosis, and syphilis; late descent of testicles; high viscosity of semen; autoimmunity as a result of trauma, vasectomy, or infection; low volume

Ductal obstructions: Resulting from epididymitis or infection of ejaculatory ducts; congenital absence of ducts

Transport-related factors: Hypospadias; ejaculatory problems; impotence

Factors affecting either male or female

Stress: Physical or psychic; long-term psychiatric problems

Nutritional deficiencies: Malnutrition such as anorexia nervosa and starvation; vitamin, mineral, or fat deficiencies

Substances: Exposure to toxins, including alcohol, nicotine, metals such as lead, dyes such as aniline dyes, drugs such as narcotics, quinine, hormonal agents, and antineoplastic drugs, radiation

Congenital anomalies: Chromosomal abnormalities (such as Turner's and Klinefelter's syndromes)

Disease processes: Dysfunctions or disturbances of thyroid, adrenal, or pituitary gland; diabetes mellitus; anemia; chronic nephritis; severe cardiac disturbances; infections; immune responses

Causes of infertility in the couple

Sexual problems: Unconsummated relationships; infrequent intercourse; sexual dysfunction; vaginismus; suboptimum technique

Other problems: Discordant relationships; immunologic reaction

Diagnostic Studies and Findings

Semen analysis (split ejaculate): Standards for fertility are volume of 2 to 6 ml semen per ejaculation; semen liquefication 30 or less minutes; semen pH 7.2 to 7.8; 20 to 300 million sperm per milliliter; 60% to 80% of sperm actively motile; 60% or more of sperm normally shaped

Vaginal examination: Cervical examination in midcycle; cervix not opened; lack of copious mucus; lack of spinnbarkeit and arborization

Transvaginal ultrasound: Produce images of pelvic organs

Tubal patency determination: Hysterosalpingography may indicate obstruction of tube if radiopaque dye fails to spill into peritoneum

Diagnostic endoscopy: Laparoscopy or culdoscopy: absence of direct observation of dye passing through fimbriated ends of fallopian tube; peritubal adhesions may be observed

Basal body temperature graph: Absence of normal biphasic pattern with sustained rise of at least 1° F during last 2 weeks of cycle

FSH and LH: Elevated with ovarian failure; suppressed with pituitary or hypothalamic disorder

Serum progesterone: Level less than 10 ng/ml indicative of abnormal luteal function; concentration of less than 3 ng/ml suggestive of anovulation

Endometrial biopsy: Findings inconsistent with cycle; premenstrual biopsy can confirm ovulation

Ultrasonography: Observation of ovarian follicle rupture

Postcoital test: Fewer than five highly motile sperm in mucus from upper cervix; inadequate spinnbarkeit and arborization suggestive of estrogen deficiency and secretory defect of cervical epithelium

Immunologic compatibility tests: Evaluation of sperm aglutination and immobilization

Other tests (female): Hysteroscopy; karyotype; T_4 level

Other tests (male): Testicular biopsy; vasography; sperm penetration assay; mucus migration test; venography; transrectal ultrasound

Multidisciplinary Plan

Surgery

Removal of myomas, polypectomy, dilation and curettage, unilateral or bilateral tuboplasty, salpingostomy, ovarian wedge resection (for patients with polycystic ovaries)

Medications

Antiinfective agents: Therapy based on culture findings

Ovulatory stimulants: Clomiphene citrate (Clomid), 50 mg qd on days 6-10 of cycle; may be repeated until conception occurs or three cycles of therapy have been completed; NOTE: Embryo reduction may be a topic of discussion[10]

Assisted Reproductive Technologies

Artificial insemination, in vitro fertilization (IVF), gamete intrafallopian transfer (GIFT), zygote intrafallopian transfer (ZIFT), embryo transfer (ET), intracytoplasmic sperm injection (ICSI)

General Management

Counseling and psychotherapy, improvement in coital technique

Comments

IVF: There is some maternal and neonatal morbidity associated with IVF. In vitro fertilization mothers have more multiple gestations, pregnancy-induced hypertension (PIH), premature labor, labor induction, and preterm deliveries than their matched counterparts in clinical studies. Infants conceived using IVF have lower birth weights, shorter gestations, longer hospitalizations, more days of oxygen therapy, more days of continuous positive airway pressure, and an increased prevalence of respiratory distress syndrome (RDS), patent ductus arteriosus, and sepsis.

GIFT: Hysteroscopic GIFT under local anesthesia (achieved by cannulating tubal ostia after hysteroscopic visualization) in patients with documented tubal patency at a previous diagnostic laparoscopy has demonstrated comparable results as laparoscopic GIFT under general anesthesia. This process can be achieved in a less costly outpatient setting and ensures advantages in terms of repeatability.

NURSING CARE

NURSING ASSESSMENT

Couple

Name; age; occupation; religion; ethnocultural influences; years of marriage; previous marriages; duration of involuntary infertility; habits; diet; health status; exposure to alcohol, nicotine, narcotics, quinine, hormones, antineoplastic agents, metals, dyes, and radiation; physical or psychic stress; use of herbs

Female

Health history: Tuberculosis; venereal disease; endometriosis; tumors; signs of endocrine dysfunction, such as delayed deep tendon reflexes, galactorrhea, visual disturbances

Gynecologic history: Menarche; frequency, duration, and amount of menstrual flow; menstrual irregularities; evidence of dysmenorrhea; mittelschmerz; increased midcycle discharge; pelvic inflammatory disease; previous surgical procedure, including pelvic operation and appendectomy

Obstetric history: Full-term deliveries; complications; abortions (reason, if elective) or premature deliveries

Conception control history: Type of contraceptives used and duration of use

Sexual history: Frequency of coitus; postcoital practices; libido; orgasm capacity; position during and after intercourse; use of lubricants; sexual involvement with other partners

Male

Health history: Tuberculosis; venereal infection; mumps; orchitis; varicocele; previous surgical procedure including orchiopexy and herniorrhaphy; hydrocele; injury to genitals

Sexual history: Frequency of coitus; technique and position; premature ejaculation; adequacy of erection; timing of coitus; sexual involvement with other partners

Male and Female Psychosocial Factors

Motivation for pregnancy; perception of and feelings related to inability to achieve conception; effect of sociocultural and familial factors related to desired pregnancy

NOTE: Because the couple-is-the-patient idea may serve to mask the very different responses, interests, and needs regarding infertility of the two people constituting the couple, it is important to dialogue with the individuals to identify important differences that may be present between the man and woman.[29]

POTENTIAL COMPLICATIONS

Failure to conceive or multiple gestation pregnancy

PATIENT PROBLEMS/NURSING DIAGNOSES & INTERVENTIONS

NIC PATIENT EDUCATION

Deficient knowledge related to lack of information about optimum sexual technique; sexual dysfunction related to altered body function

- Ensure that both partners are aware of practices that promote conception, including the following:
  - Intercourse every 2 days during fertile period
  - Woman in supine position with man astride
  - Woman's hips elevated on pillow with thighs flexed
  - Avoidance of commercial lubricants
  - Penis maintained in vagina without thrusting for short time after ejaculation
  - Woman remaining in bed with hips elevated for approximately 30 minutes after coitus
  - Woman not urinating or douching for at least 1 hour after coitus

NIC COPING ASSISTANCE

Anticipatory grieving related to potential for loss of reproductive function

Ineffective coping related to situational crises

Disturbed body image related to perceived or actual change in body structure or function

- Support couple's grief through listening and offering explanations about their reactions.
- Promote cohesiveness; avoid laying "blame" on one person.
- Help couple express their feelings when they find it difficult to do so.
- Help couple explore their feelings and eventually accept the normal ambivalence toward expectations of being a parent.
- Promote grief work with responses to grieving process of denial, isolation, depression, anger, guilt, fear, and rejection.
- Assess both partner's coping mechanisms.
- Explain consequences of prolonged stress.
- Help couple problem solve in constructive manner.
- Discuss alternatives to treatment.
- Encourage patient to express feelings about the way patient views himself or herself.
- Clarify misconceptions.
- Promote sharing of feelings with partner.
- Explore patient's personal strengths and resources.
- Promote discussion regarding resolution of altered body image.

EVALUATION/PATIENT OUTCOMES

Patient Education: Knowledge of sexual functions is increased. Patient indicates practice of optimum sexual technique. Patient relates valid information about sexual function.

Coping Assistance: Grief is resolved. Patient has expressed grief, shared concerns with partner, and planned constructively for future.

Patient uses adaptive coping behavior. Patient verbalizes feelings about infertility and altered body image and can identify personal strengths. Patient follows through with decisions and appropriate actions.

Realistic self-concept is achieved. Patient exhibits adaptive responses to altered body image through verbal statements.

BREAST DISEASE

CYSTIC BREAST CHANGES

Fibrocystic disease of the breast is the presence of singular or multiple cysts in the breast. NOTE: The College of American Pathologists formally abandoned the term *fibrocystic disease* as a histologic diagnosis in 1985.[9] Other descriptive names are used in association with cystic conditions, including benign mastopathy, chronic cystic mastitis, fibroadenosis, cystic mammary hyperplasia or dysplasia, cystic mastopathy, cyclic nodularity, blue dome cyst, Bloodgood's disease, and Schimmelbusch's disease.

Fibrocystic breast changes are the single most common condition of the breast, accounting for more than half of all surgical procedures on the female breast. It affects 10% to 25% of all women, but is not always clinically apparent and frequently is undiscovered until postmortem examination. Fibrocystic changes occur primarily in the menopause years and are a rare occurrence before adolescence and after menopause.

Controversy exists as to whether cystic changes in the breast constitute a disease process because the defining characteristics are estimated to be clinically present in 50% of women and histologically present in 90% of women.

PATHOPHYSIOLOGY

Cystic breast changes are thought to be caused by hormonal imbalance in the reproductive years, principally because of estrogen excess and progesterone deficiency during the luteal phase of the menstrual cycle. They are characterized by pain and tenderness of one or both breasts immediately before menses. The cysts may be unilateral or bilateral, firm, regular in shape, and mobile and are most common in the upper outer quadrant of the breasts. Their size may fluctuate during the cycle.

A wide variety of morphologic changes can be found, ranging from an overgrowth of fibrous stroma to a proliferation of epithelium. Four patterns of morphologic change are distinguishable: fibrosis, cyst formation, sclerosing adenosis, and duct epithelial hyperplasia.

Fibrosis is characterized by an overgrowth of stromal fibrous tissue. This type is usually unilateral and occurs most often in women from 30 to 35 years of age. The breast becomes larger before menses and then regresses with a recurrence of pain and tenderness in the next cycle.

Cystic disease is also known as Bloodgood's disease, Schimmelbusch's disease, and blue dome cyst. It is characterized by the formation of cysts, usually over 3 mm in diameter. It is thought to be caused by dilation of ducts and hyperplasia of ductal epithelium and concurrent with the menstrual cycle. This type of disease is more common in women between 45 and 55 years of age. Multiple bilateral cysts are readily palpable and usually distinguishable from the characteristic solitary focus of carcinoma.

The histologic characteristics of sclerosing adenosis are proliferation of small acini and intralobular fibrosis. It is most commonly unilateral and more common in women between 35 and 45 years of age.

Epithelial hyperplasia of the ducts are ill-defined masses found most commonly in women between 35 and 45 years of age. The more atypical the hyperplasia, the greater the risk of carcinoma. Biopsy and examination of the tissue is the only method of specifically differentiating fibrocystic disease from carcinoma. Women with fibrocystic changes have a greater risk of developing carcinoma than women without these changes.

DIAGNOSTIC STUDIES AND FINDINGS

Mammography
Ultrasonography
Stereotactic or ultrasound-guided percutaneous biopsy: Fibrosis: collagenous stroma engulfing epithelial structures and obliterating periductal and myxomatous stroma; cysts: overgrowth of stroma with cystic dilation of ducts filled with serous opaque fluid; fibroadenosis: proliferation and compression of small ducts and gland buds; epithelial hyperplasia: proliferation of epithelium lining duct, sometimes with solid masses of hyperplastic cells encroaching into lumen of duct
Needle aspiration of cyst: Varying histologic descriptions

MULTIDISCIPLINARY PLAN

Surgery

Subcutaneous mastectomy in lieu of multiple diagnostic biopsies and associated discomfort

Medication

Vitamin E, 400-800 IU PO may be useful

General Management

Local heat; support bra; avoidance of foods with methylxanthines, including tea, coffee, cola, and chocolate, which tend to stimulate cyclic adenosine monophosphate (cAMP) and increase metabolic activity in breast

NURSING CARE

NURSING ASSESSMENT

Breasts: Palpation of discrete or diffuse nodules; asymmetry; nipple discharge; irregular firmness; cyclic pain of cystic area during premenstrual period

POTENTIAL COMPLICATIONS

Misdiagnosis of benign changes that may actually be cancerous tumors

PATIENT PROBLEMS/NURSING DIAGNOSES & INTERVENTIONS

NIC COPING ASSISTANCE

Anxiety related to uncertainty of final diagnosis

- Explain rationale for tests and procedures *to allay anxiety.*
- Encourage verbalization of concerns.
- Answer patient's questions and explain disease process.

Patient Education/Continuum of Care Plan

1. Ensure that patient understands method for breast self-examination (BSE) and can demonstrate this procedure.
2. Explain that only 10% to 15% of masses are malignant and that 90% of cancers confined to breast are curable.
3. Outline a diet that avoids foods with methylxanthines.
4. Explain importance of maintaining appointments for clinical examination and mammography.

Evaluation/Patient Outcomes

Coping Assistance: Anxiety is diminished. Patient demonstrates adaptive responses to knowledge about prognosis related to fibrocystic disease.

Patient understands and monitors condition. Patient demonstrates BSE and lists progression of signs and symptoms to report to health-care provider, including increase in dimension of cyst, change in texture, lack of clearly defined margins, nipple discharge, severe pain, immobility of cysts, skin dimpling or retraction, and increasing asymmetry. Patient avoids foods with methylxanthines.

Collaborative Interventions and Related Nursing Care

Dilation and Curettage and Hysteroscopy

Description and Rationale

Dilation and curettage is the expansion of the cervix and scraping of the uterine endometrium. It is performed for diagnostic or therapeutic purposes, such as the removal of products of conception after an incomplete abortion.

Hysteroscopy is the visual inspection of the interior of the uterus through an endoscope. This procedure has not been found to be reliable in the diagnosis of tubal pathologic conditions.

NURSING CARE

Nursing Assessment

Bleeding: Vaginal hemorrhage
Pain: Pelvic and low back pain
Signs of infection: Foul odor of vaginal drainage; fever; hematuria

Potential Complications

Uterine perforation

Patient Problems/Nursing Diagnoses & Interventions

NIC Risk Management

Risk for infection related to invasive procedure

- Administer perineal care after elimination as necessary.
- Explain importance of wiping from front to back after elimination.
- If vaginal packing was used, ensure that it is removed by physician as indicated in medical plan of care.

NIC Physical Comfort Promotion

Pain related to uterine cramping

- Administer analgesics as ordered.

Patient Education/Continuum of Care Plan

1. Explain that spotting and bleeding may last a week and may be accompanied by cramping.
2. Explain signs and symptoms of infection that should be reported to physician.
3. Inform patient that coitus and douching should be avoided for 2 weeks.
4. Explain that minimal activity is preferred for a day or two.

Evaluation/Patient Outcomes

Risk Management: There are no signs of infection. Color and amount of urine are normal. Vaginal drainage decreases in amount and is not purulent.

Physical Comfort Promotion: Comfort is achieved. Patient says that she is comfortable and does not have uterine cramping.

Salpingectomy

Description and Rationale

Salpingectomy is the removal of one or both fallopian tubes. It is performed for ectopic or tubal pregnancy (see Emergency Alert box on p. 854), chronic salpingitis, and hydrosalpinx.

Nursing Care

The care of a patient undergoing salpingectomy is similar to that of a patient with a total hysterectomy, with a few exceptions:

Rh_o(D) immune globulin should be administered to an Rh-negative woman after a unilateral salpingectomy for tubal pregnancy.

The patient should understand the importance of preventing pregnancy for at least 2 months or as indicated by the physician and that reproductive ability is usually diminished, especially if a tubal pregnancy occurred as a result of acute or chronic salpingitis.

Her partner should be included in the discuss of feelings of loss and grief, especially if pregnancy was desired.

Hysterectomy and Bilateral Salpingo-Oophorectomy

Description and Rationale

Surgical removal of the uterus, both fallopian tubes, and the ovaries is most commonly done to treat malignant neoplastic disease of the reproductive tract and chronic endometriosis. Other indications for hysterectomy are an enlarged myoma, adenomyosis, and hydrosalpinx. If possible, a portion of one ovary is left to prevent symptoms of sudden menopause. The patient is under anesthesia during the procedure.

! EMERGENCY ALERT

ECTOPIC PREGNANCY

Ectopic pregnancy occurs when the fertilized ovum implants anywhere except the uterine cavity. The ovum commonly implants in the fallopian tube (95%), abdominal cavity, ovary, or cervix. Rupture usually occurs after the twelfth week of pregnancy.

Assessment

- Assess client's last menstrual period and knowledge of pregnancy; pregnancy status is often unknown.
- Perform HCG test for pregnancy.
- Assess pain and rate from mild to severe.
- Determine presence of Kehr's sign, right shoulder pain suggesting peritoneal irritation.
- Assess for abdominal rigidness, which may indicate intraperitoneal hemorrhage, shock.
- Evaluate vaginal bleeding: absent, spotty, or profuse.

Interventions

- Obtain IV access; provide fluid resuscitation as indicated.
- Monitor vital signs; hypotension is common.
- Draw samples for laboratory studies; prepare blood transfusion.
- Prepare for gynecologic consultation, surgery.

Contraindications and Cautions

Abdominal hysterectomy is preferred to vaginal hysterectomy or laparoscopic hysterectomy when the diagnosis is in question and exploration is needed, when the uterus is excessively large, when an incidental appendectomy is to be done, and when there is a history of severe pelvic inflammatory disease.

Preprocedural Nursing Care

A douche with an antiseptic solution is usually ordered the evening before or the morning of surgery, or both.

NURSING CARE

Nursing Assessment

Perineum: Vaginal hemorrhage; vaginal discharge other than serosanguineous; vaginal discharge with foul odor

Temperature: Fever

Abdomen: Diminished or absent bowel sounds; redness, pain, swelling, or drainage at site of incision of abdominal or laparoscopic procedure

Pelvic area: Congestion as evidenced by fullness, pain, or thrombophlebitis of legs

Urinary: Retention of urine, with or without overflow; burning, urgency, and frequency of urination; vaginal leakage of urine

Mental status: Emotional investment in value of uterus; signs of depression; misconceptions about procedure

Potential Complications

Paralytic ileus; pneumonia; ligation of ureter during surgery

Long-term effects associated with lack of hormone replacement (e.g., coronary artery disease, osteoporosis)

Patient Problems/Nursing Diagnoses & Interventions

NIC Tissue Perfusion Management

Ineffective renal, cerebral, cardiopulmonary, gastrointestinal, and peripheral tissue perfusion related to invasive procedure

Risk for deficient fluid volume related to NPO status

- Provide routine measures for postanesthesia recovery.
- Monitor blood pressure, temperature, pulse, and respiration every 4 hours for 24 hours, then four times a day for 2 days or as ordered.
- Avoid placing patient in high-Fowler's position and placing pressure under knees *to promote venous circulation in legs.*
- Apply antiembolic stockings as ordered *to provide intermittent compression and to prevent thrombus formation in legs.*
- Auscultate abdomen for bowel sounds every 6 to 8 hours. Permit nothing by mouth until bowel sounds are active *to prevent paralytic ileus.*
- Assist with initial ambulation as needed *to support if faintness occurs secondary to orthostatic hypotension.*
- Administer parenteral fluids as ordered, progressing to 3000 ml of fluid orally daily.
- Monitor intake and output *to ensure appropriate hydration and fluid balance.*

NIC Respiratory Management

Ineffective breathing pattern related to abdominal discomfort

- Assist with turning, coughing, and deep breathing every 2 hours or as needed, decreasing frequency as patient increases general activity *to prevent stasis of pulmonary secretions and risk of pneumonia.*
- Auscultate chest for breath sounds four times a day for 2 days and as needed thereafter *to ensure that breath sounds are clear.*

NIC Skin/Wound Management

Impaired skin integrity related to invasive surgical procedure

- Observe for drainage or hemorrhage every 2 to 4 hours, decreasing frequency as indicated.
- Change or reinforce dressing as indicated.

NIC Elimination Management

Constipation related to decreased peristalsis associated with anesthesia

Impaired urinary elimination related to neuromuscular impairment associated with anesthesia

- Progress to high-protein or high-fiber diet as ordered *to promote adequate nutritional status for wound healing.*
- Give Harris flush or insert rectal tube *for gas as indicated.*
- Give stool softeners or mild laxatives as ordered *to prevent constipation and straining at stool.*
- Maintain closed gravity drainage.

- Administer catheter care twice a day or as needed until removed.
- Promote micturition when catheter is removed *to avoid the need for recatheterization.*
- Monitor for signs of urine retention, such as small amounts of urine voided or a distended bladder.
- Encourage voiding on commode rather than bed pan *to promote complete emptying of bladder.*
- Administer catheter care twice a day or as needed until removed.

NIC COPING ASSISTANCE

Disturbed body image related to change in body structure and function

- Encourage patient's comments and questions about surgery, progress, and prognosis *to encourage understanding of same.*
- Reinforce correct information and provide factual information *to correct any misconceptions.*
- Encourage patient to talk about feelings with significant others.
- Acknowledge patient's feelings to support her in sharing this information with significant others.

NIC PHYSICAL COMFORT PROMOTION

Acute pain related to invasive surgical procedure

- Administer analgesics as ordered.
- Assist with bed bath, allowing patient to bathe or shower alone when indicated.
- Assist with moving and positioning *to promote comfort.*

PATIENT EDUCATION/CONTINUUM OF CARE PLAN

1. Explain to patient the importance of avoiding coitus or douching for 4 to 6 weeks or as indicated by physician to maintain integrity of vaginal cuff, to maintain healing process, and to prevent infection.
2. Explain to patient the importance of walking at regular intervals and to avoid sitting for prolonged periods at home or when traveling.
3. Explain abdominal incision care and signs of infection to report to physician, including redness, swelling, pain, or discharge at incision site; increase in vaginal drainage; or presence of foul odor.
4. Emphasize need to avoid heavy lifting and vigorous activities after surgery, as indicated by physician.
5. Instruct patient to maintain regular outpatient gynecologic examinations.
6. If both ovaries have been removed, explain that surgical menopause will occur and that replacement estrogen may be ordered.
7. Explain that menstruation will no longer occur and that pregnancy is no longer possible.
8. Explain importance of appropriate diet and exercise.

EVALUATION/PATIENT OUTCOMES

Tissue Perfusion and Respiratory Management: Body functioning is normal. Wound healing is normal. Vaginal drainage decreasing over 2 to 4 weeks. Bowel and bladder elimination are adequate. Ventilatory pattern has returned to presurgical state. Fluid balance is evident.

Patient resumes activities of daily living. Patient walks with erect posture. Patient avoids prolonged sitting and heavy work until physician permits them.

Skin/Wound Management: There is no infection; skin integrity is restored. There is no evidence of inflammation, swelling, pain, or discharge at abdominal site, no fever, and no purulent or odorous vaginal discharge.

Elimination Management: Urinary elimination is normal.

Coping Assistance: Patient demonstrates adaptive responses related to self-concept and body image. Patient asks appropriate questions. Patient gives correct information related to procedure and prognosis. Patient speaks appropriately about body parts that are present or absent.

Physical Comfort Promotion: Comfort is achieved. Patient says she has no lower abdominal, pelvic, or vaginal pain.

TUBAL LIGATION

Description and Rationale

Tubal ligation is tying of the fallopian tubes. Usually the procedure includes excision of a portion of the tubes to ensure that their continuity is disrupted. The procedure is done through the laparoscope with the patient under a general anesthetic. However, it can be performed through an abdominal incision, as is often done in the immediate postpartum period.

NURSING CARE

NURSING ASSESSMENT

Pain: Abdominal pain.
Signs of infection: Inflammation at site of incision; fever.

POTENTIAL COMPLICATIONS

Unlikely but possible failure of sterilization with resulting pregnancy

PATIENT PROBLEMS/NURSING DIAGNOSES & INTERVENTIONS

NIC PATIENT EDUCATION

Deficient knowledge related to lack of information about operative procedure

- Ensure that patient understands that intent of procedure is permanent sterilization.
- Reanastomosis is only up to 70% effective, complicated, and expensive.
- No hormone therapy is necessary because ovaries are not affected by procedure.

PATIENT EDUCATION/CONTINUUM OF CARE PLAN

1. Explain that sterility is considered permanent and is rarely reversible.

2. Explain that libido will not be diminished and is often increased by removal of fear of pregnancy.
3. Inform patient that ovarian function will continue because ovaries are not removed in this procedure.
4. Explain signs and symptoms of wound infection that should be reported to physician.

Evaluation/Patient Outcomes

Patient Education: Patient expresses understanding that procedure provides permanent sterilization.

References

1. AbdRabbo S, Atta A: Aspiration and tetracycline sclerotherapy for management of simple ovarian cysts, *Int J Gynaecol Obstet* 50(2):171, 1995.
2. American College of Obstetricians and Gynecologists: *Endometriosis,* Technical Bulletin 184, Washington, DC, 1993, The Association.
3. American College of Obstetricians and Gynecologists: *Uterine leiomyomata,* Technical Bulletin 192, Washington, DC, 1994, The College.
4. American College of Obstetricians and Gynecologists: *Pelvic organ prolapse,* Technical Bulletin 214, Washington, DC, 1995, The College.
5. American College of Obstetricians and Gynecologists: *Premenstrual syndrome,* Committee Opinion 155, Washington, DC, 1995, The College.
6. American College of Obstetricians and Gynecologists: *Emergency oral contraception,* Practice Pattern 3, Washington, DC, 1996, The College.
7. American College of Obstetricians and Gynecologists: *Guidelines for women's health care,* Washington, DC, 1996, The College.
8. American College of Obstetricians and Gynecologists: *Antibiotics and gynecologic infections,* Educational Bulletin 237, Washington, DC, 1997, The College.
9. American College of Obstetricians and Gynecologists: *Hormone replacement therapy,* Educational Bulletin 247, Washington, DC, 1998, The College.
10. American College of Obstetricians and Gynecologists: *Nonselective embryo reduction: ethical guidance for the obstetrician-gynecologist,* Committee Opinion 215, Washington, DC, 1999, The College.
11. Balasch J et al: Trial of routine gonadotropin releasing hormone agonist treatment before abdominal hysterectomy for leiomyoma, *Acta Obstet Gynecol Scand* 74(7):562, 1995.
12. Carter JE: Surgical treatment for chronic pelvic pain. *J Soc Laparoendosc Surg* 2(2):129, 1998.
13. Edge V, Miller M: *Women's health care,* St. Louis, 1994, Mosby.
14. Gilbert DN, Moellering RC, Sande MA: *The Sanford guide to antimicrobial therapy,* Hyde Park, Vt, 1999, Sanford.
15. Herbst AL: *Comprehensive gynecology,* ed 2, St. Louis, 1992, Mosby.
16. Hillis S, Marchbanks PA, Peterson HB: Uterine size and risk of complications among women undergoing abdominal hysterectomy for leiomyoma, *Obstet Gynecol* 87(4):539, 1996.
17. Hutchins FL: Uterine fibroids: diagnosis and indications for treatment, *Obstet Gynecol Clin North Am* 22(4):659, 1995.
18. Jennings JC: Abnormal uterine bleeding, *Med Clin North Am* 79(6):1357, 1995.
19. Kendig S, Sanford DG: *Midlife and menopause: celebrating women's health,* Washington, DC, 1998, Association of Women's Health, Obstetric and Neonatal Nurses.
20. Lando JR et al: Hormone replacement therapy and breast cancer risk in a nationally representative cohort, *Am J Prev Med* 17(3):176, 1999.
21. Lindsay SH: Menopause, naturally: exploring alternatives to traditional hormone replacement therapy, *AWHONN Lifelines* 3(5):32, 1999.
22. Lowdermilk D, Perry S, Bobak I: *Maternity nursing,* ed 5, St. Louis, 1999, Mosby.
23. Lukse MP, Vacc NA: Grief, depression, and coping in women undergoing infertility treatment, *Obstet Gynecol* 93(2):245, 1999.
24. Maiolatesi CR, Peddicord K: Methotrexate for nonsurgical treatment of ectopic pregnancy: nursing implications, *J Obstet Gynecol Neonatal Nurs* 25(3):205, 1996.
25. Munday PE: Clinical aspects of pelvic inflammatory disease, *Hum Reprod* 12(11 supplement):121, 1997.
26. Owings MF, Lawrence L: Detailed diagnoses and procedures, National Hospital Discharge Survey of 1997, *Vital Health Stat* 13(145), 1999.
27. Perper et al: Dysmenorrhea is related to the number of implants in endometriosis patients, *Fertil Steril* 63(3):500, 1995.
28. Reubinoff BE et al: Effects of hormone replacement therapy on weight, body composition, fat distribution and food intake in early postmenopausal women: a prospective study, *Fertil Steril* 64(5):963, 1995.
29. Sandelowski M: Culture, conceptive technology and nursing, *Int J Nurs Stud* 36(1):13, 1999.
30. Schaff EA et al: Methotrexate and misoprostol when surgical abortion fails, *Obstet Gynecol* 87(3):450, 1996.
31. Scholes D et al: Vaginal douching as a risk factor for cervical *Chlamydia trachomatis* infection, *Obstet Gynecol* 9(6):993, 1998.
32. Seidel HM et al: *Mosby's guide to physical examination,* ed 4, St. Louis, 1999, Mosby.
33. Stabinsky SA, Einstein M, Breen J: Modern treatment of menorrhagia attributable to dysfunctional uterine bleeding, *Obstet Gynecol Surv* 54(1):61, 1999.
34. Tucker SM et al: *Patient care standards,* St. Louis, 2000, Mosby.
35. Udoff L, Langenberg P, Adashi EY: Combined continuous hormone replacement therapy: a critical review, *Obstet Gynecol* 86(2):306, 1995.
36. Wortman M, Dagget A: Hysteroscopic myomectomy, *J Am Assoc Gynecol Laparosc* 3(1):39, 1995.

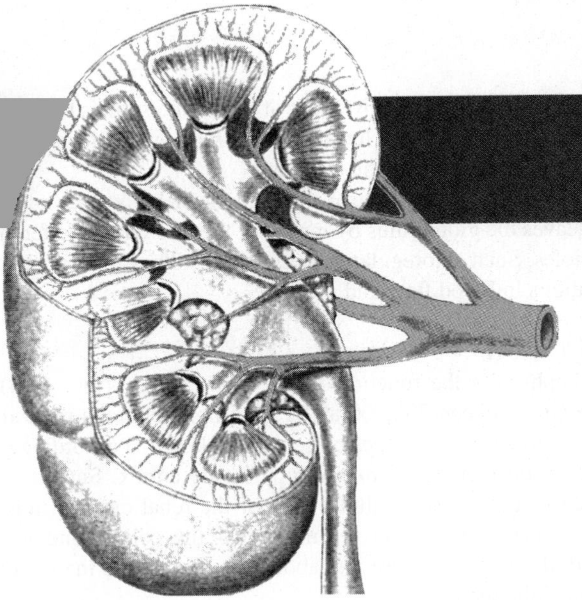

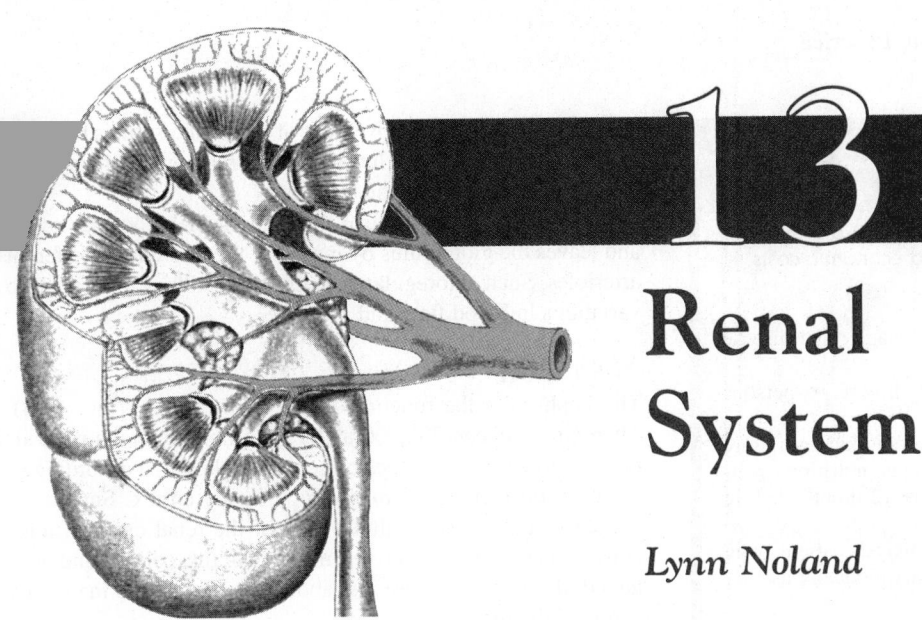

13 Renal System

Lynn Noland

Overview

The renal system functions to excrete water-soluble waste products from the body and to maintain the homeostasis of plasma, water, electrolytes, and pH.

Renal function depends on the normal and interrelated functioning of the cardiovascular, nervous, endocrine, and urinary collecting systems. The cardiovascular system delivers the blood to be filtered, sustains the hydrostatic pressure needed for filtration, and provides specialized capillaries that do the filtering. The nervous system helps regulate blood pressure, thus contributing to the first two functions.

The nervous system also controls the process of urination (see Chapter 14) and interacts with the activity of the endocrine system to affect renal function directly through aldosterone and antidiuretic hormone (ADH). The calyces, pelvis, ureters, urinary bladder, and urethra form the urinary collecting system. The urethra provides the exit for urine from the body.

Urine volume varies with food and fluid intake and extrarenal fluid losses through feces, perspiration, and respiration. A diurnal variation in volume that is associated with light-dark periods or sleep-wake patterns occurs.

The kidneys have excretory and nonexcretory functions vital to the regulation of substances essential to the human body.

Excretory functions are excretion of end products of metabolism (urea, creatinine, uric acid, phosphates, sulfates, nitrates, and phenols); excretion of excess normal fluid and electrolyte components (H_2O, Na^+, K^+, HCO_3^-, Cl^-, H^+), thus maintaining the volume, pH, and osmolality of the extracellular and intracellular fluids; and excretion of certain drugs and other substances (penicillin and metabolites of hormones).

Nonexcretory functions are secretion of renin, erythropoietin, kallikrein, and prostaglandins; metabolism of carbohydrates, lipids, plasma proteins, and peptide hormones such as insulin and glucagon; and regulation of vitamin D metabolism.

For additional information on the genitourinary system, see Chapter 14.

Anatomy, Physiology, and Related Pathophysiology

The kidneys are located in the posterior abdominal cavity in the retroperitoneal area to the right and left of the lumbar spinal column and are level with the T12 and the L1 to L3 vertebrae.

Each kidney is covered by a tough capsule, surrounded by a cushion of fat, and supported by fascia. Each kidney is partially protected by the ribs. The lower end of each kidney extends below the ribs; the right one is lower than the left (Fig. 13-1). The kidneys move downward during respiration as the diaphragm contracts.

The renal artery, vein, nerves, lymph vessels, and ureters all enter or leave the kidney on the medial surface in the indented region called the hilum or renal sinus.

Each kidney has an outer cortex, an inner medulla, and a pelvis—the area in which urine is collected (Fig. 13-2). The fluid filtered from the blood travels through the nephron to reach the large collecting ducts that form the renal pyramids in the medulla. The ducts empty into a calyx at the papilla. Interspersed between the pyramids is cortical tissue known as the "renal columns." The glomerulus, proximal and distal tubules, and most of the loop of Henle and the collecting ducts are in the medulla.

Blood Supply to the Kidneys

The renal arteries are short and wide to ensure that 20% to 25% of the resting cardiac output (about 1200 ml/min) passes through the kidneys. This volume exceeds the amount needed to meet the kidneys' oxygen needs; it permits the formation of filtrate that is needed to maintain homeostasis of the blood.

Almost 90% of the blood flows rapidly through the cortex; the rest moves slowly through the medulla. The renal artery branches into interlobar, arcuate, interlobular, and afferent arterioles, each of which leads to a glomerulus (Fig. 13-3). Only 20% of the renal blood supply is actually filtered through the glomerulus. The remaining 80% of the blood leaves the glomerulus via the efferent arteriole, which subdivides into the peritubular capillaries. These tiny vessels surround the tubules

HEALTHY PEOPLE 2010

HEALTH STATUS—CHRONIC KIDNEY DISEASE

Goal: Reduce new cases of chronic kidney disease and its complications, disability, death, and economic costs.

CHRONIC KIDNEY DISEASE

- Reduce the rate of new cases of end-stage renal disease (ESRD).
- Reduce deaths from cardiovascular disease in persons with chronic kidney failure.
- Increase the proportion of treated chronic kidney failure patients who have received counseling on nutrition, treatment choices, and cardiovascular care 12 months before the start of renal replacement therapy.
- Increase the proportion of new hemodialysis patients who use arteriovenous fistulas as the primary mode of vascular access.
- Increase the proportion of dialysis patients registered on the waiting list for transplantation.
- Increase the proportion of patients with treated chronic kidney failure who receive a transplant within 3 years of registration on the waiting list.
- Reduce kidney failure resulting from diabetes.
- (Developmental) Increase the proportion of persons with type 1 or type 2 diabetes and proteinuria who receive recommended medical therapy to reduce progression to chronic renal insufficiency.

Modified from U.S. Department of Health and Human Services: *Healthy people 2010* (conference edition, in two volumes), Washington, DC, January 2000.

NOTE: *Developmental* indicates that criteria for measurement and strategies to improve health have not as yet been specified.

and make possible the movement of water and solutes between the blood and the tubular lumen. Veins draining the kidneys follow the same pattern as the arteries.

Each nephron can control the amount of blood that enters and leaves the glomerulus by means of the afferent and efferent arterioles. Such autoregulation permits the kidney to respond to variations in blood flow and pressure.

Nephron

The nephron is the functional unit of the kidney (FIG. 13-4). There are between 700,000 and 1.2 million nephrons per kidney and three distinct types of nephrons classified according to the position their glomeruli occupy in the cortex. Superficial cortical nephrons are within 1 mm of the renal capsule; midcortical nephrons, are in the middle of the cortex; and juxtamedullary nephrons are just above the area where the cortex and medulla meet.

Each nephron is composed of a glomerulus with afferent and efferent arterioles, Bowman's capsule, proximal (convoluted) tubule, loop of Henle, and distal (convoluted) tubule. The nephrons empty into the collecting ducts. The filtrate formed follows the course of the nephron from Bowman's capsule to the collecting ducts.

The major functions of the nephron components are (1) glomerulus: filtration; (2) proximal tubule: reabsorption of sodium, potassium, chloride, bicarbonate, phosphate, glucose, amino acids, urea, and water (ADH not required) as well as secretion of hydrogen ions and some unwanted substances (toxins, drugs); (3) Henle's loop: countercurrent flow, concentration of urine; reabsorption of sodium (passively), chloride (actively), and calcium; (4) distal tubule: reabsorption of sodium,

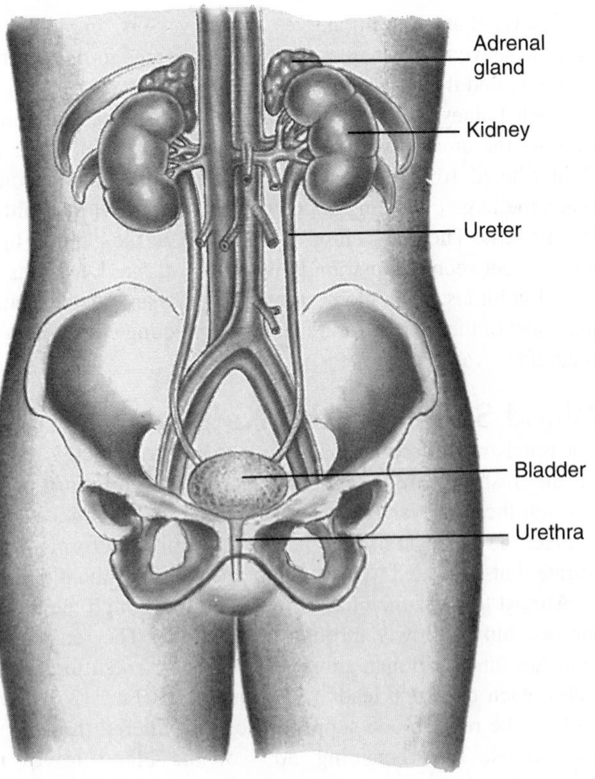

FIG. 13-1
Components of the urinary system.

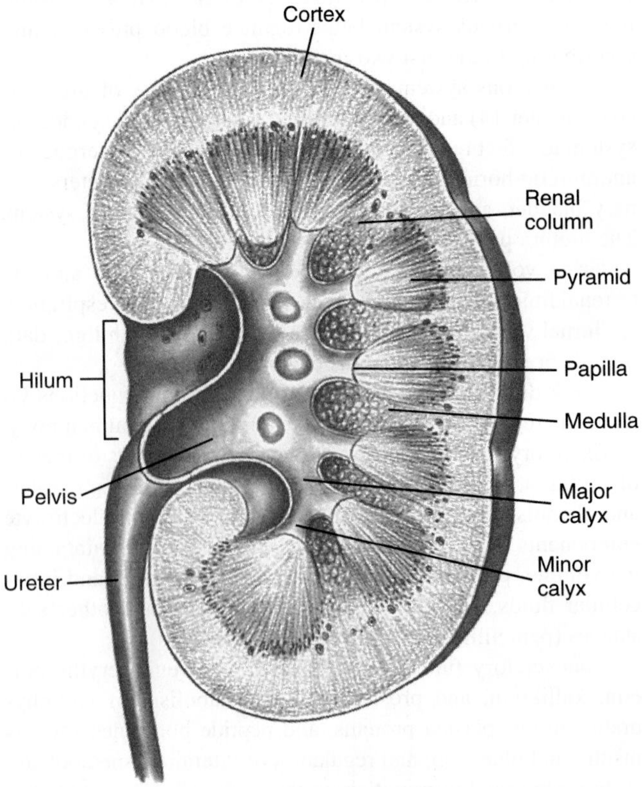

FIG. 13-2
Cross section of kidney.

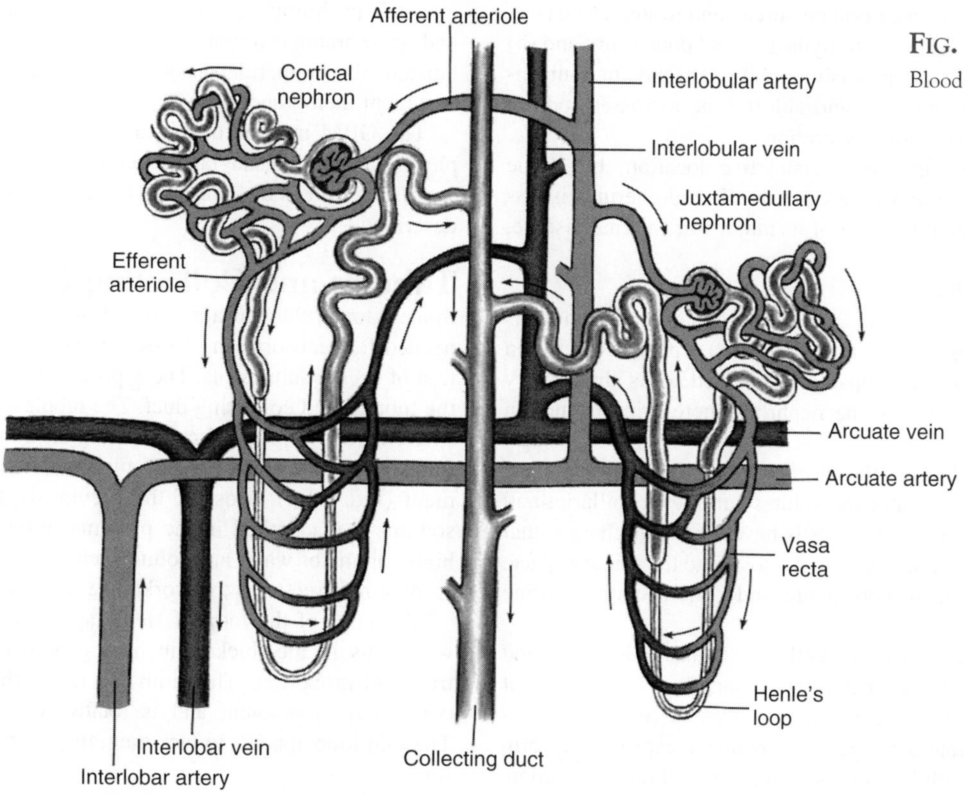

FIG. 13-3
Blood supply of nephron.

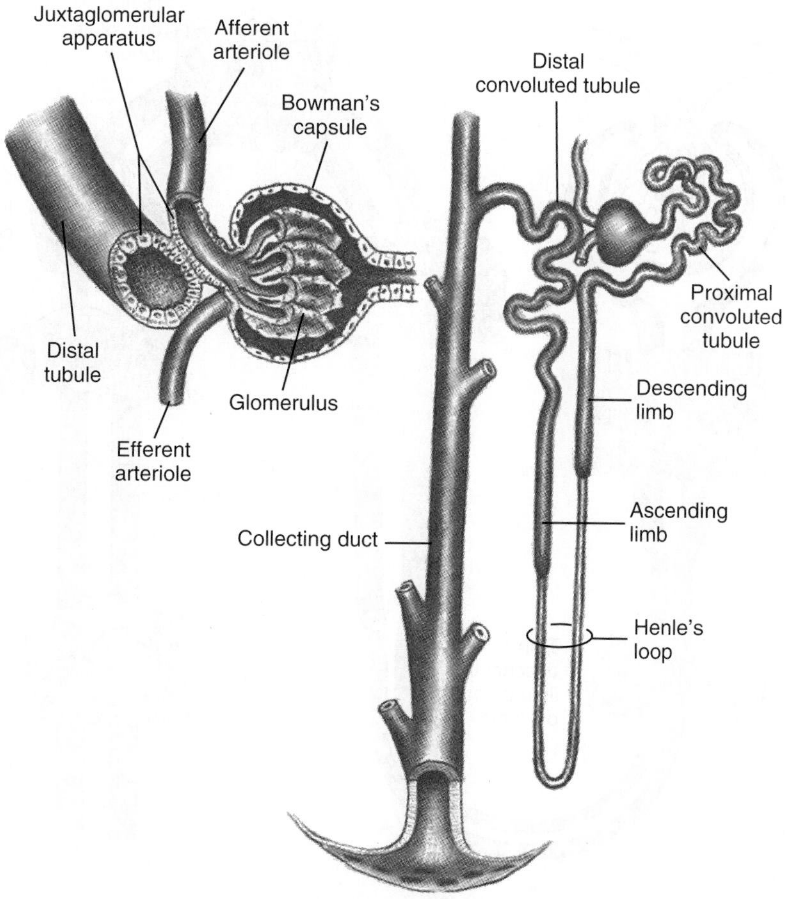

FIG. 13-4
Components of nephron.

potassium, chloride, bicarbonate, urea, and water (ADH required) as well as secretion of hydrogen and potassium; and (5) collecting duct: sodium, potassium, hydrogen, and ammonia either secreted or reabsorbed and aldosterone increases sodium reabsorption and potassium secretion.

Each nephron part has a distinctive location, histologic structure, and vascular network pattern. The glomerulus is discussed in some detail because of its major role in renal disease.

Glomerulus

The glomerulus is a fist-shaped clump of capillaries that fits loosely into a capsule (Bowman's capsule). The space between the glomerulus and the capsule is referred to as the urinary space. This is the area of the nephron where urine formation begins.

Specialized cells line the glomerulus, making possible the effective filtration of water and solutes out of the capillaries and into the urinary space. These cells have electrical charges that restrict the type of solutes that may move into the urinary space. They are discussed in more detail under the section on urine formation.

The specialized glomerular cells (epithelial, endothelial, and mesangial) can undergo pathologic changes: Proliferation of epithelial cells may fuse the foot processes (nephrotic syndrome) or obliterate the space in Bowman's capsule and form the crescents of cellular-fibrous material found on microscopic examination associated with rapidly progressive glomerulonephritis. Proliferation of endothelial cells may occlude the capillary lumen such as in hemolytic uremic syndrome. Mesangial cell proliferation occurs as part of diabetic nephropathy and membranoproliferative glomerulonephritis, causing collapse of the glomerular vessels and damage to the glomerular basement membrane (GBM).

The GBM may be damaged by deposits of immune complexes in the mesangial, subendothelial, and subepithelial spaces, as well as by damage to the glomerular cells previously described.

Tubules and Collecting Ducts

Since glomerular filtration is nonspecific, a mechanism is needed for reabsorption of essential substances and the secretion of excess substances. These processes are accomplished in the tubules and collecting duct. The tubules are composed of a single layer of epithelial cells resting on a membrane. The epithelial cells vary in form and function from segment to segment (FIG. 13-5). Most of the previously filtered water and sodium is reabsorbed in the proximal tubule. Because of the high volume of water and solute exchange, the proximal tubule is often referred to as the workhorse of the nephron.

The cells of the loop of Henle appear to be less complex, with cells in the thick limb having highly developed active transport properties. This limb can reabsorb sodium against a concentration gradient and is relatively water impermeable. The thin limb appears to lack the transport systems of the thick limb.

The distal tubule passes between the afferent and efferent arterioles of its glomerulus. In the region where the distal tubule is in close proximity to the arteriole, specialized cells, the mac-

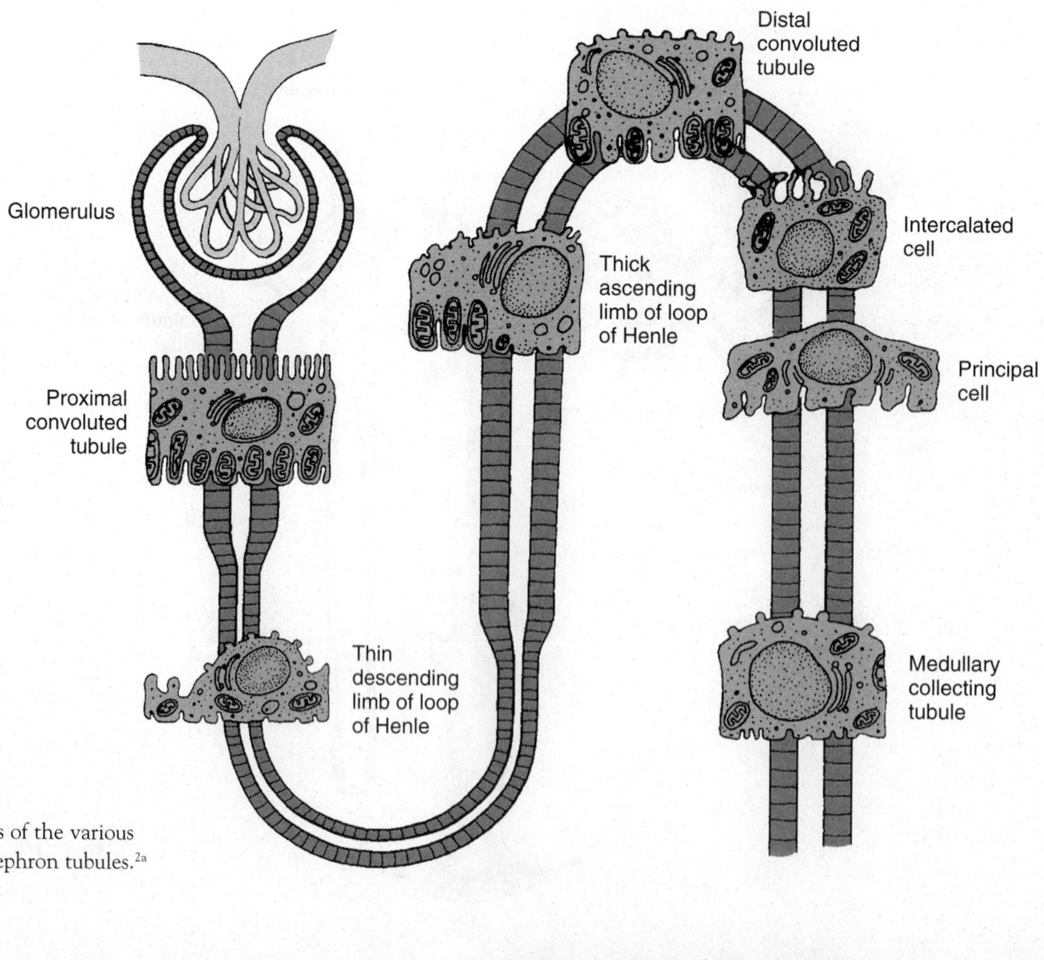

FIG. 13-5
Epithelial cells of the various segments of nephron tubules.[2a]

ula densa, are found (see "Juxtaglomerular Apparatus," p. 863). Cells here can absorb sodium ions without an equivalent amount of negatively charged particles. This segment develops both ionic and electrical gradients.

The collecting tubule has two well-defined cell types, light cells and dark cells, also known as principal and intercalated cells. These cells fill the gaps between the capillary and tubules and play a major role in the transport of water and cations and the movement of chloride, H^+, and bicarbonate. They also release prostaglandins and renin in response to certain types of intrarenal stimuli.

Renal Interstitium.

Cells that form the interstitium lie between the nephrons and their blood supply. More interstitial cells are found in the medulla than in the cortex. They are believed to affect urine concentration and prostaglandin synthesis.

Urine Formation

Glomerular Filtration.

Urine is formed when renal cells carry out the processes of filtration, reabsorption, and secretion. Urine formation begins with glomerular filtration of water and solutes. They pass from the blood through the capillary basement membrane and form a filtrate in the urinary space. Which substances actually pass across the GBM is determined by the size and electrical charge of the particle. For example, under normal circumstances, because of their size, large protein molecules are unable to move across the basement membrane. Negatively charged particles are not filtered easily either, because they are repelled by the negative electrical charge on the basement membrane.

The rate of glomerular filtration is proportional to filtration pressure. When filtration pressure falls, the pressure receptors in the afferent arteriole activate the renin-angiotensin system of the juxtaglomerular apparatus, which functions to return the afferent pressure to its optimal level.

The glomerular filtrate is isotonic, with a pH of 7.4 or equal to that of plasma. The volume of the filtrate decreases with systemic hypotension, localized renal ischemia, urine outflow obstruction, and changes in the filtering surface. Moderate reductions in glomerular filtration also occur with exercise, pain, and dehydration. Extreme reductions in glomerular filtration occur with severe hypotension. Activation of the sympathetic nervous system can inhibit urine production completely.

Glomerular filtration remains fairly constant even with a marked increase in arterial blood pressure because of the kidney's autoregulatory mechanisms.

Reabsorption and Secretion.

In the proximal convoluted tubule (PCT), 70% of the previously filtered sodium, water, and other electrolytes are reabsorbed by both active and passive transport mechanisms. They include simple diffusion—electrochemical potential gradient; convection—hydrostatic or osmotic pressure gradient; and mediated transport—facilitated diffusion, electromechanical potential gradient, and active transport, which requires free energy from metabolism. See FIG. 13-6 for a review of the three processes of urine formation.

Only a certain amount of any substance can be reabsorbed per minute. This is referred to as the "transport maximum." It is a constant value, and when the amount of a substance filtered exceeds this value, the excess is excreted in the urine. This means that the urine content of a substance commonly correlates well with dietary intake as long as the substance measured can be filtered. For example, daily sodium intake can be assessed by measuring 24-hour urine sodium excretion.

The solutes in the glomerular filtrate are threshold and nonthreshold substances. Urea, sodium, potassium, and others are nonthreshold substances, since the urine always contains at least some of each. Glucose and phosphates are threshold substances, since a certain serum level must be reached before the glomerular filtrate will contain enough that the transport maximum of the substance will be exceeded and the excess will be excreted in the urine.

As the glomerular filtrate moves through the tubules, selective reabsorption of water and solutes and selective secretion of solutes occur. A large volume of iso-osmotic glomerular filtrate is converted into a small volume of hyperosmotic urine. The composition of the glomerular filtrate triggers appropriate activities in the tubular cells. In the tubules, about 87% of the water and electrolytes, all of the glucose, and almost all of the amino acids are reabsorbed in the proximal tubules. The proximal tubule preserves metabolically important components and resists the reabsorption of nitrogenous wastes. It secretes foreign substances.

The remaining 13% of the glomerular filtrate passes through the loops of Henle and the distal tubules where variable

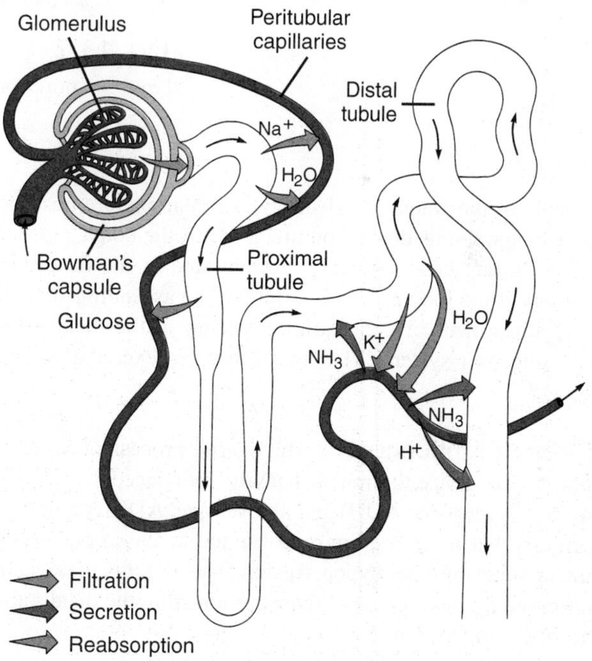

FIG. 13-6

Glomerular filtration, tubular reabsorption, and tubular secretion. The three processes by which the kidneys excrete urine. From proximal convoluted tubules, sodium and glucose are reabsorbed into peritubular capillaries by active transport. Water reabsorption by osmosis follows. From distal convoluted tubules, sodium is reabsorbed by active transport. Osmotic reabsorption of water from them occurs when ADH is present. Secretion of ammonia and hydrogen occurs from peritubular capillaries into distal tubules by active transport.[33]

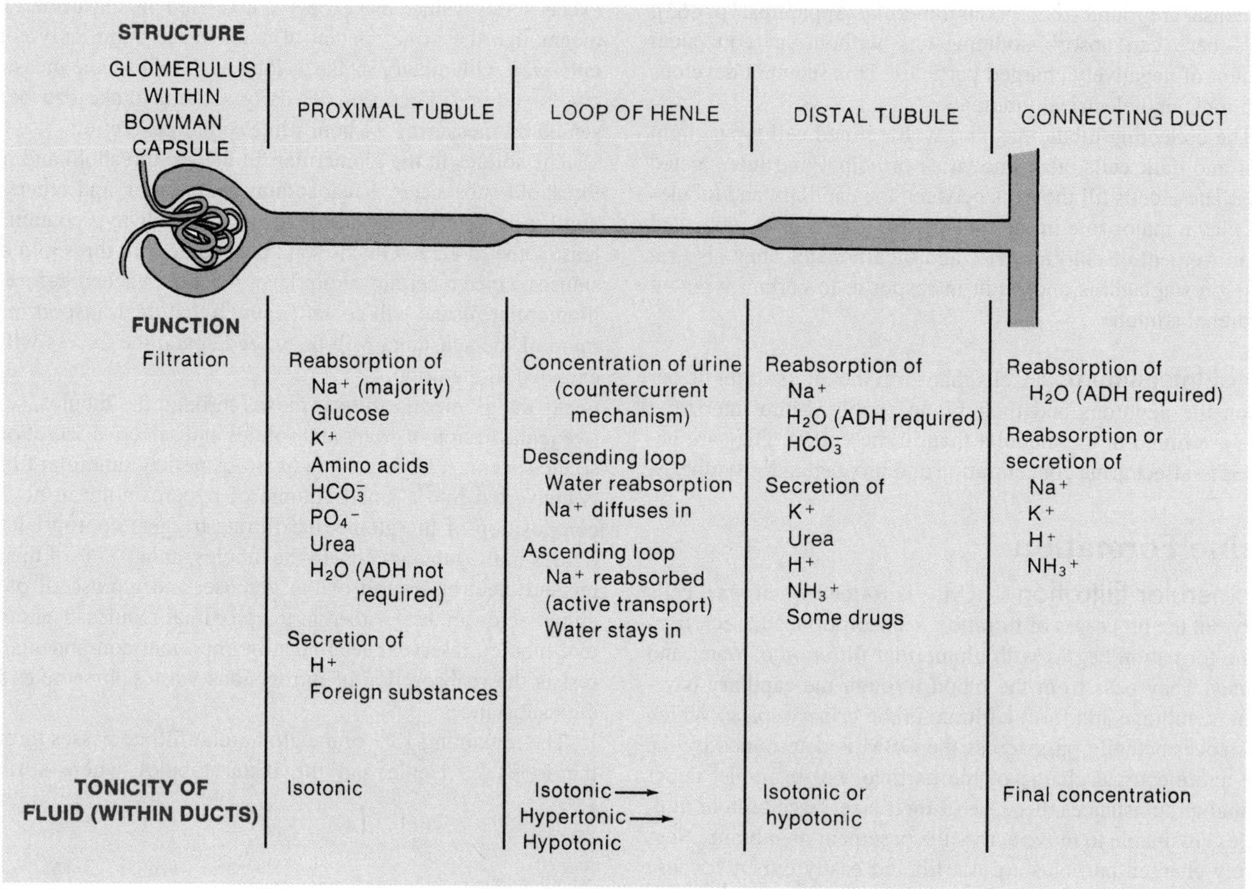

STRUCTURE
GLOMERULUS WITHIN BOWMAN CAPSULE
PROXIMAL TUBULE
LOOP OF HENLE
DISTAL TUBULE
CONNECTING DUCT
FUNCTION
Filtration
Reabsorption of Na+ (majority) Glucose K+ Amino acids HCO3- PO4- Urea H2O (ADH not required)
Secretion of H+ Foreign substances
Concentration of urine (countercurrent mechanism)
Descending loop Water reabsorption Na+ diffuses in
Ascending loop Na+ reabsorbed (active transport) Water stays in
Reabsorption of Na+ H2O (ADH required) HCO3-
Secretion of K+ Urea H+ NH3+ Some drugs
Reabsorption of H2O (ADH required)
Reabsorption or secretion of Na+ K+ H+ NH3+
TONICITY OF FLUID (WITHIN DUCTS)
Isotonic
Isotonic Hypertonic Hypotonic
Isotonic or hypotonic
Final concentration

FIG. 13-7

Process of urine formation and concentration.[37]

amounts of the water and electrolytes remaining are absorbed. The exact amounts depend on the needs of the body.

The filtrate becomes more concentrated in the descending segment of the loop and more dilute in the ascending segment. Final adjustment of concentration occurs in the distal tubule and collecting system. The final filtrate is excreted as urine (FIG. 13-7).

Hormonal Influences. The overall process of urine formation and concentration is heavily influenced by the hormones vasopressin (ADH) and aldosterone. ADH is a pituitary hormone that is released in response to decreased plasma volume or states of renal hypoperfusion. The effect is that water is conserved by the process of reabsorption from the distal tubule and collecting system.

Aldosterone, an adrenal hormone, stimulates sodium reabsorption by the collecting duct. Aldosterone is also secreted in response to reduced plasma volume and renal blood flow.

The same two stimuli also cause the juxtaglomerular apparatus of the nephron to secrete another hormone, renin. Renin activates kidney cells to form angiotensin I, which is enzymatically converted into angiotensin II, a potent vasoconstrictor. The ultimate end result of the secretion of all three hormones is to increase blood pressure and renal perfusion and reduce urine output.

Urine Concentration

Urine is considered more dilute or concentrated (specific gravity low or high) because of the final water-to-solute ratio of the filtrate in the collecting system. This filtrate is what is excreted as urine. Concentration is influenced by a number of complex mechanisms that include hormonal effects (see above), permeability of the different tubular segments to water and sodium, plasma volume/blood pressure (which influences renal blood flow), and serum osmolality (the active particles in solution expressed as osmoles per liter) (FIG. 13-8).

As is the case for most of the body's homeostatic mechanisms, urine concentration depends on the binding of cellular receptors by chemical messengers and feedback mechanisms initiated by a variety of systemic stimuli. The tonicity of body fluids ends up being controlled by the amount of water excreted by the kidneys and primarily the quantity of ADH secreted by the pituitary. The processes of baroreceptor and osmoreceptor stimulation and a more detailed description of the function of the hormones that facilitate sodium and water reabsorption are covered in Chapters 3 and 11.

Acidity and Alkalinity

The kidneys function as the slowest of the three physiologic mechanisms that maintain acid-base balance. The respiratory system controls carbon dioxide (CO_2) levels; there is an ex-

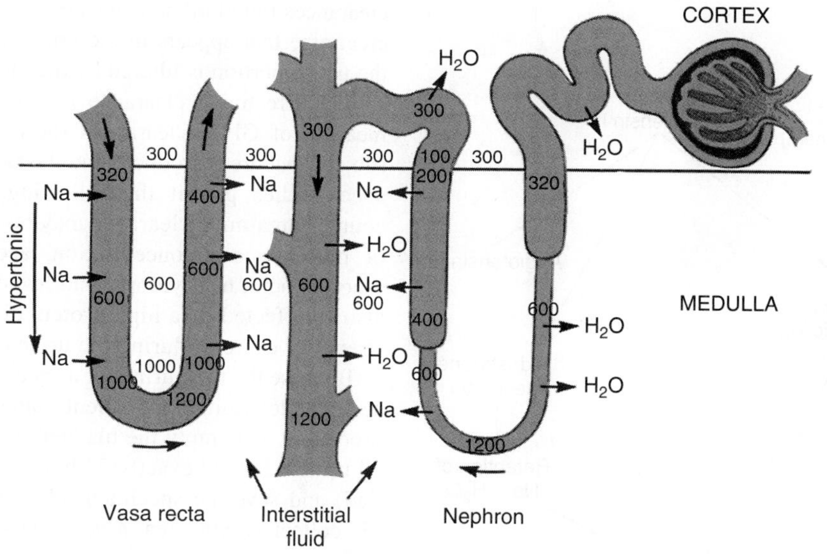

FIG. 13-8
Countercurrent mechanism for concentrating urine. Numbers represent osmotic concentration (in mOsm/kg).

Table 13-1 Sources of H^+ Ion Gain and Loss

Gain	Loss
1. Generation of H^+ ions from CO_2 in tissue capillaries	Recombination of H^+ ions and bicarbonate in pulmonary capillaries
2. Production of nonvolatile acids from the metabolism of protein and other organic molecules	Utilization of H^+ ions in the metabolism of organic anions
3. Gain of H^+ ions because of loss of bicarbonate in diarrhea or other nongastric gastrointestinal fluids	Loss of H^+ ions in vomitus
4. Gain of H^+ ions because of loss of bicarbonate in urine	Loss of H^+ ions in urine

From Vander.[36]

tracellular chemical buffering system, and the kidneys control bicarbonate levels and excrete H^+ ions in the urine. The kidneys balance H^+ ions in the same way they balance any other ion.[36] They do so to preserve acid-base homeostasis and maintain arterial pH in the required narrow range of 7.35 to 7.45. The primary gains and losses of H^+ ions are listed in Table 13-1.

The primary way that the kidney regulates H^+ ion concentration is by secreting or reabsorbing buffer (bicarbonate). They are also able to directly secrete H^+ ions in systemic acid states. Acidosis and potassium depletion enhance H^+ ion secretion. In chronic renal failure the acid residues of nitrogen metabolism accumulate, and the tubules cannot meet the demand for H^+ ion secretion. Since the tubular transport system is overwhelmed, potassium cannot be excreted and hyperkalemia results.

Juxtaglomerular Apparatus

The juxtaglomerular apparatus is composed of special epithelial cells (the macula densa cells) in the first part of the distal tubule and special myoepithelial cells in the renal afferent arteriole near the glomerulus (see FIG. 13-4). These juxtaglomerular cells respond to renal ischemia, low sodium concentration, and activity of the renal sympathetic nerves by secreting renin, which initiates the process that results in the formation of the vasopressor substance, angiotensin II.

Renin is an enzyme that acts on angiotensinogen, a glycoprotein made in the liver, to form angiotensin I. A converting enzyme formed in the lungs changes it to angiotensin II, which causes peripheral vasoconstriction and increased secretion of aldosterone. The first action elevates blood pressure by increasing peripheral resistance; the second action decreases salt and water loss and therefore increases extracellular fluid volume. Both actions cause an increase in arterial pressure, which relieves renal ischemia. The schema of the renin-angiotensin mechanism is outlined in FIG. 13-9.

The juxtaglomerular apparatus appears to play a role in the autoregulation of renal blood flow and the glomerular filtration rate (GFR) by responding either to the concentration of sodium ions or to the osmolality of the urine in the distal tubule. The conditions of the distal tubule appear to control blood flow in the afferent arteriole.

Other Renal Functions

The kidneys produce erythropoietin, which promotes differentiation, proliferation, and maturation of precursors of red blood cells in the bone marrow. Erythropoietin is produced in response to decreases in oxygen tension and renal perfusion that may arise from anemia, hypoxia, or renal ischemia.

Renal prostaglandins are synthesized in the renal cortex and medulla. They appear to be produced in response to both renal

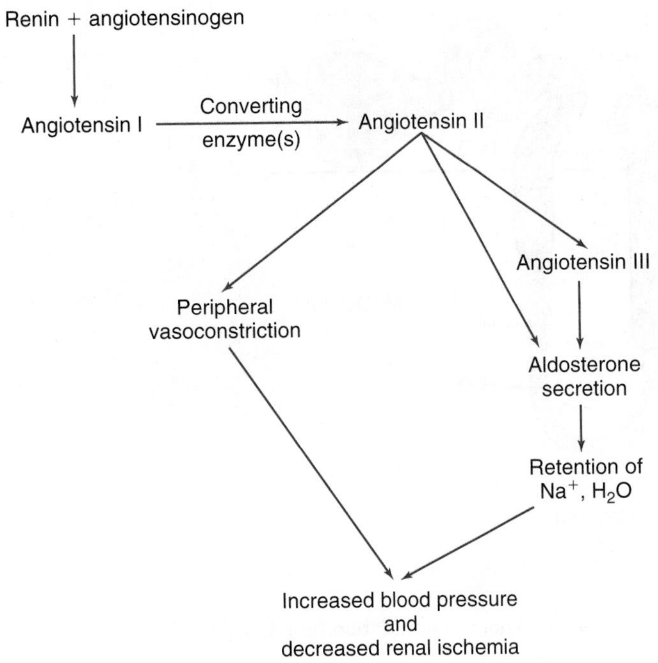

FIG. 13-9
Renin-angiotensin mechanism.

ischemia and vasoconstriction. Observations suggest that they participate in the maintenance of renal vascular resistance and GFR, especially when renal hemodynamics are altered. The complex relationships of renal prostaglandins are not yet clearly understood. It is known that their effects vary from vasodilation to vasoconstriction and that they play a major role in maintaining renal perfusion.

The kidneys have a role in the metabolism of vitamin D. Vitamin D_3 is formed in the skin, metabolized in the liver to 1-hydroxy D_3, and then metabolized by the kidney to an active form (1,25-dihydroxy D_3 and others). The 1,25-dihydroxy D_3 is produced in response to hypocalcemia or hypophosphatemia. It acts in conjunction with the parathyroid hormone to increase intestinal absorption of calcium and phosphate, mobilize calcium from bones, and increase renal tubular reabsorption of calcium and phosphate. The production of 1,25-dihydroxy D_3 is suppressed by hypercalcemia and hyperphosphatemia. Decreased production of 1,25-dihydroxy D_3 occurs in chronic renal failure and is considered significant in the development of renal osteodystrophy.

Measurement of Renal Function

The kidneys clear the plasma of unnecessary substances with such consistency that adequacy of kidney function may be determined by measuring the renal clearance of particular substances. The definition of clearance is the volume of plasma from which a substance is completely cleared by the kidneys in a specific period of time (e.g., 100 ml/min).

Clearance of creatinine is used to monitor renal function, since it is an endogenous product from muscle creatine phosphate, and its production is relatively independent of protein anabolism and catabolism. The amount of creatinine produced depends on the lean body mass, and this variation is responsible for the differences in serum creatinine levels and creatinine clearances found in men and women. While a small part of the creatinine that appears in the urine is secreted by the tubules, the major portion is filtered by the glomerulus and is not reabsorbed. Creatinine clearance is a practical, clinically useful measure of GFR. Clearances show wide variations between subjects but are reproducible in the same subject. Serial clearance studies permit the following of a patient's clinical course. Creatinine clearance may be affected by the presence of high glucose concentration, acetone, acetoacetic acid, ascorbic acid, methyldopa, and levodopa in the urine. It may also be affected by a high-protein diet before the test and by strenuous exercise during the urine collection period.

Because the total urine for a specified period is required for accurate determination, patients and staff must understand the procedure: (1) empty the bladder and mark the time; (2) save all urine; (3) void exactly 24 hours later (or the period specified) and save the specimen; (4) measure total volume; and (5) collect serum creatinine (Scr) once during the 24-hour period.

$$\text{Creatinine clearance (ml/min)} = \frac{\text{Urine creatinine (mg/dl)} \times \text{Urine volume (ml/min)}}{\text{Serum creatinine (mg/dl)}}$$

Inulin clearance is clinically useful as a measure of GFR. Inulin is freely filtered by the glomerulus and is not reabsorbed or secreted by the tubules, so that the amount filtered is the amount secreted. Inulin clearance is used when an exact measure of GFR is required.

$$\text{Inulin clearance (ml/min)} = \frac{\text{Urine inulin (mg/dl)} \times \text{Urine volume (ml/min)}}{\text{Plasma inulin (mg/dl)}} = \text{GFR}$$

Additional useful indicators of renal function are as follows:

1. **Creatinine clearance (CLcr)**
   Cockcroft Gault
   The following formula can be used if the only laboratory value available is the serum creatinine level

   $$\text{CLcr} = \frac{(140 - \text{Age}) \times (\text{Weight in kg})}{72 \times \text{Serum creatinine}}$$

   If the patient is female, multiply by 0.85.

   There are two other helpful indices that are used to evaluate renal function and to determine the etiology of dysfunction, as follows:
2. **Renal failure index (RFI)**

   $$\frac{\text{24-h Urine sodium concentration}}{\text{Urine creatinine/Serum creatinine}}$$

   A value of less than 1 = Prerenal
   A value of over 2 to 3 = Acute tubular necrosis (ATN) or postrenal
3. Fractional excretion of sodium (FE_{na})

   $$\frac{\text{24-h Urine sodium}}{\text{24-h Urine creatinine/Serum creatinine}} \times 100$$

   A value of less than 1 = Prerenal
   A value of 2 to 3 = ATN or postrenal[20,27]

Age and Renal Function

Differences in age are associated with differences in renal function that become clinically significant when a young or aged individual has an illness that places excessive demands on the kidneys.

The kidney is immature at birth. Renal blood flow and GFR of infants are low compared with those of adults. The ability to excrete sodium, potassium, water, and acid loads is limited. The kidneys continue to develop until age 1 year. Their combined weight continues to increase beyond adolescence (24 g at birth, 140 g at 6 years, 183 g at age 12 years, and 300 g for adults).

Renal blood flow decreases with age, which is partly related to a decrease in cardiac output. The loss of renal mass and functioning nephrons also decreases the effective filtering surface and GFR. Creatinine clearance is stable until the fourth decade, when it begins to decrease. Serum creatinine decreases with the decrease in muscle mass associated with aging. Therefore serum creatinine levels may overestimate GFR. To avoid overdoses of drugs in the elderly, the creatinine clearance rate is used when dosage of such drugs as digoxin is determined. Also of note is the slower rate of response in elderly patients to acute changes in fluid and electrolyte balances associated with illness. The renin-aldosterone system becomes less responsive with lowered renin levels and an associated reduction in plasma level of aldosterone. The ability to conserve Na^+ and excrete K^+ is decreased. The decrease in renal response to antidiuretic hormone and in GFR contribute to the inability to conserve water and concentrate the urine. The maintenance of Na^+, K^+, and water balance becomes exceedingly important in elderly patients.

Normal Findings

General: Temperature: normal range; blood pressure: normal range; weight: no marked increased (>2 kg); skin: warm, dry, and normal turgor; no pallor, yellowish color, excoriations, uremic frost, edema, petechiae, ecchymoses, or purpura

Eyes: No periorbital edema, conjunctival redness, retinal hemorrhages, exudates, or papilledema

Ears: Hearing normal; no tophi in ear cartilages

Mouth: No odor of ammonia; no stomatitis: ulcers, exudate, or bleeding

Neck: Parathyroid glands not palpable

Chest: Normal breath sounds, rate and rhythm; normal heart sounds, rate and rhythm

Abdomen: Normal bowel sounds; no masses; no tenderness in flank, groin, or costovertebral angle on palpation or percussion; no bruit on auscultation

Neurologic examination: No change in cognitive function, level of consciousness, or behavior; no change in superficial or deep tendon reflexes; no change in muscle action or sensation

Extremities: No edema

Abnormal Findings*

General: Lethargy, fatigue, pallor, uremic frost, consistent increase in weight, excoriation of skin from pruritus, petechiae, periorbital edema, scleral injection from soft tissue calcification, ammonia-like breath odor, stomatitis

Neck: Jugular venous distention (JVD), enlarged or irregular parathyroid glands

Chest: Cough, crackles, wheezes, tachypnea, dyspnea

Cardiovascular: Pericardial friction rub, tachycardia, arrhythmias

Abdomen/thorax: Ascites, renal artery bruits, costal vertebral angle (CVA) tenderness, palpable renal mass

Neurologic/musculoskeletal: Depressed deep tendon reflexes (DTRs), muscle weakness, confusion

Extremities: Bilateral pitting edema

⭘ These abnormal findings are present in a variety of renal disorders regardless of age but may be more debilitating in the older adult.

*⭘ = Older adult.

Conditions, Diseases, and Disorders

RENAL FAILURE

Renal dysfunction occurs along a spectrum from renal insufficiency or mild dysfunction to renal failure or reduction of function to the point of altered homeostasis. Renal failure can be categorized as either acute or chronic. Both can be caused by a variety of disease processes (described later in this chapter). The next two sections focus on acute and chronic failure.

Acute Renal Failure[7,11,14,20]

Acute renal failure (ARF) is deterioration of renal function that occurs over hours to days and results in azotemia or the accumulation of nitrogenous waste products in the blood.

Azotemia is generally accompanied by fluid, electrolyte, and acid-base disorders. ARF occurs in approximately 5% of all general hospital patients. Although it is considered reversible, it can have a 40% to 60% mortality rate.[14] This is presumed to result from the fact that the typical patient with ARF is older and often more physically vulnerable and, therefore, the typical inciting events are more common. Dehydration is more often a cause of ARF in the elderly or in very young persons than in middle-age adults. Elderly patients with multiple-system problems or preexisting renal insufficiency are particularly at risk.

The five stages of ARF are (1) onset: usually a short time from precipitating event to onset of oliguria or anuria; (2) oliguric-anuric stage: the period during which output is less than 400 ml/day (usually 8 to 15 days; if longer, the prognosis is poor); (3) early diuretic stage: extends from the time daily output is greater than 400 ml/day to the time that the blood urea nitrogen (BUN) concentration stops rising; (4) late diuretic or recovery stage: extends from the first day BUN falls to the day it stabilizes or is in the normal range; and (5) convalescent stage: extends from the day BUN is stable to the day the patient returns to normal activity and urine volume and BUN are normal. This may take several months and during this time, chronic renal failure develops in some patients.

Urine output in ARF may be diminished (oliguria; less than 400 ml/day), absent (anuria; less than 50 ml/day), or near normal.

There are prerenal, renal, and postrenal causes of ARF that include ischemia, infection, nephrotoxins, vascular and glomerular diseases, and obstruction (Fig. 13-10).

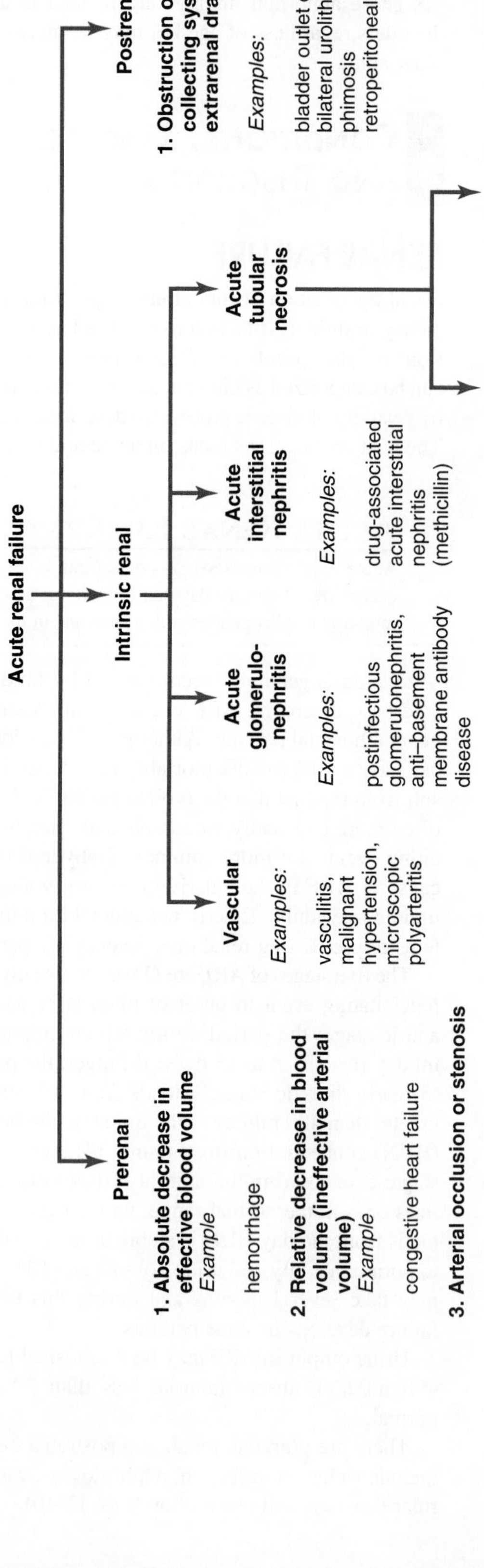

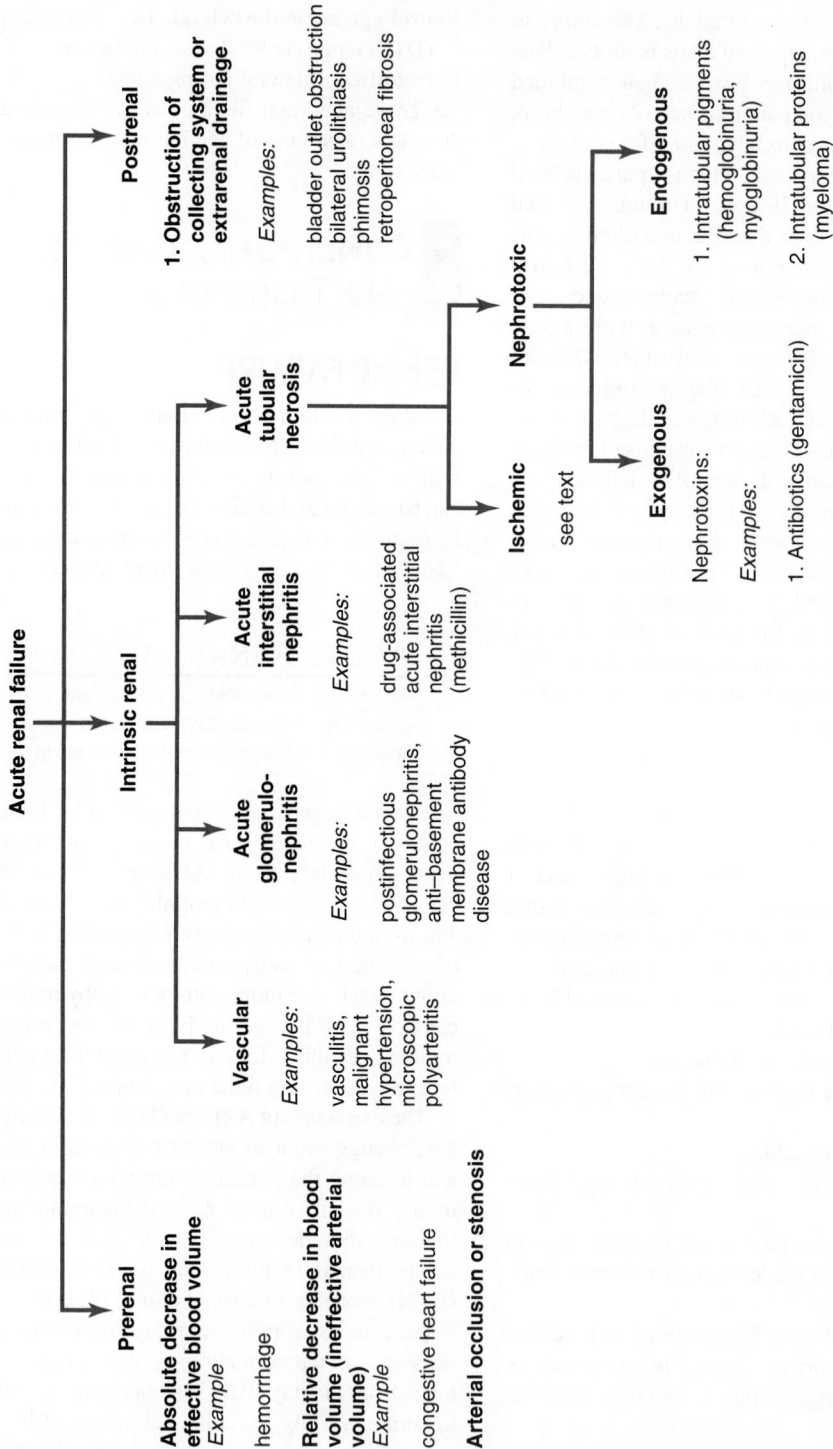

FIG. 13-10
Causes of acute renal failure.[14]

PATHOPHYSIOLOGY

Prerenal ARF is the result of decreased actual or effective blood volume. When blood volume is reduced for any reason, catecholamines and vasopressin activate the renin-angiotensin aldosterone system, which acts to preserve renal blood flow and GFR. These mechanisms are effective unless the problem persists and nephron damage results. When this occurs, signs of renal failure appear.

Intrinsic or intrarenal ARF is the result of renal parenchymal damage and can be caused by a variety of pathologic conditions. The most common cause is ATN typically from prolonged renal ischemia or nephrotoxins such as aminoglycosides or radio-contrast materials. ATN can also occur from crush injuries, rhabdomyolysis, or ethylene glycol ingestion, all of which cause tubular obstruction and damage. Diseases other than ATN that cause intrinsic ARF include acute nephritis, malignant hypertension, other medications, nonsteroidal antiinflammatory drugs (NSAIDs) such as ibuprofen, amphotericin B, ACE inhibitors, and vasculitis.

Postrenal ARF results from mechanical obstruction of urine flow and a rapid rise in proximal tubular pressure. This causes reactive renal vasodilation and ultimately a fall in GFR. The renal outcome of this sequence of events is the inability to concentrate or acidify urine normally. Causes include neurogenic bladder, tumor, and renal stones.

The current explanations for the pathogenesis of ARF include leakage of tubular fluid from damaged tubules into the interstitial areas, tubular obstructions caused by accumulation of intratubular debris or casts, glomerular abnormalities, and changes in renal hemodynamics, primarily excessive vasoconstriction (see p. 865).

Carefully managing fluid volume before, during, and after surgery helps protect renal function; using crystalloid and colloid volume replacement products and blood products helps prevent volume depletion and renal ischemia.

Attempts to maintain renal blood flow (using a low dosage of dopamine) and urine flow rate (through forced diuresis by fluid bolus and diuretics) may prevent hypovolemia from advancing to ARF. The increased urine flow helps to prevent casts and other debris from obstructing the tubules. When renal function is at risk, nephrotoxic agents such as the anesthetic methoxyflurane and the aminoglycoside antibiotics gentamicin or tobramycin should be avoided.

DIAGNOSTIC STUDIES AND FINDINGS

Urine pH: Lowered
Urine osmolality: Hyperosmotic, hyposmotic, or isoosmotic in relation to serum osmolality
Urine specific gravity: Prerenal: high; renal: low; postrenal: normal
Urine sodium: Prerenal: low; renal: increased; postrenal: normal
Urine creatinine: Prerenal: normal; renal: increased; postrenal: normal
Urine sediment: Normal or hematuria; proteinuria; double refractile fat bodies; bacteriuria; pyuria; casts
24-hour urine output: Olguric: <400 ml; nonoliguric: 1 to 2 L; diuretic phase: 2 to 3 L; recovery phase: near-normal volume
Hemoglobin (Hgb)/hematocrit (Hct): Anemia; hemoconcentration with dehydration; hemodilution with hypervolemia
Platelets: Decreased adhesiveness
White blood cell (WBC) count: Increased with infection
Serum pH: Low-acidotic
Serum bicarbonate: <22 mEq/L
Serum potassium: Hyperkalemia
Serum chloride: Normal or low, elevated
Serum sodium: Normal or low with hemodilution
Serum calcium: Low
Serum phosphate: High
Blood urea nitrogen (BUN): Increased
Serum creatinine: Increased
Ratio BUN/serum creatinine: 10:1 to 15:1; decreased urea concentration <10:1; decreased renal function >15:1
Serum osmolality: Increased
Creatinine clearance: Decreased with poor glomerular function; 50 to 84 ml/min (mild failure); 25 to 49 ml/min (moderate failure); <25 ml/min (severe failure)
Electrocardiogram (ECG): Dysrhythmias possible with hyperkalemia or hypokalemia, hypercalcemia or hypocalcemia
Kidney-ureter bladder (KUB) x-ray examination: Kidney is normal size, enlarged, or small
Renal ultrasound: Kidney size or shape may be abnormal
Intravenous urogram (IVU): Obstruction, strictures, or masses may be present
Renal scan: May reveal cysts, tumors, or impaired perfusion
Renal biopsy: May be necessary to determine cause and extent of injury

MULTIDISCIPLINARY PLAN

The goal of treatment is to prevent decreased renal perfusion from progressing to ARF. Fluids and diuretic agents may be used. The cause of the ARF is determined, if possible. Failing body systems are supported until recovery (see Emergency Alert box below). Evaluation for dialysis or transplantation may be necessary if recovery is not complete.

! EMERGENCY ALERT

ACUTE RENAL FAILURE

Acute or sudden renal failure (ARF) is a life-threatening event that requires immediate and comprehensive intervention.

ASSESSMENT

- Known renal failure history
- History of drug overdose or toxic injection that precipitated renal failure
- Laboratory values indicating renal failure

INTERVENTION

All intervention should be directed at maintaining maximum renal blood flow.

- Maintain airway, breathing, and circulation.
- Obtain IV access: Fluid replacement must be based on laboratory results *unless* patient is in shock.
- In collaboration with physician, administer medications carefully with attention to volumes.
- Record meticulously intake and output.
- Renal dialysis may be indicated.

The major complications of ARF in the oliguric-anuric stage are acidosis, hyperkalemia, infection, hyperphosphatemia, hypertension, and anemia. Hypovolemia and hypokalemia may be problems in the diuretic stage. Prompt and adequate management is essential to survival.

Medications[1]

Alkalinizing agents (for acidosis)

Sodium bicarbonate, 1-4 g/day PO, IV; 2-5 mEq/kg infused over 4-8 h

Sodium citrate and citric acid (Shohls' solution), 10-20 ml PO tid (1 mEq Na^+/ml)

Treatment for hyperkalemia

Sodium polystyrene sulfonate (Kayexalate, SPS), 15-30 g PO or enema qd-qid; give oral dose in 45-60 ml of water, syrup, or sorbital solution

- Calcium gluconate (Kalcinate), 1 g (90 mg Ca^{++}) in 10 ml IV
- Sodium bicarbonate, 2-5 mEq/kg IV infusion over 4-8 h
- Glucose 50%, 25-50 g IV, and insulin-regular, 10-15 units IV

Antihypertensive agents

Vasodilators

Sodium nitroprusside (Nipride), 0.5-10 μg/kg/min as required IV; in emergency, continuous infusion

Dopamine, 0.5-2 μg/kg/min; IV commonly given with furosemide to promote renal perfusion (dopamine dilates the renal vessels at low doses but causes vasoconstriction at other doses.)

Hydralazine, 20 mg IV for hypertensive crisis; may repeat as needed

Minoxidil, 5-10 mg PO bid for severe hypertension

Ace inhibitors

Long-acting preparations such as lisinopril or fosinopril (Monopril), 10-40 mg PO, or enalapril, 10 mg IV for acute hypertension

NOTE: Potassium and creatinine must be monitored because these drugs can cause an increase in both parameters in patients with renal disease.

Angiotensin receptor blockers

Losartan (angiotensin II receptor antagonist), 50-100 mg PO bid

Calcium channel blockers

Isradipine (dihydropyridine calcium channel antagonist), usual dosage 2.5-10 mg PO bid; maximum dosage 20 mg/day

Diltiazem (nondihydropyridine calcium channel antagonist), 180-360 mg PO usually given in divided dosages bid

Beta-adrenergic blockers

Atenolol (beta-1 selective antagonist), 25-50 mg PO qd; use with caution in diabetes and renal dysfunction

Alpha-receptor blockers

Doxazosin (alpha-receptor antagonist), 1-16 mg PO qd or qhs

Labetalol (combined alpha and beta antagonist), 200-600 mg PO bid, 2.4 g maximum

Centrally acting agents

Clonidine (Catapres), 0.1 mg PO bid or tid initially, then increase by 0.2-0.8 mg/day (maximum effective dose, 2.4 mg/day)

- May also use clonidine TTS, 0.1-0.3 mg once-a-week dermal patch; no taper required if patch is discontinued

Diuretics

Furosemide (Lasix), 20-500 mg PO qd or in divided doses; 2-10 mg/kg IV; not to exceed a rate of 4 mg/min; the dose depends on the degree of renal function; as function declines, the dose requirement increases

Bumetamide, 0.5-10 mg IV or PO

Mannitol, 25-200 g IV only; given as 5%-25% solution

Metolazone, 0.5-10 mg; rarely may use up to 150 mg PO only

Hydrochlorothiazide (HydroDIURIL, Esidrix), 25-100 mg/day PO or bid initially, then maintenance 25-100 mg/day according to patient's response (may be less effective than furosemide or bumetamide); hydrochlorothiazide not effective if GFR <30

Phosphate binders

Calcium acetate (PhosLo), 2 tabs (667 mg each) with each meal to start; 3-4 tabs per meal are usually required

Calcium carbonate, 1250 mg with meals; may use up to 12 g/24 h (NOTE: Serum calcium must be monitored as dose is increased.)

RenaGel, 403 mg, 6-12 caps total with meals, PO only

Agents used for hypovolemia: Normal saline solution, dextran, albumin

Agents used for hypotension: Vasopressors: norepinephrine and phentolamine IV

Miscellaneous

Calcitriol, 0.5-3 μg IV after dialysis

Sodium ferric gluconate, 125 mg IV for 8 doses; used for iron deficiency in place of iron dextran

Nephro-Vite (multivitamin preparation formulated for patients with renal failure), 1 tablet PO qd

Antiinfective agents

Infection is frequently a complication of ARF

Agents specific to microorganisms cultured should be used

Agents whose route of excretion is primarily renal should be omitted or used in smaller doses or at lengthened intervals, depending on GFR

Agents excreted by only the liver require no change in dosage; when partial excretion occurs via the kidney, some adjustment is needed at low GFRs

Particular care is needed in all drug administration: dosage, interval between doses, and recognition of increased sensitivity because of altered renal function[2]

General Management

Monitor and correct electrolyte and fluid abnormalities. Measure weight, potassium, creatinine/BUN, calcium, and phosphorus in particular

Dialysis, either hemodialysis or peritoneal dialysis, is used to manage fluid volume and electrolyte imbalances (see pp. 895-904); dialysis is particularly necessary with pulmonary edema, hyperkalemia, uremic pericarditis, and seizures; some nephrotoxic agents are dialyzable; hemodialysis is used in hypercatabolic patients to remove nitrogenous wastes and to control serum pH and potassium levels; peritoneal dialysis is not used in cases involving trauma, infection, immunosuppression, neutropenia, recent abdominal surgery, or severe liver disease

Continuous arteriovenous hemofiltration or continuous venovenous hemofiltration is used to remove fluid in an unstable patient, especially in an oliguric-anuric patient (see p. 905)

Fluid intake must equal amount needed to replace measurable losses in urine, nasogastric drainage, wound drainage, and estimated insensible losses; fluid overload must be avoided; daily weights reflect fluid gain or loss

Packed red blood cells may be needed if symptoms associated with anemia develop; Hgb levels should be higher than 10 g/dl

Nutritional support should include maintenance of body weight and positive nitrogen balance; a period of negative nitrogen balance and weight loss cannot be completely avoided but should be brief

Caloric intake should include 100 g of glucose per day

Excess carbohydrate intake can contribute to respiratory acidosis

Protein intake may be maintained through parenteral infusion of essential amino acids (50 to 85 g/L solutions); oral intake is started as soon as possible; desired protein intake is 0.5 to 0.6 g/kg/day or 1 to 1.5 g/kg/day if on dialysis with 70% of high biologic value; high-biologic-value proteins are those that contain essential amino acids in the proportions needed to promote growth, such as milk, eggs, and meat; serum albumin levels of 3 to 3.5 g/dl or higher are desirable; excess protein intake contributes to metabolic acidosis and increased nitrogenous wastes

Sodium intake is 0.5 to 1.0 g/day or 40 to 90 mEq/day depending on blood pressure; potassium in diet is restricted to 1500 mg/day or 60 mEq/day if hyperkalemia is present

Vitamin supplements are needed, since a limited protein diet is deficient in calcium and folic acid and low in phosphorus and the B vitamins; water-soluble vitamins are lost in dialysis

Mannitol and furosemide are infused with half-normal saline solution and 20 mEq KCl 12 hours before the use of contrast dye for radiographic purposes to prevent ARF or worsening of renal failure from contrast-induced dehydration; the infusion is titrated to maintain urine output at 200 to 400 ml/h and continued for 6 hours after procedure[14]

Phosphorous intake reduced if serum levels become elevated

Recent clinical trials show that early nutritional support improves ARF outcomes and that patients who are most ill will benefit the most[4]

Intravenous lipids may be used to maintain energy needs

Micronutrient needs are generally ill defined; since fat-soluble vitamins accumulate, they should be given twice a week. Water-soluble vitamins can be given daily

NURSING CARE

NURSING ASSESSMENT

Assessment in Acute and Chronic Renal Failure

NOTE: Those findings more typical of late chronic renal failure (ESRD) are indicated by an asterisk.

Cardiovascular-respiratory

Assess for changes indicative of volume depletion or overload: central venous pressure (CVP), rapid increase or decrease in weight, pulmonary wedge pressure change, heart rate (tachycardia), blood pressure (hypertension, hypotension, especially orthostatic changes), lungs (crackles, tachypnea, dyspnea, wheezes, Kussmaul breathing, cough, orthopnea, hyperventilation)

Assess for arrhythmias (primarily those caused by hyperkalemia or volume depletion)

*Pericardial friction rub

Neuromuscular

Assess for signs of *tetany (positive Chvostek's or Trousseau's sign because of hypocalcemia)

Assess for lethargy, orientation, lability, *increased DTRs, *insomnia, *restless leg syndrome, *other motor and sensory neuropathies, *change in level of consciousness (somnolence or coma); change in cognitive function; change in behavior; asterixis; seizures

Renal: Urine volume normal, oliguria, or anuria; nocturia; change in color or odor

Gastrointestinal: *Nausea; *vomiting; *anorexia; hematemesis; melena; *stomatitis; *metallic taste in mouth

Hematologic: Pale mucous membranes; *pallor

Skin: Bruises; *pruritus; dry skin

Skeletal: Assess for *growth retardation in children, and *osteopenia and *osteoporosis in children and adults secondary to parathyroid hyperactivity and hypocalcemia

General: Fever, headache, periorbital edema, CVA tenderness, muscle cramps, weakness, fatigue

Psychosocial: Assess family structure for available support and potential stressors; response to illness, treatment, prognosis; self-care capabilities

Nutrition: *Assess muscle wasting, decrease in tissue weight (dry weight), laboratory evidence of nutritional excess or deficit

POTENTIAL COMPLICATIONS

Myocardial infarction (MI) or CVA resulting from hypertension; pulmonary edema and respiratory failure; hyperkalemia and resultant cardiac arrhythmias; other electrolyte disorders (hypocalcemia, hyperphosphatemia); acidosis; anemia; capillary and tissue necrosis from massive edema; chronic renal failure and ESRD

PATIENT PROBLEMS/NURSING DIAGNOSES & INTERVENTIONS

NIC TISSUE PERFUSION MANAGEMENT

Ineffective tissue perfusion related to damage to nephrons from hypovolemia, ischemia, toxins, or obstruction

Deficient fluid volume related to decreased effective circulating blood volume resulting from active losses and failure of regulatory mechanisms

Excess fluid volume related to sodium and water retention

- Goal: Correct perfusion deficit, improve gas exchange, and return kidney function to normal.
- Monitor for all of the signs of renal failure listed in the assessment section (e.g., increasing BUN, creatinine, potassium) *to evaluate the kidney's ability to excrete nitrogenous wastes, excess fluids, and electrolytes.*
- Recognize blood pressure alterations consistent with renal failure, *to identify changes in fluid status.*
- Weigh daily and monitor trends, *to identify changes in fluid status.*

- Maintain accurate intake and output record. Include nasogastric drainage, emesis, etc., in intake and output (I/O).
- Weigh linens/pads *to determine corrected output.*
- Administer positive inotropic/contractility medications *to increase systemic resistance and blood pressure and thus renal blood flow.*
- Administer medications as ordered (e.g., antiarrhythmic agents, vasodilators for hypertension or vasoconstrictors for hypotension, or diuretics).
- Administer blood products as ordered *to correct anemia.*
- Administer IV erythropoietin, and iron as ordered *to correct anemia.*
- Monitor for side effects of IV iron therapy, myalgia, bone pain, and anaphylaxis.
- Restrict free water intake in the presence of serum sodium level below 130 mEq/L.
- Evaluate adverse and positive effects of medications.
- Maintain fluid balance by administering IV fluids as ordered *to maintain adequate tissue perfusion.*
- Evaluate effects of delivered fluid dose.
- Elevate head of bed as appropriate unless hypovolemic patient cannot tolerate position.
- Place in Trendelenburg position as appropriate *for hypotension or shock.*
- Insert urinary catheter *to accurately determine urine output only if patient cannot otherwise cooperate.*
- Prepare for dialysis as indicated.
- Obtain nephrology nurse consultation.
- Offer patient education regarding technical procedure and psychoemotional adjustment.

NIC Electrolyte and Acid-Base Management

Risk for imbalanced fluid volume related to altered tissue perfusion

- Monitor for abnormal serum electrolyte levels and for manifestations of electrolyte imbalance.
- Place on a cardiac monitor *to determine dysrhythmias related to increase or decrease in potassium.* Monitor for ECG changes associated with hyperkalemia (heart block, peaked T waves, fibrillation).
- Maintain patent IV access *to ensure adequate intake if necessary.*
- Consult physician on use of potassium-sparing diuretics as appropriate (spironolactone, triamterene); administer as ordered and monitor response *to determine effect of drug and side effects such as hypokalemia and ototoxicity.*
- Administer electrolytes or ions as indicated/ordered (most likely is calcium) *to maintain adequate balance.*
- Administer electrolyte-binding resins (e.g., Kayexalate) as prescribed *to prevent hyperkalemia,* usually 15 to 30 g every 4 to 6 hours in a 20% sorbitol solution.
- Administer prescribed medications *to shift potassium into cell (50% glucose and insulin, bicarbonate, and IV calcium preparations).*
- Correct acid-base balance as indicated; most commonly need to give bicarbonate *to correct acidosis.*
- Monitor for side effects of IV calcium administration (thrombophlebitis, soft tissue necrosis with extravasation).
- Monitor for neuromuscular effects of hypocalcemia (tetany, cramping, muscle twitches, altered DTRs) and for signs of overcorrection.
- Administer phosphate binders (calcium acetate or carbonate, short-term aluminum-based liquid antacid; long-term use causes aluminum toxicity).
- Monitor for signs of hyperphosphatemia (e.g., pruritus, hypocalcemia, hypomagnesemia, acidosis).
- Monitor for central nervous system (CNS) changes associated with hypocalcemia (anxiety, depression, psychosis).
- Obtain ordered laboratory specimens *to measure electrolytes and acid-base balance.*

NIC Nutrition Support

Imbalanced nutrition: less than body requirements, related to altered absorption of nutrients and restricted dietary intake

- Provide diet appropriate for patient's electrolyte imbalance (e.g., low K^+, PO_4, high CA^{++}).
- Avoid potassium-based salt substitutes.
- Provide total parenteral nutrition (TPN) *to correct catabolic state in acute disease as ordered.*
- Monitor for electrolyte imbalance due to TPN.
- Monitor food intake and dry weight; encourage food intake as prescribed or administer enteral or parenteral feedings *to ensure adequate intake within limits prescribed;* weight is assessed *to determine if weight changes are related to fluid balance or to inadequate caloric intake and the loss of muscle mass.*
- Monitor for nausea, vomiting, and anorexia; *these conditions decrease intake of needed nutrients.*
- Provide oral hygiene regularly *to improve taste in mouth.*
- Monitor laboratory data: serum protein, lipids, potassium, calcium. Refer complex problems to dietitian; team approach to managing renal diet is helpful to all concerned.

NIC Risk Management

Risk for infection related to suppressed immune response associated with azotemia

- Monitor for signs and symptoms of infection in secretions, excretions, and exudates, and assess for fever *to detect any infection early.*
- Monitor laboratory data: white blood cell count; temperature every 4 to 6 hours; levels may be only slightly increased in azotemia.
- Wash hands thoroughly and consistently; avoid exposing patient to persons with infection; ensure aseptic technique for any invasive procedure or wound care *to decrease chances for infection.*
- Encourage regular oral hygiene, hand washing, bathing, adequate rest, and nutrition *to help prevent infections.*

Risk for acute confusion related to delirium from endogenous chemical abnormalities associated with azotemia

- Monitor orientation to time, place, and person; this knowledge is lost as mental status is altered. Orient patient to reality *to decrease the possibility that disorientation is caused by isolation and lack of information.*

- Maintain safety precautions: bed rails up, sharp objects out of reach, and call bell within reach *to provide a safe environment and to prevent injury.*

NIC Self-Care Facilitation

Risk for bathing/hygiene and toileting self-care deficits related to side effects of azotemia
Ineffective therapeutic regimen management

- Assist with care as needed *to help patient return to self-care as appropriate.*
- Implement measures such as deep breathing, coughing, and turning *to prevent adverse side effects of bed rest, such as pneumonia.*

NIC Crisis Management

Ineffective coping, self and family, related to situational crisis
Interrupted family processes related to health crisis in family member

- Assess family structure and role relationships; monitor family's response to the illness, treatment, and prognosis; encourage verbalization of needs and concerns; discuss impact on roles and adaptation required; identify family strengths; assist with problem solving; support family decisions; crisis intervention may be all that is needed.
- Refer patient and family to other services as appropriate *to help resolve problems requiring time and skills beyond the nurse's capabilities.*

NIC Patient Education

Deficient knowledge related to ARF, its causes, manifestations, and treatment; need for medical follow-up; and the potential need for dialysis or transplantation in the future

- Provide patient with access to National Kidney Foundation educational materials.
- Provide opportunity for patient to talk to a nurse educator or advanced practice nurse with background in kidney disease and dialysis care.

Patient Education/Continuum of Care Plan

1. Explain the cause of the episode of ARF.
2. Explain the level of renal function after the acute phase is over.
3. Explain diet and fluid restrictions, which may continue or be lessened or discontinued.
4. Help patient practice self-observation skills, such as measuring temperature, pulse, respirations, blood pressure, I/O, daily weight, and record keeping.
5. Explain good personal hygiene.
6. Explain how to avoid infections.
7. Explain exercise and rest in the amounts advised.
8. Describe medications, if any, with name, purpose, dosage, time interval, and adverse reactions (by discussion and in writing).
9. Explain the schedule of medical follow-up.
10. Explain renal dialysis and transplantation if they are likely options for the future.

Evaluation/Patient Outcomes

Tissue Perfusion Management: Renal tissue perfusion is adequate. Renal function tests are normal or stable. Fluid balance is normal. Urine volume is normal and balances intake; there is no sign of edema, hypertension, or hypotension.

Electrolyte and Acid-Base Management: Laboratory values are within normal limits. Serum pH is normal without medications or renal replacement therapy. Serum electrolytes are normal without medications or renal replacement therapy.

Nutrition Support: Nutritional status is normal. No restrictions are required on food or fluids.

Risk Management: No infection is present. No signs or symptoms of infection are noted. No clinical evidence of immune dysfunction is seen. There is no confusion. Patient is oriented to time, place, and person.

Self-Care Facilitation: Patient has resumed self-care. Patient has no restrictions in activities of daily living (ADLs).

Crisis Management: Family has adapted to patient's illness and recovery. The family has dealt with the crisis constructively and can identify sources of help available.

Patient Education: Patient and family are knowledgeable about ARF. Patient and family can explain ARF, its causes, manifestations, and treatment; the need for medical follow-up; and the potential need for dialysis or transplantation in the future.

Chronic Renal Failure

Chronic renal failure (CRF) is a slow, insidious, and irreversible impairment of renal function. Uremia usually develops slowly.

Major causes of CRF include diabetic nephropathy, nephrosclerosis (hypertensive nephropathy), glomerulonephritis, and polycystic kidney disease. CRF can arise as primary renal disease or secondary to other systemic diseases. Primary renal disease includes glomerulonephritis, pyelonephritis, polycystic kidneys, and renal cell carcinoma. Renal problems that develop secondary to systemic disease include lupus nephritis, renal amyloidosis, myeloma kidney, nephrocalcinosis, and hereditary nephropathy, as well as diabetic nephropathy and nephrosclerosis.

Stages of CRF are identified by changes in the GFR. A reduced GFR of 25 ml/min or more is considered CRF. When the GFR is less than 25 ml/min, it is considered ESRD. Uremic symptoms are prominent in ESRD.

Patients vary greatly in their clinical picture, renal function, and performance capabilities. Criteria for evaluating the severity of established renal disease must therefore take into account the severity of the signs and symptoms, the level of impairment of the patient's renal function (GFR and serum creatinine), and the patient's performance level (what the patient says he or she is able to do). Dialysis is begun when all of these parameters suggest uremia.

PATHOPHYSIOLOGY

The various causes of failing renal function eventually lead to a final common pathway. Often the specific, initial renal insult cannot be identified.

When the kidneys fail, a variety of substances accumulate that normally are excreted. These substances include fluid, nitrogenous wastes, the so-called uremic toxins, and normal substances, such as electrolytes that may alter cellular function (i.e., enzyme pathways).

A variety of pathogenic processes can cause CRF. Infections, for example, may be localized or may accompany systemic disease. Autoimmune disorders may be caused by antigen-antibody complexes and anti–glomerular basement membrane antibodies. Metabolic disorders such as renal tubular acidosis and calcium-phosphate abnormalities may cause renal calculi. Renovascular changes may arise from occlusion, stenosis, thrombosis, diabetes mellitus, or hypertension. Urinary obstruction, renal cancer, and congenital anomalies may also end in CRF. These topics are discussed in some detail in this section.

Nephrons are permanently destroyed by various processes that occur in the course of renal disease, such as ischemia, inflammation, necrosis, fibrosis, sclerosis, and scarring. The normal nephrons remaining may respond with hypertrophy and hyperplasia. However, eventually a point is reached when renal deficits become manifest (as many as 50% of the nephrons may be lost before renal deficits are discovered). Such deficits include the inability to respond to excessive salt intake or decreased water or salt intake, a decreased synthesis of substances such as erythropoietin by the kidney, or the inability to excrete the end products of metabolism. All the organ systems are eventually affected by renal dysfunction (see box below).

Changes in renal function may be manifested by an increase or decrease in substances usually found in the body (e.g., hemoglobin, BUN, serum creatinine, sodium, potassium, calcium, and phosphate). The body's attempts to accommodate these changes eventually fail and result in pathologic mechanisms such as hypertension; pulmonary edema; altered protein, carbohydrate and fat metabolism; and osteodystrophy. Mental status, peripheral nerve conduction time, and platelet adhesiveness are also altered.

COMPLICATIONS OF CHRONIC RENAL FAILURE

- Anemia
- Hypertension
- Hyperkalemia
- Congestive heart failure
- Pulmonary edema
- Pericarditis
- Accelerated atherosclerosis
- Coagulopathy
- Peptic ulcer disease
- Osteodystrophy
- Metabolic encephalopathy
- Peripheral neuropathy
- Acidosis
- Hyperphosphatemia
- Immune dysfunction
- Sexual dysfunction
- Pruritus

DIAGNOSTIC STUDIES AND FINDINGS

Urinalysis: pH: acidic; osmolality: low; specific gravity: fixed; sediment: may contain white blood cells (WBCs), red blood cells (RBCs), normal and granular, hyaline, broad, and waxy WBC, RBC casts; 24-hour volume decreased or nonexistent; proteinuria

Complete blood count: Hgb/Hct lowered; decreased RBC survival time; platelets reduced in number with decreased adhesiveness

Blood chemistry: Decreased serum pH, bicarbonate calcium and sodium; increased creatinine, potassium, sodium, magnesium, hydrogen, and phosphate; increased serum uric acid, osmolality, BUN; decreased iron and total iron-binding capacity, percent saturation; creatinine clearance: decreased

KUB x-ray: Small, contracted kidneys, renal cysts, or mass

Renal ultrasound: Small, contracted kidneys, renal cysts or mass

MULTIDISCIPLINARY PLAN

Aggressive management of CRF should be initiated before marked decreases in renal function are noted, and it is continued until the need for dialysis or transplantation is determined. The principles guiding management are (1) treat underlying renal disease; (2) prolong the life of the native kidneys; (3) identify and prevent causes of ARF in the presence of CRF; (4) treat the complications of CRF; and (5) relieve the symptoms of uremia.

Surgery

Renal transplantation (p. 908), creation of an internal arteriovenous fistula, Gortex graft, or placement of a semipermanent double-lumen cuffed catheter in the internal jugular or superior vena cava for hemodialysis or insertion of a Tenckhoff catheter for peritoneal dialysis

Medications

Alkalinizing agents (for acidosis)

Sodium bicarbonate, 1-4 g/day PO, IV; 2-5 mEq/kg infused over 4-8 h

Sodium citrate and citric acid (Shohl's solution), 10-20 ml PO qd

Treatment for hyperkalemia

Sodium polystyrene sulfonate (Kayexalate, SPS), PO or enema, 15-30 g qd-qid; give oral dose in 45-60 ml of water, syrup, or sorbital solution

Calcium gluconate (Kalcinate), IV, 1 g (90 mg Ca^{++}) in 10 ml

Sodium bicarbonate, IV, 2-5 mEq/kg infusion over 4-8 h

Glucose 50%, IV, 25-50 g, and insulin-regular, IV, 10-15 units

Antihypertensive agents

Vasodilators

Sodium nitroprusside (Nipride), IV, in emergency, continuous infusion, 0.5-10 μg/kg/min as required

Dopamine, 1-2 μg/kg/min IV, commonly given with furosemide to promote renal perfusion (dopamine dilates the renin vessels at low doses but causes vasoconstriction at higher doses.)

Ace Inhibitors

Long-acting preparations such as lisinopril or fosinopril (Monopril), 10-40 mg PO, or enalapril, 10 mg IV for acute hypertension

Potassium and creatinine must be monitored because these drugs can cause an increase in both parameters in patients with renal disease.

Angiotensin II receptor antagonist: Losartan (angiotensin II receptor antagonist), 50 mg PO bid

Calcium channel blockers

Isradipine (dihydropyridine calcium channel antagonist), usual dosage 2.5-10 mg PO bid; maximum dosage 20 mg/day

Diltiazem (nondihydropyridine calcium channel antagonist), 180-360 mg PO usually given in divided dosages bid

Beta-adrenergic antagonist: Atenolol (beta-1 selective antagonist), 25-50 mg PO qd; use with caution in diabetes and renal dysfunction

Alpha-receptor antagonist

Doxazosin (alpha-receptor antagonist), 1-16 mg PO qd or qhs

Labetalol (combined alpha and beta antagonist), 200-600 mg bid, 2.4 g maximum/24h

Centrally acting agents

Clonidine (Catapres), PO, 0.1 mg bid or tid initially, then increase by 0.2-0.8 mg/day (maximum effective dose, 2.4 mg/day)

May also use clonidine TTS, 0.1-0.3 mg once-a-week dermal patch; no taper required if patch is discontinued

Diuretics

Furosemide (Lasix), 20-500 mg PO qd or in divided doses; IV 2-10 mg/kg; not to exceed a rate of 4 mg/min; the dose depends on the degree of renal function; as function declines, dose requirement increases; maximum daily dose 500 mg

Bumetamide, 0.5-10 mg IV or PO

Mannitol, 25-200 g IV only; given as 5%-25% solution

Metolazone, 0.5-10 mg; rarely may use up to 150 mg PO only

Hydrochlorothiazide (HydroDIURIL, Esidrix), PO, 25-100 mg/day or bid initially, then maintenance 25-100 mg/day according to patient's response; not effective if GFR is less than 30

Phosphate binders

Calcium acetate (PhosLo), 2 tabs (667 mg each) with each meal to start; 3-4 tabs per meal are usually required

Calcium carbonate, 1250 mg with meals; may use up to 12 g/24h

Renagel, 403 mg 6-12 caps with meals; PO only

Agents used for hypovolemia: Normal saline solution, dextran, albumin

Agents used for hypotension: Vasopressors: norepinephrine and phentolamine IV

Miscellaneous

Calcitriol IV, 0.5-3 μg IV after dialysis

Sodium ferric gluconate, 125 mg IV for 8 doses; used for iron deficiency in place of iron dextran

Nephro-Vite (multivitamin preparation formulated for patients with renal failure), 1 tablet PO qd

Antiinfective agents

Infection is frequently a complication of ARF and CRF

Agents specific to the microorganism cultured should be used

Agents whose route of excretion is primarily renal should be omitted or used in smaller doses or at lengthened intervals depending on GFR

NURSING CARE

Nursing Assessment

Renal: Oliguria; anuria or normal output

Cardiovascular: Pitting edema; hypertension; tachycardia; jugular venous distention; pericardial friction rub; S_4; systolic murmur

Dermatologic: Pruritus; excoriations; yellow-tan or grayish color; pallor; uremic frost; bruises; petechiae; purpura; fragile, dry skin; thin, brittle nails

Gastrointestinal: Urinelike odor on breath; metallic taste in mouth; stomatitis and gingivitis; loss of sense of smell; anorexia; nausea; vomiting and hematemesis; hiccoughs; melena; diarrhea or constipation, ascites

Neurologic: Changes in cognitive function and behavior; altered levels of consciousness; changes in motor function and proprioception; peripheral neuropathy; nocturnal leg cramping; restless leg syndromes; paresthesias of lower extremities; apathy, lethargy, and fatigue; headaches; insomnia; somnolence; hyperreflexia; tetany

Ocular: Calcification of conjunctiva (red eyes); blurred vision; periorbital edema

Reproductive: Impotence; amenorrhea; decreased libido; gynecomastia

Respiratory: Hyperventilation; Kussmaul breathing; apnea; altered lung sounds (rales, rhonchi, crackles); dyspnea; orthopnea; distant breath sounds

Musculoskeletal: Bone pain; joint swelling and pain; myalgias, osteopenia; osteoporosis

General: Insomnia; weight loss (muscle mass); weight gain (fluid accumulation); fever; chills

Psychosocial: Change in family relationships; family expresses concern about long-term implications of illness; patient denial, depression, and anger are common

Potential Complications

ESRD, immunodeficiency/frequent infections, renal osteodystrophy, iron deficiency anemia, secondary hyperparathyroidism, hypocalcemia, hyperphosphatemia, acidosis, and hyperkalemia, and all of their systemic complications; hepatitis A, B, and C; pleural effusions, pulmonary edema, congestive heart failure, moderate to severe hypertension, coagulopathies, CVA, acquired renal cysts, and renal cancer

Patient Problems/Nursing Diagnoses & Interventions

NIC Tissue Perfusion Management

Ineffective renal tissue perfusion related to nephron destruction with inability to excrete metabolic wastes

- Fluid volume excess related to failure of regulatory mechanisms
- Monitor ECG for changes; respirations (rate and depth); Chvostek's and Trousseau's signs. *Peaked T waves, prolonged PR interval, and widened QRS complex are associated with increased serum potassium; Kussmaul respirations are associated with acidosis; tetany may occur with low-calcium level. Increase or decrease in potassium*

may be associated with dysrhythmias; potassium may be lowered by vigorous diuretic therapy.

- Monitor laboratory data: serum pH, potassium, bicarbonate, calcium, magnesium, phosphate; hemoglobin and hematocrit; BUN; serum creatinine. *Levels reflect kidneys' ability to excrete nitrogenous wastes, excess fluids, and electrolytes; values also indicate kidneys' nonexcretory functions (e.g., erythropoietin production).*
- Avoid nephrotoxic drugs; kidneys' ability to excrete drugs normally is reduced.
- Administer medications with care; monitor response to drugs. Doses of medications may be less than usual, and intervals between doses may be lengthened; *monitoring determines the effectiveness of drug, dosage, and timing and aids in identifying adverse side effects.*
- Prepare for dialysis by explaining procedure to patient and family.
- Monitor weight daily, also 24-hour intake and output; assess blood pressure (standing and sitting), pulse, and respirations (including breath sounds) every 6 to 8 hours; assess mental status; monitor edema, jugular venous distention, hepatojugular reflex, and, if necessary, central venous pressure and pulmonary artery pressures *to identify altered fluid status.*
- Offer limited fluid intake over 24 hours, since the kidney's normal diurnal variation in urine output is lost; offer cool liquids that may help quench thirst. Limit volume to 1500 ml/24h in ESRD.
- Administer diuretics as ordered; monitor response *to determine the effect of drugs and observe for side effects such as hypokalemia and ototoxicity.*

NIC Nutrition Support

Imbalanced nutrition: less than body requirements, related to alterations in absorption

- Advise how to limit foods high in potassium, phosphorus.
- Monitor lipid profile and treat hyperlipidemia as ordered. If patient is taking a statin-type drug, monitor AST.
- Provide oral hygiene before meals; offer gum or sour candy *to help remove bad taste from mouth.*
- Administer antiemetics and monitor response *to determine the effect of dosage and timing and to observe for adverse side effects.*
- Monitor for hypocalcemia (serum calcium <9.0 MEq/L and hypoalbuminemia (serum albumin <3.5 g/dL); administer supplements and obtain a nutrition consult. NOTE: Calcium given with meals acts as a phosphorus binder, *not* as a calcium supplement. Give between meals to promote absorption.
- Monitor for signs of iron deficiency and treat with oral or IV iron as ordered. Be familiar with and protect against complications of iron therapy (e.g., primarily, constipation, gastric irritation, allergy).
- Nutritional supplements and vitamins should be specially formulated for patients with renal failure.

NIC Risk Management

Risk for infection related to suppressed immunity

- Monitor temperature every 4 to 6 hours; if indicated, monitor laboratory data: white blood cell (WBC) count; blood, urine, and sputum cultures; serum potassium. *Uremia may mask the usual increase in temperature and WBC count found with infection; a hypermetabolic state such as infection can cause a marked rise in the serum potassium level.*
- Wash hands thoroughly and consistently; avoid exposing patient to people with infections; ensure aseptic technique for any invasive procedure or wound care *to decrease chances of infection.*
- Encourage regular oral hygiene, hand washing, bathing, adequate nutrition, and rest; *good health habits help prevent infection.*

Risk for chronic confusion related to delirium from endogenous chemical abnormalities associated with uremia

- Assess neurologic status; orientation to person, place, and time; sleep pattern; level of consciousness; and seizure activity; *such changes reflect alterations in central and autonomic nervous system function.*
- Assess premorbid personality *to identify changes associated with uremia.*
- Observe for changes in behavior and presence of peripheral neuropathy: restless legs, burning feet, muscle cramps, other paresthesias, and dysesthesias *because metabolic changes may cause cerebral and peripheral neurologic dysfunction; demyelination of large nerve fiber and axonal degeneration may occur.*
- Orient patient to reality *to decrease the possibility that disorientation is caused by isolation and lack of information.*
- Maintain safety precautions: bed rails up, bed in low position, sharp objects out of reach, call bell in reach; institute seizure precautions if needed *to provide safe environment and prevent injury.*
- Allow extra time for patient to respond to questions and process new information; use consistent, calm, nonargumentative approach; *short-term memory loss may occur.*
- Encourage normal daytime activities and presleep relaxation training; provide periods of rest *to maintain or encourage normal sleep-rest patterns; uremia can reverse sleep-wake patterns.*

NIC Skin/Wound Management

Impaired skin integrity related to altered metabolic state the effects of uremia

- Assess for dry skin, pruritus, excoriation, and infection; *such changes may be related to decreased activity of sweat glands or desposits of calcium or phosphate crystals in cutaneous layers.*
- Assess for petechiae and purpura; *bleeding abnormalities are related to decreased number and altered function of platelets in uremia.*
- Monitor skin folds and edematous areas *because these areas are easily injured.*
- Provide meticulous care to normal and injured areas of skin *to prevent infection and to help healing.*
- Administer antipruritic drugs; vinegar or starch baths; use bland soap sparingly *to relieve pruritus.*
- Keep fingernails trimmed *to decrease injury during scratching.*

NIC Self-Care Facilitation

Bathing/hygiene and toileting related to weakness or tiredness self-care deficit

- Assess fatigue and weakness, and assist with care as needed *to respond to need for assistance.*
- Implement measures such as deep breathing, coughing, and turning regularly *to prevent adverse effects of bed rest, such as pneumonia.*
- Increase activity as tolerated *to help patient return to self-care as appropriate.*

NIC Coping Assistance

Sexual dysfunction related to altered body function from effects of uremia

Disturbed body image related to biophysical changes

- Assess patient's and spouse's response to alterations *to determine presence of problems related to libido and sexual function.*
- Allow patient and spouse or significant other to talk about their feelings; suggest the positive aspects of closeness and touching without intercourse *to help patient and spouse adjust to changes.*
- Refer patient and spouse for counseling when needed *to help resolve problems requiring time and skills beyond the nurse's training.*
- Allow patient to talk about feelings; recognize defense mechanisms such as denial, guilt, aggression, fear, displacement, regression, resentment, disbelief, and anxiety; recognize losses in psychosocial aspects of patient's life; isolation, job loss, financial instability, dependency, and altered hopes for the future may be problems; *early intervention may prevent patient distress.*
- Explain skin changes to patient (in color, easy bruising); *pallor may be caused by anemia, yellowish cast by urochrome pigment deposits in skin; black patients become more deeply pigmented, and Hispanics and Asians show pallor.*

NIC Life Span Care

Interrupted family processes related to change in health status of family member

- Monitor family's response to illness, treatment, and prognosis *to identify potential problems and strengths.*
- Encourage patient and family to discuss their needs and concerns; discuss impact of situation on roles and adaptation required *to help in adjustments indicated.*
- Assist with problem solving, and support family decisions; crisis intervention may be needed.
- Refer family to other services as appropriate *to help resolve problems requiring time and skills beyond the nurse's capability.*

Patient Education/Continuum of Care Plan

1. Explain the nature of chronic renal failure.
2. Explain the medical regimen and its rationale, including diet (restricted protein, sodium, and potassium intake), restricted fluid intake, and medications (purpose, dosage, interval, and adverse reactions).
3. Help patient learn self-observational skills (temperature, pulse, respirations, blood pressure, intake and output, and weight) and record keeping.
4. Explain avoidance of infection.
5. Explain personal hygiene, rest, and exercise.
6. Explain when to call the physician.
7. Explain the plan for medical follow-up.
8. Explain renal dialysis and transplantation.

Evaluation/Patient Outcomes

Tissue Perfusion Management: Renal tissue perfusion is adequate. Renal function tests are normal or stable. Fluid balance is normal. Urine output balances intake; there are no or minimum signs of edema.

Nutrition Support: Patient's nutritional status has improved and is maintained. Food and fluid intakes are within the limits imposed by CRF; dry weight is maintained or increased if necessary.

Risk Management: No infection is present. No signs or symptoms of infection are noted. No confusion is present. Patient is oriented to time, place, and person; alterations in sensation are not progressing; sleep pattern is normal. Mobility is not a risk if mental status is affected.

Skin/Wound Management: Skin is intact. Patient has no areas of excoriation.

Self-Care Facilitation: Patient has resumed self-care with few or no restrictions in ADLs.

Coping Assistance: Patient has accepted alterations in sexuality and has satisfactory relationships within the limits imposed by condition. Patient has adapted to any changes in body image and physical appearance that have occurred as a result of altered renal function.

Life Span Care: Patient has adapted to changes in body image associated with CRF. Patient demonstrates adjustment to altered renal function and any change in appearance. Patient and family have adapted to patient's disorder. Patient and family have dealt constructively with diagnosis and treatment regimen and can identify available sources of help. Patient and family are knowledgeable about CRF. Patient and family can explain CRF, its causes, and its manifestations; the need for medical follow-up; and the potential need for dialysis or transplantation in the future.

PYELONEPHRITIS

Pyelonephritis is an inflammatory condition of the kidney most often caused by a bacterial infection of the upper urinary tract that can be separated into an acute or chronic form. Pyelonephritis may be further classified as complicated or uncomplicated.

The chronic form is the result of repeated difficult-to-eradicate infections and is associated with chronic renal disease. This type will not be discussed.

Acute pyelonephritis (AP) may be uncomplicated, in which case it is not associated with nonreversible renal disease, only upper tract infection; it may be classified as acute complicated pyelonephritis, which may involve obstruction, or it may be a complication of any other type of renal disease. AP usually involves a clinical syndrome of dysuria, frequency, chills, flank pain, myalgias, malaise, and fatigue. Gastrointestinal symptoms are see in 10% of the cases. Note that these symptoms may not be present collectively and the patient may still have AP.

PATHOPHYSIOLOGY

Risk factors are female gender, increased age, pregnancy, intercourse, use of spermicides, postcoital micturition, instrumentation of the tract, urinary tract obstruction or anatomic abnormalities, sickle cell disease or trait, diabetes, and frequent or chronic lower urinary tract infections.

Escherichia coli is the most common causative organism, closely followed by *Klebsiella, Aerobactor, Proteus,* and *Serratia.* The medulla, the area around the loops of Henle, and the papilla are the most involved because these areas have a concentration of interstium, the tissue preferred by the offending bacteria.[20,27]

DIAGNOSTIC STUDIES AND FINDINGS

Urinalysis: RBCs, bacteriuria, WBCs, WBC casts, bacterial casts

Blood cultures: Positive if sepsis accompanies

Urine cultures: Positive for infecting organism

CBC: Increased WBC count (granulocytosis)

Ultrasound: May demonstrate obstruction (stones, enlarged kidney)

Voiding cystogram: Ureteral reflux

Intravenous pyelogram: Unnecessary in acute phase; should not be done during pregnancy; irregular outline of renal system indicates edema

MULTIDISCIPLINARY PLAN

Surgery

Surgery is indicated for certain types of obstruction. Appropriate antibacterial therapy is always combined with surgery for effective treatment.

Medications

Initial antimicrobial programs are to achieve two objectives: the regimen chosen is likely to be 99% effective against the offending organism, and accurate blood levels can be reliably achieved in a particular patient. Any antibiotic regimen that achieves these goals is acceptable; often cost is the determining factor in the selection of one over another. With the above goals in mind, several previously used drugs—ampicillin, amoxicillin, and first-generation cephalosporins—are eliminated because 20%-30% of infecting organisms are now found to be resistant to these drugs.

If it is not possible to perform a Gram's stain of the urine, initial coverage should include antimicrobials that treat gram-negative and gram-positive organisms. For example, vancomycin and gentamicin together accomplish this goal in a cost-effective manner. If only gram-negative organisms are involved, there are many options.

Drugs Used for the Most Complicated Infections

NOTE: Dose reduction or interval extension method should be used if the creatinine clearance is decreased. See American Hospital Formulary Service Drug Information for dosages in renal failure.

Otherwise use:

Imipenem-cilastatin, 250 mg-1 g IV q6h
Ceftazidime, 1 g IV, IM q8-12h
Aztreonam, 500 mg-1 g q8-12h (2 g in severe infections)
Piperacillin-tazobactam, 125-200 mg/kg in divided doses

All IV antibiotics are followed with an oral course of antibiotic with good urinary tract penetration. For example, one of the most commonly used regimens is a large dose of gentamicin, 10 mg/kg IV, followed by an oral fluoroquinolone (ciprofloxacin), 500-750 mg bid or ds.

Trimethoprim-sulfamethoxazole double strength, bid for 14 days

General Management

The goals of treatment are to eradicate the infection, relieve the symptoms, and prevent recurrence.

High normal fluid intake (3500 to 4500 ml/day) is prescribed to dilute urine, decrease burning on urination, flush out the urinary tract, and prevent dehydration (with normal renal function).

Bed rest is commonly encouraged during acute phase.

NURSING CARE

NURSING ASSESSMENT

General: Sudden onset of fever, chills, dull constant pain in flank

Renal: Hematuria; bacteriuria; pyuria; urine culture: significant growth; dysuria; nocturia; frequency; urgency; suprapubic tenderness occasionally

POTENTIAL COMPLICATIONS

Perinephric abscess, septicemia, pericarditis, chronic renal failure

PATIENT PROBLEMS/NURSING DIAGNOSES & INTERVENTIONS

NIC THERMOREGULATION

Risk for imbalanced body temperature related to effects of infection

- Monitor signs of infection. Record temperature q8h and review WBC count. Note that rigors are a sign of systemic infection and should be reported. *Their presence may indicate the need for blood cultures and IV antibiotic therapy.*
- Administer antiinfective agents as ordered, and monitor response; monitor laboratory data: urinalysis and WBC count *to determine effects of drugs and to watch for adverse side effects.*

- Encourage bed rest during acute phase of illness *to increase patient's comfort.*
- Encourage high-normal fluid intake unless contraindicated *to flush kidneys (but avoid lowering drug concentration to ineffective levels).*

NIC PHYSICAL COMFORT PROMOTION

Acute pain in flank related to distention of renal capsule
Fatigue and activity intolerance related to disease state

- Administer analgesics as needed. As swelling in the kidney decreases, pain lessens; *analgesics promote comfort.*
- Apply heat externally to painful area *to help relieve pain.*
- Provide opportunity to rest and assistance for activities of daily living (ADLs).

PATIENT EDUCATION/CONTINUUM OF CARE PLAN

1. Explain pyelonephritis: its causes, signs, symptoms, and the need to have an IV urogram to rule out any structural defect.
2. Explain antimicrobial therapy: drugs, dosage, interval, side effects, and the need to complete the course of treatment.
3. Explain the possibility of relapse or reinfection.
4. Explain measures to prevent urinary tract infection, including adequate fluid intake (2000 to 2500 ml/day for adults) to avoid dehydration, regular emptying of bladder to avoid overdistention, and good perineal hygiene and postcoital elimination for women to prevent the entrance of microorganisms from the urinary tract.

EVALUATION/PATIENT OUTCOMES

Thermoregulation: Signs and symptoms of PLN have cleared. Patient's temperature is normal; urine is clear of bacteria or pus cells; problems in urination are gone.

Physical Comfort Promotion: Patient does not experience pain.

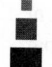

RENAL AND URINARY TRACT OBSTRUCTION

Obstructive uropathy refers to the structures or functional changes in the urinary tract that include the normal flow of urine. Obstructive nephropathy is the resultant renal parenchymal disease that occurs because of physical obstruction.[14]

Obstructive uropathy is classified as acute or chronic and high- or low-grade obstruction.

PATHOPHYSIOLOGY

There are multiple possible causes. Regardless of the etiology there is a cascade of negative renal effects that include failure of glomerular filtration and tubular transport, which may lead to permanent renal damage or failure.

Urinary tract obstruction causes a cascading series of negative renal effects. The most damaging outcome is cellular glomerular destruction caused by increased glomerular pressure. When there is tissue injury, T cells and macrophages also infiltrate the renal parenchyma, resulting in an inflammatory response and scarring of the obstructed kidney. Scarring causes further decrease in kidney function. These abnormalities generally persist to some degree even after the obstruction is relieved.[11,14,20]

Congenital causes of obstruction are renal agenesis, hypoplasia, and ectopia. Agenesis is the absence of one or both kidneys, and it may be accompanied by intrarenal and urologic abnormalities. Hypoplasia is underdevelopment of one or both kidneys, and ectopia is malposition of the kidney(s). Horseshoe kidney and gravitation of one kidney to the opposite side are the most common forms of ectopia.

Renal calculi may also cause obstruction. See p. 887 for a discussion of this disorder. Pyelonephritis may result if obstruction persists.

DIAGNOSTIC STUDIES AND FINDINGS

Radionucleide imaging: Reduced blood flow
Renal ultrasonography: Dilation of collecting system; hydronephrosis
Intravenous urogram: Calyceal clubbing is shown after injection of radiopaque dye
Serum chemistry: Increased creatinine and BUN if renal dysfunction is present
Urinalysis: Normal unless there is renal dysfunction or infection; then pyuria, casts, hematuria

MULTIDISCIPLINARY PLAN

Relief of pain; elimination of obstruction; treatment of infection

Surgery

Performed to relieve the obstruction and preserve renal function; pyeloplasty or repair of ureteropelvic junction may be indicated; nephrectomy may be necessary if the kidney is severely damaged (see "Other Kidney Surgery," p. 912)

Indications for surgery: Persistent colic, complete obstruction, large or immobile calculi

Medications

Antibiotics: Refer to treatment of pyelonephritis, p. 876

General Management

Usually conservative if the condition is not severe

NURSING CARE

NURSING ASSESSMENT

Renal: Hematuria; pyuria; reduced GFR; casts; reduced urine output
Abdomen: Kidneys may be palpable

General: Dull backache; fever with infection, hypertension, incisional drainage postoperatively; CVA tenderness with pyelonephritis

Potential Complications

Pain, urinary tract infection, hydronephrosis (engorgement/enlargement of the kidney), ARF/CRF, hypertension

Patient Problems/Nursing Diagnoses & Interventions

NIC Tissue Perfusion Management

Ineffective tissue perfusion (renal) related to increased pressure within the urine channel because of obstruction at some point in the urinary tract

- Monitor blood pressure every 6 to 8 hours, 24-hour intake and output; weigh daily; monitor laboratory data: serum creatinine, BUN, serum sodium, potassium, bicarbonate. *Postobstruction diuresis may occur; acute renal failure may develop.*

NIC Risk Management

Risk for infection related to urinary tract obstruction
Risk for altered body temperature related to infection

- Assess for signs and symptoms of urinary tract infection (fever, increased WBC count, pyuria, bacteriuria, foul-smelling urine). *Likelihood of infection is increased with obstruction.*
- Administer antiinfective agents as ordered; monitor response to drugs given *to treat any infection present.* Prepare for surgery (see "Other Kidney Surgery," p. 912).
- Administer antipyretics as ordered.

NIC Physical Comfort Promotion

Acute pain related to surgical incision

- Assess for discomfort and give analgesics as ordered *to determine the need for pain relief and to relieve discomfort.* Monitor and record response to drug *to determine effectiveness of drug, dosage, and timing and to identify any side effects.*
- Report any pain that occurs after the immediate postoperative period; *pain with fever and decreased urine output may indicate obstruction or leakage of urine into the retroperitoneal space.*

NIC Skin/Wound Management

Impaired skin integrity related to surgical incision
Delayed surgical recovery related to interruption in healing

- After surgery, monitor site of incision for drainage and signs of infection *to detect any complications promptly.* Keep area clean and dry *to avoid skin breakdown and promote healing.*
- Keep any drainage tubes patent, unkinked, and anchored *to maintain urine flow and to avoid inadvertent displacement.* Care for urethral catheter. Tubes may include a stent (a catheter inserted into the ureter), a nephrostomy tube, and a drain in the incision; drainage from the incision may continue for several days.

Patient Education/Continuum of Care Plan

1. Explain the kidney-ureter abnormality.
2. Explain possible problems: recurrent infection and obstruction.
3. Explain signs and symptoms of urinary tract infection and obstruction.
4. Explain measures to prevent urinary tract infection: adequate fluid intake to avoid dehydration, regular emptying of bladder to avoid overdistention.
5. Explain postoperative care, including care of the incision and self-monitoring skills as needed.
6. Explain plans for medical follow-up of renal function.

Evaluation/Patient Outcomes

Tissue Perfusion Management: Obstruction is relieved; renal function is normal. X-ray examination shows that hydronephrosis is lessened or has not increased; renal function tests are normal or stable.

Risk Management: No infection is present in the urinary tract. Patient has no signs or symptoms of urinary tract infection.

Physical Comfort Promotion: Patient is pain free. Patient does not complain of pain.

Skin/Wound Management: Incision is healing. No drainage, redness, swelling, or separation of incision is noted.

Congenital/Hereditary Disorders of the Kidney[11,14]

Congenital/hereditary abnormalities include renal agenesis; the absence of one or both kidneys; hypoplasia, wherein one or both kidneys are underdeveloped; as well as a number of other anatomic deviations.

A wide variety of anomalies related to the kidneys can occur. The abnormalities may be in number, volume, form, location, rotation, blood vessels, pelvis, or ureter. These errors in renal development result from failure to develop, abnormal division of the elements, fusion of the elements, or abnormal movement from the pelvis to the lumbar area. These anatomic deviations may range from minor to severe and from easily correctable to incompatible with life. Renal abnormalities are frequently associated with additional anomalies such as low-set ears, imperforate anus, genital anomalies, and abnormalities of the spinal cord and extremities. These disorders are often diagnosed during an evaluation for unexplained hypertension. Ectopia, when the kidneys and often other parts of the urological tract are malpositioned, is another common abnormality.

In ectopia one of the kidneys commonly crosses over the midline so that both are on one side. The most common form of ectopia is the horseshoe kidney, where the kidneys fuse together. Obstruction is a frequent serious complication with this abnormality. A supernumerary, or extra, kidney, rarely occurs, although duplication of the renal pelvis is common.

Pathophysiology

The malformed or displaced kidneys may be normal except for their abnormal location, rotation, or structural variation. They have increased susceptibility to trauma because they are not protected as well as a kidney in normal location. Obstruction may occur, as may infarction or infection if the normal blood supply and urinary channel are interrupted.

Diagnostic Studies and Findings

Intravenous urogram: Abnormally located or rotated kidney; extra kidney(s) or malformed kidney
CT scan/ultrasound: Same findings as above
Serum chemistry: Increased creatinine, BUN if renal dysfunction is present
CBC: Elevated WBC count if infection is present

Multidisciplinary Plan

Surgery

Correction of obstruction to blood supply or urine elimination in displaced kidney and removal of extra kidney may be indicated; function of remaining kidney tissue must be adequate
Symptom management may include control of hypertension or treatment of infection or calculi

Medications

Refer to pyelonephritis to review antimicrobial treatment

NURSING CARE

Nursing Assessment

Urinary tract: Asymptomatic; signs of infection or obstruction
General: Pain, CVA tenderness, fever, mass on abdominal examination, hypertension

Potential Complications

Pyelonephritis, renal dysfunction/failure, renal calculi, hypertension

Patient Problems/Nursing Diagnoses & Interventions

NIC Risk Management

Risk for infection related to abnormality of blood supply or urine channel

- Monitor temperature, nature of urine. *Abnormal urine channel or blood supply may increase susceptibility to urinary tract infection.*
- Administer antimicrobials as ordered. Observe for side effects, report, and document.

NIC Skin/Wound Management

Risk for impaired skin integrity

- Prepare patient for surgery (see "Other Kidney Surgery," p. 912). After surgery, assess site of incision for drainage and signs of infection *to detect complications promptly.*
- Keep area clean and dry *to avoid skin breakdown and promote healing.*
- Keep any drainage tubes patent, unkinked, and anchored *to permit continuous drainage and avoid inadvertent displacement.*
- Be alert to and report any foul-smelling urine, pus, or blood *to detect complications promptly.*

NIC Physical Comfort Promotion

Acute pain related to surgery

- Evaluate patient's need for pain relief postoperatively; administer analgesic as ordered; monitor response *to determine need for drug, promote patient's comfort, and determine effectiveness of drug, dosage, and timing; also to identify and document any side effects.*
- Adjust dose for degree of renal dysfunction.

Patient Education/Continuum of Care Plan

1. Explain the nature of the anomaly.
2. Explain the signs and symptoms of possible problems (trauma to abdomen, urinary tract infection, or urinary tract obstruction).
3. Explain measures to prevent urinary tract infection: adequate fluid intake (to avoid dehydration), regular emptying of the bladder to avoid overdistention, and good perineal hygiene to prevent the entrance of microorganisms into the urinary tract.
4. If surgery is required, explain postoperative care, including care of the incision and self-monitoring skills (intake and output, weight, temperature).

Evaluation/Patient Outcomes

Risk Management: No urinary tract infection is present. Patient's temperature and WBC count are normal; urinalysis has no bacteria or pus cells.

Skin/Wound Management: Incision has healed. Wound is closed, and no infection is present.

Physical Comfort Promotion: Patient is pain free. Patient does not complain of discomfort.

Polycystic Kidney Disease

Polycystic kidney disease (PKD) is a disorder in which the kidney tissue is replaced by grapelike clusters of cysts.

Polycystic kidney disease is a genetically transmitted disorder (autosomal dominant in adults). An infant form (autosomal recessive) occurs, but these children rarely live more than a year. The adult form of the disease has a similar onset, clinical course, and manifestations within a family. Approximately 5% to 10% of patients on dialysis have the adult form of PKD. It is important that the cysts characteristic of PKD be differentiated from tumors. Fifteen percent of patients with PKD may have an associated berry aneurysm with the possibility of subarachnoid hemorrhage. The incidence of PKD is 1 in 1000.

PATHOPHYSIOLOGY

In PKD, normal kidney tissue is replaced by grapelike clusters of cysts that enlarge over time and destroy the surrounding tissue by compression. Why cysts are formed is not clear. They may be associated with cysts in the liver. Cysts may occur anywhere along the nephron, and they are filled with a yellow or brown fluid that may be thick and cloudy and may contain urine components. Progressive fibrosis of the interstitial tissue occurs. Infection and renal stones often develop because of urinary stasis and compression. Ascending infection may become a persistent source of infection. These kidneys do not resist infection well and thus may harbor organisms; poor perfusion may prevent antibiotics from reaching pockets of infection. A perinephric abscess may form; septicemia may occur. The possibility of cystic hemorrhage is always a concern. In these cases a nephrectomy may be necessary. Hypertension and renal failure follow the onset of symptoms within 5 to 15 years.

DIAGNOSTIC STUDIES AND FINDINGS

Urinalysis: Intermittent hematuria; proteinuria; bacteria; pyuria; creatinine clearance may be decreased; creatinine and BUN may be increased

Kidney-ureter-bladder x-ray examination and renal ultrasonography: Enlarged kidneys; irregular borders, stones

Intravenous urogram: Irregular outline and distortion of calyceal pattern; presence of cysts, nephrocalcinosis, or obstruction of the collecting system

Ultrasound: Enlarged kidneys with cysts apparent

MULTIDISCIPLINARY PLAN

No specific treatment is available for PKD. Medical goals concentrate on preventing hypertension and infection to preserve renal function. Instrumentation of the urinary tract, which is occasionally followed by a urinary tract infection, should be avoided. If patients do not have symptoms, creatinine clearance and urine cultures should be obtained twice a year. Genetic counseling may be suggested for families with PKD. Renal dialysis and transplantation may be indicated when chronic renal failure ensues.

NURSING CARE

NURSING ASSESSMENT

Renal: Urgency, frequency, and dysuria with infection, hematuria, pyuria

Abdomen: Palpable kidneys, dull ache in costovertebral or loin areas or sharp colic-like CVA pain

General: Hypertension, fever

Psychosocial: Acceptance or rejection of situation by patient; change in family relationships; concerns about long-term impact of illness

POTENTIAL COMPLICATIONS

Urinary tract infection/sepsis, hemorrhage of the cyst, chronic renal failure(CRF)/end-stage renal disease (ESRD), cyst formation in other vital organs

PATIENT PROBLEMS/NURSING DIAGNOSES & INTERVENTIONS

NIC TISSUE PERFUSION MANAGEMENT

Ineffective renal tissue perfusion related to replacement of normal tissue with cysts

- Monitor intake, output, and weight if necessary *because renal insufficiency may develop.*
- Monitor blood pressure; administer antihypertensive drugs if ordered; *antihypertensives decrease effect of elevated blood pressure on already damaged kidneys.*
- Monitor laboratory data that reflect renal function *to follow any decrease in renal function.*

NIC RISK MANAGEMENT

Risk for infection related to alterations of the collecting system by cysts

- Monitor for signs and symptoms of urinary tract infection; cysts are prone to infection *because of changes caused in renal blood flow or urine flow.*
- Avoid inserting catheters or other instruments into urinary tract *to prevent nosocomial infections.*

NIC PHYSICAL COMFORT PROMOTION

Acute pain related to pressure of cysts on adjacent structures

- Administer analgesics as ordered and monitor the response.
- Monitor increases in pain, as this may mean that a cyst ruptured or is infected.

NIC COPING ASSISTANCE

Interrupted family processes related to diagnosis of a genetically transmitted disease

- Assess how diagnosis of patient's condition affects others in the family *to determine need for family counseling.*
- Provide information about genetic counseling if appropriate; some people do not want to know this information.

PATIENT EDUCATION/CONTINUUM OF CARE PLAN

1. Explain the nature of the kidney abnormality and the availability of genetic counseling.

2. Explain the need to monitor renal function and blood pressure.
3. Explain measures to prevent urinary tract infection: adequate fluid intake to avoid dehydration, regular emptying of the bladder to avoid overdistention, observation of urine.
4. Explain signs and symptoms of urinary tract infections (see "Pyelonephritis," p. 875).
5. Explain renal dialysis and transplantation as options for the future.

Evaluation/Patient Outcomes

Tissue Perfusion Management: Early decreases in renal function are recognized. Urinalysis and blood chemistries are performed every 6 months, and any change is noted.

Risk Management: Infections are treated promptly. Patient seeks medical help when signs and symptoms of urinary tract infection occur.

Physical Comfort Promotion: Patient is free from pain. Patient has no complaint of pain.

Coping Assistance: Patient and family use adaptive coping mechanisms.

GLOMERULAR DISEASES

Glomerular diseases are renal disorders that primarily affect the glomeruli. They are categorized as primary (those that only involve the kidney) and secondary (those in which the kidney is involved as part of a systemic disorder).

Both types of glomerular diseases can cause specific clinical syndromes of two major types, nephrotic and nephritic. Nephrotic syndrome is characterized by a large quantity of protein in the urine (>3.5 g/24 h), hypertension, edema, hypoproteinemia, and hyperlipidemia. Nephritic syndrome is identified by the presence of glomerular hematuria, red cell casts, and less-than-nephrotic-range proteinuria.

PRIMARY GLOMERULAR—NEPHROTIC SYNDROME

Primary glomerular diseases that cause nephrotic syndrome:
- minimal change
  - Focal segmental glomerulosclerosis
  - Membranous glomerulopathy
  - Membranoproliferative glomerulonephritis (MPGN)

PRIMARY GLOMERULAR—NEPHRITIC SYNDROME

Primary glomerular diseases that cause nephritic syndrome (nephritis):
- Acute poststreptococcal glomerulonephritis (GN)
- IgA nephritis
- Rapidly progressive GN/crescentic GN
- Antiglomerular basement membrane nephritis

Diagnosis is commonly made by renal biopsy.

See boxes on disease processes that cause nephrotic or nephritic syndrome.

The etiology of the disorders varies: infectious agent, immune complex (antigen-antibody formation) complement deposition. The treatment varies according to diagnosis. The goals of treatment, however, are similar: delay the destructive process of the disease and preserve kidney function with as few adverse effects as possible.

It is impractical to discuss all glomerular diseases; four are selected and discussed briefly here:

Acute poststreptococcal glomerulonephritis (APSGN)
IgA nephritis
Rapidly progressive glomerulonephritis (RPGN)
Focal segmental glomerulosclerosis (FSGS)

Note that the term *glomerulonephritis* is a blanket term commonly used to describe many different glomerular diseases. The definition of GN is offered later.

Since the nursing treatment plan is similar, one plan of care is presented at the end of the section for all four disorders.

GLOMERULONEPHRITIS

GN may be a primary disease of the kidneys or may develop secondary to a systemic disease, such as lupus erythematosus. GN is a disease primarily of the glomeruli caused by a variety of factors, including immunologically mediated damage (immune complex or autoantibody), vascular disorders, drug effects or toxins, and systemic diseases.

A discussion of GN is difficult because of the confusion between older definitions (used before renal biopsy was introduced) and newer terms (used afterward). Classification might be according to clinical course (acute, rapidly progressive, and chronic), histopathology (e.g., membranoproliferative), or pathogenetic mechanism (immune complexes and antibodies against renal tissue).

Four specific types of glomerular disorders are described here. Three of them are referred to as a type of GN.

ACUTE POSTSTREPTOCOCCAL GLOMERULONEPHRITIS

Acute poststreptococcal glomerulonephritis (APSGN) is an inflammation of the glomeruli that occurs after a streptococcal infection elsewhere in the body.

GN can follow a respiratory or skin infection. Several strains of group A β-hemolytic streptococci that cause GN have been isolated. In temperate zones the most common nephritogenic strain causing pharyngitis is M-type. Only about 5% of such infections are followed by APSGN. Children and young adults are affected most frequently. The incidence of APSGN decreases with age because many children (especially in urban areas) develop immunities to M-type β-hemolytic streptococci before reaching adulthood. Renal problems occur abruptly 1 to 3 weeks after the infection. Most patients (95%) recover normal renal function within 2 months. The others have irreversible damage that causes long-term problems. It is not clear whether prompt treatment of streptococcal infections prevents renal complications of APSGN.

PATHOPHYSIOLOGY

In APSGN, antibodies of the host react with circulating antigens that appear to arise from the toxic products of the infecting organism; the antibodies and antigens form immune complexes that then become lodged in the glomeruli. Both kidneys are affected by an acute, diffuse, nonsuppurative inflammation that damages the glomerular basement membrane (GBM). The kidneys respond through GBM thickening, endocapillary proliferation, scarring, necrosis, and extracapillary proliferation. The damage causes an acute interference with renal function. GN is a major cause of renal failure among patients undergoing dialysis.

DIAGNOSTIC STUDIES AND FINDINGS

Routine urinalysis: Hematuria: >0 to 5 RBCs with many dysmorphic red cells; proteinuria: >30 to 150 mg/24 hours; color change: red, red-brown; sediment: RBC casts, WBC casts, granular casts

Serum creatinine: >1.2 mg/dl (men); 1.1 mg/dl (women)

BUN: >20 mg/dl

Hemoglobin (Hgb)/hematocrit (Hct): Hgb: <15.5 ± 1.1 g (men); 13.7 ± 1 g (women); Hct: <46 ± 3.1% (men); 40.9 ± 3% (women) or normal

Complement (C3): <400 to 800 μg/ml

Circulating immune complex: >25 μg/ml aggregated human gamma globulin

Cryoglobulins: Present

Antistreptolysin O: >25 Todd units

Creatinine clearance: <85 to 125 ml/min/1.73 mm^3 (men); <75 to 115 ml/min/1.73 mm^3 (women)

Culture of throat or skin lesion: Streptococcal organism may be present early in course of disease

KUB x-ray examination: Kidneys normal size, or slight bilateral enlargement

Renal biopsy: Diffuse endocapillary proliferation with many polymorphs in glomerular tuft; immunofluorescence reveals deposits of IgG, IgM, and C3

MULTIDISCIPLINARY PLAN

The medical plan includes treating the symptoms, attempting to prevent cerebral and cardiac complications and permanent renal dysfunction, and supporting the patient through a period of decreased renal function.

Medications

Acute parenteral therapy for hypertension. Always check for need for dosage reduction in renal disease.
- Nitroprusside, 0.5-1.0 μg/kg/min, maximum 10 μg/kg/min; infuse for no more than 48 h to avoid accumulation of toxic metabolite
- Diazoxide, 1 mg/kg/min IV bolus q5-15 min or 7.5-30 mg/min infusion
- Nitroglycerin, 5-100 μg/min IV infusion
- Hydralazine, 0.5-1.0 mg/min infusion or 10-50 mg IM
- Labetalol, 2 mg/min infusion or 0.25 mg/kg
- Enalaprilat, 0.625-5.0 mg bolus given over 5 min q6h
- NOTE: For PO therapy of hypertensive emergencies, diltiazem, nifedipine, and captopril all begin to work within 15 min, but their peak effect is much later

Diuretics
- Furosemide (Lasix), 20-80 mg PO followed by second dose in 6-8 h up to 600 mg; IM, IV, 20-40 mg given slowly over 1-2 min; high dose by IV not more than 4 mg/min
- Bumetanide (Bumex) 1-2 mg PO bid not to exceed 10 mg/24 h
- Hydrochlorothiazide (HydroDIURIL, Esidrix), 25-100 mg/day or bid PO initially; then maintenance of 25-100 mg/day according to patient's response
- Sodium bicarbonate, 2-5 mEq/kg IV infusion over 4-8 h or 300 mg PO bid
- Glucose 50%, 25-50 g IV, and regular insulin, 10-15 U IV

Antiinfective agents (if infection is still present)
- Infection is frequently a complication of APSGN
- Agents specific to microorganism cultured should be used
- Agents whose route of excretion is primarily renal need to be used in smaller doses or at lengthened intervals depending on glomerular filtration rate (GFR); agents excreted by only the liver require no change; when partial excretion occurs via the kidneys, some adjustment is needed at low GFRs

Other agents as dictated by complications: Cardiac glycosides for congestive heart failure, antiinfectives if infection is still present, anticonvulsants for seizures; H_2 antagonists and proton pump inhibitors for gastritis or gastric esophageal disease (GERD), phosphate binders, erythropoietin, iron therapy if progresses to chronic renal failure

General Management

Goals are to control edema, preserve renal perfusion, treat hypertension while avoiding postural hypotension, and treat any intercurrent infection

Hemodialysis, peritoneal dialysis, continuous renal replacement therapy (CRRT) (p. 904) if indicated.

Limit sodium intake to 2 to 4 g/day; variable with urine output

Limit fluids to 500 to 1000 ml plus amount equal to volume of urine for previous 24 hours

Limit potassium intake (if hyperkalemia) or if GFR <20 ml/min

Limit protein intake (if uremic) to 0.8 to 1.08 g/kg/day, with 50% to 60% of high biologic value

Provide 2500 to 3500 calories/day

Prescribe bed rest during acute phase of illness

NURSING CARE

NURSING ASSESSMENT

General complaints: Headache; low back pain; malaise; fever, chills; weight gain, fatigue

Cardiovascular: Hypertension; edema

Potential Complications

ARF, CRF, ESRD, malignant hypertension, hypertensive encephalopathy, arrhythmias from electrolyte disorders (e.g., acidosis or hyperkalemia)

Neurologic: Seizures, change in level of consciousness (LOC) with encephalopathy

Gastrointestinal: Anorexia, nausea, vomiting, primarily with uremia

Urinary: Normal or decreased volume; dark brown or rust color[11,14,17]

Focal Segmental Glomerulosclerosis (FSGS)

FSGS is not one disease but rather it is a term for a clinicopathologic syndrome that has multiple etiologies. The most common feature is proteinuria (usually nephrotic range) and a distinctive biopsy result of clumps of glomeruli that show consolidation and scarring, as well as other glomeruli that appear normal.

The syndrome is more frequent in African-Americans, and the pathogenesis is poorly understood. The prognosis is closely linked to the degree of proteinuria. Those with massive proteinuria usually progress to ESRD within 10 years of diagnosis.

Diagnostic Studies and Findings

Urinalysis: >300 mg/dl protein on urine screen, oval fat bodies, double refractile fat bodies

Serum creatinine and BUN: Increased

Creatinine clearance: reduced

Total urinary protein: >3.5 g/24 hours

Urinary protein electrophoresis: Large quantities of albumin

Multidisciplinary Plan

Appropriate diagnosis

High-dose glucocorticoid therapy

Treatment with angiotensin converting enzyme inhibitor (ACEI)

Alternative therapy with cytotoxic drugs or cyclosporine under investigation

Prevent complications of nephrotic syndrome; appropriate treatment of hyperlipidemia, hypertension, hypoalbuminemia

Medications

Prednisone, 2 mg/kg PO qod, maximum daily dose 150 mg; continue therapy for 18-20 weeks

Omeprazole, 20-40 mg PO qhs for treatment of steroid-induced gastritis

Enalapril, 20 mg bid PO or lisinopril, fosinopril, 20-40 mg qd

General Management

Aggressive diagnosis and treatment with high-dose steroids; control sequelae: edema, hypertension, hyperlipidemia, hypoalbuminuria; frequent follow-up to monitor renal function

IgA Nephropathy

IgA nephropathy, also known as Berger's disease, is another common form of acute GN caused by deposition of immune globulin A in the mesangium.

IgA nephropathy is one of the most common forms of glomerular diseases. Why IgA is deposited in the kidney is not known. What is known is that IgA nephritis commonly follows an upper respiratory infection or, less frequently, a urinary tract infection or gastroenteritis. The infection apparently triggers the formation of immune complexes and the activation of the complement cascade, presumably through mucosal immune reaction. The disorder is more common in males in the second and third decades of life. Sixty percent of cases resolve with treatment, and up to 40% may progress to ESRD. High-dose steroid therapy is the most common form of treatment.

Diagnostic Studies and Findings

Total urinary protein: Normal to greater than 3.5 g/24 hours

Serum cretinine, BUN: Increased

Urinalysis: Oval fat bodies, double refractile fat bodies, casts, hematuria (macroscopic)

Kidney biopsy: Focal and segmental proliferative GN; IGA deposits in mesangium

Multidisciplinary Plan

The main goal is to:

Eliminate or delay progression of the disease process

Reduce proteinuria

Control hypertension

Treat appropriately [some patients have been effectively treated with omega-3 fatty acids, fish oil; others have improved on lengthy episodes of steroid (glucocorticoid) therapy]

Medications

Prednisone, 2 mg/kg qod PO, maximum dose 150 mg/24 h

Ace inhibitors: Enalapril, kisinopril, fosinopril, 20-40 mg PO

Omega-3 fatty acid as a dietary supplement[10]

Rapidly Progressive Glomerular Nephritis (RPGN)

RPGN is actually a clinical syndrome that resembles previously discussed forms of acute nephritis except that renal function is rapidly lost in weeks to months.

RPGN is also referred to as crescentic GN because of the crescent-shaped pattern of the immune complex deposits seen on biopsy. There are a number of different causes, including infection, toxins, ATN, vasculitis, or even idiopathic factors. It is accompanied by oliguria/anuria as well as other common signs of GN (e.g., hematuria, proteinuria). The prognosis depends on the cause, and the disease either improves or progresses to ESRD in 3 to 6 months.

MULTIDISCIPLINARY PLAN

Determine the etiology
Treat based on biopsy findings
Prevent complications
Prepare patient for the need for acute dialysis
Educate and support the patient and family in light of the rapidly changing clinical picture

Medications

Pharmacologic therapy is based on etiology of RPGN. In the case of idiopathic RPGN, a trial of pulse IV methylprednisolone (30 mg/kg/h) followed by alternate day PO prednisone (2 mg/kg) has become standard practice.

PATIENT PROBLEMS/NURSING DIAGNOSES & INTERVENTIONS

NIC TISSUE PERFUSION MANAGEMENT

Ineffective tissue perfusion, related to immunologic injury to kidneys
Excess fluid volume related to altered renal function

- Monitor blood pressure every 4 to 6 hours, 24-hour intake and output, and other vital signs; monitor laboratory data: serum potassium, creatinine, carbon dioxide, phosphate; BUN, Hgb, Hct, and urinalysis. *Acute renal failure may develop with azotemia, anemia, hyperkalemia, hyperphosphatemia, acidosis, and seizures.*
- Administer antihypertensive agents as ordered; administer agents to lower potassium level if needed; administer agents to lower phosphate level if ordered; administer anticonvulsant agents if ordered *to control uremic symptoms and cardiovascular complications.*
- Monitor peripheral edema; weigh daily at same time, using same scale and patient in same clothes.
- If volume excess is severe, assess pulmonary artery pressures and central venous pressure, jugular venous distention, breath sounds, and respiratory rate *to assess cardiac function and pulmonary status.*
- Limit sodium and fluid intake *to limit fluid retention.*
- Administer diuretic agents as ordered *to mobilize retained fluids.*
- Administer cardiac glycosides and ACE inhibitors if ordered *to prevent congestive heart failure.*

NIC NUTRITIO.N SUPPORT

Imbalanced nutrition: more than body requirements, related to altered renal function
Imbalanced nutrition: less than body requirements, related to proteinuria

- Encourage protein intake of 0.8 to 1 g/kg body weight per day plus the amount lost in 24-hour urine output; *excessive protein losses may occur.* Edema is a sign of hypoalbuminemia.
- Monitor food intake; monitor for anorexia, nausea, and vomiting; offer small, frequent feedings *to ensure adequate caloric intake and thus prevent metabolism of tissue protein for energy.*
- Limit protein, potassium, and phosphorus intake if uremic symptoms occur *to decrease excretory load on the kidneys and possible accumulation of potassium, phosphorus, and hydrogen ions.*
- Administer phosphate binders/calcium supplements as ordered.

NIC RISK MANAGEMENT

Risk for infection related to altered immune state

- Assess for urinary tract infection; monitor temperature; monitor WBC count; avoid exposure to individuals with infections. *Patients with GN are susceptible to urinary tract infection because of their altered immune status.*
- Administer antiinfective agents if ordered; a streptococcal infection may still be present.

PATIENT EDUCATION/CONTINUUM OF CARE PLAN

1. Explain disease process and medication/treatment regimen to individual and family.
2. Distribute teaching materials as appropriate; see enclosed National Kidney Foundation materials and address.
3. Explain the possible problems, such as urinary tract infection, renal failure, and their signs and symptoms.
4. Explain that renal dialysis and transplantation are possible future options in the event of CRF.

EVALUATION/PATIENT OUTCOMES

Tissue Perfusion Management

Patient has normal or improved renal function. Renal function tests are within normal limits. Patient's fluid intake balances output. Urine is clear; edema is gone; blood pressure is in normal range; weight is stable.

Nutrition Support: Patient's nutritional intake is adequate. Proteinuria has resolved; serum albumin and cholesterol levels are normal. Electrolytes are normal.

Risk Management: Patient is free of infection. No signs or symptoms of infection are noted.

TUBULOINTERSTITIAL DISORDERS

TUBULOINTERSTITIAL NEPHRITIS

Tubulointerstitial nephritis (TIN) is an acute, often drug-induced renal disease that involves inflammatory damage to interstitial tissue and tubules.

Damage to interstitial tissue is a frequent cause of acute and chronic renal failure. Causes of TIN include infection (e.g., streptococcal) and drug use, analgesics, antibiotics such as methicillin and ampicillin, sulfonamides, phenindione, and phenytoin). Such drugs may cause dose-related toxic reactions or nondose-related allergic reactions.

TIN also may arise from idiopathic causes. Early detection of drug reactions, infection, and urinary tract obstruction is useful. It is important to be alert to the possibility that patients who abuse over-the-counter analgesics, especially those containing acetaminofen and ibuprofen are at increased risk for TIN.

Pathophysiology

Acute inflammation of the interstitium and tubules may cause scarring and a rapid decline in renal function. The inflammatory process is usually diffuse and accompanied by edema. An immune response appears to cause acute TIN that may involve deposition of immune complex and anti–tubular basement membrane antibodies.

Chronic TIN results in a shrunken kidney with an irregular outline caused by scarring and tissue destruction. It follows a slowly progressive course with few clinical manifestations. Changes in renal hormone activity may occur, and the production of renin, erythropoietin, and vitamin D may decline. The ability to concentrate urine also decreases. Common causes of chronic TIN are anatomic abnormalities (e.g., obstruction in the urinary tract), analgesic overuse, hyperuricemia, and nephrosclerosis.

Diagnostic Studies and Findings

Urine chemistry tests: Abnormal
WBC count: Eosinophilia if drug-induced
Urinalysis: Granular and eosinophilic casts; hematuria; dilute urine (low specific gravity); mild proteinuria
Intravenous urogram: Normal or slightly enlarged kidneys; immediate, dense nephrogram; with chronic interstitial nephritis: decreased size, irregular cortex, calyceal distortion
Renal biopsy: Differentiates acute tubular necrosis from acute interstitial nephritis
Urine concentration tests: Abnormal
Serum creatinine and BUN: Increased
Creatinine clearance: Decreased
Total urinary protein: 500 to 1000 mg/24 hours

Multidisciplinary Plan

Eliminate the cause of TIN by treating infection, discontinuing the drugs associated with acute TIN, and relieving obstruction. Renal function may gradually improve. Chronic TIN requires monitoring as renal function decreases. Changes in the function of the glomeruli and tubules occur as the interstitial inflammation and scarring progress (see discussion of chronic renal failure, p. 871). Controlling blood pressure is imperative to prevent or delay progression.

Surgery

May be performed to relieve any obstruction

Medications

Antiinfective agents if needed

General Management

Dialysis if needed; nutritional support, fluid limitations, vitamin supplements as needed; see discussion of acute renal failure, p. 865

NURSING CARE

Nursing Assessment

Renal: Polyuria; nocturia
Skin: May have an allergic skin rash
General: Headache, low back pain, weight loss or gain, fever, chills, fatigue, hypertension, edema, bibasilar crackles

Potential Complications

CRF, ARF, ESRD, hypertension

Patient Problems/Nursing Diagnoses & Interventions

NIC Tissue Perfusion Management

Ineffective tissue perfusion, altered renal tissue perfusion related to damaged interstitial tissue
Deficient fluid volume related to inability to concentrate urine
Excess fluid volume related to acute renal failure associated with oliguria or anuria

- Monitor blood pressure every 6 to 8 hours; 24-hour intake and output and edema. Check laboratory data: Hgb, Hct, serum creatinine, BUN, serum potassium, phosphate, carbon dioxide; *nonoliguric renal failure may develop with hypertension, azotemia, anemia, acidosis, and increased serum potassium and phosphate.*
- Administer antihypertensive agents if needed and agents to reduce serum potassium and to reduce phosphate absorption as ordered; monitor response *to control complications of uremia and to determine effectiveness of drug, dosage, and timing.*
- Monitor state of hydration, weigh daily; measure blood pressure, pulse, and respirations every 6 to 8 hours; measure 24-hour intake and output and specific gravity *to check for inability to concentrate urine and to determine the extent of fluid loss.*
- Administer fluids as ordered; monitor response *to prevent dehydration and further decrease in renal blood flow.*
- Monitor for edema and listen to breath sounds; if fluid excess is severe, monitor central venous pressure and pulmonary artery pressures *to identify hypervolemia.*
- Administer diuretics.
- Maintain accurate intake and output to *prevent hypovolemia or hypervolemia.*

NIC Risk Management

Risk for infection related to damaged interstitium

- Monitor for signs and symptoms of urinary tract infection; administer antiinfective agents if ordered; monitor response to drug. *Renal failure alters immune response; monitoring determines effectiveness of drug, dosage, and timing.*

Patient Education/Continuum of Care Plan

1. Explain the nature of interstitial nephritis and the cause in the individual patient.
2. Explain the patient's level of renal function.
3. Explain the need for periodic medical evaluation with tests of renal function.
4. Explain likelihood of dialysis or transplantation in the future.

Evaluation/Patient Outcomes

Tissue Perfusion Management: Renal function has returned. Electrolyte balances are within normal limits; serum creatinine and BUN levels are normal. Patient's fluid intake balances output. Urine output equals intake; polyuria ceases; blood pressure is normal; weight is stable.

Risk Management: Patient is free of infection. No signs or symptoms of infection are noted.

Acute Tubular Necrosis (ATN)[7,11]

ATN is the result of toxic or ischemic injury to the renal parenchyma, causing sloughing of the tubular cells, renal obstruction, and acute renal failure.

ATN, a disease of the renal tubules, is a significant cause of acute renal failure. The most common causes are volume depletion, renal ischemia, sepsis, drug effect, multiorgan failure, surgery, and burns.

Pathophysiology[7]

ATN commonly occurs in three phases: initiation, maintenance, and recovery. The initiation phase occurs when the kidney is exposed to ischemia or a toxin that begins to cause renal injury. In this stage, renal damage is often hard to detect. In the maintenance phase, signs of significant cellular injury develop. Urine output and GFR reach their lowest levels. This phase may last from 1 week to 11 months. A common prognostic indicator is the longer the maintenance phase lasts, the greater is the likelihood of permanent renal damage. The recovery phase is the period in which renal function begins to improve as the tissue is repaired and regenerated.

If a renal biopsy is done, the most common histologic pattern is a patchy and focused loss of clumps of tubular cells. Actual necrosis of the tubule is, in fact, a rare finding.

Multidisciplinary Plan

The single most critical intervention is diagnosis of the cause and eliminating it. Symptomatic support is necessary while awaiting recovery of kidney function.

NURSING CARE

Assessment

Renal: Oliguria/anuria or normal output
General: Weight gain, edema, hypertension, dyspnea, cough

Potential Complications

CRF/ESRD, hypertension, pulmonary congestion, edema, anasarca

Patient Problems/Nursing Diagnoses & Interventions

NIC Tissue Perfusion Management

Ineffective tissue perfusion, renal, related to interruption of blood flow

Excess fluid volume or deficient fluid volume related to failure of regulator mechanisms

- Monitor blood pressure, pulse, and respirations frequently.
- Monitor abdomen, back, and extremities for anasarca or peripheral edema *to identify hypovolemia or hypervolemia.*
- Assess weight daily; assess 24-hour intake and output; assess blood pressure (sitting and standing), pulse, and respirations; monitor edema, jugular venous distention, and, as necessary, central venous pressure and pulmonary artery pressures; monitor laboratory data: urine specific gravity and protein; serum albumin and calcium; Hct *to check for altered fluid status and orthostatic hypotension.*
- Administer drugs as ordered (i.e., diuretics); monitor response to drugs *to correct fluid imbalance, to determine effectiveness of drugs, and to observe for side effects such as hypokalemia and ototoxicity.*
- Limit sodium intake as ordered; *if serum sodium levels are high, edema will be worsened by fluid retention.*
- Restrict fluid intake as ordered. *Restrictions may be necessary in cases of hyponatremia; massive edema or ascites; respiratory distress; or pleural effusion.*
- If ATN results from volume depletion, fluid boluses may be ordered to improve renal perfusion. Increase intravenous volume as ordered and monitor for signs of rebound fluid volume excess (e.g., pulmonary edema, oliguria, hypertension, cough). Discontinue causative pharmacologic agents as ordered.

NIC Electrolye and Acid-Base Management

Imbalanced nutrition: more than or less than body requirements, related to altered renal function

- Monitor serum electrolytes, especially potassium levels because levels may be lowered by vigorous diuretic therapy.
- Monitor serum CO_2 for signs of acidosis (e.g., CO_2 <20 mEq/L).
- Anticipate need for dialysis if hyperkalemia and acidosis cannot be managed otherwise.

Patient Education/Continuum of Care Plan

1. Instruct patient and family about causes of ATN and need for close follow-up after discharge.
2. Make arrangements for dialysis if indicated.
3. Explain need for close follow-up of kidney function when discharged.

Evaluation/Patient Outcomes

Tissue Perfusion Management: Kidney function is normal. Patient has normal creatinine, BUN, and creatinine clearance.

Fluid balance is normal. Urine volume is normal and there is no evidence of volume deficit or excess. Nutritional status is normal. Patient has no restrictions on food or fluid.

Electrolyte and Acid-Base Management: Electrolytes and acid-base values are within normal limits.

Renal Calculi

Renal calculi are stones formed in the kidneys, primarily in the renal pelvis, but they may also form in the ureter and bladder. Stones may resemble gravel or may be formed in the shape of the pelvis (staghorn calculus).

Calculi that pass spontaneously without discomfort present no serious health threat. However, many calculi found in the urinary tract are extremely painful and can cause obstruction and infection. Urinary calculi occur more frequently in men than in women, and some geographic areas, such as the southeastern United States, have a particularly high incidence. The peak incidence of calculus formation is in the third to fifth decades of life.

Long-term ingestion of calcium carbonate, vitamin D, antacids, megadoses of vitamin C, acetazolamide, probenecid, or triamterene can lead to stone formation. The risk can be increased by anatomic abnormalities (medullary sponge kidney), biochemical influences (cystinuria), environmental factors (diet and fluid intake patterns, climate, occupation), or hereditary diseases (PKD).

Pathophysiology

The formation of a stone is a physiochemical process involving a nidus of crystals or organic material around which the stone components form. The pH, temperature, ionic strength, and concentration of the urine affect the solubility of the stone-forming substances. Supersaturation of poorly soluble substances, absence of crystalline inhibitors, and sources of seed crystals contribute to calculus formation.

The primary components of renal calculi include calcium salts (carbonate and oxalate), uric acid, cystine, and struvite (magnesium ammonium phosphate). The stones most frequently contain calcium or uric acid.

Hypercalciuria with or without hypercalcemia may be caused by hyperparathyroidism or osteoporosis or may be idiopathic. Calcium and phosphate are more soluble when pH is low. Bacterial infection by urea-splitting organisms causes the urine to become alkaline. Stones composed of struvite are called infection stones.

Hyperuricemia occurs with idiopathic gout, renal failure, blood dyscrasias, and the use of thiazide diuretics and alkylating agents. Uric acid is less soluble in high concentrations, low urine volume, and with low urine pH.

Diagnostic Studies and Findings

KUB x-ray examination: Radiopaque stone
Renal ultrasound: Stones identified
Intravenous urogram: Filling defects; ureteral dilation; hydronephrosis
Analysis of stones: Constituents such as cystine, calcium, oxalate, and uric acid
Urinalysis: Hematuria, microscopic and macroscopic, crystals, bacteria
CBCs: Elevated WBC count if infection present

Multidisciplinary Plan

The goals of medical care are to mobilize or remove calculi, relieve effects of the calculi (pain and infection), resolve any causative factors (obstruction, infection, and metabolic abnormalities), and prevent future calculus growth. The achievement of these goals help to prevent permanent damage to the kidney and recurrence of calculi.

Surgery

10% to 20% of patients with renal calculi require a surgical procedure.
Procedures used may include pyelolithotomy, nephrolithotomy, ureterolithotomy, cystoscopy-basket extraction of calculi, and percutaneous fragmentation and extraction through a nephroscope (litholapaxy); surgical intervention is a last resort with struvite stones because recurrence is so frequent
Additional procedures: Extracorporeal shock wave lithotripsy, percutaneous lithotripsy (see p. 914)

Medications

Analgesics
- Meperidine (Demerol), 50-150 mg q3-4h, PO, subcutaneously, IM, IV
- Oxycodone (Percocet, Roxicet), 1-2 tablets PO q6h
- Codeine sulfate (generic), 15-60 mg PO qid
- Morphine sulfate, 5-15 mg q4h prn PO, subcutaneously, IM, IV

Antibiotics[29]
- Fluoroquinolones, guinolones, trimethoprim sulfisoxazole, PO
- Ancef, vancomycin/gentamicin, ceftazidime, IV

Electrolytes (used to ensure alkaline urine)
- Sodium bicarbonate, 300 mg to 1.8 g PO qd-qid, not to exceed 16 g/day

Diuretics
- Hydrochlorothiazide (HydroDIURIL, Esidrix) (to reduce idiopathic urinary calcium excretion), 50 mg PO bid

Other Drugs
- Allopurinol (Zyloprim, Alloprin), decreases uric acid production, 200-800 mg PO in divided doses if more than 300 mg dose required per day
- Cellulose sodium phosphate (ion exchange resin) (Calcibind), initially 15 g/day (5 g tid with meals) for urinary calcium >300 mg/day PO; reduced to 10 g/day (5-6 mg with main meal, 2.5 g with other two meals) when urinary calcium 150 mg/day. NOTE: There is a complicated medication regimen to be followed with this drug; please refer to a more complete discussion.
- Penicillamine (Cuprimine, Depen), combines with cystine to form a soluble compound, 250 mg PO qid

Antiinfective agents, if infection present
Potassium supplementation, 40 mEq/day PO for hypokalemia of diuretic therapy

General Management

Diet: Modifications may be required, depending on stone type; low-calcium diets (<400 mg/day) and extra-high fluid intake (3500-4000 ml/day) are helpful but difficult to maintain; patients should avoid dehydration by drinking water rather than fluids that may be high in unwanted substances (such as tea with its high oxalate content); increased fluid intake should be spread out evenly over the 24-hour period, including once during the night; low-purine diets may help decrease uric acid output; foods extremely high in purines (>150 mg/100 g) are limited; oxalate intake is usually limited to less than 50 mg/day on low-oxalate diets

Table 13-2 Summary of Diet Principles in Renal Stone Disease

Stone Chemistry	Nutrition Modification	Diet Ash Urinary pH
Calcium	Low calcium (400 mg)	Acid ash
Phosphate	Low phosphorus (1-1.2 g) (milk, cheese, egg yolk, whole grains, legumes, nuts)	
Oxalate	Low oxalate <50 mg/day (tea, chocolate, nuts, spinach)	
Struvite ($MgNH_4PO_4$)	Low phosphorus (1-1.2 g) (associated with urinary tract infection)	Acid ash
Uric acid	Low purine (organ meats, shrimp, dried beans)	Alkaline ash
Cystine	Low methionine	Alkaline ash

From Phipps, Sands, and Marek.[25]

NURSING CARE

Nursing Assessment

Urinary tract: Irritative voiding symptoms; dysuria, urgency, and urge incontinence, hematuria, crystals in urine, oliguria, or low normal output

General: Fever, rigors (with urinary tract infection); pain, at times severe, associated with renal colic (in flank or costovertebral angle radiating to groin, labia, or testicle); tenderness in the flank or costovertebral angle; nausea; vomiting

Patient Problems/Nursing Diagnoses & Interventions

NIC Physical Comfort Promotion

Acute pain related to pressure of calculus in urinary tract

- Note pattern of pain, and assess need for analgesia. *Intensified pain may indicate impaction of calculus or obstruction of urine flow; sudden relief of pain may indicate stone has passed through a narrow junction (ureteropelvic or ureterovesicle);movement of calculus may be associated with colicky pain.*
- Administer analgesic agents as ordered; monitor response to drugs *to relieve pain* and *to determine effectiveness of drug, dosage, and timing; to identify adverse reactions.*
- Apply external heat to painful flank *to relieve discomfort.*
- Assist with walking as ordered *to help passage of stone.*

NIC Elimination Management

Imbalanced nutrition: more than body requirements, related to altered metabolism of calcium, purine, or oxalan

Deficient fluid volume and impaired urinary elimination related to possible anatomic obstruction

- For calcium stones, lower calcium intake (e.g., dairy products); for uric acid stones decrease purine intake (e.g., organ meats, meat extracts, shrimp, or dried beans); lower intake of foods containing oxalate (e.g., tea, chocolate, nuts, or spinach) *to prevent formation of renal calculi.* (See Table 13-2 for review of diet modifications).
- Avoid dehydration by encouraging high-normal fluid intake (usually 3500-4000 ml/day) *to prevent high concentrations of unwanted substance in the urine.*
- Alkalinization of urine may be necessary. Administer bicarbonate as ordered.
- Strain urine if patient has symptoms of renal colic.
- Monitor intake and output.

NIC Risk Management

Risk for infection related to presence of calculus

- Monitor for fever, chills, and irritative voiding symptoms; monitor laboratory data: WBC, bacteriuria; monitor temperature q4h *to detect presence of infection.*
- Encourage high to normal fluid intake over 24-hour period *to help flush urinary tract to prevent urinary tract infection;* may also facilitate passage of calculus.
- Administer antipyretics and antibiotics as ordered.

Patient Education/Continuum of Care Plan

1. Explain the nature of renal calculi, their causes, and manifestations.
2. Explain medical management, including medications (purpose, dosage, interval, and side effects), diet (low calcium, purine, or oxalate), and fluid intake (amount, schedule, and kinds).
3. Explain medical follow-up to monitor the outcome of treatment.

Evaluation/Patient Outcomes

Physical Comfort Promotion: Pain is gone. Patient reports being free of pain.

Elimination Management: Fluid intake is adequate, and unwanted substances are avoided in the diet. Fluid intake is high normal; diet restrictions are followed correctly.

Risk Management: No signs or symptoms of urinary tract infection are noted. Temperature, urine, and WBC count are normal.

SYSTEMIC DISEASES THAT CAUSE RENAL DYSFUNCTION: DIABETES MELLITUS AND HYPERTENSION

Multiple systemic diseases affect the kidney. However, diabetes and hypertension are the most frequently seen diagnoses. These two disorders combined cause almost 70% of ESRD in the United States. They are outlined separately in the following section.

DIABETIC NEPHROPATHY

Diabetic nephropathy (DN) is the renal manifestation of diabetes mellitus; it is glomerulosclerosis, caused by lesions of the arterioles and glomeruli.

DN, or diabetic glomerulosclerosis, is an important complication of type 1 and type 2 diabetes mellitus. Approximately 30% to 40% of patients with diabetes develop DN.[19] Patients with type 2 diabetes have variable courses and may or may not develop DN. Patients with type 1 diabetes mellitus develop DN about 50% of the time.

DN is a clinical syndrome manifested by early microalbuminuria (>300 mg/24 h) and hyperperfusion (GFR >100 ml/min) followed by frank proteinuria and all of the associated complications of nephrotic syndrome. The course is progressive; there is a relentless fall in GFR and increasing azotemia until ESRD is reached in 8 to 10 years from the onset of microalbuminuria. Microalbuminuria is strongly correlated with and predictive of the clinical syndrome. Screening for microalbuminuria is a priority in the primary care of diabetics.

Patients with DN have increased morbidity and mortality. Although the survival of diabetic patients treated with dialysis or transplantation has improved somewhat in recent years, the outcomes are not nearly as good as in nondiabetic patients. Diabetic patients have particular problems with atherosclerosis, coronary artery disease, peripheral vascular disease, retinopathy, and neurologic deficits. The likelihood of their successful rehabilitation is limited but has increased in recent years.

PATHOPHYSIOLOGY

The glomeruli are affected by diffuse sclerosis and thickening of the basement membrane and mesangial areas. Nodular glomerulosclerosis may also occur. Both afferent and efferent arterioles are affected by thickened walls and hyaline deposits. The GFR decreases and azotemia occurs. The diabetic patient may appear clinically uremic at creatinine and BUN levels lower than those of the nondiabetic patient. This may be related to the diabetic patient's systemic vascular changes.

DN may not manifest clinical symptoms for years after diabetes develops. Diabetic individuals vary considerably in their susceptibility to renal failure, possibly because of genetic defects or vascular changes related to metabolism of carbohydrates, fat, and protein. Poor control of blood pressure and inadequate control of glucose levels are important factors and are known to lead to rapid progression of DN.

DIAGNOSTIC STUDIES AND FINDINGS

Blood chemistries: Increased serum creatinine, BUN, glucose, and potassium; decreased albumin; increased cholesterol and low-density lipoprotein (LDL) level
Urinalysis: Proteinuria, pyuria, or bacteriuria; hematuria; granular and hyaline casts
Creatinine clearance: Lowered values
Intravenous urogram: Kidneys may be of normal size, swollen, or small and scarred (irregular cortical surface)
Renal biopsy: Diffuse or nodular thickening of glomerular basement membrane and mesangial regions
Microalbuminuria and proteinuria: Elevated in 24-hour collection and on random specimen screens

MULTIDISCIPLINARY PLAN

Data indicate that control of blood pressure and glucose blood levels slows the deterioration of renal function. This is the mainstay of therapy for DN.

Surgery

See discussion of renal transplantation (p. 908); diabetic patients who have a renal transplant have more complications, poorer rehabilitation, and a lower survival rate than nondiabetic patients with a renal transplant; the underlying disease process cannot be corrected by renal transplantation alone.

Medications

Insulin requirements may decrease as renal degradation of the hormone decreases or may increase as resistance to insulin's effects increases; antihypertensive drugs and diuretics may be needed.

For type 2 diabetic patients, oral agents metabolized in the liver are used.

Sulfonylureas
- Glyburide, 1.25-20 mg PO daily with AM meal
- Glipizide, 5-25 mg PO before AM meal

Miscellaneous antidiabetic agents
- Metformin, 500-850 mg PO bid. **This drug can be fatal** if given to patient with renal or hepatic dysfunction. If it is used at all, it must be monitored aggressively and physician should be queried about use in this population.
- Rosiglitazone, 2-8 mg/day in divided dose; improves cell insulin sensitivity
- Acarbose, 25-50 mg PO tid initially up to 100 mg tid; alphaglucosidase enzyme inhibitor blocks carbohydrate absorption. There are many gastrointestinal side effects unless an effective dose is established gradually. Caution must be used in renal dysfunction patients.

Alkalinizing agents (for acidosis): Sodium bicarbonate, 1-4 g/day PO; 2-5 mEq/kg infused IV over 4-8 h

Treatment for hyperkalemia

Sodium polystyrene sulfonate (Kayexalate, SPS), 15 g qd-qid PO or enema; give PO dose in 45-60 ml of water, syrup, or sorbitol solution

Calcium gluconate, 1 g (90 mg Ca^{++}) in 10 ml IV

Sodium bicarbonate, 2-5 mEq/kg IV infusion over 8 h

Glucose 50%, 25-50 g IV, and regular insulin, 10-15 U IV

Antihypertensive agents

Clonidine (Catapres), 0.1 mg PO bid or tid initially; then increase by 0.2-0.8 mg/day (maximum effective dose, 2.4 mg/day)

May also use clonidine TTS, 0.1-0.3 mg once-a-week dermal patch; no taper required if patch is discontinued

Doxazosin (alpha receptor antagonist), 1-16 mg PO qd or qhs

Losartan (angiotensin II receptor antagonist), 50 mg PO bid

Labetalol (combined alpha and beta antagonist), 200-600 mg PO bid; 2.4 g maximum

Isradipine (dihydropyridine calcium channel antagonist), usual dosage 2.5-10 mg PO bid; maximum dosage 20 mg/day

Diltiazem (nondihydropyridine calcium channel antagonist), 180-360 mg PO qd usually given in divided doses bid

ACE inhibitors

Long-acting preparations such as lisinopril or fosinopril (Monopril), 10-40 mg PO, or enalapril, 10 mg IV, for acute hypertension; potassium and creatinine must be monitored because these drugs can cause an increase in both parameters in patients with renal disease

Atenolol (beta-1 selective antagonist), 25-50 mg PO qd; use with caution in diabetes and renal dysfunction

Propranolol (Inderal, nonselective beta-adrenergic blocker), 40 mg PO tid at 6-8 h intervals; increase if needed to 160-480 mg/day in divided doses; 640 mg/day may be needed

Diuretics

Furosemide (Lasix), 20-80 mg PO followed by second dose in 6-8 h up to 600 mg; 20-40 mg IM, IV given slowly over 1-2 min; high dose by IV not more than 4 mg/min and repeat in 6-8 h

Bumetanide (loop diuretic), 1-10 mg PO or IV qd; up to 20 mg may be needed in renal failure

Antiinfective agents

Infection is frequently a complication of nephropathy/CRF

Agents specific to the microorganism cultured should be used

Agents whose route of excretion is primarily renal need to be used in smaller doses or at lengthened intervals depending on GFR; agents excreted by only the liver require no change; if partial excretion occurs via the kidneys, some adjustment is needed at lower glomerular filtration rates

Phosphate-binding agents

Calcium acetate (PhosLo), 667-mg tab PO pc; 2 tabs with each meal to start; 3-4 tabs per meal usually required

Calcium carbonate, 500-1250 mg PO pc; may need up to 10-12 g/day to manage hyperphosphatemia

RenaGel, 403-mg capsule PO, 3-4 pc; may need up to 21 capsules per day

Aluminum-based antacids are no longer used routinely because they cause aluminum toxicity when used long-term. They may be used at 2-week intervals to lower phosphorus levels acutely.

Antiemetic agents

Prochlorperazine (Compazine), 5-10 mg PO tid-qid

Promethazine (Phenergan), 12.5-25 mg PO tid

Antipruritic agents

Diphenhydramine NE, 25 mg PO q6h

Hydroxyzine, 25 mg PO bid-tid

Laxatives/stool softeners

Bulk forming (Metamucil [sugarfree]), 1-2 tsp qhs

Docusate sodium (Colace, DCS), 50-200 mg/day PO

Hematinic agents

Ferrous sulfate (Feosol, Fer-Iron), 300 mg-1.2 g/day PO in divided doses

Iron polysaccharide (Nu Iron, Niferex), 150-mg capsule bid between meals and 2 h apart from calcium tablets

Iron-dextran injection (InFeD), IV, IM, varies with weight and hemoglobin level but usually given as ten 100-mg doses

Sodium ferric gluconate (Ferrlicit), 125 mg IV for 8 doses; used for iron deficiency in place of iron dextran

Vitamins

Multivitamin supplements (water-soluble vitamins)

Thiamine, 1.5 mg/day

Riboflavin, 1.8 mg/day

Niacin, 20 mg/day

Pyridoxine, 5 mg/day

Vitamin B_{12}, 3 μg/day

Vitamin C, 100 mg/day

often given in 1 capsule (Nephro-Vite)

Folic acid (Folvite), folate sodium, up to 1 mg/day PO, subcutaneously, IM, IV; maintenance: up to 0.3 mg/day

Vitamin D

Calcitriol (1,25-dihydroxycholecalciferol) (Rocaltrol), 0.25 μg/day PO; maintenance: 0.5-1 μg/day or calcitriol, 0.5-3 μg IV after dialysis

General Management

Control blood pressure and blood glucose level

See hemodialysis and peritoneal dialysis (pp. 895-904); the underlying disease process cannot be corrected by dialysis; vascular complications of diabetes cause major problems in access to vascular system for hemodialysis

Fluid intake should balance output: about 400 to 600 ml (about amount of insensible losses) plus amount equal to 24-hour urine volume unless ESRD, in which case fluid intake is not to exceed 1.5 L/day; avoid dehydration and volume excess

Nutritional modifications are made to achieve or maintain adequate nutritional status and to reduce work of diseased kidney

Weight reduction; intermediate levels of renal failure require moderate protein diets with drugs to lower LDL and triglycerides; late in course of renal failure, insulin requirements decrease, but protein, carbohydrate, and fat intake must still be controlled

Protein, 0.8-1.0 g/kg body weight/day

Sodium, 2000 mg/day

Potassium, 1500-2000 mg/day; with normal urine output (at least 800 ml/day) no restriction is needed

Calories, 35-55 kcal/kg body weight/day; calories from fat and carbohydrate are used; adequate calories must accompany protein intake to prevent use of protein for energy and weight loss; control of protein intake takes priority in nutritional management; calories from fat and carbohydrates are increased

NURSING CARE

NURSING ASSESSMENT

HEENT: Background retinopathy, decreased visual acuity, blurred vision

Renal: Oliguria or anuria; urinary retention; urinary frequency; renal tubular acidosis; microscopic hematuria, casts; leukocytes and fat bodies in urinalysis

Cardiovascular: Hypertension; postural hypotension; edema or dehydration, extra heart sounds, flow murmurs, neck vein distention

Gastrointestinal: Nausea; anorexia; thirst; weight loss; constipation; diarrhea; weight gain

Extremities: Decreased sensation, neuropathic pain, pitting edema, nonhealing leg/foot ulcers

POTENTIAL COMPLICATIONS

Myocardial infarction (MI) or cerebrovascular accident (CVA) caused by hypertension; pulmonary edema and respiratory failure; hyperkalemia and resultant cardiac arrhythmias; other electrolyte disorders (hypocalcemia, hyperphosphatemia); acidosis; anemia; peripheral vascular disease (PVD); ketoacidosis; hypoglycemia/shock as insulin requirements decrease; hyperparathyroidism and renal osteodystrophy (these occur with advanced renal failure)

PATIENT PROBLEMS/NURSING DIAGNOSES & INTERVENTIONS

NIC TISSUE PERFUSION MANAGEMENT

Ineffective tissue perfusion, renal, related to diffuse and nodular glomerulosclerosis

- Monitor vital signs, intake and output, and weight, as needed; monitor laboratory data: serum glucose, BUN, serum creatinine, creatinine clearance, and 24-hour protein excretion *to reflect status of diabetes and renal function.*
- Administer medications as ordered with care *because dosages are given in smaller amounts or at longer intervals.*
- Determine insulin dosage by serum glucose level *because urine glucose level does not accurately reflect serum glucose level owing to altered renal handling of glucose.*
- Avoid nephrotoxic drugs *becaue kidneys are less able to excrete drugs.*
- Monitor response to drugs given *to determine effectiveness of drug, dosage, and timing and to identify adverse reactions.*
- Control blood pressure: administer antihypertensives and diuretics. Restrict fluids and sodium as indicated. Blood pressure should be <130/80 mm Hg.
- Control blood glucose: administer antidiabetic agents on correct schedule to facilitate action. Blood glucose should be as close to normal as possible without causing hypoglycemia.

Excess or deficient fluid volume related to altered regulatory mechanisms

- Monitor dry weight, evaluate for signs of increasing renal failure.
- May need to administer increasing dose of diuretic (dose requirement increases as renal function declines).
- Evaluate diuretic response. There should be brisk diuresis within 30 to 45 minutes of dose.
- Hyperglycemia places patient at risk for dehydration. Monitor signs of volume deficit (hypotension, may be orthostatic; initially experiences urinary frequency and later decreased output, weight loss, decreased central venous and pulmonary wedge pressures).

NIC NUTRITION SUPPORT

Imbalanced nutrition: more than or less than body requirements, related to inability to ingest, digest, absorb, or metabolize nutrients due to biologic factors

- Monitor indications of renal failure and control of diabetic state. Make appropriate changes in therapy regimen as indicated (may require increase in antidiabetic agents, addition of or increase in phosphorus binder, or further restriction in potassium intake or dialysis).
- Monitor indicators of inadequate nutrition.
- Add iron between meals if iron deficiency anemia is diagnosed (ferritin less than 200 ng/L saturation less than 20%).
- Monitor parathyroid hormone levels; if elevated this is an indication of inadequate vitamin (D3, 125) production. Add calcitriol (Rocaltrol, Calcijex) to regimen as ordered.

NIC RISK MANAGEMENT

Risk for infection related to increased susceptibility with diabetes and chronic renal failure

- Assess for signs and symptoms of infection in secretions, excretions, and exudates; monitor and record temperature every 4 to 6 hours; monitor laboratory data: WBC, *to detect infection early.*
- Ensure aseptic technique for any invasive procedure or wound care *to decrease chance of infection.*
- Administer antimicrobials and antipyretics as ordered. Observe for and report side effects.

PATIENT EDUCATION/CONTINUUM OF CARE PLAN

1. Explain the nature of DN and CRF (see p. 889).
2. Explain the medical regimen and its rationale, including diet (restricted protein, sodium, and potassium), restricted fluid intake, and medications (purpose, dosage, interval, and adverse reactions).
3. Help the patient learn self-observational skills (temperature, pulse, respirations, blood pressure, intake and output, and weight) and record keeping.
4. Explain avoidance of infection.
5. Explain personal hygiene, rest, and exercise.
6. Explain when to call the physician.
7. Explain the plan for medical follow-up.
8. Explain renal dialysis and transplantation.

Evaluation/Patient Outcomes

Tissue Perfusion Management: Real tissue perfusion is adequate. Renal function test results are normal or stable. Fluid balance is within normal limits. Urinary output balances intake within fluid restrictions.

Nutrition Support: Nutritional status is adequate. Food restrictions are appropriate to level of renal function and diabetic needs.

Risk Management: No infection is present. No signs or symptoms of infection are noted.

RENAL DYSFUNCTION SECONDARY TO HYPERTENSION

Hypertensive Nephrosclerosis[4,26]

Severe hypertension can cause deterioration in renal function. Hypertensive nephrosclerosis is the damage to the renal arteries, arterioles, and glomeruli caused by prolonged elevated blood pressure.

Renal parenchymal disease is a major consequence of prolonged elevated blood pressure. Important factors in the development of such problems are the age at which hypertension occurs, its severity, and the presence of risk factors (e.g., race, family history of hypertension or cardiovascular disease, obesity, diabetes mellitus, smoking, and lack of exercise). Many people develop arteriosclerosis as they age; such changes are accelerated with hypertension.

Pathophysiology

A slow, variable progression of vascular changes can occur over the years. The process includes spasm, thickening, hypertrophy, and hyaline degeneration of the renal arterial system. In malignant hypertension, renal changes are rapid and include fibrinoid necrosis. The damaged kidney decreases or stops production of substances that lower blood pressure.

Diagnostic Studies and Findings

Urinalysis: Proteinuria; hematuria
Blood chemistries: BUN, serum creatinine above normal; serum potassium variable
Ultrasound and KUB x-ray examination: Small kidneys, bilaterally
Intravenous urogram: Small kidneys, bilaterally
ECG: Left ventricular hypertrophy

Multidisciplinary Plan

Goals of therapy include aggressive control of blood pressure to slow renal deterioration, delay of ESRD by conservative management, and initiation of dialysis or performance of a renal transplant at the appropriate point in the course of the disease. Drug dosages and intervals must be modified when the kidney is involved in the drug's excretion. Rates of excretion and metabolism and sensitivity to drugs may be altered. Bed rest, sodium restriction, and antihypertensive drugs are basic.

Surgery

Transplantation of donor kidney as described on p. 908.

Medications

Alkalinizing agents (for acidosis)
- Sodium bicarbonate, 1-4 g/day PO; 2-5 mEq/kg IV infused over 4-8 h or 300 mg PO bid

Treatment for hyperkalemia
- Sodium polystyrene sulfonate (Kayexalate, SPS), 15 g PO or enema qd-qid; give PO dose in 45-60 ml of water, syrup, or sorbitol solution
- Calcium gluconate, 1 g (90 mg Ca^{++}) IV in 10 ml; follow product information directions
- Sodium bicarbonate, 2-5 mEq/kg IV infusion over 8 h
- Glucose 50%, 25-50 g IV, and regular insulin, 10-15 U IV

Antihypertensive agents
- Clonidine (Catapres), 0.1 mg PO bid or tid initially; then increase by 0.2-0.8 mg/day (maximum effective dose, 2.4 mg/day)
  - May also use clonidine TTS 0.1-0.3 mg once-a-week dermal patch; no taper required if patch is discontinued
- Doxazosin (alpha receptor antagonist), 1-16 mg PO qd or qhs
- Losartan (angiotensin II receptor antagonist), 50 mg PO bid
- Labetalol (combined alpha and beta antagonist), 200-600 mg PO bid; 2.4 g maximum
- Isradipine (dihydropyridine calcium channel antagonist), usual dosage 2.5-10 mg PO bid; maximum dosage 20 mg/day
- Diltiazem (nondihydropyridine calcium channel antagonist), 180-360 mg PO qd; usually given in divided doses bid

ACE inhibitors
- Long-acting preparations such as lisinopril or fosinopril (Monopril), 10-40 mg PO, or enalapril, 10 mg IV, for acute hypertension
- Potassium and creatinine must be monitored because these drugs can cause an increase in both parameters in patients with renal disease
- Atenolol (beta-1 selective antagonist), 25-50 mg PO qd; use with caution in diabetes and renal dysfunction
- Propranolol (Inderal) (nonselective beta-adrenergic blocker), 40 mg PO bid at 6- to 8-h intervals; increase if needed to 160-480 mg/day in divided doses; 640 mg/day may be needed

Diuretics
- Furosemide (Lasix), 20-80 mg PO followed by second dose in 6-8 h up to 600 mg; 20-40 mg IM, IV given slowly over 1-2 min; high dose by IV not more than 4 mg/min and repeat in 6-8 h
- Bumetanide (loop diuretic), 1-10 mg PO or IV qd; up to 20 mg may be needed in renal failure

General Management

Dialysis by home or in-center hemodialysis, home or in-center intermittent peritoneal dialysis, or continuous ambulatory peritoneal dialysis (CAPD) may be needed if chronic renal failure develops (see pp. 895-904).

Fluid intake to balance output: about 400 to 600 ml (about the amount of insensible losses) plus amount equal to 24-hour urine volume; patient should avoid dehydration and volume excess

Nutritional modifications to achieve or maintain adequate nutritional status and to reduce work of diseased kidney

- Protein: 0.8 g/kg body weight/day
- Sodium: 2000 mg/day
- Potassium: 1500 to 2000 mg/day; with normal urine output (at least 800 ml/day), no restriction needed
- Calories: 35 to 55 kcal/kg body weight/day; calories from fat and carbohydrates used; adequate calories must accompany protein intake to prevent use of protein for energy and weight loss

NURSING CARE

Nursing Assessment

Cardiovascular: Elevated blood pressure; tachycardia; fourth heart sound; forceful apical impulse (point of maximal impulse [PMI])

Optic fundi: Retinal blood vessel changes: narrowing, hemorrhages, and exudates

Renal: Nocturia; proteinuria; hematuria

General: Headache; dizziness; fatigue; palpitations; blurred vision

Potential Complications

Arteriosclerosis, coronary artery and peripheral vascular disease, CRF, ESRD, CVA, hypertensive retinopathy, MI

Patient Problems/Nursing Diagnoses & Interventions

NIC Tissue Perfusion Management

Ineffective tissue perfusion, renal, related to damage to nephrons

- Administer medications as ordered; as renal failure progresses, dosages may be reduced and time intervals may be lengthened for drugs excreted by the kidneys. Observe response to drugs *to determine effectiveness of drug, dosage, and timing and to identify adverse reactions.*
- Monitor laboratory data: serum potassium, calcium, uric acid, bicarbonate, pH, and glucose. These substances may be altered when taking diuretics and in chronic renal failure.
- Follow ECG changes; ECG changes associated with hyperkalemia are peaked T wave, prolonged PR interval, widened QRS complex, and cardiac standstill.
- Monitor for signs of other complications of hypertension.
- Arrange for appropriate follow-up to avoid complications if possible.
- Watch for Kussmaul breathing and Chvostek's or Trousseau's signs *to identify acidosis and hypocalcemia.*
- Assess standing and lying blood pressures and pulse every 4 to 6 hours; record weight daily; calculate 24-hour intake and output *to identify increased peripheral vascular resistance, postural hypotension, and fluid retention.*

Patient Education/Continuum of Care Plan

1. Explain the nature of chronic renal failure as caused by hypertension (see p. 892).
2. Explain hypertension and its care (see Chapter 3).
3. Explain the medical regimen and its rationale, including diet (restricted protein, sodium, and potassium), restricted fluid intake, and medications (purpose, dosage, interval, and adverse reactions).
4. Teach self-observational skills (temperature, pulse, respirations, blood pressure, intake and output, and weight) and record keeping.
5. Explain avoidance of infection.
6. Explain personal hygiene, rest, and exercise.
7. Explain when to call the physician.
8. Explain the plan for medical follow-up.
9. Explain renal dialysis and transplantation as future options.

Evaluation/Patient Outcomes

Tissue Perfusion Management: Renal tissue perfusion is stable. Renal function parameters do not worsen.

Renal Artery Occlusion or Stenosis and Renal Vein Thrombosis

Renal artery occlusion is a sudden complete blockage of the renal artery or a branch of it. Stenosis is a narrowing of the artery. The renal vein or a branch of it can be blocked by an embolus or thrombus.

Renal artery problems frequently are associated with atherosclerosis (in older patients) and fibromuscular hyperplasia. Renal vein thrombosis is most frequently associated with nephrotic syndrome (NS). It also may accompany an aortic aneurysm, a hematoma, trauma, or a neoplasm that compresses the renal vein.

Pathophysiology

In renal artery occlusion, complete cessation of arterial blood flow causes an infarct, with coagulation necrosis in the kidney. If the person has a single kidney, acute oliguric renal failure ensues. Occlusion is most frequently the result of an embolism caused by mitral valve stenosis, subacute bacterial endocarditis, and mural thrombi after an MI.

Severe stenosis caused by atherosclerosis leads to ischemic atrophy and fibrosis. Decreased pressure in the arterioles stimulates the juxtaglomerular apparatus to produce an increase in renin secretion and can lead to renovascular hypertension.

A sudden, complete occlusion of the renal vein causes an infarct; the kidney swells, pressing against the capsule. If an occlusion evolves slowly, however, collateral venous circulation may develop, resulting in less impairment of renal function. Renal vein thrombosis may be associated with dehydration, sepsis, or hypercoagulable states.

Diagnostic Studies and Findings

Diagnostic Tests	Findings: Renal Artery Occlusion	Findings: Renal Artery Stenosis	Findings: Renal Vein Thrombosis
Intravenous urogram	Affected kidney is smaller, calyces are smaller, nephrogram phase is delayed		Unilateral change in kidney function when radiopaque dye is injected: enlargement, poorly visualized
Renal arteriogram	Absence of function in all or part of the kidneys as it filters radiopaque dye		
Renal venogram			Demonstrable clot
Laboratory tests			
Urine	Microscopic hematuria		Gross hematuria; proteinuria; foamy, deep yellow color
Complete blood count	Leukocytosis		
Blood chemistries	Increased lactic dehydrogenase (LDH)		Signs of nephrotic syndrome
Plasma renin activity		Increased level in renal vein	

DIAGNOSTIC STUDIES AND FINDINGS

See Diagnostic Studies and Findings table above.

MULTIDISCIPLINARY PLAN

Surgery

Embolectomies are not usually performed for renal artery occlusion, since renal damage usually has occurred by the time diagnosis is made; selected patients with renal artery stenosis may have surgical correction by percutaneous transluminal angioplasty (PTA); if a thrombus begins in the aorta and extends into the renal artery, PTA is less successful than if only the renal artery is involved; other potential options are aortorenal bypass; autogenous vascular graft; stent placement; a nephrectomy may be needed in renal artery stenosis for renovascular hypertension that does not respond to drug therapy or PTA

Medications

Anticoagulants (used for renal artery occlusion or renal vein thrombosis)
- Heparin sodium, 10,000-20,000 U initially IV, subcutaneously (68-kg man); maintenance, 8000-10,000 U q8h or 15,000-20,000 U q12h
- Warfarin (Coumadin, Panwarfin), 10-15 mg/day PO, IM, IV for 2-3 days; then maintenance dose of 2-10 mg/day

Analgesics
- Meperidine (Demerol), 50-150 mg PO, subcutaneously, IM, IV q3-4h
- Codeine sulfate (generic), 15-60 mg PO, IM, subcutaneously qid
- Morphine sulfate (generic) 5-15 mg q4h PO, subcutaneously, IV prn

Antihypertensive agents (used for renal artery stenosis)
- All available drugs may be used
- ACE inhibitors are used with caution

Lipid-lowering agents
- Atorvastatin, pravastatin, simvastatin, lovastatin, bile acid sequestrant, naicin (Niaspan); refer to product information for dosing and monitoring

General Management

Sodium, protein restriction; monitor contralateral kidney function

NURSING CARE

NURSING ASSESSMENT

Cardiovascular: In renal artery stenosis: hypertension; abdominal bruits

General: In renal artery occlusion: pain in flank or upper abdomen, few signs if infarct is small; in renal vein thrombosis: flank pain

POTENTIAL COMPLICATIONS

Complications of malignant hypertension; loss of affected kidney

PATIENT PROBLEMS/NURSING DIAGNOSES & INTERVENTIONS

NIC TISSUE PERFUSION MANAGEMENT

Excess fluid volume related to failure of regulatory mechanisms

Ineffective tissue perfusion, renal, related to altered arterial or venous flow

- Monitor vital signs every 4 to 6 hours; assess weight daily *to determine systemic effects of renal problem.*
- Evaluate degree of fluid volume excess; monitor central venous pressure and pulmonary artery pressures if appropriate; monitor blood pressure both standing and lying every 4 hours; monitor intake and output daily; monitor laboratory data: urine protein, BUN, serum creatinine, and coagulation factors (if heparin is used) *to determine effect on cardiovascular and renal function.*
- Give antihypertensive and anticoagulant agents as ordered; observe response to drugs *to determine effectiveness of drug and dosage and observe for adverse and toxic side effects.*

NIC PHYSICAL COMFORT PROMOTION

Acute pain related to altered arterial or venous flow

- Evaluate pattern of pain and determine need for analgesia; administer analgesics as ordered *to promote comfort; to determine the effectiveness of drug, dosage, and timing; and to identify adverse reactions.* Observe response to drug given. A sudden increase in pain may mean extension of the problem.

PATIENT EDUCATION/CONTINUUM OF CARE PLAN

1. Explain the nature of renal artery occlusion, renal artery stenosis, or renal vein thrombosis.
2. Explain the treatment regimen and rationale.
3. Explain follow-up medical care required.

EVALUATION/PATIENT OUTCOMES

Tissue Perfusion Management: Some function returns after renal artery occlusion. Patient's renal function tests show improvement. Medical therapy or surgery helps renal artery stenosis. Hypertension is relieved or is under control. Renal function returns completely. Renal function test results are normal or reflect degrees of impairment.

Physical Comfort Promotion: Pain is eliminated or controlled.

COLLABORATIVE INTERVENTIONS AND RELATED NURSING CARE

RENAL REPLACEMENT THERAPY

When the kidneys can no longer perform their function of filtering the blood and removing excess fluid and solutes, renal replacement therapy is required. The possibilities for treatment are one of three types of dialysis or renal transplantation.

Hemodialysis is a diffusion-driven and size-discriminatory process for the clearance of fluid and small solutes such as electrolytes and urea using a filter, a concentrated electrolyte solution, and vascular access.[1]

Hemodialysis is accomplished by gaining access to the circulatory system, pumping the blood through tiny semipermeable hollow fibers, and running a concentrated fluid on the other side of the fibers. This mimics the physical processes of diffusion/filtration and ultrafiltration that occur in the nephron. Approximately 250,000 people receive hemodialysis in the United States alone.

Peritoneal dialysis (PD) is the instillation of a concentrated salt and glucose solution (dialysate) into the peritoneal cavity with the peritoneal membrane acting as a filter. The dialysate dwells for several hours as toxic materials and fluid are filtered out of the blood and into the dialysate by diffusion and ultrafiltration. In most instances the dialysate is drained, disposed of,

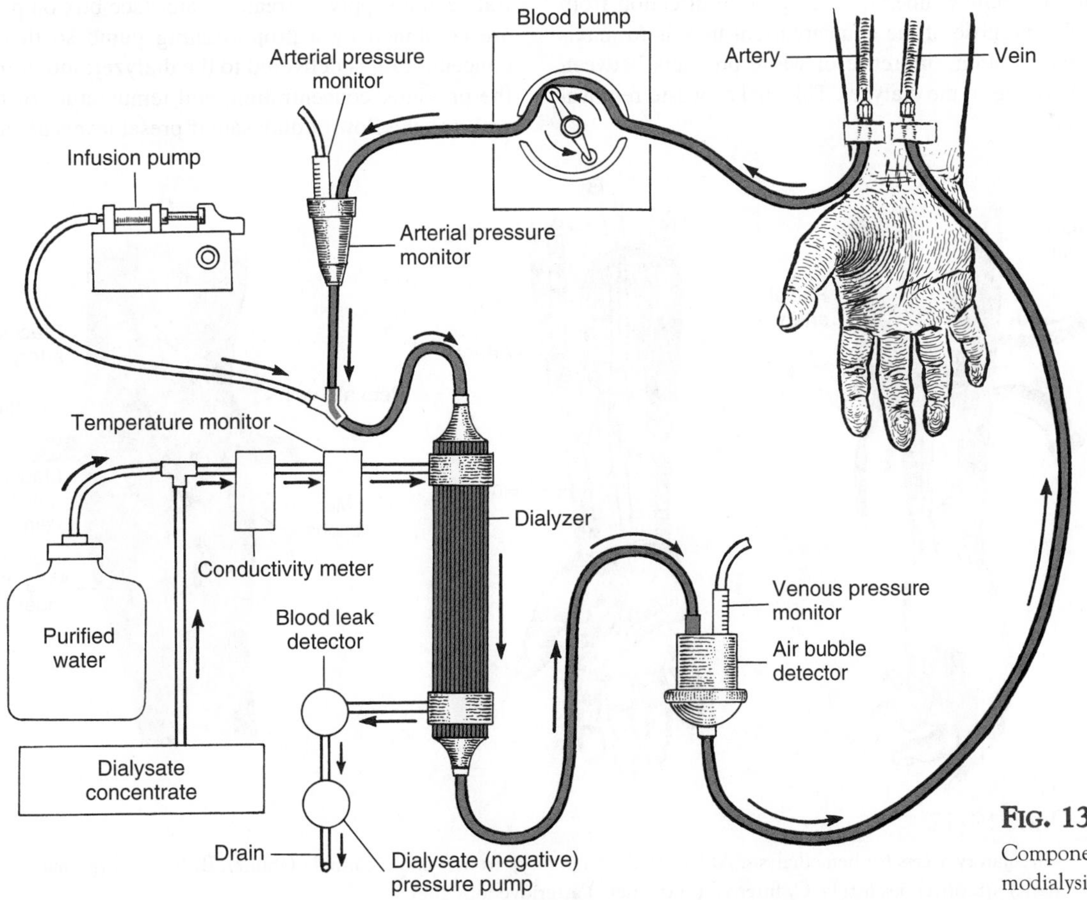

FIG. 13-11 Components of a hemodialysis system.[32]

and renewed every 4 to 6 hours. Over 70,000 people use this modality worldwide. There are three types of PD: continuous ambulatory peritoneal dialysis (CAPD); continuous cycler assisted peritoneal dialysis (CCPD); and nocturnal intermittent peritoneal dialysis (NIPD).

HEMODIALYSIS[7,9,31]

Hemodialysis involves circulating the patient's blood through semipermeable tubing that is surrounded by a dialysate solution in the artificial kidney (FIG. 13-11). It replaces part of the kidney's normal function.

Description and Rationale

To initiate hemodialysis, an access to the circulatory system is first established. This can be done with a double-lumen central catheter, a fistula (the patient's artery and vein are anastomosed directly together), or a graft (the artery and vein are connected using synthetic material, commonly Gortex or PTFE, see FIG. 13-12). There are advantages and disadvantages of each method.

Once it is clear that dialysis is necessary, the best possible hemo-access type is selected based on timing, the patient's vasculature, and the degree of morbidity.

When the access is usable, two large-bore needles are inserted. One needle allows the blood to exit the body (the arterial needle), and one returns the blood to the patient (the venous needle). The blood is pumped through the dialyzer, where it flows into multiple hollow fibers that are lined with pores, and the whole system is encased in a plastic tube. The dialysate flows around the hollow fibers in the opposite direction from the blood. The purpose of the countercurrent flow is to maximize the concentration difference of waste products between blood and dialysate in the dialyzer. This makes waste removal most efficient.

Three factors influence effective clearance of the blood by hemodialysis: blood flow rate (BFR), dialysis flow rate (DFR), and the type of dialyzer (artificial kidney) used.

Dialysis parameters are typically set as BFR, 400 ml/min and DFR, 800 ml/min.

The most commonly used dialyzer types, those that use high-flux membranes, should clear at a rate of 300 to 400 KoA (a measure of dialyzer capacity).

Hemofiltration and hemodiafiltration are alternatives to dialysis. These treatments use a convective filtration process on a continuous rather than intermittent schedule. Pressure differences in the hemofilter or a pump forces water and solutes through the highly permeable membrane in proportion to their concentrations in the blood. The ultrafiltrate formed is discarded, and, depending on the patient's condition, most of the water and solutes removed are replaced. This procedure is used increasingly in the United States for acute renal failure; in Europe, it is used with a blood pump for patients with CRF. It is a simple system that uses percutaneous access. A longer treatment time is required, thus avoiding peaks and valleys in blood chemistry values. Hemofiltration can be combined with hemodialysis in the process known as hemodiafiltration.

The actual dialysis process involves two circuits: the blood circuit and the dialysis circuit (see FIG. 13-11). The blood circuit includes an access device (cannula or internal arteriovenous fistula); arterial blood lines (with blood pressure monitor); a blood pump; a dialyzer, where diffusion, osmosis, and ultrafiltration occur; and venous lines with filter and monitors (for clots or air emboli and pressure), which return blood to the patient.

The dialysis circuit includes a supply of dialysate concentrate and a supply of treated water (see box on p. 897), which are combined by a proportioning pump so that the desired concentration is delivered to the dialyzer; monitors that detect the pressure, concentration, and temperature of the dialysate and stop the flow of dialysate if preset levels are not met; a di-

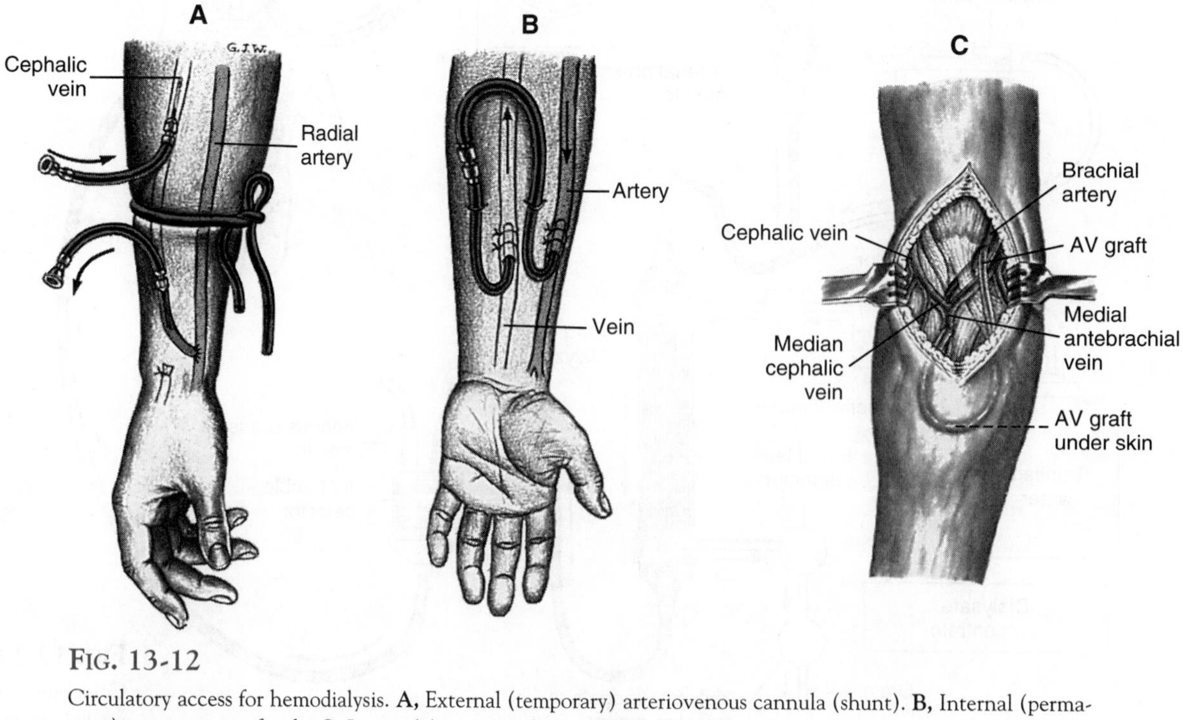

FIG. 13-12
Circulatory access for hemodialysis. **A,** External (temporary) arteriovenous cannula (shunt). **B,** Internal (permanent) arteriovenous fistula. **C,** Internal (permanent) arteriovenous graft.

alyzer, where the dialysate accepts wastes, excess electrolytes, and water; dialysate exit lines, which may have a leak detector (blood-in-effluent lines) or are monitored using Hemastix to detect the presence of blood; a negative pressure gauge on the dialysate lines that controls ultrafiltration; and a bypass circuit (not shown in FIG. 13-11) for diversion of dialysate that is not within the preset temperature, conductivity, or pressure limits.

The composition of the diluted dialysate solution is sodium, 130 to 145 mEq/L; potassium, 0 to 3 mEq/L; calcium, 2.5 to 4 mEq/L; chloride, 96 to 107 mEq/L; and acetate, 33 to 41 mEq/L. Bicarbonate is often used in place of acetate.

Blood access is achieved by means of an internal arteriovenous fistula created surgically with the patient's artery and vein, endogenous vein grafts, exogenous vein (bovine) grafts, or grafts made of artificial material such as expanded polytetrafluorethylene or by means of an external arteriovenous shunt or cannula (FIG. 13-12).

Hemodialysis treatment schedules vary with the kind of machine used and the patient's condition. Treatments are usually scheduled three times a week for 3 to 6 hours per treatment.

WATER TREATMENT

Water must be treated to remove substances toxic to the patient or harmful to the machine. Methods include filtration, softening, deionization, reverse osmosis, and distillation. Substances removed are dissolved anions or cations (sodium, chloride, iron, magnesium, manganese, copper, nitrates, fluoride, iodide) and organic materials (chloramines, pyrogens, endotoxins). Bacteria do not cross the membrane unless a leak is present. Bacterial growth in dialysate may change pH, decrease glucose concentration, and release toxins that cause chills, nausea, vomiting, and fever.

Major types of artificial kidneys are hollow fiber and flat plate. The hollow fiber kidney is increasingly used because it can be adapted to the size of the patient. In the hollow fiber kidney the blood flows through narrow filaments that are surrounded by dialysate (FIGS. 13-13 and 13-14). In the flat plate kidney the blood and dialysate flow in opposite directions in alternate

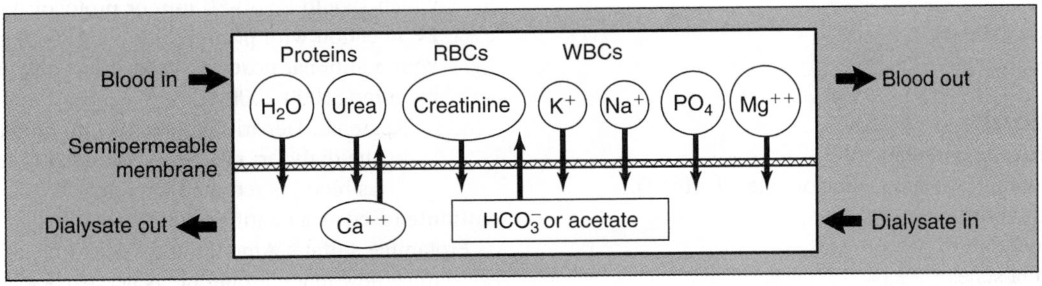

FIG. 13-13
General scheme for dialyzer design (Modified from Lancaster.[17])

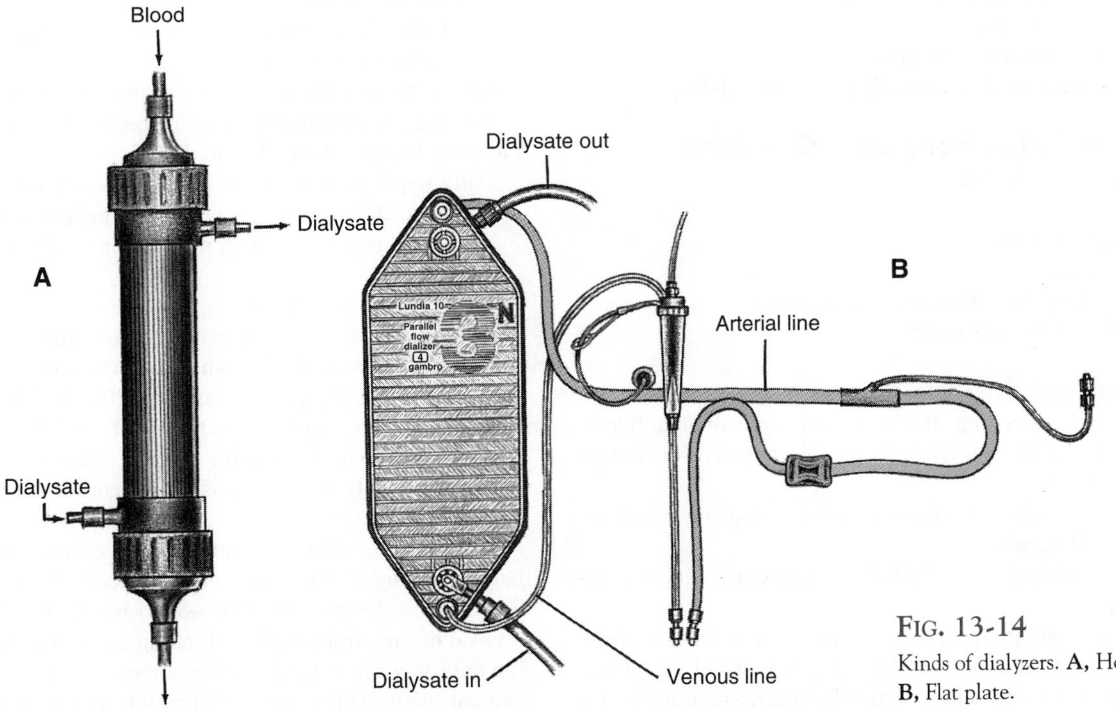

FIG. 13-14
Kinds of dialyzers. **A,** Hollow-fiber. **B,** Flat plate.

layers. Each patient's hollow fiber kidney is increasingly used multiple times (10 to 20). The kidney is either heat or chemically sterilized after dialysis to be used for the next treatment.

Hemodialysis Monitors

Each machine has visible and audible alarms that signal problems outside the preset upper and lower limits and cause portions of the system to be shut off or bypassed.

Dialysate compartment
- Temperature: Measures and controls level
- Flow rate: Reflects fluctuations in rate
- Conductivity: Detects hyperosmolality or hypoosmolality
- Pressure: Detects high or low levels
- Blood leak: Detects blood in dialysate as it leaves the machine (membrane rupture)

Blood compartment
- Pressure: Arterial and venous SP lines (stops blood pump)
- Air bubbles: Detects air in venous line (stops blood pump and clamps venous line)

Blood Access Devices

External arteriovenous shunt
Internal arteriovenous fistula
Grafts
Subclavian vein catheter
Femoral vein catheter

Indications

Need for rapid, efficient treatment
- Acute poisoning (aspirin, methanol, phenobarbital)
- Acute renal failure
- Chronic renal failure
- Severe edema states
- Hepatic coma
- Metabolic acidosis
- Hyperkalemia
- Extensive burns with prerenal azotemia
- Transfusion reactions
- Postpartum renal insufficiency
- Crush syndrome, rhabdomyolysis, and myoglobinuria

Contraindications and Cautions

Other major chronic illness
No vascular access
Hemorrhagic diathesis
Extremes of age
Inability to cooperate with treatment regimen
Inability to survive procedure

Potential Complications

Hemodynamic: Bleeding, clot formation, hypovolemia, hypervolemia, angina, dysrhythmias, anemia, hypotension, hypertension, CVA

Infectious: Vascular access site abscess, pyrogenic reactions, hepatitis B, sepsis

Metabolic: Dialysis disequilibrium syndrome, dialysis dementia

Mechanical: Membrane rupture, failure of monitors (temperature, pressure, osmolality, clot, and air bubble), loosened connections, shunt or fistula failure, hemolysis, air embolism

Multidisciplinary Plan

Anemia, hypertension, infection, peripheral neuropathy, pericarditis, renal osteodystrophy, reproductive dysfunction, and psychosocial difficulties associated with uremia continue to require treatment (see discussion of chronic renal failure, p. 871. The goal of therapy is to delay ESRD by conservative management and to begin dialysis or perform a renal transplant at the appropriate point in the course of the disease. Drug dosages and intervals must be modified when the kidney is involved in the drug's excretion. Rates of excretion and metabolism and sensitivity to drugs may be altered.[2]

Surgery

Internal arteriovenous fistula created or, rarely, external shunt inserted to provide access to arterial and venous circulation; central venous catheters may be inserted using fluoroscopy and local anesthesia

Medications

Anticoagulant agents
- Heparin sodium, systemic: As determined by clotting time, which should be 30-60 min or protocol; via intermittent IV injection with priming dose, 100 mg/kg body weight with additional doses as needed, or continuous infusion by pump (1000-2000 U/h)
  - Regional: Heparin is injected into blood line entering the dialyzer; protamine is added to exit blood line as blood is returned to patient

Antidote (used as an antiheparin agent)
- Protamine sulfate: Amount and kind of heparin used determine how much protamine is needed; each 1 mg of protamine sulfate neutralizes activity of about 90-115 U of heparin; keep patient's clotting time normal; monitor clotting time in machine and in patient; watch for heparin rebound (return of anticoagulation up to 10 h later), which may necessitate more protamine (please refer to product information)

Antihypertensive agents: Omit dosage on day of dialysis if necessary to prevent excessive hypotension during treatment

Vitamins (water-soluble, lost in dialysis)
- Daily requirements: Thiamine, 1.5 mg; riboflavin, 1.8 mg; niacin, 20 mg; pantothenic acid, 5 mg; pyridoxine, 5 mg; vitamin B_{12}, 3 μg; vitamin C, 100 mg; folic acid, 1 mg

General Management

Dietary management between dialyses includes protein (1.2 to 1.4 g/kg/day, 50% high biologic value); low sodium (500 to 3000 mg/day), low potassium (2000 to 3000 mg/day); calories (≥35 kcal/day ideal body weight); and fluid restriction (0.5-1.5 L/day, with the specific amount determined by the patient's dry weight). After dialysis the patient has normal volume relationships.

Dialysis disequilibrium syndrome may occur near the end of dialysis or after it. The condition is related to the osmotic gradient produced across the blood-brain barrier by the efficient removal of urea from the blood, but not from the brain tissue. The urea draws in water from the extracellular fluid and causes cerebral edema. Other factors that may be involved are changes in serum pH, rapid ion shift, and cardiovascular changes. The signs and symptoms of disequilibrium syndrome are headache, nausea, vomiting, agitation, twitching, confusion, and seizures. This syndrome can be prevented by slowing the rate of solute removal by dialyzing at a slower blood flow rate (100 ml/min) and for a shorter time, using a less efficient dialyzer, or using peritoneal dialysis.

Dialysis dementia, or progressive dialysis encephalopathy, is a syndrome that has emerged as experience with hemodialysis has increased. The clinical picture includes disturbed speech that occurs first during dialysis, myoclonus, dementia, or behavioral changes. It is a progressive condition that ends in death. A number of studies have implicated aluminum accumulation from the water supply or from aluminum hydroxide taken as a phosphate binder.

Dialysis-associated hepatitis B is a major concern for patients (often active carriers of the hepatitis B virus), staff (at risk because of frequent exposure to patient's blood), and families (at risk because of close contact, especially sexual, and from environmental surfaces). It should be noted that universal precautions with blood and other bodily fluids are needed to prevent spreading the hepatitis B virus (HBV). Health-care professionals and patients in dialysis units are particularly at risk because a patient with CRF may receive transfusions and may have a subclinical case of hepatitis B infection owing to impairment of the immune system.

The hepatitis B surface antigen (Hb_sAg) is a useful marker for active HBV infections. Anti-Hbs (hepatitis B surface antibody) indicates previous infection or exposure.

HBV can be found in blood and secretions containing serum or derived from serum. Oozing skin lesions, saliva, semen, and vaginal secretions can be sources of the virus. Transmission can occur by introduction of the virus-containing fluid through (1) direct percutaneous inoculation (via needles, and so forth); (2) indirect percutaneous inoculation (through minute skin abrasions); (3) absorption through mucosal surfaces (mouth, eye, and during sexual contact); and (4) transfer from environmental surfaces.

Programs to prevent the spread of HBV infections focus on identifying persons who are HB_sAg positive. Screening of all dialysis unit personnel and patients is done regularly. Such programs also include hygienic measures: safe, reliable procedures for handling laboratory specimens; procedures for hepatitis B precautions for hospitalized patients, including safe care of disposable materials, food handling, and laundry service; segregation of dialysis equipment used for patients who are HB_sAg positive; vigilant hand-washing practices; sterilization measures appropriate to the material involved; no eating, smoking, or other hand-to-mouth activity in the dialysis unit or laboratory; use of protective clothing, such as masks, goggles, gloves, aprons, shoe covers, gowns, and caps; and policy of reporting and recording any unusual exposure of HBV.

Hepatitis B vaccine is used for active immunization for preexposure prevention in high-risk populations, such as dialysis unit personnel. Hepatitis B immune globulin is used for passive immunization after exposure to HBV.

Recently, hepatitis C virus (HCV) identification has increased in the dialysis population. HCV is transmitted in the same ways as HBV and so is protected against in the same ways. Unfortunately, no HCV vaccine is available. However, recent research indicates that a treatment regimen of ribovirin and interferon appears promising as treatment.

Procedural Guidelines

Before Hemodialysis

Measure weight, temperature, pulse, respirations, and blood pressure (both lying and standing) and record for baseline

Review pretreatment BUN; serum creatinine, sodium, and potassium levels; hematocrit; be aware of HBV and HIV status of patient, if known

Check electrical status of the dialysis machine; dialysate concentration as ordered; patent, sterile tubing with all air flushed out; removal of the sterilizing agent used (formaldehyde or chlorine bleach); secure all connections; set all monitors

During Hemodialysis

Wear mask and have patient wear mask during initiation and discontinuation of dialysis; wear protective garb, goggles, apron, and gloves; use sterile technique for needle insertions and catheter connections; anchor connections securely; precautions against infection for all concerned are mandatory

Check equipment for readiness, safety, and settings of gauges; monitor vital signs, intake and output, and equipment parameters (blood flow rate, pressures, temperature, osmolality, clots, air emboli, negative pressure for ultrafiltration, and blood leaks); monitor clotting times; watch for rapid shifts in volume or electrolytes that may result in hypovolemia, angina, dysrhythmias, nausea, or muscle cramps; minimize blood loss

After Hemodialysis

Measure and record vital signs and weight after discontinuing treatment; use precautions against infection; provide routine care to access; avoid trauma to sites; avoid blood pressure readings or needlesticks in arm with shunt or fistula; check circulation; palpate thrill or auscultate venous blood flow; record BUN, serum creatinine, sodium, and potassium levels to note effects of treatment

Care Between Treatments

Encourage patient to follow diet and fluid restrictions as ordered, to take medications as ordered, and to call nurse or physician as appropriate for problems; limit weight gain to 0.5 to 1.5 kg/day between treatments; regular shunt or fistula care is required. Catheters should be taped securely; connections should be tightened and not allowed to get wet.

NURSING CARE

NURSING ASSESSMENT

Cardiovascular
- Hypervolemia: Hypertension, tachycardia, increased central venous pressure, jugular venous distention, extra heart sound (S3), lung sounds (crackles), postural edema, weight gain
- Hypovolemia: Hypotension, postural changes in blood pressure, tachycardia, flat neck veins, thirst, dry mucous membranes, weight loss, nausea, muscle cramps
- Hypertension, hypotension

Neurologic
- Dialysis disequilibrium syndrome: Headache, nausea, vomiting, agitation, twitching, confusion, and seizures
- Dialysis dementia: Disturbed speech, myoclonus, dementia: confusion or personality changes
- Intracerebral bleeding

Psychosocial: Uncooperative, angry, depressed; patient expresses concerns about family problems

General: Redness, swelling, warmth, pain at catheter, graft, or shunt exit sites, fistula at puncture site or elsewhere, fever, rigors, pruritus, restless leg syndromes, fatigue, headache

Patient Problems/Nursing Diagnoses & Interventions

NIC Tissue Perfusion Management

Excess fluid volume related to fluid accumulation since last treatment

- Monitor weight, blood pressure, intake and output, respirations, and pulse *to determine fluid status as a basis for treatment parameters.*
- Monitor laboratory values: BUN; serum creatinine; sodium, potassium, calcium, magnesium, phosphate levels; hemoglobin and hematocrit *because nitrogenous wastes and electrolytes accumulate between treatments; anemia is a continuing problem with CRF and blood losses.*
- Discuss need to limit fluid intake to 1500 ml/24 h or less

Deficient fluid volume, risk for, related to too rapid fluid removal during treatment and potential blood loss

- Monitor intake and output, weight, blood pressure, pulse, and respiration *to recognize shifts in fluid balance.*
- If possible, monitor blood clotting time *to determine effect of anticoagulant therapy.*
- Minimize blood loss by careful blood sampling, return of all blood to patient, and pressure applied to fistula puncture sites at the end of treatment *to prevent worsening of anemia of CRF.*
- Avoid weight loss greater than 3 to 4 kg during treatment *to prevent hypovolemia and its complications.*

NIC Risk Management

Risk for infection related to invasive procedure and blood transfusion requirements

- Follow universal precautions for exposure to blood and body fluids *to protect patient and nurse.*
- Use sterile technique to start and stop procedure and for shunt or fistula care *to protect patient from potential sources of infection during the procedure;* inspect shunt exit sites and fistula needle puncture sites for signs of infection *to detect infection promptly.*
- Monitor temperature and WBC count; small elevations may reflect significant infections; observe for signs of sepsis.

NIC Coping Assistance

Disturbed thought processes related to dialysis disequilibrium syndrome or to dialysis dementia

Disturbed body image related to chronic renal failure requiring dependence on a machine

Interrupted family processes related to need for dialysis

- Assess during and toward the end of treatment for headache, nausea, vomiting, or agitation, *which are associated with too rapid removal of substances during dialysis.*
- Monitor speech during dialysis; observe for myoclonus or change in behavior *because these signs of dialysis dementia first appear during dialysis.*
- Observe patient's response to chronic illness, altered renal function, other body system alterations, and the possibility of transplantation because people vary greatly in their response to such life changes.
- Recognize patient's response to having to depend on a machine *because the patient may feel helpless or hopeless, deny reality, personalize the machine, or accept it as necessary.*
- Support the patient's strengths: self-confidence, determination, and motivation to live, *since dialysis patients are not disabled in all aspects of life.*
- Be aware of changes in social involvement, and help patient develop or continue interests beyond dialysis *because the patient may participate in fewer social or recreational activities, experience lifestyle changes, or withdraw.*
- Be alert to excessive concerns with losses, to depression, to self-neglect, to noncompliance with medical regimen, and to the possibility of suicide; try to keep lines of communication open; encourage questions *because suicide is possible and the patient has access to several methods.*
- Be aware of the effect of the loss of libido, of impotence, and of decreased orgasm in the marital and sexual life of the patient *to refer patients as appropriate.*
- Try to help the patient develop realistic expectation of dialysis, *since hemodialysis does not reverse all the signs and symptoms of CRF.*
- Recognize the impact CRF with hemodialysis has on the family, *since disruption, expense, and considerable alteration in time commitments may occur.*
- Help patient and family recognize the demands of illness on the patient's and the family's needs for emotional support.
- Recognize the spouse's fears.
- Support the family's cooperation in the patient's care, and discuss with them ways to reduce domestic tension and unhappiness; recognize the patient's inability to continue his or her family role, and help the patient toward acceptance through discussion of alternatives; in home hemodialysis treatment, recognize the stresses on the family, and support them in learning about dialysis and in carrying out treatments in the home; *patient outcomes affect the family's ability to cope and vice versa.*

Patient Education/Continuum of Care Plan

1. Explain function of normal and artificial kidney.
2. Explain principles of hemodialysis.
3. Explain aseptic technique for needle insertions or shunt care. Explain care of access sites.
4. Help the patient practice self-observation skills (temperature, pulse, respiration, blood pressure, intake and output, and weight) and record keeping.
5. Explain components of the system with preparation, operation, cleaning, and storage (repair and maintenance if home hemodialysis).

6. Explain initiating dialysis, monitoring during dialysis, and discontinuing dialysis.
7. Explain emergencies related to the machine and to the patient's medical condition.
8. Explain care while off the machine: diet, fluid restrictions, medical complications, care of blood access route, medications, and prevention of infection.
9. Explain medical supervision, including help available from medical center, and schedule of return visits, and assistance from the local physician.
10. Review education plan for chronic renal failure (see p. 875).

Evaluation/Patient Outcomes

Tissue Perfusion Management: Laboratory values are within normal limits. Weight gain between treatments is in desirable range. Patient does not gain more than 0.5 to 1.0 kg/day. Treatments are done safely without hypotension. Patient does not have hypotension, nausea, or muscle cramps.

Risk Management: No infection occurs. Patient does not have signs or symptoms of infection.

Coping Assistance: Thought processes are normal. Patient does not develop the signs and symptoms associated with dialysis disequilibrium syndrome or dialysis dementia. Changes in body image are accepted. Patient and family adapt to the changes associated with CRF and hemodialysis. Patient and family have adjusted to life on hemodialysis. Patient and family have returned to work and social activities as much as possible. Family continues to use support of the health care team.

Peritoneal Dialysis[9,31]

Peritoneal dialysis (PD) involves the introduction of dialysate fluid into the abdominal cavity, where the peritoneum acts as a semipermeable membrane between the dialysate and the blood in the abdominal vessels. A machine may be used, or the fluid may be instilled and drained manually from the peritoneal cavity.

Description and Rationale

Components of PD solutions include varying amounts of glucose and electrolytes. Dextrose levels vary: 1.5% (15 g/L), 2.5% (25 g/L), and 4.25% (42.5 g/L). Electrolyte concentrations vary also: sodium—131-141 mEq/L, magnesium—0.5-1.0 mEq/l, chloride—94-102 mEq/L. Calcium is usually 3.5 mEq/L, while potassium levels are 0. Any potassium needed in the dialysate must be added at the time of use.

Additions may include insulin and heparin, 500 to 1000 U/L.

Continuous ambulatory peritoneal dialysis (CAPD) is an alternative to intermittent PD for CRF. A permanent peritoneal dialysis catheter is inserted into the abdomen; a Luer-Lok titanium connector joins the transfer set to the bag of fluid (Figs. 13-15 and 13-16).

CAPD usually involves four exchanges of 1 to 2 L each in 24 hours and dwell times of 4 to 8 hours. Dialysate in plastic bags is used. When the solution is infused, the plastic bag is folded up and concealed under the person's clothes. When the fluid is drained, that bag is discarded and a new bag is attached, and its fluid is instilled for the next cycle. CAPD is self-administered and machine free.

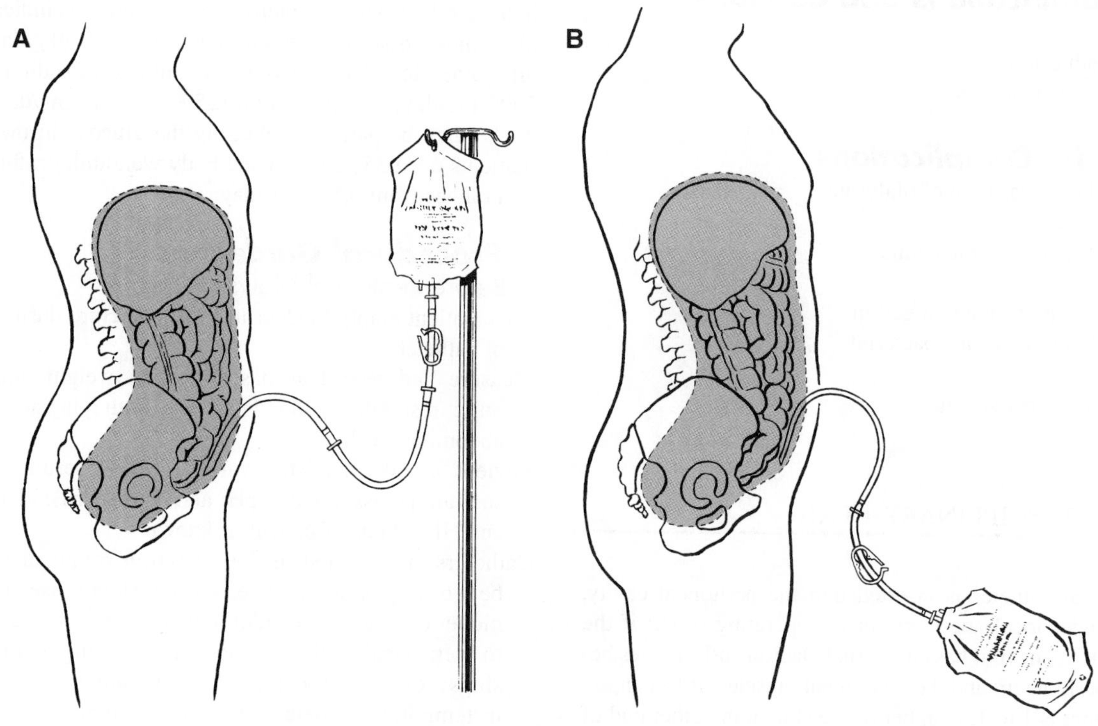

Fig. 13-15
Peritoneal dialysis. **A,** Inflow. **B,** Outflow (drains to gravity).

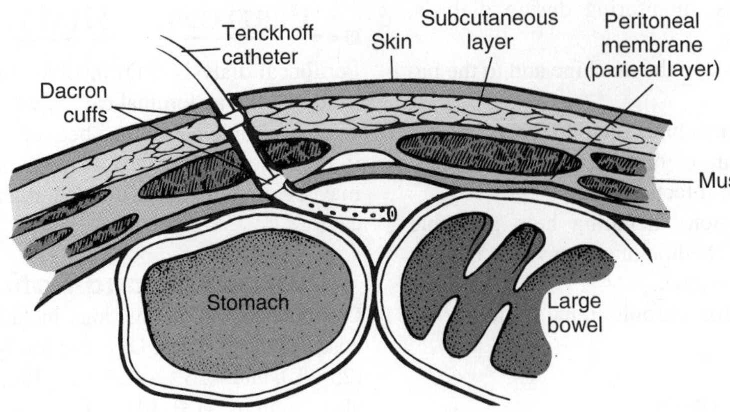

FIG. 13-16
Peritoneal catheter.[18]

Continuous cycling PD involves connecting the peritoneal catheter to an automated PD machine that performs three to seven cycles during the night while the patient sleeps. During the day, one cycle of fluid is left in the abdomen. The person is free of dialysis activities during the day, and connections are less frequent than in CAPD.

Indications

Less rapid treatment needed
Unavailability of equipment and staff for hemodialysis
Severe cardiovascular disease
Inadequate access to vascular system
Shock after cardiovascular surgery
Refusal of blood transfusion
Internal hemorrhage or risk of bleeding (because heparin cannot be administered)

Contraindications and Cautions

Peritonitis
Abdominal adhesions
Recent abdominal surgery

Potential Complications

Leakage and extravasation of dialysate
Drainage problems
Hyperglycemia, hypoproteinemia
Weight gain
Catheter exit site or tunnel infection
Peritonitis: Bacterial or nonbacterial
Bowel adhesions
Respiratory embarrassment

MULTIDISCIPLINARY PLAN

Surgery

The peritoneal catheter is inserted into the peritoneal cavity, generally under local anesthetic in the operating room; if the catheter is permanent, it has an internal Dacron cuff that lies between the peritoneum and the abdominal muscles; it has an external cuff that is 1 to 1.5 cm below the skin at the other end of a 3- to 4-cm subcutaneous tunnel (see FIG. 13-16).

Medications

Anticoagulants: Heparin may be added to dialysate to prevent fibrin formation and obstruction to the fluid flow
Antimicrobials: Used when bacterial or fungal peritonitis is diagnosed and often given by both systemic and intraperitoneal routes
Miscellaneous vitamins (water-soluble) needed to replace those lost in dialysate
Phosphorus binders: Calcium carbonate, calcium acetate, RenaGel
Vitamin (D_3, 125) (Rocaltrol), PO or IV erythropoietin: subcutaneously, weekly, or IV every dialysis
Iron supplement

General Management

Medical management of the continuing uremic problems is discussed in the section on CRF (p. 872); the use of PD causes an increased loss of blood proteins and amino acids with the fluid in the outflow; a more generous protein intake is indicated to replace these losses (suggested intake: 1.2 to 5 g/kg/day, 50% of high biologic value); restrictions continue in sodium (1500 to 2000 mg/day) and potassium (2500 to 3500 mg/day); caloric intake may be partly supplied by the glucose in the PD fluid (patients need 35 kcal/kg ideal body weight/day); fluid restriction ranges from 0.5 to 1 L/day

Procedural Guidelines

Before Peritoneal Dialysis

Have patient empty bladder to avoid puncture during insertion of catheter
Measure and record as baseline data: weight, temperature, pulse, respirations, blood pressure (both lying and standing), abdominal girth
Review blood chemistry values (BUN; serum creatinine, sodium, potassium, and pH; and hematocrit); identify HBV and HIV status of patient, if known
Catheters are inserted in the operating room; masks should be worn by patient, nurse, and physician; use sterile technique during subsequent connections of dialysis fluid to peritoneal catheter and for changing catheter dressings; observe for infection in catheter insertion site in temporary catheters and catheter tunnel site in permanent ones

CAUSES OF PERITONITIS

Peritonitis may be caused by gram-positive organisms *(Staphylococcus epidermis, S. aureus),* enterococci, gram-negative organisms *(Escherichia coli, Pseudomonas),* anaerobes *(Bacteroides, Clostridium),* and fungi *(Candida albicans, Aspergillus fumigatus, Torulopsis glabrata).*

After catheter insertion, observe for perforation of bowel (dialysate outflow stained with feces or blood) or bladder (urine pink or blood tinged)

Warm (37° C) fluid before hanging it, or use plastic bags of solution warmed in a folded heating pad set on a low setting

Add medications to dialysate as ordered; flush tubing to remove air; connect to catheter; anchor connections and tubing securely; avoid having kinks in tubing

During Peritoneal Dialysis

Measure and record intake, output, weight, temperature, pulse, respirations, and blood pressure regularly; keep accurate records of dialysis cycles (inflow, dwell, and outflow times); record strength of solutions used, additions made, and fluid balance (amounts retained or lost)

Observe for peritonitis; collect samples of dialysate for culture and sensitivity tests if it is turbid, bloody, or has an odor, as well as when it is routinely ordered (see box above)

Observe for respiratory embarrassment (manifested by dyspnea and rales), resulting from the patient's abdomen being too full of fluid or leakage of dialysate into thoracic cavity through a defect in the diaphragm

Usual Timing of an Hourly Cycle

Inflow time: 10 minutes

Dwell time: 10 to 30 minutes

Outflow time: 20 to 30 minutes

NOTE: With continuous ambulatory PD, dwell times are 6 to 8 hours

Cycle-Related Problems

Inflow problems: Obstructed catheter (clots, fibrin, omentum, or catheter malposition); leakage of fluid around catheter insertion site

Dwell time problems: Prolonged time may cause water depletion or hyperglycemia unless CAPD is method being used

Outflow problems: Kinks in tubing or catheter, catheter occluded by loops of bowel or by constipation, or fibrin

After Peritoneal Dialysis

Determine fluid balance; measure weight, temperature, pulse, respirations, blood pressure, and abdominal girth

Review postdialysis blood chemistries: blood urea nitrogen; and serum creatinine, sodium, and potassium

Care Between Peritoneal Dialysis Treatments

Encourage adequate protein intake (1.2 to 5 g/kg/day)

Restrict intake of sodium (1500 to 2000 mg/day) and potassium (2500 to 3500 mg/day)

Caloric intake at 35 kcal/kg ideal body weight should include the calories from the glucose in the dialysate solution

Fluid restrictions usually range from 0.5 to 1.5 L/day

Avoid constipation; consider use of stool softeners and laxatives as needed

Routine cleaning and dressing and avoidance of trauma at the catheter exit site are essential to prevent infection

Manage continuing uremic problems (see discussion of CRF, p. 872)

NURSING CARE

NURSING ASSESSMENT

Cardiovascular

- Hypervolemia: Hypertension, tachycardia, increased central venous pressure, jugular venous distention, extra heart sound (S3), lung sounds (crackles), postural edema, cardiomegaly, orthopnea, cough, weight gain
- Hypovolemia: Hypotension, postural changes in blood pressure, tachycardia, flat neck veins, thirst, dry mucous membranes, weight loss, nausea, muscle cramps, dizziness

Abdominal: Rigidity, tenderness, cloudy dialysate drainage, decreased or no bowel sounds; redness, tenderness, swelling around catheter site

Respiratory: Tachypnea, dyspnea, rales

General: Fever, malaise

Psychosocial: Acceptance or rejection of situation by patient; change in family relationships; concerns about long-term impact of illness

PATIENT PROBLEMS/NURSING DIAGNOSES & INTERVENTIONS

NIC TISSUE PERFUSION

Excess fluid volume related to fluid accumulation since last treatment or deficient fluid volume related to too rapid removal of body fluid during treatment

- Monitor weight and blood pressure.
- Monitor laboratory values: BUN, serum creatinine, sodium, potassium, and pH; hematocrit *to determine fluid status as a basis for treatment parameters;* nitrogenous wastes and electrolytes accumulate between treatments; anemia is a continuing problem of uremia.
- Monitor intake and output, weight, blood pressure, pulse, and respirations; note excess weight loss: markedly negative fluid balance as a result of dialysis *to recognize shifts in fluid balance and to prevent hypovolemia.*

NIC RISK MANAGEMENT

Risk for infection (peritonitis) related to invasive procedure

- Follow universal precautions for exposure to blood and body fluids *to protect patient and nurse.*
- Use sterile technique to begin and end procedure and at access site *to protect patient from sources of infection during procedure.*
- Inspect catheter insertion site for signs of infection; monitor temperature, WBCs in serum, and dialysate *to detect infection.*

NIC Nutrition Support

Imbalanced nutrition: less than body requirements, related to protein loss through peritoneum into dialysate and decreased protein intake

- Assess serum protein, calcium, and glucose regularly; monitor weight *to determine altered levels.*
- Ensure adequate protein intake (see p. 902) *to replace losses associated with PD.*
- Give calcium supplement as indicated.

Imbalanced nutrition: more than body requirements, related to caloric intake from glucose in dialysate fluid

- Limit caloric intake in diet and decrease glucose concentration in dialysate or decrease dwell time *if hyperglycemia or weight gain is a problem.*
- Limit phosphorus, potassium intake.

NIC Coping Assistance

Disturbed body image related to chronic renal failure requiring dependence on peritoneal dialysis

Interrupted family processes related to family member with CRF requiring peritoneal dialysis

- Observe patient's response to chronic illness, altered renal function, other body system alterations, and the possibility of transplantation *because patients vary greatly in their responses to such life changes.*
- Recognize patient's response to dependence on PD; try to keep lines of communication open; encourage questions *because the patient may feel helpless, hopeless, and deny reality; personalize the machine; or accept it as necessary.*
- Support the patient's strengths: self-confidence, determination, and motivation to live; *dialysis patients are not disabled in all aspects of life.*
- Be aware of changes in social involvement; help patient to develop or to continue interests beyond dialysis *because patient may participate in fewer social or recreational activities, reject lifestyle changes, and withdraw.*
- Be alert to excessive concerns with losses, depression, self-neglect, noncompliance with medical regimen, and the possibility of suicide; *suicide is possible and the patient has access to several methods.*
- Be aware of the effect that loss of libido, impotence, and decreased orgasm have on the marital and sex life of the patient, and be able to refer the patient as appropriate.
- Try to help the patient develop realistic expectations of dialysis, *since PD does not reverse all the signs and symptoms of CRF.*
- Recognize the impact of CRF with PD on the family; *disruption, expense, and considerable alterations in time commitments may occur.*
- Help patient and family recognize demands of illness on family's and patient's need for emotional support; recognize family's fears. Support family's cooperation in patient's care, and help them look at ways to reduce domestic tension and unhappiness. Recognize patient's inability to continue his or her family role, and help patient accept this through discussion of alternatives. In home PD, recognize that the family is stressed, and support them in learning about dialysis in the home. Patient outcomes affect the family's ability to cope and vice versa.

Patient Education/Continuum of Care Plan

1. Explain the nature of CRF.
2. Explain the medical regimen and its rationale, including diet (restricted protein, sodium, and potassium), restricted fluid intake, and medications (purpose, dosage, interval, and adverse reactions).
3. Explain the function of normal and artificial kidneys and the principles of PD.
4. Explain and help patient practice aseptic technique.
5. Explain components of the system, preparation, operation, cleaning, and storage (repair and maintenance if home dialysis).
6. Explain initiating dialysis, monitoring during dialysis, and discontinuing dialysis.
7. Explain emergencies related to the machine, if used, and to the patient's medical condition.
8. Explain care while off the machine: diet, fluid restrictions, medical complications, care of peritoneal access route, medications, and prevention of infection.
9. Help patient learn self-observational skills (temperature, pulse, respirations, blood pressure, intake and output, and weight) and record keeping.
10. Explain ways to avoid infection.
11. Explain personal hygiene, rest, and exercise.
12. Explain when to call the physician.
13. Explain the plan for medical follow-up.

Evaluation/Patient Outcomes

Tissue Perfusion Management: Laboratory values are within normal limits. Treatment is done safely without hypotension. Volume relationships and blood pressure are normal.

Risk Management: Peritonitis is avoided. No signs or symptoms of peritonitis are present.

Nutrition Support: Protein and caloric intake meet body requirements. Serum albumin and glucose levels are within normal limits; weight is stable. Weight gain between treatments is in desirable range. Weight is maintained at or near ideal weight.

Coping Assistance: Changes in body image are accepted. Patient and family adapt to changes associated with CRF and PD. Patient and family have adjusted to life on PD. Patient and family have returned to work and social activities as much as possible. Patient and family continue to use support of health care team.

Continuous Renal Replacement Therapies

Description and Rationale

Continuous renal replacement therapies (CRRTs) include continuous arteriovenous hemofiltration (CAVH), continuous arteriovenous hemodiafiltration (CAVHD), continuous venovenous hemofiltration (CVVH), and continuous venovenous hemodiafiltration (CVVHD). Hemofiltration therapies (CAVH, CVVH) are prescribed when fluid removal is the primary goal. Hemodiafiltration therapies (CAVHD, CVVHD) combine hemodialysis and hemofiltration and are prescribed when the goal is solute removal plus or minus fluid removal. The continuous nature of these therapies allows for a slow and gentle removal of plasma water and dissolved solutes (electrolytes, toxins, drugs) from critically ill patients with renal insufficiency or failure.

The most commonly used CRRTs are the venovenous forms, CVVHD and CVVH. Complications such as vessel thrombosis are not as frequent in the venous techniques as in the arterial therapies

There is one other CRRT, hemoperfusion, a specialty technique that is used only for toxin removal (usually acute poisoning). The toxins are eliminated by adsorption onto a substance, usually charcoal. This therapy is initiated and managed only by an expert multidisciplinary team.

Indications for CRRTs include acute renal failure or insufficiency with uremia, abnormal electrolytes, acid-base imbalance, or fluid overload in critically ill patients. These are safe and efficient therapies for patients who cannot tolerate conventional hemodialysis because of hemodynamic instability, arrhythmias, or increased intracranial pressure (ICP). Patients may not tolerate conventional hemodialysis because of the significant extracorporeal volume or the rapid fluid, electrolyte, or osmolality shifts over 2 to 4 hours. Patients who require large fluid volumes, such as parenteral nutrition, blood products, and medications, benefit from continuous fluid removal. Fluid restrictions are obsolete for patients on CRRTs. Nonrenal indications being studied include cytokine removal in sepsis and multiple organ dysfunction syndrome (MODS), fluid removal and neurohormonal changes in congestive heart failure (CHF), and myoglobin removal in rhabdomyolysis.

CRRTs involve a low-volume blood circuit with a hemofilter and an ultrafiltration collection bag. The hemofilters have semipermeable membranes that separate the blood compartment from the ultrafiltrate compartment. Either hollow fiber or flat plate hemofilters are used for CRRTs. Plasma water and mid-molecular-weight solutes (10,000 to 30,000 daltons) move from the blood compartment across the semipermeable membrane to form ultrafiltrate (UF), which drains from the hemofilter into a UF collection bag. This process is similar to the filtration process across the glomerular basement membrane in the kidney. The resulting ultrafiltrate is composed of plasma water and solutes (e.g., Na^+, K^+, Cl^-, HCO_3^-, H^+, urea, creatinine, Mg^{++}, PO_4^-, Ca^{++}, cytokines, certain drugs).

Fluid removal in CRRTs is determined by the transmembrane pressure gradient (TPG) across the hemofilter membrane. The TPG is the difference between the oncotic and hydrostatic pressure within the hemofilter system. Positive hydrostatic pressure is exerted by blood when it is pushed through the blood compartment of the hemofilter either by the patient's mean arterial pressure (MAP) in CAVH or by the set rate of the blood pump (ml/min) in CVVH. Positive hydrostatic pressure pushes fluid across the hemofilter membrane. Negative hydrostatic pressure in the ultrafiltration (UF) compartment, on the opposite side of the hemofilter membrane, is created by gravity of the UF collection bag in relation to the hemofilter. This pressure is important in determining the rate of ultrafiltration. Oncotic pressure created by RBCs, WBCs, and plasma proteins in the blood compartment prevents all of the plasma water from ultrafiltrating.

There are two mechanisms of solute removal in CRRTs: convective transport and diffusive transport. Convective transport is the movement of solutes along with fluid across a semipermeable membrane. This is the only mechanism of solute removal in CAVH and CVVH, and it is directly proportional to the amount of ultrafiltration. The larger the volume ultrafiltrated, the more solute is removed. Diffusive transport is the movement of solutes across a semipermeable membrane from an area of higher solute concentration to an area of lower concentration. In CAVHD and CVVHD a dialysate solution is infused throughout the UF compartment, countercurrent to the blood flow compartment, to create a diffusion gradient to enhance solute removal. Both convection and diffusion are mechanisms of solute removal in CAVHD and CVVHD.

PD solutions were used as dialysate in CRRTs in the past. The high dextrose concentrations of these solutions often led to hyperglycemia and additional insulin infusion therapy. New premixed dialysates made specifically for CRRTs are now used. These dialysates contain physiologic levels of sodium, potassium, calcium, magnesium, chloride, and dextrose with a lactate buffer. Common dialysate flow rates through the hemofilter are 1000 to 2500 ml/h. There is a curvilinear increase in solute removal with increases in dialysate flow rates, which plateaus around 2500 ml/h. Higher flow rates are used for hyperkalemia, drug intoxication, or rapid removal of urea.

Replacement fluid (RF) is the solution infused to maintain the prescribed hourly fluid balance. The composition of RF is determined by the patient's metabolic and electrolyte needs. Hyperalimentation, normal saline solution, bicarbonate solutions, and potassium additives are frequently prescribed replacement fluids. The amount of RF administered is calculated on an hourly basis and depends on the hourly amount of UF output, IV intake, and desired fluid balance. The RF is generally administered into the CRRT circuit via a prehemofilter. Prehemofilter RF hemodilutes the blood, which helps decrease clotting in the hemofilter.

Anticoagulation is prescribed to prevent hemofilter/circuit clotting and to maximize the clearance capability of the hemofilter. The goal is to anticoagulate the hemofilter and circuit, yet systemic anticoagulation may occur. Existing thrombocytopenia or coagulopathies may obviate the need for heparinization. Commonly used anticoagulants include heparin and trisodium citrate. If trisodium citrate is used, calcium is infused at the same time. However, most protocols require priming the hemofilter and circuit with heparinized saline solution, administering a bolus dose, and initiating a low-dose heparin infusion through a prehemofilter port in the circuit. Monitoring clotting times is required during continuous infusions of anticoagulants.

CAVH/CAVHD

Large-bore arterial and venous access sites are required for CAVH and CAVHD. The femoral artery and vein are frequently used for access, but brachial, jugular, and subclavian sites also may be used. Blood is propelled from the arterial catheter through the circuit and hemofilter and back to the patient via the venous catheter by the force of MAP created by the patient's cardiac output. CAVH/CAVHD circuits require MAPs of

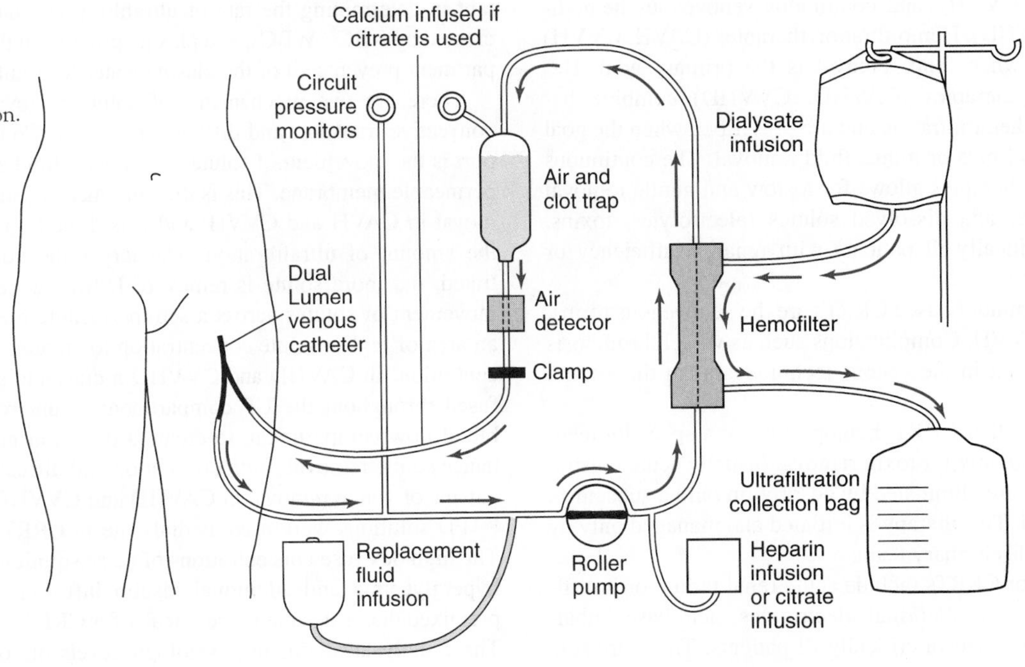

FIG. 13-17 Continuous venovenous hemodiafiltration.

at least 50 to 60 mm Hg for effective flow through the circuit and ultrafiltration.

CVVH/CVVHD

Venous access with a dual-lumen catheter is required for CVVH and CVVHD. Common access sites include the femoral, internal jugular, or subclavian veins. A pump is required for CVVH and CVVHD because arterial pressure is not available. Blood is pulled and pushed through the blood circuit and hemofilter via a roller pump (rates of 30 to 300 ml/min). The blood pump is capable of monitoring circuit pressures and has an air detector and circuit clamp for safety purposes (FIG. 13-17).

Indications

Inability to tolerate conventional hemodialysis because of hemodynamic instability, dysrhythmias, increased ICP

Acute renal insufficiency/failure with uremia, metabolic acidosis, abnormal electrolytes, symptomatic fluid overload

Sepsis, congestive heart failure, multiple organ dysfunction syndrome (MODS), rhabdomyolysis

Relative Contraindications

Inability to obtain and maintain adequate access

Hypercoagulable state with contraindication to anticoagulation

MULTIDISCIPLINARY PLAN

Medications

Additives to RF: Sodium bicarbonate, potassium chloride, etc.

Additives to dialysate: Potassium chloride

Anticoagulant

Heparin sodium: Initial dose 10-20 units/kg; continuous infusion 5 to 10 units/kg

Trisodium citrate: Infused in the front of the dialysis circuit. Its anticoagulant effect is then reversed with calcium gluconate before the blood's return to the patient. The citrate is a commercial preparation infused at 180 ml/h. The calcium is mixed as 10 g in 250 ml of normal saline and is infused at 10 ml/h. The dialysate must be bicarbonate based and calcium free.

General Management

CRRT is generally ordered by a nephrologist and is set up and monitored only by professional nursing staff trained in the technique and complications. Orders for CRRT include an hourly UF rate goal prescribed according to the patient's hemodynamic states and hemofiltration needs. Typical UF rates are 750 to 1500 ml/h. The desired hourly fluid balance is prescribed based on the patient's volume status. Fluid balance orders can range from −400 ml/h to +50 ml/h. Replacement fluid solutions are prescribed based on the patient's metabolic and electrolyte needs. The calculation that determines the hourly RF infusion rate is as follows:

$$RF = [\text{Net UF rate} + (\text{Other output}) - (\text{Total intake})] - [\text{Desired fluid balance}]$$

Monitoring the patient's pH, Na^+, K^+, Cl^-, CO_2, Mg^{++}, Ca^{++}, PO_4^-, Cr, BUN, glucose, and coagulation status is essential during CRRT. Hemodynamic monitoring required during CRRTs include blood pressure (BP), heart rate (HR), and central venous pressure (CVP).

Safety goggles, mask, and gloves must be worn by staff to protect themselves from viruses and organisms that may be transmitted via the UF. For patient safety, hemofilter circuit and access sites are monitored frequently (q1h minimum) for kinks, disconnects, leaks, and signs of clotting and air.

An assessment of the patient's nutritional needs and an understanding of the nutritional implications during CRRT help guide parenteral or enteral feeding prescriptions. Nutritional implications include vitamin, mineral, and protein losses via the UF and dextrose absorption from the dialysate.

Drug dosing for patients on CRRTs requires special attention. Guidelines for dosing take into account properties of the drugs and UF rates of the CRRT.

Mechanical Problems

Potential mechanical problems of CRRTs may involve the access catheter, hemofilter, circuit, or blood pump (CVVH). The CRRT will not work if there is an obstruction to flow from a kink or obstruction (clot, vessel wall) in the catheter. The hemofilter and circuit are monitored for leaks, ruptures, and cracks, which may result in an air embolus or hemorrhage. In CVVH the blood pump is tested and monitored to ensure that the air detector, blood leak detector, pressure transducers, and venous clamp are working.

Procedural Guidelines

Preparation for CRRTs

Assemble equipment and supplies. Prime hemofilter and circuit with heparinized saline solution to remove all air and filter preservatives. Ensure all connections are secure. Make sure the blood pump passes its self-test before use.

Before initiating therapy, monitor the patient's baseline temperature, HR, BP, CVP, weight, intake/output, creatinine, blood urea nitrogen, electrolytes, glucose, clotting times, platelet count, hematocrit, and arterial blood gas. Review the CRRT orders for RF composition, dialysate additives, anticoagulation, UF rate goal, net fluid balance, blood pump rate, laboratory monitoring, and parameters to notify the physician.

Assist with catheter insertion. Using sterile technique, check catheter patency and flow before connecting circuit to patient.

Initiation and Maintenance of CRRTs

Assemble supplies. Using sterile technique, connect circuit to the access catheters. Monitor blood flow through the circuit for air bubbles and ease of flow. Begin dialysate, heparin, and RF infusions. Establish ultrafiltration and monitor the patient's BP closely during the first 15 minutes of therapy. Secure the circuit to prevent an inadvertent disconnect or dislodgement. The blood circuit and blood pump should be kept visible at all times.

Monitor the patient's hemodynamic status and laboratory values closely. Monitor access sites for infection or bleeding. Check pulses distal to catheter sites. Monitor patient for bleeding if receiving anticoagulation.

Measure and regulate UF rate. Calculate RF rate based on the total output, total intake, and desired fluid balance hourly. Adjust height of the UF drainage bag appropriately to increase or decrease the hourly UF rate. Document accurate intake, output, and RF calculations every hour.

CVVH/CVVHD: Monitor and manage the blood pump circuit pressures. Identify and troubleshoot blood pump alarms.

Circuit Change or Discontinuation of CRRT

Discontinue infusions of dialysate, anticoagulant, and RF. Clamp UF tubing. If possible, return the blood in the circuit to the patient, then clamp the circuit tubings and the access catheters. Flush catheters with heparinized saline solution as ordered. Discard CRRT circuit and hemofilter in a biohazardous waste receptacle. Remove access catheters as ordered if the plan is to not restart therapy or convert to conventional hemodialysis. Apply pressure to catheter site for 10 minutes or longer if indicated.

NURSING CARE

Nursing Assessment

Cardiovascular

Hypervolemia: Elevated CVP. Jugular venous distention, extra heart sound (S3), lung sounds (crackles), frothy white or pink-tinged sputum, dependent or generalized edema, weight gain, dyspnea

Hypovolemia: Hypotension, tachycardia, low CVP, flat neck veins, dry mucous membranes, thirst, weight loss

Hemorrhage, coagulopathies, purpura, petechiae

Metabolic

Acidemia: Low arterial pH. Kussmaul respirations, hypotension

Alkalosis: High arterial pH, cardiac dysrhythmias, tetany

Skin: Pressure ulcers secondary to immobility/bed rest while on CRRT and with critical illness

Musculoskeletal: Limited range of motion, stiff joints, foot drop, muscle atrophy related to immobility and critical illness

Potential Complications

Air embolus; inadvertent fluid overload or fluid removal; rapid electrolyte or acid/base shifts; hypothermia; bleeding from circuit, access, or systemic; excessive hemofilter/circuit clotting; hemorrhage if catheter is dislodged

Patient Problems/Nursing Diagnoses & Interventions

NIC Tissue Perfusion Management

Acid-Base and Electrolyte Management

Ineffective tissue perfusion, renal

Excess fluid volume related to fluid accumulation caused by altered renal function or an inadvertent replacement fluid (RF) calculation error and infusion rate

Risk for deficient fluid volume related to too rapid removal of fluid (UF) caused by excess negative hydrostatic pressure in the UF bag or an inadvertent RF calculation error and infusion rate

- Monitor patient weight, intake and output, BP, HR, CVP, hourly UF rates, and oxygenation *to determine fluid status.*
- Ensure accurate calculations *to determine RF volumes every hour.*
- Monitor trends in hourly UF rates *to assess for clotting and hemofilter efficiency.*
- Monitor laboratory values: BUN, creatinine, sodium, potassium, calcium, magnesium, and phosphate *to determine electrolyte balance, accumulation of nitrogenous wastes, and solute removal efficiency; monitor CBC to detect evidence of hemorrhage.*
- Supplement electrolyte deficit as ordered.

- Correct acid-base imbalance as indicated/ordered.
- Monitor and record hourly intake and output; ensure accurate RF calculations and infusion rates *to prevent inadvertent hypovolemia from overly aggressive fluid removal.*
- Monitor BP, HR, CVP, intake and output, and hourly UF rate *to determine fluid status and note changes.*
- Alter the level of the UF bag (raise the bag) *to decrease the negative hydrostatic pressure and decrease the rate of UF removal.*
- Administer IV fluid boluses as ordered *to treat symptomatic hypovolemia.*

NIC RISK MANAGEMENT

Risk for infection related to invasive procedure
Risk for injury caused by bleeding related to inadvertent disconnect of circuit or anticoagulation therapy

- Use sterile technique whenever the circuit is accessed, including during connection and discontinuation, *to protect the patient from nosocomial contamination.*
- Inspect access sites for redness, swelling, tenderness, drainage; monitor the patient's temperature and WBC count *to detect infection.*
- Follow universal precautions for exposure to blood and body fluids *to protect patient and nurse from contamination.*
- Give site care, dressing, and tubing changes per hospital policy *to prevent infection.*
- Monitor access sites and other potential sites for bleeding; no IM or SC injections; monitor laboratory values: PT, PTT (or ACT), platelets, hemoglobin/hematocrit *to detect signs of bleeding.*
- Monitor pulses and capillary refill distal to access catheters; note any increase in edema in limbs with access catheters and record circumference changes *to detect altered perfusion.*
- Monitor for hypothermia; warm dialysate prior to hanging.

NIC IMMOBILITY MANAGEMENT

Impaired physical mobility related to presence of large-bore venous arterial catheters and connection to the hemofilter circuit

- Physical therapy and range of motion activity with caution at least tid *to prevent stiff joints, muscle atrophy, and foot drop.*
- Turn frequently and encourage patient to assist; give deep vein thrombosis prophylaxis as ordered; encourage coughing and deep breathing as appropriate and tolerated *to prevent atelectasis and other complications of bedrest.*
- Monitor skin at pressure points; float heels and elbows off pillows *to prevent skin breakdown.*
- Provide adequate nutrition. Avoid catabolic state.

PATIENT EDUCATION/CONTINUUM OF CARE PLAN

1. Explain indications and purpose for the CRRT (i.e., to decrease the extra fluid in the patient's lungs or tissues); give a simple explanation of how the therapy works and what equipment is involved.
2. Explain how the new catheter(s) will be inserted.
3. Explain that the therapy is continuous and will require bed rest and may limit movement of certain limbs.
4. Explain that the therapy is not painful but can have complications.
5. Give the patient/family an idea of the probable/average duration of therapy if known.

EVALUATION/PATIENT OUTCOMES

Tissue Perfusion Management: Fluid status is within normal limits. Absence of signs and symptoms of fluid overload or dehydration. No complications of altered perfusion occur. Patient does not develop signs or symptoms of arterial or venous occlusion and altered perfusion.

Risk Management: No infection is present. Patient shows no signs or symptoms of infection related to the access sites or circuit. No complications of bleeding occur. Patient does not develop signs or symptoms of bleeding related to inadvertent disconnect or anticoagulation.

Immobility Management: No complications of immobility occur. Patient does not develop pneumonia, deep vein thrombosis, skin breakdown, decreased range of motion, or joint stiffness.

RENAL TRANSPLANTATION

Description and Rationale

Renal transplantation (RT) is the surgical insertion of a human kidney from a living or deceased human donor into a patient with ESRD, thus restoring lost renal function. A donor may be sought when the patient's serum creatinine is around 5 mg/dl, serum blood urea nitrogen is greater than 70 mg/dl, and creatinine clearance is 15 ml/min. When successful, a transplant restores the recipient to a relatively healthy, useful life. If a transplant is unsuccessful, the patient can return to dialysis or have a second transplant.

The demand for organs far exceeds availability. In 1995 there were 31,045 patients waiting for kidneys and only 4998 available. Currently 27% of available kidneys come from living donors and the balance from cadaveric donation. Graft survival rates continue to improve as more effective immunosuppressive regimens are developed. One-year graft survival rates are now 81%.[35]

The transplantation technique is straightforward. The donated kidney is placed in the retroperitoneal area in the iliac fossa (FIG. 13-18). The donor's artery is anastomosed end-to-end or end-to-side to the recipient's hypogastric artery.

The donor's vein is anastomosed to the recipient's internal iliac vein. The donor's ureter is implanted in the recipient's bladder.

The kidney from a living related donor is flushed with a cold solution and then placed in the recipient. A cadaveric kidney may be preserved by flushing followed by cold storage or by constant perfusion with a special solution.

Transplantation is usually the treatment of choice in children. Aging patients may have problems with transplantation because of atherosclerosis or other serious systemic disorders.

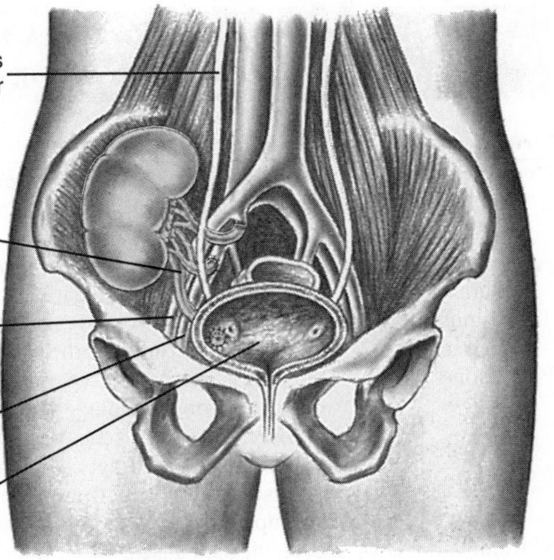

FIG. 13-18
Renal transplant.

Patients with diabetes are increasingly considered for transplantation, but the problems with the continuing diabetic condition increase complications such as infection. The use of corticosteroids exacerbates problems in glucose level control. Combined pancreas and kidney transplants are being used for the type I or insulin-dependent diabetic patient.

Criteria for Kidney Transplant

Criteria for Recipient

ESRD
Age 1 to 65 or 70 years
Absence of uncorrectable abnormalities of other major body systems, such as infection (HBV or HIV), urologic problems, severe cardiac disease, chronic pulmonary disease, preexisting cancer, or psychiatric disorder

Criteria for Living, Related Donor

Age 18 to 55 years
Excellent physical and mental health
Immunologic compatibility to recipient: A point system is used to determine histocompatabiity

Criteria for Cadaveric Donor

Age infant to 70 years
Normal renal function tests
Negative HBV and HIV
Immunologic compatibility to recipient
No systemic disease such as infection, cancer, advanced cardiovascular disease including hypertension, renal-urologic disorders, or diabetes
No hypoxia or hypotension

MULTIDISCIPLINARY PLAN

Surgery

The donor kidney is transplanted as described on p. 908; the patient is prepared with adequate dialysis for surgery (see discussion of Hemodialysis, p. 895); the uremic problems are controlled before surgery

Medications

Antiemetic agents
- Prochlorperazine (Compazine), 5-10 mg PO tid or qid
- Trimethobenzamide (Tigan, Ticon), 250 mg PO tid or qid; 200 mg IM tid or qid

Narcotic analgesic agents
- Meperidine (Demerol), 50-150 mg PO, IM, IV, q3-4h
- Codeine sulfate, 15-60 mg PO, IM, qid
- Morphine sulfate, 5-15 mg PO, IM, IV, q4h prn

Immunosuppressive agents
- Azathioprine (Imuran), 100-150 mg/day PO; 1-2 mg/kg/day determined by white blood cell level
- Antilymphocyte globulin, 5-10 mg/kg IM, IV, depending on potency of preparation, qd for 5-21 days after surgery with intermittent doses for 4 months
- Cyclophosphamide (Cytoxan, Neosar), 2 mg/kg/day PO as substitute for azathioprine in patients with liver dysfunction
- Cyclosporine (Cyclosporin A, Sandimmune), 4-8 mg/kg/day PO, IV
- Muromonab-CD3 (OKT3), 5 mg/kg/day IV bolus, for 10-14 days

Corticosteroids (used as immunosuppressive agents)
- Prednisone (Deltasone, Orasone), 20-150 mg/day PO, 0.1 mg/kg/day decreasing to 10-15 mg/day by 4 months; increase to 100-300 mg/day to treat rejection
- Mycophenolate mofetil (CellCept), 1 g PO bid

Antirejection drugs
- Methylprednisolone (Solu-Medrol, A-Methapred), 1000 mg/day IV or on alternate days for maximum dose of 3-5 g
- Muronab-CD3 (Orthoclone OKT3), IV for 5-14 days, 5 mg/day by rapid injection
- Tacrolimus (Prograf), 0.2 mg/kg individual doses PO bid

Antacids: Peptic ulcer disease may be a problem

H_2 blockers
- Ranitidine (Zantac), 150 mg PO bid; 50 mg IM, slow IV, q6-8h; maximum daily dose 400 mg

Insulin preparations (for hyperglycemia resulting from corticosteroid therapy): Highly individualized according to blood and urine glucose determinations

Other drugs (antiinfectives or antihypertensives) as needed
- Trimethoprim-sulfamethexazole (Bactrim), 1 single-strength tab qd (prophylaxis against pneumocystis pneumonia)
- Acyclovir, 200-800 mg tid (prophylaxis against cytomegalovirus [CMV] and herpes simplex virus)
- Ganciclovir or CytoGam: Prophylaxis for CMV

Indications

ESRD
Loss of solitary kidney through trauma
Inability to adjust to dialysis
No available vascular access sites for dialysis

Contraindications and Cautions

Age younger than 1 year or older than 65 years
Malignancy
Acute uncontrollable infection
Hepatic disease

Presence of antikidney antibodies
Severe psychosis
Tuberculosis or peptic ulcer disease
Chronic respiratory insufficiency
Severe atherosclerosis
Severe myocardial dysfunction

Preprocedural Nursing Care

Assess preoperative status
Explain to the patient and family what to expect during the operative and early postoperative periods

Postprocedural Nursing Care

Assess vital signs and urine output every hour gradually lengthening interval; urine begins to flow in 2 to 10 minutes after revascularization at a rate of 5 to 10 ml/min; careful fluid replacement prevents overhydration or underhydration
Anchor catheters; do not clamp them, but connect them to a closed drainage system; measure urethral and ureteral volumes and record; urine may be bloody at first; cessation of urine flow may be caused by a clot; irrigation of the urethral catheter may be needed to dislodge it; if the ureteral catheter needs irrigating, extreme care is required to avoid damage to the ureteral anastomosis
Try to maintain patency of the hemo-access in case dialysis is needed in the postoperative period

General Management

Dialysis may be needed
Fluid intake should balance output: about 400 to 600 ml (about the amount of insensible losses) plus amount equal to 24-hour urine volume; patient should avoid dehydration and volume excess
Nutritional modifications to achieve or maintain adequate nutritional status and to reduce work of diseased kidney
No dietary restrictions after gastrointestinal function returns; caloric intake may need to be restricted if appetite is increased by corticosteroids, if renal function is decreased, or if hypertension continues
Patient may need to restrict protein, sodium, and potassium and increase calories supplied by fats and carbohydrates
Routine cultures of likely places for infection (urinary tract, wound, throat, and blood) may be done, since immunosuppressive agents currently in use affect phagocytosis, cellular immunity, or humoral immunity; liver function is monitored because azathioprine can cause cholestatic hepatitis; cyclosporine may damage the kidney and liver; muromonab-CD3 causes a flulike symptom complex (Table 13-3)
Signs and symptoms of rejection are monitored; if rejection occurs and is not reversed, graft is removed and patient is returned to dialysis
Most frequent complications are related to technical problems, effects of preexisting uremia, graft rejection, and side effects of immunosuppression

NURSING CARE

Nursing Assessment

Cardiovascular: Altered pulse, respirations, blood pressure, central venous pressure, weight, intake and output associated with excess or inadequate fluid replacement

Table 13-3 Selected Side Effects of Major Immunosuppressive Drugs

Drug	Side Effects
Cyclosporine (Sandimmune)	Renal and hepatic toxicity, hypertension, hirsutism, gingival hyperplasia, nausea, vomiting, diarrhea
Azathioprine (Imuran)	Nausea, vomiting, leukopenia, anemia, thrombocytopenia, hepatic toxicity
Tacrolimus (Prograf)	Renal and hepatic toxicity, hypertension, nausea, vomiting, diarrhea, diabetes
Prednisone	Depression, euphoria, hypertension, decreased wound healing, petechiae, ecchymoses, hirsutism, acne, adrenal suppression, muscle wasting, osteoporosis, redistribution of fat (moon face, buffalo hump)
Muromonab-CD3 (Orthoclone OKT 3)	Fever, chills, nausea, vomiting, diarrhea, chest tightness, dyspnea, pulmonary edema
Mycophenolate	Myelosuppression, gastritis

! EMERGENCY ALERT

ORGAN REJECTION—RENAL

Organ rejection begins when the organ recipient's system begins to reject the transplanted organ.

Assessment

- Determine decreased urine output (cloudy/foul-smelling urine), fever, anxiety, apathy, weight gain, proteinuria, hypertension.
- Perform physical assessment to determine tenderness and/or redness over graft area.
- Evaluate pain status.
- Monitor for altered vital signs.
- Assess for compliance and side effects of medications.

Interventions

- Maintain airway, breathing, and circulation.
- During all client encounters use adequate precautions to minimize risk of infection; patient is immunosuppressed.
- Determine nature of symptoms and manage accordingly.
- Carefully monitor intake and outflow; collect excreted urine.
- Obtain IV access; monitor fluids.
- Obtain laboratory specimens.
- Provide support and reassure patient and family.

Potential Complications

Acute tubular necrosis; spontaneous rupture of graft; organ rejection; ureteral fistula or obstruction; perirenal hematoma, lymphocele, or abscess; renal artery stenosis or thrombosis; renal vein thrombosis; infection; reappearance of primary renal disease
Renal: Signs of rejection: decreased urine output, proteinuria, tenderness over graft area, fever, weight gain, hypertension, anxiety, apathy, lethargy (see Emergency Alert box above)
Urinary tract: Cloudy, foul-smelling urine
General: Fever, pain, changes in incision (red, swollen, draining, or tender), rigors, laboratory drug levels, HgB, WBCs, platelets

Psychosocial: Patient expresses guilt, concern for donor; family expresses concern about what to expect of patient after surgery

Patient Problems/Nursing Diagnoses & Interventions

NIC Tissue Perfusion Management

Deficient fluid volume or excess fluid volume related to postoperative diuresis, altered renal perfusion (acute tubular necrosis, rejection)

- Monitor blood pressure, pulse, respirations, breath sounds, central venous pressure, cardiac output, intake and output, and weight *to determine fluid status;* patient is sensitive to changes in fluid volume.
- Monitor laboratory values: BUN, serum creatinine, uric acid, sodium, potassium, calcium, magnesium, and phosphate; hematocrit and hemoglobin; urine levels of creatinine, urea, uric acid, sodium, potassium, blood, and protein *to assess functioning of new kidney.*
- Balance fluid intake with output *to avoid hypervolemia or hypovolemia.*
- Monitor dialysis access device; take no blood pressure readings or venipunctures in that arm *because dialysis may be needed in the postoperative period.*

NIC Physical Comfort Promotion

Acute pain related to surgical incision, bladder spasms

- Assess need for analgesic drugs; administer as needed; monitor response *to control surgical pain.*
- When catheter is removed, encourage patient to void frequently to avoid overdistention of the bladder; the unused bladder may spasm as it fills with urine.

NIC Risk Management

Risk for infection related to surgery, catheter in urinary tract, and immunosuppression

- Use sterile technique for wound and catheter care *to protect patient who has increased susceptibility to infection because of antirejection drugs.*
- Inspect incision *to detect changes early;* little drainage is expected.
- Monitor temperature and assess laboratory values: WBCs, urine for bacteria, pyuria, cloudy appearance, and culture results; *because signs and symptoms of infection may be masked by immunosuppression, even small increases are important.*
- Monitor visitors *to avoid exposure to persons with infections.*
- Encourage deep breathing, coughing, early ambulation *to prevent respiratory complications.*

NIC Coping Assistance

Disturbed body image related to need to accept a new body part

- Be aware that patient may feel both guilty and concerned about the donor; *mixed feelings are not unexpected.*
- Explain side effects of immunosuppressive drugs that may change appearance. Obvious changes may include alopecia, hirsutism, and redistribution of body fat (Table 13-3).

NIC Life Span Care

Interrupted family processes related to change in patient's condition

- Keep lines of communication open; assist in patient-family communication. Family is used to a chronically ill person. *Return to health may require change in family patterns.* The recipient may be perceived as too independent or not independent enough.
- Recognize the feelings of the living, related donor; before the transplant the donor may have felt like a hero or heroine; after surgery all the attention may focus on the recipient.
- Inform family of changes possible when taking immunosuppressive drugs, especially prednisone; *emotional as well as physical changes may occur in patients taking prednisone.*
- Discuss the possible need for contraception, if appropriate; *potency may return in males; ovulation, menses, and libido may return in females.*
- If patient and family do not already know others who have experienced kidney transplant, ask the family's permission to introduce them to such a patient and family. *Family-to-family assistance is often useful.*
- Refer family to professional colleagues (social workers or psychologists) when other professionals can better meet family's needs (financial concerns, occupational problems, and the need for family counseling beyond the nurse's expertise). Professional colleagues can often be helpful in meeting family needs.

Patient Education/Continuum of Care Plan

1. Preparation for discharge includes teaching the following:
   a. Self-observational skills (temperature, pulse, respiration, weight, intake and output, urine collection, and record keeping)
   b. Medications: Name, dosage, strength, schedule, purpose, and side effects
   c. Diet: Restriction, if any (patient should avoid becoming overweight)
   d. Fluids: Restriction, if any
   e. Signs and symptoms of rejection and infection
   f. Important laboratory values (serum creatinine, blood urea nitrogen level, white blood cell count, calcium, and phosphate); with an arteriovenous fistula, do not have blood pressure taken or blood drawn in that arm
2. Long-term follow-up care includes teaching the following:
   a. Medical appointment schedule for routine follow-up; plans for telephone communication between appointments
   b. Personal hygiene, prevention of infection, care of minor trauma, contraceptive device, and need for regular dental and eye examinations

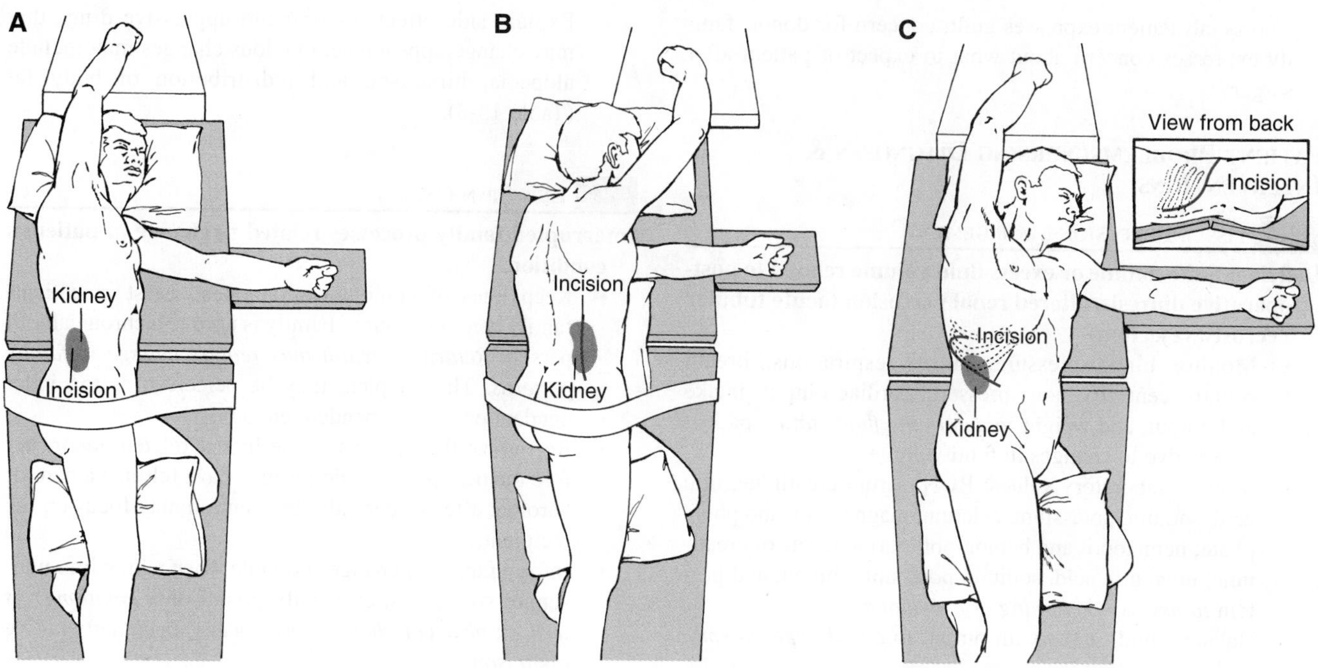

FIG. 13-19
Type of incision for kidney surgery. **A,** Flank approach. **B,** Lumbar approach. **C,** Thoracoabdominal approach.[5]

c. Body changes resulting from uremia and long-term antirejection therapy, including increased possibility of malignancies
d. Physical activity levels (daily exercise, avoidance of contact sports, and avoidance of seat belts across the hips) and return to work and other activities
e. Resources for rehabilitation (including vocational)

EVALUATION/PATIENT OUTCOMES

Tissue Perfusion Management: Fluid balance is within normal limits. No signs or symptoms of fluid overload or dehydration are present. Renal function tests are within normal limits or stable.

Physical Comfort Promotion: Patient is free of pain. Patient has no complaints of pain.

Risk Management: Patient is free of infection. Patient shows no signs or symptoms of infection in incision, urine, or elsewhere.

Coping Assistance: Body image changes are accepted. Patient and family adapt to changes associated with transplantations and immunosuppression.

Life Span Care: Patient and family adjust to life after transplant. Patient and family return to work and social activities.

OTHER KIDNEY SURGERY

Kidney surgery includes both open and closed (percutaneous) procedures. Open surgery of the kidney includes operations to obtain biopsy specimens, to remove all or part of a kidney, to repair traumatic injuries, or to implant a donated organ (FIGS. 13-19 and 13-20). Percutaneous procedures include removing renal calculi and establishing urinary drainage.

Open renal biopsy is used to obtain a specimen if the percutaneous approach is unsuccessful or if a person has a single kidney or severe hypertension or coagulopathy.

Nephrectomy is the surgical removal of the whole kidney or a part of the kidney. A partial nephrectomy usually involves the upper or lower poles of the kidney because they have well-defined blood supplies. In a simple nephrectomy the kidney (but not the adrenal gland, surrounding fat, or fascia) is removed. A radical nephrectomy refers to the removal of the kidney, adrenal gland, perirenal fat, upper ureter, and Gerota's fascia.

Nephrolithotomy is removal of a calculus through an opening in the renal parenchyma.

Pyelolithotomy is removal of a calculus through an opening in the renal pelvis.

Pyeloplasty is the procedure used to repair the renal pelvis (after hydronephrosis, for example).

Nephrostomy (open) is the creation of an opening into the kidney to provide temporary or permanent drainage when a retrograde catheter is not possible. An incision is made into the renal pelvis and out through the renal parenchyma to place a catheter that will drain the renal pelvis. The catheter is anchored in the renal pelvis; the pelvis is sutured; the distal end of the catheter extends through the kidney and exits the skin through a stab incision in the flank.

Renal transplantation. See p. 908.

Percutaneous nephrolithotomy refers to the use of a rigid or flexible nephroscope (under general anesthesia and x-ray guidance) to make a tract through the skin and other tissues to the kidney. Instruments such as a stone basket, stone grasper, or a lithotripter probe (percutaneous lithotripsy) may be used to remove stones or break them up before removal (FIG. 13-21).

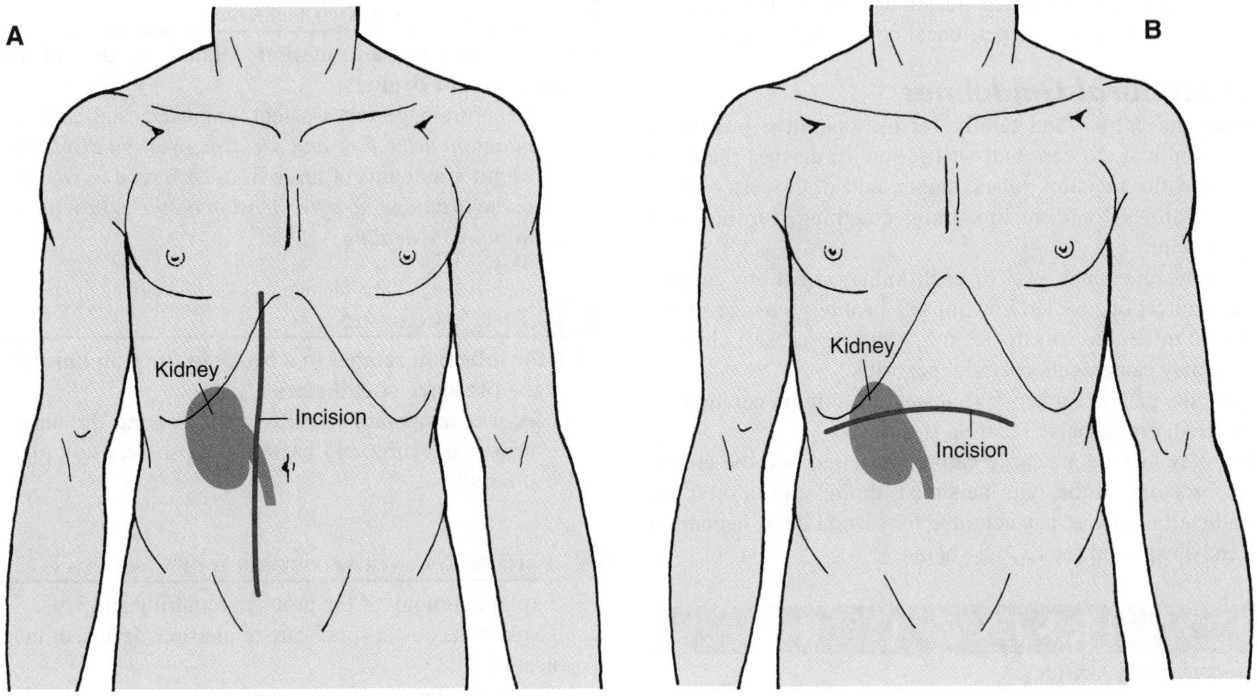

FIG. 13-20
Abdominal approaches to kidney surgery. **A,** Vertical incision. **B,** Horizontal incision.[5]

Percutaneous nephrostomy refers to the insertion of a catheter through the skin into the renal pelvis to establish temporary or permanent urinary drainage.

Indications
Staghorn calculus
Hemorrhage
Hydronephrosis
Renovascular hypertension
Neoplasms
Renal donation
Trauma
Vascular disease

Contraindications and Cautions
Nephrectomy
  Bilateral disease
  Single kidney
Percutaneous renal procedures
  Septicemia
  Urinary tract obstruction
Caution is necessary before removing a diseased kidney (even if the other one is normal) if the disorder is likely to affect the remaining kidney in the future (urolithiasis, renal vascular disease, infection, inflammatory processes).

Type of Incision Used
Flank
Lumbar
Thoracoabdominal
Abdominal

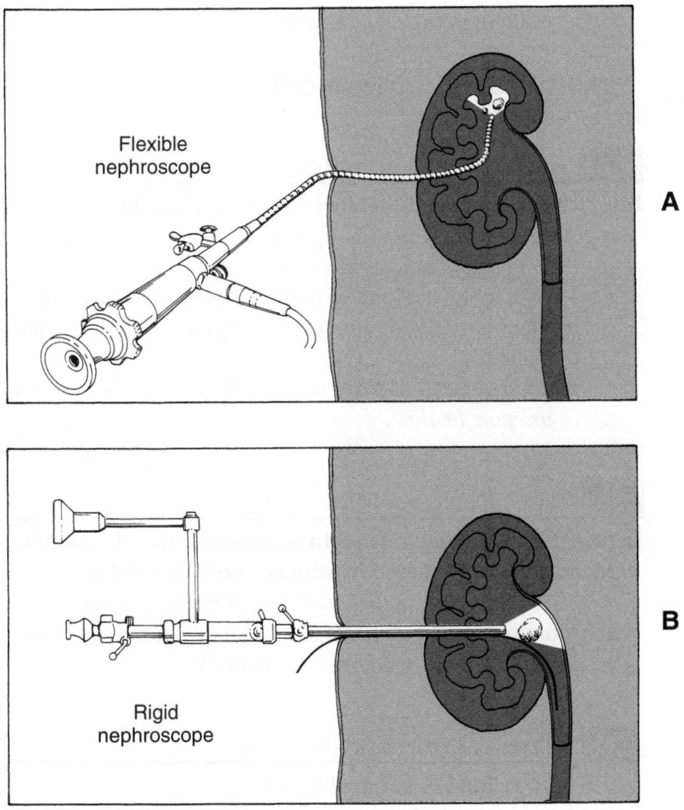

FIG. 13-21
A, Flexible nephroscope. **B,** Rigid nephroscope.[5]

The type of incision used depends on the site of the defect
The approach may be retroperitoneal or transperitoneal

Procedural Guidelines

Prepare the patient and family for the operative procedure planned and the care that will follow it; discuss the location of the incision, tubes, stents, and drains, as well as the routines for deep breathing, coughing, turning, and pain relief.
Determine functional level of each kidney; treat any urinary tract infection; bacteriuria impairs healing; leakage of infected urine into soft tissues may cause abscesses; obstruction may cause acute bacterial nephritis.
Prepare the patient for surgery: bowel and skin preparation, as ordered; preoperative sedation is used.
Tubes may include a stent (a catheter inserted into the ureter) nephrostomy tube, an incisional drain, and a urethral catheter; drainage may continue for several days; hematuria can be expected for 12 to 24 hours.

NURSING CARE

NURSING ASSESSMENT

General: Fever, incisional pain, guarding behavior
Skin incision: Redness; swelling; drainage of urine, blood
Urinary tract: Urine output from each tube or catheter (amount, character); bleeding; absence of urine

POTENTIAL COMPLICATIONS

Nephrectomy: Hemorrhage; infection; pneumothorax
Percutaneous renal procedures: Hemorrhage; infection; urinary extravasation; perirenal hematoma

PATIENT PROBLEMS/NURSING DIAGNOSES & INTERVENTIONS

NIC SKIN/WOUND MANAGEMENT

Impaired skin integrity related to surgical incision

- Assess incision site for signs of bleeding or infection *to detect complications promptly.*
- Note amount and kind of drainage from each tube; urine leakage is expected for several days after incision into the kidney.
- Keep area clean and dry *to prevent skin breakdown and to promote healing.*

NIC TISSUE PERFUSION MANAGEMENT

Deficient fluid volume related to decreased intake by mouth; increased losses caused by diuresis and hemorrhage

- Measure intake, output, and weight every 24 hours
- Monitor vital signs, hemoglobin, and hematocrit *to identify alterations in fluid status promptly.*

NIC PHYSICAL COMFORT PROMOTION

Acute pain related to surgical incision

- Assess need for analgesic drugs; administer drug as ordered; record response *to determine patient's need for drug; determine the effectiveness of timing and dosage to identify adverse side effects.*

NIC ELIMINATION MANAGEMENT

Impaired urinary elimination related to use of tubes, catheters, or drains

- Keep drainage tubes patent, unkinked, and anchored *to maintain urine flow and avoid inadvertent displacement.*
- Monitor amounts of urine from each tube *to ensure adequate drainage, to avoid tension on the suture lines, and to promote healing.*

NIC RISK MANAGEMENT:

Risk for infection related to a break in the skin barrier and to the presence of catheters

- Assess temperature, WBC count, wound drainage, and urine for pyuria and bacteriuria *to detect any infection promptly.*

PATIENT EDUCATION/CONTINUUM OF CARE PLAN

1. Explain etiology of the problem requiring surgery.
2. Explain the posthospital care of incision, drains, or tubes as needed.
3. Explain techniques for preventing recurrence of renal problems.
4. Explain any need for follow-up medical care.

EVALUATION/PATIENT OUTCOMES

Skin/Wound Management: Skin integrity is unimpaired. Incision is healed.

Tissue Perfusion Management: Fluid balance is within normal limits. Fluid intake is adequate and balances output.

Physical Comfort Promotion: No pain is present. Patient has no complaint of pain.

Elimination Management: Urinary elimination pattern is normal. All tubes, drains, and catheters are removed, or home followup is arranged.

Risk Management: No infection is present. Patient is afebrile, with normal WBC count and urinalysis.

EXTRACORPOREAL SHOCK WAVE LITHOTRIPSY

Extracorporeal shock wave lithotripsy (ESWL) is a noninvasive method used to treat renal calculi. Shock waves are carefully directed into the body through a liquid medium surrounding the body to disintegrate the calculus. The pulverized material is flushed by the normal excretion of urine.

Fluoroscopy or ultrasonography is used to pinpoint the stone's location. Radiopaque stones are seen easily; radiolucent stones are visualized by using contrast media in the renal pelvis. The patient, under general anesthesia, is positioned in the lithotripter tub filled with treated water (degassed and deionized; FIG. 13-22). After a series of 200 shock waves is delivered, fluoroscopy is used to determine the location and size of the stone fragments or gravel. The total number of

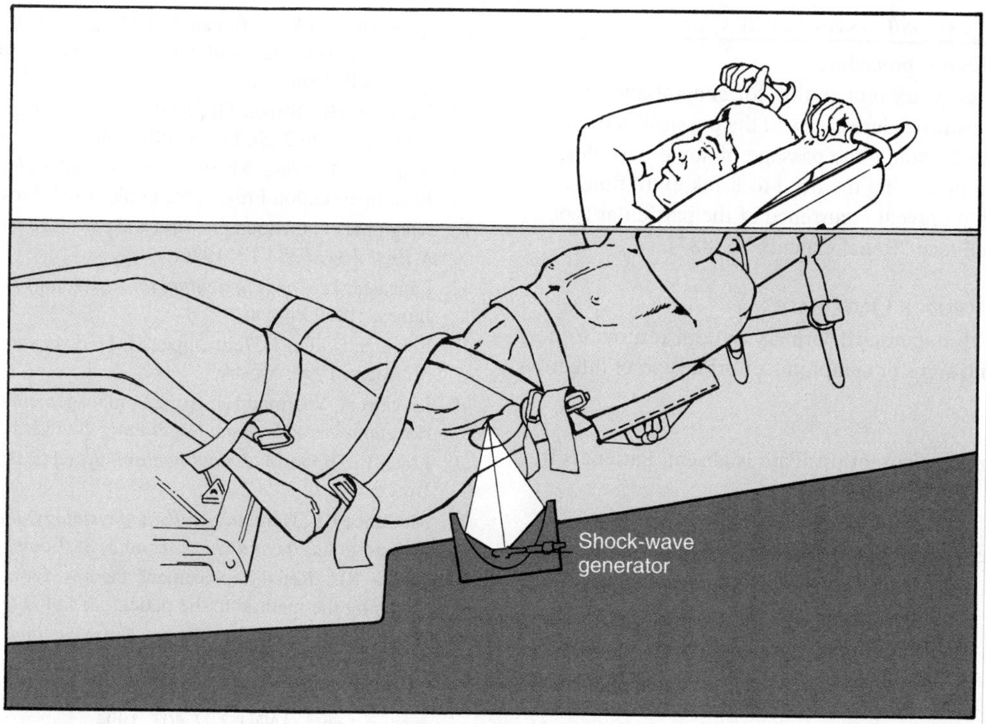

FIG. 13-22
Patient positioned for shock wave lithotripsy. Area of flank is exposed for efficient shock-wave conduction.[5]

shocks needed is related to the size of the stone; an average treatment is 1000 to 2000 shocks with a maximum of 2400 per treatment. If the gravel formed blocks the ureter, percutaneous nephrostomy may be done to promote clearance of the particles.

Contraindications and Cautions

Pregnancy
Lower ureteral stones
Bladder stones
Cardiac pacemakers
Distal ureteral obstruction
Renal artery calcifications
Bleeding diathesis

Procedural Guidelines

Explain the nature of the procedure to the patient and the family.
Prepare the patient for general anesthesia.
Any urinary tract infection is treated, and preoperative antibiotics are given if an infected stone is to be pulverized.

NURSING CARE

NURSING ASSESSMENT

Urinary tract: Hematuria for 12 to 24 hours; passage of stone particles
General: Pain of passage of stone fragments (ureteral colic); fever, dysuria, pyuria, bacteriuria, increased WBCs

POTENTIAL COMPLICATIONS

Hematuria; ureteral colic; ureteral obstruction

PATIENT PROBLEMS/NURSING DIAGNOSES & INTERVENTIONS

NIC ELIMINATION MANAGEMENT

Impaired urinary elimination related to passage of stone particles

- Assess intake and output and the nature of the urine *to identify urinary tract obstruction and to monitor the amount of hematuria.*
- Strain all urine *to observe the nature and size of particles being passed.*
- Ensure adequate fluid intake; *the extra fluid may be needed to help the passage of stone particles.*

NIC PHYSICAL COMFORT PROMOTION

Acute pain related to passage of stone particles

- Assess for pain; give analgesic drugs as ordered; monitor and record response; use nonpharmacologic methods, such as external application of heat, *to determine the need for analgesia, to provide relief, and to identify adverse side effects.*
- Help patient walk, if appropriate, *to help stones move by gravity.*

NIC RISK MANAGEMENT

Risk for infection related to tissue trauma from presence of stone

- Assess temperature every 4 hours; monitor WBCs and urinalysis for pyuria and bacteriuria *to identify urinary tract infection promptly.*

Patient Education/Continuum of Care Plan

1. Explain the ESWL procedure.
2. Explain the necessary preparation for general anesthesia.
3. Explain the postprocedure care and the possibility of hematuria for 12 to 24 hours, the passage of stone particles, the need to strain urine, and the need to drink extra fluids.
4. Explain how to prevent recurrence of the particular type of stone involved (see "Renal Calculi," p. 887).

Evaluation/Patient Outcomes

Elimination Management: Urinary pattern returns to normal. Patient has no signs or symptoms of urinary tract infection or obstruction.

Physical Comfort Promotion: Pain is absent. Patient is free of pain.

Risk Management: Infection is absent. Patient is free of infection.

References

1. Aronoff GR et al: *Drug prescribing in renal failure: dosing guidelines for adults,* ed 4, Philadelphia, 1999, American College of Physicians.
2. Baldwin IC, Elderkin TD: Continuous hemofiltration: nursing perspectives in critical care, *New Horizons* 3:738, 1995.

2a. Berne RM, Levy MN: *Physiology,* ed 2, 1988, Mosby.

3. Beto J: Which diet for renal failure? Making sense of the options, *J Am Diet Assoc* 95:8, 1995.
4. Brady HR, Wilcox CS, editors: *Therapy in nephrology and hypertension,* Philadelphia, 1999, WB Saunders.
5. Brundage DJ: *Renal disorders,* St. Louis, 1992, Mosby.
6. Brundage DJ, Swearingen PA: Chronic renal failure; evaluation and teaching tool, *ANNA J* 21:256, 1994.
7. Brenner BM, editor: *Brenner and Rector's the kidney,* ed 6, Philadelphia, 2000, WB Saunders.
8. Chow WH et al: Rising incidence of renal cell cancer in the United States, *JAMA* 281(17), May 5, 1999.
9. Daugirdas JT, Todd SI: *Handbook of dialysis,* ed 2, Boston, 1994, Little, Brown.
10. Donadio JV et al for the Mayo Nephrology Collaborative Group: The longterm outcome of patients with IgA nephropathy treated with fish oil in a controlled trial, *J Am Soc Nephrol* 10:1772, 1999.
11. Greenberg A et al: *Primer on kidney diseases,* ed 2, San Diego, 1998, National Kidney Foundation, Academic Press.
12. Hollingsworth AK: *Kidney failure: coping and feeling your best,* Atlanta, 1994, Pritchett & Hall.
13. Ignatavicius M, Workman LM, Mishler MA: *Medical surgical nursing across the health care continuum,* ed 3, Philadelphia, 1999, WB Saunders.
14. Jacobson HR, Striker GE, Klahr S: *The principles and practice of nephrology,* ed 2, St. Louis, 1995, Mosby.
15. Johnson M, Mass M: *Nursing outcomes classification (NOC),* Iowa Intervention Project, St. Louis, 1997, Mosby.
16. Klagg MJ et al: Blood pressure and end stage renal disease in men, *N Engl J Med* 334:13, 1996.
17. Lancaster L: *Core curriculum for nephrology nurses: ANNA,* New Jersey, 1995, Pitman.
18. Lewis S, Collier I, Heitkemper M: *Medical surgical nursing,* ed 4, St. Louis, 1996, Mosby.
19. Lievarrt A, Voerman HJ: Nursing management of continuous arteriovenous hemodialysis, *Heart Lung* 20:152, 1991.
20. Llach F: *Papper's clinical nephrology,* ed 2, Boston, 1993, Little, Brown.
21. McCance KL, Heuther SE: *Pathophysiology: the biologic basis for disease in adults and children,* ed 3, St. Louis, 1998, Mosby.
22. Mehta RL: Renal replacement therapy for acute renal failure: matching the method to the patient, *Semin Dialysis* 6:253, 1993.
23. Mitch WE, Klahr S, editors: *Nutrition and the kidney,* ed 2, Boston, 1993, Little, Brown.
24. Oberly ET, Compton A: Nursing interventions for rehabilitating renal patients, *ANNA J* 21:407, 1994.
25. Phipps WJ, Sands JK, Marek JF: *Medical-surgical nursing: concepts and clinical practice,* ed 6, St. Louis, 1999, Mosby.
26. Remuzzi G, Ruggenenti P, Benigni A: Understanding the nature of renal disease progression, *Kidney Int* 51:2, 1997.
27. Schrier RW: *Manual of nephrology,* ed 4, Boston, 1995, Little, Brown.
28. Schrier RW: *Renal and electrolyte disorders,* Boston, 1997, Lippincott-Raven.
29. Serio A, Fraioli A: Epidemiology of nephrolithiasis, *Nephron* 81(suppl 1):26, 1999.
30. Strohschein BL, Caruso DM, Greene KA: Continuous venovenous hemodialysis, *Am J Crit Care* 3:92, 1994.
31. Swearingen PL, Ross DG: *Manual of medical-surgical nursing care,* ed 4, St. Louis, 1999, Mosby.
32. Tanagho EA, McAnnich JW: *Smith's general urology,* ed 14, Norwalk, Conn, 1995, Appleton & Lange.
33. Thelan LA et al: *Critical care nursing: diagnosis and management,* ed 2, St. Louis, 1994, Mosby.
34. Thibodeau GA: *Anatomy and physiology,* St. Louis, 1987, Mosby.
35. United States Renal Data System: *USRDS 1994 annual data report,* Bethesda, Md, 1994, NIH, NIDDK.
36. Vander AJ: *Renal physiology,* ed 5, New York, 1995, McGraw-Hill.
37. Whaley S, Wong N: *Nursing care of infants and children,* ed 5, St. Louis, 1995, Mosby.

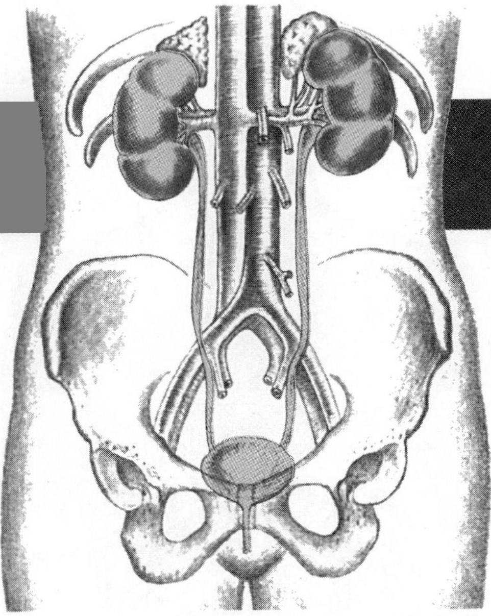

14

Genitourinary System

Mikel Gray
Kathleen Calitri Brown

OVERVIEW

Genitourinary diseases affect the kidneys, ureters, bladder, urethra, or male genitalia. Urologic disorders may result from specific disease states such as infection, hyperplasia, or neoplasia. Other disorders, such as urinary incontinence or male sexual dysfunction, are symptoms rather than specific disease states but also cause significant health problems related to the genitourinary system. For information on the renal system, refer to Chapter 13.

ANATOMY, PHYSIOLOGY, AND RELATED PATHOPHYSIOLOGY

Urinary Tract Structures

Kidneys. The kidneys are a pair of reddish brown, symmetrically shaped organs located in the retroperitoneal space, adjacent to the vertebral column at spinal levels T12 and L1 to L3 (FIG. 14-1, *A*). Because of the presence of the liver, the right kidney is lower than the left.[172] The lateral aspects of the kidneys are smooth and rounded; the medial aspects are marked by a concave surface known as the renal hilus. The renal veins, arteries, nerve plexus, and renal lymphatics are located at this hilus. The renal pelvis attaches to the kidney at the hilus before tapering into the ureters.[34,172]

The weight of the adult kidney varies from 115 to 175 g. Adult women have slightly smaller kidneys than do adult men. The kidney in the infant or young child is smaller than in the adult. However, a child's kidneys occupy a larger proportion of the child's body weight. The normal adult kidney is approximately 11 cm long, 5 to 7 cm wide, and 2 to 3.5 cm thick. The kidneys are remarkably symmetric in size and shape.[168]

A cross section of the kidneys (FIG. 14-2) reveals two distinct sections: the renal pelvis and renal parenchyma. Within the renal parenchyma, a cortex and medulla are distinguished using the unaided eye. The renal medulla is characterized by pale, striated conical structures called pyramids. The bases of these pyramids are directed toward the periphery of the kidney, and apices face the renal hilus. The renal pyramids end in papillae that project into a minor calyx. The kidneys normally contain from 8 to 18 renal pyramids that drain into 4 to 13 minor calyces. These minor calyces drain into 2 or 3 major calyces that open into the renal pelvis.[34,179]

The renal medulla is bounded by the renal cortex, which appears darker and has a granular rather than striated appearance. Cortical lobules arch over the pyramids within the medulla. Cortical columns dip between the pyramids. The renal cortex is bounded by the true renal capsule, a layer of dense connective tissue loosely adherent to the parenchyma. The kidneys are supported by the perirenal fascia and perinephric fat. The kidneys, along with the superiorly placed adrenals, are enclosed within Gerota's fascia.[34,179]

The renal fossa is bounded superiorly by the diaphragm, laterally by the abdominal musculature, and posteriorly by the quadratus lumborum muscle (FIG. 14-1, *B*).

The blood supply of the kidneys arises directly from the abdominal aorta. Typically a single renal artery enters the kidney at the renal hilus. However, duplicate renal arteries may be found and are not considered pathologic. After entering the kidney, the renal artery bifurcates into superior and inferior branches, which further divide into the interlobular arteries. These vessels and their branches provide the substantial blood supply necessary for renal function.[172]

The veins that drain the kidneys are paired with arterial vessels. The renal veins exiting the kidney empty directly into the inferior vena cava, and their number corresponds to the number of renal arteries present.[159]

Lymphatics adjacent to the renal cortex and medulla drain into para-aortic and para-vena caval lymph nodes. The sensory and motor neurons that innervate the kidneys arise from the dorsal roots of T11 and T12. Autonomic neural control of the kidneys is mediated by fibers from the vagus nerve, splanchnic nerves, semilunar ganglia, and the celiac axis.[172]

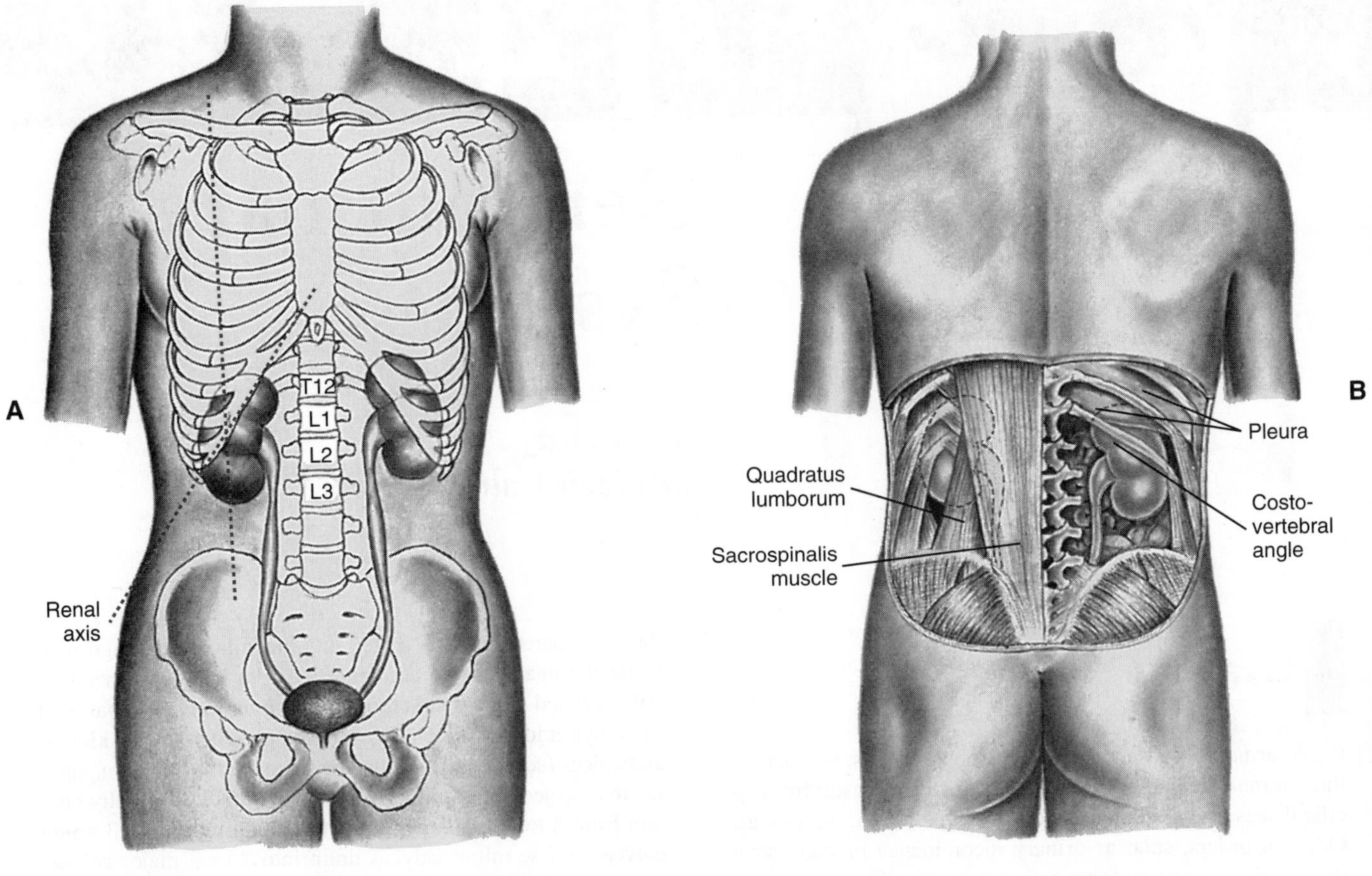

FIG. 14-1
Anatomic relation of kidneys to spinal column. A, Anterior view. B, Posterior view.

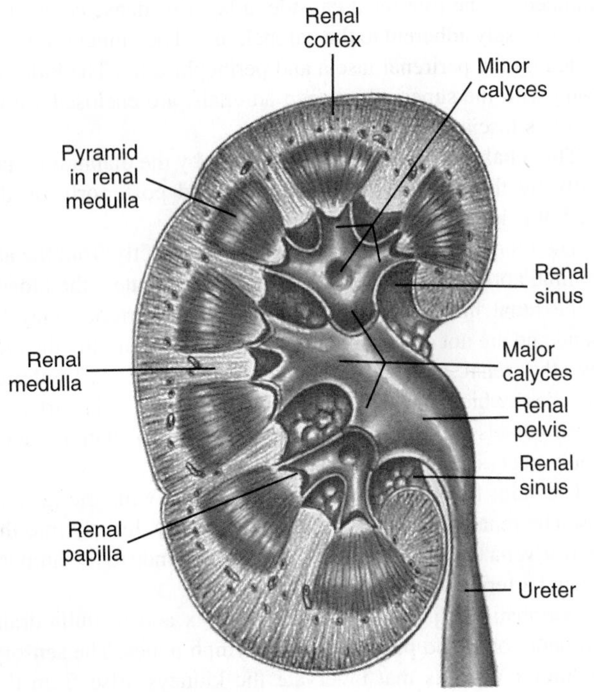

FIG. 14-2
Cross section of kidney.

The kidneys perform a number of essential functions related to the maintenance of internal homeostasis. These include maintenance of fluid and electrolyte balance and serum pH levels and excretion of the by-products of metabolism.

Renal Pelvis and Ureters. The renal pelvis and ureters are continuous, thick-walled tubes that originate at the renal hilus and implant into the bladder wall, connecting the kidneys to the bladder. The renal pelvis is a funnel-shaped structure into which the major calyces empty urine for transport to the urinary bladder. After exiting the renal hilus, the renal pelvis narrows inferomedially into the ureter.[158]

The ureters are approximately 24 to 30 cm long. The left ureter is slightly longer than the right. The course of the ureters forms an inverted S. After leaving the renal pelvis, the ureters pass medially over the psoas muscle. The ureters then progress medially to the sacroiliac joints before turning laterally to an area near the ischial spines of the pelvis. Finally, the ureters curve back laterally to insert into the bladder base at the trigone muscle.[20,158]

The internal diameter of the ureters varies from 2 to 10 mm. Three areas of anatomic narrowing have clinical implications: the ureteropelvic junction, the area where the ureters cross the iliac arteries, and the ureterovesical junction (FIG. 14-3).[158,173]

The ureters and renal pelvis share a common embryogenic origin and histologic makeup. The ureter and renal pelvis first

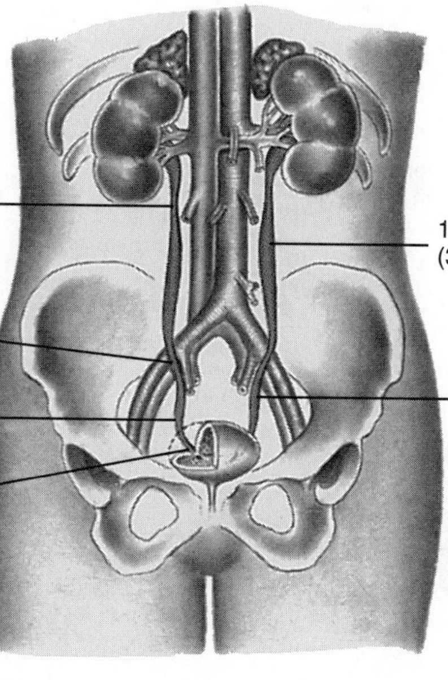

FIG. 14-3

Course of ureter with its varying internal luminal radiuses.

appear during the fourth week of life. They arise from the mesonephric duct and grow cranially to meet the metanephric cap.[158]

The ureter and renal pelvis are composed of three histologically defined layers: the external adventitia, a smooth muscle coat, and an inner mucous membrane. The adventitia is a connective tissue sheath that encircles the renal pelvis and ureters to the level of ureterovesical junction. The adventitial layer blends into the surrounding retroperitoneal tissue, providing support for the ureters. The exact arrangement of these fibers is not known. Two layers of muscle fibers, an inner longitudinal layer and an outer circular layer, have been described. However, histologic studies of ureteral smooth muscle have disputed this theory.[30] Smith[158] and Allen[5] describe the muscle fibers as arranged in bundles that are oriented in a helical or spiral fashion. The muscular tissue layer provides peristaltic activity needed to transport urine from the kidneys to the bladder. The mucous membrane lining the internal ureter is composed of transitional cell epithelium with a supportive lamina propria.[30]

The blood supply of the ureters is variable. The upper portion of the ureter and renal pelvis may receive arterial blood from branches of the renal, gonadal, or adrenal arteries. The pelvic ureters may receive arterial blood from the common iliac arteries, external iliac arteries, deferential arteries in the male, uterine arteries in the female, or the obturator artery. Blood enters the ureters via an arterial plexus located within the outer adventitial layer.[20]

Venous blood from the ureters drains into a venous plexus in the ureteral submucosa. This plexus drains into an adventitial venous plexus, which empties into veins closely paired with the arterial supply described previously.

Lymphatic drainage from the ureters is also variable. The upper ureteral and renal pelvic lymphatic channels empty into para-aortic or renal nodes. The middle and lower ureteral lymphatic channels drain into the common or external iliac nodes.[20]

The nerve supply of the ureters arises from the celiac plexus, mesenteric ganglia, and hypogastric plexus. Although the exact role of the autonomic nervous system in ureteral function remains unclear, the ureter is known to contain a rich supply of sympathetic and parasympathetic nerve receptors.[20]

The primary function of the renal pelvis and ureters is to transport urine from the kidney to the bladder. To accomplish this goal, the ureters must create a peristaltic muscular wave sufficient to drive a bolus of urine from the renal pelvis, through the ureters, and past the ureterovesical junction.[30]

Although the precise mechanisms of ureteral peristalsis remain unclear, it is influenced by mechanical, chemical, and neural stimuli. Generation of a peristaltic wave does not depend on specific neural firing. Like the muscle of the heart, ureteral smooth muscle will continue to rhythmically contract outside the body. In contrast to the heart, no specialized pacemaker has been clearly defined, although the existence of an intrinsic ureteral pacemaker is well established.[20] Multiple pacemaker cells regulating ureteral activity are thought to exist within the renal calyces. The prolonged refractory period of the smooth muscle of the renal pelvis and ureters prevents all calyceal contractions from resulting in ureteral peristaltic waves. The renal pelvis and ureters average two to six peristaltic waves each minute.[20,173]

Ureteral peristaltic waves typically arise within the renal pelvis. They travel in an antegrade direction from the renal pelvis to the ureterovesical junction. During the resting phase, the renal pelvis assumes a conical shape with an area of narrowing at the pelvic-ureteral junction. At this time both the renal pelvis and ureters maintain a low intraluminal pressure of 2 to 5 cm H_2O. Urine enters the ureter from the renal pelvis passively during the resting phase. During a peristaltic wave the pressure rises to 20 to 60 cm H_2O, sufficient to force urine past the ureterovesical junction into the bladder. Only a portion of the total renal pelvic contents is evacuated from the renal pelvis during a peristaltic wave. Once the peristaltic wave is propagated into the ureters, urine is pushed ahead of the wave through the length of the ureter and past the ureterovesical junction into the bladder.[20,158]

An increase in renal output causes greater pelvic distention, which increases both the number of peristaltic waves generated per minute and the proportion of renal pelvic contents transported to the bladder with each contraction.[158]

The ureters are also affected by neural influences. Although it has been demonstrated that the normal ureter continues to contract when removed from the body, the autonomic nervous system does influence ureteral function. The ureters are extensively innervated with alpha- and beta-receptors. Stimulation of alpha-receptors causes increased ureteral peristalsis. Stimulation of beta-adrenergic receptors results in an inhibition of ureteral peristalsis. The role of the parasympathetic nervous system in ureteral and renal pelvic function is not clearly understood. The parasympathetic nervous system is thought to potentiate ureteral peristalsis directly through the release of catecholamines.[20]

Ureteral peristalsis is also influenced by various chemical and pharmacologic agents. For example, the administration of epinephrine or catecholamines will, predictably, increase ureteral peristalsis. Increased histamine levels also stimulate ureteral peristalsis. However, the administration of serotonin, which enhances intestinal peristalsis, does not affect ureteral peristalsis. Upper ureteral dilation, which is commonly seen in

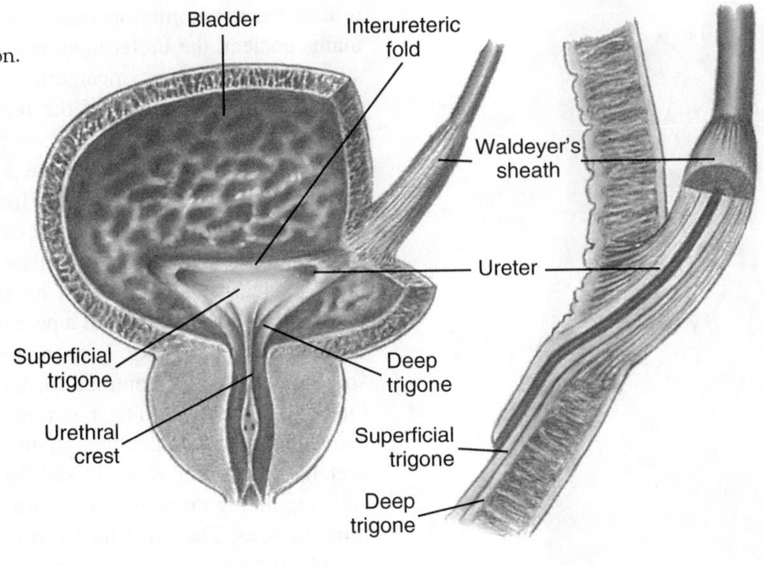

FIG. 14-4
Normal ureterovesical junction.

pregnant women, was once attributed to fluctuations in the serum levels of the sex hormones. Recent investigation has demonstrated that this dilation was caused by mechanical factors rather than hormonal influences. This hypothesis is further supported by the observation that upper ureteral dilation is not seen in women taking oral contraceptives.[158]

Ureterovesical Junction and Trigone. The ureterovesical junction is of particular interest in any discussion of genitourinary disease because of its importance in preventing vesicoureteral reflux and associated complications. The ureterovesical junction is located near the base of the bladder in the lateral aspects of the trigone muscle. The ureterovesical junction has three components important to its function: the intravesical ureter, the trigone, and the adjacent bladder wall (FIG. 14-4).[158,173]

Embryologically, the ureterovesical junction is formed in the seventh week of gestation when the caudal end of the ureter opens into the urogenital sinus. The trigone muscle is formed from the same mesonephric tissue that forms the ureter. The intravesical ureter is further connected to the bladder by a continuous connective tissue sheath. Thus, although the intravesical ureter and trigone muscle have different embryogenic origins than the bladder, the ureterovesical junction in the fully developed human functions as a single unit to allow for the passage of urine into the bladder while preventing reflux of urine into the upper tracts.[157]

The intravesical ureter enters the bladder at a hiatus in the posterior, lateral aspect of the bladder base and is approximately 1.5 cm long. It is divided into an intramural section surrounded by the detrusor muscle and a submucosal segment that travels under the bladder mucosa. The intravesical ureter terminates at an orifice that opens into the bladder vesicle.[158,173]

The histologic features of the intravesical ureter differ from upper ureteral segments in several ways. The adventitia of the intravesical ureter contains two dense sheaths. The superficial sheath is continuous with the bladder wall. The deep sheath is derived from ureteral adventitia. Between these dense sheaths is a loose connective tissue plane called Waldeyer's sheath. This sheath allows for mobility of the intravesical ureter within the adjacent bladder wall and is of surgical significance when performing ureteroneocystostomy.[173]

The arrangement of smooth muscle fibers also differs in the intravesical ureter. Unlike the upper ureters, the intravesical ureter contains longitudinally arranged fibers and is easily collapsible. The ability of the intravesical ureter to seal itself by collapsing is an important mechanism in the prevention of reflux. Muscle fibers from the intravesical ureter decussate inferiorly to fuse with the superficial trigone and medially to form Mercier's bar.[79,173]

The trigone muscle is another essential component of the ureterovesical junction. The muscle is divided into two parts, the superficial trigone and the deep trigone. The superficial trigone is continuous with muscular fibers from the intravesical ureter. It continues along the bladder base and into the proximal urethra. In the male the trigone terminates at the verumontanum. In the female the superficial trigone terminates at the bladder neck.

The deep trigone is characterized by flat, tightly bound, smooth fiber groups. It is continuous with Waldeyer's sheath along the path of the intravesical ureter. The deep trigone is rolled into a tube that is incomplete on its anterior surface. The deep trigone terminates at the bladder neck and continues into the urethra as a layer of circular smooth muscle.[57,158]

The portion of the bladder wall adjacent to the ureterovesical junction is characterized by circular and longitudinal smooth muscle fibers that secure the ureters within the vesical wall. The outer, longitudinal smooth muscle layer is the strongest, most resilient segment of the bladder wall. This strength is vital to the maintenance of continuity between the upper and lower urinary tracts.[157]

The primary functions of the ureterovesical junction are to allow efflux of urine into the bladder and to prevent reflux of urine into the ureters. During bladder filling the ureterovesical junction maintains a relatively low closure pressure, between 8 and 15 cm H_2O. This closure pressure is adequate to prevent reflux of urine from the bladder, which also fills at low pressures. However, the closure pressure is easily overcome by a ureteral peristaltic wave, which generates pressure between 20 and 60 cm H_2O. As the bladder fills and intravesical pressure rises, the

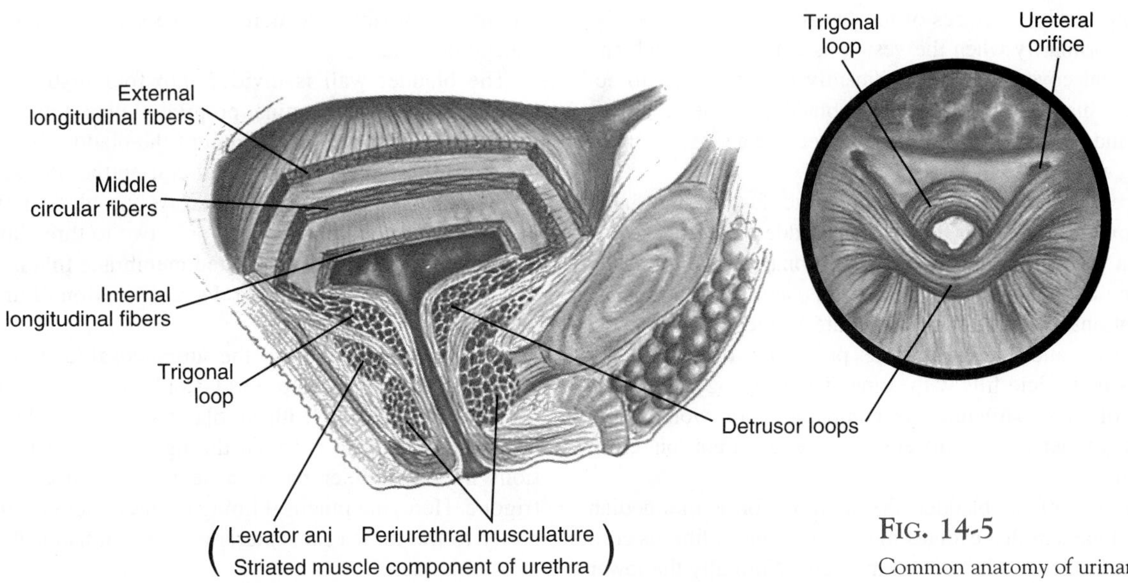

FIG. 14-5
Common anatomy of urinary bladder.

intravesical ureter becomes progressively compressed against the adjacent bladder wall. The effect of this compression is to carry the ureteral hiatus outward, thus increasing pressure of the intravesical ureter. This compensatory mechanism prevents reflux of urine even when the bladder is filled with urine. At very high volumes the compression of the intravesical ureter becomes functionally obstructed and interferes with normal ureteral peristalsis.[158,173]

During the voiding phase the ureterovesical junction must generate even greater resistance to prevent reflux into the upper urinary tract. A few seconds before intravesical pressure rises in response to a detrusor contraction, there is a sharp pressure rise within the intravesical ureter. This high closure pressure at the ureterovesical junction is maintained throughout micturition and persists for a brief period after voiding is completed. The sharp increase in pressure was once attributed primarily to the contractile activity of the adjacent bladder wall. However, studies have demonstrated that the trigone is primarily responsible for the prevention of reflux during micturition. The marked pressure rise seen immediately before a detrusor contraction is caused by an increase in the tone of the trigone, which pulls the intravesical ureter tightly closed. The trigonal contraction is maintained for approximately 20 seconds after voiding is completed. As expected, no efflux of urine into the bladder occurs during voiding.[158]

Urinary Bladder. The urinary bladder is a hollow muscular organ designed to store and expel urine produced by the kidneys. The size and shape of the bladder vary with its state of fullness and with age. When empty, the bladder assumes the shape of a tetrahedron and lies entirely within the lesser pelvis. As the bladder fills, it becomes more spheric in shape and moves upward and anteriorly toward the abdominal cavity.[148,178]

During infancy the bladder is located in the abdomen; even the bladder neck lies above the symphysis pubis. The bladder assumes its place in the pelvis shortly before puberty. The change in position is not caused by migration of the organ; rather, changes in the size and shape of the vesicle and maturation of the pelvic bone result in the change in relative location of the bladder.[173]

The bladder is characterized by two inlets and a single outlet located on the inferior aspect of the organ. Six anatomic areas are seen on gross inspection of the organ: the neck, the base or fundus, the apex, and the superior right inferolateral and left inferolateral surfaces (FIG. 14-5).[148]

The bladder neck is the lower part of the organ and is several centimeters from the lower aspect of the symphysis pubis. The bladder neck is a relatively fixed structure regardless of the volume of urine present in the vesicle or the state of the adjacent rectum. The bladder neck is pierced by the internal urethral orifice. In the male it sits directly superior to the prostate gland; in the female it sits posterior to the vaginal wall.[148]

The base of the bladder is triangular and oriented posteriorly and downward from the bladder apex. Its borders are rounded and characterized by the junction of the intravesical ureters. In the adult male the bladder is superior to the seminal vesicles and adjacent to the rectum. Denonvilliers' fascia forms an anatomic barrier between the bladder base, rectum, and the vasa deferentia. In adult women the bladder base lies in close proximity to the anterior vaginal wall. Although the female lacks any fascial borders between the bladder and adjacent vagina, the two structures are separate at this point. In contrast, the lower urethra is anatomically continuous with the anterior vaginal wall.[148]

The apex of the bladder is the uppermost surface of the organ and is oriented anteriorly toward the abdominal wall. In the empty bladder of the adult, the apex lies within the pelvis. When the bladder is filled with urine, the apex is pushed upward and anteriorly so it enters the abdominal cavity. The apex is connected to the abdominal wall via the urachus.[148,158]

The superior surface of the empty bladder is bounded laterally by a line extending from the apex to the anterior borders of the intravesical ureters. The posterior border is formed by a line extending between the external borders of the intravesical ureters. In the adult male, reflection of the peritoneum covers the superior surface. When filled, a prevesical pouch is formed that may contain a segment of the small bowel. In the adult female the superior surface of the bladder is separated from the ureters by the ureterovesical pouch.

The inferolateral surfaces of the urinary bladder can be distinguished primarily when the vesicle is empty. They lack any pelvic fascial covering and significantly change shape to accommodate bladder filling. When the bladder reaches capacity, the right and left inferolateral surfaces become a single, convex area lying adjacent to the abdominal wall.

The pelvic floor muscles, endopelvic fascia, and bony pelvis provide support for the urinary bladder. The endopelvic fascia is a unique combination of traditional fascia, primarily comprising collagen and elastin proteins, and smooth muscle. Condensations of this fascia contribute to the support of the bladder base and urethra, while providing the flexibility needed as its vesicle fills with urine. The histology and gross anatomy of these structures is comparable for women and men, but gender-related differences are apparent on close inspection.

At the apex of the bladder, the allantois forms the median umbilical ligament that evolves into the urachus, a fibrous cord that connects the bladder to the umbilicus. Normally the lower segment of the urachus remains patent, but it does not communicate with the bladder vesicle. In some cases, communication between these structures persists, or the urachus becomes filled with fluid or purulent material.[148,178]

The bladder base and proximal urethra receive support from several condensations of the endopelvic fascia, frequently referred to as "ligaments." Although these ligaments have clinical significance to the surgeon who exposes a limited portion of the fascia during a particular procedure, it is important to remember that this fascia is a functionally continuous structure with unique histologic features adapted to its functional role within the female or male pelvis.[36,129,146]

In women the bladder base rests on pubocervical fascia, and it receives indirect support from two arcus tendineus fascia (white lines) that extend from the inner surface of the pubic bones and the top of the pubic rami to the ischial spines.[36,146] These fascial structures provide significant but secondary support to the bladder base and proximal urethra, which is normally subjected to physical stress from rapid changes in abdominal pressure and occasionally owing to extraordinary physical stress produced by labor and delivery. The primary support from the bladder base is provided by the pelvic floor muscles. The anterior segment of the levator ani muscle (pubovisceral) supplies most of this support, but indirect assistance is provided by the iliococcygeus and the coccygeus (external anal sphincter).

In men puboprostatic fascia extends from the inner aspects of the symphysis pubis and pubic bones to the junction of the prostatic and membranous urethra.[129,146] Condensations of this viscera are usually called the puboprostatic ligaments in the male. Lateral support for the bladder base and urethra also arises from this fascia before it inserts into the ischial spines of the bony pelvis. Posterior to the ischial spine, pelvic fascia extends from the rectum to the pelvic side walls, providing posterior support and separating the bladder base from the rectum. As observed in the woman, the levator ani muscle provides the primary, dynamic support for the bladder base. Like the levator ani in the female, it is divided into a U-shaped segment called the pubococcygeus or pubovisceral muscle. However, in contrast to the female, the levator ani is generally thicker and narrower than in the female, and it lacks a vaginal opening, providing less flexible but more durable support according to its functional needs.

The bladder wall is divided into four distinct histologic layers: urothelium, lamina propria, tunica muscularis, and outer adventitia. The urothelium of the bladder lines the vesicle and is formed of transitional cell epithelium six to eight layers deep in the empty bladder. As the bladder fills to capacity, the urothelium becomes only two to three layers deep. The urothelium has an associated membrane that is impermeable to water, thus preventing the reabsorption of urine stored in the bladder.[104,173]

Under the urothelium is the submucosal layer, or the lamina propria. The lamina propria is only loosely attached to the urothelium and rich with areolar tissues and elastic fibers. The lamina propria is found throughout the distensible portions of the bladder but is absent in the area of the deep trigone. Here, the mucosal lining of the vesicle is attached directly to the tunica muscularis in this nondistensible portion of the bladder.[173]

Unlike its loose connection with the urothelium, the lamina propria is firmly attached to the tunica muscularis of the bladder. The tunica muscularis is composed primarily of smooth muscle and is called the detrusor. Detrusor muscle cells are arranged in bundles and interspersed within a collagenous framework. A dense autonomic plexus provides autonomic innervation for the detrusor muscle cells. The detrusor muscle is variable in thickness; three layers (inner longitudinal, middle circular, and outer longitudinal) are described. The middle circular and outer longitudinal layers consist of relatively thick muscle cells. They are most prominent in the body of the bladder and terminate at the urethral orifice. Controversy exists whether detrusor muscle bundles of the inner longitudinal layer extend into the proximal urethra. Some investigators argue that the inner longitudinal layer continues into the urethra, forming an outer longitudinal layer of smooth muscle.[60] In contrast, others note that continuity between detrusor muscle bundles and urethral smooth muscle bundles is not seen in fetal histologic specimens. They conclude that vesicle smooth muscle and urethral smooth muscle are embryologically separate.[30]

The outermost histologic layer of the bladder is the adventitia. The adventitia is composed of fibroelastic tissue and is loosely connected to the various peritoneal coverings of the bladder described previously.[104]

The blood supply of the urinary bladder arises from several sources. Arterial blood reaches the bladder from the superior, medial, and inferior vesical arteries, which are branches of the internal iliac or hypogastric artery. Small branches from the obturator and inferior gluteal muscles also supply arterial blood to the bladder. Branches from the uterine and vaginal artery supply vascular nourishment to the bladder in the female. Unlike the veins of the kidneys, those of the bladder do not follow arterial routes. Venous drainage from the bladder exits anteriorly into Santorini's plexus and laterally into a neurovascular sheath surrounded by the lateral vesical ligaments. From here venous blood from the bladder is routed into the inferior hypogastric vein.[158,167]

The lymphatic drainage of the bladder originates in the urothelium and drains into the vesical, external iliac, hypogastric, and common iliac nodes. The lymphatic channels in the urinary bladder are not clearly elucidated. Three areas of lymphatic drainage are postulated: the trigone, posterior wall, and anterior wall.[158,167]

The innervation of the bladder represents a deceptively complex discussion; the precise mechanisms of neural control of the urinary bladder are not fully understood. The sensory innervation of the urinary bladder is poorly understood. Sensory impulses from the urinary bladder are both proprioceptive and exteroceptive. Exteroceptive impulses from the bladder include pain, temperature, and touch. Proprioceptive impulses give the person an awareness of various states of vesical fullness. Morphologic studies in animals have demonstrated the presence of free nerve endings throughout the detrusor muscle with the greatest abundance in the trigone. Tension receptors and stretch receptors have also been noted in the detrusor muscle and presumably play an important role in the awareness of bladder filling. The impulses generated by the sensory receptors are thought to travel in the sensory portion of the pelvic plexus.[98,173]

The motor innervation of the bladder, like all smooth muscle, is provided by the autonomic nervous system. Parasympathetic receptors containing acetylcholine are abundant throughout the bladder body (detrusor muscle). Excitation of these receptors produces contraction of the detrusor muscle. Sympathetic receptors are also found in the bladder body and base. Beta-receptors containing norepinephrine are found principally in the body of the bladder. Excitation of these receptors causes relaxation of detrusor muscle bundles. Alpha-receptors are abundant in the bladder base and proximal urethra. Unlike the beta-receptors, they are excitatory when stimulated, causing contraction of smooth muscle bundles in the trigone and proximal urethra. Nonadrenergic, noncholinergic receptors are also found in the bladder body. They are postulated to be excitatory in nature, playing a yet undescribed role in contraction of the detrusor muscle.

Sympathetic neural signals are routed to the bladder via branches of the inferior hypogastric plexus. The spinal roots of the sympathetic component of the inferior hypogastric plexus are at T12, L1, and L2. Parasympathetic neural signals are routed to the bladder via branches of the pelvic nerve. The spinal roots of the parasympathetic component of the pelvic plexus are located in the interomedial gray matter between the dorsal and ventral horns of spinal levels S2 to S4.

Urethra. The urethra extends from the bladder to an external meatus, serves as a conduit for urine expulsion during micturition, and aids in maintaining continence during bladder filling. In the male the urethra also serves as a conduit for semen expelled at ejaculation.[173,178]

The male urethra is approximately 23 cm long and is divided into two parts: anterior and posterior (FIG. 14-6). The posterior urethra is subdivided into the prostatic and membranous urethra. The prostatic urethra is approximately 3 cm long and extends from the bladder neck to the origin of the membranous urethral segment at the apex of the prostate gland. It runs through the prostate vertically, lying nearer the anterior surface of the gland. The posterior floor of the prostatic urethra is elevated at the verumontanum. It tapers inferiorly and superiorly to form the cristae, which are mucous membrane folds that form a depression on the posterior floor known as the prostatic fossa. Secretory ducts from the middle lobe of the prostate enter the urethra at this point (FIG. 14-7).[173]

The membranous urethra is 2 to 2.5 cm long and extends from the apex of the prostate to the bulb of the penis. It pierces the area referred to as the urogenital diaphragm. Striated muscle fibers exist within the wall of the membranous urethra and significantly contribute to sphincteric function in the male. These muscle fibers are arranged in an omega-shaped pattern and are thinnest in the posterior midline. Periurethral striated muscle fibers from the pelvic floor also contribute to striated muscle sphincteric function of the urethra.[63,173] The membranous urethra is the least distensible segment, since it is anchored securely by the triangular ligament. It is the most susceptible to inflammatory urethral stricture.[173,178]

The anterior urethra tunnels the corpus spongiosum of the penis and is divided into the bulbous, pendulous, and glandular urethra. The bulbous and pendulous parts of the urethra together measure 15 cm long and extend from the distal border of the membranous urethra to the base of the glans penis. The suspensory ligament marks the border between these urethral segments. The bulbous urethra is distinguished by the orifices of the bulbourethral, or Cowper's, glands.[173]

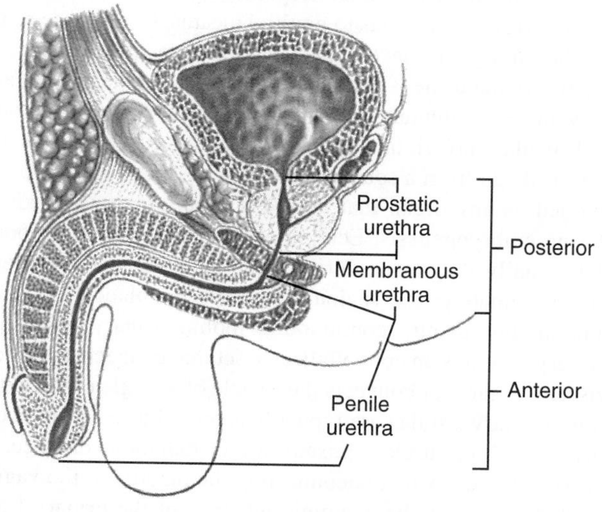

FIG. 14-6
Male urethra.

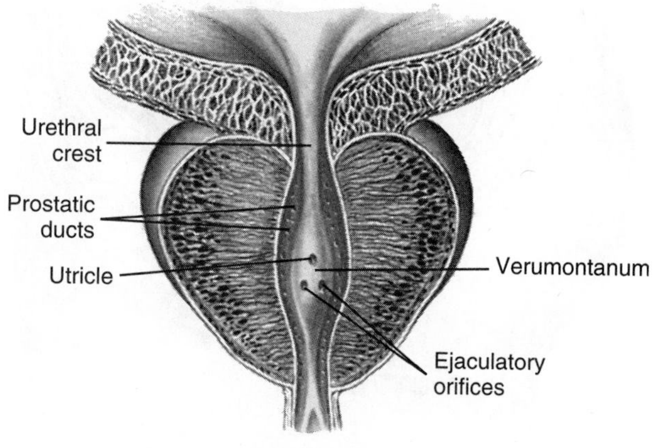

FIG. 14-7
Prostatic (posterior) urethra.

The penile urethra is the most distal segment in the male and terminates at the external meatus. Immediately before the external meatus, the penile urethra is marked by a fusiform dilation called the fossa navicularis. It originates at the corona of the glans and is 2.5 cm long. The external meatus itself is a vertical slit approximately 8 mm in diameter that lies at the summit of the glans.[173,178]

The microscope anatomy of the male urethra is characterized by an inner mucous membrane composed of columnar cell epithelium persisting throughout the posterior and anterior urethral segments to the level of the fossa navicularis. Here the urethral mucosa changes to a squamous cell epithelium near the external meatus. A submucosal layer composed of connective tissue and elastic fibers lies under the mucosa. The muscular layer of the urethra is composed primarily of smooth muscle fibers. In the prostatic urethra the smooth muscle fibers are indistinguishable from the adjacent musculature to the level of the verumontanum. Below the verumontanum, the urethral smooth fibers are arranged in an outer circular layer and an inner longitudinal layer. Striated muscle fibers have also been noted in the ventral wall of the prostatic urethra.[30,178]

The arterial blood supply of the male urethra arises from the urethral artery, which is a branch of the internal pudendal artery. Venous blood from the urethra drains into the deep vein of the penis and the pudendal plexus. The sensory innervation of the urethra is provided by branches of the pudendal nerve. Lymphatic drainage from the male urethra accompanies channels of the glans penis in the anterior segment and empties into the deep subinguinal nodes from the posterior segment.[178]

The female urethra forms a relatively short, straight path when compared with the male urethra (FIG. 14-8). In nulliparous adult women the urethra measures 3.5 to 5.5 cm. The female urethra originates at the bladder neck orifice and travels at a 16-degree angle to its external meatus at the vestibule. Striated muscle fibers within the urethral wall are densest in the middle third of the female urethra and deficient in the posterior midline. Periurethral striated muscle fibers of the levator ani also contribute to sphincteric function in the female.[60,178]

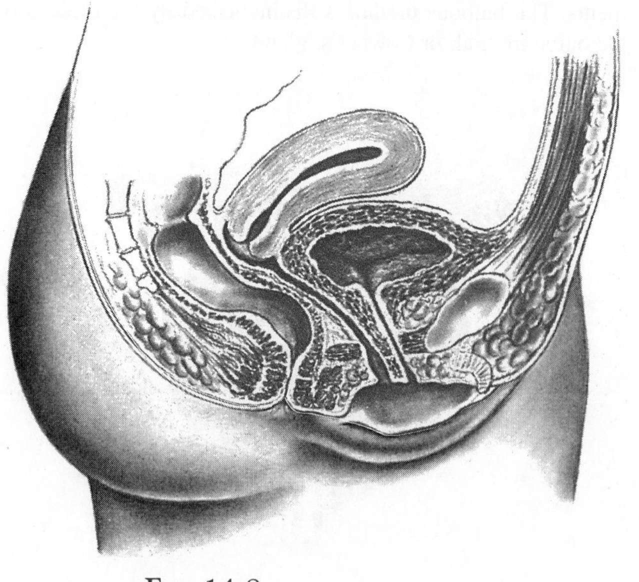

FIG. 14-8
Anatomic relations of female urethra.

Three histologic elements of the female urethra characterize its microscopic anatomy. The inner urethral lumen is lined by columnar epithelium that changes to squamous epithelium near the external meatus. The mucosal layer also contains numerous secreting glands. The muscular lining of the urethra contains an outer sheath of skeletal muscle fibers (the rhabdosphincter), an outer longitudinal layer of smooth muscle bundles, and inner circular layers of smooth muscle bundles. The lower two thirds of the female urethra is fused with the anterior vaginal wall so that the two layers of smooth muscle are indistinguishable. A spongy vascular cushion composed of an extensive venous network and arteriovenous communications lies between the urethral mucosa layer and the muscular layer of the urethral wall.[178]

Lower Urinary Tract Function

The bladder and urethra act in coordination with the pelvic floor support structures (endopelvic fascia and pelvic musculature) and act as a coordinated unit to provide continence.[61] Continence can be defined as control over bladder function, or the absence of urine loss until the individual voluntarily initiates micturition. Continence can be divided into two stages: (1) bladder filling and storage, and (2) micturition. Successful bladder filling and storage requires antegrade flow of urine from the nephron to the bladder and low-pressure storage of steadily increasing volumes of urine in the bladder despite the presence of repetitive, precipitous, and often unpredictable changes in abdominal forces acting on the bladder outlet and urethra. Successful micturition requires reversal of the resistance to urinary outflow present during micturition, accompanied by a detrusor contraction of sufficient magnitude and duration to completely evacuate urine from the bladder. Three factors, anatomic integrity of the urinary tract, neurologic modulation of bladder and urethral smooth and striated muscle, and competence of the sphincter mechanism are essential for the attainment and maintenance of continence.

Anatomic Integrity

The urinary tract can be conceptualized as a single tube extending from glomerulus to urethral meatus. Continence relies on the embryonic development and maintenance of this integrity so that urine is expelled exclusively via the urethra and only during voluntary micturition. Two conditions, ectopia and fistula, may violate this anatomic integrity, allowing urinary leakage from a source other than the urethra.[4] Ectopia is defined as any organ that develops in an abnormal position during embryogenesis. Ectopia of the ureter is a rare condition usually diagnosed during childhood. An ectopic ureter may terminate in the vagina, bypassing the bladder and urethra and producing a continuous dribbling urinary leakage. A urinary fistula is an epithelialized tract that connects to hollow visceral organs, or connects the vesicle of a single organ to the skin. Urinary fistulas are typically acquired as a result of obstructed labor, surgical misadventure, radiation, damage, or invasive tumor. A fistula connecting the bladder to the vagina or skin interrupts the anatomic integrity of the urinary tract, leading to continuous urine loss that varies from a continuous dribble superimposed on an otherwise normal voiding pattern to severe leakage replacing normal cycles of bladder filling and micturition.

Neurologic Modulation of Bladder Smooth Muscle

Urinary continence also requires control of the smooth muscle of the bladder wall, also called the detrusor. The continent person exerts voluntary control over detrusor muscle contractions.[6] This control represents the effect of multiple modulatory areas of the brain, spinal cord, and peripheral nervous system. It also reflects unique aspects of the detrusor smooth muscle when compared with that found in the upper urinary tracts or gastrointestinal system.

Modulatory areas located within the brain contribute to voluntary detrusor control.[12] A detrusor motor area is located within the superomedial area of the frontal lobes (FIG. 14-9). The detrusor motor area receives its blood supply from the middle and anterior cerebral arteries.[1] The branches of the middle and anterior cerebral arteries are the most common locations for cerebrovascular accidents in the United States, and damage to the detrusor motor area is postulated to explain the high incidence of detrusor hyperreflexia and urge incontinence following a stroke. The thalamus primarily serves as a relay center connecting the cerebral cortex with lower brain centers. It modulates the function of multiple organs, including the bladder. The extrapyramidal nervous system consists of the basal ganglia, caudate nuclei, red nuclei, substantia nigra, putamen, and globus pallidus.[1] Collectively these nuclei interact with the cerebellum and the corticospinal tracts (pyramidal system) to coordinate motor movements and to maintain the body's position in space. The basal ganglia also exert an inhibitory influence on the detrusor reflex.[12] The importance of this modulatory center upon lower urinary tract function is apparent in the case of parkinsonism, which is strongly associated with detrusor hyperreflexia.[11,14]

The cerebellum is located within the posterior fossa of the cranium. It helps coordinate voluntary movements and the ability to maintain an upright (standing) position without the need of support.[1] Although the neurologic communication between detrusor and cerebellum is not clear, detrusor hyperreflexia and cerebellar dysfunction are associated in humans.[103] Input from the hypothalamus and the limbic system are known to alter the detrusor reflex in experimental animals, but their role in modulation of the detrusor reflex in humans remains unclear.

Collectively the paired detrusor motor areas, thalamus and hypothalamus, basal ganglia, and cerebellum act together to inhibit detrusor contraction until the individual wishes to urinate. Injury to any of these areas compromises this control, resulting in hyperreflexia of the micturition reflex and urge urinary incontinence.

The brainstem represents the origin of the micturition reflex before continence mastery.[13] A micturition center is located in the dorsolateral region of the pons that coordinates detrusor and striated sphincter activity. Neurons within this area coordinate contraction of the detrusor and striated sphincter muscles, ensuring sphincter closure during bladder filling and storage and urethral opening during micturition. The significance of the pontine micturition center is illustrated in patients who experience a complete spinal cord injury causing detrusor hyperreflexia and uncoordinated contraction of the striated sphincter muscle during voiding (detrusor sphincter dyssynergia). In addition to the sphincter coordination center, the periaqueductal (paraventricular) gray matter and the L region (a collection of neurons located near the pontine micturition center) also serve as important facilitators of bladder filling and storage. In the infant the brainstem serves as the primary modulator of bladder filling/storage and micturition. In the adult it continues to play a critical role in the maintenance of continence; but it also responds to input from the higher modulatory centers in the brain described earlier.

The spinal cord influences smooth muscle function in the bladder wall through neurons found in the sympathetic and parasympathetic nervous systems.[12] Parasympathetic neurons located within sacral spinal segments 2 to 4, acting under the influence of modulatory areas in the brain and brainstem, lead to detrusor contraction during micturition by stimulating muscarinic, cholinergic receptors within the bladder wall. Stimulation of parasympathetic neurons also promotes sphincter relaxation and urethral opening, probably by a combination of inhibition of adrenergic receptors within the urethral smooth and striated muscle, and possibly by direct stimulation of smooth muscle within the endopelvic fascia causing funneling of the proximal urethra. Damage to these neurons prevents essential neurologic stimulus from reaching the detrusor, leading to areflexia (paralysis) of this muscle and subsequent urinary retention. Sympathetic neurons are located at spinal levels T10 to L2 that promote bladder storage. Stimulation of these nerves,

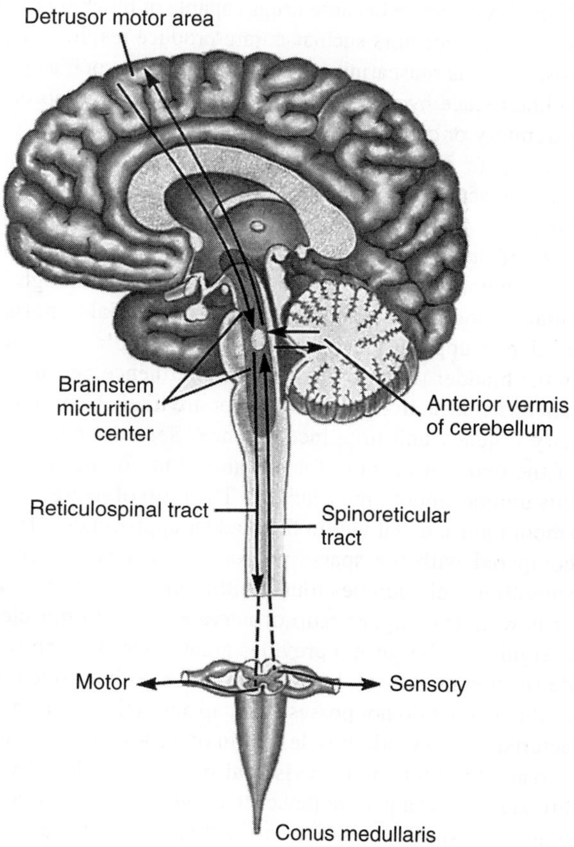

FIG. 14-9
Supraspinal and spinal innervation of the detrusor muscle.

under the influence of modulatory centers in the brainstem and brain, promote relaxation and further filling and storage, acting through beta-receptors in the bladder wall. Stimulation of alpha-receptors in the proximal urethra and bladder neck promotes urethral closure and inhibits detrusor contractions via reflex pathways within the spine.

Neurologic signals from spinal neurons communicate with the bladder via several peripheral nerves. Sympathetic stimuli reach the bladder mainly via the lumbar nerves, and parasympathetic stimuli reach the bladder primarily through the pelvic plexus. Both of these nerves contain afferent (sensory) as well as efferent (motor) axons.

Continence relies on the actions of neurotransmitters that act at neuromuscular junctions in the bladder and urethral muscle.[12] These neurotransmitters facilitate the continuous neurologic communication needed to sense bladder filling, the desire to urinate (urgency), and the act of micturition. Relatively little is known about the neurotransmitters in the brain and their influence on bladder function. Studies on animals indicate that glutamic acid may act as a primary neurotransmitter in the brain, coordinating bladder function. Other significant neurotransmitters include serotonin, gamma-aminobutyric acid (GABA), dopamine, acetylcholine, adenosine triphosphate (ATP), and nitric oxide. Within the spinal cord and periphery, preganglionic nerve synapses contain nicotinic cholinergic receptors that respond to acetylcholine. In contrast, peripheral receptors within the smooth muscles of the bladder and urethra contain muscarinic, cholinergic receptors that also respond to acetylcholine. This distinction is important from both a pharmacologic and a clinical perspective because drugs capable of blocking nicotinic cholinergic receptors such as curare produce respiratory paralysis, whereas muscarinic cholinergic blockers such as propantheline reduce hyperactive contractions without compromising respiratory or cardiac function.

Specific characteristics of the detrusor muscle and the neuromuscular junctions within the bladder wall also contribute to continence. In contrast to the skeletal muscles, most of the smooth muscle within the human is involuntary, or independent of direct neurologic control. Although involuntary smooth muscle contractions are essential to normal digestive or upper urinary tract function, a similar arrangement in the bladder wall would preclude continence because spontaneous contractions of the detrusor are likely to produce urinary urgency and urge incontinence. Several characteristics of the detrusor account for our ability to voluntarily control this unique smooth muscle.[12,13,17] The ratio of nerve ending to smooth muscle cell within the bladder approaches a 1:1 ratio, compared with the sparse proportion of nerve receptors to smooth muscle bundles found within the renal pelvis, ureter, or bowel. This higher ratio of nerve endings to muscle cells is significant because it provides greater nervous control over detrusor contractions. In addition, the smooth muscle bundles of the bladder do not possess the gap and tight junctions characteristic of smooth muscle within other visceral organs. The gap and tight junctions in visceral smooth muscle allow rapid propagation of a peristaltic contraction without nervous stimulation. A similar situation in the bladder would render continence impossible because it would be impossible to postpone a detrusor contraction once a certain bladder volume was reached.

The primary excitatory neurotransmitter of the detrusor is acetylcholine, and muscarinic cholinergic receptors are found throughout the bladder wall.[12,17] Similar receptors are found in many smooth muscles within the body, including the gastrointestinal tract, eyes, salivary glands, and arterioles. The majority of anticholinergic medications act in a nonselective manner, and they affect all of these organs. Unfortunately, this multiplicity of pharmacologic actions often produces intolerable side effects. Fortunately, additional research has resulted in identification of additional cholinergic receptor subtypes.[7] M_1, M_2, and M_3 receptors have been identified, and the urinary bladder has been found to contain primarily M_2 and M_3 receptors. Identification of these muscarinic subtypes is important because it has led to the development and testing of pharmacologic agents that may prove effective in the management of unstable (hyperactive) detrusor contractions while limiting or avoiding the often intolerable side effects associated with nonselective anticholinergics.

Other neurotransmitters modulate detrusor muscle function.[12,17] Norepinephrine acts on beta-receptors in the bladder wall, producing smooth muscle relaxation. ATP is found in nonadrenergic, noncholinergic (NANC) receptors. Stimulation of these purinergic receptors facilitates detrusor muscle contraction, but cholinergic receptors remain the predominant neurotransmitter promoting detrusor contraction. Other neurotransmitters important to the lower urinary tract include vasoactive intestinal polypeptide (VIP), substance P and the calcitonin gene-related peptide (CGRP), and nitric oxide synthase. They are postulated to regulate bladder sensations, including sensations of fullness, urgency, pressure, pain, and temperature.

Sphincter Mechanism Competence

The urethral sphincter has been traditionally defined exclusively in terms of its primary muscular components, including an internal (smooth muscle) sphincter and external (striated muscle) sphincter.[61,162] However, this conceptualization of a "dual mechanism" fails to acknowledge the significance of compressive elements of the urethral sphincter, and it does not highlight the rhabdosphincter as compared with the periurethral striated muscle. Because of these limitations, the sphincter is better defined as a single mechanism, comprising elements of compression and elements of tension, complemented by elements of support.[26] During bladder filling, these factors interact to produce a watertight seal that prevents leakage, even in the presence of physical exertion. During micturition, the sphincter mechanism rapidly changes its physical properties to provide a low-resistance conduit for urinary outflow.

Urethral softness, its mucosal secretions, and submucosal vascular cushion constitute the sphincter's compressive elements.[26,162] The epithelial mucosa of the urethra must be soft and flexible to maintain the watertight seal needed for continence. This softness is reflected during catheterization, which allows urinary outflow through the catheter's lumen while preventing leakage around the catheter. Mucosal secretions are essential for the formation of a watertight seal because they raise the surface tension of the bladder wall, filling microscopic gaps left when the epithelium closes between urination episodes. The third compressive element of the sphincter is the vascular cushion. It is a rich network of arteries and veins within the urethral submucosa; the noncompressible blood contained in this cushion effectively distributes closure pressure (tension from the smooth muscle in the urethral wall designed to prevent urinary leakage).

Although necessary for maintaining a watertight seal, the elements of urethral compression cannot prevent urinary leakage in the presence of gravity or physical exertion. In these cases, closure and the prevention of urine loss is achieved by active contraction of smooth and skeletal muscle within the urethral wall. These elements, when combined with periurethral muscle and the pelvic floor muscles, provide effective sphincter closure in the presence of significant physical or precipitous abdominal pressure rises caused by coughing or sneezing.

In men, smooth muscle bundles encircle the bladder neck, forming what has been traditionally termed the internal sphincter. This circular smooth muscle facilitates sphincter competence, and it contracts during ejaculation to prevent retrograde movement of semen into the bladder. Smooth muscle arranged in a longitudinal fashion also extends into the prostatic urethra. The rhabdosphincter is a set of specialized, Ω-shaped skeletal muscle fibers located within the membranous urethra.[22] The fibers of the rhabdosphincter are exclusively slow twitch, and they are well suited for maintaining the prolonged tone needed for continence between episodes of urination. In addition to the rhabdosphincter, periurethral striated muscle also contributes to urethral closure in men. It is a combination of slow and rapid twitch fibers that provide additional urethral closure, particularly in response to periods of intense physical exertion or sudden increases in abdominal pressure.

Smooth and skeletal muscle are also observed in the female urethra.[36,146] Circularly arranged bundles can be found at the bladder neck as they are in males, but their functional significance in the female lower urinary tract in unclear. Longitudinal smooth muscle bundles are observed at the base of the bladder that extend to the distal urethra. A rhabdosphincter comprising slow twitch muscle fibers is located in the middle third of the female urethra. In women it is usually called the sphincter urethrae.[36] Two other muscles, comprising primarily slow twitch fibers but containing some fast twitch elements, also contribute to sphincter function in the woman. The compressor urethrae originates at the perineal membrane, and the urethrovaginal sphincter extends further to encircle the vaginal wall.

The structures that support the urethra and bladder base are also critical to continence, particularly in the female. The endopelvic fascia, perineal membrane, and anal sphincter provide supplemental support to the bladder base and urethra. However, it is the levator ani that is primarily responsible for maintaining the bladder base in an intraabdominal position. This low abdominal position is significant because it provides the optimal position for urethral closure via the smooth and striated muscle of the sphincter mechanism, and because it transmits abdominal forces to the urethral lumen.

Like the detrusor, the urethral smooth muscle receives extensive neurologic innervation.[164,171] The smooth muscle of the bladder neck and proximal urethra in both genders contains an abundance of alpha-receptors. However, in contrast to the detrusor, stimulation of these receptors causes contraction of these muscle bundles and urethral sphincter closure. It has also been postulated that cholinergic innervation of urethral smooth muscle may contribute to urethral funneling during micturition. The innervation of the rhabdosphincter (sphincter urethrae in women) remains somewhat unclear. Triple innervation (somatic, parasympathetic, and sympathetic) has been observed in the rhabdosphincter of some animals, but it has not been clearly demonstrated in tissue studies of this muscle in humans.[43,164] Nonetheless, the rhabdosphincter appears to respond to alpha-blocking agents, and it probably responds to autonomic as well as somatic nervous stimuli. The periurethral and pelvic muscles, including the levator ani, receive somatic innervation from the pudendal nerve, which originates from spinal roots at sacral levels 2 to 4. The periurethral striated muscles respond to modulation from the pontine micturition center, but they can be overridden as demonstrated by contraction of the pelvic and periurethral striated muscles and interruption of urination when a person is startled during voiding. The center for this voluntary control is located in the sensorimotor nucleus of the brain that sends signals to the pelvic muscles via the pyramidal tracts.

Continence in the Adult

A description of the phases of bladder function is helpful to an understanding of the multiple neurologic and muscular elements that contribute to continence. Immediately following an episode of micturition, the bladder begins to refill with urine. During this period, the detrusor remains relaxed and the sphincter mechanism remains closed. These events are modulated by multiple areas of the brain and the brainstem that send signals to the bladder via sympathetic nuclei arising from spinal roots at T10 to L2. As the bladder continues to fill, its wall is stretched and afferent impulses signal the first urge to urinate. The management of afferent impulses by the brainstem and brain remains partially unknown, but it is likely that the thalamus and detrusor motor area play important roles. Continued bladder filling ultimately leads to increases in the frequency and amplitude (intensity) of afferent signals, causing a pressing perception of urinary urgency (the desire to urinate).[180] In addition to bladder volume, the perception of urinary urgency is influenced by the emotions, by the content of the urine, and by other extrinsic factors such as the ambient temperature. Stimulation of spinal interneurons also impacts perceptions of urgency. For example, stroking the perineal skin facilitates urgency (and micturition), whereas stimulation of the genitals is inhibitory.[171]

A combination of physiologic factors (including the intensity of urinary urgency and intravesical volume) and psychosocial factors (perception of "permission" to toilet and the availability of a toileting facility) determine when the continent person reaches a decision to urinate. The micturition reflex pathway is best described as spinobulbospinal. Voiding begins with relaxation of the pelvic muscles and by activation of the sacral parasympathetic pathways, which reflexively inhibits the urethral sphincter mechanism while activating a contraction of the detrusor. The brain removes its inhibitory influence on the brainstem via unclear mechanisms, and the brainstem stimulates detrusor contraction via activation of parasympathetic (muscarinic) receptors in the bladder wall. The brainstem also inhibits urethral sphincter tone via spinal reflex pathways. Voiding ensues and continues until the bladder is completely emptied of its contents, and the cycle starts again. Should the individual wish to discontinue voiding before complete bladder emptying, the sensorimotor cortex is used to contract the pelvic muscles, which reflexively inhibits the detrusor's contraction.

Male Genitalia

Scrotum. The scrotum is a cutaneous, fibromuscular sac that is dependent below the pubis bone and houses the testes and lower portion of the spermatic cord. The skin of the scrotum is thin and deeply pigmented and contains abundant sebaceous glands, sweat glands, and hair follicles. The cutaneous layer of the scrotum is bisected by the median ridge or raphe, which extends from the base of the penis to the anus. The skin of the scrotum is further distinguished by rugae. The rugae are formed by parallel dermal muscle fibers and are more clearly seen on younger men, particularly when the testes have retracted because of a certain stimulus. Immediately under the skin is the dartos muscle, which is composed of smooth muscle fibers and elastic tissue. The dartos is a continuation of the suspensory ligament of the penis and superficial fascia of the abdominal, inguinal, and perineal fascia. It sends a sagittal reflection inward, creating an incomplete septum between the median ridge and the radix of the penis, which form the cavities in which the testes lie.[178]

The primary functions of the scrotum are to house the testes and provide an adequate environment for the production of sperm. The structure of the dartos allows for considerable variation of scrotal size in response to a variety of stimuli, such as external temperature, physical activity level, and emotions.[8]

Testes. The testes are a pair of ovoid organs that lie in the scrotum. They receive vascular, neural, and lymphatic support from the spermatic cord; the scrotal ligament forms the single scrotal attachment for the testes. Each testis is approximately 4 to 5 cm long and 2.5 cm wide and weighs from 10.5 to 20 g. The left testis typically lies 1 cm lower than the right.[173,178]

The testes lie under three coverings: the tunica vaginalis, the tunica albuginea, and the tunica vasculosa. The tunica vaginalis arises from the peritoneum and forms a closed sac in which the testis is invaginated. The tunica albuginea is a white, fibrous covering for the testis that helps define the interior architecture of the organ. The posterior border of the tunica albuginea projects into the testis, forming an incomplete vertical septum called the mediastinum testis. From its front and lateral aspects, numerous fibrous projections extend toward the external border of the testis, dividing it into 200 to 300 lobules that contain multiple somniferous tubules. The tunica vasculosa is the third testicular covering. It consists of a plexus of blood vessels within a framework of areolar tissue extending over the internal aspect of the tunica albuginea and covering its many septa, providing a vascular supply to each lobule.[173,178]

The functional unit of the testicular cortex is the seminiferous tubule. Each lobule of the testis contains one to three (or sometimes more) seminiferous tubules that are 30 to 60 cm of tortuous length with both ends terminating in a relatively short, straight segment called the canaliculus rectus. The seminiferous tubules occupy 75% of testicular mass; their combined length is almost 1 mile.[178]

A seminiferous tubule is formed of stratified epithelium four to eight cells thick with an identifiable internal lumen. The tubules contain Sertoli's cells, spermatogenic cells, and an outer basement membrane with a fibrous tunica propria. Sertoli's cells are columnar in shape and extend radially from just within the outer basement membrane toward the tubular lumen. These interesting cells have indefinite cytoplasmic borders; spermatids and spermatocytes may be completely embedded within the cytoplasm of Sertoli's cells. Sertoli's cells are linked in tight junctions that divide the wall of the seminiferous tubule into two parts: a basal compartment containing spermatogonia and spermatocytes and a luminal compartment containing more advanced stages of testicular germ cells. The exact function of Sertoli's cells remains unclear. They are presumed to provide nourishment and succor for the germinal epithelium, help maintain the blood-testis barrier, secrete the testicular fluid seen in the lumen of the seminiferous tubules, and secrete an androgen-binding protein that promotes the accumulation of androgens in the immediate area of the germinal cell epithelium.[5]

The germinal cell epithelium of the seminiferous tubule is characterized by an ever-changing population of maturing stages of spermatic forms. The more primitive forms are found at the outer borders, and more mature forms are found nearer the inner lumen. Spermatogonia are the most immature cell form seen in the spermatic cycle. Other stages of germ cell epithelium seen in the wall of the semniferous tubules are primary and secondary spermatocytes and spermatids.[5]

The interstitial tissue within the testicular lobules is composed of Leydig's cells, blood vessels, extensive lymphatic channels, and numerous macrophages. Leydig's cells are found in small groups of 5 to 20 and compose 12% of testicular volume. These are particularly significant because they secrete testosterone, which enters the bloodstream via interstitial capillary beds or goes directly into the seminiferous tubule without going through vascular routes.[5]

The structure and function of the testes in the adult male are significantly different from those during infancy and childhood. The germinal elements of the testes have a distinct embryologic origin from the other elements of the gonads. The nongerminal cell components of the testes arise as part of the mesodermic mass that will develop into the urogenital ridge; the germ cells of the testes arise from the entoderm lining the posterior aspect of the yolk sac. Development of both the germinal cell and somatic elements of the testes begins during the fourth week of life.[109]

From their retroperitoneal position, the testes must descend caudally to the scrotal sac to mature into viable structures away from the high temperature of the internal abdomen. During the third trimester they begin moving down the posterior aspect of the abdomen, bringing their neurovascular sheath with them. By the seventh month of gestation, the testes enter the internal ring of the inguinal canal and move into their extraabdominal position at or shortly after birth. The complex factors that regulate this migration are still not fully understood.[109]

At birth the testes are composed of small tubules with poorly differentiated components and few identifiable spermatogonia. Interstitial cells are present at birth but regress over the first several weeks of life to a baseline level that persists throughout the pubescent period. During the period between 4 and 10 years of age, the seminiferous tubules slowly increase in tortuosity. Beginning around age 10 a significant increase in the size, number, and mitotic activity of the germ cell epithelium occurs. This process continues until the onset of puberty around age 12, when the interstitial Leydig's cells mature and begin to produce testosterone levels comparable with adult values and active spermatogenesis begins.[5]

The blood supply of the testes is unique, because the temperature of arterial and venous blood must be cooled approximately 2° C from abdominal levels to support spermatogenesis. Cooling arises from interactions between arterial and venous vessels in which a countercurrent heat loss mechanism occurs. In addition, the slow, nonpulsating flow of the spermatic artery aids in cooling the vascular beds of the testes.[5]

The arterial blood supply of the testes arises from the internal spermatic artery, the cremasteric artery, and the deferential, or vasal, artery. The latter are important clinically as collateral circulation of the testes. Venous blood from the testes drains into the pampiniform plexus of the spermatic cord, which empties into the internal spermatic veins.[5]

Because of the unique embryologic origins of the testes, the lymphatic drainage is not into local inguinal or pelvic lymph nodes. Rather, the extensive lymphatic channels of the testes drain into the preaortic lymph nodes.[55,173]

Three adnexa of the testes are of clinical significance; all are composed of vestiges of the embryonic structures relevant to the formation and migration of the testes and spermatic cord. The appendix testis arises in the groove between the head of the epididymis and the testicular remnant of the müllerian duct. It is subject to torsion and must be differentiated from true testicular torsion, which constitutes a urologic emergency. The appendix epididymis is a pear-shaped body attached to the epididymal head, which is a remnant of epigenitalis tubules. The organs of Giraldes are a paragenitalis remnant sometimes noted in the lower spermatic cord anterior to the head of the epididymis.[55,173]

Epididymis and Vas Deferens. The epididymis and vas deferens are the efferent routes for sperm leaving the testes after completing the spermatogenic cycle. Along with the prostate and seminal vesicles, the epididymis and vas deferens provide transport, storage, and support for maturing sperm as they migrate toward the male urethra.[178]

The epididymis is a sausage-shaped structure approximately 5 cm long that is attached to the posterolateral aspect of the testis. Three anatomic regions of the epididymis are described: the head, or globus major; the body, or corpus; and the tail, or globus minor. The epididymis contains a single compartment, so injury is likely to entirely ablate the function of the organ. The epididymis is covered by the tunica vaginalis on all except the posterior border, where a fascial reflection forms the epididymal sinus.[173]

Inside the compartment of the epididymis is a long, tortuous canal with little muscular tone but abundant cilia lining the tubular lumen folded over on itself and tightly packed so that its total length is 4 to 5 cm. The head of the epididymis is directly connected to the efferent ductules, allowing sperm leaving the testis to enter the epididymal tubules via ciliary action. At the tail the tubules have more smooth muscle in their walls as the epididymis opens into the vas deferens.[178]

The vas deferens is a firm, elastic, cylindric tube extending from the termination of the epididymal tail to the ejaculatory duct located near the base of the prostate. The initial segment of the vas deferens is tortuous, although the part of the organ more distal to the testis is straight. From its origin at the epididymal tail, the vas deferens ascends along the posterior wall of the testis adjacent to the medial aspect of the epididymis. The vas then moves upward to the posterior part of the spermatic cord, traversing the inguinal canal to the level of the deep inguinal ring. At this point, the vas deferens leaves the spermatic cord, curves around the lateral aspect of the epigastric artery, and ascends several centimeters to the external iliac artery. The vas then crosses the external iliac obliquely and enters the false pelvis where it becomes a relatively fixed structure attached to the posterior abdominal wall. From this point the vas crosses the ureter and curves at an acute angle to traverse the prostatic base and terminate at the ejaculatory duct (FIG. 14-10). The final segment of the vas deferens is characterized by a spindle-shaped dilation of the tube called the ampulla, which is approximately 10 cm long and contains several false pouches or diverticula that may or may not be clinically significant.[178]

The walls of the vas deferens comprise adventitial, muscular, and mucosal layers. The mucosa of the vas deferens comprises columnar epithelial cells, which, unlike the tubules of the epididymis, are not ciliated.[55,178] The smooth muscle of the vas deferens is divided into inner and outer longitudinal layers, separated by a middle circular layer of bundles. These smooth muscle bundles, like those of the ureter, contain gap junctions that allow rapid transmission of excitatory impulses and rapid contraction. The vas deferens serves as a conduit between the epididymis and ejaculatory duct, moving seminal fluid toward the prostatic urethra during emission. Relaxation of the circular smooth muscle of the wall of the vas deferens lengthens the vas, whereas contraction of the longitudinal smooth muscle lengthens the tube. As a result, seminal fluid is propelled in an antegrade fashion toward the prostatic urethra for ejaculation.[164] The adventitial layer of the vas deferens contains connective

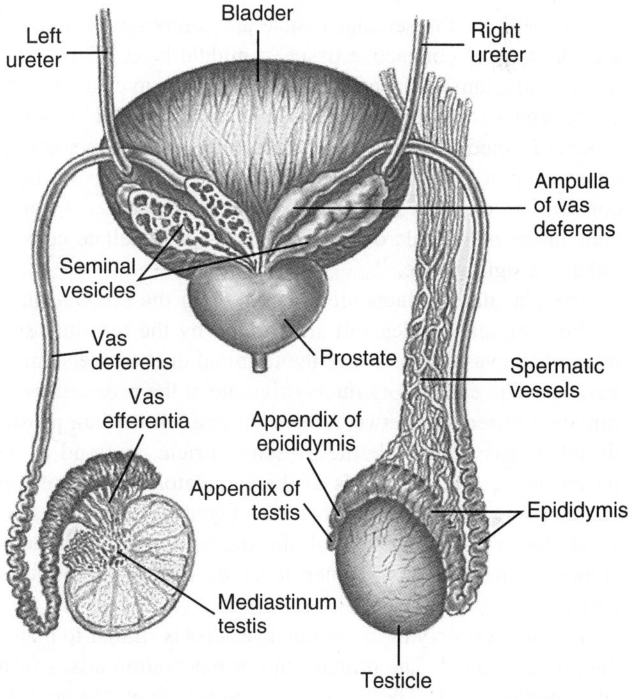

FIG. 14-10
Anatomic relation of vas deferens to bladder (posterior view).

tissue and the neural, vascular, and lymphatic supply for the vas.[173,178]

The blood supplies of the vas deferens and the epididymis are closely related. The epididymis receives arterial blood from the internal spermatic artery or the deferential artery, and the vas receives arterial blood from the deferential artery. Venous blood from the epididymis and the lower segments of the vas drain into the pampiniform plexus of the spermatic cord, which becomes the spermatic vein.[158,173]

The motor innervation of the vas deferens arises from pelvic ganglia near the seminal vesicle. Stimulation of sympathetic preganglionics causes contraction of the vas deferens and movement of seminal fluid. These adrenergic mechanisms are also responsible for contraction of smooth muscle in the bladder neck and posterior urethra, preventing the occurrence of retrograde ejaculation. Cholinergic mechanisms, mediated by parasympathetic pathways, may play an indirect or modulatory role in seminal emission and contraction of the vas deferens in the human. Other central neurotransmitters, such as gamma aminobutyric acid (GABA), prostaglandins, and bradykinins, also may play an as yet undefined modulatory role in contraction of the smooth muscle of the vas deferens.[163]

Seminal Vesicles and Ejaculatory Ducts.

The seminal vesicles are a pair of saclike structures that lie between the posterior bladder and the rectum. Each vesicle is 4 cm long; they have a pyramidal shape with the superior end oriented laterally and backward from the base. The structure of the seminal vesicles is formed by a single coiled tube that gives rise to irregularly placed diverticula connected by dense fibrous tissue. The diameter of the tube of the seminal vesicle is 3 to 4 mm, and its length is 10 to 15 cm when uncoiled. The seminal vesicles are directed to the posterior bladder surface near the implantation of the ureters and lie in close proximity to the rectum.[108,178]

The walls of the seminal vesicle are composed of an outer areolar layer of connective tissue, a middle layer of muscular tissue, and a luminal layer of mucosal epithelium characteristic of the organs for sperm transport and maturation. The muscular tunic is formed by inner circular smooth muscle fibers and an outer layer of longitudinal smooth muscle. The mucosal layer consists of columnar epithelium with an abundance of goblet cells in the diverticula of the organ and small stellate cells of unknown significance.[178]

The ejaculatory ducts are located along the median plane of the seminal vesicles and are formed by the terminal segment of the vas deferens and the terminal duct of the seminal vesicles. The ejaculatory ducts originate at the prostatic base, run anteroinferiorly between the right and left median prostatic lobes, pass alongside the prostatic utricle, and end in the posterior urethra. The walls of the ejaculatory ducts are thin and characterized by an outer fibrous layer that terminates beyond the prostatic portion of the ducts, a middle layer of smooth muscle, and an inner layer of columnar epithelial cells.[178]

The blood supply of the seminal vesicles is similar to that of the prostate gland. The primary motor innervation arises from sympathetic fibers. The lymphatic channels from the seminal vesicles drain into the hypogastric, sacral, vesical, and external iliac nodes (see FIG. 14-10).[157]

Prostate.

The prostate is a partly glandular, partly fibromuscular organ that lies at the base of the bladder and surrounds the initial 2 to 3 cm of posterior urethra. The prostate is conical with an anterior and posterior flattening; its average dimensions are 3.4 cm long, 4.4 cm wide, and 2.6 cm at its greatest thickness. The organ is securely anchored by the puboprostatic ligaments, Denonvilliers' fascia, and the adjacent pelvic floor musculature. In addition, the resilient, strong prostatic capsule provides support.[173]

The structure of the prostate can be divided into lobes,[79] anatomic aspects,[178] and zones.[121] Williams and Warwick[178] conceptualized four anatomic aspects: the base, apex, posterior surface, and anterior aspect. The prostate base is adjacent to the bladder neck. The urethra pierces the prostate at the base, near its anterior aspect. The apex of the prostate faces away from the bladder and inferior to its base; its surface is contiguous with fascia covering the superior aspect of the periurethral muscles of the pelvic floor (sometimes called the urogenital diaphragm). The posterior surface of the prostate is transversely flat and vertically convex. It is separated from the rectum by the prostatic sheath. The superior surface of the prostate is analogous to its median lobe. Its inferior border is marked by a sulcus that defines the border between the right and left lateral lobes.

The prostate also can be divided into zones (FIG. 14-11). This classification is based on examination of prostate tissue in different planes and on histologic and embryonic characteristics. There are the central zone, peripheral zone, transitional zone, and anterior fibromuscular zone. Each of the zones has distinct histologic and embryonic characteristics, and each is prone to different pathologic changes with aging. The transitional zone and peripheral zone originate from the urogenital sinus, and they experience adenomas as the man ages. Frequently, these changes cause voiding dysfunction and obstruction, the cardinal symptoms of benign prostatic hyperplasia. The peripheral zone is also the site of malignant tumors (prostatic carcinoma), although the transitional zone is not the site of carcinoma. In contrast, the central zone of the prostate is morphologically and embryonically distinct from the peripheral and transitional zones. It is probably mesogenic in origin; and its primary function is thought to be occlusion of the urethral lumen during seminal emission, thereby preventing retrograde ejaculation into the bladder.[173] Although the concept of zonal anatomy of the prostate is not new,[79] ultrasonic examination of the prostate allows identification of the peripheral and transitional zones and the fibromuscular capsule in the clinical setting.

Primarily based on digital rectal examination, clinicians have divided the prostate into lobes.[79] Intraurethral lobes, right and left lateral, anterior, and subcervical lobes have been described. Posterior and median extraurethral lobes also have been described. Enlargement of the right and left lateral prostate lobes produces the symptoms of benign prostatic hyperplasia. In contrast, the presence of asymmetric enlargement, induration or discrete nodules on the posterior lobe is highly suspicious of prostatic carcinoma. While the division of the prostate into lobes may be clinically useful when describing the findings of digital rectal examination, this classification is not based on anatomically or histologically distinct segments of the gland.[173]

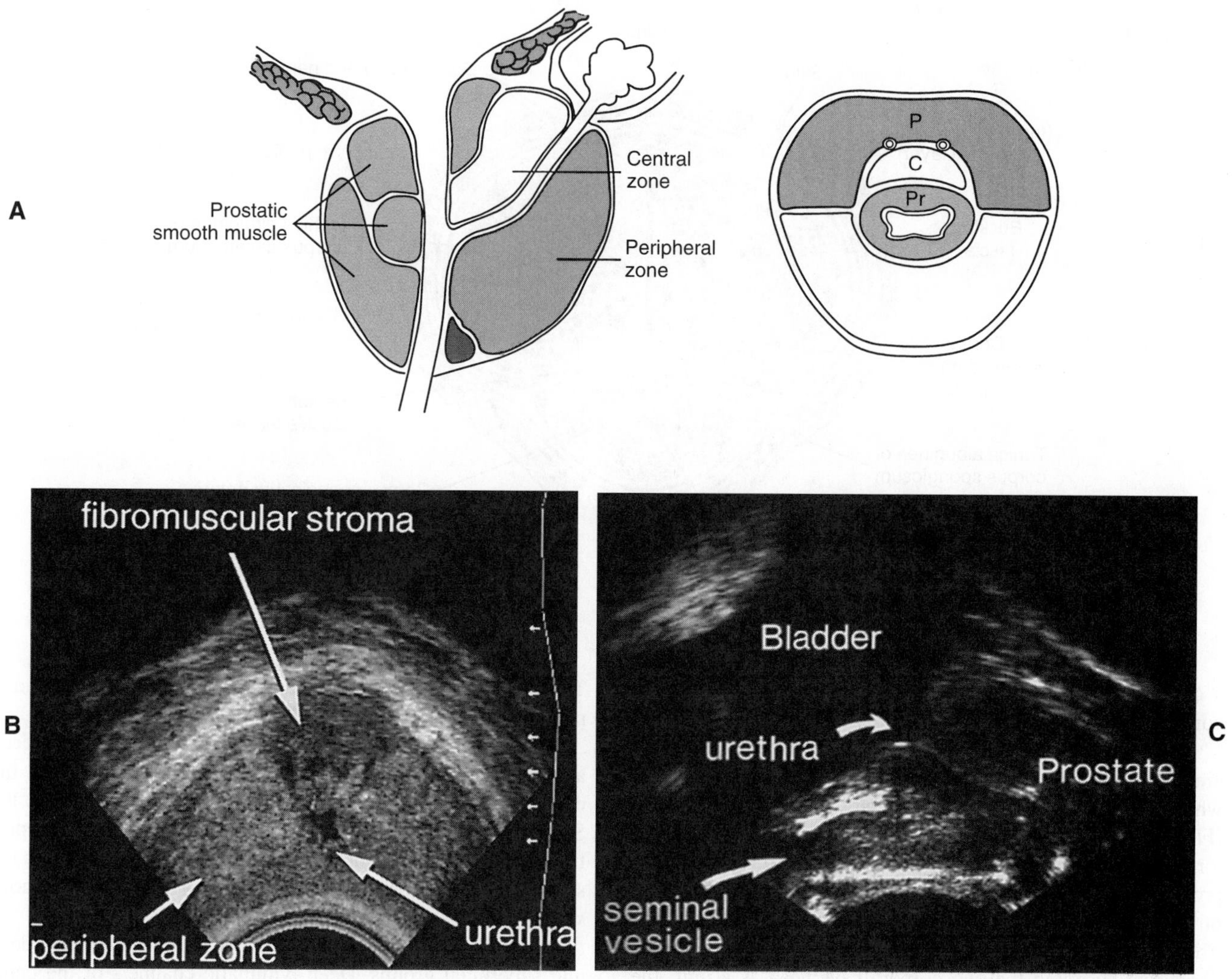

FIG. 14-11

A, Zonal anatomy of the prostate gland. B, Ultrasonic image of a normal prostate in the transverse plane; the peripheral zone and fibromuscular stroma are indicated. C, Ultrasonic image of normal prostate in the longitudinal plane. Note the anatomic relations among the bladder, proximal urethra, prostate, and seminal vesicles.

The microscopic anatomy of the prostate is characterized by glandular components and fibromuscular components. The fibromuscular capsule sends extensions into the interior of the organ, whose apices converge in the posterior urethral surface. The fibromuscular tissue is primarily nonstriated muscle with a relatively small area of skeletal muscle located ventral to and contiguous with the external urinary sphincter. The bulk of muscular tissue is located in the fibromuscular septa found throughout the gland.[178]

The glandular tissue is composed of numerous follicles with frequent papillary elevations that open into long canals seen throughout the organ. These follicles join to form 12 to 20 excretory ducts. The glandular tissue of the prostate is supported by extensions of muscular tissue and delicate areolar stroma that encapsulate a capillary plexus.

The motor and sensory innervation of the prostate gland arises from the lower segments of the inferior hypogastric plexus and the pelvic plexus. The tone of the bladder neck and prostatic smooth muscle is primarily controlled by alpha-1 receptors, which are 40 times more abundant in this area compared with other aspects of the bladder.[106] These adrenergic receptors have been subdivided into alpha-1A, alpha-1B, and alpha-1C subtypes (which are predominant in the prostatic smooth muscle).[165] These subdivisions have potential clinical significance in the search to identify a medication that selectively inhibits prostatic smooth and bladder neck tone without producing side effects of postural hypotension and nasal congestion characteristic of current alpha-blocking medications.

The arterial blood supply of the prostate is derived primarily from branches of the inferior vesical artery, as well as from the internal pudendal and middle rectal arteries. Venous blood from the prostate drains into the periprostatic space and the hypogastric vein. Lymphatic drainage exits from the periprostatic plexus located on the surface of the gland before emptying into the external, internal, and/or common iliac nodes.[55]

Penis. The penis is a cylindrically shaped organ in its flaccid state that contains two portions: a root that attaches to the perineum and a pendulous portion called the corpus, or body. The root of the penis is attached to the pelvic floor via

FIG. 14-12
Cross section of human penis.

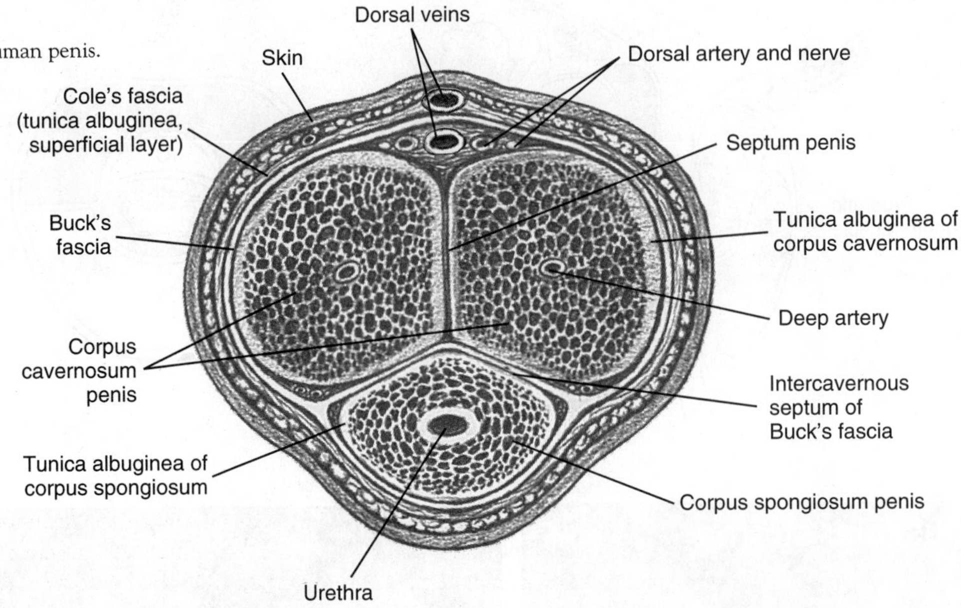

a continuation of Buck's fascia, the pubic rami (crura of the corpora cavernosa), and the suspensory ligament.[55,173]

The body of the penis contains three elongated bodies of erectile tissue that are capable of considerable enlargement when they become engorged with blood during tumescence (FIG. 14-12). The left and right corpora cavernosa form the majority of the substance of the penile body and lie in close approximation to each other. They are surrounded by an extension of the tunica albuginea containing superficial and deep layers. The superficial layer is composed of longitudinally arranged fibers that surround the two corpora cavernosa as a unit; the deep layer is composed of circularly arranged fibers that encase each corpus separately via a fibrous septum that forms two median grooves of anatomic significance. The median groove houses the corpus spongiosum and pendulous urethra; the smaller median groove houses the deep dorsal veins. The corpora cavernosa do not reach the distal end of the penis; instead, they terminate in the proximal portion of the glans.

The corpus spongiosum lies inferior to the corpora cavernosa and is pierced throughout its length by the urethra. It is smaller than the paired corpora cavernosa and is surrounded by a reflection of the tunica albuginea.[178]

The skin of the penis is characterized by its thinness, relatively dark color, and loose connection with the underlying fascia. At the distal portion of the penis, the skin is folded over on itself to form the foreskin covering the glans penis. The glans penis covers the distal portion of the corpora cavernosa and forms their terminal connection. It is pierced by the navicularis fossa of the urethra, which ends at a dorsal slit found on the interior surface of the glans.[178]

The superficial fascia of the penis is characterized by loose areolar tissue and is devoid of fat. A few fibers of dartos muscle from the scrotum are present, as are fibers from the fundiform ligament and the suspensory ligament.[178]

The arterial blood supply of the penis arises primarily from the internal pudendal artery, which branches into the dorsal arteries of the penis to supply the deep structures of the organ. The penile skin also receives arterial blood from the external pudendal and femoral arteries.[55,173]

The venous drainage of the penis can be divided into deep and superficial groups. The deep veins of the penis drain the erectile bodies via the deep dorsal veins, which empty into the Santorini's and ultimately into the hypogastric vein. The superficial veins of the penis drain venous blood from the skin via the superficial dorsal penile veins that empty into the saphenous vein.[55,173]

The lymphatic drainage of the penis is also divided into deep and superficial groups. Deep lymphatic channels of the penis are drained by the subinguinal nodes and the external iliac nodes. Superficial lymphatic channels drain into the superficial inguinal nodes.[55,173]

The nerve supply of the penis has a somatic and an autonomic component. Sensory innervation of the penile skin arises from the pudendal nerve, which has it roots in spinal segments S2 to S4. Motor innervation to the corpus spongiosum and corpora cavernosa arises from the pelvic nerves, which also have their spinal roots at S2 to S4. Sympathetic fibers from the thoracolumbar spinal cord supply the penile vessels and are particularly evident in the vascular component of the corpus spongiosum.[79]

Male Reproductive Function

Spermatogenesis and Hormonal Regulation. The testes, epididymis, vas deferens, seminal vesicles, and prostate gland function as a coordinated unit to ensure the production, maturation, and transport of sperm from the male urethra to the female vaginal tract, which is necessary for propagation of the species. Male reproductive functions are regulated by a hormonal axis that consists of certain extrahypothalamic central nervous system centers, the hypothalamus, pituitary, testes, and gonadal-sensitive end organs.[84,173]

Extrahypothalamic central nervous system centers are assumed to play an inhibitory and augmentative role in reproduction. The precise interactions by which brain centers influence the male reproductive hormonal axis are unclear, but a correlation between reproductive function and testicular function is postulated.[173]

The more clearly elucidated hormonal axis governing male reproductive function originates in the hypothalamus, where a luteinizing hormone-releasing hormone (LH-RH) is produced and travels to the median eminence of the adenohypophysis via a venous portal system. The presence of this releasing factor in the pituitary results in the direct stimulation of luteinizing hormone (LH) and is thought to stimulate the release of follicle-stimulating hormone (FSH).[55,173]

Both FSH and LH act at receptor sites in the testes to stimulate the gonadal and androgens (primarily testosterone and dihydrotestosterone). LH directly stimulates Sertoli's cells to produce testosterone and stimulate spermatogenesis. FSH is not necessary for the production of testosterone, although it does play a role in spermatogenic testicular function. FSH and LH are released sporadically in response to feedback from the hypothalamic-pituitary-gonadal hormonal axis. When blood levels of the gonadal androgens increase, the production of LH-RH in the hypothalamus is inhibited, which suppresses the production of LH by the pituitary. Conversely, decreased serum levels of gonadal androgens stimulate the hypothalamus to produce LH-RH so that more LH is produced and excreted into the systemic circulation. The feedback loop for FSH production is not entirely understood; increased levels of testosterone and estradiol exert negative feedback on the production of FSH. In addition, a substance called inhibin, which is produced in the germinal epithelium of the testes, is postulated to inhibit FSH, although its physiologic significance is unclear.[33,84]

The gonadal androgens are essential to the genesis, support, and maturation of spermatozoa. In addition to this direct role in male reproductive function, certain androgens, primarily testosterone and dihydrotestosterone, cause the development and maintenance of the secondary male sex characteristics that characterize pubescence.[33,109]

The process of spermatogenesis occurs within the seminiferous tubule in the testis and is conceptualized in three phases. During the first phase the more primitive spermatogonia enlarge and undergo mitotic divisions into primary spermatocytes that contain 92 chromosomes. The second phase is characterized by two consecutive meiotic divisions accompanied by only one duplication of chromosomes so that the final product of this phase is four spermatids that contain a haploid number of chromosomes suitable for union with the ovum. The third phase of spermatogenesis-spermiogenesis marks the transformation of spermatid to spermatozoon.[114]

The process of spermiogenesis is relatively slow; it requires 74 days to complete and is divided into four phases. The first phase is the Golgi phase, when small granules of hyaluronidase, proteases, and other substances form a single large acrosomal granule enclosed within a vesicle that attaches to the nuclear membrane at the site of the future sperm head. During the second phase a cap appears around the acrosomal vesicle. The two centrioles of the spermatid now begin to move; the proximal centriole assumes a position at the posterior pole of the nucleus opposite the acrosomal sac, and the distal centriole sprouts a flagellum consisting of two central microtubules and nine surrounding pairs of microtubules. The distal centriole will become the tail of the future spermatozoon. The third stage of spermiogenesis is the acrosomal phase, in which the developing sperm cell undergoes extensive metamorphosis so that the acrosome, nucleus, flagellum, and cytoplasm assume the characteristic appearance of the mature spermatozoon. During the acrosomal phase a mitochondrial sheath is formed to supply energy for the tail of the mature sperm when it becomes motile after ejaculation. The final stage of spermiogenesis is the maturation phase, which is characterized by the completion of the tail of the spermatozoon and the shedding of excess cytoplasm with the assistance of Sertoli's cells (FIG. 14-13).[68,114]

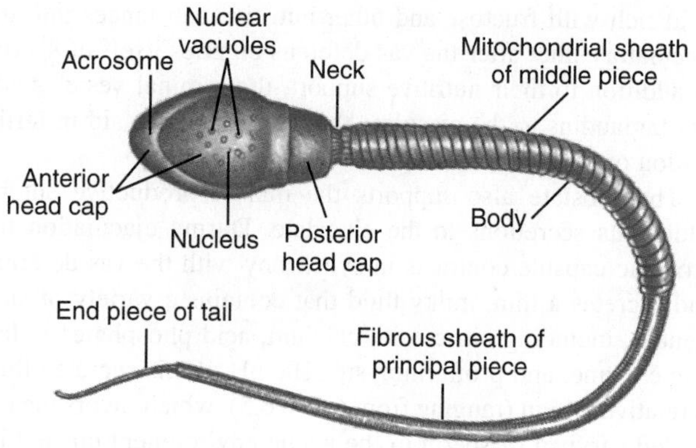

FIG. 14-13
Mature spermatozoon cell.

Transport of the sperm from the seminiferous tubule occurs via the muscular activity of the tubules and fluid movement. Although the sperm that enter the epididymis are mature in appearance, they are not yet capable of motility and not yet able to fertilize an ovum. Thus the epididymis also plays a necessary role in the maturation of sperm. The transit time of sperm through the relatively short epididymis is 12 days. The structure of the epididymis allows slow transit resulting from the slow peristaltic-like activity of the smooth muscle of the organ and the ciliary action of the efferent ductules. During the time spent within the epididymis, sperm gain the potential for motility, although a substance in the tubular fluid prevents sperm from becoming motile before ejaculation. Although the process by which this maturation occurs is not known, the epididymis is thought to play an active role under the influence of the gonadal androgens (primarily testosterone). The probable maturational functions provided by the epididymis are manipulation of the sodium ion, potassium ion, and chloride ion concentrations in the fluid in the epididymal tubule and the secretion of a variety of compounds such as glycerylphosphorylchlorine and glycoproteins, which are thought to enhance maturation of the spermatozoa.[173]

The epididymis also serves as a storage compartment for sperm. The cauda epididymidis may store sperm for a period of several weeks, although the storage time in a man who is extremely sexually active is a matter of hours.[55,173]

After exiting the epididymis the sperm enters the vas deferens in response to smooth muscle contraction associated with ejaculation. Sperm is carried into the ejaculatory ducts, where it is mixed with the nutritive secretions of the seminal vesicles. The seminal vesicles do not, as their name implies, serve as storage compartments for sperm; rather, they secrete a mucoid fluid rich with fructose and other nutritive substances into the ejaculatory duct after the vas deferens empties itself of sperm. In addition to their nutritive support, the seminal vesicles add prostaglandins to the ejaculate that are thought to aid in fertilization of the ovum.[68]

The prostate also supports the male reproductive act by adding its secretions to the ejaculate. During ejaculation the prostatic capsule contracts in synchrony with the vas deferens and secretes a thin, milky fluid that contains a variety of substances, including citric acid, calcium, acid phosphate, a clotting enzyme, and profibrinolysin. The pH of this secreted fluid is relatively high (ranging from 6.0 to 6.5), which favors the extended survival of sperm in the acidic environment created by the vaginal mucosa.[68]

The ejaculated semen thus contains fluid from the vas deferens, the seminal vesicles, and the prostate gland and mucus from the posterior urethral glands, particularly the bulbourethral gland. The pH of the semen is approximately 7.5; the prostatic secretions give the semen a milky appearance, and the seminal vesicle fluid contributes the characteristic mucoid appearance. The normal ejaculate contains 75 million to 400 million sperm cells. After ejaculation a clotting enzyme in the semen interacts with profibrinolysin contributed by the prostate to form a weak coagulum. When this dissolves, the sperm gain their maximal motility as each seeks to fertilize an ovum. Although the sperm cell can survive several months in the male genital ducts, it can survive only 12 to 24 hours in the female genital tract after ejaculation. The relatively short life of sperm in the female genital tract is primarily the result of the acidic nature of the vaginal and fallopian mucosa.[68]

Physiology of Penile Erections. Advances in knowledge concerning central and local neurotransmitters have significantly advanced our knowledge of erectile physiology. These advances have contributed to at least one oral agent available at the time of this writing, and two additional drugs are completing Phase 3 clinical trials to determine their role in the management of erectile dysfunction (impotence).

During the flaccid state, the smooth muscle of local arterioles and the corpora cavernosa maintain baseline tone under the influence of the sympathetic nervous system.[111] This tone provides ample blood flow for the nutritional needs of local tissues, but it is insufficient for penile tumescence of rigidity. Tactile, psychologic, or other stimuli trigger the release of neurotransmitters from nerve receptors within the corpora cavernosa, causing relaxation of the smooth muscle within local arterioles and the sinusoidal spaces of the corporal bodies. As a result, arterial blood flow increases, which fills the sinusoids and causes an increase in penile length and circumference. During this initial stage, tumescence occurs as the penis increases its length and circumference. Ultimately, sinusoidal filling is limited by compression of the subtunical venous plexuses between the tunica albuginea and peripheral sinusoids, as well as compression of the emissary veins. At this point, the penis achieves rigidity and intracavernous pressure reaches approximately 100 mm Hg as the erectile tissue fills the limited space allowed by its fascial coverings. Intracavernous pressure may rise to suprasystolic levels (as high as 200 mm Hg) with contraction of the ischiocavernous muscle, although this rigid erection state is transient and subsides as the muscle relaxes.

Detumescence (return to the flaccid state) occurs in three phases. In this first phase, a brief rise in intracavernosal pressure occurs with smooth muscle contraction against the closed venous system. This is followed by a longer, second phase characterized by a slow decline in intracavernosal pressure as the venous channels open and arterial blood flow returns to baseline values. At some point, venous outflow reaches its baseline state, and intracavernosal pressure falls to preerection values rapidly.

These local events are regulated by local neurotransmitters, acting under the influence of neurons in the central and peripheral nervous systems.[26] In the human, sympathetic, parasympathetic, and somatic nerves modulate penile erections. Sympathetic innervation of the corpora cavernosa arises from neural roots extending from T10 to L2. These fibers reach the penis via the superior hypogastric, inferior mesenteric, and splanchnic nerve plexuses. Parasympathetic innervation arises from sacral spinal segments 2, 3, and 4; their axons reach the penis via the pelvic plexus.

Afferent somatic pathways originate from sensory nerves in the penile skin, glans penis, urethra, and corpora cavernosum. They are carried toward the spine via the dorsal nerve, which merges with others into the pudendal nerves. The pudendal nerve enters the spine at Onuf's nucleus, found at sacral segments 2 to 4. In addition to somatic sensations (touch, temperature, pain), the dorsal nerve also carries autonomic impulses to and from the central nervous system, accounting for its modulatory role in both penile erection and ejaculation.

Similar to the bladder, erectile function is modulated by specific areas of the brain.[26,111] In the human, the medial preoptic area and the paraventricular nuclei of the hypothalamus probably act as the primary integrative centers for sexual drive and penile erection. The precise role of other areas in the brain known to influence penile erections, including the amygdala, the hippocampus, and the brainstem, are not yet understood.

Several central and peripheral neurotransmitters are important to erectile function. In the brain and brainstem, dopaminergic and adrenergic receptors promote sexual drive, and serotonergic receptors inhibit erectile activity. Within the peripheral nervous system, norepinephrine increases smooth muscle tone in the sinusoidal spaces of the corporal bodies and local arterioles, promoting detumescence and maintenance of the flaccid state. Endothelin, a potent vasoconstrictor produced by the endothelial cells of the corpora cavernosa, also promotes detumescence. Acetylcholine is released from parasympathetic (muscarinic) receptors in the corporal bodies and local arteries. However, it is not the primary neurotransmitter responsible for initiating or maintaining an erection. Instead, it acts as a secondary substance; its primary role is stimulation of the release of nitric oxide from endothelial cells. It is the release of nitric oxide from NANC receptors that increases the production of cyclic guanosine monophosphate (cGMP), which is primarily responsible for the smooth muscle relaxation essential for penile erection.

Other substances play a modulatory role in erectile activity. Testosterone was once believed essential for penile erection. It is essential to the growth and development of a normal male reproductive system, and it plays an important role in libido. However, it is not essential for the generation of an erection in an adult male with mature sexual organs.

Based on this understanding of erectile physiology, it is possible to describe three types of erections.[111] Psychogenic erections occur when sexually provocative stimuli are integrated into erectile activity as modulated by the medial preoptic area (MPOA) and the paraventricular nuclei of the hypothalamus. Activation of these areas leads to inhibition of sympathetic tone and activation of the smooth muscle relaxation under the indirect influence of acetylcholine and the direct influence of nitric oxide and GMP. Psychogenic erections are independent of testosterone, although this androgenic hormone enhances libido and subsequent sexual drive. In contrast, a reflexogenic erection is caused by tactile stimulation of the genitalia sending afferent signals to the brainstem and brain and directly activating autonomic nuclei within the spine to initiate the cascade of events leading to an erection. In contrast to the psychogenic erection, these erections are partly reliant on the presence of testosterone. Nocturnal erections are a distinctive third type; they occur during rapid eye movement (REM) sleep, but the precise mechanisms that account for their occurrence are not entirely understood.

NORMAL FINDINGS*

Kidney: Overlying skin: edema, bulges, and masses in abdomen absent; palpable only with deep inspiration; typically nonpalpable in obese or muscularly developed persons; smooth, nontender; costovertebral angle tenderness: absent; bruit over costovertebral area or upper abdominal quadrants: absent; transillumination with darkened room and fiberoptic light source: absent

Bladder: Noted as bulge in abdomen when vesicle contains 500 ml or more urine; noted as dull area under suprapubic skin when vesicle is filled with 150 ml or more urine; inspection of voiding act: steady, straight stream, no spraying, no abdominal straining; postvoid dribble absent; postvoid residual: less than 20% of total bladder volume; ✪ decreased force of stream compared with younger adult years; absent split stream, spraying, and postvoid dribble

Penis: Skin: may be darker than surrounding integument; ulcers, warts, indurated nodules: absent; foreskin: retractable over glans penis; absent in circumcised males; glans penis: hairless, sagittal slit near apex; penile shaft: absent nontender plaques beneath surface in flaccid state; erect state: even firmness and rigidity over both corpora cavernosa; straight line described between root of penis and glans penis; ✪ decreased rigidity to corpora cavernosa compared with younger adult years; lateral curvature: absent

Scrotum: Skin: rugae; hair bearing and loosely mobile; sebaceous cysts: absent; testes: firm, nontender to gentle palpation; masses: absent; ✪ testes softer to palpation than in younger adult years; epididymis: palpable as comma-shaped structure on posterior aspect of testes; no tenderness, masses, or nodules; spermatic cord: rolled between thumb and forefinger; vas deferens palpable but nontender; varicocele: absent; transillumination: no edema or solid masses that will transilluminate

Prostate: Posterior aspect of organ accessible beneath anterior rectal wall; two firm, nontender, symmetric, rounded lobes separated by median sulcus (heart shaped and 2.5 cm long): projects into rectal lumen 1 cm or less; hard, irregular nodes: absent; ✪ increased bogginess noted on digital examination; seen with benign hypertrophy of organ; asymmetric changes in lobe size or discrete nodules: absent

*✪ = Older adult.

CONDITIONS, DISEASES, AND DISORDERS

URINARY TRACT DISORDERS

CYSTITIS

Cystitis is an inflammation of the bladder wall. Many causative agents, including bacteria, viruses, fungi, chemical agents, and radiation exposure, may result in cystitis. The term is often used synonymously with urinary tract infection (UTI), although they are not strictly identical. Urinary tract infection is a nonspecific term that may be used to refer to infection anywhere in the urinary tract. Urethritis refers to inflammation of the urethra (see Chapters 15 and 16). Pyelonephritis refers to infection of the kidney and renal pelvis (see Chapter 13). Within the context of this discussion, cystitis is used in preference to the more vaguely defined concept of urinary tract infection.

The occurrence of infection in the urinary tract is second only to respiratory tract infections. Infection of the urinary bladder is the most common focus of inflammation in the urinary tract. Women are particularly prone to symptomatic bacteriuria resulting in cystitis. A study of Jamaican women revealed that 2% of those between 15 and 24 years of age had bacteriuria on culture. Stamey[161] found that the prevalence of bacterial cystitis in women increased approximately 1% to 2% during each subsequent decade of life until reaching 10% among 54- to 64-year-old women. Gaymans et al[51] corroborated these findings in a prospective study of 1758 Dutch women that revealed a 2.7% prevalence of bacteriuria among those 15 to 24 years of age and 9.3% among those 65 years of age and older. Among the general population, a woman can expect a 10% to 20% chance of having at least one episode of cystitis during her lifetime.[161]

Pregnant women and hospitalized women have an increased incidence of urinary tract infection. Among pregnant women the rate of cystitis is approximately 4% to 6%; studies have demonstrated an incidence of urinary tract infection as high as 30% among hospitalized women.[161]

In addition to a greater susceptibility to bacterial cystitis, women are more likely to have interstitial cystitis than are men. A study in Finland found that the prevalence of interstitial cystitis was 10.6:100,000 with a 10:1 preference of the disease for women.[71] Leach[103] and Raz[141] also report an incidence of 20:100,000 cases of interstitial cystitis among women, with a ratio of 10 cases in women for every case reported among men.

The incidence of cystitis among men has not been extensively studied but is generally thought to occur in only 10% as many men as women. Unlike in women, most cases of bacteriuria in men occur as a result of some known infectious focus such as bacterial prostatitis or urinary calculi.

Clearly, the most significant rate of cystitis, resulting in an alarming incidence of associated morbidity and mortality, is that associated with nosocomial urinary tract infection in the presence of an indwelling catheter. In a prospective study of 1458 patients in the United States, 131 patients acquired 136 urinary tract infections during 1474 indwelling bladder catheterizations. Among those studied, 12 deaths may have been caused by acquired urinary tract infections, and another 10 patients died with a retrospective clinical picture compatible with serious infection, although no conclusive culture data were available. Thus the authors concluded that acquisition of a nosocomial urinary tract infection was associated with a threefold increase in death rate (see Emergency Alert box).[139]

EMERGENCY ALERT

SEPTIC SHOCK

Septic shock is classified as a vasogenic shock in which severe vasodilation occurs. Commonly, septic shock results from overwhelming infection. Typically, blood volume is normal but fluids have shifted into dilated vessels. Mortality ranges from 30% to 50%.

ASSESSMENT

- Evaluate for decreased blood pressure, elevated pulse, and temperature.
- Evaluate for chills, tremors with warm, dry skin.
- Evaluate for nausea, vomiting, diarrhea.
- Evaluate decreased level of consciousness.
- Evaluate increased cardiac output, metabolic acidosis.

INTERVENTIONS

- Maintain airway, breathing, and circulation.
- Administer high-flow oxygen (10-15 L) by mask.
- Obtain intravenous (IV) access.
- In collaboration with physician, administer antibiotics and fluids.
- Collect laboratory specimens, including blood and fluid cultures.
- Administer dopamine or corticosteroids as ordered.

PATHOPHYSIOLOGY

The pathogenesis of cystitis depends on the causative agent. In this discussion cystitis is divided into three categories:

- Infectious cystitis
  - Bacterial
  - Viral
  - Fungal
  - Tubercular
  - Parasitic
- Chemotherapy- and radiation-induced cystitis
- Inflammatory lesions of the bladder
  - Cystitis cystica
  - Cystitis glandularis
  - Eosinophilic cystitis
  - Cystitis emphysematosa
  - Interstitial cystitis

Bacterial cystitis is the most common form of infectious cystitis. The most common causative pathogen in both women and men is *Escherichia coli.* Other common pathogens include strains of *Klebsiella, Enterobacter, Proteus, Pseudomonas,* and *Serratia;* gram-positive organisms such as staphylococci and streptococci are occasionally seen.[173]

The three routes of bacterial invasion into the bladder are ascension through the urethra, the hematogenous route, and via lymphatic channels; the most common is the ascending urethral pathway. Bacteria are commonly forced into the bladder without necessarily resulting in infection. The determinants of bacterial cystitis depend on the virulence and inoculum size of invasive bacteria and the adequacy of the host's defense mechanisms. Data concerning the number of bacteria needed to produce a bladder infection are based solely on animal studies, which show that an extremely large inoculum (over 1 million) is needed to produce cystitis if host defense mechanisms are not compromised. Fortunately, normal numbers of bacteria that enter the bladder through the urethra are considerably smaller (fewer than 100).[90]

The human body has two primary defense mechanisms that oppose the establishment of infection when bacteria enter the bladder. The first is the urine itself, which is bacteriostatic or bactericidal to the most common pathogens associated with cystitis, such as *E. coli* and a number of other anaerobic bacteria commonly found in urethral flora. The efficiency of this antibacterial activity depends on the size of the bacterial inoculum, the osmolality of the urine, and the concentration of urea nitrogen and ammonium in the urine. A urinary pH of 6.0 or greater adversely affects antibacterial activity, but the presence of specific antibodies in the urine such as IgA and IgG has not been shown to cause significant effects.[90]

The bladder wall is the second line of defense for bacterial invasion from the urethra, bloodstream, or lymphatic route. Inflammatory changes within the bladder wall are apparent within 30 minutes of invasion when polymorphonucleocytes (PMNs) begin to migrate to the bladder mucosa. Within 2 hours the entire mucosal lining is injected by PMNs, and significant antibacterial activity is measurable by the fourth hour. Inspection at 24 hours reveals clumps of PMNs throughout the mucosal lining, and urine culture is negative.[90]

Perhaps the most important defense against bacterial cystitis is the unobstructed flow of urine throughout the urinary tract and regular, complete evacuation of the bladder. This important concept is the basis of the rationale for clean intermittent catheterization. Regular emptying of the bladder flushes bacteria that would ultimately colonize the urine if allowed to remain within the bladder.[90]

Abnormalities that interfere with natural host defenses against urinary tract infection include the presence of residual urine, which provides an opportunity for bacteria to reproduce and overwhelm other inherent antibacterial mechanisms. Vesicoureteral reflux also compromises the body's defense mechanisms by allowing the spread of bacteria from the urine into the upper tracts and possibly into the renal parenchyma. Urinary calculi are often obstructive to urinary outflow and serve as a nidus for infection during antibiotic therapy. In addition, any disease or circumstance that interferes with the body's immune system decreases the efficiency of the bladder wall's reaction to bacteriuria.[90]

Women are particularly susceptible to bacterial cystitis for a number of reasons. Stamey[161] studied the problem of bacterial cystitis in women and concluded that much of the nomenclature used to describe the condition does not adequately define this condition. He described four bacteriurial states in women: first infection, unresolved bacteriuria during therapy, bacterial persistence, and reinfection (recurrence).

The etiology of first infection is unclear but is presumed to be similar to reinfections. Unlike recurrent episodes of cystitis, bacteria from the first infection are typically sensitive to any antibiotic and are unlikely to recur within 2 to 3 years unless other predisposing factors are present.[173]

Unresolved bacteriuria during therapy may arise from several causes. The bacteria may be resistant to the antibiotic chosen for therapy, or selection of a secondary strain may become predominant as the primary form of bacteria is eliminated. In approximately 6% of patients treated, resistant, mutant bacteria develop and proliferate. Renal insufficiency may cause inadequate concentrations of antibiotic in the urinary tract, although the correct agent has been chosen. A staghorn calculus may be large enough to support a critical mass of bacteria too great for antibiotics to resolve.[173]

True bacterial persistence may arise after 5 to 10 days of therapy, resulting in culture-proven nonsterile urine from one of two causes. Men with chronic bacterial prostatitis have a persistent focus for ascending urethral infection from the prostatic ductal system. Women or men with struvite stones in the urinary tract have a site of persistent bacteria even after antibiotic therapy.[173]

Reinfection of the bladder accounts for the majority of occurrences of bacterial cystitis among women. The most common route for bacteria to gain access to the bladder is from the urethra. The colonization of the urethra arises from the vaginal introitus and vestibule rather than from the rectum, as is commonly assumed. Longitudinal studies show that cultures of the vaginal vestibule and distal urethral mucosa are more predictive of recurrent bacterial cystitis than analysis of rectal flora. Ascending infection in the female is particularly problematic because of the relatively short, straight course of the urethra and plentiful flora in the genital area. The relationship between vaginal flora and urethral bacteria is further supported by examining the close anatomic relationship of these two structures, which are confined by the distal labia minora.[161]

The role of sexual intercourse in recurrent urinary infections has been studied repeatedly. Sexual intercourse is associated with an increased incidence of recurrent urinary tract infections, and some women specifically correlate intercourse and recurrence. It is interesting to note that nuns have a 0.4% to 1.6% incidence of urinary tract infection, which is lower than the general population, and that married women have a higher incidence than single women. Although sexual intercourse does not cause bacterial cystitis, it does promote the milking of bacteria into the bladder and can cause inner urethral injury that may result in infection among women predisposed to the condition.[161]

Changes in the urinary tract unique to pregnancy also increase a woman's likelihood for having recurring urinary tract infections or experiencing a first infection of the bladder. The primary urologic change noted with pregnancy is the "physiologic hydroureter of pregnancy," which is the reversible dilation of the ureters and renal pelvis. This dilation often begins as early as the seventh week of gestation and progresses until delivery. The right ureter is more extensively affected than the left, and ureteral peristalsis is significantly slowed after the second month of gestation so that intraureteral volume may be as great as 25 times normal.[9]

Bacteriuria is more common among pregnant women than in nonpregnant women in the same age group. The presence of ureteral dilation may play a role in this increased incidence. It is known that pregnant women with bacteriuria are at a significantly increased risk (20% to 40%) for developing pyelonephritis and that this risk is dramatically reduced by treating the bladder infection. In addition, catheterization during pregnancy is associated with increased risk of subsequent bacterial cystitis. Although the association between premature delivery and pyelonephritis is well documented, no correlation exists between bacteriuria and premature delivery.[9]

Bacterial cystitis is likely to result in urinary frequency, urgency, and dysuria. Women in particular may complain of suprapubic discomfort and a feeling of pressure in the perineal area. Nocturia and low back pain are also caused by bladder infection. Urge incontinence may take the form of detrusor instability with subsequent painful bladder "spasms" and associated leakage, or it may occur as urethral instability allowing urine passage into the posterior urethra and causing a perception of intense urgency and urinary leakage. Gross hematuria, chills, fever, and flank pain occur only occasionally in the presence of cystitis unless it is also associated with pyelonephritis. Approximately half of patients with significant bacteriuria are asymptomatic. Women with dysuria and frequency who have no bacteriuria or a colony count of fewer than 10,000/ml are typically diagnosed as having an "acute urethral syndrome."[161]

Cystitis caused by fungal infection is much less prevalent than bacterial cystitis, but its incidence and recognition have greatly increased within the past 25 years. The most common fungal infection of the bladder is candidiasis. *Candida* is endemic to the human body and can often be found in the pharynx, stomach, intestinal tract, and vaginal vault (particularly in pregnant women). The increasing incidence of candidal overgrowth is related to the use of antibiotics. Administration of antibiotics is thought to stimulate the production of *Candida albicans* by altering the pH of gastrointestinal mucosa, suppressing normal bacterial flora that competes with the fungus for food, and inhibiting polymorphonuclear phagocytosis, which helps the body guard against overgrowth.

The body's defenses against candidal infection of the urinary tract include the presence of normal bacterial flora that inhibits fungal growth and the presence of PMNs in the mucosa of the urethra and bladder, which have marked anticandidal effects. In addition, prostatic fluid in the male is fungicidal, which helps explain the relatively low incidence of candidal cystitis in males compared with females. Cell-mediated immunity and other white blood cells also help the body prevent candidiasis.[173]

Candidal cystitis often occurs in the presence of predisposing factors such as diabetes mellitus, obstructive prostatic enlargement, and pregnancy and is often noted after the patient has undergone antibiotic therapy for bacterial infection. Symptoms are similar to those of bacterial cystitis and include urgency, marked frequency, dysuria, suprapubic pain, and nocturia. Pneumaturia (the expression of gas or air through the urethra during or after micturition) may be seen. The mucosal lining of the bladder is marked by grayish white spots that result in mucosal bleeding if removed. The ureteral orifices may be affected so that cystoscopic findings may resemble tubercular infection of the bladder. In certain cases asymptomatic candidal colonization of the urine without inflammation of the bladder may be seen.[173]

Tuberculosis of the bladder results from the implantation of the tubercle bacilli into the wall, causing an uneven mix of inflamed areas interspersed with normal mucosal segments. The cystoscopic picture of the bladder may resemble interstitial cystitis or candidal infection with patches of inflamed tissue and reddened ureteral orifices. The anterior urethra is not affected by the infection, but the posterior urethra and prostate are heavily involved in men, representing progression from prostate to bladder. The trigone is relatively spared from inflammatory changes, but the dome of the bladder is extensively affected, resulting in a marked loss in capacity.[173]

The primary symptom of tubercular cystitis is marked frequency and urgency. Bladder volume rapidly decreases and may result in irreversible changes in advanced stages of the infection.[173] Urodynamic assessment in advanced cases may reveal poor compliance of the bladder wall and a functional capacity of 60 ml of urine or less.

Although schistosomiasis is relatively rare in the United States, it is relatively common elsewhere in the world. The ova of this parasite enter the bloodstream via penetration of the skin. The veins of the bladder are a popular breeding site for the parasites. The eggs are then extruded into the vesicle for further spread of the parasitic organisms. The healing of the affected areas of the bladder causes thickening and contraction of the bladder wall. Damage of the ureterovesical junction often occurs, resulting in vesicoureteral reflux. Contracted bands mar the bladder and may extend into the lower ureter. Urinary calculi may be present because of urinary stasis and presence of ova in the urine.[143]

Chemotherapy- or radiation-induced cystitis is characterized by inflammatory changes in the bladder wall in the absence of infection. The symptoms are similar to those of infectious cystitis and include urgency, frequency, and suprapubic pain. Detrusor instability and urge incontinence may occur.[78,159]

Although the bladder is relatively resistant to radiation, therapeutic doses greater than 6000 to 7000 rad over a 6- to 7-week period may result in cystitis. The bladder's tolerance to radiation is significantly compromised if schistosomiasis is present. Chemotherapy-induced cystitis may arise from systemic cyclophosphamide (Cytoxan) or intravesical antineoplastic drugs such as mitomycin. Diagnosis is made when symptoms of cystitis are reported in the presence of a normal culture and positive history of exposure to radiation or a chemotherapeutic agent.[78,159]

Cystitis cystica occurs as a result of chronic infection of the bladder or recurrent episodes of cystitis. It is characterized by cysts seen mostly near the base of the bladder and trigone. These cysts are approximately 1 cm in diameter, have a rounded shape, and may extend into the upper urinary tract. The lesions are benign, and the etiology of the condition is unknown. Because of the gross similarities between these lesions and malignancies of the bladder, biopsy is indicated to rule out cancer.[142]

Cystitis glandularis is a relatively rare, potentially premalignant lesion associated with adenocarcinoma of the bladder. This form of cystitis is particularly common among patients with a history of bladder exstrophy and pelvic lipomatosis. Biopsy is done to rule out malignancy, and follow-up examination for potential cancer of the bladder is recommended.[145]

Eosinophilic cystitis is a severe inflammatory lesion of the bladder that is thought to have an allergic etiology. The bladder mucosa is extensively invaded by eosinophils and exhibits multiple polypoid lesions. The associated signs and symptoms of cystitis are particularly severe.[142]

Cystitis emphysematosa is a rare form of bladder inflammation resulting from infection by gas-forming urinary bacteria or (more commonly) vesicoenteric fistula. The condition may also be observed after urologic instrumentation or urodynamic testing using carbon dioxide. Pneumaturia is associated with this form of cystitis.[142]

Diagnostic Studies and Findings

Urine culture and sensitivity: Greater than 100,000 colony-forming units (CFU)/ml bacterial colonies on an agar culture plate or tube indicates clinically significant bacteriuria and associated cystitis; sensitivity disks indicate bacterial sensitivity, intermediate sensitivity, or resistance to a given antibiotic agent; urine culture negative in other forms of infectious cystitis and cystitis caused by chemotherapy and radiotherapy

Urinalysis: Color: dark yellow or pinkish red, cloudy with or without sediment; nitrate/nitrite: positive in bacterial cystitis; glucose oxidase: positive in bacterial infection; catalase: positive in bacterial cystitis; microscopic examination: positive for bacteria, fungus, and parasites in the various forms of infectious cystitis; positive for eosinophils in eosinophilic cystitis; greater than 7 white blood cells (WBCs) per high-power field in infectious cystitis; red blood cells with or without gross hematuria

Cystoscopy: Red, inflamed bladder wall; reddened, swollen trigone; ureteral orifices may be inflamed; hemorrhagic patches in urothelial lining; findings for specific inflammatory lesions of the bladder described under Pathophysiology

Biopsy: Cystitis cystica: negative; cystitis glandularis: negative or positive for adenocarcinoma of bladder; eosinophilic cystitis: extensive infiltration of eosinophils into bladder tissues; interstitial cystitis: chronic inflammation with extensive invasion of lymphocytes and other white blood cells into submucosa of bladder wall

Urodynamics: Infectious cystitis: urodynamic testing typically contraindicated; tubercular cystitis: decreased functional capacity with poor compliance of bladder wall; detrusor unstable or areflexic; sensory urgency present; chemotherapy- or radiation-induced cystitis: sensory urgency with decreased functional capacity; detrusor instability may be present; compliance of bladder wall may be normal or impaired

Voiding cystourethrogram (VCUG): Cystitis emphysematosa: lucent filling defect consistent with gas in vesicle of bladder with or without extravasation of contrast material into vesicoenteric fistula

Multidisciplinary Plan

Surgery

Tubercular cystitis: In cases of advanced tubercular cystitis when bladder contraction is irreversible, augmentation

Table 14-1 Bacterial Pathogens Commonly Encountered in the Urinary Tract and Treatment Options

Pathogen	Commonly Effective Antibiotic Agents*
Escherichia coli	Trimethoprim-sulfamethoxazole, ampillicin, amoxicillin clavulanate (Augmentin), nitrofurantoin, ciprofloxacin
Pseudomonas	Carbenicillin (Geocillin), gentamicin,† ciprofloxacin
Klebsiella	Cephalexin, tetracycline, trimethoprim-sulfamethoxazole, norfloxacin
Proteus mirabilis	Ampicillin, tetracycline, trimethoprim-sulfamethoxazole, amoxicillin clavulanate, nitrofurantoin
Morganella morganii	Trimethoprim-sulfamethoxazole
Serratia	Trimethoprim-sulfamethoxazole, carbenicillin
Group D *Streptococcus*	Ampicillin, nitrofurantoin, amoxicillin clavulanate
Staphylococcus	Cephalexin, tetracycline, trimethoprim-sulfamethoxazole
Staphylococcus saprophyticus	Cephalexin, trimethoprim-sulfamethoxazole, tetracycline

*Antibiotic therapy is guided by individual culture and sensitivity reports.
†Requires parenteral administration.

cystoplasty may be employed after infection is controlled; colocystoplasty (placing an isolated segment of colon onto the bladder dome to enlarge storage capacity) or ileocystoplasty (placing an isolated segment of small bowel on the bladder dome) may be used to restore reasonable bladder storage capacity

Cystitis glandularis: Transurethral resection of lesion done because of its premalignant potential

Medications

Bacterial cystitis

Treatment of choice is oral antibiotic therapy guided by culture and sensitivity data (Table 14-1)

For first-time infections or recurrent infections, short-term therapy with oral antibiotics favored

In more severe cases or when resistant bacteria are identified, parenteral therapy is indicated

For recurrent infections, suppressive antibiotic therapy may be used for 6 months to 24 months; first choice for long-term antibiotic suppression among women with recurrent bacterial cystitis is nitrofurantoin or trimethoprim-sulfamethoxazole

Nitrofurantoin absorbed in upper intestinal tract so that it does not promote mutation of resistant strains of bacteria in intestinal tract; exerts its antibacterial effects on bacteria that have reached bladder

Trimethoprim-sulfamethoxazole will kill pathogens in vaginal vestibule, preventing bacterial invasion of bladder but does alter intestinal flora, which can lead to selection of bacteria resistant to drug

Fungal infections

Two drugs, amphotericin B and 5-fluorocystine, are indicated in cases of nonmucocutaneous infection

Amphotericin B has disadvantages of requiring parenteral administration and significant side effects such as fever, chills, nausea and vomiting, headache, vertigo, and potential nephrotoxicity with prolonged use

5-Fluorocystine may be administered orally and is effective against *Candida;* side effects include bone marrow depression, potential nephrotoxicity, and eosinophilia

Production of resistant strains of fungi is problematic

Tubercular cystitis

Drug therapy must be long term (2 years recommended), and multiple agents are often more effective than any single medication

Combination of isoniazid (INH), ethambutol, rifampin, streptomycin, para-aminosalicylic acid (PAS), cycloserine, or kanamycin is indicated

Parasitic cystitis

Drugs used for schistosomiasis have potentially dangerous side effects and are not approved by the U.S. Food and Drug Administration

Current drug of choice is nitrofurantoin given over a period of 5-7 days

Early treatment essential for prevention of irreversible urinary changes from drug

Cystitis caused by infection, chemotherapy, or radiotherapy

Other chemotherapeutic agents may be used to provide symptomatic relief; anticholinergic agents or antispasmodics such as oxybutynin and propantheline may ameliorate sensory urgency and provide greater functional capacity

Eosinophilic cystitis

Antihistamines and oral steroid agents are indicated

Antibiotic therapy will control related bacteriuria

General Management

Caffeine intake should be restricted because its mild irritative effect exacerbates frequency

Citrus juices should be restricted because their mild irritative effect exacerbates frequency

Citrus juices not effective in lowering urinary pH

Cranberry juice effective in lowering urinary pH only if taken in extremely large quantities

Plentiful fluid intake indicated to encourage movement of pathogens out of urinary tract

NURSING CARE

Nursing Assessment

Suprapubic area: Tender on palpation

Costovertebral angle: No tenderness

Voiding behavior: Frequency, urgency, dysuria, nocturia

Potential Complications

Recurrent infections, potential nephrotoxicity, potential bone marrow depression

Patient Problems/Nursing Diagnoses & Interventions

NIC Elimination Management

Impaired urinary elimination related to dysuria

- Assist patient to attain adequate fluid intake: 30 ml/kg of body weight per day.[131] *Fluids flush urinary system, enhancing removal of pathogens and toxins.*
- Instruct patient to avoid limiting fluid intake in an attempt to reduce urinary frequency. *Limiting fluid intake will concentrate urine, paradoxically increasing rather than alleviating frequency and discomfort.*
- Administer, or teach patient to self-administer, antiinfective medications as directed. *Antiinfective medications reverse bladder inflammation by assisting body in ridding itself of infections.*
- Reassure patient with instability (urge or reflex) urinary incontinence that any recurrence of leakage is temporary. *Instability incontinence often recurs with acute infection of lower urinary tract; management of inflammation will alleviate this condition.*
- Administer intravenous (IV) fluids as directed when patient cannot tolerate oral beverages because of fever and nausea. *Infection of upper urinary tracts may cause nausea and intolerance of oral beverages. Intravenous fluids are given until oral intake is tolerated.*
- Administer one-time intramuscular dose or ongoing intravenous and intramuscular medications. *UTI recurrence or persistence is minimized by complete eradication of existing infection.*

NIC Behavior Therapy

Noncompliance with medical therapy related to misbelief that resolution of symptoms indicates eradication of bacteriuria

- Teach patient who self-administers antiinfective medications to complete 3- to 10-day course as prescribed. *UTI recurrence or persistence is minimized by complete eradication of existing infection.*
- Teach patient the potential side effects of antiinfective medications and strategies to counteract or eliminate these effects. *Patients are likely to discontinue medications if unpleasant side effects occur. Simple strategies may relieve these effects, or antibiotic agents may be switched when more serious untoward effects occur* (Table 14-2).
- Instruct patient concerning signs and symptoms of hypersensitive reaction. Advise patient to discontinue drug immediately and contact his or her physician or nurse. *Hypersensitive reactions to a medication are potentially life threatening, warranting prompt treatment and a change in pharmacologic agent* (see box on p. 941).
- Advise patient who undergoes resection or other management of inflammatory bladder lesion about importance of follow-up examinations, including cystoscopic evaluation, as indicated. *Inflammatory lesions represent a variable risk for malignant degeneration; routine surveillance may be indicated until lesion is resolved.*

NIC Physical Comfort Promotion

Acute and chronic pain related to inflammation

- Encourage patient to take a warm Sitz bath with water above waist. *Warm water will relieve lower back and suprapubic discomfort.*
- Encourage intake of clear, caffeine-free fluids; discourage excessive intake of citrus beverages, coffee, or carbonated fluids. *Caffeinated, carbonated, or citrus beverages may cause mild irritation of the bladder wall, enhancing discomfort. Clear liquids may relieve this discomfort.*
- Provide external applications of heat to lower back *to relieve discomfort.*
- Administer, or teach patient to self-administer, urinary analgesics, as directed. *Urinary analgesics relieve bladder and urethral discomfort via unclear pharmacologic mechanisms.*
- Encourage patient to urinate regularly and not to attempt to refrain for long periods when acute infection occurs. *Bladder filling increases discomfort and promotes bacterial replication of retaining urine.*
- Administer, or teach patient to self-administer, nonsteroidal antiinflammatory agents as directed. *Antiinflammatory agents relieve irritative symptoms and discomfort produced by certain inflammatory lesions.*
- Prepare patient with a bladder inflammatory lesion for diagnostic cystoscopy and resection, if indicated. *Inflammatory bladder lesions may respond to fulguration or transurethral resection.*

Table 14-2 Common Side Effects of Urinary Antiinfective Drugs

Drug	Side Effect	Nursing Management
Trimethoprim-sulfamethoxazole (Bactrim, Septra)	Renal toxicity	Administer with water, maintain adequate fluid intake.
Nitrofurantoin (Macrodantin)	Nausea, gastrointestinal upset	Administer with meals or snack.
Carbenicillin (Geocillin, Geopen)	Diarrhea	Administer with Lactinex, 2 tablets, given with antibiotic.
	Nausea related to medication odor, foul taste	Administer with iced water; advise patient to swallow rapidly and avoid smelling drug; drug may need to be discontinued if intolerance is marked.
Cephalexin (Keflex)	Nausea, mild diarrhea	Administer with meals or snack.

Modified from Gray.[61]

- Administer, or teach patient to self-administer, antispasmodic agents as directed. *Antispasmodic agents reduce detrusor contractility, irritative symptoms, and enhance capacity.*

Patient Education/Continuum of Care Plan

1. Provide instruction concerning potential risk factors for cystitis, including altered urinary elimination patterns or urinary retention.
2. Provide instruction concerning prevention of recurrence of urinary tract infection, including increased fluid intake, strategies to acidify urine, and choice of materials for undergarments.
3. Provide instruction concerning expected actions and potential side effects of medications used to treat infection or alleviate symptoms associated with cystitis.

Evaluation/Patient Outcomes

Elimination Pattern: Patient drinks approximately 30 ml/kg/day or receives adequate fluids from parenteral source. Voiding frequency returns to premorbid patterns. Urge urinary incontinence resolves or returns to premorbid baseline.

Behavior Therapy: Patient completes entire antibiotic course, regardless of early symptom relief. Patient attends follow-up visits as indicated.

Physical Comfort Promotion: Dysuria is alleviated within 24 to 72 hours following institution of therapy and relieved by end of antibiotic therapy. Suprapubic and/or lower back discomfort are alleviated within 24 to 72 hours following institution of therapy and relieved by end of antibiotic therapy.

HYPERSENSITIVITY REACTIONS

Signs and Symptoms

Rash
Urticaria
Anaphylaxis
Diaphoresis
Wheezing or bronchoconstriction
Nausea or vomiting
Pounding headache
Stevens-Johnson syndrome (rare, potentially lethal sloughing of skin)

Nursing Management

Prevention

Obtain careful history of drug allergies.
Teach patient signs and symptoms of hypersensitivity response and their management.

Management of Ongoing Reaction

Stop medication immediately.
Seek emergency medical care if symptoms of wheezing or bronchoconstriction and anaphylaxis occur.
Promptly contact health care professional for management of symptoms and alternate drug therapy.
Administer steroidal antiinflammatory drugs, antihistamines, and cardiorespiratory drugs as directed for severe response with anaphylaxis.
Single-dose therapy is an alternative to short-term antibiotic therapy.
Administer parenteral medications when oral drugs are not tolerated or when pathogens are resistant to oral agents.
Administer parenteral fluids when oral fluids are not tolerated because of fever, nausea, and vomiting.
Administer suppressive antibiotic drugs for 6 to 24 months for recurrent infections.

From Gray.[61]

Interstitial Cystitis

Interstitial cystitis (IC) is a chronic, idiopathic disorder of the urinary bladder that causes reduced bladder capacity, frequency of urination, nocturia, and discomfort associated with bladder filling. Because specific diagnostic criteria have not been defined, IC is diagnosed by the presence of characteristic symptoms and the absence of physical evidence for related disorders, including acute urinary tract infection or inflammatory lesions of the bladder.[61]

The prevalence and incidence of interstitial cystitis are unknown. Approximately 20,000 to 90,000 individuals in the United States have been diagnosed with IC, but some researchers believe that as many as 450,000 Americans with the condition are undiagnosed or incorrectly diagnosed. Epidemiologic investigations are primarily limited by the lack of specific diagnostic criteria for this painful bladder condition. IC occurs most frequently in younger, white women. Its occurrence in children remains controversial, although several suspicious cases have been described.[61,85]

Several possible risk factors for IC have been identified; however, their role in the pathogenesis of bladder wall inflammation remains speculative. These include sensitivities or allergic reactions to medications, rheumatoid arthritis, food allergies, asthma, and hay fever. These risk factors are based on an unproved supposition that IC has a significant autoimmune component. Additional risk factors, abdominal cramping, irritable bowel syndrome, and spastic colon assume a significant emotional distress component associated with IC.[95]

The etiology of IC remains unclear. IC shares certain characteristics with autoimmune disorders, and antiinflammatory agents provide relief from pain in certain patients. Bladder wall biopsy specimens and blood samples have demonstrated the presence of antibodies that may attack the bladder wall, producing the characteristic pain and voiding dysfunction of IC. Other research has focused on loss of integrity of the glycosaminoglycan (GAG) layer covering the bladder and urethral epithelium. This layer comprises the mucosal film that covers the epithelial cells of the bladder lining and contributes to the lower urinary tract's impermeability to the reabsorption of urinary constituents. Still others have speculated that IC may be caused by chronic ischemia, perhaps representing one form of a reflex sympathetic dystrophy.[61]

Occult infection has been implicated as a causative factor for IC. In this scenario, an acute urethritis leads to a secondary infection of the bladder mucosa, causing denudation of the GAG layer and chronic inflammation and mast cell invasion.[117] This secondary infection would be undetectable to urine culture, and certain patients have experienced relief from IC symptoms after a prolonged course of antiinfective medications.[85] Toxic agents or medications in the urine have been speculated to cause IC, but specific substances have not been identified. Psychologic factors have been associated with the etiology of IC, but it is more likely that psychologic distress represents a response to the condition, rather than its cause.[61,140]

PATHOPHYSIOLOGY

The primary symptoms of IC are pain and voiding dysfunction.[95] The pain is frequently described as a continuous burning pain located in the suprapubic area with moderate to intense severity. Others experience recurring episodes of pain, described as bladder spasms, localized to the suprapubic and right lower quadrant of the abdomen. Other symptoms associated with IC include pelvic discomfort and pressure, and an intolerance of restrictive clothing or abdominal compression. Typically, the pain of IC is transiently relieved by urination but returns promptly as the bladder refills. In addition to bladder filling, emotional distress and sexual intercourse commonly exacerbate the pain. The pain produced by intercourse may persist for days. Acidic, caffienic, carbonated, or alcoholic beverages, as well as spicy or greasy foods or chocolates, also exacerbate IC pain in certain patients.

The discomfort of IC is chronic in nature. Patients experience only temporary, incomplete relief from narcotic analgesics, nonsteroidal antiinflammatory drugs, urinary analgesics, or antispasmodics. In contrast, the burning pain of IC may respond to amitriptylene, an agent commonly used to relieve the chronic, burning pain produced by peripheral polyneuropathies. Like other forms of chronic pain, the discomfort of IC is cyclical. Patients frequently report exacerbation of their symptoms, lasting from weeks to months, followed by periods of reduced pain and urinary frequency. These acute exacerbations of IC symptoms are frequently referred to as "attacks" or "flares"[175] and are managed symptomatically by analgesics, narcotic agents, sleeping aids, dietary modifications (primarily avoidance of irritating beverages and foods), and assertive toileting behaviors.

The voiding dysfunction produced by IC is related to bladder inflammation and pain. Urinary frequency may be severe, and many patients report diurnal frequency exceeding every half hour. Nocturia also occurs, and chronic fatigue is a frequent component of the condition. Because bladder filling typically exacerbates the condition, patients with IC are unable to postpone urination, although urge incontinence and unstable detrusor contractions do not occur.

The natural history of IC remains unclear. The long-term clinical course of IC commonly begins with a sudden onset of bladder pain, followed by frustrated attempts at relief by short course antiinfective therapy. The pain associated with IC is particularly intense during the earlier course of the condition, which may last for months or years. Persons with IC over a period of years to decades may enter a later stage characterized by a small, contracted bladder with low compliance. In this stage, voiding frequency remains, but the bladder may become relatively insensitive to pain. Ironically, even bladder augmentation or cystectomy with urinary diversion may fail to adequately relieve the pain of IC, even though these procedures are effective in alleviating associated voiding dysfunction.[61]

DIAGNOSTIC STUDIES AND FINDINGS

Urinalysis: Negative
Urine culture: Negative
Cystoscopy: Frequently negative, punctate hemorrhagic lesions of the bladder lining may be noted (glomerulations); Hunner's ulcers (larger ulcerations surrounded by linear hemorrhagic lesions) are seen in some patients
Biopsy: Absence of carcinoma in situ, other inflammatory lesions; mucosal denuding and evidence of chronic inflammation frequently observed
Urodynamics: Small bladder capacity, bladder filling produces pain and urgency; discomfort is associated with bladder filling rather than with unstable detrusor contractions

MULTIDISCIPLINARY PLAN

Surgery

Open surgery: Augmentation enterocystoplasty, urinary diversion with and without cystectomy, subtrigonal cystectomy, and substitution cystoplasty may be used to treat IC. Surgical procedures are effective in reducing the voiding dysfunction of IC, but they have not uniformly ablated the pelvic or suprapubic pain.[48]
Endoscopic laser therapy: Neodymium ablation of lesions of Hunner's ulcers may be used to relieve pain of IC.

Medications

Urinary analgesics, antispasmodics: Increase bladder capacity; produce little effect on the pain of IC
Narcotic analgesics: Transient relief from the pain of IC; the effectiveness of narcotics in managing the burning pain associated with IC is inconsistent
Nonsteroidal antiinflammatory drugs: Transient relief of the pain of IC; the effectiveness of these agents in relieving the pain of IC is inconsistent
Tricyclic antidepressants (amitryptilene [Elavil] or doxepin [Sinequan]): Reduce burning pain associated with IC with chronic administration; typically given before sleep to produce drowsiness and assist sleep patterns; anticholinergic side effect may increase bladder capacity[70]
Calcium channel antagonists (nifedipine, verapamil, diltiazem): Relaxation of vascular smooth muscle may reduce ischemia-induced pain of IC; relaxation of detrusor muscle may increase bladder capacity; immunosuppressive actions may reduce autoimmune aspects of disorder
Hydroxizine: H_1 receptor antagonist may reduce IC associated pain by blocking neuronal actions of mast cells
Pentosan polysulfate (Elmiron): Urinary analgesic effect not known; it is postulated to relieve impaired GAG layer of bladder sometimes found with IC; it also exerts weak anticoagulant effect; usually administered as 100 mg PO tid; maximum analgesia requires at least 3 months of ongoing therapy.[71,80]

L-Arginine: Nitric oxide synthase substrate has been reported to decrease pain and urgency in a subset of patients with IC when compared to placebo in a randomized controlled trial[97]; available in 500-mg capsules; the recommended dosage is 1,500 mg/day PO

Intravesical Therapies

Bladder hydrodistention/hydrodilation: Transient relief from pain of IC (6 months to 1 year) and increased bladder capacity occur in some patients; bladder distention under endoscopic control; the patient is under general or epidural anesthesia and the bladder is passively filled with sterile saline to an intravesical pressure of 60 to 80 cm H_2O; or a balloon is inserted into the bladder and filled to the halfway point between diastolic and systolic blood pressure[147]

Silver nitrate: Solution of 1:500 to 1% to 2% instilled and retained in the bladder producing transient relief from pain of IC in some patients (up to 1 year); treatment is contraindicated in patients with vesicoureteric reflux; leakage of silver nitrate into pelvis, peritoneum, or retroperitoneum may cause death

Sodium oxychlorosene (Chlorpactin): 0.4% solution is instilled into the bladder, exerting "detergent" and antimicrobial effects; transient relief from pain and voiding dysfunction of IC in certain patients (relief may last from 6 to 12 months)

Dimethyl sulfoxide (DMSO): Intravesical solution instilled into the bladder provides transient relief from pain and voiding dysfunction of IC in some patients; has antiinflammatory, analgesic, antispasmodic, and mast cell inhibitory effects[29]

Heparin: Administered as intravesical or subcutaneous form; transient relief of pain and voiding dysfunction of IC in some patients (up to 1 year), possibly due to protective effects of bladder epithelium (palliating damage to GAG layer)[137]

NURSING CARE

NURSING ASSESSMENT

Primarily based on symptom assessment (Table 14-3)

PATIENT PROBLEMS/NURSING DIAGNOSES & INTERVENTIONS

NIC PHYSICAL COMFORT PROMOTION

Chronic pain related to interstitial cystitis

Disturbed sleep pattern related to pain and urinary frequency

- Administer intravesical agents as directed, assist patient to retain agent for 30 minutes or prescribed length *to relieve chronic pain and urinary frequency of IC.*
- Teach patient to self-administer amitriptyline, calcium channel blocking agent, or hydroxyzine as directed; teach patient importance of chronic administration *to alleviate chronic, burning pain of IC and to increase bladder capacity.*
- Administer transvaginal or transrectal electrical stimulation in consultation with physician, provide 10-Hz current for work period of 4 seconds, followed by 4- to 8-second rest period, *to alleviate chronic pain of IC and enhance bladder capacity.*
- Advise patient to avoid or limit intake of bladder irritants: caffeine, alcoholic beverages, carbonated beverages, citrus juices, spicy foods or chocolates; teach person to alleviate foods or beverages one at a time *to judge its effect on IC-related pain and urinary frequency.*
- Advise patient to discontinue smoking *to alleviate vasoconstriction and bladder irritant effects that may exacerbate IC pain.*
- Advise individual to avoid strenuous exercises that may exacerbate IC pain.
- Advise patient to avoid tight-fitting clothing *to reduce abdominal constriction and associated IC pain.*
- Advise patient to apply local heat as tolerated *for temporary relief from IC pain.*
- Teach patient self-care strategies *to alleviate and cope with IC-related pain, including:*
  - Biofeedback techniques *to reduce emotional distress*
  - Biofeedback techniques *to relax pelvic muscles*
  - Assertive toileting during "attacks/flares" *for temporary pain relief*

Table 14-3 Signs and Symptoms of Interstitial Cystitis[55,175]

Characteristic Signs and Symptoms	Exclusionary Signs and Symptoms
Urinary frequency more than 5 times during 12 waking hours	Age <18 years (suspicious cases in children have been described)
Nocturia more than twice	Absence of intense urge to void when bladder filled with 10 ml of CO_2 or 150 ml of sterile water or saline
Symptoms present more than 1 year	Unstable detrusor contractions associated with symptoms of discomfort
Urgency	Duration of symptoms <9 months
Pain with bladder distention or fullness	Absence of nocturia
Pain temporarily relieved by micturition	Symptoms relieved by antiinfectives, antispasmodics
Suprapubic, pelvic, vaginal, and/or perineal discomfort	Diagnosis of bacterial cystitis or prostatitis within 3 months
Negative urine cultures	Current bladder or ureteral calculi
Cystoscopy/endoscopy: glomerulations of bladder wall	Active genital herpes
Petechiae	
Hunner's ulcer absent malignancies	
Bladder capacity <350 ml on urodynamic testing	Uterine, cervical, vaginal, or urethral cancer
	Cyclophosphamide treatment; must rule out chemical cystitis
	Tubercular cystitis
	Radiation therapy of the pelvis or diagnosed radiation cystitis
	Active vaginitis

Data from Gillenwater and Wein[55] and Wein, Hanno, and Gillenwater.[175]

Supplementation of dietary vitamin intake as indicated
Bladder retraining techniques (restricted to those with mild to moderate pain and significant urinary frequency)
Nonvigorous, low-impact exercise, including walking, yoga, swimming, *to relieve stress and promote physical fitness within limitation of chronic IC*
Teach patient to schedule amitriptyline before sleep. *Amitriptyline produces drowsiness, which assists with sleep.*

- Assist patient in exploring possibility of napping during daylight hours to supplement sleep. Pain and voiding dysfunction may prevent more than 2 hours of uninterrupted sleep, particularly during "attacks" or "symptom flares." Short naps during day may be needed *to supplement sleep and alleviate chronic fatigue.*
- Counsel family and significant others concerning need for napping as needed.
- Teach patient to administer sleep aids as directed *to promote drowsiness and uninterrupted sleep.*

NIC Elimination Management

Impaired urinary elimination related to chronic IC

- Advise the patient to avoid prolonged, severe restriction of fluid intake; *concentration of urine increases its irritating effect on bladder, rather than relieving urinary frequency.*
- Teach patient that transient restriction of fluids may be advisable when toilet access is limited.
- Teach person to identify potential bladder irritants and limit or eliminate them from diet.
- Reassure patient that assertive toileting is an appropriate and effective strategy to cope with IC-related pain.

NIC Coping Assistance

Ineffective coping related to chronic pain, fatigue, voiding frequency of IC; sexual dysfunction related to IC

- Provide name and address of Interstitial Cystitis Association (see box above right) and local IC support group *to strengthen the supportive network.*
- Encourage patient to identify and maintain diversional or recreational activities.
- Reassure patient that frequent voiding is necessary and acceptable.
- Counsel patient's family and significant others of need for frequent voiding, emotional support needed to cope with chronic pain, fatigue, and frequent voiding associated with IC.
- Encourage patient to use humor and candor when coping with chronic pain of IC. *Expressions of humor assist others in understanding symptoms and distress of IC in a positive and easily acceptable manner.*
- Reassure patient that expression of negative feelings is acceptable when coping with symptoms of IC. *Expression of negative feelings is appropriate when coping with discomfort and frustrations caused by symptoms of IC.*

INTERSTITIAL CYSTITIS ASSOCIATION

Goals

1. To share common experiences among those affected by the disease.
2. To provide information for interstitial cystitis patients and their families.
3. To foster research related to interstitial cystitis, its causes, care, and cure.

Address

PO Box 1553, Madison Square Station
New York, NY 10159

From Gray.[61]

- Reassure patient that assertive seeking of health-care providers with expertise and compassion when managing persons with IC is both appropriate and necessary. *Patients with IC are frequently misdiagnosed or undiagnosed, leading to frustration with health-care providers and unnecessary suffering.*
- Advise person that sexual intercourse, particularly when associated with prolonged pressure on abdomen and suprapubic area, may exacerbate IC pain in certain individuals under certain circumstances.
- Reassure individual that act of sexual intercourse is not the sole means to express intimacy. *Alternate expressions of sexual intimacy provide satisfaction without aggravating bladder pain.*
- Teach patient that sexual intercourse is acceptable only when *both* partners consent. *Assertiveness in avoiding sexual intercourse is necessary during intense IC-related pain.*
- Consult a therapist as indicated. Reduced ability to engage in intercourse may cause distress in marriage or intimate, sexual relationship. *Therapist can assist couple in exploring alternatives in sexual expression and in reducing estrangement related to pain, voiding dysfunction, and chronic fatigue associated with IC.*

Patient Education/Continuum of Care Plan

1. Teach patient nonpharmacologic methods to manage pain of IC.
2. Teach patient a variety of self-care strategies to manage pain, chronic fatigue, and voiding dysfunction of IC.
3. Provide a written list of foods and beverages that may exacerbate IC pain, and instruct person to eliminate these items one at a time to determine their influence on the bladder.

Evaluation/Patient Outcomes

Physical Comfort Promotion: IC related pain is reduced. Patient reports reduced pain intensity using visual analog scale, reduced frequency of pain ("bad days") using pain diary. Patient demonstrates knowledge of common bladder irritants and risks of excessive dehydration on pain. Patients demonstrates ability to identify, isolate, contract, and relax pelvic muscles as part of overall pain management program. Patient demonstrates knowledge of relationship between specific medications and sleep. Patient demonstrates knowledge of alternative strategies for sleep/rest, including short daytime naps.

Elimination Management: Patient demonstrates knowledge of fluid intake and its impact on urinary frequency and pain of IC. Diurnal voiding patterns return to normal patterns (every 2 hours or less frequently); episodes of nocturia fall to one to two episodes per night.

Coping Assistance: Patient demonstrates knowledge of Interstitial Cystitis Association and nearest support group. Patient's family demonstrates knowledge of the disease and need for "assertive" voiding habits by patient. Patient demonstrates trust in health-care providers regarding chronic IC. Patient and significant other maintain sexual relationship and demonstrate knowledge of impact of IC flares on sexual performance and readiness.

URINARY CALCULI

Urinary calculi are stones that are formed within the urinary tract.

Calculi that pass spontaneously and without discomfort present no serious threat to health. However, calculi that partly or entirely obstruct urinary outflow produce pain, comprise renal and urinary system function, and predispose the individual to urinary tract infection. The problem of urinary calculi must be addressed by urologists and nephrologists, and it often involves the gastroenterologist because of the close relationships among stone formation, metabolic predisposition involving the gastrointestinal tract, and dietary factors. A further discussion of medical aspects of urinary calculi is presented in Chapter 13. This discussion focuses on the two principal urologic complications associated with stone disease: infection and obstruction. In addition, extracorporeal, endoscopic, and surgical options for the management of obstructing calculi are presented.

The prevalence of clinically relevant urinary calculi varies because of the influence of a number of factors, including age, gender, race, geographic location, seasonal factors, fluid intake, diet, and occupation.[83,124b] Because of this variability, and particularly geographic differences, it is difficult to report meaningful prevalence or incidence numbers applicable to the general population. One study in Rochester, Minnesota, reported a 1.1/1000 incidence of symptomatic calculi in men and a 0.26/1000 incidence in women.[88] Another study conducted within a large prepaid health plan in Northern California reported an overall prevalence of 0.26/1000.[74] However, the variability in prevalence and incidence are demonstrated when published prevalence rates for North Carolina (3.0/1000) are compared with Missouri (0.4/1000).[153]

The peak incidence of stones occurs between the second and fourth decades of life, although persons who form multiple calculi often report the onset of episodes during the teenage years.[124b] In contrast, when reviewing 6000 patients requiring urologic intervention for stone disease, Gentle et al[52] found that only 12% were elderly (over 65 years of age). Many developed their first stone after age 50 years. When compared with younger patients with obstructing stones, elderly patients were more likely to have isolated hypocitraturia, and they were more likely to require parathyroid surgery for related disorders. Children are generally at low risk for obstructing stones, possibly because of greater intrinsic inhibiting factors.[128]

Men are generally more likely than women to experience obstructing calculi,[124b] but black women were found to have a higher risk than were black men.[149] Pregnant women experience hypercalciuria, but pregnancy, alone, is not a significant risk factor for stone formation. Whites are generally more likely to form stones than African-Americans, native Americans, native-born Israelis, or Africans.[124b]

Geographic location probably influences the epidemiology of stone formation via indirect factors, including climate, fluid and dietary patterns, and occupational tendencies. For example, persons who live in desert or warm tropical areas have a higher prevalence and incidence of calculi than do persons living in cooler regions.[83] Seasonal changes also influence geographic-related risks, with the warmer late spring or summer months carrying a higher risk than the autumn and winter.

The influence of water intake on the epidemiology of stone formation remains only partly understood, and it is partly shrouded in assumptions and traditions.[124b] Two factors are presumed to affect the risk of calculus formation: the volume of water consumed and the presence of trace minerals in the drinking supply. Water intake ("forcing" sufficient fluids is typically recommended in sufficient quantity to ensure urine output of 2 to 3 L/day) is postulated to reduce the risk of calculus formation because it reduces the growth time for crystals within the upper urinary tracts. Conflicting data exist concerning the effect of mineral content on stone formation; Churchill et al[31] concluded that the mineral content of water significantly altered the risk, but Shuster et al[152] failed to find any association.

Dietary habits probably interact with intrinsic factors to alter the risk for calculus formation.[73] Diets that are high in purines, oxalates, calcium, or phosphate increase the ionic concentration of these substances in the urine. Particular dietary patterns have also been associated with an increased risk for particular types of stones. For example, patients with oxalate stones may consume large volumes of Worcestershire sauce, and a vegetarian diet is associated with a higher risk of calculi during childhood.[124b]

In addition to these factors, occupation also influences the risk of stone formation. Persons who have sedentary occupations (including managers and professional occupations) are at risk for obstructing calculi compared with persons with active occupations.[83] Similarly, social status affects the risk of urolithiasis; this effect is presumed to occur because more affluent persons have more disposable income to spend on the more costly foods known to alter ionic balances in the urine.

PATHOPHYSIOLOGY

The formation of a calculus requires precipitation of a poorly soluble salt, usually with an organic matrix, from a solution (urine).[83] Precipitation occurs only when the salt supersaturates the solution. Supersaturation is defined as the presence of a higher concentration of a salt within a given fluid than the volume is able to dissolve when in equilibrium in the solid phase.

Within the urine, the potential for supersaturation is influenced by the effective concentration of particular ions. This effective concentration is different from its actual (measured) concentration. It is determined by the ionic strength of the salts within the solution and the influence of other ions. Ionic strength is a result of the magnitude of the electrical fields formed by the ions that form a specific salt (for example Ca^{++} and $C_2O_4^-$ interact to form the salt calcium oxalate). Because the urine typically contains high concentrations of many positively and negatively charged ions, multiple ion pairs may form, and precipitation of one or more of these salts may promote mineralization (stone formation) within the urinary tract.

In addition to ionic strength, precipitation of salts from the urine is influenced by temperature and pH. Because the temperature of urine within the human urinary tract remains relatively constant, the sensitivity of two common salts, calcium phosphate and uric acid, to pH becomes particularly relevant. An increase in the pH of urine with a supersaturation of calcium phosphate causes an increase in the concentration of hydroxyl (OH^-), and it causes hydrogen ion activity to diminish. As a result, the concentration of phosphate ions (PO_4^{3-}) increases, the solubility of calcium phosphate diminishes, and precipitation of calcium phosphate calculi becomes more likely. In contrast, in an acidic urine (pH 5.5 or less) more than half of uric acid exists as a dissolved salt, and less than half exists as the urate ion. Because uric acid is less soluble than the urate ion, lower pH values promote precipitation and subsequent stone formation. Clinically, these relationships are reflected in patients who tend to form calcium phosphate stones and experience an alkaline urine compared with patients who form uric acid stones and tend to have an acidic urine.

The first step in calculus formation is the birth of a crystal in the urine (precipitation). In a chemical solution prepared with distilled water as its solvent, crystals form as homogenous structures, and it is possible to accurately predict their formation when controlling for the concentrations of the salt within the fluid, temperature, and pH. Urine, however, contains many different ions capable of forming multiple salts, and it contains many foreign surfaces, such as cell membranes, that act as heterogenous nuclei for crystallization. In general, heterogenous nucleation occurs at a lower supersaturation level compared with homogenous crystallization. Because of the extremely complex and rapidly changing nature of heterogenous crystallization, it is not possible to predict the precise concentration of a salt, pH, or temperature that will produce a crystal leading to a clinically detectable stone. Nonetheless, a range of factors can be identified as likely to lead to crystallization, and this range is referred to as the formation product.

To reach clinical relevance, crystals must grow into larger stones capable of producing obstruction. Although this growth in a biologic system such as the urinary tract deviates from the identical units arranged in repetitive patterns characteristic of ideal crystals, they do posses approximately repetitive structures, or lattices, that can be observed via x-ray imaging techniques. Crystalline nuclei grow to larger stones when the urine remains supersaturated following the precipitation stage. This growth is postulated to occur at screw dislocations (imperfections with lattice formation caused by heterogenous crystallization). As the crystal continues to grow, it winds itself into a spiral whose center lies at the dislocation. In addition to this spiral type of proliferation, growth may occur when smaller crystals collide within the supersaturated urine and adhere to one another in a process called aggregation or agglomeration. Spiral growth produces a particularly dense calculus, whereas aggregated crystals are less dense and more easily disrupted using lithotripsy shock waves or similar techniques.

Although supersaturation of a salt within a solution (the urine) is essential for stone formation in the clinical setting, the urine does not need to be continuously supersaturated for a crystal to grow once it has precipitated from solution. Instead, periods of supersaturation allow intermittent growth of the calculus, and these commonly occur after the ingestion of a meal, particularly when it contains high amounts of the constituents of the precipitating salts (such as calcium or oxalate). Supersaturation also occurs when the body becomes dehydrated, or when fluid intake falls during sleep or prolonged periods of physical exertion causing high fluid loss via sweat and respiration.

In addition to supersaturation, stone formation in the human is influenced by three endogenous factors: crystal growth inhibition, particle retention, and matrix.[27] It is the interaction of these factors that explains why some individuals form clinically significant urinary calculi whereas others with similar dietary intake and crystalluria remain stone free.[54,176]

Inhibiting substances within the urine prevent crystallization, and they may reduce nucleation. Inhibitor substances are usually studied according to their ability to prevent calcium phosphate or calcium oxalate crystals; therefore, it is not possible to precisely predict their overall potency in the heterogenous and variable urine solutions produced by humans. Known inhibiting substances include pyrophosphate, citrate, magnesium, and nephrocalcin.

Crystal formation in the urine probably occurs at the papillary collecting ducts. Nevertheless, the vast majority of these crystals are flushed from the tract with the normal antegrade movement of urine, and only 5% to 10% of persons with proven crystalluria will experience clinically relevant calculi.[83] Urinary stasis, anatomic abnormalities, or adherence to the epithelium may prevent flushing of these particles from the system, predisposing the individual to crystalline growth and calculus formation. Urinary crystal retention may occur in one of two settings. The free-particle hypothesis assumes that precipitation, nucleation, and some crystal growth occur in the tubular lumen. Because of this rapid early growth, particles become entrapped in the collecting ducts of the kidney. In contrast to this hypothesis, the fixed-particle mechanism assumes that precipitation occurs in the tubular lumen, but nucleation and crystal growth occur when the particle adheres to epithelium within the urinary system. The locations of such adherence are not known; possible sites include the loop of Henle, lymphatic vessels in the renal pelvis, and distal collecting ducts. Damaged epithelium has also been postulated as a site for fixed-particle nucleation and subsequent growth.[92,93] Oxalate is toxic to the epithelium, and the debris from inflammation and cellular damage may further promote crystalline growth by providing an ideal microenvironment for aggregation, as well as spiral growth of precipitated crystals.

The availability of matrix within stones also affects the patient's predisposition to stone disease. Matrix is defined as the organic material contained within a urinary calculus. Although most stones primarily comprise mineralized crystals and small volumes of matrix, occasional calculi contain primarily matrix, usually as the result of tissue damage from urea-splitting pathogens. The precise relationship between matrix and crystalline growth remains unclear. However, most researchers agree that matrix is significant to stone formation because it acts as a ground substance promoting crystallization.[83]

Related Disorders

The most common cause of urinary calculi, idiopathic calcium urolithiasis (ICU), accounts for 70% to 80% of all stones treated in the United States.[83,124b] As implied in its name, a precise etiology of ICU has not been defined, and it may represent several different conditions. Upon metabolic evaluation, patients with ICU are frequently found to have hypercalciuria, mild hyperoxaluria, hyperuricosuria, hypocitruria, "incomplete" renal tubular acidosis, or crystal growth inhibitor deficiencies. The most commonly identified of these disorder is hypercalciuria, usually attributable to intestinal hyperabsorption of dietary calcium.

Although idiopathic calcium urolithiasis accounts for as much as 80% of all stones treated in the United States and Western Europe, a minority of patients form recurring stones as the result of specific disorders (Table 14-4). Renal tubular acidosis (RTA) is characterized by abnormal acidification within the renal tubules, leading to hyperchloremic metabolic acidosis.[64] Renal stones (nephrolithiasis) occur in approximately 70% of children with distal tubular defect and 30% who experience type 1 RTA, which is associated with a proximal tubular disorder.[83]

Cystinuria is a genetic disorder affecting amino acid metabolism, specifically, the body's ability to transport cystine, ornithine, lysine, and arginine in the gastrointestinal tract and renal tubule.[83] Because cystine is the least soluble of these acids, excessive amounts within the urine lead to supersaturation, precipitation, and calculus formation. Cystinosis is a distinctive disorder characterized by buildup of excessive cystine within the intracellular space. Although patients with cystinosis tend to excrete large volumes of cystine in the urine, they are at low risk for cystine calculi because their urine, in contrast to patients with cystinuria, remains alkaline, reducing the risk of precipitation of crystals and subsequent stone growth.

Hyperparathyroidism is the most common cause of hypercalcemia-induced urinary calculi. It is usually caused by a benign, solitary adenoma that is amenable to surgical resection without disturbing the remaining parathyroid glands.

Several uncommon metabolic disorders tend to produce highly specific stones.[83] Uric acid excretion depends on the biosynthesis of endogenous purines, or the intake of dietary purines. Disturbance of the urinary pH, such as the acidic urine associated with gout, dramatically alters the product formation of this ion, predisposing the individual to uric acid stones. Xanthine is less soluble than uric acid. Its solubility is also influenced by pH, although the magnitude of the effect is not as great as uric acid. Nevertheless, restoration of an alkaline urine inhibits the precipitation of xanthine oxidase from the urine and the subsequent risk of xanthine stones. 2,8-dihydroxyadeninuria is a rare genetic disorder characterized by abnormal purine reabsorption. The risk of urinary stones in these patients is high because adenine is converted to 2,8-dihydroxyadenine, which is insoluble over a wide range of urinary pH values. The stones formed by these patients are sometimes mistaken for uric acid, and it is important to ensure accurate analysis when dealing with a child who forms recurring radiolucent stones. Primary hyperoxaluria is also a rare, inherited disorder of glyoxylate metabolism that causes nephrocalcinosis, calcium oxalate calculi, and renal failure.

Infected renal lithiasis is defined as the occurrence and recurrence of ammonia magnesium phosphate (struvite) stones. Production of these calculi occurs after infection with a urease-producing bacterial pathogen. The most common of these organisms are *Proteus* species, but specific strains of *Klebsiella, Pseudomonas,* and *Staphylococcus* also may produce urease. Struvite calculi are frequently branched or grow into a staghorn configuration; but it is important to remember that not all branched or staghorn stones are composed of struvite.

Some drugs also predispose the individual to urinary calculi, usually owing to the limited solubility of the agent or its metabolites in solution. Table 14-5 identifies drugs that have been directly associated with an increased risk of stone formation.

Table 14-4 Disorders Associated With Urinary Calculus Formation

Urinary system disorders	Renal tubular acidosis Cystinuria Medullary sponge kidney Urinary tract infection with a urea-splitting organism
Endocrine disorders	Cushing's syndrome Hyperthyroidism Hyperparathyroidism
Joint disorders	Gouty arthritis
Enzyme disorders	Primary hyperoxaluria Xanthinuria 2,8-Dihydroxyadeninuria
Gastrointestinal disorders	Enteric hyperoxaluria Milk-alkali syndrome Extensive bowel resection with urinary diversion

Table 14-5 Drugs Associated With Urinary Calculi Formation

Drug (Brand Name)	Description of Associated Calculi
Acetazolamide (Diamox)	Nephrocalcinosis
Allopurinol (Zyloprim)	Oxypurinol stones, rarely xanthine stones
Triamterene (Dyrenium)	Calcium stones
Sulfonamides (e.g., Septra, Bactrim)	Sulfadiazine stones in acquired immunodeficiency syndrome (AIDS) patients
Laxatives	Ammonium acid urate stones with routine misuse or abuse

The presence of a urinary calculus is typically discovered when the stone becomes entrapped, resulting in the abrupt onset of acute renal or bladder colic. The most common sites of entrapment are a calyx or calyceal diverticulum, the ureteropelvic junction, the segment of ureter at or near the pelvic brim adjacent to the point where the ureter crosses the iliac vessels, the posterior pelvic portion of the ureter in women, and the ureterovesical junction. Of all the areas of anatomic narrowing, the ureterovesical junction is the most difficult for a calculus to pass.

The renal colic typically occurs at night or during the early morning hours when the patient is sedentary. The pain begins in the flank and radiates to the groin and testes in men or the labia majora and broad ligament in women. As the stone moves to the midureter, the pain radiates to the lateral portion of the flank and lower abdomen. As the calculus moves toward the ureterovesical junction, the pain associated with the initial renal colic may recur, associated with irritable voiding symptoms of urinary urgency or urge incontinence. Colic is perceived most intensely as the calculus moves or if it implants at a certain site. Movement of the stone also causes localized pain resulting from obstruction.[55,173]

Bladder colic is characterized by bladder pain that crescendoes immediately after micturition. A stabbing pain may be felt when changing position, and urinary urgency and urge incontinence are commonly associated.[55,173]

Because visceral pain such as renal colic is mediated by the autonomic nervous system via the celiac ganglia, nausea and vomiting, intestinal stasis, and ileus may occur. Patients are typically restless as they change position to reduce discomfort. Grunting respirations signaling distress may be present. The pulse and blood pressure may be elevated in response to pain. Fever is rare unless a urinary tract infection is present.[55,173]

Many urinary calculi pass spontaneously and do not require urologic intervention, but others need prompt attention. The decision to intervene surgically, endoscopically, or via extracorporeal shock wave lithotripsy is based on prevention of the most significant complications of calculi: obstruction, loss of renal function, and infection.

Obstruction of the urinary tract in the presence of calculi results in adverse changes in renal and ureteral function associated with hydronephrosis. The adverse effects of acute hydronephrosis have been studied in laboratory animals and divided into the following stages. During the first 90 minutes after the onset of obstruction, ipsilateral renal blood flow is dramatically increased and intramural pressure in both ureters rises. In the second stage, lasting from 90 minutes to the end of the fifth hour, renal blood flow to both kidneys decreases while pressure in the ureters remains high in an attempt to compensate for and overcome the obstruction. From the fifth through the eighteenth hour following acute obstruction, renal blood flow in the affected side and intraureteral pressure decrease as compensatory mechanisms are overwhelmed. Intrarenal changes on the affected side include an early rapid redistribution of blood from the medullary to cortical nephrons during the initial period after obstruction. Later, the renal plasma flow, glomerular filtration rate, and tubular function are slowed as kidney function is impaired.[55,173]

Ureteral peristalsis is also adversely affected by obstruction. The creation of acute obstruction in animal models resulted in an initial rise in ureteral pressure and the frequency of peristaltic waves. However, these compensatory mechanisms were soon overcome, resulting in dilation of the ureters and loss of smooth muscle tone and fibrotic replacement in the ureteral wall.[173]

In humans, progressive changes from hydronephrosis include renal pelvic dilation and an initial rise in kidney weight because of renal edema. Parenchymal mass decreases as a result of atrophy and adverse changes in the structure and function of the nephron. If hydronephrosis persists for 8 weeks or more, the parenchymal mass may be dramatically compromised with only a thin shell of tissue remaining around a hydronephrotic, distorted collecting system.[55,173]

Obstruction may be complicated by infection leading to pyelonephritis. In such cases the infection may become the dominant aspect of the disease, requiring immediate intervention before stone manipulation or surgical removal is attempted. Pyelonephritis is characterized by fever, chills, flank pain, and irritative voiding symptoms. Destruction of parenchymal mass by inflammatory changes and sepsis is a serious complication of the condition. Children with pyelonephritis are especially susceptible to renal scarring with subsequent loss of nephric function.[161,173]

Examination of a patient with calculous pyohydronephrosis may reveal a giant or intermediate-size hydronephrotic kidney or an atrophic kidney. The giant hydronephrotic kidney has a massively dilated collecting system with a thin shell of functioning parenchyma. The surface of the kidney is nodular and densely adherent to adjacent perirenal fat. An atrophic kidney is small because of extensive damage. Only a small mass of parenchymal tissue remains in this kidney, and progressive failure of function is likely. The intermediate-size hydronephrotic kidney is not as large as the giant kidney or as severely compromised in its function as the atrophic kidney. Microscopic examination of this type of kidney reveals more nearly normal nephrons than the other types of infected kidney, although inflammatory damage is present.[173]

Multiple factors influence the decision to attempt endoscopic manipulation or surgical removal of a urinary calculus. The patient's occupation must be considered when contemplating urologic intervention for a calculus. Persons in certain occupations (for example, a pilot) may subject themselves and others to danger if renal colic occurs during the performance of their jobs.[173]

A stone more than 4 mm in diameter is unlikely to pass through the ureter. Even smaller stones that are securely implanted into the wall of a calyx or ureter are less likely to pass and more likely to be obstructive or cause infection.

Aggressive removal of urinary calculi is considered for any patient who has a single kidney or significant renal insufficiency. Because of age and general health status, however, a patient may be a poor candidate for the anesthesia necessary for calculus manipulation.[173]

Diagnostic Studies and Findings

Kidneys, ureters, and bladder (KUB): Calcifications in urinary tract; calcium phosphate calculi are most densely radiopaque; uric acid stones are radiolucent

Intravenous pyelogram (IVP): Filling defects in conjunction with calculus; ureteral dilation on affected side if calculus is obstructive; hydronephrosis may be present with dilation of calyces and renal pelvis, clubbing of calyces in advanced cases of hydronephrosis; signs of pyelonephritis (parenchymal enlargement with impairment of excretion) if calculous pyohydronephrosis is present

VCUG: Of limited value in diagnosing bladder calculi, which are appreciated as intravesical filling defect

Retrograde pyelography: Useful in cases of radiolucent calculi that cannot be localized by routine radiographic studies or when patient is hypersensitive to intravenous injection of contrast material

Ultrasonography: Presence of calculi

Analysis of stones: Prominent constituents such as cystine, calcium, oxalate, and uric acid; provides guidance for medical therapy to prevent recurrence

Urine calcium: Elevated in patients with calcium stones or renal tubular acidosis

Urine oxalate: Elevated in patients with calcium oxalate stones

Urine uric acid: Elevated in patients with uric acid stones

Urinary pH: Acidic in patients with uric acid or cystine stones; alkaline in patients who form calcium phosphate, calcium oxalate, and struvite stones

Urine culture: Bacteriuria if infection is due to presence of calculi

Antibody-coated bacteria: Positive in pyelonephritis

Serum calcium: Elevated in hyperparathyroidism

Serum parathormone: Elevated in hyperparathyroidism

Multidisciplinary Plan

Surgery

Once the mainstay of urologic management of stones, surgical procedures are currently reserved for patients who fail to respond adequately to extracorporeal shock wave lithotripsy or endoscopic manipulation

Medications

For calcium and calcium oxalate stones: Sodium bicarbonate or citrate (inhibits urinary excretion of calcium), hydrochlorothiazide, trichlormethiazide (reduces urinary calcium excretion in patients with idiopathic hypercalciuria; may have some benefit among normocalciuric individuals), orthophosphate (decreases urinary calcium excretion), cellulose phosphate (binds calcium in the intestinal tract), potassium citrate (reduces incidence of stones in patients with hypocitruria)

For cystine stones: D-penicillamine, alpha-mercaptopropinoglycide, captopril (bind with cystine to enhance its solubility)

For uric acid stones: Allopurinol (reduces urinary excretion of urinary acid), sodium bicarbonate or citrate (raises urinary pH, favoring solubility of uric acid)

For oxalate stones: Pyridoxine (reduces urinary oxalate excretion in patients with primary hyperoxaluria), cholestyramine (binds oxalate in the intestine for fecal excretion)

General Management

Percutaneous removal of upper urinary tract stones using stone basket or by crushing stones via ultrasonic shock waves, electrohydraulic means, or laser techniques; avoids open surgery but does require invasive percutaneous access into the upper urinary tract

Extracorporeal shock wave lithotripsy uses shock waves to crush calculi into small fragments that can be passed through the urinary tract and expelled into the urine; technique is noninvasive

Chemolysis uses a chemical solution to dissolve urinary calculi by reversing environmental conditions favorable to calculi crystallization and aggregation; a percutaneous tract into the renal pelvis is established, and chemolytic solution is used to dissolve calculi

Dietary restrictions for preventive therapy

- To prevent all forms of stones: Ensure adequate fluid intake
- To prevent calcium stones: Reduction of dietary calcium indicated only in certain patients with abnormal intestinal absorption of calcium (absorptive calciuria); a moderate restriction is recommended (400 to 600 mg/day)[136]
- To prevent oxalate stones: Reduce intake of foods high in oxalates, including asparagus, beets, plums, raspberries, rhubarb, spinach, almonds, cashew nuts, cranberries, cocoa, cranberry juice, grape juice, grapefruit juice, Worcestershire sauce
- To prevent uric acid stones: Reduce intake of foods high in purines such as organ meats, lean meats, and whole grains

NURSING CARE

Nursing Assessment

Pain: Renal colic or bladder colic; may be severe; flank pain noted with pyelonephritis

Voiding behaviors: Irritative voiding symptoms

Fever: Elevated if infection is present

Nausea and vomiting: Associated with renal colic

Patient Problems/Nursing Diagnoses & Interventions

NIC Physical Comfort Promotion

Acute pain related to urinary obstruction

- Administer, or teach patient to self-administer, narcotic pain medications as directed *to reduce discomfort.*
- Minimize environmental noises and activity *to enhance pain-relieving action of narcotics and to promote rest.*
- Apply warm compresses to patient's flank *to relieve pain caused by renal colic.*
- Observe patient for sudden increase in intensity of pain, *which may indicate acute obstruction of urinary system with embedding of a stone.*
- Observe patient for acute relief from pain, *which may indicate passage of a stone through a narrow segment of system and relief from obstruction.*
- Advise patient that "anticipatory watching" is necessary before invasive or extracorporeal procedures. Reassure patient that aggressive pain management will be maintained throughout this procedure. *Approximately one half*

of all symptomatic stones pass spontaneously. Invasive or extracorporeal procedures are reserved for those calculi that produce significant obstruction and infection.

- Encourage patient to maintain adequate fluid intake (at least 30 ml/kg of body weight per day[131] and up to 3000 ml in special circumstances) *to promote flushing of he urinary system with passage of partially obstructing stones.*
- Encourage patient to ambulate as feasible *to promote passage of urinary calculi and sediment from upper to lower urinary tract.*

NIC Tissue Perfusion Management

Ineffective tissue perfusion (renal) related to mechanical reduction of blood flow

- Advise patient that urinary calculi may recur, emphasizing need for prevention and prompt management. *Urinary calculi often produce obstruction and infection that compromises renal function unless rapidly managed.*
- Teach patient to strain urine when watching for calculus to pass and to preserve stone for analysis. *Stone analysis may provide clues to an underlying, treatable metabolic disorder amenable to treatment, preventing the recurrence of calculi with coexisting obstruction and infection.*
- Teach patient to drink an adequate volume of liquids each day (30 ml/kg of body weight[131]). *Fluids dilute urine, reducing risk of urinary calculi formation.*
- Teach patient to change his or her diet or to self-administer medications, as directed. *Specific medications or dietary modifications reduce risk of stone recurrence in certain individuals.*
- Assist patient to minimize or reverse specific risk factors for urinary calculi. *Specific risk factors for urinary stones, such as immobility or urinary retention, may be modulated or removed, reducing concurrent risk for calculi in urine.*

NIC Elimination Management

Impaired urinary elimination related to urinary obstruction

Risk for infection (urinary system) related to tissue trauma of caliculi or of urine

- Perform urinalysis and urine culture studies as directed *to detect presence of coexisting urinary infection.*
- Monitor vital signs and body temperature *to detect presence of febrile urinary tract infection or urosepsis.*
- Administer, or teach patient to self-administer, antiinfective medications as directed *to eradicate urinary infection.*
- Administer, or teach patient to self-administer, prophylactic antiinfective medications as directed before invasive diagnostic or therapeutic procedures (e.g., percutaneous, nephroscopic, or ureteroscopic stone manipulation) *to prevent systemic spread of bacteria from urine.*
- Encourage adequate fluid intake (at least 30 ml/kg of body weight per day[131] and up to 3000 ml in certain circumstances) *to promote stone passage and to flush urinary system of pathogens and related toxins.*
- Reassure patient that irritative voiding symptoms are temporary. *Irritative symptoms (frequency, urgency, and nocturia) are related to obstruction and infection; symptoms are relieved as stone passes or is removed and as infection is eradicated.*
- Reassure patient experiencing urge incontinence that this condition is expected to be temporary. *Passage of urinary calculus through ureterovesical junction into bladder often produces unstable bladder contractions that are relieved as stone is passed in urine.*
- Advise patient who has undergone removal of an obstructive stone that urinary urgency and frequency will persist for a brief period following manipulation of urinary system. *Manipulating urinary system produces transient inflammation with irritative voiding symptoms. Frequency and urgency are also affected by postobstructive diuresis caused by stone removal.*

Patient Education/Continuum of Care Plan

1. Provide explanation of analysis of stone, adjunct medical therapy aimed at prevention of recurrence, and associated dietary restrictions.
2. Provide instruction concerning options of treatment should manipulation of stones be indicated.

Evaluation/Patient Outcomes

Physical Comfort Management: Renal colic pain is relieved. Patient experiences reduction in pain intensity as assessed by visual analog scale.

Tissue Perfusion Management: Patient demonstrates knowledge of risk factors for recurrent urinary calculus. Patient demonstrates relationship between fluid intake, intake of foods or beverages known to increase precipitating materials in urine, urine pH, and risk of recurring stone formation. Patient consistently takes medications to reduce risk of recurrent stone formation as directed.

Elimination Management: Urine remains free of infection (urinalysis demonstrates absence of nitrites, leukocytes). Kidneys remain infection free (absent costovertebral angle [CVA] tenderness, fever, chills). Patient maintains normal patterns of urinary elimination (diurnal frequency every 2 hours or less frequently, one episode of nocturia per night, absence of urinary leakage).

Urinary Incontinence

Urinary incontinence is the involuntary leakage of urine after the age of toilet training.

Incontinence is not a disease; it is a symptom that represents a significant health problem and may underlie a serious disease process. Urinary incontinence is a particularly appropriate area of intensive investigation and intervention for nurses who manage patients with genitourinary disease.

The problem of incontinence occurs throughout the life span and is particularly problematic for the elderly. In the United

States the National Institutes of Health have estimated that at least 13 million adults experience urinary incontinence, creating an annual cost of $10.3 billion. As many as 55% of the institutionalized elderly in this country experience chronic incontinence,[2] and approximately 70% experience intermittent episodes of urinary leakage. Approximately 15% to 30% of community-dwelling, aged persons are incontinent. Many cases of incontinence are transient, caused by infection, acute immobility, or other factors; many cases represent a chronic condition that will persist for months, years, or a lifetime if left untreated.

A Welsh study of 1060 women 18 years of age and over revealed that 45% of these women had some degree of incontinence. Symptoms consistent with stress incontinence were reported by 22% of the women, and those of urge incontinence were reported by 10%. A combination of stress and urge incontinence was reported by 14% of those surveyed. In the majority of the women, urinary incontinence was assessed as mild, but 5% related severe enough symptoms to necessitate changing clothing daily. Over 3% of the women reported that urinary incontinence significantly interfered with their daily lives, yet less than half of these had sought medical treatment for the problem.

The prevalence of urinary incontinence in men is less well documented. In the Danish population, 2% of all adults have urinary incontinence severe enough to prompt them to seek medical help. Among men over 65 years of age, 5% suffer from incontinence; among men under 50 years approximately 20% to 25% develop symptoms of obstruction and dribble after voiding because of benign prostatic hyperplasia.[69,75]

Urinary continence in childhood is typically accomplished by 5 years of age. Incontinence most often takes the form of enuresis, which is seen in 15% of all 5-year-olds.[78]

PATHOPHYSIOLOGY

Many classification schemes for urinary incontinence have been proposed. In this discussion, Wheatley's four types of incontinence[177] are used because they offer a simple, comprehensive conceptual framework for this condition. The four types of incontinence are stress urinary incontinence (SUI), instability incontinence, overflow or paradoxic incontinence, and constant or extraurethral incontinence.

Stress urinary incontinence occurs when bladder pressure exceeds urethral closure pressure, resulting in leakage of urine in the absence of a detrusor contraction. Although the condition is most common among women, it is also noted among males. The causes of stress urinary incontinence are pelvic relaxation, sphincteric incompetence, or a combination of these factors.[141,162]

Pelvic relaxation, most typically seen in women, occurs when the support structures of the pelvis lose their optimum competence, resulting in descent of pelvic organs. Cystocele describes the protrusion of the bladder into the vaginal space; rectocele describes protrusion of the rectum into the vaginal space. The often-used term *urethrocele* is a misnomer; the condition typically refers to hypermobility of the urethra associated with increased abdominal pressure seen during physical examination. Uterine prolapse occurs when the uterus descends into the vaginal space as a result of a loss of normal support mechanisms.[63] Multiparity, aging, and menopause are associated with pelvic relaxation.[177]

Childbirth via vaginal delivery is associated with pelvic relaxation, at least partly because of traction placed on the pelvic ligaments during delivery and denervation of the pelvic floor musculature.[8,160] Other causes of pelvic floor relaxation are associated with pelvic floor muscle denervation. Peripheral neuropathy, as seen in diabetes mellitus, and traumatic and iatrogenic nerve damage resulting from extensive pelvic surgery can cause pelvic floor relaxation. Obesity may exacerbate the condition.[63,162]

Although a causal relationship between pelvic relaxation and stress urinary incontinence remains unestablished, the principal pathophysiologic mechanism is probably loss of normal urethrovesical anatomy. The urethra is no longer maintained in its normal position, resulting in inefficient transmission of abdominal pressures along the urethral length. As a result, a precipitous increase in abdominal pressure is not transmitted to the urethral sphincteric mechanism, resulting in a temporary condition when bladder pressure exceeds urethral closure pressure and urinary leakage occurs.

Intrinsic sphincter deficiency (ISD) also causes stress urinary incontinence. Damage to the neuromuscular components of the urethra results from any process that causes denervation of the pelvic floor musculature of smooth muscle of the proximal urethra. Iatrogenic damage resulting from radical prostatectomy or transurethral resection of the prostate may cause ISD and stress urinary incontinence. Multiple antiincontinence procedures or Y-V plasty in men or women also may result in incontinence.[178] Pelvic trauma or metabolic conditions resulting in peripheral neuropathy affecting the pelvis may result in stress urinary incontinence as a result of sphincteric incompetence.[63]

Stress urinary incontinence in a woman may represent a combination of ISD and pelvic relaxation. Stress incontinence in a man is caused by ISD alone.

Instability incontinence is the condition of urinary leakage that occurs when the detrusor contracts at inappropriate times. The concept of instability arises from Hodgkinson, Ayers, and Drukker's description of dyssynergic detrusor activity among women with urinary incontinence.[76] Other terms have been used to describe the condition. Detrusor hyperreflexia is often used synonymously with instability. Nonetheless, the term is defined by the International Continence Society as the occurrence of an uninhibited detrusor contraction in the presence of a known neurologic disease. Other terms, such as detrusor hyperactivity or overactivity, are less commonly used.

Detrusor instability is associated with disease or trauma of the central nervous system. Diseases of the brain typically result in loss of volitional control over detrusor activity with preservation of coordination between the striated sphincter mechanism and detrusor activity. Such diseases include cerebrovascular accidents, parkinsonism, and brain tumors affecting the frontal lobes or cerebellum. Incontinence is preceded by a feeling of urgency followed by an unstable bladder contraction with relaxation of the sphincteric mechanism and evacuation of the bladder. Bladder emptying often is efficient, so urinary tract infections are not typically associated with this condition. The nursing diagnosis associated with this form of incontinence is urge urinary incontinence.

Instability incontinence also is associated with neurologic abnormality of the spinal cord above the level of the sacral micturition center (S2-4).[177] Spinal cord injury is the most commonly noted lesion. Nontraumatic lesions include those seen in multiple sclerosis or other demyelinating diseases. Incontinence is not preceded by any sensation of urgency. A detrusor contraction is triggered by bladder filling or other stimulus, and the person is aware of the incontinence via perception of urinary leakage. Detrusor contraction is often associated with contraction of the pelvic floor and rhabdosphincter. This condition is called detrusor-sphincter dyssynergia and is associated with urinary retention, urinary tract infection, and upper tract deterioration.[63] The nursing diagnosis for this form of instability incontinence is reflex urinary incontinence.

Nonneuropathic conditions also are associated with detrusor instability. Bladder outlet obstruction has been associated with instability incontinence among men with benign prostatic hyperplasia. Irritative bladder disorders caused by bacterial, viral, fungal, or parasitic infection of the bladder have been labeled as a cause of instability incontinence.[177] Although these conditions are associated with increased sensations of bladder filling, little evidence supports the supposition that they cause detrusor instability.[15] Instability incontinence is associated with bladder irritation caused by bladder calculi and carcinoma of the urothelial lining of the vesicle. The leakage of urine into the posterior urethra seen in stress urinary incontinence has been speculated to cause instability of the detrusor.[177] Indeed, detrusor instability is often seen among women with stress urinary incontinence, and the condition is often relieved by surgical correction of the stress incontinence. Nonetheless, other investigators have failed to confirm this association, and the relation between detrusor instability and urinary leakage into the posterior urethra remains unclear.[141]

The underlying cause of many cases of instability incontinence is unclear, and the condition is termed idiopathic. Such instability may arise from a psychogenic or behavioral source, or it may be due to subtle neuropathy yet to be elucidated.

Overflow or paradoxic incontinence is the leakage of urine in the presence of a large residual. The nursing diagnosis associated with this form of incontinence is urinary retention. The two causes of overflow incontinence are deficient detrusor function and bladder outlet obstruction.[178] Deficient detrusor function may result from a variety of causes. Neurologic lesions of the sacral micturition cord such as that noted in myelomeningocele cause an autonomous neurogenic bladder with detrusor areflexia, lack of sensations of urgency, and overflow incontinence. Other central nervous system disorders associated with overflow incontinence are cauda equina syndrome, multiple sclerosis, tabes dorsalis, and poliomyelitis. Peripheral nervous system trauma or abnormalities that compromise parasympathetic innervation of the detrusor muscle also result in overflow incontinence. Examples are herpes zoster, extensive pelvic surgery, pelvic trauma, and diabetes mellitus.[177]

Other factors that result in overflow incontinence and detrusor areflexia are the result of chronic overdistention. The "nurse's bladder," "teacher's bladder," or "librarian's bladder" arises from overdistention of the bladder because of perceived inability to interrupt work for micturition. Acute illness and immobility may also result in deficient detrusor function. Severe constipation or fecal impaction is associated with temporary detrusor failure and overflow incontinence. Certain patients may suffer from urinary retention because of hysterical conversions.

Patients with overflow incontinence may not be aware of their inability to empty the bladder. Symptoms of deficient detrusor function are urgency, frequency, nocturia, and a dribbling, intermittent stream. Urinary tract infection is commonly an associated condition. Low back pain and vague abdominal discomfort may be the result of bladder enlargement.

Bladder outlet obstruction is also a cause of overflow incontinence. Types of bladder outlet obstruction include prostatic enlargement owing to inflammation, benign hypertrophy, or adenocarcinoma. Internal sphincter dyssynergia, bladder neck hypertrophy, and bladder neck contracture are particularly prevalent in men with highly stressful lifestyles and may lead to overflow incontinence. Urethral stricture in a man or urethral distortion in a woman may obstruct normal bladder emptying and lead to incontinence.[177]

Patients with bladder outlet obstruction are acutely aware of their problem because of high pressures generated by the detrusor during micturition. Symptoms of bladder outlet obstruction include frequency, nocturia, and poor urinary stream. A dribble after voiding is often noted.

Constant or extraurethral incontinence results when the normal sphincteric mechanism is bypassed, causing failure of urinary storage that is continuous. The causes of extraurethral incontinence are urinary fistula, ectopia, or surgical creation of a conduit for evacuation of urine. Congenital ectopic defects of the urinary tract, including urethral duplication, epispadias, and exstrophy, are relatively rare and may be associated with severe urinary leakage that may persist even after surgical leakage.[61] Ureteral ectopia is a more common congenital defect and results in a continuous, dribbling discharge superimposed on a normal voiding pattern if the orifice bypasses normal sphincteric mechanisms.[177]

Urinary fistula is most commonly noted among adult women. A fistula is created when tissue between the bladder or urethra and an adjacent structure erodes; the normal sphincteric mechanism is bypassed, resulting in urinary leakage. A fistula between the bladder and vagina is termed vesicovaginal fistula; a fistulous tract between the urethra and vagina is termed urethrovaginal fistula. Symmonds reviewed 800 cases of urinary fistulas seen at the Mayo Clinic over a 30-year period and found that the leading cause of fistula was pelvic surgery. Hysterectomy was the most common procedure associated with the condition. Other causes of fistula include penetrating trauma, radiation therapy, and obstetric complications.[166] In the Mayo Clinic study, only 5% of the patients reviewed developed fistula as a result of obstetric complications. Nonetheless, childbearing is thought to account for the largest incidence of fistulous tracts worldwide.[173]

Diagnostic Studies and Findings

VCUG: Stress incontinence: pelvic descent below pubis; urethral excursion and leakage of contrast material with abdominal strain; instability incontinence: normal or trabeculated narrowing of membranous urethra noted with micturition in presence of detrusor-sphincter dyssynergia; diverticulae, vesicoureteral reflux may be noted in presence of detrusor-sphincter dyssynergia; overflow/paradoxic incontinence: large capacity, poor filling of proximal urethra with bladder outlet obstruction; failure of bladder neck funneling with detrusor-sphincter dyssynergia; urethral narrowing with stricture; constant extraurethral incontinence: leakage of contrast material through fistulous tract or from ectopic structure

Urodynamic testing: Stress incontinence: normal capacity, sensations, and compliance; stable detrusor; explosive flow with low-pressure detrusor contraction during micturition; normal electromyographic (EMG) findings; instability incontinence: decreased functional capacity; early sensations; normal compliance; unstable detrusor and/or urethra; EMG findings normal or indicative of detrusor-sphincter dyssynergia; overflow incontinence with deficient detrusor function: large capacity, delayed sensations, abnormally compliant; with detrusor hypotonic or areflexic: urinary stream poor or absent, large residual present after voiding; bladder outlet obstruction: normal or enlarged capacity; sensations may be delayed; compliance normal or impaired owing to detrusor hypertrophy; detrusor contraction is high pressure with poor urinary flow; constant incontinence: normal or impaired urine storage with large fistulous tract

IVP: Constant incontinence: ureteral duplication with ectopic opening below bladder neck or outside urinary tract; extravasation of contrast material in fistula

Retrograde urethrogram (RUG): Presence of urethral stricture

Cystoscopy-urethroscopy: Stress incontinence: normal findings in pelvic relaxation or open bladder neck with sphincteric damage; overflow incontinence: large capacity in deficient detrusor function; localization of obstruction in some cases; constant incontinence: ectopia or fistulous tract

Urinalysis and urine culture: Instability incontinence: normal findings or presence of bacterial infection

Bladder biopsy: Instability incontinence: normal findings or presence of transitional cell carcinoma or carcinoma in situ

MULTIDISCIPLINARY PLAN

Surgery

Stress Incontinence

Vesicourethral suspension; over 100 procedures described in literature; commonly performed types include Marshall-Marchetti-Krantz, Stamey or Raz needle suspension, Burch's colposuspension

Artificial urinary sphincter for stress incontinence caused by ISD; cuff of device placed at bladder neck or proximal urethra, abdominal reservoir positioned, pump mechanism placed in scrotum or fascia of labia

Suburethral sling surgery for stress incontinence caused by ISD and pelvic relaxation with urethral hypermobility

Suburethral glutaraldehyde cross-linked collagen (GAX collagen) injections for ISD without coexisting urethral hypermobility

Overflow Incontinence

Transurethral resection of enlarged prostate; open prostatectomy or radical prostatectomy in certain cases

Correction of urethral stricture by internal urethrotomy or urethral dilation

Correction of female distortion by open surgical reconstruction

Constant Extraurethral Incontinence

Removal or repair of ectopic structures

Open surgical repair of urinary fistula

Medications

To affect detrusor contractility

- Autonomic drugs
  - Propantheline, up to 150 mg/day in 3 divided doses
  - Oxybutynin, 5 mg bid to tid
- Central nervous system drugs
  - Imipramine, 1.5-2 mg/kg in single dose at bedtime
- Spasmolytic agents
  - Dicyclomine, 10-20 mg tid or qid
  - Hyoscyamine, 0.125-0.25 mg tid-qid

To increase detrusor activity and tone

- Autonomic drugs: Bethanechol, 15-30 mg tid or qid

To increase bladder neck tone

- Autonomic drugs: Norephedrine or ephedrine (Sudafed S.A.), 1 tablet bid

To decrease bladder neck tone

- Autonomic drugs
  - Terazosin, 2-10 mg at hs
  - Doxazosin, 2-8 mg at hs

To decrease external muscle tone

- Central nervous system drugs: Baclofen, 5-20 mg tid

NURSING CARE

NURSING ASSESSMENT

Bladder

- Suprapubic tenderness associated with cystitis; suprapubic and lower abdominal distention in overflow incontinence

Vaginal vault

- Bulge in anterior wall in cystocele associated with pelvic relaxation; discharge in vesicovaginal or ureterovaginal fistula or ureteral ectopia in the vagina or uterus
- Pale, friable mucosa, tender to touch

Minimum assessment for urinary incontinence[2]

- History (including current patterns of urinary elimination; duration of urinary leakage; exacerbating and alleviating factors; urologic, neurologic, reproductive systems review)
- Focused physical examination (perineal inspection including vaginal rectal examination and integument, focused neurologic examination, functional assessment for mobility, dexterity, cognition)
- Urinalysis (culture and sensitivity testing only when suspicion of urinary tract infection is raised by urinalysis)
- Postvoid urinary residual measurement (strongly recommended)
- Bladder log (voiding diary) for at least 24 hours (strongly recommended)

Patient Problems/Nursing Diagnoses & Interventions

NIC Elimination Management

Impaired urinary elimination
Stress urinary incontinence related to urethral hypermobility or intrinsic sphincter deficiency
Urge urinary incontinence related to sensory urgency and detrusor instability
Reflex urinary incontinence related to detrusor hyperreflexia with vesicosphincter dyssynergia
Urinary retention related to bladder outlet obstruction or deficient detrusor contraction strength
Total urinary incontinence related to urinary fistula or ureteral ectopia
Functional urinary incontinence related to altered mobility, dexterity, cognitive deficit, or limited toilet access

- Provide patient with appropriate urinary containment system (pad, dribble pouch, continent brief, incontinent briefs, or other device) *to contain urinary leakage until a definitive management program can be instituted.*
- Encourage patient to drink an adequate volume of fluids (30 ml/kg of body weight per day[131]) *to prevent concentration of urine and intensification of irritative voiding symptoms.*
- Assist patient in identifying and modifying intake of food and beverages that aggravate irritative symptoms. *Caffeinic, carbonated beverages, and certain spicy foods or chocolates may produce mild bladder irritation, aggravating symptoms of urinary incontinence.*
- Encourage patient who smokes to stop. *Cigarette smoke may act as a mild bladder irritant, aggravating symptoms of urinary incontinence.*

Stress incontinence care

- Teach patient to identify, isolate, and contract pelvic muscles and to perform pelvic (Kegel) exercises using principles of physiotherapy[41] *to strengthen periurethral striated muscles.*
- Perform electrostimulation therapy *to supplement success of pelvic muscle exercises in individual with profound weakness of pelvic muscles.*
- Teach female patient to use vaginal cones *to strengthen periurethral muscles.*
- Administer, or teach patient to self-administer, alpha-sympathomimetic agents or imipramine as directed (see box above right). *Alpha-sympathomimetics increase urethral sphincter resistance, alleviating or ablating stress incontinence.*
- Administer, or teach patient to self-administer, topical or systemic estrogens as directed. *Estrogen replacement therapy may alleviate stress incontinence and related irritative bladder symptoms by its trophic effects on urethral mucosa.*
- Place, or assist physician or nurse specialist to place, pessary, and teach patient to care for device. *Pessary device may alleviate or relieve stress incontinence by mechanically restoring more normal urethrovesical anatomy.*
- Prepare patient for surgical repair of stress incontinence as indicated. *Surgical repair of stress incontinence restores urethrovesical anatomy to nearly normal.*

Drugs Used for Stress Incontinence

Alpha-Sympathomimetics:

Ephedrine, pseudoephedrine, phenylpropanolamine
Over-the-counter preparations: Sudafed, Sudafed S.A. capsules, Dexatrim without caffeine capsules (preparations with antihistamines are avoided; generic substitutes are available)
Prescription preparations: Entex L.A., Ornade Spansule
Action and administration: Increases tone of urethral smooth muscle and rhabdosphincter; taken only during daytime hours and may be taken before physically demanding activities (exercise, walking) exclusively
Side effects: Tachycardia, hypertension, anxiety, nervousness, insomnia

Tricyclic Antidepressant

Prescription preparations: Imipramine (may be used with estrogens)
Action: Alpha-sympathomimetic action increases tone of urethral smooth muscle and rhabdosphincter; anticholinergic effect relaxes detrusor and increases functional capacity in cases of SUI mixed with unstable detrusor
Administration: 10-25 mg PO, tid to qid; administered over a 24-hour period; individual is gradually withdrawn from drug using tapered doses
Side effects: Drowsiness, urinary retention, dry mouth, constipation, mydriasis (mild), hypertension

From Gray.[61]

- Prepare patient with stress incontinence caused by sphincter mechanism incompetence for periurethral injection of bulking agent. *Urethral bulking agents alleviate stress incontinence by promoting coaptation of urethral surfaces.*
- Prepare patient with stress incontinence caused by sphincter incompetence for implantation of artificial urinary sphincter, as directed. *Artificial urinary sphincter is a mechanical device that performs a function similar to intrinsic sphincter mechanism.*
- Prepare female with sphincter incompetence causing stress incontinence for suburethral sling as directed. *Suburethral sling is a procedure in which a segment of fascia or synthetic material is placed around urethra, promoting closure of sphincter mechanism.*

Urge incontinence care

- Institute a timed voiding schedule based on results of a voiding diary *to encourage voluntary bladder evacuation before unstable contractions cause leakage.*
- Administer, or teach patient to self-administer, antispasmodic or anticholinergic medications as directed *to suppress unstable bladder contractions and to enhance bladder capacity* (see box on p. 955).
- Combine pharmacotherapy with a timed voiding schedule. *Pharmacotherapy for instability (urge) incontinence increases bladder capacity and suppresses unstable contractions. Nonetheless, these contractions will inevitably occur if bladder is allowed to overfill.*
- Teach patient to manipulate fluid intake. Ensure that patient obtains an adequate daily fluid intake (30 ml/kg

DRUGS USED TO TREAT INSTABILITY (URGE OR REFLEX) INCONTINENCE

ANTICHOLINERGICS

Preparations: Dicyclomine (Bentyl), flavoxate (Urispas), hyoscyamine (Levsin or Levsinex), propantheline (Pro-Banthine), oxybutynin (Ditropan, sometimes called "classic" Ditropan, Ditropan XL)

Action and administration: Nonselective anticholinergic/antispasmodic drugs increase bladder capacity and threshold volume for unstable (overactive) bladder contractions

Side effects: Dry mouth, mydriasis, blurred vision, urinary retention, constipation, flushing and heat intolerance, confusion in certain cases (particularly when administered at higher doses or when given to elderly patients); (Ditropan XL associated with less severe dry mouth than classic Ditropan in randomized clinical trial; effect due to reduction of metabolite of oxybutynin in Oros preparation associated with systemic side effects)[67]

MUSCARINIC RECEPTOR ANTAGONIST

Preparations: Tolterodine (Detrol)

Action and administration: Pharmacologically nonselective antispasmodic with actions similar to anticholinergics; however, drug shows physiologic and clinical evidence of uro-selectivity when comparing affinity of parotid muscarinic receptors and when asking patients to rate severity of dry mouth compared with oxybutynin (classic Ditropan)[1,184]

Side effects: Dry mouth, dyspepsia, headache, urinary retention

of body weight per day[131]), while avoiding intake of large volumes of fluids with meals or before bedtime *to avoid acute large intake of fluid and unstable contractions.*

- Institute bladder drill therapy consisting of regimen to increase time interval between toiletings to a goal of every 3 hours. *Bladder drill therapy is a behavioral technique designed to gradually enhance capacity and diminish urge incontinence.*
- Institute electrostimulation therapy alone or in combination with bladder drill therapy. *Electrostimulation therapy is a technique that inhibits unstable bladder contractions and sensations of urgency and enhances capacity. Bladder drill therapy probably supplements this approach to therapy. Electrostimulation therapy may enhance bladder capacity and inhibit unstable contractions by reflex inhibition of pelvic plexus or by other, unknown actions.*
- Administer, or teach patient to self-administer, antispasmodic medications, and teach patient to perform self-intermittent catheterization using a clean technique, as directed. *Antispasmodic medications can be used to "pharmacologically paralyze" detrusor muscle. Intermittent catheterization is used to ensure regular, complete evacuation of urine.* Acceptance of this regimen is limited by occurrence of side effects from relatively high doses of anticholinergic medications and acceptability of intermittent catheterization among individuals with normal urethral and bladder sensations.
- Insert and indwelling urethral or suprapubic catheter, as directed. Teach patient to care for catheter and drainage bags. *Indwelling catheter represents a "last option" for patient with instability (urge) incontinence; however, it may be necessary for patient with limited dexterity or with limited family or other ongoing caretakers.*

Reflex incontinence care

- Administer, or teach patient to self-administer, antispasmodic medications, and teach patient to perform clean, intermittent catheterization. *Antispasmodics are used to suppress all bladder contractions, and intermittent catheterization is used to provide regular, complete bladder evacuation.* Acceptability of this program is enhanced by absence of urethral and bladder sensations and is limited when upper extremity dexterity is compromised.
- Apply condom catheter to male patient who is to be managed by "reflex voiding program" for instability (reflex) leakage. Teach patient and family to change catheter routinely (daily or twice daily) and to inspect penile skin for integrity with each change. *Condom drainage is a realistic option for males who are unable to perform self-catheterization.* The long-term safety of reflex voiding program is affected by presence and severity of detrusor-sphincter dyssynergia.
- Administer, or teach patient to self-administer, alpha-sympathomimetic blocking agents *to reduce urethral resistance and obstruction caused by detrusor-sphincter dyssynergia; condom is used to contain urinary leakage.*
- Prepare male patient who is unable to perform catheterization for transurethral sphincterotomy, as directed. *Sphincterotomy is incision of striated sphincter mechanism providing relief of bladder outlet obstruction caused by detrusor-sphincter dyssynergia*
- Prepare patient for insertion of urethral stent device, as directed. *Urethral stents are inserted under endoscopic guidance and used to reduce urethral resistance caused by detrusor sphincter dyssynergia.*
- Prepare patient with instability (reflex) incontinence, who is capable of self-catheterization, for augmentation enterocystoplasty or continent urinary diversion, as directed. *Augmentation enterocystoplasty is surgical anastomosis of detubularized bowel or stomach with bladder muscle. It reduces detrusor contractility and enhances bladder capacity; catheterization is required for bladder evacuation. Continent urinary diversion is creation of urinary reservoir and continent abdominal stoma, using bowel or stomach. It is reserved for particularly small or hostile bladders not amenable to less extensive reconstruction. Continent urinary diversion also requires intermittent catheterization for evacuation of urine.*
- Insert indwelling urethral or suprapubic catheter, as directed. Teach patient to care for catheter and drainage bags. *Indwelling catheter represents "last option" for patient with instability (reflex) incontinence; however, it may be necessary for patient with limited dexterity and limited family or other ongoing caretakers.*

Urinary retention care

- Teach patient technique of double voiding. Instruct patient to urinate and sit on the toilet for 3 to 5 minutes, followed by second episode of urination. *Double voiding may relieve mild to moderate urinary retention caused by minimally compromised detrusor contractility.*

- Administer, or teach patient to self-administer, cholinergic agonist (such as bethanechol chloride) alone or in combination with alpha-antagonist, as directed, *to stimulate bladder sensations, to enhance contractility, and to reduce urethral resistance.* A cholinergic agonist is of limited therapeutic benefit for patients with compromised detrusor contractility. It is probably most helpful for patients with compromised contractility coexisting with altered sensations of bladder filling.
- Teach patient with urinary retention to perform intermittent catheterization after consultation with physician. *Intermittent catheterization provides regular, complete bladder evacuation, preventing bladder overdistention and urinary system distress.*
- Place intermittent or long-term, indwelling urethral or suprapubic catheter, as directed, *to provide chronic urinary drainage.*
- Teach patient with indwelling catheter to care for catheter and to routinely clean collection bags used for drainage of urine. *Routine cleaning of drainage bags prevents overgrowth of pathogens, reducing likelihood of symptomatic infection.*

Total incontinence care

- Assist patient in selecting and applying a urinary containment device *to minimize effects of continuous urinary leakage.*
- Provide patient with extraurethral incontinence caused by surgically created stoma with proper pouching system after consultation with the enterostomal therapy (ET) nurse.
- Prepare patient for surgical correction of fistula or urinary ectopia *to provide definitive repair of extraurethral leakage.*
- Administer, or assist physician in administering, a sclerosing agent (such as tetracycline in saline suspension) *to ablate extraurethral leakage by progressive scarring and closure of fistulous tract.*

Functional incontinence care

- Assist patient with compromised mobility to attain and use assistive devices, as indicated, *to minimize time needed to ambulate to toilet.*
- Assist patient to remove any environmental barriers *to maximize access to toilet.*
- Assist individual with compromised dexterity to alter clothing to minimize need for manipulating buttons, zippers, or similar devices, *minimizing time required to remove clothing for toileting.*
- Assist individual with compromised dexterity to obtain and use assistive devices, as indicated, *to maximize ability to manipulate clothing for toileting.*
- Begin prompted voiding program for individual with impaired cognitive ability.

NIC SKIN/WOUND MANAGEMENT

Impaired skin integrity related to urinary leakage

- Teach patient to perform routine skin care for all skin areas routinely exposed to urinary leakage. Routine care consists of daily washing, with thorough drying, and applying skin barrier or moisture barrier. Skin that is exposed to particularly severe leakage or skin affected by ammonia contact dermatitis is dried under a blow dryer turned to lowest (warm) setting for 10 to 15 minutes each day. *Routine skin care minimizes risk of altered skin integrity.*
- Apply antifungal cream to skin affected by monilial rash, as directed. *Monilial rash often compromises skin routinely exposed to urinary leakage.*

NIC PSYCHOLOGIC COMFORT PROMOTION

Disturbed body image related to biophysical change

- Teach patient that urinary incontinence is a treatable condition and that failure of one treatment strategy does not imply that leakage is "intractable" or "incurable." *Urinary incontinence is often defined as an insignificant problem that is untreatable or as an inevitable process of aging or certain surgical procedures. Avoidance of social situations and personal shame are encouraged by these misperceptions.*
- Provide patient with name and address or telephone number of continence support group, such as Help for Incontinent People, Inc (HIP). *Advocacy groups provide support, advice, and assistance for individuals learning to live with and overcome urinary incontinence.*

PATIENT EDUCATION/CONTINUUM OF CARE PLAN

1. Provide instruction on technique of medication regimens and need for continuous therapy in neuropathic bladder cases.
2. Provide list of signs and symptoms of urinary tract infection and other conditions requiring medical attention.
3. Provide instructions for intermittent catheterization technique of care of long-indwelling Foley catheter.
4. Provide instruction about relationship of incontinence to fluid intake, various medications, and compliance with medical and nursing strategies for prevention.
5. Provide information on support groups (see box on p. 957).

EVALUATION/PATIENT OUTCOMES

Elimination Management: Continence is alleviated or restored; patient experiences fewer or absence of urinary leakage episodes assessed by bladder log or weighed pad test. Normal urinary elimination patterns are restored, patient experiences diurnal voiding frequency every 2 hours or less often, nocturia limited to one to two episodes per night. Urinary residual volumes remain less than 200 ml.

Skin/Wound Management: Perineal skin integrity is maintained or restored. Patient demonstrates knowledge of preventive skin management program.

Psychologic Comfort Promotion: Patient demonstrates knowledge of national support group and nearest local support group. Patient maintains or returns to desired social activities

PATIENT ADVOCACY AND SUPPORT GROUPS FOR INCONTINENCE

National Association for Continence (NAFC)	
Executive Director:	Nancy Muller
Address:	PO Box 544 Union, South Carolina 29379
Simon Foundation For Continence	
Director:	Cheryl Gartley
Address:	PO Box 835 Wilmette, Illinois 60091

From Gray.[61]

(e.g., community or church activities, recreational or sporting activities). Body image is intact.

PROSTATE DISORDERS

Benign Prostatic Hyperplasia

Benign prostatic hyperplasia (BPH) is the progressive enlargement of the prostate gland. The symptoms of BPH are caused by bladder outlet obstruction and its sequelae. In the majority of males, BPH is a quality of life disorder. In unusual cases, BPH produces a significant obstructive uropathy and compromised renal function.[3]

BPH is the most common neoplastic growth in men past the fifth decade of life.[70,76] Histologic evidence of BPH can be found in men as young as 25 to 30 years of age, and its incidence increases steadily, affecting 50% of men over age 60 years, and 90% of men 85 years and older. The prevalence of symptomatic BPH is not known, partially due to differences in evaluation of the symptoms that constitute the condition. In one study combining digital rectal examination and a symptom score,[50] the prevalence of symptomatic BPH was 138/100,000 among men in their fifties, and 400 per 100,000 among octogenarians.

No risk factors for BPH have been identified.[172,179] Sexual activity (or celibacy), cigarette smoking, alcohol use, or social factors have not been associated with an increased incidence in the development of BPH. A congenital absence of androgens, or the enzyme needed to convert testosterone to dihydrotestosterone, prevents normal prostate development and subsequent BPH.[165] Orchiectomy also prevents normal prostate development and BPH, and diabetes mellitus may or may not reduce the risk of prostatic enlargement.

Serious complications or death due to BPH are rare. The incidence of significant renal insufficiency is low, as is the presence of urinary infection or bladder calculi. The mortality rate directly attributable to BPH is approximately 1.8 per 100,000.[3] There is no clear relationship between BPH and prostate cancer.[56] Nonetheless, an increased risk for prostate cancer has been reported among men with BPH,[10] although this relationship may be limited to "atypical patterns" of hyperplasia, rather than classic, benign prostatic enlargement.[55]

As the number of elderly men living in the United States continues to grow, so will the prevalence of BPH. Approximately 1 in 4 men with symptoms of BPH will seek relief by the age of 80 years. More than 300,000 procedures are performed each year for BPH, and the condition produces an annual cost of approximately $4.5 billion.[2,77]

Pathophysiology

The etiology and natural history of BPH remain unclear, although significant progress has been made in understanding certain elements of the pathogenesis of prostate enlargement.[165] Prostatic hyperplasia is influenced by the presence of the hormones testosterone and dihydrotestosterone. The prerequisites for prostatic enlargement are aging, androgen receptors, and a functioning testis capable of producing testosterone for conversion to dihydrotestosterone. Luteinizing hormone is released from the hypothalamus and acts on Leydig's cells to produce testosterone. Ninety-five percent of testosterone is produced by the testes; 5% arises from the adrenal glands.

The majority of testosterone produced by the testes and adrenals is bound to an androgen-binding protein in the serum and remains physiologically inactive. A small portion of circulating testosterone (approximately 2%), however, remains unbound and can be converted to dihydrotestosterone by the prostate. An enzyme, 5α-reductase, is required to convert testosterone to dihydrotestosterone. After diffusing into the prostate, testosterone is converted into dihydrotestosterone by this enzyme, resulting in release of local growth factors and proliferation of prostatic tissue. Testosterone ablation or inhibition of 5α-reductase will arrest prostatic hyperplasia and reduce the size of the prostate gland.[165]

Nonetheless, the actions of the androgens testosterone and dihydrotestosterone and the enzyme 5α-reductase, alone, do not explain the association of BPH with aging.[174] In the aging male, the serum concentrations of both bioavailable and bound testosterone is diminished, and these effects would be expected to hinder, rather than produce, hyperplasia of the prostatic stroma. The relation between prostatic hyperplasia and aging is partly explained by an increase in nuclear androgen receptors that compensates for the reduction in circulating androgens. In addition, other local factors, including epidermal growth factor, insulin growth factor, basic fibroblast growth factor, and nerve growth factor, influence prostatic hyperplasia by mechanisms that have not yet been defined.[165]

It is the presence of voiding dysfunction, rather than enlargement of the prostate gland per se, that causes men to seek treatment. The voiding dysfunction associated with BPH is divided into two symptom types, obstructive and irritative. Obstructive voiding symptoms related to BPH include a slow or intermittent urinary stream, hesitancy when initiating urination, postvoid dribbling, and feelings of incomplete bladder evacuation. Irritative voiding symptoms include the urgency to urinate, frequency of urination, and nocturia.[2,165]

The initial symptoms of BPH are primarily obstructive and include a slowing of the urinary stream, hesitancy to initiate urination, and a postvoid dribbling. This effect is partly explained by a reduction in the cross-sectional area of the urethra as it passes through the prostate. Obstruction of the bladder outlet also arises from increased smooth muscle tone at the prostate and bladder neck, causing poor funneling of the proximal urethra during micturition. This smooth muscle of the prostate and proximal urethra is richly innervated by alpha-receptors, and alpha antagonistic drugs partially block this tone. During the early stages of BPH, the detrusor muscle hypertrophies and the symptoms of BPH may subside. If the magnitude of bladder outlet obstruction increases, however, compensatory hypertrophy of the detrusor also causes trabeculation of the detrusor muscle, diverticulae, and hypertrophy of the trigone.[157,172]

When the hyperplasia of BPH progresses, obstructive symptoms are exacerbated, and the person is prone to episodes of acute urinary retention. Acute urinary retention is characterized by the inability to urinate. It is a relatively common complication of BPH, occurring in as many as 54% of a group of British men undergoing treatment for prostate enlargement. Acute urinary retention is a medical emergency and potent incentive for prompt management of prostatic hyperplasia.

The pathophysiology of the irritative symptoms associated with BPH is less well defined than the obstructive symptoms. The hypertrophic detrusor muscle may be more sensitive to the neurotransmitters responsible for bladder contraction, or the process of chronic obstruction may cause changes in the function of the sensory nerves of the bladder. Sensory nerve enlargement of the bladder had been noted in experimental studies of animal models and humans, and stimulation of nerve growth factor caused by obstruction may contribute to these neurologic changes in the bladder muscle.[165]

In some patients with BPH, irritative voiding symptoms may be related to unstable detrusor contractions. Denervation changes in the neuromuscular units of the detrusor muscle oc-

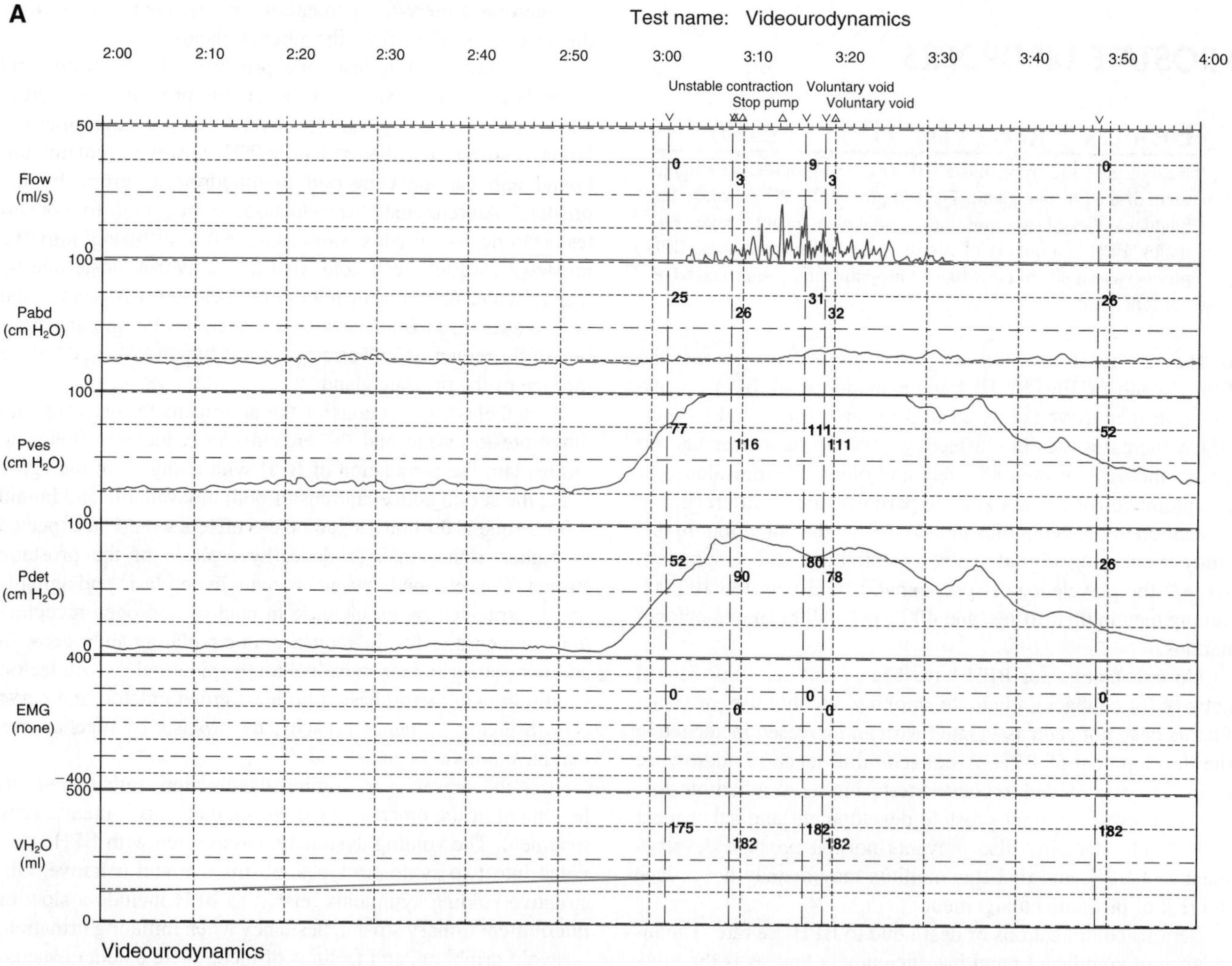

FIG. 14-14

Voiding pressure study of prostatic outlet obstruction. **A,** Urodynamic tracing demonstrates high voiding pressure (maximum detrusor contraction pressure [Pdet] is 96 cm H_2O, but maximum flow is only 9 ml/sec). **B,** Abrams-Griffith nomogram comparing detrusor contraction pressure (Pdet on Y axis) versus flow rate (flow on X axis) is consistent with bladder outlet obstruction. **C,** Fluoroscopic image with real-time tracing shows high detrusor contraction pressure, with diminished flow. Note incomplete funneling of the bladder neck, poor filling of the prostatic urethra, and trabeculation of the bladder, indicating significant obstruction.

Continued

cur with obstruction, and there is some evidence that these changes cause hyperactive (unstable) contractions of the bladder. An unstable contraction in a man with bladder outlet obstruction and BPH is likely to cause an immediate urgency to urinate, frequency of urination, and nocturia. Nonetheless, because of the obstruction, the man is unlikely to experience urge incontinence. Rather, he is likely to experience the irritative symptoms (urgency, frequency, and nocturia) of BPH, as well as obstructive symptoms.

In some patients, severe, prolonged obstruction may lead to decompensation of detrusor muscle contraction strength. The bladder wall becomes increasingly noncompliant, and detrusor contractions become less efficient, causing larger postvoid urinary residual volumes, a high risk of urinary infection, vesicoureteral reflux, or compromised renal function.[157] Fortunately, these cases of severe obstruction and upper urinary tract decompensation are uncommon, and BPH remains primarily a disorder that affects the quality of life.

Diagnostic Studies and Findings

Prostate-specific antigen: Abnormally high values raise suspicion of prostate cancer

Serum creatinine: Abnormally high values indicate compromised renal function or renal failure

Urinalysis/urine culture and sensitivity: Nitrites and white blood cells on dipstick and white blood cells and bacteriuria and pyuria on microscopic examination raise suspicion of urinary tract infection; a urine culture is obtained when urinalysis raises suspicion of urinary tract infection

Uroflowmetry: Identifies abnormal voiding patterns; diminished maximum and mean flow rate indicate the possibility of bladder outlet obstruction; the uroflow does not differentiate abnormal flow caused by poor detrusor contraction strength from abnormal flow caused by obstruction

Pressure-flow study: Provides the best evaluation of bladder outlet obstruction; diminished maximum and mean flow rate with elevated intravesical voiding pressures indicate bladder outlet obstruction; results from a voiding pressure study may be plotted on one or more voiding pressure nomograms, allowing comparison with age-matched males with and without symptomatic BPH (Fig. 14-14)

Postvoid residual volume: Elevated postvoid residual volume is not diagnostic of BPH, but larger volumes may indicate a greater need for treatment, and reduction in residual volumes can be used to determine the effects of treatment[3]

Intravenous pyelogram: Not recommended for routine evaluation of BPH; occasionally helpful when prostatism is complicated by hematuria, calculi, urinary tract infection

Cystoscopy: Not indicated for routine evaluation of BPH, or to determine the need for treatment; used as an adjunctive modality during invasive endoscopic procedures (e.g., transurethral resection of the prostate gland)

Transrectal ultrasound of the prostate: Not indicated for the routine evaluation of BPH; used as an adjunctive modality to define the anatomy of BPH; presence of potentially malignant tumors, cysts, or other unexpected anatomic findings (Fig. 14-15)

B

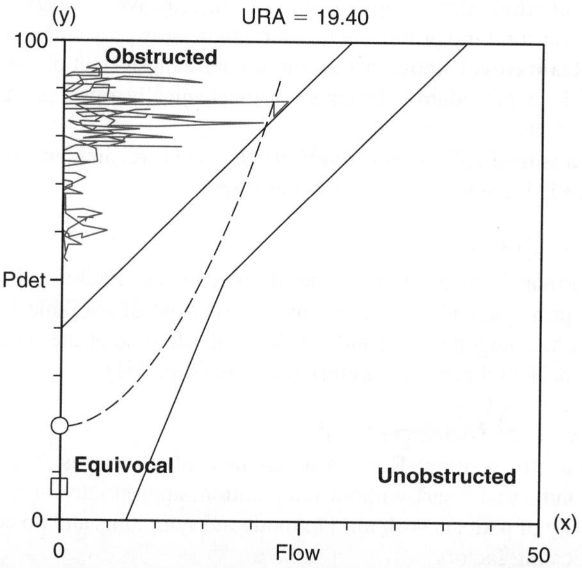

C

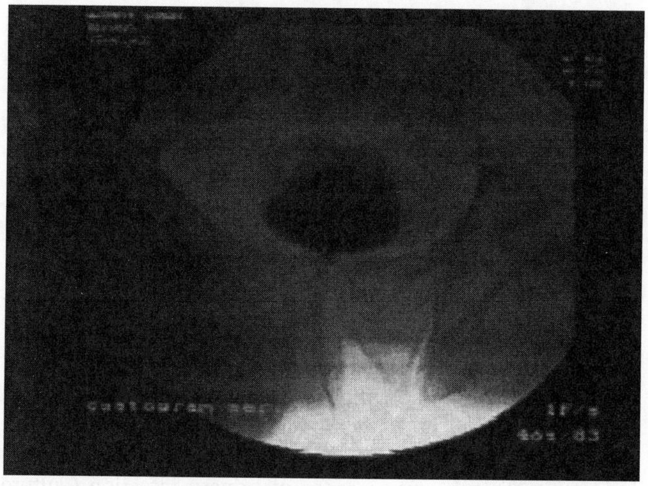

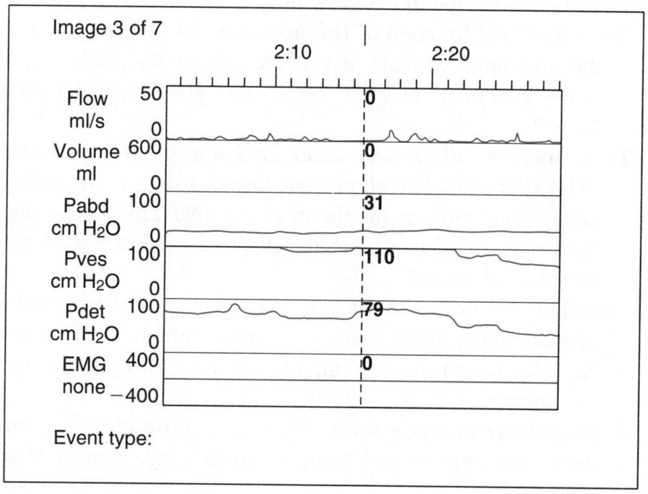

Fig. 14-14, cont'd
For legend see previous page.

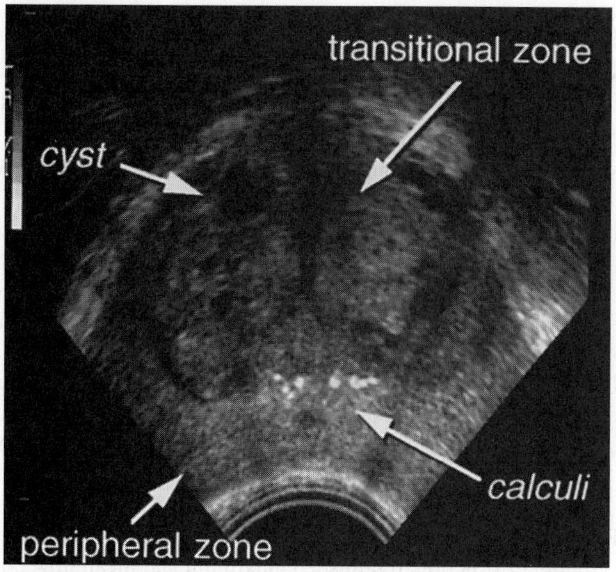

FIG. 14-15
Ultrasonic image of the prostate demonstrating BPH. Note that the transitional zone has become enlarged and is detectable on this image, as in the peripheral zone. A cyst and prostatic calculi also are indicated.

MULTIDISCIPLINARY PLAN

(See Table 14-11 on pp. 984-985)

Surgery and Transurethral Procedures

Open prostatectomy: Removal of the prostate from a suprapubic approach; the prostatic capsule is left intact; typically reserved for severe enlargement (glands larger than 60 to 80 g)

Transurethral prostatic resection (TURP): Resection of prostatic tissue under endoscopic control; the outcomes for TURP are considered the "gold standard" for prostatectomy; the efficacy of all other modalities are compared with this technique

Transurethral vaportrobe: Ablation of prostatic tissue using a "roller ball" type of device with electrocautery energy.

Transurethral incision of the prostate (TUIP): Incision of the prostatic capsule using electrocautery endoscopic knife; generally reserved for prostate glands smaller than 40 g[165]

Transurethral ultrasonic laser incision of the prostate (TULIP): Ablation of prostate tissue using a side-firing neodymium:yttrium-aluminum-garnet (Nd:YAG) laser and ultrasonic imaging to ensure adequate penetration of the prostatic adenoma[23]

Visual laser ablation of the prostate (VLAP): Ablation of the prostate under direct endoscopic visualization. A side-firing Nd:YAG laser is used to provide the energy for prostate tissue ablation.[23]

Contact laser prostatectomy: Ablation of prostatic tissue under endoscopic control using a direct-firing, contact laser fiber

Interstitial laser therapy: Application of laser energy into the prostate without interrupting the integrity of the urothelium; the energy is applied via transrectal, transperineal, or transurethral routes

Transurethral ultrasonic aspiration: Application of ultrasonic energy fragmenting tissues high in water content (such as the prostate) while preserving tissues with greater collagen content (such as the bladder neck and membranous urethra) followed by aspiration of the fragmented tissue[165]

Transurethral needle ablation (TUNA): Application of radiofrequency energy (of lower level than laser energy) capable of ablating prostate tissue; the procedure is performed using a 22 French catheter and 2-cm needles with special shields to protect urethral and rectal tissues; the procedure is performed under endoscopic visualization and using ultrasonic imaging to determine the depth of needle placement[29]

High-intensity focused ultrasonography (HIFU): Ablation of prostate tissue using focused ultrasonic energy applied via a transrectal probe surrounded by a condom and degassed water[21]

Cryotherapy: Rapid cooling/freezing of prostatic tissue via a transurethral route; more commonly used for prostate cancer[165]

Hyperthermia: Application of microwave energy via transurethral or transrectal routes to destroy prostate tissue[101]

Intraurethral stent: Placement of a wire mesh stent under endoscopic control designed to mechanically open prostatic urethra[61]

Transurethral balloon dilation: No longer recommended for BPH due to poor long-term efficacy[49]

Medications

Hormonal agents: Finasteride, a 5α-reductase inhibitor, is the principal endocrine agent used to manage BPH (Table 14-6)

Alpha antagonists: Reduce smooth muscle tone at the bladder neck and prostatic urethra (see box on p. 961)

General Management

Watchful waiting: Routine assessment of symptoms (every 6 months to 1 year) without intervention; appropriate for a majority of patients with mild to moderate symptoms and no complicating factors

NURSING CARE

NURSING ASSESSMENT

Minimum Evaluation of BPH[3]

History: Including duration of symptoms, patterns of urine elimination, episodes of acute urinary retention, previous prostate evaluation; **all** patients should complete an International Prostate Symptom Score (see box on p. 961); a voiding diary/bladder log is strongly recommended

Physical examination: Including digital rectal examination for prostate size, symmetry between lateral lobes, evidence of induration, discrete nodules

Serum prostate-specific antigen (optional): To determine need for further evaluation for prostate cancer

Serum creatinine: To assess renal function

Urinalysis: To rule out presence of urinary infection (culture and sensitivity obtained only when history, physical assessment, and/or urinalysis raises index of suspicion)

Table 14-6 Hormonal Agents Used to Treat Benign Prostatic Hyperplasia

Agent	Pharmacologic Action	Side Effects
Antiandrogen agents: Flutamide, Casodex	Selectively block androgenic receptors	Gastrointestinal upset, impaired libido (uncommon), erectile dysfunction, gynecomastia
Progestins: Megestrol acetate, hydroxyprogesterone caproate	Inhibits production of leutinizing hormone, production of testosterone, dihydrotesterone	Gastrointestinal upset, heat intolerance, flushing, reduced libido, erectile dysfunction
5α-Reductase enzyme inhibitors: Finasteride	Inhibits conversion of testosterone to dihydrotestosterone without reduction in serum levels of testosterone	Loss of libido, erectile dysfunction (rare), gynecomastia (uncommon), decreased ejaculatory volume

Data from Grayhack and Kozlowski.[66]

ALPHA-ADRENERGIC BLOCKERS USED TO TREAT BPH

Agents

Nonselective alpha-adrenergic blockers (block $alpha_1$- and $alpha_2$-adrenergic receptors):
- Phenoxybenzamine, 5-10 mg PO bid

Short acting, selective $alpha_1$-adrenergic blockers:
- Prazosin, 1-5 mg PO bid

Long acting, selective $alpha_1$-adrenergic blockers:
- Terazosin, 1-10 mg PO daily (HS)
- Doxazosin, 1-12 mg PO daily (HS)
- Tamsulosin, 0.4 mg daily

Pharmacologic Action

Phenoxybenzamine blocks $alpha_1$- and $alpha_2$-adrenergic receptors in the bladder neck, prostatic urethra, and distant sites; all other agents selectively block $alpha_1$-adrenergic receptors in the bladder neck, prostatic urethra, and other sites

Side Effects

General: Postural hypotension, tachycardia, drowsiness, prolonged fatigue, rhinitis, flulike syndrome

Specific: Postural hypotension associated with prazosin administration may be intensified with hyponatremia, the therapeutic dosage range of alfuzosin for BPH has not been established

From Lepor.[105]

INTERNATIONAL PROSTATE SYMPTOM SCORE

Voiding Dysfunction Items:

1. Over the past month, how often have you had a sensation of not emptying your bladder completely after you finished urinating?
2. Over the past month, have you had to urinate again less than 2 hours after you finished urinating?
3. Over the past month, how often have you found you stopped and started again several times when you urinated?
4. Over the past month, how often have you found it difficult to postpone urination?
5. Over the past month, how often have you had a weak urinary stream?
6. Over the past month, how often have you had to push or strain to begin urination?

These questions are answered on a Likert type of scale of 0-5; a response of 0 indicates not at all, 1 indicates less than 1 time in 5; 2 indicates less than half of the time, 3 indicates about half of the time, 4 indicates more than half of the time, and 5 indicates almost always

7. Over the past month, how many times did you most typically get up to urinate from the time you went to bed at night until the time you got up in the morning?

This item is answered on a scale of 0-5; 0 indicates no episodes of nocturia, and 5 indicates 5 episodes or more each night

Quality of Life Item

If you were to spend the rest of your life with your urinary condition just the way it is now, how would you feel about that?

This item is answered on a scale of 0-6; 0 indicates that the respondent would be delighted with his condition and 6 indicates that the person would feel terrible about his condition

From AHCPR Guideline.[3]

Patient Problems/Nursing Diagnoses & Interventions

NIC Elimination Management

Urinary retention related to BPH

Impaired urinary elimination, related to bladder outlet obstruction

Risk for infection related to urinary stasis

- Teach patient the signs and symptoms of acute urinary retention. *Acute urinary retention is a common complication of BPH and constitutes a medical emergency.*
- Advise patient of risk factors for acute urinary retention, including over-the-counter decongestants or diet pills, prescription antidepressants, anticholinergics, calcium channel blockers, antispasmodics, antiparkinsonian agents, and antipsychotics. *Decongestants and diet pills contain an alpha-adrenergic agonist that creates a risk of acute urinary retention by increasing smooth muscle tone of prostate, bladder neck, and proximal urethra. Other agents listed increase risk of acute urinary retention by relaxing detrusor muscle contractions.*
- Instruct man with BPH to drink no more than 8 to 12 ounces with meals, to sip beverages throughout the day, and to avoid intake of large amounts of fluid over a short period of time. *Intake of large bolus of fluid over brief period of time will rapidly fill bladder and increase risk of an episode of acute urinary retention.*
- Advise patient to warm up before attempting to urinate. *Micturition is more difficult when body is coping with cold weather.*

- Advise patient who is unable to urinate despite repeated attempts to drink a cup of warm tea or coffee and to attempt urination while sitting in tub of warm water or while showering under warm water. Instruct patient to ensure privacy while attempting to void and to urinate while in tub or shower, rather than attempting to transfer to toilet. *Drinking warm coffee or tea acts as a mild bladder irritant, increasing desire to void. A warm sitz bath or tub bath assists patient in relaxing pelvic muscles and voiding. Transferring to toilet is avoided because this action may jeopardize attempts at toileting.*
- Counsel patient who remains unable to void after 6 to 8 hours of attempts to seek immediate care from his primary health-care provider, immediate care center, urologist, or local hospital emergency department. *Acute urinary retention is a medical emergency, requiring prompt care to avoid bladder rupture and subsequent infection.*
- Teach patient with significant postvoiding urinary residual volumes (typically greater than 100 ml or 25% of bladder capacity) to double void by urinating, resting on toilet for 2 to 3 minutes, and voiding again. *Double voiding may promote more complete bladder evacuation.*
- Teach patient to perform intermittent self-catheterization as directed. Role for self-catheterization in men with BPH is limited, primarily because of technical difficulties inserting catheter past significantly enlarged prostate. *Nonetheless, self-catheterization is sometimes used as a temporary measure to ensure regular, complete bladder evacuation until more definitive treatment can be completed.*
- Insert indwelling catheter as directed. *An indwelling catheter provides continuous urinary drainage for individual who has experienced acute urinary retention.* It is considered a temporary measure before definitive management of prostatic obstruction.
- Teach patient to self-administer medications to reduce obstruction associated with BPH as directed. Alpha-adrenergic blockers or 5α-reductase enzyme inhibitors are used to inhibit smooth muscle tone at bladder outlet or reduce prostate size, respectively. *Both agents reduce chronic obstruction and urinary retention associated with BPH and resulting risk of acute urinary retention.*
- Prepare patient for prostatectomy as directed. Consult physician concerning method of prostate tissue removal for this patient. Multiple methods of prostate tissue removal are used to relieve the symptoms of BPH. (See Table 14-11, pp. 984-985).

Bladder outlet obstruction care

- Teach patient with mild to moderate symptoms of BPH a fluid management program, emphasizing adequate intake of fluid (30 ml/kg of body weight per day). *Avoiding fluids will concentrate the urine, exacerbating irritative voiding symptoms.*
- Instruct man with symptoms of BPH to avoid or limit intake of caffeinic beverages, alcoholic drinks, coffee, tea, aspartame, chocolates, or spicy foods. *The substances act as mild bladder irritants, increasing irritative symptoms of BPH.*
- Teach patient with chronic urinary retention to perform intermittent catheterization as directed. Intermittent catheterization has a limited role in BPH, primarily due to technical difficulties catheterizing man with significant BPH and risk for infection and bleeding with difficult catheterization. *Nonetheless, it may be used as a temporary measure to alleviate significant urinary retention in select patients.*
- Teach patient the signs and symptoms of urinary tract infection and pyelonephritis. Advise him to promptly seek care if urinary tract infection occurs. *Although rare, significant urinary tract infection can occur in patient with BPH and retention of urine.*

PATIENT EDUCATION/CONTINUUM OF CARE PLAN

1. Teach patient to self-administer alpha-adrenergic antagonists, including dosage, administration, and special considerations when taking these medications for relief of symptoms of BPH.
2. Teach patient to self-administer finasteride, including dosage, administration, and side effects.
3. Assist patient who elects watchful waiting to design program of routine evaluation in consultation with physician. Emphasize importance of follow-up care for this evolving condition.
4. Assist patient who elects invasive removal of prostate tissue with schedule for routine follow-up evaluation. Remind patient that benign prostate tissue may recur over a period of years, necessitating reevaluation and, possibly, repeated treatment.
5. Counsel person undergoing treatment for BPH to schedule routine follow-up evaluation of prostate, including digital rectal examination and prostate-specific antigen test for prostate cancer.

EVALUATION/PATIENT OUTCOMES

Elimination Management: Acute urinary retention is prevented or promptly managed. Patterns of urine elimination are alleviated; reported diurnal frequency returns to every 2 hours or less often, nocturia is reduced to two episodes or less. Lower urinary tract symptoms as evaluation by the International Prostate Symptom Score are reduced by at last 2 to 3 points.

PROSTATITIS

Prostatitis is the inflammation of prostatic acini and surrounding tissue that is particularly pronounced in the periurethral portion of the gland.

Inflammation of the prostate is commonly divided into four types: acute bacterial, chronic bacterial, nonbacterial, and prostatodynia. Each form of prostatitis has a distinctive clinical presentation and is managed differently.[161]

Prostatitis is most commonly observed in males after the onset of pubescence, but rare cases of the disease have been reported among children and infants. Nonbacterial prostatitis (also named prostatosis) is the most common form of the disease. Acute and chronic bacterial prostatitis is less commonly seen. Rarer forms include viral, fungal, parasitic, and allergic prostatitis.[78]

PATHOPHYSIOLOGY

Acute bacterial prostatitis is caused by the ascent of bacteria via the urethra or the hematogenous route. Acute infection may be precipitated by urethral instrumentation or prostatic massage in the presence of chronic bacterial prostatitis. Common causative pathogens include *E. coli, Proteus, Klebsiella, Pseudomonas,* and *Enterobacter.* An acute episode of prostatic infection is characterized by a sudden onset of fever, chills, myalgia, arthralgia, and general malaise. These symptoms rapidly progress to localized discomfort in the perineal area or low back associated with irritative voiding symptoms, including urgency, frequency, nocturia, dysuria, and a persistent burning sensation in the urethra after micturition. Pain in the prostate results in varying degrees of functional bladder outlet obstruction that may cause significant urinary hesitancy or even acute urinary obstruction.[79,173]

Histologic examination of prostatic tissue will reveal diffuse glandular inflammation with edema and hyperemia of the stroma. Abscesses are common and may hemorrhage in severe cases. Polymorphonucleocytes, bacteria, and cellular debris are present within the acini of the gland. Rectal palpation of the prostate reveals an exquisitely tender organ. Vigorous massage is contraindicated because of the associated pain and the danger of bacteremia. Acute bacterial cystitis is typically associated so that urine culture provides an excellent clue to the causative prostatic pathogen. An objective diagnosis of acute bacterial prostatitis is made in the presence of evidence of inflammation on expressed prostatic secretions (over 10 leukocytes per high-power field), positive bacterial culture of this expressed prostatic secretion, positive bacterial cystitis, and an abnormal rectal examination.[79,173]

Chronic bacterial prostatitis commonly occurs as a result of ascending infection from the urethra. The condition may arise following an inadequately treated episode of acute bacterial prostatitis, or it may occur via hematogenous arterial invasion. However, the precise etiology of chronic bacterial prostatitis remains unclear.[158]

The clinical symptoms of chronic bacterial prostatitis vary widely. Some men have no symptoms of prostatitis other than recurrent urinary tract infections or asymptomatic bacteriuria. More commonly, men with prostatitis note recurring irritative voiding symptoms such as urgency, frequency, dysuria, nocturia, and urethral irritation. Perineal pain, postejaculatory pain, hematospermia, and a mucoid urethral discharge may also be noted.[55,173]

Rectal palpation of the prostate may reveal the presence of prostatic calculi or may be unremarkable. Histologic examination of the prostate shows moderate inflammatory changes that are less localized than in acute infections. Objective diagnosis of chronic bacterial prostatitis requires the presence of inflammatory cells on microscopic examination of expressed secretions, a positive culture of these secretions, and a nontender gland on rectal examination.[55,173]

Unlike acute bacterial prostatitis, the chronically infected prostate is relatively resistant to antibiotic treatment because of the poor absorption of non–lipid-soluble substances into the prostatic fluid. The chronically infected prostate has deficient levels of prostatic antibacterial substance. Prostatic calculi may also lower antibiotic susceptibility by serving as a nidus for persistent infection. Thus even extended periods of oral antibiotics may not cure chronic bacterial prostatitis.[55,173]

Nonbacterial prostatitis is the most common form of symptomatic prostatic inflammation. Although the causative agent of nonbacterial prostatitis has not been identified, *Chlamydia* has been implicated as a possible pathogen. Unfortunately, cultures are difficult to obtain, so verification of this suspicion requires further investigation.[42]

Nonbacterial prostatitis is an idiopathic inflammation of the prostate. Its symptoms are similar to those of chronic, bacterial prostatitis, and they include perineal discomfort and lower urinary symptoms such as hesitancy, poor force of urinary stream, intermittency, and urgency. Diagnosis requires objective documentation of past UTI or evidence of inflammatory cells obtained by expressed prostatic secretion. Some authors have advocated combining this diagnosis with that of prostatodynia,[123] but newer insights into these syndromes suggest differing etiologies and treatments.[110,186] Specifically, patients with true nonbacterial prostatitis may be successfully managed with antibiotic therapy, whereas those without objective evidence of infection should not be diagnosed as having nonbacterial prostatitis, nor are they likely to benefit from antibiotic therapy.

The term *prostatodynia* has been used to describe men who experience perineal discomfort, as well as lower urinary tract and/or ejaculatory symptoms.[110] The pain associated with prostatodynia is usually localized to the perineum and lower abdomen. In addition, these men may complain of discomfort in the testes or the tip of the penis. The pain is typically characterized as burning, and it may be transiently exacerbated by urination, ejaculation, physical exertion, or fatigue. Lower urinary tract symptoms associated with prostatodynia include dysuria, diurnal frequency, nocturia, urgency, poor force of urinary stream, intermittency, and feelings of incomplete bladder emptying. Ejaculatory symptoms include discomfort during or following ejaculation.

Prostatodynia is an ill-defined and poorly understood condition. It is often misdiagnosed as prostatitis, and as many as one third of men are treated with antibiotics, usually without success.[32a] Although the etiology remains unclear, a growing body of evidence suggests that pelvic floor dysfunction rather than an inflammation is the underlying cause of the perineal discomfort and the voiding and ejaculatory dysfunction associated with prostatodynia.[186]

Other forms of prostatitis occur rarely and include viral prostatic inflammation following an upper respiratory infection, tubercular prostatitis, or mycotic prostatitis from blastomycosis, coccidioidomycosis, histoplasmosis, and candidiasis. Symptoms are similar to bacterial prostatitis with the presence of perineal area pain and inflammation of the prostate associated with irritative voiding symptoms.[173]

Complications of prostatitis include acute urinary retention, bladder neck contracture, and obstruction in the presence of chronic inflammation. Cystitis is typically associated with the condition, and epididymitis is not uncommon. Pyelonephritis and bacteremia may be associated with acute infection.[42,173]

DIAGNOSTIC STUDIES AND FINDINGS

Urine tests: Examination of the urine is recommended using a "three-glass" technique; the patient is asked to void 10 to 15

Table 14-7 Laboratory Findings in Prostatitis

Prostatitis Type	Urine Culture (Midstream Collection)	Expressed Prostatic Secretion (EPS) Findings
Acute bacterial prostatitis	Positive for UTI (pathogen consistent with that affecting prostate)	Typically deferred because of risk of systemic spread
Chronic, bacterial prostatitis	Positive for UTI	WBC, bacteria
Chronic nonbacterial prostatitis	Negative	WBC, no bacteria
Prostatodynia	Negative	Negative

ml in a cup and switch to a second cup, without interrupting the stream, in which he will collect 2 to 3 ounces (midstream specimen); the patient is cautioned not to squeeze out the last several drops; the prostate is then gently milked or massaged to obtain expressed prostatic secretions (EPS); the midstream urine and the EPS are analyzed to establish an accurate diagnosis; Table 14-7 lists the urine and EPS findings characteristic of the various types of prostatitis

Semen examination: Less accurate than EPS testing; semen may be analyzed for WBC and cultured

Blood tests: Blood cultures may be obtained in patients with acute systemic sepsis related to acute bacterial prostatitis

Symptom score: The NIH Chronic Prostatitis Symptom Index should be administered to men with chronic nonbacterial prostatitis or prostatodynia (FIG. 14-16)

Pelvic muscle EMG: Increased baseline tone in cases of prostatodynia (typically combined with biofeedback-assisted pelvic muscle reeducation)

Urodynamics: Completed to exclude other conditions with similar symptoms such as bladder neck dyssynergia, detrusor sphincter dyssynergia

MULTIDISCIPLINARY MANAGEMENT

Acute Bacterial Prostatitis

Medications

Antiinfective agents to eradicate prostatic infection; dual-agent broad-spectrum antibiotics covering gram-positive and gram-negative pathogens (such as ampicillin and gentamycin) may be administered parenterally in severe cases; sensitivity-guided parenteral antiinfective drugs are administered based on results of urine culture, or possibly EPS or blood culture; parenteral agents are generally administered until the patient remains afebrile for 48 hours

Oral medications of choice for acute bacterial prostatitis include the fluoroquinolones (ciprofloxacin, enoxacin, norfloxacin, or ofloxacin) and trimethoprim-sulfamethoxazole[123]; they may be administered initially in patients with mild to moderate cases of acute bacterial prostatitis, or they may be given after initial parenteral therapy; they should be administered for 30 days

Antipyretics may be administered as indicated for infection and antiemetics for nausea

Narcotic analgesics may be required for pain control during the early stages of the disease

General Management

Urethral instrumentation (catheterization) should be avoided; a suprapubic catheter should be placed if acute urinary retention occurs[107,173]

Chronic Bacterial Prostatitis

Surgery

Transurethral resection of infected prostatic tissue may relieve symptoms in certain cases; particularly if prostatic calculi serve as a focus for infection[122]

Medications

Sensitivity-guided antiinfective therapy determined by culture of urine and EPS; oral medications for chronic bacterial prostatitis must be selected that are able to penetrate the fatty fluid contained in the acini of the prostate; they include the fluoroquinolones (ciprofloxacin, enoxacin, norfloxacin, or ofloxacin) and trimethoprim-sulfamethoxazole given over a 30- to 120-day period[123]

Nonsteroidal antiinflammatory drugs are the analgesic of choice for the discomfort associated with chronic bacterial prostatitis

Intraprostatic injection of antibiotics[182,183] or antibiotics combined with xylocaine[118] may provide relief from chronic bacterial prostatitis in selected patients

General Management

Alcohol intake often exacerbates the discomfort associated with chronic bacterial prostatitis; intake should be limited to 2 to 3 ounces per day or eliminated from the diet all together

Foods that contain chili powder, curry, or other "hot" spices may exacerbate the discomfort associated with prostatitis; they should be individually eliminated from the diet to determine their effect on the patient's symptoms

Nonbacterial Prostatitis

Medications

Empiric pharmacotherapy using fluoroquinolones or trimethoprim-sulfamethoxazole is administered *only* to patients with evidence of prior UTI and significant WBCs in the EPS; otherwise, they should be classified as prostatodynia and treated accordingly[123]; doxycycline or trimethoprim-sulfamethoxazole may be administered for a 1-week trial

Prostatodynia

Medications

Antiinfective agents are generally *not* indicated in these patients unless there is specific evidence of prostatic infection reflected in urine or EPS analysis

Alpha-adrenergic blocking agents (doxazosin, terazosin, tamsulosin) may be administered to reduce urethral outlet resistance and associated lower urinary tract symptoms[14];

Pain or Discomfort

1. In the last week, have you experienced any pain or discomfort in the following areas?
   a. Area between rectum and testicles (perineum)
      Yes (1) No (0)
   b. Testicles
      Yes (1) No (0)
   c. Tip of penis (not related to urination)
      Yes (1) No (0)
   d. Below your waist, in your pubic or bladder area
      Yes (1) No (0)
2. In the last week have you experienced:
   a. Pain or burning during urination?
      Yes (1) No (0)
   b. Pain or discomfort during or after sexual climax (ejaculation)?
3. How often have you had pain or discomfort in any of these areas over the last week?
   Never (1)
   Rarely (2)
   Sometimes (3)
   Often (4)
   Usually (5)
   Always (6)
4. Which number best describes your AVERAGE pain or discomfort on the days that you had it, over the last week?
   ←(1) (2) (3) (4) (5) (6) (7) (8) (9) (10)→
   NO PAIN — PAIN AS BAD AS YOU CAN IMAGINE

Urination

5. How often have you had a sensation of not emptying your bladder completely after you finished urinating, over the last week?
   Not at all (0)
   Less than one time in five (1)
   Less than half the time (2)
   About half the time (3)
   More than half the time (4)
   Almost always (5)
6. How often have you had to urinate again less than 2 hours after you finished urinating, over the last week?
   Not at all (0)
   Less than one time in five (1)
   Less than half the time (2)
   About half the time (3)
   More than half the time (4)
   Almost always (5)

Impact of Symptoms

7. How much have your symptoms kept you from doing the things you usually do, over the last week?
   None (0)
   Only a little (1)
   Some (2)
   A lot (3)
8. How much did you think about your symptoms over the last week?
   None (0)
   Only a little (1)
   Some (2)
   A lot (3)

Quality of Life

9. If you were to spend the rest of your life with your symptoms just the way they have been during the last week, how would you feel about that?
   Delighted (0)
   Pleased (1)
   Mostly satisfied (2)
   Mixed (about equally satisfied and dissatisfied) (3)
   Mostly dissatisfied (4)
   Unhappy (5)
   Terrible (6)

Scoring:
PAIN SUBSCALE: Total items 1-4
URINARY SYMPTOMS: Total items 5 and 6
QUALITY OF LIFE: Total items 7-9

FIG. 14-16
NIH Chronic Prostatitis Symptom Index.

higher dosages are frequently needed to obtain significant symptom relief[123] (refer to BPH discussion, p. 957)

General Management

Patients should be referred to a continence nurse specialist, continence nurse practitioner or other health-care provider for pelvic floor muscle training

Transrectal electrical stimulation may provide relief for the discomfort associated with prostatodynia

Alcohol intake often exacerbates the discomfort associated with prostatodynia; intake should be limited to 2 to 3 ounces per day or eliminated from the diet all together

Foods that contain chili powder, curry, or other "hot" spices may exacerbate the discomfort associated with prostatodynia; highly spiced foods should be individually eliminated from the diet to determine their effect on the patient's symptoms

NURSING CARE

NURSING ASSESSMENT

Prostate

Acute bacterial prostatitis: Digital rectal examination (DRE) contraindicated

Chronic bacterial prostatitis/nonbacterial prostatitis: Enlarged, firm gland, moderately to extremely tender to palpation

Prostatodynia: Discomfort associated with insertion of finger beyond hypertonic anal sphincter; generalized tenderness includes prostate

Pain: Location: perineal pain (52%), testicular (40%), tip of penis (42%); suprapubic (56%)[110]; usually described as burning with moderate intensity

Voiding symptoms: Urgency, diurnal frequency, nocturia, hesitancy, poor force of stream, intermittency of stream, feelings of incomplete emptying, dysuria

Ejaculatory symptoms: Pain with or following ejaculation, difficulty achieving ejaculation
Bowel elimination symptoms: Constipation, discomfort when straining for bowel movement

Patient Problems/Nursing Diagnoses & Interventions

NIC Physical Comfort Promotion

Pain related to prostatic inflammation

- Teach nonpharmacologic pain reduction strategies, including application of local heat, sitz baths *to encourage local blood flow and transient relief from discomfort.*
- Perform gentle prostate massage or enable patient to obtain this service for chronic bacterial or chronic nonbacterial prostatitis *to relieve congestion and related prostatic discomfort.* NOTE: Prostatic massage is contraindicated in acute bacterial prostatitis because of risk of systemic infection, and it is not indicated in prostatodynia because prostatic infection is not present.
- Advise patients that urination may relieve discomfort of prostatitis. *Urination often provides transient relief because it promotes local blood flow and reduces irritative lower urinary tract symptoms.*
- Teach patients to manage and avoid constipation using a combination of dietary means (fluid and fiber), recreation to encourage gastrointestinal peristalsis, and stool softeners as indicated. *Constipation and associated rectal distension reduce local blood flow and exacerbate pain associated with prostatitis; straining to defecate also increases this discomfort.*
- Advise patient that highly spiced foods or alcohol may exacerbate pain associated with prostatitis.
- Assist patient with prostatodynia to undergo biofeedback-assisted pelvic floor reeducation or electrical stimulation in association with physician. *Because prostatodynia represents a pelvic pain disorder associated with pelvic muscle dysfunction rather than an infection of the prostate[123,186]; therapy to address local pain and pelvic muscle hypertonicity is indicated.*
- Teach patient to select and take nonsteroidal antiinflammatory drug obtained over the counter or via prescription in consultation with physician. *These drugs provide transient relief from discomfort associated with prostatitis; however, higher doses may be indicated to achieve relief.*

NIC Elimination Management

Urinary retention (increased risk for) related to blockage from inflamed edematous prostate

- Monitor fluid intake and urinary output in patient with acute bacterial prostatitis and percuss the bladder *to assess for signs of urinary retention and bladder overdistension.*
- If suprapubic catheter is placed in patient with acute bacterial prostatitis, monitor intake and output *to assess patency of tube and prevent urinary retention.* Securely tape tube *to prevent kinking and blockage of urinary outflow.*
- Advise patient experiencing difficulty with urination to drink a cup of caffeinated coffee or hot tea and to stand in warm shower in an attempt to urinate. Patient is further advised to urinate in shower rather than transferring to toilet. *Caffeine in coffee or hot tea acts as bladder irritant, and warm shower encourages local blood flow while providing transient relief of prostatic discomfort, promoting urination.*

NIC Behavior Therapy

Noncompliance with medical therapy related to lack of understanding about need for long-term therapy

- Teach rationale for long-term antibiotic therapy. *Long-term treatment is needed to achieve therapeutic levels within fatty fluid of prostatic acini.*
- Advise patient to continue antiinfective therapy for 30-120 days as prescribed *to achieve optimum results and to reduce the risk of rebound infection.*[123]

Patient Education/Continuum of Care Plan

1. Provide information concerning prostate's resistance to short-term antibiotic therapy and risk for recurrence of symptoms when long-term antibiotic therapy is not completed.
2. Educate patient about different etiologies of inflammatory prostatitis compared with prostatodynia.

Evaluation/Patient Outcomes

Physical Comfort Promotion: Pain and symptom impact of prostatitis is alleviated as assessed by NIH Chronic Prostatitis Symptom Index. Prostatic infection is resolved; urine and EPS are free from pathogens. Patient adheres to medical care regimen; all antibiotics are taken according to prescribed schedule.

Elimination Management: Acute urinary retention is prevented or promptly managed. Urinary residual volumes are less than 200 ml.

Behavior Therapy: Patient understands rationale and commits to long-term antibiotic therapy.

SEXUAL FUNCTION DISORDERS

Epididymitis

Epididymitis is defined as any inflammation of the epididymis; it may be caused by bacteria, viruses, parasites, chemicals, or trauma. Epididymitis is divided into three categories: nonspecific, specific, and traumatic. Complications from this condition include orchitis, testicular infarction, and sterility.[79,173]

Epididymitis is the most common of all intrascrotal lesions. It is almost always unilateral and must be differentiated from testicular torsion, tumor, or trauma. An estimated 600,000 cases occur in the United States each year. In men under 35 years of age, epididymitis is most often associated with sexually transmitted disease. It accounts for 20% of all inpatient admissions in military urology practices. In men over 35 years of age, gram-negative rods associated with some abnormality of the urinary tract or performance of some urologic procedure constitute the most common presentation of the condition. Epididymitis is rare in prepubertal boys.[82]

Pathophysiology

Epididymitis occurs most frequently as a result of reflux of urine or some pathogenic agent through the posterior urethra, prostatic ducts, or seminal vesicles. In rare instances the causative pathogen may reach the epididymis via retrograde lymphatic pathways from the wall of the vas deferens or via hematogenous or metastatic routes. In its earlier stage, epididymitis occurs as a type of cellulitis associated with local pain and edema. In the acute stage the entire hemiscrotum becomes a single erythematous, exquisitely painful mass often associated with an inflammatory hydrocele produced by the tunica vaginalis. Later changes include peritubular fibrosis and occlusion of the epididymis that may result in sterility.[133,158]

Nonspecific epididymitis refers to a group of common pathogens that typically gain access to the organ via urethral-vasal reflux in the presence of infected urine. Bladder outlet obstruction requiring the individual to strain to void is a predisposing factor to this condition. Nonspecific epididymitis is a common complication of prostatitis, urethral stricture disease, and seminal vesiculitis. Occasionally a nonspecific epididymitis arises from a septic focus such as a pharyngitis. Reflux of sterile urine into the epididymis has been reported to result in inflammation,[78,173] although others dispute this possibility.[57] Strenuous exercise has also been connected with nonpyrogenic epididymitis.[173]

Nonspecific epididymitis also occurs as a complication of certain urologic procedures, particularly transurethral resection of the prostate and urethral catheterization. Postprocedure epididymitis may occur as late as several months following instrumentation because of the persistence of subclinical amounts of bacteria in the urine. It is significant to note that the rate of epididymitis following transurethral resection of the prostate has dropped from 20% to 4% following the institution of routine prophylactic antibiotics after the procedure. Vasectomy has been advocated as a prophylactic measure for men undergoing prostatectomy, but the efficacy of this intervention remains unproven.[78]

Traumatic epididymitis (also referred to as epididymo-orchitis) arises from straining, with reflux of urine into the organ. The etiology of this form of epididymitis remains unclear. Some argue that the trauma only inflames an already present subclinical inflammation of the epididymis, whereas others propose that the trauma lessens resistance to some more distant foci of infection, allowing invasion of pathogens into the area.[55,173]

Specific epididymitis refers to a group of known pathogens that invade the epididymis from a urinary focus or via the hematogenous route. The causative organisms most commonly associated with sexually transmitted epididymitis are *Neisseria gonorrhoeae* and *Chlamydia trachomatis* among heterosexual males and *E. coli* among homosexual males. Prompt, aggressive treatment of these sexually transmitted diseases helps curtail the incidence of subsequent epididymitis as demonstrated by the decreasing incidence of gonococcal epididymitis.[82]

Syphilitic epididymitis may occur more often than has been suspected. This form of epididymal inflammation is typically asymptomatic and connected with the second stage of the disease. Diagnosis of syphilitic epididymitis is presumptive and established when other evidence of syphilis is present while urinary tract infection, prostatitis, and urethritis are absent.[82,173]

Many forms of specific epididymitis have been reported that have spread to the organ via the hematogenous route. In cases of brucellosis, epididymitis may be the initial symptom of the condition. Meningococcal septicemia, pneumococcal pneumonia, *Haemophilus influenzae,* and other bacterial diseases have been associated with epididymal invasion. Various parasites such as amebae, *Schistosoma,* and fungi are known to invade the epididymis.[82]

Tubercular epididymitis arises from involvement of the prostate and is one of the few painless forms of the disease. Tuberculosis of the epididymis produces a thickened, beaded organ on palpation and leads to occlusion of the epididymal lumen.

The most common complication of epididymitis is orchitis, so the term *epididymo-orchitis* is used. Infertility is a serious long-term complication of epididymitis. Sterility among men with chronic or recurrent bilateral epididymitis is 40%, and men with unilateral epididymitis have a 25% chance of infertility. Recurrences of epididymitis are particularly likely when the underlying disease process (e.g., prostatitis) remains unresolved.[78]

Diagnostic Studies and Findings

White blood cell count: Generally between 20,000 and 30,000 in an acute episode[144]
Urinalysis: Signs of infection may be present
Urine culture: Reveals associated bacterial cystitis if present
Urethral discharge culture: Reveals associated gonococcal or chlamydial urethritis
Prostatic secretion culture: Reveals associated prostatitis
Doppler stethoscope: Good blood flow rules out torsion of testis
Testicular radionuclide scan: Good blood flow rules out torsion of testis

Multidisciplinary Plan

Surgery

Epididymectomy rarely indicated as a therapeutic measure in chronic or tubercular epididymitis[41]

Medications

Mild to moderate cases: Oral antiinfective agents, which may be guided by culture and sensitivity data when appropriate; analgesics (nonsteroidal antiinflammatory drugs [NSAID]) used to manage pain and control fever
Severe cases: Hospitalization and broad-spectrum antibiotics; combination of ampicillin and aminoglycosides given pending results of blood culture
Very severe cases: Spermatic cord block with lidocaine or procaine hydrochloride; use of steroids has been advocated but

any beneficial antiinflammatory activity is outweighed by potential side effects[177]

Antiemetic agent may be required to control associated nausea and vomiting during acute epididymitis; antipyretics may be indicated for associated fever; administration of antiemetics justified to prevent progression of nausea to a severe state that threatens fluid and electrolyte balance

General Management

Urethral discharge may be copious and is managed by regular cleansing of meatus with hydrogen peroxide[107]

NURSING CARE

Nursing Assessment

Scrotum

Initial stages of epididymitis: Scrotal skin is reddened or normal in appearance; as infection progresses, scrotal skin becomes red and hot to touch

Varicocele a common finding

Moderate to severe cases: Significant edema of epididymis and adjacent structures (including testis) causes a large mass in affected hemiscrotum so epididymitis cannot be distinguished; overlying skin dry, flaky, and without its normal rugose appearance; spontaneous rupture may occur; mass is exquisitely tender

Elevation of scrotum may result in relief from pain (Prehn's sign)[78]

Testis: Testis on affected side may be painful and enlarged; masses or induration possible

Abdomen: Lower quadrant pain perceived on affected side

Nausea and vomiting: Vomiting may be severe during acute period

Patient Problems/Nursing Diagnoses & Interventions

NIC Physical Comfort Promotion

Acute pain related to inflammation of epididymis

- Support scrotum using athletic supporter, towel placed gently underneath scrotum, or Bellevue bridge *to relieve congestion and discomfort.*
- Provide analgesics as directed, or instruct patient to self-medicate using prescribed narcotic analgesic or NSAID as directed *to relieve discomfort.*
- Provide bed rest during acute period *to prevent inadvertent trauma and to promote comfort.*
- Advise patient that sexual activity or strenuous physical activity is contraindicated even in mild cases. *These activities exacerbate discomfort associated with epididymitis and should be avoided.*

NIC Electrolyte and Acid-Base Management

Risk for deficient fluid volume related to vomiting

- Assess and curtail oral intake in patient with significant nausea and vomiting *to reduce fluid and electrolyte loss.*
- Document intake and output, including frequency and amount of vomitus, *to evaluate fluid volume deficit.*
- Administer antiemetics as directed.
- Administer parenteral fluids as directed *to correct fluid volume deficit and electrolyte imbalance.*

NIC Psychologic Comfort Promotion

Fear related to potential for malignancy and subsequent infertility

- Reassure patient that epididymitis is not a malignant process, and that mass effect is caused by inflammation.
- Reassure patient that spermiogenesis is expected to recuperate following resolution of infection.

Patient Education/Continuum of Care Plan

1. Provide instructions on risk factors associated with epididymitis: prostatitis, urethritis (particularly gonococcal and chlamydial), cystitis, and unusually strenuous physical activity.
2. Emphasize need for follow-up care aimed at identifying underlying causes of epididymitis in certain cases.
3. Provide information on signs and symptoms and the natural history of epididymitis and importance of seeking care promptly.

Evaluation/Patient Outcomes

Physical Comfort Promotion: Scrotal pain is alleviated within 24 to 72 hours of instituting antibiotic and analgesic therapy and entirely resolved within 7 to 10 days. Scrotal swelling is alleviated, and the ipsilateral and contralateral epididymis testes are nontender upon gentle palpation.

Electrolyte and Acid-Base Management: Vomiting is curtailed; dehydration is prevented or promptly reversed.

Serum electrolytes remain within normal limits.

Patient is able to tolerate fluid intake.

Psychologic Comfort Promotion: Patient demonstrates knowledge of cause of epididymitis and anticipated outcomes regarding fertility potential.

Erectile Dysfunction

Erectile dysfunction (impotence) is the inability to achieve or sustain an erection sufficient for sexual performance.[132]

Pathophysiology

From a purely mechanical perspective, an adequate erection must achieve adequate tumescence and rigidity for penetration to be defined as "sufficient for sexual performance." Three types of erections occur in the male with normal erectile function. Psychogenic erections occur in response to visual, auditory, tactile, gustatory, or olfactory stimuli and are processed by modulatory centers in the brain that ultimately produce penile tumescence and rigidity. Reflexogenic erections, in contrast, are modulated by the spinal cord in response to autonomic or tactile stimuli, and nocturnal erections occur during specific stages of sleep. Erectile dysfunction (ED) primarily implies difficulty achieving or sustaining psychogenic erections as a component of intentional sexual activity. ED is considered clinically relevant when it occurs during at least 50% of attempts at sexual activity.

The prevalence of men with clinically relevant ED in the United States is nearly 25 million.[124a] As of 1995, estimated global prevalence was 152 million.[11] Based on projected growth in the population and the proportion of older men, it is estimated that this global prevalence will be 322 million by 2025. When a group of 1709 community-dwelling men in New England was questioned about any episode of erectile failure, 17% reported minimal impotence, 25% reported moderate problems, and 10% reported complete impotence (never able to achieve an erection adequate for sexual performance), equaling a 52% overall prevalence.[44a] ED prevalence is also influenced by age; approximately 39% of men in the fourth decade of life reported any level of ED, including a 5% prevalence of complete impotence, whereas 67% of men in the seventh decade of life reported any level of ED, including 15% who reported complete erectile failure.

As pointed out in the physiology section of this chapter, erectile function represents a combination of local neurovascular events, modulated by multiple areas of the central nervous system, and more indirectly influenced by the endocrine system. Therefore, it is not surprising that further epidemiologic research into ED has revealed a wide variety of risk factors. Table 14-8 lists risk significant factors associated with ED based on epidemiologic research.

Although aging itself does not cause impotence, aging does play a role as a risk factor for ED.[168] Older men experience several age-related changes in the erectile tissue of the penis; they include an increase in alpha-1 adrenergic factors promoting detumescence and the flaccid stage of erectile function, a decrease in acetylcholine-induced smooth muscle relaxation, and a reduction in nitric oxide immunoreactive nerves. Endocrine factors affecting erectile function include a reduction in total and free (bioavailable) testosterone, an increase in circulating estradiol levels, a diminution of luteinizing hormone pulse frequency, and higher serum prolactin levels. These changes probably produce an indirect effect on erectile frequency because they alter libido (the desire to engage in sexual activity). Collectively, these age-related changes are reflected in a reduced number of nocturnal erections when compared with younger men, an increased arousal period, and a slowed refractory time (interval between successful erections). Nonetheless, it is also important to note that none of these changes produces ED, and many otherwise healthy men are capable of successful erections into the eighth and ninth decades of life.

Table 14-8 Risk Factors for Erectile Dysfunction

Condition	Magnitude of Risk
Aging	39% prevalence at age 40 years 67% prevalence at age 70 years
Atherosclerosis	40% of ED in men aged ≥50 years
Heart disease	39% in men treated for heart disease
Hypertension (impact of medications used to treat high blood pressure significant)	15% of men treated for hypertension
Cigarette smoking	Odds ratio for ED 1.5 compared with nonsmokers
Diabetes mellitus	28%-50% prevalence (time since onset more significant age)

Cardiovascular conditions constitute a major risk factor for ED.[124a] Atherosclerotic changes leading to peripheral vascular disease compromises arteriolar function and probably affects the vascular sinusoids of the corpora cavernosa. Coronary artery disease also increases the risk of ED, as does hyperlipidemia. Our knowledge of the influence of essential hypertension on erectile function is confounded by the use of antihypertensive drugs, which are known to act as independent risk factors.

Long-term cigarette smoking also affects erectile function.[86] Over the short term, nicotine causes a transient rise in circulating epinephrine and norepinephrine. Although norepinephrine promotes detumescence and maintenance of the flaccid stage of erectile phase, smoking is not associated with transient impotence. However, long-term smoking is associated with significant morphologic changes in local arterioles and cavernosal tissue. These include enhanced platelet and leukocyte adherence to local vessels, increased release of substances associated with inflammation such as cytokines, thrombogens, chemotactins, and mitogens. The adherent platelets and leukocytes also release vasoconstrictors, which include thromboxane A_2 and serotonin. This concentration of vasoconstrictors upsets the normal balance between vasodilating and constricting paracrine substances, and it has been found that long-term smoking reduces nitric oxide synthase activity in animals.[181]

Smoking also increases the risk of ED because of its role in atherosclerotic disease and its deleterious effects on the endothelium throughout the vascular system.[86] As a result, the compliance of the penile corporal tissue is compromised, and the elasticity of the tunica albuginea is reduced, adversely affecting both the arterial inflow required for an erection and the venous occlusion needed to sustain that erection.

Diabetes mellitus is associated with peripheral polyneuropathies, autonomic polyneuropathies, and large and small vessel angiopathies.[111] Each of these factors may increase the risk of ED among men with diabetes mellitus, and the relative contribution of each remains unclear. Although the pathophysiologic mechanisms leading to the high incidence of ED among these patients is unclear, it is known that nitric oxide release from nerve receptors and the local endothelium is impaired. In addition to these direct contributors, depression, hypertension, increased triglyceride levels, and diminished sensory innervation are also postulated to influence the risk of ED.

Many other conditions are known to produce ED. However, they account for a much smaller portion of impotence compared with the prevalence of ED attributed to cardiovascular disease, hypertension, diabetes mellitus, or a history of smoking. For example, multiple endocrine disorders have been found to increase the risk for ED (Table 14-9).[6] Although it is known that a man is able to achieve and sustain an erection independent of testosterone, it is also clear that deficiency of circulating androgens reduces libido (the desire for sexual activity), the frequency of sexual fantasies, and the frequency of spontaneous erections and morning erections. Primary hypogonadism predisposes the man to ED because of its deleterious effects on the

Table 14-9 Hormonal Disorders Associated With ED

Condition	Effect of Erectile Function
Primary hypogonadism Klinefelter's syndrome Prepubertal testicular trauma Prepubertal orchitis Prepubertal orchiectomy	Indirectly affects erectile function; patients have poorly developed secondary sex characteristics and eunuchoidal body habitus, hypotrophic testes, short penile length, small prostate, diminished libido
Secondary hypogonadism Idiopathic *hypogonadotropic hypogonadism* Hyperprolactinemia Hemochromatosis Pituitary adenomas Cushing's syndrome	Loss of libido, diminished endurance and assertiveness; gynecomastia occurs, but secondary sex characteristics generally well developed; prostate size and penile length are normal
Thyroid disorders Hyperthyroidism Hypothyroidism	Hyperthyroidism: Increased testosterone but bioavailable (free) testosterone levels reduced in combination with increased circulating estradiols reduce libido Hypothyroidism: Hyperprolactinemia suppresses testosterone secretion from testis with loss of libido and secondary hypogonadism
Morbid obesity	Excessive conversion of testosterone to estradiols in adipose tissue causes secondary hypogonadism
End-stage renal disease	Multiple factors contribute to ED, including erythropoietin deficiency, hyperprolactinemia, hyperestrogenism and deficiency of FSH and LH

development of the penis, prostate, and secondary male characteristics, as well as its impact on libido. Secondary endocrine disorders, including Cushing's syndrome, hyperthyroidism and hypothyroidism, hyperprolactinemia, and morbid obesity produce secondary testosterone deficiencies and/or hyperestrogenism leading to a loss of libido and secondary ED.

Hemachromatosis is an inherited disorder characterized by excessive absorption of iron from the gastrointestinal system.[170] Deposition of this excessive iron produces many adverse effects, including suppression of FSH and LH secretion from the pituitary with secondary hypogonadism. ED generally occurs in the third to fourth decade of life.[6]

Men with end-stage renal disease are also at high risk for ED.[102] Several endocrinologic factors probably contribute to this risk, including erythropoietin deficiency, hyperprolactinemia, diminished FSH and LH production, and anemia. Exogenous supplementation frequently improves erectile function and libido by increasing testosterone, FSH, and LH and by correcting anemia.

Neurologic disorders produce ED through their effects on the spinal or brain centers that modulate erectile activity.[111] Spinal cord lesions affecting suprasacral segments (above S1-S2) are associated with a loss of psychogenic erections, although reflexogenic erections are typically preserved. Nevertheless, these patients experience clinically relevant ED because they are unable to produce and sustain the purposeful, sustained erections required for sexual performance. In contrast, patients with sacral spinal cord injuries may be able to produce a psychogenic erection, even though they are unable to produce a reflex erection.

Multiple sclerosis is a chronic, systemic neurologic disorder characterized by inflammatory lesions (plaques) affecting many sites within the central nervous system. Goldstein, Siroky, and Sachs[58] reported a 71% prevalence of ED in a small sample of men with multiple sclerosis, and it has been reported to occur in as many as 91% of men at some point during the course of their disease.[108] Neurologic evaluation of men with ED and multiple sclerosis demonstrates a variety of contributing lesions, affecting the suprasacral spinal segments and the peripheral nerves responsible for parasympathetic innervation of the penis and cavernosal tissue. In addition to these neurologic deficits, secondary psychologic, emotional, and functional disturbances, as well as changes in brain function, also influence erectile and sexual function among patients with long-term symptoms.[13a]

Other neurologic disorders affecting the brain and central nervous system are also associated with ED. Cerebrovascular accident (CVA) (stroke) is known to negatively affect multiple aspects of sexual function, including libido, frequency of intercourse, ejaculatory function, and erectile function,[96] but the precise mechanisms that lead to ED remain unclear. Parkinsonism is known to affect both motor and autonomic nervous systems, including urinary, bowel elimination, and erectile function.[155] A neurologic cause of ED is likely, as demonstrated by somatosensory-evoked response testing[44] and by changes in erectile function observed during administration of apomorphine, a D_2-receptor agonist, and levodopa.[87,135] Multiple system atrophy, a disease of progressive neuronal atrophy often confused with parkinsonism, has also been associated with ED, although the contributing factors are not yet understood.[17]

Chronic disease increases the risk of ED owing to direct effects on erectile function or indirect effects, including depression, fatigue, and functional limitations.[111] Chronic diseases frequently associated with ED include cancer, chronic obstructive pulmonary disease,[89] acquired immunodeficiency syndrome (AIDS), and advanced liver disease.

Pelvic or penile trauma may produce ED, usually as a result of local nerve damage or injury to the cavernosal tissue. Nerve entrapment has been attributed to an increased risk of ED among long-distance cyclists,[7] and bony injury with subsequent denervation is postulated to produce the high prevalence of ED

Table 14-10 Commonly Used Medications Associated With ED

Drug Classification	Examples
Antidepressants	Tricyclics (e.g., amitriptyline) Selective serotonin reuptake inhibitors (SSRIs) (e.g., fluvoxamine) Monoamine oxidase inhibitors (MAOIs) (e.g., phenelzine)
Antimanic agents	Lithium
H_2 Antihistamines	Cimetidine, ranitidine
Nonsteroidal antiinflammatory drugs (NSAIDs)	Indomethacin, naproxen
Diuretics	Thiazide-like diuretics (chlorothiazide) Potassium-sparing diuretics (spironolactone)
Calcium channel blockers	Verapamil, nifedipine
Cardiac glycosides	Digoxin
Antianxiety agents	Diazepam, flurazepam
Antiepileptic agents	Phenytoin, primidone
Beta-adrenergic blockers	Propranolol
Alpha-adrenergic agonists (decongestants)	Ephedrine, pseudoephedrine
Antineoplastic (hormonal) agents	Leuprolide, goserelin

following pelvic fracture.[116] Local tissue damage is a more unusual cause of posttraumatic ED; however, cases of penile retraction with tissue damage or scarring following local trauma with tissue destruction have been reported.[154a]

Two disorders directly affecting the penis are associated with ED. Peyronie's disease is the formation of a fibrous plaque within the cavernosal tissue of the penis. When erect, these plaques may produce ED by producing an abnormal curvature of the penis or because of associated pain.[4] Priapism is a painful, prolonged erection due to incomplete evacuation of blood from the cavernosal tissue (low flow) or abnormally high arterial inflow into the penis (high flow). Although most cases of priapism are transient and attributable to specific treatment for ED, it also occurs as a complication of systemic diseases such as sickle cell anemia or as an idiopathic event. Priapism usually constitutes a urologic emergency, and approximately 50% of men with normal erectile function experience ED after a clinically relevant episode of priapism.[19]

Numerous prescription and over-the-counter medications have been associated with ED owing to their effects on the neurovascular events essential for an erection and their indirect effects on libido and ejaculatory function.[154] Table 14-10 lists some of the most common causative agents. In addition to these medications, excessive intake of alcohol, and the misuse or abuse of recreational agents, including the opiates, marijuana, cocaine, barbiturates, and the hallucinogens such as heroin, have also been shown to cause transient or ongoing loss of erectile function.[108]

Surgical procedures produce ED by a variety of mechanisms, including local or central denervation, alteration of local blood flow, or hormonal balance. Multiple abdominopelvic surgeries, such as radical prostatectomy and those requiring removal of the bladder or rectum and surgical resection of associated cancer followed by urinary or fecal diversion, result in ED because of unavoidable denervation.[22,18,185]

Traditionally ED has been subdivided into psychogenic and organic causes. Although many cases of ED can be attributed to psychogenic causes, it must be remembered that virtually all cases produce secondary psychosocial distress. Impotence from psychogenic causes is particularly common among younger men, but it may occur in all age groups. In young men, psychologic issues leading to ED frequently focus on sexual abuse issues, paraphilia (unusual sexual fantasies), gender identity issues, and homoerotic fantasies in the man who defines himself as strictly heterosexual.[119] Among older men, death of a spouse, deterioration of a relationship or divorce, serious vocational problems, or a change in the partner's health status are common contributing factors.

Diagnostic Studies and Findings

Serum testosterone: Low in impotence with dysfunction of hypothalamic-pituitary-gonadal axis

Serum prolactin: High when testosterone is abnormally low

Serum FSH: Abnormal when impotence is result of abnormality of hormonal axis

Serum LH: Abnormal when impotence is result of abnormality of hormonal axis

Glucose tolerance test: Abnormal in cases of diabetes mellitus

Sacral evoked responses: Increased bulbocavernous latency in diabetic males with autonomic neuropathy

Urodynamic testing: Abnormal sensations of bladder filling on cystometrogram and abnormal urecholine supersensitivity test in males with autonomic neuropathy

Penile systolic blood pressure: Low in cases of vascular impotence

Penile pulse volume recording: Abnormal in cases of vascular impotence

Dynamic infusion cavernosometry and cavernosography: Presence of venous leakage (failure to sustain); presence of arterial insufficiency (failure to fill); presence of neuropathic or psychogenic disorders (failure to initiate an erection)

Nocturnal penile tumescence: Absent nocturnal erections when underlying cause of impotence is primarily organic rather than psychogenic[104]

Snap-gauge testing: Breakage of three pressure-sensitive plastic bands indicates sufficient pressure for penetration; inability to break bands during sleep study indicates erectile dysfunction

Multidisciplinary Plan

Surgery

Corrective surgery for arterial occlusion may improve ED in certain cases

Revascularization of the penis, accomplished by isolating the epigastric artery and reanastomosing it directly to a corporal body, has shown efficacy in selected cases of ED[91]

A penile prosthesis may be implanted to mimic erectile function; inflatable devices are generally preferred because they

ORAL MEDICATIONS USED TO TREAT ERECTILE DYSFUNCTION — Box 14-1

SILDENAFIL CITRATE (VIAGRA)

Actions: Enhances nitric oxide activity by inhibiting phosphodiesterase type 5, which denigrates GMP in cavernosal tissue. The drug enhances the potential for an erection; it will not produce an erection without tactile and/or psychogenic stimuli.

Dosage: 50-100 mg PO no more than once daily

Side effects: Headaches, facial flushing, dizziness, nausea or indigestion, transient bluish haze to vision

Contraindications: Sildenafil citrate must never be administered to men taking nitrates (including those using nitroglycerine tablets sublingual prn); commonly used nitrates include the following:

- Erythrityl (Cardilate)
- Isosorbides (Iso-Bid, Isordil, Isotrate, Sorbitrate, Timecelles)
- Nitroprusside (Nitropress)
- Amyl nitrate
- Nitroglycerines (Nitrostat, Nitro-Bid, Nitro-Dur, Nitrolingual, Nitrodisc, Transderm-Nitro, Nitrogard)

INJECTABLE AGENTS USED TO TREAT ERECTILE DYSFUNCTION — Box 14-2

PREPARATIONS: INTRAURETHRAL ALPROSTADIL (MUSE), INTRACAVERNOSAL ALPROSTADIL (CAVERJECT)

Actions: Relaxes smooth muscle of cavernosal tissue and local arterioles, promoting erectile activity

Dosage: Intraurethral dose 500 mcg; intracavernosal dose: 2.5-10 μg; both preparations require considerable titration for maximum efficacy

Side effects: Pain within urethra or at injection site, hypotension, dizziness, priapism

allow both flaccid and erect states; semirigid devices are also available[47,130]

Medications

Sildenafil citrate (Viagra), a selective GMP/phosphodiesterase inhibitor, may be administered for ED in men who do not have severe cardiac disease and who are not taking nitrates in any form (Box 14-1)[59]

Trazodone has been used to treat ED, but its modest efficacy and its side effects, including drowsiness and nausea, limit its utility[124]

Yohimbine, an alpha-adrenergic antagonist, is frequently used to treat ED. However, randomized, placebo-controlled trials of high-dose yohimbine have not shown it to be effective when compared with placebo[100]

Two oral agents, phentolamine mesylate and apomorphine, are under investigation to determine their role in the management of ED[135,169]

Testosterone replacement is indicated for men with ED associated with documented primary or secondary hypogonadism and abnormally low free and/or total testosterone serum levels. Oral preparations are avoided because of the potential for hepatotoxicity. Intramuscular injections may be used, but transdermal agents are generally preferred

- Testoderm or Androderm patches are commercially available with a prescription from a physician or nurse practitioner.
- Prostaglandin E_1 (alprostadil) may be injected into the corpora cavernosa (Caverject) or given intraurethrally (MUSE) to achieve an erection (Box 14-2). Papaverine, phentolamine, and prostaglandin E_1 have been injected as single agents or in combination to achieve erections.[111] However, neither papaverine, phentolamine, nor any combination of these agents is approved by the U.S. Food and Drug Administration (FDA) for use in the management of ED.

General Management

Education and reassurance are effective in cases of occasional erectile failure owing to anxiety or cognitive dissonance.

Patients with significant psychologic issues must be referred to a qualified mental health care provider.

Treatment of contributing medical disorders may improve or restore erectile function without the need for additional management of ED; adjustment or alteration of prescriptive or over-the-counter medications may alleviate or correct ED.

Recreational drugs or smoking should be discontinued; reduced alcohol consumption may alleviate or correct ED; alcoholism must be treated when present.

A vacuum erection device (VED) combines a vacuum chamber that establishes blood flow into the cavernosal tissue with a restrictive device (ring), which is then placed on the base of the penis to maintain the erection until sexual activity is completed; this device may be left in place for 30 minutes.

Pelvic muscle exercises have been shown to improve erectile function.[12]

NURSING CARE

Nursing Assessment

History: Including a detailed review of sexual practices, essential to characterize ED and to differentiate clinically relevant ED from occasional erectile failure owing to anxiety or cognitive dissonance

Physical examination: Evaluation of male secondary sex characteristics; cardiovascular and peripheral vascular assessment; neurologic assessment, including bulbocavernosus reflex testing; perineal and penile sensations, pelvic muscle tone; scrotal examination, including testicular size and consistency; palpation of shaft for evidence of Peyronie's plaque

Laboratory testing: Urinalysis and serum testosterone (preferably morning measurement) should be performed routinely; serum LH, FSH, prolactin when indicated

External genitalia

- Normal appearance of penis, scrotum, perineal area, and hair distribution except in cases of primary hypogonadism
- Normal phallic size (stretched length should be at least 9.3 cm) except in cases of primary hypogonadism or penile trauma or cancer with tissue loss or resection

Bilaterally descended testes; testes will be small and soft in cases of primary or secondary hypogonadism

Palpation of penis will reveal hardened Peyronie's plaque; photograph obtained during erection useful to document and evaluate curvature[108]

Digital rectal examination: Loss of anal sphincter tone with absent or diminished bulbocavernosus reflex with sacral spinal cord injury, cauda equina syndrome, severe local neuropathy; absent or markedly diminished perineal or penile sensation with advanced peripheral polyneuropathies, spinal cord injury, disk problems

Peripheral pulses: Decreased or absent in cases of vascular impotence associated with advanced peripheral vascular disease

Neurologic examination: Abnormal with underlying neurologic disease, including CVA, multiple sclerosis, spinal cord injuries, or related disorders

Patient Problems/Nursing Diagnoses & Interventions

NIC Coping Assistance

Sexual dysfunction related to erectile dysfunction
Situational low self-esteem related to sexual dysfunction

- Encourage male patient to seek evaluation and treatment of ED. *Erectile dysfunction is a significant quality of life disorder affecting both the patient and his partner. It can almost always be alleviated or corrected with proper evaluation and treatment.*
- Assist male patient in altering behaviors, such as cigarette smoking, excessive alcohol intake, or drug abuse, that cause or increase risk of ED.
- Consult with physician or nurse practitioner concerning alterations to drug regimens to reduce or correct ED. *Multiple pharmacologic agents cause ED; deletion of specific drugs or substitution of alternative agents may alleviate or correct ED.*
- Teach male patient the dosage, administration, and side effects (including contraindication to nitrate use) of oral medications used to treat ED. *When used properly, oral agents provide effective and attractive alternative for management of ED. If misused, the drug can produce serious adverse effects, including death.*
- Advise patient using oral sildenafil that the agent enhances potential for an erection only when combined with psychogenic and related stimuli. *Unlike intracavernosal or intraurethral agents, sildenafil does not produce an erection without additional stimulation.*
- Teach male patient to insert intraurethral pellet as directed. Teach proper technique for urethral insertion, including assumption of a sitting position, placement of the delivery device, occlusion of the urethra immediately following insertion, and massage of the urethra until the drug is absorbed. *When used properly, intraurethral prostaglandin E_1 provides an effective and attractive alternative for the management of ED. If misused, the drug can produce serious adverse effects, including urethral burning, dizziness, and syncope.*
- Teach male patient to self-inject vasodilating agent as directed. Teach proper techniques for self-injection, dosage, frequency of injections, and potential side effects, including priapism. *Self-injection therapy has potentially harmful effects unless correct dose of drug is injected into proper place on body at safe intervals.*
- Teach any male patient who attains an erection using a self-injection technique to recognize and manage priapism. *Priapism, a prolonged painful erection, is a potential of pharmacologic erection therapy. Treatment of the condition is necessary to prevent tissue ischemia and damage.*
- Teach male patient who performs self-injection therapy to wear a barrier device (condom) whenever engaging in intercourse with multiple partners. *Self-injection therapy subtly compromises skin integrity at site of injection. Barrier device is used to prevent spread of sexually transmitted diseases.*
- Teach patient to use vacuum erection device as directed. *Vacuum erection device uses a vacuum to draw blood into penis and constricting device to trap blood until intercourse is completed.*
- Teach patient who uses vacuum erection device to remove restriction (tourniquet) device promptly after intercourse is completed *to prevent ischemia and tissue damage.*
- Empathy and opportunities to express feelings are indicated as patient reintegrates self-concept following change in body image.
- Male sexuality is deeply rooted in ideals of social, athletic, physical, and sexual performance. Any circumstance that significantly alters self-concept and threatens self-esteem may adversely affect sexual function. Chronic disease, creation of a surgical stoma, and physical changes resulting from neurologic disease or spinal cord trauma significantly challenge any man's self-image.
- Psychologic or psychiatric counseling is often a useful adjunct and may be suggested to patient after a sufficiently trusting relationship has been established *to reestablish positive, realistic self-concept.*

Patient Education/Continuum of Care Plan

1. Provide written instructions about oral medication for ED when appropriate, including list of contraindicated nitrates. Emphasize importance of *not* sharing medication with anyone.
2. Instruct significant other concerning ED management plan whenever feasible.
3. Provide education and written instructions about management of priapism for patient who uses intraurethral or intracavernosal injection therapy for ED.
4. Advise patient of variety of options for management of ED.

Evaluation/Patient Outcomes

Coping Assistance: Impotence is resolved. Patient reports ability to engage in satisfying sexual activity. Complications of treatment are avoided or promptly treated. Patient demonstrates knowledge of significant risks and contraindications for therapy and strategy for their management.

Collaborative Interventions and Related Nursing Care

Bladder Neck Suspension

Bladder neck suspension is a broad term used to describe more than 100 surgical procedures performed to correct stress urinary incontinence caused by pelvic descent and urethral hypermobility. Fixation of the urethrovesical junction can be accomplished through a suprapubic, vaginal, or combined approach. For the Marshall-Marchetti-Krantz procedure the surgeon approximates periurethral fascia to the cartilage of the posterior symphysis pubis. A retropubic colposuspension (Burch procedure) requires fixation of the urethrovesical junction to Cooper's ligament. The anterior urethropexy requires placement of absorbable sutures to anchor the urethrovesical junction to the periosteum of the symphysis bone.[41]

Needle suspensions are performed through the vagina. A U-shaped vaginal incision is made, and the vagina and urethra are carefully separated. The urethra is then moved to an intraabdominal position by ligature carriers that are inserted into the abdominopelvic cavity via two small (3 to 5 cm) incisions in the lower abdomen. The Stamey procedure requires mobilization of tissue lateral to the urethra to fixate the urethrovesical junction; the Raz procedure uses four sutures for fixation.[41,57]

The suburethral sling is used to correct stress incontinence caused by pelvic descent and urethral hypermobility and, in certain circumstances, to correct leakage caused by sphincter mechanism incompetence. A fascial sling (obtained from the rectis abdominis or fascia lata from the thigh) or a Gore Tex strip is placed around the proximal third of the urethra through a vaginal incision. The tension of the sling is minimized to avoid obstruction of the outlet.[41,57]

Contraindications and Cautions

Bladder neck suspension is indicated for stress incontinence caused by pelvic descent and urethral hypermobility. Detrusor instability may or may not be corrected by bladder neck suspension. Bladder neck suspension is contraindicated in cases of incontinence caused by intrinsic sphincter deficiency without coexisting urethral hypermobility.

Preprocedural Nursing Care

1. Teach all patients who undergo bladder neck suspension about the high risk for urinary retention (typically transient) or for infection following surgery.
2. Discuss with the patient who experiences stress and urge incontinence that detrusor instability may or may not resolve following surgery. Reassure the patient that persistent instability (urge) incontinence will be managed by medications, electrostimulation therapy, bladder drill, or other management techniques.
3. Inform the patient with an abdominal procedure or pubovaginal sling that hospitalization is required for approximately 5 days. Inform the patient undergoing a vaginal or needle procedure that hospitalization for approximately 3 days is required.
4. Advise the patient undergoing a vaginal procedure that a vaginal pack will be placed during surgery and removed approximately 24 hours following the procedure.
5. Consult with the surgeon concerning self-intermittent catheterization instruction before surgery. Explain to the patient that intermittent catheterization is used to provide regular, complete bladder emptying until postoperative urinary retention is resolved.

NURSING CARE

Nursing Assessment

Abdomen: Redness, edema, and drainage at wound site if abdominal approach used

Perineum: Vaginal discharge; pain if wound infection present

Voiding behaviors: Decreased force of urinary stream; perceptions of incomplete bladder emptying or acute urinary retention

Pain: Dysuria; pelvic pain; incisional or abdominal pain

Patient Problems/Nursing Diagnoses & Interventions

NIC Elimination Management

Impaired urinary elimination related to obstruction of urinary outflow

- Monitor indwelling catheter for patency *to prevent acute overdistention and disruption of delicate surgical repair.*
- Remove indwelling catheter as directed (as early as first postoperative day for certain patients and as late as 1 month postoperatively for others). Carefully monitor patient for urination and urinary residual volumes. *Urinary retention may occur after catheter removal, possibly because of postoperative edema and inflammation.*
- Institute an intermittent catheterization program in consultation with physician *to avoid overdistention for the patient with postoperative distention.*

NIC Physical Comfort Promotion

Acute pain related to surgical trauma or bladder distention

- Assess the character, location, and duration of pain. *Incisional pain is perceived as a dull, boring, and prolonged pain, whereas bladder spasms produce a cramping pain with a sudden onset and relatively short duration.*
- Administer analgesics or narcotic medications as directed *to relieve incisional pain.*
- Administer anticholinergic or antispasmodic medications as directed *to relieve discomfort produced by bladder spasms.*
- Monitor catheter for patency. *Catheter blockage produces bladder overdistention, bladder spasms, and suprapubic discomfort.*
- Minimize noise, bright lighting, and environmental distractions during immediate postoperative period *to minimize pain.*

Patient Education/Continuum of Care Plan

1. Reassure patient that urinary retention experienced following bladder neck suspension is expected to be temporary.
2. Patient teaching before surgery should include a specific plan to manage postoperative urinary retention.

3. Advise patient to avoid heavy lifting or strenuous exercise for at least 6 weeks after surgery.

EVALUATION/PATIENT OUTCOMES

Elimination Management: Altered urinary elimination patterns are improved. Urodynamics are normal. Marshall test is negative. Postvoid residual is 20% of total bladder volume or less.

Physical Comfort Promotion: Pain is minimized. Patient receives adequate relief of pain and spasms from medication.

SUBURETHRAL INJECTION OF GLUTARALDEHYDE CROSS-LINKED COLLAGEN

Description and Rationale

GAX collagen is a bulking substance comprising types I and III bovine collagen. In addition, a very small amount of glutaraldehyde is added to inhibit the action of the enzyme collagenase, an enzyme that breaks down collagen in the body. Suburethral injections of GAX collagen may be used for women and men with stress urinary incontinence caused by ISD. Collagen is indicated for women who have ISD but no urethral hypermobility; those with both conditions are typically managed by a suburethral sling. All men with stress urinary incontinence are potential candidates for GAX collagen, because urethral hypermobility affects women exclusively.

GAX collagen is injected via transurethral or transperineal access, under endoscopic control (FIG. 14-17). A cystoscope is used to identify the urethral sphincter mechanism, and a specially designed needle is advanced through the working port for injection of collagen. Several injection sites are identified, and collagen is injected until the urethral lumen is closed. Repeated injections may be required to gain continence. In some cases, a perineal approach may be used to inject collagen. The urethra is visualized, the sphincter mechanism is identified, and the needle is inserted until its movement just beneath the urethral mucosa is appreciated. GAX collagen is then injected until the urethral coaptation occurs.

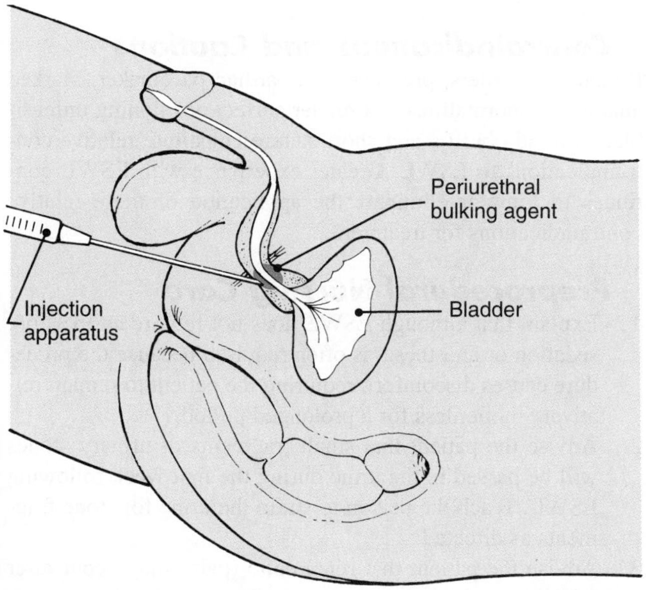

FIG. 14-17

Transperineal injection of a urethral bulking agent in a male. (From Gray.[61])

Contraindications and Cautions

1. Hypersensitivity to GAX collagen may occur. A subdermal skin test is required before suburethral injection of collagen.
2. GAX collagen injections will not correct stress urinary incontinence caused by urethral hypermobility.
3. Repeated injections of GAX collagen may be required, particularly in males with urethral scarring following radical prostatectomy.
4. The long-term efficacy of GAX collagen (more than 7 years) has not been determined.
5. GAX collagen injections will not alleviate or cure urge incontinence.

Preprocedural Nursing Care

1. Inject 0.5 ml of Xyderm via a subdermal technique into the forearm to test for hypersensitivity to bovine collagen. Teach the patient the signs and symptoms of a positive response (local redness, itching, induration). Monitor the site after 72 hours and after 30 days.
2. Inform the patient that GAX collagen is injected under local, spinal, or general anesthesia. Consult the physician and anesthesiologist about the method of anesthesia for that patient.
3. Inform the patient that transient urinary retention may occur, but that prolonged retention is unlikely unless she or he is experiencing retention requiring self-catheterization before the procedure or unless the individual voids exclusively by abdominal straining.
4. Teach the patient to perform self-intermittent catheterization to manage transient urinary retention before the procedure.
5. Advise the patient that repeated injections of GAX collagen may be required.
6. Inform the patient that the long-term effectiveness of GAX collagen has not been established and that repeated injections may be required.

MULTIDISCIPLINARY PLAN

Medications

Antiinfective medications may be administered before and after collagen injection.

Analgesics may be administered after the procedure.

General Management

An indwelling catheter may be placed temporarily (some urologists avoid catheterization to reduce the risk of extrusion of the collagen through the injection sites).

Intermittent catheterization is preferred for management of transient urinary retention.

NURSING CARE

NURSING ASSESSMENT

Forearm: Redness, itching, induration, indicating hypersensitivity to GAX collagen
Perineum: Urethral discharge
Voiding behaviors: Decreased force of urinary stream; acute urinary retention
Pain: Dysuria; pelvic pain

PATIENT PROBLEMS/NURSING DIAGNOSES & INTERVENTIONS

NIC ELIMINATION MANAGEMENT

Impaired urinary elimination related to suburethral or transperineal injection of GAX collagen

- Monitor indwelling catheter for patency and urinary output. An indwelling catheter may be left in place for a brief period after collagen injection. *Occlusion of catheter increases pain and may increase risk of urinary tract infection.*
- Remove catheter as directed and monitor patient for spontaneous voiding. *Transient urinary retention may occur after collagen injection.*
- Assist patient who is unable to spontaneously urinate to perform self-catheterization. Prolonged urinary retention is rare, unless individual has experienced this condition before procedure.

NIC PHYSICAL COMFORT PROMOTION

Acute pain related to endoscopic instrumentation and suburethral or transperineal injections

- Teach patient to self-administer urinary or systemic analgesics as directed. Transient discomfort after collagen injection may occur.
- Advise patient that a warm sitz bath or warm shower may relieve discomfort associated with collagen injection.

PATIENT EDUCATION/CONTINUUM OF CARE PLAN

1. Remind patient that repeated injections may be required. Reabsorption of collagen may occur, or reduction of urethral edema may be associated with recurrence of urinary incontinence.
2. Teach patient to recognize signs and symptoms of urge incontinence and to seek care for this condition if it occurs.
3. Advise patient that repeated treatment may be necessary within 2 to 5 years. The long-term efficacy of collagen is not known, and recurrent urinary leakage has been noted within 2 to 5 years.

EVALUATION/PATIENT OUTCOMES

Elimination Management: Stress urinary incontinence is alleviated or ablated. Transient urinary retention is resolved.

Physical Comfort Promotion: Pain is minimized. Patient receives adequate relief of urethral and pelvic discomfort from analgesics and warm sitz baths or showers.

EXTRACORPOREAL SHOCK WAVE LITHOTRIPSY

Extracorporeal shock wave lithotripsy (ESWL) uses shock waves to reduce calculi to smaller particles capable of spontaneous transport and excretion from the urinary tract. Shock waves used for ESWL differ from ultrasonic waves in several significant aspects. Ultrasonic sound waves create a sinusoidal pattern with gentle peaks and valleys, whereas shock waves create a single positive-pressure front with several frequencies, a sharp onset, and a gradual decline. When transmitted through degassed water or water-containing viscera, these waves lose only a small portion of their original energy without producing significant tissue damage. As these shock waves pass through a urinary stone, the stone is shattered; with repeated application, the stone is pulverized into sand.

ESWL is performed in a specially designed stationary or mobile suite (the latter is usually situated in the cab of a large truck) containing a large reservoir of degassed water (bath) or other medium for the transmission of shock waves, fluoroscopic or ultrasonic imaging equipment capable of locating the stone within a three-dimensional perspective, and a mobile chair for placing a body in the bath.

The anesthesia is usually required for ESWL; the urinary calculus is located by ultrasound or fluoroscopy, and repeated applications of shock waves are used to pulverize the stone. A nephrostomy tube or ureteral catheter is often placed to prevent urinary obstruction as the fragments of the stone pass down the ureter to the bladder.

The advances in the technology of lithotripsy have led to second-generation units that use a minibath or membrane to deliver shock waves to a urinary stone. The spark gap generator used in the original ESWL units has also been modified so that shock waves can be generated from a piezoceramic (piezoelectric), a 10-mg lead azide pellet, or an electromagnetic shock wave generator (FIG. 14-18).[55]

Contraindications and Cautions

Bleeding disorders, presence of a cardiac pacemaker, marked anatomic abnormalities that render correct positioning unfeasible, extreme obesity, and short stature constitute relative contraindications to ESWL. Greater experience with ESWL continues to limit or eliminate the application of these relative contraindications for treatment.

Preprocedural Nursing Care

1. Explain that although ESWL does not require an incision, sedation or anesthesia is often required because the procedure causes discomfort, requiring the patient to remain relatively motionless for a prolonged period.
2. Advise the patient that small fragments of urinary stones will be passed in the urine during the first week following ESWL. Teach the person to strain the urine for stone fragments as directed.
3. Advise the patient that renal colic (pain) may occur after ESWL, particularly when a large stone burden is pulverized.
4. Reassure the patient that aggressive pain management will be maintained until all stone fragments are passed.

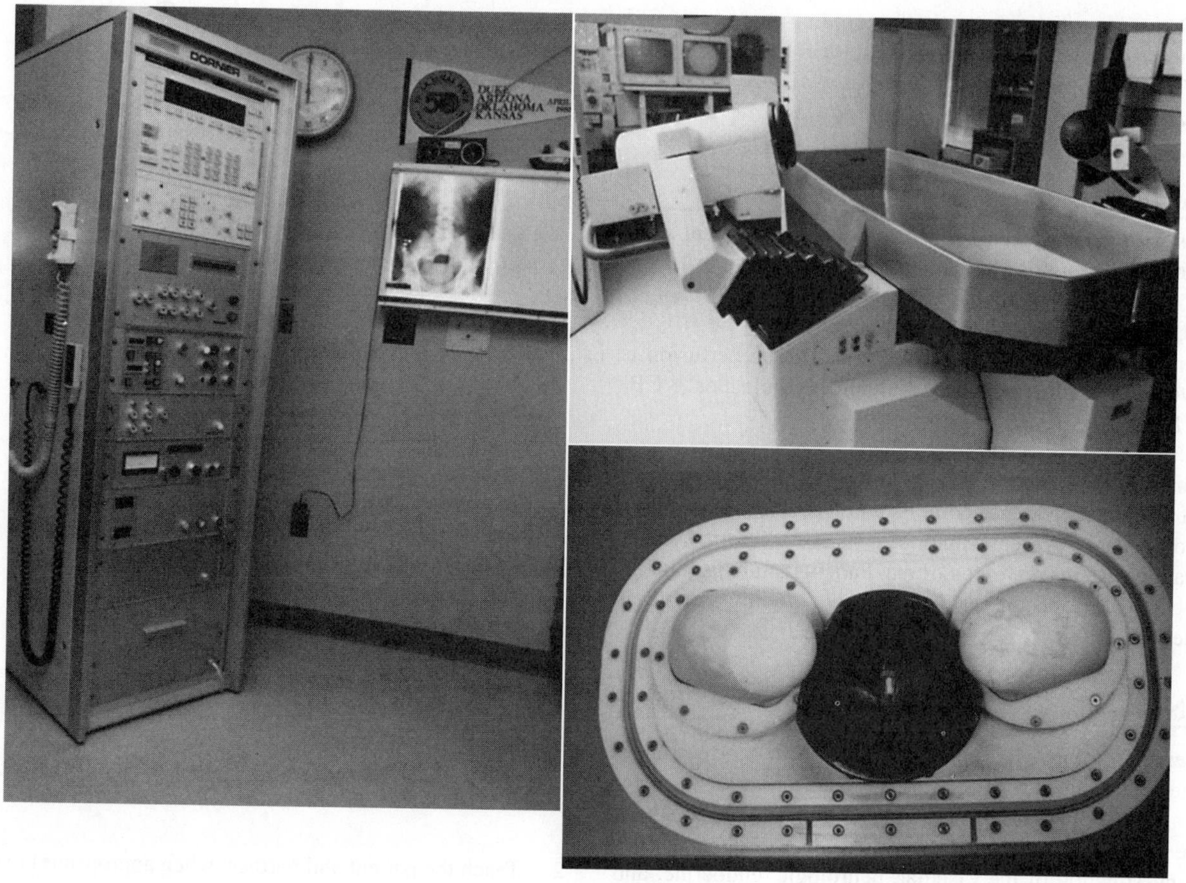

FIG. 14-18
A, ESWL control panel and x-ray (see stones in left kidney and marker on right kidney). **B,** Tub for extracorporeal shock wave lithotripsy (ESWL). **C,** Source of impulse located in bottom of tub.

NURSING CARE

NURSING ASSESSMENT

Urinary output and voiding behavior: Passage of stone particles; dysuria; bladder colic
Pain: Renal colic
Temperature: Fever

PATIENT PROBLEMS/NURSING DIAGNOSES & INTERVENTIONS

NIC TISSUE PERFUSION MANAGEMENT

Ineffective peripheral tissue perfusion (renal) related to mechanical reduction of blood flow

- Question patient concerning use of any anticoagulant medications (including aspirin) before ESWL, and obtain any history of bleeding or clotting disorders. *ESWL causes trauma to renal tissue as stone fragments are pulverized and transported to bladder. Uncontrolled bleeding disorders may produce significant hematuria unless adequately managed before ESWL.*
- Monitor patient for hematuria following ESWL *to prevent occurrence of excessive bleeding.*
- Teach patient to monitor urine at home for resolution (or persistence) of hematuria. Instruct patient to call physician should persistent hematuria occur. *Because most patients undergo ESWL as an outpatient procedure, teach self-monitoring for potential complications.*

NIC ELIMINATION MANAGEMENT

Acute pain related to urinary obstruction
Impaired urinary elimination related to urinary obstruction

- Assess pain for character, location, duration, and intensity. *Obstructing fragments produce a renal colic type of pain; bladder spasms produce a sharp cramping pain in the suprapubic area with dysuria.*
- Prepare patient for additional endoscopic, ESWL, or percutaneous procedures, as directed, *to relieve obstruction and discomfort produced by residual fragments.*
- Administer, or teach patient to self-administer, analgesic or narcotic medications, as directed, *to relieve discomfort of renal colic.*
- Administer, or teach patient to self-administer, urinary analgesics or antispasmodic drugs, as directed, *to relieve discomfort produced by bladder spasms or inflammation.*
- Encourage patient to maintain an adequate intake of fluid (at least 1500 ml per day) *to assist in elimination of stone fragments.*

- Reassure patient that irritative voiding symptoms and urinary frequency experienced after ESWL are transient. *Passage of stone fragments and relief of obstruction produce some urinary tract inflammation and diuresis.*

Patient Education/Continuum of Care Plan

Discuss with patient techniques for preventing recurrent stone formation, including drugs, diet, and fluid intake.

Evaluation/Patient Outcomes

Tissue Perfusion Management: Renal tissue perfusion is improved. X-ray films of kidneys, ureters, and bladder (KUB) and IVP are normal.

Elimination Management: Comfort level is maintained. Patient does not experience pain. Patient learns to self-administer medications to prevent pain or spasms as necessary. Urinary elimination patterns return to normal. Patient maintains fluid intake of at least 1500 ml per day. Irritative voiding symptoms subside.

Intrapenile Prosthetic Devices

Intrapenile prosthetic devices are used when pharmacologic treatment, vacuum device therapy, or vascular surgical procedures are inadequate or unacceptable for the patient seeking to restore erectile activity. Placement of the device relies on thorough investigation of the vascular, neurologic, endocrine, and psychogenic aspects of erectile dysfunction for a particular individual.

The choice of penile prosthesis is affected by the patient's and surgeon's preference and technical considerations. There are two general types of implants: semirigid and inflatable. The semirigid devices maintain a continuous state of tumescence (Fig. 14-19). The Small-Carrion device has a silicone exterior and sponge interior, and the Jonas prosthesis is composed of silicone with silver wires that can be positioned for better concealment beneath clothing.

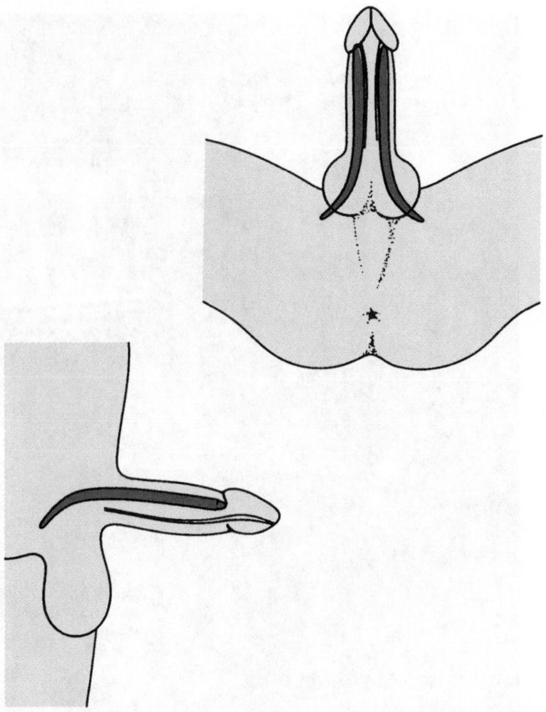

Fig. 14-19
Semirigid intrapenile prosthesis. (From Beare and Myers.[16])

The inflatable devices are capable of imitating the flaccid and tumescent penis. The Scott inflatable prosthesis consists of dual rods in the cavernosal bodies, an abdominal reservoir, and a pump mechanism (Fig. 14-20). Fluid can be baffled into the abdominal reservoir to mimic a flaccid state and into the rods to imitate an erection. The two-piece inflatable prosthesis uses the same principles as the Scott inflatable device by combining the pump and reservoir into a single piece, reducing the risk of mechanical complications. One-piece inflatable systems use a baffling system contained within each of the two rods (Fig. 14-21). An alternate, one-piece device mimics an erection by shortening a cable that is surrounded by plastic bodies (Fig. 14-22).

Contraindications and Cautions

Intrapenile prosthetic devices are contraindicated in patients with deep-rooted psychologic abnormalities underlying erectile dysfunction.

Preprocedural Nursing Care

1. Sexual counseling for the patient and his partner during preoperative and postoperative periods may be necessary.
2. Teach the patient and partner (when appropriate) to manipulate inflatable prosthetic devices before the procedure.
3. Advise the patient that the presence of an implant may carry a risk for infection during an invasive genitourinary procedure. Instruct the patient to discuss the need for antibiotic prophylaxis with his urologist before future procedures.

NURSING CARE

Nursing Assessment

Penis: Redness; edema; signs of erosion of prosthetic device
Scrotum and perineum: Hematoma for 2 to 3 weeks; edema for 24 hours postoperatively; discharge and hemorrhage from incision
Temperature: Fever
Urinary output: Normal voiding patterns; catheter drainage rarely needed

Patient Problems/Nursing Diagnoses & Interventions

NIC Physical Comfort Promotion

Acute pain related to surgical trauma

- Reassure patient that scrotal discomfort is temporary, although bruising and some scrotal swelling will persist for approximately 2 weeks.
- Administer analgesic or narcotic agents, as directed, *to relieve pain.*
- Advise patient to wear comfortable brief type of underwear *to minimize excess jostling and discomfort of the penis and scrotum.*

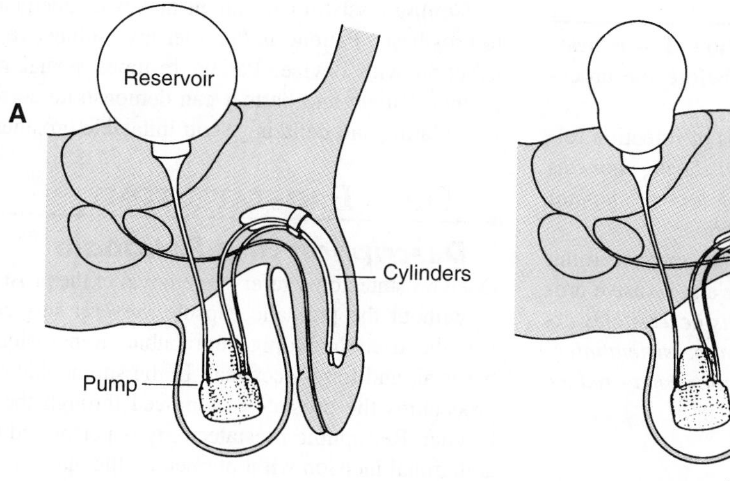

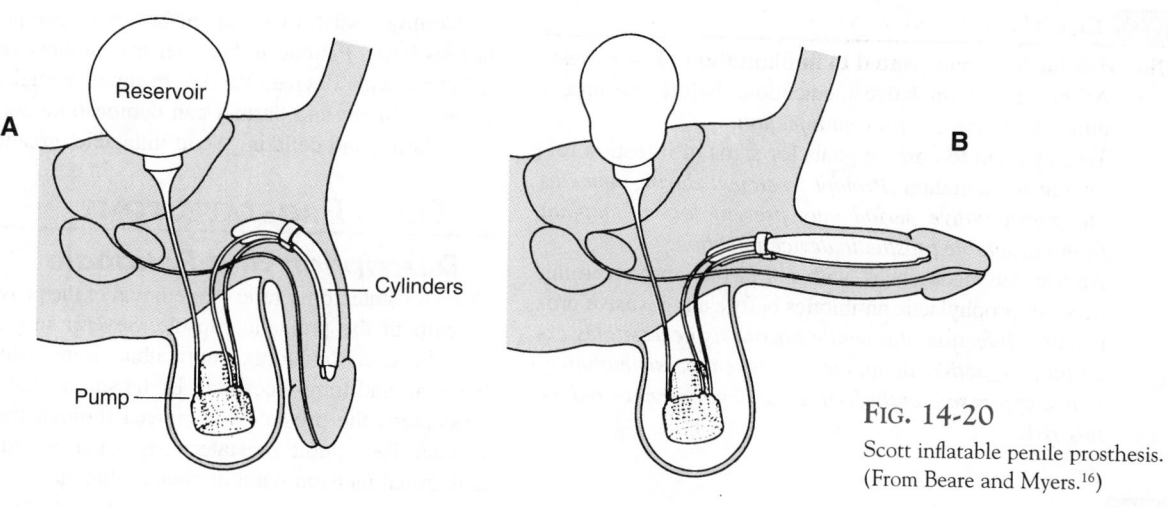

FIG. 14-20
Scott inflatable penile prosthesis. (From Beare and Myers.[16])

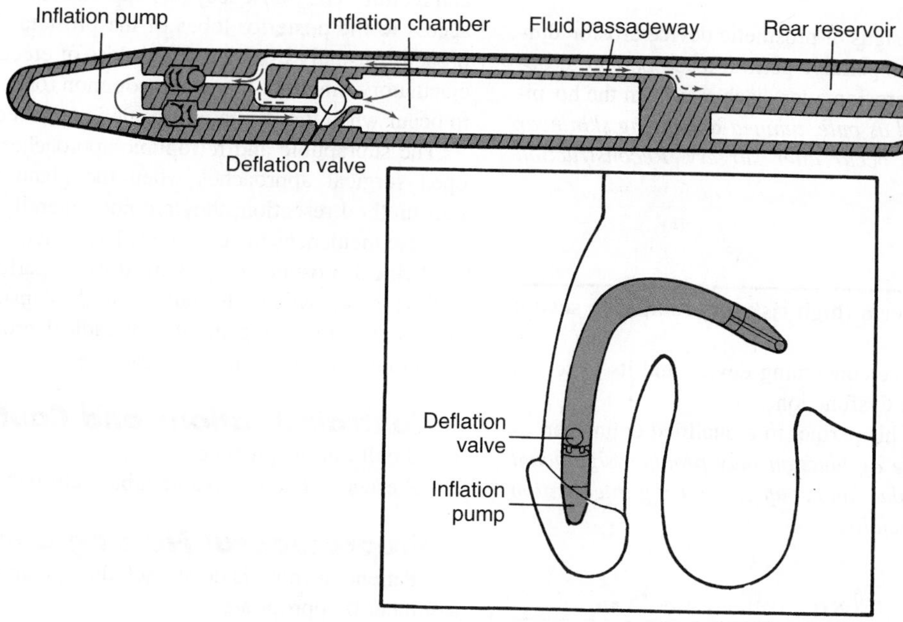

FIG. 14-21
One-piece inflatable penile prosthesis. (From Gray.[61]).

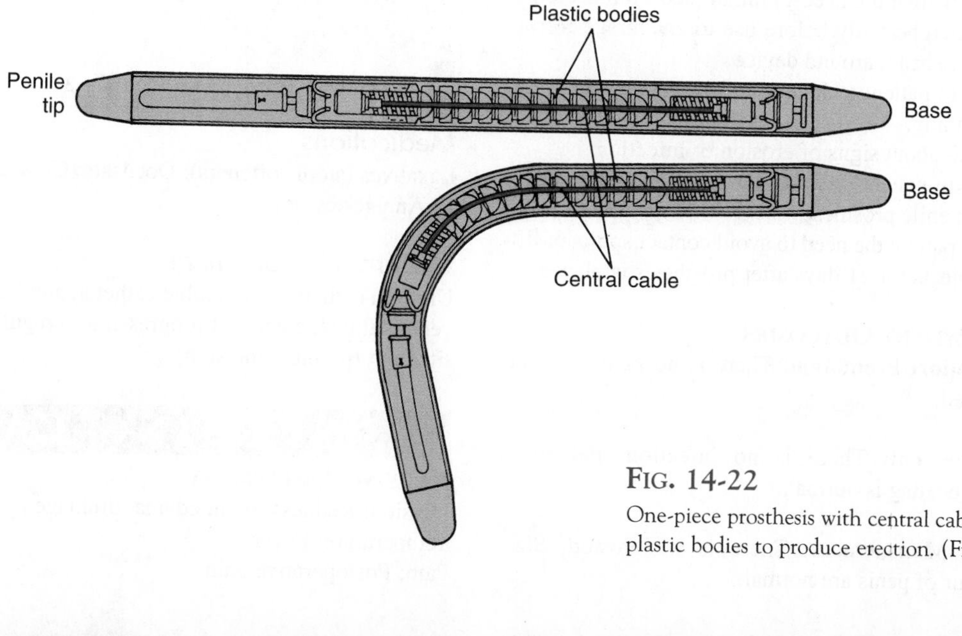

FIG. 14-22
One-piece prosthesis with central cable that shortens plastic bodies to produce erection. (From Gray.[61]).

NIC RISK MANAGEMENT

High risk for infection related to implantation of prosthesis

- Administer antiinfective medications before the procedure, as directed, *to prevent infection.*
- Teach patient to observe penis for signs of infection following implantation. *Prompt treatment during immediate postoperative period may prevent loss of implant from intractable prosthetic device infection.*
- Advise patient to check with his physician concerning need for prophylactic antibiotics before any invasive procedures. *Infection of a penile prosthesis necessitates explaining to patient about how to prevent persistent infection. Suppressive antiinfective medications may reduce this risk.*

NIC SKIN/WOUND MANAGEMENT

Risk for impaired tissue integrity related to presence of foreign body (prosthesis)

- Observe penis for signs of prosthetic device erosion during immediate postoperative period; teach patient to observe for signs of erosion after discharge from the hospital. *Erosion (noted as pale, thinned-appearing skin near glans penis) may occur after surgery. Reconstruction may be required.*

NIC COPING ASSISTANCE

Situational low self-esteem (high risk for) related to sexual dysfunction

- Provide reassurance concerning device and its expected impact on erectile dysfunction
- Refer patient and his partner to a qualified counselor, as indicated. *Erectile dysfunction may produce significant discord for individual and couple, requiring intervention by a qualified specialist.*

PATIENT EDUCATION/CONTINUUM OF CARE PLAN

1. Inform patient to abstain from sex for 21 days after surgery to allow for adequate healing if semirigid device is used.
2. Discuss with patient the need to inflate Scott inflatable penile prosthesis repeatedly before use to encourage formation of fibrous sheath around device.
3. Demonstrate to patient techniques of concealing semirigid device in clothing.
4. Inform patient about signs of erosion or infection.
5. Demonstrate to patient *and partner* inflation and deflation of inflatable penile prostheses.
6. Discuss with patient the need to avoid contact sports or lifting heavy objects for 21 days after prosthesis is placed.

EVALUATION/PATIENT OUTCOMES

Physical Comfort Promotion: There is no pain. Comfort level is maintained.

Risk Management: There is no infection. Patient is afebrile. Wound healing is normal.

Skin/Wound Management: There is no erosion. Size, color, and contour of penis are normal.

Coping Assistance: Patient makes an adequate adjustment to prosthesis. Patient *and* partner give subjective report of satisfaction with device. Patient resumes sexual relations with partner. Patient and partner can demonstrate correct technique for inflating and deflating Scott inflatable prosthesis.

OPEN PROSTATECTOMY

Description and Rationale

Open prostatectomy refers to removal of the prostate gland with or without the prostatic capsule. Several surgical approaches may be used including suprapubic, transvesical, retropubic, perineal, and transcoccygeal. In the suprapubic or transvesical procedures the prostate is removed through the cavity of the bladder. Retropubic prostatectomy is performed through a low abdominal incision without opening the bladder. The most radical of the open procedures for prostatectomy is the perineal approach in which the incision is made between the scrotum and rectum. The transcoccygeal approach allows better surgical access to the posterior lobes of the prostate. The perineal approach is usually associated with loss of erection, orgasm, and ejaculatory function. It is not uncommon for sexual dysfunction to occur when the prostatic capsule is removed.

The suprapubic and retropubic approaches may be used as open surgical approaches when the gland is too large for transurethral resection; they are not generally used for cancer. In these incidences the capsule is left intact.

Perineal prostatectomy is most often performed for cancer of the prostate when it is confined to the capsule. Some controversy exists regarding the use of radical prostatectomy when the tumor extends through the capsule.

Contraindications and Cautions

1. Small fibrous prostate
2. Presence of cancer (suprapubic, retropubic)

Preprocedural Nursing Care

1. Patient teaching is done, including potential sexual impairment if appropriate.
2. Perineum, external genitalia, abdomen, and upper halves of thighs are shaved the night before surgery.
3. Cleansing enemas are given until clear.

MULTIDISCIPLINARY PLAN

Medications

Laxatives (stool softeners): Docusate (Colace), 100 mg/day PO
Analgesics prn

General Management

Urethral catheter, suprapubic catheter, and Penrose drain; intravenous fluids; clear diet progressing to regular diet; heat lamp; sitz bath (perineal incision)

NURSING CARE

NURSING ASSESSMENT

Incision: Redness; pain; edema; drainage
Temperature: Fever
Pain: Postoperative pain

Urinary output: Amount of urinary output through urethral catheter or suprapubic catheter; presence of bright red blood; stress incontinence (may last for a few days to 6 months); urethral stricture

Other complications: Epididymitis

Sexual dysfunction: Impotence; retrograde ejaculation

Patient Problems/Nursing Diagnoses & Interventions

NIC Tissue Perfusion Management

Risk for hemorrhage related to surgical resection

- Observe urine output for color, consistency, volume, and presence of blood clots *to assess for excessive bleeding.*
- Maintain catheter traction as directed *to prevent hemorrhage.*
- Monitor vital signs *to assess for systemic signs of hemorrhage.*

NIC Risk Management

Risk for infection related to surgical trauma

- Maintain sterile urinary drainage system *to prevent infection.*
- Monitor vital signs *to assess for systemic signs of infection.*

NIC Elimination Management

Impaired urinary elimination related to potential obstruction of urinary outflow

- Assess output through urethral or suprapubic catheter for volume *to prevent urinary retention.*
- Observe catheters for kinking and presence of blood clots *to prevent urinary retention.*

NIC Coping Assistance

Disturbed body image related to altered erectile and fertility function

- Discuss implications of removal of prostatic capsule with patient and in consultation with urologist. *Likelihood of altered erectile dysfunction varies significantly with surgical techniques. Altered high risk for fertility is expected and must be discussed fully with patient.*
- Assist patient in exploring anxiety and fears related to procedure; provide factual information concerning implications of procedure as indicated. *Exploration of feelings of fear and anxiety with reassurance of objective facts related to procedure allows optimum opportunity for patient to regain positive body image.*
- Discuss alternative means of sexual expression, such as penile prosthesis, as indicated and in consultation with urologist *to reassure patient of realistic alternatives in cases where erectile dysfunction may occur.*

NIC Skin/Wound Management

Risk for impaired skin integrity related to drainage from wound

- Change dressing frequently *to prevent skin irritation from damp dressing.*
- Cleanse skin gently and pat dry or use a hair dryer *to dry skin and prevent irritation.*
- Apply moisture barrier ointments and skin sealants (Bard Protective Barrier Film; Skin Prep) *to protect the skin.*

Patient Education/Continuum of Care Plan

1. Discuss incisional care with patient.
2. Discuss skin protection techniques with patient if drainage is still continuing at time of discharge.
3. Urine color will not clear up for 4 to 8 weeks, but patient should notify physician if it changes and becomes bright red with clots.
4. Provide teaching and counseling regarding sexual concerns.

Evaluation/Patient Outcomes

Tissue Perfusion Management: No hemorrhage occurs. Urine remains clear and free of clots.

Risk Management: There is no infection. Patient remains afebrile and experiences no symptoms indicative of infection.

Elimination Management: Urinary elimination is normal. Output is adequate. Color is clear. Patient does not experience pain, burning, or bladder spasms.

Coping Assistance: Sexual functioning resumes. Patient is able to obtain an erection. Retrograde ejaculation may occur. Patient is scheduled for or has had a penile prosthesis if indicated.

Skin/Wound Management: Skin integrity is maintained. No skin irritation or breakdown occurs.

Open Urologic Surgery

Description and Rationale

Open urologic surgeries include nephrectomy, partial nephrectomy, nephrolithotomy, pyelolithotomy, ureterolithotomy, and cystectomy. The care of the patient during these procedures is similar, and all involve an open surgical incision. Surgery of the kidney is accomplished through a flank incision, whereas the operative approach for bladder surgeries is an anterior incision.

Indications for nephrectomy include calculus, hemorrhage, hydronephrosis, hypertension, neoplasms, renal donation, trauma, and vascular disease.[51] Partial nephrectomy is performed to preserve as much renal function as possible in the same conditions that may require nephrectomy. A partial nephrectomy is important when contralateral renal function is impaired. Stones in the kidney, pelvis, or ureter may be removed by an open urologic incision if newer techniques of ESWL and percutaneous ureteroscopic stone removal are ineffective.

Contraindications and Cautions

1. If the condition is bilateral, it is important to preserve total renal function.

2. Nephrostomy drainage may be required following open urologic surgeries through stents or tubes to allow for adequate healing when the potential for wound healing is suboptimal, scar tissue is significant, or reconstructive procedures require splinting.

Preprocedural Nursing Care

1. Preoperative teaching concerns the procedure, presence of catheter, and stents for surgery, and turning, coughing, and leg exercises following surgery.
2. Give nothing by mouth past midnight.

NURSING CARE

NURSING ASSESSMENT

Incision: Redness; pain; edema; drainage
Temperature: Fever
Urinary output: Amount of urinary output through nephrostomy tube or catheter; presence of bright red blood; absence of urinary output through catheter
Pain: Incisional; postoperative
Hemorrhage: Incisional; through drains, tubes, or catheter

PATIENT PROBLEMS/NURSING DIAGNOSES & INTERVENTIONS

NIC TISSUE PERFUSION MANAGEMENT

High risk for hemorrhage or infection related to surgical trauma

- Assess patient for signs and symptoms of bleeding.
- Evaluate all tube drainage for amount, color, and consistency. *Persistent bleeding is noted as bloody or serosanguineous discharge through surgical drains.*
- Observe surgical wound for color, warmth, and discharge *to assess for signs of bleeding (bloody discharge through wound with or without separation of borders) and signs of infection (purulent discharge from wound, increasing redness, warmth at operative site).*

NIC ELIMINATION MANAGEMENT

Risk for deficient fluid volume related to surgical manipulation of kidney that obstructs urine flow

Impaired urinary elimination related to surgical obstruction of drainage catheter

- Monitor intake and output, daily weights, and blood urea nitrogen (BUN) and creatinine levels *to assess for hypovolemia; poor fluid intake, rising BUN and creatinine, and rapid weight loss are potential signs of fluid volume deficit that impair healing and may compromise renal function.*
- Monitor urinary output through urethral catheter, nephrostomy tube, suprapubic catheter, or other drainage tube *to prevent urinary retention.*

NIC PHYSICAL COMFORT PROMOTION

Acute pain related to surgical trauma

- Provide analgesics as ordered.
- Provide medications to decrease detrusor contractility as ordered *to prevent bladder spasm associated with urethral or suprapubic catheterization and surgical manipulation of the lower urinary tract.*

NIC SKIN/WOUND MANAGEMENT

Risk for impaired skin integrity related to drainage from wound

- Use skin barrier (pectin wafer) around Penrose drain or stab wound *to protect skin from potential irritation from discharge.*
- Use a sterile drainage wound collection system if drainage is copious *to protect skin from discharge and to assess output.*
- Maintain sterile dressing changes *to protect skin adjacent to surgical incision from discharge.*

PATIENT EDUCATION/CONTINUUM OF CARE PLAN

1. Patient education varies with primary etiology; refer to specific discussions of urologic diseases.
2. Patient should be informed about incision care and management of any drains or tubes.

EVALUATION/PATIENT OUTCOMES

Tissue Perfusion Management: There is no hemorrhage. No bleeding or excessive serosanguineous drainage occurs.

Elimination Management: Urinary output is adequate; no retention occurs. BUN and creatinine levels are normal. Weight remains normal.

Physical Comfort Promotion: Comfort level is maintained. Patient experiences minimal pain.

Skin/Wound Management: Skin integrity remains intact. No skin breakdown occurs. There is no infection. There are no signs of redness, edema, or inflammation of incision.

PERCUTANEOUS NEPHROSCOPIC STONE REMOVAL

Description and Rationale

Percutaneous nephroscopic stone removal is a nonsurgical technique to treat urolithiasis. A nephrostomy tube is placed percutaneously into the proper calyx under fluoroscopic monitoring, and a dilator system is used to allow insertion of a nephroscope with one or more working channels. Several methods may be used to remove calculi percutaneously. A stone basket may be used to retrieve relatively small calculi. Larger stones may be first broken via ultrasonic lithotriptor, laser, or electrolysis. Remaining fragments are then removed via a stone basket or flushed from the collecting system mechanically or physiologically.

Contraindications and Cautions

1. Septicemia should be adequately controlled before percutaneous nephroscopic stone removal is attempted.

2. If obstruction is significant, a nephrostomy tube may be placed with the patient under local anesthesia to facilitate adequate pelvic drainage.

Preprocedural Nursing Care

Monitor for signs and symptoms of gram-negative septicemia and septic shock, including increased fever, pulse, respirations, and blood pressure followed by hypotension and potential cardiovascular compromise.

NURSING CARE

Nursing Assessment

Pain: Renal colic; acute flank pain
Temperature: Fever
Urinary output: Oliguria or anuria in cases of bilateral obstruction
Other complications: Nausea, vomiting, and ileus secondary to renal colic
Nephrostomy tube: Hematuria; frank bleeding

Patient Problems/Nursing Diagnoses & Interventions

NIC Tissue Perfusion Management

Risk for hemorrhage related to manipulation of kidney

- Observe flank for mass and observe nephrostomy tube for amount and characteristics of discharge (color, consistency) *to assess for hemorrhage from affected kidney and urinary transport system.*
- Monitor pulse and blood pressure *to assess for systemic signs of hemorrhage.*

NIC Elimination Management

Impaired urinary elimination related to potential obstruction of urinary outflow
Risk for infection related to surgical trauma
Acute pain related to urinary obstruction

- Observe output through nephrostomy tube for color consistency and volume *to prevent urinary retention.*
- Monitor patency of tubes and irrigate tubes as directed *to prevent urinary retention and potential infection*
- Monitor vital signs, especially temperature, for possible infection.
- Administer analgesics as ordered.

Patient Education/Continuum of Care Plan

Teach techniques for preventing recurrent stone formation, including drugs, diet, and fluid intake.

Evaluation/Patient Outcomes

Tissue Perfusion Management: Hemorrhage is absent. Urine drainage from nephrostomy tube is clear. Vital signs are within normal limits.

Elimination Management: There is no obstruction. Patient does not experience renal colic. Creatinine and BUN levels are within normal limits. Infection is absent. Patient is afebrile. Urine and blood cultures are negative. Urinary elimination patterns return to normal. No urinary retention occurs. Pain is absent. Comfort level is normal.

Transurethral Resection of the Prostate and Alternative Procedures for Prostate Tissue Ablation

Description and Rationale

Transurethral resection of the prostate (TURP) is the removal of prostatic tissue under endoscopic control. A rigid cystoscope is inserted into the urethra, and the prostatic urethra is identified. A resectoscope is inserted, and tissue is removed by a small loop with electrocautery energy (Fig. 14-23). Blood, tissue, and other debris are irrigated with a glycine or sorbitol solution. The resected prostate tissue is collected and sent for pathologic analysis. The glycine or sorbitol solutions allow electrocauterization of bleeding vessels in the prostatic bed without damage to adjacent tissue. The area of resection varies with each patient but typically encompasses the bladder neck and prostatic urethra. The resection frequently extends to the urethra just above the verumontanum.[57,61]

Multiple alternative procedures for prostatic tissue ablation have been described. Some have gained relatively widespread use, whereas others are in earlier stages of clinical investigations. Table 14-11 summarizes alternative approaches for prostate tis-

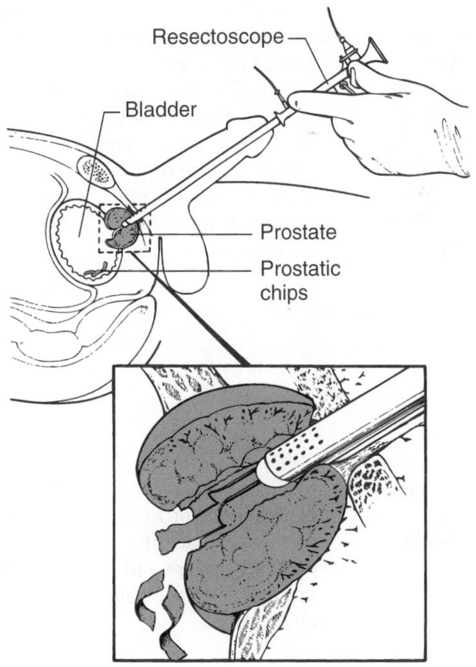

Fig. 14-23

Continuous irrigation of the bladder requires a three-way Foley catheter that allows simultaneous infusion and drainage of an irrigating solution (normal saline) through the bladder. The solution is infused rapidly into the bladder, and the bedside drainage bag is assessed for evidence of excessive bleeding and then drained every 1 to 2 hours. (From Beare and Myers.[16])

Table 14-11 Alternative Procedures for Prostate Tissue Removal (All Procedures Are Compared With TURP)*

Procedure	Description	Advantages	Disadvantages	Postprocedural Care†
Transurethral vaportrode (Fig. 14-24)	Resection of prostatic tissue under direct, endoscopic visualization. Tissue is removed using a "roller ball" or "roller bar" and electrocautery energy.	• Superior visualization of prostate • Less risk of bleeding • Possibly less risk of transurethral resection (TUR) syndrome • Procedure may be performed as outpatient • Prostate tissue available for pathologic analysis to determine presence of prostate cancer • Additional equipment costs are relatively low	None yet identified	Indwelling catheter for 24 h; patient may experience some hematuria for several days; passage of scabs with transient hematuria in 7-10 days
Transurethral incision of the prostate (TUIP)	Incision of the prostatic capsule under direct endoscopic visualization. A small cutting loop and electrocautery energy are used to incise the prostatic capsule.	• Local anesthesia may be used to reduce risk of spinal or general anesthesia • Reduced hospital stay (1-2 days shorter when compared with TURP) • Less risk of bleeding, retrograde ejaculation, bladder neck contracture • Lower risk of TUR syndrome • Additional equipment relatively inexpensive	• Limited to smaller glands • Marked enlargement of median lobe comprises relative contraindication • Risk of incontinence, erectile dysfunction similar to TURP • Prostate tissue not available for pathologic analysis	Brief hospital stay may be necessary; indwelling catheter for 24 h; three-way irrigation not typically required, but catheter is placed under gentle traction
Laser prostatectomy (laser prostatectomy, transurethral incision of the prostate, visual laser ablation of the prostate [VLAP])	Ablation of prostate tissue using laser energy (Nd:YAG). The visualization technique varies; VLAP is generally preferred because of the ability to visualize the prostate using direct endoscopy.	• Hospitalization not required • Low risk of bleeding • Less risk of retrograde ejaculation • Reduced mortality rate	• Prolonged period of tissue slough (7 days; may persist up to 30 days) • Postoperative discomfort and irritation occur with prolonged edema • Long-term efficacy as compared with TURP has not been established • Prostate tissue not available for pathologic analysis • Additional equipment costs are significant	Indwelling (suprapubic or urethral) catheter for at least 7 days; postprocedure discomfort may occur during period of edema and tissue slough
Intraurethral stent insertion (Fig. 14-25)	A medical-grade steel is placed in the prostatic urethra to widen the prostatic urethra and mechanically alleviate obstruction.	• Less risk of bleeding • No risk of TUR syndrome • Procedure is reversible (limited window of opportunity)	• Does not correct bladder neck obstruction • Occasionally causes discomfort requiring removal • Urethral tissue may fail to reepithelialize around stent, necessitating removal	Performed as outpatient; suprapubic catheter up to 30 days after insertion; initial irritative voiding symptoms may require antispasmodic therapy

*References 23, 37, 38, 39, 61, 101, 112, 113, 150, 151, 165.

†Refined nursing care plans may not be available, primarily because of a lack of clinical experience with these techniques.

Procedure	Description	Advantages	Disadvantages	Postprocedural Care†
Interstitial laser therapy	Ablation of prostate tissue using a transurethral, transrectal, or transperineal approach. Prostatic size and location are determined using ultrasonic techniques. Laser energy is used to ablate prostate tissue without disrupting integrity of rectal or urethral wall.	• Similar to laser prostatectomy • Preservation of urothelium may reduce postprocedure discomfort, irritative voiding symptoms	• Degree of postprocedure discomfort has not been determined • Tissue not available for pathologic analysis	Indwelling catheter, otherwise unknown
Transurethral ultrasonic aspiration	Destruction of prostate tissue, using ultrasonic energy (0-700–micron vibration) at an excursion rate of 39 kHz; maximum power 100 W. Prostatic size and location are determined using ultrasound imaging.	• Lower risk for significant bleeding • Incontinence rate may be reduced • Impotence risk is comparable to TURP	• Procedure will not correct significant bladder neck hypertrophy obstruction	Indwelling catheter for 18-24 h; in-hospital stay 2-3 days
Transurethral needle ablation of the prostate (TUNA)	Ablation of prostatic tissue under indirect endoscopic visualization (the surgeon will see the prostatic urethra, but does not see the needles penetrate the prostatic capsule). Low-level radiofrequency energy is used to heat the prostate, causing tissue destruction.	• Lower risk of significant blood loss • Lower risk of postprocedure irritative voiding symptoms • Lower risk of impotence • Lower risk of retrograde ejaculation	• Tissue not available for tissue analysis • Prolonged time for symptom improvement (>1 month) • Transient urinary retention, approximately 3 days (range 1-21 days) • Urethral stricture may occur	Hematuria and dysuria persist for 2-3 days; indwelling catheter may be left in place for 7-10 days
High-intensity focused ultrasound (HIFU)	Coagulative destruction of prostate tissue using high-intensity, focused ultrasonic energy. The ultrasonic energy is delivered via a transrectal route, and the prostate is localized using ultrasonic imaging techniques.	• Less risk of bleeding • Low postoperative discomfort • No risk of TUR syndrome	• Transient retention lasting 6 days (range 1-42 days) • Hematospermia, mild hematuria • Urinary tract infection • Moderate symptom improvement only	PSA values are transiently elevated (12-24 h); suprapubic catheter for 6-7 days; symptom improvement generally requires 6 months
Transurethral microwave thermotherapy (TUMT)	Microwave (radiating heat energy) is used to destroy prostate tissue while conductive cooling is used to prevent urethral injury. The microwave energy is delivered via a 20 French balloon type of catheter, and a temperature probe is then placed to measure anterior rectal wall temperature.	• Performed as an outpatient • Less risk of significant bleeding • No risk of TUR syndrome • Low risk of retrograde ejaculation	• Multiple treatments may be required • Rectal wall injury may occur • Long-term efficacy (>12 months postprocedure) has not been established • Effect of therapy on the bladder neck is not known	PSA values are transiently elevated following procedure (up to 3 months); transient urinary retention occurs, and suprapubic catheter drainage is required
Cryotherapy	Prostate tissue is destroyed by rapid freezing. A cryotherapy probe is inserted into the prostate, and the adjacent tissue is rapidly cooled to −180° to −190° C.	• Less risk of bleeding • Reduced risk of TUR syndrome	• Risk of impotence and incontinence may be significant when compared with TURP • Urethrorectal, urethrocutaneous fistulae may occur • Tissue not available for pathologic analysis	Indwelling catheter for several weeks; sloughing of tissue will occur during this period; primarily used for prostate cancer

sue removal. It is important to remember that the nursing management of the majority of these alternative procedures has not been adequately defined, primarily because of a lack of clinical experience.

Because BPH is typically a quality-of-life condition, prostate tissue ablation is indicated when voiding dysfunction symptoms are significant, and the patient chooses this treatment rather than watchful waiting or pharmacotherapy. Prostatic tissue destruction also is indicated when BPH is associated with acute urinary retention, compromised renal function, or urinary tract infection.[3]

Contraindications and Cautions

1. Prostatic tissue ablation is contraindicated in the presence of a urinary tract infection or when acute prostatitis is present.
2. Physical conditions such as ankylosis of the hip or irreversible scrotal hernia may interfere with positioning of the patient for TURP, and alternative procedures may be considered.

Preprocedural Nursing Care

1. Discuss the technique of prostatic tissue destruction with the urologist before the procedure. Advise the patient of the procedure and anticipated outcomes based on this discussion.
2. Advise the patient that prostate tissue destruction may affect aspects of sexual function, including libido, antegrade ejaculations, erectile function, and fertility. Counsel him to consult his urologist to discuss specific concerns related to the incidence and nature of these potential complications.
3. Reassure the patient that the incidence of erectile dysfunction following prostate tissue destruction for BPH is relatively low. Advise the patient to discuss specific concerns with his urologist because the relative risk varies according to the technique used for prostatectomy.

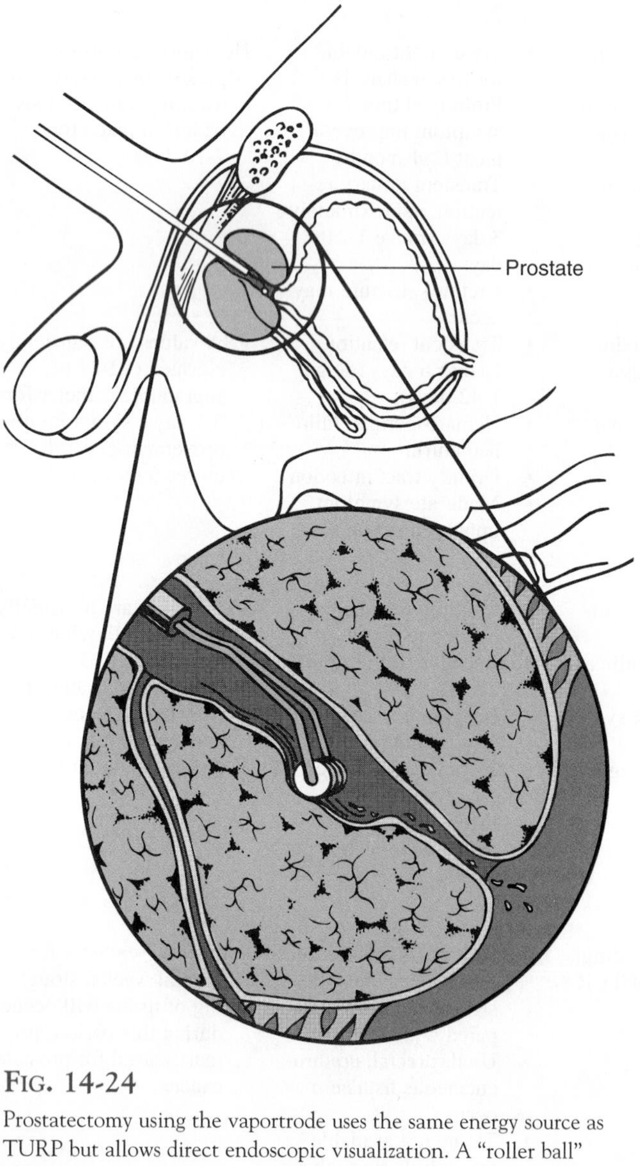

FIG. 14-24
Prostatectomy using the vaportrode uses the same energy source as TURP but allows direct endoscopic visualization. A "roller ball" blade device is used to ablate prostatic tissue.

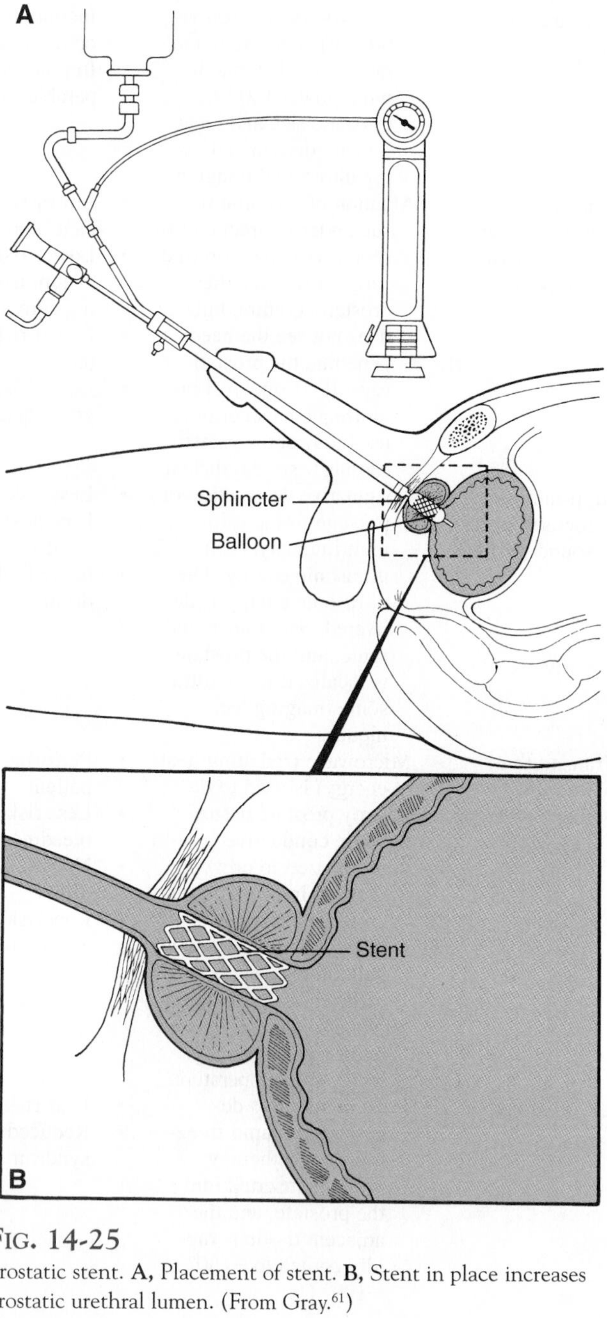

FIG. 14-25
Prostatic stent. **A,** Placement of stent. **B,** Stent in place increases prostatic urethral lumen. (From Gray.[61])

Multidisciplinary Plan

Medications

Antiinfective medications: Commonly administered before and after prostatic tissue ablation. An aminoglycoside may be given intravenously before and for 12 to 24 hours after the procedure.
Systemic urinary analgesics, anticholinergics, or antispasmodics administered as indicated for pain.

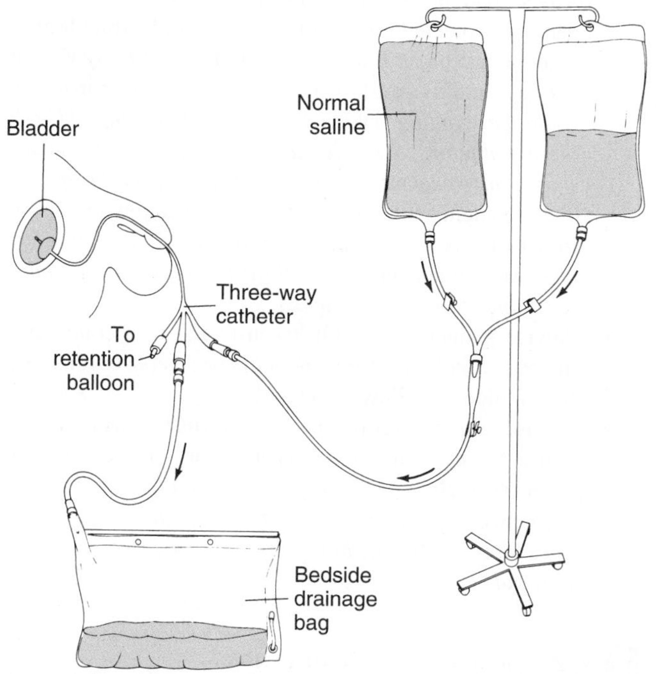

Fig. 14-26

Continuous irrigation of the bladder requires a three-way Foley catheter that allows simultaneous infusion and drainage of an irrigating solution (normal saline) through the bladder. The solution is infused rapidly into the bladder, and the bedside drainage bag is assessed for evidence of excessive bleeding and then drained every 1 to 2 hours. (From Beare and Myers.[16])

General Management

A three-way indwelling catheter with continuous irrigation required following TURP (Fig. 14-26); Variable periods of indwelling catheter drainage required following alternative procedures (see Table 14-11)

NURSING CARE

Nursing Assessment

Bladder and prostate: Urinary output, presence of clots; flow rate of irrigation following TURP, character of output, volume of fluid in irrigating bags and catheter drainage bag
Significant blood loss (TURP associated with greatest risk): Changes in serum hematocrit and hemoglobin; changes in vital signs; rapid pulse with increased blood pressure followed by declining blood pressure with severe loss; presence of large quantities of bright red blood and clots in catheter drainage bag
Temperature: Fever
Transurethral resection (TUR) syndrome (TURP carries greatest risk): Acute confusion; restlessness; bradycardia, tachypnea; hyponatremia

Patient Problems/Nursing Diagnoses & Interventions

(See Table 14-11 for differences in care with alternative procedures.)

NIC Tissue Perfusion Management

Ineffective tissue perfusion related to bleeding from prostatic urethra
Risk for ineffective tissue perfusion related to deep vein thrombosis of lower extremities

- Maintain three-way indwelling catheter with continuous irrigation *to remove debris and clots from bladder and to prevent blockage of urinary outflow.*
- Maintain gentle traction on catheter *to prevent excessive bleeding from operative site* (Fig. 14-27).
- Obtain serum hemoglobin and hematocrit as directed; compare preoperative and postoperative values. *Signifícnt hemorrhage may occur from prostatic bed following TURP.*

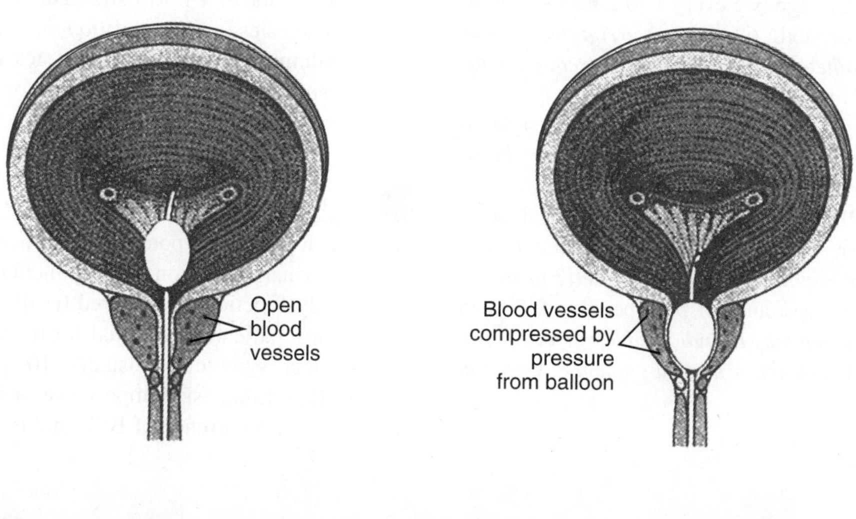

Fig. 14-27

Gentle traction is maintained against prostatic vascular bed to prevent excessive bleeding after transurethral resection. (From Beare and Myers.[16])

- Remove indwelling catheter as directed (typically 36 to 72 hours after TURP). Assist patient in saving urine from each voiding episode. The "string of bottles" obtained after catheter removal is used *to monitor resolution of hematuria from prostatic bed.*
- Reinsert indwelling catheter as directed if marked hematuria persists or if significant hematuria occurs. *Reinsertion of catheter with gentle traction may be required to prevent persistent bleeding from operative site.*
- Reassure patient that pink-tinged urine and flecks of dark blood may occur for 10 to 14 days. *Dark flecks of blood and pink-tinged urine (indicating minimal bleeding mixed with urine) indicate spontaneous release of scabs from the operative site.*

Deep vein thrombosis care

- Assist the patient in applying antiembolic stockings before TURP, and in wearing them for 1 week postoperatively. *TURP requires prolonged positioning of legs in stirrups, increasing the risk of deep vein thrombosis of the legs; antiembolic stockings encourage venous return from the lower extremities.*
- Raise foot of bed 20 to 30 degrees during first postoperative day *to encourage venous return from legs.*
- Teach patient to perform passive leg exercises until catheter is removed and he is able to walk. *Contraction of leg muscles before ambulation will encourage venous return.*
- Maintain adequate fluid intake (30 ml/kg of body weight per day). *Dehydration increases risk of deep vein thrombosis of legs.*

NIC Elimination Management

Urinary retention related to debris and blood clots from operative site, scarring and contracture at operative site

Risk for TUR syndrome related to fluid absorption and electrolyte imbalance following TURP*

Impaired urinary elimination related to postoperative urethral obstruction

- Maintain continuous irrigation with three-way catheter for 24 hours after TURP. *Continuous bladder irrigation removes clots and debris from bladder, preventing catheter occlusion and retention.*
- Select a large drainage bag for catheter (at least 2000 ml). *Drainage bag will fill rapidly during irrigation.*
- Empty catheter drainage bag every 1 to 2 hours or more frequently as indicated. *Continuous irrigation causes rapid filling of catheter drainage bag, and frequent emptying is required to prevent retention.*
- Irrigate catheter gently with saline, or assist physician in completing irrigation as indicated. *Irrigation may be required to remove larger blood clots.*
- Monitor urine elimination patterns after removal of indwelling catheter. *Urinary retention may occur after catheter removal, requiring prolonged catheter drainage.*
- Advise patient of importance of postoperative follow-up care. *Urethral dilation may be indicated to correct or prevent bladder neck contracture and subsequent obstruction.*
- Monitor patient for signs and symptoms of TUR syndrome (acute confusion, restlessness, bradycardia, tachypnea, vomiting, dilutional hyponatremia) after transurethral surgery. *TUR syndrome is an uncommon but potentially fatal complication of TURP.*
- Maintain adequate fluid intake (30 ml/kg of body weight per day) using oral and parenteral fluid as available. *Maintenance of adequate hydration may reduce risk of TUR syndrome.*
- Promptly consult physician if signs or symptoms of TUR syndrome occur. TUR syndrome is managed with fluid replacement and supportive care; *the condition can be fatal without prompt intervention.*
- Advise patient that transient urinary frequency and urgency is expected after catheter removal. Instruct him to maintain adequate fluid intake (30 ml/kg of body weight per day) and to avoid or limit intake of bladder irritants. *Irritative voiding symptoms occur following TURP; these symptoms are related to surgical trauma, endoscopic instrumentation, and the indwelling catheter.*
- Teach patient with stress incontinence following TURP to perform pelvic muscle exercises. *Pelvic muscle exercises strengthen the periurethral muscles and minimize or ablate stress urinary leakage.*
- Advise patient to consult his urologist or a continence nurse specialist if stress incontinence persists for more than 6 months following TURP.
- Advise patient with persistent urge (instability) incontinence to seek care from his urologist or a continence nurse specialist. *Persistent urge incontinence requires aggressive behavioral or pharmacologic therapy if it does not resolve within 1 to 2 weeks after catheter removal.*

NIC Physical Comfort Promotion

Acute pain related to prostatic tissue resection, endoscopic instrumentation

- Administer anticholinergic or antispasmodic medications as directed. *These medications prevent unstable (hyperactive) bladder contractions or spasms, which may occur following TURP, causing intermittent, cramping pain.*
- Advise patient that mild dysuria (discomfort with urination) may occur after catheter removal. Provide adequate fluid intake, a warm sitz bath, warm shower, or urinary analgesics (as directed) *to minimize dysuria.*
- Administer systemic analgesics as indicated *to reduce generalized pain and discomfort related to prostatectomy.*

Patient Education/Continuum of Care Plan

1. Teach patient the potential complications of TURP, including urinary retention, urinary incontinence, persistent erectile dysfunction, and altered fertility potential.
2. Inform patient of potential for regrowth of BPH with subsequent symptoms (usually 10 years or more after a TURP). Emphasize importance of routine prostate evaluations for recurrence of BPH and for prostate cancer.

---

*Not a NANDA diagnosis.

EVALUATION/PATIENT OUTCOMES

Tissue Perfusion Management: Decline in International Prostate Symptom Score indicates relief of bothersome symptoms of BPH.

Elimination Management: Significant bleeding is avoided or promptly managed. TUR syndrome is prevented or promptly managed. Urinary residual volumes and urinary flow variables indicate relief from obstruction.

Physical Comfort Promotion: Patient is comfortable. Pain is managed.

TRANSURETHRAL SURGERY

Transurethral surgeries consist of transurethral resection of bladder tumors (TURBT), transurethral sphincterotomy, and transurethral bladder neck incision.

Description and Rationale

Transurethral resection of bladder tumors is the removal of superficial, malignant bladder tumors with a resectoscope, under endoscopic control. Postoperative bleeding may be significant when multiple tumors are resected, and the risk of TUR syndrome may be comparable to that for TURP. TURBT may or may not be combined with intravesical chemotherapy. Transurethral resection is initially preferred when managing a bladder tumor; laser ablation of the tumor may be performed following initial pathologic analysis of resected tissue and bladder cancer staging.

Transurethral sphincterotomy is the incision of the striated urethral sphincter under endoscopic control. It is reserved for males with detrusor sphincter dyssynergia who agree to manage their bladders by condom catheter containment after the procedure. The incision required for an adequate sphincterotomy is significant, and life-threatening postoperative bleeding may occur. Women are not appropriate candidates for a transurethral sphincterotomy because there is no adequate condom device to contain the urinary leakage that inevitably occurs after transurethral sphincterotomy.

Transurethral incision of the bladder neck is a single incision of the circular smooth muscle at the bladder neck under endoscopic visualization. The incision is relatively small, and the postprocedure bleeding is minimal, as is the risk of TUR syndrome.

Preprocedural Nursing Care

1. The role of transurethral resection of bladder tumors as a diagnostic and therapeutic measure is emphasized before initial treatment.
2. Patients are counseled that pathologic analysis will require several days.
3. Patients undergoing transurethral sphincterotomy are counseled that dribbling incontinence (stress urinary incontinence due to iatrogenic intrinsic sphincter deficiency) is expected to occur after the procedure, and a condom catheter will be required to contain urinary leakage.
4. Patients undergoing transurethral sphincterotomy or bladder neck incision are advised of the risk of retrograde ejaculation and altered fertility potential.

MULTIDISCIPLINARY PLAN

Medications

Preoperative and postoperative antibiotic agents as ordered
Anticholinergic or antispasmodics may be required to manage bladder spasms
Analgesic medications as needed

General Management

An indwelling catheter is required following TURBT; a three-way irrigation system may be indicated in special cases
A three-way irrigation system is required after transurethral sphincterotomy; typically for 2 to 3 days postoperatively
An indwelling catheter is required after bladder neck incision

NURSING CARE

NURSING ASSESSMENT

Bladder and urethra: Urinary output, presence of clots and bright red bleeding in urine; significant bleeding (particularly following transurethral sphincterotomy) with signs of hypovolemic shock (rapid pulse with increased pressure followed by falling blood pressure and bradycardia)
Temperature: Fever
TUR syndrome (TURBT carries greatest risk): Acute confusion; restlessness; bradycardia, tachypnea; hyponatremia

PATIENT PROBLEMS/NURSING DIAGNOSES & INTERVENTIONS

NIC **TISSUE PERFUSION MANAGEMENT**

Ineffective peripheral tissue perfusion (bladder or urethral) related to interruption of arterial venous flow

- Maintain indwelling catheter as directed; assess urinary output for presence of blood and clots, and assess catheter for patency. *Significant bleeding may occur after transurethral surgery, causing hypovolemia and catheter obstruction.*
- Maintain three-way irrigation as directed (required after transurethral sphincterotomy) with adequate flow rate to maintain pink-tinged urine for at least 24 hours. Do not reduce the irrigation to "keep open rate" for at least 24 hours after transurethral sphincterotomy. Significant bleeding frequently occurs after a transurethral sphincterotomy, and brisk irrigation is required *to maintain catheter patency and prevent filling of the bladder with clots.*
- Assist patient in obtaining adequate fluid intake, using parenteral or oral routes as indicated. *Postoperative bleeding causes fluid loss from body that must be replaced.*
- Evaluate patient's serum hematocrit and hemoglobin as indicated; promptly inform physician if these values are significantly abnormal as compared with preoperative values.
- Monitor vital signs (blood pressure, pulse, respiration) for signs of significant blood loss or impending hypovolemic shock.

NIC ELIMINATION MANAGEMENT

Urinary retention related to debris and blood clots from operative site, scarring and contracture at operative site

Risk for TUR syndrome related to fluid absorption and electrolyte imbalance following TURP*

- Maintain continuous irrigation with three-way catheter or indwelling catheter as directed. *Continuous catheter drainage with or without bladder irrigation provides drainage of clots or debris from bladder, preventing catheter occlusion and retention.*
- Empty catheter drainage bag every 1 to 2 hours or more frequently as indicated when bladder irrigation is required after transurethral surgery. *Continuous irrigation causes rapid filling of catheter drainage bag, and frequent emptying is required to prevent retention.*
- Irrigate catheter gently with saline, or assist physician in completing irrigation as indicated. Irrigation may be required *to remove larger blood clots.*
- Monitor urine elimination patterns after removal of indwelling catheter. *Urinary retention may occur after catheter removal, requiring prolonged catheter drainage.*
- Monitor patient for signs and symptoms of TUR syndrome (acute confusion, restlessness, bradycardia, tachypnea, vomiting, dilutional hyponatremia) following transurethral surgery. *TUR syndrome is an uncommon but potentially fatal complication of transurethral surgery.*
- Maintain adequate fluid intake (30 ml/kg of body weight per day) using oral and parenteral fluid as available. *Maintenance of adequate hydration may reduce the risk of TUR syndrome.*
- Promptly consult physician if signs or symptoms of TUR syndrome occur. *TUR syndrome is managed with fluid replacement and supportive care; the condition can be fatal without prompt intervention.*

PATIENT EDUCATION/CONTINUUM OF CARE PLAN

1. Encourage patient to maintain adequate fluid intake.
2. Explain to patient and family the importance of promptly reporting any signs and symptoms associated with TUR syndrome, including confusion, restlessness, slow heart rate, rapid breathing, and vomiting.
3. Report to urologist any signs of incontinence, urinary tract infection (burning, urgency), or inability to void.
4. Reinforce importance of continuing outpatient care.

EVALUATION/PATIENT OUTCOMES

Tissue Perfusion Management: Adequate fluid volume is maintained. Vital signs are within normal limits. Hematocrit and hemoglobin are within normal range

Elimination Management: TUR syndrome is prevented or promptly managed. Patient voids without difficulty

URINARY DIVERSION

Description and Rationale

A urinary diversion is any one of a number of surgical procedures that establish an unimpeded flow of urine, usually through a stoma. It is possible to divert the urine at any level in the urinary tract.

Supravesical Diversions

Diverting the urine at the level of the kidney is done by nephrostomy or pyelostomy. A nephrostomy is a high urinary diversion involving the placement of a catheter through the renal pelvis and into the renal calyces. Indications for placement of a nephrostomy tube are complete obstruction of the ureter, bypassing a urinary fistula, or irrigation of the renal pelvis. A nephrostomy tube is placed intraoperatively during a pyeloplasty or as an emergency procedure for the relief of kidney or ureteral obstruction.[57] Percutaneous placement of a nephrostomy tube under radiographic or ultrasound control has largely replaced the more traditional method of placement. The dePezzer or mushroom catheter, the Malecot or batwing catheter, or a small-lumen Foley catheter with a 5-ml balloon are used as nephrostomy tubes.[138]

Because of the problems associated with long-term nephrostomy drainage (infection, stone formation, intermittent hematuria, frank renal hemorrhage, or accidental dislodgment of the tube), it is typically used only as a temporary method of diversion.[173]

A pyelostomy is an opening into the renal pelvis made by catheter placement or by the creation of a stoma. Tube pyelostomy diversion carries equal risk as a nephrostomy; therefore tubeless diversion is substituted whenever possible. A cutaneous pyelostomy is performed infrequently but is designed for children requiring a high urinary diversion. Because children have less subcutaneous fat and a relatively mobile kidney, it is a comparatively simple technical procedure.

Ureterostomy, another type of supravesical urinary diversion, is done with a tube or stoma. A cystoscope may be used to pass a ureter catheter up the ureter into the renal pelvis if the ureter is unobstructed or only partially obstructed. A diversion where the ureter is anastomosed to the skin is called a cutaneous ureterostomy.[134] Ureterostomy is appropriate in a patient with thickened dilated ureters when more aggressive urinary diversion surgery is not feasible. A ureterostomy forms a small, flush, pale pink stoma. It is difficult to manage; urinary reflux and infections are common. One or two stomas may be present.[24]

Ureteroenterocutaneous Diversions

It is possible to isolate any segment of the healthy intestinal tract caudal to the jejunum for use as a conduit for urine. The isolated intestinal segment serves as a conduit to bridge the gap from ureter to skin when the bladder must be removed or bypassed. Invasive transitional cell carcinoma of the bladder is the most frequent reason for cystectomy in the adult patient.[57]

Urinary diversion using a segment of small intestine is the most common form of permanent urinary diversion (FIG. 14-28). Bricker's operation was first described in 1950; it creates an ileal conduit by isolating a 15- to 20-cm segment of the terminal ileum close to the ileocecal valve.[156] The distal end of the isolated segment is brought out through the right lower abdominal quadrant and everted to form a budded stoma. The ureters are excised from the bladder and implanted near the proximal end of the conduit, which is sutured closed. The conduit is isoperistaltic; urine flows in the same direction as peristaltic

*Not a NANDA diagnosis.

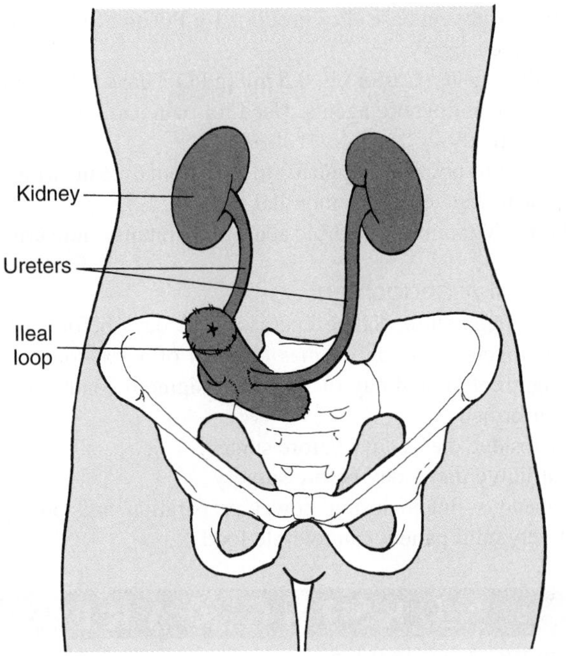

FIG. 14-28
Urinary diversion (ileal conduit). (From Gray.[61])

waves of the intestine. The ileal conduit is not a storage area; urine passes through quickly without residual.[40]

Jejunum may be used for small bowel permanent diversion if the ileum has been damaged by radiation. Patients with jejunal conduits are prone to a particular electrolyte imbalance called jejunal conduit syndrome, which is characterized by hypochloremic metabolic acidosis with hyperkalemia and hyponatremia.

The principal indications for small bowel urinary diversion are bladder cancer and severe neuropathic bladder dysfunction.[57] Long-term complications of the small bowel diversions are particularly prevalent after the first 5 years. Upper tract deterioration is significant and is associated with the bacteriuria and reflux that characterize the ileal or jejunal conduit.

A segment of large bowel may be isolated to form a urinary conduit. The primary advantage of using a segment of large intestine rather than small is the ability to create a nonrefluxing ureterointestinal anastomosis by tunneling the ureters into the submucosa of the colon. Nonetheless, the large bowel conduit leaves the patient with a stoma and continuous urinary incontinence. In addition, because obstruction at the ureteroenteric anastomosis is a serious complication, the large bowel conduit is used only in select cases.[57]

The ideal urinary diversion has not been developed. It would be an antirefluxing, continent diversion without the electrolyte disturbances that result from urine in prolonged contact with intestinal mucosa. This ideal diversion would have a reservoir with a functional capacity requiring catheterization only two or three times daily.

Continent Urinary Diversion

A continent urinary diversion provides the patient with an internal reservoir for urine and eliminates the need for an external appliance. There is an abdominal stoma and the patient performs clean intermittent catheterization through the stoma to empty the internal reservoir of urine.

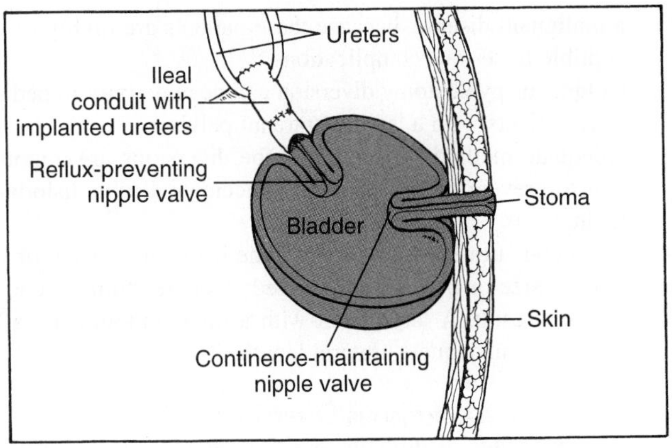

FIG. 14-29
Kock pouch. (From Belcher.[18])

A reservoir for urine constructed from the small intestine was first devised in the 1960s. The urinary Kock pouch involves isolating a 60- to 7-cm segment of the ileum (FIG. 14-29). The mesentery and its blood supply to this isolated segment of ileum is left intact. The middle 40 cm of this segment is split open and folded back on itself to form a reservoir to hold urine. The entrance and exit to this reservoir have a nipple valve constructed by intussusception or telescoping back of the intestine on itself. The ureters are implanted into the proximal nipple valve in an attempt to prevent urine from refluxing up to the kidneys. The distal nipple valve ends in a right-sided abdominal stoma and makes the stoma continent of urine. The reservoir expands in volume with time, and the patient ultimately catheterizes the stoma four or five times a day using an 18 to 26 French catheter. The patient wears an absorptive pad or adhesive strip over the stoma to collect the mucus it secretes. In addition, reservoir irrigations are performed at least once daily using a 50- to 60-ml catheter tip or bulb syringe to remove the mucus that has accumulated in the reservoir.[25,46,53]

The ileocecal reservoir is another continent urinary diversion that was developed in the late 1970s. The distal 20 cm of ileum, a segment of the cecum, and part of the ascending colon are isolated, and continuity of the gastrointestinal tract is restored. The ureters are anastomosed into the ascending colon with an antirefluxing tunneling method similar to the one used in the construction of a sigmoid conduit. The ileum forms the outflow tract with a nipple valve for continence and a right lower quadrant abdominal stoma. The cecum and ascending colon form the reservoir for urine. The patient catheterizes the stoma and irrigates the reservoir as with the Kock reservoir.[115]

Continent urinary diversions are an attempt to provide the patient with a more acceptable form of urinary diversion and to make the adjustment to the presence of a stoma easier. Careful patient selection is important. Long-term consequences have yet to be studied.

Contraindications and Cautions

Supravesical Diversions

1. Nephrostomy or pyelostomy tube drainage is discouraged in patients with bilateral ureteral obstruction as a result of

a malignant disease, because these patients are highly susceptible to serious complications.[57]
2. Cutaneous pyelostomy diversion can be done only in pediatric patients with a large extrarenal pelvis.
3. Adequate methods of securing tube diversions are important to prevent kidney damage or accidental tube dislodgment.
4. Cutaneous ureterostomy is not done if the ureters are of a normal size or poorly vascularized, because stomal stenosis may result. A large adult with a thick abdominal wall may have inadequate ureteral length.[138]

Ureteroenterocutaneous Diversions

1. Obesity makes it difficult to construct a good stoma because of tension on the mesentery, which can lead to a flush or retracted stoma and the development of either stomal necrosis in the early postoperative phase or subsequent stomal stenosis.
2. A sigmoid conduit is avoided in patients with severe diverticulosis or inflammatory bowel disease.[173]
3. A sigmoid conduit is not advised for the patient needing radical cystectomy and irradiation for bladder cancer, because the altered blood supply to the rectum and the sigmoid colon may negatively affect healing.[57]

Continent Urinary Diversions

1. The noncompliant patient with a tendency toward psychologic or social problems or the patient with already compromised renal function should not have a continent urinary diversion.
2. The need for postoperative radiation therapy may be related to a higher rate of failure.
3. The patient must be highly motivated to avoid wearing an external appliance.
4. Nipple valve failures can render the diversion incontinent of urine and necessitate a second surgical procedure to revise the intussusception.
5. Electrolyte disorders may result from urine in prolonged contact with intestinal mucosal lining.
6. Risk of malignancy from urine in prolonged contact with intestinal mucosa has not been fully evaluated.

Preprocedural Nursing Care

1. Intensive bowel preparation is started 2 to 3 days before surgery.
2. Preoperative stoma site selection is done by an ET nurse.
3. Preoperative teaching and consultation with an ET nurse is important.
4. The patient talks to an ostomy visitor if appropriate.

MULTIDISCIPLINARY PLAN

The following medical plan is for ureteroenterocutaneous diversions.

Medications

Antiinfective agents

Neomycin (Mycifradin), 1 g PO q4h for 4 doses; then 1 g q6h until NPO for surgery (begins 3 days before surgery)

Erythromycin base (Erythrocin), 1 g PO q4h for 3 doses before surgery

Laxative agents: Castor oil, 0.5 ml/kg PO 3 days before surgery

Analgesic/antipyretic agents: Used for pain and fever prn postoperatively

Mycostatin powder: Applied to peristomal skin with each pouch change prn for monilial rash

Vitamin: Vitamin C (ascorbic acid) to maintain acidic urine pH

General Management

Bowel preparation: Saline enemas for 2 days before surgery; neomycin retention enemas (200 ml of a 1% solution) the night before and day of surgery if sigmoid conduit is to be performed

Low-residue diet 2 days before surgery

Clear liquid diet 1 day before surgery

Intravenous fluids during bowel preparation and postoperatively until patient can tolerate food

NURSING CARE

NURSING ASSESSMENT

Incision: Redness, pain, edema, drainage

Hemorrhage: Incisional drains, sumps; urethral catheter (promotes drainage of operative site)

Urinary output: Amount and color; mucus normal in ileal/sigmoid conduit

Sexual dysfunction (male): Erectile dysfunction; ejaculatory incompetence—if prostate removed

Stoma: Viability; mucocutaneous border; edema

Peristomal skin: Intact; erythematous; signs of monilial infection; maceration

Intestine: Paralytic ileus, intestinal obstruction, abdominal distention, constipation; nasogastric suctioning prolonged owing to intestinal anastomosis

PATIENT PROBLEMS/NURSING DIAGNOSES & INTERVENTIONS

NIC ELIMINATION MANAGEMENT

Impaired urinary elimination related to obstruction of urinary diversion device

Constipation related to ileus or segmental resection and anastomosis in GI tract

- Assess stoma color and suture line *to recognize any change in viability or mucocutaneous separation.*
- Provide appropriate pouching system with antireflux valve and spout. Connect to bedside drainage and check frequently to prevent tubing from kinking *to prevent urine pooling on skin or refluxing from pouch to stoma.*
- Monitor amount and color of urine. If no urine is present, check all drainage sites (sumps, urethral catheter, Penrose drain) for urine *to determine if there has been an ileal-ureteral leakage or decreased renal function.*
- Arrange for ET nurse to assess stoma and drainage system and *to provide appropriate pouching system.*
- Obtain all urine specimens for urinalysis or culture and sensitivity by catheterizing ileal stoma (exception: monitoring urine pH).
- Monitor patient for first bowel movement.

- Auscultate abdomen for bowel sounds each shift.
- Observe for signs of paralytic ileus or intestinal obstruction.
- Monitor patient for signs and symptoms of peritonitis, which would indicate a leakage or failure of the intestinal reanastomosis: fever, abdominal pain, rebound tenderness, drop in blood pressure, or shallow respirations.

NIC Tissue Perfusion Management

Impaired peripheral tissue perfusion related to immobility
Hemorrhage related to surgery or surgical resection

- Assess blood pressure every 4 hours for 5 to 6 days or until removal of nasogastric suctioning and intravenous fluids.
- Apply antiembolic stockings. Remove and reapply daily *to prevent venous stasis and thrombophlebitis.*
- Auscultate abdomen for bowel sounds; note any signs of abdominal distention.
- Assess stoma for color (i.e., blood supply). Ileal conduit stoma should be bright red and moist; ureterostomy stoma is pale or dark pink.
- Assist patient with progressive ambulation.
- Encourage patient to turn every 2 hours and to perform leg exercises.
- Observe all drains, sumps, and catheters for amount, color, and consistency of drainage.
- Monitor intake and output; weigh daily.
- Observe incisional dressing *for color and amount of drainage.*
- Monitor color, consistency, and amount of drainage from nasogastric tube, sumps, urethral catheter, and stoma output *to prevent hypovolemic shock.*
- Monitor vital signs for shock.

NIC Risk Management

Risk for infection related to tissue trauma of incision

- Provide antibiotics as ordered.
- Observe incision for signs of infection: redness, edema, pain, and drainage. Assess patient's skin (under the arms and breasts, groin, perineum) *for monilial infections associated with prolonged antibiotics, intense bowel preparation, and moisture.*

NIC Respiratory Management

Ineffective breathing pattern related to post-anesthetic hypoventilation

- Assist patient in turning, coughing, and deep breathing *to counteract effects of general anesthesia.*
- Auscultate chest for breath sounds four times each day.
- Provide analgesics and splinting of abdomen when encouraging patient to deep breathe and cough.

NIC Physical Comfort Promotion

Acute pain related to surgical trauma

- Provide analgesics as ordered.
- Assist patient in finding comfortable positions.

NIC Coping Assistance

Disturbed body image related to presence of stoma and pouch
Sexual dysfunction related to altered body structure

- Provide an opportunity for patient and partner to discuss implications of surgery, stoma, and external pouch.
- Explore patient's and partner's feelings regarding presence of stoma and pouch.
- Discuss presence of pouch and inability of detecting it under clothing and how to manage embarrassing leakages and odor.
- Assess patient and partner's readiness to discuss sexual matters.
- Discuss sexual implications of presence of stoma, such as feelings of attractiveness, desirability, and worth.
- Explain separate nerve pathways for sexual excitement, erection, ejaculation, and orgasm *to point out effect of cystectomy on erections only.*
- Mention sexual counseling, alternative methods of sexual expressions, and penile prosthesis or external devices to aid in achieving erections *to assist patient in resuming sexual activity that is fulfilling for him.*

NIC Skin/Wound Management

Risk for impaired skin integrity related to creation of urinary stoma
Impaired skin integrity related to effects of urine on peristomal skin

- Change pouch whenever it appears to be leaking under faceplate or when there is an overt leakage.
- See box on pouch change procedure, p. 994.
- Assess skin integrity frequently because *rash can occur under the tape or faceplate and on any part of skin where pouch lies. Causes of skin rashes may be a leaking appliance, perspiration, allergies to tape, or hair follicle irritation.*
- Use lamp with a 60-watt bulb 1 foot away from skin or hair dryer set on cool *to dry skin.*
- Powder skin on which the pouch lies. *Avoid cornstarch powders, which encourage the growth of monilia.*
- Advise patient to make or buy a pouch cover.
- Ulcerated area on stoma may occur if stomal opening of pouch is too small or activities are causing faceplate to rub or cut into stoma.
- Evaluate patient's activities: *a different faceplate size or shape may be needed.*
- Decrease size of stomal opening in faceplate; use skin sealant *to waterproof skin. Waterlogged skin between opening of faceplate and stoma can occur if too much skin is exposed between stoma and faceplate and urine pools on unprotected skin.*
- Urinary yeast infection on skin surrounding stoma may extend beyond faceplate.
- Apply nystatin (Mycostatin) powder to area, blow off excess powder, and seal this in with a thin coat of a skin sealant. Apply pouch in usual manner.
- Advise patient to drink sufficient fluids and add buttermilk or yogurt to diet *to help restore normal gut flora.*

PROCEDURE FOR URINARY POUCH CHANGE

1. Assemble all supplies.
   a. To clean the skin, paper towels, washcloths, or towels may be used. Several of these should be rolled into "wicks" that can be placed on top of the stoma to absorb urine while keeping the peristomal skin unencumbered. Tampons can also be used as wicks. Premoistened towelettes should not be used.
   b. Pouch—a urinary pouch with a precut opening for the stoma should be sized large enough to bypass any creases or dimples in the skin around the stoma. A pouch that needs to be cut out before application should be cut to avoid any creases or dimples in the immediate peristomal area. Check for creases or dimples while the patient is sitting and when he or she is lying down. The outer diameter of the pouch's adhesive faceplate may be trimmed to avoid umbilicus, rib cage, incisions, hip bones, pubic areas, or folds at the waist.
   c. Karaya powder
   d. Skin sealant—protects the skin from the macerating effects of urine and the stripping effects of tape or adhesive. Most skin sealants are a liquid copolymer with alcohol as the vehicle for spreading it. Skin sealants come in spray form, dab-on applicators, or wipes.
   e. Tape—such as Micropore or paper tape. Some patients prefer waterproof tape.
   f. Plastic bag for disposal of used pouches
2. Take off old pouch by unsticking the skin from the pouch's adhesive faceplate. Dispose of used pouch.
3. Wash the stoma and peristomal skin free of mucus and urine with warm water only and let dry.
   a. Soap may leave a residue on the skin and prevent the next pouch from adhering.
   b. Traces of cement or adhesives may be on the skin. Rough cleansing to remove these may do damage to the peristomal skin.
4. Examine the peristomal skin for any signs of redness or irritation. Apply a light dusting of karaya powder to irritated skin.
   a. If the peristomal skin needs to be shaved, use a dry razor over powdered skin. Brush away excess karaya powder.
   b. If irritation is severe, a skin barrier in wafer form may be added to the pouch's adhesive faceplate. Urine will melt the skin barrier and decrease the pouch's seal, but a pouch's adhesive faceplate should not be applied directly over severely irritated skin.
5. Apply a skin sealant to peristomal skin. Keep the stoma "wicked" to absorb urine.
   a. In the presence of skin irritation, a skin sealant will cause a momentary stinging sensation.
   b. If karaya powder was applied to irritated skin, the skin sealant will seal in the karaya powder and, once dry, will provide a skin surface to which the pouch can adhere.
6. Center pouch over stoma and apply to dry skin.
   a. Try to avoid creating any wrinkles or creases in pouch's adhesive faceplate that will encourage urine leakage.
   b. The pouch may be angled straight down or medially for an ambulatory patient to facilitate emptying.
7. Close the pouch's spout.
8. Use the tape to picture-frame the pouch's adhesive faceplate and increase the pouch's wearing time.
9. Check the pH of the urine from the first drops of urine in the freshly changed pouch.
   a. Do not touch the pH paper to the stoma or the skin, since this will give an inaccurate reading.
   b. An acidic urine pH should be maintained, since alkaline urine is more likely to have a foul odor, create crystals on or around the stoma, predispose the patient to kidney stone formation, and provide a medium for infection. An adequate fluid intake or ascorbic acid (vitamin C, 500 mg) four times a day will acidify urine. Acidic urine has a pH of 6.0 or less.

- Urine crystals may form on the stoma or around the stoma base if patient has alkaline urine and a predisposition for stone formation.
- Swab vinegar on stoma when changing pouch *to help dissolve crystals.*
- Insert vinegar into pouch while patient is wearing it. For a minor formation, insert twice a day; for an excessive formation, insert four times a day.
- Remove antireflux valves *to allow vinegar to come into contact with stoma.*
- Monitor urine pH and provide instructions for maintaining an acid urine, including increased fluid intake and ascorbic acid (vitamin C).

PATIENT EDUCATION/CONTINUUM OF CARE PLAN

1. Demonstrate to patient how to empty pouch when it is one-third to one-half full.
2. Show patient use of bedside drainage bag at night.
3. Demonstrate to patient pouch change procedure (see box above). This includes treatment of minor peristomal skin irritations and monitoring urine pH.
4. Explain fluid intake requirements—10 to 12 glasses a day to acidify urine.
5. Review dietary considerations in terms of urine odor; fish, eggs, asparagus, and spicy foods can cause a temporary increase in urine odor.
6. Define routine follow-up care for patient with a urinary diversion, including correct method of obtaining urine for culture (see box on p. 995).
7. Provide patient with ostomy supply and supplier information and availability of community support groups, such as United Ostomy Association.[40]

EVALUATION/PATIENT OUTCOMES

Elimination Management: Bowel elimination is normal. Patient experiences a return to presurgical bowel habits.

PROCEDURE FOR OBTAINING A URINE CULTURE FROM ILEAL-SIGMOID CONDUIT (SINGLE-LUMEN CATHETERIZATION)

1. Explain procedure to patient.
   a. Catheterizing the stoma is painless because ureteroenterocutaneous stomas have no sensory nerve endings.
   b. Patient should be aware that no urine for culture should be obtained from the pouch itself. This specimen needs to be obtained sterilely.
2. Assemble supplies for reapplying the pouch once the specimen is obtained.
3. Set up equipment for obtaining a urine specimen on a sterile field:
   a. Catheter (may be a 12 or 14 French straight catheter)
   b. Betadine swabs (three)
   c. Sterile, water-soluble lubricant
   d. Sterile urine cup
   e. Dry, sterile gauze
   f. Sterile gloves
4. Take off the old pouch.
5. Drape patient with Chux to keep him or her dry.
6. Wipe stoma free of mucus with gauze.
7. Put on sterile gloves.
8. Swab the stoma three times with the Betadine swabs.
9. Let urine run over the stoma to wash away Betadine *or* wipe stoma free of Betadine with dry, sterile gauze. Introducing Betadine into the specimen will kill the bacteria for which the culture is checking.
10. Lubricate the tip of the catheter with water-soluble lubricant.
11. Gently insert the catheter into the stoma about 1½ to 2 inches. Do not force or poke. It is desirable to pass catheter beneath fascia level if possible.
12. Wait until about 5 ml of urine passes through the catheter into the sterile urine cup. To facilitate obtaining specimen, instruct the patient to sit up or turn on one side.
13. Remove the catheter.
14. Reapply the pouch.

Tissue Perfusion Management: Tissue perfusion is normal. Stoma is red, healthy, moist, and viable. Blood pressure and pulse are within normal limits.

Risk Management: There is no infection or hemorrhage. Temperature is within normal range. There are no signs or symptoms of infection or bleeding. Incision is healed.

Respiratory Management: Breathing pattern remains normal. Patient's respiratory status is managed appropriately. Breath sounds remain clear.

Physical Comfort Promotion: Patient resumes activities of daily living. Patient returns to presurgical activities, including work and recreational interests. Patient does not change his or her style of dress.

Coping Assistance: Body image is not disturbed. Patient adapts to presence of stoma and external pouch. Patient recognizes that adaptation is a continuous process.

Skin/Wound Management: Skin integrity is maintained. Peristomal skin is intact. There are no signs of irritation. Pouch seal is appropriate (3 to 5 days). Women return to presurgical sexual pattern. Men experiencing sexual dysfunction receive counseling regarding erectile dysfunction.

REFERENCES

1. Abrams P et al: Tolterodine, a new muscarinic agent: as effective but better tolerated than oxybutynin in patients with an overactive bladder, *Br J Urol* 81:801, 1998.
2. Agency for Health Care Policy and Research Urinary Incontinence in Adults Guideline Panel: *Urinary incontinence in adults,* Rockville, Md, 1992, U.S. Department of Health and Human Services.
3. Agency for Health Care Policy and Research Benign Prostatic Hyperplasia Guideline Panel: *Benign prostatic hyperplasia: diagnosis and treatment,* Rockville, Md, 1994, U.S. Department of Health and Human Services.
4. Akkus E et al: Structural alterations in the tunica albuginea of the penis: impact of Peyronie's disease, ageing, and impotence, *Br J Urol* 79:47, 1997.
5. Allen TD: The non-neurogenic neurogenic bladder, *J Urol* 116:638, 1977.
6. Anawalt BD, Bremner WJ: Endocrinology of male sexual dysfunction. In Hellstrom WJG, editor: *The handbook of sexual dysfunction,* San Francisco, 1999, American Society of Andrology.
7. Andersen KV, Bovim G: Impotence and nerve entrapment in long distance amateur cyclists, *Acta Neurol Scand* 95:233, 1997.
8. Anderson RS: A neurogenic element to genuine urinary stress incontinence, *Br J Obstet Gynaecol* 91:41, 1984.
9. Andriana RT, Carson CC: Urolithiasis, *Clin Symp* 38:3, 1986.
10. Armenian HK et al: Relationship between benign prostatic hyperplasia and cancer of the prostate: a prospective and retrospective study, *Lancet* 2:115, 1974.
11. Ayta IA, McKinlay JB, Krane RJ: The likely worldwide increase in erectile dysfunction between 1995 and 2025 and some possible policy consequences, *BJU Int* 84:50, 1999.
12. Ballard DJ: Treatment of erectile dysfunction: can pelvic muscle exercises improve sexual function? *J Wound Ostomy Continence Nurs* 24:255, 1997.
13. Bannister R: *Brain and Bannister's clinical neurology,* Oxford, UK, 1992, Oxford University Press.

13a. Barak Y et al: Sexual dysfunction in relapsing-remitting multiple sclerosis: magnetic resonance imaging, clinical, and psychological correlates, *J Psychiatry Neurosci* 21:225, 1996.

14. Barbalias GA, Nikiforidis G, Liatsikos EN: Alpha-blockers for the treatment of chronic prostatitis in combination with antibiotics, *J Urol* 159:883, 1998.
15. Barrington FJF: The nervous mechanisms of micturition of the cat, *Q J Exp Physiol* 54:177, 1931.

16. Beare PG, Myers JL: *Principles and practice of adult health nursing,* St. Louis, 1990, Mosby.
17. Beck RO, Betts CD, Fowler CJ: Genitourinary dysfunction in multiple system atrophy: clinical features and treatment in 62 cases, *J Urol* 151:1336, 1994.
18. Belcher A: *Cancer nursing,* St. Louis, 1992, Mosby.
19. Benchekroun A et al: Priapism in adults, *Ann Urol* 32:103, 1998.
20. Bergman H, editor: *The ureter,* New York, 1981, Springer-Verlag.
21. Bihrle R et al: High intensity focused ultrasound for the treatment of benign prostatic hyperplasia: early United States clinical experience, *J Urol* 151:1271, 1994.
22. Bjerre BD, Johansen C, Steven K: Sexological problems after cystectomy: bladder substitution compared with ileal conduit diversion: a questionnaire of male patients, *Scand J Urol Nephrol* 32:187, 1998.
23. Boone TB, Gilling PJ, Husmann DA: Ureteropelvic junction disruption following blunt abdominal trauma, *J Urol* 150:33, 1993.
24. Broadwell DC, Jackson BS, editors: *Principles of ostomy care,* St. Louis, 1982, Mosby.
25. Brogna L, Lakaszawaski M: Nursing management: in the continent urostomy, *J Enterostom Ther* 13:139, 1986.
26. Burnett AL: Neurophysiology of erectile function and dysfunction. In Hellstrom WJG, editor: *The handbook of sexual dysfunction,* San Francisco, 1999, American Society of Andrology.
27. Burns JR, Finlayson B: Why some people have stone disease and others do not. In Roth RA, Finlayson B: *Stones: clinical management of urolithiasis,* Baltimore, 1983, Williams & Wilkins.
28. Catalona WJ et al: Potency, continence and complication rates in 1870 consecutive radical retropubic prostatectomies, *J Urol* 162:433, 1999.
29. Childs SJ: Dimethyl sulfone (DMSO) in the treatment of interstitial cystitis, *Urol Clin North Am* 21:85, 1994.
30. Chisholm GD, Williams ID, editors: *Scientific foundations of urology,* St. Louis, 1982, Mosby.
31. Churchill ND et al: Urolithiasis: a study of drinking water hardness and genetic factors, *J Chronic Dis* 33:727, 1980.
32. Collins MM, O'Leary MP, Barry MJ: Prevalence of bothersome genitourinary symptoms and diagnoses in younger men on routine primary care visits, *Urology* 159:1224, 1998.
32a. Collins MM et al: How common is prostatitis? A national survey of physician visits, *J Urol* 159:1224, 1998.
33. Crockett AT, Urry DL, editors: *Male infertility: workup, treatment and research,* New York, 1977, Grune & Stratton.
34. Crouch JE: *Functional human anatomy,* ed 4, Philadelphia, 1985, Lea & Febiger.
35. DeGroat WC: Innervation of the lower urinary tract: an overview. Twentieth annual meeting of the Society for Urodynamics, Dallas, May 1, 1999.
36. DeLancey JOL: Functional anatomy of the female pelvis. In Kursh ED, McGuire EJ, editors: *Female urology,* New York, 1994, JB Lippincott.
37. de la Rosette JJMHC, Froeling FMJA, Debruyne FMJ: Clinical results with microwave thermotherapy of benign prostatic hyperplasia, *Eur Urol* 23:68, 1993.
38. de la Rosette JJMHC et al: Transurethral microwave thermotherapy (TUMT) in benign prostatic hyperplasia: placebo versus TUMT, *Urology* 44:58, 1994.
39. Dixon CM: Transurethral needle ablation of benign prostatic hyperplasia, *Urol Clin North Am* 22:441, 1995.
40. Dobkin KA: Nursing care of a patient with ileal conduit, *J Urol Nurs* 4:340, 1985.
41. Doughty D, editor: *Urinary and fecal incontinence: nursing management,* St. Louis, 1991, Mosby.
42. Drach GW: Prostatitis: man's hidden infection, *Urol Clin North Am* 2:499, 1975.
43. Elbadawi A et al: Immunohistochemical and ultrastructural study of rhabdosphincter component of the prostatic capsule, *J Urol* 158:1819, 1997.
44. Eterkin C et al: The value of somatosensory potentials and bulbocavernosus reflex in patients with impotence, *Acta Neurol Scand* 71:48, 1985.
44a. Johannes CB et al: Incidence of erectile dysfunction in men 40 to 69 years old: longitudinal results from the Massachusetts Male Aging Study, *J Urol* 163:460, 2000.
45. Fitzmaurice H et al: Micturition disturbance in Parkinson's disease, *Br J Urol* 57:652, 1985.
46. Reference deleted in proofs.
47. Furlow WL: Use of the inflatable penile prosthesis in erectile dysfunction, *Urol Clin North Am* 8:181, 1981.
48. Gallaway NTM, Irwin PP: Interstitial cystitis: surgical management of interstitial cystitis, *Urol Clin North* 21:145, 1994.
49. Ganabathi K et al: Prospective urodynamic evaluation of the efficacy of prostatic balloon dilatation, *Neurourol Urodyn* 11:483, 1992.
50. Garraway M, Collins G, Lee R: High prevalence of benign prostatic hyperplasia in the community, *Lancet* 38:469, 1991.
51. Gaymans R et al: A prospective study of urinary tract infections in a Dutch general practice, *Lancet* 2:674, 1976.
52. Gentle DL et al: Geriatric urolithiasis, *J Urol* 158:2221, 1997.
53. Gerber A: The Kock continent ileal reservoir: an alternative to the conventional urostomy, *J Enterostom Ther* 12:15, 1985.
54. Gill WB, Silvert MA, Roma MJ: Supersaturation levels and crystallization rates from urines of normal humans and stone formers determined by a ^{14}C-oxalate technique, *Investig Urol* 12:203, 1974.
55. Gillenwater JY, Wein AJ: Summary of the national institute of arthritis, diabetes, digestive and kidney diseases workshop on interstitial cystitis, *J Urol* 140:203, 1987.
56. Gillenwater JY et al: Doxazosin for the treatment of benign prostatic hyperplasia in patients with mild to moderate essential hypertension: a double blind, placebo controlled, dose-response multicenter study, *J Urol* 154:110, 1995.
57. Glenn JF: *Urologic surgery,* New York, 1991, JB Lippincott.
58. Goldstein I, Siroky MB, Sachs DS: Neurologic abnormalities in multiple sclerosis, *J Urol* 128:541, 1982.
59. Goldstein I et al: Oral sildenafil in the treatment of erectile dysfunction. Sildenafil Study Group. *N Engl J Med* 338:1397, 1998.
60. Gosling JA: The structure of the bladder and urethra in relation to function, *Urol Clin North Am* 6:31, 1979.
61. Gray ML: *Genitourinary disorders,* St. Louis, 1992, Mosby.
62. Gray ML, Campbell F: Extraurethral urinary incontinence, *J Wound Ostomy Continence Nurs* (in press).
63. Gray ML, Dougherty MC: Urinary incontinence: pathophysiology and treatment, *J Enterostom Ther* 14(4):152, 1987.
63a. Gray M et al: Urinary diversions: perspectives on nursing care, *Perspectives 2000* 10(74):40, 2000.
64. Gray M, Rayome RG: Urinary system disorders. In Luckman J: *Adult health nursing,* Philadelphia, 1997, WB Saunders.
65. Gray M, Rayome RG, Moore KN: The urethral sphincter: an update, *Urol Nurs* 15(2):40, 1995.
66. Grayhack JT, Kozlowski JM: Benign prostatic hyperplasia. In Gillenwater JY et al, editors: *Adult and pediatric urology,* ed 3, St. Louis, 1996, Mosby.

67. Gupta SK et al: Quantitative characterization of therapeutic index: application of mixed-effects modeling to evaluate oxybutynin dose-efficacy and dose-side effects relationship, *Clin Pharmacol Ther* 65:672, 1999.
68. Guyton AC: *Medical physiology,* Philadelphia, 1978, WB Saunders.
69. Hald T, Bradley WE: *The urinary bladder: neurology and dynamics,* Baltimore, 1982, Williams & Wilkins.
70. Hanno PM: Diagnosis of interstitial cystitis, *Urol Clin North Am* 21:63, 1994.
71. Hanno PM: Analysis of long-term Elmiron therapy for interstitial cystitis, *Urology* 49:93, 1997.
72. Hegde SS, Eglen RM: Muscarinic receptor subtypes modulating smooth muscle contractility in the urinary bladder, *Life Sci* 64:419, 1999.
73. Hesse A, Seiner R: Current aspects of epidemiology and nutrition in urinary stone disease, *World J Urol* 15:165, 1997.
74. Hiatt RA et al: Frequency of urolithiasis in a prepaid medical program, *Am J Epidemiol* 115:255, 1982.
75. Hinman JF, editor: *Benign prostatic hypertrophy,* New York, 1983, Springer-Verlag.
76. Hodgkinson CP, Ayers MA, Drukker BH: Dyssynergic detrusor dysfunction in apparently normal females, *Am J Obstet Gynecol* 87(6):717, 1963.
77. Holtgrewe HL et al: Transurethral prostatectomy: practice aspects of the dominant operation in urology, *J Urol* 141:248, 1989.
78. Hurst JW, editor: *Medicine for the practicing physician,* ed 2, Boston, 1988, Butterworth.
79. Hutch JA, Rambo ON: A study of the anatomy of the prostate, prostatic urethra, and the urinary sphincter system, *J Urol* 104:443, 1970.
80. Hwang P et al: Efficacy of pentosan polysulfate in the treatment of interstitial cystitis: a meta-analysis, *Urology* 50:39, 1997.
81. International Continence Society: *The standardization of terminology of lower urinary tract function,* Glasgow, Scotland, 1984, The Society.
82. Ireton RC, Berger RE: Prostatitis and epididymitis, *Urol Clin North Am* 11:83, 1984.
83. Jenkins AD: Calculus formation. In Gillenwater JY et al, editors: *Adult and pediatric urology,* St. Louis, 1996, Mosby.
84. Jenkins AD, Turner TT, Howards SS: Physiology of the male reproductive system, *Urol Clin North Am* 5:437, 1978.
85. Jensen H, Nielsen K, Fromodt-Moller C: Interstitial cystitis: review of the literature, *Urol Int* 44:189, 1989.
86. Jeremy JY, Mikhailidis DP: Cigarette smoking and erectile dysfunction, *J R Soc Health* 118:151, 1998.
87. Jiminez-Jiminez FJ et al: Fluctuating penile erection related to levodopa therapy, *Neurology* 52:210, 1999.
88. Johnson CM et al: Renal stone epidemiology: a 25 year study in Rochester, Minn, *Kidney Int* 16:624, 1979.
89. Kass I, Updegraff K, Muffly RB: Sex in chronic obstructive pulmonary disease, *Med Aspects Hum Sex* 6:33, 1972.
90. Kay D: Host defense mechanisms in the urinary tract, *Urol Clin North Am* 2:407, 1975.
91. Kedia KR: Vascular disorders and male erectile dysfunction, *Urol Clin North Am* 8:153, 1981.
92. Khan SR, Hackett RL: Hyperoxaluria, enzymuria and nephrolithiasis, *Contrib Nephrol* 101:190, 1993.
93. Khan SR, Hackett RL: Role of organic matrix in urinary stone formation: an ultrastructural study of crystal matrix interface of calcium oxalate monohydrate stones, *J Urol* 46:239, 1993.
94. Khan Z, Starer P, Bohla A: Urinary incontinence in female Parkinson disease patients: pitfalls of diagnosis, *Urology* 33:486, 1989.
95. Koizol JA: Epidemiology of interstitial cystitis, *Urol Clin North Am* 21:7, 1994.
96. Korpelainen JT, Nieminen P, Myllyla VV: Sexual functioning among stroke patients and their spouses, *Stroke* 30:715, 1999.
97. Korting GE et al: A randomized double blind trial of oral L-arginine for treatment of interstitial cystitis, *J Urol* 161:558, 1999.
98. Krane RJ, Siroky MB: *Clinical neurology,* Boston, 1979, Little, Brown.
99. Krane RJ, Siroky MB, Goldstein I, editors: *Male sexual dysfunction,* Boston, 1983, Little, Brown.
100. Kunelius P, Hakkinen J, Lukkarinen O: Is high dose yohimbine hydrochloride effective in the treatment of mixed-type impotence? A prospective, randomized, controlled double blind crossover study, *Urology* 49:441, 1997.
101. Laduc R, Bloem FAG, Debruyne FMJ: Transurethral microwave thermotherapy in symptomatic benign prostatic hyperplasia, *Eur Urol* 23:274, 1993.
102. Lawrence IG et al: Erythropoietin and sexual dysfunction, *Nephrol Dial Transplant* 12:741, 1997.
103. Leach GE: Urodynamic manifestations of cerebellar ataxia, *J Urol* 128:348, 1982.
104. Leeson CR, Leeson TS: *Histology,* ed 4, Philadelphia, 1981, WB Saunders.
105. Lepor H: Alpha blockade for the treatment of benign prostatic hyperplasia, *Urol Clin North Am* 22:375, 1995.
106. Lepor H, Shapiro E: Characterization of the alpha 1 adrenergic receptor in human benign prostatic hyperplasia, *J Urol* 132:1226, 1984.
107. Lerner J, Khan Z: *Manual of urologic nursing,* St. Louis, 1982, Mosby.
108. Libertino JA, editor: *International perspectives in urology,* vol 5, Baltimore, 1982, Williams & Wilkins.
109. Lipschultz LI, Howards SS, editors: *Infertility in the male,* ed 2, St. Louis, 1991, Mosby.
110. Litwin MS et al: The National Institutes of Health chronic prostatitis symptom index: development and validation of a new outcome measure, Chronic Prostatitis Collaborative Research Network. *J Urol* 162:369, 1999.
111. Lue TF: Physiology of penile erection and pathophysiology of erectile dysfunction and priapism. In Walsh PC et al, editors: *Campbell's urology,* Philadelphia, 1998, WB Saunders.
112. Madersbacher S et al: Tissue ablation in prostatic hyperplasia with high-intensity focused ultrasound, *Eur Urol* 23:39, 1993.
113. Madersbacher S et al: Tissue ablation in benign prostatic hyperplasia with high intensity focused ultrasound, *J Urol* 152:1956, 1994.
114. Mann R, Lutwak-Mann C: *Male reproductive function and semen,* Berlin, 1981, Springer-Verlag.
115. Mansson W: The continent caecal reservoir for urine, *Scand J Urol Nephrol Suppl* 85:1, 1984.
116. Mark SD et al: Impotence following pelvic fracture urethral injury: incidence, etiology and management, *Br J Urol* 75:62, 1995.
117. Maskell R: Are fastidious organisms an important cause of dysuria and frequency? The case for. In Asscher AW, Brumfitt W, editors: *Microbial diseases in nephrology,* London, 1986, John Wiley & Sons.
118. Mayersak JS: Transrectal ultrasonography directed intraprostatic injection of gentamycin-xylocaine in the management of the benign painful prostate syndrome: a report of a 5 year clinical study of 75 patients, *Int Surg* 83:347, 1998.

119. McCullough AR, Fine JL: Psychosexual issues in the man, woman and couple. In Hellstrom WJG, editor: *The handbook of sexual dysfunction,* San Francisco, 1999, American Society of Andrology.
120. McConnell JD: Hormonal treatment, *Urol Clin North Am* 22:387, 1995.
121. McNeal J: Pathology of benign prostatic hyperplasia, *Urol Clin North Am* 17:477, 1990.
122. Meares EM: Chronic bacterial prostatitis: role of transurethral prostatectomy (TURP) in therapy. In Weidner W et al, editors: *Therapy of prostatitis,* Munich, 1986, Verlag.
123. Meares EM: Prostatitis and related disorders. In Walsh PC et al, editors: *Campbell's urology,* ed 7, Philadelphia, 1998, WB Saunders.
124. Meinhardt W et al: Trazodone: a double blind trial for treatment of erectile dysfunction, *Int J Impot Res* 9:163, 1997.
124a. Melman A. Gingell, JC: The epidemiology and pathophysiology of erectile dysfunction, *J Urol* 161:5, 1999.
124b. Menon M, Parkular BC, Drach GW: Urinary lithiasis: etiology, diagnosis and medical management. In Walsh PC et al, editors: *Campbell's urology*, ed 7, Philadelphia, 1998, WB Saunders.
125. Messing E, Stamey TA: Interstitial cystitis: early diagnosis, pathology and treatment, *Urology* 12(4):381, 1978.
126. Mikuma N et al: Magnetic resonance imaging of the male pelvic floor: the anatomical configuration and dynamic movement in healthy men, *Neurourol Urodyn* 17:591, 1998.
127. Simonis LA et al: Erectile dysfunction due to a hidden penis after pelvic trauma, *Int J Impot Res* 11:53, 1999.
128. Miyake O et al: Possible causes for the low prevalence of pediatric urolithiasis, *Urology* 53:1229, 1999.
129. Myers RP et al: Anatomy of radical prostatectomy as defined by magnetic resonance imaging, *J Urol* 159:2148, 1998.
130. Narayan P, Lange P: Semirigid penile prosthesis in the management of erectile impotence, *Urol Clin North Am* 8:169, 1981.
131. National Academy of Sciences, Food and Nutrition Board: *Recommended daily allowances,* ed 9, Washington, DC, 1980, The Academy.
132. NIH Consensus Conference: *Impotence 1992* 10:4, December 7-9, 1992.
133. Nistal M, Paniagua R: *Testicular epididymal pathology,* New York, 1984, Thieme Medical Publishers.
134. Noorgard JP, Pedersen EB, Djurhuus JC: Diurnal antidiuretic hormone levels in enuretics, *J Urol* 134:1029, 1985.
135. O'Sullivan JD, Hughes AJ. Apomorphine induced penile erections in Parkinson's disease, *Mov Disord* 13:536, 1998.
136. Pak CYP et al: Dietary management of idiopathic calcium urolithiasis, *J Urol* 131:850, 1984.
137. Parsons CL: The therapeutic role of polysaccharides in the urinary bladder, *Urol Clin North Am* 21:93, 1994.
138. Phipps WJ, Long BC, Woods NF, editors: *Medical-surgical nursing: concepts and clinical practice,* ed 4, St. Louis, 1991, Mosby.
139. Platt R et al: Mortality associated with nosocomial urinary-tract infection, *N Engl J Med* 307:637, 1982.
140. Ratliff TL, Klutke CG, McDougall EM: The etiology of interstitial cystitis, *Urol Clin North Am* 21:21, 1994.
141. Raz S, editor: *Female urology,* Philadelphia, 1983, WB Saunders.
142. Resnick MI, Older RA, editors: *Diagnosis of genitourinary disease,* New York, 1982, Thieme Medical Publishers.
143. Riley TW et al: Use of radioisotopic scan in evaluation of intrascrotal lesions, *J Urol* 116:472, 1976.
144. Rose BD: *Pathophysiology of renal disease,* ed 2, New York, 1987, McGraw-Hill.
145. Rud T et al: Factors maintaining urethral pressure in women, *Investig Urol* 17:343, 1980.
146. Sampselle CA, DeLancey JOL: Anatomy of female continence, *J Wound Ostomy Continence Nurs* 25:63, 1998.
147. Sant GR, LaRock DR: Standard intravesical therapies for interstitial cystitis, *Urol Clin North Am* 21:73, 1994.
148. Sarma KP: *Tumors of the urinary bladder,* London, 1969, Butterworth.
149. Sarmina I, Spirnak JP, Resnick MI: Urinary lithiasis in the black population: an epidemiological study and review of the literature, *J Urol* 138:1417, 1987.
150. Shulman CC, Vanden Bossche M: Hypothermia and thermotherapy of benign prostatic hyperplasia: a critical review, *Eur Urol* 23:53, 1993.
151. Shulman CC et al: Transurethral needle ablation (TUNA): safety, feasibility, and tolerance of a new office procedure for treatment of benign prostatic hyperplasia, *Eur Urol* 24:415, 1993.
152. Shuster J et al: Water hardness and urinary stone disease, *J Urol* 128:422, 1982.
153. Sierakowski R et al: The frequency of urolithiasis in hospital discharge diagnoses in the United States, *Investig Urol* 15:428, 1978.
154. Sikka SC: Drug, environment and chemical exposures in the realm of sexuality. In Hellstrom WJG, editor: *The handbook of sexual dysfunction,* San Francisco, 1999, American Society of Andrology.
154a. Simonis LA et al: Erectile dysfunction due to a "hidden" penis after pelvic trauma, *Int J Impot Res* 11:53, 1999.
155. Singer C, Weiner WJ, Sanchez-Ramos JR: Autonomic dysfunction in men with Parkinson's disease, *Eur Neurol* 32:134, 1992.
156. Slade DKA: Interstitial cystitis: a challenge to urology, *Urol Nurs* 9:5, 1989.
157. Smith AD: Causes and classifications of impotence, *Urol Clin North Am* 8:79, 1981.
158. Smith DR: *General urology,* ed 11, Los Altos, Calif, 1984, Lange Medical.
159. Smith PH, Prout GR, editors: *Bladder cancer,* London, 1984, Butterworth.
160. Snooks SJ et al: Perineal nerve damage in genuine stress incontinence, *Br J Urol* 57:522, 1985.
161. Stamey TA: *Pathogenesis and treatment of urinary tract infections,* Baltimore, 1980, Williams & Wilkins.
162. Staskin DR et al: Pathophysiology of stress incontinence, *Clin Obstet Gynaecol* 12:357, 1985.
163. Steers WD: Physiology of the vas deferens, *World J Urol* 12:281, 1994.
164. Steers WD: Physiology and pharmacology of the bladder and urethra. In Walsh PC et al, editors: *Campbell's urology,* ed 7, Philadelphia, 1998, WB Saunders.
165. Steers WD, Zorn B: Benign prostatic hyperplasia, *Dis Mon* 41:437, 1995.
166. Symmonds RE: Incontinence: vesicle and urethral fistulae, *Clin Obstet Gynecol* 27:499, 1984.
167. Tejada IS, Goldstein I, Krane RJ: Local control penile erection: nerves, smooth muscle and endothelium, *Urol Clin North Am* 15:9, 1988.
168. Tenover JL: Aging and male sexual function. In Hellstrom WJG, editor: *The handbook of male sexual dysfunction,* San Francisco, 1999, American Society of Andrology.
169. Traish A et al: Phentolamine mesylate relaxes penile corpus cavernosum tissue by adrenergic and non-adrenergic mechanisms, *Int J Impot Res* 10:215, 1998.

170. Tweed MJ, Roland JM: Hemachromatosis as an endocrine cause of subfertility, *Br Med J* 316:915, 1998.

171. Van Arsdalen K, Wein AJ: Physiology of micturition and continence. In Krane RJ, Siroky MB, editors: *Clinical neuro-urology,* Boston, 1991, Little-Brown.

172. Walsh PC et al: Tissue content of dihydrotestosterone in human prostatic hyperplasia is not abnormal, *J Clin Invest* 72:1772, 1983.

173. Walsh PC et al, editors: *Campbell's urology,* ed 6, Philadelphia, 1992, WB Saunders.

174. Weidman CL, Northcutt RC: Endocrine aspects of impotence, *Urol Clin North Am* 8:143, 1981.

175. Wein AJ, Hanno PM, Gillenwater JY: Interstitial cystitis: an introduction to the problem. In Hanno PM et al, editors: *Interstitial cystitis,* New York, 1990, Springer-Verlag.

176. Werness PG, Bergert JH, Smith LH: Crystalluria, *Crystal Growth* 53:166, 1981.

177. Wheatley JK: Causes and treatment of bladder incontinence, *Compr Ther* 9:27, 1983.

178. Williams P, Warwick R: *Gray's anatomy,* ed 37, New York, 1989, Churchill Livingstone.

179. Wilson JD: The pathogenesis of benign prostatic hypertrophy, *Am J Med* 68:745, 1980.

180. Wyndaele JJ: The normal pattern of perception of bladder filling during cystometry studies in 38 young healthy volunteers, *J Urol* 160:479, 1998.

181. Xie Y et al: Effect of long-term passive smoking on erectile function and penile nitric oxide synthase in the rat, *J Urol* 157:1121, 1997.

182. Yamamoto M et al: Chronic bacterial prostatitis treated with intraprostatic injection of antibiotics, *Scand J Urol Nephrol* 30:199, 1996.

183. Yavascaoglu I et al: Percutaneous suprapubic transvesical route: a new and comfortable method of intraprostatic injection, *Urol Int* 60:229, 1998.

184. Yono M et al: Pharmacologic effects of tolterodine on human isolated urinary bladder, *Eur J Pharmacol* 368:223, 1999.

185. Zenico T et al: Sexual dysfunction after excision of the rectum, *Acta Urol Belg* 57:213, 1989.

186. Zermann DH et al: Neurourological insights into the etiology of genitourinary pain in men, *J Urol* 161:903, 1999.

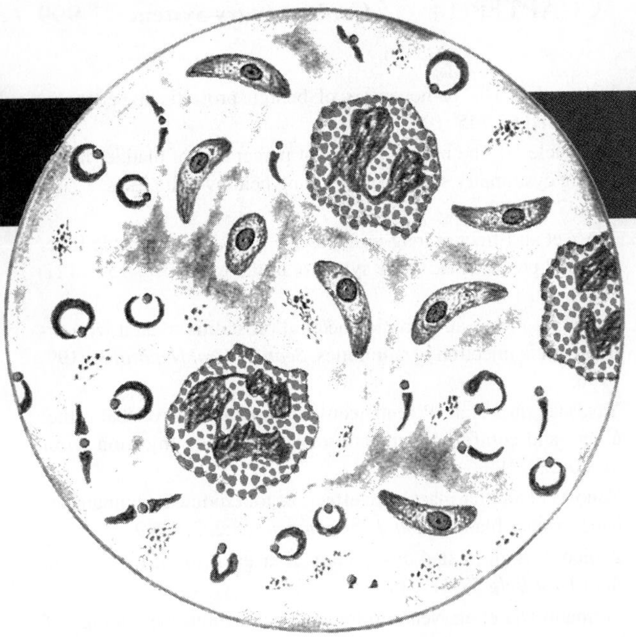

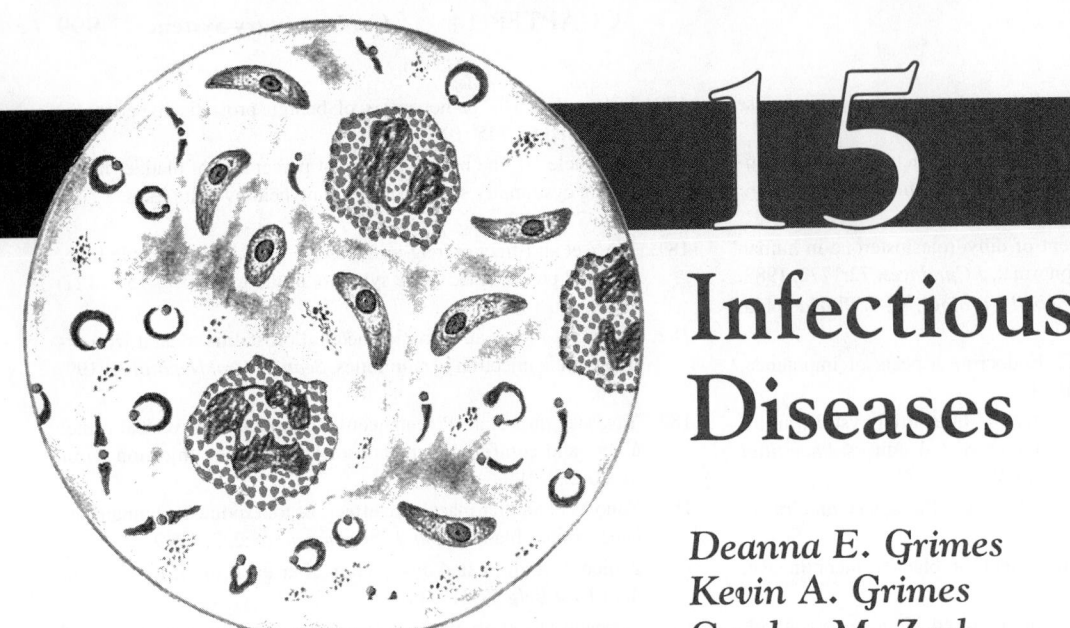

15 Infectious Diseases

Deanna E. Grimes
Kevin A. Grimes
Carolyn M. Zack

Overview

At the beginning of the nineteenth century, no infectious disease was controlled in America. Major efforts in environmental sanitation, advances in immunization and antibiotic therapy, and application of antimicrobial technology to disease agents have resulted in control of many of the dreaded infectious diseases of the past. Today, most health professionals in the United States never see cases of the major killers, such as yellow fever, cholera, typhus, smallpox, malaria, polio, and plague. They see, however, new killers, such as acquired immunodeficiency syndrome (AIDS) and increasing numbers of cases of hepatitis, tuberculosis, and sexually transmitted diseases. Vaccine-preventable diseases, such as measles and mumps, persist despite the availability of vaccines. Antibiotic-resistant organisms flourish, and new infectious disease agents are being identified (Table 15-1). Misuse of antimicrobial therapy has created new strains of pathogens that are resistant to previously effective therapy. Table 15-2 lists some of the documented drug-resistant pathogens and the body systems most often affected. In addition, many of the major killers, such as cholera and yellow fever, continue to cause death in other parts of the world, necessitating a vigilant attitude toward infectious diseases everywhere (see box on p. 1002).

Because all infectious diseases have characteristics in common, this overview discusses the following aspects:

Stages of infection
Pathogenic agents
Chain of transmission

Stages of Infection

The infection process, from transmission of a pathogenic agent to infectious disease, results from a complex interaction between organisms, an environment conducive to transmission, and a susceptible human host. Once transmission has occurred, more than one outcome is possible. The first is contamination of a body surface or object with a pathogenic agent. The process may stop there if host first-line defenses, such as intact skin and mucous membranes, block the infectious agent from invading host tissue; however, the organism may invade and begin replicating, a condition called colonization. This period is referred to as the latent phase (or incubation phase) in the infection process. Further host defenses, such as inflammatory and immune responses, may fight off the multiplying pathogens during the latent phase, before they have an opportunity to produce damage in host tissue. At the other extreme, the pathogen or its products may begin destructive action on undefended host tissue, resulting in a disease stage in the infection process. By definition, infectious disease is the pathophysiologic response of the host, resulting from the action of the pathogen (or its products) in host tissue or from the host responses to eliminate the pathogen. This pathophysiologic response is generally symptomatic. An asymptomatic response is called a subclinical infection.

Symptoms of infectious disease need not be present for a host to transmit the pathogen. A person, with or without symptoms, may harbor an infectious agent in sufficient quantities to shed the organism in body secretions, excretions, or exudates. Organisms may be shed during the incubation phase before symptomatic disease, during the course of a subclinical infection, or during convalescence following symptomatic disease. In all cases a person who is capable of transmitting organisms in the absence of discernible infectious disease is called a carrier.

Pathogenic Agents

Most of the multitude of microorganisms in our environment are not harmful to the host with a normal immune system. These organisms have coexisted with humans in complex, mutually beneficial relationships. Nonetheless, many organisms are pathogenic (disease producing). Pathogens are parasites that maintain themselves at the expense of their human host, thus producing disease.

Table 15-1 Emerging Infectious Disease in the United States

Infectious Disease	Pathogen	Significance
Hantavirus pulmomary syndrome	Hantavirus spp.	Outbreaks since 1993; 50% mortality rate
Cryptosporidiosis	*Cryptosporidium parvum*	Largest outbreak of waterborne illness in U.S. history; over 400,000 ill and 4400 hospitalized in Milwaukee
Coccidioidomycosis (Valley fever, San Joaquin Valley fever)	*Coccidioides immitis*	Marked increase since 1991 in desert areas of California, affecting all segments of the population
Toxic shock syndrome (TSS)	*Streptococcus pyogenes* (Group A beta-hemolytic streptococci), *Staphylococcus aureus*	Streptococcal TSS has emerged since 1987; staphylococcal TSS associated with tampon usage
Lyme disease	*Borrelia burgdorferi*	Transmitted by deer ticks; cases reported in 47 states; disease often goes undiagnosed and untreated, leading to chronic disability
Legionnaires' disease	*Legionella* spp.	First recognized outbreak in 1976 among attendees at a convention; high mortality; the organism is widespread in the environment in surface and potable waters, with the potential for producing single-source outbreaks
AIDS	Human immunodeficiency virus (HIV)	688,200 reported cases in the United States alone; epidemic continues unabated; modes of transmission make prevention difficult; therapy now extends life of infected persons
Hepatitis C	Hepatitis C virus	Identified in 1975; the principal cause of transfusion-related hepatitis
Hemorrhagic colitis	*Escherichia coli* 0157:H7 (enterohemorrhagic *E. coli* [EHEC])	Outbreak in 1993 from a single source of undercooked hamburger resulted in death of at least four children; outbreaks continue
Chagas' disease	*Trypanosoma cruzi*	Once considered an "exotic" tropical infection; the parasite is now known to be transmitted in blood donated from travelers to areas where the disease is endemic
Leishmaniasis	*Leishmania* spp.	12,000,000 people are infected worldwide, with 400,000 new cases reported annually; has been diagnosed in military personnel returning from the Persian Gulf conflict

Data from Benenson[3] and Centers for Disease Control and Prevention.[7]
*Emerging infectious diseases are diseases of infectious origin whose incidence in humans has increased within the past two decades or threatens to increase in the near future.

Table 15-2 Super Bugs: New Strains of Pathogens Resistant to Therapy

Drug-Resistant Pathogens	Body System Affected
Mycobacterium tuberculosis (multidrug-resistant: MDR-TB)	Respiratory
Streptococcus pneumoniae (multidrug-resistant)	Respiratory
Staphylococcus aureus (methicillin-resistant: MRSA; vancomycin-resistant: VRSA)	Respiratory, circulatory, musculoskeletal, skin
Staphylococcus epidermidis (VRSE), (MRSE)	Skin
Bordetella pertussis	Respiratory (whooping cough)
Neisseria gonorrhoeae	Genitourinary
Salmonella spp.	Gastrointestinal, circulatory, urinary
Enterococcus spp. (multidrug resistant, including vancomycin-resistant: VRE)	Urinary, circulatory, wound, respiratory, central nervous system
Enterobacter spp.	Urinary, wound, respiratory, circulatory
Pseudomonas aeruginosa	Wounds, eye, ear, circulatory, musculoskeletal, respiratory
Klebsiella spp.	Respiratory, urinary, wound, circulatory
Acinetobacter spp.	Respiratory, urinary, wound, circulatory
Other gram-negative organisms developing drug resistance: *Citrobacter freundii, Escherichia coli, Morganella morganii, Providencia* spp., *Serratia* spp.	Multiple body systems

Data from Murray et al[26] and Centers for Disease Control and Prevention.[10,11]

The microorganisms pathogenic to humans are classified, in order of decreasing size, as protozoa, fungi and yeasts, bacteria, rickettsiae, chlamydiae, mycoplasmata, viruses, and prions. A larger group of organisms, also parasitic to humans, are the helminths, or worms.

The likelihood of a pathogen producing infectious disease and the type of disease elicited are influenced by characteristics of the organism. The first is the organism's infectivity: its ability to invade and multiply in the host. Invasiveness is promoted by a variety of pathogen-produced enzymes that either protect

HEALTHY PEOPLE 2010

Health Status—HIV

Goal: Prevent HIV infection and its related illness and death.

- Reduce AIDS among adolescents and adults.
- Reduce the number of new AIDS cases among adolescent and adult men who have sex with men.
- Reduce the number of new AIDS cases among females and males who inject drugs.
- Reduce the number of new AIDS cases among adolescent and adult men who have sex with men and inject drugs.
- (Developmental) Reduce the number of cases of HIV infection among adolescents and adults.
- Increase the proportion of sexually active persons who use condoms.
- (Developmental) Increase the number of HIV-positive persons who know their serostatus.
- Increase the proportion of substance abuse treatment facilities that offer HIV/AIDS education, counseling, and support.
- (Developmental) Increase the number of state prison systems that provide comprehensive HIV/AIDS, sexually transmitted diseases, and tuberculosis (TB) education.
- (Developmental) Increase the proportion of inmates in state prison systems who receive voluntary HIV counseling and testing during incarceration.
- Increase the proportion of adults with TB who have been tested for HIV.
- (Developmental) Increase the proportion of adults in publicly funded HIV counseling and testing sites who are screened for common bacterial sexually transmitted diseases (STDs) (chlamydia, gonorrhea, and syphilis) and are immunized against hepatitis B virus.
- Increase the proportion of HIV-infected adolescents and adults who receive testing, treatment, and prophylaxis consistent with current Public Health Service treatment guidelines.
- Reduce deaths from HIV infection.
- (Developmental) Extend the time between an initial diagnosis of HIV infection and AIDS diagnosis to increase years of life of an individual infected with HIV.
- (Developmental) Increase years of life of an HIV-infected person by extending the time between an AIDS diagnosis and death.
- (Developmental) Reduce new cases of perinatally acquired HIV infection.

Modified from U.S. Department of Health and Human Services: *Healthy people 2010* (conference edition, in two volumes), Washington, DC, January 2000.

NOTE: *Developmental* indicates that criteria for measurement and strategies to improve health have not as yet been specified.

the pathogen from host defenses or dissolve connective tissue to facilitate spread in the host. The second characteristic refers to the organism's pathogenicity, or ability to produce disease. This in turn relies on the pathogen's speed of reproduction, extent of tissue damage, or production of a toxin. The third characteristic is its mode of action. Some pathogens cause direct cellular damage leading to cellular necrosis and death. Others, such as viruses, interfere with cellular metabolism. Still others produce toxins that stimulate local or systemic reaction. The fourth characteristic, virulence, refers to the potency of the pathogen in producing severe disease. Closely related to virulence is the toxigenicity of some pathogens. Agents vary in the amount and destructive potential of the toxins they produce. Some bacteria secrete water-soluble antigenic exotoxins that are quickly distributed by the blood, causing potentially severe systemic and neurologic manifestations. Diseases associated with exotoxins are tetanus, botulism, and diphtheria. Endotoxins make up the cell wall of some bacteria and cause local inflammation and destruction of host tissue. They are weakly toxic, are relatively stable, and are not antigenic. Diseases associated with endotoxins include staphylococcal food poisoning and cholera.

A final characteristic, antigenicity, is the ability of a pathogen to induce an antibody response in the host. Pathogens vary according to this characteristic. Some have intrinsic antigens (proteins, polypeptides, or polysaccharides) that cause the host to produce antibodies against the antigen.

Chain of Transmission

The ability of a pathogenic agent to produce infectious disease in humans depends on the agent's characteristics plus an intact chain of transmission. The chain includes a host reservoir, mode of escape from the reservoir, environment conducive to transmission of the pathogen, entry into a new host, and susceptibility of the new host to the infectious disease.

Reservoir. A reservoir is a person, animal, plant, soil, or organic substance, alone or in combination, in which an infectious agent lives and multiplies. The agent depends on the reservoir for its reproduction and consequent survival. Humans are the only reservoir for some pathogens, whereas other pathogens require an intermediate animal or chain of animal or inanimate reservoirs. The human, as a reservoir for an infectious agent, may have a symptomatic infectious disease, may have a subclinical infectious disease, or may be a carrier of the agent.

Escape. The organism escapes from the reservoir at the site of the multiplication of the organism. Portals of exit may be the genitourinary tract, the gastrointestinal tract, the oral cavity, the respiratory tract, open lesions, or mechanical escape of blood. There may be more than one portal of exit for any one disease process. The duration of escape coincides with the period of communicability and varies with each disease. Generally, there is an inverse relationship between the length of the communicable period and the infectivity of the organism. Highly infectious organisms such as the influenza virus have a short duration of escape, whereas the less infective *Mycobacterium tuberculosis* has a long duration of escape.

The portal of exit of an organism determines its mode of transmission and is therefore an important consideration for health-care workers in contact with infectious agents.

Transmission. The organism may have a single or multiple routes of transmission. In general, the organism may be

YOU CAN HELP PREVENT THE FURTHER DEVELOPMENT OF MULTIDRUG-RESISTANT ORGANISMS

Drug-resistant organisms have developed from misuse/abuse of antimicrobial therapy. **How has this occurred?** Effective antimicrobial therapy eliminates or suppresses a significant proportion of microbes, thus allowing the body's natural defenses to control the remaining pathogens. Incomplete therapy merely exposes the microorganisms to the antimicrobial without eliminating or sufficiently suppressing them. Thus the surviving microorganisms are those that have developed resistance to the drug. These survivors are able to transfer this resistance, not only to their progeny but to other adult microorganisms with similar cell structures. For example, vancomycin-resistant enterococci (VRE) can transfer the gene that confers high-level resistance to other gram-positive bacteria such as *Staphylococcus aureus.*

What can you do to stop the proliferation of drug-resistant pathogens? Educate all of your patients and their families about the importance of taking antibiotics and other antimicrobial medications only when prescribed by a physician or a nurse practitioner. Instruct them verbally and in writing to take the medication exactly as prescribed for as long as prescribed, even if symptoms are resolved before the medication has been completed. The only acceptable reason for not completing the prescribed therapy is an adverse reaction to the medication, which should be reported to the physician at once. Further, instruct your patients to *never* share their medications with another person, even with a member of one's family, and to *never* take medication prescribed for a previous infection. In addition, instruct that antibiotics *should not* be taken for nonbacterial infections, such as the common cold. We are all responsible for controlling the escalating problem of drug resistance. We all will suffer if the "super bugs" continue to develop.

transmitted *directly* through person-to-person contact or *indirectly* through an animate or inanimate vehicle of transmission. Direct contact occurs when there is actual physical contact between the source and the victim as is the case with sexual, fecal-oral, or mucous droplet transmission. Indirect transmission requires that the organism survive outside the human on or in animate or inanimate vehicles. Animate vehicles include animals and vectors. Inanimate vehicles are air, food, water, milk, soil, fomites, or biologic materials. If an inanimate vehicle has the potential of infecting many persons, it is called a common vehicle.

Entry. Portal of entry into a new host corresponds frequently with the portal of exit from the reservoir. Entry may be by ingestion, by inhalation, by percutaneous injection, through the mucous membranes, or across the placenta. The duration of the exposure and the numbers of organisms necessary to start the infectious process in the new host vary with each disease.

Host Susceptibility. Susceptibility refers to those host conditions that increase the probability that disease may develop in the host. Susceptibility is affected by specific resistance factors such as the immunologic responses and nonspecific body defenses against disease agents, both of which are discussed in the next section. Host susceptibility is also affected by general human characteristics such as age, sex, ethnic group, and heredity; behaviors regarding eating and personal hygiene;

Table15-3 Chain of Transmission of Infectious Disease

Transmission Chain	Factors
Agent	Bacteria, rickettsiae, fungi, chlamydiae, mycoplasmata, viruses, helminths, protozoa, prions
Reservoir (where agent lives and multiplies)	Humans (frank cases, subclinical cases, carriers) Inanimate organic matter Animals
Portal of exit	Genitourinary tract, gastrointestinal tract, respiratory tract, oral cavity, open lesions, blood
Transmission	Direct: person to person (fecal-oral, sexual, droplet) Indirect: through a vehicle (animate: animal or vector; inanimate: food, water, soil, milk, air, intravenous therapy or catheters)
Modes of entry	Ingestion, inhalation, percutaneous injection, transplacental entry, mucous membranes
Susceptible host	Specific immune reactions Nonspecific body defenses Host characteristics: age, sex, ethnic group, heredity, behaviors Environmental; general health status

geographic and environmental living conditions; and general health status, including nutritional status, hormonal balance, and the presence of concurrent disease. All of these factors either determine the type of pathogenic agent to which the person is exposed or determine the extent of the host response and resistance to the pathogens (Table 15-3).

Control. Control of infectious disease relies on procedures aimed at breaking the chain of transmission at one or more of its links. The point of the chain most amenable to control varies with the organism and its reservoirs, the disease process, and available technology. Control measures may be directed to killing or altering the virulence of the agent, destroying nonhuman reservoirs and vectors, isolating the infected persons, using precautions with infected body fluids and contaminated inanimate objects, and altering host resistance, defenses, and immunity.

Effective control is also based on monitoring of disease occurrence to facilitate early intervention (see box on p. 1004). Certain diseases must be reported to the local health authority. These are identified in the overview table presented for each disease discussed in this chapter.

ANATOMY, PHYSIOLOGY, AND RELATED PATHOPHYSIOLOGY

Physiology of the Human Response to Infection

Certain anatomic and physiologic characteristics of the human operate to increase resistance to infectious diseases and to fight the infectious process once it occurs. These characteristics can be considered as lines of defense against pathogenic agents.

SPECTRUM OF DISEASE OCCURRENCE

Characteristics of the organism and mode of transmission are the two most important factors in how often a particular infectious disease occurs and how many people are affected.

Sporadic disease is the occasional, irregular appearance of cases in a population over a given period.

Endemic disease occurs at a constant rate affecting about the same number of people in a population over a given period.

Epidemic disease is a definite increase over its expected endemic pattern.

Pandemic disease is an epidemic occurring over a very wide area and usually affecting a large proportion of the population.

Some diseases also demonstrate predictable seasonal, yearly, or geographic variation in occurrence.

From Grimes.[25]

The first line of defense against infection is external and consists of mechanical barriers, chemical barriers, and the body's own population of microorganisms.

The two internal barriers come into play when the external line of defense is breeched. Operating as the second line of defense, the inflammatory response is aimed at preventing an invading pathogen from becoming established, reproducing, and invading other tissues. The third line of defense is the immune response, which is activated after the inflammatory response. Although inflammation and immune response are two events, they cannot always be easily separated because both events involve many of the same processes and cellular components. In addition to these defenses, the human characteristically responds to an infectious process with a change in body temperature.

First Line of Defense: Barriers

Every surface of the body that is exposed in any way to the environment is involved in first-line defense.

Mechanical Barriers. Certain anatomic characteristics prevent the invasion of microorganisms. These include the intact skin and mucous membranes and oil and perspiration on the skin. Ciliary action in the respiratory tract, reflexes such as coughing and sneezing, and peristalsis in the gastrointestinal tract act to remove an organism before its penetration into tissue. The flushing action of body secretions such as tears, saliva, and mucus further protects against invasion. Compromise in any of these barriers increases susceptibility to invasion of infectious agents.

Chemical Barriers. In addition to the mechanical barriers, the chemical composition of body secretions is protective. The pH of saliva, vaginal secretions, urine, and digestive secretions prevents or inhibits growth of some microbes. Bile acts to decrease the surface tension, causing changes in the cell wall of some bacteria. This renders the organisms more digestible by other digestive enzymes. Oil and sweat secretions contain chemicals that are bactericidal to some microbes.

Normal Flora. The normal flora of microorganisms on the skin and mucous membranes and in the intestinal and vaginal tracts protect against invasion of pathogenic agents through a mechanism termed microbial antagonism. The importance of this mechanism in controlling the replication of pathogenic organisms becomes evident when the normal flora are disturbed during antibiotic therapy. Extensive penicillin therapy, for example, may precipitate the growth of *Candida albicans,* normally controlled by the normal flora bacteria in the vaginal tract.

Some indigenous flora are themselves pathogenic under certain conditions. They can be responsible for infection when the immune system is impaired, the skin or mucous membranes are breeched, or the flora are displaced from their natural habitat to another area of the body. This latter event is explained by the fact that the normal flora are tissue specific—that is, a particular type of bacteria normally colonizes a particular type of tissue, adhering to specific receptors on epithelial cells. As a result, the normal composition of flora varies from one part of the body to another.

Displacement of indigenous flora to another area is a common cause of nosocomial (hospital-acquired) infection, such as urinary tract infection from enteric bacteria following catheterization.

Components of Internal Defense

The second and third lines of defense (the inflammatory response and the immune system) share several components. These components include the lymphatic system, leukocytes, and a multitude of chemicals, proteins, and enzymes that facilitate the internal defense systems (see Chapter 16 for an in-depth review of these components).

Second Line of Defense: The Inflammatory Response

Once a microorganism penetrates the first line of defense and invades cells, the inflammatory response is initiated. Inflammation is a local reaction to cell injury of any type, whether from physical, chemical, or thermal damage or microbial invasion. As a response to microbial injury, inflammation is aimed at preventing further invasion by walling off, destroying, or neutralizing the invading organism. Repair is also an integral part of inflammation, and in "clean" injuries, which do not involve microbes, repair is the primary beneficial result.

The early inflammatory response is protective, but it can continue for sustained periods of time in some infections. The production of new leukocytes (particularly phagocytic leukocytes) may be stimulated for weeks or months in some infections, as reflected in an elevated white blood cell (WBC) count (particularly neutrophils and monocytes) for prolonged periods. However, sustained inflammation can become chronic and result in the destruction of healthy tissues. Extensive necrosis from persistent inflammation can actually increase tissue susceptibility to the infectious agent or provide an ideal setting for invasion by other pathogens.

The inflammatory response is limited to vascularized tissues, because the molecular and cellular components of inflammation are delivered via blood vessels. Inflammation develops in a series of interrelated steps that involve blood vessels, fluid and cellular blood components, the lymphatic system, and the surrounding connective tissue.

Stages of Inflammatory Response.

The complex mechanisms of the inflammatory response can be divided into three interdependent stages: cell response to injury, vascular response, and phagocytosis.

The cellular response to injury is the same regardless of the method of injury. A number of metabolic changes occur within the injured cell. The injured cell swells because it can no longer pump out sodium ions. Nearly all cells contain specialized sacs called lysosomes that contain a multitude of enzymes capable of digesting portions of the cell if its metabolic activity has been severely disrupted. The resulting cellular atrophy reduces metabolic demands on the cell. Cell death occurs if metabolism can no longer be maintained, and enzymes are released to dissolve the cellular contents and stimulate the inflammatory process in surrounding tissue.

The vascular response occurs shortly after injury. The arterioles, venules, and capillaries in the surrounding area dilate, producing a localized hyperemia. This increases the filtration pressure of the blood and capillary permeability, causing fluid exudate to leak from the blood vessels into the interstitial spaces. Proteins, enzymes, and other chemical components in the exudate attract more fluid into the interstitial spaces, producing edema in an effort to wall off the inflamed area from uninvolved tissues.

Inflammatory exudate serves the important function of transporting phagocytic cells into the injured area. As fluid leaks from the blood, blood flow in the area slows, allowing leukocytes to collect (marginate) along the vascular endothelium. Leukocytes, particularly neutrophils and monocytes, emigrate through the endothelium to the injured tissue, attracted by chemicals released by the injured cells.

Phagocytosis is the process of engulfing, digesting, and thus destroying infectious agents and other material. This is done primarily by circulating macrophages, the majority of which are neutrophils and monocytes that are dispatched to an injured area in fluid exudate. Some macrophages reside in tissue and are found in lymph nodes, bone marrow, lungs (alveolar macrophages), spleen, liver (Kupffer's cells), and other organs. Phagocytes also perform the essential "housekeeping" chore of cleaning up dead cells and other debris.

Intracellular phagocytosis occurs at the site of tissue invasion, but it also extends into lymphatic and blood circulation if infection becomes systemic. The intracellular activity of phagocytosis stimulates release of chemicals that induce lysis of the leukocytes. These dead leukocytes, together with dead organisms and fluid from the blood, make up the inflammatory exudate.

Patterns of Inflammation.

Both local and systemic symptoms of inflammation can occur. Heat, redness, swelling, and pain are local reactions to inflammation that may vary considerably in severity. The first three characteristics result from response of the vasculature to injury. Pain is produced partly from pressure of the exudate against nerve endings in the surrounding tissue, but prostaglandins and possibly other chemicals also play some role in causing pain.

Several types of inflammatory exudates are produced. Serous exudate, which typically occurs in early inflammation, contains only plasma and proteins. Mucinous or catarrhal exudate contains increased secretions from inflamed mucous membranes and may include both live and dead organisms. Fibrinous exudate forms on tissue, particularly mucous membranes, when large amounts of fibrinogen are extravasated into the tissue. Purulent exudate, such as pus, contains both live and dead leukocytes, live and dead microorganisms, serous exudate, and liquefied digestive products of necrotic tissue. Some inflammatory conditions produce combinations of exudates. The characteristic fibrinopurulent exudate of diphtheria results from necrosis of the mucous membrane in the throat.

Inflammation and its exudates may remain localized, may permeate the tissue, or may spread throughout the body via the blood or lymph. An abscess is an example of a localized infection and inflammation with purulent exudate. Leukocytes form a wall around the organisms. The abscess deepens as more leukocytes are drawn into the area, more organisms are killed, and more necrotic tissue is dissolved. The exudate may eventually be autolyzed and resorbed by the body, in which case the inflammation and infection are resolved. Resolution may leave a cavity, ulcer, or scar tissue. Calcification around the exudate occurs in some instances, such as in tuberculosis, walling off the live infectious agents inside the tissue. Rupture of the abscess and drainage into other tissues can spread the infection to other areas of the body.

Systemic symptoms can include fever and chills, diaphoresis, malaise, and nausea and vomiting. The inflammatory process also causes changes in blood components, such as an increased number of leukocytes or a change in the type of leukocytes.

Chronic inflammation may result from a low-grade inflammatory response that fails to elicit an acute response. Agents most often responsible for chronic inflammation are those that cannot penetrate deeply or spread rapidly, such as *M. tuberculosis,* the treponemata that cause syphilis, some viruses, fungi, and many helminths. Inadequate specific immune response or a hyperimmune response can also lead to chronic inflammation, such as occurs in autoimmune disorders.

Chronic inflammation is marked by tissue infiltration with macrophages, lymphocytes, and plasma cells rather than neutrophils. Exudates are not generally formed, although some types of chronic inflammatory disorders are characterized by certain types of exudates. Rheumatoid arthritis, for example, is accompanied by synovial effusions, an exudate into the joint. A proliferation of fibroblasts results in greater formation of scar tissue that sometimes replaces normal connective tissue or other tissue. Some chronic inflammations result in formation of granulomas, which are 1- to 2-mm lesions caused by the massing of macrophages surrounded by lymphocytes around an infectious agent. A dense membrane of connective tissue may encapsulate the lesion, as occurs in tuberculosis.

Several factors affect the outcome of the inflammatory process. Age, nutritional status, and general health greatly affect the individual's ability to mount an effective inflammatory response. Agent factors, such as virulence and size of inoculum, can overcome even an aggressive host defense and promote spread of the organism. In addition, some pathogens are effective intracellular parasites and are capable of surviving and multiplying in phagocytes. These include some viruses, *M. tuberculosis,* and *Rickettsia.* The immune response, the third line of defense, is activated to combat invaders that survive phagocytosis.

Third Line of Defense: The Immune Response

The first and second lines of defense are nonspecific—that is, they operate against all infectious agents in the same manner. In contrast, the immune system responds in a very specific manner to individual pathogens, as long as the organism has antigenic characteristics. Generally speaking, antigens are either proteins, large polysaccharides, or large lipoprotein complexes that stimulate antibody production. Not all microorganisms are antigenic, but some are bound by complement or other host-produced substances to form an antigen that elicits an immune response.

The immune system has several unique characteristics:

Self- or nonself-recognition: It normally recognizes host cells as nonantigenic and therefore responds only to foreign agents as antigens. In autoimmune diseases, there is a breakdown in this distinction, and the immune system attacks host cells as if they were antigens.

Antibody production: It produces specific antibodies that target specific antigens for destruction; it can produce new antibodies in response to new antigens.

Memory: It remembers antigens that have invaded the body in the past, allowing a quicker response to subsequent invasion by the same antigen.

Self-regulation: It monitors its own performance, turning on when antigens invade and turning off when infection is eradicated, preventing destruction of healthy tissue.

An immune response is triggered after foreign materials have been cleared from an area of inflammation. After phagocytes digest the pathogens, antigenic material appears on their surface. Phagocytes, primarily macrophages, serve as antigen-presenting cells to introduce the pathogen to lymphocytes. Recognition of the antigen as "nonself" by receptors on lymphocytes in blood, lymph, or tissue exudate sets up a chain of responses to destroy or neutralize the antigen. Two types of immune responses can occur: cell-mediated immunity and humoral immunity. These processes begin with the differentiation of lymphocytes into B or T cells. These two types of responses overlap and interact considerably, but the distinction is useful in understanding how the immune system is activated.

Cell-Mediated Immune Response.

The cellular immune response is activated with the invasion of intracellular pathogens, such as viruses, mycobacteria, fungi, and protozoa, and it is a component of the host response to tumors and tissue transplants. Cell-mediated immunity, directed primarily by T cells, results from cell interaction with antigens expressed on phagocytes. T cell receptor binding to the antigen causes T cells to differentiate into subsets and proliferate. Helper T cells initiate the cell-mediated response by releasing interleukin-2, which stimulates the production of cytotoxic T cells. Cytotoxic T cells kill the antigen directly by releasing lymphokines, an event that also attracts more macrophages to the area. Suppressor T cells slow or halt the activity of other T cells.

Cell-mediated immunity is the basis for many skin tests, such as the tuberculin test. Cellular immunity cannot be transferred passively to another person.

Humoral Immune Response.

Humoral (antibody-mediated) immunity protects against many gram-positive and certain gram-negative bacteria. Antibody production also aids in neutralizing viruses, enhances phagocytosis, and activates the complement system. B cells, the antibody-producing lymphocytes, are responsible for humoral immunity.

Humoral immunity can be initiated in two ways. Some antigens are not recognized by T cells (T-independent antigens) and stimulate B cells directly. Most antigens, however, will bind to T cells (T-dependent antigens), and the helper T cells act to stimulate B cells. In either case, the stimulated B cells differentiate into antibody-producing plasma cells and memory B cells. Antibodies appear on the surface of plasma cells and bind to antigen. Once antigens are immobilized, cytotoxic T cells are activated and eradication of the pathogen begins. Suppressor T cells halt the humoral response after the infection is resolved.

The amount and type of antibody produced depend on the nature and amount of antigen present, the site of the antigen stimulus, and the number of previous exposures to the same antigen. The initial antibody production, the primary response occurs the first time a particular antigen invades the body (from 1 to 7 days after initial exposure to the antigen). Depending on the nature of the antigen and the efficiency of antibody production, the response peaks in 1 to 10 weeks. Antibody titers can usually be detected within 10 days of exposure.

Memory B cells allow a more efficient humoral response on subsequent exposure to the same antigen (the secondary response). The memory cells generate more rapid, prolific, and sustained response, producing higher antibody titers that are usually detectable in a shorter period of time and for a longer duration.

The strength and persistence of the humoral immune response are determined by maintaining a correct balance between helper and suppressor T cells. Helper T cells must be present in sufficient numbers to stimulate B cell production of antibodies, and the correct proportion of T suppressor cells is needed to shut off the immune response. An imbalance can result in inadequate production of antibodies, leading to immune deficiency states, or the unchecked overstimulation of the immune response, resulting in autoimmune disorders. The normal helper-to-suppressor ratio is 2:1, whereas a 1:1 ratio is typical in AIDS patients.

The humoral immune response is more rapid than the cell-mediated response and is more frequently a factor in resistance to acute bacterial infections. Humoral immunity can be transmitted to another person, either by inoculation or by maternal transfer via the placenta or breast milk.

Immunoglobulins.

Immunoglobulins are the protein molecules that compose antibodies. There are five major classes of immunoglobulins that are able to combine in an endless number of ways to produce antibodies specific against a particular antigen. When the humoral immune response is initiated, more than one class may be activated. Table 15-4 summarizes the characteristics of the immunoglobulin classes.

Immunoglobulins perform four major functions:

1. Immunoglobulins directly attack antigens, destroying or neutralizing them through the processes of agglutination (clumping the antigens together to inactivate them), precipitating the toxins out of solution, neutralizing antigenic substances, and lysing the organism's cell wall.

Table 15-4 Immunoglobulin Classes

Immunoglobulin	Characteristics	Functions
IgG	Accounts for about 80%-85% of antibodies in normal serum; most abundant in blood but also found in lymph, cerebrospinal, synovial, and peritoneal fluid and breast milk; the only immunoglobulin that crosses placenta and provides temporary immunity in neonate	Develops slowly during primary response, appearing about 1 wk or more after IgM, then reaches a peak in 1-3 wk or longer after IgM peaks; may persist for years; highest concentration during secondary immune response; activates complement system; involved in opsonization; attacks antigens directly
IgM	Accounts for about 5% of antibodies in normal serum	First antibody to form during viral or bacterial infection; usually peaks 1-2 wk after clinical symptoms appear; highest concentration during primary response; is increased in chronic infections; binds with viral and bacterial antigens in the circulation, which activates the complement cascade
IgA	Accounts for about 15% of antibodies in normal serum; found in blood and secretions (tears, saliva, colostrum, respiratory tract, stomach, and accessory organs)	Secretory antibody; increased in chronic infections and chronic inflammation
IgE	Accounts for <1% of antibodies in normal serum; found also in tissues	Sensitizing antibody; triggers release of histamine; involved with certain allergic disorders, especially atopic diseases; increased in parasitic diseases
IgD	Accounts for <1% of antibodies in normal serum	Function unclear, but increases in chronic infection

From Grimes.[25]

Table 15-5 Types of Acquired Immunity

Type of Immunity	How Acquired	Length of Resistance
NATURAL		
Active	Natural contact and infection with the antigen	May be temporary or permanent
Passive	Natural contact with antibody transplacentally or through colostrum and breast milk	Temporary
ARTIFICIAL		
Active	Inoculation of antigen	May be temporary or permanent
Passive	Inoculation of antibody or antitoxin	Temporary

From Grimes.[25]

2. Immunoglobulins activate the complement system.
3. Immunoglobulins activate anaphylaxis by releasing histamine in tissue and blood.
4. Immunoglobulins stimulate antibody-mediated hypersensitivity.

Acquired Immunity. Immunity refers to the presence of or acquisition of antibodies. Immunity can be acquired as a result of exposure to a specific antigenic agent or pathogen. Acquired immunity may be gained by natural means through inadvertent contact with an antigen (active) or antibodies (passive). Artificial immunity is intentionally induced through inoculation of antigen (active) or antibodies (passive) (Table 15-5). Active immunity, whether naturally or artificially induced, produces physiologically identical immune responses (see Immunizations, p. 1076).

Body Temperature Response

A change in body temperature is a characteristic systemic symptom of infectious diseases. The causes of fever in infectious diseases are discussed here. Fever patterns associated with specific infectious diseases are described with each disease.

Causes of Fever in Infectious Diseases. Body temperature is normally maintained within a range around 98.6° F (37° C) with predictable variations within any 24-hour period that coincide with metabolic activity. Fever, a sustained temperature above normal, can be caused by abnormalities of the hypothalamus, brain tumors, dehydration, or toxic substances affecting the temperature-regulating center of the hypothalamus. Certain substances, either directly or indirectly, can cause the "set point" of the hypothalamic thermostat to rise. This results in activation of the hypothalamus to signal body mechanisms to conserve heat and to increase heat production. Substances that cause these effects are called pyrogens. In infectious diseases the endotoxins of some bacteria and the extracts of normal leukocytes (interleukins) are pyrogenic. They act to raise the "thermostat" in the hypothalamus, thus raising the body temperature.

Fever is not a failure of the body to regulate temperature. During the fever response, temperature is merely regulated at a higher level than normal. Four stages of the fever process can be observed. The first is a prodromal period, with no notable change in temperature but with nonspecific symptoms of discomfort. A chill accompanies the second stage when the body temperature is being raised toward the higher thermostat setting.

The third stage, flush, occurs when the temperature reaches the new setting. During the fourth stage, body temperature returns to normal, which causes sweating.

Distinct patterns of fever onset and resolution and characteristic temperature curves are associated with different infectious diseases. Fever onset may be abrupt or gradual. A persistent elevation may be maintained throughout the disease, or there may be remissions at specific times of the day or certain days in the illness. Fever associated with some diseases follows a "saddle back" curve with a high fever initially, followed by a few days of remission and then another high elevation. A habitual fever is a low-level fever present in some diseases for years. Intermittent fevers have predictable cycles of paroxysms and remissions. Relapsing fevers are those that recur after apparent recovery. Fevers may resolve suddenly or gradually.

For each degree Fahrenheit of temperature elevation there is a 7% increase in body metabolism, necessitating fluid and calorie supplements to meet metabolic needs.

A fever that goes too high may damage cells irreversibly. Temperature elevation to 104° F (40° C) may cause delirium and convulsions, particularly in children. Fever above 106° F (41.1° C) can cause irreparable damage, impairing regulation of the hypothalamic control center, which results in inability to lower temperature.

NORMAL FINDINGS

Refer to specific chapters in this book to obtain normal findings pertinent to each body system.

DIAGNOSTIC STUDIES AND FINDINGS

Culture of specimen and direct examination of the culture: To identify organism by its characteristics

Microscopic examination of specimen prepared through a variety of chemical or staining procedures: To identify microscopic organisms

Examination of the specimen for antigen/antibody reactions: To identify the antigen or toxin in the specimen

Serology: Immunologic tests applied to serum to identify circulating antibodies to the organism.

CONDITIONS, DISEASES, AND DISORDERS

CENTRAL NERVOUS SYSTEM INFECTIOUS DISEASES

MENINGITIS

Meningitis is an inflammation of the meninges covering the brain and spinal cord. The inflammation may result from an acute infection of the meninges caused by the invasion of bacteria, viruses, fungi, or parasitic worms into the tissues or from the iatrogenic introduction of a substance that is irritating to the meninges. The forms of meningitis discussed in this section are those caused by bacterial and viral invasion occurring commonly in adults (Table 15-6).

Table 15-6 Overview of Meningitis

	Meningococcal Meningitis	Pneumococcal Meningitis	Viral Meningitis (Aseptic)
Occurrence	Endemic and epidemic; worldwide; greatest during winter and spring; greatest in males, in children and teens, and in persons in crowded living conditions, such as college dormitories or military barracks	Endemic; greatest in infants, elderly persons, and alcoholics; follows pneumococcal pneumonia	Worldwide; epidemics, seasonal outbreaks, and sporadic cases associated with other viral infections
Etiologic agent	*N. meningitidis,* with many subgroups	*S. pneumoniae,* many serotypes	Most viruses (e.g., mumps, herpes, and polio) produce the syndrome
Reservoir	Humans	Humans; many carriers	Humans
Transmission	Direct contact with droplets from respiratory passages of infected persons and carriers	Direct and indirect contact with discharges from respiratory passages	Not transmitted at this stage
Incubation period	2-10 days; usually 3-4 days	Not well known	Depends on virus and associated viral disease
Period of communicability	Until organism is not present in discharges: within 24 hours of treatment with antimicrobials	Until organism is not present in respiratory discharges: 24-48 hours after antibiotic treatment	
Susceptibility and resistance	Susceptibility to clinical disease is low; many carriers; group-specific immunity of unknown duration follows infection	Infants and elderly most susceptible; immunity for specific type persists for years	Children, elderly and immunocompromised patients, and those unimmunized against vaccine-preventable viral diseases
Report to local health authority	Mandatory case report	Only epidemics; no individual case reports	Yes, in endemic areas

Data from Benenson.[3]

Meningococcal meningitis is an acute communicable inflammation of the meninges caused by *Neisseria meningitidis.* It frequently occurs in epidemic form.

Pneumococcal meningitis is an acute inflammation of the meninges caused by *Streptococcus pneumoniae.* The meningitis frequently results from an extension of a primary infection in the upper respiratory tract. Patients infected with *S. pneumoniae* have a high risk of fatality.

Viral (aseptic or serous) meningitis is an acute meningeal inflammation that occurs as a sequela to many viral diseases. The condition is usually self-limited and benign.

PATHOPHYSIOLOGY

Bacterial Meningitis

Bacteria causing the type of meningitis being considered here are inhaled in mucous droplets from infected persons or carriers. The bacteria invade the respiratory passages and are disseminated by way of the blood to meninges of the brain and spinal cord. The respiratory phase is generally subclinical in meningococcal meningitis, although organisms present in respiratory secretions can be transmitted to another host. The respiratory phase is usually symptomatic in pneumococcal meningitis. The bacteremia produced during dissemination causes toxic manifestations. In the case of meningococcus the organism penetrates and damages vascular endothelium. This results in petechial and purpuric lesions of the skin.

Bacteria in the meninges elicit an inflammatory response and the production of an exudate in the subarachnoid space. Cerebrospinal fluid may be thin or thick and have plaquelike accumulations and high leukocytosis, with the majority of the leukocytes being neutrophils. In untreated disease the cerebrospinal fluid may achieve a thickness that interferes with its circulation and reabsorption. An internal or external hydrocephalus may result. Extension of the bacteria into brain tissue may produce a bacterial encephalitis.

Meningococcal infections may be so severe in the systemic stage that they produce an acute meningococcemia that leads to death or adrenal infarction and acute adrenal insufficiency (see Emergency Alert box). Meningococcemia may become chronic, with toxic symptoms persisting intermittently for weeks or months. Recurrent meningitis is usually of the pneumococcal form and is frequently associated with an undetected skull fracture.

Symptomatic and asymptomatic infection with bacterial meningitis results in a protective immune response of unknown duration.

Viral Meningitis

Aseptic (viral, serous, or nonsuppurative) meningitis is a syndrome generally associated with an existing systemic viral disease, the most common one being mumps. Inflammation and lymphocytic infiltration of the meninges occur with a wide gradient in clinical severity, depending on the infectious agent. Toxic and meningeal symptoms are usually less severe than in suppurative meningitis; cerebrospinal fluid leukocytes are fewer and consist primarily of lymphocytes. This form may also progress to clinical encephalitis. The disease is usually self-limited with complete recovery, although patients may experience muscle weakness and malaise during a prolonged convalescence.

DIAGNOSTIC STUDIES AND FINDINGS[26]

Cerebrospinal fluid (CSF) examination

- **Gross appearance:** Bacterial: turbid; viral (aseptic): clear
- **Leukocytes:** Bacterial: 500 to 20,000/mm^3; viral: 10 to 500/mm^3
- **Cell types:** Bacterial: neutrophils; viral (aseptic): lymphocytes
- **Protein:** Bacterial: elevated; viral: normal or elevated
- **Glucose:** Bacterial: low to normal; viral (aseptic): normal

CSF culture and microscopic examination: Positive for *N. meningitidis* or *S. pneumoniae;* negative suggests viral origin

CSF antigen/antibody tests: Positive for *N. meningitidis* or *S. pneumoniae*

Gram's stain of scrapings from petechial skin lesions: Positive for *N. meningitidis*

Respiratory secretions culture: Positive for *N. meningitidis* or *S. pneumoniae*

Blood culture: Positive for *N. meningitidis* or *S. pneumoniae*

Serology: Antibodies present for *N. meningitidis, S. pneumoniae,* or specific virus

Urine: Antigen/antibody tests: positive for *N. meningitidis* or *S. pneumoniae*

MULTIDISCIPLINARY PLAN[3,26]

Medications

Antiinfective agents for pneumococci: Penicillin, chloramphenicol, vancomycin

> **! EMERGENCY ALERT**
>
> **MENINGITIS**
>
> An acute infectious process that is an inflammation of the meninges of the spinal cord and brain. The infection carries a mortality ranging between 10% and 30% for bacterial meningitis.
>
> **ASSESSMENT**
>
> - Assess for fever, headache.
> - Assess for nuchal rididity.
> - Assess for mental alterations, changes in behavior, level of consciousness.
> - Assess for increased intracranial pressure.
> - Assess for shock, signs of adrenal insufficiency.
>
> **INTERVENTIONS**
>
> - Maintain airway, breathing, and circulation; intubation and ventilation may be indicated if respiratory status is inadequate.
> - Obtain intravenous (IV) access; in collaboration with physician, administer antibiotics, anticonvulsants, and antipyretics as indicated.
> - Manage shock.
> - Assist physician with lumbar puncture to evaluate cerebrospinal fluid.
> - Obtain laboratory studies, including blood cultures.

Antiinfective agents for meningococci: Ceftriaxone, ciprofloxacin

All of above are administered by rapid IV infusion; therapy should continue for 5 days after temperature is normal and clinical signs have cleared. The patient may be given rifampin before hospital discharge

Antiinfective agent for herpes viral meningitis: Acyclovir IV; PO for prophylaxis; no specific treatment for other viruses

Analgesics prescribed for headache and muscle pain (nonnarcotic); benzodiazapines or barbiturates may be given for seizures

Immunologic agents prescribed for prevention of bacterial meningitides

Meningococcal polysaccharide vaccine used against group A, C, Y, and W-135 for patients over 2 years at risk for epidemic disease; group A serotype given to children 3 months to 2 years; routine immunization of the public is not recommended

Pneumococcal polysaccharide vaccine given to patients at high risk for pneumococcal pneumonia and subsequent systemic complications such as immunocompromised persons, chronically ill persons, and the elderly

Antiinfective agents for meningococcal contacts: Rifampin (rifamycin, others), 600 mg bid (adults) for 2 days, or ciprofloxacin, 500 mg PO in a single dose

Sulfadiazine, 1 g bid for 3 days for mass prophylaxis during meningococcal epidemics or for close patient contacts if strain is proven susceptible

Osmotic agents (e.g., dexamethasone) for cerebral edema

General Management

Endotracheal intubation

Ventilatory assistance

IV therapy and dopamine if shock is present

Fluid restriction to two thirds of daily needs if renal failure is present

Control of intracranial pressure

Close monitoring for early diagnosis of patient contacts

NURSING CARE

Nursing Assessment

See Nursing Care for meningitis and encephalitis, p. 1011.

ENCEPHALITIS

Encephalitis is an inflammation of the tissues of the brain and spinal cord, resulting in altered function of various portions of these tissues. Encephalitis is frequently accompanied by signs of systemic infection. Clinical disease manifestations range from mild to severe to death, and disease may be followed by temporary or permanent neurologic sequelae or complete recovery.

Similar to meningitis, encephalitis may result from at least four causes: a toxemia accompanying an infectious disease, an allergic response to microbial antigens, direct invasion of central nervous system tissue by pathogens as a primary focal infection, or direct invasion of central nervous system tissue secondary to hematogenous dissemination from a primary focal infection elsewhere in the body. Direct invasion, either primary or secondary, is usually caused by a virus, a great many of which are capable of producing encephalitis.

The majority of viruses producing encephalitis as a primary focal infection are transmitted by mosquitoes and are discussed together. Encephalitides occurring secondary to other viral diseases are discussed as infectious encephalitis. A rarer form of meningoencephalitis caused by direct invasion of an ameba is also discussed (Table 15-7).

Infectious viral encephalitides are acute inflammations of the central nervous system that are associated with and sequelae to systemic viral infections; they are commonly caused by the genus *Herpesvirus.*

Mosquito-borne viral encephalitides are a group of acute inflammatory diseases of the brain, spinal cord, and meninges caused by a variety of viruses transmitted to humans through bites from infected mosquitoes.

Amebic meningoencephalitis is an acute and severe inflammation of the brain and meninges caused by invasion of the tissues by a free-living ameba usually found in water, soil, and decaying vegetation. The disease is frequently fatal.

PATHOPHYSIOLOGY

Infectious Viral Encephalitis

A variety of directly transmittable viruses are capable of producing encephalitides either as a concomitant to or as a sequela of clinical viral diseases (e.g., measles, mumps, rubella, and chickenpox) or as a result of a subclinical viral infection, such as herpes. In both cases the pathologic manifestations of the encephalitis may result from a postinfection autoimmune response to the virus or from direct invasion of the central nervous system by the virus. Timing of the onset of central nervous system manifestations in relationship to the associated disease symptoms and the ability to isolate the virus from cerebrospinal fluid allow differentiation between postinfection and direct invasion encephalitis.

Disease onset may be acute or insidious, and disease severity may be mild to severe depending on the virus and the distribution, location, and concentration of the neuronal lesions. Mumps virus usually produces a more benign disease, whereas herpes encephalitis is frequently fatal. Permanent neurologic sequelae are also more common in herpes infections.

Mosquito-Borne Viral Encephalitis

A variety of viruses capable of infecting animals and birds can be carried to humans by vector mosquitoes that feed on infected animals. The virus, injected into humans from a mosquito bite, rapidly localizes in the central nervous system and produces congestion, edema, and small hemorrhages in the brain. Neuronal lesions with nerve cell necrosis and destruction and foci of cellular infiltration are widespread throughout the brain and spinal cord. Disease severity depends on the virus and on host resistance factors. Generally, older persons are more severely affected and have the highest fatality. Disease onset may be acute or insidious, depending on the virus involved.

An antibody response can be seen within 7 days. Duration of the disease is variable, depending on the virus. The virus cannot be recovered from blood, secretions, or discharges and is therefore not communicable from person to person.

Table 15-7 Overview of Encephalitis

	Infectious Viral Encephalitis	Mosquito-Borne Viral Encephalitides (Equine and St. Louis Encephalitis)	Amebic Meningoencephalitis
Occurrence	Worldwide; epidemic and sporadic; associated with other viral diseases	Warm, moist climates; summer and early fall when mosquitoes are most common	Worldwide, but rare; greatest in young persons, in warm climates, and during summer
Etiologic agent	A variety of viruses, commonly the *Herpesvirus*	A variety of diseases, each caused by a different virus	*Naegleria fowleri; Acanthamoeba culbertsoni*
Reservoir	Humans	Birds, rodents, bats, reptiles, and amphibians; differing for each virus	Amebae that are free-living in water and soil
Transmission	Direct contact with droplets from respiratory passages or other excretions harboring the virus	Bite of infective mosquitoes	Water infected with *N. fowleri* forced into nasal passages while swimming; *Acanthamoeba* enters a skin lesion
Incubation period	Depends on viral disease	5-15 days	3-7 days or longer
Period of communicability	Depends on viral disease	Not communicable person to person; mosquitoes are infective for life	Not communicable person to person
Susceptibility and resistance	Depends on viral disease	Highest susceptibility to clinical disease is infancy and old age; in endemic areas, adults are immune to local strains of virus because of subclinical infections	Unknown; immunosuppressed persons are susceptible to infection with *Acanthamoeba*
Report to local health authority	In select endemic areas	Mandatory case report	Only for means of surveillance

Data from Benenson.[3]

Amebic Meningoencephalitis

Two types of ameba, *Naegleria* and *Acanthamoeba,* are capable of producing meningoencephalitis in humans. *Naegleria* infection is caused when water containing the pathogen is forced into the nasal passages, usually by diving or swimming in water containing large amounts of organic matter. The organism colonizes and invades the mucosa, travels along olfactory nerves to the meninges and brain, and produces a severe and rapidly fatal fulminating pyogenic meningoencephalitis. *Acanthamoeba* colonizes a skin lesion and travels to the central nervous system along peripheral nerves to produce a meningoencephalitis with a more insidious onset and prolonged course. Immunologic investigations have shown many people to have a natural antibody against these organisms, suggesting that more subclinical than clinical infections may occur.

DIAGNOSTIC STUDIES AND FINDINGS[26]

CSF examination: Viral: 50-500/mm^3 leukocytes (predominately lymphocytes), many red blood cells (RBCs), normal glucose, elevated proteins (50 to 150 mg/dl); mosquito-borne: 50 to 500/mm^3 leukocytes (usually lymphocytes), rare to have RBCs; normal to high glucose, elevated protein; amebic: polymorphonuclear leukocytes, RBCs, low to normal glucose, elevated protein

Culture and/or microscopic examination of CSF: All: negative for bacteria; viral: virus can sometimes be isolated; mosquito-borne: virus can sometimes be isolated; amebic: mobile amebae can be visualized by microscopic examination

Serology: Viral and mosquito-borne: fourfold increase in antibody titer between early disease and convalescence.

Examination of biopsied brain tissue: Viral: positive for specific viruses

Hematology (WBC): Mosquito-borne: range from 10,000 to 66,000/mm^3, depending on virus

MULTIDISCIPLINARY PLAN[3]

Medications

Antiinfective Agents

Amebic meningoencephalitis: Combination of the following drugs (individual dose calculation)
- Amphotericin B (Fungizone), IV
- Miconazole (Monistat), IV
- Rifampin (rifamycin, others), PO

Mosquito-borne: No specific treatment

Infectious viral encephalitides: No specific treatment except for herpes infections: acyclovir IV, acyclovir PO, for prophylaxis

General Management

Endotracheal intubation; assisted ventilation; suction; sedatives for hyperexcitability and seizures; IV fluids and electrolytes; nasogastric tube feedings

NURSING CARE

NURSING ASSESSMENT

History

Meningitis: Recent upper respiratory or ear infection; contact with person with rhinitis or meningitis; pneumonia and otitis media frequently precede pneumococcal meningitis; living in crowded condition

Encephalitis: Viral: systemic viral infection; mosquito-borne: exposure to mosquitoes; amebic: swimming and diving in fresh water

Subjective symptoms

Meningitis: Severe throbbing headache, muscle pains, stiff neck, backache, chills, expressions of fear; malaise and irritability in chronic meningococcemia

Encephalitis: Severe frontal headache, nausea and vomiting, dizziness, fever and chills, prostration

Body temperature

Meningitis: 38° to 41° C (100.4° to 106° F), starting in systemic phase; flushed, hot, dry skin; perspiration; intermittent low-grade fever in chronic meningococcemia

Encephalitis: 39° to 41° C (102.2° to 106° F); may be acute-onset fever accompanying CNS symptoms or a 1- to 4-day prodromal period with fever and chills before CNS symptoms

Vital signs

Meningitis: Pulse may be slow as intracranial pressure increases; BP increases with intracranial pressure

Encephalitis: Tachypnea, tachycardia

Level of consciousness

Meningitis: Alert early in disease but may show delirium progressing to deep coma later

Encephalitis: Alterations in consciousness—mild listlessness progressing to confusion, stupor, and eventual coma; may be extremely irritable; bizarre behavior with temporal lobe involvement of herpes encephalitis; seizures

Neurologic status

Meningitis: Reflex changes: absence of abdominal reflexes, absence of cremasteric reflexes in male, alteration of tendon reflexes; resistance to neck flexion; Brudzinski's sign positive (attempted flexion of neck will elicit flexion of knees and hips); Kernig's sign positive (limitation in angle at which a straight leg may be raised with patient supine)

Encephalitis: Focal neurologic signs, aphasia, olfactory hallucinations; nuchal rigidity (if meningeal irritation); weakness, accentuated deep tendon reflexes, extensory plantar response; ataxia, spasticity, tremors; herpes encephalitis: may be a flaccid paralysis and depression of tendon reflexes with spinal cord involvement and bowel and bladder paralysis; postinfectious encephalitis: motor signs may not be manifest

Fluids and electrolytes

Meningitis: Poor skin turgor; decreased urine output

Encephalitis: Excess or deficient urine output

Musculoskeletal status

Meningitis: Chronic meningococcemia: swelling and pain in large joints (especially knees and ankles)

Skin

Meningitis: Meningococcemia: petechial and purpuric lesions preceded by a rash resembling measles on trunk and extremities (recurring with chronic meningococcemia); large ecchymotic lesions on face and extremities in severe disease

Potential Complications

Loss of consciousness, delirium, coma; shock; renal failure; loss of cranial nerve function (blindness, deafness); myocarditis, pericarditis

Bacterial Meningitis
Internal hydrocephalus; cranial nerve function deficits that lead to blindness and deafness; arthritis, myocarditis, pericarditis, and neuromotor and intellectual deficits; adrenal insufficiency

Viral Meningitis
Clinical encephalitis: muscle weakness and malaise during prolonged convalescence

Infectious Encephalitis
Permanent neurologic sequelae are more common in herpes infections

Mosquito-Borne Viral Encephalitis
Motor and mental disabilities (e.g., seizures, hydrocephalus, and mental retardation), more likely in infants and children

Amebic Meningoencephalitis
Severe and rapidly fatal fulminating pyogenic meningoencephalitis

Patient Problems/Nursing Diagnoses & Interventions

NIC Risk Management

Risk for infection related to pathogen in CSF and respiratory secretions

- Administer antiinfective agent as soon as ordered *to prevent complications and decrease risk of transmission of infection.*
- Employ droplet precautions (see Box 15-4, p. 1087) for 24 hours after initiation of antibiotic therapy for bacterial meningitis *to prevent transmission of infection* (in addition to standard precautions [see Box 15-2, p. 1086]).
- Encourage patient contacts to be examined and immunized or treated prophylactically *to prevent further occurrences of infection.*

NIC Neurologic Management

Ineffective cerebral tissue perfusion related to inflammation and edema of brain and meninges

Risk for injury related to altered consciousness

Self-care deficit (bathing/hygiene, dressing/grooming, feeding, toileting) related to CNS alterations

- Continually supervise patient who has convulsions or is delirious; place patient in a room near the nurses' station or arrange for a sitter.
- Pad bed and provide restraints for delirious patients; keep side rails up; prevent aspiration or injury during convulsions.
- Monitor vital signs and neurologic findings every 5 to 30 minutes for patient with increased intracranial pressure; report changes to physician immediately.
- Monitor patient carefully, particularly after lumbar puncture.
- Have patient lie flat for 4 to 6 hours or as ordered after lumbar puncture *to prevent headache associated with alterations in CSF pressure.*
- Monitor for signs of increased intracranial pressure throughout course of disease (e.g., slowing of pulse, in-

creased blood pressure [BP], altered consciousness, arrhythmic breathing, altered pupillary response, and facial weakness); report changes to physician immediately.
- Administer hypertonic agents or steroids, as prescribed, *to lower intracranial pressure.*
- Provide bed rest and limit unnecessary movement of patient.
- Instruct patient to exhale while turning or moving in bed.
- Elevate patient's head slightly; prevent unnecessary movements of head and neck; avoid neck flexion that increases intracranial pressure; use log roll to turn patient.
- Position patient to avoid knee or hip flexion *to prevent muscle straining that could increase intracranial pressure.*
- Assist patient with all activities and movements; provide all feedings and hygiene measures *to conserve the patient's energy.*
- Maintain indwelling catheter *to empty bladder of unconscious patient.*
- Administer stool softeners as prescribed (avoid enemas) *to reduce straining.*
- Maintain quiet environment *because excessive stimuli may induce seizures.*
- Time nursing procedures so as to provide periods of relaxation and/or sedation; avoid unnecessary stimuli *to prevent excitation and possible seizures.*
- Provide clear, concise explanations to a confused patient; interpret environment to patient to orient him or her; put calendars in the room and provide other cues *to lessen disorientation and to clarify impaired sensory perceptions.*
- Evaluate patient during convalescence for motor, sensory, and intellectual impairment *to refer for rehabilitation.*

NIC Electrolyte and Acid-Base Management

Risk for deficient fluid volume related to fever and vomiting
Risk for excess fluid volume related to excess secretion of antidiuretic hormone (ADH)
- Monitor intake and output, urine specific gravity, serum electrolytes, and weight.
- Monitor BP for decrease associated with bleeding.
- Administer frequent oral or continuous IV fluids *to prevent dehydration.* (Administer IV fluids carefully to prevent overload if fluid retention is likely.)
- Limit IV fluids to two thirds of needs if signs of fluid retention occur.
- Administer osmotic agents as prescribed *to decrease fluid overload.*

NIC Respiratory Management

Ineffective breathing pattern related to altered consciousness
Ineffective airway clearance related to neuromuscular dysfunction
- Monitor depth and rate of respirations, breath sounds, and blood gas levels *to detect altered oxygenation.*
- Support breathing with oxygen and/or mechanical ventilation, as necessary.
- Maintain patent airway; oxygenate before suctioning; limit suctioning to 10 to 15 seconds for apneic patients; perform endotracheal care.

NIC Thermoregulation

Hyperthermia related to infection
- Carefully monitor body temperature and intervene accordingly.
- Administer antipyretics, as ordered.
- Bathe with tepid water or alcohol *to reduce high fever.*
- Adjust room temperature *to facilitate body heat loss.*
- Remove excess clothing and bedding *to ensure body heat loss.*
- Encourage adequate fluid intake or administer IV fluids *to compensate for fluid loss associated with elevated body temperature.*
- Encourage adequate nutritional intake *to compensate for increased metabolic needs associated with fever.*

NIC Tissue Perfusion Management

Ineffective peripheral tissue perfusion related to interruption of altered venous flow
- Monitor peripheral circulation, pulses, purpura *to detect signs of increased vascular permeability.*
- For patients with no signs of elevated intracranial pressure, frequently change position and administer range-of-motion exercises *to stimulate peripheral circulation and to prevent contractures and pressure ulcers.*

NIC Physical Comfort Promotion

Acute pain related to inflammation of meninges and brain
- Administer analgesics as prescribed. (Do not give narcotics or sedatives that will depress vital functions of patients with increased intracranial pressure.)
- Place blanket roll under knees (in absence of elevated intracranial pressure) *to relieve pain in back.*
- Darken room and provide ice pack for head *to relieve headache.*

NIC Psychologic Comfort Promotion

Fear related to understanding of severity of condition
- Allow patient and significant others to verbalize fears.
- Instruct patient and family regarding disease course, diagnostic procedures, and treatments. Inform patient that symptoms are temporary and recovery is usually complete *to relieve fear of unknown.*

Patient Education/Continuum of Care Plan[25]

1. Inform patient of diagnostic procedures that may be performed.
   a. Neurologic assessment and eye examination
   b. Cultures of blood, CSF, and respiratory secretions to identify causative organism
   c. Serologic tests of blood to identify viral antibodies
   d. Lumbar puncture to obtain spinal fluid for analysis

2. Instruct the patient to lie flat for 24 hours following lumbar puncture and to report change in symptoms.
3. Explain purposes of antibiotic therapy to patients receiving antibiotic therapy. Discuss dosage, time, rationale, route of administration, and side effects for each prescribed drug. Antiinfective therapy for bacterial meningitis must be continued as prescribed for 5 days after temperature returns to normal. Exacerbation of symptoms should be reported to physician immediately.
4. Instruct patients who have positive sputum cultures about respiratory isolation procedures.
5. Explain to patient and family that convalescence is of variable duration, depending on severity of disease. Patients should allow adequate time for recovery before resuming full activities. Exacerbation of symptoms should be reported to physician immediately.
6. Recovery is usually complete in meningitis; however, neurologic sequelae do occur. Patient should be evaluated during convalescence for functional and neurologic deficits and should participate in rehabilitation if prescribed.
7. Sequelae of encephalitis include mental deterioration, paralysis, and possible convulsive disorders, particularly in children. Families should be informed of the need for periodic evaluation and long-term physical therapy and of potential resources to help them cope with a handicapped family member.
8. Prophylactic measures should be initiated for close patient contacts. Patient contacts should be evaluated medically for early detection and treatment of bacterial meningitis.
9. Amebic meningoencephalitis can be prevented by swimming in chlorinated pools only. Mosquito-borne encephalitis can be prevented by environmental control of mosquitoes, particularly through elimination of stagnant pools of water (where mosquitoes breed), and by wearing protective clothing, screening living quarters, and using repellents.

Evaluation/Patient Outcomes

Risk Management: Patient is free of infection and complications of meningitis and encephalitis; CSF findings: less than 30 cells per cubic millimeter; glucose, protein, and pressures are normal; color is clear; CSF and blood cultures are negative for bacteria.

Infection is not transmitted to patient contacts, including hospital personnel.

Neurologic Management: Neurologic signs are normal; pupils are equal and reactive to light; neck flexion is unimpaired; straight legs may be raised from the bed from a prone position; reflexes are normal.

Patient is alert, responds appropriately to questions and environmental stimuli, is oriented to person, place, and time and has memory of recent and past events.

Affect is appropriate to environmental stimuli.

Cognition, ability to problem solve, and concentration are intact.

Seizures have been avoided, or no injury has resulted from seizures.

Patient is able to walk and perform all functions without residual weakness or impairment.

Patient with residual limitation in physical or mental function has been referred for appropriate therapy during convalescence.

Electrolyte and Acid-Base Management: Patient shows no excessive thirst or weight loss.

Serum electrolyte levels are within normal limits.

Fluid intake and output are balanced.

Skin turgor is good.

Urine specific gravity is within normal limits (1.01 to 1.025).

Respiratory Management: Breathing patterns are normal.

Blood gas levels (O_2 saturation, CO_2, and Po_2) are normal.

Aspiration and pneumonia have been avoided.

Thermoregulation: Body temperature is maintained within normal range (35.8° to 37.3° C).

Flushing, chills, and seizures are absent.

Tissue Perfusion Management: Vital signs are within normal limits; shock has been avoided.

Skin is warm and normal color.

No petechiae or purpura are present.

Physical Comfort Promotion: Patient is free of pain; alternates periods of activity and rest; sleeps 3 to 4 hours at a time.

Psychologic Comfort: Fear of disease and disability is reduced; patient is able to sleep.

Patient and significant others trust care providers, are participating in treatment, and have realistic expectations of recovery.

Family of a disabled person has been given an opportunity to express concerns and has been referred for counseling and/or to a support group.

VACCINE PREVENTABLE INFECTIOUS DISEASES

The infectious diseases presented in this section are preventable with routine immunization. An overview of all of the diseases is presented in Table 15-8 on pp. 1016-1017.

Chickenpox

Chickenpox (varicella) is an acute, highly communicable viral disease common in childhood and young adulthood. It is characterized by a sudden-onset fever, mild malaise, and a skin eruption that is maculopapular for a few hours and vesicular for 3 to 4 days, leaving a granular scab.

Pathophysiology

The varicella-zoster (V-Z) virus, a herpesvirus, enters the body by way of the respiratory mucous membranes and produces systemic disease and skin lesions. The lesions are generally superficial unilocular vesicles. Lesions generally occur in successive crops with several stages of maturity present at one time. They are generally more abundant on covered areas of the body; however, they may appear everywhere, including the scalp, conjunctivae, and upper respiratory tract.

Lesions have been found in the lungs, liver, spleen, adrenal glands, and pancreas. Disease is severe in those with deficiencies in cell-mediated immunity. After recovery the virus is believed to remain in the body in an asymptomatic latent stage, possibly localized in the dorsal root ganglia.

Reactivation of the infection with the V-Z virus can occur later in life or during time of altered immune status. It leads to the disease manifestation of herpes zoster, in which there is a localized eruption of grouped vesicles on an erythematous base. The vesicles are restricted to the skin areas supplied by sensory nerves of a single or associated group of dorsal root ganglia.

Diagnostic Studies and Findings

Microscopic examinations of specimen of vesicular fluid: Visualization of V-Z virus during first 3 days after eruption

Giemsa-stained scrapings from lesions: Multinucleated giant cells are visualized

Multidisciplinary Plan[3]

Medications

Acyclovir (Zovirax) or vidarabine (ara-A) may be helpful for immunocompromised or older persons if administered early in the disease

Varicella vaccine within 96 h of exposure

Varicella vaccine for prevention (see Immunizations, p. 1076)

General Management

Relief of pruritus; management of fever; treatment of complications; encephalitis (see p. 1010), viral pneumonia (see Chapter 4)

NURSING CARE

Nursing Assessment

History: Exposure within past 2 to 3 weeks to person with chickenpox

Subjective symptoms: Headache, anorexia, malaise, chills

Body temperature: Fever: 38° to 39° C (100.4° to 103° F) during prodrome

Respiratory status: Coryza during prodrome

Skin and mucous membranes: Lesions in various stages of development; may have lesions on buccal mucosa, palate, or conjunctivae

Potential Complications

Secondary infections; pneumonia; conjunctival ulcers; encephalitis, meningitis; Guillain-Barré syndrome; Reye's syndrome

Patient Problems/Nursing Diagnoses & Interventions

NIC Risk Management

Risk for infection (patient contacts) related to virus in respiratory secretions and in skin lesions.

- Observe airborne and contact precautions until all lesions have crusted (see Boxes 15-3 and 15-5, p. 1087).
- Refer high-risk patient to physician for prophylactic treatment with varicella-zoster immune globulin *to lessen risk for infection.*

NIC Skin/Wound Management

Impaired skin integrity related to lesions

- Bathe or encourage patient to bathe regularly *to remove exudate.*
- Apply calamine lotion or cornstarch *to relieve itching.*
- Caution patient against scratching lesions *to prevent spread of exudate and potential scarring and introduction of bacteria into lesions.*

NIC Thermoregulation

Hyperthermia related to infection

- Monitor body temperature *to detect fever.*
- Administer antipyretics, as ordered.
- Bathe with tepid water or alcohol *to reduce high fever.*
- Adjust environmental temperature *for patient's comfort.*
- Remove excess clothing and bedding *to ensure heat loss.*
- Encourage adequate fluid intake or administer IV fluids *to compensate for fluid loss associated with elevated body temperature.*

Patient Education/Continuum of Care Plan[25]

1. Chickenpox is usually a benign condition with complete recovery. However, complications do occur. Report to physician any symptoms appearing during convalescence, such as a secondary rise in fever, headache, or respiratory or neurologic symptoms.
2. Chickenpox is communicable 1 to 2 days before onset of rash until lesions have crusted over. The disease is transmitted by droplets of respiratory secretions. Incubation period is 2 to 3 weeks.
3. Avoid trauma or scratching of lesions to prevent secondary infection and scars. Daily bathing without irritating soaps is encouraged.
4. Manage fever by taking antipyretic agents and tepid sponge baths, wearing minimal clothing, and maintaining a cool environment. Avoid giving children aspirin because it has been implicated in Reye's syndrome.
5. Manage itching with applications of calamine lotion or cornstarch. Avoid greasy lotions and creams. Maintain a cool environment to relieve itching associated with perspiration.
6. Encourage intake of foods and fluids as tolerated. Popsicles and soft drinks may appeal to young children.
7. Immunocompromised patient contacts should be referred to a physician for prophylactic treatment with varicella-zoster immune globulin.

Evaluation/Patient Outcomes

Risk Management: Infection has not been transmitted. Patient contacts and health personnel have not acquired chickenpox. Immunocompromised patient contacts have received varicella-zoster immune globulin.

Table 15-8 Overview of Vaccine-Preventable Infectious Diseases

	Chickenpox	Diphtheria	Mumps (Infectious Parotitis)	Pertussis (Whooping Cough)
Occurrence	Worldwide; in metropolitan areas 90% of the population has had chickenpox by age 15 years, and 95% by young adulthood	Formerly a prevalent disease; rare in United States with immunization; affects unimmunized children under 15 years and adults	Occurs commonly in winter and spring; one third of those exposed have subclinical infections; incidence decreasing with immunization	Common in children; worldwide; decline in incidence in areas with active immunization programs; cases increasing in United States in recent years in adults
Etiologic agent	Varicella-zoster (V-Z) virus, a member of the herpesvirus group	*Corynebacterium diphtheriae,* with many toxigenic strains	A type of paramyxovirus; antigenically related to parainfluenza viruses	*Bordetella pertussis,* the pertussis bacillus
Reservoir	Humans	Humans	Humans	Humans
Transmission	Direct and indirect contact with droplets from respiratory passages; an extremely contagious disease	Direct or indirect contact with exudate from mucous membrane lesions of infected persons or carrier; raw milk may also be a vehicle	Direct contact with saliva droplets from infected person	Direct contact with droplets from respiratory passages
Incubation period	2-3 weeks; commonly 13-17 days	2-5 days; occasionally longer	12-25 days; commonly 18 days	6-20 days; commonly 7 days
Period of communicability	1-2 days before onset of rash and until lesions have crusted over (not more than 6 days after first appearance of vesicles)	Variable; until bacilli have disappeared from discharges and lesions (usually in 2 weeks); a carrier may shed bacilli for 6 months	6 days before parotid symptoms to 9 days after; most communicable 48 hours before parotid swelling	7 days after exposure to 3 weeks after onset; highly communicable in early catarrhal stage before cough; not communicable after 3 weeks for nonhousehold contacts even though cough may persist
Susceptibility and resistance	General; one attack confers long immunity; second attacks are rare; recurs as herpes zoster	Unimmunized children most susceptible; infants born of immune mothers have passive immunity for 6 months; recovery from clinical disease confers temporary immunity	General; immunity is lifelong and develops after clinical and subclinical disease; placental transfer of antibodies occurs	General; nonimmunized children under 5 years most susceptible; no passive immunity from mother; attack confers prolonged, but not lifetime immunity
Report to local health authority	Case report required in most states	Case report required	Case report required in some areas	Case report required

Data from Benenson.[3]

Skin/Wound Management: Patient is free of secondary bacterial infection of skin and mucous membranes; skin is free of lesions and scars. Crusts are shed. Skin is warm and moist, and natural color returns to skin and mucous membranes. Patient is not observed scratching lesions.

Thermoregulation: Body temperature is maintained within normal limits; comfort and safety are maintained. Body temperature is between 36° and 38° C (96.8° and 100.4° F) oral. Pulse and respirations are within normal limits. Skin is cool to touch and free of excess perspiration; patient's clothing and bedding are dry. Patient is free of headache and malaise associated with fever. Reye's syndrome is prevented.

DIPHTHERIA

Diphtheria is an acute communicable disease in which a bacterial toxin affects the mucous membranes of the respiratory tract. The disease is manifest as fibrinopurulent exudative membranes, commonly on the tonsils and pharynx but also on the larynx, nasal passages, skin, conjunctivae, and genitalia, and as systemic symptoms resulting from toxin dissemination.

PATHOPHYSIOLOGY

Corynebacterium diphtheriae, widely available in the nasopharynx of carriers and persons with inapparent infection, in-

Poliomyelitis	Rubella (German Measles)	Measles (Rubeola)	Tetanus
Worldwide; commonly in summer and early autumn; highest in children and adolescents but does affect nonimmune adults; U.S. incidence rare with immunization	Worldwide and endemic; most common in winter and spring; primarily a disease of children but does occur in unimmunized adolescents and adults	Worldwide; endemic and epidemic occurrences; seen more in adolescents and adults since routine immunization of children	Worldwide; occurs sporadically and affects all ages; rare in United States with immunization; common among agricultural workers, parenteral drug abusers, and elderly
Poliovirus, types 1, 2, and 3; all are paralytogenic	Rubella virus	Measles virus, a type of paramyxovirus	*Clostridium tetani,* the tetanus bacillus (an anaerobic pathogen)
Humans, particularly children with subclinical infections	Humans	Humans	Intestines of humans and animals
Direct and indirect contact with respiratory discharges and feces; fecal-oral route more common than respiratory transmission	Direct or indirect contact with nasopharyngeal secretions of infected persons; transplacental transmission leads to congenital rubella syndrome	Direct or indirect contact with nasal secretions from infected persons; highly communicable	Tetanus spores enter body through a wound (usually puncture wound) contaminated with soil and feces; necrotic tissue favors the growth of the anaerobic bacillus
3-35 days: commonly 7-14 days	14-23 days: commonly 16-18 days	Commonly 10 days; 7-18 days until fever; 14 days until rash	3-21 days; commonly 10 days
Highly communicable during first days after onset of symptoms; virus is in throat secretions in 36 hours and in feces in 72 hours after infection and remains 1 week in throat and 6 weeks in feces	From 1 week before and 4 days after appearance of rash; highly communicable; infants with congenital rubella syndrome may shed virus for months after birth	A few days before fever to 4 days after appearance of rash	Not directly transmitted
General; paralytic infections are rare and risk increases with age; infection confers long-term immunity; second attacks are result of another virus type	General; infants born with passive immunity from mother lasting 6-9 months; one attack confers lifetime immunity for most, but reinfections (mostly asymptomatic) have been documented	General; acquired immunity from infection is permanent; artificial active immunity may not be permanent; infants born to mothers with antibodies retain immunity for 6-9 months	General; recovery from tetanus does not confer permanent immunity; temporary active immunity provided by tetanus toxoid
Case report required	Case report required	Case report required in most states	Case report required

vades and multiplies in the nasopharynx of susceptible persons. The pathogen produces a toxin that is disseminated by the blood and lymph throughout the body. The toxin first causes necrosis of the local tissue, resulting in a fibrinopurulent exudative membrane characteristic of this disease. The membrane appears as grayish membrane patches surrounded by a red zone of inflammation on the tonsils, pharynx, larynx, nasal mucosa, or skin. Edema is present in adjacent and underlying tissue and in the cervical lymph nodes. Laryngeal edema and the extension of the membrane into the trachea, bronchial tree, and alveoli may result in suffocation. Nasopharyngeal diphtheria and laryngeal diphtheria are the most severe types. Nasal diphtheria is mild and marked by one-sided nasal excoriations and discharge. Cutaneous diphtheria lesions are variable and may resemble impetigo.

Disseminated toxin inhibits protein synthesis primarily in the heart, peripheral nerves, and muscle tissue. Effects of toxin absorption appear early and include fatty degeneration, edema, and interstitial fibrosis in the myocardium and in the myelin sheath of peripheral nerves. Damage to peripheral nerves results in peripheral motor and sensory palsies. The spleen and kidneys also may be affected.

Potential Complications

Otitis media; peritonsillar abscess; peripheral motor or sensory paralysis; toxemia; myocarditis; pharyngeal or respiratory paralysis; pneumonia; diphtheria is completely preventable with active immunization (see p. 1077).

No care plan is provided here because the disease is so rare today.

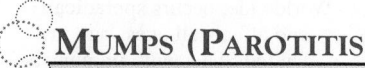

MUMPS (PAROTITIS)

Mumps (parotitis) is an acute, communicable systemic viral disease characterized by localized unilateral or bilateral edema of one or more of the salivary glands, with occasional involvement of other glands.

PATHOPHYSIOLOGY

The paramyxovirus invades and multiplies in the parotid gland or the superficial epithelium of the upper respiratory passages, enters the blood, and subsequently localizes in glandular or nervous tissue. Interstitial tissue edema and infiltration with lymphocytes occur in the affected gland. Cells of the glandular ducts degenerate, producing an accumulation of necrotic debris, resulting in plugging of the ducts or tubules. The parotid and testes are the glands most frequently involved, but mumps may also affect the pancreas, other salivary glands, ovaries, breast, and thyroid. Testicular atrophy follows mumps orchitis, but sterility is rare. The intensity of symptoms in mumps is variable; at least 30% of infections are asymptomatic. Elevated cerebrospinal fluid protein concentrations are common even in the absence of clinical symptoms of meningoencephalitis. Glucose levels may be depressed.

DIAGNOSTIC STUDIES AND FINDINGS[26]

Culture of specimen of saliva or urine: Saliva positive for virus up to 9 days after onset of infection; in urine up to 2 weeks after infection onset

Serology: Fourfold increase in antibody titer between acute and convalescent stages

MULTIDISCIPLINARY PLAN

Medications

Steroids for treatment of orchitis
Analgesics for pain
Active immunization for prevention (see p. 1077)

General Management

Relief of pain with heat or cold applications; fluid diet until patient tolerates solid food; support of scrotum

NURSING CARE

NURSING ASSESSMENT

History: Inadequate immunization for mumps; exposure within 2 to 3 weeks to person with mumps

Subjective symptoms: Feeling hot or chilled; headache; pain in parotid glands, testes, or other glands (tender to touch); parotid pain is aggravated by eating

Body temperature: 38° to 39° C (100.4° to 102.2° F) for 3 to 4 days; higher if orchitis is present

Head and neck: Variable parotid swelling lasting up to 1 week; severe parotid pain aggravated by eating, particularly sour substances; parotid gland (or other glands) tender to touch; hooked lobe of parotid gland (extending under earlobe) can be palpated

Testes: Swollen and tender to touch; patient has severe pain

Breast: Inflammation and pain associated with mastitis

Abdomen: Pain from pancreatitis or oophoritis

POTENTIAL COMPLICATIONS

Signs of meningitis or encephalitis; pericarditis

PATIENT PROBLEMS/NURSING DIAGNOSES & INTERVENTIONS

NIC RISK MANAGEMENT

Risk for infection (patient) related to inadequate secondary deafness

Risk for infection (patient contacts) related to virus in saliva

- Monitor for signs indicating complications of mumps. Refer to physician *for early diagnosis and medical management.*
- If patient is hospitalized, employ droplet precautions (Box 15-4, p. 1087) for 9 days after onset of swelling *to prevent transmission to others.*
- Ensure that patient contacts are immunized for mumps.

NIC PHYSICAL COMFORT PROMOTION

Acute pain related to glandular edema

- Administer analgesics, as prescribed, *to relieve pain.*
- Give liquid or soft diet, as prescribed, *to minimize pain with swallowing.* Allow patient to drink from a straw *to minimize mouth movement, which is painful.*
- Apply warm or cold compresses, whichever is more comfortable to patient, *to relieve pain.*
- Support scrotum with small pillow or an adhesive tape bridge between the thighs (or nest of cotton for infant) *to relieve pressure on testes.*

NIC THERMOREGULATION

Hyperthermia related to infection

Anxiety related to fear of sterility

- Monitor body temperature *to detect fever.*
- Administer antipyretics, as ordered.
- Bathe patient with tepid water or alcohol *to reduce high fever.*
- Adjust environmental temperature *for patient's comfort.*
- Remove excess clothing and bedding *to ensure heat loss.*
- Encourage adequate fluid intake *to compensate for fluid loss associated with elevated body temperature.*
- Inform patient that testicular atrophy does not result in impotence and that sterility is extremely rare *to allay anxiety regarding effects of orchitis.*

PATIENT EDUCATION/CONTINUUM OF CARE PLAN[25]

1. Mumps is transmitted by direct contact with saliva of infected persons. It is communicable from 6 days before parotid swelling to 9 days after. Disease onset is between 2 and 3 weeks after exposure to infection.
2. Transmission of the infection to others can be prevented by hand washing and avoiding contact with respiratory secretions.
3. Mumps can be prevented by active immunization.
4. Manage fever with antipyretics, tepid sponge baths, minimal clothing, and a cool environment. Avoid chilling. Avoid giving children aspirin. Encourage intake of fluids and food as tolerated. Popsicles and soft drinks may appeal to young children.
5. Manage other symptoms with analgesics for pain, soft bland foods and liquid diet, scrotal support for testicular pain, and local application of warm or cold compresses.
6. Report the following complications to physician: headache, photophobia, hearing disturbance, stiff neck, joint pain, kidney pain, convulsions, or disturbance in gait.
7. Contacts should be referred to a physician for active immunization.
8. Convalescence is usually complete with no residual disability; testicular atrophy does not result in impotence, and sterility is extremely rare.

EVALUATION/PATIENT OUTCOMES

Risk Management: Patient is free of infection and complications of mumps. There are no signs of glandular edema or pain. Body temperature is normal. There are no signs of complications.

Infection is not transmitted to patient contacts. Appropriate isolation procedures are implemented on hospitalized patients soon after infection is confirmed. Patient demonstrates behavior to prevent transmission of pathogens to others. Patient's contacts are adequately immunized for mumps.

Physical Comfort Promotion: Patient obtains relief from pain. Facial expression is calm and relaxed. Posture is normal. Muscles are relaxed when patient is resting and motionless. There is no pain in any glandular area. Patient has not developed distress mannerisms. Oral intake is adequate.

Thermoregulation: Body temperature is maintained within normal range; comfort and safety are maintained. Body temperature is between 36° and 38° C (96.8° to 100.4° F). Pulse and respiration are normal. Skin is cool to touch and free of excess perspiration. Patient's clothing and bedding are dry. Patient is free of headache and malaise associated with fever.

PERTUSSIS (WHOOPING COUGH)

Pertussis (whooping cough) is an acute communicable bacterial infection of the mucous membranes of the tracheobronchial tree, characterized by paroxysms of repeated and violent coughing. Paroxysms are terminated by a prolonged, high-pitched inspiratory whoop and the expulsion of clear, tenacious mucus. This disease is most severe in children under 1 year of age.

PATHOPHYSIOLOGY

The toxigenic *Bordetella pertussis* bacillus enters the respiratory passages by airborne droplets of respiratory secretions from persons with asymptomatic infections or with clinical disease. The organism reproduces in the mucous membranes of the trachea, bronchi, and bronchioles, producing a toxin that causes necrosis to the ciliated mucosa. There are three stages of the disease: catarrhal, paroxysmal, and convalescent. A serous exudate is produced initially in the catarrhal stage, lasting 1 to 2 weeks. This is followed by a viscid mucopurulent exudate that is irritating to the mucosa. The exudate, which is difficult to expel, initiates severe spasmodic coughing (paroxysms), frequently followed by vomiting, that may persist for 1 to 2 months. Coughing may also be initiated by toxin stimulation to the central nervous system.

Local necrosis of the tracheal and bronchial epithelium is extensive, with an inflammatory infiltrate. Unexpelled mucous plugs may produce areas of atelectasis and emphysema. Paratracheal and bronchial lymphadenopathy may be present. Edema, congestion, and hemorrhage may occur in lung tissue, and edema and petechial hemorrhages are commonly found in brain tissue. These pathologic findings result from anoxia during the prolonged paroxysms of coughing. Paroxysms may also result in complications resulting from increased intraabdominal and intraocular pressure during paroxysms.

The convalescent stage is characterized by a cessation of whooping and vomiting with a gradual decrease in the number of paroxysms over a 2- to 3-week period. Some patients develop exacerbations of paroxysms of cough, whooping, and vomiting during subsequent respiratory infections.

DIAGNOSTIC STUDIES AND FINDINGS

Microscopic examination of stained nasopharyngeal secretions during catarrhal stage: Positive for *B. pertussis*
WBC count: Leukocytes: 15,000 to 40,000/mm^3; may be as high as 175,000 to 200,000/mm^3
Differential WBC count: 90% lymphocytes

MULTIDISCIPLINARY PLAN[3]

Medications

Antiinfective agents: Shorten the period of communicability but do not reduce symptoms unless given in incubation period; erythromycin (Erythrocin)
Corticosteroids: Hydrocortisone sodium succinate (Solu-Cortef)
Active immunization: for prevention for those under 7 years of age (see p. 1077)
Prophylaxis for case contacts: Erythromycin for 14 days

General Management

Suction of respiratory secretions; ventilatory assistance, if needed; oxygen administration; parenteral fluid and electrolyte therapy; small, frequent feedings; postural drainage following paroxysms

NURSING CARE

Nursing Assessment

History: Inadequate immunization for pertussis; exposure to pertussis during past 3 weeks

Respiratory status

- Catarrhal stage: Normal respirations: dry, hacking cough
- Paroxysmal stage (after 1 or 2 weeks): paroxysms of cough (40 to 50 per 24 hours in severe cases), followed by high-pitched inspiratory whoop; vomiting frequently follows paroxysm
- Convalescent stage: Paroxysms and vomiting become gradually less frequent and prolonged

Mucous membranes

- Catarrhal stage: Serous rhinorrhea, sneezing, lacrimation, conjunctivitis
- Paroxysmal stage: Tenacious mucus; epistaxis

Skin: Color may be cyanotic following paroxysms; loss of turgor because of dehydration

Body temperature: Normal or low-grade fever; elevated in secondary infection

Activity patterns: Exhaustion following paroxysms

Potential Complications

Venous engorgement of face and neck during paroxysms; scleral hemorrhages and periorbital edema may be present; anoxic convulsions; umbilical or inguinal hernia complications; rectal prolapse; secondary bacterial infection (otitis media, pneumonia)

Patient Problems/Nursing Diagnoses & Interventions

NIC Risk Management

Risk for infection (patient) related to inadequate secondary defenses

Risk for infection (patient contacts) related to pathogen in respiratory secretions

- Collect nasopharyngeal specimen for examination. *Incorrect collection and handling of specimens may destroy the pathogen or contaminate the specimen with environmental organisms, interfering with accurate diagnosis and treatment. Improper handling can also contaminate the health-care worker.*
- Administer antiinfective agents as soon as prescribed *to prevent severe disease and death.*
- Monitor temperature and respiratory status *to detect signs of secondary infection for early treatment.*
- Employ droplet precautions for 5 days after onset of antimicrobial therapy (see Box 15-4, p. 1087) *to prevent transmission to health-care workers, other patients, and patient contacts.*
- Refer patient contacts to physician to ensure that they are examined, treated, and immunized.
- Ensure that case of pertussis is reported to local health authority.

NIC Respiratory Management

Ineffective airway clearance related to tenacity of mucus

Ineffective breathing pattern related to coughing spasms

- Place infant on lap with infant's head down during paroxysms *to drain secretions.*
- Suction pooled secretions if necessary *to maintain patent airway.*
- Provide moist air *to liquify secretions.*
- Assess patient's skin color and behavior *to detect symptoms of anoxia.*
- Provide oxygen by mask *to restore breathing after paroxysms.*
- Assist respiration, if necessary, *to maintain oxygen.*
- Monitor breathing for signs of atelectasis or pneumonia *to report to physician for intervention.*

NIC Electrolyte and Acid-Base Management

Risk for deficient fluid volume related to severe vomiting and inability to swallow

- Assess skin turgor and urinary output *for signs of dehydration.*
- Give frequent, small liquid feedings or parenteral fluids if vomiting is excessive *to maintain adequate fluids and electrolytes.*

NIC Thermoregulation

Hyperthermia related to infection

- Monitor patient's body temperature *to detect fever.*
- Administer antipyretics, as ordered.
- Bathe patient with tepid water or alcohol *to reduce high fever.*
- Adjust environmental temperature *for patient's comfort.*
- Remove excess clothing and bedding *to ensure heat loss.*
- Encourage adequate fluid intake *to compensate for fluid loss associated with elevated body temperature.*

Patient Education/Continuum of Care Plan[25]

1. Pertussis is transmitted by direct contact with droplets from respiratory passages. It is communicable from 7 days after exposure to 3 weeks after disease onset (highly communicable during early catarrhal stage). Disease onset is between 7 and 12 days from exposure to the infection.
2. Transmission of the infection to others can be prevented by hand washing, avoiding inhalation of respiratory secretions, and disinfecting items contaminated with respiratory secretions.
3. Pertussis can be prevented by active immunization.
4. Manage fever with antipyretics, tepid sponge baths, minimal clothing, and a cool environment. Avoid chilling. Avoid giving children aspirin. Encourage intake of fluids and food, as tolerated. Popsicles and soft drinks may appeal to young children.
5. Manage other symptoms: moist air in environment, frequent liquids and soft foods, and bed rest.
6. Report the following symptoms of complications to physician: convulsions, rise in fever, recurrence of respiratory symptoms, whooping, or vomiting.
7. Contacts should be referred to a physician for early diagnosis, treatment, and prophylaxis, with a booster dose of pertussis vaccine.
8. Convalescence is slow, with gradual cessation of whooping and vomiting over a 2- to 3-week period. Subsequent respiratory infections predispose to recurrence of symptoms.

Evaluation/Patient Outcomes

Risk Management: Patient is free of infection and complications of pertussis. Blood leukocyte count is normal. Bacterial culture is negative. Breathing patterns are normal. Body temperature is normal.

Infection is not transmitted. Patient contacts are free of infection. Children are immunized for pertussis. Infection is reported to local health department.

Patient does not experience injury. Patient experiences no injury associated with seizures.

Respiratory Management: Airway is patent and aspiration of secretions is avoided. Patient does not aspirate secretions during paroxysms of coughing and returns to normal coughing and breathing patterns during convalescence.

Patient demonstrates normal respiratory pattern, oxygen intake, and blood gas levels. Skin, nails, lips, and earlobes are warm, with natural color. Breathing pattern, rhythm, rate, and depth are regular. Oxygen saturation, carbon dioxide, Po_2, and Pco_2 are normal.

Electrolyte and Acid-Base Management: Skin turgor is good. Secretions are thin. Urine output equals intake. Urine specific gravity is normal.

Thermoregulation: Body temperature is maintained within normal range; comfort and safety are maintained.

Body temperature is between 36° and 38° C (96.8° to 100.4° F). Pulse and respiration are normal. Skin is cool to touch and free of excess perspiration. Patient's clothing and bedding are dry. Patient is free of headache and malaise associated with fever.

Poliomyelitis

Poliomyelitis is an acute communicable systemic viral disease affecting the central nervous system with variable severity ranging from subclinical infection, to a nonfebrile illness, to an aseptic meningitis, to paralytic disease, and possibly to death.

Pathophysiology

Three immunologically distinct polioviruses produce poliomyelitis, an infection that occurs 100 times more frequently in a subclinical form than in clinical disease. The polioviruses are all enteroviruses; that is, they multiply in the intestinal tract and can be recovered from the feces of cases and subclinical cases. Transmission of the virus is primarily by the fecal-oral route and sometimes by direct contact with respiratory secretions.

Once in a susceptible host, the virus multiplies in the lymphoid tissue of the throat and ileum, producing follicular necrosis. A transient viremia follows with subsequent viral invasion of the central nervous system, producing cell damage primarily in the anterior horn cells of the spinal cord, in the medulla and pons, in the midbrain, and in the motor area of the precentral gyrus. Damage may be reversible at this point, with complete recovery, or it may progress to necrosis and phagocytosis of the neurons, resulting in clinical disease concomitant with the extent and concentration of neuron destruction.

Clinical paralysis results when there is extensive damage to motor neurons associated with any one functional motor group. Skeletal muscle fiber groups atrophy rapidly from absence of innervation from associated destroyed motor neurons. Paralysis is characteristically asymmetric, involving the lower extremities and muscles of respiration and swallowing.

Clinical poliomyelitis may be seen in three phases: a systemic stage, a phase of central nervous system involvement, and the paralytic stage. The onset of the systemic phase is acute, with low-grade fever, headache, nausea, abdominal tenderness, occasional vomiting, and the presence of a mild tonsillitis or pharyngitis. These symptoms subside within 24 to 36 hours, and the infectious process is terminated for about 80% of patients.

Within 1 to 4 days, a small percentage of patients manifest signs of the second phase with a higher fever, frontal headache, vomiting, strained anxious expression on the face, dermal hypersensitivity, and hyperhidrosis, particularly around the head and neck. The symptoms may end here or progress to the paralytic stage, with nuchal and spinal stiffness from spasm of back and hamstring muscles, positive spinal fluid findings, hypertension, and paralysis.

Paralysis may affect different parts of the body depending on the area of central nervous system damage, giving rise to the differentiation of types of paralysis as spinal, spinobulbar, bulbar, ataxic, encephalitic, or meningitic. Complications are associated with the areas of muscle paralysis or weakness and the effect on body functioning.

Potential Complications

Motor paralysis, including respiratory, oral, facial, ocular, and urinary bladder paralysis

Poliomyelitis is completely preventable with active immunization (p. 1077). No care plan is provided here because of the rareness of this disease.

Rubella (German Measles)

Rubella (German measles) is a mild, febrile, highly communicable viral disease characterized by a diffuse punctate macular rash. Symptoms in the prodromal period include low-grade fever, coryza, malaise, headache, lymphadenopathy, and conjunctivitis. Infection during the first trimester of pregnancy may lead to infection in the fetus and may produce a variety of congenital anomalies: the congenital rubella syndrome.

Pathophysiology

Rubella is a usually mild disease caused by a specific virus that invades and is present in nasopharyngeal secretions, blood, urine, and feces. The virus is transmitted primarily through contact with nasopharyngeal secretions of persons with clinical and subclinical infections 7 days before to 5 days after the appearance of the rash. The virus may also be transmitted transplacentally, producing active infection in the fetus. This may result in death to the fetus or congenital damage (congenital rubella syndrome). Infants born with congenital rubella syndrome generally have the virus in their nasopharyngeal secretions, stools, and urine for up to 1 year after birth, indicating the presence of a chronic infection.

In acquired rubella the virus invades the lymph glands from the nasopharynx, producing lymphadenopathy. It subsequently enters the blood, stimulating an immune response that is responsible for the development of the rash. Once the rash appears, the virus can no longer be found in the blood, and prodromal symptoms of a viremia subside. The disease is generally mild, particularly in children. Complications are rare.

Congenital rubella syndrome is a much more serious manifestation, affecting about 25% of infants born to mothers who were infected with rubella virus during their first trimester. Infection later in the pregnancy carries a lesser risk for congenital damage. The syndrome is characterized by a variety of permanent or transitory defects. including cataracts, microphthalmia, microcephaly, mental retardation, deafness, patent ductus arteriosus, arterial or ventral septal defects, congenital glaucoma, retinopathy, purpura, hepatosplenomegaly, neonatal jaundice, and bone defects. There is a high risk for death during the first 6 months, generally from congenital heart disease and sepsis.

Diagnostic Studies and Findings[3,26]

Culture of pharyngeal secretions (also blood, urine, or stool): Positive for rubella virus in pharyngeal secretions 7 days before rash in postnatal rubella; virus present up to 1 year following birth in congenital rubella syndrome; decreasing with age

Serology: Fourfold increase in antibody titer between acute and convalescent stages indicates recent infection: one-time elevated titers suggest immunity

Multidisciplinary Plan

Medications

Acquired Rubella

Antipyretics for temperature control
Antibiotic treatment of otitis media, an infrequent complication
Active and passive immunization for prevention (p. 1077)

NURSING CARE

Nursing Assessment

History: Inadequate immunization for rubella; exposure to person with symptoms of rubella within the past 2 to 3 weeks

Body temperature
- 37° to 38° C (99° to 100.4° F) during 1- to 5-day prodrome in adult and adolescent; subsiding after rash appears
- Elevated temperature with rash in children

Respiratory status: Coryza, sore throat, cough during prodrome

Head and neck
- Postauricular, postcervical, and occipital lymphadenopathy (small, shotty, and occasionally tender nodes can be palpated during prodrome and a few days after rash fades)
- Mild conjunctivitis and headache possible later complication

Skin
- Light pink to red, discrete macular rash, rapidly becoming papular; appearing on the first day of the rash on face and trunk and by the second day on the upper and lower extremities; rash fades within 3 days
- Purpura is a rare complication, appearing several days to several weeks after the rash

Oral cavity: Reddish spots, pinpoint or larger, on soft palate during prodrome or on first day of rash (Forchheimer spots)

Potential Complications

Self-limiting polyarthritis with inflammation and pain in proximal interphalangeal and metacarpophalangeal joints of hand and knee and ankle joints (begins within 5 days of rash and persists for more than 2 weeks); symptoms of complicating encephalitis very rare, usually during first few days after rash; hemorrhagic manifestations

Nursing Diagnoses/Patient Problems & Interventions

NIC Risk Management

Risk for infection (patient contacts) related to virus in pharyngeal secretions
- For acquired rubella: Isolate child from pregnant women. Select nursing personnel who are not at risk for rubella infection to care for patient *to prevent perinatal infections and their congenital sequelae.*
- If patient is hospitalized, employ droplet precautions (see Box 15-4 on p. 1087) for 7 days after rash.
- Ensure adequate immunization of patient contacts.
- Administer immune globulin, as indicated, for unimmunized persons exposed to rubella *to increase their resistance to these infections.*

NIC Thermoregulation

Hyperthermia related to infection
- Monitor body temperature *to detect fever.*
- Administer antipyretics, as ordered.
- Bathe with tepid water or alcohol to *reduce high fever.*
- Adjust environmental temperature *for patient's comfort.*
- Remove excess clothing and bedding *to ensure heat loss.*
- Encourage adequate fluid intake *to compensate for fluid loss associated with elevated body temperature.*

Patient Education/Continuum of Care Plan[25]

1. Rubella is transmitted by direct or indirect contact with nasopharyngeal secretions and transplacentally. It is communicable from 1 week before to 4 days after onset of rash; infants with congenital rubella may shed virus for months. Disease onset is between 14 and 23 days from exposure to the infection.
2. Transmission of the infection to others can be prevented by control of contact with respiratory secretions and by hand washing.
3. Rubella can be prevented by active immunization.
4. Manage fever with antipyretics, tepid sponge baths, minimal clothing, and a cool environment. Avoid chilling. Avoid giving children aspirin. Encourage intake of fluids and food as tolerated. Popsicles and soft drinks may appeal to young children.
5. Report the following symptoms of complications to a physician: inflammation and pain in joints, severe headache, altered consciousness, bleeding, or bruising.

6. Contacts should be referred to a physician for active or passive immunization.
7. Inform female patients that pregnant women should not be given rubella vaccine and that women should avoid pregnancy for 3 months after receiving rubella vaccine.
8. Convalescence should be uneventful.

EVALUATION/PATIENT OUTCOMES

Risk Management: Patient is free of infection and complications of rubella. Joints are not inflamed or tender. There are no signs of encephalitis or purpura. Lymph nodes are not palpable. Skin is free of rash. Hospital personnel and patient contacts are free of infection. They are immunized for rubella or have received immune globulin.

Thermoregulation: Body temperature is maintained within normal range; comfort and safety are maintained. Body temperature is between 36° and 38° C (96.8° and 100.4° F). Pulse and respiration are normal. Skin is cool to touch and free of excess perspiration. Patient's clothing and bedding are dry. Patient is free of headache and malaise associated with fever.

MEASLES (RUBEOLA)

Rubeola (hard measles or red measles) is an acute, highly communicable viral disease manifest as a prodromal fever, conjunctivitis, coryza, bronchitis, Koplik's spots on the buccal mucosa, and a characteristic red, blotchy rash. The rash appears on the third to seventh day on the face, becomes generalized, lasts 4 to 7 days, and sometimes ends in a brawny desquamation.

PATHOPHYSIOLOGY

The virus of rubeola (measles) is a paramyxovirus that can be found in the blood, urine, and pharyngeal secretions of infected persons. It is transmitted directly and indirectly through contact with respiratory secretions of infected persons during the catarrhal phase of the illness (from 4 days before to 5 days after the onset of the rash). The virus invades the respiratory epithelium and multiplies there. It spreads by way of the lymph system, producing a primary viremia. The virus then spreads in leukocytes to the reticuloendothelial system. The infected reticuloendothelial cells necrose, an increased amount of virus is released, and a reinvasion of leukocytes with a secondary viremia results. With the secondary viremia the entire respiratory mucosa becomes infected, producing upper respiratory symptoms.

Within a few days after the occurrence of generalized involvement of the respiratory tract, Koplik's spots appear on the buccal mucosa and a dermal rash develops. The virus appears to invade the cells of the epidermis and oral epithelium, producing histologic changes and stimulating a cell-mediated immune response manifested by the rash. The onset of the rash, following respiratory prodrome, coincides with the production of serum antibodies. Uncomplicated disease lasts 7 to 10 days.

DIAGNOSTIC STUDIES AND FINDINGS[3,26]

Culture of secretions from nasopharynx, conjunctiva, blood, or urine: Positive for measles virus

Serology: Detects long-lasting antibodies; therefore useful for determining immune status; significant increase in antibodies between acute and convalescent stages is diagnostic of recent infection; lack of antibodies indicates susceptibility

MULTIDISCIPLINARY PLAN

Medications

Antiinfection therapy for secondary infections only
Antipyretics for temperature control
Active immunization for prevention (p. 1077)
Active immunization for postexposure prophylaxis (within 72 hours of exposure)

NURSING CARE

NURSING ASSESSMENT

History: Inadequate immunization status (see p. 1077 for update on assessing immunization status of those previously immunized for measles); exposure to person with measles (rubeola) during past 8 to 14 days
Subjective symptoms: Headache; feels hot or chilled
Body temperature: Up to 40° C (104° F) during prodrome; decrease in 3 to 5 days (when rash appears)
Respiratory status: Hacking cough; coryza within 24 hours of fever, increasing in intensity until rash appears, gradually subsiding within 5 to 10 days
Eyes: Periorbital edema; conjunctivitis, subsiding with appearance of rash; photophobia
Head and neck: Lymphadenopathy
Oral cavity: Koplik's spots on buccal mucosa, most often opposite second molars; appear 2 to 4 days after onset of prodrome; resemble tiny grains of bluish white sand surrounded by inflammatory areola
Skin: Irregular macules appear on face and neck and in front of and behind ears 3 to 4 days after onset of prodrome; rash rapidly becomes maculopapular, spreading to trunk and extremities within 24 to 48 hours; at this time it begins to fade from face; rash is brownish pink and irregularly confluent; petechiae or ecchymoses may be present in severe cases; rash fades in 4 to 7 days, leaving a brownish desquamation

POTENTIAL COMPLICATIONS

Symptoms of encephalitis, a rare complication, within 2 days to 1 week of onset of rash; secondary elevation of temperature; headaches; seizures; altered state of consciousness; secondary bacterial infections (otitis, pneumonia); viral pneumonia; delayed subacute sclerosing panencephalitis; symptoms of secondary acute appendicitis; severe lethargy or prostration after onset of rash may indicate a secondary bacterial infection; dyspnea may indicate secondary bacterial infection; acute thrombocytopenic purpura with hemorrhage may be a complication

PATIENT PROBLEMS/NURSING DIAGNOSES & INTERVENTIONS

NIC RISK MANAGEMENT

Risk for infection (patient) related to inadequate secondary defenses

Risk for infection (patient contacts) related to virus in nasal secretions

- Collect specimen. *Incorrect collection and handling of specimens may destroy the pathogen or contaminate the specimen with environmental organisms, interfering with accurate diagnosis and treatment. Improper handling can also contaminate health-care workers.*
- Monitor systemic and local responses suggesting bacterial infection with a pathogen (elevated body temperature, localized inflammatory response, pain); report findings. *Early detection of bacterial infection and treatment with antiinfective agents may prevent dissemination of the pathogen, severe disease, and death.*
- Initiate airborne precautions for duration of illness (see Box 15-3, p. 1087).
- Use protective isolation procedures as indicated. Prevent patient exposure to infected visitors or staff. Limit visitors, if necessary, *to limit the exposure of patients to additional pathogens.*
- Participate in the follow-up of patient contacts *to ensure that all patient contacts are examined, treated, and immunized.*
- Report to the local health authority as required by law *to facilitate public health monitoring and control of outbreaks.*

NIC THERMOREGULATION

Hyperthermia related to infection

- Administer antipyretics, as ordered.
- Bathe with tepid water or alcohol *to reduce high fever.*
- Adjust environmental temperature *for patient's comfort.*
- Remove excess clothing and bedding *to ensure heat loss.*
- Encourage adequate fluid intake *to compensate for fluid loss associated with elevated body temperature.*

NIC NEUROLOGIC MANAGEMENT

Disturbed sensory perception (visual) related to viremia

- Assess patient for photophobia. Dim lights if photophobia is present *to prevent pain.*
- Cleanse eyelids with warm water *to remove crusts or secretions.*

PATIENT EDUCATION/CONTINUUM OF CARE PLAN[25]

1. Rubeola is transmitted by direct or indirect contact with nasal secretions. Virus remains viable in air for more than 2 hours. It is communicable from a few days before fever to 4 days after appearance of rash.
2. Transmission of the infection to others can be prevented by avoidance of contact with respiratory secretions of infected persons.
3. Rubeola can be prevented by active immunization.
4. Manage fever with antipyretics, tepid sponge baths, minimal clothing, and a cool environment. Avoid chilling. Avoid giving children aspirin. Encourage intake of fluids and food as tolerated. Popsicles and soft drinks may appeal to young children.
5. Manage other symptoms: dim lights if photophobia is present; employ bed rest.
6. Report the following symptoms of complications to physician: secondary rise in fever, pain in ear, abdominal pain, nosebleeds, bruising, shortness of breath, coughing, headache, seizures, or alterations in alertness.
7. Contacts should be referred to a physician for active immunization within 72 hours of exposure or immune globulin up to 6 days after exposure.
8. Convalescence in uncomplicated disease lasts 7 to 10 days. Recovery is usually complete.

EVALUATION/PATIENT OUTCOMES

Risk Management: Patient is free of infection and complications of measles. Cultures of body secretions, excretions, and exudates are negative for colonized pathogens. WBC count is within normal limits. There are no signs of injury associated with complications.

Infection is not transmitted to patient's contacts. Patient care staff members wash hands after providing care to each patient and follow airborne precautions (see Box 15-3, p. 1087) with all patients. Appropriate isolation procedures are implemented for hospitalized patients soon after infection is confirmed. Patient or family describes transmission of pathogen, demonstrates proper procedures for handling infective materials, and demonstrates proper hand-washing and other behaviors necessary to prevent transmission. All patient contacts are adequately immunized.

Thermoregulation: Body temperature is maintained within normal range; comfort and safety are maintained. Patient's body temperature is between 36° and 38° C (96.8° and 100.4° F). Pulse and respiration are normal. Skin is cool to touch and free of excess perspiration. Patient's clothing and bedding are dry. Patient is free of headache and malaise associated with fever.

Neurologic Management: Patient is not confused or frightened by environmental stimuli; visual function returns to normal. Pupils are normal and reactive. Patient is calm and rests comfortably during acute illness. There is no startle response to environmental stimuli. During convalescence the patient correctly identifies letters on Snellen's eye chart at a distance of 20 feet.

TETANUS

Tetanus (lockjaw) is an acute neurointoxication induced by the tetanus bacillus growing anaerobically at the site of an injury. It is manifested as tonic rigidity and painful, intermittent tonic spasms of the masseter and cervical muscles and muscles of the trunk and extremities. Abdominal rigidity, a position of opisthotonus, generalized spasms induced by sensory stimuli, and a facial expression known as risus sardonicus are characteristic. Fatality is high.

PATHOPHYSIOLOGY

Tetanus spores enter through a trivial or extensive injury to the skin. The anaerobic organism multiplies in the wound, even after the injury has healed, producing a lethal toxin. The toxin (tetanospasmin) reaches the central nervous system by the bloodstream or by passages along peripheral motor nerves. The toxin binds with central nervous system tissue and spinal motor ganglia. There it interferes with the release of an inhibitory transmitter and induces a hyperexcitability of motor neurons, resulting in tonic rigidity and spasms of facial, cervical, masseter, respiratory, abdominal, and extremity muscles. The bound toxin cannot be neutralized by an antitoxin.

The permanency of pathologic changes in the central and peripheral nervous system in patients who recover has not been determined. Neonatal tetanus generally leaves no permanent neurologic sequelae. Central nervous system findings in fatal cases range from mild congestion to definite hemorrhage, areas of demyelination, gliosis, and tissue necrosis in the cerebral hemispheres.

Potential Complications

Anoxia resulting from respiratory involvement
Asphyxial convulsions
Hemorrhage and rupture of striated muscles

Tetanus is completely preventable with active immunization and passive immunization for wound management (see p. 1076). No care plan is provided here because of the rareness of this condition.

GASTROINTESTINAL INFECTIOUS DISEASE

A wide range of gastrointestinal (GI) infectious diseases are caused by pathogens that are ingested in contaminated food or water or by contact with feces from an infected person.

The following are presented in three sections:

1. Food poisoning caused by pathogens that have already multiplied in the food at the time of ingestion:
   - Staphylococcal food poisoning
   - Botulism
   - Food poisoning: enteric infections
     - *Bacillus cereus*
     - *Clostridium perfringens*
     - *Vibrio parahaemolyticus*
2. Acute gastroenteritis produced by bacteria and viruses that multiply in the gastrointestinal tract after ingestion:
   - *Campylobacter*
   - *Escherichia coli*
   - *Shigella*
   - Norwalk virus
   - Rotavirus
3. *Salmonella* gastroenteritis (salmonellosis)

Food Poisoning

Food poisoning is the generic term applied to illnesses acquired through consumption of food or water contaminated with chemicals, bacteria and bacterial toxins, or organic poisons naturally present in some edible substances.

The food poisonings caused by bacteria and bacterial toxins are discussed here. In all cases disease is produced in the host shortly after ingestion of food containing bacteria that have already multiplied in the food. These diseases are not directly communicable. If the bacteria have produced a toxin in the food, the resulting disease in the host is intoxication, as in staphylococcal food poisoning and botulism. If the bacterial cells are antigenic, they produce an infection in the host, such as those caused by *B. cereus, C. perfringens,* and *V. parahaemolyticus* (Table 15-9).

Staphylococcal Food Poisoning

Staphylococcal food poisoning is an enteric intoxication of acute onset. Symptoms are severe nausea, intestinal cramps, vomiting, diarrhea, prostration, and occasionally subnormal temperature and hypotension. The intensity of the disease depends on the quantity of the ingested toxin and host susceptibility. The duration of the illness is 1 to 2 days, and recovery is generally complete.

Pathophysiology

The ingested enterotoxin acts on the abdominal viscera, creating a sensory stimulus that reaches the vomiting center of the brain by way of the vagus and sympathetic nerves. The action of the enterotoxin on the gastric mucosa produces a patchy hyperemia, erosions, petechiae, and a purulent gastric exudate. Diarrhea results from inhibition of water absorption from the intestinal lumen and from increased transport of fluid into the lumen.

Botulism

Botulism is a severe neurointoxication with a wide range of neurologic symptoms and severity of symptoms. In the United States 10% of cases under treatment result in death, primarily from respiratory failure. Three types of botulism have been recognized: food-borne, wound, and infant botulism.

Pathophysiology

Clostridium botulinum, a spore-forming anaerobe capable of withstanding boiling, produces a potent toxin in anaerobic conditions. A common source of botulinal toxin is improperly processed canned foods. Less commonly, *C. botulinum* enters the body through a wound and produces toxin in traumatized, necrotic tissue. Ingestion of *C. botulinum* spores does not result in toxin production in adults and children but does cause toxin production in the bowel lumen of some infants, producing infant botulism.

The botulinal toxin is hematogenously disseminated to peripheral cholinergic synapses, where it becomes irreversibly bound. This action blocks the release of acetylcholine, producing impaired autonomic and voluntary neuromuscular transmission and muscular paralysis. Gradual recovery occurs over a period of weeks from the regeneration of terminal motor neurons to reinnervate noncontracting muscle fibers.

Intestinal stasis predisposes to the colonization of any ingested viable spores of *C. botulinum.* Additional toxin is produced in vivo, prolonging the course of the disease.

Food Poisoning: Enteric Infections

The three enteric infections discussed here are all caused by ingestion of food contaminated with specific bacteria that have already multiplied in the food. Disease occurs in the host shortly after ingestion of the food and manifests as symptoms of gastroenteritis.

Table 15-9 Overview of Food Poisonings

	Staphylococcal Food Poisoning	Botulism	*Clostridium perfringens*	*Vibrio parahaemolyticus*	*Bacillus cereus*
Occurrence	Widespread and frequent: one of the principal acute food poisonings in the United States	Worldwide; sporadic; family-grouped cases occur	Widespread and frequent in countries with cooking practices that favor growth of organism	Sporadic cases and outbreaks occur in warm months of the year	Worldwide; rare in the United States
Etiologic agent	Several enterotoxins of staphylococci; stable at boiling temperature	Toxins produced by *C. botulinum* in anaerobic conditions; destroyed by boiling	Type A strains of *C. perfringens* (*Clostridium welchii*)	*V. parahaemolyticus* (many types)	*B. cereus,* an aerobic spore former that produces two enterotoxins—one heat stable, causing vomiting, and one heat labile, causing diarrhea
Reservoir	Humans; cows with infected udders; dogs and fowl	Soil, marine sediments, and intestinal tract of animals and fish	Soil and gastrointestinal tract of humans and animals	Marine silt, coastal waters, fish, and shellfish	Soil; commonly in rice and other raw, dried, or processed foods
Transmission	Ingestion of food containing staphylococcal toxin, which formed while food was held at room temperature	Ingestion of food in which toxin has formed, such as home-canned vegetables, fruits, and meats; onions and potatoes cooked and held at room temperature; feeding raw honey to infants	Ingestion of food, especially meat, contaminated by soil or feces; spores survive normal cooking temperatures, germinate, and multiply during cooking and reheating	Ingestion of raw or undercooked contaminated seafood, food contaminated with seawater, and by handling seafood	Ingestion of food that has been kept at ambient temperatures after cooking, such as rice dishes, permitting multiplication of the organism
Incubation period	30 minutes to 8 hours; usually 2-4 hours	12-36 hours	6-24 hours; usually 10-12 hours	4-96 hours; usually 12-24 hours	1-6 hours for disease causing vomiting; 6-24 hours for disease causing diarrhea
Period of communicability	Noncommunicable	Noncommunicable	Noncommunicable	Noncommunicable	Noncommunicable
Susceptibility and resistance	General; no immune response	General; no immune response	General; no resistance develops from exposure	General	Unknown
Report to local health authority	Prompt report of outbreaks	Report of cases and outbreaks	Prompt report of outbreaks	Report of outbreaks	Report of cases and outbreaks

Data from Benenson.[3]

C. perfringens generally causes a mild intestinal infection characterized by sudden onset of abdominal colic, nausea, and diarrhea. Fever and vomiting are rare.

V. parahaemolyticus is a moderately severe intestinal infection characterized by sudden-onset abdominal cramps and watery diarrhea lasting 1 to 7 days. Nausea, vomiting, fever, and headache may be present.

B. cereus food poisoning is a gastrointestinal infection characterized by sudden-onset nausea and vomiting or colic and diarrhea, lasting no longer than 24 hours.

PATHOPHYSIOLOGY

C. perfringens, a spore former widely distributed in feces, soil, and water, multiplies rapidly in foods that have been cooled and reheated. The organism produces an enterotoxin in the intestinal tract within 6 to 24 hours after ingestion. The enterotoxin acts on the epithelial layer of the ileum, increasing the secretion of sodium, chloride, and fluid, and inhibiting the absorption of glucose.

V. parahaemolyticus multiplies in uncooked, contaminated seafood. When ingested, the pathogen directly invades intestinal tissue to produce necrosis, ulceration, possible hemorrhage, and granulocytic infiltration of the mucosa. Disease intensity ranges from asymptomatic to severe; duration ranges from 2 hours to 10 days.

The spores of *B. cereus* survive cooking and multiply in food held at room temperature. One type of enterotoxin that is heat stable attacks the gastric mucosa. Another type, which is heat labile, affects the intestinal mucosa. Thorough reheating of food destroys the heat-labile enterotoxin but not the enterotoxin that causes vomiting.

DIAGNOSTIC STUDIES AND FINDINGS[3]

Culture of stomach contents, feces, or suspected food: More than 10^5 enterotoxin-producing staphylococci per gram of specimen; positive for *C. botulinum;* more than 10^5 spores of *C. perfringens* or *B. cereus* per gram of specimen; or positive for *V. parahaemolyticus*

Serum: Positive for botulinal toxins; circulating toxins found in about one third of hospitalized patients with botulism

MULTIDISCIPLINARY PLAN

Medications for Botulism

Trivalent (ABE) botulinal antitoxin (not used for infants) administered IV as soon as possible after onset of symptoms; obtained from Centers for Disease Control and Prevention (CDC)

Antiinfective agents: Penicillin for wound botulism; agent-specific, antiinfective agents for secondary bacterial infection

General Management

For botulism
- Gastric lavage initially
- Mechanical ventilation in the event of respiratory paralysis
- Suction of secretions
- Intubation of tracheostomy
- Nasogastric feedings
- IV fluid and electrolytes
- Must be reported to local health authority immediately
- All patient contacts known to have eaten the same food should have gastric lavage, high enemas, and cathartics and should be kept under close medical supervision

For staphylococcal poisoning and enteric infection: Oral fluids if tolerated; IV fluids and electrolytes if needed

NURSING CARE

NURSING ASSESSMENT

See Assessment Considerations table on p. 1028.

POTENTIAL COMPLICATIONS

Staphylococcal Food Poisoning
Dehydration, particularly in infants and older adults; prostration, particularly in infants and older adults

Botulism
Respiratory failure; death

Enteric Infections
Dehydration, particularly in infants and older adults, prostration, particularly in infants and older adults

PATIENT PROBLEMS/NURSING DIAGNOSES & INTERVENTIONS

NIC ELECTROLYTE AND ACID-BASE MANAGEMENT

Deficient fluid volume related to vomiting and diarrhea
- Monitor fluid and electrolyte balance, intake and output, urine specific gravity, moisture of skin and mucous membranes, skin turgor, frequency of vomiting and diarrhea, vital signs, and weight loss. *Fluids, sodium, and potassium lost through diarrhea and vomiting must be replaced.*
- Encourage small amounts of oral fluids as tolerated. Administer IV fluids and electrolytes as prescribed *to maintain adequate intake and replace those lost in vomitus and diarrhea.*

NIC ELIMINATION MANAGEMENT

Diarrhea related to pathogens and toxins in the intestinal tract
- Collect fecal specimen. *Incorrect collection and handling of specimens may destroy the pathogen or contaminate the specimen with environmental organisms, interfering with accurate diagnosis and treatment. Improper handling can also contaminate the health-care worker.*
- Monitor frequency and characteristics of stool *to detect complications.*
- Provide air circulation and room deodorization.
- Wash hands frequently *to prevent transmission of organisms* to other patients or health care workers. Lubricate the patient's anal opening frequently *to prevent skin irritation.*

NIC RESPIRATORY MANAGEMENT

For botulism: ineffective airway clearance related to neurologic effects of botulinal toxins
Ineffective breathing pattern related to neurologic effects of toxins
- Monitor cough and gag reflexes *to detect and report loss of patency of airway.*
- Suction secretions *to prevent aspiration.*
- Have tracheostomy tray available for emergency use. Provide tracheostomy care *to maintain patent airway.*
- Assess ability to swallow *to prevent aspiration of oral fluids or food.*
- Monitor for signs of respiratory paralysis and oxygen insufficiency; initiate mechanical ventilation and oxygen as prescribed *to assist breathing to ensure adequate oxygen intake.*
- Monitor patient on respirator for signs of hyperventilation or hypoventilation *to prevent or detect early signs of respiratory acidosis or alkalosis.*

Assessment Considerations

Assessment	Staphylococcal Food Poisoning	Botulism	Enteric Infections
History	May have eaten within past 7 hours at a picnic or large gathering where food has been sitting unrefrigerated	Consumption of home-canned food within past 36 hours	Ingestion within past 24 hours of high-risk food (see Table 15-9)
Subjective symptoms	Weakness; prostration	Vertigo and neurologic symptoms	Nausea and abdominal pain
Gastrointestinal concerns	Acute-onset nausea, vomiting, intestinal cramps, and diarrhea	Vomiting, diarrhea, and constipation	If incubation period (time from food ingestion to symptom onset) has been short, patient will be vomiting; if long, patient will have severe diarrhea Acute-onset nausea, abdominal cramping, and diarrhea in *C. perfringens* infections Diarrhea may be watery and bloody and persist up to 7 days in *V. parahaemolyticus* infections Acute-onset nausea and vomiting or colic and diarrhea in *B. cereus* infections
Vital signs	Subnormal temperature; hypotension	Normal	Usually normal
Head and neck		Abrupt onset, bilateral and symmetric: ptosis, blurred vision, diplopia, dry mouth, dysphagia, dysphonia, dysarthria, and nasal regurgitation	
Respiratory concerns		Paralysis of muscles of respiration	
Large muscles		Symmetric flaccid paralysis; motor disturbances but no sensory disturbances	

NIC IMMOBILITY MANAGEMENT

Impaired physical mobility related to neurologic effects of toxins

- Position in proper body alignment *to prevent contractures and footdrop.*
- Assist with range-of-motion exercises *to prevent joint stiffness.*
- Turn every 2 hours *to prevent skin pressure sores and pooling of secretions.*
- Provide total hygienic care as needed *to prevent skin breakdown.*

NIC NEUROLOGIC MANAGEMENT

Disturbed sensory perception (visual) related to neurologic effects of toxins

Impaired verbal communication related to neurologic effects of toxins

- Interpret environment and stimuli for patient whose vision is altered *to minimize injury.*
- Explain that condition is not permanent *to relieve fear associated with vision changes.*
- Minimize stimuli *to prevent confusion.*
- Anticipate patient's needs and provide necessary care. Explain that loss of speech is not permanent *to relieve anxiety of patient who cannot communicate.*

PATIENT EDUCATION/CONTINUUM OF CARE PLAN[25]

Provide patient with the following instructions:

1. These conditions are transmitted by contaminated food and can be prevented by proper food handling.
2. Cooked foods should not be held at room temperature; they should be kept hot (140° F) or should be refrigerated. Reheating should be done rapidly and completely.
3. All seafood should be cooked at a temperature above 60° C (140° F) for 15 minutes.
4. Keep all seafood, raw or cooked, adequately refrigerated before eating.
5. Handle cooked seafood to avoid its contamination with raw seafood or with contaminated seawater.
6. All persons should wash hands thoroughly following defecation and before handling food.
7. Destroy all canned food and containers from same batch that contained the *C. botulinum* by burying deep in soil or boiling 3 minutes before discarding. Commercial canned

foods should be submitted for laboratory examination. Contaminated cooking utensils should be sterilized by boiling for 3 minutes before reuse.

8. No questionable canned food should ever be tasted. Foods containing *C. botulinum* do not necessarily have "off" odors or a spoiled taste.
9. Recommended processing times and temperatures for home canning must be followed to ensure killing of all *C. botulinum* spores. This information is available through state agricultural extension services.
10. Home canned vegetables and meats should be boiled for 3 minutes to destroy botulinal toxin.
11. Honey must not be given to infants under 1 year of age.
12. Fluids should be encouraged, and food may be eaten when tolerated.
13. Report the following symptoms of complications to a physician: vomiting and diarrhea persisting beyond 1 to 2 days; alteration in consciousness; loss of skin turgor, particularly in infants and children, fever, absence of urination; and severe prostration.
14. Explain that food poisonings are self-limiting.

EVALUATION/PATIENT OUTCOMES

Electrolyte and Acid-Base Management: Fluid and electrolyte balance is maintained. Patient's skin turgor is good. Urine output equals intake. Urine specific gravity is normal. Measurements of sodium, potassium, chloride, magnesium, and calcium in blood are normal.

Elimination Management: Patient returns to normal pattern of bowel elimination. Patient's stools are soft, formed, and normal colored. Abdomen soft; bowel sounds normal. Patient tolerates regular diet. Weight returns to normal. Stool specimens are negative for any pathogen.

Respiratory Management: Airway is patent and aspiration of secretions is avoided. Patient's airway is open. Secretions are thin and easily coughed up by patient. Patient swallows without difficulty. Breathing is quiet.

Patient demonstrates normal respiratory pattern, oxygen intake, and blood gas levels. Patient's respiratory rate is normal. Respirations are of normal depth. There is no dyspnea. Skin and mucous membranes are warm and moist with normal color. Oxygen saturation, CO_2, Po_2, and Pco_2 are normal.

Immobility Management: Patient maintains function, comfort, and skin integrity and demonstrates increasing strength and movement. Patient moves extremities and changes position in bed. During convalescence, patient sits, stands, and walks without signs of contractures, foot drop, or pain.

Neurologic Management: Patient is not confused or frightened by environmental stimuli; visual function returns to normal. There are no startle responses to environmental stimuli. During convalescence, the patient correctly identifies letters on Snellen's eye chart from a distance of 20 feet. Pupils are normal and reactive.

Patient communicates needs; speech returns to normal. Health-care workers and visitors respond to patient's nonverbal cues. Patient speaks audibly during convalescence.

ACUTE BACTERIAL AND VIRAL GASTROENTERITIS

Gastroenteritis is the inflammation of the stomach and intestines. It can be caused by bacterial enterotoxins or bacterial or viral invasion. Symptoms include anorexia, nausea, vomiting, abdominal discomfort, or diarrhea.

Many forms of acute gastroenteritis are caused by ingestion of food and water contaminated with pathogenic agents or by fecal-oral transmission directly or indirectly from an infected person. These infections differ from the food poisonings previously discussed in the following ways:

The pathogenic agents causing these diseases invade, colonize, and multiply in the human intestinal tract.

The incubation periods are slightly longer, ranging from 1 day to several weeks.

Direct and indirect fecal-oral transmission is possible.

Acquired immunity of varying duration results from many of these infections.

In addition, the predominant manifestation of these diseases is acute-onset diarrhea of varying intensity and duration. The bacterial- and viral-caused gastroenteritises discussed here are usually self-limited diseases (Table 15-10). This is not a complete list of all pathogens causing diarrhea.

Campylobacter enteritis is an acute bacterial intestinal infection lasting from 1 to 10 days and is considered to be an important cause of "traveler's diarrhea." Prolonged illness may occur.

Escherichia coli diarrhea is an acute infection of the colon. Disease is severe or mild depending on whether the strain of *E. coli* causing disease is enterohemorrhagic, enterotoxigenic, enteroinvasive, or enteropathogenic.

Shigellosis (bacillary dysentery) is an acute bacterial infection of the large intestine with severity ranging from asymptomatic infection to fulminating diarrheal disease and death.

Epidemic viral gastroenteritis is usually a self-limited, mild gastric and intestinal infection lasting 24 to 48 hours. Disease often occurs in outbreaks.

Rotavirus gastroenteritis is a sporadically occurring gastric and intestinal infection of infants and young children ranging in severity from asymptomatic to severe disease and occasionally death.

PATHOPHYSIOLOGY

Bacterial and viral agents that produce gastroenteritis produce pathologic conditions in one of four ways:

Toxigenic agents, such as some *Shigella* strains and enterotoxigenic *E. coli,* release an enterotoxin that acts on the small intestine to produce a local inflammation and a secretory diarrhea with rapid loss of electrolytes.

Invasive pathogens, such as *Shigella, Campylobacter,* and invasive strains of *E. coli,* penetrate the small or large intestine, producing cellular destruction, necrosis, and potential ulceration. The diarrheal stools in these conditions frequently contain leukocytes and erythrocytes.

Some pathogens, such as the rotaviruses and enteropathogenic *E. coli,* attach to the mucosal epithelium without invasion. They destroy cells of the intestinal villi, resulting

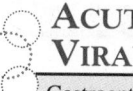

Table 15-10 Overview of Acute Bacterial and Viral Gastroenteritis

	Campylobacter Enteritis	*Escherichia coli* Diarrhea	Shigellosis (Bacillary Dysentery)	Epidemic Viral Gastroenteritis	Rotavirus Gastroenteritis
Occurrence	Worldwide; common-source outbreaks occur; highest in warmer months; common cause of "travelers' diarrhea"	Worldwide; common-source-outbreaks occur; high in areas of poor sanitation and during warm months; common cause of "travelers' diarrhea"	Worldwide; highest in children under 10 years old; outbreaks common in crowded living conditions, day care	Worldwide and common; epidemics and outbreaks occur; affects infants and adults	Worldwide; sporadic and in outbreaks; highest in infants and young children
Etiologic agent	*Campylobacter jejuni* and *Campylobacter coli*	Enterohemorrhagic (EHEC) Enterotoxigenic, invasive, or enteropathogenic strains of *E. coli*	Four different groups of *Shigella* bacteria, with many strains	Many viruses; Norwalk virus most common	Many types of rotaviruses
Reservoir	Domestic and wild animals and birds	Humans, who are often asymptomatic; cattle	Humans	Humans	Humans
Transmission	Ingestion of water, food, or raw milk contaminated with organism from feces; contact with infected animals or infants; fecal-oral	Ingestion of food, including undercooked beef, water and baby formula contaminated with feces; transmitted to infant during delivery; fecal-oral, by hand	Direct or indirect fecal-oral transmission from infected person or carrier, usually by hand	Fecal-oral route; food-borne and waterborne transmission	Fecal-oral; possibly fecal-respiratory
Incubation period	2-5 days; range: 1-10 days	Enterohemorrhagic: 3-8 days (usually 3-4) Enterotoxigenic: 10-72 hours Enteroinvasive: 10-18 hours Enteropathogenic: 9-12 hours	12-96 hours; usually 1-3 days	Usually 24-48 hours; range: 10-50 hours	24-72 hours
Period of communicability	Several days to weeks throughout course of infection; usually 2-7 weeks; carriers are rare	Duration of fecal excretion of organism, possibly weeks	During acute infection to 4 weeks after illness; carrier state may persist for months	During acute stage and up to 48 hours after diarrhea stops	During acute stage and as long as virus is shed (up to 30 days)
Susceptibility and resistance	General; immune mechanisms not understood	Infants very susceptible; travelers to developing countries; duration of acquired immunity unknown	General; more severe in children and elderly and debilitated individuals; strain-specific antibodies develop	General; short-term (14 weeks) immunity may follow infection with specific serotypes	By age 3 years most individuals have acquired antibodies against most serotypes
Report to local health authority	Report cases	Report epidemic only	Report cases	Report epidemic only	Report epidemic only

Data from Benenson.[3]

in malabsorption of electrolytes and the potential for electrolyte imbalance.

Enterohemorrhagic strains of *E. coli* elaborate a toxin that can cause severe intestinal hemorrhage and, if absorbed, produces hemolytic-uremic syndrome and thrombotic thrombocytopenic purpura.

The general effect of all of the above pathologic conditions is to increase gastrointestinal motility and to increase the secretory rate of fluids and electrolytes into the intestines. The result may be rapid dehydration, electrolyte imbalance, circulatory failure, and death. Fluid and electrolyte loss in other forms of gastroenteritis may develop more gradually or may not occur at all. Infants, small children, and debilitated individuals are at greater risk for severe dehydration.

The attachment of the pathogens to the mucosa may be altered by nonspecific resistance factors in the host:

The normal bacterial flora of the intestinal tract prevents attachment by competing for attachment sites or by production of volatile organic acids. If the normal flora is diminished as a result of antibiotic therapy or malnutrition, this host defense is ineffective.

The pH of the gastrointestinal tract impedes the growth of some microbes. Altering the pH through the ingestion of antacids reduces the effectiveness of this defense.

Normal gastrointestinal motility purges the intestinal tract of many pathogens, and interference with this function increases the risk for invasion of pathogens.

Specific immune responses of varying duration occur in the host following infection with *Shigella,* parvovirus-like agents, rotavirus, and *E. coli.*

DIAGNOSTIC STUDIES AND FINDINGS[26]

Diagnosis of these conditions relies on culture, isolation, and identification of the pathogen in a fecal specimen or a specimen obtained by a rectal swab.

Culture and direct examination of bacterial colonies: Positive for *Campylobacter, E. coli,* and *Shigella.*

Microscopic examination: Visualization of motile *Campylobacter;* visualization of fecal WBCs associated with shigellosis.

Serotyping: Differentiates serotypes of *E. coli* and *Shigella* spp.

Immunologic techniques: Identify rotavirus and Norwalk virus

MULTIDISCIPLINARY PLAN[3]

Medications

Agents that suppress intestinal motility are not given for bacterial gastroenteritis

For shigellosis

Antiinfective agents: Trimethoprim-sulfamethoxazole (Septra, Bactrim), ciprofloxacin or ofloxacin

For *E. coli* diarrhea caused by entertoxigenic and enteroinvasive strains

Antiinfective agents: Trimethoprim-sulfamethoxazole or doxycycline, or ciprofloxacin or norfloxacin

Treatment for EHEC has not been determined

General Management

IV fluids and electrolyte replacement

For shock: Rapid infusion of 20 to 30 ml/kg of lactated Ringer's solution, isotonic saline, or similar isotonic solution given within an hour

For complete rehydration after circulation is restored: Glucose electrolyte solution (oral or IV hypotonic electrolyte solutions in amounts equal to estimated fluid loss)

NURSING CARE

NURSING ASSESSMENT

History: Travel to another country; ingestion of questionable food or water during past week; eating food contaminated by person with diarrheal disease during past week; eating undercooked beef

Subjective symptoms: Myalgia, headache, malaise, prostration

Gastrointestinal status

Campylobacter: Days 1 and 2: nausea, vomiting, abdominal pain; days 2 to 4 (maybe 10): foul-smelling or liquid diarrhea; sometimes 20 to 30 stools per day; blood in stools after day 4; day 7: ulcerative colitis may occur

E. coli diarrhea: Day 1: vomiting; day 2 (lasting 7 to 10 days): mucous and bloody diarrhea or profuse watery diarrhea without blood or mucus

Infection with EHEC presents with bloody diarrhea, progressing rapidly to circulatory collapse and death

Shigellosis: Day 1: nausea, abdominal pain, colic, vomiting, painful diarrhea; days 2 to 5: stools contain blood, pus, and mucus; rectal irritation and tenesmus

Epidemic viral gastroenteritis: Day 1 (lasts 24 to 48 hours): nausea, vomiting, diarrhea, abdominal pain

Rotavirus gastroenteritis: Day 1: vomiting for 48 hours; days 2 to 8: watery diarrhea; rectal bleeding may occur

Body temperature

Campylobacter: 38° to 41° C (100.4° to 105° F); febrile convulsions

E. coli diarrhea: Low-grade fever on day 1 or 2

Shigellosis: Days 1 to 5: 38° to 41° C (100.4° to 105° F)

Epidemic viral gastroenteritis: Low-grade fever

Rotavirus gastroenteritis: Day 1: usually low-grade fever (up to 39° C [102° F])

Respiratory status: Rotavirus gastroenteritis: pharyngeal exudate, cough, and rhinitis

POTENTIAL COMPLICATIONS

Dehydration

Circulatory failure and death

Fluids and electrolyte imbalance

Campylobacter: Anytime during disease: poor skin turgor, dry mucous membranes, faint pulse, hypotension

E. coli diarrhea: Anytime during disease: poor skin turgor, dry mucous membranes, faint pulse, hypotension

Shigellosis: Days 2 to 5: loss of turgor, oliguria, hypotension, weak pulse, shock

Epidemic viral gastroenteritis: Usually no alteration in fluid balance

Rotavirus gastroenteritis: Days 2 to 8: severe dehydration possible

PATIENT PROBLEMS/NURSING DIAGNOSES & INTERVENTIONS

NIC ELECTROLYTE AND ACID-BASE MANAGEMENT

Risk for deficient fluid volume related to vomiting and diarrhea

- Monitor for symptoms of dehydration and electrolyte imbalance (e.g., oliguria and loss of skin turgor) *to detect early signs of dehydration for early intervention.*
- Measure fluid output (emesis, urine, and diarrhea); measure intake *to determine if intake compensates for output.*
- Monitor blood pressure, temperature, pulse, and respirations *to detect symptoms of circulatory collapse early.*
- Administer liquids frequently as tolerated *to maintain adequate intake.*
- Administer electrolytes as prescribed *to replace those lost during diarrhea.*

- Provide patient with oral glucose electrolyte solution as soon as patient can take oral fluids. *Oral fluids can usually be tolerated once electrolyte balance is corrected.*
- Gradually add clear fluids and soft foods (milk and cream products should be avoided at first; apple juice and clear soda [7-Up] are usually well tolerated). *Clear carbohydrates (fluids and foods) are easier to tolerate with nausea.*

NIC Elimination Management

Diarrhea related to pathogenic activity in GI tract

- Obtain stool specimens for culture *to identify pathogen.*
- Measure watery diarrhea output *to estimate rapidity of fluid loss.*
- Cleanse perianal area and lubricate after each diarrheal stool *to prevent irritation of skin.*
- Provide adequate air circulation, room deodorization, and privacy *to control odors and prevent embarrassment.*

NIC Thermoregulation

Hyperthermia related to infection

- Monitor temperature *to detect fever.*
- Sponge with tepid water *to reduce temperature.*

NIC Risk Management

Risk for infection (patient contacts) related to presence of pathogen in stool

- Collect fecal specimen. *Incorrect collection and handling of specimens may destroy the pathogen or contaminate the specimen with environmental organisms, interfering with accurate diagnosis and treatment. Improper handling of specimens can also contaminate the health-care worker.*
- Use standard precautions until three fecal cultures are negative for infecting *Shigella* organism; use standard precautions for duration of illness for others *to prevent transmission to health-care workers, other patients, and patient contacts* (see Box 15-2, p. 1086).
- Report shigellosis to local health authority; *reporting is required by law to facilitate public health monitoring and control of outbreaks.*

Patient Education/Continuum of Care Plan[25]

Provide patient with the following instructions:

1. These conditions are transmitted by food or water contaminated with organisms from feces of infected person.
2. They are communicable while the organisms are in the feces (usually from onset of diarrhea until up to 7 weeks).
3. Disease onset is between 1 to 7 days from exposure to the infection.
4. Transmission of the infection to others can be prevented by thorough hand washing before eating and after bowel movements, changing diapers, or handling feces.
5. For patients cared for at home, teach family:
   a. Signs of dehydration and importance of prompt medical attention should dehydration occur
   b. Measurement of intake and measurement or estimation of output
   c. Maintenance of oral fluid intake equal to output
   d. Types of clear, high-glucose oral fluids that may be tolerated (apple juice, mildly carbonated beverages, such as 7-Up)
   e. Scrupulous hand washing; avoidance of food contamination
6. Persons with *Shigella* infections should not be permitted to handle food or provide child care until two successive fecal samples or rectal swabs are free of *Shigella* organisms.
7. Child day-care programs should provide for:
   a. Frequent hand washing of workers
   b. Separate areas for food preparation and diaper changing
   c. Separate rooms for children of different age groups
   d. Routine exclusion of children with diarrhea
8. Most acute gastroenteritis can be prevented by:
   a. Thorough hand washing after toileting, handling feces, or contact with animals
   b. Thorough cooking of all food derived from animals, and avoidance of recontamination within the kitchen after cooking
   c. Using pasteurized milk and chlorinated water
   d. Maintaining food at hot or cold temperatures
9. Report the following symptoms of complications to physician:
   a. Dry mucous membranes, loss of skin turgor, listlessness or change in level of consciousness, or absence of urination
   b. Continuation of diarrhea or blood in urine or stool
   c. Increase in colic or pain
   d. Increase in fever or convulsions
10. Food supplies should be protected from fly contamination. Travelers to areas where water supply is not chemically treated or protected from sewage contamination should boil all water used in cooking, drinking, or making ice.

Evaluation/Patient Outcomes

Electrolyte and Acid-Base Management: Fluid and electrolyte balance is maintained. Blood pressure and pulse are normal. Skin turgor is good. Mucous membranes are moist. Urine output is equal to intake. Blood levels of sodium, potassium, chloride, magnesium, and calcium are normal. Urine specific gravity is normal. Secretions are thin.

Elimination Management: Patient returns to normal pattern of bowel elimination. Stools are soft, formed, and brown. Abdomen is not distended. There is no cramping.

Thermoregulation: Body temperature is within normal range; comfort and safety are maintained. Body temperature is between 36° and 38° C (96.8° and 100.4° F). Pulse and respiration are normal. Skin is cool to touch and free of excess perspiration. Patient's clothing and bedding are dry. Patient is free of headache and malaise associated with fever.

Risk Management: Infection is not transmitted to patient's contacts. Patient care staff members wash hands after providing care to each patient and follow standard precautions with all patients.

Patient has information to prevent further episodes of food-borne gastroenteritis. Patient or family describes transmission of the pathogen. Patient or family demonstrates proper procedures for handling infective materials and proper hand washing and other behaviors necessary to prevent transmission.

Salmonella Gastroenteritis (Salmonellosis)

Salmonellosis is manifested by an acute gastroenteritis and sometimes a septicemia. It is frequently classified as a food poisoning because of the short incubation period following ingestion of food contaminated with *Salmonella.* The greater the number of organisms present in the food, the shorter the incubation period (Table 15-11).

Pathophysiology

Salmonella organisms ingested in contaminated food or water invade and multiply in deep mucosal layers of the stomach and small intestine. The inflammatory response produces a gastroenteritis if the *Salmonella* is not *Salmonella typhi* or *Salmonella paratyphi.* The mesenteric lymph nodes become edematous, and the Peyer's patches show edema and superficial ulceration. The disease may be contained here, or the organism may invade beyond the lymph system and be disseminated into the vascular circulation, producing a septicemia or lesions in other organs.

Several nonspecific host defenses affect the type and severity of clinical disease produced by *Salmonella.* Gastric acidity impedes *Salmonella* growth, and persons with hypochlorhydria or achlorhydria or who have had gastric surgery are more susceptible to infection. Normal intestinal peristalsis, intact mucous membranes, and the normal intestinal flora all act to prevent invasion. Anything interfering with these defenses increases the risk for more severe infection.

Cellular and humoral immunity also appears to interfere with invasion of *Salmonella,* and persons with an impaired immune system are more susceptible to systemic disease with *Salmonella.* In addition, systemic focal lesions most commonly appear in those tissues that are damaged or devitalized or in those persons with altered immune systems.

Table 15-11 Overview of Salmonellosis

Occurrence	Worldwide; classified as a food-borne disease; small outbreaks in institutions; 5 million cases per year in United States; increasing
Etiologic agent	2000 serotypes of *Salmonella,* a bacterium
Reservoir	Humans and domestic and wild animals, particularly chickens
Transmission	Ingestion of food contaminated with feces from an infected person or animal; ingestion of meat and animal products, including eggs; handling infected animals; fecal-oral contact
Incubation period	6-72 hours; usually 12-36 hours
Period of communicability	Throughout infection; days to weeks; temporary carrier state may continue up to 1 year
Susceptibility and resistance	General; increased risk for those with achlorhydria, antacid therapy, gastrointestinal surgery, immunosuppression, and sickle cell disease
Report to local health authority	Mandatory case report

Data from Benenson.[3]

Diagnostic Studies and Findings

Culture, isolation, and identification of fecal specimen: Positive for *Salmonella* during first week

Microscopic examination of fecal specimen: Positive for WBCs

WBC: 10,000 to 15,000 WBC/mm^3

Multidisciplinary Plan[3]

Medications

Antiinfective agents: Used only if systemic disease is present
- Ciprofloxacin, chloramphenicol (Chloromycetin)
- Ampicillin
- Trimethoprim-sulfamethoxazole: For organisms resistant to above drugs

Corticosteroids: Prednisone

General Management

IV fluids and electrolytes; bed rest; hyperalimentation; treatment of complications; avoidance of antispasmodics, laxatives, and salicylates

NURSING CARE

Nursing Assessment

History: Ingestion of undercooked meat or eggs; chicken is a common source

Onset: Acute abdominal symptoms

Gastrointestinal status:
- Acute onset: Abdominal pain, diarrhea, nausea, and vomiting, persisting for several days
- Stool is greenish brown, slimy, watery, and foul smelling; may contain mucus, blood, or WBCs
- Bloody diarrhea more common in children

Body temperature: Low-grade fever to 41° C (105° F); chills; lasting 2 to 7 days

Skin: May have rose spots on trunk

Potential Complications

Intestinal perforation and hemorrhage; endocarditis; meningitis; pneumonia; pyelonephritis; osteomyelitis, especially in those with sickle cell disease; cholecystitis; hepatitis

Fluids and electrolytes: Dehydration: loss of skin turgor, dry mucous membranes, prostration, circulatory collapse, and death are possible, especially in infants

Neurologic system: Vertigo

Respiratory system: Possible cough

Sensory system: May have slight deafness or otitis media

Septicemia with localized infection: Symptoms depend on site of systemic lesions; symptoms of appendicitis, cholecystitis, peritonitis, otitis media, meningitis, pneumonia, osteomyelitis, pyelonephritis, cystitis, and endocarditis

Septicemia without localized infection: Intermittent fever; chills; anorexia; weight loss

Patient Problems/Nursing Diagnoses & Interventions

NIC Risk Management

Risk for infection (patient contacts) related to presence of *Salmonella* in stool and urine

- Collect blood, stool, or urine specimen. *Incorrect collection and handling of specimens may destroy the pathogen or contaminate the specimen with environmental organisms, interfering with accurate diagnosis and treatment. Improper handling can also contaminate the health-care worker.*
- Administer antiinfective therapy as ordered. Initiate universal blood and body secretion precautions and other isolation procedures as indicated. *Antiinfective therapy and isolation procedures should be initiated as soon as possible to prevent transmission to health-care workers, other patients, and patient contacts.*
- Employ standard precautions (see Box 15-2, p. 1086) for duration of diarrhea with salmonellosis *to prevent transmission.*
- Use protective isolation procedures as indicated. Prevent patient exposure to infected visitors or staff. Limit visitors, if necessary *to limit the exposure of patients to additional pathogens.*
- Participate in follow-up of patient contacts *to ensure that they are examined and treated.*
- Report all *Salmonella* infections to the local health authority. *Reporting is required by law to facilitate public health monitoring and control of outbreaks.*
- Teach safe food handling practices, proper hygiene, nutritional and fluid requirements, and hand washing after defecating or handling raw foods or feces *to prevent recurrence of infection.*

NIC Thermoregulation

Hyperthermia related to infection

- Monitor body temperature *to detect fever.*
- Administer antipyretics, as ordered.
- Bathe with tepid water or alcohol *to reduce high fever.*
- Adjust environmental temperature *for patient's comfort.*
- Remove excess clothing and bedding *to ensure heat loss.*
- Encourage adequate fluid intake *to compensate for fluid loss associated with elevated body temperature.*
- Do not administer aspirin. *High risk exists for GI hemorrhage with these conditions.*

NIC Elimination Management

Diarrhea related to infection in intestinal tract

Constipation related to invasion of *Salmonella* in intestinal mucosa

Urinary retention related to *Salmonella* in urinary tract

- Measure output *to replace fluids equal to output.*
- Apply heating pad to abdomen *to help cramping (antispasmodic agents should be avoided).*
- Use room deodorizers and adequate ventilation.
- Obtain stool specimen for culture *to detect pathogen present.*
- Wash and lubricate skin around anal opening frequently *to prevent irritation and skin breakdown.*
- Observe stool *to detect blood.*
- Monitor for signs of perforation and hemorrhage *for immediate medical intervention.*
- Check for and prevent abdominal distention. *Unresolved distention adds to the risk of perforation of the intestines.*
- Administer small low enema or glycerin suppositories, as ordered (do not give laxatives), *to relieve distention.*
- Monitor for bladder distention. Measure output *to detect urinary retention.*
- Catheterize if necessary *to empty bladder.*

NIC Electrolyte and Acid-Base Management

Risk for deficient fluid volume related to vomiting and diarrhea

- Assess for symptoms of dehydration (e.g., oliguria and loss of skin turgor) *to intervene early.*
- Give oral fluids as tolerated *to maintain adequate intake.*
- Administer IV fluids and electrolytes as prescribed *to provide for rehydration.* (Once circulation is stabilized, the initial rate of IV infusion and type of IV electrolytes may be altered.)
- Measure all fluid output (emesis, urine, diarrhea). Measure all intake *to ensure that fluid intake compensates for output.*

Patient Education/Continuum of Care Plan[25]

Provide patient with the following information:

1. This condition is transmitted by contaminated food or direct fecal-oral route
2. This condition is communicable as long as the infective organism is in the feces or urine, which may persist for up to 1 year.
3. Transmission of infection to others can be prevented by hand washing after defecating and urinating and through proper disposal of excretions so as not to contaminate food or water supply.
4. Follow enteric isolation procedures.
5. This disease can be prevented by eating thoroughly cooked food and shellfish, screening food from flies, and other methods listed below.
6. Manage fever with antipyretics, tepid sponge baths, minimal clothing, and by maintaining a cool environment. Avoid chilling and aspirin. Encourage intake of fluids and food as tolerated. Popsicles and soda may appeal to young children.
7. Manage other symptoms with bed rest; avoid laxatives or antispasmodics.
8. Report the following to a physician: signs of dehydration, any bleeding, or recurrence of symptoms.

Important:

9. Scrupulous hand washing after defecation and before and after preparing food is necessary.
10. Family and close contacts should be examined and treated if specimens from them are positive for any *Salmonella* bacilli.
11. All foods of animal origin, including eggs, must be thoroughly cooked; cross-contamination of cooked and uncooked foods must be avoided; and foods must be refrigerated below 8° C (46° F) to avoid infection with *Salmonella.*
12. Frozen meat, particularly poultry, should be defrosted in the refrigerator.
13. All milk should be pasteurized, and water should be chlorinated.
14. Children should be protected from handling pet turtles and should be taught to wash hands after touching any animal.

EVALUATION/PATIENT OUTCOMES

Risk Management: Patient is free of infection and complications of *Salmonella.* Vital signs are within normal limits. Blood, stool, or urine cultures are negative for *Salmonella.* Blood count is within normal limits. Hemorrhage has been avoided.

Infection is not transmitted to patient's contacts. Patient care staff members wash hands after providing care to each patient and follow standard precautions with all patients. Patient or family describes transmission of the pathogen and demonstrates proper procedures for handling infective materials and proper hand washing and other behaviors necessary to prevent transmission. Infection has been reported to local health department. Patient contacts have been examined and treated. Patient completes full course of antiinfective therapy.

Thermoregulation: Body temperature is maintained within the normal range; comfort and safety are maintained. Body temperature is between 36° and 38° C (96.8° and 100.4° F). Pulse and respiration are normal. Skin is cool to touch and free of excess perspiration. Patient's clothing and bedding are dry. Patient is free of headache and malaise associated with fever.

Elimination Management: Patient returns to normal pattern of bowel elimination. Patient eats without nausea, vomiting, or abdominal distention. Stools are soft, formed, and brown. Abdomen is soft and nondistended. No cramping or pain occurs.

Patient experiences relief from constipation. Patient has bowel movement at least every 3 days. Stools are soft and pass easily.

Urine is eliminated and patient resumes normal voiding pattern. There is no bladder distention. Urine output equals fluid intake.

Electrolyte and Acid-Base Management: Fluid and electrolyte balance are maintained. Skin turgor is good. Mucous membranes are moist. Urine output is normal. Secretions are thin. Blood levels of sodium, potassium, chloride, magnesium, and calcium are normal. Urine specific gravity is normal.

HEPATITIS

VIRAL HEPATITIS

Viral hepatitis refers to several distinct infections of the liver, each caused by a different hepatitis virus. Depending on the etiologic agent, the diseases differ in their mode of transmission and in their immunologic, pathologic, and clinical characteristics. Treatment is similar for each disease, but prevention and control vary greatly.

To date, six types of primary hepatitis viruses have been identified. These are hepatitis A, B, C, D, E, and G. Hepatitis G is rare, accounting for about 0.3% of acute viral hepatitis. Little more is known at this time. Hepatitis types A to E are summarized in Table 15-12. Hepatitis can also occur as a secondary infection during the course of diseases associated with cytomegalovirus, Epstein-Barr, herpes simplex, varicella-zoster, coxsackievirus B, and rubella viruses.

PATHOPHYSIOLOGY

Although the etiologic agents, mode of transmission, and course of the disease vary with each type of hepatitis, the pathologic condition produced in the liver is similar with all types. The similarities in pathologic findings for each type are presented first, followed by the variations.

The hepatitis virus, regardless of its type, invades, replicates, and produces damage only in the liver. Inflammation and mononuclear cell infiltration in the parenchyma and portal ducts, hepatic cell necrosis, proliferation of Kupffer's cells, cellular collapse, and accumulation of necrotic debris in the lobules and portal ducts all act to produce architectural changes in the lobules and portal ducts. The result is disturbance in bilirubin excretion.

Cellular regeneration and mitosis are usually concurrent with hepatocyte necrosis; complete regeneration usually occurs within 2 to 3 months. Failure of the liver cells to regenerate while the necrotic process progresses results in a severe, fulminant, frequently fatal hepatitis. This occurs more often in hepatitis B. Continuation of the inflammatory response and necrosis, also more common in types B, C, and E, result in active chronic or persistent chronic hepatitis. In active chronic hepatitis the necrotic process, fibrosis, and architectural destruction continue throughout the hepatic lobes and portal ducts. In persistent chronic hepatitis the inflammatory process is limited to the portal tracts with little or no evidence of hepatocellular necrosis. All types of hepatitis may be present with or without icterus and may have a clinical severity ranging from subclinical infection to acute fulminating disease. All types stimulate an antibody response specific to the type of virus causing the disease.

The identification of serologic markers for type-specific virus antigens and antibodies has been important in the diagnosis, prevention, and control of viral hepatitis. The standard nomenclature and abbreviation with characteristics and implications are presented here for easy reference (Table 15-13).

Hepatitis A virus (HAV) is acquired by ingestion of the HAV in food, water, or uncooked shellfish contaminated with feces containing the virus or by direct fecal-oral transmission. The virus localizes in the liver, replicates, enters the bile, and is

Table 15-12 Overview of Viral Hepatitis

	Hepatitis A	Hepatitis B	Hepatitis C	Hepatitis D	Hepatitis E
Occurrence	Worldwide; sporadic and epidemic, with a tendency toward cyclic recurrence; outbreaks in institutions	Worldwide; endemic; highest in young adults, homosexual men, heterosexuals with multiple sex partners, parenteral drug users, and health-care and public safety workers	Worldwide; 20% of cases of hepatitis; since screening of blood donors <2% associated with transfusions	Worldwide; occurs epidemically and endemically in populations at risk for HBV infection	Epidemic and sporadic cases, particularly in developing countries; highest in young adults; rare in children or elderly
Etiologic agent	Hepatitis A virus (HAV)	Hepatitis B virus (HBV)	Hepatitis C virus (HCV)	A viruslike particle (HDV, or the delta agent); coinfects with HBV	Viruslike particle (HEV)
Reservoir	Humans and captive primates	Humans and possibly captive primates	Humans; experimentally transmitted to chimpanzees	Humans, chimpanzees	Unknown; possible nonhuman reservoirs
Transmission	Person to person by fecal-oral route; contaminated food, water, shellfish	Direct and indirect contact with blood and serum-derived fluids such as vaginal secretions, saliva, and semen; sexual contact; perinatal	Parenteral; person-to-person and sexual and perinatal transmission have not been defined	Similar to HBV, including sexual contact	Contaminated water; person to person by fecal-oral route
Incubation period	15-50 days; average: 28-30 days	45-180 days; average: 60-90 days	2 weeks to 6 months; commonly 6-9 weeks	2-10 weeks	15-64 days; average: 26-42 days
Period of communicability	Latter half of incubation period to 1 week after onset of jaundice	During incubation period and throughout clinical course of disease; carrier state may persist for years	From 1 or more weeks before symptom onset, indefinitely during chronic and carrier states	Throughout acute and chronic disease	Not known; detected in stool 14 days after onset of jaundice
Susceptibility and resistance	General; usually affects children and young adults; immunity after infection probably lasts for life	All age groups; disease is mild in children; lifetime immunity follows infection if antibody to HBsAg develops and HBsAg is negative	General; all age groups; degree of immunity following infection is unknown	All persons susceptible to hepatitis B (HB), HBV carriers; disease is severe in children	Unknown; no explanation for epidemics among young adults; pregnant women in third trimester susceptible to fulminating disease
Report to local health authority	Mandatory case report	Mandatory case report	Mandatory case report	Mandatory case report	Mandatory case report

Data from Benenson[3] and Centers for Disease Control and Prevention.[8]

carried to the intestinal tract, where it is shed in the feces. Fecal shedding occurs late in the incubation period, usually before onset of clinical symptoms. Antibodies develop during acute disease and later during convalescence. Hepatitis A does not lead to chronic disease or the carrier state.

Hepatitis B virus (HBV) is viable in blood and in secretions containing serum (oozing cutaneous lesions) or derived from serum (e.g., saliva, semen, and vaginal secretions). Transmission may be by one of five routes: (1) direct percutaneous inoculation of infective serum or plasma by needle or transfusion of infective blood or blood products; (2) indirect percutaneous introduction of infective serum or plasma, such as through minute skin cuts or abrasions; (3) absorption of infective serum or plasma through mucosal surfaces, such as those of the mouth or eye; (4) absorption of other potentially infective secretions, such as saliva or semen through mucosal surfaces, as might occur during vaginal, anal, or oral sexual contact; and (5) transfer of infective serum or plasma via inanimate environmental surfaces

Table 15-13 Standard Nomenclature, Abbreviations, and Characteristics of Hepatitis Virus Antigens and Antibodies

Abbreviation	Term	Characteristics and Implications
HAV	Hepatitis A virus	Etiologic agent
Anti-HAV	Antibody to HAV	Detectable at onset of symptoms and persists for lifetime; probably confers lifetime immunity
IgM	Immunoglobulin M (antibody to HAV)	The anti-HAV is present early in the infection; it represents current infection and is used to establish the diagnosis; serum levels drop during convalescence and disappear in 4-6 months
IgG	Immunoglobulin G (antibody to HAV)	The anti-HAV that develops late in the infection and persists for years; its presence in serum indicates past infection and present immunity
HBV	Hepatitis B virus	Etiologic agent of hepatitis B (HB)
HBsAG	Hepatitis B surface antigen	Surface coat of HB virus; large quantities detectable in serum 2-7 weeks before and during acute clinical disease, during chronic disease, and in carriers; its presence indicates infectious blood
HBeAg	Hepatitis B antigen	Soluble antigen that correlates with HBV replication; indicates a high titer of HBV in serum and consequent infectivity of serum; it rises 2-7 weeks before clinical disease onset and usually drops before acute disease; its persistence is associated with progression to chronic hepatitis; found only in HBsAg-positive serum
HBcAg	Hepatitis B core antigen	Part of HB virus; found in liver cells; cannot be detected in sera with present technology
Anti-HBs	Antibody to HBsAG	Rises in serum during convalescence; its presence indicates immunity to HBV from past infection, passive antibody from HBIG, or active immune response from HBV vaccine
Anti-HBe	Antibody to HBeAg	Its presence in serum of person with continuing levels of HBeAg suggests chronic presence of HBV and infectivity of blood
Anti-HBc	Antibody to HBcAg	Appears at disease onset and increases during clinical disease, peaks during convalescence, and persists for years; presence indicates current or past infection with HBV
IGM anti-HBc	IGM antibody to HBcAg	Presence indicates current or recent infection with HBV; positive for 4-6 months after infection
IG	Immunoglobulin	Formerly called immune serum globulin (ISG) or gamma globulin; given before and within 2 weeks after exposure to HAV and HCV
HBIG	Hepatitis B immune globulin	Contains a higher titer of HB immune globulins than does IG; preferred for use after exposure to HBV
HB vaccine	Hepatitis B vaccine	Inactivated vaccine prepared from carriers of HBsAg; stimulates production of anti-HBs; series of three injections recommended for those at risk for hepatitis B
HCV	Hepatitis C virus	Etiologic agent of hepatitis C
Anti-HCV	Antibody to HCV	Presence indicates acute or chronic infection; positive antibody test with negative test for HCV-RNA antigen may indicate clearance of infection
HDV	Hepatitis D virus	Etiologic agent of delta hepatitis; may only cause infection in presence of HBV infection
HDAg	Delta antigen	Detectable in early, acute delta infections
Anti-HDV	Antibody to delta antigen	Indicates past or present infection with delta antigen
HEV	Hepatitis E virus	Etiologic agent of hepatitis E
Anti-HEV	Antibody to HEV	IgM rises during acute infection and declines during convalescence; IgG rises during acute infection and persists, possibly conferring immunity

Data from Benenson[3] and Centers for Disease Control.[5,12,18]

or possibly vectors. Fecal transmission of HBV does not occur. HBV may be transmitted transplacentally, or the infant may become contaminated at birth with the mother's infective blood.

HBV is composed of three antigens: the core antigen (HbcAg), an outer surface antigen (HbsAg), and a soluble antigen (HbeAg). HBV antigens infect the blood within 30 to 60 days of exposure to HBV and are at their peak before disease onset. They persist for varying lengths of time, and their presence is useful for determining the course of the disease and the carrier state. Antibodies specific for the antigens develop at different times during convalescence. Detection of serum antibodies is useful for predicting the course of the disease and for determining immune status.

Hepatitis C virus (HCV) is a parenterally transmitted hepatitis virus causing a disease similar to hepatitis B (i.e., prolonged incubation period, insidious onset, and potential chronicity). A test for the antibody has recently been developed and is used for screening blood donors and for confirming infection.

Hepatitis D virus (HDV), a viruslike particle called the delta agent, is pathogenic only with HBV, causing coinfection with the HBV or superimposing infection on an inapparent HBV carrier state. Prolongation or an increase in severity of an HBV infection may be attributable to the delta agent.

Hepatitis E virus (HEV) is an enterically transmitted hepatitis virus that causes disease with a clinical course similar to hepatitis A (i.e., shorter incubation period, acute onset, and complete recovery). Disease may be more severe in pregnant women, particularly in the third trimester. A serologic test for HEV antibodies has been developed but is not currently available in the United States.

DIAGNOSTIC STUDIES AND FINDINGS[3,26]

Liver Function Tests

Serum enzymes: Asparate aminotransferase (AST, SGOT) and alanine transaminase (ALT, SGPT): elevated during clinical disease, indicators of liver damage, peak at onset of jaundice and fall during recovery, persisting for months; alkaline phosphatase; elevated; lactic dehydrogenase (LDH): elevated; creatine phosphokinase (CPK): normal

Serum bilirubin: Elevated

Prothrombin time: Normal; elevated only in severe fulminating hepatitis

VDRL: False positive

Hepatitis A

Examination of stool specimen: Positive for HAV 2 weeks before illness to several days after onset of symptoms, then is negative; HAV may be absent from stool by time patient is hospitalized

Serology: Fourfold rise in anti-HAV antibodies between early disease and convalescence; identification of IgM antibodies during early disease indicates present infection; peak at 3 months and then drop; IgG peaks after clinical disease and persists for life; high IgG levels indicate past infection and present immunity

Hepatitis B

Serum antigen tests: Detect HBeAg and HBsAg in serum 1 to 2 weeks after exposure and 2 to 7 weeks before onset of clinical disease; peak and begin to drop during clinical disease; HBsAg remains in serum of chronic carriers for life; positive tests indicate present infection or carrier state; positive test in carrier with disease symptoms may misdiagnose infection with other hepatitis viruses; HBcAg cannot be detected with present technology

Serum antibody tests: Anti-HBc increases during clinical disease and peaks during convalescence; indicates past or present infection; may be detected in person who has received immunoglobulin (IG); anti-HBe begins rising during convalescence; both persist and gradually decrease over time; anti-HBs rises rapidly during late convalescence and persists; carriers are always HBeAg positive and/or HBsAg positive and anti-HBs negative

Hepatitis C

Serum antigen tests: Detect HCV serum antibody; used to detect anti-HCV in blood donors

Hepatitis D: Serum antibody: to detect anti-HDV

Hepatitis E: Diagnosis by exclusion of other causes of hepatitis; tests are available in research laboratories only

MULTIDISCIPLINARY PLAN[3,5,12,18]

Medications

There is no direct chemotherapeutic treatment for acute viral hepatitis; however, supportive medications may be used for fulminating hepatitis

Alpha interferon is used for treatment of chronic hepatitis B; interferon or interferon with ribavirin is used for hepatitis C.

Immunologic Agents

Hepatitis A: Hepatitis A vaccine (Havrix) provides protection within 14 to 30 days of administration: for persons over 18 years of age: 1440 EL.U. per dose in two doses (second dose 6-12 months after the first)

Immunologic agent for rapid, but short-term protection: Immune globulin (IG), 0.02 ml/kg in a single dose intramuscularly (IM)

Immunologic agent for prolonged travel: Immune globulin (IG), 0.06 ml/kg IM in a single dose

Hepatitis B: Preexposure prophylaxis against HBV for high-risk persons (e.g., health-care workers, hemodialysis patients, multiple sexual partners, and household and sexual contacts of HBV carriers) (Table 15-14)

For postexposure prophylaxis see Table 15-15.

General Management

For nonfulminating hepatitis: Hospitalization for those with bilirubin concentrations greater than 10 mg/dl or greater than 10 times normal and for those with a prolonged prothrombin time; bed rest until symptoms subside; diet as tolerated; small, frequent, low-fat, high-carbohydrate feedings may be better tolerated; symptomatic treatment for nausea (avoid chlorpromazine); symptomatic treatment for pain (acetaminophen preferred over aspirin); avoid all unnecessary medications, particularly sedatives

For fulminating hepatitis: Hospitalization and bed rest; low-protein diet; 20 to 30 mg protein per day; enemas; discontinue any sedatives; IV fluids and electrolytes; central venous pressure line; nasogastric tube feedings; urinary catheter; fresh frozen plasma to correct coagulation defects

NURSING CARE

NURSING ASSESSMENT

History: Sexual contact with multiple or unknown partners; homosexual contact; household contact with person with hepatitis; injection drug abuse; unimmunized for HB; blood transfusion (prior to 1992 in United States); tatoos or body piercing

Onset: Within 2 to 7 weeks of exposure for HA; within 6 weeks to 6 months for HB; within 2 weeks to 6 months for HC

Preicteric Phase (3 to 10 Days)

Subjective symptoms: Malaise, weakness, dull headache, anorexia, intermittent nausea and vomiting, myalgias, chills; right, upper quadrant abdominal pain

Body temperature: 38° to 40° C (100.4° to 104° F) for hepatitis A; low-grade fever or normal for hepatitis B and C

Skin: For hepatitis B; urticarial pruritic hives, maculopapular lesions, or fleeting, irregular patches of erythema in some patients; multiple forearm pricks in drug users; exacerbation of acne; excoriations with severe pruritus

Musculoskeletal status: For hepatitis B: mild to moderate non-deforming polyarticular arthritis (migratory, affecting elbows, wrists, knees, and small joints of hands)

Abdomen: Bowel sounds normal; slightly enlarged, tender liver (9-13 cm), edges smooth, regular, and firm

Table 15-14 Recommended Doses of Currently Licensed Hepatitis B Vaccines

Group	Recombivax HB* Dose (μg)	Recombivax HB* (ml)	Engerix-B* Dose (μg)	Engerix-B* (ml)
Infants of HBsAg†-negative mothers and children <11 years	2.5	(0.25)	10	(0.5)
Infants of HBsAg-positive mothers; prevention of perinatal infection	5	(0.5)	10	(0.5)
Children and adolescents 11-19 years	5	(0.5)	20	(1.0)
Adults ≥20 years	10	(1.0)	20	(1.0)
Dialysis patients and other immunocompromised persons	40	(1.0)‡	40	(2.0)§

From Centers for Disease Control and Prevention.[5]
*Both vaccines are routinely administered in a three-dose series. Engerix-B has also been licensed for a four-dose series administered at 0, 1, 2, and 12 months.
†*HBsAg,* Hepatitis B surface antigen.
‡Special formulation.
§Two 1.0-ml doses administered at one site in a four-dose schedule at 0, 1, 2, and 6 months.

Table 15-15 Postexposure Prophylaxis Recommendations

HEPATITIS B PROPHYLAXIS FOLLOWING PERCUTANEOUS OR PERMUCOSAL EXPOSURE

Exposed Person	Treatment When Source Is Found to Be: HBsAg-Positive	HBsAg-Negative	Source Not Tested or Unknown
Unvaccinated	HBIG × 1* and initiate HB vaccine†	Initiate HB vaccine†	Initiate HB vaccine†
Previously vaccinated known responder	Test exposed for anti-HBs 1. If adequate,‡ no treatment 2. If inadequate, HB vaccine booster dose	No treatment	No treatment
Known nonresponder	HBIG × 2 or HBIG × 1 + 1 dose HB vaccine	No treatment	If known high-risk source, may treat as if source were HBsAg-positive
Response unknown	Test exposed for anti-HBs 1. If inadequate,‡ HBIG × 1 + HB vaccine booster dose 2. If adequate, no treatment	No treatment	Test exposed person for anti-HBs 1. If inadequate,‡ HB vaccine booster dose 2. If adequate, no treatment

*HBIG dose 0.06 ml/kg IM.
†HB vaccine dose—see Table 15-4.
‡Adequate anti-HBs is 10 milli-international units.
Data from Centers for Disease Control and Prevention.[5,14]

Icteric Phase (Bilirubin Greater Than 2.5 mg/dl; Lasts 1 to 3 Weeks)

Subjective symptoms: Nausea and vomiting frequently abate and appetite returns, but symptoms may worsen; malaise continues

Skin: Jaundice with or without pruritus may be present or absent; can be observed under the tongue

Eyes: Scleral icterus

Urine: Dark

Stools: May be clay colored

Vital signs: Normal, although there may be a bradycardia with severe hyperbilirubinemia

Body temperature: Normal or low grade

POTENTIAL COMPLICATIONS

Fulminant hepatitis with encephalopathy
- Level of consciousness
  - Patient becomes lethargic and somnolent with personality changes; may show mild confusion, sexual or aggressive activity, loss of usual inhibitions
  - Lethargy may alternate with excitability, euphoria, or unruly behavior
  - Worsening of the condition leads to stupor and eventual coma
  - An early sign is asterixis (the irregular flapping of forcibly dorsiflexed, outstretched hands)
- Circulatory system: Prothrombin time is prolonged; abdominal bleeding; epistaxis; prolonged bleeding from puncture sites; blood in vomitus, stool, or urine; easy bruising

Chronic hepatitis infection

Hepatic carcinoma

PATIENT PROBLEMS/NURSING DIAGNOSES & INTERVENTIONS

NIC RISK MANAGEMENT

Risk for infection (patient contacts) related to presence of HAV in feces and HBV and HBC in blood and body fluids

Ineffective tissue perfusion related to hemorrhage

Risk for acute confusion related to encephalopathy

- Collect fecal or blood specimens as required. *Specimens must be handled correctly so as not to destroy or transmit the virus.*
- Employ contact precautions for 7 days after onset of jaundice for hepatitis A. Employ standard precautions for all patients (see Box 15-2, p. 1086).
- Ensure that all patient contacts, including health-care personnel, are protected against hepatitis.
- Monitor and report signs of bleeding. Provide care as warranted by bleeding *for early detection and intervention for coagulation and bleeding problems.*
- Monitor and report signs of encephalopathy as were described under Nursing Assessment.
- Monitor and report progression of icterus.
- Provide care as warranted by patient's level of consciousness. *These are severe signs of the progression of the disease; these patients require protection from injury and may require life support.*

NIC ACTIVITY AND EXERCISE MANAGEMENT

Activity intolerance related to decreased energy metabolism by liver

- Maintain bed rest during acute symptoms *to conserve energy and avoid unnecessary stress to the liver.* (Patients activities need not be limited during convalescence.)
- Do necessary tests and procedures at one time *to allow for uninterrupted rest.*

NIC NUTRITIONAL SUPPORT

Imbalanced nutrition: less than body requirements, related to anorexia, nausea and vomiting, and altered digestion of food

- Encourage frequent small feedings as patient tolerates; largest meal in morning. *Anorexia frequently worsens as day progresses.*
- Provide high-carbohydrate, low-fat feedings *to provide easily digested meals.*
- Administer nasogastric tube feedings for patients with hepatic encephalopathy and coma; administer IV fluids for patients with persistent vomiting or for those with hepatic encephalopathy, as ordered, *to avoid aspiration while ensuring adequate intake of food and fluids.*
- Offer hard candy *to soothe nausea.*

NIC ELECTROLYTE AND ACID-BASE MANAGEMENT

Deficient fluid volume related to failure of regulatory mechanisms

- Monitor fluid intake and output and laboratory values *to detect fluid and electrolyte imbalance.*
- Provide frequent high-carbohydrate fluids, as tolerated, during acute symptoms *to compensate for fluid loss with vomiting and diarrhea.*

PATIENT EDUCATION/CONTINUUM OF CARE PLAN[25]

1. Educate patient about disease and disease transmission. Emphasize self-limited nature of most episodes of hepatitis but need for follow-up of liver function tests and serum HBsAg.
2. Follow-up serology in 1 or 2 months is necessary for all hepatitis B patients to determine the presence or absence of HBsAg.
3. Patients should follow precautions with blood and secretions until they are determined to be free of HBsAg. Close personal contacts should be examined and receive HBIG or HB vaccine.
4. HBV carriers should be aware that their blood and secretions are infectious. Close contacts of HBV carriers should receive HB vaccine. Carriers should not share razors or toothbrushes and must be cautious in handling cuts and lacerations. HBV carriers and patients with a history of HCV should not donate blood.
5. Patients caring for themselves at home during acute stage of disease should avoid alcohol and any nonprescribed medications, particularly sedatives and aspirin.
6. Severity of symptoms can determine patterns for bed rest and diet. Frequent, small feedings of low-fat, high-carbohydrate foods may be better tolerated; however, it is not necessary to limit diet in any way.
7. Liver function tests should be monitored until normal.
8. Hepatitis A patients must wash hands thoroughly following toileting, must disinfect articles soiled with feces (boil 1 minute), and must not prepare foods for others during symptomatic disease. They should avoid sharing items such as eating utensils, toothbrushes, and toys.
9. Sexual activity should be avoided during acute stage of hepatitis B and C. Ideally hepatitis B patients should not resume sexual activity until tests for HBsAg are negative or until partner has received HB vaccine or HBIG if HB vaccine is unavailable.

EVALUATION/PATIENT OUTCOMES

Risk Management: Infection is not transmitted. Patient returns for examination to determine when serum HBsAg and HBeAg tests are negative. Close, personal contacts of hepatitis patients have received HBIG and HB vaccine or IG vaccine for hepatitis A.

Patient is knowledgeable about need for follow-up, means of preventing transmission to others, and convalescent self-care. Items listed in Patient Education/Continuum of Care Plan are met.

Infection resolves without complications. There is no icterus. Patient has full appetite and energy and has no right upper quadrant abdominal pain. Urine and stool are normal colored. There are no changes in personality or level of consciousness. SGPT (ALT), SGOT (AST), alkaline phosphatase, LDH, serum bilirubin, and prothrombin time are all within normal limits.

Activity and Exercise Management: Patient achieves adequate rest during active disease and returns to preillness level of activity during convalescence. Extended periods of uninterrupted sleep are experienced. Patient has gradually increasing amounts of energy without relapses of extreme fatigue.

Nutritional Support: Adequate calorie intake and nutritional status are maintained; weight is stable. Patient has full appetite and energy. Weight is at preillness state. RBC counts are normal.

Electrolyte and Acid-Base Management: Fluid and electrolyte balance is maintained. Fluid intake equals output. The urine is straw colored. Specific gravity, sodium, and albumin levels are within normal limits. Skin turgor is normal; no ascites or edema.

INFECTIOUS DISEASES OF THE HEMATOLYMPHATIC SYSTEM

The infectious diseases grouped here produce either primary pathologic findings in the lymphatic system or disseminated infection with lymphadenopathy as part of the clinical picture (Table 15-16).

MONONUCLEOSIS

Mononucleosis is an acute viral infectious disease that produces a generalized lymph node hyperplasia and is characterized by fever, exudative pharyngitis, lymphadenopathy, and splenomegaly.

PATHOPHYSIOLOGY

The Epstein-Barr virus (EBV) is transmitted in saliva by prolonged direct contact, probably through kissing with salivary exchange. The pathogen invades B lymphocytes in lymphatic tissue and stimulates the development of a surface membrane antigen on the infected lymphocytes. T lymphocytes actively proliferate in response to the antigen and produce a generalized lymph node hyperplasia. Atypical T lymphocytes infiltrate the spleen, tonsils, lungs, heart, liver, kidneys, adrenal glands, central nervous system, and skin. The circulating T cells are not infective and therefore do not produce necrosis in these systems. Their infiltration causes enlargement, particularly of the spleen, and disturbs functioning of those organs.

The severity of the disease varies from asymptomatic disease (usually in children) to severe systemic and localized organ involvement. Lymphadenopathy, splenomegaly, and exudative pharyngitis are characteristic. More serious manifestations of the disease include hepatitis, pneumonitis, and central nervous system involvement. Possible sequelae include Burkitt's lymphoma, nasal pharyngeal carcinoma, and other malignancies.

Saliva remains infective for 18 months despite the development of EBV-specific antibodies early in the disease. The virus can be cultured from the throats of 10% to 20% of normal, healthy adults, suggesting that the disease may be contracted from asymptomatic viral shedders.

Potential Complications

Splenic rupture; hemolytic anemia; agranulocytosis; thrombocytopenic purpura; pericarditis; orchitis; encephalitis; seizures; Guillain-Barré syndrome; hepatitis

DIAGNOSTIC STUDIES AND FINDINGS[3,26]

Differential white blood cell count: Lymphocytes and monocytes greater than 50% with more than 10% being atypical lymphocytes; decreased platelets

Leukocyte count: Normal early in disease; rises to 12,000 to 20,000/mm^3 in second week; occasionally rises to 50,000/mm^3

Table 15-16 Overview of Hematolymphatic Infectious Diseases

	Mononucleosis	Cytomegalovirus Infections	Toxoplasmosis
Occurrence	Worldwide; highest in adolescents and young adults in developed countries; asymptomatic infection in children	Worldwide; many asymptomatic infections; congenital infection may be severe	Worldwide; common in humans, mammals, and birds; many asymptomatic infections; congenital infection may be severe
Etiologic agent	Epstein-Barr virus (EBV), one of the herpesviruses	Cytomegalovirus (CMV)—one of the herpesviruses	*Toxoplasma gondii,* a protozoan
Reservoir	Humans and possibly primates	Humans	Cats; other mammals and birds are intermediate hosts
Transmission	Direct contact with saliva; through blood transfusions	Direct contact with secretions and excretions (blood, urine, saliva, semen, breast milk, and cervical secretions) and transplacentally	Transplacental if mother has active infection; eating infective meat; water contaminated with cat feces
Incubation period	4-6 weeks	Unknown; 3-8 weeks following transplantation or transfusion; in neonate, 3-12 weeks following delivery-produced infection	Unknown; probably 5-23 days depending on mode of transmission
Period of communicability	Prolonged; pharyngeal excretion may persist for years; 15%-20% of EBV antibody-positive adults are long-term oropharyngeal carriers	Virus excreted in saliva and urine for months to years	Not directly transmitted except transplacentally; cysts in infected meat remain infective as long as meat is edible and uncooked
Susceptibility and resistance	General; infection confers a high degree of resistance	General; fetuses, immunosuppressed individuals, organ allograft recipients, and those with other chronic disease have more severe symptoms	General, but risk for infection increases with age; immunity after infection persists indefinitely
Report to local health authority	No	No	In some states

Data from Benenson.[3]

Serology: Elevated heterophile antibody titer (with compatible mononucleosis symptoms) is sufficient for diagnosis; rapid forms of test are monospot, monoscreen, or monotest.

Liver function tests: Serum transaminases (AST [SGOT], ALT [SGPT]): all elevated in hepatic involvement; bilirubin: elevated if there is hepatic involvement

MULTIDISCIPLINARY PLAN[1,3]

Surgery

For splenic rupture: surgical removal of the spleen

Medications

Corticosteroids: Sometimes used for severe neurologic complications, airway obstruction, thrombocytopenic purpura, or hemolytic anemia

General Management

Bed rest during acute stage; saline throat gargle; aspirin or acetaminophen for sore throat and fever

NURSING CARE

NURSING ASSESSMENT

See p. 1044.

CYTOMEGALOVIRUS INFECTIONS

Cytomegalovirus infections are extremely common viral infections that are ordinarily asymptomatic. Clinical disease in the adult resembles mononucleosis. Congenital and perinatal acquired infections are serious in the neonate and lead to irreversible central nervous system damage.

PATHOPHYSIOLOGY

The cytomegalovirus (CMV), with several antigenically related strains, is a member of the herpesvirus group and has characteristics common to other herpesviruses. Like the Epstein-Barr herpesvirus, CMV produces a frequently asymptomatic mononucleosis type of infection in children and adults. CMV is similar to herpes types 1 and 2 in that it remains latent in body tissue and has the potential for producing recurrent infection. CMV, like herpes 1 and 2, also crosses the placental barrier and is shed in cervical secretions. Therefore it has the potential for producing congenital infection with severe congenital anomalies and perinatal infection acquired during vaginal delivery. Like Epstein-Barr and herpes 2, the CMV is suspected of having oncogenic properties.

CMV can be found in all body secretions, including saliva, blood, urine, semen, cervical secretions, and breast milk, even in the presence of CMV-specific antibodies. Transmission requires prolonged direct contact with secretions. Although the exact mechanism for postnatal transmission is not known, sexual, oral, blood transfusion, and renal and bone marrow transplant transmission are modes of transmission.

Regardless of the mode of transmission, CMV may invade the cells of most tissues in the body. An inflammatory response with focal tissue destruction, areas of calcification, and hyperplasia of the reticuloendothelial system develops. These lesions occur widely, particularly in the brain, liver, lungs, kidney, and spleen.

A humoral and cell-mediated anti-CMV antibody response occurs. The response does not appear to alter the course of the spread of the virus from cell to cell or alter the presence of the virus in body secretions. Nor do circulating maternal antibodies in the fetus appear to impede the infectious process or the development of congenital anomalies.

The disease may be asymptomatic, or there may be symptoms of liver and lung involvement or a mononucleosis-like syndrome. There is no evidence of chronic organ impairment in acquired CMV infections. Primary or reactivation infection can be severe and life threatening in the immunosuppressed individual.

DIAGNOSTIC STUDIES AND FINDINGS[26]

Culture of specimen of urine, saliva, throat washings, blood, or biopsy tissue (lung, kidney, spleen, liver, brain, and retina): Positive for specific cytopathic effect of CMV; presence of CMV in infant's urine at birth suggests congenital infection

Microscopic examination of biopsy of liver tissue: Histologic evidence of typical inclusion bodies

Serology: Elevated IgM titer in adults suggests current infection. Elevated IgG suggests current or past infection.

Serum transaminase (AST): Elevated in CMV hepatitis

Platelets: May be as few as 5000/mm^3

Differential WBC count: Increase in lymphocytes, many atypical

Differential diagnosis: heterophil agglutination: Negative in CMV (positive in mononucleosis)

MULTIDISCIPLINARY PLAN[1]

Medications

Ganciclovir, foscarnet, acyclovir (alone or in combination) for treatment of CMV retinitis and other severe disease manifestations; dosages vary depending on the severity of the infection and the immune status of the patient

For bone marrow transplantation recipients: Ganciclovir plus CMV hyperimmune globulin

General Management

Transfusion of packed RBCs for anemia

Transfusion of platelet-rich plasma for thrombocytopenia

Antipyretics for fever in CMV mononucleosis-like syndrome

Experimental live CMV vaccines currently being evaluated for prevention

Infants born of antibody-free mothers should not receive breast milk from women serologically positive for CMV antibodies, because the virus may be in the milk

NURSING CARE

NURSING ASSESSMENT

See p. 1044.

Potential Complications

To immunocompromised: Progressive pneumonitis, hemolytic anemia, purpura, GI ulceration, hepatitis, pericarditis, retinitis, and neurologic changes

To neonate infected in utero: Neurologic defects (e.g., microcephaly, psychomotor retardation, and severe mental retardation)

Toxoplasmosis

Toxoplasmosis is a systemic protozoan infection, ranging from subclinical to severe to chronic. Four different clinical syndromes can be identified, depending on where the pathogen localizes in the body. Transplacental transmission results in congenital toxoplasmosis, which may be fatal to the fetus or neonate.

Pathophysiology

Toxoplasmosis, like the CMV infections, may be congenital or acquired. Unlike CMV, there is not a risk for perinatal acquired toxoplasmosis. Both forms of toxoplasmosis may be present, with clinical patterns ranging from subclinical infection to severe generalized infection (with neurologic and sensory sequelae) to death. Both may occur in latent or recurring forms under conditions of reduced host defenses.

The pathogen producing toxoplasmosis, *Toxoplasma gondii,* is a protozoan that is pathogenic to animals and humans and can multiply only in living cells. This parasite exists in three forms: trophozoites, tissue cysts, and oocysts. Trophozoites are capable of invading, multiplying in, and necrotizing all host cells. Trophozoites can remain viable extracellularly in body secretions such as peritoneal fluid, breast milk, urine, saliva, or tears for a few hours to days. They cannot survive drying, heating, freezing, or contact with digestive juices.

Tissue cysts are formed within host cells. A surrounding membrane produced by the pathogen encapsulates up to 3000 organisms. This enables the parasites to maintain their viability for the life of the host in spite of circulating host antibodies. Tissue cysts are responsible for recurrent infection in humans and for transmission of the pathogen from animal reservoirs. Tissue cysts also cannot survive freezing, drying, or heating.

Oocysts are a form in the life cycle of *T. gondii* that occurs only in cats. Oocysts, are discharged in the feces of infected cats. Oocysts sporulate in 1 to 21 days in environmental temperatures of 4° to 37° C (39° to 99° F). They can remain infectious in the soil for 1 year.

Transmission of *T. gondii* can occur by one of two modes: by ingestion of tissue cysts in uncooked meat or ingestion of sporulated oocysts by hands or food contaminated with cat feces, or by transplacental transmission of trophozoites in maternal circulation during acute infection acquired by the mother during the pregnancy.

In ingestion-acquired toxoplasmosis the capsule surrounding ingested cysts is digested by gastric juices. This permits viable trophozoites to invade intestinal mucosa and to disseminate throughout the body by way of blood and the lymphatics. They invade cells, producing inflammation and necrosis. The spleen, liver, brain, lung, myocardium, and eye are most frequently involved. The development of cysts and tissue calcifications may impair organ functioning.

An early antibody response destroys many parasites before they form tissue cysts and supports cyst formation by the remainder. Thus the infection is limited to its mild or subclinical form for the majority of infected persons. Failure of an immune response, as is the case with immunosuppressed patients or those with debilitating disease, is more likely to result in progressive, life-threatening infection with multiple organ involvement and extensive damage.

Transplacentally transmitted *T. gondii* is disseminated to every organ in the developing fetus, particularly in the brain, heart, lungs, adrenal glands, striated muscle, and eye. Focal necrotic and inflammatory lesions are produced with cyst formation and calcification. Extensive destruction may occur in the central nervous system, leading to microcephalus, hydrocephalus, or varying degrees of central nervous system (CNS) impairment.

Infection in the eye produces edema and necrosis of the retina. Chorioretinitis may be manifested within weeks after birth or at some time later in life when the latent infection becomes reactivated.

Maternal infection early in the pregnancy is usually associated with fetal death or severe disease at birth. Infection later in pregnancy results in less severe or no manifestations at birth. Only 11% of maternal infections result in infants damaged at birth. The majority, 60% of infants, are not affected; 29% have subclinical infections that are manifest as neurologic or sensory defects as the infant develops.

Diagnostic Studies and Findings[26]

Microscopic examination of tissue sections or smears: Identification of trophozoites present during acute infection; identification of cysts does not differentiate between acute or chronic infection

Serology: IgM antibodies appear during the first 2 weeks of illness, peak in 4 to 8 weeks, and then decline to undetectable levels; IgG antibodies (1:4) appear within 1 to 2 weeks after acute infection, reach high titers (over 1:1000) in 6 to 8 weeks, and then gradually decline over months or years to titers of 1:4 to 1:64; false-positive results may follow blood transfusions; fourfold rise in titers or slow decline after the peak is diagnostic; may be false negative in immunosuppressed persons

Imaging by computed tomography (CT) scan or magnetic resonance imaging (MRI): Positive for lesion

Multidisciplinary Plan[3]

Medications

Treatment for active chorioretinitis, myocarditis, or other organ involvement: pyrimethamine (Daraprim) combined with sulfadiazine and leucovorin (to avoid bone marrow depression) for 4 weeks; dosages vary depending on age of patient, disease severity, and immune status

In early pregnancy to prevent transplacental transmission: Spiramycin; immunocompromised pregnant women are treated additionally with pyrimethamine and sulfadiazine

General Management

To prevent spread, reject leukocyte or organ donors who are antibody positive

NURSING CARE

NURSING ASSESSMENT

See Assessment Considerations table below.

POTENTIAL COMPLICATIONS

Spontaneous abortion; microcephalus, hydrocephalus, or other CNS impairment in neonate; chorioretinitis; multiple organ involvement in immunocompromised patients; encephalitis

PATIENT PROBLEMS/NURSING DIAGNOSES & INTERVENTIONS

NIC RISK MANAGEMENT

Risk for infection (patient contacts) related to methods of transmission of CMV and mononucleosis

Risk for injury related to splenomegaly and to antiinfective agents prescribed for toxoplasmosis

- Employ standard precautions for all patients (see Box 15-2, p. 1086).
- Women of childbearing age or who are pregnant should wash hands thoroughly after handling diapers of neonates with congenital CMV *to prevent acquiring CMV infection.*
- Monitor for signs of neurologic or purpuric complications *to detect splenic rupture.*
- Protect patient from activity *to reduce risk of splenic rupture.*

NIC THERMOREGULATION

Hyperthermia related to infection with mononucleosis, CMV, or toxoplasmosis

- Monitor body temperature.
- Bathe patient frequently *to lower body temperature and to remove perspiration.*
- Administer oral fluids freely *to compensate for increased needs.*
- Maintain comfortable environmental temperature with freely circulating air.
- Administer antipyretics, as ordered.

Assessment Considerations

	Mononucleosis	Cytomegalovirus Infection	Toxoplasmosis
History	Contact with person with mononucleosis	Immunosuppression	Exposure to cat feces; immunosuppression
Subjective symptoms	Fatigue, anorexia, chills, retroorbital headache, photophobia, dysphagia	Fatigue, nausea, myalgia, headache, photophobia	Fatigue and malaise 6 to 10 days preceding other symptoms; headache; photophobia
Body temperature	Marked elevation (1 to 2 wk) 38° to 41° C (100.4° to 105.8° F), peaks in afternoon	Low-grade fever lasting 2 to 5 weeks	Fever up to 41° C (105.8° F)
Eyes	Periorbital edema	Retinitis	Chorioretinitis: blurred vision, pain, loss of central vision
Throat	Painful, exudative tonsillitis (white or greenish gray), pasty membrane with bad odor; inflammation and tonsillar edema may be severe	No involvement	No involvement
Oral cavity	Bleeding gums, palatine petechiae	No involvement	No involvement
Lymph nodes	Cervical, submandibular, and axillary node discrete enlargement and tenderness	No involvement	Generalized lymphadenopathy: firm, smooth, discrete, movable enlarged nodes; tenderness, or may be painless
Abdomen	Splenomegaly; hepatomegaly	Splenomegaly; hepatomegaly	Splenomegaly
Skin	Jaundice, macular rash, or purpura	Rubelliform rash	Generalized bright red or pink maculopapular rash, blanching on pressure
Respiratory	Symptoms of pneumonia	Cough or symptoms of pneumonia	Coarse rales, cough, dyspnea, cyanosis
Neurologic	Meningitis or encephalitis	Sensory and motor weakness, pyramidal tract signs	Encephalitis: convulsions, ataxia, vomiting, confusion
Other		Myocarditis	Symptoms of myocarditis
Congenital		Jaundice, petechial rash; hepatosplenomegaly; lethargy; microcephaly; respiratory distress; retardation; chorioretinitis; seizures	Hydrocephalus or microcephalus; convulsions; pneumonitis; jaundice, purpura, petechial or maculopapular rash; bilateral chorioretinitis; hepatomegaly, splenomegaly

From Grimes.[25]

NIC ACTIVITY AND EXERCISE MANAGEMENT

Activity intolerance related to fatigue from mononucleosis, CMV, or toxoplasmosis

- Encourage bed rest during acute symptomatic disease *to conserve energy.*
- Assist patient in developing a realistic plan for returning to work or school during convalescence following mononucleosis. *Prolonged malaise accompanying these diseases may be unanticipated.*

NIC RESPIRATORY MANAGEMENT

Ineffective breathing pattern related to pneumonitis of mononucleosis, CMV, or toxoplasmosis

- Assess ventilation to include evaluation of breathing rate, rhythm, and depth: chest expansion; presence of respiratory distress (e.g., dyspnea, shortness of breath, nasal flaring, pursed-lip breathing, prolonged expiratory phase, use of accessory muscles, or adventitious sounds) *to detect pneumonitis, which is a potential complication of these infections, particularly in the immunocompromised.*
- Maintain patient in position that facilitates ventilation (head of bed in semi-Fowler's position or patient sitting and leaning forward on overbed table) *to facilitate lung expansion for improved air exchange.*
- Instruct patient in proper pulmonary hygiene routines *to promote easy effective breathing, facilitate removal of secretions from tracheobronchial tree, and minimize pulmonary congestion, which could lead to superinfections.*
- Assess patient for tiring in relation to attempts to breathe.
- Assist ventilation, if necessary. Administer O_2 *to provide adequate intake of* O_2.
- Protect patient from known sources of secondary infection, *which is common with these patients.*
- Administer antiinfectives as prescribed *to control progression of the pneumonitis.*

NIC NEUROLOGIC MANAGEMENT

Disturbed sensory perception (visual) related to chorioretinitis of CMV and toxoplasmosis

- Provide a safe environment for patients with chorioretinitis. Assist patient with interpreting environment, personal care, and ambulation as needed. Refer for rehabilitation for vision loss *to prevent injury.*

PATIENT EDUCATION/CONTINUUM OF CARE PLAN[25]

Instruct patients with infectious mononucleosis or CMV:

1. Although complete bed rest is usually unnecessary during acute disease or convalescence, patient caring for himself or herself at home should be encouraged to rest as symptoms dictate. Convalescence may be as long as 3 to 4 weeks.
2. The patient with splenomegaly should avoid heavy lifting, contact sports, or any activity that may increase risk of injury to spleen. Active children must be protected from injury.
3. Report to physician any jaundice, excess bruising or bleeding, or symptoms of abnormal central nervous system functioning.
4. EB virus is transmitted by contact with saliva; CMV is transmitted by contact with all body secretions and excretions.

Instruct patients with toxoplasmosis:

1. Patients treated with pyrimethamine (which depresses bone marrow) should have peripheral blood cell and platelet counts twice a week during therapy. Explain medication regimen, particularly use of folinic acid or baker's yeast to counteract effects of pyrimethamine.
2. Immunocompromised persons and pregnant women can avoid exposure by cooking all meat to 60° C (140° F), washing fruits and vegetables, washing hands thoroughly after handling uncooked meat, wearing gloves while working in soil, and avoiding cat feces. Children's sandboxes should be kept free of cat feces.
3. Infants born with asymptomatic toxoplasmosis should be evaluated periodically for visual problems and developmental delays.
4. Refer families of infants with congenital toxoplasmosis to counseling, support, or rehabilitation resources as needed. Provide information about resource and its services and how to access resource.
5. The congenital anomalies do not represent a hereditary defect.
6. There is not a risk for congenital toxoplasmosis in subsequent pregnancies. The risk is present only when toxoplasmosis is acquired during the pregnancy.

EVALUATION/PATIENT OUTCOMES

Risk Management: Infection will not be transmitted. Patient demonstrates behavior to prevent transmission of pathogens to others. Health-care team washes hands after providing care to each patient and follows standard precautions with all patients. Health-care staff remain free of signs of infection.

Patient does not experience injury. Patient's spleen is nonpalpable and nontender. Leukocyte, lymphocyte, and platelet counts, bilirubin level, and serum transaminase (SGOT, SGPT) levels are normal.

Patient self-administers antiinfective agents as prescribed. Patient completes full course of antiinfective therapy. No preventable drug interactions or allergic reactions are experienced. If untoward reactions are experienced, the patient discontinues drug and contacts physician immediately.

Thermoregulation: Body temperature is maintained within normal range; patient comfort and safety are maintained. Patient's body temperature is between 36° and 38° C (96.8° and 100.4° F). Pulse and respiration are normal. Skin is cool to touch and free of excess perspiration. Patient's clothing and bedding are dry. Patient is free of headache and malaise associated with fever.

Activity and Exercise Management: Patient achieves adequate rest to conserve energy during active disease and returns to preillness level of activity during convalescence. Patient maintains bed rest during acute disease, with gradual return of activity. No fatigue with exertion during convalescence.

Respiratory Management: Patient demonstrates normal respiratory pattern, oxygen intake, and blood gas levels. Bronchovesicular breath sounds are heard throughout patient's lungs. There are no areas of decreased breath sounds or consolidation. Respiratory rate is normal. CO_2, Po_2, and Pco_2 are normal.

Neurologic Management: Patient is not confused or frightened by environmental stimuli during time of alteration in vision; visual function returns to normal. Persons with vision loss are aware of counseling, support, or rehabilitation resources and have phone numbers and names of people to contact at those services.

LYME DISEASE

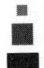

Lyme disease is a multisystem, multistage, inflammatory disease caused by a spirochete that is transmitted by the bite of a tick. If untreated in early infection, the disease becomes chronic and mimics other rheumatic diseases. It usually occurs in stages characterized by different clinical manifestations and by exacerbations and remissions (see box below, right). The most common early sign is erythema migrans, an annular skin lesion that appears at the site of a tick bite. Systemic symptoms and neurologic, cardiac, or arthritic involvement occur in varying combinations over months to years.

PATHOPHYSIOLOGY

The spirochete *Borrelia burgdorferi* is introduced into the skin by the bite of an ixodid tick. The spirochete produces an endotoxin, which causes initial vascular and cellular inflammation. Later pathologic changes appear to result from the immune response to the pathogen. The pathogen can remain localized in the initial lesion or can invade and replicate in any tissue. The spirochete has been cultured from blood, skin, CSF, and joint fluid and has been observed in specimens of skin, myocardial, retinal, and synovial lesions.

POTENTIAL COMPLICATIONS

Aseptic meningitis or encephalitis; chorea; cerebellar ataxia; cranial or peripheral neuropathies; heart block; congestive heart failure; congenital infection

FACTS ABOUT LYME DISEASE

Occurrence: Most commonly reported vector-borne infectious disease in the United States; endemic foci according to geographic areas where the tick vectors occur; i.e., along Atlantic coast (Massachusetts to Maine), upper Midwest (Wisconsin, Minnesota), and west (California, Oregon); also occurs in Canada, Europe, former Soviet Union, China, and Japan; seasonal variation depends on the life cycle of ticks in different geographic regions

Etiologic agent: B. burgdorferi, a spirochete; three different subgroups have been identified in Europe

Reservoir: Certain ixodid ticks that feed on deer and small mammals such as rats; tick genus varies with geographic location

Transmission: Tick bite; experimental transmission in animals does not occur until the tick has been attached for 24 or more hours

Incubation period: 3-32 days until onset of erythema migrans; earlier stages may be asymptomatic

Period of communicability: No person-to-person transmission; rare reports of congenital transmission but no evidence of adverse pregnancy outcomes

Susceptibility and resistance: General; reinfection has occurred in those treated with antibiotics during early disease

Report to local health authority: Mandatory case report required

Data from Benenson.[3]

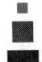

DIAGNOSTIC STUDIES AND FINDINGS[26]

Culture of specimen of blood: Positive for spirochete

Microscopic examination of stained specimen of skin taken from outside the periphery of erythema migrans (EM) Positive for spirochete

Serology: Elevation of antibody titers (serologic tests are not reliable by themselves for diagnosis; they are not sensitive in early disease stages, leading to many false-negative results; in addition, the tests cross-react with the antibodies to other pathogens with similar antigens, such as the spirochetes associated with syphilis, leptospirosis, and periodontal disease)

MULTIDISCIPLINARY PLAN[22]

Medications

Doxycycline, 100 mg PO bid for 21 days, or
Amoxicillin, 500 mg PO qid for 21 days

SIGNS AND SYMPTOMS OF LYME DISEASE

One or more of the following may be present at different times during the infection:

EARLY INFECTION

Rash: Erythema migrans (EM)
Migratory muscle and joint pain
Headache
Stiff neck
Significant fatigue/malaise
Fever
Facial paralysis (Bell's palsy)
Meningitis
Conjunctivitis (less common)
Myocarditis (less common)

LATE INFECTION

Arthritis
Central nervous system pathologic conditions such as encephalitis, confusion (less common)
Skin pathologic conditions

Data from Grimes[25] and Centers for Disease Control and Prevention.[22]

For children under 9 years and pregnant and lactating women: Amoxicillin 50 mg/kg/day in divided doses
For penicillin allergy: Erythromycin or cefuroxime axetil
Duration of treatment with all of the above depends on the stage of disease
Immunologic agent for persons at risk for prolonged exposure to tick-infested areas: lyme disease vaccine (LYMErix), 0.5 ml, IM, in three doses, 0; 1 month, 12 months
Treatment of localized EM is 2 weeks; for early disseminated disease, 3-4 weeks; for arthritis, 4 weeks
Other antiinfective regimens are suggested for neurologic and cardiac pathologic conditions

General Management

Antiinflammatory drugs; joint aspiration, surgical joint lining removal

NURSING CARE

Nursing care varies depending on the stage in the disease and the body system affected when the infected person presents to the health care providers. See related chapters in this book. Providing support during the diagnosis is important.

Patient Education/Continuum of Care Plan[25]

1. Instruct patient to take entire course of antibiotic as prescribed.
2. Instruct patient and family that relapses may occur and recurrence of symptoms should be reported to health-care provider so that antibiotic therapy can be resumed immediately.
3. Instruct public to avoid tick-infested areas and to check body surfaces every 3 to 4 hours for attached ticks if working or playing in infested areas.
4. Instruct public to remove any ticks promptly and carefully without crushing. Apply tweezers or forceps close to the skin and, using gentle traction, remove tick from the skin. Protect hands with gloves or tissue. Swab bite area with an antiseptic after removing the tick.

RESPIRATORY INFECTIOUS DISEASES

The respiratory infectious diseases discussed in this section are the acute and chronic respiratory pathologic conditions that are caused by a specific pathogenic agent that is transmitted by inhalation or by direct contact with infectious respiratory secretions. These include influenza, tuberculosis, histoplasmosis, and legionellosis (legionnaires' disease).

Nonspecific lower respiratory infections such as pneumonia are discussed in Chapter 4. Nonspecific upper respiratory infections such as pharyngitis and tonsillitis are discussed in Chapter 9.

INFLUENZA

Influenza is a generalized, acute, febrile disease associated with upper and lower respiratory infection; it is characterized by a severe and protracted cough, fever, headache, myalgia, prostration, coryza, and mild sore throat.

Pathophysiology

Influenza viruses A, B, or C, each with many mutagenic strains, are inhaled in aerosolized mucous droplets shed from infected persons. The viruses are deposited on and penetrate the surface of upper respiratory tract mucosal cells, producing cell lysis and destruction of the ciliated epithelium. Viral neuraminidase decreases the viscosity of the mucosa, thus facilitating the spread of virus-containing exudate to the lower respiratory tract. An interstitial inflammation and necrosis of the bronchiolar and alveolar epithelium result, filling the alveoli with a purulent exudate.

Regeneration of epithelium, following necrosis and desquamation, slowly begins after the fifth day of illness. Regeneration reaches a maximum within 9 to 15 days, at which time mucus production and cilia begin to appear. Before complete regeneration the compromised epithelium is prone to secondary bacterial invasion, resulting in bacterial pneumonia usually caused by *Staphylococcus aureus.*

The initial invasion of the virus can be aborted at the portal of entry if virus-specific secretory antibodies (IgA) are present in mucous secretions and if virus-specific serum antibodies are adequate.

The disease is usually self-limited. Acute symptoms last 2 to 7 days and are followed by a convalescent period of about a week. The disease is important because of its cyclic epidemic and pandemic nature and because of the high mortality associated with pulmonary complications resulting from secondary bacterial pneumonia. This risk is highest in elderly and chronically diseased persons.

Diagnostic Studies and Findings

Tissue culture of nasal or pharyngeal secretions: Positive for influenza virus
Antigen/antibody tests of secretions: Direct identification of viral antigens

FACTS ABOUT INFLUENZA

Occurrence: Worldwide in pandemics, epidemics, localized outbreaks, and sporadic cases; highest in winter in temperate zones
Etiologic agent: Three types of viruses (A, B, and C), each with many strains
Reservoir: Humans; some mammals suspected as sources of new strains of viruses
Transmission: Direct transmission by inhalation of virus in airborne mucous discharge
Incubation period: 24-72 hours
Period of communicability: 3 days from onset of symptoms
Susceptibility and resistance: Universal; infection produces immunity to a specific strain of virus, but duration of immunity depends on antigenic drift in strain
Report to local health authority: Mandatory case report

Data from Benenson.[3]

Table 15-17 Recommended Dosage for Amantadine and Rimantadine Treatment and Prophylaxis

Antiviral Agent	Age: 1-9 yrs	10-13 yrs	14-64 yrs	≥65 yrs
AMANTADINE*				
Treatment	5 mg/kg/day up to 150 mg† in two divided doses	100 mg twice daily‡	100 mg twice daily	≤100 mg/day
Prophylaxis	5 mg/kg/day up to 150 mg† in two divided doses	100 mg twice daily‡	100 mg twice daily	≤100 mg/day
RIMANTADINE§				
Treatment	NA	NA	100 mg twice daily	100 or 200¶ mg/day
Prophylaxis	5 mg/kg/day up to 150 mg† in two divided doses	100 mg twice daily‡	100 mg twice daily	100 or 200¶ mg/day

From Centers for Disease Control and Prevention.[20]

NOTE: Amantadine manufacturers include: Dupont Pharma (Symmetrel—syrup); Solvay Pharmaceuticals (Symadine—capsule); Chase Pharmaceuticals and Invamed (Amantadine HCL—capsule); and Copley Pharmaceuticals, Barre National, and Mikart (Amantadine HCL—syrup). Rimantadine is manufactured by Forest Laboratories (Flumandine—tablet and syrup).

*The drug package insert should be consulted for dosage recommendations for administering amantadine to persons with creatinine clearance U50 mL/min.

†5 mg/kg of amantadine or rimantadine syrup = 1 tsp/22 lb.

‡Children ≥ 10 years of age who weigh <40 kg should be administered amantadine or rimantadine at a dose of 5 mg/kg/day.

§A reduction in dose to 100 mg/day of rimantadine is recommended for persons who have severe hepatic dysfunction or those with creatinine clearance <10 mL/min. Other persons with less severe hepatic or renal dysfunction taking >100 mg/day of rimantadine should be observed closely, and the dosage should be reduced or the drug discontinued, if necessary.

¶Elderly nursing-home residents should be administered only 100 mg/day of rimantadine. A reduction in dose to 100 mg/day should be considered for all persons ≥65 years of age if they experience possible side effects when taking 200 mg/day.

NA = Not applicable.

Serology: Fourfold increase in antibody titer between acute and convalescent stages

MULTIDISCIPLINARY PLAN[20]

Medications

Antiinfective agents: See Table 15-17 for recommended dosages for amantadine and rimantadine treatment and prophylaxis of influenza virus A

Agent-specific antiinfective agents for bacterial complications or for patients with chronic pulmonary disease

Antipyretics: Acetylsalicylic acid (ASA), 600 mg PO q4h for adults; acetaminophen for children

Adrenergic agents: Phenylephrine (Neo-Synephrine), 0.25%, 2 drops in each nostril for nasal congestion

Antitussive agents: Terpin hydrate with codeine, 5-10 ml PO q3-4h for adults for cough

Active immunization: Vaccine must be repeated yearly in the fall for viral strain expected in the winter; recommended for any person over 6 months who, because of age or medical condition, is at risk for complications of influenza; this includes residents of nursing homes and chronic care facilities and health-care providers in contact with high-risk patients; children under 12 should receive only split-virus vaccine

AGE GROUP	DOSAGE	NO. OF DOSES	ROUTE
6-35 months	0.25 ml	1 or 2	IM
3-8 years	.5 ml	1 or 2	IM
9-12 years	.5 ml	1	IM
>12 years	.5 ml	1	IM

General Management

Oxygen and IV fluid and electrolytes for complications

NURSING CARE

NURSING ASSESSMENT

History: Failure to receive influenza vaccine within the present season; exposure to person with influenza

Subjective symptoms: Prostration; myalgia (particularly in back and legs); anorexia and malaise; headache; photophobia; and retrobulbar aching

Body temperature: Sudden-onset fever (38° to 40° C [100.4° to 104° F]) that gradually falls and rises again on the third day

Head and neck: Conjunctivitis and anterior cervical lymphadenopathy may be present; flushed face

Respiratory status

Initial (mild at first): Sore throat, substernal burning; nonproductive cough; coryza

Advanced: Severe and productive cough; erythema of soft palate, posterior hard palate, tonsillar pillars, and posterior pharynx; increased respiratory rate

POTENTIAL COMPLICATIONS

Primary viral pneumonia: Dyspnea, cyanosis, hemoptysis, crepitant and subcrepitant rales

Secondary bacterial pneumonia: Same as for viral pneumonia plus purulent or bloody sputum

PATIENT PROBLEMS/NURSING DIAGNOSES & INTERVENTIONS

NIC RISK MANAGEMENT

Risk for infection (patient and patient contacts) related to presence of virus in nasopharyngeal secretions

- Collect pharyngeal specimen. *Incorrect collection and handling of specimens may destroy the pathogen or contaminate the specimen with environmental organisms, interfering with accurate diagnosis and treatment. Im-*

proper handling can also contaminate the health-care worker.

- Administer vaccine or antiviral agent as prescribed. *Antiviral agents decrease severity of influenza.*
- Protect patient from exposure to bacteria. Monitor for a subsequent increase in temperature accompanied by chest pain, dyspnea, hemoptysis, purulent sputum, or ear pain; report findings. *Early detection of secondary infection and treatment with antiinfective agents may prevent dissemination of the pathogen, severe disease, and death.*
- Initiate droplet precautions for duration of illness *to prevent transmission to health-care workers, other patients, and patient contact* (see Box 15-4, p. 1087).
- Use protective isolation procedures as indicated. Prevent patient exposure to infected visitors or staff. Limit visitors, if necessary, *to limit the exposure of patients to additional pathogens.*
- Participate in follow-up of high-risk patient contacts *to ensure that patient receives flu vaccine or antiviral agent.*

NIC THERMOREGULATION

Hyperthermia related to infection

- Monitor body temperature *to detect fever.*
- Administer antipyretics, as ordered.
- Bathe with tepid water or alcohol *to reduce high fever.*
- Adjust environmental temperature *for patient's comfort.*
- Remove excess clothing and bedding *to ensure heat loss.*
- Encourage adequate fluid intake *to compensate for fluid loss associated with elevated body temperature.*

NIC RESPIRATORY MANAGEMENT

Ineffective breathing pattern related to infectious process in respiratory epithelium

- Administer decongestants, as prescribed, *to reduce edema in air passages.*
- Provide cool, humidified air *to liquify secretions.*
- Suction, if necessary, *to remove secretions.*
- Monitor for signs of viral or bacterial pneumonia *to intervene early with antiinfectives.*
- Provide oxygen, as prescribed, *to ensure an adequate supply of oxygen.*
- Encourage as much fluids as patient can tolerate (3000 ml for adult) *to liquify secretions.*
- Administer IV fluids, as prescribed, *to provide additional fluids required during infection.*
- Encourage bed rest *to decrease demands on respiratory system.*

PATIENT EDUCATION/CONTINUUM OF CARE PLAN[25]

1. Maintain bed rest for 2 or 3 days after temperature returns to normal.
2. Force fluids.
3. Continue to take antibiotics for duration, as prescribed, for bacterial complications.
4. Report symptoms of secondary infection (e.g., ear pain, purulent or bloody sputum; chest pain, and increase in temperature) to physician.
5. High-risk persons should be encouraged to receive influenza vaccine before start of flu season.
6. Side effects of amantadine prophylaxis include nausea, dizziness, nervousness, insomnia, and impaired concentration. These disappear when drug is stopped. These and other side effects, particularly in persons at risk for impaired renal function, should be reported to a physician.

EVALUATION/PATIENT OUTCOMES

Risk Management: Infection is prevented in persons experiencing risk factors. High-risk persons are vaccinated or are receiving antiviral agent. Patient's sputum cultures are negative; body temperature is normal; leukocyte count and sedimentation rate are normal.

Infection is not transmitted. All patient contacts are adequately immunized or examined and treated with antiviral agent.

Thermoregulation: Body temperature is maintained within the normal range; comfort and safety are maintained. Patient's body temperature is between 36° and 38° C (96.8° and 100° F) orally; pulse and respirations are within normal limits; skin is cool to touch and free of excess perspiration. Patient's clothing and bedding are dry.

Respiratory Management: Patient demonstrates normal respiratory pattern and blood gas levels. Patient's breathing patterns are normal; blood levels (O_2 saturation, CO_2, and PaO_2) are normal; skin is warm and normal colored. Patient shows no signs of pneumonia, and secretions are clear and thin. There is no cough.

TUBERCULOSIS

Tuberculosis (TB) is a chronic pulmonary and extrapulmonary infectious disease acquired by inhalation of a dried-droplet nucleus containing a tubercle bacillus into the alveolar structure of the lung; it is characterized by stages of early infection, which may progress to active, infectious TB disease or to latency, and a potential for recurrent postprimary disease (see box on p. 1050).

PATHOPHYSIOLOGY

Tuberculosis infection is different from tuberculosis disease (also called active tuberculosis). Tuberculosis infection is characterized by the presence of *Mycobacterium tuberculosis* and certain other mycobacteria in the tissue of a host. The other mycobacteria (e.g., *Mycobacterium africanium, Mycobacterium bovis*) are rare in developed countries. The term *tuberculosis disease* refers to the condition that results when invasion of tissue by the mycobacterium results in pathologic changes in tissue. *M. tuberculosis* is capable of remaining viable in host tissue for long periods of time. When tissue invasion has occurred but pathologic change has not occurred, individuals are considered to be tuberculosis infected. Tuberculosis disease occurs when that infection leads to pathologic changes (see Emergency Alert box on p. 1050).

Tuberculosis infection and disease occur in stages: (1) initial infection, (2) latency, and (3) active disease, which can either

FACTS ABOUT TUBERCULOSIS

Occurrence: Worldwide; after a period of decline in the United States, incidence has increased; recent outbreaks have occurred among homeless, migrants, persons with human immunodeficiency virus (HIV) infection and health-care workers and in correctional facilities
Etiologic agent: M. tuberculosis and, occasionally, other mycobacteria; drug-resistant strains are an increasing problem
Reservoir: Humans; *M. bovis* in diseased cattle
Transmission: Inhalation of airborne droplets from the sputum of persons with tuberculosis disease; infrequently by ingestion or skin penetration
Incubation period: An immune response can be demonstrated 4-12 weeks after exposure; once one has been infected, disease can occur at any time during one's lifetime
Period of communicability: As long as bacilli are in sputum: some are intermittently communicable for years
Susceptibility and resistance: All are susceptible; Highest is in children less than 3 years; adolescents, young adults, those over 65 years, the HIV infected, silicone and asbestos workers, the malnourished, and other immunosuppressed individuals
Report to local health authority: Mandatory case report

Data from Benenson.[3]

EMERGENCY ALERT

SCREENING FOR TUBERCULOSIS

Because the incidence of TB in the United States is increasing, careful assessment and proactive intervention are required.

RISK FACTORS/ASSESSMENT

- Cough: Nonproductive initially then purulent secretions, possible rhonchi, hemoptysis, hoarseness
- Fever, malaise, chills, night sweats
- Weight loss
- Exposure to person with TB, skin test with purified protein derivative (PPD) is positive
- History of travel or living outside United States
- Homelessness
- History of spending time in prison
- HIV infection, cancer chemotherapy, malnutrition, chronic disease, corticosteroid therapy
- History of injection drug use

INTERVENTIONS

- Mask patient immediately to provide respiratory isolation; the goal is to minimize the spread of airborne droplets.
- Move patient to properly ventilated (reverse flow ventilation, if possible) area or away from groups of people.
- Instruct patient to cover mouth with tissue when coughing.
- Ensure adequate respiratory function, provide oxygen and support as indicated.
- Collect sputum specimens for laboratory examination.
- Obtain chest radiograph as ordered.
- Initiate medication therapy as ordered.
- Discuss need for screening with family, friends, etc.

follow initial infection or recur as postprimary disease after a period of latency. Transmission resulting in the initial infection is usually by inhalation of minute droplet particles coughed or sneezed into the air by a person whose sputum contains the tubercle bacilli. Less commonly, transmission may occur by ingestion or by invasion of the skin or mucous membranes. The initial (primary) infection develops when tubercle bacilli invade tissue at the portal of entry (usually the middle zones of the lungs), multiply there over 3 weeks, and create an inflammatory lesion. Once the bacteria have invaded, they enter the lymphatic system and are carried to the nearest group of lymph nodes, where they also produce inflammatory lesions. In addition, hematogenous dissemination of the bacilli results in subclinical bacteremia and the production of inflammatory lesions throughout the body. Individuals who are in the initial stage of infection are not capable of transmitting the organism to others.

The sites and the extensiveness of the systemic lesions depend on the numbers of disseminated bacilli and the speed with which the host produces an immune response. These early lesions at the portal of entry and in the lymph nodes and hematogenously disseminated lesions are referred to as the primary complex.

The extent of inflammatory response at the sites of tissue invasion increases with the number of invading bacilli. Nonspecific cellular resistance permits some phagocytosis of tubercle bacilli, producing suppuration and necrosis in the central portion of the lesion. Bacilli continue to replicate at the periphery of the lesion. This initial or primary infection stage is generally symptomless.

Within 3 to 12 weeks a cellular and humoral immune response can be detected by a skin test. *Mycobacterium*-specific lymphocytes and antibodies stimulate a fibroblastic response at the periphery of the lesion, resulting in a dense connective tissue enclosure and the formation of a noncaseating granuloma. The focal lesions continue to harbor viable tubercle bacilli, with the potential for reactivation under conditions of decreased host resistance. This period is called latency.

The specific immune response results in successful encapsulation of the lesions in 90% to 95% of infected persons. All but about 5% of those will remain free of tuberculosis disease for the rest of their lives. However, the immune response does not preclude reinfection with subsequent exposure. Conversion from latency to the postprimary stage of active disease is associated with human immunodeficiency virus (HIV) infection, other severe disease, age greater than 65 years, and immunosuppressive therapies. HIV infection is particularly likely to facilitate conversion from latency to tuberculosis disease. Individuals with latent *M. tuberculosis* infection who are coinfected with HIV are thought to convert to active tuberculosis at a rate of 7% to 10% a year.

Reactivated disease following latency accounts for most of the active tuberculosis diagnosed today. It occurs most frequently in aged persons, in the immunosuppressed, and in persons with chronic and debilitating disease. Untreated reactivated disease has a variable course with many exacerbations and remissions. Complications caused by excessive cavitation are common.

For the 5% to 10% of infected persons whose host responses are inadequate to contain the initial infection, active disease progresses in the portal-of-entry lesion or in all lesions in the body. Necrosis and cavitation continue in the lesions, forming caseation. The lesions may rupture, spreading necrotic residue and bacilli throughout the tissue and throughout the body. Disseminated bacilli establish new focal lesions that progress through stages of inflammation, noncaseating granulomas, and caseating necrosis.

The disease symptoms vary with the body tissue affected. Extrapulmonary tuberculosis in the meninges, blood vessels, kidneys, bones, joints, larynx, skin, intestines, lymph nodes, peritoneum, or eyes is much less common than pulmonary tuberculosis.

Diagnostic Studies and Findings[8,10]

Sputum culture: Positive for *M. tuberculosis* in active disease; will not be positive during latency; new polymerase chain reaction (PCR) test detects organism in 24 hours

Drug sensitivity studies: Reported as sensitive, intermediate and resistant, indicating the effectiveness of the drug against the strain of *M. tuberculosis*

Microscopic examination of acid-fast stained specimen of sputum (CSF, urine, or blood in extrapulmonary disease): Positive for acid-fast bacilli

Histologic examination or culture of tissue in extrapulmonary disease: Positive for *M. tuberculosis*

Skin tests: intradermal infection of antigen (Mantoux test: five tuberculin units of purified protein derivative [PPD] infected intradermally): Test is read in 48 to 72 hours; a positive reaction (see box at right) indicates past infection and presence of antibodies; does not indicate active disease; nonspecific reactions during first 48 hours can be overlooked; if reaction is negative and if person has not had a skin test in some time, a second test may be performed 1 week later, if the second test is negative, the patient is considered not infected; if the second test is positive, the person should be considered to be positive, but not to have a recent infection

Pleural needle biopsy: Positive for granulomas of tuberculosis; giant cells indicating caseation necrosis

Chest radiograph examination: Findings may show calcification at the original site, enlargement of hilar lymph nodes, parenchymal infiltrate representing extension of the original site of infection, or the appearance of pleural effusion or cavitation; not diagnostically definitive of TB

Multidisciplinary Plan[8,10]

Medications

Prophylaxis for persons infected with *M. tuberculosis* who are skin test positive and who do not have active disease to prevent active disease: Isoniazid, 300 mg in a daily dose in adults and 10 to 15 mg/kg in children with the daily dose to not exceed 300 mg/dose; therapy is maintained for 6 months in immunocompetent adults, 9 months in children, and 12 months in HIV-infected persons; rifampin prophylaxis is sometimes used for close contacts of individuals with isoniazid-resistant *M. tuberculosis;* isoniazid therapy is

SUMMARY OF INTERPRETATION OF TUBERCULOSIS SKIN TEST RESULTS

1. An induration of 5 mm is classified as positive in:
   - Persons who have human immunodeficiency virus (HIV) infection or risk factors for HIV infection but unknown HIV status;
   - Persons who have had recent close contact* with persons who have active tuberculosis (TB);
   - Persons who have fibrotic chest radiographs (consistent with healed TB).
2. An induration of 10 mm is classified as positive in all persons who do not meet any of the criteria above but who have other risk factors for TB, including:

   High-risk groups—
   - Injecting-drug users known to be HIV seronegative;
   - Persons who have other medical conditions that reportedly increase the risk for progressing from latent TB infection to active TB (e.g., silicosis; gastrectomy or jejunoileal bypass; being 10% below ideal body weight; chronic renal failure with renal dialysis; diabetes mellitus; high-dose corticosteroid or other immunosuppressive therapy; some hematologic disorders, including malignancies such as leukemias and lymphomas; and other malignancies);
   - Children <4 years of age.

   High-prevalence groups—
   - Persons born in countries in Asia, Africa, the Caribbean, and Latin America that have high prevalence of TB;
   - Persons from medically underserved, low-income populations;
   - Residents of long-term–care facilities (e.g., correctional institutions and nursing homes);
   - Persons from high-risk populations in their communities, as determined by local public health authorities.
3. An induration of 15 mm is classified as positive in persons who do not meet any of the above criteria.
4. Recent converters are defined on the basis of both size of induration and age of the person being tested.
   - 10-mm increase within a 2-year period is classified as a recent conversion for persons <35 years of age;
   - 15-mm increase within a 2-year period is classified as a recent conversion for persons 35 years of age.
5. PPD skin-test results in health-care workers (HCWs)
   - In general, the recommendations in sections 1, 2, and 3 of this table should be followed when interpreting skin-test results in HCWs.

   However, the prevalence of TB in the facility should be considered when choosing the appropriate cut-point for defining a positive PPD reaction. In facilities where there is essentially no risk for exposure to *Mycobacterium tuberculosis* (i.e., minimal- or very low-risk facilities), an induration of 15 mm may be a suitable cut-point for HCWs who have no other risk factors. In facilities where TB patients receive care, the cut-point for HCWs with no other risk factors may be 10 mm.

From Centers for Disease Control and Prevention.[8]

*Recent close contact implies either household or social contact or unprotected occupational exposure similar in intensity and duration to household contact.

Table 15-18 Dosage Recommendations for the Initial Treatment of Tuberculosis in Children* and Adults

	Dosage Schedule					
	Daily Dose (Maximum Dose)		Two Doses per Week (Maximum Dose)		Three Doses per Week (Maximum Dose)	
Drug	Children	Adults	Children	Adults	Children	Adults
Isoniazid	10-20 mg/kg (300 mg)	5 mg/kg (300 mg)	20-40 mg/kg (900 mg)	15 mg/kg (900 mg)	20-40 mg/kg (900 mg)	15 mg/kg (900 mg)
Rifampin	10-20 mg/kg (600 mg)	10 mg/kg (600 mg)	10-20 mg/kg (600 mg)	10 mg/kg (600 mg)	10-20 mg/kg (600 mg)	10 mg/kg (600 mg)
Pyrazinamide	15-30 mg/kg (2 g)	15-30 mg/kg (2 g)	50-70 mg/kg (4 g)	50-70 mg/kg (4 g)	50-70 mg/kg (3 g)	50-70 mg/kg (3 g)
Ethambutol	15-25 mg/kg	15-25 mg/kg	50 mg/kg	50 mg/kg	25-30 mg/kg	25-30 mg/kg
Streptomycin	20-40 mg/kg (1 g)	15 mg/kg (1 g)	20-40 mg/kg (1.5 g)	20-40 mg/kg (1.5 g)	20-40 mg/kg (1.5 g)	20-40 mg/kg (1.5 g)

From Centers for Disease Control and Prevention.[10]
*Persons less than 12 years of age.

not recommended for persons over 35 years of age unless they are at high risk of developing active tuberculosis because the risk of isoniazid-related hepatitis outweighs the benefits of preventive therapy in this group.

Treatment for active disease: The pharmacologic treatment of active tuberculosis is based on multidrug therapy for extended periods of time; the current recommendations for treatment are contained in Table 15-18; the success of these regimens is entirely dependent on patient compliance; if the patient does not adhere to the schedule, his or her infection will not be eliminated; in addition, the growth of drug-resistant strains of *M. tuberculosis* will be encouraged, making the eradication of the disease even more difficult; unfortunately, because of the length and complexity of anti-TB drug therapy, noncompliance is widespread (up to 25%); failure to follow the drug regimen is found in all population groups and social classes; the best method for assuring compliance with the drug regimen is directly observed therapy, a system whereby a public health representative is physically present while the patient takes each scheduled dose of the medications; because of the cost of directly observed therapy, alternative drug regimens have been devised that involve taking higher doses less frequently; these alternative regimens are shown in Table 15-19; treatment of patients with HIV disease may vary from these regimens.

Multidrug-resistant tuberculosis (MDRTB): Usually defined as resistant to both isoniazid and rifampin, MDRTB is increasingly found in the United States; often resistance is found to other antituberculosis drugs as well; treatment of MDRTB is very complex and depends on the number and nature of the drugs to which the organism is resistant; there are currently nine second-line anti-TB drugs used in treating MDRTB; the treatment usually must be individually tailored for the strain of the organism and for the patient's tolerance profile; it should only be treated by or in consultation with someone who is familiar with the treatment of MDRTB

Corticosteroids: May be used in conjunction with the anti-infective agents for overwhelming and life-threatening disease

Surgery

Intervention for complications

Resectional procedures for persisting cavitary lesions (less common since antimicrobial therapy)

Surgical intervention for massive hemoptysis, spontaneous pneumothorax, abscess drainage, intestinal obstruction, or ureteral stricture

General Management

After stabilization most patients can be effectively managed on an outpatient basis with monitoring for compliance with drug taking, drug side effects, and patient response to the drug therapy

Skin testing: Identify recent converters to TB skin tests; trace their contacts to identify persons with active disease; isoniazid therapy for 1 year for recent converters and for close household contacts of persons with active disease (not routine for those over 35); TB skin testing is recommended for children at school entry and again at age 14

BCG vaccine: For children and infants who are at high risk for contact with active cases, who are skin test negative, and who are not immunosuppressed (benefits of BCG vaccine are controversial); receiving the vaccine results in a positive skin test

NURSING CARE

Nursing Assessment

History: Close contact with a person with TB or previous positive TB skin test; immunosuppression or chronic disease

Subjective symptoms: History of weight loss, anorexia, and generalized weakness and fatigue

Body temperature: Slight continued elevation with chills and night sweats

Respiratory status

Initial: A nonproductive cough; later mucopurulent secretions

Advanced: Hemoptysis; dyspnea on exertion and at rest; rales over apex of lung; chest pain with respiratory

Table 15-19 Regimen Options for the Treatment of Tuberculosis in Children and Adults

			Initial Treatment Phase		Continuation Treatment Phase		
Option	Indication	Total Duration of Therapy	Drugs*	Interval and Duration	Drugs*	Interval and Duration	Comments
1	Pulmonary and extrapulmonary TB in adults and children	6 mo	INH RIF PZA EMB or SM	Daily for 8 wk	INH RIF	Daily or two or three times wkly† for 16 wk‡	• EMB or SM should be continued until susceptibility to INH and RIF is demonstrated. • In areas where primary INH resistance is <4%, EMB or SM may not be necessary for patients with no individual risk factors for drug resistance.
2	Pulmonary and extrapulmonary TB in adults and children	6 mo	INH IF PZA EMB or SM	Daily for 2 weeks then two times wkly† for 6 wk	INH RIF	Two times wkly† for 16 wk‡	• Regimen should be directly observed. • After the initial phase, EMB or SM should be continued until susceptibility to INH and RIF is demonstrated, unless drug resistance is unlikely.
3	Pulmonary and extrapulmonary TB in adults and children	6 mo	INH RIF PZA EMB or SM	3 times wkly† for 6 mo§			• Regimen should be directly observed. • Continue all four drugs for 6 mo.‖ • This regimen has been shown to be effective for INH-resistant TB.
4	Smear- and culture-negative pulmonary TB in adults	4 mo	INH RIF PZA EMB or SM	Follow option 1, 2, or 3 for 8 wk	INH RIF PZA EMB or SM	Daily or two or three times wkly† for 8 wk	• Continue all four drugs for 4 mo. • If drug resistance is unlikely (primary INH resistance <4% and patient has no individual risk factors for drug resistance), EMB or SM may not be necessary and PZA may be discontinued after 2 mo.
5	Pulmonary and extrapulmonary TB in adults and children when PZA is contraindicated	9 mo	INH RIF EMB or SM	Daily for 8 wk	INH RIF	Daily or two times wkly† for 24 wk‡	• EMB or SM should be continued until susceptibility to INH and RIF is demonstrated. • In areas where primary INH resistance is <4%, EMB or SM may not be necessary for patients with no individual risk factors for drug resistance.

From Centers for Disease Control and Prevention.[10]

**EMB*, Ethambutol; *INH*, isoniazid; *PZA*, pyrazinamide; *RIF*, rifampin; *SM*, streptomycin.

†All regimens administered intermittently should be directly observed.

‡For infants and children with miliary TB, bone and joint TB, or TB meningitis, treatment should last at least 12 months. For adults with these forms of extrapulmonary TB, response to therapy should be monitored closely. If response is slow or suboptimal, treatment may be prolonged on a case-by-case basis.

§Some evidence suggests that SM may be discontinued after 4 months if the isolate is susceptible to all drugs.

‖Avoid treating pregnant women with SM because of the risk for ototoxicity to the fetus.

NOTE: For all patients, if drug susceptibility results show resistance to any of the first-time drugs, or if the patient remains symptomatic or smear- or culture-positive after 3 months, consult a TB medical expert.

movement if pleura is involved; hoarseness with involvement of larynx; dysphagia with pharyngeal involvement; sibilant and sonorous rhonchi

Potential Complications

Extrapulmonary disease, cavitation and destruction of lungs

Extrapulmonary TB

Depends on the system involved; the onset of symptoms is generally insidious, as is the onset of pulmonary TB

Cardiovascular system: TB pericarditis precordial chest pain, fever, and pericardial friction rubs, jugular venous distension, hepatic congestion, ascites, and peripheral edema

Gastrointestinal status:

TB peritonitis: Abdominal pain simulating that of appendicitis; abdominal distension; anorexia, vomiting, and weight loss; night sweats; abdominal tenderness when palpated; ascites

TB of GI tract: Symptoms depend on area involved; may have GI bleeding, pain; constipation, or diarrhea; partial or complete obstruction

Systemic status: Miliary TB: more severe symptoms of respiratory involvement: dyspnea, hyperventilation, and cough; hypoxemia; spontaneous unilateral or bilateral pneumothorax (manifested by sudden chest pain and breathlessness) and fever; painful, nodular cutaneous lesions (which may ulcerate) may be present

Neurologic status: TB meningitis: headache, vomiting, fever, and anorexia; alterations in intellectual function, diminishing levels of consciousness, and neurologic deficits; CSF leukocytes of 100 to 400 cells/mm^3 and increase in protein

Lymph nodes: TB lymphadenitis: palpable enlargement of supraclavicular and cervical lymph nodes

Musculoskeletal status: Osteoarticular TB: pain in joints, aggravated by movement; swelling, minimal erythema, and tenderness to palpation; limitation of motion and gross deformities (most common in vertebral column, hip, and knee joints)

Genitourinary (GU) status: TB of GU organs: urgency, frequency, dysuria, hematuria, and pyuria; salpingitis with lower abdominal pain and infertility; amenorrhea; abnormal vaginal discharge or bleeding

Patient Problems/Nursing Diagnoses & Interventions

NIC Risk Management

Risk for infection (patient contacts) related to viable *M. tuberculosis* in respiratory secretions

Risk for infection (chronic in patient) related to noncompliance with therapy

- Obtain specimen for culture. *Incorrect collection and handling of specimen may destroy or contaminate specimen, thus interfering with diagnostic results.*
- Use airborne precautions until antimicrobial therapy is successfully initiated and three sputum specimens are negative *to prevent transmission of organism* (see Box 15-3, p. 1087).
- Use standard precautions until wounds stop draining for patients with external TB lesions *to prevent transmission of organism* (see Box 15-2, p. 1086).
- Teach hospitalized patient to cough and sneeze into paper tissue and to dispose of tissues properly *to prevent transmission of organism.*
- Report to local health authority.
- Instruct patient regarding the prescribed therapy *to ensure that patient takes medication as prescribed;* see Patient Education/Continuum of Care Plan

NIC Respiratory Management

Ineffective breathing pattern related to necrosis of lung tissue

- Monitor breathing *to detect dyspnea and signs of pneumothorax.*
- Initiate respiratory assistance as needed. Observe sputum for hemoptysis to *detect signs of complications.*
- Assist immobile patient to turn, cough, and deep breathe every 2 to 4 hours *to prevent pooling of secretions.*

Patient Education/Continuum of Care Plan[25]

1. Teach care of sputum if discharged patient still has positive sputum cultures.
2. Teach patient hand washing and good hygiene.
3. Drug therapy must be continued uninterrupted for designated time period. Explain dosage, frequency of administration, and purpose of prolonged treatment to the patient.
4. Explain medication's toxic and side effects:
   a. INH: Infrequent toxic effects—peripheral neuropathy, convulsions, ataxia, dizziness, optic neuritis; older patients may experience a drug-related hepatitis with fatigue, malaise, and anorexia
   b. Ethambutol: Reduced visual acuity with inability to perceive the color green
   c. Streptomycin: Skin rash, fever, malaise, vertigo, and deafness; gastrointestinal disturbances and central nervous system symptoms
   d. PAS: Toxic reactions more common with this drug and include symptoms of hypersensitivity, hepatic damage, gastrointestinal disturbances, and renal failure
   e. Rifampin: Red-orange–colored urine common; jaundice, nausea, anorexia, vomiting, diarrhea, cramps, occasional central nervous system disturbances, and hypersensitivity reactions; may interfere with actions of oral contraceptives
   f. Ethionamide: Gastrointestinal irritation and symptoms of hepatotoxicity
   g. Pyrazinamide: Hepatoxicity
   h. Cycloserine: Central nervous system effects, including seizures, somnolence, and muscle twitching
5. Discuss with patient the need to report side effects to physician immediately.
6. Emphasize to patient the need for periodic reculturing of sputum during period of therapy—monthly until cultures are negative, then every 3 months for duration of therapy.
7. Patient must report to the physician: hemoptysis, chest pain, difficulty in breathing, hearing loss, or vertigo.
8. Discuss with patient the need to maintain adequate fluid and caloric intake.

9. Household and close contacts should be examined at time of treatment of patient and again in 2 to 3 months.

Evaluation/Patient Outcomes

Risk Management: Infection is not transmitted to patient's contacts. Contacts do not convert to a positive skin test. Patient demonstrates behavior to prevent transmission of pathogens to others or to prevent contamination of the environment.

Patient is free of infection and complications of TB. Sputum cultures are consistently negative. Chest roentgenograms show a reduction in the size of cavities and decrease in the thickness of cavity walls. Body temperature is normal. Patient does not experience chills or night sweats. Serum alkaline phosphatase levels, hematocrit, hemoglobin, and leukocyte count are normal. Urine does not contain erythrocytes. Patient does not manifest the extrapulmonary symptoms described under Nursing Assessment.

Patient self-administers antiinfective agents as prescribed Patient completes full course on antiinfective therapy. No preventable drug interactions or allergic reactions are experienced. If untoward reactions are experienced, patient discontinues the drug and contacts physician immediately.

Respiratory Management: Patient demonstrates normal respiratory pattern, oxygen intake, and blood gas levels. Patient does not experience dyspnea, cough, or pain on breathing.

Histoplasmosis

Histoplasmosis is a pulmonary and systemic infection, similar to tuberculosis, resulting from inhalation of the spores of *Histoplasma capsulatum,* which are frequently found in the soil. Infection is common, but overt clinical disease is rare. Five clinical forms of the disease have been recognized (see box above, right).

Pathophysiology

Spores of *H. capsulatum,* a fungus, are inhaled when soil containing them is disturbed. A lesion is formed within the lung parenchyma, where the spores convert to a yeast phase and are phagocytosed by macrophages. Lesions may also be formed in the lymph nodes as a result of migration of yeast-laden macrophages to those areas. Dissemination and lesion formation may also occur in the spleen, liver, and eye. These primary lesions become necrotic at the center, build up a fibrotic capsule, and frequently calcify. In most cases where calcification occurs, there is no reactivation of the infection and the host manifests no symptoms except an immune response to histoplasmin.

Four other clinical forms of the disease are possible: acute benign respiratory disease, acute disseminated disease, chronic disseminated disease, and chronic pulmonary disease. In acute benign respiratory disease the primary pulmonary lesion remains active, resulting in a spreading infiltration pneumonia. In acute disseminated disease, inflammatory and necrotic lesions may result in septic type of fever, hepatosplenomegaly, severe prostration, and death. Chronic disseminated histoplasmosis results when there is extensive invasion by yeast-laden macrophages via the reticuloendothelial system to bone marrow, spleen, liver, and lungs. The inflammatory and necrotic reaction in those tissues is subacute but progressive and may eventually result in death. Chronic pulmonary histoplasmosis is manifest as a progressive emphysema. Fluid-filled cysts surrounded by chronic inflammation progress through stages of caseation necrosis and cavitation, continuing to disseminate the yeast through pulmonary tissue.

The clinical symptoms are quite varied but are generally more severe in infants, immunosuppressed persons, and chronically debilitated persons.

FACTS ABOUT HISTOPLASMOSIS

Occurrence: Worldwide; higher in eastern and central United States; increases with age to 15 years; no differences by sex; outbreaks in groups with common exposure
Etiologic agent: H. capsulatum (a fungus)
Reservoir: Soil around chicken houses, caves harboring bats, and around starling, blackbird, and pigeon roosts and decaying trees
Transmission: Inhalation of airborne spores
Incubation period: 3-14 days after exposure, commonly 10 days
Period of communicability: Not transmitted from person to person
Susceptibility and resistance: General; inapparent infections are common and result in increasing resistance; this is an opportunistic infection in immunocompromised persons
Report to local health authority: In some states

Data from Benenson.[3]

Diagnostic Studies and Findings[26]

Culture and examination of respiratory exudate, blood, bone marrow, or exudate from ulcerated lesions: Positive for *H. capsulatum;* results are frequently erratic, necessitating the culture of many specimens
Serology: Increase in antibodies within 3 to 4 weeks; fourfold increase suggests disease progression; agglutinins greater than 1:8 or 1:16 have suggestive diagnostic value
Imaging with MRI, CT scan, chest roentgenogram: Transient parenchymal pulmonary infiltrates resembling lobar pneumonia in acute phase; progressively enlarging areas of necrosis with or without cavitation in chronic disease

Multidisciplinary Plan[1,3]

Medications

Antiinfective agents
- Amphotericin B (Fungizone), 30-40 mg/kg IV for disseminated infection in immunocompromised
- Ketoconazole, 400 mg/day (up to 800 mg) PO for 6-12 months (approved for treatment of immunocompetent)
- Itraconazole, 200-400 mg/day PO for 6-12 months

Corticosteroids: May be mixed with the infusion to minimize the side effects of amphotericin B

Antihistamines: Diphenhydramine (Benadryl), added to IV to control side effects

NURSING CARE

NURSING ASSESSMENT

History: Outdoor exposure to fungus; immunosuppression
Subjective symptoms: Malaise, weakness; anorexia
Acute pulmonary histoplasmosis
- Pleural and substernal chest pain
- Dry or productive cough with metallic tone, suggesting tracheobronchial obstruction
- Low-grade fever
- Erythema multiforme, erythema nodosum
- May have complicating symptoms of pericarditis

Chronic pulmonary histoplasmosis
- Purulent sputum; hemoptysis; increasing signs of pulmonary insufficiency
- Chronic low-grade fever
- Erythema multiforme, erythema nodosum
- May have complicating symptoms of pericarditis

Acute disseminated histoplasmosis
- High fever
- Enlarged liver or spleen

Chronic disseminated histoplasmosis
- Symptoms of pneumonia
- Purpura
- Symptoms of endocarditis
- Symptoms of GI ulcer, hepatitis, and peritonitis
- Ulcerated lesions resembling epidermoid cancer in larynx, mouth, nose, or pharynx

POTENTIAL COMPLICATIONS

Blindness associated with ocular disease; pneumonia; progressive emphysema; septic type of fever; hepatosplenomegaly; severe prostration; death

PATIENT PROBLEMS/NURSING DIAGNOSES & INTERVENTIONS

NIC RISK MANAGEMENT

Risk for injury related to chemotherapeutic agent

- Monitor for cyanosis, change in pulse, respiratory rate, and signs of renal dysfunction *to detect signs of amphotericin toxicity.*
- Administer antihistamines and corticosteroids, as prescribed, *to prevent and control allergic reaction to amphotericin.*
- Encourage fluids high in potassium if nausea and vomiting persist *to replace lost potassium.*
- Use small-gauge needle for IV line. Agitate IV bag every 15 to 20 minutes while chemotherapeutic agent is administered *to evenly distribute drug and fluid in bag and in IV line.* Give infusion over 5 to 6 hours *to prevent phlebitis associated with amphotericin.*
- Reposition patient frequently during prolonged, painful IV infusions. Provide diversional activities *to promote patient comfort.*
- Administer analgesics before IV administration, as prescribed, *to decrease pain from drug therapy.*

Other related nursing diagnoses for progressive disease: Ineffective breathing pattern, hyperthermia, decreased cardiac output, activity intolerance, and impaired oral mucous membranes.

PATIENT EDUCATION/CONTINUUM OF CARE PLAN[25]

1. Inform patient that medical follow-up for 1 year after treatment to prevent relapses is necessary.
2. Inform patient that reinfection can be prevented by avoiding infected sites, wearing a protective mask, or sterilizing site with 3% formalin solution.

EVALUATION/PATIENT OUTCOMES

Risk Management: Patient is free of signs of infection and complications of treatment. Patient's sputum cultures are negative. Body temperature is normal. There is no cough, dyspnea, sputum, or hemoptysis. There are no lesions in mouth, larynx, pharynx, or nose. There is no purpura, erythema multiforme, or erythema nodosum. Patient has energy to carry out all daily activities. Patient does not have abdominal pain, is able to eat all desired foods, and is not jaundiced. There are no signs of phlebitis, renal dysfunction, electrolyte imbalance, pain, or neuritis.

Patient does not experience reinfection. Patient states intent to see physician on a regular basis for 1 year after hospitalization. Patient states methods to use to avoid reexposure.

LEGIONELLOSIS (LEGIONNAIRES' DISEASE)

Legionellosis (legionnaires' disease) is an acute bacterial infection so named because it caused an outbreak of pneumonia at a convention of American Legionnaires at a Philadelphia hotel (see box below). The acute disease is a patchy pulmonary infiltrate and consolidation, with a high fever, malaise, myalgia and headache, nonproductive cough, and a high risk for respiratory failure and death.

FACTS ABOUT LEGIONELLOSIS (LEGIONNAIRES' DISEASE)

Occurrence: Europe, United States, and Canada; first recognized in 1977; sporadic cases and outbreaks in summer and autumn
Etiologic agent: L. pneumophila (a bacterial species with 18 serogroups; serogroup 1 associated with disease)
Reservoir: Unknown but probably environmental; organism survives in hot and cold tap water and distilled water for months
Transmission: Common source, airborne transmission suspected
Incubation period: 2-10 days, commonly 5-6 days
Period of communicability: No documented person-to-person transmission
Susceptibility and resistance: General; rare in those less than 20 years; greatest in males, smokers, immunosuppressed persons and persons over 50 years of age
Report to local health authority: In some states

Data from Benenson.[3]

PATHOPHYSIOLOGY

Inhalation of *Legionella pneumophila* causes two distinct clinical syndromes: Pontiac fever, which resembles influenza, and legionnaires' disease, with pathologic changes characteristic of lobar pneumonia. In the latter there is a cellular exudate consisting of polymorphonuclear leukocytes and macrophages with extensive necrosis of the exudate and alveolar septa. Bronchi are clear of the necrotic process. Rarely is a purulent sputum produced. The disease progresses rapidly during the first 4 to 6 days of clinical illness.

DIAGNOSTIC STUDIES AND FINDINGS[3,26]

Culture of blood, sputum, bronchial or tracheal aspirates, pleural fluid, and lung tissue: Positive for *L. pneumophila*
Examination of stained smear of respiratory specimens: Positive for *L. pneumophila*
Antigen/antibody test of specimen of urine: Positive for *L. pneumophila* antigen
Serology: Fourfold or greater rise in antibody titer to 1:128 within 21 days of onset of illness
Chest radiograph examination: Shows patchy pattern of pneumonia and small pleural effusions
WBC Count: 10,000-15,000/mm^3
Sedimentation rate: Markedly elevated
Others: Hematuria, proteinuria, and laboratory evidence of liver dysfunction and electrolyte abnormalities

MULTIDISCIPLINARY PLAN[1-3]

Medications

Antiinfective Agents

Erythromycin, 0.5-1 q6h for adults (15 mg/kg q6h for children) IV or PO for 21 days
Ciprofloxacin or azithromycin for persons allergic to erythromycin
Rifampin (rifamycin, others), as adjunct therapy for seriously ill patients

General Management

Assisted ventilation, oxygen therapy, temporary renal dialysis, and IV fluids and electrolytes

NURSING CARE

NURSING ASSESSMENT

Body temperature: 38° to 41° C (100.4° to 105.8° F) within a day
Subjective symptoms: Anorexia, malaise, myalgia, chills, abdominal pain, headache
Respiratory status: Nonproductive cough, dyspnea, tachypnea, pluritic chest pain, and rales or rhonchi
Digestive status: Diarrhea, sometimes vomiting
Cardiovascular status: Tachycardia, symptoms of shock
Neurologic status: Confusion, slurring of speech, and falling (infrequent symptoms)

POTENTIAL COMPLICATIONS

Renal failure, bacteremic shock, and respiratory failure resulting in death to 15% of patients

PATIENT PROBLEMS/NURSING DIAGNOSES & INTERVENTIONS

NIC THERMOREGULATION

Hyperthermia related to infection

- Monitor body temperature *to detect fever.*
- Administer antipyretics as ordered.
- Bathe with tepid water or alcohol *to reduce high fever.*
- Adjust environmental temperature *for patient's comfort.*
- Remove excess clothing and bedding *to ensure heat loss.*
- Encourage adequate fluid intake *to compensate for fluid loss associated with elevated body temperature.*

NIC RESPIRATORY MANAGEMENT

Ineffective breathing pattern related to pneumonia

- Assess ventilation to include evaluation of breathing rate, rhythm, and depth: chest expansion; presence of respiratory distress, such as dyspnea, nasal flaring, pursed-lip breathing, prolonged expiratory phase, and use of accessory muscles *to detect signs of respiratory failure for immediate intervention.*
- Assess patient for tiring from exertion in relation to attempts to breathe; assist ventilation, if necessary. Administer oxygen *to maintain circulating oxygen.*
- Maintain patient in position with head of bed in semi-Fowler's position or patient sitting and leaning forward over overbed table. *These positions facilitate respiration by decreasing abdominal pressure on diaphragm.*
- Instruct patient in proper pulmonary hygiene routines such as postural drainage. *These will promote easy, effective breathing and facilitate removal of secretions from tracheobronchial tree and minimize pulmonary congestion, which could lead to superinfections.*

PATIENT EDUCATION/CONTINUUM OF CARE PLAN[25]

To prevent reinfection:

1. Decontaminate implicated sources of infection by chlorination or super-heating of water supply.
2. Cooling water towers and misters should be drained and cleaned when not in use.

EVALUATION/PATIENT OUTCOMES

Thermoregulation: Body temperature is maintained within the normal range; comfort and safety are maintained. Body temperature is between 36° and 38° C (96.8° and 100.4° F) orally. Pulse and respirations are within normal limits. Skin is cool to touch and free of excess perspiration. Patient's clothing and bedding are dry. Patient is free of headache and malaise associated with the fever. Patient experiences no injury associated with seizures. Body fluids are adequate. Serum electrolytes are within normal limits. Urine output and specific gravity are normal.

Respiratory Management: Patient demonstrates normal respiratory pattern, oxygen intake, and blood gas levels.

Table 15-20 Overview of Streptococcal Throat, Scarlet Fever, and Rheumatic Fever

	Streptococcal Throat	Scarlet Fever	Rheumatic Fever
Occurrence	More common in temperate zones; may be endemic, epidemic, or sporadic in occurrence; highest in late winter or spring; ages 3-15 years most often affected; no sex or racial difference		Increase in outbreaks since 1984
Etiologic agent	*Streptococcus pyogenes* (group A streptococcus of approximately 80 serologically distinct types)	Three erythrogenic toxins	GABHS
Reservoir	Humans	Humans	Humans
Transmission	Direct contact with mucous droplets from patient or carrier; may follow ingestion of contaminated food	Sequela to streptococcal throat	Sequela to streptococcal throat
Incubation period	1-3 days	2-4 days (range: 1-7 days)	3-35 days after clinical strep throat (average: 19 days)
Period of communicability	Untreated, uncomplicated cases: 10-21 days; complicated: weeks to months; antibiotic treated: 24-48 hours	Not communicable	Not communicable
Susceptibility and resistance	General: many develop antitoxic and/or antibacterial immunity to one of the types of streptococci through inapparent infection	Permanent acquired immunity from active disease with type of toxin; second attacks due to different toxin	Persons who have suffered one attack are predisposed to a recurrent episode following group A streptococcal upper respiratory infections
Report to local health authority	Epidemics only	Epidemics only	Case report in some states

Data from Benenson.[3]

Bronchovesicular breath sounds are heard throughout lungs. There are no areas of decreased breath sounds or consolidation. Respiratory rate is normal. CO_2, Po_2, and Pco_2 are normal.

Streptococcal Throat, Scarlet Fever, Rheumatic Fever

Streptococcal throat is an acute exudative tonsillitis or pharyngitis caused by group A beta-hemolytic streptococci (GABHS). Coincident or subsequent otitis media or peritonsillar abscess may be present. Rheumatic fever, chorea, scarlet fever, and acute glomerulonephritis are possible sequelae (Table 15-20).

Scarlet fever is a group A beta-hemolytic streptococcal disease characterized by a skin rash. It occurs when the infecting strain of streptococcus produces a toxin, causing a sensitivity reaction in the infected host. Clinical characteristics may include those of streptococcal sore throat plus enanthem, strawberry tongue, and exanthem.

Rheumatic fever is a sequela of group A streptococcal infection of the upper respiratory tract, occurring in about 2.8% of those having a streptococcal throat infection. The condition is thought to result from an altered immune reaction to the streptococcus organism. Rheumatic heart disease is a potential complication.

Pathophysiology

Infection with group A streptococci results in a number of related clinical disease entities, such as streptococcal throat, scarlet fever, and erysipelas, as well as nonsuppurative complications, such as nephritis and rheumatic fever. The type of disease resulting from group A streptococci depends on the site of tissue invasion, the antigenic characteristics of the infecting strain of streptococcus, and the immune status of the host. There are approximately 75 serologically distinct strains of group A streptococci, producing a variety of enzymes and at least three different erythrogenic toxins. These antigenic characteristics determine the type of enzyme-specific and toxin-specific antibodies produced by the host. A host with adequate antibodies against a particular serotype with or without antitoxic immunity may not develop clinical disease if reinfected with the same serotype. A person with antitoxic immunity resulting from previous group A infections but with no antibodies against a particular invading serotype may develop a clinical streptococcal throat. A person with no antitoxic immunity and no antibodies against an invading toxigenic group A streptococcus may develop clinical scarlet fever.

Streptococcal Throat

Streptococcal throat (septic sore throat) results when the streptococcus invades and remains in the lymphoid tissue of the oropharynx, rapidly producing inflammation with edema, erythema, and infiltration with polymorphonuclear leukocytes. The mucosal surfaces, particularly over the tonsils, become ulcerated, releasing a mucopurulent exudate. Cervical lymphadenopathy is present. Severity of symptoms increases with age. Untreated, uncomplicated disease lasts a few days to a week. The streptococcus may invade surrounding tissue producing suppurative complications.

Scarlet Fever

Scarlet fever (SF) results if the invading streptococcus releases an erythrogenic toxin stimulating a sensitivity reaction in the host. Dilation of small capillaries and toxic injury of the vascular epithelium may be widespread in the body, particularly in the liver, myocardium, and kidneys. The pathologic changes are most visible on the skin, with an erythematous rash and desquamation, and in the oral cavity, with the strawberry tongue and an enanthem. Hepatocellular damage and destruction of red cells may result in jaundice, increased bilirubin, mild anemia, and increased number of reticulocytes. In rare situations, toxins may be disseminated in the bloodstream, producing a severe toxic illness. Streptococcus may invade adjacent tissue and the bloodstream, producing a severe septic scarlet fever and/or toxic scarlet fever. Both are extremely rare because of antibiotic treatment of early disease.

Rheumatic Fever

Rheumatic fever (RF) is a delayed complication of upper respiratory infection with group A streptococci, producing nonsuppurative inflammatory lesions in connective tissue of the heart, joints, subcutaneous tissues, and central nervous system. Symptoms may be present in all or some of those systems. The exact causal mechanism is not known. The following have been hypothesized: (1) there is direct tissue invasion by group A streptococci or by cell wall antigens of the microorganism; (2) streptococcal enzymes, particularly streptolysins S or O, induce tissue injury; (3) antigen-humoral antibody reactions localize in affected tissue; and (4) an autoimmune reaction is operative. The autoimmune theory is supported by the detection of heart-reactive antibodies (HRAs) in the sera of patients with rheumatic heart disease.

Cardiac connective tissue lesions show early fragmentation of collagen fibers, cellular lymphocytic infiltration, and fibrin deposits. These changes are followed by the development of the Aschoff's nodule, a perivascular locus of inflammation with an area of central necrosis surrounded by large mononuclear and polymorphonuclear leukocytes. Cardiac findings include pericarditis, myocarditis, and left-sided endocarditis. Valvular lesions cause thickening and deformity of the valves, resulting in valvular stenosis and insufficiency. Carditis may result in long-term disability or death.

Joint lesions are characterized by a fibrinous exudate over the synovial membrane and a serous effusion without joint destruction. Subcutaneous nodules form that resemble the Aschoff's nodules described previously.

A later neurologic sequela of rheumatic fever is Sydenham's chorea. The latent period for this condition may be so long as to occur in the absence of laboratory changes associated with rheumatic fever.

Diagnostic Studies and Findings[3]

Culture of specimen of pharyngeal secretions: Identification of GABHS by colonial morphology and hemolysis of blood agar

Antigen/antibody test on specimen of pharyngeal secretions (Rapid Strep Test): Positive for streptococcal antigens in 1 to 2 hours

Serology: Rise in titers between acute and convalescent disease

C-reactive protein (CRP): Normally not present in serum; presence of CRP in serum is diagnostic of rheumatic fever

Erythrocyte sedimentation rate: Elevated in rheumatic fever

Electrocardiogram (ECG): Elongation of PR interval in rheumatic fever

Multidisciplinary Plan[2,3]

Medications

Antiinfective agents

- Penicillin G benzarhine (Bicillin), 1,200,000 U IM one time for adults
- Oral penicillin, 125-250 mg bid for 10 days, *or*
- Penicillin G procaine (Wycillin), 600,000 U IM for 10 days for severe scarlet fever
- Erythromycin (Erythrocin, others), 250 mg PO qid for 10 days for patients allergic to penicillin or clindamycin 300 mg tid
- Aminoglycocides for endocarditis

Antipyretic agents

- Aspirin for treatment of polyarthritis of rheumatic fever
- Antipyretics for management of fever

Corticosteroids

- Prednisone (Deltasone, others), 40-60 mg/day for 2-3 weeks for treatment of carditis, *or*
- Methylprednisolone sodium succinate (Solu-Medrol), IV, in severe cases; decrease to complete withdrawal in 3 weeks

To prevent recurrent streptococcal infections in postrheumatic fever patients: Antiinfective agents; penicillin G benzathine (Bicillin), 1,200,000 U IM q4wk during and following convalescence for at least 5 years, or sulfisoxazole or sulfadiazine, PO, for those allergic to penicillin

General Management

- Bed rest during febrile stage of all streptococcal diseases; bed rest for 3 weeks for patients without carditis; for an additional month after carditis is detected
- Nonstimulating environment and sedation for patients with chorea
- Fluid therapy as indicated
- Treatment of heart failure with O_2, salt restriction, diuretics, and digitalis

NURSING CARE

Nursing Assessment

See Assessment Considerations table on p. 1060.

Potential Complications

Streptococcal Throat

Peritonsillar cellulitis and abscess; retropharyngeal abscess; sinus purulence; otitis media; mastoiditis; meningitis; cervical lymphadenitis; pneumonia; periorbital abscess; septicemia; toxin dissemination leading to rheumatic fever or nephritis

Scarlet Fever

Severe disseminated toxic illness; septicemia; hepatic damage; extremely high temperature and rapid pulse; hemmorrhage

Rheumatic Fever

Valvular heart disease; congestive heart failure; persistent arthritis

Patient Problems/Nursing Diagnoses & Interventions

NIC Risk Management

Risk for infection (secondary) related to complications of streptococcal throat

Risk for infection (patient contacts) related to GABHS in pharyngeal exudate

- Collect pharyngeal secretions for culture *for diagnosis of* Streptococcus *organisms and proper interventions.*

Assessment Considerations

Assessment	Streptococcal Throat	Scarlet Fever	Rheumatic Fever
History	Contact with person with sore throat	Contact with person with sore throat	Untreated sore throat within past month; previous episode or family history of RF
Subjective symptoms	Pain on swallowing, headache, anorexia, malaise, chills; abdominal pain in children	Pain on swallowing, headache, anorexia, malaise, chills; abdominal pain in children	Malaise, abdominal pain
Body temperature	38°-39.6° C (100.4°-103.2° F)	38°-39.6° C (100.4°-103.2° F)	Low-grade fever; 38° C (100.4° F)
Cardiovascular	Rapid pulse	Rapid pulse	Insidious onset of symptoms of carditis within 3 weeks: cardiac enlargement, pericardial friction rubs, congestive heart failure, signs of effusion, tachycardia, gallop rhythm, and diastolic and possibly systolic murmurs Three types of murmurs associated with acute carditis: (1) high-pitched blowing holosystolic apical murmur of mitral regurgitation, (2) low-pitched apical middiastolic flow murmur, (3) high-pitched decrescendo diastolic murmur of aortic regurgitation heard at the secondary and primary aortic areas Mitral and aortic stenotic murmurs associated with chronic rheumatic valvular disease
Head and neck	Enlarged, tender cervical lymph nodes; suppurative complications (mastoiditis, otitis media, periorbital abscess, sinus empyema)	Enlarged, tender cervical lymph nodes; suppurative complications (mastoiditis, otitis media, periorbital abscess, sinus empyema)	
Oropharynx	Edema, erythema (fiery red to dull red), and petechiae of uvula, tonsils, and posterior oropharynx Confluent, easily removable mucopurulent exudate May be suppurative complications	Edema, erythema (fiery red to dull red), and petechiae of uvula, tonsils, and posterior oropharynx Confluent, easily removable mucopurulent exudate May be suppurative complications	
Oral cavity		Tongue is inflamed and heavily coated at first; after the rash appears, the papillae become swollen and appear as red bumps on a gray background (strawberry tongue); within a few days the tongue peels, first at the tip and margins; by day 6 the tongue is completely denuded, beefy red, moist, and glistening (raspberry tongue); tongue returns to normal by the end of the second week Enanthem: for a few days around the time of rash's appearance on the skin there may be a hemorrhagic rash on the soft palate and anterior pillars of the fossae	
Respiratory	Complications: symptoms of pneumonia	Complications: symptoms of pneumonia	

From Grimes.[25]

Assessment	Streptococcal Throat	Scarlet Fever	Rheumatic Fever
Skin		Erythematous and punctate rash appearing within 2 days of streptococcal throat, becoming generalized rapidly; appearing first on upper chest and back and then on lower back, upper extremities, abdomen, and lower extremities Extensiveness of rash is variable; it may be better felt (like sandpaper) than seen Petechiae may precede rash on lower extremities; more common in skin folds Desquamation may develop between 5 days and 4 weeks after appearance of the rash, starting on neck, upper chest, back, fingertips, or toes; skin peels in large sections, particularly on palms and soles Flushing of cheeks with circumoral pallor	One to two dozen firm, painless, variable in size (3 mm to 2 cm), subcutaneous nodules; usually over bony prominences and tendons; lasting 1 to 2 weeks Nonpruritic, erythematous macular eruption on the trunk or proximal extremities (erythema marginatum); lesions appear to be a vasomotor phenomenon, moving over the skin with a tendency to advance at the margins and clear at the center; individual lesions clear within hours, but the process persists intermittently for weeks or months
Neurologic	Complications: symptoms of meningitis	Complications: symptoms of meningitis	Symptoms of chorea: involuntary, purposeless, rapid motions; irritability; emotional lability; weakness; restlessness or fretfulness, gradually increasing in intensity over 2 weeks, reaching a plateau, and gradually subsiding
Musculoskeletal		Tender, slightly inflamed; edematous joints possible	Acute onset of mild to severe symptoms of polyarthritis: heat, swelling, redness, and severe tenderness affecting mainly the knees, ankles, elbows, and wrists; migratory, with multiple joint involvement at one time; inflammation subsides in each joint in 1 to 2 weeks; entire episode subsides in 4 weeks
Abdomen		Liver may be slightly enlarged and tender	

- Administer antibiotics, as prescribed, *to prevent progression to SF or RF.*
- Maintain droplet precautions (see Box 15-4, p. 1087) of hospitalized patients for 24 hours after antibiotic therapy is initiated *to prevent transmission to others.*

NIC Thermoregulation

Hyperthermia related to infectious process

- Monitor body temperature *to detect fever.*
- Administer antipyretics.
- Bathe with tepid water or alcohol *to reduce high fever.*
- Encourage adequate fluid intake *to compensate for increased demands associated with elevated body temperature.*

NIC Activity and Exercise Management

Activity intolerance related to cardiovascular complications of RF and SF

- Maintain complete bed rest for SF and RF patients. Provide all care, including hygiene and feeding, *to conserve patient energy and prevent complications by relieving stress on cardiovascular system.*

NIC Physical Comfort Promotion

Impaired oral mucous membrane related to exudative infectious process of GABHS and inflammatory response to toxin in SF

- Assess pharyngeal area *to detect hyperemia and exudate that may interfere with swallowing.*
- Provide frequent oral fluids and oral hygiene. Provide high humidity in room. Lubricate lips and nares *to promote comfort for patient.*

Patient Education/Continuum of Care Plan[25]

1. Oral antibiotics must be taken for prescribed length of time. Follow-up throat cultures may be necessary.
2. Compliance with prescribed long-term antibiotic therapy is necessary to minimize risk for recurrence of rheumatic fever with subsequent streptococcal infections.
3. Upper respiratory infections should be diagnosed and treated promptly in postrheumatic fever patients.
4. Continued rest during convalescence is necessary for postrheumatic fever patients.
5. Medical monitoring for cardiac complications is necessary after rheumatic fever.

6. Persons with residual rheumatic valvular disease must follow an antimicrobial regimen whenever they undergo dental or surgical procedures that would increase their risk for bacteremia.

Evaluation/Patient Outcomes

Risk Management: Infection is not transmitted. All patient contacts are examined and treated for infection.

Patient self-administers antiinfective agents as prescribed. Patient completes full course of antiinfective therapy. No preventable drug interactions or allergic reactions are experienced. If untoward reactions are experienced, patient discontinues drug and contacts physician immediately.

Complications are prevented. Patient's pulse rate is normal. ECG is normal. No murmurs are auscultated. There is no limitation of joint movement. Patient can move all joints without pain. Patient exhibits purposeful movement, indicating no signs of chorea.

Thermoregulation: Body temperature is maintained within the normal range; comfort and safety are maintained. Patient's body temperature is between 36° and 38° C (96.8° and 100.4° F). Pulse and respiration are normal. Skin is cool to touch and free of excess perspiration. Patient's clothing and bedding are dry. Patient is free of headache and malaise associated with the fever.

Activity and Exercise Management: Patient achieves adequate rest during active disease and returns to preillness level of activity during convalescence. Patient maintains bed rest during acute disease with gradual return of activity. Patient does not experience fatigue on exertion.

Physical Comfort Promotion: Patient's mucous membranes return to prepathogenic state. Patient's mucous membranes are moist, with natural color. There is no edema, inflammation, or exudate in oropharynx. Exanthem and enanthem of scarlet fever are not present.

SEXUALLY TRANSMITTED DISEASES

The term *sexually transmitted diseases (STDs)* refers to a large group of disease syndromes that can be transmitted sexually, irrespective of whether the disease has genital pathologic manifestations. STD is more encompassing than the previously used "venereal disease" categorization. The STDs, similar to other infectious diseases, can be classified as to their etiologic agent or according to their disease manifestations. The following pathogens are known or thought to be sexually transmitted:

Bacteria: *Neisseria gonorrhoeae; Chlamydia trachomatis; Mycoplasma hominis; Ureaplasma urealyticum; Treponema pallidum; Gardnerella vaginalis; Haemophilus ducreyi; Shigella; Calymmatobacterium granulomatis*

Viruses: Herpes simplex virus; *Papillomavirus;* hepatitis A, B, C, and D viruses; molluscum contagiosum virus; cytomegalovirus; HIV

Protozoa: *Trichomonas vaginalis; Entamoeba histolytica; Giardia lamblia*

Fungi: *Candida albicans*

Ectoparasites: *Phthirus pubis; Sarcoptes scabiei*

The list of disease syndromes produced by the listed pathogens is equally extensive. Many pathogens produce multiple disease syndromes, and many of the disease syndromes may be caused by more than one pathogenic agent. The STDs are grouped in this section according to disease manifestations patients are most likely to present to health-care providers (Table 15-21). It must be noted that patients with symptoms of a sexually transmitted disease frequently have multiple sexually transmitted diseases and should be evaluated accordingly.

Gonorrhea and Nongonococcal Urethritis

Gonorrhea (clap, strain, gleet, dose, jack) is an inflammation of the columnar and transitional epithelium caused by the gonococcus. Symptoms, course of disease, and severity differ between males and females. Chronic and severe complications may result from untreated infections. Nongonococcal urethritis is a sexually transmitted urethritis in males (cervicitis and salpingitis in females) caused by an agent other than the gonococcus, most commonly *C. trachomatis.*

The diseases discussed in this section are manifest as urethritis or cervicitis with an inflammatory pyogenic exudate. Salpingitis and other related sequelae may be present (Table 15-22).

Pathophysiology

In gonococcal infections the gonococcus attaches to and penetrates columnar epithelium, producing a patchy inflammatory response in the submucosa with a polymorphonuclear exudate. Affected areas in the male are the urethra, Littre's and Cowper's glands, the prostate, seminal vesicles, and the epididymis. Affected areas in the female include the Bartholin's and Skene's glands, the urethra, the cervix, and the fallopian tubes. The stratified and transitional squamous epithelia are resistant to the gonococcus; therefore the bladder, upper urinary tract, preputial sac, vulva, vagina, and uterus are infrequently involved. The only exception is prepubescent girls who are susceptible to a gonococcal vulvovaginitis before changes occur in the vaginal epithelium that accompany puberty. In both sexes primary infections may also affect the pharynx, conjunctivae, and anus.

Direct extension of the infection occurs by way of lymph vessels. In the female, extension most frequently occurs unilaterally or bilaterally to the fallopian tubes, bypassing the uterus. It appears that some cell surfaces of gonococci have greater ability to attach to fallopian tube mucosa. Thus not all gonococcal cervicitis leads to salpingitis. Direct extension in the male most frequently occurs to the epididymis.

Localized infection in any of the above areas may produce cysts and abscesses. The infection may infrequently resolve without treatment if an adequate cellular immune response develops and if there is adequate drainage of the purulent exudate containing the organism. More commonly, the inflammatory exudate is replaced with fibroblasts, and fibrous tissue fills the inflamed tissue. Hardening of the fibrous tissue causes strictures of the lumen of the urethra, epididymis, or fallopian tubes.

Table 15-21 Sexually Transmitted Disease Categories According to Disease Manifestations

Disease Manifestations	Sexually Transmitted Disease
Urethritis, cervicitis with an inflammatory pyogenic exudate, salpingitis, and related sequelae; proctitis	Gonorrhea; nongonococcal urethritis (*Chlamydia*)
Ulcerative lesions with systemic dissemination of pathogen	Syphilis; lymphogranuloma venereum; herpes
Ulcerative lesions only	Chancroid; granuloma inguinale (donovanosis)
Nonulcerative lesions	Molloscum contagiosum; condylomata acuminata
Vulvovaginitis	Trichomoniasis; candidiasis; bacterial vaginosis (*G. vaginalis* vaginitis)
Systemic infections without lesions	Cytomegalovirus; hepatitis; AIDS
Enteric infections	Giardiasis; *Campylobacter* enteritis: shigellosis; amebic dysentery; salmonellosis; *Mycobacterium avium-intracellulare* (MAI); *Cryptosporidium; Isospora*
Pubic infestations	Scabies; pediculosis
Congenital and perinatal infections and anomalies	Syphilis; gonorrhea; *Chlamydia;* herpes; *Candida* infections; trichomoniasis; AIDS; cytomegalovirus; hepatitis B; genital warts; bacterial warts, bacterial vaginosis

Table 15-22 Overview of Sexually Transmitted Diseases Manifested With Urethritis or Cervicitis

	Gonorrhea	Nongonococcal Urethritis, Cervicitis (*Chlamydia*)
Occurrence	Worldwide; highest in 15- to 30-year-olds of both genders; decreasing in United States	Worldwide; three times more common than gonorrhea
Etiologic agent	*N. gonorrhoeae,* the gonococcus	*C. trachomatis,* less commonly *U. urealyticum, Treponema vaginalis, C. albicans*
Reservoir	Humans	Humans
Transmission	Contact with exudates from mucous membranes of infected persons, usually by direct sexual contact	Direct contact with exudates either sexually or during birth
Incubation period	2-7 days	Range 7-10 days for *C. trachomatis*
Period of communicability	Months, if untreated	Unknown
Susceptibility and resistance	Universal; antibodies are not protective against reinfection	Universal; no acquired immunity
Report to local health authority	Mandatory case report	Case report required in most states

Data from Benenson.[3]

Complete or partial occlusion of the fallopian tubes results in sterility or increased risk for ectopic pregnancy.

Infection with gonorrhea does result in a short-lived cellular immune response and a longer-lasting humoral immune response, neither of which protects against future infections.

Nongonococcal urethritis and cervicitis are most frequently caused by strains of *C. trachomatis* that are pathogenic to columnar epithelium in a manner similar to *N. gonorrhoeae.* Symptomatic manifestations are generally less severe than with gonorrhea, with many subclinical infections. Infection with *C. trachomatis* stimulates a cellular and humoral immune response, neither of which is protective against future infections.

Diagnostic Studies and Findings[3,26]

Culture of exudate from urethra, vagina, fallopian tubes, pharynx, or anus: Positive for *N. gonorrhoeae* or *C. trachomatis.*

Microscopic examination of stained exudate: Gonorrhea positive: detection of gram-negative diplococci; chlamydia positive: detection of *C. trachomatis.*

Enzyme-linked immunosorbent assay (ELISA): Detects *C. trachomatis* antibody reaction in specimen and detects *N. gonorrhoeae* in urethral and voided urine specimens.

Genetic probe: Positive for RNA of *C. trachomatis* or *N. gonorrhoeae* in specimen

Leukocyte esterase test of first-void urine: 10 or fewer WBCs per high-power field confirms presence of urethritis

All patients with gonorrhea or *Chlamydia* infection should be tested for syphilis and counseled and tested for HIV

Multidisciplinary Plan[16]

Medications

Antiinfective Agents

Uncomplicated gonococcal infections in adults and presumption of coexisting *Chlamydia* infection

- Ceftriaxone, 125 mg IM single dose *or*
- Cefixime, 400 mg PO single dose *or*
- Ciprofloxacin, 500 mg PO single dose *or*
- Ofloxacin, 400 mg PO single dose plus doxycycline hyclate (Vibramycin), 100 mg PO bid for 7 days *or*

HEALTHY PEOPLE 2010

Health Status—Sexually Transmitted Diseases

Goal: Promote responsible sexual behaviors, strengthen community capacity, and increase access to quality services to prevent sexually transmitted diseases (STDs) and their complications.

Bacterial STD Illness and Disability

- Reduce the proportion of adolescents and young adults with *Chlamydia trachomatis* infections.
- Reduce gonorrhea.
- Eliminate sustained domestic transmission of primary and secondary syphilis.

Viral STD Illness and Disability

- Reduce the proportion of adults with genital herpes infection.
- (Developmental) Reduce the proportion of persons with human papillomavirus (HPV) infection.

STD Complications Affecting Females

- Reduce the proportion of females who have ever required treatment for pelvic inflammatory disease (PID).
- Reduce the proportion of childless females with fertility problems who have had an STD or who have required treatment for PID.
- (Developmental) Reduce HIV infections in adolescent and young adult females ages 13 to 24 years that are associated with heterosexual contact.
- Reduce congenital syphilis.
- (Developmental) Reduce neonatal consequences from maternal STDs, including chlamydial pneumonia, gonococcal and chlamydial ophthalmia neonatorum, laryngeal papillomatosis (from HPV infection), neonatal herpes, and preterm birth and low birth weight associated with bacterial vaginosis.

Personal Behaviors

- Increase the proportion of adolescents who abstain from sexual intercourse or use condoms if currently sexually active.
- (Developmental) Increase the number of positive messages related to responsible sexual behavior during weekday and nightly prime-time television programming.

Community Protection Infrastructure

- Increase the proportion of tribal, state, and local STD programs that routinely offer hepatitis B vaccines to all STD clients.
- (Developmental) Increase the proportion of youth detention facilities and adult city or county jails that screen for common bacterial STDs within 24 hours of admission and treat STDs (when necessary) before persons are released.
- (Developmental) Increase the proportion of all local health departments that have contracts with managed-care providers for the treatment of non–plan partners of patients with bacterial STDs (gonorrhea, syphilis, and chlamydia).

Personal Health Services

- (Developmental) Increase the proportion of sexually active females age 25 years and under who are screened annually for genital chlamydia infections.
- (Developmental) Increase the proportion of pregnant females screened for STDs (including HIV infection and bacterial vaginosis) during prenatal health-care visits according to recognized standards.
- Increase the proportion of primary-care providers who treat patients with STDs and who manage cases according to recognized standards.

Modified from U.S. Department of Health and Human Services: *Healthy people 2010* (conference edition, in two volumes), Washington, DC, January 2000.

NOTE: *Developmental* indicates that criteria for measurement and strategies to improve health have not as yet been specified.

Azithromycin, 1 g PO single dose, *or*
Doxycycline, 100 mg PO bid for 7 days
Pharyngeal gonococcal infection
Ceftriaxone, 125 mg IM single dose, *or*
Ciprofloxacin, 500 mg PO once
Disseminated gonococcal infection (DGI)
Ceftriaxone, 1 g IM or IV, q24h, *or*
Ceftizoxime, 1 g IV, q8h, *or*
Adult gonococcal ophthalmia: Ceftriaxone, 1 g IM single dose
Uncomplicated *Chlamydia* infection only
Doxycycline, 100 mg PO bid for 7 days, *or*
Azithromycin, 1 g PO in a single dose
Ofloxacin, 300 mg PO bid for 7 days
Erythromycin base, 500 mg PO qid for 7 days, *or*
Erythromycin ethylsuccinate, 800 mg PO qid for 7 days

The above therapy, recommended by the Centers for Disease Control and Prevention (CDC) in 1998, is not all inclusive. Consult CDC 1998 recommendations for treatment of infants and children and for alternative therapies. The recommendations are based on the increase in infections with antibiotic-resistant *N. gonorrhoeae,* such as penicillinase-producing *N. gonorrhoeae* (PPNG), tetracycline-resistant *N. gonorrhoeae* (TRNG), and strains with chromosomally mediated resistance to multiple antibiotics. They also consider the high frequency of concurrent *Chlamydia* infections with gonorrhea. All sexual partners of patients with gonorrhea or *Chlamydia* infection should be examined and treated. Quinolones, tetracyclines, and oflaxicin are contraindicated during pregnancy.

NURSING CARE

Nursing Assessment

For Gonorrhea and Nongonococcal Urethritis and Cervicitis *(Chlamydia)*

History: Unprotected sexual contact (vaginal, anal, or oral) with an infected person; multiple sexual partners or unknown partner; history of previous STD

Subjective symptoms

Male: May be asymptomatic; dysuria; severe pain of epididymitis; urinary retention with prostatitis

Female: Usually asymptomatic, dysuria or urinary frequency; pelvic inflammatory disease (PID) (pelvic pain, low back pain, dyspareunia, menstrual irregularity, constipation, malaise)

Male and female: Rectal infection (anal pruritus, burning, or tenesmus); pain with defecation; pharyngeal infection, sore throat

Genitalia

Male: Purulent yellow-white discharge from urethra (clearer discharge with *Chlamydia*); inflammation around meatus; swelling and severe pain in scrotum with epididymitis

Female: Leukorrhea, usually goes unnoticed

Pelvis (with PID): Female: Rebound tenderness; normal bowel sounds progressing to ileus in untreated persons; nausea and vomiting

Pharyngeal infection: Usually asymptomatic or inflamed with visible exudate; red, dry tongue

Rectal infection: Bloody or mucous diarrhea; purulent discharge

Eyes: Purulent discharge from conjunctiva

Systemic manifestations of disseminated disease: Painful vesicular pustular skin lesions on an erythematous base; petechial skin lesions; symptoms of septicemia, endocarditis, meningitis, arthritis

Body temperature: Low-grade fever, higher with systemic manifestations, PID, or epididymitis

Potential Complications

Recurrent, noninfectious urethritis; acute or chronic pelvic inflammatory disease peritonitis; Reiter's syndrome (reactive arthropathy); amnionitis during pregnancy; disseminated infection in neonate; ophthalmia neonatorum; pneumonia in neonate; postpartum endometriosis

See Patient Problems/Nursing Diagnoses & Interventions, p. 1074.

Syphilis

Syphilis (lues) is a chronic systemic infection of the vascular system, generally transmitted by sexual contact. It is characterized by a primary lesion, a secondary eruption involving skin and mucous membranes, long latency periods, and late seriously disabling lesions of skin, bone, viscera, CNS, and cardiovascular system.

Syphilis is one of several sexually transmitted diseases that have both ulcerative lesions and systemic dissemination. Others are herpesvirus infections and lymphogranuloma venereum (Table 15-23).

Pathophysiology

Syphilis is a systemic infection of the vascular system characterized by five distinct stages: incubation, primary and secondary stages, latency, and late syphilis. Incubation begins with the penetration of *T. pallidum* into intact mucous membranes or abraded skin. Some of the pathogens remain at the site of invasion, whereas others migrate, within hours, to regional lymph nodes, where some remain while others are disseminated throughout the body. *Treponema* can invade and multiply in any organ system, producing lesions wherever the concentration of the microorganism is the greatest. During this incubation period, blood containing the *Treponema* organisms is infectious.

Vascular pathologic manifestations are the consequence of treponemal tissue invasion at all stages. The inflammatory response in the endothelial tissue, endothelial swelling, and an obliterative endarteritis of terminal arterioles and small arteries results in eventual tissue necrosis.

The primary stage is characterized by a single lesion at the site of initial invasion containing the *Treponema* and appearing 10 to 90 days after infection. The lesion is firm and hard as a result of intense cellular infiltration accompanied by serum accumulation in connective tissue. The lesion heals spontaneously within 1 to 5 weeks (average of 2 to 3 weeks). A satellite lesion, or bubo, may develop in an inguinal lymph node.

The secondary stage begins as the primary lesion is resolving, lasts 2 to 6 weeks, and is manifested with parenchymal, systemic, and mucocutaneous symptoms that indicate treponemal pathologic manifestations throughout the body. *Treponema* can be recovered from all skin and mucous membrane lesions.

A period of latency, ranging from 1 to 40 or more years, follows the secondary stage. During the first year of latency there may be recurrence of secondary stage manifestations. Subclinical infection with progressive arterial damage continues for some number of infected persons.

About one third of infected, untreated persons manifest symptoms of late syphilis with clinical evidence of degenerative lesions of the cardiovascular and central nervous systems, the skin, and the viscera. These lesions, called gummas, are granulomatous lesions consisting of a necrotic, coagulated center with obliterative endarteritis of small vessels in the tissue. Lesions of late syphilis, including open gummas on the skin, do not contain *Treponema.* They are therefore not infectious.

Disease manifestations of late syphilis depend on the area of arterial lesions and the extent of circulatory insufficiency. Central nervous system disease may be asymptomatic, meningovascular, or parenchymatous. Parenchymatous neurosyphilis can be seen clinically as paresis (resulting from progressive cortical neuron degeneration) or tabes dorsalis (resulting from posterior column degeneration).

Cardiovascular symptoms frequently result from aortic necrosis with resultant aortic insufficiency.

The immune response in syphilis is not completely understood. Humoral antibodies develop early and persist in untreated persons, but they do not seem to alter the course of the disease. The cell-mediated immune response increases during latency. This may account for the lack of progression to late syphilis for a large portion of untreated persons. Antibody levels will gradually decrease in persons treated in primary and secondary stages.

Congenital transmission of *Treponema* may occur at any time during pregnancy, but the fetus does not develop an inflammatory response to the pathogen until around the fifteenth week of gestation. Treatment of infected pregnant women before the fifteenth week may prevent damage to the fetus. Evidence of congenital syphilitic damage includes early malformations, observed at birth or during the first 2 years of life, and later evidence of developmental deformities. Infants with congenital syphilis born to untreated or inadequately treated mothers will have active infection and must be treated.

Table 15-23 Overview of Sexually Transmitted Diseases With Ulcerative Lesions and Systemic Dissemination

	Syphilis	Anogenital Herpes	Herpes Type 1	Lymphogranuloma Venereum
Occurrence	Worldwide; increasing in incidence; highest in persons 20-30 years old of both genders; increasing in neonates	Worldwide; increasing rapidly; highest in persons 15-30 years old; 20%-30% of U.S. adults have herpes simplex virus type 2 (HSV-2) antibody	Worldwide; 70%-90% of adults have antibodies against herpes simplex virus type 1 (HSV-1); primary infection probably occurs by age 5 years	Worldwide; higher in tropical and subtropical climates
Etiologic agent	*T. pallidum,* a spirochete	HSV-2	HSV-1	Several strains of *C. trachomatis*
Reservoir	Humans	Humans	Humans	Humans
Transmission	Direct contact with exudates from lesions on skin and mucous membranes; body fluids and secretions (saliva, semen, blood, vaginal discharges) of infected people, usually during sexual contact; blood transfusion from infected donor during early disease; and congenital	Direct contact with saliva or secretions from mucous membranes and lesions; congenital	Contact with saliva of carriers and active lesions; may be transmitted sexually	Direct contact with open lesions
Incubation period	10 days to 12 weeks; usually 3 weeks	2-12 days; average of 6 days	2-12 days	3-30 days
Period of communicability	Variable; during primary and secondary stages and in mucocutaneous recurrences; 2-4 years if untreated	Transient shedding of virus in absence of lesions probably occurs; 7-12 days with lesion	During lesions; virus in saliva found as long as 7 weeks after recovery of lesions; transient shedding of virus is common	Variable; weeks to years as long as lesions are present
Susceptibility and resistance	Universal, although only 30% of exposures result in infection; no natural immunity; infection leads to gradually developing resistance to new infections	Universal; immune response does not prevent recurrence	Universal susceptibility	General susceptibility; resistance is not clear
Report to local health authority	Mandatory case report	No	No	In some states

Data from Benenson[3] and Centers for Disease Control and Prevention.[16]

Diagnostic Studies and Findings[26]

Microscopic examination of specimen of exudate or cells from lesions or regional lymph nodes: Positive for *T. pallidum* during primary and secondary stages

Detection of antigen in specimen through treponemal antigen/antibody test: Reported as nonreactive, borderline, or reactive; these tests become reactive earlier in primary stage and are used to confirm a previously reactive, rapid plasma reagin (RPR), which may have been positive due to other conditions

Serology (Venereal Disease Research Laboratory [VDRL]; [RPR]): Increase in nonspecific antibodies 1 to 3 weeks after appearance of the chancre or 4 to 6 weeks after infection; tests become nonreactive in 6 to 12 months after treatment of primary syphilis, 12 to 18 months after treatment of secondary syphilis; serologic tests may not revert to nonreactive if treatment is delayed beyond 2 years.

Persons with early syphilis should be tested for other STDs and counseled and tested for HIV.

Multidisciplinary Plan[16]

Medications

Antiinfective Agents

Primary, secondary, or early syphilis of less than 1 year's duration: Penicillin G benzathine, 2.4 million U IM single dose

Of more than 1 year's duration: Penicillin G benzathine (Bicillin), 7.2 million U total; 2.4 million U IM/wk for 3 successive weeks

Patients allergic to penicillin

Tetracycline (Achromycin; others) 500 mg PO qid for 15 days for infections of less than 1 year and 30 days for infections of longer duration, *or*

Doxycycline, 100 mg PO bid for 2 weeks for infections of longer duration (pregnant women should not receive tetracycline or doxycycline)

Penicillin-allergic pregnant women should be skin tested and desensitized and then treated with penicillin in a hospital setting (no alternative drug therapies to penicillin are currently effective for treating syphilis in pregnancy, congenital syphilis, or neurosyphilis)

Neurosyphilis

Aqueous crystalline penicillin G, 18-24 million U/day administered 3-4 million U q4h IV for 10-14 days, *or*

Procaine penicillin, 2.4 million U IM/day plus probenecid, 500 mg PO qid, both for 10-14 days

NURSING CARE

NURSING ASSESSMENT

For Syphilis

History: Unprotected sexual contact (vaginal, anal, or oral) with an infected person; multiple sexual partners or unknown partner, previous STD

Primary Stage: Within 10 to 90 Days After Exposure (Average of 21 Days); Lasts 1 to 5 Weeks

Genitalia: Single painless papule erodes to become a hard, painless, indurated chancre without an exudate; located at site of inoculation, usually on glans penis of male and on cervix or external genitalia of female; may be seen on scrotum, anus, rectum, lips, tongue, tonsils, nipples, and fingers; abraded ulcer exudes serous fluid teeming with *T. pallidum* organisms

Lymph nodes: Hard, nonfluctuant, painless, enlarged inguinal lymph nodes

Secondary Stage: Within 6 to 12 Weeks After Infection, Lasting a Few Days to 1 Year

Subjective symptoms: Malaise, headache, anorexia, nausea, aching in bones, fatigue, neck stiffness; fever; anemia; jaundice

Skin

Lesions, recurring local or generalized, papulosquamous, macular, papular, or pustular rash; bilateral and symmetric, beginning on trunk and proximal extremities, frequently on soles of feet and palms of hands; lesions are 3 to 10 mm, nonpruritic, and contain *T. pallidum* organisms

Condylomata lata: Lesions on moist areas coalesce and erode to produce painless, moist, pink to grayish white, raised plaques

Alopecia: Nonscarring, temporary hair loss in patches on head and eyebrows

Mucous membranes: Mucous patches: silver-gray superficial erosion surrounded by red periphery on mucous membranes

Gastrointestinal status: Epigastric pain or vomiting associated with ulceration

Latent Stage: Lasts a Few Years Through the Remainder of Person's Life

May have relapses of mucocutaneous symptoms of secondary stage early in latency; otherwise, no symptoms

Late Stages (Tertiary Syphilis): Benign Tertiary Syphilis of the Skin, Bone, and Viscera (3 to 10 Years After Infection)

Gumma lesions (a chronic granulomatous reaction, causing lesions, ulcers, or tumors); lesions are of varying sizes, appear anywhere on the body, and do not contain *T. pallidum;* they may occur in palate, nasal septum, and other submucosal tissue, causing disfigurement; gumma lesions in bones cause pain

Cardiovascular Syphilis (10 to 25 Years After Initial Infection)

Aortic valvular insufficiency, thoracic aneurysm, narrowing of coronary ostia

Neurosyphilis (May Be Asymptomatic or Symptomatic)

Meningovascular symptoms: Focal neurologic signs depending on area of lesions; seizures; parenchymatous symptoms: paresis; personality changes, ranging from minor to severe psychosis; alteration in intellect and judgment; hyperactive reflexes; tabes dorsalis; ataxia, areflexia, paresthesias, bladder disturbance, impotence; sharp, tearing pain; trophic joint changes; optic atrophy with small, irregular pupils that are not reactive to light but respond normally to accommodation

POTENTIAL COMPLICATIONS

CNS and cardiovascular disease of tertiary syphilis; congenital syphilis with congenital anomalies; fetal or neonatal death

PATIENT PROBLEMS/NURSING DIAGNOSES & INTERVENTIONS

See p. 1074.

HERPESVIRUS INFECTIONS

Herpes simplex is a systemic viral infection characterized by a localized primary lesion, latency, and a tendency to localized recurrence. Two serologically distinct herpes viral agents, 1 and 2, generally produce distinct clinical syndromes. Herpes simplex virus type 2 (HSV-2) is most often implicated in genital herpes (see Table 15-23).

PATHOPHYSIOLOGY

Two antigenically distinct herpes simplex viruses (HSV), types 1 and 2, are responsible for herpes infections. Both are capable of producing infection in epithelial tissue anywhere in the body, but HSV-1 is most often associated with oral, labial, ocular, or skin herpes, whereas HSV-2 is implicated in 90% of genital, anal, and perianal herpes or oral herpes associated with genital, oral, or sexual transmission. Infections caused by both types of HSV are discussed in this section because of the potential for sexual transmission of both agents and because both produce essentially the same pathologic findings.

All HSV infections have two characteristics in common: once present in tissue, HSV produces a chronic infection initiated with active self-limiting tissue destruction. The lesions heal, but the organism continues to be viable in the body in the presence of circulating antibodies and in the absence of symptomatic disease.

There is a latent period during which the genome of the virus is present in tissue in a nondestructive form. Infectious virions cannot be recovered until the virus becomes reactivated and produces recurrent infectious disease. Active infection, either initial or recurrent, need not be symptomatic.

Initial infection refers to the first infection with the HSV type. Initial infection with HSV-1 usually occurs by age 4 years and is manifest as a clinical or subclinical gingivostomatitis. Initial infection with HSV-2 usually occurs during the ages of sexual activity and is usually manifested by clinical or subclinical genital herpes.

The organism is transmitted by close contact with saliva or genital secretions of persons with active clinical or subclinical infections either directly or by hand.

The transmitted virus invades and replicates in the epithelial cells of mucous membranes or traumatized skin. Polymorphonuclear cells infiltrate, forming a thin-walled intradermal vesicle on an erythematous base. Multiple grouped vesicles can be visualized at the sites of tissue inoculation. The superficial epithelium collapses and sloughs, leaving single shallow ulcers, or the vesicles may coalesce into large painful ulcers. Crusting may occur on nonmucous membrane ulcers. All ulcers spontaneously granulate without scarring in about 12 days in initial infections.

The virus may enter the lymphatic system, producing localized lesions there. Rarely, the virus is disseminated to visceral organs, particularly the liver, adrenal glands, lungs, or central nervous system, producing discrete focal areas of necrosis in epithelial tissues in those organs. The virus may also be spread to other external body sites by autoinoculation.

Cellular immune response and nonspecific host defenses appear to inhibit dissemination. Circulating humoral antibodies develop but do not appear to be protective against reinfection or recurrent infection.

After the primary infection, the HSV travels along sensory nerve pathways to a sensory nerve ganglion where it remains in a latent stage. The viral DNA is stored in ganglion neurons in the absence of other viral products. The virus is not pathogenic in this form. It appears that the transient viral shedding may occur during this stage.

The exact mechanism for reactivation of the virus to produce recurrence of lesions is not known. Recurrence of HSV lesions is generally in the area of initial inoculation. Genital recurrence is usually associated with HSV-2 and is usually less severe, lasting 4 or 5 days. Genital recurrence is common in women with asymptomatic cervical lesions. Oral HSV-1 infections frequently recur on the lips. Recurrence of either type may be triggered by another infectious disease, menstruation, emotional stress, and immunosuppression.

Potential Complications

Neuralgia, meningitis, encephalitis, ascending myelitis, urethral stricture, lymphatic suppuration, spontaneous abortion, cervical cancer, congenital herpes infection

Diagnostic Studies and Findings[3,26]

Virus tissue culture of specimen from base of vesicles: Identification of type 1 or type 2 viral cytopathogenic effect in tissue culture

Microscopic examination of stained smear from base of vesicles: Direct identification of multinucleated giant cells with intranuclear inclusions

Serology: Fourfold increase in antibody titer in paired sera; difficult to differentiate type 1 from type 2

Persons with a new infection with herpes should be examined for syphilis, gonorrhea, Chlamydia, *and HIV*

Multidisciplinary Plan[16]

Medications

Antiinfective Agents

For first clinical episode of genital herpes: Initiated within 6 days of onset of lesions: acyclovir, 200 mg PO, five times per day for 7-10 days, or 400 mg PO, three times per day for 7-10 days, or famciclovir, 250 mg PO, three times per day for 7-10 days, or valacyclovir 1 g PO 2 times per day for 7-10 days

For severe infections: Acyclovir 5-10 mg/kg q8h IV for 5-7 days or until clinical resolution

For proctitis: Acyclovir, 400 mg PO, five times per day for 10 days

Recurrent episodes: Acyclovir, 200 mg PO, five times per day for 5 days, or acyclovir, 800 mg PO, three times per day for 5 days, or acyclovir 400 mg PO tid for 5 days

Suppressive therapy: Acyclovir, 400 mg PO bid, or valacyclovir, 250 mg PO two times per day or 500 mg PO once per day or 1000 mg PO once per day

NURSING CARE

Nursing Assessment

See Nursing Care on p. 1069.

Lymphogranuloma Venereum

Lymphogranuloma venereum is a systemic, disabling bacterial infection that begins with a small, painless evanescent erosion on the penis or vulva. Regional lymph nodes undergo suppuration, spreading the inflammatory process into adjacent tissue. The disease is disseminated further by the lymph system. There are usually systemic symptoms of lymphadenitis and serious complications in untreated individuals.

For an overview of lymphogranuloma venereum see Table 15-23.

Pathophysiology

Lymphogranuloma venereum is a systemic infection produced by mucosal invasion of a number of closely related strains of *Chlamydia.* The disease has three stages: a primary lesion, regional and disseminated lymphadenitis, and late complications resulting from progression of the regional lymphadenitis.

A primary transient nodular or vesicular lesion forms at the site of inoculation. Dissemination of the organism to regional lymph nodes (primarily inguinal lymph nodes) results in lymph node lesions that are initially similar to the inoculation lesion. Satellite lesions are formed in the lymph node, surrounded by a narrow layer of epithelioid cells. Spread of the inflammation throughout the nodes causes the nodes to become matted together and form a large abscess. These abscesses develop in one or more areas along the lymphatic system. Untreated, the abscesses may rupture through the skin or other epithelial surfaces to produce chronic draining sinuses or fistulas. If the condition is not treated, it progresses, producing complications resulting from the impaired lymph and draining sinuses.

DIAGNOSTIC STUDIES AND FINDINGS[3]

Cell culture of lesion exudate or bubo aspirate: Positive for *C. trachomatis*

Serology: Fourfold rise in antibody titer between early infection and convalescence; nonspecific, because it detects antibodies against all *C. trachomatis* strains; this agent can cause a false-positive RPR test for syphilis

These patients should be examined for other STDs, as well.

MULTIDISCIPLINARY PLAN[16]

Surgery

Aspiration of fluctuant lymph nodes as needed (incision and drainage or excision is contraindicated)

Strictures or fistulas may require surgery

Medications

Antiinfective agents: doxycycline, 100 mg PO bid for 21 days, or erythromycin base, 500 mg PO qid for 21 days

NURSING CARE

NURSING ASSESSMENT

For Herpes Type 1, Herpes Type 2, and Lymphogranuloma Venereum (LV)

History: Unprotected sexual contact (vaginal, anal, or oral) with an infected person; multiple or unknown sexual partners; previous herpes lesions

Subjective symptoms

- Herpes 1 and 2: Burning or pruritus in areas of lesions; fever in initial infection; malaise
- LV: Fever, chills, headache, joint pains, anorexia, abdominal pain, urinary retention

Oral cavity

- Herpes 1 and 2: Multiple vesicular and ulcerative lesions on labial and buccal mucosa, tongue, and larynx; erythema of gums; excessive salivation; infection heals in 7 to 10 days; recurrent infections rare in mouth
- LV: May have lesions in mouth as described under genitourinary/rectal below

Lips: Herpes 1: recurrent "cold sore" or "fever blister" preceded by 1 or 2 days of paresthesia; lesions crust and heal within 3 to 10 days

Genitourinary/rectal

- Herpes 2: Asymptomatic or extensive vesicular lesions with deep ulceration and marked hyperplasia and erythema of cervix, labia, fourchette, and clitoris (sometimes vagina); may extend to anal area, buttocks, and thighs; dysuria, leukorrhea, and marked genital tenderness; scattered vesicles over glans, prepuce, and shaft of the penis (lesions heal in 10 days); urinary retention; urethritis may occur without genital lesions; anal lesions possible
- LV: 2- to 3-mm painless, discrete, superficial vesicle or nonindurated ulcer at site of inoculation (frequently unnoticed); usually on glans or shaft of penis in males and on labia, vagina, or cervix in females; may be in rectum; rectal inoculation initially produces bloody discharge and tenesmus, and mucopurulent discharge, cramps, and diarrhea later; complications may include elephantiasis of prepuce, penis, scrotum, or vulva; perianal abscess; rectovaginal, rectovesical, and ischiorectal fistulas; rectal stricture 1 to 10 years after infection

Lymph nodes

- Herpes 1: Enlarged and palpable cervical lymph nodes
- Herpes 2: Bilateral lymphadenopathy of inguinal lymph nodes in 50% of initial genital infections
- LV: 7 to 30 days after primary lesion: initially a firm, tender, discrete, movable inguinal lymph node, which later becomes indolent, fixed, and matted; may be unilateral or bilateral; may subside spontaneously or proceed to form an abscess that may rupture to produce a draining sinus or fistula; female lymph node involvement may be mainly in the pelvic nodes with extension to rectum and rectovaginal septum

Skin: Herpes 1 and 2: clustered vesicular lesions anywhere on body; deep burning; skin edema

Eyes: Herpes 1 and 2: keratitis and conjunctivitis (unilateral or bilateral); periauricular lymphadenopathy

POTENTIAL COMPLICATIONS

Genital elephantitis; perianal abscesses and fistulas; rectal stricture, obstruction, rupture; peritonitis

See Patient Problems/Nursing Diagnoses & Interventions on p. 1074.

CHANCROID AND GRANULOMA INGUINALE

Chancroid, also called "soft sore" or "soft chancre," is an acute, localized, autoinoculable bacterial infection of the genitalia. Necrotizing ulceration occurs at the site of inoculation, frequently accompanied by suppuration of regional lymph nodes. Systemic dissemination does not occur.

Granuloma inguinale (donovanosis) is a mildly communicable, chronic and progressive, autoinoculable bacterial infection of the skin and mucous membranes, external genitalia, inguinal and anal regions, face, and oral cavity. Lesions first appear as small, painless papules or vesicles that become ulcerated and slowly develop into bleeding granulomatous masses. The disease may be difficult to differentiate from carcinoma (Table 15-24).

PATHOPHYSIOLOGY

Although both chancroid and granuloma inguinale are manifest as ulcerative lesions, their pathophysiologies differ.

Chancroid

In chancroid the transmitted pathogenic bacteria initially invade genital skin or mucous membranes at sites traumatized by sexual

Table 15-24 Overview of Sexually Transmitted Diseases With Ulcerative Lesions Without Systemic Manifestations

	Chancroid	Granuloma Inguinale (Donovanosis)
Occurrence	Most common in tropical and subtropical climates; more often diagnosed in males than in females	Most common in tropical and subtropical climates and in 20-40 year-old men
Etiologic agent	*H. ducreyi,* a bacterium	*C. granulomatis*
Reservoir	Humans	Humans
Transmission	Direct sexual contact with exudate from lesions; autoinoculation to other areas	Direct sexual contact with lesions or with organism in rectum of nondiseased carriers
Incubation period	3-14 days	1-16 weeks
Period of communicability	Until lesions heal (can be weeks)	Duration of open lesions
Susceptibility and resistance	General, but highest in uncircumcised males; no evidence of resistance, although women may have more subclinical infections	Susceptibility is variable; no evidence of immunity
Report to local health authority	Mandatory case report	Mandatory case report

Data from Benenson[3] and Centers for Disease Control and Prevention.[16]

contact. A preexisting abrasion facilitates invasion. A small papule is formed, surrounded by a zone of erythema. This erupts to form a shallow and painful ulcer.

A purulent exudate results from the extensive necrotic process. The ulcers may enlarge and continue to erode and destroy tissue, or they may become secondarily infected and produce even more rapid destruction of tissue. Fresh lesions may occur from autoinoculation. Extragenital lesions may occur on fingers, tongue, lips, breasts, and eyelids.

Lymphatic dissemination results in a unilateral or bilateral painful inguinal adenitis within 7 to 10 days of the primary lesion. The enlarged lymph gland (bubo) softens, becomes fluctuant, and may rupture spontaneously.

Granuloma Inguinale

The transmission of granuloma inguinale is less well understood. The pathogenic bacterium can be found in the rectum of nondiseased patients, suggesting that the organism may be part of the normal gastrointestinal flora of some persons. Lesions may result from autoinfection, possibly following trauma to the genitalia. The pathogen in the lesions is transmitted sexually, but repeated exposure seems to be necessary for transmission. The disease is rare in heterosexual partners of infected persons. Clinical disease is highest in men who have sex with men.

The organism invades endothelial cells and forms a small, painless papule or nodule at the site of dermal invasion. The epithelium overlapping the lesion softens, erodes, ulcerates, and then produces a gradually enlarging granulomatous ulcerating lesion that bleeds easily. Pronounced marginal epithelial proliferation may simulate early epitheliomatous changes of cancer. The raised mass of granulation tissue looks more like a tumor than an ulcer. Single or multiple lesions may coalesce, or lesions may spread to contiguous tissue. Lesions have variable clinical appearances depending on the area where they are located, mode of spread, tissue resistance, and texture of the skin.

The lesions heal by fibrosis at the same time that tissue destruction is occurring in expanding lesions. Resultant scarring may produce urethral occlusion. The inguinal swelling that is sometimes seen with this disease is not a lymphadenopathy, but rather a subcutaneous granuloma.

Diagnostic Studies and Findings

Chancroid: Culture or microscopic examination of exudate from bulbo or lesions; positive for *H. ducreyi* bacilli; tests to rule out other causes of ulcers, particularly syphilis and herpes

Granuloma inguinale: Microscopic examination of scrapings from ulcer margins; Donovan's bodies can be visualized; *tests to rule out carcinoma; examination for other STDs*

Multidisciplinary Plan[3,16]

Surgery

Chancroid: Fluctuant lymph nodes should be aspirated through adjacent normal skin (incision and drainage or excision of nodes is contraindicated)

Medications[16]

Antiinfective Agents

Chancroid
- Erythromycin base, 500 mg PO qid 7 days, *or*
- Azithromycin, 1 g PO single dose
- Ceftriaxone, 250 mg IM single dose
- Ciprofloxacin, 500 mg PO bid for 3 days

Granuloma inguinale
- Trimethoprim-sulfamethoxazole, 1 double-strength tablet PO bid for 3 weeks *or*
- Doxycycline, 100 mg PO bid for 3 weeks

NURSING CARE

Nursing Assessment

For Chancroid and Granuloma Inguinale

History: Unprotected sexual contact (vaginal, anal, or oral) with an infected person; multiple or unknown sexual partners; history of previous STD

Subjective symptoms: Chancroid: pain

Genitalia

Chancroid: 1 to 10 primary lesions; inflamed macule, papule, or pustule; irregularly shaped and of variable size (1 mm to 2 cm); surrounded by a zone of inflammation; erupts to produce a sharply circumscribed, nonindurated ulcer with a granulating base and ragged edges; abundant, purulent exudate; location: frenulum, prepuce, coronal sulcus, glans and shaft of penis, and urinary meatus in males; cervix, vagina, fourchette, labia, and perianal area in females

Variations in clinical appearance of lesions

Follicular pustules rupture and form ulcers

Dwarf chancroid lesions look similar to herpes lesions

Transient chancroid lesion resolves quickly but is followed by an inguinal bubo

Papular chancroid starts as an ulcer but becomes raised

Giant chancroid frequently follows rupture of inguinal abscess and grows rapidly

Phagedenic chancroid, a small lesion, rapidly extends and becomes necrotic and destructive

Granuloma inguinale: Single or multiple, indurated, sharply defined but irregular papules or nodules; erode to form a beefy, exuberant granulomatous, heaped, clean ulcer, progressing slowly and coalescing with adjacent lesions; serous exudate; location: glans, prepuce, urethra, shaft of penis, and perianal area in males; labia and fourchette in females; lesions bleed easily; if secondarily infected, may have odorous necrotic exudate

Variations in clinical appearance

Oral lesions are painful and resemble malignancies

Vaginal and cervical ulcers produce profuse, purulent discharge and irregular bleeding

Cervical ulcers are soft, friable, irregular, and not well fixed to tissue; resemble cancer

Male genital ulcers may be hypertrophic and verrucose, destructive and necrotic, discoid (buttonlike), or chronic and indolent

Inguinal ulcers and ulcers on female genitalia are generally fleshy and exuberant

Anal ulcers are hypertrophic and verrucose or chronic and indolent

Inguinal area

Chancroid: single, unilateral (can be bilateral), tender, and unilocular lymphadenopathy with overlying erythema; suppuration and rupture of fluctuant nodes in 5 to 10 days may occur, leaving a single, large ulcer

Granuloma inguinale: rarely any inguinal involvement; may have a subcutaneous granuloma that suppurates and mimics a lymphadenopathy

Potential Complications

Chancroid

Phimosis and urethral fistulas in males; females frequently asymptomatic; associated with increased risk for HIV infection

Granuloma inguinale

Hematogenous spread of the pathogen to bones, joints, and liver is rare but has been reported; lymphatic spread questionable; secondary infection and expanding necrosis in untreated lesions may result in complete genital erosion

See Patient Problems/Nursing Diagnoses & Interventions on p. 1074.

Molluscum Contagiosum and Condylomata Acuminata

Molluscum contagiosum is a viral disease of the skin that results in pearly pink to white papules with a central exudative pore. Multiple lesions appear on the genitalia and clear spontaneously in 6 to 9 months. Children develop lesions on skin elsewhere on the body.

Condylomata acuminata constitute one of the four major categories of virus-produced warts; this category occurs primarily on the genitalia or perineum. The warts appear as single or multiple, soft pink to brown, elongated lesions, usually in clusters and sometimes as large cauliflower-like masses (Table 15-25).

Pathophysiology

The viruses of both these diseases invade superficial layers of the epidermis and infect single epithelial cells and stimulate the cells to divide. In the case of condylomata there is excessive proliferation of the cells of the stratum spinosum, constituting the bulk of the wart. Microscopic examination of the infected cells shows aggregates of the virus particles. In the case of molluscum contagiosum, a central pore containing the virus and exudative material develops in the papules.

Both molluscum papules and genital warts appear as multiple lesions on the external genitalia. Genital warts may also be

Table 15-25 Overview of Sexually Transmitted Diseases With Nonulcerative Lesions

	Molluscum Contagiosum	Condylomata Acuminata (Anogenital Warts)
Occurrence	Worldwide	Worldwide
Etiologic agent	A member of the poxvirus group	Human papillomavirus (HPV)
Reservoir	Humans	Humans
Transmission	Direct sexual contact and indirect contact	Direct sexual contact; childbirth
Incubation period	2-7 weeks	1-20 months (usually 2-3 months)
Period of communicability	Unknown; probably as long as lesions persist	Unknown; probably as long as lesions persist
Susceptibility and resistance	Usually occurs in small children	General; increases in immunosuppressed
Report to local health authority	No	No

Data from Benenson.[3]

found in the vagina and cervix of females and anterior urethra of males. Perineal and anal warts in females are generally caused by spread, whereas anal warts in males are associated with anal coitus. Genital warts that resemble skin warts suggest hand-to-genital transmission of another category of skin warts.

The papules of molluscum contagiosum clear spontaneously in 6 to 9 months as a result of an immune response. Warts sometimes clear spontaneously, which suggests an immune response.

DIAGNOSTIC STUDIES AND FINDINGS[3]

Microscopic examination of material in core of molluscum lesion: Pathognomonic molluscum inclusion bodies can be visualized

Condylomata: Biopsy necessary for definitive diagnosis to rule out malignancy; rule out condylomata lata of syphilis with serologic test for syphilis

MULTIDISCIPLINARY PLAN[16]

Surgery

Alternative therapies for warts may include cryotherapy, electrosurgery, or surgical removal (scissors, curette, or carbon dioxide laser) no treatment should be initiated on cervical warts until results of a Papanicolaou smear are available

Molluscum lesions may resolve spontaneously or be removed by curettage after cryoanesthesia or cryotherapy or by the use of caustic chemicals

Medications

Keratolytic agents: Condylomata acuminata: podophyllin, 10%-25% in compound tincture of benzoin to wart only; to be washed off in 1-4 hr; four weekly treatments (not to be used during pregnancy or with urethral, oral, cervical, or anorectal warts) or trichloroacetic acid (TCA) or bichloroacetic acid (BCA) 80%-90%; apply to wart and allow to dry until a white "frosting" develops; repeat weekly

NURSING CARE

NURSING ASSESSMENT

For molluscum and condylomata

History: Sexual contact with infected person; multiple or unknown sexual partner; previous STD

Anogenital area

- Molluscum contagiosum: Multiple, distinct, dome-shaped papules, 1 to 10 mm, pearly pink to white, with a central pore containing a cheeselike white exudate; may be surrounded by red or scaling skin
- Condylomata (warts): Multiple or single, soft pink to brown, elongated lesions, usually in cluster, may be in large masses; painless

POTENTIAL COMPLICATIONS

Secondary infection and bleeding of warts; malignant transformation, particularly in cervix and urinary bladder; laryngeal warts in neonate

See Patient Problems/Nursing Diagnoses & Interventions on p. 1074.

VULVOVAGINITIS

Vulvovaginitis is an inflammation of superficial mucous membranes of the vulva and vagina caused by a number of microorganisms that are frequently part of the normal vaginal flora in adult women. The inflammation is accompanied by a purulent exudate with characteristics that differ with causative agents. The etiologic agents most frequently associated with vulvovaginitis are *T. vaginalis* (a protozoan), *C. albicans* (a yeast form of fungus), and bacteria such as *G. vaginalis, Corynebacterium vaginale,* and *Haemophilus vaginalis.* They are responsible for trichomoniasis, candidiasis, and bacterial vaginoses, respectively (Table 15-26). In addition, the inflammation can be caused by mechanical irritants, contact allergens, and ectoparasites (pinworms, lice) (Table 15-27).

PATHOPHYSIOLOGY

The presence of estrogen in women supports a normal flora of microorganisms in the vagina and anterior urethra. Under certain conditions imbalance occurs in the normal flora. Certain opportunistic organisms colonize on the superficial mucosal layers and produce patches of inflammation and exudate that contain large numbers of the pathogens. The infection rarely extends beyond the endocervix. There is a wide range in severity of infections. Many are asymptomatic. The organism may be transmitted to a male sexual partner who may or may not develop symptomatic urethritis. Reinfection of the female from untreated males is common.

Certain physiologic changes in the host support the pathogenic growth of different organisms. Trichomoniasis is exacerbated during and after menstruation, whereas bacterial infections such as *G. vaginalis* vaginitis are not associated with hormonal changes during the menstrual cycle. *G. vaginalis* vaginitis is associated with an altered vaginal pH; the organism usually does not grow in the normal acid secretions. Yeast infections, such as candidiasis, are greatly exacerbated preceding menstruation, during pregnancy, and in women taking oral contraceptives. Candidiasis is also exacerbated by the elimination of normal flora bacteria with antibiotic therapy or with any other condition that compromises skin or mucous membrane defenses.

Whereas *Trichomonas* and *Gardnerella* rarely extend beyond the vulvovaginal or anterior urethral area, *Candida* has the potential for producing infection anywhere in the body where normal defenses are altered. *Candida* is part of the normal gastrointestinal, oral, and cutaneous flora of many persons, and it may become pathogenic in those areas. Severe infection with invasion and abscess formation, particularly in the gastrointestinal tract, may lead to hematogenous dissemination of the yeast to other organs. The organism may also be introduced to internal organs through surgical procedures, catheters, or implanted devices and produce multiple microabscesses in infected tissue. The areas most commonly infected are the central nervous system (particularly the meninges), lungs, peritoneum, heart (myocardium, pericardium, and endocardium), endometrium, eyes, ears, joints, oral cavity, esophagus, skin, and nails. Deep tissue infection is more common in patients with neoplastic disease. Cutaneous infections are more commonly associated with skin

Table 15-26 Vulvovaginitis Caused by a Pathogen

	Trichomoniasis	Candidiasis	Bacterial Vaginosis
Occurrence	Worldwide: highest in females 16-35 years; often accompanies other STDs	Worldwide; fungus is part of normal flora in 50% of women 15-45 years; most common cause of vaginitis	Worldwide; bacteria are part of normal vaginal flora in many asymptomatic women
Etiologic agent	*T. vaginalis,* a protozoan	*C. albicans,* a fungus (yeast); occasionally other species of *Candida*	*G. vaginalis, H. vaginalis, C. vaginale, M. hominis*
Reservoir	Humans	Humans	Humans
Transmission	Direct and indirect contact with vaginal and urethral discharges	Direct and indirect contact with secretions from mouth, skin, vagina, and rectum of infected persons and carriers; transmitted to infant during vaginal delivery	Direct contact with vaginal and urethral discharges
Incubation period	4-20 days; average is 7 days	2-5 days in thrush in newborn	Variable
Period of communicability	Duration of infection; may last for years	Duration of lesions	Duration of infection
Susceptibility and resistance	General, but clinical disease is mainly in females: exacerbated during menstruation and pregnancy	Many persons have organism but few acquire infection; exacerbated during pregnancy, before menstruation, with oral contraceptives, and antibiotic therapy	General, but clinical disease is only in females; many women have the organism, but not all acquire symptomatic infections; results from changes in vaginal pH
Report to local health authority	No	No	No

Data from Benenson[3] and Centers for Disease Control and Prevention.[16]

Table 15-27 Vulvovaginitis of Noninfectious Origin

Etiology	Epidemiology	Signs and Symptoms	Diagnostic Studies	Medical Plan
Postmenopausal vaginitis (atrophic vaginitis)	Occurs because of decreased estrogen levels	Thin watery discharge; burning and itching	Direct visual examination	Atrophic changes cannot be reversed but can usually be prevented with hormone therapy
Allergic or irritative vaginitis owing to thermal, chemical, and physical causes	Thermal sources: douching with excessively hot water, wearing nylon undergarments Chemical sources: douche solutions, hygiene sprays, soaps, detergents on undergarments, poor personal hygiene Physical sources: retained tampon, diaphragm, toilet paper, condom, or pessary	Redness, burning, and itching of excoriated skin Increase in type and amount of secretions; rash; burning and itching Foul-smelling, serosanguineous, or purulent discharge	Direct visual examination; wet smear; detailed history; bimanual examination	Avoidance of source; secondary infection should be treated according to cause; oral antihistamines for allergic vaginitis, local cortisone ointment; wearing cotton undergarments

injury or continual wetting of the skin. *Candida* infections may involve multiple organs and tissue simultaneously, a particular risk for immunosuppressed individuals.

Vaginal candidiasis may be transmitted to the infant during delivery. A common manifestation of such an infection in the newborn is thrush, an infection in the oral cavity. Creamy white, curdlike patches consisting of desquamated epithelial cells, leukocytes, bacteria, keratin, necrotic tissue, and food debris are formed on the oral mucosa. Scraping of the patches leaves a raw, bleeding, painful surface.

DIAGNOSTIC STUDIES AND FINDINGS[3,16,26]

Trichomoniasis: Culture of vaginal secretions (urethral discharge): positive for *T. vaginalis;* microscopic examination of saline wet mount of vaginal secretions or Papanicolaou smear: visualization of motile protozoa

Candidiasis: Culture of vaginal secretions: positive for *C. vaginale* in symptomatic women; because *Candida* is part of normal oral flora, culture is not useful in thrush; microscopic examination of Gram's stain or KOH wet mount preparation of vaginal secretions: visualization of yeast cells or pseudohyphae

Bacterial vaginosis: Culture of vaginal secretions: positive for *G. vaginalis, M. hominis,* or other bacteria in symptomatic women; microscopic examination of Gram's stain or KOH wet mount preparation of vaginal secretions: identification of "clue" cells; or vaginal pH of 4.5 or higher

MULTIDISCIPLINARY PLAN[16]

Medications

Antiinfective agents for trichomoniasis

Metronidazole (Flagyl), 2 g PO single dose, *or*

Metronidazole, 500 mg bid for 7 days (contraindicated during the first trimester of pregnancy; asymptomatic women and their sexual partners should be treated to prevent sexual transmission)

Antiinfective agents for vulvovaginal candidiasis

Butoconazole (2% cream), 5 g intravaginally at hs for 3 days, *or*

Terconazole, 80-mg suppository, *or* 5 g 0.8% cream intravaginally at hs for 3 days *or* 0.4% 5 g for 7 days

Clotrimazole 1% cream, 5 g intravaginally at hs for 7-14 days, *or*

Clotrimazole (vaginal tablets, 100 mg), 2 tablets intravaginally for 3 days, *or*

Clotrimazole (vaginal tablets, 100 mg), 1 tablet intravaginally for 7 days

Clotrimazole, 500 mg vaginal tablet in one application

Miconazole nitrate (vaginal suppository, 200 mg), intravaginally at hs for 3 days, *or*

Miconazole (vaginal suppository, 100 mg or 5 g 2% cream), intravaginally at hs for 7 days, *or*

Nystatin, or other combinations not included here 100,000-unit vaginal tablet, 1 tablet for 14 days

Tioconazole 6.5% ointment, 5 g intravaginally in a single application

Antiinfective agents for bacterial vaginosis

Metronidazole (Flagyl), 500 mg PO bid for 7 days (contraindicated during pregnancy), *or*

Clindamycin, 300 mg PO, bid for 7 days (not necessary to treat male sex partners or asymptomatic women)

(Others not included here)

NURSING CARE

NURSING ASSESSMENT

For Vulvovaginitis

History: Pregnancy or oral contraceptive use

Vulva and vagina

Trichomoniasis: Inflammation of vaginal walls and endocervix; punctuate hemorrhagic lesions; painful coitus; copious loose "frothy" discharge with an odor; one third of patients have yellow-green discharge with bubbles

Candidiasis: Severe perivaginal pruritus; pale or erythematous labia; labial excoriations; erythema extending into vagina and toward anus; tiny papulopustules beyond main area of erythema; discharge thick and adherent (containing curds) or thin and loose; no odor

Bacterial vaginosis: Milder symptoms; less erythema; mild or moderate discharge; thin white or grayish white discharge; uniformly adheres to vaginal wall; 25% have gas bubbles in discharge; fishy or aminelike odor to discharge

Lymph nodes: Trichomoniasis: may be inguinal lymphadenopathy

Urinary

Trichomoniasis: dysuria or frequency

Candidiasis: dysuria

POTENTIAL COMPLICATIONS

Candida hematogenous spread to CNS, lungs, peritoneum, heart, endometrium, eyes, ears, joints; a risk for immunocompromised persons; transmission to neonate at time of delivery

Bacterial vaginosis: May cause premature rupture of membranes in pregnant women (not proven)

PATIENT PROBLEMS/NURSING DIAGNOSES & INTERVENTIONS

For gonorrhea and nongonococcal urethritis; syphilis; herpesvirus infections; lymphogranuloma venereum; chancroid and granuloma inguinale; molluscum contagiosum and condylomata acuminata; and vulvovaginitis

NIC RISK MANAGEMENT

Risk for infection (patient contacts) related to presence of pathogens in lesions or secretions or exudates from cervix, urethra, eyes, pharynx, or anus

Risk for infection (patient complications) related to extension or dissemination of disease if untreated or inadequately treated

- Collect specimen for laboratory examination; collect blood for serology for syphilis, herpes, or *Chlamydia for definite diagnosis and treatment.*
- Use standard precautions (see Box 15-2, p. 1086) when handling specimens and examining patient; *lesions and mucous membrane exudates are infectious.*
- Examine and treat patient contacts to *prevent reinfection of patient.*
- Serologically screen all pregnant women for syphilis at least once during pregnancy. Rescreen high-risk women during third trimester and again at delivery (testing the mother's blood). Administer antiinfectives as prescribed. *Syphilis is transmitted to the fetus. Adequate treatment of the mother before the fifteenth week will prevent damage to fetus. High-risk women are at risk for reinfection during the pregnancy. Infants born of infected mothers are at risk for active infection and severe anomalies.*
- Reexamine and treat pregnant women with history of STDs before delivery.
- Counsel all pregnant women to be tested and treated for HIV infection
- Examine newborn for symptoms and administer prophylactics for eyes. *A neonate may become infected on any mucous membrane during a vaginal delivery if mother has a cervical infection.*
- Ensure that pregnant women with *Candida* organism are treated during last trimester *to prevent transmission to neonate during vaginal delivery.*
- Report to local health authority if not previously reported by physician or laboratory; *it is required by law.*
- Administer antiinfectives or teach patient to take as prescribed. *Early treatment can prevent complications and transmission of STDs.*
- Counsel patient to return for follow-up *to ensure cure.*
- Monitor immunocompromised persons for signs of disseminated infection with herpes and *Candida. Immunocompromised persons are at greater risk for serious systemic disease.*
- Monitor body temperature and symptoms of PID and dissemination of gonorrhea and *Chlamydia. Early detection of infection and treatment with antiinfective agents*

may prevent dissemination of the pathogen, severe disease, and fertility problems.

- Monitor for symptoms of complications of tertiary syphilis if patient has been infected over 1 year *to initiate supportive care, as needed.*

Patient Education/Continuum of Care Plan[25]

General instructions

1. Sexual activity should be avoided until treatment is completed and follow-up examinations of secretion or exudates is negative for pathogens and when herpes lesions are present.
2. Sexual contacts must be examined and treated, even if asymptomatic.
3. Antiinfective agents must be taken for full prescribed course to avoid treatment failure, chronic infection, and complications.
4. If tetracycline is administered, it must be taken for full prescribed course. It should be taken 1 hour before or 2 hours after meals. The patient should avoid dairy products, antacids, iron, other mineral-containing preparations, as well as sunlight.
5. Condoms may provide protection from future infections.
6. Counsel patients and their partners to be tested for HIV.

Specific instructions

7. For gonorrhea or *Chlamydia:* Patients should return for reexamination 4 to 7 days after completion of treatment. Care should be taken with vaginal or urethral discharges to avoid contamination of eyes.
8. For syphilis: All sexual partners should be referred for examination and treatment (sexual contacts up to 3 months preceding primary infection, up to 6 months preceding secondary stage, and up to 1 year preceding latent stage). Treated patients should return for follow-up serologic tests 3 and 6 months after therapy (1, 2, 3, 6, 9, and 12 months, if HIV positive). A systemic reaction (e.g., fever, chills, headache, or tachycardia) 1 to 2 hours after onset of antibiotic treatment is attributable to endotoxin release from dying spirochetes. The condition is benign and self-limited. Bed rest and aspirin help.
9. For herpes: Pregnant women should inform physician of history of genital herpes. Annual Papanicolaou smears are recommended. Recurrent episodes of lesions are less painful and less extensive than initial episode. The virus probably cannot be transmitted when there are no lesions present, but this is still being investigated. Proper hand washing following toileting is important to prevent autoinoculation.
10. For lymphogranuloma venereum: The sequelae of untreated lymphogranuloma venereum are serious. Patient must complete prescribed antibiotic regimen and return for evaluation 3 to 5 days after treatment is begun and weekly or biweekly until infection is entirely healed.
11. For chancroid: Sex partners should be examined and treated as soon as possible. Sexual contacts 2 weeks before or after onset of chancroid lesions must be treated. Females may be asymptomatic; however, they should be treated. In chancroid the prepuce should remain retracted during therapy and lesions should be cleaned three times daily. Retraction is contraindicated if there is preputial edema.
12. For granuloma inguinale: The patient should return for evaluation within 3 to 5 days of beginning therapy and weekly or biweekly thereafter until all lesions are healed. Total healing of granuloma inguinale takes 3 to 5 weeks. If treatment is stopped prematurely, lesions may become reactivated.
13. For molluscum and condylomata (warts): Follow-up examination should take place 1 month after treatment for molluscum so new lesions can be removed. Follow-up examinations should be done weekly until all warts have been resolved. All women with anogenital warts should have a Papanicolaou smear. Patients should be informed of the recurrent nature of these conditions.
14. For vulvovaginitis: Recurrent infections are common. Patient should return for treatment if symptoms recur. Alcohol should be avoided until after 3 days following metronidazole therapy. See instruction number 4 regarding tetracycline. Vaginal suppositories for candidiasis should be stored in a refrigerator. Treatment should continue during menstruation. Sanitary pads can be worn to protect clothing. Teach patient to wipe from front to back when toileting. Instruct patient not to douche routinely to avoid removal of normal vaginal flora. Instruct patient to avoid using sprays, soaps, powders, and deodorants; to wear cotton undergarments to permit free airflow to the perineum and to avoid trapping moisture; to wash undergarments in mild detergent and to rinse them twice; to avoid sharing towels and washcloths with others; and to use water-soluble lubricants, if necessary, before intercourse.

Evaluation/Patient Outcomes

Risk Management: Infection is not transmitted to others or back to patient after treatment. Patient contacts are examined and treated. Newborn is free of signs of infection (no lesions, nonreactive serology, and absence of other symptoms). Healthcare workers have used adequate precautions.

Infection is resolved before extension or dissemination. Absence of signs of secondary or tertiary syphilis; CSF is normal. Follow-up serologic tests for syphilis indicate decreasing antibody titers. For gonorrhea or *Chlamydia:* body temperature, urination, and bowel movements are normal. Patient reports absence of nausea and vomiting, dysuria, pain, dysmenorrhea, abnormal menstrual bleeding, and other signs of complications. There is no exudate. Cultures are negative for gonococcus or *Chlamydia.* Patient has been tested for other STDs. For LV: lymph nodes are not swollen, hot, or tender. Mucopurulent exudate no longer drains from lesions or sinuses. Body temperature is normal. Rectum and anal opening are patent. There is no abdominal distention or cramping. Defecation is normal. For chancroid: lesions are healed without scarring. Patient verbalizes intent to return for follow-up. For herpes: no signs of CNS disease or infection of visual organs.

Patient has knowledge to self-administer antiinfectives as prescribed. Patient describes medication regimen and intent to take antiinfectives for length of time prescribed.

Patient has information to prevent further episodes of an STD and to prevent transmission of this STD. Patient verbalizes intent to avoid sexual contact until lesions are healed, describes correct use of condom, and verbalizes intent to return for follow-up.

Collaborative Interventions and Related Nursing Care

Immunizations

Immunization is the action of artificially stimulating an immune response in a host. Two methods are available. The first method is active immunization, in which an antigen in the form of a vaccine is injected to stimulate the person to produce antibodies against the infectious agent. The second method is passive immunization, in which antibodies, produced in another host, are injected in the form of immune globulins, antitoxins, or antisera. Clinical considerations for active and passive immunization, general recommendations for administration of vaccines, and a schedule for administration of vaccines for the diseases discussed in the section on vaccine-preventable infectious diseases are presented here.

Clinical Considerations for Active and Passive Immunization

Active Immunization. Vaccines used for active immunization are prepared from bacteria or viruses, or their derivatives, that have been modified to stimulate antibody production without causing disease. Modification is accomplished by inactivation or killing of the organism or by alteration of the organism so it retains its antigenicity while losing its virulence (attenuated).

Inactivated vaccines must be given in multiple first doses to stimulate an adequate antibody response, and a periodic booster must be given to maintain serum antibody levels. Attenuated vaccines stimulate lifetime antibody levels with one administration.

Routine immunizations are given according to a schedule that facilitates administration at a time earliest in life when the vaccine will be effective. The health-care provider administering the immunization should fully inform the patient or parent of the reason for the immunization, the schedule, side effects that may occur, and actions to take in the event of side effects. Informed consent must be obtained (Tables 15-28 to 15-30).

HEALTHY PEOPLE 2010

Health Status—Immunizations and Infectious Diseases

Goal: Prevent disease, disability, and death from infectious diseases, including vaccine-preventable diseases.

Diseases Preventable Through Universal Vaccination

- Reduce or eliminate indigenous cases of vaccine-preventable disease.
- Reduce chronic hepatitis B virus infections in infants and young children (perinatal infections).
- Reduce hepatitis B.
- Reduce bacterial meningitis in young children.
- Reduce invasive pneumococcal infections.
- Reduce hepatitis A.
- Reduce meningococcal disease.
- Reduce Lyme disease.
- Reduce hepatitis C.
- (Developmental) Increase the proportion of persons with chronic hepatitis C infection identified by state and local health departments.
- Reduce tuberculosis.
- Increase the proportion of all tuberculosis patients who complete curative therapy within 12 months.
- Increase the proportion of contacts and other high-risk persons with latent tuberculosis infection who complete a course of treatment.
- Reduce the average time for a laboratory to confirm and report tuberculosis cases.
- (Developmental) Increase the proportion of international travelers who receive recommended preventive services when traveling in areas of risk for select infectious diseases: hepatitis A, malaria, and typhoid.
- Reduce invasive early onset group B streptococcal disease.
- Reduce hospitalizations caused by peptic ulcer disease in the United States.
- Reduce the number of courses of antibiotics for ear infections for young children.
- Reduce the number of courses of antibiotics prescribed for the sole diagnosis of the common cold.
- Reduce hospital-acquired infections in intensive care unit patients.
- Reduce antimicrobial use among intensive care unit patients.
- Achieve and maintain effective vaccination coverage levels for universally recommended vaccines among young children.
- Maintain vaccination coverage levels for children in licensed day care facilities and children in kindergarten through the first grade.
- Increase the proportion of young children who receive all vaccines that have been recommended for universal administration for at least 5 years.
- Increase the proportion of providers who have measured the vaccination coverage levels among children in their practice population within the past 2 years.
- Increase the proportion of children who participate in fully operational population-based immunization registries.
- (Developmental) Increase routine vaccination coverage levels of adolescents.
- Increase hepatitis B vaccine coverage among high-risk groups.
- Increase the proportion of adults who are vaccinated annually against influenza.
- Increase the proportion of adults vaccinated against pneumococcal disease (one dose).

Vaccine Safety

- Reduce vaccine-associated adverse events.
- Eliminate vaccine-associated paralytic polio (VAPP).
- Increase the number of persons under active surveillance for vaccine safety via large-linked databases.

Modified from U.S. Department of Health and Human Services: *Healthy people 2010* (conference edition, in two volumes), Washington, DC, January 2000.

NOTE: *Developmental* indicates that criteria for measurement and strategies to improve health have not as yet been specified.

Table 15-28 Clinical Considerations for Commonly Administered Immunizations

Disease	Vaccine/Route	Recommendation	Contraindications*	Adverse Reactions	Less Severe Reactions	Passive Immunization
Tetanus	Toxoid (detoxified toxin)/IM; administered with diphtheria and pertussis as DTaP; given to those over 7 years as Td	Ideally begin first of 4 infant doses at 2-3 months of age; tetanus toxoid given every 10 years to adults; can be given to persons infected with HIV	Encephalopathy within 7 days of previous dose; anaphylactic reaction to vaccine	Rare neurologic reactions, including neuritis and transverse myelitis	Fever within 24-48 hours; soreness at injection site; urticaria, malaise	Immune globulin following injury for those without active immunization
Diphtheria	Toxoid/IM; same as tetanus	Same as tetanus	Same as tetanus	Same as tetanus	Same as tetanus	Antitoxin for unimmunized contacts with an active case
Pertussis	Acellular vaccine contains inactivated pertussis toxin/IM; same as tetanus	Same as tetanus; not given after 7 years of age	Same as tetanus	Less than with earlier vaccines; febrile seizures Rare CNS disturbances	Fever, drowsiness	No longer recommended
Measles (Rubeola)	Live attenuated virus/subcutaneous; administered with mumps and rubella as MMR	First dose given after 12 months of age because of maternal antibodies; second dose at age 4-12 years	Anaphylactic reaction to egg ingestion or to neomycin; pregnancy; severe, symptomatic immunodeficiency	Rare CNS reactions—encephalitis	Anorexia, malaise, rash, fever within 7-10 days	Immune globulin for unimmunized contacts of active cases; given within 6 days of exposure
Mumps	Same as measles	Same as measles	Same as measles	Rare encephalomyelitis	Brief, mild fever	Not recommended
Rubella	Same as measles	Same as measles	Same as measles	Transient arthralgia and arthritis within 2 weeks in older children	Mild rash lasting 1-2 days	Not recommended
Polio	Live attenuated virus: trivalent oral polio vaccine (TOPV)/oral or inactivated vaccine (IPV)/subcutaneous	Ideally, begin first of 4 infant doses at 2 months of age; inactivated vaccine recommended for persons who are immune compromised and for first and second infant doses	TOPV: HIV or household contact of person with HIV; IPV: anaphylactic reaction to neomycin streptomycin, or polymyxin B	Rare paralysis within 2 months of administration of TOPV	None	None

Data from Centers for Disease Control and Prevention.[4,6,9,13,15,17,21,23]

*Moderate or severe illness with or without fever is a contraindication for all immunizations.

Continued

Table 15-28 Clinical Considerations for Commonly Administered Immunizations—cont'd

Disease	Vaccine/Route	Recommendation	Contraindications*	Adverse Reactions	Less Severe Reactions	Passive Immunization
Influenza	Inactivated virus/IM	Vaccine must be readministered yearly; recommended for persons infected with HIV/AIDS	Anaphylactic reaction to ingested eggs	Hypersensitivity	Soreness at administration site; fever, malaise, myalgia persisting for 1-2 days	None
Haemophilus influenzae type b (Hib)	Bacterial polysaccharide conjugated to protein/IM	Ideally, begin primary series of three doses at 2 months of age	Previous anaphylactic reaction to the vaccine	None identified	None identified	None
Hepatitis B	Inactivated viral antigen/IM	Recommended for infants before hospital discharge and adults at risk for infection, including those with HIV	Anaphylactic reactions to common baker's yeast	Anaphylactic reactions	None identified	Hepatitis B immune globulin (HBIG) for postexposure prophylaxis
Varicella	Attenuated live virus/subcutaneous	Single dose can be given anytime after 12 months of age; give to children and adults who have not had a prior infection	Not available at this time	Rare: encephalitis, ataxia, Stevens-Johnson syndrome, pneumonia, herpes zoster	Rash within 2 weeks of administration	Varicella zoster immune globulin (VZIG) for postexposure prophylaxis for immunocompromised persons, susceptible pregnant women, and perinatally exposed infants

Data from Centers for Disease Control and Prevention.[4,6,9,13,15,17,21,23]

*Moderate or severe illness with or without fever is a contraindication for all immunizations.

Table 15-29 Recommended Childhood Immunization Schedule*— United States, January–December 2001

Vaccine	Age: Birth	1 mo	2 mo	4 mo	6 mo	12 mo	15 mo	18 mo	24 mo	4-6 yr	11-12 yr	14-18 yr
Hepatitis B†		Hep B #1										
			Hep B #2				Hep B #3				Hep B	
Diphtheria and tetanus toxoids and pertussis§			DTaP	DTaP	DTaP		DTaP			DTaP	Td	
H. influenzae type b¶			HiB	HiB	HiB	Hib						
Inactivated polio**			IPV	IPV		IPV				IPV		
Pneumococcal†† conjugate			PCV	PCV	PCV	PCV						
Measles-mumps; rubella§§						MMR				MMR	MMR	
Varicella¶¶							Var				Var	
Hepatitis A***											Hep A in selected areas	

From Centers for Disease Control and Prevention.[19]

▭ Range of recommended ages for vaccination.

⬭ Vaccines to be given if previously recommended doses were missed or were given earlier than the recommended minimum age.

▬ Recommended in selected states and/or regions.

* This schedule indicates the recommended ages for routine administration of currently licensed childhood vaccines as of November 1, 2000, for children through age 18 years. Additional vaccines may be licensed and recommended during the year. Licensed combination vaccines may be used whenever any components of the combination are indicated and the vaccine's other components are not contraindicated. Providers should consult the manufacturer's package inserts for detailed recommendations.

† **Infants born to hepatitis B surface antigen (HBsAg)-negative mothers** should receive the first dose of hepatitis B vaccine (Hep B) by age 2 months. The second dose should be administered at least 1 month after the first dose. The third dose should be administered at least 4 months after the first dose and at least 2 months after the second dose, but not before age 6 months. **Infants born to HBsAg-positive mothers** should receive Hep B and 0.5 ml hepatitis B immune globulin (HBIG) within 12 hours of birth at separate sites. The second dose is recommended at age 1-2 months and the third dose at age 6 months. **Infants born to mothers whose HBsAg status is unknown** should receive Hep B within 12 hours of birth. Maternal blood should be drawn at delivery to determine the mother's HBsAg status; if the HBsAg test is positive, the infant should receive HBIG as soon as possible (no later than age 1 week). **All children and adolescents (through age 18 years)** who have not been immunized against hepatitis B should begin the series during any visit. Providers should make special efforts to immunize children who were born in or whose parents were born in areas of the world where hepatitis B virus infection is moderately or highly endemic.

§ The fourth dose of diphtheria and tetanus toxoids and acellular pertussis vaccine (DTaP) may be administered as early as age 12 months, provided 6 months have elapsed since the third dose and the child is unlikely to return at age 15-18 months. Tetanus and diphtheria toxoids (Td) is recommended at age 11-12 years if at least 5 years have elapsed since the last dose of diphtheria and tetanus toxoids and pertussis vaccine (DTP), DTaP, or diphtheria and tetanus toxoids (DT). Subsequent routine Td boosters are recommended every 10 years.

¶ Three *Haemophilus influenzae* type b (Hib) conjugate vaccines are licensed for infant use. If Hib conjugate vaccine (PRP-OMP) (PedvaxHIB or Com-Vax [Merck]) is administered at ages 2 and 4 months, a dose at age 6 months is not required. Because clinical studies in infants have demonstrated that using some combination products may induce a lower immune response to the Hib vaccine component, DTaP/Hib combination products should not be used for primary immunization in infants at ages 2, 4, or 6 months unless approved by the Food and Drug Administration for these ages.

** An all-inactivated poliovirus vaccine (IPV) schedule is recommended for routine childhood polio vaccination in the United States. All children should receive four doses of IPV at age 2 months, age 4 months, between ages 6 and 18 months, and between ages 4 and 6 years. Oral poliovirus vaccine should be used only in selected circumstances (*1*).

†† The heptavalent pneumococcal conjugate vaccine (PCV) is recommended for all children ages 2-23 months. It is also recommended for certain children ages 24-59 months (*2*).

§§ The second dose of measles, mumps, and rubella vaccine (MMR) is recommended routinely at age 4-6 years but may be administered during any visit, provided at least 4 weeks have elapsed since receipt of the first dose and that both doses are administered beginning at or after age 12 months. Those who previously have not received the second dose should complete the schedule no later than the routine visit to a health-care provider at age 11-12 years.

¶¶ Varicella vaccine (Var) is recommended at any visit on or after the first birthday for susceptible children, (i.e., those who lack a reliable history of chickenpox [as judged by a health-care provider) and who have not been immunized)]. Susceptible persons age ≥13 years should receive two doses given at least 4 weeks apart.

*** Hepatitis A vaccine (Hep A) is recommended for use in selected states and/or regions, and for certain high-risk groups. Information is available from local public health authorities (*3*).

Additional information about the immunization schedule is available on the National Immunization Program World Wide Web site, *http://www.cdc.gov/nip,* or by telephone, (800)232-2522 (English) or (800)232-0233 (Spanish).

Table 15-30 Recommendations for Tetanus Prophylaxis in Wound Management

History of Tetanus Immunization	Clean Minor Wounds: Toxoid (Detoxified Toxin; Td)*	Clean Minor Wounds: Tetanus Immune Globulin (TIG)	All Other Wounds: Toxoid (Detoxified Toxin; Td)*	All Other Wounds: Tetanus Immune Globulin (TIG)
Uncertain history or <three doses	Yes	No	Yes	Yes
Three or more doses†				
Last dose within past 5 years	No	No	No	No
Last dose 5-10 years ago	No	No	Yes	No
Last dose over 10 years ago	Yes	No	Yes	No

Data from Centers for Disease Control and Prevention.[4]

*For children under 7 years, administer DTP (or DT if pertussis vaccine is contraindicated).

†If *only* three doses of fluid toxoid have been administered, a fourth dose of toxoid, preferably an absorbed toxoid, should be given.

Passive Immunization. Active immunization is preferred to passive in most situations. Passive immunization with serum antitoxins prepared in animals or with human immune globulins is recommended only for those situations where active immunization procedures have not been developed; exposure has already occurred, leaving insufficient time for active immunization; or concurrent active and passive immunization is required for immediate and future protection.

The use of human immune globulins for passive immunization is preferred to use of serum antitoxins from animals. The risk for anaphylaxis-like reactions and serum sickness is greater when prepared animal sera are used. Anaphylaxis-like reactions affect principally the cardiovascular and respiratory systems, producing dyspnea, asthma, respiratory decompensation, and possible death. These reactions occur in minutes to a few hours after administration of the serum, and they range from mild to severe. The much more common serum sickness reactions develop in 7 to 12 days after injection of the serum, producing mild to severe symptoms of fever, urticaria, or arthralgia. The severity of the symptoms depends on the type of serum and the route of administration (IV administration leads to more severe reactions). Individuals previously sensitized to the serum may react within 1 to 3 days of receiving the serum.

Multiple-Dose Vaccines. Some vaccines must be administered in more than one dose for full protection. If the intervals between doses are longer than recommended, there is usually not a reduction in final antibody levels. It is therefore unnecessary to restart an interrupted series or to add extra doses.

Simultaneous Administration of Certain Vaccines. Most of the widely used vaccines can be safely and effectively administered simultaneously. Inactivated vaccines can be administered simultaneously at different sites unless the person is known to have experienced past side effects to one or more of the vaccines. In that case the vaccines should be administered on separate occasions. An inactivated vaccine and a live attenuated virus vaccine can be administered simultaneously at different sites.

Hypersensitivity to Vaccine Components. Vaccine antigens produced in systems or with substrates that contain allergenic substances may cause hypersensitivity reactions and possible anaphylaxis. Antigens grown in eggs of chickens or ducks should not be given to anyone with a history (or questionable history) of allergy to eggs. Influenza vaccine antigens, although produced from viruses grown in eggs, are highly purified and are associated with only rare hypersensitivity reactions. Influenza vaccine should not be administered to anyone with a history of anaphylactic reaction to eggs.

No hypersensitivity reactions have been reported from administration of live attenuated measles, mumps, or rubella (MMR) vaccine prepared from viruses grown in cell cultures.

Vaccines that contain preservatives or trace amounts of antibiotics, as indicated on the package insert, should not be given to any person with a history of hypersensitivity to those substances.

Because national immunization recommendations change regularly, see Box 15-1 for ways to access current information

RESOURCE—IMMUNIZATION RECOMMENDATIONS **Box 15-1**

National immunization recommendations change regularly. To obtain updated information, please access the Centers for Disease Control and Prevention's website: *www.cdc.gov/publications/ACP-list.htm* or *www.immunize.org* or obtain updated statements for the Advisory Committee on Immunization Practices (ACP) at (800) 232-2522

Contraindications for Immunization

Altered immunity: Severely immunosuppressed persons should not receive live attenuated virus vaccines (MMR, TOPV) because of the risk for multiplication of the virus within those persons. MMR should be given to asymptomatic HIV-infected children. Also, individuals living in the same household with a severely immunocompromised person should not be given oral polio vaccine (OPV) because vaccine viruses are excreted and may be transmitted to other persons. These persons should be given inactivated polio vaccine (IPV). Killed or inactivated vaccines, such as the influenza vaccine, are safe for HIV-infected persons.[6]

Severe febrile illnesses: Although the presence of mild illnesses does not preclude vaccination, immunization should be deferred for those with severe febrile illnesses.

Pregnancy: Attenuated virus vaccines, particularly measles, mumps, and rubella (MMR), should not be given to pregnant women or women who may become pregnant within 3 months of the vaccination. OPV and yellow fever vaccines may be given if there is a high risk for acquired infection. There is no contraindication for administration of inactivated viral vaccines, bacterial vaccines, or toxoids to pregnant women. Influenza vaccine can be given safely.

Recent administration of immune globulin: Live attenuated virus vaccines should not be administered within 3 months of passive immunization. Similarly, immunoglobulins should not be administered for at least 2 weeks after a vaccine has been given. These precautions reduce the risk that high serum levels of immunoglobulins would prevent the development of active acquired immunity.

All adverse reactions to vaccines must be reported to the local or state health authority since the passage in 1988 of the Vaccine Adverse Event Reporting System.

DPT or single-antigen pertussis vaccine is contraindicated if any of the following events occurred after the patient received a vaccine containing pertussis antigen:

- Allergic hypersensitivity
- Fever of 40.5° C (104.9° F) or higher within 48 hours
- Collapse or shocklike state within 48 hours
- Persistent, inconsolable crying lasting 3 hours or more or an unusual, high-pitched cry occurring within 48 hours
- Convulsion(s) with or without fever occurring within 3 days of receipt of pertussis vaccine
- Encephalopathy (with generalized or focal neurologic signs or alterations in consciousness) occurring within 7 days
- Children with a history of seizure or other neurologic disorders should be evaluated before vaccine administration

Health-care workers are at risk for many vaccine-preventable diseases and should be protected (Table 15-31).

Isolation Precautions

Isolation precautions have been designed to prevent the spread of microorganisms among hospitalized patients, personnel, and visitors. Most of the infectious diseases discussed in this chapter have the potential for being transmitted to others. For infections that can be transmitted, the recommended hospital isolation precautions are specified in this chapter in the sections on Patient Problems/Nursing Diagnoses & Interventions.

Recommendations for isolation precautions in hospitals have been revised by the Centers for Disease Control and Prevention together with the Hospital Infection Control Practices Advisory Committee. The revised guideline contains two tiers of precautions. The first tier, standard precautions, contains precautions that apply to all hospitalized patients irrespective of their infectious status. The second tier, transmission-based precautions, are used for patients known or suspected of being infected with pathogens that can be transmitted by airborne or droplet transmission or by contact with dry skin or contaminated surfaces.[24]

Standard precautions combine universal (blood and body fluid) precautions (designed to reduce the risk of transmission of blood-borne pathogens) and body substance isolation (designed to reduce the risk of transmission of pathogens from moist body substances). Standard precautions apply to blood, all body fluids, secretions, and excretions except sweat regardless of whether they contain visible blood, nonintact skin, and mucous membranes (Box 15-2, p. 1086).

Transmission-based precautions are designed for patients known or thought to be infected with highly transmissible pathogens for which additional precautions beyond standard precautions are needed to interrupt transmission in hospitals. There are three types of transmission-based precautions: airborne precautions, droplet precautions, and contact precautions. They may be combined together for diseases that have multiple routes of transmission. When used either singularly or in combination, they are to be used in addition to standard precautions.

Airborne precautions reduce the risk of transmission of small airborne droplet nuclei of evaporated droplets suspended in the air or dust particles containing infectious agents. Microorganisms transmitted by the airborne route can be widely dispersed by air currents and may become inhaled by or deposited on a susceptible host within the same room or over a longer distance from the source patient. Airborne precautions incorporate special air handling and ventilation systems (Box 15-3, p. 1087).

Droplet precautions reduce the risk of transmission of large droplets containing infectious agents from the conjunctivae or the mucous membranes of the nose or mouth. Such droplets are generated when the infected host or carrier coughs, sneezes, or talks or during procedures such as suctioning and bronchoscopy. Because large droplets do not remain suspended in air and travel only short distances, they only can be transmitted by close contact between source and recipient (Box 15-4, p. 1087).

Contact precautions reduce the risk of transmission of microorganisms by direct or indirect contact. Direct contact involves skin-to-skin contact and physical transfer of organisms from one person to another. Indirect contact involves contact of a susceptible host with a contaminated intermediate object in the environment (Box 15-5, p. 1087).

The revised guideline also lists specific clinical syndromes or conditions that are highly suspicious for infection and identifies appropriate transmission-based precautions to use on a temporary basis until a diagnosis can be made; these precautions also are to be used in addition to standard precautions.

Text continued on p. 1088.

Table 15-31 Immunizing Agents and Immunization Schedules for Health-Care Workers (HCWs)*

Generic Name	Primary Schedule and Booster(s)	Indications	Major Precautions and Contraindications	Special Considerations
IMMUNIZING AGENTS STRONGLY RECOMMENDED FOR HEALTH-CARE WORKERS				
Hepatitis B (HB) recombinant vaccine	Two doses IM 4 weeks apart; third dose 5 months after second; booster doses not necessary.	**Preexposure:** HCWs at risk for exposure to blood or body fluids.	On the basis of limited data, no risk of adverse effects to developing fetuses is apparent. Pregnancy should *not* be considered a contraindication to vaccination of women. Previous anaphylactic reaction to common baker's yeast is a contraindication to vaccination.	The vaccine produces neither therapeutic nor adverse effects on HBV-infected persons. Prevaccination serologic screening is not indicated for persons being vaccinated because of occupational risk. HCWs who have contact with patients or blood should be tested 1-2 months after vaccination to determine serologic response.
Hepatitis B immune globulin (HBIG)	0.06 ml/kg IM as soon as possible after exposure. A second dose of HBIG should be administered 1 month later if the HB vaccine series has not been started.	**Postexposure** prophylaxis: For persons exposed to blood or body fluids containing HBsAg and who are not immune to HBV infection—0.06 mL/kg IM as soon as possible (but no later than 7 days after exposure).		
Influenza vaccine (inactivated whole-virus and split-virus vaccines)	Annual vaccination with current vaccine. Administered IM.	HCWs who have contact with patients at high risk for influenza or its complications; HCWs who work in chronic care facilities; HCWs with high-risk medical conditions or who are age 65 years.	History of anaphylactic hypersensitivity to egg ingestion.	No evidence exists of risk to mother or fetus; when the vaccine is administered to a pregnant woman with an underlying high-risk condition, influenza vaccination is recommended during second and third trimesters of pregnancy because of increased risk for hospitalization.
Measles live-virus vaccine	One dose SC; second dose at least 1 month later.	HCWs† born during or after 1957 who do not have documentation of having received 2 doses of live vaccine on or after the first birthday **or** a history of physician-diagnosed measles or serologic evidence of immunity. Vaccination should be considered for all HCWs who lack proof of immunity, including those born before 1957.	Pregnancy; immunocompromised persons, § including HIV-infected persons who have evidence of severe immunosuppression; anaphylaxis after gelatin ingestion or administration of neomycin; recent administration of immune globulin.	MMR is the vaccine of choice if recipients are likely to be susceptible to rubella and/or mumps as well as to measles. Persons vaccinated during 1963-1967 with a killed measles vaccine alone, killed vaccine followed by live vaccine, or with a vaccine of unknown type should be revaccinated with 2 doses of live measles virus vaccine.
Mumps live-virus vaccine	One dose SC; no booster.	HCWs† believed to be susceptible can be vaccinated. Adults born before 1957 can be considered immune.	Pregnancy; immunocompromised persons§; history of anaphylactic reaction after gelatin ingestion or administration of neomycin.	MMR is the vaccine of choice if recipients are likely to be susceptible to measles and rubella as well as to mumps.

vaccine		women, who do not have documentation of having received live vaccine on or after their first birthday **or** or laboratory evidence of immunity. Adults born before 1957, **except women who can become pregnant** can be considered immune.	sons†; history of anaphylactic reaction after administration of neomycin.	malformations in the offspring of women pregnant when vaccinated or who become pregnant within 3 months after vaccination is negligible. Such women should be counseled regarding the theoretical basis of concern for the fetus. MMR is the vaccine of choice if recipients are likely to be susceptible to measles or mumps, as well as to rubella.
Varicella zoster live-virus vaccine	Two 0.5 ml doses SC 4-8 weeks apart if 13 years of age.	Indicated for HCWs† who do not have either a reliable history of varicella or serologic evidence of immunity.	Pregnancy, immunocompromised persons, § history of anaphylactic reaction following receipt of neomycin or gelatin. Avoid salicylate use for 6 weeks after vaccination.	Vaccine is available from the manufacturer for certain patients with acute lymphocytic leukemia (ALL) in remission. Because 71%-93% of persons without a history of varicella are immune, serologic testing before vaccination is likely to be cost-effective.
Varicella-zoster immune globulin (VZIG)	Persons <50 kg: 125 u/10 kg IM; persons 50 kg: 625 u.	Persons known or likely to be susceptible (particularly those at high risk for complications, e.g., pregnant women) who have close and prolonged exposure to a contact case or to an infectious hospital staff worker or patient.		Serologic testing may help in assessing whether to administer VZIG. If use of VZIG prevents varicella disease, patient should be vaccinated subsequently.
BCG VACCINATION				
Bacille Calmette Guérin (BCG) vaccine (tuberculosis)	One percutaneous dose of 0.3 ml; no booster dose recommended.	Should be considered only for HCWs in areas where multidrug tuberculosis is prevalent, a strong likelihood of infection exists, and comprehensive infection control precautions have failed to prevent TB transmission to HCWs.	Should not be administered to immunocompromised persons,§ pregnant women.	In the United States tuberculosis-control efforts are directed toward early identification, treatment of cases, and preventive therapy with isoniazid.
OTHER IMMUNOBIOLOGICS THAT ARE OR MAY BE INDICATED FOR HEALTH-CARE WORKERS				
Immune globulin (hepatitis A)	Postexposure—One IM dose of 0.02 ml/kg administered 2 weeks after exposure.	Indicated for HCWs exposed to feces of infectious patients.	Contraindicated in persons with IgA deficiency; do not administer within 2 weeks after MMR vaccine, or 3 weeks after varicella vaccine. Delay administration of MMR vaccine for 3 months and varicella vaccine for 5 months after administration of IG.	Administer in large muscle mass (deltoid, gluteal).

Modified from Centers for Disease Control and Prevention.[14]

*Persons who provide health care to patients or work in institutions that provide patient care (e.g., physicians, nurses, emergency medical personnel, dental professionals and students, medical and nursing students, laboratory technicians, hospital volunteers, and administrative and support staff in health-care institutions).

†All HCWs (i.e., medical or nonmedical, paid or volunteer, full time or part time, student or non-student, with or without patient-care responsibilities) who work in health-care institutions (e.g., inpatient and outpatient, public and private) should be immune to measles, rubella, and varicella.

§Persons immunocompromised because of immune deficiency diseases, HIV infection, leukemia, lymphoma or generalized malignancy or immunosuppressed as a result of therapy with corticosteroids, alkylating drugs, antimetabolites, or radiation.

HBsAg, hepatitis B surface antigen; *HBV,* hepatitis B virus; *HIV,* human immunodeficiency virus; *IM,* intramuscular; *MMR,* measles, mumps, rubella vaccine; *SC,* subcutaneous.

Continued

Table 15-31 Immunizing Agents and Immunization Schedules for Health-Care Workers (HCWs)—cont'd

Generic Name	Primary Schedule and Booster(s)	Indications	Major Precautions and Contraindications	Special Considerations
Hepatitis A vaccine	Two doses of vaccine either 6-12 months apart (HAVRIX), or 6 months apart (VAQTA).	Not routinely indicated for HCWs in the United States. Persons who work with HAV-infected primates or with HAV in a research laboratory setting should be vaccinated.	History of anaphylactic hypersensitivity to alum or, for HAVRIX, the preservative 2-phenoxyethanol. The safety of the vaccine in pregnant women has not been determined; the risk associated with vaccination should be weighed against the risk for hepatitis A in women who may be at high risk for exposure to HAV.	
Meningococcal polysaccharide vaccine (tetravalent A, C, W135, and Y)	One dose in volume and by route specified by manufacturer; need for boosters unknown.	Not routinely indicated for HCWs in the United States.	The safety of the vaccine in pregnant women has not been evaluated; it should not be administered during pregnancy unless the risk for infection is high.	
Typhoid vaccine, IM, SC, and oral	*IM vaccine:* One 0.5-ml dose, booster 0.5 ml every 2 years. *SC vaccine:* two 0.5 ml doses, 4 weeks apart, booster 0.5 ml SC or 0.1 ID every 3 years if exposure continues. *Oral vaccine:* Four doses on alternate days. The manufacturer recommends revaccination with the entire four-dose series every 5 years.	Workers in microbiology laboratories who frequently work with *Salmonella typhi.*	Severe local or systemic reaction to a previous dose. Ty21a (oral) vaccine should not be administered to immunocompromised persons† or to persons receiving antimicrobial agents.	Vaccination should not be considered an alternative to the use of proper procedures when handling specimens and cultures in the laboratory.

(smallpox)	a bifurcated needle; boosters administered every 10 years.	cultures with vaccinia, recombinant vaccinia viruses, or orthopox viruses that infect humans.	nancy, in persons with eczema or a history of eczema, and in immunocompromised persons† and their household contacts.	HCWs who have direct contact with contaminated dressings or other infectious material from volunteers in clinical studies involving recombinant vaccinia virus.
OTHER VACCINE-PREVENTABLE DISEASES				
Tetanus and diphtheria (toxoids [Td])	Two IM doses 4 weeks apart; third dose 6-12 months after second dose; booster every 10 years.	All adults.	Except in the first trimester, pregnancy is not a precaution. History of a neurologic reaction or immediate hypersensitivity reaction after a previous dose. History of severe local (Arthus-type) reaction after a previous dose. Such persons should not receive further routine or emergency doses of Td for 10 years.	Tetanus prophylaxis in wound management.
Pneumococcal polysaccharide vaccine (23 valent).	One dose, 0.5-ml, IM or SC; revaccination recommended for those at highest risk 5 years after the first dose.	Adults who are at increased risk of pneumococcal disease and its complications because of underlying health conditions; older adults, especially those age 65 who are healthy.	The safety of vaccine in pregnant women has not been evaluated; it should not be administered during pregnancy unless the risk for infection is high. Previous recipients of any type of pneumococcal polysaccharide vaccine who are at highest risk for fatal infection or antibody loss may be revaccinated 5 years after the first dose.	

Modified from Centers for Disease Control and Prevention.[14]

*Persons who provide health care to patients or work in institutions that provide patient care (e.g., physicians, nurses, emergency medical personnel, dental professionals and students, medical and nursing students, laboratory technicians, hospital volunteers, and administrative and support staff in health-care institutions).

†All HCWs (i.e., medical or nonmedical, paid or volunteer, full time or part time, student or non-student, with or without patient-care responsibilities) who work in health-care institutions (e.g., inpatient and outpatient, public and private) should be immune to measles, rubella, and varicella.

§Persons immunocompromised because of immune deficiency diseases, HIV infection, leukemia, lymphoma or generalized malignancy or immunosuppressed as a result of therapy with corticosteroids, alkylating drugs, antimetabolites, or radiation.

HBsAg, hepatitis B surface antigen; *HBV,* hepatitis B virus; *HIV,* human immunodeficiency virus; *ID,* intradermal; *IM,* intramuscular; *MMR,* measles, mumps, rubella vaccine; *SC,* subcutaneous.

Continued

STANDARD PRECAUTIONS — Box 15-2

To be used for the care of all patients

Hand Washing

1. Wash hands after touching blood, body fluids, secretions, excretions, and contaminated items, regardless of whether gloves are worn. Wash hands immediately after gloves are removed, between patient contacts, and when otherwise indicated to avoid transfer of microorganisms to other patients or environments. It may be necessary to wash hands between tasks and procedures on the same patient to prevent cross-contamination of different body sites.
2. Use a plain (nonantimicrobial) soap for routine hand washing.
3. Use an antimicrobial agent or waterless antiseptic agent for specific circumstances as defined by the infection control program of the institution.

Gloves

Wear gloves (clean nonsterile gloves are adequate) when touching blood, body fluids, secretions, excretions, and contaminated items; put on clean gloves just before touching mucous membranes and nonintact skin. Change gloves between tasks and procedures on the same patient after contact with material that may contain a high concentration of microorganisms. Remove gloves promptly after use, before touching noncontaminated items and environmental surfaces, and before going to another patient. Wash hands immediately.

Mask, Eye Protection, Face Shield

Wear a mask and eye protection or a face shield to protect mucous membranes of the eyes, nose, and mouth during procedures and patient-care activities that are likely to generate splashes or sprays of blood, body fluids, secretions, and excretions.

Gown

Wear a gown (a clean nonsterile gown is adequate) to protect skin and prevent soiling of clothing during procedures and patient-care activities that are likely to generate splashes or sprays of blood, body fluids, secretions, or excretion or cause soiling of clothing. Select a gown that is appropriate for the activity and amount of fluid likely to be encountered. Remove a soiled gown as promptly as possible and wash hands.

Patient-Care Equipment

Handle used patient-care equipment soiled with blood, body fluids, secretions, and excretions in a manner that prevents skin and mucous membrane exposures, contamination of clothing, and transfer of microorganisms to other patients and environments. Ensure that reusable equipment is not used for the care of another patient until it has been appropriately cleaned and reprocessed and single-use items are properly discarded.

Environmental Control

Ensure that the hospital has adequate procedures for the routine care, cleaning, and disinfection of environmental surfaces, beds, bed rails, bedside equipment, and other frequently touched surfaces. Ensure that these procedures are being followed.

Linen

Handle, transport, and process used linen soiled with blood, body fluids, secretions, and excretions in a manner that prevents skin and mucous membrane exposures, contamination of clothing, and avoids transfer of microorganisms to other patients and environments.

Occupational Health and Blood-Borne Pathogens

1. Never recap used needles or otherwise manipulate them using both hands or use any other technique that involves directing the point of a needle toward any part of the body; rather, use either a one-handed "scoop" technique or a mechanical device designed for holding the needle sheath. Do not remove used needles from disposable syringes by hand, and do not bend, break, or otherwise manipulate used needles by hand. Place used disposable syringes and needles, scalpel blades, and other sharp items in appropriate puncture-resistant containers located as close as possible to the area of use. Place reusable syringes and needles in a puncture-resistant container for transport to the reprocessing area.
2. Use mouthpieces, resuscitation bags, or other ventilation devices as an alternative to mouth-to-mouth resuscitation methods in areas where the need for resuscitation is predictable.

Patient Placement

Place in a private room a patient who contaminates the environment or who does not (or cannot) assist in maintaining appropriate hygiene or environmental control.

Data from Garner and the Hospital Infection Control Practices Committee.[24]

AIRBORNE PRECAUTIONS — Box 15-3

In addition to standard precautions, use airborne precautions for patient known or suspected to be infected with microorganisms transmitted by airborne droplet nuclei that can be widely dispersed by air currents (e.g., *M. tuberculosis*).

PATIENT PLACEMENT

Place patient in a private room with a monitored negative air pressure, 6 to 12 air changes per hour, and appropriate discharge of air outdoors or monitored high-efficiency filtration of room air before the air is recirculated. Keep the patient in the room with the door closed.

RESPIRATORY PROTECTION

Wear respiratory protection when entering the room of a patient with known or suspected infectious pulmonary tuberculosis. Susceptible persons should not enter the room of patients known or thought to have measles (rubeola) or chickenpox (varicella). Susceptible persons should wear respiratory protection.

PATIENT TRANSPORT

Limit the movement and transport of the patient from the room to essential purposes only. If transport or movement is necessary, place a surgical mask on the patient.

Data from Garner and the Hospital Infection Control Practices Committee.[24]

DROPLET PRECAUTIONS — Box 15-4

In addition to standard precautions, use droplet precautions for a patient known or thought to be infected with microorganisms transmitted by droplets that can be generated by the patient during coughing, sneezing, talking, or the performance of procedures.

PATIENT PLACEMENT

Place the patient in a private room or in a room with a patient who has active infection with the same microorganism, but with no other infection. If this is not possible, maintain separation of patients by at least 3 feet. The door may remain open, and special ventilation is not necessary.

MASK

Wear a mask when working within 3 feet of the patient.

PATIENT TRANSPORT

Limit the movement and transport of the patient from the room to essential purposes only; mask the patient during transport, if possible.

Data from Garner and the Hospital Infection Control Practices Committee.[24]

CONTACT PRECAUTIONS — Box 15-5

In addition to standard precautions, use contact precautions for patients known or suspected of being infected with important microorganisms that can be transmitted by direct (skin to skin) contact or indirect contact with a contaminated object in the environment.

PATIENT PLACEMENT

Place the patient in a private room, if possible, or in a room with a patient infected with the same microorganism but with no other infection. If these options are not available, consult with the infection control practitioner in the institution.

GLOVES AND HAND WASHING

In addition to wearing gloves as specified under standard precautions, wear gloves (clean, nonsterile gloves are adequate) when entering the room. While providing care, change gloves after having contact with infective material. Remove gloves before leaving the patient's room, and wash hands with an antimicrobial agent or a waterless antiseptic agent. After removing gloves and washing hands, do not touch potentially contaminated environmental surfaces in the patient's room.

GOWN

In addition to wearing a gown as outlined under standard precautions, wear a gown (a clean, nonsterile gown is adequate) when entering the room if the patient is incontinent or has diarrhea, an ileostomy, a colostomy, or wound drainage not contained by a dressing. Remove the gown before leaving the patient's environment. After removing the gown, ensure that clothing does not contact potentially contaminated environmental surfaces.

PATIENT TRANSPORT

Limit the movement and transport of the patient from the room to essential purposes only. If the patient does leave the room, ensure that precautions are maintained.

PATIENT-CARE EQUIPMENT

If possible, dedicate the use of noncritical patient-care equipment to a single patient or to a cohort of patients infected with the same pathogen.

Data from Garner and the Hospital Infection Control Practices Committee.[24]

REFERENCES

1. Bartlett JG: *Pocket book of infectious disease therapy,* Baltimore, 1993, Williams & Wilkins.
2. Beers M, Berkow R, editors: *The Merck manual of diagnosis and therapy,* ed 17, Whitehouse Station, NJ, 1999, Merck Research Laboratories.
3. Benenson AS, editor: *Control of communicable diseases manual,* ed 16, Washington, DC, 1995, American Public Health Association.
4. Centers for Disease Control and Prevention: Update on adult immunization: recommendations of the Immunization Practices Advisory Committee (ACIP), *MMWR Morb Mortal Wkly Rep* 40(RR-12):1, 1991.
5. Centers for Disease Control and Prevention: Hepatitis B virus: a comprehensive strategy for eliminating transmission in the United States through universal childhood vaccination: recommendations of the Advisory Committee on Immunization Practices (ACIP), *MMWR Morb Mortal Wkly Rep* 40(RR-13):1, 1991.
6. Centers for Disease Control and Prevention: Use of vaccines and immune globulins in persons with altered immunocompetence: recommendations of the Immunization Practices Advisory Committee (ACIP), *MMWR Morb Mortal Wkly Rep* 42(RR-4): 1, 1993.
7. Centers for Disease Control and Prevention: *Addressing emerging infectious disease threats: a prevention strategy for the United States,* Atlanta, 1994, U.S. Department of Health and Human Services, Public Health Service.
8. Centers for Disease Control and Prevention: *Core curriculum on tuberculosis: what the clinician should know,* Atlanta, ed 4, 2000, U.S. Department of Health and Human Services, Public Health Service, *www.cdc.gov,* 2001.
9. Centers for Disease Control and Prevention: General recommendations on immunization: recommendations of the Advisory Committee on Immunization Practices (ACIP), *MMWR Morb Mortal Wkly Rep* 43(RR-1):1, 1994.
10. Centers for Disease Control and Prevention: Guidelines for preventing the transmission of *Mycobacterium tuberculosis* in health-care facilities, 1994, *MMWR Morb Mortal Wkly Rep* 43(RR-3):1, 1994.
11. Centers for Disease Control and Prevention: Recommendations for preventing the spread of vancomycin resistance, *MMWR Morb Mortal Wkly Rep* 44(RR-12):1, 1995.
12. Centers for Disease Control and Prevention: Prevention of Hepatitis A through active or passive immunization: recommendations of the Advisory Committee on Immunization Practices (ACIP), *MMWR Morb Mortal Wkly Rep* 48(RR-12):1, 1999.
13. Centers for Disease Control and Prevention: Poliomyelitis prevention in the United States: introduction of a sequential vaccination schedule of inactivated poliovirus vaccine followed by oral poliovirus vaccine: recommendations of the Advisory Committee on Immunization Practices (ACIP), *Morb Mortal Wkly Rep MMWR* 46(RR-3):1, 1997.
14. Centers for Disease Control and Prevention: Immunization of health care workers: recommendations of the Advisory Committee on Immunization Practices (ACIP) and the Hospital Infection Control Practices Advisory Committee (HICPAC), *MMWR Morb Mortal Wkly Rep* 46(RR-18):1, 1997.
15. Centers for Disease Control and Prevention: Pertussis vaccination: use of acellular pertussis vaccines among infants and young children: recommendations of the Advisory Committee on Immunization Practices (ACIP), *MMWR Morb Mortal Wkly Rep* 46(RR-7):1, 1997.
16. Centers for Disease Control and Prevention: 1998 guidelines for treatment of sexually transmitted diseases, *MMWR Morb Mortal Wkly Rep* 47(RR-1): 1, 1998.
17. Centers for Disease Control and Prevention: Measles, mumps, and rubella: vaccine use and strategies for elimination of measles, rubella, and congenital rubella syndrome and control of mumps: recommendations of the Advisory Committee on Immunization Practices (ACIP), *MMWR Morb Mortal Wkly Rep* 47(RR-8):1, 1998.
18. Centers for Disease Control and Prevention: Recommendations for prevention and control of hepatitis C virus (HCV) infection and HCV-related chronic disease, *MMWR Morb Mortal Wkly Rep* 47(RR-19):1, 1998.
19. Centers for Disease Control and Prevention: Recommended childhood immunization schedule—United States, 2001, *MMWR Morb Mortal Wkly Rep* 50(1):7, 2001.
20. Centers for Disease Control and Prevention: Prevention and control of influenza: recommendations of the Advisory Committee on Immunization Practices (ACIP), *MMWR Morb Mortal Wkly Rep* 48(RR-4):1, 1999.
21. Centers for Disease Control and Prevention: Prevention of varicella: update recommendations of the Advisory Committee on Immunization Practices (ACIP), *MMWR Morb Mortal Wkly Rep* 48(RR-6):1, 1999.
22. Centers for Disease Control and Prevention: Recommendations for the use of Lyme disease vaccine: recommendations of the Advisory Committee on Immunization Practices (ACIP), *MMWR Morb Mortal Wkly Rep* 48(RR-7):1, 1999.
23. Centers for Disease Control and Prevention: Recommendations of the Advisory Committee on Immunization Practices: revised recommendations for routine poliomyelitis vaccination, *MMWR Morb Mortal Wkly Rep* 48(27):590, 1999.
24. Garner JS, the Hospital Infection Control Practices Advisory Committee: Guidelines for isolation precautions in hospitals. II. Recommendations for isolation precaution in hospitals, *Am J Infect Control* 24(1):32, 1996 (or *www.cdc.gov*).
25. Grimes DE: *Infectious diseases,* St. Louis, 1991, Mosby.
26. Murray PR et al: *Manual of clinical microbiology,* ed 6, Washington, DC, 1995, ASM Press.

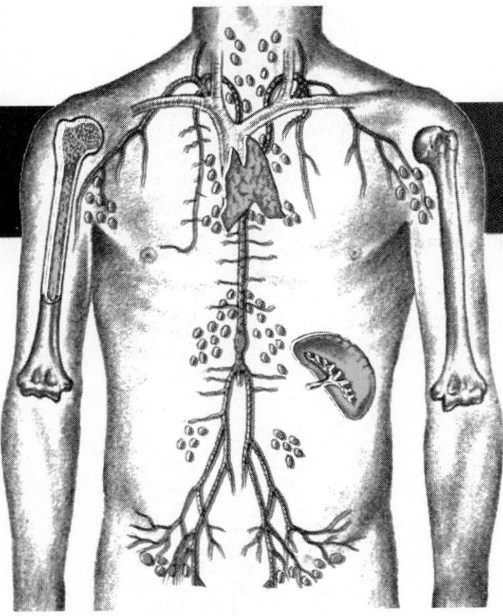

16 Immunologic System

Christine Miaskowski

Overview

The immune system is a highly specialized group of cells and tissues that protects the host. One role of the immune system is defense against invasive microorganisms. A second function is to maintain homeostasis by removing damaged cellular elements from the circulation. In addition, the immune system serves as a surveillance network to guard against the development, growth, and dissemination of tumor cells.

If the immune response is too weak or too vigorous, a disruption in homeostasis results. Certain hypersensitivity reactions and autoimmune diseases can occur when the regulatory cells of the immune system do not adequately control effector cell activities. Similarly, a depression in immune reactivity caused by regulatory or effector cell dysfunction can result in host susceptibility to recurrent infections and malignant disease.

Knowledge of basic immunology is increasing at a rapid rate and has had a profound influence on various aspects of medical and surgical practice. Immunodulatory agents are being widely used to augment immune function in cancer patients and persons with immunodeficiency disease. Histocompatibility matching and the development of pharmacologic agents that selectively depress immune reactivity have had a major impact on organ transplantation. Since a number of diseases, such as cancer, rheumatoid disorders, and certain hematologic and gastrointestinal problems, have been associated with immunologic changes, therapies involving immunologic manipulation may soon play a pivotal role in all clinical specialty fields.

Anatomy, Physiology, and Related Pathophysiology

Cellular Components and Their Anatomic Organization

The cellular constituents of the immune system include granulocytes, mononuclear phagocytes, and lymphocytes (Fig. 16-1). White cells are grouped into these three general categories on the basis of cell structure, functional activities, and stem cell derivation.

Granulocytes, that is, basophils or mast cells, eosinophils, and neutrophils, are derived from a common bone marrow progenitor cell, the myeloblast. Basophils comprise 0.5% to 1% of the circulating white blood cell (leukocyte) population. Mast cells, tissue counterparts of the blood basophil, are found adjacent to smooth muscle in the perivascular and peribronchiolar tissues. Mast cells and basophils are important sources of mediators, such as histamine in allergic reactions. Eosinophils make up 1% to 3% of peripheral blood leukocytes. They accumulate at sites of anaphylaxis, may influence the host response to parasitic infections, and play a lesser role in phagocytosis. Neutrophils make up as much as 70% of the blood leukocyte population. Neutrophils are active phagocytic cells that leave the vascular compartment and rapidly accumulate within the tissue spaces at sites of inflammation.

Mononuclear phagocytes, all originally derived from the bone marrow monoblast, are distributed throughout the body. Monocytes comprise approximately 5% of the circulating leukocyte population. Following a brief interval in the blood, monocytes migrate into the tissues, where they mature into macrophages. Macrophages are present in the brain (microglial cells), spleen, and lymphoid tissues. They also line the lung alveoli, the blood sinusoids of the liver (Kupffer's cells), and most extravascular tissue spaces. Mononuclear phagocytes help protect the host from invasive organisms, clear tissue debris from sites of tissue injury, may serve as surveillance cells in antitumor host defense, and may be important in the recognition and processing of antigen; antigen may be necessary for induction of specific immunologic responses.

Lymphocytes play a key role in the development of acquired immunity. All lymphocytes (T, B, and null cells, which do not have surface markers identifying them as either B or T lymphocytes) are derived from a common bone marrow progenitor cell. Certain immature lymphocytes leave the bone marrow and populate the thymus, where under the influence of thymic hormones they proliferate and differentiate into mature T lymphocytes. Other immature lymphocytes proliferate and differentiate

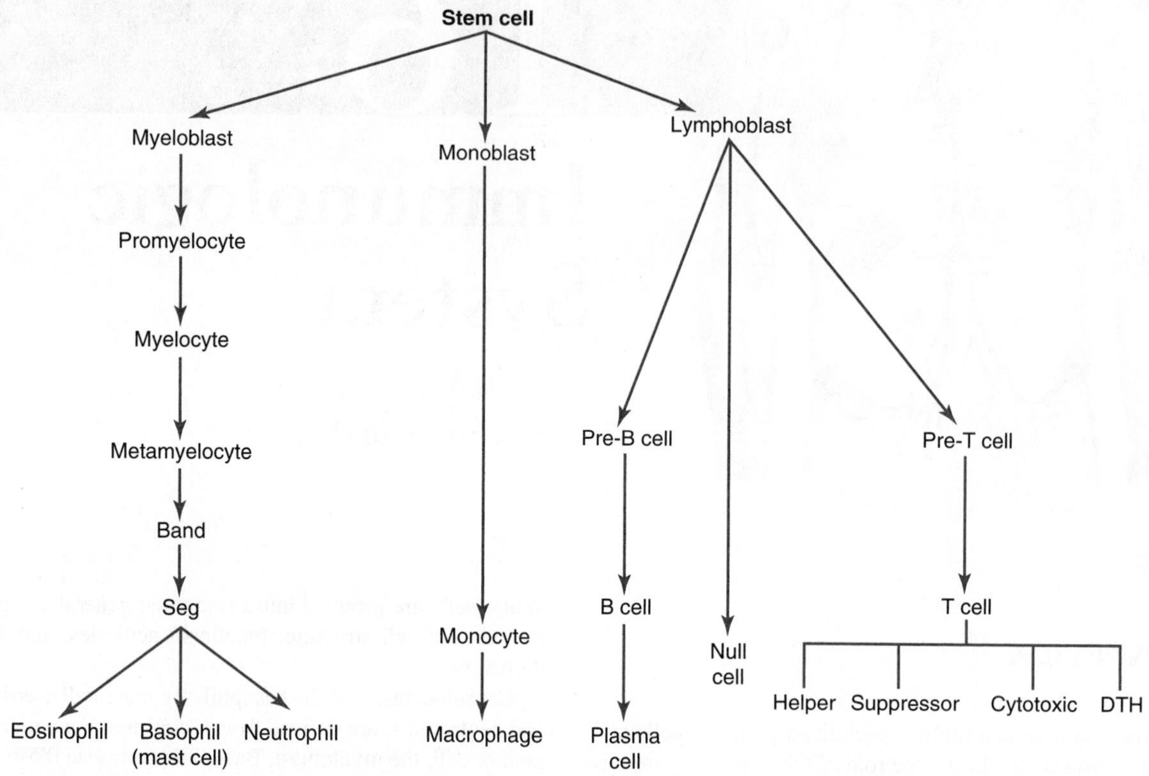

FIG. 16-1
Leukocyte development. All peripheral white blood cells are thought to be derived from common pluripotent bone marrow stem cells that can differentiate into myeloblasts, monoblasts, or lymphoblasts. Replication of these differentiated stem cells serves to replenish blood and tissue leukocyte populations. Mature leukocytes protect host against invasive organisms, participate in removal of particulate material from circulation, and serve as a surveillance network to guard against development and dissemination of tumor cells. *DTH*, delayed-type hypersensitivity.

into mature B lymphocytes. In birds this maturation takes place in an organ called the bursa of Fabricius. No mammalian bursal equivalent tissue has been identified. It is thought that B cell maturation in humans may take place in the bone marrow or in the lymphoid tissues lining the gastrointestinal tract.

After maturation, T and B lymphocytes are released into the circulation and populate the peripheral lymphoid tissues, including the spleen, lymph nodes, and tonsils. Mature lymphocytes are also localized in lymphoid tissues directly associated with the mucosal surfaces of the body. Such organized tissues comprise the appendix, Peyer's patches of the ileum, and bronchial-associated lymphoid tissue. The major organs housing the cellular elements of the immune system are illustrated in FIG. 16-2.

Nonspecific Immune Mechanisms

Physical and Chemical Barriers.

The first line of defense against invasive organisms is provided by intact skin and mucous membranes. These structures not only serve as a physical barrier to invasion but also provide a chemically unsuitable milieu to support microbial growth.

Microbial Factors.

Resident normal flora of the skin and mucous membranes also provide a defense against colonization with pathogenic bacteria. These resident microorganisms suppress growth of infectious agents by competing for essential nutrients, producing growth-inhibiting substances, and altering pH. When normal flora are reduced by antibiotic treatment, a person is more susceptible to infection with pathogenic microorganisms.

Inflammatory Response.

When a microorganism transcends the physical, chemical, and microbial barriers afforded by the host, or the body is injured by mechanical or chemical means, an inflammatory response is generated. At the onset of inflammation a rapid vasodilation occurs. Within minutes, blood neutrophils accumulate along the endothelial cells of vessels at the site of injury, migrate to the junctional zones between the vascular endothelial cells, and extravasate into the tissue spaces. Neutrophils within an inflammatory site represent the first line of cellular defense against invasive microorganisms.

If neutrophils do not neutralize (ingest and destroy) the inflammatory focus within a few hours, monocytes and lymphocytes begin to accumulate at the site of tissue injury. These cells attempt to localize the inflammatory response, providing a cellular barrier against the migration of the infectious organism into the lymphatic compartment, blood vessels, or neighboring tissues. When neutrophils, lymphocytes, and monocytes neutralize the inflammatory focus (phagocytose and respond with specific humoral and cell-mediated phenomena), granulation tissue is laid down and inflammation subsides. If the acute inflamma-

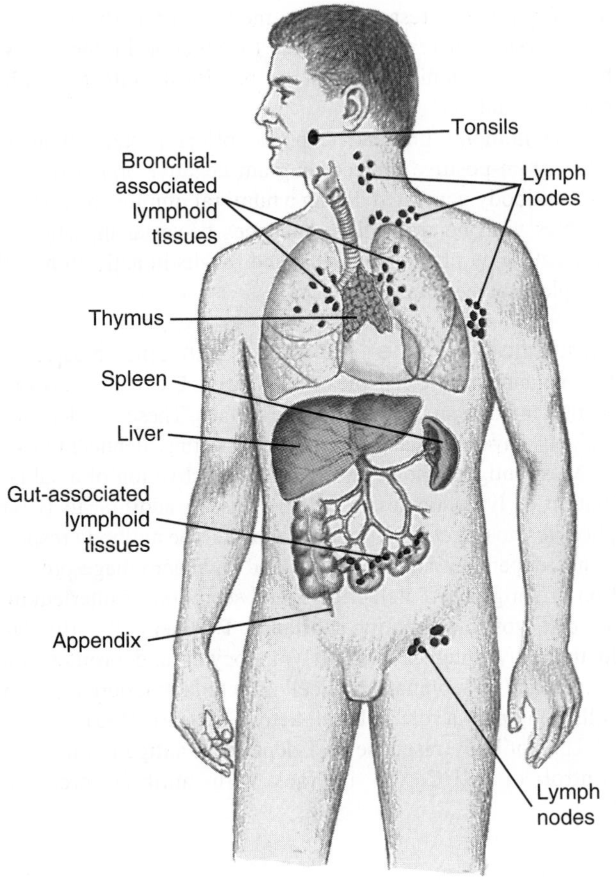

FIG. 16-2
Organization of immune system. Cellular constituents of immune system are derived from bone marrow stem cells. On maturation, these cells are released into peripheral blood and subsequently populate organized tissues of the lymphorecticular system.

tory response is unsuccessful at eliminating the infectious agent, or if tissue repair is incomplete, chronic inflammation results.

The persistence of an infectious agent during chronic inflammation results in granuloma formation. Granulomatous lesions are characterized by accumulations of lymphocytes and macrophages surrounding a central core of foreign material. Fibrotic tissue laid down on the periphery of the granuloma acts as a physical barrier that separates the lesion from surrounding normal tissues.

Accompanying the cellular responses that occur during inflammation are elevations in serum levels of certain proteins. These acute phase proteins, which include C-reactive protein and serum amyloid A protein, are used clinically to detect the presence of an infectious or inflammatory process. C-reactive protein may play a protective role by activating the complement pathway and influencing certain leukocyte responses. Large increases in the serum concentrations of globular proteins and fibrinogen may also accompany episodes of infection, inflammation, and tissue necrosis. In vitro, an elevation in the levels of these plasma proteins increases the aggregation and precipitation of erythrocytes suspended in plasma. This phenomenon, manifested in the laboratory as an elevation in erythrocyte sedimentation rate (ESR), is indicative of an ongoing inflammatory process.

Table 16-1 Humoral and Cell-Mediated Immune Responses

	Humoral	Cell-Mediated
Effector cells	B lymphocytes	T lymphocytes and macrophages
Regulatory cells	T helper cells and T suppressor cells	T helper cells and T suppressor cells
Effector mechanisms	Elaboration of antibody	Generation of factors that are directly toxic to target cells
Host protection	Against many gram-positive and certain gram-negative bacteria	Against mycobacteria, fungi, protozoa, and tumors

Specific Immune Mechanisms

Antigenicity. An antigen (or immunogen) is a substance capable of evoking an immune response. To qualify as an antigen a molecule must be recognized as foreign by the immune system. Antigens present on bacteria, viruses, molds, and pollens can induce a detectable immune response.

Similarly antigens found on mammalian cells and tissues can be immunogenic. Autologous antigens are tissue determinants that under normal conditions do not evoke an immune response. When these self-antigens are altered by infectious or inflammatory processes, the immune system recognizes its own tissues as "foreign" and produces an autoimmune response. Alloantigens are genetically determined antigens that discriminate individuals within a given species. Red cells, for example, have on their surface a number of determinants, including A, B, and Rh antigens, that may precipitate an immunologic reaction following the transfusion of incompatible blood. Similarly human leukocyte antigens (HLAs), present on the surface of all nucleated cells, have a profound influence on allograft survival. The human major histocompatibility complex (MHC) is a genetic region on chromosome 6 that codes for these human alloantigens. Gene products of the HLA-A, HLA-B, and HLA-C loci appear on all nucleated cells, whereas HLA-D region products are found primarily on lymphocytes, macrophages, epidermal cells, and sperm.

Induction of a Specific Immune Response. Antigen specific responses are designated as either humoral or cell-mediated immunity (Table 16-1). Humoral immunity is mediated by B lymphocytes that synthesize and secrete γ-globulins in response to antigenic challenge. Cell-mediated immune mechanisms involve the participation of effector T lymphocytes and macrophages. Humoral immunity can be transferred from an immune to a nonimmune host with cell-free globulin-bearing serum, whereas cell-mediated immunity is transferred with sensitized cells. Although the body's response to an antigenic challenge usually involves both cell-mediated and humoral immune mechanisms, one response may predominate.

A specific immune mechanism involves the participation of T and B lymphocytes that have been genetically programmed to recognize and interact with unique antigenic determinants on a foreign material. A specific immune response is triggered after the clearance of foreign materials from an inflammatory site, the lymph, or the vascular compartment by tissue macrophages. These phagocytic cells internalize and degrade the foreign antigens. The processed antigens are reexpressed on the macrophage surface in a highly immunogenic form for presentation to lymphocytes that continuously circulate through the lymphoid organs. Recognition of antigen by specific receptors on lymphocytes results in their stimulation and sequestration within the tissue.

Humoral Immunity. When confronted with an antigen, B lymphocytes synthesize and secrete specifically reactive γ-globulins called antibodies or immunoglobulins. On first exposure to a given antigen, a primary humoral immune response is evoked. This response occurs after a lag period of 1 to 7 days during which only trace amounts of specific antibody can be detected. During this induction period, antigen is processed and specific clones of B lymphocytes are stimulated to divide and differentiate ultimately into two different cell types. The first type, plasma cells, synthesizes and secretes antibodies. Other B lymphocytes, memory cells, remain quiescent until secondary exposure to a given antigen.

The secondary, or anamnestic, response that occurs after subsequent exposure to a particular antigen has a short lag period, produces high levels of antibody, and is more sustained than the primary response. This memory property of the immune system increases resistance to infection in persons who have been immunized against, or previously infected with, a particular antigen.

The humoral immune response offers protection against many gram-positive and certain gram-negative organisms. Specific antibody generated during a humoral immune response facilitates viral neutralization, enhances bacterial ingestion and destruction by phagocytic cells, and results in activation of the complement system.

Regulation of the Humoral Immune Response. Certain antigens are capable of stimulating B cells directly or after presentation on the macrophage surface. These T-independent antigens have a primary structure of repeating identical units.

Most antigens, however, require the activation of a subpopulation of lymphocytes, T helper cells, in addition to B lymphocytes, to effect an antibody response. The antibody response to a T dependent antigen is initiated by macrophage presentation of antigen to T helper cells and secretion of interleukin 1, a T cell growth-promoting substance. T helper cells, stimulated in this way, interact with B lymphocytes and promote their growth and differentiation. B cell growth factor, derived from T cells, may play a role in B cell activation (FIG. 16-3).

The antibody response to T-dependent antigen is under the control of MHC. To interact with antibody-presenting

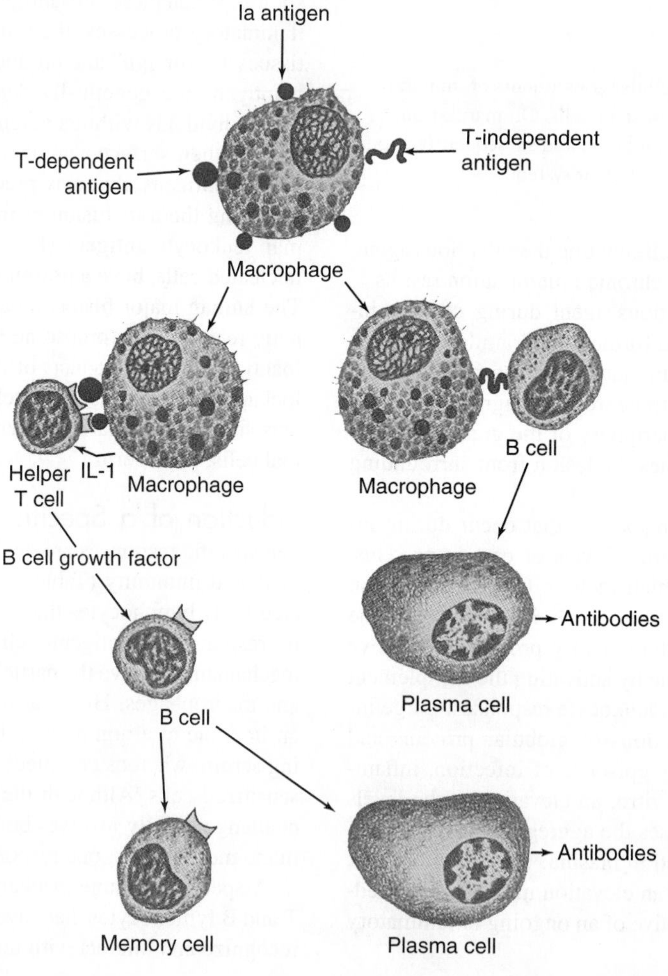

FIG. 16-3
Humoral immune responses. Antibody response to T-dependent antigens involves interaction between macrophages, T cells, and B cells. Macrophages ingest foreign materials, reexpress processed antigen on their surface, and present it in context of Ia molecule to T helper cells. T helper cells facilitate B lymphocyte proliferation and differentiation. On primary exposure to given T-dependent antigen, memory cell generation occurs, although little antibody is generated. During anamnestic response, plasma cells synthesize large quantities of specific antibody. Humoral response to T-independent antigens may be a macrophage-dependent or independent process. This response generally produces only antibody of IgM class and has little or no memory. *IL-1*, Interleukin 1.

macrophages, helper T cells have to recognize and bind self-antigens, called Ia antigens, on the macrophage surface. These self-antigens are coded for by genes of the HLA region. Similarly, T cell binding to B lymphocytes involves their recognition of a genetically determined marker on the B cell surface.

In addition to T lymphocytes that provide help in the induction of an immune response, certain other T lymphocytes depress immune reactivity. Suppressor T cells have an important role in homeostatic control because they maintain the humoral immune response at a level appropriate for the stimulus. Suppressor T cells are activated during the generation of all immune responses. They limit the immune response by acting at the level of the helper T cell or B lymphocyte (FIG. 16-4). The modulatory activity of suppressor T cells may be mediated by direct cell-to-cell contact or, alternatively, may involve the release of suppressor factors.

The relative numbers and functional reactivities of helper and suppressor cells determine the strength and persistence of an immune response. When the delicate balance between T helper and T suppressor cell populations is disrupted, autoimmune or immunodeficiency disease may result. Since helper and suppressor T lymphocytes have distinct surface markers and can be readily discriminated in the laboratory, immune function can be estimated by measuring the T helper/T suppressor cell ratio. Normally a person has roughly twice as many T helper cells as T suppressor cells. In contrast, patients with acquired immunodeficiency syndrome (AIDS) may demonstrate a T helper/T suppressor cell ratio of 1:1 or less.

Biologic Activities of Immunoglobulins.

The γ-globulin–bearing or antibody-bearing fractions of serum are referred to as immunoglobulins. The immunoglobulins are a highly heterogenous population of proteins, not a singular molecular species. Currently five physiochemical classes of immunoglobulins are recognized: IgG, IgM, IgA, IgE, and IgD.

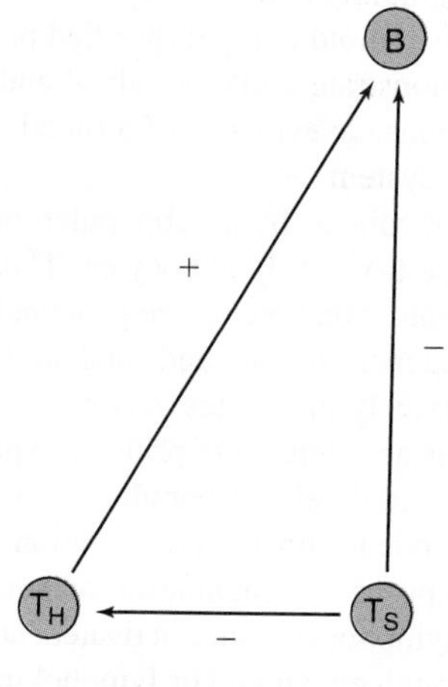

FIG. 16-4
Regulation of humoral immune responses. Generation of humoral immune response is facilitated by interaction of T helper (T_H) lymphocytes with antigen-specific B cells. This response can be down-regulated by T suppressor (T_S) lymphocytes that act at the level of either the T helper or B lymphocyte.

Immunoglobulin molecules are made up of a four-chain polypeptide (protein) unit consisting of two identical high–molecular weight (heavy) chains and two identical low–molecular weight (light) chains. The immunoglobulins have been assigned to their respective classes on the basis of their heavy chains: gamma (γ), mu (μ), alpha (α), epsilon (ε), and delta (δ). There are two different light chain types: kappa (κ) and lambda (λ). A schematic representation of a structural unit of immunoglobulin is shown in FIG. 16-5, *A*. The five major immunoglobulin classes is shown in FIG. 16-5, *B*.

IgG is the predominant serum antibody and represents a large proportion of the immunoglobulin found in internal secretions (for example, pleural, synovial, and peritoneal fluids). Specific IgG is produced only in small amounts late in the primary immune response, but it is the major antibody generated during a secondary challenge with antigen. IgG can neutralize toxins produced by various strains of bacteria and induces the agglutination of infectious organisms, facilitating their uptake by phagocytic cells. In addition, IgG has opsonic activity and can activate the complement system resulting in the lysis of certain strains of bacteria. IgG is thought to play a crucial role in neonatal host defense, because it is the only immunoglobulin class to be transferred across the placenta.

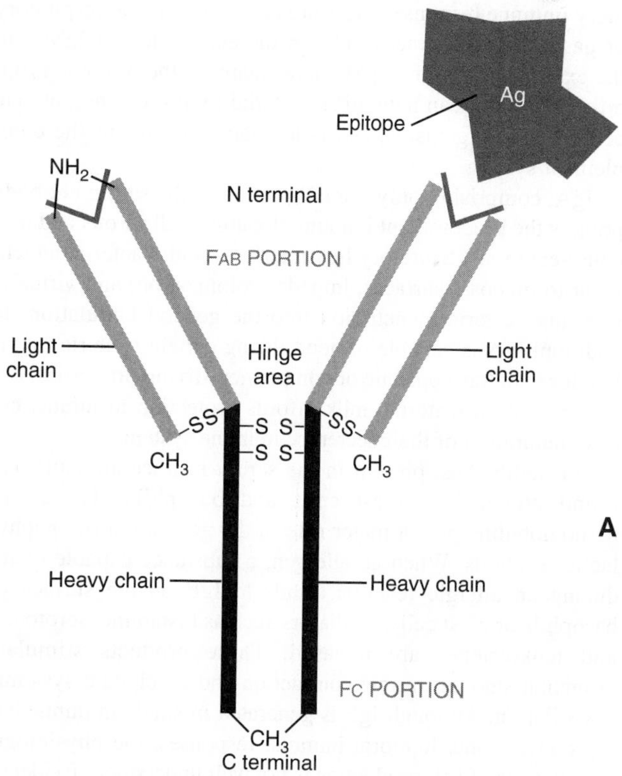

FIG. 16-5
A, Structure unit of immunoglobulin. The FAB (antigen-bindery fragment) binds to antigens (Ag) specifically. This antigen-binding ability is primarily due to the behavior of the light chains. The hinge area gives the immunoglobulin molecule flexibility. The angle of the arms of the Y can range from 0 to 180 degrees. The FC (crystalline fragment) end of the antibody can bind to other immune cells, phagocytic cells, platelets, and components of the complement system[8a].

Continued

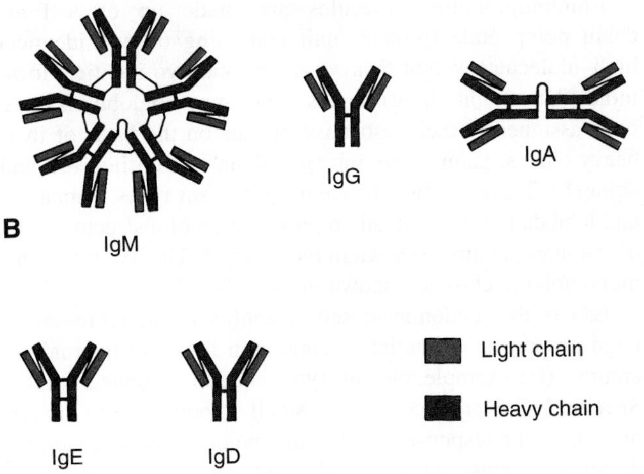

FIG. 16-5

B, Classes of antibodies. Antibodies are classified into five major groups: immunoglobulin M (IgM), immunoglobulin G (IgG), immunoglobulin A (IgA), immunoglobulin E (IgE), and immunoglobulin D (IgD). Notice that each IgM molecule comprises five Y-shaped basic antibody units, IgA of two basic antibody units, and the others of a single basic antibody unit.[38a]

IgM, comprising approximately 10% of the serum immunoglobulins, is the first antibody to appear during the primary immune response. Exposure to antigen via the respiratory or gastrointestinal tract results in the elaboration of IgM into the external secretions. IgM shares many of the biologic properties of IgG: it can neutralize bacterial toxins, can agglutinate certain microorganisms, and is a potent activator of the complement system.

IgA, comprising only a small portion of the serum antibody pool, is the predominant immunoglobulin in all serous and mucous secretions. Secretory IgA interferes with bacterial attachment to mucosal surfaces, impedes colonization, and virtually prevents bacterial penetration into the general circulation. In addition, IgA is capable of neutralizing certain bacteria toxins but does not have opsonic or complement-fixing properties. Secretory IgA in maternal milk affords protection to infants before maturation of their secretory immune system.

IgE antibodies, present in the serum in trace amounts, are found attached to mast cells and basophils. These immunoglobulins play a major role in the generation of anaphylactic reactions. When an allergen, a substance capable of inducing an allergic reaction, binds to IgE on the surface of basophils or mast cells, mediators such as histamine, serotonin, and leukotrienes are released. These products stimulate bronchial smooth muscle contraction and precipitate systemic vasodilation. Although IgE is generated in small amounts during conventional humoral immune responses, the physiologic significance of IgE production is not well understood. Evidence suggests that IgE may afford protection against parasitic infections by facilitating eosinophil recognition and destruction of the parasite.

IgD is only a minor component of the serum immunoglobulin pool and is not found in appreciable amounts in external or internal secretions. The biologic function of IgD has not been elucidated, but it may play a role in antigen-triggered lymphocyte differentiation.

Cell-Mediated Immunity. Whereas humoral immune mechanisms afford protection against many gram-positive and certain gram-negative organisms, cell-mediated immunity is important during host infection with intracellular pathogens such as mycobacteria, fungi, viruses, and protozoa. Cell-mediated reactions are also elicited as a component of the host response to tumors and tissue transplants.

Cell-mediated immune responses are characterized as either delayed-type hypersensitivity (DTH) or cytotoxic T lymphocyte (CTL) reactions (FIG. 16-6). CTL reactions play a major role in host defense against tumors, virally infected cells, and allogenic tissue transplants, whereas DTH reactions are activated by host infection with intracellular pathogens.

Generation of a DTH response involves the participation of macrophages, T helper cells, and DTH-effector T cells. During a primary infection the organisms are ingested by macrophages that process and reexpress antigen on their surface for presentation to helper cells. T helper cells, stimulated by antigen presentation and macrophage release of interleukin 1, induce proliferation of a pool of antigen-specific DTH-precursor T cells. The major portion of these cells remain quiescent until secondary challenge with antigen.

On secondary exposure an anamnestic response develops. Macrophages present processed antigen to antigen-specific T helper cells that rapidly stimulate large numbers of DTH-effector T cells, previously generated by clonal expansion. The activated DTH-effector cells release factors, called lymphokines, that stimulate other cells, particularly macrophages. Most tissue macrophages are incapable of killing intracellular pathogens; however, macrophages activated by exposure to lymphokines are avidly bactericidal.

The duration and magnitude of a DTH response are regulated by T suppressor cells. In general, a secondary DTH reaction can be demonstrated within a few hours of antigen challenge, peaks at 24 to 48 hours, and gradually recedes as the inflammatory focus is eliminated. A person's capacity to generate a secondary DTH response can be measured by intradermal injection with a battery of skin test antigens. If, for example, persons with normal immunity and a history of tuberculosis are tested with purified tuberculoid antigen (purified protein derivative [PPD]), they demonstrate a classic wheal and flare reaction. This positive response is evidence of a functionally intact cell-mediated immune system.

CTL reactions are mediated by a subpopulation of T lymphocytes known as cytotoxic T lymphocytes. These lymphocytes have surface receptors that recognize genetically different MHC markers on allogeneic tissues and mediate tissue rejection. Similarly cytotoxic lymphocytes recognize tumor- and virus-infected host cells as foreign. On primary exposure to genetically different or altered cells, a population of cytotoxic T precursor cells is expanded with the participation of T helper cells. On secondary exposure an anamnestic response is generated. The cytotoxic T lymphocyte, once activated, attaches to its target and lyses it, through enzymatic or lymphokine reactions. CTL reactions, like all classic immune responses, can be downregulated by T suppressor cells.

The recognition and destruction of tumor- and virus-infected target cells are not limited to cytotoxic T lymphocytes. Other categories of effector cells include mononuclear phagocytes and natural killer cells.

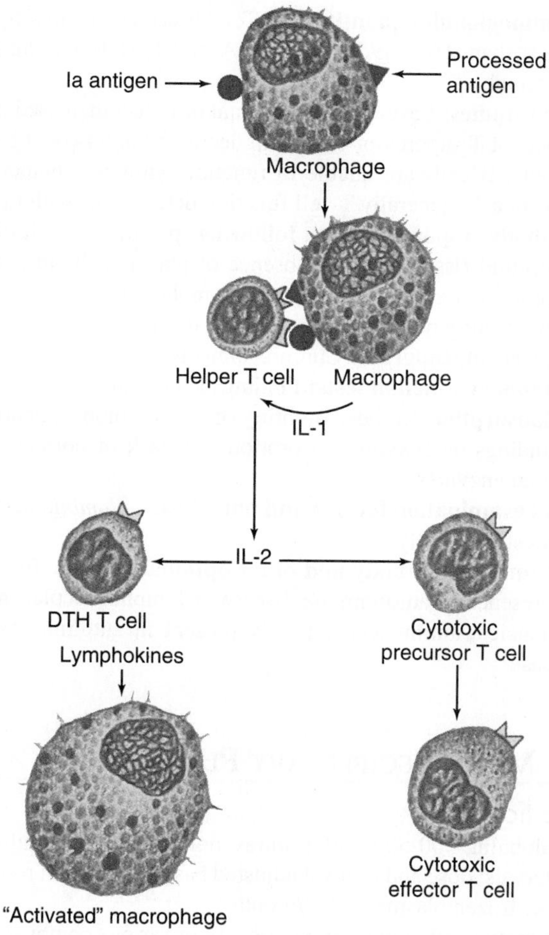

FIG. 16-6

Cell-mediated immune reactions are initiated by macrophage presentation of processed antigen to helper T lymphocytes. Stimulated T helper cells release interleukin 2 (*IL-2*) that activates DTH and cytotoxic T lymphocytes. Targets, such as tumor or virus-infected cells, are lysed directly by cytotoxic T cells. Following infection with intracellular pathogens, activated macrophages are the major effector cell population generated. *IL-1*, Interleukin 1.

Natural killer (NK) cells, often called null cells, are large granular lymphocytes that do not bear the classic markers found on B or T lymphocyte surfaces. They bind to and lyse target cells using either an antibody-dependent or independent mechanism. Target cell lysis by NK cells that requires antibody is described as antibody-dependent cell-mediated cytotoxicity (ADCC). Killing by NK cells occurs naturally and is not enhanced by immunization. Although NK cells do not have immunologic memory, their functional activities can be modified. Interferons, protein products of stimulated lymphocytes, increase NK killing of target cells. In contrast, certain prostaglandins depress NK function.

Mononuclear phagocytes can kill target cells directly or by an ADCC mechanism. Peripheral blood monocytes and resident tissue macrophages exhibit low levels of antitumor activity. Following activation with T lymphocyte–derived products such as interferon-γ, macrophage lysis of tumor- and virus-infected target cells increases.

Because immunization is not generally required for the activities of NK and mononuclear phagocytic cells, these populations are thought to play an important host defense role in early stages of infection and tumor growth, before CTL effector cells are generated. Interferon, shown experimentally to increase both NK cell and macrophage cytotoxic activities, is being used to treat certain malignancies and immunodeficiency disorders.

Complement System. The complement system is comprised of a series of proteins that when activated serve to amplify an immune response. Activation of the complement system leads to the elaboration of potent inflammatory mediators, facilitates particle opsonization and clearance, and may result in the direct lysis of altered mammalian cells and certain bacteria. The complement system may be activated by a number of immunologic and nonimmunologic stimuli.

Although the complement system protects the host against infectious organisms and may play a role in tumor cell destruction, the uncontrolled activation of this system would result in inflammatory changes and lytic destruction of host tissues. These potentially devastating effects are modulated by a number of control proteins, including C1 inhibitor, factors H and I, C4 binding protein, S protein, anaphylatoxin inactivator, and inhibitors of the membrane attack complex.

NORMAL FINDINGS

Since certain alterations in immune status appear to be genetically determined, a family history of recurrent infections, malignancies, allergies, immunodeficiency, and autoimmune disease should be elicited.

A detailed patient history is an essential component of the immune status profile. In addition to documentation of the patient's age, race, sex, and ethnic background, the following information should be obtained:

Past history—allergies, childhood and recurrent infections, malignancy, autoimmune disease, primary disorders known to suppress immune function, immunization profile, medications (prescription and over-the-counter)

Social, occupational, and nutritional habits

Abnormal signs and symptoms—fever, diaphoresis, rashes, joint pain, unusual masses, lymphadenopathy, overt signs of infection, poor wound healing, eczema, hepatosplenomegaly

Because immunologic and inflammatory disease can involve many organ systems, a complete physical examination is warranted. Particular attention should be paid to signs of infection (abscesses, persistent lesions, and so on), inflammatory tissue changes, wheezing, joint swelling, and skin integrity.

Alterations in vital signs may indicate the presence of an ongoing inflammatory process. (Geriatric patients, however, frequently demonstrate a reduced febrile response to infection.)

Liver: Usually located completely under rib cage; may be palpated just below right costal margin with deep inspiration

Spleen: Not generally palpable

Thymus: Can be detected only by radiologic examination; size varies with age (between birth and 20 years, thymic mass increases; after age 20, thymus progressively decreases in size until age 60, when thymic involution is complete)

Lymph nodes (head and neck, axillary, inguinal, epitrochlear): Generally not palpable; small, nontender nodes may be found in cervical or inguinal chain of persons with history of local infection

CONDITIONS, DISEASES, AND DISORDERS

IMMUNODEFICIENCY DISEASES

COMMON VARIABLE IMMUNODEFICIENCY (ACQUIRED HYPOGAMMAGLOBULINEMIA)

Common variable immunodeficiency (CVID) is an immune disorder of unknown cause that predominantly affects the B cell system. The clinical features include severe depression or absence of plasma cell.[36]

The immunologic feature of acquired hypogammaglobulinemia that is shared with the X-linked form is the marked depression or absence of all five classes of globulin. Consequently, recurrent bacterial infections are observed in this disorder. Other common features include malabsorption syndromes (usually resulting from *Giardia lamblia* infestation) and an increased incidence of autoimmune and lymphoreticular malignancies. A predilection for autoimmune and neoplastic disease in first-degree relatives of these patients suggests a hereditary influence.

CVID is distinguished by the presence of defective B lymphocytes and a higher-than-normal incidence of abnormalities in T cell immunity. Patients with CVID may manifest hyperplasia of lymphoid tissue, including the tonsils, nodes, and spleen. Acquired hypogammaglobulinemia occurs in both sexes equally and at any age, with symptoms appearing from age 15 to 35 years. Genetic studies demonstrated an autosomal recessive mode of inheritance in certain families in which abnormal lymphocyte metabolism is inherited. However, in most cases no clear genetic transmission can be demonstrated.

PATHOPHYSIOLOGY

The cause of acquired hypogammaglobulinemia is an intrinsic defect in B cell antibody production. In addition, excessive suppressor T cell activity may inhibit B cell functioning. In some cases, helper T cell activity may be inadequate to assist B cells to make antibody.

DIAGNOSTIC STUDIES AND FINDINGS

B cell quantitation and function: B cells low, normal, or increased; cells clonally diverse and relatively immature; fail to respond to most antigens and mitogens by differentiating into plasma cells; in some patients B cells synthesize but do not secrete immunoglobulin

Immunoglobulin quantitation: Total less than 300 mg/dl; IgG less than 250 mg/dl; serum IgA and IgM levels are subnormal

T cell studies: Levels may be normal or reflect increased numbers of T suppressor cells with decreased numbers of helper cells; B cells are unable to function without T helper cell feedback; generally T cell function deteriorates with time

Antibody response: Absent following specific immunization

Lymphoid tissue biopsy: Absence of plasma cells in B cell–dependent areas; hyperplasia of lymphoid tissue

Chest roentgenogram: Chronic lung disease

Sinus roentgenogram: Chronic sinusitis

Pulmonary function tests: Findings abnormal

Malabsorption studies: Blunting of villi on biopsy; abnormal findings on D-xylose absorption test; lack of normal intestinal enzymes

Stool examination for ova and parasites: *G. lamblia* detected most frequently

Antinuclear antibody and other optional studies: To detect presence of autoimmune disease or lymphoreticular malignancies; antinuclear antibody present in autoimmune disease

MULTIDISCIPLINARY PLAN

Medication

γ-Globulin, 300-500 mg/kg intravenously (IV) at monthly intervals; dose and interval adjusted based on clinical response

Fresh-frozen plasma, 1-2 U/month

Antibiotics, often given continuously in various combinations

Metronidazole, 750 mg tid for 10 days for malabsorption associated with *Giardia* infection

General Management

Pulmonary physical therapy and pulmonary rehabilitation in presence of chronic lung disease; chest x-ray examination and pulmonary function tests to determine adequacy of treatment; dietary restriction for secondary enzymatic deficiencies resembling celiac disease; treatment of associated autoimmune disorders (see specific condition)

NURSING CARE

NURSING ASSESSMENT

Respiratory status: Vital signs and respiratory status; monitor rate, rhythm, and quality of respirations, presence of cyanosis, adventitious breath sounds, and restlessness; monitor results of pulmonary function studies, arterial blood gas studies, and chest roentgenograms

Recurrent infection (usually chronic): Evidence of infection at sites of invasive procedures; breaks in skin integrity, particularly over pressure ulcers and oral mucosa; evidence of conjunctivitis; evidence of central nervous system (CNS) infection; joint pain and swelling; ear pain, discharge, diminished hearing; temperature; monitor laboratory data (white blood cell [WBC] count and differential, erythrocyte sedimentation rate, C-reactive protein, urinalysis, cultures)

Gastrointestinal status: Monitor intake and output, weight, and electrolytes for imbalances; chronic diarrhea (i.e., assess

frequency, volume, consistency, and pattern of bowel movements); monitor stool for ova and parasites
Lymphatic system: Lymphadenopathy; splenomegaly
Presence of concomitant autoimmune disease: Signs and symptoms associated with systemic lupus erythematosus; dermatomyositis; hemolytic anemia; rheumatoid arthritis–like disorder; idiopathic thrombocytopenic purpura; hypothyroidism; Graves' disease; pernicious anemia
Presence of concomitant neoplastic disease: Signs and symptoms associated with leukemia, lymphoma, gastric carcinoma, and skin cancers

Potential Complications

Sepsis; pneumonia; osteomyelitis; conjunctivitis; sinusitis; pharyngitis; otitis

Patient Problems/Nursing Diagnoses & Interventions

NIC Respiratory Management

Impaired gas exchange related to recurrent sinopulmonary infections and/or chronic lung disease

- Position patient for optimal chest excursion, usually with head elevated 30 to 60 degrees. Resting arms on padded overbed table may increase comfort for patients with chronic lung disease.
- Teach and encourage patient to cough and deep breathe every 2 hours.
- Turn patient frequently to move secretions.

NIC Elimination Management

Diarrhea related to giardiasis or enzymatic deficiencies

- Assist with toileting activities, as necessary, *to prevent skin breakdown.*
- Gradually increase intake, beginning with liquids and nonstimulating foods.

NIC Nutrition Support

Imbalanced nutrition: less than body requirements, related to malabsorption

- Provide gluten-free diet, when necessary.
- Provide small, frequent feedings as tolerated.
- Encourage family members to provide patient's favorite foods within diet parameters.
- Provide dietary supplements.
- Determine the need for parenteral nutrition if oral intake is deficient.

NIC Risk Management

Risk for infection related to compromised immunologic system

- Maintain optimal nutritional status and fluid intake.
- Maintain body hygiene.
- Limit environmental stress.
- Promote pulmonary toilet; breathing exercises, postural drainage, and chest physical therapy.
- Maintain normal sleep and rest patterns.
- Protect patient from physical injury.
- Restrict contact with family and health-care providers who have infectious diseases.

Patient Education/Continuum of Care Plan

1. Discuss with patient the techniques to prevent recurrent pulmonary infection: prophylactic antibiotics, breathing exercises, postural drainage, and chest physiotherapy.
2. Stress to patient the importance of compliance with regular follow-up examinations for γ-globulin level and clinical evaluation.
3. Give patient a list of risk factors associated with infection, and discuss signs and symptoms to report.
4. Explain to patient the principles of gluten-free diet.
5. Explain to patient the importance of adhering to medication regimen.
6. Refer patient for genetic counseling to explain inheritance pattern and to dietitian for diet plan.
7. Stress to patient the importance of wearing medical alert identification.

Evaluation/Patient Outcomes

Respiratory Management: Patient's respiratory rate and rhythm are within normal limits. Arterial blood gas levels are normal. Cyanosis, restlessness, and adventitious breath sounds are absent.

Elimination Management: Consistency and volume of patient's bowel movements are normal. Intake and output are balanced. Weight is stable. Electrolytes are within normal limits.

Nutrition Support: Weight is within normal range. Patient chooses and consumes a gluten-free diet.

Risk Management: Culture findings are negative. Urinalysis findings are negative. Ig G levels are within therapeutic range. Patient maintains mobility. Patient remains alert and oriented. Patient's skin is intact. Patient shows no manifestations of infection.

Selective IgA Deficiency

Selective IgA deficiency is the presence of serum IgA in quantities less than 5 mg/dl while other immunoglobulins are present in normal amounts.[7]

Selective IgA deficiency is the most common immunodeficiency disease. In the United States the incidence is approximately 1 in 700. Although the disease is most commonly detected during the first decade of life, patients often survive until the sixth or seventh decade. It cannot be diagnosed before 1 year of age because infants may not produce IgA until then.

As discussed previously, IgA is the predominant immunoglobulin of external secretions. Therefore bacterial infections of the respiratory, gastrointestinal, and urogenital tracts are the major clinical manifestations associated with this disorder.

Many affected persons are asymptomatic. Autoimmune disease develops in 25% of those affected. Recently IgG subclass deficiencies were reported in association with IgA deficiency.

Morbidity is associated with recurrent sinopulmonary infections, autoimmune disease, and rarely, neoplastic disease. Spruelike disease may also complicate the disease course.

PATHOPHYSIOLOGY

The immunopathogenesis of this disorder is unclear. The presence of normal numbers of IgA B cells suggests that the underlying defect involves decreased synthesis or release of IgA. However, lymphocyte culture studies have demonstrated that IgA B cells synthesize but do not secrete immunoglobulin. Therefore the underlying defect probably occurs in the transformation of the IgA B lymphocyte to the plasma cell. T suppressor mechanisms may influence this process. The presence of antibodies to IgA in as many as 44% of cases of IgA deficiency implies that an autoimmune process is involved as well. See p. 1094 for a description of the role of IgA.

A genetic predisposition has also been postulated. Autosomal recessive and autosomal dominant modes of inheritance have been implicated. IgA deficiency appears with greater-than-normal frequency in families with a variety of immunodeficiency diseases. In addition, the presence of HLA-A1, HLA-B8, and HLA-DW3 is associated with IgA deficiency and autoimmune disease.

Whatever the cause, the lack of secretory IgA antibody promotes the attachment of infectious microbes at the mucosal surfaces and explains the occurrence of gastrointestinal, urogenital, and sinopulmonary infections. In addition, IgA probably acts to prevent absorption of other foreign proteins such as those in the diet. Its absence may explain the spruelike syndrome associated with selective IgA deficiency.

The deficiency of IgA may not be primary. Instead it may follow the administration of certain drugs such as phenytoin or penicillamine. In this case the decreased serum levels may result from induction of T suppressor cells that interfere with B cell maturation.

DIAGNOSTIC STUDIES AND FINDINGS

Ig quantitation: IgA level less than 5 mg/dl; IgG, IgM, IgD, and IgE normal or increased
Immunization: Normal antibody response
B cell quantitation: Normal numbers of B cells, including IgA-bearing lymphocytes
T cell studies: Normal findings
Chest roentgenograms: Pneumonia
Sinus roentgenograms: Sinusitis
Pulmonary function tests: Findings abnormal
Gastrointestinal studies: Findings abnormal in celiac disease; abnormal D-xylose absorption
Antinuclear antibody: Positive findings in presence of autoimmune disease

Differential diagnoses that must be excluded include chronic mucocutaneous candidiasis, Nezelof syndrome, and drug-induced IgA deficiency

MULTIDISCIPLINARY PLAN

Because no replacement therapy is yet available, treatment is aimed at management of recurrent infections and serial assessment for the presence of autoimmune and neoplastic disease.

Medications

Antibiotic therapy according to system involved and culture results

General Management

Gluten-free diet for celiac disease
Chest physical therapy, breathing exercises, postural drainage, and oxygen therapy as prophylaxis or for treatment of chronic pulmonary disease
Serial sinus and chest roentgenograms and pulmonary function tests to follow the disease course and determine adequacy of treatment
Follow-up for, and treatment of, concomitant and autoimmune or neoplastic disease as needed
Administration of IgA-deficient blood products to prevent future antigen-antibody reaction

NURSING CARE

NURSING ASSESSMENT

Recurrent infection: Sinusitis; pneumonia; gastrointestinal infections; genitourinary infections
Presence of concomitant autoimmune disease: Signs and symptoms associated with systemic lupus erythematosus, rheumatoid arthritis, dermatomyositis, pernicious thyroiditis, anemia, Sjögren's syndrome, allergic conditions.

PATIENT PROBLEMS/NURSING DIAGNOSIS & INTERVENTIONS

The majority of IgA-deficient patients are asymptomatic; the rest may seek treatment for infections. See Acquired Hypogammaglobulinemia, p. 1096 for sinopulmonary or gastrointestinal infections, and Chapter 15 for other infections.

DISORDERS OF COMPLEMENT

Disorders of complement occur as a result of a primary deficiency or dysfunction of one or more complement components that results in an increased susceptibility to infection.

In acquired complement disorders, particularly immune complex disease, activation of complement and subsequent inflammatory mediator involvement may cause increased tissue damage.

The classical and alternative complement systems play an integral role in the amplification of nonspecific host defense mechanisms to invading organisms and in clearance of circulating immune complexes from the serum.

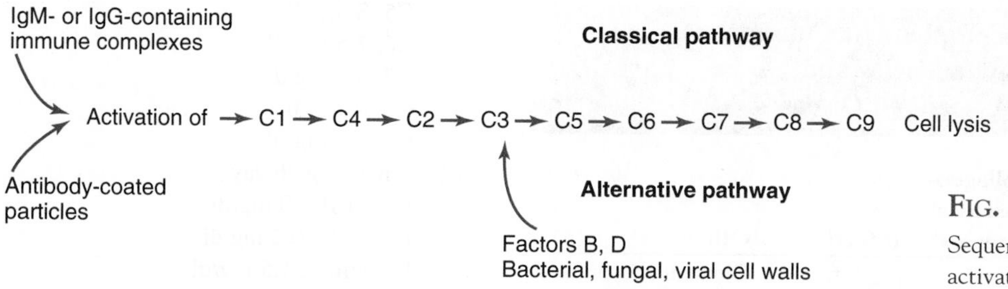

FIG. 16-7
Sequence of complement activation.

Complement proteins are present in the serum in inactive form, and activation leads to biologic activity. Activation occurs in a cascade fashion and is regulated by four complement proteins.

Primary complement disorders account for less than 1% of primary immunodeficiencies. Deficiency or dysfunction has been identified for each of the classical complement components; none have been identified in the alternative pathway. Certain of these disorders, especially those late in the cascade, have a benign clinical course, but as many as 5% of these patients have severe *Neisseria* infections.

In contrast, defects involving key complement components that regulate the complement cascade or components early in the cascade may be associated with severe, recurrent infections or autoimmune diseases.

Secondary complement deficiencies arise when a disease process causes decreased synthesis or triggers increased consumption. With increased activation, as occurs in immune complex disease, tissue damage often occurs because of the inflammatory mechanisms modulated by complement.

PATHOPHYSIOLOGY

A brief schema of the sequence of activation of the complement cascade is shown in FIG. 16-7.

With deficiency or dysfunction in one of the classical complement components, activation of the normal cascade can occur only to the deficient component. Activation of the remainder of the pathway theoretically should not occur. However, because the classical and alternative pathways share the same terminal components, activation through a different regulatory point in the cascade can compensate for the deficiency.

Deficiencies in the C1, C4, and C2 proteins are the most commonly reported. C2 deficiency occurs in 1 in 10,000 persons. Persons with these deficiencies may be in good health and usually do not have difficulties with recurrent infections. When infections do develop, bacterial rather than viral organisms are involved. In addition, as many as 50% of persons with C2 deficiency have autoimmune disease, particularly systemic lupus erythematosus and juvenile rheumatoid arthritis.

Clinically, C3 is one of the most important complement components because of its place in the complement cascade, and C3 deficiency is the most severe disorder identified. Patients with this abnormality have recurrent, fulminant, pyogenic bacterial infections. C3 deficiency may result from a genetic defect in production. Some persons, including those with nephritic factor, have serum factors that continuously activate and thus deplete C3. Other persons lack C3bI, a regulatory protein that prevents continuous consumption of C3 once the alternative pathway is activated.

Terminal complement component deficiencies (C5 through C9) have also been identified. Many affected persons are asymptomatic. Others may manifest an increased incidence of infection with *Neisseria gonorrhoeae* and *Neisseria meningitidis.* Although persons with C9 deficiency have been identified, this abnormality has not been associated with clinical disease. These persons show normal resistance to infection with bacterial, viral, and fungal organisms.

In C5 dysfunction all levels of complement components including C5 are normal, but serum chemotactic and opsonic activities are reduced because of a defect in C5 activity. Clinical features of C5 dysfunction resemble those of C5 deficiency. Susceptibility to recurrent infections, particularly of the skin and gastrointestinal tract, is increased.

C1 inhibitor deficiency is also known as hereditary angioedema. C1 inhibitor is a regulatory protein that controls activation of C1. Continuous activation of C1 with resultant depletion of C2 and C4 may be due to a failure of this control protein to "turn off" primary pathway activation once initiated. Possibly deficiency of C1 inhibitor, which also inhibits kinin activation, allows kinin formation with subsequent vascular permeability and tissue edema, leading to angioedema.

Association of primary complement disorders with various autoimmune diseases is common (Table 16-2), although the cause is unknown.

Secondary disorders of complement have multiple pathophysiologic mechanisms. The degree of complement disorder will vary with the severity of the underlying disease process. In extreme protein-deficiency states, decreased synthesis results in overall depression of the total complement component quantities, resulting in inadequate host defense.

Various disease states may result in increased complement consumption. In fulminant bacterial infections, complement is consumed and production cannot meet demand.

Complement activation is an integral component of the pathophysiology of diseases associated with circulating immune complexes. With involvement of complement, and resultant inflammatory response, tissue damage occurs. Degree of complement activation correlates with activity of disease and is often monitored as an indicator of disease activity or response to therapy.

The following are some of the factors associated with secondary disorders of complement:

Decreased synthesis
- Asplenia

Table 16-2 Complement Component Deficiencies and Associated Diseases

Component	Collagen-Vascular Diseases*	Infections†	Other
Clq	+	+	Glomerulonephritis; immunodeficiencies
Clr	+	+	Glomerulonephritis
Cls	+	+	
C4	+	−	
C2	+	+	Glomerulonephritis
C3	+	+	Nephritis
C5	+	+	
C6	+	+	
C7	+	+	
C8	+	+	
C9	−	+	
I‡	−	+	
H‡	−	−	Hemolytic-uremic syndrome
Properdin‡	−	−	
C1INH‡	+	+	Hereditary angio-edema

*A variety of autoimmune diseases have been described.
†A variety of infective organisms have been identified.
‡Control proteins.

- Sickle cell disease
- Protein-deficient states: Cirrhosis; malnutrition; severe burns; anorexia nervosa
- Newborns (up to 6 months)

Increased consumption
- Acute nephritis
- Partial lipodystrophy
- Immune complex diseases, especially systemic lupus erythematosus
- Bacteremia, endotoxins
- Dialysis (renal, plasmapheresis, heart-lung)

DIAGNOSTIC STUDIES AND FINDINGS

History: Recurrent bacterial infections, autoimmune disease
Physical examination: Dependent on disease process
Laboratory findings: Serum complement protein levels*

Classical pathway†
- C1q, 7 mg/dl
- Clr, 3.4 mg/dl
- Cls, 3.1 mg/dl
- C2, 2.5 mg/dl
- C3, 160 mg/dl
- C4, 50 mg/dl
- C5, 8 mg/dl
- C6, 7.5 mg/dl
- C7, 5.5 mg/dl
- C8, 8 mg/dl
- C9, 5.8 mg/dl

Alternative pathway
- Factor B, 20 mg/dl
- Factor D, 0.2 mg/dl
- Properdin, 1.5 mg/dl

Control proteins
- C1q inhibitor, 12.5 mg/dl
- C3b inactivator (factor I), 2.5 mg/dl
- Anaphylatoxin inactivator, 5 mg/dl
- C4 binding protein, 25 mg/dl
- S protein, 50 mg/dl
- Factor H, 50 mg/dl

CH50, 20 to 40 units/ml*

*C3, C4, and CH50 assays are available in most laboratories. Reference laboratories generally perform other assays. Numbers will be decreased in specific complement deficiency. With control protein abnormalities, succeeding component will be depressed.
†Detects quantity and not functional capacity. Ranges vary among laboratories.

MULTIDISCIPLINARY PLAN

No therapy is available for direct treatment of complement disorders. With primary complement disorders, aggressive management of infections is indicated. Management of hereditary angiodema is discussed elsewhere in this text.

In secondary complement disorders, management of the disease process should restore normal complement levels. The reader is referred elsewhere in this text for management of individual diseases.

ACQUIRED IMMUNODEFICIENCY SYNDROME

Acquired immunodeficiency syndrome (AIDS) is a condition characterized by dysfunction of cell-mediated (i.e., T cell) immunity.[5,8] The progressive decrease in the CD4 helper subset of T lymphocytes results in the clinical manifestations of immunosuppression and susceptibility to numerous opportunistic infections (e.g., *Pneumocystis carinii* pneumonia [PCP]) and neoplasms (e.g., Kaposi's sarcoma).

In 1981 the initial cases of AIDS were reported. By 1982 the syndrome was being identified in certain high-risk groups (i.e., homosexual men, IV drug users, hemophiliacs, and Haitians). In 1983, the human immunodeficiency virus (HIV) was discovered, and by 1985 a blood test was available that could identify individuals infected with HIV before they developed AIDS. With the advent of the blood test, most clinicians began to think about the spectrum of HIV disease, which ranges from asymptomatic seropositivity to full-blown AIDS.

Infection with HIV has reached epidemic proportions worldwide. Recent estimate suggest that 10 million people worldwide are infected with HIV or related retroviruses.

In the United States, approximately 700,000 Americans are infected with HIV. In 1997 approximately 230,000 Americans were living with AIDS. Estimates of the number of Americans

*Indicative of classical pathway integrity; measures the dilution of serum required to lyse 50% of a standard number of antibody-coated sheep red blood cells; normal values determined within each laboratory.

who will develop AIDS were scaled down in the 1990s. However, in the United States, there is a rapid increase in the number of AIDS cases in women.

Dramatic increases in the efficacy of antiretroviral therapies, particularly those that contain protease inhibitors, changed the course of the epidemic and improved the prognosis of patients with HIV/AIDS. However, patients with HIV disease who present with symptoms warrant a systematic evaluation of the body system that is involved. Clinical conditions associated with various body systems in persons who are infected with HIV include the following:

Pulmonary system: *P. carinii* pneumonia; bacterial, mycobacterial, and viral pneumonias; Kaposi's sarcoma; non-Hodgkin's lymphoma; interstitial pneumonitis

Central nervous system: Toxoplasmosis; central nervous system lymphoma; AIDS dementia complex; cryptococcal meningitis; HIV myelopathy

Peripheral nervous system: Inflammatory polyneuropathies; sensory neuropathies; mononeuropathies

Musculoskeletal system: Arthritis; myopathies

Ear, eye, nose, and throat: Sinusitis; retinitis

Oral cavity: Oral candidiasis; hairy leukoplakia; gingival disease; aphthous ulcers

Gastrointestinal system: Esophagitis; hepatic disease; biliary disease; enterocolitis

Endocrine disorders: Disorders of the adrenal gland

Integumentary system: Herpes simplex; herpes zoster; *Staphylococcus* infections; bacillary angiomatosis

HIV-related malignancies: Kaposi's sarcoma; non-Hodgkin's lymphoma; primary lymphoma of the brain; cervical cancer

Gynecologic manifestations: Vaginal candidiasis; cervical dysplasia; pelvic inflammatory disease

Populations at Risk

In 1993, the Centers for Disease Control and Prevention expanded the AIDS definition (see box below). The modes of transmission of HIV are similar to those of hepatitis B. The risk

CDC AIDS CASE DEFINITION FOR SURVEILLANCE OF ADULTS AND ADOLESCENTS

Definitive AIDS Diagnoses (With or Without Laboratory Evidence of HIV Infection)

1. Candidiasis of the esophagus, trachea, bronchi, or lungs
2. Cryptococcosis, extrapulmonary
3. Cryptosporidiosis with diarrhea persisting >1 month
4. Crytomegalovirus disease of an organ other than the liver, spleen, or lymph nodes
5. Herpes simplex virus infection causing a mucocutaneous ulcer that persists longer than 1 month; or bronchitis, pneumonitis, or esophagitis of any duration
6. Kaposi's sarcoma in a patient <60 years of age
7. Lymphoma of the brain (primary) in a patient <60 years of age
8. *Mycobacterium avium-intracellular* complex or *Mycobacterium kansasii* disease, disseminated (at a site other than or in addition to lungs, skin, or cervical or hilar lymph nodes)
9. *P. carinii* pneumonia
10. Progressive multifocal leukoencephalopathy
11. Toxoplasmosis of the brain
12. CD4 lymphocyte count below 200 cells/μl or a CD4 lymphocyte percentage below 14%
13. Pulmonary tuberculosis
14. Recurrent pneumonia
15. Invasive cervical cancer

Definitive AIDS Diagnoses (With Laboratory Evidence of HIV Infection)

1. Coccidioidomycosis, disseminated (at a site other than or in addition to lungs or cervical or hilar lymph nodes)
2. HIV encephalopathy
3. Histoplasmosis, disseminated (at a site other than or in addition to lungs or cervical or hilar lymph nodes)
4. Isosporiasis with diarrhea persisting >1 month
5. Kaposi's sarcoma at any age
6. Lymphoma of the brain (primary) at any age
7. Other non-Hodgkin's lymphoma of B cell or unknown immunologic phenotype
8. Any mycobacterial disease caused by mycobacteria other than *Mycobacterium tuberculosis,* disseminated (at a site other than or in addition to lungs, skin, or cervical or hilar lymph nodes)
9. Disease caused by extrapulmonary *M. tuberculosis.*
10. *Salmonella* (nontyphoid) septicemia, recurrent
11. HIV wasting syndrome

Presumptive AIDS Diagnoses (With Laboratory Evidence of HIV Infection)

1. Candidiasis of esophagus: (a) recent onset of retrosternal pain on swallowing and (b) oral candidiasis
2. Cytomegalovirus retinitis: A characteristic appearance on serial ophthalmoscopic examinations
3. Mycobacteriosis: Specimen from stool or normally sterile body fluids or tissue from a site other than lungs, skin, or cervical or hilar lymph nodes, showing acid-fast bacilli of a species not identified by culture
4. Kaposi's sarcoma: Erythematous or violaceous plaquelike lesion on skin or mucous membrane
5. *P. carinii* pneumonia: (a) a history of dyspnea on exertion or nonproductive cough of recent onset (within the past 3 months), and (b) chest x-ray evidence of diffuse bilateral interstitial infiltrates or gallium scan evidence of diffuse bilateral pulmonary disease, and (c) arterial blood gas analysis showing an arterial oxygen partial pressure of <70 mm Hg or a low respiratory diffusing capacity of <80% of predicted values or an increase in the alveolar-arterial oxygen tension gradient, and (d) no evidence of a bacterial pneumonia
6. Toxoplasmosis of the brain: (a) recent onset of local neurologic abnormality consistent with intracranial disease or a reduced level of consciousness; and (b) brain imaging evidence of a lesion having a mass effect or the radiographic appearance of which is enhanced by injection of contrast medium, and (c) serum antibody to toxoplasmosis or successful response to therapy for toxoplasmosis
7. Recurrent pneumonia: (a) more than one episode in a 1-year period and (b) acute (new symptoms, signs, or radiologic evidence not present earlier) pneumonia diagnosed on clinical or radiologic grounds by the patient's physician
8. Pulmonary tuberculosis: (a) apical or miliary infiltrates and (b) radiographic and clinical response to antituberculosis therapy

EMERGENCY ALERT

AIDS—ACQUIRED IMMUNODEFICIENCY SYNDROME

An infection caused by the human immunodeficiency virus (HIV) that is most commonly transmitted through sexual contact, IV drug use, and from mother to unborn child.

ASSESSMENT

- Verify or determine HIV status, AIDS status.
- Rule out opportunistic infections as patient is immunosuppressed
- Assess for change in level of consciousness, stability of vital signs, and nutritional status.
- Rule out potentially life-threatening infections such as *P. carinii,* cryptococcal meningitis, cerebral toxoplasmosis.
- Rule out thrombocytopenia, granulocytopenia.

INTERVENTIONS

- Administer oxygen as indicated by either nasal cannula or mask.
- Obtain clinical evaluation and perform indicated intervention directed at determining cause(s).
- Obtain IV access; in collaboration with physician, administer fluids and medications as appropriate.
- Protect client with altered level of consciousness from injury.
- Provide support and reassure patient and family.

of sexual transmission varies with particular sexual practices; anal intercourse is associated with the highest risk.

In the United States, 42% of AIDS cases are reported in gay or bisexual men and 25% are heterosexual intravenous drug users. The remainder of the cases occur in infants of infected mothers, heterosexual contacts of infected individuals, and recipients of contaminated blood or blood products. Among risk groups, the most rapid percentage increases are among young gay and bisexual men and heterosexual men and women, especially blacks and Latinos.

The number of women with AIDS is increasing rapidly. The two major risk factors for women are intravenous drug use and heterosexual contact with an infected partner. The increased incidence of AIDS in women has been associated with an increase in the number of perinatally infected children.

The rate of progression to symptomatic disease is variable (see Emergency Alert box above). Once clinical symptoms develop, outcomes are variable. With improvements in treatments, patients are living longer with the disease.

PATHOPHYSIOLOGY

HIV can infect all cells that express the CD4 antigen. Once the virus enters the cell, it causes cell death by an unknown mechanism. The cell primarily infected is the CD4 (helper-inducer) lymphocyte. The CD4 cell directs other cells of the immune system. Other immune cells are also infected by HIV, including B lymphocytes and macrophages.

The defect in B cells is mainly due to disordered CD4 lymphocyte function. Macrophages act as a reservoir for HIV and serve to disseminate it to other organ systems (e.g., central nervous system). In addition, the virus can act directly on glial cells and oligodendrocytes that may express CD4 antigen and cause neurologic effects.

Clinical findings of HIV disease are consistent with profound immunosuppression. Because T cell–mediated immunity is important in tumor surveillance and in defense against intracellular pathogens such as viruses, protozoa, mycobacteria, and fungi, deregulation within this component of the body's defensive network results in the development of characteristics of AIDS, such as the following:

- Cutaneous anergy
- Leukopenia
- Lymphopenia
- Decreased T cell function and reactivity
- Reduced or absent T helper cells
- Increased percentage of T suppressor cells
- Depressed natural killer cell activity
- Depressed interferon production by peripheral blood leukocytes
- Normal or increased immunoglobulin levels
- Abnormal immunoglobulin function in some cases
- Normal phagocytic function

DIAGNOSTIC STUDIES AND FINDINGS

Enzyme-linked immunosorbent assay (ELISA): Repeated reactivity with confirmation by a second assay such as Western blot

Polymerase chain reaction (PCR): Detection of HIV

White blood cell (WBC) count: Depressed

Lymphocyte count: Depressed

T cell studies: T cell numbers and function depressed; delayed hypersensitivity skin test shows decreased or absent response to cutaneous recall antigens (anergy); T helper/T suppressor cell ratio reversed (less than 0.5)

Absolute CD4 lymphocyte count: Most widely used predictor of HIV progression; risk of opportunistic infections high with CD4 less than 200 cells/μl

B cell studies: B cell numbers and function normal or increased; immunoglobulin levels normal or increased

Beta$_2$-microglobulin cell surface protein: Indicative of macrophage-monocyte stimulation; levels less than 3.5 mg/dl associated with rapid progression of disease

p24 antigen: Indicates active HIV replication

Natural killer cell activity: Usually depressed

Complement: Normal to increased

Cultures: Polymicrobial (fungal, viral, protozoal, and bacterial) infections

Tissue biopsy: Kaposi's sarcoma; *P. carinii* pneumonia; lymphoreticular malignancies

Viral titers: Document exposure to herpes simplex, hepatitis, Epstein-Barr virus, cytomegalovirus (CMV); elevated titers may explain panhypergammaglobulinemia

Chest roentgenogram: Used in initial evaluation of respiratory complaints; pneumonia, pneumonitis, pulmonary infiltrates detected (causative agents determined via culture, bronchoscopy with brushings, or biopsy)

Gallium scan: Useful in early detection of interstitial pneumonias

Table 16-3 Staging System of Kaposi's Sarcoma

Stage	Description
I	Cutaneous, locally indolent
II	Cutaneous, locally aggressive with or without regional lymph nodes
III	Generalized mucocutaneous or lymph node involvement
IV	Visceral

SUBTYPES

A. No systemic signs or symptoms
B. Systemic signs: 10% weight loss or temperature greater than 100° F orally, unrelated to identifiable source of infection, and lasting more than 2 weeks

Generalized: More than upper or lower extremities alone; includes minimal gastrointestinal disease defined as more than five lesions and larger than 2 cm in combined diameters

From Friedman-Klein and Laubenstein.[15]

Stool for ova and parasites: Variety of parasites, including *G. lamblia* and *Cryptosporidium*

Neurologic work-up, cerebrospinal fluid analysis, brain computed tomography (CT) scan, brain biopsy, electromyography, nerve conduction studies, ophthalmic examination, electroencephalogram, magnetic resonance imaging (MRI): Indicated for evaluation of changes in mentation and fever of unknown cause; variety of AIDS-associated disorders may be detected, including progressive multifocal leukoencephalopathy, cryptococcal meningitis, encephalitis, organic brain syndrome, and toxoplasmosis

Staging work-up for Kaposi's sarcoma: Skin: photographs and biopsies of representative lesions; nodes: biopsy of accessible nodes, CT scan of abdomen and pelvis; gastrointestinal tract: endoscopy, colonoscopy, and gastrointestinal contrast studies; lung: bronchoscopy (if chest roentgenogram shows abnormalities); liver: CT scan or radioisotope scan; bone: bone scan when alkaline phosphatase level is elevated (Table 16-3).

Bronchoscopy: *P. carinii* pneumonia (PCP); cryptococcal pneumonia

Sputum induction: PCP, cryptococcal pneumonia

Pulmonary function tests: Useful in early detection of interstitial pneumonias

Serologic antigen test: Cryptococcosis

Bone marrow biopsy: Histoplasmosis disseminated in bone marrow

Acid fast bacillus (AFB) stain: Confirmation of *Mycobacterium tuberculosis*

Endoscopy: Disseminated CMV in the gastrointestinal tract; *Candida* esophagitis

Barium swallow: *Candida* esophagitis

KOH preparation of yeast: Confirmation of oral thrush

Lumbar puncture: Cryptococcal meningitis

Ophthalmic examination: Disseminated CMV causing retinitis

MULTIDISCIPLINARY PLAN

The goals include rapid detection and treatment of opportunistic infections and neoplastic disease, management of signs and symptoms, and prevention of complications from treatment. The ultimate object for treatment of AIDS is reconstitution of the immune system. However, all attempts to correct the underlying immune defect, including bone marrow transplantation, have been unsuccessful.

Treatment for individual AIDS patients varies considerably and depends on the degree of immunosuppression and systemic involvement.

Surgery

Placement of a venous access device, such as a Hickman catheter, to facilitate frequent blood drawing, total parenteral nutrition, transfusions, and administration of chemotherapy

Surgical intervention for treatment of malignancies in certain cases

Medications

The development of antiretroviral therapy (i.e., drugs that suppress HIV infection itself rather than its complications) is an important development in the management of HIV disease. In addition, other medications are used to treat the opportunistic diseases associated with AIDS.

Antiretroviral therapy: Necleoside analogues

- Zidovudine (AZT), 500 to 600 mg PO daily in two or three divided doses
  - Adverse reactions: Anemia, neutropenia, nausea, malaise, headache, insomnia
- Didanosine (ddl), 125 to 300 mg PO bid
  - Adverse reactions: Peripheral neuropathy, pancreatitis, dry mouth, hepatitis
- Zalcitabine (ddC), 0.375 to 0.75 mg PO tid
  - Adverse reactions: Peripheral neuropathy, aphthous ulcers, hepatitis
- Stavudine (d4T), 20 to 40 mg PO bid
  - Adverse reactions: Peripheral neuropathy, hepatitis, pancreatitis
- Lamivudine (3TC), 150 mg PO bid
  - Adverse reactions: Rash, peripheral neuropathy

Antiretroviral therapy: Protease inhibitors

- Saquinavir (Invirase, hard gel capsule), 600 mg PO q8h; (Fortovase soft gel capsule) 1200 mg PO q8h
  - Adverse reactions: Rash, nausea and vomiting, diarrhea, abdominal pain, increased liver function tests (LFTs)
- Ritonavir, 600 mg PO bid or 400 mg PO bid in combination with other protease inhibitors
  - Adverse reactions: Asthenia, nausea and vomiting, circumoral paresthesias, peripheral paresthesias, altered taste
- Indinavir, 800 mg PO q8h
  - Adverse reactions: Nausea, vomiting, diarrhea, mild elevations in bilirubin, increased aspartate transaminase (AST) and alanine transaminase (ALT)
- Nelfinavir, 750 mg PO tid
  - Adverse reactions: Diarrhea, abdominal pain, flatulence, rash, nausea

Antiretroviral therapy: Nonnucleoside reverse transcriptase inhibitors (NNRTIs)

Nevirapine, 200 mg PO daily for 2 weeks and then 200 mg PO bid

Adverse reactions: Rash

Delaviridine, 400 mg PO q8h

Adverse reactions: Headache, fatigue, nausea, vomiting, diarrhea, increased LFTs, rash, pruritis

Kaposi's sarcoma

Limited cutaneous disease: Observation, intralesional vinblastine

Adverse reactions: Inflammation, pain at the injection site

Extensive or aggressive cutaneous disease: Systemic chemotherapy (e.g., liposomally encapsulated doxorubicin); interferon-α for patients with CD4 greater than 200 cells per microliter and no constitutional symptoms; radiation therapy to ameliorate edema.

Adverse reactions: Bone marrow suppression, peripheral neuritis, flulike syndrome

Visceral disease: Combination chemotherapy (e.g., daunorubicin, bleomycin, vinblastine)

Adverse reactions: Bone marrow suppression, cardiac toxicity, fever

Prophylaxis against PCP

Trimethoprim-sulfamethoxazole, 1 double-strength tablet, daily or three times weekly

Adverse reactions: Nausea, neutropenia, anemia, hepatitis, rash

Dapsone, 100 mg PO daily or 50 mg PO bid

Adverse reactions: Nausea, neutropenia, anemia, hepatitis, rash, methemoglobin

Treatment of PCP

Trimethoprim-sulfamethoxazole, 15 mg/kg/day PO or IV for 14 to 21 days

Adverse reactions: See above

Pentamidine, 3 to 4 mg/kg/day IV for 14 to 21 days

Adverse reactions: Hypotension, hypoglycemia, anemia, neutropenia, pancreatitis, hepatitis

Trimethoprim, 15 mg/kg/day PO with dapsone, 100 mg/day PO for 14 to 21 days

Adverse reactions: See above

Primaquine, 15 to 30 mg/day PO and clindamycin, 600 mg PO q8h for 14 to 21 days

Adverse reactions: Hemolytic anemia in glucose-6-phosphate dehydrogenase (G6PD) deficient patients, methemoglobinemia, neutropenia, colitis

Atovaquone, 750 mg PO tid with meals for 21 days

Adverse reactions: Rash, fever, headache, nausea, diarrhea, elevated liver enzyme levels

Candidiasis

Oral *Candida:* Clotrimazole troches, 10 mg dissolved orally five times daily, or nystatin 100,000 swish and swallow five times a day, or ketoconazole, 200 mg per day, or fluconazole, 100 mg per day.

Esophageal *Candida:* Fluconazole, 100 to 200 mg daily or ketaconazole, 200 mg bid for 14 to 21 days

Adverse reactions: Clotrimazole: nausea, vomiting; nystatin hypersensitivity; ketoconazole; hepatotoxicity, nausea, vomiting, diarrhea, abdominal pain, headache; fluconazole: nausea, vomiting, diarrhea, abdominal pain, rash, increased liver enzyme levels, headache

Cryptococcus

Amphotericin B, 0.6 mg/kg/day IV with or without flucytosine, 100 mg/kg/day PO in four divided doses for 2 weeks, followed by fluconazole, 400 mg PO daily for 4 weeks, then 200 mg PO daily

Adverse reactions: Amphotericin: nephrotoxicity, fever, chills, nausea, vomiting, anorexia, headache, joint pain

Cryptosporidium

Paromomycin, 1.5 to 2.25 g/day divided into 3 to 6 times per day for 10 to 14 days

Adverse reactions: Nausea, diarrhea, abdominal cramps

Cytomegalovirus

Ganciclovir: 5 mg/kg/IV bid for 10 days followed with 6 mg/kg daily five times a week or foscarnet 60 mg/kg IV q8h for 14 to 21 days followed with 90 to 120 mg/kg IV daily

Adverse reactions: Ganciclovir: granulocytopenia, thrombocytopenia, skin rash, phlebitis, fatigue, nervousness; foscarnet: nausea, diarrhea, anemia, thrombocytopenia, fever, acute renal failure, seizures, hypercalcemia/hypocalcemia, hypokalemia, hypomagnesemia, hyperphosphatemia/hypophosphatemia, genital ulcers

Herpes simplex

Acyclovir, 200 mg five times a day for 10 to 14 days

Adverse reactions: Arthralgias, diarrhea, headache, nausea, vomiting, dizziness

Mycobacterium avium-intracellulare complex

Azithromycin, 500 mg PO daily, or clarithromycin, 500 mg PO bid, with either ethambutol, 25 mg/kg PO daily, or rifabutin, 300 mg PO daily

Adverse reactions: Azithromycin: nausea, vomiting, abdominal discomfort, diarrhea; clarithromycin: headache, nausea, vomiting, abdominal discomfort, taste changes; ethambutol: headache, confusion, hyperuricemia, nausea, vomiting, abdominal pain; rifabutin: neutropenia, leukopenia, rash, discolored urine

Toxoplasmosis

Sulfadiazine, 1 to 1.5 g PO q6h, plus pyrimethamine, 50 to 100 mg PO, plus folinic acid, 10 mg PO; alternative treatment is clindamycin, 600 to 1200 mg IV or 450 to 600 mg PO q6h, pyrimethamine, 50 to 100 mg PO daily, plus folinic acid, 10 mg PO daily

Adverse reactions: Sulfadiazine: nausea, anorexia, diarrhea, headache, peripheral neuropathy, impaired folic acid absorption, leukopenia, thrombocytopenia, methemoglobinemia, crystalluria, photosensitivity; pyrimethamine megaloblastic anemia, thrombocytopenia, leukopenia, anorexia, vomiting, ataxia, tremors, increased liver enzymes, hypersensitivity reaction; folinic acid: allergic sensitization; clindamycin: rash, nausea, vomiting, diarrhea, pseudomembranous colitis

General Management

Chest physiotherapy, postural drainage, positioning, and oxygen therapy in conjunction with antimicrobial therapy if needed for pulmonary infections

Reduction of risk factors for infection: Malnutrition, exposure to infectious sources or invasive procedures such as contaminated equipment, frequent venipuncture, or Foley catheterization

Maintenance of adequate hydration, particularly during acute febrile episodes and with administration of nephrotoxic medications or with individuals who have chronic diarrhea

Maintenance of optimal nutritional status with high-calorie, high-protein diet, use of supplemental feedings such as Osmolite and Ensure if needed; total parenteral nutrition if necessary

Physical therapy for immobilized patients; regular program of rest and exercise for ambulatory patients

Administration of analgesics as needed to minimize discomfort and pain; assistance with alternative therapies and selection of distracting measures

Support services as appropriate: Social workers, clergy, psychologist, psychiatrist, clinical nurse specialist, support groups, involvement of significant others (partner and family) in care

NURSING CARE

Nursing Assessment

As noted earlier, the signs and symptoms of AIDS vary greatly. Clinical manifestations depend on the degree of immunosuppression and the opportunistic infections and neoplasms that develop secondarily. Nonspecific complaints may also occur and are usually exacerbated as the disease progresses. The multiple problems associated with AIDS are included in assessment.

Respiratory status: Rate, rhythm, and regularity of respirations; use of accessory muscles, adventitious breath sounds; cough, shortness of breath (SOB), cyanosis, wheezing, hemoptysis

Neurologic status: AIDS dementia complex

- Cognitive: Memory impairment, poor concentration, slowed thought processes, confusion
- Motor: Unsteady gait; weakness, especially lower extremities; decreased hand coordination; tremors; seizures
- Behavioral: Decreased animation, withdrawal, depression, emotional liability, psychosis
- Pain: Location, onset, duration, intensity, aggravating and relieving factors
- Other: paresthesias, paralysis, headache, nuchal rigidity, altered consciousness, coma

Ocular status: Cotton wool exudate, photophobia, blurred vision, papilledema, diplopia, proptosis, visual field deficits, blindness

Skin and mucous membrane integrity

- Oral/esophageal: White to gray-white patches, may appear hairy if dried; red to purple-brown lesions, macular, nodular, or plaquelike; gingivitis
- Perioral or lips: Corners of mouth, red fissures, crusted; hepatic vesicles
- Skin: Pink-purple to brown lesions, may appear as bright red subconjunctival mass, vesicles, diaphoresis, rash, dryness, delayed wound healing
- Lymphadenopathy: Nodes not fixed or hard

Gastrointestinal status: Loss of appetite; difficulty chewing or swallowing; retrosternal pain; nausea, vomiting; unintentional weight loss, 10% in 1 to 2 months; abdominal cramping/pain; diarrhea, at least two stools per day for 1 month, intractable; rectal: bleeding, fissures, itching, pain

Hematologic status: Splenomegaly, petechiae, purpura, easy bruising, epistaxis, gingival bleeding

Systemic status: Night sweats, severe fatigue, elevated temperature

Nutritional status: Height, weight, caloric intake, total protein, serum albumin

History: Hepatitis, sexually transmitted diseases, frequent viral illnesses, amebiasis, exposure to contaminated needles, IV drug use, recipient of blood or blood products (1978-1984), multiple sex partners, sexual preference, alcohol use, support system, work/productive activities, fatigue, stress factors, previous losses, coping patterns, self-concept, conceptualization of illness

Potential Complications

Septic shock, disseminated intravascular coagulation

Patient Problems/Nursing Diagnoses & Interventions

NIC Respiratory Management

Impaired gas exchange related to altered alveolocapillary membrane changes caused by *P. carinii*

- Maintain patent airway at all times.
- Encourage patient to report cough and progressive dyspnea on exertion.
- Obtain sputum specimens as needed *to determine appropriate antibiotic therapy.*
- Monitor results of pulmonary function studies.
- Provide preprocedural teaching before bronchoscopy, lung biopsy, CT scans, pulmonary function tests, and other procedures *to decrease anxiety and ensure informed consent.*
- Provide chest physiotherapy and postural drainage as indicated *to open airways and mobilize secretions.*
- Instruct patient in breathing exercises such as pursed-lip or diaphragmatic breathing and encourage patient to perform them *to decrease respiratory effort required.*
- Instruct patient in relaxation techniques *to prevent hyperventilation from anxiety caused by shortness of breath.*
- Instruct patient in energy conservation measures during activities of daily living (ADLs) *to decrease respiratory effort required.*
- Encourage patient to stop smoking *to increase resistance to respiratory infections.*
- In collaboration with physician, determine need for mechanical ventilation if respiratory status worsens or if patient becomes uncomfortable.

NIC Nutrition Support

Imbalanced nutrition: less than body requirements, related to protracted diarrhea, malabsorption, or anorexia

- Determine need for dietary changes, enteral feedings, and total parenteral nutrition.

- Provide vitamin supplements for deficiencies.
- In collaboration with physician, provide prescribed therapy such as antiemetic agents 30 to 60 minutes before meals *to alleviate nausea and aid patient's food tolerance.*
- Provide small, frequent, high-calorie, high-protein feedings *to help patient take in more calories, tolerate food, and regain and maintain weight.* Encourage patient to eat. Have favorite foods brought from home.
- Provide or encourage patient to perform frequent oral hygiene *to prevent oral infection and offer comfort.* Correct stomatitis.
- Monitor intake and output, daily weight, laboratory values, and skin integrity *to monitor nutritional status.*

NIC Elimination Management

Diarrhea related to chemotherapy or gastrointestinal infection

- Monitor vital signs for evidence of hypovolemia.
- Monitor for signs and symptoms associated with fluid and electrolyte imbalance *to determine appropriate replacement therapy.*
- Monitor perianal skin condition and provide skin care after every stool *to prevent breakdown;* provide application of skin barrier or fecal incontinence bag if necessary.
- In collaboration with physician, administer and assess effectiveness of prescribed antibiotics and antidiarrheal agents *to determine whether treatment is adequate or changes in regimen are needed.*

NIC Skin/Wound Management

Risk for impaired skin integrity related to malnutrition, Kaposi's sarcoma, frequent venipunctures, immobility, or side effects of chemotherapy

- Monitor lesions for signs of infection, desquamation, and other abnormal changes *to prevent further skin breakdown.*
- Provide or encourage patient to perform meticulous hygiene in involved areas *to maintain integrity.*
- For stomatitis: Perform regular oral care, avoid acidic oral fluids, provide topical viscous anesthetic, and serve bland foods at medium temperatures *to alleviate pain and discomfort.*
- Provide or encourage use of mild, hypoallergenic, nondrying soaps for skin cleansing and massage with oils and lotions.
- Soak feet and hands in warm water and apply isopropyl alcohol afterward *to prevent or treat fungal infections.*
- If Kaposi's lesions are present, assess response to chemotherapy; note changes in size, color, and configuration *to determine if therapy is adequate.*
- Avoid trauma to the skin. Do not allow more than 2-hour periods of immobilization. Assist with position change *to prevent pressure sores.*
- Encourage mobility within functional limits *to facilitate circulation to extremities and pressure points.*
- Implement pressure sore care as indicated.
- Use appropriate beds and appliances such as egg-crate mattresses *to allow pressure relief.*

NIC Physical Comfort Promotion

Chronic pain related to neoplasm, sites of infections, or peripheral neuropathy

- In collaboration with physician, provide appropriate antiinflammatory and analgesic agents. Assess effectiveness and note side effects *to determine whether therapy is relieving patient's pain.*
- Use alternative therapies such as massage and relaxation *to minimize patient's perception of pain.*

NIC Cognitive Therapy

Disturbed thought processes related to memory deficits, impaired judgment or orientation

- Reorient as needed. Identify self when interacting with patient.
- Use clear, direct terms, giving one direction at a time.
- Redirect misinterpretations of stimuli. Keep conversation reality centered.
- Provide items in environment *to maintain orientation.*
- Post schedule of activities. Label and keep familiar objects, such as pictures, nearby.
- Give positive reinforcement for participation in activities.
- Assist family in dealing with changes. Enlist family's aid in maintaining reality-based behavior.
- Ensure calm environment and quiet, undisturbed rest periods *to allow patient the opportunity to relax.*

NIC Activity and Exercise Management

Risk for activity intolerance related to weakness, fatigue, side effects of therapy, dyspnea, fever, malnutrition, or fluid and electrolyte imbalances

- Assist with ADLs as needed.
- Encourage regular exercise and rest as tolerated. Confer with physical or occupational therapist *to determine optimal approach.*
- Teach patient energy conservation measures and evaluate response to instruction.
- Monitor tolerance for visits and phone calls. Suggest limits as appropriate *to conserve energy and reduce environmental factors of intolerance.*
- In collaboration with physician, provide appropriate treatment for underlying causes of activity intolerance such as pain, infections, sleeplessness, or malnutrition. Assess effectiveness *to determine if treatment is adequate.*

NIC Psychologic Comfort Promotion

Body image disturbance related to weight loss, Kaposi's lesions, or side effects of chemotherapy

Anxiety related to diagnosis, poor prognosis, hospitalization, perception of unknown threat, knowledge deficit

- Provide atmosphere of individual acceptance.
- Provide opportunities for patient to express feelings.
- Avoid false reassurances but encourage hope. Inform patient of current research findings *to stimulate positive mental attitude.*

- Engage in honest, consistent communication with patient.
- Provide accurate information about AIDS and related treatment. Include information about diagnostic procedures *to ease fear of the unknown.*
- Increase simplicity, concreteness, and repetitions in communications *to ensure that patient hears, absorbs, and understands information.*
- Explain features of immediate environment *to allow patient self-control.*
- Keep door open and light on at night, visit frequently, and use touch as appropriate *to decrease feelings of isolation and loneliness.*
- Assist patient in identifying signs and symptoms of anxiety. Discuss coping measures with the patient, and encourage patient and significant others to use them.
- Encourage patient to participate in care as much as possible *to promote feelings of self-control.*
- Involve hospital and community resources *to assist patient and significant others where appropriate.*
- Encourage patient to use available resources *to decrease feelings of isolation.*
- Acknowledge change in body image but focus on identifying strengths and accomplishments. Praise appropriately and emphasize functions that have stabilized or improved.
- Have family and significant others bring in clothes, pajamas from home, and personal toileting items and suggest use of makeup for Kaposi's sarcoma lesions, especially facial lesions.
- Encourage patient to participate in AIDS support groups *to increase socialization and feelings of acceptance.*

NIC RISK MANAGEMENT

Risk for infection related to immune deficiency, disease process, effects of chemotherapy, malnutrition, frequent venipunctures, immobility, and environmental pathogens

Risk for injury related to visual, auditory, or tactile changes caused by CNS, HIV, or opportunistic infection

Risk for injury related to decreased circulating hemostatic mechanisms

- Observe strict aseptic technique for all invasive therapies and procedures.
- Initiate neutropenic precautions per hospital protocol whenever necessary (usually when absolute neutrophil count is less than 1000).
- Restrict contact with visitors and health-care providers who have infectious diseases.
- Maintain thorough hand washing before and after patient contact.
- Provide clean environment.
- Protect patient from physical injury.
- Limit environmental stress.
- Promote hygiene and oral care measures.
- Maintain optimal nutritional status and fluid intake.
- Maintain normal sleep and rest patterns.
- Maintain needed items, and approach patient within the patient's field of vision.
- Protect eyes using patches and eye medication to prevent injury.
- Maintain objects, furniture, and materials required for self-care or feeding in same place if patient's vision is severely diminished or absent *to allow patient control over activities.* Assist as needed.
- Provide alternate method of communication if hearing is impaired.
- For patient with mental confusion:
  - Reorient frequently and remind to call for assistance.
  - Check status every 30 minutes and as needed.
  - Restrain as appropriate.
- Implement safety precautions for patients with low platelet counts (less than 50,000) *to decrease risk of bleeding.*
  - Avoid using toothbrushes, use electric razors, do not take rectal temperatures, use side rails and fall precautions, avoid IM injections, avoid use of aspirin, and use stool softeners to prevent rectal bleeding.
- Instruct patient, family, and significant others on safety precautions.

PATIENT EDUCATION/CONTINUUM OF CARE PLAN

1. Explain to patient the disease process, methods to prevent transmission, and importance of obtaining current factual information.
2. Discuss with patient the need to follow safe sex guidelines.
3. Give patient information about and assist patient with methods to observe for signs and symptoms of opportunistic infections and cancer complications.
4. Discuss with patient ways to reduce risk of infection (see box on p. 1108):
   a. Maintenance of home environment
   b. Avoidance of persons with infections
   c. Prevention of injury to skin
   d. Promotion of personal hygiene measures
   e. Management of activity, rest, stress, and nutrition
   f. Avoidance of high-risk sex behaviors, use of recreational drugs, use of alcohol and tobacco products
   g. Importance to adhering to medication schedule
5. Provide patient with information about financial resources and community support: self-help groups, psychologic or psychiatric referrals, home aid, hot lines, or legal resources.
6. Discuss with patient the importance of regular follow-up care, the need to inform all health-care givers about diagnosis, and the need to refrain from donating blood.
7. Stress to patient the need to wear medical alert identification.
8. Demonstrate to patient and have patient and significant other caregiver demonstrate necessary procedures, such as total parenteral nutrition (TPN), IV, or aerosol medication administration.

EVALUATION/PATIENT OUTCOMES

Respiratory Management: Arterial blood gas levels are within normal range. There are no symptoms associated with respiratory distress.

BODY SUBSTANCE ISOLATION (BSI) PRECAUTIONS

All patients are considered infected.

In Hospital

1. The door to the patient's room need not be closed.
2. Gloves must be worn only if in *direct* contact with specimens, linen, and items or surfaces exposed to blood or body fluids. Gloves need *not* be worn if one is merely conversing with the patient or walking into the room.
3. A mask must be worn if secretions may be aerosolized onto the face during suctioning, oral hygiene, and other procedures. A mask should be worn if a health-care worker with a respiratory infection must enter the room of a severely immunosuppressed patient.
4. Protective eyewear should be worn if aerosolization of secretions or blood may contact the conjunctiva (as during suctioning or blood drawing).
5. A moisture-resistant gown must be worn if clothing is likely to become contaminated with blood or body fluids, as during bathing of the patient, linen changes, some specimen collections, or dressing changes.
6. Proper isolation technique must be used. Gown and gloves must be removed in the room when used.
7. Specimens must be bagged.
8. Special care in handling contaminated needles is essential. Never recap needles, because most needle-stick injuries occur this way. Needles must be disposed of in a puncture-resistant container, which should be sealed before being taken from the room.
9. Hand washing must be performed in the room before and after contact with the patient.
10. Contaminated nondisposable items must be cleaned with soap and water and bagged for autoclaving, wearing personal protective equipment. Items that cannot be autoclaved must be washed with soap and water, 10% bleach solution, or other solution recommended in the hospital procedure manual.
11. A private room may be given to patients unable to maintain scrupulous hygiene (those with intractable diarrhea, incontinence, or central nervous system infections leading to altered sensorium).
12. Usually no precautions are needed when handling food trays.
13. Disposable resuscitation equipment (Ambu-bags, airways, and so on) must be available at all times.
14. Postmortem handling of the body must include the use of personal protective equipment.

At Home

1. Disposable gloves must be worn by family members who come in direct contact with the patient's blood and body fluids.
2. Linen and clothing soiled with secretions or excretions should be washed separately with 10% bleach solution (¼ cup bleach to 1 gallon of water).
3. Dishes and eating utensils do not require separate handling but should be washed in hot, soapy water.
4. Dry waste contaminated with blood or body fluids must be disposed of in a separate container and bagged securely.
5. Any needles used for the administration of medication must be placed in an impervious container before disposal.
6. Meticulous hand washing before and after contact with the patient is essential.

Nutrition Support: Albumin and total protein levels are within normal limits. Weight is approaching normal for patient's height and build.

Elimination Management: Frequency and consistency of stools are within normal limits for patient. Frequency of stools is reduced, and soft consistency returns.

Skin/Wound Management: Dermatologic signs and symptoms are improved or controlled. Skin integrity is intact. Circulation to affected part is uncompromised.

Physical Comfort Promotion: Patient reports that pain is reduced to a tolerable level or resolved. Patient can now perform activities because pain is controlled.

Cognitive Therapy: Patient is oriented and communicates appropriately.

Activity and Exercise Management: Patient participates in ADLs. Patient uses energy conservation measures.

Psychologic Comfort Promotion: Patient verbalizes understanding of own anxiety and demonstrates methods to manage it.

Patient participates in own hygiene and grooming. Patient verbalizes realistic expectations. Patient acknowledges personal strengths.

Risk Management: New infectious processes are prevented or minimized. There is no WBC elevation or shift in differential. Sites of infection are stable or healing as evidenced through assessment.

Injury is prevented or minimized. There are no falls or other injuries. Patient requests assistance with movement when needed. Patient uses visual and hearing aids appropriately.

There are no ecchymoses, petechiae, hematomas, or signs of internal bleeding.

INFLAMMATORY DISEASES

Wegener's Granulomatosis

Wegener's granulomatosis is a multisystem disorder of unknown cause characterized by vasculitis of small arteries, arterioles, and capillaries; necrotizing granulomatous lesions of both upper and lower respiratory tract and glomerulonephritis.[10,21,25]

Wegner's granulomatosis occurs in a male-to-female ratio of 1:1. It may appear at any age, with a peak incidence in the fourth and fifth decades of life.

Wegener's granulomatosis usually develops over 4 to 12 months. The majority of the patients present with upper or lower respiratory tract symptoms or both. The lung is affected initially in 40% of the patients, and eventually 80% of patients will have lung involvement, including cough, dyspnea, and hemoptysis. The disease is usually diagnosed before the patient experiences renal involvement. The kidneys are affected in 75% of the patients with Wegener's granulomatosis. Additional symptoms associated with this syndrome include fever, malaise, and weight loss.

Early recognition and treatment of this disease is essential to avoid renal failure. Patients are usually treated with cyclophosphamide and prednisone or methotrexate and prednisone.

Pathophysiology

Any organ may become involved with granuloma formation and vasculitis. Although the immunopathogenesis remains an enigma, these manifestations suggest that delayed-type hypersensitivity or cell-mediated reactions may be involved. Immune complex deposition may also occur.

Histologic features include widespread necrotizing vasculitis of small arteries, venules, arterioles, and some capillaries, together with granuloma formation. Almost all patients have pulmonary involvement. Paranasal sinuses and the nasopharynx demonstrate granuloma formation. Pansinusitis may result in erosion of adjacent bones and septum perforation. Sinuses often become secondarily infected with bacteria. Saddle-nose deformity may be observed as well. Diffuse, bilateral, nodular lesions that tend to cavitate are found in lung tissue. Renal findings include necrotizing angiitis, focal glomerulonephritis with thrombosis of glomerular capillaries, crescent formation, glomerular and interstitial necrosis and granuloma formation, progressing to renal failure.

Diagnostic Studies and Findings

Serum test for cytoplasmic antinuclear antibodies (ANCA): A cytoplasmic pattern (cANCA) is observed and is caused by antibodies to serine proteinase

Biopsy of affected tissue: Granuloma formation; vasculitic lesions

Complete blood count: Mild anemia (normochromic, normocytic); lymphocytosis in presence of superimposed infection

Erythrocyte sedimentation rate: Elevated during active disease

Serum protein electrophoresis: Mild hypergammaglobulinemia (especially IgA)

Renal status: Proteinuria, hematuria, and granular or cellular casts

Differential diagnoses include other vasculitides, connective tissue diseases, infectious and noninfectious granulomatous diseases, pulmonary neoplasia, and lymphomatoid granulomatosis.

Multidisciplinary Plan

Medications

Antineoplastic agents: Used as immunosuppressant; cyclophosphamide (Cytoxan), 1-2 mg/kg/day PO; dosage adjusted to maintain total WBC at greater than 3000/mm^3, treatment continued 1 year after remission is achieved

Corticosteroids: Prednisone; may be added to above regimen if disease course is fulminant; 60 mg recommended as starting dose and should be continued until cyclophosphamide produces therapeutic effect (within 14 days); prednisone should then be tapered and eventually discontinued unless disease course accelerates.

In patients without life-threatening disease, may use methotrexate 20 mg/week with prednisone as the initial treatment

NURSING CARE

Nursing Assessment

Respiratory status: Respiratory rate and rhythm; auscultate lungs for presence of adventitious sounds; monitor blood gases; monitor chest roentgenograms; paranasal sinus pain; purulent or blood rhinorrhea; nasal mucosa ulceration; septal perforation; saddle-nose deformity; serous otitis media; epistaxis; chronic cough, pleurisy; dyspnea; chest pain; hemoptysis

Physical comfort: Perform a pain assessment including description, location and radiation, intensity, aggravating and relieving factors, previous treatments and effectiveness, and associated symptoms (e.g., weight changes, changes in mood, sleep disturbances)

Renal status: Blood urea nitrogen, serum creatinine, blood pressure, urinalysis results, presence of edema, hematuria, intake and output balance, and rapid weight gain; NOTE: Hypertension is usually not present

Skin integrity: Texture, lesions, temperature, moisture, color, vascularity, and vasculitis dermatitis

Ocular status: Degree of visual impairment; mild conjunctivitis; episcleritis; granulomatosis sclerouveitis; ciliary vessel vasculitis, proptosis

Potential Complications

Renal failure, pulmonary hemorrhage, bladder cancer or lymphoma (from cyclophosphamide treatment)

Patient Problems/Nursing Diagnoses & Interventions

NIC Respiratory Management

Impaired gas exchange related to alveolar capillary membrane changes

- Position patient for optimal chest excursion *to facilitate ventilation.*
- Encourage deep breathing and coughing *to move secretions.*
- Assist with ADLs *to conserve patient's energy.*
- In collaboration with physician, institute other interventions (such as oxygen therapy) for related conditions. Assess effectiveness.

NIC Physical Comfort Promotion

Acute pain related to sinusitis, headache, ocular inflammation, or dermatitis

- In collaboration with physician, administer appropriate analgesic and antiinflammatory agents. Assess effectiveness and note side effects.
- Use warm or cold compresses as patient desires *to increase eye or sinus comfort.*
- Maintain low lighting and noise level *to reduce stimuli.*
- Provide soothing baths and application of lotion *to promote increased skin comfort.*

NIC Tissue Perfusion Management

Ineffective renal tissue perfusion related to exchange problems

- Provide fluids of choice to amount allowed.
- Monitor dietary intake. Provide six small feedings *to meet caloric needs when food tolerance decreases.*
- In collaboration with physician, institute appropriate interventions related to treatment of glomerulonephritis (diet, fluids); assess effectiveness.

NIC Communication Enhancement

Disturbed sensory perception (visual) related to altered status of eyes caused by conjunctivitis, episcleritis, or proptosis

- Orient patient to location of personal items and furniture; maintain these items in the same position.
- Remind patient to call for assistance with ambulation or unfamiliar activities *to prevent accidents.*
- Arrange food and liquids so spillage does not occur.
- Institute safety precautions *to prevent falls.*

NIC Skin/Wound Management

Risk for impaired skin integrity related to altered circulation

- Provide or encourage patient to maintain meticulous hygiene in involved areas.
- Turn and reposition every 2 hours. Use devices to reduce pressure.

Patient Education/Continuum of Care Plan

1. Provide and discuss with patient information about cyclophosphamide and steroid therapy or methotrexate.
2. Stress to patient the importance of regular follow-up visits with physician and importance of regular eye examinations.
3. List significant changes for patient to report: visual impairment, hematuria, oliguria, pyuria, sinusitis, hemoptysis, dyspnea, and vasculitis.
4. Remind patient of the importance of medical alert identification.

Evaluation/Patient Outcomes

Respiratory Management: Lungs are clear on auscultation; no respiratory distress or sinusitis is observed.

Physical Comfort Promotion: Patient states comfort is increasing and pain is under control.

Tissue Perfusion Management: Patient's intake and output are balanced. Patient's vital signs and weight are stable. Patient takes diet and fluids allowed.

Communication Enhancement: Patient states vision has returned to normal. No presence of infection is observed. No injuries occurred.

Skin/Wound Management: Patient's skin color and turgor are good. No lesions are present.

Polyarteritis Nodosa (Periarteritis Nodosa)

Polyarteritis nodosa, a multisystem inflammatory disorder of unknown cause, is characterized by necrotizing inflammation of segments of small arteries.[20,22,31]

Polyarteritis nodosa occurs from infancy to old age and affects two to three men for every woman. The onset and clinical presentation of this disorder vary greatly, depending on the location of the arteries affected and the severity of the involvement. Widespread lesions may involve arteries of the heart, abdominal mesentery, kidneys, muscles, and vasa vasorum. Involvement of the central nervous system and pulmonary tissue is unusual.

Although the cause remains an enigma, some evidence suggests that this type of vasculitis may result from immune complex deposition in tissues following exposure to an infectious antigen. The findings of hepatitis B surface antigen (HBsAg) or hepatitis C surface antigen (HBeAg) in the sera of 30% to 50% of these patients further suggests that this may be true.

Drugs have been implicated as causes. Suspected agents include sulfonamides, penicillin, phenytoin, arsenicals, thiouracil, iodides, thiazides, and parenteral methamphetamine.

The prognosis of polyarteritis nodosa is guarded. Renal involvement denotes rapid disease progression. Death often occurs from renal failure, myocardial infarction, heart failure, infection, or gastrointestinal bleeding. However, with early diagnosis and treatment, the 5-year survival rate is 60 to 90%.

Pathophysiology

The inciting agent that leads to inflammation within the blood vessels is unknown. The inflammatory process is characterized by early infiltration of polymorphonuclear leukocytes. New lesions are often surrounded by older lesions characterized by cells that respond late in the inflammatory reaction—monocytes, lymphocytes, and plasma cells. This suggests that the inflammatory process involved in polyarteritis is chronic, although subjected to repeated insults, perhaps by antigen that is continuously available.

Chronic inflammation within the vessel walls leads to obliteration and ischemia of involved tissues as the lesion evolves.

Finally, the vessel is replaced by fibrous tissue. Blood supply to major organs and other structures diminishes. Tissue ischemia and infarction are the notable outcomes.

Diagnostic Studies and Findings

No specific laboratory tests exist for polyarteritis nodosa. The abnormalities observed depend largely on the organ systems affected. Differential diagnoses include systemic lupus erythematosus, trichinosis, heart failure, and infection.

White blood cell count: Elevated owing to neutrophilia

Erythrocyte sedimentation rate: Elevated during acute phase

Serum complement: Normal or elevated

Angiography: Detects characteristic aneurysms at bifurcation points of arteries in kidneys, mesentery, liver, pancreas, and so on (acute), or narrowing and thrombosis of involved arteries (late)

Tissue histologic studies: Necrotizing inflammation of segments of medium and small arteries; aneurysms at areas of arterial bifurcation; invasion of tissue by polymorphonuclear leukocytes and monocytes

Multidisciplinary Plan

Medications

Corticosteroids: Prednisone, 40-60 mg to start; titrate to effect and taper gradually

Antineoplastic agents: Used as immunosuppressants; use controversial (e.g., cyclophosphamide, 2 mg/kg/day) but has been successful in some cases, particularly when corticosteroid therapy has failed

NURSING CARE

Nursing Assessment

Renal status: Development of glomerulonephritis, renal failure, and hypertension; monitor blood urea nitrogen, creatinine, hemoglobin, hematocrit, blood pressure, urinalysis results, presence of edema and rapid weight gain, and symptoms associated with hypertension (headache, visual disturbances)

Gastrointestinal status: Abdominal pain, anorexia, nausea, vomiting, and findings compatible with gastrointestinal ulceration or hemorrhage, appendicitis, cholecystitis, hepatitis, or pancreatitis

Cardiovascular status: Myocardial and pleural changes, including changes in serial electrocardiograms (ECGs) and chest roentgenograms; auscultate chest for presence of a pericardial friction rub or adventitious breath sounds; monitor serial cardiac enzyme levels; monitor for signs and symptoms of congestive heart failure, pericarditis, myocardial infarction, asthma, bronchitis, and pneumonia

Skin integrity: Ecchymosis, purpura, ulcerations, gangrene, and vasculitic lesions; cutaneous nodules in extremities along the course of arteries; livedo reticularis

Musculoskeletal system status: Muscle weakness and myalgias

Physical comfort: Headache, testicular pain, and dysuria

Potential Complications

Renal failure, myocardial infarction, congestive heart failure, bowel infarction, gastrointestinal bleeding, seizures, pneumonia

Patient Problems/Nursing Diagnoses & Interventions

NIC Tissue Perfusion Management

Ineffective tissue perfusion related to interruption of flow or exchange problems

Renal, related to glomerulonephritis, glomerulosclerosis, or failure

Gastrointestinal, related to ulceration, hemorrhage, infarction, perforation, or cholecystitis

Cardiopulmonary, related to myocardial ischemia infarction, congestive heart failure, or bronchitis

Peripheral, related to muscle and subcutaneous changes

Cerebral, related to occlusion and stenosis

- Monitor intake and output.
- Provide restricted diet and fluids as allowed.
- Palpate abdomen *to detect areas of tenderness or pain.*
- Perform Hemoccult or guiaic test of stool *to check for gastrointestinal blood loss.*
- Report significant findings to physician.
- Monitor vital signs.
- Report significant findings to physician.
- Position patient for optimum chest excursion and comfort.
- Teach and assist patient with stress-reducing measures.
- Plan care with patient to schedule periods of rest. Assess response to increasing activities.
- Monitor lesions for signs of infection and other abnormal changes.
- Provide meticulous skin care using mild, nondrying hypoallergenic soaps for cleansing.
- In collaboration with physician, provide appropriate treatment for lesions as ordered. Assess effectiveness.
- Protect skin from further injury: use paper or cloth tape; apply dressings loosely; avoid venipunctures.
- Gently massage skin *to promote circulation to area.*
- Perform mental status examination *to assess level of consciousness and overall mentation.*
- Perform ophthalmic examination of fundus and disc *to determine presence of cerebral edema.*
- Provide for patient's safety *to prevent injury.*

NIC Immobility Management

Impaired physical mobility related to muscle weakness

- Provide progressive physical and occupational therapy. Encourage patient's participation.
- Provide for patient's safety *to prevent injury.*
- Assist with activities of daily living as needed.

NIC Physical Comfort Promotion

Acute and chronic pain related to tissue and organ ischemia resulting from vasculitis

- In collaboration with physician, provide appropriate analgesic agents. Assess effectiveness and note side effects.
- Teach and assist patient with alternative pain-relieving techniques: visual imagery or music therapy.
- Position patient for comfort, using pressure-reducing or support materials.

Patient Education/Continuum of Care Plan

1. Teach patient methods of self-assessment, and emphasize importance of reporting significant changes to physician. Teach patient to monitor patient's blood pressure, pulse, weight, proteinuria, edema, intake, and output. Instruct patient to report dyspnea, unexplained weight gain, proteinuria, oliguria, hematuria, hypertension, abnormal changes in the eyes, paresis, new pain, and melena.
2. Give patient information about medications, and stress importance of not stopping medications without physician's knowledge.
3. Outline diet for patient to follow. Arrange consultation for patient when needed.
4. Provide patient with information about needed rest, alternating with increasing activity as tolerance improves.
5. Teach patient alternative methods for pain relief: relaxation techniques, biofeedback, and guided imagery.
6. Teach patient to keep a log of disease course, treatments, and other disease-related information. Stress to patient the importance of keeping follow-up medical appointments.
7. Teach patient to carry medical identification (especially if patient is taking steroids).

Evaluation/Patient Outcomes

Tissue Perfusion Management: Renal function is maintained. Patient's intake and output are balanced. Weight and blood pressure are within patient's normal limits; patient follows restricted dietary and fluid plan.

- Gastrointestinal function is maintained. Nausea and vomiting are absent; no presence of bleeding is noted; normal bowel pattern is achieved.
- Cardiopulmonary status is within normal limits. Patient's vital signs are stable; no ectopic rhythms are present; heart and breath sounds are normal.
- Peripheral circulation is normal. Patient's skin is warm and dry, with good turgor. No lesions or discoloration are present.
- Central nervous system is intact. Patient is alert and oriented, without complaints of headache or visual disturbances.

Immobility Management: Patient performs ADLs without limitation.

Physical Comfort Promotion: Patient's body posture and face are relaxed; patient states that comfort is achieved.

Giant Cell Arteritis (Temporal Arteritis)

Giant cell arteritis is an inflammatory disorder of unknown etiology that affects large and medium-sized arteries, especially those branching from the proximal aorta that supply the neck and the extracranial structure of the head and arms.[23,40]

Giant cell arteritis affects persons of both sexes usually older than 50 years of age. It is twice as common in women as in men. This disease is rarely seen in blacks. Any artery or the aorta may be involved, but the diagnosis is often made through biopsy of the temporal artery. Patients initially show nonspecific systemic signs, including fever. Morning headaches are frequent. Other clinical findings are related to the arteries involved.

Although the etiology is unknown, the disease may have some basis in immunologic dysfunction similar to that of other vasculitides such as polyarteritis nodosa. Cellular and humoral mechanisms reactive against elastic arterial tissue may play a role.

The prognosis for giant cell arteritis is good, particularly when major vessels are uninvolved. The disease tends to be self-limited in 2 to 5 years, but the threat of blindness makes treatment imperative. Patients respond dramatically to corticosteroid therapy with remission of clinical manifestations and lowering of the erythrocyte sedimentation rate, which can be serially monitored for recurrence of inflammatory episodes.

Pathophysiology

Giant cell arteritis is distinguishable from other vasculitides because small vessels such as arterioles and capillaries are not involved. Histologic characteristics include the accumulation of histiocytes, epithelioid cells, multinucleated giant cells, lymphocytes, and plasma cells in the interna and media adjacent to the internal elastic lamina of medium-sized arteries. The elastic lamina is fragmented and may be absent in some areas. In large arteries and the aorta the media tends to be inflamed, with fragmentation of the elastic fibers. The intima is thickened more than would be expected from age alone. The lesions are spotty and do not involve long stretches of arteries. Thrombosis may occur at inflammation sites.

Diagnostic Studies and Findings

Giant cell arteritis should be suspected in any elderly person who has a fever of unknown origin and an elevated erythrocyte sedimentation rate. It is often associated with polymyalgia rheumatica.

Erythrocyte sedimentation rate: Greater than 50 mm/hr
Temporal artery biopsy: Positive; demonstrates lymphocyte infiltration and giant cells in vessel wall
Muscle enzyme: Normal
Electromyography: Normal
Muscle biopsy: Normal
Complete blood count: Anemia, normochromic, normocytic
γ-Globulin: Diffuse increased, α-globulin increased

MULTIDISCIPLINARY PLAN

Medications

Corticosteroids: Prednisone, 60 mg PO tapered for 2 to 4 weeks until symptoms abate and erythrocyte sedimentation rate returns to normal; maintenance dose 10 mg or less PO qd until disease is controlled clinically; alternate-day therapy not successful; can be discontinued eventually in most patients; monitor for side effects associated with steroid therapy

NURSING CARE

NURSING ASSESSMENT

Cerebrovascular perfusion status: Visual acuity, mental status, level of consciousness, and motor function; monitor vital signs; temporal artery for warmth, redness, tenderness, or diffuse headache; diplopia and vision loss (acute or insidious); transient ischemic attacks, cranial nerve palsies, and signs and symptoms of stroke

Cardiovascular status: Myocardial ischemia and infarction; monitor for angina; monitor serial electrocardiograms; ascultate heart for rate, rhythm and regularity of pulse; monitor cardiac enzyme levels; and monitor vital signs

POTENTIAL COMPLICATIONS

Blindness, aortic aneurysm

PATIENT PROBLEMS/NURSING DIAGNOSES & INTERVENTIONS

NIC TISSUE PERFUSION MANAGEMENT

Ineffective tissue perfusion related to interruption of arterial flow

Cerebral
- Position for comfort. Usually the head is elevated 30 to 60 degrees on bed rest.
- Assess effectiveness of administered analgesics.
- Encourage and assist with ambulation as needed.

Cardiopulmonary
- Position patient for comfort *to ease respirations and chest pain.*
- Assist patient with learning stress-reducing activities.

NIC COMMUNICATION ENHANCEMENT

Disturbed sensory perception: visual related to altered status of the ophthalmic and retinal arteries
- Familiarize patient with immediate surroundings.
- Maintain safety precautions *to prevent injuries.*
- Encourage self-care. Assist with only those activities that patient is unable to perform because of other incapacities.

PATIENT EDUCATION/CONTINUUM OF CARE PLAN

1. Provide patient with information about steroid therapy. Stress to patient the importance of not stopping medications without notifying physician.
2. List signs and symptoms that patient must report to physician concerning recurrence of disease process, especially any eye changes.
3. Discuss with patient the self-limiting aspect of the disease process.
4. Stress to patient the need to wear medical alert identification, to inform all health-care workers about treatment, and to keep appointments for follow-up care.

EVALUATION/PATIENT OUTCOMES

Tissue Perfusion Management: Patient has no redness, warmth, or tenderness over temporal artery site; patient reports no headache, is alert, and is oriented, with good motor activity and coordination. Patient reports no chest pain; electrocardiogram (ECG) shows no ectopy; vital signs are stable.

Communication Enhancement: Patient reports no blurring of vision, diplopia, or diminished vision; patient uses safety precautions in presence of diminished vision.

POLYMYALGIA RHEUMATICA

Polymyalgia rheumatica is a well-defined inflammatory disorder of the proximal muscles that usually affects women more than men older than 50 years of age. It is a self-limiting condition.[11,19,29]

Polymyalgia rheumatica is accompanied by a highly elevated erythrocyte sedimentation rate and is often diagnosed on the basis of a rapid clinical response to corticosteroid therapy. The onset may be acute or insidious and is associated with pain and morning stiffness in the back and neck, as well as in the pelvic and shoulder girdles.

PATHOPHYSIOLOGY

The origin and pathogenesis of polymyalgia rheumatica are unknown. Although elevation of the erythrocyte sedimentation rate is indicative of an inflammatory process, and despite the severe pain associated with the muscle involvement, findings of muscle examinations are normal.

DIAGNOSTIC STUDIES AND FINDINGS

Erythrocyte sedimentation rate: Elevated (often greater than 100 mm/hr)
Red blood cells (RBCs): Anemia (normochromic, normocytic)
Corticosteroid challenge: Rapid, dramatic response
Creatine phosphokinase: Normal, to distinguish from polymyositis
Muscle biopsy: Normal; to distinguish from polymyositis
Serum protein electrophoresis: Normal; to distinguish from myeloma
Rheumatoid factor: Normal; along with absence of synovitis, to distinguish from arthritis

MULTIDISCIPLINARY PLAN

The goal of the treatment plan is to induce a remission of the disease using low-dose corticosteroid therapy.

Medications

Corticosteroids: Prednisone, 10 mg/day, or equivalent low-dose corticosteroid; although some patients are able to discontinue drug after several months, most require prolonged maintenance therapy with small doses

Nonsteroidal antiinflammatory drugs: May be added to control mild discomfort that may occur while corticosteroids are being tapered

NURSING CARE

NURSING ASSESSMENT

Musculoskeletal system status: Bilateral pain and stiffness to pectoral and pelvic girdles, increasing at night and in the early morning; muscle weakness

Physical comfort: Perform a pain assessment including description, location and radiation, intensity, aggravating and relieving factors, previous treatments and effectiveness, and associated symptoms (e.g., weight changes, changes in mood, sleep disturbances); evaluate for fever and fatigue

POTENTIAL COMPLICATIONS

None

PATIENT PROBLEMS/NURSING DIAGNOSES & INTERVENTIONS

NIC PHYSICAL COMFORT PROMOTION

Chronic pain related to proximal muscle involvement

- Administer hot or cold thermal therapy to affected muscles.
- Perform limited range-of-motion exercises as tolerated *to combat stiffness and prevent atrophy from immobilization.*

PATIENT EDUCATION/CONTINUUM OF CARE PLAN

1. Give patient information about prednisone; discuss its importance and side effects, as well as the need to continue medication.
2. Teach patient that temporal (giant cell) arteritis may be a complication of the disease. Alert patient to associated symptoms to report, including headache, scalp tenderness, and any vision changes.
3. Teach patient the importance of medical alert identification.

EVALUATION/PATIENT OUTCOMES

Physical Comfort Promotion: Patient reports increasing ability to use shoulder and pelvic muscles without pain. Erythrocyte sedimentation rate is within normal limits.

SARCOIDOSIS

Sarcoidosis is a multisystem granulomatous disorder of unknown cause.[4,26,34]

In the United States approximately 34 cases of sarcoidosis per 100,000 persons are diagnosed each year. Cases are equally distributed between both sexes. Although all races and age groups may be affected, sarcoidosis occurs most commonly in adults, especially blacks younger than 40 years of age.

The prognosis of sarcoidosis varies depending on the degree of systemic involvement and the intensity of steroid therapy. Sarcoidosis may be staged according to international standards that are based on chest roentgenograms of patients with pulmonary involvement, the major clinical finding (Table 16-4).

The disease is fatal in about 5% of patients. Current research focuses on determining the immunologic pathogenesis of the disease through detailed studies of immune function of cells derived from sarcoid tissue.

PATHOPHYSIOLOGY

Recent data suggest that the pathophysiology of sarcoidosis involves a process in which macrophages initiate cellular responses to some unknown antigen. The macrophage releases various factors (e.g., interleukin 1) that cause accumulation and proliferation of helper T cells. In addition, B lymphocytes are stimulated to produce immunoglobulins, fibroblasts proliferate, and suppressor T cells predominate. These immunologic responses result in the formation of granulomas in affected organs, depression of delayed-type hypersensitivity reactions to common antigens, and an increased synthesis of immunoglobulins.

DIAGNOSTIC STUDIES AND FINDINGS

Differential diagnoses include tuberculosis, mediastinal lymphoma, and other granulomatous lung diseases.

T cells: Decreased circulating cells

Bronchoalveolar lavage fluid: Increased macrophages and helper T cells

Table 16-4 Staging, Prognosis, and Treatment of Sarcoidosis

Stage	Chest Roentgenogram	Prognosis	Corticosteroid Therapy
1	Bilateral hilar adenopathy	Resolves in 60% of cases	None
2	Bilateral hilar adenopathy with parenchymal pulmonary infiltration	Resolves in 46% of cases	Yes, to decrease pulmonary fibrosis and relieve symptoms
3	Advanced parenchymal pulmonary infiltration with nodular densities	Resolves in 12% of cases	Same as stage 2

Delayed-type hypersensitivity skin test: Absence of response (anergy)
Chest roentgenogram: Varies from prominent hilar lymphadenopathy to diffuse pulmonary infiltrates with fibrosis
Serum protein electrophoresis: Polyclonal hypergammaglobulinemia: usually increased IgG, but IgA and IgM may also be elevated
Kviem test: Intradermally injected saracoid tissue suspension; positive in 60% to 80% of cases
Tissue biopsy: Noncaseating granulomas
C-reactive protein: Elevated in associated acute arthritis
Erythrocyte sedimentation rate: Elevated in associated acute arthritis

MULTIDISCIPLINARY PLAN

Medications

Corticosteroids: Prednisone in doses adjusted to relieve symptoms and reverse fibrosis of pulmonary tissue
Optic agents: Methylcellulose eyedrops and assorted ophthalmic ointments to treat ocular manifestations
Antidysrhythmic agents: For ventricular ectopy
Treatment of arthritis manifestations varies depending on their severity; salicylates used first, followed by nonsteroidal antiinflammatory agents, and finally corticosteroids, including intraarticular injections

General Management

Chest physiotherapy, breathing exercises, postural drainage, and oxygen therapy as necessary for prophylaxis or as treatment for chronic pulmonary disease
Serial sinus and chest roentgenograms and pulmonary function studies as necessary to follow disease course and determine adequacy of treatment
See Chapter 6

NURSING CARE

NURSING ASSESSMENT

Respiratory status: Respiratory rate, rhythm, and quality; hemoptysis, cough, adventitious breath sounds, or dyspnea; decreased vital capacity and signs and symptoms of infection
Skin and mucous membrane integrity: Small skin nodules over face, neck, and extremities; vitiligo; alopecia; erythema nodosum
Ocular status: Blurred vision; lacrimation; ocular pain; conjunctival infection; uveitis; Sjögren's syndrome; iritis
Reticuloendothelial system status: Lymphadenopathy; bilateral hilar adenopathy; mediastinal or peripheral lymphadenopathy; splenomegaly with or without anemia, leukopenia, and thrombocytopenia
Cardiovascular status: Signs and symptoms associated with decreased cardiac output: hypotension, dyspnea, edema, jugular venous distention, and rales; dysrhythmias, including bundle-branch block or ventricular ectopy

POTENTIAL COMPLICATIONS

Congestive heart failure, ventricular arrhythmias, pulmonary failure, pericardial effusion

PATIENT PROBLEMS/NURSING DIAGNOSES & INTERVENTIONS

NIC RESPIRATORY MANAGEMENT

Impaired gas exchange related to pulmonary fibrosis, infection, restrictive disease, or parenchymal lesions

- Monitor results of pulmonary function studies.
- Obtain sputum specimens for culture *to determine presence of secondary pulmonary infection(s).*
- Reinforce teaching related to proper positioning, body mechanics, and breathing exercises.
- Institute chest physiotherapy.

NIC TISSUE PERFUSION MANAGEMENT

Decreased cardiac output related to dysrhythmias or congestive heart failure

- Monitor electrocardiograms for rate, rhythm, and ectopy.
- Report significant electrocardiographic irregularities and other abnormal assessment data to physician.
- Position for increased comfort, usually with head elevated.
- Adjust patient's activity *to reduce oxygen demands and provide rest periods.*
- Assess response to oxygen therapy and other interventions.

NIC PHYSICAL COMFORT PROMOTION

Chronic pain related to ocular discomfort, arthralgias

- In collaboration with physician, institute appropriate interventions and administer analgesics based on underlying cause of pain. Assess effectiveness, and note side effects.

PATIENT EDUCATION/CONTINUUM OF CARE PLAN

1. Give information to patient about, and discuss importance of, prescribed medications.
2. Provide information related to system involvement: assessment and reporting of signs and symptoms.
3. Teach the importance of chest physiotherapy.
4. Teach signs and symptoms of infection.
5. Teach about the avoidance of risk factors associated with infection.
6. Teach the principles of good nutrition.
7. Teach the importance of medical alert identification.

EVALUATION/PATIENT OUTCOMES

Respiratory Management: Patient's chest roentgenogram shows clear or improved lung fields. Patient's respiratory pattern and breath sounds are within normal limits.

Tissue Perfusion Management: Patient's ECG shows no ectopy. Vital signs are within patient's normal limits.

Physical Comfort Promotion: Patient reports no eye, muscle, or chest discomfort. Patient's position and face are relaxed.

REITER'S SYNDROME

Reiter's syndrome is a relatively common, chronic, multisystem inflammatory disease characterized by the development of seronegative arthropathy that affects the lower extremities and may be associated with urethritis, conjunctivitis, or mucocutaneous disease involving the penis, oral mucosa, palms, and soles.[1,3,6]

Reiter's syndrome has been a subject of worldwide research since the discovery of its link with HLA-B27 in 80% of patients in 1973. This finding suggested a genetic predisposition. A search for the environmental factor or factors that act as inciting agents ensued. Although such an agent remains elusive, current data suggest that enteric infection may play a role. Microbes that have been implicated include *Shigella flexneri, Shigella dysenteriae,* and *Yersinia enterocolitica.* Venereal infections with *Chlamydia* and *Mycoplasma* have also been associated with Reiter's syndrome.

Based on this evidence, it is theorized that patients with a specific genetic background (HLA-B27) may develop Reiter's syndrome following infestation by a variety of microbes. Research continues with the goals of improving its recognition, defining etiologic factors, and ultimately finding a cure.

The incidence of Reiter's syndrome is difficult to assess for a variety of reasons. Current research indicates that this disease occurs primarily in white males throughout the world. Although it may be detected at any age, it is usually diagnosed in the third decade. Reiter's syndrome may be the most common inflammatory arthropathy detected in young men. The pathogenesis of Reiter's syndrome is unknown.

DIAGNOSTIC STUDIES AND FINDINGS

Differential diagnoses include infective arthritis, psoriatic arthropathy, and ankylosing spondylitis.

History: Recent history of dysentery or venereal disease combined with inflammatory monarthropathy or oligoarthropathy, urethritis, cervicitis, and ocular and cutaneous inflammatory changes.

Roentgenograms of musculoskeletal system: Fluffy periosteal proliferation of lower extremity joints

Leukocytosis: Mild

Erythrocyte sedimentation rate: Variable from 1 to 130 mm/hr

HLA typing: HLA-B27 (this test is costly and unnecessary and is usually performed only as an academic endeavor)

MULTIDISCIPLINARY PLAN

The goals of the treatment plan include management of signs and symptoms and early detection of disabling complications. This disease has no cure, and current treatment is empiric and inadequate.

Medications

Nonsteroidal antiinflammatory agents: To treat synovitis and arthralgias; any agent may be tried; one clinician reports success with indomethacin (Indocin), 25-50 mg tid, and phenylbutazone (Butazolidin), 100 mg tid or qid

Antibiotics: Tetracycline may be given for 3 months to patients with Reiter's syndrome associated with *Chlamydia trachomatis*

Corticosteroids:

Methylprednisolone (Medrol), 40-80 mg intralesionally for arthropathy, tendinitis, and so on.

Steroid eyedrops or subconjunctival ointments for conjunctivitis

Analgesics and nonsteroidal antiinflammatory agents: To reduce pain associated with arthritis and ocular inflammation

Optic agents: Methylcellulose eyedrops for symptomatic relief of ocular discomfort

General Management

Physical therapy for arthritis complications

NURSING CARE

NURSING ASSESSMENT

Musculoskeletal system status: Arthritis, particularly of weight-bearing joints; tendinitis, especially of Achilles tendon; plantar fasciitis; back pain such as sacroiliitis and ankylosing spondylitis; costochondritis, often manifested as pleuritic chest pain; dactylitis; degree of physical immobility

Genitourinary system status: Urethritis; cervicitis; cystitis; balanitis; dysuria, pyuria, hematuria, and fever

Physical comfort: Pain assessment, including description, location and radiation, intensity, aggravating and relieving factors, previous treatments and effectiveness and associated symptoms; fatigue and malaise

Ocular integrity status: Conjunctivitis; uveitis

Skin integrity: Keratoderma blennorrhagica (thick keratotic lesions of palms and soles); balanitis circinata: painless, superficial lesions of coronal margins of prepuce and adjacent glands; nails: subungual, corny material that accumulates under and may lift nail plate, which becomes yellow and thickened

Cardiovascular status: Electrocardiogram for increased PR interval, heart block, ST segment changes, and abnormal Q waves, palpitations; transient murmurs; pericardial rub; and aortic regurgitation

POTENTIAL COMPLICATIONS

Pericarditis; aortic regurgitation

PATIENT PROBLEMS/NURSING DIAGNOSES & INTERVENTIONS

NIC IMMOBILITY MANAGEMENT

Impaired physical mobility related to arthritis

- In collaboration with physician, provide nonsteroidal antiinflammatory agents. Assess effectiveness.
- Encourage patient to rest joints during periods of acute inflammation. Otherwise, encourage program of regular exercise, including range-of-motion exercises, as tolerated. Confer with physical or occupational therapist *to determine other beneficial interventions.*
- Provide assistive devices as needed.

NIC Physical Comfort Promotion

Acute and chronic pain related to inflammatory conditions of eye, genitourinary tract, and joints

- In collaboration with physician, provide analgesic agents as ordered. Assess effectiveness and note side effects.
- In collaboration with physician, institute other appropriate measures relative to system involved. Assess effectiveness.

NIC Skin/Wound Management

Risk for impaired skin integrity related to mucocutaneous manifestations

- Monitor lesions for signs of infection, dissemination, and other abnormal changes.
- Provide or encourage patient to perform meticulous hand and foot care with special attention to nail integrity.
- Provide mild, nondrying, hypoallergenic soaps for skin cleaning and encourage their use.
- Assess effectiveness of treatment of lesions.

NIC Elimination Management

Impaired urinary elimination related to urethritis or cystitis

- Monitor intake and output.
- In collaboration with physician, administer appropriate antiinfective agents. Assess effectiveness and note side effects.

NIC Tissue Perfusion Management

Risk for decreased cardiac output related to carditis

- In collaboration with physician, institute appropriate measures based on assessment. Assess effectiveness of specific interventions.

Patient Education/Continuum of Care Plan

1. Teach importance of reporting symptoms associated with significant complications of Reiter's syndrome: spondylitis, uveitis, and cardiopulmonary disease.
2. Teach that use of a condom during sexual activity will limit exposure to venereal disease, which could exacerbate Reiter's syndrome.
3. Teach importance of physician follow-up to monitor disease course. Physician should also be consulted for management of acute episodes.
4. Teach facts about and importance of prescribed medications.
5. Teach importance of keeping a log of disease course, treatments, and other disease-related information.
6. Teach importance of using medical alert identification.

Evaluation/Patient Outcomes

Immobility Management: Patient performs ADLs without difficulty. Patient uses assistive devices as necessary to maintain mobility. Patient maintains daily exercise program.

Physical Comfort Promotion: Patient has relaxed body posture and facial expression; patient verbalizes no eye or other pain.

Skin/Wound Management: Patient's skin is warm, with good color and turgor; patient performs daily skin care and maintains nails.

Elimination Management: Patient's intake and output are balanced; patient reports no frequency, burning, or urgency.

Tissue Perfusion Management: Patient's vital signs are stable, and ECG pattern exhibits normal sinus rhythm.

Sjögren's Syndrome

Sjögren's syndrome is a chronic autoimmune disorder of unknown etiology that affects primarily the lacrimal and salivary glands.[13,32,37,38]

The major symptoms of Sjögren's syndrome are keratoconjunctivitis and xerostomia, which result from decreased lacrimal and salivary gland secretion, respectively. The syndrome is often associated with other connective tissue diseases, especially rheumatoid arthritis, systemic lupus erythematosus, and progressive systemic sclerosis (scleroderma). Raynaud's phenomenon is manifested by 20% of patients with Sjögren's syndrome. Middle-age women with a mean age of 50 years constitute 90% of Sjögren's syndrome patients. All races may be affected. There is evidence that sex hormones play an etiologic role in the disease, and research in this area continues.

Pathophysiology

Biopsy specimens from glandular lesions demonstrate infiltration by lymphocytes, plasma cells, and macrophages, which replace secretory acinar tissue. Anti–salivary duct antibodies have been observed. The factors precipitating such autodestruction of host tissue are unknown. Destruction of tissue results in decreased secretion by involved glands. In addition, dryness of the nose, pharynx, and tracheobronchial tree may occur.

Diagnostic Studies and Findings

Differential diagnoses include Felty's syndrome, Raynaud's phenomenon, chronic thyroiditis, hepatomegaly, chronic active hepatitis, gastric achlorhydria, acute pancreatitis, adult celiac disease, polymyositis, drug-induced xerostomia, irradiation xerostomia, diabetes, sarcoidosis, salivary duct stones, and mumps.

Salivary scintigraphy: Decreased uptake, concentration, and excretion of intravenous ^{99m}Tc pertechnetate by major salivary glands; measured by means of sequential scintiphotographic technique

Sialography: Dilations and other changes such as atrophy within intrasalivary duct system

Labial salivary gland biopsy: Infiltration of tissue by lymphocytes, plasma cells, and macrophages; replacement of acinar tissue

Schirmer's test: Decreased tear production; less than 15 mm of filter strip wetted

Complete blood count: Mild anemia; leukopenia

Erythrocyte sedimentation rate: Elevated
Serum protein electrophoresis: Hypergammaglobulinemia
Rheumatoid factor: Elevated (90%)
Antinuclear antibody: Greater than 1:80 (70%) anti–salivary duct antibodies, thyroid antibodies, gastric-parietal cell autoantibodies

MULTIDISCIPLINARY PLAN

The goals of the treatment plan are to provide palliative measures and to prevent complications of this chronic disorder.

Medications

Corticosteroids: Prednisone; dose titrated for relief of *severe* symptoms; usually administered only late in course of disease when symptoms are unrelieved by supportive approaches
Artificial saliva preparations
Optic agents: Artificial tears (0.5% methylcellulose eyedrops) as needed

General Management

Avoidance of sour or sweetened drinks or candies; mouth rinses of 1% methylcellulose; oral hygiene with frequent brushing, flossing, and fluoride rinses; regular dental examinations; regular conjunctival cultures to detect ocular infections

NURSING CARE

NURSING ASSESSMENT

Oral cavity status: Xerostomia; dental caries (multiple); oral candidiasis; dysphagia; difficulty chewing; changes in phonation, adherence of food to buccal mucosa; hoarseness; fissures and ulcerations of tongue, buccal mucosa, and lips; frequent ingestion of liquids with meals
Ocular status: Conjunctivitis; foreign body sensation; "grittiness"; burning; accumulation of thick, ropy strands at inner canthus; decreased tearing; redness; photosensitivity; eye fatigue; pruritus; filmy sensation that interferes with vision; (late) corneal ulceration, vascularization, and opacification
Vaginal status: Dry membranes; dyspareunia
Respiratory status: Nasal mucosal dryness; epistaxis; bronchitis; pneumonia

Potential Complications
Pleuritis; renal tubular acidosis; pancreatitis

PATIENT PROBLEMS/NURSING DIAGNOSES & INTERVENTIONS

NIC SKIN/WOUND MANAGEMENT

Impaired tissue integrity related to irritants

Eyes
- Administer 0.5% methylcellulose eyedrops as needed *to maintain moisture at conjunctival surface.* Observe effect.
- Obtain regular cultures of eye *to determine presence of infection.*
- Stress importance of wearing protective glasses, especially out-of-doors, *to prevent tissue injury.*
- Instruct in use and care of contact lenses, if ordered, *for protection.*

Mouth and nose
- Provide items for frequent oral hygiene: for brushing, for flossing, and for rinsing.
- Stress importance of regular mouth care and use of artificial saliva.
- Provide fluids and sugarless gum or candies *to stimulate salivary secretion.*

Vagina
- Avoid use of tampons during menstrual period.
- Use water-soluble lubricant to relieve dyspareunia.

PATIENT EDUCATION/CONTINUUM OF CARE PLAN

1. Provide information and discuss with patient the use of artificial tears or saliva and vaginal lubricants.
2. Stress to patient the need for routine oral hygiene throughout the day.
3. List and demonstrate for patient the method of assessing for signs and symptoms of increasing severity of condition.
4. Discuss with patient the need for regular follow-up care.
5. Discuss with patient the use of protective eye covering and the use of nighttime humidification.

EVALUATION/PATIENT OUTCOMES

Skin/Wound Management: Patient's eyes are clear. Patient uses medication appropriately. Patient reports increased eye comfort. Patient's oral cavity is pink, moist, and clean. Patient breathes nasally without discomfort. Patient reports no dyspareunia.

AMYLOIDOSIS

Amyloidosis is a syndrome characterized by deposition of amyloid (proteinaceous material) in tissues.[17,24]

Amyloidosis occurs as an acquired or hereditary disorder and may be a primary disease or be associated with a variety of other illnesses. Although its etiology is unknown, at least two observations suggest that amyloidosis represents immunologic dysfunction: the presence of immunoglobulin proteins in amyloid deposits and the syndrome's increased incidence in inflammatory, infectious, and neoplastic diseases.

The term *amyloid,* which means starchlike, is a misnomer. The syndrome is actually characterized by the diffuse deposition of insoluble proteinaceous material in the extracellular matrix of one or more organs. The accumulation of amyloid encroaches on parenchymal tissues and compromises organ function. Clinical manifestations of amyloidosis vary widely and depend on the organs involved and the severity with which they are affected. Specific immunotherapy to treat the underlying cause of organ failure is lacking, so treatment is restricted to management of signs and symptoms. For this reason amyloidosis is usually fatal. Renal failure and cardiac diseases are the most frequent causes of death.

Types of Generalized Amyloidosis

Primary generalized amyloidosis (PGA) occurs in the absence of associated diseases, although most patients exhibit some type of plasma cell dyscrasia. PGA accounts for 50% to 60% of all cases of amyloidosis. Deposits of amyloid are found in mesenchymal tissues of the heart, tongue, carpal tunnel, gastrointestinal tract, peripheral nerves, skin, joints, and skeletal muscle. Although this type of amyloidosis may occur as early as the second decade, the mean age at diagnosis is approximately 60 years. Men are affected more often than women, and whites more than nonwhites. Virtually all patients with classic PGA demonstrate a monoclonal immunoglobulin in their serum or urine and bone marrow plasmacytosis.

Multiple myeloma–associated amyloidosis (MMA) accounts for approximately 30% of cases. In roughly 15% of myeloma patients, clinical findings are consistent with a diagnosis of amyloidosis. Serum and urine paraproteins are found. The clinical symptoms, age at diagnosis, and sexual predilection are similar to PGA. Amyloidosis contributes to early morbidity in myeloma disease.

Secondary generalized amyloidosis (SGA), detected in 10% of the patients, occurs as a result of a variety of long-term or poorly controlled inflammatory, infectious, or neoplastic diseases. Adult and juvenile rheumatoid arthritis may be the most frequent predisposing factor. SGA is also reported in other inflammatory conditions, including ankylosing spondylitis, Reiter's syndrome, psoriatic arthritis, chronic rheumatic heart disease, dermatomyositis, scleroderma, Behçet's disease, and systemic lupus erythematosus.

Neoplastic diseases associated with the development of amyloidosis include gastrointestinal, pulmonary, and genitourinary carcinomas, non-Hodgkin's lymphomas, malignant melanomas, and most frequently, hypernephroma and Hodgkin's disease. Chronic, systemic infections are a significant factor associated with worldwide distribution. Such infectious diatheses include tuberculosis, pyelonephritis, osteomyelitis, inflammatory bowel disease, and chronically infected burns.

In addition to the above types, amyloidosis is also described as a hereditary illness detected with increased frequency in various countries and some well-defined areas of the United States. Neuropathic, nephropathic, and cardiopathic syndromes have been described.

Pathophysiology

Only limited insight has been gained into the pathogenesis of this syndrome. Histologic staining techniques and electron microscopy have provided some clues. Fibers formed from laterally aggregated protein fibrils have been detected in amyloid deposits. Some of these fibrils are apparently derived from free immunoglobulin light chains. In addition, amyloid deposits are further constructed of globular glycoprotein subunits (pentagonal, or "P," components) absorbed from the serum into the fibrillar units.

An explanation for the deposition of the proteinaceous substance has not yet been found. Whatever the reason, accumulation of amyloid in extracellular spaces results in pressure atrophy and eventual necrosis and destruction of underlying tissue. Organ dysfunction and failure are responsible for clinical manifestations. Amyloid deposition occurs in the following areas:

Articular: Glenohumeral junction; synovial villi
Neurologic: Dural blood vessels; autonomic ganglia; spinal nerve roots; peripheral nerves
Renal: Glomeruli; arteriolar walls; tubular basement membranes
Cardiac: All layers of the cardiac walls (predominantly myocardium); conduction tissue; intramural coronary arterioles
Pulmonary (any area): Upper nasal passages; vocal cords; tracheobronchial submucosa; parenchyma
Gastrointestinal (any area): Gingiva; tongue; oropharyngeal muscles; liver; voluntary muscles of upper third of esophagus; diffuse esophageal infiltrates; small bowel
Integumentary: Face; upper trunk

Diagnostic Studies and Findings

Tissue biopsy: Apple-green birefringence of Congo red-stained tissue specimens under polarization microscopy; tissue from organ suspected to be infiltrated with amyloid preferred, but rectal biopsy findings positive in approximately 80% of cases of generalized amyloidosis
Serum and urine electrophoresis: Paraproteins detected in presence of associated plasma cell dyscrasia
Bone marrow aspiration and biopsy: Plasmacytosis in presence of associated multiple myeloma

Multidisciplinary Plan

The goals of therapy in amyloidosis are to prevent further deposition of amyloid material and to promote or accelerate its resorption.

Surgery

Serial biopsies to determine regression of amyloid deposition

Medications

Antineoplastic agents: May be used to reduce the serum concentration of amyloid precursor light chains if underlying B cell dyscrasia is present

General Management

Plasmapheresis may interrupt dissemination of amyloid precursor light chains
Family and patient counseling to assist in coping with fatal illness
Supportive approaches for complications
- For congestive heart failure: Conservative management; avoid use of digitalis unless closely monitored in hospital setting (usually cardiac amyloid is unresponsive to treatment with digitalis)
- For neuropathic hypotension: Elastic stockings
- For malabsorption syndromes: Broad-spectrum antibiotics
- For macroglossia: Supplemental gastrostomy feeding; tracheostomy for upper airway obstruction
- For respiratory tract amyloidosis: Bronchoscopy with curettage of amyloid deposits
- For renal failure: Dialysis

NURSING CARE

NURSING ASSESSMENT

Respiratory status: Rate, rhythm, and quality of respirations; auscultate lungs and note adventitious breath sounds; note the use of accessory muscles of respiration; for respiratory distress, bronchiectasis, airway obstruction, and wheezing

Cardiovascular status: Signs and symptoms of decreased cardiac output, including hypotension, dyspnea, edema, jugular venous distention, rales and pulse irregularities; restrictive cardiomyopathy on low-voltage electrocardiogram; chest pain, signs and symptoms of myocardial infarction, and conduction disturbances

Renal status: Renal insufficiency, including level of blood urea nitrogen and creatinine, creatinine clearance, blood pressure, urinalysis, presence of edema and rapid weight gain, and intake and output; for proteinuria and idiopathic nephrotic syndrome

Physical comfort: Perform a pain assessment, including description, location and radiation, intensity, aggravating and relieving factors, previous treatments and effectiveness, and associated symptoms (e.g., weight changes, changes in mood, sleep disturbances); fever and fatigue

Skin integrity: Skin color, temperature, and the presence of lesions (i.e., waxy, indurated papules and purpura, skin thickening, "orange-peel" skin)

Gastrointestinal status: Dysphagia, impaired esophageal peristalsis; gastric accumulation, motility disturbances, hemorrhage, obstruction, achlorhydria, and vitamin B_{12} deficiency; signs and symptoms of small bowel impairment, including diarrhea, constipation, malabsorption, hemorrhage, protein-losing enteropathy, perforation and ischemic necrosis, and hepatomegaly

POTENTIAL COMPLICATIONS

Myocardial infarction; airway obstruction; restrictive cardiomyopathy; renal failure; gastrointestinal hemorrhage

PATIENT PROBLEMS/NURSING DIAGNOSES & INTERVENTIONS

NIC RESPIRATORY MANAGEMENT

Impaired gas exchange related to amyloid deposition in pulmonary tissue

- Maintain open airway at all times.
- In collaboration with physician, institute appropriate interventions, relative to type and severity of pulmonary compromise. Assess effectiveness.
- Be prepared to institute measures for respiratory arrest as symptoms increase.

NIC TISSUE PERFUSION MANAGEMENT

Decreased cardiac output related to amyloid deposition in cardiac structures and subsequent myopathy and ischemia

Ineffective renal tissue perfusion related to amyloid deposition in kidneys

- Monitor electrocardiogram for rate, rhythm, and ectopy. Note in particular presence of ischemia, infarction, and conduction abnormalities.
- Report significant electrocardiographic changes and other abnormal assessment data to physician.
- In collaboration with physician, institute appropriate interventions (such as oxygenation) relative to type and severity of cardiac compromise. Assess effectiveness and note side effects of medications.
- Adjust patient's activity and provide rest periods *to reduce oxygen demands.*
- Report significant abnormal findings to physician.
- Institute dialysis in event of renal failure.

NIC NUTRITION SUPPORT

Imbalanced nutrition: less than body requirements, related to amyloid deposition in gastrointestinal tract

- Assess degree of malnutrition: note presence of hypoalbuminemia, hypoproteinemia, negative nitrogen balance, protein and calorie deficit, and weight loss.
- Assist physician in determining underlying cause of malnutrition, such as malabsorption, dysphagia, and impaired esophageal peristalsis.
- Provide and encourage patient to maintain nutritionally balanced diet. Determine need for parenteral nutrition *to maintain nutritional balance.*
- Weigh patient weekly *to detect weight loss.*

NIC PHYSICAL COMFORT PROMOTION

Chronic pain related to arthritis, cardiac ischemia, or gastrointestinal distress

- In collaboration with physician, administer appropriate analgesics. Assess effectiveness and note side effects.
- Position for maximum comfort.

NIC SKIN/WOUND MANAGEMENT

Risk for impaired skin integrity related to amyloid deposition in dermis

- Protect skin from injury or infection.

PATIENT EDUCATION/CONTINUUM OF CARE PLAN

1. Teach patient facts about the importance of managing signs and symptoms and frequent physician follow-up.
2. Teach patient care and methods of self-assessment relative to systems involved.
3. Refer patient and family for counseling to assist in coping with this potentially fatal illness.
4. Teach patient the importance of medical alert identification.

EVALUATION/PATIENT OUTCOMES

Respiratory Management: Patient's rate, rhythm, and pattern of respirations are within normal limits. Patient's breath sounds are normal.

Tissue Perfusion Management: Vital signs are within patient's normal limits. ECG reveals no ectopy. Patient's intake and output are balanced. Patient weight is stable. No edema is reported.

Nutrition Support: Patient takes diet and fluids without difficulty. Patient has no nausea, diarrhea, or constipation.

Physical Comfort Promotion: Patient reports increased comfort level. Patient's body posture and face are relaxed.

Skin/Wound Management: Patient's skin is warm and dry, with good turgor. Lesions are present but are without induration.

Systemic Lupus Erythematosus

Systemic lupus erythematosus (SLE) is a chronic, multisystem, autoimmune disorder characterized chiefly by antibody formation directed against autologous tissues and serum factors.[18]

SLE has no cure. Although its origin remains elusive, increasing evidence suggest that multiple factors—genetic, hormonal, immunologic, and possibly viral—may play a role in the onset and perpetuation of the disease.

In the United States approximately 500,000 persons have this disease. Although virtually anyone may be affected, SLE has a predilection for women of childbearing age. Nine times more women than men are affected. Three times as many blacks as whites have SLE. Late-onset (sixth decade or later) SLE accounts for 12% of cases.

SLE was once considered a fatal illness of young women, but 85% of patients now survive longer than 15 years after diagnosis. This improved prognosis reflects advances in the diagnosis and treatment of the disease. Patients with central nervous system involvement and renal failure have poorer prognoses. Complications, especially infections, associated with the long-term use of steroids used to control the disease also significantly contribute to early mortality.

Despite the significant improvements in the treatment of SLE, it can be a serious and potentially life-threatening illness. Because of this, as well as the recognition that SLE is a prototype of autoimmune disease, it has been a subject of worldwide research.

The cause of SLE remains unknown, but several etiologic factors have been proposed. It is unlikely that any single factor is the cause. Most researchers conclude that SLE is probably caused by an unknown inciting agent coupled with a genetic "lupus diathesis."

Drugs

During the past 30 years many drugs have been implicated in the development of a reversible lupuslike syndrome that includes elevated antinuclear antibody (ANA) titers and well-defined clinical features. Perhaps certain drugs alter tissues to such a degree as to make them act as immunogenic stimuli. Both hydralazine and procainamide can bind to and alter the physical properties of DNA, perhaps enhancing its immunogenicity. There may also be some correlation between an individual's ability to metabolize certain drugs and a predisposition for SLE.

The following outline lists drugs thought to induce lupuslike syndromes. Once these drugs are discontinued, clinical manifestations disappear:

Definite: Hydralazine; procainamide; isoniazid; chlorpromazine; methyldopa; quinidine

Possible: Phenytoin; captopril; cimetidine; propranolol; penicillamine; propylthiouracil; practolol; acebutolol; lithium carbonate

Unlikely: Griseofulvin; phenylbutazone; oral contraceptives; gold salts; allopurinol; reserpine; penicillin

Pathophysiology

The pathogenesis of SLE is characterized by the development of antibodies directed against "self" tissues, cells, serum proteins, or all of these. The presence of autoantibodies reflects a loss of tolerance, or autoimmunity, and constitutes a serious defect in the regulatory components of the immune system. The T lymphocytes are the primary group of white cells responsible for control of the immune response. In SLE the number of T suppressor cells is decreased. In addition, T suppressor cell activity is inhibited. Polyclonal hypergammaglobulinemia occurs as a result, because B cells proliferate unrestrained by normal suppressor mechanisms.

In most SLE patients, antibodies develop directed against native, double-stranded DNA, as well as other antigens. The combination of autoantibodies and autoantigens, or immune complexes, may circulate or be deposited within capillary plexuses, near basement membranes, and in other tissues such as glomeruli, renal interstitia, serosal (pleural, pericardial, or peritoneal) membranes, the choroid plexus, and the vasculature of the lungs. Immune complex formation triggers the inflammatory response, which is the primary mechanism by which tissue destruction and subsequent clinical disease occur. Chronic deposition of immune complexes leads to chronic destruction of the host tissue. *The intensity and location of the inflammatory process dictate the severity of the clinical response and organ involvement, respectively.*

Diagnostic Studies and Findings

A variety of autoantibodies may be detected by serologic assay. Some of these are listed in Table 16-5.

ANA: Positive in titers greater than 1:80

Table 16-5 Autoantibodies in Systemic Lupus Erythematosus

Autoantibody	Clinical Manifestations
Antinuclear Anti–double-stranded DNA (ds-DNA)	Nephritis; vasculitis; pleuritis; pericarditis; synovitis; peritonitis
Antineuronal	Cerebritis; organic brain syndromes; peripheral neuropathies
Anticoagulant	Coagulopathies
Anti-RBC	Anemia
Anti-WBC	Leukopenia; lymphopenia; immunosuppression; infection
Antiplatelet	Thrombocytopenia
Anti–basement membrane	Dermatitis; nephritis

Anti–double-stranded DNA antibody (ds-DNA): Positive in titers greater than 1:80

Rapid plasma reagin (RPR) test: Falsely positive

Fluorescent treponemal antibody absorption (FTA-ABS): Negative

Complement (C3 and C4): Decreased during flares, indicative of acute inflammation; otherwise within normal limits

Skin or muscle biopsy: Evidence of inflammation with or without tissue necrosis; deposits of immunoglobulin and complement at dermal-epidermal junctions

Kidney biopsy: Focal or diffuse proliferative nephritis; also membranous or interstitial disease

Complete blood count: Pancytopenia or selective deficits; lymphopenia during flare

C-reactive protein: Elevated during flares, indicative of acute inflammatory state

Erythrocyte sedimentation rate: Elevated during flares, indicative of acute inflammatory state

Coombs' test: Positive in presence of hemolytic anemia because of autoantibody production against erythrocytes

Coagulation profile: Prolonged prothrombin time and partial thromboplastin time if circulating anticoagulant antibodies are present

Rheumatoid factor (RF) (anti-IgG antibody): Usually positive in titer greater than 1:40

Circulating immune complexes: Present during flares

Urinalysis: Abnormal casts and sediment associated with renal damage

Antibodies to single-stranded DNA (ss-DNA): May be present in ANA-negative lupus and associated with congenital heart block in lupus patients' neonates

The 1982 revised classification of SLE is based on the 11 criteria defined below. For the purpose of identifying patients in clinical studies, a person should be said to have SLE if any 4 or more of the 11 criteria are present, serially or simultaneously, during any interval of observation.

Malar rash: Fixed erythema, flat or raised, over malar eminences, tending to spare nasolabial folds

Discoid rash: Erythematous raised patches with adherent keratotic scaling and follicular plugging; atrophic scarring may occur in older lesions

Photosensitivity: Skin rash as result of unusual reaction to sunlight, based on patient history or physician's observation

Oral ulcers: Oral or nasopharyngeal ulceration, usually painless, observed by physician

Arthritis: Nonerosive arthritis involving two or more peripheral joints, characterized by tenderness, swelling, or effusion

Serositis: Pleuritis—convincing history of pleuritic pain or rub heard by a physician or evidence of pleural effusion—*or* pericarditis—documented by electrocardiogram, rub, or evidence of pericardial effusion

Renal disorder: Persistent proteinuria greater than 0.5 g/day or greater than 3+ if quantitation not performed *or* cellular casts—may be red cell, hemoglobin, granular, tubular, or mixed

Neurologic disorder: Seizures in absence of offending drugs or known metabolic derangements (such as uremia, ketoacidosis, or electrolyte imbalance) *or* psychosis in absence of offending drugs or known metabolic derangements

Hematologic disorder: Hemolytic anemia with reticulocytosis *or* leukopenia—less than 4000/mm^3 total on two or more occasions—*or* lymphopenia—less than 1500/mm^3 on two or more occasions—*or* thrombocytopenia—less than 100,000/mm^3 in absence of offending drugs

Immunologic disorder: Positive LE cell preparation *or* anti-DNA—antibody to native DNA in abnormal titer—*or* anti-Sm—presence of antibody to Sm nuclear antigen—*or* false-positive serologic test for syphilis known to be positive for at least 6 months and confirmed by *Treponema pallidum* immobilization or fluorescent treponemal antibody absorption test

Antinuclear antibody: Abnormal titer of antinuclear antibody by immunofluorescence or equivalent assay at any point in time and in absence of drugs known to be associated with "drug-induced lupus" syndrome

MULTIDISCIPLINARY PLAN

The goals of the treatment plan include management of signs and symptoms, induction of remission, prevention of untoward complications of therapy, and early recognition of "flares."

Surgery

Joint replacement may be indicated if chronic synovitis and pain have been problematic.

Medications

Nonsteroidal antiinflammatory agents: Acetylsalicylic acid (aspirin) may be given in a daily oral dose of 3 to 6 g for adults. Indomethacin (Indocin) is given orally, 25 to 50 mg three or four times a day for adults. The patient should be monitored for evidence of gastrointestinal bleeding.

Antiinfective agents: Hydroxychloroquine (Plaquenil), 200 to 400 mg orally twice a day for adults, or chloroquine, 250 mg orally daily to twice weekly for adults, is given. The patient should be started on therapy slowly. Gastrointestinal intolerance may occur when full doses are used initially. The beneficial effect of these drugs is usually demonstrated within a month or two. Nonsteroidal antiinflammatory agents should be continued until this time. Retinal toxicity may occur at higher doses, so patients should receive pretreatment and annual ophthalmic examinations.

Corticosteroids: Prednisone (Orasone, Deltasone, Meticorten) is given orally in low doses (15 mg/day), moderate doses (16 to 40 mg/day), or high doses (41 to 120 mg/day). The amounts listed above may be given in divided doses to provide more sustained antiinflammatory action. Alternate-day dosage may be instituted as maintenance therapy.

Methylprednisolone (Solu-Medrol) is given intravenously for acute crisis in a dose of up to 1000 mg/day for adults. Central nervous system involvement (psychosis, grand mal seizures) requires 35 to 40 mg methylprednisolone intravenously every 6 hours. The dose should be doubled if no response is attained in 48 hours.

Topical steroids include hydrocortisone (Cortaid), fluocinonide (Lidex), betamethasone dipropionate (Diprosone), flurandrenolide (Cordran), betamethasone valerate (Valisone), and fluocinolone acetonide (Synalar).

Antineoplastic agents: Azathioprine (Imuran) is given in an oral dosage of 150 mg/day to 25 mg thrice weekly for adults. The patient should be monitored for pancytopenia, gastrointestinal distress, skin rash, hepatic toxicity, and hyperuricemia. Cyclophosphamide (Cytoxan) is given at 150 mg/day to 25 mg thrice weekly for adults. The patient should be monitored for pancytopenia, cardiotoxicity, gastrointestinal distress, hemorrhagic cystitits, and hyperuricemia. Chlorambucil (Leukeran) is given orally as 10 mg/day to 2 mg thrice weekly for adults. The patient should be monitored for pancytopenia, exfoliative dermatitis, and hyperuricemia.

Other medications: A variety of antiinfective agents may be used to treat infections associated with SLE or immunosuppressive therapy. Treatment of renal disease includes the use of antihypertensive agents and aluminum derivatives. Raynaud's phenomenon may respond to biofeedback or sympatholytic drugs such as guanethidine, nifedipine, reserpine, and tolazoline. Intraarticular steroid injections may prove useful in the alleviation of synovitis and joint pain.

General Management

Plasmapheresis (see p. 1148) has been shown to decrease circulating immune complexes and autoantibodies. To circumvent a rebound effect, a brief course of cytotoxic medication, often cyclophosphamide intravenously, may be administered after the plasmapheresis series.

Peritoneal dialysis or hemodialysis may be indicated in the treatment of renal insufficiency or failure.

A balanced diet with salt restriction should be followed.

Table 16-6 Frequency of Clinical Symptoms in Systemic Lupus Erythematosus

Symptom	Percent
Fever	83
Weight loss	62
Arthritis, arthralgia	90
Skin	74
Butterfly rash	42
Photosensitivity	30
Mucous membrane lesions	12
Alopecia	27
Raynaud's phenomenon	17
Purpura	15
Urticaria	8
Renal	53
Nephrosis	18
Gastrointestinal	38
Pulmonary	47
Pleurisy	45
Effusion	24
Pneumonia	29
Cardiac	46
Pericarditis	27
Murmurs	23
Electrocardiographic changes	39
Lymphadenopathy	46
Splenomegaly	15
Hepatomegaly	25
Central nervous system	32
Psychosis	15
Convulsions	15
Cytoid bodies	11

From Schur.[35]

NURSING CARE

Nursing Assessment (Table 16-6)

Respiratory status: Respiratory rate and rhythm; auscultate lungs for the presence of adventitious breath sounds; dyspnea; respiratory distress; pain with inspiration

Cardiovascular status: Irregularities of apical pulse, murmurs; tachycardia; bradycardia

Neurologic status: Orientation, judgment, intellectual functioning; headaches; depression; seizures; psychoses

Renal status: Hypertension, weight gain, anorexia, and nausea; urinalysis results, including blood urea nitrogen, serum creatinine, hemoglobin, hematocrit, creatinine clearance, and urine and serum electrolytes; monitor for hematuria, cellular casts, proteinuria, and azotemia

Musculoskeletal system status: Degree of limitation; joint integrity; presence of pain, deformity, and muscular atrophy

Potential Complications

Cardiomegaly, renal failure, pleurisy, interstitial fibrosis, pericarditis, sepsis

Patient Problems/Nursing Diagnoses & Interventions

Because of the multiple systemic effects of SLE, nursing care must be structured to cope with the patient's individual requirements. Therefore nursing care often varies greatly, ranging, for example, from minor application of topical steroids to aggressive pulmonary toilet for an intubated patient. The following is meant to provide a generalized perspective. Refer to other chapters for a detailed approach to systems involved.

NIC Respiratory Management

Ineffective breathing pattern related to fatigue and pulmonary involvement

- Maintain bed rest with head elevated during acute phase *to conserve oxygen.*
- Provide chest physiotherapy and postural drainage *to treat or prevent pneumonia.*
- Teach deep breathing exercises and encourage patient to perform exercises as often as needed *to increase pulmonary function.*
- Monitor chest roentgenograms and sputum culture *to detect pneumonia.*

NIC Tissue Perfusion Management

Decreased cardiac output related to alterations in mechanical/electrical factors caused by disease

Ineffective cerebral and renal tissue perfusion related to exchange problems

- Auscultate for pericardial friction rub. Monitor for subjective distress: syncope, palpitations, and dyspnea.
- Monitor electrocardiographic results.
- Monitor for presence of peripheral edema.
- Assess patient's ability to cope.
- Assess for suicidal ideation.
- Work with patient to identify resources for support and coping mechanisms that have proved helpful in past.
- Provide emotional support and attempt to limit patient's fears through frequent explanations of tests and procedures.
- Encourage visits by family and friends.
- If orientation is a problem in the hospital, provide familiar articles from home. Provide clock and calendar *to orient patient to time.*
- Maintain patient's safety.
- Encourage participation in local chapter of Lupus Foundation.
- Monitor specific gravity *to determine ability to concentrate urine.*
- Modify diet as indicated *to prevent azotemia.*
- Monitor for symptoms of electrolyte and intake and output imbalance.

NIC IMMOBILITY MANAGEMENT

Impaired physical mobility related to general weakness and joint involvement

- Perform range-of-motion exercises as tolerated *to maintain joint integrity.*
- In collaboration with physician, administer analgesics according to appropriate and regular time schedules. Assess patient's response.
- Administer thermal therapy to muscles and joints *for pain control.*
- Confer with physical or occupational therapist *to determine other beneficial interventions.*

NIC SKIN/WOUND MANAGEMENT

Impaired skin integrity related to integumentary manifestations

- Monitor skin lesions for signs of infection.
- In collaboration with physician, administer topical steroidal or antiinfective creams and ointments as indicated. Assess response.
- Provide hypoallergenic, nondrying soaps and mild shampoos.
- Encourage use of sunscreen products if patient is photosensitive.

NIC NUTRITION SUPPORT

Imbalanced nutrition: less than body requirements, related to anorexia, electrolyte imbalance, or chemotherapy side effects

- Encourage balanced diet with supplements if indicated.
- Encourage weight reduction diet for patients who have gained weight while taking steroids.
- Low-sodium, high-potassium diet may be indicated for patients receiving steroids.
- Encourage intake of vitamin supplements for patients who are pregnant or dieting.

NIC RISK MANAGEMENT

Risk for infection related to altered immune system or steroid therapy

- Monitor temperature and vital signs for evidence of fever or sepsis.
- Maintain body hygiene.
- Promote pulmonary toilet: breathing exercises, postural drainage, and chest physical therapy.
- Maintain normal sleep and rest patterns.
- Protect patient from physical injury.
- Provide clean environment.
- Restrict contact with family and health-care providers who have infectious diseases.
- Wash hands thoroughly before and after contact with patient.

PATIENT EDUCATION/CONTINUUM OF CARE PLAN

1. Teach patient the side effects of medications.
2. Teach patient the importance of avoiding contact with persons who may expose patient to infection.
3. Teach patient the importance of frequent assessment for signs and symptoms associated with infection. While steroids are being given, many of these findings are masked, so the slightest change in temperature, wound characteristics, or other parameters should be reported immediately.
4. Teach patient the importance of skin care. Tell patient to avoid dryness and use of irritant soaps, shampoos, chemical coloring, or permanent waving of hair. Encourage use of hypoallergenic makeup and wearing wig if there is hair loss. Teach photosensitive patients to avoid sun exposure: limit outdoor activities between 10 AM and 4 PM; wear long sleeves, pants, and hats; and use sunscreen products with a sun protection factor of at least 15.
5. Teach patient methods to cope with arthralgias and myalgias: range-of-motion exercises, balance between rest and exercise, use of analgesics and nonsteroidal antiinflammatory agents, joint supports at night, contacting Arthritis Foundation.
6. Teach patient the importance of regular follow-up by physician and need for blood tests.
7. Teach patient the importance of recognizing factors that lead to a flare: psychologic and physical stress, use of drugs that induce a lupuslike syndrome, abrupt cessation of medications, and photosensitivity.
8. Teach patient warning signs of a flare: fever, chills, excessive fatigue and malaise, nausea, muscle weakness, increased joint pain, chest pain, oliguria, and dysuria—essentially, exacerbation of an old symptom or development of a new one.

9. Teach patient the importance of maintaining a balanced diet; include restrictions associated with medications.
10. Teach family planning. Pregnancy is usually allowed during remissions with close monitoring. Barrier contraceptives such as a condom or diaphragm are recommended.
11. Teach patient the importance of keeping a log of disease course, treatments, and other disease-related information.
12. Teach patient the importance of obtaining up-to-date information about SLE.
13. Teach patient to carry medical alert identification.
14. Direct patient to available resources.

EVALUATION/PATIENT OUTCOMES

Respiratory Management: Patient's respiratory pattern and breath sounds are within normal limits. Patient performs respiratory toilet.

Tissue Perfusion Management: Patient's vital signs are normal. No ectopy is noted on ECG. Patient is alert and oriented; judgment, mental acuity, and behavior are within patient's normal parameters.

Patient's intake and output are balanced. Findings of kidney function studies are within normal limits.

Immobility Management: Patient returns to baseline ability to perform ADLs. Patient reports decreased fatigue and no discomfort with movement.

Skin/Wound Management: Patient's skin is warm and dry, with good turgor and color.

Nutrition Support: Patient maintains balanced diet and takes supplements as indicated.

Risk Management: Patient shows no signs or symptoms associated with infection.

ALLERGIC DISORDERS

ATOPIC DISEASE

The term *allergy* was initially used to describe "altered reactivity" and has evolved over the years to refer broadly to any immunologic reaction to a foreign substance that produces detrimental consequences to the body. It is often used interchangeably with atopy.

Atopy is an abnormal immune response mediated by IgE antibody produced against substances that normally occur in the environment. Atopic diseases include anaphylaxis, allergic rhinoconjunctivitis, allergic asthma, atopic dermatitis, gastrointestinal allergy, and occasionally urticaria or angioedema. Allergy to a drug or an insect bite or sting can cause anaphylaxis or hives by an immunologic IgE mechanism in persons with or without other allergic symptoms (atopic or nonatopic).

Atopy appears in approximately 20% of the population and is thought to be inherited through genes linked to HLA antigen haplotypes. The expression of atopy has been linked to multiple factors, including hormonal changes, antigen exposure, and concurrent illness. Expression of symptoms can occur at any time during life and varies from mild to life threatening in severity.

PATHOPHYSIOLOGY

The genetic defect is thought to be in T suppressor cell modulation, which allows increased or unmodulated production of IgE antibody.

The antigens precipitating the IgE response are restricted to either complete protein antigens with specific carrier and antigenic determinants or low-molecular-weight substances that function as haptens by combining with serum or tissue proteins to form a complex. Antigens may be inhaled (tree, grass, or weed pollens; mold spores; dust; animal proteins), ingested (food, drugs), injected (venom, drug), or touched.

On initial exposure the antigen (allergen) is processed by a macrophage and then presented to the appropriately responsive T lymphocyte. Interaction then occurs with B lymphocytes, which, when stimulated, develop into mature plasma cells and secrete the antigen-specific IgE antibody.

Only a very small amount of IgE antibody circulates in the serum. Most IgE is found fixed to the surface of mast cells (fixed in tissue) or basophils (circulating). There may be 5000 to 500,000 IgE molecules on a single mast cell. A mast cell may have a large variety of antigen-specific IgE antibodies on its surface.

Mast cells and basophils contain several potent chemical mediators of inflammation, including histamine, arachidonic acid metabolites such as prostaglandins and leukotrienes C, D, or S, eosinophil chemotactic factors of anaphylaxis (ECF-A), and platelet activating factor (PAF). Mediators may exert a direct pharmacologic effect or release or activate other mediators potentiating the response. Mediators initiate a sequence of physiologic events in various organ systems that result in such responses as vasodilation, enhanced vasopermeability, smooth muscle contraction, and increased mucus production (FIG. 16-8).

On reexposure and entry the antigen binds to IgE antibodies. This causes degranulation of the mast cell and release of the mediators that initiate the pathophysiologic responses. Symptoms of atopic disease are the result of tissue response to the mediators. Symptoms may be generalized (anaphylaxis) or localized (e.g., in bronchi, conjunctiva, nasal membranes, skin, or gut). This mechanism of tissue reaction occurs immediately on exposure to the antigen and is identified as a type I anaphylactic or immediate hypersensitivity reaction by the Gell and Coombs classification.

Mast cell mediators are responsible for both the well-known "classic" allergic response, in which symptoms occur immediately on exposure, as well as the less well known–late phase response, in which symptoms begin hours after allergen exposure and result from tissue inflammation and damage.

Anaphylactoid reactions mimic allergic reactions and clinically may be identical to IgE-mediated responses. However, no IgE is involved and symptoms result from direct action on mast cells that causes release of chemical mediators (occurs with dextran and radiocontrast media), prostaglandin activation (occurs with acetylsalicylic acid and some nonsteroidal antiinflammatory agents), or complement activation (occurs with aggregated IgG). The exact trigger mechanism and pathways of

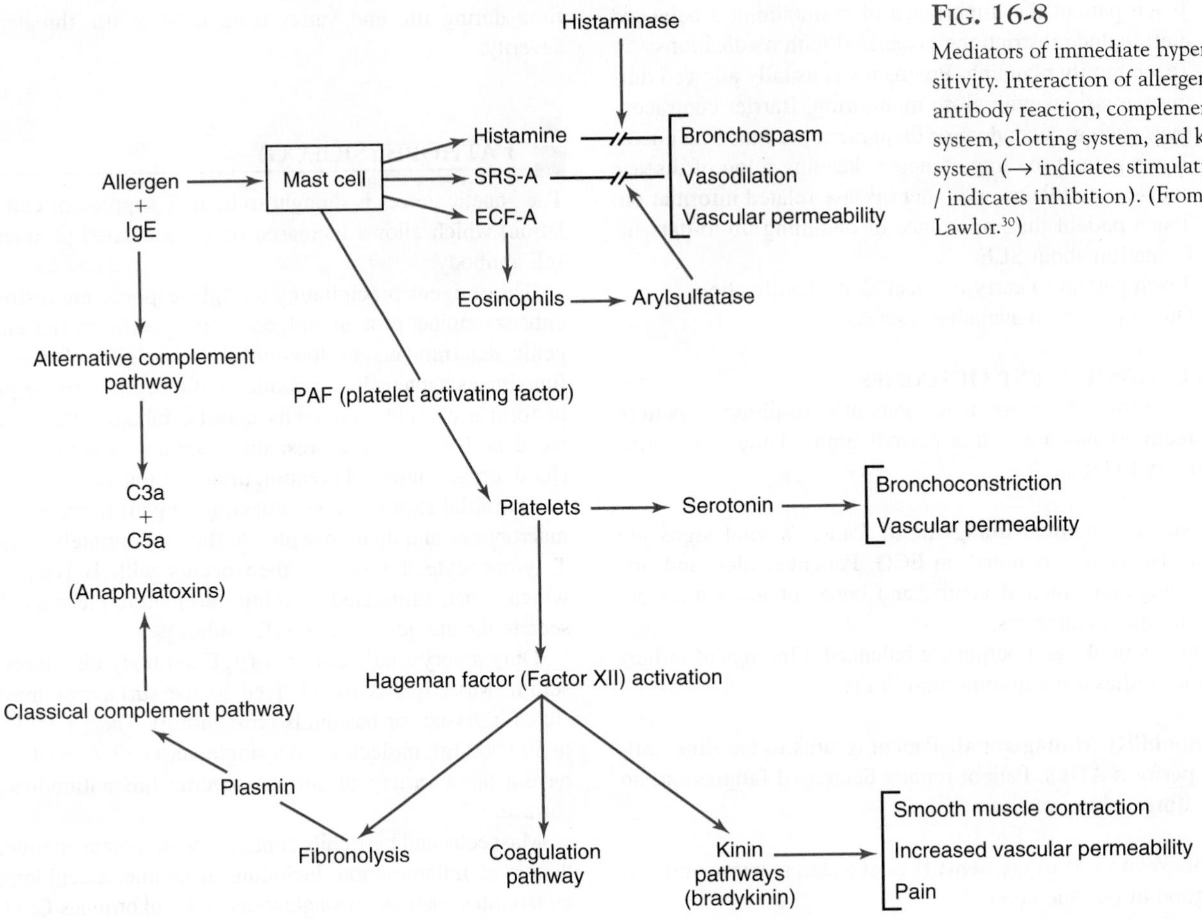

FIG. 16-8 Mediators of immediate hypersensitivity. Interaction of allergen-antibody reaction, complement system, clotting system, and kinin system (→ indicates stimulation; / indicates inhibition). (From Lawlor.[30])

inflammatory responses are not fully understood. However, these reactions are treated in the same manner as anaphylactic reactions. The only clinical difference is that, because IgE is not involved, skin testing is of no value and reactions can occur with the first exposure; prior sensitization is not required.

DIAGNOSTIC STUDIES AND FINDINGS

A thorough history is by far the most important diagnostic tool. The physical examination focuses on all areas of potential atopic manifestations. Laboratory studies may be useful in supporting the diagnosis and in monitoring response to therapy but are not in themselves diagnostic.

History: Onset, nature, and progression of symptoms; aggravating and alleviating factors; frequency, time, and duration of symptoms; complete environmental history, including occupational, chemical, smoking, animal, and hobby exposures; household description, including heating and cooling systems, pets, and bedding; past medical history; medications; family history, including atopic history

Physical examination: Skin; external ear canal and tympanic membrane; conjunctiva; nasal membranes; nasooropharynx; chest

Laboratory studies

Complete blood count: Within normal limits

Differential: May have eosinophil percentage, up to 5%

Eosinophil count: Within normal limits or increased up to 10% (up to 700 cells/mm^3), but range of normal is wide and increases may also occur in other diseases that have similar symptoms

Smears for eosinophils: Generally predominate in secretions (up to 90% of total) during symptomatic periods

Total serum IgE levels: Within normal limits or increased (up to 700 U/ml), but there is wide range of normal and increases can also occur in other diseases

Skin testing: Demonstrates presence of specific IgE antibody; most reliable test for allergy; reliable correlation for inhalants, much less reliable for foods; false-positive findings may result from irritant response; false-negative findings may result from poor skin response or antihistamines; findings must correlate with history; drug may be hapten or metabolite; testing currently limited to penicillin, horse serum, insulin, and egg-based vaccines

Radioallergosorbent test (RAST): Demonstrates presence of specific circulating IgE antibody; less reliable than skin testing (not as sensitive; difficulty in standardization of test and reproducibility of tests among reference laboratories)

Provocative testing: Specific antigen challenges performed under controlled conditions to demonstrate clinical reactivity

Elimination testing: Demonstration of clinical sensitivity to antigen by removing and then reintroducing it while monitoring clinical symptoms

MULTIDISCIPLINARY PLAN

The goals of the treatment plan include symptom management through medications, environmental control, and immunotherapy. Specific plans are discussed with each disease.

Medications

Medications are used to prevent the tissue response and resultant symptoms. The choice of medication is to some extent organ specific, since the tissue response differs in specific organ systems, and these are discussed with the specific allergic disease.

Antihistamines: Six classes of older antihistamines are available, as well as newer histamine$_1$ (H_1) antihistamines; topical preparations should be avoided because of potential for sensitization; they may be given orally or intramuscularly depending on preparation and with dose adjustments to any patient older than 3 months, including pregnant women (who may receive selected antihistamines, including chlorpheniramine)

Cromolyn sodium

Intal, via Spinhaler or metered dose inhaler, q6h or as needed before exposure for adult and child older than 6 years

Nebulizer solution, 1 ampule via nebulizer q6h or as needed before exposure for adult and child older than 2 years

Nasalcrom, 1 spray q4-6h or as needed before exposure for adult and child older than 6 years

Opticrom, 1 drop in each eye as above

Immunotherapy recommended for inhalant antigens (e.g., tree, grass, and weed pollens) and venoms, but not for foods

Desensitization for insulin and penicillin requires special protocols performed under close supervision and is done only when medically indicated

Environmental Control

Environmental control is the preferred method of treatment because complete avoidance of the offending allergen affords total relief of symptoms. The following is a representative list of allergens and possible measures:

Tree, grass, and weed pollens—air-conditioning, closing bedroom or car windows during pollen season (times of pollination depend on geographic area)

Mold spores—removal of source (such as plant dirt), application of mold retardant solutions for damp areas (for example, crawl spaces, bathrooms), air filtration by a high-efficiency particulate-arresting (HEPA) filter or electrostatic air cleaner.

House dust and mites—plastic mattress casing, removal of carpets, damp dusting and face masks while dusting, air filtration

Epidermals (feather, animal protein)—removal of source

Foods—avoidance

Drugs—avoidance

Stinging or biting insects—avoidance

NURSING CARE

NURSING ASSESSMENT

Allergic responses may involve one or more organ systems, and symptoms may range from mild to severe. Symptoms may be episodic or perennial depending on exposures. Assessment must also discriminate among possible concurrent diseases. Specific assessment is discussed with each allergic disease.

PATIENT PROBLEMS/NURSING DIAGNOSES & INTERVENTIONS

Because of the variable expression of atopic disease, the following is included as part of the comprehensive overview of the disease. Specific interventions are addressed with discussion of each disease.

NIC RISK MANAGEMENT

Risk for injury related to exposure to antigen
Risk for infection related to depressed immune system

- Obtain complete allergy history and record in appropriate places.
- Emphasize potential harm of repeat exposure.
- Identify and teach patient the measures to institute if patient is reexposed to antigen.
- Emphasize need for medical alert identification.
- Assess for signs and symptoms of concurrent infection.
- Maintain optimal nutritional intake.
- Maintain appropriate rest patterns.
- Monitor use of medications *to control or eliminate symptoms.*

NIC ACTIVITY AND EXERCISE MANAGEMENT

Risk for activity intolerance related to medication side effects

- Modify activity prescriptions based on status of current symptoms, including fatigue.
- Encourage full activity schedule for growth and developmental age. Make appropriate medication adjustments and apply environmental control measures.

NIC PATIENT EDUCATION

Ineffective health maintenance related to lack of knowledge

- Assess patient's and family's knowledge of disease process, relationship to symptoms, and methods of preventing or controlling symptoms.
- Provide education *to achieve optimum level of health.*

PATIENT EDUCATION/CONTINUUM OF CARE PLAN

1. Review disease process with patient to assess accuracy of patient's understanding.
2. Review with patient medication use and expected response to therapy.
3. Teach patient self-responsibility for allergen identification and avoidance measures.
4. Direct patient to support and educational groups.

EVALUATION/PATIENT OUTCOMES

Specific criteria are identified with discussion of each atopic disease. The following are general outcome measures for any atopic disease.

Risk Management: Symptoms are resolved in response to therapeutic measures.

Activity and Exercise Management: Patient performs activities appropriate for growth and developmental age.

Patient Education: Patient and family describe allergy, medical plan of care, environmental control, and other self-care measures.

ALLERGIC RHINITIS/ALLERGIC RHINOCONJUNCTIVITIS

Allergic rhinitis/allergic rhinoconjunctivitis is a complex of symptoms resulting from an antigen–IgE antibody reaction occurring in the nasal membranes, conjunctiva, or nasopharynx. The antigen is generally inhaled and deposited on the mucous membrane surface. Symptoms may also result from injected or ingested antigen transported to the site.[33,42]

Approximately 18.6 million infants, children, and adults in the United States have seasonal or perennial allergic rhinitis. An estimated $224 million is spent annually for physician services and $300 million for medications, and some 28 million days each year are lost because of restricted activity or absence from school or work.

Symptoms may develop as early as infancy but can occur at any time throughout the life span. A positive family history may be obtained in the majority of cases. Without intervention, symptoms may remain constant, increase, or diminish over time.

PATHOPHYSIOLOGY

With antigen-antibody linkage, mast cell degranulation and chemical mediator release occur, resulting in slower ciliary action, stimulation of mucosal glands, vasomotor instability, leukocyte infiltration (primarily eosinophilic), and tissue edema because of vasodilation and capillary permeability. Histamine is the major mediator of the inflammatory response, although other mediators such as ECF-A, prostaglandins, and leukotrienes participate.

With prolonged exposure, basement membrane destruction and foam cell formation occur. More chronic and irreversible changes include hyperplasia and thickening of the mucosal epithelium, mononuclear cellular infiltration, and connective tissue proliferation.

Symptoms generally result from inhalant allergen exposure or occasionally, especially in infants, from food ingestion. The inflammatory response may be confined to the nasal membranes or extend to the conjunctiva or oropharynx. Symptoms begin immediately on exposure and may be prolonged because of the late-phase reaction.

DIAGNOSTIC STUDIES AND FINDINGS

Skin tests: Positive responses that correlate with history

Sinus roentgenogram: Within normal limits; may be necessary to rule out other diseases such as cysts, nasal polyps, infective rhinitis, and structural defects

CT scan of sinuses: Rules out other diseases and structural defects

MULTIDISCIPLINARY PLAN

The goal of the treatment plan is to block symptoms, maintain optimum function, and prevent sequelae such as fatigue, infections, serous otitis, and restricted activity.

Medications

Antihistamines: May be used prn or around-the-clock; long-acting compounds generally best; tolerance avoided by using different antihistamines; often combined with decongestants

Cromolyn sodium: Used prn before known antigen exposure (cat, dog, dusting) but more effective around-the-clock; short half-life often requires doses q4-6h or concomitant nocturnal antihistamine

Sympathomimetic agents

Topical decongestants: Over-the-counter; should not be used for more than 3 consecutive days; useful for severe acute symptoms until other medications take effect

Oral decongestants: Agents available (phenylephrine, phenylpropanolamine, pseudoephedrine); may be obtained over-the-counter or by prescription; age-dependent dosage; may be used from 3 months of age; often used in combination with antihistamines and in long-acting preparations for decreased dosage schedule; must be used with caution in patients with hypertension or glaucoma; blood pressure monitoring needed

Corticosteroids

Topical: Excellent for controlling more severe symptoms; must be used on regular basis

Flunisolide (Nasalide), 1 spray q8h for adult or child older than 6 years

Beclomethasone (Vancenase, Beconase), 2 sprays q8h for adult or child older than 12 years

Dexamethasone phosphate (Decadron Phosphate Turbinaire), 2 sprays q8h for adult; 1-2 sprays bid for child older than 6 years

Oral: Rarely used since advent of topical agents; should be considered only when symptoms are severe and other measures have failed

Ocular: Because of side effects, even short-term use severely restricted and closely monitored

Antiinfective agents: Used for secondary bacterial infections; synthetic penicillins, sulfa, or erythromycin generally recommended and should be used for 10 days to 2 weeks

Analgesic agents: Used to reduce symptoms of pressure headache until appropriate medications achieve symptom control

Environmental Control

Allergic rhinitis responds dramatically to removal of allergen; see p. 1127 for control of antigen exposure

Immunotherapy

Allergic rhinitis responds well to appropriately designed immunotherapy program

General Management

Increased fluid intake to liquify secretions and counter loss from obligatory mouth breathing; steam or topical nasal saltwater solutions to decrease irritability and help loosen secretions

NURSING CARE

NURSING ASSESSMENT

The goal of assessment is to confirm extent and severity of organ involvement and establish a baseline for later evaluation.

Conjunctival inflammation: Hyperemia; edema (chemosis) involving either palpebral or bulbar membranes; secretions in palpebral fissures; superficial keratitis; edema; hyperplasia of papillae

Facial changes: Dark discoloration in orbital-palpebral groove beneath lower eyelids ("allergic shiners"); adenoidal facies consisting of elongated maxilla, narrow chin, gaping expression, possible dental malocclusion, and transverse crease across top of nose

Nasal membrane inflammation: Swollen, wet, pale turbinates; mucosal edema; glistening, clear, watery or serous drainage; more variability in chronic disease

Oropharyngeal inflammation: Nasal secretions; erythema; edema; high-arched palate; overbite

Tympanic membrane involvement: Bulging or retracted; prominent bony landmarks or none present; membrane thick, dull, or wrinkled, with gray, pink, amber, slightly yellow, or deep blue color; injected; evidence of fluid levels or bubbles

POTENTIAL COMPLICATIONS

Respiratory infections; ear infection

PATIENT PROBLEMS/NURSING DIAGNOSES & INTERVENTIONS

NIC RESPIRATORY MANAGEMENT

Ineffective breathing pattern related to inflammatory response

- Assess for obligatory mouth breathing, paroxysmal nocturnal dyspnea, snoring, or sleep apnea that may contribute to "allergic fatigue."
- Elevate head of bed to 45 degrees *to facilitate mucus drainage.*
- Humidify air as needed.
- Monitor medication schedule *to block symptoms adequately.*
- Assess environment for presence of offending allergens and remove if possible.
- Emphasize importance of nasal breathing.

NIC SELF-CARE FACILITATION

Impaired home maintenance related to lack of knowledge

- Discuss chronicity of disease process and reinforce need to prevent symptoms through medications and environmental control.

NIC RISK MANAGEMENT

Risk for infection related to inadequate primary defense

- Maintain adequate nutritional intake and appropriate rest.
- Discuss rationale for adequately controlling symptoms and self-monitoring for secondary infections.

PATIENT EDUCATION/CONTINUUM OF CARE PLAN

1. Assess patient's current knowledge of disease process and reinforce concept of self-care and self-management of the disease.
2. Assess patient's current knowledge of medications, side effects, and rationale for use of medications, and reinforce concepts of prophylaxis and prevention of symptoms.
3. Teach patient the importance of environmental control measures and patient's responsibility for implementing recommended measures.
4. Teach patient the importance of monitoring symptom response to therapies, recording any difficulties, new symptoms, and untoward effects, and communicating this on an ongoing basis to those prescribing the therapies.

EVALUATION/PATIENT OUTCOMES

Respiratory Management: Patient exhibits normal breathing pattern, and there is no evidence of dyspnea.

Self-Care Facilitation: Patient can identify all recommended therapies and provide information related to self-management. Patient engages in normal work, school, or recreational activities without restrictions.

Risk Management: There is no evidence of infection.

ANAPHYLAXIS

Anaphylaxis results from a systemic IgE-mediated antigen-antibody response. It is an immediate and often life-threatening event in which massive release of mediators triggers a sequence of events in target organs throughout the body, resulting in a variety of symptoms that may include respiratory embarrassment or circulatory collapse.[14,16]

As with other IgE antigen-antibody reactions, prior sensitization to the antigen must have occurred for anaphylaxis to take place. Anaphylactoid reactions and blood transfusion reactions are mediated by a non-IgE mechanism with the same final common pathway as IgE-mediated reactions. Reactions must be differentiated from vasovagal reactions, syncopal attacks, myocardial infarctions, insulin reactions, hysterical reactions, and shock or respiratory obstruction from other causes.

A systemic reaction is any organ involvement away from the site of antigen deposition. Reactions are classified as mild, moderate, or severe and may involve the respiratory tract cardiovascular system, gastrointestinal tract, or skin (Table 16-7). Symptoms may progress in minutes from mild to severe, or severe reaction may occur without warning. Reactions may occur up to 2 hours after exposure. Reactions that occur immediately are the most life threatening. Resolution of symptoms may be immediate or take several days. Resolution depends on the

Table 16-7 Potential Symptom Complex of Anaphylaxis

Target Organ	Mild	Moderate	Severe
General status (prodromal)	Malaise; sense of illness	Greater malaise and sense of illness	Deep malaise and strong sense of illness
Skin	Hives; erythema; tingling; warm sensation; itching	Generalized urticaria; flushing; generalized pruritus; periorbital edema	Cyanosis; pallor
Upper respiratory tract	Nasal congestion; sneezing; rhinorrhea; conjunctivitis	Profuse congestion and rhinorrhea	Periorbital edema; obligatory mouth breathing
Upper airway	Fullness in mouth or throat	Edema of tongue, larynx, and pharynx; hoarseness	Stridor; completely occluded airway
Lower airway	Cough	Bronchospasm; dyspnea; cough; wheezing; air trapping	Severe dyspnea; hypoxia; respiratory arrest
Gastrointestinal tract	Cramping	Nausea; vomiting; increased peristalsis	Dysphagia; intense abdominal cramping; diarrhea
Cardiovascular system	Tachycardia	Hypotension; syncope	Coronary insufficiency; cardiac dysrhythmias; shock; circulatory collapse
Central nervous system	Anxiety	Intense anxiety; confusion	Seizures; coma

severity of the reaction, the promptness of medical intervention, and any complications occurring during the reaction. Early recognition and rapid intervention may prevent progression to severe reactions.

PATHOPHYSIOLOGY

A history of atopic disease is often not elicited from patients with anaphylaxis. Previous exposures to the offending antigens may or may not have caused an untoward reaction.

Anaphylactoid reactions, through direct mast cell destabilization, immune complex aggregation, or prostaglandin-activating mechanisms, may also cause the release of mediators that results in a systemic reaction clinically similar to anaphylaxis (see Emergency Alert box). The following are some mechanisms that have been proposed for anaphylactoid reactions:

Direct mediator release (agents such as dextran and radiopaque dyes)

Immune complex aggregation (agents such as γ-globulin administered intramuscularly or intravenously)

Cytotoxic antibody transfusion reactions (agents such as whole blood and cryoprecipitate)

Prostaglandin-induced (agents such as aspirin and nonsteroidal antiinflammatory agents)

Anaphylaxis may result from injection of antigen (subcutaneous, intravenous, or intramuscular drugs or venom stings), although enough antigen may be absorbed from the gut (ingested food or drug) or from the respiratory tract (inhaled antigen) to precipitate the reaction. The antigen is distributed via the bloodstream and fixes to IgE antibody on mast cells and basophils, triggering mediator release. On reexposure to antigen and its subsequent linkage with IgE antibody, mediator release occurs and affects the end-organ responses (Table 16-8).

Almost any drug may precipitate an anaphylactic reaction. Subcutaneous, intramuscular (IM), and intravenous routes provide sufficient antigen for overwhelming systemic reactions. Anaphylaxis produced by insect venom may account for more than 100 deaths annually. Foods may generate an anaphylactic reaction, particularly in adults, although this is not common. The following are some common antigens of anaphylaxis:

Drugs: Proteins (presumably complete antigens), foreign serum, vaccines, allergen extracts, enzymes

Nonprotein drugs (presumably haptens): Penicillin and other antibiotics, sulfonamides, local anesthetics, hormones

Venoms: Hymenoptera (honeybee, wasp, hornet, yellow jacket), deerfly, fire ant

Foods: Legumes (especially peanuts), nuts, berries, seafood, egg albumin

> **! EMERGENCY ALERT**
>
> **ANAPHYLACTIC SHOCK**
>
> Anaphylactic shock is classified as a vasogenic shock in which severe vasodilation occurs. Anaphylactic shock is an antigen-antibody reaction when a sensitized person is exposed to an antigen. Common allergies are to stings, shellfish, and medications. A relative hypovolemia results from intervascular fluid shifting.
>
> **ASSESSMENT**
>
> - Signs of respiratory distress, bronchospasm, wheezing, airway obstruction, respiratory arrest.
> - Edematous tongue.
> - Skin may be warm and dry or present with urticaria or edema.
> - Dysrhythmias or cardiopulmonary arrest may occur.
>
> **INTERVENTIONS**
>
> - Maintain airway, breathing, and circulation
> - Administer high-flow oxygen (10-15 L) by mask.
> - Obtain intravenous access; in collaboration with physician administer epinephrine 0.1-0.5 ml of a 1:10,000 solution; may repeat as indicated.
> - If further medication is indicated, in collaboration with physician administer aminophylline, Benadryl, and/or corticosteroids.

Table 16-8 Physiologic Response to Mediators

Mediator	Effect	End-Organ Response
Histamine	Vascular permeability	Edema of larynx, gut, and airways; urticaria
Leukotrienes	Vascular smooth muscle relaxation	Decreased peripheral volume; decreased peripheral resistance
Kallikrein	Vasodilation and vascular engorgement	Decreased blood pressure; bronchospasm
Platelet activating factor	Increased bronchial smooth muscle tone	Rhinorrhea; bronchorrhea
Others	Mucous gland secretion; irritability of peripheral nerve endings; intestinal smooth muscle tone	Pruritus; gut motility; rhinorrhea; bronchorrhea

Diagnostic Studies and Findings

The diagnosis is based on a history of signs and symptoms of anaphylaxis immediately after exposure to a likely offending agent, as well as supportive laboratory data.

Complete blood count: Within normal limits or increased hematocrit value resulting from hemoconcentration

Blood chemistries: Within normal limits unless myocardial or renal damage has occurred owing to circulatory collapse

Chest roentgenogram: Normal appearance or hyperinflation with or without atelectasis; pulmonary edema

Electrocardiogram: Normal unless myocardial damage or hypoxemic changes are present

Skin tests: Must be done at least 4 weeks after anaphylactic episode to ensure adequate repopulation of IgE antibody; requires extreme caution; usefulness limited to egg-based vaccines, venom, foods, horse serum, insulin, and penicillin

Multidisciplinary Plan

The goal of the treatment plan is swift, aggressive management of symptoms. Establishment of an airway and maintenance of blood pressure are crucial. Therapy is individualized based on organ involvement and severity of reaction.

Medications

Medications used to counteract effects of mediator release, block additional mediator release, and protect organ system involved; continued until all symptoms have completely resolved; given over sufficient time to prevent further symptom development; withdrawn with careful monitoring

General Management

Maintained until all symptoms of anaphylaxis are resolved
- Airway with suctioning as appropriate
- Endotracheal tube or tracheostomy if indicated
- Arterial blood gas monitoring
- Treatment of acidosis
- Volume replacement and vasopressors
- Intake and output
- Monitor electrocardiograms
- Treat dysrhythmias if present

Complete drug allergy history before administration of any new drug

Human serum preparations preferred, if antiserum indicated

Skin testing for vaccines, venoms, antivenoms, insulin, and penicillin

Use of pretreatment protocols and close monitoring required in the special circumstances when patients at risk must be exposed (to radiologic contrast media, insulin, or penicillin)

NURSING CARE

Nursing Assessment

Because of multisystem involvement, anaphylactic or anaphylactoid reactions may initially have a variety of manifestations.

Laryngeal involvement: Hoarseness; stridor; use of accessory muscles; difficulty in speech

Respiratory status: Dyspnea; substernal tightness; use of accessory muscles; cough

Bronchospasm: Mucus production; rales; wheezing; decreased breath sounds; anxiety; inability to lie supine; evidence of air trapping or atelectasis on chest roentgenogram

Pulmonary edema: Wet rales at base; frothy clear or blood-streaked secretions

Respiratory arrest: No air movement

Cardiovascular status: Hypotension; weak, thready pulse; tachycardia; oliguria; mental confusion; dysrhythmias; cardiac arrest

Neurologic status: Anxiety; malaise; sense of illness; mental confusion; obtundation; coma

Skin integrity: Pruritus; erythema; flushing; urticaria; angioedema; cyanosis; pallor

Gastrointestinal status: Nausea; vomiting; diarrhea; gastrointestinal cramping

Respiratory status: Rhinorrhea; congestion; sneezing; conjunctivitis; tearing

Potential Complications

Respiratory arrest, cardiopulmonary arrest

Patient Problems/Nursing Diagnoses & Interventions

NIC Respiratory Management

Risk for ineffective breathing pattern related to tracheobronchial obstruction

Impaired gas exchange related to alveolar-capillary membrane changes

- Maintain endotracheal tube or tracheostomy, if instituted. Suction carefully.
- Monitor for mouth breathing and rhinorrhea.
- Maintain 45-degree elevation of patient's head if possible.
- Assess for laryngeal involvement, including stridor, hoarseness, and difficulty in swallowing or speech.

- Be prepared for respiratory arrest management.
- Administer oxygen at indicated rate.
- Monitor fluid replacement, and assess for pulmonary overload.

NIC Tissue Perfusion Management

Ineffective tissue perfusion (cardiopulmonary, cerebral, peripheral, and gastrointestinal) related to exchange problems

- Report signs of hypotension.
- Place in supine position to promote venous return.
- Use safety measures if confused.
- Monitor parenteral fluids carefully *to prevent overload.*
- Be prepared to institute cardiopulmonary resuscitation.
- In conjunction with physician, administer antihistamines as indicated.
- In conjunction with physician, administer epinephrine, fluids, or vasopressors as indicated.

NIC Risk Management

Risk for injury: anaphylaxis, related to exposure to inciting agent

- Obtain complete drug allergy history before administering new drug.
- Put label noting allergic drug history in all appropriate places.
- Closely monitor patient for 30 minutes after administering new drug.

Patient Education/Continuum of Care Plan

1. Reassure patient during procedures.
2. Explain to patient the reason for each procedure.
3. Explain to patient the relationship of symptoms to anaphylactic reaction.
4. Explain to patient the absolute necessity of avoiding causative agent.
5. Discuss with patient the need for follow-up care and for allergy testing when indicated.
6. Explain to patient the need to carry or wear medical alert identification and to inform other health-care personnel.
7. Stress to patient the importance of avoiding any medications without first checking with physician.
8. Teach patient self-administration of epinephrine and subsequent measures, including oral administration of antihistamine and seeking immediate medical care.

Evaluation/Patient Outcomes

Respiratory and Tissue Perfusion Management: Patient is symptom free. Patient expresses feeling of well-being. There is no evidence of urticaria or angioedema or subjective complaint of pruritus or swelling. There is no evidence of rhinoconjunctivitis, asthma, pulmonary edema, or laryngeal edema. Blood pressure and pulse rate are normal. There is no evidence of hypoxia.

Risk Management: Patient can identify triggering agent and explain all appropriate avoidance measures.

Food Allergy

Food allergy is an IgE-mediated hypersensitivity disease. It may be manifested in the respiratory, integumentary, or gastrointestinal system as rhinitis, asthma, atopic dermatitis, urticaria, nausea, vomiting, diarrhea, or cramps or may result in anaphylaxis. An adverse food reaction is any untoward symptom complex resulting from food ingestion.

Adverse reaction to food is a complex diagnostic problem. There are various causes for adverse food reactions. True food allergy is mediated by IgE antibody (type 1 hypersensitivity reaction) in sensitized individuals on exposure to the offending antigen. Antibody-antigen linkage occurs and results in mediator release and symptoms.

Food intolerance is any abnormal physiologic response to an ingested food or food additive that is nonimmunologic in nature. Other immunologic mechanisms have been identified in adverse food reactions, including IgA deficiency, cytotoxic responses (type II), immune complex formation (type III), and cell-mediated reactions (type IV). Adverse reactions to food may have multiple origins, with a variety of nonimmunologic mechanisms resulting in a clinically abnormal host response. An idiosyncratic response in an individual may result in an anaphylactoid reaction, as with ingestion of monosodium glutamate. A metabolic defect such as lactose enzyme deficiency may cause foods to be improperly digested, or a metabolic problem such as diabetes may result in an abnormal response. Toxic responses to spoiled food are well known. Pharmacologic properties such as those of caffeine may exert a direct untoward effect. All these reactions are well documented and reproducible in controlled settings.

Other clinical syndromes are ascribed to foods or food additives, but this cannot be substantiated by reproducible, objective studies. Although anecdotal evidence exists to support a relationship between food ingestion and behavior, other causal relationships have not been adequately ruled out. Tension-fatigue syndrome, hyperactivity syndrome, and psychiatric disorders such as mood swings are among the many disorders identified as being linked to food. Similar reports linking foods to rheumatoid arthritis or vasculitis and other physical syndromes also have not been substantiated. Other causes of vomiting, diarrhea, and stool abnormalities must also be excluded.

The prevalence of food allergy is unknown. Estimates range from 0.1% to 7% of the population, with a male/female ratio of approximately 2:1. If one sibling has a documented food allergy, a 50% probability of food hypersensitivity exists in other siblings. Anaphylactic episodes are most common in adults but may occur at any age. Nonimmunologic-mediated adverse food reactions have a much higher prevalence than immunologic reactions.

In exquisitely sensitive persons merely inhaling the antigen in cooking odors can precipitate a massive allergic reaction. Reactions are often dose related and may vary with time in the same individual. The foods most commonly associated with allergic reactions are milk, eggs, wheat, and soybeans in children, and fish, shellfish, peanuts, nuts, and seeds in adults, although virtually any food may cause an allergic response. Families of foods may share allergenic features, and thus cross-reactivity among those foods (for example, shellfish) is more common.

Because of absorption characteristics, the reaction may be immediate or delayed up to 2 hours after ingestion.

PATHOPHYSIOLOGY

As with other responses mediated by IgE antibody–antigen interaction, prior exposure with sensitization in the atopic individual must occur. On reexposure, antigen-antibody linkage occurs with resultant mediator release. For reasons unknown, one end-organ may be affected with a localized response, as in urticaria, or loss of sensitivity may occur with time.

Why different individuals become sensitized to particular food is also unknown. Allergenicity of the protein correlates with its heat-labile or enzyme-resistant properties. Although cooking or digestion may alter the protein, rendering it less allergenic, the altered protein may still precipitate an allergic response. An alteration in the original protein may contribute to false-negative skin test findings if the unaltered food is used as the test antigen.

The gastrointestinal tract plays an important role in food allergy. The gut normally reaches maturity by 2 years of age. Before maturation there is a greater likelihood of absorption of food protein before complete digestion. Increase in absorption of potentially antigenic substances may also occur in IgA deficiency, malabsorption disease, and chronic inflammatory bowel diseases and after viral, parasitic, or bacterial diseases when the normal protective barriers have been damaged. These clinical syndromes may also contribute to adverse food reactions by decreasing normal flora, decreasing digestive enzymes, bile salts, and other secretions, reducing peristalsis, and interfering with cell renewal.

When the gut mucosal wall is damaged, protein may be absorbed and may precipitate IgE and IgG involvement or immune complex formation. Increased immunologic reactivity involving IgG and immune complex formation may result in enteropathies. Aspiration of milk in infancy may stimulate an IgE host defense response.

Genetic factors, amount of food ingested, food-drug interactions, contaminants, infections, pharmacologic properties, and nonimmunologic mechanisms have all been identified as contributing to adverse food reactions (Table 16-9).

Because of the multiple pathophysiologic mechanisms involved, clinical manifestations of adverse food reactions are widely variable (see Table 16-9). Depending on the mechanisms, amount, and duration of exposure, symptoms may vary from episodic to chronic and from mild to severe, and consequences may be reversible or irreversible.

Table 16-9 Adverse Reactions to Foods

Type	Mechanism	Food (Examples)	Host Response
TYPE I HYPERSENSITIVITY			
Food allergy	IgE antibody–antigen linkage	Shellfish; nuts	Urticaria; angioedema; rhinitis; bronchospasm; nausea; vomiting; diarrhea; anaphylaxis
METABOLIC REACTIONS			
Enzyme deficiencies	Lactase deficiency	Milk	Bloating; diarrhea; cramps
	Glucose-6-phosphate dehydrogenase (G6PD) deficiency	Fava beans	Hemolytic anemia
	Phenylketonuria	Nutrasweet	Central nervous system changes
Severe chronic inflammatory bowel disease	Loss of enzymes through diarrhea and decreased production	Saccharides	Bloating; diarrhea; cramps; malabsorption
Medication interactions	Monoamine oxidase inhibitors	Cheese	Hypertensive crisis
Celiac disease	Probable type IV reaction	Wheat	Bloating; diarrhea; malabsorption
Gallbladder disease	Decreased bile salts	Fats	Bloating; indigestion; diarrhea; cramping
Diabetes	Decreased insulin	Sugar	Hyperglycemia
Cystic fibrosis	Inadequate pancreatic function	Fats; proteins	Fatty, foul-smelling stools; malabsorption
NATURAL PHARMACOLOGIC AGENTS			
Psychoactive agents	Direct sympathetic stimulation	Caffeine; theobromine	Central nervous system stimulation
Vasoactive amines (e.g., tryptamine, tyramine)	Direct action on end-organ or autonomic stimulation	Cheese; chocolate	Headaches
FOOD CONTAMINATION BY INFECTIOUS AGENTS, MICROBES, AND TOXINS			
Bacteria; viruses; parasites; fungi	Endotoxins; neurotoxins; toxic alkaloids; damage to gut wall	Contaminated foods	Nausea; vomiting; diarrhea; bloating; weight loss; liver dysfunctions; headaches; fever; chills
NATURAL TOXIC AGENTS			
Licorice	Sodium retention	Licorice	Hypertension
Glycoalkaloids	Probable direct blood vessel effect	Green potatoes; lima beans	Angioedema; urticaria

Continued

Table 16-9 Adverse Reactions to Foods—cont'd

Type	Mechanism	Food (Examples)	Host Response
ANAPHYLACTOID REACTIONS			
Chemical mediator release	Direct action on mast cell	Strawberries; tomatoes	Urticaria; angioedema; diarrhea
Nonimmunologic	Unknown	Tartrazine (FD & C yellow #5)	Urticaria; angioedema; rhinitis; asthma
	Unknown	Sodium metabisulfite	Urticaria; angioedema; rhinitis; asthma; anaphylaxis
	Unknown	Monosodium glutamate	Headache; flush; asthma
TYPES II, III, AND IV HYPERSENSITIVITY			
Immune complexes with food antigen	Complement activation	After acute viral gastroenteritis	Diarrhea; cramping
Weiner's syndrome	IgG-antigen complexes; also type IV reaction	Milk	Respiratory symptoms; failure to thrive
Enteropathies	IgG precipitating antibodies	Milk; soy	Gastrointestinal bleeding; malabsorption; diarrhea; cramping
IgA deficiency	Failure to regulate antigen absorption	Variable	Malnutrition; diarrhea; increased with severity of disease

DIAGNOSTIC STUDIES AND FINDINGS

Diagnostic studies are chosen based on the presentation of the adverse food reaction. The history is by far the most important diagnostic tool. The physical examination focuses on the clinical presentation.

Laboratory tests are chosen based on the suspected mechanisms of the adverse food reaction. Cytotoxic testing, sublingual testing, and red blood cell lysis have no proven efficacy in diagnosis and should not be employed.

History: Frequency, duration, and seasonality of symptoms; onset, severity, progression, and nature of symptoms; timing between ingestion and symptom onset; amount and nature of provoking food; concomitant illnesses; nutritional history; drug history; atopic history; infectious disease history.

Physical examination: Skin; upper and lower respiratory tract; gastrointestinal tract; oropharynx; weight and height; growth and development; general appearance; vital signs; muscle mass and amount of subcutaneous tissue; texture and amount of hair; hepatomegaly

Laboratory tests

Type I hypersensitivity

Skin tests: May have false positives or negatives; not diagnostic; must be used in conjunction with challenge tests

Radioallergosorbent test (RAST): May be less sensitive and has more limited panel than skin tests; may also have false positives or negatives; not diagnostic; must be used in conjunction with challenge tests

Total serum IgE: Not specific indicator, not helpful

Eosinophil count: Not specific indicator, not helpful

Elimination diets: Aid in diagnosis by symptom response; used in conjunction with rechallenge; strict elimination diets difficult and cannot be used for more than 7 days

Food rechallenge: Confirms diagnosis; not to be used if there is history of anaphylaxis

Types II, III, and IV hypersensitivity

Biopsy of involved tissue: Demonstrates presence of IgG, IgM, complement activation, or T cell involvement

Hemagglutination: May be present in persons without disease or absent in persons who have disease

IgA deficiency: IgA level—wide range of normal (80 to 350 mg/dl); may be low normal or depressed

Natural pharmacologic agents

Diet diary and elimination diet: Correlates symptoms with suspected agents

Food rechallenge: Confirms diagnosis

Food contamination by infectious agents: Stool cultures—document infectious agent

Natural toxic agents: Diet diary and elimination diet—correlate symptoms with suspected agent

Food rechallenge: Confirms history

Anaphylactoid reactions

Diet diary and elimination diet: Correlate symptoms with suspected agent

Food rechallenge, unless systemic reaction: Confirms history

Metabolism: Disease-specific work-up (refer to discussion of specific disease elsewhere in text)

MULTIDISCIPLINARY PLAN

The goal of the treatment plan is to eliminate the offending food, thus preventing recurrence of symptoms. Types I, II, III, and IV hypersensitivity reactions to natural pharmacologic agents and natural toxic agents, and anaphylactoid reactions respond completely to elimination of the offending food. Often symptoms are time limited and resolve without therapy.

Medications

Based on severity and nature of symptoms, organ system involved, and mechanisms of reaction (Table 16-10).

Table 16-10 Medications Used in Treatment of Adverse Food Reactions

Mechanism	Potential Organ Involvement	Class of Medication
Type I hypersensitivity	Skin	Antihistamines
Anaphylactoid reactions	Upper respiratory tract	Sympathomimetic agents
Penicillin, drug contamination	Lower respiratory tract	Bronchodilators
Glycoalkaloids	Upper airway; gastrointestinal tract; multiorgan	Corticosteroids
Types II, III, and IV hypersensitivity (IgG-mediated, immune complex, and T cell sensitization, respectively)	Gastrointestinal tract Skin; respiratory tract	Topical or oral corticosteroids Nonsteroidal antiinflammatory agents
Infectious agents (bacterial, fungal, parasitic, viral)	Multisystemic response; gastrointestinal tract	Antiinfective agents
Metabolic reactions (enzyme deficiencies [cystic fibrosis], chronic inflammatory bowel disease)	Gastrointestinal malabsorption; protein-calorie deficiencies	Enzyme replacement; see specific therapy for disease process

General Management

Based on nature and severity of symptoms and mechanisms of adverse drug reactions; goal of supportive therapy is to facilitate healing process

Restriction of activity while symptoms are acute

Use of anaphylaxis kit

Breast-feeding with some maternal dietary restriction and delay in introduction of new foods to prevent or minimize food allergy in infants

NURSING CARE

NURSING ASSESSMENT

Response to therapy is based on the underlying mechanism, degree, and length of exposure. The symptom complex may vary among individuals

Type I hypersensitivity, anaphylactoid reactions, reactions to glycoalkaloids
- Laryngeal involvement: Hoarseness; stridor; use of accessory muscles; difficulty in speech
- Respiratory status: Dyspnea; substernal tightness; use of accessory muscles; cough; rhinorrhea; congestion; sneezing; tearing; conjunctivitis
- Bronchospasm: Mucus production; rhonchi; wheezing; decreased breath sounds; anxiety; inability to lie down; evidence of air trapping or atelectasis on chest roentgenogram
- Skin integrity: Pruritis; erythema; flushing; urticaria, angioedema; cyanosis; pallor
- Gastrointestinal status: Nausea; vomiting; bloating, diarrhea; cramping; distention
- Anaphylaxis: All of the above

Immunogenic (type II [IgG], type III [circulating immune complexes], type IV [T cell sensitization] IgA deficiency)
- Gastrointestinal status: Nausea; vomiting; bloating; distention; diarrhea; cramping; gastrointestinal bleeding; malabsorption; failure to thrive; hepatomegaly
- Skin integrity: Vasculitic lesion; contact dermatitis; hair thinning
- Musculoskeletal system status: Muscle mass loss; subcutaneous tissue loss
- See IgA deficiency assessment

Infective agents
- Gastrointestinal status: Nausea; vomiting; bloating; distention; diarrhea; cramping; gastrointestinal bleeding; malabsorption
- Systemic status: Fever; arthralgias; malaise

Reactions to natural pharmacologic agents
- Psychoactive agents
  - Central nervous system stimulation: Palpitations; anxiety; tachycardia; irritability
- Vasoactive amines
  - Central nervous system: Vascular headaches; migraines

Metabolic reactions (cystic fibrosis, diabetes, phenylketonuria, glucose 6-phosphate dehydrogenase deficiency, chronic inflammatory bowel disease, celiac disease, gallbladder disease)
- See specific disease process
- Gastrointestinal status: Nausea; vomiting; diarrhea; cramps; bloating; flatulence; fatty, foul-smelling stools; presence of occult blood in stool; failure to thrive; malnutrition; hepatomegaly; protuberant abdomen
- Skin integrity: Sparse hair; lanugo
- Musculoskeletal system status: Loss of muscle mass; subcutaneous tissue

PATIENT PROBLEMS/NURSING DIAGNOSES & INTERVENTIONS

The nursing diagnosis and interventions are based on the mechanism of the adverse food reaction and the severity of symptoms.

NIC NUTRITION SUPPORT

Imbalanced nutrition: less than body requirements, related to inability to digest food or absorb nutrients

- Obtain complete history of adverse food reactions, and put labels specifying history in appropriate places.
- Maintain elimination diet.
- Assess dietary intake for caloric and nutritional requirements.
- Teach alternative choices for balanced diet.
- Arrange dietary consultation.
- Monitor intake, output, and weight.
- Provide fluid supplementation.

- Teach patient self-care measures, such as reading labels, alternative choices, and his or her role in management of disease process.

See Anaphylaxis for altered cardiopulmonary and cerebral tissue perfusion (p. 1130).

Patient Education/Continuum of Care Plan

1. Assess patient's current knowledge of disease process and reinforce concept of self-care and self-management of disease.
2. Explain to patient that disease is a chronic one, and reinforce the need to prevent symptoms through avoidance of foods that cause them.
3. Teach patient the importance of monitoring response of symptoms to therapies; recording any difficulties, new symptoms, and cause-effect relationships noted; and communicating this on an ongoing basis to those prescribing therapies.
4. Emphasize to patient the importance of carrying appropriate identification and sharing information with significant others.
5. For patients at risk of anaphylaxis, teach self-administration of epinephrine and subsequent measures to take.

Evaluation/Patient Outcomes

Nutrition Support: Patient is symptom free. Patient's intake, output, and weight are stabilized. Patient can identify causative food and explain appropriate measures to avoid it.

Drug Allergy

An adverse drug reaction is any noxious or unintended effect of a drug. True drug allergy is mediated by IgE antibody–antigen interaction. Adverse reactions may also be mediated by other immunologic mechanisms.

Adverse drug reactions have steadily increased with the increase in available pharmacologic preparations. Drug allergy is one of the most common iatrogenic problems.

The incidence of adverse reactions is unknown. Three percent of hospitalizations are attributed to adverse drug reactions, and approximately 15% to 30% of hospitalized patients have an adverse drug reaction. Hospitalized patients sometimes receive 10 or more drugs, which obviously increases the risk of adverse drug reaction. The contribution of most additives or contaminants in adverse reactions is unclear, although idiosyncratic responses to tartrazine, sodium metabisulfite, and sodium benzoate have been well described.

Symptoms may affect any organ system of the body and may have a short or protracted course. Symptoms may range from mild to severe, and resolution of symptoms depends on the initiating mechanisms, amount of drug, and host response.

Drug and host factors can influence the development of an adverse drug reaction:

Drug factors
- Nature of drug: Class; weight; size; metabolites; ability to bind as hapten to protein (generally low molecular weight [500-1000])
- Route of administration: IV, IM, subcutaneous, oral, topical (in descending order of risk)
- Degree of exposure: prolonged course, high doses, and intermittent exposures increase risk; risk increases in first 2 to 3 weeks of therapy

Host factors
- Age: Adult at greater risk than child, probably because of total exposure and greater need for drugs
- Sex: No difference except that women at greater risk with muscle relaxants and chymopapain
- Atopic history: No greater incidence but appears to be associated with more severe reactions
- Genetic: May contribute by influencing metabolic pathways or increased mediators
- Prior drug reactions: Increased tendency with new drugs

Underlying disease state: May compromise immunologic mechanisms or alter metabolic pathways

Pathophysiology

Adverse drug reactions may be classified according to mechanisms of reaction (Table 16-11)

Non–drug-related reactions of the psychogenic type generally occur only with fear of pain, as with the intramuscular or subcutaneous route of administration. Coincidental symptoms are more easily distinguished with knowledge of disease symptoms.

Adverse drug reactions that any patient may experience are the most common and most predictable. Overdosage results in toxic pharmacologic effects of the drug and occurs most commonly in pediatric or geriatric populations with dosage miscalculations or with failure to recognize concurrent drug or host factors that delay the metabolism and excretion of the drug.

Side effects vary among patients and with drugs. They are most commonly seen with drugs that directly or indirectly affect the central nervous system or gastrointestinal system.

Drug interactions are complex, and thoughtful analysis is required before administration of more than one drug. Drug interactions may potentiate, decrease, or negate the desired therapeutic effects and may place the patient at risk of overdose.

Disease-associated effects generally result in toxic overdose as a result of decreased metabolism or excretion. In gastrointestinal diseases, drugs may be poorly absorbed, resulting in lack of therapeutic response.

Intolerance is a common problem. Many patients exhibit increased side effects or gastrointestinal sensitivity to numerous drugs at normal doses.

Idiosyncratic responses of an anaphylactoid nature are nonimmunologic. Direct action on mast cells resulting in release of chemical mediators, prostaglandin activation, or IgG aggregation result in clinical symptoms similar to IgE antibody hypersensitivity. The following are some mechanisms of anaphylactoid reactions:

- Mast cell degranulation (e.g., codeine, morphine, radiocontrast media)
- Prostaglandin-induced reactions (e.g., dextran and other plasma expanders, aspirin, nonsteroidal antiinflammatory agents, tartrazine)
- Immune complex aggregation (e.g., intramuscular or intravenous γ-globulin)
- Cytotoxic antibody transfusion reactions (e.g., mismatched blood transfusions)

Table 16-11 Adverse Drug Reactions

Reaction	Mechanism	Example
NON–DRUG RELATED (SYMPTOMS DISSIMILAR TO EXPECTED PHARMACOLOGIC EFFECTS)		
Psychogenic	Vasovagal	Syncope; anxiety
Coincidental symptoms	Disease process itself	Viral rash with antibiotics
DRUG-RELATED IN ANY PATIENT (SYMPTOMS SIMILAR TO EXPECTED PHARMACOLOGIC EFFECTS)		
Overdose	Increased intake, lowered metabolism, overdose, decreased liver excretion, toxic pharmacologic effect	Digoxin toxicity in elderly
Side effects	Undesirable pharmacologic effect of drug, often unavoidable with normal dose	Sleepiness with antihistamine
Secondary effects	Indirectly related to primary pharmacologic action	Vaginal infection after orally administered antibiotics
Drug interactions	Alter normal physiology of host, e.g., changes in absorption, metabolism, excretion; additive effects	Erythromycin changes liver metabolism and thus slows metabolism of theophylline
Disease-associated effects	Decreased absorption, metabolism, excretion; alteration in metabolic pathways	Digoxin toxicity
DRUG-RELATED IN SUSCEPTIBLE PATIENTS (SYMPTOMS, EXCEPT FOR INTOLERANCE, DISSIMILAR TO EXPECTED PHARMACOLOGIC RESPONSE)		
Intolerance	Quantitatively greater effect at normal dosages	CNS excitation with pharmacologic dose of adrenergic drug
Idiosyncracy	Qualitatively abnormal response that is different from pharmacologic effects (nonimmunologic)	Adverse response to local anesthetics
Genetic	Lack of enzyme or metabolic pathway	Hemolytic anemia in G6PD deficiency
Anaphylactoid	Nonimmunologic	Aspirin-induced bronchospasm
Allergy	IgE antigen-antibody interaction	Penicillin allergy
Cytotoxic	Cytotoxic antibody-mediated against cell membranes with involvement of complement, IgG, and IgM	Coombs' test–positive hemolytic anemia
Immune complex	Drug–IgG, IgM–drug immune complexes, complement	Serum sickness, drug-induced lupus
Cell-mediated	T lymphocyte sensitization	Fixed drug eruption, photosensitivity eruptions

In anaphylactoid reactions, prior exposure is not required, the host response may be variable over time, reactions can be produced with minute quantities, and the reaction resolves after the drug is discontinued.

Allergic, IgE antibody mechanisms account for a large proportion of adverse drug reactions because of the frequency with which drugs that fall in this category are prescribed. Some examples are penicillin and synthetic penicillins, sulfonamide antibiotics, sulfonylurea hypoglycemics, thiazide diuretics, carbonic anhydrase inhibitors, insulin and other hormones, egg-based vaccines, enzymes including chymopapain, antitoxins, and allergen extracts. The drug may act directly, it may bind with serum or tissue protein as a hapten, or a metabolite of the drug may be the offending antigen.

The allergic response requires prior exposure, can be reproduced by agents with cross-reacting structures, and can be produced by minute quantities. The reaction resolves after the drug is discontinued.

In cytotoxic, or type II, hypersensitivity, IgG or IgM antibody activates complement that results in damage to cell membranes. A drug may act as a hapten by binding to a cell surface, a drug-antibody complex may be absorbed to the cell surface, or a drug may change or modify a cell membrane leading to cell destruction.

In circulating immune complex, or type III, hypersensitivity, drug or drug hapten bound to protein may bind with antibody, forming circulating immune complexes.

In cell-mediated reactions, or type IV hypersensitivity, T lymphocytes are sensitized, resulting in skin or organ damage. A drug may elicit symptoms through more than one mechanism, for example, penicillin allergy or serum sickness.

In allergic, cytotoxic, immune complex and cell-mediated reactions the evolution of symptoms often suggests an immunologic mechanism, although the exact mechanism may be impossible to establish and the diagnosis is commonly made on clinical grounds.

Certain medications have been associated with induction of ANA. This may lead to a clinical picture of rashes or arthritis-like symptoms.

DIAGNOSTIC STUDIES AND FINDINGS

There are no simple, rapid, and predictable in vitro tests, nor is there safe and reliable in vivo testing for most adverse drug reactions. Demonstration of IgE antibody is limited to selected cases. No test is available for non–drug-related reactions, drug-related intolerance, or anaphylactoid adverse drug reactions. The clinical history is the most important tool in diagnosing adverse drug reactions.

Drug history: All drugs taken by patient within last 2 weeks, including over-the-counter preparations; time between exposure and symptom onset (delay of 7 to 10 days is common); route of administration and duration of treatment; prior drug exposure; onset, progression of severity, and nature of symptoms; clinical course after drug is discontinued; concomitant diseases; infectious disease history

Table 16-12 Medications Used in Treatment of Adverse Drug Reactions

Mechanism	Potential Organ Involvement	Categories of Medications
Type I hypersensitivity, anaphylactoid reactions	Skin Upper and lower respiratory tract Upper airway Gastrointestinal tract	Antihistamines Sympathomimetic agents Bronchodilators Corticosteroids
Type II, cytotoxica	Gastrointestinal tract, skin	Rarely immunosuppressive agents (e.g., azothiaprine, cyclophosphamide, nonsteroidal antiinflammatory agents)
	Renal	Corticosteroids
	Hematologic	Oral corticosteroids
Type III, immune complex	Vascular, skin, kidney, heart, liver	Nonsteroidal antiinflammatory agents
Type IV, cell-mediated	Skin	Antihistamines, topical corticosteroids

Skin testing: Limited because of lack of knowledge of true antigen-inducing response; available only for penicillin, toxoids, antisera, insulin, adrenocorticotropic hormone (ACTH), egg-based protein; must be done under strict protocol with close supervision

Patch testing: Useful in diagnosing contact sensitivity to topical preparation only

RAST: Not generally useful for drug allergy; useful for chymopapain

Enzyme assays: See specific enzyme deficiency disease, G6PD

Eosinophil levels: May be elevated in inflammatory tissue response

Anti-DNA (12%): May be elevated (single stranded) in certain drug-induced reactions

ANA (1:20): Speckled or homogeneous pattern

Complete blood count with differential: Leukocytosis in serum sickness

Erythrocyte sedimentation rate: May be elevated in inflammatory tissue response

Direct challenge: Can confirm suspected drug but is generally not done because of potential morbidity and mortality

Multidisciplinary Plan

The goal of the treatment plan is to eliminate the offending drug and thus prevent further symptoms. Most symptoms respond quickly to removal of the offending drug and resolve without therapy. Choice of medications and supportive therapy is dependent on the nature and severity of symptoms, organ system involved, and mechanism of the reactions.

Medications

See Table 16-12.

General Management

Forcing fluids to increase renal clearance of drug

Plasmapheresis to remove circulating immune complexes

Hemodialysis or peritoneal dialysis in severe overdose to remove drug rapidly

Emesis or stomach lavage to remove drug in overdose

Patient with allergic drug reaction should not receive that drug or cross-reacting one, if possible

If drug must be given, informed consent and administration under strict protocol necessary

Always check history before administering a new drug

NURSING CARE

Nursing Assessment

Adverse drug reactions have multiple mechanisms. Coincidental symptom assessment varies, because it is based on manifestations of the disease process. Drug-related reactions of overdose toxicity, side effects, intolerance, and secondary effects are related to specific drugs, and knowledge of the drug mechanisms makes it possible to identify potential symptoms. In immunologic mechanisms, organ system involvement may also be variable. The reader is referred elsewhere in this text for specific organ assessment.

Type I hypersensitivity, anaphylactoid reactions: See section on anaphylaxis

Type II, cytotoxic
- Hematologic status: See assessment for hemolytic anemia, thrombocytopenia, agranulocytosis
- Renal status: See assessment for interstitial nephritis

Type III, immune complex
- Serum sickness
- Drug fever: Systemic—low-grade fever, malaise
- Drug-induced lupus: See lupus assessment
- Vasculitis: See vasculitis assessment

Type IV, cell mediated: Contact dermatitis; photosensitivity eruptions

Potential Complications

Respiratory arrest, cardiopulmonary arrest

Patient Problems/Nursing Diagnoses & Interventions

Nursing interventions are based on the mechanisms and the organ involved. Refer to the discussion of the specific organ involved for the nursing diagnosis and nursing interventions.

NIC Risk Management

Risk for injury related to adverse antibody-antigen interaction

- Obtain complete drug allergy history before administering new drug.

- Put labels concerning allergic drug history in appropriate places.
- Closely monitor patient for 30 minutes after administering new drug intramuscularly, subcutaneously, or intravenously.
- Maintain emergency equipment and drugs, and be prepared to use them.
- Maintain high index of suspicion with patients receiving any medications.
- Monitor patient for development of new symptoms during course of medication therapy and for 2 weeks after drug administration ends.

PATIENT EDUCATION/CONTINUUM OF CARE PLAN

1. Explain to patient the relationship of symptoms to adverse drug reaction.
2. Explain to patient the absolute necessity of avoiding use of causative agents.
3. Explain to patient the need to carry appropriate identification and to share information when necessary.
4. Provide information to patient on medical alert identification.

EVALUATION/PATIENT OUTCOMES

Risk Management: Patient is symptom free. Patient can identify causative drug and explain appropriate avoidance measures.

ANGIOEDEMA (AND URTICARIA)

Angioedema is soft tissue swelling in submucosal or subcutaneous tissues as the result of increased local vascular permeability and serum transudation. Urticarial lesions occur in the upper stratum corneum of the dermis, whereas angioedema lesions occur in the deeper subcutaneous tissues.[27,28,43]

Urticaria (discussed in detail in Chapter 7) and angioedema have the same pathophysiologic features. Urticaria is more common; angioedema may be associated with urticaria or may occur independently. Why some patients have urticaria and others have angioedema is not known.

Angioedema may occur anywhere on the skin, but the periorbital area, lips, throat, tongue, larynx, area around joints, and tips of the extremities are the most common sites. Urticaria and angioedema may occur at any age, and as much as 20% of the population may be affected with acute, self-limited episodes. Episodes greater than 6 weeks in duration are defined as chronic. Symptoms may be mild or life threatening, and death may result from laryngeal involvement.

PATHOPHYSIOLOGY

With antigen-antibody linkage, mast cell or basophil degranulation and chemical mediator release occur. Histamine and other mediators interact with receptors along the lymphatic, capillary, and venule walls, resulting in dilation, engorgement, and increased capillary permeability with a perivascular mononuclear cell infiltrate in which eosinophils may predominate. This inflammatory response usually resolves within 6 hours after insult, although in soft tissues nonpitting edema may be more diffuse and reabsorption of fluid may take up to several days. Complaints of burning pain or tightness are more commonly associated with angioedema than is pruritus.

Other immunologic mechanisms may precipitate the same pathophysiologic response.

Physical or environmental factors may also trigger or exacerbate urticaria and angioedema (Table 16-13). In addition, urticaria and angioedema may occur in different disease states (Table 16-14). In as many as 60% of cases, no causative agent can be identified.

DIAGNOSTIC STUDIES AND FINDINGS

History: Exceptionally important onset; distribution; aggravating and ameliorating factors; time sequencing; food history; past, current, and infective history; contactant or insect exposures; family and atopic history; occupational, hobby, and environmental history; travel.

Drug history: Any medications, including over-the-counter and oral contraceptive preparations, may precipitate urticaria and angioedema

Clinical examination: All areas of potential involvement: periorbit, oropharynx, joints, tips of extremities

Tests: See Table 16-15

Table 16-13 Mechanisms of Angioedema

Mediator	Example	Proposed Mechanism
IMMUNOLOGIC		
Circulating immune complexes	Autoimmune phenomena	Activation of complement cascade
Cytotoxic antibodies	Transfusion reactions	Activation of complement cascade
Antigen-antibody complexes	Serum sickness reactions; malignancies	Activation of complement cascade
Drugs—directly or as haptens	Opiates; muscle relaxants; dextran	Direct mast cell degranulation
Foods—directly or as haptens	Tomatoes; strawberries; citrus fruits	Direct mast cell degranulation
Chemicals—directly or as haptens	Radiocontrast media; thiamine; bile salts	Direct mast cell degranulation
Drugs	Aspirin; indomethacin	Alteration of arachidonic acid metabolism
Chemical additives	Tartrazine	Alteration of arachidonic acid metabolism

Continued

Table 16-13 Mechanisms of Angioedema—cont'd

Mediator	Example	Proposed Mechanism
NONIMMUNOLOGIC		
Pressure	Tight garments; sitting	Unknown
Vibratory	Electric shavers; steering wheels	Unknown; autosomal dominant; genetically transmitted
Solar (five types)	Exposed areas	Unknown except for type IV, production of erythrocytic protoporphyria
Aquagenic	Water contact, regardless of temperature	Unknown
Heat	Direct contact	Unknown
Cholinergic	Heat exposure; emotional stress; vigorous exercise	Release of acetylcholine from cholinergic sympathetic nerve fibers
Cold	Delayed onset (30 minutes to 4 hours)	Autosomal dominant inheritance
	Exposed areas, immediate response	Unknown
	Associated with underlying disease	Presence of abnormal proteins with cold-dependent properties: cold hemoglobins, cryofibrinogens, cold agglutinins, cryoglobulins

Table 16-14 Diseases Associated With Angioedema

Type	Proposed Mechanisms
Systemic mastocytosis	Accumulation of mast cells that spontaneously or easily degranulate in dermis, bone marrow, and gastrointestinal tract
Infections: viral parasitic (infectious mononucleosis, hepatitis), rarely bacterial	Circulating antigen-antibody complexes with activation of complement cascade
Endocrinopathies: hyperthyroidism, pregnancy, menses	Unknown
Hereditary angioedema	Autosomal dominant, genetically inherited deficiency or malfunction of C1 esterase inhibitor with activation of complement cascade
Malignancies	In addition to antigen-antibody complexes, interference with C1 esterase inhibitor and resultant activation of complement cascade
Psychogenic	Rarely primary but may be exacerbating factor through hormonal and neural secretory mediators

MULTIDISCIPLINARY PLAN

The goal of the treatment plan is to prevent symptoms of angioedema. Obviously, with removal of the causative agent, no further therapy is necessary.

Medications

Antihistamines are the drugs of choice.

Drugs Used in Hereditary Angioedema

Hormones: Danazol (Danocrine), 200 mg tid; androgen derivative; contraindicated in children and pregnancy

Hemostatic agents

Aminocaproic acid, 3.5 mg qid for adults; antifibrinolytic agent, plasminogen inhibitor

Transexamic acid, 1 g tid for adults before dental procedures, etc.

Blood products: Fresh-frozen plasma during acute attacks

Drugs Used in Urticaria and Angioedema

Antihistamines*

Cyproheptadine (Periactin), 4-8 mg PO q6h

Chlorpheniramine (Chlor-Trimeton), 2 mg/kg/24 h PO in 4 divided doses

Clemastine (Tavist), 1.34 or 2.68 mg PO q8-12h

Diphenhydramine (Benadryl), 25-100 mg PO q6h or 5 mg/kg/day

Doxepin (Sinequan), 10-30 mg PO q8-12h

Histamine receptor antagonists*

Cimetidine (Tagamet), 300 mg PO q6h

Ranitidine (Zantac), 150 mg PO q12h

Famotidine (Pepcid), 20 mg PO q12h

Hydroxyzine (Atarax), 25 mg PO q6h to maximum total of 400 mg

Adrenergic agents

Appear to be of limited value in long-term therapy but may be employed for control of acute symptoms

Epinephrine

Aqueous (Adrenalin), 0.2-0.3 ml subcutaneously q30min or 0.01 mg/kg

Long-acting (Sus-Phrine), 0.1-0.3 ml subcutaneously q4-6h or 0.005 mg/kg (maximum dose 0.15 ml)

Ephedrine (Bronkaid), 20-50 mg q4h or 3 mg/kg/24 h in 4 divided doses

Corticosteroids

May be used if symptoms are unresponsive to above therapy but should be limited to lowest possible dose and alternate-day therapy with monitoring of side effects

Prednisone (Deltasone, Orasone, Liquid Pred), 2 mg/kg/day up to 100 mg

*Available in syrup form; dosage calculated by patient's weight.

Table 16-15 Diagnostic Tests for Urticaria and Angioedema

Condition Suspected	Test*
Atopic: food or drug (inhalent or contactant) sensitivity	Elimination of offending agent; daily symptom diary; challenge with suspected foods; skin tests to food or selected drugs; total serum IgE determination; eosinophil count; skin tests or radioallergosorbent tests of suspected antigens
Cutaneous vasculitis or systemic collagen vascular disease	Immunoglobulin analysis; antinuclear antibody; rheumatoid factor; cryoglobulins; cryofibrinogens; complete complement profile; skin biopsy with immunofluorescence
Hereditary angioedema	C4; C2; C3; total hemolytic complement (CH50); C1 esterase inhibitor (immunochemical and functional assays)
Physical urticaria	
Dermatographia	Firm stroke on skin with tongue blade
Cold	Ice cube test; cryoglobulins; cryofibrinogens; VDRL test
Cholinergic urticaria	Exercise challenge; methacholine skin test
Solar urticaria	Exposure to various wavelengths of light; protoporphyrin and coproporphyrin determinations
Pressure urticaria and angioedema	Application of pressure with weights for 10 minutes
Vibratory angioedema	Vibratory stimulation of skin for 4 minutes
Aquagenic urticaria	Tap-water challenge at various temperatures
Infections	Appropriate cultures and x-rays; stool for ova and parasites; hepatitis B antigen and antibody
Urticaria pigmentosa	Test for dermatographia; skin biopsy
Malignancy with angioedema	Total hemolytic complement (CH50); C1; C1-esterase inhibitor
Idiopathic urticaria	Skin biopsy with immunofluorescence

From Fineman.[12]
*General screening consists of complete blood count, urinalysis, and erythrocyte sedimentations rate determination.

Topical agents

Sun blockers with sun protection factor of at least 15 (Total Eclipse [15-18], Super Shade [15], Coppertone [15], Pre Sun [20]); used to block ultraviolet light in solar urticaria

Mild analgesics for pain associated with swelling

General Management

Cool compresses to reduce periorbital edema; restricted activity during acute episodes; endotracheal tube placement or tracheostomy for extensive laryngeal involvement

NURSING CARE

Nursing Assessment

Because angioedema may have multiorgan involvement, careful assessment should be made of all potential organ systems.

Laryngeal involvement: Hoarseness; stridor; use of accessory muscles; difficulty in speech
Skin integrity: Concurrent urticaria
Ocular status: Periorbital edema
Gastrointestinal status: Nausea; vomiting; diarrhea; gastrointestinal swelling
Oropharyngeal status: Swelling of lip, tongue, and uvula
Articular status: Swelling at tips of extremities, in soft tissue, and around joints

Potential Complications

Respiratory arrest, cardiopulmonary arrest

Patient Problems/Nursing Diagnoses & Interventions

NIC Respiratory Management

Ineffective breathing pattern related to allergic response

- Maintain endotracheal tube or tracheostomy if instituted.
- Assess for presence of laryngeal involvement, including stridor, hoarseness, and difficulty in speech or swallowing. Record if present.

NIC Risk Management

Risk for injury related to allergic response

- Obtain complete history of drug allergies before administering new drug.
- Put labels indicating allergic drug history in all appropriate places.
- Closely monitor patient for 30 minutes after administering each new drug.

Patient Education/Continuum of Care Plan

1. Explain to patient the relationship between symptoms and exposure to causative agent.
2. Explain to patient the necessity of avoiding use of causative agent.
3. Explain to patient the need, if appropriate, to carry appropriate identification and to share information when necessary.
4. Provide patient with information on medical alert identification.
5. Teach patient self-administration, if appropriate, of epinephrine and subsequent measures, including oral administration of antihistamine and seeking immediate medical care.

Evaluation/Patient Outcomes

Risk Management: Patient is symptom free, bowel sounds and elimination pattern are normal with no evidence of soft tissue swelling or joint restriction.

Respiratory Management: There are no subjective feelings of tightness or swelling, hoarseness, or difficulty in swallowing, speech, or air movement.

Patient can identify triggering agent and explain appropriate avoidance measures. Patient can identify appropriate medications to use, dosage, and length of therapy if symptoms occur.

Patient can identify nondrug therapeutic measures to institute if symptoms occur.

Collaborative Interventions and Related Nursing Care

Bone Marrow Transplantation

Description and Rationale

Bone marrow transplantation (BMT) is the treatment of choice for patients with severe aplastic anemia who are younger than 50 years of age and have a compatible donor. Marrow transplantation is also a treatment modality for severe immunodeficiency disorders and is being used with increasing success in the treatment of patients with leukemia, lymphoma, and selected solid tumors.

Bone marrow is harvested in the operating room with the donor under general or spinal anesthesia. Multiple aspirations from the posterior iliac crests are performed; if necessary the anterior iliac crests and sternum may be used. A small volume of bone marrow is collected with each aspiration and placed into tissue culture medium containing heparin. This solution is filtered through stainless steel screens to remove bone chips, fat globules, and clots and then is transferred to a blood transfusion bag.

The amount of bone marrow aspirated depends on a number of factors: the donor's weight, the concentration of cells in donated marrow, and the processing procedures employed before the marrow is transfused. If no special processing is done, the volume of marrow obtained is approximately 10 to 15 ml/kg of the recipient's body weight. In the typical adult a volume of 500 to 750 ml of blood and marrow contains 10 to 20 $\times 10^9$ nucleated marrow cells.

After harvesting, the marrow is either administered intravenously to the recipient through a central venous access device such as a Hickman or Raaf catheter or is cryopreserved and stored for future use. In the latter case, which occurs only with autologous bone marrow transplantation, the harvested marrow may be treated before cryopreservation to eliminate any occult tumor cells that may be present, especially in lymphohemopoietic malignancies. Ex vivo treatment with 4-hydroperoxycyclophosphamide (4-HC), an analog of cyclophosphamide, is one method used to treat the marrow. More recently, immunologic approaches using monoclonal antibodies are being tested in clinical trials for diseases such as T cell lymphoma and common acute lymphocytic leukemia (ALL).

Until recently most marrow transplants have involved donors of two types: an identical twin or an HLA-matched, mixed lymphocyte culture (MLC)–compatible sibling. A syngeneic transplant, using marrow from an identical twin, is ideal because the donor is matched with the recipient at all genetic loci.

Transplantation using marrow from anyone other than an identical twin or the patient himself or herself is called an allogeneic transplant. In most allogeneic bone marrow transplants a sibling who matches at HLA-A, HLA-B, HLA-C, and HLA-D loci is the donor. The HLA loci are on a small chromosomal region of the sixth chromosome; these loci are usually inherited as a unit known as a haplotype. Each parent has two haplotypes, and a child inherits one haplotype from each parent. A 25% probability exists that two siblings will be HLA identical.

A partially matched donor (such as a sibling, parent, or uncle) may be selected when no HLA-identical sibling is available, or an HLA-identical unrelated donor may be used. The chances of finding an unrelated HLA-identical donor are 1:50,000. Preliminary reports using partially matched or unrelated identical donors are encouraging, but further investigation in this area is needed.

A third form of bone marrow transplantation, the autologous graft, involves use of the patient's own marrow. As with the identical twin situation, in this circumstance no clinically significant graft-versus-host disease (GVHD) will occur. However, with autologous grafts, tumor cells may be present in marrow harvested during remission; therefore attempts to purge marrow of occult tumor cells before cryopreservation are being investigated. Autologous bone marrow transplants are now being completed on a regular basis. The results from this type of transplant are encouraging.

The rationale for bone marrow transplantation is to replace defective or missing host hemopoietic stem cells with healthy stem cells. In the treatment of neoplasm the transplant is done after therapy designed to rid the patient of the tumor. The patient's normal bone marrow is destroyed with high-dose therapy, and the transplant is designed to repopulate the patient's hemopoietic system.

Graft-Versus-Host Disease

GVHD presumably results from the attack of host tissue by immunocompetent donor T lymphocytes. In acute cases the peak onset occurs 30 to 50 days after the transplant. In chronic cases the onset occurs 100 days after the transplant. Tables 16-16 and 16-17 give two systems for the clinical staging of GVHD.

Conditioning Regimen

Pretransplant conditioning regimens include high-dose chemotherapy with or without radiotherapy. The purposes of condi-

Table 16-16 Proposed Clinical Stage of Graft-Versus-Host Disease According to Organ System

Stage	Skin	Liver	Intestinal Tract
+	Maculopapular rash over 25% of body surface	Bilirubin 2-3 mg/dl	Greater than 500 ml diarrhea/day
++	Maculopapular rash over 25%-50% of body surface	Bilirubin 3-6 mg/dl	Greater than 1000 ml diarrhea/day
+++	Generalized erythroderma	Bilirubin 6-15 mg/dl	Greater than 1500 ml diarrhea/day
++++	Generalized erythroderma with bullous formation and desquamation	Bilirubin greater than 15 mg/dl	Severe abdominal pain with or without ileus

From Thomas.[39]

tioning are to eliminate defective stem cells, to provide immunosuppression to minimize the possibility of rejection, and to eliminate any residual malignant cells.

The conditioning regimen used before bone marrow transplantation varies depending on the disease being treated. The use of multiple-day chemotherapy may or may not be preceded or followed by local or total body irradiation (TBI).

Preprocedural Nursing Care

Immediate concerns are related to the conditioning regimen using chemoradiotherapy. The patient, family, donor, and significant others are instructed in the procedure, its course, and complications.

Radiation. Dose varies, in general from 800 to 1200 cGy. For example, 1000 cGy may be given in fractionated doses (250 cGy per day). Single-dose whole body irradiation may be used. Typical side effects include nausea, vomiting, diarrhea, erythema of the skin, and parotitis. These side effects are usually of short duration when moderate fractionated radiotherapy is used. With the exception of erythema of the skin, they usually resolve within 7 days.

Chemotherapy. Side effects are usual after administration of chemotherapeutic agents. These side effects will vary with the agent used but may include nausea, vomiting, stomatitis, diarrhea, electrolyte imbalances, renal dysfunction, and pancytopenia. Symptoms of side effects specific to each agent must be known, observed for, reported, and treated.

Multidisciplinary Plan

Infusion of bone marrow is used to restore defective or missing stem cells. For autologous marrow, blood bags containing approximately 50 ml of cryopreserved marrow are thawed quickly, one at a time, in a basin of warm water at approximately 100°F. The contents of the blood bag are removed using a 50-ml syringe with a 16-gauge needle and then administered rapidly through a central line (double-lumen Raaf catheter or Hickman catheter). A solution of 0.9 normal saline is infused during the procedure. Epinephrine, diphenhydramine, and hydrocortisone are kept at the bedside.

For a syngeneic or allogeneic donation, a standard type of blood bag containing fresh bone marrow just obtained from a donor is transported from the operating room. The donated marrow is administered slowly (over a period of 4 hours) through a right atrial catheter without a filter.

Table 16-17 Overall Clinical Grading of Severity of Graft-Versus-Host Disease

Grade	Degree of Organ Involvement
I	+ to ++ skin rash; no gut involvement; no liver involvement; no decrease in clinical performance
II	+ to +++ skin rash; + gut involvement or + liver involvement (or both); mild decrease in clinical performance
III	++ to +++ skin rash; ++ to +++ gut involvement or ++ to ++++ liver involvement (or both); marked decrease in clinical performance
IV	Similar to grade III with ++ to ++++ organ involvement and extreme decrease in clinical performance

From Thomas.[39]

NURSING CARE

Nursing Assessment

Fluid overload: Increased respiratory rate; dyspnea; rales, rhonchi

Micropulmonary emboli: Shortness of breath; chest pain; increased heart rate

Reaction to white cells in marrow: Chills; fever; urticaria; chest pain

Hematuria: Hemastix-positive urine normal for first 24 hours after bone marrow transplant

Bacterial contamination of marrow: Hypotension; fever; shaking chills

Engraftment: No evidence of hematologic recovery 2 to 4 weeks after bone marrow transplant

Infection: Fever; pain; redness; swelling of any site; wound drainage; cough; dyspnea; sore throat; headache; dysuria; frequency; urgency; positive blood culture findings; change in mental status

Anemia: Decreased red blood cell count, hematocrit, and hemoglobin level; excessive fatigue

Stomatitis: Oral soreness; dryness; burning or tingling; taste changes; erythema; ulcerations or patches on oral mucosa

Thombocytopenia: Petechiae; purpura; bleeding from any body orifice or site of catheter; hemoptysis; hematemesis, hematuria; hematochezia; seizures; change in mental status

Nutritional status: Anorexia; decreased weight; nausea; vomiting; diarrhea

Psychosocial status: Anger, depression; frustration; anxiety

GVHD: Mild maculopapular rash; generalized erythroderma with desquamation; increase in serum bilirubin, serum glutamic oxaloacetic transaminase (SGOT), or alkaline phosphatase; abdominal cramping; diarrhea (green, watery); hematochezia

Veno-occlusive disease (VOD): Sudden weight gain; right upper quadrant pain; jaundice; hepatomegaly; ascites; encephalopathy

Potential Complications

Hypervolemia, pulmonary emboli, sepsis

Patient Problems/Nursing Diagnoses & Interventions

NIC Fluid Management

Risk for excess fluid volume related to marrow infusion

- Monitor rate of infusion carefully *to decrease incidence of overload and to ensure completion of administration within 4 hours to prevent destruction of cells.*
- Assess vital signs and response to administration of marrow every 5 to 10 minutes during infusion, then every 30 minutes for 2 hours *to detect early signs of volume excess.*

NIC NUTRITION SUPPORT

Imbalanced nutrition: less than body requirements, related to nausea, vomiting, or inability to ingest nutrients because of chemotherapy

- Maintain calorie count, intake and output, and weight record *to ensure required nutrients are taken* (33 to 38 kcal/kg, 1.5 g protein/kg and 2500 to 3000 ml fluid).
- Eliminate predisposing factors for nausea and vomiting when possible; collaborate with physician to determine best time and type of medication most effective *to prevent onset of symptoms.*
- Arrange dietary consultation *to adjust dietary and fluid intake.*
- Consider use of behavioral relaxation techniques.
- Provide frequent oral hygiene.
- Instruct patient to avoid quick movements while nauseated.
- Encourage patient to eat or drink when not nauseated regardless of the time.
- Encourage patient to eat slowly and chew thoroughly.
- Suggest high-protein, high-calorie diet.
- Suggest small, frequent, low-fat meals.
- Encourage patient to drink liquids (clear, cool beverages or soups) slowly through a straw before, not during, meals.
- Provide patient with beverages or foods that may curb nausea; carbonated beverages such as cola or ginger ale; dry crackers or toast; tart foods such as lemons or sour pickles; ice pops and gelatin desserts.
- Instruct patient to avoid favorite foods during periods of nausea.
- Instruct patient to avoid lying flat for at least 1 hour after eating.
- Administer TPN when ordered if the patient is unable to ingest food or fluids; monitor electrolytes, urine glucose, proteins, and ketones.

NIC RISK MANAGEMENT

Risk for infection related to leukopenia

- Maintain protective environment. (Reverse isolation protocols vary among centers from simple protective isolation to sterile laminar airflow rooms.)
- Monitor white blood cell count and absolute granulocyte count daily.
- Monitor vital signs every 4 hours.
- Check skin and mucous membranes.
- Inspect all body orifices daily for redness, swelling, and pain.
- Auscultate lungs every 8 hours for increased or decreased breath sounds, rhonchi, and rales.
- Inspect site of insertion of venous access device for redness, swelling, and pain.
- Assess patient for complaints of dysuria and frequency.
- Note any change from patient's baseline vital signs, behavior, or appearance.
- Encourage turning, coughing, and deep breathing exercises.
- Maintain integrity of skin and mucous membranes. (Skin care measures vary among centers from use of povidone-iodine to use of antibacterial soap.)
- Maintain meticulous mouth care. (Mouth care varies among centers.)
- Use strict aseptic technique when changing dressings.
- Use strict aseptic technique in intravenous preparation and administration.
- Avoid bladder catheterization.
- Avoid administering enemas and suppositories and taking rectal temperatures.
- Encourage patient to use deodorant rather than antiperspirant. (Axillary sweat glands are blocked by antiperspirants, which may promote infection.)
- Obtain surveillance cultures of throat, urine, stool, skin, and other areas as ordered. (Need for surveillance cultures to detect colonization before infection is controversial.)
- Maintain dietary restrictions as ordered. (Efficacy of bacteria diets has not been established.)
- Eliminate stagnant water in patient's room.
- Do not allow fresh-cut flowers or plants in patient's room.
- Limit number of visitors, and screen them for infection, recent vaccinations, or exposure to communicable diseases.
- Provide mask, gloves, and gown for patient when patient leaves room.
- Obtain culture and sensitivity tests and Gram's stain of all potential sites of infection per physician's order.
- Administer antibiotics on schedule per physician's order.
- Control fever with tepid sponge baths and acetaminophen.
- Maintain adequate nutrition and hydration of patient.
- Administer colony-stimulating factors as ordered.

NIC TISSUE PERFUSION MANAGEMENT

Ineffective tissue perfusion (bladder) related to local effect of cyclophosphamide

Decreased cardiac output related to effects of cyclophosphamide

Risk for injury related to thrombocytopenia

- Begin intravenous hydration 4 hours before cyclophosphamide administration and continue for 24 hours after therapy. Intravenous fluids should be administered 1½ to 2 times maintenance rates.
- Perform continuous bladder irrigations using three-way Foley catheter if ordered. If patient can void every hour to eliminate toxic products of cyclophosphamide that irritate bladder lining, catheter is unnecessary.
- Monitor urine for blood every 4 hours.
- Maintain accurate intake and output records.
- Check results of ECG for decreased voltage and transient changes. ECG is taken daily while patient is treated with high-dose cyclophosphamide.
- Monitor heart function continuously during drug administration *to check for cardiotoxicity.*
- Monitor platelet count regularly. *Risk of bleeding is high when platelet count is less than 10,000 cells/mm^3.*
- Inspect skin and mucous membranes daily. Monitor for increased bruising tendencies, petechiae, bleeding gums, and epistaxis.

- Test stool, urine, and emesis for occult blood.
- Note any changes in patient's vital signs or behavior. *Changes may indicate intracranial hemorrhage.*
- After invasive procedures such as bone marrow aspiration and biopsy, monitor site frequently for any oozing of blood.
- Avoid giving intramuscular or subcutaneous injections.
- Avoid taking rectal temperatures and administering rectal suppositories and enemas.
- Encourage adequate fluid intake and use of stool softener *to prevent constipation and straining.*
- Avoid invasive procedures.
- Place sign indicating bleeding precautions over patient's bed.
- Administer medroxyprogesterone acetate as ordered *to control menses.*
- Instruct patient to avoid cutting, bruising, or bumping self. Eliminate sharp objects in environment.
- Instruct patient to use electric razor rather than hand razor.
- Instruct patient to wear shoes or slippers—no bare feet while walking.
- Instruct patient to use soft-bristled toothbrush. If platelet count is less than 20,000/mm³, use toothette rather than a toothbrush.
- Flossing may be contraindicated. Instruct patient to discontinue if bleeding occurs.
- Instruct patient to avoid use of toothpicks.
- Teach patient to avoid use of aspirin and products containing aspirin.
- Teach patient to avoid use of all beverages containing alcohol.
- Instruct patient to avoid blowing nose forcefully or sneezing forcefully.
- If epistaxis occurs, keep patient in sitting position. Application of ice helps to constrict small vessels. Local application of pressure may control bleeding. Nasal packing may be indicated if these measures fail.
- Bleeding in oral cavity may be controlled with iced saline mouth rinses.
- Administer irradiated platelet transfusions rapidly as ordered. (Families are encouraged to find donors for blood products.) Monitor posttransfusion platelet counts.

NIC ACTIVITY AND EXERCISE MANAGEMENT

Activity intolerance related to anemia, disruption of sleep, or anxiety

- Administer irradiated red blood cell transfusions as ordered.
- Monitor hemoglobin levels and hematocrit values regularly.
- Arrange nursing care so patient has uninterrupted periods of rest and sleep, especially during the night.
- Encourage progressive activity program as tolerated.
- Encourage patient to verbalize feelings and concerns.
- Explain reasons for fatigue.

NIC SELF-CARE FACILITATION

Impaired oral mucous membrane related to conditioning regimen or infection

- Implement nursing care for stomatitis based on assessment using grading system developed by Capizzi et al[7a]
  - Grade 1: Generalized erythema of oral mucosa
  - Grade 2: Isolated small ulcerations or white patches
  - Grade 3: Confluent ulcerations with white patches covering more than 25% of oral mucosa
  - Grade 4: Hemorrhagic ulcerations
- For grade 1 or 2 stomatitis:
  - Perform oral hygiene regimen every 2 hours while awake and every 6 hours during night, as follows:
    - Use normal saline mouthwash if crusts are absent. (One teaspoon of salt in 1 L of sterile water may be used.) If crusts and debris are present, use either one part hydrogen peroxide* diluted† with three parts water‡ or sodium bicarbonate solution (1 teaspoon mixed in 8 ounces of water‡). Perform mouth care every 2 hours while patient is awake. Alternate either hydrogen peroxide or bicarbonate solution with normal saline. Rinse with normal saline after the use of either.
    - Floss gently with unwaxed dental floss every 24 hours; discontinue if bleeding occurs.
    - Brush, using soft toothbrush and nonabrasive toothpaste, after each meal and before sleep.
    - Remove dentures or partial plates. Replace only for meals. Keep meticulously clean.
    - Apply water-soluble lip lubricant four times a day and as needed.
  - Use measures for oral pain per physician's order Suggestions are:
    - Dyclonine (Dyclone) 0.5% or 1% (available in spray or gargle), 5 to 10 ml every hour
    - Viscous lidocaine (Xylocaine) 2%, 10 ml every 2 hours
    - Hydrocortisone (Orabase) or carbamide peroxide (Gly-Oxide) applied to affected sites
    - "Stomatitis cocktail": Equal parts viscous lidocaine (Xylocaine), diphenhydramine (Benadryl) elixir, and magnesium and aluminum hydroxide mixture (Maalox), 30 ml every 2 to 4 hours
    - One part diphenhydramine (Benadryl) elixir mixed with one part kaolin and pectin (Kaopectate), every 2 to 4 hours
  - Implement dietary measures, including the following:

---

*Hydrogen peroxide should not be used if the patient has fresh granulation tissue.

†Hydrogen peroxide solutions should be prepared immediately before use, because hydrogen peroxide decomposes rapidly in water.

‡Sterile water or normal saline should be used for mouthwash or dilution of agents when patients are immunosuppressed. Whether using nonsterile solutions for dilution increases the number of infections is unknown.

Instruct patient to avoid abrasive foods such as toast, apples, and celery.
Encourage intake of pureed, bland foods.
Instruct patient to avoid tart or acid foods, hot beverages, or iced drinks.
Instruct patient to avoid spices and vinegar.
Instruct patient to avoid alcohol.
Arrange for dietary consultation.
Discourage smoking.
Recommend use of artificial saliva for xerostomia. No comparative research of various agents is available.

- For grade 3 or 4 stomatitis:
  Obtain samples from suspicious area and culture—one culture for bacteria and one for fungus—per physician's order.
  Institute oral hygiene regimen:
    Alternate antifungal or antibacterial suspension with warm saline mouthwash every 2 hours while patient is awake and every 4 hours during night.
    Do not floss.
    Brush gently using toothettes or cotton-tipped applicators.
    Remove dentures or bridge. Do not replace for meals.
    Apply lip lubricant every 2 hours.
  In addition to local measures as indicated for grade 1 and 2 stomatitis, systemic analgesics may be indicated, especially before eating.
  Liquid diet may be indicated. If not, use pureed diet. See other dietary measures as indicated for grade 1 and 2 stomatitis.
  Discourage smoking.

NIC ELIMINATION MANAGEMENT

Diarrhea related to effects of total body irradiation on gastrointestinal mucosa or GVHD

- Administer antidiarrheal agents as ordered.
- Maintain adequate hydration.
- Suggest bland, low-residue diet that is high in potassium.
- Instruct patient in meticulous perianal skin care.
- Apply soothing lubricant to perianal area after each bowel movement.

NIC SKIN/WOUND MANAGEMENT

Risk for impaired skin integrity related to chemoradiotherapy or GVHD

- Assess skin integrity every 8 to 24 hours.
- Assess level of pain and pruritus, and administer analgesics and antihistamines as needed.
- Provide meticulous skin care, including daily bath with povidone-iodine and normal saline or other antibacterial solution. Oatmeal baths may be indicated for pruritus.
- Apply creams or lotions on intact skin *to minimize breakdown.*
- Explain need to prevent scratching. Use mittens if necessary on infant or child.
- Use gowns and linens washed in nondetergents *to prevent skin reactions.*
- Use flotation type of bed for patient with extensive skin involvement.
- Use bed cradle *to prevent linens from touching skin if patient has extensive skin involvement.*
- Assist patient frequently with turning and active or passive range-of-motion exercises.
- Provide meticulous perianal skin care.
- Observe and record frequency, amount, character, and presence of frank or occult blood for all stools.
- Teach patient to perform perianal care after each stool.
- Monitor closely for dehydration, electrolyte imbalance, and weight change.
- Administer replacement fluids containing electrolytes as ordered.
- Auscultate bowel sounds every 8 hours *to monitor for development of ileus.*
- Monitor bilirubin and SGOT levels daily.
- Measure abdominal girth twice a day.
- Position patient on left side *to decrease pressure on liver.*
- When ordered, permit nothing by mouth *to allow bowel to rest.*
- Reinstate oral feedings with iso-osmotic, low-fat, lactose-free beverages, as ordered, increasing to allowed diet when tolerated.

NIC PSYCHOLOGIC COMFORT PROMOTION

Anxiety related to uncertain outcome of treatment or severity of responses to chemoradiotherapy

- Encourage patient and significant others to express feelings and concerns and to ask questions *to dispel misconceptions.*
- Assist patient to use relaxation techniques, such as visual imagery, *to reduce anxiety.*
- Reinforce and restate information given to patient and significant others *to promote understanding.*
- Encourage patient and significant others to discuss hopes for positive outcome.
- Reassure that patient will not be alone and that care and treatment will be given when needed.
- Recognize and discuss use of positive coping methods.

PATIENT EDUCATION/CONTINUUM OF CARE PLAN

1. Teach patient self-care procedures: central line care, heparin flush, administration of TPN, and use of volumetric pump, when required; oral hygiene and skin care measures; hand-washing technique; use of incentive spirometer; temperature taking; urine and stool testing method for presence of blood; use of safety measures; and measurement of weight, intake, and output.
2. Teach patient to assess for signs or symptoms of infection, GVHD, veno-occlusive disease, renal involvement, anemia, and bleeding; teach patient when to report signs or symptoms.
3. Explain to patient the diet for optimum nutritional status. (Ideally patient must be able to tolerate 1000 calories a day to be discharged.)

4. Teach patient measures to prevent occurrence of infection. Precautions are more rigid during the first 3 months after bone marrow transplantation and are relaxed as the year progresses.
   a. Wear face mask when outside home.
   b. Avoid contact with young children who attend school.
   c. Avoid contact with anyone who has a cold or illness.
   d. Avoid crowds; go to grocery stores, theaters, restaurants, and other public places when they are not crowded.
   e. Avoid restaurant food for the first 3 months.
   f. Wear a mask. (Walks can be taken without wearing a mask, but one should be carried in case of contact with other pedestrians.)
   g. Wash hands well before eating, after using the toilet, and after contact with someone who has a cold.
   h. Avoid contact with any pets in living quarters for the first 3 months. Do *not* clean litter boxes or come in contact with animal feces.
   i. Avoid contact with plants and flowers.
   j. Do not swim in private or public pool for the first year after bone marrow transplant.
   k. Maintain good dental hygiene.
   l. Do not have immunizations without physician's approval.
   m. Take prophylactic antibiotics as prescribed.
5. Discuss with patient the routine measures for him or her to practice daily to minimize occurrence of complications.
6. Discuss with patient the daily maintenance of home environment, equipment, and supplies.
7. Emphasize to patient the importance of ongoing health and mental health care.

EVALUATION/PATIENT OUTCOMES

Fluid Management: Patient's vital signs remain stable; lung sounds are clear on auscultation.

Nutrition Support: Patient's weight is maintained or loss is less than 5% of original body weight; patient takes required nutrients and fluids, or patient maintains TPN without difficulty—no nausea, vomiting, or diarrhea is present.

Risk Management: Patient's vital signs are within normal limits; skin and mucous membranes are clear, warm, and with good turgor; lungs are clear; patient remains oriented.

Tissue Perfusion Management: Patient's intake and output are balanced; patient voids without difficulty; urine is clear, light yellow.

Patient's ECG shows normal sinus rhythm without changes; cardiac rate and rhythm are within normal range.

Patient shows no evidence of bruising, petechiae, or bleeding; platelet count is normal; patient remains infection free.

Activity and Exercise Management: Patient tolerates activity with minimal fatigue and feels rested.

Self-Care Facilitation: Signs and symptoms of stomatitis have been minimized. Patient tolerates oral intake with minimal/absent discomfort.

Elimination Management: Stool consistency and pattern of elimination are within normal limits.

Skin/Wound Management: No lesions or breaks are present; patient demonstrates skin and oral care.

Psychologic Comfort Promotion: Patient discusses feelings and responses freely. Patient remains relaxed, participates in care, and uses grooming techniques to enhance appearance. Patient makes plans to effect lifestyle changes.

CORTICOSTEROIDS

Synthetic corticosteroids are pharmacologic agents that mimic the effects of the major endogenous glucocorticoid, cortisol. They are used in the treatment of many immunologic diseases because of their potent antiinflammatory and immunosuppressive effects. Corticosteroids exert their widespread effects by initially binding to a specific cytoplasmic receptor protein that is present on most cells. This complex then enters the nucleus, where alteration in the rate of synthesis of specific proteins occurs.

Synthetic corticosteroids should be used with caution in persons with hepatic disease or hypoalbuminemia or in patients who are receiving phenytoin, barbiturates, or rifampin. Lower-dose therapy is recommended in these cases. In addition, care should be exercised in prescribing steroid therapy for persons who are predisposed to or have known histories of diabetes, osteoporosis, peptic ulcer disease, infections, hypertension, psychosis, or coronary artery disease.

A major concern with the use of corticosteroid therapy is suppression of the hypothalamic-pituitary-adrenocortical axis (HPAA) (Table 16-18). Exogenous steroids provide negative feedback to this mechanism, which promotes total body homeostasis via the regulation of cortisol production. Therefore suppression of the HPAA results in widespread systemic manifestations. To limit this untoward effect, steroids are administered in as low a dosage as possible to control the disease for which they are being prescribed. However, to control acute exacerbations of many inflammatory disorders, corticosteroids are usually prescribed initially in relatively high doses (greater than 40 mg daily), so HPAA suppression is unavoidable. Once the disease is under control, the dosage is lowered at a rate of 2.5 to 5 mg per week. *Gradual* tapering of the dosage of corticosteroids is necessary, because the body cannot respond quickly to changes in cortisol levels owing to the initial suppression of the natural HPAA feedback mechanisms. It may take as long as 12 months for adaptation to occur when the patient has received high-dose therapy for a month or more. Although useful in controlling many clinical manifestations, steroid therapy is not without inherent dangers. Because these agents exert such widespread systemic effects, their adverse effects are diverse and often complicate the course of the disease for which they are being used.

The type and severity of side effects are dose dependent and related to the duration of therapy. Although alternate-day

Table 16-18 Comparison of Various Glucocorticoids With Hydrocortisone

Glucocorticoid	Antiinflammatory Potency	Equivalent Potency (mg)	Sodioum-Retaining Potency	Duration of HPAA Suppression (hours)
Hydrocortisone	1.0	20	2	12
Cortisone	0.8	25	2	12
Prednisolone	4.0	5	1	24-36
Prednisone	3.5	5	1	24-36
Methylprednisolone	5.0	4	0	24-36
Triamcinolone	5.0	4	0	24-36
Paramethasone	10.0	2	0	24-36
Betamethasone	25.0	0.60	0	More than 48
Dexamethasone	30.0	0.75	0	More than 48

therapy (single doses every other day) has been associated with fewer side effects, it is not recommended for control of acute disease.

γ-GLOBULIN THERAPY

γ-Globulin administration is indicated as replacement therapy for immunodeficiency diseases affecting the humoral or antibody-mediated immune system. Recurrent, severe, sinopulmonary infections are hallmark clinical manifestations of the humoral immunodeficiency diseases. The frequency and severity with which these infections occur assist the clinician in evaluating the effectiveness of γ-globulin therapy. γ-Globulin is also used to provide passive immunity against a variety of infectious agents, such as the hepatitis virus.

For the past 30 years, human immune serum globulin (HISG) has been available for intramuscular administration. Its use has effectively limited both the severity and frequency of infections in antibody immune deficient patients. The usual dose of HISG ranges from 100 to 200 mg/kg/month. Only IgG is present in significant quantities in HISG.

Although untoward side effects are uncommon, rare anaphylactic reactions to the intramuscular injections have been reported. Patients who have such reactions should be treated immediately with epinephrine and antihistamines. Later, therapy may resume, but HISG from a different manufacturer should be used following a skin test of HISG from the new lot.

Long-term monthly injections produce local pain. HISG is slowly degraded within the injection sites. The risk of entering the intravenous compartment in infants and malnourished patients is high. In addition, large doses of γ-globulins require multiple injections.

Recently, modified preparations of intravenous immune serum globulin (Gamimmune N, Intraglobin) have been available. Data indicate that these products are effective as replacement therapy. Larger doses of γ-globulin may be delivered with greater efficacy. Serum levels of IgG are reached early and maintained longer. In addition, minimum side effects are associated with its administration.

Doses of intravenous γ-globulin preparations range from 100 to 300 mg/kg/month to maintain IgG serum levels at a minimum of 200 mg/dl. The therapy is usually well tolerated, although chills, fever, and transient leukopenia have been reported. Several researchers indicate that intravenous γ-globulin therapy is highly superior, in terms of clinical efficacy, to intramuscularly administered immunoglobulin. Intravenous γ-globulin therapy appears to be useful for the treatment of patients who require large doses of immunoglobulin, debilitated patients who might not tolerate monthly intramuscular injections, and Wiskott-Aldrich patients who are prone to hemorrhage. It is used routinely in all bone marrow transplant patients and in all patients who have immunoglobulin deficiencies. Research to prolong platelet half-life is underway.

γ-Globulin is used for passive immunization in bone marrow transplant patients to provide passive immunity against a variety of infectious and viral agents. It is also used to protect against the hepatitis virus in the immunocompetent host.

IMMUNOTHERAPY

Immunotherapy has a role in the treatment of allergic and immune deficiency diseases, some autoimmune disorders, and cancer. In allergic diseases immunotherapy is used to hyposensitize the patient. (Desensitization is discussed elsewhere.) In immunodeficiency disease the aim is to restore absent or deficient products; for example, in X-linked hypogammaglobulinemia, treatment involves administration of γ-globulin. Patients with autoimmune disorders such as systemic lupus erythematosus may benefit from therapeutic plasmapheresis (a type of immunotherapy), with removal of circulating immune complexes. (Immunodeficiency and autoimmune disorders are discussed elsewhere.) Immunotherapy in the treatment of cancer, whether it is the sole form of treatment or used as adjunct therapy, is currently being investigated. There are now some forms of immunotherapy available for the oncology patient. Cancer immunotherapy is manipulation of the immune system to control or eliminate the growth of neoplastic cells.

PLASMAPHERESIS

Apheresis is the separation of the whole blood into its various components by passage through automated centrifugation devices or membrane filters. After fractionation, certain blood constituents are discarded, while others are returned to the donor. Apheresis can be performed as a therapeutic protocol or to obtain donor blood products.

Plasmapheresis is the procedure by which plasma is selectively removed from whole blood. This experimental therapeutic manipulation is employed in certain diseases to remove an abnormal constituent from the plasma or replenish a deficient

Table 16-19 Disorders Treated With Therapeutic Plasma Exchange

Disorder	Rationale
Autoimmune hemolytic anemia	Removal of antiplatelet antibodies
Myasthenia gravis	Removal of antibodies directed at acetylcholine receptor
Goodpasture's syndrome	Removal of anti–basement membrane antibodies
Multiple sclerosis	Removal of putative antimyelin antibodies
Systemic lupus erythematosus	Removal of circulating immune complexes
Amyloidosis	Removal of immunoglobulin
Thrombotic thrombocytopenic purpura	Replenishment of plasma factor

Table 16-20 Complications of Therapeutic Plasma Exchange

Complication	Nursing Care
Trauma or infection at site of vascular access	Keep entry site clean and dry; inspect regularly for signs of infection
Disequilibrium syndrome (nausea, diaphoresis, lightheadedness, tachycardia, and hypotension resulting from hypovolemia)	Monitor fluid balance and vital signs closely; administer fluids as needed; offer patient orange juice or saltines
Hypokalemia, hypocalcemia (which may predispose to cardiac irregularities)	Monitor electrolyte balance and replace electrolytes as needed
Bleeding owing to temporary depletion of platelets and clotting factors	Maintain safe environment; observe for signs of bleeding or bruising
Temporary paresthesias, muscle twitching, nausea, and vomiting owing to administration of citrated plasma	Provide comfort measures and reassurance; add calcium gluconate to replacement fluids
Anemia owing to hemolysis	Replace erythrocytes in combination with fluids or plasma
Increased risk of infection owing to depletion of certain plasma proteins	Observe for signs of infection
Transient peripheral edema owing to fluid shifts	Symptoms are transient, and no further treatment is warranted
Hypothermia owing to infusion of cool fluids	Provide extra blankets; prewarm replacement fluids

plasma factor. During therapeutic plasma exchange, patient plasma is removed and the cellular elements of the blood are reinfused following reconstitution with normal plasma or a suitable colloidal substitute.

Although not many well-controlled scientific studies concerning the therapeutic efficacy of plasmapheresis have been performed, it is being employed to treat a number of immunologic and nonimmunologic disorders. Conditions commonly treated with plasma exchange are outlined in Table 16-19.

Patients treated with plasmapheresis may expect to experience only temporary clinical improvement. Since therapeutic plasma exchange is designed to relieve the manifestations of a clinical disease process without affecting the underlying disorder, repeated treatments are usually indicated. Patients undergoing therapeutic plasma exchange to remove plasma antibodies of circulating immune complexes are treated concomitantly with immunosuppressive drugs to retard the recovery of immunoglobulin levels.

Although plasmapheresis is generally believed to be a benign procedure, a number of complications are associated with this treatment. These untoward effects and suggested patient management are described in Table 16-20.

REFERENCES

1. Amor B: Reiter's syndrome: diagnosis and clinical features, *Rheum Dis Clin North Am* 24(4):677, 1998.
2. Austin HA, Balow JE: Natural history and treatment of lupus nephritis, *Semin Nephrol* 19(1):2, 1999.
3. Barth WF, Segal K: Reactive arthritis (Reiter's syndrome), *Am Fam Physician* 60(2):499, 1999.
4. Belfer MH, Stevens RW: Sarcoidosis: a primary care review, *Am Fam Physician* 58(9):2041, 1998.
5. Brennan C, Porche DJ: HIV immunopathogenesis, *J Assoc Nurses AIDS Care* 8(4):7, 1997.
6. Bryant GA: Reiter's syndrome, *Orthop Nurs* 17(1):57, 1998.
7. Burrows PD, Cooper MD: IgA deficiency, *Adv Immunol* 65:245, 1997.

7a. Capizzi RL et al: Methotrexate therapy of head and neck cancer: improvement in therapeutic index by the use of leucovorin "rescue," *Cancer Res* 30:1782, 1970.

8. Chopra KF, Tyring SK: Current antiretroviral therapy in the treatment of HIV infection, *Semin Cutan Med Surg* 16(3):224, 1997.

8a. Copstead LC, Banasik JL: *Pathophysiology: biological and behavioral perspectives.* Phildelphia, 2000, WB Saunders.

9. Crane M et al: The interdisciplinary team's approach to lupus nephritis, *Lupus* 7(9):660, 1998.
10. de Groot K, Gross WL: Wegener's granulomatosis: disease course, assessment of activity and extent and treatment, *Lupus* 7(4):285, 1998.
11. Evans JM, Hunder GG: Polymyalgia rheumatica and giant cell arteritis, *Clin Geriatr Med* 14(3):455, 1998.
12. Fineman S: Urticaria and angioedema. In Lawlor GJ, editor: *Manual of allergy and immunology,* Boston, 1981, Little, Brown.
13. Fox RI et al: Evolving concepts of diagnosis, pathogenesis, and therapy of Sjèogren's syndrome, *Curr Opin Rheumatol* 10(5):446, 1998.
14. Freeman TM: Anaphylaxis: diagnosis and treatment, *Prim Care* 25(4):809, 1998.
15. Friedman-Klein AE, Laubenstein LS, editors: *AIDS: the epidemic of Kaposi's sarcoma and opportunistic infections,* New York, 1984, Masson.
16. Gavalas M, Sadana A, Metcalf S: Guidelines for the management of anaphylaxis in the emergency department, *J Accid Emerg Med* 15(2):96, 1998.
17. Gillmore JD, Hawkins PN, Pepys MB: Amyloidosis: a review of recent diagnostic and therapeutic developments, *Br J Haematol* 99(2):245, 1997.
18. Godfrey T, Khamashta MA, Hughes GR: Therapeutic advances in systemic lupus erythematosus, *Curr Opin Rheumatol* 10(5):435, 1998.

19. Gross WL: New concepts in treatment protocols for severe systemic vasculitis, *Curr Opin Rheumatol* 11(1):41, 1999.
20. Guillevin L, Lhote F: Treatment of polyarteritis nodosa and microscopic polyangiitis, *Arthritis Rheum* 41(12):2100, 1998.
21. Harman LE, Margo CE: Wegener's granulomatosis, *Surv Ophthalmol* 42(5):458, 1998.
22. Hunder G: Vasculitis: diagnosis and therapy, *Am J Med* 100(2A):37S, 1996.
23. Hunder GG: Giant cell arteritis, *Lupus* 7(4):266, 1998.
24. Husby G: Treatment of amyloidosis and the rheumatologist: state of the art and perspectives for the future [editorial], *Scand J Rheumatol* 27(3):161, 1998.
25. Jaffe IA:Wegener's granulomatosis and ANCA syndromes, *Neurol Clin* 15(4):887, 1997.
26. Krzystolik M, Power WJ, Foster CS: Diagnostic and therapeutic challenges of sarcoidosis, *Int Ophthalmol Clin* 38(1):61, 1998.
27. Kumar SA, Martin BL: Urticaria and angioedema: diagnostic and treatment considerations, *J Am Osteopath Assoc* 99(3 suppl):S1, 1999.
28. Kwong KY, Maalouf N, Jones CA: Urticaria and angioedema: pathophysiology, diagnosis, and treatment, *Pediatr Ann* 27(11):719, 1998.
29. Labbe P, Hardouin P: Epidemiology and optimal management of polymyalgia rheumatica, *Drugs Aging* 13(2):109, 1998.
30. Lawlor G, editor: *Manual of allergy and immunology,* Boston, 1981, Little, Brown.
31. Lhote F, Guillevin L: Polyarteritis nodosa, microscopic polyangiitis, and Churg-Strauss syndrome: clinical aspects and treatment, *Rheum Dis Clin North Am* 21(4):911, 1995.
32. Oxholm P, Prause JU, Schidt M: Rational drug therapy recommendations for the treatment of patients with Sjögren's syndrome, *Drugs* 56(3):345, 1998.
33. Rusznak C, Devalia JL, Davies RJ: Advances in the pharmacological treatment of allergic rhinitis, *Curr Probl Dermatol* 28:102, 1999.
34. Rybicki BA et al: Epidemiology, demographics, and genetics of sarcoidosis, *Semin Respir Infect* 13(3):166, 1998.
35. Schur P: *The clinical management of systemic lupus erythematosus,* New York, 1983, Grune & Stratton.
36. Spickett GP et al: Common variable immunodeficiency: how many diseases? *Immunol Today* 18(7):325, 1997.
37. Sumida T: Sjögren's syndrome, *Intern Med* 38(2):165, 1999.
38. Tabbara K, Sharara N: Sjögren's syndrome: pathogenesis, *Eur J Ophthalmol* 9(1):1, 1999.
38a. Thibodeau GA, Patton KT: *Anatomy & physiology,* ed 4, St Louis, 1999, Mosby.
39. Thomas ED: Bone marrow transplantation, *N Engl J Med* 292:896, 1975.
40. Tovilla-Canales JL: Ocular manifestations of giant cell arteritis, *Curr Opin Ophthalmol* 9(6):73, 1998.
41. Unawe BR, Benacerraf B: *Textbook of immunology,* Baltimore, 1984, Williams & Wilkins.
42. Van Cauwenberge P, Watelet JB, Bachert C: New insights in the pathogenesis of allergic rhinitis, *Curr Probl Dermatol* 28:95, 1999.
43. Wagner WO: Angioedema: frightening and frustrating, *Cleve Clin J Med* 66(4):203, 1999.

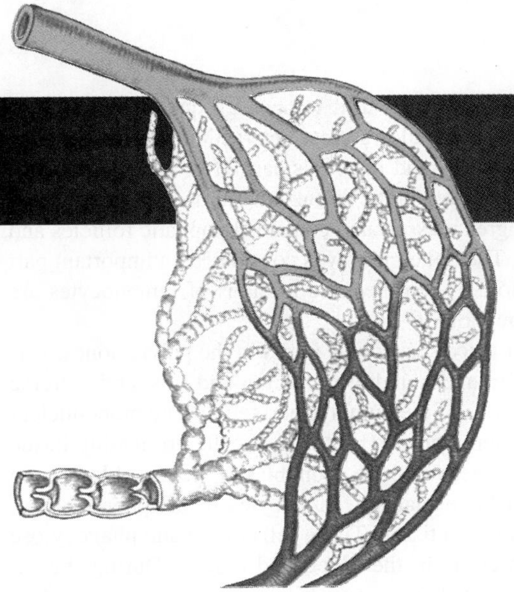

17 Hematolymphatic System

Anne Elizabeth Belcher

Overview

The hematolymphatic system is composed of blood and blood-forming organs, the bone marrow, the spleen, the liver, and the lymphatics.

Blood, which circulates continuously through the heart and vascular system, performs numerous vital functions, such as (1) transporting oxygen and absorbed nutrients to cells; (2) transporting waste products, including carbon dioxide, to the kidneys, skin, and lungs; (3) transporting hormones from their origin in the endocrine glands to other tissues; (4) protecting the body from life-threatening microorganisms; and (5) regulating body temperature by heat transfer.

Major characteristics of blood include color (arterial blood is bright red; venous blood is dark red); viscosity (blood is three to four times thicker than water); reaction (the pH is 7.35 to 7.4); and volume (adults have approximately 70 to 75 ml/kg of body weight, or 5 to 6 L).

The four physiologic disturbances likely to occur in the hematologic system are decreased number of cells, overproduction of normal or abnormal cells, defects in the clotting mechanism, and disorders of the spleen. Causative factors may be idiopathic (unknown) or one of the following: dietary deficiencies, malabsorption, drug toxicity, metabolic disorders, hemorrhaging, infection, malignancy, genetic predisposition, or immunologic defects.

The lymphatic system also has numerous functions, including transporting lymph; producing lymphocytes and antibodies; phagocytosis; and absorbing fats and fat-soluble matter from the intestine.

The lymphatic system includes peripheral lymphatics, regional nodes, main lymphatic ducts, and the thoracic duct. The major characteristics of the lymphatic system are the formation of lymph, which is regulated by exchange of fluid between capillaries and tissue spaces, and its function as a muscle pump, which is responsible for the movement of lymph. The amount of lymphoid tissue and the distribution of lymph nodes are related to age. The two basic physiologic disturbances that can occur in the lymphatic system—enlargement of nodes and swelling of soft tissues—are usually caused by infection, inflammation, neoplasm, or obstruction.

Anatomy, Physiology, and Related Pathophysiology

Blood, a suspension of particulate matter in an aqueous solution of colloid and electrolytes, serves as a medium of exchange for body cells between themselves and the exterior. It also has protective properties that benefit the body and the blood itself. The liquid portion, plasma, is a suspension of colloid, electrolytes, proteins, and numerous other substances. The particulate matter includes red blood cells (RBCs) (erythrocytes), white blood cells of several types (leukocytes), and platelets (thrombocytes). All of these cells are believed to be derived from a single stem cell, which divides and matures to produce three distinct types of cells with different functions, properties, and characteristics.

Erythrocytes, of which there are approximately 5 million/mm^3 of blood, have as their principal functions transporting oxygen (which attaches to hemoglobin, the iron-containing substance of the cell) to the tissues; transporting carbon dioxide to the lungs; and maintaining normal blood pH through a series of intracellular buffers. Normal hemoglobin level is 15 g/100 ml of blood. Erythrocytes are produced in the red bone marrow and found in the ribs, sternum, skull, vertebrae, and bones of the hands, feet, and pelvis. Numerous nutrients are needed for normal cell formation, including iron, vitamin B_{12}, folic acid, and pyridoxine. The young reticulocytes released from the bone marrow circulate for 4 days while maturing into adult erythrocytes. The average life span of an erythrocyte is 115 to 130 days; dead cells are eliminated by phagocytosis in the mononuclear phagocyte system, particularly in the spleen and liver.

The size and shape of the erythrocyte are ideal for its function as a carrier of gases. It is a small disk with the unique characteristics of biconcavity and reversible deformability. The flattened, biconcave shape provides a surface area–to–volume ratio that is optimal for the diffusion of gases into and out of the cell. Reversible deformity enables the cell to alter its shape to squeeze through the microcirculation and then return to normal.

Hemoglobin is composed of a simple protein called globulin (consisting of two alpha chains and two beta chains of amino acids) and a red compound called heme, which contains iron and porphyrin. Normal adult hemoglobin is called hemoglobin A (Hb A). The total hemoglobin of normal healthy adults is usually composed of 98% to 99% Hb A, with a small percentage of a fetal form of hemoglobin (Hb F). Each erythrocyte contains 200 to 300 million molecules of hemoglobin, which combine chemically with oxygen to form oxyhemoglobin. Hemoglobin also combines with carbon dioxide. These two capacities enable the blood to carry oxygen to the tissues and carbon dioxide to the alveoli and thus to the atmosphere.

Total iron in the body ranges from 2 to 6 g, two thirds of which is contained in hemoglobin; the rest is stored in the bone marrow, spleen, and liver. Iron is obtained from such rich dietary sources as liver, oysters, lean meats, kidney beans, green leafy vegetables, apricots, and raisins.

When hemoglobin is phagocytosed in the liver or spleen, it breaks down into its heme and globin factors. The heme's iron is reused by the liver to make fresh hemoglobin, whereas the porphyrin is converted into bilirubin that is excreted by the body in feces and urine.

Leukocytes, of which there are approximately 5000 to 10,000/mm^3 of blood, are divided into three major categories: granulocytes, lymphocytes, and monocytes. Granulocytes, which make up 70% of all white blood cells (WBCs), are produced by the bone marrow and function according to the type of granule: (1) polymorphonuclear leukocytes (PMNs or neutrophils), whose main function is to fight bacterial infections through a process of phagocytosis (foreign particulate matter, or breakdown products from cells, is also digested); these cells are present during the early, acute phase of an inflammatory reaction; (2) eosinophils, which have a similar phagocytic function and are particularly important in digesting bacteria; they appear to play a role in combating allergic reactions; and (3) basophils, which contain many enzymes believed to play a role in combating acute systemic allergic reactions.

Lymphocytes, which are mainly produced in the lymph nodes, make up about 25% of the leukocytes. They are primarily concerned with producing antibodies and maintaining tissue immunity. Monocytes, which are derived from components of the mononuclear phagocyte system, are responsible for the phagocytosis of dead erythrocytes, and leukocytes in the blood. They are also important in the processing of antigenic information.

There are approximately 250,000 to 500,000 thrombocytes/mm^3 of blood. Formed in the bone marrow, they maintain capillary integrity, initiate coagulation, and retract clots.

The lymphoid system includes lymph nodes, spleen, thymus, lymphoid tissue associated with mucosal surfaces, and bone marrow. Lymph nodes, the most numerous component, are present in virtually every area of the body. The most familiar nodes are those palpable in the neck and groin. They serve as filters along the course of lymphatic channels and have a rich blood supply, which is important in transporting lymphocytes. The spleen is a mass of lymphoid and mononuclear phagocyte cells found under the ribs in the upper left quadrant of the abdomen. Its structure allows close interaction among lymphocytes, macrophages, and materials carried in the bloodstream. The thymus is located in the thorax anterior to the upper part of the heart and great vessels and contains lymphatic follicles and lymphocytes. The bone marrow is considered an important part of the lymphoid system because millions of lymphocytes are scattered throughout it.

In an adult active marrow is found in the pelvic bones, vertebrae, cranium and mandible, sternum and ribs, and extreme proximal portions of the humerus and femur. The mononuclear phagocyte system consists of a line of cells originating in the bone marrow; these include monoblasts, promonoblasts, and monocytes in bone marrow; monocytes in peripheral blood; and macrophages in tissue. These cells ingest and phagocytose unwanted materials in the blood and organs. During the inflammatory process, they engulf and digest foreign protein particles, microorganisms, debris from injured or dead cells, injured or defective erythrocytes, and dead neutrophils. This system is also the main line of defense against bacteria in the bloodstream; it cleanses the blood by removing a variety of cells.

Monocytes and macrophages secrete colony-stimulating factor (CSF), which is necessary for the formation and growth of colonies of macrophages and granulocytes in the bone marrow. The macrophages also secrete prostaglandin E, which inhibits colony-forming cells. They may also indirectly regulate erythrocyte differentiation by producing erythropoietin, which stimulates erythrocyte production in the bone marrow.

The various lymphatic channels in the body drain fluid from organs and tissues, conduct it centrally, and introduce it into the bloodstream via a large vein in the thorax. Many lymphocytes are found in the lymph and are recycled for variable periods of time.

Normal Findings

Erythrocyte: Biconcave disk when viewed laterally; appears to have lighter center and to be thicker on outer perimeter
Reticulocyte: Young, nonnucleated cell formed in bone marrow; stain gray-blue
Granulocyte: Neutrophil (PMN): faint, pink, acidophilic granules; eosinophil: refractive, eosinophilic granules; basophil: large blue granules
Lymphocyte: Single, round nucleus; cytoplasm has faintly basophilic, heavily clumped nuclear chromatin pattern
Monocyte: Folded or indented nucleus; often looks lobulated; has clumped nuclear chromatin pattern; cytoplasm is bluish gray or light sky blue
Thrombocyte: Nucleate, disk-shaped fragments of megakaryocytes of the lymphoid system
Lymph nodes: Not normally palpable in adults
Spleen: Located in the left upper outer quadrant; not normally palpable
Thymus: Reticular framework densely infiltrated with lymphocytes arranged in pattern of cortex and medulla
Lymphoid tissue associated with mucosal surfaces—that is, gastrointestinal and respiratory tracts: May be distributed diffusely or in nodular aggregates

Bone marrow: Myeloid tissue located only in the ribs, sternum, and at the ends of long bones

COMMON ABNORMAL FINDINGS

Changes in erythrocyte count (usually decreased)
Changes in hemoglobin concentration
Changes in hematocrit (usually decreased)
Changes in mean corpuscular volume (MCV), mean corpuscular hemoglobin (MCH), and mean corpuscular hemoglobin concentration (MCHC)
Changes in leukocyte count (decreased or elevated)
Changes in thrombocyte count (usually decreased)
Presence of Hb S (sickle cell test)
Changes in prothrombin time (PT) and partial thromboplastin time (PTT)

CONDITIONS, DISEASES, AND DISORDERS

ERYTHROCYTIC DISORDERS

Two basic pathophysiologic processes can be used to classify all disorders of red blood cells: inadequate numbers of circulating cells (anemia) and increased numbers of circulating cells (polycythemia). Anemias result from insufficient production or defective synthesis, increased destruction, or loss of erythrocytes. Polycythemia results from idiopathic causes or as a compensatory mechanism in response to tissue hypoxia.

Although not a disease per se, anemia is the primary manifestation of many abnormal states, including dietary deficiencies of iron, vitamin B_{12}, and folic acid; hereditary disorders; bone marrow damaged by toxins, radiation, or chemotherapy; renal disease; malignancy; chronic infection; overactive spleen; or bleeding from a tract or organ. The incidence of anemia is high; as much as 50% of the world's population suffers from anemia at any one time.

The major physiologic effect of anemia is to reduce the oxygen-carrying capacity of the blood; thus the symptoms of anemia are the result of tissue hypoxia.

POSTHEMORRHAGIC ANEMIA

Posthemorrhagic anemia is a disorder of decreased hemoglobin in the blood caused by traumatically induced hemorrhage.

Acute posthemorrhagic anemia develops as the result of the rapid loss of large quantities of erythrocytes during a hemorrhage, that is, traumatic severance of blood vessels, rupture of an aneurysm, or arterial erosion by a cancerous or ulcerative lesion. The severity of symptoms and the prognosis depend on the rate of bleeding, site of bleeding, and volume of blood loss. The rapid loss of less blood is more dangerous than is the slower loss of more blood.

In general, a 20% loss of total blood volume results in vascular insufficiency; a 30% loss causes circulatory failure, shock, and coma; and with a 40% loss, death is imminent, unless there is immediate and extensive blood value replacement.

PATHOPHYSIOLOGY

Within 24 hours after the hemorrhage, fluids move from the interstitium into the blood vessels, and plasma volume expands. Although this mechanism maintains adequate blood volume, it decreases the viscosity of the blood, which flows faster and with greater turbulence than normal blood. This increased blood flow in the heart can cause ventricular dysfunction, cardiac dilation, and heart valve insufficiency. Hypoxia causes arterioles, capillaries, and venules to dilate, also speeding blood flow. The heart must pump harder and faster to prevent congestion from the rapid venous return. Congestive heart failure may result.

The rate and depth of respiration increase as the body attempts to provide more oxygen in the remaining erythrocytes. Cardiac output increases to handle the increased venous return and to speed the oxygen-carrying erythrocytes to hypoxic tissue cells. The hemoglobin in these erythrocytes releases oxygen faster than usual at the tissue level. If the usual compensatory mechanisms are overcome, the person experiences dyspnea, palpitations, dizziness, and fatigue.

During the first hours after a hemorrhage, peripheral blood vessels constrict so that available blood flows primarily to the vital organs. The kidneys sense the decrease in blood flow and, in the effort to improve kidney perfusion, the renal renin-angiotensin response is activated, resulting in salt and water retention. Because the hemoglobin concentration has been reduced, the skin, mucous membranes, lips, nail beds and, conjunctivae become pale. Vasoconstriction and loss of plasma volume distort the erythrocyte count, hemoglobin level, and hematocrit, which appear high when they are actually quite low.

Restoration of a normal hemoglobin level can take 6 to 8 weeks.

Chronic blood loss anemia, which is caused by bleeding peptic ulcers, menstrual disorders, bleeding hemorrhoids, or gastrointestinal neoplasms, results in continuous loss of erythrocytes and iron. Symptoms and laboratory findings are identical to those of iron deficiency anemia.

DIAGNOSTIC STUDIES AND FINDINGS

Erythrocytes: 6.1/mm³ (initial); 4.7/mm³ (after fluid volume increase)
Hemoglobin: 16.5 g/dl (initial); 14.5 g/dl (after fluid volume increase)
Hematocrit: 50% (initial); 40% (after fluid volume increase)
Reticulocyte count: Increased mean corpuscular volume (MCV): slightly low

MULTIDISCIPLINARY PLAN

Surgery

If indicated to control source of bleeding

Medications

Hematinic agents: Iron supplements when dietary therapy is insufficient: ferrous sulfate (Feosol), 200 mg tid PO with meals

General Management

Initial intravenous (IV) fluids are noncolloid, contain electrolytes; followed by plasma, packed red blood cells, or both, as needed to correct cell deficit

Whole blood may be administered, after typing and crossmatching, to correct fluid volume and cell deficit as needed

Oxygen by nasal catheter or mask to maintain sufficient oxygenation of circulating blood volume

Sedation and rest to reduce patient's energy expenditure

Oral fluids as tolerated to maintain adequate tissue hydration and renal perfusion

Diet high in protein and iron as basis for erythropoiesis

NURSING CARE

NURSING ASSESSMENT

Cardiovascular function: Apical and peripheral arterial pulses, heart sounds, orthostatic blood pressure; rapid, thready pulse and hypotension present; central venous pressure and pulmonary artery pressure; blood loss

Respiratory function: Respiratory rate and character: initial rapid, deep respirations may later become shallow

Neurologic function: Level of consciousness and orientation: restlessness, dizziness, syncope, severe headache, disorientation

Integument: Trunk and extremities: evidence of pallor, diaphoresis, coolness

Fluid and electrolyte balance: Intake and output: decreased urinary output likely to occur; complaints of thirst

POTENTIAL COMPLICATIONS

Response to fluid therapy: avoid circulatory overload, observe for changes in cardiac and/or respiratory function; reaction to blood/blood components; recurrent bleeding

PATIENT PROBLEMS/NURSING DIAGNOSES & INTERVENTIONS

NIC TISSUE PERFUSION MANAGEMENT

Decreased cardiac output related to decreased circulatory volume

Deficient fluid volume related to blood loss

Ineffective peripheral tissue perfusion related to vasoconstriction

- Place patient on bed rest in semi-Fowler's position *to reduce cardiac workload and enhance systemic circulation.*
- Anticipate patient's needs *to reduce cardiac workload.*
- Provide warm environment *to prevent shivering and vasoconstriction.*
- Avoid stress (e.g., expression of strong emotions, overexertion, coughing, straining at stool) *to reduce cardiac workload.*
- Protect patient from injury (e.g., put up side rails) *to avoid accidents and to decrease risk of further blood loss.*
- Discourage smoking, which causes vasoconstriction of peripheral vessels and increased cardiopulmonary activity.
- Encourage exercise, including range of motion, *to promote peripheral circulation.*
- Apply ice bag and manual pressure or dressing over site of blood loss *to constrict damaged vessel or tissue and prevent further blood loss.*
- Elevate and immobilize affected body part when possible *to promote blood return to the heart and reduce blood loss at site of damage.*
- Administer intravenous fluids, including blood/blood components, as ordered; monitor patient's response to therapy to replace lost fluid volume.
- Increase oral fluid intake as tolerated *to maintain tissue hydration and renal perfusion.*

PATIENT EDUCATION/CONTINUUM OF CARE PLAN

1. Encourage patient to avoid overexertion, fatigue, and emotional states because they place a strain on cardiovascular system that may result in respiratory distress, cardiac damage, or impaired peripheral arterial circulation.
2. Discuss the need to report to physician serious symptoms, such as pain, dyspnea, extreme fatigue, and blood in urine or feces, because they may signal recurrent internal bleeding.
3. Support patient in maintenance of normal bowel elimination to avoid strain on cardiovascular system.
4. Discuss importance of regular exercise to maintain adequate peripheral circulation and cardiac and respiratory tone.
5. Plan with patient how to maintain a diet high in iron and protein, with adequate fluid intake, to promote production of erythrocytes and ensure adequate fluid volume.

EVALUATION/PATIENT OUTCOMES

Tissue Perfusion Management: Vital signs are within normal limits. Respirations, blood pressure, and pulse are within normal limits. Patient's vitality is maintained. Patient is mentally alert, with good concentration and attentiveness. Patient experiences no malaise, fatigue, or weakness. Color of skin and mucous membranes is good. Skin, nails, lips, and earlobes are warm and moist and have a natural color. Body hydration is normal. There is no edema or thirst. Urinary output balances with fluid intake.

IRON DEFICIENCY ANEMIA

Iron deficiency anemia is caused by an inadequate supply of iron needed to synthesize hemoglobin.

Iron deficiency anemia, which is high in incidence worldwide and the most prevalent anemia, is caused by inadequate absorption or excessive loss of iron. The disease occurs most frequently in women, young children, and the elderly in underdeveloped countries.

The principal cause of iron deficiency anemia in adults is acute or chronic bleeding secondary to trauma; excessive menses; gastrointestinal tract bleeding (usually chronic and occult) caused by peptic ulcer, hiatal hernia, diverticulosis, or cancer; or blood donation. Another cause is inadequate dietary intake of foods high in iron. A third cause is defective absorption caused by malabsorption syndromes, clay eating (pica), chronic diarrhea, high intake of cereal products with low intake of animal protein, and partial or complete gastrectomy.

PATHOPHYSIOLOGY

Iron deficiency anemia is a chronic, microcytic, hypochromic anemia; in other words, the erythrocytes are small and pale because of a low hemoglobin level. Although the total erythrocyte count is only moderately reduced, the serum iron level may drop dramatically.

DIAGNOSTIC STUDIES AND FINDINGS

Hemoglobin level: As low as 3.6 g/dl
Total erythrocyte count: Rarely below 3 million cells/dl
Mean corpuscular hemoglobin (MCH): Less than 27 pg
Mean corpuscular hemoglobin concentration (MCHC): 20 to 30 g/dl
Serum iron level: As low as 10 μg/dl
Hematocrit: Male: less than 47 mg/dl; female: less than 42 mg/dl
Total iron-binding capacity (TIBC): Increased
Serum ferritin level (one of the forms in which iron is stored in the body): Decreased

MULTIDISCIPLINARY PLAN

Medications

Hematinic agents: To increase iron available in the blood
- Ferrous sulfate (Feosol), 0.75-1.5 g PO in divided doses tid with meals
- Ferrous gluconate (Fergon), 200-600 mg PO tid
- Ferrous fumarate, 200 mg PO tid to qid
- Iron dextran (Imferon), 100 to 250 mg/dl

Ascorbic acid: As indicated

General Management

Diet high in iron-rich foods to correct nutritional deficiency—including red meats, organ meats, kidney beans, whole-wheat products, spinach, egg yolks, carrots, and raisins

NURSING CARE

NURSING ASSESSMENT

Cognitive, sensory, and motor function: Cognitive/behavioral changes such as irritability, decreased concentration; complaints of headache, numbness and tingling in limbs, sensitivity to cold, fatigue, dizziness
Cardiovascular function: Pulse: tachycardia may be present
Respiratory function: Respirations: complaints of dyspnea on exertion
Integument: Brittle hair and nails (spoon shaped)
Gastrointestinal function: Trophic glossitis (tongue inflamed and smooth), stomatitis, dysphagia

PATIENT PROBLEMS/NURSING DIAGNOSES & INTERVENTIONS

NIC ACTIVITY AND EXERCISE MANAGEMENT

Ineffective cardiopulmonary tissue perfusion related to decreased hemoglobin
Fatigue related to anemia
Impaired physical mobility related to sensoriperceptual impairments

- Provide safe environment *to prevent injury.*
- Assist patient with ambulation and change in position as needed *because sense of balance, sensation, and position may be altered.*
- Help patient to concentrate on safe movements in activities of daily living *to avoid injury.*
- Help patient plan balance between rest and activity *to reduce cardiac workload and conserve energy.*
- Encourage patient to discuss feelings related to fatigue and its impact on quality of life.

NIC FLUID MANAGEMENT/NUTRITION SUPPORT

Imbalanced nutrition: less than body requirements, related to defective absorption
Impaired oral mucous membrane related to iron deficiency

- Encourage diet high in iron *to correct deficiency.*
- Remove dentures if indicated in the presence of oral infection; initiate dental consultation as needed.
- Provide soft food and nonirritating fluids *to decrease discomfort and irritation.*
- Provide small, frequent feedings if indicated.
- Provide frequent mouth care if indicated *to remove irritating secretions.*

NIC SKIN/WOUND MANAGEMENT

Impaired skin integrity related to decreased tissue perfusion
Disturbed tactile sensory perception related to decreased tissue perfusion

- Maintain warm, clean, dry environment *to decrease sensitivity to cold.*
- Wash hair with care *to avoid irritation of scalp.*
- Provide nail care *to avoid damage.*

PATIENT EDUCATION/CONTINUUM OF CARE PLAN

1. Discuss the need for correct oral hygiene, including regular dental care, to prevent irritation and infection of oral cavity.
2. Assist patient in maintenance of a diet high in iron to promote production of healthy erythrocytes.
3. Discuss factors in ongoing self-medication with iron supplements, including proper timing, dilution-enhancing and dilution-reducing absorption; and awareness of change in stool color.
4. Discuss the importance of continuing all prescribed therapy, even when patient is feeling well.
5. Encourage use of bowel regimen.

6. Discuss general hygienic measures (e.g., proper care of hair and nails) to prevent damage and loss.
7. Discuss general safety precautions to prevent injury from dizziness or fatigue.

Evaluation/Patient Outcomes

Activity and Exercise Management: Patient can easily ambulate. Patient avoids contact with stable and moving objects. There is no reported dizziness. Activities of daily living are accomplished without fatigue. Patient has sufficient energy to carry out activities of daily living. Patient participates in regular exercise as tolerated.

Fluid Management/Nutrition Support: Daily intake includes essential food groups. Patient's diet includes foods high in iron.

Skin/Wound Management: General body cleanliness and health are maintained. Hair and nails are clean and not brittle. Mouth is clean, with no ulceration or other oral irritation. Skin is dry and warm to touch, without evidence of damage or irritation.

Vitamin B_{12} (Pernicious Anemia) and Folate Deficiencies

Vitamin B_{12} and folic acid deficiencies, which disrupt the formation of the precursors of DNA, result in abnormal maturation of RBCs.

Pathophysiology

The primary cause of impaired absorption of vitamin B_{12} is intrinsic factor deficiency. Because the parietal cells of the gastric mucosa secrete this factor, deficiency can occur in patients who have had a total gastrectomy or small bowel resection involving the ileum. Pernicious anemia is considered an autoimmune disease that occurs when intrinsic factor secretion fails because of gastric mucosal atrophy. Its onset is insidious, has a familial tendency, and usually begins during middle age or later.

Persons whose diets are inadequate in dairy products and meat, such as strict vegetarian diets, may develop a B_{12} deficiency. Conditions such as tapeworm, overgrowth of intestinal bacteria, and diverticula also may impair absorption.

Because folate stores in the body are limited, maintenance of adequate intake is essential; the diet must contain green leafy vegetables, whole-grain and fortified cereals, yeast, and fruit. Mechanisms that can lead to deficiency include malabsorption syndromes, alcohol abuse, liver disease, and anorexia. Drugs that interfere with the absorption of folic acid include the anticonvulsants and such folic acid antagonists as oral contraceptives, broad-spectrum antibiotics, hydroxyurea, and methotrexate.[9]

Diagnostic Studies and Findings

Erythrocyte count: Below 3 million/dl; elevated MCV and concentration (MCHC, decreased WBC count and MCH)
Bone marrow biopsy: Increased number of megaloblasts
Bilirubin: Unconjugated forms; usually elevated
Serum vitamin B_{12}: Deficient
Serum folate: Low
Gastric analysis: Scanty secretions, elevated pH, and no free hydrochloric acid
Therapeutic trial with parenteral vitamin B_{12}: Large numbers of reticulocytes in blood 4 to 5 days after injection
Hemoglobin: Decreased to 4 to 5 g/dl

Multidisciplinary Plan

Medications

Vitamin derivatives

Cyanocobalamin (vitamin B_{12}) 30-100 μg/day intramuscularly (IM) for 5 days, followed by weekly doses until Hct corrects; must be continued for life by patients who have had pernicious anemia or noncorrectable malabsorption

Folic acid (Folvite), up to 1 mg/day PO; given IM to patients with malabsorption

Hematinic agents: To correct nutritional deficit; ferrous sulfate (Feosol) or ferrous gluconate (Fergon), 0.3 g tid with meals PO as needed

Digestants: To enhance metabolism of vitamins

Hydrochloric acid (HCl), 4-10 ml PO well diluted in water tid with meals during first weeks of vitamin B_{12} therapy

General Management

Blood transfusions to correct anemia; nutritious diet, including fish, meat, milk, and eggs, to enrich diet deficient in vitamins; bed rest as needed for rest, recovery, and safety; physical therapy to prevent complications from impaired motor function

Nursing Care

Nursing Assessment

Cognitive, sensory, and motor function: Numbness and/or tingling of hands and feet, weakness, fatigue; disturbed coordination, such as "wobbly" legs, poor balance; irritability, depression, poor memory, impaired judgment

Integument: Pallor, jaundice, waxy appearance of skin; presence of petechiae and/or purpura

Gastrointestinal function: Weight loss; constipation; diarrhea; smooth beefy red tongue; indigestion, anorexia, sore mouth

Respiratory function: Dyspnea

Cardiovascular function: Tachycardia; blood pressure: wide pulse pressure; palpitations

Patient Problems/Nursing Diagnoses & Interventions

NIC Activity and Exercise Management

Ineffective cardiopulmonary tissue perfusion related to immature RBCs
Fatigue related to anemia
Impaired physical mobility: sensoriperceptual impairments, related to ineffective tissue perfusion
Disturbed sensory perception related to ineffective tissue perfusion, decreased erythrocytes, and decreased hemoglobin

- Provide a safe environment; help patient concentrate on safe conduct of tasks of daily living *to avoid injury.*
- Place patient on bed rest with side rails up as needed *to promote safety.*
- Assist with ambulation; encourage the patient to use an assistive device such as a walker or cane *to avoid falls.*
- Plan periods of rest and activity *to avoid complaints of dyspnea, palpitations, or fatigue.*

NIC Fluid Management/Nutrition Support

Imbalanced nutrition: less than body requirements, related to impaired absorption

Impaired oral mucous membrane related to vitamin deficiency

- Encourage diet high in vitamins, iron, and protein *to promote production of healthy erythrocytes.*
- Offer small, frequent feedings *to prevent digestive overload.*
- Provide frequent oral hygiene *to promote nutritional intake and prevent irritation/infection of oral mucosa.*

NIC Skin/Wound Management

Impaired skin integrity related to impaired tissue perfusion

Disturbed tactile sensory perception related to impaired tissue perfusion as a result of anemia

- Maintain skin hygiene *to prevent risk to skin integrity.*
- Avoid trauma to skin; for example, use electric razor, soft toothbrush.
- Apply heat with caution *to avoid thermal burn.*
- Use bed cradle or footboard on bed *to prevent pressure on lower legs and feet.*
- Maintain warm environment *to optimize tissue perfusion.*

Patient Education/Continuum of Care Plan

1. Discuss precautions in use of heat-therapy devices such as heating pads or hot compresses (patient may have impaired sensitivity to heat and pain), as well as general safety measures.
2. Emphasize general hygiene, that is, skin and oral care.
3. Practice physical therapy activities and general exercise (patient may have possible neurologic damage as a result of the disease).
4. Discuss the importance of a diet high in vitamin B_{12}, the use of maintenance therapy with vitamin B_{12}, and the need to maintain this lifelong treatment.

Evaluation/Patient Outcomes

Activity and Exercise Management: There is no evidence of physical injury. There is no evidence of skin damage or physical sign of an injury. Patient is oriented, calm, and able to provide self-care. Patient participates in regular exercise as tolerated. Vital signs are within normal limits. Respirations, pulse, and blood pressure are within normal limits. Patient has sufficient energy to carry out activities of daily living.

Fluid Management/Nutrition Support: Daily intake includes adequate fluid and the essential food groups. Patient's diet is high in iron, protein, and vitamins. Mouth is free of irritation, with pink and moist mucosa.

Skin/Wound Management: Color of skin and mucous membranes is good. Skin, nails, lips, and earlobes are warm and moist and have a natural color. There is no discoloration.

Aplastic Anemia

Aplastic anemia is the term most frequently used to describe a decrease in the number of circulating erythrocytes caused by a failure of the bone marrow. It is usually accompanied by agranulocytosis and thrombocytopenia, in which case the condition is referred to as pancytopenia.

Pathophysiology

In half of all diagnosed cases of aplastic anemia, the cause is unknown; in the other half, it results from exposure to a specific toxin. The myelotoxins are (1) agents that always cause damage when given in large doses: radiation (e.g., x-rays, radium, and radioactive isotopes), benzene and its derivatives, alkylating agents, and antimetabolites; (2) agents that sometimes cause failure: chloramphenicol (Chloromycetin), sulfonamides, phenytoin, and others; and (3) suspicious agents such as streptomycin, chlorophenothane (DDT), and carbon tetrachloride. The disease also may be immunologic in origin or the result of a severe disease, such as liver failure. There is some evidence that this anemia may be a sequela of viral infection such as Epstein-Barr virus, cytomegalovirus, or hepatitis B.

Diagnostic Studies and Findings

Erythrocyte count: Usually less than 1 million/mm^3; reticulocyte count also low

Leukocyte count: May be less than 2000/mm^3

Serum iron: Elevated

Total iron-binding capacity: Normal or slightly reduced

Platelet count: Less than 30,000/mm^3

Bone marrow biopsy: Marrow fatty with few developing blood cells

Multidisciplinary Plan

General Management

Immediate removal of the causative agent; blood transfusions as needed to replace cells; prevention and treatment of complications such as infection and bleeding with such therapies as antibiotics, corticosteroids, and bone marrow transplantation

NURSING CARE

Nursing Assessment

Sensory and motor function: Complaints of progressive fatigue and lassitude; activity intolerance

Respiratory function: Complaint of dyspnea

Immunologic function: Complaints of fever, "sniffles," sore throat, pain and burning with urination
Gastrointestinal function: Ulcerations on oral mucous membranes; evidence of severe anorexia, such as weight loss
Vascular function: Petechiae or ecchymosis; bleeding from nose, gastrointestinal (GI) tract; hematuria; "seeping" from injection sites

Potential Complications

Profuse bleeding or hemorrhage; infection or septicemia

Patient Problems/Nursing Diagnoses & Interventions

NIC Activity and Exercise Management

Ineffective cardiopulmonary tissue perfusion related to decreased hemoglobin
Fatigue related to anemia
Impaired physical mobility related to anemia

- Provide safe environment *to avoid tissue injury.*
- Assist patient with ambulation; encourage patient to use an assistive device such as a walker or cane as indicated.
- Place patient in upright position when in bed if dyspneic when lying in flat bed position.
- Plan rest periods to balance with activity *to conserve energy.*
- Assist with activities of daily living as needed.

NIC Risk Management

Risk for infection related to inadequate circulating WBCs

- Maintain reverse isolation if indicated *to avoid exposure to pathogens.*
- Administer antibiotics as prescribed; give injections only if necessary and apply pressure afterward *to promote vascular constriction and clotting.*
- Encourage mobility, turning, coughing, deep breathing, and increased intake of fluids *to reduce susceptibility to infection.*
- Encourage intake of foods high in fiber *to avoid constipation and bowel irritation.*
- Handle patient gently when assisting with activities of daily living *to avoid trauma.*

Patient Education/Continuum of Care Plan

1. Assist patient to maintain a balance between rest and activity.
2. Discuss with patient how to avoid infection, especially of respiratory or urinary tract.
3. Discuss with patient how to avoid trauma (e.g., use soft toothbrush and electric razor) to prevent bleeding.
4. Plan with patient a self-assessment for bleeding, what signs and symptoms to report, and first aid for bleeding.

Evaluation/Patient Outcomes

Activity and Exercise Management: Physical appearance of patient indicates sufficient rest and activity. Patient has good concentration and coordination. Patient walks, bicycles, or performs some other type of exercise. Patient carries out activities of daily living.

Risk Management: Patient's surroundings are safe. Patient uses safety precautions and avoids trauma. There is no evidence of physical injury. Patient does not have cuts, abrasions, or other signs of injury. No petechiae or ecchymoses are found. Patient does not have an infection. Oral temperature is 37° C (98.6° F). There is no evidence of inflammation, purulent drainage, pain, or aching. Vital signs are within normal limits. Respirations, pulse, and blood pressure are within normal limits.

Hemolytic Anemia

Hemolytic anemia is a disorder in which the rate of erythrocyte destruction is greatly accelerated. The most common types of hemolytic anemias in industrialized countries are the immunohemolytic anemias.

Pathophysiology

Hemolytic anemia is the result of either an intracorpuscular defect or an extracorpuscular factor. This causes a shortened life span for the erythrocytes, abnormally large numbers of erythrocytes being destroyed by cells of the mononuclear phagocyte system, and inadequate replacement of lost cells by the bone marrow.

Intracorpuscular defects include a deficiency in glucose 6-phosphate dehydrogenase (G6PD) and hereditary spherocytosis. Extracorpuscular factors include trauma, such as burns or surgery; chemical agents such as lead poisoning; immune response; infectious organisms, such as infectious hepatitis, mononucleosis, miliary tuberculosis; systemic diseases, such as Hodgkin's disease, leukemia, systemic lupus erythematosus; isoimmune reactions, such as fetalis erythroblastosis; autoimmune disorders; and paroxysmal hemoglobinurias.

Factors such as trapping of cells in the liver or spleen, drug toxicity (e.g., methyldopa, penicillins), and mechanical injury (e.g., thrombotic thrombocytopenia purpura, hemolytic-uremic syndrome, disseminated intravascular coagulation, valve hemolysis, vasculitis) may cause the hemolysis.

In immunohemolytic anemia, immune system components attack their own RBCs. There are two types: the warm antibody type is frequently associated with excessive immunoglobulin G (IgG) antibody; these antibodies are most active at 37° C (98.6° F) and may be stimulated by chemicals, drugs, or other autoimmune disorders. The cold antibody type is commonly associated with a Raynaud-like response and with fixation of complement proteins on immunoglobulin M (IgM), which best occurs at 30° C (86° F).

Diagnostic Studies and Findings

Red blood cell count: Normocytic anemia
Reticulocyte count: Increased
Red blood cell fragility: Increased

Erythrocyte life span: Shortened
Bilirubin level: Increased
Lactic dehydrogenase: Elevated
Fecal and urinary urobilinogen: Increased
Bone marrow biopsy: Hyperplasia
Ultrasound/gallbladder studies: Cholelithiasis

MULTIDISCIPLINARY PLAN

Surgery

Splenectomy if steroids fail to arrest erythrocyte destruction by the spleen

Medications

Corticosteroids to suppress such extracorpuscular factors as inflammation; prednisolone (Delta-Cortef, others), 10-20 mg qid
Immunosuppressive therapy with cyclophosphamide (Cytoxan) and azathioprine (Imuran) if steroid therapy fails
Osmotic diuretics to prevent acute tubular necrosis (mannitol, urea)
Antiemetics

General Management

Elimination of causative factors; blood component therapy; plasma exchange therapy; parenteral fluids; diet enriched with protein and iron

NURSING CARE

NURSING ASSESSMENT

Fluid and electrolyte balance: Intake and output: decreased urinary output; urine color, quantity, specific gravity, pH
Gastrointestinal function: Enlargement of liver or spleen; complaints of nausea, evidence of vomiting; weight changes
Integument: Jaundice
Thermoregulation: Chills and fever
Motor function: Complaints of weakness and fatigue
Comfort: Complaints of back or abdominal pain

POTENTIAL COMPLICATIONS

Acute renal failure

PATIENT PROBLEM/NURSING DIAGNOSES & INTERVENTIONS

NIC ACTIVITY AND EXERCISE MANAGEMENT

Fatigue related to anemia
Impaired physical mobility related to activity intolerance

- Provide safe environment *to diminish risk for injury.*
- Assist with ambulation; encourage patient to use an assistive device such as a walker or cane *to promote safe mobility.*
- Plan for periods of rest balanced with activity *to prevent fatigue.*

NIC FLUID MANAGEMENT/NUTRITION SUPPORT

Imbalanced nutrition: less than body requirements, related to abdominal distention
Nausea related to decreased GI motility
Impaired urinary elimination related to decreased renal perfusion

- Monitor fluid intake and output *to provide adequate hydration without causing circulatory overload.*
- Offer carbonated beverages, ice chips, and other fluids of patient's choice *to promote satiety and avoid distention.*
- Provide oral hygiene as indicated *to promote comfort and enhance appetite.*
- Provide balanced diet rich in iron and protein *to promote erythropoiesis.*
- Give small, frequent feedings, avoiding fatty foods *to prevent distention or satiation.*
- Offer antiemetics as prescribed *to avoid nausea.*

NIC SKIN/WOUND MANAGEMENT

Impaired skin integrity related to jaundice

- Provide frequent skin hygiene, including lubrication and antipruritic solutions, *to prevent dryness and irritation.*
- Maintain cool room temperature with adequate humidity *to enhance patient's comfort.*
- Advise patient to avoid scratching skin *to avoid abrasions.*

NIC PHYSICAL COMFORT PROMOTION

Acute pain related to abdominal distention
Ineffective thermoregulation related to altered immune function

- Provide warmth when chilling occurs, analgesia and other pain relief measures as needed and/or prescribed *to promote comfort.*
- Administer antipyretics as needed and prescribed *to reduce fever.*
- Have blankets, extra clothing, and external sources of warmth available if chilling occurs.

PATIENT EDUCATION/CONTINUUM OF CARE PLAN

1. Assist patient in finding a balance between rest and exercise.
2. Discuss with patient the need for a well-balanced diet.
3. Help patient to identify comfort measures.

EVALUATION/PATIENT OUTCOMES

Activity and Exercise Management: Patient activity level is normal. Patient exercises regularly, uses assistive devices as needed, and rests when tired.

Fluid Management/Nutrition Support: Body hydration is normal. Skin turgor and color are good. Patient has thin secretions. Balance between intake and output is maintained; absence of nausea and vomiting.

Daily intake includes essential food groups. Patient's diet is especially high in iron and protein.

Skin/Wound Management: Skin and mucous membranes have good color. Skin, nails, lips, and earlobes are warm and moist and have a natural color. Patient maintains general body cleanliness. Patient's skin is clean, and patient does not complain of itching.

Physical Comfort Promotion: Patient reports feeling comfortable. No complaints of back or abdominal pain. Temperature within normal limits.

Sickle Cell Disease

Sickle cell disease occurs in persons who are homozygous for hemoglobin S (Hb S), an abnormality of the beta chains that is sensitive to changes in RBC oxygen content.

Sickle cell disease is the result of a genetic mutation that is transmitted from parent to child. Between 45,000 and 75,000 black people in the United States have the disease, and 2.5 million carry the trait. The incidence of the trait is less than 1%, and the disease is nonexistent in nonblacks.

Pathophysiology

The erythrocytes of persons with sickle cell anemia contain more Hb S than Hb A, which causes them to assume a sickle or crescent shape when exposed to decreased oxygen tension. These "sickled" cells are then easily destroyed as they enter smaller blood vessels in the body. The sickle cell trait is usually a mild condition found in heterozygous carriers, who have few or no symptoms.

The exact cause of sickling crises is unknown, but two factors have been identified: hypoxia caused by low oxygen tension (such as climbing to high altitudes, exercising strenuously, or inadequate oxygenation during anesthesia) and elevated blood viscosity caused by a concentration of cells and dehydration resulting from such factors as vomiting, diarrhea, diaphoresis, or diuretics. Occlusion of the microcirculation occurs in the presence of sickling, with resultant hypoxia, which causes more sickling. Anoxia leads to infarction and thrombosis in tissues and organs such as the brain, kidneys, bone marrow, liver, and spleen.

Persons with sickle cell disease experience episodes of crisis (see Emergency Alert box at right,) which are sudden in onset and can occur as often as weekly or as infrequently as once a year. Repeated occlusions of progressively larger vessels result in numerous clinical manifestations (Fig. 17-1).

The average life span of an RBC that contains 40% or more of Hb S is approximately 20 days; this reduced life span results in hemolytic anemia.

Many patients die during childhood from cerebral hemorrhage or shock; however, with appropriate supportive care, many individuals survive into their 30s and 40s. Progressive renal damage, which eventually causes uremia, is the usual cause of death.

Diagnostic Studies and Findings

Stained blood smear: Sickle cell observed

Hemoglobin electrophoresis: Less than 40% Hb S indicates sickle cell trait; 85% to 95% Hb S indicates sickle cell disease

Hematocrit: Low

Reticulocyte count: Elevated

Erythrocyte life span: Less than 20 days

Leukocyte count: Above normal

! EMERGENCY ALERT

SICKLE CELL DISEASE—CRISIS

Sickle cell disease is a genetic disorder affecting black people, in which sickle-shaped cells clump together, preventing oxygen and other products from reaching microcirculation, leading to more hypoxia and sickling. The causes are unknown, but factors thought to precipitate a crisis are hypoxia, infection, and dehydration. Tissue necrosis can result if prolonged.

Assessment

- Pain in extremities, joints, abdomen
- Weakness, pallor
- Cardiac dysfunction: dysrhythmias, murmurs
- Dyspnea, chest pain, cyanosis
- Altered level of consciousness
- Decreased urinary output
- Signs of infection

Interventions

- Administer oxygen as prescribed; 10-12 L/min by mask.
- Manage pain with medications as prescribed and comfort measures.
- Administer intravenous (IV) fluids as prescribed and oral fluids as tolerated.
- Provide restful environment.
- Remove constrictive clothing.
- Encourage patient to keep extremities extended to promote venous return.
- Do not raise bed knee gatch.
- Elevate the head of the bed (no more than 30 degrees).
- Keep room temperature warm (at or above 72° F).
- Check circulation in extremities frequently (pulse oximetry, capillary refill, peripheral pulses).

Multidisciplinary Plan

The plan of care is generally supportive: rest, oxygen, intravenous fluids and electrolytes, sedatives, and analgesics.

NURSING CARE

Nursing Assessment

See Fig. 17-1.

Respiratory function: Breath sounds; cyanosis, signs of dyspnea, chest pain; signs/symptoms of pneumonia

Cardiovascular function: Vital signs, particularly pulse and blood pressure; signs/symptoms of myocardial infarction, congestive heart failure, cerebrovascular accident

Gastrointestinal function: Bowel sounds; complaints of nausea; enlargement of liver and spleen

Integument: Pale, cyanotic skin; leg ulcers

Musculoskeletal integrity: Peripheral pulses; joint swelling, disproportionately long arms and legs, small stature

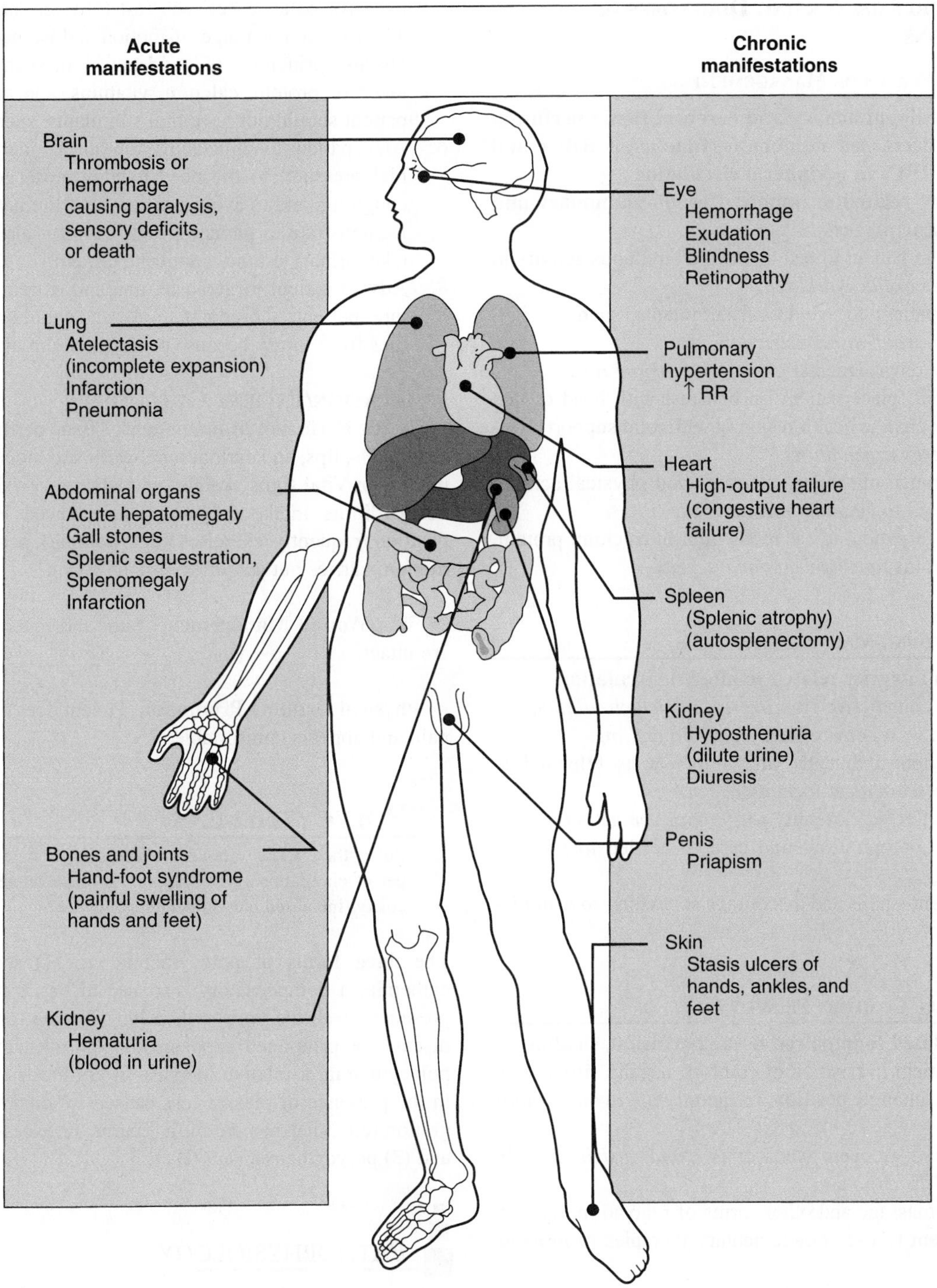

FIG. 17-1
Clinical manifestations of sickle cell disease. (From Belcher.[1])

Developmental status: delayed sexual maturity

Genitourinary function: Body weight; intake and output; edema; decreased concentration, abnormal color, content and odor of urine; test for protein; priapism

Comfort: Pain in chest, abdomen, bones (particularly extremities with moderate activity); headache; joint swelling or abnormal alignment

Neurologic function: Confusion, change in level of consciousness; pupillary responses, reflexes

POTENTIAL COMPLICATIONS

Cerebral hemorrhage; tissue necrosis and infection; anemia; myocardial infarction; congestive heart failure

Patient Problems/Nursing Diagnoses & Interventions

NIC Tissue Perfusion Management

Ineffective cardiopulmonary and cerebral tissue perfusion related to decreased number of functional RBCs and sickling of RBCs in peripheral circulation

Risk for injury related to impaired cardiopulmonary and cerebral tissue perfusion

- Encourage patient to rest and avoid strenuous activity *to decrease cardiac workload.*
- Advise patient to avoid oral stimulants, such as cigarettes, *to avoid vasoconstriction.*
- Decrease environmental stimuli *to promote rest.*
- As needed, place patient on bed rest with head of bed elevated; change position slowly with joint support *to reduce energy expenditure.*
- Initiate range-of-motion exercises and physical activity as tolerated *to maintain muscle tone.*
- Encourage patient to eat foods high in calcium, protein, and vitamins *to enhance bone integrity.*

NIC Skin/Wound Management

Impaired skin integrity related to altered circulation

- Remove constrictive clothing *to enhance circulation.*
- Maintain warm environment *to avoid chilling.*
- Turn patient frequently and ambulate as tolerated *to avoid pressure ulcer formation.*
- Elevate affected extremity *to enhance venous return.*
- Provide appropriate wound care as needed *to promote healing.*
- Cut patient's nails and discourage scratching *to avoid injury.*

NIC Physical Comfort Promotion

Acute pain related to impaired tissue perfusion, sickling

- Place patient in position of comfort, usually sitting with support; change position frequently *to avoid venous stasis.*
- Give small, frequent feedings *to avoid gastric and abdominal distention.*
- Provide massage and other forms of relaxation; encourage patient to use complementary therapies *to promote comfort.*

Patient Education/Continuum of Care Plan

1. Alert patient to the need for family testing to determine the presence of Hb S; genetic counseling is available for carriers.
2. Explain how to avoid sickle cell crises: avoid high altitudes, flying in unpressurized planes, dehydration, cold temperatures, iced liquids, and vigorous exercise; use stress reduction methods.
3. Explain to patient that young pregnant women have a high risk for developing pulmonary and/or renal complications.
4. Practice range-of-motion exercises and encourage regular physical activity to prevent bone demineralization. Explain need for balance between rest (physical and mental) and activity, such as range-of-motion and isometric exercises.
5. Discuss principles of good nutrition, such as the importance of protein, calcium, vitamins, and adequate fluids; patient should not have oral stimulants, such as cigarettes.
6. Alert patient to signs and symptoms of increased intracranial pressure, to the need to blow nose gently, to avoid coughing, and to avoid straining on elimination.
7. Demonstrate to patient how to monitor his or her oral intake, urinary output, and urine protein.
8. Advise patient to avoid trauma and extremes in temperature; patients should not smoke and should protect extremities from injury because of impaired circulation.

Evaluation/Patient Outcomes

Tissue Perfusion Management: Tissue perfusion adequate. Skin, nails, lips, and earlobes are warm and moist and have natural color. Vital signs, weight, and laboratory values are within normal limits. Intake and output are balanced. Patient changes position frequently, exercises (e.g., walking), performs range of motion; carries out activities of daily living.

Skin/Wound Management: Skin and mucous membranes are intact.

Physical Comfort Promotion: Patient does not complain of pain and appears comfortable.

Polycythemias

Polycythemia is a term used to describe an increase in the number of circulating erythrocytes. It is characterized by hyperviscosity (increased blood thickness).

The three forms of polycythemia are (1) secondary polycythemia, a compensatory response to tissue hypoxia in the presence of chronic obstructive lung disease, congenital heart disease, or prolonged exposure to high altitudes; (2) relative polycythemia, a relative increase in erythrocyte concentration in the presence of plasma loss caused by fluid loss and dehygration (e.g., diarrhea, vomiting, burns, or excessive diuretics); and (3) polycythemia vera (PV).

Pathophysiology

PV is a chronic disorder with excessive production of erythrocytes, myelocytes, and megakaryocytes in the bone marrow. It is thought to originate from abnormal cell production at the stem cell level. The excessive hematopoiesis may be linked to a heightened responsiveness to such regulatory molecules as interleukin 3. PV progenitor cells may also have an increased sensitivity to insulin-like growth factor. Although the onset is usually insidious, the patient may have a long survival if the excessive proliferation of red blood cells and platelets can be controlled. Unfortunately, patients with PV may develop acute leukemia, myelofibrosis, or other conditions. The clinical course evolves through a series of stages: asymptomatic (splenomegaly and isolated erythrocytosis and thrombocytosis); erythrocytotic phase (patient generally symptomatic); inactive phase; postpolycythemic myeloid metaplasia (PPMM with bone marrow fibrosis, enlarging splenomegaly, and cytopenias); and acute myeloid leukemia. Transformation of PV to acute leukemia occurs in 25% to 50% of patients who enter the PPMM phase.

DIAGNOSTIC STUDIES AND FINDINGS

Erythrocyte count: Elevated, as high as 8 to 12 million/mm^3
Thrombocytes: Elevated, more than 400,000/mm^3
Leukocytes: Elevated, more than 12,000/mm^3
Serum erythropoietin: Low
Bone marrow biopsy: Hypercellularity; abnormal marrow proliferative capacity

MULTIDISCIPLINARY PLAN

Surgery

Splenectomy (as a last resort with persistent splenomegaly)

Medications

Mylosuppressive agents

Busulfan (Myleran), 4-6 mg/day PO for 4-8 weeks; stop when blood counts are normalized or platelet count is less than 300,000/mm^3
Hydroxyurea, 30 mg/kg PO for 1 week, then 15-20 mg/kg
Recombinant interferon-α therapy
Radioactive phosphorus (^{32}P), 2.3 mCi/m^2 IV every 12 weeks as needed (limit 5 mCi per dose) for elderly patients
Anagrelide (platelet inhibitor)
Low-dose aspirin

Antacids
Antipruritic agents

General Management

Phlebotomy to maintain hematocrit equal to or below 45%

NURSING CARE

NURSING ASSESSMENT

Cardiovascular function: Ruddy complexion, dusky redness of oral mucosa, conjunctival plethora (beefy red coloration); blood pressure: hypertensive with complaints of dizziness, headache, and sense of "fullness" in head; vital signs, including peripheral pulses
Respiratory function: Respiratory rate; breath sounds; chest pain, dyspnea, hemoptysis
Gastrointestinal function: Bowel sounds; enlargement of liver and spleen; weight; epigastric distress; bleeding (e.g., in feces), emesis
Integument: Sweating, complaints of pruritus
Skeletal integrity: Signs/symptoms of secondary gout
Neurologic function: Level of consciousness, pupillary responses, reflexes; visual abnormalities; weakness, paresthesias

POTENTIAL COMPLICATIONS

Thrombosis such as cerebrovascular accidents, myocardial infarctions, deep vein thrombosis; may also occur in such unusual sites as hepatic veins, mesentery, and femoral veins or arteries
Hemorrhage ranging from epistaxis to gastrointestinal hemorrhage
Neurologic changes such as transient ischemic attacks, confusional states, cerebral infarction, cerebral hemorrhage
Erythromelalgia evidenced by burning pain, redness, and warmth of toes and fingers; may progress to cyanosis and tissue necrosis
Acute leukemia

PATIENT PROBLEMS/NURSING DIAGNOSIS & INTERVENTIONS

NIC TISSUE PERFUSION MANAGEMENT

Ineffective cardiopulmonary, cerebral, and gastrointestinal tissue perfusion related to increased numbers of RBCs

- Maintain warm environment *to avoid vasoconstriction.*
- Encourage patient to plan for balance between activity and rest *to optimize tissue perfusion.*
- Encourage patient to change position frequently, with emphasis on sitting, *to enhance lung expansion.*
- Ambulate as tolerated *to enhance cardiopulmonary function.*
- Encourage patient to perform range-of-motion and isometric exercises *to promote circulation.*
- Avoid application of heat or cold, constrictive clothing, and pressure in the popliteal area, *which can impair circulation.*
- Encourage deep breathing and coughing *to promote removal of secretions.*
- Discourage such oral stimulants as smoking *to prevent vasoconstriction.*
- Teach relaxation exercises and other stress management techniques.
- Administer medications as ordered (e.g., anticoagulants, analgesics and antacids, particularly for abdominal pain).
- Recommend balanced diet while avoiding sodium-rich foods *to reduce fluid retention.*
- Avoid foods that are acidic or gas forming *to avoid distention and flatus.*
- Offer small, frequent feedings with focus on bland foods and carbonated beverages *to relieve gastric distress.*

NIC SKIN/WOUND MANAGEMENT

Impaired skin integrity related to pruritus and sweating

- Encourage patient to bathe in warm water; may add one-half box of cornstarch, followed by gentle toweling, *to soothe irritated skin.*
- Teach patient to dry skin gently *to avoid irritation.*
- Suggest distraction therapy such as music, imagery, and relaxation *to minimize discomfort.*

NIC IMMOBILITY MANAGEMENT

Risk for injury related to weakness and parasthesias
Impaired physical mobility related to weakness and parasthesias

- Provide a safe environment *to reduce risk for injury.*

- Prescribe bed rest and joint rest as needed *to reduce inflammation and irritation.*
- Encourage range-of-motion exercises as tolerated *to enhance circulation.*
- Remind patient not to compress knees and to avoid crossing legs or dangling legs over side of bed *to avoid venous stasis.*
- Encourage use of elastic support hose *to promote peripheral venous return.*
- Assist patient with ambulation; encourage use of an assistive device such as a walker or cane *to prevent injury.*
- Encourage patient to use electric razor and soft-bristled toothbrush, to avoid constipation, and to prevent nosebleed *to prevent injury.*
- Provide massage, warm compresses, and other interventions *to relieve pain and increase mobility.*

Patient Education/Continuum of Care Plan

1. Encourage patient to protect extremities from injury, such as heat, cold, or pressure.
2. Assist patient to do range-of-motion and isometric exercises safely and correctly.
3. Advise patient to avoid trauma and protect body parts, to use safety precautions, and to use a soft toothbrush.
4. Encourage patient to handle stress in a healthy way and to balance rest with exercise.
5. Advise patient of the need to stop smoking and to avoid other oral stimulants.
6. Advise patient of the need for dietary modification, that is, to use low-sodium, low-acid, and low-gas-forming foods, foods high in alkaline, and foods low in purines.
7. Discuss with patient the signs and symptoms of bleeding and thrombus formation, as well as interventions and the need to report findings.

Evaluation/Patient Outcomes

Tissue Perfusion Management: Vital signs are within normal limits. Blood pressure is within normal limits.

Skin/Wound Management: Color of skin and mucous membranes is good. Skin, nails, lips, and earlobes are warm and moist. There is no evidence of bleeding.

Immobility Management: Frequent change of position is achieved. Patient walks, sits, stands, and performs range of motion.

LEUKOCYTIC DISORDERS

Neutropenia

Neutropenia is a term used to describe a lower-than-normal number of circulating neutrophils in the blood. Febrile neutropenia is the presence of both neutropenia and fever, even if other signs and symptoms of infection are not present. This condition can quickly become life threatening if not diagnosed and treated quickly.

Pathophysiology

Neutropenia is most often the result of drug toxicity or hypersensitivity from large-dose, long-duration drugs such as antineoplastic agents, radiation therapy, benzenes, certain tranquilizers (chlorpromazine HCl [Thorazine]), antithyroid agents (propylthiouracil), anticonvulsants (phenytoin), and antibiotics (chloramphenicol). It may also develop during the course of such diseases as tuberculosis, uremia, aplastic anemia, and multiple myeloma.

The onset and duration of cancer chemotherapy-induced neutropenia are dependent on the drug; white blood cells are most often affected 7 to 14 days after the drugs are administered. The immunosuppressive effect can last up to 8 weeks. The expected nadir—the point at which the WBC count is lowest—indicates the patient's time for greatest risk for infection. The longer neutropenia is present, the greater the risk for infection.

The most common site of infection in the patient with neutropenia is the gastrointestinal tract. Other sites include the respiratory tract, skin, and urinary tract.

Diagnostic Studies and Findings

Leukocyte count: Leukopenia (500 to 3000 WBC/mm^3)
Absolute neutrophil count: 1000/mm^3 or less

Multidisciplinary Plan

Medications

Broad-spectrum antibiotics

Colony-stimulating factors: Granulocyte colony-stimulating factor (G-CSF); granulocyte-macrophage colony-stimulating factor (GM-CSF)

Acetaminophen for bone pain and flulike symptoms

General Management

Isolation; granulocyte transfusions

NURSING CARE

Nursing Assessment

Energy level: Complaints of fatigue and weakness

Thermoregulation: Temperature: observe for high fever, severe chills, tachycardia, cough, nasal congestion; restlessness, irritability; recent exposure to contagious disease

Gastrointestinal function: Ulcerative lesions of pharyngeal and buccal mucosa; complaints of sore throat, dysphagia; abdominal pain, tenderness, or distention; change in bowel habits; vomiting; perirectal mucosal damage

Urinary function: Urine: quantity, color, odor; burning with urination; frequency, hesitancy, or difficulty emptying the bladder; perineal itching

Integument: Skin, eyes, nose, and ears; redness, tenderness, ulceration

Respiratory function: Breath sounds; cough, character of sputum, patient complaint of chest pain

POTENTIAL COMPLICATIONS
Septic shock

PATIENT PROBLEMS/NURSING DIAGNOSES & INTERVENTIONS

NIC ACTIVITY AND EXERCISE MANAGEMENT

Activity intolerance related to fatigue, weakness
Ineffective cardiopulmonary tissue perfusion related to impaired transport of oxygen across alveolar membrane associated with respiratory infection

- Anticipate patient's needs when on bed rest or restricted activity (e.g., place objects within reach) *to avoid excess energy expenditure.*
- Encourage patient to balance rest with activity *to optimize energy level.*
- Assist with ambulation; encourage patient to use an assistive device such as a walker or cane *to promote safety and to prevent injury while promoting activity.*

NIC NUTRITION SUPPORT

Imbalanced nutrition: less than body requirements, related to mucositis, dysphagia, abdominal pain
Impaired oral mucous membrane related to infection and/or treatment

- Provide frequent oral care for mucositis *to promote hygiene and comfort.*
- Apply ice collar to neck *to reduce pharyngeal pain and swelling.*
- Offer bland, soft foods in frequent, small feedings *to reduce buccal irritation.*
- Use stool softeners as needed to avoid constipation; avoid enemas and straining to have bowel movement.

NIC THERMOREGULATION

Deficient fluid volume related to fever
Risk for infection related to decreased WBCs
Ineffective thermoregulation

- Institute reverse isolation.
- Avoid or limit exposure to fresh flowers, pets, persons with infections.
- Encourage a diet high in protein, vitamins, and calories.
- Encourage fluid intake, 2 to 3 L/day.
- Monitor intake and output.
- Teach good hand-washing technique.
- Encourage daily bath or shower; follow with gentle toweling and application of lotion to skin.
- Use cooling methods as needed (e.g., alcohol rub, tepid bath).
- Provide oral hygiene, skin care, and perineal hygiene.

PATIENT EDUCATION/CONTINUUM OF CARE PLAN

1. Discuss with patient the use of frequent, thorough oral hygiene to treat or prevent oral and pharyngeal infection.
2. Explain the need for a diet high in protein, vitamins, and calories with soft, bland foods.
3. Encourage a balance between rest and activity to prevent fatigue and generalized weakness.
4. Explain the need to avoid crowds, people with infectious diseases, and cold or hot environments; also teach signs and symptoms of infection and appropriate interventions.
5. Teach patient self-injection of G-CSF or GM-CSF.

EVALUATION/PATIENT OUTCOMES

Activity and Exercise Management: Vitality is maintained. There is no evidence of malaise, fatigue, or weakness. Patient performs activities of daily living.

Nutrition Support: Patient consumes daily intake of essential food groups. Diet is high in protein, vitamins, and calories. Mouth is clean and free of ulceration.

Thermoregulation: Vital signs are within normal limits.

LEUKEMIAS

Leukemias are a group of usually fatal cancers that involve the blood-forming organs of the blood-forming tissues of the bone marrow, spleen, and lymph nodes. These may be acute or chronic and are characterized by the abnormal proliferation of leukocytes and their precursors.

Leukemias represent 2% of all newly diagnosed cases of cancer and 4% of all cancer deaths. Although survival rates have improved each decade, mortality is still high, especially for adults with acute leukemias. Most cases of leukemia occur in adults over the age of 55.

For inexplicable reasons, the incidence of leukemias is increasing. Several factors are under study: chronic, repeated exposure to relatively small doses of radiation; exposure to certain chemicals; presence of primary immune deficiency diseases; possible viral etiologic factors; and a genetic predisposition, such as among siblings or in children with Down syndrome.

PATHOPHYSIOLOGY

The major effects of leukemia on the body result from the proliferation of large numbers of abnormal, immature leukocytes; accumulation of these cells within the lymph nodes; and eventual infiltration of these cells into tissues throughout the body. If the patient lives long enough, all organs become involved in the leukemia process.

Leukemias are classified according to the following criteria:

Type of cell and tissue involved: The major types of cells are lymphocytes and myelocytes. Acute leukemias may be classified as lymphoblastic or myeloblastic because of the prevalence of immature cell forms. Lymphocytic leukemias cause hyperplasia of the lymphoid tissue, whereas myelocytic leukemias cause hyperplasia of the bone marrow and spleen. Ninety per cent of all leukemias are lymphocytic.

Course and duration of disease: Acute forms of leukemia have a rapid onset, with progression to death within days or months if not diagnosed and treated. Chronic forms have a gradual onset and a slower course. Chronic leukemias are more common in persons 25 to 60 years of age.

Adult acute myeloid leukemia (AML) affects the blasts that are developing into granulocytes. AML results from acquired genetic damage to DNA of the cells in the bone marrow or exposure to high doses of radiation, benezene, or certain chemotherapeutic agents. The disease progresses rapidly and is often difficult to diagnose because the early signs and symptoms may be similar to the flu or other common illnesses. There is a tenfold increase in incidence from age 30 (1/100,000) to age 70 (1/10,000). AML is of equal incidence in men and women. Age at diagnosis affects both treatment and prognosis, though prognosis is generally poor overall. A bone marrow transplant may improve the patient's longevity.

Adult acute lymphocytic leukemia (ALL) results from an acquired genetic injury to the DNA of a single cell in the bone marrow, which results in the uncontrolled growth of lymphoblasts. Unlike other types of leukemia, ALL occurs at different rates in different locations; that is, there are higher rates in more developed countries and in higher socioeconomic groups. ALL occurs most often in the first decade of life but increases in frequency again in older age; there is a predilection for males and whites. The subtypes are L1 (small), L2 (large) (more frequently seen in adults), and L3 (large with other features). The immunophenotypes are B lymphocytic lineage, which account for 85% of cases, and T lymphocytic lineage.

Chronic myelogenous leukemia (CML) permits the development of mature leukocytes that can function normally, resulting in a less severe early course of disease. CML is diagnosed more often in adults than in children and demonstrates an acquired genetic abnormality called the Philadelphia chromosome (translocation of chromosome material between 9 and 22). The prognosis is generally poor and is worse if there is no Ph^1 chromosome. CML may develop as a result of high-dose radiation for lymphoma. Its onset is usually insidious, with the patient describing vague complaints for months or years. Development of a blastic crisis (accelerated phase) indicates more acute disease.

Chronic lymphocytic leukemia (CLL) refers to a malfunction in the production of B cells or T cells that have reached a relatively mature developmental stage; this malfunction more often occurs in the production of B cells. This is the only leukemia with a possible genetic predisposition. CLL is found most often in persons 50 to 70 years of age. The incidence increases with age. It is the most common of the leukemias in Western countries. Two thirds of those diagnosed with CLL are men. The course of the disease is 4 to 10 years; conversion to the acute form is rare.

Diagnostic Studies and Findings

Leukocyte count: Elevated 20,000 to 100,000/mm^3

Bone marrow aspiration and biopsy: Marrow full of leukemic blast cells

Cell markers: T-11 protein, enzyme terminal deoxynucleotidyl transferase (TdT), common acute lymphoblastic leukemia antigen (CALLA)

Coagulation variables: Decreased levels of fibrinogen and other coagulation factors; increased clotting time, elevated PTT

Cytogenic analysis: Presence of Philadelphia chromosome

Polymerase chain reaction (PCR): Alternation in DNA caused by chromosome breakage in CML

Multidisciplinary Plan

Medications

Dosages are based on protocol and body surface area.

Phases of drug therapy

- Induction therapy: Intensive combination chemotherapy at time of diagnosis; goal is rapid, complete remission
- Consolidation therapy: Occurs early in remission; goal is cure; another course of drugs used in induction or a different combination of drugs; may be single course of therapy or regularly repeated courses over 1 to 2 years
- Maintenance therapy: May be repeated for months to years after induction and consolidation; goal is to maintain remission

Antitumor antibiotics: Daunorubicin (rubidomycin, Cerbidine), doxorubicin (Adriamycin, Rubrex), mitoxantrone (Novantrone), idarubicin (Idamycin)

DNA repair enzyme inhibitors: Etoposide (VP-16, VePesid), teniposide (VM-26, Vumon), topotecan (Hycamptamine)

DNA synthesis inhibitors: Carboplatin (Paraplatin)

DNA damaging agents: Cyclophosphamide (Cytoxan), ifosfamide (Ifex)

Antimetabolites: 5-Azacytidine (Mylosar), cytarabine (cytosine arabinoside, Ara-C, Cytosar) 2-chlorodeoxyadenosine (cladribine), fludarabine (Fludara), hydroxyurea (Hydrea), 6-mercaptopurine (Purithenol), methotrexate (Mexate), 6-thioguanine (thioguanine)

Vinca alkaloids: Vincristine (Oncovin), vindesine (Eldisine)

Enzymes that prevent cells from surviving: L-Asparaginase (Elspar), PEG-L-Asparaginase (pegaspargase, Oncaspar)

Synthetic hormones: Prednisone, prednisolone, dexamethasone

Biologic response modifiers: Interferon-α (Roferon-A, Intron A)

Immunotoxins

General Management

Intravenous immune globulin therapy (IVIG) for recurrent infections

Epoetin alfa (Epogen or Procrit), 50-100 U/kg tid to increase production of RBCs

Cytokines: Granulocyte colony-stimulating factor (G-CSF); granulocyte-macrophage colony-stimulating factor (GM-CSF)

Leukapheresis: Removal of excessive white cells from blood

Antibiotic and antibacterial, antifungal, and antiviral therapy

Radiation therapy

Blood component therapy

Bone marrow transplantation: Stem cell, autologous, allogenic

NURSING CARE

Nursing Assessment

Neurologic function: Complaints of progressive fatigue, headache; papilledema, scleral hemorrhage; level of consciousness, pupillary responses, reflexes; ability to communicate

Respiratory function: Breath sounds; complaints of shortness of breath when active

Immunologic function: Mild fever, frequent minor infections, inability to tolerate warm temperatures; enlargement of lymph nodes

Musculoskeletal function: Complaints of bone and joint aching and swelling; range of motion and strength

Integument and mucous membranes: Petechiae, ecchymoses, nosebleed; pallor of skin, conjunctiva, nail beds, palmar creases, and around mouth; excessive sweating; drainage on dressings and around IV sites; vaginal bleeding

Gastrointestinal function: Anorexia, weight loss; complaint of pain on left side of abdomen as result of enlarged spleen; sore throat; abdominal distention after meals; bleeding gums; occult blood in stool; enlargement of liver

Cardiovascular function: Orthostatic hypotension, complaints of palpitations; tachycardia, murmurs and bruits

Renal function: Hematuria; urine specific gravity and pH

Potential Complications

Tumor lysis syndrome; leukemic infiltration of meninges or central nervous system

Patient Problems/Nursing Diagnoses & Interventions

NIC Activity and Exercise Management

Ineffective cardiopulmonary tissue perfusion related to tachycardia, hypotension

Fatigue related to anemia

- Provide a safe environment; help patient concentrate on safe conduct of tasks of daily living *to reduce risk of injury.*
- Place patient on bed rest with side rails up as needed *to protect from injury.*
- Assist with ambulation; encourage the patient to use an assistive device such as a walker or cane *to conserve energy.*
- Plan periods of rest and activity *to avoid complaints of dyspnea, palpitations, or fatigue.*
- Administer blood component therapy as ordered *to replace missing components.*
- Place ice/cold pack and topical agents on wound sites when there is bleeding or serosanguinous drainage *to promote clotting and prevent blood loss.*
- Count and weigh sanitary pads or tampons *to quantify blood loss.*
- Administer oral contraceptives as prescribed to stop menses.
- Assist patient with daily bathing *to prevent fatigue.*
- Encourage mobility, turning, coughing, deep breathing, and increased intake of fluids *to enhance cardiopulmonary function.*
- Handle patient gently when assisting with activities of daily living.

NIC Fluid Management/Nutrition Support

Imbalanced nutrition: less than body requirements, related to anorexia, hepatomegaly, mucositis

Impaired oral mucous membranes related to side effects of medications

Risk for deficient fluid volume related to decreased platelets

- Encourage diet high in vitamins, minerals, protein, and calories *to restore nutritional balance.*
- Offer small, frequent feedings *to enhance appetite and prevent distention.*
- Provide frequent oral hygiene *to maintain patient comfort.*
- Weigh patient daily *to monitor nutritional status.*
- Discourage smoking and oral stimulants *to decrease irritation.*
- Offer oral anesthetic or antiemetic agents before meals *to decrease buccal irritation and nausea.*
- Offer analgesics as needed for abdominal discomfort.
- Encourage adequate intake of fluid *to increase circulating volume.*
- Encourage intake of foods high in fiber *to avoid straining at stool and reduce risk of tissue damage.*
- Offer stool softener, laxatives *to prevent/manage potential constipation and to avoid straining at stool.*
- Avoid raw fruits and vegetables *to avoid irritation of colon.*

NIC Skin/Wound Management

Impaired skin integrity related to bleeding

Disturbed tactile sensory perception related to CNS irritation

- Maintain skin hygiene *to avoid risk to skin integrity.*
- Avoid trauma to skin; for example, use electric razor, soft toothbrush *to avoid bleeding from cuts or abrasions.*
- Apply heat and cold with caution *to avoid burns or dermal ulcers.*
- Maintain warm environment *to provide neutral thermal environment.*

NIC Risk Management

Risk for infection related to decreased WBCs

- Initiate protective isolation *to protect from pathogens.*
- Administer antibiotics as prescribed; give injections only if necessary and apply pressure afterward *to enhance clotting.*
- Teach patient and family proper hand-washing techniques *to reduce risk for infection.*
- Screen visitors for contagious infectious disease.
- Use cool sponge baths, alcohol rubs, and antipyretic drugs as needed *to promote comfort.*
- Avoid such invasive procedures as injections, rectal temperatures, urinary catheters *to reduce risk for bleeding and infection.*
- Instruct patient to avoid picking or blowing the nose *to avoid bleeding and tissue damage.*

Patient Education/Continum of Care Plan

1. Advise patient to avoid situations in which patient is likely to contract infection, such as inclement weather or crowds.

2. Plan with patient and/or family a well-balanced diet, especially high in vitamins, minerals, protein, calories, and fluids.
3. Instruct the patient to observe for and report signs and symptoms of infection, bleeding, and anemia.
4. Discuss ways to avoid tissue damage (e.g., use soft toothbrush, blow nose gently, avoid constipation, use electric razor).
5. Discuss nonanalgesic pain measures (e.g., complementary therapies).
6. Encourage patient to avoid smoking and oral stimulants.
7. Teach patient and/or family care of venous access device.

EVALUATION/PATIENT OUTCOMES

Activity and Exercise Management: Ambulation is safe. Activities of daily living are accomplished safely. No complaints of fatigue, dyspnea on exertion. Vital signs are stable.

Fluid Management/Nutrition Support: Daily intake of food and fluids is sufficient. Mouth is clean and moist. Weight is stable or increased as needed.

Skin/Wound Management: Skin is dry and warm to touch. There is no evidence of bruising. Skin is clean and free of wounds.

Risk Management: Daily intake and output are balanced; Temperature is within normal limits. There are no pathogenic organisms in blood, wound, or urine cultures.

MULTIPLE MYELOMA

Multiple myeloma is characterized by an abnormal malignant growth of plasma cells, development of single or multiple abnormal plasma cell tumors within the bone marrow, destruction of bone throughout the body, and later dissemination of the disease into the lymph nodes, liver, spleen, and kidneys.

PATHOPHYSIOLOGY

The onset of multiple myeloma is usually gradual and often insidious. Many patients experience a presymptomatic period of 5 to 20 years, during which the individual may have recurrent bacterial infections, especially pneumonia. This increased susceptibility to infection is believed to be related to disturbed antibody formation caused by plasma cell abnormalities. Ninety percent of patients have multiple sites of involvement at the time of diagnosis. Other variations are described as solitary, localized (a few neighboring sites), or extramedullary (involvement of tissues such as skin, muscle, or lung).

Myeloma results from an acquired injury to the DNA of a single cell in the B lymphocyte developmental sequence that is destined to become plasma cells. In patients with myeloma, plasma cells are often seen in abnormally large numbers. These cells may gather in only one bone and form a plasmacytoma; in most cases, this tumor spreads to many bones, including the pelvis, ribs, vertebrae, scapulae, sternum, and skull. Large amounts of monoclonal immunoglobulin (Ig) are made for no purpose and are secreted into the blood; changes in the amount of this protein usually parallel disease progression or regression. In about 75% of cases, a smaller piece of the Ig is made by the myeloma cells (the light chain), enters the blood, and is rapidly excreted in the urine; it is often called Bence Jones protein. This protein can cause renal damage.

Myeloma cells also secrete cytokines that stimulate cells that erode bone; lytic spots (holes) develop in the bone, which is thinned and can break with the normal stresses of walking or lifting, as well as with coughing and minor falls.

Eighty per cent of cases occur in persons over the age of 60, with African-Americans having a significantly higher incidence and more men affected than women.

DIAGNOSIS STUDIES AND FINDINGS

Total blood count: Pancytopenia
Total serum protein: Elevated
Blood urea nitrogen: Elevated
Serum calcium: Elevated
X-rays, scanning, and magnetic resonance imaging (MRI): Diffuse bone lesions, demineralization, and osteoporosis, "Swiss cheese" appearance
Bone marrow aspiration: Large numbers of malignant plasma cells
Blood and urine analyses: Monoclonal immunoglobulin and Bence Jones protein

MULTIDISCIPLINARY PLAN

Medications

Agents may be used alone or in combination: melphalan (Alkeran)—most commonly used; cyclophosphamide (Cytoxan); dexamethasone (Decadron, Dexacort); doxorubicin (Adriamycin, Rubex); idarubicin (Idamycin); interferon-α (Roferon A, Intron A); prednisone; vincristine (Oncovin); cytokines

General Management

Autologous stem cell transplantation
Allogeneic stem cell transplantation from HLA-matched donor in patients 30 to 50 years
Bisphosphonates (potent inhibitors of bone resorption): pamidronate (Aredia); clodronate
Erythropoietin for treatment of anemia
Aggressive hydration
Radiation therapy

NURSING CARE

NURSING ASSESSMENT

Skeletal system: Complaints of bone pain that worsens with movement; evidence of pathologic fracture, signs of osteoporosis; height: patient may lose stature with deformities; gait, coordination, and stability; posture and body alignment
Renal function: Intake and output; evidence of calculi (e.g., flank pain, renal colic); hematuria
Neurologic function: Spinal cord compression (e.g., motor function, sensory function, reflexes); headache

Immunologic function: Signs/symptoms of infection (e.g., urinary, bronchial, lung)
Cardiopulmonary function: Vital signs: dyspnea; bleeding (e.g., urine, stools, gums, skin); complaints of fatigue; evidence of pallor

Potential Complications

Infections; hypercalcemia; spinal cord compression; hyperviscosity; amyloidosis; acute myelogenous leukemia

Patient Problems/Nursing Diagnoses & Interventions

NIC Activity and Exercise Management

Impaired physical mobility related to weakness, pathologic fractures
Activity intolerance related to weakness

- Encourage patient to balance activity with rest *to conserve energy.*
- Assist patient with ambulation; encourage use of an assistive device such as a walker or cane *to prevent injury.*
- Provide range-of-motion exercises and assistance with turning *to maintain mobility.*
- Decrease number of environmental barriers, such as chairs, tables, and rugs, *to prevent injury.*
- Provide a trapeze for increased mobility in bed *to assist with movement in bed.*
- Help patient turn in bed at least every 2 hours while maintaining proper alignment; log roll as needed *to prevent circulatory/pulmonary stasis.*
- Support spinal area with brace or traction as needed *to avoid injury.*
- Apply heat and massage to relieve pain.
- Offer analgesics and complementary therapies as needed *to increase mobility while providing comfort.*

NIC Nutrition Support

Imbalanced nutrition: less than body requirements, related to anorexia

- Encourage well-balanced diet *to optimize nutritional status.*
- Offer laxatives and stool softeners *to avoid constipation/impaction.*
- Suggest small, frequent feedings *to avoid distention and to promote adequate nutritional intake.*

NIC Risk Management

Risk for infection related to decreased WBCs
Ineffective tissue perfusion related to decreased platelets

- Provide protective isolation *to protect from pathogens.*
- Screen visitors *to avoid contagious-infectious diseases.*
- Teach patient and family proper hand washing technique *to prevent manual transmission of microbes.*
- Administer antibiotics as prescribed.
- Encourage patient to turn, cough, deep breathe *to prevent cardiopulmonary stasis and to maintain respiratory function.*
- Provide skin, perineal, and oral hygiene *to prevent development of skin irritation and portal for infection.*
- Handle patient gently *to avoid trauma and bleeding.*
- Give injections only if necessary; apply pressure after injection for several minutes *to promote hemostasis.*

NIC Elimination Management

Impaired urinary elimination related to renal calculi

- Provide adequate hydration of 3000 to 4000 ml per day *to prevent urinary stasis.*
- Encourage patient to eat diet low in calcium and phosphorus *to prevent formation of calculi.*
- Offer urine-acidifying juices; avoid bicarbonates and carbonated beverages.

Patient Education/Continuum of Care Plan

1. Discuss the need for good body mechanics, safety measures, and assistive devices.
2. Plan with patient for pain management, which includes analgesics and complementary therapies.
3. Discuss the importance of adequate nutrition and hydration.
4. Teach patient and family signs and symptoms of possible complications that should be reported to the physician (i.e., infection, hypercalcemia, pathologic fractures, spinal cord compression).

Evaluation/Patient Outcomes

Activity and Exercise Management: There is no evidence of physical injury. Patient expresses and manifests comfort when ambulating.

Nutrition Support: Diet is adequate in quantity and well balanced. Weight remains stable.

Risk Management: Color of skin and mucous membranes is good. Vital signs are within normal limits. There is no evidence of infection.

Elimination Management: Body hydration is normal. There is a balance between intake and output.

THROMBOCYTIC DISORDERS

Thrombocytopenia

Thrombocytopenia refers to a decrease in the number of platelets below the level needed for normal coagulation. It may occur as a result of treatments or conditions that suppress bone marrow activity or through processes that limit platelet formation or increase the rate of platelet destruction.

The thrombocytopenias that affect adults are autoimmune thrombocytopenic purpura (previously know as idiopathic thrombocytopenic purpura or ITP), thrombotic thrombocytopenic purpura, and chemotherapy-induced thrombocytopenia.

PATHOPHYSIOLOGY

Autoimmune thrombocytopenic purpura is a condition in which platelets are destroyed prematurely (survival time decreases from 8 to 20 days to 1 to 3 days) in spite of normal or even elevated levels of platelet production by the bone marrow. It is believed to result from the development of autoantibodies to platelet-membrane antigens. The antibody-coated platelets are destroyed primarily in the spleen. This disorder is most common among women between the ages of 20 and 40 and among individuals with a preexisting autoimmune disorder such as systemic lupus erythematosis.

Thombotic thrombocytopenic purpura is a rare disorder in which platelets clump in the microcirculation, leaving insufficient numbers of platelets in the systemic circulation. There is inappropriate clotting, yet the blood fails to clot properly when the patient experiences trauma. The underlying cause seems to be an autoimmune reaction in endothelial cells.

Chemotherapy-induced thrombocytopenia results from high-dose treatment regimens and cumulative thrombocytopenia, a dose-limiting toxicity associated with many chemotherapeutic regimens.

DIAGNOSTIC STUDIES AND FINDINGS

Platelet count: Decreased
Megakaryocytes: Increased numbers in bone marrow
Antiplatelet antibodies: Detectable levels in peripheral blood

MULTIDISCIPLINARY PLAN

Surgery
Splenectomy

Medications
Corticosteroids; immunoglobulin (IV); anti-D (Rho) globin in Rh^+ patients (IV); intravenous immune globulin therapy; azathioprine; low doses of chemotherapeutic agents (such as the antimitotic agents and cyclophosphamide for autoimmune thrombocytopenic purpura); attenuated androgens (danazol); platelet aggregation inhibitors such as aspirin, alprostadil (Prostin VR), and plicamycin (for thrombotic thrombocytopenic purpura); thrombopoietic growth factor—oprelvekin (Neumega) (for prevention of severe thrombocytopenia after myelosuppressive chemotherapy)

General Management
Platelet transfusions; plasma exchange therapy

NURSING CARE

NURSING ASSESSMENT
Integument and mucous membranes: Petechial rash or ecchymoses on arms, legs, neck, and upper chest; epistaxis; bleeding from gums and nose
Sensory and motor function: Signs/symptoms of increased intracranial pressure; headache, nerve pain, parasthesias
Gastrointestinal function: Melena, hematemesis, occult blood in stool, emesis
Renal function: Hematuria
Cardiovascular function: Tachycardia
Respiratory function: Shortness of breath and complaints of dyspnea
Gynecologic function: Vaginal bleeding

POTENTIAL COMPLICATIONS
Cerebrovascular accident

PATIENT PROBLEMS/NURSING DIAGNOSES & INTERVENTIONS

NIC SKIN/WOUND MANAGEMENT
Impaired nasal and vaginal tissue integrity related to decreased platelets
Impaired tissue integrity related to bleeding
Impaired oral mucous membrane related to treatment
- Position patient with head forward and elevated, and press nostrils together gently; press nostrils *to stop bleeding.*
- Provide perineal hygiene *to promote comfort.*
- Count perineal pads and weigh them *to determine amount of blood loss.*
- Protect patient from injury by assisting with ambulation; use assistive devices (walker, cane) *to avoid injury.*
- Handle patient gently *to avoid trauma.*
- Avoid injections or use of sharp objects such as razor, *which may cause bleeding.*
- Apply ice pack and/or manual pressure over any site of bleeding *to control bleeding.*
- Provide mouth care with soft toothbrush *to minimize tissue trauma.*
- Encourage patient to eat soft foods and chilled liquids *to avoid trauma.*
- Apply bed cradle and lightweight clothing *to avoid skin irritation.*
- Maintain oral and perineal hygiene; remove patient dentures.

NIC TISSUE PERFUSION MANAGEMENT
Ineffective renal, gastrointestinal, and cerebral tissue perfusion related to decreased platelets
- Teach patient to report presence of discolored urine.
- Teach patient to report presence of blood in stool or on tissue paper after bowel movement or in vomitus *to identify blood loss.*
- Avoid use of rectal thermometer or enema tube *to prevent trauma and potential for rectal bleeding.*
- Encourage high-fiber foods and increased fluids *to prevent constipation, impaction, straining at stool, and potential for bleeding.*

NIC RESPIRATORY MANAGEMENT
Impaired gas exchange related to alveolar-capillary membrane changes resulting from decreased platelets
- Place patient on bed rest in semi-Fowler's position as needed *to enhance cardiopulmonary function.*

- Dress patient warmly and maintain warm room temperature *to enhance vasodilation.*
- Remove constrictive clothing *to facilitate chest expansion.*
- Discourage smoking and use of oral stimulants *to avoid vasoconstriction and dyspnea.*
- Monitor patient's rest and activity *to identify and minimize energy-inefficient activities.*

Patient Education/Continuum of Care Plan

1. Explain the need to stop smoking.
2. Assist patient in avoiding trauma.
3. Discuss with patient the need to detect report signs and symptoms of bleeding.

Evaluation/Patient Outcomes

Skin/Wound Management: Skin is intact, and free of discoloration. Patient is able to ambulate safely. Bowel and bladder elimination are normal. Patient is alert, oriented, and appropriate in communication.

Tissue Perfusion Management: Vital signs are within normal limits. There is no evidence of bleeding.

Respiratory Management: Patient is adequately oxygenated, and there is no evidence of dyspnea.

Disseminated Intravascular Coagulation Syndrome

Disseminated intravascular coagulation syndrome (DIC) is the term used to describe abnormal activation of coagulation pathways that result in bleeding and clotting.

The incidence is about 1 in 1000 hospital admissions. DIC is a life-threatening condition with a mortality rate of 70%.

Pathophysiology

States of physiologic disequilibrium that precipitate this syndrome include cancer of the prostate, breast, colon, pancreas, lung, or stomach and leukemia; a history of cancer treatments; liver disease; acute pancreatitis; recent blood transfusions or hemolytic transfusion reactions; sepsis (usually a gram-negative infection); or pregnancy, which is the most common cause.

The result of this disequilibrium is a systemic activation of coagulation and fibrinolysis, with diffuse intravascular fibrin formation and deposition of fibrin in the microcirculation. As a consequence of these processes, clots accumulate in the body's capillaries of vascular organs such as the brain, liver, kidneys, heart, and spleen; these small clots inhibit oxygenation of these organs, resulting in hypoxia and ischemia, which results in anaerobic metabolism.

Clotting factors are used at a rate that exceeds their replenishment, with circulating thrombin waiting in the intravascular spaces for fibrinogen. The excessive thrombin formation greatly decreases the availability of the inhibitor antithrombin III.

Diagnostic Studies and Findings (Fig. 17-2)

Prothrombin time/international normalized ratio (PT/INR): Prolonged (greater than 15 seconds)
Activated partial thromboplastin time (PTT): Prolonged
Thrombin time: Prolonged
Platelet count: Less than 50,000/mm^3

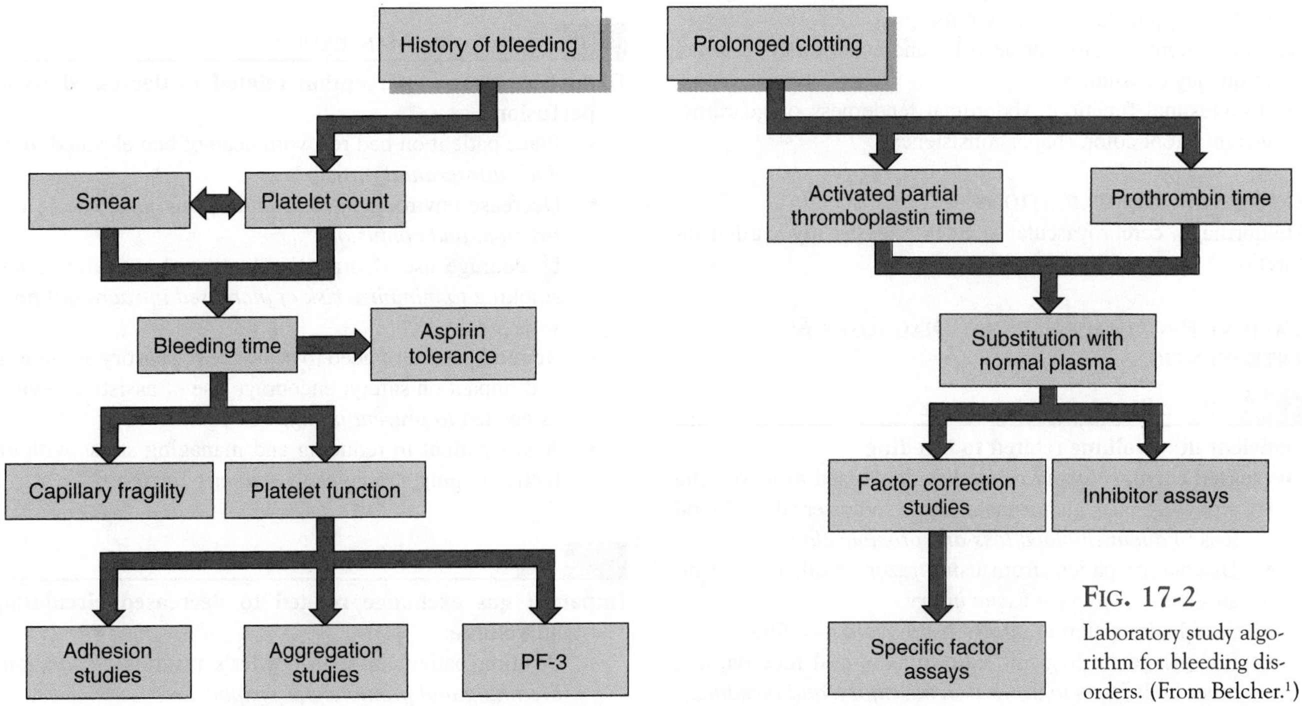

Fig. 17-2 Laboratory study algorithm for bleeding disorders. (From Belcher.[1])

Fibrinogen level: Decreased (less than 150 mg/dl)
Antithrombin III level: Decreased
Fibrin degradation products (most sensitive indicator): Elevated (greater than 40)
Plasminogen levels: Decreased

MULTIDISCIPLINARY PLAN

The best treatment is prevention. If DIC occurs in spite of preventive efforts, the focus should be on the treatment of the underlying cause or disease process.

Medications

IV antibiotic therapy; anticoagulants such as heparin in early phase; cryoprecipitated clotting factors in later phase; ε-aminocaproic acid; cardiotonic and vasoconstricting drugs; antidysrhythmic drugs

General Management

Strict adherence to aseptic technique; transfusion of blood products

NURSING CARE

NURSING ASSESSMENT

Vascular function: Bleeding from many sites (i.e., nose, gums, sites of infection), stool, urine, emesis, and sputum for presence of occult and observable blood; petechiae, purpura, and ecchymosis; skin color and temperature; apical, brachial, carotid, radial, femoral, and tibial pulses
Neurologic function: Strokelike signs/symptoms (e.g., decreased movement and strength of extremities); altered level of consciousness, orientation, and pupillary reaction; dizziness
Respiratory function: Dyspnea; tachypnea, cyanosis, pallor
Basilar rales, rhonchi, high-pitched bronchial sounds
Cardiovascular function: Tachycardia; dysrhythmias, gallop rhythm; hypotension, narrow pulse pressure
Renal function: Oliguria; urine color and consistency of urine; frequency of voiding
Gastrointestinal function: Abdominal tenderness or guarding; weight; stool color, shape, consistency

POTENTIAL COMPLICATIONS

Hemorrhage; cerebrovascular accident; sepsis; myocardial infarction

PATIENT PROBLEMS/NURSING DIAGNOSES & INTERVENTIONS

NIC TISSUE PERFUSION MANAGEMENT

Deficient fluid volume related to bleeding
Decreased cardiac output related to decreased fluid volume

- Apply ice pack and/or manual pressure over site of blood loss *to diminish blood loss and promote clotting.*
- Discourage patient from using razor or other sharp instruments *to prevent tissue injury.*
- Avoid administering injections *to avoid bleeding.*
- Provide gentle hygienic care to skin, oral mucosa, and other body parts *to avoid trauma, injury, and bleeding.*

> **! EMERGENCY ALERT**
>
> **DISSEMINATED INTRAVASCULAR COAGULATION (DIC)**
>
> A serious complication in which the blood clotting mechanism is accelerated, resulting in diffuse intravascular fibrin formation that settles in microcirculation.
>
> **ASSESSMENT**
> - Obtain patient's history. DIC is generally precipitated by acute hemorrhage as in shock, abruptio placentae, incompatible blood transfusion, leukemia, carcinoma.
>
> **INTERVENTIONS**
> - Maintain airway, breathing, and circulation.
> - Administer high-flow oxygen (10-15 L) by mask.
> - Obtain IV access, laboratory studies, and fluid resuscitation as indicated.
> - Prepare to provide replacement of clotting factors, platelets, fresh frozen plasma, packed cells.
> - In collaboration with physician, administer heparin therapy.

- Maintain patient in semi-Fowler's position with legs elevated as necessary *to maximize venous return and promote adequate cardiac output.*
- Encourage patient to avoid straining at stool *to prevent gastrointestinal bleeding.*

NIC ELIMINATION MANAGEMENT

Impaired urinary elimination related to decreased fluid volume

- Use Foley catheter as needed *to monitor urine production.*

NIC NEUROLOGIC MANAGEMENT

Disturbed sensory perception related to decreased tissue perfusion

- Place patient on bed rest with head of bed elevated *to reduce intracranial pressure.*
- Decrease environmental stimuli *to minimize stress, distraction, and confusion.*
- Discourage use of oral stimulants such as caffeine and smoking *to minimize risk of increased intracranial pressure.*
- Remind patient of need to be aware of sensory alterations and impact on safety; encourage use of assistive devices as needed *to prevent injury.*
- Assist patient in reducing and managing stress with effective coping strategies *to minimize anxiety.*

NIC RESPIRATORY MANAGEMENT

Impaired gas exchange related to decreased circulating blood volume

- Position patient in semi-Fowler's position *to facilitate breathing and promote chest expansion.*

- Encourage patient to take frequent deep breaths *to reduce hyperventilation.*
- Provide oxygen therapy as prescribed *to reduce cardiopulmonary workload and to enhance tissue oxygenation.*
- Help patient maintain a balance between rest and activity *to decrease oxygen requirement.*
- Maintain a warm environment *to avoid shivering and increased oxygen requirement.*

PATIENT EDUCATION/CONTINUUM OF CARE PLAN

1. Discuss with patient and family signs and symptoms of DIC that should be reported immediately to the health-care provider.
2. Have patient learn to self-administer heparin therapy.
3. Assist patient and family in avoiding mechanical trauma such as from a hard toothbrush, blade razor, vigorous nose blowing, or contact sports.

EVALUATION/PATIENT OUTCOMES

Tissue Perfusion Management: Vital signs are within normal limits. Fluid balance is maintained.

Elimination Management: Bowel and bladder elimination are normal.

Neurologic Management: Neurologic function is within normal limits. Patient is oriented, alert, and calm.

Respiratory Management: Respiratory function is within normal limits.

HEMOPHILIA

Hemophilia is a disorder characterized by impaired coagulability of the blood and a tendency to bleed.

The incidence of hemophilia, an X-linked recessive trait, is 1 in 10,000. Hemophilia A (classic hemophilia) is the result of a deficiency of factor VIII; it accounts for 80% of cases and is, with rare exceptions, a disease of males. Hemophilia B (Christmas disease) is the result of a deficiency of factor IX; it accounts for 20% of cases.

All daughters of hemophiliac males become carriers; the sons of a female carrier have a 50% chance of being hemophiliac, and the daughters have a 50% chance of becoming carriers. Homozygous females with hemophilia (father a hemophiliac, mother a carrier) are extremely rare. In patients with hemophilia who have no family history of the disease it is thought that the disease is the result of a new mutation.

Other less common forms of hemophilia include hemophilia C, a hemorrhagic susceptibility transmitted as an autosomal dominant trait and caused by a lack of clotting factor XI; calpriva, a bleeding tendency caused by a serum calcium deficiency; vascular hemophilia, also called angiohemophilia; and von Willebrand's disease, an autosomal dominant trait in both males and females with factor VII_{VWF} and VIII_{AHC} deficiency and a platelet adhesion defect.

Prior to transfusion therapy, few persons with hemophilia A survived more than 3 years from birth; with the advent of blood transfusions and factor VIII, many persons with hemophilia become adults.

> **EMERGENCY ALERT**
>
> **HEMOPHILIA**
>
> Hemophilia is a genetic disorder affecting males that causes bleeding that results from the absence of a clotting factor.
>
> **ASSESSMENT**
> - Bleeding gums, epistaxis
> - Hemarthrosis causing joint immobility
> - Severe bruises with minor trauma
> - Bleeding history
> - Other pain
>
> **INTERVENTIONS**
> - Monitor vital signs.
> - Administer oxygen as needed to maintain comfort and adequate oxygen saturation.
> - Elevate any affected joint, apply gentle pressure to bleeding site, immobilize the area, and apply ice.
> - Obtain IV access and provide hydration.
> - Prepare to administer fresh frozen plasma.
> - Aspirate joint if needed.

PATHOPHYSIOLOGY

The degree of bleeding experienced by the patient is related to the amount of factor activity and the severity of the injury. When factor activity levels are below 1%, spontaneous bleeding, hemarthrosis, and deep tissue bleeding occur. When levels are 5% or higher, bleeding usually results from trauma or surgical procedures and occurs because of the absence of or deficiency in a specific clotting factor. The patient forms platelet plugs at the site of bleeding, but the deficiency in clotting factor impairs this response, especially the capacity to form a stable fibrin clot. This results in abnormal bleeding, which may be mild to severe.

DIAGNOSTIC STUDIES AND FINDINGS

Prothrombin time INR (PT/INR): Normal
Partial thromboplastin time (PTT): Prolonged
Bleeding time: Normal; prolonged in von Willebrand's disease

MULTIDISCIPLINARY PLAN

General Management

Replacement of deficient factor
- For hemophilia A, cryoprecipitate containing 8 to 100 U of factor VIII per bag at 12-hour intervals until bleeding stops
- For hemophilia B, plasma or factor IX concentrate given every 24 hours until bleeding stops

Treatment for development of antibody inhibitors against the specific coagulation factor

Immunosuppressive agents

Plasmapheresis to remove the inhibitor
Prothrombin complexes that bypass the inhibitor
Synthetically produced desmopressin (DDAVP) administered IV to increase factor VIII activity level

NURSING CARE

Nursing Assessment

Vascular function: Hypotension, tachycardia, hyperpnea; bleeding from nose, gums, and infection sites; petechiae, purpura, and ecchymosis; menorrhagia; hemarthrosis with pain and deformity, especially in hip and knee; hematuria or melena; abdominal girth

Neurologic function: Signs of disorientation or confusion; convulsions, projectile vomiting; decreased reflexes, including pupillary

Potential Complications

Cerebrovascular accident; hemorrhage

Patient Problems/Nursing Diagnoses & Interventions

NIC Tissue Perfusion Management

Deficient fluid volume related to blood loss

Ineffective (peripheral) tissue perfusion related to decreased fluid volume

- Administer blood therapy as prescribed *to control bleeding.*
- Observe patient for adverse reactions to therapy.
- Observe for signs/symptoms of hepatitis such as jaundice, clay-colored stool, mahogany-colored urine, nausea, and abdominal distention.
- Apply cold pack to affected joint or traumatized area *to control bleeding.*
- Administer analgesics as prescribed to relieve joint pain.
- Assist patient *to avoid trauma such as falls, bumps.*
- Do not administer injections unless absolutely necessary *to avoid bleeding.*

NIC Neurologic Management

Disturbed sensory perception related to decreased tissue perfusion

- Place patient on bed rest with head elevated *to reduce intracranial pressure and unnecessary activity.*
- Protect patient's head with helmet and pad side rails if necessary *to protect from injury.*
- Discourage oral stimulants such as caffeine and smoking, *which might increase intracranial pressure.*
- Remind patient to ambulate safely; encourage use of assistive devices such as a walker or cane *to avoid injury.*

Patient Education/Continuum of Care Plan

1. Teach patient to self-administer blood products.
2. Discuss the need to avoid injury such as that caused by contact sports, use of use of sharp objects.
3. Discuss the need to report signs and symptoms of bleeding to health-care provider.
4. Encourage the patient to seek genetic counseling.

Evaluation/Patient Outcomes

Tissue Perfusion Management: Vital signs are within normal limits. Gastrointestinal function is normal with no evidence of bleeding or hepatitis. Renal function is normal; no evidence of bleeding. Skin and skeletal structure are within normal limits without evidence of bleeding or swelling of joints.

Neurologic Management: Neurologic function is within normal limits. Patient is oriented, alert, and calm.

Malignant Lymphomas

Malignant lymphomas are solid tumors of the lymphoid system.

The proliferation of committed lymphocytes occurs in lymphoid tissue throughout the body, including the lymph nodes and spleen. There are two major categories of malignant lymphomas among adults: Hodgkin's disease and non-Hodgkin's lymphomas, which include indolent or nodular lymphomas (small lymphocyte, mantle cell, follicular cell) and the aggressive or diffuse lymphomas (large B cell, lymphoblastic, peripheral T cell, Burkitt's).

Pathophysiology

The etiology of most lymphomas is unclear but is related to a genetic or chromosomal abnormality developing in a single normal lymphocyte in the body. Hodgkin's disease (HD) is a chronic and progressive form of cancer that primarily affects adults in the mid-to-late 20s and then persons over the age of 50. Men are affected twice as often as women. The disease is characterized by the abnormal proliferation of histiocytes called Reed-Sternberg cells, which eventually replace the normal cellular structure of the lymph nodes and cause areas of necrosis and fibrosis to develop. Possible causes of HD include viral infections and previous exposure to alkylating chemical agents.

HD initially affects one lymph node and then travels via lymphatic channels to nodes throughout the body. It may also appear in the liver, lungs, bone, and bone marrow. Staging of HD is based on microscopic appearance of the lymph nodes, extent and severity of the disease (Fig. 17-3), and prognosis (see Table 17-1 for one method of staging). The prognosis for untreated patients is about 5 years; those diagnosed in stage I or II have a 95% cure rate, whereas those in stage III or IV have a poor prognosis.

Lymphosarcoma and reticulum cell sarcomas account for about 40% of malignant lymphomas. Early widespread dissemination is common, with oropharyngeal lymphoid tissue, the gastrointestinal tract, and bone frequently affected. Other organs that may be involved are the skin and the nervous system. These lymphomas usually progress in a less systematic and predictable manner, and most consist of malignant B cells. The

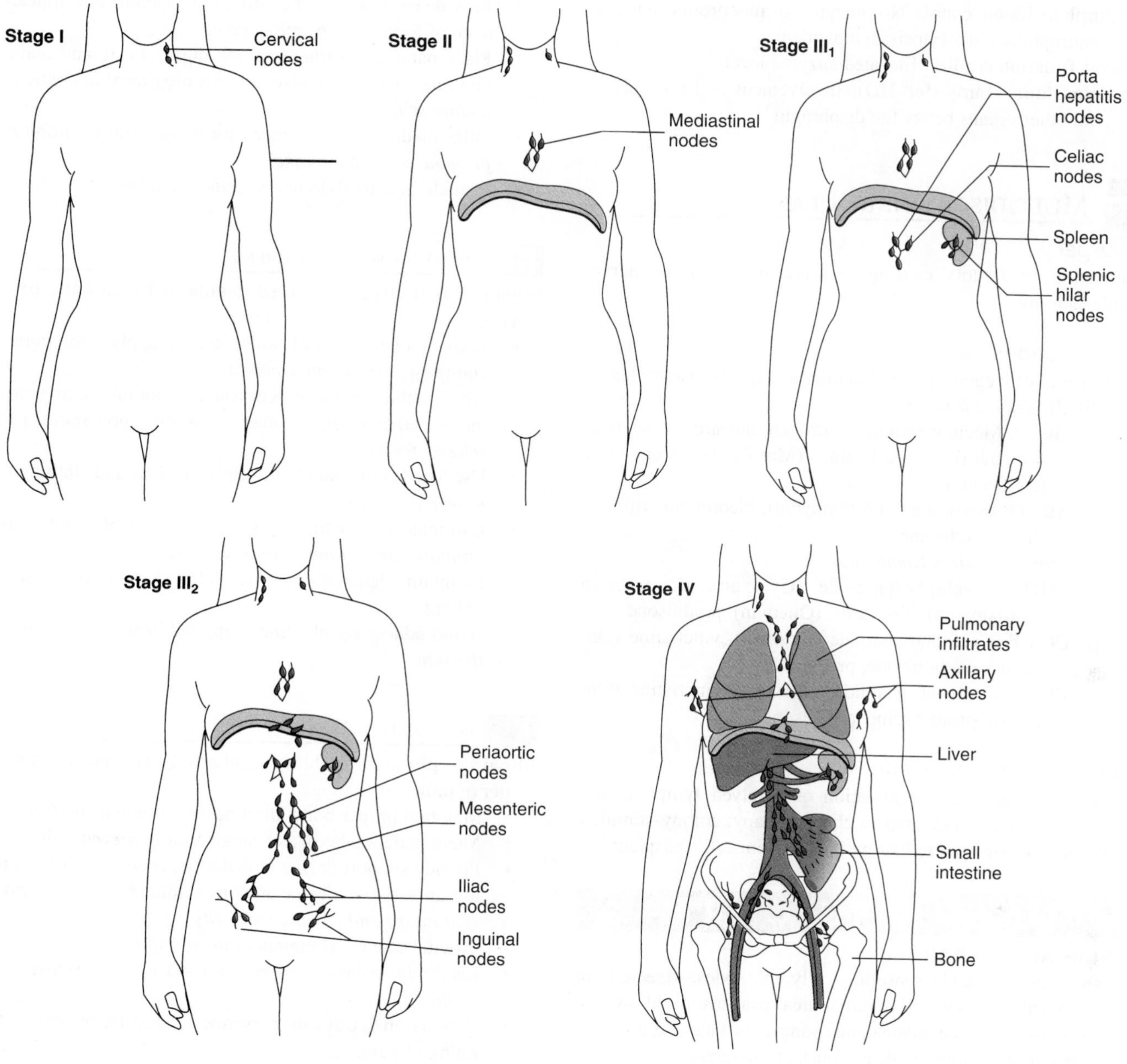

FIG. 17-3

Nodal involvement by stage in Hodgkin's disease. (Based on modified Ann Arbor staging system.) (From Belcher.[1])

prognosis for patients with non-Hodgkin's lymphomas is generally poorer than for HD.

Diagnostic Studies and Findings

Lymph node biopsy: Presence of Reed-Sternberg cells (HD) or malignant B cells

Bilateral bone marrow biopsies: Malignant cells

Roentgenogram and computed tomography (CT) of chest: Mediastinal or hilar lymphadenopathy

Abdominal CT and ultrasonography: Lymphadenopathy

Lumbar puncture: Presence of malignant cells

Table 17-1 Staging of Hodgkin's Disease

Stage*	Definition
I	Single lymph node region
II	Two or more node regions limited to one side of the diaphragm
III	Disease on both sides of the diaphragm but limited to the lymph nodes and spleen
IV	Involvement of the bones, bone marrow, lung parenchyma, pleura, liver, skin, gastrointestinal tract, central nervous system, renal, and other sites

From Belcher.[1]

*All stages are subclassified as A or B to describe the absence (A) or presence (B) of systemic symptoms.

Complete blood count: Normocytic normochromic anemia; neutrophilic leukocytosis; lymphopenia
Liver function studies: Elevated enzyme levels
Staging laparotomy (for HD): Involvement of liver, spleen, and other organs below the diaphragm

MULTIDISCIPLINARY PLAN

Surgery

Excision of tumors causing pressure on organ or nerve; splenectomy

Medications

Antineoplastic agents in combination therapy, for example:

For Hodgkin's disease

MOPP: Mechlorethamine (nitrogen mustard), vincristine (Oncovin), procarbazine (Matulane), prednisone (Deltasone)

ABVD: Doxorubicin (Adriamycin), bleomycin, vinblastine, dacarbazine

For non-Hodgkin's lymphomas

CHOP: Cyclophosphamide (Cytoxan), doxorubicin (Adriamycin), vincristine (Oncovin), prednisone

COMP: Cyclophosphamide (Cytoxan), vincristine (Oncovin), methotrexate, prednisone

COPP: Cyclophosphamide (Cytoxan), vincristine (Oncovin), procarbazine, prednisone

General Management

Wide-field megavoltage radiation of involved lymph nodes; combination radiotherapy and chemotherapy; colony-stimulating factors; bone marrow or peripheral stem cell transplant

NURSING CARE

NURSING ASSESSMENT

Skin integrity: Painless swelling of lymph nodes, especially in cervical, axillary, and inguinal area; pruritus, night sweats, malaise; jaundice; edema and cyanosis of face and neck; irregular fever, high-grade or constant low-grade

Sensory and motor function: Bone pain, nerve pain (especially in lower back and extending down one or both legs), fatigue, numbness, and tingling; impaired mobility

Respiratory function: Cough, "sniffles," stridor; dyspnea, chest pain, palpitations; laryngeal paralysis; hoarseness; recent upper respiratory infections

Gastrointestinal function: Splenomegaly, hepatomegaly, abdominal distention; weight; anorexia, abdominal discomfort, nausea, vomiting, indigestion

PATIENT PROBLEMS/NURSING DIAGNOSES & INTERVENTIONS

NIC NUTRITION SUPPORT

Imbalanced nutrition: less than body requirements, related to enlarged spleen and liver, anorexia

- Provide small, frequent feedings of high-calorie, high protein foods and fluids *to increase nutritional intake while minimizing feeling of fullness.*
- Assist patient with oral care *to enhance appetite.*
- Provide environmental control, that is, odors and appearance of food, *to enhance appetite.*
- Place patient in sitting position during meal, and maintain this position for several hours after meal *to decrease feeling of fullness.*
- Offer medications as needed for nausea and vomiting *to promote adequate intake.*
- Provide heat to abdomen *to relieve discomfort.*

NIC SKIN/WOUND MANAGEMENT

Impaired skin integrity related to enlarged nodes and pruritis

- Bathe patient in cool water and/or apply cool, moist compresses *to enhance comfort.*
- Apply calamine lotion, cornstarch, sodium bicarbonate, medicated powder, or other antipruritic preparations *to relieve itching.*
- Use a bed cradle and lightweight blankets and clothing *to relieve pressure.*
- Lubricate skin with baby oil, bath oil, or body lotion *to promote comfort and relieve dryness.*
- Maintain adequate humidity and cool room *to decrease itching.*
- Avoid adhesives, alkaline soap, and heat, *which irritate the skin.*

NIC IMMOBILITY MANAGEMENT

Impaired physical mobility (potential) related to bone, nerve pain

- Maintain proper body alignment *to promote comfort.*
- Move patient's body as a single unit *to prevent injury.*
- Provide support during ambulation; encourage patient to use an assistive device such as a walker or cane *to prevent injury and enhance mobility.*
- Provide safe environment *to avoid injury.*
- Encourage balance between rest and activity *to maximize mobility.*
- Provide analgesics as prescribed based on patient self-rating of pain.

NIC THERMOREGULATION

Risk for infection related to decreased WBCs
Ineffective thermoregulation related to impaired immune response

- Encourage patient to drink large volumes of fluid *for hydration.*
- Maintain protective isolation *to protect from pathogens.*
- Administer antibiotics as ordered *to treat infection.*
- Bathe patient in cool water *to reduce fever.*
- Cover patient with lightweight linens and clothing *to promote comfort and avoid chilling.*
- Maintain cool room temperature *for patient's comfort.*

NIC RESPIRATORY MANAGEMENT

Ineffective breathing pattern related to infection, enlarged nodes

- Place patient in sitting position *to enhance chest expansion.*

- Remove constrictive clothing *to relieve pressure on chest.*
- Encourage deep breathing and coughing *for alveolar expansion.*
- Administer oxygen therapy as prescribed and needed *to maximize tissue oxygenation.*
- Plan rest periods *to conserve energy.*
- Provide emergency equipment on standby.

Patient Education/Continuum of Care Plan

1. Discuss the need to avoid scratching and to care for skin with care to avoid skin damage and infection.
2. Practice with patient and family correct body alignment, use of assistive devices, and provision of safe environment.
3. Assist patient in pain management strategies, including analgesics and nonpharmacologic interventions.
4. Emphasize the importance of respiratory hygiene.
5. Emphasize the importance of a well-balanced diet and adequate hydration.
6. Plan with patient for dealing with probable sterility caused by treatment, (i.e., sperm banking, freezing of ova).

Evaluation/Patient Outcomes

Nutrition Support: Patient has adequate nutritional and fluid intake.

Skin/Wound Management: Skin has healthy color and is free of lesions or other irritation.

Immobility Management: There is no evidence of physical injury. Patient ambulates without difficulty.

Respiratory Management/Thermoregulation: Vital signs are within normal limits.

Collaborative Interventions and Related Nursing Care

Blood Transfusions

Infusion of blood and blood products may be lifesaving for the patient with anemia or thrombocytopenia. The transfusion immediately increases the body's ability to receive oxygen and to enhance blood clotting. Types of transfusions are red blood cells, platelets, plasma, cryoprecipitate, and granulocyte.

Contraindications and Cautions

1. Hemolytic reactions are caused by blood type or Rh incompatibility. The reaction can be severe, with DIC and circulatory collapse.
2. Bacterial reactions result from infusion of contaminated blood, usually a gram-negative organism.
3. Allergic reactions are seen most often in patients with a history of allergy.
4. Febrile reactions occur in patient with anti-WBC antibodies, which develop after multiple transfusions.
5. Circulatory overload results from too rapid an infusion or too great a quantity of blood, usually whole blood.
6. Transfusion-associated graft-versus-host disease can occur in immunosuppressed and immunocompetent patients; in the former donor T lymphocytes attack host tissues; in the latter, the host and donor share similar human leukocyte antigens.

Preprocedural Nursing Care

A physician's order is needed to administer blood or blood products: type of product, volume, and special conditions must be ordered. The nurse verifies the order and evaluates the patient's need for transfusion. A blood specimen is obtained for typing and crossmatching. The procedure and frequency of it are specified by institutional policy. A 19-gauge needle or larger (unless needleless system), a blood filter, and Y tubes or straight tubing sets are used. Normal saline is the preferred solution. Medications are never added to transfusions. Two registered nurses together check the physician's order, the patient's identity, and the match between the institutional identification band name and number with those on the blood product tag. The blood bag label and attached tag and the requisition slip are checked for ABO and Rh type compatibility. The expiration date is also checked. The product is inspected for cloudiness, discoloration, or gas bubbles. The patient may receive premedication per physician order or institutional policy. Vital signs are monitored before and throughout the course of the transfusion.

Multidisciplinary Plan

Medications and other interventions are administered as needed in response to transfusion reactions.

NURSING CARE

Nursing Assessment

Hemolytic reaction: Chills and fever; tachycardia, chest pain; dyspnea, cyanosis, tachypnea; hypotension; nausea and vomiting; hematuria or oliguria; headache, backache; apprehension, sense of impending doom

Febrile reaction: Chills and fever, sensations of cold; tachycardia; tachypnea

Allergic reaction: Urticaria, itching; bronchospasm; anaphylaxis

Circulatory overload: Hypertension; bounding pulse; distended jugular veins; dyspnea, cough, hemoptysis; confusion, restlessness

Transfusion-associated graft-versus-host disease: Thrombocytopenia; anorexia, nausea, vomiting; chronic hepatitis; weight loss; recurrent infection

Patient Problems/Nursing Diagnoses & Interventions

NIC Risk Management

Risk for injury related to reaction to transfusion

- Discontinue blood transfusion immediately if reaction occurs.
- Notify physician and blood bank.
- Send remaining blood and patient blood sample to laboratory for testing.

- Administer intravenous fluids *(to maintain patency of line),* oxygen therapy, and medications as prescribed or via protocol (i.e., vasopressors, epinephrine, sedatives, bronchodilators, corticosteroids, analgesics, antiemetics).
- Monitor vital signs, central venous pressure.
- Insert Foly catheter as needed.
- Use cooling measures as needed.

PATIENT EDUCATION/CONTINUUM OF CARE PLAN

Instruct patient to report signs and/or symptoms listed in Assessment.

EVALUATION/PATIENT OUTCOMES

Risk Management: Color of skin and mucous membranes is normal. Vital signs are within normal limits. Patient has normal body hydration. Daily fluid output is equal to fluid intake. There is no evidence of physical injury.

BONE MARROW TRANSPLANTATION

For a discussion of bone marrow transplantation, see Chapter 16.

SPLENECTOMY

Although it serves various important functions, the spleen can be surgically removed from adults without harm. Hypersplenism, the destruction of excessive numbers of blood cells by the spleen, is a major reason for its surgical removal. Another frequent indication is splenic rupture with severe hemorrhage, often caused by trauma. The procedure is relatively simple unless the spleen is greatly enlarged or surrounded by adhesions.

MULTIDISCIPLINARY PLAN

Surgery

Removal of the spleen by abdominal or laparoscopic incision

General Management

Parenteral therapy, analgesia, intake and output

NURSING CARE

NURSING ASSESSMENT

Vascular function: Signs and symptoms of hemorrhaging and shock; amount and color of drainage

Gastrointestinal function: Abdominal distention and discomfort; gastric discharge

Metabolic activity: Elevated temperature

Pulmonary function: Decreased breath sounds; splinting with respirations; tachypnea; evidence of atelectasis

Immunologic function: Infection secondary to wound contamination

Comfort: Pain at surgical site

POTENTIAL COMPLICATIONS

Atelectasis; pneumonia; abdominal distention; abscess formation

PATIENT PROBLEMS/NURSING DIAGNOSES & INTERVENTIONS

NIC TISSUE PERFUSION MANAGEMENT

Risk for deficient fluid volume related to intravascular hypovolemia, fever, nasogastric drainage, and paralytic ileus

Ineffective peripheral or gastrointestinal tissue perfusion related to hemorrhaging

- Administer intravenous fluids, including blood, as ordered *to maintain adequate fluid volume.*
- Measure intake and output *to assess balance.*
- Check surgical incision *to determine its condition.*
- Apply ice bag and manual pressure or dressing over surgical site *to control bleeding.*
- Estimate blood loss *to determine need for replacement.*
- Apply cool, damp cloth to the face of febrile patient *to promote heat loss by evaporation.*
- Bathe the patient in cool water, apply ice bag or alcohol, and cover with lightweight blankets and clothing *to reduce fever.*
- Maintain cool room temperature.
- Increase fluid intake, especially iced liquids.
- Monitor amount, color, and consistency of drainage.
- Ambulate when possible *to promote gastric motility.*

NIC RISK MANAGEMENT

Risk for infection related to wound contamination

- Monitor temperature, pulse, respirations, and breath sounds *for early indications of infection.*
- Have patient turn, cough, and deep breathe and use incentive spirometry at regular intervals *to maintain ventilatory function.*
- Change dressing, using sterile technique.
- Encourage fluids, monitor intake and output, and assess urine *to prevent urinary tract infection.*

NIC PHYSICAL COMFORT PROMOTION

Pain related to surgical incision

- Identify patient's preferred pain relief measures; implement when feasible.
- Apply abdominal binder *for support of dressing and wound.*
- Apply warmth, such as with a heating pad, to abdominal area.
- Administer medications, such as neostigmine (Prostigmin) and mild analgesics, as ordered *to relieve distention.*
- Observe for increased complaints of pain, nausea, vomiting, diarrhea, and abdominal distention, *which indicate dehiscence and obstruction.*
- Evaluate effectiveness of pain relief measures.

PATIENT EDUCATION/CONTINUUM OF CARE PLAN

1. Demonstrate to patient care of the surgical incision.
2. Discuss the importance of gradually increasing level of activity.

3. Emphasize the importance of a well-balanced diet, exercise, rest, and other healthful behaviors.

Evaluation/Patient Outcomes

Tissue Perfusion Management: Color of the skin and mucous membranes is good. Skin, nails, lips, and earlobes are warm and moist and have a natural color.

Risk Management: Vital signs are within normal limits. Respirations, pulse, blood pressure, and temperature are within normal limits.

Physical Comfort Promotion: Patient has the physical appearance of comfort. Patient has calm, relaxed facial expression. Posture is normal, and patient expresses comfort.

References

1. Belcher AE: *Cancer nursing,* St. Louis, 1992, Mosby.
2. Erickson JM: Anemia, *Semin Oncol Nurs* 12:2, 1996.
3. Hawkins R: Disseminated intravascular coagulation, *Clin J Oncol Nurs* 3:127, 1999.
4. Knoop T: Polycythemia vera, *Semin Oncol Nurs* 12:70, 1996.
5. Leukemia Society of America: *Acute lymphocytic leukemia,* New York, 1997, The Society.
6. Leukemia Society of America: *Acute myelogenous leukemia,* New York, 1998, The Society.
7. Leukemia Society of America: *Myeloma,* New York, 1998, The Society.
8. Leukemia Society of America: *Chronic myelogenous leukemia,* New York, 1999, The Society.
9. Deleted in proofs.
10. Nunez AM, Liebman MC: Febrile neutropenia, *ONS Supplement,* p 9, 1999.
11. Rust DM, Wood LS, Battiato LA: Oprelvekin: an alternative treatment for thrombocytopenia, *Clin J Oncol Nurs* 3:57, 1999.
12. Sheridan CA: Multiple myeloma, *Semin Oncol Nurs* 12:59, 1996.

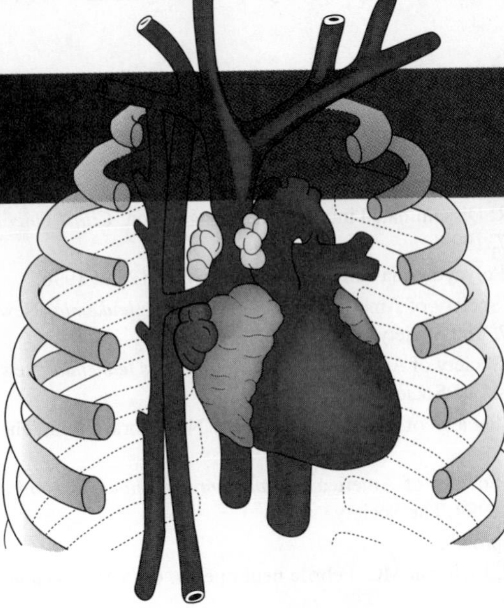

18 Neoplasia

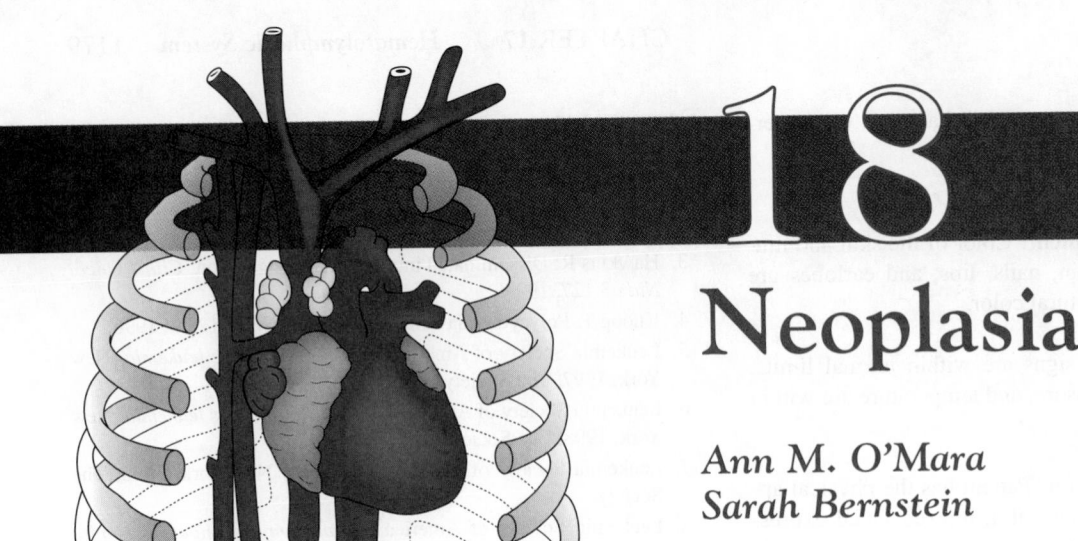

Ann M. O'Mara
Sarah Bernstein

OVERVIEW

Cancer is the second most common cause of death in the United States, killing about 552,200 people annually. An estimated 1,220,100 new cases of cancer are diagnosed in the United States every year, and this number does not include carcinoma in situ and basal and squamous cell skin cancers. Earlier diagnosis and treatment of certain cancers and better health practices have improved the outlook for people with cancer. Six out of 10 people whose cancer was diagnosed in 2000 will be alive 5 years later.[1]

Cancer is a universal disease that affects people without regard to race, sex, socioeconomic status, or culture; however, different forms of cancer strike specific age, racial, and sexual groups. For example, cancer incidence increases rapidly with aging; some researchers believe that anyone who lives long enough will eventually develop cancer. Social and environmental factors are thought to explain racial differences in cancer. Both incidence and mortality are higher in African-Americans than in whites and in men than in women. The sites in men that are associated with the greatest mortality are the lung, colon and rectum, and prostate. In women the leading sites are the breast, lung, and colon and rectum (FIG. 18-1).

Cancer is probably caused by many interacting factors (initiators and promoters) rather than by a single one, and its development appears to be a multistep process. Some causative agents have been found, and others are suspected. One predisposing factor is chronic irritation, such as frequent, prolonged exposure to sunlight or sustained alcohol consumption. Some benign lesions, such as leukoplakia of the oral cavity, colon and rectal polyps, and pigmented moles, may undergo malignant transformation. People whose cancer is already diagnosed are at risk for later development of the disease at the same or another site. Environmental carcinogens that have been identified include cigarette smoke, asbestos, uranium, asphalt, and aniline dye. Iatrogenic factors that have been implicated are radiation and drugs, for example, diethylstilbestrol (DES), certain cancer chemotherapeutic agents, radioisotopes such as phosphorus (^{32}P) and radium, and immunosuppressive drugs.

Recent research findings have demonstrated the increasing role genetic factors are playing in the etiology of cancer. All cancer cells demonstrate genetic alterations or mutations. Of particular interest are the two types of growth-control genes called *oncogenes* or proto-oncogenes and *anti-oncogenes* or tumor suppressor genes. As their names suggest, oncogenes code for proteins that stimulate growth, and anti-oncogenes code for proteins that block the action of growth-promoting factors.[13,17]

Most genetic alterations are found only within the cancer cells, not elsewhere in the body, and are labeled sporadic or somatic. In addition, there is another category of mutations that are found within both the cancer cells and throughout the body, are considered hereditary or germ-line in origin, and can be passed on to offspring. Most cancers are sporadic, accounting for 85% of all cancers. In either hereditary or sporadic cancers an array of proto-oncogenes and/or anti-oncogenes has been implicated in the initiation and promotion of the particular malignant tumor. For hereditary cancers, BRCA1 and BRCA2 have been found to be responsible in the development of breast and ovarian cancers and at least four mutator genes may account for approximately 70% to 80% of hereditary nonpolypoid colorectal cancer.[13,17]

ANATOMY, PHYSIOLOGY, AND RELATED PATHOPHYSIOLOGY

In describing the nature and possible causes of cancer, it is important to understand that cancer cells, unlike normal cells, proliferate without organization and often without differentiation. Certain stimuli are believed to initiate this process, which subsequently overpowers the normal control mechanism. The results are uninhibited growth (autonomy), lack of differentiation (anaplasia), and uncontrolled motility, permitting spread to other parts of the body (metastasis) via blood or the lymphatic system.

Normal cell division occurs in a pattern of sequential events referred to as the *cell cycle*. There are five stages of this cycle, which include resting phase (G_0), postmitotic phase (G_1), synthesis (S), premitotic phase (G_2), and mitosis (M). During mitosis, the actual growth phase, cytoplasmic and nuclear separation, occurs within the cell, which results in two identical

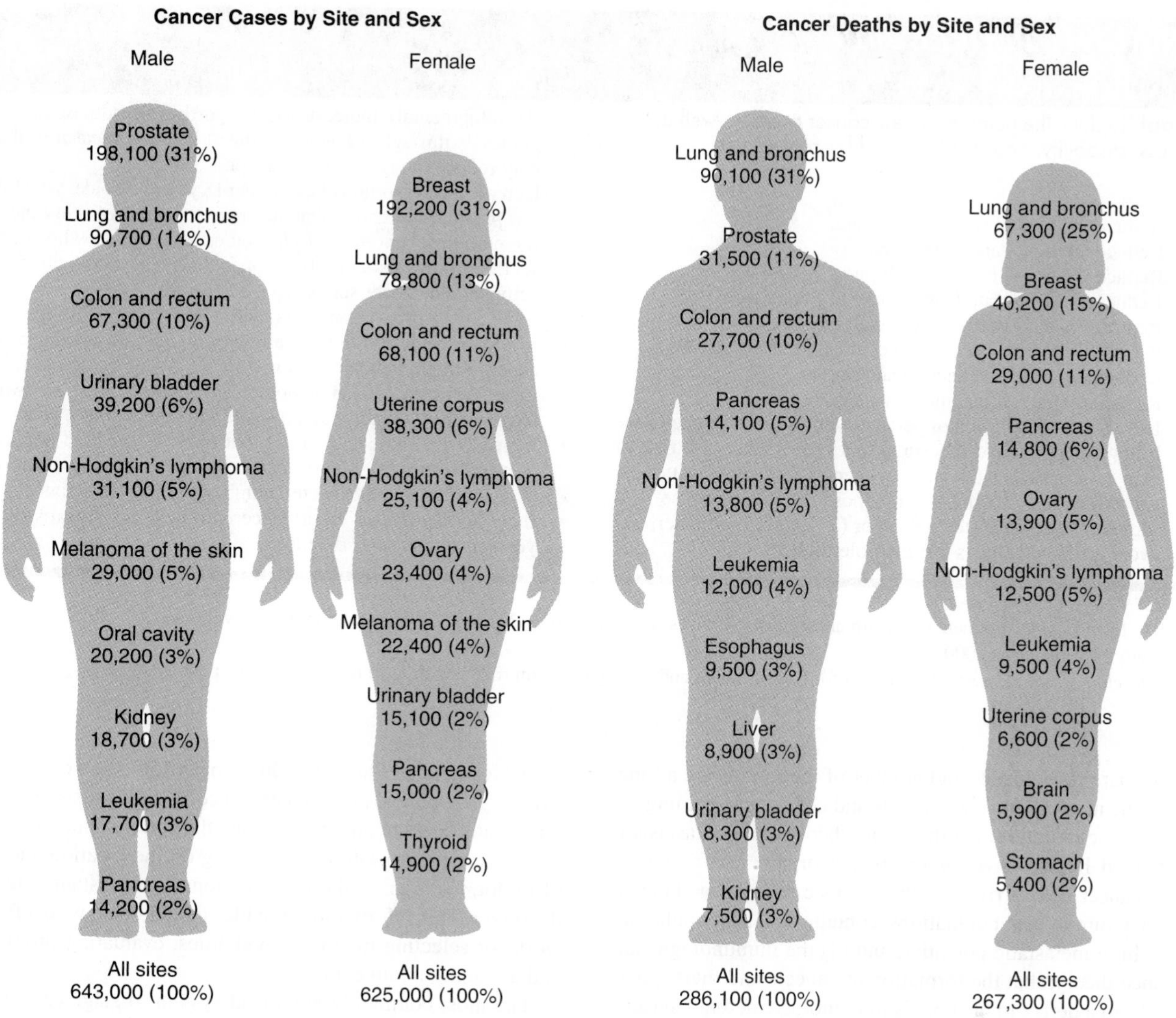

FIG. 18-1

Cancer incidence and deaths by site and sex—2001 estimates. (*Excluding basal squamous cell skin cancer and carcinoma in situ.) (Data from American Cancer Society: *Cancer facts and figures*, Atlanta, 2001, The Society. *www.cancer.org* and National Cancer Institute: *surveillance, epidemiology, and end results* [SEER]).

daughter cells containing the full complement of genetic information found in the parent cell.

Neoplasia, a group of "new growth" cells, is the result of cells' unresponsiveness to the normal mechanisms of growth control. Cancer cells exhibit changes in the cytoplasm, including enzyme alterations, chromosome changes, and the production of new proteins via an active anabolic process; mitochondrial changes, increased energy production to meet the neoplasm's increased rate of glucose utilization and lactic acid production; and nuclear changes in which DNA is altered.

Unique characteristics of neoplasms include their having more cells in active reproduction at a given time than do normal tissues, a shorter cell cycle time, and increased doubling time.

Neoplasms are described as benign or malignant. Benign tumors have little or no invasive activity, are generally encapsulated, usually grow more slowly, and are rarely fatal. Malignant tumors not only invade surrounding tissues but also produce metastases. If untreated, these tumors usually result in death.

The primary site of a malignant neoplasm is its place of origin, which is sometimes discovered after a secondary or metastatic site has been identified and diagnosed. The secondary site has characteristics similar to those of the primary site. Some people have additional primary sites, which may be different types of cancer presenting different signs and symptoms at the same time (e.g., breast and ovarian cancers).

The malignant neoplasm's ability to invade surrounding tissues and to colonize distant sites is called *metastasis*. This may occur via direct extension, wherein the neoplasm expands, invades, and destroys normal adjacent tissue. The most frequent routes are penetration of the lymphatic system and bloodstream, which enable cancer cells to disseminate throughout the body. Another less common route is penetration of body cavities, for example, dissemination through the cerebrospinal fluid or transabdominal spread within the peritoneal cavity.

There are numerous theories regarding the process of cancer invasion and metastasis. Some of these are (1) the mechanical

HEALTHY PEOPLE 2010

HEALTH STATUS—CANCER

Goal: Reduce the number of new cancer cases as well as the illness, disability, and death caused by cancer.

CANCER

- Reduce the overall cancer death rate.
- Reduce the lung cancer death rate.
- Reduce the breast cancer death rate.
- Reduce the death rate from cancer of the uterine cervix.
- Reduce the colorectal cancer death rate.
- Reduce the oropharyngeal cancer death rate.
- Reduce the prostate cancer death rate.
- Reduce the rate of melanoma cancer deaths.
- Increase the proportion of persons who use at least one of the following protective measures that may reduce the risk of skin cancer: avoid the sun between 10 AM and 4 PM, wear sun-protective clothing when exposed to sunlight, use sunscreen with a sun protective factor (SPF) of 15 or higher, and avoid artificial sources of ultraviolet light.
- (Developmental) Increase the proportion of adolescents in grades 9 through 12 who follow protective measures that may reduce the risk of skin cancer.
- Increase the proportion of adults age 18 years and older who follow protective measures that may reduce the risk of skin cancer.
- Increase the proportion of physicians and dentists who counsel their at-risk patients about tobacco use cessation, physical activity, and cancer screening.
- Increase the proportion of women who receive a Pap test
- Increase the proportion of adults who receive a colorectal cancer screening examination.
- Increase the proportion of women age 40 years and older who have received a mammogram within the preceding 2 years.
- Increase the number of states that have a statewide population-based cancer registry that captures case information on at least 95% of the expected number of reportable cancers.
- Increase the proportion of cancer survivors who are living 5 years or longer after diagnosis.

Modified from U.S. Department of Health and Human Services: *Healthy people 2010* (conference edition, in two volumes), Washington, DC, January 2000.

NOTE: *Developmental* indicates that criteria for measurement and strategies to improve health have not as yet been specified.

theory, that the incidence and number of metastases are a function of the number and size of cells and cell groups gaining access to the circulation; (2) the "soil" theory, that metastasis is determined by the environment of the organs and tissues in which cancer cells arrive; (3) the intrinsic cellular factors theory, that tumor cell populations contain cell subpopulations with a high metastatic potential; and (4) the immunologic surveillance theory, that the formation of cancers and their spread result from a defect in the body's immunologic defense system.

The four types of cancer are carcinomas, usually solid tumors that arise from epithelial cells; sarcomas, derived from muscle, bone, and fat and other connective tissues; lymphomas, originating in lymphoid tissue; and leukemias, cancers of the hematologic system.

Some cancers can be prevented; for example, the risk of lung cancer can be virtually eliminated if a person stops smoking, and skin cancer can be prevented by avoiding overexposure to direct sunlight. These are both examples of primary prevention, a process by which people avoid carcinogens. Secondary prevention is a process used to diagnose a cancer or its precursor as soon as possible after it develops. Breast self-examination and testicular self-examination are examples of secondary prevention (Table 18-1).

The National Cancer Institute provides a description of the signs and symptoms that may indicate cancer. Alterations in eating habits, loss of appetite, difficulty in swallowing, or increased constipation or diarrhea should be evaluated. The presence of a lump or nodule anywhere in or on the body (especially if it is painless and slowly increasing in size), bleeding from orifices, unexplained recurrent pain or fever, steady weight loss, and repeated infections are typical signs and symptoms of cancer that must be assessed. The nurse must stress primary and secondary prevention through public education, screening, and early detection activities.

A biopsy of the suspected lump or lesion is the only definitive way of diagnosing cancer. Once the diagnosis has been made and before treatment is begun, the patient undergoes a series of staging procedures, depending on the location and type of tumor, to describe the local, regional, and distant extent of the tumor. This information provides the clinician with a framework for selecting treatment modalities, evaluating prognosis, and assessing treatment outcomes.

The most commonly employed system to stage cancer that is recommended by the American Joint Committee on Cancer is the TNM system. *T* describes the size of the tumor, *N* describes the number of lymph nodes, and *M* defines the absence or presence of distant metastasis. In conjunction with the TNM system is a system using Roman numerals I to IV. At the low end is stage I, which usually describes localized or well-defined disease, and at the high end is stage IV describing disseminated or metastatic disease. Some cancers use different systems; for example, the Dukes classification system is used in staging colon cancer. As the patient undergoes these staging procedures, the role of the nurse is one of educating the patient and family and assisting in preparing the patient for the test.

PSYCHOSOCIAL ASPECTS OF CANCER

Cancer evokes deep fears of pain, suffering, dependence, disfigurement, and death. Indeed, the fear of the disease is often so strong that a person may delay examination and diagnosis in hopes that the signs or symptoms will go away. This lag time between awareness of a problem and seeking medical attention can affect the impact of therapy and the prognosis. Thus awareness of attitudes toward cancer and efforts to influence them in a more hopeful direction through education are an important part of the nurse's role.

Table 18-1 Summary of Recommendations for the Early Detection of Cancer in Asymptomatic Persons at Average Risk

Examination	Sex	Age	Periodicity
Sigmoidoscopy	M and F	50 yr and older	1 examination every 5 yr
Stool occult blood test	M and F	50 yr and older	Annual
Digital rectal examination	M and F	40 yr and older	Annual
Prostate-specific antigen blood test*	F	50 yr and older	Annual
Papanicolaou (Pap) and pelvic examinations	F	Women who have been sexually active or are age 18 yr or older	Annual; after 3 or more satisfactory, consecutive, normal annual examinations, the Pap test may be performed less frequently at the discretion of the physician
Endometrial tissue sample	F	At menopause; women at high risk†	At menopause
Breast self-examination†	F	20 yr and older	Monthly
Clinical breast examination	F	20-39 yr	Every 3 yr
		40 yr and older	Annual
Mammography	F	40 yr and over	Annual
Health counseling†	M and F	20-40 yr	Every 3 yr
Cancer checkup§	M and F	40 yr and older	Annual

Data from National Cancer Institute[14a] and U.S. Preventive Services Task Force.[19b]
*Offered to men who have at least a 10-year life expectancy and to younger men who are at high risk.
†History of infertility, obesity, failure to ovulate, abnormal uterine bleeding, or estrogen therapy.
‡To include counseling about tobacco control, sun exposure, diet and nutrition, risk factors, sexual practices, and environmental and other occupational exposures.
§To include examination for cancers of the thyroid, testicles, prostate, ovaries, lymph nodes, oral cavity, and skin.

Variables that have been identified as shaping attitudes toward cancer are life experiences, especially those related to this disease; parental and cultural values and attitudes toward illness; society's emphasis on youth, health, and beauty; social pressures for early sexual experience, smoking, and other harmful behaviors; and portrayals of people with cancer in the mass media. Positive experiences and hopeful presentations of cancer and its treatment will give the individual, group, or community a clear perspective on the value of prevention, early diagnosis, and treatment.

Myths and Erroneous Beliefs

The following myths regarding cancer should be dispelled or at least clarified:

"Cancer is contagious." There is no clear evidence that this is true, although a human leukemic virus has been identified and some cancers do seem to occur with greater frequency in family members.

"All cancer patients have pain." Pain is highly variable and is related to the type, size, and location of the malignancy and the patient's pain tolerance.

"The treatment is worse than the disease because of disfiguring surgery and side effects of chemotherapy." This may be true for patients who are asymptomatic or relatively free of symptoms at the time of diagnosis.

"Sexual activity and other aspects of normal life must be forfeited." This is certainly not true if the patient and significant others are willing to consider modifications in lifestyle.

"Cancer is a death sentence." There are hundreds of thousands of cured cancer patients (almost 60% of people with cancer) in the United States today. With early diagnosis and treatment, most people with cancer could live long and productive lives.

Some common concerns of cancer patients are fear of alienation from family, friends, or health-care providers; mutilation, particularly if surgery is the treatment of choice; vulnerability, dependence, or lack of control; and mortality. The emotional responses of a patient to these and other concerns related to the disease may be feelings of hopelessness, helplessness, guilt, denial, apathy, hostility, self-blame, withdrawal, and a sense of unreality. The nature and severity of these behaviors depend on the patient's usual behavior, attitudes toward illness in general and cancer in particular, the site of the disease, therapeutic options, and the expected outcome. All of these factors must be recognized as influencing the response of the patient and family.

Coping Strategies

The nurse and other health-care providers should assess the patient's coping style, evaluate its effectiveness, and intervene when there is increasing distress or a continuing problem.

General nursing interventions that have been identified as helpful to cancer patients during the various stages of the illness include maintaining hope while avoiding false optimism; using a gentle, unhurried manner; expressing caring and concern; and focusing on the patient's strengths rather than weaknesses.

Many patients find self-help groups useful in dealing with the effects of cancer and its treatment. The value of receiving help from another person who has undergone a similar experience is well documented. The functions of such groups are to provide special information and successful coping techniques to people with similar problems, encouragement to maintain prescribed regimens, normalization of a behavior, and education of health-care professionals and the public about cancer patients' special needs. The most useful aspects of this approach to coping are believed to be the modeling aspects ("You can do it—I did it!") and the observation that helping someone else benefits the helper.

The family of the cancer patient may also need the assistance of health-care team members. Factors to be assessed when determining the impact of cancer on the family include the age of the patient and other family members, family dynamics, communication style, family background, and practical matters of concern to the patient and family. Specific nursing interventions that are of value to the family are as follows:

- Assessing and understanding cultural values about disease and treatment
- Giving the patient quality care
- Communicating frequently with the family
- Listening to the family
- Making the family comfortable, such as by orientation to the institutional setting and policies
- Referring the family to other members of the health-care team as appropriate
- Using touch to comfort family members as appropriate
- Preparing the family for home care of the patient
- Doing small things that are important to the family, such as rearranging a mealtime to permit a special dinner from home

Additional coping strategies that patients and their families may wish to learn about and use include relaxation exercises, meditation, imagery, self-hypnosis, music therapy, and humor. The nurse may serve as teacher or provide referral to resources for instruction in these techniques.

As previously mentioned, disfigurement is a particular concern of cancer patients. A change in body image may be actual (as with mastectomy) or perceived (as with hysterectomy). The visibility of the alteration may not affect the patient's reaction to it; perhaps of more significance is the function of the part or system and the patient's emotional attachment to it.

Another area of concern to patients and their families that may be less readily discussed is sexuality and feelings regarding gender and gender role identity. Many beliefs (cultural, religious, personal, and societal) affect a person's ability to deal with an alteration in sexuality. The following have been identified as especially influential:

- The duty of a man to satisfy a woman and vice versa
- The man as the aggressor and the woman as the passive recipient
- The obsession of both sexes with performance
- The use of sexual intercourse for procreation

These beliefs, as well as the other attitudes regarding masculine and feminine behaviors, may confuse and depress both the patient and partner. In addition, the symptoms of cancer, such as fatigue, malaise, fever, discharge, and odor, may adversely affect libido and the patient's general view of his or her sexuality. This is further complicated by hospitalization, with the resultant lack of privacy.

The nurse's role in this sensitive area is to assess the patient's readiness to discuss sexual concerns, identify appropriate resources, provide oral and written information that will assist the patient in understanding sexual concerns and possible solutions, and respect the patient and partner's need for privacy.

Complementary and Alternative Therapies

Therapies outside the traditional medical and surgical methods for treating cancer are gaining increasing attention from researchers and clinicians. Originally labeled as unproven or questionable methods of cancer treatment, complementary and/or alternative therapies pose special challenges for both patient and nurse. Some of these methods, which are touted as providing a high probability of cure, include various machines and devices, drugs and chemicals, nutritional approaches, and psychologic techniques. Other methods, which do not make these same claims, involve behavioral, psychologic, social, and spiritual approaches to health.[8]

Cancer patients, as well as patients with other chronic or debilitating diseases, are especially susceptible to claims made by practitioners of methods touted as curative. On the other hand, a number of therapies pose the potential for helping patients while they undergo standard medical and/or surgical therapy. The nurse's role in this domain includes assessing the presence of feelings of helplessness and hopelessness in the patient and pressure from family and friends to "keep trying," providing open communication with the patient and family regarding these issues, and providing information about and opportunities to discuss alternative therapies. See Chapter 2 for a discussion of complementary and alternative medicine.

In response to the many controversies surrounding complementary and/or alternative therapies, Congress, in 1992, mandated the establishment of the Office of Alternative Medicine (OAM), which later became the National Center for Complementary and Alternative Medicine as part of the National Institutes of Health (NIH). The express purpose of the Center is to facilitate and conduct research, as well as to disseminate information on complementary and/or alternative therapies.

Informed Consent

The issue of informed consent often presents dilemmas for both the patient and the nurse, especially if experimental therapy is being recommended. The nurse should serve as both teacher and advocate for the patient, who may need further explanation of the proposed procedure or protocol, answers to specific questions, or an opportunity to "think out loud." The consent process should include, at the least, the basic steps of explanation of the medical condition, explanation of the nature and purpose of the procedure or protocol, and explanation of the risks, alternatives, and consequences of the procedure or protocol.

If consent is to be informed, there must be a patient of legal age and sound mind; a patient capable of cognition and reason; voluntariness; lack of coercion, deceit, or fraud; the right to refuse; comprehensible language; satisfactory answers to the patient's questions; and assurance of privacy and confidentiality.

Whatever the issue, the nurse should assess the patient's comprehension of the consent form, notify the physician if the patient is confused or ambivalent (unless a nursing procedure or protocol is being proposed), respect the individual's freedom of choice, and promote the patient's autonomy and independence in decision making.

Palliative and End of Life Care

Many people are living longer with cancer and its sequelae, prompting increased attention to hospice and palliative care. Optimally, palliative care begins at the time of a patient's diagnosis by managing the physical and psychosocial problems that occur during the disease continuum. Hospice provides support and care for patients and their families in the terminal stages of cancer. The hospice movement has been particularly useful to patients and their families who desire terminal care at home by providing palliative care, as well as end of life care.

Meeting the psychosocial needs of the cancer patient and family is one of the greatest challenges facing the nurse. The roles of counselor, teacher, consultant, and resource person are used to their maximum to enhance the patient's and family's coping with this complex of diseases and therapies.

Normal Findings

For assessment of a specific body system, see that chapter. Each site-specific cancer will highlight important assessment findings.

Conditions, Diseases, and Disorders

Primary Carcinoma of the Lung

Carcinoma of the lung is an uncontrolled growth of anaplastic cells in the lung. Types are epidermoid (squamous cell), adenocarcinoma, small cell undifferentiated (oat cell), and large cell undifferentiated.

Lung cancer varies significantly in its presentation, natural history, and response to treatment. Consequently, lung tumors are generally referred to as non–small cell and small cell. Within these two classifications are found cell types with some similarities. For example, squamous cell carcinomas, adenocarcinomas, and large cell carcinomas are considered non–small cell lung tumors, whereas tumors characterized by cells that contain large nuclei and very little cytoplasm (previously called oat cell) are considered small cell.

Carcinoma of the lung is the leading cause of death from cancer in men and women in the United States.[1] The incidence among women is steadily increasing, and more African-Americans than whites develop the disease. More than 90% of people with lung cancer die of it.

Approximately 80% of lung tumors are linked to cigarette smoking. The people at highest risk began smoking in their teens, inhale deeply, and smoke at least half a pack a day. People who quit smoking have a gradual decline in risk, eventually reaching levels similar to those of nonsmokers. Passive smoking or sidestream smoke contains as many carcinogens, if not more, than inhaled smoke.

Another etiologic factor in the development of lung carcinoma is occupational exposure to such substances as asbestos, uranium, nickel, and chromate. Air pollutants have not yet been proved a cancer risk factor, but the incidence of the disease is higher in urban populations (see box above).

Facts About Lung Cancer

Incidence: An estimated 169,500 new cases among men and women during 2001. The incidence rate in men is declining significantly from the high rate of 86.5 per 100,000 in 1984 to 69.1 in 1997. The rapid increase in women seen in the early 1990s has slowed to 43.1 per 100,000.

Mortality: An estimated 157,400 deaths in 2001. From 1990 to 1997, mortality from lung cancer declined significantly among men (−1.7% per year) while rates for women increased.

Risk factors: Cigarette smoking remains the strongest risk factor. Risk also increases with exposure to certain industrial substances, such as arsenic, certain organic chemicals, and asbestos, particularly for persons who smoke, and radiation exposure from occupational, medical, and environmental sources. Nonsmokers exposed to sidestream cigarette smoke are at an increased risk.

Early detection: Because of the asymptomatic nature of early lung cancer, it is difficult to detect it in the initial stage. If smokers stop smoking when early precancerous cellular changes have occurred, damaged bronchial lining tissues frequently return to normal. Smokers who continue to smoke may form abnormal cell growth patterns leading to cancer. Diagnosis is based on the chest x-ray findings, analysis of the types of cells contained in sputum, and fiberoptic examination of the bronchial passages.

Treatment: The type of lung cancer and its particular stage determine the treatment modality. Surgery is the treatment of choice for localized cancers. When the disease has spread, radiation and chemotherapy are often used in combination with surgery. Chemotherapy alone or in combination with radiation therapy is the treatment of choice in small cell lung cancer, with a large percentage of patients experiencing remission.

Data from American Cancer Society[1] and National Cancer Institute.[14a]

Pathophysiology

The length of time from a person's initial exposure to a carcinogen to the onset of lung cancer ranges from 10 to 30 years. A lesion not detected on x-ray but found by sputum cytologic study and by fiberoptic bronchoscopy can be surgically resected and is potentially curable. This is not generally true of a lesion first found on a chest roentgenogram; the smallest detectable tumor on a roentgenogram is 1 cm.

The major histologic types of lung cancer are divided into two categories.

Non–small cell lung cancers (NSCLCs) are usually not as aggressive as small cell lung cancers for early stage disease. However, with respect to surgery, they have a limited potential response to treatment for early stage disease. Several facts should be noted:

1. Squamous cell (epidermoid) tumors are the most common, comprising 35% of all lung tumors. Ninety percent occur

in men. These tumors tend to be centrally located and often produce bronchial obstruction.

2. Adenocarcinoma is often located peripherally; it is a common scar carcinoma that arises in an area of fibrosis at the site of previous pulmonary damage. This cancer is less often associated with smoking than are the other types. These tumors frequently spread through the submucosal lymphatics to regional lymph nodes and often metastasize to the brain and other distant organs by vascular invasion.
3. Large cell undifferentiated tumors may appear in any area of the lung. This type tends to disseminate early in its course and is associated with a poor prognosis. Giant cell and clear cell carcinomas are subtypes.

Small cell lung cancer (SCLC), also called oat cell cancer, comprises 10% of lung tumors. It is the most aggressive cancer, with lymphatic and distant metastases usually present at the time of diagnosis. Paraneoplastic syndromes are more common with this type. It tends to be highly sensitive to both chemotherapy and radiation therapy.

All types may have lymphatic metastasis early in the disease's course, beginning in the bronchial and mediastinal nodes and extending upward to supraclavicular nodes and downward to nodes below the diaphragm and to the liver and adrenal glands. Distant metastasis via the bloodstream to brain, bones, and contralateral lung may occur.

A chronic cough and wheezing are the most common early symptoms; other symptoms are fatigue, chest tightness, and aching joints. Late but clinically significant signs include hemoptysis, clubbing of the fingers, weight loss, and pleural effusion. Invasion of the superior vena cava causes edema of the neck and face. Phrenic nerve involvement results in paralysis of the diaphragm. A superior sulcus tumor involving the brachial plexus may manifest as shoulder and arm pain and paresthesias.

The chest lesion may be relatively asymptomatic, with the chief complaint caused by metastatic disease. Metastasis to the brain may result in headache, unsteady gait, and other neurologic signs. Weight loss, jaundice, or anorexia may occur with liver involvement. Localized bone pain or pathologic fractures may accompany skeletal involvement.

Paraneoplastic syndromes may be associated with lung cancer, particularly small cell lung cancer. For example, syndrome of inappropriate antidiuretic hormone (SIADH, low serum sodium) or Cushing's syndrome from ectopic adrenocorticotropic hormone production occurs in some patients with small cell cancer. Other syndromes include hypercalcemia, resulting from the production of ectopic parathormone-like substance (squamous cell cancer); carcinomatous neuropathy and myopathy; dermatomyositis; and hypertrophic pulmonary osteoarthropathy. Because the lung cancer is the underlying cause, chemotherapy provides the most significant improvement.[14]

Diagnostic Studies and Findings

Sputum cytologic study: Positive for malignant cells
Chest x-ray examination: Presence of tumor; invasion of chest wall or mediastinum
Computed tomogram (CT) of chest: Precise delineation of nodule, its density, and presence of calcium; invasion or compression of vascular structures; abnormal mediastinal lymph nodes
CT of upper abdomen: Metastatic disease in liver or adrenal glands
Magnetic resonance imaging (MRI): Invasion or compression of vascular structures by tumor
Fluoroscopy: Paralysis and phrenic nerve involvement
Bronchoscopy with bronchial brushing and biopsy: Presence of malignant cells
Mediastinoscopy and mediastinotomy: Presence of malignant cells in mediastinal lymph nodes
Transthoracic or transbronchial fine-needle aspiration: Presence of malignant cells
Thoracentesis: Presence of malignant cells
Scalene or supraclavicular node biopsy: Presence of malignant cells in palpable lymph nodes
Pulmonary function tests: Reduction of 50% in predicted forced vital capacity (FEV_1), maximum voluntary ventilation (MVV), or vital capacity (VC)
Arterial blood gas analysis: PaO_2 under 65 torr; $PaCO_2$ over 45 torr
Ventilation and perfusion radionuclide scanning: Little or no function in lung tissue to be resected
Abdominal CT or ultrasound: Metastatic disease to liver
CT or MRI of brain: Metastatic disease to brain
Bone scan: Metastatic disease to bone

Multidisciplinary Plan

Surgery

Thoracotomy: An exploratory surgical incision of the chest wall during which a biopsy specimen is collected; ribs are spread and pleura is opened
Limited pulmonary resection (segmental, wedge)
Lobectomy: Removal of a lobe of the lung and regional node dissection
Pneumonectomy: Surgical removal of an entire lung
Extended resection: En bloc removal of portions of the chest wall, vertebral body, left atrium, and/or diaphragm
Resection of subcarinal, lobar, and mediastinal nodes
Surgical excision of solitary metastatic disease to brain
Review the discussion of thoracic surgeries in Chapter 4

Radiation Therapy

External beam
Interstitial/endobronchial brachytherapy
Prophylactic cranial irradiation for small cell lung cancer

Chemotherapy

For Advanced NSCLC

The following combinations, including cisplatin with one or more other agents, have been used to achieve similar survival outcomes: vinblastine, mitomycin, vinorelbine, paclitaxel, and gemcitabine.[11]
Carboplatin, paclitaxel
Ifosfamide

Vindesine
Etoposide

For Small Cell Lung Cancer

CAV: Cyclophosphamide, doxorubicin (Adriamycin), vincristine
CEA: Cyclophosphamide, etoposide, doxorubicin (Adriamycin)
ICE: Ifosfamide, carboplatin, etoposide [VP-16]
EP or EC: Etoposide [VP-16], cisplatin, or carboplatin
CODE: Cisplatin, vincristine, doxorubicin (Adriamycin), etoposide

Other Therapies

Endobronchial laser therapy
Sclerosis for treatment of malignant pleural effusions

The prognosis for people with lung cancer correlates with tumor cell type. Those with well-differentiated squamous cell cancer have the best chance of survival; those with undifferentiated small cell cancer have the poorest. Peripheral tumors are more curable than central lesions. The presence of lymph node and distant metastases reduces the chance of cure. The stage of disease, patient's performance status, and immunologic state of the patient are important prognostic signs. Patients with gross supraclavicular adenopathy, a malignant pleural effusion, massive local extension, or distant metastases usually survive less than 1 year.

NURSING CARE

Nursing Assessment

Respiratory function: Chronic cough, nonproductive or productive; wheezing; chest tightness; hemoptysis; dyspnea; hoarseness; change in sputum amount or odor; orthopnea; tachypnea; frequent upper respiratory tract infections; abnormal resonance; dullness on percussion; clubbed fingers; shoulder and arm pain with paresthesia (Pancoast's syndrome); pale; cyanosis
Cardiovascular function: Chest pain; chest tightness
Neurologic function: Headaches; mental status changes related to brain metastasis or increased intracranial pressure
Endocrine function: SIADH with hyponatremia
Gastrointestinal function: Abdominal discomfort; elevated liver function tests; enlarged liver related to liver metastasis
Comfort level: Fatigue; shoulder and arm pain with paresthesia; bone pain related to bone metastasis
Nutritional status: Weight loss; anorexia; nausea and/or vomiting; decreased serum protein levels; dysphagia
Psychosocial status: Fear, anxiety

Potential Complications

Superior vena cava syndrome

Patient Problems/Nursing Diagnoses & Interventions

NIC Nutrition Support

See Comprehensive Care Plan, p. 1237

NIC Respiratory Management

Ineffective airway clearance related to bronchial obstruction secondary to tumor invasion
Ineffective breathing pattern related to discomfort and lack of pulmonary expansion

- Place patient in sitting position and change position frequently *to enhance breathing.*
- Encourage coughing and deep breathing with splinting of chest *to relieve congestion.*
- Ambulate patient as soon as possible *to increase circulation and chest expansion.*
- Encourage fluids *to liquify secretions.*
- Administer oxygen therapy as prescribed *to maintain adequate tissue oxygenation.*
- Anticipate patient's needs *to decrease unnecessary energy expenditure.*
- Discourage smoking *to decrease pulmonary workload.*

NIC Activity and Exercise Management

Activity intolerance related to generalized weakness

- Provide progressive increase in activity as tolerated to slowly increase the number of and endurance for activities (as tolerance allows) *to promote as much independence as possible.*
- Provide oxygen as needed *to decrease work of breathing during activity.*
- Instruct patient and family in use of equipment *to ensure proper use and decrease frustration of users.*
- Keep frequently used objects within reach for patient's convenience and *to decrease oxygen demand.*
- Problem solve with patient to determine methods of conserving energy while performing tasks (e.g., sit on stool while shaving; dry skin after bath by wrapping in terrycloth robe instead of drying skin with a towel *to use less oxygen, thereby producing less carbon dioxide.*

Patient Education/Continuum of Care Plan

1. Discourage smoking by the patient and family or significant others.
2. Explain how to cough productively and to perform breathing exercises and other respiratory therapy as prescribed to maintain pulmonary function.
3. Help patient ambulate, and instruct patient in the use of assistive devices such as canes and walkers to maintain mobility.
4. Explain how to self-administer medication for pain to maintain comfort.
5. Inform patient of the need for adequate nutrition (high-calorie, high-protein diet) to maintain energy.
6. Inform patient of the signs and symptoms of complications or adverse reactions to chemotherapy, radiation therapy, or both so that they can be treated immediately.
7. Help patient identify resources and support systems to help in rehabilitation and maintenance of quality of life.
8. Alert patient to the signs and symptoms of recurrence or metastatic disease, such as shoulder or arm pain, superior vena cava syndrome, liver disease, and central nervous

FACTS ABOUT COLORECTAL CANCER

Incidence: An estimated 135,400 new cases among men and women during 2001. Incidence declined significantly about 1.6% per year from 1985 through 1997.

Mortality: An estimated 56,700 deaths (48,100 from colon cancer, 8,600 from rectal cancer) in 2001, accounting for about 10% of cancer deaths. Mortality rates for colorectal cancer have also declined for men and women over the past 20 years.

Warning signs: Rectal bleeding, blood in the stool, changes in bowel habits (constipation or diarrhea), change in diameter of stool.

Risk factors: Familial polyposis of the colon or rectum, inflammatory bowel disease, and villous adenomas of the colon. A high fat and/or low-fiber diet, physical inactivity, and inadequate intake of fruits and vegetables may also play a role. Studies indicate that estrogen replacement therapy and nonsteroidal, antiinflammatory drugs, including aspirin, may reduce risk.

Data from American Cancer Society[1] and National Cancer Institute.[14a]

system changes, so that they can be treated as soon as possible.

EVALUATION/PATIENT OUTCOMES

Respiratory Management: Airway is patent. Breathing occurs without secretions. Breath sounds are clear in all areas. Lungs are clear on chest x-ray. Breathing is less labored.

Activity and Exercise Management: Activities of daily living are accomplished with minimal fatigue and dyspnea. Patient identifies methods to conserve energy.

CANCERS OF THE COLON AND RECTUM

Cancer of the colon and rectum is an uncontrolled growth of anaplastic cells in the colon or rectum. Types are adenocarcinoma, carcinoid tumor, leiomyosarcoma, and lymphoma (see box above).

PATHOPHYSIOLOGY

The most common symptom of colorectal cancer is rectal bleeding, followed by changes in bowel pattern (constipation or diarrhea), excessive flatus, distention, cramps, obstruction, and unexplained anemia. The presence of symptoms depends on the location of the tumor. Left-sided colonic lesions present as altered bowel habits, decreased stool caliber (pencil-like), urgency to defecate, vague abdominal pain, and hemorrhoids. Right-sided colonic lesions may manifest as unexplained iron deficiency anemia and gastrointestinal (GI) tract bleeding. Tumors of the sigmoid are characterized by obstruction from napkin ring growth. Rectal tumors are evidenced by gross rectal blood and tenesmus with a feeling of incomplete evacuation.

The majority of colorectal cancers are adenocarcinomas; others are carcinoid tumors, leiomyosarcomas, and lymphomas. Regional lymph nodes are involved in at least half of the patients. Most colon cancers spread to periaortic nodes. Anal carcinomas spread into perineal nodes. Distant metastasis is most often to the liver and lungs.

The 5-year survival rate for patients with localized disease is 88% for colon tumors. This rate is reduced by half with regional or distant involvement. The earlier the diagnosis and treatment, the more curable the cancer. Even with a large tumor and invasion of adjacent structures, the prognosis is favorable if appropriate treatment is provided. Only the presence of distant metastases precludes the possibility of cure.

DIAGNOSTIC STUDIES AND FINDINGS

Digital rectal examination: Palpation of suspect lesion

Fiberoptic colonoscopy: Visualization and biopsy of suspect lesion

Barium enema: Visualization of suspect lesion

Fecal occult blood test (FOBT): Presence of blood may be indicative of ulcerating malignancy

Carcinoembryonic antigen (CEA): Elevated

Hematocrit: Lower than normal as the result of blood loss

Vaginal examination: Presence of fistula

CA19-9: Elevated

MULTIDISCIPLINARY PLAN

Surgery

Local excision of well-differentiated rectal cancers

Resection of primary colon lesion with all mesentery that contains lymph nodes to which tumor is likely to spread; end-to-end anastomosis (is only curative treatment)

En bloc resection of colon, small bowel, bladder, uterus, and/or ovaries

Surgical bypass for inoperable obstructing tumors, with creation of fecal stoma

Review discussion of abdominal surgeries for the GI tract in Chapter 10

Radiation Therapy

Intraoperative radiation therapy

Radiation seeds

External beam therapy for inoperable obstructing rectal tumors

Transanal irradiation

Postoperative adjuvant therapy with radiation sensitizers for tumors dissecting the bowel wall or with positive lymph nodes

Palliation

Chemotherapy

Adjuvant regimen of 5-fluorouracil (5-FU) with leucovorin or levamisole[18]

Radiation sensitization with 5-FU and metronidazole

Endoscopic Laser Therapy

For small rectal tumors

NURSING CARE

Nursing Assessment

Gastrointestinal function

General: Change in bowel habits; blood in stool; abdominal pain; flatulence; indigestion; diminished or absent bowel sounds

Right colon: Dull, vague abdominal pain radiating to the back, dark/mahogany red blood in stool; weakness; liquid stool

Left colon: Cramps; gas pains; decrease in caliber of stool; bright red bleeding; constipation; rectal pressure; incomplete evacuation of stool

Transverse: Palpable masses; obstruction; bloody stool

Rectal: Bleeding; diarrhea; abdominal and/or low back pain; incomplete evacuation

Nutritional status: Anemia, weight loss, nausea, vomiting, anorexia, fatigue

Psychosocial status: Fear, anxiety

Potential Complications

Total bowel obstruction

Patient Problems/Nursing Diagnoses & Interventions

NIC Physical Comfort Promotion

See Comprehensive Care Plan, p. 1237.

NIC Elimination Management

Constipation related to colorectal obstruction by tumor
Diarrhea related to colorectal obstruction by tumor

For constipation

- Ambulate patient frequently, and encourage moderate physical exercise *to enhance GI motility.*
- Encourage increased intake of high-bulk foods and fluids; give fresh fruits, prune juice, hot coffee, and warm liquids *to increase GI motility.*
- Place patient in sitting position *to relieve abdominal pressure.*
- Give stool softeners and laxatives *to enhance elimination.*
- Administer enemas *to cleanse bowel.*
- Measure intake and output *to monitor hydration and quantity of feces.*
- Provide fluids so intake equals output *to prevent dehydration.*
- Cover patient with warm blankets *to prevent loss of body heat.*
- Encourage adequate rest *to decrease energy expenditure.*

For diarrhea

- Discourage oral stimulants, which increase GI motility.
- Discourage intake of high-bulk foods, which increase GI motility.
- Give tea, carbonated beverages, clear-liquid or full-liquid diet *to maintain hydration.*
- Refrain from giving hot or iced liquids, enemas, or laxatives, which irritate bowel.
- Refrain from inserting rectal tube or taking rectal temperatures, which irritate bowel.
- Be alert for complaints of pain caused by abdominal cramping or anal irritation, which may be precursors to diarrhea.

NIC Electrolyte and Acid-Base Management

Deficient fluid volume related to blood loss through rectum

- Apply ice bag to rectal area *to enhance vasoconstriction.*
- Change patient's position slowly *to avoid vascular trauma.*
- Cover patient with warm blankets *to maintain warmth and comfort.*
- Maintain complete bed rest if bleeding is severe *to avoid excessive blood loss.*
- Elevate foot of bed *to maintain blood flow to vital organs.*
- Refrain from giving enemas or laxatives, inserting rectal tube, or taking rectal temperature *to avoid tissue trauma and bleeding.*

Patient Education/Continuum of Care Plan

1. Inform patient of the need to maintain adequate GI function.
2. Instruct patient in pain relief measures.
3. Explain bowel changes (e.g., bleeding) patient should report.
4. Instruct patient in care of an ostomy if present.
5. Help patient plan an adequate and appropriate diet.
6. Help patient contact resources and support groups, such as the United Ostomy Association.

Evaluation/Patient Outcomes

Elimination Function: Bowel elimination is normal. Stools are soft and formed. Abdomen is soft and not distended. Bowel sounds are normal.

Electrolyte and Acid-Base Management: There is no evidence of rectal bleeding. Vital signs are within normal limits. Stool occult blood test results are negative. Blood counts are within normal limits. Patient reports usual energy and activity levels.

Carcinoma of the Breast

Carcinoma of the breast is an uncontrolled growth of anaplastic cells in the breast. Carcinoma of the breast includes the following histologic types: infiltrating ductal, infiltrating lobular, tubular, medullary, mucinous, and inflammatory. In addition, Paget's disease, sarcomas, papillary carcinomas, and invasive cribiform constitute the remaining malignant tumors of the breast.

Although the incidence of lung cancer is increasing, the breast remains the most common site of cancer in women between ages 25 and 75 years. Each year breast cancer is diagnosed in approximately 182,800 women in the United States. While lung cancer is the leading cause of cancer deaths for all women, breast cancer is the leading cause of cancer death in women ages 40 to 44 years. One of every nine women will be diagnosed with breast cancer during her lifetime. Elderly women

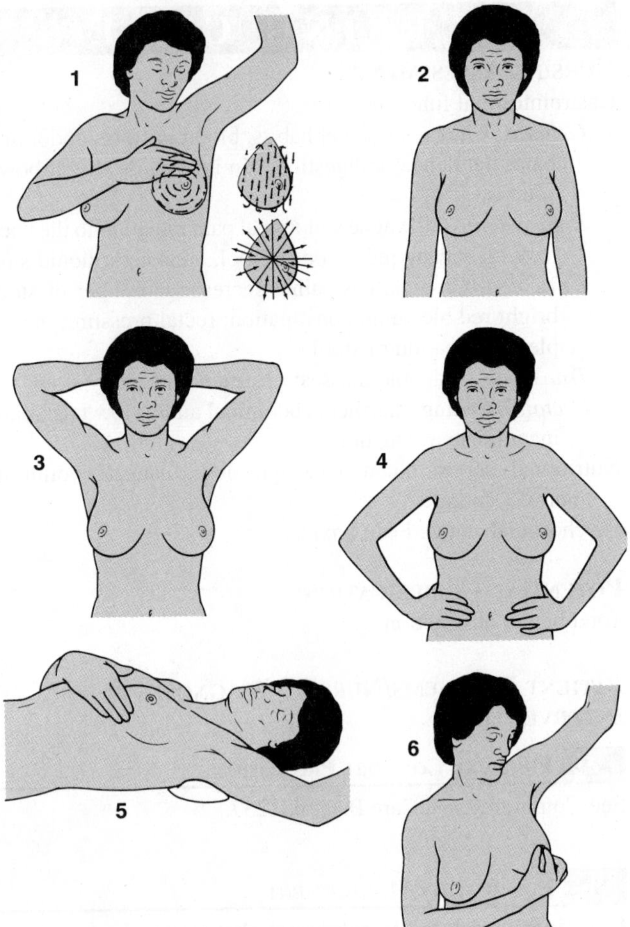

FIG. 18-2

Breast self-examination and patient instruction. (1) While in the shower or bath, when the skin is slippery with soap and water, examine your breasts. Use the pads of your second, third, and fourth fingers to firmly press every part of the breast. (While examining your left breast, use your right hand, and use your left hand to examine your right breast.) Check for any lump, hard knot, or thickening of the tissue. (2) Look at your breasts in the mirror. Stand with your arms at your side. (3) Raise your arms overhead and check for any changes in the shape of your breasts, dimpling of the skin, or any changes in the nipple. (4) Next, place your hands on your hips and press down firmly, tightening the pectoral muscles. Observe for asymmetry or changes, keeping in mind that your breasts probably do not exactly match. (5) Feel your breasts while lying down. When examining your right breast, place a folded towel under your right shoulder and put your right hand behind your head. Using the pads of the fingers on your left hand, examine the entire breast using small circular motions in a spiral or in an up-and-down motion so that the entire breast area is examined. Repeat the procedure using your right hand to examine your left breast. Repeat pattern of palpation under the arm. (6) Finally, gently squeeze the nipple of each breast between your thumb and index finger to check for any discharge.[7a]

(those over age 65 years) have twice the incidence of breast cancer of younger women. Breast cancer also develops infrequently in men. Symptoms and treatment are the same for men and women.[1]

Most breast lesions are first detected by a woman during breast self-examination (FIG. 18-2) or by her sexual partner. The possibility for cure is 85% for women with localized disease at the time of diagnosis. Half of breast cancers are in the upper outer quadrant, 20% in the central portion, 20% in the medial quadrants, and 10% in the lower outer quadrant.

Risk factors that have been cited in the incidence of breast cancer include previous breast cancer, a family history of breast cancer, nulliparity, or a first pregnancy after age 30 years. Irradiation, particularly as therapy for postpartum mastitis or as multiple chest fluoroscopies, is believed to contribute to breast cancer development. Obesity and total fat content in the diet, especially animal fat, may be factors. Total lifetime exposure to endogenous estrogen is a major risk factor. This disease is more common among white women, but the incidence among African-Americans is rising (see the box on p. 1191 for general information on breast cancer).

PATHOPHYSIOLOGY

Most breast malignancies occur in the upper outer quadrant. More than 75% of breast cancers are invasive ductal carcinomas, usually presenting as a single, unilateral, solid, irregular, poorly delineated, nonmobile, painless mass. This type grows as a fibrotic, stellate mass with long tentacled extensions that radiate from a central dense core, invading and distorting surrounding breast structures.

The mean diameter of a lesion detected by a woman on breast self-examination (BSE) is 3 to 3.5 cm, a size associated with a greater than 50% incidence of occult axillary lymph node metastases.

DIAGNOSTIC STUDIES AND FINDINGS

Mammogram: Solid nodule with ill-defined borders; clustered microcalcifications (FIG. 18-3 compares tumor size by mammography, BSE, and chance)

Thermography: Thermal "hot spot"

Biopsy

Lesion: Evidence of malignant cells

Axillary lymph nodes: Evidence of malignant cells

Sentinel lymph node biopsy: Identifies the first node in the lymph node chain before the disease proceeds to higher levels of nodes within the chain. If negative for disease, axillary node dissection is not necessary.

Estrogen receptors and progestin receptors: <3 fmol/mcp receptor negative tumor; >10 fmol/mcp receptor positive tumor

CEA: Elevated in metastatic liver disease

FACTS ABOUT BREAST CANCER

Incidence: An estimated 192,200 new invasive cases of breast cancer are expected to occur among women in the United States during 2001. Breast cancer occurs rarely in men, with about 1500 new cases expected to be diagnosed in 2001. After increasing about 4% per year in the 1980s, breast cancer incidence rates in white women are continuing to increase slightly.

Mortality: An estimated 41,200 deaths (40,800 women, 400 men) in 2000; breast cancer ranks second among cancer deaths in women. From 1990 to 1997, mortality rates declined significantly with the largest decreases in younger women, both white and African-American.

Warning signs: Breast changes that persist, such as a lump, thickening, swelling, dimpling, skin irritation, distortion, retraction, scaliness, pain, or tenderness of the nipple.

Risk factors: Over age 50 years: Personal or family history of breast cancer; never had children; first childbirth after age 30 years; biopsy-confirmed atypical hyperplasia; early menarche; late menopause; recent use of oral contraceptives or postmenopausal estrogens; higher education and socioeconomic status. Research about BRCA1 and BRCA2 susceptibility genes, the complex characteristics of these genes, and their contribution to the development of breast cancer is in progress.

Early detection: It is recommended that women age 40 years and older have an annual mammogram, an annual clinical breast examination performed by a health-care professional, and perform monthly BSE. Women ages 20 to 39 years should have a clinical breast examination performed by a health-care professional every 3 years and should perform monthly BSE. Most breast lumps are not cancers, but only a tissue biopsy can confirm a diagnosis. All suspicious lumps should be biopsied for a definitive diagnosis.

Treatment: Based on the medical situation and the patient's preferences, treatment may involve lumpectomy and removal of the lymph nodes under the arm; mastectomy and removal of the lymph nodes under the arm; radiation therapy; chemotherapy; or hormone therapy. Often, two or more methods are used in combination. For early stage disease, long-term survival rates after lumpectomy plus radiotherapy are similar to survival rates after modified radical mastectomy. High-dose chemotherapy with bone marrow transplant or stem cell rescue is a new treatment under study for special cases of breast cancer.

Data from American Cancer Society[1] and National Cancer Institute.[14a]

S phase index: >5% to 8%
Ploidy: Aneuploid DNA

MULTIDISCIPLINARY PLAN

Surgery

Lumpectomy: Wide excision and removal of tumor and margin of healthy tissue
Partial mastectomy: Simple excision of tumor and wider margin of healthy tissue
Quadrantectomy: Removal of one quarter of breast
Mastectomy
- Subcutaneous: Removal of all breast tissue while preserving overlying skin and nipple-areolar complex
- Total (simple): Complete removal of breast tissue and tail of Spence
- Modified radical: Removal of breast and axillary lymph nodes

Breast reconstruction

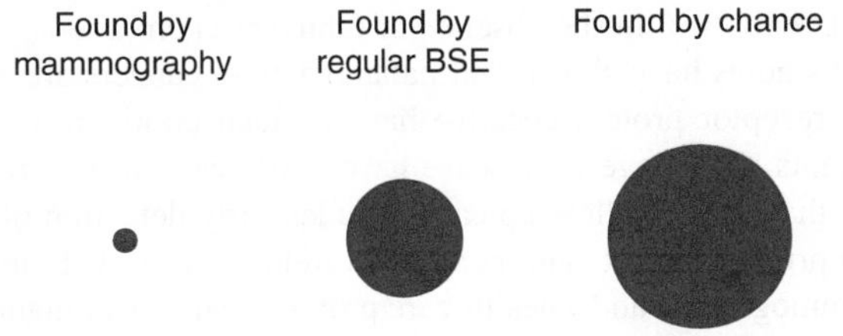

FIG. 18-3
Comparison of tumor size when found by different methods.

Radiation Therapy

Brachytherapy: Implantation of radioactive sources
Teletherapy: Use of external beam (photon or electron)
Regional node irradiation

Adjuvant Therapy

Combination Chemotherapy

CMF: Cyclophosphamide, methotrexate, 5-FU
CMFVP: CMF with vincristine and prednisone
CA: Cyclophosphamide, doxorubicin (Adriamycin)
CAF: Cyclophosphamide, doxorubicin (Adriamycin), 5-Fu

Antiestrogen Therapy (Ablative)

Tamoxifen citrate

Estrogens (Additive)

Diethylstilbestrol
Ethinyl estradiol

Androgens (Additive)

Fluoxymesterone
Testosterone
Methyltestosterone

Progestins (Additive)

Megestrol acetate
Medroxyprogesterone acetate

Aromatase Inhibitors

Anastrozole
Letrozole
Vorozole

Monoclonal Antibody

Herceptin

Bone Marrow Transplant

Autologous bone marrow transplantation (ABMT)
Peripheral blood progenitor cell (stem) transplant

Patients with stage I tumors and no involvement of axillary nodes have a 10-year survival rate of greater than 80%; those with stage II tumors have a greater than 60% 10-year survival rate; if the lymph nodes are involved, the 10-year survival rate is 30% to 40% in the absence of adjuvant chemotherapy. Recent studies have shown that patients whose cancers are estrogen receptor protein negative have a much poorer prognosis. Patients with stage IV disease have a 10-year survival rate of less than 10%. Follow-up care includes early detection of second primary breast cancers and recurrent disease. BSE, annual mammography, and a health-care professional's examination of the intact breast and nodes are important. Rehabilitation is an essential intervention after primary treatment.[10]

NURSING CARE

NURSING ASSESSMENT

Breast and lymphatics: Most common symptoms: mass (hard, irregular, nontender) or thickening in the breast or axilla; restricted mobility of lesion; dimpling or puckering of the skin or nipple; change in size, shape, or texture of breast (asymmetry); serosanguinous, bloody, or watery nipple discharge; local or regional spread: redness, ulceration, edema, or dilated veins; peau d'orange skin changes; enlarged axillary lymph nodes; metastatic disease: enlarged supraclavicular cervical lymph nodes

Respiratory function: Abnormal chest x-ray with or without pleural effusion

Gastrointestinal function: Abnormal liver function tests

Fluid and electrolyte function: Elevated alkaline phosphatase level; elevated calcium level

Psychosocial status: Fear, anxiety, withdrawal, avoidance of physical intimacy, restlessness, fight-or-flight-behavior; indecision

Pain: Localized at site of surgical incision or radiation

PATIENT PROBLEMS/NURSING DIAGNOSES & INTERVENTIONS

NIC PHYSICAL COMFORT PROMOTION, DECISIONAL CONFLICT

See Comprehensive Care Plan, p. 1237.

NIC SKIN/WOUND MANAGEMENT

Risk for impaired skin integrity related to surgery, node dissection, or radiation therapy

- Cleanse skin frequently *to prevent infection.*
- Apply warm, moist compresses *to promote circulation and drainage.*
- Apply antibiotic ointment and sterile dressing *to prevent infection.*
- Expose draining area to air (depending on patient's immunocompetence) *to promote healing.*
- Elevate arm to *enhance venous return.*
- Observe for increased or change in drainage character, skin changes (color, dimpling), swelling, or skin lesions *to detect infection or further breakdown of skin.*

NIC COPING ASSISTANCE

Disturbed body image related to alteration in or loss of breast

- Help patient to identify personal meaning of loss of breast *to clarify fears, concerns, and needs.*
- Encourage patient to discuss change in body with husband or significant other *to use social support.*
- Refer patient to appropriate resources (i.e., health-care providers, support group) *to provide external support.*

PATIENT EDUCATION/CONTINUUM OF CARE PLAN

1. Explain how to care for skin overlying breast *to prevent infection and ulceration.*
2. Explain how to assess the body for further breast disease or evidence of spread by performing BSE.
3. Explain use of nonpharmacologic interventions *for coping with pain and fear.*
4. Provide information about resources and support systems, such as Reach to Recovery of the American Cancer Society.

EVALUATION/PATIENT OUTCOMES

Skin/Wound Management: Skin is intact and free of infection. Skin is clean, dry, and warm with normal color and turgor. No evidence of lymphedema is seen. Affected arm is equal in size and diameter to unaffected arm.

Coping Assistance: Patient identifies issues related to loss of breast.

CANCERS OF THE URINARY TRACT

CARCINOMA OF THE BLADDER

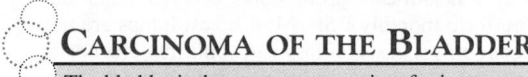

The bladder is the most common site of urinary tract malignancy.

Bladder cancer accounts for 4% to 5% of cancers in the United States. Incidence is highest in white men, average age 65 years. White men are twice as likely as African-American men and have a 3:1 ratio to white women to be diagnosed with bladder cancer.[12]

Risk Factors

The exact genetic events that cause the transformation of the normal bladder cell to a cancerous one are not well known, but there are four hypotheses: cigarette smoking, occupational exposure to industrial chemicals, ingestion of other physical agents, and exposure to *Schistosomas haemotobium.*

Cigarette smoking accounts for as much as 50% of bladder cancer in men and 31% in women. Reducing the use of tobacco and tobacco products, especially among young people, would likely lower the incidence of this cancer as aging occurs. Occupational exposure to agent arylamine(s) from the synthetic textile dye agency, the rubber industry, hair dyes, and as paint pigment is most strongly related to bladder cancer. Occupational exposure to dust or fumes of dyes, rubber, leather and its products, paint, and organic chemicals such as benzidine may be factors in bladder cancer development, with a 6- to 20-year latent period from the time of exposure to tumor transformation.[10]

Physical agents such as coffee, alcohol, saccharin, and phenacetin are linked to bladder cancer in mice and weakly in humans. *S. haemotobium* is a parasite rarely found in the

FACTS ABOUT BLADDER CANCER

Incidence: An estimated 54,300 new cases among men and women during 2001. Rates for women have remained constant, with rates decreasing for men.
Mortality: An estimated 12,400 deaths in 2001. If detected early, the 5-year survival rate is 94%.
Warning signs: Hematuria followed by marked urgency and dysuria.
Risk factors: Smokers are two times more likely to develop bladder cancer than nonsmokers.
Early detection: Cystoscopy is the primary method for detecting bladder cancer.
Treatment: In over 90% of bladder cancer cases, surgery, either alone or in combination with chemotherapy and/or radiation therapy, is used.

Data from American Cancer Society[1] and National Cancer Institute.[14a]

United States but common in African countries, especially Egypt, and a risk factor for bladder cancer.[12]

Signs and Symptoms

The most frequent sign of bladder cancer is hematuria, although some patients are asymptomatic until urethral obstruction occurs. Women are more likely to have been treated with antibiotics for urinary tract infection for hematuria believed to be hematuric cystitis.

The second most common symptom complex is marked urgency, dysuria, and frequency with small volumes of urine. Low back pain may be indicative of sacral or lumbar metastases.

PATHOPHYSIOLOGY

Ninety percent of bladder tumors are transitional cell carcinoma, 6% to 7% are true squamous cell carcinoma, and only 1% to 2% are glandular cancer. Some of these tumors are undifferentiated. Depth of invasion (stage) is more important than grading in predicting prognosis.

Lymph node involvement is present in half of the patients with deep muscle infiltration and has a poor prognosis. The disappointing long-term survival rate of patients with deeply invasive tumors has led to an integrated form of therapy in which irradiation is followed by cystectomy.

The bladder is also the site for contiguous spread of cancer from lesions of neighboring viscera, especially the uterine cervix and the prostate.

DIAGNOSTIC STUDIES AND FINDINGS

Urine culture: Sterile urine in patient with symptoms of cystitis
Excretory urography: Tumor or evidence of ureteral or urethral obstruction
Cystoscopy with selected bladder biopsies and urinary tract cytologic studies: Tumor visualization; presence of malignant cells
Bimanual abdominal examination: Firm or hard nodularity
Cystoscopic retrograde ureteropyelography: Tumor visualization; evidence of obstruction
Flow cytometry: More than 15% of cells above diploid level or clearly aneuploid tumor cell line with greater or less than half the number of chromosomes usually found
Renal arteriography: Evidence of obstruction or increased tumor vascularization
Renal ultrasound: Local extent and degree of bladder wall involvement by tumor
CT and MRI of abdomen and pelvis: Extent of local tumor; identification of pelvic lymph node metastases
Chest and skeletal x-ray examinations, bone scan, liver function studies: Evidence of metastatic disease
CEA: Elevated
Autocrine motility factor (AMF): Increased in widely metastatic disease

MULTIDISCIPLINARY PLAN

Surgery

Noninvasive Bladder Cancer

Endoscopic resection and fulguration; laser therapy

Invasive Bladder Cancer

Radical cystectomy with urinary diversion
Refer to discussion of urinary diversion in Chapter 14, p. 990

Radiation Therapy

Preoperative, before radical cystectomy
Control of hemorrhage and bony metastases

Chemotherapy

Noninvasive Bladder Cancer

Intravesical instillation with bacillus Calmette-Guérin (BCG), thiotepa, doxorubicin or mitomycin C, interferon alpha-2a as a secondary treatment after intravesical failure

Invasive Bladder Cancer

Combination regimens
- CISCA: Cyclophosphamide, doxorubicin, cisplatin
- CMV: Cisplatin, methotrexate, vinblastine
- MVAC: Methotrexate, vinblastine, doxorubicin (Adriamycin), cisplatin
- PC: Paclitaxel and carboplatin

Single agents: Gemcitabine, paclitaxel

RENAL TUMORS

Renal cancer is an uncontrolled growth of anaplastic cells of the kidney. Types include hypernephroma, parenchymal tumors, papillary tumors, and nephrotic carcinomas.

Renal cell carcinoma (also called *hypernephroma* or *adenocarcinoma*) occurs in the parenchyma of the kidney and is the most common type of renal cancer, accounting for 90% of all kidney cancers and 3% of all adult malignancies. Wilms' tumors are usually diagnosed in children under age 5 years and account for 4% of kidney cancers. Renal cell cancer (RCC) is twice as common in men as in women and rarely occurs in people under age 35 years.

In early stage RCC the presenting symptoms are intermittent, painless hematuria. In advanced disease the classic triad of symptoms of hematuria, palpable flank mass, and flank pain are noted.[2]

Risk Factors

The etiology of RCC is unclear. Many epidemiologic studies indicate tobacco as a significant risk factor. Studies report an increased risk of 1.5:2.2 for tobacco users. A genetic link has been discovered. Patients with Lindau–von Hippel disease have a higher incidence of RCC, as do patients with acquired cystic disease.

PATHOPHYSIOLOGY

Renal cell carcinomas have been characterized by a mixture of clear, granular, or spindlelike sarcomatoid cells arranged in solid, cystic, tubular, or papillary patterns. Renal carcinomas locally invade the capsule and can create their own blood supply, often spreading to the renal vein and vena cava. The most common sites for RCC metastasis are lung, bone, liver, and brain. RCC has the unusual ability to regress spontaneously.[12]

Thirty-five percent of patients have metastases at the time of diagnosis. The prognosis is best when the disease is found early. Local recurrence occurs infrequently; therefore metastatic disease and nodal spread are the causative factors of failure in this population.

DIAGNOSTIC STUDIES AND FINDINGS

Urinalysis: Red blood cells
Intravenous retrograde pyelogram: Filling defect
Renal ultrasound: Presence of a solid or cystic mass
Abdominal CT scan: Shows density and size of tumor, extent of local invasion, vena caval or renal vein involvement, and location of metastasis
Nuclear bone scan: Highlight areas of potential or suspected bone metastatsis
Renal MRI: Renal vein or vena cava involvement

MULTIDISCIPLINARY PLAN

Surgery

Radical nephrectomy (abdominotransperitoneal or thoracoabdominal approaches)
Lymphadenectomy (controversial)
Palliative nephrectomy for bleeding and pain control
Resection of solitary metastatic site, such as in brain or liver
Bilateral tumors
  Nephrectomy of larger tumor and partial nephrectomy for smaller lesion in bilateral disease
  Bilateral nephrectomies and chronic hemodialysis or peritoneal dialysis; later transplantation
Nephroureterectomy for renal pelvis carcinomas
Refer to discussion of other kidney surgery, p. 912

Radiation Therapy

Used in treatment of local recurrences or symptomatic bony tumor
Postoperative irradiation for residual or recurrent tumor

Biologic Response Modifiers

Combination regimens: Interferon alpha-2a (rIFNa2) with interleukin-2 (rIL-2)
Single-agent regimen: Interleukin-2 (IL-2)

Improved survival rates (5-year survival of 65% for early hypernephroma) have been attributed to thoracoabdominal nephrectomy with node dissection and earlier diagnosis of "incidental" carcinomas. Reports of spontaneous regression prompted investigational therapy with biologic response modifiers.

NURSING CARE

NURSING ASSESSMENT

Hematologic function: Anemia; hypovolemic shock
Urinary function: Hematuria; dehydration; renal failure; urinary obstruction (from blood clots or tumor)
Pain: Low back or pelvic pain, leg edema; chronic aching pain, renal colic, nerve pain
Nutritional status: Weight loss; nausea and or vomiting
Psychosocial status: Fear of incontinence; altered sexuality and fertility, pain, death; anxiety; grieving

PATIENT PROBLEMS/NURSING DIAGNOSES & INTERVENTIONS

NIC PHYSICAL COMFORT PROMOTION AND COPING ASSISTANCE

See Comprehensive Care Plan, p. 1237.

NIC ELIMINATION MANAGEMENT

Impaired urinary elimination related to disease and/or treatment

- Inspect urine for blood; check with Hemoccult *to detect bleeding.*
- Encourage adequate rest and exercise *to avoid stress-related distention.*
- Increase patient's fluid intake *to enhance renal circulation and flush bladder.*
- Apply heating pad or hot water bottle to abdomen as ordered *to relax abdominal muscles.*
- Catheterize patient only if necessary *to avoid infection associated with catheterization.*

NIC ELECTROLYTE AND ACID-BASE MANAGEMENT

Deficient fluid volume related to potential blood loss and urine flow disruption related to urinary stasis from blood clots

- Observe characteristics (particularly color) and amount of urine *to determine need for fluid and blood component replacement.*
- Monitor vital signs at frequent intervals during episodes of gross hematuria *to detect shock early.*

- Encourage patient to drink large volumes of fluid *to prevent dehydration.*
- Administer IV fluids as prescribed *to replace lost fluid volume.*
- Observe for signs and symptoms of worsening fluid volume deficit, including decreased urine output, concentrated urine, output greater than intake, weakness, and changes in mental status, *to determine the need for rapid infusions of large volumes of IV fluids and blood components.*

Patient Education/Continuum of Care Plan

1. Emphasize the need for adequate fluid intake, exercise, and rest.
2. Encourage oral fluids and foods that cause alkaline urine such as fruits, vegetables, and milk. Avoid tobacco and foods and fluids that irritate the bladder, such as alcohol, tea, and spices.
3. Explain that, to reduce the incidence of urinary tract infections, female patients should:
   a. Void after sexual intercourse to reduce the number of bacteria that may be introduced into the urethra.
   b. Avoid bubble baths.
   c. Wear cotton undergarments.
4. Discuss pain-relieving measures, such as exercise, warmth, safety, and medication.
5. Instruct the patient in self-care if the patient has undergone urinary diversion.
6. Provide the patient with information and referrals as needed for sperm banking, sexual counseling, and reconstructive/implant surgery.

Evaluation/Patient Outcomes

Elimination Management: Urinary function is normal. Patient does not complain of urgency, frequency, or dysuria. No evidence of hematuria is present.

Electrolyte and Acid-Base Management: Hydration is normal. Patient is able to maintain adequate intake by mouth, and electrolyte levels are within normal limits.

CANCERS OF THE MALE REPRODUCTIVE SYSTEM

Cancer of the Prostate

Cancer of the prostate is a malignant tumor arising from the parenchyma of the prostate gland.

Prostate cancer is the most common cancer in men in the United States, accounting for 41% of all newly diagnosed cancer in men.[15] African-American men have the highest incidence of prostate cancer and tend to develop it at an earlier age than white men, and their mortality rate is higher. In men over age 85 years the incidence may be as high as 89%.

Most prostatic cancers are adenocarcinomas discovered by a physician during rectal examination, which should be done yearly on all men over age 50 years. These slow-growing tumors arise in the posterior portion of the prostate and eventually involve the entire gland. They spread via the lymphatics throughout the pelvic region and into the pelvic bones.

FACTS ABOUT PROSTATE CANCER

Incidence: An estimated 198,000 new cases during 2001. African-American men have twice the incidence rate as white men. Improved detection methods, particularly the use of the prostate-specific antigen screening test, have resulted in a 50% increase in incidence rates.

Mortality: Prostate cancer is the second leading cause of cancer death in men, with an estimated 31,500 deaths in 2001.

Warning signs: The signs and symptoms of prostate cancer often mimic benign prostatic hypertrophy. These include weak or interrupted urine flow, nocturia, dysuria, and hematuria.

Risk factors: Age remains the strongest risk factor, with over 80% of all prostate cancers diagnosed in men over age 65 years. There appears to be a geographic distribution of prostate cancer. Northwestern Europe and North America have a higher incidence, and the disease is considered rare in the Near East, Africa, Central America, and South America. The role of dietary fat as an etiologic factor is under study.

Early detection: Beginning at age 50 years an annual prostate-specific antigen screening (PSA) test and a yearly digital rectal examination is recommended. Men with known risk factors should begin testing at age 45 years. Should either test reveal any abnormalities, a transrectal ultrasound should be performed.

Treatment: There are a number of options available to men diagnosed with prostate cancer. These include hormone therapy, chemotherapy, surgery, or radiation therapy.

Data from American Cancer Society[1] and National Cancer Institute.[14a]

The influence of endogenous hormones, especially dihydrotestosterone, is the only factor clearly associated with the promotion and development of prostate cancer. Other possible etiologic factors include genetic influences; dietary fat; exposure to certain viruses, pathogens, or industrial chemicals; and urbanization.

Pathophysiology

Most prostatic cancers are adenocarcinomas. These slow-growing tumors arise in the posterior portion of the prostate, are usually multifocal, and eventually involve the entire gland. They spread via the lymphatics throughout the pelvic region and into the pelvic bones. Hematogenous spread involves the lungs, liver, kidneys, and bones (vertebrae, pelvis, femur, and ribs). By the time of diagnosis, most of these cancers already have invaded the base of the bladder, seminal vesicles, or perivesicular fascia or have moved laterally into the levator ani muscles.

The rest of these tumors are ductal (transitional and squamous cell carcinoma, endometroid cancer, and sarcoma). Acinar dysplasia has been characterized as prostatic intraepithelial neoplasia (PIN), a premalignant lesion.

Grading of the tumors—as well, moderately, or poorly differentiated—correlates with the prognosis. Early symptoms resemble those of benign prostatic hypertrophy and include weak urinary stream, urinary frequency, dysuria, and difficulty in starting and stopping urination. Some patients initially report pain in the lower back, pelvis, or upper thighs. Bilateral ureteral obstruction with renal insufficiency is not uncommon at the time of diagnosis. Symptoms associated with advanced disease also include fatigue and weight loss.

Diagnostic Studies and Findings

Digital rectal examination: 50% of palpable prostatic nodules are cancer
Excretory urogram: Bladder outlet involvement; ureteral obstruction or displacement
Closed or open fine-needle biopsy via perineal or transrectal route: Presence of malignant cells
Transrectal ultrasonography: Prostatic lesions seen
Pelvic CT: Local extensions; nodal involvement
MRI: Capsular penetration; seminal vesicle involvement
Lymphangiography: Paraaortic and pelvic node involvement
Prostate-specific antigen: Elevated in localized disease; clinical recurrence
Prostatic acid phosphatase: Elevated in localized disease

Multidisciplinary Plan

Surgery
Transurethral resection
Radical prostatectomy
Bilateral orchiectomy
Refer to Chapter 14 on p. 980 for care of patient with open prostatectomy

Radiation Therapy
External beam; interstitial implant

Chemotherapy
Single Agent Regimens
Estramustine
Goserelin acetate implant
Nilutamide
Prednisone

Combination Regimens
Estramustine and vinblastine
FL: Flutamide with leuprolide acetate
FZ: Flutamide with goserelin acetate
Mitoxantrone with prednisone
Bicalutamide with leuprolide *or* goserelin acetate
PE: Paclitaxel with estramustine

Hormonal Therapy
Diethylstilbestrol (Stilphostrol), conjugated estrogens (Premarin), estradiol, estramustine phosphate
Medical adrenalectomy: Aminoglutethimide, ketoconazole, spironolactone, glucocorticoids
Antiandrogens: Cyproterone acetate, flutamide, megestrol acetate
GnH agonist: Leuprolide acetate, goserelin acetate

NURSING CARE

Nursing Assessment
Urinary and renal function: Weak urinary stream; frequency; dysuria; difficulty starting and stopping urination; renal insufficiency as evidenced by decreased output, elevated specific gravity, blood urea nitrogen, creatinine
Comfort level: Pain in lower back, pelvis, or upper thighs
Psychosocial status: Expressed fears of incontinence, altered sexuality, pain, death
Hematologic function: Anemia
Hydration: Poor skin turgor; edema of scrotum and extremities; dry oral mucosa
Neurologic function: Spinal cord compression as evidenced by constipation, urinary retention, low back pain, change in gait, foot drop

Potential Complications
Complete urethral obstruction

Patient Problems/Nursing Diagnoses & Interventions

NIC Physical and Psychologic Comfort Promotion
See Comprehensive Care Plan, p. 1237.

NIC Elimination Management
Impaired urinary elimination related to presence of tumor surrounding urethra
- Be alert for patient's complaints of frequency, pain, and urination difficulties *to monitor the presence of infection or obstruction.*
- Encourage adequate rest and activity *to decrease stress on urinary system.*
- Increase patient's fluid intake *to flush renal system.*
- Catheterize patient only if necessary *to eliminate urine retention.*

Patient Education/Continuum of Care Plan
1. Emphasize the need for adequate fluid intake, exercise, and rest.
2. Explain the use of alternative pain-relieving measures such as exercise, warmth, and medication.
3. Tell the patient to notify the physician or nurse if signs and symptoms of renal insufficiency appear (provide instructions in writing).
4. Discuss alternate expressions of sexuality, the value of sexual counseling, and the possibility of recovering some or all of sexual function after treatment ends.

Evaluation/Patient Outcomes
Elimination Management: Urinary function is normal. Patient has no complaints of urgency, frequency, or dysuria. Patient able to start and stop urine stream.

TESTICULAR CANCER

Testicular cancer is a rare form of cancer but is the most common cancer in young men ages 15 to 35 years. With the advent of tumor markers (indicating the presence of disease and enabling the physician to monitor its response to treatment), refined surgery, and effective chemotherapy, the cure rate is as high as 90%.[4]

The etiologic factors of testicular cancer are unknown, although its occurrence is higher in men with cryptorchidism (undescended testis) or atrophic testis. Men with either of these conditions have a 40 times greater likelihood of developing cancer than do those with normal testes. When orchiopexy (surgical descent of the cryptorchid testis) is performed on the male child before age 2 years, the likelihood of his developing cancer is virtually eliminated. Testicular cancer is more common in white males than in African-American males in the United States. There is also a higher incidence in the higher socioeconomic classes. Men whose mothers took exogenous hormones during pregnancy also have a higher incidence of testicular cancer.

Early detection is best accomplished by testicular self-examination (TSE) and is recommended for patients with a prior history of testicular malignancy. The American Cancer Society recommends males ages 15 through 40 years be instructed and encouraged to perform monthly TSE.[4]

The first sign of the disease is usually a small, hard, painless lump in the testicle. Symptoms reported include a sensation of heaviness in the testicle, sudden fluid accumulation in the scrotum, and perineal pain or discomfort.

Some men report a history of trauma, mumps, or orchitis; episodic testicular pain; low back, groin, or abdominal ache; and breast enlargement or tenderness. If symptoms persist after antibiotic therapy for suspected epididymitis, the physician should suspect testicular cancer.

PATHOPHYSIOLOGY

Most testicular tumors are of germ cell origin and are malignant. The basic categories are the seminoma and heterogeneous, nonseminomatous germ cell tumor. Paraaortic lymph node involvement, ureteral obstruction, and pulmonary metastases may be present at diagnosis.

Dramatic responses to single agent and combination drug chemotherapy have made even advanced cases of testicular cancer curable. Radiation therapy is still used for seminomas but has been replaced by chemotherapy for nonseminomatous tumors. Tumor markers (alpha-fetoprotein [AFP] and human chorionic gonadotropin [hCG]) are useful not only in early diagnosis but also in follow-up monitoring for recurrent disease.[15]

DIAGNOSTIC STUDIES AND FINDINGS

Palpation of testes: Presence of mass
Transillumination: Detection of intrascrotal lesion
Excretory urography: Displacement of ureters or kidney
Abdominal CT and ultrasound and lymphangiogram: Areas of abnormality seen
Serum alpha-fetoprotein (AFP): Elevated
Human chorionic gonadotropin (hCG): Elevated
Chest x-ray examination, CT, and whole-lung CT: Evidence of metastatic disease
Radical inguinal orchiectomy (biopsy): Presence of malignant cells

MULTIDISCIPLINARY PLAN

Surgery

Inguinal exploration and orchiectomy; bilateral retroperitoneal lymph node dissection

Radiation Therapy

External beam

Chemotherapy

BEP: Bleomycin, etoposide, cisplatin
EP: Etoposide and cisplatin
PVB: Cisplatin, vinblastine, bleomycin
VIP: Vinblastine or etoposide and ifosfamide, cisplatin and mesna

NURSING CARE

NURSING ASSESSMENT

Scrotum: Small, hard painless lump in testis; sensation of heaviness; swelling
Breasts: Enlargement or tenderness
Comfort level: Perineal pain or discomfort; low back, groin, or abdominal ache
Psychosocial status: Withdrawal, anxiety, fear of altered sexuality, infertility, pain, death

PATIENT PROBLEMS/NURSING DIAGNOSES & INTERVENTIONS

NIC PHYSICAL AND PSYCHOLOGIC COMFORT PROMOTION

See Comprehensive Care Plan, p. 1237.

NIC COPING ASSISTANCE

Disturbed body image related to changes in scrotum from tumor or surgery

- Respect patient's need for period of denial *to allow patient to cope.*
- Respect patient's individual coping style because patient may have used his coping style to deal effectively with other crises.
- Assist patient in expressing such feelings as anger *to allow patient to "defuse" some of his anxiety.*
- Encourage patient to talk about alterations when he is able to do so *to help patient view problem realistically.*
- Explore patient's feelings about impact of alterations on personal appearance *to determine need for disguising the change.*
- Provide information about treatment options *to enable patient to make realistic and individualized decisions* on sexuality (removal of testicle during adulthood has no

impact on sexuality), control of pain, and prognosis *to decrease patient's fears.*
- Assist patient to identify coping skills used successfully in the past *to facilitate problem solving.*
- Encourage patient to ask questions and express feelings *to relieve patient's anxiety and help patient put thoughts into perspective.*

NIC Skin/Wound Management

- Review care plan in Part III, Perioperative Nursing.

Patient Education/Continuum of Care Plan

1. Explain about the availability of testicular implants.
2. Discuss the testes' ability to compensate for loss of function in one testis so that male characteristics are not adversely affected.
3. Provide information about sperm banking and sexual counseling.
4. Stress the importance of follow-up evaluation for the rest of the patient's life.

Evaluation/Patient Outcomes

Coping Assistance: Patient describes feelings related to altered body image. Patient is able to look at and touch scrotum. Patient can describe self as person with unique body configuration.

GYNECOLOGIC CANCERS

Cancer of the uterus, both endometrial and cervical (including in situ), accounts for 15% of all female cancers. Although increasing in incidence, cancers of the female genital organs—uterus, ovaries, vulva, and vagina—also have an increasing rate of survival.[1]

Cancer of the Cervix

Cancer of the uterine cervix is a neoplasm that can be detected in the early, curable stage by the Papanicolaou (Pap) smear test.

Cancer of the uterine cervix has its highest incidence in women who are age 35 years or older, began sexual activity in puberty, and have had multiple partners. Other risk factors include low socioeconomic status, poor prenatal and postnatal care, and in utero exposure to diethylstilbestrol (DES). Women in urban, industrialized areas and white or Jewish women have a lower incidence of the disease than do those in rural, underdeveloped areas and nonwhites. Celibate women and those in religious groups that encourage male circumcision and monogamy also have a lower incidence. Women with multiple genital infections such as herpes, *Trichomonas* infection, and gonorrhea are at greater risk

Multiple studies have been done on the causal relationship of detecting human papilloma virus (HPV) and cervical cancer. It is thought that the HPV interacts with specific genes that control cell growth and cause loss of proliferation control, resulting in uncontrolled growth[7] (see box).

FACTS ABOUT CERVICAL CANCER

Incidence: An estimated 12,900 invasive cervical cancers are expected to be diagnosed in 2001. Noninvasive cervical cancer is about four times as common as the invasive type. For the past decade the incidence of invasive cervical cancer had been dropping. Considered a precancerous condition, cervical carcinoma in situ is now more frequent than invasive cancer among women under age 50 years.

Mortality: African-American women are twice as likely as white women to succumb to cervical cancer. In 2001 an estimated 4400 women will die.

Warning signs: Watery vaginal discharge, abnormal vaginal bleeding or spotting. In advanced disease the woman may complain of pain in the pelvis, hypogastrium, flank, or leg.

Risk factors: First intercourse at an early age, multiple sex partners, and genital infections with human papillomavirus; cigarette smoking.

Early detection: A yearly PAP test with a pelvic examination in women who are, or have been, sexually active or who have reached age 18 years is recommended. When three or more consecutive examinations reveal no abnormalities, the PAP test may be performed less frequently at the discretion of the physician.

Treatment: Surgery, alone or in combination with radiation, is the treatment for invasive cancer. Cryotherapy, electrocoagulation, or local surgery can be used for carcinoma in situ.

Data from American Cancer Society[1] and National Cancer Institute.[14a]

Improved general and genital hygiene and cytologic screening with the Pap smear have contributed to decrease the mortality of invasive cervical cancer. However, the incidence of carcinoma in situ is increasing and is affecting a younger population.

Changes in cells of the cervical epithelium may be present for 10 years before invasive cancer develops. However, a Pap smear can detect even the earliest changes, so regular Pap tests, as well as manual pelvic examinations, are the most important means of reducing mortality from cervical cancer.

Pathophysiology

Abnormal bleeding is the most common presenting sign of cervical cancer. The bleeding initially may be a thin, watery, blood-tinged vaginal discharge that progresses to spotting and frank bleeding. Other signs and symptoms include prolonged or intermittent menstrual periods, "contact" bleeding after intercourse or douching, and anemia in the presence of chronic blood loss. Advanced disease is evidenced by odor; pain in the lower back, legs, and groin; lower extremity edema; difficulty voiding, urgency, or hematuria (invasion of the bladder); and rectal tenesmus and rectal bleeding (invasion of the rectum). Cervical cancer rarely occurs during pregnancy but should be ruled out in the presence of unexplained bleeding.

When symptoms appear, the cancer has usually progressed beyond its early stages. Squamous cell carcinoma accounts for 95% of all invasive tumors diagnosed, and adenocarcinomas account for most of the rest. Clear cell carcinoma develops in the cervix and vagina of women exposed in utero to DES. Invasive carcinoma of the cervix spreads by direct extension to the vaginal wall, laterally into the parametrium toward the pelvic wall, and anteroposteriorly into the bladder and rectum. Metastases to the pelvic lymph nodes are more common than those to distant nodes.

DIAGNOSTIC STUDIES AND FINDINGS

Cervical examination and biopsy via colposcopy: Presence of visible mass, malignant cells, or both
CT of the abdomen: Involvement of retroperitoneal lymph nodes
MRI: Estimated tumor volume
Lymphangiography followed by fine-needle aspiration biopsy: Presence of malignant cells
Supraclavicular node biopsy: Presence of malignant cells
Chest x-ray examination, excretory urography, cystoscopy, and proctosigmoidoscopy: Evidence of spread of tumor
Complete blood cell count: Anemia
Serum chemistries: Elevated blood urea nitrogen (BUN), creatinine, aspartate amino transferase (AST), alanine amino transferase (ALT), total bilirubin levels

MULTIDISCIPLINARY PLAN

Surgery

Conization; cryotherapy or laser ablation; abdominal or vaginal radical hysterectomy and pelvic node dissection; pelvic exenteration; see Chapter 12, Female Reproductive System, for medical interventions and related nursing care

Radiation Therapy

External beam; intracavity

Chemotherapy

Cisplatin-based therapy either in combination with other chemotherapeutic agents or alone is the only chemotherapeutic agent proved efficacious in cervical cancer.

NURSING CARE

NURSING ASSESSMENT

Perineal area: unusual bleeding or vaginal discharge, prolonged or intermittent menstrual periods, "contact" bleeding after intercourse, skin irritation or excoriation, malodorous discharge
Hematologic function: Anemia, fatigue
Renal function: Difficulty voiding, urgency, hematuria
Intestinal function: Rectal tenesmus, bleeding
Comfort level: Pain in lower back, legs, and groin; lower extremity edema

POTENTIAL COMPLICATIONS

Massive vaginal hemorrhage, renal failure

PATIENT PROBLEMS/NURSING DIAGNOSES AND INTERVENTIONS

NIC PHYSICAL COMFORT PROMOTION

See Comprehensive Care Plan, p. 1237.

NIC SKIN/WOUND MANAGEMENT

Impaired skin integrity related to vaginal discharge

- Change dressings or pads frequently; maintain dry, clean linen and dry skin; provide clean clothing *to maintain cleanliness and enhance patient's comfort.*
- Observe quality and quantity of drainage *to determine status of infection.*
- Administer antibiotics as ordered *to combat infection.*
- Administer perineal care as indicated *to promote comfort and remove drainage from skin.*

NIC ACTIVITY AND EXERCISE MANAGEMENT

Fatigue related to blood loss and anemia

- Help patient and significant others understand the physiologic basis for fatigue and that it will diminish on improvement or correction of the anemia *to help patient better tolerate the fatigue.*
- Encourage patient to discuss feelings related to fatigue *to relieve patient's anxiety (which can cause fatigue).*
- Encourage patient to identify behaviors associated with fatigue, such as emotional lability and irritability, *to help patient distinguish these temporary behaviors that are caused by the anemic condition.*
- Help patient plan periods of rest and activity *to achieve adequate levels of energy for activities of daily living.*

NIC ELIMINATION MANAGEMENT

Impaired urinary elimination related to pressure of tumor on urethra

- Encourage increased oral fluid intake.
- Encourage adequate rest and exercise *to maintain general well-being.*
- Encourage patient to ambulate often *to promote circulation and urinary elimination.*
- Catheterize only if necessary *to avoid infection.*

NIC COPING ASSISTANCE

Disturbed body image related to actual or potential alteration in female structure

- Encourage patient to discuss feelings and concerns with health-care providers and significant others *to alleviate anxiety.*
- Help patient identify, label, and express feelings about the significance of the female genitalia, treatment modalities, and anticipated prognosis *to allow patient to deal with specific issues.*

- Promote acceptance of a positive, realistic body image *so patient can resume pre-illness lifestyle.*

Patient Education/Continuum of Care Plan

1. Emphasize the need to maintain perineal hygiene.
2. Explain the use of alternative nonpharmacologic comfort measures, such as the use of heat, positioning, relaxation exercises, guided imagery, and distraction.
3. Assist the patient in planning periods of activity and rest, which will enable her to accomplish activities of daily living and recreational activities.
4. Explain the importance of drinking large quantities of water and nonacidic fluids, of voiding when she feels the urge, and of using warmth and other individually effective techniques to stimulate voiding.
5. Refer the patient to support groups, sexual counselors, and other community programs that will be helpful to her in maintaining a positive self-image.

Evaluation/Patient Outcomes

Skin/Wound Management: Perineal area is clean and odor free. Perineal area is normal in color. Patient reports feeling of cleanliness and comfort in perineal area.

Activity and Exercise Management: Patient expresses no fatigue. Patient is able to coordinate rest and activity so that she can carry out activities of daily living and enjoy recreational activities.

Elimination Management: Urinary function is normal. Patient maintains a balance between intake and output. Patient voids without difficulty.

Coping Assistance: Patient's body image is realistic. Patient verbalizes realistic sense of self and body.

Other Gynecologic Cancers

Malignant diseases occur in all parts of the female reproductive system. They include cancers of the uterine endometrium, the vagina, the vulva, the ovaries, and the fallopian tubes, as well as gestational trophoblastic neoplasms.

Endometrial Cancer

Endometrial cancer is the most common gynecologic cancer in women, occurring primarily in postmenopausal women. Etiologic factors include infertility, late menopause (after age 52 years), obesity, diabetes, and hypertension. The use of tamoxifen or estrogen replacement therapy (without progestins) places a woman at higher risk for endometrial cancer. A diet high in animal fat is another risk factor that affects hormone metabolism. Other etiologic factors are endometrial hyperplasia, polycystic ovarian disease, history of irregular menses, and a history of breast, colon, or ovarian cancer. Cancer of the endometrium occurs 70% more often in white women than in African-American women. The benefits of maintaining an ideal weight and careful management of estrogen therapy for menopause should be emphasized.[7,21]

The most common initial symptom is intermenstrual, postcoital, or postmenopausal bleeding. The diagnosis of endometrial cancer is based on histologic tissue examination.

The most common treatment for each stage disease is a total hysterectomy and bilateral salpingo-oophorectomy with more extensive surgery if the disease has spread. External radiation is added to the treatment plan when the cancer extends beyond the fundus. The most commonly used systemic therapy for recurrent endometrial cancer is synthetic progestational agents; response rates are 30% to 37%.[10]

The 5-year survival rate for patients with early endometrial cancer is greater than 83%. The cure rate drops to 26% when the cancer has metastasized to distant sites.

Vaginal Cancer

Vaginal carcinoma is rarely a primary lesion and occurs in both menopausal and postmenopausal women. Risk factors include DES exposure in utero, prior radiation to a field including the vagina, and increasing age. The primary signs and symptoms are vaginal spotting and discharge, pain, groin masses, and changes in urinary pattern. Treatment is based on the stage of the disease. Premalignant lesions may be treated with local excision, carbon dioxide laser, or topical chemotherapy. A partial or total vaginectomy may be performed depending on the extent of the disease.[2]

Radiation therapy consists of intracavity irradiation combined with total pelvic external irradiation. Radical surgery includes complete vaginectomy, pelvic node dissection, and anterior exenteration as indicated. Grafting may be used to avoid vaginal stenosis, especially in younger patients. Survival at 5 years after diagnosis for all stages ranges from 42% to 56% (stage I, 65% to 100%; stage II, 42% to 75%).[10]

Vulvar Cancer

There is an increasing incidence of vulvar intraepithelial neoplasia (VIN) and carcinoma in situ (CIS) in older women. Vulvar cancer occurs most commonly in women who are between age 50 and 70 years and in lower socioeconomic strata. Symptoms include vaginal discharge, pruritus, and bleeding.

The leukoplakic changes (whitish, plaquelike, or ulcerated lesions) that precede carcinoma can be eliminated by simple vulvectomy. Once carcinoma develops, invasion of the inguinal nodes and the lower vagina is common.

Surgery for this form of cancer may be preventive to remove precancerous lesions (hemivulvectomy or local excision with a wide margin of normal tissue), curative (radical vulvectomy), or palliative (extent depends on the patient's symptoms).

The 5-year survival rate is 90% to 98% for women with early, localized lesions but is much lower when nodal or distant metastasis is present.[7]

Ovarian Cancer

Ovarian cancer is the fifth leading cause of death in women in the United States. The incidence of ovarian cancer is greater among women who are single, nulliparous, and infertile; the incidence is lower among women who use oral contraceptives.[2] The peak incidence is between age 50 and 59 years.

These tumors do not usually produce symptoms until intraabdominal metastasis has occurred, with outward signs such as ascites. Therefore the mortality is high; only 44% of patients survive the disease. When symptoms do occur, they include increasing abdominal girth, weight loss, abdominal pain, dysuria or urinary frequency, and constipation.

Treatment of ovarian cancer consists of hysterectomy and bilateral salpingo-oophorectomy. Radiation therapy and chemotherapy may be used in conjunction with surgery or when the cancer is inoperable.

Cancer of the Fallopian Tube

Fallopian tube cancer is the rarest of the gynecologic malignancies. It is difficult to diagnose, and diagnosis is usually made at time of surgery. Most are adenocarcinomas and detected in women between the ages of 40 and 60 years. The most common symptoms are pelvic pain, abnormal vaginal bleeding, and a heavy, watery vaginal discharge. Colicky pain may be associated with bleeding.[10]

Removal of the uterus, fallopian tubes, ovaries, and omentum is the usual treatment. Radiation and chemotherapy have been used postoperatively with some success. Survival rates are as high as 90% with early disease, although the overall 5-year survival rate is 38%.

Gestational Trophoblastic Disease (GTD)

The gestational trophoblastic neoplasms include hydatidiform mole, invasive mole (chorioadenoma destruens), and choriocarcinoma. Molar pregnancy, the most common of these tumors, occurs in approximately 1 in 1000 pregnancies in the world. These neoplasms can also develop after aborted, ectopic, or normal delivery.[7]

The measurement of human chorionic gonadotropin (hCG) by the b subunit radioimmunoassay test is essential for diagnosis, monitoring of therapy, and follow-up. Early diagnosis is facilitated by amniography and ultrasonography. Treatment of GTD is based on staging.

Hydatidiform mole is treated with suction curettage when preserving fertility is desirable. Postevacuation monitoring of hCG levels is done at 48 hours, weekly for 3 consecutive weeks, and then monthly for 6 to 12 months or until hCG is undetectable. During this time pregnancy should be avoided. If fertility is not desired, total abdominal hysterectomy is the treatment of choice when the mole is in situ.

Locally invasive mole or choriocarcinoma is diagnosed by elevated hCG levels, pelvic angiography, ultrasonography, and curettage. If fertility is desired, intermittent courses of single-agent chemotherapy, such as methotrexate with citrovorum rescue or actinomycin D, yield a cure rate of 100%. When fertility is not desired, hysterectomy is the treatment of choice.

Metastasis is most common with choriocarcinoma; the most frequent sites are the lung, vagina, oral cavity, gastrointestinal tract, central nervous system, and liver. The treatment of choice is chemotherapy with a single agent or a combination of drugs. Surgery or adjunctive radiation therapy may be required. The overall survival with metastasis is still good, although the prognosis is poor with metastases to the liver or brain.

NURSING CARE

Nursing Assessment

Vaginal bleeding: Excessive or prolonged; serosanguineous discharge with associated pruritus
Pain: Back, abdominal, and pelvic pain; guarding of abdominal or pelvic area; pelvic pressure
Fear: Depression, anger, withdrawal, expressions of fear
Psychosocial status: Loss of appetite, change in sleep patterns, and activity level

Potential Complications

Ascites

Patient Problems/Nursing Diagnoses & Interventions

Nursing Care of the Woman With Endometrial Cancer

NIC Physical and Psychologic Comfort Promotion

See Comprehensive Care Plan, p. 1237.

NIC Tissue Perfusion

Deficient fluid volume related to postmenopausal bleeding

- Observe characteristics and amount of blood loss *to determine need for fluid and blood component replacement.*
- Monitor vital signs at frequent intervals during episodes of heavy bleeding *to detect shock early.*
- Encourage patient to drink large volumes of fluid *to prevent dehydration.*
- Monitor patient's input and output and urine specific gravity *to detect renal dysfunction.*
- Administer IV fluids as prescribed *to replace lost fluid volume.*
- Monitor laboratory reports *to detect development of anemia.*
- Observe patient for signs and symptoms of worsening fluid volume deficit, including decreased urine output, concentrated urine, output greater than intake, weakness, and change in mental status, *to determine need for large volumes of IV fluids and rapid infusion of blood components.*

Evaluation/Patient Outcomes

Tissue Perfusion: Laboratory findings are normal. Hematocrit and albumin levels are within normal limits.

Nursing Care of the Woman With Vaginal Cancer

NIC Psychologic Comfort Promotion

See Comprehensive Care Plan, p. 1237.

NIC Coping Assistance

Ineffective sexuality patterns related to presence of tumor or alterations in structure and lubrication related to treatment

- Assist patient to identify current and potential changes in sexual structure and function.
- Encourage patient to identify and use support systems for exchange of thoughts and feelings with significant other and with other women who have the same or similar experiences.
- Encourage patient to vent her feelings about potential loss of uterus and resultant sexual dysfunction.
- Assess the patient's understanding and level of comprehension regarding the function of the uterus in relation to

sexual response cycle and the potential impact of therapy on sexual function.
- See nursing care of the patient with endometrial cancer, p. 1201.

Evaluation/Patient Outcomes

Coping Assistance: Sexual function is normal. Patient has identified alternate methods of achieving sexual satisfaction.

Nursing Care of the Woman With Vulvar Cancer

NIC Psychologic Comfort Promotion

See Comprehensive Care Plan, p. 1237.

NIC Skin/Wound Management

Impaired skin integrity related to pruritus, presence of a lump or mass, and bleeding or discharge

- Cleanse patient's skin *to prevent infection.*
- Apply antibiotic ointment and sterile dressing if indicated *to prevent or treat infection.*
- Expose draining area to air if possible *to promote healing.*
- Observe for increased discharge, skin changes, swelling, and lesions *to detect complications early.*

Evaluation/Patient Outcomes

Wound/Skin Management: Skin is intact and free of infection in area of disruption. Skin is clean, dry, and warm, with normal color and turgor.

Nursing Care of the Woman With Ovarian Cancer

NIC Physical and Psychologic Comfort Promotion

See Comprehensive Care Plan, p. 1237.

NIC Elimination Management

Altered patterns of urinary elimination related to pressure of tumor on bladder as evidenced by urinary frequency, dysuria, incontinence, infection, and/or retention

- Measure patient's intake and output *to monitor for fluid balance.*
- Inspect urine for bleeding *to detect evidence of infection or bladder wall irritation.*
- Inspect abdomen for distention *to determine effectiveness of bladder emptying.*
- Encourage patient to ambulate as tolerated *to promote urinary elimination.*
- Instruct on usefulness of warm tub baths *to promote urinary elimination.*
- Catheterize only as necessary *to avoid infection.*

Patient Education/Continuum of Care Plan

See section under Gynecologic Cancers on p. 1200.

Evaluation/Patient Outcomes

Elimination Management: Urinary function is normal. Patient does not complain of urgency, frequency, or dysuria. There is no evidence of hematuria.

CANCERS OF THE HEAD AND NECK

Cancers of the head and neck are found in the larynx, oral cavity, pharynx, or salivary glands. Although fewer than 5% of all cancers are neoplasms of the head and neck, they are important to understand because surgical treatment may result in extensive cosmetic deformities and may impair such vital functions as eating and speaking.

The most common site is the larynx, followed by the oral cavity, pharynx, and salivary glands. Etiologic factors for oral and laryngeal cancers include wood dust (nasal cavity cancer); chronic irritation; poor oral hygiene; prolonged heavy use of alcohol, snuff, or tobacco, and Epstein-Barr virus (associated with nasopharyngeal cancer).

Pathophysiology

Most head and neck cancers grow as malignant ulcerations on surface mucosa. The infiltrative, endophytic lesions are more aggressive and difficult to control than the less common elevated, fungating, exophytic growths. The signs and symptoms depend on the location and are as follows:

Oropharynx: "Silent" area; dysphagia; local pain, pain on swallowing, referred pain to ear, enlarging cervical mass

Hypopharynx: Another "silent" area; dysphagia, painful swallowing of food, referred ear pain, or neck mass

Nasopharynx: Bloody nasal discharge; obstructed nostril; neurologic problems such as facial pain, diplopia, or hoarseness; conductive deafness

Nose and sinuses: Bloody nasal discharge, nasal obstruction, diplopia, facial pain or swelling

Parotid and submandibular glands: Painless local swelling, hemifacial paralysis

Larynx: Persistent hoarseness, pain, referred ear pain, dyspnea, stridor, dysphagia

Multidisciplinary Plan

The goals of treatment for head and neck cancers are eradication of both clinically demonstrated disease and microscopic subclinical disease; maintenance of adequate physiologic function by reversal dysfunction and posttreatment dysfunction in the special senses, chewing and swallowing, respiration, and speech; and socially acceptable cosmesis, including sufficient surgical, radiation, plastic surgical, and prosthesis rehabilitation.

Treatment decisions involve a multidisciplinary approach with emphasis on such factors as age, general physical condition, other morbidity (such as extensive dental disease, premalignant mucosa, leukoplakia, erythroplasia, or second primary lesion), habits and lifestyle, occupation, and the patient's desires.

Surgery and radiation therapy (see p. 1233 [surgery], p. 1230 [radiation]) are the major curative modalities. Chemotherapy is employed as adjuvant therapy or sequentially before radiation or surgery (see p. 1222). Speech therapy is used for speech and swallowing rehabilitation.

More than 75% of head and neck cancer patients whose treatment fails have the first recurrence in areas above the clavicles. The most common failure pattern is recurrent primary tumor with neck metastasis and subsequent carotid erosion or rupture. Distant metastasis to the lung, bone, and elsewhere occurs in long-term survivors of local or regional disease. Intercurrent disease such as alcoholism or chronic lung disease, accidents, and suicide account for 10% to 30% of deaths.

CANCERS OF THE ORAL CAVITY

Cancers of the oral cavity are neoplasms that may invade the tongue, buccal mucosa, and hard palate.

Although easily detected, oral cancers are generally discovered late; 80% to 90% are 2 cm or more in diameter at the time of diagnosis.

PATHOPHYSIOLOGY

Identified carcinogens in oral cancer include cigarettes, ethyl alcohol, snuff, chewing tobacco, and products of the textile industry and of leather manufacturing (see box below).

Although relatively accessible to self-examination, dental evaluation, and routine physical examination, delays in the diagnosis of oral cavity cancer result from lack of unique symptomatology (painless lesion); confusion with traumatic, inflammatory, or infectious lesions; or patient delay because of fear and the false hope that the tumor will eventually disappear. The oral cavity and oropharynx are, after the larynx, the most common sites for squamous cell carcinoma of the head and neck. Patients tend to be males in their fifties and sixties, but the number of females is growing. There is also a downward trend in the age group most affected, since chewing tobacco and snuff dipping have become more common practices among women in rural areas and among young boys. Oral cancers are almost always squamous cell carcinoma. The oropharynx, which includes the lymphoid tissue of the palatal and lingual tonsils, can also be the site of lymphoma.

These lesions tend to be poorly delineated, often spread submucosally, and are not confined by the anatomic midline. Deep muscle involvement of the tongue or pterygoid musculature is an ominous finding. The invasion of bony structures—that is, mandible, palate, maxilla, maxillary sinus, or spine—is serious in terms of both prognosis and treatment morbidity. Surgical treatment of a primary tumor that extends across the midline is much more debilitating than one that has remained localized.

Nodal metastases are relatively uncommon with oral cancer but are more frequent when the site of the primary lesion extends farther into the oropharynx or when the lesion grows toward the midline. To some extent this feature (along with a higher incidence of poorly differentiated lesions) accounts for oropharyngeal tumors having a worse prognosis than that of oral cancer.

Early lesions have a good chance for cure, whereas second primary lesions are a problem, especially in oral cancer. The addition of nodal disease, an advanced primary lesion, or a recurrence after previous treatment significantly decreases the chance for survival and adds a substantial risk for distant (usually pulmonary) metastasis. The overall 5-year survival rate for oral cavity tumors is in the 50% range; for oropharyngeal cancers it is about 35%. Tumors at the base of the tongue and pharyngeal walls and those that involve bone are particularly deadly. More than 80% of persons with oral cancer who die of their disease die of uncontrolled local disease rather than distant metastasis.

The most common sign of oral cancer is the presence of a lesion, often a white spot or sore in the oral cavity or oropharynx, that is slow healing. Other complaints include difficulty with dentures, persistent ulcerations, and blood-tinged sputum. Complaints of difficulty in swallowing or in speech indicate more extensive disease.

FACTS ABOUT ORAL CANCER

Incidence: An estimated 30,100 new cases in 2001. It is most frequently seen in men over age 40 years, and the incidence is more than twice as high in men as in women. Rates declined significantly (−2.5%) during 1992-1996.

Mortality: An estimated 7800 deaths in 2001.

Warning signs: An easily bleeding, nonhealing oral sore; a lump or thickening; a red or white patch that persists. Dysphagia, difficulty in chewing or moving tongue or jaws are often signs of advanced disease.

Risk factors: Smoking cigarettes, cigars, or pipes as well as using smokeless tobacco; excessive use of alcohol.

Early detection: The dental community has taken a major role in the early detection of oral cancer by including a screening examination in routine visits.

Treatment: Surgery, alone or in combination with radiation, is the treatment of choice. For advanced cases, chemotherapy may be useful as an adjunct to surgery.

Data from American Cancer Society[1] and National Cancer Institute.[14a]

DIAGNOSTIC STUDIES AND FINDINGS

Biopsy: Areas of redness or inflammation lasting longer than 2 weeks; presence of malignant cells

Mandible x-ray examination and/or bone scan: Presence of bone involvement

CT: Parapharyngeal, spinal, carotid artery, or pterygoid muscle involvement

Endoscopy and examination under anesthesia: Evaluation of the extent of primary lesion site and possibility of synchronous second primary lesions

MULTIDISCIPLINARY PLAN

Surgery

Transoral, intraoral, or transcervical resection and reconstruction

Total laryngectomy

Modified or radical neck dissection (FIG. 18-4)

Mandibular resection and reconstruction

CO_2 laser excision

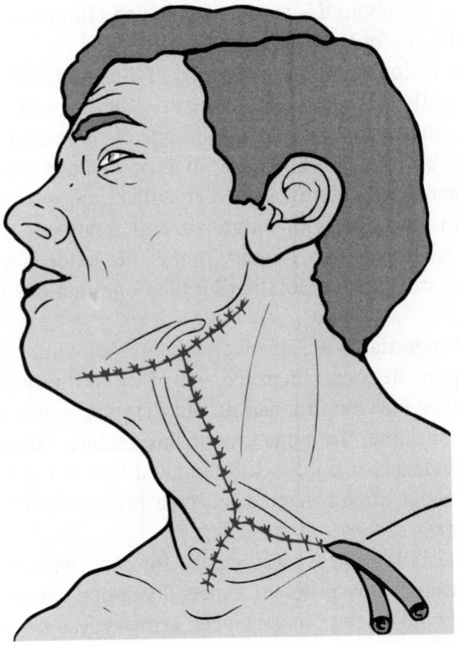

FIG. 18-4
Radical neck incision with suction tubing in place.[11a]

Radiation Therapy
External beam; external and interstitial implant

Chemotherapy
Controversial role as adjunctive therapy

NURSING CARE

NURSING ASSESSMENT

Oral cavity: Leukoplakia; erythroplakia; chronic, nonhealing ulcer; localized pain; dysphagia; excessive secretions; difficulty with denture fit
Lymphatic function: Enlarged nodes
Nutritional status: Weight loss, dehydration
Pain: Localized or referred

PATIENT PROBLEMS/NURSING DIAGNOSES & INTERVENTIONS

NIC **PHYSICAL COMFORT PROMOTION AND COPING ASSISTANCE**

See Comprehensive Care Plan, p. 1237.

PATIENT EDUCATION/CONTINUUM OF CARE PLAN

1. Emphasize the need for adequate oral hygiene and dietary management.
2. Discuss signs and symptoms of progressive disease or side effects of treatment that should be reported to the physician.

CANCER OF THE LARYNX

Cancers of the larynx arise from the epithelial lining of the laryngeal mucous membrane.

Carcinoma of the supraglottic larynx (epiglottis, aryepiglottic folds, arytenoids, and false cords) has a lower incidence than glottic carcinoma; 60% to 65% of laryngeal carcinomas occur in the glottic larynx (true vocal cord). Ninety percent occur in men, with the highest incidence in those between ages 60 and 70 years. Identifying the early warning sign of progressive hoarseness, caused by a change in the phonating edge of the vocal cord, has led to 5-year survival rates of nearly 80% for localized lesions.[1]

Early cancer can be treated by radiation therapy or surgery. Extensive lesions, which cause necrosis of cartilage or glottic extension, require total laryngectomy.

DIAGNOSTIC STUDIES AND FINDINGS

Indirect mirror examination: Presence of lesion on larynx
Direct laryngoscopy and biopsy: Presence of tumor, vocal cord fixation, occult extension, malignant cells
Anterior-posterior laryngeal tomography: Subglottic extension of disease
Pulmonary function studies: Assessment of preoperative pulmonary status
Chest x-ray examination: Identification of associated pulmonary functional disease, coexistent lung cancer

MULTIDISCIPLINARY PLAN

Surgery
Total laryngectomy: Removal of the entire larynx, hyoid bone, cricoid cartilage, two or three tracheal rings and strap muscles connected to larynx; requires permanent opening in neck for trachea and laryngectomy tube insertion.
Hemilaryngectomy: Usually one true and one false vocal cord removed; temporary tracheostomy is performed; patient's voice returns, although sounds hoarse
Supraglottic laryngectomy: Epiglottis or false vocal cords removed; permanent tracheostomy is performed; patient retains voice

Chemotherapy
For advanced disease, cisplatin with 5 FU[6]

Radiation Therapy
External beam

NURSING CARE

NURSING ASSESSMENT

Respiratory function: Dyspnea, stridor, hemoptysis, excessive secretions
Comfort level: Pain referred to ear (otalgia), dysphagia
Communication: Hoarseness, loss of speech

Patient Problems/Nursing Diagnoses & Interventions

NIC Physical Comfort Promotion and Nutrition Support

See Comprehensive Care Plan, p. 1237.

NIC Respiratory Management

Ineffective breathing pattern related to airway obstruction by tumor

Ineffective airway clearance related to tumor and upper airway secretions or laryngectomy tube

- Place patient in sitting position *to enhance chest expansion.*
- Encourage deep breathing *to ensure effective ventilation.*
- Suction airway as necessary *to remove secretions.*
- Provide standby emergency equipment (oxygen and tracheostomy tray) in case of acute obstruction.
- Provide tracheostomy care as indicated (see Chapter 9).
- Feed patient slowly with small, frequent feedings *to avoid choking.*
- Give clear-liquid, full-liquid, pureed, or soft foods as tolerated *to avoid choking.*
- Have suction equipment available in case of aspiration.

NIC Communication Enhancement

Impaired verbal communication related to altered anatomy and/or function due to presence of tumor or response to therapy

- Maintain open communication by call light in patient's reach at bedside and use of pad and pencil or Magic Slate.
- Ask questions that require a "yes" or "no" answer.
- Wait for patient to write responses.
- Assist with use of artificial larynx if applicable.
- Support activities of speech therapist to develop esophageal speech.
- Recommend support group.

NIC Health System Management

Impaired home maintenance related to need for permanent laryngectomy care

- Review convalescent care of tracheostomy patient (see Chapter 9).
- Refer to local chapter of American Cancer Society for recommending vendors who supply laryngectomy appliances.

Patient Education/Continuum of Care Plan

1. Explain methods of maintaining respiratory function, such as deep breathing, coughing, and use of oxygen; provide a list of emergency resources.
2. Discuss the value of speech therapy, and put the patient in touch with support groups, such as the Lost Cord Club.
3. Explain the use of various methods of managing pain.

Evaluation/Patient Outcomes

Respiratory Function: Patient maintains normal respiratory function. Patient is able to cough up secretions. Patient does not aspirate food or fluid.

Communication Enhancement: Patient is able to communicate need. Patient uses normal structures or artificial devices as needed to speak clearly and distinctly.

Home System Management: Patient is independent in care of laryngectomy. Patient identifies two resources for obtaining laryngectomy appliances.

CANCERS OF THE DIGESTIVE ORGANS AND ENDOCRINE GLANDS

Cancers of the esophagus and stomach account for 4% of all cancers. Unfortunately, many of the early symptoms of these diseases (dysphagia, epigastric discomfort, anorexia, and weight loss) are nonspecific, and therefore affected people often delay seeking treatment. Approximately 6% of cancers detected in the United States affect the digestive and endocrine glands. Some are easily detected because of their location and secretory patterns, whereas others are more difficult to diagnose. The 5-year survival rate varies from 1% for pancreatic carcinoma to 95% for localized thyroid cancer.[2]

Esophageal Cancer

Carcinomas of the esophagus are neoplasms that usually arise from squamous epithelium and are epidermoid in type.

Esophageal cancer usually occurs in people age 50 years or older and predominantly in men. It is also more common in the African-American population. There are indications that esophageal cancers are related to tobacco and alcohol use, nutritional deficiencies, and environmental carcinogens. The highest frequency of esophageal cancers is found in the Caspian Sea area, Transkei in southern Africa, and northern China.

Some of the suggested environmental or nutritional factors in the development of esophageal cancer include nitrosamines or fungi contaminating pickled vegetables or in grains; chronic addiction to morphine, particularly in areas where opium is eaten; tobacco residue; silica fragments associated with millet bran (northern China); and abuse of alcohol. In associating the suggested carcinogens with esophageal cancer, alcoholism is the one that has a clear relationship with epidermoid carcinoma of the esophagus. Chronic inflammation of the esophagus is also associated with a higher incidence of carcinomas. There is also an association between cancer of the esophagus and squamous cell carcinoma of the oropharynx or larynx, which is probably a result of exposure of the oral cavity, respiratory tract, and esophagus to the same carcinogenic factors. An increased incidence of esophageal cancer occurs among persons with achalasia.

Pathophysiology

Approximately 50% of esophageal cancers are at the esophagogastric junction (these cancers are generally adenocarcinoma and arise from the stomach rather than the esophagus); 25% are in the upper thoracic esophagus; 17% are in the lower esophagus; and 8% are in the cervical esophagus. Two thirds of these are squamous cell carcinomas. Adenocarcinomas are the second most common type.

Squamous cell carcinoma begins as a small mucosal patch that eventually grows, ulcerates, and protrudes into the lumen. Local extension to the recurrent laryngeal nerve or tracheobronchial tree is common. Unfortunately, local extension of the cancer is often present at the time of diagnosis. Metastasis to the local lymph nodes includes those around the hilum of the lung and in the neck. Metastases to the abdominal lymph nodes of the celiac axis occur. Metastases to the liver, lungs, kidney, and bone occur with decreasing frequency. Submucosal spread of the carcinoma does occur. Satellite lesions occur several inches away from the primary lesion.

Carcinoma of the bronchus or stomach often metastasizes to the esophagus. Mediastinal lymph node metastasis from other organ carcinomas may lead to esophageal involvement and symptoms of obstruction. Breast carcinomas may metastasize to the esophagus. Primary adenocarcinoma of the esophagus is rare and should be considered the result of Barrett's esophagus or of spread from an adenocarcinoma of the stomach cardia.

Dysphagia is the most common complaint of persons with esophageal cancer. It is usually first noticed with the ingestion of bulky foods, later with soft foods, and finally with liquids. Weight loss, regurgitation, and aspiration pneumonitis may also be noted. The most prevalent symptoms in persons without dysphagia are odynophagia (pain on swallowing) and symptoms of gastroesophageal reflux. Signs and symptoms of advanced disease include cervical adenopathy; chronic cough; choking after eating; hemoptysis, hematemesis, or both; and hoarseness. Pain is an unusual symptom and indicates local extension.

Diagnostic Studies and Findings

Esophageal x-ray examination: Irregular, ragged mucosal pattern with luminal narrowing

Esophagoscopy with brush biopsy: Presence of lesion with malignant cells in biopsy specimen

Multidisciplinary Plan

Surgery

Esophagogastrectomy
- Left chest for lesions in lower esophagus
- Laparotomy and right thoracotomy or transhiatal approach for higher lesions
- Transhiatal approach for lesions at thoracic inlet and cervical esophagus; stomach as esophageal replacement

Radiation Therapy

External beam for squamous cell lesions above aortic arch; palliation for obstructive symptoms, pain control

Chemotherapy

Preoperative cisplatin-based chemotherapy alone or in combination with radiation therapy; used alone for palliation with locally recurrent or metastatic disease; used with radiation therapy (without surgery) for palliation of dysphagia

NURSING CARE

Nursing Assessment

Nutritional status: Dysphagia, initially with solids and progressing to liquids; difficult or painful swallowing; sensation of food taking longer to go through segments of the chest (i.e., to reach the stomach) described by the patient; anorexia; weight loss; regurgitation

Comfort level: Odynophagia

Patient Problems/Nursing Diagnoses & Interventions

NIC Physical Comfort Promotion and Nutrition Support

See Comprehensive Care Plan, p. 1237.

Patient Education/Continuum of Care Plan

See Comprehensive Care Plan, p. 1237.

Gastric Cancer

Gastric carcinoma refers to malignant neoplasms and tumors found in the stomach. Adenocarcinomas that arise from normal or metaplastic mucosa cells are the most common. Benign neoplasms of the stomach are rare and include leiomyomas and polyps.

The incidence of gastric cancers has significantly decreased in western Europe and the United States. The American Cancer Society estimated that approximately 21,900 new cases occurred in 2000. In the 1940s gastric cancer was the most common malignant disease in the United States.[1] No apparent change in the incidence of gastric cancer has occurred in Japan, where it accounts for 60% of all cancers in men and 40% of all cancers in women.

Many questions exist about the decline in gastric cancer. The answers to those questions would provide valuable clues in the early diagnosis, treatment, and ultimately prevention of gastric carcinomas. In addition, interesting geographic variations exist. Gastric cancer is higher in the north central and northeast regions of the United States. It is more common in urban than in rural areas in England, but this is not true in the United States. Although it is very common in Japan, gastric cancer is less common in Japanese persons in Hawaii, and the incidence decreases with each generation.

Genetic factors may play a role in the development of gastric cancer. Gastric cancers are more frequent in certain families and in persons with type A blood. Gastric cancer is more common in African-Americans than whites and in men than in women. Hereditary nonpolyposis colon cancer (HNPCC or Lynch syndrome) and familial adenomatous polyposis are inherited genetic disorders that slightly increase the risk of stomach cancer in families affected by these inherited gene mutations.[1]

Long-term infection with *Helicobacter pylori* may lead to chronic atrophic gastritis, a possible precancerous change in the stomach's lining. Although the vast majority of patients who carry this bacterium never develop cancer, patients with adenocarcinoma of the stomach do have a higher rate of infection than people without this cancer.[1]

The role of dietary factors has been studied to identify foods or soil contaminants that may lead to gastric cancers. Starches, pickled vegetables, and salted fish and meats have been associated with gastric cancers. However, whole milk, fresh vegetables, vitamin C, and refrigeration are inversely associated with gastric cancers. Nitrates, which are converted into nitrites, are commonly found in the diet. Compounds formed with nitrites (nitrosamines and nitrosamides) have been carcinogenic in animals. Although not confirmed as a carcinogen in humans, nitrite-forming bacteria are increased in the upper gastrointestinal tract of people with hypochlorhydria and achlorhydria after gastric surgery. Hypochlorhydria and achlorhydria are often found in patients with pernicious anemia and atrophic gastritis. The reduced acid appears to support or allow colonization of the stomach by the bacteria.

Cold temperatures inhibit the conversion of nitrates to nitrites. Better refrigeration and decreased use of nitrates as food additives might explain the decreased incidence of gastric cancers.

Gastric cancer appears to be higher in individuals with late-onset immunoglobulin deficiency. Patients with celiac sprue with reduced IgA are at greater risk for gastric cancer. Other factors associated with gastric cancer are gastric ulcers, atrophic gastritis, gastric polyps, and pernicious anemia.

Pathophysiology

The carcinoma found in the stomach is epithelial growth arising from the mucosal membrane. Microscopically the cells resemble intestinal metaplasia and contain goblet cells characteristic of the intestines. The parietal and chief glands of the stomach are seldom seen in gastric tumors. Adenocarcinomas in the stomach have been classified in several ways.

First, according to cellular or extracellular characteristics, carcinomas are referred to as papillary, colloid or mucinous, medullary, and signet ring. Papillary refers to cells forming glandular structures in a papillary form. When excessive mucin secretion and extracellular aggregates are present, the adenocarcinoma is referred to as colloid or mucinous. Medullary is a solid band or a mass of undifferentiated cells. The signet ring adenocarcinoma refers to a well-differentiated adenocarcinoma with large amounts of intracellular mucinous material that compresses the nucleus to an unusual location.

Second, an adenocarcinoma of the stomach may be classified histologically according to the degree of cell differentiation—from well differentiated to poorly differentiated.

Unfortunately, the preceding two classifications and their parts are not mutually exclusive. Various cellular characteristics and degrees of differentiation may occur within a tumor. The third classification system reflects the biologic behavior of the tumor and defines gastric carcinomas as intestinal or diffuse. The intestinal type is a glandular tumor, and the diffuse type is composed of single cells or small groups of cells.

The fourth system is an expansion of the intestinal and diffuse definitions and classifies cancers in the stomach as expanding or infiltrating. The expanding (intestinal) type is characterized by a group of cells that are similar, maintain a coherent relationship, and push aside other cells as they grow. The infiltrative (diffuse) class is characterized by deep, wide infiltration by individual tumor cells.

The intestinal type of gastric cancer is associated with intestinal metaplasia and gastritis. The carcinoma tends to be circumscribed, and spread of the disease is through the bloodstream. The liver is a common site of metastasis. The diffuse type of carcinoma is less circumscribed, spreads by way of the lymphatics, and may take the form of linitis plastica, which is a diffuse fibrosis and thickening of the gastric wall.

The most common site of carcinoma is the lower half of the stomach. An exception occurs when gastric atrophy is a precursor to the cancer, and then the lesion tends to be in the upper portion of the stomach.

In early gastric cancers the disease is confined to the mucosa and submucosa. The symptoms with early gastric cancers may be vague and nonspecific and include complaints of epigastric discomfort or indigestion and occasional vomiting, belching, or postprandial fullness. The only observation that can lead to an early diagnosis is a positive stool occult blood test result.

Advanced gastric cancer denotes involvement of the muscular layer of the stomach with invasion of the pancreas, esophagus, colon, duodenum, gallbladder, liver, or adjacent mesenteries. Metastases, local and distant, are common.

Gastric ulcers have been associated with gastric cancers. This may be a diagnostic issue. Previously radiologically diagnosed gastric ulcers have later been found to be carcinomas. Occasionally a benign gastric ulcer has a focal carcinoma at a margin. Also, malignant cells may be found at the base of the ulcer and at the margin. Most physicians routinely perform a biopsy of gastric ulcers during endoscopy to rule out the presence of gastric carcinoma.

Gastric atrophy and pernicious anemia are associated with achlorhydria. Achlorhydria is a precursor of gastric cancer. Gastric polyps are often found in atrophic mucosa. A polyp may be benign or malignant, and the recommended treatment is removal through an endoscope and histologic examination. Approximately 10% of gastric polyps are malignant.

Diagnostic Studies and Findings

Hematocrit: Slightly below normal; patient may have macrocytic or microcytic anemia secondary to decreased iron or vitamin B_{12} absorption

Stool for occult blood: Positive for blood

Upper GI series (barium swallow): Polypoid mass; ulceration surrounded by mass; thickened, fibrosed gastric wall

CT: Thickness of gastric wall; presence of metastasis (may assist in differentiating between benign and carcinogenic lesion)

Endoscopy and cytologic studies: Biopsy and cytology specimens examined for cancer cells; can visualize lesion

Liver function studies: Abnormal findings may indicate metastasis

Endoscopic ultrasound: Estimates how far cancer has spread into wall of stomach, nearby tissues, lymph nodes

MULTIDISCIPLINARY PLAN

Surgery

Exploratory celiotomy: Initial intervention in all patients with gastric cancer except those with peritoneal metastases, documented liver metastases, or other distant metastases; if tumor is regionally localized, resection of primary tumor, as well as actual and potentially involved regional lymph nodes, is done; postoperative staging of the tumor is completed and further treatment decisions are made

Distal subtotal gastric resection

Proximal subtotal gastric resection

Total gastrectomy: Includes resection of adjacent organs involved by local extension, such as body and tail of pancreas, portion of liver, transverse colon, or duodenum and head of pancreas

Palliative resection

Radiation Therapy

Palliation of obstruction, particularly in the cardia, or of chronic bleeding

Chemotherapy

Single agent palliation with 5-fluorouracil

Combination chemotherapy

- 5-Fluorouracil, nitrosourea, mitomycin C, doxorubicin,
  - FAM: 5-fluorouracil, doxorubicin (Adriamycin), mitomycin C
- 5-Fluorouracil, semustine (methyl CCNU)

The prognosis for patients with gastric cancer is poor because almost two thirds have findings at the time of diagnosis that limit the possibility of survival. Nodal involvement is a significant prognostic factor. Patients with a short history of symptoms have a poorer prognosis than do those with a longer history. Patients with ulcer syndrome do better than those with the more common symptoms of indigestion.

NURSING CARE

NURSING ASSESSMENT

Nutritional status: Loss of appetite, anorexia; feeling of fullness with minimum intake; distaste for meats; weight loss; persistent midepigastric pain; dysphagia; vague epigastric discomfort; vomiting, hematemesis; belching; postprandial fullness

Physical examination: Tenderness in midepigastrium; rebound tenderness; abdominal guarding; mass in epigastrium (late stage); enlarged liver; positive supraclavicular nodes; ascites (loss of albumin into gastric lumen); acanthosis nigricans (rare); signs of metastasis: myeloid metaplasia or primary central nervous system (CNS) disease

PATIENT PROBLEMS/NURSING DIAGNOSES & INTERVENTIONS

NIC NUTRITION SUPPORT

See Comprehensive Care Plan, p. 1237.

PATIENT EDUCATION/CONTINUUM OF CARE PLAN

1. Ensure that patient understands the rationale for combination therapies of surgery, chemotherapy, and radiation therapy in the treatment of gastric cancers. Provide written information in the form of do's and don'ts during chemotherapy and radiotherapy, sequence of treatment, and potential side effects.
2. Explain the importance of regular follow-up endoscopies.

DIGESTIVE GLAND TUMORS

Carcinomas of the digestive glands are neoplasms that may involve the pancreas, liver, or gallbladder.

Carcinoma of the gallbladder, with its insidious onset, may be diagnosed only during surgery for presumed acute cholecystitis. The only possibility of cure is with complete removal of the gallbladder; often a partial hepatectomy is also required because of early liver invasion. Mortality is as high as 75%; the 5-year survival rate is about 4%.

Carcinoma of the liver is usually metastatic; primary tumors constitute only 1% of hepatic cancer. One primary tumor, hemangiosarcoma of the liver, is a rare disease thought to be caused by vinyl chloride exposure. The risk of hepatocellular carcinoma is about 40 times greater in patients with ethanol-induced cirrhosis. Early signs and symptoms of hepatic cancer are often absent or insidious and slow to localize (FIG. 18-5). The most common complaints are vague upper abdominal pain

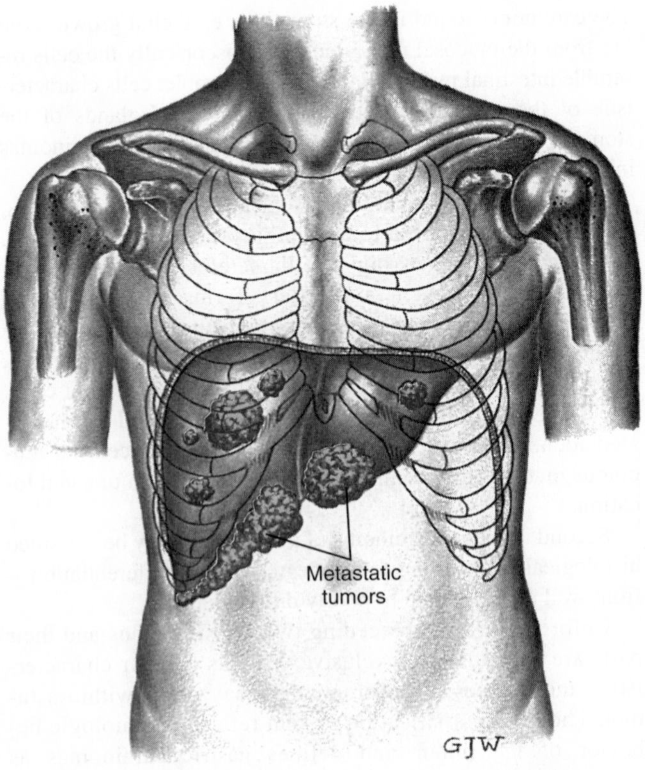

FIG. 18-5
Hepatic carcinoma (liver cancer).

and generalized weakness. Other indications of liver involvement are anemia, anorexia, jaundice, weight loss, pain, and respiratory distress. Obstruction of the portal vein, sometimes occurring suddenly, may cause splenomegaly, esophageal varices, and ascites. Patients may also have fever of unknown origin and dependent edema. Diagnosis is based on laboratory data obtained from a liver profile, scanning, angiography, and biopsy.

The only possibility for cure is lobectomy to remove the diseased tissue. In some major medical centers, liver transplantation is being used as an alternative procedure for eligible patients. If surgery is contraindicated by the extent of the disease or the patient's condition, radiation therapy and chemotherapy via implantable infusion pump may be used. The prognosis is poor, and few patients are alive 5 years after the initial diagnosis.

Over the past 20 years, rates of pancreatic cancer have declined in men and have remained approximately constant in women.[1] As in liver and gallbladder disease, the onset is insidious and the diagnosis is made late in the course.[19]

Because of the vagueness of the signs and symptoms, few pancreatic tumors are diagnosed at a curable stage. Surgery (Whipple's procedure), radiation therapy, and chemotherapy are treatment options than can extend survival and/or relieve symptoms in many patients but are not likely to produce a cure (FIG. 18-6, Whipple procedure). The prognosis is extremely poor; only 20% of patients are still alive 1 year after diagnosis.[1]

Salivary gland tumors grow slowly and are often diagnosed late. Complete excision, although difficult to accomplish without producing facial nerve damage, is important to prevent recurrence. If the tumor cannot be removed surgically, radiation therapy may be used to shrink it.

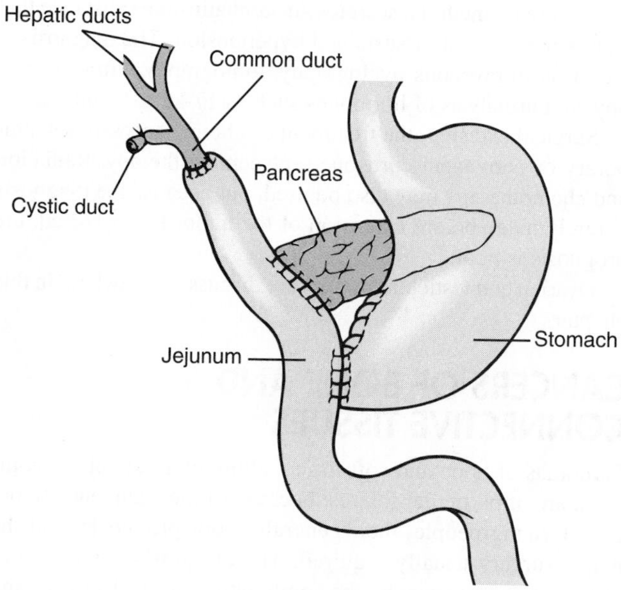

FIG. 18-6
Whipple procedure or radical pancreaticoduodenectomy. This surgical procedure involves resection of the proximal pancreas, adjoining duodenum, distal portion of the stomach, and distal portion of the common bile duct. An anastomosis of the pancreatic duct, common bile duct, and stomach to the jejunum is done.[7b]

DIAGNOSTIC STUDIES AND FINDINGS

Biliary (Gallbladder)

Serologic studies: Increased levels of alkaline phosphatase, bilirubin, CEA, and CA19-9

Liver

Liver function tests: Elevations noted with alkaline phosphatase, asparate aminotransferase, and alanine aminotransferase

Alpha-fetoprotein (AFP): Elevated; useful as a marker for monitoring response to therapy

Abdominal ultrasound, CT of abdomen and lungs, MRI: All useful in obtaining information on presence, location, and size of tumor

Needle biopsy under ultrasound: Obtain tissue sample for biopsy

Pancreas

CT: Location and size of tumor

Endoscopic retrograde cholangiopancreatogram (ERCP): Determines blockage of pancreatic ducts; in presence of blockage, percutaneous biliary drainage tube may be inserted to facilitate drainage

Fine-needle aspiration biopsy: Used in place of surgery to obtain tissue sample for biopsy

Laparoscopy: Identifies metastatic sites

MULTIDISCIPLINARY PLAN

Biliary (Gallbladder)

Surgery

Liver transplants attempted but survival remains limited because of high relapse rate; certain subsets of patients (depending on location of tumor) may have longer survivals

Chemotherapy

Mitomycin and 5-FU are the most common but response is very poor

Liver

Surgery

Treatment of choice for localized, early disease; liver transplantation has not been promising because of high incidence of recurrence in new liver

Radiation Therapy

Tumor may be controlled, with potential for cure

Chemotherapy

Regional perfusion of the liver via the hepatic artery or portal vein using one or more of the following drugs: 5-fluorodeoxyuridine, 5-FU, cisplatin, streptozotocin, etoposide, mitomycin-C, folinic acid, and mitoxantrone[9]

Systemic administration of 5-FU and leucovorin[9]

Pancreas

Surgery

If disease is confined or localized, either a total pancreatectomy or a Whipple procedure (pancreaticoduodenectomy) is done to remove tumor; location and size of tumor tend to cause biliary and/or gastric outlet obstructions; several different palliative procedures (biliary bypass cholecystojejunostomy or a choledochojejunostomy, gastroenterostomy) may be performed[19]

Radiation Therapy

Palliation of obstruction and symptoms in advanced cases

Chemotherapy

Single agents

5-FU; mitomycin C; streptozocin, ifosfamide; doxorubicin; gemcitabine for locally unresectable or metastatic disease[19]

Combination chemotherapy

SMF (streptozocin, mitomycin C, 5-FU)

NURSING CARE

Nursing Assessment

For all three cancers, onset of symptoms is gradual, insidious, and similar, unless otherwise noted.

Gastrointestinal function: Dull abdominal pain, right upper quadrant (liver), epigastric fullness, increased girth (liver), obstructive jaundice

Nutritional status: Weight loss, anorexia, fatigue, hypoglycemia (islet cells)

Elimination patterns: Episodes of constipation or diarrhea (liver); occult blood in stools (pancreas)

Potential Complications

Ascites

Patient Problems/Nursing Diagnoses & Interventions

NIC Physical Comfort Promotion and Nutrition Support

See Comprehensive Care Plan, p. 1237.

Patient Education/Continuum of Care Plan

See Comprehensive Care Plan, p. 1237.

Endocrine Gland Tumors

Carcinomas of the endocrine gland are neoplasms that may occur in the parathyroid, thyroid, or adrenal glands.

Because they are so rare, only a brief overview of the pathophysiology, incidence, and signs and symptoms is presented here.

Parathyroid tumors are rare. When they do occur, they produce excessive amounts of parathyroid hormone, which causes bony deformities and renal calculi. These tumors are treated by surgical excision.

Carcinoma of the thyroid has its highest incidence (37% of endocrine cancers) in people ages 25 to 44 years. It occurs most frequently in women and in whites. Those at high risk are people who as children received radiation therapy to the neck for such conditions as hypertrophy of the tonsils, adenoids, or lymphatic tissue; enlarged thymus gland; or skin disorders such as acne.

The initial sign of a thyroid tumor is a lump in the gland, which may first be palpated during a routine physical examination. More extensive local involvement causes hoarseness, dysphagia, or dyspnea. Thyroid scanning, ultrasonography, and biopsy are used to diagnose the lesion, which is most commonly papillary carcinoma of the thyroid, a slow-growing, easily removed tumor. Even without total surgical eradication, many patients live 10 to 15 years with few symptoms. The 5-year survival rate is 97% for patients with localized disease and 86% if the disease has spread. Spread is usually to adjacent cervical lymph nodes.

Undifferentiated thyroid cancers are more likely to cause tracheal compression and metastasis to cervical lymph nodes. For these patients, treatment is lobectomy or total thyroidectomy and en bloc dissection of lymph nodes. Radioactive iodine (I^{131}) and radiation therapy may also be used.

Neoplasms of the adrenal glands cause changes in body functioning, depending on the affected component. Cortical neoplasms may alter the body's sex characteristics and cause complex steroidal changes, such as Cushing's syndrome. Medullary neoplasms may precipitate attacks of hypertension. The median age for occurrence is 40 years, although people of any age may be affected. The tumors may be benign or malignant and may be linked with a specific pituitary tumor.

Signs and symptoms, such as pain, distention, and hemorrhage, are usually noted at a late stage, when local extension obstructs or destroys the kidneys. Pheochromocytoma, a tumor of the adrenal medulla, secretes an adrenalin-like substance that causes paroxysmal or sustained hypertension. The diagnosis is based on intravenous pyelography, tomography, ultrasonography, and urinalysis of hormones such as 17-ketosteroid.

Surgical excision, the treatment of choice, necessitates temporary or permanent cortisone replacement therapy. Radiation and chemotherapy may also be used, but because the diagnosis is rarely made before extension of the tumor has occurred, the prognosis is poor.

Ovarian and testicular tumors are discussed elsewhere in this chapter.

CANCERS OF BONE AND CONNECTIVE TISSUES

Sarcomas of bone and soft tissue, although relatively uncommon, are of particular interest because of their tendency to occur in young people, their generally poor prognosis, and the major surgery usually required. The prognosis has been improved in recent years by the combination of local surgery and chemotherapy. In addition, in many patients the primary tumor can be successfully treated by more conservative surgical procedures combined with high-dose radiation therapy. However, 60% to 65% of bone cancers are metastatic from other primary lesions and thus are more difficult to treat successfully.

Bone Sarcomas

Bone cancer is a skeletal malignancy occurring as a primary sarcomatous tumor in an area of rapid growth.

People at high risk for the development of bone sarcomas are those with Paget's disease of bone, Ollier's disease, multiple exostoses, retinoblastoma, or previous high-dose radiation therapy to bone. Osteosarcoma and Ewing's sarcoma occur most commonly in people under age 20 years. This is in contrast to reticulum cell sarcoma, fibrosarcoma, and chondrosarcoma, which occur later in life but with a much wider age distribution.

Pathophysiology

The patient's complaints are initially subtle and intermittent, with gradually increasing severity. An initially painless mass is the most common symptom; others include pain, functional deficit, or pathologic fracture. The pain is usually described as mild and brief and is often associated with a minor injury. It may increase in severity but is often reported as being a localized, dull ache. It usually does not increase with activity or decrease with rest but may be greater at night. This pain rarely responds to simple analgesic medication but requires narcotics for relief.

There may not be any symptoms; if they are present, they are dependent on the size, site, and patterns of local infiltration. The site and extent of pathologic fractures dictate the severity of symptoms. Metastases to regional lymph nodes are uncommon, but systemic illness may be related to pulmonary, visceral, and subcutaneous tissue involvement.

Diagnostic Studies and Findings

Roentgenograms of involved bones and soft tissues: Visualization of suspect lesion
Chest roentgenogram: Evidence of metastasis
Bone scan: Evidence of primary lesion or metastasis
CT: Evidence of cortical bone destruction
Blood studies: Increased alkaline and acid phosphatase; increased calcium indicative of bone disease and demineralization
Urine study: High calcium excretion secondary to hypercalcemia
Open or needle biopsy: Histologic evidence of malignancy

Multidisciplinary Plan

Surgery*

Amputation with limb salvage to degree possible
- Foot and ankle: Below-knee amputation or knee disarticulation
- Proximal tibia: Thigh amputation
- Distal femur: Hip disarticulation
- Proximal end of femur: Modified hemipelvectomy

En bloc resection for low-grade malignant lesions; reconstruction with bone autografts, cadaver hemografts, or metal or plastic devices

Chemotherapy

Antineoplastic agents

Preoperative and postoperative systemic chemotherapy for osteogenic sarcoma; high-dose methotrexate (amethopterin; Mexate) with leucovorin rescue; doxorubicin (Adriamycin) by intraarterial perfusion; cisplatin, ifosfamide, etoposide, carboplatin
Systemic chemotherapy for metastatic disease
Biologic response modifiers (interferon)

Radiation Therapy

Osteosarcoma is a radioresistant tumor, whereas Ewing's sarcoma is radiosensitive.

Disease-free survival rates for patients whose osteogenic sarcoma is treated with surgery and chemotherapy appear to be greater than 50% at 5 years. Among patients with localized Ewing's sarcoma, the disease-free survival at 5 years is 50% after chemotherapy and radiation therapy.

*See Chapter 6 for postoperative nursing diagnoses and interventions.

NURSING CARE

Nursing Assessment

Musculoskeletal function: Presence of mass, functional deficit, pathologic fracture
Pain: Mild and fleeting, dull and aching, increased at night, not affected by activity or rest, need for narcotics to obtain relief
Systemic function: Fever; malaise, easy fatigability; anorexia; weight loss

Patient Problems/Nursing Diagnoses and Interventions

NIC Physical Comfort Promotion

See Comprehensive Care Plan, p. 1237.

NIC Immobility Management

Impaired physical mobility related to pressure of tumor, pain
- Assist patient with ambulation; control distance *to avoid injury and fatigue.*
- Have patient use walker, cane, or wheelchair as needed as assistive devices *to promote mobility.*
- Minimize environmental barriers *to avoid falls.*
- Encourage use of involved limb *to maintain function.*

NIC Activity and Exercise Management

Activity intolerance related to systemic effects of disease and treatment
- Ambulate patient, or seat patient in armchair *to promote circulation.*
- Encourage moderate physical exercise, adequate rest, and performance of range-of-motion exercises *to maintain activity level and avoid immobility.*

- Balance nutritional intake; supplement protein *to increase strength.*
- Observe for increased nutritional requirements and weakness as indications of advancing disease.

Patient Education/Continuum of Care Plan

1. Discuss the principles of safe ambulation: wide supportive stance; well-fitting, low-heeled shoes; good body mechanics; and weight bearing on unaffected side.
2. Plan pain relief measures with activities to enhance patient self-care.

Evaluation/Patient Outcomes

Immobility Management: Patient is mobile and able to tolerate activity. Patient walks independently or with assistive device.

Activity and Exercise Management: Patient can tolerate activities of daily living.

Soft Tissue Sarcomas

Soft tissue sarcomas are neoplasms that arise in soft tissue, parenchymatous organs, or hollow viscera and include fibrosarcoma, malignant fibrous histiocytoma, liposarcoma, rhabdomyosarcoma, leiomyosarcoma, angiosarcoma, synovial sarcoma, mixed mesenchymal sarcoma, Kaposi's sarcoma, and unclassified or spindle cell sarcoma.

Only among children are soft tissue tumors, especially rhabdomyosarcoma, relatively frequent.

Pathophysiology

A painless mass is the most common initial symptom. Masses in the thigh area are suspect because of the high number of sarcomas occurring there. Advanced local disease is rare except for large tumors arising in the retroperitoneal or pelvic areas. Lymph node metastases are uncommon except in patients with rhabdomyosarcoma, high-grade synovial sarcoma, and epithelioid sarcoma.

Rhabdomyosarcoma arises from the embryonic mesenchymal cells that form striated muscle. It may develop in almost any body site; the most common primary sites are the head and neck, extremities, genitourinary tract, trunk, and orbit. The prognosis depends on the primary site and the stage of the disease (histologic grade), which is in turn based on extent of disease and resectability. Genitourinary lesions generally have the most favorable prognosis, and extremity tumors have one of the worst prognoses.

Kaposi's sarcoma (KS), the malignancy most frequently associated with acquired immunodeficiency syndrome (AIDS), is recorded as the syndrome's initial clinical manifestation in approximately 25% of cases. The epidemic form (EKS) affects primarily homosexual men and may be of greater incidence than just noted because subsequent malignant and infectious complications (after initial diagnosis) are not reported to the Centers for Disease Control and Prevention.

The initial manifestations of EKS include nodular, macular, or papular lesions on the skin and mucosal surfaces; fever; weight loss; malaise; anorexia; and diarrhea. The lesions are frequently located on the trunk, arms, head, neck, and oral cavity. Lesions on the head and neck can be especially disfiguring and can cause symptoms of obstruction or compression. Fifty percent of patients with EKS have visceral involvement, particularly of the GI tract. Pulmonary involvement can lead to progressive respiratory dysfunction and failure. Lymph nodes are often affected; involvement in the brain, liver, pancreas, adrenal glands, spleen, heart, and testes has been noted. Therapy for EKS remains experimental and controversial, with chemotherapy, radiotherapy, and immunotherapy used with varying degrees of success.

Diagnostic Studies and Findings

Radiographic study of affected part (CT, xerography, arteriography): Visualization of suspect lesion and vasculature

Chest tomography or chest CT: Evidence of metastasis

Excisional, incisional, or needle biopsy: Histologic evidence of malignancy

Multidisciplinary Plan

Surgery

Radical surgical excision: Amputation, muscle group resection, radical local excision

Chemotherapy

Antineoplastic agents

Vincristine sulfate (Oncovin), 2 mg/m^2 for children, 1.4 mg/m^2 for adults Doxorubicin (Adriamycin), 60-75 mg/m^2 at intervals of 21 days or 30 mg/m^2 on each of 3 successive days repeated every 4 weeks

Cyclophosphamide (Cytoxan), 40-50 mg/kg IV or individual doses over several days, then adjusted to lower maintenance dosage; PO 1-5 mg/kg qd

Cisplatin (Platinol), 50-80 mg/m^2 IV every 3 weeks or by individually determined dosage

Radiation Therapy

External beam

NURSING CARE

Nursing Assessment

Pain: In area of tumor

Body contours: Painless mass

Sensory and motor function: Peripheral neuralgia, paralysis

Patient Problems/Nursing Diagnoses & Interventions

NIC Physical Comfort Promotion

See Comprehensive Care Plan, p. 1237.

NIC **Immobility Management**

Impaired physical mobility related to peripheral neuralgia, paralysis

- Assist patient with ambulation; control distance *to avoid stress and fatigue.*
- Use walker, cane, or wheelchair as needed for added support.
- Minimize environmental barriers *to prevent injury.*
- Encourage use of involved limb *to maintain tone.*
- Test for impaired coordination as evidence of further dysfunction.

Patient Education/Continuum of Care Plan

1. Explain the principles of safe ambulation.
2. Discuss the management of disease-related pain.

Evaluation/Patient Outcomes

Immobility Management: Patient is mobile and able to tolerate activity. Patient walks independently or with assistive device.

Cancers of the Central Nervous System

Tumors of the CNS are neoplasms of the brain or spinal cord.

Tumors of the CNS account for more than 2% of annual cancer deaths. Eighty percent of CNS tumors involve the brain, with as many as half of these metastatic from primary cancers of the lung, breast, kidney, melanoma, and GI tract; the other 20% involve the spinal cord.

Pathophysiology

The majority of CNS tumors are gliomas, which are peculiar because they rarely spread beyond the CNS. There are no known etiologic factors, although childhood tumors are believed to be developmental in origin.

Spinal cord tumors are gliomas (23%), meningiomas or schwannomas (56%), or miscellaneous other forms such as epidermoid and dermoid cysts, hemangioblastomas, and chordomas. These tumors produce symptoms in the body below the level of tumor location in the cord: difficulty in walking, postural disturbances, back pain, and changes in sensation and muscle power. The pain of a spinal cord tumor is worse at night.

Spinal tumors in adults are divided as follows:

Intramedullary

1. Ependymoma and astrocytoma: Most common; usually extend over many spinal cord regions; most have slow, progressive onset with sensory loss of pain and temperatures; caudal region tumors may result in bowel, bladder, and sexual dysfunction
2. Oligodendroglioma
3. Hemangioblastomas

Extramedullary

1. Intradural tumors: Include meningioma, neurofibroma, and congenital lesions; thoracic spine is frequent site; slow, gradual onset; local and radicular pain may be present
2. Extradural tumors: Include metastic carcinoma, lymphoma, and multiple myeloma; rapid onset of symptoms; local pain at area of tumor and along spinal nerve dermatomes; increased pain with bed rest, movement, and straining

The more common adult brain tumors are as follows[16]:

Astrocytoma: The most common in the adult and frequently described as low- or high-grade tumors. They are infiltrative, invading surrounding normal tissue, and cannot be surgically removed.

Oligodendroglioma: Grow more slowly than astrocytoma, usually of a mixed histology.

Meningioma: A slow-growing tumor arising from the dural covering of the brain. While benign histologically, it can be malignant by location where it is impossible to remove and can eventually cause death.

Diagnostic Studies and Findings

Brain Tumors

Brain scan: Increased uptake of isotope in the tumor

Cerebral angiography: Increased or obstructed cerebral blood flow

Positron emission tomography (PET): Details sites of glucose metabolism in the brain under various conditions

Skull x-ray examination: Erosion of posterior clinoid process or presence of intracranial calcifications

CT and MRI: Identification of vascular tumors, shifts in midline structures, changes in cerebral ventricular sizes

Electroencephalogram (EEG): Marked focal slowing; rhythmic, periodic, and high-voltage slowing

Dural sinus venography: May indicate narrowed sinuses and interference with cranial drainage

Echoencephalogram: Shifts in midline structures

Stereotaxic biopsy: Identification of cell type

Ophthalmoscopic examination: Papilledema

Spinal Tumors

Spinal x-ray examination: Presence of vertebral column lesions and bony destruction

Myelography (with contrast medium): Identification of size, boundaries, and level of tumor

Cerebrospinal fluid (CSF) sampling: Elevated protein levels; Froin's syndrome (xanthochromatic CSF with large amounts of protein, rapid coagulation, and absence of an increased number of cells)

Electromyogram (EMG): Useful in differential diagnosis

Queckenstedt's test: Positive finding

CT: Location of lesion

Spinal angiograms: Differentiation of vascular lesions from tumors

PET: Location of lesion

MULTIDISCIPLINARY PLAN

Brain Tumors

Surgery
Craniotomy for supratentorial tumor excision
Craniectomy for infratentorial tumor excision
Transsphenoidal for excision of pituitary tumor
Shunting procedures to treat secondary complications of hydrocephalus
Implantation of Omaya reservoir for administration of intraventricular chemotherapy
Stereotactic-guided craniotomy

Radiation Therapy
External beam, brachytherapy, with implantation of radioactive seeds by stereotaxic techniques directly into tumor bed

Chemotherapy
Corticosteroids: Dexamethasone, 10-20 mg/day PO, IV
Agents dependent on type of tumor; must be able to cross blood-brain barrier
Carmustine (BCNU) for astrocytomas

Spinal Cord Tumors

Surgery
Laminectomy

Radiation Therapy
Postoperative external beam; palliative relief of cord compression

Chemotherapy
Corticosteroids: Dexamethasone, 10-20 mg IV qid

Despite therapeutic advances, CNS tumors have high morbidity and mortality. About 40% of people with brain tumors can return to a useful life, and another 30% gain good palliation. The neoplasms vary in their aggressiveness and consequently their prognosis. The earlier the diagnosis, the better are the patient's chances for maximum restoration of function.

Table 18-2 Localizing Signs and Symptoms of Brain Tumors

Frontal lobe	
Anterior portion	Disturbances in mental function
Posterior portion	Motor system dysfunction; convulsions; aphasia (dominant hemisphere)
Parietal lobe	Sensory deficits (contralateral); paresthesia; hyperesthesia; astereognosis; loss of two-point discrimination; finger agnosia; convulsions; visual field defects; defects in speech and recognition (dominant hemisphere)
Temporal lobe	Psychomotor convulsions; visual field defects; auditory disturbances; Wernicke's aphasia (dominant hemisphere)
Occipital lobe	Headaches; convulsions with visual aura; visual field deficit
Cerebellar tumors	Nystagmus; ataxia; unsteady gait; dysmetria; problems with rapid alternation movements
Brainstem and cranial nerve tumors	Hemiparesis; nystagmus; extraocular nerve palsies; facial paralysis; depressed corneal reflex; hearing loss, tinnitus; problems swallowing, drooling; vertigo, dizziness; ataxia; vomiting

NURSING CARE

NURSING ASSESSMENT
Increased intracranial pressure: Early headache; nausea and vomiting; decreased level of consciousness; failing vision; changing pupillary response
Localizing signs and symptoms of brain tumors (Table 18-2).
Localizing signs and symptoms of spinal cord tumors (Table 18-3).

PATIENT PROBLEMS/NURSING DIAGNOSES AND INTERVENTIONS

NIC NEUROLOGIC MANAGEMENT

Disturbed sensory perception (visual) related to brain tissue compression
- Arrange environment *to minimize barriers and avoid injury.*

Table 18-3 Localizing Signs and Symptoms of Spinal Cord Tumors

Cervical tumors	
C4 and above	Sensory: Vertigo Motor: Quadiparesis, atrophy of sternocleidomastoid muscles; dysphagia; dysarthria; tongue deviation; respiratory insufficiency and/or failure Other: Occipital headaches; nuchal rigidity; down-beat nystagmus; papilledema
C4 and below	Sensory: Paresthesia; Horner's syndrome (ipsilateral pupillary constriction, ptosis, and anhidrosis) Motor: Weakness, muscle fasciculation; muscle atrophy Other: Shoulder and arm pain
Thoracic tumors	Sensory: Hyperesthesia band immediately above level of lesion Motor: Spastic paresis of lower extremities; positive Babinski's sign; lower motor neuron deficits Other: Sphincter impairment
Lumbar tumors	Sensory: Localized loss in legs and saddle area Motor: Foot drop; diminished or absent patellar and Achilles reflexes Other: Severe low back pain with radiation down legs; perianal and bladder discomfort; decreased libido; impotence; bladder disturbances

- Illuminate room adequately *to enhance visibility.*
- Place objects within site and reach *to facilitate self-care.*
- Provide frequent patient contact *to monitor needs.*
- Encourage expression of feelings, listen attentively, and offer feedback *to lower anxiety.*
- Reduce demands placed on patient *to avoid added stress.*
- Observe for irritability or unusual behavior as evidence of difficulty with coping.

NIC Activity and Exercise Management

Risk for injury related to increased intracranial/cord pressure and subsequent effects on balance, gait

- Maintain complete bed rest *to avoid falls.*
- Provide quiet *to reduce stimulation.*
- Lower bed height *to avoid injury if patient leaves bed.*
- Subdue room lighting *to reduce stimulation.*
- Elevate patient's head, and change position slowly *to avoid increased intracranial pressure.*
- Discourage oral stimulants *to avoid increased intracranial pressure.*
- Refrain from jarring bed and performing nonessential procedures *to keep patient calm.*
- Place padded side rails up; place airway or padded tongue blade on bed for use in case of seizure *to avoid injury.*
- Inspect eyes for pupillary response, and observe for papilledema as evidence of increasing intracranial pressure.
- Observe for confusion, lethargy, restlessness, vomiting, and complaints of headache and nausea as signs of increasing pressure.
- Palpate pulse rate and rhythm, and monitor volume *to determine adequacy of cardiovascular function.*

NIC Elimination Management

Impaired urinary elimination related to urinary sphincter disturbances

Risk for constipation related to disruption of innervation to bowel

- Measure postresidual voids *to determine need for more frequent catheterization.*
- Encourage fluid intake with even distribution throughout the day, and decrease patient's fluid intake at night *to maintain renal function and prevent infection.*
- Discourage intake of caffeinated beverages *to avoid bladder irritation.*
- Encourage fluids *to facilitate formation of soft stool.*
- Encourage a diet high in fiber and roughage *to maintain soft stool.*
- Administer stool softeners as prescribed *to facilitate elimination.*
- Stimulate rectal sphincter with digital stimulation and/or suppository *to initiate reflex peristalsis and evacuation.*

Patient Education/Continuum of Care Plan

1. Explain ways of adjusting to potential visual changes.
2. Emphasize the need to avoid injury.
3. Emphasize need to maintain adequate fluid and fiber in the diet.
4. Refer patient and family to appropriate community resources.

Evaluation/Patient Outcomes

Neurologic Management: Patient compensates for altered visual perception. Patient has environment arranged to facilitate mobility, self-care, and safety.

Activity and Exercise Management: Patient compensates for alterations in balance and gait. Patient rests quietly in bed as necessary. Patient's vital signs and neurologic status remain stable.

Elimination Management: Patient demonstrates normal urinary elimination. Intake and output are stable. Bladder is nondistended. Postvoid residual catheterization is less than 100 ml. Patient demonstrates normal bowel elimination. Bowel evacuation pattern is regular. No evidence of constipation or fecal impaction is present.

CANCERS OF THE SKIN

Basal Cell and Squamous Cell Carcinoma

Basal cell carcinoma is a malignant, epithelial cell tumor that begins as a papule and enlarges peripherally. Squamous cell carcinoma is a slow-growing malignant tumor of squamous epithelium.

Skin cancer is the most common human malignancy. An estimated 1.3 million cases are discovered each year. The vast majority are the highly curable basal cell and squamous cell carcinomas. Malignant melanoma, the most serious skin cancer, is diagnosed in about 51,400 persons annually, with the incidence increasing at the rate of 4% per year.[1] The reason for the increasing incidence of all skin cancers is believed to be a widespread change in lifestyle, with greater exposure of successive generations to sunlight, specifically ultraviolet radiation (see box on p. 1216).

Other less common but clinically significant skin cancers include Bowen's disease (squamous cell carcinoma in situ), Kaposi's sarcoma, lymphangiosarcoma, dermatofibrosarcoma protuberans, leiomyosarcoma, and mycosis fungoides.

Pathophysiology

Basal cell and squamous cell cancers are more common among persons with lightly pigmented skin and those living at latitudes near the equator. Basal cell carcinoma is slightly more common in men than in women, and its incidence is higher in persons over age 40 years. Now it is being seen in a younger population, perhaps because people are spending more time in the sun.[1] Squamous cell carcinoma is also more common in men, with the average age of onset at 60 years. Additional risk factors are excessive exposure to the sun and occupational exposure to

FACTS ABOUT CANCERS OF THE SKIN

Incidence: Over 1.3 million cases per year of basal cell or squamous cell cancer. Both of these cancers are highly curable. An estimated 51,400 new cases of melanoma, a more virulent skin cancer, will be diagnosed in 2001, and its incidence has been increasing about 4% per year since 1973. Whites are 10 times more likely to develop skin cancer.

Mortality: Of the 9800 estimated deaths, 7800 will be attributed to malignant melanoma.

Warning signs: A change in size or color of a mole, bump, or nodule or other darkly pigmented growth or spot. A bump or nodule that scales, oozes, or bleeds. A change in sensation, itchiness, tenderness, or pain.

Risk factors: Fair complexion (blonde hair, blue eyes) and overexposure to ultraviolet radiation, occupational exposure to coal tar, pitch, creosote, arsenic compounds, or radium. This is considered a highly preventable disease by avoiding the sun's ultraviolet rays between 10 AM and 3 PM. In addition, protective clothing should be worn and sunscreens should be used.

Early detection: Monthly skin self-examination for all adults is recommended, and suspicious lesions should be promptly evaluated.

Treatment: Surgery is used in 90% of early skin cancers. Other therapies for basal and squamous cell skin cancers are radiation therapy, electrodesiccation, and cryosurgery. Surgery, including lymph node removal, is often the treatment for malignant melanoma.

Data from American Cancer Society[1] and National Cancer Institute.[14a]

coal, tar, pitch, creosote, arsenic compounds, and radium. Black persons, because of their heavy skin pigmentation, are at low risk for developing these skin cancers.

Basal cell carcinoma often presents as a single, small, firm, dome-shaped, flesh-colored nodule with raised edges and pearly white borders. Small, red, focal lesions (telangiectatic vessels) are often prominent and seen through the thin epidermis. The lesion may resemble a pimple that has failed to heal, with an ulcerated and bleeding center. The most common form, noduloulcerative cancer, occurs frequently on the face, especially the cheeks, forehead, eyelids, and nasolabial folds. Invasion is usually local, although metastatic disease may occur rarely. Untreated, the tumor will invade such vital structures as blood vessels, lymph nodes, nerve sheaths, cartilage, bone, lungs, and the dura mater. The histologic appearance of the tumor is that of small undifferentiated basal cells with minimum nuclear atypia. Recurrence indicates initial incomplete tumor destruction; however, 90% to 95% of patients are considered cured after surgery or radiation therapy.

Squamous cell carcinoma is a scaly, slightly elevated lesion with or without a cutaneous horn. This tumor occurs frequently on the hands and forearms, as well as on the head and neck region, especially the ears, lower lip, scalp, and upper face. It is found most often in sun-damaged skin previously affected by actinic keratoses. These are erythematous, scaly lesions found especially on the face, shoulders, and dorsa of the hands. With complete tumor destruction the prognosis is excellent. Tumors more difficult to treat are those arising in an old, unstable thermal burn scar (Marjolin's ulcer); a chronically ulcerated area at the site of a chronic sinus tract (such as that caused by osteomyelitis); or a site of prior radiation damage. Squamous cell carcinoma can metastasize, with 2% to 3% spreading to regional lymph nodes or the lung. Primary tumors of the lip metastasize at a rate greater than 10%. The cure rate for this cancer is 75% to 80% when treated with surgery or radiation therapy.

DIAGNOSTIC STUDIES AND FINDINGS

Physical examination: Careful inspection, particularly of lesions showing biologic activity, such as change in size, shape, or color; bleeding and ulceration seen in more advanced lesions

Incisional or total excisional biopsy: For histologic confirmation of malignancy

MULTIDISCIPLINARY PLAN

Surgery

Scalpel excision with wide margin of skin and subcutaneous tissue; may be supplemented with split-thickness graft, adjacent flaps, distant pedicles, or free graft

Chemosurgery (Moh's procedure)

Cryosurgery

Electrodesiccation and curettage

Lasers: The carbon dioxide laser

Medications

Antineoplastic agents: 5-FU, topical application to skin bid for several weeks

General Management

Radiotherapy by beam electron and superficial x-rays, especially for cancers around face

Lesions greater than 20 cm in diameter, those in such critical areas as the central third of the face, recurrent lesions, and lesions with histologic signs of sclerosis are associated with a poor prognosis. Treatment for cure at the time of initial therapy and frequent examination for at least 2 years are essential.

NURSING CARE

NURSING ASSESSMENT

Skin integrity: Raised, hard, red or red-gray, pearly lesion on forehead, eyelid, cheek, nose, preauricular fold, or lip; scaly, slightly elevated lesion with irregular border; ulceration

NIC SKIN/WOUND MANAGEMENT

Impaired skin integrity related to presence of tumor

- Bathe patient in warm water or apply warm, moist compress *to maintain cleanliness.*
- Clean skin with agents appropriate to therapy *to prevent infection.*
- Maintain dry skin *to avoid irritation and infection.*

- Use paper or transparent tape over dressings *to avoid irritation.*
- Observe lesions for change in shape, size, and color and bleeding.

Patient Education/Continuum of Care Plan

See Comprehensive Care Plan, p. 1237.

1. Explain the importance of having regular physical examinations and self-examination.
2. Explain about the need for careful protection of the skin with use of sunscreens, avoidance of excessive exposure to sun, and limited exposure to ionizing radiation.

Evaluation Patient Outcomes

Skin/Wound Management: Skin is healed. Skin integrity is maintained without infection or ulceration.

Malignant Melanoma

Malignant melanoma is a skin cancer composed of melanocytes.

Melanoma accounts for approximately 4% of skin cancer cases but causes 79% of skin cancer deaths. The American Cancer Society estimates about 51,400 new melanomas will be diagnosed in 2001. About 7800 people in the United States are expected to die of melanomas during 2001. This skin cancer is more common in whites and in persons over age 60 years. The incidence is higher in men than in women.[1] This cancer develops from melanocytes that migrate into the skin, eye, CNS, and mucous membranes during fetal development.[15]

The exact cause of malignant melanoma is unknown. A hereditary factor is involved in 6% to 7% of patients. Two important environmental factors are sun exposure and geographic latitude. Intense, intermittent exposure during childhood and adolescence increases the risk for melanoma in later life.[15] Other theories suggest ultraviolet light exposure or an autoimmunologic effect.[10]

Malignant melanoma is easily recognized in its early stages and should be suspected in any patient with a history of change in a preexisting nevus or with a new pigmented lesion that has irregularities such as the following:

Various shades of brown and black plus red, white, or blue and the half tones of pink or gray

Notching or indentation of the border and pigment streaming from the lesion's edge

Loss of skin markings or development of a nodule, especially with erosion or ulceration

Bleeding of mole or change in color, size, or thickness

Pathophysiology

The four distinct forms of malignant melanoma, in order of decreasing incidence, follow:

Superficial spreading melanoma (70%) occurs anywhere on the body surface. The average patient age is 50 years. The lesion has a haphazard combination of colors and irregular shapes.

Nodular melanoma (15%) also occurs anywhere on the body surface and has a wide age distribution. It may be small and usually is darkly pigmented. Invasion is usually into the dermis, with resultant lymph node metastasis.

Acral (extremity) lentiginous melanoma (10%) occurs on palms, soles, nail beds, and mucous membranes. It is usually flat to slightly raised with an irregular pigment pattern and border.

Lentigo malignant melanoma (5% to 10%) is a slowly evolving lesion occurring on exposed surfaces (especially face and hands) of elderly people. It usually undergoes many color changes.

Diagnostic Studies and Findings

Routine laboratory tests: CBC, lactate dehydrogenase, BUN, PTT, liver enzyme studies, urine analysis, serum creatinine, blood chemistries[10]

Chest x-ray[10]

Nuclear bone scan: If bone pain is present

Other essential studies such as CT or MRI: Guided by symptomatology[15]

Total excisional biopsy: Deep margin to include subcutaneous fat preferred; performed to determine presence, type, and stage of malignancy

Prognosis is poorer with increased depth of invasion, lymphatic and vascular invasion, high number of mitotic figures per high-power microscopic field, little or no lymphocytic infiltration at the tumor base, and ulceration. The overall prognosis is better in women.

Multidisciplinary Plan

Surgery

Wide, deep excision of primary lesion; regional lymph node dissection

Medications

Antineoplastic agents

Combination regimens

CVD: Cisplatin, vinblastine, dacarbazine

CVD + IL-21: Cisplatin, vinblastine, dacarbazine, interleukin-2, interferon-alpha

Dacarbazine, carmustine, cisplatin, tamoxifen

Single-agent regimens

Dacarbazine (DTIC), aldesleukin

Biologic response modifiers: Interferon-alpha, interleukin-2

Radiation Therapy

For palliation of metastases

NURSING CARE

Nursing Assessment

Skin integrity: Dark brown or black pigmentation; scaliness; oozing, ulceration, and bleeding of nevus; spread of pigment beyond normal border; change in sensation; itchiness; tenderness or pain; enlarged regional lymph nodes

ABCD RULE FOR EARLY DETECTION OF MELANOMA

ASYMMETRY

Most true moles tend to be symmetric. Melanomas tend to be asymmetric (one half does not match the other half).

BORDER

Most true moles have a clear-cut border. Melanomas tend to have a notched, scalloped, or indistinct border.

COLOR

True moles may be dark or light, but they usually are uniform in color. Early melanomas have an uneven or variegated color (may range from various hues of tan and brown to black, with red and white intermingled).

DIAMETER

Most melanomas, once they have A, B, and C characteristics, have a diameter greater than 6 mm. Moles tend to be smaller. A sudden or continued increase in the size of a mole should be reported.

PATIENT PROBLEMS/NURSING DIAGNOSES & INTERVENTIONS

NIC SKIN/WOUND MANAGEMENT

Impaired skin integrity related to presence of lesion

- Bathe patient in warm water or apply warm, moist compresses *to maintain cleanliness.*
- Apply sterile dressings with antibiotic ointments as prescribed *to prevent infection.*
- Observe lesion(s) for change in shape, size, color, and presence of bleeding *to detect progressive disease.*

PATIENT EDUCATION/CONTINUUM OF CARE PLAN

See Comprehensive Care Plan, p. 1237.

1. Emphasize the need for regular physical examinations and self-examination (see box above).
2. Inform the patient of the need for meticulous skin care and assessment and the importance of avoiding ultraviolet light.

EVALUATION/PATIENT OUTCOMES

Skin/Wound Management: Patient's skin is healed. Skin integrity is maintained.

ONCOLOGIC EMERGENCIES

Oncologic emergencies arise from the impact advanced cancer has on body functioning. As many as 20% of patients develop one or more of these emergency conditions in the course of their illness. Among the most serious but most treatable acute conditions that can occur are hypercalcemia, obstruction of the superior vena cava, spinal cord compression, and cardiac distress. Other oncologic emergencies include pleural effusions, sepsis, disseminated intravascular coagulation (DIC), syndrome of inappropriate antidiuretic hormone (SIADH), and tumor lysis syndrome.

Hypercalcemia

Hypercalcemia occurs when the bones release more calcium into the extracellular fluid than can be excreted in the urine (above the normal calcium level of 9 to 11 mg/dl). This occurs most frequently in patients with cancer of the breast, lung, prostate, or multiple myeloma.

The most common cause of hypercalcemia is thought to be tumors producing parathyroid hormone or a substance with the same physiologic effects. This causes increased resorption of calcium from bone, increased intestinal absorption of calcium, and reduced renal excretion. Bony metastasis from any malignant primary tumor is also a causative condition. Other causes are tumor production of vitamin D–like substances and osteoclast-activating factors, dehydration, and immobilization.

Excessive calcium can cause bradycardia, increased cardiac contractility, depression of the CNS and peripheral nervous system (mild lethargy that may progress to coma), fatigue, muscle weakness, anorexia, nausea and vomiting, confusion, or irritability. Interference with reabsorption of water from the distal tubules leads to nocturia, polyuria, dehydration, polydipsia, and pruritus.

Acute hypercalcemia is treated initially with intravenous saline solution. Furosemide may also be given intravenously to encourage diuresis. Careful recording of intake and output, monitoring of electrolyte levels, and frequent cardiopulmonary assessment are necessary. Pamidronate (Aredia) is given over 4 to 24 hours intravenously. This may be repeated every 2 to 3 weeks as needed. Other agents that may be employed include etidronate, calcitonin, biphosphates, plicamycin, and gallium nitrate (Ganite).

Steroid administration and restriction of dietary calcium are thought to be of little therapeutic value. Orally administered phosphates and calcitonin injections may be used. Use of vitamin D, thiazides, absorbable antacids, and estrogens should be avoided.

External Compression of the Superior Vena Cava

Compression of the superior vena cava can occur slowly or quickly, owing to pressure from an adjacent tumor mass or enlarging lymph node. Most patients with superior vena cava syndrome have bronchogenic cancer; other causes of this syndrome are lymphoma, breast cancer, and GI tract metastases.

Prompt diagnosis and treatment are needed to relieve the distressing symptoms, which are progressive shortness of breath, cough, distention of neck veins, and edema of the face and hands. Dilated veins may appear on the upper chest wall. The patient may complain of headache and visual disturbances.

The patient must be kept in the Fowler's position. Diuretics may be of some help. However, the obstruction must be relieved to prevent cerebral anoxia, hemorrhage, or strangulation. Radiation therapy is the treatment of choice for this. If the obstruction is not accessible, chemotherapeutic agents such as cyclophosphamide (Cytoxan) can produce good results.

Spinal Cord Compression

Compression of the spinal cord is extremely dangerous because of the possibility of a permanent neurologic deficit. The usual cause of compression is a tumor, such as lymphoma or cancer of the breast, lung, or prostate, that metastasizes to the bony vertebral body and grows into the epidural space.

Pain, localized in the spinal region or radicular, is almost always an early symptom. The pain may be constant and aggravated by movement or coughing. Relief is usually obtained with opioids in combination with nonsteroidal antiinflammatory drugs (NSAIDs) or with steroids. Bed rest is recommended, and transfer and position change should be done using multiple personnel.

A careful neurologic examination should be performed to check motor and sensory function and the autonomic nerve tracts. Imaging studies, MRIs, x-rays, or myelograms should be done immediately to localize the destruction and determine its extent. The prognosis appears to be related to the patient's ability to walk at the time of diagnosis; if he or she is unable to do so, motor function is not recoverable, even with emergency radiotherapy or laminectomy.

Severe or prolonged cord compression can lead to extremity paralysis and loss of sphincter control, which is manifest as difficulty starting urination or as bowel incontinence. A prompt and thorough nursing assessment of the patient's bowel, bladder, and sexual function and any recent changes noted by the patient can assist in assessing the severity of dysfunction and facilitate earlier treatment, thus saving function.

Treatment must be prompt. Corticosteroids, such as dexamethasone, in high doses reduce swelling and inflammation around the cord. Surgical decompression or radiotherapy may be required. Early diagnosis is important for recovery.

Cardiac Tamponade

Cardiac tamponade results from excessive amount and pressure of fluid on the pericardial sac, which is a response to metastasis or direct invasion by tumor. The normal diastolic filling is impaired, and stroke volume is reduced. If tamponade is untreated, circulatory collapse occurs.

Signs and symptoms depend on how quickly the fluid accumulates. Frequent signs of tamponade include rapid and weak pulse, distended neck veins during inspiration (Kussmaul breathing), pulsus paradoxus (inspiratory decrease in arterial blood pressure exceeding 10 mm Hg from baseline), ankle or sacral edema, pleural effusion, lethargy, and altered consciousness.

The diagnosis is confirmed with echocardiography and pericardiocentesis; the latter also provides immediate symptomatic relief. Palliative measures, such as surgical construction of a pericardial window, may also be taken; total pericardectomy is usually not practical. Newer techniques include catheter drainage of fluid and instillation of a sclerosing agent, such as tetracycline or bleomycin. Radiation therapy with an external beam is effective with sensitive tumors.

Pleural Effusion

See Chapter 4.

Sepsis

Sepsis is a serious condition exemplified by inadequate tissue perfusion that results from bacterial invasion of the circulatory system. The most common causative agents, gram-negative bacteria, release an endotoxin from their cell walls, which causes increased capillary permeability and leakage. This in turn causes stagnation of blood, lactic acidosis, a decrease in the circulating blood volume, and decreased cardiac output. Sepsis is the most common cause of death in neutropenic patients. Signs and symptoms of sepsis include fever, chills, restlessness, confusion, tachycardia, hypotension, decreased pulses, cool clammy skin, decreased urinary output, and bleeding from one or more sites, which may be caused by DIC.

The diagnosis is confirmed by positive blood culture findings, the presence of infiltrates on a chest roentgenogram, depressed or elevated white blood cell (WBC) levels, metabolic acidosis via arterial blood gas analysis, and a prolonged prothrombin time and partial thromboplastin time. Interventions include monitoring of vital signs, arterial blood gas values, and hemodynamic stability; performance of blood cultures as needed; administration of antibiotics; temperature reduction with such measures as antipyretics, ice packs, and a hypothermia blanket; and fluid volume replacement. Prompt and thorough assessment of the patient during the neutropenic phase with continued education of the patient and his or her family could assist in decreasing patient/family anxiety and facilitate prompt interventions should this crisis occur.

Disseminated Intravascular Coagulation (DIC)

DIC is an imbalance of normal coagulation always secondary to an underlying cause, such as the release of tissue thromboplastin from tumor cells (e.g., lung and prostate cancers); sepsis, infection; hemolytic transfusions; or hepatic failure. The pathophysiology is based on the uncontrollable triggering of the internal or external pathway of the clotting cascade, resulting in accelerated coagulation and the formation of excessive thrombin. As long as coagulation occurs, the fibrinolytic system is activated, so that clotting and bleeding continue at a life-threatening pace. Signs and symptoms of DIC include systemic bleeding, ranging from petechiae to hematuria to an acute GI hemorrhage; organ dysfunction (e.g., pulmonary emboli, thromboemboli in the extremities, renal failure); decreased blood pressure and pulse; cool, clammy skin; anemia; pallor; and shortness of breath. A diagnosis of DIC is confirmed by the presence of prolonged thrombin time, prothrombin time, and partial thromboplastin time; decreased platelets; decreased fibrinogen; and elevated fibrin split products. Appropriate interventions include such medical therapies as antibiotics, chemotherapy, heparin, and blood products. Heparin use remains controversial because of the lack of clinical trials and the potential of increasing the patient's bleeding risk. The nurse should continuously monitor sites and amount of bleeding and laboratory values, assess adequacy of tissue perfusion, and prevent or minimize bleeding.

Syndrome of Inappropriate Antidiuretic Hormone (SIADH)

Antidiuretic hormone, which is normally released from the posterior pituitary in response to increased plasma osmolarity or decreased plasma volume, may be abnormally produced or stimulated as a result of tumor secretion (e.g., small cell lung cancer, lymphoma, and pancreatic and prostate cancers); stimulation by such drugs as vincristine and cyclophosphamide; viral or bacterial pneumonia; or neurologic trauma. The results of this abnormal production or stimulation are excessive water retention and hyponatremia. Signs and symptoms of SIADH include confusion, irritability, weakness, lethargy, headache, hyporeflexia, nausea, vomiting, anorexia, diarrhea, and weight gain without edema. Diagnosis is confirmed by a serum sodium level of less than 130 mEq/L, serum osmolarity of less than 280 mOsm/kg H_2O, and a urine sodium level of more than 20 mEq/L. Medical interventions may include chemotherapy, antibiotics, hypertonic saline solution (3% to 5% sodium chloride), diuretics, demeclocycline, and discontinuation of the causative agent. The nurse should also maintain an accurate intake and output record, restrict fluids as necessary, monitor laboratory reports of fluid and electrolyte balance, and provide safety measures for weak and confused patients.

Tumor Lysis Syndrome

The metabolic imbalance tumor lysis syndrome is caused by the rapid release of such intracellular components as potassium, phosphorus, and uric acid. The patient's risk of developing tumor lysis syndrome increases with the presence of bulky tumors that have a high growth fraction. The syndrome usually begins 1 to 5 days after the initiation of chemotherapy for non-Hodgkin's lymphomas and leukemia. Signs and symptoms include oliguria, anuria, urine crystals, flank pain, hematuria, cardiac dysrhythmias, muscular cramps, tetany, and confusion. The diagnosis is confirmed by elevated serum BUN, creatinine, potassium, phosphorus, and uric acid levels and by decreased serum calcium levels. Medical orders may include administering allopurinol (IV or PO) and calcium supplements, giving intravenous fluids with sodium bicarbonate for 3 to 5 days after initiating chemotherapy, or earlier in patients at higher risk, while maintaining a urine pH greater than 7, and preparing the patient for peritoneal dialysis or hemodialysis if needed.

Metastatic Disease and Terminal Stage of the Disease

Metastases are the major cause of death from cancer. The likelihood of a person with cancer developing metastatic disease is increased by the presence of a primary tumor of extended duration; high mitotic rate; trauma, such as tumor biopsy; dead tumor cells; heat; radiation; and chemotherapeutic agents. A metastasis is a tumor that is distant from the primary tumor and occurs as a result of seeding throughout a body cavity, such as the peritoneal or thoracic cavity; mechanical transport via instruments or gloved hands; lymphatic spread; and hematogenous spread. The most common sites of metastases are as follows:

The lung, from such primary sites as the colorectum, breast, renal system, testes, and bones

The liver, from such primary sites as the lung, colorectum, breast, and renal system

The CNS, from such primary sites as the lung and breast

Bone, from such primary sites as the lung, breast, renal system, and prostate

NURSING CARE

Nursing Assessment

Respiratory function: Cough; hemoptysis; wheezing; fever; dyspnea; chest pain; hoarseness; enlargement of neck with venous distention; clubbing of fingers; chest expansion asymmetry; cyanosis; breath and voice sounds, rales, rhonchi

Metabolic function: Nonspecific abdominal complaints, such as increasing distention, right upper quadrant mass; weight loss; anorexia; nausea and vomiting; signs and symptoms of cirrhosis such as spider angioma and gynecomastia

Central nervous system function: Headaches; nausea and vomiting; disturbances in mental, motor, and/or sensory function; focal or generalized convulsive activity; visual field, speech, or auditory defects; vertigo; confusion; fatigue; dizziness; ataxia; nystagmus; depressed corneal reflex; facial paralysis (see Table 18-2)

Musculoskeletal function: Pain; disturbances in sensory and/or motor function; urinary urgency, difficulty initiating urination, retention, and overflow incontinence; contralateral loss of temperature and pain sensation; ipsilateral loss of motor function, touch, and position sense (see Table 18-3)

Communication: Difficulty with speech and hearing

Psychosocial status: expressions of fear regarding disease progression and prognosis; anxiety; depression; anger

The nurse should include in his or her ongoing assessment of a person with cancer an emphasis on early detection of signs and symptoms of metastatic disease. This requires a knowledge of usual sites of spread for specific cancers, as well as sensitivity to patient complaints, changes in laboratory values, and observable alterations in function that indicate metastatic spread.

The nurse should query the patient as to the presence of advance directives (see box below).

Nursing diagnoses and interventions appropriate to each of the common metastatic sites follow.

Patient Problems/Nursing Diagnoses & Interventions

NIC Tissue Perfusion Management

Ineffective tissue perfusion (cardiopulmonary and peripheral) related to pulmonary metastases

- Identify hoarseness *to detect involvement of recurrent laryngeal nerve.*
- Report signs and symptoms of pleural effusion; have access to chest drainage equipment *to detect involvement of*

ADVANCE DIRECTIVE

An advance directive is a legal document executed by a competent person, which designates durable power of attorney for health care decisions when the person is no longer competent. Laws govern specific procedures for each state.

- Determine if a living will or durable power of attorney exists and for what situations.
- Be aware that items such as CPR, intubation, use of medications, and heroic procedures may be included in the document, and therefore withheld from the patient.
- Generally supportive care, pain management, and nutritional support are not included in living wills and are to be provided.

viscera or parietal pleura. Thoracotomy may be needed to prevent or treat pneumothorax.
- Report fever and hemoptysis indicating pneumonitis or abscess formation in the lung to the physician.
- Administer medications as needed with analgesics *to relieve chest pain.*
- Provide oxygen therapy as needed *to relieve dyspnea.*
- Report enlargement of neck with venous distention indicative of compression or invasion of superior vena cava.
- Document and report clubbing of fingers indicative of hypertrophic pulmonary osteoarthropathy.
- Position patient comfortably with head elevated *to promote chest expansion.*
- Encourage coughing and deep breathing *to clear and maintain patent respiratory tract.*
- Administer vaporized air *to moisten secretions and oxygen to ensure adequate tissue perfusion.*
- Suction airway as needed *to relieve obstruction caused by secretions.*
- Encourage adequate rest *to decrease respiratory work load.*
- Remove constrictive clothing *to relieve pressure on chest.*
- Discourage smoking *to decrease respiratory distress.*
- Monitor blood studies *to determine adequate oxygenation.*
- Be alert for complaints of cyanosis, dyspnea, wheezing, confusion, and fatigue *to monitor increasing respiratory distress.*
- Monitor respiratory rate, rhythm, and pulse *to assess for adequacy of cardiopulmonary function.*

NIC Risk Management

Risk for injury related to CNS metastases
- Raise and pad side rails and tape padded tongue blade to head of bed *to protect patient during convulsion.*
- Maintain patient on bed rest *to avoid falls or other trauma.*
- Provide quiet environment with subdued lighting *to relax patient.*
- Remove furniture, rugs, and other barriers *to minimize environmental danger.*
- Inspect patient for abnormal body movements *to monitor seizure activity.*
- Observe for confusion, decreased pupillary response, and reduced level of consciousness *to detect increased intracranial pressure.*

NIC Immobility Management

Impaired physical mobility related to CNS or peripheral nervous system metastases
Activity intolerance related to generalized weakness
- Provide patient support when ambulating (e.g., walker, three-point cane) *to maintain mobility.*
- Provide range-of-motion exercises (active and/or passive) *to avoid muscle contractures.*
- Assess patient for altered gait and position sense *to determine need for further assistance.*
- Observe for signs of thrombophlebitis (i.e., calf pain, calf redness, Homans' sign, swelling, and warmth) *to detect and report to physician this common complication of immobility.*
- Use antiembolic stockings *to prevent venous stasis.*
- Reposition patient every 2 hours if on bed rest *to prevent skin breakdown.*
- Observe response to activity *to determine extent of tolerance.*
- Identify factors contributing to intolerance (e.g., stress, side effects of drugs) *to plan interventions to counteract their effect.*
- Assess patient's sleep patterns *to document a causative factor of weakness.*
- Plan rest periods between activities *to reduce fatigue by providing additional rest.*
- Perform activities for patient until he or she is able to perform them *to meet patient's need without causing fatigue.*

NIC Elimination Management

Impaired urinary elimination related to CNS or peripheral nervous system metastases
- Assess voiding pattern, palpate bladder, and monitor intake and output *to determine need for intermittent catheterization.*
- Devise intermittent catheterization schedule *to avoid incontinence.*
- Encourage fluid intake with even distribution during the day and decreased intake at night *to maintain renal function while avoiding nighttime incontinence.*
- Discourage use of caffeine beverages *to avoid their diuretic-like effect.*

NIC Communication Enhancement

Impaired verbal communication related to CNS metastases
- Listen carefully and speak clearly *to patient to enhance ability to communicate.*
- Provide paper and pencil, chalkboard, or erasable board *to provide alternate methods of communication.*

NIC Psychologic Comfort

See Comprehensive Care Plan, p. 1237.

Patient Education/Continuum of Care Plan

See Comprehensive Care Plan, p. 1237.

1. Teach patient and family to avoid stress, exposure to environmental pollution, and others' infections.
2. Plan for periods of activity, balanced with rest.
3. Alter environment as necessary to enhance patient safety.
4. Provide a varied, attractive, and balanced diet.
5. Explain alternative nonmedication pain management strategies, such as guided imagery, relaxation, and distraction.
6. Encourage patient to ambulate, using assistive devices as needed.

7. Enhance communication with active listening and assistive devices as needed.
8. Explain ways of adjusting to potential visual changes.
9. Emphasize the need to avoid injury.
10. Emphasize the need to maintain adequate fluid and fiber in the diet.
11. Refer patient and family to appropriate community resources.
12. Use bladder training strategies as needed to avoid incontinence.
13. Encourage continued expression of fears and use of problem-solving techniques to deal with patient's fears in a realistic manner.

Evaluation/Patient Outcomes

Tissue Perfusion Management: Patient maintains optimal cardiopulmonary and peripheral tissue perfusion. Skin, nails, lips, and earlobes are warm, moist, and of natural color. Respirations, pulse, blood pressure, and temperature are within normal limits.

Risk Management: Patient is free of injury. Patient does not complain of pain. Patient's facial expression and body are relaxed.

Immobility Management: Patient ambulates frequently. Patient uses assistive devices as needed.

Patient compensates for any altered visual perception. Patient has environment arranged to facilitate mobility, self-care, and safety. Patient compensates for alterations in balance and gait. Patient rests quietly in bed as necessary. Patient's vital signs and neurologic status remain stable.

Patient performs usual activities without fatigue or dyspnea. Patient performs self-care activities.

Elimination Management: Patient demonstrates normal urinary elimination. Intake and output are stable. Bladder is nondistended. Postvoid residual catheterization is less than 100 ml.

Patient demonstrates normal bowel elimination. Bowel evacuation pattern is regular. No evidence of constipation or fecal impaction is present.

Communication Enhancement: Patient is able to communicate. Patient speaks without difficulty or uses assistive devices effectively. Patient is able to hear those speaking to him or her.

Collaborative Interventions and Related Nursing Care

Blood Component Therapy

The goal of blood component therapy is to administer only the components needed by the patient. This minimizes transfusion reactions and increases the number of patients who can benefit from a single unit (Table 18-4).

The infusion of granulocytes as a blood replacement product is no longer the standard of care since the development of granulocyte colony stimulating factors (G-CSF). (See discussion of biologic response modifiers for more information regarding G-CSF.)

Platelets are usually given to patients with thrombocytopenia and bone marrow depression resulting from chemotherapy or radiation therapy. Platelet concentrates are obtained through platelet pheresis of a single donor or prepared from units of platelets collected from as many as four to 10 donors. Blood is removed from the donor into a machine with a centrifuge bowl, where platelets are separated, and red blood cells and plasma are then returned to the donor. The procedure takes 1½ to 2 hours. Pheresis donors may give as many as 12 units of platelets at a time. The platelets should be administered within 24 hours.

Anemia in the cancer patient may be treated by two methods: infusion of packed red blood cells (PRBCs) or, in the case of chronic anemia, epoetin alfa (Procrit), a red blood cell production stimulator taken subcutaneously or by intravenous bolus. The target hematocrit range of treatment is 36% to 40% and takes 2 to 8 weeks to achieve. Once the target range is obtained, a maintenance dose is then required.

Infusion of PRBCs is an immediate treatment for anemia-induced symptoms of fatigue, pallor, hypotension, headaches, and irritability. Patients are transfused based on review of their hemoglobin (less than 8.0 g/100 ml) and/or patient symptoms related to anemia. For review of transfusion procedures, see Chapter 17.

The nurse is an essential member of the team involved in this therapy; it is often the nurse who identifies the patient's need for blood components, recruits donors, obtains the blood components from the donors, and administers the therapy to the patient.

Chemotherapy

Description and Rationale

Chemotherapy is a relatively new cancer treatment modality; the first patient was treated with nitrogen mustard in 1942. The use of chemical agents is especially important in the treatment of systemic disease. Researchers continue to discover drugs that kill cancer cells without causing extensive damage to normal tissues. In addition, combinations of chemotherapeutic agents and the combination of chemotherapy with other treatment modalities have increased the cancer cure rate.

Chemotherapy is used to cure patients, prolong life, increase the disease-free interval, and palliate symptoms, thus improving the quality of life.

Chemotherapeutic agents are highly toxic, attacking all rapidly dividing cells, both normal and malignant. Thus the contraindications and cautions are a reflection of the patient's pretreatment condition, stage of disease, response to therapy, and allergies or sensitivities. The nurse involved in drug administration and monitoring of the patient's responses must have a comprehensive baseline assessment to use in evaluating the patient's condition and ability to tolerate the treatment.

The selection of chemotherapeutic agents used in a disease treatment plan is based on the following key items:

1. The drug selected is known to be effective in this disease.
2. When multiple drugs are used, they act synergistically.
3. The drugs used have different side effect profiles.

Table 18-4 Blood Component Therapy

Component	Indications	Special Considerations
PACKED RED BLOOD CELLS (PRBCs)		
	Hemoglobin is <8.0 g. Patient is symptomatic. Active bleeding occurs.	Type and cross-match procedure is necessary. Infuse over 2-4 hours. Monitor for transfusion reaction (fever, chills, urticaria).
Leukocyte-poor PRBCs: Leukocytes are removed during transfusion.	Patient has experienced febrile transfusion reactions. Patient is at risk for alloimmunization.	Infuse through a special filter (Pall).
Washed PRBCs: Blood is washed with 1000 ml normal saline solution and repacked before transfusion.	Patient has known severe allergic reaction to plasma and leukocytes.	Infuse at 20-30 gtt/min until completion of unit. Unit expires within 24 hours of washing.
PLATELET CONCENTRATES		
	Platelet count is <20,000. Active bleeding occurs. Platelets are given before minor procedures or surgery.	ABO compatibility is preferred but not necessary. 1-hour or 24-hour posttransfusion increments are monitored to determine effectiveness. Splenomegaly, DIC, fever, and sepsis may increase demand. Monitor for transfusion reactions. Prophylaxis is done with diphenhydramine, acetaminophen, and hydrocortisone.
Random-donor platelets (RDPs): Several units (6-10) harvested from whole blood are pooled into one bag.	Patient has had no prior transfusions. Patient has had no reactions or alloimmunization.	Units expires about 4 hours after pooling.
Leukocyte-poor RDPs: Leukocytes are removed before or during transfusion.	Patient is at risk for alloimmunization. Patient has experienced febrile transfusion reactions.	Unit is either centrifuged and leukocytes mechanically trapped (Leukotrap) or special filter (Pall) is used for infusion.
Single-donor platelets (SDPs): Platelets are collected by pheresis from one donor.	Patient is refractory to RDPs. Patient is at risk for alloimmunization.	Try to match ABO/Rh of patient. Usually transfuse with special filter (Pall). Unit expires within 24 hours of collection.
HLA-matched platelets: Platelets are collected by pheresis from a donor whose HLA typing closely matches patient's type.	Patient is refractory to RDPs and SDPs. Patient is at risk for alloimmunization.	Patient must have been HLA typed. Unit expires within 24 hours of collection.
Resuspended platelets: Plasma is removed from pooled units, and an equivalent amount of normal saline solution is added.	Patient has experienced severe reaction to platelet concentrates despite prophylaxis.	Prophylaxis is usually needed.
FRESH FROZEN PLASMA	Patient has had multiple PRBC transfusions. Abnormal coagulation factors are evident.	Provide ABO-compatible component. Transfuse immediately after thawing.
IRRADIATED COMPONENTS		
Gamma radiation delivered to blood components inactivates lymphocytes within product.	Severely immunocompromised patients are at risk for graft-versus-host disease.	Component is not radioactive. Component should be labeled as being irradiated. RBCs and platelets are not affected.

From Otto.[15]

These items refer to the mechanism of action of a drug. Chemotherapeutic agents can be cell-cycle phase specific or cell-cycle phase nonspecific. This specificity allows the medications to work either at a particular phase of the cell cycle, or the medication will work no matter what phase the cancer cell is currently in. This premise also allows for the cells to have a rest period in the schedule, allowing the normal cell to regenerate and repair normal tissue.[3]

The most commonly used chemotherapeutic agents and the common side effects are listed in Table 18-5. Many others are being developed and tested for possible therapeutic value.

Depending on the drug's pharmakokinetics, chemotherapy may be administered by a variety of routes: intravenous, oral, central venous catheter, venous access via an implantable access device, intraarterial, intraperitoneal, intrapleural, intrathecal, topically, or via ventricular reservoir. The intramuscular and subcutaneous routes are rarely used. In recent years, use of intraarterial and venous access lines (see Table 18-6) has become important because of the ease of access to the arterial or venous system for drug delivery, increased patient comfort, and the addition of external or internal pump systems for more continuous infusion of drugs.

CLINICAL TRIALS

A clinical trial is a research study conducted in humans and designed to answer specific scientific questions using scientifically controlled methods.

Of the 1,250,000 newly diagnosed cancer patients in the United States each year, fewer than 50,000 patients participate in federally sponsored therapeutic clinical studies.

Clinical trials study a variety of items, including chemotherapeutic agents, biologic agents, monoclonal antibodies, vaccine development, surgical interventions, radiation therapy, mechanical devices, or psychometric tools.

Clinical trials are defined as "phases."

A phase I clinical trial is the first time an agent has been used in a human being. The purpose of the study is to determine the toxicities of the agent and to determine the maximum tolerated dose of that agent.

A phase II trial is to determine the effectiveness of an agent in one or more types of cancer. The trial is designed to employ the dose, schedule, and route of administration that has been determined in the phase I study. The primary goal is to detect any antitumor effect.

A phase III trial is to compare an agent with other therapies to demonstrate if the agent or other therapy is more effective than standard therapy. The results are used to make recommendations for general use and Food and Drug Administration (FDA) approval. A phase III trial is only necessary if a dramatic effect is not seen in a phase II trial.

Therapeutic trials usually involve patients with refractory, incurable cancer, since there is no assurance of direct personal benefit.

To assure patients' safety, each clinical trial has an action plan (protocol) that explains how it will work. These plans are first reviewed and approved by the internal review board (IRB) at the institution(s) that are administering the trial.

Potential benefits to patients include high-quality cancer care and the opportunity to help others and improve cancer treatment.

Possible disadvantages include the possibility that the experimental treatment may not improve the patient's status or may not work for a particular person. Costs may also impact the patient, as not all insurance companies will cover experimental treatment costs. All potential side effects, benefits, costs, and risks must be fully explained to any potential patients and provided to the patient in writing, known as "informed consent."

Clinical trials are an excellent opportunity for the oncology nurse. The nurse can review the pros and cons of clinical trials with the patient and family and also assist the patient with enrollment. Calls from nurses requesting information are encouraged and welcomed.

For more information on clinical trials, nurses, physicians, and patients may call 1-800-4-CANCER or access the National Cancer Institute's websites:
http://www.nci.nih.gov
http://cancertrials.nci.nih.gov
http://cancernet.nci.nih.gov

Table 18-5 Toxic Side Effects of Chemotherapy

Chemotherapeutic Agent	Myelosuppression	Mucositis	Nausea and Vomiting	Alopecia	Vesicant (V)/ Irritant (I)	Allergic Reaction	Other Specific Toxicities
Aminoglutethimide (Cytadren)	+	−	+	−	−	−	Skin rash; sensory alterations, including lethargy, visual blurring, vertigo, ataxia, and nystagmus; hyponatremia, hyperkalemia, cortisol insufficiency
Actinomycin D (Cosmegan)	+	+	+	+	+ (V)	0	Diarrhea
Amsacrine (M-AMSA)	+	0	+	0	+ (V)	0	Flulike syndrome, venoocclusive disease, hepatotoxicity
5-Azacytidine	+	+	+	0	0	0	Hepatotoxicity
Busulfan (Myleran)	+	0	±	0	0	0	Pulmonary fibrosis
Bleomycin (Blenoxane)	±	+	±	+	0	+	Pulmonary toxicity, skin rash
Camptothecin-11 (CPT-11)	+	−	+	+	−	−	Diarrhea, pulmonary toxicity
Carboplatin (Paraplatin)	+	0	+	0	0	0	Pigmentation at injection site, hepatotoxicity, neurotoxicity, renal toxicity, pulmonary toxicity
Cannustine (BCNU)	+	+	+	0	+ (I)	0	Hepatotoxicity
Chlorambucil (Leukeran)	+	0	±	0	0	0	
Chlorodeoxyadenosine	+	0	0	0	0	0	Neurotoxicity, renal toxicity
Cisplatin (Platinol)	+	0	+	0	0	+	Nephrotoxicity, peripheral neuropathy, ototoxicity

From Bender, Yasko, and Strohl.[3]

+, Common; ±, infrequent; 0, uncommon; −, no effect.

Chemotherapeutic Agent	Myelosuppression	Mucositis	Nausea and Vomiting	Alopecia	Vesicant (V)/ Irritant (I)	Allergic Reaction	Other Specific Toxicities
Cladribine (Leustatin)	+	–	+	–	–	–	Fever, rash, diarrhea, constipation, cough, shortness of breath, tachycardia, edema
Cortisone	+	–	–	–	–	–	Gastric irritation, hyperglycemia, sodium and water retention, hypokalemia, hypocalcemia, behavioral changes
Cyclophosphamide (Cytoxan)	+	0	+	+	0	0	Sterile hemorrhagic cystitis, heart failure
Cytarabine (Cytosar, Ara-C)	+	+	+	+	0	0	Hepatotoxicity
Dacarbazine (DTIC) (Daunomycin)	+	0	+	0	+ (I)	+	Hypotension
Diethylstilbestrol (DES)	0	0	+	0	0	0	Congestive heart failure
Doxorubicin (Adriamycin)	+	+	+	+	+ (V)	0	Cardiotoxicity, diarrhea
Estramustine (Emcyt)	+	–	+	–	+ (V)	0	Diarrhea, hepatotoxicity, hypocalcemia, hypophosphatemia, gynecomastia, congestive heart failure, thrombophlebitis, rash
Etoposide (VePesid)	+	0	+	+	+ (I)	±	Hepatotoxicity, neurotoxicity, hypotension
Floxuridine (FUDR)	+	+	+	+	0	0	Diarrhea, rash
Fludarabine (Fludara)	+	+	+	–	–	–	Pulmonary toxicity, pericardial effusion, neurotoxicity
5-Fluorouracil (5-FU)	+	+	±	±	0	0	Diarrhea, photosensitivity
Fluoxymesterone (Halotestin)	0	0	+	0	0	0	Masculinization
Gemcitabine (Gemzar)	+	–	+	–	–	–	Flulike symptoms
Hexamethylmelamine	+	0	+	±	0	0	Peripheral neuropathy
Hydroxyurea (Hydrea)	+	+	+	+	0	0	
Idarubicin (Idamycin)	+	+	+	+	0	0	Cardiomyopathy
Ifosfamide (Ifex)	±	0	±	+	0	0	Hematuria, neurotoxicity, hemorrhagic cystitis
L-Asparaginase (Elspar)	0	0	+	0	0	+	Major organ failure
Lomustine (CCNU)	+	+	+	±	0	0	Hepatotoxicity
Megestrol acetate Megace)	0	0	0	+	0	0	Fluid retention
Mechlorethamine (nitrogen mustard)	+	0	+	+	+ (V)	0	
Melphalan (Alkeran)	+	±	±	+	0	0	Rare pulmonary toxicity, secondary malignancy
6-Mercaptopurine (6-MP)	+	+	+	0	0	0	Hepatotoxicity
Methotrexate (MTX, Amethopterin)	+	+	±	±	0	0	Nephrotoxicity
Mithramycin (Mithracin)	+	+	+	0	+ (V)	0	Hemorrhagic tendency
Mitomycin (Mutamycin)	+	+	+	+	+ (V)	0	Nephrotoxicity, pulmonary toxicity
Mitotane (Lysodren)	–	–	+	–	–	–	Diarrhea, neurotoxicity, skin irritation or rash
Mitoxantrone (Novantrone)	+	+	+	+	0	0	Drug fever, diarrhea, increased liver enzymes
Oxaliplatin	+	–	+	–	–	–	Peripheral neuropathy
Oxymethalone (Anadrol-50)	0	0	+	0	0	0	Hepatotoxicity
Paclitaxel (Taxol)	+	0	+	±	0	±	Sensory neuropathy

Continued

Table 18-5 Toxic Side Effects of Chemotherapy—cont'd

Chemotherapeutic Agent	Myelosuppression	Mucositis	Nausea and Vomiting	Alopecia	Vesicant (V)/ Irritant (I)	Allergic Reaction	Other Specific Toxicities
Pentostatin (Nipent)	+	–	+	+	+ (V)	–	Nephrotoxicity, hepatotoxicity, mental status changes, pulmonary toxicity, severe conjunctivitis
Prednisolone	0	0	0	0	0	0	Steroid side effects
Prednisone	0	0	0	0	0	0	Steroid side effects
Procarbazine (Matulane)	+	±	+	0	0	0	Monoamine oxidase inhibitor
Semustine (Methyl CCNU)	+	+	+	0	0	0	
Streptozocin (Zanosar)	+	0	+	±	+ (I)	0	Nephrotoxicity
Tamoxifen (Nolvadex)	±	0	+	0	0	0	
Taxotere (Docetaxel)	+	–	–	+	–	+	Rash, fluid and electrolyte imbalance, peripheral edema, pleural effusion
Teniposide (Vumon)	+	–	+	+	+ (I)	+	Hypotension, hepatoxicity, cardiac arrhythmias, peripheral neuropathy
6-Thioguanine (6-TG)	+	+	+	0	0	0	Hepatotoxicity
Thiotepa	+	–	+	–	–	+	Sexual dysfunction, secondary malignancies, dizziness, headache, fever
Uracil mustard	+	0	+	±	0	0	
Vinblastine (Velban)	+	+	+	±	+ (V)	0	Neurotoxicity
Vincristine (Oncovin)	0	0	0	+	+ (V)	0	Neurotoxicity
Vindesine (Eldisine)	+	±	+	+	+ (V)	–	Peripheral neuropathy, constipation, rash, diarrhea
Vinorelbine (Navelbine)	+	+	+	+	+ (V)	–	Neurotoxicity, diarrhea, hepatotoxicity, injection site reaction, sexual/reproductive dysfunction

From Bender, Yasko, and Strohl.[3]
+, Common; ±, infrequent; 0, uncommon; –, no effect.

Table 18-6 Venous Access Devices

CVC Type	Site(s)	Uses	Special Considerations
Nontunneled peripheral	Basilic, cephalic, or medial cubital veins	Medications, blood products; may be able to draw blood depending on catheter size	Need to verify blood return for vesicant drugs, requires q8h flushing
Central line	Subclavian, femoral, internal jugular veins	Blood drawing, medication or blood infusion, hemodynamic monitoring	Temporary catheter
PICC lines	Basilic, cephalic, or medial cubital veins	Medications, PPN, blood products, blood sampling	Requires special training of RN for insertion
Tunneled	Subclavian, internal or external jugular, cephalic or femoral veins	Long-term IV access	Dacron cuff allows fixation at exit site and promotes security of catheter
Implanted port (single or double)	Subclavian, internal or external jugular, cephalic veins (access may be in chest, antecubital or under rib cage)	Ports may be used as IVs or for fluid sampling (ascites) or direct chemoinfusion into tumor site	Patients enjoy freedom to swim, bathe, etc. once port is deaccessed; flush monthly and prn
Groshong*	Subclavian, internal or external jugular, cephalic or femoral veins	Long-term IV access	Requires weekly flushing; has two-way valve—does not require clamping
Pheresis	Subclavian, internal or external vein, femoral or jugular vein	Apheresis/hemodialysis	Large-bore catheter, precautions needed to prevent bleeding; temporary catheter

Data from Camp-Sorrell.[5]
*Bard Access Systems, Salt Lake City, UT.

Venous Access Devices

Table 18-6 is a summery of the most common venous access devices (VADs) used in the cancer patient population. Please refer to your institution policy and procedure manual for directives on flushing and site care.

NURSING CARE

NURSING ASSESSMENT

Gastrointestinal function: Nausea and vomiting; diarrhea; constipation; stomatitis; esophagitis; anorexia; intake and output

Dermatologic status: Alopecia; dermatitis; changes in skin color; extravasation; hyperpigmentation of nail beds; rash; jaundice; pruritus

Hematologic function: Fatigue and dyspnea (anemia); petechiae; ecchymoses; frank bleeding (thrombocytopenia); fever; chills; hypotension (leukopenia); dehydration

Reproductive function: Sterility; amenorrhea; decreased libido

Renal function: Edema; blood studies related to renal function, e.g., BUN, serum creatinine, creatinine clearance, electrolytes

Urinary function: Hemorrhagic cystitis, as evidenced by hematuria, burning during urination, backache; nephrotoxicity, as evidenced by renal failure (decrease or absence of urinary output)

Neurologic function: Ototoxicity (vertigo, tinnitus, loss of hearing); peripheral neuropathies, as evidenced by muscle weakness; numbness and tingling; jaw pain; absence of deep tendon reflexes

Musculoskeletal function: Myalgia; muscle weakness; osteoporosis; gout

Respiratory function: Pulmonary fibrosis, as evidenced by dyspnea, chest pain, or cyanosis

Cardiac function: Congestive heart failure, as evidenced by exertional dyspnea, cough, rales, electrocardiogram changes

Psychosocial status: Fear; depression; anger; anxiety

PATIENT PROBLEMS/NURSING DIAGNOSES & INTERVENTIONS

NIC ELIMINATION MANAGEMENT

Constipation related to impaired intestinal motility
Diarrhea related to intestinal irritation
Impaired urinary elimination related to drug-induced nephrotoxicity

- Offer fluids and foods high in fiber and bulk *to stimulate motility.*
- Offer stool softener or laxatives *to stimulate motility.*
- Avoid enemas because they may traumatize the intestinal mucosa.
- Offer clear liquids *to prevent dehydration.*
- Offer antidiarrheal agent, such as Kaopectate or diphenoxylate (Lomotil), per physician's order *to control diarrhea.*
- Maintain good perineal care *to avoid irritation and discomfort.*
- Test stools for occult blood *to identify evidence of blood.*
- Record number and consistency of stools *to monitor need for further intervention.*
- Force fluids *to maintain renal blood flow.*
- Administer diuretics as ordered *to enhance renal excretion.*
- Encourage foods high in potassium *to prevent diuretic-related hypokalemia.*
- Administer normal saline solution and mannitol before cisplatin therapy per physician's order *to maintain fluid and electrolyte balance.*
- Administer allopurinol as prescribed with high fluid intake *to prevent uric acid accumulation in kidneys.*
- Encourage patient to empty bladder frequently, especially at night, *to avoid stasis, inflammation, and infection.*
- Provide adequate hydration to maintain renal function.

NIC SKIN/WOUND MANAGEMENT

Impaired oral mucous membrane related to poor oral hygiene, preexisting dental disorders, or drug-induced irritation
Impaired skin integrity related to drug-induced changes, extravasation

- Encourage good oral hygiene *to promote comfort and prevent infection.*
- Discourage spicy or hot foods *to avoid irritation or pain.*
- Offer topical agents *for relief of pain (lidocaine or dyclonine)* per physician's order *to soothe irritated membranes.*
- Apply K-Y jelly to lips *to maintain moisture.*
- Offer popsicles *for hydration and comfort.*
- Use oral assessment guide *to monitor changes in voice, ability to swallow, and condition of lips, tongue, mucous membranes, gingiva, teeth, and saliva to evaluate response to interventions.*
- Discourage alcohol, tobacco, difficult-to-chew foods, and highly acidic beverages *to avoid irritation of mucous membranes.*
- Administer nystatin oral suspension or suppository or clotrimazole (Mycelex) troche per physician's order *to combat infection.*
- Have patient postpone dental work if possible, brush teeth gently, and use toothettes *to avoid further trauma.*

For alopecia

- Help patient plan for wig, scarf, or hat before hair loss *to maintain self-esteem.*
- Offer tourniquet or ice cap preventive therapy based on policy and diagnosis *to decrease hair loss.*
- Have patient wash and comb remaining hair gently *to decrease hair loss.*
- Reassure patient that hair will grow back after therapy *to lessen patient anxiety and worry.*

For dermatitis

- Use cornstarch, Alpha Keri, calamine lotion, or other agent *to relieve itching.*
- Warn against overexposure to sun *to avoid further irritation.*
- Keep skin clean and dry *to avoid infection.*

For changes in color of skin or nail beds

- Assure patient that discoloration will fade with time *to lessen patient anxiety and worry.*

- Use nail polish according to patient's wishes *to mask discoloration.*

For jaundice

- Monitor hepatic enzymes *to determine liver function.*
- Assess skin and sclera daily for evidence of increase or decrease in discoloration.

For extravasation

- Observe for early signs—pain or burning sensation at or above IV site (as reported by patient), blanching, redness, swelling, slowing of infusion, and absence of blood return—*to detect problem before tissue damage occurs.*
- Stop infusion, aspirate remaining drug from needle, inject antidote, apply topical ointment, heat, or cold as dictated by protocol *to prevent tissue damage.*

NIC Respiratory Management

Impaired gas exchange related to anemia, pulmonary fibrosis, cardiotoxicity

- Have patient change position slowly *to conserve energy.*
- Encourage adequate rest *to conserve energy.*
- Observe patient for dyspnea and increased weakness as evidence of further dysfunction.
- Administer oxygen therapy as needed *to increase oxygenation of tissues.*
- Monitor hemoglobin and hematocrit *to determine effect of therapy.*
- Administer transfusions as ordered *to increase red blood cell count.*
- Monitor respiratory function with pulmonary function test *to detect changes in status.*
- Note limitation of lifetime dosage of bleomycin *to prevent irreversible toxicity.*
- Assist with pulmonary function studies *to detect changes in status.*
- Observe for dyspnea; report to physician as ordered for further interventions.
- Monitor heart rate, blood pressure, and ECG *to detect cardiac dysfunction.*
- Limit cumulative dosage of doxorubicin *to prevent irreversible toxicity.*

NIC Risk Management

Risk for infection related to leukopenia/bone marrow suppression

Ineffective peripheral tissue perfusion related to bleeding

- Warn patient to avoid crowds and people with cold, flu, or cold sore *to prevent exposure to pathogens.*
- Use sterile technique whenever needed *to prevent infection.*
- Initiate reverse isolation as indicated *to protect patient from pathogens.*
- Monitor temperature and leukocyte count; observe skin temperature, color, and odor *to detect signs of infection.*
- Encourage careful hygiene *to prevent infection.*
- Discourage fresh-cut flowers, which may carry microorganisms.
- Avoid using indwelling catheters or performing rectal procedures or examination *to prevent infection.*
- Administer antibiotics as prescribed *to treat infection.*
- Protect patient from injury (e.g., use precautions when shaving with razor blade, do not permit cluttered environment, and do not administer rectal suppositories) *to avoid trauma.*
- Have patient avoid using aspirin and aspirin products, *which increase clotting time.*
- Avoid giving injections; if they are necessary, apply pressure at site for 3 to 5 minutes afterward *to prevent bleeding.*
- Use toothettes for oral care *to avoid trauma to mucosa.*
- Monitor petechiae, ecchymoses, and stools for blood.
- Evaluate neurologic status *to identify intracranial bleeding.*
- Have nasal packing available should bleeding occur.
- Administer platelet transfusions as necessary *to control bleeding.*
- Monitor vital signs *to detect bleeding early.*
- Support patient in ambulation *to prevent injury related to weakness.*

NIC Coping Assistance

Sexual dysfunction related to drug-induced changes in hormonal status

Ineffective coping related to stress of dealing with treatment

- Help patient explore alternatives for sterility, such as sperm banking, hormonal therapy during treatment, and postponement of conception and childbearing, *to be proactive in dealing with changes in sexuality.*
- Refer to sexual counselor as needed *to deal with dysfunction.*
- Assess coping behavior; determine its effectiveness for patient *to determine need for new strategies.*
- Reassure patient that mood changes are temporary and dose related *to reduce anxiety.*
- Allow independence in self-care *to maintain patient self-esteem and promote effective coping.*
- Maintain supportive, nonjudgmental attitude *to foster patient coping.*
- Encourage use of resources, such as support groups, *to assist patient in coping.*

NIC Neurologic Management

Disturbed sensory perception (auditory) related to drug-induced neurotoxicity

- Monitor hearing with baseline and periodic audiograms *to detect early hearing loss.*
- Speak clearly and in normal tone of voice *to enhance hearing.*
- Assess patient for numbness and tingling in extremities *to detect paresthesias.*
- Prohibit smoking and have patient observe placement of feet and hands *to promote safety.*

NIC Immobility Management

Impaired physical mobility related to drug-induced gout, osteoporosis, myelotoxicity

- Monitor calcium level *to determine bone status.*

- Provide safety measures *to prevent injury.*
- Be alert for complaint of pain over bony area; if patient has such a complaint, maintain bed rest until roentgenograms are taken for fracture to detect injury.
- Use assistive devices for ambulation *to enhance tolerance of activity.*
- Encourage range-of-motion exercise *to maintain mobility.*
- Position patient in proper anatomic alignment *to avoid stretching, pressure, or fracture.*

Patient Education/Continuum of Care Plan

See Comprehensive Care Plan, p. 1237.

1. Encourage maintenance of adequate nutrition and hydration.
2. Emphasize the need for self-regulation of medication to control nausea, vomiting, constipation, diarrhea, itching, urinary distress, and oral irritation.
3. Discuss the warning signs of bleeding and infection that the patient should report to a physician.
4. Discuss the need for thorough personal hygiene and oral care.

Evaluation/Patient Outcomes

Elimination Management: Bowel elimination is normal. Patient experiences no constipation, diarrhea, or distention. Urinary elimination is normal. Patient expresses no complaints of urinary distress. Intake and output are balanced.

Skin/Wound Management: Oral mucous membranes are healthy. Mucous membranes, lips, tongue, and gingiva are of normal color and moisture. Patient has clean teeth, moist saliva, ability to swallow, and a normal voice.

Skin is healthy and intact. Patient expresses no complaints of itching. There is no evidence of rash or changes in pigmentation. Patient's hair is healthy.

Respiratory Management: Gas exchange and peripheral tissue perfusion are adequate Patient expresses no complaints of fatigue or weakness. Patient has warm, pink skin and normal respirations, pulse, and blood pressure. There are no signs or symptoms of bleeding or cardiac dysfunction. The ECG findings are normal.

Risk Management: Infection is absent. Patient has normal temperature, normal WBC count, and cool, dry skin.

Coping Assistance: Sexual function is normal. Patient has satisfactory libido and has made plans for dealing with possible sterility. Patient is able to cope with stress of therapy. Patient discusses fears, anger, and sadness. Patient has made progress in problem solving.

Neurologic Management: Hearing and sense of touch are normal. Patient is able to hear speaker and is aware of body sensations.

Immobility Management: Physical mobility is normal. Patient is able to ambulate without assistance.

Biologic Therapy

Description and Rationale

Biologic therapy is now considered the fourth cancer treatment therapy and can be used either alone or in combination with chemotherapy, surgery, or radiation. Biologic therapy and biologic response modifier (BRM) therapy are agents that change the response of the host to the tumor cells.

The rationale for the use of BRMs in cancer care is based on animal studies and clinical observations such as the following:

- Postoperative patients are often found to have malignant cells in circulating blood and in operative wound washings but may never receive a diagnosis of cancer.
- Among transplant patients who receive immunosuppressant therapy, cancer occurs at a rate at least 80 times that of the general population.
- Rapidly progressive recurrent cancer sometimes appears 10 to 20 years after cure.
- Patients with congenital or acquired immunologic deficiencies have a greater incidence of cancer than does the general population.

The types of immunotherapy are classified as active and passive.

Active therapy involves administration of an antigen to stimulate the patient's immune system, with subsequent development of immunity (antibody). The response may be *specific* or *nonspecific.* Specific active immunotherapy stimulates an immune response to a tumor-associated antigen. Nonspecific immunotherapy stimulates the immune response to a wide variety of antigens, including tumor-associated antigens.

Passive immunotherapy involves the direct transfer of transient immunity from person to person and may also be specific or nonspecific.

Nonspecific Active Immunotherapy

One group of nonspecific active immunologic agents is the cytokines, which include interferon, interleukin-2 (IL-2), and tumor necrosis factor.

Interferon has three major types:

- Alpha (derived from leukocytes)
- Beta (derived from fibroblasts)
- Gamma (immune- or lymphocyte-derived).

Interferons have been observed to inhibit viral replication and produce a possible direct antiproliferative effect on the tumor. This effect may be augmentation or induction of host-effector mechanisms such as natural killer cell activity or the induction of membrane antigens on tumor cells, which produces immune recognition. The tumors most responsive to interferon are hematologic, including non-Hodgkin's lymphomas, cutaneous T cell lymphoma, and chronic myelogenous and hairy cell leukemias.

Lymphokines such as interleukin-1 (IL-1) and IL-2 cause T cell proliferation, activation of the lytic mechanisms of lymphokine-activated killer (LAK) cells, emigration of lymphoid cells from the peripheral blood, and the release of other lymphokines, such as tumor necrosis factor (TNF) and gamma interferon, and of other hormones, such as corticotropin, cortisol, and growth hormone. Toxicity is a major deterrent to the use of IL-2; the patient may experience chills and fever, nausea and vomiting, diarrhea, cutaneous erythema, weight gain, anemia, hypotension, tachycardia, and hepatic and renal dysfunction and capillary leak syndrome. IL-2 has demonstrated responses in renal cell cancer and malignant melanoma.

Nonspecific Passive Immunotherapy

The nonspecific passive immunologic agents include the cytokines and lymphokine-activated killer (LAK) cells. LAK cells (e.g., natural killer cells) lyse the tumor.

Specific Passive Immunotherapy

Monoclonal antibodies (MoAbs) are the result or the genetic fusing of cancer cells with leukocytes to produce specific antibodies, which provide passive immunity and serve as carriers of cytotoxic agents to malignant cells. For example, they are labeled with such isotopes as I^{131} to seek occult tumor deposits throughout the body. Monoclonal antibodies may also activate complement, a stage in the immune response that leads eventually to cell death. Two MoAbs have been approved for clinical use by the FDA: muromonab-CD3 (Orthoclone OKT3), a MoAb targeted to the CD3 receptor of human T cells for the treatment of acute reaction in renal transplant patients, and satumomab pendetide (OncoScint CR/OV) to aid in the detection of colorectal and ovarian cancers. Great care must be used in the infusion of MoAbs because they have the potential for causing anaphylaxis. MoAbs have a mouse lymphocyte derivation and are seen by the human body as a foreign protein. The nurse delivering the product should be prepared for a potential emergency situation.[3]

Colony-Stimulating Factors

One of the most exciting and promising developments of recent years in the area of supportive care has been the identification and use of hematopoietic colony-stimulating factors (CSFs). It is believed that CSFs could ameliorate or even eliminate the major hazard of cancer treatment, including neutropenia and thrombocytopenia. CSFs are involved in all aspects of hematopoiesis, including proliferation, differentiation, maturation, and functional activation. They may be categorized by (1) the number of blood cell lines affected (e.g., multilineage, such as IL-3 and hemopoietin-1, or single lineage, such as erythropoietin) or (2) biologic function.

The major endogenous human CSFs are produced in the hematopoietic microenvironment of the bone marrow by T lymphocytes, monocytes and macrophages, endothelial cells, and fibroblasts. Each CSF binds to and activates its unique, high-affinity protein receptor on the surface membrane of target cells. Receptors for granulocyte CSF (G-CSF) are found predominantly on the mature elements of the neutrophil line, whereas receptors for granulocyte-macrophage CSF (GM-CSF) are found predominantly among early cells. Macrophage CSF (M-CSF) receptors predominate on the mature cells of the monocyte and macrophage series.

Both G-CSF and GM-CSF sustain the viability and potentiate the functions of neutrophils. GM-CSF also stimulates production of such cytokines as tumor necrosis factor and interleukin-1. M-CSF enhances the production of monocytes of colony-stimulating activity, interferon, and tumor necrosis factor (TNF). IL-3 may regulate the functions of mature eosinophils and monocytes.

CSFs have been studied in leukopenic persons with AIDS, in cancer patients receiving chemotherapy, and in bone marrow transplant patients.

The standard dosage for the cancer patient receiving myelosuppressive chemotherapy is 5 μg/kg/day. Side effects are rare, but patients should be monitored for an allergic or anaphylactic reaction, redness at the site of the injection, cardiac transient supraventricular arrhythmia (noted in patients with a preexisting cardiac condition), and mild bone pain that responds well to NSAIDs or mild opioid therapy.[20]

Nursing management of patients receiving CSF therapy includes pretreatment assessment, patient and family education, monitoring for side effects and toxicities, and implementing specific instructions depending on the treatment protocol.

RADIATION THERAPY

Description and Rationale

The goal of radiation in the treatment of cancer is the local destruction of malignant cells or their reproductive capability, with minimum damage to normal tissue. This treatment modality is used in the prevention, treatment, and palliation of cancer, either alone or with chemotherapy or surgery. Radiation therapy can be administered either externally or internally.

Ionizing radiation is the form used in cancer treatment because it causes cellular damage or alteration. Some examples of such radiation are x rays, gamma rays, electrons, and beta particles. Cells exposed to ionizing radiation undergo the following stages of reaction:

- Physical stage: The cells' molecules become agitated and excited
- Physiochemical stage: The agitated molecules break into stable molecules and chemically active substances
- Chemical stage: Chemical reactions take place inside the cell, causing changes in nuclear DNA
- Biologic stage: DNA alterations occur, with consequent cell death

The substances used most for radiation therapy include the following:

- X rays: The higher the voltage, the deeper the penetration; for example, high voltage is used for bladder cancer and low voltage is used for superficial tumors such as skin cancers
- Radioactive elements, such as radium and cobalt, which occur in nature
- Radioactive isotopes, such as iodine, gold, and phosphorus, which are produced in atomic reactors

External radiation, the treatment of choice for such cancers as early laryngeal cancer, early retinoblastoma, and some brain tumors, is delivered by x ray or radioisotope via sophisticated equipment with refined delivery, such as the linear accelerator. External radiation is also used as adjuvant therapy and for palliation through reduction of tumor mass.

Internal radiation, including temporary or permanent implants, intracavitary or interstitial instillation, or parenteral or oral administration. Specific uses for these forms of therapy are as follows:

- Implants (such as radon, iodine, and gold seeds) sutured into the tumor via tubes or needles

Intracavitary or interstitial instillation via "seeding" with radioactive gamma ray–emitting beads such as radium or cesium; "afterloading" with an applicator that provides channels through which to place the radioisotope may be used to reduce exposure; used in cancers of the head and neck, breast, prostate, and gynecologic cancers. (Figs. 16-7 and 16-8)

Radioactive isotopes administered orally or parenterally for thyroid cancers

Radioactive isotopes administered orally or parenterally for thyroid cancer, chronic leukemia, or myeloma

The nurse involved in the care of patients receiving internal irradiation should avoid radiation damage by adhering to the principles of **time** (by being efficient but brief), **distance** (by standing as far as possible from the source), and **shielding** (by wearing a lead apron or using other precautions as determined by the radiation safety officer).

Radiosensitive cells—those most likely to be adversely affected by radiation—include relatively undifferentiated and rapidly dividing cells such as those of genes, the mucosa of the GI tract, and lymphoid tissue. The most radioresistant cells are those originating from the connective tissue. At the cellular level the degree of sensitivity is related to the degree of cell differentiation, rate of mitosis, and mitotic potential. The degree of vascularity and oxygenation are also important in determining tissue responsiveness.

The side or toxic effects of radiation therapy depend on the site of irradiation, the volume of tissue irradiated, the total dosage delivered, and the time frame within which it is administered. Although newer technology has increased the therapist's ability to treat the cancer more precisely, surrounding or underlying healthy tissue may still be damaged.

The dose of radiation that can be delivered to any tumor is limited by the radiation tolerance of the adjacent normal tissues. One method of improving the therapeutic ratio is fractionation of treatment, or dividing the total dosage of radiation into multiple doses. This allows four processes to occur: repair of sublethal tissue damage, repopulation of clonogenic cells, reassortment of cells in the cell cycle, and reoxygenation of hypoxic cells. The best results are achieved with predetermined doses given five times a week for 4 to 6 weeks.

Before initiating therapy the therapist may localize the treatment portals with a simulator, such as an x-ray machine that produces the geometric factors of actual therapy or CT scanning that defines both the tumor-bearing volume and critical normal structures. The information obtained is used to produce, with computer assistance, an individualized treatment plan.

In combining surgery with radiation, the relative merits of preoperative or postoperative radiation for many cancers are still a matter of controversy. The use of chemotherapy with radiation requires careful monitoring of peripheral blood counts and observation for exacerbation of drug-induced disorders, such as severe dysuria (cyclophosphamide), enhanced mucositis (methotrexate), or carcinogenesis, such as leukemia. Actinomycin D and doxorubicin produce a recall phenomenon in which reactions appear in previously irradiated tissues when the drug is given as late as 1 year after the patient's radiation exposure.

NURSING CARE

Nursing Assessment

Gastrointestinal function: Nausea and vomiting, anorexia, taste changes, esophagitis, diarrhea, xerostomia, mucositis, radiation tooth decay, perianal irritation

Genitourinary function: Urinary frequency, vaginal discharge, amenorrhea, impotence

Skin: Hair loss; dry desquamation; reddened area; dry, itchy feeling; moist desquamation—blistering and sloughing of skin surface

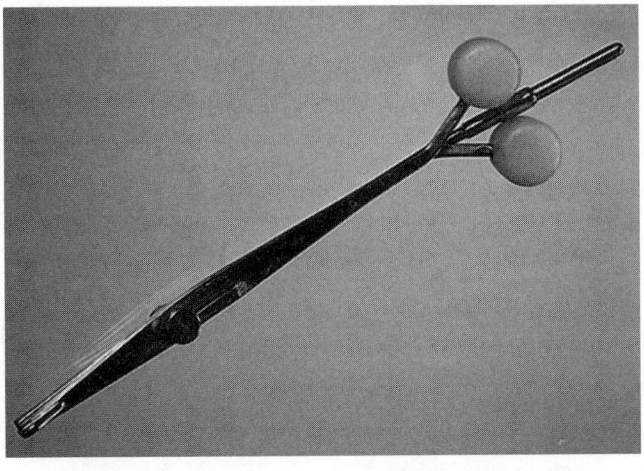

Fig. 18-7

Applicator for gynecologic implant.[3]

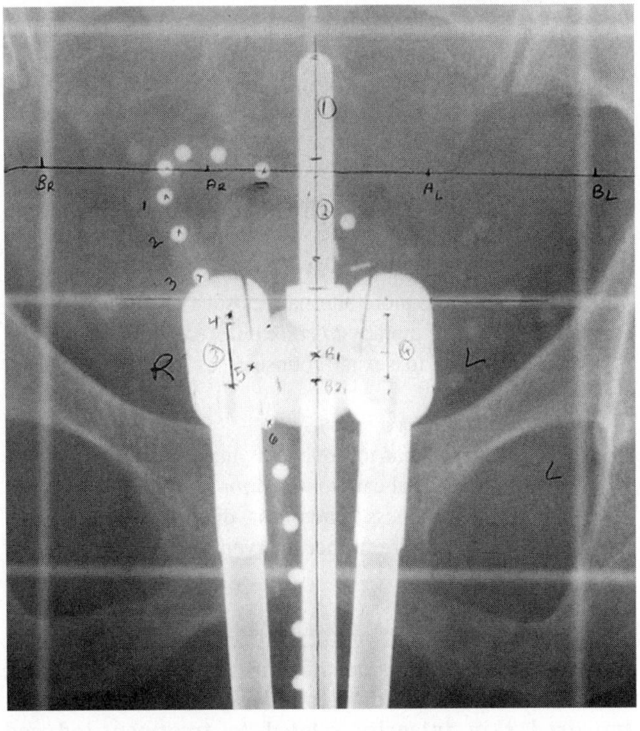

Fig. 18-8

Simulation film of gynecologic implant.[3]

Central nervous system function: Headache, irritability, confusion, restlessness
Neuromuscular function: Transient paresthesia, paresis or paralysis, fatigue
Cardiovascular function: Pneumonitis—dry, hacking cough; dyspnea; pericarditis; chest pain; ECG changes; myocarditis; friction rub
Hematopoietic function: Anemia, infection, bleeding

Patient Problems/Nursing Diagnoses & Interventions

NIC Elimination Management

Diarrhea related to gastrointestinal irritation
Impaired urinary elimination related to bladder irritation

- Encourage clear liquids and low-residue diet *to increase comfort.*
- Offer antidiarrheal agents per physician's order *to control intestinal irritability.*
- Maintain good perineal care *to prevent pain, infection, and patient's fear of eating caused by painful bowel movement.*
- Test stools for occult blood *to identify intestinal bleeding.*
- Record number and consistency of stools *to monitor effect of therapy.*
- Observe for dehydration and electrolyte imbalances *to determine need for further intervention.*
- Force fluids *to maintain renal and bladder hydration.*
- Encourage patient to empty bladder completely *to avoid distention.*
- Administer urinary antiseptics as prescribed *to reduce inflammation.*
- Observe for signs of infection, such as burning, cloudy urine, hematuria, and fever, *to determine the need for antibiotics and other interventions.*

NIC Coping Assistance

Sexual dysfunction related to treatment-induced changes in hormonal status

For sterility

- Help patient explore alternatives such as sperm banking and hormonal therapy *to counteract sterility.*
- Refer patient to sexual counselor as necessary *to treat impotence.*

For vaginal discharge

- Encourage patient to douche as needed and to perform thorough perineal care *to maintain hygiene.*
- Observe for redness, tenderness, discharge, or drainage, which may require further intervention.

NIC Skin/Wound Management

Impaired oral mucous membrane related to mucositis, xerostomia, or radiation tooth decay
Impaired skin integrity related to treatment-induced changes

- Encourage good oral hygiene with use of dental floss or Water Pik *to prevent infection and promote healing.*
- Discourage spicy or hot foods and dry, thick foods, *which increase discomfort.*
- Offer topical relief of pain with lidocaine ointment, Aspergum, or ice chips *to promote comfort.*
- Apply K-Y jelly to lips *to maintain moisture.*
- Offer popsicles *to increase comfort and hydration.*
- Offer artificial saliva *to moisten mucosa.*
- Encourage increased fluid intake with meals *to maintain hydration.*
- Use mouth irrigations or sprays, such as half-strength hydrogen peroxide and saline solution, for oral hygiene.
- Encourage use of sugarless lemon drops or mints *to promote feeling of freshness.*
- Discourage smoking, alcohol, and ginger ale, which irritate mucosa.
- Assess mouth for dryness, lesions, bleeding, discharge, and tooth decay *to determine need for specific interventions.*
- Consult with dentist as needed for dental care, including fluoride therapy, *to prevent further irritation and infection.*

For alopecia

- Help patient plan for wig, scarf, turban, or hat before hair loss *to avoid scalp damage.*
- Have patient gently wash and comb remaining hair *to avoid further hair loss.*
- Reassure patient that hair will grow back after therapy unless whole brain radiation is used.

For dermatitis

- Observe irradiated area daily *to monitor for inflammation or other reactions.*
- Apply baby oil or ointment as prescribed: lanolin or Aquaphor *to maintain moisture.*
- Keep reddened area dry and aerated *to avoid infection.*
- Use cornstarch, A and D ointment, or hydrocortisone ointment *to relieve dryness and itching.*

For moist desquamation

- Provide saline soaks, exposure to air, topical vitamins, steroids, or antibiotic ointments *to enhance healing.*
- Avoid the use of adhesive tape, *which irritates the skin.*
- Assist patient with bathing *to maintain markings.*
- Have patient avoid excessive heat; sunlight; tight, restrictive clothing; and soap, *which further irritate damaged skin.*
- Provide special skin care to tissue folds such as buttocks, perineum, groin, and axilla, *which may be sites of infection.*
- Avoid application of deodorant or aftershave lotion to treated area, *as these may irritate the skin.*
- Avoid use of soaps, heating pad, or sun exposure *to prevent impairment.*

NIC Immobility Management

Impaired physical mobility related to fatigue and impaired motor function

- Plan frequent rest periods *to avoid fatigue.*
- Assist with ambulation and remove environmental barriers *to avoid injury.*
- Assess reflexes, tactile sensation, and movement in extremities, and report abnormal findings *to detect complications.*

- Observe for Lhermitte's sign (sensation of electric shock running down back and over extremities), *which is indicative of cervical cord compression.*

NIC Tissue Perfusion Management

Ineffective cardiopulmonary tissue perfusion related to pneumonitis, pericarditis, myocarditis, anemia, bleeding

- Auscultate lungs, and report signs of pleural rub *to assess pulmonary status.*
- Observe for cough, dyspnea, and pain on inspiration as evidence of respiratory dysfunction.
- Treat with antibiotics and steroids as prescribed *to reduce irritation and treat infection.*
- Auscultate heart, and report signs of friction rub, dysrhythmias, or hypertension *to detect complications.*
- Observe for chest pain and weakness, *which are indicative of cardiac dysfunction.*
- Monitor ECG reports *to monitor cardiac status.*
- Administer drugs as prescribed *to counteract dysrhythmias.*
- Encourage adequate rest; alternate rest and activity periods *to avoid stress on respiratory system.*
- Observe patient for dyspnea and increased weakness as signs of further anemia.
- Administer oxygen therapy as needed *to increase oxygenation of tissues.*
- Monitor hemoglobin and hematocrit *to determine effectiveness of therapy.*
- Administer transfusions as ordered *to increase circulating RBCs.*

Patient Education/Continuum of Care Plan

See Comprehensive Care Plan, p. 1237.

1. Discuss the need for skin care such as maintenance of dye markings, avoidance of soap and other ointments, and avoidance of sunbathing or heat applications.
2. Emphasize the need to avoid injury to the skin.
3. Explain the maintenance of adequate nutrition.
4. Explain the patient's "radioactive state," if present, and precautions to be taken.
5. Discuss the management of fatigue and the maintenance of mobility.

Evaluation/Patient Outcomes

Elimination Management: Bowel elimination is normal. Patient has no diarrhea. Urinary elimination is normal. Patient makes no complaints of urinary distress. Intake and output are balanced.

Coping Assistance: Sexual function is normal. Patient has satisfactory libido and has made plans for dealing with possible sterility, absence of vaginal discharge, or lack of erectile ability.

Skin/Wound Management: Oral mucous membranes are healthy. Mucous membranes, lips, tongue, and gingiva are of normal color and moisture. Patient has clean teeth, moist saliva, an ability to swallow, and a normal voice. Skin is healthy and intact. Patient makes no complaints of itching. There is no evidence of rash or blistering or redness.

Immobility Management: Physical mobility is normal. Patient is able to ambulate without assistance.

Tissue Perfusion Management: Cardiopulmonary tissue perfusion is adequate. Patient makes no complaints of chest pain, cough, or dyspnea. Complete blood cell count is within normal limits.

Surgery

Surgical procedures utilized in oncologic care include biopsies, surgical staging, resection of tumors, and reconstruction.

Surgery has historically been the treatment of choice for most cancers. A decision to use this therapy is based on analysis of various data, including a thorough history and physical examination; laboratory, radiologic, and other specialized procedures; and biopsy-obtained proof of cancer.

A radical surgical approach to operable tumors is no longer routinely used because of an increased variety of surgical procedures and more sophisticated disease staging. The current treatment of choice is excision of the primary tumor and enough surrounding tissue and lymph nodes to offer maximum protection against local recurrence. These are termed curative resections. Palliative resections may be done when there is spread to distant, previously (preoperatively) undetected sites.

A tumor is considered inoperable if it is large or in a difficult-to-reach place or if there is evidence of extensive local growth or metastasis.

Staging operations such as laparotomy may be performed to determine appropriate therapy. Secondary operations may be done for local recurrence. "Second-look" operations may be performed in the absence of chemical evidence of recurrent disease, but the effectiveness of this procedure for finding recurrent disease is questionable.

Distant metastasis (e.g., pulmonary or hepatic) may respond to direct surgical resection. Indirect ablative procedures such as adrenalectomy and hypophysectomy may be useful in the palliation of hormonally sensitive cancers of the breast or prostate. Other indirect palliative procedures include cordotomy for relief of intractable pain and ostomy to relieve GI obstruction.

Reconstructive surgery of the head and neck, breast, and extremities has become an important aspect of cancer rehabilitation in recent years. For example, the development of maxillofacial prosthodontics has enabled people treated with radical neck dissection to regain cosmetic appearance and the ability to eat and drink in a more natural manner. Breast reconstruction is an option for women whose disease and treatment enable the surgeon to implant a prosthesis or to transplant tissue from other areas of the body.

Whatever the surgery, the patient's nutritional status, both preoperatively and postoperatively, has been found to be significant in the amount of surgery that can be tolerated, recovery from the surgical procedure, and wound healing.

NUTRITIONAL SUPPORT

Patients with cancer must deal not only with the metabolic effects of the disease on their nutritional status, but also with the effects of treatment. In addition, an inability to eat or difficulty with eating may affect the patient psychologically because nutrition is not only a basic human need but often a source of social interaction. Patients with cancer who experience anorexia, nausea and vomiting, mucositis, changes in taste, and difficulty swallowing face the challenge of eating when they least want to or are least able, yet have the greatest need to do so. It has been shown through numerous research studies that a poor nutritional status adversely affects the patient's ability to tolerate both cancer and its treatment.

The body of the person with cancer responds to the increased demand for glucose, which is required by both normal and cancer cells because of the increased rate of gluconeogenesis. This is the synthesis of glucose by the liver and renal cortex from noncarbohydrate sources such as lactate and amino acids. When protein is broken down to provide amino acids for gluconeogenesis, muscle wasting results. Progressive muscle wasting is called cachexia and gives the patient a characteristic appearance of emaciation.

Fat metabolism is also adversely affected in persons with cancer. Fat stored in the form of fatty acids is mobilized from adipose tissue and released into the bloodstream for use as fuel. This process, which is controlled by the inhibitory effects of insulin, is compromised in persons with cancer, so that body stores of fat are depleted as the disease progresses.

Persons with cancer also exhibit deficiencies in such vitamins as A, C, and thiamine. Iron deficiency may also occur. Fluid and electrolyte imbalances include hypercalcemia, hyperuricemia, hyperphosphatemia, and hyperkalemia. These alterations result from either the direct or indirect effects of tumors, such as paraneoplastic syndromes.

Poor nutrition also adversely affects immunocompetence by decreasing the size of the lymphoid tissues, including the spleen, lymph nodes, and thymus. There is a resulting decreased function of B cell and T cell lymphocytes, which is directly correlated with the degree of malnutrition and which produces a delayed hypersensitivity response.

Local effects of cancer, such as the presence of tumors that adversely affect chewing, swallowing, and peristalsis, can alter the patient's nutritional status. Obstruction, pain, and distention affect the patient's ability to digest and metabolize food.

As discussed earlier, the treatment modalities—surgery, chemotherapy, radiation therapy, and BRMs—also compromise the patient's nutritional status. Thus the nurse must assess the patient's nutritional status at frequent intervals to obtain a baseline measure and to identify the need for aggressive intervention. Clinical observation, including the identification of concurrent health problems (diabetes, hypertension, malabsorption), psychosocial factors (home environment, methods of food preparation, patient's body image), and physical assessment provide the data needed to monitor the patient's nutritional status. Examination of the patient's hair, teeth, gums, and general muscle tone can provide early signs of nutritional deficiencies.

Dietary evaluation is also useful and includes a 24-hour food diary, a complete dietary history with food allergies and preferences, direct observation of dietary intake, and evaluation of nutrient composition. Biochemical measurements include such laboratory values as serum albumin, serum transferrin, and urine urea nitrogen levels and total lymphocyte count. Anthropometric measurements include the patient's midarm muscle circumference (MAMC), triceps, skin fold thickness (SFT), subscapular skin fold thickness (SST), and weight-for-height measurements.

Nutritional interventions for the person with cancer have been shown to decrease the morbidity and mortality of cancer by preventing weight loss, increasing response to therapy, minimizing the side effects of treatment, and improving quality of life. The type of nutritional support required by the patient is based on his or her functional abilities and limitations, severity of the nutritional deficiency, potential for complications, duration of therapy, cost, and psychologic effect.

Nutritional support may include oral, enteral, and parenteral nutritional management. The oral route is preferred because it is more natural and least invasive. Oral nutritional support may range from the addition of sauces and gravies to foods to more complex interventions such as dietary supplements. The patient with anorexia may benefit from frequent small meals and snacks. Foods high in protein and calories are recommended, such as cheese, fish, poultry, milkshakes, peanut butter on crackers, and prepackaged puddings.

If the patient has mucositis or taste alterations, a high-calorie bland diet may be helpful. The patient should avoid seasoning and liquids with high acidity such as orange and lemon juices. Use of a topical analgesic, good mouth care, and avoidance of commercial mouthwashes reduce oral discomfort. Cold foods such as popsicles and ice cream have a numbing effect, which patients tolerate better than warm or hot foods.

Psychosocial support is also critical. Both the patient and family should be encouraged to try a variety of strategies and to be supportive of one another because this is a difficult and challenging problem. The patient's appetite can be enhanced by occasionally eating at the table with family and friends in an attractive environment. Using small plates, eating more often, and decreasing exposure to strong food odors may also be helpful. Antiemetics and artificial saliva can be used to control the symptoms of gastrointestinal irritation.

Multiple high-calorie high-protein foods may be helpful to the patient; however, some are not well tolerated by patients with lactose intolerance, and the patient should be monitored for any intolerance to the supplement.

The enteral route via a feeding tube may be needed by patients who are anoretic, hypermetabolic, or unconscious and by those who have a mechanical impairment. Parenteral feeding is indicated only for patients with totally nonfunctioning GI tracts, those who require bowel rest, or those who cannot tolerate enteral nutritional support.

Patients with functioning GI tracts who are not able to ingest adequate nutrients to meet their metabolic demands should be considered candidates for enteral feeding. These include patients with anorexia; cachexia; cancers of the head or neck, esophagus, stomach; CNS disease, which impairs swallowing; and intractable diarrhea.

Tube feedings may be administered by the nasogastric, nasoduodenal, nasojejunal, esophagostomy, gastrostomy, and jejunostomy routes (FIG. 18-9). The most common routes involve

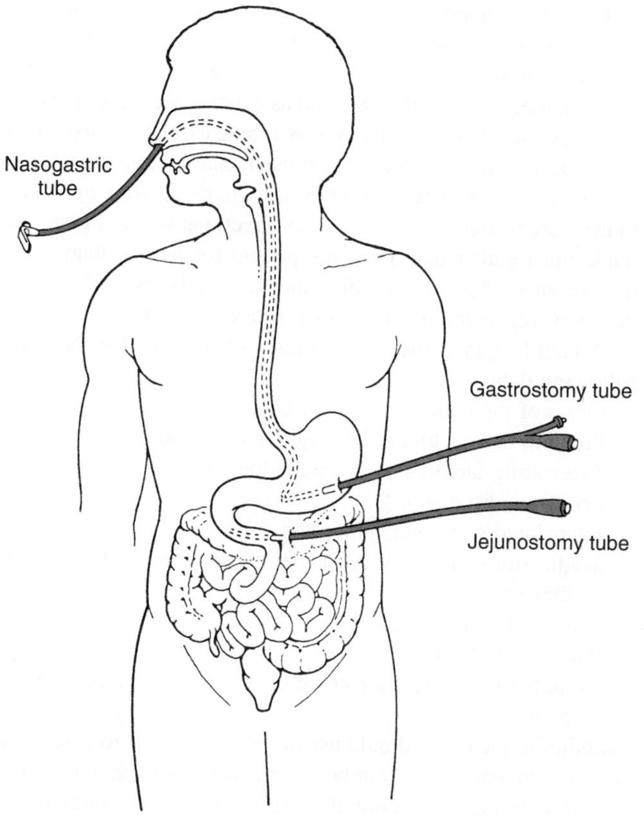

FIG. 18-9
Three routes for tube feeding.

passage of a small, flexible feeding tube through the nose into the stomach or intestine. Feeding ostomies such as the gastrostomy require a surgical percutaneous insertion and are preferred for long-term nutritional support. The cervical esophagostomy is a surgically created, skin-lined canal extending from the border of the neck to the area below the cervical esophagus; the feeding tube is passed through this opening to the stomach for each feeding and then removed.

Aspiration may occur more often with gastric feedings because only the gastroesophageal sphincter is functioning to prevent gastric reflux, whereas the intestinal feedings use both the gastroesophageal and pyloric sphincters to prevent reflux. When feedings are improperly selected or administered, nausea, diarrhea, and cramps can occur.

The volume and concentration of the nutriment provided by tube feeding should meet the needs of the individual patient and should be compatible with the size of the tube, the location of the tube, and the patient's tolerance of formula strength and rate of administration. Feedings may be delivered by bolus or gravity, as well as via enteral pump. The position of the tube and gastric residual should be checked frequently. The patient should be monitored for the development of dumping syndrome, aspiration, weight loss, and diarrhea; each of these conditions requires evaluation of the formula and infusion rate for changes.

The patient may also complain of thirst, taste deprivation, and the inability to satisfy the appetite, as well as a sense of altered body image. The patient may be permitted to chew gum or suck on hard candies, drink fluids, and eat soft, bland foods. Referral to a support group may help the patient to accept the alterations in the social and aesthetic aspects of eating.

Complications of tube feedings may be mechanical, such as nasal irritation and erosion, esophagitis or pharyngitis, or tube dislocation or occlusion; GI, such as abdominal distention, nausea and vomiting, constipation or diarrhea; respiratory (aspiration pneumonia); or metabolic, such as hyperglycemia, hypokalemia, hyperkalemia, hypernatremia, and dehydration. The nurse and patient should monitor the feedings to identify problems early and intervene before serious alterations occur. Because many patients receive enteral feedings in the home, a caregiver and the patient should be taught general care of the patient and the tube to ensure safe and effective therapy.

Parenteral nutrition (also called hyperalimentation) supplies all of the essential nutrients by intravenous infusion. Total parenteral nutrition (TPN) and peripheral parenteral nutrition (PPN) supply all of the daily requirements for protein and calories directly into the patient's bloodstream and is indicated for such patients as those with cancers of the GI tract, other obstructions, radiation enteritis, and intractable diarrhea.

PPN is delivered via peripheral veins, most often those of the arm or the external jugular vein. Limitations of peripheral infusion include provision of limited calories, vein irritation, and limited usefulness for long-term therapy. TPN uses central lines into a major vein such as the superior vena cava, providing for a large amount of calories and protein as well as high dextrose and amino acid concentrations, and useful for long-term therapy. Central lines used for TPN include ports, triple-lumen catheters, Broviac, Hickman, PICC, and Groshong catheters (FIG. 18-10). When central infusion is used, the solution must be tapered down by rate and concentration to discontinue therapy without inducing profound hypoglycemia.

TPN contains glucose, amino acids, and fats to provide both immediate and long-term energy. Patients receiving TPN may have a multilumen central venous catheter inserted so that there is access for the administration of medications and blood drawing.

TPN and PPN may be given continuously or by cycling, with cycling at night used most often for patients receiving therapy at home. Cycling enables the patient to be mobile during the day but does require an ability to tolerate a high-volume load. Programmable pumps are used to prevent or minimize hypoglycemia and hyperglycemia. Ambulatory patients benefit from the use of the portable pump, which is worn as a waist pack.

The nurse should assess the patient's lifestyle, home environment, family and support systems, body image, and perceptions about TPN to plan for the optimal acceptance of and adaptation to the therapy. Daily monitoring of vital signs, weight, and laboratory values enables the nurse to determine the need for adjustment of formula or rate of administration before the patient's discharge. Follow-up visits in the home are important and ensure the patient's compliance and tolerance of TPN or PPN.

The nurse's role in nutritional support is critical and includes comprehensive assessment, monitoring, and patient education to maintain the person with cancer in optimal nutritional status.

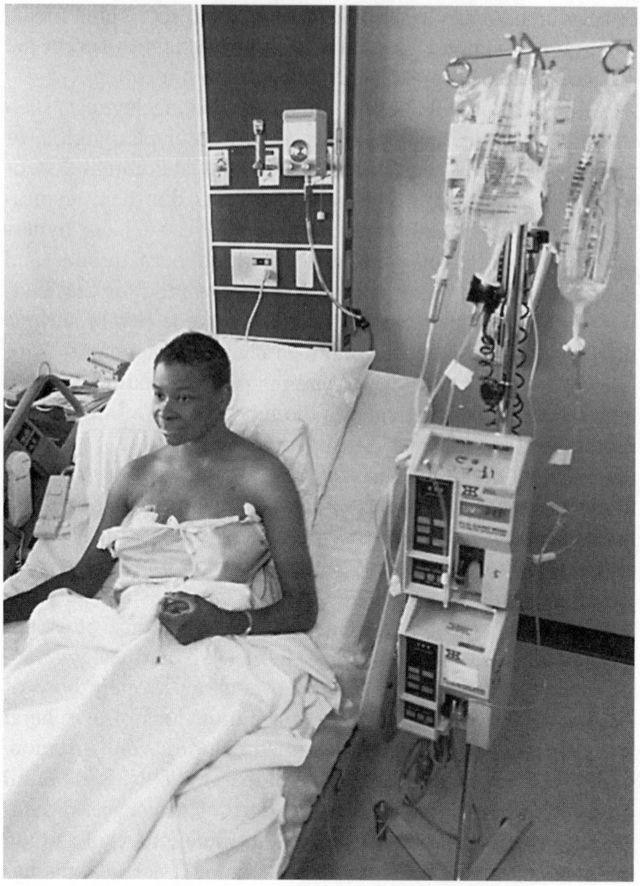

FIG. 18-10
Hickman-Broviac catheter. This patient has a Hickman-Broviac catheter for venous access. Note the catheter's lift over the right breast, with a protective dressing and tape to prevent dislodgment. The patient is receiving multiple intravenous infusions via the catheter.

PAIN MANAGEMENT

Persons with cancer may experience pain at any point during the course of their disease and its treatment. Of the 4 million people throughout the world who die of cancer each year, 70% experience pain as a primary symptom. Unfortunately, many persons believe that pain is an early symptom of cancer and do not seek diagnosis until pain occurs. Pain is (almost without exception) a late symptom of cancer and indicates the presence of tumor obstruction, pressure on nerves, invasion of bone, phantom sensation, peripheral neuropathy, postherpetic neuralgia, mucositis, or incisional irritation.

It is estimated that 85% of patients with cancer pain can be managed effectively with appropriate therapy. The American Cancer Society, the American Pain Society, the World Health Organization, the Oncology Nursing Society, and many other organizations consider pain control to be a major issue in the management of the person with cancer. If not relieved, pain contributes to nausea, vomiting, anorexia, and insomnia. In addition, anxiety, fear, and depression contribute to and interfere with the patient's ability to cope with pain and diminish an individual's quality of life, however long that life may be.

One of the many challenges facing the nurse who cares for the patient with pain is the assessment of that pain. The nurse must accept the definition of pain as whatever the person experiencing the pain says that it is and as existing wherever the person says that it does. This is frustrating to many nurses and physicians, who may doubt the presence and nature of the patient's pain when there are no physiologic parameters by which to measure it. Because there are no direct measures of pain, the nurse must gather data from the patient for use in diagnosing the presence of pain, describing its characteristics, and making decisions regarding the most appropriate interventions.

A pain history gathered from the patient should include the following data:

- Onset of the pain (when it started)
- Precipitating factors (what triggers the pain)
- Alleviating factors (what lessens the pain)
- Location of the pain
- Associated signs and symptoms
- Medications taken by the patient and the extent to which they provide relief
- Pain quality and intensity
- Patient's view of the pain
- Actions that have either helped or not helped to relieve the pain

In addition, the nurse should use observation skills to assess the patient's appearance; motor behavior; affective behavior; verbal behavior; brainstem automatic responses, such as increase in heart rate, respirations, and blood pressure; spinal cord reflex responses; and nonverbal pain clues. The psychosocial dimensions of the pain must also be explored. These include personality, cultural, and religious factors; the patient's interpretation of pain; the patient's prior experience with pain; and the physical environment in which the patient is experiencing the pain.

General guidelines for the use of pain relief measures are as follows:

1. Use a variety of pain relief measures.
2. Use pain relief measures before the patient's pain becomes severe.
3. Include pain relief measures that the patient believes will be helpful.
4. Determine the patient's ability or willingness to participate actively in the use of pain relief measures.
5. Rely on patient behavior that indicates pain severity rather than on known physical stimuli.
6. Encourage the patient to try a pain relief measure at least two times before abandoning it as ineffective.
7. Keep an open mind about what may relieve the patient's pain, including nonpharmacologic measures.
8. Keep trying to relieve the pain; do not become discouraged and stop working with the patient.

Chemical means of pain management include the use of narcotics and nonnarcotics. Nonnarcotic analgesics of value in the treatment of cancer pain are acetaminophen, aspirin, and nonsteroidal antiinflammatory drugs (NSAIDs) such as ibuprofen, indomethacin, and naproxen. One potential drawback of aspirin is its antiplatelet effect, which can create problems in the myelosuppressed patient. Acetaminophen could be a problem in patients with impaired liver function. Both aspirin and the NSAIDs are generally well tolerated but have the potential for causing GI ulceration, renal toxic effects, and inhibition of platelet aggregation. If a nonnarcotic agent does not have a therapeutic effect initially, the dose should be increased before trying another type of drug. When a ceiling is reached with a nonnarcotic agent, a moderately potent narcotic such as oxycodone or codeine can be added. Some persons with cancer benefit from such a combination. NSAIDs should be considered in combination with opioid therapy to potentiate opioid effectiveness.

Narcotics (opioids) used in the management of cancer pain include morphine, hydromorphone, methadone, oxycodone, and fentanyl. Sustained-release opioids in an oral form, such as MS Contin, Roxanol SR, or OxyContin, has been found to be of particular value in the management of patients who require opioid therapy for an extended period. Patients with chronic, *stable,* cancer pain have had positive results using transdermal fentanyl (Duragesic). The administration of narcotics via intravenous and epidural infusion has enhanced the analgesic effect of the opioids. The need for around-the-clock dosing has been noted, so that fixed dosing schedules with adequate doses for pain relief provide more constant blood levels and predictable pain relief. Some patients experience breakthrough pain that requires additional dosing, but the fixed dosing schedule should be maintained.

Side effects of narcotics that require nurse monitoring and intervention include constipation, nausea, vomiting, and sedation. Respiratory and CNS depression are a rare occurrence in chronic opioid use.

The following medications may be used in conjunction with opioid therapy, but should not replace it. The nurse should be familiar with the medications outlined in this section and use the appropriate drug for the appropriate indication.

Analgesic potentiators include the phenothiazine derivatives such as promethazine (Phenergan), prochlorperazine (Compazine), chlorpromazine (Thorazine), hydroxyzine pamoate (Vistaril), diazepam (Valium), lorazepam (Ativan), and diphenhydramine (Benadryl). Also used are stimulants such as cocaine, methylphenidate (Ritalin), dextroamphetamine, and caffeine.

For neuropathic pain, tricyclic antidepressants such as desipramine, nortriptyline, amitriptyline (Elavil), imipramine (Tofranil), and doxepin (Sinequan) may be used either alone or in combination with anticonvulsants: phenytoin, carbamazepine, valproate, clonazepam, and gabapentin.

Another category of drugs that may be used, but is not recommended in cancer pain management, includes the narcotic agonists and antagonists such as nalbuphine (Nubain), butorphanol (Stadol), pentazocine (Talwin), and buprenorphine (Buprenex).

One particular medication not recommended in cancer pain management is meperidine (Demerol) because of its ceiling effect and side effect profile.

Patient self-control methods include distraction, massage, relaxation, biofeedback, hypnosis, and imagery. Many patients respond positively to the opportunity for self-care in the management of their pain and perceive such self-control measures to enhance the effectiveness of other prescribed pain interventions.

Pain technology includes the use of the following:

1. External pumps for the intravenous, epidural, and intrathecal administration of narcotic analgesics
2. Implantable pumps for the intravenous, epidural, and intrathecal administration of narcotic analgesics
3. Patient-controlled analgesia, particularly for the management of acute pain, such as postoperative pain
4. Transcutaneous electrical nerve stimulation (TENS)
5. Continuous subcutaneous infusion (CSCI) with an ambulatory infusion pump

In each instance the nurse must develop the technical skills needed to initiate and monitor the therapy and to teach the patient and family the use and maintenance of the system. Each of these technologies has expanded the options for the patient with pain and has increased the degree of self-control experienced.

Other interventions for pain include (1) anesthetic procedures such as nerve blocks, trigger point injections, and the use of nitrous oxide; (2) neuroaugmentive therapies such as counterirritation, rubbing, TENS, and percutaneous nerve stimulation; (3) neuroablative procedures such as cordotomy; and (4) physiatric supportive measures such as the use of a prosthesis, physical therapy, and occupational therapy.

The nurse's unique contributions to pain management are placement as the key link between the patient and the health-care team, the amount of time spent with the patient, the ability to assess the patient's response to pain and its management, and the role of patient and family educator. In addition, the nurse has the ability to articulate a concise pain assessment, use equinalgesic charts for dosage guidelines, and anticipate and address patient, family, and health-care provider misconceptions about pain management. For instance, many patients and their families experience opioid phobia, the irrational and undocumented fear that the appropriate use of narcotics causes addiction. This fear of addiction among both health-care providers and the public seems to be a major reason for the undertreatment of pain. The nurse must understand and be able to articulate the differences between addiction, tolerance, and physical dependence to use pain management strategies appropriately and to enable patients and their families to accept the therapeutic value of drugs such as the narcotics.

Comprehensive Care Plan for the Patient With Cancer

Physical Comfort Promotion

Nursing Assessment

Comfort level: Onset, duration, location, intensity, quality, pattern of pain

Patient Problems/Nursing Diagnoses & Interventions

NIC Physical Comfort Promotion

Pain related to tumor pressure and/or metastatic disease

Interventions for all patients

- Involve patient in selection of other pain measures *to enhance comfort and patient's participation in care.*
- Administer analgesic as prescribed *to relieve pain.*
- Assist with and teach use of patient-controlled analgesic device if ordered.
- Instruct patient to request analgesic before pain becomes severe *to avoid inconsistent control of pain.*

- Evaluate effectiveness of pain relief measures *to determine need for further intervention.*
- Position patient comfortably *to relieve pressure.*
- Exercise patient's limbs gently in range of motion *to maintain muscle tone.*
- Massage gently *to relax muscles.*
- Monitor pain character, intensity, and frequency *to evaluate effect of analgesic and determine need for change in amount, route, or frequency of administration.*
- Teach patient to use relaxation, guided imagery, and diversional activities *to enhance analgesic effect or to decrease need for analgesic.*
- Use massage, heat, or cold as appropriate *to increase comfort.*

Colorectal cancers
- Change patient's position frequently; increase movement if tolerated *to relieve distention.*
- Discourage smoking, which may increase distention.
- Give small, frequent feedings *to prevent further distention.*
- Encourage decreased intake of gas-forming foods *to prevent further distention.*
- Refrain from giving iced liquids and carbonated beverages, *which increase cramping.*
- Avoid use of straws and swallowing air *because this causes gas formation in GI tract.*
- Give nonprescription drugs, such as simethicone, *to relieve flatus.*
- Encourage moderate physical activity *to relieve pressure on abdomen.*
- Remove restrictive clothing *to relieve pressure on abdomen.*
- Inspect abdomen for distention *to determine need for further intervention.*
- Auscultate abdomen for abnormal bowel sounds *to assess effect of therapy.*
- Restrict liquids at mealtime; give warm liquids after meals *to relax abdomen.*
- Encourage decreased intake of fatty foods *to decrease formation of flatus.*
- Give bland foods *to relieve GI irritation.*
- Apply heat to abdomen *to relax abdomen and relieve cramping.*
- Apply warm, moist compress to rectal area or provide sitz bath *to relax anal sphincter.*
- Increase fluid intake to 2000 ml daily *to maintain soft stool.*
- Encourage decreased intake of high-bulk food *to relieve GI distention.*

Breast cancer
- See general nursing interventions.

Urinary tract cancers
- Demonstrate use of pillow *to support flanks,* exercises *to relax muscles,* and massage *to relieve discomfort*
- Administer bladder antispasmodics as ordered *to relieve bladder spasms.*

Prostate cancer
- Place patient in whirlpool bath or apply heat *to relax muscles.*
- Provide safety measures (e.g., physical support when patient moves in bed or walks, use of assistive devices such as a walker) *to avoid injury.*

Testicular cancer
- Discuss pain-relieving measures such as scrotal support, analgesics, and massage.
- Implement (as feasible) patient preferences *to further patient comfort.*
- Review care of postoperative pain (Part III, Perioperative Nursing).

Cervical cancer
- Give small, frequent feedings *to avoid abdominal distention.*
- Place patient in sitting position *to relieve abdominal pressure.*
- Insert rectal tube as indicated *to relieve flatus.*

Other gynecologic cancers
- Demonstrate exercises and use of pillow *to splint abdomen to relax back and pelvic muscles.*

Oral cancers
- Apply ice or cold compress to nose, face, or throat *to relieve irritation.*
- Provide frequent oral hygiene, including warm saline throat irrigations, *to decrease mucosal dryness because patient often breathes through mouth.*
- Instruct patient not to blow nose *because this may trigger bleeding.*
- Place basin nearby so that patient will spit out secretions rather than swallow them *to avoid further irritation of mucosa.*
- Apply heat to face, particularly over sinuses, *to relieve sinus headache pain.*

Laryngeal cancer
- Apply heating pad, hot water bottle, or warm, moist compress *to relieve pain.*
- Maintain warm room temperature *to avoid irritation caused by cold air.*

Esophageal cancer
- Place the head of the patient's bed on 4-inch blocks *to prevent reflux esophagitis.*
- Provide antacids at bedside *so that patient can medicate self when indigestion occurs*
- Assess patient for evidence of mouth filling with fluid refluxing from esophagus, for dysphagia, and for heartburn (which increases when the patient lies down) as evidence of esophagitis, *which requires aggressive medical management.*
- Administer solution of meat tenderizer *to relieve food impaction, which may be a cause of pain.*
- Observe for evidence of GI bleeding, such as hematemesis or melena, *which indicates severe esophageal irritation.*

Digestive gland tumors
- Teach strategies to relieve pain (i.e., back pain is often relieved by sitting up and bending forward or lying curled in a fetal position).
- Monitor diet *to determine if certain foods increase or decrease patient pain or GI discomfort.*
- Offer patient frequent baths, lotions, and ointments *to soothe skin and decrease itching.*

Bone sarcomas
- Change patient's position slowly *to avoid stretching and pressure.*
- Provide whirlpool or use heat applications *to promote relaxation and healing.*
- Provide safety *to avoid further injury to patient.*
- Discuss "phantom" pain with patient (amputee) and significant other.

Soft tissue sarcomas
- Change patient's position slowly *to avoid additional discomfort.*
- Support affected part(s) *to prevent strain.*
- Place patient in whirlpool or use heat applications *for muscle relaxation.*
- Provide safety measures *to avoid injury.*

Metastatic disease
- Maintain body alignment *to prevent muscular stretching.*
- Position patient with support (e.g., pillows), change position slowly, and support joints *to avoid fractures and decrease pressure.*

EVALUATION/PATIENT OUTCOMES

Physical Comfort Promotion: Pain is not reported. Patient expresses comfort and freedom from pain, identifies strategies to relieve pain, and states when pain is not relieved.

Nutrition Support

NURSING ASSESSMENT

Nutritional status: Change in weight, usually loss over short period of time; nausea and/or vomiting; decreased serum protein; anemia; anorexia; fatigue

Gastrointestinal function: Diminished or absent bowel sounds

PATIENT PROBLEMS/NURSING DIAGNOSES & INTERVENTIONS

NIC NUTRITION SUPPORT

Imbalanced nutrition: less than body requirements

Interventions for all patients
- Assess dietary habits and needs *to help individualize the patient's diet.*
- Weigh patient weekly to note any weight gain (an indication of improved nutrition) or loss *to intervene quickly with nutritional supplements and fluids.*
- Monitor albumin and lymphocytes *to determine if visceral protein needed for the immune system is adequate.*
- Assess psychologic factors (e.g., depression, anger) *to identify the effect of psychologic factors that may decrease food and fluid intake.*
- Provide high-protein diet *to support immune system.*
- Administer vitamins as ordered *to supplement diet.*
- Administer antiemetics before meals *to reduce nausea that may interfere with eating.*
- Offer antiemetics as prescribed *to provide relief from vomiting and nausea.*
- Arrange pleasant surroundings; provide appealing selection of foods; encourage family and friends to bring in food of patient's choice; and provide attractive meal tray *to enhance patient's appetite.*
- Postpone feeding when patient is fatigued; *patient is more likely to eat when rested.*
- Give patient small, frequent feedings *to avoid distention.*
- Feed patient slowly and provide rest periods *to avoid tiring patient.*
- Observe and record food intake, and measure body weight daily *to monitor nutritional status.*
- Elevate patient's head *to promote comfort.*
- Encourage deep breathing *to relieve feeling of nausea.*

Lung cancer
- Provide oxygen to patient while eating as ordered *to reduce dyspnea* by reducing the work of breathing.
- Encourage oral care before meals *to remove taste of sputum that may reduce appetite.*
- Position patient to facilitate breathing, *thereby improving appetite.*
- Provide frequent small feedings *to lessen fatigue.*
- Provide soft foods and liquids *to lessen energy required to eat, thereby reducing oxygen requirement.*

Head and neck cancers
- Provide and teach patient thorough oral hygiene—such as frequent brushing with soft toothbrush and baking soda and use of oral gavage or Water Pik and nonalcohol-based mouthwashes—*to prevent halitosis and prevent infection of surgical site.*
- Offer artificial saliva for the patient who experiences decreased production of saliva.
- When oral feeding is begun, assess for swallowing and gagging abilities.
- Refrain from offering the patient hot or iced fluids, *which may irritate the mucous membranes.*
- Have suction equipment available *to remove excessive secretions.*

Esophageal cancer
- Assess patient to determine those foods patient can and cannot swallow *to select and prepare edible foods.*
- Provide a diet that omits alcohol, spices, or foods at extreme temperatures and includes bland foods *to prevent irritation of the esophageal mucosa.*
- Teach the patient to eat slowly, chew food thoroughly, and arch back while swallowing *to increase amount ingested.*
- Have patient eat while sitting in the upright position and remain sitting after meal *to avoid regurgitation or aspiration.*
- Have patient avoid eating 1 to 2 hours before bedtime *to avoid heartburn or reflux esophagitis.*
- Have patient sip half a glass of water after each meal *to cleanse the esophagus.*

Gastric cancer
- Assess whether patient is experiencing discomfort or indigestion, vomiting, belching, postprandial fullness, or weakness as evidence of tumor pressure and obstruction.
- Offer medications that relieve abdominal distention and flatulence *because these symptoms tend to adversely affect appetite.*
- Provide frequent small feedings each day.

Digestive gland cancers
- Ask patient if he or she is experiencing anorexia, constipation, bloating, flatulence, or other signs and symptoms

of GI distress as evidence of tumor pressure and possible disease progression.
- Encourage the patient to eat frequent small meals *to increase intake.*
- Offer medications that relieve abdominal distention and flatulence *because these symptoms tend to adversely affect appetite.*

Metastatic disease and terminal stage of the disease
- See interventions for all patients.

Chemotherapy
- Administer antiemetic (5-HT_3 receptor antagonists, prochlorperazine, thiethylperazine, trimethobenzamide, mitoclopramide, intravenous dexamethasone, or d-9 tetrahydrocannabinol [THC]) prophylactically before chemotherapy and on a regular schedule after therapy per physician order *to decrease incidence of nausea and vomiting.*
- Assess need to withhold food and fluids for 4 to 6 hours before treatment *to decrease gastric irritation.*
- Provide frequent mouth care *to promote patient's comfort.*
- Provide clean environment with fresh air and no odors *to reduce noxious stimuli.*
- Administer intravenous therapy as ordered *to maintain fluid and electrolyte balance.*
- Use relaxation techniques, guided imagery, self-hypnosis, and distraction as indicated *to reduce nausea.*
- Offer bland or pureed foods *to facilitate swallowing.*
- Have patient avoid spicy foods, alcohol, and tobacco *to decrease irritation.*
- Offer antacids *to counteract gastric acid.*
- Encourage patient to eat by explaining need to maintain strength.
- Offer small, frequent feedings *to avoid distention.*
- Do not rush meals, *so that patient will increase intake.*

Radiation therapy
- Administer antiemetic as needed *to control incidence of nausea and vomiting.*
- Plan rest periods before and after meals *to enhance patient's appetite.*
- Provide small, bland, frequent feedings and increased fluids *to maintain nutrition and hydration.*
- Offer frequent mouth care *to promote comfort and appetite.*
- Provide clean environment with fresh air and no odors *to decrease noxious stimuli.*
- Administer intravenous therapy as ordered *to maintain hydration.*
- Encourage patient to eat high-calorie, high-protein diet *for maximum nutrition.*
- Do not rush meals *to increase intake.*
- Use enteral feeding tube or TPN if necessary *to maintain nutritional balance.*

EVALUATION/PATIENT OUTCOMES

Nutrition Support: Nutritional status has improved. Weight loss has diminished, or weight gain is present. Patient is eating a balanced diet. Albumin equals 3.2 to 4.5 g/dl. Lymphocytes equal 2100 or 35% to 40%/mm^3 blood. Nausea and vomiting are controlled.

Coping Assistance

NURSING ASSESSMENT

Psychosocial status: Fear, anxiety, withdrawal, avoidance of physical intimacy, restlessness, fight-or-flight behavior, grieving

PATIENT PROBLEMS/NURSING DIAGNOSES AND INTERVENTIONS

NIC COPING ASSISTANCE

Decisional conflict related to treatment options
Anticipatory grieving related to potentially poor prognosis
Ineffective coping (potential for, individual) related to advanced disease state

Interventions for all patients with a diagnosis of cancer
- Give nonjudgmental explanation of alternatives *to enable patient to select option consistent with values and expectations.*
- Use objective, factual materials such as reports *to enable patient to select option consistent with values and expectations.*
- Encourage patient to discuss options with family or significant others *to enable patient to select option consistent with values and expectations.*
- Provide sufficient time for making decisions.
- Help patient identify previously helpful coping skills *to use in present situation.*
- Teach patient newer coping skills *to add to choices.*
- Deal with distorted perceptions and misinformation *to dispel misconceptions.*
- Encourage patient's use of such comfort measures as music, religious practices, and presence of family and friends *to distract self from focusing on fears.*
- Provide information as appropriate to the patient's level of readiness to learn.
- Initiate referral, as appropriate, for outside services in the home such as home care nursing and hospice.
- Initiate referral, as appropriate, for psychosocial support (social worker, support group) to the patient and family *to deal with this potentially life-threatening disease.*

EVALUATION/PATIENT OUTCOMES

Coping Assistance: Course of action is selected and implemented. Patient expresses that informed decision is consistent with personal values. Patient is able to focus on need for further treatment and/or follow-up. Concerns are refocused toward resuming activities of daily living.

Psychologic Comfort Promotion

NURSING ASSESSMENT

Psychosocial status: Expressed fears of loss of physical functioning (activities of daily living, sexual, bladder, communication); pain, death, nature of disease, abandonment; restlessness; withdrawal

PATIENT PROBLEMS/NURSING DIAGNOSES AND INTERVENTIONS

NIC PSYCHOLOGIC COMFORT PROMOTION

Fear related to nature of cancer; pain; death; abandonment; loss of physical and mental functioning

Interventions for all cancer patients

- Validate sources of fear with patient *to guide therapeutic interventions.*
- Assist patient to identify coping skills used successfully in the past *to facilitate problem solving.*
- Encourage patient to ask questions and express feelings *to relieve anxiety and help patient put thoughts into perspective.*
- Encourage patient to talk about specific fears and feelings about fears *to help patient clarify what fears are.*
- Provide accurate information about control of physical functioning, sexuality, control of pain, and prognosis *to decrease patient's fears.*
- Analyze patient's appetite, sleep patterns, and activity level *to determine etiology (physiologic or psychologic).*
- Assess presence and quality of support system *to determine if there are persons available to assist patient.*
- Monitor changes in patient's communication with others (e.g., silence or withdrawal), *which may indicate anger or depression.*
- Encourage patient to use physical expression of fears *because physical activity can be used as a way of expressing fears and anger.*
- Assist patient in identifying information, support groups, and other resources of value *to solve problems that cause patient to be fearful.*

EVALUATION/PATIENT OUTCOMES

Psychologic Comfort Promotion: Fears have been reduced. Concerns are refocused toward resuming activities of daily living. Patient acknowledges fears of loss of control of physical functioning (activities of daily living, sexual, bowel, bladder, communication), potential for suffering, death, but concerns are refocused toward resuming activities of daily living.

PATIENT EDUCATION/CONTINUUM OF CARE PLAN[19A]

Blood Component Therapy

Ensure that the patient and/or significant other knows and understands the following:

Importance of maintaining position of extremity during transfusion

Importance of reporting symptoms of reaction: rash, flushed feeling, chills, shortness of breath, chest pain

Importance of not changing the flow rate

Chemotherapy and Biologic Therapy

1. With help of audiovisual aids, explain how drugs work and expected therapeutic effects of chemotherapy/biotherapy treatment.
2. Provide patient and/or significant other(s) with written material regarding name of drug, action of drug, and potential side effects.
3. Explain method, frequency, and duration of administration of each drug.
4. Provide verbal and written material regarding management of side effects/toxicity.
5. Instruct patient regarding early side effects, such as nausea and vomiting, and side effects that will be delayed such as myelosuppression.
6. Discuss side effects that are reversible.
7. Instruct patient regarding side effects to report to physician.
8. Give written information on how and where to reach health care personnel if necessary.
9. Involve significant other(s) in care planning as much as possible.
10. Assess patient's ability to provide for own physical and daily living needs; arrange home health providers as needed.
11. Assess availability of transportation to follow-up appointments; assist with arrangements as needed.
12. Facilitate patient joining a community support group for continuing psychosocial and emotional counseling and support.
13. Plan for sufficient, clean space for storage of medical supplies.
14. Arrange for durable medical equipment as needed.

Radiation Therapy

External Radiation/Teletherapy

1. Explain radiation therapy procedures and pretreatment and posttreatment events.
2. Explain the need for time, distance, and shielding precautions.
3. Explain the need to avoid persons with infections, especially URIs.
4. Discuss symptoms of infection to report to physician.
   a. Cold, flu, elevated temperature
   b. Diarrhea and frequency of or burning on urination
   c. Reddened, painful skin areas
   d. Mouth redness, swelling, ulceration, bleeding, increased salivation
5. Emphasize importance of maintaining nutritious diet and fluid intake to 3000 ml/day unless contraindicated.
   a. Take six to eight small meals daily.
   b. Avoid eating immediately before or after treatment.
6. Explain that radiation effects continue for 10 to 14 days after last treatment; tell patient signs of healing will not be seen until 18 to 21 days after last treatment.
7. Explain the need for daily oral hygiene—in the morning, after meals, and at bedtime—to keep mouth fresh and clean.
8. Discuss the following symptoms to report to physician.
   a. Mucositis
   b. Nausea and vomiting
   c. Inability to eat
   d. Increasing headache or tiredness
   e. Severe diarrhea
   f. Increasing redness, swelling, pain, or pruritus at site of therapy
9. Emphasize importance of follow-up outpatient care.
10. Teach name of medication, dosage, time of administration, purpose, and side effects.
11. Explain need to avoid taking over-the-counter medications without physician approval.
12. Assess ability to provide for own physical care and daily living needs; arrange home-health providers as needed.
13. Assess availability of transportation to follow-up appointments; assist with arrangements as necessary.

14. Plan for sufficient, clean storage space for medical supplies.

Internal Radiation/Brachytherapy (Implants)

1. Explain that patient is not a source of danger from radioactivity to family or others if precautions are followed.
2. Discuss importance of continued activity balanced with periods of rest *to enhance well-being.*
3. Stress importance of continuing follow-up care with physician.

Gynecologic implants

1. Discuss methods *to eliminate constipation prn.*
2. Instruct patient to notify physician of vaginal bleeding (slight spotting is expected).
3. Discuss signs and symptoms of UTI to report.
4. Instruct patient to use water-soluble lubricant during intercourse (when physician approves resumed sexual activity).
5. Instruct patient in use of vaginal dilator prn.

Prostate implants

1. Instruct patient to strain all urine for dislodged seeds (small radioactive seeds are implanted).
2. Instruct patient in safe retrieval of seeds with tweezers and foil, need to return to radiation therapy physician.
3. Instruct patient to report changes in urine elimination pattern and/or hematuria.
4. Instruct patient to wear condoms during sexual activity.

Head and neck implants

Instruct patient to report increased difficulty swallowing or controlling secretions to physician.

General

1. Patient is no longer a source of radiation exposure once discharged; however, if seeds are implanted, pregnant women and young children should stay several feet away for first 2 months.
2. Assess patient's ability to provide for own physical and daily living needs; arrange home health providers prn.
3. Assess availability of transportation to follow-up appointments; assist with arrangements as necessary.

REFERENCES

Chapter opener illustration from Ignatavicius DD, Workman ML, Mishler MA: *Medical-surgical nursing across the health care continuum,* ed 3, vol 1, Philadelphia, 1999, WB Saunders.

1. American Cancer Society: *Cancer facts and figures,* The Society, *www.cancer.org.,* 2001.
2. Baird SB et al: *Cancer nursing: a comprehensive textbook,* ed 2, Philadelphia, 1996, WB Saunders.
3. Bender CM, Yasko JM, Strohl RA: Nursing management: cancer. In Lewis C, Heitkemper M, Dirksen S, editors: *Medical-surgical nursing,* ed 5, St. Louis, 2000, Mosby.
4. Brock D: Male genital cancers. In Varricchio M et al, editors: *A cancer source book for nurses,* ed 7, Atlanta, 1997, American Cancer Society.
5. Camp-Sorrell D: *Access device guidelines: recommendations for nursing and education,* Pittsburgh, 1996, Oncology Nursing Press.
6. Carew JF, Shah JP: Advances in multimodal therapy for laryngeal cancer, *CA Cancer J Clin* 48:211-228, 1998.
7. Di Saia PJ, Creasman WT: *Clinical gynecologic oncology,* ed 5, St. Louis, 1997, Mosby.

7a. Dirksen SR, Lewis SM: Nursing management: breast disorders. In Lewis C, Heitkemper M, Dirksen S, editors: *Medical-surgical nursing,* ed 5, St. Louis, 2000, Mosby.

7b. Elrod R: Nursing management: Liver, biliary tract, and pancreas problems. In Lewis C, Heitkemper M, Dirken S, editors: *Medical-surgical nursing,* ed 5, St. Louis, 2000, Mosby.

8. Ernst E, Cassileth BR: The prevalence of complementary/alternative medicine in cancer: a systematic review, *Cancer* 83:777-782, 1998.
9. Groen KA: Primary and metastatic liver cancer, *Semin Oncol Nurs* 15:48-57, 1999.
10. Groenwald SL et al: *Cancer nursing: principles and practice,* ed 4, Boston, 1997, Jones & Bartlett.
11. Harwood KV: Non-small cell lung cancer: an overview of diagnosis, staging, and treatment, *Semin Oncol Nurs* 14:285-294, 1996.

11a. Hickey MM, Hoffman LA: Nursing management: upper respiratory problems. In Lewis C, Heitkemper M, Dirksen S, editors: *Medical-surgical nursing,* ed 5, St. Louis, 2000, Mosby.

12. Lind J: Urinary tract cancers. In Varrichio C et al, editors: *A cancer source book for nurses,* ed 7, Atlanta, 1997, American Cancer Society.
13. Lynch HT, Fusaro RM, Lynch JF: Cancer genetics in the new era of molecular biology, *Ann NY Acad Sci* 833:1-28, 1997.
14. Martin VR, Comis RL: Small cell lung cancer: an "updated" overview, *Semin Oncol Nurs* 14:295-302, 1996.

14a. National Cancer Institute, *www.cancernet.nci.nih.gov,* 2001.

15. Otto SE: *Oncology nursing,* ed 3, St. Louis, 1997, Mosby.
16. Owens B: Central nervous cancer. In Varricchio C et al, editors: *A cancer source book for nurses,* ed 7, Atlanta, 1997, American Cancer Society.
17. Peters J, Dimond E, Jenkins J: Clinical applications of genetic technologies to cancer, *Cancer Nurs* 20:359-377, 1997.
18. Saddler DA, Ellis C: Colorectal cancer, *Semin Oncol Nurs* 15:58-69, 1999.
19. Sauter PK, Coleman J: Pancreatic cancer: a continuum of care, *Semin Oncol Nurs* 15:36-47, 1999.

19a. Tucker M et al: *Patient care standards,* ed 7, St. Louis, 2000, Mosby.

19b. U.S. Preventive Services Task Force: *Guide to clinical preventive services,* ed 2, Baltimore, 1996, Williams & Wilkens.

20. USP DI/Micromedex: *Oncology drug information,* ed 3, Versailles, 2000, World Color Book Services.
21. Walczak JR, editor: Gynecologic cancers, *Semin Oncol Nurs* 6(3):190-198, 206-214, 1990.

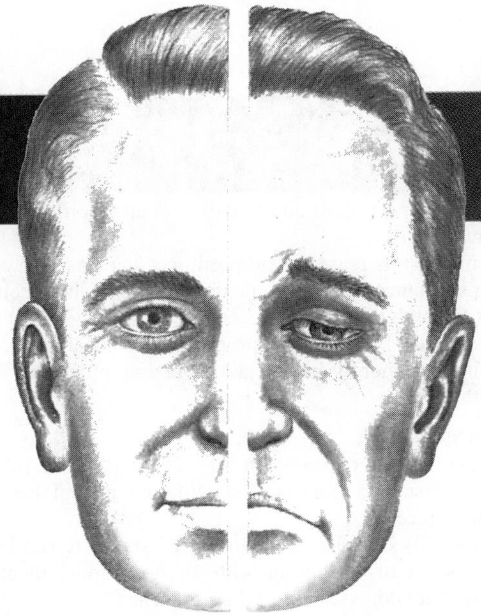

19 Mental Health

Georgia Griffith Whitley
Kim Hart

OVERVIEW

Mental health is an elusive concept with diverse definitions. Not all theorists identify the same personality traits as indicators of healthy functioning, but their definitions are not necessarily contradictory. The diversity is related to the complexity of human beings and the beliefs each theorist has about human nature. Theorists recognize that biologic, social, cultural, and psychologic influences all contribute to healthy personality functioning, but each theorist emphasizes one dimension over the others.

Characteristics of healthy personality functioning compiled from psychoanalytic, interpersonal, and cognitive theories include positive self-identity; awareness of oneself as a psychologically separate individual; responsibility for oneself and one's own actions; acceptance of emotions and ability to correct faulty ones; constructive use of cognitive processes; achievement of satisfying interpersonal relationships; and autonomy, which includes use of self-supports; and flexibility to adapt to change. The list is not exhaustive, and characteristics are not in order of importance, but all are indicators of mental health. When personality growth and development go awry because of genetic, psychologic, social, cultural, or biologic influences, the person may become mentally ill. A mental illness is often further complicated by physical consequences, posing terrific challenges for the nurse. Characteristics of the nurse, essential to successful interaction and therapy for the person with mental illness, are empathy, warmth, genuine concern, respect, ability to communicate, immediate and constructive confrontation that supports behavioral changes, and occasional self-disclosure relevant to the concerns and interests of the patient.[47] Topics that are integral to current clinical practice are discussed in this chapter. It is important to note that each psychiatric diagnosis is representative of a specific set of symptoms or a syndrome. Each individual presents a unique expression of the disorder. Some psychiatric disorders may overlap, or coexist, resulting in more than one diagnosis. Topical areas discussed in this chapter include eating disorders, substance use/dependence, schizophrenia, mood disorders, anxiety disorders, personality disorders, sleep disorders, suicide, crisis, and violence.

CONDITIONS, DISEASES, AND DISORDERS

EATING DISORDERS

Eating disorders are characterized by a persistent pattern of aberrant eating or dieting behavior. Specifically, the behaviors include extreme restriction of food intake or bingeing, sometimes associated with purging. These patterns of eating behaviors are associated with significant emotional, physical, and relational sequelae. An estimated 5 million people in the United States are affected by eating disorders each year. The majority of eating disorders affect females between the ages of 12 and 20. These disorders can be difficult to differentiate from normal variations in eating patterns. Although effective treatments are available, as many as 50% of persons with eating disorders do not disclose symptoms and may even conceal them.[13] Suicide occurs in 2% of the eating-disorder population.[23,24,41] Diagnoses are generally made by clinicians on the basis of specific criteria from the *Diagnostic and Statistical Manual of Mental Disorders* (DSM-IV).[5,78] The three general categories of eating disorders are **anorexia nervosa, bulimia nervosa,** and **binge eating disorder.** A major issue in eating disorders is attaining a sense of control of the self and of the environment.[5,41,78] Through dieting and weight loss these persons believe they will experience control, autonomy, and competence.

PATHOPHYSIOLOGY/PSYCHOPATHOLOGY

Eating is a source of anxiety for persons with anorexia nervosa or bulimia nervosa. Some persons with anorexia never engage in binge eating and purging because of a strong self-discipline; those with binge/purging behaviors are more likely to exhibit

HEALTHY PEOPLE 2010

Health Status—Mental Health and Mental Disorders

Goal: Improve mental health and ensure access to appropriate, quality mental health services.

Mental Health Status Improvement

- Reduce the suicide rate.
- Reduce the rate of suicide attempts by adolescents.
- Reduce the proportion of homeless adults who have serious mental illness (SMI).
- Increase the proportion of persons with SMI who are employed.
- (Developmental) Reduce the relapse rates for persons with eating disorders including anorexia nervosa and bulimia nervosa.

Treatment Expansion

- (Developmental) Increase the number of persons seen in primary health care who receive mental health screening and assessment.
- (Developmental) Increase the proportion of children with mental health problems who receive treatment.
- (Developmental) Increase the proportion of juvenile justice facilities that screen new admissions for mental health problems.
- Increase the proportion of adults with mental disorders who receive treatment.
- (Developmental) Increase the proportion of persons with co-occurring substance abuse and mental disorders who receive treatment for both disorders.
- (Developmental) Increase the proportion of local governments with community-based jail diversion programs for adults with SMI.

State Activities

- Increase the number of states and the District of Columbia that track consumers' satisfaction with the mental health services they receive.
- (Developmental) Increase the number of states, territories, and the District of Columbia with an operational mental health plan that addresses cultural competence.
- Increase the number of states, territories, and the District of Columbia with an operational mental health plan that addresses mental health crisis interventions, ongoing screening, and treatment services for elderly persons.

Modified from U.S. Department of Health and Human Services: *Healthy people 2010* (conference edition, in two volumes), Washington, DC, January 2000.

NOTE: *Developmental* indicates that criteria for measurement and strategies to improve health have not as yet been specified.

impulse, out-of control, and chaotic behaviors, and some have substance use problems.

As the disorders develop, personal relationships tend to become more superficial and distant. Social contacts are avoided because of the fear of being invited to eat and being discovered; purging is also performed out of view of others. The patients are preoccupied with food, meal planning (especially for others), their own caloric intake throughout the day, and methods to avoid eating. Eating, whether it is normal, in tiny quantities, or as much as 10,000 calories, becomes a private endeavor rather than a socially enjoyable activity. The model child, who is a high achiever and a people pleaser, becomes defiant, aggressive, and irritable when the anorexic or bulimic pattern becomes well ingrained.

Anorexia that develops in prepubertal children can have severe and irreversible physical consequences. Growth may be interrupted and can result in short stature if starvation is not reversed before the closure of the epiphyses. Delayed puberty can result in sterility and even incomplete development of secondary sex characteristics. Children and adolescents can be more difficult to diagnose than adults because of the wide variability in the rate, timing, and magnitude of both height and weight gain during puberty. They may present with failure to make expected weight gains during a period of growth in height. Children may become more rapidly emaciated because of differences in fat distribution, making smaller weight loses more significant. Since determination of expected weight gain can be difficult, some clinicians use a measure of body mass index (BMI) to assess body size of children and adolescents.[90]

Researchers have found that disturbances in brain neurotransmitters such as serotonin, dopamine, norepinephrine, and the endogenous opioids are present in anorexia and bulimia. Impaired functioning of neurotransmitters can affect behavior including eating behaviors. It is unknown whether some disturbances in the neurotransmitters and other hormonal and neuroendocrinologic abnormalities reflect an underlying biologic abnormality or are secondary to the eating disorders.[78]

Eating disorders, such as anorexia nervosa and bulimia nervosa, should be differentiated from other mental disorders, such as depression, schizophrenia, hysteria, obsessive-compulsive disorder, and substance abuse. In these disorders weight loss does not involve a fundamental drive for thinness; instead weight loss occurs because the person has a lack of interest in food, has a fear of germs, or experiences delusions. However, secondary psychopathologic factors such as depression, anxiety, and obsessive-compulsive disorder can accompany the eating disorders. It is also possible that some secondary psychopathologic conditions are due to the effects of starvation rather than specifically to bulimia or anorexia.

Physiologic disorders can also be differentiated from eating disorders based on information gleaned from the patient's history, physical examination, and laboratory and other tests. Physiologic conditions include chronic wasting caused by tumors and hypothalamic diseases and endocrine disorders such as thyroid abnormalities, diabetes mellitus, Addison's disease, gastrointestinal disorders, and malignancies. Persons with eating disorders generally do not seek treatment from a physician concerning weight loss; they usually complain about medical disorders such as amenorrhea or gastrointestinal, sleep, and concentration disturbances. Occasionally they seek treatment for emotional disorders.

The onset of anorexia nervosa and bulimia nervosa occurs primarily in adolescents and young adults and rarely in persons over age 40 years. The disorders occur predominantly in industrialized societies such as Europe, Japan, Australia, and the United States, where food is abundant and thin bodies are ideal.[13] This phenomenon has been referred to as a *maladaption of societal cultural beliefs and practice.* Cultural beliefs about female beauty seem to have resulted in eating disorders, threatening the fertility, physical heath, and even the life of affected individuals.[10] Eating disorders were thought to occur mainly in whites, formerly almost exclusively in the upper social classes; now they also occur in other ethnic groups and other socioeconomic levels. Persons who have first-degree biologic relatives with eating disorders are at greater risk for the disorders.

The psychologic profile of a person with anorexia nervosa is a young girl who displays a negative self-worth, perfectionism, and possibly obsessive-compulsive personality disorder. Her parents may have eating disorders or be preoccupied with dieting. In the home, adverse comments made by family members about eating, appearance, or weight may also be a factor. The profile of a person with bulimia nervosa is one who tends to have been obese as a child with obese parents. Typically, this person is female, and she may have experienced early menarche. The tendency toward obesity in childhood brings about social consequences and often encourages dieting, which may lead to bulimic behavior. Substance abuse is common in these persons, and it may be a parental issue as well.[33,41]

Various theories regarding the cause of eating disorders exist. **Psychoanalytic theory** emphasizes the relationship between weight control in anorexia nervosa and the desire to minimize or suppress sexual development and adult sexuality. Some theorists point out the strong perfectionistic tendencies of persons with this disorder, as well as the frequent co-occurrence of obsessive-compulsive tendencies or disorder as a related causative factor. **Cognitive and behavioral theorists** point to the media images of thinness as the model for acceptable body image. Significant abnormalities have been identified in all major **neuroendocrine pathways and neurotransmitter systems** of persons with anorexia.[78] Twin studies showing that when one twin has anorexia, the other identical twin has a higher rate of anorexia than in fraternal twins suggest a **genetic predisposition** to anorexia.[106] In considering the various theories of causation, the question of whether the identified factors are causative of or resultant from anorexia nervosa must be considered.

Treatment of persons with eating disorders occurs mainly in outpatient settings. A team approach is used to attend to both psychologic and physical disturbances brought on by weight loss and altered eating patterns. The team usually consists of a pediatrician or an internist, a nutritionist, a psychotherapist, and a psychiatrist. A variety of therapies are used, often in combination. Therapies typically include individual and group cognitive behavior treatment, family therapy, psychoeducational group treatment, nutritional therapy, and pharmacotherapy. Innovative nurse therapists may be involved in meal therapy, a process of treating patients within the psychosocial context of a family meal in the patient's home.[41]

Inpatient treatment programs have largely closed as a result of poor insurance reimbursement. Hospitalization may occur when a person with anorexia nervosa or bulimia nervosa shows evidence of severe medical or psychologic complications (see Emergency Alert box, p. 1246). The patient may deny being in any physical danger or deny the need for hospitalization, even when emaciated. Psychiatric evaluation and assessment of the risk of suicide should be routine because suicidal behavior is not uncommon.[13] To decrease resistance, the protective nature of and the reasons for hospitalization should be emphasized. Patients need to believe that the staff is interested in helping them deal with problems in their lives other than the eating disorder alone. If eating is resisted, high-protein, high-calorie nasogastric tube feedings may be prescribed. A desirable target weight should be discussed with the patient. Daily weight gains of ¼ to ½ pound are generally acceptable for the emaciated patient, and weight stabilization (without binge/purge behaviors) is expected for the patient with bulimia. Patients with severe anorexia nervosa need close supervision when refeeding is started to observe for signs of gastric bloating, edema, and in rare cases, heart failure. Gastrointestinal motor dysfunction as a consequence of malnutrition can cause the refeeding process to be slow.[13] In place of or following acute hospitalization for eating disorders, patients may be treated in intensive outpatient treatment programs, regular outpatient programs, or partial hospitalization programs. The majority of patients in this country are now treated in outpatient settings.[41] This is primarily due to the type of reimbursement available to patients.

Various therapies are available, with psychotherapy ranging from psychoanalytic, cognitive and behavioral, group, and family types. In addition, educational, nutritional, and pharmacologic approaches are used. Nurses play various roles in these therapies and programs. Staff nurses care for patients in the acute medical and psychiatric settings and may participate in or manage outpatient programs. Advanced practice nurses may function as primary care providers for persons or groups or as managers of programs.

ANOREXIA NERVOSA

Anorexia nervosa is a formidable eating disorder in which preoccupation with dieting and thinness leads to excessive weight loss.

These individuals exhibit an intense fear of gaining weight and a significant disturbance in perception of body shape and size. The National Institute of Mental Health estimates the lifetime prevalence of anorexia nervosa in women to be 0.5%, with most cases occurring in adolescent and young adult women.[78] The prevalence among men is about one tenth that among women. Even after treatment, approximately 30% to 50% of persons relapse, requiring repeated hospitalizations.

Diagnostic criteria included in the DSM-IV[5] are as follows:

1. Body weight less than 85% of that expected for age and height.
2. Failure to make expected weight gain during period of growth (puberty), leading to body weight less than 85% of that expected.
3. Denial of ill health related to low body weight and fear of gaining weight.
4. Absence of at least three consecutive menstrual cycles.

   NOTE: Amenorrhea is diagnosed when a woman's menstrual cycle occurs only after hormone administration (estrogen).

The diagnosis of anorexia nervosa includes two subtypes of the disorder that describe two behavioral patterns.

Persons with the **restricting type** maintain their low body weight by restricting food intake, fasting, or sometimes by excessive exercising. Persons with the **binge eating/purging type** regularly engage in episodes of bingeing and purging with intermittent periods of restricting food. Purging is accomplished through self-induced vomiting or the misuse of emetics, laxatives, diuretics, or enemas. Some individuals may not binge eat but may purge after the consumption of small amounts of food. Physical characteristics and consequences of anorexia nervosa include amenorrhea (resulting from abnormally low serum levels of estrogen), hypotension, bradycardia, hypothermia, dry skin, hypercarotenemia (pale yellow-red pigmentation of the skin, pseudojaundice), lanugo, acrocyanosis (hands and sometimes feet are persistently cold, blue, and sweaty), atrophy of the breasts, prolonged QT interval, bone loss (assessed by bone densitometry), hypoglycemia, hyponatremia (possibly resulting from increased water intake), lethargy, and constipation.[5,13,41] Mortality rates for anorexia nervosa are significant. Persons suffering from this disorder have a mortality rate of 6% to 7% after 10 years and 18% to 20% after 20 to 30 years.[23,40]

Bulimia Nervosa

Persons suffering with bulimia nervosa regularly engage in discrete periods of overeating followed by attempts to compensate by purging (vomiting that is self-induced or by use of emetics, or by misuse of laxatives, enemas, or diuretics). The bingeing and purging behavior is often followed by intense feelings of guilt and shame.

The person with bulimia may not be visibly underweight and may even be slightly overweight. A typical binge involves discrete eating of amounts of food definitely in excess of what most persons would eat under similar circumstances. The prevalence of bulimia nervosa is estimated to be between 3% and 8%.[5,13,36,41]

Diagnostic criteria included in the DSM-IV[5] are as follows:

1. Recurrent episodes of binge eating followed by compensatory behaviors of:
   Purging, method used by 80% to 90% of persons with bulimia
   Use of laxatives or diuretics
   Excessive exercise
   These behaviors must occur at least twice a week for 3 months or longer.
2. Binge eating in secrecy characterized by rapid consumption of food sometimes in excess of 10,000 calories. There is a sense of lack of control over eating during the episode.
3. Self-evaluation reveals an excessive emphasis on body shape and size, a desire to lose weight, and a fear of gaining weight.

The diagnosis of bulimia nervosa includes two subtypes of the disorder that describe two behavioral patterns. The **purging type** of person describes regular self-induced vomiting or the misuse of laxatives, diuretics, or enemas during the current episode. The **non–purging type** of person uses different inappropriate compensatory behaviors, such as fasting or excessive exercise after bingeing, during the current episode. Physical characteristics and consequences of bulimia include normal or slightly overweight, depressive symptoms or mood disorder, substance use, hypokalemia, hyponatremia and hypochloremia (metabolic alkalosis, elevated serum bicarbonate), diarrhea and metabolic acidosis (prolonged and frequent use of laxatives), loss of dental enamel and increased frequency of cavities, enlarged parotid and salivary glands, scars or calluses on the dorsal surface of the hand (hand used to induce vomiting), menstrual irregularity, esophageal tears, gastric rupture (rare), and cardiac arrhythmia.[5,13,51] The long-term outcome for persons suffering from bulimia is unknown. The mortality rate for bulimia nervosa is estimated to be 0% to 3%.[51]

> **! EMERGENCY ALERT**
>
> **EATING DISORDERS**
> **ANOREXIA NERVOSA AND BULIMIA NERVOSA**
> - Dehydration and fluctuating electrolyte imbalances can lead to cardiac arrhythmias and sudden death.
>
> **BULIMIA NERVOSA**
> - Obesity can lead to hypertension, hyperlipidemia, elevated cholesterol, diabetes, gallbladder disease, and cancer, which cause disabilities and death.

Binge Eating Disorder

Binge eating disorder is a term used to describe compulsive, uncontrolled eating. The term was officially introduced in 1992 and is used to describe persons who engage in frequent eating binges consuming large amounts of food, but unlike persons with bulimia, do not purge after eating.

Binge eating disorder is often associated with obesity. Binges are followed by intense feelings of guilt and shame. Up to 40% of persons who are obese are thought to be binge eaters. Binge eating disorder is not an officially recognized eating disorder in the DSM-IV, but it is included in the category titled "Eating Disorders Not Otherwise Specified." Physical characteristics and consequences of binge eating disorder include weight fluctuations, obesity, hypertension, high cholesterol, heart disease, diabetes, gallbladder disease, and depression/antisocial behavior.

Diagnostic Studies and Findings

Computerized tomography (CT scan), magnetic resonance imaging (MRI): To screen for intracranial tumors and other brain lesions

Complete blood count: To screen for anemia and infections

Sequential multiple analyzer with computer (SMAC): To screen for abnormalities; if electrolytes are abnormal, repeat electrolyte tests once a day until stable

Serum thyroid-stimulating hormone (TSH), serum thyroxine (T_4), and serum triiodothyronine (T_3): To rule out abnormal thyroid function

Electrocardiogram: To screen for anomalies

Chest x-ray examination: To assess lung and heart conditions

Urinalysis: To screen for urinary and systemic abnormalities

Bone density test: To assess bone loss

MULTIDISCIPLINARY PLAN

Medications[13]

Fluoxetine (Prozac), 60 mg/day PO for bulimia nervosa even without depression
Desipramine, up to 300 mg/day
Imipramine, up to 300 mg/day
Vitamin supplementation
Calcium, 1000-1500 mg/day
Multivitamin (including 400 IU vitamin D)

General Management

Outpatient or inpatient care with multidisciplinary care team including internist, nutritionist, nurse therapist, psychotherapist, and psychiatrist
Individual counseling, group therapy, family therapy
Consultation with dietitian to provide diet in divided feedings progressing in caloric content and texture of food based on patient's tolerance
Nutrition therapy with high-protein, high-calorie nasogastric tube feedings if indicated by condition

NURSING CARE

NURSING ASSESSMENT

Signs and symptoms of anorexia, bulimia, and binge eating disorders vary from person to person; no one experiences all of those listed.

Eating patterns: Times and amounts eaten, food preferences, and concerns about eating

Emotional status: Anxiety, depression, lability of mood, irritability, anger; previous and current coping skills, including substance abuse; capacity for dealing with events and relationships; feelings about self and body; sense of lack of control about treatment plan; sense of helplessness in relation to life

Thought processes: Denial of hunger; fear of eating and weight gain; mistrust of self and others; low self-esteem; shame at being discovered bingeing and purging; sense of failure even when successful; perfectionism; rejection of feminine role; fear of psychosexual maturation; fear of physical changes, especially the development of secondary sexual traits; lack of interest in sex and opposite sex; impairment in concentration and cognition

Family: Knowledge of eating disorders and interactions with patient

Physical Assessment

Associated with anorexia
- Malnourished appearance
- Dulled reflexes
- Hypotension
- Decreased body temperature
- Hair loss
- Loss of muscle mass

Associated with bulimia
- Loss of skin turgor; dehydration
- Persistent vomiting; bloody vomitus
- Tooth decay

POTENTIAL COMPLICATIONS

Cardiac arrhythmias; death; self-destructive behavior

PATIENT PROBLEMS/NURSING DIAGNOSES & INTERVENTIONS

Nursing care should be implemented selectively based on severity and type of symptoms and behaviors.

NIC NUTRITION SUPPORT

Imbalanced nutrition: less than body requirements, related to distorted drive for thinness and distorted body image and inability to ingest or digest foods or absorb nutrients due to biologic, psychologic, or economic factors

- Have dietitian discuss nutritional plan and rationale and body's nutritional needs and provide appropriate nutritional counseling.[15] Encourage patient (as able) to assume responsibility for planning well-balanced meals *to increase sense of control and decrease anxiety about eating.*
- If patient has been on starvation diet, be alert for gastric dilation if refeeding is rapid. To prevent this, a 1200- to 1500-calorie, liquid diet (e.g., Ensure), divided into frequent feedings, may be prescribed initially.
- Inform patient that abdominal discomfort or bloating will be experienced with increased food intake and symptoms will disappear. Encourage patient to eat slowly *to learn to taste and enjoy food.*
- *To prevent vomiting,* permit patient's use of bathroom only if accompanied by staff for 1 to 2 hours after eating.
- Explain nasogastric feedings and rationale in matter-of-fact yet sensitive, supportive manner *to decrease loss-of-control feelings.* (Nasogastric feedings may be prescribed if patient does not gain weight or electrolyte balance is viewed as unsafe.) After each instillation of high-protein, high-calorie fluid (e.g., Ensure), observe patient for at least 30 minutes *to prevent vomiting.* If patient is willing, allow drinking of food instead of instilling it in tube.
- As patient begins to gain weight or stabilize weight, help patient deal with anxiety (which sometimes reaches panic level). Remain with patient (especially when eating), and demonstrate slow, deep relaxation breathing *to decrease anxiety.* Reinforce relaxation technique.
- Administer medication as prescribed. Explain purpose of medication and its effects and side effects *to increase compliance with treatment.*
- Explain that, as caloric intake is increased, the amount will not make patient fat *to assure patient that metabolism is slowed as a protective mechanism during a starvation diet.*
- Avoid power struggles over food to prevent reenactment of food struggles at home.
- Encourage good oral hygiene *to prevent oral disease from vomiting and malnutrition.*
- Begin to help patient identify role low weight plays in patient's life *(e.g., as way of avoiding dealing with frightening adolescent and adult issues).* Continue to explore meaning of weight loss, expectation and reality of weight loss, and restrictions in areas of life resulting from preoccupation with food *to increase self-awareness.*

- Monitor patient's weight as prescribed, but prevent patient from indiscriminate frequent self-weighing. Remain nonjudgmental about weight gains and losses. (Weight monitoring will continue with less frequency.)
- When appropriate, encourage participation in occupational therapy *to develop skills and learn to view tasks as enjoyable.*
- Encourage patient to implement and evaluate new behaviors *to determine appropriateness of choices.*
- Discuss with patient how to meet own needs *to develop self-support and how to ask others to meet needs rather than meeting only theirs to develop social support.*
- As patient is physically able, encourage participation in occupational therapy *to learn skills and to engage in enjoyable activities.*
- Help patient begin to identify and reinforce strengths. Help patient assess abilities and accomplishments realistically, using problem-solving approach. Encourage acceptance of abilities and choices patient makes *to begin to feel positive about self and to develop realistic self-expectations, including an acceptance of limitations and mediocre performance.*
- Encourage patient to wear loose clothing *to avoid focus on body size and weight.* Encourage patient to give "skinny" wardrobe away *to avoid longing for thinness and relapsing.* Suggest new lifestyle for patient in nonthreatening way.
- Begin to correct patient's distorted perceptions about body size. Assist patient in perceiving body size correctly and accepting appearance.
- Encourage patient to accept positive self-appraisals and take pride in appearance.
- As female patient gains more mature-appearing body or stabilization of weight, explore meaning of sexuality and feminine role *to assist in dealing with sexual identity issues including menses.*
- Encourage self-acceptance.

NIC BEHAVIOR THERAPY

Powerlessness related to lifestyle of helplessness

- Convey to patient that treatment plan is developed to help and protect and not to control.
- Encourage patient to drink at least 2000 ml of fluid (variety of fluids, not just water) per day for proper hydration. Monitor and record intake and output.

NIC COPING ASSISTANCE

Ineffective coping related to dysfunctional cognitions and maladaptive behaviors

Disturbed body image related to cognitive perception

- Begin to develop safe, trusting relationship with patient *to promote security.* Continue to develop relationship through working and termination phases.
- Explain treatment plan explicitly *to allay anxiety and decrease resistance.* Review plan with patient and invite participation at regular intervals.
- Assist patient in identifying emotions that precede bingeing and past alternatives to bingeing and fasting.
- Assist patient in identifying and participating in healthy coping strategies such as relaxation techniques, reinterpretation of thoughts and emotions, problem solving, and diversionary activities (e.g., watching television, listening to the radio, talking with friends, reading) *to develop alternatives to dysfunctional eating and to develop enjoyable, relaxing behaviors.*
- If patient denies eating problem, encourage patient to examine difficulties in other areas of life and eventually to relate these to preoccupations with eating *to deal with less anxiety-provoking areas than eating.*
- Help patient begin to identify fears associated with starving, bingeing, and purging *to eventually identify issues dealing with loss of control.*
- Correct misconceptions about bingeing-purging behaviors (e.g., laxatives will not prevent absorption of calories). Assist patient to use problem-solving approach to examine issues and *to assess possible consequences of choices.*
- Encourage patient, when able, to make decisions about the treatment regimen *to provide a sense of control and to increase self-confidence.*
- Begin to role-play with patient about how to become assertive with others and, as able, with parents to share needs with others. Emphasize that patient can assume responsibility for self and is not responsible for happiness or discomfort of others.
- Help patient to practice assertiveness skills, and critique them together *to learn how to assess own behavior realistically.*
- As patient is physically able, encourage participation in recreational therapy *to learn social skills in group activities.*
- Help patient identify wants and needs and choose not to binge and purge or starve.
- Assist patient in developing beginning skills in how to function in ambiguous situations *to learn how to deal with conflict and unclear situations (e.g., by negotiating, assessing importance of issue, or clarifying issue with others).*

NIC LIFE SPAN CARE

Interrupted family processes related to inability to accept or express needs of members.

- Assess family's knowledge of eating disorder and interaction patterns with patient.
- Discourage family from discussing patient's dietary intake, bringing in food, or phoning during mealtimes *to avoid power struggles about eating.*
- Assist parents in understanding illness without blaming each other.
- In family sessions help parents and patient become aware of any unhealthy interactions.
- Help family members begin to alter their interactional patterns as necessary (e.g., by speaking for self only and not for others and by responding to one another's messages) *to foster relationships that encourage autonomy of family members.*

Other related nursing diagnoses: Risk for deficient fluid volume related to imbalanced nutrition and purging

behaviors; risk for impaired skin integrity related to malnutrition; constipation related to laxative abuse and inadequate fiber intake; anxiety related to self-concept; disturbed sleep pattern related to malnourishment; social isolation related to discomfort with others.

Patient Education/Continuum of Care Plan

1. Encourage patient to participate in a self-help eating disorder group.
2. Ensure that patient verbalizes knowledge of problem-solving techniques to correct misconceptions of self and performance.
3. Discuss with patient the need to continue practice of assertiveness skills and techniques to increase a sense of control.
4. Review patient's social and physical activity plans for the time after discharge.
5. Ensure that patient verbalizes an understanding of well-balanced, weight-maintenance diet and of the need for continued contacts with a dietitian regarding diet.
6. Review with patient the adverse effects of starving, bingeing, and purging behaviors.
7. Encourage patient to comply with the medical regimen and with the continued psychotherapy after discharge.

Evaluation/Patient Outcomes

Nutrition Support: Patient establishes healthy eating habits to achieve normal body weight. Patient verbalizes knowledge of maintenance diet and expected average weight. Patient states that preoccupation with food has decreased.

Behavior Therapy: Patient verbalizes an increased sense of control over self. Patient practices beginning assertive behavior skills. Patient views weight-maintenance diet as evidence of self-control.

Coping Assistance: Patient begins to implement problem-solving approach to increase coping ability. Female patient practices problem-solving approach to deal with issues such as the feminine role, sexuality, and social interactions with others. Patient demonstrates a beginning acceptance of body image. Patient verbalizes body size accurately and states a beginning acceptance of a more mature-appearing body. Patient wears clothing that is appropriate for body shape.

Life Span Care: Patient and family demonstrate increased efforts to clarify and resolve issues, verbalize increased satisfaction in interactions, and develop beginning skills in identifying and resolving issues.

SUBSTANCE USE DISORDERS

Substance use disorders are characterized by exposure to chemical substances, including legal and illegal drugs or toxins that lead to abuse.

The 1998 National Household survey on Drug Abuse (NHSDA) reported an estimated 13.6 million people in the United States were current users of illicit drugs.[67] The National Institute on Drug Abuse (NIDA) estimated the total economic cost of drug and alcohol abuse to be $245.7 billion in 1992. The costs included substance abuse treatment (health-care costs) and prevention, lost earnings and costs associated with reduced job productivity, and costs associated with drug-related crime. The U.S. government assumes these costs (46%), as well as drug abusers and their families (44%). The NIDA reports that in 1995 there were nearly 1.9 million admissions to publicly funded substance abuse treatment centers. Of those admissions, 54% were treated for alcohol abuse, and 46% were treated for illicit drug abuse. Men made up about 70% of those in treatment, and women made up about 30%.[74]

Chemical substances can be taken by any route of administration, can affect cognition and mood, and can adversely affect health. Some substances are obtained legally such as over-the-counter and medically prescribed drugs; others are obtained illicitly. A number of terms are used to describe excessive drug use. **Substance abuse** is a term that describes drug-using behavior despite real or potential harm that might result from that drug use. **Intoxication** occurs in both cases of abuse and dependence as a result of exposure to a substance that impairs the person's ability to function psychologically and physically. **Tolerance** refers to an acquired resistance to the effects of a drug. The drug dosage must be increased progressively to reproduce the initial desired physical and psychologic effects. **Withdrawal** is a drug-specific set of symptoms that may cause illness when abruptly stopping the use of that drug, especially after prolonged heavy use. **Drug dependence** is the result of a person's inability to control use of a drug. **Compulsivity** refers to the tendency of persons who are unable to discontinue use of a drug even though intoxicated; that is, they develop behavioral or psychologic changes directed toward obtaining the substance(s) that affect the central nervous system.[5,37]

If the person abstains from use for at least 1 month, he or she may be designated as being in early remission; if the person abstains for 12 months or more, he or she is designated as being in sustained remission. The remission may be "full," meaning the person has met none of the criteria for dependence or abuse, or it may be "partial," meaning the person has not met the full criteria for dependence or abuse, but one or more criteria for dependence have been met.[5]

Substance use and dependence most commonly begin during adolescence and young adulthood. The reasons for becoming involved with chemical substances are many and include influence of peers, rebellion against parents and society, and attempts to bolster self-esteem. Most young adults are able to discontinue use as they take on the responsibilities of adulthood, but some may become chronic abusers and often engage in polydrug abuse.

Substance use disorders may also be associated with relief of pain, especially when pain is severe and chronic, among immature, easily frustrated persons, those with psychic disorders, and those with countercultural lifestyles. Viewing substances as a way of coping with life stresses and experiences is a factor in brief, limited episodes of use to continued chronic use/dependence.[5]

Because chemical substances affect the central nervous system, use/dependence may cause transient or permanent brain dysfunction and other medical problems. Deterioration of physical health is caused in part by malnutrition, poor personal hygiene, and inattention to signs and symptoms of illnesses.

Infections such as hepatitis, tetanus, septicemia, and abscesses can occur from substances administered with contaminated needles and syringes. In addition, the transmission of acquired immunodeficiency syndrome (AIDS) has become an increasing threat to substance users. Because the potency and purity of illicitly obtained substances are seldom known, fatal overdose and toxic reactions occur. The mood-altering effects of substances may cause erratic, impulsive, aggressive, violent, and other irresponsible behaviors that cause problems and injury to the user or to others (see Emergency Alert box). Relationships with family and friends become disturbed and are sometimes severed. Drug habits, including alcohol, drain the financial resources of families. The user may also engage in criminal behaviors to support the substance dependency or violate laws when in an intoxicated drug state (e.g., burglaries, automobile accidents). Changes may occur in occupational, social, interpersonal, and academic functioning. Table 19-1 lists some commonly used types of chemical substances, their uses, and their intoxication and withdrawal effects. Nicotine, cannabis, and alcohol use have been selected for further discussion because of the prevalence of their use.

Nicotine

Use of tobacco products is the leading preventable cause of death in the United States. It is estimated that smoking accounts for at least 30% of all cancer deaths and may account for one of every five deaths each year as a result of a substantially increased risk of cardiovascular disease. The Centers for Disease Control and Prevention (CDC) Tobacco Information and Prevention Source (TIPS) has reported that exposure to second-

Table 19-1 Effects of Intoxication and Withdrawal of Substances

Drug	Usual Route of Administration	Use
OPIATES		
Opium	Oral; sniffed; smoked	Analgesic, antidiarrheatic
Morphine	Oral; injected	Analgesic
Diacetylmorphine (heroin)	Injected; sniffed; smoked	Analgesic (illegal)
Hydromorphone (Dilaudid)	Oral; injected	Analgesic
Meperidine (Demerol)	Oral; injected	Analgesic
Propoxyphene (Darvon)	Oral; injected	Analgesic
Codeine	Oral; injected	Analgesic; antitussive
Methadone	Oral; injected	Detoxification of opiates
DEPRESSANTS		
Alcoholic beverages (e.g., liquor, beer, wine)	Oral	Tension relief; analgesic
Sedative-hypnotics		Anesthetic; anticonvulsant; sedation
Barbiturates		
Amobarbital (Amytal)	Oral; injected	
Secobarbital (Seconal)	Oral; injected	
Pentobarbital (Nembutal)	Oral; injected	
Other		
Meprobamate (Equanil, Miltown)	Oral	Antianxiety; sedation
Diazepam (Valium)	Oral; injected	Antianxiety; anticonvulsant
Glutethimide (Doriden)	Oral	Hypnotic
Chloral hydrate (Noctec and others)	Oral	Hypnotic
STIMULANTS		
Cocaine	Oral; smoked; sniffed; injected	Local anesthetic
Amphetamine (Benzedrine, Dexedrine)	Oral; injected	Narcolepsy; attention deficit disorder, weight control
Phenmetrazine (Preludin)	Oral	Weight control
HALLUCINOGENS		
Lysergic acid diethylamide (LSD)	Oral	None
Phencyclidine (PCP)	Oral; smoked; injected	Animal tranquilizer
Mescaline	Oral	None
Psilocybin	Oral	None
CANNABIS SATIVA		
Marijuana, hashish	Oral; smoked	Stimulant and sedative (illegal drug)

hand smoke is thought to be responsible for approximately 3000 lung cancer deaths per year.[103] Smoking is the most common cause of lung cancer. The chance of developing lung cancer is 25 times greater for heavy smokers than for nonsmokers. Lung cancer is considered an epidemic in the United States. In 1997 there were an estimated 178,100 new cases: 98,300 males and 79,800 females. The death rate from lung cancer is higher in women than any other cancer.[61]

A 1996 National Household Survey on drug abuse reported an estimated 62 million (29%) people in the United States were current smokers and 6.8 million used smokeless tobacco.[70] Among youths ages 12 to 17 years, an estimated 20%, 4.5 million, were current smokers. The prevalence of smoking in U.S. high school students increased from 27.5% in 1991 to 36.4% in 1997.[76] Among adults, men had somewhat higher rates of smoking than women, but rates of smoking were similar for males and females ages 12 to 17 years.

It is estimated that between 80% and 95% of alcoholics smoke cigarettes. Approximately 70% of alcoholics are heavy smokers (more than 30 cigarettes per day), in contrast to just 10% of the general population. Persons who smoke are 10 times more likely to develop alcoholism than are nonsmokers. Alcohol and nicotine are both thought to activate release of dopamine in the brain, which ultimately contributes to reinforcement of addictive behaviors. Furthermore, alcohol and nicotine create a cross-tolerance of adverse effects of these drugs. Alcohol's sedating effects may mitigate aversive effects of nicotine such as increased heart rate, facilitating continued or increased use of tobacco. Conversely, nicotine's stimulating effects can mitigate alcohol-induced loss of mental alertness. The long-term effects of abuse of these two drugs are devastating to the body. There is a dramatically increased risk of developing mouth or throat cancer. Risk of developing cardiovascular disease, lung disease, gastrointestinal (GI) disease and liver disease are increased as well.[68]

Intoxication Effect	Withdrawal Effect
OPIATES	
Euphoria with tranquility; emotional lability; drowsiness; clouding of consciousness; psychomotor retardation; slow, shallow respirations; constricted pupils; decreased muscle tone; with circulatory collapse and cyanosis, dilated pupils; coma; possible death	Runny nose; watery eyes; severe anxiety to panic; gooseflesh; hot and cold flashes; yawning; irritability; loss of appetite; muscle cramps; tremors; nausea and vomiting; tachycardia; hypertension; increased respirations and temperature; insomnia; after 24 hours, diarrhea and dehydration; symptoms peak 48 to 72 hours after last dose
DEPRESSANTS	
Slurred speech; lack of coordination; unsteady gait; talkativeness; euphoria or depression; emotional lability; impaired attention or memory	Hyperactivity; tremors; psychomotor agitation; hypertension; tachycardia; irritability or depression; impaired attention and memory; illusions (misinterpretation of stimuli); hallucination, auditory, tactile, or visual; disorientation; delusions; delirium; orthostatic hypotension; convulsions
Slurred speech; irritability; impaired attention, memory, and judgment; emotional lability; talkativeness; lack of coordination; confusion; tremors; cold, clammy skin; dilated pupils (with barbiturates, constricted pupils)	Nausea and vomiting; weakness; hypertension; tachycardia; orthostatic hypotension; gross tremors; agitation; disorientation; anxiety; nightmares; visual hallucinations; hyperthermia; delirium; convulsions; coma
STIMULANTS	
Euphoria; psychomotor agitation; mood lability; hypervigilance; chest pain; tachycardia; hypertension; dilated pupils; perspiration or chills; impaired judgment; psychotic symptoms; insomnia; tremors; confusion; convulsions; possible death	Fatigue; depression; disturbed sleep; apathy; cravings; possible agitation after prolonged use
HALLUCINOGENS	
Tachycardia; hypertension; hyperthermia; dilated pupils; hyperreflexia; nausea; visual hallucinations; extreme emotional lability; poor time perception; feeling of depersonalization; psychic numbness; psychosis; violent outbursts; amnesia; convulsions; possible death	None reported; flashbacks occur episodically long after use of PCP, with catalepsy, agitation, and unpredictable violent outbursts
CANNABIS SATIVA	
Panic; depression; disorientation; hallucinations; delusions; flashbacks; psychotic symptoms; apathy; impaired attention, judgment, and coordination; increased appetite	Uncertain if clinically significant; irritability; insomnia; loss of appetite; tremors; perspiration; nausea

More than 4000 chemicals are found in the smoke of tobacco products such as cigarettes, cigars, and pipes. Nicotine is the primary component that acts on the brain and is recognized as one of the most frequently used addictive drugs. Since nicotine was identified in the early 1800s, it has been extensively studied and has been shown to have a number of complex and even unpredictable effects on the brain and body. Nicotine has been shown to have an effect on levels of the neurotransmitter dopamine, which is associated with feelings of pleasure. Smokers have been found to have 40% less of a brain enzyme, monoamine oxidase B (MAO B), which is thought to break down dopamine. The pharmacokinetic properties of nicotine increase its abuse potential. Inhalation of smoke containing nicotine produces a rapid distribution of nicotine to the brain and peak drug levels within 10 seconds of inhalation. The acute effects dissipate within a few minutes, causing the smoker to continue dosing frequently to maintain the drug's pleasurable effects.[61,77]

Acute withdrawal from nicotine can elicit a range of symptoms including mood change (irritability, frustration, anger, anxiety), depression, drowsiness, fatigue, restlessness, difficulty concentrating, and increased hunger. Approximately 50% of persons who smoke regularly experience physical withdrawal symptoms when they quit. Established criteria for the diagnosis of nicotine withdrawal are listed in the DSM-IV and include use of nicotine daily for at least several weeks and abrupt reduction or cessation of nicotine use followed by four or more of the following symptoms (within 24 hours): dysphoric or depressed mood; insomnia; irritability, frustration, or anger; anxiety; or difficulty concentrating.

Addiction to nicotine is a chronic disorder. The smoker may attempt to quit several times before being successful. Interventions involving both medications and behavioral treatments are thought to increase cessation rates. The primary medication therapy used to treat nicotine addiction is nicotine replacement. There are four types of nicotine replacement products available. Nicotine gum and nicotine patches are available over the counter. The gum (Nicorette) is available in 2-mg and 4-mg dosages. The higher dose is recommended for heavy smokers (30 or more cigarettes per day). Typically, a person will use up to 15 pieces of gum per day. The recommended dose for nicotine patches is 1-mg per cigarette smoked per day. Nicotine nasal spray and nicotine inhalers are available by prescription. All types of nicotine replacement therapies are equally effective and are thought to double a smoker's chance of successfully stopping. The Food and Drug Administration (FDA) recently approved use of the antidepressant bupropion (Zyban) for individuals having difficulty with symptoms associated with smoking cessation. The nurse's role is important in the education of individuals with nicotine addiction. Any opportunities for education of clients about the treatments to aid in smoking cessation should be taken. In addition to medications such as Zyban or nicotine replacement, acupuncture, hypnosis, and behavioral therapy are sometimes used for nicotine addiction.[27,37,60]

Marijuana

Marijuana is the most commonly used illicit drug in the United States. Data from the 1996 NHSDA reported more than 68.6 million people in the United States (32%) age 12 years and older had tried marijuana at least once in their lifetime, and almost 18.4 million (8.6%) had used marijuana in the last year.[73] Marijuana dependence leads to more than 120,000 people seeking treatment per year for marijuana addiction.

Marijuana is a green or gray mixture of dried shredded flowers and leaves of the hemp plant *Cannabis sativa.* It is typically smoked as a cigarette or in a pipe. Some users also mix marijuana into foods or use it to brew tea. The active chemical in marijuana is Δ-9-tetrahydrocannabinol (THC). Short-term effects of marijuana use include euphoria, difficulties with short-term memory and learning, distorted perception, difficulty with problem solving, loss of coordination, tachycardia, anxiety, and panic attacks. The chemical THC is thought to change the way in which sensory information gets to the hippocampus, a component of the brain's limbic system that is involved in learning, memory, and the integration of sensory experiences. Marijuana smoke is highly irritating to the nasopharynx and the bronchial lining and therefore can increase the risk of chronic cough and lung diseases. Marijuana smoke contains large amounts of known carcinogens and may increase the risk of lung cancer. Marijuana is not regarded as a hallucinogen; however, it is often mixed with other hallucinogenic drugs. The use of this drug is not known to cause physical dependence, although a psychologic compulsive dependence is not uncommon.[5,37,73]

Heroin

Heroin is the most commonly abused drug of the opiate classification. It is illegal, rapid acting, and highly addictive. It is processed from morphine, a naturally occurring substance extracted from the seed of particular varieties of poppy plants. Heroin may be smoked, snorted, or injected, and because street-bought heroin is often mixed with other substances, users who are not certain of the strength commonly overdose. The Drug Abuse Warning Network (DAWN) collects data on drug-related hospital emergency department episodes from 21 metropolitan areas. In 1996 DAWN estimated that 14% of all drug-related emergency department episodes involved heroin.[71] The 1996 National Household Survey on Drug Abuse reported that 2.4 million people had used heroin at some time in their life, and more than 200,00 people were current users. Heroin use has been increasing at all age levels, especially among persons age 12 to 25 years.[71]

A number of medications are used to aid patients in the very difficult withdrawal process. Methadone, a synthetic opiate that blocks the effects of heroin and associated withdrawal symptoms, has been utilized for more than 30 years. A newer medication, levo-α-acetylmethadol (LAAM), also a synthetic opiate, has fewer side effects and is known to block the effects of heroin for up to 72 hours. Naloxone and naltrexone act as heroin antagonists with long-lasting effects ranging from 1 to 3 days. A newer drug, buprenorphine, is awaiting FDA approval and may be even more useful because it does not cause the same level of physical dependence as methadone and other synthetic opiates.[71]

Inhalants

Inhalants are chemical vapors that can be inhaled into the lungs, causing intoxication. They are readily available products that are inexpensive, easily purchased, and most commonly found around the home. The most common substances used include the aliphatic and aromatic hydrocarbons found in gasoline, glue, paint thinners, and spray paints; the halogenated hydrocarbons found in cleaners, typewriter correction fluid, and spray-can propellants; and other volatile compounds containing esters, ketones, and glycol. Often, mixtures of compounds are inhaled. All compounds are capable of producing intoxication, and abuse dependence. A variety of methods are used to inhale chemical vapors, including inhalation from the container or from aerosols sprayed in the mouth or nose and placement of the substance in a plastic bag and inhaling the gases. Also, a rag may be soaked with the substance and then applied to the mouth and nose.

Use of inhalants often starts early in adolescence as a cheap, accessible substitute for alcohol and other drugs. The NHSDA reported that in 1996 5.9% of 1.3 million adolescents (ages 12 to 18 years) reported use of inhalants at least once in their lifetime.[67] A national survey of drug use in 1997 by NIDA showed that use of inhalants was highest in eighth graders (21%), followed by tenth graders (18.3%), and finally twelfth graders (16.1%).[72]

The use of inhalants can produce behavioral and psychologic changes in a person, such as aggressiveness, apathy, and poor judgment, and physical changes, such as dizziness, incoordination, slurred speech, unsteady gait, tremor, weakness, stupor, or coma. The irreversible side effects include hearing loss (toluene paint sprays, glues, dewaxers, trichloroethylene cleaning fluids, correction fluids), peripheral neuropathies or limb spasms (hexane glues, gasoline, nitrous oxide, whipping cream, gas cylinders), central nervous system or brain damage (toluene paint sprays, glues, dewaxers), bone marrow damage (benzene gasoline), and heart failure and death (fluorocarbons, butane-type gases).

The serious but possibly reversible side effects include liver and kidney damage (toluene and chlorinated hydrocarbons, correction fluids, dry-cleaning fluids), and hypoxia (organic nitrates and methylene chloride, varnish removers, paint thinners).[75]

Chemical Dependency Among Nurses

Chemical dependency among nurses is a problem that has received increasing attention and study in the United States. Estimates of incidence of substance abuse among nurses vary between 3% and 20% but are generally thought to mirror the general population.[24,65,87,105] Drug-related disciplinary cases referred to state boards of nursing annually average 62%, with some states being much higher.

There are a number of factors that contribute to substance-related disorders among nurses with above-average performance. These factors include personal and job stress; easy accessibility provided by available drugs on drug carts in the work setting; knowledge of drugs that leads nurses to believe their knowledge protects them from dependency; a focus on the needs of others, often at the expense of meeting personal needs; vulnerability and denial of vulnerability, such as a belief that healers must not be weak; familial risk factors; a history of parental drug or alcohol abuse in childhood; personal or familial depressive illness; and assumption of parental roles by the nurse during childhood. External risk factors include major hospitalization within 5 years before addiction, recent health problems, diagnosis or treatment for mental illness, sexual trauma, lack of knowledge about chemical dependency, graduating in the top third of the nursing class, holding an advanced degree, high degree of respect of peers, and holding a demanding, responsible position.

The chemically dependent nurse may be one who came from a chaotic, even pathologic, family with mental illness or drug and/or alcohol abuse or who has experienced victimization and development of a low self-esteem. In a study of 115 drug-dependent nurses, 51% reported a prior history of mental illness, primarily depression (84%). More than half of the participants of the study reported suffering from abuse (49% refused to comment about victimization) that contributed to development of low self-esteem.[65]

Burns[18] asserted that the chemically dependent nurse focuses on her knowledge of medication and the ability to relieve pain and distress. The nurse may have very little knowledge concerning the addictive nature of medications or substance abuse in general. Furthermore, it was reported that only 57% of nursing programs require curricular content related to substance abuse. The required number of hours ranged from 1 to 5. Coleman et al[24] did a study of drug use in 588 nursing, medical, and pharmacy students entering their respective programs and followed their drug habits over a 3-year period. The study focused primarily on differences in drug use between nursing and pharmacy students. Drug use among nursing students increased over the 3-year period, while pharmacy students remained relatively stable by comparison. The pharmacy students received an entire course on drug and alcohol abuse, and there was a greater emphasis on drug and alcohol education throughout compared with the nursing curriculum, which was deficient in drug and alcohol education.

State nurses' associations began to develop peer assistance programs for nurses in about 1980. Before the assistance programs, impaired nurses were abandoned by employers through dismissals or forced resignations, without referrals for treatment. Nurse managers in some institutions still have a long way to go in terms of supporting chemically dependent nurses and encouraging them to get treatment.[105] Formal assistance programs have been developed in many states to serve as a confidential alternative to the usual disciplinary procedures. The programs serve to guide impaired nurses into treatment and to provide professional and public understanding of the disease through education.

! EMERGENCY ALERT

SUBSTANCE USE DISORDERS

The mood-altering and cognition-altering effects of substance abuse may cause:

- Erratic, aggressive, violent, impulsive, and other irresponsible behaviors
- Actions that cause injury to the self or others
- Withdrawal states that must be treated as medical emergencies to avoid death

ALCOHOL

Alcohol abuse/dependence consists of a pattern of use that leads to impairment in social, legal, and occupational performance experienced from continued alcohol consumption or from actual intoxication. Evidence of alcohol intoxication is impaired ability to function physically and psychologically, with signs such as slurred speech, unsteady gait, emotional outbursts, impaired judgment and memory, transient amnesia or "blackouts," and in higher doses, coma and death.

Alcohol dependence is more serious and includes the criteria for substance dependence such as tolerance, withdrawal, ingesting more than intended, and continued use despite its harmfulness to self. Typically a patient may deny having a drinking problem. This discussion focuses on alcoholism as an addiction or compulsion to drink alcohol. Use of alcohol is accepted at social gatherings and business meetings and as part of cultural and religious celebrations such as marriages and births. Alcohol use in the United States is widespread and affects all socioeconomic groups.

The incidence of alcoholism in the United States is estimated to be 10.5 million people, with a lifetime prevalence of approximately 13.6%.[20] Nearly one fifth of patients treated in general medical practices report drinking at levels considered dangerous and may be at risk for developing alcohol dependence. Two types of alcoholism are identified. Type I affects men and women equally and is generally characterized as a milder form of alcoholism. It is associated with life and environmental stresses. Type II is associated with binge drinking and is thought to be more common in men. A genetic predisposition is thought to be more common among type II alcoholics. Although alcohol dependency appears to be more common among men than among women, data on women may not be accurate because it is suspected that women are more isolated, private drinkers.[37] There is some variance among racial and ethnic groups. Whites have the highest rate of alcohol use (56%) compared with Latinos (45%) and African-Americans (41%). Native Americans have been reported to have higher rates of alcoholism.[20]

Some families may be dysfunctional before a member becomes alcohol dependent; in others, dysfunction may be caused by the effect of alcoholism. Drinking alcoholic beverages (e.g., beer, wine, spirits) and occasional drunkenness may be accepted initially by family members as normal social behavior. As the frequency and amount of use increases, problem drinking begins to have detrimental effects on the drinker and family members. The drinker's personality changes with severe mood swings; he or she may be arrested for driving while intoxicated (blood alcohol levels above 0.05 g/dl with legal definitions ranging from 0.08 to 1.10 g/dl in various states) or other infractions of law, and engage in mental and physical abuse, especially of family members. Family relationships deteriorate, and family members feel trapped between the sober and intoxication phases of the alcoholic. They experience shame, anger, confusion, and guilt. Family conversations are increasingly focused on the alcohol-dependent behavior and issues related to it. Family members unconsciously engage in enabling behaviors to protect the family reputation and keep the family secret. Such behaviors include making excuses to friends and employers, attempting to keep the alcoholic out of trouble, and sometimes buying liquor for the alcoholic. The person with a drinking problem offers alibis for his or her behavior or is unwilling to discuss it. If the spouse threatens to leave or no longer make excuses, the alcohol-dependent person may promise never to touch another drop. These promises are usually broken. The family members may be locked into dysfunctional behaviors, including denial, or may sever their relationship with the drinker.

PSYCHOPATHOLOGY/PATHOPHYSIOLOGY

Among the many reasons for dependence on alcoholic beverages are low self-worth, feelings of inadequacy, stress, family- and work-related problems, economic difficulties, and feelings of social inadequacy. In some instances alcohol dependency is secondary to mental disorders such as early behavioral problems in children, personality disorders (e.g., antisocial personality disorder), anxiety disorders (e.g., panic disorders, social phobias), schizophrenia, and major depression. Mentally ill persons who are not capable of seeking out, or are resistant to, professional intervention may use alcohol to self-medicate their psychiatric symptoms and eventually become dependent.[119]

Genetic factors have been implicated in the development of alcoholism. Close relatives of alcohol-dependent persons have a three to four times greater risk for alcoholism than those with no close alcohol-dependent relatives. The risk for alcoholism is higher for identical twins than for fraternal twins or same-sex siblings in families with alcoholism.[5] If the child with alcoholic parents is adopted by nonalcoholic parents, the risk to the child for developing an alcohol problem is related to the alcoholism of the biologic parents. The opposite was found in that a child of nonalcoholic parents adopted into the home of alcoholic parents was unlikely to show increased alcohol use as an adult. Persons with a genetic predisposition for developing alcoholism may not necessarily do so because of environmental influences on their behaviors.

Attention must be given to the abuse of multiple drugs, because a person found to be dependent on one substance is probably also dependent on others that potentiate or inhibit the effects of the first. Although it is common for patients to deny use or minimize the amount they consume, a nonjudgmental attitude will help the nurse elicit the necessary information. Obtaining accurate information on the use of legal and illegal substances is important in all inpatient and outpatient settings, such as medical-surgical, pediatric, and psychiatric settings.

A person who withdraws from alcohol use (usually following chronic intake) is likely to experience withdrawal symptoms referred to as tremors (the shakes) that occur within 3 to 6 hours and peak within 36 hours after the last drink. The early symptoms include tremors, nervousness, tachycardia, agitation, increased blood pressure, nausea, lack of appetite, and restless sleep. A person who develops a more severe withdrawal syndrome exhibits psychomotor agitation and may suffer from acute auditory hallucinations that progress to disorientation, delusions, visual or tactile hallucinations, severe delirium and agitation, fever, perspiration, and seizures. It is estimated that less than 5% of persons who develop alcohol withdrawal progress to this stage.[5,37] DSM-IV criteria for alcohol withdrawal include:

Cessation of alcohol use that has been heavy and prolonged.

Two or more of the following within several hours to a few days after cessation of use: autonomic hyperactivity (tachycardia, diaphoresis); increased hand tremor; insomnia; nausea or vomiting; transient visual, tactile, or auditory hallucinations or illusions; psychomotor agitation; anxiety; and grand mal seizures.

Withdrawal symptoms cause significant impairment and distress and affect ability to function. These symptoms are not due to a general medical condition or disorder.

Chronic alcohol abuse can lead to numerous physical and mental disabilities and consequences, including:

Cardiovascular system: Anemia, hypertension, tachycardia, dysrhythmias, cardiomegaly, edema

Liver: Hepatomegaly, edema, ascites, and cirrhosis

Gastrointestinal (GI) system: Gastritis; esophagitis and/or esophageal varices; duodenal and gastric ulcers; nausea; malabsorption syndrome; colitis; cancer of GI system.

Neurologic system: Fatigue; unsteady gait; depression, irritability; memory and learning deficits; severe head trauma from falls; tremors; polyneuropathy that typically begins in feet; degeneration of cerebellum; Wernicke's encelaphalopathy; Korsakoff's syndrome; decreased testosterone levels and erectile dysfunction; and immune impairment and infection.

Fetal alcohol syndrome or spontaneous abortion.

Detoxification support is provided through a variety of interventions, including pharmacologic. Pharmacologic support is helpful in relieving the symptoms of acute withdrawal, and in preventing seizures the goal should be to maintain a moderate level of sedation. Medications should be administered in adequate amounts and frequency. When the patient is stabilized, medication should be tapered over 3 to 5 days.

Diazepam (Valium, 5 to 20 mg q6h) and chlordiazepoxide (Librium, adults 5 to 100 mg PO, stat and q6h) are administered during the acute stage. The elderly or adolescents should receive 5 mg PO, stat and q6h during the acute stage to prevent or decrease serious alcohol withdrawal symptoms, including grand mal seizures. Intramuscular administration is generally avoided because of the slow and erratic absorption. The antianxiety drug is gradually discontinued within a short time in favor of nonpharmacologic approaches to rehabilitation. The drug acts to reduce anxiety and seizure level and promote drowsiness and hypotension. If the patient becomes somnolent, the dose should be reduced. Patients with impaired liver function may require the lesser hepatically metabolized benzodiazepines, lorazepam 10 mg q4h or oxazepam 15 to 30 mg PO tid/qid, to reduce symptoms of alcohol withdrawal with low sedation.

Phenobarbital is also sometimes used for detoxification. It is safe, predictable, and has a longer active countereffect than benzodiazepines. An initial dose of 60 to 120 mg is given orally or intramuscularly, followed by 60 mg q4h until the patient is stabilized. Then a 30-mg dose is given qid, and then bid until tapered off.

Clonidine may be used as an adjunct to benzodiazepines to suppress cardiovascular signs of withdrawal and to control anxiety. It is given in doses of 0.3 to 0.6 mg/kg orally q6h or in the form of a patch. Tigan or Atarax may be given for nausea and vomiting, and Imodium may be given for diarrhea.

Vitamin B, pyridoxine, folate, and especially thiamine, should be given to any patient in withdrawal. Megadose, multivitamin, and multimineral supplements (such as Tropagen, 1 tablet PO twice daily with meals) should be administered. Because of malnutrition generally seen in alcoholism, improvement in nutritional status is essential to prevent or decrease chronic medical disorders. To prevent precipitation of Wernicke's syndrome, intravenous glucose solutions should not be administered before thiamine.[20]

After the patient has gone through detoxification, benzodiazepines and any type of sleeping pill are generally discontinued. Buspirone may be used in highly anxious patients. Antidepressant medications may be used for patients with a diagnosis of depression.

Disulfiram (Antabuse) is frequently prescribed for the prevention of further alcohol abuse. This medication acts to inhibit hepatic aldehyde-NAD oxidoreductase, an enzyme in the pathway that metabolizes alcohol. The patient is instructed that consuming alcohol while taking this medication will cause physical illness resulting from an accumulation of toxic metabolites in the body. Symptoms would include flushing, palpitations, shortness of breath, nausea, and vomiting lasting up to an hour. Effects of this drug last for up to 72 hours after the most recent dose; therefore disulfiram cannot be easily stopped to allow for an unplanned binge.[20,37]

Alcohol addiction causes devastating physical, emotional, and social complications at some point during the course of the disease. As tolerance develops with compulsive use, tolerant persons may function well with blood alcohol levels that would have profound effecs in nontolerant persons. The chronic effects of alcohol abuse include serious damage to many body systems. The alcoholic may suffer physical deterioration of bone marrow and cardiovascular, hepatic, pancreatic, gastrointestinal, genitourinary, and neurologic systems.

Korsakoff's syndrome is a neurologic complication of chronic alcoholism that includes dementia (especially loss of recent memory), amnesia, and psychosis with a poor prognosis for cognitive recovery. Generally, nutritional deficiencies are a contributing factor. This is also the case in **Wernicke's encephalopathy,** which is manifested by delirium with cranial nerve dysfunction. Typically a thiamine deficiency is identified and treated with improvement of symptoms. Symptoms include changes in mental status and paralysis of extraocular eye movements (disconjugate gaze).[5,37]

Diagnostic Studies and Findings

Blood studies: Complete blood count; prothrombin time; blood alcohol level; blood glucose

Urine studies: Urinalysis; urine toxicology for other drugs of abuse

Imaging studies: CT scan of head to screen for head trauma; chest x-ray to screen for pulmonary infection and cardiac disease

Electrocardiogram: To screen for cardiomyopathy
Stool evaluation: For occult blood

MULTIDISCIPLINARY PLAN

Medications

Benzodiazepines
- Diazepam (Valium) 5-20 mg q6h, PO/IM/IV
- Chloridazepoxide (Librium), 5-100 mg PO/IM/IV stat and q6h; not to exceed 300 mg qd
- Lorazepam, 10 mg PO q4h or oxazepam 15-30 mg PO tid/qid

Phenobarbital, 60-120 mg PO or IM followed by 60 mg q4h until patient is stabilized; decrease dosage to 30 mg qid, then bid until drug can be discontinued as indicated by patient's response
Clonidine, 5 mcg/kg PO q2h to suppress cardiovascular signs of withdrawal and to control anxiety
Buspirone (BuSpar), 5 mg PO tid to control anxiety
Trimethobenzamide (Tigan), 250 mg PO tid/qid or hydroxyzine (Atarax) 25-100 mg tid/qid for nausea
Vitamin therapy: Vitamin B, pyridoxine, folate, thiamine
Mineral supplements
Disulfiram (Antabuse), 250-500 mg PO od for 1 to 2 weeks; decrease to 125-500 mg od until fully recovered

NURSING CARE

NURSING ASSESSMENT

Emotional status: Anxiety; emotional lability; depression, types of situations and interactions that trigger alcohol intake and coping strategies
Thought processes: Denial of alcoholism; guilt; shame; sense of inadequacy; impairment of judgment and memory; suicidal ideation (correlation exists between alcoholism and suicide)
Physical status: Type of drinking pattern established; duration and amount of last alcohol consumed; irritability to psychomotor agitation; demanding behavior; memory lapses (blackouts); tachycardia; hypertension; increased respirations; tremors; fatigue; nausea and vomiting; anorexia; abdominal cramps; insomnia; elevated temperature; illusions; hallucinations (most frequently visual, sometimes auditory); seizure potential; fluid intake and output and nutritional intake
Social and occupational interactions: Argumentativeness with family, friends, and co-workers; aggressiveness with others; tardiness at work; work absences because of "not feeling well"; sensitivity to criticism; mistakes at work
Family: Knowledge the patient's family has about the patient's alcoholism and the family's enabling behaviors

POTENTIAL COMPLICATIONS

Multibody system deterioration: Hepatic failure; GI hemorrhage; metabolic encephalopathy
Korsakoff's syndrome: Dementia, amnesia, psychosis
Wernicke's encephalopathy: Changes in mental status; paralysis of extraocular eye movements (disconjugate gaze); conusion, delirium, coma

PATIENT PROBLEMS/NURSING DIAGNOSES & INTERVENTIONS

NIC BEHAVIOR THERAPY

Alcohol withdrawal* related to decreased intake of alcohol following chronic use

- Minimize the number of people attending the patient *to prevent excitement; provide quiet environment to decrease stimuli and decrease possibility of agitation, anxiety, and belligerence caused by central nervous system (CNS) stimulation during withdrawal.*
- Administer benzodiazipines as prescribed (because of patient's tolerance to sedative effects of alcohol, larger doses are needed than for nonalcoholic patients) *to prevent agitation and seizures.*
- Explain reasons for and effects of medicine *to increase the patient's acceptance of the treatment.*
- Evaluate the effects of medicine.
- Provide physical protection in bed, such as side rails, bed in low position, and mechanical restraints, if needed, *to protect patient from harm.*
- Explain to patient the psychologic and physiologic effects of alcoholism and the effects alcohol has on patient's relationships with self and others *to help patient become aware of harmful effects in all areas of his or her life.*
- Correct patient's misconceptions about physiologic, psychologic, and social effects of alcoholic beverages.
- If suicidal ideation exists, assess its seriousness.
- Maintain light in the room, especially at night, *to decrease the possibility that the patient might misinterpret environmental stimuli.*

NIC TISSUE PERFUSION MANAGEMENT

Excess fluid volume related to effects of alcoholic beverages

- Avoid forcing fluids to prevent overhydration, *because alcohol initially exerts antidiuretic effects.*
- Monitor blood pressure, pulse, and respirations every 15 minutes until stable and then as ordered *to detect changes resulting from agitation and other complications of withdrawal.*
- Monitor temperature every 4 hours *to detect signs of infection.*
- Observe for infection (e.g., of respiratory tract) resulting from impaired immune system.

NIC NUTRITION SUPPORT

Imbalanced nutrition: less than body requirements, related to lack of interest in food

- Help to ensure adequate nutrition in collaboration with the physician and dietitian *to counteract the effects of inadequate diet and malabsorption of nutrients.*
- Offer bland food if gastric distress. Antacids may be prescribed *to decrease distress.*
- Administer vitamins as ordered with meal *to decrease nutritional deficits.*

---

*Non-NANDA nursing diagnosis.

- Explain to patient the essentials of a nutritionally balanced diet, the adverse effects of alcohol on the digestion and absorption of food, and the importance of compliance *to prevent or alleviate malnutrition and the effects of alcoholism.*

NIC Coping Assistance

Ineffective coping related to maladaptive behaviors of alcoholism

- Establish a supportive, nonjudgmental relationship *to promote a decrease in patient's denial and guilt about excessive drinking of alcohol.*
- Assist patient to identify feelings of anxiety and relate them to stress-producing situations *to encourage patient's awareness of his or her maladaptive coping mechanisms.*
- Help patient identify healthy methods for coping with anxiety instead of relying on alcohol. Methods include problem solving, relaxation techniques (e.g., slow, deep breathing), and diversionary activities (e.g., physical exercise and watching television).
- Explain and practice assertiveness skills and evaluation of effects of skills *to increase patient's self-esteem.*
- Encourage patient to learn to ask for support and to deal with positive and negative responses.
- Assist patient in developing skills to refuse alcohol in social situations *to help in learning to socialize without the use of alcohol.* Refer patients to Alcoholics Anonymous *to obtain support for nondrinking behavior and to prevent relapse.*
- Correct patient's misconceptions about physiologic, psychologic, and social effects of alcohol.
- Encourage patient to examine consequences of drinking behavior on self, family, and social and work functioning and to identify alternative behaviors to increase patient's sense of adequacy when engaged in nondestructive behaviors.

NIC Life Span Care

Disabled family coping related to alcoholism

- Explain that alcoholism is a disease and describe the psychologic, physiologic, and social effects of alcoholism.
- Assist patient and family to identify interaction patterns *to discuss the expectations each has, and to discuss each family member's willingness to meet these expectations.*
- Assist each family member in beginning to identify differences and to learn to negotiate disagreements *and accept conflicting views among family members.*
- Help family members to understand the disease *so that they will not blame themselves, believing that they caused the abuse and the alcoholism.*
- Refer family for counseling, if indicated.
- Recommend attendance at Al-Anon for spouse and Al-Ateen for children *to help them deal with painful feelings, such as guilt, anger, and despair, and to help them accept responsibility only for their own behaviors and not those behaviors of the problem drinker.*

Other related nursing diagnoses: Impaired physical mobility related to cognitive and perceptual impairment; bathing/hygiene self-care deficit related to depressed mood

Patient Education/Continuum of Care Plan

1. Review with patient that alcoholism is a chronic disorder and that recovery is a lifelong endeavor.
2. Ensure that patient accepts responsibility for his or her own behavior and sobriety.
3. Reinforce patient's active participation in Alcoholics Anonymous and other aftercare programs.
4. Ensure that patient understands the need to practice healthy coping behaviors for dealing with anxiety and life problems related to family, friends, and work.
5. Elaborate on the need for social supports and the development of self-supports.

Evaluation/Patient Outcomes

Behavior Therapy: Recovery from withdrawal symptoms of alcohol is uncomplicated. Patient has minimal signs or symptoms of alcohol withdrawal with no agitation or seizures. Patient recovers with no physical harm to self. Patient verbalizes knowledge of the physical, psychologic, and social effects of consuming alcoholic beverages.

Tissue Perfusion Management: Patient evidences normal fluid balance and vital signs. Patient has adequate intake and output with normal electrolyte balance. Patient maintains stable vital signs with no evidence of infection.

Nutrition Support: Patient is cognizant of well-balanced diet. Patient lists essentials of nutritionally balanced diet and acknowledges the adverse effects of alcohol on nutrition. Patient participates in choosing meals.

Coping Assistance: Patient is aware of healthy coping strategies for stress-producing situations. Patient practices relaxation techniques and engages in physical exercise. Patient practices assertiveness skills and evaluates their effects on self and others. Patient practices refusal of alcoholic beverages in social situations. Patient begins to attend Alcoholics Anonymous meetings and lists dates, times, and places of meetings, as well as the name and phone number of his or her sponsor in the program.

Life Span Care: Family demonstrates ability to obtain support from community agencies and verbalizes knowledge of alcoholism and of enabling behaviors. Patient and family verbalize knowledge of alcohol and its adverse effects on their relationships. Family expresses knowledge of enabling behaviors and responsibilities related to alcoholism. Spouse attends Al-Anon meetings.

Cocaine

Cocaine is one of the oldest known drugs. Pure cocaine has been an abused substance for more than 100 years, and the coca leaves have been ingested for thousands of years. Pure cocaine was first extracted from the leaf of the *Erythroxylon coca* bush, which grew primarily in Bolivia and Peru, in the middle of the nineteenth century. In the early part of this century it was the main stimulant drug used in many tonics and elixirs including the original Coca-Cola.[69] At present, cocaine is taken intravenously, or intranasally, and crack, a street name given to the freebase form of cocaine processed from the powdered form, is smoked. Crack has become a popular form of this drug because it is inexpensive to produce and to buy.

Pathophysiology/Psychopathology

A report from the NHSDA estimated that 1.5 million people in the United States age 12 years and older, were current cocaine users.[67] Additional data sources from the Office of National Drug Control Policy have taken into account users underrepresented in the NHSDA and estimate the number of cocaine users in the United States to be 3.6 million. The age group of adults ages 18 to 25 years has the highest rate of cocaine use, and women are as commonly represented among abusers as men. Crack cocaine is a serious problem in the United States, and the NHSDA estimated the number of crack users to be about 604,000 in 1997.

Although classified as a narcotic, cocaine is a central nervous system stimulant similar in action to amphetamine and has almost the same criteria for a clinical disorder. The euphoria with persistent cravings produced by cocaine makes it very appealing and can lead to tolerance in hours to days. The level of response varies with differences in genetics and with previous experience with cocaine or similar drugs. Cocaine acts in the brain's reward centers to block reuptake of neurotransmitters dopamine and norepinephrine. These two excitatory neurotransmitters then continually stimulate the reward centers. In high doses the effects of cocaine on bodily drives are very strong. Cocaine is mainly metabolized by the liver. Whether physical dependence exists is questionable because it does not produce severe symptoms experienced with other substances; however, the psychologic cravings for the substances are strong. Patterns vary from occasional to episodic to chronic or almost daily use, with low to high doses of cocaine.[37]

Diagnostic Studies and Findings

Sequential multiple analyzer with computer (SMAC): To screen for systemic abnormalities
Thyroid-stimulating hormone, T_4, T_3: To rule out thyroid disorder
Chest x-ray: To screen for cardiopulmonary disease
Electrocardiogram: To screen for substance-induced heart disorder
Urinalysis: To screen for urinary and systemic abnormalities
Urine toxicology: To screen for substance abuse

Multidisciplinary Plan

Medications

Medications are not currently available that are specific for the treatment of cocaine addiction. Several newly emerging compounds are being investigated at this time.

Selegiline, a promising anticocaine drug, has been in multisite phase III clinical trials to evaluate a transdermal patch and a time-released pill.
Disulfiram (Antabuse) is sometimes used and has been effective in reducing cocaine abuse.
Antidepressant therapy to treat symptoms of depression or chlordiazepoxide (Librium) to decrease anxiety may be used.
If bipolar disorder exists, lithium may be prescribed to counter the euphorigenic effects of cocaine and the disorder.[74]

NURSING CARE

Nursing Assessment

Emotional status: Depression, anxiety, sense of worthlessness, irritability, sense of emptiness
Physiologic status: Pattern and amount of cocaine use, including type of cocaine, route of administration, and time of last dose: cardiac dysrhythmia; hypertension; hyperthermia; sleep disturbances; restlessness, tremors, agitation
Thought processes/activities: Suicidal ideation, denial, impaired concentration and judgment, psychomotor agitation
Social and occupational interactions: Deterioration in social behavior, interpersonal difficulties, impairment in occupational or student role; types of discomforts patient has in various social and occupational situations
Family: Knowledge of patient's drug use and quality of family relationships

Potential Complications

Cocaine intoxication: Convulsions, CNS depression
Toxic psychosis: With CNS stimulation (tachycardia, hypertension, cardiac arrhythmias, sweating, hyperpyrexia, and convulsions
Lethal overdose: Death usually results from respiratory failure

Patient Problems/Nursing Diagnoses & Interventions

NIC Behavior Therapy

Cocaine withdrawal* related to decreased intake of cocaine after long-term use or overdose

- Restrict visitors during the first week of hospitalization *to prevent stimulation and possible stresses associated with visitors and to prevent reintroduction of drugs.*
- Obtain urine specimens at intervals, as ordered, for drug testing.
- Administer medication as ordered *to decrease severe symptoms associated with termination or overdose of cocaine.* Evaluate the effects. As patient is able to comprehend, provide patient with information of effects and adverse effects of medicines.
- Encourage patient to identify negative experiences with drug use rather than only euphoric, positive aspects *to begin self-awareness of problems arising from abuse.*
- Provide information on cocaine and other substances as indicated *to increase patient's knowledge of effects and adverse consequences and to correct misconceptions.*

---

*Non-NANDA nursing diagnosis.

NIC Coping Assistance

Ineffective coping related to maladaptive reactions to life experiences

- Establish supportive, nonjudgmental relationship *to promote trust and comfort.*
- Assist patient in identifying stress-provoking situations *to help increase awareness of areas of discomfort.* Help patient identify healthy coping strategies *to reinforce strengths.*
- Practice assertiveness skills with patient, rather than reliance on cocaine, *to increase patient's self-confidence and comfort in social and work situations.* Techniques include role-playing and confrontation with feedback in group therapy setting.

NIC Nutrition Support

Imbalanced nutrition: less than body requirements, related to lack of interest in food

- Ensure adequate nutrition in collaboration with physician and dietitian *to counteract effects of inadequate diet.*
- Provide a bland diet and antacids as ordered *to decrease gastric discomfort.*
- Explain essentials of a nutritionally balanced diet *to prevent or alleviate malnutrition.*

NIC Life Span Care

Dysfunctional family processes related to effects of substance abuse

- Talk with family about cocaine and its consequences *to provide information and correct misconceptions.*
- Help patient and family members to identify and discuss problem areas, including feelings of anger, and help them begin *to resolve difficulties to improve relationships and develop realistic expectations of each other.*
- Refer family members for counseling, if indicated, and self-help groups such as Al-Anon or Nar-Anon *to learn how to deal with effects of patient's substance use.*

Patient Education/Continuum of Care Plan

1. Encourage patient to follow through with medical treatment.
2. Ensure that patient verbalizes understanding of healthy coping strategies for dealing with stress.
3. Reinforce use of self-supports and supports from others, including active participation in self-help groups such as Cocaine Anonymous.
4. Support patient's plans to implement a relapse-preventive lifestyle.

Evaluation/Patient Outcomes

Behavior Therapy: Patient has an uncomplicated termination from cocaine. Patient demonstrates drug-free state verbally, and urine tests during hospitalization are drug free. Patient demonstrates knowledge of effects and consequences of cocaine dependence. Patient describes psychologic and physiologic effects and consequences of cocaine use. Patient discusses effects of cocaine use on self and significant others.

Coping Assistance: Patient demonstrates evidence of practicing healthy coping techniques for dealing with stress-producing situations. Patient practices relaxation techniques. Patient practices assertiveness skills and evaluates their effects on self and others. Patient practices techniques for avoiding cocaine-related situations. Patient develops an enjoyable non-drug-related activity schedule to manage free time.

Nutrition Support: Patient participates in meal planning and eats regular, well-balanced meals. Patient verbalizes knowledge of good nutrition. Patient chooses and eats nutritionally balanced meals.

Life Span Care: Patient demonstrates participation in relationships with family. Patient participates in dealing with conflicts in the family and in shared activities.

Schizophrenic Disorders

An individual who is out of touch with reality, experiencing distorted perceptions of the environment and internal cues, as well as significant impairment in functioning, may be experiencing a psychotic episode. A psychotic episode may include symptoms such as hallucinations, delusions, and social/occupational withdrawal. Because some distortions in reality (e.g., delirium) can occur as a result of general medical conditions, a complete history and review of systems is indicated in patients experiencing an acute psychotic episode. Nursing observations are key in ruling out other diagnoses that may cause acute psychosis. Assessment of the psychotic patient is done through a mental status examination, which includes three main categories: observation, conversation, and formal testing (Box 19-1).

Possible nonpsychiatric causes of acute psychosis include metabolic disorders, electrical (seizure) disorders, neoplastic diseases, degenerative (chronic) brain diseases, arterial (cerebrovascular) diseases, mechanical diseases (acute physical structures of the brain), infectious diseases, nutritional diseases, and drug toxicity.[34]

Mental Status Examination — Box 19-1

Observation

Appearance: Dress, hygiene, grooming, physical health
Behavior: Eye contact, posture, gait, activity level
Level of consciousness (LOC): Awareness and orientation

Conversation

Mood and affect: Range, stability and congruency
Speech: Rate, volume, clarity, rhythm
Thought processes: Flow, organization, content, preoccupations

Testing

Suicidal/homicidal thoughts: Ideation, plan, intent, means
Memory: Remote, recent, and immediate; abstract thinking; judgment; insight; reasoning; and intellectual status
Perceptions: Hallucinations, illusions, and delusions

From Farrell, Harmon, and Hastings.[34]

Schizophrenia and manic-depressive disorder are the major causes of prolonged psychosis seen in psychiatric patients. Distinguishing between these two major causes can be difficult, and some persons who exhibit a mixture of symptoms are given a DSM-IV diagnosis of **schizoaffective disorder.** A diagnosis of schizophrenia is made if a person exhibits continuous signs of marked behavioral impairment in the areas of work, social relationships, and self-care activities for at least 6 months, including a minimum of 1 month of psychotic symptoms such as delusions, hallucinations, grossly disorganized affect, and disorganized speech. The subtypes of schizophrenia identified in the DSM-IV are **paranoid type,** characterized by persecutory or grandiose delusions and, commonly, auditory hallucinations but less cognitive impairment; **disorganized type,** involving odd, silly, childlike behavior and severe disintegration of the personality, as well as incoherent speech; **catatonic type,** presenting predominately as an intense psychomotor disturbance; **undifferentiated type,** which has some aspects of each of the subtypes but does not clearly meet the criteria for any of them; and **residual type,** which is the diagnosis used if the person has had at least one acute episode of schizophrenia and is now free of positive symptoms (delusions, hallucinations, disorganized speech, and grossly disorganized catatonic behavior) but has some negative symptoms (affective flattening, alogia, and avolition). When the symptoms are similar to schizophrenia except for a (shorter) duration of 1 month to less than 6 months with no "decline in functioning," the condition is diagnosed as **schizophreniform disorder.**[5]

The symptoms developed are the best solutions the person is capable of at the time to restore a sense of equilibrium. The presentation of schizophrenia that follows is not specific to a diagnostic type but deals with dysfunctional behaviors that are common to persons with schizophrenia.

Schizophrenia is a disorder in which a person exhibits psychotic symptoms, including disturbances in perceptions, thought, affect, and psychomotor behaviors during an acute phase. The person's social and psychologic abilities are impaired. Characteristic symptoms are generalized into two broad categories: positive and negative.[5] Two or more of the positive symptoms, reflecting an excess or distortion of normal function, disordered speech/thoughts, delusions, hallucinations, disorganized or catatonic behavior, must be present.[5,37]

Persons with schizophrenia have great difficulty communicating because their flow of thoughts is loose and disordered. A seemingly unrelated thought or idea may follow an initial thought or idea. Although any of the single topics or ideas may make sense, when put together they seem disordered and even unrelated. It is not a disordered speech but a disordered thought process that results in disordered speech. As the condition evolves, language may reveal even more bizarre thought processes, and the person can eventually lose the ability to communicate.

A patient with schizophrenia who loses the ability to effectively communicate has difficulty expressing needs, ideas, or intentions to others. These terms may be defined as follows. **Derailment** is speech that goes off the point or subject. **Tangentiality** is a failure to reach a goal or stick to a point. **Incoherence** is speech that is not logically connected. *Word salad* is a group of disconnected words. A **neologistic word** is an invented word that has specific meaning to the person with schizophrenia.

A person who has a disordered thinking process will exhibit disordered behavior. The overall appearance and dress may be sloppy, eccentric, or bizarre. An extreme of disordered behavior is **catatonic behavior,** which is a marked decrease in the ability to react to the environment, sometimes an apparent disconnection or complete unawareness of what is happening in the immediate environment.

Delusions are false beliefs or misrepresented perceptions or experiences that are a major defining characteristic of psychosis in persons with schizophrenia. **Grandiose delusions** are perceptions of importance in which persons may believe they have special powers. Persons with **persecutory delusions** have paranoid beliefs that others intend to do harm to them. **Referential delusions** include the beliefs that common events (song passages, comments of people in the room) refer to self.

Hallucinations are false sensory perceptions with no apparent external stimulus. They are sensory experiences that are not perceptible to other nonpsychotic individuals. **Auditory hallucinations** are the most frequent form of perceptual disturbance; voices may be negative, insulting, or commanding, or especially in chronicity, voices may be friendly and helpful. **Visual hallucinations** occur occasionally in the acute phase and involve seeing nonexistent things such as insects or people.

The negative symptoms, which reflect a diminution or loss of normal functions, include flattened affect, alogia, avolition, and anhedonia. These symptoms can be difficult to detect early in the illness, but as the disease progresses, they often lead to withdrawal and social isolation.[34,37] These negative symptoms are defined as follows: **flattened affect,** the loss of expressiveness that includes emotional distance and lack of human response; **blunting,** a reduction of affective, emotional expression; **alogia,** the tendency of patients with schizophrenia to use brief and seemingly empty phrases or the tendency to speak very little in general; **avolition,** the lack of motivation for work or other goal-directed activities; and **anhedonia,** the inability of the person to take pleasure from the performance of acts that would ordinarily be pleasurable.

The onset of schizophrenia may be slow and insidious or sudden. In some persons the onset is preceded by a significant external event such as loss of a friend, marriage, or leaving home; in others, the onset is not related to an identifiable external event. External events, if identified, are insufficient to evoke a psychosis if the internal processes such as relatedness to self and environment are not impaired. Impairments reduce the person's ability to cope with social and psychologic experiences, such as processing information received from others and social problem solving. Community-based services are the preferred treatment for this type of chronic mental illness. Involving patients' families in psychoeducational and support groups increases their ability to cope with the stresses and stigma of having a mentally ill family member.[108]

Substance abuse is a major concern with patients who have schizophrenia regardless of whether they are taking antipsychotic medications. It is not known with precision how or if substance abuse causes persistent psychosis or alters the course of the illness. Alcohol and substance abuse/dependence may be as high as 47% to 60% among persons with schizophrenia. Alcohol abuse is most frequent (approximately 37%), followed by marijuana and cocaine. Alcohol has been known to increase or decrease the rate of metabolism of antipsychotic medications. Acute alcohol consumption stimulates a hepatic enzyme that can increase the metabolism of persons taking antipsychotic medications and reduces their plasma levels. In contrast, chronic liver dysfunction can decrease the rate of metabolism of antipsychotic medications, causing accumulation of levels and toxicity. Alcohol and antipsychotic medication can also lower the seizure threshold. Marijuana can cause an escalation of positive and negative symptoms and an increase in the side effects of antipsychotic medication. Cocaine abuse may cause an exaggeration of positive symptoms, a tendency for paranoid behaviors, and possibly a higher rate of depression and suicide. The use of nicotine is also significant in patients with schizophrenia (80%).[56]

Nurses caring for patients with a mental illness that presents with psychosis and agitation must be concerned about violent behavior. Although patients with schizophrenia are not always violent, there is an increased risk for aggressive and even assaultive behavior in this patient population. It is estimated that 10% to 15% of these patients become physically assaultive, especially after hospitalization, and as many as 30% to 35% engage in fear-inducing behaviors. Recent data suggest that atypical antipsychotics (see medications) may be more effective in reducing violent behavior, as well as risk of suicide.[91]

Schizophrenia is a chronic disorder in which the person may appear cold, distant, and apathetic. Response to therapy is extremely slow, and obvious signs of success are few. Nurses often find it easier to withdraw from the eremitic schizophrenic than to experience a sense of helplessness, hopelessness, and inadequacy in dealing with the patient. The nurse needs to establish small goals with the patient, such as having the patient speak to him or her, share an activity, or ask to have a need or want met. If unrealistic goals are established, the nurse is bound to experience frustration and hopelessness. If the goal is attainable, specific, and immediate, the nurse's frustration is reduced.

It can be difficult for nurses to separate the patient from the label of the diagnosis that is carried into the clinical setting. This diagnostic label is often used to explain every aspect of the behavior, often stripping patients of the identity they once knew. Thus a psychiatric hospitalization itself may adversely affect a patient's sense of self. The therapeutic role of the psychiatric nurse involves reflecting on the aspects of the mentally ill person that are positive parts of the whole person and helping the patient hold on to them as a separate entity from that of the diagnosis. The development of the nurse-patient relationship can be paramount to patient outcomes.[44]

The onset of schizophrenia in men appears in their late teens or early twenties, whereas onset in women is typically in their late twenties to early thirties. Schizophrenia is more rare but has occurred in younger and older persons. The disease is almost equally distributed between males and females. Genetic background appears to be significant in predicting overall risk of schizophrenia. A person with two schizophrenic parents has nearly a 50% risk of contracting the disease. Studies of twins have shown a much higher prevalence among monozygotic (identical) twins (60% to 70%) than among dizygotic twins (0 to 15%).[37,79]

Prevalence rates are similar throughout the world; however, pockets of higher prevalence have been reported in specific areas. The overall prevalence rate is estimated to be 0.5% to 1% of the population in the United States.[5,37,85] Although some persons recover completely, a majority have residual effects of the schizophrenic process. Among this majority group, some have acute relapses, some maintain a stable course, and others gradually worsen with severe disabilities. It is a very lonely disease that results in depression for 60% of those afflicted, with 10% to 13% of persons with schizophrenia committing suicide and 20% to 40% making suicide attempts.[46,85] Some risk factors for suicide include being less than age 30 years and male, experiencing depressive symptoms, and being unemployed.[37,79]

> **! EMERGENCY ALERT**
>
> **SCHIZOPHRENIC DISORDERS**
>
> **ASSESSMENT**
>
> - May be agitated, aggressive, frightened, and dangerous to self or others.
> - May abuse substances such as prescribed, illegal, and over-the-counter-medications, and/or alcohol.
>
> **INTERVENTIONS**
>
> - Provide safe quiet environment to decrease stimuli and make frequent, brief contacts with patient.
> - Monitor for side effects and therapeutic effects of psychotropic medications.

PSYCHOPATHOLOGY/PATHOPHYSIOLOGY

During the past decade the focus of causation of schizophrenia has centered on neurobiologic and genetic factors. The genetic component of schizophrenia has emerged as an important factor. Genetic influences are illustrated by the "at risk" statistic, which indicates that for the person with two parents who have schizophrenia, the risk of development of the illness is 50%. In addition, first-degree relatives of persons with schizophrenia are 10 times as likely to develop schizophrenia as the general population.[5] Twin studies have illustrated the influence of genetic factors.[62] Despite these strong genetic links, there are no decisive theories that explain the role of genetics in the occurrence of schizophrenia.

Neuroanatomic factors of the brain have been studied with the hope of unlocking the mystery of causation of schizophrenia. Computed tomography (CT) scans have revealed that males with schizophrenia have larger lateral ventricles than nonschizophrenic males, but it is not known whether this is a cause or an effect, or if it is either. Studies of regional blood flow and metabolic activities of the brain have shown some abnormalities but no conclusive causative findings.

Specific enzymes and neurotransmitters have been studied in detail for causality in schizophrenia. The dopamine hypothesis evolved after scientists noted that the antipsychotic drugs act by blocking the activities of postsynaptic dopamine receptors in the brain. Based on this finding, scientists proposed that schizophrenia was caused by hyperdopaminergic activity in the brain. The process has proven to be more complicated than was first described. It was identified that the most recently developed medications for schizophrenia, the atypical antipsychotics, not only affect dopamine receptors but also specifically target serotonin. Despite continuing research on neurotransmitters and the causation of schizophrenia, the dopamine hypothesis is tentative and controversial. Several additional avenues of research involving neurotransmitters and schizophrenia are ongoing.

Some researchers believe that schizophrenia may be related to viral infections, autoimmune disturbances, and other pathophysiologic factors. The potential impact of pathophysiologic causes is compelling and merits continuing investigation. Social and environmental factors must also be examined to assess whether stressors interact with genetic and biologic susceptibilities to produce the disorder.

Management includes the use of antipsychotic drugs, which have been used for nearly 50 years to control psychotic symptoms in patients with this disorder. These drugs have very unpleasant side effects, and noncompliance among schizophrenic patients in taking these medications is common. Furthermore, there is evidence that these patients often suffer from memory and attention deficits and need a consistent means of reminding them about taking their medications.[50]

Conventional neuroleptics were the first pharmacologic treatment for acute psychoses and have been in use since the release of chlorpromazine (Thorazine) in 1952. Although significant side effects have been a problem, the developments of antipsychotic medications have given hope and functional lives to many patients with schizophrenia. These medications work by blocking dopamine transmission in the brain. They appear to be most effective in blocking the positive symptoms of psychoses (hallucinations, delusions, and agitation), typically with no effect or enhancement of negative symptoms.[109] Commonly used antipsychotic medications are Thorazine, Haldol, Prolixin, Trilafon, Mellaril, Navane, and Loxitane.

Side effects of these medications include orthostatic hypotension; extrapyramidal symptoms (EPS); and neuroleptic malignant syndrome (NMS), a potentially fatal disorder that has been reported with antipsychotic medicines. Major clinical manifestations of NMS are muscular rigidity, tachycardia, diaphoresis, labile blood pressure with hypotension and hypertension, cardiac dysrhythmia, dyspnea, hyperpyrexia, and coma.

Atypical antipsychotic medications have been available since the late 1980s. These antipsychotics are different because of their antagonist effect on several neurotransmitters: serotonin, dopamine, and histamine. These drugs are less likely to cause the side effects associated with the typical antipsychotics and are known to be effective for both positive and negative symptoms of schizophrenia. **Clozapine** is used in schizophrenia that is refractory to conventional antipsychotic drug treatment. Initially, it held promise as a new antipsychotic medication with the ability to affect both positive and negative symptoms; however, a major side effect in some patients is agranulocytosis, which is life threatening. Other side effects include EPS in some patients (although usually of short duration), sedation, enuresis, and a lowered seizure threshold. It is the most prescribed antipsychotic drug in the United States.

Risperidone, like clozapine, improves positive and negative symptoms of schizophrenia but has not been associated with agranulocytosis. For this reason it is often used as a first-line treatment for schizophrenia. Side effects include lowered seizure threshold, akathisia, weight gain, difficulty with concentration, and hypotension.[109]

Olanzapine is a newer antipsychotic effective for both positive and negative symptoms, with a low risk of EPS or agranulocytosis. The most common side effects include somnolence, agitation, asthenia (weakness), nervousness, and weight gain.[17,38,91,109]

DIAGNOSTIC STUDIES AND FINDINGS

SMAC: To screen for systemic abnormalities
Thyroid function tests
Syphilis serology
Electrocardiogram: To rule out cardiomyopathy
Computed tomography: To rule out brain abnormalities
Routine urinalysis
Urine toxicology screen: To rule out substance abuse

MULTIDISCIPLINARY PLAN

Medications

Typical antipsychotic drugs (phenothiazines)
- Chlorpromazine (Thorazine), 100 mg or 20-2000 mg qd, PO/IM
- Haloperidol (Haldol), 2-5 mg or 1-100 mg qd, PO/IM
- Fluphenazine (Prolixin), 2 mg or 2-40 mg qd, PO/IM
- Perphenazine (Trilafon), 10 mg or 8-64 mg qd, PO/IM
- Thioridazine (Mellaril), 100 mg or 50-800 mg qd, PO
- Thiothixene (Navane), 4 mg or 5-60 mg qd, PO/IM
- Loxapine (Loxitane), 10 mg or 20-250 mg qd, PO/IM

Atypical antipsychotic drugs
- Clozapine (Clozaril), 50 mg or 50-900 mg qd, PO
- Risperidone (Risperdal), 2-6 mg qd, PO
- Olanzapine (Zyprexia), 5-20 mg qd, PO

NURSING CARE

NURSING ASSESSMENT

Thought processes: Disturbance in orientation to person, place, and time; retarded thought processes; impaired ability to process incoming information; blocking of thoughts; autistic thinking (i.e., inability to distinguish between reality and fantasy); suspiciousness; distorted, illogical thinking; false beliefs, such as of being persecuted or poisoned; projection (i.e., disowning aspects of self while ascribing them to something or someone in environment); poor judgment; distractibility; fear of rejection and of interpersonal and physical closeness; lack of trust; vulnerability to stress

Perception: Appearance of listening to voices observed as movement in vocal cords and lips, head, and face; ability to process incoming stimuli; environment or persons may be perceived as threatening

Affect: Anxiety, loneliness, depression, apathy, colorless speech and monotonous voice, incongruity between emotional responses and idea, hostility

Activities: Withdrawal from relationships and contact with others; impairment in goal-directed activity; purposeless movement such as pacing and mannerisms; unpredictable behavior that may be related to delusions or hallucinations; agitation, fear, and potential violence; impairment or absence of social skills; poor work history; substance abuse

Self-care: Neglectfulness; lack of motivation; impairment in bathing, grooming, and hygiene

Nutrition: No awareness of hunger or thirst; apathy to food at mealtime; fear of eating (e.g., belief that food is poisoned)

Sleep pattern: Disturbed sleep patterns; reluctance to go to bed at night or inability to awaken in morning

Physical/Behavioral status: Evidence of substance abuse, inattention to physical health

Side effects of medications

- Typical antipsychotic medications (phenothiazines)
  - Orthostatic hypotension
  - Neuroleptic malignant syndrome (NMS): Diaphoresis; muscular rigidity; tachycardia, labile blood pressure with hypotension and hypertension, cardiac dysrhythmia; dyspnea, hyperpyrexia
- Atypical antipsychotic medications
  - Decreasing leukocyte count
  - Lowered seizure threshold
  - Akathisia
  - Weight gain
  - Somnolence
  - Difficulty with concentration
  - Agitation, nervousness
  - Asthenia (weakness)
  - Hypotension

Potential Complications

Related to medications: agranulocytosis, coma; injury to self or others

Patient Problems/Nursing Diagnoses & Interventions

NIC Communication Enhancement

Impaired social interaction related to social withdrawal

Disturbed sensory perception (auditory) related to altered sensory reception, transmission, and/or integration

- Begin to establish a trusting relationship *to provide sense of security for patient, starting with one-on-one interactions.*
- Visit patient frequently for brief periods *to demonstrate concern and to decrease fears of interpersonal closeness.*
- Tell patient when you are leaving and let him or her know when you will return.
- Avoid pushing a nonverbal patient to respond to questions *to prevent further withdrawal.*
- Comment on neutral subjects, such as patient's immediate environment (e.g., items in room, activities of others in room, pictures in a shared magazine).
- As you and patient are able to tolerate longer periods together, increase time gradually *to help patient begin working on issues.*
- If patient becomes increasingly agitated and distracting techniques are unsuccessful, medication may be administered in collaboration with physician *to decrease agitation.* Briefly explain reason for medication.
- Assist patient to develop social skills *to help patient interact, initiate a conversation, or make requests because these skills are often impaired.*
- Attend a small inpatient counseling session with the patient.
- Explain to patient that others have responsibilities for interactions and that patient is responsible only for his or her own behavior. Assist patient to elaborate on and build on strengths *to encourage patient to identify and accept skills.*
- Help patient to attend and participate in occupational therapy as prescribed *to promote skills and interests.*
- As patient is able to tolerate interactions with others, encourage recreational therapy *to gain skills in various activities, to expend energy through exercise, and to learn leisure activities.*
- Include outpatient meetings in the discharge plan.
- Establish trust through frequent, brief interactions, eventually encouraging patient to talk about fears, hallucinations, and other concerns.
- Approach in a calm, nonthreatening manner with low to moderate voice tone.
- Express reality regarding patient reports of hallucinations and delusions; continue to present a nonthreatening reality, engaging patient in reality-based topics and activities, *to increase awareness of actual versus irrational events and to promote socialization.*
- Assist and encourage patient's attending to self-care needs *to increase self-esteem, to provide a structured routine, and to encourage peer acceptance.*

NIC Risk Management

Risk for self-directed and other-directed violence related to agitated behavior patterns, paranoid delusions, vigilance and scanning, and hallucinations

Disturbed thought processes related to non–reality-based thinking

- Prevent violence and promote safety of patient and others.
- Provide frequent time away from stimulation of others, brief nonconfrontational interactions, and prn medications.
- Promote opportunities for rest and relaxation and ventilation of feelings.
- Present nonthreatening reality but enforce reality.
- Praise efforts made to refrain from impulsivity, from angry outbursts, and for compliance with medication regimen.
- Engage patient and family in treatment plan.
- Orient patient, as needed, to person, place, and time *to correct disorientation.*
- Avoid increasing patient's anxiety by approaching in a calm, low-key manner.
- Reduce environmental stimuli that are distracting *to decrease suspiciousness and guardedness.*
- Listen attentively to patient, listening for themes, feeling tones, or reality-oriented phrases or thoughts *to increase patient's willingness to relate to another human being.* Do not pretend understanding, but comment on understandable conversation.

- Assist patient, as he or she is able, to elaborate on reality-oriented ideas.
- Assist patient in correcting misconceptions about environment, self, and experiences through recall of events and use of problem solving.
- Do not encourage patient to repeat false beliefs by arguing or agreeing with him or her. To avoid reinforcing ideas of reference and delusions, "I find that hard to believe" may be an appropriate comment.
- Assist patient in examining what he or she was experiencing before delusional thoughts began. Attempt to assist patient in identifying thoughts and feelings toward self *to determine if patient was feeling threatened.* Gradually assist patient to recognize and correct delusional content of thoughts and feelings.
- When patient shows signs of anxiety or expresses discomfort, change topic *to decrease anxiety.* If patient is able to discuss an anxiety-provoking topic, help patient to identify feelings (awareness of feelings will evolve slowly).
- Administer medication as ordered. If you suspect patient is not swallowing tablets, concentrates may be administered.
- Briefly explain reason for medication, as well as its effects and side effects.
- Observe patient closely *to detect effects and side effects of medication,* and report to physician for dose adjustments as needed. Check vital signs as indicated.
- As patient is able to comprehend, describe effects and side effects of medication and reasons for medication *to increase potential for compliance.*

NIC NUTRITION SUPPORT

Imbalanced nutrition: less than body requirements, related to psychologic factors

- When a patient is suspicious of food, emphasize that food is nutritious and has not been tampered with; have patient participate in choosing foods and liquids *to decrease suspicousness.*
- Obtain patient's attention and suggest eating. If necessary, direct patient to take each mouthful (e.g., "Take a spoonful. Now eat it.").
- Offer fluids between meals to maintain hydration.
- Explain the ingredients and importance of good nutrition when patient is able to process information.

NIC SELF-CARE FACILITATION

Disturbed sleep pattern related to psychologic factors

- If patient has fears about going to sleep, assist him or her in talking about them *to begin to correct misconceptions.*
- Offer warm milk *to assist sleeping.*
- Encourage slow, deep breathing while focusing on the number "1" *to promote relaxation.*
- If helpful, turn the radio to soothing music at a low volume *to decrease panic or fears.*
- Discourage naps during the day *to enhance restful sleep at night.*

PATIENT EDUCATION/CONTINUUM OF CARE PLAN

1. Reinforce problem-solving techniques and social skills.
2. Assist patient in identifying and verbalizing strengths.
3. In conjunction with a community liaison, assist patient in establishing contact with a continuing care program in the community and in initiating participation.
4. Provide written information about medications, dosage, route, frequency, and when to contact care provider.
5. Educate patient regarding the need for continuing care from community providers.

EVALUATION/PATIENT OUTCOMES

Communication Enhancement: Patient participates in social activities with staff and other patients, spends less time alone in unit, and states that he or she enjoys participating in some planned and unplanned activities.

Patient no longer hallucinates, and states he or she no longer hears voices.

Risk Management: Patient no longer has psychotic symptoms. Patient is oriented to person, place, and time. He or she begins to use problem-solving methods to correct misconceptions. Patient verbalizes knowledge of effects and side effects of medicine and plans to comply with medication regimen.

Nutrition Support: Patient participates in choosing well-balanced meals, is no longer suspicious of food, eats food at mealtime, and verbalizes knowledge of nutritionally balanced food.

Self-Care Facilitation: Patient sleeps through the night, practices relaxation techniques before bedtime, and verbalizes that he or she is sleeping well during the night and is awakening refreshed.

MOOD DISORDERS

Mood is an emotional reaction that is sufficiently intense to affect a person's entire psychic state. **Mood disorders,** also known as *affective disorders,* are common psychiatric disorders characterized by disturbances in regulation of emotion, ranging from intense elation and irritability to severe depression. The major mood disorders include the **depressive disorders**

! EMERGENCY ALERT

MOOD DISORDERS

BIPOLAR DISORDERS: MANIC PHASE

- May be a danger to self or others due to agitation and decreased judgment.
- May not comply with treatment regimen or voluntary admission to hospital.
- May not attend to basic physical needs.

DEPRESSIVE DISORDERS

- Suicidal ideation and attempts are common.
- Lack of interest and energy often interfere with activities of daily living and adequate food and fluid intake.
- Sleep pattern disturbances may be severe.

(unipolar), the **bipolar disorders** (bipolar), mood disorders that result from a medical condition, and substance-induced mood disorders. The two major moods are manic and depressive episodes, whereas a person with a unipolar disorder has experienced at least one or more episodes of depression with no manic phase. The focus of this discussion will be on bipolar and depressive disorders. The manic and depressive manifestations of the disorders are compared in the Emergency Alert box.[5,37]

Bipolar Disorders

In the bipolar disorders, the **manic phase** is characterized by grandiosity, excessive excitement, flight of ideas, and psychomotor overactivity; the **depressive phase** is characterized by a sense of despair, retarded thinking, and psychomotor retardation or agitation.[5]

Manic behavior is excessive mental and physical activity. Thought is accelerated and expansive; mood is labile with rapid sequences of euphoria, irritability, depression, elation, and rage. Physical activity is excessive with boundless energy, little need for sleep, constant motion, and assaultiveness in response to limit setting. Persons in manic states have pressured speech and flight of ideas and are self-indulgent, impatient, humorous, extroverted, friendly, impulsive, and distractible. They appear to have unlimited self-confidence and self-assurance as they propel their energy outward into the environment. The levels of mood disturbance vary from mild to severe with psychotic features[5] (see Emergency Alert box, p. 1264).

The **bipolar I disorder** has at least one or more frank manic to psychotic or mixed episodes and usually one or more major depressive episodes. **Bipolar II disorder** has one or more major depressive periods and at least one hypomanic episode. When the bipolar disorder episodes occur at least four times within a 1-year period, the diagnosis includes the specifier of rapid-cycling.[5] The phases must be separated by either a period of remission or by a distinct switch to the opposite polarity. For a mixed episode, the period must be for at least 1 week, with rapidly alternating moods of depression and mania occurring nearly every day.

In the **hypomanic episode** the mood is elevated and grandiose, and the person is very talkative, has flight of ideas, pressured speech, and decreased need for sleep. This distinctly observable period lasts for at least 4 days.

In **cyclothymic disorder,** numerous fluctuating symptoms of mania and depression are present for at least 2 years, but the severity does not achieve the criteria of a major depressive or manic episode.[5]

Although depression affects women twice as often as men, bipolar disorders occur at the same rate in both sexes. Persons with a first-degree biologic relative who has been diagnosed with depression have a 4% to 24% chance of developing bipolar I disorder and a 1% to 5% chance of developing bipolar II disorder. It is estimated that 10% to 15% of adolescents with recurrent major depressive disorder will go on to develop bipolar I disorder.[5]

In 20% to 30% of patients the first episode of the disorder is likely to occur before age 20 years, and the incidence rises until age 35 years. The highest prevalence is in persons between ages 18 and 44 years, with women having an earlier onset than men. The onset of each phase can be sudden, especially in mania; symptoms can escalate within a few hours. However, both phases can have slower onsets. The episodes in bipolar disorders often occur irregularly but may also alternate regularly, such as with seasonal patterns of mania in the spring and summer and with depression in the fall and winter.[5] Episodes may be separated by symptom-free periods or may follow each other with no appreciable interval between them. The average duration of episodes in bipolar disorders ranges from 4 to 13 months (the longer duration generally occurred before the availability of current medications). Modern treatment methods, including medications, have obscured the phases and blurred the development of symptoms.[97]

The prevalence of bipolar disorders is underestimated in the population because of inconsistencies in the diagnostic classifications used among investigators and clinicians in the same or between countries. Without a detailed history of the patient's previous symptoms, caregivers will be unable to accurately identify the chronic, cyclic nature of the disorders. The lifetime prevalence rate for bipolar disorders is estimated to be between 0.3% and 1.6% in the adult population.[5] The National Institute of Mental Health (NIMH) estimates that at least 2.3 million people in the United States suffer from bipolar illness.[79]

Psychopathology/Pathophysiology

The cause of bipolar disorders is unknown. There is widespread belief that the disease is due to some genetically determined biochemical abnormality of the brain. Twin studies reveal that when one monozygotic twin has bipolar I disorder, the likelihood that the other twin will have it is very high, approaching 90% to 100%.[40] For fraternal twins the rate is approximately 20%. First-degree relatives of persons with bipolar I disorder have occurrence rates of 4% to 24%, occurrence rates of bipolar II disorder of 1% to 5%, and occurrence rates of major depressive disorder of 4% to 24%.[5]

In looking for biochemical abnormalities of the brain, scientists have noted that there are recognizable differences in the brain metabolism of persons with mania than in so-called normal persons. Also of note are the suspected abnormalities of serotonin and dopamine in depressive disorders. In addition, there are identifiable differences in patterns of urinary and plasma catacholamines in persons with bipolar disorder and persons with unipolar depression. Longitudinal studies are indicated to identify the time of occurrence of structural and functional abnormalities, whether before, during, or after the illness, and whether there is a return to normal during remission.

Sleep deprivation has been identified clinically as a precipitating factor in manic episodes. Sleep deprivation can cause a rapid shift from depression to mania and has been related to manic states that occur after jet lag, after the death of a family member, and during the postpartum period. Manic episodes may also be precipitated by physical illnesses such as infectious diseases, thyroid and other endocrine disorders, and neurologic disorders.

In the past much attention was paid to psychologic theories as an etiologic factor in bipolar illnesses. The current thinking is that environmental and psychosocial factors play a role in the precipitation of an episode in an individual who was genetically predisposed to the illness.

Hypomania is a pathologic state that is less severe than mania. The person has intensified energy, a stable elated mood, self-indulgence, distractibility, pressured speech, poor judgment, and increased motor activity. Hypomanic persons radiate good health, appear tireless, and are humorous and friendly to the point of being unacceptably personal with others. Their intolerance to limit setting is observed as irritability or anger.[5]

Mania or acute mania is a more intense and disturbed level in which propriety and discretion are absent. Persons in this state tease and joke, often making others the butt of their jokes. Their good humor can change rapidly to vicious anger. They flit from one activity to another without completing anything. They may talk incessantly because impulses are expressed in words, with flight of ideas proceeding to incoherence and clang association (mental association between dissociated ideas made because of similarity of sounds of words used to describe the ideas). These persons have delusions of grandeur concerning their wealth and power and have lost control of their behavior, but they do not have severe disturbances of self-identity as in schizophrenia.[37]

Persons with delirious mania or psychosis evidence all of the symptoms of the previous levels plus loss of contact with reality. Speech is incoherent, activity is constant and purposeless, and delusions and hallucinations are present. At times incontinence of urine and feces occurs.[43] Interactions with manics, and less so with hypomanics, are stressful to others because of their exploitative behaviors, which include manipulating the self-esteem of others by praise and deflation; striking exploitatively at vulnerable areas; projecting responsibility onto others; testing limits of rules by trying to extend them; and alienating others, especially family members.

Family members dealing with the difficulties of supporting a loved one with bipolar disorder are often in need of support themselves. Educational needs are typically of greatest importance initially. Family members need knowledge about the chronic, cyclic nature of bipolar disorders, the symptoms, and treatment. Because of the inherited nature of the disorder, genetic counseling may be requested or even recommended. They also need support and coping skills to lessen the stressfulness of family life. When able, the patient should participate in family sessions to help correct communication difficulties and to develop problem-solving skills. Patients with supportive, knowledgeable families are more likely to comply with the treatment regimen than those with no families or nonsupportive ones.[37]

Mood stabilizers are the preferred pharmacologic agents for management of bipolar disorders. They are used to treat and prevent mania. Antidepressants can provoke manic episodes in bipolar patients if used alone but may be used in combination with an effective mood stabilizer. Lithium, Tegretol, and Depakote are mood stabilizers that are most commonly used.[28,37,97,99]

Diagnostic Studies and Findings

SMAC: To rule out abnormalities in various systems, including serum electrolytes; repeat serum electrolytes after lithium therapy is started

Complete blood count: To rule out infections before lithium therapy; follow-up to assess elevated white blood cell count resulting from lithium therapy or infection

Thyroid function tests: To assess for abnormal thyroid; repeat after beginning lithium therapy every 6 to 12 months

Lithium levels: To obtain baseline before lithium therapy (normal values) and after therapy is initiated

Electrocardiogram: To obtain baseline level and to rule out cardiac disease; after lithium therapy to assess changes resulting from therapy

Pregnancy (test in women during childbearing years: To rule out pregnancy before initiating lithium therapy to prevent abnormality in fetus, especially in the first trimester

Urinalysis: To screen for infection or systemic abnormalities

Urine toxicology: To screen for substance abuse

Multidisciplinary Plan

Medications

Lithium carbonate (Lithane, Eskalith), 300 mg PO qid or 600 mg PO tid
  Monitor serum levels

Divalproex (Depakote), 500-1500 mg daily PO

Carbamazepine (Tegratol), 400-1200 mg daily; similar to Depakote in tolerance and side effects

NURSING CARE

Nursing Assessment

The mental and physical activities of manic persons vary with the severity of the mood disturbance.

Physical activity: Hyperactivity (moving rapidly from one activity to another, bustling about, restlessness, pacing, fidgeting); limited ability to complete tasks owing to distractibility; eyes bright; face flushed; head erect; animated facial expression; increased metabolism; unrestrained playfulness and mischievousness; uninhibited activity (e.g., singing, dancing); expansive gesturing; dramatic self-expression in movement; colorful appearance (wearing bright colors, jewelry); telephone abuse (calls at all hours); acting out of impulses; sexual acting out without discretion; alcohol abuse; giving money and possessions away; assaultiveness, especially when requests are denied and limits are set; violation of rules; abusiveness; destruction of belongings or bedclothes; violent motor excitement in severely disturbed patients, which may be directed toward self or others

Thought processes: Enhanced sensory acuity (stimulated by other people, objects, and environment); flight of ideas (skipping from one idea to another without completing any); distractibility; expansive, vivid, intense thoughts; impaired judgment; intact memory and orientation to person, place, and time (except when severely disturbed); lack of motivation to change based on feeling well; self-confidence, self-centeredness; enthusiasm; self-will; overvaluing of abilities and performance; projection of responsibility onto others; loose associations evidenced in incoherence; paranoid ideation (emerges from anger); arrogance; haughtiness; vengeful ideas; criticism of others; delusions of grandeur (false beliefs of power, wealth, achievements; wish-fulfilling type); clang association of thoughts (words with similar sounds but no relation of meaning, such as ring, ding, and ling); loss of contact with reality; clouded consciousness; visual and auditory hallucinations when severe

Communication: Loquacity to logorrhea; pressured, rapid speech, speaking with vigor, excitement, animation, emphasis; flowery, witty, loud, lewd, or pompous speech; superficial content; manipulative (pleas and threats, praise and deflation, ingratiating manner, excuses, bargaining, demanding, deception, verbal abuse, trying to extend limits)

Affect: Labile mood (elation, euphoria, exhilaration, irritability, anger, laughter, cheerfulness, tearfulness, tremulousness, depression, sadness)

Social interactions: Appearance of warmth and lability, entertaining, humorous affect; joking, making others the butt of joke; fear of interpersonal intimacy; meddling; interference with and intrusion in others' interaction; attempts to dominate others; exploitation of others' vulnerable areas; destructiveness in group interactions; group interactions may heighten hyperactivity; may abuse substances

Self-care: Obliviousness concerning infections and other physical illness as disturbance increases; neglect of personal needs and grooming

Nutrition: Decrease in appetite but no major weight loss; dehydration possible with hyperactivity

Family: promises to partner made and broken; demeaning of family with anger and blame; family conflicts and instability; spouse perceives patient as spiteful, lacking in understanding and knowledge of condition, and as having diminished self-esteem

Medication side effects

Lithium: Thirst, polyuria, diarrhea, thyroid abnormalities, weight gain

Divalproex: Prolongation of anticoagulant effects if patient is taking Coumadin

Potential Complications

Violence, self-directed or directed to others

Patient Problems/Nursing Diagnoses & Interventions

NIC Communication Enhancement

Impaired social interactions related to hyperactivity, social influences, and biochemical factors

Impaired verbal communication related to flight of ideas

- Provide quiet, nonstimulating environment *to prevent escalation of excitement.*
- If patient is highly excited, restrict patient from the general patient population areas *to avoid stimulation and the possibility of aggression toward others and abuse by other patients.*
- Explain restrictions simply and make use of distractibility.
- Permit patient on unit for brief periods as excitement decreases *to adapt to stimulation and less structure.*
- Begin to develop a supportive relationship through consistent, frequent interpersonal exchanges.
- Administer medication as prescribed *to begin treatment of mania.*
- Be certain patient swallows oral medication; to set limits, do not allow patient to bargain to take medication later.
- Monitor for effects and possible adverse reactions to medication *to prevent toxicity.*
- Explain the effects and the side effects of medication when condition stabilizes and patient is able to hear instruction *to increase compliance.*
- Discuss the importance of maintenance dose of medication and ongoing compliance (be aware that patient is concerned about losing sense of well-being).
- As excitement begins to decrease, involve patient in gross motor activities such as walking and exercise. Be aware that activities often increase excitement rather than produce tranquility and fatigue.
- To set firm, consistent limits on behavior, give short explanation as needed. Staff members need to understand and conform to uniform limits. Encourage patient, when able, to set own limits on behavior, consistent with treatment goals.
- Allow patient opportunity to express anger about restriction in an appropriate way; if anger is inappropriate, use distraction to change focus.
- Gradually help integrate patient into general unit milieu; be alert for overstimulation.
- As patient is able, assist to identify frequency, duration, and type of patient's mood changes *to learn to detect subtle changes and patterns indicating mood disturbances.*
- Explain illness and treatment to patient *to deal with chronicity and cyclic nature of illness and to increase self-awareness and compliance with treatment regimen.*
- When patient's speech is pressured, rapid, and loud, respond in soft, assertive voice, make short statements, and speak slowly *to help calm patient.*
- Respond to appropriate humor, but be careful not to escalate excitement and hostility.
- When patient is able, explore inappropriate humor. For example, when humor is inconsistent with content, assist patient to express himself or herself directly.
- When patient makes requests, indicate what you will and will not do in interactions and in the treatment plan *to maintain consistent limits.*
- Schedule frequent brief sessions with patient during an acute manic episode (e.g., 15 minutes) *to begin to develop a relationship.* Increase length of sessions as excitement decreases and patient is able to respond.
- When patient verbally strikes out at you, help patient identify underlying feelings. If patient continues, communicate your discomfort and let patient know that you will leave if abuse continues. Leave if patient does not stop.
- Practice assertiveness skills with patient *to assist patient to gain a sense of control and influence.*

NIC Risk Management

Risk for self-directed or other-directed violence related to manic state excitement

- Be alert for possible physical aggression against other patients, staff, or self. If patient is in general unit area, remove from situation, giving short, firm directions *to provide a "time out."*

- Use distraction before aggression escalates.
- Protect patient from other patients' aggressiveness and pranks *to prevent him or her from being verbally or physically abused.*
- If necessary, obtain an order for medication as needed (e.g., haloperidol) *to decrease aggressiveness.*
- Evaluate patient for suicide potential. If patient is suicidal, institute precautions.
- Encourage patient, when able, to identify and accept angry feelings and to increase self-understanding.
- Encourage use of a problem-solving approach *to relate feelings to events that evoked them and develop appropriate ways to resolve issues.*
- Help patient to attend occupational therapy activities and recreational activities when ready and as prescribed.
- Provide opportunities to talk about activities *to resolve problem areas.*
- Encourage patient to identify enjoyable activities.
- Direct patient to appropriate activities, such as punching bag or exercise, *to discharge energies.*

NIC Nutrition Support

Imbalanced nutrition: less than body requirements, related to hyperactivity

- When patient is highly excited, provide food in small unbreakable containers or finger foods *to eat while standing or pacing.* If necessary, provide food in liquid form.
- Ensure that patient's fluid intake is more than 1000 ml *to prevent lithium toxicity.*
- Explain to patient the importance of good nutrition with normal sodium and fluid intake.
- If oral intake of fluids is to be restricted before medical treatments, such as surgery or laboratory tests, inform physician *so intravenous fluids can be given to prevent dehydration and lithium toxicity.*
- Have dietitian provide additional information on diet as needed.

Other related nursing diagnoses: Disturbed thought processes related to altered mental status; ineffective coping related to labile mood; self-care deficit (bathing/hygiene and dressing/grooming) related to labile mood; disturbed sleep pattern related to excessive excitement; interrupted family processes related to family's lack of understanding of the illness.

Patient Education/Continuum of Care Plan

1. Teach patient about the cyclic nature of the illness and the importance of adherence to the treatment regimen.
2. Provide written materials that present the effects and side effects of medications, the need for regular lithium blood level tests, and behavioral symptoms and signs that should be reported to the care provider.
3. Provide teaching and written materials about the importance of good nutrition, sodium intake, and fluid intake.
4. Assist with linkages to continuing care.

Evaluation/Patient Outcomes

Communication Enhancement: Patient attains persistent mood level nearing healthy state for self. Patient sits quietly for periods. Patient accepts realistic limits and delays. Patient verbalizes knowledge of illness and treatment and makes plans to continue treatment regimen after discharge. Patient states major effects and adverse effects of medications.

Risk Management: Patient demonstrates decrease in aggressiveness and verbalizes beginning awareness of angry feelings and beginning skills in resolving issues. Patient carries on normal conversations with others and speaks in a well-modulated manner. Patient practices assertiveness skills to deal with events and communicates needs directly. Patient continues to work on listening skills with others.

Nutrition Support: Patient demonstrates knowledge of adequate nutrition, including adequate daily sodium and fluid intake.

Depressive Disorders

Depression is an abnormal mood state in which a person characteristically has a sense of hopelessness, helplessness, worthlessness, and despair; morbid thoughts; and psychomotor retardation or agitation.

This mood state may be indicative of a first episode or of a recurrent episode of depression. The symptoms experienced occur as a result of the disorder and not from the effects of a substance, medical condition, or loss of a loved one within the previous 2 months. There is a period of at least 2 weeks during which there is a depressed mood, which usually includes the loss of interest in nearly all activities (anhedonia). Depression may occur as the polarity of mania in the bipolar disorder. It frequently occurs as a unipolar disorder, in which the person experiences depressive symptoms with no manic episodes.[5,37]

The common diagnostic categories of unipolar depression identified in the DSM-IV follow.

Major depressive disorder is a single episode consisting of severe symptoms of depression and loss of interest and pleasure in self and environment nearly every day for most of the day for at least 2 weeks. Loss of energy, feelings of worthlessness and hopelessness, decreased ability to think or concentrate, and psychomotor retardation or agitation are some symptoms that are present. The person has no manic episode and has only one major depressive episode with a return to premorbid functioning. Untreated depression typically last for 6 months or more.

Major depressive disorder is a recurrent condition in which the person has two or more major depressive episodes with a separation between episodes of at least 2 months, and with no previous manic states.

Dysthymic disorder in the adult is a chronic, milder depressive disturbance than major depressive disorder. Duration is almost every day for most of the day for at least 2 years (duration for children or adolescents is at least 1 year). There is a poor appetite or overeating, sleep disturbances, fatigue, low self-esteem, feelings of hopelessness, and poor concentration. It is estimated that up to

50% of dysthymic persons eventually develop major depression.[5,37,42] Some specifiers for the most recent disorder include moderate, severe with psychotic features, severe without psychotic features, in partial or full remission, and chronic.

For patients with recurrent seasonal depressive episodes or bipolar disorders, the specifier "with seasonal pattern" may be included. The time of year is a feature of this, with depression most frequently occurring in the fall or winter and alleviating in spring.[5]

Women are twice as likely as men to be affected by a unipolar depressive illness. The disorder is one and one-half to three times more common among first-degree biologic relatives than it is in the general population. Depression is a serious and frequent complication of heart attack (20% to 50%), stroke (30% to 50%), rheumatoid arthritis (42%), and cancer (50%).[5,37,55,79] The elderly are especially susceptible to depression, with nursing home residents showing a prevalence as high as 25%.[89] Depressive symptoms in the elderly are often missed and incorrectly attributed to organic disorders. Because mild depression evidenced in sulkiness, withdrawal from social activities, and restlessness is common among adolescents because of maturation crises, the more severe depressions may not be identified.[5]

Depression is the single most frequently occurring psychiatric condition in the general population. Because of social and occupational discrimination, people are resistant to seeking treatment for depression and other psychiatric conditions; therefore many go undiagnosed and untreated. The onset of depression appears to be occurring in younger persons, and 19 million people in the United States who are age 18 years and older are affected each year. Major depression is the leading cause of disability in the United States, costing more than 30 billion dollars per year. The suicide rate is approximately 15% and is estimated to be as much as 50% higher in the depressed elderly.[96] The onset of depression usually occurs in the twenties, but it may begin in childhood, in infancy, or in old age.[55,79]

PSYCHOPATHOLOGY/PATHOPHYSIOLOGY

Studies of mood disorders in families show that there is consistent concordance within families. First-degree relatives of persons with mood disorders are two to three times more likely to be affected by a mood disorder than the general population. Adoption and twin studies also support the theory of an underlying genetic component for depressive disorders. The most widely published neurotransmitter hypothesis in relation to causation of depression involves the serotonin hypothesis. This postulates that a decrease of available serotonin in the brain causes depression. This theory is supported by the success of the selective serotonin reuptake inhibitors (SSRIs). The norepinephrine hypothesis postulates that a deficit in norepinephrine at receptor sites in the brain also contributes to the occurrence of depression and is validated by the effectiveness of the monoamine oxidase inhibitors (MAOIs) and the tricyclic antidepressant medications, which increase the availability of catacholamines, specifically norepinephrine, at the postsynaptic receptor sites. Other neurotransmitters that are being explored in relation to their role in depression include γ-aminobutric acid (GABA) and dopamine. GABA, the major inhibitory neurotransmitter, is being explored for its role in the inhibition of brain excitability, and dopamine is being explored in relation to decreased dopaminergic activity in depression, specifically psychomotor retardation.[9]

Mild depression is often undiagnosed. Those with severe depression are easier to identify. Symptoms of **mild depression** include unpleasant feelings about self and the environment; self-sacrificing, especially in relation to giving to others; inhibition of normal pleasurable activities; inhibition of spontaneous behavior; extra effort needed to concentrate; preoccupation with trivial failures and underestimating ability; pessimistic outlook toward life; self-reproach and irritability for not living up to an ideal standard; dependence on others for gratification; and somatic symptoms.[5] Symptoms of **severe depression** include utter despair and hopelessness, sense of emptiness, unrelieved sense of guilt and feeling of worthlessness, severe immobility or agitated behavior that is purposeless and lacks conscious control, catastrophic expectations, lack of interest in self and environment, retarded thought processes to process and respond to stimuli, retardation of bodily processes, preoccupation with bodily functions, and delusional thinking that becomes severe when contact with reality is greatly impaired or lost.

Family members may feel sympathy and be supportive of the depressed person, but as the depression continues and even deepens, the family may become discouraged. All of their help does nothing to lift the person's mood. Because the depressed person makes known his or her feelings of helplessness, despair, and emptiness, family members may begin to experience similar feelings. Family members require knowledge about depression and their ill member in particular. They also need emotional support and guidance through family therapy, which includes the patient, to learn to communicate with each other and cope with their concerns.[37]

Pharmaceuticals have evolved into a major treatment approach for persons with depression. Since the 1950s antidepressants have been evolving and improving the quality of life of persons suffering from depressive disorders. The biggest improvement in these drugs has been in the side-effect profiles. All antidepressant medications are based on the theory that depression results from decreased amounts of the neurotransmitters serotonin or norepinephrine in the brain. The first generation of antidepressants, the MAOIs, block monoamine oxidase (an enzyme that breaks down the neurotransmitters serotonin and norepinephrine). The tricyclics block the reuptake of these neurotransmitters by neurons. As the neurotransmitter serotonin became a focus in depression, the SSRIs were developed and because of their safety profile, now dominate the pharmaceutical market for antidepressant use.[37,55,99] Full antidepressant effect may take up to 4 weeks or more. Caution must be taken when there is a possibility of pregnancy, as well as when the patient is on other medications.

Seasonal affective disorder (SAD), is a nonpsychotic depression that occurs in the winter months, especially at high altitudes. It is most prevalent in women (60% to 90%) and young adults. It is a cyclic disorder in which episodes begin in the fall or winter and improve in the spring. Therapeutic lighting, which is about 5% to 20% brighter than indoor lighting, is prescribed by knowledgeable clinicians and administered in the home.

Diagnostic Studies and Findings

SMAC: To screen for general medical causes for depression
Thyroid function tests: To rule out abnormal thyroid, especially in depressed women age 50 years and over
Electrocardiogram: To rule out cardiopathy; this is particularly important with most antidepressant medications
Urinalysis: To rule out urologic problems and other medical disorders

Multidisciplinary Plan

Medications

MAOIs
Phenelzine (Nardil), 45-90 mg/day
Tranylcypramine (Parnate), 30-60 mg/day
Isocarboxazid (Marplan), 30-50 mg/day

Tricyclics and heterocyclics
Amitriptyline (Elavil), 25-300 mg/day
Doxepin (Sinequan), 25-300 mg/day
Imipramine (Tofranil), 25-300 mg/day
Trimipramine (Surmontil), 50-300 mg/day
Desipramine (Norpramin), 25-300 mg/day
Nortriptyline (Pamelor), 30-100 mg/day
Protriptyline (Vivactil), 15-60 mg/day
Clomipramine (Anafranil), 75-300 mg/day
Amoxapine (Asendin), 50-600 mg/day
Maprotiline (Ludiomil), 100-225 mg/day
Side effects of tricyclic and heterocyclic antidepressants can be serious, including cardiac toxicity (arrhythmias), delirium, seizures, memory loss, disorientation, and agitation; less serious side effects include sedating and drying (dry mouth) effects, constipation, and weight gain

Aminoketones
Wellbutrin, 200-450 mg/day
Common side effects include headache, restlessness, tremors, insomnia, and nausea

SSRIs
Fluoxetine (Prozac), 10-40 mg/day
Fluvoxamine (Luvox), 50-300 mg/day
Paroxetine (Paxil), 10-50 mg/day
Sertraline (Zoloft), 50-200 mg/day

Serotonin-norepinephrine reuptake inhibitor (SNRI)
Effexor, 75-375 mg/day

Serotonin-receptor modulator (SRM)
Traxodone (Desyrel), 150-600 mg/day
Nefazodone (Serzone), 300-600 mg/day
These drugs, although more expensive, have been shown to have a wide therapeutic range and a greater margin of safety; the most common side effects include nausea, diarrhea, insomnia, anxiety, restlessness, tremor, and sexual dysfunction

General Management

Behavioral therapy
Phototherapy for SAD
Electroconvulsive therapy (ECT) if unresponsive to antidepressants or if severe suicidal risk; or for acute mania and catatonia; considered as safe or safer than drug therapy.
Tyramine-restricted diet if taking MAOIs
Nutritional consultation

NURSING CARE

Nursing Assessment

The severity and types of symptoms vary with each patient, with no one symptom experienced by all persons with depression.

Affect: Extreme sadness, despair, painful dejection, tearfulness, irritability, anxiety, feeling of emptiness
Activities: Low energy; fatigue; lack of ability or motivation to perform tasks; slow movements; eyes downcast and avoidance of eye contact; agitated, purposeless behavior evidenced by pacing and restlessness; substance abuse (e.g., alcohol)
Self-care: Lack of interest and energy to perform activities of daily living such as bathing, dressing, and hygiene
Nutrition: Lack of appetite or interest in food (occasionally increased appetite); indigestion; weight loss, usually not critical but may be when condition is very severe or psychotic; evidence of malnutrition or obesity
Bowel elimination: Constipation
Sleep pattern: Inability to fall asleep, especially with anxiety, or waking early in morning; restless sleep; hypersomnia, occasionally through most of the day, owing to fatigue or withdrawal
Power and control: Sense of lack of power or control; decreased coping strategies; inability to identify own strengths; hopelessness, usually greatest when awakening in the morning; helplessness; feeling that nothing the patient can do will make a difference
Self-harm: Seriousness of suicidal risk, suicidal thoughts and threats, previous self-harming behavior, statements indicating intent and development of a plan
Thought processes: Morbid thoughts; worry; narrow and repetitive range of thoughts; forgetfulness and inability to concentrate; self-rejection and criticism of self and others; somatic complaints; delusions about body and environment, especially bizarre in severe depression; negative view of self, environment, and the future; failures exaggerated; achievements disowned; paranoid ideation
Communication: Impaired ability to process and respond to verbal stimuli, slow thinking, slow speech, low voice, monotonous tone, limited ability to concentrate
Social interactions: Withdrawal from social interactions and activities because of sense of unworthiness, limited social skills, loneliness, apathy concerning others
Side effects of monoamine oxidase inhibitors: Dry mouth; agitation, anxiety, insomnia; decreased heart rate, hypotension; dizziness, syncope, blurred vision; urinary hesitancy, sexual dysfunction; weight gain; peripheral neuropathy
Side effects of monoamine oxidase inhibitors in conjunction with consumption of tyramine-rich foods (e.g., strong cheeses, salami, sauerkraut): Elevated blood pressure, headache, restlessness
Side effects of tricyclics and heterocyclics: Dry mouth, constipation, weight gain; arrhythmias secondary to cardiotoxicity; disorientation, agitation, memory loss; delirium; seizures
Side effects of aminoketones: Headache, nausea; restlessness, tremors, insomnia

Side effects of serotonin-norepinephrine reuptake inhibitors: Nausea, diarrhea; anxiety, restlessness, tremors, insomnia; sexual dysfunction

Potential Complications

Hypertensive crisis with MAOIs or tyramine-rich foods, sleep deprivation due to depression, injury to self or others, substance abuse as self-medication for depression

Patient Problems/Nursing Diagnoses & Interventions

Nursing care should be implemented based on severity of symptoms and presenting behaviors.

NIC Risk Management

Risk for self-directed violence related to sense of hopelessness and depression

- Institute suicide precautions: Safe environment, removal of harmful objects, and close observation *to prevent suicide attempts.*
- Begin to establish trusting, supportive relationship *to let patient know you care and are concerned.*
- Schedule frequent, brief therapeutic periods daily *so they are tolerable to patient and nurse;* schedule longer sessions as depression lifts and patient is able to tolerate more *to develop relationship.*
- Speak slowly, using short sentences, *to increase patient's ability to attend to and comprehend words.* As patient is able, assist patient *to identify abilities and communicate hopes for the future to reinforce resources.*
- Continue close observation as depression lifts or as depression deepens *because patient has energy to attempt suicide;* observe for verbal and nonverbal clues to self-harm.
- Administer medication as ordered.
- Briefly describe the medicine's effects and side effects initially.
- When patient has improved, teach effects of medications and importance of compliance *to counteract depressive symptoms.*

NIC Coping Assistance

Ineffective coping related to inadequate coping methods

- When patient is agitated, accept pacing and inability to sit still.
- To let patient know of your presence, say, for example, "I am here and want to help you."
- Discuss and assist patient with diversionary techniques when restless, such as an activity *to decrease emotional discomfort;* encourage patient to practice the techniques *to help strengthen patient's healthy strategies for dealing with inappropriate feelings.*
- Practice relaxation exercises, such as slow, deep breathing while focusing on the number 1, *to promote relaxation and sense of control.*
- Help patient to identify positive attributes about self and about achievements *so that patient can begin to accept self realistically and develop a positive self-view.*
- Identify patient's own resources and social support system of family, friends, and community resources *to reinforce strengths.*
- Assist patient in developing interests and social skills *to increase self-confidence.*
- Practice with patient how to ask for and accept help *to increase sense of control.*
- Practice with patient how to accept others' refusals *to give help without the patient's feeling rejected, guilty, or self-critical to reinforce the idea that refusals are not rejection of patient.*
- Role-play assertiveness techniques *to give patient sense of control and to let others know needs and desires.*

NIC Behavior Therapy

Disturbed thought processes related to psychologic conflicts and psychomotor retardation

- To interrupt ruminations, suggest diversionary activities if attempts fail *to help patient appropriately focus on topics.*
- Assist patient in monitoring subject change to make decisions about changing subject a conscious choice.
- Encourage patient to think about self and experiences realistically *to identify and accept positive attributes.*
- Assist patient in identifying relationship between incorrect thoughts and feelings of depression.
- Help patient identify the stimulus or event *to examine inappropriateness of faulty thinking about behavior and self to correct misinterpretations and negative views of self.*
- Discuss and practice role-playing and problem-solving approach to problematic events and evaluate the possible consequences of alternative solutions *to learn effective methods to resolve issues.*
- Help patient to anticipate problems that may be encountered after discharge *to identify possible responses to issues and consequences of each solution.*

Other related nursing diagnoses: Impaired verbal communication related to delusional thinking; self-care (bathing/hygiene and dressing/grooming) deficit related to lack of interest in self; imbalanced nutrition: less than body requirements related to lack of appetite; constipation related to retarded body processes; impaired urinary elimination related to retarded body processes; disturbed sleep pattern related to severe depression; powerlessness related to lack of interest in self or environment; social isolation related to sense of worthlessness; interrupted family processes related to depression

Patient Education/Continuum of Care Plan

1. Provide patient with written instructions regarding therapeutic effects and possible side effects of medications and phone number of health-care provider.
2. Assist patient in verbalizing understanding of depression and the importance of the treatment regimen.
3. Provide liaison for informal and formal support systems for the patient, including contact persons, addresses, and phone numbers.
4. Review the use of problem-solving and cognitive-thinking techniques to aid in the use of resources and self-support.

EVALUATION/PATIENT OUTCOMES

Risk Management: Patient demonstrates relief of symptoms of suicidal thoughts and threats. Self-harming behavior is absent. Patient states no plan to do self harm.

Coping Assistance: Patient demonstrates increased coping skills. Patient practices increased ability to identify needs, to ask others for help, and to use self-support procedures in a more self-confident manner. Patient uses increased social skills in interactions with others.

Behavior Therapy: Patient demonstrates increased ability to correct impaired thinking. Patient expresses an increased awareness of the relationships among experiences, thoughts, and depressive feelings. Patient practices use of problem-solving approach to correct misconceptions about self and the future.

ANXIETY DISORDERS

Anxiety is an integral part of human existence. It may be a feeling of uneasiness, impending threat, or overwhelming danger. Anxiety is a subjective experience that can be inferred by observing a person's behavior and physiologic responses and by subjective reports. Apprehension, dread, and intense alertness to an unspecified source of danger are symptoms of anxiety.

Anxiety may be mild or severe responses to an unmet expectation. In mild anxiety the person becomes alert and is able to observe more of himself or herself and of his or her environment, which may occur when a person is late or misses an appointment. In moderate anxiety the person is selectively inattentive to stimuli outside a narrow field, as might be experienced when taking a difficult examination. Learning can occur in these levels of anxiety. The anxious person uses defense mechanisms as the primary method of managing the anxiety; however, as the level of anxiety increases, the person becomes more disorganized and the perceptual field more narrow. When a person experiences severe anxiety, such as witnessing an accident, the focus is on specific detail. When in a state of panic, the person experiences a state of awe, doom, and possibly terror. The disorganization of the personality causes the person to lose control; no learning occurs unless anxiety is reduced because of reduced perception of stimuli and because of responses that are mainly automatic relief behaviors. Unlike fear, which is a response to an actual object or event, anxiety is a response to no specific source or actual object.[37]

Anxiety disorders are classified in the DSM-IV according to their characteristic diagnostic criteria. These disorders share several common features, including hyperarousal, a morbid sense of fear, and a hyperactive autonomic nervous system (shortness of breath, rapid heart rate, diaphoresis, dry mouth, and polyuria).[5] Some anxiety disorders have additional features that distinguish them.

Panic disorder is characterized by the presence of recurrent panic attacks, which are episodes of intense fear with autonomic hyperarousal that come on suddenly and peak within 10 minutes, possibly lasting for hours. There is intense fear or discomfort accompanied by several physiologic symptoms, including tachycardia, diaphoresis, tremors, shortness of breath, choking sensations, chest pain, nausea, dizziness, and fear of losing control or of dying. The term *panic disorder* is not used interchangeably with *panic attack.* Panic disorder can be chronic with a waxing and waning course. Typical onset is between late adolescence and mid-thirties, but onset can occur late in life.

Agoraphobia is a fear of being in certain situations (usually many) in which escape might be difficult or embarrassing. There is the perception that help might not be available and one is helpless and powerless. An example would be traveling in an airplane or in a bus. Agoraphobia may or may not occur in the context of panic disorder.

Obsessive-compulsive disorder (OCD) presents with obsessions (recurrent and persistent ideas, thoughts, or impulses that cannot be ignored) perceived as alien to the person's nature and compulsions (repetitive, purposeful, and intentional behaviors performed in response to an obsession) that cause distress and are time consuming. This condition usually begins in adolescence or early adulthood but is known to take a chronic course and often persists into later life.

Posttraumatic stress disorder (PTSD) typically occurs after an extreme and frightening event (accident, crime, war experience, or a natural disaster). The event is replayed and reexperienced through dreams, hallucinations, and flashbacks. Individuals exhibit numbing of feelings, increased arousal, impairment of function, and general anxiety symptoms for more than a month. This disorder can occur at any age.

Acute stress disorder is similar to PTSD. The individual experiences a traumatic event, and exhibits the same symptoms as PTSD. The disturbance lasts for a minimum of 2 days and a maximum of 4 weeks and occurs within 4 weeks of the traumatic event.

Phobias are persistent fears of a specific situation or even an object. Social phobia is a profound fear of public speaking or performance situations in which embarrassment might occur. Specific phobias almost always involve an object (insects) or situation (elevators). Specific phobias develop at an early age but may persist into adulthood and remain significant in the elderly. Specific phobias can develop in the elderly after a traumatic life experience (crime) or especially as health deteriorates and independent living become an issue.

Anxiety due to a general medical condition is an anxiety disorder that has been determined by a physician to be caused by an underlying medical condition. There are a number of medical illnesses that are known to be associated with particular anxiety disorders. Determining the cause of anxiety can be clinically challenging, particularly in the elderly. In addition to one of many medical conditions, stimulants (caffeine) or side effects of medications can precipitate anxiety. Medical illnesses that commonly cause anxiety include cardiovascular conditions (stroke, arrhythmias, coronary artery disease, and heart failure), pulmonary conditions (asthma, chronic obstructive and restrictive diseases, and pulmonary embolism), neurologic conditions (demyelinating diseases, epilepsy, migraine, delirium, and dementia), depression, renal dysfunction or failure, cancer, electrolyte imbalances, and endocrine disorders (thyroid).[5,11,112]

Substance-induced anxiety disorder is the clinical presentation of an anxiety disorder that is judged to be due to the effects of a substance, such as a medication, a toxin, or a drug of abuse. The disturbance must not be better accounted for by a

! EMERGENCY ALERT

ANXIETY DISORDERS

- Patients taking antianxiety medications must be instructed not to operate motor vehicles or other machinery if they are experiencing sedation, a common side effect of these medications.
- Patients taking antianxiety medications must be instructed in the serious and possibly life-endangering effects of abrupt cessation of these medications.

mental or medical condition. Anxiety disorders can be associated with intoxication of substances or even withdrawal from them.

Generalized anxiety disorder (GAD) is an expressed feeling of persistent and excessive anxiety or dread that is present for at least 6 months or more and is not associated with drugs or illness. This is a diagnosis of exclusion and generally affects adults.[5]

The most common psychiatric disorders associated with sleep disturbances are anxiety and depression. At least 25% of patients who report chronic insomnia have a known anxiety disorder. These patients have difficulty with sleep onset (prolonged sleep latency), with awakenings, decreased deep sleep (slow-wave sleep), and decreased rapid eye movement (REM) sleep.[64] Sleep disturbances are common in the adult population. A multitude of factors can cause variation in sleep, because it is a complex physiologic process. The aging process itself complicates sleep, with alterations in sleep architecture that progress through life. The elderly often have secondary physical conditions and chronic pain, disrupting sleep further. More than 50 million people in the United States have chronic sleep disorders, and of those who report insomnia, 50% have been diagnosed with a psychiatric illness.

Insomnia leading to excessive daytime sleepiness may affect quality of life, job performance, cognitive ability, and concentration. Chronic insomnia should be evaluated, with treatment directed at the underlying cause. A number of pharmacologic sleep agents are used to treat insomnia (see Medications), as well as behavior modification strategies stressing good sleep hygiene. Long-term use of sedative/hypnotic medication may lead to decreased efficacy, as well as dependence, and eventual withdrawal is recommended. Some patients may benefit from the use of a placebo to maintain a nightly ritual.[98]

Low-to-moderate levels of anxiety are common in the general population; in fact, without it people would be unlikely to be productive or creative. It is proportionate to a given threat and is used constructively to alter a situation or object. The incidence of pathologic anxiety, which is disproportionate to a threat and can paralyze a person, can be difficult to measure because proper diagnosis may not be established, or there is a lack of boundaries between psychiatric disorder categories. The lifetime prevalence of any type of anxiety disorder in the general population is 24.9%. The most common anxiety disorder is phobia, with a lifetime prevalence of 10% to 13%. Panic disorder, agoraphobia, and GAD range from 5% to 6%, and OCD occurs in approximately 2.6% of the population. The development of PTSD in persons exposed to serious danger is 3% to 58%, depending on the trauma experienced.[5,35,63] Panic disorder, OCD, PTSD, social phobia, and GAD affect more than 16 million adults in the United States.[79]

Gender differences occur among the various types of anxiety disorders. The lifetime prevalence of a generalized anxiety disorder is 6.6% in young to midlife adult women and 3.6% in young to midlife adult men. These women are more likely than men to develop panic disorder (5% versus 2%) and agoraphobia without panic (7% versus 3.5%).[63] Obsessive-compulsive disorder is equally common in men and women.[5]

In the elderly population it has also been reported that women are twice as likely as men to develop an anxiety disorder and that being married lowers a person's risk for developing anxiety. Anxiety disorders in the elderly are estimated to be 13.7% to 15%, with phobic disorders being the most common (10% to 12%).[53]

PSYCHOPATHOLOGY/PATHOPHYSIOLOGY

The biology of anxiety disorders is mainly obscure, although it appears that heterogeneous factors are involved. First-degree biologic relatives of people with an anxiety disorder have a greater chance of developing an anxiety disorder than those without such a relative.[5] Biochemical factors, including neurotransmitters, appear to play a role in anxiety disorders. For example, an excess of serotonin is found in persons with obsessive-compulsive disorder. Brain imaging techniques suggest increased metabolism in the orbitofrontal regions in patients with OCD.[35] Hormones and other biochemicals such as cortisone seem to be involved, but specifics are often lacking or inconsistent.

Psychologic and interpersonal factors that predispose a person to anxiety disorders include early psychic trauma such as separation anxiety in childhood, pathogenic parent-child relationships, pathogenic family patterns, disturbed interpersonal relationships, and loss of social supports. Other experiences that may contribute to the disorders include threats to one's values, stressors that interfere with achievement of important goals, and exhaustion of adaptive coping resources.[5]

Neurobiologic theories of the cause of anxiety disorders have gained much credibility in recent years. Several neurochemicals and neurohormones are activated in the limbic system during anxiety states as a response to the activation of the autonomic nervous system. It has been postulated that excessive secretion of norepinephrine, a stimulating neurotransmitter, is a factor in anxiety disorders. Concomitantly, it has been postulated that GABA, a regulatory neurotransmitter normally released in the brain to dampen the response to norepinephrine, is present in low levels or that fewer GABA receptors are present in persons who experience anxiety disorders. Because some anxiety disorder are responsive to antianxiety medications that affect GABA and some are responsive to selective serotonin reuptake inhibitors, the role of serotonin dysfunction in anxiety disorders is also under investigation.

Genetic studies of twins and of adolescents and children with first-degree relatives with anxiety disorders suggest familial patterns of these disorders. In a study by Torgersen,[104] monozygotic twins were shown to be five times as likely to develop panic disorder as dizygotic twins. Lenane[54] found that

25% of the children and adolescents in their study had a first-degree relative with obsessive disorder. It may be hypothesized that these individuals have a genetic vulnerability that predisposes them to an anxiety sensitivity.

Psychodynamic theories have postulated that anxiety disorders occur when the ego attempts to deal with psychic conflict and emotional tension. This anxiety is initially created by birth trauma and originates in separation from the mother. If developmental tasks are achieved, the individual matures and becomes adept at handling anxiety; if not, anxiety disorders may result.

Cognitive theory proports that anxiety disorders derive from a cognitive process that occurs when a threat is perceived and the anxious person exaggerates the threat through faulty cognitions. These faulty cognitions are described as overgeneralization and all-or-none perceptions, which distort cognitions and cause intense anxiety and impaired social functioning.[9]

Diagnostic Studies and Findings

SMAC: To screen for various medical conditions
Complete blood count: To rule out infection and other medical disorders
Thyroid function tests: To screen for thyroid dysfunction
Electrocardiogram (ECG): To screen for cardiomyopathy
Routine urinalysis: To screen for urologic problems and other medical conditions

Multidisciplinary Plan

Medications

Benzodiazepines: Can cause physical dependence, and abrupt withdrawal can cause return of symptoms of anxiety and, rarely, seizures; discontinuation of benzodiazepines must be done slowly over several weeks
- Alprazolam (Xanax), 0.25-0.5 mg PO initial dose that may be increased up to a dose of 4 mg (anxiety, and 4-10 mg (panic)
- Clonazepam (Klonopin), 2.5 mg PO initial dose may be increased up to a dose of 6 mg (anxiety) and 20 mg (seizures)
- Chlordiazepoxide (Librium), 10 mg PO/IM/IV initial dose may be increased up to a dose of 25-200 mg (anxiety, alcohol withdrawal, psychosis)
- Diazepam (Valium), 5 mg PO/IM/IV initial dose may be increased up to a dose of 40 mg (anxiety, psychosis, status epilepticus)
- Estazolam (ProSom), 1-2 mg PO used as hypnotic
- Flurazepam (Dalmane), 15-30 PO mg used as hypnotic
- Lorazepam (Ativan), 0.5-1 mg PO/IM/IV initial dose may be increased up to 10 mg (anxiety, psychosis)
- Oxazepam (Ativan), 0.5-1 mg PO/IM/IV initial dose may be increased up to 10 mg (anxiety, psychosis)
- Oxazepam (Serax), 15-30 mg PO initial dose may be increased up to 120 mg (anxiety, anxiety with depression, alcohol withdrawal)
- Prazepam (Centrax), 10-20 mg PO initial dose may be increased up to 60 mg (anxiety)
- Quazepam (Doral), 2 mg PO initial dose used as hypnotic, may be increased up to 30-50 mg
- Temazepam (Restoril), 15-30 mg PO used as hypnotic
- Triazolam (Halcion), 0.125-0.25 mg PO used as hypnotic

Barbiturates: Rarely used; overdose is serious, causing confusion, drowsiness, irritability, hyporeflexia, and potential for coma, respiratory depression, and death
- Phenobarbital (Luminal), 100-200 mg
- Secobarbital (Seconal), 100-300 mg
- Pentobarbital (Nembutal), 100-200 mg
- Butabarbital (Butisol), 50-100 mg
- Amobarbital (Amytal), 100-200 mg

Nonbenzodiazepine: Buspirone (BusPar), 10-60 mg/day PO
Beta-blocker: Propranolol (Inderol), 10-40 mg/day (used for social phobia when symptoms of autonomic arousal are severe)
SSRIs (e.g., Prozac, Luvox, Paxil, Zoloft): Used to treat panic disorder—they are more commonly used than benzodiazepines—also used for OCD (higher cases) and agoraphobia
Zolpidem (Ambien) and zaleplon (Sonata), 5-10 mg PO; to treat insomnia, especially chronic insomnia
Antihistamines: Infrequently used as sedative/hypnotic; not usually recommended for the elderly
- Diphenhydramine (Benadryl), 25-100 mg/day, PO
- Ethchlorvynol (Placidyl), 25-100 mg/day, PO

OCD may be more successfully treated with an SSRI, such as fluoxetine (Prozac), or clomipramine (Anafranil), a tricyclic antidepressant; often the dosage of antidepressant medications may be higher to control symptoms of OCD[11,35,94]

General Management

Psychotherapy
Electroconvulsive therapy (ECT): For extremely depressed patients with anxiety, especially if the response to the medications is not adequate and there is concern about suicidal behavior
Cognitive behavior therapy (CBT): For panic disorder with or without agoraphobia, GAD, or social phobia; treatment is focused on educating patients about the cognitive, physiologic, and behavioral aspects of their disorder and how to deal with their thoughts and behaviors by confronting their fears; in OCD, patients are exposed to triggers for their obsessive thoughts and then prevented from performing rituals in a form of CBT known as exposure and response prevention; specific phobias are treated by brief repeated exposures; patients suffering from PTSD can be very difficult to treat successfully, but often maginal exposure to the traumatic event combined with stress management procedures is recommended[37,49,113]
Patients with OCD may need protection from scrutiny from others and protection from self-harm related to the rituals
All staff needs to be informed regarding patients' phobias so that exposure can be regulated
Protocols need to be in place for both patients and staff for persons with panic disorders
Social exposure needs to be explicitly planned for persons with agoraphobia
Depression is a frequent coexisting disorder in persons with anxiety disorders

NURSING CARE

NURSING ASSESSMENT

Affect: Anxiety, apprehension; dread; terror; tearfulness; sobbing; irritability; anger; helplessness; frustration; sometimes laughter; nervousness

Thought processes: Decreased cognitive abilities; scattering of thoughts or focus on details; preoccupation with self, behavior, and bodily functions; lack of confidence in abilities; low self-esteem; worry; anticipation of adversity; jealousy; envy of others; lack of control to effect or influence outcome; impaired sense of responsibility for self and behavior; sense of worthlessness and rejection by others; distractibility; indecisiveness; vacillation, especially in conflict; forgetfulness; somatization

Communication: Stuttering; blocking; rapid, pressured speech; selective inattention to messages; frequent requests (e.g., for water, medication, information on physician's visit, or laboratory tests); repetitive questioning about treatments, procedures, activities; petty complaining

Physical status: Dizziness; light-headedness; hyperventilation; chest pain; difficulty breathing; palpitation; perspiration; weakness, heartburn; flushing or pallor of face; tachycardia; muscle ache, especially in the neck and back; jitteriness; tremulousness; restlessness to agitation; pacing; dry mouth; dilated pupils; blurred vision; darting eyes; headache; accident proneness; impaired sexual functioning

Nutrition: Increased (occasionally decreased) appetite; nausea; belching

Bowel and bladder elimination: Diarrhea or occasionally constipation; urinary urgency and frequency

Sleep pattern: Insomnia; difficulty falling asleep; restless or interrupted sleep

Social interactions: Discomfort interacting with others because of fear of rejection or humiliation; decreased social activities because of fear of failure, especially in competitive activities

Side effects of benzodiazepines: Sedation, possible amnesia

POTENTIAL COMPLICATIONS

Patients with PTSD may experience flashbacks and panic states, which require immediate nursing interventions; patients with PTSD may self-medicate with alcohol and over-the-counter, prescription, and illegal drugs.

PATIENT PROBLEMS/NURSING DIAGNOSES & INTERVENTIONS

NIC PSYCHOLOGIC COMFORT PROMOTION

Anxiety related to a sense of uneasiness and tension

- Provide a nondemanding, comfortable environment *to decrease stressors.*
- Begin to establish a supportive, safe relationship *to prevent threats to self-esteem.*
- Allow temporary dependence.
- Remain with patient during panic attack *to decrease terror.*
- Acknowledge painfulness of patient's feelings *to convey understanding of his or her sense of helplessness.*
- Listen to patient's somatic complaints initially and slowly help patient relate complaints to anxiety level *to connect somatic symptoms with anxiety.*
- Inhibit patient's ventilation of feelings if escalation to a nonconstructive level occurs; change focus (e.g., to comfort measures, such as offering juice) *to decrease overwhelming discomfort.*
- Assist patient in breathing slowly and deeply; breathe with patient as needed *to demonstrate technique.*
- Briefly explain that breathing slowly at regularly scheduled times and when anxiety increases will help patient *to learn to relax and increase the oxygen supply and energy.*
- Administer medication as ordered. Elaborate on effects and side effects of medication, including need for gradual discontinuation of medication *to promote informed participation in and compliance with medical regimen.*
- Encourage patient to monitor his or her own restlessness and engage in diversionary activities, such as exercise, walking, and table tennis, *to decrease anxiety and to develop a sense of control over feelings.*
- Encourage patient to identify and realistically accept strengths and weaknesses *to develop self-supports.*

NIC BEHAVIOR THERAPY

Disturbed thought processes related to psychologic conflicts

- Speak calmly, using patient's name frequently, *to obtain patient's attention.*
- Give clear, concise directions *to ensure that patient is able to comprehend.*
- Assist patient to identify any thoughts he or she had just before anxiety experience *to connect cognition to anxiety.*
- Begin to help patient to correct misconceptions about experiences before anxiety using problem-solving approach *to alter emotional reaction of anxiety.*
- Encourage patient to become aware of automatic thoughts when anticipating negative experiences and to examine evidence *to learn to monitor own thoughts.*
- Invite patient to reframe events (e.g., to think of his or her boss as a "purring kitten" instead of a "growling lion" and to redefine anxiety as a pleasant, exciting sensation) *to learn to think positively and decrease anxiety.*
- Help patient to anticipate realistically possible negative and positive outcomes of anxiety-evoking events *to learn how to implement remedial actions, as needed.*
- Assist patient to accept abilities *to influence events.*
- Assist patient in setting realistic goals *to prevent a decrease in self-confidence by failure to achieve unrealistic goals.*
- Encourage patient to ask for help in work and home situations *to prevent patient from viewing self as weak or incompetent.*

NIC COMMUNICATION ENHANCEMENT

Impaired verbal communication related to psychologic barriers

- Initially answer repetitive questions simply and concisely *to help patient decease anxiety.*

- Inform patient of plans and schedules and write them down so patient can refer to the paper *to assist in remembering, thereby increasing a sense of security.*
- As patient is able, help identify anxiety when patient questions repetitively, has petty complaints, stutters, and blocks *to increase awareness of emotional state.*
- Suggest that patient speak more slowly when stuttering. Encourage patient to breathe slowly and deeply to increase energy, decrease stuttering and blocking, and be able to complete sentences.
- Inform patient that saying "I stutter when I get excited or uncomfortable" to others may help him or her to decrease stuttering and embarrassment.
- State matter-of-factly that patient will remember blocked material later *to acknowledge patient's strength and abilities.*
- Practice assertiveness skills with patient through role-playing *to increase self-confidence in interactions and social activities.*
- Encourage visitation of family members, as appropriate, and determine typical family processes.
- Discuss existing social support mechanisms for the family and assist family members *to use existing support.*
- Assist patient to accept positive feelings about interactions with others, and help patient examine interactions in which he or she expects rejection or disapproval *to identify evidence and correct misperceptions.*

Other related nursing diagnoses: Imbalanced nutrition: more than body requirements, related to overeating when tense; impaired urinary elimination related to anxiety; diarrhea or constipation related to anxiety; disturbed sleep pattern related to anxious state; social isolation related to dread of social interactions; interrupted family processes related to anxiety

Patient Education/Continuum of Care Plan

1. Teach patient about anxiety disorder and about therapeutic effects and side effects of antianxiety medications, including precautions related to sedation and abrupt termination of these medications.
2. Practice with patient self-management strategies to decrease anxiety, such as problem solving, relaxation techniques, and diversionary activities, which include physical and social activities.
3. Engage in rehearsal activities for dealing with issues to be faced after discharge.
4. Establish a linkage for continuity of care.

Evaluation/Patient Outcomes

Psychologic Comfort Promotion: Patient evidences relief of severe symptoms. Patient verbalizes relationship between anxiety and physical sensations. Patient lists major effects and side effects of medication, including danger of abrupt discontinuation. Patient develops system to ensure accurate self-administration of medication as prescribed after discharge. Patient practices relaxation techniques and engages in diversionary activities to relieve anxiety. Patient schedules appointment with provider to continue treatment plan after discharge.

Behavior Therapy: Patient demonstrates use of problem-solving methods to correct faulty thoughts. Patient practices problem-solving approach to resolve issues and correct automatic, incorrect thoughts. Patient verbalizes a beginning awareness and acceptance of strengths.

Communication Enhancement: Patient evidences increased confidence in communicating with others. Patient practices assertiveness skills and realistically evaluates consequences of interactions. Patient can express self and verbalizes feeling less anxiety when interacting with others.

Personality Disorders

Personality is a descriptive term that illustrates complex patterns of thinking and behaving that have developed from childhood and may be based on how a person interprets the self, others, and the world. Personality disorders are a category of conditions in which a person maintains enduring personality traits that are inflexible and maladaptive. These traits are rigid patterns of perceiving, thinking, and relating to the world and self, even in the face of disastrous consequences. The inflexibility of the personality may not be apparent until adaptations to environmental changes are expected or the person experiences subjective pressures.[5]

A very difficult feature is the tendency for people with personality disorders to view their behavior as normal, appropriate, and comfortable, even when it is out of line with societal expectations. There is clearly an inability to see things from another person's point of view or to realize how others view them. Frequently, the person is right and others are wrong. Personality disorders are not recognized as often as other psychiatric illnesses because persons maintain ability to function and seldom enter the mental health care system, but instead are labeled as difficult, manipulative, or hostile. Those who do seek treatment are often diagnosed with an acute mental illness (such as depression), and the personality disorder is subsequently observed.[107]

Personality disorders occur in at least 10% of the general population and usually become recognizable by adolescence or early adulthood. Persons with a personality disorder display behaviors that are characteristic of their long-term functioning, with an enduring pattern of thinking, feeling, and behaving that is fairly stable over time.[5,107] The DSM-IV lists 11 different personality disorders, which are grouped into three clusters, based on their similarities. Cluster A includes the **paranoid, schizoid,** and **schizotypal** personality disorders, which are associated with displays of odd or eccentric behavior. Persons with these disorders tend to be uncomfortable around people and lack social skills. These diagnoses may occur alone or in combination with psychotic disorders. Cluster B includes the **antisocial, borderline, histrionic,** and **narcissistic** disorders that make the person appear dramatic, emotional, or erratic. This group of personality disorders is most often associated with affective disorders and substance abuse. Cluster C includes the **avoidant, dependent,** and **obsessive-compulsive** personality disorders, in which the person appears anxious and fearful. The fear prevents persons from setting or attaining goals because of anxiety about rejection or criticism. These diagnoses are often associated with anxiety disorders.[58]

Personality disorders are typically associated with young and middle-age adults and are thought to be less severe as the person ages. Researchers suggest, however, that although impulsivity decreases with age, dependent and obsessive-compulsive behaviors remain constant or increase.[22] There is thought to be an increased rate of depression among the elderly (see Depression in Mood Disorders in the Elderly, p. 1298), and the suicide rate in elder males, 85 years and older, is three to five times higher than in any other age group.[80]

It should be pointed out that some behaviors seen in the elderly population are developed as a result of age-related social and biologic factors, which require adaptation of the elderly person. Extreme concerns about the potential for crime and abuse by others, for example, might be viewed as paranoia, when it may be reasonable for the vulnerable elderly person.[93]

Cluster A Personality Disorder—Odd and Eccentric

Those of the paranoid type are distrusting, suspicious, argumentative, and humorless. It is estimated that paranoid personality disorder occurs in up to 2.5% of the general population.[37]

A schizoid personality type is socially distant, unmotivated by interactions with others, and appears to lack emotion. A key feature is the absence of concern about either criticism or praise from others and the withdrawal of the individual into a cold, silent self. A schizoid personality can be difficult to distinguish from early symptoms of schizophrenia. With time, the schizoid personality remains stable or develops as a schizophrenic progressing to psychosis and development of negative symptoms.[37]

Schizotypal personality typically exhibits eccentric behavior with unusual perceptual distortions, and odd thinking and speech. Behavior is viewed as bizarre and disordered, but the individual maintains ability to function and is not psychotic. It does not usually develop into schizophrenia and is estimated to occur in up to 3% of the population, men more commonly than women.[37,107]

Cluster B Personality Disorder—Dramatic and Emotional

Antisocial personality types are impulsive, manipulative, dishonest, and often violent. The individual lacks remorse for having mistreated or stolen from others. There is difficulty in the workplace (possibly associated with violence), troubled relationships, and even criminal behavior. The prevalence is estimated to be 3% in males and 1% in females.[37]

Borderline personality exhibits labile mood swings and manipulative, power-seeking behavior. This behavior is difficult, demanding, and emotional. Emotions are difficult to control and impulsive, fueled by an unstable self-image and feelings of emptiness and anger. Suicide attempts are common. Women are more often affected than men, and it estimated that 2% of the population meet the criteria for diagnosis.[37]

Histrionic personality disorder is dramatic and theatrical. The person is emotional and self-consumed. The focus is on displays of inappropriate sexually seductive or provocative behavior or use of physical appearance to accomplish the goal of being the center of attention. The histrionic personality type is uncomfortable in situations where the person is not the center of attention. The prevalence of this personality disorder is estimated to be 2% to 3% of the general population.[37]

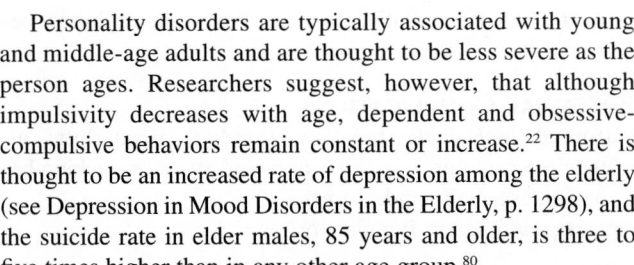

> **! EMERGENCY ALERT**
>
> **BORDERLINE PERSONALITY DISORDER**
>
> **Assessment**
> - Persons with this disorder may exhibit impulsivity, emotional lability, hostility, and rage.
> - Behaviors may include self-mutilation, sexual acting out, substance abuse, and illegal acts.
> - Suicide attempts are common.
>
> **Interventions**
> - Provision of a safe, quiet environment is essential.

The narcissistic personality type has a grandiose sense of self-importance and is preoccupied with demanding admiration, attention, recognition, and power. This personality type overestimates his or her abilities and importance and is insensitive toward anyone other than the self. This disorder is more common in men and affects approximately 1% of the general population.[37,107]

Cluster C Personality Disorder—Anxiety and Fear Based

Avoidant personalities have a very poor self-image, limiting contact with people because of anxiety and sensitivity about being criticized. There is a history of extreme shyness in childhood that increases in adolescence and young adulthood, a time when shyness most often decreases. It is equally common in males and females and estimated to be found in less than 1% of the general population.[37]

Mental health care professionals, because of the need for support and attention, frequently see dependent personalities. Dependent persons are passive, submissive, seemingly helpless, and overcompliant, regardless of cost. Decision making is difficult and usually done with the help of another. These persons feel unable to function alone and are willing to do what others want even if they disagree. They are unable to express disagreement and go along to ensure that others will care for them.

Obsessive-compulsive personality disorder (OCPD) describes a person who is extremely rigid, controlling, and detail oriented. Persons with OCPD are perfectionists who are consumed with order and conformity, lacking flexibility or the ability to negotiate. They differ from persons with obsessive-compulsive disorder (OCD) because their entire life is controlled by their rigid behavior. A person with OCD may show symptoms only in response to a specific fear (obsession) that triggers a compulsive behavior. These two disorders can overlap, however, in that both may share patterns of rigidity or tendencies to hoard things, and a person can have characteristics of both disorders. The prevalence of OCPD is approximately 1%, with males affected twice as often as females.[37,107]

Pathophysiology/Psychopathology

It is generally assumed that personality disorders are developed during a troubled childhood, as a healthy personality is developed during a healthy and happy childhood. Issues of violence and abuse, abandonment, excessive criticism or adoration, substance abuse, and neglect are apparent. The tendency for any of the personality disorders to cluster in families does not exclude genetic predisposition, but most experts place the greatest significance on environmental factors.[37]

Persons with personality disorders do manifest some biologic markers that may be indicative of a genetic tie. Impaired eye tracking behavior, often demonstrated in schizophrenic persons, has been noted in those with schizotypal personality disorder. Disturbances in the level of neurotransmitters, especially serotonin, suggest a possible biologic link to aggressive and even suicidal cluster B behaviors.[58]

MULTIDISCIPLINARY PLAN

Medications

Cluster A disorders: Often treated with low-dose antipsychotics (see Schizophrenia) or antidepressants (see Mood Disorders).

Cluster B disorders: Treated with SSRIs (see Mood Disorders), because they are generally linked to mood disorders.

Fluoxetine, at doses of 20-80 mg/day, has been shown to reduce affective instability, impulsivity, overt aggressiveness, and self-mutilation

Cluster C disorders: Treated with anxiolytics (see Anxiety Disorders) or antidepressants (see Mood Disorders)

General Management

Psychoanalysis, psychodynamic or interpersonal therapy, cognitive behavior therapy, and client-centered therapy; transitional objects and phenomena (e.g., blankets, teddy bears, toys, clothes, found objects [rock or stone], cars, or words, songs, movements, and mannerisms)

NURSING CARE

NURSING ASSESSMENT

Physical status: Personal grooming, appropriateness of dress, nutritional status, and physical activity level; a history of physical illnesses and complaints with attention to any history of epilepsy, progressive neurologic disorder, head trauma, hormonal imbalance, mental retardation, substance abuse, sleep disorders, or mania; specific observations, such as manner of speech, ability to make eye contact, facial tension, and increased perspiration

Emotional status: Demanding, hostile behavior, aggressive behavior; poor impulsive control; highly fearful, anxious, or suspicious behavior; thoughts of harming self or others; low or highly inflated self-esteem; or highly critical behavior; describe mood and capacity for empathy or motivation

Cognitive status: Ability to interpret internal and external stimuli, ability to problem solve, understand abstract ideas, tell the truth, and remain focused on a topic; memory loss, delusions, hallucinations, presence or absence of a value system, any odd beliefs or magical thinking that may influence behavior

Social interactions: Ability to relate to others; patient prefers to be alone or with others; the role of friends and family in patient's life; manipulative, hostile, abusive, or exploitive behavior toward others

POTENTIAL COMPLICATIONS

Self-mutilation/suicide: Impulsivity, radical mood shifts, altered perceptions, low self-worth, and attention-seeking behavior, especially under stress

Aggression/violence: Impulsivity, rage

PATIENT PROBLEMS/NURSING DIAGNOSES & INTERVENTIONS

Cluster A—Odd and Eccentric

NIC BEHAVIOR THERAPY

Disturbed thought processes related to difficulties in interpreting internal and external stimuli

Anxiety related to feelings of inadequacy and insecurity

Social isolation related to feelings of inadequacy and insecurity

- Provide opportunities to discuss delusional thoughts or ideas.
- Help patient correct distortions in perceptions, thought processes, and definitions of an event, using problem-solving approach.
- Begin to develop trusting, interpersonal relationship with patient without being too nurturing or overinvolved *to prevent increasing fears.*
- Involve patient in treatment plan by having patient identify how he or she wants you and other staff members to help him or her *to avoid trying to anticipate needs.*
- Communicate routines and expectations in a matter-of-fact way *to provide structure for patient.*
- Administer medication ordered by physician *to decrease disturbing symptoms;* observe for adverse reactions.
- Show genuine interest in patient; listen attentively.
- Express unconditional acceptance of patient in interactions.
- Use a calm, reassuring approach.
- Clearly state expectations for behavior, reinforce behavior, as appropriate.
- Explain procedures and medications, providing factual, necessary information.
- Provide (transitional) objects that symbolize safeness.
- Encourage verbalization of feelings, perceptions and fears

Cluster B—Dramatic and Emotional

NIC RISK MANAGEMENT

Risk for other-directed violence related to projection of hostile feelings onto others

Risk of self-directed violence related to acting out of tensions and feelings

Risk for self-mutilation related to intolerance of stress and frustration

- Remove potential weapons from environment (sharps and ropelike objects).
- Monitor safety of objects being brought into the environment by visitors.

- Instruct visitors and other caregivers about relevant patient safety issues.
- Place patient with potential for self-harm with a roommate *to decrease isolation and opportunity to act on self-harm thoughts, if appropriate.*
- Assign a single room to a patient with potential for violence toward others.
- Encourage patient to describe events that lead to impulsive behaviors, including thoughts and actions in events, *to help patient become aware of personal contributions in events.*
- Be alert to patient's omissions of own behaviors and focus on others *to prevent patient from projecting difficulties onto others.*
- Encourage patient to identify and evaluate consequences of impulsive behaviors *to learn, for example, how they achieved or did not achieve desired outcome.*
- Assist patient to examine and evaluate possible alternative behaviors *to achieve a satisfying outcome.*
- Ask patient what help he or she wants in controlling or preventing impulsive behaviors *to increase self-responsibility.*
- If patient is unable to control impulsivity, use diversionary techniques (such as escorting patient to quiet area, taking him or her for a walk, or changing subject) *to prevent or interrupt unacceptable behaviors.*
- After patient is calm, encourage discussion of details regarding the issues and patient's feelings about using a problem-solving approach for dealing with situations and *to examine possible consequences of alternative responses.*
- Inform patient about which behaviors are permitted and set limits consistently *to provide a sense of security to communicate clearly to patient what behaviors will not be permitted.*
- Be alert to self-destructive acts; take suicide threats and minor suicidal acts seriously, even if manipulative. If indicated and if in collaboration with physician, institute suicide precautions.
- Medicate as needed for uncontrollable behavior and hostility; explain to patient the medication's effects and possible side effects.
- Be alert to potential substance abuse.

NIC Coping Assistance

Ineffective coping related to poor judgment and impaired problem solving
Disturbed personal identity related to sense of inadequacy and insecurity
Chronic low self-esteem related to manipulation of others, which evokes counterattacks, disagreements, and competitive behaviors
Impaired social interaction related to sense of being special, denial of responsibility for behavior, and demanding behaviors

- Use calm, reassuring approach.
- Appraise the impact of patient's life situation on roles and relationships.
- Encourage verbalization of feelings, perceptions, and fears.
- Appraise and discuss alternative responses to situation.
- Provide an atmosphere of acceptance.
- Provide factual information concerning diagnosis and treatment.
- Evaluate patient's decision-making ability and seek to understand the patient's perspective of a stressful situation.
- Acknowledge patient's spiritual and cultural background.
- Encourage the use of spiritual resources, if desired.
- Explore patient's previous achievements of success.
- Explore reasons for self-criticism.
- Assist patient in identifying positive responses from others.
- Appraise patient's needs/desires for social support.
- Provide appropriate social skills training.

Cluster C—Anxiety and Fear Based

NIC Coping Assistance

Anxiety related to feelings of emptiness and loneliness
Chronic low self-esteem related to feelings of inadequacy and insecurity
Ineffective coping related to poor judgment and inadequate problem solving
Impaired social interaction related to feelings of inadequacy and insecurity

- Show genuine interest in patient; listen attentively.
- Express unconditional acceptance of patient in interactions.
- Use a calm, reassuring approach.
- Clearly state expectations for behavior and reinforce behavior, as appropriate.
- Explain procedures and medications, providing factual, necessary information.
- Provide (transitional) objects that symbolize safeness.
- Encourage verbalization of feelings, perceptions, and fears
- Appraise the impact of patient's life situation on roles and relationships.
- Encourage verbalization of feelings, perceptions, and fears.
- Provide an atmosphere of acceptance.
- Provide factual information concerning diagnosis and treatment.
- Evaluate patient's decision-making ability and seek to understand patient's perspective of a stressful situation.
- Acknowledge patient's spiritual and cultural background.
- Encourage the use of spiritual resources, if desired.
- Explore patient's previous achievements of success.
- Explore reasons for self-criticism.
- Assist patient in identifying positive responses from others.
- Appraise patient's needs/desires for social support.
- Provide appropriate social skills training.

Patient Education/Continuum of Care Plan

1. Teach patient the value of open communication and clear, definite expectations.
2. Emphasize the importance of clearly defined limits and structure for the patient.

3. Assist patient to identify and minimize negative behaviors and to increase effective coping strategies.

Evaluation/Patient Outcomes

Behavior Therapy: Patient begins to practice problem-solving approach and decreases impulsive behaviors. Patient states major effects and adverse effects of medications and a knowledge of accurate self-administration of medications. Patient makes plans to comply with treatment plan after discharge. Patient will not act on anxious thoughts, but will seek nurse when needed. Patient will be able to identify a positive attribute to the personality. Patient will be able to identify and discuss negative behaviors with nurse or therapy group.

Risk Management: Patient will remain safe, will not harm self or others. Patient will verbalize the plan for dealing with impulsive urges to inflict harm, including alternative behaviors. Patient will be able to maintain control of anger and will discuss feelings and needs without threatening or aggressive behavior.

Coping Assistance: Patient will be able to determine basic needs, and make requests in a calm, thoughtful manner. Patient evidences reduction in symptoms and an increased ability to use adaptive coping strategies. Patient verbalizes a decrease in uncomfortable feelings and an increase in sense of control.

Sleep Disorders

Our health is promoted by healthy sleep, and we need to become aware of its peril and promise:[30] The field of sleep is relatively new as a science and discipline. This field includes the study and treatment of conditions that involve abnormal **physiology** and abnormal **behavior.** Sleep disorders fall into the realm of multiple disciplines, including psychiatry, neurology, pulmonology, and otolaryngology. In recent years, the field has gained its own identity, with dedicated sleep specialists who diagnose and treat sleep disorders full-time. The Academy of Sleep Medicine now offers board certification in this discipline. Disorders such as insomnia, narcolepsy, restless legs syndrome (RLS), periodic leg movement disorder (PLMD), and obstructive sleep apnea syndrome (OSAS) have diverse presentations and treatment plans. Although this field has been traditionally underrepresented in medical and nursing education (see Sleep-Disordered Breathing in Chapter 4), the prevalence of sleep disorders and the impact they have on daytime neurobehavioral function mandate inclusion in any review of physical and mental health assessment.

The impact of **excessive daytime sleepiness** in our society is massive when viewed in terms of safety and economic cost. For example, it is estimated that drowsy drivers may account for as many as 56,000 motor vehicle accidents, claiming more than 1500 lives each year. Indeed, sleepiness secondary to sleep indebtedness contributed to both the *Exon Valdez* and *Challenger* disasters.[30]

The patient with a sleep complaint will usually present with one of the following three symptoms: acute or chronic inability to sleep adequately; chronic fatigue, sleepiness, or tiredness during wakefulness; or an abnormal behavior during sleep. Nurses can provide valuable insight into the recognition of sleep disorders in the acute and ambulatory care setting by including a sleep history as part of their overall physical and mental health assessment of any patient, regardless of the underlying condition.

A number of terms are commonly used in sleep medicine.[3] **Rapid eye movement (REM), dream sleep,** is a dramatic physiologic state during which the brain is active but there is generalized muscle atonia. **NREM sleep** consists of sleep stages 1 to 4, with 3 and 4 characterized as the deepest stages of sleep. **Apnea** refers to the cessation of airflow for at least 10 seconds. **Hypopnea** is a reduction in airflow during sleep, an event not meeting strict definition of apnea. **Polysomnograms, or sleep studies,** are the electrophysiologic recording of multiple biologic parameters during sleep. **Respiratory disturbance index (RDI)** is the number of apnea and hypopnea events per hour observed during a sleep study.

Obstructive sleep apnea syndrome (OSAS) is repetitive collapse of the upper airway during sleep, typically associated with loud snoring. These events contribute to sleep disruption and cardiovascular changes. Typical manifestations include daytime sleepiness and an increased incidence of adverse cardiovascular consequences. **Central sleep apnea** is a less common condition in which cessation of breathing is of central origin and not related to upper airway collapse. It is most commonly seen in stroke and congestive heart failure (Cheyne-Stokes respiration).

Hypersomnia or **excessive daytime sleepiness (EDS)** pertains to the subjective and objective propensity to fall asleep during wakefulness. **Dyssomnia** is a condition in which there is an abnormality in the amount, quality, or timing of sleep. **Insomnia** is difficulty with initiating or maintaining sleep. **Parasomnia** is an abnormal physiologic behavioral event during sleep (sleepwalking). In **REM behavior disorder (RBD),** the usual REM-associated muscle paralysis is absent, so that an individual acts out the dream he or she is having. Punching and kicking are common. **Sleep hygiene** addresses practices that affect sleep quality or behavior (e.g., caffeine intake, daytime napping).

Narcolepsy is a sleep disorder of unknown cause characterized by EDS and sleep attacks, cataplexy, sleep paralysis, and hypnagogic hallucinations. **Cataplexy** is a sudden episode of loss of muscle function. It is frequently triggered by sudden emotional reactions (laughing, anger). **Sleep paralysis** refers to the temporary inability to talk or move when falling asleep or waking up. **Hypnogogic hallucinations** are vivid, often frightening dreamlike experiences that occur while dozing or falling asleep.

Restless leg syndrome (RLS) is a disorder in which a person experiences unpleasant sensations in the legs, such as creeping, crawling, tingling, pulling, or painful sensations, which can impede sleep initiation. **Periodic limb movement disorder (PLMD)** is characterized by involuntary leg movements or jerking during sleep that occur every 10 to 60 seconds.

Most adults sleep 7 to 8 hours per night. Even in healthy asymptomatic individuals there can be considerable variability in the timing, quantity, and structure of that sleep. Sleep physiology also changes with age. The human brain has three states of existence: wakefulness, REM sleep, and NREM sleep. Sleep is characterized by a transition through these states in an orderly cycle. The sleep cycle is characterized by the transition from wakefulness and progressing through NREM stages to REM sleep. The first REM sleep usually occurs about 90 minutes after sleep onset. This sleep cycle repeats approximately four to five times per sleep period. The NREM stages 3 and 4 (referred to as slow wave or deep sleep) are most prominent during the first two sleep cycles. REM sleep periods, however, progressively lengthen, with the greatest concentration of REM sleep occurring in the early morning hours just before awakening.

Sleep state organization is in part age dependent. In infancy REM sleep may constitute 50% of total sleep time. REM stage sleep remains a relatively constant percentage of total sleep time after infancy. On the other hand, slow wave sleep (stages 3 and 4) is most prominent during childhood and progressively declines with aging and is completely absent in the elderly.

Sleep disorders are classified by the American Psychiatric Association DSM-IV and the American Academy of Sleep Medicine (AASM).[5] There are numerous disorders, and diagnoses may often overlap (e.g., insomnia resulting from RLS). The International Classification of Sleep Disorders, designated by the AASM, classifies most insomnia as intrinsic or extrinsic dysomnias. Narcolepsy, OSAS, RLS, and PLMD are classified as intrinsic dysomnias.[3,26]

In recent epidemiologic studies, it was estimated that one third of adults experience occasional or persistent sleep disturbances.[26] The National Center on Sleep Disorders Research (NCSDR), part of the National Heart, Lung & Blood Institute (NHLBI) of the National Institute of Health (NIH), reports that approximately 40 million people in the United States suffer from sleep disorders, most commonly insomnia, OSAS, narcolepsy, RLS, and PLMD.[66] Insomnia is the most prevalent of the sleep disorders. Although insomnia is the complaint of inadequate sleep, it is typically classified according to the nature of the sleep disruption or the duration of the insomnia complaint. As many as 10% of patients seen in the primary care setting complain of severe insomnia, and it is reported 1.3 times more often in women than in men. Of an estimated 12% to 25% of healthy elderly patients who complain of insomnia, one in six receives treatment for it. At least 40% of patients with insomnia also have a psychiatric diagnosis (especially anxiety disorders), and 10% to 15% are chronic substance abusers.[52]

The prevalence of OSAS in the adult male population is 4% to 9%, and the prevalence is 2% in women, until after menopause, when prevalence rates eventually equal those of men.[26,30,59] Those at risk for the development of OSAS are individuals who develop obesity (especially loud snorers), individuals with certain craniofacial abnormalities, and hypertensive adults.[30,83]

Although narcolepsy is estimated to affect as many as 200,000 people in the United States, fewer than 50,000 of these individuals are recognized because narcolepsy is often misdiagnosed as depression, epilepsy, or drug reaction. It affects as many men as women, and symptoms are usually noted during the teen or young adult years.[66] Those at risk for development of narcolepsy are persons with a genetic predisposition[83] and those who have suffered serious head injury.

Most individuals with RLS also have or develop PLMD. The symptoms of RLS and PLMD can occur at any age; however, the incidence of PLMD increases markedly, to approximately 30%, after age 65. It is estimated that 5% to 8% of adults and children develop RLS. Primary or idiopathic RLS is thought to have a genetic component, and secondary RLS can develop in pregnancy, end-stage renal disease, iron deficiency anemia, and following gastrectomy.[66,88]

PATHOPHYSIOLOGY/PSYCHOPATHOLOGY

Several neurotransmitters are thought to play a part in the sleep-wake cycle of the human brain. Although there are many theories regarding the role of sleep, it remains a central nervous system function of essential but unknown purpose. The function of the sleep-wake cycle appears to be related to an individual's memory and ability to perform cognitively. Many areas of the brain are involved in the sleep-wake cycle. The forebrain and the medulla appear to drive NREM sleep, and REM sleep is thought to be a function of a system of neurons and neurotransmitters that demonstrate antagonistic roles to turn REM "on" and "off." The sleep-wake cycle is also influenced by the suprachiasmatic nucleus of the hypothalamus, which acts as a sleep-wake pacemaker, also known as the internal body clock or circadian rhythm.[83]

The developing neural structures governing the sleep of infants are immature, and infants may sleep up to 20 hours per day. A circadian rhythm is usually developed by age 3 years. Growth hormone secretion, in children, is known to reach peak levels during sleep. Children may sleep 8 to 12 hours per night. The average adult sleeps 4 to 9 hours per night. The aging process facilitates a gradual decline in sleep efficiency and total sleep time, as well as the amount of deep (states 3 and 4 NREM) sleep. The elderly may have a variety of chronic illnesses that interfere with sleep because of symptoms such as pain and breathing difficulties.[26]

The cause of insomnia is related to the nature of the sleep disruption. It is usually subclassified as difficulty falling asleep, frequent or sustained awakenings, early morning awakenings, or persistent sleepiness despite sleep of adequate duration. Insomnia can be transient (situational or stress related), short term (lasting up to 3 weeks), or chronic (lasting for months or years). It may be primary (no apparent cause) or secondary (related cause identified). Mood and anxiety disorders (see Anxiety and Sleep) are the most common psychiatric illnesses related to insomnia. Alcohol, commonly consumed to promote sleep, can have a rebound effect after the initial sedation. Sleep maintenance may be affected by sympathetic arousal, due to release of catecholamines, when blood alcohol levels decrease. Substance abuse, including tobacco and caffeine, is associated with insomnia because of stimulant effects on the central nervous system.[64]

Obstructive sleep apnea occurs as a result of mechanical and structural airway collapse, associated with relaxation of the muscles of the throat and tongue during sleep. The person may have a narrow airway as a result of excess tissue in the oropharynx. It is possible to have a genetic predisposition to the development of OSAS because of inherited physical traits, such as certain craniofacial features (large tonsils, narrow palate/jaw). Obesity is a major causative factor in the development of OSAS, and symptoms may improve dramatically in some individuals after significant weight loss. Patients are encouraged to attempt to attain a body mass index that is within a more healthy range.[30]

Although narcolepsy was the first major sleep disorder to be discovered and characterized, its cause is unknown. The usual neural mechanisms that induce the sleep-wake cycles are impaired or altered, and the narcoleptic is unable to control the constant "sleep attacks" experienced regardless of the time of day. The narcoleptic struggles to stay awake and can fall asleep in the middle of a sentence, while eating, or during almost any activity. The individual passes directly from wakefulness to REM sleep and typically awakens again after 10 to 20 minutes, feeling refreshed, but gets sleepy again and again during the course of the day. Narcolepsy appears to have a genetic component, and it is estimated that 8% to 12% of those affected have a close relative with the disease.[30,66]

Restless leg syndrome is a relatively common sleep disorder that is associated with many factors and diseases; however, the cause is unknown. Many persons have a family history of RLS, but it is also associated with the later months of pregnancy, anemia (low iron), caffeine intake, and certain chronic diseases (renal failure, diabetes, rheumatoid arthritis, and peripheral neuropathy).[66] Most individuals with RLS also develop PLMD and frequently present with a complaint of insomnia. The reverse is not the case, however; PLMD is not as frequently associated with development of RLS, but more often with other sleep disorders such as OSAS, narcolepsy, insomnia, and other REM disorders. As is the case with RLS, the cause of PLMD is unknown.[26]

Diagnostic Studies and Findings

Polysomnogram (PSG) or sleep study
Multiple sleep latency test (MSLT)
Complete blood count (CBC) and ferritin level
Human lymphocyte antigen (HLA) B-27 testing: May be indicated

Multidisciplinary Plan

Surgery

Continuous positive airway pressure (CPAP): The most common and effective treatment for moderate to severe OSAS is CPAP. Positive pressure is delivered through a sealed nasal mask to effectively maintain patency of the upper airway during sleep. Titration of CPAP is done in the sleep laboratory (see Chapter 4).

Removal of the tonsils or adenoids or repair of other structural deformities (narrow palate or mandibular malalignment): Not uncommon but may be more successful in children and in adults with primary snoring (without apnea) than in adults with OSAS

Uvulopalatopharyngoplasty (UPPP): A procedure used to remove excess oropharyngeal tissue (tonsils, uvula, and even part of the soft palate); less than 50% of patients demonstrate benefit from this surgery, and long-term side effects/benefits are unknown

Laser-assisted uvulopalatoplasty (LAUP): To remove uvula and excess soft palate; thought to be less effective.[66,83]

> **! EMERGENCY ALERT**
>
> **SLEEP DISORDERS**
>
> - Benzodiazepines are contraindicated in patients with OSAS, should be avoided in pregnancy, and should be used with extreme caution in patients with a history of substance/alcohol abuse
> - Proceed with caution when administering any hypnotic medication to an elderly person because of problems with decreased clearance and comorbid conditions that increase the likelihood of respiratory depression and altered mental status.
> - OSAS patients hospitalized for surgery or any procedure requiring sedation or anesthesia must be carefully monitored with pulse oximetry. Proper maintenance of the airway is crucial to positive outcome.

Medications[115]

Benzodiazepines

Estazolam (ProSom), 1-2 mg single dose
Flurazepam (Dalmane), 15-30 mg single dose
Quazepam (Doral), 7.5-15 mg single dose
Temazepam (Restoril), 7.5-30 mg single dose
Triazolam (Halcion), 0.125-0.25 mg is a short-acting benzodiazepine and is the least likely to cause daytime sedation[52]

Nonbenzodiazepines (nonbarbiturates)

Zaleplon (Sonata), 5-10 mg q hs
Zolpidem (Ambien), 5-10 mg q hs
Rarely used:
Chloral hydrate (Noctec), 500-2000 mg single dose
Ethchlorvynol (Placidyl) 500-1000 mg single dose[52]

Stimulants

Premoline, 150 mg/day (may be contraindicated because of hepatic toxicity)
Methylphenidate, 100 mg/day
Dextroamphetamine, 100 mg/day
Methamphetamine, 80 mg/day

The pharmacologic treatment of RLS and PLMD is more complicated because no one drug is effective for all patients; other measures are employed initially (see General Management), and medications are reserved to control symptoms of more severe cases

Iron replacement: May be given to those identified with an iron deficiency anemia

Benzodiazepines: May be used (see Benzodiazepines), especially clonazepam (Klonopin), 1.5-2.0 mg/day, in some patients

Dopamine agonists: Others may benefit from the use of these, such as carbidopa (Sinemet), 25-100 mg, or levodopa (Madopar), 100-400 mg, taken in divided doses before bedtime

Opioids: Sometimes used in patients with severe painful and unrelenting symptoms[89]

Because no manufacturers have received U.S. Food and Drug Administration approval for the use of their drugs in

RLS or PLMD, drugs and dosages may vary with practitioners

General Management

Behavior therapy: Focus on eliminating behaviors considered incompatible with sleep, such as lying in bed and worrying, by encouraging the patient to leave the bedroom at these times

Good sleep hygiene

Limit or stop use of nicotine, caffeine, and alcohol.

Have regular bedtime and wake times, even on weekends and days off from work.

Get regular exercise before early evening.

Write a "worry list" that can be updated before bedtime and keep separate from the bed.

Use bedroom only for sleep and sexual relations—no reading, TV, or eating in bed.

Try to limit time in bed to 8 hours.

Try to avoid naps. If nap is necessary, limit to 30 minutes per day.

Eat meals on a regular basis, no heavy meals before bedtime (only light snacks).

Get regular exposure to sunlight, especially in late afternoon.

Continuous nasal positive airway pressure (CPAP)

NURSING CARE

Nursing Assessment

Monitor sleep pattern, noting any physical (apnea) or psychologic circumstances that interrupt sleep.

Interview Questions

Do you have difficulty falling asleep at night? If so, how often, and does anything you have tried help?

Do you wake up during the night? If so, do you know why and how often, and are you able to get back of sleep?

Do you snore? If so, has your bed partner noticed that you sometimes stop breathing?

Do you have excessive fatigue or sleepiness during the day, and do you fall asleep at various times during the day?

Has your sleepiness interfered with activities, work, chores, or ability to drive?

Have you ever fallen asleep while driving an automobile? If so, have you caused an accident?

Potential Complications

Excessive daytime sleepiness—especially when operation of motor vehicles or dangerous machinery is involved

Patient Problems/Nursing Diagnoses & Interventions

NIC Self-Care Facilitation

Disturbed sleep pattern associated with physiologic or psychologic sequelae

- Plan care activities according to patient's sleep-wake cycle.
- Administer medications and determine effects of medications on sleep pattern. Adjust medication to support patient's sleep-wake cycle.
- Adjust environment to promote sleep.
- Encourage proper sleep hygiene.
- Instruct patient and family about sleep disorder, medications necessary for symptom control, use of CPAP equipment, and measures taken *to promote healthy sleep/lifestyle.*
- Encourage involvement in sleep disorder support group.

Patient Education/Continuum of Care Plan

1. Teach patient techniques for good sleep hygiene.
2. Validate that patient understands how to control symptoms based on causative factors/nature of disorders.
3. Refer to support groups (e.g., AWAKE for OSAS patients).
4. Instruct patient to take prescribed medications as ordered.
5. Instruct patient in use and troubleshooting of CPAP machine.
6. Instruct patient not to drive a car or operate machinery when sleep deprived.

Evaluation/Patient Outcomes

Self-Care Facilitation: Patient will demonstrate knowledge of sleep disorder and understanding of treatment. Patient will understand the need to maintain treatment consistently and notify health professionals of sleep disorder status whenever acute care is needed. Patient will demonstrate proper sleep hygiene. Patient will verbalize concerns about medications, behavioral therapy techniques, or CPAP. Patient will agree not to operate an automobile or other dangerous machinery until properly treated.

SUICIDE, CRISIS, VIOLENCE

High risk for suicide, crisis, and violence are presented in this section. Suicide, crisis, and violence are not actual classifications of mental disorders in the DSM-IV but do have serious implications for mental health. Crisis intervention and clinical data keeping can be traced back to the early 1940s and the work of Lindeman, who reported a landmark study on the grief process after assisting survivors of a large fire in Boston.[2] Services for suicide prevention and crisis intervention for the general population began to evolve in the 1950s. Preventive strategies are emphasized. In high risk for self-harm the immediate goal is prevention of suicide; in crisis intervention a primary goal is the prevention of the maladaptation of mental illness. Alternative effective coping responses are sought when intervening in these conditions.[37]

Psychosocial and environmental problems may play a part in the development of dysfunctional responses. DSM-IV takes into account such problem categories as primary support group, health problems or loss of family members, occupational or housing problems, extreme poverty, and legal system difficulties (e.g., arrests). These factors may exacerbate a mental disorder or may be caused by a disorder. Therapeutic interventions are directed toward fostering adaptive rather than maladaptive responses. Adaptation is the ability to mobilize the resources needed to make changes in the self or in the external environment to cope effectively with stress. Maladaptation is the inability to mobilize the necessary resources to manage stress.[5]

SUICIDE

Suicide is a self-harming act intended to terminate one's life. It is more common than homicide, but it is not always a psychiatric problem. Although most persons who commit suicide have a history of psychiatric illness, some do not. There is growing pressure leading to legal physician- and nurse-assisted suicide for mentally competent individuals who are terminally ill.[114]

Suicide potential refers to a person's risk level for completing a suicide. A patient who is rational, has a **suicide plan,** and has the means to carry out that plan is at very high risk for completing suicide. There may be up to five levels of suicidal thought leading to action. Persons with **suicidal ideation** are preoccupied with thoughts of terminating their lives without acting on the thoughts. These thoughts may even by expressed through artwork, writing, or verbally. **Suicide threats** are direct verbal or written expressions of intent to commit suicide. **Suicide gestures** are self-directed actions that result in no injury or minor injury. Usually the person does not intend to end his or her life but rather tries to make the gesture look suicidal in purpose. **Suicide attempt** refers to an unsuccessful self-destructive act that is apparently intended to result in death, and **completed suicide** is the cessation of life resulting from self-destructive behavior. Persons may indicate suicidal wishes directly or indirectly by behavior such as making a final will or by saying that they wish to die. Some suicides may occur based on unplanned high-risk actions.[12]

Assisted suicide occurs when the person commits suicide with the help of someone else, usually a physician or nurse, who supplies the means. **Euthanasia** refers to an act of killing or permitting a death for reasons of mercy. The physician, or nurse, provides the means and carries out the act.[14,116] The term suicide does not explain the cause of death but only the mode of death or the presence of life-threatening thoughts and acts.

Intent to commit suicide is a determination by the person to end his or her life. The degree of intent is difficult to assess accurately because people exaggerate or deny their intent to kill themselves. Some persons may state a strong desire to commit suicide to manipulate others, with no intention of committing suicide. Others deny their intentions even though they have well-formulated plans and a serious intent to kill themselves. Health professionals must take the perspective of the person with suicidal ideation and behaviors rather than superimpose their own beliefs on the person, regardless of whether the behaviors are manipulative ploys or serious attempts in response to mild or severe stressors. All suicidal thought and acts must be taken seriously and responded to appropriately (see Emergency Alert box).

In 1997 suicide was the eighth leading cause of death for all ages in the United States, claiming more than 30,000 people. It was the third leading cause of death for young people ages 15 to 24 years. In 1997 there were three suicides in the United States for every two homicides committed, and there were twice as many deaths due to suicide as deaths due to human immunodeficiency virus (HIV)/AIDS. The most common method was by the use of firearms, accounting for 58% of all suicides. It is estimated that there are 8 to 25 attempted suicides for each completion.[81]

! EMERGENCY ALERT

SUICIDE

ASSESSMENT

- Assess thoroughly for suicidal ideation, plan, compulsions, delusions, or common hallucinations.

INTERVENTIONS

- Provide a safe physical environment and close supervision.
- Contract with the patient that she or he will inform the nurse of suicidal danger to self.

Death by suicide is four times more common in men than in women and is much more common in whites and Native Americans than among African-Americans, Hispanics, or Asians. White men accounted for 72% of all completed suicides in 1997. It is also more prevalent among men of certain age groups. The highest rate of suicide continues to be among white men over age 85 years with a rate of 65.3 deaths/100,000 people in that age group, although suicide is not the leading cause of death in this group. The completed suicide rate among adolescents ages 15 to 19 years was 9.5/100,000 with a gender ratio (male/female) of 5 : 1, and among young adults ages 20 to 24 years it was 13.6/100,000 with a gender ratio (male/female) of 7 : 1.[81]

Persons who are chronically or terminally ill may be a higher risk for suicidal ideation. The overall suicidal risk is, however, reported to be much lower than might be expected, with 5% of suicides occurring in chronically ill patients.[45] Many cancer patients become depressed after the diagnosis is made, making detection of suicide risk an important component of care.[37]

Separation from or the death of a loved one, divorce, and the loss of health, money, or a job are powerful factors in suicide. Persons who come to believe that life has no meaning or who believe there is no longer a purpose in their life may be at risk for suicide. A decrease in social support systems often creates the potential for severe depression in late life irrespective of personality or intrapsychic conflicts. Family support, concern, and acceptance are vitally important to an older person.[31]

The elderly make up approximately 13% of the population, but they account for 20% of all suicides. Suicide rates among the elderly are highest for those who are divorced, widowed, or never married. It is estimated that nearly 5 million of the 32 million elderly (age 65 years and older) in the United States suffer from depression. Most elderly suicide victims have visited their primary care provider within a month of completing the suicide. Many of these individuals may not understand that depression is not a normal part of the aging process.[82]

PSYCHOPATHOLOGY/PATHOPHYSIOLOGY

Although many factors may contribute to the complex act of suicide, it is clearly associated with psychiatric illnesses. More than 90% of persons who commit suicide have a diagnosable psychiatric illness. Depression and alcohol abuse are associated most frequently with completed suicide.[45] Patients with a history of bipolar disorder may have a 25% to 50% higher incidence of suicide attempt during their lifetime, with women attempting more often than men, but men having a higher rate of completed suicide. Schizophrenic persons, who are less likely to tell others of their intention to commit suicide, have an 8% lifetime risk of suicide completion and more than 30% risk for suicide attempt. Alcohol and substance abuse are also strongly related to suicide potential. Researchers suggest that alcohol and/or drug ingestion are often related to impulsive and violent suicides, especially when the substance abuse occurs in persons suffering from a personality disorder.[37]

Young people who are at risk for suicidal thoughts and behaviors are typically those who suffer from psychiatric disorders (especially mood disorders), substance abuse, sexual abuse, bullying, and deteriorating family relationships. The breakdown of a relationship with a friend or relative is often a precipitating factor to self-harm in this patient population.[8] There is also concern that young people learn suicidal behaviors from suicidal peers, family members, and even the media. Suicide information and "advice" have reportedly been available on the Internet. Sensational accounts in the media of adolescent suicides have led to copycat attempts by other teens seeking the same notoriety. Nearly 65% of teen suicides are accomplished with guns as the tool of destruction because they are not difficult for teens to obtain.[16]

Suicide is commonly viewed in American society as wrong, even criminal. Research has demonstrated that many nurses express unsympathetic and even hostile feelings toward suicidal patients.[57] Preconceived ideas and attitudes can make it difficult for the nurse to communicate with the suicidal person in an understanding and empathetic manner.[57] This , at a time when the suicidal patient is most in need of attention and therapeutic interpersonal interaction, can influence outcome in a less than positive way.

Peplau, a leader in psychiatric nursing, developed the psychodynamic nursing theory, which focused extensively on the therapeutic nurse-patient relationship. Peplau believed the formation of a therapeutic relationship was critical to maintaining a lifeline to the suicidal patient. As four phases of the psychodynamic relationship evolve, the nurse is attaining a bond of trust with the patient, moving through various roles—stranger, resource person, teacher, leader, surrogate, and counselor—to attempt to redirect energy from a negative to a positive direction.[48]

Theories about suicide involve social, psychologic, and biologic explanations. Socially, suicidal individuals are disconnected, with a sense of hopelessness about life's direction, leading to negative and impulsive behaviors. Psychologic theories are numerous and generally focus on the relationship of suicidal behavior to the psychiatric diagnosis. Biologic research with neurotransmitters has linked depression with low levels of serotonin in the brain. There is much interest in the relationship of serotonin and suicide, because suicide and depression are closely related.[37]

Although the environment should be made as safe as possible by removing any materials suicidal patients might use to harm themselves, it is may not be possible to stop a person who is determined to commit suicide. The importance of developing a concerned, supportive interpersonal relationship with the patient cannot be overemphasized. Most suicide attempts occur after a person has verbally communicated suicidal ideation and sometimes suicide plans, but patients who typically exhibit impulsive behaviors often act without a stated plan.[37]

When working with suicidal patients, even when they are manipulative, nurses need to be aware of and manage their own feelings while empathizing with the patients' point of view. Nursing care should be implemented selectively based on seriousness of symptoms and presenting behaviors. In the clinical setting, it is helpful to initiate a contract with the patient not to act on suicidal thoughts for a specified period, allowing more time to establish a relationship with the patient. The potential for self-harm is ever present in the suicidal patient, however, and it may not always be possible to protect patients from harming themselves.

Diagnostic Studies and Findings

SMAC: To screen for systemic abnormalities
Complete blood count: To rule out infection and other medical disorders
Thyroid function tests: To screen for thyroid abnormalities
ECG: To screen for cardiopathy
Urinalysis: To rule out urologic disorders and other medical conditions
Toxicology screen: To screen for drug use
Blood alcohol level: To determine possibility of intoxication

Multidisciplinary Plan

Medications

Antidepressants: Tricyclics or serotonin reuptake inhibitors
Anxiolytics
Antipsychotics

General Management

Suicide precautions
- Remove sharp objects, such as scissors, knives, and mirrors, from the patient's possession or access

Check for and remove any toxic substances, such as drugs and alcohol, and secure any unit medications
Remove potentially dangerous clothing articles, such as belts, neckties, or stockings
Close supervision, even one-to-one supervision, may be necessary
Seclusion if deemed necessary for patient's protection
Electroconvulsive therapy: To prevent completion of suicide act if the threat of suicide is strong and the patient does not respond to medication
Psychotherapy: To promote the use of a therapeutic relationship focusing on the patient's personal and social circumstances that precipitate or perpetuate suicidal thoughts
- Cognitive behavior therapy techniques: To deal with frustration and anger[37]
- Life review therapy: To remember the past, analyze important aspects, and then put it all in perspective[31]

NURSING CARE

NURSING ASSESSMENT

Violence: Instability or changes in life situation; thoughts that life is not worthwhile; presence, duration, and strength of self-harm thoughts; contemplation of ways of harming or killing self; development of well-formulated plans; strength of motive or serious intent to follow through with plans; availability of chosen suicide method; factors, such as family, religion, and additional stress, that may push person toward or deter suicide; previous thoughts and attempts of suicide along with intent and lethality of attempts or ideas; loss of significant other through suicide

Power and control: Hopelessness; inability to influence or alter interpersonal or life situation

Affect: Sadness or depression; inappropriate feelings such as laughter; anger; distress; tranquility once decision and plan are finalized

Thought processes: Negative view of the future; humiliation (e.g., feeling of being a failure); perceived or actual recent losses, stressors, or changes; ambivalence; fantasies about how others may react (e.g., "They'll be sorry"); vengeful thoughts; delusions or auditory hallucinations of sin, self-punishment, and atonement

Communication: Comments such as saying good-bye instead of good night, "I wont be seeing you again," or "Next time you see me, I'll be riding in a hearse"; informing family or spouse of whereabouts of important papers, such as insurance papers, bankbooks, and will; threats of suicide as a cry for help or to manipulate interactions

Activities: Making or changing will; increasing life insurance; visiting or phoning relatives and friends for intense conversations; giving away prized possessions; demonstrating increased concern or care for others; buying tools needed to implement suicide, such as a gun, rope, or prescription refills; acting out behavior; writing a farewell note

Social interactions: Perceived or actual lack of support from others; loss of valued relationships through separation, divorce, death, or romantic breakups

Family: Dysfunctional patterns of interactions such as conflict, arguments, and blaming; others not perceiving and responding to needs or wishes

POTENTIAL COMPLICATIONS

Physical harm to self

PATIENT PROBLEMS/NURSING DIAGNOSES & INTERVENTIONS

NIC RISK MANAGEMENT

Risk for self-directed violence related to despair and hopelessness

- Determine history of suicide attempts.
- Institute suicide precautions *to protect patient from harming self.*
- Encourage patient to make a verbal no-suicide contract.
- Determine whether there is a specific suicide plan.
- Place patient in the least restrictive environment that allows for necessary level of observation.
- Demonstrate concern for welfare of patient.
- Refrain from negative criticism.
- After initial suicide precautions are instituted, continue to observe for dangerous items in patient's environment and assess possible need for protective window coverings.
- Facilitate support of patient by friends and family, providing appropriate instructions regarding precautions.
- Instruct family that suicidal risk increases for severely depressed patients as they begin to feel better.
- Begin to establish supportive relationship with patient *to demonstrate respect, concern, and worth of patient.*
- Provide psychiatric counseling as needed; include discussion of signs and symptoms of depression.
- Escort patient during off-ward activities, as appropriate.
- While suicide precautions are in effect, engage patient in simple activities, such as exercises or looking at magazines, *to promote the relationship and encourage interest in the environment.*
- Continue close observation with knowledge of patient's whereabouts when on unit.
- Convey a sense of hope in patient's abilities and in his or her future.
- Evaluate patient's condition frequently at first and at least once a day *to determine his or her mood and potential for self-harm.*
- Observe for changes in patient's mood, such as calmness or tranquility, as a possible prelude to suicide.
- Allow patient to keep more possessions as deemed safe and as precautions become less stringent *to provide reasonable restrictions that promote the well-being of patient.*
- Administer medication with a simple explanation, including a description of possible side effects, such as orthostatic hypotension and drowsiness. When condition improves, explain to patient the effects and side effects of medication, and leave patient opportunities to ask questions *to encourage knowledge and participation in treatment plan during and after hospitalization.*

NIC COPING ASSISTANCE

Disturbed thought processes related to psychologic conflicts.

Ineffective coping related to feelings of powerlessness and hopelessness

- Assess patient's abilities to think logically and to problem solve.
- Assist patient in identifying meaning of suicide threats (or attempts) and what patient expected to happen to himself or herself and others *to help patient become aware of experiences that led to self-harm behaviors.*
- Examine losses and stressors that evoked self-harm behaviors *to begin a problem-solving approach to correct illogical thoughts and to identify alternative behavior.*
- Help patient recall and identify reasons for living *to examine experiences when life was better than it is currently.*

- Avoid reinforcing delusions and hallucinations; assist patients in examining experiences before delusions or hallucinations *to help patient gradually connect thoughts and feelings with development of false beliefs and perceptions.*
- Assist patient in anticipating future issues and in developing methods other than suicide for handling them.
- Assess patient's coping strategies *to assist patient in dealing with stressors and life situations.*
- Examine appropriateness of patient's emotional responses to events, using a problem-solving approach, *to reinforce healthy adaptive behavior.*
- When patient shows signs of increased tension, encourage slow, deep breathing *to help decrease tension.* Encourage patient to practice relaxation techniques daily.
- Explain and practice assertiveness skills *to begin to increase patient's confidence in self and to learn how to let others know of his or her needs.*
- Encourage patient to identify his or her social skills.
- Help patient deal with uncomfortable feelings in social situations *to begin to develop healthy coping strategies.*
- Assist patient in identifying social inadequacies, and encourage patient *to begin to correct these;* provide names of community resources *to assist with correcting social inadequacies after discharge and to increase social supports.*

Other related nursing diagnoses: Powerlessness related to perceived lack of control over environment; impaired verbal communication related to lack of willingness to discuss personal concerns; social isolation related to feelings of unease when interacting with others; interrupted family processes related to multiple conflicts among members

Patient Education/Continuum of Care Plan

1. Instruct patient/family to remove firearms and any stockpiles of medications from the home.
2. Instruct family on how to act in the best interest of the suicidal patient and work with mental health care providers.
3. Instruct patient to call if patient is feeling the urge to self-harm of if feeling alone/abandoned.[37]

Evaluation/Patient Outcomes

Risk Management: Patient evidences reduced potential for self-harm. Patient makes no suicide attempts and verbalizes the desire to live and reasons for living. Patient states accurate information about actions of medications and treatment plan and knowledge of self-administration after discharge.

Coping Assistance: Patient demonstrates increased ability to think logically about problem areas. Patient states beginning knowledge of experiences contributing to hopelessness. Patient begins to demonstrate constructive behaviors and is using problem-solving techniques to correct misconceptions and to consider alternative solutions. Patient demonstrates coping skills. Patient develops skills and practices appropriate coping strategies for dealing with issues. Patient practices assertiveness behaviors and evidences increased self-assurance.

Crisis

A crisis is an event that causes stress and forces the individual to respond or adapt in some way. A crisis is not necessarily good or bad, and the outcome can be negative or positive. A crisis can affect an individual, a family, or even an entire community.

A **situational crisis** is an event that may threaten or challenge an individual. A serious accident, illness, or loss of a loved one, are examples. A **maturational crisis** is a stage in an individual's life requiring adjustment and adaptation to new life changes and challenges. An example of this is midlife crisis. A **cultural crisis** occurs when a person must adjust and adapt to a new culture or return to a culture after having adjusted to another. A **community crisis** is typically a natural disaster or criminal act that affects an entire community.[37]

There are four stages an individual progresses through in a crisis. In the first phase, the situation or threat results in anxiety. Coping mechanisms are used to reduce anxiety, but if that does not occur, the second phase is manifest. In the second stage anxiety increases and coping mechanisms decrease. During the third phase, the individual uses every means available to attempt to control the situation and escalating anxiety level. If the individual reaches the fourth phase, the anxiety level has escalated to a level of panic, disorganization, and crisis.[2,37] As anxiety and tension increase, the ability to find a solution decreases and the sense of helplessness increases. It is accepted generally as a normal response produced by a threatening event rather than a pathologic state.

Posttraumatic stress disorder (PTSD) is an anxiety disorder that may develop in response to a traumatic event. Persons who develop PTSD persistently reexperience the stressful event, in very distressing ways, such as flashbacks or dreams. Victims persistently avoid any stimuli associated with the trauma, although they appear unable to recall important aspects of the event. There is often a detachment or estrangement from loved ones or friends and a general numbing of responsiveness.[5,92]

The person may be in a vulnerable state because of efforts to deal with hazardous events before the crisis reaction. Despite being in a state of moderate anxiety or depression, the person is able to mobilize resources to cope, although possibly at a reduced level, with the initial stressors. However, when an overpowering experience (the precipitant) occurs, it produces the disorganizing effect of a crisis reaction. For example, the initial stressor may be a surgical procedure that produces a vulnerable state, and the crisis-precipitating event may be the knowledge that the excised tumor was cancerous. Sometimes a person experiences just one stressor of sufficient force to precipitate the crisis. Crisis is typically self-limiting and lasts approximately 4 to 6 weeks[2] (see Emergency Alert box, p. 1288).

Two types of crisis have been differentiated on the basis of the person's previous life experiences: an exhaustion crisis and an acute crisis. In exhaustion crisis the person has coped effectively under emergency conditions for a long time and reaches a point of exhaustion when all energy and resources have been spent. In acute crisis the person is overwhelmed by an explosive release of emotions in response to a sudden external change. Too much has happened unexpectedly and rapidly for the person to assimilate and integrate the excess stimuli. Nursing interventions for these two types of crisis differ. A person in

! EMERGENCY ALERT

CRISIS

ASSESSMENT

- Emotional state of disorganization and scattered thinking may cause failure of previously used problem-solving methods with perceived loss of control.

INTERVENTIONS

- Assist patient to decrease anxiety and offer concrete, succinct verbal assistance.
- Assist with problem solving as necessary.
- Intervene in physical problems such as exhaustion, attempting to deal with emergency conditions over an extended time as necessary.

exhaustion crisis is unable to gain control over emotions and is apathetic to interpersonal contact or intervention techniques. A benign, supportive environment is essential for the person to regain energy slowly before attempting to deal with the crisis. A person in acute crisis is open to change and highly motivated to accept help in resolving it.[37]

Crisis situations occur episodically throughout a person's lifetime because of normal developmental stages and the demands associated with anticipated life situations. In addition, unanticipated crisis situations occur during the life span. Many crises do not come to the attention of health-care professionals but are resolved with the help of family, friends, or the clergy. Because crises are time limited, the person may successfully deal with them or maladaptively resolve them so that precrisis functioning level is not regained.

Posttraumatic stress disorder is commonly associated with crisis attributable to disaster (natural disaster, such as a tornado, or manmade disaster, such as a school shooting). In the United States as many as 5.2 million people have PTSD during the course of a given year.[79]

From birth to death a person is exposed to crisis situations that are anticipated and predictable or unanticipated and accidental. Anticipated crises, which are described as maturational or developmental, are somewhat inconsistent with the assumptions of crisis theory that threatening events are external rather than internal. Unanticipated crises are unexpected traumatic events that may occur at any stage of life.

Unanticipated events may affect individuals, communities, and countries. They include natural catastrophic events, such as tornadoes, floods, and earthquakes, and man-made catastrophes, such as economic depressions, unemployment, and bank failures. Loss of a job and money creates a crisis not only for the person experiencing the loss but also for the family members, who are suddenly faced with changes in lifestyle and status.

Loss or threatened loss of a loved one through an untimely death or reduced capacity to function because of an accident or illness creates havoc for all involved. Although death of any loved person is stressful, the loss of a child or young adult is especially shocking to survivors. Unanticipated traumatic stress occurs in "victim crisis," in which physically or emotionally aggressive acts are perpetrated on a person. These include persecution of an individual or group and violent crimes such as assault, rape, and murder. The crisis situation can have a lifelong effect because of the intense emotional trauma and possible irreversible physical disability such as paralysis or loss of an extremity. The person may have flashbacks in which the violence or aggressiveness of the precipitating event is reexperienced. This can happen in persons who have successfully resolved the crisis issues.

In some instances a preexisting psychopathologic condition, such as schizophrenia or anxiety disorder, in a person or family is a contributing variable to a crisis reaction. The person's lowered tolerance to stressors, personal and social resources, and inadequate coping skills impair his or her ability to resolve crises successfully.

It is estimated that approximately 30% of men and women who have spent time in war zones develop PTSD. Although PTSD can develop at any age, it is more common in women than in men, occurring frequently after violent personal assaults, such as rape, mugging, or domestic violence. It is also common for other anxiety disorders, depression, or alcohol or other substance abuse to accompany PTSD.[79]

PSYCHOPATHOLOGY

Individuals deal with stress or crisis based on factors such as cognitive perception of the situation, environmental and situational support, and coping mechanisms. Many issues play a part in the balance of these factors. Among these issues are age, cultural background, education, and psychologic development. Furthermore, particular strengths or weaknesses influence the onset of crisis, as well as its resolution.[2,37]

In cognitive or learning framework, crisis is considered to be a result of sensory overload that interrupts the cognitive processes of perceiving, thinking, decision making, and evaluating. The overload may be related to a perceived or actual bombardment with stressful stimuli the person is unable to process logically. The person's definition of the situation determines whether it is interpreted as a crisis or as a challenging experience. Thus the person's definition also determines the person's response and methods of dealing with the situation. Intervention is directed toward correcting cognitive distortions, learning new skills to resolve the problem, unlearning inappropriate thinking patterns, and reinforcing gratifying patterns of behavior.[25,95]

Environmental and situational support involves the availability of resources and the person's ability to turn to others for support. It is dependent on the presence of established relationships and the willingness of those to whom the person turns to provide support. A meaningful relationship provides nurturance and support, with vital assurance of availability and assistance in dealing with crisis. Social isolation or loss of meaningful relationship increases an individual's vulnerability to stress and crisis development.[2]

Coping mechanisms are defensive actions developed over time in each person to reduce anxiety and maintain emotional stability. Coping mechanisms reflect a person's usual reaction to a problem or stressful situation. Because each person has different life experiences, each develops different coping mechanisms that work to reduce anxiety when faced with a problem.[2]

Generally persons experiencing crises have healthy personalities, and interventions are focused on the current crisis situation. Even when an underlying psychopathologic condition exists, interventions remain issue oriented to alleviate the crisis situation; the patient can be referred later to other resources for further help. If treatment is continued to deal with problems other than those related to the crisis, interventions are no longer viewed as crisis ones.[2]

General goals of crisis intervention are to reinforce interpersonal assets, to resolve the crisis event, to connect with social supports in the family or in the community, and to integrate the crisis experience into the personality. A minimum expectation of crisis intervention is the person's return to a precrisis level of functioning.

Three general approaches are useful in crisis intervention. The first is the free discharge of emotions such as despair, anxiety, and anger. If anger is the only emotion expressed, it may be nonconstructive when used to deny fear and emotional pain, but it is constructive when it counteracts the feelings of helplessness. A second approach is the enhancement of the patient's cognitive processes, thus providing a sense of control and an intellectual understanding of the crisis. The patient is helped to remember details of the event, including painful ones, and to correct misconceptions. A third approach allows the patient to experience security and hope through a supportive relationship to reduce anxiety (which leads to increased disorganization of the personality). It requires helping the person examine alternative ways of coping. The supportive approach is particularly useful in exhaustion crisis, when the person must regain energy before beginning to deal with the crisis. These approaches overlap to some extent, and all three are useful with a given patient depending on his or her needs at different phases of crisis intervention.[2]

Crisis intervention in hospitalized psychiatric wards may be stressful because these patients are often easily provoked into disruptive and even dangerous behaviors. Many times chemical, physical, and environmental restraint is utilized. Because the use of seclusion, with or without restraints, can negatively affect patients, the use of a less restrictive measure might be more beneficial to the patient and staff. Removal from stimuli (often combined with medication) has been found to be effective in eliciting cooperation from even the most difficult of psychiatric patients.[19]

Diagnostic Studies and Findings

SMAC: To screen for general medical conditions
Complete blood count: To screen for infection and other medical conditions
Thyroid function tests: To rule out thyroid disorders
Urinalysis: To screen for urologic disorders and other medical conditions

Multidisciplinary Plan

Medications

Anxiolytics
Antidepressants
Medications to manage symptoms (e.g., antacids, acetaminophen)
Psychobehavioral therapy
Suicide precautions

NURSING CARE

Nursing Assessment

Type and nature of crisis: Anticipated or unanticipated; precipitating event, duration of crisis, and coping abilities; suicidal ideation; basis for physical complaints such as headache and abdominal pain; level and source of helplessness and aspects of events that provoked those feelings; interpersonal assets and current state of social supports
Affect: Severe anxiety to panic; depression; anger; apathy; tearfulness to convulsive crying; feeling of alienation; emptiness; motionless state; temporary lowered self-esteem
Thought processes: Paralysis of cognitive processes; impaired recall of crisis event; misinterpretation of events; forgetfulness; blocking; confusion; indecisiveness; frustration; conflicting thoughts; denial; guilt; psychophysiologic symptom complaints; suicidal or homicidal thoughts
Power and control: Helplessness; hopelessness; vulnerability; lack of control
Activities: Paralysis or aimless, automatic behavior; agitation; tremors; stiffness of body as if trying to hold self together; clenched fists; contorted facial features; limpness of body, sometimes with impaired balance; impaired performance of tasks; regressive childlike behaviors such as tantrums
Sleep pattern: Impaired sleep; inability to sleep; restless sleep; hypersomnia
Nutrition: Change in eating pattern, such as overeating or inability to eat; picking at food; nausea; vomiting
Social interactions: Withdrawal from social support network; loosening of ties with loved ones

Potential Complications

Need for services of health care/social services network if lack of other supportive network for client (family, friends, social groups, religious affiliation, community resources)
Panic disorder or other anxiety states, psychotic episode, or serious physical illnesses such as heart attack or stroke if needs unmet during initial crisis

Patient Problems/Nursing Diagnoses & Interventions

NIC Coping Assistance

Anxiety related to situational or maturational crises
Ineffective coping related to situational or maturational crises
Powerlessness related to overwhelming situation
Social isolation related to alterations in mental status

For patient in acute crisis:

- Convey concern and caring through temporarily taking charge of activities (e.g., direct patient to comfortable chair and provide comfort measures such as drink and tissues) *to reduce panic and loss of control.*
- Provide the patient with opportunities to express emotions in his or her own way (as long as they are nondestructive) within a safe, supportive relationship.

- Increase use of cognitive processes by helping patient review details of stressful events and, if appropriate, by providing factual information related to the event *to correct misperceptions and to expand patient's perspective.*
- Assist patient to examine alternative choices and possible consequences of each choice.
- Encourage patient to identify social supports in the family and community.
- Help patient deal with initial reactions to the crisis situation such as emotional upsets and to accept and integrate the crisis experience into his or her personality.
- Provide quiet, calm environment *to avoid increasing anxiety.*
- Address patient by name and speak calmly in concise sentences *to obtain patient's attention.*
- If exhaustion crisis is present, be supportive and giving *to help patient regain energy.*
- Encourage patient to express feelings *to discharge emotions rather than to keep them inside.*
- If patient is crying, help to identify and clarify feelings (e.g., despair, anger, or hopelessness) during or after this expression; for example, say "Tell me what you're feeling as you're crying" *to become aware of meaning of emotions.*
- Administer medication if ordered and as needed to relieve emotional discomfort. Briefly inform patient of effects and side effects, such as drowsiness and lightheadedness. More fully discuss effects and side effects when patient is calm if medication is to be continued. Emphasize the need for medical follow-up care.
- Acknowledge physical signs of discomfort and ask patient to identify emotional experience *to connect bodily sensation with feeling state.*
- When patient is able, identify previous painful emotions and successes in dealing with them *to reinforce positive coping techniques.*
- Encourage the use of relaxation techniques, such as slow, deep breathing, diversionary activities, and sharing feelings with others, *to help patient develop ways to deal with current feelings.*
- If patient is in hospital, encourage participation in occupational therapy as ordered *to provide diversionary activity and learn new skills.* (If there is no physical or emotional contraindication, recreational therapy may also be ordered to reduce anxiety, expend excess energy, and teach new skills.)
- Clarify perceptions of issues and events before the crisis.
- When patient with exhaustion crisis is able, identify various stressors along with their patterns, and explore coping strategies used in the past. Reinforce healthy methods for dealing with those stressors *to support successful behaviors and increase patient's confidence in his or her abilities.*
- If crisis is developmental, identify specific issues and assist patient to resolve them *to learn to deal with developmental tasks and accept self.* If crisis was unanticipated, assist patient to begin to resolve issues related to both crisis and underlying conflict reactivated because of crisis events *to understand meaning of current crisis and integrate this new understanding into the personality.*
- In problem solving, help patient explore possible consequences of various choices *to evaluate potential impact of decisions.*
- Provide factual information as appropriate (e.g., knowledge of crisis phases, tasks of developmental stage, and factors related to crisis situation) *to alter and broaden patient's perspective on issues.*
- Assist patient in identifying behaviors that contributed to or exacerbated the threatening situation (e.g., accumulation of large debts before loss of employment) *to help patient become aware of noneffective forms of behavior.* Help patient anticipate similar future events and identify ways of coping *to increase a sense of security and decrease apprehension about recurrence of crisis.*
- Assist patient in beginning to deal with long-term impact of crisis events, such as cancer, changes in body image (e.g., facial disfigurement and mastectomy), and birth of an imperfect baby.
- Help patient identify relationship between physical symptoms and emotional state *to increase understanding of his or her maladaptive coping strategies.*
- Convey to patient a realistic sense of optimism and hope that alternative ways of viewing and dealing with issues exist.
- Assist patient in recalling and accepting previous and current successful coping strategies *to increase confidence in his or her abilities and a sense of control over self.*
- Explain use of assertiveness skills and practice these with patient *to increase self-concept and abilities to be direct in making requests of others.*
- Help patient identify persons viewed as supportive *to begin to reconnect with significant others.*
- Discuss how supportive person(s) can be helpful now and how patient can share problems *to encourage patient to use available resources.*
- If useful, ask patient to role-play, sharing problems and asking for help, *to increase confidence in asking for support.*
- If patient is in an emergency room or a community agency and alone, arrange to have someone drive him or her home (if he or she will not be hospitalized). If patient lives alone, encourage staying at someone else's home or having someone stay with patient *to alleviate fears of being alone and to reduce stress.*
- Facilitate patient and family communication with each other. *When one person experiences a crisis episode, family and friends who have a close relationship with that person are likely to share in the crisis reactions. Because a crisis often loosens close relationships, each person may suffer alone rather than support each other.*
- Identify community resources; write down names, addresses, and phone numbers; and encourage patient to use them *to obtain immediate emergency services,* as needed.

Other related nursing diagnoses: Disturbed sleep pattern related to high level of anxiety; interrupted family processes related to crisis.

Patient Education/Continuum of Care Plan

1. Provide written materials for all resources and support systems needed by patient during crisis.
2. Assist patient in making appropriate contacts and arrangements as necessary and appropriate for dealing with crisis.
3. Encourage patient to move toward independence in coping with crisis situation as appropriate.
4. Teach essential information about medications and provide written materials as needed.

Evaluation/Patient Outcomes

Coping Assistance: Patient experiences reduction in anxiety level. Patient participates in treatment plan during hospitalization. Patient expresses knowledge of effects and side effects of medications. Patient verbalizes decrease in anxiety and demonstrates skill in relaxation methods. Patient demonstrates adaptive coping skills. Patient uses problem-solving skills to examine issues and to promote adaptive behaviors. Patient experiences increased sense of control over own abilities and activities. Patient expresses sense of hope and realistic view to deal with issues. Patient practices assertiveness techniques to tell others of needs and to request help from others. Patient demonstrates decrease in social isolation. Patient initiates contact with and receives support from significant others. Patient makes initial contact for assistance from community agency.

Violence

The term violence often refers to an act of physical injury, a state in which an individual exhibits behaviors that can be physically harmful either to the self or others. However, because mental injury must also be considered, the term **abuse** can be used interchangeably with it.

The **victim** is the recipient of violence or abuse. Violence and abuse involve harmful acts resulting in physical and/or psychologic injury that have varying ability for recovery to a prior state of well-being. **Interpersonal or family violence** refers to acts of violence in traditional family and significant other relationships that have similar dynamics. Further acts of abuse may include noncompliance with health recommendations or difficulty in the management of existent medical conditions of victims. **Domestic violence** is usually described as spousal or partner abuse, or battering syndrome. **Spousal rape** is forced sexual intercourse against the victim's will.[21]

Elder abuse involves the physical or mental injury of an elder by a parent or caregiver. **Elder sexual abuse/battery** involves sexual assault or touching of an elder against his or her will, which may or may not involve **rape,** the act of forced sexual intercourse. **Negligence** is the failure of a parent or caregiver to provide adequate supervision, food, clothing, shelter, or medical care to a dependent child or elder.[100,101]

Acts of violence are common in American society, as well as societies around the world. Because millions of violent injuries occur every year, victims of violence are commonly seen in health-care settings. Injuries that are violent in nature often raise suspicion for interpersonal abuse, but it can be very difficult for health-care providers to address the topic with their patients. Issues such as cultural influences and beliefs can make intervention complicated and difficult. Even when there is an attempted intervention, many victims deny abuse or refuse help, making it arduous for nurses or physicians to be effective in their intervention.

Nurses themselves may become victims of abuse in the health care or home care setting. Often, a patient's behavior is excused when the patient is ill and stressed, and many nurses tolerate verbal and physical abuse, assuming patients are behaving in a manner that is atypical or aberrant in comparison with behavior that is expected when in a state of well-being. Nurses are encouraged to remain tolerant and empathetic with patients, always cognizant of physical, social, and psychologic needs. The question of how well nurses are equipped to deal with violence and abuse when it is directed at them, or when it is their responsibility to maintain a safe environment for the safety of others, should be more thoroughly addressed.

More than half of women who are murdered in the United States are killed by their male partner. Patterns of domestic abuse occur repetitively in the lives of 8% to 17% of women in the United States every year. Accurate prevalence rates are hindered by variations in the way domestic violence is defined and by many problems in detection and underreporting. As many as 6 out of every 100 married couples admit to the occurrence of at least one violent act (kicking, biting, hitting with a fist, and threatening to use or using a knife or gun) during their marriage. It is estimated that $44 million is spent each year on medical care of abused women, and there are at least 175,000 lost days of work.[21,86,100,111]

Elder abuse is becoming increasingly more common as older adults are living longer and becoming more dependent on others, mainly family members, as caregivers. An estimated 4% to 5% (one and a half million) of elderly adults are abused annually, suffering at the hands of a partner/spouse or family members. Only one in eight cases of elder abuse is reported, whereas one in three cases of child abuse is reported. Many elders are reluctant to report abuse because of dependence on the caregiver.[21,84,101]

Violence occurs frequently in the health-care workplace and is thought to be an increasing phenomenon. It may, however, be grossly underreported because of the perception that violence within health care is so often tolerated and is part of the job. Although homicides occur, the majority of violence against nurses is nonfatal in nature. More than 85% of nonfatal workplace violence occurs in service-oriented work environments such as

! EMERGENCY ALERT

VIOLENCE

Assessment

- Violence is most commonly directed at children, women, and elders.
- Assessment for violence should be a part of every health assessment.

Interventions

- An essential component of intervention is ensuring the safety of the victim.
- Health care professionals must follow all legal requirements when caring for a victim of abuse.

health care. Health-care providers, mainly nurses, are at least 16 times more likely to encounter on-the-job nonfatal assaults than workers of other professions.[32,118]

Psychopathology

Men and women can be victims of domestic abuse, although it is far more common for a woman to be the victim. Domestic violence permeates all socioeconomic levels. The abuser has an anger control problem, tends to be controlling in the relationship, and blames others for any personal problems, failures, and certainly for the violent acts inflicted on the spouse. Persons living in an abusive relationship may have been abused as children. Violent men are thought to be three times more likely to be alcohol or substance abusers. Substance and alcohol abuse is also prevalent in women and children who are victims of family violence. Abused victims suffer from low self-esteem and appear isolated from family and friends and completely dependent on the abusive spouse.[21,84]

Although the elderly are physically and psychologially abused, often abuse occurs in the form of neglect. There are no national standards for measuring how well the elderly person is being cared for. Many of the elderly at risk are those living in long-term care facilities. Most commonly, victims are women, age 75 years or older, and suffering from chronic physical and even mental illnesses. Abusers are usually family members, often stressed with the demands of family and job responsibilities in addition to the responsibility of care of the elder. The more dependent the elder is on others as caretakers, the higher the risk for physical or emotional abuse or neglect, failure to provide medical needs, and exploitation by threatening the elder into signing over assets.[84]

Health professionals are at increased risk for workplace violence for many reasons, including a 24-hour open-door policy for patient access with unrestricted movement of the public, availability of drugs and money in hospital settings, increased prevalence of weapons among patients and visitors (a factor of the community in which the health-care workplace is located), the current cost-cutting focus and widespread downsizing within the health-care industry that largely affects nurse staffing levels, and working alone during the night or early morning hours.[32] In addition, the clinical specialty areas that have been identified as being higher risk include psychiatric mental health, emergency department, long-term care, and home care nursing.[117]

Nurses are involved in many aspects of care of women and elders who are abused. Nursing education directed at primary prevention of family violence reduces or attempts to control the causative factors associated with the violence or abuse. By identifying families at high risk for abuse, nurses assist the family in planning efforts to modify those risk factors. This might include improving the family's coping skills, which would increase self-esteem and sense of competence as a caregiver. Issues of mental illness and substance abuse as they relate to the violence may be addressed. Discussions about adult or older adult development, stress management, and counseling services may be beneficial. It is important for the nurse to consider interventions that serve to change the perception of the family that violence is an acceptable way to resolve conflicts.

Secondary prevention incorporates early detection and treatment in family violence that has occurred. It is most important to protect the victim from further abuse and attempt to break the cycle of abuse that is currently taking place. This often involves reporting the violence to authorities and removing the victim from the abusive home setting. Action should also be taken to institute counseling or psychiatric care for the abuser. Tertiary prevention should provide a continuum of supportive and rehabilitative services to violent families to prevent further abuse and neglect.[101]

The Occupational Safety and Health Administration (OSHA) and the National Institute for Occupational Safety and Health (NIOSH) have developed guidelines for creating a safer workplace for nurses, but they are not enforceable standards and instead serve as advisory guidelines. It would be beneficial to nurses to be educated about violence in the workplace, as well as how to deal with potentially violent individuals, while in training. However, many nurses become educated only after a violent incident has occurred, and it is only then that issues such as staffing and security are addressed. The American Nurses Association reports that many state nurses associations continue to move legislation forward to protect against workplace violence in health care.[4,32,82]

Diagnostic Studies and Findings

Blood chemistry studies: For evidence of malnutrition, dehydration

Blood toxicology studies: For evidence of substance abuse

Urinalysis: For evidence of bleeding or infection

Vaginal cultures: For evidence of trauma, infection, sperm

X-ray examination: For evidence of acute as well as "old" fractures

CT scan of head: For evidence of subdural hematoma, brain hemorrhage, or contusions, even without external signs of injury (shaken baby syndrome)

Multidisciplinary Plan

General Management

Establish and implement safe environment

Domestic violence: Screen women using questions that focus on perception of interpersonal relationships and interactions; use a set protocol developed for the health-care setting that dictates acute management of the victim of violent abuse; collect evidence of and carefully document injuries; provide initial crisis intervention (see Crisis) as appropriate

Follow state laws and adult protective services statutes; provide for safety needs; use the interdisciplinary team for patient and family teaching and support[84]

Manage the chronically angry patient by setting limits; offer psychologic/psychiatric consultation to provide assistance to guide strategies for limit setting[102]; ensure that health professionals are aware of the increased incidence of abusive patient behaviors in certain clinical specialty areas—psychiatric mental health, emergency room, long-term care setting, and home health care; establish and institute a protocol in those areas to ensure availability of backup security support; screen patients for weapons to prevent possible violent situations and injuries in known high-risk geographic locations (e.g., urban emergency departments)[7,117]; evaluate a violent or potentially violent episode that has occurred to be sure that it was properly documented and steps are taken to prevent reoccurrence[117]

NURSING CARE

Nursing Assessment

Domestic Abuse

General appearance: Contusions, bruises, abrasions, lacerations, scars, burns

Affect: Anxious, frightened, depressed, passive, embarrassed, ashamed, avoids eye contact, looks to partner to answer questions (partner may be possessive, smothering, and controlling)

Multiple injuries with or without history of significant trauma: Evidence of current or old fractures or dislocations; unexplained bruises, welts, scratches, bite marks, burns, or lacerations; injuries inconsistent with history; women may have injuries on breasts, arms, abdomen, chest, neck, face, and genital area

Eyes, ears, nose, and mouth: Bruising, bleeding, burns, abrasions, missing teeth

Head: Localized absence of hair due to hair pulling, burns

Elder Abuse

General appearance: Poor hygiene, inappropriate dress; lack of glasses, teeth, or hearing aid despite evidence of need; evidence of malnutrition

Affect: Confused, fearful, depressed, poor eye contact, looks to caregiver for answers or approval

Injuries with or without history of significant trauma: Fractures, current or evidence of old fractures; muscle wasting, severely limited range of motion, contractures; bruises, welts, scratches, bite marks, burns, contusions, or lacerations; injuries inconsistent with history

Signs of internal bleeding, abdominal distension, or fecal impaction

Potential Complications

Serious or life-threatening injury, long-term psychologic trauma, including PTSD

Patient Problems/Nursing Diagnoses & Interventions

NIC Risk Management

Risk for injury related to violence

Disturbed body image/situational low self-esteem related to physical or psychologic abuse/trauma

- Stay with patient during physical examination.
- Reassure patient that she or he is in a safe place.
- Encourage continued discussion of battering or sexual abuse.
- Take proper legal action as stipulated by state (notify authorities).
- Take steps to inform protective services.

NIC Coping Assistance

Ineffective coping related to physical or psychologic trauma

- Encourage patient to verbalize fears, anger, guilt, rage, helplessness.
- Provide crisis counseling.
- Assist in developing social support systems, community resources (shelters, job training programs, parenting classes).
- Discussion of strategies for anger control with abuser and partner, with focus on intervention strategy.
- Discussion of short-term and long-term physical/psychologic effects of child, partner, or elder abuse.
- Talk to patient about the abuse and the fact that it is not the patient's fault, the patient is the victim, and he or she needs protection and support.
- Adult victims can identify behaviors used to try to prevent assault and be encouraged to feel more like a survivor than a victim.
- Encourage decision making and individual expression of needs.

Patient Education/Continuum of Care Plan

1. Teach patient to assess personal situation.
2. Teach patient coping techniques to deal with potential abusive situations.
3. Teach patient to develop a "safety plan" for dealing with abuse and violence.
4. Teach patient about available protective services and resources.

Evaluation/Patient Outcomes

Risk Management: Patient will state that he or she feels safe in the health-care environment. Patient will communicate details of abuse. Patient will give details of past injuries. Patient will accept treatment for injuries. Steps will be taken to provide protection and remove patient from danger. Patient will cooperate with protective measures.

Coping Assistance: Patient will verbalize the fact that he or she does not deserve abusive treatment; Patient will agree to let others help, care, and protect. Patient will not return to abusive home until it is deemed safe by protective services. Patient will become more knowledgeable about available resources. Patient will participate in self-care needs and demonstrate interest in self-care. Patient will verbalize concern for body image and bodily functions. Patient will verbalize fears concerning potential for future injury and show interest in protecting self. Patient will allow interdisciplinary team to provide assistance with home situation and follow through on plan.

References

1. Academy for Eating Disorders (AED): Binge eating disorder, 1999.
2. Aguilera D: Crisis intervention. In Fortinash K, Holoday-Worret P, editors: *Psychiatric mental health nursing,* ed 2, St. Louis, 2000, Mosby.
3. American Academy of Sleep Medicine (AASM): International classification of sleep disorders, *www.aasm.org/,* 1999.

4. American Nurses Association (ANA): Department of state government relations 1998 safety and quality initiatives, *www.ana.org/,* 1998.
5. American Psychiatric Association: *Diagnostic and statistical manual of mental disorders,* ed 4, Washington, DC, 1994, The Association.
6. Amey S: Transitional objects, phenomena, and relatedness: understanding and working with individuals with boarderline personality disorder, *J Am Psychiatric Nurses Assoc* 2(5):143, 1996.
7. Anderson L, Clarke J: De-escalating verbal aggression in primary care settings, *Nurse Pract* 21(10):95, 1996.
8. Anderson M: Waiting for harm: deliberate self-harm and suicide in young people—a review of the literature, *J Psychiatric Ment Health Nurs* 6:91, 1999.
9. Antai-Otong D: *Psychiatric nursing: biological and behavioral concepts,* Philadelphia, 1995, WB Saunders.
10. Baker C: Cultural relativism and cultural diversity: implications for nursing practice, *Adv Nurs Sci* 20(1):3, 1997.
11. Bakey A, Levy J, Fernandez F: Diagnosis and management of anxiety in the geriatric patient, *Clin Geriatr* 6(8):10, 21, 1998.
12. Barbee M, Bricker P: Suicide. In Fortinash K, Holoday-Worret P, editors: *Psychiatric mental health nursing,* St. Louis, 1996, Mosby.
13. Becker et al: Eating disorders, *N Engl J Med* 340(14):1092, 1999.
14. Billings J: A review of physician-assisted suicide, *J Holist Nurs* 14(3):206, 1996.
15. Blegen M, Tripp-Reimer T: Implications of nursing taxonomies for middle-range theory development, *Adv Nurs Sci* 19(3):37, 1997.
16. Bloch D: Adolescent suicide as a public health threat, *J Child Adolesc Psychiatr Nurs* 13(1):26, 1999.
17. Boritz-Wintz C: Nursing management of psychotropic drug reactions, *Nurs Clin North Am* 33(1):217, 1998.
18. Burns C: A retroductive theoretical model of the pathway to chemical dependency in nurses, *Arch Psychiatr Nurs* 12(1):59, 1998.
19. Canatsey K, Roper J: Removal from stimuli for crisis intervention: using the least restrictive methods to improve the quality of patient care, *Issues Ment Health Nurs* 18:35, 1997.
20. Carter-Martin A, Schaffer S, Campbell R: Managing alcohol related problems in the primary care setting, *Nurse Pract* 24(8):14, 1999.
21. Champion J: Family violence and mental health, *Nurs Clin North Am* 33(1):201, 1998.
22. Clarkin J, Abrams R: Personality disorders in the elderly, *Curr Opin Psychiatr* 11:131, 1998.
23. Clarkin-Watts A: Eating disorders. In Fortinash K, Holoday-Worret P, editors: *Psyciatric mental health nursing,* St. Louis, 1996, Mosby.
24. Coleman E et al: Assessing substance abuse among healthcare students and the efficacy of educational interventions, *J Prof Nurs* 13(1):28, 1997.
25. Crompton N: Crisis theory and crisis management: the way forward, *Ment Health Nurs* 16(5):16, 1996.
26. Czeisler C, Richardson G: Disorders of sleep and circadian rhythms. In Fauci A et al, editors: *Harrison's principles of internal medicine,* ed 14, New York, 1998, McGraw-Hill.
27. Dale L, Hurt R, Hays J: Drug therapy to aid in smoking cessation, *Postgrad Med* 104(5):75, 1998.
28. Davis K, Mathew E: Pharmacologic management of depression in the elderly, *Nurse Pract* 23(6):16, 1998.
29. DeBattista C, Glick I: Pharmacotherapy of personality disorders, *Curr Opin Psychiatry* 8:102, 1995.
30. Dement W, Vaughan C: *The promise of sleep,* New York, 1999, Delacorte Press Random House.
31. Devons C: Suicide in the elderly: how to identify and treat patients at risk, *Geriatrics* 51:67, 1996.
32. Elliott P: Violence in health care: what nurse managers need to know, *Nurs Manage* 28:38, 1997.
33. Fairburn C et al: Risk factors for anorexia nervosa, *Arch Gen Psychiatry* 56:468, 1999.
34. Farrell S, Harmon R, Hastings S: Nursing management of acute psychotic episodes, *Nurs Clin North Am* 33(1):187, 1998.
35. Frisch N, Frisch L: The client experiencing anxiety. In Frisch N, Frisch L, editors: *Psychiatric mental health nursing,* Albany, NY, 1998, Delmar.
36. Frisch N, Frisch L: The eating disorders. In Frisch N, Frisch L, editors: *Psychiatric mental health nursing,* Albany, NY, 1998, Delmar.
37. Frisch N, Frisch L, editors: *Psychiatric mental health nursing,* Albany, NY, 1998, Delmar.
38. Frisch L, Wilson W: Pharmacology in psychiatric care. In Frisch N, Frisch L, editors: *Psychiatric mental health nursing,* Albany, NY, 1998, Delmar.
39. Gitlin M: Pharmacotherapy of personality disorders: conceptual framework and clinical strategies, *J Clin Psychopharmacol* 13(5):343, 1993.
40. Goodwin F, Jamison K: *Manic-depressive illness,* New York, 1990, Oxford University Press.
41. Grothaus K: Eating disorders and adolescents: an overview of a maladaptive behavior, *J Child Adolesc Psychiatr Nurs* 11(3):146, 1998.
42. Hagerty B: Advances in understanding major depressive disorder, *J Psychosoc Nurs* 33(11):27, 1995.
43. Hagerty B: Mood disorders: depression and mania. In Fortinash K, Holoday-Worret P, editors: *Psychiatric mental health nursing,* St. Louis, 1996, Mosby.
44. Hall B: The psychiatric model: a critical analysis of its undermining effects on nursing in chronic mental illness, *Adv Nurs Sci* 18:16, 1996.
45. Hall R, Platt D, Hall R: Suicide risk assessment: a review of risk factors for suicide in 100 patients who made severe suicide attempts, *Psychosomatics* 40:18, 1999.
46. Harkavy-Friedman J et al: Suicidal behavior in schizophrenia: characteristics of individuals who had and had not attempted suicide, *Am J Psychiatry* 156(8):1276, 1999.
47. Holoday-Worret P: Foundations of psychiatric mental health nursing. In Fortinash K, Holoday-Worret P, editors: *Psychiatric mental health nursing,* St. Louis, 1996, Mosby.
48. Howk C et al: Psychodynamic nursing (Hildegard E. Peplau). In Tomey A, Alligood M, editors: *Nursing theorists and their work,* ed 4, St. Louis, 1998, Mosby.
49. James I, Blackburn I: Psychological approaches to anxiety disorders, *Curr Opin Psychiatry* 10:481, 1997.
50. Jarboe K, Schwartz S: The relationship between medication noncompliance and cognitive function in patients with schizophrenia, *J Am Psychiatr Nurses Assoc* 5(2):S2, 1999.
51. Keel P, Mitchell J: Outcome in bulimia nervosa, *Am J Psychiatry* 154:313, 1997.
52. Kirkwood C: Management of insomnia, *J Am Pharm Assoc* 39(5):688, 1999.
53. Krasucki C, Howard R, Mann A: Anxiety and its treatment in the elderly, *Int Psychogeriatr* 11(1):25, 1998.
54. Lenane M: Family therapy for children with obsessive-compulsive disorder. In Patton M, Zohar J, editors: *Current treatment of*

obsessive-compulsive disorder, Washington, DC, 1991, American Psychiatric Press.

55. Lesseig D: Primary care diagnosis and pharmacologic treatment of depression in adults, *Nurse Pract* 21:72, 1996.
56. Littrell K, Littrell S: Schizophrenia and comorbid substance abuse, *J Am Psychiatr Nurses Assoc* 5(2):S17, 1999.
57. Long A, Long A, Smyth A: Suicide: a statement of suffering, *Nurs Ethics* 5(1):1998.
58. Marcus P: Personality disorders. In Fortinash K, Holoday-Worret P, editors: *Psychiatric mental health nursing,* St. Louis, 1996, Mosby.
59. Mauri M: Sleep and the reproductive cycle, *Health Care Women Int* 11:409, 1990.
60. Mayo Clinic Nicotine Dependance Center: *Bupropion (Zyban) as a smoking cessation tool* (ed 2) (brochure), 1999, Mayo Press.
61. McCance K, Huether S: *Pathophysiology,* ed 3, St. Louis, 1998, Mosby.
62. McKenna P: *Schizophrenia and related syndromes,* New York, 1994, Oxford University Press.
63. Merikangas K, Swendsen J: Genetic epidemiology of psychiatric disorders, *Epidemiol Rev* 19(1):144, 1997.
64. Mosier W, Nelson AS, Walgren K: Wanted: a good night's sleep, *Adv Nurse Pract* 5:31, 1998.
65. Mynatt S: A model of contributing risk factors to chemical dependency in nurses, *J Psychosoc Nurs* 34(7):13, 1996.
66. National Heart Lung & Blood Institute (NHLBI)/National Institutes of Health (NIH): National center on sleep disorders research, *www.nhlbi.nih.gov/,* 1999.
67. National Household Survey on Drug Abuse (NHSDA), Substance Abuse and Mental Health Services Administration (SAMHSA): Highlights, *www.samhsa.gov/oas/NHSDA/98SummHtml/NHSDA98Summ-01.htm,* 1998.
68. National Institute on Alcohol Abuse and Alcoholism (NIAAA), National Institutes of Heath; Alcohol alert, vol 39, *http://silk.nih.gov/silk/niaaa1/publicatoin/aa39.htm,* 1998.
69. National Institute on Drug Abuse (NIDA), National Institutes of Health: Cocaine abuse and addiction, *www.nida.nih.gov/researchreports/Cocaine/cocaine2.html,* 1999.
70. National Institute on Drug Abuse (NIDA), National Institutes of Health: INFOFAX: Cost to society, *www.nida.nih.gov/Infofax/costs.html,* 1999.
71. National Institute on Drug Abuse (NIDA), National Institutes of Health: INFOFAX: Heroin: abuse and addiction, *www.nida.nih.gov/Reports/Heroin/heroin2.html.html,* 1999.
72. National Institute on Drug Abuse (NIDA), National Institutes of Health: INFOFAX: Inhalants 013, *www.nida.nih.gov/Infofax/inhalants.html,* 1999.
73. National Institute on Drug Abuse (NIDA), National Institutes of Health: INFOFAX: Marijuana, *www.nida.nih.gov/Infofax/marijuana.html,* 1999.
74. National Institute on Drug Abuse (NIDA), National Institutes of Health: INFOFAX: Treatment trends, *www.nida.nih.gov/Infofax/treatmenttrends.html,* 1999.
75. National Institute on Drug Abuse (NIDA), National Institutes of health: Inhalant abuse, *www.nida.nih.gov/researchreports/Inhalants/Inhalants2.html,* 1999.
76. National Institute on Drug Abuse (NIDA), National Institutes of Health: Nicotine addiction, *www.nida.nih.gov/researchreports/nicotine/nicotine2.html,* 1999.
77. National Institute on Drug Abuse (NIDA), National Institutes of Health: NIDA notes: facts about nicotine and tobacco products, vol 13, issue 3, *www.nida.nih.gov/NNVol13N3/tearoff.html,* 1999.
78. National Institute of Mental Health: Annual report on the rare diseases and conditions research activities of the National Institutes of Mental Health (NIMH), *www.nimh.gov.com,* 1997.
79. National Institute of Mental Health: The numbers count, NIH 99-4584, *www.nimh.nih.gov/publicat/,* 1999.
80. National Institute of Mental Health: Suicide among the elderly, *www.nimh.nih.gov/research/suielderly,* 1999.
81. National Institute of Mental Health: Suicide facts, *www.nimh.nih.gov/research/suifact,* 1999.
82. National Institute for Occupational Safety and Health: Violence in the workplace, *www.cdc.gov/niosh/violence/,* 1996.
83. Nelyan T, Reynolds C, Kupfer D: Sleep disorders. In Hales R, Yudofsky S, Talbott J, editors: *The American psychiatric press textbook of psychiatry,* ed 3, Washington, DC, 1998, American Psychiatric Press.
84. Nieves-Khouw F: Recognizing victims of physical and sexual abuse, *Crit Care Nurs Clin North Am* 9(2):141, 1997.
85. O'Brien S: Health promotion and schizophrenia: the year 2000 and beyond, *Holist Nurs Pract* 12:38, 1998.
86. Poirier L: The importance of screening for domestic violence in all women, *Nurse Pract* 22(5):105, 1997.
87. Pullen L, Green L: Identification, intervention and education: educational curriculum components for chemical dependency in nurses, *J Contin Educ Nurs* 28(5):211, 1997.
88. Restless Legs Syndrome Foundation (RLS): Medical bulletin, *www.rls.org/,* 1999.
89. Reynolds C: Depression: making the diagnosis and using SSRIs in the older patient, *Geriatrics* 51:28, 1996.
90. Robin A, Siegel P: Differences between child, adolescent, and adult eating disorders, *Int J Eat Disord* 24:422, 1998.
91. Robinson L, Littrell S, Littrell K: Managing aggression in schizophrenia, *J Am Psychiatr Nurses Assoc* 5(2):S9, 1999.
92. Saleh M: Disasters and crises: challenges to mental health counseling in the twenty-first century, *Education* 116:519, 1996.
93. Segal D et al: Personality disorders in community-dwelling older adults, *J Ment Health Aging* 4(1):171, 1998.
94. Sherr J: Psychopharmacology and other biologic therapies. In Fortinash K, Holoday-Worret P, editors: *Psychiatric mental health nursing,* St. Louis, 1996, Mosby.
95. Simington J, Cargill L, Hill W: Crisis intervention, *Clin Nurs Res* 5(4):376, 1996.
96. Surgeon General's Call to Action to Prevent Suicide, 1999: At a glance: suicide among the elderly; suicide in the United States, *www.surgeongeneral.gov/library/calltoaction/fact1&2,* 1999.
97. Swann A: Selection of a first-line mood stabilizing agent, *Curr Opin Psychiatry* 11:71, 1998.
98. Tablowski P, Cooke MS, Thoman E: A procedure for withdrawal of sleep medication in elderly women who have been long-term users, *J Gerontol Nurs* 9:20, 1998.
99. Terpstra T, Terpstra T: Treating geriatric depression with SSRIs: what primary care practitioners need to know, *Nurse Pract* 22(9):118, 1997.
100. Thobaben M: Caring for interpersonal violence survivors, *Home Care provider* 2(4):162, 1997.
101. Thobaben M: Survivors of violence or abuse. In Frisch N, Frisch L, editors: *Psychiatric mental health nursing,* Albany, NY, 1998, Delmar Publishers.
102. Thomas S: Assessing and intervening with anger disorders, *Nurs Clin North Am* 33(1):121, 1998.

103. Tobacco Information and Prevention Source (TIPS), Centers for Disease Control: Healthy people 2000 midcourse review and 1995 revisions, *www.cdc.gov/tobacco/hpl2000.htm*, 1995.
104. Torgersen S: Genetic factors in anxiety disorders, *Arch Gen Psychiatry* 40:1085, 1983.
105. Torkelson D, Anderson R, McDaniel R: Interventions in response to chemically dependent nurses: effect of context and interpretation, *Res Nurs Health* 19:153, 1996.
106. Treasure J, Holland A: Genetic vulnerability to eating disorders: evidence from twin and family studies, In Remschmidt H, Schmidt M, editors: *Anorexia nervosa,* Toronto, 1990, Hogrefe & Huber.
107. Trimpey M, Davidson S: Nursing care of personality disorders in the medical surgical setting, *Nurs Clin North Am* 33(1):173, 1998.
108. Tuck I et al: The experience of caring for an adult child with schizophrenia, *Arch Psychiatr Nurs* 11(3):118, 1997.
109. Tugrul K: Newer antipsychotic agents: impact on quality of life and alternative applications, *J Am Psychiatr Nurses Assoc* 4(4):S35, 1998.
110. U.S. Department of Health and Human Services: *Healthy People 2010* (conference edition, in two volumes), Washington, DC, 2000, The Department.
111. US Department of Health and Human Services (DHHS), Surgeon General: Mental health: a report of the surgeon general, *www.surgeongeneral.gov/library/mentalhealth/,* 1999.
112. Valente S: Diagnosis and treatment of panic disorder and generalized anxiety in primary care, *Nurse Pract* 21:26, 1996.
113. Valente S: Anxiety and panic disorders in older adults, *Home Health Care Manage Pract* 11(4):49, 1999.
114. Volker D: Assisted suicide and the domain of nursing practice, *J Nurs Law* 5(1):39, 1998.
115. Wagner J, Wagner ML, Hening WA: Beyond benzodiazepines: alternative pharmacologic agents for the treatment of insomnia, *Ann Pharamcother* 32(6):680, 1998.
116. White B: Assisted suicide and nursing: possibly compatible? *J Prof Nurs* 15(3):151, 1999.
117. Whitley G, Jacobson G, Gawrys M: The impact of violence in the health care setting upon nursing education, *J Nurs Educ* 35(5):211, 1996.
118. Williams M, Robertson K: Workplace violence, *Crit Care Nurs Clin North Am* 9(2):221, 1997.
119. Wu L, Kouzis A, Leaf P: Influence of comorbid alcohol and psychiatric disorders on utilization of mental health services in the national comorbidity survey, *Am J Psychiatry* 156(8):1230, 1999.

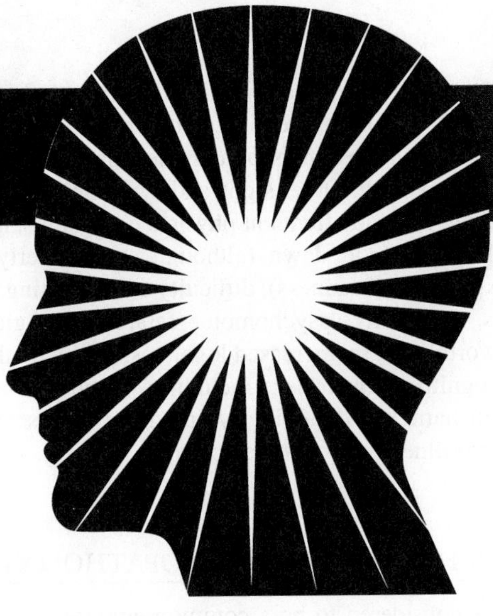

20 Mental Health Disorders in the Elderly

Gertrude K. McFarland

Overview

By the year 2030, 20% of people in the United States will be over age 65 years; by the year 2050, 5% will be over age 85, the fastest growing segment of the elderly.[22] Women experience different mortality rates than men. Women outnumber men at age 65 years and over, and the gap widens with advancing age. Elderly women are also at greater economic risk and are more likely to be widowed and living alone than elderly men.

Normal aging is a process that eventually leads to noticeable changes in the body. Not all changes, however, are due to the normal aging process. One or two chronic diseases are present in 70% of adults over 80.[22] Among the common mental health disorders are depression, dementia, anxiety, alcohol-related problems, and prescription/over-the-counter drug misuse.

Although the underlying mechanisms of the aging process are poorly understood, a number of theories have been proposed.[20] Biologic theories include genetics (aging process is encoded in genes); glycosylation (glucose changes associated with tissue changes in aging); eversion or cross-linkage (changes in collagen structure associated with aging); immune system (decreased immune competence and altered regulation of immune system); and free radical theory (role of oxygen free radicals).

Researchers have identified specific cognitive capabilities that are subject to age-related decline.[120] Aging is associated with a slowing in information processing, with a decline noted especially in secondary memory. "Consequently, aging appears to exert a profound effect in the acquisition and retrieval of new information in secondary memory."[120] Although some age-related decline in selective attention tasks are reported, divided attention tasks are noted to decline more consistently. Some aspects of intellectual functioning decline with age (e.g., fluid abilities or abilities to solve novel problems). Word recognition memory can be affected by age, as may auditory processing of speech comprehension and problem solving. Although a cumulative degeneration of brain tissue exists with normal aging, the effects are not noticeable in most persons under ordinary circumstances unless other stressors are added. Disease and pathologic conditions, however, can lead to a rapid decline in cognitive functioning.

The elderly are confronted with a number of issues, losses, and transitions with which they have to cope and to which they have to adapt. Successful adaptation, in turn, can contribute to preserving mental health. Issues faced by elderly persons include dealing with aging; alterations in autonomy; major life transitions, such as retirement; death of significant others; changes in the body; physical illness; meeting sexual needs; engaging in meaningful activities; using available resources maximally; and dealing with one's own impending death. Elderly with different personality types will respond differently to these life events and experience different consequences.[120] "Patterns characterized by better adjustment earlier in life may well lead to more positive outcomes later in life."[120]

A number of social/psychologic theories of aging have been proposed.[20] Disengagement theory views aging as inevitable disengagement and mutual withdrawal with decreasing interactions of older persons with others. Activity theory, on the other hand, espouses that those elderly who are active, socially involved, and productive will remain the most satisfied. Continuity theory proposes that elderly people will continue engaging in behavior patterns established in younger years. In symbolic interactionism, the social world and subjective reality is constructed by means of interacting with other persons. The theory of life events and stress postulates that key events associated with aging are important to health. The minority group theory holds that the aged as a cohort experience many of the same types of discrimination as minorities. Developmental theory addresses stages of life, with the last stage centering on ego-integrity or despair. Many elderly, despite facing losses, transitions, and challenges, remain psychologically robust.

CONDITIONS, DISEASES, AND DISORDERS

MOOD DISORDERS IN THE ELDERLY

Mood disorders[2] comprise depressive disorders, bipolar disorders, and mood disorder based on etiology.

Depressive disorders[2] include (1) major depressive disorder, characterized by the presence of one or more depressive episodes (includes five or more of the following symptoms: depressed mood, diminished pleasure in activities, suicidal ideation, difficulty concentrating or thinking, psychomotor retardation or agitation, weight loss, sleep disturbance, fatigue, feelings of worthlessness and guilt, symptoms that can cause impaired occupational and social functioning), with at least 2 weeks of depressed mood or loss of pleasure or interest but no evidence of manic, mixed, or hypomanic episodes; (2) dysthymic disorder, characterized by presence of depressed mood for 2 years and other symptoms of depression but not of a major depressive episode and no evidence of manic, mixed, or hypomanic episodes; and (3) depressive disorder not otherwise specified, characterized by depressive features but does not meet, for example, criteria for major depressive disorder, dysthymic disorder, and no evidence of manic, mixed, or hypomanic episodes.

Bipolar disorders[2] include (1) bipolar I disorder, characterized by one or more manic episodes (elevated mood, talkative, flight of ideas, grandiosity, psychomotor agitation, reduced need for sleep, involvement in pleasurable activities with potential adverse outcomes, impaired occupational and/or social functioning) or mixed episode (has characteristics of both depressive and manic episodes, impaired occupational and/or social functioning) along with major depressive episodes; (2) bipolar II disorder, characterized by one or more major depressive episodes and one or more hypomanic episodes (similar to manic episodes except that social and occupational functioning are not as markedly impaired); (3) cyclothymic disorder, characterized by 2 years of hypomanic and depressive symptoms but not actual manic episodes or major depressive episodes; and (4) bipolar disorder not otherwise specified, characterized by bipolar features that do not meet criteria for bipolar I, bipolar II, or cyclothymic disorders.

Mood disorder based on etiology[2] includes (1) mood disorder due to a general medical condition characterized by mood disturbance caused by a general medical condition; (2) substance-induced mood disorder, characterized by mood disturbance caused by drug abuse, a medication, or a toxin; and (3) mood disorder not otherwise specified, characterized by mood disturbance not readily meeting criteria or other diagnosis.

DEPRESSION

Depression can refer to a mood state, symptom, syndrome, or disease.[37] Depression in the elderly can be construed from a categorical perspective (as in the *Diagnostic and Statistical Manual of Mental Disorders,* ed 4, [DSM-IV]) or from a functional perspective (as impaired role relationships) or as a unitary phenomenon (as from mild to severe).[11] Without meeting the typical *DSM-IV* criteria for a depressive disorder, the elderly nevertheless often suffer from depressive symptoms. In the elderly, lack of pleasure or interest in usual activities may be one of the first signs of depression. Other signs and symptoms of depression in the elderly include frequent physical complaints, lack of energy, feeling blue and down (although some elderly may minimize expression of sadness), difficulty concentrating, sleep disturbances, irritability, psychomotor retardation, agitation, feelings of worthlessness, increased loneliness, onset of alcohol problems, cognitive impairment including memory loss, and deliberate self-harm.[6] Overlapping symptoms of depression and actual physical illness may also be common.

PATHOPHYSIOLOGY/PSYCHOPATHOLOGY

Depression is considered to be a common emotional problem among the elderly and in this population is both underdiagnosed and undertreated.[112] The rates of depression vary depending on the definition used and the setting.[85] About 15% of community-dwelling elderly manifest depressive symptoms, and 3% manifest a major depressive disorder.[85] In primary care clinics, 10% to 12% of the elderly have a major depression and about 20% have depressive symptoms, whereas in nursing homes 12% to 16% experience a major depressive disorder and from 30% to 40% manifest depressive symptoms.[85] Depression will increase in magnitude as the elderly population increases. Twenty one percent (or 65 million people) are projected to be 65 years of age and over by 2030.[36] Also, as more elderly reach their 80s and 90s, late-onset depression, which may be associated with neurologic or cardiovascular disease, may increase.

Factors contributing to depression in the elderly can be predisposing or precipitating.[6,66] Genetic, neurobiologic, physiologic, and biochemical factors may contribute to the etiology of depression in the elderly.[6,11] A genetic link to major depression has been identified, although this becomes weaker in late-life depression. Neurotransmitter changes in the elderly may contribute to a predisposition to depression, as can dysregulation of the hypothalamic-pituitary-adrenal axis, dysregulation of the thyroid axis, and desynchronization of circadian rhythms. Structural brain changes—neurodegenerative changes possibly subcortical in location—may predispose some elderly to depression. Major health problems and specific diseases can also predispose the elderly to depression.

Personality, psychosocial factors, and environmental stressors may also play a role in predisposing or precipitating depression in the elderly.[6,11,112] Personality dysfunction, lifelong inability to achieve intimacy, lack of social support, and childhood sexual abuse have all been implicated in the development of depression in the elderly. Actual or threatening life events—such as the loss of significant others, major illness of self or significant other, severe financial problems, loss of one's home—can also play a role in the development of depression. Depression in all ages, including the elderly, is more prevalent in women.

Suicide is a great risk in depressed elderly, especially for elderly who are chronically ill with a debilitating disease; acutely ill elderly with impairment of activities of daily living (ADLs); the widowed, divorced, or isolated; and substance abusers. Most persons visit their primary care physician within the month before suicide with their depressive symptoms being unrecognized and untreated.[88]

Diagnostic Studies and Findings

Diagnosis and recognition of depression in late life may be more difficult than earlier in life for a number of reasons: symptoms of depression may be attributed to the aging process; the actual symptoms of depression may be different from those in younger persons (i.e., more somatic complaints); the elderly are less likely to acknowledge depressed mood; there may be more concern over the presence of actual medical conditions; the presence of dementia and stroke may compromise accurate reporting of symptoms; there may be a lack of understanding of depression; and there may be a fear of expense of treatment.[88]

Comprehensive interview and complete physical and mental examination[37]: To determine (a) presence of depression; (b) presence of depression occurring secondary to physical illness (either as a direct physiologic effect or as the medical condition acting as a psychologic precipitant of depression), for example, conditions of the cardiovascular system such as congestive heart failure, cardiac arrhythmias, and myocardial infarction; conditions of the central nervous system such as cerebrovascular accident, multiinfarct dementia, Alzheimer's disease, Parkinson's disease, acquired immunodeficiency syndrome (AIDS), dementia, tumors, meningiomas, and epilepsy; autoimmune conditions such as rheumatoid arthritis; conditions of the endocrine system such as hyperparathyroidism, hypoparathyroidism, hypothyroidism, and diabetes mellitus; other conditions such as anemia, infectious disease, malnutrition, and chronic pain syndrome; (c) presence of depression that may be masked by somatic ailments; and (d) presence of depression occurring as a result of use of medications that can precipitate depression such as digitalis, clonidine, propranolol, phenylbutazone, opiates, benzodiazepines, barbiturates, alcohol, sulfonamides, progesterone, and corticosteroids

Survey of medications: To determine both over-the-counter and prescribed medication use

Nutritional survey: To determine adequacy of current dietary intake

Routine diagnostic procedures: To determine presence of coexisting medical condition; this can include electrocardiogram (ECG), blood count, urinalysis, B_{12} level, liver function tests, levels of folate, T_4, thyroid-stimulating hormone, glucose, electrolytes, blood urea nitrogen (BUN), creatinine, and VDRL test

Neuropsychologic testing[37]: To differentiate conditions such as depression and dementia (e.g., dementia syndrome of depression [pseudodementia]), syndrome of depression as part of organic process in dementia of the Alzheimer's type

Electrophysiologic and psychometric evaluation[37]: To differentiate depression (with early morning awakening) from sleep disorders of the elderly such as primary insomnia

Psychometric assessment for depression[37,66]: Self-report tools can be used to determine presence of depression (e.g., Beck Depression Inventory, Geriatric Depression Scale, Zung Self-Rating Depression Scale, Profile of Mood States, Multiscore Depression Inventory, Center for Epidemiological Studies Depression Scale [CES-D]); structured interview tools can be used to determine presence of depression (e.g., Structured Interview Guide for the Hamilton Rating Scale for Depression, Diagnostic Interview Schedule); projective tests can be conducted by psychologists to determine presence of depression (e.g., Rorschach, Thematic Apperception Test)

Multidisciplinary Plan

Medications*

Physiologic changes and decreased capacity to adapt are associated with changes in pharmacokinetics. Because of pharmacodynamic and pharmacokinetic changes, the elderly may experience increased sensitivity to psychotropic medications and their side effects. Because there is no uniformity in the aging process, the response and sensitivity of the elderly to medications is variable. In general, however, the elderly may be more vulnerable to the side effects of medications (e.g., anticholinergic side effects).[112] In the elderly it is important to start with reduced initial dosing of a number of medications such as antidepressants.

Because major depressions are often recurrent, maintenance drug treatment may be necessary after remission of the depression. After the first episode of major depression, medications should be maintained for 6 months; after the second episode or more, 12 months.[88] Before initiating drug therapy with antidepressants in the elderly, a very careful assessment is necessary along with regular evaluation for efficacy when treatment is prolonged.

Selective serotonin reuptake inhibitors (SSRIs): For example, fluoxetine, sertraline, paroxetine, fluvoxamine

Tricyclic antidepressants (TCAs): For example, desipramine and nortriptyline[70,131]

Other antidepressants: For example, trazodone, bupropion, venlafaxine, mirtazapine, and nefazodone[70,131]

Other Treatment

Electroconvulsive therapy (ECT): To treat severely depressed elderly not responsive to other treatments, including pharmacotherapy[14,80]; effect of depression on quality of life, functional deficits, and severity of symptoms such as weight loss may lead to increased use of ECT in the elderly[80]

General Management

Individual therapy: To assist elderly in mastery of the present through therapy that is time limited, structured, and goal oriented

Individual cognitive behavior therapy: Useful in treating acute major depression by focusing on changing faulty thought patterns[16,138,144]

Individual insight psychotherapy: To resolve previous intrapsychic and interpersonal conflicts and fear of dependence for elderly with a mild depression

Supportive psychotherapy: To provide support, specific directives, and counseling for elderly patients with severe depression

Group therapy: To provide support and counseling

*References 17, 25, 27, 54, 70, 112, 131.

Mutual support group: To encourage exchange of information, sharing of emotions, and problem solving[16]; the elderly patient observes that others share similar experiences
Day treatment: To provide a structured daytime treatment milieu
Music, dance, art therapy: To focus thoughts and feelings on something pleasant, encourage interpersonal interactions, and enhance expression of feelings
Group exercise training program[13]: To reduce depressive symptoms and to promote a sense of self-esteem and well-being by actively participating in three supervised aerobic exercise sessions per week for 10 weeks

NURSING CARE

Nursing Assessment

Risk factors for depression in the elderly: Alcoholism; chronic illness; chronic pain; physiologic factors; previous suicide attempts; use of multiple medications
Psychosocial stressors and risk factors: Being a caregiver of a cognitively impaired dependent; extreme isolation; family stress; inadequate social support; lack of adequate finances; loss of significant other; loss of social network; loss of social stability; major life transitions; marital breakdown; retirement; institutionalization; presence of multiple concurrent crises
Symptoms of depression: Anxiety; change in sleep patterns; depressed mood; diminished ability to concentrate; expressions of helplessness, worthlessness, hopelessness; fatigue; feelings of failure; irritability; lack of appetite; lack of interest in activities that were a source of pleasure; lack of motivation; loss of interest in life; loss of weight; low self-esteem; multiple somatic complaints; restlessness; thoughts of suicide; withdrawal from others
Denial of presence of depression and/or nonclassic symptoms of depression: Resistance to express depressive feelings; denial of depressed feelings; increased somatic complaints; avoidance of mental health care; sleeplessness; difficulty discussing suicidal thoughts; mental illness viewed as stigma
Side effects of medications
  Selective serotonin reuptake inhibitors (SSRIs): Gastrointestinal upset, sexual dysfunction, insomnia, agitation, sedation[70,88]
  Tricyclic antidepressants (TCAs): Cardiac toxicity, constipation/bowel obstruction, dry mouth, lack of ability to eat, orthostatic hypotension, potential for falls, decreased memory, delirium, confusion[112]
  Bupropion: Seizures
  Venlafaxine: Increased blood pressure, headache, nausea[112]

Potential Complications[17,25]

Suicide potential because the elderly have the highest suicide rate and are at a very high risk for completed suicide
  Stressful events (e.g., losses, abuse/misuse of medications, illness, abuse)
  Behavioral changes (e.g., unkempt appearance, lack of appetite, insomnia)
  Feelings and thoughts (e.g., hopelessness, anger, inability to concentrate)
  Presence of suicidal thoughts
  Presence of suicidal plan, resources, and time
Comorbitities and complex physical health problems that may mask signs and symptoms of depression (e.g., dementia)
Symptoms of cardiovascular disease; use extreme caution before administering TCAs because TCAs can have major electrophysiologic effects in the elderly[25]
Presence of glaucoma or incipient glaucoma: if present do not administer medications with anticholinergic effects such as tricyclic antidepressants[17]

Patient Problems/Nursing Diagnoses & Interventions

NIC Risk Management

Risk for self-directed violence related to depression

- Develop supportive and nurturing therapeutic relationship with patient *because this will become the basis for future social integration.*
- Collaborate with interdisciplinary team to maintain safe environment free of potential of self-harm: one-to-one observation may be required when patient is preoccupied with thoughts of suicide.
- Collaborate with interdisciplinary team to develop treatment plan for physical and mental disorders *to treat conditions that may contribute to depression.*
- Stress importance of treatment, including medication regimen, in hospital and compliance with medication regimen after hospitalization. *Early diagnosis, referral, and treatment is critical in resolving depression because elderly are generally responsive to treatment and lack of treatment can lead to lethal consequences.*
- Be an empathetic listener, present a sense of optimism, and convey hope.
- Help patient examine alternative actions to his or her problems *to overcome a sense of hopelessness and ineffectuality.*
- Have patient engage in meaningful activities within his or her level of coping and capabilities *because such activities can distract from problems and be therapeutic.*
- Alleviate isolation and reduced independence caused by immobility and/or sensory deprivation.

NIC Coping Assistance

Ineffective coping related to depression

- Use cognitive therapy strategies *to help patient view situation in an alternative, more positive manner and to replace faulty perceptions with more valid ones.*
  Assist patient in examining distortions.
  Discuss basic assumptions behind beliefs.
  Help patient change thoughts from negative to positive.
  Systematically reinforce positive input thought patterns.
- Have patient record pleasant and unpleasant thoughts in a daily diary.
  Have patient record sleep time and other activities.
  Discuss diary with patient, commenting on performance, encouraging expression of feelings, and dis-

cussing problem solving *to solve problems that can be changed and to instill hope.*

- Facilitate recovery from depression by helping elderly women through phases of redefining the self.[114,115]
- Facilitate grief work *to assist patient in resolving emotions related to multiple and major losses so frequently experienced by the elderly.*
- Assist patient in examining remaining relationships after death of a significant person and in developing new relationships *to maintain social contacts for companionship, support, and intimacy.*
- Engage patient in life review reminiscence to experience pleasures of previous life experiences by recalling them *to combat depression and increase patient's self-esteem.*
- Acknowledge progress made by patient.
- Use humor when appropriate *because humor can reduce stress and is life affirming.*
- Encourage social contacts *to reduce social isolation and develop sense of self-worth.*
- Help patient focus on the here and now.
  Explore present situation and problems.
  Assist patient in forming alternative and more positive views.
  Engage patient in problem solving, setting realistic expectations
- Explore reality with patient and assist in developing strategies to deal with stressors *to focus on and cope with reality.*
  Examine patient's strengths and potential.
  Examine current life stressors.
  Explore coping strategies previously used by patient.
  Assist patient in examining alternative coping strategies to deal with current stressors.
  Have patient try out new behavior in a supportive environment.
- Use behavioral strategies *to help patient focus on present behavior that can be changed and thus foster a sense of self-control and mastery.*
  Use role play to have patient model new behavior.
  Develop verbal contract with patient to try out new behaviors.
  Have elderly patient examine own goals to determine whether too much is expected of self.
  Have elderly patient compare self with others of same age to help patient realize that he or she is not alone in what is being experienced.
- Instill hope *so that patient will once again feel that there is the prospect of regaining power over his or her life.*
  Determine presence and meaning of stressful life events, medical problems, and mental disorders.
  Examine with patient coping strategies used in past to deal with stressors and those that could be currently applied.
  Promote social support: identify adequacy of patient's social support system; determine functioning of social support system.
  Increase patient's sense of personal control.
  Enhance patient's ability to perform ADLs.
  Build on patient's spiritual and religious strengths.
- Engage elderly patient in group *to deal with stressors and solve problems* (e.g., adjusting to retirement, dealing with loneliness).
- Use psychoeducational group therapy to *increase knowledge of depression and coping skills, decrease anxiety and depressive symptoms, and enhance self-esteem, social support, and interpersonal relationships.*[101]
- Use cognitive behavior group therapy or focused visual imagery group therapy *to decrease cognitive impairments in elderly depressed patients with mild to moderate cognitive limitations.*[138]
- Encourage healthy lifestyle habits *because improved self-care can restore a sense of mastery, independence, and coping with depression*
  Encourage balanced diet.
  Encourage use of good sleep habits.
  Encourage balanced rest/sleep and activity/exercise pattern.
- Encourage family and significant others to be involved in elderly patient's recovery from depression. *Family and significant others can offer social support that can protect elderly from depression.*
- Engage elderly patient and family in family therapy *to help patient strengthen social support and enhance social networks and resources. Depression can have a negative impact on family relationships.*
- Enhance socialization by working with patient *to develop or restore a social network by involving patient in activity groups.*[112]

Patient Education/Continuum of Care Plan

Develop patient educational programs on prevention, diagnosis, and treatment of depression.

1. Teach patient about nature, symptom, causes, and treatment of depression, including medications and their side effects.
2. Teach importance of continuing prescribed medication regimen and self-monitoring for occurrence of side effects.
3. Teach patient self-help strategies in coping with depressed mood and depression. For example, "Do not set yourself difficult goals or take on a great deal of responsibility."
   a. Break large tasks into small ones, set some priorities, and do what you can as you can.
   b. Do not expect too much from yourself too soon because this will only increase feelings of failure.
   c. Try to be with other people; it is usually better than being alone.
   d. Participate in activities that can make you feel better.
   e. Try mild exercise, going to a movie, a ball game, or participating in religious or social activities.
   f. Don't overdo it or get upset if your mood is not greatly improved right away. Feeling better takes time.
   g. Do not make major decisions, such as changing jobs, getting married, or getting divorced, without consulting others who know you well and who have a more objective view of your situation. In any

case, it is advisable to postpone decisions until your depression has lifted.

h. Do not expect to snap out of your depression. People rarely do. Help yourself as much as you can, and do not blame yourself for not being up to par.

i. Remember, do not accept your negative thinking. It is part of the depression and will disappear as your depression responds to treatment.[92]

4. Refer to multidisciplinary psychiatric home care for depressed elderly, including professional nursing care and interventions.[35,36]
   a. Provide support to caregiver of depressed elderly person.
   b. Assist caregiver in dealing with own feelings.
   c. Assist caregiver in coping with role change and stressors.
   d. Teach elderly person and caregiver about depression and treatment and care-related tasks.
   e. Observe patient for recurring symptoms of depression.
   f. Monitor patient's medication compliance.
   g. Teach and support coping skills.
   h. Promote healthy lifestyle for caregiver and patient.
   i. Refer to community support service.
5. Refer to extended family or community resources *to deal with travel barriers to facilitate receiving Agency for Health Care Policy and Research (AHCPR) guideline follow-up treatment for depression.*[49]
6. Refer to and encourage participation in community activities and groups *to facilitate socialization, meeting new friends, and social support.*
7. Refer to community resources as needed (e.g., day care, senior citizens center).

Evaluation/Patient Outcomes

Risk Management: Patient will not harm self; partial or complete remission of symptom of depression will occur.

Coping Assistance: Patient will experience partial or complete remission of characteristics of depression, achieve optimal functioning, engage in activities of daily living, experience enhanced functioning in social and occupational roles, experience an increase in quality of life, experience restored hope and a sense of optimism about the future, and achieve a sense of pleasure from living.

DELIRIUM, DEMENTIA, AND AMNESTIC AND OTHER COGNITIVE DISORDERS IN THE ELDERLY

Delirium, dementia, and amnestic and other cognitive disorders include the disorders of (a) delirium, (b) dementia, (c) amnestic disorders, and (d) other cognitive disorders.[60,93,113]

Delirium is characterized by rapid onset (usually over a few hours to a few days) and lasts a few hours to several weeks. Signs and symptoms of delirium include altered consciousness; reduced attention span and/or ability to shift attention; altered awareness; reduced awareness of environment; changed cognition; some memory deficits especially for recent events; disorientation to time, place, and person; disorganized thinking; incoherent speech; altered perception; delusions; hallucinations, often visual; multifocal myoclonus; sleep disturbances; strong emotional reactions; and altered behavior. Symptoms develop rapidly over a short period of time and often fluctuate. Symptoms are often worse in the afternoon or at night.

There are three subtypes of delirium[93,113]: (1) quiet delirium, in which the patient can be drowsy, withdrawn, and lethargic; (2) agitated delirium, in which the patient can be agitated, irritable, have psychomotor hyperactivity, and signs of sympathetic nervous system activity; and (3) mixed type, in which the patient can exhibit unpredictable swings between the quiet and agitated types. In acute delirium the patient may be combative, appear flushed, have dilated pupils, sweat, experience a rapid heart rate and elevated blood pressure, and manifest a fever. In severe delirium, there is multiple-level impairment in nervous system metabolism. Stupor and coma can follow extreme drowsiness. Other signs and symptoms associated with delirium can include fear and anxiety, irritability, anger, euphoria, apathy or depressed mood, and labile emotions. Overall, in delirium there is a rapid change in cognition, disorientation, and confusion developing over hours or days.[93] Delirium can be caused by certain medical conditions, substance use, medication use, or toxin exposure that create a general upset in brain metabolism.

In elderly medical patients who are hospitalized, 10% to 22% suffer from delirium, which can increase to 30% after admission.[93] Increased rates of delirium in elderly following admission can result from removal from familiar surroundings, stress of hospitalization, addition of medications, use of physical restraints, loss of weight, catheterization, and other iatrogenic events in the hospital.[93] The incidence of postoperative delirium is 5% to 10% and is particularly high following hip replacement and cardiac surgery. Delirium is a common and frequent psychopathologic condition in later life, after age 60. After the age of 80, it is even more common. With the increasing number of older persons, delirium will continue to increase.[60]

It is critical that delirium be recognized and properly diagnosed in the elderly because it is often one of the first signs of an underlying medical problem that, if not treated, can lead to irreversible brain damage or even death. Delirium in the elderly is also associated with lengthier hospitalizations; decrease in functional abilities; increased needs for rehabilitation, home health care, and/or nursing home care; and caregiver burden.[60] From 14% to 56% of elderly patients with delirium have been reported to die.[60]

Delirium can be difficult to diagnose from other conditions such as cognitive disorders, depression, Lewy body dementia, and chronic dementia. Delirium must be differentiated from dementia. This can be difficult because demented patients can also be delirious, and delirious patients may have some underlying dementia. Misdiagnosis also occurs commonly in patients with delirium who present with symptoms of depression. Delirium must be differentiated from mental disorders presenting with a functional confusional state. With proper diagnosis and treatment, however, there can be full recovery from delirium.

Delirium includes (1) delirium due to a general medical condition, characterized by delirium resulting from the physiologic effects of a general medical condition; (2) substance-induced delirium, characterized by delirium resulting from the effects of substance withdrawal or substance intoxication, (3) delirium due to multiple etiologies, characterized by delirium caused by more than one etiology; and (4) delirium not otherwise specified, characterized by delirium that does not meet diagnostic criteria of other diagnostic categories of delirium.

Dementia is characterized by multiple cognitive deficits, including impaired memory and one or more of the following: disturbed executive functioning, agnosia, apraxia, aphasia, and impaired occupational or social functioning, caused by a medical condition, substance use, or a combination of these factors.[2] Dementia includes (1) dementia of the Alzheimer's type (see Chapter 5); (2) vascular dementia, characterized by multiple cognitive deficits, including memory impairment; one or more of the following cognitive disturbances: disturbed executive functioning, agnosia, apraxia, and aphasia; impaired occupational or social functioning; and evidence of cerebrovascular disease; (3) dementia due to human immunodeficiency virus (HIV) disease, characterized by dementia resulting from HIV; (4) dementia due to head trauma characterized by dementia from head trauma; (5) dementia due to Parkinson's disease (see Chapter 5); (6) dementia due to Huntington's disease, characterized by dementia resulting from the effects of Huntington's disease; (7) dementia due to Pick's disease, characterized by dementia resulting from the effects of Pick's disease; (8) dementia due to Creutzfeldt-Jakob disease, characterized by dementia from the physiologic effects of Creutzfeldt-Jakob disease; (9) dementia due to other general medical conditions, characterized by dementia from the physiologic effects of medical conditions other than those listed in this section; (10) substance-induced persisting dementia; (11) dementia due to multiple etiologies; and (12) dementia not otherwise specified, characterized by a dementia that does not fit criteria of any of the other categories of dementia. Eleven percent of elderly over 65 years old are diagnosed with dementia; Alzheimer's disease is the most common type.[140] Vascular dementia, caused by cerebral blood flow disruption, is less common than dementia of the Alzheimer's type.

Amnestic disorders[2] include (1) amnestic disorder due to a general medical condition, characterized by memory impairment with the inability to learn new information or recall information already learned, impaired social or occupational functioning, and caused by the physiologic effects of a medical condition; (2) substance-induced persisting amnestic disorder, characterized by memory impairment with the inability to learn new information or recall information already learned, impaired social or occupational functioning, and caused by substance use; and (3) amnestic disorder not otherwise specified, characterized by memory disturbance and does not meet criteria of the other amnestic disorders.

Other cognitive disorders[2] include cognitive disorder not otherwise specified, characterized by cognitive dysfunction caused by physiologic effect of a general medical condition that does not readily fit into any of the above diagnostic categories.

DELIRIUM

Delirium is characterized by altered consciousness; reduced attention span and/or ability to shift attention; altered awareness; reduced awareness of environment; changed cognition; some memory deficits, especially for recent events; disorientation to time, place, and person; disorganized thinking; incoherent speech; altered perception; delusions; hallucinations, often visual; multifocal myoclonus; sleep disturbances; strong emotional reactions; and altered behavior.

PATHOPHYSIOLOGY/PSYCHOPATHOLOGY

In the elderly, delirium usually results from multiple factors.[93] Predisposing factors can include polypharmacy, dementia, severe illness, hearing or vision impairment, sleep deprivation, dehydration, alcohol abuse, cognitive impairment, immobility, infections, and fever. Precipitating factors can include noxious insults, such as surgery; serious illness; taking additional medications, especially psychoactive medications; malnutrition; and use of physical restraints, bladder catheterization, and other iatrogenic events.[60]

Biologic/genetic theories can offer an explanation for delirium in the elderly.[64,93,113] Diffuse impairment in neurotransmission and in cerebral oxidative metabolism can result in delirium.[93] Delirium can, in part, also represent a stress reaction with increased effects or levels of glucocorticoids.[93] Decreased homeostatic regulation and changes in drug metabolism and brain neurochemistry can predispose the elderly to delirium.[93] Any medication or acute insult can precipitate delirium. Predisposing and precipitating factors are interrelated and contribute to delirium in the elderly in substantive, independent, and cumulative ways.[60]

Delirium can be caused by (a) a number of medical conditions and disorders (fever; septicemia; pulmonary or urinary tract infections; HIV; encephalitis; myocardial infarction; arrhythmia; congestive heart failure; hypoxia; transient ischemic attack; stroke; seizure disorders, including nonconvulsive seizures; intracranial infections; subdural hematomas; meningitis; brain tumors; organ failure; organ transplantation; hypothyroidism; hyponatremia; hypoglycemia; hypercalcemia; thiamin deficiency; dehydration; burns; sleep deprivation; sensory overload or underload); (b) substance use (substance withdrawal, such as alcohol, benzodiazepines, sedatives, or hypnotics); (c) medications (e.g., anticholinergic medications, tricyclic antidepressants, antipsychotics [thioridazine], benzodiazepines [diazepam], antiepileptics, sedatives, digitalis, analgesics [nonsteroidal antiinflammatory agents (NSAIDs)], lithium, dopamine-activating drugs, antihistamines, antiarrhythmics, calcium blockers, diuretics, digitalis, antibiotics, asthma drugs, laxatives)[64]; or (d) toxins. Prescription drug intoxication is a very common cause of delirium in the elderly. The most important causes are infections, cardiovascular disease, and medication effects.

The elderly are more vulnerable to delirium for a number of reasons. Age-related cell loss may occur, for example, in brain centers. Age-related physiologic changes can occur, such as decreased cerebral blood flow. Sensory changes can also occur in the elderly (e.g., hearing impairment). Finally, the elderly tend to suffer from more chronic medical conditions and are often prescribed medications or self-medicate themselves.

Psychologic/CulturalTheories

Environmental and psychologic factors can be contributing factors in delirium.

DIAGNOSTIC STUDIES AND FINDINGS[93,109,113,141]

Agitated delirium is more easily recognized than quiet delirium. Differential diagnosis is important to distinguish delirium from such conditions as Lewy body dementia and depression.[93]

History from significant other/caregiver
Complete physical examination
Complete neuropsychiatric evaluation: To determine factor(s) contributing to delirium[141]
Cognitive tests (e.g., High Sensitivity Cognitive Screen, Delirium Severity Scale, Confusion Rating Scale, NEECHAM Confusion Scale, Delirium Rating Scale, Organic Brain Syndrome Scale, Mini-Mental State Examination, Global Accessibility): To diagnose for presence of delirium.
Frontal lobe release signs
Papilledema
Thyroid function tests
Laboratory tests such as blood counts, blood levels of ammonia, glucose, urea nitrogen, electrolytes
Urinalysis
Blood gas studies
X-ray examination, especially chest x-ray examination, because pneumonia can be a common cause
Other studies as necessary
Computed tomography (CT) scan
Magnetic resonance imaging (MRI)
ECG
Lumbar puncture
Electroencephalogram (EEG): To determine generalized slowing of EEG trace, which, however, can also be seen in dementia and generalized aging.
Toxin screen

MULTIDISCIPLINARY PLAN[93,141]

Medications

Antipsychotics: To treat highly agitated delirious patients, especially with unknown etiology
Short-acting benzodiazepines (e.g., oxazepam; lorazepam): To treat delirious patients for withdrawal and to decrease extrapyramidal side effects

Other Treatment

Treat cause of delirium (e.g., treat medical conditions as infections, cardiovascular disease; remove or adjust medications; treat substance-related disorders; remove exposure to toxins)
Treat comorbid psychiatric symptoms (e.g., depression)

General Management

Supportive measures (e.g., good nutrition and fluid intake; multivitamins; careful monitoring of vital signs); offer psychosocial support; treat sensory deficits (e.g., glasses; hearing aids); avoid polypharmacy; avoid sedative-hypnotics, if possible, except benzodiazepines to treat withdrawal symptoms; increase observation to monitor physical deterioration and/or behaviors dangerous to self

NURSING CARE

NURSING ASSESSMENT[51,93,109]

Information from family and significant others regarding changes in physical health; medications currently taken, including over-the-counter medications; any history or current substance abuse; any exposure to toxins; patient's usual lifestyle; any change in behavior; any assistance needed currently
Changes in behavior and functional status
Nature of and speed of symptom onset
Level of awareness and presence of any fluctuation in awareness
Level of consciousness and any fluctuation
Cognitive impairment and any fluctuation
Presence of delusions or hallucinations
Emotional state (e.g., presence of fear, anxiety, anger, depressed mood, labile mood)
Nature of speech and verbal ability
Presence of any motor symptoms
Monitor laboratory values, signs and symptoms of physical illness, effects of medications to assist in determining treatment response
Monitor carefully all medications prescribed or taken on own by patient

POTENTIAL COMPLICATIONS

Dementia: Delirium is an important risk factor for dementia, and delirium may either lead to brain injury predisposing or causing dementia in the elderly or be an important marker for subclinical dementia[93,109]
Delirium: Poor nutrition, falls, pressure sores, urinary incontinence, infections[93]
Note that delirium is also an important marker for very poor health outcomes, including death[109]

PATIENT PROBLEMS/NURSING DIAGNOSES & INTERVENTIONS*

NIC RISK MANAGEMENT

Acute confusion related to delirium

- Collaborate with interdisciplinary team *to treat causes of delirium.*
- Collaborate with interdisciplinary team *to eliminate toxic or pharmacologic causes of delirium.*
- Capitalize on and use patient's strengths in planning care.
- Maintain patient's safety.
  - Use safety mechanisms such as call lights and safety rails as needed.
  - Clear clutter in patient's environment *to prevent falls.*
  - Provide constant and close observation as needed *to detect physical condition or behaviors that are harmful.*
  - Provide constant reorientation.
  - Administer medications, always being aware of potential effects.
  - Use restraints only if absolutely necessary: Observe frequently while restraints are used *because use of*

*References 15, 23, 51, 89, 93, 128.

physical restraints can increase delirium in the elderly.

Ascertain that patient's visual or hearing impairments are corrected.

- Create safe, comfortable, calm, consistent *environment to minimize stress, to augment patient's psychologic coping mechanisms, to help patient remain oriented, and to reduce potential for self-harm. Because patient experiences changed cognition and perception, level of consciousness, and/or confusion, it is very important to use interventions to help patient remain oriented as much as possible.*

    Provide moderate lighting; avoid high-intensity lighting or low lighting.
    Use soft colors.
    Reduce noise in environment.
    Use relaxation tapes as appropriate.
    Provide calendars, night-lights, clocks, schedule for the day.
    Keep patient in same surroundings with consistent physical layout *to foster a sense of security.*
    Have family bring in familiar objects and possessions and make allowances for personal belongings *to increase a feeling of security.*
    Develop structured, predictable routine.
    Plan periods of increased activity and cognitive stimulation within tolerance.
    Avoid sensory overload or sensory understimulation.
    Decorate with seasonal decorations.
    Assign consistent staff to patient.
    Increase staff-patient interaction as tolerated.
    Offer one-to-one contact as needed.
    Convey emotive empathy *because it has been shown to be beneficial in caring for the elderly.*[89]
    Convey warmth as well as kind firmness.
    Call patient by name and refer to self and others by name.
    Explain necessary information in a simple way: repeat as necessary.
    Use nonverbal communication to reinforce (e.g., pointing to object).
    Make every effort to understand patient's communications.
    Speak very slowly, enunciating words carefully.
    Keep choices at a minimum: present only one task at a time.
    Clarify perceptions, and validate accurate perceptions.
    Orient to time, place, person, and situation as often as needed.
    Offer orientation at beginning of each interaction with patient.
    Consistently reinforce reality.
    Use statements that are simple and direct.

- Deal with irritability and agitation calmly.
- Use distraction to prevent escalation rather than confrontation or argument.
- Acknowledge patient's feelings.
- Within tolerance and ability encourage patient to verbalize feelings.
- Minimize agitation and disruptive behavior.
    Determine precipitating factors.
    Adhere to personal routine.
    Keep apart from agitated patients.
    Use distraction.
- Manage and reduce anxiety.
- Negotiate for voluntary compliance *because forcing compliance can lead to resistance.*
- Encourage family members, friends, and other persons familiar to patient to visit. *Significant others can have a calming influence, as for example on the anxious or agitated delirious patient. They can support the patient's communication, provide orientation, and offer support.*
- Refer patient to community resources such as a community health nurse.

NIC Self-Care Facilitation

Self-care deficit related to perceptual or cognitive impairment

- Maintain patient's health.
    Maintain fluid intake and output.
    Provide for adequate nutrition.
    Encourage regular exercise such as walking.
    Implement strategies to help patient sleep: keep interruptions during nighttime at minimum, and facilitate nighttime sleep by measures such as massage and warm milk at bedtime and restricting daytime sleep *because sleep problems are common in delirium.*
    Offer pain therapy as needed.
- Assist with ADLs as needed.
    Have family assist patient with ADLs when possible.
    Give simple, clear instructions to patient to aid in meeting ADLs.

Patient Education/Continuum of Care Plan[23,60,93]

1. Explain to patient and family reason(s) for delirium, stressors that may have contributed to the delirium, and any planned ongoing treatments.
2. Teach family about risk factors predisposing elderly patient to delirium (e.g., malnutrition, iatrogenic events, use of physical restraints, bladder catheterization, more than three new medications added to treatment of regimen)[60]
3. Teach patient and family to seek health care from a consistent primary health-care provider who is familiar with patient's needs for medication to monitor medications prescribed and taken, to observe for side effects of medications, and to discard old medications when no longer needed.
4. Teach patient and family to monitor changes in cognition, level of awareness, or consciousness and to report them to medical personnel immediately.
5. Teach patient and/or family about preventive measures—good nutrition, hydration, use of eyeglasses and hearing aids as needed, use of nonpharmacologic sleep aids, reassurance from significant others.

EVALUATION/PATIENT OUTCOMES[23]

Risk Management: The patient will exhibit less confusion; sustain no injury; manifest improved cognition, level of awareness, and level of consciousness; and experience diminished risk for predisposing factors of delirium.

Self-Care Facilitation: Patient maintains physical health and can perform some ADLs.

ANXIETY DISORDERS IN THE ELDERLY

Anxiety disorders[2] comprise the following:

Panic disorder without agoraphobia is characterized by recurring panic attacks (period of sudden intense apprehension, terror, or fearfulness, often along with sense of doom); anxiety sensitivity (AS), or fear of anxiety-related sensations, is believed to play a role in panic attacks and panic disorders.

Panic disorder with agoraphobia is characterized by recurrent agoraphobia (anxiety about or avoidance of situations/places where escape is difficult or help is not available in case of panic attack) and panic attacks.

Agoraphobia without history of panic disorder is characterized by paniclike symptoms but no actual panic attacks along with agoraphobia.

Specific phobia is characterized by clinically significant anxiety provoked by a specific feared situation or object, often along with avoidance.

Social phobia is characterized by extreme anxiety provoked by exposure to social situation, often along with avoidance.

Obsessive-compulsive disorder is characterized by obsessions causing significant anxiety and compulsions designed to neutralize the anxiety.

Posttraumatic stress disorder (PTSD) is characterized by reexperiencing a very traumatic event.

Acute stress disorder is characterized by reexperiencing a very traumatic event but occurring right after that event.

Generalized anxiety disorder (GAD) is characterized by 6 months of excessive persistent anxiety; often a chronic condition with periodic remissions followed by exacerbations with a situational stressor as trigger.

Anxiety disorder due to a general medical condition is characterized by anxiety due to physiologic effect of a general medical condition.

Substance-induced anxiety disorder is characterized by anxiety caused by a physiologic effect of drug abuse, medication, or toxin exposure.

Anxiety disorder not otherwise specified is characterized by anxiety and cannot be categorized into any of above diagnoses.

ANXIETY

Anxiety, a key symptom in anxiety disorders, is a subjective feeling of "apprehensive anticipation of future danger or misfortune accompanied by a feeling of dysphoria or somatic symptoms of tension."[97]

Anxiety is characterized by (a) cognitive symptoms—apprehension, distractability, fearfulness, irritability, nervousness, worry; (b) behavioral symptoms—hyperkinesis, phobias, pressured speech, repetitive motor acts, startle response, avoidance; and (c) physiologic symptoms—chest tightness, hyperventilation, light-headedness, muscle tension, palpitations, paresthesias, sweating, and urinary frequency. In the elderly, anxiety often manifests itself in physiologic arousal, including restlessness, sleep disturbances, motor tension, or overt behavioral responses, including exaggerated startle response and compulsions. Anxiety occurs on a continuum, ranging from mild to moderate to severe to panic. Anxiety can be adaptive (mild to moderate levels), which can prepare the person for, or help the person to avoid, noxious situations. Or, anxiety can be maladaptive ranging from severe to extreme panic. Anxiety can exist as a chronic pathologic condition resulting in occupational and social malfunctioning.[40]

Types of anxiety include the following:

Situational anxiety: Short-lived anxiety to a stressful stimuli that can also be affected by the elderly patient's self-esteem

Phobic anxiety: Situational anxiety to a stressful stimuli in which avoidance is used as the method of coping

Anticipatory anxiety: Anxious apprehension or worry occurring before the dreaded object or situation is encountered, often associated with panic attacks

Free-floating anxiety: Pattern of indiscriminate anxiety with no close temporal link to precipitating stimuli and often a part of generalized anxiety disorder

Traumatic anxiety: Anxiety occurring in persons who survive tragic and unanticipated experiences

Anxious depression: Anxiety in which patients exhibit both anxiety and depression. Comorbidity between general anxiety disorder and depression is common.[39] "Anxious depression is the most common clinical presentation of anxiety in older people. Up to 70% of older people with GAD have coexistent major depression."[39]

Anxiety secondary to medical conditions: Anxiety is an overt symptom of these conditions

Anxiety can also be classified as (a) state anxiety (anxiety associated with a specific stimulus that remits once the stressor is reduced or eliminated) or (b) trait anxiety (a persistent feature of the person's personality).

PATHOPHYSIOLOGY/PSYCHOPATHOLOGY

Many elderly experience a high quality of life in their later years. For others, old age becomes fraught with anxiety and feelings of loneliness and worthlessness. Real-life problems, the loss of significant others, diminished financial resources, isolation, diminishing physical and/or mental health, and vulnerability to crime can be challenging and take their toll. Self-esteem and a sense of security can be threatened, resulting in anxiety.[124]

Symptoms of anxiety severe enough to warrant treatment occur in more than 17% of men and more than 25% of women over the age of 55.[18] However, actual anxiety disorders are less common in the elderly than they are in younger persons.[39] Among the elderly, GADs and phobias are the most common anxiety disorders. In persons over 65 years of age, 5.5% suffer from panic disorders, phobic disorders, and obsessive-compulsive disorders, and 2.2% suffer from generalized anxiety disorders.[40]

"Major depression is present in up to 70% of older people with generalized anxiety disorder and in quite a few people with phobias and PTSD."[40] Most anxiety disorders in the elderly started in younger years and have persisted. Late life–onset anxiety is frequently associated with either medical problems or depression. Late-onset agoraphobia without panic can start after a traumatic experience such as a mugging, medical illness, fall, or house fire. Late-life onset of panic disorders or obsessive-compulsive disorders is rare, but these conditions can persist into old age from younger years. The incidence of PTSD in late life is unclear. PTSD can impair the elderly person's coping ability and prevent the elderly from successfully engaging in late-life developmental stages.[134]

Feelings of anxiety in the elderly (older than 65 years of age) are quite common and appear to be present in about 20% of the elderly.[48] Feelings of anxiety in the elderly are associated with many medical conditions, drug reactions, dementia, mood disorders, anxiety disorders, psychotic symptoms, dissatisfaction with the social network, and being female.[48] A level of anxiety that interferes negatively with ADLs can lead to hospitalization.

Psychologic Models

Psychoanalytic/psychodynamic theory views anxiety as signaling danger and as a defense against unacceptable impulses; anxiety can also be viewed as originating during a child's separation from the mother, which in later life can reemerge when a satisfying person is not available.

Classical conditioning theory proposes that phobias arise because of conditioning and relief of anxiety by avoidance, which serves as a reinforcer.

Cognitive behavioral theory, the most accepted theory today, combines cognitive and conditioning paradigms. According to this theory, patients misinterpret sensations as those in normal anxiety responses and create catastrophic thoughts about these sensations, such as panic attacks.[124]

Vulnerability-stress model proposes that vulnerability factors, such as low educational level, female gender, extreme previous trauma, and external locus of control; stressors, such as physical illness and loss of significant other; and network-related factors, such as size of social network, play a role in the development of anxiety disorders.[10].

Biologic Models

Four neurotransmitter systems appear to be involved in the biochemistry of anxiety disorders and anxiety states: the serotonergic system, the γ-aminobutyric acid system, the noradrenergic system, and the mesocortical dopaminergic system. There may be a physiologic basis, for example, for panic attacks (i.e., the locus ceruleus is implicated, increased parahippocampal activity has been documented); panic disorders may be linked to a mendelian gene; the serotonergic neurotransmitter system is implicated in obsessive-compulsive disorder.[124].

Diagnostic Studies and Findings

Comprehensive history, physical examination, and drug and alcohol inventory: To determine presence of physical illnesses and conditions often presenting with prominent symptoms of anxiety (e.g., alcoholism, medication side effects or toxicity [e.g., from steroids, antihistamines, neuroleptics, analgesics, digitalis]), use of medications such as stimulants, withdrawal from central nervous system (CNS) depressant drugs, caffeine-related disorder, angina pectoris, cardiac arrhythmias, myocardial infarction, pain, congestive heart failure, chronic obstructive pulmonary disease, asthma, pulmonary embolism, hypoxemia, hyperinsulinism, hypoglycemia, hyperthyroidism, hypothyroidism, premenstrual tension, monosodium glutamate allergy, cerebral arteriosclerosis, brain tumor, dementia, delirium, seizure disorders, epilepsy, pancreatic tumor.[7] Anxiety is sometimes the first symptom of an impending medical disorder (e.g., anemia, hypoglycemia, hyperthyroidism).[94] However, in the elderly, somatic complaints are often the presenting symptom of anxiety.

Symptom-focused tests (e.g., ECG, blood gas studies or pulse oximetry, computed tomographic scanning, serum electrolytes, urinalysis, thyroid function studies, folate levels, vitamin B_{12} levels, blood glucose level, complete blood count): To rule out CNS, acute cardiovascular diseases, or other medical conditions and to assist in determining origins of anxiety disorder[7,44]

Comprehensive mental examination: To determine presence of anxiety and anxiety disorders, acuteness or chronicity and degree of impaired functioning, and to examine for dementia, psychosis, and depression[111]

History of mental illness and conditions: To determine previous episodes of anxiety disorders because a number of these can be recurrent

Psychologic instruments (e.g., Brief Social Phobia Scale [BSPS], Social Avoidance and Distress Scale [SADS], Fear of Negative Evaluation Scale [FNES], Social Anxiety Scale [SAS], Hamilton Anxiety Scale, Penn State Worry Questionnaire, Zung Anxiety Scale, State Trait Anxiety Inventory, Beck Anxiety Inventory): To evaluate specific types of distress and to document the presence and clinical course of anxiety[44,116]

Multidisciplinary Plan

Medications[7,39,40]

Antidepressant medications: To treat elderly with generalized anxiety disorders and depression or elderly with anxiety secondary to depression; elderly with anxious depression may need benzodiazepines (e.g., lorazepam) for a short time

Selective serotonin reuptake inhibitors (SSRIs) (e.g., fluoxetine, sertraline): To treat posttraumatic stress disorder, social phobia, panic disorder, and obsessive-compulsive disorder in the elderly

Tricyclic antidepressants (e.g., imipramine): To treat agoraphobia associated with panic disorder (but effect of these drugs is less clear if panic disorder is not present), panic attack, or obsessive-compulsive disorder

Buspirone: To treat elderly with generalized anxiety disorders and anxiety associated with general medical conditions because it has fewer side effects than benzodiazepines

Benzodiazepines (e.g., lorazepam, alprazolam): To treat elderly with generalized anxiety disorder, obsessive-compulsive disorder, social phobia; side effects include ataxia, sedation, and confusion; can be associated with tolerance, withdrawal, and abuse problems

Psychologic Treatment

Dynamic psychotherapy: To treat elderly with mild anxiety[72]

Cognitive therapy: To treat elderly with panic disorder; may also be used to treat generalized anxiety disorder, posttraumatic stress disorder, and social phobia[39,40]; this treatment helps elderly modify interpretation of situations that cause anxiety by modifying and controlling negative thoughts and attitudes

Exposure therapy: To treat agoraphobia without panic and obsessive-compulsive disorders[39,40]; treatment helps elderly face fears by exposing patients in a gradual manner to the feared object or situation

Behavioral therapy, muscle relaxation, and breathing exercises: To treat elderly with anxiety disorders[7,72]

Other Treatment

Treat medical conditions, pain, and psychiatric disorders associated with anxiety

General Management

Carefully monitor medication regimen: Elderly patients should not be suddenly switched from benzodiazepine to buspirone because buspirone has a 2-week delayed onset of action and does not suppress benzodiazepine withdrawal symptoms

Physical therapy: To teach muscle relaxation techniques

Music therapy: To help patient deal with anxiety when faced with the unknown, such as before surgery

NURSING CARE

Nursing Assessment

Appropriateness of level of anxiety to experience and situation of elderly person because elders can have realistic fears of situations or objects[7,40]

Patient's description of current symptoms and life circumstances, changes, stressors

Presence of risk factors for anxiety: Adaptation stressors (e.g., relocation to nursing home); chronic pain; diet (e.g., caffeine intake); environmental stressors; financial stressors; general loss of health; impaired role performance caused by major illness (e.g., cancer); impending surgery; loss of friends and family; role stressors

Physiologic symptoms of anxiety[7]: Complaints of physical symptoms; facial grimacing; hypervigilance (e.g., irritability, low concentration level); motor restlessness; muscle tension (e.g., clenching of fists); pacing; sleep disturbance; sweating; tachycardia

Subjective symptoms of anxiety: Uneasiness, unrealistic apprehension, worry

Beck Anxiety Inventory: A self-administered tool that can be used to detect anxiety[24]

Depressive symptoms because anxious depression is common in elderly

Use of prescribed or over-the-counter medications

Effect of anxiety on daily functioning

Strategies used by patient to cope with anxiety

Resources available to patient (e.g., significant others, spiritual resources, problem-solving skills)

Potential Complications

Suicide potential because "symptoms of anxiety have been associated with suicide, which has its highest prevalence in the elderly"[111]

Medication use and side effects/toxicity, especially for symptoms characteristic of anxiety (e.g., toxicity from stimulants or withdrawal from depressants such as alcohol or benzodiazepines)[40]

Side effects of benzodiazepines in the elderly, which can include significant cognitive impairment, psychomotor impairment, drowsiness, confusion, gait instability, falls and fractures, memory loss, paradoxical excitement, benzodiazepine dependence[40,72]; in the elderly, "benzodiazepines are overused and antidepressant medications and behavioral therapies are underused"[40]

Medical conditions so that they are not misdiagnosed as an anxiety disorder[40]

Functional impairment—social, recreational, occupational—due to inadequately treated or untreated anxiety disorders in the elderly

Patient Problems/Nursing Diagnoses & Interventions

NIC Psychologic Comfort Promotion

Anxiety related to perceived threats to self-esteem and personal sense of security

- Collaborate with interdisciplinary team to treat conditions contributing to anxiety.
- Use strategies to reduce sleep disturbance *because in the elderly anxiety often manifests itself in physiologic arousal.*[97]
- Use therapeutic listening skills to demonstrate acceptance of patient as he or she describes the experience of anxiety.
- Encourage patient to discuss anxiety-provoking situations with others: openly discuss issues surrounding the anxiety. *Elderly patients may prefer somatic descriptors for their feelings of anxiety and may see emotional problems or mental illness as stigmatizing.*[124] *It is important that open discussion about stressors and issues surrounding anxiety occur because this is therapeutic.*[7]
- Develop supportive relationship with patient *because providing reassurance and support to patient is an important strategy to reduce anxiety: the reduction of severe anxiety to a lesser, more manageable level is the first goal.*[40,72]
- Assist patient in identifying and recognizing sources of threat. *Unexaggerated appraisal of potential or actual sources of threat are important in anxiety reduction.*
    - Have patient keep anxiety diary. *"By rating their anxiety several times each day and noting all their symptoms and thoughts, patients can expose previously unrecognized stressors and clarify the negative thinking processes that are often associated with anxiety."*[7]

- Assist in exploring link between source of threat, manifestations of anxiety, and consequences of anxious state.
- Determine with patient whether there are any secondary gains from anxious state.
- Assist patient in exploring ways to remove or manage source of threat.
- Help patient develop an action plan to deal with anxiety.
- Teach relaxation techniques (e.g., breathing exercises, diaphragmatic breathing, exercise, back rubs, massage, imagery, meditation, prayer, relaxation therapy, therapeutic touch).
- Offer stress inoculation training *to reduce anxiety reaction by modification of cognitions.*[72]
- If elderly person is still employed, teach strategies to manage work-related stress.
- Have patient list goals and eliminate nonattainable goals.
- Assist patient in achieving goal(s):
  - Subdivide tasks into manageable parts.
  - Have patient establish a priority list of tasks, including realistic time requirements to accomplish them.
  - Have patient begin with tasks that can readily be achieved.
  - Have patient look at ways his or her work environment can be organized.
  - Encourage patient to learn to say "no" to additional tasks.
  - Teach patient to break up stressful projects/tasks by doing something relaxing and to use imagery to envision peaceful places.
- Offer encouragement and support.
- Instruct patient about importance of balancing work, exercise, recreation, sleep.
- Encourage support from clergy or other spiritual advisor *because prayer and spiritual beliefs can be a very supportive resource for the elderly patient.*[124]
- Use cognitive behavioral therapy strategies *to correct faulty appraisal of threat, to decrease tension and anxiety, and to decrease avoidance.*
- Use reengagement strategies, such as reexposure of desensitization, especially in patients with phobias, *to assist patient in coping with sources of threat. Anxiety can usually be overcome with gradual and repeated exposure to the source of threat.*[24]
- Offer relaxation books and tapes.
- Encourage and teach breathing exercises, guided imagery, progressive muscle relaxation.
- Use distraction techniques *in order for patient to focus on some routine task or detail to deal with high anxiety level.*[7]
- Use role play *to help patient learn coping skills and adaptive responses.*[7]
- Encourage development and maintenance of strong social support network and system. *Role stress and dissatisfaction with social network can lead to stress and anxiety. Social support can be a buffer to reduce impact of stressors on well-being.*[48]
- When appropriate, refer patient to group psychotherapy or family therapy.
- Encourage involvement in hobbies and recreational events.
- Have patient exercise regularly. *Aerobic forms of exercise are associated with reduction in anxiety, with exercise duration needing to be at least 20 minutes to reduce state and trait anxiety.*
- Encourage patient to limit intake of caffeine-containing beverages and other stimulants such as diet pills.

Patient Education/Continuum of Care Plan

1. Teach patient about cause, manifestation, and treatment of anxiety. Refer to self-help books on coping with anxiety.[24]
2. Teach patient to monitor self for signs and symptoms of anxiety.
3. Teach patient about both positive and negative aspects of anxiety. On the one hand, anxiety is a normal emotion serving useful arousal in helping person cope with a dangerous threat. On the other hand, it can become maladaptive and self-defeating if person repeatedly avoids experiences that do not need to be avoided or has such intense feelings and thoughts that they interfere with daily living. Explain to patient that "pessimistic or helpless thoughts may lead to more anxiety and more avoidance behavior and, thus, to still more negative thinking."[24]
4. Teach patient self-control strategy for worry. (1) Closely observe your thinking during the day and learn to identify the antecedents of worry; (2) establish a daily half-hour worry period that takes place at the same time and in the same place; (3) postpone worrying until your worry period, but jot down the worries beforehand if necessary; (4) use the daily worry period to think intensively about your current concerns and to generate possible solutions; and (5) replace worrisome thoughts with focused attention on a task at hand or on anything else in your immediate environment.[24]
5. Encourage family involvement in treatment and follow-up.
6. Refer to anxiety disorder support groups to facilitate support and the recovery process.[116]
7. Refer elderly patient to case managers, home health care, or more supportive living arrangements because increasing frailty can decrease level of independence and increase anxiety.[7]

Evaluation/Patient Outcomes

Psychologic Comfort Promotion: Patient will experience reduced or eliminated symptoms of severe anxiety (e.g., severe apprehension, severe worry, painful sense of helplessness and worthlessness, severe feeling of diffuseness, purposeless activity, reduced range of perception, lack of clear comprehension of immediate situation, ineffective functioning, tachycardia, hyperventilation, urinary frequency, nausea, dizziness, headache, insomnia).

SLEEP DISORDERS IN THE ELDERLY

Sleep disorders[2] include four major categories: (1) primary sleep disorder, (2) sleep disorder related to another mental disorder, (3) sleep disorder due to a general medical condition, and (4) substance-induced sleep disorder.

Primary sleep disorders include both dyssomnias and parasomnias. Dyssomnias are disturbances in the quality, the amount, or the timing of sleep that are not caused by a medical diagnosis, substance abuse, or another psychiatric diagnosis. Examples of dyssomnias include primary insomnia, primary hypersomnia, narcolepsy, breathing-related sleep disorder, and circadian rhythm sleep disorder. Parasomnias are disturbances in physiologic or behavioral events that are associated with sleep, sleep stages, or sleep-wake transitions that are not caused by a medical diagnosis, substance abuse, or another psychiatric diagnosis. Examples of parasomnias include nightmare disorder, sleep terror disorder, and sleepwalking disorder. Dyssomnia: primary insomnia is characterized by difficulties in starting or maintaining sleep, inadequate/insufficient sleep, or nonrestorative sleep and daytime fatigue that lasts minimally 1 month and causes changes in mood or concentration level, distress, or impaired functioning in such areas as occupational or social roles.[2] Primary insomnia is not due to the physiologic effects of a medical condition, substance use, or abuse, nor does it occur solely during the course of a mental disorder or another sleep disorder. Dyssomnia breathing-related sleep disorder is characterized by sleep disruption with insomnia or excessive sleepiness caused by a sleep-related breathing condition, such as central sleep apnea syndrome or obstructive sleep apnea syndrome, and is not caused by substance abuse, medical condition, or mental disorder. The incidence of sleep apnea is estimated to be 20% to 40% in the elderly and is often missed.

Sleep disorder related to another mental disorder includes both insomnia related to another mental disorder and hypersomnia related to another mental disorder. Insomnia related to another mental disorder is a condition directly caused by a mental disorder other than substance abuse and is characterized by difficulty in falling and staying asleep during the night that lasts at least a month and results in feelings of daytime fatigue and impaired functioning.

Sleep disorder due to a general medical condition is a sleep disturbance caused by a physiologic consequence of a medical condition that results in impaired daytime functioning. Insomnia type is predominantly characterized by insomnia.

Substance-induced sleep disorder is characterized by a sleep disturbance caused by physiologic effects of a substance (toxin, medication, drug abuse) resulting in impaired daytime functioning. Insomnia type is predominantly characterized by insomnia.

INSOMNIA

Insomnia is a chronic inability to sleep or to remain asleep throughout the night.

PATHOPHYSIOLOGY/PSYCHOPATHOLOGY

Sleep is important biologically and clinically; it is essential for health, well-being, and a satisfactory quality of life.

> Sleep is of great importance for health and the quality of life. There is a strong association between sleep disorders and illnesses or early death. Mortality is at least 1.6 to 2 times higher among elderly persons with sleep disorders than in those who sleep well, and the excess mortality is related to the predominant causes of death, such as heart disease, stroke, cancer, and suicide. . . . However, poor sleep is not only associated with shortened life expectancy. It also shows a negative interaction with many somatic and psychiatric diseases and symptoms, as well as causing a deterioration in the quality of life. . . . there is a tendency towards an increase in sleep problems with increasing age, especially after the age of 75 years.[4]

The physiologic need for sleep is controlled by the daily circadian rhythm and total quantity of sleep.[87] Most persons sleep between 4 and 12 hours per night, with those sleeping less than 4 to 5 hours considered short sleepers and those requiring more than 9 to 10 hours, long sleepers, and the average adult requiring 7 to 8 hours of sleep.[118] Whether the person's sleep is adequate can be determined by whether he or she feels rested and refreshed when waking up.[118] The normal sleep cycle includes (a) alert/wakeful state; (b) readiness for sleep; (c) alpha state; (d) nonrapid eye movement phase of sleep (NREM), including stage 1—characterized by light sleep, being easily aroused, having fleeting thoughts; stage 2—characterized by transitional sleep, having fragmented and short thoughts, being unaware of environment; stage 3—characterized by deeper sleep, relaxed muscles, decreased and stable pulse, deeper and more regular breathing, decreased temperature; and stage 4—(physically restorative sleep) characterized by deep sleep, difficulty in being awakened, few body movements; and rapid eye movement phase of sleep (REM)—(occurs after about 45 minutes of movement through previous phases) (mentally restorative sleep, important for memory, adaptation, problem solving, and learning) characterized by bursts of CNS activity and aroused state of body; muscle and eye movements; irregular and often increased heart rate, breathing, and blood pressure; and dreaming.[118,119] One sleep cycle usually takes about 90 minutes to complete. During sleep, the brain waves become slower and higher, becoming their slowest (deep slow-wave sleep) during stages 3 and 4, whereas during REM sleep the brain waves become more shallow and are of mixed frequency.[118,119] Primary insomnia can represent a lifetime disorder or a trait characteristic; primary insomnia can develop following a period of severe stress.

Sleep disturbances/disorders affect about one third of the adults in the United States, with insomnia (insufficient, inadequate; and/or nonrestorative sleep resulting in daytime fatigue and impaired functioning in general activities of daily living) being the most common complaint.

Poor sleep is reported by 10% of elderly men and by 20% of elderly women; frequent awakenings are reported by 21% and 27%, respectively; and difficulty in falling asleep after awakening is experienced by 22% and 41%, respectively. Compared with the younger population, who are often troubled by difficulties in falling asleep in the evening, elderly persons more often experience frequent awakenings and an increased length of time before falling asleep again. Their total sleep is shortened even though they spend more time in bed, and they have a smaller proportion of slow-wave sleep.[4] The incidence of poor sleep is even higher among institutionalized elderly, with up to 94% experiencing disturbed sleep.[29] Sleep pattern disturbances are so common among the elderly that often the misperception exists that poor sleep is part of the "normal aging process.

Problems in the elderly can include less total sleep time, less time in deeper sleep stages, difficulty falling asleep, and early morning awakening.[87] Factors that can play a role in sleep disturbances include genetic factors; medical illness or conditions (e.g., cardiovascular disease, stroke, pulmonary disease, neurologic disease, arthritis, diabetes, cancer, asthma, gastrointestinal disease, pain, nocturnal polyuria syndrome); psychiatric disorders (e.g., clinical depression, anxiety disorder, Alzheimer's disease, dementia); medications or substances (e.g., caffeine, nicotine, herbal remedies, alcohol, antidepressants, anticholinergics, diuretics, antihypertensives); poor sleep habits (e.g., daytime napping, irregular sleep-wake times); and primary sleep disorders (e.g., circadian rhythm problems, restless legs syndrome, periodic limb movement disorder, sleep apnea, REM behavior disorder).[4,9,87]

Chronologic age per se is not necessarily correlated highly with major sleep problems. Although mild deterioration in sleep quality can often be seen in the elderly, significant sleep problems and difficulties in daytime functioning due to sleepiness are not part of the "normal aging process."[87] Although the elderly may require the same amount of total nighttime sleep as younger persons, they often achieve less total nighttime sleep. Although REM sleep may be preserved, non-REM sleep may be reduced. The older person may spend more time in bed with more time being awake in bed, but less time sleeping in one stretch without waking up, may be fatigued, and may be less alert and nap during the daytime.[41,42] The type of sleep may change with advancing age (e.g., greater number of sleep stage shifts, increased number of awakenings, more transitional sleep [stage 1]), with lighter sleep (i.e., less deep slow-wave sleep [stages 3 and 4]), less tolerance for phase shifts in the sleep-wake schedule and shortened REM sleep latency but unchanged percentage of REM sleep, increase in abnormal breathing events, increase in frequency of leg movements, and report of poorer subjective quality of sleep.[29,42] Overall, the elderly retire to bed earlier, wake up earlier, wake up more frequently during the night, and find it harder to go back to sleep. Ineffective sleep or lack of adequate sleep in the elderly can lead to apathy, decreased facial expression, depression, reduced attention span, lack of coordination, fatigue, burning of eyes, muscle tremor, and skeletal muscle weakness. Lack of sleep and overuse of sedatives can result in falls or accidents. Sleep apnea can have serious systemic effects such as hypertension.[87] Sleep deprivation can result in cognitive impairment, as well as increased sleepiness. It is important to understand that sleep is a very complex phenomenon and can be affected by numerous factors, especially other psychiatric disorders.

Diagnostic Studies and Findings

Personal and family history of sleep disorders: To determine onset, duration, severity, and characteristics of sleep problem

Complete history and physical examination: To determine presence of any medical condition, sleep-related breathing conditions, use of medications or drugs that may be the cause of insomnia[9]

Complete mental status examination: To determine presence of any psychiatric disorder (e.g., mood disorders, substance abuse, anxiety disorder, cognitive disorders such as dementia, substance-related disorders) that may be causing insomnia

Blood alcohol, toxin, or medication levels: To determine presence of substance potentially causing insomnia

Polysomnography: To assess both the nature and the severity of the insomnia and assess the discrepancy between subjective complaints and actual sleep problems experienced[9]

Wrist actigraphy: A home monitoring system to assess for sleep disorders[9]

Sleep assessment tools (e.g., Sleep Impairment Index, sleep diary): To measure nature and severity of insomnia[83,84]

Multidisciplinary Plan

Surgery/Other Treatment

Referral to sleep disorder center especially for sleep-related breathing disorders: Surgery may be useful in treating certain sleep-related disorders (e.g., obstructive sleep apnea)

Continuous nasal–positive airway pressure (CPAP): To treat central sleep apnea along with having the patient quit smoking and lose weight

Acupuncture: To treat sleep disorders by means of a possible analgesic component[4]

Low energy emission therapy (LEET): To treat sleep disorders by means of an amplitude-modulated electromagnetic field[4]

Light therapy/bright light therapy: To treat insomnia in the elderly by means of bright light[4,83]

Medications

Pharmacologic approaches to treatment of sleep disturbances in the elderly are affected by age-related drug kinetics and dynamic changes. The elderly may experience altered drug distribution, slowed drug metabolism caused by decreased liver function, reduced drug elimination caused by reduced renal function, and thus longer half-lives of medications.[29] Use of hypnotics needs to be carefully evaluated, since they are not risk free in the elderly. Antihistamines purchased over the counter can lead to urinary retention, constipation, or confusion in the elderly.

Pharmacologic management of primary sleep disorders contributing to insomnia[87]

- Dopaminergic agents, benzodiazepines, opiates: To treat restless legs syndrome
- Dopaminergic agents: To treat periodic limb movement disorder
- Clonazepam: To treat REM-behavior disorder
- Melatonin: To treat sleep problems in melatonin-deficient elderly[4]

Pharmacologic management of insomnia[4,41,45,68,104]

- Sedatives: Untoward side effects can occur in the elderly, as well as potential development of tolerance and dependence with use of certain sedatives (e.g., barbiturates and SSRI antidepressants suppress REM sleep; benzodiazepines suppress stages 3 and 4 sleep and REM; flurazepam and other long-lasting sedatives can lead to impaired cognition and increased risk of falls in the elderly and should be avoided); tolerance can develop toward barbiturates; rebound insomnia after withdrawal of short–half-life benzodiazepines can occur; minimal use is recommended in the elderly because chronic use can lead to chronic sleep disturbance; sedatives may be prescribed for 2 months (the ideal use, however, is 14 days or less), then gradually discontinued by one quarter the dose every 2 weeks; useful sedatives/hypnotics in the elderly initiate sleep rapidly, maintain sleep during normal sleeping hours, and result in little sedative activity or other side effects during normal waking hours; there is no hypnotic available that is completely risk free in elderly patients

Antidepressants: Trazodone, which has few anticholinergic effects and does not depress respiration, is useful as a hypnotic in the elderly[104]; sedative effects of tricyclic antidepressants (e.g., imipramine, clomipramine) may improve sleep in the elderly, but side effects can include blurred vision, orthostatic hypotension, urinary retention, and dry mouth[4]

Benzodiazepines (e.g., triazolam, oxazepam, lorazepam, clonazepam): The most commonly used hypnotics; will increase total sleep time and sleep efficiency, especially in first months of treatment; adverse effects can include weakness, vertigo, confusion, fatigue, sexual and memory impairment[4,104]

Miscellaneous medications (e.g., zolpidem, zopiclone, chloral hydrate): Zolpidem has few of the usual benzodiazepine side effects; however, cognitive disturbances and dependency have been reported; zopiclone has fewer side effects than benzodiazepines, but bitter taste, cognitive disturbances, and dependency have been reported[4,104]

Discontinue use of offending medications or caffeine if insomnia linked to medication use

Reduce or alter use of stimulants

Analgesics (e.g., aspirin or Motrin): For pain control and management because pain can lead to insomnia

Avoid use of antihistamines for sedation in the elderly because of potential side effects of urinary incontinence and dizziness.[104]

General Management

Treatment of underlying cause of insomnia based on accurate assessment, which is critical in care of elders (e.g., treat medical disorders and conditions such as fecal or urinary incontinence, psychiatric disorders, especially mood disorders, anxiety disorders, substance abuse disorder)

Dementia management

Relaxation therapy for anxiety management and to wean patients from sleep (hypnotic) medication dependence[77]

Elimination of toxic substances

Aromatherapy

Regular exercise program

Biofeedback: To increase patient's awareness of internal state of arousal that allows for a degree of influence over his or her own level of arousal

Cognitive behavior therapy: To modify time spent in bed and reduce stimuli (stimulus control procedures), alter erroneous attitudes about sleep (cognitive therapy component), and information about aging and sleep (educational component)

NURSING CARE

Nursing Assessment[9,34,87]

Quality and amount of sleep: Have patient complete 24-hour sleep-wake log or diary for 1 to 4 weeks; examine log or diary for factors contributing to insomnia[9]; use checklist to observe elderly client's sleep-wake pattern over 24 hours; family member can be taught to use checklist[9]

Perceived sleep quality and patterns[34]

Complaints of insufficient nighttime sleep

Meaning of sleep-wake experience for patient; patient often bases this on actual length of nighttime sleep, number of awakenings, and quality or depth of sleep

Regularity of bedtime

Degree of difficulty and time needed to fall asleep at bedtime

Difficulty in staying asleep during the night, including number of awakenings

Number of interruptions with consequent incomplete sleep cycles

Arousability from sleep

Early morning awakenings

Daytime fatigue

Daytime distress/impairment in performing other activities of daily functioning

Duration of sleep difficulty

Total sleep time

Assess risk and etiologic factors

- Presence of medical or psychiatric disorders
- Presence of primary sleep disorders
- Use of and timing of medication administration
- Amount and timing of caffeine intake before bedtime
- Alcohol use before bedtime
- Type, duration of pain, or discomfort
- Degree of immobility caused by physical illness
- Lifestyle patterns, including degree of regular physical exercise
- Poor sleep habits
- Presence of nocturia or incontinence
- Unnecessary awakening (e.g., for vital signs, medications, blood draws)
- Late-life events that are stressors (e.g., loss of significant other)
- Emotions/emotional discomfort such as presence of depression or anxiety; worries such as finances or health; disturbing dreams[42]
- External environmental factors such as noise, uncomfortable temperature, sleep partner's snoring, too much light

Sleep difficulty as described by bed partner

Structured sleep history questionnaire,[42] sleep questionnaire,[118,119] Pittsburgh Sleep Quality Index, 2-week sleep-wake log: To obtain information about sleep history

Sleep pattern disturbance

- Major defining characteristics: Complaints of difficulty in falling asleep; early awakening; sleep latency; difficulty in staying asleep at night/interrupted sleep; patient complaint of not feeling well rested[67]
- Other minor defining characteristics: Agitation; mood alteration; napping during day or daytime sleepiness; frequent yawning; thick speech; physical signs such as slight hand tremor, mild nystagmus, ptosis of eyelid, expressionless face; irritability; listlessness; lethargy; disorientation

Potential Complications

Chronic insomnia (nonrestorative inadequate sleep for over 1 month) and resulting complications—patients with dementia now needing nursing home care; dependence on sedatives; increased alcohol consumption; depression; decreased quality of life[107]

Chronic sleep medications (hypnotic) use, which can result in drug dependence, reduced sleep efficiency, and impaired functioning[77]

Potential drug interactions because many elderly use nonprescription sleep products, along with medications for other medical conditions and experience increased sensitivity to medications[126]

Patient Problems/Nursing Diagnoses & Interventions

NIC Self-Care Facilitation

Disturbed sleep pattern related to emotional state and poor sleep hygiene practices in elderly patient with insomnia

- Have patient record sleep-rest activity pattern over a period of 1 week: use of such tools as the modified sleep chart to record information may be useful. *Baseline information is critical in determining potential factors causing sleep pattern disturbance because underlying problems such as a psychiatric disorder should be treated by the interdisciplinary team.*[42]
- Examine sleep record *to determine factors interrupting sleep.*
- Have patient monitor daytime napping *to assess personal effects on nighttime sleep and daytime quality of life. Napping does not seem to disturb a number of aspects of nighttime sleep, and findings regarding sleep latency (time it takes to fall asleep at night) and number of awakenings during the night are not conclusive.*[42]
- Encourage patient to describe personal meaning of sleep *because this can affect his or her response to its disruption.*
- Explain normal sleep pattern and changes that can be expected with increasing age and conditions present. *For example, in high stress, illness, or hospitalization, the need for sleep may increase, especially for the elderly.*
- Control environment *to reduce environmental factors and facilitate uninterrupted, quality sleep*[43]: reduce noise level; use "white noise" to promote sleep; maintain consistent temperature: avoid extreme temperatures; reduce bright lights; suggest use of earplugs.
- Reduce level of anxiety *because anxiety can contribute to sleep disturbances.*
- Determine presence and nature of stressor and assist patient in reducing stress level. *Stressors may be present in patients with recent onset insomnia: the stressor can have an effect on the duration and severity of the sleep disturbance and its management.*
- Carefully monitor intake of substances such as stimulants *because they can affect sleep:* do not offer caffeinated beverages past afternoon; instruct patient to avoid drinking alcohol close to bedtime *because it can interfere with sleep maintenance;* encourage patient to avoid drinking excessive fluids in the evening, and encourage patient to void before going to bed *to decrease need to void during night;* administer diuretics minimally 4 hours before bedtime *to decrease need to void during night.*
- Use behavioral treatment approaches: use stimulus control *to avoid pairing anxiety on the part of patient with either bedtime ritual or sleep environment;* teach patient that sleep—besides sexual activity that is conducive to sleep—is the only behavior allowed in bed[119]; teach patient not to go to bed until sleepy; teach patient not to stay in bed very long (i.e., over 10 minutes) after waking up during the night, but to get up, do something boring and/or relaxing, and then return to bed only when sleepy again.
- Engage patient in circadian repatterning[43]: encourage sleep restriction *to decrease sleep-onset time and wakings in the night while increasing overall sleep time;* do not vary time in going to bed; do not spend excessive time in bed per night (e.g., over 8½ hours); do not vary time getting up in the morning; do not sleep-in/sleep late as a way to make up for poor night's sleep; do not stay in bed a long time after waking up from sleep even if during the middle of the night.
- Teach patient good sleep habits and practices *to increase restorative nighttime sleep*[87]: minimize irregular sleep-wake routines; engage in a regular bedtime routine *because a regular bedtime routine will help patient feel calm, fall asleep more quickly, awaken less often, feel more refreshed in the morning, and feel more satisfied with his or her sleep;* avoid heavy exercise close to bedtime, but daily regular exercise is helpful; go to bed to sleep only when sleepy; do not stay in bed a long time after waking up from sleep even if during the middle of the night; work through attitudes viewing sleep as a chore or struggle; avoid clock watching: remove clock if necessary to reduce performance anxiety; establish regular wake times in the morning.
- For elderly with cognitive impairments, provide a regular and predictable bedtime routine and cues, which is extremely important for these elderly.[29]
- Teach patient relaxation strategies *to reduce cognitive or somatic arousal.*[43]
- Teach patient relaxation procedures (progressive muscle relaxation, autogenic training) *to reduce somatic arousal such as muscle tension.*[43]
- Offer autogenic training *because linking of relaxing somatic sensations, for example, warmth and visual images, can promote deep relaxation.*[119]
- Teach attention-focusing procedures (meditation, thought stopping) *to reduce cognitive arousal or intrusive thoughts.*[43]
- Encourage patient to maintain social network and receive social support from significant others. *Social support can serve as a buffer from negative effects of emotionally charged and negative events and thus lessen impact of these events on patient's sleep.*
- In collaboration with physician, administer medications (e.g., pain medication for pain before bedtime, nitroglycerine for angina, bronchodilators for bronchospasm, tricyclic antidepressants for depression).
- For institutionalized elderly patients, selectively use techniques to promote relaxation, provide for orientation, and promote sleep[104]: offer calming music; reduce light in sleeping areas; reduce nighttime noise and disruptions; offer taped ocean sounds or other white noise;

use large clocks and calendars on walls; have patient engage in deep breathing; promote environment conducive to meditation; offer light snack before going to bed; collaborate with spiritual advisor to encourage prayer or meditation; engage in bedtime routine; offer back rubs/massage[34]; assist with personal hygiene at bedtime.

- Examine hospital environment for possible causes of nighttime awakenings (e.g., noise, discomfort/pain, incontinence, interruptions from caregivers). *The number of times elderly patients wake up during the night increases during hospitalization.*
- For surgical patients preoperatively, enhance patient's knowledge about surgery and postoperative experience; encourage verbalization of fears and anxiety; and enhance patient's coping skills, such as how to cope with confusion should it occur. *Preoperative psychiatric interventions play a part in preventing postoperative psychosis.*
- For surgical patients, both preoperatively and postoperatively, (a) protect patient's sleep patterns; (b) eliminate unessential caregiver interventions during sleep time; (c) control factors in environment that can disrupt sleep such as noise, uncomfortable bedding; (d) build on patient's own personal sleep routines; and (e) understand particular patient's physiologic and psychologic state. *Sleep disturbances are associated with postoperative psychosis and can also delay tissue repair and recovery.*

Patient Education/Continuum of Care Plan

1. Increase awareness of patient and family of importance of sleep and increased need for sleep during times of stress.
2. Instruct patient to try to avoid tobacco, alcohol, and caffeine[119] if at all possible: If patient does drink alcohol at home, for example, have patient avoid drinking close to bedtime because it can interfere with sleep maintenance.
3. Assist patient in developing program of balance in daytime activities (e.g., social activities, exercise).
4. Instruct patient in use of progressive relaxation (tensing and relaxing of muscle groups) and other techniques that help patient relax at home. Progressive relaxation, for example, has been found to decrease time for sleep onset and nocturnal awakenings, increase sound sleep, result in feeling more refreshed, and increase subjective feelings of experiencing more satisfactory sleep.
5. Have family assist patient in ensuring that home environment can be made secure for nighttime (e.g., use of security system).
6. Instruct patient and family to avoid regular use of hypnotic agents (i.e., do not use more than twice per week).[87] Data are lacking that document better sleep from long-term use of hypnotics in the elderly.[9] Common problems in the elderly using hypnotics regularly include cardiovascular disease, balance disturbance, and nocturnal micturition.[4] Supervise reduction of hypnotic in hypnotic-dependent insomnia.[83]
7. Refer to sleep disorder specialist if insomnia persists and excessive daytime sleepiness is experienced.

Evaluation/Patient Outcomes

Self-Care Facilitation: Patient falls asleep easily; does not experience early awakening; does not have difficulty in staying asleep at night; feels energetic; and feels rested on waking up from sleep.

SCHIZOPHRENIA AND OTHER PSYCHOTIC DISORDERS IN THE ELDERLY

Schizophrenia and other psychotic disorders include (1) **schizophrenia,** characterized by active-phase symptoms (disorganized speech, negative symptoms, disorganized behavior, hallucinations, delusions) lasting minimally 1 month, with the disturbance itself lasting at least 6 months; types include residual type, undifferentiated type, catatonic type, paranoid type, and disorganized type; (2) **schizophreniform disorder,** characterized by symptoms similar to schizophrenia but lasting only from 1 to 6 months with less decline in functioning; (3) **schizoaffective disorder,** characterized by both mood episodes and active-phase schizophrenic symptoms; (4) **delusional disorder,** characterized by nonbizarre delusions lasting at least 1 month; (5) **brief psychotic disorder,** characterized by psychotic disturbance with a short duration of at least 1 day and no more than 1 month; (6) **shared psychotic disorder,** characterized by delusions similar to those suffered by someone else; (7) **psychotic disorder due to a general medical condition,** characterized by psychotic symptoms, especially prominent delusions and/or hallucinations caused by physiologic effects of a medical condition; (8) **substance-induced psychotic disorder,** characterized by psychotic symptoms caused by medications, toxins, or drug abuse; and (9) **psychotic disorder not otherwise specified,** characterized by psychotic disturbance that cannot be classified into any of the above categories.[2]

Schizophrenia affects about 1% of the elderly but accounts for a major portion of mental health care expenses.[96] Although it is particularly difficult to establish the actual incidence of schizophrenia in the elderly, the reported rates appear underestimated.[94] In fact, the number of elderly patients with schizophrenia is expected to increase because of increasing longevity and decreased mortality because of more effective treatment options.[96] Late-life schizophrenia falls into two groups—the group of patients with schizophrenia manifested early in life who are now elderly and those patients who developed symptoms of schizophrenia late in life. In the elderly with early-onset schizophrenia, about 20% will experience a marked decline and may need long-term institutionalization and protective living arrangements.[96] However, another 20% to 30% of these patients experience marked improvement or even recovery, possibly associated with changed role expectations and age-related neurobiologic changes with decreasing psychotic symptoms. Research findings show "substantial heterogeneity associated with symptom manifestation and course of illness associated with aging in schizophrenia."[50]

Although the onset of schizophrenia is typically early in life (late teens to mid-30s), late-onset schizophrenia, after age 45, does occur.* Women have a high rate of late-onset schizophre-

*References 1, 2, 5, 94, 142, 143.

nia. These patients also tend to have a better work history, and more have been married compared with patients with early-onset schizophrenia. Signs and symptoms include a higher frequency of hallucinations that are often auditory. There are also visual, tactile, olfactory, and paranoid delusions that are often bizarre and less disorganization and negative symptoms.[1] Addonizio[1] found that "persecutory delusions, organized delusions and running commentary, and abusive auditory hallucinations were more common in late-onset cases." In those with late-onset schizophrenia who are older than age 60 years, sensory deficits appear to play a role. Schizophrenia, paranoid type,[2] tends to manifest itself later in life, with delusions (often centered around a theme) of the persecutory or grandiose type being the most common symptom. Mistrust, anger, hostility, anxiety, and aloofness are common in the patient who is paranoid. Risk of fatalities in elderly persons with schizophrenia includes suicide (the incidence is higher than in the general population), infection (often attributed to poor hygiene), and accidents (elderly patients with schizophrenia have more lethal accidents than younger patients).

For those elderly patients for whom schizophrenia has been a lifelong chronic condition, stressors encountered in late life may lead to exacerbations of the illness with the person becoming more noncommunicative, withdrawn, and paranoid. They may also exhibit problems with affect and orientation. Furthermore, their lifelong social support system may decline in old age, leaving them more vulnerable to becoming institutionalized or homeless. On the other hand, the outcome of the schizophrenic process in late life can be variable, with the potential for improvement and, in some elderly patients, complete remission.

Although psychotic disorder due to a general medical condition can occur at any age, the elderly are more prone to medical illnesses and chronic medical conditions. Examples of medical conditions[2] in which the pathophysiology can lead to psychotic symptoms include cerebrovascular disease, deafness, hyperthyroidism, renal disease, hepatic disease, and neoplasms.

SCHIZOPHRENIA

Schizophrenia is characterized by active-phase symptoms (e.g., disorganized speech, negative symptoms, disorganized behavior, hallucinations, delusions) lasting minimally 1 month with the disturbance itself lasting at least 6 months.

PATHOPHYSIOLOGY/PSYCHOPATHOLOGY

Psychologic, Sociocultural Theories and Factors

Childhood trauma, early childhood maladjustment, female gender, premorbid schizoid and paranoid traits, adverse factors such as living alone and being socially isolated, and deafness may play a role in late-onset schizophrenia.[94,96]

Biologic/Genetic Theories

Much effort is being put into researching a genetic link for schizophrenia. There tends to be an increased risk of schizophrenia among relatives.[94] Progressive brain structure changes soon after onset of schizophrenia have been found in recent studies.[50] Changes in ventricular size and in specific brain structures have been noted. Recent findings are pointing to possible neurodevelopmental anomalies that may lead to or interact with subsequent neuronal changes.[50] Neurochemical deficits have also been cited (e.g., serotonergic and noradrenergic deficits are noted in elderly cognitively impaired persons with schizophrenia).[50] Nonspecific brain abnormality has been noted on brain imaging in patients with late-onset paranoid disorders.[1] Although it has been suggested that late-onset schizophrenia is a neurodegenerative condition,[96] recent studies show that "the brains of patients with schizophrenia do not exhibit high levels of the classical manifestations of neurodegenerative change."[50] An association has been reported between visual and hearing impairments and late-life schizophrenia and paranoid disorder.[1]

DIAGNOSTIC STUDIES AND FINDINGS

Computed tomographic (CT) scans: To detect brain tumors that may present with schizophrenia-like psychosis[1]

Physical examination and laboratory tests (e.g., TSH, T_4, serologic tests for neurosyphilis): To rule out any physical condition that may present with schizophrenia-like psychosis

Mental status examination/neuropsychologic assessment (e.g., Hierarchic Dementia Scale, Paired Associate Subtest of the Wechsler Memory Scale; Mini-Mental State Examination): To evaluate presence of symptoms indicative of mental illness and to evaluate cognitive functioning[142,143]

Hearing tests: To detect hearing impairment

Vision screening: To detect visual impairment

Abnormal involuntary movement scale: To detect presence of movements indicative of tardive dyskinesia

Diagnostic criteria and tools (*DSM-IV*, ICD-10, Carpenter, Research Diagnostic Criteria [RDC], Schneider, Langfeldt, New Haven Schizophrenia Index, Feighner, Taylor and Abrams, PSE9-CATEGO4, Diagnostic Interview Schedule): To assess for presence of symptoms indicative of schizophrenia

Zung Self-Rating Depression Scale (SCS): To assess for presence of depressive symptoms in schizophrenia[6]

MULTIDISCIPLINARY PLAN

Medications

For elderly with schizophrenia, antipsychotic medications are relatively effective, but lower dosages are used. The selection of a specific antipsychotic is based on the patient's previous response to the medication, potential adverse effects from drug interactions with the preexisting medication regimen, and the side-effect profile of the medications. Start elderly patients with low dosages, increase dosage incrementally, and monitor for adverse effects and symptom response. Polypharmacy is also a problem in the elderly, and the prescription of multiple medications with sedative and anticholinergic effects should be avoided.[61]

Atypical (newer) antipsychotic medications[61,140]: Often these are now first-line agents in the treatment of the elderly

Dibenzodiazepines (e.g., clozapine [Clozaril]; olanzapine [Zyprexa]): Clozapine is used only for treatment of treatment-resistant patients with chronic schizophrenia; granulocytosis may occur in the elderly, so a weekly complete blood count (CBC) check is needed before more drug is dispensed

Common side effects include limited EPS, sedation, enuresis, benign fevers, lowered seizure threshold

Benzisoxazole (e.g., risperidone [Risperdal]): Side effects of risperidone include hypotension, lowered threshold for seizures, gain in weight, lack of concentration, and akathisia

Conventional antipsychotic medications[140]: The elderly may experience increased side effects from these medications

Phenothiazines (e.g., chlorpromazine [Thorazine]; fluphenazine [Prolixin]; thioridazine [Mellaril]; trifluoperazine [Stelazine])

Dibenzoxazepine (e.g., haloperidol [Haldol])

Thioxanthenes (e.g., chlorprothixene [Taractan]; thiothixene [Navane])

Common side effects include extrapyramidal symptoms (EPS), acute dystonia, tardive dyskinesia, neuroleptic malignant syndrome

Other Treatment

Bilateral ECT supplementing clozapine: To treat patients with refactory schizophrenia[62]

General Management

Psychosocial interventions (e.g., cognitive behavioral treatment): To treat elderly patients with schizophrenia especially because of high risk of medication side effects and drug-drug interactions[96]

Psychiatric inpatient treatment: To treat psychotic decompensation or acute psychotic phase of illness, provide safety to patient, and stabilize symptoms[86]

Extended hospitalization: To provide care to patients with treatment-resistant chronic schizophrenia who may be a danger to self or others and unable to care for self[86]

Room and care homes: To provide private rooms, meals, supervised medications for long-term support and maintenance

Day treatment: Nursing homes with a psychologic treatment program; to provide general care and mental health services to patients unable to meet ADLs and live in other settings

Group family psychosocial education: To decrease family caregiver burden, increase caregiver health, and increase knowledge of interacting with and caring for relatives with schizophrenia[145]

NURSING CARE

Nursing Assessment[50,94,96,145]

History from family members if patient is too paranoid to be cooperative

Underlying feelings as delusions and hallucinations described during initial interview

Degree of insight

Medication inventory to assess for adverse drug effects, drug interactions, proper dosages

History of substance abuse, which is increasing in elderly with schizophrenia

Depressive symptoms

Comorbid medical illness[94]

Presence of cognitive and sensory deficits and ability to comply with therapeutic regimen

Level of social interactions, available social network, and social isolation

Patient's strengths

Risk factors predicting poor long-term outcome[50]: Progressive functional impairment, progressive cognitive impairment, poor social and occupational functioning, increased hospitalizations, poor response to neuroleptic treatment, poorer premorbid adjustments, lower educational levels, multiple severe symptom exacerbations, delays in starting antipsychotic medications, severe positive symptoms

Potential Complications[94]

Potential for suicide: The risk of suicide is elevated in patients with schizophrenia (10% actually commit suicide) and is correlated with previous attempts, poor premorbid social or occupational functioning, suicidal ideation, depressive symptoms, psychomotor agitation, sexual difficulties, and family history of depression[127]

Increased risk of adverse reactions to antipsychotic medications (e.g., extrapyramidal symptoms from traditional antipsychotics such as chlorpromazine and haloperidol)[94]

Tardive dyskinesia (TD) linked to antipsychotic use: There is a higher incidence of TD in the elderly[94]

Potential toxic effects of anticholinergic drugs such as benztropine and procyclidine used to treat extrapyramidal symptoms; these toxic effects can include agitation, delirium, and hypotension

Potential orthostatic hypotension linked to adverse cardiovascular effects of antipsychotics; falls and potential injury can result[94]

Patient Problems/Nursing Diagnoses & Interventions

NIC Risk Management

Disturbed thought processes related to perceptual alterations, psychologic conflicts, anxiety in patient with late-onset schizophrenia

- In collaboration with psychiatrist, administer antipsychotic medications *to relieve symptoms such as hallucinations and paranoid delusions. It is important to monitor antipsychotic medication regimen for therapeutic effect, side effects (e.g., extrapyramidal symptoms, anticholinergic effects, tardive dyskinesia), and drug interactions.*
- Monitor changes in functioning *to determine responsiveness to medication treatment and presence of physical illness. Patients with schizophrenia tend to underreport medical symptoms and overestimate physical well-being. They are more likely to manifest physical illness by behavioral changes such as mood changes and exacerbations of symptoms and changes in performance of ADLs.*
- Ascertain that any sensory deficits are referred to the appropriate professional and corrected.

- Use a kind, firm, matter-of-fact approach *to allow patient to set pace for development of relationship.*
- Avoid being too friendly or too reassuring *because closeness may be perceived as very threatening by patient*
- Allow patient to set limits on degree of closeness in relationship *because this will reduce threat that he or she may perceive from interaction. Isolation is often used by patient to cope with fear of closeness or to keep from being flooded with too much stimulation. Patients are often unable to deal with too much intimacy. As trust increases, ability to tolerate interpersonal closeness will increase.*
  - Do not invade the patient's personal space.
  - Avoid lengthy interactions with patient.
  - Watch for cues to determine tolerance of patient for length and frequency of interaction.
- Create a therapeutic milieu that is safe, predictable, and with moderate sensory stimulation *because elderly patients with schizophrenia have reported phantom sights and sounds if not enough sensory stimulant is present.*
- Explain all procedures and schedule changes.
- Keep appointments made with patient.
- Assist with ADLs if patient is too withdrawn to care for self.
- Provide feedback as patient begins to assume responsibilities for ADLs.
- Build trust with patient. *Building trust is critical because patient may not want help, blames others for problems, is angry and often noncooperative.*
- Use consistent one-to-one interactions.
- Use same staff to work with patient initially.
- Be honest in all interactions with patient.
- Use active listening skills.
- Use communication techniques.
- Keep communication simple.
- Communicate empathy.
- Use short, frequent contacts with patient.
- Accompany patient on walks without making demands for conversation.
- Assist patient in managing delusions.
  - After initial assessment, avoid frequently focusing and asking patient questions about his or her delusions.
  - Listen to patient without comment: determine what need delusions are meeting; provide feedback on feelings generated by delusions.
  - Do not communicate disapproval of patient as a person.
  - Do not confront validity of patient's thinking or debate validity of delusions.
  - Raise doubts and questions about patient's perspective.
  - Point out reality when appropriate: validate reality-based aspects of delusions.
  - Set parameters on behaviors based on altered perceptions.
  - Do not personalize accusations.
  - Evaluate stressors that triggered delusions. *These strategies will avoid reinforcing delusions and minimize threat and avoid increasing anxiety.*
- Allow patient to express feelings as anger within acceptable parameters (e.g., no injury to self or others), *recognizing that such feelings are often reactions to perceived threat. It is important to have patient learn to describe feelings with words.*
- Use interventions to decrease anxiety. *It is very important that patient is not threatened in any way and that confrontational efforts are not used to remove delusions and hallucinations because that will only increase patient's reliance on them.*
- Enhance self-esteem: assist patient in developing positive perceptions; give positive feedback on appropriate behavior.
- Recognize and build on patient's strengths: permit patient to make as many decisions as capable *because this will enhance cooperation and constructive behavior.*
- Assist patient in developing interpersonal skills *to reduce loneliness, reduce relapse, improve clinical outcome, and improve quality of life.*[117]
  - Teach social skills for maintaining and supporting social network.
  - Teach coping strategies and problem-solving skills.
  - Teach patient skills to use positive reappraisal reframing experiences and emotions.
  - Use role play and modeling as skill-building experiences.
- Assist patient in developing, building on, and expanding social-functioning skills.
- Engage in reality-based activities that focus on the here and now.
- Offer opportunity to engage in group activities but do not force patient to do so.
- Offer opportunities to get involved in predictable activities.
- Assist patient in identifying and participating in activities found to be enjoyable.
- Encourage involvement of family or significant other in total treatment regimen. *Family involvement can reduce recidivism and readmissions.*[53]
- Offer support to family in their attempts to interact with patient. *Lack of social support can affect compliance with therapeutic regimen.*
- Encourage participation in support groups and family psychoeducation interventions *to educate family about illness, to offer family support, to increase problem-solving skills, and to offer crisis intervention.*[28]
- Assist patient in setting realistic goals and acquiring skills needed to meet them (e.g., social interaction skills, communication skills, assertive behavior skills, problem-solving techniques). Goals and aspirations may need to be modified to adjust to current personal strengths and limitations and community resources available.
- Develop with patient a satisfactory structure of daily activities that can be followed when he or she is living in the community.
- Assist patient to build on and expand social network in community.
- Assist patient and significant others to identify and use community resources such as self-help groups, support groups for family caregivers, community case managers,

psychoeducational groups, other community mental health rehabilitation services, respite options for caregivers, housekeeping assistance, transportation services, and financial resources.

Patient Education/Continuum of Care Plan

1. Teach patient and family about importance of need for antipsychotic medication compliance. Noncompliance with therapeutic regimen is a problem with potential for relapse and institutionalization.[96] Medication compliance and outpatient follow-up by a community psychiatric mental health nurse can increase medication compliance.
2. Teach patient and family about the risk of relapse in late-life schizophrenia if antipsychotic medications are suddenly withdrawn. If decreased dosage or elimination of antipsychotic medication is desired, careful supervision by a health professional will be needed, because a graduated taper of antipsychotic will be required and only in those elderly outpatients with a stable chronic condition.
3. Teach elderly patient and significant others to observe for signs of TD. This is very important because being elderly is one of the risk factors for developing TD for patients on antipsychotic medications.
4. Teach elderly patient on antipsychotic medications and significant others to observe for extrapyramidal side effects.
5. Teach patient not to discuss delusions openly with persons other than close friends to prevent negative reactions from others.
6. Teach patient to develop better life skills and to overcome and cope with other psychiatric symptoms.
7. Reduce barriers to outpatient participation in therapeutic, rehabilitative regimen.[5]
   a. Help patient establish good relationship with mental health team.
   b. Monitor and reduce medication side effects.
   c. Monitor compliance with medication regimen.
   d. Assist patient in developing insight into schizophrenia, including ability to question own perception, accept reality of illness, and necessity of treatment.
   e. Encourage family member to offer support. *Insight about schizophrenia enhances successful rehabilitation. Insight is enhanced by patient's compliance with medication regimen, family support, and cognitive efforts*
8. Encourage support and involvement of family and significant other in patient's discharge planning and use of community treatment options such as support groups for family caregivers to increase caregiver coping skills, improve care provided, and enhance psychologic well-being.[139]

Evaluation/Patient Outcomes

Risk Management: The patient will exhibit and feel less conflicted and anxious, live in least restrictive community setting, and function optimally within capabilities

SOMATOFORM DISORDERS IN THE ELDERLY

Somatoform disorders* are disorders in which patients have recurrent multiple bodily complaints that cannot be explained on a physiologic basis but that are not under voluntary control. There are frequent visits to physicians with requests for physical examinations and treatment, which can increase health-care utilization and costs. Somatoform disorders affect patient functioning and quality of life. Somatization—generally a maladaptive coping strategy—ranges from severe disability from a somatoform disorder to temporary nonpathologic daily experience of physical symptoms related to temporary stress. Continuous stress along with maladaptive responses can result in chronic somatization and a somatoform disorder. Onset and persistence of somatization can be related to the severity of psychopathology and the degree to which a patient has an unfavorable view of personal health.

Somatoform disorders[2] comprise a number of disorders. **Somatization disorder,** or **hysteria,** is characterized by sexual, gastrointestinal, pseudoneurologic symptoms and pain extending over a number of years. The physical symptoms that are expressed often involve multiple body systems, and an early onset, usually before the age of 30, as well as a chronic course. Health care is often sought from multiple physicians. No actual physical signs can be determined for the complaints, nor is there evidence of structural or laboratory abnormalities. These patients may undergo invasive procedures, treatment with medications, hospitalization, and/or surgery.

Undifferentiated somatoform disorder is characterized by physical complaints over 6 months or more that are unexplained but cannot be diagnosed as another somatization disorder.

Conversion disorder is characterized by unexplained symptoms related to sensory functions or voluntary motor functions. Onset is usually late childhood to early adulthood and rarely in old age. Duration is short, and patients show indifference to the nature of symptoms.

Pain disorder is characterized by the symptom of acute or chronic pain with an important role being played by psychologic factors in the onset, severity, and maintenance of the pain. The pain leads to occupational, social, and/or other distress or impairment in daily functioning. **Hypochondriasis** is characterized by fear of and preoccupation with having a serious illness based on misinterpretation of one or more bodily functions or bodily signs or symptoms. The fear continues for at least 6 months despite medical evaluation and support. The complaint can be without an organic abnormality or can be an exaggeration of an existing pathologic condition; the complaint is not delusional, but the patient is unaware of the underlying conflicts presented by the symptoms. Anxiety and depression are often present; distress or impaired social, occupational, and other daily functioning exists. The disorder is associated with considerable personal distress, with functional impairment, and with a long-term morbidity.

Body dysmorphic disorder is characterized by preoccupation with an exaggerated or an imagined defect in one's physical appearance.

---

*References 2, 8, 21, 56, 73, 78, 79, 121, 133.

Somatoform disorder not otherwise specified is characterized by somatoform symptoms but does not meet criteria of any of the disorders.

PATHOPHYSIOLOGY/PSYCHOPATHOLOGY*

Psychologic/Cultural Theories

Somatoform disorders are a frequent class of problems in primary care medicine and are diagnosed in about 10% to 20% of primary care patients. Because of remaining stigma, psychiatric patients frequently present with new complaints about a chronic medical condition or report a new physical symptom. Somatoform disorders are prevalent in psychiatric settings, and differential diagnosis is important. The prevalence of somatoform disorders varies by type; these disorders are more prevalent in women, although some studies do not support the belief that females experience somatoform disorders more commonly than males. Somatization disorders occur in about 2% to 3% of women. Undifferentiated somatoform disorder is a common somatoform disorder that is more prevalent in women. Conversion disorders rarely are first reported in old age, are more common in women, and more prevalent in persons of lower socioeconomic status and in those with less education. Hypochondriasis is experienced by 10% to 20% of the population from time to time. About 2% of patients obtaining cosmetic surgery have body dysmorphic disorder.

Older persons are more likely to suffer from actual physical symptoms than younger persons. However, in the elderly, a psychiatric disorder may be masked by physical systems as, for example, in depression. The elderly are also more likely to complain about physical symptoms than talk about emotional distress. In addition, about 10% to 20% of elderly assess their health to be poorer than it actually is. The physical symptoms in somatoform disorders, over which the patient has no conscious control, are real for the patient. They function to relieve or to prevent anxiety, serve to achieve a secondary gain in that expected role responsibilities may be temporarily waived and attention may be given by others to the patient, enhance interaction with others by means of the symptoms, serve to identify with a deceased significant other, manipulate and control others' behavior, or cope with guilt by self-punishment. Somatoform disorders, such as hypochondriasis, are more frequently identified in the elderly and can be associated with depression or anxiety disorders. Selective attention and excessive concern about an organ system by patients with hypochondriasis leads to more anxiety, which can then lead to additional physical signs and symptoms. However, care must be taken to rule out actual physical illnesses that can coexist or develop at any time in the elderly. In those with conversion disorder, the symptoms may be a means of social communication, precipitated by life stressors that activate intrapsychic conflicts.

Psychosocial factors and family factors can play a part in somatization disorders. Families of origin of these patients may be dysfunctional. In such families, members find it difficult to express feelings and conflicts openly. In times of stress, a child may become ill with the focus of the family then shifting away from the stressor or conflict and onto the child's illness. The expression of physical symptoms in response to stress in patients with somatization disorder may be also a learned pattern within their families of origin.[129]

Psychosocial stressors can precipitate the symptoms. For example, hypochondriasis can be precipitated by a major life event. Childhood sexual abuse, neglect, or physical abuse can be a factor. Defense mechanisms can play a role in elderly who develop hypochondriasis. For example, symptoms can be used to avoid role expectations or excuse failure, shift anxiety from threatening psychologic conflict to bodily part, relieve guilt or punish self for anger and hostility toward a significant other, or experience social isolation and withdraw to a focus on self and bodily function. A number of psychologic theories are proposed for hypochondriasis—disturbed object relations, dynamics of guilt, conflicted dependency needs, repressed displaced hostility, a perceptual disorder with somatosensory amplification—"a tendency to experience bodily and visceral sensations as intense, noxious and disturbing. It consists of heightened attentional focus on bodily sensations, selective focus on weak and infrequent bodily sensations, and a tendency to misinterpret these as evidence of illness."[98] In conversion disorder, an internal conflict is kept out of awareness, thereby reducing anxiety. Pain disorders can be associated with psychologic factors or with psychologic factors and a medical condition.[21] From 25% to 50% of community-residing elderly experience pain: the elderly commonly suffer from physical conditions associated with pain. Many elderly with chronic pain also suffer from depression.

Cultural factors may also play a role.[57] Somatoform disorders vary in prevalence and form in different ethnocultural groups. Cultural-specific symptoms are recognized. Somatic symptoms can have different levels of meaning in different cultures. For example, the expression of physical symptoms for psychosocial distress can be a culturally normative expression. In some cultures, emotional states, such as depression, are primarily manifested through physical symptoms.

Biologic/Genetic Theories

Recent studies of somatization disorders point to a possible biologic basis. For example, higher levels of physiologic arousal—heart rate, cortisol, finger pulse volume—have been noted. "The perception of interoceptive signals is influenced by physiological arousal. The amplification and misinterpretation of physiological signals may, in turn, be one of the main processes in the development of somatoform symptoms."[108] "Increased levels of physiological activity as well as changes of the activity of the HPA axis may affect the adequate interoception of physiological signals."[108] A familial pattern seems evident in somatization disorder, but whether this is a genetic or a learned pattern is not clear. However, an age-related biologic change affecting pain perception by the elderly has not been established.[21]

DIAGNOSTIC STUDIES AND FINDINGS*

Medical and psychiatric history: Conduct a thorough and complete history because somatoform disorders are

*References 21, 32, 38, 69, 73, 75, 78, 79, 90, 98, 102, 133, 135.

*References 38, 69, 79, 90, 108, 121.

diagnosed, in part, in retrospect; this should include interviews with family members, friends, and an examination of old medical records; it should be noted that it is not uncommon for physical complaints to be attributed to a somatoform disorder, only to later be found to have a physical basis; therefore, the patient's physical complaints should not be lightly dismissed

Complete medical examination: To rule out any general medical condition, or new symptoms of an actual chronic condition that could account for the person's complaints of physical signs or symptoms and fear of having a disease, which is especially important in the elderly; tests must be scheduled and then not postponed because that can increase the patient's sense of not being taken seriously and increase insecurity

Neurologic examination and testing: To differentiate between neurologic condition (e.g., diabetic neuropathy, multiple sclerosis, Parkinson's disease, brain tumors) and conversion disorder

Psychologic tests (e.g., Minnesota Multiphasic Personality Inventory; Whiteley Index; Illness Behavior Questionnaire; Illness Attitude Scale; Composite International Diagnostic Interview; RAND Short Form Health Survey; Somatic Symptom Index; Hopkins Symptom Checklist; Diagnostic Interview Schedule; Schedules for Clinical Assessment in Neuropsychiatry; Somatosensory Amplification Scale): To assist in screening for somatoform disorders

Complete mental examination: To rule out any other major psychiatric disorder, especially depression, and to differentiate among the types of somatoform disorders. In patients with hypochondriasis, fear of illness is more prominent than actual physical complaints, the latter being more frequent in somatization disorder; mood disorder and anxiety disorders are frequently associated with hypochondriasis, especially in the elderly

MULTIDISCIPLINARY PLAN[21,78,79,98]

Medications[21,78,79,98]

Pharmacologic treatment: To treat specific comorbid psychiatric disorders (e.g., use of anxiolytics for patients with symptoms of anxiety or anxiety disorders; use of antidepressants for patients with symptoms of depression; set-dose analgesic medication to treat patients with pain disorder; use of trazodone to treat sleep disorders associated with somatoform disorders)

Selective serotonin reuptake inhibitors: To treat hypochondriasis and body dysmorphic disorder

Avoid medications with major side effects, medications that are addictive, or medications used unsuccessfully by patient

Other Treatment[21,78]

Treat specific physical (e.g., analgesics or acupuncture to treat pain) or mental disorder (e.g., antidepressants to treat depression) that may actually occur along with the somatoform disorder

Avoid invasive diagnostic or treatment procedures unless an actual objective physical basis exists

Schedule regular office visits not based strictly on a new complaint

Conduct partial physical examination for each new symptom, but avoid large-scale work-ups and referrals to subspecialists unless actual physical basis exists

Avoid hospitalizations except to special psychiatric units for treatment of somatization disorders

Hypnotherapy to treat symptoms of patients with conversion disorder.

General Management

Refer for psychiatric consultation

Cognitive-educational approach: To treat patients with hypochondriasis by providing reassurance about the benign nature of their symptoms and correcting myth and misperceptions about the actual anatomy and physiology of the body

Cognitive-behavioral interventions: To treat patients with hypochondriasis and other somatoform disorders by assisting them in reducing reliance on physical symptoms for control and coping with emotions and learning new ways of processing perceptions; such behavioral techniques can be used as attention training, cognitive behavior group therapy, exposure to feared event, thought stopping, desensitization, implosion, imaginal flooding

Operant conditioning: To assist patients with pain disorder to reduce focus on pain and engage in activities that they have avoided because of the pain

Group therapy: To help patient reduce the need to rely on somatic complaints

- Supportive self-help groups: To provide social support
- Specific focused groups: To teach patient about somatoform disorder and to provide mutual support
- Cognitive group therapy: To treat patients with dysmorphic disorder

Psychotherapy: To help patients with somatization disorders to become aware that psychologic factors are playing a role in the illness, understand the basis for the condition, and resolve underlying emotional distress and problems

Supportive brief psychotherapy: To treat patients with conversion disorder or undifferentiated somatoform disorder.

NURSING CARE

NURSING ASSESSMENT*

Health history to obtain health-related information that is relative to current health concern

Signs and symptoms indicative of somatoform disorders

Depression and anxiety disorders, which are frequently associated with somatoform disorders

Ongoing monitoring of physical symptoms and laboratory tests to determine emergence of any physical evidence of symptoms described and actual illness

Ongoing monitoring of mental status to determine emergence of any emotional problem or potential psychiatric disorder and to determine comorbidity between somatoform disorder and other mental disorders such as anxiety disorders or depression

Suicide potential

*References 21, 38, 57, 58, 69, 75, 79, 133.

Attitudes about physical illness: Do physical symptoms interfere with ADLs and social or occupational functioning?
Potential secondary gains (e.g., use of exaggerated complaints to gain attention and comfort from others)
How long these physical symptoms have persisted
Environmental stressors that may precipitate physical symptoms
Activities of daily living
Level of social and occupational functioning
Social network and presence of strengths
Strengths of patient's family and any evidence of dysfunctional interactions
Presence of emotional themes: Patient's ability to express dependency needs and feelings of anger, for example
Stressors and life circumstances that occurred before beginning of physical illness
Strengths, strategies for coping with stressors, and interpersonal resources; self-identification limitations
Patient's understanding of connection between physical symptoms and emotions or intrapsychic stress
Consequences of physical illness on ADLs, social functioning, or family functioning

NOTE: When assessing patient, avoid discounting evidence of actual underlying physical illness requiring actual medical or surgical intervention; be aware, however, that "patients with somatization are at high risk for iatrogenic harm and unnecessary medical costs because multiple tests and procedures are ordered in a futile attempt to discover occult organic disease"[133]; differential diagnosis in psychiatric settings is very important to differentiate somatoform disorders from other psychiatric illness, otherwise inappropriate pharmacotherapy or other treatment could be initiated.

POTENTIAL COMPLICATIONS

Overmedication or drug interactions because the patient may have been followed by several physicians; Suicide potential because elderly with hypochondriasis and other somatoform disorders may also be depressed; Comorbidity—depression and anxiety disorders—because comorbidity of somatoform disorders and affective disorders is strongly predictive of psychosocial dysfunction

PATIENT PROBLEMS/NURSING DIAGNOSES & INTERVENTIONS*

NIC COPING ASSISTANCE

Ineffective coping related to inadequate coping skills along with use of physical symptoms to deal with underlying conflict, dependency needs, and anxiety

- Establish a therapeutic nurse-patient relationship. Permit patient to ventilate about physical complaints *to prevent patient from becoming defensive and looking to someone else to describe physical symptoms to and to establish rapport with patient so that he or she feels understood. Accepting patient's feelings is important. A supportive nurse-patient relationship can itself reduce symptoms of somatization and is critical in bringing about change.*
- Interact with patience and communicate acceptance *so that fears of rejection and abandonment are minimized and patient is free to express such emotions as anger.*
- Set and adhere to time limits for one-to-one *interaction so ability to bring up new complaints at close of session is minimal.*
- Do not imply to patient that it is all in "his or her head." *Disregard for patient's physical complaints impedes development of interpersonal trust and establishment of a therapeutic relationship.*
- Collaborate with patient to identify strategies to constrain or deal with "the disease" (e.g., pacing activities of daily living). *Patient's perception of a nurse-patient alliance against "their disease" is important.*
- Initially, provide nurturing and support to meet patient's dependency needs. *Psychologic defenses should be supported until a therapeutic nurse-patient relationship is established and more appropriate coping strategies can be developed.*
- Gradually withdraw attention and time given to patient's complaints of physical symptoms, and encourage patient to become less dependent and more independent.
- Use approach that discourages and does not reinforce somatic complaints.
- Normalize the distress but do not encourage prolonged discussion of physical symptoms (e.g., "Others may find your symptoms distressing"). *This approach legitimizes the complaint while allowing for discussion of actual anxiety or stress.*
- Encourage patient to remain with one primary physician or psychiatrist and to respect and follow primary physician's medical treatment guidelines.
- Be alert to emergence of physical symptoms indicative of actual physical illness.
- Matter-of-factly state that symptoms will be reported to physician. *A determination of an organic basis for the complaint should always be made to ensure patient's health and safety.*
- Initially, have patient use chart to document both stressful life events and occurrence of physical symptoms.
- Determine nature of secondary gains, such as obtaining attention or avoidance of need to deal with actual life demands or stressors, from physical symptoms expressed by patient. *Pain complaints may be used to manipulate significant others.*
- Model open communication when interacting with patient *to encourage patient to express feelings and concerns.* It is essential that patient learn to identify feeling states and be able to express feelings to others.
- Discuss anger with patient and encourage him or her to express anger appropriately.
- Develop realistic goals with patient, which may focus on symptom reduction and increased functioning because "cause" may not be a realistic goal.
- Teach patient assertive communication skills *to help patient express needs without relying on physical symptoms.*
- Teach patient conflict resolution skills.
- Involve family and significant others *to evaluate support and system's influence on patient's use of symptoms as a coping strategy.*

*References 21, 30, 69, 79, 100, 133, 137.

- Explore with family and significant others impact of patient's illness and strategies for dealing with it.
- Use behavior therapy techniques:
  - Have staff and significant others consistently reduce reinforcing physical symptoms by, for example, not rushing patient to physician each time there is a complaint.
  - Do not reward continual complaining.
  - Teach and encourage patient to use self-help treatments for symptoms so that control of symptoms is in patient's hands (e.g., use of heating pads).
  - Have patient begin to focus on actual psychosocial problems that are currently faced.
  - Encourage more open and appropriate expression of emotional distress.
  - Use praise for movement away from physical complaints and more functional expression of emotional distress.
- Use cognitive behavior group therapy:
  - Use informational interventions.
  - Teach self-monitoring of thoughts and behaviors.
  - Assist with cognitive restructuring.
  - Encourage exposure to avoided situations.
  - Encourage response prevention.
  - Engage in developing schedule.
- Teach patient to use techniques such as meditation, relaxation techniques, exercise, and imagery *to deal with emotions such as fear and anxiety.*
- Help patient link physical symptoms with actual emotions felt. For example, patient can be taught about physiologic aspects of anxiety.
- Help patient reframe physical complaints and focus on link of symptoms with real stressors currently being faced.
- Give feedback to patient about how overuse of complaints about physical symptoms can negatively affect relationship with others, and teach patient to use social skills if necessary.
- Use positive reinforcers *to give feedback when patient is not ruminating about physical symptoms and for actual use of adaptive coping skills.*
- Use anticipatory guidance in working with patient *to help patient prepare for potential changes and related stress.*
- Use role play for patient *to gain actual experience with use of adaptive techniques when faced with stressful situations.*
- Encourage participation in activities in which patient does not focus on complaints of pain or other symptoms

PATIENT EDUCATION/CONTINUUM OF CARE PLAN[30,58,78,91]

1. Teach patient and significant other about specific somatoform disorder from which patient is suffering. It is important for patient to know that physical complaints are not actually part of an organic disease and to understand that link between physical symptoms and emotional distress.
2. Teach patient and family members patterns of interactions that do not rely on physical symptoms to deal with stress and anxiety. It is critical to involve family and significant others in examining patient's lifestyle and helping him or her achieve more adaptive coping skills.
   a. Encourage caring and supportive family atmosphere.
   b. Encourage family members to communicate openly and honestly, including expression of feelings.
   c. Encourage respect among patient's family members for differences of opinion.
   d. Teach patient and family members conflict resolution strategies.
   e. Teach patient and family flexible problem-solving strategies.
   f. Discuss with patient and family the need for balance between needs for belonging and needs for separation.
   g. Help patient and family identify community resources that may be helpful when faced with multiple stressors.
3. Teach patient and family strategies to adapt to ongoing life changes.
4. Refer to community resources and activities from which patient can meet social needs and reassurance.
5. Refer to outpatient geriatric evaluation and management unit (GEM). Outpatient GEMs have lowered the use of outpatient services by those elderly who score higher on measures of somatization.

EVALUATION/PATIENT OUTCOMES

Coping Assistance: The patient will be able to recognize and express feelings; avoid reliance on physical symptoms to cope with stressors; experience reduced anxiety; and recognize link between stressors, emotions, and expression of physical symptoms. Patient demonstrates use of more adaptive coping strategies to meet personal needs and to deal with life stressors.

SUBSTANCE-RELATED DISORDERS IN THE ELDERLY

Substance-related disorders include two groups, substance use disorders and substance-induced disorders.*

Substance use disorders include substance dependence and substance abuse. **Substance dependence** is characterized by a pattern of substance use that is maladaptive, leads to clinically significant distress or impairment, and is manifested by three or more of the following criteria within 12 months: tolerance; withdrawal; much time spent on obtaining, using, and recovering from substance; substance taken in larger amounts over longer time periods; unsuccessful efforts to reduce or stop use of substance; altered or reduced social, recreational, and/or occupational roles and activities resulting from substance use; and continued use of substance despite recognition of negative physical or psychologic effects.

Substance abuse is characterized by a pattern of substance use that is maladaptive, leads to clinically significant distress or impairment, and is manifested by one or more of the following criteria within 12 months: major occupational, social, and/or academic role failure caused by recurrent substance use; engaging in activities that are physically hazardous when im-

*References 2, 31, 55, 59, 99, 105, 106.

paired by substance use; legal problems related to substance use; and continued substance use despite major interpersonal or social problems linked to substance use.

Substance-induced disorders include (1) **substance intoxication,** characterized by substance-specific syndrome caused by ingestion of or exposure to substance that is reversible; effect on CNS caused by the substance during or shortly after its use and leading to maladaptive psychologic or behavioral changes; and (2) **substance withdrawal,** characterized by substance-specific syndrome caused by the reduction of or cessation of a specific substance after long-term, heavy use or maladaptive psychosocial changes resulting from the substance-specific syndrome. Mild withdrawal symptoms from alcohol, sedatives, hypnotics, and anxiolytics include anxiety, sleep disturbance, depressed mood, difficulty concentrating, psychomotor agitation, and periods of panic, with some patients also manifesting tachycardia, tachypnea, transient diastolic or systolic hypertension, and increased temperature.[125] Severe withdrawal syndrome can be life-threatening (e.g., seizures, delirium tremens). A postwithdrawal syndrome may present in patients detoxified from abuse of benzodiazepines.

The term *substance* as used in the DSM-IV refers to drugs of abuse, as well as medications and toxins. Substance-related disorders[2] include those disorders that are related to (1) exposure to toxic substances (e.g., heavy metals, carbon monoxide, antifreeze, nerve gas, or rat poison); (2) over-the-counter or prescribed medications (e.g., corticosteroids, anesthetics, muscle relaxants, or chemotherapeutic agents); and (3) 11 classes of substances described in detail in the DSM-IV that include (a) alcohol; (b) sedatives, hypnotics, and anxiolytics; (c) cocaine; (d) amphetamine or similarly acting sympathomimetics; (e) hallucinogens; (f) opioids; (g) nicotine; (h) inhalants; (i) cannabis; (j) phencyclidine (PCP) or similarly acting arylcyclohexylamines; and (k) caffeine. Similar features are shared by (a) and (b). Similar features are also shared by (c) and (d).

In the elderly,[31] body composition changes, and there is less lean body mass, total body water, and serum albumin, and more total body fat. Other functional, structural, and compositional changes occur that can affect how drugs are metabolically handled and how the elderly person responds to the substance. The elimination half-life of many substances may rise in the elderly, and the elderly may become more sensitive to drugs, requiring less dosage or amount for the same effect. In the elderly, similar amounts of alcohol result in higher blood alcohol concentration because of changes in body composition.[105] Medical complications of alcohol-related disorders in the elderly include pancreatitis, peptic ulcers, gastritis, gastrointestinal bleeding, peripheral neuropathy, hepatitis, cirrhosis, malnutrition, anemia, increased infections, hypercortisolemia, delirium tremens, and withdrawal seizures. Alcoholism in the elderly can be a life-threatening illness. Other problems in the elderly linked to substance-related disorders include injuries due to affected gait, cognition, and balance; a decline in functional abilities; impaired driving ability; depression; memory impairment; delirium tremens; cerebellar degeneration; peripheral or autonomic neuropathies; muscle weakness; malnutrition; hypocalcemia; hypokalemia; hypomagnesemia; orthostatic hypotension; hypertension; sexual dysfunction; incontinence; suicide; and risk of cancer (especially of the esophagus, head, or neck).[105,125]

Although illicit drug use is generally uncommon in the elderly, the prevalence of substance-related disorders (i.e., misuse of prescription and over-the-counter drugs, as well as alcohol) is predicted to increase significantly as the baby boom generation ages.[99] Of note, however, is a recent identification of the emergence of a cohort of elderly illicit drug abusers.[55] The prevalence rate of substance-use disorders in a geriatric psychiatry outpatient clinic is 20%, significantly higher than previously predicted.[59] The Center for Substance Abuse Treatment calls alcohol abuse and prescription drug abuse and misuse among elderly over 60 an invisible epidemic, the current prevalence being 17%.[106] Between 5% and 12% of elderly men and 1% and 2% of elderly women are problem drinkers.[55] Between 60% and 78% of the elderly use prescription medications.[105]

Psychoactive drugs have high abuse potential in the elderly, and prescription drug use problems develop frequently in later life. In the elderly, substance dependence can be more problematic because tolerance decreases with age.[59] Complications of benzodiazepine misuse can include new memory problems, increased depression or anxiety, changes in psychomotor functioning, and risk of falling.[105] Polypharmacy is also a danger in the elderly. For example, drug interactions with alcohol occur. Acute ingestion of alcohol can potentiate medication side effects, and chronic alcohol ingestion can reduce drug efficacy.[105]

PATHOPHYSIOLOGY/ PSYCHOPATHOLOGY[55,110,125]

The incidence of chronic illnesses increases in the elderly along with increased treatment with prescribed medications, especially tranquilizers, analgesics, and hypnotics, as well as use of over-the-counter medications by the elderly themselves, especially analgesics and laxatives. Polypharmacy is a problem.[125] That is, the use of multiple medications either concurrently or intermittently is common in the elderly. This increases the potential for either inadvertent or intentional misuse of medications and the potential for the emergence of substance-related disorders in the elderly. Frequently misused drugs that can lead to substance-related disorders in the elderly include alcohol, medications that have an addictive potential such as opioid analgesics, barbiturates, and benzodiazepines. Elderly persons with substance-related disorders are more likely to be male. Gender differences occur across culture, with elderly men having a higher incidence of alcohol-related disorders than women. More alcohol abuse is reported among elderly of lower socioeconomic status.

Alcohol use disorders in the elderly are more common than previously recognized: for example, 8% to 23% among hospitalized elderly, 15% among the elderly in emergency departments, and 6% to 10% among the elderly seen in primary care settings.[105] From 11% to 33% of elderly suffering from alcohol use disorders (AUD) develop late-onset AUD.[105] Three major types of elderly with alcoholism have been identified. Elderly persons with early-onset alcoholism have abused alcohol most of their adult lives and are survivors; many of their cohorts have died. These patients manifest symptoms of chronic alcoholism and are often physically ill. Personality disturbances, difficult interpersonal relationships, and diminished support systems are common. The elderly person with late-onset alcoholism generally begins drinking past the age of 40, often in response to a stressor, such as the death of a loved one. Social drinking may develop. Late-onset alcoholism is often due to depression, loneliness, or boredom. The elderly person with intermittent alcoholism uses alcohol to relieve stress with binges during high-stress periods.

Little data are available on the illicit use of drugs other than alcohol among the elderly. Opiate abuse, for example, is often not visible because it occurs among a group of urban elderly who are often isolated. Elderly persons are much more likely than younger persons to abuse prescription drugs, for example, sedatives and hypnotics, and are much less likely to abuse illicit drugs. In institutionalized elderly, for example, the rate of use of hypnotics and long-acting benzodiazepines is greater than in the general population of elderly. One study reported that in their sample of addicts who were elderly, 35% abused benzodiazepines; 12%, oral opiates; and 4%, marijuana.[125]

The problem of substance-related disorders is often underestimated in the elderly because the elderly (a) may use small but frequent quantities of the substance, (b) may present with nonspecific physical complaints that can obscure the symptoms, and (c) can be misdiagnosed because of similar symptom presentation as physical conditions. There can also be present a lack of awareness among health-care providers regarding the possibility of substance-related disorders in the elderly. The elderly often are not working or driving and may live alone, so they are less likely to be noticed.

Similar stages of addiction occur regardless of the drug abused.[125] Stage 1 is characterized by patient euphoria, bingeing, attempts to reduce or cease use of drug, and some shame. The patient's family seeks opinions from friends and other family members. Stage 2 is characterized by patient resentment, alternating times of use and abstinence, and unwillingness to travel places without a sure supply of the drug. The patient's family engages in enabling behaviors. Stage 3 is characterized by the patient engaging in unreasonable behaviors; blaming others; paranoia; beginning interpersonal, legal, and/or occupational problems. The patient's family often isolates the patient. Stage 4 is characterized by the patient demonstrating a high degree of resentment and blame, emotional withdrawal, guilt, depressed mood, anger, physical illness, suicidal behavior, and increasing social problems. Family members become increasingly angry and depressed. Marital separation may occur. Stage 5 is characterized as the stage of addiction. The patient feels hopeless, is continuously intoxicated, and admits defeat. The family basically gives up on the patient. Stage 5 is either death or "the bottom," in which case the patient is willing to try anything to get better.

Psychologic, Cultural, and Environmental Factors[110,125]

A number of psychologic, cultural, and environmental factors and stressors can contribute to the occurrence of substance-related disorders in the elderly.[110,125] These include cultural attitudes toward aging, burden of caregiving, multiple losses such as loss of income, death of spouse and/or significant others, loss of permanent home with relocation of residence, retirement, and other role changes. Such factors as social class, age, ethnicity, gender, occupation, religious affiliation, and culture may increase risk in some persons.[110] Social isolation, depression, and boredom can lead to drinking and alcohol-related disorders. Alcohol abuse can occur in patients with major depression or dementia. Social learning theory suggests that behavioral patterns of alcohol consumption can be learned in families and thus transmitted across the generations. Environmental factors, including modeling the substance abusive behavior by significant others, stressors from significant others, subcultural expectations and norms, and availability of substances, are risk factors for substance abuse disorders.[110]

Biologic/Genetic Theories[110,125]

Candidate genes, especially for alcoholism, have been identified, and advances are being made in molecular genetics.[110] Genetics may play a direct or indirect role in the development of substance use disorders.

Physiologic changes and risk factors occurring in the elderly can contribute to the occurrence of substance-related disorders.[110,125] These changes include increased susceptibility to drug-drug interactions and increased biologic sensitivity leading to toxic effects. Slower biotransformation and excretion of substances can occur as a result of altered substance absorption, distribution, and/or elimination. In the elderly, for example, there is a smaller volume of distribution for a substance like alcohol; thus, after ingesting the same amount as a young person, the elderly one demonstrates a higher blood level. Also, the ability to metabolize alcohol can be lowered in those elderly patients who use sedatives or hypnotics at the same time as alcohol. The rate of both elimination and absorption is decreased in the elderly, so more CNS effects from, for example, barbiturates, that also last longer, result. In the elderly, there is an increasing neuropharmacodynamic effect resulting from alcohol abuse, as well as the fact that in the elderly with chronic alcoholism, neuropsychologic deficits are magnified. Decreased absorption and metabolism can lead to the accumulation of medications such as benzodiazepines. In relation to opioid analgesics, the elderly experience slower onset of action because the absorption rate is lowered, longer action because of a reduction in liver function, and more adverse effects because of receptor sensitivity changes. If an elderly person is prescribed a potentially addictive medication over time, tolerance, withdrawal, and substance-related disorder can result. A biologic vulnerability to addiction and a strong genetic component have been noted as a cause for substance-related disorders. Finally, other factors that can contribute to the occurrence of substance-related disorders include psychiatric comorbidities such as mood and anxiety disorder, physical illness, chronic pain, decreased mobility, sensory deficits, and short-term memory deficits. Studies suggest that elderly addicts frequently have another mental health disorder that is affected by the substance-related disorder and affects the substance-related disorder.

DIAGNOSTIC STUDIES AND FINDINGS[103,105,106,110]

Alcohol and drug use history from patient and others: To determine type and amount of the substance being consumed and effects of substance use

Addiction history from patient and others: To obtain information about the patient's drug addiction from a variety of persons; for the elderly, determine if an "at-risk" drinker or "problem drinker"

Family history: To determine presence of history of substance-related disorders among family members

Complete physical examination: To determine signs and symptoms and consequences of substance-related disorder; to determine signs and symptoms and presence of other physical conditions, some of which can obscure in the elderly a diagnosis of substance use disorder (e.g., pulmonary embolism, diabetes, hypothyroidism, hyperthyroidism, urinary tract infection, myocardial infarction)

Liver function studies (e.g., serum glutamic-oxaloacetic transferase [SGOT] or transpeptidase): To determine presence of hepatic damage caused by substances such as long-term alcohol use, as well as to monitor abstinence

Serum toxicologic studies and urinary drug screen: To determine presence of substance-related disorders caused by toxin exposure

Complete blood count: To determine presence and any effects from substance abuse; elevated mean corpuscular volume (MCV) often suggests alcohol abuse, and heavy alcohol use can result in anemia and/or suppression of blood lines

Complete mental examination: To determine signs, symptoms, and effects of substance-related disorder (the presenting symptoms of a substance-related disorder may mimic other mental disorders); to determine presence of other mental disorders[125]

Routine initial screening and rescreening: To determine presence of substance use disorders when elderly experience life transitions

CAGE, Michigan Alcoholism Screening Test (MAST), Alcohol Use Disorders Identification Test (AUDIT), Cyr Wartman Screens: To screen for an alcohol-related disorder

Drug Abuse Screening Test (DAST), CAGE AID: To detect alcohol and drug use

Inventory of Drug-Taking Situations (IDTS): To assess antecedents to drug or alcohol use

Chemical dependency screening tools (e.g., Manitoba Drug Dependency Screen): To detect presence of chemical dependency

Clinical Institute Withdrawal Assessment for Alcohol Scale (CIWA), Modified Selective Severity Assessment Scale (MSSA): To assess withdrawal during detoxification

Drug Taking Confidence Questionnaire (DTCQ): To evaluate situation-specific coping self-efficacy in high-risk situation in alcohol or drug users

MULTIDISCIPLINARY PLAN[71,105,125]

Treatment

Detoxification programs: To manage withdrawal phase of substance-related disorder

Hospitalization for benzodiazepine withdrawal: To treat benzodiazepine withdrawal, which in the elderly can be severe

Methadone maintenance program: To treat the elderly opiate user

In-patient treatment of alcohol withdrawal: Symptoms include increased prodromal symptoms of tremor, tachycardia, agitation, diaphoresis; delirium; hallucinations including auditory, tactile, or visual that are often threatening; delusions that are often paranoid; generalized seizures; in the elderly, the risk for complicated and severe alcohol withdrawal may be increased by chronic comorbid conditions, susceptibility to adverse effects of drug treatment, and limited physiologic reserve[71]

- Thiamine immediately
- Short-acting benzodiazepines: Used prn to treat withdrawal
- Parenteral fluids and electrolytes: To treat dehydration and restore electrolyte abnormalities
- Potassium chloride: To treat potassium deficit and prevent cardiac arrhythmias
- Magnesium sulfate: To treat magnesium depletion
- Elemental phosphorus: To treat hypophosphatemia
- Vitamin K: To treat increased prothrombin time
- Folic acid
- Water-soluble vitamin supplement
- Valium or Librium: As a prophylactic anticonvulsant

Treat complications of alcohol withdrawal

- Determine origin of and treat fever
- Free water restriction of hypertonic sodium chloride solution: To treat hyponatremia
- 5% Dextrose: To treat hypoglycemia
- Sedation and potassium and magnesium supplements: To treat alkalosis
- Prednisone: To treat alcoholic hepatitis
- Folic acid: To treat folate deficiency
- Treat underlying cause of hematologic disorders

Thiamine, folic acid, niacin: To treat patients with alcohol-related disorder who have history of poor nutrition

Supportive emergency measures: 1 g ascorbic acid intravenously (IV), IV ephedrine sulfate and antihistamines; to maintain blood pressure and treat shock in severe alcohol-disulfiram reactions

Medications

Propranolol or clonidine: To treat withdrawal symptoms not controlled by benzodiazepines

Antidepressants: To treat persistent depressive symptoms in alcoholics; suicide can be a serious problem in the elderly depressed alcoholic patient

Anxiolytics: To treat symptomatic anxiety in patients with alcohol-related disorders

Risperidone: In low doses to treat severe agitation

General Management

Inpatient treatment program: To provide a structured program, free from access to substance, designed to assist patient to cease use/abuse of substance(s)

- Tapering and cessation of problem drug
- To reduce or eliminate such potentially drug-related side effects/toxic effects as sleep disturbances, falls, depression, confusion, memory loss, incontinence, anxiety, poor hygiene
- Structured supervised environment: To provide alcohol-free facility for elderly alcoholics with cognitive disorders

Outpatient-based treatment program: To provide treatment and counseling to elderly patient on an outpatient basis

Self-help groups (e.g., Alcoholics Anonymous (AA) [12-step model]): To obtain support from other persons recovering from alcoholism
Long-term residential treatment program (e.g., halfway house): To provide ongoing shelter, support, and counseling
Individual psychotherapy: To help elderly patient focus on the here and now, deal with problems resulting from substance abuse, help develop insight, and prevent relapse
Family therapy: To assist elderly patient and family in developing insight into the process of substance-related disorders and family interactions
Group therapy: To assist elderly patient in confronting problem, to enhance self-esteem, to instill hope, to build interpersonal skills, and to enhance knowledge about substance abuse
Disulfiram (Antabuse): To treat chronic alcoholism by deterring patient from ingesting alcohol; used with great care in the elderly; Antabuse interferes with normal metabolism of alcohol and is given to deter further drinking because even a small amount of alcohol while on Antabuse can result in an unpleasant reaction; Antabuse is contraindicated in patients with selected psychosis or myocardial disease; also, the patient must be reliable to avoid alcohol even in disguised forms (e.g., cough and cold mixtures, aftershave lotions, sunscreens, back-rub lotions, sauces, mouthwashes, certain medications), must be motivated and socially stable, and must not be depressed or suicidal
Naltrexone: Anonsel ectitopioid antagonist used as an adjunct to alcoholism treatment to treat alcohol dependence; decreases desire to drink alcohol and alcohol consumption and prevent relapse; can cause severe nausea

NURSING CARE

NURSING ASSESSMENT*

History of substance-related disorders
Quantity and frequency of alcohol or medication use
History and current use of over-the-counter and prescribed medications
Presence of and causes for polypharmacy and potential or actual drug misuse
Degree of denial of presence of substance-related disorder or misinformation provided about alcohol or drug use[125]
Accuracy in reporting current medications and medication side effects
History of falls or accidents
Current physical symptoms and conditions
Use of multiple refills, use of different pharmacies, use of multiple physicians without checking with primary health-care provider
Self-medicating by use of over-the-counter drugs or borrowing medications from friends or family
Characteristics of health care being provided to patient (e.g., Was patient given clear instructions about prescribed medications and their side effects? Was adequate follow-up provided to patient?)
Degree of social change or impairment: The elderly often do not exhibit the degree of social disturbances that younger persons do, nor do they engage in criminal behaviors or drive while intoxicated; they are often no longer employed in an occupation and may live alone; therefore their use and abuse of substances may be more difficult to detect
Presence of social contexts in which there is access to substance and its use is accepted; for some elderly alcohol abusers, the tavern is the only social outlet
Presence of social isolation, loneliness, loss, and boredom, as well as degree of social isolation and extent of becoming housebound
Social network available to patient and role others play in substance use
Attitudes of significant others toward presence of substance-related disorder
Lack of role or purpose in life
Housing problems, legal problems, marital problems, social problems
Changes in physical health or patterns; it is important to note that the elderly alcohol abuser is unlikely to ask for direct help in coping with alcohol problem but will indirectly present with medical problems (falls, seizures, trauma, chest pain, malnutrition), psychologic problems (aggression, depression, hallucinosis); legal problems (offensive behavior, assault); or social problems (family disturbances, self-neglect)
- Failure to thrive
- Poor nutrition
- Self-neglect
- Poor hygiene and self-care
- Unexpected reaction to medications
- Insomnia
- Incontinence
- Tremors
- Peripheral neurologic damage
- Lack of exercise
- Nonadherence to prescribed health-care regimen
- Gastrointestinal disturbances
- Pain
- Difficulty in performing activities of daily living
- Falls
- Chest pain

Changes in emotions and mental health
- Low self-esteem
- Loss of motivation or ambition
- Conflicts about dependency needs after loss of love object[125]
- Hostility toward and subsequent guilt related to loss of love object[125]
- Labile mood
- Personality changes
- Irritability
- Threats of violence
- Depressed mood
- Anxiety
- Phobias
- Cognitive changes
- Memory loss
- Impairment in sensory functions
- Confusion
- Paranoid ideation
- Hallucinations (auditory, visual)
- Suicidal ideation and potential

*References 12, 22, 33, 55, 59, 105, 123, 130.

Potential Complications

Life-threatening emergency substance-induced side effects in the elderly (e.g., from misuse of prescription drugs, over-the-counter medications, or alcohol[33,130])

Acute dystonia and associated laryngeal spasm or neuroleptic malignant syndrome (adverse effect of antipsychotic medication)

Seizures, delirium, or serotonin syndrome (adverse effect of psychotropic medications)

Cardiac conduction delay and bundle branch block (adverse effect of excessive use of tricyclic agents)

Cardiovascular collapse (from tricyclic overdose)

Sinoatrial node dysfunction and sudden cardiac death or lithium toxicity (side effect of lithium carbonate)

Agranulocytosis and severe anemia (side effects of psychotropic medication)

Hyperandrenergic crisis (combining monoamine oxidase [MAO] inhibitors with foods high in tyramine)

Wernicke's encephalopathy, intoxication, withdrawal, delirium tremens (from excessive alcohol consumption over time)

Nephrotoxicity from long-term analgesic abuse

Note that substance-related disorders can be difficult to diagnose in the elderly.[59] Beware of barriers such as the elderly person hiding the condition from health-care professionals, inaccurate self-reporting, misinterpretations of symptoms by professionals for the aging process with usual social markers that may no longer be relevant in the elderly (e.g., work difficulties); "DSM-IV criteria may not apply to many older adults who have reduced role obligations at work, school, or home and who may not experience the legal, social, or psychological consequences specified by the criteria"[106]; assess for atypical presentation of symptoms, which may mimic signs and symptoms of psychiatric or medical conditions

Dangerous drug interactions in the elderly (e.g., alcohol and sedative hypnotics)

Combination of depression and alcohol disorders in the elderly and potential for suicide: Affective disorders combined with alcohol abuse or the most common conditions in elderly committing actual suicide[12]

Patient Problems/Nursing Diagnoses & Interventions*

NIC Coping Assistance

Ineffective coping related to biopsychosocial problems

- Establish caring, trusting therapeutic relationship with patient. *This is important in structuring interventions to help elderly patient increase awareness of problem, achieve behavioral change, and enhance coping skills.*[3]
- Discuss impact of substance-related disorder on physical health of patient and provide corrective interventions.
- Provide information about the negative consequences of alcohol and substance use.
  - Teach importance of adequate nutrition and use of resources (e.g., Meals on Wheels).
  - Assist patient in coping with sleep disturbances.
  - Assist patient in dealing with concerns about sexual dysfunction.
- Assist patient in decreasing anxiety present. *Anxiety is frequently present in patient with a substance-related disorder and is often the reason substance was prescribed and used in the first place.*[125]
- Assist patient in developing adaptive strategies to express anger (e.g., participation in sports, exercise, verbal expression).
- Determine extent to which patient is using denial, minimizing substance-related disorder, or rationalizing.
- Assist patient in working through defenses such as denial and accepting presence of substance-related disorder. *Patients with substance-related disorders often deny existence of problem and refuse to seek or accept treatment. They often complain about a number of psychiatric symptoms but do not complain about being an addict. Overcoming denial is the first step in treatment.*
- Emphasize importance of personal responsibility.
- Involve multidisciplinary team and patient's social network.
- Refer patient to alcohol counselor and AA to assist patient in recognizing substance abuse problem. *The recovered alcoholic is an invaluable asset to treatment team to assist patient in recognizing existence of problem and that recovery is possible.*
- Begin by using the least intrusive way of confronting patient with problem, relying on more confrontational measures if there is no change in recognition of problem and willingness to engage in treatment.
- Encourage assistance from elderly patient's social network in helping patient recognize existence of problem and become motivated to change his or her lifestyle. *It is very important to confront and work through enabling and codependency behaviors in significant others.*
- Assist patient in eliminating or altering those stressors contributing to substance-related disorder. *"Stress, isolation, various losses, loneliness, and onset of illness have all been related to late-onset drug use."*[99]
- Assist patient in developing more adaptive coping strategies to deal with these stressors.
- Maximize patient's motivation for abstinence.
- Educate patient and family about substance-related disorders by printed material, counseling, videotapes, and literature.
- Build on patient's strengths, such as recreational skills, in identifying and developing more adaptive coping skills.
- Place great emphasis on patient for assuming responsibility for own self and own behavior.
- Assist patient in rebuilding a lifestyle that is free of substance abuse.
- Explore with elderly patient the constructive use of free time and involvement in pleasant activities.
- Encourage patient to develop friendships with persons who do not abuse substances.
- Explore with patient ways to deal with mundane tasks of life on a regular basis.
- Encourage family members to interact with patient and reestablish positive relationships.
- Offer social skills training to help patient deal more effectively with environment (e.g., communication skills,

---

*References 55, 99, 103, 122, 123, 125.

assertive communication skills, problem solving, refusal skills).

- Use role play to have patient cope with potential high-risk situations that can be encountered after treatment to develop useful coping strategies and enhance perceived self-efficacy. *Increased perceived self-efficacy lowers relapse vulnerability.*
- Enroll in integrated drug and alcohol intervention.[122]
- Enhance engagement and enhance motivation: build rapport-use reflective listening; encourage self-motivational ideas; encourage a healthy lifestyle and abstinence; and use cognitive restructuring to change attitudes about lifestyle change.
- Provide feedback and training in basic skills: provide feedback on effects of substance use; help patient set achievable goals and monitor own progress; provide tips on harm reduction; and encourage enrollment in self-help groups.
- Assist patient to plan ahead: help patient identify antecedents and high-risk situations leading to substance use; teach patient problem-solving and coping skills to deal with high-risk situations, including obtaining support from others; explore options for engaging in alternative activities that are pleasant; and role play drug and alcohol refusal skills.
- Assist patient in preventing setbacks and coping with relapses: discuss motivation strategies; discuss strategies to prevent setback and relapse; and teach patient and family to maintain contact with health-care professionals.
- Refer to appropriate therapies (e.g., alcohol counselor, individual counseling, family counseling, cognitive therapy, individual supportive psychotherapy, group psychotherapy, family therapy).
- Refer to community services (e.g., AA, Al-Anon, Ala-Teen, social services, Adult Children of Alcoholics, Senior Citizens Center). *Continuing support after rehabilitation is important for elderly substance users. Community services and groups can offer elderly patient the support needed to abstain from substance abuse. Self-help groups can help patient learn more adaptive ways to handle stress, maintain sobriety, and incorporate adaptive coping skills into lifestyle.*[3]

Patient Education/Continuumof Care Plan[26,33,103,105,106]

1. Teach patient, family, and significant others about causes, course, and effects of substance use. Use printed matter to reinforce content taught (e.g., AA literature).
2. Teach patient and family changes that occur in normal aging and their impact on the effect of substance abuse. "Treatment outcomes may improve when older patients receive age-specific treatment."[105]
3. Teach patient and significant others about the importance of compliance with the prescribed medical regimen.
4. Teach patient and significant others about potential drug interactions with substance that is abused, such as alcohol-drug interactions.
5. Teach patient and significant other importance of outpatient treatment recommendations such as the importance of attending AA meetings and other peer support groups.
6. Teach patient and family about recommendations that were set by the National Institute on Alcohol Abuse and Alcoholism for low-risk drinking for the elderly (e.g., for men not over one drink per day; for women less than one drink per day).
7. Teach patient and significant other the importance of prevention (e.g., avoid requesting long-term prescriptions of hypnotics or sedatives).
8. Teach patient and significant others the importance of good nutrition.
9. Support public policy that examines and reduces availability of over-the-counter medications such as analgesic mixtures containing caffeine or codeine and two analgesic components.
10. Link patient to needed supportive resources and monitor patient after discharge to prevent relapse and potential negative consequences (e.g., elderly men with alcohol use disorder can become homeless[26]). Older homeless men have a higher incidence of alcohol use disorders.
11. Counsel patient about hazards of driving or other dangerous activities while drinking or using drugs.

Evaluation/Patient Outcomes

Coping Assistance: The patient will accept the fact that a substance-related disorder is present, develop self-awareness related to the problem, abstain from use of substance, develop coping skills to deal with stressors, and increase quality of life and lead a healthier lifestyle.

SEXUAL DISORDERS IN THE ELDERLY

Sexual disorders include **sexual dysfunctions, gender identity disorders, sexual disorder not otherwise specified,** and **paraphilias.** Sexual dysfunctions[2] are disorders in which patients experience a disturbance in the processes and changes that are part of the sexual response cycle—desire (phase of fantasies and sexual desire), excitement (phase of subjective sexual pleasure and physiologic changes), orgasm (peaking of sexual pleasure with release of sexual tension), and resolution (phase of muscle relaxation and sense of well-being)—or in which the patient experiences pain during sexual intercourse and that leads to interpersonal or other distress. Subtypes of sexual dysfunctions, indicating etiologies, for example, include (a) those due to psychologic factors, in which the onset, severity, and maintenance of the sexual dysfunction are due to psychologic factors only; and (b) those due to combined factors, in which the onset, severity, and maintenance of the sexual dysfunction are due to psychologic factors and a medical condition or substance use.

Sexual dysfunctions[2] include (1) **sexual desire disorders**: (a) hypoactive sexual desire disorder, characterized by lack of desire or fantasies for sexual activity and causing interpersonal and/or personal distress; (b) **sexual aversion disorder,** characterized by active avoidance of sex with partner and causing interpersonal and/or personal distress; (2) **sexual arousal disorders**: (a) female sexual arousal disorder, characterized by inability to maintain lubrication, swelling, and sexual excitement responses and causing interpersonal and/or personal distress; (b) male erectile disorder, characterized by inability to attain or maintain an adequate erection and causing personal and/or interpersonal distress;

(3) **orgasmic disorders:** (a) female orgasmic disorder, characterized by delay or absence of orgasm and causing personal and/or interpersonal distress; (b) male orgasmic disorder, characterized by delay or absence of orgasm and causing personal and/or interpersonal distress; (c) premature ejaculation, characterized by onset of ejaculation and orgasm with little sexual stimulation before penetration and causing personal and/or interpersonal distress; (4) **sexual pain disorders:** (a) dyspareunia, characterized by genital pain during coitus and causing personal and/or interpersonal distress; (b) vaginismus, characterized by involuntary perineal muscle contraction on penetration of vagina and causing personal and/or interpersonal distress; (5) **sexual dysfunction due to a general medical condition,** characterized by sexual dysfunction caused by physiologic effects of a medical condition and causing personal and/or interpersonal distress; (6) **substance-induced dysfunction,** characterized by sexual dysfunction caused by effects of a substance and causing personal and/or interpersonal distress; and (7) **sexual dysfunction not otherwise specified,** which includes those sexual dysfunctions that cannot be classified into any of the other categories.

Pathophysiology/Psychopathology

Psychologic, Cultural, and Environmental Theories and Factors

A number of psychologic, cultural, and environmental factors can contribute to sexual dysfunction in the elderly.[65,82] Untreated depression and anxiety can be contributing factors. Stressors encountered by the elderly, such as major changes and losses, can lead to anxiety and depression and can lead to sexual dysfunction. Negative withdrawal from pleasurable activities by those elderly who become bored with life and/or their partner can contribute to sexual dysfunction. Self-esteem can be lowered because of a negative body image as a result of the aging process, especially in elderly women; the lowered self-esteem can lead to feelings of being sexually unattractive. The interpersonal relationship with the partner is important, because a distressing relationship can lead to sexual dysfunction.

> Marital conflict, relationship imbalances, commitment issues, intimacy and communication problems, lack of trust, mismatches in sexual desires, boredom, and poor sexual techniques are just some of the common sources of sexual dissatisfactions. . . . In older people these factors may be amplified by anger and resentment that may have built over the years, as well as by feelings of entrapment and resignation if the option to leave the relationship no longer seems viable.[82]

Sexual activity, especially in widows, may be restricted because of the lack of available partners. In restricted environments, such as nursing homes, inappropriate sexual behaviors may be exhibited, especially by men, because often no normal outlets exist to fulfill sexual needs, and there is usually a lack of privacy in such institutions. Stereotypes may also contribute to sexual dysfunctions in the elderly (e.g., the elderly have no sexual desires, sexuality in the elderly is shameful, the elderly are sexually undesirable).[129] The fact is that sexuality remains important to elderly men and women.[52]

Biologic/Genetic Theories

Elderly men and women, if they are in good health, have been sexually active earlier in life, and have an interested partner, maintain an interest and capacity for being active sexually into their seventies, eighties, and even nineties.[82] Physical changes do occur in the reproductive system of elderly men and women, and some elderly couples entirely give up sexual intercourse and display their physical affection in other ways.

In elderly men, there is a decline of testosterone production along with a decline in libido; reduced secondary sexual characteristics, muscle loss, lowered aggressiveness; decreased penile sensitivity and a decline in penile erectile function; reduced sperm production; and reduced prostate secretions.[52,82] The most common sexual complaint of elderly men is impotence, which may have a psychologic basis in part but is often due to loss of vascular function or loss of neurologic function. This loss of function can be the result of medical conditions such as diabetes or thyroid disease, or drugs such as alcohol, nicotine, or antihypertensive drugs. In general, in elderly men a longer time period is needed during the excitement phase, including a need for more direct stimulation of the penis.[52] There is a decrease in the firmness of the erection; erectile dysfunction (ED) is common in elderly men. Contributing factors for ED include psychogenic factors such as performance anxiety or stressful relationships, iatrogenic factors such as medications, vascular causes, and neurogenic disorders.[136] In the orgasm phase, the ejaculatory experience is reduced in intensity and a decrease is noted in ejaculatory demand, as well as a decline in seminal volume. The resolution phase lengthens as age increases.

In elderly women, libido gradually declines.[52] The four stages of sexual response likewise gradually change as the woman ages. In the excitement phase vaginal lubrication may be reduced as is genital engorgement and the clitoris requires more stimulation. Less expansion and less vasocongestion in the vagina occurs during the plateau phase. Fewer contractions occur during orgasm, and in resolution vasocongestion is lessened.

Many of the changes in elderly women are related to menopause and menopausal symptoms that occur around the age of 45 to 50 years.[52,82] Estrogen levels become nearly depleted over time, the ovaries and breasts atrophy, the vagina and external genitals become smaller, and the vaginal wall thins and loses elasticity and lubrication, becoming more lax. During intercourse, variation in vaginal size is diminished. Along with a decline of vaginal secretions and stickier secretions, these changes can cause vaginal discomfort and painful intercourse. Dyspareunia is a common sexual problem in elderly women. Vaginismus is also a common problem in elderly women. Atrophic vaginitis can also occur, with tender vaginal walls becoming raw and bleeding with the possibility of infection, as well as dyspareunia. In elderly women, orgasm itself can even be painful. In general, older women may experience decreased sexual function (e.g., less sexual interest, less responsiveness, less coital frequency, dyspareunia).[52]

The use of certain medications can result in sexual dysfunction in the elderly. For example, antidepressants, lithium, illicit drugs, and antipsychotics can lead to sexual dysfunction. Chronic alcohol use can lead to impotence. Other medications that can alter the sexual response include antihypertensives, diuretics, antihistamines, nicotine, and chemotherapeutic agents.

The physiologic effects of certain medical conditions or treatments can lead to sexual dysfunction in elderly men and women.

Examples include diabetes; hypothyroidism, hyperthyroidism; vascular disease, including venous leakage, penile vascular disease, penile arterial occlusive disease, hypertension, arrhythmias, coronary artery disease; neurologic diseases and mental disorders such as dementia, depression, anxiety disorders, Parkinsonism, multiple sclerosis, Alzheimer's disease; sexually transmitted diseases; carcinomas of the reproductive system; and diseases such as tuberculosis, liver malfunction, infections, urinary incontinence, and renal failure. Conditions such as dyspnea, osteoarthritis, and rheumatoid arthritis can interfere with sexual activity and may require altered sexual techniques. AIDS can also contribute to sexual dysfunction in the elderly. The risk for contracting AIDS exists for the elderly[132] because (1) the immune system may be compromised in the elderly; (2) blood transfusions can spread AIDS; and (3) changes in vaginal tissue may increase the risk for women engaging in unprotected sex for contracting AIDS from infected partners. Surgery on sexual organs or pelvic irradiation can also affect sexual functioning. In addition, medical conditions in the elderly can negatively affect the elderly person's body image and lead to feeling less attractive sexually.

Diagnostic Studies and Findings

Sexual history: To determine nature and basis for sexual dysfunction

Evaluation of endocrine factors: To determine part played by hormones in sexual dysfunction

Complete medical and gynecologic examination: To rule out presence of medical conditions or substances that cause sexual dysfunction

Complete medication review: To rule out medication-induced sexual dysfunction

Laboratory studies

Diagnostic intracavernosal injection of vasodilator: To evaluate erectile failure in men[52]

Multidisciplinary Plan

Surgery/Other Treatment

Plastic surgery intervention: To correct physical changes that occur in some women after a period of abstinence and assist them in becoming able to be sexually active again

Dilation procedure: Use of graduated series of dilators to treat vaginismus in some women

Penile prosthetic implant or new tumescence techniques for men: To correct, for example, neurogenic impotence caused by such conditions as diabetes mellitus and to treat male erectile disorder

Vacuum/constriction devices: To treat male erectile dysfunction[19,52]

Penile prosthesis surgery: To treat male erectile dysfunction[19,52]

Penile vascular surgery: To correct vascular lesions[19]

Medications

Dose reduction or discontinuation of medications causing sexual dysfunctions.[52]

Estrogen creams or lubricants: To treat vaginal discomfort and lack of vaginal lubrication in elderly women[82]

Self-injection of vasoactive drug: Medications such as papavarine to treat male erectile disorder[52]

PGE (Caverject): Drug injected into penis to treat erectile dysfunction[52]

Medicated Urethral System for Erections (MUSE): A suppository of PGE put into the urethra to treat erectile dysfunction[52]; alprostadil: intrapenile injection to treat impotence secondary to neuropathy, vasculogenic, psychogenic, and mixed etiology

Estrogen replacement therapy: For beneficial effect on urogenital tissue in women[82]

Depo-injections of testosterone or testosterone patches (Testdoderm) to the scrotum: To treat hypoactive sexual desire disorder in men and to improve libido[19,52]

Trazodone: To treat psychogenic erectile dysfunction[19]

Yohimbine: To treat psychogenic erectile dysfunction in men

Sildenafil citrate (Viagra): To treat erectile dysfunction in men[95,136]

SSRIs, antiandrogens, estrogens, gonadotropin-releasing hormone Gn-RH analogues: To treat hypersexual paraphilic behavior in the elderly in nursing homes[76]

General Management

Treatment of medical conditions known to cause sexual dysfunction

Sex therapy: To enhance communication, knowledge about sexual function and activity between two partners and enhance their ability to enjoy sexual pleasure (e.g., simple counseling, individual therapy, couples therapy, group therapy)

Forced ejaculation or body work therapy: To treat male orgasmic disorder

Stop-start technique: To treat premature ejaculation

Standard sex therapy techniques: To treat female orgasmic disorder

Psychotherapy: To treat sexual dysfunctions that have no organic basis or have a combined etiology

Individual therapy or couples therapy: To treat sexual dysfunctions in men or women in which the causes are psychosocial

Psychotherapy and cognitive imagery: To identify psychologic factors such as developmental factors, traumatic events, or relationship issues and treat dyspareunia

NURSING CARE

Nursing Assessment

Presence of physical factor(s) or medical condition(s) that can affect sexual functioning.

Knowledge about aging process and effect on reproductive system and sexual activity

Present medication uses that can affect sexual functioning

Evidence of current substance abuse

Amount of caffeine or alcohol consumed

Risk factors for sexual dysfunction: Use of medications, use of tobacco; conditions such as increased blood pressure; medical or psychiatric problems

Sexual history: Early sexual experiences; history of sexual experiences and any trauma encountered; attitudes, values, beliefs, and feelings about sex; importance of sexual activity to patient; relationship with partner; expression of sexual needs and preferences in the relationship; level and type of sexual

activity desired; previous sexual problems; current sexual habits and patterns
Presence of life changes and/or stressors
Nature of family interactions and ways of dealing with stressors and crisis
Interpersonal relationship with partner
Opportunity or lack of opportunity for patient to express sexual needs
Self-image, self-esteem body image

Potential Complications

Sexual abuse (evidence includes fear or refusal of pelvic or rectal examination, hematomas on inner thighs, diminished rectal or vaginal sphincter tone, sexually transmitted disease; abuser is often a family member); particularly at risk for sexual abuse are women with dementia who are physically and/or financially dependent

Patient Problems/Nursing Diagnoses & Interventions

NIC Coping Assistance

Sexual dysfunction related to psychosocial factors and aging process

- Examine own sexual attitudes and prejudices toward sexual activity in the elderly, and become professionally informed about subject of sexuality among the elderly.
- Bring up topic of sexuality and have patient express sexual difficulties and dysfunction in own words along with own interpretation of experience.
- Listen nonjudgmentally to patient discuss own values, religious beliefs, and cultural and environmental factors that influence his or her perspective about human sexuality.
- Encourage expression of feelings such as fear and anxiety.
- Encourage communication between patient and partner about sexual concerns when they are ready to do so.
- Involve partner of patient in plan of care where appropriate.
- Dispel myths that sexual activity in the elderly is abnormal.
- Use active listening *to provide a trusting, nonthreatening, nonjudgmental atmosphere to help patient freely talk about sexual problems that may be somewhat embarrassing.*
- *Dispel any myths or misinformation about sexual functioning in the elderly: tailor information to needs of patient.*
- *Teach patient and partner about physical changes that take place throughout sexual response phases as one gets older.*

Discuss ways to minimize effects of these changes (e.g., use of lubricants, use of different sexual techniques, and other ways to express intimacy and love).

- Encourage elderly female to use estrogen creams *to reduce vaginal discomfort during intercourse.*
- Enhance patient's self-esteem.
- Assist patient in identifying psychosocial stressors that may affect patient's sexual functioning and activity.
- Teach elderly patient that intercourse does not have to result in ejaculation to be satisfying.
- Encourage patient and partner to use tactile stimulations and close physical contact and intimacy *to enhance sexual pleasure even if orgasm is not achieved.*
- Encourage patient and partner to rely on patience and affection *to increase pleasure during prolonged period of stimulation.*
- Refer patient to other members of multidisciplinary team for specific therapy as needed (e.g., sex counselor, couples therapy, sex therapist, group therapy).
- Teach healthy lifestyle practices (e.g., low-fat diet, avoid tobacco, avoid unnecessary medication).[52]
- Refer to appropriate community resources.

Patient Education/Continuum of Care Plan

1. Teach patient and partner about male and female aging process and changes in reproductive system and in phases of sexual intercourse.
2. Teach patient the importance of regular self-examination.
3. Teach elderly women that lubrication can be a very important sexual aid.
4. Teach patient to refrain from such substances as alcohol and high caffeine intake because both can diminish sexual performance.
5. Teach elderly patient about strategies to enhance sexual pleasures and alternate ways to express intimacy.
6. Teach patient communication skills to increase ability to express self assertively to partner about sexual needs and preferences.

Evaluation/Patient Outcomes

Coping Assistance: The patient will understand factors contributing to the sexual dysfunction, describe ways to enhance relationship and sexual pleasure with partner, experience an improved sexual relationship with partner, experience less sexual dysfunction, feel sexually more attractive to partner, and enjoy more sexual pleasure.

References

1. Addonizio GC: Late paraphrenia, *Psychiatr Clin North Am* 18(2):335, 1995.
2. American Psychiatric Association: *Diagnostic and statistical manual of mental disorders,* ed 4, Washington, DC, 2000, The Association.
3. ANA: *Standards of addictions nursing practice with selected diagnoses and criteria,* Kansas City, Mo, 1988, ANA.
4. Asplund R: Sleep disorders in the elderly, *Drugs Aging* 14:91, 1999.
5. Baier M, Murray R: A descriptive study of insight into illness reported by persons with schizophrenia, *J Psychosoc Nurs Ment Health Serv* 37:14, 1999.
6. Baldwin R: Depressive illness. In Jacoby R, Oppenheimer C, editors: *Psychiatry in the elderly,* ed 2, Oxford, 1997, Oxford University Press.
7. Banazak D: Anxiety disorders in elderly patients, *J Am Board Fam Pract* 10:280, 1997.

8. Barsky A et al: A prospective 4- to 5-year study of DSM-III-R hypochondriasis, *Arch Gen Psychiatry* 55:737, 1998.
9. Beck-Little R, Weinrich S: Assessment and management of sleep disorders in the elderly, *J Gerontol Nurs* 24:21, 1998.
10. Beekman A et al: Anxiety disorders in later life: a report from the longitudinal aging study Amsterdam, *Int J Geriatr Psychiatry* 13:717, 1998.
11. Blazer DG, Koenig HG: (1996). Mood disorders. In Busse EW, Blazer DG, editors: *Textbook of geriatric psychiatry,* ed 2, Washington, DC, 1996, American Psychiatric Press.
12. Blixen C, McDougall G, Suen L: Dual diagnosis in elder discharged from a psychiatric hospital, *Int J Geriatr Psychiatry* 12:307, 1997.
13. Blumenthal J et al: Effects of exercise training on older patient with major depression, *Arch Intern Med* 159:2349, 1999.
14. Brandt B, Ugarriza D: Electroconvulsive therapy and the elderly client, *J Gerontol Nurs* 22:14, 1996.
15. Brannstrom B: Care of the delirious patient, *Dement Geriatr Cogn Disord* 10:416, 1999.
16. Bright J, Baker K, Neimeyer R: Professional and paraprofessional group treatment for depression: a comparison of cognitive behavioral and mutual support interventions, *J Consult Clin Psychol* 67:491, 1999.
17. Buffum M, Buffum J: The psychopharmacologic treatment of depression in elders, *Geriatr Nurs* 18:144, 1997.
18. Burke W, Folks D, McNeilly D: Effective use of anxiolytics in older adults, *Clin Geriatr Med* 14:47, 1998.
19. Burnett A: Erectile dysfunction: a practical approach for primary care, *Geriatrics* 53:34, 1998.
20. Busse E: The myth, history, and science of aging. In Busse EW, Blazer DG, editors: *Textbook of geriatric psychiatry,* ed 2, Washington, DC, 1996, American Psychiatric Press.
21. Busse E: Somatoform and psychosexual disorders. In Busse EW, Blazer DG, editors: *Textbook of geriatric psychiatry,* ed 2, Washington, DC, 1996, American Psychiatric Press.
22. Cobbs E, Ralapati A: Health of older women, *Med Clin North Am* 82:127, 1998.
23. Cole M: Delirium: effectiveness of systematic interventions, *Dement Geriatr Cogn Disord* 10:406, 1999.
24. Danton WG, Altrocchi J, Antonuccio D: Nondrug treatment of anxiety, *Am Fam Physician* 49(1):161, 1994.
25. Davis K, Mathew E: Pharmacologic management of depression in the elderly, *Nurse Pract* 23:16, 1998.
26. DeMallie D, North C, Smith E: Psychiatric disorders among the homeless: a comparison of older and younger groups, *Gerontologist* 37:61, 1997.
27. DeVane C, Pollock B: Pharmacokinetic considerations of antidepressant use in the elderly, *J Clin Psychiatry* 60:38, 1999.
28. Dixon L: Services to families of adults with schizophrenia: from treatment recommendations to dissemination, *Psychiatr Serv* 50:233, 1999.
29. Dowling G: Part 5, Sleep problems in older adults, *Am Nurse* 27(3):24, 1995.
30. Downes-Grainger E et al: Clinical factors associated with short-term change in outcome of patients with somatized mental disorder in primary care, *Psychol Med* 28:703, 1998.
31. Downes-Grainger E et al: Drugs and the elderly, *J R Soc Health* 118:7, 1998.
32. Eisemann M: Childhood experiences and personality traits in patients with motor conversion symptoms, *Acta Psychiatr Scand* 98:288, 1998.
33. Elseviers M, DeBroe M: Analgesic abuse in the elderly, *Drugs Aging* 12:391, 1998.
34. Ersser S: Measuring the sleep patterns of older people, *Nurs Times* 95:46, 1999.
35. Farran C et al: Psychiatric home care for the elderly, *Home Health Care Serv Q* 16:77, 1997.
36. Farran C et al: Psychiatric home care of elderly persons with depression: unmet caregiver needs, *Home Health Care Serv Q* 11:57, 1998.
37. Fernandez F et al: The management of depression and anxiety in the elderly, *J Clin Psychiatry* 56(suppl 2):20, 1995.
38. Fink P et al: Somatization in primary care, *Psychosomatics* 40:330, 1999.
39. Flint A: Management of anxiety in late life, *J Geriatr Psychiatry Neurol* 11:194, 1998.
40. Flint A: Anxiety disorders in late life, *Can Fam Physician* 45:2672, 1999.
41. Floyd J: The use of across method triangulation in the study of sleep concerns in healthy older adults, *Adv Nurs Sci* 16(2):70, 1993.
42. Floyd J: Another look at napping in older adults, *Geriatr Nurs* 16(3):136, 1995.
43. Floyd J: Sleep promotion in adults, *Ann Rev Nurs Res* 17:27, 1999.
44. Folks D, Fuller W: Anxiety disorders and insomnia in geriatric patients, *Psychiatr Clin North Am* 20:137, 1997.
45. Folks D, Burke W: Sedative hypnotics and sleep, *Clin Geriatr Med* 14:67, 1998.
46. Fontaine KL, Fletcher JS: *Essentials of mental health nursing,* ed 3, Redwood City, Calif, 1995, Addison-Wesley.
47. Foreman MD, Wykle M: Nursing standard-of-practice protocol: sleep disturbances in elderly patients, *Geriatr Nurs* 16(5):238, 1995.
48. Forsell Y, Winblad B: Feelings of anxiety and associated variables in a very elderly population, *Int J Geriatr Psychiatry* 13:454, 1998.
49. Fortney J et al: The impact of geographic accessibility on the intensity and quality of depression treatment, *Med Care* 37:884, 1999.
50. Friedman J et al: Cognitive and functional changes with aging in schizophrenia, *Soc Biol Psychiatry* 46:921, 1999.
51. Frisch N, Frisch L: *Psychiatric mental health nursing,* Albany, NY, 1998, Delmar Publishers.
52. Gentili A, Mulligan T: Sexual dysfunction in older adults, *Clin Geriatr Med* 14:383, 1998.
53. George R, Howell C: Clients with schizophrenia and their caregivers' perceptions of frequent psychiatric rehospitalizations, *Issues Ment Health Nurs* 17:573, 1996.
54. Gerson S et al: Pharmacological and psychological treatments for depressed older patients; a metaanalysis and overview of recent findings, *Age Ageing* 7:1, 1999.
55. Ghodse A: Substance misuse by the elderly, *Br J Hosp Med* 58:451, 1997.
56. Gureje O, Simon G: The natural history of somatization in primary care, *Psychol Med* 29:669, 1999.
57. Gureje O et al: Somatization in cross-cultural perspective: a WHO study in primary care, *Am J Psychiatry* 154:989, 1997.
58. Hiller W, Rief W, Fichter M: How disabled are patients with somatoform disorders? *Gen Hosp Psychiatry* 19:432, 1997.
59. Holroyd S, Duryee J: Substance use disorders in a geriatric psychiatry outpatient clinic: prevalence and epidemiologic characteristics, *J Nerv Ment Dis* 185:627, 1997.
60. Inouye S: Predisposing and precipitating factors for delirium in hospitalized older patients, *Dement Geriatr Cogn Disord* 10:393, 1999.

61. Jeste D et al: Conventional vs newer antipsychotics in elderly patients, *Am J Geriatr Psychiatry* 7:70, 1997.
62. Kales H, Dequardo J, Tandon R: Combined electroconvulsive therapy and clozapine in treatment-resistant schizophrenics, *Progress in Neuropsychopharmacol Biol Psychiatry* 23:547, 1999.
63. Kaneda Y: Usefulness of the Zung self-rating depression scale for schizophrenics, *J Med Invest* 46:75, 1999.
64. Karlsson I: Drugs that induce delirium, *Dement Geriatr Cogn Disord* 10:412, 1999.
65. Kellett J: Psychosexual disorders. In Chiu E, Ames D: *Functional psychiatric disorders of the elderly,* Cambridge, 1994, University Press.
66. Kick S: An education intervention using the Agency for Health Care Policy and Research depression guidelines among internal medicine residents, *Int J Psychiatry Med* 29:47, 1999.
67. Kim M, McFarland G, McLane A: *Pocket guide to nursing diagnoses,* ed 6, St. Louis, 1996, Mosby.
68. Kirkwood C: Management of insomnia, *J Am Pharm Assoc* 39:688, 1999.
69. Kirmayer L, Taillefer S: Somatoform disorders. In Turner S, Hersen M, editors: *Adult psychopathology and diagnosis,* ed 3, New York, 1997, John Wiley & Sons.
70. Koenig H: Late life depression: how to treat patients with comorbid chronic illness, *Geriatrics* 54:56, 1999.
71. Kraemer K, Conigliaro J, Jaitz R: Managing alcohol withdrawal in the elderly, *Drugs Aging* 14:409, 1999.
72. Krasucki C, Howard R, Mann A: Anxiety and its treatment in the elderly, *Int Psychogeriatr* 11:25, 1999.
73. Kroenke K et al: A symptom checklist to screen for somtaoform disorders in primary care, *Psychosomatics* 39:263, 1998.
74. Lecomte T et al: Efficacy of a self-esteem module in the empowerment of individuals with schizophrenia, *J Nerv Ment Dis* 187:406, 1999.
75. Lenze E et al: Psychiatric symptoms endorsed by somatization disorder patients in a psychiatric clinic, *Ann Clin Psychiatry* 11:73, 1999.
76. Levitsky A: Pharmacologic treatment of hypersexuality and paraphilias in nursing home residents, *J Am Geriatr Soc* 47:231, 1999.
77. Lichstein K et al: Relaxation to assist sleep medication withdrawal, *Behav Modif* 23:379, 1999.
78. Martin R, Yutzy S: Somatoform disorders. In Hales R, Yudofsky S, editors: *Synopsis of psychiatry,* Washington, DC, 1996, American Psychiatric Press.
79. Martin R, Yutzy S: Somatoform disorders. In Hales R, Yudofsky S, Talbott J, editors: *Textbook of psychiatry,* ed 3, Washington, DC, 1999, American Psychiatric Press.
80. McCall W et al: Pretreatment differences in specific symptoms and quality of life among depressed inpatients who do or do not receive electroconvulsive therapy: a hypothesis regarding why the elderly are more likely to receive ECT, *J ECT* 15:193, 1998.
81. McCloskey JC, Bulechek GM, editors: *Nursing interventions classification (NIC),* ed 3, St. Louis, 2001, Mosby.
82. Meston D: Aging and sexuality, *West J Med* 167:285, 1997.
83. Morin C, Mimeault V, Gagne A: Non-pharmacological treatment of late life insomnia, *J Psychosom Res* 46:103, 1999.
84. Morin C et al: Behavioral and pharmacological therapies for late life insomnia, *JAMA* 281:991, 1999.
85. Mulsant B, Ganguli M: Epidemiology and diagnosis of depression in late life, *J Clin Psychiatry* 60 (suppl 20):9, 1999.
86. Munich RL, Sledge WH: Treatment settings: providing a continuum of care for patients with schizophrenia or related disorder. In Gabbard GO, editor: *Treatments of psychiatric disorders,* ed 2, vol I, Washington, DC, 1995, American Psychiatric Press.
87. Neubauer D: Sleep problems in the elderly, *Am Fam Physician* 59:2551, 1999.
88. NIH Consensus Development Panel on Depression in Late Life: Diagnosis and treatment of depression in late life, *JAMA* 268(8):1018, 1992.
89. Norman K: The role of empathy in the care of dementia, *J Psychiatr Ment Health Nurs* 3:313, 1996.
90. Noyes R, Happel R, Yagla S: Correlates of hypochondriasis in a nonclinical population, *Psychosomatics* 40:461, 1999.
91. O'Donnell J, Toseland R: Does geriatric evaluation and management improve the health behavior of older Veterans in psychological distress? *J Aging Health* 9:473, 1997.
92. Office of Scientific Information: *Plain talk about depression,* Bethesda, Md, 1994, National Institute of Mental Health.
93. O'Keeffee S: Delirium in the elderly, *Age Ageing* 28:5, 1999.
94. Owen P, Castle D: Late onset schizophrenia, *Drugs Aging* 15:81, 1999.
95. Padma-Nathan H: A new era in the treatment of erectile dysfunction, *Am J Cardiol* 84:18N, 1999.
96. Palmer B, Heaton S, Jeste D: Older patients with schizophrenia: challenges in the coming decade, *Psychiatr Serv* 50:1178, 1999.
97. Palmer B, Jeste D, Sheikh J: Anxiety disorders in the elderly: DSM-IV and other barriers to diagnosis and treatment, *J Affect Disord* 46:183, 1997.
98. Papageorgiou C, Wells A: Effects of attention training on hypochondriasis: a brief case series, *Psychol Med* 28:193, 1998.
99. Patterson T, Jeste D: The potential impact of the baby boom generation on substance abuse among elderly persons, *Psychiatr Serv* 50:1184, 1999.
100. Peters S et al: Patients with medically unexplained symptoms: sources of patients' authority and implications for demands on medical care, *Soc Sci Med* 46:559, 1998.
101. Phoenix E, Irvine Y, Kohr R: Sharing stories: group therapy with elderly depressed women, *J Gerontol Nurs* 23:10, 1997.
102. Piccinelli M, Simon G: Gender and cross cultural differences in somatic symptoms associated with emotional distress: an international study in primary care, *Psychol Med* 27:433, 1997.
103. Poldrugo F: Integration of pharmacotherapies in the existing programs for the treatment of alcoholics: an international perspective, *J Addict Dis* 16(4):65, 1977.
104. Rajput V, Bromley S: Chronic insomnia: a practical review, *Am Fam Physician* 60:1431, 1999.
105. Reid M, Anderson P: Geriatric substance use disorders, *Med Clin North Am* 81:999, 1997.
106. Reid M, Anderson P: Report describes epidemic of alcohol abuse and misuse by older Americans, *Psychiatr Serv* 49:983, 1998.
107. Reynolds C, Buysse D, Kupfer D: Treating insomnia in older adults, *JAMA* 281:1034, 1999.
108. Rief W, Shaw R, Fichter M: Elevated levels of psychophysiological arousal and cortisol in patients with somatization syndrome, *Psychosom Med* 60:198, 1998.
109. Rockwood K et al: The risk of dementia and death after delirium, *Age Ageing* 28:551, 1999.
110. Ross S, Chappel J: Substance use disorders: difficulties in diagnoses, *Psychiatr Clin North Am* 21:803, 1998.
111. Sadavoy J, LeClair J: Treatment of anxiety disorders in late life, *Can J Psychiatry* 42:28S, 1997.
112. Salzman C: Practical considerations for the treatment of depression in elderly and very elderly long term care patients, *J Clin Psychiatry* 60:30, 1999.
113. Sandberg O et al: Clinical profile of delirium in older patients, *J Am Geriatr Soc* 47:1300, 1999.

114. Schreiber R: Understanding and helping depressed women, *Arch Psychiatr Nurs* 10:165, 1996.
115. Schreiber R: Clueing in: a guide to solving the puzzle of self for women recovering from depression, *Health Care Women Int* 19:269, 1998.
116. Segee P et al: Demographics, treatment seeking, and diagnoses of anxiety support group participants, *J Anxiety Disord* 13:315, 1999.
117. Semple S et al: Self perceived interpersonal competence in older schizophrenic patients, *Acta Psychiatr Scand* 100:126, 1999.
118. Shaver JLF, Landis CA: Part 1, Understanding the behavior of sleep, *Am Nurse,* October, 1994.
119. Shaver JLF, Landis CA: Part 3, Helping people manage primary insomnia, *Am Nurse* 27(1):22, 1995.
120. Siegler I et al: Psychological aspects of aging. In Busse EW, Blazer DG, editors: *Textbook of geriatric psychiatry,* ed 2, Washington, DC, 1996, American Psychiatric Press.
121. Simon G, Gureje O: Stability of somatization disorder and somatization symptoms among primary care patients, *Arch Gen Psychiatry* 56:90, 1999.
122. Sitharthan T et al: Integrated drug and alcohol intervention: development of an opportunistic intervention program to reduce alcohol and other substance use among psychiatric patients, *Aust N Z J Psychiatry* 33:676, 1999.
123. Sklar S, Turner N: A brief measure for the assessment of coping self-efficacy among alcohol and other drug users, *Addiction* 94:723, 1999.
124. Smith SL, Sherrill KA, Colenda CC: Assessing and treating anxiety in elderly persons, *Psychiatr Serv* 46(1):36, 1995.
125. Solomon K et al: Alcoholism and prescription drug abuse in the elderly: St. Louis University grand rounds, *J Am Geriatr Soc* 41(1):57, 1993.
126. Sproule B et al: The use of nonprescription sleep products in the elderly, *Int J Geriatr Psychiatry* 14:851, 1999.
127. Stephens J, Richard P, McHugh P: Suicide in patients hospitalized for schizophrenia, *J Nerv Ment Dis* 187:10, 1999.
128. Stuart G, Laraia M: *Principles and practice of psychiatric nursing,* ed 6, St. Louis, 1998, Mosby.
129. Townsend M: *Psychiatric mental health nursing,* ed 2, Philadelphia, 1996, FA Davis.
130. Tueth M, Zuberi P: Life threatening psychiatric emergencies in the elderly: overview, *J Geriatr Psychiatry Neurol* 12:60, 1999.
131. Unutzer J et al: Patterns of care for depressed older adults in a large staff model HMO, *Am J Psychiatry* 7:235, 1999.
132. Varcarolis E: *Foundations of psychiatric mental health nursing,* ed 3, Philadelphia, 1998, WB Saunders.
133. Walker E: Medically unexplained physical symptoms, *Clin Obstet Gynecol* 40:589, 1997.
134. Weintraub D, Ruskin P: Posttraumatic stress disorder in the elderly: a review, *Harvard Rev Psychiatry* 7:144, 1999.
135. Whitney JD: Somatization. In McFarland GK, Thomas MD: *Psychiatric mental health nursing application of the nursing process,* St. Louis, 1991, Mosby.
136. Wierman M: Advances in the diagnosis and management of impotence, *Adv Intern Med* 44:1, 1999.
137. Wilhelm S et al: Cognitive behavior group therapy for body dysmorphic disorder, *Behav Res Ther* 37:71, 1999.
138. Wilkinson P: Cognitive therapy with elderly people, *Age Ageing* 26:53, 1997.
139. Winefield H, Barlow J, Harvey E: Responses to support groups for family caregivers in schizophrenia, *Aust N Z J Ment Health Nurs* 7:103, 1998.
140. Wintz C: Nursing management of psychotropic drug reactions, *Nurs Clin North Am* 33:217, 1999.
141. Wise M, Gray K: Delirium, dementia, and amnestic disorders. In Hales R, Yudofsky S, editors: *The American Psychiatric Press synopsis of psychiatry,* Washington, DC, 1996, American Psychiatric Press.
142. Yassa R, Suranyi-Cadotte B: Clinical characteristics of late-onset schizophrenia and delusional disorder, *Schizophr Bull* 19(4):701, 1993.
143. Yassa R et al: The prevalence of late-onset schizophrenia in a psychogeriatric population, *J Geriatr Psychiatry Neurol* 6:120, 1993.
144. Zaretsky A, Segal Z, Gemar M: Cognitive therapy for bipolar depression: a pilot study, *Can J Psychiatry* 44:491, 1999.
145. Zhang M et al: Group psychoeducation of relatives of schizophrenic patients, *Psychiatry Clin Neurosci* 52:S344, 1998.

PART III

PERIOPERATIVE NURSING

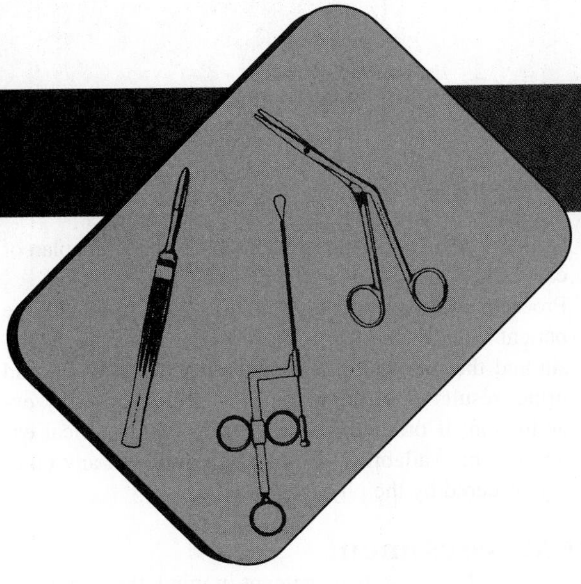

21

Perioperative Nursing Care

Marsha A. Miller
Shelley A. Carroll
Sheila Gleeson

OVERVIEW

The purpose of this chapter is to outline the important aspects of nursing care in the perioperative period. Rather than focusing on specific invasive procedures and/or surgical interventions that have already been covered in this text, this chapter will define general principles that guide the care of patients during the perioperative phase of their care.

Patient care during the perioperative phase demands knowledge of and skill in perioperative care and also requires an in-depth understanding of related disease processes that have brought the patient to seek treatment.

With the advances in surgical and anesthetic technology, and improved intraoperative monitoring techniques such as mass spectrometry, pulse oximetry, transesophageal echocardiography, hemodynamic monitors, electroencephalograms (EEGs), cell savers, and pharmacologic advances, virtually all patients are candidates for intervention regardless of their preexisting health status. Perioperative nursing must encompass all specialties to meet the needs of this diverse patient population.

Perioperative nurses *do practice nursing.* The Association of periOperative Registered Nurses (AORN) defines the perioperative nurse in the following statement:

Perioperative nurse is defined as the registered nurse who, using the nursing process, designs, coordinates, and delivers care to meet the identified needs of patients whose protective reflexes or self-care abilities are potentially compromised because they are having operative or other invasive procedures. Perioperative nurses possess and apply knowledge of the procedure and the patient's intraoperative experience throughout the patient's care continuum. The perioperative nurse assesses, diagnoses, plans, intervenes, and evaluates the outcome of interventions based on criteria that support a standard of care targeted toward this specific population. The perioperative nurse addresses the physiological, psychological, sociocultural, and spiritual responses of the individual that have been caused by the prospect or performance of the invasive procedure.[6]

In 1999 the AORN Perioperative Nursing Data Set (PNDS) was recognized by the American Nurses Association as useful to nursing practice. It describes four domains, 29 outcomes in five categories, 64 nursing diagnoses, and 127 nursing interventions.[4]

The conceptual model of the PNDS consists of four domains. These are the three domains of nursing concern (safety, physiologic responses, and behavioral responses of the family and individual), as well as the structural elements of the perioperative environment or health system. The domains of nursing concern consist of patient outcomes, nursing diagnoses, and interventions, whereas the health system includes benchmarks and desired outcomes, report cards, and structural elements.[4]

Perioperative nurses should be familiar with the American Hospital Association Bill of Rights and the interpretation pertinent to the agency,[1] as well as the tenets of the American Nurses Association Code for Nurses.[2]

The ongoing coordination and organization of resources to provide a consistent response to fiscal realities and patient needs is known as case management. It reflects a dynamic process that focuses on the patient and the clinical system. Case management goals include the achievement of timely, measurable, cost-effective, intraoperative resource utilization; the redesign of delivery systems; and the promotion of informed decision making by the patient and all health-care providers.[7,19]

As with the nursing process in other nursing arenas, there are overlapping steps of the perioperative nursing process. Intervention, evaluation, and discharge planning occur during the assessment and planning phases. Ongoing assessment and planning occur during the intervention phases, ensuring optimal outcomes for each patient.

Perioperative nursing not only incorporates the assessment, planning, implementation, and evaluation steps of the nursing process, but also allows for multiple nursing roles. Perioperative nurses may function as clinical practitioners, educators, managers, consultants, and/or researchers. They may practice in hospitals, clinics, ambulatory surgery centers, physicians offices, industry, or other patient environments.[25] The practice of perioperative nurses may be less visible than other specialties to patients and nursing colleagues, but it is still the practice of nursing.

PREOPERATIVE NURSING ASSESSMENT AND CARE

Function of Preoperative Nursing Assessment

The primary function of preoperative nursing assessment is to ensure that all pertinent medical and psychosocial data regarding each patient are available to perioperative personnel before the induction of anesthesia. Data necessary for each procedure may include an informed consent, documentation of specific drug allergies, documentation of the patient's medical history and physical examination, and results of pertinent laboratory studies. Before general anesthesia for elective procedures, the perioperative nurse confirms that the patient has had nothing to eat or drink during the previous 6 to 8 hours.

The nursing diagnosis most pertinent to preoperative care is anxiety related to the situation. A preoperative assessment reveals the patient's concerns, which frequently include fear of death, disfigurement, or permanent injury; fear of pain and unknown outcome; and the possibility of impaired mobility postoperatively. Interventions include providing a calm environment and the opportunity to be with significant family member(s). In addition, it is essential that the perioperative nurse convey a caring concern while completing routine preoperative checks. Addressing the physical and emotional needs of the patient's spouse, family, and friends includes providing factual information regarding the impending invasive procedure and anesthesia and estimating the length of the procedure and the recovery period. Nursing intervention related to family members provides them with additional information about whom to call in the postanesthesia care unit (PACU) after the procedure, the PACU visiting policy, the location of the family waiting areas, and the location of the hospital cafeteria or nearest restaurant. The preoperative nurse answers questions from the patient, friends, and family.

Preoperative Teaching

From the outset, an important goal of preoperative teaching is to return the patient to his or her environment with the skills and abilities to achieve optimal outcomes. Preoperative teaching is designed to reinforce the importance of postoperative pulmonary toilet and early postoperative ambulation; it is also designed to provide information about postoperative pain management alternatives. In the immediate preoperative period, explanations should be brief and easily understood. The nursing objective is to eliminate or minimize anxiety related to the impending procedure and to the postoperative period.

Patient Safety

Before each procedure the perioperative nurse ensures the patient's safety:

1. Consult the schedule to determine the procedure to be performed.
2. Consult the preference cards to determine the surgeon's specifications: patient position, instruments, draping materials, sutures, special equipment, and supplies.
3. Collaborate with the scrub nurse on the patient's plan of care.
4. Proceed to the preoperative holding area to review the patient's chart. Check for informed consent for anesthesia and the procedure; laboratory results on blood and urine; results of electrocardiogram and chest x-ray examination, if ordered; current history and physical examination; availability of ordered blood; and any other data ordered by the physician.

Patient Assessment

With the concepts of case management in mind, the perioperative nurse introduces himself or herself and begins the patient assessment.

Patient Identification

1. Ask the patient to state his or her name.
2. Verify the identification band.
3. Check for consistency between the patient's description of the procedure on the consent form and the procedure listed on the physician's notes, verifying the side as appropriate.
4. Observe the patient's skin condition at the operative site and over the rest of the patient's body. Note any bruises, lacerations, or abrasions. Inspect incisions from previous procedures, and verify these with the patient.
5. Consult with the patient regarding his or her usual activity level.
6. Evaluate for limitation of motion, deformities, or other musculoskeletal considerations.
7. Note previous implants or prostheses on the perioperative record.
8. Document congenital anomalies or missing extremities.
9. Assess sensory functions, and note any impairments.
10. Consult with the patient regarding his or her surgical history.
11. Discuss with the patient any necessary accommodations to be made after discharge and initiate referrals as necessary.

Patient Data

Review patient data, and ascertain whether the values are within normal limits.

1. Review the patient's chart, and note deviation from the standard in laboratory values, x-ray examination, electrocardiogram, or other studies, as ordered.
2. Obtain vital signs, either on the nursing unit before transporting the patient to the preoperative holding area or in the preoperative area.
3. Document the patient's blood pressure, temperature, pulse, and respiration.
4. Report any deviations or abnormal findings to the appropriate physician.

Physical Status

Evaluate the cardiovascular status of the patient:

1. Check the patient's pulse for rate, rhythm, and irregularities.
2. Review the electrocardiogram, and report any abnormalities to the physician.
3. Document the location of arterial and central lines on the perioperative record.

Evaluate the respiratory status of the patient:

1. Note the patient's skin color.
2. Assess the patient's breath sounds.
3. Review the patient's laboratory values of arterial blood gases, and report any abnormalities to the physician.
4. Document the location of chest tubes, if present.

Evaluate the renal status of the patient:

1. Note the patient's urinalysis and renal function studies. Review the results of input and output documentation for balance.
2. Check the patient's weight, and document the weight on the chart.
3. Verify that the patient has had nothing to eat during the previous 6 to 8 hours.
4. Document the total parenteral nutrition line, if present.

Question the patient regarding allergies:

1. Elicit the details of the patient's allergic reaction to certain medications.
2. Ask the patient about side effects after ingesting foods.
3. Evaluate the patient's environmental allergies, including specific reference to latex.
4. Incorporate allergies to chemicals (such as iodine) into the plan of care.

Ascertain details of any controlled substance use or abuse:

1. Question the patient about the use of drugs, alcohol, or tobacco products.
2. Observe the patient for skin integrity.
3. Review the patient's medical record.
4. Check the patient's laboratory studies and admission assessment.

Psychosocial Status

Observe the psychosocial status of the patient during interaction with the patient, family, and caregivers:

1. Question the patient regarding his or her perception of the surgery.
2. Communicate any overreaction or inappropriate response to the surgeons and anesthesia personnel.
3. Question the patient about his or her expectations for the intraoperative period.
4. Reassure the patient that optimal care will be given and that he or she will not be left alone.
5. Address the concerns of the patient, and give additional information, as needed.

Analyze the patient's knowledge of the proposed intervention:

1. Incorporate the patient's verbal and nonverbal communication skills and hearing status into the nursing care plan.
2. Estimate the patient's level of knowledge as the prospective procedure is being discussed, and assist the patient to obtain more information if the patient's knowledge is not adequate.
3. Arrange for an interpreter if the patient's understanding is hampered because of a language barrier. Interpreters may often be family members, operating room staff, or other hospital personnel.
4. Elicit information from the designated family member, guardian, or agent, who is acting on the patient's behalf, if the patient demonstrates a lack of understanding because of mental impairment.

Ascertain the religious preference and ethnicity of the patient:

1. Discuss the wishes of the patient and family members regarding ceremonies and clergy.
2. Document specific requests on the patient's chart and care plan.
3. Clarify any other cultural beliefs that may influence care.
4. Assess own cultural and religious values in relation to those of the patient, and modify the plan of care to reflect the patient's beliefs.

Perioperative Nursing Care Plan

Formulate nursing diagnoses to guide the patient's care providing a generic perioperative nursing care plan based on the most frequent nursing diagnoses:

1. Interpret and prioritize assessment data to meet the needs of the patient.
2. Select the diagnoses based on scientific knowledge, current nursing practice, and interaction with the patient and family.
3. Document the diagnoses on the perioperative record, and communicate this information to members of the health-care team.[25]

Develop realistic outcome statements for the patient, including maintenance of skin integrity and freedom from infection (Table 21-1, *A* and *B*):

1. Take into account the behavior patterns and physical status of the patient.
2. Address the patient's education needs, as well as his or her comfort and safety.
3. Develop criteria for measurement of goals based on laboratory data, vital signs, and symptom alleviation or improvement.
4. Identify tasks and procedures to be used in achieving outcomes.
5. Document goals on the perioperative record, and inform other members of the health-care team.
6. Prioritize goals with the patient, considering Maslow's hierarchy of needs.[23]
7. Organize priorities in a logical sequence, taking into account the immediate and the long-term goals.
8. Interact with other departments to provide needed services to support the patient after discharge.

Anticipate and procure equipment and supplies before they are needed:

1. Consider the availability of instruments and potential scheduling conflicts affecting equipment and supplies.
2. Obtain necessary equipment from the appropriate departments.
3. Check and operate electrical equipment and powered surgical instruments according to the manufacturers' instructions.

Table 21-1A Perioperative Nursing Data Set Nursing Care Plan: Immediate Preoperative

Nursing Diagnosis	Interventions	Outcome Criteria	Outcome Statement
Risk of injury	• Confirms identity before the invasive procedure. • Verifies allergies. • Verifies presence of prosthetics or corrective devices. • Notes sensory impairments. • Verifies surgical site. • Verifies surgical procedures. • Verifies consent. • Verifies NPO status. • Evaluates for signs and symptoms of physical injury. • Evaluates for signs and symptoms of skin and tissue injury as a result of transfer or transport. • Performs surveillance.	• Patient's skin remains intact, nonreddened, and free of blistering. • Patient will maintain or improve baseline neuromuscular function. • Patient verbalizes comfort related to transfer/transport activities.	The patient is free from signs and symptoms of physical injury. The patient is free from signs and symptoms of injury related to transfer/transport.
Risk of anxiety related to knowledge deficit and stress of surgery	• Assesses coping mechanisms based on psychological status. • Determines knowledge level based on psychological status. • Identifies individual values and wishes concerning care. • Identifies psychosocial status. • Assesses readiness to learn based on psychological status. • Includes family members and support person in perioperative teaching.	• Patient verbalizes or indicates · decreased anxiety and an ability to cope, · understanding of procedure and sequence of events, · that questions have been answered, and · expected outcomes. • Patient verbalizes concern about decisions being discussed and participates in decision making.	The patient participates in decisions affecting his or her plan of care. The patient demonstrates knowledge of psychological responses to invasive procedure.
Risk for acute/chronic pain	• Assesses pain control. • Identifies cultural and value components related to pain. • Implements pain guidelines. • Evaluates response to pain management interventions.	• The patient demonstrates adequate pain management and verbalizes relief of pain/discomfort.	The patient demonstrates and/or reports adequate pain control throughout the perioperative period.

From Beyea.[6a]

4. Remove any piece of equipment from the operating room that does not function properly, and report it to the appropriate personnel.
5. Know the location, contents, and operation of the defibrillator and emergency cart.
6. Ensure that adequate numbers and types of personnel are available for the patient's transfer and care.
7. Use equipment and supplies in a cost-effective manner.
8. Document the judicious use of supplies and equipment to demonstrate cost-effective and appropriate patient care, thereby allowing for accurate reimbursement.

Direct professional and paraprofessional personnel to assist with implementation of patient care:

1. Take into account the preparation level of each person when assigning patient care responsibilities.
2. Maintain certification in cardiopulmonary resuscitation in the event that intervention is needed, and to meet institutional and regulatory requirements.

Control the environment to ensure optimal patient care:

1. Decrease sensory stimuli, especially during induction and emergence from anesthesia. The room should be as quiet as possible.
2. Decrease the risk for infection by limiting traffic to a minimum.
3. Maintain appropriate temperature and humidity of the room where care is administered.
4. Know the disaster plan evacuation routes and procedures for removing the patient from the room while the intervention is in progress.
5. Keep the corridors free from obstructions at all times.

Collaborate with biomedical personnel to contain hazards:

1. Verify initial safety testing, performance testing, and routine preventive maintenance on all equipment.
2. Follow standard procedures for care and use of electrical hazards: check plugs, cords, and connections; observe delicate handling of cords and connections; secure cords to prevent tripping; avoid passing heavy equipment over cords; and remove and repair defective equipment.
3. Follow standard procedures for use of volatile liquids, ionizing radiation sources such as x-rays, and nonionizing radiation sources such as lasers.
4. Properly dispose of biohazardous waste in clearly marked containers.
5. Confine sharp objects and syringes to prevent injury.

Table 21-1B Perioperative Nursing Data Set Nursing Care Plan: Intraoperative

Nursing Diagnosis	Interventions	Outcome Criteria	Outcome Statement
Risk for infection	• Implements aseptic technique. Classifies surgical wound. Assesses susceptibility for infection. • Performs skin preparations. • Protects from cross-contamination. • Monitors for signs and symptoms of infection. • Minimizes length of invasive procedure planning care. • Administers prescribed prophylactic treatments. • Initiates traffic control. • Administers care to invasive device sites. • Administers care to wound sites. • Dresses wound at completion of procedures.	• Monitors for signs and symptoms of infection. • Surgery is performed using aseptic technique and in a manner to prevent cross-contamination.	The patient is free from signs and symptoms of infection.
Risk for impaired skin integrity related to immobilization, pressure, and/or shearing forces	• Identifies physical alterations that may affect procedure-specific positioning. • Positions the patient. • Implements protective measures to prevent skin or tissue injury due to thermal, chemical, or mechanical sources. • Evaluates the patient for signs and symptoms of injury to skin and tissue. • Uses supplies and equipment within safe parameters. • Evaluates the patient for signs and symptoms of injury as a result of positioning.	• Skin remains smooth, intact, nonreddened, nonirritated, and free of bruising, other than surgical incision.	The patient is free from signs and symptoms of physical injury.
Risk of injury related to surgical environment, extraneous objects, and equipment (ie, laser, electrical, use of x-rays/radiation)	• Implements protective measures to prevent injury due to electrical sources. • Implements protective measures to prevent injury due to laser sources. • Implements protective measures to prevent injury due to radiation sources. • Records devices implanted during invasive procedure. • Performs required counts. • Evaluates for signs and symptoms of laser, electrical, and radiation injury.	• Skin remains smooth, intact, nonreddened, nonirritated, and free of bruising. • Sensation, motions, and function are maintained or improved from baseline.	Patient is free from signs and symptoms of laser, electrical, and radiation injury.
Risk of hypothermia	• Implements thermoregulation measures. • Monitors body temperature.	• Core body temperature remains within expected range.	The patient is at or returning to normothermia at the conclusion of the immediate postoperative period.

From Beyea.[6a]

6. Define maintenance and cleaning programs.
7. Verify regular inspections of the steam, electrical, vacuum, hydraulic, ventilation, plumbing, and emergency generator systems.
8. Report any situations requiring intervention between inspections.
9. Use good body mechanics and application of work-simplification principles to decrease the chance of personal injury.

Transport the patient in a safe and timely manner into the procedure room:

1. Confirm the patient's identity, both by verbal response and by comparison to the identification bracelet. If the patient cannot identify himself or herself, the identification should be provided by a family member or the health-care professional accompanying the patient.
2. Select the appropriate mode of transport based on the patient's condition. The patient may be transported in a bed, on a gurney, in a wheelchair, or may walk into the room.
3. Document the mode of transport on the patient's record.
4. Determine the number and qualifications of transport personnel.
5. Reassure the patient and provide any comfort measures needed during transport.

Assess the needs of the patient and the family regarding protocols:

1. Explain the routine procedures to the patient and to the family, if they have not been previously instructed. Determine the complexity of the teaching based on the patient's attention span and anxiety level.
2. Instruct the patient in coughing and deep breathing. Give suggestions for enhancing the patient's comfort while the patient is performing those activities.
3. Question the patient about his or her understanding, and ask for a return demonstration.

4. Review the routine of the postanesthesia care unit, and address relevant discharge questions.
5. Document patient and family teaching on the perioperative record.

Record Keeping

Records and forms are established by the facility to safeguard patient confidentiality, to document informed consent for surgical and invasive procedures, and to provide for communication among health-care personnel.[25] Electronic documentation is being used with increasing frequency.

The Joint Commission on Accreditation of Healthcare Organizations requires that records be kept of each operation, including preoperative diagnoses, procedures performed, a description of the findings, the number and types of specimens removed, the postoperative diagnoses, and the names of participating personnel.[19]

The Association of PeriOperative Registered Nurses Standards, Recommended Practices, and Guidelines states that documentation of all nursing activities is important for clear communication and collaboration between health-care team members and continuity of patient care (see box at right).[5]

The incorporation of the AORN Perioperative Nursing Data Set (PNDS) into perioperative nursing records will allow for a system to quantify, code, and computerize just what it is that perioperative nurses do when they care for patients. This, in turn, will lead to recognition of and reimbursement for their influence on perioperative patient outcomes.[6]

AORN, INC., STANDARDS, RECOMMENDED PRACTICES, AND GUIDELINES 2001

Document the following:
- Identification of persons providing perioperative patient care; name, title, signature of person responsible for the care
- Description of the patient's overall skin condition on arrival and discharge from the perioperative suite
- Perioperative patient care planning, including baseline physical, emotional, psychosocial, and cultural data
- Presence and/or disposition of sensory aids and prosthetic devices
- Placement of the dispersive pad for the electrosurgical unit, identification number and settings of the unit
- Use of temperature-regulating devices and documentation of the patient's body temperature on arrival and discharge from the perioperative area
- Placement of electrocardiogram electrodes, blood pressure cuff, pulse oximetry, temperature probe, and all other invasive and noninvasive monitoring devices
- Patient positioning and/or repositioning devices and supports
- Administration of blood or blood products, medications, and solutions used during the perioperative period
- Specimens and cultures taken
- Location and solution used for skin prep
- Location and type of drains, catheters, and packing and dressing materials
- Placement of tourniquet cuffs, including identification of the unit, pressure settings, and inflation and deflation times
- Placement and location of implants, including the manufacturer name, lot and serial numbers, type and size of implant, and expiration date if indicated
- Placement of radioactive implants including location, time, number, and type of material
- Sponge, sharp, and instrument counts
- Use of intraoperative fluoroscopy and x-ray examination
- Laser used, including type, number, surgeon's name, lens used, length of time, and wattage used
- Wound and anesthesia classification
- Patient discharge time and status, method of transport, receiving area
- Any significant occurrences during the perioperative period
- Communication with family members or significant others and patient or family teaching provided

From AORN, Inc.[5]

INTRAOPERATIVE NURSING CARE

ASEPSIS

Infection Control

The perioperative nurse is knowledgeable in the principles and practices of infection control. According to *Alexander's Care of the Patient in Surgery:*

> Infection control practices should focus on prevention. Transmission of infection involves a chain of events, including presence of a pathogenic agent, reservoir, portal of exit, transmission, portal of entry and host susceptibility. Prevention occurs where there is a break in the chain of transmission. Infection control practices involve both personal and administrative measures. Personal measures include fitness for work and application of aseptic principles. Administrative measures include provision of adequate physical facilities, appropriate surgical supplies, and operational controls (FIG. 21-1).[25]

Each facility determines policies for proper operating room attire and standard precautions to comply with infection control practices (Fig. 21-2).[29]

The use of barriers and precautions when handling sharps and hand washing should be addressed in the policies at each facility.

Sterilization and Disinfection

To ensure consistent, high-quality care for all surgical patients, regardless of the venue in which the care is rendered, principles of disinfection and sterilization must be followed. Instruments are decontaminated after use, mechanically washed, ultrasonically cleaned (to decrease the bioburden), and reassembled. The perioperative nurse is aware of preventive maintenance of equipment and of regular testing of equipment with chemical and biologic indicators.

Sterilization results in the destruction of all microorganisms on inanimate surfaces, including spores. Sterilization methods include dry heat, steam under pressure, hydrogen peroxide, plasma, and chemical means. Selection of a sterilization method is dependent on the composition of the material to be

A

B

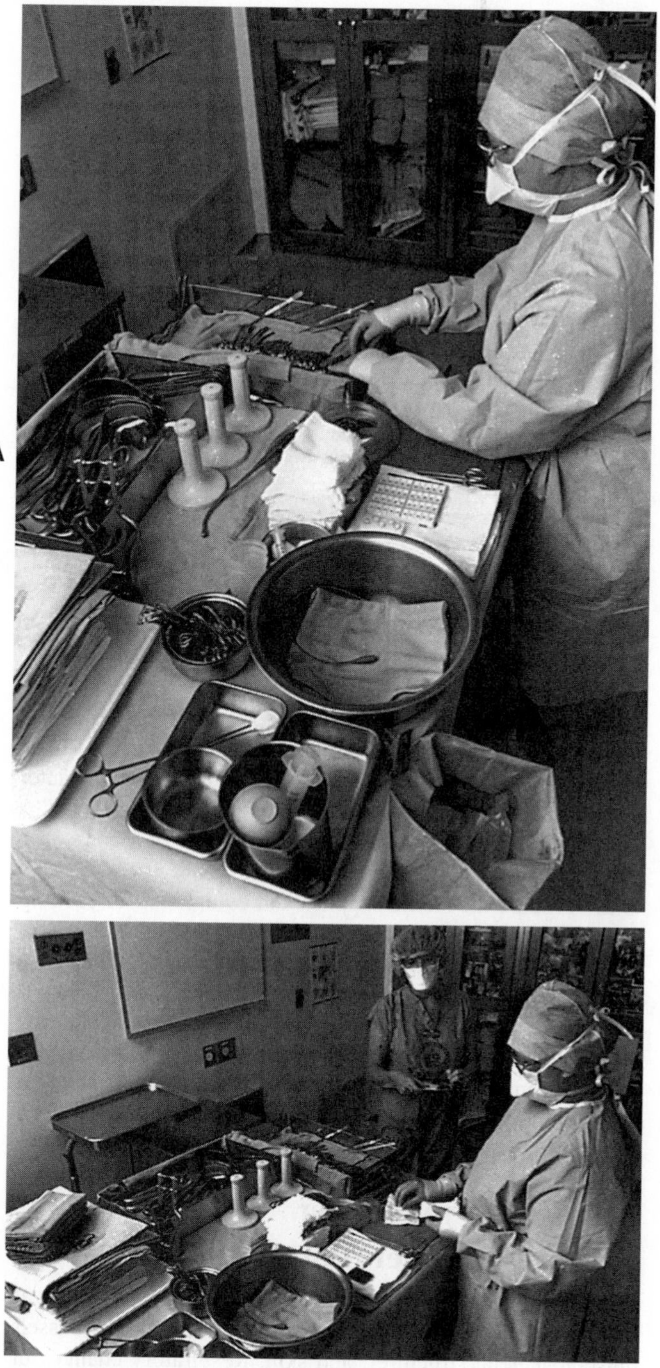

FIG. 21-1
A, Scrub nurse prepares instrument table. **B,** Scrub nurse and circulating nurse count sponges, instruments, and needles before surgical procedure begins.

sterilized, required turnover time for the item, and considerations for personnel and patient safety.

High-level disinfection may be used for items that are not suitable for the sterilization process or those that are not required to be sterile. Selection of a disinfectant is based on the need for high-, intermediate-, or low-level action; compatibility with the materials to be disinfected; chemical properties of the disinfectant; time required for the disinfection process; and ease of use. Activated glutaraldehyde and *ortho*-phthalaldehyde are commonly used for disinfection of heat-sensitive medical devices. Various compounds may be used for different environmental surfaces and purposes. Phenols and hypochlorites are often used on operating room surfaces.[25]

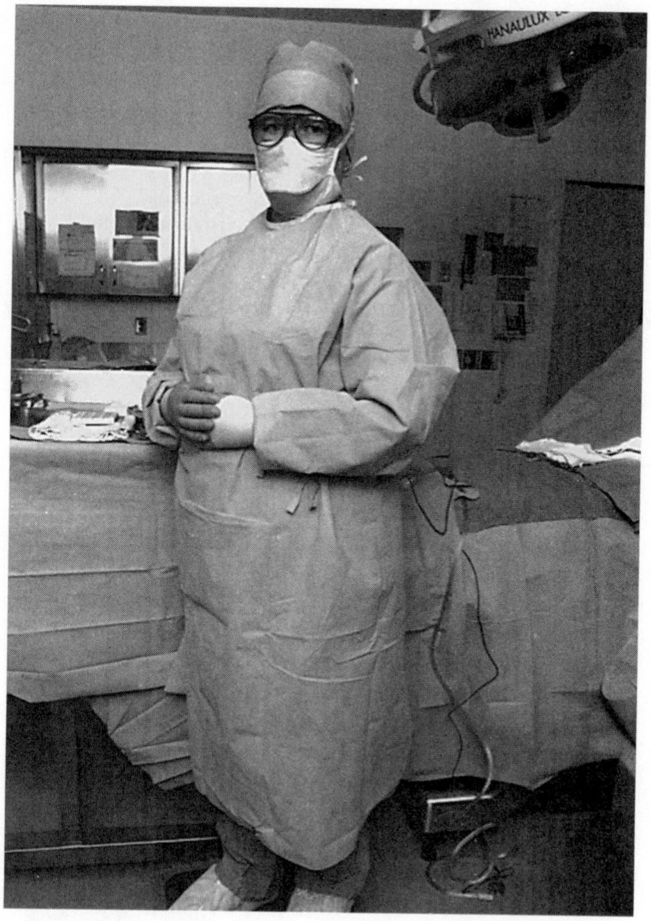

FIG. 21-2
Scrub nurse is properly attired for surgical procedure.

The AORN Standards, Recommended Practices, and Guidelines include the rationale and interpretive statements that serve as a foundation for the practice of aseptic technique in the operating room (see box, p. 1344).[5] *Alexander's Care of the Patient in Surgery* states that "the goal of each aseptic technique is to optimize primary wound healing, prevent surgical infection, and minimize the length of recovery from surgery."[25]

WOUND HEALING

Surgical wounds can be classified as clean, clean-contaminated, contaminated, or infected. Wound types consist of those with no tissue loss, those with tissue loss, and those caused by underlying disease. Wounds with no tissue loss are primary closures and heal by first intention. Wounds with tissue loss, such as burns or traumatic injuries, heal by second intention or granulation.[25] Conditions that contribute to delayed wound closure are heavy contamination of the wound or removal of an inflamed organ.

The three phases of wound healing begin with an inflammatory response lasting 1 to 4 days. Vasoconstriction and clot formation maintain hemostasis and provide protection from contamination. During this edematous phase, leukocytes,

AORN, INC., STANDARDS, RECOMMENDED PRACTICES, AND GUIDELINES 2001

MAINTAINING A STERILE FIELD

- Scrubbed persons function within a sterile field.
- Sterile drapes should be used to establish a sterile field.
- Items used within a sterile field should be sterile.
- All items introduced onto a sterile field should be opened, dispensed, and transferred by methods that maintain sterility and integrity.
- A sterile field should be maintained and monitored constantly.
- All personnel moving within or around a sterile field should do so in a manner to maintain the sterile field.
- Policies and procedures for maintaining a sterile field should be written, reviewed annually, and readily available within the practice setting.[5]

REQUIREMENTS FOR DEVELOPING A SURGICAL CONSCIENCE

1. Knowledge of the principles of asepsis.
2. The nurse's self-discipline in inspecting and regulating his or her hygiene, dress, and nursing practice, always giving attention to breaks in technique.
3. Ability to anticipate the need for services based on knowledge of the patient, the procedure being performed, the preferences of the surgical team, and where and how to obtain necessary supplies.
4. Good communication skills to determine the needs of patients and team members and to identify and correct breaks in technique.
5. Maturity to overcome personal preference and prejudice to provide optimum patient care, regardless of the surgical procedure, the patient's circumstances, or other surgical personnel.

From Kneedler and Dodge.[21]

macrophages, and basal cells migrate into the area. When fibroblasts are formed, the second stage of wound healing begins. This reconstructive phase lasts from 5 to 20 days, while collagen forms fibers that strengthen the connective tissue. The maturation phase of wound healing process may last for months or years. Complications of wound healing, if they should occur, include fistulas, hematomas, infections, wound disruptions, adhesions, or keloids. Wound healing is influenced by patient factors, such as nutritional status, weight, and the presence or absence of underlying disease, as well as environmental asepsis (see box above) and surgical tissue-handling technique. The selection of needles, sutures, and suturing, stapling, and skin closure techniques affects wound approximation and healing, as does the judicious use of intraoperative antibiotics.[21]

Surgical Conscience

According to Kneedler and Dodge[21]:

> A surgical conscience means attention to aseptic principles during the perioperative period. It involves constant inspection, monitoring, and regulation of the surgical patient, environment, personnel, and equipment. The nurse anticipates the patient's and the surgical team's needs and gives unselfish, vigilant care to the patient.

A surgical conscience can be considered fully developed when the operating room nurse's attention to sterile technique and aseptic practices becomes automatic. It requires awareness of what is occurring at all times during the intraoperative period, even when attention is directed to other activities (see box above, right).[21]

Preparation for Surgery

The skin of the patient and the members of the surgical team requires disinfection before the surgical procedure begins. The selection of an antimicrobial agent is made to remove dirt and transient microorganisms from the skin, reduce the number of resident microorganisms, and leave an antimicrobial residue on the skin surface, while minimizing skin irritation. Commonly used agents include povidone-iodine, chlorhexidine, alcohol, and hexachlorophene.

Before the application of the chosen antimicrobial agent, the patient's skin may be prepared by shaving, clipping, or using a depilatory.

The skin of the surgical team is scrubbed, using a brush and nail cleaner or a foam preparation for the length of time determined by the facility.[21]

Prepare the sterile field using the principles of asepsis:

1. Comply with operating room attire policy.
2. Procure the sterile supplies and equipment for each operative procedure (see FIG. 21-1, *A*).
3. Inspect supplies for package integrity and evidence of sterilization (FIG. 21-3).
4. Distribute supplies to the field aseptically.
5. Create a sterile operative field by using appropriate draping materials.
6. Monitor and correct aseptic practice during the procedure.

Positioning the Patient

Patient Considerations

Positioning has five major effects on the surgical patient: it affects respiration, circulation, peripheral nerves and vessels, musculoskeletal structures, and skin. Respiratory changes include disturbance of the ventilation-perfusion ratio, decreased stretchability of lung tissue, redistribution of inspired air, and mechanical restriction of lung expansion. Anesthesia is the primary cause of circulatory changes. Major vessels are dilated, lowering the blood pressure and leading to dependent pooling and decreased circulatory return. The medulla is depressed, compensatory mechanisms are hindered, and muscle tone is decreased. Effects on peripheral nerves from poor positioning include compromised blood supply or ischemia from stretching, hyperextending, compressing, or twisting. Because anesthesia reduces or eliminates the patient's normal defense mechanisms, care must be taken to safeguard the patient against inadvertent injury. Even patients who have normal range of motion can be compromised because of overzealous movement of extremities during positioning. Two factors to

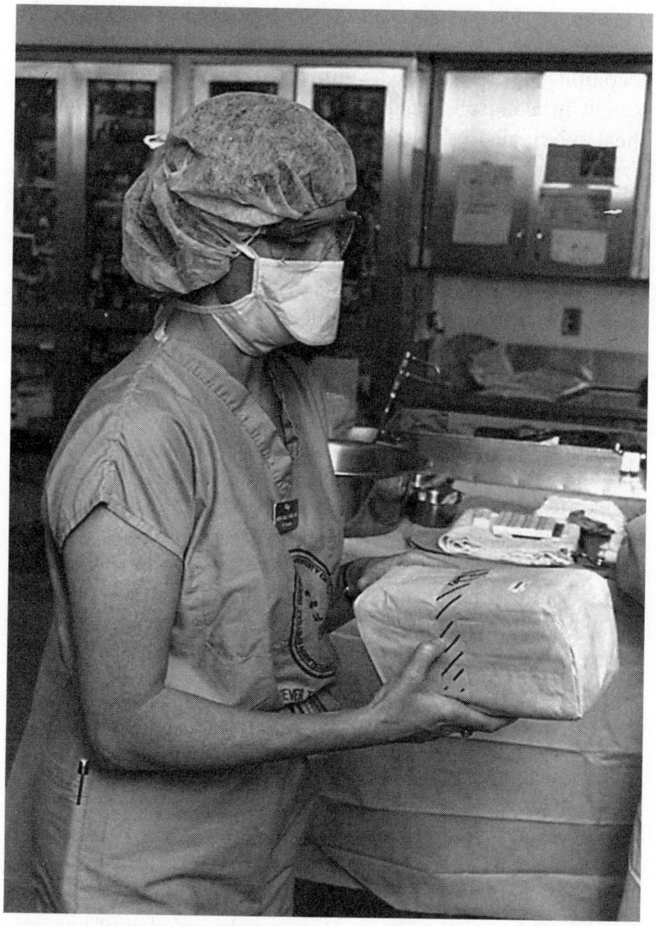

FIG. 21-3
Circulating nurse checks the integrity of the package of towels.

consider in relation to skin integrity are the location of bony prominences and the duration of pressure (FIG. 21-4). Decreased tissue perfusion can lead to ischemia, and shearing forces can lead to patient injury. Patients frequently cross their legs in the moments just before the induction of anesthesia; limbs should be checked for proper alignment after induction. Factors to be considered include the patient's age, weight, general health status, distribution of weight, blood pressure, nutrition, and duration of immobility.

Supine

Supine or dorsal recumbent position, with the patient lying on his or her back, is the position most commonly used. Careful placement of the extremities is important to avoid injury. The most common injury occurs to the brachial plexus when the arm is abducted greater than 90 degrees. Special attention must be paid to the elbows and fingers to prevent their contact with hard surfaces, and padding is essential to prevent pressure on bony prominences. Both the vital capacity and tidal volume are decreased, and obese patients experience a 40% to 50% increase in respiratory effort. Circulation is affected less in the supine position than in the other positions; however, the mean arterial pressure is decreased, and there is an increased volume of blood in the heart and lungs, when compared with sitting or standing.[21]

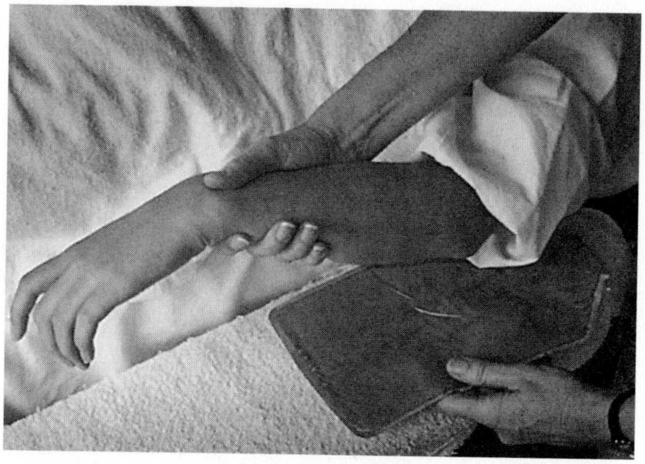

FIG. 21-4
Placement of gel pad to prevent injury during intraoperative period.

Trendelenburg's

Trendelenburg's position is a variation of the supine position, with the patient's head positioned down. More respiratory changes occur; tidal volume and vital capacity are further decreased. Shift of the abdominal viscera impedes free movement of the diaphragm, and intrathoracic pressure is increased. The patient should be moved slowly from supine to Trendelenburg's position to allow for gradual changes. The perioperative nurse must be constantly vigilant to prevent pressure on the patient's toes from the Mayo stand or instrument table.[21]

Reverse Trendelenburg's

Reverse Trendelenburg's position, with the head up, must also be accomplished slowly. The respiratory function is affected less; however, circulation is affected more. The legs may be wrapped to prevent pooling of blood; however, it is important to avoid compression of the peroneal nerve at the head of the fibula.[25]

Lithotomy

Lithotomy position, lying on the back with the legs flexed, decreases respiratory effectiveness because the diaphragm is restricted. Pulmonary blood volume is increased, and vital capacity and tidal volume are decreased. Pressure from thigh flexion causes circulatory pooling in the lumbar area. The effects of this position are exacerbated if the patient is placed into Trendelenburg's position as well. The leg supports must be carefully chosen and applied securely to the operating room bed. The hands should be positioned across the chest or on armboards to prevent digital damage when the foot of the bed is lowered. The timing of leg movement is coordinated with the anesthesiologist. Two members of the surgical team move the legs simultaneously to prevent sacroiliac dislocation, and special consideration is given to patients with hip prostheses. Padding is applied to the knee area to prevent peroneal nerve damage.[21]

Modified Fowler's

Modified Fowler's, or sitting, position is physiologically best for respiratory function. Venous pooling, sometimes leading to hypotension, is the primary systemic circulatory effect. The ischial tuberosities bear the majority of the patient's weight, creating the potential for pressure areas and sciatic nerve damage. Judicious use of padding can help to prevent such occurrences.[25]

Lateral

Side-lying or lateral position decreases respiratory efficiency because the body's weight is on the lower chest. This position interferes with intercostal breathing and results in decreased respiratory efficiency, vital capacity, and tidal volume.[25] Pooling in the dependent limbs occurs when the abdominal vessels are compressed. Peripheral nerve injuries can occur when scrupulous attention is not given to arm position. If the legs are allowed to lie in contact with each other during the operation, there is a potential for skin abrasions or friction injuries. Lateral position is best accomplished by a team of four health-care workers. The patient's flank is positioned over the kidney rest (bridge) on the operating room bed, and then the bridge of the operating room bed is raised slowly. The bottom leg is flexed, while the top leg remains straight. Padding is placed between the legs, around the ankles, and elsewhere if deemed necessary. The arm on the bottom is positioned at an angle slightly less than 90 degrees from the body, and the elbow, wrist, and hand are padded and secured to the armboard. A soft roll is placed at the apex of the scapula to prevent brachial compression. The arm on the top is secured to a padded support or to an elevated armboard. The body is secured with tape, braces, or sandbags.

Prone

Prone or face-down position requires the patient to be anesthetized on the stretcher before being turned over on the abdomen. Respiration is restricted because of the weight of the body on the abdomen; the blood pressure may fall. Body rolls that support the patient from the acromioclavicular joint to the iliac crest are placed on the operating room bed. The move is accomplished using four health-care workers and turning the patient in a logroll manner. Careful attention to the endotracheal tube and to the monitoring devices is essential during turning. Arms may be secured at the sides of the operating room bed or to padded armboards extending alongside the head. Care is taken to move the arms down and forward to avoid hyperextending the shoulder joints. The body rolls are adjusted to provide support, to allow full excursion of the lungs, and to prevent encroachment on the female breasts. The male genitalia are checked for impingement. The knees are padded, and a pillow is placed under the ankles to prevent the toes from coming in contact with the mattress.

Jackknife

Jackknife (Kraske) position is the most precarious surgical position. Because of reduced negative intrathoracic pressure, the respiratory system is severely compromised. Blood pooling in the extremities is the most common circulatory effect and is caused by obstruction at the break in the operating room bed. Other concerns are the same as those for the patient in prone position.[21]

Determine the position of the patient by the need for adequate exposure of the operative site, accessibility to the patient's airway and monitoring devices, and considerations for the patient's safety.

1. Employ knowledge, planning, and teamwork when positioning the patient.
2. Understand the consequences of improper positioning and body alignment, using your knowledge of anatomy and physiology.
3. Before moving the patient, lock both the operating room bed and the stretcher for patient safety.
4. Identify equipment used for patient positioning.

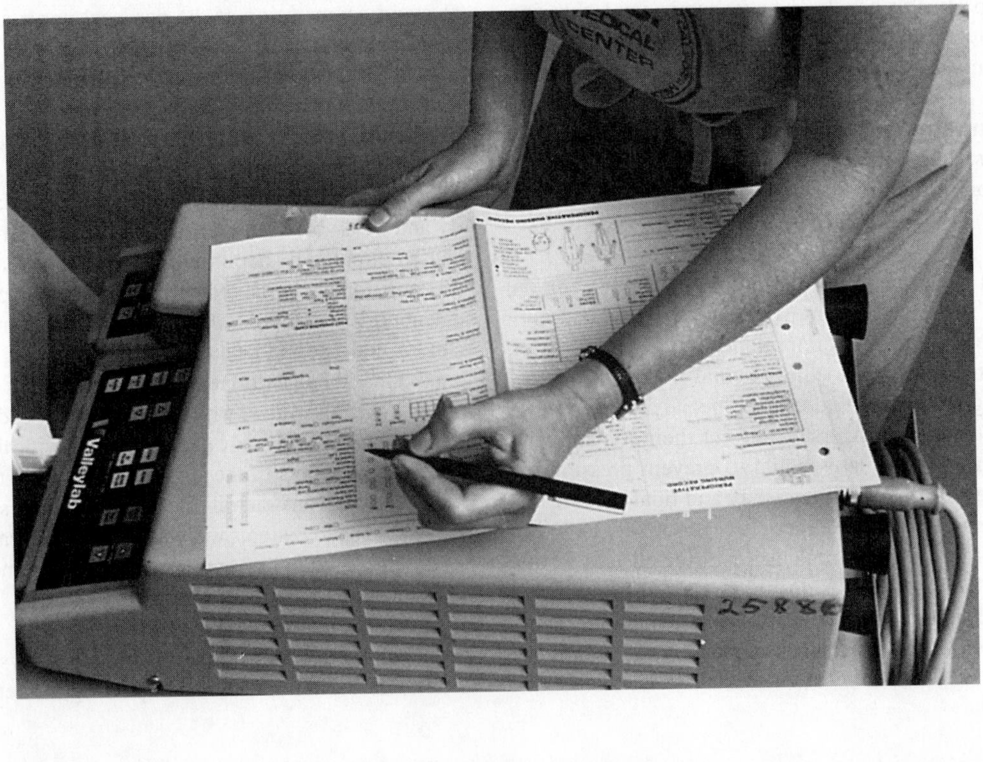

FIG. 21-5 Circulating nurse performs intraoperative documentation.

Monitoring the Patient

The perioperative nurse is responsible for maintaining an awareness of the physiologic monitoring devices used during the procedure:

1. Observe the electrocardiogram, the pulse oximeter, and the patient's skin color. Note and document any changes.
2. Watch the patient for behavioral changes, such as restlessness or a change in the level of consciousness. Communicate this information to the appropriate personnel.
3. Monitor fluid intake, and calculate blood loss.
4. Operate patient monitoring devices according to the manufacturer's instructions.
5. Complete documentation of the patient intervention (FIG. 21-5).

Conclusion of the Procedure

The steps taken to conclude any operative or invasive procedure must be followed closely to ensure a smooth transition to recovery. Call the appropriate postoperative care unit to give a preliminary report on the patient's status before completion of the procedure.

Control materials used on the patient:

1. Count sponges, sharps, and instruments as delineated in the policy and procedure manual of the facility.
2. Relate result of counts to the surgical team.
3. Implement corrective actions if the counts are incorrect, including notifying the surgeon and the x-ray department and filling out the risk management report.

Administer medications to the patient:

1. Document drug, dosage, and route of administration on the perioperative record.
2. Observe the patient for reactions, complications, side effects, and efficacy.

Postoperative Evaluation

Reassess the patient during the postoperative evaluation:

1. Correlate changes in the health status of the patient with the nursing diagnoses.
2. Review laboratory data and patient signs and symptoms.
3. Revise the patient care plan to reflect this evaluation.
4. Reevaluate patient outcomes.
5. Measure and document patient responses to the interventions.

Patient Transfer

Conclude the procedure and transfer the patient to the stretcher for transport:

1. Provide a clean gown to maintain the patient's dignity and privacy.
2. Perform a skin assessment, giving special attention to areas that are dependent or are under the dispersive electrode pad.
3. Keep the safety strap in place until all personnel are ready to transfer the patient to the stretcher.
4. Place the stretcher adjacent to the bed with the wheels locked.
5. Determine the patient position on the stretcher after assessing the patient for responsiveness.
6. Determine airway maintenance, proper body alignment, and availability and security of tubes, drains, lines, and monitoring devices.
7. Transfer the patient slowly and smoothly to the stretcher with concern for patient safety, good body mechanics, and coordination of team members.

Anesthesia

The anesthesiologist reports on the surgical procedure and anesthetic management. The perioperative nurse adds, validates, and verifies important information for the postoperative care of the patient. Baseline data included in the report are the patient's name; age; preoperative and postoperative diagnoses; surgical procedure; anesthesia agents and technique; intraoperative information; primary language; preoperative level of consciousness; medical history; allergies; airway status; catheters, drains, lines; blood loss; nursing considerations; and special symptoms that are observed.[25]

Inhalation Anesthetics and Their Physiologic Effects

Inhalation anesthetic agents are used to render patients unconscious and insensible to noxious stimuli. Generally, these agents are used in conjunction with intravenous sedative or narcotic agents to achieve surgical anesthesia. This concept of "balanced" anesthesia uses the lowest effective dose of inhalation agents, which reduces the possibility of administering an overdose. The physiologic effects of inhaled anesthetics, besides producing anesthesia, are important considerations for the nurses providing care to postoperative patients because all organ systems are affected by these agents.

The five major inhalation anesthetic agents that are used alone to create surgical anesthesia are halothane, enflurane (Ethrane), isoflurane (Forane), desflurane (Suprane), and sevoflurane (Ultrane). Nitrous oxide is also used as an anesthetic gas; however, it cannot be used alone because it is less potent than the others. To anesthetize an average person for surgery, the partial pressure of nitrous oxide necessary in the alveoli (and therefore in the blood and brain) is 105%—enough to eliminate oxygen from the mixture of the inspired gases used to deliver anesthesia. Therefore nitrous oxide is used in conjunction with another inhalational agent or with narcotics. Although the exact mechanism by which inhalation agents produce the anesthetic state is not completely understood, all of them produce known physiologic effects that often last into the recovery period; these effects may be observed in the PACU.

Respiratory Effects

Inhalational anesthetics alter gas exchange, affecting both $PaCO_2$ and PaO_2, and they also affect the muscles of respiration and airway protection.

Gas Exchange

The overall respiratory effect of the inhalation agents is profound respiratory depression. This occurs in a dose-dependent way, eventually producing respiratory arrest if the inspired concentration becomes high enough. Tidal volume is greatly reduced, predisposing the patient to respiratory acidosis via alveolar hypoventilation. All inhalation agents cause tachypnea during induction of anesthesia and during any increase in delivered concentration to increase anesthetic depth if patients are allowed to breathe spontaneously. Even though the respiratory rate is increased, it does not compensate for the decrease in tidal volume because the dead space ventilation does not change. The effect of this respiratory depression results in increased $Paco_2$. In the central nervous system (CNS) inhalation agents depress the ventilatory response to increases in $Paco_2$. The combined effects result in (1) "resetting" to a higher level the $Paco_2$ necessary to stimulate breathing and (2) a decreased response to additional CO_2 that may occur during surgery.

Oxygenation is impaired (Pao_2 may decrease) during anesthesia from a number of effects of the inhalation anesthetics. First, there is alveolar hypoventilation, as described previously. In addition, the regular resting breathing pattern is altered. When a person is awake, there is a periodic "sigh" that entails taking a breath two to three times the normal tidal volume. This serves to reexpand any alveoli that have collapsed because of immobility. If this were not done, eventually the atelectasis would cause an increase in the blood "shunted" past nonventilated alveoli, which decreases overall oxygenation and results in a fall in Pao_2. This sigh mechanism is eliminated by inhalational anesthetics in patients who are breathing spontaneously, further predisposing to atelectasis and hypoxemia. All patients who are anesthetized, whether being ventilated mechanically or breathing spontaneously, are prone to atelectasis due to the fact that they are either supine or in other positions even less favorable to adequate alveolar expansion. Normally, in the awake state, the response to atelectasis (besides the sigh) is pulmonary vasoconstriction, which diverts pulmonary capillary blood away from the atelectatic portion of the lung. Inhalational anesthetics blunt this response also, further creating a right-to-left pulmonary shunt, thereby increasing arterial hypoxemia. Effects that work to decrease oxygenation explain why it is important to increase the inspired oxygen concentration during and after surgery, until all of the effects of the inhalation anesthetics have resolved.

Mechanics of Breathing

Inhalation anesthetics affect the muscles of breathing and those used for airway protection. As the muscles of the tongue become anesthetized, patients tend to develop upper airway obstruction. Maintaining a patent airway during recovery from anesthesia not only is necessary for efficient gas exchange, but also facilitates the elimination of anesthetic gases. As the anesthetic concentration is increased during the induction of anesthesia, use of the accessory muscles to assist ventilation progressively decreases—an event that normally occurs in unanesthetized individuals as hypoventilation is sensed. The diaphragm continues to function unless very high concentrations (anesthetic overdose) are reached. As patients recover from anesthesia, they recover their ability to use accessory respiratory muscles if necessary.

Inhalation anesthetics also depress the airway protective reflexes; if patients vomit during anesthesia, they may not be able to cough efficiently enough to clear any material that enters the trachea. Pulmonary aspiration of the gastric contents, if allowed to occur, remains a serious consequence of the unprotected airway.

The mechanisms used by the body to clear secretions from the tracheobronchial system, particularly the cilia, are impaired by the use of inhalation anesthetics. Patients who produce sputum preoperatively often require tracheal suctioning during surgery and into the postoperative period in the PACU.

Special Respiratory Considerations

Halothane is the inhalation agent most commonly used in children because it is least irritable to the airway. This is an important consideration because it is generally easier to induce anesthesia in children by having them breathe an inhalational agent through a mask than it is to start an intravenous line. In addition, halothane, unlike the other inhalation agents, appears not to stimulate respiratory secretions, making its use valuable in patients with obstructive pulmonary disease who are prone to produce sputum. Isoflurane and desflurane, on the other hand, cause the greatest airway irritation, and induction with these agents may occasionally be characterized by coughing, breath holding, and laryngospasm. Although halothane is often chosen, all inhalation anesthetics are bronchial smooth muscle dilators and are effective in reducing wheezing from asthma during anesthesia and surgery.

Cardiovascular Effects

Inhalation anesthetics affect each of the following parameters of the cardiovascular system: myocardial contractility, blood pressure, peripheral vascular resistance, coronary artery blood flow, and heart rate. They do not, however, have equal effects on each parameter at the same anesthetic dose. In patients with preexisting myocardial disease these effects are more pronounced.

All inhalation agents are myocardial depressants. In addition, they all produce hypotension (in the absence of surgery), and all decrease coronary blood flow. Both enflurane and isoflurane cause a larger fall in peripheral vascular resistance than halothane. Fortunately, myocardial oxygen consumption during anesthesia is reduced so that the coronary blood flow, although reduced, is sufficient to meet the metabolic needs of the myocardium. As with the respiratory effects, these cardiovascular effects are dose-dependent. The higher the anesthetic concentration, the lower the blood pressure and the more profound the myocardial depression.

Enflurane, isoflurane, sevoflurane, and particularly desflurane, often cause an increase in heart rate, whereas halothane does not. When enflurane and isoflurane are combined with small doses of intravenous narcotics, the increase in heart rate associated with these agents is not as great. The increased heart rate associated with increasing the inspired concentration of desflurane is often accompanied by a slight increase in blood pressure. The mechanism of these changes is not yet understood.

Halothane "sensitizes" the myocardium to the effects of catecholamines, an effect not shared by the other inhalation anesthetics.

Cardiovascular reflexes, including tachycardia in response to hypotension and bradycardia in response to vagal or baroreceptor stimulation, remain intact; however, these reflexes are reduced or depressed during anesthesia with any of the inhalation agents.

Because patients are brought to the PACU before all the inhalation agents have had time to be eliminated from the body, many of the effects on the cardiovascular system described above may be seen in the PACU. It is particularly important to remember that during the early postoperative period, patients' compensatory cardiovascular reflexes remain depressed. Hypotension will need early intervention because the patients' sympathetic nervous system may be unable to respond appropriately if inhalation agents remain in their bodies—even if they remain in minimal concentrations.

Circulatory Effects on Other Body Systems

Cerebral

All of the inhalational agents blunt the ventilatory response to rising P_{CO_2}. Carbon dioxide is a potent cerebral vasodilator, and its presence in the circulation in higher-than-normal concentrations increases cerebral perfusion. In addition, inhaled anesthetic gases tend to inactivate the cerebral metabolic control (autoregulation) of its own circulation; therefore no compensation is made for the increased cerebral perfusion secondary to hypercarbia. These agents also act directly on cerebrovascular smooth muscle. The combination of all of these effects increases the intracranial blood volume and the intracranial pressure of the patient under anesthesia.

Gastrointestinal

Hepatic blood flow is reduced when patients are anesthetized with inhalational agents. The reduced hepatic blood flow affects the metabolism of all other drugs given during the anesthetic period and the initial recovery phase. This is an important consideration for nurses in the PACU because dosages of analgesics must be titrated, keeping in mind the patient's preexisting sedation and impaired ability to metabolize drugs effectively.

Renal

Inhalational anesthetics increase renal vascular resistance and decrease renal cortical blood flow. Consequently the glomerular filtration rate is decreased and the urine output volume is reduced during anesthesia, perhaps by as much as 60% to 70%. The decrease in renal blood flow and the fall in blood pressure seen during inhalation anesthesia combine to activate the renin-angiotensin system. In addition, stimulation of the sympathetic nervous system is associated with release of antidiuretic hormone (ADH), contributing further to a decrease in urine volume during anesthesia.

Skeletal Muscles

All inhalation anesthetics cause skeletal muscle relaxation. If muscle relaxation is required for optimal surgical conditions (i.e., for abdominal surgery), however, intravenous muscle relaxants are used. The concentration of inhaled anesthetics necessary to create surgical relaxation is in the lethal dose range and would likely cause severe cardiovascular depression or collapse.

Cutaneous Circulation

Inhalation agents cause cutaneous vasodilation. This direct effect interferes with temperature regulation because heat loss through the skin is increased. As a result of this effect, and from surgical incisions that expose body cavities to the ambient environment, most patients have some degree of hypothermia when they are admitted to the PACU. Interestingly, patients in whom finding venous access preoperatively may be difficult will usually exhibit many potential intravenous (IV) sites soon after inhalation anesthesia is started because of peripheral vasodilation.

BALANCED ANESTHESIA

As mentioned previously, inhalational anesthetics are almost always used in conjunction with other agents to achieve optimal surgical conditions. This concept of "balanced anesthesia" uses the minimal dose of each agent to achieve the desired surgical conditions. Other than the inhalation agents, almost all of the additional anesthetic agents are administered intravenously. Barbiturates, narcotics, benzodiazepines, and neuromuscular blocking agents are the classes of drugs used most often in combination with inhaled gases to produce balanced anesthesia.

Barbiturates

The most commonly used drug in this class is thiopental sodium. It is administered intravenously at the beginning of surgery to induce anesthesia. Thiopental is an ultrashort-acting barbiturate that depresses the central nervous system, producing hypnosis and anesthesia without analgesia. The peak effect of an induction dose is achieved within 1 minute after intravenous administration, and the effect is gone after 5 to 10 minutes. This, like all barbiturates, is a potent respiratory depressant. Methohexital (Brevital) is an ultrashort-acting IV anesthetic agent that is two to three times more potent than thiopental.

Propofol

Propofol (a substituted isopropylphenol) is an intravenous induction agent that may have some advantages over thiopental and other barbiturates. Like thiopental, it is rapidly cleared from the plasma, so the duration of action is short. The clearance of propofol from the plasma exceeds hepatic blood flow, so metabolism of the drug occurs to some extent in the plasma itself and is therefore not dependent on liver and renal function. Clinical experience indicates that propofol causes less nausea than barbiturates, and its rapid elimination prevents the feeling of a "hangover" that often accompanies recovery from anesthesia induced by thiopental. In addition, propofol can be used as an anesthetic itself when given by continuous infusion. When used in this manner, recovery from general anesthesia is accomplished more quickly and without the unpleasant side effects (nausea, vomiting, and residual sedation) that often accompany recovery from other agents. Propofol has gained popularity in recent years and is frequently used in outpatient surgical settings to facilitate rapid recovery in patients who are going home the day of surgery.

Narcotics (Opioids)

Morphine sulfate, fentanyl, and sufentanil are the narcotic agents most commonly used to supplement general and regional anesthesia. All are analgesics, and that is the main reason for their use. All narcotics cause respiratory depression in a dose-related manner. Morphine is longer acting than fentanyl and sufentanil. Morphine and fentanyl are commonly used postoperatively for pain relief and intraoperatively as part of a balanced anesthetic.

Benzodiazepines

Diazepam (Valium) and midazolam (Versed) are the most commonly used drugs in this class; recently, however, the use of midazolam has exceeded that of diazepam because it is shorter acting and because it is an excellent amnestic agent. These agents are also anticonvulsant. The dose of these agents should be decreased in the elderly or debilitated patient. These agents are respiratory depressants, and when used in combination with narcotics, severe respiratory depression may occur.

Neuromuscular Blocking Agents

Neuromuscular blocking agents are used in surgery as an adjunct to general anesthesia to provide an optimal surgical environment and to minimize the need for other potent anesthetic agents. Skeletal muscle relaxation is essential during abdominal and thoracic procedures and is often used during a variety of other surgeries to eliminate patient movement.

Muscle relaxants are divided into two general categories: depolarizing and nondepolarizing (competitive) agents. The most commonly used depolarizing muscle relaxant is succinylcholine (Anectine). After IV injection, succinylcholine binds with the acetylcholine receptor site at the neuromuscular junction, causing depolarization, then muscular contraction—seen clinically as fasciculations. Unlike acetylcholine, however, succinylcholine is not metabolized by acetylcholinesterase. The motor end plate remains depolarized and so is unable to accept subsequent stimuli until succinylcholine is eventually metabolized by serum pseudocholinesterase. The duration of action of a standard dose of succinylcholine is approximately 3 to 5 minutes. The primary use for succinylcholine is to facilitate tracheal intubation immediately after induction of anesthesia. Because succinylcholine is not metabolized by acetylcholinesterase, its effects cannot be reversed. Competitive blocking agents can be reversed pharmacologically. The commonly used blocking agents are pancuronium, *d*-tubocurarine, and vecuronium. After IV injection these agents combine with acetylcholine receptors; however, they do not cause depolarization of the motor end plate. When enough receptor sites are blocked, the normal neurotransmitter, acetylcholine, cannot activate enough receptors to raise the end plate potential for excitation and so neuromuscular blockade ensues. Generally, the duration of action of nondepolarizing muscle relaxants varies between 30 and 60 minutes, depending on the dose and the specific agent used. The onset of action of these agents is approximately 3 to 5 minutes, depending on the dose. They are primarily used for surgical relaxation rather than intubation. They can, however, be used for tracheal intubation when succinylcholine is contraindicated.

Nursing considerations in the immediate postoperative period for patients who have received neuromuscular blocking agents primarily concern the evaluation of respiratory function. Incomplete recovery from the effect of neuromuscular blocking agents is manifested as discoordinated breathing, that is, asymmetric chest movement resulting in inadequate tidal volumes. The patient may complain of "weakness" and an inability to breathe. A reliable test to determine whether the effects of the neuromuscular blocking agents have been fully reversed is to ask the patient to lift his or her head off the bed and keep it elevated for 5 seconds. A person with normal muscle tone, in the absence of neck injury, will be able to perform this maneuver. If it is determined that the patient is still experiencing the effects of neuromuscular blockade, an anticholinesterase agent may be administered.

Table 21-2 Centroneuraxis Narcotic Bolus

Drug	Bolus Dose (mg)	Onset (min)	Duration (h)
EPIDURAL ROUTE			
Morphine	1-10	30-60	6-24
Fentanyl	0.025-0.15	4-20	2.6-4
SUBARACHNOID ROUTE			
Morphine	0.1-0.5	15	8-24

Reversal Agents

Anticholinesterase agents are given to reverse the effects of neuromuscular blockers. The two most commonly used drugs in this class are edrophonium (Tensilon) and neostigmine (Prostigmin). The action of these drugs is to combine with cholinesterase to prevent the metabolism of acetylcholine. The acetylcholine plasma level increases, which allows the acetylcholine to compete with the neuromuscular blocker and bind with its receptor sites. The muscarinic effects of the increased plasma levels of acetylcholine include bradycardia, bronchospasm, and excessive salivation. Because the bradycardia may be hemodynamically significant, anticholinergic agents are administered in conjunction with the anticholinesterase agent. Atropine and glycopyrrolate are the anticholinergic agents most frequently used to avoid bradycardia when reversing the effects of neuromuscular blockers. The nurse in the immediate postoperative phase must be able to assess the adequacy of the patient's breathing and to recognize the need for airway support if the patient is still suffering from the effects of neuromuscular blocking agents.

REGIONAL ANESTHESIA

Regional anesthesia includes a variety of techniques that use local anesthetic drugs. They can be used on any part of the CNS and every type of nerve fiber. Local anesthetics affect the nerve cells by preventing the transport of sodium across the cell membrane, which prevents depolarization and impulse conduction.

Local anesthetics are pharmacologically classified as amides or esters (Table 21-2). Esters are rapidly metabolized in the plasma; their half-life is short. One of the metabolic degradation products is *p*-aminobenzoic acid, which is associated with allergic reactions in sensitive individuals. Amides are metabolized by the liver and have longer half-lives. Patients with severe liver dysfunction are at greater risk for adverse reactions. Adverse reactions are manifested as CNS toxicity, cardiovascular toxicity, or hypersensitivity reactions.

Central Nervous System Reactions

Early symptoms of blurred vision, nystagmus, and numbness of the tongue may progress to seizures and CNS depression.

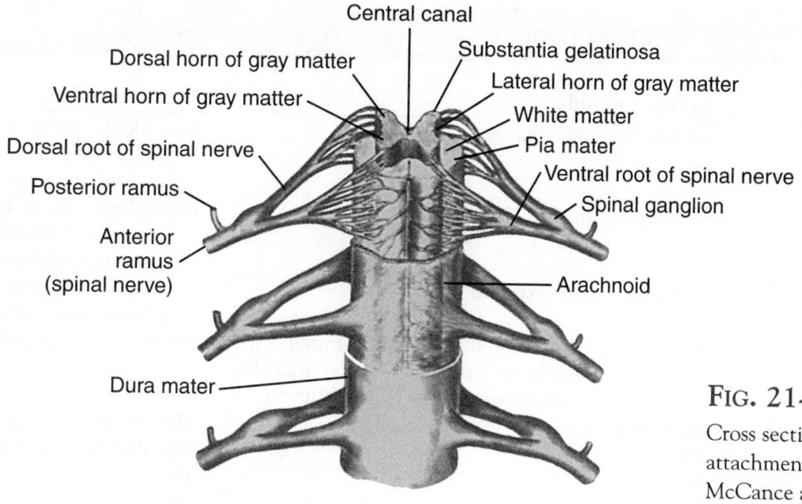

FIG. 21-6
Cross section of spinal cord showing attachments of spinal nerves. (From McCance and Huether.[24])

Treatment is supportive and includes airway management, hyperventilation, and intubation, if necessary. Intravenous diazepam is indicated if seizures do not respond to supportive measures.

Cardiovascular Reactions

Myocardial depression and hypotension may occur. Toxic doses slow the myocardial conduction as evidenced by prolongation of the PR interval and duration of the QRS and sinus bradycardia. Cardiac dysrhythmias are usually short lived; however, they may progress to life-threatening situations that require cardiopulmonary resuscitation (CPR). Hypotension is treated with the administration of intravenous fluids, Trendelenburg's position, and if the patient is not responsive, the IV administration of phenylephrine or ephedrine.

Hypersensitivity Reactions

Allergic reactions are rare. The treatment for anaphylactic reactions is symptomatic and supportive. Bronchoconstriction is treated with epinephrine. Hypotension is treated with the administration of fluids and vasopressor support, as indicated. Urticarial reactions respond to the administration of diphenhydramine; with severe or prolonged reactions the administration of steroids may be necessary.

Methods of Regional Administration

Local infiltration is the injection of a local anesthetic drug, either intradermally or subcutaneously, which produces anesthesia within the site of injection.

Intravenous regional is the IV injection of an anesthetic solution into a limb (usually the arm). Before injection the limb is exsanguinated using an Esmarch bandage, and the vein is occluded with a tourniquet. The effects of the anesthetic last until the tourniquet is deflated. Maximum recommended tourniquet time is 2 hours. After deflation of the tourniquet the local anesthetic is flushed into the venous system. At this time the patient is at risk for toxic reactions; however, such reactions are rare.

In peripheral nerve blocks the local anesthetic is injected at the proximity of a peripheral nerve. The onset of anesthetic effect is rapid and, depending on the drug used, can last for several hours.

Plexus nerve blocks are the injection of a local anesthetic near a nerve plexus. The most common sites are the brachial plexus, the lumbar plexus, and the cervical plexus.

Central nerve blockade includes subarachnoid (spinal) and epidural, including caudal blocks. It is useful to review the anatomy of the spinal cord and meninges. The subarachnoid space contains the cerebrospinal fluid (CSF), spinal nerves, and blood vessels that supply the spinal cord. The epidural space that surrounds the dura mater contains spinal nerve roots, fat, lymphatics, and blood vessels. Caudal blocks use the sacral canal, which contains the terminal portion of the dural sac and a venous plexus—a part of the valveless vertebral venous plexus (FIG. 21-6).

Physiologic Effects of Centroneuraxis Blocks

Centroneuraxis blocks cause sympathetic blockade, as well as motor blockade and sensory analgesia. With pharmacologic sympathetic blockade the normal physiologic compensatory response to changes in blood pressure is obliterated. Venous dilation of the affected blood vessels results in a decrease in blood pressure. The block also interferes with autoregulation of blood pressure, heart rate, myocardial contractility, and vascular resistance. It is important to remember that sympathetic blockade is present at higher levels than sensory blockade—which is higher than motor blockade.

Sensory and motor blocks can be anxiety provoking for patients. High thoracic motor blocks can interfere with movement of the intercostal muscles. Cervical motor blocks interfere with the movement of the diaphragm, and that leads to use of the accessory muscles of respiration. Cervical sensory blocks of C3 to C5 interfere with phrenic innervation, which can block cardiac accelerator fibers.

Spinal anesthesia is the administration of local anesthetic drugs into the subarachnoid space. The drug may be given as a single injection or, with the use of subarachnoid catheters, as a continuous spinal injection. Contraindications to the use of spinal anesthesia include allergy to local anesthetics, increased intracranial pressure, coagulopathy or anticoagulation therapy, sepsis, infections at or near the site of injection, and chronic back pain or deformities.

Table 21-3 Side Effects of Epidural Opioids and Local Anesthetic Agents

Side Effect	Spinal Opioids	Local Anesthetics
Cardiovascular	Minor heart rate changes	Low block (below T_{10}) Sympathetic blockade Postural hypotension
	Usually not postural hypotension	High block (above T_4) Sympathetic blockade Postural hypotension
	Vasoconstrictor response intact	Cardioaccelerator block ↓ heart rate, inotropic drive
Respiratory	Respiratory depression may occur 30 minutes to 16 hours (can be as long as 24 hours) after the injection or after discontinuing the infusion	Respiratory depression may occur immediately after injection
Central nervous system sedation	May be marked	Mild or absent depending on agent or dose
Nausea and/or vomiting	Yes	Yes (usually accompanies hypotension)
Urinary retention	Yes	Yes
Pruritis	Yes	No
Motor blockade and/or weakness	No	Yes, depending on concentrations used

From Fulk and Hadely.[14]

Table 21-4 Differences Between Local Anesthetic Analgesia and Opioid Analgesia

	Opioid Analgesics	Local Anesthetics
Mechanism	Opioid receptors	Nerve roots C fibers A delta fibers
Pathways	Mu pain modulation	Pain Sensory Sympathetic Motor

Complications of spinal anesthesia include hypotension secondary to the sympathetic block. This is self-limiting because the blood pressure returns to normal as the block recedes.

Spinal headaches can result from a small leak of the CSF through the dura. The headache is usually resolved by increasing fluid intake (intravenously or by mouth), by bed rest, and by analgesics. Occasionally the use of an epidural blood patch is necessary to stop the leak.

Epidural anesthesia consists of the administration of local anesthetics into the epidural space. These can be given as a bolus; however, usually they are given through a catheter for repeated injections. The added advantage is that the catheters may be left in place postoperatively for pain management in the form of continuous narcotic infusions or narcotic infusions combined with local anesthetic (Tables 21-2 to 21-4).

Contraindications are the same as for spinal anesthetics. The most serious complication is the inadvertent injection of the drug into the subarachnoid space. Because more drug is needed for epidural anesthesia, this could lead to an unintentional total spinal block. The treatment is supportive until the block recedes. The patient may require intubation with ventilatory support and treatment of the accompanying hypotension. Hypotension secondary to sympathetic blockade is usually less severe than with spinal anesthesia.

Nursing Assessment for Regional Anesthesia

Assessment of the level of motor and sensory block
Hemodynamic monitoring
High risk for fluid volume deficit secondary to venous dilation of sympathetic block
Psychosocial concerns or anxiety secondary to fear of permanent damage
Skin integrity secondary to immobility
Safety related to decreased sensation

POSTOPERATIVE COMPLICATIONS

PULMONARY COMPLICATIONS

Pulmonary complications can be life threatening in the immediate postoperative period. Many complications can be avoided when the care is approached in a collaborative manner with the anesthesiologist. Communication of intraoperative report and preexisting medical conditions may help prevent many complications.

Airway Obstruction

The most common and easily relieved cause of airway obstruction is pharyngeal obstruction by the tongue in an unconscious patient. It can usually be relieved by a chin lift or modified jaw thrust, or by inserting either a nasal or an oral airway until the obstruction is relieved as the patient arouses.

Laryngeal spasm also causes airway obstruction. The presence of mechanical irritants near the glottis by secretions or blood causes the larynx to close. Initial treatment is administration of 100% oxygen by positive-pressure mask. This continuous positive airway pressure (CPAP) is usually sufficient to terminate the laryngospasm. If the complete obstruction continues, it may be necessary to administer a small dose of succinylcholine while hand ventilating the patient by CPAP mask with 100% oxygen. Succinylcholine will relax the vocal cords sufficiently to open the airway and allow ventilation. If an ade-

SOURCES OF LARYNGEAL STIMULATION CAUSING LARYNGOSPASM

Blood
Secretions
Vomitus
Chemical mucosal irritation
Attempted intubation with insufficient anesthesia
Attempted extubation under light anesthesia
Suctioning
Surgical stimulation

From Fetzer-Fowler.[12]

quate airway cannot be established, the patient must be intubated, using direct laryngeal visualization. If the larynx cannot be visualized and the trachea cannot be intubated, an emergency cricothyroidotomy will relieve the obstruction and permit ventilation (see box above).

Airway swelling may also be a cause of postoperative airway obstruction. Glottic edema may be caused by irritation from traumatic intubation, surgical manipulation, excessive coughing on the endotracheal tube, or allergies to the materials used in the endotracheal tube. Subglottic edema is seen in small children because of anatomic differences in their airway. In small children the larynx is made up of loose areolar tissue and the cricoid ring is the narrowest part of the larynx.

The treatment of both glottic and subglottic edema is administration of warm humidified oxygen by mask, nebulized racemic epinephrine, and, if edema is unrelieved, dexamethasone intravenously or by inhaler.

Hypoxemia

Hypoxemia can be defined as decreased arterial oxygen tension. With the advent of pulse oximetry it is easy to identify; however, the cause may be difficult to find. Common causes of hypoxemia in the postanesthetic period are low concentrations of inspired oxygen, hypoventilation, and ventilation-perfusion mismatch, including intrapulmonary right-to-left shunts.

As a rule, all patients who have had general anesthesia should have supplemental oxygen; in rare instances, oxygen is contraindicated.

Hypoventilation is defined as reduced alveolar gas exchange, resulting in an increase in arterial carbon dioxide levels. Causes include the respiratory depressant effects of anesthetics and narcotics, poor respiratory muscle function secondary to inadequate reversal of muscle relaxants, or previous pulmonary disease. Postoperative respiratory depression, resulting from narcotics, can be reversed with small doses of Narcan without affecting the pain-relieving properties of the narcotics.

Respiratory muscle function may be affected by incomplete reversal of neuromuscular blocking agents. Muscle relaxants may need to be pharmacologically reversed. Factors that interfere with reversal of neuromuscular blocking agents include inadequate renal excretion of the drug secondary to renal failure; use of antibiotics, such as gentamicin, neomycin, or clindamycin, which potentiate the neuromuscular blockade; and respiratory acidosis, which limits or prevents the antagonism of the neuromuscular blocking agent.

Surgical causes for hypoventilation include incisions of the upper abdomen or thorax, gastric dilation, and tight restrictive dressings. Obesity is also a factor in hypoventilation because total lung volume and functional residual capacity are reduced. Treatment is directed toward the underlying cause for the hypoventilation. If pain is the cause for splinting in patients with upper abdominal or thoracic incisions, regional nerve blocks or small doses of narcotics may be warranted.

Patients with preexisting pulmonary disease are at high risk for postoperative pulmonary complications.

By its nature the physiologic process of respiration is not static but dynamic. Oxygenation of venous blood is accomplished by ventilation of the alveoli with air and perfusion of the pulmonary capillaries with blood. Oxygen diffuses from the alveoli into the pulmonary circulation. Carbon dioxide diffuses from the capillaries into the alveoli and is exhaled. In normal healthy individuals there are physiologic variations of ventilation and perfusion. Disease states can alter this ratio in different ways. Right-to-left shunts occur when blood reaches the arterial system without passing through ventilated areas of the lung. At rest, normal physiologic shunting is between 2% and 5% of cardiac output.

Postoperatively the most common cause of increased right-to-left shunting is atelectasis. Atelectatic portions of the lung are perfused; however, they are not ventilated because of the alveolar collapse. Atelectasis may be caused by secretions and hypoventilation.

Pneumothorax may be caused by central line placement, incidental surgical manipulation, or tears in the pleura or regional anesthesia (i.e., intercostal nerve blocks). Pneumothorax causes hypoxemia because of atelectasis and intrapulmonary shunting. A small pneumothorax of less than 20% (in a healthy individual with no mechanical ventilation) usually resorbs spontaneously. A pneumothorax of greater than 20%, or a pneumothorax in any patient who is mechanically ventilated should be treated with the insertion of chest tubes.

Postoperative pulmonary edema is a rare but life-threatening complication of general anesthesia. Causes may be cardiac or noncardiac. Treatment for cardiac pulmonary edema is directed toward improving left ventricular function. Noncardiac pulmonary edema is related to injury of the capillary membrane. In the postanesthetic period it may be caused by aspiration, blood transfusion reaction, or upper airway obstruction (see box, p. 1354). Pulmonary edema following upper airway obstruction is probably caused by reduction in interstitial hydrostatic pressure. A dramatic pressure difference between the interstitium and capillary causes transudation of fluid through the membrane. Unilateral pulmonary edema may be present postoperatively if, during surgery, the patient has been placed in a lateral position. The dependent lung receives most of the perfusion, while the superior lung receives most of the ventilation. The increase in hydrostatic pressure of the dependent lung causes unilateral pulmonary edema. Treatment for noncardiac pulmonary edema is directed at supporting gas exchange across the interstitium until the alveolar-capillary membrane can be stabilized.

Pulmonary embolism caused by either thromboemboli or fat emboli are rare postoperative complications. The thrombi block the pulmonary artery, which leads to areas of the lung that are ventilated but are not perfused. This increases physiologic dead space and shunting (see Pulmonary Embolism on p. 191).

DISEASE STATES ASSOCIATED WITH NONCARDIAC PULMONARY EDEMA (NCPE)

Sepsis
Fat or air embolism
Smoke inhalation
Pancreatitis
Oxygen toxicity
Inhaled chemical-induced lung injury
Near-drowning
Transfusion reaction
High-altitude rapid ascent
Postreexpansion of lung
Uremia
Postradiation of pulmonary system
Aspiration of gastric contents
Drug ingestion
Interstitial viral pneumonia
Disseminated intravascular coagulation
Craniocerebral trauma
Traumatic pulmonary contusion

From Fetzer-Fowler.[12]

Aspiration of gastric contents is prevented in the normal, awake individual by the gastroesophageal and pharyngoesophageal sphincters. General anesthetics and narcotics may depress these protective mechanisms, putting patients at risk for aspiration. The degree of injury to the lung parenchyma is related to the pH of the fluid and the volume aspirated. Gastric pH of less than 2.5 causes chemical pneumonitis, local edema, and inflammation. Preventive measures include maintenance of nothing by mouth (NPO) status, use of H_2 blockers, and antacids. Patients at high risk for aspiration include those with intestinal obstruction, increased intraabdominal pressure, pregnancy, obesity, hiatal hernia, and emergency surgery when NPO status cannot be verified.

PAIN

Virtually all patients undergoing surgical manipulation have acute pain afterward. Postsurgical cellular and tissue damage excites nociceptors (pain-sensitive nerve fibers). Injury is believed to stimulate the release of neurotransmitters that serve as algesic substances. They include prostaglandins, histamine, serotonin, bradykinin, and arachidonic acid. Prostaglandins lower the nociceptive threshold.

After stimulation of the nociceptors, pain impulses are relayed via the afferent nerve fibers through the dorsal horn of the spinal cord. Thinly myelinated A delta and unmyelinated C fibers transmit to the neuraxis. A delta nociceptive fibers transmit sharp pain. A delta fibers transmit impulses that pass to the anterior and anterolateral horns to provoke segmental reflex responses. These responses are responsible for increased muscle tone, skeletal muscle spasm, increased oxygen consumption, and lactic acid production. C nociceptive fibers transmit burning, dull aching types of pain.

Other impulses are transmitted to higher centers via spinothalamic and spinoreticular tracts that initiate suprasegmental and cortical responses. Suprasegmental reflex response further increases oxygen consumption, sympathetic tone, and endocrine function. Cortical responses are concerned with integration and perception of pain. The individual psychologic response of increased apprehension and anxiety further increases hypothalamic stimulation. These emotional responses appear to facilitate nociceptive transmission in the spinal cord and lower the pain threshold.

High-dose narcotics may delay the transmission of stimuli through A delta and C fibers. The reflex phenomena of muscle spasm associated with pain are not modified by narcotics.

Many complex theories of pain perception have been suggested. The current belief is that pain has a sensory and a reactive component. Three current theories on pain perception involve specificity, pattern, and gate. The specificity theory suggests that specific fibers conduct specific sensations that terminate at specific sites in the CNS. Pattern theory suggests that after initiation of painful impulses a pattern-generating mechanism can be established in the dorsal horn, causing pain perception even though no stimuli are present. The gate theory suggests that pain impulses can be modulated in the brain or spinal cord.

Opioid receptors are located in the midbrain and dorsal horn. The highest concentrations are found in the limbic system, substantia gelatinosa, and laminae I, II, and V of the dorsal horn. The term *opioid* refers to drugs that are derivatives of opium or are synthetically made to produce similar effects. Opioids are used primarily for analgesia; they react with specific opioid receptors. Opioids are chemically similar to the naturally occurring peptides, the enkephalins, the endorphins, and the dynorphins.

There are four major categories of opioid receptors in the CNS. Mu receptors mediate supraspinal analgesia, feelings of well-being, morphinelike physical dependence, and respiratory depression. Kappa receptors are responsible for sedation with minimal respiratory depression. Sigma receptors cause dysphoric states with rapid thoughts and altered visual and auditory perceptions. Delta receptors cause alterations in affective behavior.

Drugs can interact with opioid receptors in different ways. Opioid agonists are drugs that stimulate the opioid receptors, causing analgesia. Opioid antagonists are drugs that reverse the effects of the opioid agonists. Opioid agonist-antagonists are drugs that act as agonists at some receptors and antagonists at other sites.

Morphine remains the standard by which all analgesics are measured (Table 21-5).

Fentanyl and its derivatives, sufentanil and alfentanil, are frequently used during anesthesia. The onset of action following IV administration is very rapid, and the incidence of incomplete amnesia, hypotension, and hypertension is less than with morphine. Fentanyl and its derivatives are sometimes used postoperatively when rapid control of pain is warranted. Fentanyl can also be used via the epidural route for patients allergic to morphine.

Remifentanil is a new ultrashort-acting synthetic opiod that is chemically related to fentanyl.

Adverse Effects of Pain

Cardiovascular System

The increased stimulation of sympathetic neurons causes tachycardia, increased stroke volume, and increased cardiac work, increasing myocardial oxygen consumption. Hypercoagulation

Table 21-5 Equipotency of Narcotics

Morphine (mg)	Demerol (mg)	Dilaudid (mg)	Fentanyl (micrograms)
1			12.5
1.33	10		
2			25.0
2.5		0.5	
3.325	25		
4			50.0
5		1.0	
6			75.0
6.65	50		
7.5		1.5	
8			100.0
10	75	2.0	125.0

and decreased mobility increase the risk of deep vein thrombosis and pulmonary embolism.

Respiratory System

Pain associated with upper abdominal or thoracic surgery causes spasm and splinting of the abdominal and intercostal muscles, decreasing the ability to cough and breathe deeply. It also decreases the vital capacity and inspiratory capacity, as well as the functional residual capacity. Surgery on peripheral parts of the body does not appear to alter lung volumes.

Nursing Assessment of Pain

Pain is a subjective experience for patients. The North American Nursing Diagnosis Association (NANDA) defines pain as "a state in which an individual experiences and reports the presence of severe discomfort or an uncomfortable sensation." A patient's rights include an adequate assessment and treatment of pain.

It is sometimes difficult for the nurse to understand the severity and quality of the patient's pain. To objectify the pain as much as possible, it is helpful to obtain as much objective data as possible. In all cases it is important to determine the site of the pain, as well as its type. Using a visual analog scale or verbal integer scale of 0 to 10, with 0 being no pain and 10 being the worst pain imaginable, gives a clear picture of the intensity of the pain and enables the nurse to determine the effects of pain management therapy. Objective signs of pain are the sympathetic responses of tachycardia, hypertension, diaphoresis, and pallor, as well as grimacing facies and a splinting respiratory pattern. In the immediate postanesthetic period, these signs may be the first indication of the patient's pain. Judicious use of narcotics at this time can stall the deleterious sympathetic effects of pain. To objectify pain levels for infants, toddlers, and children, see the pediatric pain and discomfort scale (Table 21-6).

The traditional method of pain management postoperatively is intramuscular or IV narcotic administration. Narcotics are administered at the request of the patient or when objective assessment deems it necessary. However, this method is frequently inadequate because the pain may be too intense or the treatment may come too late. Following intramuscular administration, the absorption of the drug is variable, which delays

Table 21-6 Pediatric Pain and Discomfort Scale

Observation	Criteria	Points
Blood pressure	±10% preop	0
	>20% preop	1
	>30% preop	2
Crying	Not crying	0
	Cries, but responds to TLC*	1
	Cries, but does not respond to TLC	2
Movement	None	0
	Restless	1
	Thrashing	2
Agitation	Patient asleep or calm	0
	Mild	1
	Hysterical	2
Posture	No special posture	0
	Flexing legs and thighs	1
	Holding scrotum and groin†	2
Complains of pain (where appropriate by age)	Asleep, or states no pain	0
	Cannot localize	1
	Can localize	2

From Wilson and Graves.[35]
**TLC,* tender loving care.
†Used to assess analgesic effectiveness following orchiopexy.

the effectiveness of the drug. Following IV administration of narcotics, the uptake of the drug is more rapid and more predictable. However, intermittent boluses of narcotic will result in peaks and troughs of plasma concentration. At peak levels, pain perception may be obliterated; however, an increased risk for respiratory depression exists. At trough levels, the plasma concentration may be too low for analgesia.

Ketorolac is a nonsteroidal antiinflammatory drug (NSAID). It provides pain relief effectively for the postsurgical patient and is often used in combination with opioids. Its onset is slower than opiods (75 minutes), but it lasts longer, thereby providing a longer period of pain relief.

With patient-controlled analgesia (PCA), patients can administer a small dose of narcotic when pain occurs. PCA pumps can be programmed to deliver narcotics at a basal rate hourly, as well as allowing the patient to self-administer predetermined doses at set time intervals. Studies have shown that patients using PCA maintain plasma concentrations at a consistent level. Patient acceptance and satisfaction are high with PCA.

Epidural and subarachnoid narcotics have a significant advantage over other types of pain management. They produce prolonged, intense segmental analgesia without the deleterious side effects of respiratory depression or sympathetic disturbance. These narcotics affect the nociceptive pathways in the dorsal horn by interacting with the mu opiate receptors. They do not affect proprioception or motor and sensory function. Epidural narcotics can be administered in a bolus, a continuous drip, or a combination of both; they also can be mixed with local anesthetics. Following administration of a narcotic into the epidural space, epidural narcotics cross into the spinal fluid and into the epidural veins, where vascular absorption occurs.

Subarachnoid narcotics are administered as a bolus injection. Analgesia tends to be more profound; however, this route is also associated with a higher incidence of side effects. The incidence of respiratory depression peaks between 6 and 10 hours after injection. Pruritus occurs in approximately 10% of patients receiving spinal narcotics. Naloxone (Narcan) is the narcotic antagonist of choice to reverse these unwanted side effects. With doses of 1 to 2 μg/kg there is little effect on the analgesia. Narcan has a high affinity for all opioid receptors; however, its affinity for mu receptors is generally higher than for kappa or delta receptors. The incidence of nausea, vomiting, and urinary retention is similar to that for patients receiving parenteral narcotics (see Table 21-3).

Cardiovascular Complications

Hypotension

Hypotension is frequently seen in the immediate postoperative phase of recovery. The most common cause is hypovolemia secondary to fluid volume depletion. This can be the result of blood loss, third space fluid shifts, or unreplaced insensible fluid losses. The treatment consists of replacement of the fluid volume losses, institution of Trendelenburg's position, and, if the patient is unresponsive, small doses of a vasopressor, such as ephedrine or Neo-Synephrine, administered IV.

Hypotension may also be secondary to residual myocardial depression from the anesthetic or, more seriously, from perioperative myocardial ischemia or infarction. Prompt differential diagnosis and treatment are essential because hypotension leads to hypoperfusion of vital organs. Cardiac hypoperfusion leads to further ischemia and damage. Patients at risk for cardiac disease, or those who have had myocardial infarctions in the past, are at greater risk than the general population for perioperative myocardial infarction. Patients who have had infarctions more than 6 months previously have reinfarction rates of 1.9% to 8%. Patients with a more recent history—less than 3 months since infarction—have reinfarction rates as high as 37%. Patients having perioperative myocardial infarctions have mortality rates from 36% to 70% (see box above, right).

Surgical causes of hypotension include bleeding at the surgical site or at sites of central venous catheter insertion. Inadvertent puncture of the pleura can lead to pneumothorax or hemothorax.

Hypertension

Hypertension is common in the early postanesthesia phase. The most common causes are pain, hypercapnia, hypoxemia, or fluid volume overload. Treatment of these causes usually resolves the hypertension. If the condition is unresolved, the administration of antihypertensive medications is necessary. Hypertension is usually transient, and drug therapy is necessary for a few hours. Drugs frequently used are short-acting beta-blockers, such as propranolol, labetalol, and esmolol. Nitroprusside is used because it is fast acting and because its results are rapidly reversed after the drug is discontinued. If the patient is at risk for myocardial ischemia, nitroglycerin may be administered IV or nifedipine may be given sublingually. Hydralazine is sometimes used; however, its onset of action is slow compared with that of newer antihypertensive drugs, and it causes a reflex tachycardia that may be detrimental to patients with increased cardiac risk factors.

PATIENTS AT RISK FOR PERIOPERATIVE MYOCARDIAL INFARCTION

- History of myocardial infarction within the last 6 months
- Preexisting coronary artery disease or diffuse multivessel disease
- History of disabling angina
- Congestive heart failure
- Severe preoperative myocardial ischemia
- Fluid and electrolyte imbalance
- Debilitated health
- Elderly
- Undetected medical problems
- Diabetes
- Obesity
- Emergency surgery
- Abdominal, intrathoracic, and vascular surgery
- Prolonged anesthesia time

Hypothermia

The incidence of iatrogenic hypothermia is between 60% and 80% of all postoperative patients. Hypothermia is defined as a core body temperature of less than 36° C. Metabolic heat production and thermoregulation are depressed with general anesthetics. Regional anesthetics can cause hypothermia by depressing regional thermal sensations, vasoconstriction, and shivering. Shivering-like activity occurs in approximately 40% of postanesthesia patients. However, not all patients who shiver are hypothermic, suggesting that hypothermia is just one cause of the mechanism of shivering. Shivering increases the metabolic rate and therefore increases oxygen consumption, as well as carbon dioxide production. If the patient also has some degree of respiratory depression, the deficit in oxygen supply may lead to anaerobic metabolism and lactic acidosis. This is especially dangerous for patients at risk for cardiac ischemia.

Shivering also exacerbates pain. Treatment is preventive, as well as supportive. Patients who shiver should have supplemental oxygen and external warming.

A focused thermal environment (i.e., Bair Hugger) can be placed over the patient postoperatively. The temperature is set to high, medium, or low. The patient's temperature should be taken hourly to document rewarming. Meperidine in small doses (25 to 30 mg) is helpful in decreasing shivering.

Hyperthermia

Malignant hyperthermia (MH) is a rare but potentially fatal complication of general anesthesia. The onset of symptoms usually occurs during the induction of anesthesia but in rare instances may occur in the PACU. It is an inherited disorder that is triggered by anesthetic agents. In patients who are genetically predisposed to MH, the triggering agent interferes with the reentry of calcium into the sarcoplasmic reticulum.

This hypercalcemic state activates metabolic pathways that deplete adenosine triphosphate, causing metabolic acidosis, membrane destruction, and cellular death. Dantrolene sodium is given intravenously as soon as a diagnosis of MH is made. Dantrolene sodium acts by decreasing the amount of calcium released from the sarcoplasmic reticulum. Treatment is supportive, correcting hypoxemia and acidosis, reducing fever,

Table 21-7 Antiemetics Used After Anesthesia

Drug	Adult Dose (mg)	Action	Side Effect/Contraindications
Dolasetron mesylate (Anzemet)	12.5 mg	Antinauseant Antiemetic	Electrocardiogram interval changes
Prochlorperazine (Compazine)	5-10 IM	Antiemetic Neuroleptic	Increased incidence of dystonia Contraindicated for patients with bone marrow depression
Droperidol (Inapsine)	0.625-1.25 IV	Antiemetic Neuroleptic Antagonizes emetic effect of opioids that act on CTZ	Drowsiness Extrapyramidal symptoms Potentiates other CNS depressants
Promethazine HCl (Phenergan)	25-50 IM, IV, or PO	Antihistamine Antiemetic Thought to depress CTZ in medulla	CNS depression Disturbed coordination
Metoclopramide (Regian)	10 IV over 1-2 min	Cholinergic Antiemetic Increased CTZ threshold enhances gastric emptying	Contraindicated in seizure disorders
Scopolamine patch	Transdermal patch releases 0.5 mg over 3 days Applied to skin preoperatively	Anticholinergic	CNS depression Disorientation Urinary retention

monitoring electrolytes, and assessing renal function for acute tubular necrosis secondary to myoglobinuria.

Nausea and Vomiting

Postoperative nausea and vomiting can be caused by anesthetics and opioids that affect the vestibular portion of the inner ear, the chemoreceptor trigger zone (CTZ), and vomiting centers in the brain. Other causes for postoperative nausea and vomiting include increasing intracranial pressure, severe dehydration, and fluid and electrolyte imbalance. Factors that influence the incidence of postoperative nausea and vomiting include the use of general anesthesia by mask technique, patient history of motion sickness, or previous postoperative nausea and vomiting, intraabdominal surgery, prolonged anesthesia, and obesity.

Treatment is preventive, supportive, and pharmacologic (Table 21-7). Patients at high risk for aspiration are pretreated with drugs that increase the pH of gastric contents or that facilitate gastric motility. Nasogastric tubes can be used to empty gastric contents. The use of antiemetics intraoperatively and postoperatively reduces the incidence of nausea and vomiting. Vigilant nursing observation is the primary means of preventing aspiration in the PACU.

NURSING CARE

POSTANESTHESIA PATIENT

NURSING ASSESSMENT

Respiratory status

Signs of upper airway obstruction, stridor, retractions, asynchronous or asymmetric chest movement

Laryngospasm, high-pitched squeaky respirations with partial to total airway obstruction

Diminished breath sounds, evaluate inspiratory and expiratory wheezing, rales, rhonchi, or any abnormality

Residual neuromuscular blockade; weak inspiratory effort; inability to lift head; or inadequate muscle strength

Cardiovascular status: Cardiac output has returned to baseline as indicated by blood pressure, cardiac rate and rhythm, and, if present, central venous pressures and pulmonary artery pressures

Neurologic status: Arouses easily to name; follows simple instructions; mobility at preoperative level

Pain and discomfort: Level of pain tolerable to patient

Incision/wound site: Bleeding, integrity, drainage

Gastrointestinal status: Abatement of nausea or vomiting

Genitourinary status: Absence of bladder distention

Musculoskeletal status: Absence of sensory, motor, or perceptual deficits

Primary disease states: Evaluation and maintenance of therapy for primary medical disease.

PATIENT PROBLEMS/NURSING DIAGNOSES & INTERVENTIONS

NIC RESPIRATORY MANAGEMENT

Ineffective breathing pattern
Impaired gas exchange
Ineffective airway clearance

- Assess upper airway for signs of obstruction.
- Assess rate and depth of respirations, as well as chest movement; note air exchange at nose and mouth.
- Continuously monitor oxygen saturation; administer oxygen per physician's order *to maintain saturation greater than 95%.*
- Suction oropharynx, as necessary, *to prevent potential aspiration of gastric contents.*
- Position patient *to maximize respiratory pattern;* if patient is awake, raise head of bed to 30 degrees; if there is partial airway obstruction or high risk for aspiration, place the patient on his or her side.
- Identify factors contributing to airway obstruction, such as inhalational anesthetics, narcotics, and muscle relaxants.

- Identify surgical interventions that may alter breathing pattern and contribute to upper airway obstruction.
- Maintain patient in proper alignment *to facilitate opening of the upper airway:* chin lift, jaw thrust, and hyperextension of the head; if obstruction is unrelieved by these measures, insert nasal or oral airway; if obstruction remains unrelieved, notify physician; patient may need to be endotracheally intubated.
- If mechanical ventilation becomes necessary, provide care and monitoring consistent with accepted guidelines.
- Observe closely because patients are at risk for atelectasis and right-to-left shunt, secondary to anesthetic agents; immobility during prolonged surgical procedure; physiologic splinting caused by pain, especially high abdominal or thoracic surgical sites; and preexisting disease states (see Atelectasis, Chapter 4).
- Assess breath sounds to determine areas of hypoventilation and the possibility of interstitial pulmonary edema; if endotracheal tube is present, determine that the tube is in the correct position; *absence of breath sounds on the left side may indicate right mainstem intubation.*
- Position patient *to maximize expansion of the lungs.*
- Encourage patient to deep breathe and cough; begin use of incentive spirometry *to facilitate maximum expansion of the lungs.*
- Administer narcotics *to decrease splinting and anxiety.*
- Identify primary disease states that may contribute to impaired gas exchange; initiate treatment according to prescribed orders.
- Monitor arterial blood gases *to assess level of hypoxia and hypercarbia.*
- Monitor end-tidal carbon dioxide levels *to follow course of hypercarbia.*
- Anticipate potential ventilation problems by having emergency equipment at hand to mask-ventilate patient with positive pressure.
- Assess patient to determine if patient is able to mobilize secretions; if patient is unable, assist patient to cough by splinting area of surgery with pillows or blankets; note characteristics of cough and secretions; suction if necessary.
- Turn patient *to mobilize secretions;* provide chest physical therapy, as needed.
- Administer nebulized medications as prescribed by physician *to dilate bronchioles; assist with expectoration of secretions.*

NIC TISSUE PERFUSION MANAGEMENT

Decreased cardiac output
Risk for imbalanced fluid volume

- Monitor vitals signs at least every 15 minutes *to assess for signs of left ventricular failure secondary to ischemia; fluid volume deficit; fluid volume overload; primary disease state; hypoxia; and myocardial depression secondary to inhalational agents;* continuously monitor electrocardiogram (ECG) rhythm for tachycardia, bradycardia, dysrhythmias, and signs of cardiac ischemia.
- Assess for symptoms of decreased cardiac output, including hypotension, tachycardia, pallor, or diaphoresis.
- Monitor hemodynamic parameters, if present, *to evaluate patient's clinical status.*
- Review patient's preoperative history and ECG *to determine level of preexisting cardiac disease;* note if patient has taken routinely prescribed medications the morning of surgery.
- Evaluate urine output hourly if Foley catheter is present; if there is no Foley catheter present, palpate bladder *to check for bladder distention.*
- Monitor vital signs at least every 15 minutes *to assess for hypovolemia secondary to blood loss, insensible fluid loss, or relative hypovolemia caused by vasodilation secondary to autonomic nerve blocks.*
- Monitor intake and output, mindful of the type of surgical procedure; crystalloid, colloid, and blood replacement; surgical drains; and wound dressings.
- Administer crystalloids and colloids, as ordered, *to maintain cardiac output, as well as renal, cerebral, and all other tissue perfusion.*
- Initiate Trendelenburg's position *to increase preload.*
- Administer vasoactive drugs, as ordered, *to improve cardiac contractility and peripheral vascular resistance.*
- Monitor electrolytes and hematocrit *to evaluate blood and fluid loss and the effectiveness of replacement therapy.*
- Monitor urine output hourly if Foley catheter is present; note specific gravity of urine *to determine concentration of urine.*

NIC PHYSICAL COMFORT PROMOTION

Acute pain

- Assess location of pain *to differentiate surgical pain from other types of pain, including cardiac, bladder, headache, spasm, pressure areas from surgical positioning, or restrictive dressings.*
- Using a visual or verbal analog scale (VAS), ask patient to rate pain from 0 to 10 *to objectify level of pain.* Record the results clearly *to assist in regular assessment and follow-up.* This allows nurse to assess effectiveness of pain-relieving medications.
- Provide medications *to alleviate pain.*
- Provide a calm, nurturing atmosphere for patient.
- Assure patient that you will continue to provide pain medications until pain is at a tolerable level.
- Position patient in a comfortable position.
- If using patient-controlled analgesia, teach patient to administer medications whenever he or she has pain; assure patient that he or she will not be able to overdose because of safety features programmed into computer.
- Observe patient for nonverbal signs of pain, including restlessness, agitation, grimacing, hypertension, tachycardia, and diaphoresis; keep in mind that these signs can indicate hypoxia or hypercarbia; sedating a patient who is hypoxic or hypercarbic is contraindicated.
- Determine if patient has been taking pain-relieving medications preoperatively; if so, this may increase patient's tolerance to narcotics, causing him or her to require higher-than-average doses of narcotics.

NIC SKIN/WOUND MANAGEMENT

Impaired skin integrity related to incision from surgical procedure or insertion sites of drainage devices

- Assess visible incision site for approximation of wound edges, dehiscence, evisceration, drainage, erythema, and edema.
- Monitor incision site and dressing for any changes in the type, color, amount, or consistency of any drainage *to identify any unexpected changes.*
- Reinforce dressing as needed, and notify physician if drainage is excessive.
- Keep skin clean and dry around incision/dressing *to prevent erosion of skin from moisture/drainage.*
- Position patient in a normal anatomic position that protects incisional site from pressure, friction, or restraint *to protect from trauma.*
- Reposition patient periodically to relieve constant pressure on skin surfaces and bony prominences *to maintain skin integrity.*
- Monitor color, warmth, sensation, and pulses of affected extremity of surgical procedure *to identify any decrease in circulation.*
- Place cold or ice pack on surgical site, if ordered, *to prevent or reduce edema.*
- Observe insertion site of drainage tubes or catheters *to ensure they are secure.*
- Secure catheters and tubes *to prevent pulling sensation and tension on tissue or dislodgement.*
- Monitor drainage tubes and collection devices *to identify excess blood loss.*
- Label each drainage tube if there are more than one *to allow for accurate assessment of output from each system.*
- Note the amount and describe characteristics of drainage from each drainage tube separately *to identify correct source of unexpected volume, color, or consistency.*
- Ensure that catheters and tubes are patent and not kinked *to promote optimal drainage and prevent pressure on wound from backflow of drainage.*
- Encircle drainage site on a cast, and note date and time *to determine extension of bleeding.*
- Position patients with external fixator devices in a manner that prevents pressure or friction on the device *to prevent trauma to surrounding skin.*
- Check insertion site of chest tubes and surrounding area for air leaks *to avoid pneumothorax.*
- Ensure patency of chest tubes and avoid any blockage to underwater-seal system *to avoid a tension pneumothorax.*
- Maintain closed water-seal drainage for chest tubes lower than patient's chest *to prevent backflow of drainage into chest.*
- Observe water-seal drainage system of chest tubes for normal fluctuations when patient inhales (fluid level rises during inhalation and falls during exhalation) *to identify normal function of sealed drainage system.*

EVALUATION/PATIENT OUTCOMES

Respiratory Management: Airway is patent. Patient's respirations are normal; no signs of upper airway obstruction. Patient's breathing is coordinated between thorax and abdomen; accessory muscles of respiration are not used. Patient's breath sounds are clear to auscultation. Oxygen saturation is greater than 95% when breathing room air; if not, supplemental oxygen is administered.

Tissue Perfusion Management: Cardiovascular function has returned to preoperative level. Patient's blood pressure has returned to within 20 mm Hg of baseline for at least 30 minutes. There are no changes in the ECG readings, and there is an absence of dysrhythmias. Patient's heart rate is between 60 and 100 beats per minute. For children, the heart rate should be ±20 beats per minute from preoperative baseline. Patient's skin is warm and dry, peripheral pulses are present at preoperative level, and capillary refill time is less than 3 seconds. Patient's urine output is greater than 30 ml/h for adults and 0.5 ml/kg/h for children. Patient's sensory and motor blockade has receded following regional anesthesia.

Physical Comfort Promotion: Comfort and pain levels are satisfactory for patient. Patient shows an absence of nonverbal signs of pain: restlessness, anxiety, or grimacing. Patient verbalizes comfort level. If using patient-controlled analgesia for pain management, patient is able to correctly self-administer and understands mechanism for use. If using conventional pain management, patient is able to identify when to request pain medications.

Skin/Wound Management: Incision site is intact. Drainage amount, color, and consistency from incision site, drainage tubes, and catheters are within normal limits. Drainage tubes and catheters are secure, patent, and there is no backflow. Skin is warm with color indicative of adequate tissue perfusion. There is no evidence of a potential pressure ulcer.

REFERENCES

1. American Hospital Association: *Patient's bill of rights,* Chicago, 1992, The Association.
2. American Nurses Association: *The code for nurses with interpretive statements,* Kansas City, 1985, The Association.
3. AORN, Inc: *Perioperative nursing process.* Denver, 1990, The Association.
4. AORN, Inc: *Perioperative nursing data set: the perioperative nursing vocabulary* (Beyea, SC, editor), Denver, 2000, The Association.
5. AORN, Inc: *Standards, recommended practices and guidelines 2001 with official AORN statements,* Denver, 2001, The Association.
6. AORN, Inc: *The PNDS in action: perioperative documentation,* Denver, 2001, The Association.

6a. Beyea SC: The ideal state for perioperative nursing, *AORN J,* 73:5, 2001.

7. Botsford J: *Care-tracing: case management in the OR,* presented at the 42nd Annual AORN Congress, Atlanta, March 8, 1995.
8. Capuuno TA: Clinical pathways: practical outcomes. *Nurs Manage* 26:1, 1995.
9. Drain CB, Shipley CS: *Recovery room: a critical care approach,* Philadelphia, 1987, WB Saunders.
10. Drasner K, Katz JA, Schapera A: Control of pain and anxiety. In Wood K, editor: *Principles of critical care medicine,* New York, 1991, McGraw-Hill.

11. Dripps RD, Echenhogg JE, Vandam LD: *Introduction to anesthesia,* ed 8, Philadelphia, 1989, WB Saunders.
12. Fetzer-Fowler SJ: Managing sympathetic blockade in the post anesthesia care unit. *J Post Anesth Nurs* 9(1):34, 1994.
13. Firestone LL: *Clinical anesthesia procedures of the Massachusetts General Hospital,* ed 3, Boston, 1988, Little, Brown.
14. Fulk C, Hadely JC: Something new for pain: new trends in epidural analgesia. *J Post Anesth Nurs* 5:1, 1990.
15. Goodman AG, Gilman LS: *The pharmacological basis of therapeutics,* ed 8, New York, 1990, Macmillan.
16. Grimaldi PL: A glossary of managed care terms, *Nurs Manage* 27(suppl 10):5, 1996.
17. Gruendemann BJ, Fernsebner B: *Comprehensive perioperative nursing,* Boston, 1995, Jones & Bartlett.
18. Hudak C, Gallo BM, Morton PG: *Critical care nursing: a holistic approach,* New York, 1998, JB Lippincott.
19. Joint Commission on Accreditation of Healthcare Organizations: *2001 hospital accreditation standards,* Oakbrook Terrace, Ill, 2001, The Commission.
20. Kleinbeck SVM: Developing nursing diagnoses for a perioperative care plan: a classroom research project, *AORN J* 49:1613, 1989.
21. Kneedler J, Dodge G: *Perioperative patient care,* ed 3, Boston, 1994, Jones & Bartlett.
22. Litwack K: *Core curriculum for perianesthesia nursing practice,* Philadelphia, 1998, WB Saunders.
23. Maslow AH: *Motivation and personality,* New York, 1970, Harper & Row.
24. McCance KM, Huether S: *Pathophysiology: the biologic basis of disease in adults and children,* ed 2, St. Louis, 1994, Mosby.
25. Meeker MH, Rothrock JC: *Alexander's care of the patient in surgery,* ed 11, St. Louis, 1999, Mosby.
26. Miller RD: *Anesthesia,* ed 4, New York, 1994, Churchill Livingstone.
27. Miller RD, Stocking RK: *Basics of anesthesia,* ed 3, New York, 1994, Churchill Livingstone.
28. Morgan GE, Mikhail MS: *Clinical anesthesiology,* Norwalk, Conn, 1992, Appleton & Lange.
29. Rothrock JC: *Perioperative nursing care planning,* ed 2, St. Louis, 1996, Mosby.
30. Schroeter K: Pain management: ethical issues for the perianesthesia nurse, *J Perianesth Nurs* 14(6):393, 1999.
31. Stein RS: The perioperative nurse's role in anesthesia management. *AORN J* 62:794, 1995.
32. Thelan LA, Davie JK, Urden LD: *Textbook of critical care nursing: diagnosis and management,* St. Louis, 1994, Mosby.
33. Warren JJ, Bickford C: ANA recognized nursing data sets, classification systems, nomenclatures, *Briefing book,* nursing vocabulary summit conference, Nashville, Tenn, June 10-13, 1999.
34. Way LW: *Current surgical diagnosis and treatment,* ed 8, Norwalk, Conn, 1988, Appleton & Lange.
35. Wilson TA, Graves SA; Pediatric considerations in a general postanesthesia care unit, *J Post Anesth Nurs* 5:1, 1990.

PART IV

DIAGNOSTIC STUDIES AND LABORATORY VALUES

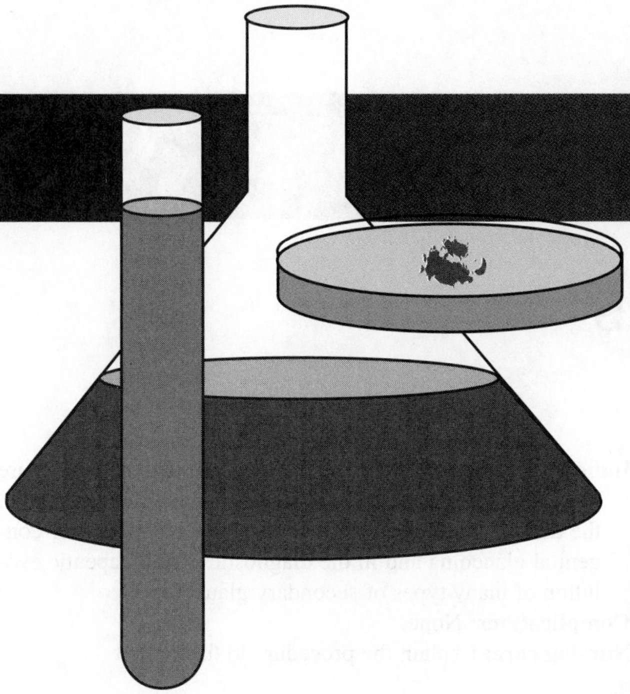

22

Care of the Patient Undergoing Diagnostic Studies and Laboratory Tests

Joan LaBarr
James Hill
Nikky Chahon

Diagnostic Studies

VISUALIZATION STUDIES

Direct Ophthalmoscopy

Description: The examiner uses an ophthalmoscope to view the retinal surface and inner structures of the eye. The pupils are usually dilated, and examination takes place in a dark room. Retinal structures and vessels are magnified 15 times.

Indications: Used for diagnosis and visualization of the optic disk, arteries, veins, retina, choroid, and media and for evaluation of significant ocular and systemic disease. About half of the fundus may be seen.

Complications: Caution should be used when dilating the pupil of a patient with a shallow anterior chamber to avoid precipitating an attack of angle-closure glaucoma. Soft contact lenses should be removed before pupil dilation, and dilation should not be performed if an implanted intraocular lens was placed during cataract surgery.

Nursing care: Indicate both the duration of effect of the medication used to dilate the pupil and the limitation in vision. Instruct the patient to arrange transportation and to wear sunglasses if going outside after pupils are dilated.

Indirect Ophthalmoscopy

Description: The examiner wears a head-mounted binocular instrument. The patient is supine, usually with dilated pupils. The examiner stands 30 inches away and holds a convex lens over the patient's eye for focusing. The image is magnified four to five times; a greater visual field can be viewed than with direct ophthalmoscopy. A scleral depressor (blunt rod) may be used to compress the eyeball so ora serrata (tissue behind the iris) can be viewed.

Indications: Permits detection and evaluation of minimal elevations of the sensory retina and retinal pigment epithelium, which are not evident with direct ophthalmoscopy. Useful in the detection of opacities in the media.

Complications: None.

Nursing care: Assure the patient that mild or no discomfort will be experienced if a scleral depressor is used. Inform the patient about side effects of the medication.

Gonioscopy

Description: A corneal contact lens (goniolens) is placed over an anesthetized cornea to permit viewing of anterior chamber angles with a microscopic lens, mirror, or contact lens combined with a prism, because the opaque sclera and corneoscleral limbus prevent direct inspection of the angle of the anterior chamber.

Indications: Assists in distinguishing between angle-closure glaucoma and open-angle glaucoma. It has also been used in the development of an effective surgical procedure for congenital glaucoma and in the diagnostic and therapeutic evolution of many types of secondary glaucoma.

Complications: None.

Nursing care: Explain the procedure to the patient.

Slit Lamp Examination

Description: The examiner views the corneal layers, anterior chamber, lens, and anterior vitreous through a microscope that magnifies these structures up to 20 times. A thin slit of light permits scrutiny of anterior structures for lesions or trauma.

Indications: Used to detect the depth of the abnormality.

Complications: None.

Nursing care: Explain the procedure to the patient.

Pupil Dilation

Description: Short-acting, topical medication is used for pupil dilation to facilitate examination of the fundus with direct or indirect ophthalmoscopy. Mydriatic (adrenergic) drugs such as phenylephrine 2.5% (Neo-Synephrine, Mydfrin) dilate the pupil but do not inhibit accommodation. Mydriatic drug may be combined with cycloplegic drug (which inhibits accommodation) such as tropicamide 0.5% (Mydriacyl) to enhance and maintain pupil dilation.

Indications: Diagnosis and evaluation of significant ocular and systemic disease.

Complications: May be contraindicated for patients with a shallow anterior chamber, certain intraocular lens implants, or vascular hypertension or who are taking monoamine oxidase (MAO) inhibitors or tricyclic antidepressants.

Nursing care: Remove contact lenses before instillation. Warn the patient that blurred vision and photophobia may last for 3 to 6 hours after examination. Instruct patient to arrange transportation and to wear sunglasses if going outside during this period.

Lacrimal System Testing

Description

Basic secretion test: Topical anesthetic is administered to the eyeball before filter paper is placed in the lateral portion of the lower eyelid. The anesthesia reduces lacrimal output to allow measurement of the tear production of accessory glands in the eyelid.

Dacryocystography: A radiopaque medium such as Pantopaque is injected through the punctum and canaliculus into the lacrimal sac, followed by roentgenography.

Dacryoscintigraphy: Sodium pertechnetate (^{99m}Tc) in a dilute solution is instilled in each conjunctival sac, followed by a seinogram taken with a gamma camera to indicate its passage through the lacrimal drainage system.[18]

Dye disappearance: A dye, 0.25% to 2% fluorescein in alkaline solution or rose bengal, is instilled topically into the conjunctival sac to stain the Bowman's membrane and the stroma of the cornea. The stain can be intensified if a 2% cocaine ophthalmic solution is instilled into the eye or if the eye is illuminated with a cobalt blue filter to stimulate fluorescence.

Rose bengal staining: A drop of 1% or 2% solution is placed in the conjunctival sac. The 2% solution demonstrates loss of corneal and conjunctival epithelium in keratoconjunctivitis sicca; the 1% solution is valuable in demonstrating conjunctival and corneal epithelial cell loss and degeneration. Patients with a deficiency of the aqueous portion of tears have punctate staining of the lower two thirds of the cornea and bright red staining of the bulbar conjunctiva in the area corresponding to the palpable aperture.

Schirmer's test: A strip of filter paper, 3.5 × 0.05 cm, is placed in the conjunctival cul-de-sac of the lower lid for 5 minutes. A 10- to 15-mm length of paper wetted with tears is considered normal. More than 25 mm of moistened paper indicates excessive tearing.

Indications: Used to determine the adequacy and patency of the lacrimal system; it can demonstrate obstruction or overproduction of tears.

Fluorescein is instilled in the eye for a variety of diagnostic tests. It demonstrates breaks in the epithelium and the dilution that occurs when anterior aqueous humor escapes from a postoperative fistula, penetrating wound, or conjunctival bleb following glaucoma surgery. It is also used to demonstrate areas of contact between the lens and the cornea and sclera in the fitting of contact lenses. The rate of disappearance through the nasolacrimal passages (normally 1 minute) estimates their patency.

Rose bengal dye is usually used to demarcate devitalized conjunctival epithelium in keratoconjunctivitis sicca, because it stains devitalized cells better than fluorescein does.

Complications: Dyes stain soft contact lenses, so the lenses should be removed before the dye is instilled; lenses should not be reinserted until all evidence of dye is gone. Because it is possible for fluorescein to become contaminated with *Pseudomonas* spp., it should be instilled with either a single-dose container or a strip of sterile filter paper saturated with the dye.

Nursing care: Explain the procedure to the patient.

Provocative Testing

Description: Used for patients with mildly elevated intraocular pressure (IOP), those who have optic nerve changes or field defects without elevated IOP, and those with shallow anterior chambers and compromised anterior angles. Their results are not definitive but may distinguish potentially glaucomatous persons from others.

Water drinking test: In the morning, the fasting patient drinks approximately 1 L of water as fast as possible (within 2 to 4 minutes). The IOP is measured before and at 15-minute intervals for 45 minutes. Normal eyes show an IOP increase of 3 to 5 mm Hg. An increase of 8 mm Hg is indicative of glaucoma.

Dark room test (for narrow-angle glaucoma): The patient sits in a dark room for 60 minutes to dilate pupils. An IOP increase of 7 to 8 mm Hg is indicative of iris bunching into and blocking anterior angle flow.

Mydriatic testing: One eye is dilated at a time (under careful supervision), and the pupil is constricted when the test is ended. IOP increase of 8 mm Hg is indicative of glaucoma.

Indications: These tests are indicated in patients with an intraocular pressure of 21 mm Hg or more, a coefficient outflow of less than 0.18, a ratio of intraocular pressure to coefficient outflow facility greater than 100, optic nerve changes suggestive of glaucoma, and field changes suggestive of glaucoma.[18]

Complications: None.

Nursing care: Explain the study to the patient. Encourage the patient to have eyes tested periodically for glaucoma.

Visual Field Screening

Description

Central field tangent screen: Central vision covers approximately 50 degrees of the patient's central vision, 25 degrees in each direction from the central fixation point. A black screen (1 m^2) is placed 1 m from the eye. Blind spots are outlined by using a 1- to 3-mm white target placed on a board. A normal blind spot is 13 to 18 degrees temporal from central fixation. Abnormal isolated spots (scotomas) or confluent areas can be identified. Nasal areas are usually lost first.

Automated perimetry: Various automatic machines (such as Goldmann perimeter) measure both central and peripheral fields.

Indications: Method of assessing function of retinal periphery by measuring the peripheral field of vision. It is indicated as part of a routine vision screening or as part of a diagnosis of visual problems or deterioration.

Complications: None.

Nursing care: Explain the study to the patient.

Otoscopy

Description: Inspection of the external auditory canal and middle ear. The largest speculum that will fit comfortably in the patient's ear is inserted to a depth of 1 to 1.5 cm to inspect the auditory canal from the meatus to the tympanic membrane.

Indications: Any discharge, scaling, excessive redness, lesions, foreign bodies, or cerumen can be noted. The tympanic membrane is inspected for landmarks, color, contours, and perforations. The direction of the light can be varied to see the entire tympanic membrane and anulus.[28]

Complications: None.

Nursing care: Explain the procedure to the patient.

Rhinoscopy

Description: Inspection of the nasal cavity using a nasal speculum and a light. The patient's head should be held erect to examine the vestibule and inferior nasal turbinate and tilted back to visualize the middle meatus and turbinate.[28]

Indications: Color, discharge, masses, lesions, and swelling of the turbinates may be noted, and the septum inspected for alignment, perforation, bleeding, and crusting.

Complications: None.

Nursing care: Explain the procedure to the patient.

Rigid Endoscopy of Pharynx

Description: An instrument producing bright illumination is held in the patient's mouth to visualize the nasopharynx when the instrument is turned upward, and the hypopharynx and larynx when the instrument is turned downward.

Indications: Detection of abnormalities of the oropharynx or nasopharynx and evaluation of symptoms of infection or abscess.

Complications: None.

Nursing care: Explain the procedure to the patient.

Laryngoscopy (Direct, Suspension, Indirect)

Description

Direct laryngoscopy: Direct examination of the larynx under local or general anesthesia, performed by introducing a laryngoscope into the patient's mouth over the tongue; the tongue is raised, the patient's neck is slowly extended, and the laryngoscope is passed over the posterior portion of the epiglottis and raised to expose the vocal cords. The method can be used for biopsy or excision of a polyp.

Suspension laryngoscopy: Essentially the same as direct laryngoscopy, but an attachment holds the laryngoscope so the examiner can use both hands; usually used in conjunction with a microscope, which provides magnification and binocular vision.

Indirect laryngoscopy: The most common way to examine the larynx; usually performed in the physician's office; the patient sits upright in a chair, and a laryngeal mirror is used to visualize the larynx.

Indications: Hoarseness, burning in throat, dysphagia, dyspnea, muffled voice.

Complications: None except that the gag reflex is abolished. The usual care must be taken to prevent aspiration.

Nursing care: Explain the procedure to the patient. Observe the patient for respiratory distress for the first 2 to 4 hours. If the patient had a local (topical) anesthetic administered before the procedure, be aware that the gag reflex may be absent until the anesthetic wears off, so fluids should be withheld until the gag reflex returns. Humidified oxygen provides additional moisture to the patient's airway.

Videolaryngoscopy

Description: Videolaryngoscopy is the standard of practice when a laryngeal pathologic condition is suspected. A rigid 90-degree telescope is used to perform a transoral examination of the larynx, and a flexible fiberoptic scope is used to perform a transnasal examination. The rigid scope is used more frequently because it offers greater ease of examination and produces a video image of higher resolution. It provides the luxury of repeated reviews and closer scrutiny of the laryngeal examination without repeated manipulation of the patient and may enhance the identification of less obvious laryngeal lesions. This study may also assist with identification of decreased subtle vocal cord mobility that may otherwise be missed.

Indications: Hoarseness, burning in throat, dysphagia, dyspnea, muffled voice.

Complications: None except that the gag reflex is abolished. The usual care must be taken to prevent aspiration.

Nursing care: Explain the procedure to the patient. Observe the patient for respiratory distress for the first 2 to 4 hours. If the patient had a local (topical) anesthetic administered before the procedure, be aware that the gag reflex may be absent until the anesthetic wears off, so fluids should be withheld until the gag reflex returns. Humidified oxygen provides additional moisture to the patient's airway.

Fiberoptic Bronchoscopy

Description: This procedure, performed with the patient under local anesthesia, permits direct inspection of the larynx, trachea, and bronchi. The flexible fiberoptic bronchoscope is the preferred instrument because it is better tolerated by patients and permits improved visualization of distal subsegmental airways. The fiberoptic bronchoscope, which has an external diameter between 3 and 6 mm, is inserted through the patient's nose or mouth. Conscious sedation may be used for this procedure if necessary.

Indications: Collection of secretions for cytologic or bacteriologic examination; tissue biopsy for examination; cells and secretions via a brush biopsy technique that involves using a small brush inserted through the bronchoscope to brush the tissue walls. Location and biopsy of tumors; bleeding locations; removal of foreign bodies or heavy, blocking, mucous plug secretions; implantation of radioactive gold seeds for tumor treatment.

Complications: Bronchospasm, increased sputum production, productive mild bronchitis, sore throat, hoarseness.

Nursing care: The patient should receive nothing by mouth for 8 hours before the procedure and is usually given a preprocedure sedative medication. Any dental prostheses should be removed. In the examination area, the patient's mouth, throat, and tongue will be sprayed with a topical anesthetic. An oxygen catheter is placed and remains in one nostril throughout the procedure. Lidocaine jelly is generally used as the bronchoscope lubricant; this helps to decrease the patient's cough and gag reflexes. After the procedure the patient should be carefully watched and positioned until the full gag and swallowing reflexes return. Patency of the patient's airway and the swallowing reflex should be evaluated, and the patient should be assessed for severe complications such as bronchospasms.

Mediastinoscopy, Mediastinotomy, Thoracoscopy

Description: Surgical endoscopy procedures in which a biopsy is taken from a tumor in the upper mediastinum, the pleura, or the lung. They are also used to determine if metastasis has occurred.

Mediastinoscopy: The incision is made in the suprasternal notch, and the scope is passed through that incision to biopsy tissue from the upper mediastinum.

Mediastinotomy: The incision is made above the third rib along the sternal border. Lung biopsy may also be done by this technique.

Thoracoscopy: Done to obtain a biopsy from a peripheral lesion of the lung or pleura. The incision site, along the lateral or anterior chest wall, depends on the location of the lesion.

Indications: Diagnosis of primary or secondary mediastinal disease; evaluation of metastasis to mediastinal modes in primary lung carcinoma.

Complications: Hemorrhage, pneumothorax, infection, left recurrent laryngeal nerve damage.

Nursing care: For all procedures the patient receives a general anesthetic; therefore all preoperative procedures apply. Postoperatively the patient should be observed for pneumothorax, cardiac dysrhythmias, and bleeding. A chest tube is frequently used after the thoracoscopy procedure.

Esophagogastroduodenoscopy (EGD)

Description: Permits visual examination of the esophagus, stomach, and upper duodenum. Dentures are removed. A local anesthetic is sprayed into the mouth and throat. A fiberoptic endoscope is passed through the mouth and swallowed. Saliva may need to be suctioned if it doesn't flow out the side of the mouth adequately. A mouth guard should be used to protect the teeth and the endoscope. The patient's head is repositioned throughout the procedure to facilitate movement of the endoscope. Conscious sedation may be used for this procedure if necessary.

The procedure is contraindicated in patients with recent ulcer perforation, large aortic aneurysms, cardiac disease or a recent myocardial infarction, and Zenker's diverticulum.

Indications: Useful in diagnosing inflammatory disease, varices, ulcers, tumors, structural abnormality, and Mallory-Weiss tears.

Complications: Complications include the following: cervical esophagus perforation (pain on swallowing and neck movements); thoracic esophagus perforation (substernal or epigastric pain that increases with respirations and trunk movements); diaphragmatic esophageal perforation (shoulder pain and dyspnea); gastric perforation (abdominal or back pain, cyanosis, fever, or pleural effusion).

Other signs of complications include difficulty in swallowing, persistent pain, fever, black stools, or hematemesis.

Nursing care: Give nothing by mouth for 6 to 12 hours before the procedure; during an emergency procedure a nasogastric tube is used to aspirate gastric contents. Explain the procedure to the patient and ensure that a signed consent form is obtained. Before the procedure, have the patient remove any dentures or partial plates. Monitor pain, blood pressure, pulse, temperature, and respirations. Anxiety and fear of the procedure are expected, and the patient should be given emotional support before and throughout the procedure; sedatives and analgesics may be used to help the patient relax. Fluids and foods should be withheld until the gag reflex returns.

Colonoscopy

Description: The patient is placed in the left lateral decubitus position, and a well-lubricated colonoscope is inserted through the anus. Air is inserted to help the physician visualize the mucosa and to facilitate advancement of the colonoscope. Occasionally position changes are required to assist advancement of the scope at the descending-sigmoid colon junction and splenic flexure. Barium studies should be made after the colonoscopy; thorough bowel preparation is required for good visualization of mucosa. Specimens for cytologic and histologic examination may be obtained as well as for biopsy.

Contraindications to the procedure include pregnancy, ischemic bowel disease, acute diverticulitis, peritonitis, toxic megacolon of ulcerative colitis, fulminant granulomatous colitis, and irradiation colitis.

Indications: Used to examine the colon and rectum to diagnose inflammatory bowel disease, including ulcerative colitis and granulomatous colitis. Polyps can be removed through the colonoscope. The colonoscope is also helpful in diagnosing or locating the source of lower gastrointestinal bleeding. A biopsy of lesions suspected to be malignant may also be performed; biopsies may also be advisable for patients with ulcerative colitis or Crohn's disease.

Complications: Complications include perforation of the bowel. Signs and symptoms include abdominal pain and distention, rectal bleeding, fever, and mucopurulent drainage. If the bowel is fixed—secondary to irradiation, surgical adhesions, or inflammatory disease—the physician may have difficulty during the procedure.

Nursing care: Bowel preparation is required for visualization of the mucosa. Colon electrolyte lavage preparations may be used. Patients need instructions for mixing the solution. Avoid all solid food and sugar the day of the prep.

Alternatively, the bowel may be cleansed with laxatives and enemas; be careful in patients with ulcerative colitis and granulomatous colitis because laxatives can exacerbate the disease (special protocols are required for this patient group). Avoid soapsuds enemas in all patients, because this irritates the mucosa. Fluid and electrolyte problems may occur in elderly patients who receive high-volume enemas; ensure that patients are alerted to potential effects.

The procedure is uncomfortable and embarrassing, so be supportive. Let the patient know that flatus is from air inserted during the procedure and cannot be controlled. A sedative may be given to help the patient relax; because midazolam or diazepam may be used, ensure that the patient is appropriately monitored during the procedure.

Proctosigmoidoscopy

Description: Examination of the sigmoid colon, rectum, and anal canal. The sigmoidoscope and proctoscope may be rigid metal instruments or flexible scopes inserted to visualize the mucosa; a biopsy may be performed. Examination usually includes a digital examination of the anus and anal canal.

Patients often dread the proctosigmoidoscopy examination because of the embarrassing and uncomfortable positioning and the discomfort caused by the rigid instrument. Patients are placed in a knee-chest position on a tilting table. Although the procedure can be done with the patient in a left lateral position, it is important to elevate the right buttock;

GUIDELINES FOR CONSCIOUS SEDATION

Definition

Conscious sedation is the condition produced by the administration of a drug or combination of drugs to relieve pain or anxiety during diagnostic or therapeutic procedures. The patient receiving conscious sedation has an altered level of consciousness, but should retain the ability to maintain and protect a patent airway as well as to respond appropriately to verbal commands and physical stimuli. Because the administration of drugs to produce conscious sedation can have the unintended effect of compromising a patient's protective reflexes, these guidelines are intended to ensure the performance of safe and effective diagnostic and therapeutic procedures. These guidelines do not apply to the use of "deep sedation" or in the routine management of postoperative pain.

Deep sedation is a medically controlled state of depressed consciousness or unconsciousness from which the patient is not easily aroused. Deep sedation may be accompanied by a partial or complete loss of protective reflexes, including the inability to maintain a patent airway independently and to respond purposefully to physical stimulation or to verbal commands. The state and risks of deep sedation may be indistinguishable from those of general anesthesia.

Requirements for All Patients Receiving Conscious Sedation

Personnel

A physician and a registered nurse/licensed vocational (LVN/LPN) nurse, who are familiar with basic life support and emergency airway management including bag and mask ventilation, must be in attendance or immediately available until the procedure is completed. One health care provider should have the primary responsibility of monitoring the patient's vital signs and level of consciousness and must remain with the patient until there is satisfactory recovery from the acute effects of the sedation agents (i.e., vital signs and level of consciousness have returned to *baseline*). In case of an airway emergency, a clearly defined plan for obtaining assistance with airway management must be activated.

In circumstances where a painful dressing change procedure is routinely performed by the nursing staff, the personnel requirement can be met by a single registered nurse and either a second registered nurse or a licensed vocational nurse, provided the responsible physician (or physician designee) is *immediately available.*

Equipment (required and immediately available)

1. Oxygen source
2. Equipment for oxygen administration (nasal cannula, masks)
3. Self-inflating resuscitation bag
4. Functioning suction source
5. Crash cart
6. Emergency airway equipment (masks, airways, and laryngoscopes with blades)
7. Telephone
8. Electrical outlet connected to emergency power supply
9. Monitoring equipment, including electrocardiogram, pulse oximeter, sphygmomanometer, and cuff and/or automated blood pressure monitor

Other Requirements

1. Supplemental oxygen should be administered to all patients during conscious sedation unless pulse oximetry data indicate satisfactory oxygenation.
2. Intravenous access should be secured in all adult patients. For pediatric patients, the skilled personnel and equipment to start an IV should be immediately available.
3. Agents to reverse effects of drugs immediately available (naloxone and flumazenil).

Medications for Conscious Sedation

The following sedatives and narcotics may be administered for the purpose of conscious sedation only by a physician, or by a registered nurse under the direct supervision of a physician, in the manner prescribed. The agents listed below shall be titrated to effect in accordance with the monitoring standards described below. The following schedule can be modified according to the judgment and practice of the prescribing physician. All routes of administration are intravenous unless otherwise specified.

Medications

Adults

Agents	Dose	Frequency
Diazepam	1-2 mg	q3-10min
Midazolam*	0.25-1 mg	q1-5min
Fentanyl	Loading dose up to 1 mcg/kg then 12.5-50 mcg	q5-10min
Morphine	1-3 mg	q2-15min
Meperidine	12.5-25 mg	q2-15min
Droperidol	0.625-1.25 mg	q5-10min

Pediatrics

Agents	Dose	Frequency
Diazepam	0.05-0.1 mg/kg (max dose 0.25 mg/kg)	q3-10min
Midazolam*	**IV** 0.04-0.08 mg/kg **PO** 0.3-0.5 mg/kg **Intranasal** 0.25 mg/kg **Rectal** 0.3-0.5 mg/kg	q3-5min
Fentanyl	0.5 mcg/kg	q5-10min
Morphine	0.05 mg/kg	q5-10min
Meperidine	0.5 mg/kg (max dose 2 mg/kg)	q5min
Pentobarbital	**IV** 1-2 mg/kg (max dose 6 mg/kg)	q5min
	IM 2-6 mg/kg	one time
	PO/PR 5 mg/kg	one time
Chloral Hydrate	50 mg/kg PO or PR	25 mg/kg prn once

*See midazolam guidelines in hospital formulary

GUIDELINES FOR CONSCIOUS SEDATION—cont'd

In pediatric sedation, note that benzodiazepines may be associated with disinhibition. Pentobarbital occasionally can produce paradoxical excitement. Small doses of opiates can ameliorate these effects.

Conscious Sedation Antagonists (Reversal Agents)

ADULTS

Agents	Dose	Frequency
Naloxone	40-400 μg	q5-10min
Flumazenil	0.2 mg	q1min up to 1 mg

PEDIATRICS

Agents	Dose	Frequency
Naloxone	2-10 μg/kg	q5-10min

Any patient receiving reversal agents should be monitored for at least 2 hours after administration of reversal agent to detect potential resedation. Flumazenil is not approved for pediatric patients (oversedation is not commonly associated with benzodiazepine administration in pediatric patients).

RESTRICTION ON AGENTS TO BE ADMINISTERED

The following medications, when administered intravenously, are for the provision of deep sedation and general anesthesia and are not appropriate for conscious sedation. Furthermore, they should only be administered by a physician trained in airway management, including endotracheal intubation and/or under the direct supervision of an anesthesiologist:

1. Neuromuscular blocking agents (e.g., succinylcholine, vecuronium)
2. Intravenous anesthetics
   a. Sodium thiopental
   b. Methohexital
   c. Propofol
   d. Ketamine
   e. Alfentanil
   f. Sufentanil
3. Fentanyl oralets

NPO STATUS

The following are the guidelines for NPO status for otherwise healthy patients:

1. Patients less than 2 years old; NPO for 2 hours; clear liquids up to 2 hours before procedure; solids up to 6 hours before procedure.
2. Patients greater than 2 years old; NPO for 4 hours; clear liquids up to 4 hours before procedure; solids up to 6 hours before procedure.

PREPROCEDURE PATIENT EVALUATION

An appropriate medical history and physical examination must be performed and written in the chart prior to the procedure. An assessment of the patient's preprocedure responsiveness to verbal and physical stimuli and vital signs should be performed. For the patient who is scheduled for an elective procedure, the availability and appropriateness of transportation following the procedure should be verified prior to the administration of conscious sedation. Prior to the procedure, patients must be given written discharge instructions, including the names and phone numbers of medical center staff to contact in the event of an emergency.

MONITORING DURING PROCEDURE

The objective of monitoring the patient during conscious sedation is to ensure the adequacy of ventilation, oxygenation, and circulatory function. The following guidelines for monitoring are considered a minimum standard that is required for any patient receiving conscious sedation. Departments and units where conscious sedation is performed may develop their own specific guidelines that delineate requirements for monitoring of special patient populations that exceed the minimum standards below.

1. Electrocardiographic monitoring should be available and used in selected patients (e.g., with cardiac and pulmonary disease) if clinically possible.
2. Blood pressure every 5 minutes (manually or with automated device) if clinically possible; heart rate and respiratory rate every 15 minutes.
3. Continuous pulse oximetry (SpO_2).
4. Assessment of adequacy of ventilation (observation of chest excursion, measuring respiratory rate, or, if possible, the detection of end-tidal carbon dioxide) at least every 15 minutes.
5. Responsiveness to verbal and physical stimuli should be assessed 5 minutes after administration of any agent and at least every 15 minutes thereafter.

DOCUMENTATION DURING PROCEDURE

Valid consent must be obtained and documented in the medical record as required by Medical Center policy prior to the beginning of the procedure and the administration of any sedative agents. The record should contain:

1. Procedure performed
2. Personnel involved
3. Record of vital signs and responsiveness to verbal and physical stimuli at least every 15 minutes or more frequently if indicated (heart rate or ECG rhythm, if used, BP, SpO_2, respiratory rate)
4. Time and dosage of medications administered
5. Documentation of any abnormal ECG rhythm, blood pressure 30% below or above baseline, SpO_2 of less than 90%, or respiratory rate less than 10 breaths per minute and any other complications.

POSTSEDATION MONITORING AND RECOVERY CRITERIA

Following completion of the procedure, the patient must be monitored and vital signs assessed using the same parameters and protocol as described in *Monitoring During the Procedure* until the patient meets the following recovery criteria.

1. All patients should be monitored until their vital signs and responsiveness to verbal and physical stimuli have returned to their preprocedure baseline.
2. Outpatients undergoing procedures with conscious sedation, including those in the emergency department, should be stable enough to safely return home.

Continued

GUIDELINES FOR CONSCIOUS SEDATION—cont'd

3. Outpatients undergoing elective procedures and who are discharged home must be accompanied by a responsible adult.
4. Inpatients must be able to return to their preprocedure level of care and monitoring.

For pediatric and neonatal patients, age-specific recovery criteria should be established by each group of practitioners involved in conscious sedation.

Evidence that the patient has met recovery criteria must be clearly documented in the patient's medical record.

Reporting of Adverse Events

All cases in which the following events occur will be reported by the physician and/or nursing staff using the Confidential Report of Incident and, if appropriate, the Adverse Drug Reaction Report form.

1. All cases in which naloxone or flumazenil is administered
2. All cases in which *new* assisted ventilation is required
3. All unanticipated hospital admissions or increased level of care
4. All cases in which the oxygen saturation (SPO_2) is <90% for more than 5 minutes, including recovery period, or 80% at any time
5. All cases in which there is hemodynamic instability defined as a 30% change from baseline in blood pressure or heart rate and/or the occurrence of new atrial or ventricular dysrhythmias

Evaluation of New Agents for Conscious Sedation

When a new agent for conscious sedation is added to the hospital formulary, the guidelines for its use will be established by the Pharmacy and Therapeutics Committees following the basic principles set forward in this document.

most physicians prefer to use a tilting table and the knee-chest position for best visualization.

A proctoscope may be used to examine the rectum and anus, but when a sigmoidoscope is removed slowly, the rectum and anal canal can be viewed, thereby eliminating the need for a proctoscope.

Indications: Changed bowel habits, rectal bleeding, weight loss, anemia, stools positive for occult blood.

Complications: Complications include possible bowel perforation (see the discussion of colonoscopy); decreased blood pressure, pallor, diaphoresis, and bradycardia are signs of vasovagal stimulation and require immediate notification of the physician.

Nursing care: Preparation varies with the expected diagnosis: Clear liquid diets for 48 hours and a small sodium biphosphate enema may be used. Tell the patient what to expect.

Cystoscopy and Panendoscopy

Description: The cystoscope and panendoscope are instruments that allow direct visualization of the bladder and urethra. Cystoscopy and panendoscopy may be performed while the patient is under general or spinal anesthesia; in other cases, a local anesthetic, such as lidocaine jelly, is used.

The patient is placed in the lithotomy position. Sterile equipment is used; surgical gowns, gloves, and masks are typically worn. A single sheath through which both the cystoscope and panendoscope will be passed is inserted into the bladder via the urethra, with adequate lubrication. A telescope is then passed through the sheath while the bladder is being filled with fluid. Using a fiberoptic system within the cystoscope, the urologist visualizes the internal architecture of the bladder, including the bladder neck, urothelial lining, and ureteral orifices. Bladder tumors, trabeculation, and inflammatory changes within the internal mucosa are assessed via cystoscopy. A panendoscope is used to view the bladder neck, prostatic urethra (in a male), external urinary sphincters, and anterior urethra.

Fluid is infused into the bladder throughout the procedure. Infusion is stopped and the bladder drained when it becomes filled with 300 to 500 ml of fluid.

Cystoscopic and panendoscopic examination may be combined with radiographic diagnostic studies such as a retrograde pyelogram or with therapeutic procedures, such as transurethral resection of a bladder tumor or the prostate.

Indications: Hematuria, dysuria, tumor or polyp removal or biopsy.

Complications: Mild dysuria and transient hematuria should disappear within the first 48 hours after the procedure. The patient usually should be able to void normally after a routine cystoscopic examination, although some burning may be experienced.

Nursing care: If a general or spinal anesthetic is used, the patient will be sent to the postanesthesia care unit after the procedure and should be closely monitored for potential postanesthesia complications, such as a low-grade fever (≤38° C [101° F]). This may occur for 24 to 48 hours after the procedure. Instruct the patient to notify the physician if this occurs, because sepsis may occur. If the patient experiences burning with urination, suggest sitz baths and increased fluid intake, unless contraindicated. Explain to the patient that only minimal discomfort will be experienced following the procedure.

Pelvic Endoscopy

Description: Visualization and examination of pelvic and abdominal viscera with a high-intensity fiberoptic or video light source inserted via a laparoscope through the abdominal wall and into the peritoneum.

Indications: The procedure is performed when hysterosalpingography suggests tubal abnormality and the patient does not become pregnant. It is also performed before certain surgical procedures, such as a tuboplasty, and may reveal the presence of unsuspected tubal or ovarian disease, such as peritubal adhesions and endometriosis.

Complications: Bowel perforation; bleeding.

Nursing care: Because a general anesthetic is used, the patient will be sent to the postanesthesia care unit after the procedure and should be monitored for potential complications.

Colposcopy

Description: Examination of the cervix and vagina with a colposcope—a stereoscopic binocular microscope with various levels of magnification.

Indications: Dysplasia; to elevate the vascular pattern, intercapillary distance, surface pattern, color, tone, opacity, clarity, demarcation, and extent of a lesion. To differentiate between inflammatory atypia and neoplasms or between invasive and noninvasive cervical lesions, and to enable follow-up.

Complications: None.

Nursing care: Prepare the patient (in the lithotomy position) for a vaginal examination. Show her the colposcope and explain that it will not be inserted into the vagina. A vaginal speculum is used to expose the vagina and cervix, and the colposcope then focuses on the cervix, allowing careful examination, outlining of the lesion, and biopsy and specimen removal. Inform the patient that she may have slight vaginal bleeding if specimens were taken, and suggest that she wear a sanitary pad until the bleeding subsides. Provide emotional support and allow patient to voice any concerns related to procedure or findings.

Culdoscopy

Description: Visual examination of female pelvic viscera by means of an endoscope inserted through the posterior vaginal fornix. The patient is usually sedated, but a general anesthetic is not used. The procedure is performed with the patient in the knee-chest position. If necessary, CO_2 may be instilled into the peritoneal cavity to allow better visualization of the pelvic organs.

Indications: Investigation of infertility. It determines gross anatomic and pathologic conditions (i.e., congenital abnormalities or the sequelae of traumatic or inflammatory processes).

Complications: None.

Nursing care: Tell the patient that once the endoscope is removed, she will be required to exhale as forcefully as possible to push out intraperitoneal air; this maneuver will minimize shoulder pain caused by trapped CO_2 when she sits up.

Hysteroscopy

Description: Direct visual examination of the cervical canal and uterine cavity through a hysteroscope, a fiberoptic instrument; procedure most often performed with the patient under spinal anesthesia.

Indications: To examine the endometrium, secure a specimen for biopsy, remove an intrauterine device, or excise cervical polyps.

Complications: Perforation of the uterus (usually at the fundus), bleeding, infection.

Nursing care: The patient should be maintained in a flat position for 8 hours after the procedure to recover fully if spinal anesthesia is used. Provide routine postanesthesia care, and advise the patient to rest during the next 24 hours and to avoid heavy lifting to prevent uterine hemorrhage.

Laparoscopy

Description: With the patient under general anesthesia, the abdominal and pelvic organs are visualized and examined with a laparoscope inserted through a small incision in the abdominal wall; the abdomen is insufflated with CO_2 to enhance visualization. The procedure usually lasts 10 to 15 minutes.

Indications: Therapeutic procedures may also be performed, including removal of peritubular adhesions, sterilization through fulguration of oviducts, laser treatment for endometriosis, cholecystectomy, and appendectomy.

Complications: Bleeding from a puncture injury, misplacement of gas, thermal burns.

Nursing care: Provide routine presurgical and postanesthetic care. Inform the patient that he or she may experience a sore throat from intubation and a sore chest from insufflation of the abdomen. These sensations usually disappear within 48 hours. Shoulder pain caused by trapped CO_2 may also be experienced.

Arthroscopy

Description: Insertion of a specially designed endoscope through an incision at a certain joint, often the knee. By means of lenses and lights on the scope, the tissues are examined. The arthroscope also permits the removal of loose bodies, pieces of torn cartilage, and biopsy of the synovium if desired. The procedure is performed in an outpatient surgical or operative suite, often as a 23-hour stay procedure.

Indications: To determine the condition of the joint, tissues, cartilage, meniscus (of knee), and ligaments. It is most frequently performed on the knee and shoulder, and less often on the hip, elbow, ankle, and other joints.

Complications: Possible joint swelling after the procedure and at times some bleeding into the joint. Infection is also possible.

Nursing care: Explain to the patient about the skin preparation, application of a tourniquet to decrease blood flow, sterile draping, and administration of a local anesthetic to one or more areas before insertion of the arthroscope into the joint. After the procedure, instruct the patient about applying a compression dressing and ice around the joint to lessen bleeding and edema. Caution the patient to avoid excessive joint use for 24 to 48 hours, but explain that weight bearing is permitted after knee arthroscopy. Use of other joints varies with the purpose and extent of the arthroscopic repair or procedure done. Instruct the patient about signs of infection, restrictions or limitations of joint use, and the return physician's appointment. Mild analgesics (no aspirin) may be prescribed for postprocedural discomfort or pain.

BODY FLUID EXAMINATION

Sputum Examination (Direct Method)

Description: The microbiologic evaluation of sputum is vitally important in the evaluation of the respiratory system. The two laboratory procedures commonly performed with sputum examination are microscopic Gram's stain and culture and sensitivity.

Direct method: Voluntary coughing to produce sputum specimen. With this procedure, early morning specimens are sent on 3 consecutive days if tuberculosis (TB) is suspected. Ensure that a sputum and not a saliva specimen has been obtained.

Sputum induction: This technique may be used if voluntary coughing does not produce a specimen. With this technique the patient is instructed to breathe for several minutes using a heated, nebulized mist of distilled water or a sodium chloride solution. Following this nebulization the sputum collection technique as described is performed.

Indications: Evaluation of pneumonias, suspected malignancies.

Complications: None.

Nursing care: The sputum should be collected in a wide-mouthed, sterile container with a tightly fitting lid and should be transported immediately to the laboratory.

Instruct the patient to brush teeth and gargle before the collection of the specimen. Instruct the patient to spit out any postnasal secretions. Instruct the patient to take a deep breath to the lungs' full capacity and then to exhale the air with an expulsive deep cough. The specimen should be coughed directly into the sterile, wide-mouthed container. Instruct patient not to touch inside the sputum container or cover. Note and document the color, consistency, odor, and amount of the sputum. Number the specimens serially for each of the 3 days.

Sputum Examination (Indirect Method)

Description: One of two indirect methods may be used.

Nasotracheal suctioning: This technique is used to obtain specimens from the trachea via a catheter that has been passed transnasally. Causes some patient discomfort.

Endotracheal suctioning: Used to obtain specimen from trachea via a catheter that has been passed through an endotracheal tube.

Indications: Evaluation of pneumonias or suspected malignancies.

Complications:

Nasotracheal suctioning: Hypoxemia; dysrhythmias; blood pressure (BP) changes.

Transtracheal aspiration: Subcutaneous or mediastinal emphysema and cervical infections at the site of the aspiration.

Nursing care: For both types, ensure that emotional support is provided, and that appropriate preprocedure or postprocedure care is given.

Nasotracheal and endotracheal suctioning: Assist the patient to a sitting position. The nurse, physician, or respiratory therapist passes a catheter through the patient's nose or an endotracheal tube into the trachea to suction tracheobronchial secretions. Oxygen may be administered during the procedure. Cardiac response and the patient's oxygenation should be monitored.

Pleural Fluid Examination (Diagnostic Thoracentesis)

Description: A needle is inserted through the chest wall into the pleural space to remove pleural fluid.

Indications: May be performed therapeutically to drain fluid and relieve lung congestion and also diagnostically to collect pleural fluid for examination in patients with symptoms of inflammation, infection, or malignancy.

Complications: Hemothorax, pneumothorax, air embolism, subcutaneous emphysema, hypotension, hypoxemia, acute fluid shifts.

Nursing care: Instruct the patient regarding the procedure. Advise the patient not to move suddenly, cough, or breathe deeply during the procedure. Record baseline vital signs. Assist with positioning the patient comfortably, and provide emotional support during the procedure. After the procedure, monitor the patient's vital signs and respiratory status for any complications.

Gastric Analysis (Basal Gastric Secretion Test)

Description: Measures basal secretion under fasting conditions; stomach contents aspirated through a nasogastric tube, with the patient in supine, left lateral decubitus, and right lateral decubitus positions.

Histamine may be injected to stimulate flow. Normal values of gastric secretions are 0.2 to 3.8 mEq/h for females; 1 to 5 mEq/h for males. High values may indicate a duodenal or jejunal ulcer; depressed values may indicate gastric carcinoma or benign gastric ulcer; absence of gastric secretion indicates pernicious anemia; markedly high levels indicate Zollinger-Ellison syndrome.

Indications: Indicated for patients with anorexia, weight loss, and epigastric pain.

Complications: Dysrhythmias may develop during intubation.

Nursing care: The patient must be relaxed and isolated from sensory stimulations of foods. (Gastric acid secretions are increased by external factors, including the sight and smell of food and psychologic stress.) The patient should have nothing to eat for 12 hours and not smoke for 8 hours before the test. The following drugs should be withheld for 24 hours: antacids, anticholinergics, cholinergics, alcohol, H_2 blockers, reserpine and adrenergic blockers. Adrenocorticosteroids should be held for approximately 12 hours before the test.

To prevent contamination of gastric contents with saliva, the patient should be instructed to expectorate excess saliva rather than swallow it.

Check the location of the nasogastric tube for placement by aspirating gastric contents. Paroxysms of coughing or cyanosis may indicate a tube in the trachea. Clamp the tube during removal to prevent aspiration from fluids in the lumen. Sore throat following intubation may be treated with soothing lozenges, viscous lidocaine (Xylocaine), or benzocaine (Cetacaine) spray.

Gastric Acid Stimulation Test

Description: Normally follows basal gastric secretion test. A drug, usually pentagastrin, is given to stimulate gastric acid output; specimens are collected every 15 minutes for 1 hour. Normal values are 11 to 21 mEq/h for females and 18 to 28 mEq/h for males.

Indications: Clinical diagnosis of the following is indicated by certain results of gastric acid secretion:

Duodenal ulcers: High values
Zollinger-Ellison syndrome: Markedly high values
Gastric carcinoma: Low values
Pernicious anemia: Achlorhydria (low acid levels are considered normal in patients over 60 years of age)

Complications: Side effects of pentagastrin include abdominal pain, nausea, vomiting, flushing, transitory dizziness, faintness, and numbness of extremities. Check the patient's history for hypersensitivity to pentagastrin.

Nursing care: Same as for gastric analysis. Tell the patient that the collection of specimens every 15 minutes is normal.

Gastric Lavage

Description: The procedure includes an early morning suctioning of gastric contents after a nasogastric tube has been properly placed. The timing of the procedure is early morning because it is assumed that the patient swallows sputum at night while sleeping and in the early morning with morning coughing. The gastric contents are sent to the laboratory for sputum analysis.

Indications: This technique, although infrequently used, may be helpful in the diagnosis of patients with suspected tuberculosis or lung cancer.

Complications: None.

Nursing care: The patient should be given nothing by mouth after midnight. In the early morning, a nasogastric (NG) tube is inserted through the patient's nose. Suction is applied to the NG tube with a large syringe, and the gastric contents are removed. The contents are placed in a specimen container and are sent immediately to the laboratory. The NG tube is removed.

Peritoneal Fluid Analysis

Description: Examines a sample of peritoneal fluid obtained by paracentesis. Normally, peritoneal fluid is sterile, odorless, clear to pale yellow, and less than 50 ml in volume, with no red blood cells, bacteria, or fungi. Normal values: white blood count—less than 300 mg/μl; protein—0.3 to 4.1 g/dl; glucose—70 to 100 mg/dl; amylase—138 to 404 U/L; ammonia—less than 50 μg/dl. Alkaline phosphatase: male age over 18 years—90 to 239 U/L; female under 45 years—76 to 196 U/L; female age 45 years or older—87 to 250 U/L.

Indications: To determine the composition of ascitic fluid, to assist in diagnosis of hepatic or other systemic disease, or to detect abdominal trauma.

Complications: Perforation of abdominal organs or vessels. Signs include those for hemorrhage and shock, increasing pain, and abdominal tenderness.

Patients with severe hepatic disease should be observed for signs of hepatic coma. Observe the patient for mental changes, drowsiness, and stupor.

Nursing care: Record baseline vital signs, weight, and abdominal girth measurement for comparison with posttest results. Consent forms are generally required. The patient should void immediately before the procedure to prevent injury to bladder when the trocar is inserted. The patient is usually sitting with feet flat on the floor or on a footstool with the back supported; if the patient cannot tolerate this, use a high-Fowler's position.

Provide emotional support to the patient before and during the procedure.

Check vital signs every 15 minutes during the procedure and compare with baseline values; note signs of dizziness, pallor, perspiration, and increased anxiety. Rapid aspiration of peritoneal fluid may induce hypovolemia and shock; in such a case, slow the rate of aspiration.

After the test has been completed, monitor vital signs frequently (every 30 minutes for 2 hours; every hour for next 4 hours; every 4 hours for 24 hours). Weight and abdominal girth should be measured and compared with the baseline.

Cover the site with a sterile dressing. If the site continues to drain, requiring frequent dressing changes, consider application of a skin barrier and a pouch for collection of drainage and accurate measurement of output.

Monitor urinary output for 24 hours and observe for hematuria. Observe the patient closely for signs of hypovolemic shock if large amounts were aspirated. Assess aspiration site for signs of infection.

Cytologies

Description: Body secretions collected and examined for cells, which are stained and evaluated; examples are the Papanicolaou smear and examinations of cervical discharge, sputum, gastric washings, pleural fluid, and urinary washings

Indications: Suspected malignancies, infection, inflammation.

Complications: None, usually.

Nursing care: Explain the purpose of the test and tell the patient what to expect. Assist with individual procedures.

Cerebrospinal Fluid Studies

Description

Lumbar puncture: Insertion of a needle into the lumbar subarachnoid space to obtain cerebrospinal fluid for examination and to detect spinal subarachnoid block. The needle is inserted in the L3-L4 interspace.

Lateral cervical puncture: Insertion of a needle into the C1-C2 interspace through to the subarachnoid space to obtain cerebrospinal fluid. The needle is inserted perpendicular to the neck with the patient in a supine position.

Cisternal puncture: Insertion of a short-beveled needle immediately below the occipital bone into the cisterna magna to obtain cerebrospinal fluid. It can be inserted simultaneously with lumbar puncture to demonstrate subarachnoid block.

Ventricular puncture: Insertion of a ventricular needle (in adults and older children) through burr holes into the lateral ventricle.

Indications: The lumbar puncture, or spinal tap, is a common neurologic test performed to measure cerebrospinal fluid pressure, remove cerebrospinal fluid for visualization and laboratory analysis, inject medications (e.g., spinal anesthesia, intrathecal injection of antibacterial agents) or contrast media, and determine the degree of subarachnoid block by means of spinal dynamics.

A cisternal puncture may be performed if a subarachnoid block is present, if a lumbar puncture is contraindicated, to reduce intracranial pressure, to perform encephalography, and to introduce air or a contrast medium for myelography.

A ventricular puncture is indicated if a lumbar or cisternal puncture is contraindicated, for injection of contrast medium into an infant's ventricles to determine the type of hydrocephalus, for removal of cerebrospinal fluid, for injection of air or oxygen to localize a tumor, and as a preliminary to ventricular drainage.

Complications: Infection, leakage of cerebrospinal fluid, dysuria, headache, nausea, and vomiting. Signs of meningeal irritation are increased intracranial pressure and convulsions.

Nursing care: Position the patient on a firm surface and maintain the spine in a horizontal position. Assist in obtaining a manometer reading of cerebrospinal fluid pressure. A sterile manometer is attached to the needle used in lumbar puncture, and the pressure is measured. A pressure above 200 cm H_2O is considered abnormal.

Keep the patient flat in bed (or on side) for 4 to 6 hours after the procedure. Force fluids, unless contraindicated. Monitor vital signs and neurologic signs frequently. The procedure should be performed with extreme caution when intracranial pressure is elevated. Provide emotional support to the patient as indicated. Provide pain medication as necessary if headache develops.

Vaginal Smears

Description: Vaginal examination is performed, and vaginal secretions are placed on a slide with 1 drop of normal saline placed on one side and 1 drop of 10% to 20% potassium hydroxide (KOH) on the other side.

Indications: *Trichomonas vaginalis* can be observed at the saline end of the slide, and *Candida albicans* at the KOH side; other organisms can also be identified with this procedure.

Complications: None.

Nursing care: Prepare the patient for a vaginal examination and assist with the procedure. Provide emotional support because the patient may fear results.

FECAL EXAMINATION

Fecal Fat

Description: Qualitative (random sample) and quantitative (72-hour collection) tests are used. Qualitative tests identify undigested muscle fibers and various fats, and quantitative tests can confirm steatorrhea. Fecal lipids normally are less than 20% of excreted solids or less than 7 g/24 hours.

A Sudan stain can be made on a sample to test for presence of fat.

Indications: Steatorrhea—excessive secretions of fecal lipids—may be observed in some malabsorption syndromes.

Complications: None.

Nursing care: Have the patient avoid alcohol ingestion for 72 hours before and during stool collection, and maintain a high-fat diet, 100 g/day for 72 hours before and during collection.

Avoid use of waxed collection containers because wax can become incorporated into the stool and distort results. Each specimen should be labeled appropriately and sent to the laboratory as soon as collected.

During the test, inform patient to avoid use of azathioprine, kanamycin, bisacodyl, cholestyramine, neomycin, colchicine, aluminum hydroxide, calcium carbonate, potassium chloride, and mineral oil because they inhibit absorption of fats or affect chemical digestion, producing inaccurate results.

Fecal Urobilinogen

Description: Determines the amount of urobilinogen (result of breakdown of bilirubin by intestinal flora) excreted in urine and feces.

Random stool specimen required. Normal values are 50 to 300 mg/24 h. Low levels may indicate hepatocellular jaundice from cirrhosis or hepatitis or extrahepatic disorders such as tumors obstructing bile flow. Low levels are also seen in aplastic anemia with depressed erythropoiesis. Elevated levels are found in hemolytic jaundice, thalassemia, and hemolytic pernicious anemia.

Indications: May be used as an indicator of hepatobiliary and hemolytic disorders.

Complications: None.

Nursing care: May be a 2-hour afternoon specimen or a 24-hour collection. If possible, avoid the following for 2 weeks before stool collection: broad-spectrum antibiotics, which inhibit bacterial growth in the colon and may inhibit fecal urobilinogen levels; sulfonamides, which react with the reagents used in the test; and salicylates, which in large doses can raise fecal urobilinogen levels. Stool container must be light resistant because urobilinogen breaks down to urobilin on exposure to light.

Fecal Occult Blood

Description: Procedure consists of a patient collecting small samples from three separate stool specimens. Their color may indicate the site of bleeding (e.g., melena is common with esophageal or gastric bleeding; a dark maroon color may indicate a lesion below the ligament of Treitz; and bright red may be from a low rectal carcinoma or hemorrhoids).

Complications: None.

Nursing care: With guaiac-impregnated pad tests (Hemoccult), discuss with the patient how to collect the stool specimen. Have the patient avoid red meats, poultry, fish, turnips, and horseradish for 48 to 72 hours before the test begins and throughout the collection period.

Withhold iron preparations, bromides, iodides, rauwolfia derivatives, indomethacin, colchicine, salicylates, and phenylbutazone for 48 hours before collection begins and throughout the test. If the patient is taking steroids, accuracy of the test may be affected. Do not collect during menses because false-positive results may be obtained. Ascorbic acid can interfere with the accuracy of the test and should be withheld 48 hours before the collection period begins.

ROENTGENOGRAMS

Chest Roentgenogram (X-Ray)

Description: Gives information regarding the anatomic location and abnormalities of the heart, great vessels, and lungs. Routine views in a cardiac series are posterior-anterior (PA), lateral, right anterior oblique (RAO), and left anterior oblique (LAO). Roentgenograms are also used to determine the position of the heart (normal is situs solitus: left thoracic heart); cardiothoracic size (normal is less than 50% of the internal dimensions of the thorax); cardiac silhouette (thorax, aorta, ventricular chambers, atrial chambers, pulmonary artery); presence of calcifications (visualized in great vessels and on valves); lung fields (used to determine normal distribution of pulmonary blood flow); increase in pulmonary congestion; presence of pulmonary hypertension; pleural effusions; pneumothoraces; and presence of fractures.

The normal chest roentgenographic examination includes PA and lateral views (as shown in FIG. 22-1). In young,

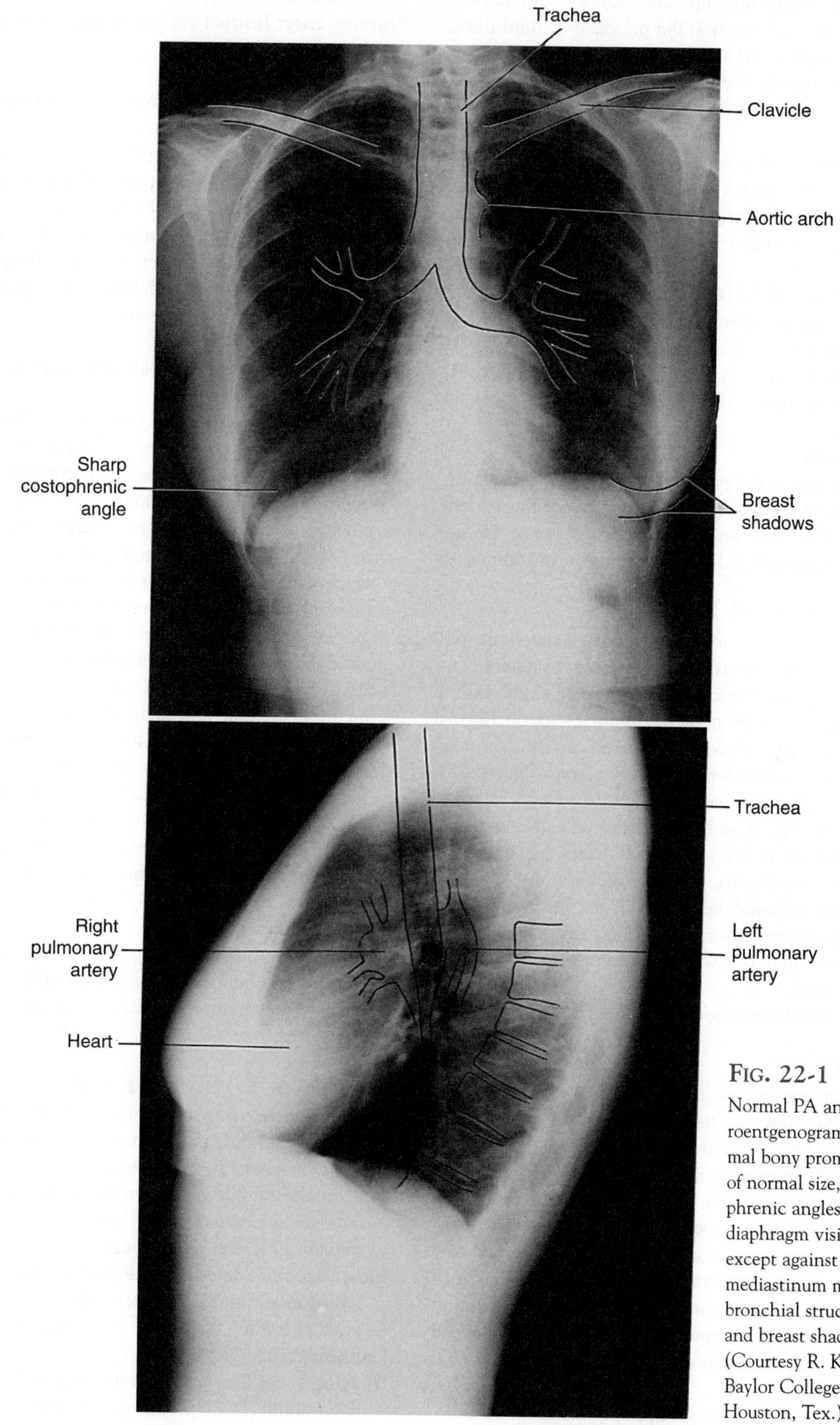

FIG. 22-1
Normal PA and lateral chest roentgenogram. Note no abnormal bony prominences, heart of normal size, sharp costophrenic angles, lung fields clear, diaphragm visible throughout except against heart border, mediastinum midline with bronchial structures visible, and breast shadows. (Courtesy R. Keith Wilson, MD. Baylor College of Medicine, Houston, Tex.)

healthy individuals or in asymptomatic persons only the PA view is used for screening. A lateral view should be obtained if disease is suspected or if the individual is over age 40 years. Chest roentgenograms in the upright position are preferred over those taken in the supine position so that the abdominal viscera do not push up on the diaphragm.

Indications: Chest roentgenograms are evaluated for normal structure, position, and outlines; the presence of fluid lines; foreign bodies; infiltration; and abnormal shadows. An anterior oblique view may be used to visualize the thymus in patients with immune disorders.

Complications: None.

Nursing care: Explain the procedure. Inquire if the patient is or may be pregnant. All neck jewelry or garments containing metal clasps, buttons, or ornaments must be removed. The patient should be wearing a hospital gown.

Musculoskeletal Films

Description: Examination of musculoskeletal tissues by means of roentgenographic exposure.

Indications: To determine injury, fracture, degeneration, inflammation, or neoplasm in one or more musculoskeletal tissues.

Complications: None.

Nursing care: Explain to the patient the purpose of the examination. Caution radiologic technicians to move the patient carefully and to support the joints above and below the affected tissues to prevent additional discomfort or trauma.

Sella Turcica/Skull Films

Description: Simple roentgenographic study of the skull. AP and lateral views are most frequently ordered to detect configuration, density, and vascular markings of skull. Initial roentgenographic evaluation of the pituitary gland begins with high-quality skull films that focus on the sella turcica, the bony structure in which the pituitary gland is located.

Indications: Skull films provide important data about vascular abnormalities, the shape and size of the cranial and facial bones, the presence of fractured skull bones, degenerative changes (i.e., bone erosion), unusual calcifications (e.g., tumors or chronic subdural hematomas), the position of the pineal body, investigation for cranial masses, Cushing's disease work-up, hypopituitary work-up, and precocious puberty.

Complications: None.

Nursing care: Instruct the patient regarding the procedure.

Spinal Films

Description: Simple roentgenographic study of different spinal regions: cervical, thoracic, lumbar, or sacral. Anterior, posterior, and lateral views are most common.

Indications: Spinal roentgenograms are taken when there has been trauma, pain, or sensory or motor impairment to the back or vertebral column. Roentgenograms of the spine usually include anterior, posterior, and lateral views to pinpoint fractures of the irregularly shaped vertebrae. Abnormal findings of spinal roentgenography include vertebral dislocation or fracture, bone erosion, unusual calcification, collapsed vertebrae and wedging, spondylosis, and spurs.

Complications: None.

Nursing care: Instruct the patient regarding the procedure.

Mastoid Films

Description: Roentgenograms of temporal bone. If mastoiditis is present, characteristic findings are clouding of the mastoid air cells and decalcification of bony walls between the cells.

Indications: A thick purulent discharge from the ear, low-grade temperature, a dull ache behind the ear.

Complications: None.

Nursing care: Instruct the patient regarding the procedure.

Sinus Films

Description: Roentgenograms taken to diagnose sinusitis by determining clouding or possible fluid levels in sinuses. The usual views include Waters' view (orbits, frontal and maxillary sinuses, and nasal septum); Caldwell's view (frontal sinuses, ethmoid air cells between each orbit, nasal septum, and petrous portion of temporal bone); and the lateral view (sphenoid sinus and posterior wall of frontal sinuses).

Indications: Headache, facial pain, low-grade temperature, a feeling of fullness or pressure in the face or sinus area.

Complications: None.

Nursing care: Instruct the patient regarding the procedure.

Mammography, Xeromammography

Description: Mammography is soft tissue roentgenography of the breast with low-energy roentgenographic and high-contrast film. Xeromammography is the use of a dry photoelectric process to make roentgenograms of soft tissues of the breast. The roentgenographic image is recorded on an electrostatically charged plate. The image is transferred to plastic-coated paper by pressing the plate and the paper together and exposing them to heat. All of this is performed automatically in a commercial processor.

Indications: The American Cancer Society's guidelines (2000) recommend that a woman get her first mammogram between the ages of 35 and 40; between the ages of 40 and 50, mammograms are recommended every other year, depending on the advice (and annual breast examination) of a physician; and annual mammograms are recommended after the age of 50. If a breast has been resected, the woman should have an annual mammogram of the other breast regardless of age.

Complications: None.

Nursing care: Ensure that the patient does not have powder, lotion, or ointment on her breasts. Explain the procedure and provide information to decrease anxiety about the outcome of the test.

Kidneys, Ureters, Bladder (KUB)

Description: Roentgenographic film of kidneys, ureters, and bladder without contrast material. It is important as a scout film when performing an intravenous pyelogram and as a diagnostic study to determine the presence of radiopaque calculi, or to evaluate lower intestinal obstruction, soft tissue masses, or bowel perforations.

Indications: To determine the size and location of kidneys and radiopaque stones; to detect abnormal gas patterns in the gastrointestinal (GI) tract; stool impaction.

Complications: None.

Nursing care: Preparation is not standardized. An intravenous pyelogram (IVP) preparation is used when KUB is performed as part of this extensive roentgenographic study. In other situations, no preparation is indicated.

CONTRAST STUDIES

Contrast Radiography

Description: Examination of an area of the body with a contrast medium during a roentgenographic study. Different types of contrast medium are used depending on the tissues involved and the radiographic techniques. A nonabsorbable medium, such as barium sulfate, is given by mouth, stoma, or rectum for gastrointestinal studies. Iodine-based contrast media, or dyes, can be injected or instilled intravascularly or through a tube or catheter.

Single-contrast intestinal studies use barium alone, whereas double-contrast studies use barium and air.

In addition to roentgenography (passage of radiation through the patient to create a roentgenogram), cineradiography, fluoroscopy, and video are used in many of these procedures. Cineradiography is a rapid-sequence roentgenographic procedure that films motion; fluoroscopy is the projection of roentgenograms onto a screen or fluoroscope, permitting continuous observation of motion.

Indications: Examination of soft and bony tissues of the body; diagnosis of certain pathologic conditions that requires the visualization of details not revealed by plain film radiography.

Complications: Barium retained in the intestine may harden and cause an obstruction or fecal impaction. Before giving iodine-based contrast, check for hypersensitivity to iodine, seafood, and contrast media. Symptoms of an allergic reaction include nausea, vomiting, flushing, urticaria, sweating, and (rarely) anaphylaxis. An intraductal injection may be accompanied by tachycardia and fever.

Nursing care: Barium as a contrast material precludes effective use of fiberoptic endoscopy for several hours and of arteriography for 24 to 48 hours.

For most patients, clear liquids before and forced fluids after a barium procedure, along with ambulation, are sufficient to clear the barium from the intestine. Healthy patients may take a mild laxative. Inform the patient of the need to clear all the barium. The nurse may need to examine the patient's stools to ensure this is happening, especially if the patient is debilitated. Inform patients that stools will initially be very light in color, darkening as the barium is eliminated.

The patient with a colostomy should be instructed to irrigate after the barium procedure is concluded and to repeat the irrigation the next morning. If upper gastrointestinal series or small bowel follow-through has been performed, the patient should irrigate after the last delayed spot film (approximately 6 hours after ingestion). The patient with an ileostomy should never receive a laxative or an enema before or after a barium study.

Warn patient due to receive an intravascular injection of iodine-based contrast that it can cause a sudden warm or burning, flushed feeling, which passes in seconds.

Ventriculography

Description: A ventriculogram depends on the injection of air or positive-contrast medium via a ventricular puncture directly into the lateral cerebral ventricles. The procedure is performed in the operating room under strict aseptic technique. Following the ventricular puncture, cerebrospinal fluid is gradually removed and replaced with air or a positive-contrast medium, and roentgenograms are taken.

Indications: Indications for a ventriculogram include determination of patency of the ventricular system, localization of a brain tumor, and detection of cerebral anomalies.

Complications: Nausea and vomiting, headache, increased intracranial pressure, respiratory distress, seizures, air embolus, shock.

Nursing care: General anesthesia may be required for young pediatric patients. Observe for signs and symptoms of intracranial or subdural hematoma (especially in patients with noncommunicating hydrocephalus). Frequently monitor vital signs and neurologic signs. Keep the patient flat in bed for 24 to 48 hours after the procedure. Encourage fluids. Keep accurate intake and output records. Institute seizure precautions for 24 hours after the procedure.

Barium Swallow

Description: Examination of the pharynx and esophagus with a fluoroscope after barium sulfate ingestion.

Indications: Used to diagnose or detect hiatal hernia, achalasia, diverticulum, varices, strictures, ulcers, tumors, motility disorders, and polyps.

Complications: Retained barium may harden and cause an impaction or obstruction.

Nursing care: Required fasting after midnight. Once the mixture is ingested, the patient is placed in various positions. The esophagus is also examined fluoroscopically during swallowing of the solution. Barium swallow is contraindicated in patients with an intestinal obstruction. Ensure evacuation of barium, as described under Contrast Radiography.

Upper Gastrointestinal and Small Bowel Series (UGI and SB Series)

Description: Fluoroscopic examination of the esophagus, stomach, and small intestine after ingestion of barium sulfate: as barium passes through the system, fluoroscopy outlines mucosal contours. Spot films are used to record significant findings. Follow-up spot films after 6 hours can provide some evaluation of gastrointestinal motility. The procedure is contraindicated in patients with intestinal perforations and intestinal obstructions.

Indications: Useful in detecting or diagnosing hiatal hernias, diverticula, varices, ulcers, strictures, tumors, regional enteritis (also called granulomatous ileitis or Crohn's disease), and motility disorders.

Complications: Retained barium may cause a fecal impaction or obstruction.

Nursing care: The patient is given nothing by mouth past midnight, and a mild laxative may be ordered. The patient should also increase fluid intake and maintain a low-residue diet for 2 to 3 days before the test. Smoking should be avoided from midnight before the test and throughout the procedure. Anticholinergics and narcotics are withheld for 24 hours before the study if intestinal motility is of concern. Ensure evacuation of barium as described under Contrast Radiography.

Oral Cholecystography (OCG)

Description: Roentgenographic examination of the gallbladder. Contrast medium is given the evening before the test. Iopanoic acid is usually used, but other commercial contrast media are available. The abdomen is examined fluoroscopically to evaluate gallbladder opacification. Spot films are taken of significant findings. Fat stimulus may also be used during the roentgenographic procedure. Fluoroscopy is then used to observe emptying of the gallbladder. Spot films are taken, as indicated.

The procedure is not performed in the presence of severe renal or hepatic disease or jaundice.

Indications: Evaluation of gallbladder disease.

Complications: Diarrhea commonly occurs; nausea, vomiting, and abdominal cramps, or dysuria occurs in rare cases.

Nursing care: The diet before the test includes a lunch meal containing fats and a fat-free evening meal. Check the patient for allergies to iodine, seafood, or contrast media before giving tablets—iopanoic acid, 3 g, given as one tablet with a total of 240 ml (8 ounces) of water. Check any emesis or diarrheal stools for undigested tablets.

Barium Enema

Description: Instillation of barium sulfate or barium sulfate and air through the anus into the large intestine. A barium enema should precede a barium-swallow upper gastrointestinal series with small bowel follow-through. Once this was the most effective means of identifying colon carcinomas above the level of sigmoid colon; colonoscopy examinations are now effectively used for visualization of the entire large intestine.

Barium enemas are contraindicated in patients with fulminant inflammatory bowel disease, toxic megacolon, suspected perforations, and suspected obstructions. Caution should be used for patients with acute inflammatory bowel disease, ischemic bowel disease, acute fulminant bloody diarrhea, and pneumatosis cystoides intestinalis.

Indications: Used as one method of diagnosing colorectal cancer and inflammatory bowel disease. It will also detect polyps, diverticula, and other changes in the colon and rectum.

Complications: Retained barium may cause fecal impaction or obstruction.

Nursing care: Careful bowel preparation is necessary to cleanse the bowel of fecal material. An ileostomy patient has no large intestine and requires only clear liquid for 24 to 48 hours as a "bowel" preparation; the site of the colostomy will determine the preparation.

Patients with suspected inflammatory bowel disease (ulcerative colitis or granulomatous colitis) should not be given a routine preparatory kit for barium enemas. The condition can be greatly exacerbated by irritants and may require surgical intervention; check with the physician.

Evacuation of barium from the bowel should be ensured, as described under Contrast Radiography.

Intravenous Cholangiography (IVC)

Description: Provides better visualization of the biliary ducts than does oral cholangiography, which is useful in gallbladder disease. IVC involves roentgenographic and tomographic studies after intravenous infusion of a contrast medium. Fluoroscopy spot films are made every 10 minutes until visualization of the bile ducts is satisfactory, which may take 25 to 40 minutes; tomograms are then made. Films and tomograms are repeated 2 to 2½ hours later, when maximal opacification of the gallbladder has occurred. (This would be unnecessary in patients with cholecystectomies.) Delayed films of the gallbladder may be taken at 4 and 24 hours. IVC should precede any barium studies, because retained barium clouds roentgenograms.

Indications: Generally indicated in patients with right upper quadrant or epigastric pain after cholecystectomy. Pain suggests biliary tract disease.

Complications: Hypersensitivity reactions.

Nursing care: The diet should be low residue the day before the test with an evening meal high in simple fats (milk, cream, eggs, butter); the patient should be given nothing to eat after midnight. Mild cathartics may be ordered. Check with the patient for a history of hypersensitivities to iodine, seafood, and contrast media. A fatty meal may be given so that, with fluoroscopy, emptying may be viewed.

Hypotonic Duodenography

Description: Barium sulfate and air instilled through an intestinal catheter for fluoroscopic examination of the duodenum. Intravenous infusion of glucagon or intramuscular injection of propantheline bromide is used to induce duodenal atony. A catheter is inserted through the nose and into the stomach while the patient is sitting or in a supine position under fluoroscopy; a catheter is advanced into the duodenum.

Administration of anticholinergics is contraindicated in the presence of severe cardiac disorders or glaucoma.

Indications: Demonstrates small duodenal lesions and tumors at the head of the pancreas.

Complications: Retained barium may cause fecal impaction or obstruction.

Nursing care: Explain the procedure to the patient. Ensure the evacuation of barium from the bowel as described.

Percutaneous Transhepatic Cholangiography

Description: Fluoroscopic examination of biliary ducts after the injection of iodinated contrast medium directly into the biliary tree. The liver is punctured by a thin, flexible needle, and contrast medium is injected as the needle is slowly withdrawn. Contrast medium slowly flows through the biliary ducts, outlining the biliary tree. The catheter used to inject the dye is sometimes left in place to drain the biliary tree.

Percutaneous transhepatic cholangiography is contraindicated in patients with cholangitis, severe ascites, uncorrectable coagulopathy, and hypersensitivity to iodine.

Indications: Helps to distinguish between obstructive and nonobstructive jaundice. The procedure helps to determine the location, the extent, and often the cause of mechanical obstruction of the biliary tree.

Complications: Hypersensitivity reactions, peritonitis, bleeding.

Nursing care: Check with the patient for a history of hypersensitivity to iodine, seafood, or contrast media. Check the patient for normal bleeding, clotting, prothrombin times, and platelet count.

The patient should remain in bed for 6 hours after the procedure. Check vital signs frequently (every 15 minutes for 1 hour, every 30 minutes for the next 2 hours, every hour for 4 hours after that, and then every 4 hours). Check the injection site for bleeding, swelling, and tenderness. Check for signs of peritonitis: chills, a temperature of 38.9° to 39.4° C (102° to 103° F), abdominal pain, tenderness, distention, nausea, and vomiting.

Postoperative Cholangiography or T Tube Cholangiography

Description: Contrast medium is injected through a T tube, and the flow of medium outlining the biliary tree can be visualized with fluoroscopy. This is performed 7 to 10 days following a cholecystectomy or common bile duct exploration in which a T tube has been left in the common bile duct to facilitate drainage.

Indications: To evaluate the patency and size of ducts and to identify calculi, strictures, neoplasms, or fistulas in the ductal system.

Complications: Sepsis, hypersensitivity reactions.

Nursing care: Some physicians have the T tube clamped for 24 hours before the procedure to eliminate air bubbles in the tube. A cleansing enema to evacuate the large intestine may be ordered. Check with the patient for allergies to iodine, seafood, and contrast media.

The T tube may be removed after the procedure if no stones are obstructing the common duct. A sterile dressing is applied. Note the amount and characteristics of any drainage. If frequent dressing changes are required, consider application of a sterile skin barrier and drainable pouch. Monitor the patient for signs and symptoms of peritonitis.

Endoscopic Retrograde Cholangiopancreatography (ERCP)

Description: Fluoroscopic examination of the pancreatic duct and hepatobiliary ductal system by injection of a contrast medium into the duodenal papilla. Endoscopy is performed and the duodenal papilla located. A cannula filled with contrast medium is passed through the endoscope, into the duodenal papilla and ampulla of Vater. The pancreas is visualized first with injection of dye and then fluoroscopically; then the cannula is repositioned for injection of additional contrast medium, allowing for visualization of the hepatobiliary tree. Tissue biopsy or fluid for histology may be obtained before the endoscope is removed. Some centers are able to perform sphincterotomy and to snare and remove stones.

ERCP is contraindicated in patients with acute pancreatitis, pancreatic pseudocysts, strictures or obstruction of the esophagus or duodenum, cholangitis, infectious disease, or cardiorespiratory disease.

Indications: To diagnose cancer of the duodenal papilla, pancreas, or biliary ducts; to detect calculi or stenosis of ducts; and to evaluate obstructive jaundice.

Complications: Cholangitis and pancreatitis may develop. Signs of cholangitis include fever, chills, and hyperbilirubinemia; late symptoms may include hypotension and gram-negative septicemia. Pancreatitis may be indicated by upper left quadrant pain, tenderness, elevated serum amylase, and transient hyperbilirubinemia.

Nursing care: Assess the patient for a history of hypersensitivity to iodine, seafood, or contrast media.

Frequent vital sign checks are indicated when the procedure is completed (every 15 minutes for 4 hours; every hour for the next 4 hours; and then every 4 hours for 48 hours). Check for voiding, because urinary retention may be a side effect of anticholinergics. Monitor the patient for bleeding after the procedure and for signs and symptoms of cholangitis or pancreatitis.

Splenoportography (Splenic Portography)

Description: Cineradiographic study of the splenic veins and portal system. It generally provides a cleaner definition of the venous system than does superior mesenteric arteriography (which offers the advantage of outlining the splenic and portal veins during reverse blood flow and has fewer complications). Splenoportography may result in excessive bleeding, requiring transfusions and occasionally a splenectomy.

Splenic pulp pressure is measured before the dye is injected by attaching a spinal manometer filled with normal saline to a sheath inserted in the spleen. Normal splenic pulp pressure is 50 to 180 mm H_2O (or 3.7 to 13.2 mm Hg). Contrast medium is injected into the splenic pulp.

This procedure is contraindicated in patients with ascites, uncorrectable coagulopathy, splenomegaly secondary to infection, hypersensitivity to iodine, or markedly impaired liver or kidney function.

Indications: Used to diagnose or assess portal hypertension and to stage cirrhosis.

Complications: Hypersensitivity reactions, bleeding.

Nursing care: Assess the patient for a history of allergies to iodine, seafood, or contrast media. Frequent assessment of vital signs is required after the procedure (every 15 minutes for 1 hour, every 30 minutes for the next 2 hours, and then every hour for 4 hours). Check for bleeding, swelling, and tenderness at the site of injection.

The patient should remain on the left side for 24 hours to minimize risk of bleeding. An additional 24 hours of bed rest is recommended. Hematocrit levels may be obtained every 8 to 12 hours until values have stabilized.

Intravenous Pyelogram (IVP), Intravenous Urogram, Excretory Urogram

Description: Contrast-enhanced roentgenographic study that provides detailed anatomic information about the urinary tract. Clues to kidney function are provided by assessment of the organ's ability to concentrate and excrete contrast material. Information concerning the transport of urine through the ureters is provided by use of sequential films after a contrast medium is injected. Compression over ureters may be used to provide additional detail. Assessment of bladder function is made by obtaining films of the vesicle filled with contrast material (after asking the patient to void). IVP is performed after adequate preparation and after a KUB is done.

The patient is placed in a slight Trendelenburg's position or supine, and contrast material is injected intravenously. Serial films of kidneys, ureters, and the bladder are obtained over a period of time. The entire examination requires approximately 30 minutes. A nephrotomogram may be performed as part of the IVP to provide a more detailed reproduction of anatomic detail by focusing on a specific plane of the kidney rather than a nonspecific picture of the entirety of the kidneys.

Because of the risk of hypersensitivity reactions and potential renal failure secondary to IVP, a number of relative contraindications should be considered before performing the study. These include (1) a history of allergic reaction when given intravenous iodine-bound contrast material and (2) patients at higher risk for dehydration, including elderly persons and patients with severe diabetes mellitus, multiple myeloma, renal insufficiency, or only one functioning kidney.

Indications: Evaluation of renal masses, cysts, ureteral obstruction, retroperitoneal tumors, renal trauma, and bladder abnormalities; evaluation of renal disease and hypertension.

Complications: Hypersensitive reactions and acute renal failure. Observe for allergic reactions such as flushing of skin, urticaria, rhonchi, dyspnea, shortness of breath, and hypotension. Acute renal failure is a rare but serious complication of IVP.

Nursing care: Explain procedure to the patient, and tell him or her that sequential or serial films are normal. Assess the patient for a history of allergies to iodine, seafood, or contrast media. After procedure, encourage increased fluid intake to ensure excretion of contrast. Observe urinary output (at least 30 ml/h) while ensuring adequate fluid intake.[14]

Whitaker and Pfister Tests

Description: The Whitaker test is performed by placing a nephrostomy tube percutaneously into the pelvis of the affected kidney. A urethral catheter is also placed to measure bladder pressure. Sterile water, saline, or radiographic contrast material is perfused through the nephrostomy tube via a pump at a specific rate. Continuous pressure monitoring is used to detect the presence of ureteral obstruction with the bladder empty and full.

The Pfister test is similar to the Whitaker test, except that a 20-gauge spinal needle is used in place of a nephrostomy tube, and intermittent rather than continuous pressure monitoring is used to assess ureteral obstruction.

Indications: Performed to assess ureteral obstruction when other methods (IVP, Lasix-enhanced renogram) fail to diagnose clearly or to rule out any obstruction.

Complications: Bleeding and infection.

Nursing care: Vital signs should be monitored regularly for the first 24 hours after testing. Temperature is an important parameter in the assessment of febrile urinary tract infection (UTI). Elderly patients may not become febrile with a UTI and should have other vital signs monitored carefully.

Retrograde Pyelogram (RPG)

Description: Provides a detailed anatomic description of the ureter and renal pelvis. It is performed in conjunction with cystoscopy because it requires placement of a 4 or 5 French ureteral catheter within the ureter to be studied. Radiographic contrast material is then injected into the collecting system via gravity infusion or by syringe, and roentgenographic images are obtained.

Indications: Evaluation of renal disease, obstruction, trauma, or in patients who are not candidates for IVP because of insufficient blood flow.

Complications: Pyelonephritis and overdistention of renal collecting system, which may result in extravasation of contrast medium leading to pain and fever. The reaction is typically transient; effects should disappear within 48 hours.

Nursing care: The patient should be closely observed for signs of infection (flank pain, fever, chills) for a 24- or 48-hour period after testing.

Retrograde Urethrogram (RUG)

Description: Provides a detailed description of urethral anatomy. It is made by injecting contrast material in a retrograde manner into the urethra. The patient is typically placed in a supine position, and oblique films are taken.

Indications: Evaluation of trauma or stricture.

Complications: Urethritis, cystitis.

Nursing care: The patient should be encouraged to force fluids for a 24-hour period after testing. Mild dysuria should cease within 24 hours of testing. Inform patients that sitz baths may help. Watch for signs of infection.

Cystogram, Voiding Cystourethrogram (VCUG)

Description: Provides a detailed picture of bladder anatomy; also, vesicoureteral reflux is assessed by visualizing the area over the ureters and right and left renal pelves. A voiding cystourethrogram provides information given by a cystogram along with images of the urethra during the voiding phase of bladder function. A cystogram is performed by infusing a roentgenographic medium intravesically under fluoroscopic monitoring. A voiding cystourethrogram is made in the same manner. Urethral images during voiding are obtained by removing the catheter and asking the patient to void while under the fluoroscope.

Indications: Assessment of bladder function.

Complications: Because cystogram and VCUG require placement of an indwelling catheter, cystitis is a potential complication.

Nursing care: The patient should be encouraged to force fluids for 24 hours following testing. Urinary frequency or mild dysuria should disappear completely within 24 hours.

Hysterosalpingography

Description: Injection of radiopaque contrast material, such as ionized oil or water-soluble material, through the cervix so that it fills the cervical canal and body of the uterus, flows through the fallopian tubes, and spills into the peritoneal cavity. The procedure should be performed no sooner than 6 weeks after delivery, abortion, or dilation and curettage.

The patient should be screened for *contraindications* to the procedure, including active pelvic inflammatory disease, vaginitis, cervicitis, pregnancy, or severe systemic illness.

Indications: Most commonly, to determine whether infertility is caused by an anatomic defect. It can also be used to confirm tubal occlusion and investigate the cause of dysmenorrhea, postmenopausal bleeding, or repeated abortion.

Complications: Rare; uterine or tubal inflammation, allergic reaction to contrast material.

Nursing care: The patient may experience pelvic pain resulting from spillage of contrast material; manage, as indicated, with pain medication. If indicated by the physician, assist the patient to walk for 30 minutes after the procedure until another film is taken. Observe for signs of infection.

Myelogram

Description: A roentgenographic procedure in which a needle is inserted into a disk space below the spinal cord, and 2 to 6 ml of spinal fluid is removed. A radiopaque solution is injected and distributed to the various tissues and structures to be examined, and roentgenograms are taken frequently. A water-soluble radiopaque solution is absorbed into the cerebrospinal fluid rather rapidly, but an oil-based solution must be removed by tilting the patient while observing the image monitor until the solution moves to the needle tip, from which it is withdrawn into a syringe. It is important that all or most of the solution be removed because even small amounts of retained solution may lead to persistent postmyelogram headaches and possibly adhesive arachnoiditis.

Indications: Aids in the diagnosis of spinal stenosis or obstruction within the spinal canal caused by a ruptured or herniated nucleus pulposus. It also detects distortion of spinal cord, spinal nerve roots, and the subarachnoid space.

Complications: Complications vary depending on whether a water-soluble agent, metrizamide (Amipaque), or an oil agent, iophendylate (Pantopaque), is used. With metrizamide, the patient may have nausea, vomiting, or headache and possible seizures, chest pain, dysrhythmias, and speech disorders. With iophendylate, common complications include headache, meningeal and nerve root irritation, and adhesive arachnoiditis.

Nursing care: The patient is allowed a clear liquid breakfast and then is given nothing by mouth. Any possible allergy to iodine is determined, and a mild sedative (diazepam, 10 mg) may be given. The patient must lie flat in bed for 8 to 12 hours if oily iophendylate was used, and fluids are forced to replace the cerebrospinal fluid. After the use of metrizamide the head of the patient's bed may be raised and fluids forced. If the patient complains of a headache, lowering the bed to the flat position is usually sufficient to relieve the pain. Mild analgesics may be ordered for persistent pain. Observe the patient for the other side effects already described.

Diskogram

Description: A roentgenographic procedure similar to a myelogram, in which radiopaque solution is injected into a disk space (L3 to L5 areas), and roentgenograms are taken.

Indications: To determine the condition of the disk spaces.

Complications: Possible development of diskitis.

Nursing care: Explain to the patient that a radiopaque solution will be injected into the disk, and roentgenograms will be taken. After the procedure, neurologic checks are performed, and mild analgesics may be required for pain. Monitor vital signs frequently.

Arthrogram

Description: Through use of a radiopaque solution, fluoroscopy, and multiple roentgenograms, any tissues not normally seen by roentgenograms are visualized. A needle is inserted into the joint; its position is verified by fluoroscopic examination. A radiopaque solution is injected into the joint, and the needle is removed. The site is sealed with collodion. The patient is asked to move the joint through its range of motion while roentgenograms are taken. The radiopaque solution is usually rapidly absorbed into the joint fluids.

Indications: To outline the structures of the joint capsule being studied and to aid in the diagnosis of injuries to the joint muscles, ligaments, cartilage, or bursa.

Complications: Joint swelling after the procedure, soreness or pain, and crepitus (noise on joint movement).

Nursing care: Explain to the patient that skin around the joint will be cleansed with an antiseptic and that a local anesthetic will be administered. After the procedure, instruct the patient in applying a compression bandage and ice around the joint to lessen edema. Explain that the joint should be held at rest for 12 or more hours and that use is then dependent on the findings of the arthrogram. Mild analgesics can be prescribed for pain.

ELECTRODIAGNOSTIC STUDIES

Electrocardiogram (ECG)

Description: Electrical representation of myocardial activity. It is used to determine the presence of abnormal transmission of heart impulses through the conduction tissue of heart muscle (see Chapter 3 for normal findings).

Indications: Chest pain; to evaluate cardiac disturbance; for routine diagnostic study during physical examinations and preoperatively.

Complications: None.

Nursing care: Explain the procedure. Ensure electrical safety measures, and provide privacy during the procedure.

Ambulatory Electrocardiography (Holter Monitor)

Description: A portable recorder, worn by the patient, records cardiac activity continuously while the patient is going about usual activities.

Indications: Used to detect ECG rhythm disturbances that may occur over an extended period of time, to evaluate effectiveness of antidysrhythmic drug therapy and to evaluate chest pain episodes. It is also capable of recording ECGs over a 24- to 48-hour period.

Complications: None.

Nursing care: Explain the procedure. Instruct the patient in the care of electrodes at home and about the importance of keeping a diary of symptoms or activities at times designated by the physician.

Electrophysiologic Studies (EPS, Cardiac Mapping)

Description: Involves insertion of a catheter via a central vein into the right atrium and right ventricle (right heart catheterization).

Indications: To detect atrioventricular conduction disturbances, diagnose syncope, and assist in selection of antidysrhythmic agents.

AV interval (atrioventricular): Conduction time from the low right atrium through the AV node to the His bundle. Normal is 60 to 125 msec.

HV interval (His-ventricle): Conduction time from the proximal His bundle to the ventricular myocardium. Normal is 35 to 55 msec.

PA interval: Conduction time from the beginning of the P wave to the beginning of the A defection. Normal is 20 to 40 msec.

Sinus node disease: Sinus node exit block; depression of sinus node automaticity.

Atrioventricular block: Mobitz type II block.

Intraventricular block: Bifascicular block.

Tachycardias: Supraventricular tachycardia with a rate of more than 200 beats per minute associated with symptoms, or with recurrent bouts that are refractory to therapy.

Accessory pathway tachycardia: Wolff-Parkinson-White syndrome.

Ventricular tachycardia: Tachycardia caused by irritable ventricular foci firing repetitively.

Unexplained syncope: Cardiac arrest patients resuscitated from sudden cardiac death.

Contraindications include dysrhythmias that will be difficult to treat because of an underlying cardiac disorder (e.g., acute myocardial infarction, class IV heart failure, severe aortic stenosis).

Complications: Dysrhythmias, phlebitis, pulmonary emboli, hemorrhage, cardiac perforation.

Nursing care: Ensure that informed consent is obtained. Explain that the procedure will last 1 to 3 hours and that the patient will be awake and may feel slight pressure. Instruct the patient to report any discomfort. Permit nothing by mouth for 6 hours before the procedure. After the procedure, check vital signs every 15 minutes for 1 hour, then every 4 hours for 24 hours. Check the insertion site for bleeding every 30 minutes to 1 hour for 8 hours.

Electroencephalogram (EEG)

Description: An EEG provides a graphic record of brain wave activity. Generally, between 17 and 21 electrodes are attached with collodion to the patient's head at corresponding areas over the prefrontal, frontal, temporal, parietal, and occipital lobes. After the electrodes are attached, the patient is instructed to remain quiet with the eyes closed and is informed of the need to refrain from talking or moving unless otherwise required (the patient is asked to hyperventilate for a short period during the test to accentuate abnormalities).

The brain waves recorded during an EEG are called alpha, beta, delta, and theta rhythms. *Alpha* rhythms occur in the adult at 8 to 13 cycles/sec and are most prominent in the occipital leads. Apprehension and anxiety can decrease the frequency of the alpha waves. *Beta* wave forms are prominent in the frontal and central areas and occur at a rate of 18 to 30 cycles/sec. Beta rhythm indicates normal activity, when an individual is alert and attentive with the eyes open. *Delta* waveforms indicate serious brain dysfunction or deep sleep. This rhythm occurs at a rate of less than 4 cycles/ sec. *Theta* waveforms occur at a rate of 4 to 7 cycles/sec and come primarily from the temporal and parietal areas. Theta rhythm indicates drowsiness or emotional stress in adults.

Indications: Seizure activity, coma, brain tumor, or infection.

Complications: None.

Nursing care: Stimulants such as coffee, tea, chocolate, cola, and smoking are not permitted for 8 hours before the procedure. The adult patient should have minimal sleep (i.e., 4 to 5 hours) the night before the procedure. Explain to patient that if taking anticonvulsant medications, the medications should be continued. Hair should be washed before test. After the test ensure that paste is removed from patient's hair; some paste is water-soluble, but some requires acetone for removal.

Electromyogram (EMG)

Description: Surface electrodes or monopolar electrodes measure and record electrical properties of skeletal muscle and nerve conduction. Electrical activity is picked up by a needle electrode inserted into the muscle and displayed on an oscilloscope. For example, EMG needles, hooked wire electrodes, and pediatric ECG surface electrodes may be placed directly into the external urinary sphincter, or they may be placed over the perianal sphincter to measure the activity of pelvic floor musculature, including the response of the urinary sphincter to bladder filling and storage and to micturition.

Indications: The diagnosis of myopathies and muscle responses to electrical stimuli may be performed in the patient's room, depending on the number of muscles to be studied.

Complications: Rare; hematoma at the injection site.

Nursing care: Explain to the patient that a small needle will be inserted into one or more muscles to be studied and that the muscle will be stimulated with a small electrical impulse. The results will be recorded on a graph. Explain to the patient that the procedure may cause some minor discomfort when the needle is inserted but otherwise is not painful.

Nerve Conduction Velocity Determination

Description: Study of nerve conduction velocity calculated by division of the distance between proximal and distal points by the time required for the electrical stimulus to travel between those two points.

Indications: To diagnose neuromuscular problems.

Complications: None.

Nursing care: Explain that this study may be performed in conjunction with the electromyogram (EMG) and uses the same machine.

Electrocochleography

Description: Permeatal transtympanic electrode placement in contact with the promontory of the cochlea to record acoustically evoked potentials from the cochlea. Three distinct evoked potentials can be recorded: cochlear microphonic potential, summating potential, and vestibulocochlear nerve compound action potential.

Indications: Measures auditory function; aids in the differential diagnosis of auditory disorders (i.e., vestibulocochlear nerve disorders); provides the prognosis for auditory disorders.

Complications: Potential vertigo, middle ear infection, perilymph leak.

Nursing care: Explain the procedure to the patient.

Electronystagmography

Description: Graphic recording and measuring electrical potentials of eye movements during spontaneous, positional, or calorically-evoked nystagmus. Intensity, frequency, and speed of the fast and slow components of nystagmus are recorded.

Indications: To assess and evaluate neurologic disorders.

Complications: None.

Nursing care: Patient's eyes must be open during the procedure.

Plethysmography

Description: Measures venous flow in limbs by recording changes in volume and vascular resistance. There are two types: digital plethysmography (to evaluate digital pulse volume) and venous occlusion plethysmography (to evaluate arterial responses to temporary block of the venous system). A pneumatic cuff is applied to a limb to occlude venous return. Two electrodes are applied to the limb, and a very weak electrical current is passed through it. The resistance of the limb to the current is measured and recorded on graph paper.

Indications: Used to detect deep vein thrombosis in the leg and to screen patients at high risk for thrombophlebitis.

Complications: None.

Nursing care: Explain the procedure, and assist the patient into a position to promote venous drainage of the limb to be studied.

ULTRASOUND STUDIES

Ultrasonography

Description: The ultrasound machine uses high-frequency waves (5000 to 20,000 Hz) to detect vibrations reflected from soft tissues of varying density. The vibrations (echoes) are converted into electrical potential and displayed on an oscillograph. The A-scan machine registers varying acoustic densities as spikes on linear tracing; the B-scan registers a two-dimensional "picture."

Doppler ultrasonic techniques measure the movement of red blood cells by measuring the change in sound frequency that occurs when sound waves are bounced off the cells. Doppler devices are used to evaluate the patency of arteries and veins. Duplex ultrasonic devices combine an ultrasonic scanner to provide two-dimensional images of vascular structures with a Doppler device.

Ultrasonography is a painless procedure that is useful in evaluating soft tissues and does not involve the use of roentgen rays. A transducer, which is able to transmit and to receive high-frequency sound waves, is placed against the patient's body. The sound waves, which cannot be heard by the human ear, are bounced off the tissues inside the body. Tissues of different densities echo the sound in different ways. The echoes are received by the machine and are translated into an image on a TV screen.

In dehydrated patients, ultrasound can fail to define boundaries between organs and tissue structures because of a deficiency of body fluids.

Indications: Ultrasonography is useful for assessment of almost all body systems.

Head and neck: For the eye ultrasonography is useful for diagnosing intraocular tumors, retinal detachment, and fibrous tissue proliferation. The examiner holds the probe (attached to machine) over the patient's eyelid. For the thyroid, ultrasonography reveals diffuse or localized enlargements of the gland and differentiates between cystic or solid lesions.

Chest: Ultrasound has limited usefulness in evaluation of the lungs because sound beams are not transmitted well by air-containing tissue. Ultrasonographic examination is useful to detect pericardial effusion and fluid-containing or solid tissue lesions.

Breast: Ultrasound mammography is used to differentiate cystic and solid breast lesions. It is also used to evaluate women for whom roentgenographic mammography is contraindicated (e.g., pregnant, age under 25 years).

Gastrointestinal

Gallbladder and biliary system: Ultrasonography of the gallbladder and biliary system can be used if cholecystography is inconclusive or does not adequately visualize the gallbladder. It is useful in confirming cholelithiasis, diagnosing acute cholecystitis, and distinguishing between obstructive and nonobstructive jaundice. Sincalide, a hormonal analogue, may be given to cause the gallbladder to contract and expel bile. It allows an evaluation of gallbladder function.

Liver: Ultrasonography of the liver is indicated for patients with jaundice of unknown cause, because it helps to distinguish between obstructive and nonobstructive jaundice. It can be used in a screening or diagnostic test for hepatocellular disease and hepatic metastases. It can also be used after abdominal trauma to detect a hematoma and define cold spots found on liver scans in the presence of severe ascites. Ultrasonic examination may be combined with placement of a biopsy needle to evaluate masses or obtain specimens for culture.

Spleen: Ultrasonography of the spleen is used to demonstrate splenomegaly, to evaluate changes in splenic size, to evaluate the spleen following abdominal trauma, and to clarify cold spots found on scans of the spleen. Computed tomography (CT) scans often provide more information on splenomegaly than ultrasonography does.

Pancreas: Ultrasonography of the pancreas is used to detect anatomic abnormalities such as pseudocysts and pancreatic carcinomas. It detects alterations in size, contour, and parenchymal texture of the pancreas.

Renal and genitourinary tracts: Ultrasonography of these tracts is a noninvasive way to identify a dilated collecting system; calculi; cysts; perirenal collections of blood, pus, lymph, or urine; solid masses; and kidney size.

Ultrasonography of kidneys: The patient is placed in the prone position. An outline of the kidneys is obtained and marked on the skin. Serial scans are made 1 to 2 cm apart perpendicular to the longitudinal axis. Obtaining additional views with the patient in a supine position helps elucidate the kidneys' position relative to other abdominal organs.

Ultrasound-guided biopsy of kidney: Ultrasonic examination may be combined with placement of a biopsy needle to define makeup of a renal or juxtarenal mass. Routine ultrasonographic examination of the affected kidney is completed first. The mass is then located and marked on the skin. With use of sterile drapes, gloves, and a local anesthetic, the biopsy needle is placed into the mass, and a tissue sample is withdrawn. Aspiration of a renal cyst may be performed the same way.

Ultrasonography of bladder and ureters: Ultrasonography of a distended bladder provides some detail of vesical outline and may be used to evaluate the diverticulum. Abdominal ultrasonography detects the presence of ureteral dilation, although normal ureters may not be completely visualized. It is typically combined with examination of the kidneys.

Ultrasonography of testes: This is used to differentiate solid and cystic masses. In addition, torsion of the testes is assessed by Doppler ultrasound techniques, which assess both testicular structure and blood flow.

Vascular: Ultrasonography detects anatomic abnormalities of blood vessels, including aneurysms, dissections, and arteriovenous fistulas. It is used to evaluate vascular patency and measure blood flow. It identifies emboli, atherosclerotic plaques, and other causes of vascular obstruction.

Aorta: Ultrasonography can determine the presence and size of aortic aneurysms, which occur most commonly at the abdominal aorta. Evidence of an aortic aneurysm greater than 5 cm or one that is significantly enlarging is an indication for surgical intervention.

Cerebrovascular and carotid arteries: Ultrasonography can examine the cerebral and carotid arteries for the presence of anatomic anomalies, emboli, and plaques that may obstruct blood flow to the brain. In certain cases ultrasonography can provide more accurate information about vascular abnormalities than can arteriograms. Because carotid ultrasonography is noninvasive and not risky to patients, it is used for long-term follow-up of endarterectomy patients. It is recommended for patients with neurologic symptoms such as headache, dizziness, syncope, confusion, hemiparesis, paresthesia, and acute speech or visual abnormalities.

Peripheral arteries: Doppler ultrasonography can evaluate arterial blood flow to extremities and identify causes of impaired flow. Most peripheral arterial occlusions are the result of plaque formation in atherosclerosis.

Ankle pressure: Doppler can evaluate arterial blood flow to the lower extremities by measuring ankle and brachial systolic blood pressures. The ankle/brachial index is calculated by dividing ankle pressure by brachial pressure. In normal individuals the index is usually greater than 1. Values significantly below 1 indicate impaired flow to the legs.

Peripheral veins: Ultrasonography of peripheral veins can identify venous insufficiency and thrombosis. Thrombophlebitis causes thrombus formation within the venous system. Pulmonary emboli most often come from femoral or iliac veins or the inferior vena cava. Venous duplex ultrasonography to identify venous thrombus has gained acceptance over traditional methods, such as venography, because it is accurate, noninvasive, and comparatively risk free.

Complications: Bleeding with ultrasound-guided biopsies.

Nursing care: Explain the procedure to the patient. For gastrointestinal ultrasonography, the patient is allowed nothing by mouth (NPO) 8 to 12 hours before the procedure to reduce bowel gas. For gallbladder ultrasonography give the patient nothing to eat for 8 to 12 hours before the procedure. The patient should have a fat-free meal the evening before the test (which allows bile to accumulate in the gallbladder). For ultrasound-guided biopsy of solid organs, the patient is kept NPO for 8 to 12 hours before the procedure.

Side effects of sincalide include abdominal cramping, tenesmus, nausea, dizziness, sweating, and flushing; sincalide should not be given during pregnancy.

For bladder ultrasonography, because of the necessity of distending the bladder to evaluate it, the patient will wish to void immediately after the examination, or unclamp the Foley if appropriate.

Barium can interfere with sound waves. Ultrasound studies should be performed before studies or procedures that use barium.

Explain to the patient that the gel used for ultrasound is water soluble and easily washed off.

Echocardiogram

Description: Ultrasonographic technique of evaluating internal structures and motion of the heart. Sound waves reflected from cardiac structures are received by a transducer and converted to real-time images.

There are several modes: M-mode, or one-dimensional; two-dimensional; cross-sectional; real-time motion; and Doppler, in which continuous-wave combined with pulse ultrasound gives an image of the heart pulse and indicates the direction of blood flow within the heart.

Indications: Echocardiograms are used to determine internal dimensions of ventricles, the size and motion of the intraventricular septum and posterior wall of the left ventricle, valve motion and anatomy, the presence of pericardial fluid, the direction of blood flow, and the presence of blood clots and myomatous tumors. Echocardiograms are also used in cardiac stress testing and to evaluate patients with chest pains. Ultrasonography demonstrates decreased heart wall motion when myocardium is ischemic.

Complications: None.

Nursing care: Explain the procedure to the patient.

Transthoracic echocardiography (TTE): Noninvasive technique using a transducer applied to the chest or abdominal wall. The quality of images is limited by the ribs, sternum, lungs, and subcutaneous fat, which interfere with the sound waves. In addition, the quality of the test is decreased in obese patients. The procedure is painless.

Transesophageal echocardiography (TEE): An ultrasound transducer is placed into the esophagus by endoscopy. It provides a view of the heart unobstructed by the tissues that limit TTE. High-resolution images of the heart can be obtained. The procedure is contraindicated in patients with esophageal pathologic conditions.

Complications: Esophageal perforation or bleeding, cardiac dysrhythmias.

Nursing care: Explain the procedure to the patient. The patient should be NPO at least 4 hours. Remove dental prosthetics. Obtain IV access. Measure baseline vital signs. Monitor cardiac rhythm, vital signs, and oxygen saturation during the procedure. The patient may be given a sedative. Observe patient for 1 hour after procedure.

BIOPSIES

Brain Biopsy

Description: Removal of a small brain tissue sample, usually accomplished during intracranial surgery.

Indications: Useful in the evaluation of neurologic disorders.

Complications: Bleeding, infection.

Nursing care: Frequent monitoring of vital signs and neurologic signs.

Thyroid Biopsy

Description: Sterile aspiration of thyroid tissue. It is often performed to help determine if surgery is needed because it is a relatively simple, effective way of ascertaining if a thyroid nodule is malignant.

Indications: Differentiates between benign and malignant nodules; assists in the diagnosis of subacute thyroiditis in atypical cases, Hashimoto's disease, or multinodular goiter.

Complications: Puncture of the esophagus or trachea.

Nursing care: Support during the procedure; assessment for esophageal or tracheal puncture after the procedure.

Lung Biopsy

Description and indications: Lung biopsy may be performed in one of four ways. The purpose of all techniques is to obtain a tissue sample for histologic evaluation.

Transbronchial biopsy: This biopsy is taken with the fiberoptic bronchoscope from the bronchial area of concern.

Nursing care: See the discussion under fiberoptic bronchoscopy, p. 1366.

Percutaneous needle biopsy with aspiration: In this procedure fluids and cells are aspirated into the syringe through a long, 18- to 20-gauge needle inserted percutaneously under fluoroscopic control into the suspected lesion. When the needle is in the lesion, the syringe is generally rotated to obtain a tissue specimen. This procedure is used most often if malignancy is suspected. A contraindication to needle aspiration is a patient who cannot hold his or her breath when required.

Nursing care: The procedure is performed with the patient under local anesthesia after the skin has been disinfected and a sterile field has been prepared. The patient is instructed to hold his or her breath for 15 to 30 seconds during the procedure. The aspirated material is sent for cytologic examination and for stains and cultures of microorganisms. The major postprocedural complication is pneumothorax. Therefore careful respiratory assessment is indicated.

Percutaneous biopsy with a cutting needle: Three procedure options are possible: a punch biopsy with a Vim-Silverman needle; a high-speed drill biopsy with a trephine-lung biopsy drill; or a suction excision biopsy with an Abrams' needle or a modification of the Abrams' needle. The cutting needle procedure is indicated when the patient has diffuse pulmonary infiltrates. These techniques have significant complications and therefore are not usually done until other diagnostic procedures have failed to identify the problem.

Nursing care: These procedures are performed with the patient under local anesthesia and after a sterile field has been prepared. Major complications include hemorrhage and pneumothorax. Careful postprocedural assessment is indicated.

Open lung biopsy or exploratory thoracotomy: This is an invasive procedure used to confirm a suspected diagnosis of lung or chest disease by obtaining lung specimens. The chest is opened through a standard thoracotomy incision, and the lung is inspected and a biopsy performed. An open lung biopsy is indicated only after other investigative procedures have not clearly identified the patient's problem.

Nursing care: General anesthesia is used. Ensure that informed consent is obtained. A chest tube connected to water-seal drainage is used for 1 to 2 days after surgery because of the surgically induced pneumothorax. Several days of postprocedural chest roentgenograms are normally ordered. The procedure may have several major complications, including postoperative respiratory failure, empyema, and chronic bronchopleural fistula.

Pleural Biopsy

Description: A small tissue sample is taken by a special biopsy needle from the parietal pleura. It may be necessary to collect tissue samples from several different spots. Although some authorities advocate pleural biopsy every time a thoracentesis is performed, others claim that it should be done only when granulomatous disease or malignancy is suspected.

Indications: Evaluation of pulmonary disease.

Complications: Rare, but include pneumothorax, hemothorax, and intercostal nerve injury.

Nursing care: Position the patient as for thoracentesis and provide support during the procedure. Monitor vital signs and assess the patient for symptoms of complications.

Lymph Node Excision and Scalene Node Biopsy

Description: Excision of a peripheral lymph node or biopsy of a palpable scalene node. The incision and biopsy are performed in the supraclavicular scalene region.

Indications: Performed to assess immunologic function in suspected immunodeficiency diseases and to stage certain malignancies.

Complications: Bleeding, erythema, infection at site.

Nursing care: Provide an occlusive dressing. Check the surgical site for bleeding, erythema, or purulent drainage.

Bone Marrow Aspiration and Biopsy

Description: Needle biopsy of marrow performed after entering the marrow cavity of the sternum, iliac crest, posterosuperior iliac spine, spinous process, rib, or tibial head. Bone marrow cellularity is determined.

Indications: Evaluation of the immune and hematolymphatic systems, useful in differential diagnosis of thrombocytopenia, leukemia, granulomatous disease, and aplastic, hypoplastic, or megaloblastic anemias.

Complications: Bleeding, infection, or pain at the site.

Nursing care: Exert immediate pressure over the biopsy site. Apply an occlusive dressing. Check the biopsy site for bleeding, erythema, or purulent drainage. Maintain bed rest for 1 hour. Administer analgesics as needed.

Muscle and Nerve Biopsy

Description: Removal of a small muscle or nerve tissue sample for histologic, histochemical, ultrastructural, or biochemical studies.

Indications: Aids in the diagnosis of myopathies, such as muscle atrophy, degeneration, or inflammation, and determines the extent of damage to myelinated and unmyelinated nerve fibers.

Complications: Mild soreness or stiffness of muscle or nerve that has undergone biopsy.

Nursing care: Explain to the patient that the procedure will be performed with the patient under local anesthesia in the operating suite. After the procedure, encourage the patient to move the affected area and to walk (if the leg or foot is involved) to prevent stiffness. Provide analgesics, if required. Monitor for bleeding or infection at the site. If sutures are used, remove them in 7 to 10 days.

Synovial Biopsy

Description: Biopsy of the synovium by means of a special needle. The biopsy specimen is sent for histologic examination.

Indications: Aids in the differential diagnosis of various forms of arthritis.

Complications: Joint effusion or hemorrhage into the joint.

Nursing care: Explain to the patient that the biopsy is performed after the skin is cleansed with antiseptic solutions and a local anesthetic is administered (occasionally a synovial biopsy is taken during open surgery). After the procedure, apply a small compression dressing and an elastic bandage around the joint. Caution the patient to restrict joint use for 24 hours to prevent hemorrhage or effusion.

Bladder, Prostate, Urethra Biopsies

Description: Biopsy specimens from a bladder, urethra, or prostate may be obtained with a cystoscopic/panendoscopic system. A resectoscope, which uses an electrically activated wire loop or a tubular cold knife, is positioned over the lesion, and a specimen is obtained. The bladder must be relatively full when a specimen is obtained to prevent inadvertent damage to normal mucosal folds. Transrectal or transperineal needle biopsies are often taken in conjunction with cystoscopic examination.

A transperineal biopsy is performed by injecting a local anesthetic into the skin of the perineum, over the area where the needle will enter. A finger in the rectum is used to guide the needle toward the area in question. The procedure may be repeated several times to ensure an adequate biopsy.

A transrectal biopsy requires no anesthesia. Preparation includes cleansing enemas to decrease the likelihood of introducing intestinal bacteria into the bloodstream or prostatic tissue. Prophylactic antibiotics are also indicated. When obtaining the specimen, the tip of the needle is placed on the examining finger and advanced gently to an area over which the biopsy is to be obtained. The needle is then pushed, and a biopsy is taken. The procedure may be repeated several times.

Indications: Hematuria, pain, suspected malignancy.

Complications: Hematuria. The primary complication of transrectal biopsy (the more commonly performed of the two techniques described) is sepsis from perforation of the bowel.

Nursing care: Postprocedural care is similar to that of routine cystoscopic examination. Mild dysuria may be seen with hematuria during the first 48 hours following the procedure. If a general anesthetic is used, low-grade fever may occur over the first 24 to 48 hours after the procedure. Hematuria may recur 5 to 7 days after the procedure. The patient should be assured that the lesion is healing and that such hematuria is normal. The patient should not experience dysuria or a significant frequency of urination at this time. Fever and chills must be reported to the physician at once. A prophylactic antibiotic regimen must be adhered to after the transrectal needle biopsy.

Renal Biopsy

Description: In a renal biopsy a small piece of tissue is obtained via a special needle (percutaneous) or through a surgical incision (open). Roentgenography of the kidney, ureter, or bladder; intravenous urography, and ultrasonography may be used to locate the kidney for biopsy.

The absolute contraindications to renal biopsy are a solitary kidney (except posttransplant, when a biopsy must be performed on a transplanted kidney to evaluate for rejection) or for irreversible hemorrhagic tendencies. The relative contraindications are an uncooperative patient, a suspected renal tumor or cysts, gross sepsis, very small kidneys, horseshoe kidney, ectopic kidney, severe hypertension, massive obesity, severe spinal deformity, and pregnancy.

Indications: Indications include persistent proteinuria, nephrotic syndrome, unexplained hematuria, controlled therapeutic trials of new drugs, and evaluation of rejection transplant.

Complications: Bleeding from the biopsy site (i.e., microscopic or gross hematuria, perirenal hematoma, retroperitoneal hematoma, arteriovenous fistula in the kidney, passage of clots, ureteric colic from a clot); hypotension; anemia; local infection; pain; perforation of other nearby structures.

Nursing care: Before the procedure, prepare the patient for the possibility of pain during the procedure. The patient should cooperate by holding his or her breath, on command. Explain that 24 hours of bed rest is needed after the biopsy, and that some hematuria is normal in the first 24 hours.

Record baseline vital signs. Review the chart for hemoglobin and hematocrit levels, platelet count, prothrombin time, and bleeding and clotting times. Review the type and crossmatch report for 2 units of blood. Review the outcome of any test for pregnancy.

Explain the reason for the biopsy and the need for observation after the biopsy. Explain that for several days the patient should avoid contact sports, lifting or heavy exercise, and swimming. Normal activities can be resumed gradually after 48 to 72 hours. Explain the need to call the physician if there is any hematuria after the first 24 hours, draining from the biopsy site, persistent fever, or pain.

Measure output carefully and collect the voidings individually. Watch for hematuria. Check for microscopic hematuria, which is invariably present in the first two specimens. The urine may appear pink. Report profuse or persistent hematuria. If no hematuria occurs in the first 24 hours, bathroom privileges can be instituted for the next 24 hours.

A tight dressing is applied to the biopsy site. Check the dressing for bleeding. Apply external pressure for 30 minutes by having the patient lie prone with a sandbag placed directly on the biopsy site. Measure blood pressure, pulse, and respirations every 15 minutes for 4 hours and then every 4 hours for 24 hours.

Ensure adequate hydration of 1000 to 2000 ml to ensure a good urine flow. Monitor the hematocrit 3 to 6 hours after biopsy. Any decrease from the prebiopsy level suggests perirenal bleeding.

Give a nonaspirin analgesic agent for mild pain after the anesthesia wears off, as ordered by the physician. Report severe lower back or flank pain.

Brush Biopsy of Renal Pelvis and Calyces

Description: A ureteral catheter with a steel guidewire is placed using a cystoscope as a guide. The catheter is then removed, and a steel or nylon brush is inserted to the level of the lesion to obtain a biopsy. The specimen is then smeared on slides and prepared with a 95% ethanol solution. After the specimen is obtained, the renal pelvis is irrigated with normal saline.[9]

Indications: Allows urologist to obtain a tissue biopsy from the renal pelvis or calyces without an open surgical incision to assist in the diagnosis of renal disease.

Complications: Irritation of the renal system because of manipulation.

Nursing care: Postprocedural care is similar to that of routine cystoscopic examination. A low-grade fever may be noted. Flank pain secondary to ureteral manipulation is not uncommon and should disappear within 48 hours. Fever greater than 38.3° C (101° F) and severe flank pain should be reported to physician. Remember that elderly patients may not become febrile even with sepsis.

Skin and Tissue Biopsy

Description: The lesion is marked, and the area is infiltrated with lidocaine. A small circular punch or scalpel is used to obtain tissue to determine cell structure.

Indications: For evaluation of abnormal lesions or tissue. The biopsy can be incisional (surgical excision of tumor section), excisional (removal of entire growth), or aspiration (removal of small tumor plug or fluid). Frozen section involves freezing questionable tissue removed during surgery for microscopic study.

Complications: Infection, bleeding at site.

Nursing care: Cleanse the site with an antibacterial solution. Give the patient information regarding the procedure. Apply direct pressure over the area to stop the bleeding (sutures may be used for areas larger than 3 cm). Apply a bandage.

Liver Biopsy

Description: Percutaneous biopsy of liver tissue. With the patient lying down, a needle is inserted into the liver, and a small amount of tissue is withdrawn to establish a pathologic and microscopic picture of the liver cells.

Indications: Abnormal liver function; hepatomegaly or hepatosplenomegaly of unexplained origin; suspected malignancy of the liver; suspected systemic or infiltrative disease, such as sarcoidosis; routine evaluation for rejection in a transplanted liver.

Complications: Hemorrhage, pneumothorax, peritonitis.[29]

Nursing care: Permit nothing by mouth after midnight before the biopsy. Have the patient void before the biopsy. Record baseline vital signs. Review the chart for hemoglobin and hematocrit levels, platelet count, and bleeding and clotting times. After the biopsy, instruct the patient to lie on the right side to keep pressure on the site. Monitor the vital signs frequently for 4 to 6 hours. Postbiopsy protocols regarding bed rest and activity vary; ensure familiarity with institutional procedures.

Cervical Biopsy

Description: Biopsy of cervical epithelium and shallow layer of underlying stroma to diagnose malignant invasion.

Indications: Suspicious Papanicolaou smear.

Complications: Bleeding.

Nursing care: Prepare the patient for a vaginal examination. After the procedure, give the patient a perineal pad, and inform her that spotting will occur for 24 hours or so.

Endometrial Biopsy

Description: Biopsy of endometrial uterine lining. It is generally performed on the first day of menses of premenopausal patients and anytime in postmenopausal patients. A tissue specimen may be obtained by a Gravlee jet washer (isotonic saline solution is forced through an intrauterine cannula, flushing endometrial cells into an external collecting reservoir) or a Nova curette (a curette attached to a syringe scrapes the endometrium, and cell samples are drawn into the syringe).

Indications: Suspected endometrial carcinoma.

Complications: None.

Nursing care: Prepare the patient for a vaginal examination. Explain that she may experience cramping because of dilation of the cervix during the procedure. Teach and assist her with relaxation and breathing techniques. Give the patient a perineal pad after the procedure. Ensure that menstrual data are noted on the laboratory specimen slip for the pathologist.

Cervical Conization (Cone Biopsy)

Description: Surgical removal of cervical tissue in the shape of a cone for diagnosis or for treatment of cervical infection or carcinoma in situ. It is performed by a physician with a cold knife scalpel. The procedure is frequently called cold knife conization (CKC) or cryosurgery.

Indications: Treatment of cervical infection or carcinoma in situ.

Complications: Bleeding.

Nursing care: After the procedure assist the physician with removal of vaginal packing, usually within 24 hours. Give perineal care with an antiseptic solution and change the perineal pad every 4 hours and as needed. Instruct the patient to avoid coitus, douching, or tampons for 6 weeks or until directed by the physician; report excessive bleeding (if it lasts longer than 7 to 10 days); avoid constipation; maintain good perineal hygiene; and report signs of infection to physician.

RADIOISOTOPE STUDIES AND SCANS (SCINTIGRAPHY)

Brain Scan

Description: Intravenous injection of a small amount of radioactive substance (e.g., technetium-99 pertechnetate). The head is then scanned with a special sensing device to pick up areas of concentrated uptake.

Indications: Assessment of neurologic disease, brain tumors, headache, coma, intracerebral hemorrhage.

Complications: None.

Nursing care: Obtain a careful history regarding any existing allergies, particularly to iodine. Assure the patient that the procedure is painless, the radioactive substance is harmless, and there will be no aftereffects.

Cisternography

Description: Injection of a radioisotope into the subarachnoid space through a cisternal or lumbar puncture. The head is then scanned at regular intervals to determine the amount of time it takes for the radioisotope to clear from the circulating cerebrospinal fluid.

Indications: To assess the circulation of the cerebrospinal fluid.

Complications: As for cisternal or lumbar puncture.

Nursing care: As for cisternal or lumbar puncture.

Thyroid Uptake and Scan

Description: Tracer doses of ^{131}I, ^{123}I, or ^{99m}Tc pertechnetate are given. A scanner is then passed over the gland to record graphically the amount of radioisotope taken up by the gland over a period of time (e.g., 6, 8, or 24 hours). Pregnancy is a contraindication.

Indications: Not used for routine screening, but rather to answer specific questions regarding the localization of functioning or nonfunctioning thyroid tissue; it gives evidence of gland size and function.

Complications: None.

Nursing care: Assess for dietary intake of iodine, for administration of iodine-containing medications, and for the use of antithyroid drugs before the test, because test results may be affected by any ingestion of these.

Ventilation/Perfusion Lung Scan

Description: A scanning device records the pattern of pulmonary radioactivity after the inhalation or intravenous injection of gamma ray–emitting radionuclides (e.g., xenon-133), thus providing visual images of the distribution of blood flow in the lungs.

Indications: The major indications for this procedure are to evaluate whether the patient has pulmonary thromboembolism and to study preoperative lung function.

Complications: None.

Nursing care: Explain the procedure to the patient.

Breast Scan (Breast Scintigraphy)

Description: Evaluation of breast image after intravenous injection of radioisotope.[30]

Indications: Used as second-line imaging study in patients with dense breast tissue that prevents accurate evaluation by mammography. Also helpful in staging of breast cancer patients.

Contraindications: Patients who are pregnant or lactating.

Complications: None.

Nursing care: Explain the procedure to the patient. Assure the patient that because tracer amounts of radioisotope are used radiation exposure is very low. Assess for menstrual cycle.

Scanning should be avoided during menstruation because the incidence of false-positives increases.

Bone Scan

Description: Roentgenographic procedure in which a radioisotope, usually technetium-99 pertechnetate is injected intravenously. The radioisotope is picked up on a special scanning camera as it is passed over the musculoskeletal tissues of the body from head to foot, and a picture of the isotope's distribution in the bony tissues is produced. The scan takes about 1 hour and is painless.

Indications: Aids in the diagnosis of bony metastatic lesions and traumatic, inflammatory, or infectious conditions of musculoskeletal tissues. The scan will show the injured or diseased tissues as darker or "hot" areas on the scan pictures as much as 3 to 6 months earlier than roentgenograms can reveal the condition.

Complications: None usually, although infrequently a hematoma, redness, or edema may develop at the site of the injection.

Nursing care: Explain to the patient that the radioisotope will be injected intravenously 1 to 3 hours before the scan is to be performed and that he or she will be required to drink several glasses of water or tea during the waiting period to aid in excreting the radioisotope that is not absorbed by bone tissue. After the procedure, check the injection site for redness or edema, and inform the patient to check it at home if the procedure is performed on an outpatient basis.

Liver or Spleen Scan

Description: Injection of a radioactive colloid (e.g., technetium-99m labeled albumin), which concentrates in the reticuloendothelial cells through phagocytosis. Kupffer's cells in the liver take up to 80% to 90%, spleen takes 5% to 10%, and bone marrow takes 3% to 5%.

Indications: Used to screen patients for hepatic metastases, cirrhosis, and hepatitis. It also assists in identifying focal lesions such as tumors, cysts, and abscesses and may demonstrate splenic infarct, hepatomegaly, and splenomegaly.

Complications: None.

Nursing care: The patient will need to know he or she will be asked to lie very still and placed in several positions. The patient also should know that the procedure will not be painful, with the exception of the intravenous injection.

Some patients will have a reaction to a stabilizer added to the colloid; observe for anaphylaxis or for pyogenic response.

Do not schedule the patient for more than one radionuclide scan on one day. Radionuclides administered in other studies may interfere with liver-spleen imaging.

Renal Scans (DTPA, DMSA)

Description: Provides a functional assessment of glomerular filtration rate (GFR) and effective renal plasma flow (ERPF). The DTPA scan also provides an assessment of the ureters and bladder. A DMSA scan provides an assessment of individual kidney function.

Other radionuclides such as 33I hippurate and radioxenon have been used for renal scans,[12] but are no longer widely used.

The DTPA scan is used primarily to assess upper urinary tract obstruction. Radionuclide is injected in an intravenous bolus, and sequential images are obtained. A 30-second film is taken to assess cortical blood flow; a 1-minute image and two images are obtained at 5, 10, 15, and 20 minutes. The bladder and ureters are included in the DTPA scan. It assesses GFR and ERPF and provides differential renal function.

Indications: To assess urinary tract obstruction. Because the radionuclide used is affected by diuretics, furosemide is typically given, and the change in renal excretion rate is quantified. Delays in excretion indicate obstruction.[12]

The DMSA scan is useful in assessing functional renal cortical mass,[12] the radionuclide used in DMSA scanning is taken up by renal tubule so that functional cortical mass can be quantified. As with the DTPA scan, an intravenous bolus of radioisotope is administered, and delayed images are obtained. It is indicated in cases of suspected renal scarring, assessment of segmental renal ischemia, and suspected intrarenal mass.

Complications: None.

Nursing care: Requires no preparation. Patients are exposed to significantly less radiation than is required by IVP; however, because a radioisotope is injected and excreted by the kidneys, the patient may continue to excrete radionuclide after the study is completed. Pregnant caregivers are advised not to empty or measure waste products during the initial 24 hours after testing.

Nuclear Cystogram (Radionuclide Cystogram)

Description: Performed in a manner similar to roentgenographic cystography except that normal saline with a dose of a pertechnetate radionuclide is used instead of an iodine-bound contrast solution. Like roentgenographic cystography, the study requires no preparation.

An indwelling catheter is passed into the bladder via the urethra. Normal saline is infused into the bladder, and radionuclide is injected into the solution during bladder filling. It may be performed in place of a roentgenographic cystogram because the patient is exposed to less radiation; however, a nuclear cystogram does not provide the anatomic detail seen with standard cystography.

Indications: Measures certain parameters of bladder function.

Complications: Cystitis.

Nursing care: The patient should be encouraged to force fluids for a 24-hour period following the test and informed that mild dysuria and urinary frequency should disappear completely within this time period.

^{125}I Fibrinogen Uptake (Radioactive Fibrinogen Uptake, RFU)

Description: A noninvasive procedure involving the injection of a small amount of a radioisotope and then the passing of a scanning camera over the involved area beginning 2 hours later. The procedure is used to detect the presence or enlargement of a deep vein thrombosis. Serial readings are taken on successive days following administration of the radioisotope, at 24 hours, but patients can be studied daily for

7 to 14 days. A 20% increase in uptake in one area over a 24-hour period is considered positive.

Indications: Deep vein thrombosis.

Complications: None.

Nursing care: Explain the procedure to the patient.

White Blood Cell Scan (WBC Scan)

Description: White blood cell scan is a nuclear medicine test using radioisotope tagged WBCs to identify areas of presumed infection that cannot be found by cultures or other scans. A 50-ml volume of blood is drawn from the patient and tagged. The WBCs are isolated, tagged, and reinjected in 24 hours. The scan is then performed.

Indication: Fever of unknown origin. A patient is thought to have an infection but the source cannot be identified.

Complications: Possible inflammation at the injection site.

Nursing care: Explain the procedure and provide a supportive atmosphere.

COMPUTED TOMOGRAPHY AND MAGNETIC RESONANCE IMAGING SCANS

Computed Tomography (CT)

Description: CT scanning was introduced in the early 1970s. CT scans use a roentgen ray beam and a computer to provide very accurate images of thin cross sections (0.8 to 1.3 cm) of the body.[3]

The CT scanner has many advantages: it is safe and painless; there is a very small amount of radiation exposure; data can be collected in early stages of the dysfunction; and it reduces the need for more invasive diagnostic procedures.

During the CT scan procedure the patient lies on a table with the body part to be studied inside the scanner's opening. The scanner then is moved to various angles and rotated slowly around the patient's body as repeated roentgenograms are taken. This information is recorded on a computer printout, and film prints (i.e., hard copy) of these visual images are taken. The scan usually is completed in 10 to 45 minutes. Cross-sectional, horizontal, or sagittal plane roentgenographic images are translated by a computer and displayed on an oscilloscope. These images are much sharper, more sensitive, and clearer than conventional roentgenograms. The CT scan takes pictures of small layers or "slices" of the tissues being examined (FIGS. 22-2 and 22-3).

CT scanning is contraindicated during pregnancy.

Indications: Useful in diagnosing disorders of multiple body systems.

Brain: Head trauma, cerebrovascular disturbances, hydrocephalus, abnormal brain development, identification of space-occupying lesions, metastatic tumors, and brain abscesses.

Endocrine: CT of sella turcica, adrenal glands, and abdomen is indicated in the following: presence of adrenal adenoma, diabetes-related tumors, Cushing's disease work-up, hypopituitary work-up, and precocious puberty work-up.

Eye: Diagnosis of eye disorders. It contrasts orbital contents and tumors because of difference in tissue density.

Respiratory system: Identifies exact morphologic characteristics of a chest lesion.

Renal and genitourinary systems: Determines kidney size, cysts, abscesses, masses, hematomas, and collecting system dilation. It is particularly valuable in defining abnormalities of the renal parenchyma. It provides an estimate of the density of masses and has

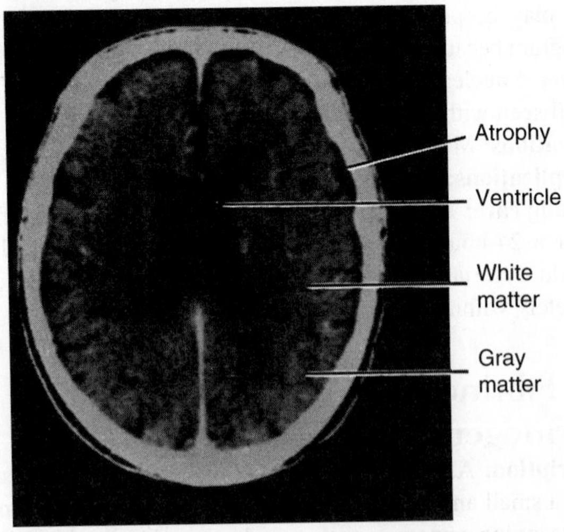

FIG. 22-2
CT scan printouts. CT brain scan differentiates between gray and white brain matter. (From Ballinger.[2])

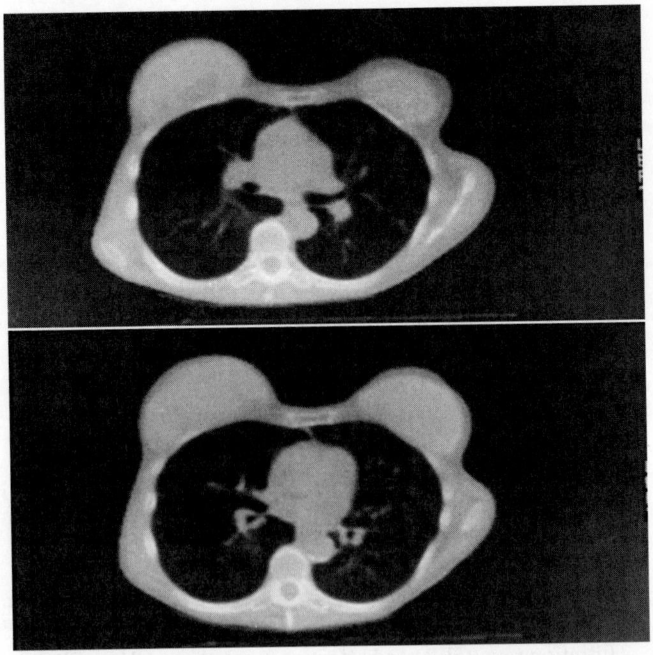

FIG. 22-3
CT scan of female patient. On this transverse scan through upper chest, bilateral breast shadows are evident. Heart, pulmonary arteries, and main bronchi are also visible. (Courtesy R. Keith Wilson, MD. Baylor College of Medicine, Houston, Texas.)

the potential to differentiate solid tissue masses from cystic or hemorrhagic structures. Varying densities are displayed as Hounsfield units: normal renal parenchyma measures 80 to 100 Hounsfield units, and density of a cyst is lower, whereas solid tumors have a density similar to that of renal parenchyma. CT scanning is also used in evaluation of adrenal masses. It is a useful technique for evaluating masses (tumors) of pelvic contents and lymphatic enlargement that may be the result of metastatic invasion. Pelvic abscesses may be elucidated by CT scanning of that area; it may elucidate any mass effect that causes distortion of the bladder.

Gastrointestinal system: In the biliary tract and liver CT scanning can be used to identify focal points found on nuclear scans as solid, cystic, inflammatory, or vascular. A biopsy may be necessary to distinguish between metastatic or primary tumors or to rule out malignancy. CT scanning can also identify hematomas after abdominal trauma. It is used to determine if the cause of jaundice is obstructive or nonobstructive.

CT scanning and ultrasonography are both effective in biliary tract and liver diagnosis. A CT scan proves to be better in obese patients or patients whose liver is located high under the rib cage because bone and excessive fat hinder ultrasound transmission. Contrast medium is also used during CT scanning to intensify vascular structures and liver parenchyma, aiding in visualization of the biliary tract. A general CT scan of the abdomen is valuable in defining the relationship of organs and identifying the presence of tumors. In the pancreas, CT scanning is used to diagnose pancreatic carcinoma and pancreatitis and to distinguish between pancreatic disorders and disorders of the retroperitoneum.

Complications: None, unless the patient experiences a reaction to the contrast.

Nursing care: Explain to the patient that he or she will lie flat on a narrow table, which will be moved inside a round opening of the scanner. The scanner will make a loud clicking sound as it moves around and along the patient. The scan will take 10 to 60 minutes, depending on whether or not some parts only or the entire body is scanned. The patient must lie still without moving during the scan. A radiopaque solution may be given to outline the blood vessels more clearly if needed, although the majority of CT scans are made without such an agent. Occasionally a sedative may be required to calm a nervous or restless patient.

If contrast medium is to be used, assess the patient for allergies to iodine, seafood, or contrast media. Barium studies should be made at least 4 days before the CT scan, or barium obscures the film. The contrast media excreted in bile used in earlier diagnostic studies may interfere with biliary tree detection.

The patient is given nothing to eat past midnight before the test, depending on hospital procedure.

Positron Emission Tomography (PET)

Description: Intravenous injection of deoxyglucose with radioactive fluorine. The head is scanned, and a color-composite picture is obtained. Various shades of colors indicate levels of glucose metabolism.

Indications: Assists in the diagnosis and differentiation of neurologic disorders.

Complications: None.

Nursing care: Same as for a CT scan.

Magnetic Resonance Imaging (MRI)

Description: MRI, also termed nuclear magnetic resonance (NMR) imaging, is a technique of tomography based on the magnetic behavior of protons (hydrogen nuclei) in body tissues.[7,10] The scanner produces images when protons are placed in a strong external magnetic field and then are subjected to short computer-programmed pulses of additional energy in the form of radiofrequency waves. When placed in the magnetic field, positively charged nuclei and negatively charged electrons align uniformly. Short pulses of radiofrequency waves are then applied, which tip the atoms out of their magnetic alignment, causing uniform spinning (resonance) of the nuclei. When the radiofrequency wave is stopped, the atoms realign uniformly with the magnetic field and emit tissue-specific signals that are based on realignment time and the relative proton density (water content) of nuclei. These signals are then monitored, processed, and displayed as a high-resolution image by the MRI computer.

Indications: MRI is indicated for detecting a variety of neurologic disorders, including central nervous system (CNS) malignancies. CNS degenerative disorders (e.g., Alzheimer's disease), brain edema, spinal cord edema, spinal lesions, ischemic-infarcted areas of the CNS, arteriovenous malformations, congenital anomalies, and hemorrhagic areas of the CNS and spinal cord.[15]

MRI is an excellent aid for the diagnosis of musculoskeletal conditions because MRI clearly differentiates various types of tissues such as bones, fat, and muscles. It produces clear images of soft tissues such as tumors, nucleus pulposus, and blood vessels. Individual cells may be defined. It also aids in the detection of renal masses, especially in distinguishing simple cysts from those complicated by hemorrhage. It is used to detect and stage neoplasms.

Complications: None.

Nursing care: The patient should be instructed that MRI is a painless and noninvasive procedure with no known risks. Explain to the patient that he or she will lie flat on a narrow table inside a round opening of a large magnet and should lie still during the scan. Many patients find the MRI to be claustrophobic. The nurse can prepare the patient for this, and explain the use of imagery, which may help the patient tolerate the examination better. A description of the equipment and procedure should be given. The patient also should be informed that a soft humming sound and the on-off pulses of the radiofrequency waves will be heard. Provide earplugs. The patient should be instructed to remove all metal objects because the strong magnetic field may damage jewelry and watches. Some facilities may have an open MRI scanner that is free standing and may prevent claustrophobia in some patients.

A careful assessment of any existing ferromagnetic implants (e.g., pacemakers, metallic orthopedic devices) or known foreign bodies (e.g., metallic splinters or fragments) must be made before the procedure because these objects produce image deformation. MRI also may move some metallic devices (e.g., metal intracranial aneurysm clips); therefore patients with such implants or foreign bodies cannot be exposed to MRI.

SKIN ASSESSMENT/TESTING

The following studies are commonly used for diagnostic purposes.

Scrapings

Description: The area is cleansed with alcohol and air dried so that superficial fine dry scale is apparent. The scale is scraped with a sharp scalpel and gathered on a glass slide or in a blood collection tube. Nail and hair clippings are also used. Scrapings are covered with 10% KOH (potassium hydroxide) and examined microscopically for the presence of mycelia in fungal infections. The fungus appears as branching, threadlike elements.

Indications: Fungal conditions of skin.

Complications: None.

Nursing care: Explain the procedure to the patient.

Diascopy, Side Lighting, Wood's Light, Gram's Stain, Culture, Electron Microscopy, Cytology

Description

Diascopy: The lesion is covered with a glass slide or piece of clear plastic to determine whether dilated capillaries or extravasated blood is causing redness of lesion.

Side lighting: A beam of light is directed from the side over the lesion to reveal minor elevations or depressions in the lesion. This helps determine the configuration and degree of eruption.

Wood's light: The skin is viewed in a darkened room under ultraviolet light with wavelength of 360 nm ("black light"). Certain disease-producing fungi and bacteria show a characteristic color.

Gram's stain: Exudate from the lesion is smeared onto a glass slide and stained with gentian or crystal violet. The violet is washed off, and the smear is flooded with iodine solution, which is then washed off. The smear is then flooded with 95% alcohol and counterstained with safranin red dye. The stain will differentiate gram-negative from gram-positive bacteria based on their ability to pick up one or both of the two stains.

Culture: For pustular lesions a swab sample is placed in a broth culture medium. For chronic bacterial and fungal infections, a biopsy specimen is used for culturing. Cultures are incubated or refrigerated and observed for fungal or bacterial growth.

Electron microscopy: A glass slide smear of vesicular fluid or crusted tissue is viewed under an electron microscope to determine the presence of a virus.

Cytology: Cellular material is scraped from the base of the vesicle and stained with Wright's or Giemsa stain, or a clean glass slide is touched to the surface of the lesion so the cells can adhere to it. The cells are sprayed with a fixative and viewed microscopically after staining. Multinucleated giant cells are present in herpes simplex, herpes zoster, and varicella. Pemphigus is diagnosed by the presence of typical acantholytic cells.

Indications: Dermatologic lesions.

Complications: None.

Nursing care: Explain the procedure to the patient.

Patch Test

Description: The suspected allergen is applied to the skin under a nonabsorbent adhesive patch and left for 48 hours. A positive test consists of erythema with some induration and occasional vesicle formation. Some reactions do not occur until after the patch is removed from the site.

Indications: Sensitivity to allergens.

Complications: None, although itching or burning may occur.

Nursing care: Instruct the patient to leave the patch on, to keep the area dry, and to return for site inspection in 48 hours. Instruct the patient to remove the patch if itching or burning develops before 48 hours and to return for inspection of the site. Reinspect at 72 hours.

Thermography

Description: Measures and plots areas of localized elevation of skin temperature over inflammatory or malignant lesions; takes photographs of infrared radiation (heat) coming from any part of the body. For breast thermography the patient is placed in a draft-free room at a temperature of about 20° C (68° F). Clothing above the waist is removed, and the patient waits for about 15 minutes until the skin cools before infrared photographs are taken.

Indications: Presence of dermatologic lesions that are inflamed or suspected of being malignant.

Complications: None.

Nursing care: Explain to the patient that the room will be cool. Provide reassurance, especially if the test is being done because of suspected malignancy.

Allergy Skin Testing

Description: An antigen is introduced by scratching or pricking the skin surface or by intradermal injection.

Indications: Sensitivity to allergens.

Complications: Erythema at site; hypersensitivity, including anaphylaxis.

Nursing care: Check for erythema at the site of antigen introduction 20 minutes after administration. Observe for potential anaphylactic reactions following antigen introduction. Antihistamines may be administered as a comfort measure.

Schick Test

Description: This is a test to determine the presence or absence of a significant quantity of diphtheria antitoxins in the blood. The presence of these antitoxins indicates an immunity to diphtheria.

Indications: For susceptibility to diphtheria.

Complications: None.

Nursing care: Draw 0.1 ml of purified diphtheria toxin dissolved in human serum albumin into a tuberculin syringe. In a second syringe draw up 0.1 ml of inactivated diphtheria toxoid to be used as a control in the other arm (to rule out any sensitivity to culture proteins). Attach 26- or 27-gauge 1.25-cm (1/2-inch) needles to both syringes. Clean the volar surfaces of both forearms. Intradermally inject the toxin in one forearm and the toxoid in the other forearm. Carefully record which was injected in each arm. Examine the areas at 24 and 36 hours.

A positive reaction is indicated when the site of the toxin injection begins to redden in 24 hours. The redness, swelling, and tenderness continue until it reaches maximum size—usually 3 cm in diameter at the end of 1 week. The skin at the injection site may flake, and the center may appear as a dark pigmented spot. The area of the toxoid injection should show no reaction. With a negative result there is no flaking or erythema at either injection site.

Tuberculin Skin Testing

Description: Two types of tuberculin are currently being used for testing: old tuberculin (OT) and purified protein derivative (PPD). The PPD is the preferred tuberculin preparation because its strength is standardized and tests with the same dose are comparable.

Contraindications for testing include patients with known active TB infection, and previous BCG vaccine, because they will demonstrate a positive reaction to the PPD.

Indications: Provides evidence of whether the tested individual has been infected, either past or present, with *Mycobacterium tuberculosis* or has had contact with someone who has TB.

Complications: None.

Nursing care: Each type of multiple puncture unit is slightly different; usually an intradermal injection is administered. Carefully read the manufacturer's instructions regarding the administration of the test. A positive reaction for all brands consists of the formation of separate papules at each of the puncture sites or a large papule over the entire area. Refer to the manufacturer's instructions regarding specific interpretation, reading of results, and documentation.

Testing for Fungal Diseases

Description: For patients suspected of having coccidioidomycosis, skin tests are available from lysates of both the mycelial (coccidioidin) and the spherule (spherulin) forms. Skin tests with either form are highly specific and become positive 3 to 4 weeks after infection and 12 to 20 days after the onset of clinical illness. An intradermal injection is given.

Indications: Respiratory or other systemic symptoms that may indicate infection with coccidioidomycosis.

Complications: None.

Nursing care: Explain the purpose of the test to the patient. Observe the injection site for a reaction: erythema, swelling, or hardening at the site.

Delayed-Type Hypersensitivity (Anergy) Testing (Cell-Mediated Immunity Testing)

Description: Measures the capacity to generate a delayed-type hypersensitivity (DTH) response. The patient is injected intradermally with four common soluble recall antigens (for example, PPD, *Candida* spp., *Trichophyton* spp., and tetanus) and examined for induration and erythema after 48 hours. Most young, healthy persons respond positively to at least one antigen. Reactivity may decline with age and with protein- and calorie-deficiency states.

Indications: Suspected immunodeficiency or protein-calorie deficiency.

Complications: None.

Nursing care: Check for local erythema and induration at 48 hours.

ARTERIOGRAPHIC (ANGIOGRAPHIC) AND VENOGRAPHIC STUDIES

Arteriography or venography consists of the infusion of a radiopaque substance into the arterial or venous system, followed by a series of roentgenograms that allow visualization of the vessel systems and assist in the diagnosis of any abnormalities.

Arteriography and venography may be used in many body systems. In addition to those described here, selective arteriography may also be performed to localize possible tumors of the parathyroid, adrenal, and pancreatic glands, and a procedure similar to arteriography may be used to perform serial venous sampling to obtain hormone levels.

Cerebral Arteriography

Description: Cerebral arteriography requires the infusion of a radiopaque substance into the cerebral arterial system; during infusion of the contrast medium, a series of roentgenograms is taken for visualization of the extracranial and intracranial vessels. To outline the anterior, middle, and posterior cerebral arteries and returning venous circulation, the injection is made into the carotid system. If visualization of the vertebral-basilar system in the posterior fossa is needed, the injection is made into the vertebral artery.[3]

There are two approaches (open or closed) to performing the arteriography. The *open* method is performed in the operating room and involves the surgical exposure of the internal carotid before injection of the contrast substance. After the procedure, the incision is sutured and dressed. The actual procedure and aftercare are the same as those for the closed method. The *closed* method involves injection of the contrast medium directly into the carotid or vertebral arteries or indirectly (injection of the carotid or vertebral vessels by way of the femoral, brachial, subclavian, or axillary artery).[3] Following the injection a series of roentgenographs is taken for visualization of arterial and venous circulations.

Contraindications include the following: anticoagulant therapy, age, recent embolic or thrombotic occurrences, sensitivity to the contrast medium, and severe liver, thyroid, or kidney disease.

Indications: Identification of cerebral circulatory anomalies (e.g., aneurysm, hematoma) and their site and size, and visualization of cerebral arteries and veins.

Complications: Complications generally occurring during or shortly after the procedure include seizures, stroke, allergic reactions (to dye), thrombosis, hemiparesis, visual disturbances, pulmonary emboli, and dysphasia.

Nursing care: Observe the puncture site for hematoma or hemorrhage. Frequently monitor vital signs and neurologic signs during and after the procedure. (Make sure that baseline neurologic data and vital signs are documented before the procedure.) Observe for signs of allergic dye reactions.

Fluorescein Arteriography (and Photography)

Description: A 10% solution of sodium fluorescein injected into the antecubital vein is relayed to retinal arteries in 10 to 16 seconds and to veins in 25 seconds. The pupils are dilated with short-acting cycloplegics in combination with a mydriatic. An ophthalmoscope with a blue filter can show the entire diameter of a vessel, whereas ordinary ophthalmoscopy provides only a surface view.

Photography. Black-and-white film with appropriate filters should be used in a camera that takes rapid-sequence photographs from 9 to 30 seconds after injection of fluorescein. The patient and examiner are seated at a table opposite each other, each looking into the camera.

Indications: Eye disorders.

Complications: Subcutaneous leakage of dye causes local burning. A patient may experience a brief hot flash or nausea. A temporary yellowish discoloration of sclera may occur until the dye is excreted in the urine (within 48 hours).

Nursing care: Inquire about previous allergies to fluorescein (the allergic response is usually hives and itching). Inform the patient what to expect in terms of the effects of mydriatic or cycloplegic medications. Inform the patient about possible scleral discoloration.

Cardiac Catheterization

Description: An invasive procedure involving insertion of a radiopaque catheter via the peripheral artery or vein into the heart. It is used to determine the anatomy of heart chambers, valves, great vessels, and coronary arteries; ventricular wall thickness and motion; hemodynamic functions of the heart by pressure recordings of heart chambers and great vessels and pressure gradients across the valves; ventricular function and cardiac output; degree of valve competence; and intracardiac oxygen saturations. It also selectively visualizes the heart, coronary arteries, and great vessels by recording serial roentgenograms (angiograms). It is usually performed as an outpatient procedure; the patient should recover for 6 to 8 hours after the procedure.

Indications: Symptoms of angina pectoris, myocardial infarct, or other cardiac dysfunction.

Complications: Myocardial infarction, dysrhythmias, hematoma, or hemorrhage at the insertion site. Vascular obstruction distal to insertion site secondary to thrombus or hematoma formation; reaction to contrast medium, infection, pulmonary edema, cardiac tamponade.

Nursing care: Ensure that informed consent is obtained. Explain that the procedure will last 2 to 4 hours, that the patient may feel pressure during insertion of the catheter and a hot flushing sensation or nausea with injection of contrast medium, that the patient may also experience a salty taste when dye is injected, that the patient should cough when instructed by the physician, and that the patient will receive medication if chest pain occurs and may be given nitroglycerin to dilate coronary vessels. Determine any allergies or hypersensitivity to shellfish, iodine, or other contrast media. Obtain baseline vital signs and peripheral pulses. After the procedure check the vital signs every 15 minutes for 1 hour, every 30 minutes for 2 hours, and every hour for 4 hours or until stable. Keep the patient flat in bed for 6 to 8 hours with a pressurized dressing over the puncture site. Check the dressing and surrounding area for bleeding, pain, and swelling. Check the peripheral pulses, color, warmth, and feeling of the extremities distal to the insertion site. Give pain medication as indicated. Encourage fluid intake for first 6 to 8 hours to assist in the elimination of contrast medium.

Digital Vascular Imaging (DVI) (Digital Subtraction Arteriography)

Description: An invasive procedure using a computer system and fluoroscopy with an image intensifier to permit complete visualization of the arterial supply to a specific area.

Indications: Carotid and renal artery disease, pulmonary embolism, aneurysms, thrombotic and embolic disease of the great vessels, coarctation of the aorta.

Complications: Dysrhythmias, reaction to contrast medium, infection, bleeding at site.

Nursing care: Ensure that informed consent is obtained. Explain that the procedure will last 1 to 2 hours and that the patient will be requested to hold his or her breath for 10-second intervals. Digital vascular imaging can be done on an outpatient basis and may cause certain sensations. After the procedure, check the vital signs immediately and as ordered. Check the site for bleeding. Instruct the patient to observe the site for infection and/or bleeding and to drink a minimum of 1 L of fluid on the day of the procedure.

Scintigraphy

Radionuclide Arteriography

Description: Gives information regarding myocardial perfusion and contractility through the use of radionuclide imaging. The procedure involves injecting a radioisotope and passing a scanning camera over the patient repeatedly.

Indications: Poor myocardial perfusion or contractility.

Complications: None.

Nursing care: Explain the procedure to the patient. Ensure that informed consent is obtained. Reassure the patient that the radiation exposure involved is less than with a chest roentgenogram; caution the patient to remain quiet and still during the study. Encourage the patient to use imagery if it is helpful.

Technetium-99m Pyrophosphate Myocardial Imaging

Description: Tracer isotope is injected 2 to 3 hours before the procedure, and scanning takes 30 to 60 minutes, during which time a scanning camera is passed repeatedly over the patient in several positions: anterior, left anterior oblique, right anterior oblique, and left lateral.

Indications: To detect recent myocardial infarction and the extent of its damage; "hot spots" appear within 12 hours of the infarct and disappear after 1 week.

Complications: None.

Nursing care: Explain the procedure to the patient. Ensure that informed consent is obtained. Inform the patient that he or she may eat lightly before the study but should not smoke or drink alcoholic or caffeine-containing beverages for 3 hours before the test.

Thallium-201 Imaging

Description: "Cold spot" myocardial imaging used in conjunction with a bicycle ergometer or treadmill stress ECG test to diagnose ischemic heart disease.

Indications: To assess myocardial perfusion (myocardial blood flow) and to evaluate the patency of grafts after bypass surgery; also used in conjunction with exercise stress testing (EST) in the diagnosis of coronary artery disease (stress imaging).

Complications: None.

Nursing care: If performed in conjunction with EST, instruct the patient to avoid tobacco, alcohol, or unprescribed medication for 24 hours before the study and to take nothing by mouth for 3 hours before the test. NOTE: If chest pain, shortness of breath, or a drop in blood pressure develops, stress imaging should be stopped.

Scintigraphic Blood Pool Imaging (Multiple-Gated Blood Pool Imaging, Multiple-Gated Acquisition [MUGA] Scanning)

Description: Involves injection of human serum albumin or red blood cells (RBCs) tagged with the isotope technetium-99m pertechnetate. A scintillation camera records several pass images of the isotope as it passes through the ventricle. Imaging can be "gated" to systolic and diastolic events of the cardiac cycle. The normal left ventricular ejection fraction is 55% to 65%. The procedure is contraindicated in pregnancy.

Indications: Used to evaluate regional and global ventricular performance and to detect aneurysms of the left ventricle and areas of hypokinesis and dyskinesis.

Complications: None.

Nursing care: Explain the procedure to the patient. Ensure that informed consent is obtained. Determine if the patient is pregnant. The patient may eat and drink before the procedure. Inform the patient that the blood-labeling agent is given intravenously.

Pulmonary Arteriography

Description: A radiopaque dye is injected rapidly into the pulmonary circulation by various routes: one or more systemic veins, or the chambers of the heart, or directly into the pulmonary arteries. After the rapid injection a series of roentgenograms is taken.

Indications: To detect pulmonary emboli and a variety of congenital and acquired thromboembolic lesions.

Complications: Hematoma development; occasionally, frank hemorrhage or thrombus formation; infection at the catheter insertion site.

Nursing care: Before the procedure, determine any allergies to radiopaque dye. After the procedure the patient must be observed for hematomas or inflammation around the injection site, absence of peripheral pulses, or complaints of numbness or pain.

Vena Caval Catheterization

Description: In vena caval catheterization a radiopaque catheter is introduced into the vena cava through the femoral vein. The catheter is guided into the vena cava with fluoroscopic assistance. Venous samples are obtained from different sites along the vena cava for catecholamine determination.

Patients with pheochromocytoma should receive alpha-blockers before the procedure to prevent catecholamine release and hypertensive crisis.

Indications: The procedure is performed to assist the surgeon in localizing the pheochromocytoma and to rule out bilateral or multiple tumors.

Complications: Pulmonary embolus, hematoma formation at the catheter insertion site.

Nursing care: Before the procedure, give alpha-blockers as prescribed. Have a cardiac arrest cart available. A physician or nurse should accompany the patient with a supply of intravenous phentolamine.

After the procedure, assess vital signs every 15 minutes for an hour, every 30 minutes for another hour, and every hour twice after that. Observe the affected extremity for color, temperature, edema, and pedal pulses to observe for postoperative loss of perfusion, and compare with unaffected extremity. Observe for hematoma formation, and notify the physician if any occurs or if pulses disappear. Keep the patient flat in bed for 4 hours with no hip flexion.

Celiac and Mesenteric Arteriography

Description: Contrast medium is injected into the celiac, superior mesenteric, or inferior mesenteric artery for visualization of the vasculature. Superselective arteriography permits a detailed visualization of a particular area. As the contrast medium is injected, serial roentgenograms outline abdominal vessels in arterial, capillary, and venous phases of perfusion.

A radiologist inserts a needle into the femoral artery. A guide wire is passed through the needle into the aorta, and the needle is then removed. An arteriographic catheter is inserted over the guidewire, and placement is checked roentgenographically and fluoroscopically before the guide wire is removed. The catheter, under fluoroscopy, is advanced into one of the three arteries; placement is checked, and an automatic injection of contrast medium is attached. A rapid sequence of serial films is taken as the medium is injected. The catheter is repositioned for superselective visualization.

Indications: Can be used for locating gastrointestinal bleeding and for treating bleeding by either infusion of vasopressin at the site or injection of embolic material to form a clot. The embolic material includes aminocaproic acid (Amicar) clot or gelatin sponge (Gelfoam). It is also used to evaluate cirrhosis and portal hypertension, vascular damage after abdominal trauma, intestinal ischemia, and vascular abnormalities. It may be used in evaluating tumors (distinguishing between benign and malignant) when other tests are inconclusive.

Complications: Bleeding, hematoma formation, or infection at the catheter's insertion site.

Nursing care: Assess the patient for sensitivities to iodine, seafood, and contrast media. Blood work should include hemoglobin, hematocrit, clotting time, prothrombin time, activated partial thromboplastin time, and platelet count. The patient should remain flat in bed for at least 12 hours. Check the puncture site frequently for bleeding and hematoma; a sandbag may be used for 2 to 4 hours to provide some pressure.

Monitor the vital signs as ordered—usually every 15 minutes for 1 hour, every 30 minutes for 2 hours, and then every hour for 4 hours or until the patient is stable. Depending on the patient's reactions to the test and the potential problems of bleeding, this pattern may change. Monitor the peripheral pulses by observing vital signs. Compare pulses in each foot. Also observe the leg (of the puncture site) for color and temperature and compare with the alternate leg.

Notify the physician about continued or excessive bleeding, changes in the peripheral pulse and temperature, and color changes. Also notify the physician if vital signs change significantly, or if there is stinging pain or sensation at the femoral site. This may mean that blood is irritating subcutaneous tissues. Check thigh for swelling.

Renal Arteriography and Venography

Description: Provides information concerning arterial and venous blood supply to the kidneys.

Arteriography: A preprocedure antianxiety or narcotic injection is given. The patient is taken to a radiologic suite, and an additional local anesthetic is given in the area over the femoral artery. The patient is placed in a supine position, and a femoral puncture is performed. An opaque catheter is then passed from the femoral artery to the aorta and into the desired renal artery under fluoroscopy. A radiopaque contrast material is then injected into the renal artery. (If passage into the aorta via the femoral artery is not feasible, the axillary artery may be used as an alternative.)

Rapid roentgenographic images are used to assess the three phases of the arteriogram: the arterial phase lasts 2 to 4 seconds and provides a detailed outline of the principal renal arteries; the nephrogenic phase is seen as a marked opacification of the renal parenchyma, lasting 15 to 20 seconds; and the venous phase is of limited value because of the kidney's ability to extract and excrete contrast material (principally useful in assessing arteriovenous shunting).

Digital subtraction arteriography (DSA) is a method of imaging that allows visualization of the kidney's arteries using a significantly smaller dose of contrast material than does the standard technique. It has the advantage of being rapid and relatively noninvasive compared with standard techniques, so it can be performed on an outpatient basis with an IVP. Limitations include poorer visualization of peripheral renal artery branches.[20]

Venography: To perform this procedure, a percutaneous catheter is placed into the right femoral vein and advanced to the opening of the renal vein. Contrast material is injected, and the catheter is then directed upward to enter the contralateral (right) renal vein. The procedure is repeated. Imaging may be enhanced by injecting 6 to 10 μg of epinephrine into the renal artery followed by renal venography 10 seconds later.

Indications: Indications for arteriography include palpable renal masses, potential renovascular hypertension, and renal trauma: it is also used to determine the suitability of renal donors.[9]

Indications for venography include renal vein thrombosis, renovascular hypertension, elucidation of renal cell carcinoma, and various congenital abnormalities of the renal veins.

Complications: The two major complications are bleeding at the site of the arterial puncture and allergic reactions to the contrast material.

Nursing care: Pedal pulses and capillary filling of the nail beds of the foot should be assessed before the procedure. After the renal arteriogram is completed, the femoral puncture site should be assessed regularly (every 1 to 2 hours) for hematoma or external bleeding. Assessment of capillary refill and the affected foot's appearance is indicated; compare to unaffected side. Vital signs and signs of allergic reaction with the contrast material should be assessed frequently (every 1 to 2 hours). Signs of allergic reaction include pruritus, wheezing, dyspnea, and flushed skin.

Phlebography (Venography)

Description: Invasive procedure used to identify and locate venous thrombi. It involves injection of a radiopaque dye (technetium-99 microaggregated albumin) into the venous system of the affected extremity followed by serial roentgenograms. Abnormal filling of the vein indicates a positive finding that thrombosis exists.

Indications: Deep vein thrombosis.

Complications: Reaction to the contrast media, subcutaneous infiltration of dye, embolism caused by dislodgment of the thrombus.

Nursing care: Explain that the procedure may take from 30 minutes to an hour and that a warm flushed sensation may be felt with the injection of the dye. No preprocedure fasting is required.

Lumbar Venography

Description: Injection of contrast medium to visualize the epidural venous plexus. The catheter is inserted percutaneously into the femoral vein and then guided into the internal iliac vein or ascending lumbar vein.

Indications: When performed for neurologic or musculoskeletal conditions, lumbar venography aids in outlining the blood supply to or through a tumor or other structure under study and thereby aids in the preoperative assessment and determination of possible operative treatment. The study can be made as an outpatient procedure.

Complications: Bleeding, hematoma formation, infection at the catheter's insertion site.

Nursing care: Monitor the site for signs of hemorrhage or infection. Immobilize the affected extremity for 12 hours after the procedure.

Lymphangiography

Description: Radiopaque medium introduced via a tiny catheter into the peripheral lymphatics to allow visualization of the deep femoral, iliac, and periaortic lymph nodes. Dye is injected locally into the hands and feet via small incisions, and roentgenograms are taken immediately after the injection and 24 hours later.

Indications: Swelling of lymph nodes; suspected malignancy, such as lymphoma, Hodgkin's disease.

Complications: Hypersensitive reaction to the contrast material; inflammation at the injection sites.

Nursing care: Inform the patient about the procedure. Ensure that informed consent is obtained. Have patient void before procedure and alert patient that procedure will take several hours. Encourage fluids after the procedure to flush the dye. Inform the patient that a bluish tint to the skin and urine will disappear within a few weeks. Remind patient to return in 24 hours for additional films.

BLOOD STUDIES

Blood studies are key diagnostic indicators and are used to assist in the diagnosis of almost every body system. Following are some descriptions of blood studies that require special nursing care used for hematolymphatic, immune, and neoplastic disorders. Also included is a discussion of arterial blood gas analysis.

The following blood studies are used to diagnose a wide variety of disorders:

Red cell count: Determines the number of red blood cells (RBCs) in 1 mm^3 of blood

White cell count: Determines the number of white blood cells (WBCs) in 1 mm^3 of blood

Differential count: Determines the percentage of various types of WBCs

Platelet count: Determines the number of platelets in 1 mm^3 of blood

Hemoglobin concentration: Determines the amount of hemoglobin in a given volume of blood

Hematocrit: Determines the percentage of blood composed of RBCs

Mean corpuscular volume (MCV): Determines the size and volume of each RBC

Mean corpuscular hemoglobin (MCH): Determines the hemoglobin content in RBCs of average size

Mean corpuscular concentration (MCHC): Determines the amount of hemoglobin in packed RBCs (hemoglobin of 100 ml RBCs)

Reticulocyte count: Determines the effectiveness and speed of RBC production and the responsiveness of bone marrow to decreased circulating RBCs

Erythrocyte life span determination: Estimates the rate at which RBCs tagged with chromium-51 disappear from circulation; the patient and a normal subject with comparable blood type are injected with tagged cells

Erythrocyte fragility test: Measures the rate at which RBCs burst in hypotonic solutions of varied concentrations

Direct Coombs' test: Detects autoantibodies against RBCs, which can cause cellular damage. The patient's RBCs are mixed with Coombs' serum, which is a solution containing antibodies against human antibodies. If the RBCs are not coated with the patient's antibodies against RBCs, agglutination (clumping) does not occur

Indirect Coombs' test: Used to identify antibodies to RBC antigens

Serum iron level: The amount of iron found in a sample of blood

Bleeding time: Measured by making a small stab wound in the earlobe or forearm; the time it takes for the bleeding to stop is noted, and a measurement is made of the rate at which a clot is formed; the patient must not take aspirin for at least 5 days before the test; the patient is also advised not to drink alcoholic beverages before the test

Coagulation time: The time required for blood to form a solid clot on a foreign surface such as glass test tube

Capillary fragility: Determined by the tourniquet test; positive or negative pressure is applied to various areas of the body, and the relative number of petechiae is noted

Therapeutic trial with parenteral vitamin B_{12}: Requires that the patient be given intramuscular injections of vitamin B_{12} for 10 days; blood work and the patient's subjective feeling of well-being are evaluated

Schilling test: Measures the absorption of radioactive vitamin B_{12} before and after parenteral administration of intrinsic factor; it may be a three-stage procedure and involves 24-hour urine collection

Bilirubin test: Requires that a venous sample be collected for measuring the total amount of bilirubin; differentiation of conjugated and unconjugated levels can also be determined

Serologic tests: Frequently used to help determine the causative pathogens in fungal diseases and atypical pneumonia; the outcome of the test depends on the development of antibodies to the organism in the patient's serum that can be detected by agglutination, complement fixation, or precipitation reactions when the serum is exposed to a specific antigen; examples are the fungal antibody tests that detect coccidioidomycosis, blastomycosis, and histoplasmosis

HLA typing: Requires that a venous blood specimen be collected for use in the identification of HLA-A, HLA-B, HLA-C histocompatibility antigens; it is used for screening patients and potential donors for tissue transplantation

Immunofluorescence (IF): Measured after the serum or tissue specimen is viewed microscopically; an indirect IF test demonstrates that the serum of a patient with pemphigus or bullous pemphigoid contains specific antibodies that bind to different areas of the epithelium; in the direct IF test, a skin sample shows characteristic patterns for specific diseases

In vitro leukocyte function tests: Used to evaluate patients with recurrent infections and suspected immunodeficiency diseases; normal values are determined in each laboratory

Lymphocyte stimulation: Requires that lymphocytes be incubated with a particular antigen or mitogen (polyclonal activator), and the cell proliferation determined; alterations may be seen in genetic or acquired immunodeficiency states

Cytotoxicity: Lymphocytes are incubated with tumor cells or virally infected cells, and target cell lysis is measured; in the absence of any antibody, natural killer (NK) cell function is measured; if the donor has been sensitized to a target cell in vivo, a secondary cytotoxic T lymphocyte (CTL) response can be determined

Chemotaxis: Phagocytic cells are incubated in a chamber that permits cells to migrate through a filter toward a chemoattractant; when samples from the patient are incubated with standard chemotactic factors, chemotactic capabilities of phagocytic cells are assessed; alternatively one can incubate normal phagocytes with patient serum to test the ability of that serum to generate chemotactic factors

Phagocytosis: Particle uptake assays measure phagocytic cell function or the opsonizing capacity of the patient's serum; to assess phagocyte function, the patient's monocytes or neutrophils are incubated with test particle in the presence of normal human serum; to examine opsonization, normal phagocytic cells are incubated with particles in the presence of the patient's serum; phagocytosis can be assessed by direct visualization or use of radiolabeled particles

Bactericidal activity: Phagocytic cells are incubated with appropriately opsonized bacteria and then washed and lysed; the number of live intracellular bacteria is then determined

NBT dye reduction: Phagocytic cells are incubated with particles in the presence of oxidized (NBT); on stimulation of respiratory burst activity, reducing equivalents are generated and NBT is converted into deep blue insoluble precipitate; NBT dye reduction does not occur in certain patients with genetic phagocytic cell defects

Chemiluminescence: Phagocytes are incubated with opsonized particles, and light emission is measured in a spectrophotometer; during phagocytosis, normal monocytes and neutrophils generate highly unstable oxygen intermediates that emit light during decay to the ground state; chemiluminescence is reduced in patients with certain phagocyte dysfunctions

Tumor Markers

Acid phosphatase
- Increased in prostatic cancer
- Increased in some primary bone malignancies, multiple myeloma

Alkaline phosphatase
- Increased in metastatic cancer to bone and liver, osteogenic sarcoma, myeloma, and Hodgkin's lymphoma with bone involvement

Alpha-fetoprotein (AFP)
- Increased in hepatocellular cancers; choriocarcinoma; teratoma; embryonal cell tumors of testis and ovary; some pancreatic, stomach, colon, and lung tumors

Carcinoembryonic antigen (CEA)
- Increased in colon cancer
- Also seen in lung, pancreas, hepatobiliary, stomach, breast, cervix, endometrial, and ovary

Chorionic gonadotropin (beta subunit) (B-HCG)
- Increased in hydatidiform mole, choriocarcinoma, testicular teratoma
- Ectopic HCG production by some cancers of pituitary gland, stomach, pancreas, lung, colon, and liver

Prostate-specific antigen (PSA)
- Increased in prostate cancer, also increased in benign prostate hypertrophy and prostatitis

CA19-9
- Increased in pancreatic cancer; gastric, colon, and some bladder cancers
- More sensitive than CEA for pancreatic cancer

CA125
- Increased in nonmucinoid ovarian carcinomas; also increased in endometrial, pancreatic, lung, breast, and colon cancers
- Increased in benign processes: menstruation, pregnancy, endometriosis, pelvic inflammatory disease (PID), and peritoneal irritation

CA15-3
- Used in management of breast cancer; also increased in cancers of lung, stomach, uterus, and pancreas

Hormones

Adrenocorticotropic hormone (ACTH)
- Increased in ectopic-ACTH–producing tumors (especially small-cell lung cancer), adrenal carcinoma, adenoma, thymic and pancreatic cancer

Antidiuretic hormone (ADH)
- Increased in brain tumors, lung cancer (most common), prostate cancer, adrenal cancer, and Hodgkin's disease

Calcitonin
- Increased in medullary carcinoma of thyroid, some lung and breast tumors, colon cancer, and GI malignancies

Estrogens, total
- Increased in estrogen-producing ovarian tumors, some testicular tumors, and adrenal cortical tumors

Estrogen (Estradiol) receptor assay
- 60% of breast cancer characterized by estrogen receptors

Glucagon
- Decreased in some pancreatic tumors

Growth hormone (GH)
- Increased in ectopic secretion by some stomach and lung tumors

Parathyroid hormone (PTH)
- Increased in squamous cell or epidermoid lung cancers and renal cell cancers

Progesterone receptor assay
- May be useful in predicting tumors likely to respond to hormonal manipulations

17-Ketogenic steroids
- Increased in adrenal adenoma and carcinoma, ectopic ACTH syndrome

17-Ketosteroids
- Increased in adrenal tumors, testicular tumors, interstitial cell tumors, androgenic ovarian tumors

Testosterone
- Increased in some adrenocortical tumors, gonadotropin-producing extragonadal tumors

Enzymes

Amylase
- Increased in some lung and ovarian tumors

Amylase isoenzymes
- Increased in some bronchogenic or serous ovarian tumors

Lactate dehydrogenase (LDH) and LDH isoenzymes
- Increased in malignant processes, acute leukemia, and non-Hodgkin's lymphoma

Serum γ-glutamyl transpeptidase (SGGT)
- Increased in some cases of renal cell cancer and liver metastases, also in melanoma, breast and lung cancer

Table 22-1 Hormone Tests

Hormone	Stimulation	Suppression
Antidiuretic hormone (ADH)	Water deprivation Nicotine	Saline infusion Pitressin
Growth hormone (GH)	Insulin tolerance test Arginine tolerance test Levodopa Exercise stimulation test	Glucose tolerance test
Thyroid-stimulating hormone (TSH)	Thyrotropin-releasing hormone (TRH)	Triiodothyronine Thyroxine
Prolactin (PRL)	Insulin tolerance test Chlorpromazine TRH	Levodopa
Adrenocorticotropic hormone (ACTH)	Insulin tolerance test (hypoglycemia will occur) Corticotropin-releasing hormone (CRH)	Dexamethasone Metyrapone
Luteinizing hormone (LH)	Luteinizing-releasing hormone (LRH)	Testosterone Estrogen
Follicle-stimulating hormone (FSH)	Clomiphene	
Triiodothyronine (T_3)	TSH	T_3
Thyroxine (T_4)		T_4
Cortisol	ACTH CRH Insulin tolerance test Arginine tolerance test	Dexamethasone Metyrapone
Aldosterone	ACTH	Salt loading/volume expansion Spironolactone
Norepinephrine	Histamine Tyramine Glucagon	Phentolamine
Progesterone	Human menopausal gonadotropin (HMG) Human chorionic gonadotropin (HCG)	Provera Progesterone
Testosterone	HMG HCG	Testosterone
Parathyroid hormone (PTH)	PTH infusion	Calcium infusion
Glucose	Glucagon	Insulin tolerance test Tolbutamide
Insulin	Glucose tolerance test (GTT) Leucine Fructose	Prolonged fast
Gastrin	Pentagastrin Calcium infusion High-protein, high-carbohydrate meal	Cimetidine

Serum aspartate transaminase (AST)
- Increased in liver metastases

Serum alanine transaminase (ALT)
- Increased in some liver cancers

Immunoglobulins

IgA
IgO
IgE
IgG
IgM

Endocrine Studies of Hormones

Provocative endocrine tests are classified as either stimulation or suppression studies. Evaluation of secretory reserve by a *stimulation* test is useful for diagnosing hypofunction and for detecting impaired secretory reserve. *Suppression* tests are useful for diagnosis of hyperfunction because the hyperfunctioning gland by definition is not operating under normal control mechanisms.

Table 22-1 lists tests according to the hormone being evaluated. These tests are associated with specific procedures dependent on the laboratory capabilities of the institution. Injection of some hormones (e.g., TRH) may produce a warm, flushed feeling. The nursing care includes education of the patient about the purpose, procedure, and possible side effects and support of the patient during the procedure. The insulin tolerance test will cause profound and purposeful hypoglycemia, requiring a nurse in attendance at all times. When the physician terminates the test, intravenous glucose (10 D/W; 20 D/W; 50 D) is infused immediately and is followed by a high-protein meal.

Arterial Blood Gas Analysis

Description: Arterial blood gas analysis is the most direct method to assess the patient's oxygen and blood gas status.

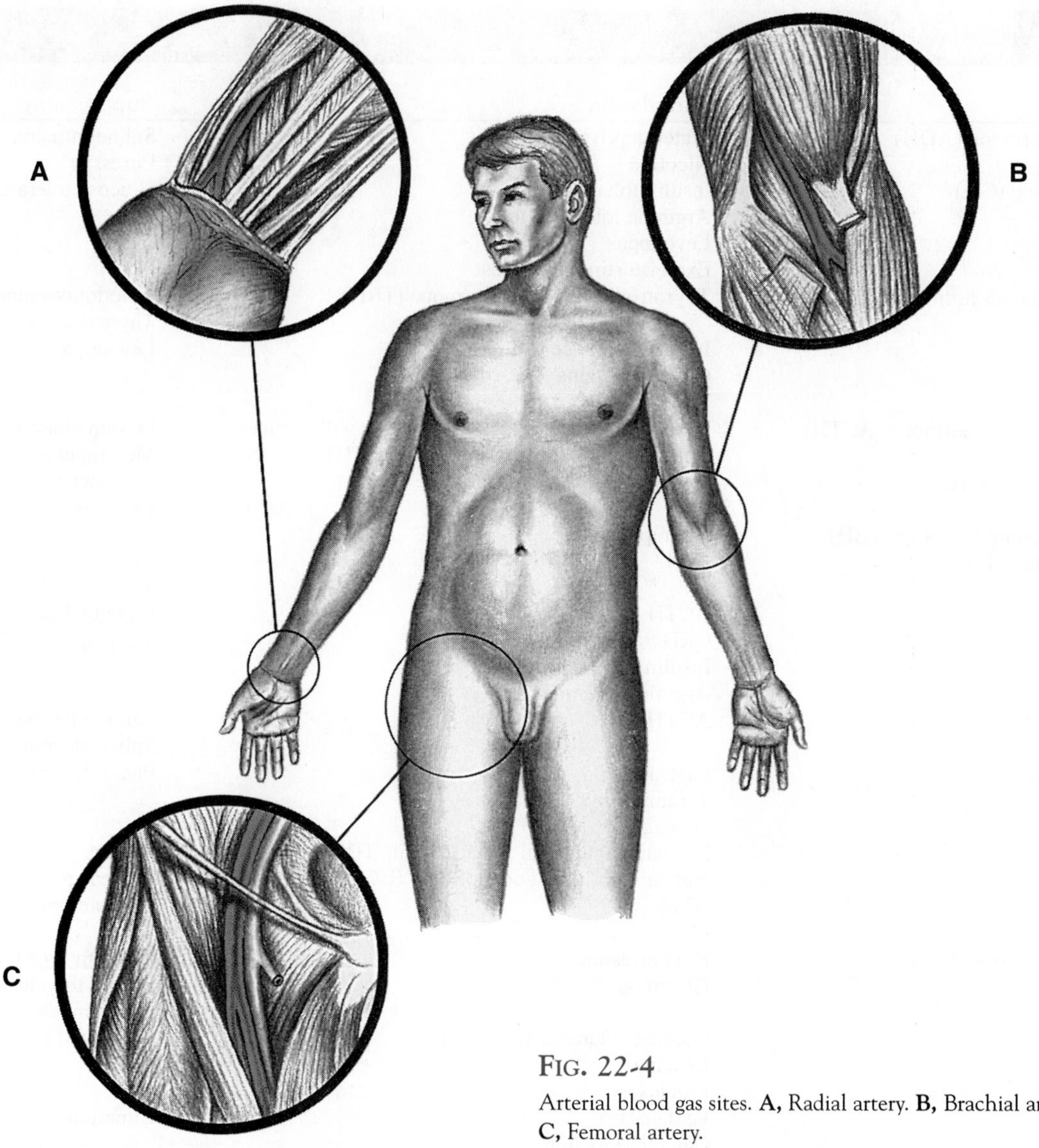

FIG. 22-4
Arterial blood gas sites. **A,** Radial artery. **B,** Brachial artery. **C,** Femoral artery.

Indications: The procedure is indicated for any patient who is seriously ill or injured, whose respiratory status and metabolic balance are in question. Most commonly, arterial blood gases are required for patients with hypoxemia or desaturation secondary to altered ventilatory patterns from any cause.

Arterial blood gas collection procedure

1. Gather the equipment: an ABG syringe with dry heparin with a 20- or 21-gauge needle (21- or 23-gauge for children); rubber stopper or Luer-Lok cap, alcohol swab or iodophor preparation, gauze pads, and basin with crushed ice and water.
2. Position the patient in either a sitting or supine position and explain the procedure.
3. Locate the arterial puncture site: possible sites include the radial artery, brachial artery, and femoral artery (FIG. 22-4). Vessel criteria include the following:
   a. Collateral blood flow: The radial artery has excellent collateral flow: the brachial artery has reasonable collateral flow; and the femoral artery has no collateral blood flow.
   b. Vessel accessibility: It is easier to palpate, stabilize, and puncture superficial vessels than it is to work with deep ones. The more distal an artery, the more superficial it is.
   c. Periarterial tissue: Muscles, tendon, and fat are reasonably insensitive to pain. Bone periosteum and nerves are very sensitive. Therefore choose a site that avoids close sensitive structures or parallel veins. The sites of choice are first, radial; second, brachial; and third, femoral.
4. When using the radial artery, perform Allen's test. This will evaluate the collateral blood supply. The technique is as follows:
   a. Instruct the patient to close his or her fist tightly.
   b. Obliterate both radial and ulnar arteries simultaneously.
   c. Instruct the patient to relax the hand (not fully); watch for blanching of the palm and fingers.
   d. Remove obstructing pressure from only the ulnar artery and observe for capillary refill and

flush of the hand (within 15 seconds). This refill response, which is a positive Allen's test, verifies that the ulnar artery alone is capable of supplying the entire hand.

e. If the Allen's test is negative, do not use the radial artery for arterial puncture.

f. If the patient is unconscious or uncooperative, a similar response to the closed fist can be obtained by placing the patient's hand up in the air until blanching occurs; obliterate the arteries, lower the hand, and release pressure over the ulnar artery.

NOTE: The remaining procedure assumes that the radial artery has been chosen for arterial puncture:

5. Donning gloves, palpate the radial artery to locate a spot where maximum pulsation is felt.
6. Clean the area with an iodophor preparation, then with an alcohol swab.
7. With one hand locate the radial pulse proximal to the area cleaned. This will provide landmark information. Keeping the fingers of one hand on the pulse, insert the heparinized needle and syringe into the radial artery distal to the palpating fingers. The angle between the needle and the artery should be approximately 45 degrees. This makes the hole through the arterial wall oblique so that the muscle fiber will seal the hole as soon as the needle is removed.
8. When the artery is punctured, the pulsating blood will push up the hub of the syringe. Do not make more than two attempts at any one site.
9. Obtain a sample of approximately 1 ml.
10. After the blood is obtained, remove the needle, apply gauze, and use firm and continuous pressure over the site for a minimum of 5 minutes. If the patient is taking anticoagulants, pressure must be maintained for a much longer period.
11. Remove all air bubbles from the syringe (this will affect blood gas results).
12. Place the syringe in an iced container and send it to the laboratory. The ice will decrease the alterations of the true pH, oxygen, and carbon dioxide levels of the specimen.

Blood Gas Analysis[19,26]

Step-by-step analysis

1. pH (hydrogen ion concentration): Assess patient's acid-base status
   - Normal = 7.35 to 7.45
   - Acidosis = Less than 7.35
   - Alkalosis = Greater than 7.43 (when pH is normal, but when $Paco_2$ and HCO_3^- are both abnormal, compensation is probably occurring)
2. $Paco_2$ (carbon dioxide tension): Evaluates the patient's ventilation
   - Normal = 35 to 45 mm Hg
   - Hyperventilation (hypocarbia) = Less than 34 mm Hg; this means that there is excessive loss of carbon dioxide
   - Abnormal value indicates there may be respiratory compensation for a metabolic problem
   - Decreased values may be caused by hyperventilation or ventilation-perfusion inequality
   - To evaluate for respiratory acidosis and alkalosis and for compensation caused by metabolic acidosis and alkalosis
3. $Paco_2$ in relation to pH
   - $\uparrow Paco_2 + \downarrow pH$ = Acidemia of respiratory origin
   - $\uparrow Paco_2 + \uparrow pH$ = Respiratory retention of carbon dioxide to compensate for metabolic alkalosis
   - $\downarrow Paco_2 + \uparrow pH$ = Alkalosis of respiratory origin
   - $\downarrow Paco_2 + \downarrow pH$ = Respiratory elimination of carbon dioxide to compensate for metabolic acidosis
4. Bicarbonate (HCO_3^-): This is the metabolic component
   - Normal = 16 to 24 mEq/L (infant), 21 to 28 mEq/L (arterial, children and adults), 22 to 27 mEq/L (venous, children and adults)
   - Alkalosis = Greater than 26 mEq/L
   - Acidosis = Less than 22 mEq/L
   - A normal value indicates that there are no primary metabolic problems and that there is no metabolic compensation for a respiratory problem
5. HCO_3^- in relation to pH: To evaluate for metabolic acidosis and alkalosis and for compensation caused by respiratory acidosis and alkalosis
   - $\downarrow HCO_3^- + \downarrow pH$ = Acidemia of metabolic origin
   - $\downarrow HCO_3^- + \uparrow pH$ = Renal retention of hydrogen ion or elimination of HCO_3^- to compensate for respiratory alkalosis
   - $\uparrow HCO_3^- + \uparrow pH$ = Alkalosis of metabolic origin
   - $\uparrow HCO_3^- + \downarrow pH$ = Renal retention of HCO_3^- or elimination of hydrogen ion
6. Pao_2 and O_2 saturation
   - Pao_2 saturation: Normal = 80 to 95 mm Hg; 60 to 70 mm Hg (newborn)
   - O_2 saturation: Normal = 95% to 99%
   - These values may be abnormal because of hypoventilation, shunting, ventilation-perfusion inequality, or a reduction of inspired oxygen

Acid-base imbalance[25]

Alkalosis

Respiratory

- $\downarrow Paco_2 + \downarrow HCO_3^-$ = Patient attempting to compensate
- $\downarrow Paco_2$ + Normal HCO_3^- = No patient compensation

Metabolic

- $\uparrow HCO_3^- + \uparrow Paco_2$ = Patient attempting to compensate
- $\uparrow HCO_3^-$ + Normal $Paco_2$ = No patient compensation

Clinical signs of alkalosis: Dizziness, tingling of fingers and toes, muscle weakness or muscle spasm, muscle twitching, sweating, cardiac dysrhythmia, shallow respirations, nausea or vomiting, tachypnea, tremor, or convulsion

Fluid and electrolyte imbalances (contributing to alkalosis)

- $\downarrow$ Serum sodium
- $\uparrow$ Serum chloride

↓ Serum chloride (if alkalosis is caused by gastric suctioning)
↓ Potassium

Acidosis

Respiratory

↑ $Paco_2$ + ↑ HCO_3^- + = Patient attempting to compensate

↑ $Paco_2$ + Normal HCO_3^- = No patient compensation

Metabolic

↓ HCO_3^- + ↓ $Paco_2$ = Patient attempting to compensate

↓ HCO_3^- + Normal $Paco_2$ = No patient compensation

Clinical signs of acidosis: Headache, slowness in responding to questions, hand tremor when patient is instructed to extend arms, confusion, drowsiness, Kussmaul breathing, nausea or vomiting, tremor, confusion, tachycardia, coma

Fluid and electrolyte imbalances (contributing to acidosis)

↓ Serum sodium
↓ Serum chloride
↑ Serum potassium

Complications[11]: Hematoma from multiple attempts at puncture or from inadequate pressure to the site after arterial stick; ischemia of an extremity secondary to thrombus after the procedure; adjunct nerve damage secondary to incorrect technique.

Nursing care: Explain the procedure fully before attempting technique. Assist the physician in administering a local anesthetic if indicated before obtaining arterial blood gases. Following procedure, apply direct pressure over the puncture site for at least 5 minutes to prevent hematoma or ecchymosis. Carefully and systematically analyze the blood gas results according to the assessment guidelines. Monitor the patient's response to actual or potential blood gas acid-base imbalances to include the following:

Mental state: Depression or stimulation of the central nervous system

Respiratory status: Breathing pattern and depth and quality of respiration

Cardiovascular response: Pulse rate, rhythm, and quality

Fluid and electrolyte status: Disorders, such as vomiting and diarrhea, that could cause the imbalance; the patient's responses secondary to fluid and electrolyte imbalances

URODYNAMIC STUDIES

Uroflowmetry

Description: Determines the rate, time, and volume of urinary flow. This study requires no catheterization; the patient voids into a device that measures the characteristics of bladder elimination. Results are displayed in graph form.

Indications: Aids in the diagnosis and description of ureteral, urethral, and bladder function.

Complications: None.

Nursing care: The patient should force fluids and refrain from voiding for 2 hours before testing in order to have at least 300 ml of urine in the bladder.

Urethral Pressure Studies

Description: These studies measure urethral resistance to urinary outflow. The catheter is pulled through the urethra at a given rate while water or carbon dioxide is infused through several side ports. A specialized catheter may be placed at the external urinary sphincter to measure the urethral response to bladder filling/storage and micturition.

Indications: Aids in the diagnosis of bladder disorders.

Complications: Cystitis.

Nursing care: Instruct the patient to watch for signs of cystitis (frequency of urination and mild dysuria), which should disappear within the first 24 hours after testing.

Cystometry

Description: Evaluates the two phases of bladder function: filling/storage and expulsion/micturition. One or more catheters are placed in the bladder urethrally or suprapubically. The bladder is then filled with liquid contrast material (water or a roentgenographic material) or carbon dioxide. The patient is asked to report sensations of an urgency to void or of bladder fullness. The study is completed by asking the patient to void voluntarily.

Indications: Bladder, micturition disorders.

Complications: Cystitis.

Nursing care: Instruct the patient to watch for signs of cystitis (frequency of urination, dysuria), which should disappear within the first 24 hours after testing.

Cystometry With Pharmacologic Testing

Description: Two comparative cystometrograms are performed before and 30 minutes after administration of a certain drug. The most commonly used drugs are bethanechol chloride (Urecholine) and propantheline bromide (Pro-Banthine).

Indications: Bethanechol is used to assess "denervation" (neuropathic changes in bladder function) as opposed to functional voiding abnormalities. Propantheline is used to assess the clinical response of detrusor overactivity to an anticholinergic agent.

Complications: Bethanechol may cause nausea and vomiting, hypotension, and shock. Atropine is given subcutaneously as an antidote if needed. Propantheline may cause hypotension, hypertension, tachycardia, angina, and atrial or ventricular fibrillation; physostigmine salicylate is given parenterally as an antidote if needed.

Nursing care: Vital signs should be monitored every 15 to 30 minutes for a 2-hour period after testing.

Loopogram

Description: Water-soluble contrast material is instilled into the urostomy stoma via a small catheter and observed under fluoroscopy; a roentgenogram is taken. The loop is then drained and the catheter removed: a 10-minute procedure.

Indications: Assesses length and emptying ability of the ileal/sigmoid conduit; also assesses presence of stricture, reflux angulation, or obstruction.

Complications: None.

Nursing care: Provide the patient with a replacement urinary pouch, because it will be removed during the test.

MISCELLANEOUS STUDIES

Echoencephalogram

Description: An echoencephalogram is a noninvasive diagnostic technique that records sonic pulses from cerebral structures by reflection of ultrasonic impulses directed through the patient's skull and back toward the source. These pulses are then recorded and projected onto an oscilloscope screen.[3]

The procedure is performed by placing an ultrasonic transducer on the skull's midaxis in the temporoparietal region. The waves produced are called M-echos, which then are recorded and projected on a screen to provide a graphic representation of the distance from the reflecting surface to the source of the ultrasonic beam.[22] Pictures of these M-echo waves may become a permanent part of the patient's record. The procedure takes only several minutes, and the reliability of the results depends on the skill of the technician. Abnormal shifts of the midline structures are recorded in millimeters, and a shift of 3 mm or more in the adult is considered abnormal.

Indications: Useful in determining ventricular size and cerebral midline shifts.

Complications: None.

Nursing care: Explain the procedure to the patient.

Testing for *Helicobacter pylori*

Description: *Helicobacter pylori* is a gram-negative bacterium associated with gastritis, gastric and duodenal ulcers, and gastric cancer. *H. pylori* resides in the gastric mucus and the mucosal cells of the stomach and duodenum. There are a variety of diagnostic tests for *H. pylori.*

Endoscopy with biopsy: Specimens of gastric mucus or mucosa are obtained via endoscopy for urease testing, histology, or culture (see discussion of esophagogastroduodenoscopy [EGD]).

Urease testing: Biopsy specimen is placed in solution with urea and phenol red. The solution turns pink in the presence of urease, an enzyme produced by *H. pylori.*

Breath test: The patient swallows a dose of urea with radioactive carbon-14 or nonradioactive carbon-13. Urease will break down the urea into carbon dioxide and ammonia. The isotopic CO_2 concentration in the breath is measured to determine the presence of *H. pylori.*

Immunoassay: Blood tests to measure serum antibodies to *H. pylori.* They are very accurate and easily performed. Most commonly tested is the anti-*Helicobacter pylori* immunoglobulin G (IgG) antibody.

Indications: Diagnose *H. pylori* infection in patients with gastritis, gastric or duodenal ulcers, or gastric cancer.

Complications: See discussion of EGD.

Nursing care: Explain the procedure or test to the patient. For endoscopy see discussion of EGD. No fasting is required for the blood test.

Tonometry

Description: Several types of instruments (tonometers) measure intraocular pressure; all of them indent the globe and measure the force (or weight) necessary to cause the indentation.

Schiøtz's tonometer: This hand-held instrument has a curved footplate that is rested on the cornea. A local anesthetic is instilled into each eye. The patient lies supine and is asked to stare straight ahead. The examiner holds the lids open. As the tonometer is placed on the corneal surface, a scale reading is taken from the instrument and converted with a chart to pressure in millimeters of mercury.

Applanation tonometer: This machines measures the force required to flatten rather than indent the central cornea. It is more accurate than Schiøtz's tonometer. A spring tension knob records the pressure, and a local anesthetic is used.

Noncontact tonometer: This machine uses a rapid puff of air to exert and register pressure. It does not require any anesthetic and is very accurate except in higher-pressure ranges. It cannot be used for patients with corneal edema or those with irregular optic interface.

Indications: For measurement of intraocular pressure; for routine screening of glaucoma and diabetes; for assessment of penetrating injuries.

Complications: None; a risk of cross-contamination exists if the tonometer is not sterilized between patients.

Nursing care: Sterilize the tonometer before each use. Inquire about corneal injuries or abrasions. Assure the patient that no discomfort will be experienced.

Caloric Test

Description: Stimulation of the semicircular canals by introduction of either water or air (above or below body temperature) into the external auditory canal. Water below body temperature causes endolymphatic fluid to flow in a downward direction when directed against the tympanic membrane. The injection of cold water into the ear causes maximal stimulation of the semicircular canals and causes nystagmus and falling reactions in 10 to 20 seconds in the normal individual. Warm caloric tests have given reactions opposite to those induced by cold water tests. Specific tests include the following.

Caloric test for vestibular function: Cold or hot water is injected into the external auditory canal with the patient lying down and the head elevated at 30 degrees. The patient is observed for nystagmus.

Hallpike caloric test: Hot or cold water is injected into the external auditory canal. The time interval from the beginning of water flow to the end of visible nystagmus is recorded.

Nelson caloric test: Small amounts of ice water are injected into the external aural canal while the patient is in a supine position with the head tilted 30 degrees forward or in a sitting position with the head tilted 60 degrees backward. The patient is observed for nystagmus.

Indications: The caloric test indicates whether the labyrinth is reacting normally and is hypoactive or hyperactive, or whether no labyrinthine response is present.[15] In patients who complain of dizziness, vertigo, unsteadiness, or nystagmus, it is important to know whether the labyrinth is functioning normally.

Complications: None.

Nursing care: Maintain bed rest, with the head of the bed elevated 20 to 30 degrees until subjective symptoms disappear. The patient is given nothing by mouth 6 hours before the procedure.

Specific Audiometric and Hearing Testing

Description: The following are some of the tests used to determine hearing loss.

Weber's test: The handle of a lightly vibrating tuning fork is placed in the middle of the forehead. Tones should normally be heard equally in both ears.

Rinne test: When a softly struck tuning fork is placed alternately behind the ear on the mastoid process, and then in front of the same ear, the normal ear hears a tuning fork about twice as long by air conduction as by bone conduction.

Schwabach's test: The examiner and patient hear tones equally when a tuning fork is alternately placed on the patient's and the examiner's mastoid processes.

Pure tone test: A series of tones is volume calibrated at different frequencies (400 to 3000 Hz). The speech threshold represents the loudness at which a person with normal hearing can perceive a tone. Both air and bone conduction are measured for each ear, and the results are graphed. With normal hearing, the line is plotted at 0 dB.

Speech audiometry: A normal-hearing person hears and correctly repeats 95% of words spoken by the examiner.

Impedance audiometry: Disorders of the middle ear are detected, thereby determining the degree of tympanic membrane and middle ear mobility. An impedance audiometer is used. One end is a probe with three small tubes inserted into the external canal, and the other end attaches to an oscillator. One tube delivers a low tone of varying intensity, the second contains a microphone, and the third has an air pump. A normal tympanic membrane reflects minimal sound waves and produces a low-voltage curve on the graph.

Tympanometry: A tympanometer, with the impedance audiometer, measures the tympanic membrane's compliance with air pressure variations in the external canal and determines the degree of negative pressure in the middle ear.

In addition to these tests, patients may be tested to differentiate sensory (cochlear) hearing losses from neural (acoustic nerve) hearing losses. These tests include recruitment, sensitivity to small increases in intensity, and pathologic adaptation.

Recruitment is the ability to hear loud sounds normally despite a hearing loss or an abnormal increase in the perception of loudness. This is absent in neural hearing losses and present in sensory hearing losses. It can be demonstrated by having the patient compare the loudness of sounds in the affected ear with the loudness of sounds in the normal ear. In sensory hearing losses the sensation of loudness in the affected ear increases more with each increment in intensity than it does in the normal ear. In neural hearing losses the sensation of loudness in the affected ear increases less with each increment in intensity than in the normal ear. This is called *decruitment.*

Sensitivity to small increments in intensity can be determined by having a patient listen to a continuous tone of 20 dB and then briefly and intermittently increasing the intensity. Patients with neural hearing losses, as well as those with normal hearing, cannot detect small changes in intensity. On the other hand, a patient with a sensory hearing loss can easily perceive these changes.

Pathologic adaptation, or tone decay, is found when a person cannot continue to hear a constant tone above the hearing threshold. The findings are mildly abnormal with sensory losses and severely abnormal with neural losses.

Indications: To diagnose hearing impairment.

Complications: None.

Nursing care: Explain the procedure to the patient.

Pulmonary Function Testing (Table 22-2)

Simple Spirometer

Description: The simple spirometer is a basic office tool used to measure the presence and severity of disease in large and small airways and to distinguish between obstructive and restrictive patterns. It is most commonly used to measure vital capacity (VC), inspiratory capacity (IC), expiratory reserve volume (ERV), tidal volume (VT), inspiratory reserve volume (IRV), forced expiratory flow between 200 and 1200 ml of forced vital capacity ($FEF_{200\text{-}1200}$), and forced expiratory flow, 25% to 75% ($FEF_{25\%\text{-}75\%}$). There are two types of spirometers: volume and flow. Both types are usually computerized. Two of the most common are the water seal and dry rolling seal spirometers. The volume measurement spirometer is most common. As the person exhales or inhales into the mouthpiece, water or air already in the spirometer is displaced, causing the pen to touch the rotating drum and record the pattern. The presence and severity of respiratory dysfunction are determined by comparing observed values with those predicted for a normal person considering age, gender, height, weight, and race.

Spirometer With Gas Dilution

Description: The spirometer with gas dilution is used to measure the following:

FRC (functional residual capacity)
RV (residual volume)

Table 22-2 Pulmonary Function Tests*

Test	Description	Significance
LUNG VOLUME TEST†		
VC = Vital capacity (VC = ERV + VT + IRV)	This capacity test combining more than one lung volume is the maximum amount of air that can be expired slowly and completely following a maximum inspiration. Response values of this test, as well as all other pulmonary function tests, are directly dependent on patient's effort. From VC other pulmonary function values may be calculated, including ERV, IRV, VT, and IC.	A decrease in VC may be caused by a loss of distensible lung tissue, as seen in bronchiolar obstruction, pulmonary edema, pneumonia, atelectasis, pulmonary restriction, surgery, pulmonary congestion, or by depression of the respiratory center in the brain.
FRC = Functional residual capacity (FRC = ERV + RV)	This capacity test combining more than one lung volume is the volume of air remaining in the lungs at the end of normal expiration. Open- or closed-circuit techniques of body plethysmography are used to measure concentration of a gas (either helium or nitrogen); from this the FRC can be calculated. This is actually calculated measurement of airway resistance.	The values help to differentiate obstructive from restrictive diseases. An increased FRC represents hyperinflation, which is seen with bronchiolar obstruction, emphysema, or asthma. An increased FRC results in muscular and mechanical inefficiency. A decreased FRC may be seen in diseases that occlude the alveoli such as pneumonia, and in fibrosis, asbestosis, or silicosis.
ERV = Expiratory reserve volume	This single-volume calculation is the maximum amount of air that can be exhaled following a resting expiratory level.	Although the ERV (approximately 25% of VC) has no diagnostic value, it must be calculated so that the RV can be calculated.
IRV = Inspiratory reserve volume	This single-volume calculation is the maximum amount of air that can be inspired following a normal inspiration.	
RV = Residual volume (RV = FRC − ERV)	This single-volume measurement is the volume of air remaining in the lungs at the end of maximal expiration. This is measured indirectly by subtracting the ERV from the FRC.	This value helps to differentiate restrictive from obstructive diseases. An increased RV indicates that despite maximal expiratory effort the lungs still contain an abnormally large amount of air. This may be seen in patients with emphysema or chronic bronchial obstruction. The RV usually decreases with restrictive lung disease.
IC = Inspiratory capacity (IC = VT + IRV)	This calculated measurement is a capacity test involving more than one lung volume. It is the largest volume of air that can be inspired in one breath from the resting expiratory level.	IC normally composes approximately 75% of the VC. Changes in the IC usually parallel increases or decreases in VC. Other than its use in postoperative care, this value is not commonly measured.
TLC = Total lung capacity (TLC = FRC + IC) or (TLC = VC + RV)	This capacity test combining more than one lung volume is the volume of air contained in the lung at the end of a maximal inspiration. The TLC is a derived calculation.	TLC differentiates obstructive from restrictive diseases. It may be decreased in pulmonary edema, atelectasis, neoplasms, pulmonary congestion, pneumothorax, or thoracic restriction. TLC may be increased in bronchiolar obstruction with hyperinflation and in emphysema.
RV/TLC ratio = Residual volume/total lung capacity ratio (RV/TLC × 100)	This is a statement of the fraction of the TLC that can be defined as RV, expressed as a percentage.	Values greater than 35% are seen in patients with emphysema or chronic air trapping.
VENTILATION TESTS		
VT = Tidal volume	This single-volume measurement is the volume of air inspired or expired during each respiratory cycle. This is measured at the bedside by a simple spirometer for 1 minute. The total is then divided by the rate (the number of breaths per minute) to determine the average VT.	Decreased or increased VT may occur in various pulmonary disorders. VT should be considered in relation only to arterial blood gases and respiratory rate and minute volume.
VE = Minute volume	This is the total volume of air inspired or expired in 1 minute. It is determined by measuring the inspired or expired air over several minutes and dividing by the number of minutes. It may also be measured easily at the bedside by simple spirometry.	This value must be considered in conjunction with arterial blood gases. VE increases in response to hypoxia, hypercapnia, acidosis, and exercise. It is most commonly used in exercise testing.

*Normal values for pulmonary tests vary depending on the patient's age, gender, weight, and race.
†To best interpret these tests, see FIGS. 22-5 and 22-6.

Continued

Table 22-2 Pulmonary Function Tests*—cont'd

Test	Description	Significance
VD = Respiratory dead space	This is the volume of the lungs that is ventilated but not perfused by pulmonary capillary blood flow. This includes the conducting airways, or anatomic dead space, and the nonfunctioning alveoli, or alveolar dead space.	The measurement of VD provides important information regarding the status of the functional lung capacity. It is used primarily for exercise testing.
VA = Alveolar ventilation VA = (VT − VD) f f = respiratory rate	This is the volume of air that participates in gas exchange in the lungs.	The adequacy of VA can be determined only by arterial blood gas studies. It is used primarily for exercise testing.
PULMONARY SPIROMETRY TESTS		
FVC = Forced vital capacity	This is the volume of air that can be expired forcefully and rapidly after maximal inspiration. The measurement is made directly by spirometer.	The FVC is normally equal to the VC. FVC may be reduced in chronic obstructive diseases, whereas the VC may appear close to normal. The FVC is decreased in restrictive diseases also. The test's validity depends largely on the individual's effort and cooperation.
FEV_T = Forced expiratory volume timed	This is the volume of air expired over a given interval during the performance of an FVC. The interval (T) is stated as a subscript to FEV. For example, $FEV_{0.5}$ indicates the interval is 0.5 second, and in FEV_1 the interval is 1 second. FEV_T is a calculated measurement by spirometer. After 3 seconds, FEV should equal FVC.	FEV_T is the most common screening test for detection of obstructive airway disease, in which the finding is a reduced response.
FEV% = FEV_T/FVC ratio × 100 (usually FEV_1/FVC%)	This is the percentage of the measured FVC that a given FEV_T represents.	By measuring the expiratory flow over time the severity of obstruction can be assessed. FEV% or a reduced ratio is decreased in obstructive lung disease. It usually remains within normal limits for persons with restrictive disease unless there is some type of secondary problem.
$FEF_{25\%-75\%}$ = Forced expiratory flow, 25% to 75% or MMEF = Maximum midexpiratory flow rate	This is the average flow during the middle 50% of an FEV. It was previously known as the maximum midexpiratory flow rate (MMEF or MMF). Its reported value provides a picture of peripheral airway resistance. This value is then compared with the VC.	This measures the average flow rate over a given interval. It is an index of the status of the medium-sized airways. Decreased flow rates, when compared with the VC, are seen in early stages of obstructive diseases such as emphysema.
PEFR = Peak expiratory flow rate	This is the maximum flow rate attainable at any time during an FEV.	This measurement is of questionable diagnostic value. Children with asthma have a decreased PEFR.
F-V loop = Flow-volume loop	This is a graphic analysis of the maximum forced expiratory flow volume (MEFV) followed by a maximum inspiratory flow volume (MIFV). This technique uses a forced expiratory vital capacity followed by a forced inspiratory vital capacity. It is actually another way to display the forced vital capacity. Curves, reported as continuous loops on spirometric graphs, have distinctive sizes and shapes.	The inspiratory flow may show evidence of upper airway obstruction. With obstructive disease the flow is reduced out of proportion to the volume. In restrictive disease the flow and volume are proportionally decreased, or the flow may be better than would be expected for the volume. As the flow-volume loop is examined, the shapes of the inspiratory and expiratory sides are analyzed.
MVV = Maximum voluntary ventilation	This is the largest volume of air that can be breathed per minute by voluntary effort. The actual testing period lasts 10 to 15 seconds.	The MVV measures the status of respiratory muscles, the resistance offered by airways and tissues, and the compliance of the lung and thorax. This measurement depends greatly on the individual's effort.
GAS EXCHANGE		
DLCO = Diffusing capacity of CO	The diffusing capacity rate of the lung provides a measure of the lung's gas exchange mechanism. It assesses the amount of functioning pulmonary capillary bed in contact with functioning alveoli. A common way to measure this is the *single-breath Krogh method:* The patient deeply inhales	The test is used primarily to differentiate various disease processes and for patient care monitoring.

*Normal values for pulmonary tests vary depending on the patient's age, gender, weight, and race.
†To best interpret these tests see FIGS. 22-5 and 22-6

Test	Description	Significance
DLCO = Diffusing capacity of CO—cont'd	(from the residual volume level) a mixture of air containing 0.3% carbon monoxide and 10% helium gas, holds his or her breath for 10 seconds, and then exhales. The carbon monoxide levels are then remeasured.	
R_{AW} = Airway resistance G_{AW} = Airway conductance	R_{AW} is the pressure difference required for a unit flow change. G_{AW} is the flow generated per unit of pressure drop in the airway. It is the reciprocal of R_{AW}. Measurements are made with a body plethysmograph. They are taken at the same time as FRC.	R_{AW} increases in an acute asthmatic attack, emphysema, or other obstructive diseases. The calculations are most useful in evaluation of the qualitative response to various bronchodilators.

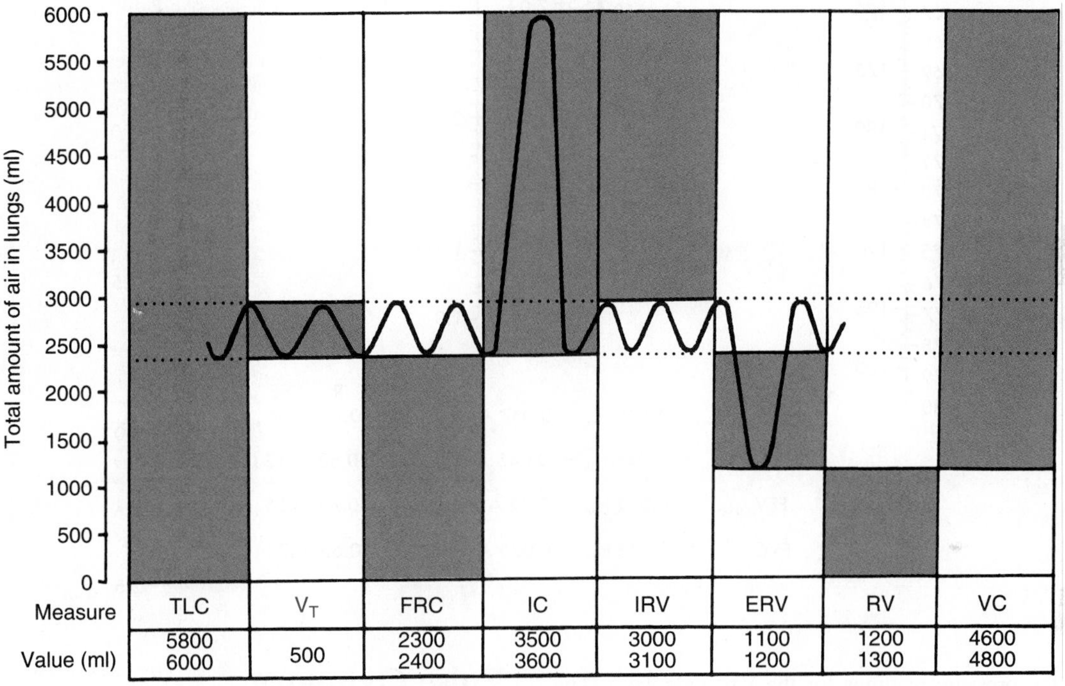

FIG. 22-5

Lung volume measurements. All values are approximately 25% less in women. *TLC*, Total lung capacity; *VT*, tidal volume; *FRC*, functional residual capacity; *IC*, inspiration capacity; *IRV*, inspiratory reserve volume; *ERV*, expiratory reserve volume; *RV*, residual volume; *VC*, vital capacity.

RV/TLC ratio (residual volume/total lung capacity)

DLCO (oxygen diffusing capacity of the lung)

The purpose of the technique is to measure the rate of diffusion. The measurement of lung volumes is by either the helium-dilution technique or the nitrogen-washout technique. In the helium-dilution technique the patient rebreathes a known concentration of diluted helium through the spirometer mouthpiece until the helium concentration in the spirometer and the patient's lungs are equal. The helium concentration in the spirometer and the volume of gas can then be used to calculate the patient's FRC. In the nitrogen-washout technique the patient breathes 100% O_2 from one source and exhales the expired gas into the spirometer.

Plethysmography

Description: Plethysmography is used to measure the following:

R_{AW} (airway resistance)

G_{AW} (airway conductance)

VTG (thoracic gas volume)

FRC (VTG = FRC shutter is closed at end of expiration)

The plethysmograph is an airtight chamber in which the patient sits. The patient is seated in the airtight chamber, is fitted with nose clips, and is instructed to breathe through the mouthpiece, which is connected to a transducer. To calculate VTG, the patient is instructed to pant into the mouthpiece while keeping the cheeks rigid and glottis open. This

FIG. 22-6
Spirometric standards for males and females.
(From Morris, Roski, and Johnson.[17])

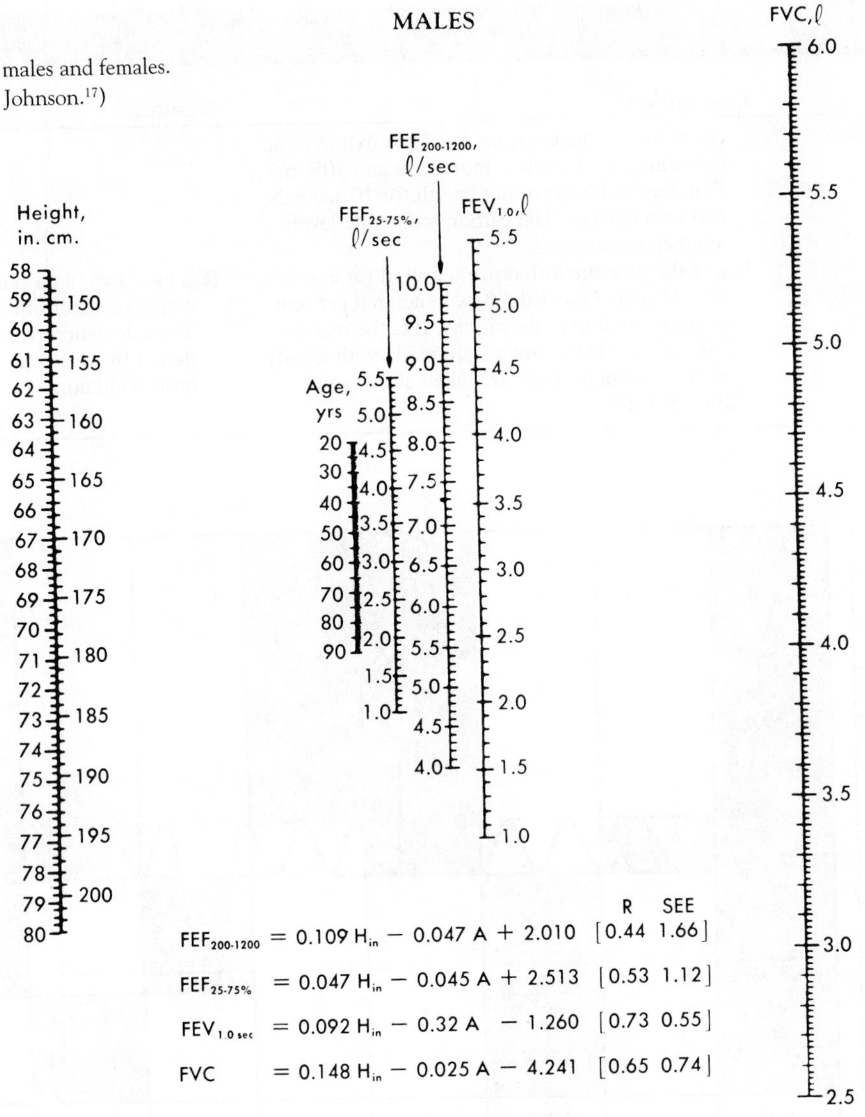

		R	SEE
$FEF_{200\text{-}1200}$	$= 0.109\ H_{in} - 0.047\ A + 2.010$	0.44	1.66
$FEF_{25\text{-}75\%}$	$= 0.047\ H_{in} - 0.045\ A + 2.513$	0.53	1.12
$FEV_{1.0\,sec}$	$= 0.092\ H_{in} - 0.32\ A - 1.260$	0.73	0.55
FVC	$= 0.148\ H_{in} - 0.025\ A - 4.241$	0.65	0.74

provides the pressure readings for the VTG calculator. The R_{AW} and G_{AW} may be mathematically calculated as the patient breathes rapidly and shallowly.

Resting Energy Expenditure

Description: Measurement of oxygen consumption and carbon dioxide production via expired gas analysis provides a means of calculating an approximation of a person's energy expenditure and caloric requirements. Measurements can be performed on spontaneously breathing or mechanically ventilated patients usually using a commercially manufactured metabolic cart. Data are usually collected for a short time period (15 to 30 minutes) and extrapolated for the energy requirement (Kcal/day) needs in 24 hours.

Indications: To determine a patient's caloric requirements. The final result is an estimation of the patient's energy needs at rest and adjustments needed to account for the patient's activity and stress level.

Complications: No known complications.

Nursing care: The patient must be resting during the test and not be experiencing pain or discomfort for accurate results.

Pulse Oximetry

Description: Pulse oximetry is a noninvasive means of determining oxygen saturation. The principles of operation that are used to obtain this value are spectrophotometry (measurement of light) and plethysmography (measurement of blood flow through tissue). Plethysmography senses the arterial pulse wave as it passes through the tissue. Sensing the arterial pulse wave, the oximeter can then determine the change in light absorption at that time and calculate the arterial oxygen saturation.

Indications: Frequently used to assess a patient's oxygen saturation level.

Complications: No known complications.

Nursing care: Visualize the waveform to verify accuracy.

Exercise Stress Test (EST)

Description: Examines cardiovascular and pulmonary response to exercise. It is also used to detect and quantify ischemic heart disease, to determine patients considered at risk, and to determine cardiovascular fitness preceding exercise programs. The test consists of raising, in gradual incre-

FIG. 22-6 cont'd

Spirometric standards for males and females. (From Morris, Roski, and Johnson.[17])

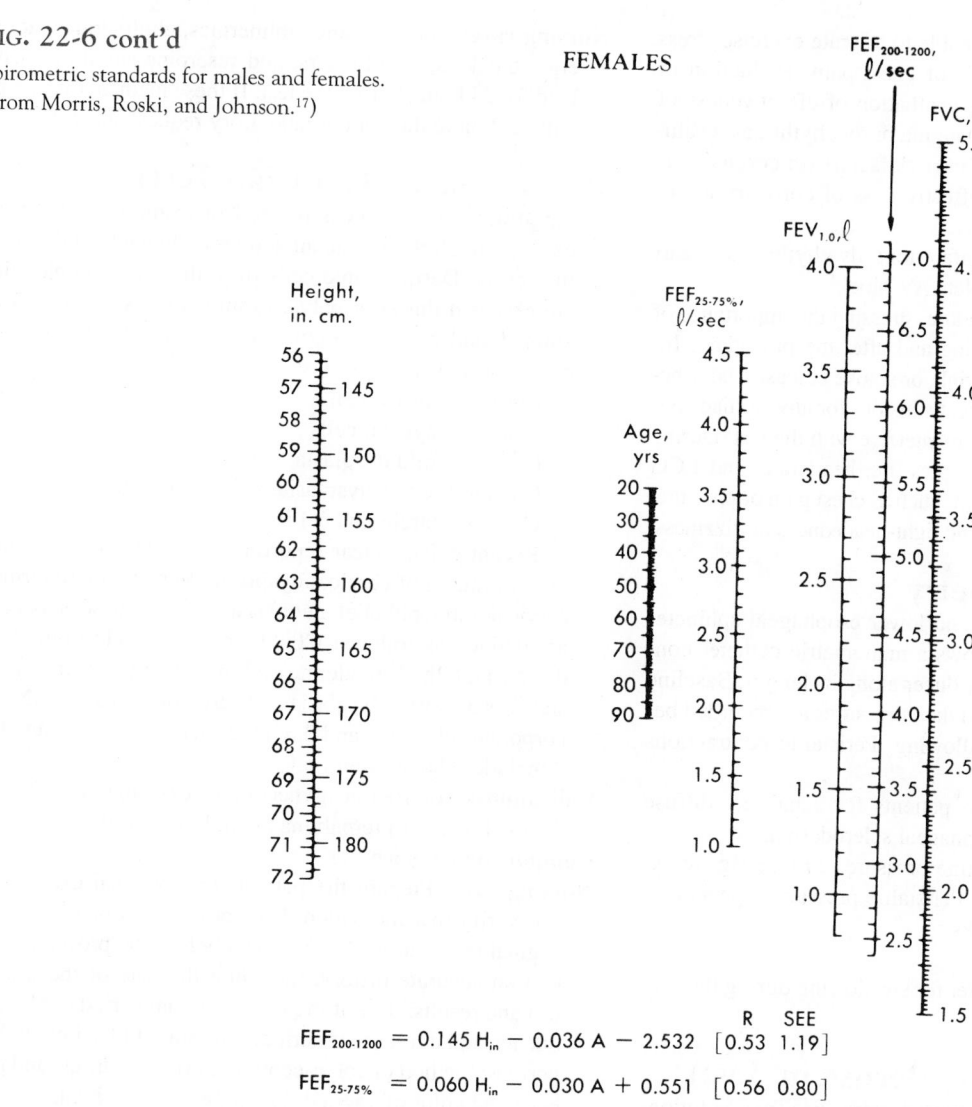

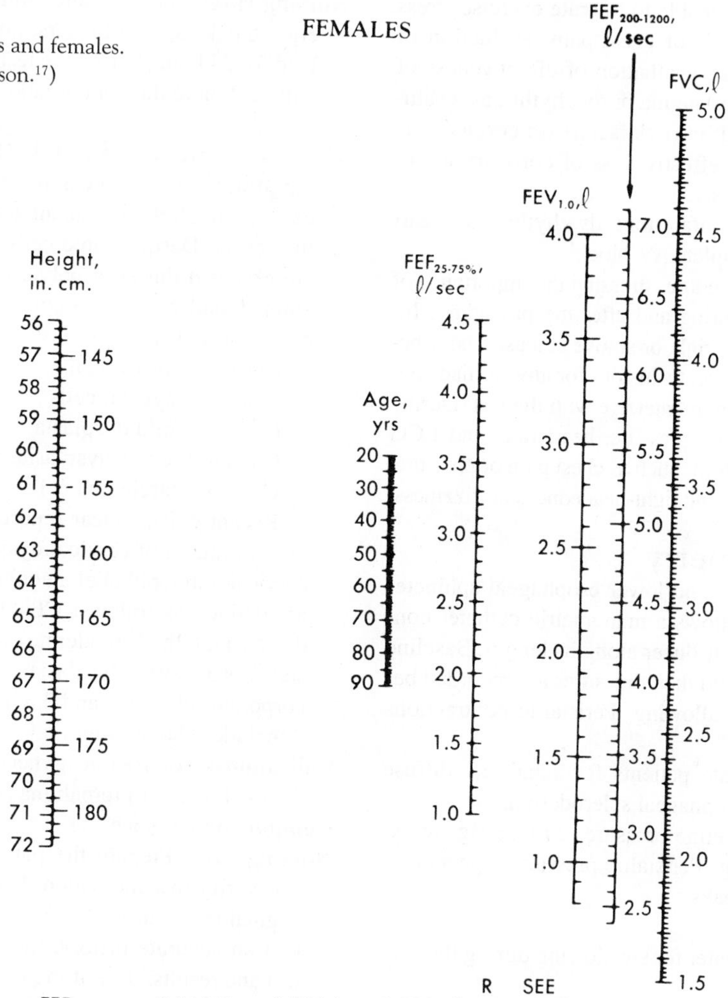

	Equation	R	SEE
$FEF_{200\text{-}1200}$	$= 0.145\,H_{in} - 0.036\,A - 2.532$	0.53	1.19
$FEF_{25\text{-}75\%}$	$= 0.060\,H_{in} - 0.030\,A + 0.551$	0.56	0.80
$FEV_{1.0\,sec}$	$= 0.089\,H_{in} - 0.025\,A - 1.932$	0.73	0.47
FVC	$= 0.115\,H_{in} - 0.024\,A - 2.852$	0.71	0.52

ments, the exercise level on a motorized treadmill or bicycle ergometer while the ECG is being monitored. Blood pressure and heart electrical activity are also measured, and expired gases can be collected, O_2 consumption and saturation monitored, and samples collected for blood gas determinations. Key end points during exercise may define physiologically the causes of the patient's symptoms.

Indications: Differential diagnosis of chest pain; determination of workload level (exercise) when symptoms of ischemia occur; evaluation of therapy for angina; evaluation of patients who have multiple risk factors for coronary artery disease; evaluation of exercise-induced dysrhythmias.

Complications: Recent myocardial infarction (4 to 6 weeks) (but such patients may perform submaximal EST before discharge from hospital); rapid ventricular or atrial dysrhythmia; heart failure; severe aortic stenosis; blood pressure greater than 170/100 mm Hg before the onset of exercise; complete AV block.

Nursing care: Explain the procedure, stressing the need for the patient to report any symptoms during and after the procedure. Instruct the patient to dress comfortably in shorts or gym clothes and tennis shoes. Instruct the patient not to eat for 1 hour before the test. During the procedure, monitor blood pressure, heart rate, ECG changes such as ST elevation or depression, and dysrhythmias. Observe for symptoms such as chest pain or pressure, shortness of breath, or fatigue.

Chemical Stress Test (Persantine Stress Test)

Description: Examines cardiovascular response to a pharmacologic agent that stresses the heart. Persantine (dipyridamole) and adenosine vasodilate the coronary arteries and cause blood to shunt away from partially occluded coronary vessels. Dobutamine stresses the heart by increasing the strength of heart muscle contraction. With these agents areas of the heart at risk for ischemia and infarction can be identified by ECG, ultrasonography, or radionuclide imaging. Chemical stress testing is accurate, and testing can be done safely under controlled conditions.

Indications: Patients who are unable to tolerate exercise stress testing. Differential diagnosis of chest pain; evaluation of stress-induced dysrhythmias; evaluation of effectiveness of pharmacologic treatments of angina or dysrhythmias; evaluation of patients having multiple risk factors for coronary artery disease; evaluation of effectiveness of coronary artery bypass grafting or angioplasty.

Complications: Myocardial infarction; dysrhythmias; heart failure; severe angina; complete AV block.

Nursing care: Explain the procedure, stressing the importance of reporting any symptoms during and after the procedure. Instruct the patient not to eat, drink, or smoke at least 1 hour before the test. Evaluate the patient's history for any cardiac conditions or medications that may interfere with the test. During the procedure, monitor blood pressure, heart rate, and ECG changes. Observe for symptoms such as chest pain or pressure, shortness of breath, fatigue, and light-headedness or dizziness.

Esophageal Manometry

Description: Measures upper and lower esophageal sphincter pressure. The patient swallows a manometric catheter containing a small pressure transducer along its length. Baseline measurements are taken, and then pressures are recorded before, during, and after swallowing. Peristaltic contractions are recorded.

Indications: Used to evaluate patients for achalasia, diffuse esophageal spasm, and esophageal scleroderma.

Normal values are baseline pressure, 20 mm Hg; relaxation pressure, 18 mm Hg. Peristaltic pressure appears as a series of high-pressure peaks.

Complications: None.

Nursing care: Provide ice water for swallowing during the procedure.

Acid Perfusion Test (Bernstein Test)

Description: Evaluates esophageal mucosa. Two solutions (saline and acidic) are dripped through a nasogastric tube. The presence of pain with the acidic solution indicates esophagitis. The test is contraindicated in patients with esophageal varices, congestive heart failure, acute myocardial infarction, and other known cardiac disorders.

Indications: Patients with gastric reflux often have symptoms of epigastric or retrosternal pain that radiates to the back or arms. The test is used to distinguish between the chest pain of esophagitis and the chest pain of cardiac disorders.

Complications: None.

Nursing care: If the patient continues to complain of pain or burning after the test, antacids may help relieve discomfort.

Esophageal Acidity Test (pH Monitoring)

Description: Evaluates competence of lower esophageal sphincter by measuring intraesophageal pH with an electrode attached to a manometric catheter.

Indications: Will indicate gastric reflux. Normal value: pH of esophagus is 6.0 or higher. The 24-hour monitoring involves the patient writing down all the activities performed during that period.

Complications: None.

Nursing care: Antacids, anticholinergics, cholinergics, adrenergic blockers, H_2 blockers, and reserpine should be withheld for 24 hours before the test. If these medications are not withheld, note this on the laboratory request sheet.

Papanicolaou Test (Pap Test)

Description: Simple smear method of examining exfoliative cells, particularly malignant and premalignant conditions of the cervix. Desquamated cells from the cervical epithelium are obtained during a pelvic examination, stained, and examined under a microscope. Histologic classification includes class 1 through class 5.

Class 1—normal cells
Class 2—atypical cells
Class 3—mild dysplasia
Class 4—severe dysplasia, suspicious cells
Class 5—carcinoma cells

Recently, Pap smear reporting has changed to recognize the continuum of cervical dysplasia. Reports are in terms of cervical intraepithelial neoplasia (CIN). These subclasses are defined as follows: CIN 1: mild and mild-to-moderate dysplasia; CIN 2: moderate and moderate-to-severe dysplasia; CIN 3: severe dysplasia and carcinoma in situ. CIN 1 incorporates classes 2 and 3, CIN 2 includes class 3, and CIN 3 includes classes 4 and 5.

Indications: For routine gynecologic examination screening for malignant or premalignant conditions of the cervix.

Complications: None.

Nursing care: Prepare the patient for a vaginal examination and verify that the patient has not douched or inserted any vaginal medications for 24 hours before the procedure. Obtain an accurate history, including the date of the last Pap test and results; date of the last menstrual period (LMP); frequency and duration of periods; amount of bleeding with the periods; method of contraception; hormonal drugs; and presence and color of vaginal discharge, pain, or itching.

Tubal Insufflation (Rubin's Test)

Description: Assesses patency of fallopian tubes by insufflation with carbon dioxide, which is introduced through a tight-fitting cannula inserted through the cervical os at pressures up to 200 mm Hg. If the tubes are open, gas enters the abdominal cavity, and recorded pressure falls below 180 mm Hg. High-pitched bubbling can be heard through the abdominal wall with the stethoscope as gas escapes from the tubes. Shoulder pain from diaphragmatic irritation also indicates that gas has escaped into the abdominal cavity. Kymographic tracing shows pressure changes and may indicate tubal obstruction, spasm, or a leak in the system.

Indications: Inability to conceive.

Complications: None.

Nursing care: Be prepared to assist the patient with the cramping pain, dizziness, nausea, and vomiting that may occur after the procedure. Explain that shoulder pain (if present) is caused by an insufflation of gas and will subside. Mild analgesics may be taken if necessary.

Erectile Dysfunction Studies

Description and indications: Monitors nocturnal penile tumescence; snap-gauge devices are designed to determine whether cases of erectile dysfunction are caused by psychogenic or organic disease and to assess the efficiency of an erection. Endocrine disorders that may affect erectile activity are investigated by determining serum levels of FSH, LH, and testosterone and by physical examination. Vascular disorders are diagnosed via dynamic infusion cavernosgraphy and cavernosometry, which reproduces an erection via mechanical means, or by vascular studies of the arterial or venous supplies of the penis—including internal pudendal arteriography, venography, or penile blood pressure or pulse volume assessment. Neurologic disorders that may contribute to erectile dysfunction are diagnosed by a variety of methodologies, including physical examination, electromyography, nerve conduction, and evoked potential studies. The effect of drugs on erectile dysfunction may be determined by altering drug regimens and observing the effects on tumescence.

Complications: None.

Nursing care: Provide a supportive atmosphere and explain the procedure to the patient.

Normal Laboratory Values

CEREBROSPINAL FLUID STUDIES

Appearance: Crystal clear, colorless
Pressure (lateral recumbent): 50 to 180 mm H_2O
Protein
  Lumbar
    6 months and up: Approximately 15 to 50 mg/dl
    Ventricular CSF protein is generally lower
  Cisternal: 15 to 25 mg/dl
  Ventricular: 6 to 15 mg/dl
Cell count
  No RBCs
  0 to 5 WBCs
  0 to 10 cells/mm^3 (all lymphocytes and monocytes)
Glucose
  50 to 80 mg/dl (60% to 70% of plasma glucose)
A/G rates: 8 : 1 (albumin to globulin)
Serologic studies
  Complement fixation: nonreactive
  Treponema pallidum immune adherence: Nonreactive
  Treponema immobilization test: Nonreactive
Gram's stain: Negative for organisms
Culture and sensitivity: No growth of organisms
Electrolytes
  Sodium: 141 mEq/L
  Potassium: 3.3 mEq/L
  Chloride: 110 to 125 mEq/L
Bilirubin: Negative
Cholesterol: 0.2 to 0.6 mg/dl
Creatinine: 0.5 to 1.2 mg/dl
Urea: 7 to 15 mg/dl
Urea nitrogen: 10 to 15 mg/dl
Uric acid: 0.5 to 4.5 mg/dl
pH: 7.32 to 7.35
Specific gravity: 1.007
Glutamine: 6 to 15 mg/dl (enzymatic)
IgG index: 0.3 to 0.7
IgG: 0% to 11% of total protein
Lactic acid
  Control group with no CNS disorder: 0.6 to 2.2 mEq/L (0.6 to 2.2 mmol/L; 10 to 20 mg/dl)
LDH
  Fluid LDH activity normally much less than plasma LDH activity; normal spinal fluid LDH levels are about 10% of serum levels
Myelin basic protein: <4 ng/ml CSF is normal
Oligoclonal bands: Normal CSF: no demonstrable oligoclonal bands
Protein electrophoresis (normal range depends on methodology)
  Gamma: 3% to 13%
  Beta: 7.3% to 17.9%
  $Alpha_2$: 3% to 12.6%
  $Alpha_1$: 1.1% to 6.6%
  Albumin: 56.8% to 76.9%
  Prealbumin: 2.2% to 7.1%
  CSF albumin: 13.4 to 23.7 mg/dl
  Total protein: 15 to 50 mg/dl
  Beta-gamma ratio: 1.67 to 2.3
  Oligoclonal bands: Absent
FTA-ABS: Nonreactive
Cryptococcal antigen titer: Negative
VDRL: Nonreactive
Mycobacteria culture: No growth
Counterimmunoelectrophoresis: Negative
India ink preparation: No *Cryptococcus* identified

BLOOD STUDIES

CBC

RBC
  Male: 4.7 to 6.1 million/mm^3
  Female: 4.2 to 5.4 million/mm^3
Hemoglobin (Hgb)
  Male: 14 to 18 g/dl or 8.7 to 11.2 mmol/L (SI units)
  Female: 12 to 16 g/dl or 7.4 to 9.9 mmol/L
  Elderly: Values may be slightly decreased
Hematocrit (Hct)
  Male: 42% to 52%
  Female: 37% to 47% (pregnancy <33%)
  Elderly: Values may be slightly decreased
RBC indices
  MCV: 80 to 95 μm^3
    (mean corpuscular volume)
  MCH: 27 to 31 pg
    (mean corpuscular hemoglobin)
  MCHC: 32 to 36 g/dl
    (mean corpuscular hemoglobin concentration)
WBC and differential
  Total: 5000 to 10,000/mm^3
  Differential
    Neutrophils: 55% to 70%
    Lymphocytes: 20% to 40%
    Monocytes: 2% to 8%

Eosinophils: 1% to 4%
Basophils: 0.5% to 1%

Platelets
150,000 to 400,000 mm³ or 150 to 400 × 10^9/L

Reticulocyte Count

0.5% to 2%

Prothrombin Time (PT)

11 to 12.5 seconds; 85% to 100%
(should include use of international normalized ratio [INR] value to ensure uniform results)

Partial Thromboplastin Time (PTT)

60 to 70 seconds

Activated Partial Thromboplastin Time (APTT)

30 to 40 seconds

Erythrocyte Sedimentation Rate (ESR) (Westergren Method)

Males age <50: 0 to 15 mm/h
Males age ≥50: 0 to 20 mm/h
Females age <50: 0 to 25 mm/h
Females age ≥50: 0 to 30 mm/h

Zeta Sedimentation Ratio

Age <50: <55%
Age 50 to 80: 40% to 60%

Fibrinogen (Plasma)

200 to 400 mg/dl

Fibrin Split Products

<10 μg/ml

Erythrocyte Fragility Test

Hemolysis starts at 0.45% to 0.39% saline solution
Hemolysis complete at 0.33% to 0.30% saline solution

Erythrocyte Life Span Determination

Approximately 120 days
Half-life: 27 to 86 days

Lymphocyte Populations (%)

Total B cells: 5% to 11%
Total T cells: 75% to 90%
T helper cells (T_4 positive): 40% to 58%
T suppressor/cytotoxic cells (T_8 positive): 19% to 30%

Bone Marrow Differential Cell Counts (%)

Erythroblasts: 22.5%
Myeloblasts: 1.0%
Promyelocytes: 3.0%
Eosinophils: 4.0%
Basophils: <0.5%
Monocytes: 2.0%
Myelocytes: 15.0%
Metamyelocytes: 15.0%
Stab cells: 15.0%
Segmented cells: 7.0%
Lymphocytes: 7.5%
Reticular cells: 6.5%
Plasmacytes: 1.0%
Megakaryocytes: <0.5%

Chemistry

Acid phosphatase
0.11 to 0.6 μg/L

Albumin
Serum quantitative (age 1 to 31): 3.5 to 5 g/dl with A/G ratio greater than 1; after age 40, normal range gradually decreases
4 to 5.5 g/dl (electrophoresis)

Aldolase
3.0 to 8.2 Sibley-Lehninger μg/dl or 22 to 59 mU at 37° C (SI units)

Alkaline phosphatase
30 to 85 international milliunits (ImU)/ml

Ammonia
Varies somewhat between laboratories; 11 to 35 μmol/L

Amylase
56 to 190 IU/L (may be slightly increased in normal pregnancy and in the elderly)

Bile acids
Whole blood, serum, or plasma
Positive: >10 cholesterol monohydrate or calcium bilirubinate crystals per slide
Suspicious: 1 to 9 cholesterol monohydrate or calcium bilirubinate crystals per slide

Bilirubin
Direct (conjugated): Up to 0.4 mg/dl

BUN
Age 1 to 40: 5 to 20 mg/dl; gradual slight increase subsequently occurs

Calcium
Serum
Ionized: 3.9 to 4.8 mg/dl for one formula available
Total (up to age 30): 8.2 to 10.5 mg/dl; decreases very slightly in older years

Creatinine
Serum
Men: Up to 1.2 mg/dl
Women: Up to 1.1 mg/dl

Electrolytes
Sodium: 135 to 145 mEq/L
Potassium: 3.5 to 5 mEq/L
Chloride: 97 to 107 mEq/L
Bicarbonate: 22 to 29 mEq/L

Folate
>2 mg/ml

Glucose
60 to 115 mg/dl (normal range increase with age over 50)

Oral glucose tolerance (serum or plasma)
Fasting: 60 to 115 mg/dl (normal range increases with age over 50)
30 minutes: 30 to 60 mg/dl above fasting
60 minutes: 20 to 50 mg/dl above fasting
120 minutes: 5 to 15 mg/dl above fasting
180 minutes: Fasting level or below 2-hour postprandial

Ages 0 to 50: 70 to 140 mg/dl
Ages 50 to 60: 70 to 150 mg/dl
Ages 60 and up: 70 to 160 mg/dl

Haptoglobin
40 to 180 mg/dl (values are method dependent)

Iron
Total: 42 to 135 mg/dl
Binding capacity: 218 to 385 mg/dl
Saturation: 20% to 50%

Lactose
Lactic acid (lactate)
Venous: 5 to 20 mg/dl
Arterial: 3 to 7 mg/dl
Lactose intolerance
Increase of blood glucose <20 mg/dl over fasting level, with symptoms, is considered abnormal; evidence for lactase deficiency: >30 mg/dl is normal

Lipase
Method dependent

Lipid profile
Total: 400 to 800 mg/dl
Cholesterol: 100 to 210 mg/dl
Triglycerides (at 95th percentile)
White men
Ages 25 to 29: Up to 250 mg/dl
Ages 35 to 54: Up to 320 mg/dl
Ages 55 to 64: Up to 290 mg/dl
Ages 65 and older: Up to 260 mg/dl
White women
Ages 35 to 39: Up to 195 mg/dl
Ages 55 to 64: Up to 250 mg/dl
Lipoproteins
High density (HDL)
Men, ages 15 to 34: 30 to 65 mg/dl
Women: 35 to 80 mg/dl
Low density (LDL)
White men, ages 35 to 39: Up to 190 mg/dl
Phospholipids: 150 to 380 mg/dl
Fatty acids: 9 to 15 mmol/L

Magnesium: 1.2 to 1.9 mEq/L
Mucoprotein: 80 to 200 mg/dl
Osmolality: 280 to 300 mOsm/kg H_2O
Phenylalanine: >3 mg/dl
Phosphorus: 2.5 to 4.5 mg/dl

Protein
Serum
Total: 6 to 8 g/dl
Albumin: 3.5 to 5 g/dl with A/G ratio >1
Globulin: 2.3 to 3.5 g/dl
Electrophoresis
Albumin: 58% to 74%; 4 to 5.5 g/dl
Alpha-1: 2% to 3.5%; 0.15 to 0.25 g/dl
Alpha-2: 5.4% to 10.6%; 0.43 to 0.75 g/dl
Beta: 7% to 14%; 0.5 to 1 g/dl
Gamma: 8% to 18%; 0.6 to 1.3 g/dl

Prostate specific antigen (PSA): <4 ng/ml

Uric acid
Serum
Male: 3.4 to 7 mg/dl or slightly higher
Female: 2.4 to 6 mg/dl or slightly higher

Vitamins

Vitamin A
Serum
15 to 60 μg/dl
Vitamin A tolerance: Fasting 3 hours or 6 hours after 5000 μg: 15 to 60 μg/dl
Vitamin A/kg/24 hours: 200 to 600 μg/dl; fasting values are higher

Vitamin B_{12}
Serum
160 to 950 pg/ml
Unsaturated vitamin B_{12} binding capacity: 1000 to 2000 pg/ml

Vitamin C
Serum or plasma: 0.2 to 2 mg/dl

Zinc
Whole blood, serum, or plasma: 0.66 to 1.1 μg/ml

Blood Enzymes

Cardiac enzymes
Creatine phosphokinase (CPK)
Males: 55-170 U/L
Females: 30-135 U/L
CPK-MB (isoenzyme): 0 to 7 U/L
AST: 5 to 40 IU/L
Lactate dehydrogenase (LDH)
Isoenzymes (method dependent)
LDH_1: 22% to 36%
LDH_2: 35% to 46%
LDH_3: 13% to 26%
LDH_4: 3% to 10%
LDH_5: 2% to 9%
LDH (specific for heart, kidney, blood cells): 0.17 to 0.27 of total LDH
Glucose-6-phosphate dehydrogenase (G6PD): 140 to 280 U/billion cells
γ-glutamyltransferase serum: 5 to 40 IU/L
ALT: 5-35 U/L
Troponin-cardiac specific: 0-2 ng/ml

BLOOD GAS VALUES

Whole Blood

pH
Arterial range: 7.35 to 7.45 (average 7.4)
Venous range: 7.32 to 7.35
Mixed venous: 7.36

PCO_2
Arterial range: 35 to 42 mm Hg (average 40 mm Hg)
Venous range: 35 to 50 mm Hg
Mixed venous: 46 mm Hg

PO_2
Arterial range: 80 to 95 mm Hg (average 95 mm Hg)
Mixed venous: 40 mm Hg

HCO_3^-
Arterial range: 24 to 28 mEq/L
Venous range: 24 to 28 mEq/L
Mixed venous: 24-28 mEq/L

SO_2
Arterial range (average 97%): 95% to 99%
Venous range (average 75%): 70% to 75%
Pulmonary artery: 75%
Mixed venous: 75%
O_2 content
Arterial range: 17 to 21 ml/dl or 17 to 21 vol%
Venous range: 10 to 16 ml/dl or 10 to 16 vol%
Mixed venous: 15 ml/dl
CO_2 content
Arterial range: 22 to 29 mEq/L
Venous range: 23 to 30 mEq/L
Mixed venous: 26 mEq/L

Plasma

CO_2 content
Arterial range: 21 to 30 mEq/L
Venous range: 24 to 34 mEq/L

Hemoglobin

CO saturation (carboxyhemoglobin)
Nonsmoker: 0% to 2%
Smoker: 3% to 5%
Heavy smoker: 9% to 10%

Drug Levels

Digoxin
Therapeutic: 1 to 2 ng/ml
Toxic: 3 ng/ml
Underdigitalization: <0.5 ng/ml
Digitoxin
Therapeutic: 10 to 30 ng/ml
Toxic: >35 ng/ml

ENDOCRINE AND HORMONAL STUDIES

Blood or Serum

Adrenocorticotropic hormone (ACTH)
8 AM: <140 pg/ml
4 PM: 10 to 50 pg/ml
Aldosterone
Normal salt diet
Supine: 5.4 to 9.8 ng/dl
Upright: 8.9 to 58 ng/dl
Low salt diet: 2 to 4 times above values
Androstenedione: <250 ng/dl
Calcitonin: <150 pg/ml; usual basal fasting level is about 20 to 100 pg/ml, depending on assay
Catecholamines
Supine
Epinephrine: 0.5 to 20 μg/24 hours
Norepinephrine: 15 to 80 μg/24 hours
Dopamine: 65 to 400 μg/24 hours
Metanephrine: 24 to 96 μg/24 hours
Normetanephrine: 75 to 375 μg/24 hours
VMA: 1.8 to 7 mg/24 hours
Standing
Epinephrine: 20 to 109 pg/ml
Norepinephrine: 169 to 515 pg/ml
C-peptide
Fasting: 0.9 to 4.2 ng/ml
Nonfasting: 1.5 to 9.0 ng/ml
Dehydroepiandrosterone (11-deoxycortisol)(DHEA)
Adult male: 270 to 1400 mg/dl
Adult female: 200 to 800 ng/dl
DHEA sulfate (serum)
Adult male: 130 to 550 μg/dl
Premenopausal female: 60 to 340 μg/dl
Postmenopausal female: <130 μg/dl
17-Hydroxysteroids
Male: 3 to 10 mg/24 hours
Female: 2.5 to 10 mg/24 hours
Free thyroxine
Approximately 0.7 to 1.8 ng/dl (varies among laboratories)
Gastrin
Fasting: 50 to 170 pg/ml
Postprandial: 95 to 140 pg/ml; usually <250 pg/ml
Glucagon: 20 to 100 pg/ml
Growth hormone: <10 ng/ml
Human chorionic gonadotropin: <3 mIU/ml (nonpregnant)
Insulin
Fasting level: up to 25 μU/ml with slight differences in upper limit of normal among laboratories
Karyotyping: Sex chromosomes: XX or XY
Luteinizing hormone
Male: 7 to 24 mIU/ml; normal ranges vary among laboratories
Female:
Follicular phase: 6 to 27 mIU/ml
Midcycle: 35 to 154 mIU/ml
Luteal: 5 to 17 mIU/ml
Older adult: postmenopausal women: 29 to 96 mIU/ml
Parathyroid hormone
Dependent on individual laboratory, calcium result; the calcium value is related to the parathyroid hormone value by some laboratories on a two-dimensional graph or nomogram to ascertain abnormality
Phenylalanine: <20 mg/dl
Progesterone
Male: 13 to 97 ng/dl
Older adult: 7 to 33 ng/dl
Female
Follicular: 95 ng/dl
Luteal: 1130 ng/dl
Progesterone receptor assay: <5 fmol/mg protein is negative
Prolactin: 2 to 37 ng/ml
Hydroxyprogesterone
Adult female
Early cycle: 100 ng/dl
Late cycle: 80 to 300 ng/dl
Renin
Age 20-39: 0.1-4.3 ng/ml/ hours
Upright: Age >40: 0.1-3.0 ng/ml/ hours
Somatomedin C: 0.4 to 2.0 U/ml
Somatostatin: 10 to 80 pg/ml
Testosterone
Male: 300 to 1100 ng/dl
Female: 20 to 100 ng/dl

Triiodothyronine
Approximately 80 to 200 to 230 ng/dl with some variation among laboratories; increase occurs in pregnancy
Thyroglobulin
About 1 to 20 ng/ml; mean values of 5.1 to 9.5 ng/ml
Thyroid-stimulating hormone (TSH)
Upper limit of normal varies among laboratories from about 5.4 μU/ml to approximately 10 μU/ml
Thyroxine
5.5 to 11.5 μg/dl
Pregnancy: Approximately 5.5 to 16 μg/dl
Thyroxine-binding globulin
Variability among laboratories exists; 10 to 28 μg/ml; increased in pregnancy
Transferrin
Approximately 200 to 360 mg/dl with some variation among laboratories
Alpha-fetoprotein
Up to approximately 40 ng/ml for serum (interlaboratory differences exists); maternal serum increases to maximum of 500 ng/ml at week 32, and ranges are stratified by weeks of gestation
Chorionic somatomammotropin
Varies with duration of gestation; may reach 10 μg/ml
Creatine: 0.2 to 0.8 mg/dl; increased in pregnancy
Creatinine
Adult female: 0.8 to 1.8 g/24 hours; creatinine excretion decreases with advanced age as muscle mass diminishes
Creatinine clearance
Male: 85 to 125 ml/min/1.73 m^2
Female: 75 to 115 ml/min/1.73 m^2
Dihydrotestosterone: None detectable
Estradiol
Menstruating female
Early cycle: 20 to 170 pg/ml
Midcycle: 70 to 500 pg/ml
Late cycle: 45 to 340 pg/ml
Patient taking oral contraceptives: 12 to 50 pg/ml
Postmenopausal female: 1 to 5 ng/dl
Adult male: 13 to 42 pg/ml
Estriol
Nonpregnant female less than 0.5 ng/ml
Pregnant female: Estriol increases until term and then decreases
30 to 32 weeks: 2 to 12 ng/ml
33 to 35 weeks: 3 to 19 ng/ml
36 to 38 weeks: 5 to 27 ng/ml
39 to 40 weeks: 10 to 30 ng/ml
Estrogens, total
Menstruating female: 15 to 80 μg/24 hours
Postmenopausal female: less than 20 μg/24 hours
Male: 6 to 40 ng/ml
Estrone
Menstruating female
Early in cycle: 50 to 300 pg/ml
Midcycle: 100 to 600 pg/ml
Late cycle: 80 to 450 pg/ml
Menopausal female: 0 to 30 pg/ml
Calcium
Varies with diet; based on average calcium intake of 600 to 800 mg/24 hours, excretion may be 100 to 250 mg/24 hours
On a diet of 400 to 800 mg of calcium daily, others set the upper limit at 200 mg calcium in a 24-hour urine collection
Free cortisol
Male: 11 to 84 μg/24 hours
Female: 10 to 34 μg/24 hours
FSH
Male: 3 to 11 IU/24 hours
Female: 5 to 50 IU/24 hours
Older adult: postmenopausal women: 2 to 3 times adult values
Hydroxyprolines
See individual laboratory reference ranges; excretion on meat-free, gelatin-free diet is approximately 10 to 50 mg/24 hours
Follicle-stimulating hormone
Follicular phase: 5 to 20 IU/24 hours
Luteal phase: 5 to 15 IU/24 hours
Midcycle: 15 to 60 IU/24 hours
Menopause: 50 to 100 IU/24 hours
Luteinizing hormone
Follicular phase: 2 to 25 IU/24 hours
Ovulatory phase: 30 to 95 IU/24 hours
Luteal phase: 2 to 20 IU/24 hours
Postmenopausal: 40 to 110 IU/24 hours
Pregnanediol
Proliferative phase: 0.5 to 1.5 mg/24 hours
Luteal phase: 2 to 7 mg/24 hours
Menopause: 0.2 to 1 mg/24 hours
10 to 12 weeks pregnant: 5 to 15 mg/24 hours
12 to 18 weeks pregnant: 5 to 15 mg/24 hours
18 to 24 weeks pregnant: 15 to 33 mg/24 hours
24 to 28 weeks pregnant: 20 to 42 mg/24 hours
28 to 32 weeks pregnant: 27 to 47 mg/24 hours

IMMUNOLOGIC STUDIES

Serum immunoglobulin levels
IgG: 600 to 1600 mg/dl
IgM: 50 to 250 mg/dl
IgA: 80 to 350 mg/dl
IgE: <125 ng/dl
IgD: 0 to 30 mg/dl
Macroglobulins, total
Whole blood, serum, or plasma: 53 to 375 mg/dl
Autoantibody titers
Anti-DNA
Low levels of antibody or none; units and reference range depend on laboratory and method
Antinuclear antibody (ANA): Negative at 1:20 dilution
Rheumatoid factor (RF): Negative
Sjögren's antibody: Negative
Nonspecific indicators of inflammation
C-reactive protein (CRP): <6 μg/ml
C3 complement (serum): 800 to 1800 μg/ml
Circulating immune complexes
Clq binding assay
<25 μg/ml aggregated human γ-globulin (AHGG) equivalents
Raji cell assay; 0 to 12 μg/ml AHGG equivalents

γ-Globulin
Serum: 0.5 to 1.6 g/dl
Globulins (total)
Serum: 2.3 to 3.5 g/dl

URINE STUDIES

Urinalysis
Albumin: <20 mg/dl
Bilirubin: Negative
Color: Clear, golden yellow
Glucose: Negative
Hemoglobin: Negative
Ketones: Negative
Microscopic urinalysis
Bacteria: Negative
Casts: 0 to 4 hyaline casts per low-power field
Crystals: Interpreted by physician
Mucous threads: Negative
Red blood cells: 0 to 5 per high-power field
Squamous epithelial cells: Seen on voided specimen in females; negative on voided specimen in males; negative for catheterized specimens
White blood cells: 0 to 5 per high-power field
Calcium
24 hours: 100 to 250 mg/day (diet dependent; based on average calcium intake of 600 to 800 mg/24 hours)
Chloride: 110 to 250 mEq/24 hours
Creatinine: Men: 1 to 2 g/24 hours: women: 0.8 to 1.8 g/24 hours
Glucose: Up to 100 mg/24 hours
Osmolality: 250 to 900 mOsm/kg
Protein: 30 to 150 mg/24 hours (method dependent)
pH: 4.5 to 8.0
Phosphorus: 0.9 to 1.3 g/day (diet dependent)
Potassium: 26 to 123 mEq/24 hours (markedly intake dependent)
Sodium: 27 to 287 mEq/24 hours (diet dependent; output is lower at night)
Specific gravity: 1.003 to 1.029 (range in SI units)
Urea nitrogen: 6 to 17 g/24 hours
Cystine: Random sample negative
Fructose: 30 to 65 mg/24 hours
Galactose: 10 mg/dl
Uric acid: 250 to 750 mg/24 hours
Urea nitrogen: 6 to 17/24 hours
Mucin: 100 to 150 mg/24 hours

REFERENCES

1. Anderson KN, Anderson LE, Glanz WD, editors: *Mosby's medical, nursing, and allied health dictionary,* ed 5, St. Louis, 1999, Mosby.
2. Ballinger PW, Frank ED: *Merrill's atlas of radiographic positions and radiologic procedures,* ed 9, St. Louis, 2000, Mosby.
3. Bates B: *A guide to physical examination and history taking,* ed 8, Philadelphia, 2000, JB Lippincott, Williams & Wilkins.
3.a. Borer W, Rakel RE, editors: *Conn's current therapy 2000,* Philadelphia, WB Saunders.
4. Davis JE, Mason CB: *Neurologic critical care,* New York, 1979, Van Nostrand Reinhold.
5. Emmett JL. Witten DM: *Clinical urography.* Philadelphia, 1990, WB Saunders.
6. Fishman AP, editor: *Pulmonary diseases and disorders,* ed 3, New York, 1998, McGraw-Hill.
7. George RB et al, editors: *Chest medicine: essentials of pulmonary and critical care medicine,* ed 2, Baltimore, 1990, Williams & Wilkins.
7.a. Gitlin N, Jensen DM, editors: *Clinics in liver disease,* vol 3, Philadelphia, 1999, WB Saunders.
8. Harrison JH et al: *Campbell's urology,* ed 7, Philadelphia, 1997, WB Saunders.
9. Hickey J: *The clinical practice of neurological and neurosurgical nursing,* ed 4, Philadelphia, 1996, JB Lippincott.
10. Kelalis PP, King LR, Belman AB: *Clinical pediatric urology,* ed 3, Philadelphia, 1992, WB Saunders.
11. Kendall AR, Karafin R: *Urology: Goldsmith's practice of surgery,* Philadelphia, 1983, Harper & Row.
12. Kim MJ, McFarland GK, McLane AM: *Pocket guide to nursing diagnoses,* ed 7, St. Louis, 1997, Mosby.
13. Kintzel K, editor: *Advanced concepts in clinical nursing,* ed 4, Philadelphia, 1992, JB Lippincott.
14. Lerner J, Khan Z: *Mosby's manual of urologic nursing,* St. Louis, 1996, Mosby.
15. Merritt HH: *A textbook of neurology,* ed 9, Philadelphia, 1995, Lea & Febiger.
16. Miller LG, Kazemi H: *Manual of clinical pulmonary medicine,* New York, 1997, McGraw-Hill.
17. Morris JF, Roski WA, Johnson LC: Spirometric standards for healthy nonsmoking adults, *Am Rev Respir Dis* 103:57, 1971.
18. Newell FM: *Ophthalmology: principles and concepts,* ed 7, St. Louis, 1992, Mosby.
19. Pagana KD, Pagana TJ: *Diagnostic testing and nursing implications: a case study approach,* ed 4, St. Louis, 1994, Mosby.
20. Pagana KD, Pagana TJ: *Mosby's diagnostic and laboratory test reference,* ed 4, St. Louis, 1999, Mosby.
20.a. Pizzarello DJ, Witcofski RL, editors: *Medical radiation biology,* ed 2, Philadelphia, 1982, Lea & Febiger.
21. Robinson S, Russo P, editors: *Providing respiratory care: nursing photobook,* Springhouse, Pa, 1979, Intermed Communications.
22. Sanderson RG, Kurth CC: *The cardiac patient,* ed 2, Philadelphia, 1983, WB Saunders.
23. Seidel HM et al: *Mosby's guide to physical examination,* ed 3, St. Louis, 1995, Mosby.
24. Stell PM: *Stell and Maran's head and neck surgery,* ed 3, Boston, 1993, Oxford.
25. Tucker SM et al: *Patient care standards: collaborative practice planning guides,* ed 6, St. Louis, 1995, Mosby.
26. Williams ID, Johnston JH: *Paediatric urology,* ed 2, London, 1982, Butterworth.
27. Wilson JD et al, editors: *Harrison's principles of internal medicine,* ed 14, New York, 1998, McGraw-Hill.
28. Youmans JR, editor: *Neurological surgery,* ed 3, Philadelphia, 1990, WB Saunders.

PART V

NURSING DIAGNOSES, OUTCOMES, AND INTERVENTIONS

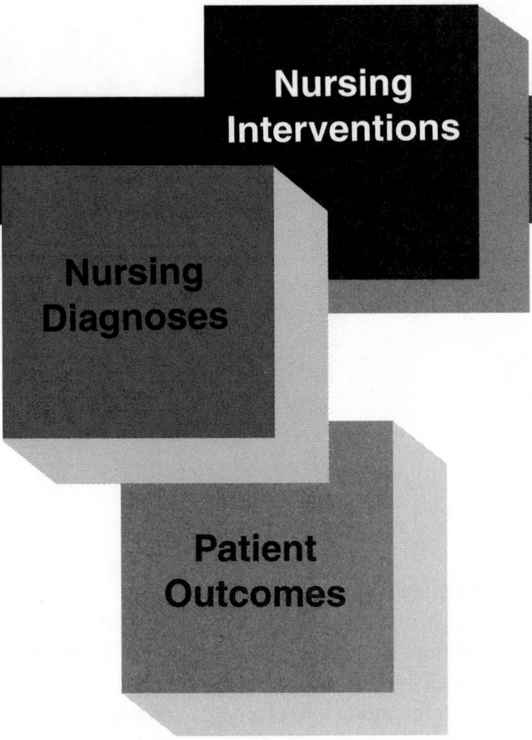

23

NANDA Nursing Diagnoses, Outcomes, and Nursing Interventions

Priscilla LeMone
Roxanne W. McDaniel
Peggy L. Payne

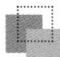

Health Perception–Health Management

Disturbed Energy Field

Disturbed energy field occurs when there is a disruption of the flow of energy surrounding a person's being that results in a disharmony of the body, mind, or spirit.[5,6]

Related Factors[5]

Physiologic changes

Illness
Injury
Pain
Pregnancy
Trauma

Situational/maturational changes

Anxiety
Developmental difficulties
Fear
Grieving
Perioperative experiences
Perinatal experiences

Defining Characteristics[5]

Disruption of the field (vacant/hold/spike/bulge)
Movement (wave/spike/tingling/dense/flowing)
Sounds (tones or words)
Temperature changes (warmth or coolness)
Visual changes (image or color)

Expected Patient Outcomes and Nursing Interventions With Rationale[1-4]

Experience a multidimensional effect, as evidenced by:

Describes a sense of physiologic, emotional, and spiritual well-being
Experiences repatterning of imbalanced areas
Verbalizes relaxation, comfort, and a sense of well-being

- Prepare the patient and environment for and provide therapeutic touch.
- Provide privacy
- Give preparatory explanation of therapeutic touch to the patient, emphasizing the patient's ability to discontinue at any time.
- Await the verbalization of understanding and acceptance by the patient before commencing therapeutic touch.
- Assist the patient to a position of comfort.
- Focus initially on self-centering and own internal energy.
- Scan the patient's body from head to feet with palms of hands about 3 inches away from the body.
- Sense variations indicative of energy imbalance including temperature variations, heaviness, lightness, tingling, absence of feeling.
- Perform vigorous hand movements from head to toe over the patient.
- Move hands in a sweeping motion from head to feet.
- Shake hands to remove congestion from field.
- Ensure that energy is flowing over legs and feet; if not, continue to move hands to facilitate energy flow.
- Place hands at rest over the patient's solar plexus (just above the waist) upon completion of therapeutic touch while focusing on the flow of healing energy to the patient.
- Provide a period of rest for the patient.

During the process of applying therapeutic touch the nurse focuses on creating a state of balance and harmony while sensing or passively visualizing the free flow of energy to the patient with the intent of facilitating healing. This process takes a great deal of energy and concentration by the nurse, who must have a great degree of self-awareness, sensitivity, and skill. The healing process is one of balancing or centering and "unruffling" or clearing the energy field and directing the transfer of energy to the patient. An important part of the specialized training is knowing when to discontinue the energy flow to achieve the best outcome for the patient. The effects of therapeutic touch on the patient are a sense of relaxation and balance.

Effective Therapeutic Regimen Management

Effective therapeutic regimen management is a pattern of regulating and integrating into daily living a program for treatment of illness and its sequelae that is satisfactory for meeting specific life goals.[4]

Related Factors[1,3]

Capacity and motivation to provide self-care
Perceived health status
Readily available resources
Supportive relationships with health-care providers, family, and/or friends

Defining Characteristics[4]

Appropriate choices in daily activities to meet treatment goals
Illness symptoms within expected range
Verbalized desire to manage the treatment of illness
Verbalized desire to reduce risk factors for progression of illness and sequelae

Expected Patient Outcomes and Nursing Interventions With Rationale[1-3,5-6]

Interact with health-care personnel to develop a realistic plan of care, as evidenced by:

Expresses desire to establish self-management behaviors
Expresses willingness to learn regimen-specific tasks

- Assist patient with identification of benefits of following prescribed therapeutic regimen.
- Determine the existence of potential barriers to integration of regimen into daily living.
- Help patient identify values and preferences in the process of developing goals and strategies.

Effective management of a complex therapeutic regimen may require a daily struggle with economic, social, and emotional components. Diet, exercise, taking medications, and monitoring body sensations and symptoms require attention and vigilance.

Implement therapeutic regimen in daily living program, as evidenced by:

Demonstrates ability to perform regimen-specific tasks
Monitors symptoms related to illness and/or treatment
Reallocates personal and economic resources to manage demands of therapeutic regimen

- Evaluate self-management skills and provide feedback.
- Teach self-monitoring of symptoms and response to treatment (e.g., teach use of daily log).
- Provide written information about availability and access to community resources.

Decision making within a self-care frame of reference increases self-confidence in one's ability to engage in self-management tasks. Recording decisions and the outcomes of decisions provides an ongoing record of success and feedback with respect to adequacy of resources, identified self-care systems, and self-care actions.

INEFFECTIVE THERAPEUTIC REGIMEN MANAGEMENT

Ineffective therapeutic regimen management is a pattern of regulating and integrating into daily living a program for treatment of illness and the sequelae of illness that is unsatisfactory for meeting specific health goals.[9]

Related Factors[9]

Complexity of therapeutic regimen and/or health-care system
Cultural or family health values and beliefs
Decisional conflicts
Excessive demands on individual or family
Knowledge deficit
Lack of access to health promotion resources
Lack of desire for self-care
Lack of economic resources
Lack of social support
Mistrust of regimen or health-care providers
Perceived barriers to meeting health goals
Perceived benefits to meeting health goals
Perceived lack of competency in carrying out therapeutic regimen
Perceived seriousness of illness
Perceived susceptibility
Powerlessness

Defining Characteristics[9]

Acceleration of illness symptoms
Choices in daily living that do not support the treatment goals
Verbalized desire to manage the treatment and prevent sequelae
Verbalized difficulty with integrating therapeutic regimen into daily living
Verbalized inability or lack of desire to reduce risk factors

Expected Patient Outcomes and Nursing Interventions With Rationale[1-8,10-12]

Make appropriate daily choices for effectively meeting goals of the treatment program, as evidenced by:

Manages illness symptoms
Takes actions to integrate treatment regimen into daily routine
Verbalizes ways that can integrate, without difficulty, treatment regimen into daily routine and lifestyle

- Assess patient's perception of and knowledge about the illness, the severity of the illness, potential complications, the long-term impact on lifestyle, and the treatment regimen resources needed to manage illness; *illness-related factors can influence the outcomes of an illness crisis; a baseline is needed for intervention.*
- Teach patient about nature of illness and the related treatment regimen, including expected outcomes and any potential complications.
- Teach patient about and/or refer patient to appropriate community resources in regard to equipment needs, transportation needs, services, housing needs and adaptations, and financial support available, *to maximally match patient's needs with what is available in the community to meet the health-care needs.*
- Encourage patient to identify strengths that will promote adherence to treatment regimen.
- Encourage patient to identify barriers that affect adherence to treatment regimen and then approach barriers specifically.
- Assess patient's emotional response to illness and treatment regimen: level of anxiety, degree of stress, level of depression, level of anger, and phase of grieving; *degree of emotional response can have an effect on learning and adaptive functioning and can influence the energy level needed to deal with the illness and engage in the therapeutic treatment regimen.*
- Assist patient to work through emotional responses *to reduce emotional response levels so patient can use energies to cope with illness and with the demands of the therapeutic treatment regimen.*

- Assess how patient views the illness, the benefits that can be achieved from the treatment regimen, and the barriers to engaging in the treatment regimen.
- Discuss with patient outcomes and consequences of nonadherence to treatment regimen.
- In collaboration with the interdisciplinary team and the patient, plan a comprehensive but realistic treatment regimen that takes into account the patient's individual situation.
- Encourage patient to draw from resources available: family, friends, neighbors, health-care professionals, support groups, and community financial and health-care resources. *Social and environmental factors can facilitate the management of illness-related symptoms and the participation in treatment regimen.*
- Assess patient's (1) previous life experiences, including any experience with illness and the health-care system; and (2) coping strategies used by the patient and his or her family and significant other in dealing with stressful situations; *prevous coping strategies can be useful in dealing with current illness and treatment regimen demands.*
- Have patient list coping strategies used previously and current strengths useful in dealing with stressful situations.
- Encourage patient to use coping strategies and strengths in dealing with current illness demands.
- Teach patient new coping strategies, such as stress management techniques.
- Assess patient's values and beliefs especially as related to current illness and its meaning for patient.
- Assess patient's spiritual resources. *Spiritual resources can be useful in helping patient understand meaning of illness situation for self and in developing strengths in coping with the illness and its impact on his or her lifestyle.*
- Use behavioral contracting interventions and contracts for patients *to achieve selected outcomes.*

INEFFECTIVE FAMILY THERAPEUTIC REGIMEN MANAGEMENT

Ineffective family therapeutic regimen management is a pattern of regulating and integrating into family processes a program for treatment of illness and the sequelae of illness that is unsatisfactory for meeting specific health goals.[5]

Related Factors[5]

Complexity of health-care system
Complexity of therapeutic regimen
Decisional conflicts
Economic difficulties
Excessive demands made on individual or family
Family conflict

Defining Characteristics[5]

Acceleration of illness symptoms
Inappropriate family activities to meet treatment goals
Lack of attention to illness and its sequelae
Verbalized desire to mange the illness treatment
Verbalized difficulty with integrating treatment into family activities
Verbalized lack of action to reduce risk factors for illness progression

Expected Patient Outcomes and Nursing Interventions With Rationale[1-4,6,7]

Effectively manage therapeutic regimen, as evidenced by:

Participates in the development of a plan to engage in required activities
Verbalizes willingness to learn regimen-specific tasks and provide care
Provides appropriate personal and health care for family member

- Provide verbal and written regimen-specific instructions to family members. *Having the necessary knowledge, skill, and resources to provide required care is essential to competent family care giving.*
- Teach family members to keep a written record of patient's responses to regimen.
- Facilitate family understanding of the illness. *Knowing a family, understanding the meaning of the therapeutic regimen to a patient and family members, and using their values and preferences in developing and selecting individualized care strategies provide a foundation for family success in meeting the day-to-day challenges of integrating a therapeutic regimen into daily living.*
- Identify and respect family members' coping mechanisms.[6]
- Refer family members to support groups, as appropriate.[6]
- Use telephone contact to provide support and assistance to homebound family caregivers.[1]

Patient takes part in daily activities and life experiences, as evidenced by:

Family provides opportunities for patient to take part in usual life experiences
Patient participates in family, school, and community activities appropriate for developmental level and functional abilities
Family demonstrates same expectations for ill family member as for well members

- Promote normalization by assisting family members in providing normal life experiences. *Normalization is a common strategy used by families to facilitate an ill member's adaptation to a chronic illness.*
- Assist family in serving as an advocate for the ill family member in the school and health-care systems.

INEFFECTIVE COMMUNITY THERAPEUTIC REGIMEN MANAGEMENT

Ineffective community therapeutic regimen management is a pattern of regulating and integrating into community processes programs for treatment of illness and the sequelae of illness that are unsatisfactory for meeting health-related goals.[5]

Related Factors

Designation as health provider shortage area
Economic status of the community
Geographic location of the community (e.g., rural or urban)

Defining Characteristics[1,5]

Deficits in advocates for aggregates
Deficits in community activities for secondary and tertiary prevention
Deficits in people and programs accountable for illness care of aggregates
Illness symptoms above the norm expected for the number and type of population
Health-care resources insufficient for the incidence or prevalence of illness(es)
Unavailable health-care resources for illness care
Unexpected acceleration of illness(es)

Expected Community Outcomes and Nursing Interventions With Rationale[1-4]

Effectively manage the therapeutic regimen, as evidenced by:
Decrease in incidence of infectious illnesses in the community
Decrease in prevalence of chronic illnesses in the community
Culturally competent care provided for targeted aggregate populations
Health programs and resources available to aggregates at risk
Community health-care resources and facilities accessible, available, and affordable

- Identify preventive activities, based on knowledge of the natural history of specific illnesses, *which can be used to control the further spread of the disease.*
- Analyze host-age-environment factors, including populations at risk; available primary, secondary, and tertiary preventive measures; consideration of community resources, cost, facilities, and personnel; and significance in relation to other community needs.
- Implement activities to control the illness, including breaking the chain of transmission, encouraging immunization, and carrying out case finding.
- Provide education for individuals and aggregates about infection control.
- Evaluate effectiveness of the epidemiologic control plan *to ensure continual improvement in the process and to serve as a basis for future control measures.*
- Provide activities for primary prevention of chronic illnesses. *Interventions and teaching that help control communicable disease, decrease accidents and increase safety, control stress, and emphasize adequate perinatal care all help prevent certain chronic illnesses.*
- Implement screening programs for such illnesses as diabetes mellitus, hypertension, cancer, and glaucoma *to provide secondary prevention through early detection and treatment.*
- Provide interventions to maximize remaining functional capacity and to assist individuals with chronic illnesses to live within their limitations.
- Provide care that is sensitive to the values, beliefs, and health cultures of various cultures *to increase minority health and satisfaction with the health-care system.*
- Facilitate community empowerment by designing programs that are specific to group needs.
- Provide health education programs and materials that are culturally sensitive to minority aggregates.
- Serve as advocate for minority health.
- Focus health planning on problems within the community, such as violence, the needs of the elderly, domestic abuse, drug addiction, child abuse, people with AIDS, and the homeless.
- Involve the community as partners in population-based health-care planning *to bring about change by solving health-related problems before they develop.*
- Collaborate with community leaders and providers in mobilizing resources and in developing community initiatives that address problem areas.
- Advocate policy development to improve the health-care system of the community.
- Be actively involved in federal, state, and local health-care legislation *because the political arena is where health-care decisions are made.*

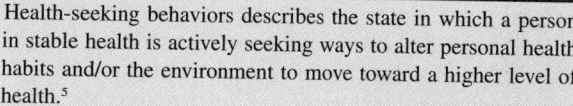

HEALTH-SEEKING BEHAVIORS (SPECIFY)

Health-seeking behaviors describes the state in which a person in stable health is actively seeking ways to alter personal health habits and/or the environment to move toward a higher level of health.[5]

Related Factors

Cultural beliefs and norms
Desire to maintain functional status
Fear of disease or illness
Fear of pain
Increased awareness of optimum health through public education
Personal and family values
Professional prescription, advice, or encouragement

Defining Characteristics[5]

Expressed concern about effect of current environmental conditions on health status
Expressed desire to have increased control over health practices
Expressed desire to seek a higher level of wellness
Verbalized lack of knowledge of community wellness resources
Verbalized lack of knowledge of healthy behaviors

Expected Patient Outcomes and Nursing Interventions With Rationale[1-3,4,6]

Demonstrate health-seeking behaviors, as evidenced by:
Verbalizes desire for and assistance with change in a specific health-related behavior
Describes current health, health beliefs and values; health behaviors; and goals for change
Requests information about available community support and resources

- Assess current health status, using information from health history and health-behavior and health-risk assessment instruments, *to establish a baseline against which further assessments can be made.*

- Assess verbal and behavioral cues to health values *to identify lifestyle and cultural health-related practices that may either facilitate or serve as barriers to change.*[7-8]
- Mutually develop a plan for change that includes time-oriented goals and specific strategies for change *to provide flexibility in the health plan and to develop strategies for change that are supportive of optimal well-being.*
- Provide information about available community support and resources *to facilitate use of available resources in meeting goals for change.*

Demonstrate commitment to health behavior change, as evidenced by:
Focuses on change in one specific health behavior
Meets short-term goals as specified in the health plan

- Develop a written nurse-patient contract, including the health behavior change to be made, how the change will be accomplished, who will be a part of the change, the time frame for attaining the change, and the consequences of meeting or not meeting the goals. *Formalizing a personal commitment through a contract often facilitates motivation to change, provides direction for change, and allows active participation in change.*[6]
- Develop a time frame or implementation of the desired health behavior change *to allow progress toward healthier behaviors over time in reasonable steps.*

Maintain health behavior change, as evidenced by:
Evaluates and revises plan for change as needed
Verbalizes satisfaction with health behavior change
Verbalizes increased well-being

- Maintain regular contact with the patient *to monitor progress toward goals and provide positive reinforcement for meeting goals.*
- Assist the patient to evaluate progress by comparing records of previous behavior to present behavior *to serve as positive reinforcement for change and to identify barriers and facilitators of desired change.*
- Support self-efficacy and problem-solving skills *to assist in long-term maintenance of the desired change.*
- Review and make changes in the plan, if appropriate, at regular intervals. *The targeted health-related behavior may be fully integrated, changes in lifestyle or values may have occurred, or a new change may be desired.*[6]

INEFFECTIVE HEALTH MAINTENANCE

Ineffective health maintenance is the inability to identify, manage, and/or seek out help to maintain health.[6]

Related Factors[6,8]

Dysfunctional grieving
Ineffective family coping
Ineffective individual coping
Lack of ability to make deliberate and thoughtful judgments
Lack of access to health promotion resources
Lack of or significant alterations in ability to communicate (verbal, written, gestures)
Lack of material resources
Perceptual or cognitive impairments
Spiritual distress

Defining Characteristics[6]

Inability to take responsibility for meeting basic health practices
Impairment of personal support system
Lack of ability to adapt to changes in internal or external environment
Lack of equipment, financial, or other necessary resources
Lack of knowledge of basic health practices
Verbalized interest in improving health behaviors

Expected Patient Outcomes and Nursing Interventions With Rationale[1-5,7-10]

General Public

Receive consistent, accurate information, as evidenced by:
Meets public health goals

- Use mass media (TV, electronic media, newspapers), printed material, closed-circuit television, and interactive teaching methods *to reach diverse populations and accommodate different learning styles and educational levels.*
- Encourage primary health-care providers to provide verbal reinforcement to public in health-care visits *to maximize effectiveness of media presentations and increase motivation to act.*
- Engage target population and community leaders in needs assessment activities *to clarify community's perceptions of health and illness, identify unmet needs, and assist in tailoring of education, programs to local needs and resources.*
- Include indigenous care providers and local health experts in rural or cultural communities in the planning and implementation of programs *to enhance community acceptance and facilitate consistency of information and approach.*
- Provide health education/teaching in the primary language of target group *to increase understanding and utilization of information.*
- Provide health teaching in culturally acceptable format (e.g., use elders, older health-care providers for teaching health counseling in American Indian groups in which age confers respect, leadership roles) *to bridge cultural barriers.*
- Make health information/service available where large numbers of target population gather (e.g., AIDS information and condoms in colleges) *to maximize exposure and decrease access barriers.*
- Use social marketing techniques for promotion, e.g., payroll stuffers, invitations, or contests, *to motivate individuals to participate.*

High-Risk Individuals

Assume responsibility for primary health maintenance, as evidenced by:
Identifies personal health goals
Identifies factors contributing to altered health maintenance
Identifies males specific plan to alter targeted behavior
Identifies multiple personal reinforcers

Uses community resources

- Use health appraisal techniques that elicit patient's perceptions of health *to facilitate identification of personal health values and goals.*
- Use pertinent health risk appraisal/inventory to assist patient to identify personal health risks related to lifestyle, family history, ethnicity, gender, and age, *to increase awareness of personal vulnerability, which motivates health behavior change.*
- Assist patients to list factors they perceive are interfering with their ability to meet personal health goals *to identify the factors most significant to the patient.*
- Help patient identify personal strengths and resources *to establish foundation for planning and enhance perceptions of ability to make desired changes.*
- Engage patient in "brainstorming" of possible strategies to effect desired behavior change *to increase creativity and avoid tendency for repetition of unsuccessful strategies.*
- Negotiate setting of both short-term and long-term goals *to provide opportunity for observable successes and strengthen competence in self-regulation of behavior.*
- Have patient list perceived benefits and disadvantages for specific behavior(s) targeted *to clarify outcome expectations that influence motivation.*
- Break the complexities of the behavior(s) desired into smaller, more manageable parts *to enhance perceptions of efficacy and avoid overwhelming patient.*
- Ask patients to rank-order target behaviors according to their beliefs that they can carry them out and sequence behaviors, beginning with ones patient feels most confident with, *to increase probability that patient will incorporate changes.*
- Develop written contract with patient for behavior change using patient-identified rewards and consequences *to promote patient control, provide self-reinforcements, and increase commitment to plans.*
- Schedule health maintenance counseling with other primary care appointments when possible *to decrease inconvenience and financial barriers to patient.*
- Make audiovisual educational materials available where patient uses other primary care services *to convenience patient and increase perceived validity of information being offered.*
- Include lay or traditional healers in planning where appropriate *to ensure development of a culturally acceptable plan and provide another professional source of encouragement, reinforcement for plan.*
- Consider relaxation training for anxiety if present *to reduce unpleasant physiologic arousal that inhibit self-efficacy.*
- Use small group discussion and support groups *to provide support and verbal persuasion.*
- Encourage participation in reference groups where patient can align with perceived powerful individuals, institutions *to enhance own sense of control and provide vicarious success.*
- Follow up with telephone calls and letters *to provide verbal encouragement for plan and provide visual reminders that increase chances for behavior change.*

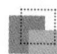

INEFFECTIVE PROTECTION

Ineffective protection is the state in which an individual experiences a decrease in the ability to guard self from internal or external threat, such as illness or injury.[7]

Related Factors

Abnormal blood profiles
Alcohol or drug abuse
Cancer
Chronic maladaptive stress
Coagulation disorders
Disorientation
Drugs
Extremes of age
Graft rejection
Graft versus host disease
Immobility
Inadequate sleep
Infection
Invasive devices
Radiation therapy
Surgery

Defining Characteristics[7]

Anorexia
Altered clotting
Chills
Cough
Dyspnea
Fatigue
Impaired healing
Insomnia
Itching
Pressure ulcers
Weakness

Expected Patient Outcomes and Nursing Interventions With Rationale[1-6,8,9,11]

Demonstrate measures to maintain protective defenses, as evidenced by:

Maintains cleanliness and safety
Symptoms of infection, bleeding, or discomfort are absent
Vital signs and laboratory data remain within normal limits

- Assess for risk factors and side effects of disease and therapy.
- Assess protective mechanisms (e.g., immune, hematopoietic, integumentary, sensorimotor).
- Teach strategies to promote personal and environmental cleanliness.
- Monitor vital signs and laboratory values. 10
- Institute safety precautions.

Injury must be avoided because of compromised protective mechanism.

Demonstrate measures to restore protective defenses, as evidenced by:

Eats balanced diet
Maintains normal rest/sleep/activity pattern

Discomfort is reduced

- Monitor weight.
- Monitor dietary and fluid intake.
- Teach measures to conserve energy (e.g., pacing of ADLs).
- Provide comfort for symptoms (e.g., chills, fever, myalgias).

Immune function is supported through sleep, nutrition, and energy conservation and avoidance of discomfort.

Demonstrate measures to promote protective defenses, as evidenced by:

Manages stress

Reports increased well-being

- Initiate stress management techniques (e.g., relaxation exercises, coping strategies, exercise). *Stress may depress immune function.*
- Provide nurse presence. *Presence nurtures and supports.*

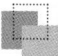

NONCOMPLIANCE (SPECIFY)

Noncompliance is the extent to which a person's behavior coincides or fails to coincide with a health-promoting or therapeutic plan agreed upon by the person (and/or family, and/or community) and a health-care professional. In the presence of an agreed-on, health-promoting or therapeutic plan, a person's behavior may be fully, partially, or nonadherent and may lead to clinically effective, partially effective, or ineffective outcomes.[9]

Related Factors[9]

Health-care plan

Cost
Complexity
Duration
Intensity

Individual factors

Cultural influences
Health beliefs
Individual's value system
Knowledge and skill relevant to the regimen behavior
Motivational forces
Personal and developmental abilities
Spiritual values

Health-care system

Access and convenience of care
Communication and teaching skills of the provider
Credibility of provider
Financial flexibility of plan
Individual health coverage
Patient-provider relationships
Provider continuity and regular follow-up
Provider reimbursement of teaching and follow-up
Satisfaction with care

Network

Involvement of members in health plan
Perceived beliefs of significant others
Social value regarding plan

Defining Characteristics[9]

Behavior indicative of failure to adhere (by direct observation or by statements of patient or significant other)

Evidence of development of complications

Evidence of exacerbation of symptoms

Failure to keep appointments

Failure to progress

Objective tests (e.g., physiologic measures, detection of physiologic markers)

Expected Patient Outcomes and Nursing Interventions With Rationale[1,3-5,7,8,11-13]

Engage in behaviors consistent with goals of therapeutic regimen, as evidenced by:

Sets goals and priorities consistent with therapeutic regimen

Accurately performs specific health-related behavior(s)

Identifies barriers to carrying out desired health behavior(s)

Verbalizes plan to deal with restraining factors/situations

Identifies sources of support, resources

- Assist the patient and family to identify barriers to compliance *so that barriers can be altered or regimen revised.*
- Engage patient in values clarification strategies *to identify motivation and to increase consistency between beliefs and actions.*
- Encourage the patient and family to discuss the solutions they believe will be most effective *to recognize family competence and avoid stereotypical interventions.*
- Encourage self-monitoring *to make specific behavioral patterns and the antecedent variables more observable.*[7]
- Assess patient's and family's beliefs about their ability to carry out the required behaviors *to assess self-efficacy and identify where competence may be augmented.*[7]
- Adjust prescribed regimen and interventions to patient's lifestyle, culture, spiritual beliefs, value system, and circumstances where possible *to decrease the lifestyle changes being requested of the patient and to demonstrate that patient's needs are recognized.*[12,13]
- Provide opportunities to patient and family to discuss their concerns about therapeutic regimen *to validate feelings and provide verbal encouragement.*
- Include patient-designated support persons in treatment planning *to improve communication and increase motivation for support and involvement in implementation of plan.*
- Sequence strategies from easiest to more complex, setting short- and long-term goals, *to avoid overwhelming patient and provide for successes to enhance self-efficacy.*
- Develop written contract with patient and support persons for specifics regarding therapeutic plan *to signify importance of plan and to provide a written reminder.*
- Assist patient to make a list of relevant, accessible resources in the community *to provide support for implementation of treatment.*
- Inform patient and family about relevant lay support groups *to provide opportunity for vicarious performance information and to access the expertise of others living with chronic illness.*
- Devise a graphic representation of results, such as a chart, *to provide visual reinforcement of success and enhance positive outcome expectations.*

- Ensure that patient education is provided in the patient's primary language *because the primary language is most influential in processing information.*

Report that the health-care system recognizes and provides for individual needs and abilities, as evidenced by:

Actively participates in negotiation of goals, priorities, regimen
Freely expresses feelings, beliefs, requests
Keeps appointments
Uses available resources
Reports noncompliance, with expectation of further negotiation or assistance
Verbalizes satisfaction with health-care providers

- Ascertain which family members or significant others patient wants to include in treatment decision making *to empower patient and recognize cultural norms.*
- Ask the patient what assistance he or she requires to enhance compliance *to encourage involvement in treatment decision making and to promote congruence of perceptions, goals in the patient-provider relationship.*
- Offer patient and support persons training in assertive techniques that can be used in interactions with health-care providers *to increase input to treatment decisions and make needs known to providers.*
- Collaborate with other health-care providers involved with patient to coordinate and simplify medication regimens and treatment plans *to ensure consistency in approach, avoid contradictory advice, and decrease complexity.*
- Schedule follow-up or home health-care opportunities with same provider *to ensure continuity in care and increase opportunity for tailoring of interactions.*[6]
- Assess cultural preferences and beliefs *to ensure negotiation of therapeutic regimen that accommodates patient's cultural norms.*[10]
- Assess patient's beliefs in the efficacy of the therapeutic plan, that desired outcomes are contingent upon adherence, *to determine outcome expectations, correct misinformation, and align nurse-patient perceptions.*[2,13]

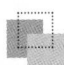

RISK FOR FALLS

Risk for falls is the state of increased susceptibility to falling that may cause physical harm.[6]

Risk Factors—Adults[1,3,6,9]

Age 65 or over
Female sex (if elderly)
Living alone
Lower limb prosthesis
Previous history of falls
Use of assistive devices (e.g., walker, cane) or wheelchair

Physiologic

Acute illness
Bowel or bladder urgency or incontinence
Chronic illnesses (e.g., anemia, arthritis, vascular disease, cancer)
Decreased strength or function in one or both lower extremities
Deficits in vision, hearing, and/or proprioception
Fatigue
Impaired balance, gait, physical mobility
Orthostatic hypotension
Postoperative status
Postprandial blood glucose changes
Sleep disturbances

Cognitive

Cognitive impairment
Wandering

Environmental

Cluttered environment
Slippery showers and tubs
Unfamiliar, dimly lit room
Use of throw or scatter rugs
Weather conditions (e.g., snow, ice, and wet floors)

Medications

ACE inhibitors
Alcohol
Antianxiety agents
Antihypertensives
Diuretics
Hypnotics
Narcotics
Sedatives
Tricyclic antidepressants

Risk Factors—Children[6]

Age less than 2 years, or in males less than 1 year
Bed location near window without window guards
Lack of automobile restraints
Lack of gate on stairs
Lack of parental supervision
Infant unattended on bed, sofa, changing table

Expected Patient Outcomes and Nursing Interventions With Rationale[2,4,5,7,8,10]

Diminished or absent risk for falls in the health-care facility and at home, as evidenced by:

Verbalizes understanding of risk for falls
Takes necessary precautions to prevent falls
Uses assistive devices correctly
Does not fall or decreases number of falls

- Teach client (if able to understand instruction) and family members to use the call light, ask for assistance with getting out of bed, toileting, keep floors clear of clutter, and keep the bed at a low position. *A major cause of falls is trying to get out of bed unassisted, especially when attempting to meet elimination needs.*
- Assess all patients for risk for falls, especially those who are older, cognitively impaired, have multiple comorbidities, use assistive devices, or have a history of falls. *Although all patients are at risk for falls, these factors increase risk.*
- Identify patients at risk in the acute care, residential, or long-term care facility by using a risk assessment to identify indicators for possible falls and institute a fall prevention program by a method such as placing an orange dot on the patient's wristband, on the call light terminal in the nurses' station, and/or on the spine of the chart. Post a sign in the patient's room to alert all care

providers. Use a bed sensor if the patient is assessed at greatest risk. *The number of falls increases with the number of risk factors. The "spot the dot" program has proven to be effective in alerting all health-care providers to patients who are at risk for falls.*

- Provide assistance to the patient who uses a wheelchair, walker, or cane for mobility. *The use of assistive devices for mobility increases the risk for falls.*
- Provide an initial orientation to the health-care facility for all patients, and provide ongoing orientation to patients who have cognitive deficits or alterations in orientation *to avoid disorientation when in a new environment and increase awareness of surroundings.*
- Provide interventions in the health-care facility *to decrease the risk for falls:*

  Lock the wheels of beds, stretchers, and wheelchairs when moving or transferring patients.
  Place call bell, TV control, light cord, telephone, and personal belongings within easy reach of patients who must remain in bed or are immobile.
  Maintain bed in low position.
  Avoid use of restraints.
  Use a night-light.
  Evaluate effects and interactions of medications, especially diuretics, laxatives, and antihypertensives.
  Encourage patients to use glasses and hearing aids; ensure glasses are clean and hearing aids are functioning.
  Adjust (if possible) height of toilet seat.
  Assist patients with an unsteady gait with transferring and ambulation.
  Assist with toileting at regular, scheduled intervals.
  Keep rooms free of clutter and floors dry and glare-free.
- Teach patient and caregivers how to reduce risk from falls at home:

  If patient lives alone, refer for a Lifeline or other telephone alert system.
  Do not wax floors or use scatter rugs.
  Do not place objects on stairs.
  Use a night-light, and turn on lights when moving through rooms.
  Wear shoes or slippers with nonskid soles.
  Place nonskid decals or tape on the bottom of tubs and showers.
  Install hand rails on stairs and hand grips in bathrooms.
  Do not sit or stand quickly *to prevent dizziness and falls from orthostatic hypertension.*
  Take medications such as diuretics at a time of day that causes the least interference with sleep at night.

No accidental falls with injury in infants and children, as evidenced by:[5]

Caregivers verbalize and practice safety promotion activities

- Teach home safety for infants and children to prevent falls *because falls are one of the leading causes of infant and child injury and death. Babies roll and crawl, toddlers and children explore and climb.*

  Keep crib rails up and securely fastened.
  Use a sturdy highchair.
  Use a federally approved car seat or car booster chair. (Do not buy used car seats.)
  Strap child securely in grocery or shopping carts.
  Install safety locks on windows and lock windows securely if toddler can climb on window sill.
  Install a safety gate at the top and bottom of stairs.
  Keep floor clear of articles that might cause the child to trip and fall (e.g., rugs, cables, wires, toys).
  Clean up spills immediately.
  Install nonskid decals or tape in bathtubs or showers.

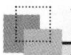

RISK FOR INFECTION

Risk for infection is the state in which a person or group is at increased risk for being invaded by pathogenic organisms.[6]

Risk Factors*

Pathophysiologic

Agranulocytosis
Altered cough, blink, or sneeze reflex
Altered enzyme activity
Altered normal protective flora
Altered peristalsis
Broken or burned skin or tissue
Chronic illness
Comatose state
Decreased ciliary action
Decreased hemoglobin
Decreased or changes in pH of secretions
Dysfunction of the thymus and lymphatic system
Immunosuppression
Impaired oxygenation
Inadequate acquired immunity
Leukopenia
Malnutrition or dehydration
Premature rupture of amniotic membranes
Spinal cord injury
Stasis of body fluids
Traumatized tissue

Developmental/behavioral

Abuse of alcohol, nicotine, drugs
Extremes of age
IV drug use
Lack of knowledge
Poor hygiene
Unsafe sexual practices

Treatment-related

Chemotherapy
Contaminated equipment and/or supplies
Dialysis
Fetal monitoring
Immobility
Inadequate or prolonged use of antibiotics
Invasive procedures
IV infusions
Organ transplant
Pharmaceutical agents
Radiation therapy
Surgical treatment

---

*References 1, 3, 5, 6, 9, 10.

Environmental

Contaminated food or water
Crowded living conditions
Exposure to pathogens from foreign travel, occupation, living conditions
Homelessness
Inadequate community immunization levels
Inadequate control of vectors
Inadequate sanitation

Defining Characteristics*

Anorexia
Fatigue
Increased serum levels of antibodies
Loss of weight
Manifestations of infection (e.g., chills, fever, malaise, purulent drainage, pain, leukocytosis)
Night sweats
Presence of pathogens or their eggs in any body tissue, excretion, or secretion
Productive cough
Redness or swelling

Expected Patient Outcomes and Nursing Interventions With Rationale[1-4,7-10]

No presence of infection in person experiencing risk factors, as evidenced by:

Verbalizes knowledge of risk
Receives recommended immunizations
Describes health habits that increase resistance to infection
Decrease in incidence of infection in the community

- Assess for the presence of risk factors. *Host susceptibility for infection increases with impaired defenses, altered immune response, disease, extremes of age, and lack of immunization. Host behaviors, such as unsafe sexual practices, sharing needles, and unsafe food handling, increase the risk for exposure to pathogens.*
- Instruct person on the risks associated with the altered life state or life stage and discuss behaviors to increase resistance to infection. *Adequate nutrition, hydration, rest, stress reduction, personal and environmental hygiene, cessation of smoking, control of alcohol use, and cessation of drug use may improve host resistance.*
- Discuss behaviors to reduce exposure to environmental pathogens. These include safe sexual practices, avoidance of sharing needles, proper food handling, and avoidance of vectors in the environment.
- Provide community education for safe food handling, water purification, and avoidance of vectors that normally carry pathogens.
- Support public health programs aimed at environmental sanitation; report to public health officials any infractions against sanitation codes. *Control of the environment is the most expedient way to prevent transmission of pathogens to large numbers of people.*
- Immunize persons of all ages who are inadequately immunized. Participate in community immunization programs to provide immunizations to high-risk populations. *Even distribution of immunized persons in the community decreases risk for outbreaks and epidemics of vaccine-preventable diseases.*

Infection is prevented in person experiencing treatment/hospital-related risks, as evidenced by:

Demonstrates behavior that reduces risk for infection during and after treatments
Vital signs and WBC are within normal limits
Cultures of body secretions, excretions, and exudates are negative for pathogens
Self-administers antiinfective agents, as prescribed
Surgical wounds heal without signs of infection
Invasive lines are discontinued as soon as possible
Discharge from the hospital in a timely manner

- Provide preprocedure instruction and postprocedure assistance to encourage deep breathing, coughing, ambulation, bladder emptying, and asepsis of invasive site. *Infection is associated with pooling of respiratory secretions, alterations in blood circulation, distention of the urinary bladder, and contamination of sites of invasion.*
- Turn frequently, and provide skin care to immobilized patients *to ensure circulation to compromised tissue.*[2]
- Monitor vital signs, changes in WBC count, and body secretions, excretions, and exudates for signs of infection. Obtain specimens as ordered. Report abnormalities to physician for early intervention.
- Monitor hydration and electrolyte balance, and ensure adequate fluid and food intake *to improve resistance to infection.*
- Teach patient and caregiver signs and symptoms of infection *in order for them to report the signs and symptoms. Delay in treatment can result in severe and life-threatening disease.*
- Administer antiinfectives as ordered and instruct patient or caregiver on the proper use of antiinfective agents. *Some foods and beverages alter the effectiveness of some antibiotics. Therapeutic drug levels are maintained with proper timing of drug administration. Antiinfective agents must be taken for the recommended time to prevent the development of drug-resistant organisms.*
- Observe and report signs of superinfection in patients receiving antimicrobial therapy. *These drugs may destroy protective normal flora organisms, thus facilitating the growth of opportunistic organisms.*
- Avoid invasive procedures, if possible, *because they interfere with primary defenses.*
- Use strict aseptic technique when performing invasive procedures and when caring for sites of invasion *to decrease the risk of introducing pathogens from the hospital environment.*
- Discontinue invasive lines in a timely manner *to decrease risk for colonization of pathogens at the insertion site.*
- Wash hands before and after contact with patient *to remove organisms before they can colonize the skin.*
- Prevent contamination of dressings and casts with urine or feces *to prevent transfer of normal flora organisms to a compromised part of the body.*

---

*References 1, 3, 5, 6, 9, 10.

- Use protective isolation procedures as indicated. Prevent patient exposure to infected visitors and staff. Limit visitors, if necessary. Ensure that patient care staff do not work when they have an infectious disease. Discharge patient as soon as possible from the hospital. *All of the above are necessary to prevent hospital-acquired infections.*

Infection is not transmitted to patient's contacts, as evidenced by:

Care staff practice standard precautions and hand washing and remain free of signs of infection

Appropriate isolation procedures implemented on hospitalized patients soon after infection is confirmed

All patient contacts adequately immunized or examined and treated for infection

Demonstrates behavior to prevent transmission of pathogens to others or to the environment

Infections are reported to the local health department and the incidence of communicable infections decreases in the hospital and in the community

- Monitor all patients for signs of infection and report findings so that prompt treatment can be initiated. Use standard precautions and other isolation procedures as indicated. *Both interventions decrease opportunity for transmission of pathogens.*
- Participate in follow-up of patient contacts *so that they can be treated or counseled to take appropriate preventive measures.* Administer immune globulin, as prescribed, to nonimmunized persons exposed to hepatitis B *to decrease the severity of the infection, if transmitted.*
- Instruct patient or caregiver in precautions for handling infective secretions, excretions, or exudates *to prevent transmission.* Discuss with patient the behaviors necessary to prevent transmission of STDs and foodborne infections.
- Report to the local health authority those infections that must be reported by law.
- Protect pregnant nursing personnel from contact with selected infections (rubella, cytomegalovirus, toxoplasmosis, herpes).
- Ensure that high-risk patient care staff have been immunized against hepatitis B virus, rubella, tetanus, and other vaccine-preventable conditions.
- Participate in educating patient care staff regarding pathogen transmission *to ensure that staff protect themselves adequately while caring for all patients.*
- Educate pregnant women to prevent or seek early treatment for infections that can be transmitted to the fetus *to prevent fetal infections and their sequelae.*
- Participate in public education programs regarding safer sexual practices *to help prevent the spread of AIDS and other STDs.*

RISK FOR INJURY

Risk for injury is the state in which an individual is at risk of injury as a result of environmental conditions interacting with the individual's adaptive and defensive resources.[5]

Risk Factors[4,5]

External

Biologic (e.g., immunization level of community, microorganism)

Chemical (e.g., pollutants, poisons, drugs, pharmaceutical agents, alcohol, caffeine, nicotine, preservatives, cosmetics, and dyes)

Mode of transport or transportation

Nutrients (e.g., vitamins, food types)

People or provider (e.g., nosocomial agents, staffing patterns, cognitive, affective, and psychomotor factors)

Physical (e.g., design, structure, and arrangement of community, building, and/or equipment)

Internal

Abnormal blood profile (e.g., leukocytosis/leukopenia)

Alcohol withdrawal

Altered clotting factors

Biochemical, regulatory function (e.g., sensory dysfunction)

Decreased hemoglobin

Developmental age (physiologic, psychosocial)

Immune-autoimmune dysfunction

Malnutrition

Physical (e.g., broken skin, altered mobility)

Psychologic

Sickle cell disease

Thalassemia

Thrombocytopenia

Tissue hypoxia

Expected Patient Outcomes and Nursing Interventions With Rationale[1-3,6]

Diminished or absent risk for injury from falls, as evidenced by:

Verbalizes understanding of risks for falls

Takes necessary precautions to prevent injury from falls

- Assess all patients for mobility and risk for falls. *Fall are more likely in patients who are weak, debilitated cognitively impaired, depressed, dizzy, confused, or ex perience changes in elimination patterns.*
- Implement fall precautions for patients at risk: post sign in the patient's room, and place a designated color arm band on the patient *to increase the awareness of health care providers and visitors.*
- Lock the wheels of beds, stretchers, and wheelchair when moving or transferring patients *to prevent acciden tal falls during transfers.*
- Provide a thorough orientation to the hospital or long term care facility to the patient on admission and as nec essary thereafter *to avoid disorientation.*
- Place call bell, TV controls, light cord, telephone, an patient's belongings in easy reach of patients confined t bed or who are immobile. *Reaching to get needed iten may precipitate a fall.*
- Leave side rails up, using half or three-quarters rails, ar maintain bed in low position. *Confused or disoriente patients are likely to climb over full rails and fall; falli from a higher distance is more likely to produce an i jury.*
- Use a night-light in all health-care and home settings.
- Assist patients at risk to the bathroom for toileting a the shower for hygiene.

- Avoid use of restraints. *Patients who fall while trying to get out of restraints can have serious injuries, because they often fall head first.*
- Evaluate interactions and effects of medications. *Patients taking multiple medications and those taking antihypertensives, sedatives, hypnotics, diuretics, and narcotics are at risk for falls.*
- Encourage patients to wear glasses and hearing aids; keep glasses clean.
- Encourage patients to use assistive devices such as canes and walkers when ambulating.
- Teach methods to reduce orthostatic hypotension:
  Change positions slowly.
  When awakening, first sit on the side of the bed, then stand.
  Rest in a recliner rather than in bed during the day.
  Avoid prolonged sitting or standing.
  NOTE: *Dizziness from orthostatic hypotension is a major cause of falls in the elderly.*
- Teach home safety:
  Do not use scatter rugs on the floor.
  Do not wax floors.
  Do not place objects on stairs.
  Make sure lights are on when walking through rooms.
  Wear slippers or shoes with rubber soles.
  If patient lives at home alone, refer for a Lifeline or other call device.
  Place nonslip tape or decals on the bottom of tubs and showers.
  Install hand rails on stairs, and hand grips in bathrooms.

See Risk for Trauma, Risk for Suffocation, Risk for Aspiration, and Risk for Poisoning for other interventions to decrease the risk for injury.

Risk for Perioperative-Positioning Injury

Risk for preoperative-positioning injury is the state in which the patient is at risk for injury as a result of the environmental conditions found in the perioperative setting.[6]

Risk Factors[6]

Disorientation
Edema
Emaciation
Immobilization
Muscle weakness
Obesity
Sensory/perceptual disturbances from anesthesia

Expected Patient Outcomes and Nursing Interventions With Rationale[1-5]

No injury related to perioperative positioning, as evidenced by:
Absence of respiratory injury related to positioning or hypoxia

- Preoperatively, have patient demonstrate turning, deep-breathing exercises, and the use of the incentive spirometer if applicable.
- Note presence of cough.
- When placing the patient in lithotomy position, place the legs *to cause minimal restriction of diaphragmatic movement.*
- When placing the patient in lateral position, ensure that the location of the upper arm contributes to proper intercostal breathing.
- When placing the patient in prone or jackknife position, ensure that the selection and location of body rolls allow for proper chest expansion *to promote maximal respiratory movement while in the position required for the operative procedure.*

No perioperative positioning injury, as evidenced by:
Is free from circulatory compromise

- Assess baseline data for coagulopathy.
- Determine patient activity level and positioning requirements.
- Provide cardiovascular supports *to prevent pooling of blood in dependent extremities, to aid in enhancing circulatory return,* and *to promote efficient peripheral circulation and venous return of blood to the central circulation.*

No perioperative positioning injury, as evidenced by:
Is free from injuries to nerves or peripheral vessels

- Based on patient condition, select appropriate safety measures such as pads and supports.
- Ensure there are adequate personnel to move the patient safely.
- Move the patient with careful attention to proper body alignment.
- Avoid overextension of joints.
- Pay scrupulous attention to arm positioning *to avoid peripheral nerve injuries.*
- Place padding at knee area in lithotomy position *to prevent compression damage to the peroneal nerve.*
- Place a soft roll at the apex of the scapula *to prevent brachial compression when in lateral position* and *to preserve the integrity of the neurovascular system.*

No preoperative positioning injury, as evidenced by:
Is free from musculoskeletal trauma

- Assess preoperative range of motion.
- Encourage patient participation in positioning and elicit comfort level before the induction of anesthesia.
- Ensure proper alignment of the limbs after induction.
- Avoid overzealous movement of the extremities during positioning.
- Give special consideration while moving patients with prostheses.
- Pad ischial tuberosities when in lithotomy position or modified-Fowler's position *to prevent pressure on sciatic nerves.*
- Move legs simultaneously into and out of lithotomy position *to prevent sacroiliac dislocation.*
- Pay careful attention to the fingers when adjusting the foot of the operating room bed for lithotomy position *to prevent digital damage.*
- When positioning the patient prone, avoid hyperextending the shoulder joints when moving the arms.
- When positioning the patient prone, ensure the knees are padded and a pillow is placed under the ankles *to prevent pressure on the toes from the mattress.*

- Adjust body rolls for prone position *to prevent encroachment on the breasts.*
- Ensure there is no impingement on the male genitalia when in prone position *to provide support for the musculoskeletal system.*

No perioperative positioning injury, as evidenced by:
Is free from impaired tissue or skin integrity

- Assess for contributory factors such as allergy, nutrition, and existing disease processes.
- Consider duration of pressure and location of bony prominences and/or other areas at risk.
- Lift, rather than slide, the patient *to prevent shearing force injuries.*
- To prevent skin abrasions or friction injuries, position the legs so they are not in contact with each other when in lateral position *to maintain tissue and skin status.*

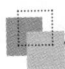

Risk for Poisoning

Risk for poisoning is the accentuated risk of accidental exposure to or ingestion of drugs or dangerous products in doses sufficient to cause poisoning.[6]

Risk Factors[6]

External

Availability of illicit drugs potentially contaminated by poisonous additives
Chemical contamination of food or water
Dangerous products placed or stored within reach of children or confused people
Flaking, peeling paint (especially lead-based) or plaster in presence of young children
Large intake of illicit drugs or alcohol
Large supplies of drugs in home
Medicines stored in unlocked cabinets accessible to children or confused people
Paint, lacquers, etc., in poorly ventilated areas or without effective protection
Presence of atmospheric pollutants
Presence of poisonous vegetation
Unprotected contact with heavy metals or chemicals

Internal

Cognitive or emotional difficulties
Insufficient finances
Lack of proper precautions
Lack of safety or drug education
Reduced vision
Verbalization of occupational setting without adequate safeguards

Expected Patient Outcomes and Nursing Interventions With Rationale[1,3,4,7]

Diminished or absent risk for poisoning, as evidenced by:
Verbalizes risks for poisoning
Takes necessary precautions to prevent poisoning
Verbalizes knowledge of emergency measures for accidental poisoning

- Conduct thorough assessment of the home environment, noting potential substances for poisoning, such as cleaning agents, paints and paint thinners, fertilizers, insecticides, gasoline, oil, medications in cabinets, medications in purses, faulty or unrepaired furnace and/or dirty fireplace chimney (carbon monoxide sources), and peeling paint (especially in older homes and apartments). *All of these agents may cause poisoning. The ingestion of lead from lead-based paint is a common source of poisoning for infants and preschool children. Iron toxicity, from iron in medications and over-the-counter vitamin and mineral tablets is a serious and potentially lethal type of childhood poisoning.*
- Assess the numbers and types of medications taken by elderly, confused, or disoriented patients. *Interactions of multiple medications may cause poisoning.*
- Identify environmental and workplace risks for poisoning.
- Teach parents to keep cleaning agents, gardening agents, medications, and any other hazardous materials securely locked in a place out of reach of children.
- Teach parents to:
  - Keep the phone number of the poison control center readily available.
  - Place Mr. YUK stickers on poisonous materials and medications, and teach children not to touch anything with such a label.
  - Keep syrup of ipecac on hand for accidental ingestion of poisonous materials *to induce vomiting after contacting the poison control center.*
  - Have furnaces checked and fireplace chimneys cleaned on a regular schedule.
  - Install carbon monoxide detectors.

NOTE: *Children are most vulnerable for poisoning between the ages of 1 and 3 years, but accidental deaths from poisoning can occur at any age.*

- Teach patients to:
  - Keep medications out of the reach of children.
  - Maintain a system of taking medications that prevents taking more than is prescribed (such as using day and time dispenser boxes).
  - Never share prescription medications.
  - Request large-print labels if vision is decreased.
  - Never mix alcohol with medications unless approved by the health-care provider
  - Never use food from cans that are bulging or leaking
  - Boil home-canned vegetables before eating; discard if contents are discolored, foamy, or have a bad odor
  - Store perishable items in the refrigerator.

NOTE: *These activities decrease the risk of poisoning in the home.*

Risk for Suffocation

Risk for suffocation is the accentuated risk of accidental suffocation (inadequate air available for inhalation).[3]

Risk Factors[3]

External

Children inflating rubber balloons
Children inserting small objects into their mouths or nose
Children left unattended in bathtubs or pools
Children playing with plastic bags

Discarded or unused refrigerators or freezers without doors removed
Household gas leaks
Infant sleeping on stomach
Large mouthfuls of food
Long miniblind cords
Low-strung clothesline
Pacifier hung around infant's head
Pillow placed in an infant's crib
Propped bottle placed in an infant's crib
Smoking in bed; falling asleep while smoking
Use of fuel-burning heaters not vented to outside
Vehicle running in closed garage

Internal

Cognitive or emotional difficulties
Disease or injury process
Lack of safety education
Lack of safety precautions
Reduced motor abilities
Reduced olfactory sensation

Expected Patient Outcomes and Nursing Interventions With Rationale[1-2,4]

Diminished or absent risk for suffocation, as evidenced by:

Verbalizes knowledge of risks for suffocation
Takes necessary precautions to prevent suffocation
Demonstrates proper techniques for the Heimlich maneuver and CPR

- Conduct a thorough assessment of the home environment, noting hazards such as large plastic bags, cribs with wide slats, pillows in cribs, pacifiers on a string, pull toys with long strings, miniblind cords that can be reached by children, abandoned large appliances such as refrigerators and freezers. *All of these items have the potential to induce suffocation in infants and small children.*
- Conduct a thorough assessment of the home environment for potential hazards such as gas leaking from pilot lights or burners of gas stoves, carbon monoxide leaking from furnaces, kerosene fumes from portable heaters, holes in automobile mufflers. Assess for working carbon monoxide and smoke detectors. Assist with finding resources for repairs as necessary. *Eliminating potential hazards and installing safety devices help reduce the risk of suffocation.*
- Teach parents to:

  Avoid giving infants and small children foods that can be inhaled, such as nuts, popcorn, hard candy, pieces of hotdog, grapes.
  Prevent small children from playing with rubber balloons.
  Have old appliances hauled away immediately.
  Keep garage door openers out of children's reach.
  Keep automobile trunks locked.
  Place infants on their side or back to sleep.
  Teach children water safety at an early age.
  Never leave young children unattended in the bathtub.
  Perform the Heimlich maneuver and CPR.

  NOTE: *As the primary caregivers, parents are responsible for maintaining the safety of their children.*

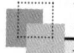

RISK FOR TRAUMA

Risk for trauma is the accentuated risk of accidental tissue injury (e.g., wound, burn, fracture.)[3]

Risk Factors[3]

External

Children playing with matches, candles, cigarettes, sharp-edged toys
Contact with intense cold
Contact with rapidly moving machinery, industrial belts, or pulleys
Defective appliances
Driving at excessive speeds
Driving under the influence of alcohol or drugs
Faulty electrical plugs or frayed wires
Guns or ammunition stored unlocked
High-crime neighborhood and vulnerable patients
Highly flammable children's toys or clothing
Inadequately stored combustibles or corrosives (e.g., matches, oily rags, lye)
Knives stored uncovered
Litter or liquid spills on floors or stairways; highly waxed floors
Misuse or nonuse of necessary headgear for cyclists
Nonuse or misuse of seat restraints
Obstructed passageways
Overexposure to sun, sun lamps, and radiotherapy
Overloaded electrical outlets and/or fuse boxes
Play or work near vehicle pathways (e.g., driveways, laneways, railroad tracks)
Playing with fireworks or gunpowder
Pot handles facing toward front of stove
Snow or ice on stairs, walkways
Unscreened fires, fireplaces, or heaters
Unsupervised bathing of young children

Internal

Balancing difficulties
Cognitive or emotional difficulties
History of risk-taking behavior
Insufficient finances to purchase safety equipment or effect repairs
Lack of safety education
Lack of safety precautions
Poor vision and/or hearing
Reduced hand-eye coordination
Reduced large or small muscle coordination
Reduced temperature and/or tactile sensation
Weakness

Expected Patient Outcomes and Nursing Interventions With Rationale[1,2,4]

Diminished or absent risk for trauma, as evidenced by:

Verbalizes understanding of risks for trauma
Takes necessary precautions to prevent injury from trauma

- Assess patient for cognitive function, risk-taking behaviors, use of alcohol or drugs, vision, and hearing. *People who are cognitively impaired, take risks, use alcohol or drugs, or have impaired sight or hearing are at increased risk for trauma.*
- Teach patient, family, and/or caregivers to:
  - Use good lighting and glasses, and decrease safety barriers (such as slick floors and throw rugs) *to improve ability to see and decrease chance of falls or automobile accidents.*
  - Test temperature of water before showers, baths, or washing dishes *to reduce risk of burns.*
  - Keep stairs, walks, and driveways clear of ice and snow.
  - Keep guns in locked cabinets or closets.
  - Install and maintain smoke detectors.
  - Install safety devices, such as higher commodes and hand grips, in the bathroom.
  - Use bright tape to mark edges of steps and stove knobs *to reduce the risk of falls and burns.*
  - Discourage driving at night if vision is decreased or cognitive function is impaired.
  - Keep emergency numbers for the police and fire department by the phone.
  - Practice evacuation routes in case of fire.
  - Have fire extinguishers readily available in the garage and kitchen.
  - Report abuse or neglect from caregivers.
  - Never allow anyone to smoke in bed.
  - Wear seatbelts.
- Teach parents to:
  - Teach children never to play with matches.
  - Keep matches and cigarette lighters out of reach.
  - Teach home fire safety drills.
  - Never leave infants or toddlers unattended on a bed or couch.
  - Teach how to safely cross streets.
  - Teach the dangers of strangers.
  - Take older children, interested in guns, to a firearms safety program.
  - Teach farm children about the safe use of machines and care of animals.
  - Ensure that screens and windows are securely fastened.
  - Ensure that children wear helmets when riding bikes or skateboarding.
  - Discuss the dangers of substance abuse, and driving under the influence of alcohol or drugs with adolescents.
  - Discuss the legal and safety aspects of wearing seat belts when driving the car.
  - Provide role models of ways to resolve conflict without use of guns, knives, or physical abuse
  - Ensure that day-care providers and schools are safe environments, with safety-conscious caregivers and teachers

  NOTE: *As primary caregivers, parents are responsible for the safety of their children.*

REFERENCES

Health Perception–Health Management

1. Gordon M: *Manual of nursing diagnosis,* ed 9, St. Louis, 2000, Mosby.

Disturbed Energy Field

1. Collins SB: Nursing diagnosis and energy field disturbance, *Beginnings* 15(4):4, 1995.
2. Hover-Kramer D: Touch therapies in the perioperative environment: human connecting for enhanced healing, *Semin Periop Nurs* 7(2):101, 1998.
3. McCloskey JC, Bulechek GM, editors: Therapeutic touch. In *Nursing interventions classification (NIC),* ed 3, St. Louis, 2001, Mosby.
4. Mornhinweg GC: Energy field disturbance: a validation study. In Rantz MR, LeMone P, editors: *Classification of nursing diagnoses: proceedings of the twelfth conference, North American Nursing Diagnosis Association,* Glendale, Calif, 1997, Cinahl Information Systems.
5. North American Nursing Diagnosis Association: *Nursing diagnoses: definitions and classification 2001-2002,* Philadelphia, 2001, The Association.
6. Rogers M: *An introduction to the theoretical basis of nursing,* Philadelphia, 1970, FA Davis.

Effective Therapeutic Regimen Management

1. Cameron C: Patient compliance: recognition of factors involved and suggestions for promoting compliance with therapeutic regimen, *J Adv Nurs* 24(2):244, 1996.
2. Glasgow RE et al: Quality of life and associated characteristics in a large national sample of adults with diabetes, *Diabetes Care,* 20(4):562, 1997.
3. Lubkin IM: *Chronic illness: impact and interventions,* ed 4, Boston, 1999, Jones & Bartlett.
4. North American Nursing Diagnosis Association: *Nursing diagnoses: definitions and classification 2001-2002,* Philadelphia, 2001, The Association.
5. Orem DE: *Nursing: concepts of practice,* ed 5, St. Louis, 1995, Mosby.
6. Taylor CA, Keller ML, Egan JJ: Advice from affected persons about living with human papillomavirus infection, *Image J Nurs Sch* 29(1):27, 1997.

Ineffective Therapeutic Regimen Management

1. Cameron C: Patient compliance: recognition of factors involved and suggestions for promoting compliance with therapeutic regimen, *J Adv Nurs* 24(2):244, 1996.
2. DeGeest S, von Renteln-Kruse W, Steeman E et al: Compliance issues with the geriatric population: complexity with aging, *Nurs Clin North Am* 33(3):467, 1998.
3. Hsu JW, Chao MC, Tsai PL et al: Influence of referral source on return compliance of adolescents, *J Adolesc Health* 23(2):110, 1998
4. Kane K: Help patients help themselves, *Practice Nurse* 16(10):628, 1998.
5. Lowry DA: Issues of non-compliance in mental health, *J Adv Nurs* 28(2):280, 1998.
6. Lubkin IM: *Chronic illness: impact and interventions,* ed 4 Boston, 1999, Jones & Bartlett.
7. McCloskey JC, Bulechek GM, editors: Health system guidance. In *Nursing interventions classification (NIC),* ed 3, St. Louis, 2001 Mosby.
8. McGann E: Medication compliance in adults with asthma, *Am J Nurs* 99(3):45, 1999.

9. North American Nursing Diagnosis Association: *Nursing diagnoses: definitions and classification 2001-2002,* Philadelphia, 2001, The Association.
10. Orem DE: *Nursing: concepts of practice,* ed 5, St. Louis, 1995, Mosby.
11. Paskett ED, McMahon K, Tatum C et al: Clinic-based interventions to promote breast and cervical cancer screening, *Prev Med* 27(1):120, 1998.
12. Pender NJ: *Health promotion in nursing practice,* ed 3, Stamford, Conn, 1996, Appleton & Lange.

Ineffective Family Therapeutic Regimen Management

1. Chang BL: Cognitive-behavioral intervention for homebound caregivers of persons with dementia, *Nurs Res* 48(3):173, 1999.
2. Johnson M, Maas M, Moorhead S, editors: Caregiver performance: direct care. In *Nursing outcomes classification (NOC),* ed 2, St. Louis, 1997, Mosby.
3. Knafl KA, Deatrick JA: How families manage chronic conditions: an analysis of the concept of normalization, *Res Nurs Health* 9(3):215, 1986.
4. Lubkin IM: *Chronic illness: impact and interventions,* ed 4, Boston, 1999, Jones & Bartlett.
5. North American Nursing Diagnosis Association: *Nursing diagnoses: definitions and classification 2001-2002,* Philadelphia, 2001, The Association.
6. McCloskey JC, Bulechek GM, editors: Family involvement; Family mobilization. In *Nursing interventions classification (NIC),* ed 3, St. Louis, 2001, Mosby.
7. Schumacher KL, Stewart BJ, Archbold PG: Conceptualization and measurement of doing family caregiving well, *Image J Nurs Sch* 30(1):63, 1998.

Ineffective Community Therapeutic Regimen Management

1. Clemen-Stone S, McGuire SL, Eigsti DG: *Comprehensive community health nursing: family, aggregate, and community practice,* ed 5, St. Louis, 1998, Mosby.
2. Flynn BC: Communicating with the public: community-based nursing research and practice, *Public Health Nurs* 15(3):165, 1998.
3. Laffrey SC, Kulbok PA: An integrative model for holistic community health nursing, *J Holist Nurs* 17(1):88, 1999.
4. McCloskey JC, Bulechek GM, editors: Environmental management: community; Health policy monitoring. In *Nursing interventions classification (NIC),* ed 3, St. Louis, 2001, Mosby.
5. North American Nursing Diagnosis Association: *Nursing diagnoses: definitions and classification 2001-2002,* Philadelphia, 2001, The Association.

Health-Seeking Behaviors (Specify)

1. Andrews MM, Boyle JS: *Transcultural concepts in nursing care,* ed 3, Philadelphia, 1999, Lippincott-Raven.
2. *Clark CC: Wellness self-care by healthy older adults,* Image: J Nurs Sch 30(4):351, 1998.
3. McCloskey JC, Bulechek GM, editors: health education; Self-modification assistance. In *Nursing interventions classification (NIC),* ed 3, St. Louis, 2001, Mosby.
4. McFarland GK, McFarlane EA: *Nursing diagnosis and intervention: planning for patient care,* ed 3, St. Louis, 1997, Mosby.
5. North American Nursing Diagnosis Association: *Nursing diagnoses: definitions and classification 2001-2002,* Philadelphia, 2001, The Association.
6. Pender NJ: *Health promotion in nursing practice,* ed 3, Stamford, Conn, 1996, Appleton & Lange.
7. Sowell RL, Seals B, Moneyham L et al: Barriers to health-seeking behaviors for women infected with HIV, *Nursingconnect* 9(3):5, 1996.
8. White JC, Dull VT: Health risk factors and health-seeking behavior in lesbians, *J Womens Health* 6(1):103, 1997.

Ineffective Health Maintenance

1. Borum ML: Does age influence screening for colorectal cancer? *Age Ageing* 27(4):509, 1998.
2. Casaneda DM, Bigatti S, Cronan TA: Gender and exercise behavior among women and men with osteoarthritis, *Womens Health* 27(4):33, 1998.
3. Gerard MJ, Frank-Stromborg M: Screening for prostate cancer in asymptomatic men: clinical, legal, and ethical implications, *Oncol Nurs Forum* 25(9):1561, 1998.
4. Maddox MA: Reminder interventions increased women's use of mammography and Pap smear screening (commentary), *Evidence-Based Nurs* 1(2):59, 1998.
5. McCloskey JC, Bulechek GM, editors: Health education. In *Nursing interventions classification (NIC),* ed 3, St. Louis, 2001, Mosby.
6. North American Nursing Diagnosis Association: *Nursing diagnoses: definitions and classification 2001-2002,* Philadelphia, 2001, The Association.
7. Pender NJ: *Health promotion in nursing practice,* ed 3, Stamford, Conn, 1996, Appleton & Lange.
8. Scarlach AE, Midanik LT, Runkle MC et al: Health practices of adults with elder care responsibilities, *Prev Med* 26(2):155, 1997.
9. Siddorov J, Christianson M, Girolami S et al: Patient outcomes: a successful tobacco cessation program led by primary care nurses in a managed care setting, *Am J Managed Care* 3(2):207, 1997.
10. Williams SJ, Drew J, Wright B et al: Health promotion workshops for seniors: predictors of attendance and behavioral outcomes, *J Health Educ* 29(3):166, 1998.

Ineffective Protection

1. Auduino RC, DuPont HL: Diarrhea in the critically ill: is it causing or complicating severe illness? *J Crit Illness* 13(5):320, 1998.
2. Brook I, Frazier HE: Aerobic and anaerobic microbiology of infection after trauma, *Am J Emerg Med* 16(6):585, 1998.
3. Goldman DA, Cunningham RS: Infection management in the ambulatory setting for the adult patient with acute leukemia, *Dev Support Cancer Care* 2(3):87, 1998.
4. Johns A: Overview of bone marrow and stem cell transplantation, *J Intraven Nurs* 21(6):356, 1998.
5. Kellum JA, Decker JM: The immune system: relation to sepsis and multiple organ failure, *AACN Clin Issues: Adv Pract Acute Crit Care* 7(3):339, 1996.
6. McCloskey JC, Bulechek GM, editors: Infection control; Infection protection; Surgical precautions; Surveillance: safety. In *Nursing interventions classification (NIC),* ed 3, St. Louis, 2001, Mosby.
7. North American Nursing Diagnosis Association: *Nursing diagnoses: definitions and classification 2001-2002,* Philadelphia, 2001, The Association.
8. Schuman P: Mucosal candidiasis among women living with human immunodeficiency infection, *Home Healthcare Consult* 5(4):36, 1998.
9. Taylor C, Lillis C, LeMone P: *Fundamentals of nursing: the art and science of nursing care,* ed 4, Philadelphia, 2001, JB Lippincott.
10. Volker D: Fever of unknown origin, *Nurse Pract Forum* 9(3):170, 1998.
11. Witek-Janusek L, Stoddard J, Mathews HL: Trauma-induced immune dysfunction: a challenge for critical care, *Dimens Crit Care Nurs* 17(4):187, 1998.

Noncompliance (Specify)

1. Branden PS: Contraceptive choice and patient compliance: the health care provider's challenge, *J Nurse Midwifery* 43(6):471, 1998.
2. Brus H, van de Laar M, Taal E et al: Determinants of compliance with medication in patients with rheumatoid arthritis: the importance of self-efficacy expectations, *Patient Educ Counsel* 36(1):57, 1999.
3. Cameron C: Patient compliance: recognition of factors involved and suggestions for promoting compliance with therapeutic regimen, *J Adv Nurs* 24(2):244, 1996.
4. Crespo-Fierro M: Compliance/adherence and care management in HIV disease, *J Assoc Nurses AIDS Care* 8(4):43, 1997.
5. DeGeest S, von Renteln-Kruse W, Steeman E et al: Compliance issues with the geriatric population: complexity with aging, *Nurs Clin North Am* 33(3):467, 1998.
6. Hsu JW, Chao MC, Tsai PL et al: Influence of referral source on return compliance of adolescents, *J Adolesc Health* 23(2):110, 1998.
7. Lowry DA: Issues of non-compliance in mental health, *J Adv Nurs* 28(2):280, 1998.
8. Moore SM, Ruland CM, Pashkow FJ et al: Women's patterns of exercise following cardiac rehabilitation, *Nurs Res* 47(6):318, 1998.
9. North American Nursing Diagnosis Association: *Nursing diagnoses: definitions and classification 2001-2002,* Philadelphia, 2001, The Association.
10. Racelis MC, Lombardo K, Verdin J: Impact of telephone reinforcement of risk reduction education on patient compliance, *J Vasc Nurs* 16(1):16, 1998.
11. Sowell RL, Seals B, Moneyham L et al: Barriers to health-seeking behaviors for women infected with HIV, *Nursingconnections* 9(3):5, 1996.
12. Spector RE: *Cultural diversity in health and illness,* Stamford, Conn, 1996, Appleton & Lange.
13. Sung JC, Nichol MB, Venturini F et al: Factors affecting patient compliance with antihyperlipidemic medications in an HMO population, *Am J Managed Care* 4(10):1421, 1998.

Risk for Falls

1. Clemson L, Cumming RG, Rowland M: Case control study of hazards in the home and risk of falls and hip fractures, *Age Ageing* 25(2):97, 1996.
2. Gillespie LD, Gillespie WJ, Cumming R et al: Interventions for preventing falls in the elderly (Cochrane Review). In *The Cochrane Library,* Issue 3, Oxford, 2000, Update Software.
3. Kiely DK, Kiel DP, Burrows AB et al: Identifying nursing home residents at risk for falling, *J Am Geriatr Soc* 46(5):551, 1998.
4. McCloskey JC, Bulechek GM, editors: *Nursing interventions classification (NIC),* ed 3, St. Louis, 2001, Mosby.
5. Murray RB, Zentner JP: *Health promotion strategies through the life span,* ed 7, Upper Saddle River, NJ, 2001, Prentice Hall.
6. North American Nursing Diagnosis Association: *NANDA Nursing diagnoses: definitions and classification 2001-2002,* Philadelphia, 2001, The Association.
7. Rawsky E: Review of the literature on falls among the elderly, *Image J Nurs Sch* 30(1):47, 1998.
8. Rogers PD, Bocchino NL: Restraint-free care: is it possible? *Am J Nurs* 99(10):27, 1999.
9. Steinberg M, Lyketsos CG, Steele C et al: Falls in the institutionalized elderly with dementia: a pilot study, *Ann Long Term Care* 6(5):153, 1998.
10. Stolley JM, Lewis A, Moore L et al: Risk for injury: falls. In Maas ML, Buckwalter KC, Hardy MD et al: *Nursing care of older adults: diagnoses, outcomes and interventions,* St. Louis, 2001, Mosby.

Risk for Infection

1. Bond G: Infection control in the perioperative setting, *Semin Periop Nurs* 8(1):24, 1999.
2. Krasner D: The AHCPR pressure ulcer infection control recommendations revisited, *Ostomy Wound Manage* 45(suppl 1A):88S, 1999.
3. Leaper DJ: Defining infection, *J Wound Care* 7(8):373, 1998.
4. McCloskey JC, Bulechek GM, editors: Infection control; Infection protection. In *Nursing interventions classification (NIC),* ed 3, St. Louis, 2001, Mosby.
5. McKenzie SB, Laudicina RJ: Hematologic changes associated with infection, *Clin Lab Sci* 11(4):239, 1998.
6. North American Nursing Diagnosis Association: *Nursing diagnoses: definitions and classification 2001-2002,* Philadelphia, 2001, The Association.
7. Watanakunakorn C, Wang C, Hazy J: An observational study of hand washing and infection control practices by healthcare workers, *Infect Control Hosp Epidemiol* 19(11):858, 1998.
8. West K, Cohen M: Standard precautions: a new approach to reducing infection transmission in the hospital setting, *J Intraven Nurs* 20(6S):7, 1997.
9. Witek-Janusek L, Stoddard J, Mathews HL: Trauma-induced immune dysfunction: a challenge for critical care, *Dimens Crit Care Nurs* 17(4):187, 1998.
10. Volker D: Fever of unknown origin, *Nurse Pract Forum* 9(3):17, 1998.

Risk for Injury

1. Ackley BJ, Ladwig GB *Nursing diagnosis handbook: a guide for planning care,* St. Louis, 1999, Mosby.
2. Carpenito LJ: *Handbook of nursing diagnosis,* ed 8, Philadelphia, 1999, JB Lippincott.
3. McCloskey JC, Bulechek GM, editors: Fall prevention; Surveillance: safety. In *Nursing interventions classification (NIC),* ed 3, St. Louis, 2001, Mosby.
4. McFarland GK, Wasli EL, Gerety EK: *Nursing diagnoses and process in psychiatric mental health nursing,* ed 3, Philadelphia, 1997, JB Lippincott.
5. North American Nursing Diagnosis Association: *Nursing diagnoses: definitions and classification 2001-2002,* Philadelphia, 2001, The Association.
6. Taylor C, Lillis C, LeMone P: *Fundamentals of nursing: the art and science of nursing care,* ed 4, Philadelphia, 2001, JB Lippincott.

Risk for Perioperative-Positioning Injury

1. Alexander CM: Perioperative ulnar nerve injury, *Curr Rev Post Anesthesia Care Nurses* 17(20):171, 1995.
2. Daley MD: The best is yet to be: positioning and the geriatric surgical patient, *Today's Surg Nurse* 19(5):13, 1997.
3. Green S: Positioning the patient for surgery, *Br J Theatre Nurs* 6(5):35, 1996.
4. Hoshowsky VM: Surgical positioning, *Orthop Nurs* 17(5):55, 1998.
5. McCloskey JC, Bulechek GM, editors: Positioning: intraoperative; Skin surveillance. In *Nursing interventions classification (NIC),* ed 3, St. Louis, 2001, Mosby.
6. North American Nursing Diagnosis Association: *Nursing diagnoses: definitions and classification 2001-2002,* Philadelphia, 2001, The Association.
7. Scott EM: Research focus: hospital acquired pressure sores as an indicator of quality: a research programme centred in the operating theatre, *Br J Theatre Nurs* 8(5):19, 1998.

8. Taylor C, Lillis C, LeMone P: *Fundamentals of nursing: the art and science of nursing care,* ed 4, Philadelphia, 2001, JB Lippincott.

Risk for Poisoning

1. Ackley BJ, Ladwig GB: *Nursing diagnosis handbook: a guide for planning care,* St. Louis, 1999, Mosby.
2. Babl FE, Kharsch S, Woolf A: Airway edema following household bleach ingestion, *Am J Emerg Med* 16(5):514, 1998.
3. Jones AL: Initial management of poisoned patients in the out-of-hospital environment, *Prehosp Immediate Care* 2(3):141, 1998.
4. McCloskey JC, Bulechek GM, editors: Environmental management: safety. In *Nursing interventions classification (NIC),* ed 3, St. Louis, 2001, Mosby.
5. Meert KL, Heidemann SM, Sarnaik AP: Outcome of children with carbon monoxide poisoning treated with normobaric oxygen, *J Trauma-Injury Infect Crit Care* 44(1):149, 1998.
6. North American Nursing Diagnosis Association: *Nursing diagnoses: definitions and classification 2001-2002,* Philadelphia, 2001, The Association.
7. Taylor C, Lillis C, LeMone P: *Fundamentals of nursing: the art and science of nursing care,* ed 4, Philadelphia, 2001, JB Lippincott.

Risk for Suffocation

1. Ackley BJ, Ladwig GB: *Nursing diagnosis handbook: a guide for planning care,* St. Louis, 1999, Mosby.
2. McCloskey JC, Bulechek GM, editors: Airway management; Environmental management: safety. In *Nursing interventions classification (NIC),* ed 3, St. Louis, 2001, Mosby.
3. North American Nursing Diagnosis Association: *Nursing diagnoses: definitions and classification 2001-2002,* Philadelphia, 2001, The Association.
4. Taylor C, Lillis C, LeMone P: *Fundamentals of nursing: the art and science of nursing care,* ed 4, Philadelphia, 2001, JB Lippincott.

Risk for Trauma

1. Ackley BJ, Ladwig GB: *Nursing diagnosis handbook: a guide for planning care,* St. Louis, 1999, Mosby.
2. McCloskey JC, Bulechek GM, editors: Environmental management: safety. In *Nursing interventions classification (NIC),* ed 3, St. Louis, 2001, Mosby.
3. North American Nursing Diagnosis Association: *Nursing diagnoses: definitions and classification 2001-2002,* Philadelphia, 2001, The Association.
4. Taylor C, Lillis C, LeMone P: *Fundamentals of nursing: the art and science of nursing care,* ed 4, Philadelphia, 2001, JB Lippincott.

FUNCTIONAL HEALTH PATTERN

2

Nutritional-Metabolic[1]

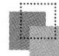

ADULT FAILURE TO THRIVE

Adult failure to thrive is progressive functional physical and cognitive deterioration; the individual's ability to live with multisystem diseases, cope with ensuing problems, and manage his or her care is remarkably diminished.[4,6]

Related Factors[1,4,6]

Apathy
Depression
Fatigue

Defining Characteristics[1,4,6]

Altered mood
Apathy
Cognitive decline
Consumption of minimal to no food at most meals
Decreased participation in activities once enjoyed
Decreased social skills and social withdrawal
Decreased verbal communication with staff, family, friends
Dehydration
Difficulty in reasoning, decision making, and concentration
Difficulty performing simple self-care tasks
Fatigue
Feelings of sadness
Frequent exacerbations of chronic health problems
Inadequate nutritional intake
Incontinence of bowel and bladder
Lack of attention to physical cleanliness or appearance
Neglect of home environment and/or financial responsibilities
Physical decline
Verbalized desire for death
Verbalized lack of appetite
Weight loss

Expected Patient Outcomes and Nursing Interventions With Rationale[2,3,5,7,8]

Increase nutritional intake, as evidenced by:
Eats adequate amounts and types of food
Increases and maintains weight to normal for age and height

- Assess factors contributing to decreased nutrition, such as depression. *Depression may cause decreased appetite.*[3]
- Provide small, attractively prepared snacks and meals, served in a pleasant environment.
- Provide "comfort foods." *"Comfort foods" are asso ated with pleasant memories and may encourage intak*
- Encourage the patient to:
  Choose a variety of foods (see FIG. 23-1).
  Eat at least 50% of food served at each meal.
  Take liquid supplements as necessary *to provide ad quate caloric intake.*
- Instruct family or significant others on strategies, such verbal cuing, to encourage eating. *Verbal cuing is effe tive in improving nutritional status.*[2]

Maintain physical and cognitive functioning, as ev denced by:
Takes part in usual activities of daily living
Provides self-care
Engages in social activities

- Identify factors that may contribute to decreased cog tive or physical function, such as infection or depressic *Change in mental acuity or fatigue may be an indicat of underlying physical or mental pathology.*
- Refer for psychotherapy and possible medication for d pression.[2]
- Provide cognitive therapy for depressed patients.
- Encourage reminiscence about past experiences. *Rem niscence enhances coping.*[7]
- Encourage patient to participate in a planned program exercise.[5]
- Provide activities that facilitate interaction with others a regular basis.
- Involve patient in family and social activities.
- Encourage patient to maintain contact with family a significant others.
- Provide physical touch for patients. *Touch helps soci relatedness.*[2]
- Provide positive reinforcement when patient interac with others or participates in activities. *Reinforceme supports patient's efforts.*

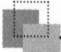

DEFICIENT FLUID VOLUME

Deficient fluid volume is the state in which an individual experi ences decreased intravascular, interstitial, and/or intracellula fluid. This refers to dehydration, water loss alone withou changes in sodium.[5]

Related Factors[5,6]

Active fluid volume loss (e.g., hemorrhage)
Diarrhea
Failure of regulatory mechanisms

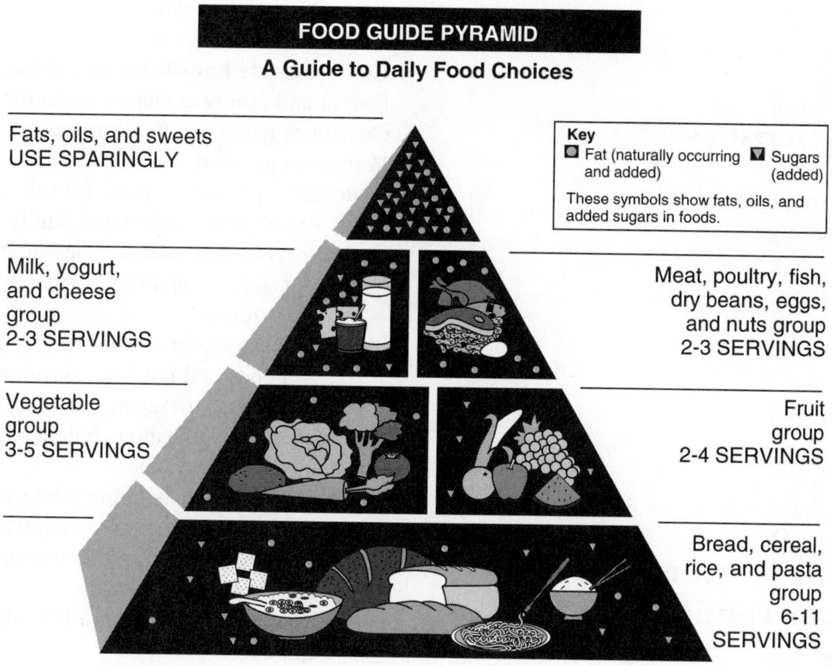

Food Group	Suggested Daily Servings	What Counts as a Serving?
Breads, cereals, and other grain products Whole-grain Enriched	**6-11** servings from entire group *(Include several servings of whole-grain products daily.)*	• 1 slice of bread • 1/2 hamburger bun or English muffin • a small roll, biscuit, or muffin • 3 to 4 small or 2 large crackers • 1/2 cup cooked cereal, rice, or pasta • 1 ounce of ready-to-eat breakfast cereal
Fruits Citrus, melon, berries Other fruits	**2-4** servings from entire group	• A whole fruit such as a medium apple, banana, or orange • A grapefruit half • A melon wedge • 3/4 cup of juice • 1/2 cup of berries • 1/2 cup of cooked or canned fruit • 1/2 cup dried fruit
Vegetables Dark-green leafy Deep-yellow Dry beans/peas (legumes) Starchy Other vegetables	**3-5** servings from entire group *(Include all types regularly: use dark-green leafy vegetables and dry beans and peas several times a week.)*	• 1/2 cup of cooked vegetables • 1/2 cup of chopped raw vegetables • 1 cup of leafy raw vegetables, such as lettuce or spinach
Meat, poultry, fish and alternates (eggs, dry beans and peas, nuts and seeds)	**2-3** servings from entire group	Amounts should total 5 to 7 ounces of cooked lean meat, poultry, or fish a day. Count 1 egg, 1/2 cup cooked beans, or 2 tablespoons peanut butter as 1 ounce of meat.
Milk, cheese, and yogurt	**2** servings from entire group *(3 servings for women who are pregnant or breast-feeding and for teens; 4 servings for teens who are pregnant or breast-feeding)*	• 1 cup of milk • 8 ounces of yogurt • 1 1/2 ounces of natural cheese • 2 ounces of processed cheese
Fats, sweets, and alcoholic beverages	Avoid too many fats and sweets. If you drink alcoholic beverages, do so in moderation.	

FIG. 23-1
Food Guide Pyramid.

Fever with poor intake
Overdiuresis
Vomiting

Defining Characteristics[2,4,6]

Changes in mental status
Decreased pulse volume or pressure
Decreased skin or tongue turgor
Decreased urine output
Decreased venous filling
Elevated hematocrit
Hypotension
Increased body temperature
Increased urine concentration
Tachycardia
Weakness
Weight loss

Expected Patient Outcomes and Nursing Interventions With Rationale[1-4]

Maintain adequate fluid and electrolyte balance, as evidenced by:
Elastic skin turgor
Moist mucous membranes
Absence of thirst
Balanced intake and output
Blood pressure and pulse within normal limits
Serum osmolality within normal limits
Hemoglobin and hematocrit within normal limits
Urine specific gravity and osmolality within normal limits

- Measure vital signs. Observe for hypotension, including postural hypotension; pulse will be elevated.
- Measure central venous pressure or pulmonary capillary wedge pressure. *These reflect the pressure of the circulating blood volume and will be decreased.*
- Assess capillary refill time. *Refill time will be >5 seconds, indicating the reduced blood volume requiring more time for the capillaries to fill.*
- Measure intake and output *to monitor the fluid balance.*
- Weigh patient *to monitor fluid balance.*
- Measure abdominal girth when ascites is present.
- Monitor electrolytes, especially potassium, sodium, calcium, and magnesium.
- Measure urine specific gravity.
- Monitor hemoglobin (Hgb) and hematocrit (Hct).
- Assess oral mucous membranes.
- Assess skin turgor.
- Administer intravenous or oral fluids as ordered by physician.
- Administer electrolytes as ordered.
- Administer regulating hormones as ordered (e.g., insulin, vasopressin) *to retain fluids. Insulin is given to counteract polyuria associated with diabetes mellitus. Vasopressin is given to replace antidiuretic hormone to treat diabetes insipidus.*
- Orient patient when confusion or disorientation occurs.
- Maintain safety when patient is sitting or standing. *Observe for postural hypotension or confusion.*
- Provide oral care.
- Provide skin care.

Communicate knowledge of self-care, as evidenced by:
Patient and family explain reasons for fluid deficit
Consumes foods and fluids to prevent recurrence
Verbalizes purpose, dosage, and side effects of medications ordered by physician; plans for follow-up care

- Assess what patient and family already know.
- Provide information concerning:
  - Cause of this fluid deficit and how to prevent recurrence
  - Reasons for treatments
  - Foods and fluids to consume
  - Purpose, frequency of administration, and side effects of medications ordered by physician for patient to take at home
- When patient is going home to receive total parenteral nutrition as ordered by physician, have family demonstrate how to change tubing and fluid bags, and what to do when problems arise.
- Review the plan for follow-up *to ensure their understanding.*

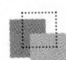

RISK FOR DEFICIENT FLUID VOLUME

Risk for deficient fluid volume is a state in which an individual is at risk for experiencing vascular, extracellular, or intracellular dehydration.[5]

Risk Factors[2,4-6,8]

Altered intake
Excessive loss through diarrhea, vomiting, diaphoresis
Excessive loss through drainage
Extremes of age
Extremes of weight
Inability to access, take in, or absorb fluids
Increased urinary output
Lack of knowledge of adequate intake of fluids
Medications
Metabolic states
Psychotic state

Expected Patient Outcomes and Nursing Interventions With Rationale[1,3,6,7]

Maintain fluid and electrolyte balance, as evidenced by:
Stable weight
Vital signs within normal limits
Elastic skin turgor
Moist mucous membranes
Balanced intake and output
Sodium and potassium levels within normal limits

- Weigh patient and compare with previous values.
- Measure vital signs. Observe for hypotension, includin postural hypotension, elevated pulse, and fever.
- Measure intake and compare with output.
- Monitor electrolytes, especially potassium, sodium, an magnesium.
- Assess oral mucous membranes, *which may become dr from fluid loss.*

- Assess skin turgor (*skin may lose its elasticity and become tented with fluid loss*).
- If patient can have oral fluids, keep fluids at the bedside within patient's reach and encourage fluid intake.
- If patient is unable to take oral fluids, use other routes: intravenous (crystalloids, colloids, or total parenteral nutrition), nasogastric, or gastrostomy.
- Provide oral care *to moisten the mucous membranes.*
- Provide skin care *to replace moisture to the skin.*
- Administer medications (e.g., antiemetics, antidiarrheals, or antipyretics) as ordered *to prevent fluid loss.*
- Evaluate therapeutic, side, and adverse effects of medications.

Communicate knowledge of fluid balance, as evidenced by patient and family explaining:

Actions to prevent actual loss
Foods and fluids to consume
Foods and fluids to avoid
Medications and treatments for home use
Plan for follow-up care

- Assess what patient and family already know.
- Provide information to prevent a fluid deficit:
  - Over-the-counter antiemetics or antidiarrheals
  - Actions to use to prevent actual deficit
  - Reasons for treatments
  - What foods and fluids to consume
  - What foods and fluids to avoid

Family members need to know the types of fluid replacements to use. For example, milk and milk products should be withheld from individuals with diarrhea. Clear liquids, such as ginger ale, apple juice, beef broth, and popsicles, are the fluids of choice. Family members need to know the purpose, frequency of administration, and side effects of medications to be taken. They can keep a record of the intake and output to evaluate fluid balance.

Excess Fluid Volume

Excess fluid volume is a state in which an individual experiences increased isotonic fluid retention.[7]

Related Factors[7]

Compromised regulatory mechanisms
Excessive fluid intake
Excessive sodium intake
Ineffective heart pump
Renal insufficiency

Defining Characteristics[2-4,6-8]

Altered electrolytes
Anasarca
Anxiety
Ascites
Auscultation of S_3 heart sound
Blood pressure alterations
Central venous pressure changes
Change in mental status
Change in respirations
Crackles
Decreased hemoglobin and hematocrit
Edema
Increased jugular vein distention
Intake greater than output
Oliguria
Orthopnea
Pulmonary congestion on x-ray
Pulmonary wedge pressure changes
Restlessness
Shortness of breath
Urine specific gravity changes
Weight gain
Wheezes

Expected Patient Outcomes and Nursing Interventions With Rationale[1,4-6,9]

Regain fluid balance, as evidenced by:

Stable weight
Absence of edema
Intake equal to output
Clear breath sounds
Vital signs within normal limits

- Measure vital signs. *Observe for hypertension and a full bounding pulse.*
- Measure central venous pressure or pulmonary capillary wedge pressure; note increases in pressures.
- Weigh patient *to monitor fluid balance,* note weight gains *that may represent fluid excess.*
- Measure intake and output; note increase in intake or decrease in output.
- Assess mental status; *confusion, irritability, depression, and restlessness result from decreased sodium;* ensure safety of patient.
- Auscultate lungs for breath sounds; *crackles indicate fluid in alveoli, which may be caused by left-sided heart failure.* Dyspnea also may be observed.
- Auscultate heart sounds for S_3, ventricular gallop.
- Assess for ascites by measuring abdominal girth, presence of shifting dullness on percussion of the abdomen, or fluid wave on palpation of the abdomen.
- Palpate for edema in feet and lower legs when patient is sitting or walking, and sacral area if patient is confined to bed; observe for jugular vein distention; *these may be indications of right-sided heart failure.*
- Monitor laboratory data for lowered values from hemodilution (e.g., hemoglobin, hematocrit, sodium, potassium, magnesium, albumin, blood urea nitrogen, creatinine, serum osmolarity, urine osmolarity).
- Restrict fluids and sodium as ordered.
- Alleviate thirst with tart candy or chewing gum.
- Administer diuretics, inotropics, or colloids as ordered.
- Encourage range-of-motion exercises, either passive or active.
- Assist patient to change positions, and provide skin care *to prevent skin breakdown.*
- Apply elastic stockings and support edematous extremities with pillows *to prevent venous stasis.*
- Position patient in semi-Fowler's position and administer oxygen as ordered when breathing becomes labored as a

result of fluid in the lungs *to improve respirations and oxygenation.*
- Assist with activities of daily living *to conserve patient energy.*

Communicate knowledge of self-care, as evidenced by:
Patient and family explain reasons for fluid volume excess and symptoms of recurrence
Makes dietary alterations; understands medications and treatments for home use
Plans for follow-up care
- Assess knowledge of patient and family regarding cause, treatment, and prevention of fluid volume excess.
- Provide instruction as needed related to:
  Preventing further fluid volume excesses
  Reasons for any dietary alterations and how to implement them
  The therapeutic use of medications, along with dosage, time of administration, and side effects
  Symptoms to watch for indicating a recurrence of the fluid volume excess
  Plan for follow-up care

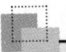

RISK FOR IMBALANCED FLUID VOLUME

Risk for imbalanced fluid volume is a risk of a decrease, increase, or rapid shift from one to the other of intravascular, interstitial, and/or intracellular fluid. It refers to the loss of or excess of intravascular, interstitial, and/or intracellular fluid. It refers to the loss or excess or both of body fluids or replacement fluids.[5]

Risk Factors[5]

Surgical procedures
Syndrome of inappropriate antidiuretic hormone secretion
Uncontrolled diabetes insipidus

Expected Patient Outcomes and Nursing Interventions With Rationale[1-4,6,7]

Maintain balanced fluid volume, as evidenced by:
Clear lung sounds
Blood pressure, pulse, and respirations maintained within normal range
Hemodynamic findings within normal ranges
Urine output of a minimum of 30 ml per hour
- Monitor for excessive or inadequate use of blood, blood products, intravenous fluids, irrigation fluids, and volume expanders.
- Monitor fluid loss, especially in patients who have coexisting diseases, artificial urinary drainage systems, severe or persistent vomiting and diarrhea, or excessive bleeding, *which may result in hypovolemic shock.*
- Monitor blood pressure, pulse, and respirations, noting abnormal findings of decreased blood pressure; weak, thready, rapid pulse; and an increase in respiratory rate, *which indicate a loss of fluid volume through hemorrhage, shock, or third-spacing, or in response to metabolic acidosis.*
- Monitor lung sounds, noting crackles and wheezes. Assess for dyspnea, cyanosis, decreased skin turgor, and pulmonary edema. *These manifestations indicate a fluid overload, with possible left ventricular failure.*
- Monitor the rate of intravenous fluid administration, pulses, and jugular vein distention. Use a microdrip and infusion pump for patients at risk for fluid volume excess. *Fluid overload may be manifested by full, bounding pulses and jugular vein distention. Other manifestations include increased respiratory rate, tachycardia, either hypotension or hypertension, and edema.*
- Monitor trends in central venous pressure (CVP) *to determine the presence of a fluid deficit or excess. CVP is the pressure of blood in the right atrium or vena cava, and provides information about blood volume, vascular tone, and the effectiveness of the heart as a pump.*
- Monitor hemodynamic values, with normal readings as follows:[2]

Pulmonary artery systolic	20 to 30 mm Hg
Pulmonary artery diastolic	12 mm Hg
Mean pulmonary artery	20 mm Hg
Pulmonary artery wedge pressure	4 to 12 mm Hg
Right atrium	2-6 mm Hg
Right ventricle	20 to 30 mm Hg (systolic)
	2 to 6 mm Hg (end diastolic)

Hemodynamic monitoring allows early recognition of cardiogenic shock or altered fluid volume balance and provides information about the patient's response to drugs used during surgery or treatment.
- Monitor urinary output, and compare intake with output. *Urinary output is one of the most valuable indicators of the adequacy of renal perfusion.*

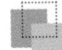

EFFECTIVE BREASTFEEDING

Effective breastfeeding is the state in which a mother-infant dyad or family exhibits adequate proficiency and satisfaction with breastfeeding process.[5]

Related Factors[5]

Basic breastfeeding knowledge
Infant gestational age greater than 34 weeks
Maternal confidence
Normal breast structure
Normal infant oral structure
Support source

Defining Characteristics[5]

Adequate infant elimination patterns for age
Appropriate infant weight for age
Effective mother/infant communication patterns
Infant eager to nurse
Infant content after feeding
Mother positions infant to promote a successful latch-on response
Regular and sustained infant suckling and swallowing
Signs and/or symptoms of oxytocin release
Verbalized satisfaction with the breastfeeding process

Expected Patient Outcomes and Nursing Interventions With Rationale[4]

Maintain breastfeeding, as evidenced by:

Infant gains weight appropriately

Mother expresses satisfaction with breastfeeding

(In addition to the breastfeeding interventions and rationale described under Ineffective Breastfeeding, the following interventions and activities may be used.)

- Provide lactation counseling.[4]
  - Determine knowledge base about breastfeeding.
  - Educate parent(s) about infant feedings for informed decision making.
  - Provide information about advantages and disadvantages of breastfeeding.
  - Correct misconceptions, misinformation, and inaccuracies about breastfeeding.
  - Determine mother's desire and motivation to breastfeed.
  - Provide support of mother's decision.
  - Give parent(s) recommended educational material, as needed.
  - Inform parent(s) about appropriate classes or groups for breastfeeding (e.g., La Leche League).
  - Evaluate mother's understanding of infant's feeding cues (e.g., rooting, sucking, and alertness).
  - Determine frequency of feedings in relationship to baby's needs.
  - Monitor maternal skill with latching infant to the nipple.
  - Evaluate newborn suck/swallow pattern.
  - Demonstrate suck training, as appropriate.
  - Instruct on relaxation techniques, including breast massage.
  - Encourage ways of increasing rest, including delegation of household tasks and suggest ways of requesting help.
  - Instruct on record keeping of length and frequency of nursing sessions.
  - Instruct about infant stool and urination patterns, as appropriate.
  - Evaluate adequacy of breast emptying with feeding.
  - Evaluate quality and use of breastfeeding aids.
  - Determine appropriateness of breastfeeding aids.
  - Determine appropriateness of breast pump use.
  - Provide formula information for temporary low supply problems.
  - Monitor skin integrity of nipples.
  - Recommend nipple care, as needed.
  - Monitor ability to correctly relieve breast congestion.
  - Evaluate understanding of plugged milk ducts and mastitis.
  - Instruct on problems to report to health-care practitioner.
  - Instruct on how to relactate, as appropriate.
  - Encourage continued lactation on return to work or school.
  - Discuss signs of readiness to wean.
  - Discuss options for weaning.
  - Discuss alternative methods of feeding.
  - Instruct about contraception.

INEFFECTIVE BREASTFEEDING

Ineffective breastfeeding is the state in which a mother, infant, or child experiences dissatisfaction or difficulty with the breastfeeding process.[5]

Related Factors[5,8,9]

Breast engorgement
Inadequate letdown
Infant anomaly
Interruption in breastfeeding
Knowledge deficit
Maternal anxiety or ambivalence
Maternal breast anomaly
Nipple soreness or cracks
Nonsupportive partner or family
Poor infant sucking reflex
Prematurity
Previous breast surgery
Previous history of breastfeeding failure
Supplemental feedings with artificial nipple

Defining Characteristics[5]

Actual or perceived inadequate milk supply
Arching and crying at the breast
Fussiness and crying within the first hour after breastfeeding
Inability to attach correctly
Insufficient emptying of each breast per feeding
Insufficient opportunity for breast suckling
No observable signs of oxytocin release
Nonsustained suckling at the breast
Observable signs of inadequate infant intake
Resistance to latching on

Expected Patient Outcomes and Nursing Interventions With Rationale[1-4,6,7,10]

Be able to satisfactorily breastfeed, as evidenced by:

Infant gains weight appropriately.

Mother expresses satisfaction with and continues breastfeeding.

- Assess the breasts and nipples *to determine presence or absence of related factors that may interfere with breastfeeding.*
- Assess maternal knowledge and understanding of breastfeeding *to individualize teaching.*
- Assess support person network *because social support is an important factor in successful breastfeeding.*
- Discourage supplemental bottle feedings, *which can interfere with the baby's desire to breastfeed and increase the risk of allergies in the baby.*
- Provide information to the mother about the proper techniques of breastfeeding:
  - Wash the hands before beginning to feed the baby *to prevent transmission of pathogens.*
  - Put the newborn to breast as soon as possible after birth *to stimulate the letdown reflex, which triggers*

the flow of milk. The letdown reflex is the contraction of the mammary glands, forcing milk forward into the nipples, in response to the release of oxytocin from the posterior pituitary gland. This reflex is triggered by the infant sucking at the breast, by the sound of a baby crying, or by the mother thinking about the baby.

Position the baby so his or her entire body is turned toward the breast.

Hold the breast with the thumb on the upper portion and the rest of the fingers cupping the breast. Lightly stroke the baby's lips with the nipple.

Direct the nipple straight into the baby's mouth, including as much of the areola as possible *so that as the infant sucks, the ducts under the areola (where milk is stored) are compressed by the baby's jaws.*

Do not set limits on the amount of time the baby should nurse; hold the baby at one breast as long as the baby is sucking well; when the breast is empty, gently burp the baby and switch to the second breast. *It may take up to 3 minutes for the letdown reflex to occur.*

Alternate the breast offered first at each feeding.

Lift the breast slightly or compress the breast tissue away from the baby's face during feeding *to prevent blocking the flow of air into the baby's nose.*

Break suction before removing the baby from the breast by inserting a finger into the baby's mouth next to the nipple *to prevent trauma to the nipple.*

After feeding, wash the nipples with warm water *to prevent milk from drying on the breast and causing soreness. Soap is drying, and should not be used.*

During the first few days, nurse every 1½ to 3 hours *to ensure a good supply of milk and prevent trauma to the nipple from too vigorous sucking by a hungry baby.*

Encourage feeding on demand.

Drink four to six 8-ounce glasses of fluid each day, and increase caloric intake by about 500 calories per day *to maintain a milk supply.*

Consult a health-care provider or lactation specialist if problems occur.

- Provide information to women with nipple inversion:

  Use special exercises or breast shields *to increase nipple protractility.*

  Apply ice to nipple a few minutes before beginning breastfeeding *to improve nipple erection.*

  Use a breast pump before beginning breastfeeding *to increase nipple prominence.*

- Provide information to women with inadequate letdown:

  Massage breasts before beginning breastfeeding *to move milk down through the lactiferous sinuses.*

  Feed the baby in a quiet, private place.

  Take a warm shower or apply warm packs to the breasts before beginning breastfeeding *to relax and stimulate letdown.*

  Drink water, juice, or a beverage without caffeine before and during breastfeeding.

  Avoid overfatigue by resting when the baby slee breastfeeding lying down, and having quiet ti alone.

  Allow the baby at least 10 to 15 minutes per side *trigger the letdown reflex.*

  Use breast-alternating methods by either using a d ferent breast for each feeding or switch brea several times during a single feeding.

- Provide information to women with sore nipples:

  Make sure baby is positioned correctly.

  Change breastfeeding positions and/or altern breasts several times with each feeding.

  Do not let the baby sleep with the nipple in his or h mouth *to avoid trauma to the nipple.*

  Break suction with a finger before removing the ba from the breast.

  Nurse more frequently.

  Apply ice to nipples and areola a few minutes befo beginning breastfeeding.

  Clean nipples with warm water, and allow nipples air dry.

  Use ventilated shields if clothing rubs nipples.

  Change breast pads frequently.

  Nurse long enough to completely empty the breast

- Provide information to women with cracked nipples:

  Use interventions as for sore nipples.

  Temporarily stop nursing on the affected breast a hand express milk until cracks heal.

  Maintain a balanced diet with adequate protein a vitamin C *to promote healing.*

  Consult a health-care provider if signs of infecti occur.

- Provide information to women with breast engorgeme and/or plugged ducts:

  Nurse every 1½ to 3 hours around the clock.

  Wear a well-fitted support bra at all times.

  Take a warm shower or apply warm compresses *trigger letdown.*

  Massage breasts and then hand express some milk *soften breasts.*

  Breastfeed long enough to empty breasts.

  Alternate starting breast.

  Maintain good nutrition and an adequate fluid intak

INTERRUPTED BREASTFEEDING

Interrupted breastfeeding is a break in the continuity of th breastfeeding process as a result of inability or inadvisability put baby to breast for feeding.[3]

Related Factors[3]

Contraindications to breastfeeding
Maternal employment
Maternal or infant illness
Need to abruptly wean infant
Prematurity

Defining Characteristics[3]

Lack of knowledge regarding expression and storage of brea milk
Maternal desire to maintain and provide breast milk
Separation of mother and infant

Expected Patient Outcomes and Nursing Interventions With Rationale[1,2,4-6]

Demonstrate effective methods of breast milk collection and storage, as evidenced by:

Mother verbalizes knowledge of expression and storage of her breast milk

- Assess mother's desire to continue breastfeeding, feasibility of resuming breastfeeding, and infant's ability to breastfeed. *Maternal desire to continue breastfeeding is associated with breastfeeding success; some conditions (such as infant cleft palate) may preclude breastfeeding; the infant must demonstrate the ability to breastfeed for resumption following an interruption.*
- Assess the mother's knowledge of and ability to perform techniques of breast milk expression.
- Teach the mother how to collect breast milk:
  - Prepare the breasts with warm soaks, light massage, and gentle stroking *to maximize the production of milk.*
  - Wash hands carefully before beginning to express milk *to prevent contamination of milk.*
  - Place the plastic milk-collecting bottle just under the nipple of the right breast. Have the woman place her right hand on her right breast with her right thumb on the top of the breast on the edge of the areola and the fingers of that hand under the breast. Using the fingers, press inward toward the chest wall and slide the hand forward in a milking motion. Move the thumb and fingers around the breast, repeating the technique. Repeat for the left breast. *Collecting bottles should be clean and made of plastic to preserve antibodies in the milk. Milk is expressed by pressure on the collecting ducts.*
  - Discuss using a breast pump if manual expression is difficult, considering factors of ease of use, efficiency, potential for breast trauma, and cost. *The pump should be clean, free of contamination, easy to use, and capable of completely emptying the breast. It should not cause trauma to the breast.*
    - Begin slowly, increasing time over the first week.
    - Express milk on a regular basis, at least five times in 24 hours, and pump a total of at least 100 minutes per day. *Milk forms in response to being used; if the breasts are completely empty they will completely fill again*
    - Refrigerate the milk if it will be used in 24 hours, or freeze the milk if it will be used at a later time. *Breast milk, like cow's milk, will spoil if it is not refrigerated or frozen.*

Ineffective Infant Feeding Pattern

Ineffective infant feeding pattern is a state in which an infant demonstrates an impaired ability to suck or coordinate the suck/swallow response.[5]

Related Factors[5]

Anatomic abnormality
Neurologic impairment or delay
Oral hypersensitivity
Prematurity
Prolonged NPO

Defining Characteristics[5]

Inability to coordinate sucking, swallowing, and breathing
Inability to initiate or sustain an effective suck

Expected Patient Outcomes and Nursing Interventions With Rationale[1-4,6]

Be able to effectively suck and coordinate the suck/swallow response, as evidenced by:

Gains weight appropriately
Progresses to a normal feeding pattern

- Assess infant's root, gag, suck, and swallow reflexes *to determine if infant has the necessary oral reflexes for successful oral feeding.*
- Assess the infant's feeding patterns and weight gain, including feeding volume, duration, and effort during feeding; respiratory rate and effort; signs of fatigue during or after feeding; weight gain, and trends in intake and output (including number and type of stools and number of wet diapers).
- Assess the infant's environment during feeding and minimize bright lights and noise *to decrease physiologic stress.*
- Monitor intravenous fluids as prescribed, *which are used to prevent hypoglycemia and supply fluids until respirations have stabilized.*
- Provide gavage feedings, preferably of the mother's milk, as prescribed for infants born before 32 to 34 weeks gestation *because the gag reflex is not intact and the infant is unable to coordinate sucking and swallowing before this time.*
- Offer a pacifier during gavage feedings. *Nonnutritive sucking helps strengthen the gag reflex, prepares the infant for bottle feeding, provides oral satisfaction, and helps the infant remember how to suck.*
- Aspirate, measure, and replace stomach secretions before each feeding. Report stomach contents of more than 2 ml. *Stomach secretions of more than 2 ml before a feeding indicate the infant is receiving more formula than can be digested in the time allowed. Feedings may be cut back to ensure better digestion and decrease the risk of regurgitation and aspiration.*
- Initiate breastfeeding if at all possible, using milk expressed by the mother, as soon as possible.
- Initiate nipple feeding when the infant is in a quiet-alert state, and allow appropriate time for nipple feeding.
- Monitor infant's weight gain and caloric intake, *which is necessary for metabolism, activity, digestion, and growth.*
- Encourage parent(s) to take part in feeding process *to promote bonding and psychosocial development of the infant and family members.*
- Teach parents methods of infant feeding.

- Refer, as appropriate, to a neonatal nutritionist, physical or occupational therapist, or lactation specialist.

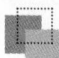

HYPERTHERMIA

Hyperthermia is a state in which an individual's body temperature is elevated above normal body temperature range.[4]

Related Factors[2,4,5]

Dehydration
Illness or trauma
Inability to perspire
Inappropriate clothing
Increased metabolic rate
Infection
Medications/anesthesia
Prolonged exposure to hot environment
Vigorous activity

Defining Characteristics[2,4]

Body temperature above normal range
Flushed, warm skin
Increased respiratory rate
Seizures
Tachycardia

Expected Patient Outcomes and Nursing Interventions With Rationale[1-3]

Regain normal body temperature, as evidenced by:
Body temperature within normal range

- Measure core body temperature.
- Assess for shivering and complaint of chills.
- Assess neurologic status: level of consciousness, mental status, motor and sensory status.
- Assess for signs of hyperthermia: visual disturbances, headache, nausea and vomiting, muscle flaccidity, hot, dry skin, delirium, seizures.
- Assess heart rate and rhythm for abnormalities.
- Monitor respirations. *Hyperventilation may occur initially, but ventilation may be impaired by seizures and hypermetabolic state.*
- Inspect and palpate skin for color and temperature.
- Monitor complete blood count, especially leukocytes, hemoglobin, and hematocrit.
- Administer antipyretics as ordered *to reduce fever.*
- Promote surface cooling by removal of clothing and use of fans.
- When fever is over 104° F (40° C) use alcohol, tepid baths, immersion, or local ice packs to groin and axilla.
- Use hypothermia blanket when patient's temperature is greater than 105° F (40.5° C) or when fever is caused by hypothalamic dysfunction.
- Administer medication (e.g., diazepam, chlorpromazine) *to control shivering and seizures.*
- Administer supplemental oxygen as ordered.
- Administer medications (e.g., antibiotics for infections, dantrolene for malignant hyperthermia, beta-blockers for thyroid storm) *to treat underlying conditions.*
- Administer fluids and electrolytes orally or parenterally.
- Encourage frequent rest periods *to decrease metabo demand.*
- Provide a high calorie diet.
- Provide frequent oral hygiene.
- Teach patient and family the value of fever (up to an o temperature of 104° F [40° C]) in increasing immu system function.
- Teach use of antipyretics as most effective way to redu fever to below 104° F (40° C) when caused by infecti or inflammation.
- Teach use of nondrug methods to reduce fever.
- Discuss importance of adequate fluids *to prevent deh dration.*
- Review signs and symptoms of hyperthermia and wh to call physician.

HYPOTHERMIA

Hypothermia is the state in which an individual's body tempera ture is reduced below normal range.[6]

Related Factors[2,6]

Aging
Consumption of alcohol
Decreased metabolic rate
Illness or trauma
Inability to shiver
Malnutrition
Prolonged exposure to cold environment

Defining Characteristics[3,6]

Cool skin
Cyanotic nail beds
Pallor
Piloerection
Shivering
Slow capillary refill
Tachycardia

Expected Patient Outcomes and Nursing Interventions With Rationale[1-5]

Regain normal body temperature, as evidenced by:
Oral temperature of 98.6° F

- Assess temperature using low-recording thermometer necessary.
- Monitor heart rate, respiration, and blood pressure for ir creases *as the patient's temperature rises.*
- Monitor signs of hypothermia: shivering, cool skin, pil erection, pallor, slow capillary refill, cyanotic nail bed decreased mentation.
- Monitor arterial blood gases *for respiratory acidosis.*
- Auscultate lungs *for crackles and rhonchi.*
- Control shivering when patient has cerebral edema.
- Perform passive warming (e.g., set room temperatur between 70° F and 75° F (21.1° C to 24.0° C), laye clothing and blankets, cover patient's head with a ca or towel); allow patient to rewarm at his or her ow pace.
- Perform active rewarming: cover patient with warme cotton blankets or a forced warm air blanket; use radiar

heat lights as available. As ordered, apply hydrothermic blankets, administer heated and humidified oxygen, and carefully administer heated intravenous fluids.
- Perform active core rewarming techniques as ordered (e.g., colonic lavage, hemodialysis, peritoneal lavage, extracorporeal blood rewarming, bladder irrigations).

Passive rewarming prevents heat loss via radiation and evaporation. Head cover is important because 60% of body heat is lost through the top of the head. Gradual rewarming limits complications associated with hypothermia. Active rewarming enhances heat gain by radiation, conduction, convection, and evaporation, whereas active core rewarming techniques increase heat gain by conduction.

RISK FOR IMBALANCED BODY TEMPERATURE

Risk for imbalanced body temperature is a state in which an individual is at risk for failure to maintain body temperature within normal range.[5]

Risk Factors[2,5,6]

Dehydration
Exposure to extremes of environmental temperature
Extremes of age
Extremes of weight
Illness or trauma affecting temperature regulation
Inactivity or vigorous activity
Inappropriate clothing for environmental temperature
Medications

Expected Patient Outcomes and Nursing Interventions With Rationale[1-4]

Maintain normal body temperature, as evidenced by:
Body temperature within normal limits
Demonstrates behaviors for monitoring and maintaining body temperature

- Monitor vital signs: temperature, pulse, blood pressure, and respiratory rate.
- Monitor laboratory data (e.g., leukocytes) suggestive of infection or inflammation.
- Determine cause of risk for altered temperature.
- Assess patient for signs of hypothermia: cool skin, piloerection, pallor, slow capillary refill, cyanotic nail beds, decreased mentation.
- Assess patient for hyperthermia: visual disturbances; headache; nausea and vomiting; muscle flaccidity; hot, dry skin; delirium.
- Adjust bedding and clothing as appropriate for patient's temperature.
- Administer antipyretics as ordered *to lower elevated body temperature.*
- Apply external cooling measures, cooling blankets, ice packs to groin and axilla *to lower elevated body temperature.*
- Provide adequate nutrition and fluid. Administer intravenous fluids at room temperature.
- Teach family members how to recognize signs of changing temperature and interventions to maintain expected temperatures.

INEFFECTIVE THERMOREGULATION

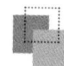

Ineffective thermoregulation is a state in which an individual's temperature fluctuates between hypothermia and hyperthermia.[3]

Related Factors[1,3,4,5]

Aging
Fluctuating environmental temperature
Prematurity
Trauma or illness

Defining Characteristics[3]

Body temperature fluctuates between hypothermia and hyperthermia

Expected Patient Outcomes and Nursing Interventions With Rationale[1,2,6]

Maintain normal body temperature, as evidenced by:
Body temperature within normal range

- Assess neurologic status: level of consciousness, mental status, motor and sensory status. *Changes in neurologic status may be evident as thermoregulation changes, with lethargy associated with hypothermia and delirium associated with hyperthermia.*
- Assess vital signs: temperature, pulse, blood pressure, and respirations. *Changes in vital signs reflect the body temperature, with a decrease in heart rate, blood pressure, temperature, and respiration during hypothermia and an increase in vital signs during hyperthermia. Monitoring of signs of hypothermia and hyperthermia may help to determine the cause of the thermoregulatory imbalance.*
- Assess for signs of hypothermia: difficult arousal, irritability, lethargy, cyanotic nail beds, slow capillary refill time, pallor, cool skin, bradycardia. Additional signs for premature infant: poor feeding, increase or decrease in spontaneous activity, weak cry, decreased muscle tone.
- Assess for signs of hyperthermia: visual disturbances; headache; nausea and vomiting; muscle flaccidity; hot, dry skin; delirium.
- Adjust bedding and clothing as appropriate for patient's temperature.
- Adjust environmental temperature to infant's needs using an incubator or radiant warmer; avoid drafts and cold environments; keep infant clothed in undershirt, diaper, gown, and hat.
- Administer intravenous fluids at room temperature.
- Administer electrolytes and medications as ordered *to restore or maintain body function.*
- Teach family members how to recognize signs of changing temperature and interventions *to maintain expected temperatures.*

IMBALANCED NUTRITION: LESS THAN BODY REQUIREMENTS

Imbalanced nutrition: less than body requirements is a state in which an individual takes in nutrients insufficient to meet metabolic demands.[12]

Related Factors*

AIDS
Altered level of consciousness
Altered oral mucous membranes
Anorexia nervosa
Bulimia
Cancer; treatment for cancer
Decreased absorption of nutrients (e.g., cirrhosis, cystic fibrosis, celiac disease)
Depression
Difficulty in ingesting sufficient calories
Difficulty in swallowing
Inadequate income
Infection
Medication effects or side effects
Mental disorders
Prematurity
Social isolation
Surgery

Defining Characteristics†

Abdominal pain
Altered ability to taste and/or smell
Amenorrhea
Anorexia
Aversion to eating
Binge-purge cycle
Body weight 20% or more under ideal for height and frame
Chronic sputum production
Decreased midarm circumference
Decreased serum albumin
Decreased serum transferrin or iron-binding capacity
Decreased lymphocyte count
Decreased triceps skinfold
Dry, scaly, inelastic skin
Dysphagia
Electrolyte imbalance
Excessive hair loss
Immediate satiety when eating
Lack of information about nutrition
Lack of interest in eating
Loss of weight with adequate food intake
Painful, inflamed oral cavity
Perceived inability to ingest food

Expected Patient Outcomes and Nursing Interventions With Rationale[2,5-10,15]

Attain adequate nutrition, as evidenced by:
Achieves recommended weight for age, height, and gender
Expected bone and tooth development
Clear skin and eyes
Firm muscles
Triceps skinfold: men, 12.5 mm; women, 16.5 mm
Midarm circumference: men, 29.3 cm; women, 25.8 cm
Serum albumin: 3.5 to 5 g/dl or 53% of total protein
Lymphocytes: 1800 to 3000/mm^3 or 30% of leukocytes
Prompt healing
Growth of 3 to 5 inches annually for children
Energy to perform activities of daily living

- Weigh patient *to establish a baseline against which the outcome can be measured.*
- Auscultate bowel sounds *to determine the presence of peristalsis.*
- Assess for possible causes of inadequate nutrition: nausea, vomiting, fatigue, mouth pain, tooth decay, loose teeth, bleeding gums, sores in mouth, dry mouth, ill-fitting dentures, inability to taste or swallow. Make referrals as needed for evaluation and treatment.
- Monitor daily calorie count *to determine calorie intake.*
- Assess skinfold measurements: *triceps skinfolds reflect fat stores; midarm circumference reflects protein stores.*
- Monitor serum albumin and leukocytes: *low values may be indicators of malnutrition.*
- Reduce nausea and pain as ordered before patient's meals.
- Determine number and type of medications patient takes.
- Provide nutrients: proteins (including albumin), carbohydrates, fats, vitamins (A, B complex, C, and K), and minerals (iron, zinc, and copper).
- Provide foods in the form appropriate for patient: general diet, mechanical soft, blenderized, formula via nasogastric or gastrostomy tube, or total parenteral nutrition via subclavian vein as ordered by physician.
- Consider patient's food preferences as governed by personal choices and cultural and religious preferences.
- Provide oral care before meals *to moisten and refresh mucous membranes and tongue.*
- Provide rest before meals if fatigue interferes with eating.
- When patient feeds self:
  - Serve food at its appropriate temperature.
  - Ensure patient is comfortable and can reach necessary utensils for eating.
  - Provide adaptive/assistive devices.
- When patient is fed by mouth:
  - Serve food at its appropriate temperature.
  - Ensure patient is comfortable.
  - Allow patient sufficient time between bites.
  - Talk with patient during the meal.
- When patient is fed by nasogastric (NG) or nasoduodenal tube:
  - Ensure proper placement of tube.
  - Add blue or green food coloring to feeding *to detect aspiration.*
  - Ensure feeding at room temperature.
  - Flush tube periodically with full-strength cranberry juice or cola followed by water *to prevent obstruction.*
- When nasogastric tube is used:
  - Aspirate gastric contents *to determine amount of the last feeding still in stomach.*
  - If aspirated contents is less than 50 ml, proceed with the feeding.
- When continuous feeding is used:
  - Refill feeding bag every 4 hours.
  - Check gravity drip rate or pump rate every hour.
- When patient is fed by total parenteral nutrition:

---

*References 1, 4, 5, 9, 12, 13.
†References 1, 3, 4, 11, 12, 14.

Check infusion rate every hour or infusion pump rate every hour.
Monitor blood glucose and urinary glucose and acetone every 6 hours *to detect hyperglycemia:* treat hyperglycemia with insulin as ordered.
Change dressing daily using sterile technique *to prevent infection;* inspect insertion site for redness and edema.
Monitor temperature every 4 hours *to detect fever.*

Identify factors that contribute to inadequate nutritional intake, as evidenced by:

Identifies strategies to improve nutrition
Uses referrals to health team members as needed

- Problem-solve with patient and family to identify socioeconomic factors contributing to inadequate nutrition.
- Determine with patient and family appropriate strategies to use to solve problems (e.g., lack of money or transportation).
- Use referrals to other members of the health-care team as needed (dietitian, social worker, community health nurse).
- Discuss with patient perceptions of factors interfering with ability or desire to eat.
- Assess for eating disorders (e.g., anorexia nervosa and bulimia nervosa).
- Assess for depression.
- Discuss with patient strategies useful to improve nutrition.
- Refer patient for additional therapy as needed.

Gain knowledge of nutritional needs, as evidenced by patient and family explaining:

Reason for altered nutrition
Actions to avoid it
Types of menus to be used
Any necessary dietary alterations (foods to include and avoid)
Community agencies to be contacted for assistance
Medication program to be followed: state dosage, action, and side effects of prescribed drugs; over-the-counter drugs to avoid

- Assess learning needs of patient and family.
- Determine their understanding of the reason for altered nutrition.
- Teach types of menus to be used.
- Teach foods to avoid.
- Determine their understanding of the plan for follow-up treatment.
- Teach them reason for vitamin and mineral supplements to be taken.
- Provide them with names and phone numbers of personnel in community agencies.

To maintain weight gain, patients and families need a follow-up plan that will support their independence in making appropriate lifestyle changes to maintain adequate weight. Interactive teaching styles that encourage active participation of patients and family contribute to more positive outcomes.

IMBALANCED NUTRITION: MORE THAN BODY REQUIREMENTS

Imbalanced nutrition: more than body requirements is a state in which an individual takes in nutrients that exceed metabolic needs.[11]

Related Factors[11]

Excessive intake in relation to metabolic need

Defining Characteristics*

Concentrating food intake at the end of the day
Eating in response to cues other than hunger
Eating in response to external cues
Pairing food consumption with other activities
Sedentary activity level
Triceps skinfold more than 15 mm in men and 25 mm in women
Weight 20% greater than ideal for height and frame

Expected Patient Outcomes and Nursing Interventions With Rationale[3,6-9]

Attain optimum weight for age, height, and gender, as evidenced by:

Verbalizes desire to attain optimum weight
Establishes short-term and long-term weight loss goals
Maintains a food diary
Verbalizes understanding of proper nutrition while losing weight
Uses support people and support groups in following plan for weight loss

- Weigh patient *to establish a baseline against which the outcome can be measured.*
- Determine patient's desire to reduce body weight, *because this is a strong motivating factor.*
- Assess patient's knowledge of the hazards of obesity, and provide information as necessary.
- Determine patient's recommended body weight for age, height, and gender *to establish a realistic outcome.*
- Assess patient's triceps skinfold measurements, *which indicate fat stores.*
- Establish with the patient a realistic plan to include reduced food intake and increased energy expenditure. A goal of 1 to 2 pounds per week weight loss is a suggested starting point.
- Analyze with the patient reasons for past failures at weight loss *so that these might be avoided or reduced.*
- Ask the patient to keep a diary of what, when, where, and with whom he or she eats and the hunger level and feelings at the time, *to evaluate changes that need to be made in lifestyle.*
- Ask the patient to post the goal for weight loss in a strategic location so that it will be remembered. The refrigerator or pantry door is a common location selected, *so the patient can be reminded of the goal when tempted to eat additional calories.*
- Discuss eating a balanced diet using as a guide the Food Guide Pyramid (see FIG. 23-1) or counting calories or fat grams, *so that nutritional needs can be maintained during weight loss.*
- Reward patient for attaining short-term goals, and encourage patient to use an internal reward system when goals are accomplished.

*References 1, 2, 4, 6, 11, 12.

- Ask patient to identify people from whom support can be sought, and provide a list of support groups for weight loss.

Communicate what is required to maintain optimum body weight, as evidenced by:

Verbalizes reason for obesity
Designs a dietary plan for weight reduction
Follows an exercise plan for weight reduction
Plans for follow-up care

- Discuss ways to maintain optimum weight by evaluating the lifestyle changes that have occurred and strategies to maintain them.
- Set a plan for follow-up monitoring of weight maintenance.
- Provide guidance in developing an exercise program as an adjunct to the diet plan *to facilitate weight loss.*[5,10]

Risk For Imbalanced Nutrition: More Than Body Requirements

Risk for imbalanced nutrition: more than body requirements is a state in which an individual is at risk of taking in nutrients that exceed metabolic needs.[4]

Risk Factors[2,4,5]

Concentrating food intake at the end of the day
Dysfunctional psychologic conditioning in relation to food
Eating in response to cues other than hunger
Eating in response to external cues
Excessive food intake during early infancy, adolescence, and middle age
Frequent, closely spaced pregnancies
Hereditary predisposition
Higher baseline weight at beginning of each pregnancy
Low income
Pairing food consumption with other activities
Parental obesity
Rapid transition across growth percentiles
Using food as a reward or comfort measure
Using solid food as the major food source before 5 months of age

Expected Patient Outcomes and Nursing Interventions With Rationale[1,3,6]

Maintain recommended weight for age, height, and gender as evidenced by:

Verbalizes desire to maintain weight
Follows recommended diet, incorporating sound nutrition (see Fig. 23-1)

- Measure weight and height to calculate body mass index [wt/(ht)²] *to obtain a baseline from which to plan strategies for meeting goals.*
- Calculate growth percentiles for infants and children.
- Discuss the relationship between food intake, exercise, and obesity *so that the patient can understand how decreasing intake and increasing exercise can reduce obesity.*
- Discuss the risks of obesity—increased incidence for diabetes mellitus, hypertension, and atherosclerosis—*so that the patient can learn the potential long-term consequences of being overweight.*
- Determine motivation for changing eating habits *to help in selecting positive rewards for meeting goals to maintain recommended body weight.*
- Determine recommended weight *so that realistic goals can be set.*
- Develop a method for patient to keep daily record of intake *to track progress toward the goals set.*
- Determine with the patient desirable, realistic weekly weight loss goals, *because patient participation improves compliance.*
- Encourage patient to write down realistic weekly goals for food intake and exercise and to display them where they can be reviewed frequently.
- Encourage patient to identify support persons in his or her environment who can give encouragement and support in attaining these goals.
- Determine stressors (job, finances, family, school) and coping mechanisms, sources of social support, and relaxation techniques.

Impaired Dentition

Impaired dentition is a disruption in tooth development or eruption patterns or structural integrity of individual teeth.[4]

Related Factors[1,4]

Barriers to self-care or professional care
Bruxism
Chronic use of tobacco, coffee or tea, red wine
Chronic vomiting (e.g., bulimia)
Dietary habits
Excessive intake of fluorides
Excessive use of abrasive cleaning agents
Genetic predisposition
Ineffective oral hygiene
Nutritional deficits
Premature loss of primary teeth
Selected prescription medications
Trauma

Defining Characteristics[3-5]

Dental caries
Enamel erosion
Excessive plaque or calculus
Halitosis
Incomplete eruption for age
Loose teeth
Malocclusion or tooth misalignment
Missing teeth
Premature loss of primary teeth
Toothache
Tooth enamel discoloration
Tooth fracture(s)
Worn down or abraded teeth

Expected Patient Outcomes and Nursing Interventions With Rationale[2,6,7]

Maintain normal tooth development and eruption patterns and structural integrity of individual teeth, as evidenced by:

Follows proper techniques for oral hygiene
Regularly visits dental provider
Verbalizes nutritional risks for dental caries

- Teach proper oral hygiene measures, including tooth brushing and flossing techniques, *to regain and maintain plaque-free teeth and decrease risk of dental caries.*
- Teach importance of regular dental screenings *to detect and treat developmental or eruption problems, and to detect and provide early treatment for dental problems.*
- Encourage adequate nutrition during pregnancy and childhood *to facilitate normal growth and development of primary and secondary teeth.*
- Teach parents to avoid putting an infant to bed with a bottle of milk or sweetened liquid, to give children water or milk rather than sweet drinks, and to eliminate sweets that are clinging (e.g., taffy or caramel) or have prolonged contact with teeth (e.g., hard candy, chewing gum). *The formation of dental caries in children is associated with a high sugar intake.*
- Refer to a dental professional.

Impaired Oral Mucous Membrane

Impaired oral mucous membrane is a state of disruption of the lips and soft tissue of the oral cavity.[5]

Related Factors[5]

Aging-related loss of connective, adipose, or bone tissue
Barriers to self-care or professional care
Chemotherapy
Cleft lip or palate
Dehydration
Ineffective oral hygiene
Infection
Immunosuppression
Lack of or decreased salivation
Malnutrition or vitamin deficiency
Mechanical (e.g., ill-fitting dentures, braces, endotracheal or nasogastric tubes)
Medication side effects
NPO for more than 24 hours
Radiation therapy
Surgery of the oral cavity
Trauma (e.g., drugs, noxious agents, alcohol, heat)

Defining Characteristics[2,3,5]

Bleeding
Desquamation
Difficult speech
Difficulty eating or swallowing
Diminished or absent taste
Edema
Fissures
Geographic tongue
Gingival hyperplasia
Gingival or mucosal pallor
Gingival recession, pockets deeper than 4 mm
Halitosis
Oral lesions or ulcers
Oral pain or discomfort
Purulent drainage or exudates
Smooth atrophic, sensitive tongue
Stomatitis
White patches or plaques, spongy patches, or curdlike exudate
Xerostomia (dry mouth)

Expected Patient Outcomes and Nursing Interventions With Rationale[1-4]

Intact oral mucous membranes, as evidenced by:

Ability to chew and swallow without difficulty
Moist oral mucous membranes
Absence of halitosis

- Inspect oral cavity daily for inflammation, lesions, discolorations, bleeding, dryness.
- Ask patient to describe usual oral care habits and date of last dental visit. Encourage brushing or cleaning of dentures after meals, daily flossing, and annual dental visits.
- Determine patient's ability to provide own oral care. When providing oral care for patient, avoid use of hydrogen peroxide and lemon and glycerin swabs. Recommended solutions are normal saline or sodium bicarbonate (½ teaspoon sodium bicarbonate, ½ teaspoon salt in 1 quart warm water). Oral care for the unconscious patient is performed with the patient in a side-lying position and the head of the bed elevated at least 30 degrees. Rinsing is done using a large syringe and oral suction. Change position of oral airway or orotracheal tube every 8 hours. *Hydrogen peroxide can damage oral mucosa, is distasteful, and may promote bacterial growth. Lemon in swabs can decalcify teeth, and glycerin contributes to tooth decay.*
- Monitor nutritional and fluid status to determine adequacy.
- Determine if medication (e.g., anticholinergics) side effects could be contributing to dry mouth.
- Discourage smoking and use of alcohol.
- Stimulate saliva with chewing gum or hard candy.

Malnutrition and dehydration predispose patient to altered oral mucous membranes. Side effects of many medications, smoking, and alcohol can cause dry mouth requiring increased efforts to keep mouth moist, such as chewing gum or hard candy. Keeping lips moist may prevent drying and promote comfort.

- Keep lips well lubricated using lanolin or vitamin A and D ointment.
- If patient's platelet count is low or if patient takes an anticoagulant drug, use a soft-bristle brush or Toothette to clean teeth.
- If mouth is severely inflamed use frequent, gentle mouth care.

- Topical anesthetic agent (viscous lidocaine) may be needed *to reduce pain.* Also modify diet to soft, pureed, or liquid *to prevent trauma or pain to mouth.*

Explain self-care, as evidenced by:

Patient and family state reasons for alteration in oral mucous membrane.
Plan for dental hygiene for all family members
Medications and treatment for home use
Plan for follow-up care

- Assess what the patient and family already know.
- Provide information about:
  Reasons for alteration in oral mucous membrane
  Importance of dental hygiene for all family members
  Review of medications and treatments ordered for home use
  Plan for follow-up care

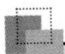

IMPAIRED SKIN INTEGRITY

Impaired skin integrity is a state in which an individual has altered epidermis and/or dermis.[4]

Related Factors[4,5]

Altered circulation
Altered fluid status
Altered immune status
Altered metabolic state
Altered nutritional state (e.g., obesity, emaciation)
Altered sensation
Altered skin turgor
Chemical substances
Extremes of age
Hypothermia or hyperthermia
Immobility
Mechanical forces (e.g., shearing forces, pressure, restraint)
Moisture (from excretions or secretions)
Psychogenic factors
Radiation
Skeletal prominence

NOTE: Risk should be determined by the use of a risk assessment tool (e.g., Braden scale).[1]

Expected Patient Outcomes and Nursing Interventions With Rationale[2,3,6,7]

Intact skin, as evidenced by:

Skin lesion clean and healing

- Assess wound (stage I–IV) and surrounding skin as a baseline. (stages I and II relate to *skin* integrity; Stages III and IV relate to *tissue* integrity.)
- Assess skin for color changes, redness, swelling, warmth, pain, sensation, signs of infection.
- Note odors from skin lesion.
- Monitor patient's continence status and minimize exposure of the site of skin impairment and other areas to moisture from incontinence, perspiration, or wound drainage.
- Monitor laboratory data (e.g., hemoglobin, hematocrit, albumin, glucose, blood urea nitrogen (BUN), creatinine, liver enzymes, arterial blood gases) for evidence of malnutrition or chronic conditions that could affect the skin.
- Note drugs (e.g., corticosteroids) taken by patient and their effect on wound healing.

Laboratory data are monitored to detect abnormalities (e.g., renal failure, liver failure, anemia, diabetes mellitus) that might affect the skin or perfusion. Certain drugs, (e.g., corticosteroids) make the skin more susceptible to impairment. Patients taking these drugs need to be especially protective of their skin.

- Determine attitudes and reactions of patient and significant others to skin lesion.
- Encourage verbalization about feelings and discuss effect of lesion on self-esteem.

A positive mental attitude can improve immune function and increase motivation for healing. Thus discussions of feelings toward skin lesions can further the wound healing efforts.

- Provide wound treatment based on stage and drainage, using gauze, polyurethane film, hydrocolloid, foam, adsorptive dressing, hydrogel, or enzymatic therapy.
- Debride and clean wound as ordered.
- Ambulate patients if possible.
- When in bed turn every 2 hours; use lateral, prone, and dorsal sides if possible.
- Have patient perform active range of motion or instruct family to perform passive range of motion.
- Position off pressure ulcer.
- Use pressure-relieving therapy bed.
- Keep pressure off skeletal prominences by positioning patients with pillows and/or foam devices, or pressure-relieving mattresses.
- Use lifting devices and/or sheets to position patients *to prevent shearing force on skin.*
- Do not massage skin over bony prominences.
- Prevent head of bed from being elevated more than 30 degrees (semi-Fowler's position) for long periods *to prevent pressure on the sacrum.*
- Use underpads or briefs that absorb moisture and leave quick drying surface toward skin if continuously moist.
- Avoid use of donuts or rubber rings.
- Provide adequate nutrition with increased calories and proteins, supplemental iron and vitamin C, and increased fluids (2 to 3 liters per day) *to promote healing.*

Communicate care of impaired skin after discharge and action to prevent recurrence, as evidenced by patient and family explaining:

Cause and prevention of altered skin integrity
Medications and treatment for home use
Dietary intake to promote wound healing
Plan for follow-up care

- Assess what patient and family need to learn.
- Provide information concerning:
  Prevention of skin integrity alterations
  How to change dressing and apply topical medicatio
  Purpose, frequency of administration, and side effect of medication
  Dietary intake to promote wound healing
  How to achieve comfort and relieve pain
  Notification of physician if skin impairmer continues

The nurse instructs the patient and family on actions to prevent skin impairment and to continue treatment of the impaired skin after discharge. Time should be made for the family and patient to perform return demonstrations on dressing changes and to ask questions about the treatment schedule.

RISK FOR IMPAIRED SKIN INTEGRITY

Risk for impaired skin integrity is a state in which an individual's skin is at risk of being adversely altered.[4]

Risk Factors[1,2,4]

Altered circulation
Altered immunity
Altered metabolic state
Altered nutritional state (e.g., obesity, emaciation)
Altered pigmentation
Altered sensation
Altered skin turgor
Chemical substances
Extremes of age
Hypothermia or hyperthermia
Immobility
Mechanical forces (e.g., shearing forces, pressure, restraint)
Moisture (from excretions/secretions)
Psychogenic factors
Radiation
Skeletal prominence
NOTE: Risk should be determined by the use of a risk assessment tool (e.g., Braden scale).

Expected Patient Outcomes and Nursing Interventions With Rationale[3,5,6]

Maintain intact skin, as evidenced by:
Skin dry with natural color
Moist, adequate turgor with intact skin
Reports intake of balanced diet
Patient and family verbalize behaviors required to maintain skin integrity

- Assess patient using a risk assessment scale or by determining the presence of the following risk factors: incontinence, immobility, inactivity, poor nutrition, edema, or diminished sensation.
- Inspect skin daily for reddened areas, bruises, blisters, excoriation, changes in tactile sensation, edema *to identify potential areas of skin breakdown early.*
- Palpate skin for elastic turgor and moisture.
- Monitor laboratory data (e.g., hemoglobin, hematocrit, albumin, glucose, blood urea nitrogen, creatinine, liver enzymes) for evidence of malnutrition or chronic conditions that could affect the skin. *Laboratory values are monitored to detect abnormalities, such as renal failure, liver failure, anemia, or diabetes mellitus, that might affect the skin or perfusion.*
- Monitor drugs (e.g., corticosteroids) taken by patient for effect on skin integrity. *Certain drugs, (e.g., corticosteroids) make the skin more susceptible to impairment. Patients taking these drugs need to be especially protective of their skin.*
- Keep skin clean and dry *to remove bacteria and prevent maceration.*
- Use underpads to absorb moisture and change as needed *to keep moisture away from skin.*
- Lubricate dry skin with lotion.
- Provide balanced diet and adequate fluids, including sufficient calories and proteins for tissue growth.
- When itching is a problem, encourage individuals not to scratch; *pressing the area or applying ice decreases the sensation and does not damage skin.* A cool environment is soothing as opposed to a warm environment. Other soothing measures include lubricating the skin with oil or lotion and taking a tub bath containing oatmeal powder, potassium permanganate, or cornstarch at 32° to 38° C (89.6° to 100.4° F). When other methods are unsuccessful, give antihistamine as ordered by physician.
- Inform individuals with altered pigmentation to wear long-sleeved shirts or blouses and hats *to shield from the sun.*
- Instruct children and adults playing and working in the sun to wear protective clothing, to apply sun screen, and to limit exposure time.
- Inform individuals receiving radiation to blot their skin rather than rub it.

Maintain circulation to the skin, as evidenced by:
Warm skin
Strong peripheral pulses

- Inspect skin for color, palpate peripheral pulses and skin temperature, and assess capillary refill *to assess adequacy of circulation.*
- Encourage patient to ambulate if possible.
- Have patient perform active range of motion, or have family perform passive range of motion when active is not possible *to stimulate circulation.*
- Keep pressure off skeletal prominences by positioning patient with pillows or mattress overlays.
- Prevent head of bed from being elevated 30 degrees (semi-Fowler's position) for long periods.
- Provide extra protection for heels such as foam or sheepskin boots. Remove boots at least three times daily to inspect skin.
- When patient is in bed, reposition him or her every 2 hours using lateral, dorsal, and prone positions if possible.
- Use lifting devices when repositioning *to avoid shearing of skin against linens.*
- Teach patient and family members how to reposition patient.
- Avoid massaging skin over bony prominences, *which can cause deep tissue trauma.*
- Avoid use of donuts or rubber ring around areas of skin that become reddened.
- When feet and ankles swell, use support stockings and periodic leg elevation. Reduction in sodium and fluids may also be indicated *to decrease swelling.*
- Do not massage legs; *this practice can dislodge a thrombus and create an embolus.*

- Teach patient and family to inspect skin daily and to take actions when abnormalities are noted; *such actions may include keeping pressure off the involved area, keeping area clean and dry, and proving a balanced diet or one high in protein.*
- Ask family to return demonstrate proper skin care.
- Teach patient and family when to call physician if symptoms worsen.

IMPAIRED TISSUE INTEGRITY

Impaired tissue integrity is a state in which an individual experiences damage to mucous membranes or corneal, integumentary, or subcutaneous tissue. It is a state in which an individual has altered body tissue.[2]

Related Factors[2]

Altered circulation
Chemical, thermal, mechanical, or radiation irritants
Fluid volume deficit or excess
Impaired physical mobility
Knowledge deficit
Nutritional deficit or excess

Defining Characteristics[2]

Damaged or destroyed tissue

Expected Patient Outcomes and Nursing Interventions With Rationale[1,3,4]

Regain tissue integrity, as evidenced by:

Intact subcutaneous tissue
Skin color and temperature consistent with unaffected tissue
For cornea, vision returned to previous status, without photophobia

- Inspect area of impaired integrity for redness, edema, purulent exudate, granulation tissue.
- Assess peripheral pulses and capillary refill supplying affected area.
- Assess sensation of affected area.
- Assess lesion for depth and classify pressure ulcers into stage III or stage IV. *Stage III is full thickness skin loss involving damage to and necrosis of subcutaneous tissue that may extend down to but not through the underlying fascia. The ulcer appears as a deep crater with or without undermining of adjacent tissue. Stage IV is full thickness loss with extensive destruction, tissue necrosis, or damage to muscle, bone, or supporting structures.*
- Monitor patient's continence status and minimize exposure of the skin impairment site to moisture of incontinence, perspiration, and wound drainage.
- Monitor laboratory data (e.g., hemoglobin, hematocrit, albumin, glucose, blood urea nitrogen [BUN], creatinine, liver enzymes, arterial blood gases) for evidence of malnutrition or chronic conditions that could affect the skin.
- Determine attitudes and reactions of patient and significant others to skin lesion.
- Encourage verbalization about feelings and discuss effect of lesion on self-esteem.

A positive mental attitude can improve immune function an increase motivation for healing. Thus, discussions of patient feelings toward skin lesions can further the wound healing efforts.

- Provide wound treatment based on stage and drainage using gauze, polyurethane film, hydrocolloid, foam, ac sorptive dressing, hydrogel, or enzymatic therapy.

Topical treatments act to stimulate tissue granulation, debrid the wound, and prevent loss of plasma and fluids from th wound, and systemic antiinfectives treat or prevent infection c the wound.

- Debride and clean wound as ordered.
- Ambulate patient if possible.
- When patient is in bed, turn every 2 hours; use latera prone, and dorsal sides if possible *to decrease pressur on skin.*
- Have patient perform active range-of-motion exercises c instruct family to perform passive range of motion.
- Position off pressure ulcer.
- Use pressure-relieving therapy bed.
- Keep pressure off skeletal prominences by positionin patients with pillows and/or foam devices, or pressure relieving mattresses.
- Use lifting devices and/or sheets to position patient *t prevent shearing force on skin.*
- Do not massage skin over bony prominences.
- Prevent head of bed from being elevated more than 3 degrees (semi-Fowler's position) for long periods.
- Use underpads or briefs that absorb moisture and leav quick drying surface toward skin if continuously moist.
- Avoid use of donuts or rubber rings.
- Provide nutrients: proteins, including albumin; carbo hydrates; fats; vitamins A, B complex, C, and K; an minerals: iron, zinc, and copper, *to promote collage synthesis.*

Corneal Tissue

- Examine the cornea.
- Maintain patches over eyes when there is no drainag from the eye.
- Administer atropine or scopolamine as ordered *to dilat pupil, thereby resting ciliary body and iris.*
- Administer topical or systemic steroids and antibiotics a ordered *to reduce inflammation.*

Communicate care of impaired tissue after discharge an action to prevent recurrence, as evidenced by patient an family explaining:

Causes and prevention of impaired tissue integrity
Medications and treatments for home use
Dietary intake to promote wound healing
Plan for follow-up care

- Instruct patient and family on the following:
  - Care of the lesion
  - Purpose and side effects of medications
  - How to prevent tissue damage
  - Plans for follow-up care

The nurse instructs the patient and family on actions to preven tissue impairment and to continue treatment after discharge Time is needed for the family and patient to perform return demonstrations of dressing changes and to ask questions abou treatment schedules, nutrition, administration of medications, and side effects.

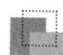

IMPAIRED SWALLOWING

Impaired swallowing is an abnormal functioning of the swallowing mechanism associated with deficits in oral, pharyngeal, or esophageal structure or function.[11]

Related Factors[2,4,11]

Achalasia
Cerebral palsy
Cerebrovascular accident
Congenital heart disease
Cranial nerve involvement
Decreased or absent gag reflex
Developmental delay
Failure to thrive
Gastroesophageal reflux disease
History of tube feeding
Laryngeal abnormalities
Mechanical obstruction (e.g., edema, tracheostomy tube, tumor)
Nasal, nasopharyngeal, or oral cavity defects
Prematurity
Protein calorie malnutrition
Respiratory disorders
Tracheal, laryngeal, esophageal defects
Traumatic head injury

Defining Characteristics[6,10,12]

Pharyngeal phase impairment:
Abnormal pharyngeal phase swallow study
Altered head positions
Choking, coughing, or gagging
Delayed swallow
Inadequate laryngeal elevation
Multiple swallows
Nasal reflux
Recurrent pulmonary infections
Refusal of food
Esophageal phase impairment:
Abnormal esophageal phase swallow study
Acidic breath
Complaints of "something stuck"
Heartburn or epigastric pain
Hyperextension of head during or after meals
Nighttime coughing or awakening
Regurgitation of gastric contents
Repetitive swallowing or ruminating
Vomiting
Oral phase impairment:
Abnormal oral phase swallow study
Coughing, choking, gagging before a swallow
Drooling
Food pushed out of mouth
Inability to clear oral cavity
Incomplete lip closure
Lack of tongue action to form bolus
Nasal reflux
Piecemeal deglutition
Pooling in lateral sulci
Weak suck resulting in inefficient nippling

Expected Patient Outcomes and Nursing Interventions With Rationale[1,5,9,12,14]

Swallow food and fluids safely, as evidenced by:
Does not gag
Does not regurgitate food or fluids
Does not aspirate food or fluids

- Consult with speech therapist, dietitian, patient, and family to develop a plan for improving swallowing.
- Assess mental status, concentration, orientation.
- Auscultate breath sounds.
- Inspect oropharynx for inflammation, altered oral mucosa, adequacy of oral hygiene.
- Assess gag and couch reflexes. (If reflexes are absent, use food tube or parenteral route for food and fluids.)
- Assess ability to swallow by observing patient swallow own saliva; then water.

Before the patient with impaired swallowing eats or drinks, the nurse makes several assessments. Assess patient's mental status for alertness. Auscultate breath sounds before patient eats or drinks to document baseline respiratory status. Inspect oropharynx to detect any problems that may hamper swallowing, such as inflammation. Test gag and cough reflexes because these are protective reflexes to help prevent aspiration.

- Collaborate with speech therapist and dietitian in planning management of swallowing difficulties.
- Progress slowly from clear liquids, to full liquids, to pureed food, to soft diet, to regular diet.
- Avoid mixing food textures.
- Ensure temperature of food and fluid is appropriate.
- Position patient in a 90-degree sitting position during meals *to facilitate peristalsis.*
- Have suction equipment at bedside ready for use if needed.
- When feeding liquids, add green or blue food coloring during initial feedings *to determine aspiration.*
- Minimize distractions while eating or drinking.
- Encourage patient to chew food completely before attempting to swallow and to wear properly fitting dentures when applicable *to facilitate swallowing.*
- When one side of the patient's face is paralyzed, food is placed in the unaffected side. Check affected side of mouth for food lodged in cheek during and after eating.
- When fatigue impairs swallowing, provide rest periods before and during meals as needed.
- If swallowing appears difficult, massage throat *to stimulate the laryngopharyngeal muscle.*
- Observe for signs of swallowing problems (e.g., coughing, choking, spitting up food, drooling, watering eyes, nasal discharge, gurgling voice).
- Perform Heimlich maneuver as needed.
- Monitor for signs of aspiration, such as obstruction of upper airway, fever, crackles, or decreased breath sounds.

Maintain adequate nutrition and hydration, as evidenced by:
Stabilization of weight

Fluid intake of 2000 ml daily, elastic skin turgor, moist mucous membranes
- Weigh patient.
- Measure intake.
- Consult with dietitian, patient, and family regarding daily caloric requirements and food and fluid preferences.
- Provide small frequent meals.
- Provide for or perform oral care before and after meals.
- Record amount of food and fluids taken.
- Praise patient and family for attaining goal.

Monitoring weight changes is an objective way to determine if nutrition is sufficient. The dietitian confers with the patient and family to create meal plans that meet preferences and textures appropriate for patient's ability to swallow. Small frequent meals will prevent fatigue, both mental and physical. Oral care before meals is refreshing and enhances appetite; after meals it ensures removal of any food remaining in the mouth. It also provides an opportunity to assess the moisture of mucous membranes, an indicator of adequate hydration. The amount of fluid drunk and percentage of food eaten are recorded to monitor adequacy of nutritional intake and evaluate the progress toward swallowing goals. Adequate intake prevents weight loss and decreases risk of muscle wasting.

Demonstrate ability to assist with eating and take action when swallowing difficulties arise, as evidenced by:

Patient and family members select nutritious foods

Family members demonstrate Heimlich maneuver and state their plan of action if patient chokes
- Teach patient and family about food selection and preparation.
- Supervise family members feeding patient.
- Teach Heimlich maneuver to family members for use in an emergency.
- Teach use of suction when necessary.

The patient and family need knowledge of how to assist the patient to eat at home. When the patient requires feeding, the family should practice in the hospital. To prevent choking, the family members must know how to perform the Heimlich maneuver on the patient. If a suction machine will be required at home, the family members need instruction on how to use it. The family may require instruction on what foods to serve and how to prepare them. Finally, they need to know the plan for follow-up care.

LATEX ALLERGY RESPONSE

Latex allergy response is an allergic response to natural latex rubber products.[8]

Related Factors[8]

Multiple surgical procedures or mucosal instrumentation involving latex

No immune mechanism response

Occupational exposure to latex

Personal or family history of allergies

Defining Characteristics[8]

Irritant reactions:
- Blisters
- Chapped or cracked skin
- Erythema

Type I reactions: Immediate

Type IV reactions:
- Delayed onset (hours)
- Eczema
- Irritation
- Reaction to additives causes discomfort (e.g., thiurams, carbinates)
- Redness

Expected Patient Outcomes and Nursing Interventions With Rationale[1,7,9]

No exposure to latex, as evidenced by:

Latex-sensitized person completely avoids exposure to latex allergens.
- Teach which health-care products are commonly made of latex: natural latex rubber gloves, blood pressure cuffs, stethoscopes, tourniquets, electrode pads, airways, endotracheal tubes, syringe plungers, bulb syringes, rubber aprons, urinary catheters, wound drains, IV injection ports, adhesive tape, ostomy pouches, wheelchair cushions, crutch pads.
- Teach which office and household products are commonly made of latex: erasers, rubber bands, dishwashing gloves, balloons, condoms, diaphragms, baby bottle nipples, pacifiers, rubber toys and balls, racquet handles, tricycle and bicycle handle grips, tires, hot water bottles, shoe soles, carpet, rubber cement, underwear elastic.
- Teach to avoid eating avocado, banana, European chestnut, almond, cherry, peach, nectarine, kiwi, papaya, tomato, and potato produce. *These items may have molecular structures analogous to latex, and cross-sensitivity may occur in highly sensitized persons.*
- Advise to wear a medical identification bracelet; place allergy band on patient.
- Post sign indicating latex precautions for hospitalized patients.
- Advise to carry autoinjectable epinephrine and teach patient and family how to administer *to counteract acute allergic response.*
- Advise to consult with physician for alternatives to beta-blockers that are prescribed for other conditions.
- Advise to negotiate in advance with health-care providers, agencies, and institutions for latex-safe health and dental care.

Latex-safe precautions and guidelines are followed, as evidenced by:

No exposure to latex, as evidenced by:

Health-care providers follow latex-safe precautions and guidelines.
- Wash hands between glove changes and after use and avoid touching objects or latex-sensitized persons with latex gloves or unwashed hands. *Glove powder readily rubs off or leaches into sweat, accumulating on the hands.*
- Never use latex gloves in the presence of latex-sensitive patients, and do not use powdered gloves in general.
- Wear low-allergen, powder-free gloves. *These gloves decrease allergen exposure and reduce the incidence of al*

lergic reactions and occupational asthma among sensitized workers.

- Identify sensitized patients and deliver all levels of care (including emergency care) using nonlatex medical devices in an environment that is free of latex contamination.
- Follow recommendations of the American Nurses Association to protect patients and personnel from latex allergy in all health-care settings:

  Eliminate the unnecessary use of latex gloves and implement the use of low-allergen, powder-free latex gloves in all other settings.

  Convene a multidisciplinary latex allergy task force to develop patient care guidelines specific to (1) ensuring the environment is free of contamination, (2) identifying and teaching latex-sensitive patients and those at risk, (3) establishing an inventory of nonlatex alternatives for latex medical devices, (4) developing procedures to identify and resolve problems with medical devices, and (5) reporting allergic events related to latex medical devices to the Food and Drug Administration MedWatch program.

  Develop multidisciplinary latex allergy occupational health guidelines that will (1) ensure a contamination-free workplace; (2) educate personnel about latex allergy and related hand care and about adherence to standard precautions; (3) provide task-appropriate, powder-free, low-allergen gloves; (4) facilitate early detection, diagnosis, and tracking of personnel with hand dermatoses or latex allergy symptoms; (5) accommodate latex-sensitized personnel safely in the workplace; (6) assist disabled employees to obtain rehabilitation services; and (7) direct disabled employees to compensatory benefits when rehabilitation is not possible.

RISK FOR LATEX ALLERGY RESPONSE

Risk for latex allergy response is the state in which an individual is at risk for allergic response to natural latex rubber products.[8]

Risk Factors[8]

Allergies to bananas, avocados, tropical fruits, kiwi, chestnuts
Allergies to poinsettia plants
Conditions needing continuous or intermittent catheterization
History of allergies and asthma
History of reactions to latex (e.g., balloons, condoms, gloves)
Multiple surgical procedures, especially from infancy (e.g., for spina bifida)
Professions with daily exposure to latex (e.g., medicine, nursing, dentistry)

Expected Patient Outcomes and Nursing Interventions With Rationale[1-7,9]

Health-care providers follow proper precautions, as evidenced by:

Health-care providers follow safety precautions to protect self and others

- Wash hands between glove changes and after use and avoid touching objects or latex-sensitized persons with latex gloves or unwashed hands. *Glove powder readily rubs off or leaches into sweat, accumulating on the hands.*
- Never use latex gloves in the presence of latex-sensitive patients, and do not use powdered gloves in general.
- Wear low-allergen, powder-free gloves. *These gloves decrease allergen exposure and reduce the incidence of allergic reactions and occupational asthma among sensitized workers.*

No use of latex products by at-risk persons, as evidenced by:

At-risk person completely avoids direct contact with all latex products

- Teach that persons at risk may develop severe reactions, including anaphylaxis, and that there is currently no treatment.
- Teach that natural rubber latex exposure occurs through contact with skin or mucous membranes and by inhalation, ingestion, parenteral injection, or wound inoculation, with the most prominent source of latex allergen exposure being latex medical gloves.
- Teach that synthetic latexes are not involved in latex allergies.
- Teach that early diagnosis and latex avoidance are essential because *continued exposure can lead to advanced allergic symptoms that disrupt careers and everyday living, and create serious barriers to health care.*

Avoid hand dermatitis, as evidenced by:

Health-care staff follow guidelines for avoiding glove-associated hand dermatitis

- Advise to seek early differential diagnosis for hand dermatitis that includes patch testing for glove chemical allergy and latex allergy testing. *Hand dermatitis, endemic among glove users, frequently is associated with latex allergy response.*
- Teach to avoid using oil-based hand care products or medications to treat skin conditions. *Oil-based products increase the risk of exposure to allergens and microorganisms.*
- Establish policy that hospital housekeeping staff and food service workers do not wear latex medical gloves, *because these increase staff exposure to allergens and can contaminate the environment and food with allergens.*

NAUSEA

Nausea is an unpleasant, wavelike sensation in the back of the throat, epigastrium, or throughout the abdomen that may or may not lead to vomiting.[5]

Related Factors[2,4,5]

Chemotherapy
Excessive alcohol intake
Ingestion of spoiled food or poisons
Irritation to the gastrointestinal system
Migraine headache
Motion sickness
Noxious odors

Pregnancy
Renal calculi
Severe pain
Side effect of medications
Surgical anesthesia

Defining Characteristics[5]

Cold, clammy skin
Gastric stasis
Increased salivation
Precedes or accompanies retching and vomiting
Swallowing movements
Tachycardia
Reports "sick to stomach"

Expected Patient Outcomes and Nursing Interventions With Rationale[1-4]

Decreased or absent nausea, as evidenced by:
Verbalizes decreased nausea
Does not retch or vomit

- Identify factors precipitating nausea.
- Explain the possible causes to women with pregnancy-induced nausea. *Pregnancy-induced nausea, believed caused by gestational hormones, is a common occurence in pregnant women.*
- Teach the patient to avoid temperature extremes in foods, foods high in fat or fiber, highly spiced foods, and caffeine. *Tepid, bland foods and fluids are usually better tolerated.*
- Keep environment free of food odors, and noxious odors and sights. *Eliminating cues, such as odors, can help reduce nausea.*
- Encourage the patient to eat small, frequent meals with dry foods such as crackers and toast and to remain sitting upright for 1 hour after eating.
- Provide or encourage oral hygiene before meals.
- Teach patient to take slow, deep breaths and to swallow *to help decrease nausea.*
- Administer prescribed antiemetics on a regular schedule.
- Administer prescribed pain medications on a regular basis. *Nausea is often a component of the experience of pain.*
- Suggest the use of acupressure to prevent nausea. *Applying pressure to the distal aspect of the wrist with an elastic band has been effective in reducing nausea.*

RISK FOR ASPIRATION

Risk for aspiration is the state in which an individual is at risk for entry of gastrointestinal secretions, oropharyngeal secretions, or solids or fluids into tracheobronchial passages.[5]

Risk Factors[5,7]

Decreased gastrointestinal motility
Delayed gastric emptying
Depressed cough and gag reflexes
Facial, oral, neck surgery or trauma
Gastrointestinal tubes
Impaired infant sucking or swallowing reflexes
Impaired swallowing
Incomplete lower esophageal sphincter
Increased intragastric pressure
Increased gastric residual
Lack of knowledge about risks, especially for young children
Medication administration
Presence of tracheostomy or endotracheal tube
Reduced level of consciousness
Situations hindering elevation of upper body
Tube feedings
Wired jaws

Expected Patient Outcomes and Nursing Interventions With Rationale[1-2,6]

Diminished or absent risk for aspiration, as evidenced by:
Verbalizes understanding of risks for aspiration
Takes necessary precautions to prevent aspiration
Demonstrates ability to perform Heimlich maneuver
Swallows and digests oral, nasogastric, or gastric feedings without aspiration
Maintains patent airway and clear lung sounds

- Monitor respiratory rate and depth, as well as lung sounds. Note abnormal findings, such as cough, dyspnea, cyanosis, crackles, wheezes, *which may indicate aspiration and airway obstruction.*
- Monitor bowel sounds and abdominal distention *because absence of bowel sounds and increasing abdominal distention may indicate an ileus or bowel obstruction, resulting in vomiting with the risk of aspiration.*
- Have suction equipment at the bedside for patients with tracheostomies, endotracheal tubes, decreased strength, or autonomic disorders *to provide immediate treatment for airway obstruction.*
- Elevate the head of the bed during feeding and for 30 to 45 minutes afterward *to help food and fluids move downward into the stomach and small intestine, decreasing risk of regurgitation and aspiration.*
- Feed patients slowly, allowing adequate time for chewing and swallowing. Assess oral cavity to ensure food does not collect in the mouth. Request dietary consult for foods that the patient likes and can most easily swallow.
- If patients are elderly, or have had a cerebrovascular accident, assess gag and swallowing reflexes before initiating food and fluids *to decrease risk of choking with aspiration*
- Teach parents:
  - To position infant on back or side for sleeping
  - To keep all small objects out of reach
  - To remove all plastic bags
  - To make sure toys do not have small removable parts
  - To avoid giving small children nuts, gum, hot dogs, popcorn, fruits with pits, or whole grapes
  - How to provide back blows and chest thrusts to infants for emergency airway obstruction
  - How to perform the Heimlich maneuver for children with emergency airway obstruction

These nursing interventions are focused on maintaining safety and managing emergency airway obstruction for infants and children, thereby decreasing the risk of aspiration.

- For patients with feeding tubes:

  Following placement, ensure accurate determination of location of feeding tube by x-ray. *X-ray determination of placement, especially of small-bore feeding tubes, is the gold standard for safe placement.*

  Assess placement of feeding tube before each feeding and every 4 hours for patients with continuous feedings. Aspirate contents from tube and determine pH and aspirate characteristics. *Testing pH and noting aspirate characteristics are the most reliable means of determining tube placement; the earlier method of listening to sounds as air was injected into the tube is no longer accurate.*

  If assessments indicate the possibility of feeding solution in mucus coughed or suctioned from the trachea, test the mucus for glucose, *which if positive, can indicate tube displacement and aspiration of feeding solution.*

  Assess gastric residual amounts before feedings, and at least every 4 hours for continuous feedings; if aspirate amount is greater than 100 ml, follow institutional guidelines for holding feeding. *Retained feeding solution can increase intragastric pressure, resulting in increased risk for regurgitation and aspiration.*

  Maintain patient in semi-Fowler's position during feedings and for 30 to 45 minutes after feeding *to facilitate movement of feeding solution through the stomach and into the small intestine, thus decreasing risk of regurgitation and aspiration.*

- For patients with tracheostomies or endotracheal tubes:

  Request referral to a speech therapist for swallowing studies before beginning feeding; follow recommendations for inflating or deflating cuff when patient eats. *It is necessary to determine swallowing capabilities before instituting guidelines for cuff inflation.*

  Suction every 1 to 2 hours, and as needed *to maintain a patent airway.*

REFERENCES

Nutritional-Metabolic

1. Gordon M: *Manual of nursing diagnosis,* ed 9, St. Louis, 2000, Mosby.

Adult Failure to Thrive

1. Hildebrand JK, Joos SK, Lee MA: Use of the diagnosis "failure to thrive" in older veterans, *J Am Geriatr Soc* 45(9):1113, 1997.
2. Jamison MST: Failure to thrive in older adults, *J Gerontol Nurs* 23(2):8, 1997.
3. Katz IR, DiFilippo S: Neuropsychiatric aspects of failure to thrive in late life, *Clin Geriatr Med* 13(4):623, 1997.
4. Ladwig GB: Adult failure to thrive. In Ackley BJ, Ladwig GB, editors: *Nursing diagnosis handbook: a guide to planning care,* ed 4, St. Louis, 1999, Mosby.
5. Markson EW: Functional, social, and psychological disability as causes of loss of weight and independence in older community-living people, *Clin Geriatr Med* 13(4):769, 1997.
6. North American Nursing Diagnosis Association: *Nursing diagnoses: definitions and classification 2001-2002* Philadelphia, 2001, The Association.
7. Puentes WJ: Incorporating simple reminiscence techniques into acute care nursing practice, *J Gerontolog Nurs* 24(2):14, 1998.
8. Wood P, Vogen BD: Feeding the anorectic client: comfort foods and happy hour, *Geriatr Nurs Am J Care Aging* 19(4):192, 1998.

Deficient Fluid Volume

1. Ackley BJ, Ladwig GB: *Nursing diagnosis handbook: a guide for planning care,* St. Louis, 1999, Mosby.
2. Fann BD: Fluid and electrolyte balance in the pediatric patient, *J Intraven Nurs* 21(3):153, 1998.
3. McCloskey JC, Bulechek GM, editors: Hypovolemia management. In *Nursing interventions classification (NIC),* ed 3, St. Louis, 2001, Mosby.
4. Metheny NM: *Fluid and electrolyte balance: nursing considerations,* ed 3, Philadelphia, 1996, Lippincott-Raven.
5. North American Nursing Diagnosis Association: *Nursing diagnoses: definitions and classification 2001-2002,* Philadelphia, 2001, The Association.
6. Porth CM: *Pathophysiology: concepts of altered health states,* ed 5, Philadelphia, 1998, JB Lippincott.

Risk for Deficient Fluid Volume

1. Ackley BJ, Ladwig GB: *Nursing diagnosis handbook: a guide for planning care,* St. Louis, 1999, Mosby.
2. Fann BD: Fluid and electrolyte balance in the pediatric patient, *J Intraven Nurs* 21(3):153, 1998.
3. McCloskey JC, Bulechek GM, editors: Hypovolemia management. In *Nursing interventions classification (NIC),* ed 3, St. Louis, 2001, Mosby.
4. Metheny NM: *Fluid and electrolyte balance: nursing considerations,* ed 3, Philadelphia, 1996, Lippincott-Raven.
5. North American Nursing Diagnosis Association: *Nursing diagnoses: definitions and classification 2001-2002,* Philadelphia, 2001, The Association.
6. Parobek V, Alaimo I: Fluid and electrolyte management in the neurologically-impaired patient, *J Neurosc Nurs* 28(5):322, 1996.
7. Phippen ML, Wells MP: *Patient care during operative and invasive procedures,* Philadelphia, 2000, WB Saunders.
8. Porth CM: *Pathophysiology: concepts of altered health states,* ed 5, Philadelphia, 1998, JB Lippincott.

Excess Fluid Volume

1. Ackley BJ, Ladwig GB: *Nursing diagnosis handbook: a guide for planning care,* St. Louis, 1999, Mosby.
2. Cirolia B: Understanding edema: when fluid balance fails, *Nursing* 26(2):66, 1996.
3. Ennen KA, Komorita NI, Pogue N: Validation of the defining characteristics of the nursing diagnosis Fluid Volume Excess. In Rantz MJ, LeMone P, editors: *Classification of nursing diagnoses: proceedings of the twelfth conference, North American Nursing Diagnosis Association,* Glendale, Calif, 1997, Cinahl Information Systems.
4. Gosling P: Fluid balance in the critically ill: the sodium and water audit, *Care Crit Ill* 15(1):11, 1999.
5. McCloskey JC, Bulechek GM, editors: Hypervolemia management. In *Nursing interventions classification (NIC),* ed 3, St. Louis, 2001, Mosby.
6. Metheny NM: *Fluid and electrolyte balance: nursing considerations,* ed 3, Philadelphia, 1996, Lippincott-Raven.

7. North American Nursing Diagnosis Association: *Nursing diagnoses: definitions and classification 2001-2002,* Philadelphia, 2001, The Association.
8. Porth CM: *Pathophysiology: concepts of altered health states,* ed 5, Philadelphia, 1998, JB Lippincott.
9. Toto KH: Fluid balance assessment: the total perspective, *Crit Care Nurs Clin North Am* 10(4):383, 1998.

Risk for Imbalanced Fluid Volume

1. Ackley BJ, Ladwig GB: *Nursing diagnosis handbook: a guide for planning care,* St. Louis, 1999, Mosby.
2. Fairchild SS: *Perioperative nursing: principles and practice,* ed 2, Boston, 1996, Little, Brown.
3. McCloskey JC, Bulechek GM, editors: Fluid monitoring. In *Nursing interventions classification (NIC),* ed 3, St. Louis, 2001, Mosby.
4. Metheny NM: *Fluid and electrolyte balance: nursing considerations,* ed 3, Philadelphia, 1996, Lippincott-Raven.
5. North American Nursing Diagnosis Association: *Nursing diagnoses: definitions and classification 2001-2002,* Philadelphia, 2001, The Association.
6. Phippen ML, Wells MP: *Patient care during operative and invasive procedures,* Philadelphia, 2000, WB Saunders.

Effective Breastfeeding, Ineffective Breastfeeding

1. Ackley BJ, Ladwig GB: *Nursing diagnosis handbook: a guide for planning care,* St. Louis, 1999, Mosby.
2. Bell KK, Rawlings NL: Promoting breast-feeding by managing common lactation problems, *Nurse Pract* 23(6):102, 1998.
3. Lawrence RA: *Breastfeeding: a guide for the medical profession,* ed 4, St. Louis, 1994, Mosby.
4. McCloskey JC, Bulechek GM, editors: Breastfeeding assistance; Lactation counseling. In *Nursing interventions classification (NIC),* ed 3, St. Louis, 2001, Mosby.
5. North American Nursing Diagnosis Association: *Nursing diagnoses: definitions and classification 2001-2002,* Philadelphia, 2001, The Association.
6. Olds SB, London ML, Ladewig PW: *Maternal newborn nursing: a family and community-based approach. Clinical handbook,* ed 6, Upper Saddle River, NJ, 2000, Prentice Hall Health.
7. Pillitteri A: *Maternal and child health nursing: care of the childbearing and childrearing family,* ed 3, Philadelphia, 1999, JB Lippincott.
8. Svedulf CI, Engberg IL, Berthold H et al: A comparison of the incidence of breast feeding 2 and 4 months after delivery in mothers discharged within 72 hours and after 72 hours post delivery, *Midwifery* 14(1):37, 1998.
9. Tarkka M, Paunomen M, Laippala P: Factors related to successful breast feeding by first-time mothers when the child is 3 months old, *J Adv Nurs* 29(1):113, 1999.
10. Whelan A, Lupton P: Promoting successful breast feeding among women with a low income, *Midwifery* 14(2):94, 1998.

Interrupted Breastfeeding

1. Ackley BJ, Ladwig GB: *Nursing diagnosis handbook: a guide for planning care,* St. Louis, 1999, Mosby.
2. Lawrence RA: *Breastfeeding: a guide for the medical profession,* ed 4, St. Louis, 1994, Mosby.
3. North American Nursing Diagnosis Association: *Nursing diagnoses: definitions and classification 2001-2002,* Philadelphia, 2001, The Association.
4. Olds SB, London ML, Ladewig PW: *Maternal newborn nursing: a family and community-based approach. Clinical handbook,* ed 6, Upper Saddle River, NJ, 2000, Prentice Hall Health.
5. Pillitteri A: *Maternal and child health nursing: care of the childbearing and childrearing family,* ed 3, Philadelphia, 1999, JB Lippincott.
6. Richie JF: Immature sucking response in premature babies: cup feeding as a tool in increasing maintenance of breast feeding, *Neonat Nurs* 4(2):13, 1998.

Ineffective Infant Feeding Pattern

1. Ackley BJ, Ladwig GB: *Nursing diagnosis handbook: a guide for planning care,* St. Louis, 1999, Mosby.
2. Carpenito LJ: *Handbook of nursing diagnosis,* ed 8, Philadelphia, 1999, JB Lippincott.
3. Lawrence RA: *Breastfeeding: a guide for the medical profession,* ed 4, St. Louis, 1994, Mosby.
4. McCloskey JC, Bulechek GM, editors: Lactation counseling. In *Nursing interventions classification (NIC),* ed 3, St. Louis, 2001, Mosby.
5. North American Nursing Diagnosis Association: *Nursing diagnoses: definitions and classification 2001-2002,* Philadelphia, 2001, The Association.
6. Pillitteri A: *Maternal and child health nursing: care of the childbearing and childrearing family,* ed 3, Philadelphia, 1999, JB Lippincott.

Hyperthermia

1. Ackley BJ, Ladwig GB: *Nursing diagnosis handbook: a guide for planning care,* St. Louis, 1999, Mosby.
2. Brickell KS: Hyperthermia: physiology, signs, symptoms, prevention, and intervention, *J Sports Chiropract Rehabil* 12(4):155, 1998.
3. LeMone P, Burke KM: *Medical surgical nursing: critical thinking in client care,* ed 2, Upper Saddle River, NJ, 2000, Prentice Hall Health.
4. North American Nursing Diagnosis Association: *Nursing diagnoses: definitions and classification 2001-2002,* Philadelphia, 2001, The Association.
5. Nowak TJ, Handford AG: *Essentials of pathophysiology: concepts and applications for health care professionals,* ed 2, Boston, 1999, McGraw-Hill.

Hypothermia

1. Ackley BJ, Ladwig GB: *Nursing diagnosis handbook: a guide for planning care,* St. Louis, 1999, Mosby.
2. Garrett JM: Hypothermia—is it cold in here? *Today's Surg Nurse* 19(6):17, 1997.
3. Lee CL: Action-stat! Hypothermia, *Nurs* 26(1):33, 1996.
4. LeMone P, Burke KM: *Medical surgical nursing: critical thinking in client care,* ed 2, Upper Saddle River, NJ, 2000, Prentice Hall Health.
5. McCloskey JC, Bulechek GM, editors: Hypothermia treatment. In *Nursing interventions classification (NIC),* ed 3, St. Louis, 2001, Mosby.
6. North American Nursing Diagnosis Association: *Nursing diagnoses: definitions and classification 2001-2002,* Philadelphia, 2001, The Association.

Risk for Imbalanced Body Temperature

1. Ackley BJ, Ladwig GB: *Nursing diagnosis handbook: a guide for planning care,* St. Louis, 1999, Mosby.
2. Holzclaw B: Perioperative problems: threats to thermal balance in the elderly, *Semin Periop Nurs,* 6(1):42, 1997.
3. McCloskey JC, Bulechek GM, editors: Temperature regulation. In *Nursing interventions classification (NIC),* ed 3, St. Louis, 2001, Mosby.
4. McKensie NE: Upping the body's thermostat: learning to maneuver the peaks and valleys of body temperature, *Nurs* 28(10):41, 1998.

5. North American Nursing Diagnosis Association: *Nursing diagnoses: definitions and classification 2001-2002,* Philadelphia, 2001, The Association.
6. Nowak TJ, Handford AG: *Essentials of pathophysiology: concepts and applications for health care professionals,* ed 2, Boston, 1999, McGraw-Hill.

Ineffective Thermoregulation

1. Ackley BJ, Ladwig GB: *Nursing diagnosis handbook: a guide for planning care,* St. Louis, 1999, Mosby.
2. Eliopoulos C: *Gerontological nursing,* ed 4, Philadelphia, 1997, JB Lippincott.
3. North American Nursing Diagnosis Association: *Nursing diagnoses: definitions and classification 2001-2002,* Philadelphia, 2001, The Association.
4. Nowak TJ, Handford AG: *Essentials of pathophysiology: concepts and applications for health care professionals,* ed 2, Boston, 1999, McGraw-Hill.
5. Porth CM: *Pathophysiology: concepts of altered health states,* ed 5, Philadelphia, 1998, JB Lippincott.
6. LeMone P, Burke KM: *Medical surgical nursing: critical thinking in client care,* ed 2, Upper Saddle River, NJ, 2000, Prentice Hall Health.

Imbalanced Nutrition: Less Than Body Requirements

1. Andris DA: Total parenteral nutrition in surgical patients, *MEDSURG Nurs* 7(2):76, 1998.
2. Collins S, Myatt M, Golden B: Dietary treatment of severe malnutrition in adults, *Am J Clin Nutr* 68(1):193, 1998.
3. Evans-Stoner N: Nutrition assessment: a practical approach, *Nurs Clin North Am* 32(4):637, 1997.
4. Holmes S: Food for thought . . . undernutrition remains a significant cause for concern in hospitals, *Nurs Stand* 12(46):23, 1998.
5. Kamel HK, Thomas DR, Morley JE: National deficiencies in long-term care: part II. Management of protein energy malnutrition and dehydration, *Ann Long Term Care* 6(8):250, 1998.
6. Keithley JK, Swanson B: Minimizing HIV/AIDS malnutrition, *MEDSURG Nurs* 7(5):256, 1998.
7. Lidington I: Malnutrition in the community, *Pract Nurse* 15(1):23, 1998.
8. McCloskey JC, Bulechek GM, editors: Weight gain assistance; Total parenteral nutrition (TPN) administration. In *Nursing interventions classification (NIC),* ed 3, St. Louis, 2001, Mosby.
9. McCormak P: Undernutrition in the elderly population living at home in the community: a review of the literature, *J Adv Nurs* 26(5):856, 1997.
10. McFarland GK, Wasli EL, Gerety EK: *Nursing diagnoses and process in psychiatric mental health nursing,* ed 3, Philadelphia, 1997, JB Lippincott.
11. Morley JE, Thomas DR, Kamel H: Nutritional deficiencies in long-term care: part I. Detection and diagnosis, *Ann Long Term Care* 6(5):183, 1998.
12. North American Nursing Diagnosis Association: *Nursing diagnoses: definitions and classification 2001-2002,* Philadelphia, 2001, The Association.
13. Palmer D: The persisting problem of malnutrition in healthcare, *J Adv Nurs* 28(5):931, 1998.
14. Ziegler PJ, Khoo CS, Sherr B et al: Body image and dieting behaviors among elite figure skaters, *Int J Eat Disord* 24(4):421, 1998.
15. Weber J, Kelley J: *Health assessment in nursing,* Philadelphia, 1998, JB Lippincott.

Imbalanced Nutrition: More Than Body Requirements

1. Adami GF, Meneghelli A, Scopinaro N: Night eating and binge eating disorder in obese patients, *Int J Eat Disord* 25(3):335, 1999.
2. Adami GF, Gandolfo P, Campostano A et al: Body image and body weight in obese patients, *Int J Eat Disord* 24(3):299, 1998.
3. Ammon PK: Individualizing the approach to treating obesity, *Nurse Pract* 24(2):27, 1999.
4. Cutting TM, Fisher JO, Grimm-Thomas K et al: Like mother, like daughter: familial patterns of overweight are mediated by mothers' dietary disinhibition, *Am J Clin Nutr* 69(4):608, 1999.
5. Dallas M: Exercise walking for obesity management in older adult women, *Issues Aging* 20(2):8, 1997.
6. Executive summary of the clinical guidelines on the identification, evaluation, and treatment of overweight and obesity in adults, *J Am Diet Assoc* 98(10):1178, 1998.
7. Golarn M, Weizman A, Apter A et al: Parents as the exclusive agents of change in the treatment of childhood obesity, *Am J Clin Nutr* 67(6):1130, 1998.
8. Lovejoy JC: The influence of sex hormones on obesity across the female life span, *J Womens Health* 7(10):1247, 1998.
9. McCloskey JC, Bulechek GM, editors: Weight reduction assistance. In *Nursing interventions classification (NIC),* ed 3, St. Louis, 2001, Mosby.
10. Mertens DJ, Kavanagh T, Campbell RB et al: Exercise without dietary restriction as a means to long-term fat loss in the obese cardiac patient, *J Sports Med Phys Fitness* 38(4):310, 1998.
11. North American Nursing Diagnosis Association: *Nursing diagnoses: definitions and classification 2001-2002,* Philadelphia, 2001, The Association.
12. Weber J, Kelley J: *Health assessment in nursing,* Philadelphia, 1998, JB Lippincott.

Risk for Imbalanced Nutrition: More Than Body Requirements

1. Executive summary of the clinical guidelines on the identification, evaluation, and treatment of overweight and obesity in adults, *J Am Diet Assoc* 98(10):1178, 1998.
2. Jones SL, Moulton MA, Moulton P et al: Self-esteem differences as a function of race and weight preoccupation: findings and implications, *Womens Health Issues* 9(1):50, 1999.
3. McCloskey JC, Bulechek GM, editors: Weight management. In *Nursing interventions classification (NIC),* ed 3, St. Louis, 2001, Mosby.
4. North American Nursing Diagnosis Association: *Nursing diagnoses: definitions and classification 2001-2002,* Philadelphia, 2001, The Association.
5. Thomas D: An unhealthy obsession with body image, *Pract Nurse* 17(4):252, 1999.
6. Weber J, Kelley J: *Health assessment in nursing,* Philadelphia, 1998, JB Lippincott.

Impaired Dentition

1. Appollonio I, Carabellese C, Frattola A et al: Influence of dental status on dietary intake and survival in community-dwelling elderly subjects, *Age Ageing* 26(6):445, 1997.
2. Bowsher J: Current issues in dental health care, *Practice Nurse* 14(9):569, 1997.
3. Milosevic A: Dental erosion in children: current understanding, *Community Pract* 71(4):142, 1998.
4. North American Nursing Diagnosis Association: *Nursing diagnoses: definitions and classification 2001-2002,* Philadelphia, 2001, The Association.
5. Slavkin HC: What's in a tooth? . . . the development of the human dentition, *J Am Dent Assoc* 128(3):366, 1997.

6. Von Burg MM, Sanaders BJ, Weddell JA: Baby bottle tooth decay: a concern for all mothers, *Pediatr Nurs* 21(6):515, 1995.
7. Watson MR, Gibson G, Guo I: Women's oral health awareness and care-seeking characteristics: a pilot study, *J Am Dent Assoc* 129(12):1708, 1998.

Impaired Oral Mucous Membrane

1. Ackley BJ, Ladwig GB: *Nursing diagnosis handbook: a guide for planning care,* St. Louis, 1999, Mosby.
2. Lawson W: Erythematous oral lesions: when to treat, when to leave alone, *Consultant* 38(7):1749, 1998.
3. Madeya M: Oral complications from cancer therapy, part 2: nursing implications for assessment and treatment, *Oncol Nurs Forum* 23(5):808, 1996.
4. McCloskey JC, Bulechek GM, editors: Oral health restoration. In *Nursing interventions classification (NIC),* ed 3, St. Louis, 2001, Mosby.
5. North American Nursing Diagnosis Association: *Nursing diagnoses: definitions and classification 2001-2002,* Philadelphia, 2001, The Association.

Impaired Skin Integrity

1. Bergstrom N, Braden B, Laguzza A et al: The Braden scale for predicting pressure sore risk, *Nurs Res* 36(4):205, 1987.
2. Lait M, Smith L: Wound management: a literature review, *J Clin Nurs* 7(1):11, 1998.
3. McCloskey JC, Bulechek GM, editors: Pressure ulcer care. In *Nursing interventions classification (NIC),* ed 3, St. Louis, 2001, Mosby.
4. North American Nursing Diagnosis Association: *Nursing diagnoses: definitions and classification 2001-2002,* Philadelphia, 2001, The Association.
5. Pieper B, Sugrue M, Weiland M et al: Occurrence of skin lesions/conditions in ill persons, *Dermatol Nurs* 9(2):91, 1997.
6. U.S. Department of Health and Human Services: *Pressure ulcers in adults: prediction and prevention,* AHCPR Publication No. 92-0047, Rockville, Md, 1992, Agency for Health Care Policy and Research, Public Health Service.
7. U.S. Department of Health and Human Services: *Treatment of pressure ulcers,* Rockville, Md, 1994, Agency for Health Care Policy and Research, Public Health Service.

Risk for Impaired Skin Integrity

1. Ayello EA: Predicting pressure ulcer sore risk. In *Try this: best practices in nursing care for older adults,* New York, 1999, Hartford Institute for Geriatric Nursing, Division of Nursing.
2. Harries-Digloria D, Pye CG: Risk for impaired skin integrity: incorporation of the risk factors from the AHCPR guidelines. In Rantz MJ, LeMone P, editors: *Classification of nursing diagnoses: proceedings of the eleventh conference, North American Nursing Diagnosis Association,* Glendale, Calif, 1995, Cihahl Information Systems.
3. McCloskey JC, Bulechek GM, editors: Pressure management; Pressure ulcer prevention. In *Nursing interventions classification (NIC),* ed 3, St. Louis, 2001, Mosby.
4. North American Nursing Diagnosis Association: *Nursing diagnoses: definitions and classification 2001-2002,* Philadelphia, 2001, The Association.
5. Pieper B, Weiland M: Pressure ulcer management within 72 hours of admission in a rehabilitation setting, *Ostomy Wound Manage* 43(8):14, 1997.
6. Pieper B, Sugrue M, Weiland M et al: Presence of ulcer prevention methods used among patients considered at-risk versus those considered not-at-risk, *J WOCN* 24(4):191, 1997.

Impaired Tissue Integrity

1. McCloskey JC, Bulechek GM, editors: Wound care. In *Nursing interventions classification (NIC),* ed 3, St. Louis, 2001, Mosby.
2. North American Nursing Diagnosis Association: *Nursing diagnoses: definitions and classification 2001-2002,* Philadelphia; 2001, The Association.
3. U.S. Department of Health and Human Services: *Pressure ulcers in adults: prediction and prevention,* AHCPR Publication No. 92-0047, Rockville, Md, 1992, Agency for Health Care Policy and Research, Public Health Service.
4. U.S. Department of Health and Human Services: *Treatment of pressure ulcers,* Rockville, Md, 1994, Agency for Health Care Policy and Research, Public Health Service.

Impaired Swallowing

1. Ackley BJ, Ladwig GB: *Nursing diagnosis handbook: a guide for planning care,* St. Louis, 1999, Mosby.
2. Davies S: Dysphagia in acute strokes, *Nurs Stand* 13(30):49, 1999.
3. Hatlebakk JG, Casteel DO: Dysphagia in the elderly: diagnostic approach and clinical management, *Clin Geriatr* 6(12):16, 1998.
4. Neurological and vascular disorders: swallowing disorders, *Rehabil RD Progress Reports* 35:172, 1998.
5. Killen J: Understanding dysphagia: interventions for care, *MEDSURG Nurs* 5(2):99, 1996.
6. Logemann JA: The evaluation and treatment of swallowing disorders, *Curr Opin Otolaryngol Head Neck Surg* 6(6):395, 1998.
7. Mann G, Hankey GJ, Cameron D: Swallowing function after stroke: prognosis and prognostic factors at 6 months, *Stroke* 30(4):744, 1999.
8. McCloskey JC, Bulechek GM, editors: Swallowing therapy. In *Nursing interventions classification (NIC),* ed 3, St. Louis, 2001, Mosby.
9. McHale JM, Phipps MA, Horvath K et al: Expert nursing knowledge in the care of patients at risk of impaired swallowing, *Image: J Nurs Sch* 30(2):137, 1998.
10. Murray KA, Brzozowski LA: Swallowing in patients with tracheotomies, *AACN Clin Issues: Adv Practice Acute Crit Care* 9(3):416, 1998.
11. North American Nursing Diagnosis Association: *Nursing diagnoses: definitions and classification 2001-2002,* Philadelphia, 2001, The Association.
12. O'Loughlin G, Shanley C: Swallowing problems—assessment and management, *Geriaction* 15(2):21, 1997.
13. Travers PL: Poststroke dysphagia: implications for nurses, *Rehabil Nurs* 24(2):69, 1999.
14. Smithard DG, O'Neill PA, Park C et al: Can bedside assessment reliably exclude aspiration following acute stroke? *Age Ageing,* 27(2):99, 1998.

Latex Allergy Response

1. American Nurses Association position statement on latex allergy, *Nevada Rnformation* 7(2):16, 1998.
2. Greer S: Living and working with latex allergies: personal perspectives from a nurse, *Semin Periop Nurs* 7(4):254, 1998.
3. Gritter M: The latex threat, *Am J Nurs* 98(9):26, 1998.
4. Harrau BO: Managing latex allergy patients, *Nurs Manage* 29(10):48N, 1998.
5. Kelly KJ, Walsh-Kelly CM: Latex allergy: a patient and health care system emergency, *J Emerg Nurs* 24(6):539, 1998.
6. McCloskey JC, Bulechek GM, editors: Latex precautions. In *Nursing interventions classification (NIC),* ed 3, St. Louis, 2001, Mosby
7. Meeropol EV: The R.U.B.B.E.R. tool: screening children for latex allergy, *J Pediatr Health Care* 12(6 part 1):320, 1998.
8. North American Nursing Diagnosis Association: *Nursing diagnoses: definitions and classification 2001-2002,* Philadelphia 2001, The Association.

9. Young MA, Myers M: Latex allergy: considerations for the care of pediatric patients and employee safety, *Nurs Clin North Am* 32(1):169, 1997.

Risk for Latex Allergy Response

1. American Nurses Association position statement on latex allergy, *Nevada Rnformation* 7(2):16, 1998.
2. Greer S: Living and working with latex allergies: personal perspectives from a nurse, *Semin Periop Nurs* 7(4):254, 1998.
3. Gritter M: The latex threat, *Am J Nurs* 98(9):26, 1998.
4. Harrau BO: Managing latex allergy patients, *Nurs Manage* 29(10):48N, 1998.
5. Kelly KJ, Walsh-Kelly CM: Latex allergy: a patient and health care system emergency, *J Emerg Nurs* 24(6):539, 1998.
6. McCloskey JC, Bulechek GM, editors: Latex precautions. In *Nursing interventions classification (NIC),* ed 3, St. Louis, 2001, Mosby.
7. Meeropol EV: The R.U.B.B.E.R. tool: screening children for latex allergy, *J Pediatr Health Care* 12(6 part 1):320, 1998.
8. North American Nursing Diagnosis Association: *Nursing diagnoses: definitions and classification 2001-2002,* Philadelphia, 2001, The Association.
9. Young MA, Myers M: Latex allergy: considerations for the care of pediatric patients and employee safety, *Nurs Clin North Am* 32(1):169, 1997.

Nausea

1. Ackley BJ, Ladwig GB: *Nursing diagnosis handbook: a guide for planning care,* St. Louis, 1999, Mosby.
2. Faries J: Controlling pain: controlling postoperative nausea, *Am J Nurs* 28(8):78, 1998.
3. Ferrara-Love R, Sekeres L, Bircher NG: Nonpharmacologic treatment of postoperative nausea, *J Perianesthesia Nurs* 11(6):378, 1996.
4. Low KG: Nausea and vomiting in pregnancy: a review of the research, *J Gender Cult Health* 1(3):151, 1996.
5. North American Nursing Diagnosis Association: *Nursing diagnoses: definitions and classification 2001-2002,* Philadelphia, 2001, The Association.

Risk for Aspiration

1. Ackley BJ, Ladwig GB: *Nursing diagnosis handbook: a guide for planning care,* St. Louis, 1999, Mosby.
2. Carpenito LJ: *Handbook of nursing diagnosis,* ed 8, Philadelphia, 1999, JB Lippincott.
3. Metheny N, Wehrle M, Wierema L et al: pH, color, and feeding tubes, *RN* 61(1):25, 1998.
4. Metheny N, Wehrle M, Wierema L et al: Testing feeding tube placement: auscultation vs. pH method, *J Parenteral Enteral Nutr* 21(5):37, 1998.
5. North American Nursing Diagnosis Association: *Nursing diagnoses: definitions and classification 2001-2002,* Philadelphia, 2001, The Association.
6. Taylor C, Lillis C, LeMone, P: *Fundamentals of nursing: the art and science of nursing care,* ed 4, Philadelphia, 2001, JB Lippincott.
7. Woolridge J, Herman J, Garrison C et al: A validation study using the case-control method of the nursing diagnosis risk for aspiration, *Nurs Diagnosis: J Nurs Lang Classification* 9(1):5, 1998.

FUNCTIONAL HEALTH PATTERN

3 Elimination[1]

Bowel Incontinence

Bowel incontinence is a change in normal bowel habits characterized by involuntary passage of stool.[10]

Related Factors[3,6,7,10]

Abnormally high abdominal or intestinal pressure
Colorectal lesions
Dietary habits
Immobility
Impaction
Impaired cognition
Inaccessible bathroom
Incomplete emptying of bowel
Inattention to urge to defecate
Laxative abuse
Loss of rectal sphincter control
Medications
Rectal sphincter abnormality
Stress
Toileting self-care deficit
Upper or lower motor nerve damage

Defining Characteristics[3,4,10]

Constant dribbling of soft stool
Fecal odor
Fecal staining of clothing and/or bedding
Inability to delay defecation
Inability to recognize urge to defecate
Rectal fullness recognized but inability to expel formed stool reported
Red perianal skin
Self-report of inability to feel rectal fullness
Urgency

Expected Patient Outcomes and Nursing Interventions With Rationale[1,2,5,9]

Decrease episodes of incontinence, as evidenced by:

Evacuates bowel contents regularly, usually every other day
Ingests foods and fluids consistent with bowel elimination program
Maintains a daily log of defecation and episodes of incontinence

- Reduce or eliminate contributing factors, when possible.
- Encourage appropriate diet, usually high fiber, *to increase volume of stools.*
- Implement bowel retraining program when bowel sounds return and ileus is resolved, if spinal cord–injured patient. *A regular time for bowel evacuation decreases incidence of incontinence.*
- Establish evacuation schedule consistent with patient and family preferences.
- Teach patient and family appropriate use of laxatives and stool softeners to aid timing of defecation.
- Instruct about use of daily log to monitor pattern of defecation.
- Teach pelvic floor exercises *to strengthen perianal muscles.*[2]

Maintain perianal skin normal in appearance, as evidenced by:

Keeps perianal area free of areas of redness, itching, and irritation

- Teach to wash, rinse, and dry area after each incontinent episode.
- Use Desitin ointment on affected area *to relieve itching or pain and to toughen skin.*

Constipation

Constipation is a decrease in a person's normal frequency of defecation accompanied by difficult or incomplete passage of stool and/or passage of excessively hard, dry stool.[9]

Related Factors[2,4,7,9]

Abdominal muscle weakness
Aluminum-containing antacids
Anticholinergics
Antidepressants
Antilipemic agents
Calcium carbonate
Calcium channel blockers
Change in usual foods and eating patterns
Decreased motility of gastrointestinal tract
Depression
Electrolyte imbalance
Emotional stress
Habitual denial or ignoring of urge to defecate
Hemorrhoids
Inadequate toileting
Insufficient fiber intake
Insufficient fluid intake
Insufficient physical activity
Iron salts
Laxative overdose

Megacolon (Hirschsprung's disease)
Mental confusion
Neurologic impairment
Nonsteroidal antiinflammatory agents
Opiates
Phenothiazides
Postsurgical obstruction
Pregnancy
Prostate enlargement
Rectocele, rectal prolapse, fissures, stricture, abscess, or ulcer
Sedatives
Sympathomimetics
Tumors

Defining Characteristics[1,2,9]

Abdominal pain or tenderness
Anorexia
Bright red blood on stool
Change in abdominal growling (borborygmi)
Change in bowel pattern
Decreased frequency or volume of stool
Distended abdomen
Dry, hard, formed stool
Feeling of rectal fullness or pressure
Headache
Inability to pass stool
Indigestion
Nausea and/or vomiting
Oozing liquid stool
Pain with defecation
Palpable abdominal or rectal mass
Percussed abdominal dullness
Presence of soft pastelike stool in rectum
Severe flatus
Straining with defecation

Expected Patient Outcomes and Nursing Interventions With Rationale[1-3,7,12,15]

Describe health behaviors that prevent constipation, as evidenced by:
Understands normal physiology of defecation
Explains importance of well-balanced diet
Describes importance of bulk and fluids in diet
Engages in daily activity

- Encourage intake of dietary fiber and bran *to keep stools soft through the mechanism of water absorption.*
- Encourage intake of 8 to 10 glasses of fluid daily *to prevent hard, dry stools.*[3]
- Encourage integrating daily exercise into lifestyle (at least 15-minute walk per day) *to maintain muscle tone in the abdominal and pelvic muscles.*
- Explore individual stimulus behaviors that are helpful in initiating a bowel movement.
- Teach the importance of responding to defecation urge when it arises naturally. *Constipation is often due to habitual neglect of afferent impulses and failure to initiate defecation.*

Initiate a bowel program to establish normal bowel functioning, as evidenced by:
Eliminates the regular use of laxatives or enemas
Describes a normal pattern of elimination for individual patient

- Establish a set routine for elimination, such as sitting on the toilet for 10 minutes after breakfast.
- Create a relaxing environment for defecation (comfortable temperature, soft music).
- Instruct on an effective position for defecation.

Use appropriate oral drug therapy to produce bowel movement within 12 to 24 hours, as evidenced by:
Takes oral laxative correctly
Understands desired effects of medication
Makes the correct decision if prescribed therapy is no longer effective

- Provide instruction for appropriate use of oral laxatives (Table 23-1).
- Assess and monitor effects of medications.
- Assess and monitor laxative and enema use.

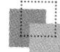

Perceived Constipation

Perceived constipation is the state in which an individual makes a self-diagnosis of constipation and ensures a daily bowel movement through use of laxatives, enemas, and/or suppositories.[9]

Related Factors[2,9]

Cultural or family health beliefs
Impaired thought processes
Lack of information about normal processes
Long-term expectations and habits

Defining Characteristics[1,2,9]

Expectation of daily bowel movement
Expected passage of stool at the same time every day
Overuse of laxatives, enemas, and/or suppositories

Expected Patient Outcomes and Nursing Interventions With Rationale[1,2,6,7]

Modify belief about need for daily evacuation, as evidenced by:
Identifies normal variations in bowel elimination

- Identify beliefs and convictions about present bowel habits. *Contradiction of erroneous beliefs may confuse patient if health beliefs and convictions are not fully explored.*
- Clarify with patient what is viewed as a normal pattern.

Express acceptance of present bowel habits, as evidenced by:
States comfort with new elimination pattern

- Support patient's efforts to monitor difference between real and perceived constipation. *Patient may need to be taught that a bowel movement every 2 to 3 days is normal.*

Decrease reliance on laxatives, as evidenced by:
Reports rarely taking laxatives
Describes variety of bulk and fiber foods eaten daily to support regular bowel habits

Table 23-1 Nonprescription Drug Therapy to Relieve Constipation[13,15]

Generic (Trade) Name	Dosage and Administration	Comments
BULK FORMING		
Psyllium hydrophilic (Metamucil, Perdiem)	Oral: 1-2 teaspoonfuls or 1 packet in a full glass of water; 1-3 times per day	Do not chew psyllium granules.
Methylcellulose (Citrucel)	Oral: 1 teaspoonful in a full glass of water; 1-3 times per day	
Methylcellulose capsules	Oral: 500 mg; 2-3 capsules	Usually taken as a single dose at bedtime.
Polycarbophil (Fibercon, Fiberall)	Oral: 1 g; 1-4 times per day	
LUBRICANT		
Mineral oil (Petrogalar, Zymenol)	Oral: 15-45 ml	Usually taken as a single dose at bedtime. Absorption of fat-soluble vitamins (A, D, E, K) may be decreased. May decrease absorption of oral contraceptives and warfarin. Do not give with docusates.
FECAL SOFTENERS		
Docusate calcium (Surfak)	Oral: 50-240 mg per day	Do not give with mineral oil.
Docusate sodium (Colace, Colax, Dialose)		
HYPEROSMOTICS		
Magnesium citrate	Oral: 240 ml	Drink increased fluids with all hyperosmotic laxatives.
Magnesium hydroxide (Milk of Magnesia)	Oral: 30-60 ml	
Magnesium sulfate (Epsom Salt)	Oral: 10-15 g in a full glass of water	
Sodium phosphates (Fleets Phosphosoda)	Oral: 20-40 ml in a full glass of water	
(Fleets Enema)	Rectal: 118 ml	
STIMULANT		
Bisacodyl (Dulcolax, Bisacolax)	Oral: 10-30 mg Rectal: 10-mg suppository	Oral, response in 6-12 hours; rectal, response in 15 minutes.
Cascara	Oral: 1-2 tablets, 5 ml cascara aromatic	
Castor oil	Oral: 15-60 ml	
Glycerin suppository	Rectal: 3-mg suppository	
Senna concentrate	Rectal: 625-mg suppository	
Sennosides (Senokot)	Oral: 15 mg	

- Encourage substitution of natural bulk and fiber from fruits, grains, and vegetables for laxative being consumed.
- Support gradual reduction of laxative use if there is heavy consumption at present or if patient needs time to relinquish or alter convictions (see Table 23-1).
- Establish a schedule with patient for gradual reduction of laxative use, if necessary.
- Provide regular times to review concerns and progress.
- Ensure adequate fluid intake of 1 to 2 quarts per day *to prevent hard, dry stools.*

Experience regular, comfortable bowel movements, as evidence by:

Attains previously identified normal elimination schedule
Notes absence of discomfort and straining at defecation
Reports absence of distention, flatus, or intense feelings of rectal fullness before defecation
Reports that stools are soft, brown, and regular in shape

- Assess willingness and interest in altering eating, fluid intake, mobility, or exercise habits.
- If multiple changes are needed, proceed slowly and establish priorities according to patient's wishes.
- Acknowledge that lifestyle changes and ensuing elimination routines may occur slowly.
- Enlist support of family or peers to assist patient with changes (if agreeable with patient).

RISK FOR CONSTIPATION

Risk for constipation is a decrease in a person's normal frequency of defecation accompanied by difficult or incomplete passage of stool and/or passage of excessively hard, dry stool.[9]

Risk Factors[2,4,9]

Abdominal muscle weakness
Aluminum-containing antacids
Anticholinergics
Antidepressants
Antilipemic agents
Calcium carbonate
Calcium channel blockers
Change in usual foods and eating patterns
Decreased motility of gastrointestinal tract
Depression
Electrolyte imbalance

Emotional stress
Habitual denial or ignoring of urge to defecate
Hemorrhoids
Inadequate toileting
Insufficient fluid and/or fiber intake
Insufficient physical activity
Iron salts
Laxative overdose
Megacolon (Hirschsprung's disease)
Mental confusion
Neurologic impairment
Nonsteroidal antiinflammatory agents
Opiates
Phenothiazides
Poor eating habits
Postsurgical obstruction
Pregnancy
Prostate enlargement
Recent environmental changes
Rectocele, rectal prolapse, fissures, stricture, abscess, or ulcer
Sedatives
Sympathomimetics
Tumors

Expected Patient Outcomes and Nursing Interventions With Rationale[2,5,7,11]

Describe health behaviors that decrease the risk of constipation, as evidenced by:
Explains importance of balanced diet and adequate fluids
Describes importance of bulk and fluids in diet
Initiates and adheres to a regular schedule for defecation

- Teach importance of balanced diet, including eating breakfast.
- Encourage intake of dietary fiber and bran *to keep stools soft through the mechanism of water absorption.*
- Teach which foods are high in fiber.
- Encourage intake of 8 to 10 glasses of fluid per day *to prevent hard, dry stools.*[3]
- Encourage daily exercise *to maintain muscle tone in the abdominal and pelvic muscles, and to stimulate peristalsis.*
- Teach stimulus behaviors that are helpful in initiating bowel movement, (e.g., warm fluids on arising, prune juice).
- Teach to respond to defecation urge when it arises naturally, *because constipation is often due to habitual neglect of afferent impulses and failure to initiate defecation.*

DIARRHEA

Diarrhea is the passage of loose, unformed stools.[7]

Related Factors[2,3,6,7]

Adverse effects of medications
Alcohol abuse
Contaminants
High stress levels and anxiety
Infectious processes
Inflammation
Laxative abuse
Malabsorption
Parasites
Radiation
Toxins
Tube feedings

Defining Characteristics[2,5-7]

Abdominal pain
At least three loose liquid stools per day
Cramping
Fluid and electrolyte imbalances
Hyperactive bowel sounds
Urgency

Expected Patient Outcomes and Nursing Interventions With Rationale[2-4]

Achieve relief of symptoms, as evidenced by:
Decreases number of stools daily; has no more than three bowel movements per day
Has formed stool that is easy to pass
States, "free of abdominal pain

- Administer antidiarrheal medication, as prescribed.
- Monitor frequency and consistency of stools.
- Teach patient and family about perianal skin care; use Desitin ointment in affected areas, *to control perianal skin excoriation and reduce spread of infectious diarrhea.*

Take prescribed medication correctly, as evidenced by:
Schedules medications as part of daily activities
Reports side effects of medications to health professionals

- Assist in integrating medications into daily routine.
- Provide instruction about use and actions of antidiarrheal medication. *Most antidiarrheal medications suppress gastrointestinal motility, thus allowing for better fluid absorption.*
- Teach to self-monitor drug effects and side effects.

Understand the mechanism of diarrhea, as evidenced by:
Describes factors associated with diarrhea
Lists changes in health practices that affect elimination pattern

- Teach about causes of diarrhea, such as antibiotics, infection, and lactose intolerance. *Diarrhea associated with antibiotics is normally relieved when the offending agent is removed.*
- Assist patient and family in identifying health behaviors that may contribute to diarrhea.
- Modify diet, cooking, or eating habits if associated with diarrhea.

IMPAIRED URINARY ELIMINATION

Impaired urinary elimination is the state in which the individual experiences a disturbance in urine elimination.[22]

Related Factors*

Constipation
Dehydration
Excess fluid volume
Fecal impaction

*References 2-4, 6, 8, 16, 17, 24, 25.

Impaired physical mobility
Incontinence
Polyuria
Urinary retention
Urinary tract infection

Defining Characteristics[11,16,18]

Diurnal urinary frequency
Dysuria
Incontinence
Nocturia
Nocturial enuresis
Split stream or spraying stream
Urinary hesitancy
Urinary infrequency
Urinary retention
Urinary urgency

Expected Patient Outcomes and Nursing Interventions With Rationale*

Exhibit behaviors that promote optimal bladder health, as evidenced by:

Maintains adequate hydration
Avoids constipation
Stops smoking or never starts smoking
Performs pelvic muscle exercises three to seven times per week, if at risk

- Assess current fluid intake using a record or log.
- Calculate recommended daily allowance of fluid, based on the formula 30 ml/kg of body weight.
- Advise of potential bladder irritants; *those at risk of urinary incontinence or sensory disturbances of the bladder should avoid or limit intake of these substances.*
- Assist to maintain adequate hydration as outlined above.
- Teach dietary sources of fiber and its role in the prevention of constipation.
- Assess current bowel elimination strategies and remind the patient with recurrent constipation to heed the urge to defecate. *Constipation has a potential association with urinary retention and recurrent urinary tract infections.*
- Advise to discontinue use of tobacco products *to reduce the risk of bladder cancer and urinary incontinence.*
- Advise women at risk for developing stress urinary incontinence that regular pelvic muscle exercise regimen may help to prevent the onset of stress incontinence.
- Advise women with stress incontinence that pelvic muscle exercises may alleviate or resolve urinary leakage by strengthening pelvic muscles.[1,7]
- Advise men who undergo radical prostatectomy that pelvic muscle exercises may alleviate or prevent stress urinary incontinence following surgery.

Resolve incontinence; contain incontinence; maintain skin integrity; reestablish normal voiding pattern, as evidenced by:

Maintains diurnal voiding pattern of 2 to 4 hours during waking hours
Limits nocturia to two times or less per night
Maintains fluid intake of 30 ml/kg of body weight

- Assess current fluid intake and urinary output.
- Ask to keep a 7-day voiding diary.
- Assess symptoms associated with alteration of urinary elimination patterns: incontinence, dysuria, urgency, hesitancy, feelings of incomplete bladder emptying.
- Assess medications that may affect urinary elimination. *The side effects of medications may exacerbate or produce incontinence.*[8,20]
- Assess strategies patient currently using to cope with altered urinary elimination patterns.
- Institute a timed voiding schedule with fluid volume control. Have patient void by the clock every 2 to 4 hours, as appropriate. Have patient keep a fluid intake and voidng diary at intermittent periods *to establish a normal voiding pattern.*[9]
- Assist to maintain adequate fluid intake *to decrease concentrated urine that may irritate the bladder and increase the risk of infection.*
- Teach to identify and avoid foods or beverages that intensify urinary urgency and predispose toward incontinent episodes.
- Instruct to individually eliminate potential irritants from the diet (coffee, citrus juices, spicy foods, or carbonated beverages) *to evaluate the effect on voiding patterns.*
- Consult a continence specialist to determine the cause of altered patterns of urinary elimination.
- Reassure that bladder control problems are *not* a part of normal aging, that they will respond to treatment, and that they may be alleviated or cured with proper care.
- Consult physician concerning referral to mental health–care professionals for altered urinary elimination patterns secondary to behavioral or psychogenic causes.
- Consult physician concerning referral to endocrinologist for altered urinary elimination patterns secondary to inappropriate antidiuretic hormone secretion or other fluid electrolyte imbalance caused by hormonal abnormality.

Prevent or resolve urinary tract infection, as evidenced by:

Obtains sterile urine culture
Exhibits no symptoms of urinary tract infection

- Assess types of urinary tract infections experienced and presence of pain and burning on urination.
- Determine if infection is associated with hematuria; fever; testicular, perineal, or scrotal pain; or vaginitis.
- Assess factors for risk of urinary tract infection: incomplete bladder emptying, sexual activity, history of urinary calculi, or history of neurogenic bladder dysfunction or incontinence.
- Assess coping strategies, including medically prescribed regimens, patient uses to deal with urinary tract infections.
- Establish voiding routine of every 2 hours as needed. Postponing voiding is contraindicated in presence of active bacterial, fungal, or parasitic cystitis.
- Encourage adequate fluid intake to avoid dehydration, *which may intensify irritating symptoms,* or overhydration, *which may reduce the urine's mechanisms against pathogens.*

*References 1, 7-9, 11, 19, 20, 24.

- Counsel concerning appropriate time to contact physician (typically 72 hours after active medication is begun) for possible alteration of medication regimen if symptoms persist.
- Advise of importance of adherence to antibiotic medication regimen *to reduce likelihood of recurrence or persistence of infection.*
- Teach principal side effects of antibiotic medications: nausea and diarrhea.
- Teach to take antibiotics with meals *to reduce nausea* and to ingest yogurt, buttermilk, or other appropriate dairy products *to restore normal intestinal flora.*
- Teach to recognize allergic reactions to medications and when to consult physician concerning discontinuing medication.
- Teach women proper perineal hygiene: wipe from urethral meatus to anal area.
- Instruct to contact physician if symptoms of infection occur.
- Consult physician concerning appropriateness of self-start therapy for recurrent urinary tract infections.
- Consult physician for appropriateness of postcoital therapy for recurrent urinary tract infections.

FUNCTIONAL URINARY INCONTINENCE

Functional urinary incontinence is the inability of a usually continent person to reach the toilet in time to avoid unintentional loss of urine.[22]

Related Factors[4,11,22]

Anxiety
Confusion
Depression
Impaired cognition
Impaired memory
Impaired vision
Neuromuscular limitations
Sleep pattern disturbance
Weakened pelvic structures

Defining Characteristics[4,11,22]

Ability to completely empty bladder
Can sense need to void
Inability to reach toilet in time after sensing urge
Loss of urine before reaching toilet
Possibly incontinent only in early morning

Expected Patient Outcomes and Nursing Interventions With Rationale[9,11,14]

Restore continence, as evidenced by:

Empties bladder regularly and completely without intermittent urinary leakage

- Assess current voiding pattern.
- Assess factors associated with incontinent episodes, including environmental factors and patient's cognitive function and physical mobility.
- Assess other forms of urinary incontinence associated with functional incontinence.
- Institute a timed voiding schedule, patterned urge toileting response program, or other toileting schedule based on the patient's status, *to reduce episodes of functional incontinence.*
- Alter environment to maximize access to toilet facilities.
- Provide bedside toilet facility or urinal.
- Provide toilet facility that may be reached with minimum number of steps and without necessity of using stairs.
- Teach to use incontinence containment devices or systems as needed *to control urinary leakage between trips to toilet.*
- Help formulate plans for bladder management during outings.

Maintain skin integrity, as evidenced by:

Keeps skin exposed to urinary leakage free from rash or lesions
Demonstrates knowledge of skin care routine for area affected by urinary leakage
States indications for contacting physician concerning skin lesions

- Assess condition of perineal skin.
- Assess strategies and products patient is using to protect skin from irritation caused by urinary leakage.
- Provide skin care to areas exposed to urinary leakage using regular hygiene routine. Wash skin with soap and water or specially formulated incontinence cleanser. Dry thoroughly using hair dryer at low or warm setting with fan at lowest speed. Use skin sealant or moisture barrier to protect skin between washings, *to protect skin from urine scalding.*
- Teach patient and family to perform skin care and to recognize common skin rashes and indications for contacting health-care professional regarding rashes, inflammation, or skin infection.

REFLEX URINARY INCONTINENCE

Reflex urinary incontinence is an involuntary loss of urine at somewhat predictable intervals when a specific bladder volume is reached.[22]

Related Factors[11,22]

Amyotrophic lateral sclerosis
Autonomic dysreflexia
Bladder diverticula
Cerebellar ataxia
Complete spinal cord injury above sacral micturition center
Hydronephrosis
Multiple sclerosis
Myelomeningocele
Spinal cord tumor
Tissue damage from radiation, inflammation, or surgery
Urinary tract infection

Defining Characteristics[11,22]

Complete emptying with lesion above pontine micturition center
Incomplete emptying with lesion above sacral micturition center
No sensation of bladder fullness

No sensation of urge to void
No sensation of voiding
Predictable pattern of voiding
Sensation of urgency without voluntary inhibition of bladder contraction
Sensations associated with full bladder
Unable to cognitively inhibit or initiate voiding

Expected Patient Outcomes and Nursing Interventions With Rationale*

Restore continence, as evidenced by:
Maintains continence between catheterizations
Remains dry at night
Uses urinary containment device or system successfully

- Monitor fluid intake and urine output to keep urine volume below 300 ml.
- Develop a schedule for fluid intake.
- Begin clean intermittent catheterization program with appropriate autonomic drugs (propantheline or oxybutynin) or spasmolytic drugs (flavoxate or dicyclomine) under physician's direction.
- Consult physician concerning altering pharmacologic regimen if incontinent episodes occur between catheterizations.
- Establish catheterization schedule according to patient's schedule, approximately every 4 to 6 hours as needed during waking hours. *Sleep is not typically interrupted for intermittent catheterization.*
- Teach catheterization using clean, rather than sterile, technique unless latter is specified by physician.
- If clean intermittent schedule is not feasible or successful, use urinary containment devices.
- Institute a reflex voiding program with containment of urine by a condom catheter for the male who is unable or unwilling to perform self-intermittent catheterization.
- Teach the male and his family to select and apply a condom catheter that is: appropriate in size, comfortable, provides adequate drainage, and adheres to penis without creating a tourniquet effect.
- Teach the patient and family to select an appropriate leg bag for urinary drainage and storage. The leg bag should have nonrubberized straps; a cloth pouch or cloth backing *to minimize skin irritation;* adequate volume; an easily opened drainage spout; an antireflux proximal opening to *preventing reflux of urine from drainage bag to condom catheter;* and durable, flexible tubing connecting the condom catheter and leg bag.
- Insert a long-term indwelling or suprapubic catheter, as directed, when alternative management strategies are proven unfeasible. Choose a Foley catheter constructed of a cystocompatible, hydrophilic material that has the lowest feasible friction coefficient.
- Choose appropriate drainage system for daytime and nighttime use. Nighttime drainage system should contain a minimum of 2000 ml.
- Use other urinary containment devices (pads, incontinence briefs), as indicated.

Prevent urinary tract infection, as evidenced by:
Exhibits no symptoms of urinary tract infection

- Encourage adequate fluid intake.
- Teach signs of urinary tract infection: sudden change in continence between catheterization, fever, flank pain, hematuria, or change in character, color, or odor of urinary output.
- Teach to clean drainage bags regularly with vinegar and water solution, *to prevent urinary tract infection.*
- Teach patient and family to assess catheter daily *to ensure adequate drainage.*
- Change catheter as needed, approximately every 30 days.

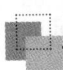

STRESS URINARY INCONTINENCE

Stress urinary incontinence is the state in which an individual experiences a urine loss of less than 50 ml, occurring with increased abdominal pressure.[22]

Related Factors*

Aging and menopause
Chronic cough
Cystocele
Enterocele
Frequent straining or heavy exercise, including long-distance running
Gravid uterus
Iatrogenic pelvic floor denervation
Multiple vaginal deliveries
Myelomeningocele
Obesity
Peripheral neuropathies
Radical prostatectomy
Rectocele
Sacral agenesis
Sphincter incompetence
Spina bifida
Trauma to pelvic support structures
Urge incontinence
Uterine prolapse

Defining Characteristics[4-8,11,22,26]

Urinary frequency (more often than every 2 hours)
Urinary leakage associated with increased abdominal pressure
Urinary leakage associated with physical exertion
Urinary leakage when bladder pressure exceeds urethral pressure in absence of detrusor contraction
Urinary urgency, frequency

Expected Patient Outcomes and Nursing Interventions With Rationale†

Maintain continence, as evidenced by:
No longer perceives urinary leakage as uncontrollable problem

- Determine causes of incontinence and any association with coughing, laughing, sneezing, abdominal strain.
- Assess urgency associated with incontinence, and identify stressors that produce these symptoms.

---

*References 9, 11, 17, 19, 21, 22.

*References 4-8, 11, 16, 18, 22, 26.
†References 1, 3-9, 11, 13, 15, 26.

- Assess frequency and severity of incontinence.
- Determine frequency of voiding, if patient is nocturic, and how often desire to void interrupts sleep.
- Monitor current fluid intake pattern.
- Assess coping strategies, including drugs or mechanical devices, patient currently employs to cope with urinary leakage.
- Assess risk factors for this patient (e.g., number of vaginal deliveries, status of estrogen production or replacement, previous surgical procedures, conditions related to peripheral neuropathies), *to help determine cause of incontinence.*
- Provide with incontinent containment device or system. Absorbent pads are usually sufficient. *Pad should provide adequate absorbency and protect clothing from urinary leakage.*
- Teach female patient to do pelvic muscle exercises *to strengthen circurrivaginal muscles (CVMs) through resistive and endurance improvement.*[7]
- Supplement a pelvic muscle exercise regimen with a referral for possible electrostimulation of the pelvic floor muscles in the female who fails to adequately respond to exercises only.[1,2]
- Teach females to use weighted vaginal cones as an alternative or supplement to pelvic muscle exercises.
- Provide females with an appropriate pessary device in consultation with or under direction of physician; teach patient care of pessary device, including appropriate hygiene and necessity of regular follow-up to change device, as indicated.
- Administer sympathomimetic medications (pseudoephedrine), as directed, *to increase smooth muscle tone of the sphincter.*
- Inform of availability of surgical options to correct stress incontinence as indicated, and encourage patient to speak with appropriate health-care professional.

URGE URINARY INCONTINENCE

Urge urinary incontinence is the state in which an individual experiences involuntary passage of urine, occurring soon after a strong sense of urgency to void.[22]

Related Factors[1,23]

Age (childhood or elderly)
Altered state of mobility
Altered thought processes
Alzheimer's disease
Anxiety
Bladder neck hypertrophy, contracture, or dyssynergia
Bladder outlet obstruction
Cerebrovascular accident
Closed head injury
Cystitis
Impaired verbal communication
Inability to reach toilet in time
Incomplete suprasacral spinal cord injury
Increased urine concentration
Lack of access to toilet
Multiple sclerosis
Parkinsonism
Prostatic enlargement, prostatitis
Sleep pattern disturbance related to nocturia
Stress incontinence

Defining Characteristics[11,18,22]

Bladder contracture or spasm
Bladder infection
Nocturia
Urinary frequency
Urinary urgency
Urinary leakage associated with marked urgency
Voiding in large amounts (more than 550 ml)
Voiding in small amounts (less than 100 ml)

Expected Patient Outcomes and Nursing Interventions With Rationale*

Restore urinary continence, as evidenced by:

States symptoms of urge incontinence are absent; or if symptoms remain, incontinent episodes are absent
Describes goals and process of timed voiding schedule with fluid intake control
Demonstrates knowledge of continence containment device
Reports dryness between intermittent catheterizations
Reports no leakage around Foley catheter

- Assess factors that predispose toward urge incontinence: neurologic disease or trauma, bladder outlet obstruction, irritative bladder disorder, stress incontinence.
- Assess associated related factors for urge incontinence: physical or cognitive impairment, environmental alterations.
- Assess access to toilet facilities and approximate transit time to nearest toilet facility, considering the patient's physical mobility limitations, if any.
- Determine current daytime urinary elimination patterns (frequency of urination, number of incontinent episodes per day).
- Assess patient for nocturia, enuresis, or incontinence before reaching toilet.
- Evaluate current fluid intake pattern (volume and time).
- Explore factors that predispose toward urge incontinence with the patient.
- Assess current coping strategies, including drugs or medical treatments, patient uses to deal with urge incontinence.
- Develop an individualized timed voiding schedule of approximately every 2 to 3 hours, progressing to every 3 to 4 hours as feasible.
- Teach patient to rapidly contract the pelvic muscles for a period of 2 to 6 seconds when precipitous episode of urgency occurs. Advise the patient to repeat this maneuver until the urgency subsides, and to promptly move to the bathroom and urinate.
- Administer anticholinergic drugs (tolterodine, propantheline, or oxybutynin) or spasmolytic drugs (flavoxate or dicyclomine) as ordered, *to inhibit smooth muscle contraction.*
- Institute bladder retraining program in consultation with physician. Instruct the patient to postpone urination for 1½ hours during waking hours even if incontinence

*References 1, 2, 4, 9, 11, 16, 20, 24, 25.

occurs in the interim. Increase time between voidings by ½ hour until a goal of 3 to 4 hours is reached.
- Combine electrostimulation of the pelvic floor muscles with bladder drill therapy, timed voiding schedules, as indicated and prescribed.
- If attempts at timed voiding and fluid control schedules and bladder drill therapy fail, consult physician concerning institution of significant pharmacologic relaxation of the detrusor muscle with intermittent catheterization schedule. Begin clean intermittent catheterization program and teach patient and family members as soon as feasible. Catheterization should be accomplished approximately every 4 to 6 hours. Sleep patterns are not usually interrupted for catheterization.
- Provide portable urinal if feasible.
- Provide bedside toilet facility for nighttime voiding needs.
- Allow patient to sit up to use toilet whenever possible.
- Bedpans or continent briefs should be employed as a final resort rather than for convenience.

Prevent urinary tract infections, as evidenced by:
Exhibits no symptoms of urinary tract infection
- Assess for history of urinary tract infections, frequency of occurrence, and any association with fever or hematuria.
- Assess coping strategies, including pharmacologic agents, patient currently uses to deal with infections.
- Determine if patient thinks that bladder is completely emptied and if patient uses specific strategies (e.g., double voiding, self-intermittent catheterization) *to ensure complete bladder emptying.*
- Assess efficiency of bladder emptying by maintaining accurate record of fluid intake and urinary output.
- Measure postvoiding residuals at least three times using straight catheter or ultrasound assessment within 5 minutes of voiding.
- Encourage adequate fluid intake.

Risk for Urge Urinary Incontinence

The risk for urge urinary incontinence involves the risk for involuntary loss of urine associated with a sudden, strong sensation of urinary urgency.[22]

Risk Factors[11,22]

Detrusor hyperreflexia
Detrusor muscle instability with impaired contractility
Effects of medications, caffeine, alcohol
Ineffective toileting habits
Involuntary sphincter relaxation
Small bladder capacity

Expected Patient Outcomes and Nursing Interventions With Rationale[2,11,23,25]

Maintain urinary continence, as evidenced by:
Has no episodes of incontinence
Describes goals and process of timed voiding schedule with fluid intake
- Assess related factors that predispose toward urge incontinence: physical or cognitive impairment, environmental alterations, neurologic disease or trauma, bladder outlet obstruction, irritative bladder disorders, stress incontinence.
- Determine if patient is in high-risk age group for condition.
- Assess access to toilet facilities and approximate transit time to nearest toilet facility, considering the patient's physical mobility limitations, if any.
- Determine current daytime urinary elimination patterns (frequency of urination, number of incontinent episodes per day).
- Ask if patient experiences nocturia, enuresis, or incontinence before reaching toilet, *to determine risk factors for urge incontinence.*
- Check current fluid intake pattern (volume and time).
- Determine specific circumstances that patient and family identify as predisposing toward urge incontinence.
- Have patient maintain timed voiding schedule of approximately every 2 to 3 hours during the day, *to decrease risk of urge incontinence.* Individualize schedule with patient and family. Progress to every 3 to 4 hours as feasible.
- Teach patient to rapidly contract the pelvic muscles for a period of 2 to 6 seconds when precipitous episode of urgency occurs. Advise the patient to repeat this maneuver until the urgency subsides, and to promptly move to the bathroom and urinate.
- Institute bladder retraining therapy regimen in consultation with physician. Instruct the patient to postpone urination for 1½ hours during waking hours. Increase time between voidings by ½ hour until a goal of 3 to 4 hours is reached.

Total Urinary Incontinence

Total urinary incontinence is the state is which an individual experiences a continuous and unpredictable loss of urine.[22]

Related Factors[11,13,18,19,22]

Bladder exstrophy
Congenital sphincter incompetence
Ectopic ureter that bypasses sphincteric mechanism
Intrinsic sphincter deficiency
Multiple antiincontinence procedures
Neurologic dysfunction causing triggering of micturition at unpredictable times
Neuropathy preventing transmission of reflex indicating bladder fullness
Surgically created stomas
Trauma to sphincter
Urethral duplication
Urinary tract infection
Urinary fistula

Defining Characteristics[11,13,18,22]

Constant urine flow at unpredictable times
Continuous urinary leakage with an otherwise normal voiding pattern
Continuous urinary leakage with failure of urinary storage

Incontinence refractory to pharmacologic or behavioral treatment
Lack of perineal or bladder filling awareness
Nocturia
Unawareness of incontinence
Unsuccessful incontinence treatments

Expected Patient Outcomes and Nursing Interventions With Rationale[1,4,11,13,18]

Contain urine, as evidenced by:
Prevents leakage around incontinent pad or brief
Maintains condom catheter system without leakage
Maintains urinary pouch system without leakage

- Determine when incontinence occurs and if patient is ever dry.
- Assess conditions that make leakage more or less severe.
- Determine if leakage is ever associated with sensation of urgency.
- Assess normal voiding patterns. Determine if continuous urinary leakage occurs in addition to "regular" voiding pattern or if incontinence is severe enough to have replaced micturition.
- Assess for urinary tract infection, and presence of hematuria or fever.
- Provide with urinary containment device or system to cope with incontinence, including pads with water-resistant backing, adult briefs, or condom catheters.
- Instruct on use of urinary pouching system for patients with total incontinence caused by surgical diversion.

Maintain skin integrity, as evidenced by:
Skin remains free from rashes, lesions, inflammation, and infection
Accurately describes skin care routine for areas exposed to constant urinary leakage
Accurately describes indications for contacting health-care professional concerning loss of skin integrity

- Assess condition of perineal skin.
- Assess strategies, including routine hygiene habits, and products patient is currently using to protect perineal skin from irritation.
- Provide skin care to areas exposed to urinary leakage using regular hygiene routine. Wash skin with soap and water or specially formulated incontinence cleanser. Dry thoroughly using hair dryer at low or warm setting with fan at lowest speed. Use skin sealant or moisture barrier to protect skin between washings, *to protect skin from urine scalding.*
- Teach patient and family to recognize common skin rashes and indications for when to contact health-care professionals.

URINARY RETENTION

Urinary retention is the state in which the individual experiences incomplete emptying of the bladder.[22]

Related Factors[11,16,18,22]

Antiparkinsonian agents
Bladder neck hypertrophy or contracture
Bladder outlet obstruction
Bladder trabeculation
Calcium channel blockers
Cannabis ingestion
Cauda equina injury or syndrome
Constipation or fecal impaction
Diabetes mellitus
Dicyclomine
Female urethral distortion
Flavoxate
Ganglionic blocking agents
Incomplete spinal cord injury
Methantheline
Multiple sclerosis
Oxybutynin
Pelvic trauma
Phenothiazines
Postpolio syndrome
Propantheline
Prostatic enlargement
Pyelonephritis
Sacral spinal cord injury
Sensory paralytic bladder
Tabes dorsalis
Tricylic antidepressants
Urethral trauma
Urethral stricture
Urinary tract infections

Defining Characteristics[11,16,18,22]

Absence of micturition with suprapubic pain or pressure
Bladder distention
Dysuria
Intermittent or poor urinary stream
Nocturia
Overflow incontinence
Postvoiding dribble
Postvoiding residual greater than 25% of total bladder volume
Sensation of bladder fullness
Small voided volumes
Urinary frequency

Expected Patient Outcomes and Nursing Interventions With Rationale[11,13,19]

Resolve urinary retention, as evidenced by:
Has no episodes of urinary frequency or nocturia
Remains free of overflow incontinence
Has postvoiding residual less than 25% of total bladder volume

- Assess current diurnal voiding patterns.
- Assess quality of voided stream.
- Determine awareness of feelings of incomplete emptying.
- Assess maneuvers (if any) patient is using to cope with urinary retention.
- Determine if patient strains or uses Crede's maneuver to assist voiding. Crede's maneuver increases bladder pressure, *which may stimulate relaxation of the sphincter to allow voiding.*

- Teach patient to double void *to enhance complete bladder emptying.* Patient should void normally, then wait on the toilet for approximately 5 minutes and attempt to void again.
- Teach patient to void using a timed schedule. Patient should void every 3 to 4 hours when awake regardless of absence of desire to urinate.
- Consult physician concerning use of medication for patients with deficient detrusor function or sphincter resistance.

Establish regular, complete bladder emptying using mechanical means, as evidenced by:

Has no overflow incontinence

- Teach patient and family members to perform intermittent catheterization (see Reflex Urinary Incontinence).
- Teach patient to keep diary or log of voided volume versus volume catheterized, and provide guidelines for returning to physician to alter catheterization schedule.
- Teach patient to maintain long-term indwelling catheter.

Prevent urinary tract infection, as evidenced by:

Urine culture remains negative

Remains free of symptoms of urinary tract infections

- Assess for presence of current urinary tract infections.
- Assess for constipation and patient's routine bowel program.
- Provide patient with bowel program, including increased fluid intake with dietary fiber and bulk, stool softeners, and/or enemas in consultation with physician. *Constipation may contribute to urinary retention.*
- Assess strategies patient uses to manage urinary tract infections.
- Teach patient to completely empty bladder on a regular basis.
- Consult physician concerning use of long-term antibiotic prophylaxis for patients with chronic urinary retention as appropriate.

References

Elimination

1. Gordon M: *Manual of nursing diagnosis,* ed 9, St. Louis, 2000, Mosby.

Bowel Incontinence

1. Beddar SAM, Holden-Bennett L, McCormick AM; Development and evaluation of a protocol to manage fecal incontinence in the patient with cancer, *J Palliative Care* 13(2):27, 1997.
2. Brown C: Pelvic floor rehabilitation: conservative treatment for incontinence . . . the Canadian Continence Foundation . . . hosted the first Canadian Multidisciplinary Professional and Consumer Conference in November 1997, entitled "Partners in Continence," *Ostomy Wound Manage* 44(6):72, 1998.
3. Dudley-Brown S: Living with ulcerative colitis, *Gastroenterol Nurs* 19(2):60, 1996.
4. Gray M: Bowel incontinence. In Ackley BJ, Ladwig GB, editors: *Nursing diagnosis handbook: a guide to planning care,* ed 4, St. Louis, 1999, Mosby.
5. Haugen V: Perineal skin care for patients with frequent diarrhea or fecal incontinence, *Gastroenterol Nurs* 20(3):87, 1997.
6. Jensen LL: Fecal incontinence: evaluation and treatment, *J WOCN* 24(5):277, 1997.
7. Loening-Baucke V: Fecal incontinence in children, *Am Fam Physician* 55(6):2229, 1997.
8. McCloskey JC, Bulechek GM, editors: *Nursing interventions classification (NIC),* ed 3, St. Louis, 2001, Mosby.
9. McFarland GK, McFarlane EA: *Nursing diagnosis and intervention: planning for patient care,* ed 3, St. Louis, 1997, Mosby.
10. North American Nursing Diagnosis Association: *NANDA nursing diagnoses: definitions and classification, 2001–2002,* Philadelphia, 2001, The Association.

Constipation, Perceived Constipation, Risk for Constipation

1. Abyad A: Constipation in the elderly: diagnosis and management strategies, *Managed Care Interface* 11(4):87, 1998.
2. Ackley BJ, Ladwig GB: *Nursing diagnosis handbook: a guide to planning care,* ed 4, St. Louis, 1999, Mosby.
3. Anti M: Water supplementation enhances the effect of high-fiber diet on stool frequency and laxative consumption in adult patients with functional constipation, *Hepatogastoenterol* 45(21):727, 1998.
4. Basta S, Anderson DL: Mechanisms and management of constipation in the cancer patient, *J Pharm Care Pain Symptom Control* 6(3):21, 1998.
5. Doenges ME, Moorhouse MF: *Nurse's pocket guide: diagnosis, interventions, and rationale,* ed 6, Philadelphia, 1998, FA Davis.
6. McCloskey JC, Bulechek GM, editors: *Nursing interventions classification (NIC),* ed 3, St. Louis, 2001, Mosby.
7. McFarland GK, McFarlane EA: *Nursing diagnosis and intervention: planning for patient care,* ed 3, St. Louis, 1997, Mosby.
8. Mead M: Drugs for constipation, *Pract Nurse* 17(1):48, 1999.
9. North American Nursing Diagnosis Association: *NANDA nursing diagnoses: definitions and classification 2001–2002,* Philadelphia, 2001, The Association.
10. Schaeffer DC, Cheskin LJ: Constipation in the elderly, *Am Fam Physician* 58(4):907, 1998.
11. Sheehy C, Hall GR: Clinical outlook. Rethinking the obvious: a model for preventing constipation, *J Gerontol Nurs* 24(3):38, 1998.
12. Turnbull G: Drug-free remedies for constipation, bloating and other "irritable bowel" problems, *Bottom Line/Health* 12(11):5, 1998.
13. United States Pharmacopeial Convention, Inc: *Volume I. Drug information for the health care professional,* Taunton, Mass, 1998, World Color Book Services.
14. Winney J: Constipation . . . and the role of nurses in assessment, management and health promotion, *Elderly Care* 10(4):26, 1998.
15. Youngkin EQ, Sawin KJ, Kissinger JF et al: *Pharmacotherapeutics: a primary care clinical guide,* Stamford, Conn, 1999, Appleton & Lange.

Diarrhea

1. Courtens AM, Abu-Saad HH: Nursing diagnoses in patients with leukemia, *Nurs Diagnosis J Nurs Language Classification* 9(2):49, 1998.
2. Hesnan KD, Ackley BJ: Diarrhea. In Ackley BJ, Ladwig GB, editors: *Nursing diagnosis handbook: a guide to planning care,* ed 4, St. Louis, 1999, Mosby.
3. Hogan CM: The nurse's role in diarrhea management, *Oncol Nurs Forum* 25(50:879, 1998.
4. McCloskey JC, Bulechek GM, editors: *Nursing interventions classification (NIC),* ed 3, St. Louis, 2001, Mosby.
5. McCray WH, Krevsky B: Diagnosing diarrhea in adults: a practical approach, *Hosp Med* 34(4):27, 1999.
6. McFarland GK, McFarlane EA: *Nursing diagnosis and intervention: planning for patient care,* ed 3, St. Louis, 1997, Mosby.

7. North American Nursing Diagnosis Association: *NANDA nursing diagnoses: definitions and classification, 2001–2002,* Philadelphia, 2001, The Association.
8. Williams MS, Harper R, Magnuson B et al: Diarrhea management in enterally fed patients, *Nutr Clin Pract* 13(5):225, 1998.

Impaired Urinary Elimination, Functional Urinary Incontinence, Reflex Urinary Incontinence, Stress Urinary Incontinence, Urge Urinary Incontinence, Risk for Urge Urinary Incontinence, Total Urinary Incontinence, Urinary Retention

1. Brown C: Pelvic floor rehabilitation: conservative treatment for incontinence . . . the Canadian Continence Foundation . . . hosted the first Canadian Multidsiciplinary Professional and Consumer Conference in November 1997, entitled "Partners in Continence," *Ostomy Wound Manage* 44(6):72, 1997.
2. Brown JS, Subak LL, Gras J et al: Urge incontinence: the patient's perspective, *J Womens Health* 7(10):1263, 1998.
3. Brubaker L, Harris T, Gleason D et al: The external urethral barrier for stress incontinence: a multicenter trial of safety and efficacy. Miniguard Investigators Group, *Obstet Gynecol* 92(6):932, 1999.
4. Chutka DS, Takahashi PY: Urinary incontinence in the elderly: drug treatment options, *Drugs* 56(4):587, 1998.
5. Davila GW, Neal D, Horbach N et al: A bladder-neck support prosthesis for women with stress and mixed incontinence, *Obstet Gynecol* 93(6):938, 1999.
6. Diokno AC: Post prostatectomy urinary incontinence . . . the Canadian Continence Foundation . . . hosted the first Canadian Multidisciplinary Professional and Consumer Conference in November 1997, entitled "Partners in Continence," *Ostomy Wound Manag* 44(6):54, 1998.
7. Dougherty MC: Current status of research on pelvic muscle straightening techniques, *J WOCN* 25(2):75, 1998.
8. Drake MJ, Nixon PM, Crew JP: Drug-induced bladder and urinary disorders: incidence, prevention and management, *Drug Saf* 19(1):45, 1999.
9. Foster P: Behavioral treatment of urinary incontinence: a complementary approach . . . the Canadian Continence Foundation . . . hosted the first Canadian Multidisciplinary Professional and Consumer Conference in November 1997, entitled "Partners in Continence," *Ostomy Wound Manage* 44(6):62, 1998.
10. Gallagher MS: Urogenital distress and the psychosocial impact of urinary incontinence on elderly women . . . including commentary by J Baggerly, *Rehabil Nurs* 23(4):192, 1998.
11. Gray M: Altered patterns of urinary elimination. In Ackley BJ, Ladwig GB, editors: *Nursing diagnosis handbook: a guide to planning care,* ed 4, St. Louis, 1999, Mosby.
12. Gray M, Petroni GR, Theodorescu D: Urinary function after radical prostatectomy: a comparison of the retropubic and perineal approaches, *Urology* 53(5):881, 1999.
13. Gulanik M, Klopp A, Galanes S et al: *Nursing care plans: nursing diagnosis and intervention,* ed 4, St. Louis, 1998, Mosby.
14. Heavner K: Urinary incontinence in extended care facilities: a literature review and proposal for continuous quality improvement, *Ostomy Wound Manag* 44(12):46, 1998.
15. Jay J, Staskin D: Urinary incontinence in women, *Adv Nurse Pract* 6(10:323, 1998.
16. Krogh RH, Bruskewitz RC: Disorders of the lower genitourinary tract, *Clin Geriatr* 6(13):19, 1998.
17. Litwiller SE, Frohman EM, Zimmern PE: Multiple sclerosis and the urologist, *J Urol* 161(3):743, 1999.
18. McCloskey JC, Bulechek GM, editors: *Nursing interventions classification (NIC),* ed 3, St. Louis, 2001, Mosby.
19. McFarland GK, McFarlane EA: *Nursing diagnosis and intervention: planning for patient care,* ed 3, St. Louis, 1997, Mosby.
20. Moore KN, Richardson VA: Pharmacology: impact on bladder function . . . the Canadian Continence Foundation . . . hosted the first Canadian Multidiciplinary Professional and Consumer Conference in November 1997, entitled "Partners in Continence," *Ostomy Wound Manage* 44(6):30, 1998.
21. Newman DK: Managing indwelling urethral catheters, *Ostomy Wound Manage* 44(12):26, 1998.
22. North American Nursing Diagnosis Association: *NANDA nursing diagnoses: definitions and classification, 2001–2002,* Philadelphia, 2001, The Association.
23. Roe B, Williams K, Palmer M: Bladder training for the treatment of urinary urge incontinence, Oxford, 1999, *The Cochrane Library.*
24. Velez JB: Behavior therapy for urge incontinence in older women, *J Fam Pract* 48(3):168, 1999.
25. Wein AJ, Rovner ES: The overactive bladder: an overview for primary care health providers, *Int J Fertil Womens Med* 44(2):56, 1999.
26. Woodtli A: Stress incontinence: clinical identification and validation of defining characteristics, *Nurs Diagnosis* 6(3):115, 1995.

4 FUNCTIONAL HEALTH PATTERN

Activity-Exercise[1]

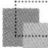

ACTIVITY INTOLERANCE

Activity intolerance is a state in which an individual has insufficient physiologic energy to endure or complete required or desired daily activities.[7]

Related Factors[3,4,7,9]

Bed rest
Climate extremes
Deconditioning (related to lifestyle)
Decreased mobility or immobility
Generalized weakness
Imbalance between oxygen supply and demand
Lack of knowledge
Lack of motivation
Lack of support
Obesity
Pain
Sedentary lifestyle

Defining Characteristics[4,7,9]

Ataxia
Avoidance of activity
Bradycardia
Decrease in activity (self-care, exercise, leisure)
Decrease in respiratory rate
Decrease in pulse strength
Dizziness, vertigo
Drooping of shoulders or head
Dyspnea
Dysrhythmia
Electrocardiographic changes reflecting dysrhythmias
Fear of activity
Inappropriate increases or decreases in blood pressure
Inappropriate tachycardia
Irregular respiratory rhythm
Lack of interest in activity
Pallor, cyanosis, flushing
Profuse diaphoresis
Syncope
Tachypnea
Verbal report of fatigue or weakness

Expected Patient Outcomes and Nursing Interventions With Rationale[1-6,8-10]

Participate in activities that enhance physiologic well-being, as evidenced by:

Maintains balance between oxygen supply and demand
Demonstrates an absence of weakness and fatigue during or after engaging in activity
Reports tolerance of activities

- Assess patient's past and present activity pattern.
- Determine past activities (self-care, exercise, and leisure) engaged in; intensity, duration, and frequency of each activity; and how these activities were tolerated, *to determine the level of activity intolerance.*
- Determine present activities and how these are tolerated.
- Determine if any physical impediments restrict or prevent participation in particular activities, *to determine appropriate activities.*[1]
- Determine if there is any change in physiologic status when engaging in activity.[2]
- Assess cardiovascular response; respiratory response; pulse rate; skin color, temperature, and moistness; posture; and equilibrium.
- Determine if there is any change in emotional status before or when engaging in activity, *to assist the patient in identifying activities that will enhance psychologic well-being.*
- Determine if patient is fearful of harming self.
- Provide patient information about activities in which to participate.
- Seek consultation with physician, exercise physiologist, and occupational and physical therapists, as necessary, *to tailor activity to the individual patient.*
- Assist patient in identifying factors that reduce activity tolerance such as inadequate sleep, medication, treatments, or environmental conditions.
- Engage immobile patients in passive exercise regimen *to increase activity tolerance.*
- Assist patient with structural limitations to adapt self-care, exercise, and leisure activities *to meet activity needs.*
- Provide assistance to patient as needed, encouraging independence in performing activities.
- Encourage patient to engage in self-care, exercise, and leisure activities that can be tolerated.

- Guide patient in increasing activity within therapeutic limits *to support an increased tolerance of activity.*

Develop activity and rest pattern supporting increased tolerance of activity, as evidenced by:

Adheres to a schedule that promotes increased activity without increasing weakness, fatigue, and untoward physiologic responses

- Discuss usual activity/rest pattern; suggest ways to modify an ineffective pattern.
- Discuss the importance of increasing activity tolerance.
- Encourage patient to participate in planning daily rest periods and activity periods *to ensure that the pattern can be integrated into the patient's lifestyle.*
- Adjust medication and treatment schedule *to support adequate rest.*
- Teach patient to monitor response to activity and to alter activity when signs and symptoms of shortness of breath or excessive fatigue are present.

Use support of family, friends, and health-care providers in adjusting activity and rest pattern, as evidenced by:

Describes the role of significant others in revising and implementing the activity and rest schedule

- Provide patient and significant others with information about importance of establishing therapeutic activity/rest pattern.
- Review schedule of daily activities of significant others and identify with them how it can be altered *to support fulfillment of patient's needs.*
- Encourage patient and significant others to participate in planning mutually agreeable daily schedule of activity/rest periods *to ensure that the pattern can be integrated into the patient's lifestyle.*
- Facilitate expression of patient and significant others' concerns regarding proposed schedule.
- Identify support available from health-care providers if need arises to revise or alter schedule *to tailor activity to the individual.*
- Encourage family and friends to support patient in efforts to meet need for activity. *Support can be essential in assisting the patient to adhere to an activity/rest pattern that will promote optimum participation.*

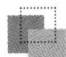

RISK FOR ACTIVITY INTOLERANCE

Risk for activity intolerance is a state in which an individual is at risk of experiencing insufficient physiologic or psychologic energy to endure or complete required or desired daily activities.[7]

Risk Factors[4,7,9]

Climate extremes
Deconditioned status (prolonged bed rest, inactivity)
Expressed concern about ability to perform the activity
Expressed lack of interest in engaging in activity or exercise
Fatigue, weakness
History of previous intolerance to activity
More than 15% overweight
Pain
Presence of chronic or progressive disease (e.g., chronic obstructive pulmonary disease, multiple sclerosis, coronary artery disease, arthritis, depression)
Refusal to participate in prescribed activities
Sedentary lifestyle

Expected Patient Outcomes and Nursing Interventions With Rationale[1-6,8-10]

Participate in activities that promote optimum well-being, as evidenced by:

Performs recommended self-care, exercise, and leisure activities daily

- Assess patient's past and present activity pattern *to determine the risk for activity intolerance.*
- Assess type, intensity, duration, and frequency of each patient activity.
- Determine physiologic response to activity.
- Determine psychologic response to activity, *to assist in identifying activities that will enhance psychologic well-being.*
- Assess risk factors for potential activity intolerance.
- Provide patient with information about desired or required daily activities.
- Assist patient in selecting activities that are enjoyable and can be integrated into lifestyle *to ensure activity can be maintained.*
- Assist patient in identifying risk factors that reduce activity tolerance.
- Encourage patient to participate in activities that promote an increase in activity tolerance within therapeutic limits.
- Identify organized activities and exercise programs in which patient might want to participate. *Participation in organized activities may be easier to maintain.*
- Encourage family and significant others to support patient and to participate in activities and exercise programs with patient. *Support can be helpful in maintaining activity.*

Appreciate the need to participate in required and desired activities, as evidenced by:

Specifies the benefits of engaging in activity
Identifies factors that could inhibit activity tolerance

- Review benefits of regularly engaging in activities that promote physical and psychologic well-being, as well as factors that could inhibit activity tolerance. *Knowledge of benefits may increase motivation.*
- Assist the patient in developing a realistic plan that includes self-care, exercise, and leisure activities.
- Encourage the patient to plan activities with persons who can support participation in activities that enhance well-being. *Support can be helpful in maintaining activity.*

AUTONOMIC DYSREFLEXIA

Autonomic dysreflexia is a state in which the individual with a spinal cord injury at T7 or above experiences a life-threatening uninhibited sympathetic response of the nervous system to a noxious stimulus.[7]

Related Factors[1,5-7]

Bladder distention or spasm
Bowel distention

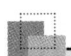

Catheter insertion or irrigation
Lack of patient and caregiver knowledge
Manipulation of the perineum
Obstructed catheter
Sexual stimulation or intercourse
Skin irritation
Traction of viscera during surgery
Uterine contractions

Defining Characteristics[1,5-7]

Chest pain and cardiac irregularities
Diaphoresis (above injury)
Pallor (below injury)
Paroxysmal hypertension (up to 240/120 or higher)
Patchy erythema (above injury)
Severe, pounding headache
Tachycardia

Expected Patient Outcomes and Nursing Interventions With Rationale[1,3-6,8,9]

Prevent or eliminate stimuli that cause hyperactive reflexes, as evidenced by:

Manages dysreflexia

- Provide dysreflexia management.[5]
  - Identify and minimize stimuli that may precipitate dysreflexia: bladder distention, infection, fecal impaction, rectal examination, suppository insertion, skin breakdown, and constrictive clothing or bed linen.
  - Monitor for signs and symptoms of autonomic dysreflexia: paroxysmal hypertension, bradycardia, tachycardia, diaphoresis above the level of injury, facial flushing, pallor below the level of injury, headache, nasal congestion, and chest pain.
  - Investigate and remove offending cause (e.g., distended bladder, fecal impaction, skin lesions, and constricting bed clothes).
  - Place head of bed in upright position, as appropriate, if hyperreflexia occurs.
  - Stay with patient and monitor status every 3 to 5 minutes if hyperreflexia occurs.
  - Administer antihypertensive agents intravenously, as ordered.
  - Instruct patient and family about causes, symptoms, treatment, and prevention of dysreflexia.

Assist with identification of symptoms and causes, and experience fewer and less severe episodes of dysreflexia, as evidenced by:

Identifies episode early
Knows when to seek further assistance from health-care professional
Understands that many health-care professionals may be unfamiliar with the syndrome
Directs care and explains interventions to staff, if necessary
Wears medical alert bracelet. *Autonomic dysreflexia is a life-threatening response.*
Blood pressure and heart rate return to normal
Maintains usual bowel and bladder elimination patterns
Headache subsides
Avoids or minimizes bowel and bladder distention
Recognizes symptoms and notifies health-care professional

- Develop awareness of signs and symptoms of dysreflexia and ensure that other staff and patients are aware of symptoms and precipitating factors.
- Assess patient for history of previous attacks of dysreflexia and possible causes.
- Assess and monitor bowel and bladder elimination patterns *to prevent distention. Bowel and bladder distention are the most common causes of dysreflexia.*[2]
- Observe urinary catheters for kinks and obstructions; ensure patency and change catheter if unable to attain patency with irrigation, *to prevent bladder distention.*
- Check cautiously for fecal impaction, if necessary, and relieve promptly with suppository or enema.
- Minimize manipulation and stimulation when performing procedures involving bladder and bowel.
- Be aware that early symptoms can include sudden pounding headache, sweating, and blotching of skin of face and thorax.
- If symptoms occur, stop any procedure being performed, notify physician immediately, and prepare to assist with treatment.
- Monitor blood pressure and pulse continuously until symptoms subside.
- Administer antihypertensive or alpha-adrenergic blockers, as ordered.
- Elevate head of bed and lower patient's legs *to counteract hypertension with orthostatic hypotension in attempt to reduce headache.*
- Remove all support hose or binders *to promote venous pooling and decrease venous return, thereby decreasing blood pressure.*
- Reassure patient and take measures to promote comfort.
- Instruct patient about syndrome *to develop awareness about possible causes and early symptoms experienced.*

RISK FOR AUTONOMIC DYSREFLEXIA

Risk for autonomic dysreflexia is the state in which there is a risk for life-threatening, uninhibited response of the sympathetic nervous system, post spinal shock, in an individual with spinal cord injury or lesion at T6 or above (has been demonstrated in patients with injuries at T7 and T8).[7]

Risk Factors[2,7]

Bladder distention
Burns
Constipation
Constrictive clothing
Cutaneous stimulations
Decongestants
Deep vein thrombosis
Distention
Ejaculation
Enemas
Epididymitis
Fractures

Gastrointestinal system pathology
Infection
Ingrown toenail
Labor contractions
Labor and delivery
Narcotic withdrawal
Ovarian cyst
Painful or irritating stimuli below the level of injury
Positioning
Pregnancy
Pressure ulcer
Pulmonary emboli
Range-of-motion exercises
Rash
Sexual intercourse
Stimulation of gastrointestinal tract
Surgical procedures
Sympathomimetics
Urethritis
Vasoconstrictors

Expected Patient Outcomes and Nursing Interventions With Rationale[2-6,8,9]

Identify stimuli that cause hyperactive reflexes, as evidenced by:

Describes stimuli that may cause dysreflexia

- Explain that bladder distention, fecal impaction, and rectal stimulation may cause dysreflexia by triggering massive vasoconstriction.
- Discuss the potential for dysreflexia with skin breakdown, infection, or constrictive clothing or bed linens.

Prevent occurrence of autonomic dysreflexia, as evidenced by:

Maintains proper hygiene regimens

- Assess and monitor bowel and bladder elimination patterns *to prevent distention. Bowel and bladder distention are the most common causes of dysreflexia.*[2]
- Teach patient to:
  Wear nonrestrictive, proper-fitting clothing.
  Avoid fall, burns, or other injuries.
  Maintain skin integrity and prevent skin breakdown.
  Wear medical alert bracelet. *Autonomic dysreflexia is a life-threatening response.*

Bathing/Hygiene Self-Care Deficit

Bathing/hygiene self-care deficit is the impaired ability to perform or complete bathing/hygiene activities for oneself.[15]

Related Factors[8,15,16,23]

Advanced age
Confusion
Decreased or lack of motivation
Delirium
Developmental delay
Environmental barriers
Excessive ritualistic behaviors
Inadequate perception of body part or spatial relationship
Lack of coordination
Musculoskeletal or neuromuscular impairment (e.g., spasticity, weakness, contractures, paralysis)
Pain
Perceptual or cognitive impairment
Phobias
Psychologic impairment (e.g., psychosis, mania, catatonia, delusions)
Severe disabling anxiety
Weakness and tiredness

Defining Characteristics[15,16,23]

Inability to dry body
Inability to get bath supplies
Inability to get in and out of bathroom
Inability to obtain or get to water source
Inability to perceive need for hygienic measures
Inability to regulate temperature or flow of bathwater
Inability to wash body or body parts

Expected Patient Outcomes and Nursing Interventions With Rationale[6,7,9,14-22]

Independently complete bathing and hygiene activities, or with assistance, as evidenced by:

Has clean, intact skin and nails; clean, combed hair; clean, brushed teeth or dentures
Remains free from offensive odors
Expresses satisfaction with self-care progress in bathing and hygiene

- Assess patient's ability to bathe and perform personal hygiene, including comprehension, awareness, cognition, and affect, *to provide data on deficits in meeting bathing and hygiene needs.*
- Ask patient about bathing habits and cultural bathing preferences, *to demonstrate respect for cultural preferences and preserve patient's self-esteem.*[6,7,14]
- Discuss daily routine with patient *to allow patient a voice in planning care.*
- Individualize bathing routine according to patient preferences, *to make bathing a calming experience, and to reduce aggression.*[9,14]
- Encourage patient to participate in bathing and personal hygiene as able, *to support and promote independence.*
- Provide privacy when bathing and performing personal hygiene.
- Prevent fatigue during bathing; seat client with feet supported. *Conservation of energy increases activity tolerance.*
- Allow patient adequate time to complete bathing and personal hygiene.
- Provide pain medication before bathing if needed, *to promote self-care.*
- Assess physical and environmental factors that may inhibit bathing, such as decreased flexibility, faucets difficult to turn, and lack of safety rails, *to identify factors*

that can be adapted to assist the patient in meeting bathing and hygiene needs.[17]

- Use adaptive bathing equipment, such as safety rails, shower chair, long-handled brushes, *to promote safety and independence and to decrease energy expenditure.*
- Respect the preference of critically ill or terminally ill patients to refuse or limit hygiene care.
- Encourage patient to do as much as possible for self, setting a realistic time frame and individualizing plan to specific related factors:
  - Lower expectations if patient becomes frustrated.
  - Avoid judgmental or disapproving responses.
  - Reward accomplishments and provide positive feedback.
  - Allow patient with ritualistic behaviors to make choices and include time for rituals.
  - Adjust routine for patient with phobia to avoid contact with feared situation.
  - Assist patient in making a chart of daily grooming and hygiene tasks to be completed in the morning and in the evening.
  - Ensure that patient with mania has a flexible schedule for hygienic measures.
- Provide assistance in bathing/hygienic measures if patient is unable, including bathing, shaving, washing hair, brushing teeth, and hand washing after toileting and before meals.

DRESSING/GROOMING SELF-CARE DEFICIT

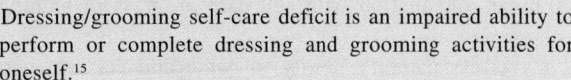

Dressing/grooming self-care deficit is an impaired ability to perform or complete dressing and grooming activities for oneself.[15]

Related Factors[8,15,16,23]

Advanced age
Confusion
Decreased or lack of motivation
Delirium
Developmental delay
Environmental barriers
Excessive ritualistic behaviors
Inadequate perception of body part or spatial relationship
Lack of coordination
Musculoskeletal or neuromuscular impairment
Pain
Perceptual or cognitive impairment
Phobias
Psychologic impairment (e.g., psychosis, mania, catatonia, delusions)
Severe disabling anxiety
Weakness or tiredness

Defining Characteristics[15,16,19,23]

Impaired ability to fasten clothing
Impaired ability to obtain or replace articles of clothing
Impaired ability to put on or take off necessary items of clothing
Inability to choose clothing
Inability to maintain appearance at a satisfactory level
Inability to pick up clothing
Inability to put on clothing on upper or lower body
Inability to put on shoes and socks
Inability to remove clothes
Inability to use assistive devices
Inability to use zippers
Refusal to dress or groom self

Expected Patient Outcomes and Nursing Interventions With Rationale*

Independently complete dressing or grooming activities, or with assistance, as evidenced by:

Dresses and grooms self to optimal potential
Accepts assistance with dressing and grooming as needed
Uses adaptive devices to dress and groom
Is appropriately clothed and neat in appearance

- Assess patient's ability to dress and groom self through observation and report, including comprehension, awareness, cognition, and affect, *to gather data on deficits in meeting dressing and grooming needs.*
- Assess factors that may interface with ability to dress or groom self, such as difficult-to-open drawers or shelves that are difficult to reach. *Adapting the environment may enhance the patient's ability to dress and groom independently.*[16]
- Encourage patient to select clothing, *to increase feelings of control.*
- Plan activities to prevent fatigue while dressing and grooming, *to conserve energy and promote self-care.*
- Provide privacy while dressing and grooming.
- Allow patient adequate time to complete dressing. *Patients with mobility or neurologic deficits require more time to complete a task.*
- Collaborate with occupational and physical therapy *to teach dressing and grooming skills.*[18]
- Select clothing that is loose-fitting; has elastic waistbands; and simple fasteners, such as Velcro fasteners, *to make dressing easier.*
- Use adaptive dressing and grooming equipment, such as grasping devices, zipper pulls, and elastic shoelaces. *Adaptive devices make dressing and grooming easier and less tiring.*
- Develop a consistent routine for dressing and grooming, *to increase normalcy and promote self-care.*[8]
- Lay clothing out in the order that it will be put on. *Simplifying dressing increases self-care ability.*[2]
- Provide cues for cognitively impaired clients when dressing and grooming.
- Teach patients who have paralysis to dress the affected side first, *for easier manipulation of clothing.*
- Respect the preference of the critically or terminally ill patient to refuse dressing and limit grooming, *to conserve energy.*
- Encourage patient to do as much as possible for self, setting a realistic time frame and individualizing plan to specific related factors:
  - Lower expectations if patient becomes frustrated.

*References 1-3, 5, 8, 13, 16, 19-22.

Avoid judgmental or disapproving responses.
Reward accomplishments and provide positive feedback.
Allow patient with ritualistic behaviors to make choices and include time for rituals.
Adjust routine for patient with phobia to avoid contact with feared situation.
Provide simple choices, such as "Do you want to wear the white shirt or the brown shirt today?"

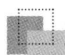

FEEDING SELF-CARE DEFICIT

Feeding self-care deficit is an impaired ability to perform or complete feeding activities.[15]

Related Factors[15,16,23]

Advanced age
Confusion
Decreased or lack of motivation
Delirium
Developmental delay
Environmental barriers
Excessive ritualistic behaviors
Musculoskeletal or neuromuscular impairment
Pain
Perceptual or cognitive impairment
Psychologic impairment (e.g., psychosis, mania, catatonia, delusions)
Severe anxiety
Weakness or tiredness

Defining Characteristics[11,12,15,16,23]

Inability to bring food from a receptacle to the mouth
Inability to chew food
Inability to complete a meal
Inability to get food onto utensils
Inability to handle utensils
Inability to ingest food in a socially acceptable manner
Inability to ingest safely
Inability to ingest sufficient food
Inability to manipulate food in mouth
Inability to open containers
Inability to pick up cup or glass
Inability to prepare food for ingestion
Inability to swallow food
Inability to use assistive devices
Refusal to feed self

Expected Patient Outcomes and Nursing Interventions With Rationale*

Independently complete feeding activity, or with assistance, as evidenced by:

Maintains adequate food and fluid intake
Maintains appropriate weight
Accepts assistance with eating and drinking when necessary
Expresses interest in overcoming limitations with eating and drinking

- Assess for cause of inability to feed self independently, including comprehension, awareness, cognition, and affect, *to assist in developing a plan specific to problems that interfere with self-care.*
- Assess patient's ability to feed self. Test gag reflex bilaterally, and note specific deficits *to prevent risk of aspiration.*
- Assess cognitive or perceptual limitations, oral-motor impairment, or ability to control hands and arms when selecting assistive devices.
- Ask for patient input on methods to facilitate eating and feeding, such as food and fluid preferences and cultural preference, *to increase food and fluid intake.*[7,11]
- Collaborate with occupational and physical therapy and dietitian. *Collaboration with interdisciplinary team members increases the client's mastery of self-care tasks.*
- Provide oral hygiene before and after meals.
- Provide a pleasant environment free of clutter, odors, and toileting devices. *A pleasant environment promotes food intake.*[17]
- Provide quiet music during mealtimes. *Quiet music may decrease anxiety and provide a more calm environment.*[4]
- Monitor eating and drinking activity at meals *to determine progress, identify problems, and offer reinforcement.*
- Ensure patient has dentures, hearing aids, and glasses in place. *Assistive devices increase opportunity for self-care.*
- Use assistive feeding devices, such as suction mats, built-up handles on utensils, and large-handled cups, *to increase independence with eating and drinking.*
- Ensure patient is seated or positioned in an upright position while eating and for 1 hour after a meal. *Gravity assists with swallowing, and aspiration is decreased when sitting upright.*
- Provide small portions of favorite foods, at proper serving temperature. *Food intake is increased when meal appeals to client and is simplified.*[11,17]
- Encourage patient to participate in feeding as able.
- Provide positive reinforcement for actively participating in eating and drinking.
- Allow adequate time to chew and swallow food.
- Choose soft foods rather than liquids for patients with dysphagia. *Choking occurs more easily with clear liquids than with solid or soft foods.*[12]
- Have suction equipment readily available. *Dysphagia increases the risk of choking.*
- Encourage patient to do as much as possible for self, setting a realistic time frame and individualizing plan to specific related factors.
  Lower expectations if patient becomes frustrated.
  Avoid judgmental or disapproving responses.
  Reward accomplishments and provide positive feedback.
  Allow patient with ritualistic behaviors to make choices and include time for rituals.
  Adjust routine for patient with phobia to avoid contact with feared situation.
  Monitor food and fluid intake and weigh weekly.
  Determine favorite foods and offer small portions to depressed patient.

*References 4, 6, 7, 14, 16, 17-22.

Offer snack foods that can be eaten while standing or moving to manic patient.

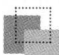

Toileting Self-Care Deficit

Toileting self-care deficit is an impaired ability to perform or complete toileting activities for oneself.[15]

Related Factors[15,16,23]

Advanced age
Confusion
Decreased or lack of motivation
Delirium
Developmental delay
Environmental barriers
Excessive ritualistic behaviors
Impaired mobility status
Impaired transfer ability
Musculoskeletal or neuromuscular impairment
Pain
Perceptual or cognitive impairment
Phobias
Psychologic impairment (e.g., psychosis, mania, catatonia, delusions)
Severe disabling anxiety
Weakness or tiredness

Defining Characteristics[15,16,23]

Inability to manipulate clothing
Inability to carry out proper toilet hygiene
Inability to flush toilet or commode
Inability to get to toilet or commode
Inability to sit on or rise from toilet or commode
Refusal to toilet self

Expected Patient Outcomes and Nursing Interventions With Rationale*

Independently complete toileting activity, or with assistance, as evidenced by:

Remains free of incontinence and/or impaction
Maintains clean and dry perianal area
Maintains adequate oral intake and output
Expresses satisfaction with use of adaptive devices for toileting
Manages toileting activities safely

- Assess ability to toilet, noting specific deficits, including comprehension, awareness, cognition, and affect, *to provide data for individualized interventions.*
- Assess patient's usual pattern of elimination.
- Ask for patient input on toileting methods and how to better provide toileting assistance, *to increase personal control.*
- Establish elimination program *to help achieve control.*
- Schedule toileting when defecation urge is strongest or voiding is likely. *The defecation urge is strongest in morning or within 1 hour after meals or warm beverages.*
- Provide privacy *to prevent suppression of elimination resulting from embarrassment.*
- Assess and remove physical barriers to toilet such as cluttered walkways. *Physical barriers can increase incontinence episodes.*
- Use assistive toileting equipment such as raised toilet seat, spill-proof urinals, support rails next to toilet, and fracture bedpans. *Assistive devices promote independence and safety.*
- Obtain a bedside commode if indicated, and avoid bedpans if possible, *to facilitate a sitting position that is more conducive to normal elimination.*
- Keep toilet paper and hand-washing items within easy reach of patient.
- Collaborate with occupational and physical therapy to help patient with transfer techniques.
- Monitor skin condition *to detect skin problems.*
- Provide skin care and linen changes after incontinence episodes *to prevent skin breakdown.*
- Assess patients with dementia for behavioral toileting cues such as pacing, restlessness, or fidgeting, and assist promptly with toileting *to reduce toileting accidents.*[10]
- Assess patient's ability to manipulate clothing for toileting, and modify clothing if necessary. *Delays in manipulating clothing may cause incontinence.*
- Encourage patient to toilet self, setting a realistic time frame and individualizing plan to specific related factors:
  - Lower expectations if patient becomes frustrated.
  - Avoid judgmental or disapproving responses.
  - Reward accomplishments and provide positive feedback.
  - Allow patient with ritualistic behaviors to make choices and include time for rituals.
  - Adjust routine for patient with phobia to avoid contact with feared situation.
  - Monitor for urinary retention and constipation in the depressed patient.
  - Avoid frequent discussion and questions about bowel movements.

*References 1, 8, 10, 13, 16, 22.

Delayed Growth and Development

Delayed growth and development is the state in which an individual demonstrates deviations in norms from his or her age group.[14]

Related Factors[13,14,16]

Effects of physical disability
Environmental and stimulation deficiencies
Inadequate caretaking
Inconsistent responsiveness by caretakers
Multiple caretakers
Prescribed dependence
Separation from significant others

Defining Characteristics[13,14,16]

Altered physical growth
Delay or difficulty in performing motor, social, or expressive skills typical of age group
Flat affect

Inability to perform self-care or self-control activities appropriate for age
Listlessness, decreased responses

Expected Patient Outcomes and Nursing Interventions With Rationale[4-6,13,14,16]

Patient will have growth and development monitored regularly, as evidenced by:

Detects developmental delays
Initiates interventions aimed at maximizing potential for development and minimizing secondary problems

- Assess anthropometrics (weight, length or height, and head circumference if less than 2 years of age) *to determine if there are deviations from normal.*
- Engage in "development surveillance": continuous, skillful observation of children during any child health encounter, soliciting input from parents, teachers, and others who have contact with the child, *to identify children at risk for deviation from normal.*
- Utilize screening tools to confirm suspicions of delay.
- Refer for further testing and treatment. *Gross and fine motor, cognitive, language, and social development, as well as health, physical growth, family dynamics, and environmental factors, are assessed in a comprehensive developmental evaluation.*

Family will demonstrate increased knowledge, confidence, and competence as caregivers, as evidenced by:

Successfully incorporates therapy and treatments into the daily routine of the family
Sets realistic goals, based on the child's strengths and abilities and the family's needs and aspirations
Decreases dependence on professional caregivers

- Evaluate family's knowledge about condition and its management. *Family must be confident and competent in use of necessary equipment, in administration of medications, and in performing medical procedures.*
- Clarify terminology and share information in a supportive and unbiased fashion.

Patient will have access to and use all necessary health services, as evidenced by:

Maintains optimal health and the absence of secondary disabilities

- Promote safety and maintenance of health and wellness.
- Teach developmentally appropriate injury prevention.
- Assist family in gaining access to health-care providers who are familiar with the special needs of individuals with altered growth and development throughout the life span. *These patients may be more vulnerable to nutritional deficits, obesity, dehydration, constipation, skin breakdown, and upper respiratory tract infection; and other special health concerns may exist related to specific disabilities (i.e., thyroid and cardiac disease are often present in patients with Down syndrome).*

Patient and family will demonstrate successful management of difficulties relating to activities of daily living, as evidenced by:

Patient attains the highest possible degree of independence in self-care.

- Assist family in dealing with difficulties in behavior, feeding, sleeping, bathing, dressing, and toileting; family dynamics, family coping strategies, family's group and individual goals, and practical limitations of the situation. *These activities will be helpful in problem solving.*

Patient will engage in comprehensive, developmentally appropriate education and rehabilitative interventions, as evidenced by:

Uses physical, occupational, and speech therapy as warranted
Uses prescribed adaptive equipment, prosthetic, or orthotic devices as needed

- Teach strategies for appropriate stimulation for infants and children *to promote motor development and language skills.*
- Work collaboratively with family and interdisciplinary team *to identify and meet health, psychologic, social, educational, and emotional needs.*
- Identify community resources. *Use of community resources can enhance development.*
- Assist family in gaining access to needed professional services, equipment, and financial resources.

Family will achieve a positive adaptation, as evidenced by:

Integrates individual with altered growth and development into the family
Successfully meets the needs of all family members
Decreases anxiety and increases confidence
Increases ability to discuss fears and concerns and to deal constructively with emotions
Demonstrates resilience, or the ability to rebound successfully from a stressful event
Uses cognitive and behavioral strategies to resolve or adapt to stressful situations

- Support family through crisis of diagnosis and later critical periods; offer anticipatory guidance *to promote positive adaptation.*
- Establish a caring, trusting relationship with the patient and family.
- Demonstrate professional competence and commitment to the patient's care.
- Encourage expression of feelings and fears, validate as normal emotional reaction to illness.
- Recognize problematic reaction and refer to appropriate professional; remain accepting and nonjudgmental.
- Advocate for the rights and needs of family, and help family develop advocacy skills.
- Support positive family relationships *to encourage cohesiveness.*
- Recognize family's strengths and skills, to enhance the family's ability *to manage the demands placed on them.*
- Encourage awareness of siblings' needs; determine meaning of illness to sibling(s), offer support group, encourage communication within the family, including verbalization of fears, questions, concerns by sibling(s).
- Celebrate family's accomplishment and successes in caring for their child.
- Encourage maintenance of a hopeful outlook.

Patient will achieve positive adaptation to disability, as evidenced by:

Achieves therapeutic goals
Behavior indicates positive self-concept

Increases understanding of disability and treatment
Is involved in management of own care

- Reinforce positive behaviors and adaptation to illness, recognizing adaptation is not static and continues throughout development.
- Encourage communication of questions and concerns; share information about disability and its impact. *Communication is necessary to clarify knowledge.*
- Encourage normalization of activities.
- Educate on health-related issues such as nutrition, exercise, physiologic functions, and sexuality *to help the patient maintain optimal health and to facilitate early recognition of health problems.*

The family will successfully adapt to the changing needs of the individual with altered growth and development throughout his or her life span, as evidenced by:

Anticipates and copes with transition periods

- Provide anticipatory guidance in recognizing changing needs as patient ages.
- Assist family in dealing with transition issues such as entering school, physical changes, adolescent sexuality and need for independence, increased involvement with peer group and changing relationships with peers, completion of school and need for alternative support systems, prevocational and vocational training, learning skills for independent living, movement out of family home, employment, guardianship, geriatric care.
- Prepare parents for the possibility of revisiting feelings of disappointment and grief as they experience life cycle transitions and again mourn for the loss of their "ideal" child.

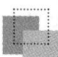

Risk for Delayed Development

Risk for delayed development occurs when an individual is at risk for delay of 25% or more in one or more of the areas of social or self-regulatory behavior, or cognitive, language, gross, or fine motor skills.[14]

Risk Factors[1,2,8-10,14]

Behavior disorders
Brain damage from accidents or shaken baby
Chemotherapy or radiation therapy
Chronic illness
Congenital or genetic disorders
Failure to thrive
Foster or adopted child
Genetic or endocrine disorders
Hearing impairment or frequent otitis media
Inadequate nutrition
Infections
Lack of, late, or poor prenatal care
Lead poisoning
Maternal age less than 15 or greater than 35 years
Mental illness, retardation, or severe learning disability
Natural disaster
Poverty
Prematurity
Seizures
Substance abuse
Unplanned or unwanted pregnancy
Violence or abuse
Vision impairment

Expected Patient Outcomes and Nursing Interventions With Rationale*

Prevent occurrence of developmental delays, as evidenced by:

Understands factors that contribute to developmental delays

- Encourage women to abstain from alcohol and drug use during pregnancy. *Exposure to drugs prenatally may affect development.*[2]
- Refer women to treatment programs for substance abuse.
- Assess medications taken by women of childbearing age. *Medications such as anticonvulsants have been shown to be teratogenic.*[15]
- Encourage women to seek prenatal care in early pregnancy.

Patient will have development monitored regularly, as evidenced by:

Detects developmental delays
Initiates interventions aimed at maximizing potential for development and minimizing secondary problems

- Assess children for development during any child health encounter, soliciting input from parents, teachers, and others who have contact with the child, *to identify children at risk for deviation from normal.*
- Use screening tools to confirm suspicions of delay.
- Refer for further testing and treatment. *Gross and fine motor, cognitive, language, and social development, as well as health, physical growth, family dynamics, and environmental factors, are assessed in a comprehensive developmental evaluation.*

Development is promoted, as evidenced by:

Optimal gross motor, fine motor, language, cognitive, social and emotional growth of preschool and school-aged children facilitated by nurse or parents/caregivers.[12]

- Provide developmental enhancement.[12]
  - Build a trusting relationship with child.
  - Establish one-on-one interaction with child.
  - Assist each child to become aware of importance as an individual.
  - Identify special needs of child and adaptations required, as appropriate.
  - Build a trusting relationship with caregivers.
  - Teach caregivers about normal developmental milestones and associated behaviors.
  - Demonstrate activities that promote development to caregivers.
  - Facilitate caregiver's contact with community resources, as appropriate.
  - Refer caregivers to support group, as appropriate.
  - Facilitate integration of child with peers.
  - Make sure body language agrees with verbal communication.
  - Encourage child to interact with others by role modeling interaction skills.

---

*References 2, 3, 7, 8, 10, 12, 15.

Provide activities that encourage interaction among children.
Assist child with sharing and taking turns.
Encourage child to express self through positive rewards or feedback for attempts.
Hold or rock and comfort child, especially when upset.
Foster cooperation, not competition, among children.
Create a safe, well-defined space for child *to explore and learn.*
Teach child how to seek help from others, when needed.
Encourage dreaming or fantasy, when appropriate.
Offer age-appropriate toys or materials.
Help child learn self-help skills (e.g., feeding, toileting, brushing teeth, washing hands, and dressing).
Listen to and discuss music.
Sing and talk to child.
Encourage child to sing and dance.
Teach child to follow directions.
Facilitate role playing of daily activities of adults in child's world (playing store and so on).
Be consistent and structured with behavior management/modification strategies.
Redirect attention, when needed.
Have child who is misbehaving "take breaks" or "time outs."
Provide opportunity and materials for building, drawing, clay modeling, painting, and coloring.
Assist with cutting out and gluing various shapes.
Provide opportunity for doing puzzles and mazes.
Teach child to recognize and manipulate shapes.
Teach child to write name/recognize first letter/recognize name, as appropriate.
Name objects in environment.
Tell or read stories to child.
Work on ordering and sequencing of letters, numbers, and objects.
Assist with spatial organization.
Teach planning by encouraging child to guess what will happen next and have child list other possible choices, and so on.
Provide opportunities for and encourage exercise and large-motor activities.
Teach child to jump over objects.
Teach child to perform somersaults.
Provide opportunity to play on playground.
Go on walks with child.
Monitor prescribed medication regimen, as appropriate.
Ensure that medical tests and/or treatments are done in a timely manner, as appropriate.

RISK FOR DISPROPORTIONATE GROWTH

Risk for disproportionate growth occurs when an individual is at risk for growth above the 97th percentile or below the 3rd percentile for age, or growth crossing two percentile channels.[14]

Risk Factors[4,11,14]

Abuse
Anorexia
Caregiver and/or individual maladaptive feeding behaviors
Chronic illness
Congenital or genetic disorders
Deprivation
Infection
Insatiable appetite
Lead poisoning
Malnutrition, poor maternal nutrition
Mental illness or retardation
Multiple gestation
Natural disasters
Poverty
Prematurity
Severe learning disability
Substance use or abuse
Teratogen exposure

Expected Patient Outcomes and Nursing Interventions With Rationale[4,11,16]

Patient will have growth monitored regularly, as evidenced by:
Identifies risks for altered growth
Detects growth delays

- Assess for exposure to toxic agents during pregnancy, such as alcohol, tetracyclines, and viruses like AIDS, *which cause harmful effects on the fetus.*
- Assess environmental factors that may inhibit normal growth.
- Assess anthropometrics (weight, length or height, and head circumference if less than 2 years of age) *to determine if there are deviations from normal.*

Parents and patient will provide proper nutrition, as evidenced by:
Describes age-appropriate nutrition for child
Provides adequate nutrition

- Assess usual eating habits.
- Assess for physical anomalies that may cause feeding problems.
- Consult with dietician to determine appropriate caloric intake.
- Provide supplemental feedings, *to increase caloric intake.*
- Provide tube feedings as appropriate for children with neuromuscular impairment.

DECREASED CARDIAC OUTPUT

Decreased cardiac output is the state in which the amount of blood pumped by the heart is inadequate to meet metabolic demands of the body.[7]

Related Factors[1,5,8]

Alteration in afterload
Alteration in preload
Inotropic changes in heart

Defining Characteristics[1,2,5,7,8]

Abnormal cardiac enzymes
Abnormal chest x-ray film (pulmonary vascular congestion)

Altered mental status
Chest pain
Cold clammy skin
Cough
Dyspnea
Dysrhythmias
ECG changes
Edema
Ejection fraction less than 40%
Elevated pulmonary artery pressures
Fatigue
Increased heart rate
Increased respiratory rate
Jugular vein distention
Mixed venous oxygen (SaO_2)
Oliguria
Orthopnea/paroxysmal nocturnal dyspnea
Rales (crackles)
Restlessness
S_3 or S_4
Skin color changes
Use of accessory muscles
Variations in blood pressure readings
Weight gain
Wheezing

Expected Patient Outcomes and Nursing Interventions With Rationale[1,3-8,9]

Maintain adequate cardiac output, as evidenced by:

Maintains normal sinus rhythm and heart rate within 20 beats of normal
Maintains blood pressure with upper limits of 140 mm Hg systolic, 90 mm Hg diastolic, and 30 to 40 mm Hg pulse pressure
Has no angina
Maintains urinary output of at least 30 ml per hour
Has warm and dry skin and peripheral pulses present and strong (normal for patient)

- Assess heart rate and blood pressure, *as indicators of cardiac output.*
- Listen to heart sounds—rate, rhythm, S_3 and S_4, rub, onset of new systolic murmur, *which can indicate onset of heart failure.*
- Observe for chest pain noting location, severity, radiation, quality, duration, and factors that precipitate and relieve the pain. *These symptoms are indicative of inadequate blood supply to the heart, which can compromise cardiac output.*
- Auscultate lungs for crackles *that may indicate fluid in the lungs.*
- Monitor cardiac rhythm continuously for changes.
- Weigh daily *to monitor fluid loss or retention.*
- Monitor arterial blood gases.
- Assess mental status for confusion, dizziness.
- Monitor cardiac enzymes.
- Monitor electrolyte values, especially potassium, *because medications often contribute to hypokalemia.*
- Titrate inotropic and vasoactive medication within defined parameters, as ordered, *to maintain contractility, preload, and afterload.*
- Measure fluid intake and urine output *to determine if there is decreased kidney perfusion.*
- Administer oxygen, as ordered, *to increase oxygen available for the myocardium.*
- Administer pain medications as ordered.
- Administer plasma volume expanders as ordered; adjust flow rate according to pulmonary artery pressures and pulmonary capillary wedge pressures.
- Administer diuretics, as ordered, *to decrease fluid overload.*
- Administer thrombolytic therapy as ordered.
- Monitor intraaortic balloon pump, as indicated.
- Restrict fluids, as ordered, *to prevent fluid retention.*
- Maintain bed rest with head of bed elevated 30 degrees and restrict activities, *to decrease workload.*
- Maintain a quiet environment and reduced stimuli, *to decrease oxygen consumption.*
- Assist with self-care or perform activities *to decrease cardiac workload.*
- Serve smaller meals of low sodium, *to decrease fluid retention,* and low cholesterol foods, *to decrease atherosclerosis.*
- Monitor bowel function, and advise patient to avoid straining with defecation. *Straining that results in the Valsalva maneuver can lead to decreased cardiac function and even death.*
- Increase activity level, as indicated by clinical status.
- Schedule rest periods between activities.

Verbalize knowledge of self-care, as evidenced by:

Explains reasons for decreased cardiac output and how to prevent it
Describes dietary alterations
Discusses exercise program and stress management activities
States medication uses and side effects
Plans for follow-up care

- Assess current knowledge of patient and family and provide information, as needed.
- Provide information concerning pathophysiology of illness, risk factors to avoid, and prevention of recurrence.
- Instruct on medication uses, side effects, and frequency of administration.
- Explain stress management techniques and physical activity program.
- Describe dietary alterations.
- Provide guidelines for resuming sexual relations and returning to work.

INEFFECTIVE TISSUE PERFUSION (SPECIFY TYPE: RENAL, CEREBRAL, CARDIOPULMONARY, GASTROINTESTINAL, PERIPHERAL)

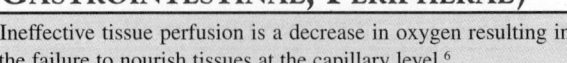

Ineffective tissue perfusion is a decrease in oxygen resulting in the failure to nourish tissues at the capillary level.[6]

Related Factors[1,6]

Altered affinity of hemoglobin for oxygen
Decreased hemoglobin concentration in blood
Hypervolemia
Hypoventilation
Hypovolemia

Impaired transport of oxygen across alveolar and/or capillary membrane
Interruption of arterial or venous flow
Mechanical reduction of venous and/or arterial blood flow

Defining Characteristics[1,6]

Renal
- Altered blood pressure outside of acceptable parameters
- Elevation in BUN/creatinine ratio
- Hematuria
- Oliguria or anuria

Gastrointestinal
- Abdominal distention
- Abdominal pain or tenderness
- Hypoactive or absent bowel sounds
- Nausea

Peripheral
- Altered sensations
- Altered skin characteristics
- Blood pressure changes in extremities
- Bruits
- Claudication
- Edema
- Skin color pale on elevation, color does not return on lowering of leg
- Skin discolorations
- Skin temperature changes
- Slow healing of lesions
- Weak or absent pulses

Cerebral
- Altered mental status
- Behavioral changes
- Changes in motor or sensory response
- Changes in pupillary reactions
- Difficulty in swallowing
- Extremity weakness or paralysis
- Speech abnormalities

Cardiopulmonary
- Abnormal arterial blood gases
- Altered respiratory rate outside of acceptable parameters
- Bronchospasms
- Capillary refill time greater than 3 seconds
- Chest pain
- Chest retraction
- Dyspnea
- Dysrhythmias
- Nasal flaring
- Sense of "impending doom"
- Use of accessory muscles

Expected Patient Outcomes and Nursing Interventions With Rationale[1-5,7,8]

Maintain tissue perfusion and cellular oxygenation, as evidenced by:

Maintains vital signs normal for patient and all pulses palpable
Skin remains warm and dry
Maintains urine output of 1500 to 3000 ml daily, or equivalent to intake
Remains alert and oriented, with recent memory intact
States no respiratory distress
Maintains hemoglobin within normal limits: 12 to 14 g/dl (women), 14 to 16 g/dl (men); partial thromboplastin time within normal limits (usually stated to be within 10 seconds of control); and arterial blood gases within normal limits: pH: 7.35 to 7.45, Po_2 80 to 95 mm Hg, Pco_2 35 to 45 mm Hg, O_2 sat: 95% to 99%

- Assess all pulses *to determine the extent of tissue perfusion.*
- Assess skin color and temperature *to determine the extent of tissue perfusion.* Inadequately perfused tissue will appear pale and feel cool to the touch.
- Assess the capillary refill *to determine if circulation is impaired.*
- Observe skin texture and the presence of hair, ulcers, or gangrenous areas on extremities.
- Inspect extremities for edema and measure circumference of extremities at the same time each day. *A thrombus or embolus may impede circulation, causing fluid to move from the intravascular to the interstitial spaces.*
- Provide meticulous foot care.
- Auscultate for systolic or continuous bruits below obstruction in extremities.
- Note characteristics of pain with or without activity.
- Monitor clotting time *to prevent bleeding.*
- Monitor hemoglobin and hematocrit *to detect blood loss and anemia.*
- Assess level of consciousness and memory.
- Assess motor and sensory changes.
- Note reports of dizziness or headache.
- Assess baseline arterial blood gases, electrolytes, BUN/creatinine, and cardiac enzymes.
- Monitor cardiac rhythm for dysrhythmias. Note complaints of chest pain or angina.
- Auscultate bowel sounds.
- Measure abdominal girth to detect edema.
- Note complaints of nausea, vomiting, and abdominal pain.
- Measure urine output. *Oliguria may be an early sign of decreased perfusion.*
- Monitor for elevated levels of BUN, creatinine, proteinuria, casts, specific gravity, and serum electrolytes.
- Assess mentation, *which may decrease as the BUN and creatinine levels rise.*
- Monitor blood pressure for elevations *from a decreased glomerular filtration rate.*
- Administer medication, as ordered (vasodilators, anticoagulants, and antilipemics), *to promote circulation.*
- Perform assistive/active range-of-motion exercises (Buerger and Buerger-Allen); *venous impairments respond to elevation of the legs; arterial impairments respond to supine or lowered positions.*
- Encourage early ambulation *to promote circulation.*
- Discourage sitting or standing for long periods, wearing constrictive clothing, crossing legs, *which may impair circulation.*
- Apply antithromboembolic stockings or Ace bandages *to promote venous return.*
- Use heating pads and hot water bottles cautiously *because ischemia may decrease sensitivity.*

- Encourage patient to quit smoking *because nicotine causes vasoconstriction.*
- Provide air mattress, sheepskin, or cradle, *to prevent skin breakdown.*
- Elevate head of bed and maintain head in midline position.
- Administer medication as ordered (e.g., corticosteroids, diuretics).
- When patient is confused, provide a safe environment.
- Administer antidysrhythmics, as ordered.
- Administer oxygen, as ordered, *to improve oxygenation to the myocardium.*
- Maintain gastric and intestinal decompression.
- Provide small, easily digested foods, when tolerated.
- Encourage rest after meals.
- Measure urine output.
- Weigh daily; a change in weight of 1 pound may represent 500 ml of fluid.
- Administer dopamine, as ordered, *to improve renal perfusion.*
- Administer corticosteroids, as ordered.

Communicate knowledge of self-care, as evidenced by:
Explains reasons for altered tissue perfusion
Describes medications and necessary lifestyle modifications

- Assess what patient and family need to know.
- Provide information concerning:
  - Changes required in activities of daily living
  - Maintaining reduction in metabolic needs
  - Appropriate exercise activities
  - Assessing skin and peripheral circulation daily
  - Meticulous foot care
  - Medication purpose, frequency of administration, and side effects
  - Safety needs associated with anticoagulant therapy
  - Maintaining a balanced diet
  - Actions to prevent recurrence of altered tissue perfusion
  - Plans for rehabilitation

DECREASED INTRACRANIAL ADAPTIVE CAPACITY

Decreased intracranial adaptive capacity is a clinical state in which intracranial fluid dynamic mechanisms that normally compensate for increases in intracranial volumes are compromised, resulting in repeated disproportionate increases in intracranial pressure (ICP) in response to a variety of noxious and nonnoxious stimuli.[4]

Related Factors[1,4]

Brain injuries
Brain tumors
Cerebral edema
Decreased cerebral perfusion
Hypotension

Defining Characteristics[1,2,5]

Baseline ICP of at least 10 mm Hg for more than 5 minutes following stimulus
Disproportionate increase in ICP following stimulus
Elevated P2 ICP waveform
Repeated increases in ICP of at least 10 mm Hg for more than 5 minutes
Volume pressure test variations
Wide amplitude waveform

Expected Patient Outcomes and Nursing Interventions With Rationale[1-3]

Intracranial pressure within normal limits, as evidenced by:
Spontaneous eye opening
Oriented to time, place, and person
Intact motor function

- Monitor changes in ICP waveforms.

Intracranial pressure monitoring provides waveforms that indicate pressures within the brain. An elevated P2 waveform may indicate actions are needed as ordered to reduce intracranial pressure.

- Monitor cerebral perfusion pressure (CPP) for normal values between 80 and 100 mm Hg.
- Assess pupil size and reactivity.

Pupillary changes of dilation and nonreactivity may indicate increased pressure on the oculomotor nerve (cranial nerve III) that controls pupillary size and reactivity.

- Monitor patient's orientation.
- Assess purposeful and nonpurposeful movement comparing left and right sides.

As pressure rises in the brain, the patient's level of consciousness declines. Consciousness is assessed by determining the client's orientation to time, place, and person. When this is not possible because of reduced consciousness, then consciousness is assessed by the amount and kind of stimulation required to get a response from the patient. These responses, in increasing order of severity, may be withdrawal from pain, flexion to pain, abnormal flexion, or abnormal extension. Abnormal flexion (decorticate posturing) with arms adducted and flexed in response to stimulation indicates high intracerebral pressure in the diencephalon. As the pressure in the cranium increases, and pushes downward, the patient's posturing may change to abnormal extension (decerebrate posturing), which indicates increased pressure in the midbrain and pons.

- Monitor arterial blood gases for hypercarbia and hypoxia.
- Monitor temperature for elevations.
- Monitor blood glucose for hypoglycemia.
- Observe for seizure activity.
- Observe for restlessness to correct cause (e.g., hypoxia, full bladder from kinked urinary catheter) or initiate sedation as ordered.

Fever, pain, agitation, external stimuli, seizures, and nursing activities such as bath, linen change, range-of-motion exercises, or position changes may increase cerebral metabolic rate of oxygen and therefore the oxygen demand. When this increased oxygen demand is not met by appropriate oxygen supply, then cerebral ischemia may result in increasing intracranial pressure.

- Monitor fluid balance and monitor for weight gain.
- Monitor effects of hemodilution or hemoconcentration on electrolytes and hematologic laboratory values.

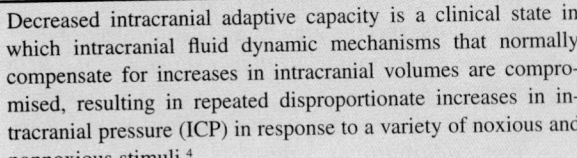

- Elevate head of the bed 30 degrees.
- Keep head in neutral position.

The head of the bed is elevated to facilitate venous return from the brain to the systemic circulation. Head alignment prevents occlusion of the jugular veins and improves venous return.

- Pace nursing care activities such as bed bath, linen change, range of motion to allow rest periods after each. Omit nursing procedures unless essential.
- Reduce external stimuli such as radio, television, noises from walls, voices of staff and visitors.
- Keep room lights dim.
- Administer oxygen as ordered to prevent hypoxia.
- Hyperventilate patient as ordered to prevent hypercarbia.
- Suction airway as little as possible; monitor ICP when suctioning. Limit suctioning to two passes of 10 seconds each.
- Maintain body temperature with decreased bed linens and hypothermia blanket.
- Administer medications as ordered, including diuretics, corticosteroids, antipyretics, neuromuscular blocking, barbiturates, anticonvulsants, antihypertensives, vasopressors.

Significant others verbalize needs for support and information

- Encourage significant others to verbalize their feelings about the patient's condition.
- Make referral to counselor, pastor, social worker, physician, or advocate as needed to meet significant others' needs.
- Provide information about the patient's condition at a level they can understand.

The patient's family and significant others need information and support during their time of waiting. Encourage them to verbalize their feeling and fears. They need information about the patient's status and what they can do to help the patient.

Deficient Diversional Activity

Deficient diversional activity is the state in which an individual experiences a decreased stimulation from or interest or engagement in recreational or leisure activities.[7]

Related Factors[1,6,7]

Activity intolerance
Apathy
Decrease in obligations
Depression or lack of motivation
Excess demands on time
Fatigue
Fear of crime
Impaired cardiopulmonary functions
Impaired mobility
Impaired senses or pain
Lack of exposure or orientation to diversional activities
Lack of knowledge of options
Lack of resources
Lack of transportation for home-based patients
Limited finances
Loneliness
Major life change (e.g., retirement, children leaving home, long-term illness)
Maturational factors (e.g., child—no toys)
Personal preference at odds with available options
Problematic time management
Social isolation
Space constraints
Unfamiliarity with routines or expectations for treatment center–based patients

Defining Characteristics[1,6,7]

Confined space
Daytime napping (seemingly unwarranted)
Disinterest in television viewing
Energy level sufficient for recreational activities but no participation in such activities
Flat affect
Frequent yawning
Hostility
Inattentiveness
No pattern of leisure activities
No post-illness substitute activities defined
Overeating or decreased eating
Perception of impossibility of leisure activities
Perception of time passing slowly
Pre-illness leisure activities impossible since illness
Refusal to attend planned recreation programs
Restlessness
Selective attendance at planned recreation programs
Statement of boredom
Statement of desire for something to do
Unavailability of resources for identified leisure activities

Expected Patient Outcomes and Nursing Interventions With Rationale[1-6,8]

Describe usual pattern of diversional activities, as evidenced by:

Indicates time free from obligations
Lists activities that are self-chosen
Relates the what, where, when, and how of diversional activities

- Assess usual activity routines before illness; *the usual pattern is a baseline for planning.*
- Assess the amount of unobligated time, leisure activities, resources used, and knowledge of recreational options.
- For persons with excessive stress and little unobligated time, suggest that they record their schedule of activities for 1 week, *which helps show time patterns.*

Identify changes in ability to engage in usual diversional activities, or identify problems perceived with usual pattern of activities, as evidenced by:

Lists changes in situation realistically
Compares present situation to past

- Assess usual activity routines since illness, hospitalization, or life change, including amount of unobligated time, leisure activities, degree of confinement, energy level, desire for activity, and mental status.

Choose one diversional activity to continue, identify a usual diversional activity that may be adapted to new

constraints, or identify a new diversional activity that may be started, as evidenced by:

Personally chooses an activity

Sees possibilities of continuation of activity within constraints

Sees an old activity in new light, or lists other interests that could be tried

Uses a problem-solving approach to change the situation

- Encourage patient to continue with activities that were meaningful. *Personal satisfaction will come with meaningful activities.*
- Encourage creativity in choices.
- Help person with busy schedule to prioritize activities.
- Encourage patient to identify activity, rather than suggesting activity. *The desire to please the nurse may preclude true choice.*
- If necessary, prompt patient thinking with suggestions of categories of activities.[4]
- Focus on the positive.
- Orient patient to options available within the system.
- Validate the patient's capabilities to engage in chosen activity with health-care team, *for realistic planning.*

Satisfactorily engage in chosen diversional activity, as evidenced by:

Lists resources needed for chosen activity

Identifies means to obtain needed resources

Engages in chosen diversional activity

Expresses satisfaction with chosen activity

- Maintain emphasis on personal choice, *to promote patient control and minimize assumptions.*[8]
- Teach time management or stress management strategies, if needed.
- Support patient in chosen activity.
- Adapt environment as necessary.
- Provide positive feedback.
- Evaluate patient's perception of chosen activity.
- Allow for change of plans if activity is unsatisfactory; *creative options do not always work as anticipated.*

DELAYED SURGICAL RECOVERY

Delayed surgical recovery is an extension of the number of postoperative days required for individuals to initiate and perform on their own behalf activities that maintain life, health, and well-being.[8]

Related Factors[8]

Chronic health conditions (e.g., diabetes mellitus, cardiovascular disease)

Complications following surgery

Dehiscence/evisceration

History of allergies and asthma

Multiple trauma

Obesity

Older age

Pathology of the problem requiring surgical treatment

Presence of infection

Defining Characteristics[8]

Difficulty in moving about

Evidence of interrupted healing of surgical area (e.g., red, indurated, draining, immobile)

Fatigue

Help required to complete self-care

Loss of appetite with or without nausea

Perception that more time is needed to recover

Postponed resumption of work/employment activities

Report of pain/discomfort

Expected Patient Outcomes and Nursing Interventions With Rationale[1-7,9-10]

Surgical recovery within normal time frame, as evidenced by:

Incision remains free of infection or other complications

Verbalizes effective pain control measures

Intake of food and fluids is sufficient to promote tissue healing

Increases mobility in incremental stages

Provides self-care activities

Returns to presurgical activities and occupation within expected time

- Provide preoperative and postoperative teaching, and predischarge teaching. *Providing preparatory procedural, sensory, and coping information has positive effects on physical recovery and rehabilitation from surgery.*
- Monitor incision for manifestations of infection, bleeding, and dehiscence or evisceration:
  - Take and record vital signs on a regular schedule
  - Monitor laboratory reports of WBCs, hemoglobin, and hematocrit
  - Monitor incision for redness, swelling, increased and/or purulent drainage, and wound edge approximation

Infection is manifested by increased body temperature and WBC count. Bleeding is evidenced by decreased hemoglobin and hematocrit. Incisional infections, which may precipitate dehiscence or evisceration, are manifested by increased pain, redness, swelling around the incision line, and drainage that is increased and/or purulent.

- Wash hands before and after patient care, and use aseptic techniques for dressing changes *to prevent transmission of infectious agents to the patient.*
- Assess pain, using a consistent scale (such as 0 for none to 10 for the worst ever experienced), and administer pain medication on a regular schedule for the first 24 to 36 hours after surgery. Supplement pain medications with other comfort measures, such as position changes and relaxation techniques. *Coping with undiminished pain requires energy. Pain also decreases the patient's ability to effectively change positions, ambulate, cough, deep breathe, and rest.*
- Monitor intake/output and food intake. *Adequate hydration and nutrients are essential for tissue healing.*
- Assist with increasing mobility as prescribed *to decrease the risk of respiratory and cardiovascular complications, such as pneumonia, atelectasis, and thrombophlebitis.*
- Provide time for verbalization of feelings of loss and changes in self-perception *to facilitate coping with change and increase ability to provide for self-care in activities of daily living and work.*

- Allow patient to be a part of decision making and goal setting throughout the surgical experience *to maintain independence and an active role in recovery.*
- Encourage use of effective coping mechanisms *to facilitate optimism about recovery and rehabilitation.*

(See Risk for Infection, Acute Pain, Imbalanced Nutrition: less than body requirements, Self-care Deficit, and Grieving for further interventions.)

Disorganized Infant Behavior; Risk for Disorganized Infant Behavior

Disorganized infant behavior is a state of disintegrated physiologic and neurobehavioral responses to the environment. Risk for disorganized infant behavior is the risk for alteration in integration and modulation of the physiologic and behavioral systems of functioning (i.e., autonomic, motor, state-organizational, self-regulatory, and attentional-interactional systems).[9]

Risk Factors[8,9]

Environmental overstimulation
Invasive or painful procedures
Lack of containment or boundaries
Oral or motor problems
Pain
Prematurity

Related Factors[8,9,12]

Caregiver factors: cue misreading or knowledge deficit
Environmental overstimulation
Feeding intolerance
Illness
Invasive or painful procedures
Malnutrition
Oral or motor problems
Pain
Physical environment inappropriateness
Prematurity
Prenatal factors: congenital or genetic disorders, teratogen or cocaine exposure
Sensory inappropriateness
Sensory overstimulation or deprivation

Defining Characteristics[2,5,8,9,14]

Abnormal response to sensory stimuli: difficult to soothe, inability to sustain alert status

Motor system

Altered primitive reflexes
Finger splay, fisting, or hands to face
Hyperextension of arms and legs
Increased, decreased, or limp tone
Jittery, jerky, uncoordinated movement
Tremors, startles, twitches

Physiologic

Bradycardia, tachycardia, or dysrhythmias
Bradypnea, tachypnea, apnea
Feeding intolerances (aspiration or emesis)
Oximeter desaturation
Pale, cyanotic, mottled, or flushed color
Regulatory problems: inability to inhibit, irritability
"Time-out signals" (e.g., gaze, grasp, hiccough, cough, sneeze, sigh, slack jaw, open mouth, tongue thrust)

State-organization system

Active-awake (fussy, worried gaze)
Diffuse/unclear sleep, state oscillation
Irritable or panicky crying
Quiet-awake (staring, gaze aversion)

Expected Patient Outcomes and Nursing Interventions With Rationale[1-4,7,10-14]

Respond and adjust positively to stimulation, as evidenced by[11]:

Experiences minimal alterations in muscle tone and extension
Experiences minimal disruption at rest and during movement
Remains calm and soothes easily
Maintains normal vital signs
Demonstrates increasing ability to adapt to stimuli
Demonstrates decreasing levels of irritability, crying, respiratory pauses, tachypnea, and color changes
Regains normal 24-hour diurnal cycles

- Assess infant for manifestations of disorganized behavior, including alterations in vital signs, sucking, and sleeping, and responses to pain and stimuli. *Full-term infants can usually regulate body systems; the premature, low-birth-weight, or ill infant may have difficulty in adapting to the extrauterine environment, especially in a neonatal intensive care unit. An infant's behavior is a reflection of central nervous system integrity and functioning.*[2]
- Conduct a neurobehavioral assessment, using a standardized scale, such as the Brazelton Newborn Behavioral Assessment Scale, *to document the behavioral and psychologic precursors of abnormal development and behavior. This is especially important in the preterm infant.*
- Conduct a neurologic assessment *to assess central nervous system function and to serve as baseline data.*
- Reduce or eliminate activities that contribute to disorganized behavior, including painful procedures, sudden moves, loud noises and bright lights, and transition from one type of bed to another, *to help the infant adjust to new experiences despite limited ability.*
- Administer pain medications as needed, including before procedures, after surgery, and when feedings are held. Consider use of a topical analgesic before heel sticks or venipunctures.
- Support the infant's own self-regulating behaviors to master the environment, such as hand grasping, foot and leg bracing, sucking on fingers, auditory and visual fixation, and postural changes, *which are behaviors the infant uses to interact with the environment.*[6]
- When moving the infant, position in a flexed prone position with head and trunk encased in the caregiver's hands; consider swaddling to maintain the position, move slowly and handle gently, and encourage sucking on a pacifier or the caregiver's finger *to allow time and position for reorganization and stabilization of the infant's regulation.*

- Position the infant in the prone or side-lying position, using blankets to maintain flexion. *to permit flexion and minimize flailing and arching.*
- Use a calm, quiet voice; shade the infant's eyes from lights, protect the infant from unnecessary touch, and either swaddle the infant or place in a nest of soft blankets *to minimize sensory input.*
- Carefully evaluate need for and timing of treatments and interventions.
- Avoid peaks of frenzy and overexhaustion.
- Maintain a calm, regular environment.
- Establish a pattern of gradual transition into sleep in the isolette or crib.

These interventions facilitate the transition to sleep and support the maintenance of sleep by providing a reliable, supportive pattern of care.

READINESS FOR ENHANCED ORGANIZED INFANT BEHAVIOR

Readiness for enhanced organized infant behavior is a pattern of modulation of the physiologic and behavioral systems of functioning (i.e., autonomic, motor, state-organizational, self-regulators, and attentional-interactional systems) in an infant that is satisfactory but that can be improved, resulting in higher levels of integration in response to environmental stimuli.[5]

Related Factors[5]

Pain
Prematurity

Defining Characteristics[5]

Definite sleep-wake states
Response to visual and auditory stimuli
Stable physiologic measures
Use of some self-regulatory behaviors

Expected Patient Outcomes and Nursing Interventions With Rationale[1-4,6-8]

Demonstrate organized infant behavior, as evidenced by:

Continues to have age-appropriate growth and development
Displays minimal or no compensatory behavior patterns

- Teach caregivers and parents to recognize behaviors used by the infant to communicate stress and needs, identifying if they are due to internal factors (such as pain from hunger) or due to external factors (such as bright lights or overstimulation by handling).
- Teach caregivers and parents to:
  - Provide eye-to-eye contact and face-to-face experiences.
  - Enhance infant's environment with bright, contrasting colors and geometric shapes.
  - When talking to the infant, use a variety of vocal tones and inflections, and call the infant by name. Avoid talking loudly.
  - Use skin-to-skin contact in a warm room; use firm, gentle touch; lay infant on a variety of textures (such as velvet, sheepskin, satin); gently massage the skin by stroking gently in a head-to-toe pattern.
  - Rock the infant; slowly change infant's position while handling or bathing.
  - Allow the infant to suck on fingers or a pacifier.
  - Feed during alert states.
  - Establish a quiet environment and stable pattern of sleep times. *These interventions are focused on supporting the interaction of the infant with the environment and increasing attachment and socialization with parents.*
  - Provide referrals for parents to community resources as appropriate.

DYSFUNCTIONAL VENTILATORY WEANING RESPONSE

Dysfunctional ventilatory weaning response is the state in which an individual cannot adjust to lowered levels of mechanical ventilator support, which interrupts and prolongs the weaning process.[6]

Related Factors*

Adverse environment
Anxiety, fear
Decreased motivation
History of multiple unsuccessful weaning attempts
History of ventilator dependence 1 week
Hopelessness
Inadequate nutrition
Inadequate social support
Inappropriate pacing of diminished ventilator support
Ineffective airway clearance
Insufficient trust in the nurse
Knowledge deficit of the weaning process, patient role
Patient perceived inefficacy about the ability to wean
Powerlessness
Sleep pattern disturbance
Uncontrolled episodic energy demands or problems
Uncontrolled pain or discomfort
Unfamiliar nursing staff

Defining Characteristics[1,3,5,6]

Adventitious breath sounds, audible airway secretions
Apprehension, agitation
Color changes, cyanosis
Decreased air entry on auscultation
Decreased level of consciousness
Deterioration in arterial blood gases from baseline
Discoordinated breathing with the ventilator
Expressed feelings of increased need for oxygen
Fatigue
Inability to cooperate or respond to coaching
Increase from baseline blood pressure
Increase from baseline heart rate
Increased concentration on breathing
Paradoxical abdominal breathing
Profuse diaphoresis
Queries about possible machine malfunction
Respiratory accessory muscle use
Respiratory rate increases from baseline
Shallow, gasping breaths
Wide-eyed look

---

*References 2, 3, 5, 6, 8, 9.

Expected Patient Outcomes and Nursing Interventions With Rationale[3-5,7-10]

Tolerate lowered levels of mechanical ventilation, as evidenced by:

Demonstrates ability to convey and receive information

Maintains baseline vital signs, cardiac rhythm, laboratory values, and mentation

Conveys comfortable and relaxed appearance

- Establish an effective communication system such as lip reading, writing, or communication board and talking tracheostomy *to reduce potential patient frustration and anxiety, to minimize negative aspects of mechanical ventilation, and to maximize patient's sense of control and energy conservation.*[5]
- Monitor for presence of altered thought process such as changes in concentration, attention, or orientation before initiating weaning process and throughout weaning process.
- Collaborate with patient's medical team to search for and treat underlying cause (e.g., fever, infection, drug therapy, fluid overload) *to optimize likelihood of successful weaning.*
- Repeat information until patient conveys understanding of explanations.
- Allow patient sufficient time to respond to information and explanations.
- Collaborate with multidisciplinary team, before weaning, to clarify whether underlying need for ventilation is resolved *to determine weaning readiness.*[2]
- Conduct baseline assessment, including vital signs, current pulmonary status, hemodynamic response, and fluid and electrolyte balance, and report abnormal findings to physician, before beginning weaning.
- Collaborate with multidisciplinary team to minimize unnecessary invasive procedures immediately before or during weaning process *to reduce potential for nosocomial infections and complications.*
- Determine patient's baseline mental status, using preestablished criteria that can be shared with other caregivers working with the patient.
- Collaborate with multidisciplinary team to determine surveillance parameters that must be continuously reviewed throughout the weaning process (e.g., oxygen saturation, heart and respiratory rate, color, signs of hypoxemia, and hypercapnia).
- Collaborate with patient's physician or pharmacist regarding drug therapy that may cause CNS depression *to ensure that the patient does not receive medication that interferes with ventilatory drive.*
- Collaborate with physician regarding use of medications *to facilitate bronchodilation and to increase diaphragm contractility.*
- Collaborate with multidisciplinary team regarding the best method for weaning patient (e.g., SIMV, CPAP, T-tube) *to maximize physiologic tolerance.*
- Prepare physical environment for potential cardiopulmonary arrest *to ensure early intervention in the event of emergency.*
- Inform patient and family regarding emergency plans *to prevent unnecessary anxiety and to build trust in health-care team.*
- Use coaching during weaning process, based on previous agreement with patient (e.g., remind patient about correct breathing during episodes of shortness of breath) *to promote patient's control of breathing.*
- Collaborate with resources, such as psychiatric consultation/liaison clinical nurse specialist for individualized stress management techniques (e.g., relaxation, imagery, and music) during weaning *to maximize potential for decreased heart and respiratory rates and to promote increased oxygen saturation.*
- Control and minimize noise and activity level in patient's bedside area, provide privacy, and allow for scheduled rest times *to decrease patient's apprehension and tension.*
- Use family as a supportive resource *to minimize patient's anxiety and fears.*
- Prepare family for a supportive role in weaning process by providing information about the unit environment and the weaning plan, by introducing caregivers and explaining their roles, and by inviting family to share issues of concern.
- Promote effective management of acute and chronic pain. Incorporate adequate periods of rest throughout the weaning process.
- During weaning trials, observe for signs of respiratory muscle fatigue: increased respiratory rate; minute ventilation; hypercarbia, with associated respiratory acidosis; altered breathing pattern; and increased discomfort.

Adhere to the weaning plan, as evidenced by:

Participates with primary nurse or registered nurse case manager in implementation of weaning plan and ongoing regimen

Communicates self-observations and concerns throughout the weaning process

- Assess the patient's cognitive ability (e.g., attention, concentration, short-term memory) to understand and remember information about the weaning process and plan.
- Obtain information from patient and family about patient's usual responses to anxiety-producing situations.[10]
- Obtain information about patient's past ability to cope with increased anxiety *to identify coping problems and to reinforce coping strengths.*
- Evaluate for behaviors indicative of psychologic dependence on ventilator, such as anticipatory anxiety, expressions of fear of dying, and blocking discussion of weaning.
- Consider use of a formal written weaning contract, mapping, or critical pathway that includes specific goals, timing of weaning interventions, expectations regarding adherence to activity or exercise protocols, patient's participation in self-care activities, role of patient and team members in achieving weaning goals, and schedule for reevaluating and revising the weaning plan.
- Include a copy of contract in patient's chart for documentation *to ensure consistency and adherence to the weaning plan.*
- Use clear and direct communication (e.g., short and simple sentences) to convey plans for the weaning process.

- Negotiate the weaning process with patient *to facilitate patient's control in decision making regarding weaning plan.*
- Ensure that a primary nurse or registered nurse case manager collaborates on a consistent basis with the patient and family and the multidisciplinary team *to facilitate successful integration of treatment approaches and evaluation of interventions.*
- Ensure that all caregivers provide consistent explanations about weaning and actual implementation *to promote trust in staff.*
- Provide information on a consistent basis about progress in reassuring manner *to convey recognition of successful weaning and to minimize unnecessary anxiety.*
- Use positive reinforcers *to convey recognition of patient's achievements and success.*
- Encourage expression of thoughts and feelings about perceptions of the weaning process.
- Encourage patient to convey perceptions of physiologic changes *to promote self-monitoring.*
- Promote active decision making in setting of realistic, attainable goals for patient's participation with self-care activities *to increase sense of personal control and to decrease stress.*

FATIGUE

Fatigue is an overwhelming sustained sense of exhaustion and decreased capacity for physical and mental work at usual level.[8]

Related Factors[1,8,11,12]

Anemia
Anxiety
Chronic disease
Depression
Disease states
Elevated temperature
Humidity
Increased physical exertion
Lifestyle
Malnutrition
Negative life events
Noise
Pregnancy
Poor physical condition
Sleep deprivation
Stress

Defining Characteristics[1,3,8,11,12]

Compromised concentration
Compromised libido
Decreased performance
Disinterest in surroundings, introspection
Drowsiness
Feelings of guilt for not keeping up with responsibilities
Inability to maintain usual routines
Inability to restore energy even after sleep
Increase in physical complaints
Increase in rest requirements
Lack of energy or inability to maintain usual level of physical activity
Lethargy or listlessness
Perceived need for additional energy to accomplish routine tasks
Tiredness
Verbalization of an unremitting and overwhelming lack of energy

Expected Patient Outcomes and Nursing Interventions With Rationale[1-7,9-13]

Has sufficient energy to engage in activities of daily living (ADLs) and fulfill role demands or adapt to decreased energy levels, as evidenced by:

Completes ADLs independently or seeks assistance to complete ADLs
Verbalizes improvement in mental outlook
Demonstrates the ability to concentrate
Participates in regular exercise program
Rests and sleeps as scheduled
Maintains an injury-free status

- Assess severity of fatigue *to establish a baseline for fatigue symptoms.*[2,9]
- Assess family patterns of living identify correlates of fatigue; *planning for energy conservation involves identification of energy-depleting factors and energy requirements of common ADLs.*
- Ensure patient has a complete history and physical examination *to identify and treat physical and mental causes.*
- Assist in establishing a plan of daily activities for effective energy use. *With careful planning to maintain energy resources and prevent energy depletion, the patient can still participate in valued activities, while delegating less valued or more energy-consuming tasks to supportive others.*[11]
- Teach strategies for energy conservation.
- Encourage patient to keep a daily journal of fatigue occurrence, feelings, and strategies used to manage fatigue. *A journal can be useful for planning strategies to manage fatigue.*[6]
- Consult with physiatrist or physical therapist to develop incremental physical exercise program.
- Teach to engage in regular exercise. *Aerobic exercise stimulates the body's endurance and energy systems and improves functional capacity.*[10]
- Enhance ability to sleep by means of mild sedatives, warm bath, massage, and quiet environment; allow for uninterrupted periods of sleep. *Adequate amounts of undisturbed sleep are necessary to replace energy stores.*
- Assess nutritional habits and alter those that contribute to fatigue. *High-quality nutrition is necessary to supply basic materials essential for energy production.*
- Administer treatments or medications to relieve other discomforts, such as pain or nausea. *Concomitant symptoms may exacerbate fatigue and/or decrease tolerance to fatigue.*
- Evaluate new or additional stressors, such as a new baby, ill family member, or financial burdens. *Prolonged stress may lead to depletion of body reserves and cause fatigue.*

- Teach stress management techniques such as controlled breathing.

Experience reduction or resolution of fatigue, as evidenced by:
Increased energy
Completes ADLs

- Regularly monitor the level of fatigue, contributing factors, and degree of adaptation to fatigue.
- Support patient's efforts to increase participation in ADLs.

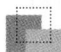

IMPAIRED BED MOBILITY

Impaired bed mobility is the limitation of independent movement from one bed position to another.[10]

Related Factors[2,10]

Decreased strength and endurance
Depression
Intolerance to activity
Musculoskeletal impairment
Neuromuscular impairment
Pain or discomfort
Perceptual or cognitive impairment
Severe anxiety

Defining Characteristics[2,10]

Impaired ability to move from supine to prone or prone to supine
Impaired ability to move from supine to sitting or sitting to supine
Impaired ability to "scoot" or reposition self in bed
Impaired ability to turn side to side

Expected Patient Outcomes and Nursing Interventions With Rationale[2,6,10,13]

Demonstrate safe, proper position in bed, as evidenced by:
Maintains proper body alignment
Prevents injury or complications

- Assess patients' risk for increased intracranial pressure (ICP), respiratory abnormalities, aspiration, pressure ulcer formation, muscle tone abnormalities, and pain levels, *to determine appropriate positioning to prevent complications.*
- For patient with increased ICP elevate the head of the bed 15 to 30 degrees *to reduce ICP, maintain cerebral perfusion pressure, cerebral blood flow, and cardiac output.*
- Assist dysphagic patients to sit upright while eating or taking medications, *to prevent aspiration.*
- Position the head of the bed at the lowest degree of elevation when moving patient, *to prevent skin shearing.*
- Position patient in proper body alignment *to prevent contractures.*
- Use pillows and rolls to support limbs and maintain proper body alignment.
- Position head and neck in neutral alignment. If indicated, place a sandbag under the pillow on one or both sides of the head to maintain head alignment.
- Position patient with hemiplegia on the affected side *to avoid circulatory impairment.*
- Perform passive range-of-motion exercises at least twice a day with those body parts that patients cannot actively range or move spontaneously, *to maintain joint mobility and muscle tone, and to prevent contractures.*
- Change body position every 2 hours.
- Apply splints as ordered, *to maintain neutral positions of limbs.*

Demonstrate proper movement in bed, as evidenced by:
Turns in bed
Exercises in bed

- Turn hemiplegic patient by moving the shoulder and arm (on side to which patient will turn) out to the side with palm facing up and flex knees with the feet flat on the bed, turn and position in correct alignment.
- Turn patient with bilateral paralysis by crossing the outside leg over the other leg and extending the arms out in front of the chest with the hands clasped together if possible; turn and position in correct alignment.
- If patient can assist with turning, instruct and assist to turn over, starting with the head, then the upper body, trunk, hips, and legs.
- To move patient to the side of the bed, have patient place both feet flat on bed, close to buttocks. Assist with movement to the side of the bed, by guiding hips.
- To move patient up in bed, have patient bend the knees with feet flat on bed. Assist patient by guiding hips to raise and move toward the head of the bed. Instruct patient to tuck the chin and lift head and shoulders off the bed, then lie back down, straightening the trunk.
- Encourage patient to perform active range of motion.
- Perform passive range-of-motion exercises at least twice a day with those body parts that patient cannot actively move. Support limbs above and below the joint being exercised. *Range-of-motion exercises maintain joint mobility and prevent contractures.*
- Teach patient to perform passive range of motion on affected limbs.
- Encourage patient to perform muscle setting and active strengthening exercises *to help maintain muscle tone and strength.*

IMPAIRED TRANSFER ABILITY

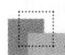

Impaired transfer ability is a limitation of independent movement between two nearby surfaces.[10]

Related Factors[3,10]

Decreased strength and endurance
Depression
Musculoskeletal or neuromuscular impairment
Pain or discomfort
Perceptual or cognitive impairment
Severe anxiety

Defining Characteristics[3,10]

Impaired ability to transfer between uneven levels
Impaired ability to transfer from bed to chair and chair to bed
Impaired ability to transfer from chair to car or car to chair
Impaired ability to transfer from chair to floor or floor to chair

Impaired ability to transfer from standing to floor or floor to standing
Impaired ability to transfer in and out of tub or shower
Impaired ability to transfer on or off a toilet or commode

Expected Patient Outcomes and Nursing Interventions With Rationale[1,3,6,13]

Demonstrate ability to transfer between two surfaces, such as bed to chair, or chair to toilet, as evidenced by:
Transfers safely between two surfaces

- Before physical therapist (PT) or occupational therapist (OT) consult, assess patient's movement abilities and strength, to determine type of transfer.
- Collaborate with PT and OT for upper and lower extremity exercise and strengthening program early in patient's mobilization. Lower extremity and trunk strength is important for weight-bearing transfers, and upper extremity strength is important for sliding transfers.
- Reinforce exercise program as outlined and encourage frequent practice.
- Instruct patients to apply appropriate equipment, such as orthotics or braces, in bed before transferring, *to maintain joint stability, immobilization, and alignment during movement.*
- Document the type of transfer, equipment, and assistance needed for transfer, *to promote consistency in transfers.*
- For weight-bearing transfers have patient wear firm, low-heeled shoes with nonskid and nonfriction soles *to prevent slipping and/or falling.*
- Recognize the normal sequence of movements for standing. Flex hips and knees; extend back; lean trunk, head, and knees over the feet; shift weight to the feet.
- Support or stabilize patient's knee(s) with one or both knees next to or encircling the patient's *to allow patient to flex the knee(s) and lean forward during transfers.*
- For sliding board transfers scoot the patient to the edge of the surface; angle one edge of the sliding board under the hip and thigh nearest the surface transferring to; encourage patient to shift weight onto both buttocks to sit on the edge of the sliding board; angle the opposite end of the sliding board onto the transfer surface; have patient assist with arms until sitting on the intended surface.
- For a patient who can assist with transfer, scoot to the edge of the bed or seat; instruct to lean forward; place one hand on surface patient is transferring from and other hand on surface transferring toward; have patient push with arms so that the hips and buttocks can swing to the desired transfer surface. Nurse should provide support or balance as needed.
- Assist patient to do a standing pivot transfer by standing in front of or to the side of patient; instruct patient to place hands on armrests or surface that client is transferring from, on nurse's shoulders, on surface toward which patient will be transferring, or on walker; have patient lean forward so weight can be shifted onto the feet; shift weight and stand erect; pivot by shifting and centering weight on the foot next to the chair or surface the patient is transferring to, so the opposite foot can be slid or pivoted and then repositioned on the floor; continue weight shifts/pivot maneuvers until the backs of the patient's legs touch the desired surface; have patient lean forward at the hips and knees to sit down, holding on to the nurse or other support.

(See Impaired Wheelchair Mobility for more information.)

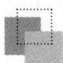

IMPAIRED WALKING

Impaired walking is the limitation of independent movement within the environment on foot.[10]

Related Factors[1,4,8,10]

Decreased strength and endurance
Depression
Intolerance to activity
Lower extremity amputation
Musculoskeletal impairment
Neuromuscular impairment
Pain or discomfort
Perceptual or cognitive impairment
Severe anxiety

Defining Characteristics[4,10]

Impaired ability to climb stairs
Impaired ability to navigate curbs
Impaired ability to walk on an incline or decline
Impaired ability to walk on uneven surfaces
Impaired ability to walk required distances

Expected Patient Outcomes and Nursing Interventions With Rationale[1,4,6-8,13]

Demonstrate safety in walking, as evidenced by:
Tolerates walking without shortness of breath, chest pain, or dizziness
Avoids falls or injuries when walking
Maintains an environment that is clear and free of obstacles

- Assess patient's baseline pulse before walking, then 5 minutes after walking. Stop walking if the pulse becomes rapid or irregular.
- Monitor patient's tolerance for walking by assessing cardiac status.
- Provide rest periods if shortness of breath, chest pain, nausea, dizziness, syncope, or other adverse effects are noted.
- Obtain appropriate number of people to assist with walking *to avoid falls and injuries.*
- Position walking assistants appropriately *to support the patient while walking.*
- Use appropriate assistive devices when walking, such as transfer belts, walkers, crutches, and canes, *to provide stability and support during walking.*
- Limit distractions and environmental clutter *to prevent injury while walking.*
- Have patient wear firm, low-heeled shoes with nonskid and nonfriction soles *to prevent slipping and/or falling.*

- Explain to patient and family the importance of proper lighting; solid floor surfaces, without throw rugs; and removing objects from the floor, *to prevent possible falls.*

Demonstrate the use of adaptive devices to increase mobility, as evidenced by:

Uses assistive devices that are appropriate for use in the patient's particular situation

- Assist patients to properly apply orthotics, immobilizers, splints, and braces before walking, *to maintain joint stability, immobilization, and alignment during movement.*
- Teach and observe proper use of appropriate assistive devices: crutches, walkers, wheelchairs, prostheses, slings, Ace bandages, *to significantly improve mobility and independent functioning.*
- Assist patients with prosthesis to correctly apply lower extremity sheaths, stump socks, liners, and prosthesis before walking. *Prostheses increase persons' functional ability to walk and cosmetically look similar to lost lower limbs. Proper use of sheaths, socks, and liners aids in appropriate fit and prevents irritation and ulcer formation.*[6]

Encourage ambulation, as evidenced by:

Promoting and assisting with walking to maintain or restore autonomic and voluntary body functions during treatment and recovery from illness or injury

- Provide exercise therapy: ambulation.[7]

  Dress patient in nonrestrictive clothing.

  Assist patient to use footwear that facilitates walking and prevents injury.

  Provide low-height bed, as appropriate.

  Place bed-positioning switch within easy reach.

  Encourage to sit in bed, on side of bed ("dangle"), or in chair, as tolerated.

  Assist patient to sit on side of bed to facilitate postural adjustments.

  Consult physical therapist about ambulation plan, as needed.

  Instruct in availability of assistive devices, if appropriate.

  Instruct patient how to position self throughout the transfer process.

  Use a gait belt to assist with transfer and ambulation, as needed.

  Assist patient to transfer, as needed.

  Provide cueing card(s) at head of bed to facilitate learning to transfer.

  Apply/provide assistive device (cane, walker, or wheelchair) for ambulation if the patient is unsteady.

  Assist patient with initial ambulation and as needed.

  Instruct patient/caregiver about safe transfer and ambulation techniques.

  Monitor patient's use of crutches or other walking aids.

  Assist patient to stand and ambulate specified distance and with specified number of staff.

  Assist patient to establish realistic increments in distance for ambulation.

  Encourage independent ambulation within safe limits.

  Encourage patient to be "up ad lib," if appropriate.

IMPAIRED WHEELCHAIR MOBILITY

Impaired wheelchair mobility is the limitation of independent operation of a wheelchair within the environment.[10]

Related Factors[5,9,10]

Amputation
Decreased strength and endurance
Depression
Intolerance to activity
Musculoskeletal impairment
Neuromuscular impairment
Pain or discomfort
Perceptual or cognitive impairment
Severe anxiety

Defining Characteristics[5,9,10]

Impaired ability to operate manual or power wheelchair on an even or uneven surface

Impaired ability to operate manual or power wheelchair on an incline or decline

Impaired ability to operate wheelchair on curbs

Expected Patient Outcomes and Nursing Interventions With Rationale[5,6,9,11,12]

Demonstrate ability to move from place to place in a wheelchair, as evidenced by:

Transfers to and from wheelchair
Moves wheelchair safely
Navigates ramps and curbs

- Instruct patients to apply appropriate equipment, such as orthotics or braces, in bed before getting into wheelchair *to maintain joint stability, immobilization, and alignment during movement.*
- Insert a padded back board, firm seat, and lumbar support in the wheelchair before patient gets into wheelchair, *to prevent pressure, provide support, and enhance comfort.*
- Remove, elevate, or swing leg rests and foot plates out of way when standing or transferring, *to allow feet to be placed flat on floor and avoid bumping, tripping, and falling.*
- Lock wheelchair brakes before transferring to or from wheelchair, *to avoid movement of chair during transfers.*
- Remove or flip up armrests if able, *to make transfers easier.*
- Instruct patient on how to operate wheelchair.
- Unlock wheelchair brakes before trying to move wheelchair.
- Encourage patient to back wheelchair into an elevator, *to allow the patient to use the control panel.*
- Instruct patient on how to navigate ramps and curbs *to prevent falls and injuries.*

Demonstrate safety in use and appropriate positioning in a wheelchair, as evidenced by:

Maintains intact skin, without pressure areas

Explains use of wheelchair components
- Explain the importance of properly fitted wheelchair *to accommodate individual physique, properly support hips and pelvis, and evenly distribute weight.*[6]
- Assist patient to position self in wheelchair with hips, knees, and ankles in 90 degrees of flexion. Make sure hips and pelvis are fully back in the chair.
- Use appropriate cushions, firm seat, and protective devices such as leather gloves, *to prevent skin breakdown in areas of high risk, such as feet, buttocks, hips, and hands.*
- Explain the importance of frequent shifts of weight while sitting in wheelchair, *to prevent skin breakdown from pressure on bony areas.*
- Assess skin for redness and pressure *to prevent skin breakdown.*
- Instruct patient on exercises to increase upper body strength.

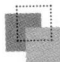

IMPAIRED PHYSICAL MOBILITY

Impaired physical mobility is a limitation in independent, purposeful physical movement of the body or of one or more extremities.[6]

Related Factors[1,5,6]

Altered cellular metabolism (e.g., hypothyroid)
Body mass index above 75th age-appropriate percentile
Cognitive impairment
Cultural beliefs regarding age-appropriate activity
Depressive mood state or anxiety
Developmental delay
Discomfort with activity
Intolerance to activity/decreased strength and endurance
Lack of knowledge regarding value of physical activity
Lack of physical or social environmental supports
Limited cardiopulmonary endurance
Medications
Musculoskeletal impairment
Neuromuscular impairment
Pain
Prescribed movement restrictions
Reluctance to initiate movement
Sedentary lifestyle or disuse or deconditioning
Sensoriperceptual impairments

Defining Characteristics[1,5,6]

Decreased reaction time
Difficulty turning
Focus on pre-illness activity
Gait changes
Limited ability to perform fine motor skills
Limited ability to perform gross motor skills
Limited range of motion
Movement-induced shortness of breath
Movement-induced tremor
Postural instability during performance of routine activities of daily living
Slowed movement
Uncoordinated or jerky movements

Expected Patient Outcomes and Nursing Interventions With Rationale[1-4,6]

Demonstrate measures to increase mobility, as evidenced by:

Performs progressive mobilization, functional activities, and appropriate transfer techniques
- Provide for progressive mobilization.
- Assist the patient to progress from active range-of-motion exercises to functional activities, as indicated. *Progressively increasing activity improves the functional abilities of the patient.*
- Teach transfer techniques.

Demonstrate maximum range of motion in all joints, as evidenced by:

Maintains range of motion and muscle mass and strength in unaffected limbs at the patient's usual level
Maintains joint mobility in affected limbs
- Teach patient to perform active range-of-motion exercises on unaffected limbs at least four times a day *to increase muscle mass, tone, and strength.*
- Perform passive range-of-motion exercises on affected limbs at least four times a day *to improve joint mobility.*

Demonstrate the use of adaptive devices to increase mobility, as evidenced by:

Uses assistive devices that are appropriate for use in the patient's particular situation
- Teach and observe proper use of appropriate assistive devices: crutches, walkers, wheelchairs, prostheses, slings, Ace bandages, *to significantly improve mobility and independent functioning.*
- Teach and observe use of appropriate assistive devices to enhance use of arms.

Use safety measures to minimize risk for injury, as evidenced by:

Complies with safety precautions that are appropriate in his or her particular situation
- Teach and observe safety precautions, such as protecting areas of decreased sensation from extremes of heat and cold.
- Instruct patient confined to wheelchair to shift position and lift up buttocks every 15 minutes.
- Instruct patient with decreased perception of lower extremity to check where limb is placed when changing positions, *to decrease the possibility of physical dangers associated with impaired physical mobility.*

Participate in a plan for integrating the mobility impairment into established lifestyle patterns, as evidenced by:

Participates actively in discussions about and shows positive responses to alternatives and modifications necessary in his or her lifestyle pattern
Accepts and uses support services that are appropriate in his or her particular situation
- Explore the patient's perceptions of mobility impairment in regard to previous lifestyle patterns, the possibility of resuming previous patterns, and willingness to accept limitations.

- Discuss alternatives, substitutions, or modifications for activities that are not achievable (either temporarily or permanently), *to enhance patient's sense of control.*
- Identify resources, special equipment, devices, and environmental modifications necessary to permit patient functioning despite physical limitations.
- Provide patient with information about available resources.
- Facilitate access to available resources by means of printed materials, telephone contacts, introductions, or written referral.
- Mobilize resources within the patient's support network.
- Refer to support services such as physical therapy, occupational therapy, and social services *to assist the patient to achieve the highest level of independence possible.*

IMPAIRED HOME MAINTENANCE

Impaired home maintenance is the inability to independently maintain a safe growth-promoting environment.[7]

Related Factors[6-8]

Change in family composition
Chronic debilitating disease
Disability caused by acute illness, injury, or congenital anomaly
Dysfunctional grieving
Impaired cognitive or emotional functioning
Impaired sensory functioning
Inadequate community resources
Inadequate dwelling and/or furnishings
Inadequate social support system
Insufficient family organization and planning
Insufficient finances or insurance
Lack of equipment and of aids for home care
Lack of socialization (role model and/or emigration)
Lack of training in adaptation of home maintenance skills
Overcrowding
Unfamiliarity with neighborhood resources

Defining Characteristics[2,6-8]

Accumulation of dirt, food waste, or hygienic waste
Apparent lack of economic resources
Community resources insufficient or unavailable
Contaminated water or inadequate sewage supply
Debts or financial crises that impede home maintenance
Difficulty in supporting personal growth of family members
Dissatisfaction with dwelling because of overcrowding or lack of personal space
Exhaustion or inability to keep up the home
Inadequate support system
Inappropriate lighting, temperature, and/or insufficient ventilation
Knowledge of home maintenance inconsistent with current environment
Lack of cooking utensils, linen, or clothes because of insufficient supply or being unwashed
Lack of knowledge about resources
Lack of necessary equipment or aids
Offensive odors
Overcrowding for available space
Presence of disease or disability necessitating adaptation of home maintenance
Presence of vermin or rodents
Repeated hygienic disorders, infestations, or infections
Requests assistance with home maintenance
Structural barriers or defects
Unrepaired defects in structure or utilities

Expected Patient Outcomes and Nursing Interventions With Rationale[1-4,6,8]

Participate in development of a feasible home maintenance plan, as evidenced by:

Identifies factors in the home environment that affect health and safety
Describes modifications to be made in home environment

- Assess home environment.
- Compare patient and family perceptions with observations.
- Identify appropriate referrals using multidisciplinary team.
- Establish realistic plan for home management involving patient and family members.
- Teach patient and family as appropriate.
- Plan and coordinate a smooth transition from inpatient to home. *Awareness of the relationship between health and the environment is necessary for planning.*

Identify factors perceived as making it difficult to maintain home, as evidenced by:

Describes home maintenance as a potential health and safety problem
States a personal standard for home maintenance

- Systematically identify factors that impede meeting household standard.
- Have family members state what factors in the home affect their health and safety. *Knowledge about how to maintain a clean, safe environment can decrease the risk of health and safety problems.*
- Increase family awareness of changed capabilities of members.

Recognize what daily maintenance realistically can be performed, as evidenced by:

Describes current roles and possible role changes that may be needed

- Discuss each member's current role.
- Discuss possible role changes.
- Differentiate factors that are esthetic from ones that negatively affect health and safety.
- Listen nonjudgmentally to realities of home situation.
- Assist family to realign roles and expectations for household maintenance standards congruent with increased patient dependency. *Accepting changes in roles can be helpful in meeting the needs of the patient and family.*

Identify and use appropriate support, as evidenced by:

Describes support system and its strengths and weaknesses
Identifies need for additional or outside help
Lists available resources in the community

- Identify members of current support system and assess their capabilities.
- Discuss community resources for daily home maintenance. *Knowledge of community resources may assist with home maintenance.*
- Mutually develop plan of care to increase supports consistent with family values.
- Assist families to seek outside assistance for respite; they may be reluctant to meet ongoing caregiver needs. *Use of community resources can enhance health and decrease caregiver burden.*

Use community resources in efficient, appropriate manner, as evidenced by:

Initiates contact with community resources

Uses community resources appropriately

- Initiate referrals to support agencies to assist with daily maintenance. *Professionals who provide in-home assistance are often in the best position to observe difficulties and to offer recommendations for assistive devices and home modifications.*[3]
- Investigate community resources for long-term maintenance.
- Increase family awareness of community resources. *Individuals are often unaware of community resources until they have a need for them.*
- Review with family how to use resources appropriately and on a continuing basis. *Community resources can contribute to the quality of life through environmental, health, and sanitation programs.*

Adapt the home and/or lifestyle to promote maximum health and safety, as evidenced by:

Removes unsafe objects and hazardous materials

Relates change to improvement of health status

Participates as able in performance of activities of daily living and home maintenance

Remains at home as long as feasible and desirable

- Discuss specific lifestyle and home changes that will promote health.
- Assess safety features of the home.
- Discuss safe arrangement of furnishings.
- Reinforce changes by discussing positive impact. Praise attempts at adaptation.
- Assist family to complete home safety assessment and follow up on deficits found.
- Assist family members to adapt to physical demands associated with caregiving.

Manage home maintenance adequately, as evidenced by:

Obtains additional support as needed

Determines and maintains a standard of cleanliness for the home

Family participates in home maintenance

Patient and family verbalize satisfaction with home situation

Maintains a safe, growth-promoting environment

- Arrange for additional support for caregiver respite *to decrease caregiver burden and prevent burnout.*
- Identify level of cleanliness necessary for safe environment.
- Counsel family members to work together to complete household tasks. *Cooperation in completing tasks can decrease workload and increase satisfaction.*
- Observe for increased level of health related to cleaner home environment. *A cleaner environment may decrease the risk and incidence of health problems such as asthma.*

IMPAIRED SPONTANEOUS VENTILATION

Impaired spontaneous ventilation is a state in which the response pattern of decreased energy reserves results in an individual's inability to maintain breathing adequate to support life.[7]

Related Factors[4,5,7]

Abdominal distention (e.g., bowel, obesity)

Activity greater than available energy

Atelectasis

Electrolyte imbalance

Hypothermia

Increased intrathoracic pressure

Increased metabolic requirements

Infection

Left ventricular dysfunction

Pulmonary edema, pulmonary embolus, pneumonia

Respiratory muscle fatigue

Uncontrolled pain

Defining Characteristics[2-4,6,7]

Apprehension

Cardiac dysrhythmias

Decreased Po_2

Decreased Sao_2

Decreased spontaneous tidal volume

Dyspnea

Increased restlessness

Increased use of accessory muscles

Increased Pco_2

Tachycardia

Tachypnea

Expected Patient Outcomes and Nursing Interventions With Rationale[1,2,4-7]

Sustain spontaneous ventilation, as evidenced by:

Maintains oxygenation of tissues (arterial-alveolar gradient less than 350, pH 7.35 to 7.45, Po_2 greater than 60, Pco_2 less than 50, Sao_2 greater than 90)

Experiences increasing level of consciousness with associated, purposeful, or nonpurposeful movement

Demonstrates synchronous use of respiratory muscles

- Conduct a thorough baseline assessment, using family and medical records as resources for obtaining medical history *to identify organs at risk because of altered oxygenation.*
- Observe for diaphragm or respiratory muscle fatigue, increased respiratory rate, minute ventilation, and hypercarbia with respiratory acidosis *to reevaluate adequacy of oxygen therapy parameters.*
- Call patient by preferred name, introduce self, and briefly explain purpose for being with patient during each contact *to decrease patient anxiety.*

- Ensure that patient has a primary nurse *to coordinate care and to monitor progress to goals.*
- Check for correct initial placement of endotracheal tube and monitor placement according to unit protocols *to maximize air entry and to maintain placement.*
- Collaborate with the multidisciplinary team to determine ventilation parameters *to ensure adequate oxygenation and to prevent ventilator-induced complications.*
- Collaborate with multidisciplinary team to develop a suction protocol with parameters for hyperoxygenation, hyperinflation, and length of stabilization period between suction catheter passes *to maximize tissue oxygenation and to prevent complications.*
- Initiate passive or active exercise *to mobilize secretions.*
- Remove secretions using sterile technique *to minimize exposure to infectious agents.*
- Monitor hemodynamic status *to detect decreased cardiac output caused by increased thoracic pressure.*
- Collaborate with the multidisciplinary team to determine timing and appropriateness for increasing ventilatory assistance until patient exhibits no spontaneous breathing effort *to allow adequate diaphragmatic rest and to prevent diaphragm muscle fatigue.*
- Observe and report indicators of airway resistance that can reduce the work of breathing, such as endotracheal tube size or uncoordinated efforts of the patient with the machine.
- Position upright or supine, based on individual tolerance, *to enhance full lung expansion and to improve cardiac output.*
- Observe breathing pattern *to determine work of breathing.*
- Use negative inspiratory pressure, positive expiratory pressure, and tidal volume as parameters to regulate activity *to prevent diaphragm fatigue, injury, and atrophy.*
- Collaborate with physician and respiratory therapist to determine timing and appropriateness of mechanically assisted muscle training (e.g., pressure support, intermittent mechanical ventilation, and inspiratory resistive training) *to maximize respiratory muscle strength.*
- Collaborate with physical therapist and physician to determine a schedule for graded manual diaphragmatic muscle exercises, incorporating principles of overload, specificity, and reversibility, *to maximize diaphragm endurance.*
- Collaborate with physician regarding use of medications *to facilitate bronchodilation and to increase diaphragm contractility.*

Meet metabolic energy requirements, as evidenced by:

Maintains nutritional intake equal to calculated requirements for nutrition

Demonstrates absence of infection

Tolerates progressive increase in activity

- Evaluate factors that contribute to increased energy expenditure, such as renal function, fluid status, cardiac status, acid-base disturbances, hepatic function, gastric bleeding, and bowel function.
- Collaborate with dietitian and physician to maintain adequate nutrition *to maximize energy resources and to prevent increased carbon dioxide production.*
- Monitor daily weight and intake and output.
- Monitor bowel function *to prevent complications, such as ileus.*
- Monitor levels of serum phosphate, potassium, calcium, and magnesium; collaborate with health team to provide replacement therapy needed, *to maintain respiratory muscle strength.*
- Observe for and report subtle signs of systemic or local infection *to conserve energy expenditure through early treatment.*
- Minimize exposure to infection by providing frequent oral hygiene, teaching family to report their exposure to possible infection or illness, and monitoring the sterility of equipment.
- Develop a therapeutic relationship *to foster patient's cooperation and participation in activity plan.*
- Monitor response to movement *to establish a baseline and observe for progress.*
- Establish a regular schedule for muscle reconditioning.
- Schedule rest periods that are congruent with patient's circadian rhythm *to facilitate adequate rapid eye movement (REM) sleep.*
- Evaluate rest and activity schedule on a daily basis; revise according to patient's tolerance.

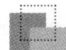

Ineffective Airway Clearance

Ineffective airway clearance is the inability to clear secretions or obstructions from the respiratory tract to maintain a clear airway.[15]

Related Factors[1,7-9,11,15,16]

Airway spasm
Allergic airways
Asthma
Chronic obstructive pulmonary disease
Excessive mucus
Exudate in the alveoli
Foreign body in airway
Hyperplasia of the bronchial walls
Infection
Neuromuscular dysfunction
Pollution
Presence of artificial airway
Retained secretions
Secondhand smoke
Secretions in the bronchi
Smoke inhalation
Smoking

Defining Characteristics[1,6,7,15]

Changes in respiratory rate and rhythm
Cough, ineffective or absent
Crackles
Cyanosis
Difficulty vocalizing
Diminished breath sounds
Dyspnea
Orthopnea
Rales
Restlessness

Rhonchi
Sputum
Wheezes
Wide-eyed look

Expected Patient Outcomes and Nursing Interventions With Rationale*

Maintain patent airways, as evidenced by:
Has clear breath sounds
Has fewer or less tenacious secretions
Has decreasing or absent dyspnea

- Auscultate lungs for rhonchi, crackles, or wheezing, *to assess lung oxygenation.*
- Monitor respiratory patterns for rate, depth, and ease of breathing, *to determine the work of breathing.*
- Assess characteristics of secretions for quantity, color, consistency, and odor.
- Monitor blood gases and/or finger oximetry *for hypoxia and hypercapnia.*
- When patient has an obstructed airway, assess patient's ability to talk; apply Heimlich maneuver as needed.
- Teach patient and family effective coughing techniques *to clear the airways without overtiring the patient.*
- Encourage patient to change positions every few hours and ambulate when possible *to increase aeration of the lungs.*
- Encourage 3 to 4 L fluids daily if not contraindicated, *to minimize mucosal drying and increase ciliary action to move secretions.*
- Remove secretions by suctioning airway as needed.
- Position patient in proper body alignment for optimal breathing pattern (head of bed up 45 degrees; if tolerated, 90 degrees) *to facilitate chest expansion.*
- If patient has unilateral lung disease, alternate semi-Fowler's position with a lateral position with unaffected lung in a dependent position ("good lung down"), *to enhance ventilation and perfusion of that lung by means of gravity and hydrostatic pressure.* (This position is contraindicated for patients with pulmonary abscess, hemorrhage, or interstitial emphysema.)
- Administer oxygen as ordered.
- Administer bronchodilators, as ordered, *to relax bronchial smooth muscles, increasing the diameter of the bronchi and thereby decreasing the work of breathing.*
- Administer corticosteroids and antibiotics, as ordered, *to reduce edema and infection.*
- Avoid suppressing cough reflex unless cough is frequent and nonproductive.
- Assist patient with oral hygiene, as needed, *to maintain comfort.*

Communicate knowledge of self-care, as evidenced by:
Explains reason for ineffective airway clearance
Describes actions to avoid ineffective airway clearance
Explains medications and treatments for home use
Plans for follow-up care

- Assess what patient and family need to learn.
- Provide information on how to prevent recurrence of airway obstruction.
- Teach patient diaphragmatic and pursed-lip breathing bronchial hygiene, and coughing techniques.
- Instruct about drugs taken at home, frequency of administration, and side effects.
- Encourage smoking cessation.
- Encourage patient to eat balanced meals with adequate fluids.
- Explain the importance of changing daily activities to decrease oxygen demands.

*References 1, 5, 6, 8, 9, 11, 13.

INEFFECTIVE BREATHING PATTERN

Ineffective breathing pattern is inspiration and/or expiration that does not provide adequate ventilation.[15]

Related Factors[2,7,15]

Anxiety
Body position
Chest cavity deformity
Decreased energy
Fatigue
Hyperventilation
Hypoventilation
Musculoskeletal impairment
Neurologic immaturity
Neuromuscular dysfunction
Obesity
Pain
Perception/cognitive impairment
Respiratory muscle fatigue
Spinal cord injury

Defining Characteristics[2,7,9,10,15]

Altered chest excursion
Assumption of three-point position
Decreased inspiratory/expiratory pressure
Decreased minute ventilation
Decreased vital capacity
Depth of breathing: adults VT 500 ml at rest; infants 6 to 8 ml/kg
Dyspnea
Increased anterior-posterior diameter
Nasal flaring
Orthopnea
Prolonged expiration phases
Pursed-lip breathing
Respiratory rate
  Adults 14 or older less than 11 or greater than 24
  Infants less than 25 or greater than 60
  Ages 1 to 4 less than 20 or greater than 30
  Ages 5 to 14 less than 15 or greater than 25
  Shortness of breath
  Timing ratio
  Use of accessory muscles to breathe

Expected Patient Outcomes and Nursing Interventions With Rationale[2,4,9,10,14]

Effective respiratory pattern without tiring patient, as evidenced by:
Has respiratory rate within normal limits

Keeps tidal volume optimal for patient, with Pa_{O_2} greater than 60 mm Hg
Maintains Pa_{CO_2} normal for patient
Experiences no dyspnea

- Monitor respiratory rate, depth, and ease of respiration, *to determine extent of respiratory distress.*
- Observe for use of accessory muscles, abdominal breathing, nasal flaring, retractions, irritability, confusion, or lethargy. *These symptoms indicate increasing respiratory difficulty and decreasing P_{O_2}.*
- Determine degree of dyspnea by counting number of words the patient can say between breaths.
- If patient is dyspneic, determine cause.
- Auscultate breathing sounds for decreased or absent sounds, crackles, and wheezes.
- Monitor patient's oxygen saturation and arterial blood gases *for hypoxia.*
- Administer oxygen, as ordered, *to decrease dyspnea.*
- Observe sputum for color, odor, and volume.
- Monitor the patient's tidal volume for a decrease.
- Review chest x-ray films *to determine severity of skeletal and lung impairment.*
- Assess emotional response that may alter breathing, such as anxiety, fear, or pain.
- Encourage patient to cough, splinting chest as necessary.
- Assist patient with weak or paralyzed intercostal or abdominal muscles with splinting intercostal muscles or applying upward pressure just below the diaphragm, *to cough effectively.*
- Medicate with analgesics before coughing or physiotherapy, *to improve ventilation.*
- Assist patient to use relaxation techniques *to control breathing rate.*
- Teach pursed-lip breathing, if indicated, *to increase oxygenation.*
- Assist patient to use most effective respiratory position, such as three-point position, *to increase exhalation phase and reduce airway collapse.*
- Encourage use of blow bottles or incentive spirometry.
- Teach use of abdominal breathing exercises *to strengthen respiratory system.*

Communicate knowledge of self-care, as evidenced by:
Patient and family explain reasons for ineffective breathing
Identifies medications and treatments for home use
Plans for follow-up care

- Assess what patient and family need to know.
- Review reasons for ineffective breathing patterns.
- Make referral for ventilatory equipment to be used in the home.
- Review reasons for medications and treatments ordered for home use.
- Review plan for follow-up care.

IMPAIRED GAS EXCHANGE

Impaired gas exchange is an excess or deficit in oxygenation and/or carbon dioxide elimination at the alveolar-capillary membrane.[15]

Related Factors[3,10,15]

Alveolar-capillary membrane changes
Ventilation-perfusion imbalance

Defining Characteristics[3,7,15]

Abnormal arterial blood gas values
Abnormal rate, rhythm, depth of breathing
Abnormal skin color
Confusion
Cyanosis (in neonates only)
Decreased or increased carbon dioxide
Diaphoresis
Dyspnea
Headache upon awakening
Hypercapnia
Hypercarbia
Hypoxemia
Hypoxia
Irritability
Nasal flaring
Restlessness
Somnolence
Tachycardia

Expected Patient Outcomes and Nursing Interventions With Rationale[3,4,7,10,12]

Maintain adequate oxygenation, as evidenced by:
Maintains P_{O_2}: 80 to 95 mm Hg (may be lower for patient with chronic obstructive pulmonary disease [COPD])
Maintains P_{CO_2}: 35 to 45 mm Hg (may be higher for patient with COPD)
Maintains O_2 saturation: 95% to 99%
Has normal level of hemoglobin: 12 to 14 g/dl (women), 14 to 16 g/dl (men)
Has normal respiratory rate: 12 to 20 breaths/min
Performs activities of daily living without becoming short of breath

- Monitor respiratory rate, depth, and effort, including use of accessory muscles, nasal flaring, and thoracic or abdominal breathing, *to determine degree of respiratory distress.*
- Auscultate breath sounds for rhonchi, crackles, and wheezes.
- Assess behavior and mental status for restlessness, agitation, confusion, and lethargy, *which indicate decreased oxygenation.*
- Monitor oxygen saturation continually via pulse oximeter *for hypoxia* and, when indicated, arterial blood gases *for hypoxia and hypercapnia.*
- Monitor complete blood count for decreases in hemoglobin and hematocrit *to assess oxygen-carrying capacity.*
- Observe skin color for paleness or cyanosis.
- Note number of words patient can say between breaths at rest and during activity, *to determine degree of dyspnea that may indicate hypoxia.*
- Position patient for maximal ventilation and perfusion. If client has unilateral lung disease, alternate semi-Fowler's position with lateral position with unaffected lung dependent ("good lung down"). If patient has bilateral lung disease, position patient on either side or semi-Fowler's position supine, changing position every few hours. *Positioning will enhance ventilation and perfusion of the lung(s).*

- Encourage patient to deep breathe and cough or use incentive spirometry every few hours while awake, *to clear airway of secretions.*
- Suction the airways when coughing is ineffective, *to stimulate the cough reflex.*
- Teach patient pursed-lip breathing *to decrease work of breathing and increase oxygenation.*
- Pace activities to patient's tolerance *to avoid increasing the oxygen demand.*
- Use sedation cautiously *to avoid respiratory depression.*
- Administer humidified oxygen as ordered, *to improve gas exchange.*
- Administer packed cells, as ordered, *to treat anemia, which impairs oxygen-carrying capacity.*
- Administer medications as ordered, such as bronchodilators, diuretics, corticosteroids, antibiotics, anticoagulants.

Communicate knowledge of self-care, as evidenced by:
Explains reasons for impaired gas exchange
States medications and treatments for home use
Plans for follow-up care

- Assess what patient and family need to know.
- Provide information about pursed-lip breathing and diaphragmatic breathing, when indicated.
- Discover reason for impaired gas exchange, and discuss how to prevent it in the future.
- State actions, side effects, dosage, and frequency of administration of all medications ordered by physician.
- Plan referral for ventilatory equipment to be used in the home.
- Alter daily activities, as necessary, *to decrease oxygen demand.*

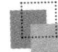

RISK FOR DISUSE SYNDROME

Risk for disuse syndrome is the state in which an individual is at risk for deterioration of body systems as the result of prescribed or unavoidable inactivity.[8]

Risk Factors[1,4,8]

Altered level of consciousness
Mechanical immobilization
Paralysis
Prescribed immobilization
Severe pain

Expected Patient Outcomes and Nursing Interventions With Rationale[1-3,5-7]

Does not experience disuse syndrome, as evidenced by:
Maintains musculoskeletal activity and cardiovascular function
Prevents respiratory complications
Plans and implements a program to maintain skin integrity
Maintains adequate nutrition and normal elimination patterns

- Consult with physiatrist or physical therapist, as appropriate.
- Implement passive and active range-of-motion exercises. *The pumping action of contracting muscles promotes venous return.*
- Instruct patient in isometric exercises, if indicated. *Isotonic, isometric, and passive muscle exercises stretch muscle fibers and also help maintain cardiac work capacity.*[2,3]
- Use a kinetic treatment table or tilt table, if appropriate, *to maintain motion, circulation, and orthostatic equilibrium and to provide stress on long bones to reduce demineralization.*
- Implement a pain management protocol, if necessary, *to allow patient to move comfortably and exercise enough in bed to achieve therapeutic goals.*
- Use antiembolism stockings or sequential compression system for legs, as ordered, *to prevent deep vein thrombus.*[5]
- Consult with physician regarding prophylactic use of anticoagulants *to prevent thrombus formation by decreasing clotting factors.*[5]
- Teach patient to move in bed without increasing intrathoracic pressure, *to decrease cardiac workload.*
- Turn and reposition patient frequently *to prevent contractures.*
- Assess lungs frequently and promote coughing and deep breathing *to mobilize secretions and prevent atelectasis.*
- Increase fluid intake, *to liquify secretions.*
- Teach use of incentive spirometer *to promote chest expansion, more complete inflation of alveoli, and better gas exchange.*
- Assess skin frequently; monitor for possible breakdown or abrasions related to traction or other devices. *Early identification of skin problems allows early intervention to limit damage.*
- Assess need for air or fluid flotation bed or provide foam mattress, *to decrease pressure and increase circulation to skin.*
- Turn and reposition patient frequently *to prevent skin breakdown from pressure.*
- Keep skin clean and dry, and keep bed linens free of wrinkles, *to prevent pressure areas and skin breakdown.*
- Encourage good nutrition *to prevent muscle and skin breakdown and to promote normal bladder and bowel elimination.*
- Encourage fluid intake of 2000 ml per day, if appropriate, *to maintain urinary output.*
- Identify previous elimination pattern *for use as a baseline of comparison.*
- Assess need for stool softener or bulk laxative and administer as needed *to increase bowel peristalsis and maintain regular soft-formed stool.*
- Ensure proper positioning and privacy *to promote elimination.*
- Assess and maximize available supports *to facilitate meeting emotional needs and stimulate intellectually.*
- Provide clock, calendar, radio, and television, *to assist in reality orientation*
- Provide frequent interactions *to maintain sensory stimulation and reality orientation.*
- Provide opportunities for patient participation in decisions regarding care, *to promote a feeling of control over the environment.*
- Assist the patient in identifying successful coping strategies.

Risk for Peripheral Neurovascular Dysfunction

Risk for peripheral neurovascular dysfunction is a state in which an individual is at risk for experiencing a disruption in circulation, motion, or sensation of an extremity.[6]

Risk Factors[2,3,5,6]

Acute compartment syndrome
Arterial occlusion
Burns
Crush syndrome
Fractures
Frostbite or snakebite
Immobilization
Mechanical compression (e.g., tourniquet, cast, brace, restraint, or dressing)
Orthopedic surgery
Trauma
Venous occlusion

Defining Characteristics[2,5,6]

Cool, mottled skin
Decreased pulses
Edema
Increased intracompartment pressure
Numbness or lessening of sensation
Pain
Pallor
Paralysis
Paresthesia (burning or tingling)
Weakness

Expected Patient Outcomes and Nursing Interventions With Rationale[1-5,7,8]

Maintain intact neurovascular status distal to the problem/injury, as evidenced by:

Has warm, pink skin, with rapid capillary refill
Demonstrates no edema
Has strong peripheral pulses and normal sensation and movement of all digits
States an absence of pain

- Assess circulatory and neurologic status in the extremity distal to the problem/injury.
- Compare extremities bilaterally and simultaneously; *early detection of circulatory and neurologic abnormalities is necessary to prevent loss of function.*
- Inspect skin for pallor, cyanosis, or mottled discoloration. *Skin changes are an excellent indicator of cardiovascular status.*
- Inspect for the presence and severity of edema by observing for swelling accompanied by taut and shining skin in the extremity. *Edema is a manifestation of excess fluid in the tissues.*
- If edema is present, describe if it is pitting or nonpitting by applying pressure with fingers; if it is dependent or unilateral. Describe the severity of the edema with the following scale:
  - 0 = none
  - +1 = trace
  - +2 = moderate
  - +3 = deep
  - +4 = very deep
- Elevate the extremity to or above heart level *to promote arterial flow and venous return thus reducing edema.*
- Perform passive or active range of motion to all joints in the affected extremity. *Muscle contraction increases venous return, keeps joints supple, and prevents contractures.*
- Assess capillary refill time by compressing nail beds or surrounding tissue and by observing the return of usual color. *Capillary refill time is an indicator of arterial perfusion and should occur within 1 to 2 seconds.*
- Assess the skin temperature using the back of the fingers *to determine arterial perfusion.*
- Palpate peripheral pulses for quality and evaluate with the following scale:[7]
  - 0 = absent
  - 1+ = diminished
  - 2+ = normal
  - 3+ = full or increased
  - 4+ = bounding
- Mark pulses that are difficult to palpate with an X with an ink pen or permanent nontoxic marker.
- Auscultate peripheral pulses with Doppler ultrasound device if pulses are difficult to evaluate; *a Doppler device magnifies sound over pulse points to assist in assessing peripheral pulses.*
- Assess for pain (character, location, intensity) at rest and with passive stretching of the muscle group.
- Have patient rate pain on a scale of 0 to 10 with 0 being "no pain" and 10 being "extreme pain"; *pain on passive stretch of the muscle passing through the compartment or pain out of proportion to what is anticipated for the type of problem or injury may be an indication of compartment syndrome.*
- With patient's eyes closed or head turned, assess for sensation in the extremities. *The presence of paresthesia (burning or tingling sensations), numbness, or decreased sense of touch may be the result of increased pressure, stretching, or lacerated nerves.*
- Determine the patient's ability to move appendages distal to the problem or injury (all fingers or all toes should be assessed) *to assess for increasing pressure, stretched, or lacerated nerves.*
- Record the above assessments on appropriate documentation tool.

Patient and/or significant other recognize and report signs and symptoms of neurovascular compromise, as evidenced by:

Describes signs and symptoms of neurovascular compromise

- Teach patient and/or significant other signs and symptoms of neurovascular compromise (as previously described). *The patient is often the first to detect subtle changes that can lead to early detection of neurovascular compromises.*
- Provide patient and/or significant other with verbal and written instructions for assessing neurovascular status;

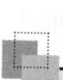

learning is enhanced by both verbal and written instruction.
- The physician should be notified immediately of abnormal neurovascular findings; *prompt treatment of circulatory and neurologic problems can result in a decreased disability or in an absence of permanent disability.*

Venous stasis is prevented, as evidenced by:
Maintains adequate venous circulation
- Encourage ambulation *to help prevent clot formation.*
- Apply compression stockings or intermittent pneumatic compression devices, as ordered, *to prevent deep vein thrombus (DVT).*[2]
- Assess for signs of DVT: pain, deep tenderness, redness, and swelling in the calf and thigh.[2]
- Measure calf and thigh circumferences *to detect differences greater that 2 cm.*
- Encourage health-promoting behaviors such as good nutrition, avoidance of nicotine, and avoidance of alcohol.

REFERENCES

Activity-Exercise
1. Gordon M: *Manual of nursing diagnosis,* ed 9, St. Louis, 2000, Mosby.

Activity Intolerance, Risk for Activity Intolerance
1. Allison M, Keller C: Physical activity in the elderly: benefits and intervention strategies, *Nurse Pract* 22(8):53, 1997.
2. Cochrane T, Davey, R, Munro J et al: Exercise, physical function and health perceptions of older people, *Physiotherapy* 84(12):598, 1998.
3. Fitts SS: Physical benefits and challenges of exercise for people with chronic renal disease, *J Ren Nutr* 7(3):123, 1997.
4. McCloskey JC, Bulechek GM, editors: *Nursing interventions classification (NIC),* ed 3, St. Louis, 2001, Mosby.
5. McFarland GK, McFarlane EA: *Nursing diagnosis and intervention: planning for patient care* ed 3, St. Louis, 1997, Mosby.
6. Nielsen KE, Nielsen DH, Lin S et al: Changes in exercise responses and tolerance following an eight week pulmonary rehabilitation program, *Cardiopulmon Phys Ther J* 8(4):3, 1997.
7. North American Nursing Diagnosis Association: *NANDA nursing diagnoses: definitions and classification* 2001–2002, Philadelphia, 2001, The Association.
8. Stofan JR, DiPietro L, Davis, D et al: Physical activity patterns associated with cardiorespiratory fitness and reduced mortality: the Aerobics Center longitudinal study, *Am J Public Health* 88(12):1807, 1998.
9. Straight LL: Activity intolerance; Risk for activity intolerance. In Ackley BJ, Ladwig GB, editors: *Nursing diagnosis handbook: a guide to planning care,* ed 4, St. Louis, 1999, Mosby.
10. Tyler DO: Activity intolerance: a clinical validation study. In Rantz MJ, LeMone P, editors: *Classification of nursing diagnoses: proceedings of the twelfth conference, North America Nursing Diagnosis Association,* Glendale, Calif, 1997, Cinahl Information Systems.

Autonomic Dysreflexia, Risk for Autonomic Dysreflexia
1. Ackley BJ: Dysreflexia. In Ackley BJ, Ladwig GB, editors: *Nursing diagnosis handbook: a guide to planning care,* ed 4, St. Louis, 1999, Mosby.
2. Ackley BJ: Risk for autonomic dysreflexia. In Ackley BJ, Ladwig GB, editors: *Nursing diagnosis handbook: a guide to planning care,* ed 4, St. Louis, 1999, Mosby.
3. Bergman SB, Yarkony RM, Stiens SA: Spinal cord injury rehabilitation: medical complications, *Arch Phys Med Rehabil* 78(suppl 3):S53, 1997.
4. Keely BR: Preventing complications: recognition and treatment of autonomic dysreflexia, *Dimens Crit Care Nurs* 17(4):170, 1998.
5. McCloskey JC, Bulechek GM, editors: *Nursing interventions classification (NIC),* ed 3, St. Louis, 2001, Mosby.
6. McFarland GK, McFarlane EA: *Nursing diagnosis and intervention: planning for patient care,* ed 3, St. Louis, 1997, Mosby.
7. North American Nursing Diagnosis Association: *NANDA nursing diagnosis: definitions and classification 2001–2002,* Philadelphia, 2001, The Association.
8. Tepper K: Management of autonomic dysreflexia in a home care setting, *Clin Excel Nurse Pract* 1(3):163, 1997.
9. Travers PL: Autonomic dysreflexia: a clinical rehabilitation problem, *Rehabil Nurs* 24(1):19, 1999.

Bathing/Hygiene, Dressing/Grooming, Feeding, Toileting Self-Care Deficit
1. Barker JC, Mitteness LS, Muller HB: Older home health care patients and their physicians: assessment of functional ability, *Home Health Care Serv Q* 17(2):21, 1998.
2. Beck C, Heacock P, Mercer SO et al: Improving dressing behavior in cognitively impaired nursing home residents, *Nurs Res* 46(3):126, 1997.
3. Bonder BR, Zadorozny C, Martin RJ: Dressing in Alzheimer's disease: executive function and procedural memory, *Clin Gerontol* 19(2):88, 1998.
4. Denney A: Quiet music: an intervention for mealtime agitation? *J Gerontol Nurs* 23(7):16, 1997.
5. Drummond AER, Miller N, Colquohoun M et al: The effects of a stroke unit on activities of daily living, *Clin Rehabil* 10(1):12, 1996.
6. Freeman EM: International perspectives on bathing, *J Gerontol Nurs* 23(5):40, 1997.
7. Gibbs KE, Barnitt R: Occupational therapy and the self-care needs of Hindu elders, *Br J Occup Ther* 62(3):100, 1999.
8. Giles GM, Ridley JE, Dill A et al: A consecutive series of adults with brain injury treated with a washing and dressing retraining program, *Am J Occup Ther* 51(4):256, 1997.
9. Hoeffer B, Rader J, McKenzie D et al: Reducing aggressive behavior during bathing cognitively impaired nursing home residents, *J Gerontol Nurs* 23(5):16, 1997.
10. Hutchinson S, Leger-Krall S, Wilson HS: Toileting: a biobehavioral challenge in Alzheimer's dementia care, *J Gerontol Nurs* 22(10):18, 1996.
11. Kayser-Jones J: Inadequate staffing at mealtime: implications for nursing and health policy, *J Gerontol Nurs* 23(8):14, 1997.
12. Kayser-Jones J, Pengilly K: Dysphagia among nursing home residents, *Geriatr Nurs Am J Care Aging* 20(2):77, 1999.
13. McKinley WO, Conti-Wyneken AR, Vokac CW et al: Rehabilitative functional outcome of patients with neoplastic spinal cord compression, *Arch Phys Med Rehabil* 77(9):892, 1996.
14. Miller M: Physically aggressive resident behavior during hygienic care, *J Gerontol Nurs* 23(5):24, 1997.
15. North American Nursing Diagnosis Association: *Definitions and classification 2001–2002,* Philadelphia, 2001, The Association.
16. Paquette M, Rodemich C: *Psychiatric nursing diagnosis care plans for DSM-IV,* Boston, 1997, Jones & Bartlett.
17. Rogers WA, Meyer B, Walker N et al: Functional limitations to daily living tasks in the aged: a focus group analysis, *Hum Factors* 40(1):111, 1998.

18. Schell ES, Kayser-Jones J: The effect of role-taking ability on caregiver-resident mealtime interaction, *Appl Nurs Res* 12(1):38, 1999.
19. Schemm RL, Gitlin LN: How occupational therapists teach older patients to use bathing and dressing devices in rehabilitation, *Am J Occup Ther* 52(4):276, 1998.
20. Skewes SM: Bathing: it's a tough job! *J Gerontol Nurs* 23(5):45, 1997.
21. Walker MF, Drummond AER, Lincoln NB: Evaluation of dressing practice for stroke patients after discharge from hospital: a crossover design study, *Clin Rehabil* 10(1):23, 1996.
22. Wilkinson JM: *Nursing diagnosis handbook with NIC interventions and NOC outcomes,* ed 7, Upper Saddle River, NJ, 2000, Prentice Hall Health.
23. Williams L: Self-care deficit. In Ackley BJ, Ladwig GB, editors: *Nursing diagnosis handbook: a guide to planning care,* ed 4, St. Louis, 1999, Mosby.

Delayed Growth and Development, Risk for Delayed Development, Risk for Disproportionate Growth

1. Aicardi J: The etiology of developmental delay, *Semin Pediatr Neurol* 5(1):15, 1998.
2. Arendt R, Angelopoulos J, Salvator A et al: Motor development of cocaine-exposed children at age two years, *Pediatrics* 103(1):86, 1999.
3. Cameron RJ: Early intervention for young children with developmental delay: the Portage approach, *Child Care Health Dev* 23(1):11, 1997.
4. Cronau H, Brown RT: Growth and development: physical, mental, and social aspects, *Prim Care* 25(1):23, 1998.
5. Dees WL, Hiney JK, Srivastava V: Alcohol's effects on female puberty: the role of insulin-like growth factor 1, *Alcohol Health Res World* 22(3):165, 1998.
6. Duck SC: Identification and assessment of the slowly growing child, *Am Fam Physician* 53(7):2305, 1996.
7. Gabriel K, Hofmann C, Glavas M et al: The hormonal effects of alcohol use on the mother and fetus, *Alcohol Health Res World* 22(3):170, 1998.
8. Hurt H, Malmud E, Braitman LE et al: Inner-city achievers: who are they? *Arch Pediatr Adolesc Med* 152(10):993, 1998.
9. Keltner BR, Wise LA, Taylor G: Mothers with intellectual limitations and their 2-year-old children's developmental outcomes, *J Intellect Dev Disabil* 24(1):45, 1999.
10. Ladwig GB: Risk for altered development. In Ackley BJ, Ladwig GB, editors: *Nursing diagnosis handbook: a guide to planning care,* ed 4, St. Louis, 1999, Mosby.
11. Ladwig GB: Risk for altered growth. In Ackley BJ, Ladwig GB, editors: *Nursing diagnosis handbook: a guide to planning care,* ed 4, St. Louis, 1999, Mosby.
12. McCloskey JC, Bulechek GM, editors: *Nursing interventions classification (NIC),* ed 3, St. Louis, 2001, Mosby.
13. McFarland GK, McFarlane EA: *Nursing diagnosis and intervention: planning for patient care,* ed 3, St. Louis, 1997, Mosby.
14. North American Nursing Diagnosis Association: *NANDA nursing diagnoses: definitions and classification 2001–2002,* Philadelphia, 2001, The Association.
15. Van Dyke DC, Bonthius NE, Bonthius DJ et al: Alcohol and anticonvulsant medication use during pregnancy: effects on the growth and development of infants and children, *Infant Young Child* 9(2):43, 1996.
16. Wetsch PA: Altered growth and development. In Ackley BJ, Ladwig GB, editors: *Nursing diagnosis handbook: a guide to planning care,* ed 4, St. Louis, 1999, Mosby.

Decreased Cardiac Output

1. Doenges ME, Moorhouse MF: *Nurse's pocket guide: diagnosis, interventions, and rationale,* ed 6, Philadelphia, 1998, FA Davis.
2. Dougherty CM: Reconceptualization of the nursing diagnosis decreased cardiac output, *Nurs Diagnosis J Nurs Language Classification* 8(1):29, 1997.
3. LeMone P, Burke KM: *Medical-surgical nursing: critical thinking in client care,* ed 2, Upper Saddle River, NJ, 2000, Prentice Hall.
4. Lessig ML, Lessig PM: The cardiovascular system. In Alspach JG, editor: *Core curriculum for critical care nursing,* ed 5, Philadelphia, 1998, WB Saunders.
5. McFarland GK, McFarlane EA: *Nursing diagnosis and intervention: planning for patient care,* ed 3, St. Louis, 1997, Mosby.
6. Morton N: Validation of the nursing diagnosis decreased cardiac output in a population without cardiac disease. In Rantz MJ, LeMone P, editors: *Classification of nursing diagnoses: proceedings of the twelfth conference, North America Nursing Diagnosis Association,* Glendale, Calif, 1997, Cinahl Information Systems.
7. North American Nursing Diagnosis Association: *NANDA nursing diagnoses: definitions and classification 2001–2002,* Philadelphia, 2001, The Association.
8. Straight LL, Ackley BJ: Decreased cardiac output. In Ackley BJ, Ladwig GB, editors: *Nursing diagnosis handbook: a guide to planning care,* ed 4, St. Louis, 1999, Mosby.
9. Taylor RD, Asinger RW: Atrial fibrillation: how best to use rate control, rhythm control, cardioversion, anticoagulation, *Consultant* 38(8):1879, 1998.

Ineffective Tissue Perfusion (Specify Type: Renal, Cerebral, Cardiopulmonary, Gastrointestinal, Peripheral)

1. Ackley BJ: Altered tissue perfusion (specify type): renal, cerebral, cardiopulmonary, gastrointestinal, peripheral. In Ackley BJ, Ladwig GB, editors: *Nursing diagnosis handbook: a guide to planning care,* ed 4, St. Louis, 1999, Mosby.
2. Alexander P, Giangola G: Deep venous thrombosis and pulmonary embolism: diagnosis, prophylaxis, and treatment, *Ann Vasc Surg* 13(3):318, 1999.
3. Elamin EM: Pulmonary embolism: update on diagnosis and management, *J Crit Ill* 14(2):91, 1999.
4. Feldman CB: Caring for feet: patients and nurse practitioners working together, *Nurse Pract Forum* 9(2):87, 1998.
5. Launius BK, Graham BD: Understanding and preventing deep vein thrombosis and pulmonary embolism, *AACN Clin Issues Adv Prac Acute Crit Care* 9(1):91, 1998.
6. North American Nursing Diagnosis Association: *NANDA nursing diagnoses: definitions and classification 2001–2002,* Philadelphia, 2001, The Association.
7. Wipke-Tevis DD: Caring for vascular leg ulcers: essential knowledge for the home health nurse, *Home Healthcare Nurse* 17(2):87, 1999.
8. Wywialowski EF: Tissue perfusion as a key underlying concept of pressure ulcer development and treatment, *J Vasc Nurs* 17(1):12, 1999.

Decreased Intracranial Adaptive Capacity

1. Hickey JV: *The clinical practice of neurological and neurosurgical nursing,* Philadelphia, 1997, JB Lippincott.
2. LeMone P, Burke K: *Medical-surgical nursing: critical thinking in client care,* Upper Saddle River, NJ, 2000, Prentice Hall Health.
3. McCloskey JC, Bulechek GM, editors: Intracranial pressure (ICP) monitoring. In *Nursing interventions classification (NIC),* ed 3, St. Louis, 2001, Mosby.
4. North American Nursing Diagnosis Association: *Nursing diagnoses: definitions and classification 2001–2002,* Philadelphia, 2001, The Association.

5. Wall BM, Philips JP, Howard JC: Validation of increased intracranial pressure and high risk for increased intracranial pressure, *Nurs Diagnosis J Nurs Language Classification* 5(2):74, 1994.

Deficient Diversional Activity

1. Ackley BJ: Diversional activity deficit. In Ackley BJ, Ladwig GB, editors: *Nursing diagnosis handbook: a guide to planning care,* ed 4, St. Louis, 1999, Mosby.
2. DeMong SA: Provision of recreational activities in hospices in the United States, *Hospice J* 12(4):57, 1997.
3. Gulick EE: Correlates of quality of life among persons with multiple sclerosis, *Nurs Res* 46(6):305, 1997.
4. Hoffman J: Alternatives: complementary therapies. Tuning in to the power of music, *RN* 60(6):52, 1997.
5. Lash AA: Quality of life in systemic lupus erythematosus, *Appl Nurs Res* 11(3):130, 1998.
6. McFarland GK, McFarlane EA: *Nursing diagnosis and intervention: planning for patient care,* ed 3, St. Louis, 1997, Mosby.
7. North American Nursing Diagnosis Association: *NANDA nursing diagnoses: definitions and classification 2001–2002* Philadelphia, 2001, The Association.
8. Patterson I, Pegg S: Leisure programs and older people in care, *Geriaction* 16(3):24, 1998.

Delayed Surgical Recovery

1. Brodie LJ, Slorman RM: Changes in health status of elderly patients following hip replacement surgery, *J Gerontol Nurs* 24(3):5, 1998.
2. Edell-Gustafsson UM, Hetta JE, Aren CB et al: Measurement of sleep and quality of life before and after coronary artery bypass grafting: a pilot study, *Int J Nurs Prac* 3(4):239, 1997.
3. Gammon J, Mulholland CW: Effect of preparatory information prior to elective total hip replacement on post-operative physical coping outcomes, *Int J Nurs Stud* 33(6):589, 1996.
4. Goodman H: Patients' perceptions of their education needs in the first six weeks following discharge after cardiac surgery, *J Adv Nurs* 25(6):1241, 1997.
5. Logsdon MC, Usui WM, Cronin SN et al: Social support and adjustment in women following coronary artery bypass surgery, *Health Care Women Int* 19(1):61, 1998.
6. McCloskey JC, Bulechek GM, editors: Incision site care; Pain management. In *Nursing interventions classification (NIC),* ed 3, St. Louis, 2001, Mosby.
7. Milisen K, Abraham IL, Broos PL: Postoperative variation in neurocognitive and functional status in elderly hip fracture patients, *J Adv Nurs* 27(1):59, 1998.
8. North American Nursing Diagnosis Association: *Nursing diagnoses: definitions and classification 2001–2002,* Philadelphia, 2001, The Association.
9. Redeker NS, Wykpisz E: Effects of age on activity patterns after coronary artery bypass surgery, *Heart Lung* 28(1):5, 1999.
10. Taylor C, Lillis C, LeMone P: *Fundamentals of nursing: the art and science of nursing care,* ed 4, Philadelphia, 2001, JB Lippincott.

Disorganized Infant Behavior, Risk for Disorganized Infant Behavior

1. Ackley BJ, Ladwig GB: *Nursing diagnosis handbook: a guide to planning care,* ed 4, St. Louis, 1999, Mosby.
2. Als H: Neurobehavioral organization of the newborn: opportunities for assessment and intervention. In Uzgiris I, editor: *New directions for child development,* San Francisco, 1991, Jossey Bass.
3. Carpenito LJ: *Nursing diagnosis: application to clinical practice,* ed 7, Philadelphia, 1997, JB Lippincott.
4. Gray K, Dostal S, Ternullo-Retta C et al: Developmentally supportive care in a neonatal intensive care unit: a research utilization project, *J Neonat Nurs* 17(2):33, 1998.
5. Keefe MR, Kotzer AM, Froese-Fretz A et al: A longitudinal comparison of irritable and nonirritable infants, *Nurs Res* 45(1):4, 1996.
6. Marshall-Baker A, Lickliter R, Cooper RP: Prolonged exposure to a visual pattern may promote behavioral organization in preterm infants, *J Perinat Neonat Nurs* 12(2):50, 1998.
7. McCloskey JC, Bulechek GM, editors: Attachment promotion. In *Nursing interventions classification (NIC),* ed 3, St. Louis, 2001, Mosby.
8. North American Nursing Diagnosis Association: *Nursing diagnoses: definitions and classification 2001–2002,* Philadelphia, 2001, The Association.
9. Pickler RH, Frankel HB, Walsh KM et al: Effects of nonnutritive sucking on behavioral organization and feeding performance in preterm infants, *Nurs Res* 45(3):132, 1996.
10. Pillitteri A: *Maternal and child health nursing: care of the childbearing and childrearing family,* ed 3, Philadelphia, 1999, Lippincott.
11. Scaridi FA, Field TM, Wheeden A et al: Cocaine-exposed preterm neonates show behavioral and hormonal differences, *Pediatrics* 97(6 part 1):851, 1996.
12. Starr NB, Hoye L: An overview of developmentally supportive care of the premature infant, *J Pediatr Health Care* 12(1):33, 1998.
13. Stevens B, Johnston C, Franck L et al: The efficacy of developmentally sensitive interventions and sucrose for relieving procedural pain in very low birth weight neonates, *Nurs Res* 48(1):35, 1999.
14. Wong DL: *Waley and Wong's nursing care of infants and children,* ed 6, St. Louis, 1999, Mosby.

Readiness for Enhanced Organized Infant Behavior

1. Ackley BJ, Ladwig GB: *Nursing diagnosis handbook: a guide to planning care,* ed 4, St. Louis, 1999, Mosby.
2. Carpenito LJ: *Nursing diagnosis: application to clinical practice,* ed 7, Philadelphia, 1997, JB Lippincott.
3. Gray K, Dostal S, Ternullo-Retta C et al: Developmentally supportive care in a neonatal intensive care unit: a research utilization project, *J Neonat Nurs* 17(2):33, 1998.
4. Marshall-Baker A, Lickliter R, Cooper RP: Prolonged exposure to a visual pattern may promote behavioral organization in preterm infants, *J Perinat Neonat Nurs* 12(2):50, 1998.
5. North American Nursing Diagnosis Association: *Nursing diagnoses: definitions and classification 2001–2002,* Philadelphia, 2001, The Association.
6. Pickler RH, Frankel HB, Walsh KM et al: Effects of nonnutritive sucking on behavioral organization and feeding performance in preterm infants, *Nurs Res* 45(3):132, 1996.
7. Pillitteri A: *Maternal and child health nursing: care of the childbearing and childrearing family,* ed 3, Philadelphia, 1999, JB Lippincott.
8. Wong DL: *Waley and Wong's nursing care of infants and children,* ed 6, St. Louis, 1999, Mosby.

Dysfunctional Ventilatory Weaning Response

1. Higgins PA: Patient perception of fatigue while undergoing long-term mechanical ventilation: incidence and associated factors, *Heart Lung* 27(3):177, 1998.
2. Jacavone J, Young J: Use of pulmonary rehabilitation strategies to wean a difficult-to-wean patient: case study, *Crit Care Nurse* 18(6):29, 1998.
3. Lysaght L: Dysfunctional ventilatory weaning response (DVWR). In Ackley BJ, Ladwig GB, editors: *Nursing diagnosis handbook: a guide to planning care,* ed 4, St. Louis, 1999, Mosby.
4. McCloskey JC, Bulechek GM, editors: *Nursing interventions classification (NIC),* ed 3, St. Louis, 2001, Mosby.

5. McFarland GK, McFarlane EA: *Nursing diagnosis and intervention: planning for patient care,* ed 3, St. Louis, 1997, Mosby.
6. North American Nursing Diagnosis Association: *NANDA nursing diagnoses: definitions and classification 2001–2002,* Philadelphia, 2001, The Association.
7. Peterson WP, Barbalata L, Brooks CA et al: The effect of tidal volumes on the time to wean persons with high tetraplegia from ventilators, *Spinal Cord* 37(4):284, 1999.
8. Vassilakopoulos T, Roussos C, Zakynthinos S: Weaning from mechanical ventilation, *J Crit Care* 14(1):39, 1999.
9. Wang M: Clinical validation of the etiology and defining characteristics of dysfunctional ventilatory weaning response. In Rantz MJ, LeMone P, editors: *Classification of nursing diagnoses: proceedings of the twelfth conference, North America Nursing Diagnosis Association,* Glendale, Calif, 1997, Cinahl Information Systems.
10. Wunderlich RJ, Perry A, Lavin MA et al: Patients' perceptions of uncertainty and stress during weaning from mechanical ventilation, *Dimension Crit Care Nurs* 18(1):2, 1999.

Fatigue

1. Ackley BJ: Fatigue. In Ackley BJ, Ladwig GB, editors: *Nursing diagnosis handbook: a guide to planning care,* ed 4, St. Louis, 1999, Mosby.
2. Cella D: The Functional Assessment of Cancer Therapy–Anemia (FACT-A) scale: a new tool for the assessment of outcomes in cancer anemia and fatigue, *Semin Hematol* 34(suppl 2):13, 1997.
3. Chung L: The clinical validation of defining characteristics and related factors of fatigue in hemodialysis patients. In Rantz MJ, LeMone P, editors: *Classification of nursing diagnoses: proceedings of the twelfth conference, North America Nursing Diagnosis Association,* Glendale, Calif, 1997, Cinahl Information Systems.
4. Cimprich B: Age and extent of surgery affect attention in women treated for breast cancer, *Res Nurs Health* 21(3):229, 1998.
5. Mast ME: Correlates of fatigue in survivors of breast cancer, *Cancer Nurs* 21(2):136, 1998.
6. McDaniel RW, Rhodes VA: Fatigue in individuals with cancer. In Yarbro CH, Frogge MH, Goodman M, editors: *Cancer nursing: principles and practice,* ed 5, Sudbury, Mass, 2000, Jones & Bartlett.
7. Mock V: Breast cancer and fatigue: issues for the workplace, *AAOHN J* 46(9):425, 1998.
8. North American Nursing Diagnosis Association: *NANDA nursing diagnoses: definitions and classification 2001–2002,* Philadelphia, 2001, The Association.
9. Piper BF, Dibble SL, Dodd MJ et al: The revised Piper fatigue scale: psychometric evaluation in women with breast cancer, *Oncol Nurs Forum* 25(4):677, 1998.
10. Schwartz AL: Patterns of exercise and fatigue in physically active cancer survivors, *Oncol Nurs Forum* 25(3):485, 1998.
11. Stuifbergen AK, Rogers S: The experience of fatigue and strategies of self-care among persons with multiple sclerosis, *Appl Nurs Res* 10(1):2, 1997.
12. Tiesinga LJ, Dassen TWN, Halfens RJG: Fatigue: a summary of the definitions, dimensions, and indicators, *Nurs Diagnosis* 7(2):51, 1996.
13. Tiesinga LJ, Dassen TWN, Halfens RJG: Validation of the nursing diagnosis fatigue among patients with chronic heart failure. In Rantz MJ, LeMone P, editors: *Classification of nursing diagnoses: proceedings of the twelfth conference, North America Nursing Diagnosis Association,* Glendale, Calif, 1997, Cinahl Information Systems.

Impaired Bed Mobility, Impaired Transfer Ability, Impaired Walking, Impaired Wheelchair Mobility

1. Colcher A: Movement disorders, *Clin Podiatr Med Surg* 16(1):127, 1999.
2. Emick-Herring B: Impaired bed mobility. In Ackley BJ, Ladwig GB, editors: *Nursing diagnosis handbook: a guide to planning care,* ed 4, St. Louis, 1999, Mosby.
3. Emick-Herring B: Impaired transfer ability. In Ackley BJ, Ladwig GB, editors: *Nursing diagnosis handbook: a guide to planning care,* ed 4, St. Louis, 1999, Mosby.
4. Emick-Herring B: Impaired walking. In Ackley BJ, Ladwig GB, editors: *Nursing diagnosis handbook: a guide to planning care,* ed 4, St. Louis, 1999, Mosby.
5. Emick-Herring B: Impaired wheelchair mobility. In Ackley BJ, Ladwig GB, editors: *Nursing diagnosis handbook: a guide to planning care,* ed 4, St. Louis, 1999, Mosby.
6. Hoeman SP: *Rehabilitation nursing: process and application,* ed 2, St. Louis, 1996, Mosby.
7. McCloskey JC, Bulechek GM, editors: *Nursing interventions classification (NIC),* ed 3, St. Louis, 2001, Mosby.
8. McDonald CM: Limb contractures in progressive neuromuscular disease and the role of stretching, orthotics, and surgery, *Phys Med Rehabil Clin North Am* 9(1):187, 1998.
9. Miles-Tapping C: Power wheelchairs and independent life styles, *Can J Rehabil* 10(2):137, 1996.
10. North American Nursing Diagnosis Association: *NANDA nursing diagnoses: definitions and classification 2001–2002,* Philadelphia, 2001, The Association.
11. Perr A: Elements of seating and wheeled mobility intervention, *OT Pract* 3(9):16, 1998.
12. Pierce LL: Barriers to access: frustrations of people who use a wheelchair for full-time mobility, *Rehabil Nurs* 23(3):120, 1998.
13. Taylor C, Lillis C, LeMone P: *Fundamentals of nursing: the art and science of nursing care,* ed 3, Philadelphia, 1997, JB Lippincott.

Impaired Physical Mobility

1. Chandler JM, Duncan PW, Sanders L et al: The fear of falling syndrome: relationship to falls, physical performance, and activities of daily living in frail older persons, *Top Geriatr Rehabil* 11(3):55, 1996.
2. DeSantis J, Engberg S, Rogers J: Geropsychiatric restraint use, *J Am Geriatr Soc* 45(12):1515, 1997.
3. Faria SH: Patient assessment: assessment of immobility hazards, *Home Care Provider* 3(4):189, 1998.
4. Ling SM, Bathon JM: Osteoarthritis in older adults, *J Am Geriatr Soc* 46(2):216, 1998.
5. North American Nursing Diagnosis Association: *NANDA nursing diagnoses: definitions and classification 2001–2002,* Philadelphia, 2001, The Association.
6. Snow T, Ackley BJ: Impaired physical mobility. In Ackley BJ, Ladwig GB, editors: *Nursing diagnosis handbook: a guide to planning care,* ed 4, St. Louis, 1999, Mosby.

Impaired Home Maintenance

1. Clemson L, Roland M, Cumming RG: Types of hazards in the homes of elderly people, *Occup Ther J Res* 17(3):200, 1997.
2. Cottrell BH, Todd NA: Patient assessment: home care concerns for the normal newborn, *Home Care Provider* 3(6):293, 1998.
3. Guerette P, Anthony P: Assistive technology for older adults: opportunities for advocacy, *Home Health Care Manage Pract* 11(3):17, 1999.
4. Jones AP: Asthma and domestic air quality, *Soc Sci Med* 47(6):755, 1998.

5. McCloskey JC, Bulechek GM, editors: *Nursing interventions classification (NIC),* ed 3, St. Louis, 2001, Mosby.
6. McFarland GK, McFarlane EA: *Nursing diagnosis and intervention: planning for patient care,* ed 3, St. Louis, 1997, Mosby.
7. North American Nursing Diagnosis Association: *NANDA nursing diagnoses: definitions and classification 2001–2002,* Philadelphia, 2001, The Association.
8. Skowronski S: Impaired home maintenance management. In Ackley BJ, Ladwig GB, editors: *Nursing diagnosis handbook: a guide to planning care,* ed 4, St. Louis, 1999, Mosby.

Impaired Spontaneous Ventilation

1. Chevron V, Menard JF, Richard JC et al: Unplanned extubation risk factors of development and predictive criteria for reintubation, *Crit Care Med* 26(6):1049, 1998.
2. Ferrin MS, Tino G: Acute dyspnea, *Adv Pract Acute Clin Care* 8(3):398, 1997.
3. Fichtelman A, Anderson B: Assessing patients' inability to sustain spontaneous ventilation from mechanical ventilator support. In Rantz MJ, LeMone P, editors: *Classification of nursing diagnoses: proceedings of the twelfth conference, North America Nursing Diagnosis Association,* Glendale, Calif, 1997, Cinahl Information Systems.
4. Lysaght L: Inability to sustain spontaneous ventilation. In Ackley BJ, Ladwig GB, editors: *Nursing diagnosis handbook: a guide to planning care,* ed 4, St. Louis, 1999, Mosby.
5. McCloskey JC, Bulechek GM, editors: *Nursing interventions classification (NIC),* ed 3, St. Louis, 2001, Mosby.
6. McFarland GK, McFarlane EA: *Nursing diagnosis and intervention: planning for patient care,* ed 3, St. Louis, 1997, Mosby.
7. North American Nursing Diagnosis Association: *NANDA nursing diagnoses: definitions and classification 2001–2002,* Philadelphia, 2001, The Association.

Ineffective Airway Clearance, Ineffective Breathing Pattern, Impaired Gas Exchange

1. Ackley BJ: Ineffective airway clearance. In Ackley BJ, Ladwig GB, editors: *Nursing diagnosis handbook: a guide to planning care,* ed 4, St. Louis, 1999, Mosby.
2. Ackley BJ: Ineffective breathing pattern. In Ackley BJ, Ladwig GB, editors: *Nursing diagnosis handbook: a guide to planning care,* ed 4, St. Louis, 1999, Mosby.
3. Ackley BJ: Impaired gas exchange. In Ackley BJ, Ladwig GB, editors: *Nursing diagnosis handbook: a guide to planning care,* ed 4, St. Louis, 1999, Mosby.
4. Anonymous: Dyspnea: mechanisms, assessment, and management: a consensus statement, *Am J Respir Crit Care Med* 159(1):321, 1999.
5. Bardana EJ, Harber P, Lockey JE: Occupational asthma: breathing easier on the job, *Patient Care* 30(3):100, 1996.
6. Brukwitzki G, Holmgren C, Maibusch RM: Validation of the defining characteristics of the nursing diagnosis ineffective airway clearance, *Nurs Diagnosis* 7(2):63, 1996.
7. Carlson-Catalano J, Lunney M, Paradiso C et al: Clinical validation of ineffective breathing pattern, ineffective airway clearance, and impaired gas exchange, *Image J Nurs Sch* 30(3):243, 1998.
8. Ciesla ND: Chest physical therapy for patients in the intensive care unit, *Phys Ther* 76(6):609, 1996.
9. Gumery L, Edenborough F, Stableforth D et al: Physiotherapy and nebuliser use in a Birmingham adult cystic fibrosis unit, *Physiotherapy* 84(3):127, 1998.
10. Hsia CC: Cardiopulmonary limitations to exercise in restrictive lung disease, *Med Sci Sports Exerc* 31(suppl 1):S28, 1999.
11. Langenderfer B: Alternatives to percussion and postural drainage: a review of mucus clearance therapies, *J Cardiopulmonary Rehabil* 18(4):283, 1998.
12. LaPier TK, Donovan C: Sitting and standing position affect pulmonary function in patients with COPD: a preliminary study, *Cardiopulmon Phys Ther J* 10(1):8, 1999.
13. McKelvie S: Endotracheal suctioning, *Nurs Crit Care* 3(5):244, 1998.
14. Mink BD: Exercise is medicine: exercise and chronic obstructive pulmonary disease: modest fitness gains pay big dividends, *Physician Sports Med* 25(11):43, 1997.
15. North American Nursing Diagnosis Association: *NANDA nursing diagnoses: definitions and classification 2001–2002,* Philadelphia, 2001, The Association.
16. Owen CL: New directions in asthma management, *Am J Nurs* 99(3):27, 1999.

Risk for Disuse Syndrome

1. Ackley BJ: Risk for disuse syndrome. In Ackley BJ, Ladwig GB, editors: *Nursing diagnosis handbook: a guide to planning care,* ed 4, St. Louis, 1999, Mosby.
2. Bamman MM, Hunter GR, Stevens BR et al: Resistance exercise prevents plantar flexor deconditioning during bed rest, *Med Sci Sports Exerc* 29(11):1462, 1997.
3. Biundo JJ, Hughes GM: Rheumatoid arthritis rehabilitation: part 1: practical guidelines on rest, ambulatory aids, and exercise programs . . . first of two articles, *Consultant* 37(11):2958, 1997.
4. Hayes KVD: Validation of risk factors for disuse syndrome. In Rantz MJ, LeMone P, editors: *Classification of nursing diagnoses: proceedings of the eleventh conference, North America Nursing Diagnosis Association,* Glendale, Calif, 1995, Cinahl Information Systems.
5. Hyers TM: Venous thromboembolism, *Am J Respir Crit Care Med* 159(1):1, 1999.
6. McCloskey JC, Bulechek GM, editors: *Nursing interventions classification (NIC),* ed 3, St. Louis, 2001, Mosby.
7. McFarland GK, McFarlane EA: *Nursing diagnosis and intervention: planning for patient care,* ed 3, St. Louis, 1997, Mosby.
8. North American Nursing Diagnosis Association: *NANDA nursing diagnoses: definitions and classification 2001–2002,* Philadelphia, 2001, The Association.

Risk for Peripheral Neurovascular Dysfunction

1. Abbott CA, Vileikyte L, Williamson S et al: Multicenter study of the incidence of and predictive risk factors for diabetic neuropathic foot ulceration, *Diabetes Care* 21(7):1071, 1998.
2. Ackley BJ: Risk for peripheral neurovascular dysfunction. In Ackley BJ, Ladwig GB, editors: *Nursing diagnosis handbook: a guide to planning care,* ed 4, St. Louis, 1999, Mosby.
3. Browne AC, Sibbald RG: The diabetic neuropathic ulcer: an overview . . . including commentary by Krasner D and Sibbald RG, *Ostomy Wound Manage* 45(suppl 1A):6S, 1999.
4. Feldman CB: Caring for feet: patients and nurse practitioners working together, *Nurse Pract Forum* 9(2):87, 1998.
5. McFarland GK, McFarlane EA: *Nursing diagnosis and intervention: planning for patient care,* ed 3, St. Louis, 1997, Mosby.
6. North American Nursing Diagnosis Association: *NANDA nursing diagnoses: definitions and classification 2001–2002,* Philadelphia, 2001, The Association.
7. Taylor C, Lillis C, LeMone P: *Fundamentals of nursing: the art and science of nursing care,* ed 4, Philadelphia, 2001, JB Lippincott.
8. Terry M, O'Brien SP, Kerstein MD: Lower-extremity edema: evaluation and diagnosis, *Wounds Compend Clin Res Pract* 10(4):118, 1998.

Sleep-Rest[1]

SLEEP DEPRIVATION

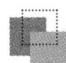

Sleep deprivation occurs when there are prolonged periods without sustained natural periodic suspension of relative consciousness.[10]

Related Factors[6,10-12]

Aging-related sleep stage shifts
Dementia
Familial sleep paralysis
Idiopathic central nervous system hypersomnolence
Inadequate daytime activity
Narcolepsy
Nightmares
Prolonged physical and/or psychologic discomfort
Sleep apnea
Sleep-related enuresis
Sundowner's syndrome
Sustained circadian asynchrony
Sustained environmental stimulation
Sustained unfamiliar or uncomfortable sleep environment

Defining Characteristics[4,9,10,12]

Acute confusion, agitation, or combativeness
Anxiety, restlessness
Apathy
Daytime drowsiness
Decreased ability to function
Hallucinations
Hand tremors
Heightened sensitivity to pain
Inability to concentrate
Mild, fleeting nystagmus
Perceptual disorders
Slowed reaction
Tiredness
Transient paranoia

Expected Patient Outcomes and Nursing Interventions With Rationale[1,3]

Regain usual sleep patterns, as evidenced by:
Describes factors that contribute to altered sleep
Participates in a plan of care to promote sleep

- Assess sleep patterns and usual bedtime rituals *to determine cause of sleep deprivation.*
- Educate patient and significant others about factors that interfere with sleep (e.g., diet, caffeine, medications, anxiety, depression). *Difficulty sleeping may be a side effect of medications or affected by caffeine intake.*
- Assess for underlying physiologic problems that may contribute to insomnia (e.g., fibromyalgia, hyperthyroidism, prostatic hypertrophy).
- Limit liquids in the evening.
- Schedule diuretics in the morning and early afternoon.
- Promote comfort, relaxation, and a sense of well-being, *to promote rest.*
- Teach relaxation strategies *to promote rest and sleep.*
- Assess for sleep apnea as indicated by loud snoring and periods of apnea.
- Promote a quiet environment *to decrease sleep interruptions.*
- Provide white noise or soothing sound generators *because these may promote greater quality and depth of sleep.*
- Encourage patient to keep a sleep diary for several weeks, *to determine the pattern of sleep deprivation.*

Approximate normal total sleep time and pattern, as evidenced by:
Has minimal awakenings during sleep
Feels rested
Has no daytime sleepiness

- Inform patient about when he or she will be awakened to prevent startling.
- Coordinate awakening with other departments (e.g., respiratory therapy, laboratory).
- Provide the opportunity for uninterrupted sleep from 1 AM to 5 AM.[1]
- Limit napping, particularly in the evening.
- Encourage moderate and low-intensity exercise *to promote sleep.*[9]
- Offer milk in the evening to promote sleep. *Milk contains L-tryptophan, which facilitates sleep.*
- Avoid use of alcohol and hypnotics to sleep.
- Encourage bedtime rituals that include quiet activities such as reading.

DISTURBED SLEEP PATTERN

Disturbed sleep pattern is a time-limited disruption of sleep (natural, periodic suspension of consciousness) amount and quality.[10]

Related Factors[1,5,8,10]

Aging-related sleep shifts
Ambient temperature, humidity

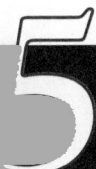

Anticipation
Anxiety
Circadian asynchrony
Daylight/darkness exposure
Delayed or advanced sleep phase syndrome
Depression
Disturbance by other individuals
Excessive stimulation
Fatigue
Fear
Fever
Frequent travel across time zones
Frequent treatments or monitoring
Gastroesophageal reflux
Grief
Lighting
Loneliness
Medications
Nausea
Noise
Noxious odors
Parent-infant interaction
Physical restraint
Shift work
Shortness of breath
Unfamiliar sleep furnishings
Urinary urgency or incontinence

Defining Characteristics[1,5,8,10]

Decreased proportion of REM, stages 3 and 4 sleep
Dissatisfaction with sleep
Early morning insomnia
Increased proportion of stage 1 sleep
Less than age-normal total sleep time
Sleep onset greater than 30 minutes
Three or more nighttime awakenings
Verbal complaint of not feeling well rested
Verbal complaint of difficulty falling asleep

Expected Patient Outcomes and Nursing Interventions With Rationale[5,7,8,11]

Experience normal sleep pattern and quality, as evidenced by:

States factors that contribute to altered sleep
Participates in a plan of care to promote sleep

- Educate patient and significant others about sleep and rest and rest needs and about factors that contribute to sleep pattern disturbances (e.g., pain, fear, stress, immobility, decreased activity, impaired oxygen transport, pregnancy, urinary frequency, medication, unfamiliar environment).
- Facilitate patient expression of emotional factors that may be interfering with normal sleep.
- Offer emotional support and continuity of care providers.
- Assess normal sleep pattern and any history of sleep disturbance or illness that may affect sleep, *because sleep patterns are unique to each individual.*
- Facilitate patient's normal bedtime rituals, *to promote normal sleep-wake cycle.*
- Assess sedative/hypnotic use or abuse.
- Promote normal sleep activity and pattern while hospitalized, *to synchronize with circadian rhythms.*
- Assess sleep effectiveness by asking patient how sleep in hospital compares with that at home.
- Limit liquids in evening *to decrease awakenings to void.*
- Schedule diuretics in the morning and early afternoon *to decrease awakenings to void.*
- Do not schedule routine procedures at night.
- Promote comfort, relaxation, and a sense of well-being; relieve pain, *to promote rest and sleep.*
- Eliminate stressful situations before bedtime; use of stress relaxation techniques may be helpful.
- Provide white noise *because this may promote greater depth and quality of sleep.*
- Minimize awakenings *to allow for at least 90-minute sleep cycles.* Continually assess need to awaken patient, particularly at night; distinguish between essential and nonessential nursing tasks.
- Organize nursing care *to allow for maximum amount of uninterrupted sleep* while ensuring close monitoring of patient's condition.
- Assist patient to maintain normal day/night cycles by decreasing lighting, noise, and sensory stimulation at night.

Total sleep time and pattern approximate normal for patient, as evidenced by:

Has minimal awakenings
States feeling rested
States an absence of daytime sleepiness
Demonstrates no signs of sleep deprivation

- Monitor physiologic parameters without awakening patient whenever possible, *to promote minimal interruption of rest and sleep.*
- Inform patient about scheduled awakenings during the night *so as not to startle patient.*
- Coordinate awakenings with other departments (e.g., respiratory therapy, laboratory, radiology).
- Minimize noise, particularly related to staff and equipment.
- Reduce level of environmental stimuli that may cause sensory overload.
- Plan nap times *to assist in equilibrating normal sleep time;* early morning naps may be beneficial in promoting REM sleep.
- Be aware of effects of commonly used medications on sleep, *becaue many sedative and hypnotic medications decrease REM sleep.*
- Do not withhold sedative and analgesic medications; rather, use drugs that minimally disrupt sleep *to complement comfort measures.* Reduce dosages gradually as medication becomes no longer necessary.
- Do not schedule diuretics near bedtime, *because they may interrupt sleep by increasing number of awakenings.*
- Offer milk in evening to promote sleep *because it contains* L-tryptophan, which facilitates sleep.
- Assess for signs of sleep deprivation (e.g., confusion, hallucinations, delusions, restlessness, combativeness,

paranoia, irritability, and decreased judgment). Be aware that the best treatment for sleep deprivation is prevention.

- Document amount of uninterrupted sleep and time awake per shift in hospitalized patients.
- Promote staff attitude that sleep is essential and should be encouraged. Assess unit for sleep-reducing stimuli and work to reduce them.
- Encourage moderate and low-intensity exercise *to promote sleep.*
- Be aware that cardiac dysrhythmias can be precipitated because of decreased arousal threshold secondary to desynchronization.
- If desynchronization occurs, plan for resynchronization by maintaining constancy in day/night pattern for at least 3 days (may require 5 to 12 days to reacclimatize).
- Plan for activities during day *to stimulate wakefulness,* and use comfort measures (position of comfort, warm blankets, back rub, etc.) *to promote sleep at night.*
- During resynchronization, assess for fatigue, malaise, and decreased ability to perform tasks.
- Administer hypnotics, as ordered, and monitor their effectiveness.

REFERENCES

Sleep-Rest

1. Gordon M: *Manual of nursing diagnosis,* ed 9, St. Louis, 2000, Mosby.

Sleep Deprivation, Disturbed Sleep Pattern

1. Ackley BJ: Sleep deprivation. In Ackley BJ, Ladwig GB, editors: *Nursing diagnosis handbook: a guide to planning care,* ed 4, St. Louis, 1999, Mosby.
2. Ackley BJ: Sleep pattern disturbance. In Ackley BJ, Ladwig GB, editors: *Nursing diagnosis handbook: a guide to planning care,* ed 4, St. Louis, 1999, Mosby.
3. Anonymous: Recognizing problem sleepiness in your patients, *Am Fam Physician* 59(4):937, 1999.
4. Bangura K: Dying for a snooze . . . sleep deprivation, *Nurs Times* 94(21):29, 1998.
5. Doenges ME, Moorhouse MF: *Nurses's pocket guide: diagnoses, interventions, and rationales,* ed 6, Philadelphia, 1998, FA Davis.
6. Hogg G: Sleep deprivation in a high-dependency unit, *Professional Nurse* 13(10):693, 1998.
7. McCloskey JC, Bulechek GM, editors: *Nursing interventions classification (NIC),* ed 3, St. Louis, 2001, Mosby.
8. McFarland GK, McFarlane EA: *Nursing diagnosis and intervention: planning for patient care,* ed 3, St. Louis, 1997, Mosby.
9. Millott MK, Berlin RM: Treating sleep disorders in patients with fibromyalgia: exercise, behavior, and drug therapy may all help, *J Musculoskel Med* 14(6):25, 1997.
10. North American Nursing Diagnosis Association: *Nursing diagnoses: definitions and classification 2001–2002,* Philadelphia, 2001, The Association.
11. Richardson SJ: Assessment techniques. A comparison of tools for the assessment of sleep pattern disturbance in critically ill adults, *Dimens Crit Care Nurs* 16(5):226, 1997.
12. Walton JC, Miller JM: Advanced practice. Evaluating physical and behavioral changes in older adults, *MEDSURG Nurs* 7(2):85-90, 1998.

6 FUNCTIONAL HEALTH PATTERN

Cognitive-Perceptual[1]

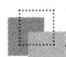

ACUTE CONFUSION

Acute confusion is the abrupt onset of a cluster of global, transient changes and disturbances in attention, cognition, psychomotor activity, level of consciousness, and/or sleep/wake cycle.[8]

Related Factors[2,3,8-10]

Acute pain
Alcohol intoxication
Anxiety
Advanced age
Dementia/Alzheimer's disease
Depression
Electrolyte abnormalities
Hyperthermia or hypothermia
Hypoxia
Organ failure
Medications
- Anticholinergics
- Antihypertensives
- Benzodiazepines
- Digoxin
- Narcotics and sedatives
- Psychotrophics

Psychoses
Street drugs
Recent major surgical procedure
Recent relocation
Sensory deprivation or overload
Shock
Sleep deprivation
Trauma

Defining Characteristics[2,7,8,11]

Alterations in level of consciousness
Alterations in psychomotor activity: restless, agitated, decreased
Inability to initiate or follow through with purposeful behavior
Inability to maintain concentration
Poorly organized delusions

Expected Patient Outcomes and Nursing Interventions With Rationale[1,3-6,9]

Demonstrate appropriate level of psychomotor activity, as evidenced by:

Decrease in risk of injury to self or others
Decrease in agitation level
Decrease in slowing or lethargy

- Assess for causes of inappropriate activity level.
  - Monitor laboratory data for acute electrolyte imbalances, abnormal hepatic and renal function *for early detection of organ failure,* and infection (especially urinary tract infection and pneumonia in the elderly.)
  - Monitor vital signs *to identify infection (febrile states), increased autonomic irritability related to withdrawal syndromes (especially withdrawal from alcohol, benzodiazepines, or narcotic analgesics); increased intracranial pressure; level of oxygenation; and pain level. These conditions contribute to agitation and acute confusion.*
  - Monitor fluid intake. *Dehydration causes electrolyte disturbances and may exacerbate cognitive problems.*
  - Monitor therapeutic medication records and therapeutic drug levels (e.g., digoxin, phenytoin, lithium) *to assess for early toxicity.*
  - Assess for elimination problems (e.g., urinary retention, fecal impaction) *especially in the demented elderly who may not be able to communicate distress.*
  - Assess level of pain especially in the elderly postoperative patient, and use appropriate interventions for pain control. *A demented patient may be unable to reliably request pain medication or use a patient-controlled analgesia pump (PCA) appropriately because of waxing and waning of acute confusion.*
- Maintain a safe environment to reduce risk of injury.
  - Place patient in room close to nurses' station whenever possible and check frequently. *Patients with acute confusion are frequently impulsive with global cognitive deficits that fluctuate widely. Increased surveillance will facilitate early assessment and treatment of organic problems and decrease risk of injury.*
  - Restrict patient's access to essential intravenous lines, endotracheal tubing, oxygen nasal prongs, and other equipment by frequently orienting patient, restricting access by concealment when appropriate, and offering patient an alternative object to hold or pull (e.g., wash cloth, safe toy).
  - Use soft limb or hard restraints sparingly and only on a time-limited basis *to protect patient from falls and self-injury, such as extubating self.*

Administer high-potency neuroleptic medication as ordered by physician (e.g., haloperidol), and minimize use of benzodiazepines *because they may worsen acute confusion. Use only in alcohol and sedative-hypnotic withdrawal.*

Demonstrate improved cognitive functioning, as evidenced by:
Increases attention and concentration
Improves orientation
Increase in recent and remote memory
Increases ability to follow commands and process new information

- Assess cognitive status on admission to the hospital and every shift (orientation, attention and concentration, memory, thought processes) *to obtain baseline information.*
  Obtain collateral information from care providers, family, and medical records *to ascertain patient's baseline cognitive functioning.*
  Use bedside mental status questions or mental status questionnaires.
- Reorient patient frequently to surroundings, routines, date and time, reason for hospitalization, and names of care providers *because short-term memory is impaired in acute confusion and disorientation will increase anxiety.*
- Use visual cues for orientation: signs in the room, signs on door, clocks, calendars, instructional signs at bedside (e.g., "Call nurse. Do not get out of bed alone.").
- Modify the environment *to decrease incidence of sensory-perceptual alterations.*
  Avoid lighting that contributes to shadows.
  Provide sensory aides (e.g., corrective lenses, hearing aids).
  Avoid overstimulation or sensory isolation.
  Maintain comfortable room temperature.
- Maintain consistent care providers *to provide consistency and decrease anxiety.*
- Communicate with patient in brief, simple, concrete language *because abstract thinking is impaired in acute confusion.*

Have improved sleep-wake cycle, as evidenced by:
Is able to rest and sleep
Regains appropriate sleep/wake patterns

- Assess for sleep deprivation.
- Maintain sleep/wake cycles (e.g., curtains open during the day to increase light, lights off at night to promote sleep).
- Allow for rest periods during the day *to decrease fatigue and overstimulation.*
- Establish a schedule for patient *to promote normal sleep/wake cycles and rest periods.*
- Continue familiar bedtime routines whenever possible.

Chronic Confusion

Chronic confusion is an irreversible, long-standing, and/or progressive deterioration of intellect and personality characterized by decreased ability to interpret environmental stimuli, decreased capacity for intellectual thought processes, and manifested by disturbances of memory, orientation, and behavior.[8]

Related Factors[3,4,8]

AIDs-related dementia
Alzheimer's disease
Cerebrovascular accident
Cerebral trauma
Korsakoff's psychosis
Medications
Multiinfarct dementia

Defining Characteristics[3-5,8,9]

Altered interpretation of stimuli
Altered personality
Clinical evidence of organic impairment
Depression
Impaired ability for abstraction and conceptualization
Impaired memory
Impaired orientation to person, place, and/or time
Impaired socialization
No alteration in consciousness
Progressive cognitive impairment
Wandering

Expected Patient Outcomes and Nursing Interventions With Rationale[3-5,8,9]

Be able to function in a structured environment, as evidenced by:
Follows an established, consistent daily routine
Interacts with caregivers and pets
Maintains emotional equilibrium

- Post a written daily routine for patient to follow. *Written directions or schedules provide additional cues to the chronically confused individual who retains the ability to read.*
- Provide a consistent caregiver(s). *Patients will experience increased security when cared for by people they recognize.*
- Provide a daily time for small group activity that is valued by patient, such as music, art, reminiscence group, selected television program, Bible therapy. *Planned activities are beneficial if they are pleasurable and incorporate the patient's culture, habits, values, manners, preferences, and occupation.*
- Place meaningful possessions (photographs, mementos, favorite furniture) in the patient's environment. *Familiar belongings promote a sense of security.*
- Avoid change in room environment, such as reassignment of patient's room, rearrangement of furniture or items, holiday decoration. *Frequent environment change may produce conflicting cues.*
- Make provision for optimal sensory input (eyeglasses are clean, hearing aid is functional, absence of cerumen impaction). *The cognitively impaired individual is at risk for misinterpretation of environment when sensory input is not accurate.*
- Provide adequate nonglare lighting. *Visual perceptions may be altered by glare or shadows.*
- Eliminate unnecessary environmental stimuli (excessive noise level, multiple conversation/activities, violent/

aggressive movies or television programs). *Disturbing visual images or loud noise can precipitate a catastrophic reaction.*

- Provide opportunity for one-to-one conversation with caregiver(s). *Providing sufficient time for interacting with patient reinforces socialization skill and a sense of self-worth.*
- Maintain eye contact, smile, and present a pleasant affect when interacting with the patient. *Verbal and nonverbal communications are important in establishing a relationship with a cognitively impaired person.*
- Encourage continued interaction with a pet (allow pet to remain with patient, allow pet to visit patient if an inpatient, or provide access to animal-assisted therapy). *Pets provide links to the past, encourage conversation, and provide a pleasurable activity option.*
- Initiate use of an observational instrument to document episodes and context of incidents of behavioral disturbance. *Documentation of behavior over time provides data to identify precursors to behavioral events.*
- Educate caregiver/staff to possible "triggers" and appropriate response (i.e., time-out, rest, distraction) to behavioral disturbance. *Early intervention may prevent or modify a behavioral disturbance.*
- Communicate new or relevant client information to other staff who see the patient. *Communication among staff is vital to the provision of continuity of care to the cognitively impaired client.*
- Maintain a level of environmental stimuli below the individual's "trigger" threshold. *Dysfunctional behavior occurs if stress levels exceed the individual's tolerance.*
- Communicate using simple one-step commands. *Complex sequenced instructions are overwhelming to the cognitively impaired individual.*
- Allow sufficient time for completion of directed task. *Sensory input/communication is slowly interpreted by the individual with dementia.*

DISTURBED THOUGHT PROCESSES

Disturbed thought processes is a state in which an individual experiences a disruption in cognitive operations and activities.[9]

Related Factors[2,3,7,9,10]

Biochemical changes
Genetic predisposition
Impaired judgment
Ineffective coping
Memory loss
Mental disorders
Physiologic/pathophysiologic changes
Psychologic conflicts
Sleep deprivation
Substance abuse

Defining Characteristics[2,8-10]

Bizarre thinking: Inappropriate use of language, inability to get to the point, overgeneralization, imputing intentions to others, use of neologisms
Changes in motor activity: Agitation, repetition
Changes in self-care: sleep, grooming, hygiene, eating
Changes in remote, recent, and immediate memory
Confabulation
Decreased affect
Difficulty concentrating
Disordered thinking
Disorientation to time, place, person, circumstances, or events
Emotional changes: sadness, mistrust, guilt, anxiety, fear, apathy, lability
Hypervigilance
Impaired ability to calculate
Impaired ability to grasp ideas, reason, or think abstractly
Inaccurate interpretation of stimuli: hallucinations, delusions, ideas of reference, obsessions
Inappropriate social behavior
Insomnia

Expected Patient Outcomes and Nursing Interventions With Rationale[1,4-7,10]

Maintain safe conditions (no injury to self or others), as evidenced by:
Remains injury-free
Demonstrates a decrease in or absence of violent behavior
Is able to control own behavior

- Maintain patient safety.
- Prevent suicide and aggression.
- Assess for suicide potential (history, plans for self-harm, verbalization of desire to die, disposal of possessions, viewing self in past tense).
- Institute suicide precautions, as indicated.
- Assess potential for aggressive behavior.
- Identify early signs of aggressive behavior.
- Remove environmental factors that contribute to aggression.
- Promote individual control.
  - Set limits on destructive behavior.
  - Encourage verbalization and safe acting-out behaviors, within limits.
  - Allow choice within constraint.
  - Use seclusion if indicated.
- Help patient set limits on own behavior.
  - Substitute verbalizations and physical activity for behavioral acting out.
  - Set incremental goals.
  - Recall and repeat successful ways of coping.

Thought and language are closely tied and interrelated. Therefore it is logical to assume that altered thought processes are reflected in the patient's language behavior. The nursing interventions are based on this link between cognitive processes and language.

Interpret reality in a realistic and constructive manner, as evidenced by:
Has clearer verbalizations
Is oriented to environment, self, time, and space
Demonstrates a decrease in or absence of delusions or hallucinations
Demonstrates an increased ability to solve problems and reason abstractly

- Explore patient's representation of reality by analyzing language behavior.
  - Listen intently to patient's verbal and nonverbal communication.
  - Analyze communication for generalization and distortions.
- Assist patient in clarifying representation of reality.
  - Clarify generalizations ("Nobody pays any attention to what I say." Clarify who, specifically. Ask, "What, specifically, do you say?") Elicit deletions in communication ("I am scared." Scared about what?) Clarify nominalistic statements. Change statements of event into statements of process ("I hate my relationship with my wife." Explore "relating" as a process versus "relationship" as an event.) Challenge distortions of control ("Steve makes me act up." Repeat statement with emphasis on "Steve makes?" Explore how that is possible.) Challenge distortions that impute intentions to others ("The doctor hates me." Analyze basis for statement: "What was said or done that makes you feel your doctor hates you?")
- Use reality orientation where indicated.
  - Orient to person, time, and place.
  - Use direct terminology, clear sentence structure. Avoid generalization. Use terms that help patient maintain individuality (e.g., "I" instead of "we"). Avoid vagueness, asides, and whispered comments. Have patient focus on real things and people.

Be able to relate to others in a positive manner, as evidenced by:
Functions as a group member
Interacts with others

- Provide group process situations that allow patients to experience relating in a controlled setting.
- Encourage validation of thoughts and feelings.
- Encourage patient to ask for wants and to express feelings.
- Help patient examine the effect of his or her behavior on others.
- Help patient recognize use of and need for personal space and distance.

Have reduced anxiety and stress, as evidenced by:
Verbalizes that he or she feels less anxious
Has decreased physical signs of anxiety and stress

- Approach in calm, nurturing manner.
  - Use calm, level voice, lower tone, familiar terms.
  - Avoid sudden movements, compose facial expression.
- Provide physical and emotional structure, as needed:

Physical structure. Environment is altered to provide for safety and comfort.

Emotional structure. A prediction of feelings and occurrences and an imaging of situations that evoke safety and comfort.

Assume responsibility for self-care, as evidenced by:
Contributes to the treatment plan
Follows through on assumed responsibility
Seeks increased responsibility for self-care

- Provide opportunity for patient to contribute to own treatment plan.
- Encourage acceptance of responsibility for actions and interactions.
- Encourage acceptance of responsibility for seeking help, following treatment plans, and changing behaviors.

ACUTE PAIN

Acute pain is an unpleasant sensory and emotional experience arising from actual or potential tissue damage caused by noxious or sensory stimuli or described in terms of such damage; sudden or slow onset of any intensity from mild to severe with an anticipated or predictable end and a duration of less than 6 months.[5]

Related Factors[5,7]

Biologic: Disease, inflammation, ischemia
Chemical: Cytotoxic agents, noxious agents, electrolyte imbalance
Physical: Trauma, extremes of temperature
Psychologic: Anxiety, fear, stress

Defining Characteristics[2,3,5,6]

Anorexia
Changes in muscle tone, from listless to rigid
Diaphoresis
Dilated pupils
Distraction behaviors
Expressions of pain (e.g., moaning, crying, sighing)
Guarding position or gestures
Grimacing
Inability to continue to work
Increased blood pressure
Increased pulse
Increased respirations
Masklike face
Protective or guarding behavior
Restlessness
Sleep disturbance
Self focus/narrow focus
Verbal or coded report of pain

Expected Patient Outcomes and Nursing Interventions With Rationale[1-3,6,8,9]

Verbalize or demonstrate an increased comfort level, as evidenced by:
Verbalizes information about the pain experience
Identifies strategies that eliminate or control pain

- Assess patient's pain status. *Nurse and patient have perceptions of pain based on past experiences, cultural influences, and other factors. The meaning of pain for each patient influences that person's response to pain.*
- Incorporate the following factors in the assessment of the patient's pain status:
  - Location/characteristics
  - Onset/duration
  - Frequency
  - Intensity, using 0 to 10 scale: 0, no pain; 10, worst pain possible
  - Quality
  - Precipitating factors

Effective pain control measures
Ineffective pain control measures
Desired interventions
Pain expression style (stoic, verbal, crying, moaning)
Movement (guarding, favoring posture)
Muscle tone
Emotional distress
Impact on quality of life
Effect of pain on daily activities
Activities affected or eliminated because of pain
Effect on sleep/wake pattern
Effect on energy level
Effect on sexual activity
Effect on relations with others
Effect on feelings of self-worth
Perception of ability to control pain

The pain assessment includes both subjective and objective data. The depth of the assessment varies according to the individual's pain status, the situation, and setting. The frequency of the assessments varies according to individual needs. The data can be recorded on a flowsheet or a graph to identify trends.

- Provide pain management interventions.[4]
- Control environmental factors that may influence the patient's response to discomfort (e.g., room temperature, lighting, and noise).
- Reduce or eliminate factors that precipitate or increase the pain experience (e.g., fear, fatigue, monotony, and lack of knowledge).
- Consider the patient's willingness to participate, ability to participate, preference, support of significant others for method, and contraindications when selecting a pain relief strategy.
- Select and implement a variety of measures (e.g., pharmacologic, nonpharmacologic, and interpersonal) to facilitate pain relief, as appropriate.
- Consider type and source of pain when selecting pain relief strategy.
- Encourage patient to monitor own pain and to intervene appropriately.
- Teach the use of nonpharmacologic techniques (e.g., biofeedback, transcutaneous electrical nerve stimulator [TENS], hypnosis, relaxation, guided imagery, music therapy, distraction, play therapy, activity therapy, acupressure, hot/cold application, and massage) before, after, and, if possible, during painful activities; before pain occurs or increases; and along with other pain relief measures.
- Collaborate with the patient, significant other, and other health professionals to select and implement nonpharmacologic pain relief measures, as appropriate.
- Provide the patient optimal pain relief with prescribed analgesics.
- Implement the use of patient-controlled analgesia (PCA), if appropriate.
- Use pain control measures before pain becomes severe.
- Medicate before an activity to increase participation, but evaluate the hazard of sedation.
- Ensure pretreatment analgesia and/or nonpharmacologic strategies before painful procedures.
- Verify level of discomfort with patient, note changes in the medical record, and inform other health professionals working with the patient.
- Evaluate the effectiveness of the pain control measures used through ongoing assessment of the pain experience.
- Institute and modify pain control measures on the basis of the patient's response.
- Promote adequate rest/sleep *to facilitate pain relief.*
- Encourage patient to discuss the pain experience, as appropriate.
- Notify physician if measures are unsuccessful or if current complaint is a significant change from patient's past experience of pain.
- Inform other health-care professionals/family members of nonpharmacologic strategies being used by the patient *to encourage preventive approaches to pain management.*
- Use a multidisciplinary approach to pain management, when appropriate.
- Consider referrals for patient, family, and significant others to support groups and other resources, as appropriate.
- Provide accurate information *to promote family's knowledge of and response to the pain experience.*
- Incorporate the family in the pain relief modality, if possible.
- Monitor patient satisfaction with pain management at specified intervals.

To treat pain effectively, the patient (and nurse) must be able to identify strategies that eliminate or control pain. Strategies that were effective in the past may be continued or adapted for the current situation. Optimal pain relief should be the goal when prescribing analgesics.[8]

Chronic Pain

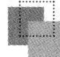

Chronic pain is an unpleasant sensory and emotional experience arising from actual or potential tissue damage or described in terms of such damage; sudden or slow onset of any intensity from mild to severe with an anticipated or predictable end and a duration of greater than 6 months.[8]

Related Factors[8,9]

Changes in activity
Chronic physical/psychosocial disability
Fatigue
Inflammation
Lack of social systems
Obesity

Defining Characteristics[3,4,8,9]

Anorexia
Atrophy of involved muscle groups
Changes in sleep patterns
Decreased socialization with others
Depression
Facial mask
Fatigue
Fear of reinjury
Guarding behavior
Protective behavior
Restlessness

Self-focusing
Weight changes

Expected Patient Outcomes and Nursing Interventions With Rationale[1,2,5-7,10]

Maintain usual activities and lifestyle with minimal disruption from pain, as evidenced by:

Verbalizes information about pain experience
Identifies activities that cause or increase pain
Identifies strategies to control pain
Avoids use of unproven remedies
Maintains or increases weight appropriate to height and frame
Verbalizes positive feelings about self

- Assess patient's pain status (see Acute Pain).
- Incorporate factors in assessment of patient's pain status (see Acute Pain).
- Implement strategies as indicated by patient condition and pain status.
  - Provide therapeutic positioning.
  - Encourage attention to proper posture and alignment.
  - Rest affected area.
  - Provide distraction.
  - Instruct patient in relaxation techniques or guided imagery.
  - Use hypnosis and biofeedback.
  - Provide music therapy, play therapy, activity therapy.
  - Use counterstimulation: pressure, massage, vibration, heat/cold, external analgesics, TENS.
  - Pace activities and plan activities ahead of time.
  - Provide touch.
- Determine realistic pain control goals with patient.
- Provide supportive environment.
- Identify emotional responses from patient.
- Assess which pain reduction strategies patient finds helpful.
- Use several pain reduction strategies.
- Attempt interventions several times before judging success.
- Include patient and family education about pain and its management.

To treat pain, the patient must be able to identify strategies that are effective in controlling pain. Any previously used interventions that were effective in controlling this pain should be continued. The nurse should consider the patient's willingness to participate, ability to participate, preferred support of significant others for method, and contraindications when selecting a pain relief strategy. Interventions unfamiliar to the patient should also be attempted and assessed using a subjective rating scale. Using more than one intervention may provide better pain control.

- Help patient to identify activities that may increase pain or precipitate pain (disease-related, treatment-related, environment).
- Discuss strategies to reduce situations that increase pain (e.g., fear, fatigue, or lack of knowledge).
- Discuss strategies to avoid these activities within patient's lifestyle.
- Encourage family members to help patient prevent painful event.
- Encourage patient to keep daily log *to monitor changes in pain and to help identify other activities that increase pain.*
- Encourage patient to report to health-care professional development of new pain or changes in his or her pain.

Activities that intensify pain should be identified. By keeping a daily diary of activities and pain ratings, the patient may be able to identify variations in pain and occurrences of new pain. Once activities that intensify pain are identified, methods to modify or reduce the activity can be explored. The importance of the activity to the individual should be addressed. If the activity has little meaning or value, the patient may readily avoid it, but interventions are needed to maintain the activity if it is meaningful to the person.

- Inform patient and family about identification of unproven remedies.
- Instruct patient in dangers of unproven remedies; *they can be life threatening, expensive, and can serve as a substitute for ongoing health care.*
- Assist patient in exploring feelings regarding unproven remedies.
- Counsel patient in determining how to respond to individuals who suggest unproven remedies.
- Provide patient with community resources *to assist in identification of unproven remedies.*
- Do not remove unharmful unproven remedies from patient *(patient may have faith in this remedy not found in other treatments).*

The nurse needs to provide information about the expense of some forms of unproven remedies and that some forms may be life threatening. The patient can then make informed decisions. It can be easy to reject current health care when pain relief is not found and an unproven remedy proclaims pain relief abilities.

- Instruct patient about effects of pain on nutrition and influence of proper nutrition on health status.
- Instruct patient on need for balanced diet *to maintain ideal weight for height and frame.*
- Obtain dietitian referral.
- Assess motivation toward obtaining proper nutrition and achievement of ideal weight.
- If underweight for height and frame, refer to Imbalanced Nutrition: Less Than Body Requirements.

Weight problems frequently occur when chronic pain is present. Many patients find that loss of appetite occurs during severe episodes of pain. Weight loss can occur also as a consequence of disease such as cancer. If a patient has decreased mobility, yet appetite is unchanged, he or she is at risk of gaining weight. Interventions for weight problems should be implemented as early as possible.

- Assess patient's perception of progress toward goal attainment.
- If the patient is unable to return to work, help identify meaningful ways to fill time and promote positive feelings of self-worth.
- Reinforce behaviors that decrease the risk of medical, social, and financial problems.
- Provide patient with positive reinforcement for activities focused away from pain.

- Assist patient in developing normalizing strategies for activities encountered in daily life.
- Educate patient on community resources for prevention or reduction of problems related to job retraining and financial assistance.
- Inform patient of importance of maintaining communications with all health professionals.
- Assess need for referrals for family or individual counseling, financial needs, or sexual concerns.
- Encourage gradual reentry into family, society, and work activities; set realistic goals for reentry.
- Assist patient in effective transition to retirement if work is no longer a realistic option.
- Use support groups.
- Provide positive reinforcement for achievements.

Chronic pain is multidimensional. It affects every aspect of life and the significant individuals in the person's life. Interventions are geared toward improving the quality of life through pain control.

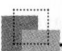

DECISIONAL CONFLICT (SPECIFY)

Decisional conflict is a state of uncertainty about courses of action to be taken when choice among competing actions involves risk, loss, or challenge to personal life values.[4]

Related Factors[4]

Conflicting or unclear values and beliefs
Equal identified consequences
Indecisive behavior pattern
Interference in decision-making process
Lack of experience
Lack of problem-solving skills
Lack of relevant information
Perceived threat to value system
Support system deficit

Defining Characteristics[4]

Delay in making decisions
Expressed concern about lack of information to make decision
Expressed distress about available choices
Expressed undesired consequences of alternatives
Physical signs of stress (restless, tachycardia, muscle tension)
Questioning of personal values and beliefs
Self-focus
Vacillation between alternative choices

Expected Patient Outcomes and Nursing Interventions With Rationale[1-3,5]

Act on an informed decision that is consistent with personal values, as evidenced by:

Verbalizes goals, alternatives, and consequences of decisions
Is able to make and follow through with a decision

- Aid patient in clarifying goals, alternatives, and potential consequences; *lack of information or clarity in these items leads to decisional conflict.*
- Help the patient clarify the likelihood of potential consequences; realign unrealistic expectations; *distortion in expectations often increases conflict (e.g., anticipating a negative consequence when the likelihood is extremely low) or regret (anticipating a positive consequence when the likelihood is extremely low).*
- With the patient, clarify the desirability of possible consequences and their priority; *unclear values contribute to decisional conflict.*
- Identify value tradeoffs implicit in making choices; *having to make tradeoffs often contributes to conflict; knowing what makes the decision difficult helps in its resolution.*
- Facilitate alternative selection consistent with personal values; *this increases satisfaction with the decision and the likelihood that the patient will follow through on the choice.*
- Teach and reinforce self-help skills required to implement the choice; *individuals have difficulty translating preferences into permanent behavior change without the resources necessary to do so.*

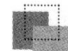

DEFICIENT KNOWLEDGE

Deficient knowledge is a state of the absence or deficiency of cognitive information related to a specific topic.[5]

Related Factors[2,5]

Altered cognitive level
Altered locus of control
Anger and hostility
Cognitive-perceptual deficits
Cultural influences
Denial regarding diagnosis or efficacy of treatment
Depression or extreme anxiety
Impaired communications
Inadequate economic resources
Irrational beliefs
Lack of formal education
Lack of motivation to learn
Lack of orientation to the future
New, complex treatment
Social isolation

Defining Characteristics[2-4]

Dependence on others for care
Development of complications
Developmental delay in children
Failure to adhere to prescribed regimen
Failure to seek needed health-care services
Inability to correctly verbalize or demonstrate material taught
Inability to make decisions about own care
Inaccurate follow-through of instruction
Inadequate performance of tasks/skills
Readmission for same problem
Request for information
Verbalization of inaccurate information
Verbalization of problem with caring for self

Expected Patient Outcomes and Nursing Interventions With Rationale[2-4]

Acquire and use adequate knowledge and skill to support needed health-care decisions and activities, as evidenced by:

Verbalizes how and why to take action or perform skill

Uses knowledge to provide self-care
Verbalizes accurate expectations of outcomes of health-care actions

- Check that communities and institutions provide freely available information through reading materials, hotlines, mass media, health fairs at work sites and schools, etc.
- At every provider/patient interaction, assess for knowledge deficit.
- Talk to patient's significant other *to obtain evidence of knowledge deficit.*
- Use patient's theories about his or her illness as a starting point for teaching, and continually seek patient's perceptions.
- During interactions, check frequently *to see if patient understands.*

Essentially all evidence of knowledge deficit is more or less indirect. With assessment, the nurse sets up situations in which the quality of the inference obtained from verbalizations or behaviors is as strong and direct as possible: ask the patient directly or set up an unobtrusive test. Because most meaningful health behaviors require knowledge, motivation, and skill, it is important in the assessment to seek evidence in each of these areas to obtain as complete a diagnosis as possible. This means data gathered must be both objective, to determine adequacy of present knowledge and behaviors, and subjective, which is the source of crucial information about the patient's motivation, sense of self-efficacy, frame of reference, and cognitive schemata.

- Simplify information to conform to patient's terms, thought patterns, and daily routines.
- Set clear learning goals with patient.
- Be accessible to patient when he or she has a question; this may require new structures of care (e.g., a diabetes education center).
- Demonstrate to patient and family how to use information.
- Reinforce correct use of information, and ensure that others in patient's natural environment do the same.
- Teach patient how to set up system of cues in the environment to remember health actions.
- Teach patient how to rehearse mentally and physically, when possible, a necessary health action.
- Teach patient how to use rewards for positive health behaviors.
- Call patient to remind him or her; show support, and see if he or she has questions.
- Make certain patient is actively involved in decisions about own care.
- Provide opportunities for patient to gain sense of control over illness.
- Offer peer support network and opportunity for patient to watch others successfully mastering health-care problems.
- Ask patient if he or she is satisfied with care.
- Use practice of knowledge and skill, perhaps with role playing, until patient feels confident and has met the standard.
- Use special teaching approaches *to deal with neurologic learning deficits.*
- After procedure, offer opportunity for reflection about what happened.
- Provide instruction in multiple modalities (visual, experimental, written, discussion) *so that patient will remember it in various ways.*
- Provide materials for patient to take *so that he or she can review and use the new knowledge.*
- Provide motivators by appealing to patient's interests and future uses of new knowledge, allowing patient to identify what is most important.

In general, nursing goals include helping the patient attain the knowledge and skills needed through the teaching and learning process. This includes assessing readiness, planning realistic goals, developing a teaching plan using appropriate multiple verbal, behavioral, and audiovisual instructional strategies, and evaluation of learning and reteaching when necessary.

Acquire knowledge and become competent in how to guide own and others' development in area of health, in how to carry out health-care activities necessary to well-being, and in how to cope adequately with health stresses, as evidenced by:

Monitors body and mental health state for signs and symptoms of illness
Acts on basis of realistic expectations in guiding development of self and others
Describes how to use verified health knowledge in daily living
Moves ahead to take health actions when satisfied they are worthwhile, including programs for self-management of disease and symptoms
Makes participatory decisions with health-care provider
Decrease in symptoms and indicators of disease state, and increase in indicators of health and well-being
Knows where to obtain sources of health-care information efficiently and does so when needed
Describes problem-solving process to deal successfully with injury, threatening diagnosis, or persistent symptom
Describes how action met personal standards of adequate coping
Developes sense of mastery and self-efficacy regarding particular health behavior
Avoids overreactions, feelings of helplessness and depression caused by inadequate knowledge and skill

- Teach with a questioning, discussion, application of knowledge, and feedback approach.
- Teach patient and family to use self-care protocols and instructional packages when appropriate.
- Teach patient how to find and use sources of knowledge and social support in the community.
- If available, help patient learn to use computerized monitoring systems (e.g., those providing diabetic persons with running summary of food and medication requirements met for the day).
- Contract with patient.
- Build on patient's developmental and learning level: this may require assistance with transferring and integrating knowledge into his or her life.

Active involvement of the patient is essential, as is practice of the thoughts and behaviors to be learned. For many, psychologic support and follow-up are important, along with a feeling of personal reward, sometimes developed through a contract with the provider, and involvement of the family. Instruction provides models for behavior, cues for correct responses, corrective feedback, and problem-solving strategies.

Impaired Environmental Interpretation Syndrome

Impaired environmental interpretation syndrome is a consistent lack of orientation to person, time, or circumstances over more than 3 to 6 months, necessitating a protective environment.[8]

Related Factors[3,8,9]

Alcoholism
Dementia
Depression
Huntington's disease
Parkinson's disease

Defining Characteristics[4-6,8,11]

Chronic confusion state
Consistent disorientation in known and new environments
Inability to concentrate
Inability to follow simple instructions
Inability to reason
Loss of occupation or social function from memory loss
Slow response to questions
Wandering

Expected Patient Outcomes and Nursing Interventions With Rationale[1,2,7,10]

Function in a structured environment, as evidenced by:
Follows a consistent daily routine
Converses with caregivers and others
Takes part in daily small group activity

- Establish a consistent daily routine schedule. *Patients compensate for inability to plan activities by developing a daily routine that becomes automatic.*
- Provide a consistent caregiver/staff member. *Patients will experience increased security when cared for by people they recognize.*
- Approach and communicate with the patient in a positive manner. *Verbal and nonverbal communication are important in establishing a relationship with a person who is cognitively impaired.*
- Provide opportunity for one-to-one conversation with caregiver(s). *Providing sufficient time for interacting with patient reinforces socialization skill and a sense of self-worth.*
- Ensure optimal sensory input (eyeglasses are clean, hearing aid is functional, absence of cerumen impaction). *The cognitively impaired individual is at risk for misinterpretation of environment when sensory input is not accurate.*
- Provide adequate nonglare lighting. *Visual perceptions may be altered by glare or shadows.*
- Eliminate unnecessary environmental stimuli (excessive noise level, multiple conversations/activities, violent/aggressive movies or television programs). *Disturbing visual images or loud noise can precipitate a catastrophic reaction.*
- Place meaningful possessions (e.g., photographs, furniture, special possessions) in the patient's environment. *Familiar belongings promote a sense of security.*
- Avoid change in room environment (e.g., reassignment of patient's room, rearrangement of furniture or items, holiday decoration). *Frequent environment change may produce conflicting cues.*
- Provide a daily time for small group activity that is valued by patient (e.g., music, art, reminiscence group, selected television program, Bible therapy). *Planned activities are beneficial if they are pleasurable and incorporate the patient's culture, habits, values, manners, preferences, and occupation.*

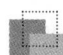

Impaired Memory

Impaired memory is a state in which an individual experiences the inability to remember or recall bits of information or behavioral skills. Impaired memory may be attributed to pathophysiologic or situational causes that are either temporary or permanent.[7]

Related Factors[2,4,7,9]

Brain trauma
Cerebral anoxia
Cerebrovascular accident
Delirium
Dementia
Electroconvulsive therapy
Encephalitis
Medications
Posttraumatic amnesia
Retrograde amnesia
Transient global amnesia
Seizure disorder
Wernicke-Korsakoff syndrome

Defining Characteristics[2,7,8]

Inability to learn or retain new information or skills
Inability to perform a behavior at a scheduled time
Inability to perform a previously learned skill
Inability to recall factual information
Inability to recall recent or past events
Observed or reported experiences of forgetting
Short and immediate-term memory deficits

Expected Patient Outcomes and Nursing Interventions With Rationale[1,3,5,6,8]

Acknowledge memory impairment and resulting limitations, as evidenced by:
Cooperates with memory assessment and testing
Verbalizes memory lapses

- Test recent memory by asking for a three-word recall after 5 minutes or asking for the hospital/facility room number or location.
- Test remote memory by asking questions such as place of birth, significant dates, names of past presidents.
- Encourage verbalization about memory deficits *to decrease anxiety about impairment and unknown outcomes.*
- Provide information about cognitive rehabilitation and expected course of recovery *because severity of traumatic brain injury will influence the type and length of memory deficits.*

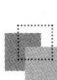

- Assist patient with realistic goal-setting for self during convalescence.
- Acknowledge emotional distress and provide encouragement. *Early stress management may help prepare the patient for emotional responses associated with a return of functional abilities.*

Participate in activities of daily living and use environmental cues to assist memory and orientation, as evidenced by:

Uses problem-solving strategies to assist memory and orientation

Uses memory aids

Follows daily schedule in plan of care

- Assist with problem-solving strategies *to cope with memory deficits.*
  - Use simple, concrete (versus abstract) communication.
  - Use repetition techniques (e.g., provide explanations, instructions, and introductions repeatedly).
  - Avoid giving explanations or instructions ahead of time.
  - Use structured. one-to-one approach *to minimize overstimulation.*
  - Use clocks and calendars.
  - Do not dispute confabulated responses but provide reality orientation.
  - Reorient throughout the day.
  - Emphasize familiar skills *to pair new learning with old learning and maximize memory during new tasks.*
- Teach augmentation of impaired memory with memory aids.
  - Teach use of a recording system, such as a notebook at the bedside for written entries and reminders.
  - Post a calendar in the room.
  - Place signs in room to aid memory (e.g., "Do not get out of bed alone. Use call light to call nurse.").
  - Provide simple instruction sheets at the bedside.
  - Use multiple modalities, especially multisensory stimuli to aid memory retention (e.g., visual, auditory, kinesthetic, etc.).
- Maintain daily care routines and schedule *to decrease confusion and disorientation and maintain consistency.*
  - Post daily schedule in room.
  - Promote regular rest periods.
  - Provide consistent caregivers whenever possible.
  - Wear name tag and remind patient frequently of caregiver's identity and purpose of interaction.
  - Keep belongings and call light in same location.
  - Use familiar objects in room to augment memory and assist with orientation to surroundings (e.g., locating own room).

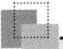

Disturbed Sensory Perception

Disturbed sensory perception occurs when an individual experiences a change in the amount or patterning of incoming stimuli accompanied by a diminished, exaggerated, distorted, or impaired response to such stimuli.[7]

Related Factors[2,4,7,8]

Altered sensory reception, transmission, and/or integration

Biochemical imbalances or sensory distortion

Electrolyte imbalance

Excessive or deficient environmental stimuli

Extreme anxiety or panic

Hypoxia

Loss and grief

Psychologic stress

Sleep deprivation

Defining Characteristics[7]

Altered communication patterns

Auditory distortions

Change in usual response to stimuli

Change in behavior pattern

Change in problem-solving abilities

Environmental overstimulation

Disorientation in time, in place, or with people

Hallucinations

Hyperesthesia or hypoesthesia

Irritability

Poor concentration

Reported or measured change in sensory acuity

Restlessness

Visual distortions

Expected Patient Outcomes and Nursing Interventions With Rationale[1,3,5,6]

Prevention

Identify related risk factors, as evidenced by:

States related factors

Recognizes self-risk profile

Uses strategies to reduce or eliminate identified risk factors

- Assess patient for risks and potential risks for alteration (see related factors); present risk profile to patient when possible.
- Provide strategies for reduction or elimination or identified related factors (e.g., altering sleep pattern to reduce sleep deprivation: altering drug habits; rearranging environment).

Identify stimuli needed for daily functioning, as evidenced by:

States source, type, amount, and patterns of usual daily stimulation

Recounts lifestyle and role patterns

- Explore source, type, amount, and patterns of stimuli needed by patient for optimum functioning.

Identify methods for maintaining adequate stimuli in environment, as evidenced by:

Verbalizes or demonstrates use for strategies for maintaining or altering environment

Lists changes planned for or already made

- Provide strategies for maintaining adequate amounts of meaningful stimuli in identified therapeutically or socially restricted environments (e.g., introducing pattern and structure in environment, orienting features, noise control, presence of familiar objects and persons).

Prevention requires careful assessment of the patient's environment for risk factors. Patient education plays a major role.

Once a pattern of defining characteristics appears and a diagnosis of disturbed sensory perception is made, the disturbance may be classified as acute or chronic.

Acute Care

Sustain no injury, as evidenced by:

No physical or reported signs of injury

- Maintain safety precautions (bed rails up; bed lowered; sharp objects out of reach; call bell in reach).

Experience decrease in or elimination of defining characteristics, as evidenced by:

Increase in ability to test reality
Becomes oriented to person, place, and time
Absence of hallucinations and delusions
Stabilization of emotions
Increases participation in care
Gives appropriate verbal feedback
Makes appropriate responses to environment
Absence of bizarre behavior
Increases in decision-making and problem-solving abilities
Lower anxiety levels

- Assess stimuli present in environment: intensity, quantity, quality, repetitiveness, movement, change, novelty, incongruity, clarity, ambiguity.
- Alter environmental factors to increase meaningful stimuli and decrease extraneous stimuli.
  Use orienting features (e.g., clocks, calendars, windows, name tags, favorite objects).
- Maintain verbal contact, eye contact, and touch.
- Reduce unnecessary traffic, personnel, and noise.
- Structure routines.
- Structure input by giving clear, concise explanations of surroundings, treatments, and procedures.
- Allow frequent short visits by significant others.
- Assist patient to orient to reality.
  Address by name; introduce self frequently and regularly; state time and place.
- Explain and allow participation, when possible, in all tasks and treatments.
- Interpret sights, sounds, and smells present in environment.
- Explain routines and policies.
- Obtain feedback or perception of events and objects; clarify misperceptions.
- Assist in clarifying reality (see Disturbed Thought Processes).

Acute alterations tend to be abrupt in onset and temporary. The degree of alteration is usually severe and dramatic in presentation of defining characteristics (e.g., sudden confusion and disorientation, rapid large mood swings, bizarre behavivor). Causes for acute alterations include trauma, drug intoxication, sudden sensory loss (blindness, deafness), acute pain, panic, and placement in intensive care units or recovery rooms.

Chronic Care

Become oriented to surroundings, as evidenced by:

Orients to person, time, and place
Recollects past and present events
Verbalizes future plans
Absence of confusion

- Use the following reality orientation techniques:
  Address by name; orient to time.
  Point out surroundings; identify self.
  Structure input with concrete, concise explanations.
  Maintain eye contact.
  Reinforce behavior that is reality oriented (e.g., responding to meaningful comments).
- Provide meaningful stimuli and reduce extraneous stimuli in environment.
  Keep clocks and calendars in view; make use of windows and outdoors.
  Observe holidays and significant occasions.
  Provide structured routines.
  Place familiar objects in plain sight.
  Structure experiences that make use of all senses.

Increase appropriate social interaction, as evidenced by:

Makes appropriate response to questions and cues
Initiates interaction
Increases interaction time
Increases meaningful interaction
Verbalizes about social events, time spent with others, and future plans

- Arrange physical environment to encourage interaction (open spaces; circles instead of rows); increase mobility with wheelchairs, walkers, and carts.
- Encourage exploration of surroundings; encourage verbalization of experiences, desires, and thoughts.
- Set up interactions with others in structural settings with defined purpose.
- Encourage reminiscence.
- Encourage decision making.
- Use small group sessions to widen interaction.

Chronic alterations are progressive in onset and are subject to recurrence because of the long-term or permanent nature of the related factors. The degree of alteration ranges from mild to severe, and defining characteristics may be subtle and ambiguous. When chronic alterations are left untreated, defining characteristics become more clear-cut and overt. Causes for chronic alterations typically include socially restricted environments (e.g., nursing homes, children's homes, prisons), declining sensory equipment, neurologic disease, chronic pain, prolonged immobility, social isolation, and chronic illness.

UNILATERAL NEGLECT

Unilateral neglect is a state in which an individual is perceptually unaware of and inattentive to one side of the body.[5]

Related Factors[3,5,6]

Neurologic illness or trauma
Perceptual deficits

Defining Characteristics[3,5,6]

Consistent failure to acknowledge affected side
Consistent inattention to affected side
Inadequate self-care
Food left on plate on affected side

Expected Patient Outcomes and Nursing Interventions With Rationale[1-4,6]

Gain realistic awareness of perceptual deficit, as evidenced by:

Verbalizes awareness of neglect

Remains free of injury

- Explain to patient that one side is being neglected; explain cause and mechanisms: repeat, as needed; encourage patient to share perceptions; provide realistic feedback; *the nurse can assist the patient to understand and acknowledge the condition by encouraging the patient to share perceptions and by providing realistic feedback.*
- Provide safe environment; regularly orient patient to environment; remove excess furniture and equipment; provide good lighting; place call bell and frequently used objects on unaffected side within easy reach; keep side rail up on affected side; *structuring the environment to decrease hazards is essential to safety.*
- Supervise or assist to transfer and ambulate *to ensure protection from injury for the affected side;* protect neglected side during activities; teach patient to assume this responsibility; teach patient to check position of limbs on affected side *to prevent unfelt trauma.*
- Note perceptual deficit on patient record and in patient's room to inform caregivers; *continuity of safe care is enhanced when all caregivers are aware of the patient's perceptual deficits.*

Exhibit adequate knowledge and skill in adaptive coping strategies, as evidenced by:

Attends to affected side in response to verbal or visual cues

Compensates for perceptual loss

Demonstrates increased self-management of ADLs

Verbalizes progress in regard to perceptual deficit

- Initially, arrange environment within patient's perceptual field *to assist compensation for perceptual deficit* (e.g., place frequently used items on unaffected side).
- After initial stress, to promote conscious attention to neglected side:
  - Place frequently used items on affected side.
  - Position patient so affected side is in view.
  - Talk to patient from affected side.
- Spend time with patient manipulating affected side and encouraging patient to use it.
  - Have patient handle ignored limbs with unaffected side.
  - Increase stimulation to affected side by touching, or massage with scented lotion.
  - Use visual and verbal communication regarding limb placement on affected side.

Verbal, visual, and tactile cues to decrease neglect of the affected side are effective in enhancing perceptual functioning.

- Teach patient to scan affected side; place clock or some frequently used item on side of deficit *to help establish pattern of scanning.*
- Use "cueing" to affected side *to increase awareness of that side:*
  - Mark red line in margin of books on affected side.
  - Attach small bells to limbs of affected side.
- Place food tray toward unaffected side; teach patient to rotate plate periodically.
- Encourage patient to perform ADLs (e.g., toothbrushing in front of mirror). Supervise and give feedback. *Activities that direct attention to the neglected side can increase awareness and use of that side.*
- Decrease confusing stimuli.
  - Avoid relocation.
  - Maintain constancy of caregivers and consistent routine for self-care.
  - Explain procedures and treatment well in advance.

An established plan of care by consistent caregivers can decrease distortions in perception and subsequent disorientation.

- Include family in rehabilitation process *so that they understand, support, and can continue it in home environment.*

Experience reduction or resolution of deficit or adaptation to deficit, as evidenced by:

Absent or reduced defining characteristics of unilateral neglect

- Assess regularly for degree of deficit, contributing factors, and adaptation to deficit; *progress toward goals is facilitated by ongoing evaluation of the effectiveness of intervention and by periodic revisions in the rehabilitation plan.*

WANDERING

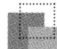

Wandering is meandering, aimless, or repetitive locomotion that exposes the individual to harm; frequently incongruent with boundaries, limits, or obstacles.[10]

Related Factors[2,8,10,12-14]

Cognitive impairment, specifically memory and recall deficits, disorientation, poor visuoconstructive (or visuospatial) ability, language (primarily expressive) defects

Cortical atrophy

Emotional state, especially frustration, anxiety, boredom, or depression (agitation)

Overstimulating or understimulating social or physical environment

Physiologic state or need (e.g., hunger/thirst, pain, urination, constipation)

Premorbid behavior (e.g., outgoing, sociable personality; premorbid dementia)

Sedation

Separation from familiar people and places

Time of day

Defining Characteristics*

Following behind or shadowing a caregiver's locomotion

Frequent or continuous movement from place to place, often revisiting the same destinations

Fretful locomotion or pacing

Getting lost

Haphazard locomotion

Hyperactivity

Inability to locate significant landmarks in a familiar setting

Locomotion that cannot be easily dissuaded or redirected

Locomotion into unauthorized or private spaces

Locomotion resulting in unintended leaving of a premise

*References 1, 3, 6, 7, 9-13, 15.

Long periods of locomotion without an apparent destination
Periods of locomotion interspersed with periods of nonlocomotion (e.g., sitting, standing, sleeping)
Persistent locomotion in search of "missing" or unattainable people or places
Scanning, seeking, or searching behaviors
Trespassing

Expected Patient Outcomes and Nursing Interventions With Rationale[1,4-9,11-15]

Maintain patient safety, as evidenced by:
Minimizes factors that might cause harm or injury to the patient
Prevents patient from wandering

- Keep outside doors securely closed.
- Provide a calm, structured environment *to decrease confusion and agitation.*
- Provide frequent reassurance and reorientation *to decrease confusion and anxiety.*
- Evaluate preferences for activities.
- Provide planned diversional activities *to keep patients involved and decrease wandering.*[4]
- Schedule routine exercise periods.
- Maintain a regular time for rest and sleep.
- Immobilize as indicated *to prevent injury to self or others.*
- Use appropriate medications if wandering individual becomes agitated. Minor tranquilizers may be useful; for severe agitation, antipsychotic medications may be needed.
- Provide in-service program for staff regarding care of patients who wander on a routine basis.[4] *In-service programs and reinforcement of information will enhance staff ability to care for patients who wander.*[4]

References

Cognitive-Perceptual

1. Gordon M: *Manual of nursing diagnosis,* ed 9, St. Louis, 2000, Mosby.

Acute Confusion

1. Ackley BJ, Ladwig GB: *Nursing diagnosis handbook: a guide for planning care,* St. Louis, 1999, Mosby.
2. Feldman J, Jaretzky A, Kaizimov N et al: Delirium in an acute geriatric unit: clinical aspects, *Arch Gerontol Geriatr* 28(1):37, 1999.
3. Granberg A, Engberg IB, Lundberg D: Acute confusion and unreal experiences in intensive care patients in relation to the ICU syndrome. Part II, *Intensive Crit Care Nurs* 15(1):19, 1999.
4. Kelley FJ: Planning care for acutely confused critically ill older persons, *Crit Care Nurs Q* 19(2):41, 1996.
5. McCloskey JC, Bulechek GM, editors: Reality orientation. In *Nursing interventions classification (NIC),* ed 3, St. Louis, 2001, Mosby.
6. McFarland GK, Wasli EL, Gerety EK: *Nursing diagnoses and process in psychiatric mental health nursing,* ed 3, Philadelphia, 1997, JB Lippincott.
7. Mentes J, Culp K, Maas M et al: Acute confusion indicators: risk factors and prevalence using the MDS data, *Res Nurs Health* 22(2):95, 1999.
8. North American Nursing Diagnosis Association: *Nursing diagnoses: definitions and classification 2001–2002,* Philadelphia, 2001, The Association.
9. Segatore M, Dutkiewicz M, Adams D: The delirious cardiac patient: theoretical aspects and principles of management, *J Cardiovasc Nurs* 12(4):32, 1998.
10. Trevisan LA, Boutros N, Petrakis IL. et al: Complications of alcohol withdrawal: pathophysiological insights, *Alcohol Health Res World* 22(1):61, 1998.
11. Walton JC, Miller JM: Evaluating physical and behavioral changes in older adults, *MEDSURG Nurs* 7(2):85, 1998.

Chronic Confusion

1. Ackley BJ, Ladwig GB: *Nursing diagnosis handbook: a guide for planning care,* St. Louis, 1999, Mosby.
2. Fontaine KL, Fletcher JS: *Mental health nursing,* ed 4, Menlo Park, Calif, 1999, Addison-Wesley.
3. Knight RG: Controlled and automatic memory processes in Alzheimer's disease, *Cortex* 34(3):427, 1998.
4. Logsdon RG, Albert SM: Assessing quality of life in Alzheimer's disease: conceptual and methodological issues, *J Mental Health Aging* 5(1):3, 1999.
5. Logsdon RG, Teri L, McCurry SM et al: Wandering: a significant problem among community-residing individuals with Alzheimer's disease, *J Gerontol B* 53B(5):P294, 1998.
6. McCloskey JC, Bulechek GM, editors: Reality orientation. In *Nursing interventions classification (NIC),* ed 3, St. Louis, 2001, Mosby.
7. McFarland GK, Wasli EL, Gerety EK: *Nursing diagnoses and process in psychiatric mental health nursing,* ed 3, Philadelphia, 1997, JB Lippincott.
8. North American Nursing Diagnosis Association: *Nursing diagnoses: definitions and classification 2001–2002* Philadelphia, 2001, The Association.
9. Willis SL, Allen-Burge R, Dolan MM et al: Everyday problem solving among individuals with Alzheimer's disease, *Gerontologist* 38(5):569, 1998.

Disturbed Thought Processes

1. Ackley BJ, Ladwig GB: *Nursing diagnosis handbook: a guide for planning care,* St. Louis, 1999, Mosby.
2. Bondy K, Maas M, McCourt A: Altered thought process: a need for conceptual clarity. In Rantz MJ, LeMone P, editors: *Classification of nursing diagnoses: proceedings of the twelfth conference, North American Nursing Diagnosis Association,* Glendale, Calif, 1997, Cinahl Information Systems.
3. Johnson B, Martin M, Guha M et al: The experience of thought-disordered individuals preceding an aggressive incident, *J Psychiatr Ment Health Nurs* 4(3):213, 1997.
4. Marlowe GS: Tackling confusion together: a case report from general practice, *Aging Ment Health* 1(3):283, 1997.
5. McCloskey JC, Bulechek GM, editors: Delusion management; Dementia management. In *Nursing interventions classification (NIC),* ed 3, St. Louis, 2001, Mosby.
6. McFarland GK, Wasli EL, Gerety EK: *Nursing diagnoses and process in psychiatric mental health nursing,* ed 3, Philadelphia, 1997, JB Lippincott.
7. Melamed E, Friedberg G, Zoldan J: Psychosis: impact on the patient and family, *Neurology* 52(7, suppl 3):S14, 1999.
8. Mentes J, Culp K, Maas M et al: Acute confusion indicators: risk factors and prevalence using the MDS data, *Res Nurs Health* 22(2):95, 1999.
9. North American Nursing Diagnosis Association: *Nursing diagnoses: definitions and classification 2001–2002,* Philadelphia, 2001, The Association.

10. Webster J: Recognition and treatment of dementing disorders in the elderly, *Clin Geriatr* 7(2):61, 1999.

Acute Pain

1. Ackley BJ, Ladwig GB: *Nursing diagnosis handbook: a guide for planning care,* St. Louis, 1999, Mosby.
2. Cheever KH: Reducing the effects of acute pain in critically ill patients, *Dimens Crit Care Nurs* 18(3):14, 1999.
3. Kuuppelomaki M, Lauri S: Cancer patients' reported experiences of suffering, *Cancer Nurs* 21(5):364, 1998.
4. McCloskey JC, Bulechek GM, editors: Analgesic administration; Pain management. In *Nursing interventions classification (NIC),* ed 3, St. Louis, 2001, Mosby.
5. North American Nursing Diagnosis Association: *Nursing diagnoses: definitions and classification 2001–2002.* Philadelphia, 2001, The Association.
6. Sandler AN: Pain control in the perioperative period, *Surg Clin North Am* 79(2):213, 1999.
7. Simon JM, Nolan L, Baumann MA: Validation of the nursing diagnoses acute pain and chronic pain. In Rantz MJ, LeMone P, editors: *Classification of nursing diagnoses: proceedings of the eleventh conference, North American Nursing Diagnosis Association,* Glendale, Calif, 1995, Cinahl Information Systems.
8. U.S. Department of Health and Human Services: *Clinical practice guideline. Acute pain management: operative or medical procedures and trauma,* (AHCPR 92-0032), Rockville, Md, 1992, Public Health Service, The Department.
9. Walker AC: Pain management in older people: lessons from the literature, *Geriaction* 17(2):13, 1999.

Chronic Pain

1. Ackley BJ, Ladwig GB: *Nursing diagnosis handbook: a guide for planning care,* St. Louis, 1999, Mosby.
2. Controlling chronic pain in older persons: highlights of new guidelines, *J Critl Ill* 13(9):587, 1998.
3. Geisser ME, Roth RS: Knowledge of and agreement with chronic pain diagnosis: relation to affective distress, pain beliefs and coping, pain intensity, and disability, *J Occup Rehabil* 8(1):73, 1998.
4. Klinger L, Spaulding SJ: Chronic pain in the elderly: is silence really golden? *Phys Occup Ther Geriat* 15(3):1, 1998.
5. Lyckholm L: Managing the chronic pain associated with terminal illness, *J Crit Ill* 13(9):539, 1998.
6. MacConnachie AM: Analgesics in the management of chronic pain, part 5: Step 3—parenteral analgesic drug therapy, *Intensive Criti Care Nurs* 15(5):58, 1999.
7. McCloskey JC, Bulechek GM, editors: Analgesic administration; Pain management. In *Nursing interventions classification (NIC),* ed 3, St. Louis, 2001, Mosby.
8. North American Nursing Diagnosis Association: *Nursing diagnoses: definitions and classification 2001–2002,* Philadelphia, 2001, The Association.
9. Simon JM, Nolan L, Baumann MA: Validation of the nursing diagnoses acute pain and chronic pain. In Rantz MJ, LeMone P, editors: *Classification of nursing diagnoses: proceedings of the eleventh conference, North American Nursing Diagnosis Association,* Glendale, Calif, 1995, Cinahl Information Systems.
10. The American Geriatrics Society: *Guidelines for the management of chronic pain in older persons,* New York, 1998, The American Geriatrics Society.

Decisional Conflict (Specify)

1. Ackley BJ, Ladwig GB: *Nursing diagnosis handbook: a guide for planning care,* St. Louis, 1999, Mosby.
2. McCloskey JC, Bulechek GM, editors: Decision-making support. In *Nursing interventions classification (NIC),* ed 3, St. Louis, 2001, Mosby.
3. McFarland GK, Wasli EL, Gerety EK: *Nursing diagnoses and process in psychiatric mental health nursing,* ed 3, Philadelphia, 1997, JB Lippincott.
4. North American Nursing Diagnosis Association: *Nursing diagnoses: definitions and classification 2001–2002,* Philadelphia, 2001, The Association.
5. Reaby LL: Breast restoration decision-making, *Plast Surg Nurs* 19(1):22, 1999.

Deficient Knowledge

1. Conley V: Beyond knowledge deficit to a proposal for information-seeking behaviors, *Nurs Diagnosis J Nurs Lang Classification* 9(4):129, 1998.
2. Laidlaw JK, Beeken JE, Whitney FW et al: Contracting with outpatient hemodialysis patients to improve adherence to treatment, *ANNA J* 26(1):37, 1999.
3. McCloskey JC, Bulechek GM, editors: Teaching: individual. In *Nursing interventions classification (NIC),* ed 3, St. Louis, 2001, Mosby.
4. McFarland GK, Wasli EL, Gerety EK: *Nursing diagnoses and process in psychiatric mental health nursing,* ed 3, Philadelphia, 1997, JB Lippincott.
5. North American Nursing Diagnosis Association: *Nursing diagnoses: definitions and classification 2001–2002,* Philadelphia, 2001, The Association.

Impaired Environmental Interpretation Syndrome

1. Ackley BJ, Ladwig GB: *Nursing diagnosis handbook: a guide for planning care,* St. Louis, 1999, Mosby.
2. Fontaine KL, Fletcher JS: *Mental health nursing,* ed 4, Menlo Park, Calif, 1999, Addison-Wesley.
3. Jennings B: A life greater than the sum of its sensations: ethics, dementia, and the quality of life, *J Ment Health Aging* 5(1):95, 1999.
4. Knight RG: Controlled and automatic memory processes in Alzheimer's disease, *Cortex* 34(3):427, 1998.
5. Logsdon RG, Albert SM: Assessing quality of life in Alzheimer's disease: conceptual and methodological issues, *J Ment Health Aging* 5(1):3, 1999.
6. Logsdon RG, Teri L, McCurry SM. et al: Wandering: a significant problem among community-residing individuals with Alzheimer's disease, *J Gerontol* 53B(5):P294, 1998.
7. McCloskey JC, Bulechek GM, editors: Environmental management. In *Nursing interventions classification (NIC),* ed 3, St. Louis, 2001, Mosby.
8. North American Nursing Diagnosis Association: *Nursing diagnoses: definitions and classification 2001–2002,* Philadelphia, 2001, The Association.
9. Schweiger JL, Huey RA: Alzheimer's disease, *Nursing* 29(6):34, 1999.
10. Volicer L, Hurley AC, Camberg L: A model of psychological well-being in advanced dementia, *J Ment Health Aging* 5(1):83, 1999.
11. Willis SL, Allen-Burge R, Dolan MM et al: Everyday problem solving among individuals with Alzheimer's disease, *Gerontologist* 38(5):569, 1998.

Impaired Memory

1. Ackley BJ, Ladwig GB: *Nursing diagnosis handbook: a guide for planning care,* St. Louis, 1999, Mosby.
2. Devasenapathy A, Hachinski VC: Cognitive impairment poststroke, *Phys Med Rehabil State Art Rev* 12(3):543, 1998.
3. Fontaine KL, Fletcher JS: *Mental health nursing,* ed 4, Menlo Park, Calif, 1999, Addison-Wesley.
4. Knight RG: Controlled and automatic memory processes in Alzheimer's disease, *Cortex* 34(3):427, 1998.

5. McCloskey JC, Bulechek GM, editors: Memory training. In *Nursing interventions classification (NIC),* ed 3, St. Louis, 2001, Mosby.
6. McFarland GK, Wasli EL, Gerety EK: *Nursing diagnoses and process in psychiatric mental health nursing,* ed 3, Philadelphia, 1997, JB Lippincott.
7. North American Nursing Diagnosis Association: *Nursing diagnoses: definitions and classification 2001–2002,* Philadelphia, 2001, The Association.
8. Webster J: Recognition and treatment of dementing disorders in the elderly, *Clin Geriatr* 7(2):61, 1999.
9. Wenden FJ, Crawford S, Wade DT et al: Assault, post-traumatic amnesia and other variables related to outcome following head injury, *Clin Rehabil* 12(1):53, 1998.

Disturbed Sensory Perception

1. Ackley BJ, Ladwig GB: *Nursing diagnosis handbook: a guide for planning care,* St. Louis, 1999, Mosby.
2. Carney AE, Moeller MP: Treatment efficacy: hearing loss in children, *J Speech Lang Hear Res* 41 (suppl 1):S61, 1998.
3. Foster J: Predicting resource use for patients with traumatic brain injury, *AACN Clin Issue Adv Prac Acute Crit Care* 7(1):168, 1996.
4. Hancock CK, Munjas B, Berry K et al: Altered thought processes and sensory/perceptual alterations: a critique, *Nurs Diagnosis* 5(1):26, 1994.
5. McCloskey JC, Bulechek GM, editors: Communication enhancement; Hearing deficit; Speech deficit; Visual deficit; Peripheral sensation management. In *Nursing interventions classification (NIC),* ed 3, St. Louis, 2001, Mosby.
6. McFarland GK, Wasli EL, Gerety EK: *Nursing diagnoses and process in psychiatric mental health nursing,* ed 3, Philadelphia, 1997, JB Lippincott.
7. North American Nursing Diagnosis Association: *Nursing diagnoses: definitions and classification 2001–2002,* Philadelphia, 2001, The Association.
8. Pichora-Fuller MK: Language comprehension in older listeners, *J Speech Lang Pathol Audiol* 21(2):125, 1997.

Unilateral Neglect

1. Ackley BJ, Ladwig GB: *Nursing diagnosis handbook: a guide for planning care,* St. Louis, 1999, Mosby.
2. Golisz KM: Dynamic assessment and multicontext treatment of unilateral neglect, *Top Stroke Rehabil* 5(1):11, 1998.
3. Hickey JV: *The clinical practice of neurological and neurosurgical nursing,* Philadelphia, 1997, JB Lippincott.
4. McCloskey JC, Bulechek GM, editors: Unilateral neglect management. In *Nursing interventions classification (NIC),* ed 3, St. Louis, 2001, Mosby.
5. North American Nursing Diagnosis Association: *Nursing diagnoses: definitions and classification 2001–2002,* Philadelphia, 2001, The Association.
6. Venneri A, Pentore R, Cotticelli B et al: Unilateral spatial neglect in the late stages of Alzheimer's disease, *Cortex* 34(5):743, 1998.

Wandering

1. Acello B: Hospital nursing: protecting the patient that wanders, *Nursing* 28(6):32, 1998.
2. Algase DL: Wandering: a dementia-compromised behavior, *J of Gerontol Nurs* 25: 10, 1999.
3. Altus DE, Matthews RM, Xaverius PK, et al: Evaluating an electronic monitoring system for people who wander, *Am J Alzheimer Dis* 15:121, 2000.
4. Cohen-Mansfield J, Werner P, Culpepper WJ et al: Evaluation of an inservice training program on dementia and wandering, *J Gerontol Nurs* 23:40, 1997.
5. Edgerly ES, Donovick PJ: Neuropsychological correlates of wandering in persons with Alzheimer's disease, *Am J Alzheimer Dis* 13:317, 1998.
6. Goldsmith SM, Hoeffer B, Rader J: Problematic wandering behavior in the cognitively impaired elderly: a single-subject case study, *J Psychosoc Nurs Ment Health Serv* 33:6, 1995.
7. Holmberg SK: Evaluation of a clinical intervention for wanderers on a geriatric nursing unit, *Arch Psych Nurs* 11:21, 1997.
8. Matteson MA, Linton A: Wandering behaviors in institutionalized persons with dementia, *J Gerontol Nurs* 22:39, 1996.
9. Meiner SE: NGNA. Wandering problems need ongoing nursing planning: a case study, *Geriatr Nurs Am J Care Aging* 21:101, 2000.
10. North American Nursing Diagnosis Association: *NANDA nursing diagnoses: definitions and classification 2000–2001,* Philadelphia, 2001, The Association.
11. Peck RL: The "ins and outs" of wandering, *Nurs Homes Long Term Care Manag* 49(8):55, 2000.
12. Riedel D, Shaw V: Nursing management of patients with brain injury requiring one-on-one care, *Rehabil Nurs* 22:36, 1997.
13. Sevier S, Gorek B: GN management. Cognitive evaluation in care planning for people with Alzheimer disease and related dementias, *Geriatr Nurs Am J Care Aging* 21:92, 2000.
14. Thomas DW: Evaluating the relationship between premorbid leisure preferences and wandering among patients with dementia, *Activ Adapt Aging* 23:33, 1999.
15. Weiner MF: Alzheimer's disease update: using what we now know to help patients, *Consultant* 39:675, 1999.

FUNCTIONAL HEALTH PATTERN 7

Self-Perception–Self-Concept[1]

ANXIETY

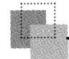

Anxiety is a vague uneasy feeling of discomfort or dread accompanied by an autonomic response; the source is often nonspecific or unknown to the individual; a feeling of apprehension caused by anticipation of danger. It is an altering signal that warns of impending danger and enables the individual to take measures to deal with threat.[7]

Related Factors[2-4,7,9,12,14]

Dietary substances
Excessive information
Exposure to toxins
Familial association/heredity
Homelessness
Interpersonal transmission/contagion
Medications
Situational/maturational crisis
Stress
Threat to or change in economic status
Threat to or change in environment
Threat to or change in health status
Threat to or change in interaction patterns
Threat to or change in role and/or role function
Threat to self-concept
Unconscious conflict about essential values/goals of life
Unmet needs

Defining Characteristics[7]

Behavioral

- Diminished productivity
- Expressed concerns caused by change in life events
- Extraneous movement (e.g., foot shuffling, hand/arm movements)
- Fidgeting
- Insomnia
- Poor eye contact
- Restlessness
- Scanning and vigilance

Affective

- Anxiety
- Anguish
- Fear/apprehension
- Feelings of inadequacy
- Focus on self
- Fright
- Increased helplessness
- Increased wariness
- Irritability
- Jitters
- Uncertainty

Physiologic

- Abdominal pain
- Anorexia
- Diarrhea
- Dilated pupils
- Dry mouth
- Facial flushing
- Fatigue
- Increased blood pressure
- Increased muscle tension
- Increased perspiration
- Increased pulse
- Increased reflexes
- Increased respiration
- Nausea
- Palpitations
- Quavering voice
- Respiratory difficulties
- Sleep disturbance
- Twitching
- Urinary frequency/urgency/hesitancy
- Weakness

Cognitive

- Blocking of thought
- Confusion
- Decreased perceptual field
- Difficulty concentrating
- Diminished ability to problem solve
- Diminished learning ability
- Fear of unspecific consequences
- Forgetfulness
- Impaired attention
- Preoccupation
- Rumination
- Tendency to blame others

Expected Patient Outcomes and Nursing Interventions With Rationale[1,3-6,8-13]

Experience reduced anxiety, as evidenced by:

Absent or reduced defining characteristics indicating presence of anxiety

- Develop constructive, positive, interpersonal relationship with patient.
  Be empathetic.

Convey unconditional positive regard.
Be congruent.
- Remain calm *so as not to increase patient's anxiety.*
  Avoid reciprocal anxiety.
  Recognize own anxiety.
  Develop control over own responses.
- Determine signs and symptoms (defining characteristics) indicating presence of anxiety; *this will assist in determining level of anxiety present.*
- Observe for perceived or actual threats *to develop some understanding about the patient's experience of anxiety.* Observe for the following:
  Personal security pattern
  Core or essence of personality
  Self-concept
  Value system, beliefs, or ideals
  Fear

Anxiety sensitivity can be present, which is a fear stemming from beliefs that sensations present in anxiety lead to harmful social, somatic, or psychologic consequences.[9]

- Listen to patient's description of state of discomfort.
- Identify maladaptive and adaptive current responses to anxiety.
- Identify strategies used by patient in past to cope with anxiety: *these can often be useful in coping with current anxiety.*
- Determine strengths and resources that are available to cope with current anxiety: problem-solving skills, decision-making skills, significant others, religion, professional assistance, recreational activities, hobbies.
- For patient with severe or extreme anxiety:
  Avoid asking patient to make decisions.
  Avoid probing for cause of anxiety.
  Avoid interpreting behavior or confrontation; *it is essential to lower anxiety when patient is at the severe or extreme level.*
  Use comfort measures (e.g., warm bath and restful environment).
  Keep in calm, nonstimulating milieu; remove any stress or threat; limit contact with other anxious patients.
  Use short, simple sentences.
  Use calm, firm tone of voice.
  Administer tranquilizers or sedatives, as prescribed.
  Observe for and institute needed protective measures.
  Use nonverbal behavior (e.g., quiet physical presence or touch) to offer reassurance.
- Intervene early *to prevent escalation of anxiety to severe or extreme levels.*
- In collaboration with psychiatrist, administer medications.
- Refer to therapist for systematic desensitization, biofeedback, or psychotherapy; *these therapies can be useful in decreasing experiences of severe or extreme anxiety.*
- Refer to self-help programs.
- Use active listening skills.
- Facilitate patient's participation in recreational and diversional activities *because these activities can decrease anxiety:*
  Sedative music
  Group singing or instrumental groups
  Simple games
  Housekeeping chores
  Grooming activities
  Routine tasks
  Walking or jogging
  Simple, concrete tasks
  Swimming
- Facilitate patient's participation in exercise (e.g., walking, jogging, swimming). *Exercise reduces anxiety. Aerobic exercise has a greater effect in reducing state anxiety. Length of exercise (16 weeks or longer) has greater effect in reducing trait anxiety. Duration of exercise (at least 21 minutes) has been shown to reduce both trait and state anxiety.*
- Encourage ventilation of feelings when patient is ready; permit crying.
- Offer brief and clear information about experiences during hospitalization; *this can prevent anxiety.*
- Use therapeutic touch, if appropriate; relaxation therapy; or imagery *because these have been found to reduce anxiety.*
- Convey attitude that there is hope and that a constructive resolution can be found.
- Prevent further escalation of anxiety by avoiding threats, indifference, rejection, judgmental attitude, impatience, unrealistic demands, insincerity, and focusing on patient's weaknesses *because these can increase feelings of insecurity and anxiety.*
- During short-term hospitalization, offer additional support and assistance in dealing with anxiety on admission, on the fifth day, and on notification of discharge.
- Mutually develop daily schedule of activities, incorporating patient's strengths, abilities, preferences, and goals.

Recognize anxiety, develop insight and use adaptive coping strategies, as evidenced by:

Verbalizes recognition of anxiety in self
Describes situations in which anxiety is increased
Uses strategies to reduce own anxiety
Uses mild anxiety for personal growth and change

- If anxiety is at mild or moderate levels, help patient to:
  Recognize presence of anxiety by providing feedback on characteristics indicating anxiety and by asking questions: "Are you uncomfortable right now?"
  Explore similarity between present and past experiences; ask questions: "Have you felt like this before? What was happening to you then? What did you do to reduce your discomfort?"
  Identify thoughts or expectations before becoming anxious.
  Identify relationship between anxiety and consequent adaptive or maladaptive responses.
  Clarify nature of threat to self.
  Develop adaptive strategies to prevent escalation of anxiety.
  Problem solve.
  Evaluate results of strategies used.
  Implement alternatives for unsuccessful results.

- Reduce any secondary gains from maladaptive strategies used in coping with anxiety.
- Permit patient to set pace in solving problems.
- Reduce negative expectations.
- Facilitate development of constructive and optimistic view of existence, especially if patient's view is distorted.
- Facilitate choice of effective, objective environmental interventions to cope with anxiety; *this is important especially if patient is already optimistic, open to new experiences, and flexible.*
- Encourage participation in new interests and hobbies.
- After establishing relationship with patient and after extreme or severe anxiety has been reduced:
  - Encourage social activities despite reluctance and fears.
  - Attend activities with patient initially; permit patient to leave if anxiety is greatly increased; gradually encourage attendance independent of staff support.
- Use role playing to deal with anxiety-provoking situations; with children, try role-play strategies using puppets, dolls, or other playthings; art; or play requiring large motor activities.
- Teach patient to do the following:
  - Recognize constructive aspects of mild or moderate anxiety in learning, growth, and movement toward self-actualization. Provide patient education pamphlets about anxiety.
  - Recognize personal characteristics that indicate presence of anxiety.
  - Recognize causes and management strategies for anxiety.
  - Examine current goals and beliefs in relation to what is actually happening.
  - Observe self and monitor management of own anxiety.
  - Develop assertive communication skills.
  - Develop problem-solving and decision-making skills.
  - Practice cognitive coping skills.
  - Use progressive muscle relaxation.
  - Increase repertoire of strategies to reduce anxiety (e.g., talking or being in presence of someone; simple, concrete tasks; walking; noncompetitive sports; professional assistance; listening to soothing music; meditating; prayer; performing deep breathing exercises and relaxation exercises).
  - Engage in progressive muscle relaxation.

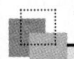

DEATH ANXIETY

Death anxiety is the apprehension, worry, or fear related to death or dying.[5]

Related Factors

Acute life-threatening illness
Death of family member or friend
Diagnosis of a terminal illness
Multiple deaths within same family

Defining Characteristics[5]

Anticipated pain
Concern about meeting creator
Concern about overworking caregiver
Deep sadness
Denial
Fear
Fear of delayed demise
Fear of developing a terminal illness
Fear of leaving family alone after death
Fear of loss of physical and/or mental abilities
Fear of premature death
Feeling doubtful about the existence of God or higher being
Negative death images
Powerlessness
Total loss of control over any aspect of own death
Unpleasant thoughts about any event related to dying
Worry about being the cause of other's grief and suffering
Worry about the impact of own death or of own mortality or impending death

Expected Patient Outcomes and Nursing Interventions With Rationale[1-4,6]

Anxiety about death is decreased, as evidenced by:
Shares feelings, needs, fears, and concerns about dying
Identifies and uses effective coping strategies
Practices anxiety-reducing strategies

- Explore the patient's knowledge of the situation, asking questions such as "What do you know about your condition?" or "What have you been told about your condition?" *to identify if the knowledge base of the patient will allow making informed decisions that will serve his or her best interests.*
- Explore the patient's perceptions of and concerns about death, asking questions such as "What are your fears and hopes?" "What do you worry about?" and "Tell me what you believe is going to happen" *to discover if the patient has unrealistic expectations or misperceptions about death.*
- Ask the patient "Tell me what or who has helped you the most in the past in dealing with problems" *to identify effective and ineffective coping methods and sources of support and strength.*
- Ask the patient "What help do you need during this time?" *to determine the adequacy of the human, financial, spiritual, and psychologic resources available to the patient.*
- Promote self-esteem by encouraging independence and control in decisions about treatments and care *to decrease feelings of powerlessness and to retain dignity in dying.*
- Encourage and support culturally appropriate spiritual rituals and practices *to provide hope and spiritual comfort.*
- Explain and assist, if necessary, with advance directives.
- Encourage life review and reminiscence *to offer affirmations of self.*
- Teach the use of visualization and imagery, focusing on pleasurable sights and sounds, *to reduce negative perceptions of death.*
- Suggest keeping a journal or leaving a legacy *to provide continuing love and support to others after death.*

- Encourage use of personal activities that facilitate calmness, such as music, aromatherapy, relaxation exercises, deep breathing, and/or massage, *to prevent or minimize anxiety.*

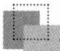

DISTURBED BODY IMAGE

Disturbed body image is a state of confusion in the mental picture of the physical self.[8]

Related Factors[2-4,8,11]

Acute physical trauma
Change in body function or structure
Cognitive-perceptual disorders
Disfigurement
Eating disorders
Family and cultural values and attitudes
Identification with others whose bodies are considered ideal
Inability to adust to normal developmental changes
Inadequate knowledge about social norms concerning appearance
Loss of body part(s)
Medication side effects
Mental disorders
Peer criticism or ostracism
Poor self-concept
Progressive deformity
Prolonged or chronic illness
Rigid ideals about appearance and body functions
Social and cultural attitudes toward disfigurement
Treatment side effects

Defining Characteristics[2-4,9,11,12]

Avoidance of looking at or touching body part
Change in ability to estimate spatial relationship of body to environment
Change in lifestyle
Change in social function
Denial of change in body boundaries
Depersonalization of a part or loss by use of impersonal pronouns
Disruption in activities of daily living
Fear of rejection by others
Feelings of grandiosity about physical size and strength
Feelings of helplessness, hopelessness regarding body change
Hiding or exposing body part
Incorporation of environmental objects into body boundary (e.g., ventilator)
Negation of awareness of reality of body change
Negative feelings about body
Overemphasis on past strength, function, or appearance
Overestimation or underestimation of body size
Overt or covert grieving
Personalization of part or loss by name
Preoccupation with change in body image or lost part
Refusal to acknowledge physical limitations
Verbalization of difficulties accepting loss or change in body function or structure
Verbalization of difficulties adjusting to limitations of body change

Expected Patient Outcomes and Nursing Interventions With Rationale[1,2,4-7,9-11]

Experience reintegration of body image, as evidenced by:
Conveys positive expression of acceptance of body change
Learns to compensate for anatomic alterations

- Encourage description of patient's perception of body image *to promote patient's understanding and accepting of reality of current situation and to obtain data to formulate an individualized plan of care,* by asking questions that explore:
  - Aspects of body that are pleasing or not pleasing
  - Perception of body changes in relation to perceived social norms
  - Integration of changes in body function or structure
  - Impact on patient of attitudes and feelings of significant others
- Explore origins of patient's perceptions or appraisal of body image as negative (as in past experiences with significant others).
- Encourage verbalization and exploration of feelings regarding the impact of missing body part or change in body image on ability to assume ADLs (family, work, social relationships).
- Encourage verbalization of feelings of concern, anger, anxiety, loss, and fear over changes in body image *to facilitate normal grieving process.*
- Encourage patient to look at, touch, and explore affected area; ask patient to verbalize feelings after doing this.
- Help patient to describe how overt body changes will be discussed with others.
- Be nonjudgmental.
- Prepare patient for possible experiences that might be encountered as consequence of physical limitations *to assist in adaptation to body changes.*
- Offer physical assistance, as needed (e.g., stoma care), when patient is unable to care for self.
- Encourage self-care activities, such as personal grooming and altering clothing *to promote perception of positive body image.*
- Assist patient to set specific self-care goals, such as exercise program to strengthen weakened muscles.
- Stress that certain physical characteristics of a person cannot be changed; emphasize the importance of learning to recognize own unique positive strengths, *to help patient achieve acceptance and a realistic appraisal of present physical self.*
- Assist significant others to understand potential impact of patient's limitations *to minimize ineffective denial and to promote family support.*
- Convey recognition of rehabilitation accomplishments *to instill hope for further gains and to promote optimism for the future.*

Reintegrate ego functions and boundaries, as evidenced by:
Increases ability to discriminate between environmental stimuli and internal stimuli
Maximizes use of remaining strengths
Resumes previous activities of daily living and lifestyle to extent that is realistically possible

- Encourage patient to verbalize feelings and anxieties over distorted perceptions of reality *to facilitate discrimination between real and unreal environmental and internal stimuli.*
- Engage patient in reality-oriented activities.
- Encourage patient to participate in all treatment modalities (pharmacologic therapy, individual or group therapies); discuss therapeutic benefits of these modalities.
- When patient has regained control of ego boundaries, encourage discussion and evaluation of possible precipitant of disturbance in body boundaries.
- Encourage patient to list strengths.
- Have patient describe perceptions of strengths, potentials, availability of social and community resources.
- Teach patient techniques and strategies for improving body image (e.g., how to dress, apply makeup, perform exercises to improve physical tone, and use cosmetic devices).
- Help patient determine the appropriate use of cosmetic services, hairpieces, wigs, and prostheses after disfiguring surgery or treatments.
- Acknowledge and give positive reinforcement whenever patient attempts to improve personal body image (e.g., improved hygiene, wearing makeup, wearing new clothes, wearing cosmetic devices after disfiguring surgery or treatment).
- Encourage participation in activities that promote increased use of body musculature (e.g., athletic games, dancing, structured exercise programs) *to enhance ego functioning for strengthening body image.*
- Offer supportive counseling *to facilitate a more rapid adjustment to change.*
- Determine need for mental health referral for evaluation for psychotherapy or antidepressant medication.
- Facilitate contact with others who have successfully adjusted to similar difficulties (people with an ostomy, laryngectomy, or mastectomy) *to convey assurance and hope for successful reintegration.*
- Encourage use of support services or reference groups in the community (e.g., self-help groups, Reach to Recovery, Voices Restored).
- Encourage patient to resume normal social activities as soon as possible, without hiding or overexposing changed body area.

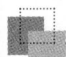

Disturbed Personal Identity

Disturbed personal identity is the inability of a person to experience an acceptable and coherent integration of sense of self and values within the context of personal, situational, and environmental stressors.[6]

Related Factors[2,3,6,8]

Being adopted
Chronic illness
Dysfunctional, abusive family life during childhood
Faulty resolution of sexual conflicts
Homelessness
Identification with inappropriate person
Inappropriate or negative role model
Negative social influence
Nonsupportive social structures and relationships
Parental deprivation
Pathologic symbiotic relationship with significant other
Unemployment
Unexpected ending of a relationship

Defining Characteristics[2,3,6,8]

Conflicting emotions about role and future goals
Conflicting emotions about sexual identity or sexual preference
Clinging, dependent behavior
Denial of significance of prior traumatic interpersonal events
Depression
Embellishment of past or present experiences
Fear of making changes
Inability to articulate feelings
Indecisiveness or inability to make decisions
Indecisiveness about sense of self, purpose, and direction in life
Overwhelming feelings
Pathologic fabrication of medical and/or social history
Uncertainty about career
Uncertainty about values
Verbal, future-oriented fantasizing
Withdrawal

Expected Patient Outcomes and Nursing Interventions With Rationale[1,2,4,5,7,8]

Develop and maintain a positive integrated sense of self and values, as evidenced by:

Describes positive attributes about self
Verbalizes acceptance of sexual identity and preference and conveys understanding of consequences associated with decisions regarding sexual preference
Responds to personal, situational, and environmental stressors without experiencing disintegration of self-identity
Demonstrates problem-solving skills and strategies that promote and maintain integration of personal identity

- Provide a therapeutic, nonjudgmental environment for discussion of concerns.
- Establish a therapeutic alliance *to encourage patient to verbalize concerns and anxieties regarding personal identity.*
- Evaluate the need for a mental health referral for the individual or family.
- Collaborate with physician regarding the need for judicious use of neuroleptics for patients with a psychosis-based identity disturbance.
- Encourage patient to verbalize anxieties concerning sexual identity and preference *to facilitate patient's gaining a healthy sense of self.*
- Have patient explore meanings of being male or female; assist patient to recognize that sexuality is only one component of personal identity.
- Emphasize that decisions associated with sexual identity and preferences are personal choices.
- Encourage patient to explore positive and negative consequences related to these choices.
- Help patient to differentiate between adaptive and maladaptive behaviors associated with sexuality.

- Teach patient principles of normal growth and development *to facilitate patient's recognition of stressors that are associated with normal developmental phases.*
- Encourage participation in peer group activities *to increase personal competency in meaningful interpersonal relationships.*
- Based on individual assessment:
  - Have patient keep a daily written record of thoughts and feelings *to promote autonomy by providing opportunity for ongoing view of self that is not solely dependent on outside feedback.*
  - Have patient draw pictures and write stories about self and family *to elicit information that might be overlooked or disconfirmed.*
  - Collaborate with patient in developing an agreed-on written treatment contract *to encourage patient responsibility in the development of problem-solving skills and strategies.*
  - Use contingency contracting (rewards or negative reinforcement) *to help the patient develop improved coping skills for maintaining integration of personal identity.*

FEAR

Fear is the response to perceived threat that is consciously recognized as danger.[9]

Related Factors[2,3,8,9,11]

Abusive relationship
Environmental stimuli
ICU environment
Intubation
Knowledge deficit
Language barrier
Learned response
Phobic stimulus
Physical or social conditions
Recurrence of life-threatening illness
Threat to safety of patient's children
Sensory impairment
Separation from support system in potentially stressful situation

Defining Characteristics[2,9]

Ability to identify object of fear
Anger
Apprehension
Change in functional ability
Concentration on the source of fear
Expressed fright/terror/dread
Fight behavior–aggression/withdrawal
Impulsiveness
Increased alertness
Increased pulse rate
Increased respiratory rate
Jitters
Panic
Verbalized vulnerability
Worry

Expected Patient Outcomes and Nursing Interventions With Rationale[1-8,10,11]

Experience absence of or reduced fear, as evidenced by:

Absence of or less diaphoresis, muscle tension, irritability, apprehension, fright, fight-or-flight behavior, and questioning
Normal heart and respiratory rate
Absence of pupil dilation
Verbalizes experiencing less fear
Good sleep

- Determine presence and level of fear. Keep in mind that patients tend to overpredict fear and exaggerate it retrospectively.
- Assist patient to recognize signs and symptoms of fear using indirect and open-ended questions.
- Help patient to identify danger that is causing fear by using indirect and open-ended questions.
- Encourage patient to verbalize feelings *to decrease intensity and duration of emotional response.*
- Provide emotional support and calm, soothing environment *to facilitate emotional coping.*
- Have patient record both episodes of fear and blocks of time when not feeling fearful. *Focusing only on fearful episodes may emphasize such experiences at the expense of episodes when fear is not experienced.*
- Assist patient in identifying major response pattern to danger (fight or flight) *to help patient develop self-understanding of response pattern.*
- Encourage verbalization, when timing is appropriate, about:
  - Perception of what is happening and degree of danger
  - Perception of ability to cope with danger
  - Questions about outcome of diagnoses and treatment
- Help patient use most appropriate coping strategies to deal with fear.
  - Facilitate realistic perception of danger.
  - Use strategies to avoid or work around danger.
  - Develop alternative resources and goals.
  - Engage patient in problem solving *to cope with danger.*
- Help patient identify strengths and adaptive skills *to cope with perceived danger and emotional responses.*
- Provide (at the level of patient understanding) factual and theoretic information about patient's illness and treatment *to facilitate understanding by the patient of his or her health status and treatment.*
- Engage in stimulus exposure or systematic desensitization, progressive muscle relaxation, visual imagery, and thought-stopping technique *to reduce and eliminate fear and related emotions.*
- Ask patient to predict experience of fear before exposure to feared event and compare with actual fear experienced *to identify discrepancies and give the patient a chance to use this information.*
- Refer for spiritual counseling or assistance from social worker.
- Avoid situations that could aggravate the fear and related feelings; give careful explanations about what is to hap-

pen to patient in the health-care setting *to decrease threat from planned procedures and treatment course.*
- Involve family and friends in patient's care.
- Encourage family and friends to offer patient emotional support.

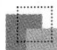

HOPELESSNESS

Hopelessness is the subjective state in which an individual sees limited or no alternatives or personal choices available and is unable to mobilize energy on own behalf.[11]

Related Factors[3-5,7,9,11]

Abandonment
Belief that stress, event, or illness is uncontrollable
Deteriorating mental or physical condition
Lifestyle of helplessness
Long-term stress
Loss of belief in transcendent values or God
Perceived significant loss
Persistent negative ideas of self, world, and future
Series of failures to reach desired goal
Sudden event that disrupts life pattern
Terminal illness

Defining Characteristics[1,3,7,11]

Absence of sense of continuity between past, present, and future
Apathy
Decreased appetite
Decreased response to stimuli
Decreased verbalization
Expressed loss of gratification from roles or relationships
Expressed psychologic discomfort (e.g., lump in throat, tenseness)
Fatigue or lethargy
Impaired decision-making ability
Inability to identify specific feelings
Increased or decreased sleep
Isolation of self from others
Lack of motivation or initiative
Lack of participation in self-care
Lack of personal goals
Nonverbal cues of withdrawal (e.g., closing eyes, turning away)
Verbal or nonverbal expressions of negative future expectations
Verbalized low self-esteem

Expected Patient Outcomes and Nursing Interventions With Rationale[1-3,5,6,8,10-12]

Maintain adequate self-care, as evidenced by:
Implements self-care activities
Recognizes unmet need
Selects appropriate self-care activity
- Assist patient in assuming responsibility for selection and implementation of self-care activities through teaching and support; *activity level affects internal sense of hopefulness.*
- Implement self-care activities *to meet needs patient is unable to meet.*
- Involve significant others in selection and implementation of self-care activities; *hope depends on interaction with significant others.*
- Provide positive reinforcement for successful attempts at self-care; *rewards encourage repetition of behaviors.*

Establish support system, as evidenced by:
Maintains sustaining relationships
Visits with significant others
Accepts assistance from others, when appropriate
- Build trust through consistency and reliability; *hope thrives in an atmosphere of trust.*
- Designate same staff, as possible, to work with patient; *for some patients, professionals are their only source of support.*
- Furnish opportunities for patient to spend time with others; gradually increase amount of time and number of persons; *the nurse can serve as the vehicle through which the patient negotiates a broader support system.*
- Identify options for increasing support system for patient.

Develop realistic self-esteem, as evidenced by:
Expresses positive self-statements
Identifies strengths and abilities
Verbalizes feelings of adequacy
- Convey unconditional positive regard; *development of self-esteem depends on repetitive positive interactions with others.*
- Assist patient to identify strengths and abilities; *identification of strengths positively influences the patient's self-esteem.*
- Assist patient to develop skills that contribute to mastery of the environment; *a positive self-esteem enables a person to seek out a new environment or deal with his or her existing environment constructively.*
- Encourage patient to carry out roles and responsibilities that reinforce positive feelings; *hopefulness is based on present opportunities for success.*

Verbalize feeling of hopefulness, as evidenced by:
Verbalizes future expectations
Verbalizes feelings of adequacy
- Observe for suicidal intent; *a negative attitude toward the future is a strong indicator of suicidal intent.*
- Encourage expression of feelings through communication; *hopelessness is abated by expression of feelings.*
- Assist patient to recognize and describe feelings of hopelessness.
- Assist patient to identify reason for living by focusing on concrete ideas and feelings.
- Assist patient to direct thoughts beyond the present to the future; *a sense of the possible and of the future is a critical element of hope.*

Control or influence self and environment, as evidenced by:
Participates in or makes health-care decisions
Sets realistic goals
Uses problem-solving skills

- Provide opportunity for patient input into health-care decisions: *patient input into care results in a sense of responsibility for outcome.*
- Teach patient to distinguish between controllable and uncontrollable events; *hopelessness is characterized by a perception of loss of control over present events and future outcomes.*
- Demonstrate and teach problem-solving skills: *control over self and environment is enhanced through expanding problem-solving capacity.*
- Assist patient to evaluate performance realistically.

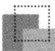

LOW SELF-ESTEEM

Low self-esteem is a state of negative self-evaluation or feelings about self or capabilities, which may be directly or indirectly expressed.[15]

Related Factors[1,2,4,7,15]

Abuse of child, spouse, elderly (physical, mental, sexual)
Chronic physical or mental illness
Cognitive-perceptual difficulties
Depression
Dysfunctional family
Early loss of parent or significant other
Excessive ridicule by others
Homelessness
Inability to adjust to alterations in body structure and/or function
Inadequate early parenting
Inadequate knowledge to cope with stressors
Loss of employment
Multiple stressors within a limited time
Neglect
Obesity
Perception of ill health
Sexual difficulties
Skin color
Traumatic developmental experiences
Unrealistic self-expectations

Defining Characteristics[4,7,11,15,17]

Attitude of superiority
Avoidance of self-disclosure
Decreased libido
Denial of problems obvious to others
Expression of shame or guilt
Evaluation of self as unable to deal with events
Grandiosity
Hesitancy to try new things or situations or ask for help
Hypersensitivity to criticism
Inattention to self-care
Lack of confidence in interactions
Lack of eye contact
Lack of participation in therapy
Projection of blame or responsibility for problems
Rationalization away or rejection of positive feedback and exaggeration of negative feedback about self
Rationalization of personal failures
School difficulties
Self-negating verbalization
Slouched or drooping position
Unassertiveness
Work difficulties
Verbalized difficulty in coping with tasks

Expected Patient Outcomes and Nursing Interventions With Rationale*

Achieve and maintain a constructive level of self-esteem, as evidenced by:

Improvement in personal appearance
Expresses appropriate mood
Increase in self-worth, self-respect, self-approval, and self-confidence
Engages in positive talk about self
Identifies and uses existing strengths, assets, and successes
Uses strategies that can promote and maintain positive level of self-esteem
Recognizes value of and uses various treatment modalities
Engages in age-appropriate activities
Interacts with family, friends, and neighbors
Takes initiative for new learning tasks
Demonstrates adequate involvement in relevant job performance
Expresses satisfaction with own achievements
Expresses satisfaction with functional ability in preferred life roles

- Demonstrate recognition of patient as a worthwhile, trusted human being by conveying genuine interest and concern.
- Monitor patient for eye contact, posture, self-care, evidence of self-neglect, and indecision.
- Evaluate and monitor the following: patient's self-description; negative feelings about self; likes and dislikes about self; strengths and weaknesses; past and current events leading to positive self-feelings or negative self-feelings; any changes planned for self; any life situations that patient does not perceive as having the power to change; perceptions of how others view patient; perceptions of ability to get along with others; feelings about self in social situations with large gatherings. *Findings from evaluation and monitoring are used to design appropriate strategies for individual enhancement of the patient's self-esteem.*
- Avoid conveying judgmental attitudes or criticism or belittling patient's feelings, actions, or ideas *to minimize reinforcement of patient's low self-esteem.*
- Maintain therapeutic environment that will foster patient's level of self-esteem. *Emphasis should be on helping patient recognize that self-respect is first related to the ability to respect self and then to respect and understand others.*
- Assist patient in expressing positive statements about self and eliminating self-derogatory statements.
  - Listen to statements.
  - Help patient to reappraise statements cognitively and to make more positive statements.
- Assist patient to examine maladaptive responses to threat to self-esteem (e.g., physical aggression, sexual acting out, substance abuse, high-risk behavior, and violence).

*References 1, 2, 4, 5, 8, 11, 12, 15, 17-21.

- Provide opportunities for patients with substance abuse to discuss positive role models who have struggled with similar problems to achieve recovery, *to lessen the stigma of illness associated with decreased self-esteem.*
- Encourage patient to identify and describe previous hopes and aspirations that may have been "buried."
- Encourage patient to accept responsibility for personal opinions and behavior and to evaluate their outcome in relation to options available.
- Encourage patient to identify disappointment and dissatisfactions. In turn, have patient develop constructive problem-solving steps, with action behaviors and realistic time frames and goals, *to lessen or correct these problem areas successfully.* Encourage patient to use this same approach when confronted with future problems.
- Offer supportive, positive, and genuine comments and feedback to patient, when appropriate; focus on specific changes in behavior and appearance when making these statements; offer positive reinforcers for actual achievements; avoid false praise.
- Assist patient to recognize the fallacies associated with "having to be perfect" to feel good; *it is important for patient to realize that he or she is as worthwhile as anyone else despite imperfections.*
- Emphasize the importance of thinking positively by teaching patient to examine and monitor own negative thoughts of self and to practice positive self-talk: "I can achieve that goal."
- Teach patient to avoid illogical thoughts that precipitate low self-esteem: thinking the worst will always happen; thinking something is a total failure; believing that a bad experience will repeat itself; focusing on negative details.
- Suggest that patient keep a journal to use as a tool to enhance thought stopping of negative thoughts and concomitant events and feelings; teach patient to generate and to record positive thoughts about self at these times.
- Have patient describe current and past successes and accomplishments *to reinforce recognition of coping skills and to foster a sense of achievement.*
- Encourage patient's recognition of current strengths, assets, and potential *to draw on these resources in dealing with new life demands.*
- Teach patient assertive techniques and communication skills: use of "I" statements; conveying clear expectations of others; using negotiation as viable tactic; using body posture, facial expression, and tone of voice consistent with verbal communication; remaining firm, yet gentle and unyielding, when appropriate; teach patient to value and accept sincere compliments; *use of assertive communication skills will assist patient in meeting own needs while preserving the integrity of others.*
- Teach patient good personal grooming skills and health habits.
- Encourage good body posture and expression of pleasant affect.
- Encourage patient to identify and participate in satisfying and rewarding experience *to enhance self-worth.*
- Encourage patient to initiate activities and to develop new interpersonal and social skills in which patient will be reasonably successful *to minimize failure and decreased self-confidence.*
- Assist patient to establish reasonable goals for self.
- Encourage patients with physical disabilities to participate in fitness programs that are designed for people with disabilities. *This environment allows them to interact with persons with similar interests and to experience positive interactions.*
- Explore with patient additional skills needed for personal competency (e.g., success at job).
- Encourage patient to reward self for personal achievements.
- Facilitate patient's participation in treatment modalities that emphasize mutual support, acceptance, and concern for others (e.g., social skills, stress management, health management, and group or family therapy) *to decrease sense of aloneness in experiencing fears and failures.*
- Encourage abused women to enroll in abused women's support groups; *women's support groups can enhance abused women's self-esteem by (1) providing knowledge about theories of violence and reducing sense of personal responsibility for the abuse; (2) replacing negative verbalizations of self-image with positive ones; and (3) recognizing the women's strengths and accomplishments.*
- Encourage women to participate in self-esteem–enhancing therapies such as women's issues groups.
- Increase opportunities to gain social support, especially for patients with chronic conditions, such as multiple sclerosis. *Social support and love can contribute to the maintenance of self-esteem.*
- Use group therapy, including support groups, to work with patients who experience similar problems *to focus realistically on their problems, diminish isolation, provide realistic support and reinforcement from other members, strengthen coping patterns, provide feedback information about the environment, and improve the patients' overall self-esteem.*
- Promote structured life review reminiscence (for elderly patients) that focuses on positive recollections and discussions of the past.
- Provide opportunities for children from dysfunctional families (e.g., families with parental substance abuse) to (1) obtain age-appropriate appraisals for their abilities on important dimensions, such as age-appropriate level of responsibility; and (2) obtain feedback and information that does not disconfirm the child's existing self-perception, *making certain that the person providing the feedback is viewed as credible by the child;* spend time engaging in activities or in an environment where the children can feel good about themselves.
- Refer for mental health services such as family therapy, when appropriate. *Families benefit from opportunities to learn how their roles enhance the patient's self-esteem and how they may unwittingly contribute to the patient's self-esteem disturbance.*
- Review appropriate social activities with patient.
- Assist patient in becoming aware of effect of constructive social experiences in building self-esteem; increase social opportunities for interactions and opportunities to gain social support, especially for patients with chronic conditions.

Chronic Low Self-Esteem

Chronic low self-esteem is a state of long-standing negative self-evaluation or feelings about self or capabilities.[15]

Related Factors[1,2,14,15,19]

Abuse, neglect, abandonment
Chronic mental illness
Chronic pain
Chronic physical illness
Family dysfunction
Institutionalization
Learned helplessness
Loss of self-control
Perceived low social or economic status
Significant early loss

Defining Characteristics[9,14,15,19]

Alienation from community resource network
Exaggeration of negative feedback or criticism
Expressed shame or guilt
Hesitancy to try new situations
Indecisiveness
Lack of success in work or relationships
Long-standing low self-evaluation
Nonassertiveness, passivity
Preoccupation with self
Rumination about past problems
Self-destructive behavior
Self-negative verbalizations
Withdrawal
(See Low Self-Esteem for other defining characteristics.)

Expected Patient Outcomes and Nursing Interventions With Rationale*

(See Low Self-Esteem for other outcomes and interventions.)

Demonstrate increasingly positive self-esteem, as evidenced by:

Increases number and type of interactions with others
Verbalizes positive statements about self
Practices and uses decision-making skills

- Conduct an assessment that includes evaluation of factors, such as substance abuse, physical abuse, and/or depression, that affect the patient's self-esteem.
- Help patient to identify lifestyle patterns that contribute to positive or negative self-esteem.
- Teach patient strategies to increase self-confidence, such as developing and expressing own opinions about specific issues, engaging in hobbies.
- Encourage patient to plan for change in small increments. *Small successes augment self-esteem.*
- Help patient to enhance decision-making skills *to increase perception and belief of ability to have control over own life.*
- Convey genuine concern and willingness to help patient and family obtain help.
- Help patient in identifying family and community resources for improving self-esteem. *Social support contributes to an individual's improved self-esteem and the perception of an increased sense of control.*
- Help family to recognize the possibility that client's improvement might be slow; *it is important for family and caregivers to have realistic expectations.*
- Collaborate with interdisciplinary colleagues for assistance in referrals for resources such as treatment for substance abuse, need for domestic violence shelter.
- Initiate referrals to mental health professional if indicated.

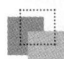

*References 5, 7, 9, 14, 16, 19.

Situational Low Self-Esteem

Situational low self-esteem is the development of a negative perception of self-worth in response to a current situation (specify).[15]

Related Factors*

Acculturation
Addition or loss of family member
Adolescent developmental crisis
Adolescent pregnancy
Being restrained
Disasters
Discrimination
Divorce or marriage
Failure in school
Financial burden
Homelessness
Hospitalization
Inability to speak (e.g., intubation)
Incontinence
Loss of body part or function
Loss of job, work, or role
Loss of material goods
Loss of pet
Loss of significant other
Obesity
Poverty
Prison term

Defining Characteristics[2,3,13,15]

Difficulty making decisions
Evaluation of self as unable to handle situations/events
Expressed shame or guilt
Indecisiveness
Verbalized negative feelings about self (e.g., helplessness, uselessness)
(See Low Self-Esteem for other defining characteristics.)

Expected Patient Outcomes and Nursing Interventions With Rationale†

(See Low Self-Esteem for other outcomes and interventions.)

Demonstrate increasingly positive self-esteem, as evidenced by:

*References 2, 3, 6, 10, 13, 15, 20.
†References 1, 2, 12, 13, 15, 17, 20.

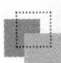

Actively seeks help in dealing with situation or event causing stress
Verbalizes positive statements about self
Realistically appraises situation and uses strategies to increase self-esteem

- Explore with patient the reason for loss, stress, or environmental factors causing low self-esteem.
- Have patient describe recollections of previous sense of positive self-esteem *to provide hope for a return to sense of constructive level of self-esteem.*
- Use psychoeducational groups for populations such as depressed women *to teach information about self-esteem and to foster the development of specific strategies for improving self-esteem.*
- Teach patient to develop strategies for coping with loss, stress, or environmental factors causing low self-esteem (e.g., problem-solving) *to increase patient's awareness of the relationship between effective coping strategies and increased self-esteem.*
- Help the patient to focus on overall strengths and capabilities, as well as the loss or alteration that has contributed to the low self-esteem. *This focus can help the client to mobilize a constructive coping repertoire.*

Risk for Situational Low Self-Esteem

Risk for situational low self-esteem is the state in which an individual is at risk for developing negative perception of self-worth in response to a current situation (specify).[5]

Risk Factors[2,5]

Behavior inconsistent with values
Body image disturbance
Developmental changes
Failures, rejections
History of abuse, neglect, abandonment, learned helplessness
Lack of recognition or reward
Loss
Physical illness or functional impairment
Powerlessness
Unrealistic self-expectations

Expected Patient Outcomes and Nursing Interventions With Rationale[1-4]

(See Low Self-Esteem, Situational Low Self-Esteem, and Risk for Relocation Stress Syndrome for other interventions with rationale.)

Demonstrate ability to maintain positive self-esteem, as evidenced by:
Verbalizes effects of current situation on self-worth
Identifies strengths and limitations
Uses effective problem-solving and decision-making skills
Asks for help when needed

- Use active listening and demonstrate respect and acceptance. *Therapeutic communication techniques are useful in enhancing self-worth and may assist in reframing the situation. They also facilitate understanding of the situational crisis, understanding of expectations, and understanding of self-response.*
- Assist patient to increase his or her personal judgment of self-worth[4] *to facilitate ability to maintain self-esteem in current situation.*
  Monitor patient's statements of self-worth.
  Determine patient's confidence in own self-worth.
  Encourage patient to identify strengths.
  Reinforce identified self-strengths.
  Convey confidence in patient's ability to handle current situation.
  Encourage patient to accept new challenges.
- Provide information about available resources and support groups, which *provide an opportunity for nonthreatening sharing of information and testing of decision-making abilities.*

Powerlessness

Powerlessness is the perception that one's own action will not significantly affect an outcome; a perceived lack of control over a current situation or immediate happening.[11]

Related Factors[1-5,11]

Authoritarian health-care system behavior
Assault on privacy
Blocking of resources
Castelike separation from persons of authority
Controlled conditions of negotiation
Excessive surveillance
Lack of individualization
Misuse of power or authority
Misuse of rewards and punishment
Monopoly of scarce or strategic resources
Stripping of personal possessions

Sociocultural
Actual or potential loss of significant other
Excessive threatening experiences
Lack of parental role model
Parental influences and styles
Peer influence
Perception of authority figures as distant or unapproachable
Repeated interpersonal problems and/or failures
Unequal power between or among persons
Unsupportive environment

Altered health status
Altered mental status
Altered physical status
Dependence on chemical substances
Frustration in obtaining pain relief
Loss of functional ability
Physical immobility
Physical restraints

Cognitive/perceptual
Altered attention span
Negative self-esteem
Knowledge deficit
Lack of ability to participate in decision making
Lack of belief in own ability

Environmental
Altered schedule

Hostile environment
Institutionalization
Lack of ability to gain a concession or do without
Lack of ability to reward a favor
Lack of available or accessible personal resources
Negative experiences with the health-care system or facilities
Overwhelming stressors
Threatening, unfamiliar technology
Unpredictable environment

Developmental

Delay or change in accomplishing developmental tasks
Loss of autonomy
Loss of independent role

Defining Characteristics[1,3-6,11]

Aimlessness
Anxiety
Asking of many questions or no questions
Expressed feelings of inadequacy
Fears about alienation from caregivers
Feelings of depression
Frustration about inability to perform previously mastered activities
Inability to influence others
Inappropriate aggression
Inappropriate, immature coping skills for age
Lack of knowledge of own illness
Loss of control over self-functioning, environment, personal behavior
Overdependence on others
Passivity
Preference for immediate rewards over long-term goals
Projection of blame on others and environment
Rationalization of behavior
Sleeplessness
Verbalized feelings of loss of control
Verbalized lack of control or influence over self, situation, or outcome
Withdrawal from activities

Expected Patient Outcomes and Nursing Interventions With Rationale[1,3-5,7-10,12,13]

Influence outcomes in current situations, as evidenced by:

Verbalizes ability to control or influence situation and outcomes
Verbalizes feelings of powerfulness and adequacy
Knowledge about control-relevant situation
Adequate role-functioning and coping skills
Goal-directed behavior
Expresses hope
Involvement in decision making
Works toward long-term goals

- Monitor powerlessness by asking these questions:
  Are perceived abilities to influence personal outcome present?
  Are there verbal expressions of having no control or influence over situation or outcome? Of feelings of loss of control and powerlessness?
  Does the patient experience characteristics such as lack of decision making? Lack of knowledge about illness and treatment? Withdrawal?
  Are environmental factors, staff behaviors, or other related factors present that can lead to a sense of powerlessness (e.g., excessive surveillance, assault on privacy, lack of individualization)?
  Does patient believe he or she has ability to accomplish a given task?

Baseline data are essential for developing an individualized plan of care.

- Make change within institutions or residential settings.
  Determine organizational barriers to patient empowerment.
  Decrease surveillance of patient unless essential for safety.
  Minimize rules and regulations; permit patient input in his or her development.
  Enhance individuality and autonomy.
  Increase patient control over rewards.
  Preserve privacy; increase territorial rights.
  Allow patient to wear own clothes.
  Prevent a castelike separation between staff and patients.
  Vary setting and routine of daily activities based on patient input. *It is important to develop a sense of partnership among health-care providers, the patient, and the patient's significant others.*
  Do not block patient's attainment and use of resources (within limits of safety).
  Do not use coercion.
  Support patient's efforts to increase resources.
  Decrease dependency on staff; encourage independent behavior.
  Maintain patient's sense of dignity; permit exploration of environment.
  Be less directive and overprotective.
  Foster personal powerfulness by putting bedside stand, call light, telephone, etc., within reach.
  Promote active involvement in appropriate decision making in activities of daily living.
  Involve patient in other decision-making opportunities and planning own care.
  Provide patient with positive and predictable events (e.g., group experiences).
  Provide opportunities for engagement in meaningful activities.
  Provide opportunities for family to participate in care.

These environmental changes help maximize the patient's ability to control events and decrease the sense of powerlessness.

- Help patient reduce feelings of powerlessness.
  Build trusting relationship.
  Be consistent and dependable.
  Use active listening.
  Encourage verbalization about feelings and concerns about feelings of powerlessness.
- Help patient recognize and describe powerlessness; identify the behavior with patient.
- Help patient separate controllable from uncontrollable events.

- Help patient identify personal preferences, wants, feelings, values, and attitudes.
- Help patient set realistic goals.
- Teach patient to problem solve and try out alternative coping strategies.
- Help patient identify and use strengths and potential: identify improvement in condition.
- Help patient improve self-esteem *because this can help patient feel capable in exerting more influence.*
- Provide situations in which patient can succeed and experience control.
- Assess patient's perception and knowledge of treatment program, encouraging expression of views before giving information.
- For those with internal locus of control, provide information that gives patient a sense of control, using different strategies of content presentation.
- For those with external locus of control, provide structured approaches, teach in small increments, and involve in determining readiness for learning.
- Help patient seek and master relevant health information.
- Provide needed information.
- Encourage patient to ask questions; reinforce right to ask questions.
- Help patient use health-care personnel.
- Restore energy imbalance.
- Allow patient to assume more complicated decision making when ready.
- Provide positive reinforcement and acknowledgement for active participation in appropriately selected therapeutic modalities, such as sensitivity training, behavior modification, brief psychotherapy, encounter groups, and community action programs, or by using interventions, such as altering perception of life situation; using behavioral rehearsal and role playing, rewarding manifestations of internality, challenging external locus of control-oriented verbalizations, examining possible outcomes of alternative approaches, and teaching assertive communication skills.
- Facilitate improvement in life circumstances: returning to work, constructive interactions with significant other, successful therapy experiences, constructive family interactions, and role models.
- Involve significant others, alerting them to importance of their reactions to the patient.
- Refer for family therapy as appropriate.
- Refer to self-help groups as appropriate.

A patient's powerlessness can be diminished by rebuilding, augmenting, or improving power resources—physical strength, psychologic stamina, support networks, self-concept, energy, knowledge, motivation, and a belief system (hope). Effective coping strategies must be preserved, augmented, and developed. Effective coping strategies result in a decrease in uncomfortable feelings, generation of hope, enhancement of self-esteem, maintenance of positive interpersonal relationships, and maintenance of or improvement in the state of coping.

Risk for Powerlessness

Risk for powerlessness is the state in which there is a risk for perceived lack of control over a situation and/or one's ability to significantly affect an outcome.[7]

Risk Factors[3,6,7,8]

Physiologic

Acute or chronic illness (hospitalization, intubation, ventilator)
Acute injury or progressive debilitating disease
Aging
Dying

Psychosocial

Absence of integrality
Decreased self-esteem
Lack of choice in living environment
Lack of control over comfort during hospitalization
Lack of health-care insurance
Lack of knowledge of illness or health-care system
Lifestyle of dependency with inadequate coping patterns
Low or unstable body image

Expected Patient Outcomes and Nursing Interventions With Rationale[1,2,5,6]

(See Powerlessness for further nursing interventions with rationale.)

Demonstrate increased self-esteem and ability to control situations and outcomes, as evidenced by:

Verbalizes self-worth
Verbalizes ability to make responsible decisions
Identifies uncontrollable situations
Expresses positive regard for self and own strengths
Takes part in health-care decision making

- Assess for feelings of self-worth, decision-making abilities, and ability to identify own strengths and weaknesses. *Power is created by personal feelings about self. When feelings of power are internalized, the person is empowered. Lack of feeling power leads to insecurity and can decrease relationships with others.*
- Provide activities that assist the patient to increase personal judgment of self-worth.[5]
  Monitor statements of self-worth.
  Determine locus of control.
  Determine confidence in own judgment.
  Reinforce identified personal strengths.
  Do not criticize or tease.
  Verbalize confidence in patient's abilities.

Every person has a desire for control. The risk for powerlessness is greater in persons who have had multiple losses and experience an injury or illness. Because powerlessness is a subjective state, the person's feelings must be validated.

- Provide opportunities for personal decision making in plan of care *to increase self-esteem and provide some measure of control over the situation.*
- Establish therapeutic relationship by spending time with the patient, providing choices, and listening. *Making choices increases autonomy. Listening demonstrates positive regard and facilitates hope.*
- Consider the patient's cultural background and values when discussing decision making. *Decision making is often culturally influenced and may differ from the nurse's belief system.*

- Encourage activities that enhance power: meditation, exercise, reminiscence, therapeutic touch, contracting, and sensation information. *These activities support belief systems, physical strength, self-concept, energy, motivation, and knowledge.*[4]
- Provide information about resources available for the underinsured or uninsured *to promote health promotion and health restoration in this population.*

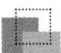

Risk for Loneliness

Risk for loneliness is a subjective state in which an individual is at risk of experiencing vague dysphoria.[12]

Risk Factors[3,9,10,12]

Affectional deprivation
Altered self-esteem
Body image disturbance
Cathectic deprivation
Impending death
Peer relationship difficulties
Physical isolation
Retirement
Shyness
Social isolation
Urinary incontinence

Expected Patient Outcomes and Nursing Interventions With Rationale[1-2,4-9,12]

Be comfortable being alone, as evidenced by:
Verbalizes reasons for feelings of isolation from others
Discusses methods to foster meaningful relationships
Identifies useful diversional activities and social supports

- Assess patient's perceptions of loneliness, causes of loneliness, and sources of support. *Loneliness is a subjective state, often caused by feeling different or the experience of loss, or lack of family relationships and friendships. Being alone does not inherently lead to feeling lonely.*[2,3,9]
- Discuss the commonality of loneliness. *A part of being human is to experience some degree of loneliness. It is often comforting to know that one is not alone in a painful experience.*[8]
- Assess patient's ability to meet physical, psychosocial, spiritual, and financial needs *because unmet needs may decrease ability to overcome loneliness.*
- Provide activities that facilitate the patient's ability to interact with others by encouraging the following[6,11]:
  - Enhanced involvement in already established relationships
  - Patience in developing relationships
  - Peer relationships (for adolescents)
  - Strong relationships with family members
  - Relationships with others who have common interests and goals
  - Social and community activities
  - Sharing of common problems with others
  - Involvement in totally new interests, hobbies, and activities
  - Changing environments, such as walking or going to movies
  - Use of alternate transportation if driving is impossible or no longer feasible
  - Developing alternate means of communication if patient has altered ability
  - Buying appliances and clothing specific to needs for those with visual or hearing deficits or surgical/traumatic disfigurements
  - Means of controlling odors (as from a colostomy) and incontinence
  - Independence in activities of daily living

All of these activities are aimed at enhancing socialization and decreasing loneliness.

- Provide support for the patient who has experienced or is anticipating a loss. *Losses that may lead to loneliness include retirement, impending death of self, death of significant other, and move to a long-term care facility.*

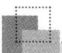

Self-Mutilation

Self-mutilation is deliberate self-injurious behavior causing tissue damage with the intent of causing nonfatal injury to attain relief of tension.[13]

Related Factors[2,5,7-9]

Adolescence
Autism
Borderline personality
Character disorder
Childhood physical or sexual abuse
Developmental delay
Family history of violence/divorce/alcoholism/self-destructive behaviors
Feelings of depression, rejection, anxiety, guilt, self-hatred, depersonalization
History of self-injurious behavior
Impulsivity
Incarceration
Institutional or foster care
Labile behavior/body image
Manipulating behaviors
Mood disorders
Loss (actual or potential) of significant relationship
Parent-child communication difficulties
Personality disorders
Psychosis
Self-esteem/body image disturbance

Defining Characteristics[13]

Abrading
Biting
Burning
Constricting a body part
Cutting/scratching
Hitting
Ingesting or inhaling harmful substances or objects
Inserting object(s) into body orifice(s)
Severing

Expected Patient Outcomes and Nursing Interventions With Rationale*

Not carry out self-mutilating activities, as evidenced by:

Decreased number of self-mutilating behaviors

Identifies when feelings of numbness, anxiety, or depersonalization are experienced

Expresses feelings being experienced

Expresses feelings of self-worth

- Assist patient to increase personal judgment of self-worth[11] *to assist in increased self-esteem and ability to withstand need to self-mutilate.*
  - Encourage to identify strengths.
  - Provide experiences that reinforce personal strengths.
  - Assist in setting realistic personal goals.
  - Assist to reexamine negative perceptions of self.
  - Explore reasons for self-criticism or guilt.
  - Monitor frequency of self-negating verbalizations.
- Help patient identify cues or triggers that precede impulsive behavior. *There are triggers that set off the need to self-mutilate. Awareness of these triggers can facilitate control over impulses.*
- Provide surveillance *to provide safety for the patient by preventing self-harm.*
  - Maintain continuous 24-hour observation.
  - Take action as necessary to stop self-mutilation.
  - Monitor for hallucinations and assure the patient that he or she will not be alone and will be safe.
  - Remove harmful objects from the environment.
- Physically hold the patient if necessary to prevent self-harm, but be cautious if reenactment of the precipitating trauma is being experienced. *Touch may be interpreted as coming from an abuser and may precipitate aggressive behavior. Explain why holding is necessary before touching the patient.*
- Take care of any self-inflicted wounds matter-of-factly *to decrease focus on attention-seeking behaviors.*
- Reinforce alternative ways of handing anxiety such as exercise, writing down feelings and putting them in a box, or verbalizing feelings.
- Teach ways to maintain self-connectness *to facilitate ability to control self-mutilation:*
  - Having a safe place for the day, going to the safe place, having an image of the safe place, wrapping self in a sheet or blanket, bathing, or applying lotion *are concrete methods of feeling, touching, and seeing self as having a boundary and being safe and secure.*
  - Set times for activities, tasks, recreation, and schoolwork. *A structured environment facilitates setting boundaries.*
- If patient is unable to control self-mutilating behavior, provide interactive supervision rather than isolation. *Isolation takes away an individual's coping abilities and may increase risk of self-mutilation.*
- Use group therapy to provide interaction with others so patient can share methods of coping with self-destructive tendencies and improving interpersonal relationships. *Through group therapy, members learn to identify behaviors that are used to cope with painful past events.*

Be able to control self-mutilating behaviors in the home environment, as evidenced by:

Reports ability to control impulses

Uses appropriate stress reduction activities

Uses community resources for counseling, education, and/or job-training skills

- Discuss activities with client and family that are feasible *to increase feelings of self-worth and being a contributing member of the family.*
- Teach stress reduction activities, such as exercise, imagery, and relaxation techniques.
- Refer patient to community services for ongoing counseling, and for needed skills or education.
- Refer family members to support groups or counseling *to provide help in understanding what self-mutilation is, how it affects the family, and learning methods of coping and support for themselves and the member who self-mutilates.*

RISK FOR SELF-MUTILATION

Risk for self-mutilation is the state in which an individual is at risk for deliberate self-injurious behavior causing tissue damage with the intent of causing nonfatal injury to attain relief of tension.[9]

Risk Factors[2-5,9]

Borderline personality disorder

Command hallucinations

Disturbed or battered child

Dysfunctional family

Feelings of depression, rejection, self-hatred, separation anxiety, guilt, depersonalization

History of physical, emotional, or sexual abuse

History of self-injury

Inability to control impulses

Inability to cope with increased tension

Mental retardation or autism

Need for sensory stimulation

Parental emotional deprivation

Psychotic state

Expected Patient Outcomes and Nursing Interventions With Rationale[1-8]

Express feelings appropriately, as evidenced by:

Names feelings being experienced

Manages anxiety

Matches expression of feeling state to person and context

- Build trust through consistency and reliability.
- Designate same staff as much as possible to work with patient.
- Create nonthreatening environment; *a sense of being safe in the environment and with people enhances ability to express feelings.*
- Assist patient to label feeling state.
- Assist patient to identify situations that precipitate feeling states.

*References 1, 3, 4, 6, 8, 10-12.

- Support use of appropriate defense mechanisms and expression of feelings *to reduce acting-out behaviors.*
- Instruct patient in the use of relaxation techniques *to reduce anxiety level.*

Experience fewer episodes of impulsive behavior, as evidenced by:
Uses resources effectively to reduce stress
Identifies consequences of behavior
Uses problem-solving skills

- Assist patient to identify perceived stressors.
- Assist patient to replace faulty interpretations of perceived stressors with reality-based interpretations.
- Explore with patient past successes in reducing stress *to capitalize use of patient's strengths.*
- Collaborate with patient in developing a plan to reduce stress; *an increase in stressors can precipitate self-mutilation.*
- Instruct patient on stress reduction techniques and assertive skills.
- Set limits on inappropriate behavior; *setting limits is helpful in differentiating appropriate behavior from inappropriate behavior.*
- Demonstrate and teach problem-solving skills.
- Assist patient to identify advantages and disadvantages of alternatives for behavior.
- Teach patient to evaluate behavior. *Increasing the patient's ability to problem solve and think through consequences expands the range of behavioral responses.*

Interact positively with family, as evidenced by:
Makes positive self-statements
Demonstrates self-differentiation
Reports satisfaction from interactions with family

- Convey unconditional positive regard.
- Facilitate an environment that will increase self-esteem.
- Assist patient in identifying positive attributes of self; *identification of strengths and repetitive positive interactions with others and the environment influence the patient's self-estimate.*
- Engage patient in values clarification, self-appraisal, and identification of ideal self *to develop a clearer sense of self-identity.*
- Point out situations in which patient overidentifies with others.
- Ascertain the extent to which the patient's self-perception is affected by his or her dysfunctional family.
- Demonstrate interpersonal skills through role play.
- Assist patient to identify positive responses from others.
- Encourage patient to carry out familial roles and responsibilities that reinforce positive feeling and interaction *to support success in and satisfaction from interaction in family.*
- Explore with patient strategies to enhance family interaction (e.g., family therapy *to decrease stressors or threats to self).*

RISK FOR SUICIDE

An individual who is at risk for suicide is at risk for self-inflicted life-threatening injury.[8]

Risk Factors[3-5,8-11]

Adolescents living in nontraditional settings (e.g., juvenile detention center, prison, half-way house, group home)
Abuse in childhood
Age: Elderly, young adult males, adolescents
Alcohol and substance use/abuse
Chronic pain
Cluster suicides
Disrupted family life
Divorce, being widowed
Economic instability
Family history of suicide
Gay or lesbian youth
Gender: male
Giving away possessions
Grief, bereavement
Guilt
Helplessness
History of prior suicide attempt
Hopelessness
Impulsiveness
Legal or disciplinary problem
Living alone
Loneliness
Loss of autonomy/independence
Loss of important relationship
Making or changing a will
Marked changes in behavior, attitude, school performance
Physical illness
Poor support systems
Presence of gun in home
Psychiatric illness/disorder (e.g., depression, schizophrenia, bipolar disorder)
Purchase of a gun
Race: Caucasian, Native American
Relocation, institutionalization
Retirement
Social isolation
Stated desire to die/end it all
Stockpiling medicines
Sudden euphoric recovery from major depression
Terminal illness
Threats of killing self

Expected Patient Outcomes and Nursing Interventions With Rationale[1-3,5-7,9,12]

Reduce risk of self-inflicted harm,[6] as evidenced by:
Maintains safety
Prevents personal injuries

- Determine whether patient has specific suicide plan identified.
- Encourage the person to make a verbal no-suicide contract.
- Determine history of suicide attempts.
- Protect patient from harming self.
- Place patient in least restrictive environment that allows for necessary level of observation.

- Demonstrate concern about patient's welfare.
- Refrain from negatively criticizing.
- Remove dangerous items from the patient's environment.
- Place patient in room with protective window coverings, as appropriate. Observe closely during suicidal crisis. Instruct patient and significant other in signs, symptoms, and basic physiology of depression.
- Instruct family that suicidal risk increases for severely depressed patients as they begin to feel better.
- Facilitate discussion of factors or events that precipitated the suicidal thoughts.
- Escort patient during off-ward activities, as appropriate.
- Provide psychiatric counseling, as appropriate.
- Facilitate support of patient by family and friends. Instruct family on possible warning signs or pleas for help patient may use.
- Refer patient to psychiatrist, as needed.

Acknowledge feelings of hopelessness and helplessness, as evidenced by:

Identifies factors that contribute to feelings of hopelessness and helplessness

Acknowledges subjective concerns or fears

- Establish therapeutic relationship.
- Conduct in-depth assessment of needs.[2]
- Explore feelings, *to identify risk factors.*
- Validate feelings and assist patient to channel feelings appropriately. *Negative feelings need to be appropriately placed and not internalized.*
- Encourage the patient to express hope, *to assist with coping.*

Acknowledge feelings of loss related to changes in lifestyle or living conditions, as evidenced by:

Acknowledges losses that accompany changes in lifestyle or living conditions

- Promote therapeutic relationship with patient *to encourage ongoing expression of feelings of distress related to changes.*
- Assess for losses that have occurred.
- Encourage patient and family to share mutual feelings and perceptions of loss, including impact of changes in lifestyle and living conditions.
- Recognize influence of past coping mechanisms on patient's current adaptation, *to assist with effective coping.*

References

Self-Perception–Self-Concept

1. Gordon M: *Manual of nursing diagnosis,* ed 9, St. Louis, 2000, Mosby.

Anxiety

1. Bakey AA, Levy JK, Fernandez F: Diagnosis and management of anxiety in the geriatric patient, *Clin Geriatr* 6(8):10, 1998.
2. Brunette M, Drake RE: Gender differences in homeless persons with schizophrenia and substance abuse, *Community Ment Health J* 34(6):627, 1998.
3. Folks DG: Management of anxiety in the long-term care setting, *Ann Long Term Care* 7(2):44, 1999.
4. Lilja Y, Ryden S, Fridlund B: Effects of extended preoperative information on perioperative stress: an anaesthetic nurse intervention for patients with breast cancer and total hip replacement, *Intensive Crit Care Nurs* 14(6):276, 1998.
5. McCloskey JC, Bulechek GM, editors: Calming technique: Preparatory sensory information. In *Nursing interventions classification (NIC),* ed 3, St. Louis, 2001, Mosby.
6. McFarland GK, Wasli EL, Gerety EK: *Nursing diagnoses and process in psychiatric mental health nursing,* ed 3, Philadelphia, 1997, JB Lippincott.
7. North American Nursing Diagnosis Association: *Nursing diagnoses: definitions and classification 2001-2002,* Philadelphia, 2001, The Association.
8. Phillips KD, Morrow JH: Nursing management of anxiety in HIV infection, *Issues in Ment Health Nurs* 19(4):375, 1998.
9. Plehn K, Peterson RA, Williams DA: Anxiety sensitivity: its relationship to functional status in patients with chronic pain, *J Occup Rehabil* 8(3):213, 1998.
10. Schweer DK, Hart LK, Glick OJ et al: The willingness of family members of critically ill adults to learn the coping technique of imagery, *J Holist Nurs* 17(1):71, 1999.
11. Taylor C, Lillis C, LeMone P: *Fundamentals of nursing: the art and science of nursing care,* ed 4, Philadelphia, 2001, JB Lippincott.
12. Thorne SE, Harris SR, Hislop TG et al: The experience of waiting for diagnosis after an abnormal mammogram, *Breast J* 5(1):42, 1999.
13. Turner JG, Clark AJ, Gauthier DK et al: The effect of therapeutic touch on pain and anxiety in burn patients, *J Adv Nurs* 28(1):10, 1998.
14. White JH, Litovitz G: A comparison of inpatient and outpatient women with eating disorders, *Arch Psychiatr Nurs* 12(4):181, 1998.

Death Anxiety

1. Ackley BJ, Ladwig GB: *Nursing diagnosis handbook: a guide for planning care,* St. Louis, 1999, Mosby.
2. Carpenito LJ: *Handbook of nursing diagnosis,* ed 8, Philadelphia, 1999, JB Lippincott.
3. Circirellli VG: Personal meanings of death in relation to fear of death, *Death Stud* 22(8):713, 1998.
4. Ireland M, Malgady RG: Thematic instrument for measuring death anxiety in children (TIMDAC), *J Pediatr Nurs* 14(1):28, 1999.
5. North American Nursing Diagnosis Association: *Nursing diagnoses: definitions and classification 2001-2002,* Philadelphia, 2001, The Association.
6. O'Gorman SM: Death and dying in contemporary society: an evaluation of current attitudes and the rituals associated with death and dying and their relevance to recent understandings of health and healing, *J Adv Nurs* 27(6):1127, 1998.

Disturbed Body Image

1. Ackley B, Ladwig GB: *Nursing diagnosis handbook: a guide to planning care,* St. Louis, 1999, Mosby.
2. Adami GF, Gandolfo P, Compostano A et al: Body image and body weight in obese patients, *Int J Eat Disord* 24(3):299, 1998.
3. Clegg A: Face value . . . disfigurement, *Nurs Times* 94(30):30, 1998.
4. Cohen MZ, Kahn DL, Steeves RH: Beyond body image: the experience of breast cancer, *Oncol Nurs Forum* 25(5):835, 1998.
5. McCloskey JC, Bulechek GM, editors: Body image enhancement. In *Nursing interventions classification (NIC),* ed 3, St. Louis, 2001, Mosby.
6. McFarland GK, Wasli EL, Gerety EK: *Nursing diagnoses and process in psychiatric mental health nursing,* ed 3, Philadelphia, 1997, JB Lippincott.

7. Norris J, Kunes-Connell M, Spelic SS: A grounded theory of reimaging, *Adv Nurs Sci* 20(3):1, 1998.
8. North American Nursing Diagnosis Association: *Nursing diagnoses: definitions and classification 2001-2002,* Philadelphia, 2001, The Association.
9. Price B: Cancer: altered body image, *Nurs Stand* 12(21):49, 1998.
10. Price B: Explorations in body image care: Peplau and practice knowledge, *J Psychiatr Ment Health Nurs* 5(3):179, 1998.
11. Thomas D: An unhealthy obsession with body image, *Practice Nurse* 7(4):252, 1999.
12. Wiseman CV, Turco RM, Sunday SR et al: Smoking and body image concerns in adolescent girls, *Int J Eat Disord* 24(4):429, 1998.

Disturbed Personal Identity

1. Ackley B, Ladwig GB: *Nursing diagnosis handbook: a guide to planning care,* St. Louis, 1999, Mosby.
2. Fontaine KL, Fletcher JS: *Mental health nursing,* Menlo Park, Calif, 1999, Addison-Wesley.
3. Goldman JB, MacClean HM: The significance of identity in the adjustment to diabetes among insulin users, *Diabetes Educa* 24(6):741, 1998.
4. McCloskey JC, Bulechek GM, editors: Self-esteem enhancement. In *Nursing interventions classification (NIC),* ed 3, St. Louis, 2001, Mosby.
5. McFarland GK, Wasli EL, Gerety EK: *Nursing diagnoses and process in psychiatric mental health nursing,* ed 3, Philadelphia, 1997, JB Lippincott.
6. North American Nursing Diagnosis Association: *Nursing diagnoses: definitions and classification 2001-2002,* Philadelphia, 2001, The Association.
7. Paquette M, Rodemich C: *Psychiatric nursing diagnosis care plans for DSM-IV,* Boston, 1997, Jones & Bartlett.
8. Robertson AE: The mental health experiences of gay men: a research study exploring gay men's health needs, *J Psychiatr Ment Health Nurs* 5(1):33, 1998.

Fear

1. Eisen A, Weber BL: Prophylactic mastectomy—the price of fear, *N Engl J Med* 340(2):137, 1999.
2. Granberg A, Engberg IB, Lundberg D: Patients' experience of being critically ill or severely injured and cared for in an intensive care unit in relation to the ICU syndrome. Part 1, *Intensive Crit Care Nurs* 14(6):294, 1998.
3. Heikkila J, Paunomen M, Virtanen V et al: Gender differences in fears related to coronary arteriography, *Heart Lung* 28(1):20, 1999.
4. Howland J, Lackman ME, Peterson EW et al: Covariates of fear of falling and associated activity curtailment, *Gerontologist* 38(5):549, 1998.
5. Kuuppelomaki M, Lauri S: Cancer patients' reported experiences of suffering, *Cancer Nurs* 21(5):364, 1998.
6. McCloskey JC, Bulechek GM, editors: Preparatory sensory information. In *Nursing interventions classification (NIC),* ed 3, St. Louis, 2001, Mosby.
7. McFarland GK, Wasli EL, Gerety EK: *Nursing diagnoses and process in psychiatric mental health nursing,* ed 3, Philadelphia, 1997, JB Lippincott.
8. Menzel LK: Factors related to the emotional responses of intubated patients being unable to speak, *Heart Lung* 27(4):245, 1998.
9. North American Nursing Diagnosis Association: *Nursing diagnoses: definitions and classification 2001-2002,* Philadelphia, 2001, The Association.
10. Northouse LL, Schafer JA, Tipton J et al: The concerns of patients and spouses after the diagnosis of colon cancer: a qualitative analysis, *J WOCN* 26(1):8, 1999.
11. Shalansky C, Ericson J, Henderson A: Abused women and child custody: the ongoing exposure to abusive ex-partners, *J Adv Nurs* 29(2):416, 1999.

Hopelessness

1. Cook JM, Ahrens AH, Pearson JL: Hopelessness: a mediator or moderator of depression in Alzheimer's disease caregivers? *J Ment Health Aging* 2(1):5, 1996.
2. Cutliffe JR: Hope, counseling and complicated bereavement reaction, *J Adv Nurs* 28(4):754, 1998.
3. Dow JS, Mest CG: Psychosocial interventions for patients with chronic obstructive pulmonary disease, *Home Healthcare Nurse* 15(6):414, 1997.
4. Johnson LH, Roberts SL: Hopelessness in the myocardial infarction patient, *Prog Cardiovasc Nurs* 11(2):19, 1996.
5. Johnson LH, Dahlen R, Roberts SL: Supporting hope in congestive heart failure patients, *Dimens Crit Care Nurs* 16(2):65, 1997.
6. Johnson LH, Roberts SL, Cheffer ND: A hope and hopelessness model applied to the family of a multitrauma injury patient, *J Trauma Nurs* 3(3):72, 1996.
7. May J, Baldwin CM: Parental voices: expression of circular hopelessness, *J Multicultur Nurs Health* 4(2):52, 1998.
8. McCloskey JC, Bulechek GM, editors: Hope instillation. In *Nursing interventions classification (NIC),* ed 3, St. Louis, 2001, Mosby.
9. McDonald ER, Hillel A, Wiedenfeld SA: Evaluation of the psychological status of ventilatory-supported patients with ALS/MND, *Palliat Med* 10(1):35, 1996.
10. McFarland GK, Wasli EL, Gerety EK: *Nursing diagnoses and process in psychiatric mental health nursing,* ed 3, Philadelphia, 1997, JB Lippincott.
11. North American Nursing Diagnosis Association: *Nursing diagnoses: definitions and classification 2001-2002,* Philadelphia, 2001, The Association.
12. Uncapher H, Gallagher-Thompson D, Osgoode NJ et al: Hopelessness and suicidal ideation in older adults, *Gerontologist* 38(1):62, 1998.

Low Self-Esteem, Chronic Low Self-Esteem, Situational Low Self-Esteem

1. Campbell JC, Soeken KL: Women's responses to battering: a test of the model, *Res Nurs Health* 22(1):49, 1999.
2. Chang AM, Mackenzie AE: State self-esteem following stroke, *Stroke.* 29(11):2325, 1998.
3. Connelly CD: Hopefulness, self-esteem, and perceived social support among pregnant and nonpregnant adolescents, *West J Nurs Res* 20(12):195, 1998.
4. Davis KB, Daniels M, See LA: The psychological effects of skin color on African Americans' self-esteem, *J Hum Behav Soc Environ* 1(2/3):63, 1998.
5. Doswell WM, Millor GK, Thompson H et al: Self-image and self-esteem in African-American preteen girls: implications for mental health, *Issues Ment Health Nurs* 19(1):71, 1998.
6. Gardner LH, Frank DI, Amankwaa L: A comparison of sexual behavior and self-esteem in young adult females with positive and negative tests for sexually transmitted diseases, *ABNF J* 9(4):89, 1998.
7. Geller J, Johnson C, Madsen K et al: Shape- and weight-based self-esteem and the eating disorders, *Int J Eat Disord* 24(3):285, 1998.
8. Herrmann MM, VanCleve L, Levisen L: Parenting competence, social support, and self-esteem in teen mothers case managed by public health nurses, *Public Health Nurs* 15(6):432, 1998.

9. Huurre TM, Komulainen EJ, Aro HM: Social support and self-esteem among adolescents with visual impairments, *J Vis Impair Blindness* 93(1):26, 1999.
10. Intili H, Nier D: Self-esteem and depression in men who present with erectile dysfunction, *Urol Nurs* 18(3):185, 1998.
11. Jones SL, Moulton MA, Moulton P et al: Self-esteem differences as a function of race and weight preoccupation: findings and implications, *Womens Health Issues* 9(1):50, 1999.
12. McFarland GK, Wasli EL, Gerety EK: *Nursing diagnoses and process in psychiatric mental health nursing,* ed 3, Philadelphia, 1997, JB Lippincott.
13. Menzel LK: Ventilated patients' self-esteem during intubation and after extubation, *Clin Nurs Res* 8(1):51, 1999.
14. Modrcin-Talbott MA, Pullen L, Ehrenberger H et al: Self-esteem in adolescents treated in an outpatient mental health setting, *Issues Compr Pediatr Nurs* 21(3):159, 1998.
15. North American Nursing Diagnosis Association: *Nursing diagnoses: definitions and classification 2000-2001,* Philadelphia, 2001, The Association.
16. Nyamathi A, Keenan C, Bayley L: Differences in personal, cognitive, psychosocial, and social factors associated with drug and alcohol use and nonuse in homeless women, *Res Nurs Health* 21(6): 525, 1998.
17. Reichenbach V: From secrecy to self-esteem: addressing incontinence can restore dignity and independence to clients, *OT Pract* 3(5):26, 1998.
18. Thompson B: Alive and kicking: increasing self-esteem among women living in deprivation, *Pract Midwife* 2(2):32, 1999.
19. Van Dongen CJ: Self-esteem among persons with severe mental illness, *Issues Ment Health Nurs* 19(1):29, 1998.
20. Wang X, Crosby LG, Harris MG et al: Major concerns and needs of breast cancer patients, *Cancer Nurs* 22(2):157, 1999.
21. Youngkin EQ, Henry JK, Gracely-Kilgore K: Women with HSV and HPV: a strategy to increase self-esteem, *Clin Excel Nurse Pract* 2(6):370, 1998.

Risk for Situational Low Self-Esteem

1. Ackley B, Ladwig G: *Nursing diagnosis handbook: a guide to planning care,* ed 4, St. Louis, 1999, Mosby.
2. Gerard M: Domestic violence: how to screen and intervene, *RN* 63(12):52, 2000.
3. Groh CJ, Whall AL: Self-esteem disturbance. In Mass ML, Buckwalter KC, Hardy MD et al: *Nursing care of older adults: diagnoses, outcomes and interventions,* St. Louis, 2001, Mosby.
4. McCloskey JC, Bulechek GM, editors: *Nursing interventions classification (NIC),* ed 3, St. Louis, 2001, Mosby.
5. North American Nursing Diagnosis Association: *NANDA nursing diagnoses: definitions and classification 2001-2002,* Philadelphia, 2001, The Association.

Powerlessness

1. Benjamin D: Powerlessness in chronic illness, *Prairie Rose* 65(4): 9a, 1997.
2. Dunn JD: Powerlessness regarding health-service barriers: construction of an instrument, *Nurs Diagnosis J Nurs Lang Classification* 9(4):136, 1998.
3. Gallagher SM: Powerlessness as a factor in health defeating behavior, *Ostomy Wound Manage* 43(2):34, 1997.
4. Gibson JM, Kenrick M: Pain and powerlessness: the experience of living with peripheral vascular disease, *J Adv Nurs* 27(4):737, 1998.
5. Johnson ME: Being restrained: a study of power and powerlessness, *Issues Ment Health Nurs* 19(3):191, 1998.
6. Keaveny ME, Zauszniewski JA: Life events and psychological well-being in women sentenced to prison, *Issues Ment Health Nurs* 20(1):73, 1999.
7. Kubsch S, Wichowski H: Restoring power through nursing intervention, *Nurs Diagnosis J Nurs Lang Classification* 8(1):7, 1997.
8. Lubkin HM: *Chronic illness: impact and interventions,* ed 4, Boston, 1999, Jones & Bartlett.
9. McFarland GK, Wasli EL, Gerety EK: *Nursing diagnoses and process in psychiatric mental health nursing,* ed 3, Philadelphia, 1997, JB Lippincott.
10. Miller JF: *Powerlessness: coping with chronic illness,* Philadelphia, 1983, FA Davis.
11. North American Nursing Diagnosis Association: *Nursing diagnoses: definitions and classification 2001-2002,* Philadelphia, 2001, The Association.
12. Thomas S, Smucker C, Droppleman P: It hurts most around the heart: a phenomenological exploration of women's anger, *J Adv Nurs* 28(2):311, 1998.
13. Tolley M: Power to the patient, *J Gerontol Nurs* 23(10):7, 1997.

Risk for Powerlessness

1. Carpenito LJ: *Nursing diagnosis: application to practice,* ed 8, Philadelphia, 2000, JB Lippincott.
2. Davidhizar RE, Giger JN: Powerlessness. In Maas ML, Buckwalter KC, Hardy MD et al: *Nursing care of older adults: diagnoses, outcomes & interventions,* St. Louis, 2001, Mosby.
3. Gibson JM, Kenrick M: Pain and powerlessness: the experience of living with peripheral vascular disease, *J Adv Nurs* 27(4):737, 1998.
4. Kubsch S, Wichowski HC: Restoring power through nursing intervention, *Nurs Diagnosis J Nurs Lang* Classification 8(1):7, 1997.
5. McCloskey JC, Bulechek GM, editors: *Nursing interventions classification (NIC),* ed 3, St. Louis, 2001, Mosby.
6. McFarland GK, Wasli EL, Gerety EK: Nursing diagnosis and process in psychiatric mental health nursing, ed 3, Philadelphia, 1997, JB Lippincott.
7. North American Nursing Diagnosis Association: *NANDA nursing diagnoses: definitions and classification 2001-2002,* Philadelphia, 2001, The Association.
8. Orne RM, Fishman SJ, Manka M et al: Living on the edge: a phenomenological study of medically uninsured working Americans, *Res Nurs Health* 23(3):204, 2000.
9. Shih S, Shih F, Chen C et al: The forgotten faces: the lonely journey of powerlessness experienced by elderly single Chinese men with heart disease in Taiwan, *Geriatr Nurs* 21(5):254, 2000.

Risk for Loneliness

1. Ackley B, Ladwig GB: *Nursing diagnosis handbook: a guide to planning care,* St. Louis, 1999, Mosby.
2. Andersson L: Loneliness research and interventions: a review of the literature, *Aging Ment Health* 2(4):264, 1998.
3. Asher SR, Gazelle H: Loneliness, peer relations, and language disorders in childhood, *Top Lang Disord* 19(2):16, 1999.
4. Bondevik M: The oldest old and personal activities of daily living: associations with loneliness, *Health Care Later Life* 2(1):14, 1997.
5. Bondevik M, Skogstad A: The oldest old, ADL, social network, and loneliness, *West J Nurs Res* 20(3):325, 1998.
6. Carpenito LJ: *Handbook of nursing diagnosis,* ed 8, Philadelphia, 1999, JB Lippincott.
7. Johnson J: Older rural adults and the decision to stop driving: the influence of family and friends, *J Community Health Nurs* 15(4):205, 1998.
8. Killeen C: Loneliness: an epidemic in modern society, *J Adv Nurs* 28(4):762, 1998.
9. Klein TM: Adolescent pregnancy and loneliness, *Public Health Nurs* 15(5):338, 1998.

10. Mahon NE, Yarcheski A, Yarcheski TJ: An empirical test of alternate explanations of loneliness in young adults, *J Nurs Sci* 2(1-6):9, 1997.
11. McCloskey JC, Bulechek GM, editors: Socialization enhancement. In *Nursing interventions classification (NIC)*, ed 3, St. Louis, 2001, Mosby.
12. North American Nursing Diagnosis Association: *Nursing diagnoses: definitions and classification 2001-2002,* Philadelphia, 2001, The Association.

Self-Mutilation

1. Alam M: Students at risk. Self-mutilation *School Nurse News* 17(1):18, 2000.
2. Bauserman SA: Treatment of persons who self-mutilate with dialectical behavior therapy, *Psychiatr Rehabil Skills* 2(2):149, 1998.
3. Clarke L, Whittaker M: Self-mutilation: culture, contexts and nursing responses, *J Clin Nurs* 7(2):129, 1998.
4. Dallam SJ: The identification and management of self-mutilating patients in primary care, *Nurse Pract* 22(5):151, 1997.
5. Favaro A, Santonastaso P: Self-injurious behavior in anorexia nervosa, *J Nerv Ment Dis* 188(8):537, 2000.
6. Favazza A: Self-mutilation. In *The Harvard Medical School guide to suicide assessment and intervention,* San Francisco, 1999, Jossey-Bass.
7. Fowler JC, Hilsenroth MJ, Nolan E: Exploring the inner world of self-mutilating patients: a Rorschach investigation, *Bull Menninger Clin* 64(3):365, 2000.
8. Green CA, Knysz W, Tsuang MT: A homeless person with bipolar disorder and a history of serious self-mutilation, *Am J Psychiatry* 157(9):1392, 2000.
9. Horsfall J: Towards understanding some complex borderline behaviors, *J Psychiatr Ment Health Nurs* 6(6):525, 1999.
10. Ingram TN: Risk for violence: self-directed or directed at others. In Maas ML, Buckwalter KC, Hardy MD et al: *Nursing care of older adults: diagnoses, outcomes and interventions,* St. Louis, 2001, Mosby.
11. McCloskey JC, Bulechek GM, editors: *Nursing interventions classification (NIC),* ed 3, St. Louis, 2001, Mosby.
12. McFarland GK, Wasli EL, Gerety EK: *Nursing diagnosis and process in psychiatric mental health nursing,* ed 3, Philadelphia, 1997, JB Lippincott.
13. North American Nursing Diagnosis Association: *NANDA nursing diagnoses: definitions and classification 2001-2002,* Philadelphia, 2001, The Association.

Risk for Self-Mutilation

1. Ackley B, Ladwig GB: *Nursing diagnosis handbook: a guide to planning care,* St. Louis, 1999, Mosby.
2. Barstow DG: Self-injury and self-mutilation: nursing approaches, *J Psychosoc Nurs Ment Health Serv* 33(2):19, 1995.
3. Clarke L, Whittaker M: Self-mutilation: culture, contexts, and nursing responses, *J Clin Nurs* 7(2):129, 1998.
4. Dallam SJ: The identification and management of self-mutilating patients in primary care, *Nurse Pract* 22(5):151, 1997.
5. Faye P: Addictive characteristics of the behavior of self-mutilation, *J Psychosoc Nurs Ment Health Serv* 33(6):36, 1995.
6. Loughrey L, Jackson J, Molla P et al: Patient self-mutilation: when nursing becomes a nightmare, *J Psychosoc Nurs Ment Health Serv* 35(4):30, 1997.
7. McFarland GK, Wasli EL, Gerety EK: *Nursing diagnoses and process in psychiatric mental health nursing,* ed 3, Philadelphia, 1997, JB Lippincott.
8. News in mental health nursing: making sense of self-mutilation, *J Psychosoc Nurs Ment Health Serv* 36(9):i, 1998.
9. North American Nursing Diagnosis Association: *Nursing diagnoses: definitions and classification 2001-2002,* Philadelphia, 2001, The Association.

Risk for Suicide

1. Arbore P: Assessing the risk for suicide in the elderly, *Home Healthcare Consultant* 5(5):23, 1998.
2. Barker P, Cutcliffe J: Creating a hopeline for suicidal people: a new model for acute sector mental health nursing, *Ment Health Care Learning Disabil* 3:190, 2000.
3. Glogoski-Williams C: Recognition of depression in the older adult, *Occup Ther Ment Health* 15(2):17, 2000.
4. Harwitz D, Racizza L: Suicide and depression, *Emerg Med Clin North Am* 18:263, 2000.
5. Jiwanlal SS, Weizel C: The suicide myth, *RN* 64:33, 2001.
6. McCloskey JC, Bulechek GM, editors: *Nursing interventions classification (NIC),* ed 3, St. Louis, 2001, Mosby.
7. McFarland GK, McFarlane EA: *Nursing diagnosis and intervention: planning for patient care,* ed 3, St. Louis, 1997, Mosby.
8. North American Nursing Diagnoses Association: *NANDA definitions and classification 2001-2002,* Philadelphia, 2001, The Association.
9. Russell D, Judd F: Why are men killing themselves? A look at the evidence, *Aust Fam Physician* 28:791, 1999.
10. Smith JE, Early JA, Green PT et al: Risk for suicide and risk for violence: a case for separating the current violence diagnoses, *Nurs Diagnosis* 8:67, 1997.
11. Smochek MR, Oblaczynski C, Lauck DL et al: Interventions for risk for suicide and risk for violence, *Nurs Diagnosis* 11:60, 2000.
12. Workman CG, Prior M: Depression and suicide in young children, *Issues Compr Pediatr Nurs* 20:125, 1997.

8 FUNCTIONAL HEALTH PATTERN

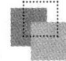

Role-Relationship[1]

ANTICIPATORY GRIEVING

Anticipatory grieving is the intellectual and emotional responses and behaviors by which individuals, families, [and] communities work through the process of modifying self-concept based on the perception of potential loss.[8]

Related Factors[2,5,8]

Growing older
HIV infection
Lack of social support
Multiple role loss
Perceived impending death of self
Perceived impending death of significant other
Perceived potential developmental or role-transition loss(es)
Perceived potential loss of significant person, significant pet, prized material possession(s), body part, body function, well-being, social role, hope for the future, future lifestyle
Uncertainty of loss

Defining Characteristics[2,5]

Altered communication patterns
Altered eating habits, sleep patterns, dream patterns, activity level, libido
Anger
Bargaining
Denial of potential loss
Denial of significance of the loss
Difficulty in taking on new or different roles
Expression of distress at potential loss
Guilt
Potential loss of significant object
Preoccupation
Resolution of grief before the reality of loss
Sense of unreality
Shame
Somatic manifestations: weakness, feeling of emptiness in stomach, tightness in throat, difficulty swallowing, sighing, fatigue
Sorrow
Stigma

Expected Patient Outcomes and Nursing Interventions With Rationale[1-7,9-10]

Participate in constructive anticipatory grief work, as evidenced by:

Discusses thoughts and feelings related to anticipated loss
Verbalizes information needs
Uses appropriate resources (e.g., friends, clergy, support groups, legal consultants, Social Security representatives)
Maintains constructive interpersonal relationships
Meets ongoing care needs
Verbalizes perception of ability to exist in the future without significant person or valued object
Makes realistic plans for dealing with future without significant person or valued object

- Encourage description of perceptions of potential loss.
- Encourage verbalization of fears and concerns.
- Determine the following:
  - Length of time since learning potential loss
  - Past experience with loss, illness, and death, as well as problem-solving and coping skills used; *past adaptation to loss influences current adaptation*
  - Cultural beliefs *because they influence the manner in which people express grief and adapt to an impending loss*
  - Spiritual beliefs; *past problem-solving abilities and personal beliefs influence current and future coping*
  - Socioeconomic background
  - Educational preparation
  - Current sources of social support (family, friends, church)
  - Disruptions in current lifestyle related to anticipated loss (finances, living arrangements, transportation)
- Assess for indications of suicidal ideation or intent.
- Recognize that patient and significant others may differ in stage of grieving they are experiencing.
- Acknowledge to patient and significant others that pattern of their past relationships with each other will be similar to their relationships as they experience anticipated loss.
- During stage of shock and disbelief:
  - Provide quiet environment.
  - Allow for constructive use of denial. *Recognize that denial and other similar mental mechanisms serve to increase the patient's or significant others' tolerance for potential overwhelming stress.*
  - Avoid reinforcement of pathologic denial.
  - Avoid confronting patient or significant others when they are experiencing distorted perceptions.
  - Provide opportunity for expression of emotions.
  - Provide assurance that it is normal to experience intense feelings and reactions.

Avoid defensive and judgmental responses to criticisms of health-care providers.

Do not encourage use of antianxiety medications. *Anxiolytics may interfere with the process of constructive grief work.*

Do not force decisions.

Enlist support from others (e.g., family, friends, clergy).

- During stage of developing awareness of potential loss:

  Encourage expression of feelings with relatives and friends, *keeping in mind that cultural patterns influence expression of feelings.*

  Facilitate contact with nursing staff and other health team members to correct misinformation about cause of loss.

  Facilitate exploration of available options.

  Support verbalizations about possible body image changes.

  Offer realistic hope for ability to cope with anticipated loss.

  Encourage and teach good health habits.

  Provide information on supportive and informational groups for patient and/or family.

  Encourage persons experiencing similar anticipated losses to consider spending time together to share mutual fears, feelings, and concerns. *Based on individual evaluation, initiate referral to formal support group to facilitate successful closure and to reduce potential for dysfunctional grieving.*

  Evaluate need for referral to resources (e.g., Social Security representatives, legal consultants, support groups).

- During stage of developing awareness of potential loss of significant other:

  Provide significant others with ongoing information of patient's diagnosis, prognosis, and plan of care *to decrease their feelings of uncertainty and anxiety.*

  Encourage significant others to describe their desires and information needs in caring for patient.

  Facilitate significant other's assistance with patient's physical care *to reduce feelings of helplessness and to decrease potential for future regret.*

  Facilitate flexible visiting hours and include younger children when appropriate.

  Help patient and significant others to share mutual fears, concerns, plans, and hopes with each other.

  Based on individual assessment, suggest the use of letter writing, audio or video taping *to provide encouragement for the patient when family and friends are unable to be physically present; the terminally ill patient can also use these forms of communication as a "legacy" for significant others (e.g., grandchildren, infants).*

  Offer hope to patient and significant others that they will have quality time together.

  Help significant others to understand the patient's verbalization of anger should not be perceived as personal attacks.

  Encourage significant others to maintain their own self-care needs for rest, sleep, nutrition, leisure activities, and time away from patient.

  Facilitate patient's and significant others' discussion of final arrangements (e.g., funeral services, burial wishes, organ donation, desire for autopsy).

  Teach patient and significant others to recognize and trust decisions that "feel" right to them in relation to their coping with impending losses.

- During period of mourning for anticipated loss:

  Help patient accept reality of impending loss.

  Provide information as sought *to minimize feelings of uncertainty and anxiety.*

  Allow patient to talk freely about anticipated loss. *There may be an increased preoccupation with the anticipated loss and an increased need to talk with others about the meaning of the potential loss.*

  Encourage expression of feelings (e.g., crying).

  Facilitate discussion of both negative and positive aspects of anticipated loss.

  Foster environment in which loss can be experienced within spiritual context.

  Provide guidance regarding availability of community resources.

- During period of mourning before death of loved one:

  Promote discussion of what to expect when death occurs *to decrease fear and anxiety about the unknown.*

  Encourage significant others and patient to share their wishes about family members being present with patient at death. Avoid judgmental responses to choices made.

  Help significant others to accept that choosing to be absent at death does not indicate a lack of love or caring for patient.

  Discuss indicators of impending death as appropriate.

  Provide comforting measures for patient; encourage significant others to assist if they wish.

  Encourage significant others to maintain verbal communication and touch with their loved one, even though patient may not respond, *to facilitate successful closure of the relationship.*

  Provide as much privacy as possible for significant others to be alone or with patient when death is imminent.

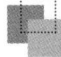

Dysfunctional Grieving

Dysfunctional grieving is the extended, unsuccessful use of intellectual and emotional responses by which individuals, families, [and] communities attempt to work through the process of modifying self-concept based upon the perception of loss.[9]

Related Factors[8,9]

Actual or perceived object loss (object loss is used in the broadest sense)

Lost objects that may include people, possessions, a job, status, home, ideals, parts and processes of the body, pregnancy

Preexisting poor self-concept

Defining Characteristics[4,9,12]

Altered: Eating habits, sleep patterns, dream patterns, activity level, libido, concentration, and/or pursuit of tasks

Anger
Crying
Denial of loss
Developmental regression
Difficulty in expressing loss
Expression of distress at loss
Expression of guilt
Expression of unresolved issues
Idealization of lost person or object
Interference with life functioning
Labile effect
Onset or exacerbation of somatic or psychosomatic responses
Overidentification with lost person, pet, or object
Prolonged interference with life functioning
Reliving of past experiences with little or no reduction (diminishment) of intensity of the grief
Repetitive use of ineffectual behaviors associated with attempts to reinvest in relationships
Sadness
Verbal expression of distress at loss

Expected Patient Outcomes and Nursing Interventions With Rationale[1-8,10,11]

Experience resolution of dysfunctional grieving, as evidenced by:
Acknowledges reality of the loss
Demonstrates emotional responses that are congruent with personal and cultural context in which loss occurred
Participates in recommended treatment modalities
Identifies alternate plans for meeting goals that were significant before the loss
Resumes or develops new social relationships and makes new emotional investments

- Avoid imposing a normative standard for manifestations and resolution of grief. *There is no specific "timetable" for successful resolution of a loss.*
- Monitor perception of current adaptation, responses from significant others, social network, life experiences, and past problem-solving and coping skills *to determine actual and potential coping strengths and deficits.*
- Evaluate influence of denial on participation with recommended treatments.
- Assess possible needs met by denial *to avoid inadvertent reinforcement of secondary gains.*
- Point out reality in nonthreatening manner without arguing with patient or significant others.
- Present patient with increasing facts.
- Defer teaching related to adaptation to loss until patient demonstrates decrease in denial.
- Monitor for suicidal ideation *to determine need for mental health referral for evaluation of need for antidepressant medication, psychotherapy, or admission to inpatient psychiatric unit for treatment.*
- Clarify and offer missing factual information *to facilitate corrections of distorted perceptions.*
- Provide opportunity for patient to describe experiences that preceded current loss *to increase awareness of thoughts and feelings associated with actual loss.*
- Encourage description of current and anticipated problems related to loss.
- Point out universality of need for normal grieving.
- Facilitate constructive working through of expression of feelings *to decrease indirect expression of grief through behavioral problems or physical illness.*
- Facilitate contact with people who can openly express feelings.
- Assist patient to reality test feelings of guilt *to minimize irrational guilt.*
- Promote therapeutic use of humor *to encourage patient to experience laughter and joy without feeling guilt.*
- Encourage patient to talk and reminisce about loss *to facilitate exploration of feelings of hurt, anger, and disappointment.*
- Convey unconditional acceptance of patient's communication of behaviors and feelings that may be viewed as socially or culturally unacceptable *to prevent grief stagnation and fixation on loss.*
- Facilitate review of positive and negative aspects of loss *to decrease ambivalence.*
- Evaluate need for referral to resources (e.g., brief psychotherapy, support groups, family therapy, spiritual counselor).
- Promote patient's recognition of past and present strengths that can be used for coping with current loss.
- Promote description of additional potential strategies for coping with current loss.
- Encourage description of future expectations.
- Offer hope for successful adaptation to loss.
- Facilitate contact with others who have successfully adapted to similar loss *to provide visible proof that grief can be resolved.*
- Provide guidance about available community resources (e.g., assertiveness training, continuing education, driver education).
- Promote coordination of resources *to help patient develop new skills, make readjustments in lifestyle, and make new emotional investments.*

Caregiver Role Strain

Caregiver role strain is the state in which an individual experiences difficulty in performing the caregiver role.[6]

Related Factors

Resources
Caregiver not developmentally ready for caregiver role
Inadequate community services
Inadequate equipment for providing care
Inadequate transportation
Insufficient finances
Insufficient information
Lack of recreational resources
Lack of respite resources
Lack of support from significant others

Roles and relationships
Change in relationship
History of family dysfunction
History of marginal family coping
Unrealistic expectations of caregiver by care receiver

Social

Alienation from family, friends, and coworkers
Insufficient recreation

Individual

Illness chronicity
Instability of care receiver's health
Problem behaviors
Psychologic or cognitive problems in care receiver

Caregiver

Addiction or codependency
Amount of activities
Inability to fulfill own or others' expectations
Ongoing changes in activities
Psychologic or cognitive problems
Twenty-four hour care responsibility
Unpredictability of care situation
Unrealistic expectations of self

Situational

Caregiver's competing role commitments
Complexity/amount of caregiving tasks
Family/caregiver isolation
Inadequate physical environment for providing care (e.g., housing, transportation, community services, equipment)
Inexperience with caregiving
Presence of abuse or violence

Expected Patient Outcomes and Nursing Interventions With Rationale[1-5,7-11]

The caregiver states appropriate informal or formal resources, as evidenced by:

Lists and describes such formal resources as the public health nurse, day care, respite care, hospice, and informal resources, such as church groups, social clubs, or neighbors

- Review caregiver's knowledge of available resources; *competency level of the caregiver can be enhanced by increasing his or her knowledge base of resources available and teaching basic caregiving skills.*
- Establish financial eligibility to obtain community resources.
- Determine caregiver's and care receiver's willingness to accept resource support.
- Evaluate current family network.
- Assist in referral process, as appropriate.

The caregiver uses stress reduction strategies, as evidenced by:

Verbalizes that stress is reduced and that stress reduction techniques are incorporated into daily routine.

- Establish a pattern of "timeout" from caregiver role.
- Provide information and access to relaxation tapes, guided imagery exercises, meditation and biofeedback techniques; *modalities must be selected appropriately to meet the unique individual needs of the caregiver.*
- Teach time management strategies.
- Encourage involvement in church and in social activities.
- Provide information, and refer caregivers to community support groups; *opportunities for caregivers with varied levels of experience to network/share information may be valuable.*
- Provide time for active listening to caregiver's concerns.
- Validate caregiver's feelings of role strain.
- Encourage consistent health monitoring for caregiver.
- Monitor for caregiver depression.

The caregiver verbalizes change in role expectations, as evidenced by:

Prioritizes role demands and experiences less role strain

- Examine usual roles within the family system; compare past, present, and future relationships within the unit; *a positive relationship between caregiver and care receiver correlates with less role strain.*
- Identify the various roles in which the caregiver engages.
- Assist the caregiver to negotiate roles with other family members.
- Educate the family about the process of caregiving; *the competency level of the caregiver can be enhanced by increasing his or her knowledge base and skill level.*
- Assist family members in dealing with the disengaged member and with the changes of status within the family unit.
- Acknowledge and validate the caregiver role; *caregivers want to be acknowledged and appreciated.*

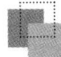

Risk for Caregiver Role Strain

Risk for caregiver role strain is the state in which a caregiver is vulnerable for felt difficulty in performing the family caregiver role.[6]

Risk Factors[1,6,7]

Addiction or codependency
Care receiver exhibits deviant, bizarre behavior
Caregiver's competing role requirements
Caregiver health impairment
Caregiver is female
Caregiver is spouse
Caregiver not developmentally ready for caregiver role (e.g., a young adult needs to provide care for middle-age parent)
Complexity/amount of caregiving tasks
Developmental delay or retardation of the care receiver or caregiver
Discharge of family member with significant home care needs
Duration of caregiving required
Family/caregiver isolation
Illness severity of the care receiver
Inadequate physical environment for providing care (e.g., housing, transportation, community services, equipment)
Inexperience with caregiving
Lack of respite and recreation for caregiver
Marginal caregiver's coping patterns
Marginal family adaptation or dysfunction before the caregiving situation
Past history of poor relationship between caregiver and care receiver
Premature birth/congenital defect
Presence of abuse or violence
Presence of situational stressors that normally affect families (e.g., significant loss, disaster or crisis, economic vulnerability, major life events)
Psychologic or cognitive problems in care receiver

Unpredictable illness course or instability in the care receiver's health

Expected Patient (Caretaker) Outcomes and Nursing Interventions With Rationale[1-5,7,8]

Identify appropriate community resources and family dynamics, as evidenced by:

Verbalizes resources for specific care needs
Identifies existing strengths and weaknesses in family dynamics
Identifies potential stressors

- Discuss range and availability of community resources appropiate for both present and future needs; *a plan for use of appropriate resources needs to be identified to diminish inappropriate decisions.*
- Discuss financial eligibility requirements for resources.
- Evaluate willingness of caregiver to accept resource support.
- Discuss and evaluate circumstances in which resources might be incorporated into the care regimen. *Competency level of the caregiver can be enhanced by increasing his or her knowledge base of resources available and teaching basic caregiving skills.*
- Evaluate family and social support network.
- Discuss and provide information about appropriate support groups.
- Encourage caregiver to participate in a support group; *opportunities for caregivers with varied levels of experience to network/share information may be valuable.*
- Identify the family relationship between caregiver and care receiver. *A positive relationship between caregiver and care receiver correlates with less role strain.*
- Identify past methods of coping with crisis.
- Offer family or individual therapy for resolution of conflict and unresolved issues.

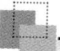

Chronic Sorrow

Chronic sorrow is a cyclic, recurring, and potentially progressive pattern of pervasive sadness that is experienced [by a patient (parent or caregiver, or individual with chronic illness or disability)] in response to continual loss, throughout the trajectory of an illness or disability.[10]

Related Factors[4,10]

Death of a loved one
Person experiencing chronic physical or mental illness or disability such as mental retardation, multiple sclerosis, prematurity, spina bifida or other birth defects, chronic mental illness, infertility, cancer, Parkinson's disease
Person experiencing one or more trigger events (e.g., crises in management of the illness, crises related to developmental stages, and missed opportunities that bring comparisons with developmental, social, or personal norms)
Unending caregiving as a constant reminder of loss

Defining Characteristics[5,10]

Expressed periodic, recurrent feelings of sadness
Expression of one or more of the following feelings: anger, being misunderstood, confusion, depression, disappointment, emptiness, fear, frustration, guilt/self-blame, helplessness, hopelessness, loneliness, low self-esteem, recurring loss, being overwhelmed
Feelings that vary in intensity, are periodic, may progress and intensify over time, and may interfere with the patient's ability to reach his or her highest level of personal and social well-being

Expected Patient Outcomes and Nursing Interventions With Rationale[1-9,11]

Accept ongoing, episodic presence of sorrow (sadness), as evidenced by:

Verbalizes that sorrow will be ongoing
Identifies triggers that intensify the experience of sorrow
Identifies personal strengths in coping with episodic sadness

- Discuss the difference between grief and chronic sorrow, and clarify that although feelings of sadness will fluctuate over the years, the sorrow will not disappear. *Grieving has a time limit and ends with adaptation to a loss, whereas chronic sorrow persists as long as the person lives.*[4]
- Discuss significant dates and milestones that may serve as triggers for the experience of greater sorrow, such as birthdays, anniversaries, high-school graduations, pregnant women. *Triggers are events that intensify feelings of sadness, guilt, anger, frustration, and fear; these occur periodically throughout the lives of people experiencing chronic loss and sorrow.*[5]
- Ask patient to describe personal strengths and methods of coping with sadness, including keeping busy, going away, taking one day at a time, joining a support group, crying, and praying, *because these activities have been found to be helpful in coping with chronic sorrow.*
- Encourage the patient to share feelings about the change or loss verbally in storytelling. *Sharing the loss as a narrative story helps put the experience in a more accepting and facilitative way*
- Use reminiscence therapy in the older patient *as a method of reviewing past experiences and effective coping methods.*
- Identify and request appropriate support for the isolated older adult without family or significant other.
- Encourage the use of spiritual support rituals that are personally and culturally relevant to the patient *to provide emotional comfort and strength.*
- Link patients and family members with appropriate community resources, such as home health, social services, and respite care.
- If sorrow is intense and debilitating, refer the patient for mental health counseling.

Dysfunctional Family Processes: Alcoholism

Dysfunctional family processes: alcoholism is the state in which the psychosocial, spiritual, and physiologic functions of the family unit are chronically disorganized, leading to conflict, denial of problems, resistance to change, ineffective problem solving, and a series of self-perpetuating crises.[8]

Related Factors[4,8]

Abuse of alcohol
Addictive personality
Biochemical influences
Family history of alcoholism
Genetic predisposition
Inadequate coping skills
Lack of problem-solving skills
Resistance to treatment

Defining Characteristics[4,8,10]

Roles and relationships

- Altered role function/disruption of family roles
- Chronic family problems
- Closed communication systems
- Deterioration in family relationships/disturbed family dynamics
- Disrupted family rituals
- Economic problems
- Family denial
- Family does not demonstrate respect for individuality and autonomy of members
- Family unable to meet security needs of its members
- Inadequate coping skills
- Inconsistent parenting/low perception of parental support
- Ineffective spouse communication/marital problems
- Intimacy dysfunction
- Lack of skills necessary for relationships
- Neglected obligations
- Pattern of rejection
- Reduced ability of family members to relate to each other for mutual growth and maturation
- Triangulating family relationships

Behavioral

- Agitation
- Alcohol, nicotine, or drug abuse
- Blaming
- Controlling communication/power struggles
- Criticizing
- Dependency
- Difficulty with intimate relationships
- Disturbances in academic performance in children or adolescents
- Disturbances in concentration
- Enabling to maintain drinking
- Harsh self-judgement
- Impaired communication
- Inability to adapt to change
- Inability to deal with traumatic experiences constructively
- Inability to express or accept wide range of feelings
- Inability to meet emotional needs of family members
- Inability to meet spiritual needs of family members
- Inadequate understanding or knowledge of alcoholism
- Ineffective problem-solving skills
- Inappropriate expression of anger
- Isolation
- Lack of dealing with conflict
- Lack of reliability
- Loss of control of drinking
- Lying
- Manipulation
- Orientation toward tension relief rather than achievement of goals
- Rationalization/denial of problems
- Refusal to get help/inability to accept and receive help appropriately
- Verbal abuse of spouse or parent

Feelings

- Anger/suppressed rage
- Anxiety or tension or distress
- Confused love and pity
- Decreased self-esteem/worthlessness
- Depression
- Dissatisfaction
- Emotional isolation/loneliness
- Failure
- Frustration
- Guilt
- Hopelessness
- Hostility
- Hurt
- Insecurity
- Lack of identity
- Lingering resentment
- Mistrust, moodiness
- Powerlessness
- Rejection
- Repressed emotions
- Responsibility for alcoholic's behavior
- Shame/embarrassment
- Unhappiness
- Vulnerability

Expected Family Outcomes and Nursing Interventions With Rationale[1-7,9,10]

Develop insights into the association of alcoholism and role relationships, communication processes, and coping mechanisms, as evidenced by:

Expedites communication within the family to share feelings and thoughts related to the impact of the alcoholic member on the family group and as individuals

Understands information about the characteristics and causes of alcoholism and corrects misinformation

- Facilitate family members in discussing and positively reinforcing adaptive coping skills in one another and in realizing that they must first help themselves by changing their own personal response
- Reinforce that family members are not responsible for the person's drinking
- Assist family members in identifying their role in enabling the alcoholic member to continue drinking (e.g., making excuses, putting to bed, bailing out of jail), and discuss strategies to avoid enabling behaviors
- Encourage the family to discuss that which has been covert in the past (e.g., avoidance, silence, denial, ignoring, distancing self, isolation) or overt (e.g., threats, hiding alcohol or car keys, crying, rigidity)

- Give examples of confusing, contradictory, and paradoxic communication, as well as broken promises that have contributed to lack of trust, consistency, predictability, and reliability
- Assist family members in expressing anger in an appropriate manner and encourage their willingness to support the alcoholic person to obtain necessary treatment
- Inform the family that the person is responsible for his or her drinking behavior and that family attempts to control the drinking prevent the person from suffering the consequences of the drinking behavior
- Identify strategies to positively change role patterns and coping mechanisms while supporting other family members to do the same
- Support the family to understand that focusing on their behavior will remove the alcoholic from the center of attention and all family roles will be challenged
- Encourage the family to commit to continued family communication sessions and to create appropriate action plans based on the development of new insights related to role relationships, communication processes, and coping skills

Encouraging verbalization of thoughts and feelings is the first step of recovery. The nurse must be aware that family members are often reluctant or unwilling to talk about issues. When only one of the family members is ready to deal with and resolve issues, it is important to be cognizant that the other family members may inhibit the willing person. The nurse must reinforce the idea that it is possible for the willing member to move toward recovery, even when other family members decline to participate.

Can be assisted to create conditions that facilitate the alcoholic family member entering into a treatment program, as evidenced by:

Verbalizes recognition and acknowledgment that alcoholism is a family problem

Commits to seek and implement appropriate interventions

- Support the family members in deciding to enable the drinking member to enter into a treatment program by determining/initiating appropriate action plans (e.g., changes in household responsibilities, contact with treatment program, child care services).
- Guide the family to locate and access child care services to facilitate the initiation and continuation of treatment because this is often a barrier to staying in treatment.
- Support the family in seeking help from and accepting assistance from competent professional caregivers and counselors, including AL-ANON, Alcoholics Anonymous, and self-help groups (e.g., ACOA [Adult Children of Alcoholics]).

In addition to interacting with the family, the nurse needs to support them in facilitating the entrance of the alcoholic person into a treatment program. Referral of family members to AL-ANON or ACOA can also facilitate their recovery. Families often benefit and are receptive to family therapy that can be provided in either an outpatient or residential setting. The nurse's role is to inform the family and explore the options they are ready to accept.

Interrupted Family Processes

Interrupted family processes are a change in family relationships and/or functioning.[8]

Related Factors[1,3,8,9]

Developmental transition and/or crisis
Family member's role reversal
Family roles shift
Informal or formal interaction with community
Modification in family finances
Modification in family social status
Power shift of family members
Shift in physical or mental health status of a family member
Situation transition and/or crises

Defining Characteristics[2,7,8]

Changes in availability for affective responsiveness and intimacy
Changes in availability for emotional support
Changes in communication patterns
Changes in effectiveness in completing assigned tasks
Changes in expressions of conflict with and/or isolation from community resources
Changes in expressions of conflict within family
Changes in mutual support
Changes in participation in decision making
Changes in participation in problem solving
Changes in patterns and rituals
Changes in power alliances
Changes in satisfaction with family
Changes in somatic complaints
Changes in stress-reduction behaviors

Expected Patient (Family) Outcomes and Nursing Interventions With Rationale[1-7,9-11]

Develop and practice positive communication among family members, as evidenced by:

Family members share feelings and thoughts related to illness, crises, traumas experienced in the family and express how these events affected the family individually and as a whole

Family members work to resolve conflict among members and develop a respectful tolerance for individual coping needs

Family members verbalize a desire to work together to resolve issues or conflicts

- Create a supportive environment *that provides safety, protects privacy, supports trust, and promotes comfort of the family unit and of individual members.*
- Provide regular contacts with the family, especially at time of crisis.
- Assess family's structural, behavioral, and interactive patterns, including boundaries, developmental stages, coping skills, role expectations, overt and covert rules, and energy output.
- Engage family members in the problem-solving process, including setting realistic goals, identifying clear behavioral objectives to be met, and anticipating possible barriers to crisis/conflict resolution.
- Expedite communication within the family *to allow members to express their feelings about the present situation or past situation.*
- Reinforce, positively, exhibition of adaptive family behaviors.

The family's cognitive capacity—their ability to appraise a situation realistically and competently and their own capabilities in relation to it—depends on their openness and their respect for each other's unique capabilities. The nurse must help the family adapt to change, deal with the crisis constructively, accomplish developmental tasks, readjust roles to accommodate situational and developmental crises, and use problem-solving techniques.

- If the crisis involves hospitalization, provide for the physical and emotional comfort of the family throughout the hospitalization. Provide liberal visitation, orientation to important areas of the unit/hospital, adequate space for family privacy, overnights as appropriate, and emotional support as indicated.
- Ascertain the religious and cultural background of the family.
- Arrange for and participate in family conferences (including the identified patient) *to teach family members how to apply what is learned and engage in problem solving about how to work through potential problems that may arise after discharge and to develop a discharge plan that may involve referral to community supports.* Ensure privacy for these conferences.
- In the community setting assume appropriate role(s) when interviewing with families in crisis. Consider among the following: support, education, guidance, role modeling, monitoring, facilitating, advocacy, and referral.

Exhibit an ability to positively negotiate issues, solve problems, or make decisions as a family or between individual family members, as evidenced by:

Family members identify goals consistent with role relationships and that focus on crisis/conflict resolution

Family members verbalize personal values that are involved in the negotiation process without judgment

Family members exhibit an ability to ask or accept help appropriately either from others in the family or from outside support resources

Family members anticipate inhibiting factors and develop strategies for coping with them

- Create a supportive environment *that provides safety, protects privacy, supports trust, and promotes comfort of the family unit and of individual members.*
- Provide regular contacts with the family, especially at time of crisis.
- Assess family's structural, behavioral, and interactive patterns, including boundaries, developmental stages, coping skills, role expectations, overt and covert rules, and energy output.
- Engage family members in the problem-solving process, including setting realistic goals, identifying clear behavioral objectives to be met, and anticipating possible barriers to crisis/conflict resolution.
- Initiate involvement of additional formal and informal supports *to assist the family to move toward crisis/conflict resolution (i.e., teaching stress reduction and coping skills, engaging extended family if authorized to do so).*
- Refer to family therapy (if indicated), social support agencies, self-help groups, financial advisors, church-affiliated supports as appropriate.
- Expedite communication within the family *to allow members to express their feelings about the present situation or past situation.*
- Reinforce, positively, exhibition of adaptive family behaviors.
- If the crisis involves hospitalization, provide for the physical and emotional comfort of the family throughout the hospitalization. Provide liberal visitation, orientation to important areas of the unit/hospital, adequate space for family privacy, overnights as appropriate, and emotional support as indicated.
- Ascertain the religious and cultural background of the family.
- Provide the family and the identified patient basic information about the nature of the illness, answer questions, and discuss strategies for managing symptoms.
- Arrange for and participate in family conferences (including the identified patient) *to teach family members how to apply what is learned and engage in problem solving about how to work through potential problems that may arise after discharge and to develop a discharge plan that may involve referral to community supports.* Ensure privacy for these conferences.
- In the community setting assume appropriate role(s) when interviewing with families in crisis. Consider among the following: support, education, guidance, role modeling, monitoring, facilitating, advocacy, and referral.
- Assist the family to identify problems and establish goals for crisis/conflict resolution.

Facilitating change within the family system is the primary goal in family work; thus a thorough knowledge of change theory is essential. The role of nursing in the care of families also includes teaching and helping families to develop adaptive skills. Family roles must be revised and strengths and weaknesses identified. Dysfunctional coping mechanisms must be replaced with effective ones. Family members can be supportive of one another by communicating needs and by adapting roles to meet reciprocal physical, emotional, spiritual, and mutual respect needs.

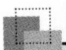

INEFFECTIVE ROLE PERFORMANCE

Ineffective role performance is the state in which the patterns of behavior and self-expression do not match the environmental context, norms, and expectations.[6]

Related Factors[2-4,6]

Knowledge

Developmental transitions
Educational level
Inadequate role preparation (e.g., role transition, skill, rehearsal, validation)
Lack of knowledge about role
Lack of knowledge about role skills
Lack of or inadequate role model
Lack of opportunity for role rehearsal
Role transition
Unrealistic role expectations

Social

Domestic violence
Family conflict

Inadequate or inappropriate linkage with the health-care system
Inadequate role socialization (e.g., role model, expectations, responsibilities)
Inadequate support system
Job schedule demands
Lack of resources
Lack of rewards
Low social economic status
Poverty
Stress and conflict
Young age, developmental level

Physiologic

Body image alteration
Cognitive deficits
Depression
Fatigue
Health alterations (e.g., physical health, body image, self-esteem, mental health, psychosocial health, cognition, learning style, neurologic health)
Inadequate/inappropriate linkage with health-care system
Low self-esteem
Mental illness
Pain
Physical illness
Postpartum depression
Substance abuse

Expected Patient Outcomes and Nursing Interventions With Rationale[1-5]

Develop role mastery, as evidenced by:

Demonstrates stable pattern of mastery of role
Expresses positive acceptance of new role
Verbalizes understanding of appropriate cognitive, instrumental, and expressive behaviors associated with role
Describes impact new role will have in assuming other role behaviors
Demonstrates use of various role supplementation strategies, with resultant ability to perform role without difficulty
Demonstrates integration of instrumental/expressive role behaviors

- Determine type of role-functioning problem patient is experiencing: role insufficiency, role distance, interrole conflict, intrarole conflict, role failure, or ineffective role transition.
- Determine transitions that may be predisposing patient to problems with role functioning: developmental, situational, or health-illness transition.
- Encourage patient to verbalize feelings, concerns, fears, and anxieties associated with assuming a particular role.
- Help patient to assess impact of new role on ability to assume present or future roles.
- Once type of role-functioning problem has been identified, use the following:
  - Role clarification *to teach patient what role entails in terms of behavior, sentiments, costs, rewards, and positive and negative reinforcement by significant others*
  - Role taking *to help patient imaginatively assume position or point of view of another person taking on new role*
  - Role modeling *to help patient enact and play out new role so that he or she can understand and emulate intricacies of behavior associated with new role*
  - Role rehearsal *to help patient fantasize, imagine, and mentally enact how encounter might take place and how new role might evolve and develop*
  - Reference groups *to expose patient to other individuals or groups who have successfully assumed mastery of new role*
- Provide therapeutic environment that allows for opportunities to learn and practice new role behaviors.
- Give patient feedback regarding failure to assume or perform expected role behaviors *to facilitate the learning of new behaviors.*
- Identify and provide appropriate role models *for patient to learn role expectations.*
- Assist patient to obtain necessary knowledge and skills for role performance.
- Have patient use role play *to practice newly acquired role behaviors.*
- Assist patient to resolve role conflicts.
- Convey recognition of approximations of expected role performance *to reinforce learning of new behaviors.*
- Be nonjudgmental *so that patient can freely engage in learning and trying out role.*
- Identify and support strengths and capabilities related to adequate role performance *to foster patient's self-awareness of abilities and self-efficacy and to support and enhance patient's belief in own self-worth.*
- Encourage self-monitoring of changes in role behavior.

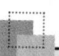

IMPAIRED PARENTING

Impaired parenting is the inability of the primary caretaker to create an environment that promotes the optimum growth and development of the child.[8]

Related Factors[2,5,8,11]

Social

Change in family unit
Father of child not involved
History of being abused
History of being abusive
Inadequate child care arrangements
Lack of family cohesiveness
Lack of, or poor, parental role model
Lack of resources
Lack of social support networks
Lack of transportation
Lack of value of parenthood
Low self-esteem
Marital conflict
Poor home environment
Poor problem-solving skills
Poverty
Relocations
Role strain or overload
Single parenthood

Social isolation
Stress (e.g., financial, legal, recent crisis, cultural move)
Unemployment or job problems
Unplanned, unwanted, or adolescent pregnancy

Knowledge

Inability to recognize and act on infant cues
Lack of cognitive readiness for parenthood
Lack of knowledge about child development
Lack of knowledge about child health maintenance
Lack of knowledge about parenting skills
Limited cognitive functioning
Low educational level
Poor communication skills
Preference for physical punishment
Unrealistic expectation for self, infant, partner

Infant or child

Altered perceptual abilities
Attention deficit hyperactivity disorder
Difficult temperament
Lack of goodness to fit (temperament) with parental expectations
Handicapping condition or developmental delay
Illness
Low birth weight
Multiple births
Not gender desired
Prolonged separation from parents
Premature birth
Separation from parent at birth
Unplanned or unwanted child

Physical or psychologic

Depression
Difficult labor and/or delivery
Disability
High number of or closely spaced pregnancies
History of mental illness
History of substance abuse or dependencies
Lack or, or late, prenatal care
Multiple births
Physical illness
Separation from infant/child
Sleep deprivation or disruption
Young age, especially adolescent

Defining Characteristics[7,8,9,11]

Infant or child

Behavioral disorders
Failure to thrive
Frequent accidents
Frequent illness
Incidence of physical and psychologic trauma or abuse
Lack of attachment
Lack of separation anxiety
Poor academic performance
Poor cognitive development
Poor social competence
Runaway

Parental

Abandonment
Child abuse/neglect
High punitiveness
Inadequate child health maintenance
Inappropriate child care arrangements
Inappropriate visual, tactile, auditory stimulation
Inconsistent behavior management
Inconsistent care
Inflexibility to meet needs of child, situation
Insecure or lack of attachment to infant
Little cuddling
Low self-esteem
Maternal-child interaction deficit
Negative statements about child
Poor or inappropriate caretaking skills
Poor parent-child interaction
Rejection or hostility to child
Statements of inability to meet child's needs
Unsafe home environment
Verbalized inability to control child
Verbalized role inadequacy and frustration

Expected Parent Outcomes and Nursing Interventions With Rationale[1-7,10-12]

Exhibit constructive and positive parenting, as evidenced by:

Verbalizes a desire to learn parenting behaviors that support infant/child/adolescent growth and development
Acquires and uses constructive and positive parenting behaviors
Demonstrates nurturing, positive behaviors toward the infant/child/adolescent

(Note: The term *child* is used with interventions to encompass all ages of children.)

- Discuss with parents their understanding of developmental milestones and needs and teach these as appropriate for level of child. *Parents may have inadequate knowledge of normal growth and development to provide constructive parenting.*
- Discuss with parents their expectations of the child and of their own role as parents within their cultural beliefs and values. *Unrealistic expectations may alter parenting behaviors; expectations are often influenced by culture.*[2,8]
- Assess for factors indicating dysfunctional parenting, including interactions with infant/child/adolescent, use of alcohol or drugs, reports of child neglect or abuse, home environment, perception of child as different or uncontrollable, social isolation. *These factors, and others may provide cues to impaired parenting.*
- Provide interventions to prevent child abuse.[10]
  - Advocate courses for high-school students on growth and development of children and parenting.
  - Help children learn effective problem-solving techniques so they are not overwhelmed as adults.
  - Foster high self-esteem in children so they are not dependent on others.
  - Help parents with responsible family planning so children are desired.
  - Help parents locate support groups in their community.

Role model ways of caring for children.
Identify parents who were abused as children and offer help to help them break the chain of child abuse.
Advocate membership in Parent Anonymous as an effective support group for parents who may be potential abusers.

Identifying parents who are potential abusers, providing information about assistance from adequate support persons, and providing parenting information are necessary for prevention.

- Provide with general parenting guidelines.[3]
  Practice open, honest dialogues. Never threaten.
  Do not lecture. Tell the child he or she is wrong, and let it go. Spend time talking about pleasant experiences.
  Compliment achievements. Make each child feel important and special.
  Verbally and nonverbally (through touch and hugs) convey to the child that he or she is loved.
  Set limits and keep them. Expect cooperation.
  Let the child help you as much as possible.
  Discipline the child by restricting activity, as in "time-out."
  Stay in control. Try not to discipline when you are angry.
  Never reprimand a child in front of another person.
  Never decide you cannot control a child's destructive behavior.
  Be a good model. Never lie to a child.
  Give each child an age-appropriate responsibility, and expect the child to complete the task.
  Share your feelings, and respect and be considerate of the child's feelings.
  Give choices and allow child freedom to choose as appropriate.
  Avoid power struggles.
- Initiate health teaching and referrals as indicated and appropriate.

Risk for Impaired Parenting

Risk for impaired parenting is the risk for inability of the primary caretaker to create, maintain, or regain an environment that promotes the optimum growth and development of the child.[7]

Risk Factors[7,9]

Social

Change in family unit
Father of child not involved
History of being abused
History of being abusive
Inadequate child care arrangements
Lack of family cohesiveness
Lack of, or poor, parental role model
Lack of resources
Lack of social support networks
Lack of transportation
Lack of value of parenthood
Low self-esteem
Marital conflict
Poor home environment
Poor problem-solving skills
Poverty
Relocations
Role strain or overload
Single parenthood
Social isolation
Stress (e.g., financial, legal, recent crisis, cultural move)
Unemployment or job problems
Unplanned, unwanted, or adolescent pregnancy

Knowledge

Inability to recognize and act on infant cues
Lack of cognitive readiness for parenthood
Lack of knowledge about child development
Lack of knowledge about child health maintenance
Lack of knowledge about parenting skills
Limited cognitive functioning
Low educational level
Poor communication skills
Preference for physical punishment
Unrealistic expectation for self, infant, partner

Infant or child

Altered perceptual abilities
Attention deficit hyperactivity disorder
Difficult temperament
Lack of goodness to fit (temperament) with parental expectations
Handicapping condition or developmental delay
Illness
Low birth weight
Multiple births
Not gender desired
Prolonged separation from parents
Premature birth
Separation from parent at birth
Unplanned or unwanted child

Physical or psychologic

Depression
Difficult labor and/or delivery
Disability
High number of or closely spaced pregnancies
History of mental illness
History of substance abuse or dependencies
Lack or, or late, prenatal care
Multiple births
Physical illness
Separation from infant/child
Sleep deprivation or disruption
Young age, especially adolescent

Expected Patient Outcomes and Nursing Interventions With Rationale[1-6,8,9]

Establish a nurturing parental role, as evidenced by:

Verbalizes parental behaviors that promote optimum growth and development of children

- Assess risk factors such as parent abused as a child, prior child abuse, history of chemical dependency, parental/family stressors, lack of support (financial, family, significant other, community), physical or mental illness.

Identifying the family at risk for impaired parenting indicates a need for teaching and referrals.
- Assess parent-child interactions that may indicate inadequate attachment or emotional bonding *to provide early interventions.*
- Discuss with parents their understanding of developmental milestones and needs and teach these as appropriate for level of child. *Parents may have inadequate knowledge of normal growth and development to provide constructive parenting.*
- Discuss with parents their expectations of the child and of their own role as parents within their cultural beliefs and values. *Unrealistic expectations may alter parenting behaviors; expectations are often influenced by culture.*
- Provide information about parenting (see Impaired Parenting).
- Provide referrals to community agencies, if available and requested.

PARENTAL ROLE CONFLICT

Parental role conflict is the state in which a parent experiences role confusion and conflict in response to crisis.[7]

Related Factors[7]

Change in marital status
Home care of a child with special needs (e.g., apnea monitoring, postural drainage, hyperalimentation)
Interruptions of family life caused by home care regimen (e.g., treatments, caregivers, lack of respite)
Intimidation with invasive or restrictive modalities (e.g., isolation, intubation)
Separation from child because of chronic illness
Specialized care centers, policies

Defining Characteristics[2,7]

Demonstrated disruption in caretaking routines
Expressed concern about perceived loss of control over decisions related to the child
Expressed concern(s) about changes in parental role, family functioning, family communication, family health
Expressed concern(s)/feeling(s) of inadequacy about providing for child's physical and emotional needs during hospitalization or in home
Reluctance to participate in usual caretaking activities even with encouragement or support
Verbalized or demonstrated feelings of guilt, anger, fear, anxiety, and/or frustrations about effect of child's illness on family process

Expected Patient Outcomes and Nursing Interventions With Rationale[1-6,8-10]

Demonstrate appropriate role behaviors in time of crisis, as evidenced by:

Verbalizes feelings of confusion and conflict regarding care of child
Demonstrates responsibility in making decisions regarding child's care
Demonstrates safe performance of necessary skills for home care
Takes active role in care of child during hospitalization and at home

- Assess usual methods of coping with stress, ability to make decisions, cultural influences on parental role behaviors, and usual parental role responsibilities *to establish a base for interventions to facilitate coping, decision making, and parental role. The way parents respond to a crisis depends on the specific crisis they are experiencing, past experiences with problem solving, and the resources available to them.*[9]
- Explore the parents' perceptions and reactions to the crisis. *Reactions to the crisis may include sadness and loss, the challenge of becoming attached while dealing with fears about the child's future, a need to maintain control while also feeling powerless, and a struggle to remain strong for others in the family.*[2]
- Provide suggestions for handling the stress of the crisis.
  - Each person experiences and responds to stress individually.
  - Talk about personal reactions to stress.
  - Reach out for support.
  - Don't rush to make decisions.
  - Anticipate life events and develop a plan for handling them.
  - Accidents increase when people are stressed.
- Explain rationale for treatments *to decrease misunderstandings and maximize parental participation.*
- Design interventions based on establishing, with parents, mutual goals and parental participation in care. Include in interventions the child's usual routines, eating and sleeping times and preferences, fears and rituals *to promote parental caregiver role and to normalize, as much as possible, the child's treatment and care.*
- Provide adequate time for learning new skills *to decrease anxiety about caring for the child at home.*
- Provide information about medical, nursing, and community support systems, including respite care *to provide the support necessary to maintain the day-to-day care necessary for children who are chronically physically or mentally ill, or physically handicapped.*

RISK FOR IMPAIRED PARENT/INFANT/CHILD ATTACHMENT

Risk for impaired parent/infant/child attachment is a disruption of the interactive process between parent/significant other and infant [child] that fosters the development of a protective and nurturing reciprocal relationship.[8]

Risk Factors[8]

Abuse of parent during childhood
Anxiety associated with the parent role
Inability of parents to meet their personal needs
Ill infant or child who is unable to effectively initiate parental contact because of altered behavioral organization
Lack of privacy
Physical barriers
Premature infant
Separation
Substance abuse

Expected Patient Outcomes and Nursing Interventions With Rationale[1,2-4,7,9,10]

Demonstrate a protective and nurturing reciprocal relationship with infant or child, as evidenced by:

Verbalizes knowledge of individualized infant/child behavioral responses

Demonstrates behaviors that indicate parent/infant attachment

- Provide interventions and teaching to promote parent/infant attachment.
  - Recognize individual differences in each infant's temperament, and explain to parents that such differences are normal.
  - Monitor new mother's patterns of behavior immediately and for a short period after birth; including calling the infant by name, how the infant is held and touched, stimulation of the awake infant, comforting techniques
  - Monitor the infant's responses to the mother, such as sucking, cooing, eye contact, grasping, or molding to the mother's body.
  - Monitor the father's attachment behaviors with the infant, called *paternal engrossment.*

The process of parenting is based on a mutual relationship between the infant and the parents, often referred to as attachment or bonding. Assessing attachment behaviors is necessary to promote this relationship.

- As soon as possible after birth, encourage parents to see and hold the infant; place the infant in close proximity to the parent's face *to establish visual contact.*
- Assess the infant with the parents present, pointing out infant behaviors such as rooting, ability to see, ability to suck, and attention to the human voice.
- Discuss with parents their expectations for the infant *to clarify misperceptions and unrealistic expectations.*
- For infants and children who are separated from their parents as a result of illness or preterm delivery, support parent/infant/child attachment by doing the following:
  - Encouraging parents to be with and touch the infant/child as much as possible
  - Supporting skin-to-skin contact
  - Encouraging parents to provide care as much as possible
- Suggest use of community agencies and support services, including contact by telephone, as needed.[9]

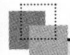

Impaired Social Interaction

Impaired social interaction is the state in which an individual participates in an insufficient or excessive quantity or ineffective quality of social exchange.[8]

Related Factors[2,3,6,8,10]

Absence of available significant others or peers
Altered physical appearance
Altered thought processes
Attention deficit disorder
Chemical addiction
Chronic illness
Inappropriate social behavior
Knowledge/skill deficit in ways to enhance mutuality
Lack of transportation
Limited physical mobility
Low self-concept
Mental retardation
Poor impulse control
Severe anxiety
Sociocultural dissonance
Therapeutic isolation

Defining Characteristics[2,3,8]

Delusional thinking
Dysfunctional interaction with peers, family, and/or caregivers
Family report of change in style of interactions
Inability to care for self
Observed use of unsuccessful social interaction behaviors
Sensory or perceptual alterations
Verbalized or observed discomfort in social situations
Verbalized or observed inability to receive or communicate satisfying sense of belonging, caring, interest, or shared history

Expected Patient Outcomes and Nursing Interventions With Rationale*

Acknowledge the existence of an impairment in social interaction and verbalize a desire to diminish the impairment, as evidenced by:

Verbalizes thoughts and feelings related to existing inability to form close interpersonal relationships with others

Verbalizes a desire to interact within a peer group

Verbalizes knowledge of rejection by others (if it exists) and identifies ways to cope

Verbalizes with others (caregivers, if inpatient) the nature of previous and/or current relationships, exploring patterns of communication and behavior that enhance and inhibit relationships

Verbalizes feelings and needs for positive, appropriate social interaction

- Explain care-related activities clearly, answering questions as accurately as possible.
- Use an interpreter when necessary.
- Involve patient and family or significant other in planning care, and encourage patient's participation in self-care on a continuing basis.
- Assist patient in identifying and using effective social-interaction behaviors (e.g., increased eye contact, using people's names when appropriate, asking questions).
- Provide non–care-related time with the patient (inpatient unit) *to encourage social interaction.* Start with one-to-one interaction, and build up to group as the patient's skills indicate.
- Give positive reinforcement for appropriate and effective interaction behaviors (verbal and nonverbal).
- Explore feelings related to interaction with others, including fears, anxieties, insecurities, needs, and wishes.
- Assist patient in the interpretation of his or her behaviors when interacting with others, including distortions, automatic thoughts, and assumptions.

---

*References 1, 2, 4, 5, 7, 9, 10.

- Assist in the development of interactive skills by the techniques of modeling, education, role play, and direct, honest, immediate feedback.

A major cause of impaired social interaction is the inability to communicate effectively. This inability can be caused partly by feelings of inadequacy. Another cause is mental impairment. The nurse must be attuned to a patient's feelings of inadequacy or the extent of mental impairment. This is often difficult because people exhibit their inadequacies by different and varying forms of communication (e.g., overtalkativeness, silence, anger, or hostility).

Identify factors that contribute to inability to interact socially and develop a plan to improve social interaction, as evidenced by:

Patient and/or family provide information concerning medical background and social background
Maintains orientation to time, place, and person
Demonstrates understanding of care-related instructions (e.g., medications, physical limitations)
Identifies behavioral goals for change
Participates in skill development specific to areas of deficit
Identifies effective coping techniques to deal with particular impairment (e.g., sociocultural differences, neurologic disorders, mental retardation, anxiety)
Remains reality based
Develops alternate means of communication if sensory impairment is present
Demonstrates problem-solving ability

- Use an interpreter when necessary.
- Involve patient and family or significant others, in planning care, and encourage patient's participation in self-care on a continuing basis.
- If delusions and/or hallucinations occur, do not focus on them; provide patient with reality-based information, and reassure patient of his or her safety.
- Give positive reinforcement for appropriate and effective interaction behaviors (verbal and nonverbal).
- Assist in finding referral sources of community support systems (if indicated), such as social services, financial counseling, home health care, mental health care, self-help groups.
- Assess for preexisting mental health problem(s) that may be reduced by the use of psychotropic medication or psychotherapy.
- Explore feelings related to interaction with others including fears, anxieties, insecurities, needs, and wishes.
- Assist patient in the interpretation of his or her behaviors when interacting with others, including distortions, automatic thoughts, and assumptions.
- Assist in the development of interactive skills by the techniques of modeling, education, role play, and direct, honest, immediate feedback.
- Educate patient and family (if indicated) on the use and side effects of psychoactive medications, as well as other symptom management strategies.

Possible causal factors related to impaired social interaction must be explored with the patient in an open, direct, and supportive manner. Problem-solving techniques should be discussed and taught to the patient, with the ultimate decision-making process focusing on the patient to promote behavioral change.

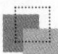

IMPAIRED VERBAL COMMUNICATION

Impaired verbal communication is the state in which an individual experiences a decreased, delayed, or absent ability to receive, process, transmit, and use a system of symbols; anything that has meaning, that is, transmits meaning.[6]

Related Factors[6]

Absence of significant others
Altered central nervous system function
Altered cerebral circulation
Altered perceptions
Altered self-esteem or self-concept
Anatomic defect (e.g., cleft palate, alteration of the neuromuscular visual system, auditory system, or phonatory apparatus)
Brain tumor or trauma
Cultural difference
Differences related to developmental age
Emotional conditions
Environmental barriers
Lack of information
Musculoskeletal weakness
Psychologic barriers (e.g., psychosis, lack of stimuli)
Physical barrier (tracheostomy, intubation)
Side effects of medication
Stress

Defining Characteristics[1,4,6]

Absence of eye contact or difficulty in selective attending
Difficulty comprehending and maintaining usual communication pattern
Difficulty expressing thought verbally (e.g., aphasia, dysphasia, apraxia, dyslexia)
Difficulty forming words or sentences (e.g., aphonia, dyslalia, dysarthria)
Disorientation
Dyspnea
Inability or difficulty in using nonverbal expressions
Inability or unwillingness to speak
Inability to speak dominant language
Inappropriate verbalization
Partial or total hearing deficit
Slurring
Speaking or verbalizing with difficulty
Stuttering

Expected Patient Outcomes and Nursing Interventions With Rationale[1-5,7]

Attend to appropriate input, as evidenced by:

Is oriented to person, place, and time
Selects and responds to relevant stimuli
Demonstrates accurate perception and absence or control of physical symptoms

- Reduce or increase environmental stimuli. *Perception and interpretation of communication are based on stimuli within the perceptual field.*
- Teach patient to identify and focus on relevant stimuli. *A person can focus consciously on only a few of the many stimuli available.*

- Assist in correction of faulty perception. *Reception and selection of appropriate stimuli depend on an individual's perception.*
- Encourage patient to seek assistance in correcting, modifying, or preventing physical conditions that interfere with communication. *Physical conditions can interfere with the ability to receive and process sensory input or generate output.*

Send concise, understandable messages, as evidenced by:
Demonstrates absence of speech impediments
Selects and organizes words appropriate to receiver and context
Speaks dominant language
Uses effective communication techniques
Uses appropriate amount of verbiage
Expresses feelings appropriately

- Use facilitative communication techniques in interacting with patient (e.g., reflection, focusing, validation). *The nurse promotes further communication and role models through use of these techniques.*
- Point out discrepancies in message sent and context within which it is sent. *Connection between message and context is explained, and perception is corrected.*
- Teach and support patient's use of appropriate communication techniques and assertive skills. *Use of effective communication techniques and assertive skills communicates sensitivity to the rights and feelings of persons involved and contributes to mutually agreed outcomes.*
- Assist patient in increasing or modifying language skills. *Words that describe intended meaning and that the other person understands must be selected.*
- Teach and encourage expression of feelings. *Appropriate expression of feelings facilitates communication.*

Send congruent nonverbal and verbal communication, as evidenced by:
Expresses congruent nonverbal behaviors
Expresses congruent verbal and nonverbal behaviors
Balances use of verbal and nonverbal behaviors

- Point out discrepancies in verbal and nonverbal behavior. *Clear communication requires congruity of verbal and nonverbal messages and consistency in meaning of nonverbal behaviors.*

Send and receive feedback, as evidenced by:
Listens actively
Examines effects of behavior on others
Asks for and receives feedback
Sends feedback to others

- Describe, demonstrate, and encourage use of active listening skills. *Listening communicates concern, interest, or acceptance.*
- Increase awareness of effects of behavior and strengths and limitations in communicating with others. *Awareness of effect on another provides opportunity for modification or correction of behavior.*
- Assist and encourage patient efforts to accept positive and negative feedback. *Feedback regulates communication by stimulating modification or correction.*
- Request patient to ask for feedback when communicating with others.

Experience gratification from communication, as evidenced by:
Reports satisfaction from communication
Reports sense of high self-esteem
Reports or shows willingness to assume responsibility for communication
Sends and receives confirmation when communicating

- Assist patient in mastering tasks appropriate for age or developmental level. *Communication involves learning a series of progressive tasks over time.*
- Encourage interaction with others.
- Teach and encourage use of stress reduction techniques. *Excessive stress can result in impaired communication.*
- Increase self-esteem.
- Help patient develop understanding of dynamics of relationships. *Communication occurs within the context of relationships, all variables of which affect the process.*
- Demonstrate and support responsibility for communication. *In successful communication both sender and receiver accept responsibility for communication.*

Relocation Stress Syndrome

Relocation stress syndrome is a state in which there is a physiologic and/or psychosocial disturbance following transfer from one environment to another.[8]

Related Factors[1-3,8,9]

Area of relocation (e.g., rural, urban, near family)
Caregiver feelings of failure
Decreased physical health
Feelings of powerlessness
History and types of previous transfers
Impaired psychosocial health status
Lack of adequate support system
Little or no preparation for the impending move
Losses involved with decision to move
Moderate to high degree of environment change
Past, concurrent, and recent losses
Type of relocation

Defining Characteristics[7,8]

Anxiety
Apprehension
Change in eating habits
Change in environment/location
Dependency
Depression
Gastrointestinal disturbances
Increased confusion
Increased verbalization of needs
Insecurity
Lack of trust
Loneliness
Restlessness
Sad affect
Sleep disturbance
Unfavorable comparison of posttransfer staff with pretransfer staff
Verbalization of being concerned/upset about transfer
Verbalization of unwillingness to relocate
Vigilance
Weight change
Withdrawal

Expected Patient Outcomes and Nursing Interventions With Rationale[1,3-7,9,11]

Adjust to relocation, as evidenced by:

Experiences decreased anxiety and grieving
Establishes new relationships
Participates in activities in the new setting
Verbalizes acceptance of changed environment

- Build relationship with patient *to foster trust, security, and support during a time of many losses.*
- Orient patient to new staff, equipment, and environment *to decrease uncertainty and anxiety.*
- Allow patient to control some aspects of the posttransfer environment (e.g., privacy, room decorations) *to increase control and autonomy.*
- Arrange for consistent caregivers and daily care routines *to facilitate continuity and predictability for the patient.*
- Teach family interventions to support the patient after relocation.
- Acknowledge patient's feelings of loss and anxiety related to relocation.
- Assist patient in identifying strengths and resources *to increase coping and problem solving in new environment.*
- Assess patient for dysfunctional grieving responses.
- Support patient in formulating realistic goals for self in the new setting *to promote a sense of mastery and to enhance self-esteem.*

RISK FOR RELOCATION STRESS SYNDROME

Risk for relocation stress syndrome is the state in which an individual is at risk for physiologic and/or psychosocial disturbance following transfer from one environment to another.[6]

Risk Factors[2,3,6,9]

Comorbidities
Decreased ability to provide self-care
Decreased physical or mental health
Dementia
Environmental change/move (physical, cultural, ethnic)
Falls
Lack of adequate support system(s)
Lack of predeparture counseling
Multiple losses
Passive coping
Powerlessness

Expected Patient Outcomes and Nursing Interventions With Rationale*

Adjust to relocation, as evidenced by:

Verbalizes decreasing anxiety over life change
Expresses ability to cope with change
Expresses satisfaction with life situation

- Ensure time to discuss the relocation with the individual and listen to concerns *to decrease anxiety.*
- Prepare individual in health-care facility for relocation *to decrease likelihood of relocation stress syndrome.*

At least 1 month before the move, tell the person that relocation is necessary *to decrease anxiety about relocation.*

Create and adhere to a schedule for relocation activities. *If an individual knows in advance about what will happen during the relocation, his or her feelings of security are enhanced.*

Send letters to family members describing the move *so they may provide support during the relocation process.*

Help the individual maintain close interpersonal relationships with family, friends, and care staff *to assist in psychosocial adaptation and to improve satisfaction with the life situation.*

- Facilitate the individual's control in the relocation by moving personal objects that define the location as "home" *to increase comfort within the setting.*
- Support an individual's voluntary decision to relocate. *Voluntary decisions provide control over the situation and have been found to have more positive outcomes.*
- Advocate for the individual in the choice of room location, room color and furnishings, packing of belongings, taking part in a resident's council, and selecting daily menus *to facilitate control over the relocation process and to enhance adjustment.*
- Provide activities significant to the individual, such as reminiscence therapy, pet ownership, religious beliefs and practices, relaxation therapy, and humor. *These activities have been found to be beneficial in preventing or decreasing the effects of relocation stress syndrome.*

*References 1, 2, 4, 5, 7, 8.

RISK FOR OTHER-DIRECTED VIOLENCE, RISK FOR SELF-DIRECTED VIOLENCE

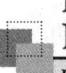

Risk for other-directed violence is the state in which an individual demonstrates behaviors that can be physically, emotionally, and/or sexually harmful to others.[8]

Risk for self-directed violence is the state in which an individual demonstrates behaviors that can be physically, emotionally, and/or sexually harmful to self.[8]

RISK FOR OTHER-DIRECTED VIOLENCE Risk Factors[4,8,10]

Availability and/or possession of weapon(s)
Body language: rigid posture, clenching of fists and jaw, hyperactivity, pacing, breathlessness, threatening stances
Cognitive impairment (e.g., learning disabilities, attention deficit disorder, decreased intellectual functioning)
Cruelty to animals
Fire setting
History of childhood abuse
History of drug/alcohol abuse
History of violence against others (e.g., hitting, kicking, spitting, scratching, throwing objects, biting, attempted rape, rape, sexual molestation, urinating/defecating on a person)
History of violence, indirect (e.g., tearing off clothes, ripping objects off walls, writing on walls, urinating or defecating on floor, stamping feet, temper tantrum, running in corridors, yelling, throwing objects, breaking a window, slamming doors, sexual advances)

History of violence of threats (e.g., verbal threats against property, verbal threats against person, social threats, cursing, threatening notes/letters, threatening gestures, sexual threats)
History of violent antisocial behavior (e.g., stealing, insistent borrowing, insistent demands for privileges, insistent interruption of meetings, refusal to eat, refusal to take medication, ignoring instructions)
History of witnessing family violence
Other factors: neurologic impairment (e.g., positive EEG, CAT, or MRI, head trauma, positive neurologic findings, seizure disorder)
Motor vehicle offenses (e.g., frequent traffic violations, use of a motor vehicle to release anger, road rage)
Pathologic intoxication
Prenatal and perinatal complication/abnormalities
Psychotic symptomatology (e.g., auditory, visual, command hallucinations; paranoid delusions; loose, rambling or illogical thought processes)

Risk for Self-Directed Violence

Risk Factors[1,8,9]

Age 15 to 19, over 45
Behavioral clues (e.g., writing forlorn love notes, directing angry messages at a significant other who has rejected the person, giving away personal items, taking out a large life insurance policy)
Conflictive interpersonal relationship
Emotional status (hopelessness, despair, increased anxiety, panic, anger, hostility)
Employment (unemployed, recent job loss or failure)
Family background (chaotic or conflictive, history of suicide)
History of multiple suicide attempts
Involvement in autoerotic sexual acts
Marital status (single, widowed, divorced)
Mental health (severe depression, psychosis, severe personality disorder, alcoholism, or drug abuse)
Occupation (executive, administrator/owner of business, professional, semiskilled)
Personal resources (poor achievement, poor insight, poorly controlled)
Physical health (hypochondriac, chronic or terminal illness)
Sexual orientation (bisexual [active], homosexual [inactive])
Social resources (poor rapport, socially isolated, unresponsive family)
Suicidal ideation (frequent, intense, prolonged)
Suicidal plan (clear and specific, lethality, method, and availability of destructive means)
Verbal clues (e.g., talking about death, "better off without me," asking questions about lethal dosages of drugs)

Expected Patient Outcomes and Nursing Interventions With Rationale[1-7,9-13]

Verbalize a lessened desire for exhibiting specific aggressive behavior and decreased feelings of anger and hostility, as evidenced by:

Verbalizes specific sources of anger, frustration, or rage
Describes current level of stress tolerance
Demonstrates a desire to control aggressive behavior
Identifies and demonstrates appropriate aids to decrease anger and hostility (physical exercise, visual imagery, relaxation techniques, appropriate verbal expressions of feelings, taking medication when indicated)
Exhibits a knowledge of physiologic or chemical causes of alterations in behavior (if appropriate)
Recognizes perceptual distortions that result from intense anger, rage, or hostility

- Provide trusting relationship with the patient *to help the patient feel more comfortable by being honest, clear, and concise during interaction.*
- Provide close supervision, and watch for early signs of agitation or increasing anxiety, such as increased motor activity and unreasonable requests or demands.
- Make short-term contracts with the patient that he or she will not harm herself or himself during a specific period. Continue negotiating until there is no evidence of suicidal ideation.
- Set limits on the patient's behavior, acknowledge and understand the patient's feelings, and invite conversation about his or her feelings.
- Encourage alternatives to violent outburst (e.g., physical expenditure of energy, by exercise, unit jobs [if inpatient], games, cleaning, discussion).
- Take the patient's feelings seriously.
- Administer and monitor effectiveness of medications prescribed to control aggressive behavior.
- Discuss reason and plan for safety and protective measures with family and significant other.
- Use positive reinforcement for no violent or suicidal behavior.

Setting limits, seclusion, and restraints (chemical and physical, which are not often used today) are all methods of controlling behavior if the patient loses control. The nurse must understand that the potentially violent patient often has low self-esteem, may be lonely, and may feel hopeless. Thus it is of utmost importance to establish trust and rapport by approaching calmly and allowing personal space.

Demonstrate self-control, as evidenced by:

Has relaxed body and muscles and no redness in the face
Maintains eye contact when communicating without a threatening stance or look
Verbalizes rationally and calmly precipitating factors to the incidents that cause anger
Verbalizes feelings of hopelessness, loneliness, and decreased self-esteem
Demonstrates and verbalizes alternatives to violent, aggressive behavior
Reports feelings of losing control to others
Allows trusted people (staff, family, friends) to approach boundaries of personal space
Demonstrates an understanding of rationale for limit setting or seclusion, if required

- Provide close supervision, and watch for early signs of agitation or increasing anxiety, such as increased motor activity and unreasonable requests or demands.
- If the patient is in an inpatient unit as a result of a suicide attempt, remove from the patient's environment anything that could be used to inflict further self-injury (e.g., razor blade, belts, glass objects, pills).

- Make short-term contracts with the patient that he or she will not harm herself or himself during a specific period. Continue negotiating until there is no evidence of suicidal ideation.
- Set limits on the patient's behavior, acknowledge and understand the patient's feelings, and invite conversations about his or her feelings.
- Encourage alternative to violent outbursts (e.g., physical expenditure of energy, by exercise, unit jobs [if inpatient], games, cleaning, discussion).
- Administer and monitor effectiveness of medications prescribed *to control aggressive behavior and help patient remain calm.*
- Establish a structured routine, and aid patient in following it.
- Assess sleep pattern, and establish a regular routine to combat sleep deprivation.
- Use short, declarative sentences when speaking to a patient who may be out of control. Speak in a firm, but not threatening, tone of voice.
- Refer the patient for appropriate assistance from a nurse therapist, psychiatrist, alcohol rehabilitation counselor, drug counselor, psychologist, social worker, etc.
- Provide patient and family with telephone numbers and other information about crisis centers, hot lines, counselors, etc.

Display no overt or covert dangerous behaviors, as evidenced by:

Avoids injuring or harming self
Avoids injuring or harming others
Verbalizes increased feelings of self-esteem
Expresses feelings in a nonviolent and nondestructive manner
Remains calm in a secure environment
Verbalizes feelings of anger and hostility rather than acting out physically
Actively participates in the prescribed treatment regimen (medications, support groups, individual therapy, hospitalization when indicated)
Verbalizes a knowledge of the supports available and demonstrates an ability to use them when needed

- Provide close supervision, and watch for early signs of agitation or increasing anxiety, such as increased motor activity and/or unreasonable requests or demands.
- If the patient is in an inpatient unit as a result of a suicide attempt, remove from the patient's environment anything that could be used to inflict further self-injury (e.g., razor blades, belts, glass objects, pills).
- Make short-term contracts with the patient that he or she will not harm herself or himself during a specific period. Continue negotiating until there is no evidence of suicidal ideation.
- Set limits on the patient's behavior, acknowledge and understand the patient's feelings, and invite conversation about his or her feelings.
- Encourage alternatives to violent outbursts (e.g., physical expenditure of energy, by exercise, unit jobs [if inpatient], games, cleaning, discussion).
- Acknowledge that you are aware of patient's potentially violent behavior.
- Administer and monitor effectiveness of medications prescribed to control aggressive behavior and maintain calm.
- Establish a structured daily routine, and aid patient in following it.
- Discuss reason and plan for safety and protective measures with family or significant other.
- Refer the patient for appropriate assistance from a nurse therapist, psychiatrist, alcohol rehabilitation counselor, drug counselor, psychologist, social worker, etc.
- Provide patient and family with telephone numbers and other information about crisis centers, hot lines, counselors, etc.
- Use positive reinforcement for no violent or suicidal behavior.

The nurse must encourage and allow verbal expressions of anger. The key to prevention of violent aggression is finding out what precipitates feeling of anger, frustration, or rage. Then, after careful discussion, the nurse and patient can find ways to decrease or eliminate the related factors and develop alternative coping mechanisms. Encouraging physical expenditure of energy by exercise, unit jobs, games, or discussion helps decrease anxiety and increase self-esteem.

SOCIAL ISOLATION

Social isolation is aloneness experienced by an individual and perceived as imposed by others or self and as a negative or threatened state.[9]

Related Factors[1-3,9,10]

Physiologic

Altered state of health
Cancer
Drug or alcohol addiction
Hospitalization or terminal illness
Incontinence (embarrassment, odor)
Obesity, anorexia, bulemia
Language disorders
Nervous system alterations
Physical handicaps
Sensory loss

Psychologic

Altered physical appearance
Delay in accomplishing developmental tasks
Emotional illness (e.g., extreme anxiety, depression, paranoia, phobias, psychoses)
Immature interests
Inability to engage in satisfying relationships

Sociocultural

Alternative lifestyle
Death of significant other
Divorce
Extreme poverty
Homelessness
Hospitalization or placement in long-term care
Inadequate personal resources
Living alone
Loss of usual means of transportation
Removal into another culture
Single parenthood
Unaccepted social values

Defining Characteristics[1,2,9]

Absence of supportive significant others
Evidence of physical and/or mental handicap
Inappropriate interests and activities for developmental age/stage
Incommunicativeness
Lack of eye contact
Preoccupation with own thoughts
Projection of hostility in voice and behavior
Repetitive, meaningless actions
Sad, dull affect
Seeking to be alone or existing in subculture

Expected Patient Outcomes and Nursing Interventions With Rationale[1-8,10-12]

Acknowledge state of social isolation and verbalize a desire and willingness to be involved with others, as evidenced by:

Expresses feelings associated with social isolation
Expresses a desire to interact with others in a positive way
Participates in and functions appropriately in group activities
Verbalizes a plan to participate in social activity

- Explore patient's perception of social isolation.
- Assess specific causes of social isolation through the use of a social history and physical assessment.

Social isolation is a subjective experience and should be validated with the patient before a diagnosis is made.

- Initiate a trusting nurse/patient relationship.
- Spend time with the patient engaged in active listening, maintaining eye contact, and when appropriate, using touch as a means of contact and comfort. (On an inpatient unit spend at least 15 minutes per shift involved in conversation with the patient.)
- Explore and help the patient identify available specific activities, groups, social outlets *to promote social interaction.*
- Positively reinforce active involvement with others. (On an inpatient unit, encourage attendance and participation in groups, social outings, social interaction at meal time or leisure time.)
- Arrange with patient for specific periods of planned socially interactive diversionary activity. Whether this is active or passive recreation depends on the patient's physical condition (e.g., cards, sports).
- Provide immediate and honest feedback about patient's behavior, especially withdrawn or alienating behaviors.
- Involve patient and family or significant other in setting goals and planning care.
- Give recognition and positive reinforcement for self-initiated and self-directed attendance at activities.
- Provide educational opportunities for patient and family *to enhance knowledge about needs and to facilitate skill development (e.g., social skills, assertiveness, communication, reading material).*

Human relationships are important to mental and physical well-being. Social isolation, the lack of human companionship, death or absence of parents in early childhood, sudden loss of love, and chronic human loneliness are significant contributors to premature death and abnormal human functioning.

Verbalize and demonstrate ways to promote meaningful relationships, as evidenced by:

Actively participates in activities on inpatient unit
Approaches others to socialize
Develops a plan to join a social peer group or activity on a regular basis
Interacts with family or significant others
Sets realistic goals and identifies realistic time schedules for achieving goals
Uses resources available through an agency (social service, home health care, psychology services, self-improvement classes) to establish realistic plan for the future

- Explore and help the patient identify specific activities, groups, social outlets available *to promote social interaction.*
- Positively reinforce active involvement with others. (On an inpatient unit, encourage attendance and participation in groups, social outings, social interaction at mealtime or leisure time.)
- Arrange with patient for specific periods of planned socially interactive diversionary activity. Whether this is active or passive recreation depends on the patient's physical condition (e.g., cards, sports).
- Provide immediate and honest feedback about patient's behavior, especially withdrawn or alienating behaviors.
- Involve patient and family or significant other in setting goals and planning care.
- Give recognition and positive reinforcement for self-initiated and self-directed attendance at activities.
- Provide educational opportunities for patient and family *to enhance knowledge about needs and to facilitate skill development (e.g., social skills, assertiveness, communication, reading material).*
- Explore available volunteer activities.

References

Role-Relationship

1. Gordon M: *Manual of nursing diagnosis,* ed 9, St. Louis, 2000, Mosby.

Anticipatory Grieving

1. Doenges ME, Townsend MC, Moorhouse MF: *Psychiatric care plans: guidelines for individualizing care,* ed. 3, Philadelphia, 1998, FA Davis.
2. Duke S: An exploration of anticipatory grief: the lived experience of people during their spouses' terminal illness and in bereavement, *J Adv Nurs* 28(4):829, 1998.
3. Ferszt GG, Heineman L, Ferszt EJ et al: Transformation through grieving: art and the bereaved, *Holist Nurs Pract* 13(1):68, 1998.
4. Fontaine KL, Fletcher JS: *Mental health nursing,* ed 4, Menlo Park, Calif, 1999, Addison-Wesley.
5. Mallison RK: Grief work of HIV-positive persons and their survivors, *Nurs Clin North Am* 34(1):163, 1999.
6. McCloskey JC, Bulechek GM, editors: Grief work facilitation. In *Nursing interventions classification (NIC),* ed 3, St. Louis, 2001, Mosby.
7. Moules NJ, Amundson JK: Grief—an invitation to inertia: a narrative approach to working with grief, *J Fam Nurs* 3(4):378, 1997.
8. North American Nursing Diagnosis Association: *Nursing diagnoses: definitions and classification 2001-2002,* Philadelphia, 2001, The Association.

9. Paquette M, Rodemich C: *Psychiatric nursing diagnosis care plans for DSM-IV,* Boston, 1997, Jones & Bartlett.
10. Stuart GW, Sundeen SJ: *Principles and practice of psychiatric nursing,* ed 5, St. Louis, 1995, Mosby.

Dysfunctional Grieving

1. Cutcliffe JR: Hope, counseling and complicated bereavement reactions, *J Adv Nurs* 28(4):754, 1998.
2. Doenges ME, Townsend MC, Moorhouse MF: *Psychiatric care plans: guidelines for individualizing care,* ed 3, Philadelphia, 1998, FA Davis.
3. Ferszt GG, Heineman L, Ferszt EJ et al: Transformation through grieving: art and the bereaved, *Holist Nurs Prac* 13(1):68, 1998.
4. Fontaine KL, Fletcher JS: *Mental health nursing,* ed 4, Menlo Park, Calif, 1999, Addison-Wesley.
5. Long A: The healing process, the road to recovery and positive mental health, *J Psychiatr Ment Health Nurs* 5(6):535, 1998.
6. McCloskey JC, Bulechek GM, editors: Grief work facilitation. In In *Nursing interventions classification (NIC),* ed 3, St. Louis, 2001, Mosby.
7. McFarland GK, Wasli EL, Gerety EK: *Nursing diagnoses and process in psychiatric mental health nursing,* ed 3, Philadelphia, 1997, JB Lippincott.
8. Moules NJ, Amundson JK: Grief—an invitation to inertia: a narrative approach to working with grief, *J Fam Nurs* 3(4):378, 1997.
9. North American Nursing Diagnosis Association: *Nursing diagnoses: definitions and classification 2001-2002,* Philadelphia, 2001, The Association.
10. Paquette M, Rodemich C: *Psychiatric nursing diagnosis care plans for DSM-IV,* Boston, 1997, Jones & Bartlett.
11. Romanoff BD, Terenzio M: Rituals and the grieving process, *Death Stud* 22(8):697, 1998.
12. Stuart GW, Sundeen SJ: *Principles and practice of psychiatric nursing,* ed 5, St. Louis, 1995, Mosby.

Caregiver Role Strain

1. Borneman R: Caring for cancer patients at home: the effect on family caregivers, *Home Health Care Manage Pract* 10(4):25, 1998.
2. Caliandro G, Hughes C: The experience of being a grandmother who is the primary caregiver for her HIV-positive grandchild, *Nurs Res* 47(2):107, 1998.
3. Cook JM, Ahrens AH, Pearson JL: Hopelessness: a mediator or moderator of depression in Alzheimer's disease caregivers? *J Ment Health Aging* 2(1):5, 1996.
4. McCloskey JC, Bulechek GM, editors: Caregiver support. In *Nursing interventions classification (NIC),* ed 3, St. Louis, 2001, Mosby.
5. McFarland GK, Wasli EL, Gerety EK: *Nursing diagnoses and process in psychiatric mental health nursing,* ed 3, Philadelphia, 1997, JB Lippincott.
6. North American Nursing Diagnosis Association: *Nursing diagnoses: definitions and classification 2001-2002,* Philadelphia, 2001, The Association.
7. Reynolds NR, Alonzo AA: HIV informal caregiving: emergent conflict and growth, *Res Nurs Health* 21(3):251, 1998.
8. Scholte op Reimer WJ, de Haan RJ, Rijnders PT et al: The burden of caregiving in partners of long-term stroke survivors, *Stroke* 29(8):1605, 1998.
9. Schumacher KI, Stewart BJ, Archbold PG: Conceptualization and measurement of doing family caregiving well, *Image J Nurs Sch* 30(1):75, 1998.
10. Vrabec NJ: Literature review of social support and caregiver burden, 1980 to 1995, *Image J Nurs Sch* 29(4):383, 1997.
11. Whitlatch C, Feinberg L, Sebesta D: Depression and health in family caregivers, *J Aging Health* 9(7):222, 1997.

Risk for Caregiver Role Strain

1. Borneman R: Caring for cancer patients at home: the effect on family caregivers, *Home Health Care Manage Pract* 10(4):25, 1998.
2. Caliandro G, Hughes C: The experience of being a grandmother who is the primary caregiver for her HIV-positive grandchild, *Nurs Res* 47(2):107, 1998.
3. Cook JM, Ahrens AH, Pearson JL: Hopelessness: a mediator or moderator of depression in Alzheimer's disease caregivers? *J Ment Health Aging* 2(1):5, 1996.
4. McCloskey JC, Bulechek GM, editors: Caregiver support. In *Nursing interventions classification (NIC),* ed 3, St. Louis, 2001, Mosby.
5. McFarland GK, Wasli EL, Gerety EK: *Nursing diagnoses and process in psychiatric mental health nursing,* ed 3, Philadelphia, 1997, JB Lippincott.
6. North American Nursing Diagnosis Association: *Nursing diagnoses: definitions and classification 2001-2002,* Philadelphia, 2001, The Association.
7. Scholte op Reimer WJ, de Haan RJ, Rijnders PT et al: The burden of caregiving in partners of long-term stroke survivors, *Stroke* 29(8):1605, 1998.
8. Whitlatch C, Feinberg L, Sebesta D: Depression and health in family caregivers, *J Aging Health* 9(7):222, 1997.

Chronic Sorrow

1. Ackley BJ, Ladwig GB: *Nursing diagnosis handbook: a guide for planning care,* St. Louis, 1999, Mosby.
2. Carpenito LJ: *Handbook of nursing diagnosis,* ed 8, Philadelphia, 1999, JB Lippincott.
3. Crookes PA: The nature of grieving, *J Cancer Care* 5(2):57, 1996.
4. Eakes GG: Chronic sorrow: the lived experience of parents of chronically mentally ill individuals, *Arch Psychiatr Nurs* 9(2):77, 1995.
5. Eakes GG, Burke ML, Hainsworth MA: Middle-range theory of chronic sorrow, *Image J Nurs Sch* 30(2):179, 1998.
6. Kagawa-Singer M: The cultural context of death rituals and mourning practices, *Oncol Nurs Forum* 25(10):1752, 1998.
7. Knafft SK, Knafft LJ: Chronic sorrow: parents' lived experience, *Holist Nurs Pract* 13(1):59, 1998.
8. Lubkin IM: *Chronic illness: impact and interventions,* ed 4, Boston, 1999, Jones & Bartlett.
9. McCamdess NJ, Conner FP: Older women and grief: a new direction for research, *J Women Aging* 9(3):85, 1997.
10. North American Nursing Diagnosis Association: *Nursing diagnoses: definitions and classification 2001-2002,* Philadelphia, 2001, The Association.
11. Romanoff BD, Terenzio M: Rituals and the grieving process, *Death Stud* 22(8):697, 1998.

Dysfunctional Family Processes: Alcoholism

1. Forgays DK: An evaluation of the relationship between family bonding characteristics and adolescent alcohol use, *J Child Adolesc Subst Abuse* 7(4):1, 1998.
2. Grant BF: The impact of family history of alcoholism on the relationship between age at onset of alcohol use and DSM-IV alcohol dependence: results from the National Longitudinal Alcohol Epidemiologic Survey, *Alcohol Health Res World* 22(2):144, 1998.
3. Johnson K, Bryant DD, Collins DA et al: Preventing and reducing alcohol and other drug use among high-risk youths by increasing family resilience, *Soc Work J Natl Assoc Soc Work* 43(4):297, 1998.

4. Lindeman M, Hokanson J, Bartek JK: The alcoholic family: a nursing diagnosis validation study, *Nurs Diagnosis J Nurs Lang Classification* 5(2):65, 1994.
5. McCloskey JC, Bulechek GM, editors: Family process maintenance. In *Nursing interventions classification (NIC),* ed 3, St. Louis, 2001, Mosby.
6. McFarland GK, Wasli EL, Gerety EK: *Nursing diagnoses and process in psychiatric mental health nursing,* ed 3, Philadelphia, 1997, JB Lippincott.
7. Murray BL: Perceptions of adolescents living with parental alcoholism, *J Psychiatr Ment Health Nurs* 5(6):525, 1998.
8. North American Nursing Diagnosis Association: *Nursing diagnoses: definitions and classification 2001-2002,* Philadelphia, 2001, The Association.
9. Paquette M, Rodemichy C: *Psychiatric nursing diagnosis care plans for DSM-IV,* Boston, 1997, Jones & Bartlett.
10. Stuart GW, Sundeen SJ: *Principles and practice of psychiatric nursing,* ed 5, St. Louis, 1995, Mosby.

Interrupted Family Processes

1. Beck CT: Postpartum depressed mothers' experiences interacting with their children, *Nurs Res* 45(2):98, 1996.
2. Carruth AK, Tate US, Moffett BS et al: Reciprocity, emotional well-being, and family functioning as determinants of family satisfaction in caregivers of elderly parents, *Nurs Res* 46(2):93, 1997.
3. Gates MF, Lackey NR: Youngsters caring for adults with cancer, *Image J Nurs Sch* 30(1):11, 1998.
4. Lubkin IM: *Chronic illness: impact and interventions,* ed 3, Boston, 1999, Jones & Bartlett.
5. McCloskey JC, Bulechek GM, editors: Family integrity promotion; Family integrity promotion: childbearing family. In *Nursing interventions classification (NIC),* ed 3, St. Louis, 2001, Mosby.
6. McFarland GK, Wasli EL, Gerety EK: *Nursing diagnoses and process in psychiatric mental health nursing,* ed 3, Philadelphia, 1997, JB Lippincott.
7. Morrissette PJ: Trouble on the farm: conflicting lifestyles and parent-adolescent discord, *J Fam Soc Work* 2(3):33, 1997.
8. North American Nursing Diagnosis Association: *Nursing diagnoses: definitions and classification 2001-2002,* Philadelphia, 2001, The Association.
9. Saunders JC: Family functioning in families providing care for a family member with schizophrenia, *Issues Ment Health Nurs* 20(2):95, 1999.
10. Schumacher KL, Stewart BJ, Archbold PG: Conceptualization and measurement of doing family caregiving well, *Image J Nurs Sch* 30(1):63, 1998.
11. Twibell RS: Family coping during critical illness, *Dimens Crit Care Nurs* 17(2):100, 1998.

Ineffective Role Performance

1. Beck CT: Postpartum depressed mothers' experiences interacting with their children, *Nurs Res* 45(2):98, 1996.
2. Caliandro G, Hughes C: The experience of being a grandmother who is the primary caregiver for her HIV-positive grandchild, *Nurs Res* 47(2):107, 1998.
3. Deatrick JA, Brennan D, Cameron ME: Mothers with multiple sclerosis and their children: effects of fatigue and exacerbations on maternal support, *Nurs Res* 47(4):205, 1998.
4. Gates MF, Lackey NR: Youngsters caring for adults with cancer, *Image J Nurs Sch* 30(1):11, 1998.
5. McCloskey JC, Bulechek GM, editors: Role enhancement. In *Nursing interventions classification (NIC),* ed 3, St. Louis, 2001, Mosby.
6. North American Nursing Diagnosis Association: *Nursing diagnoses: definitions and classification 2001-2002,* Philadelphia 2001, The Association.

Impaired Parenting

1. Ackley BJ, Ladwig GB: *Nursing diagnosis handbook: a guide to planning care,* ed 4, St. Louis, 1999, Mosby.
2. Barclay L, Kent D: Recent immigration and the misery of motherhood: a discussion of pertinent issues, *Midwifery* 14(1):4, 1998.
3. Carpenito LJ: *Nursing diagnosis: application to clinical practice,* ed 7, Philadelphia, 1997, JB Lippincott.
4. Hall LA, Sachs B, Rayens MK: Mothers' potential for child abuse: the roles of childhood abuse and social resources, *Nurs Res* 47(2):87, 1998.
5. Lesser J, Koniak-Griffin D, Anderson NL: Depressed adolescent mothers' perceptions of their own maternal role, *Issues Ment Health Nurs* 20(2):131, 1999.
6. McCloskey JC, Bulechek GM, editors: Abuse protection: child; Developmental enhancement. In *Nursing interventions classification (NIC),* ed 3, St. Louis, 2001, Mosby.
7. Nicholson J, Sweeney EM, Geller JL: Mothers with mental illness: family relationships and the context of parenting, *Psychiatr Serv* 49(5):643, 1998.
8. Niska K, Snyder M, Lia-Hoagberg B: Family ritual facilitates adaptation to parenthood, *Public Health Nurs* 15(5):329, 1998.
9. North American Nursing Diagnosis Association: *Nursing diagnoses: definitions and classification 2001-2002,* Philadelphia, 2001, The Association.
10. Pillitteri A: *Maternal and child health nursing: care of the childbearing and childrearing family,* ed 3, Philadelphia, 1999, JB Lippincott.
11. Reece SM, Harkless G: Self-efficacy, stress, and parental adaptation: applications to the care of childbearing families, *J Fam Nurs* 4(2):198, 1998.
12. Sachs B, Hall LA, Lutenbacher M et al: Potential for abusive parenting by rural mothers with low-birth-weight children, *Image J Nurs Sch* 31(1):21, 1999.

Risk for Impaired Parenting

1. Ackley BJ, Ladwig GB: *Nursing diagnosis handbook: a guide to planning care,* ed 4, St. Louis, 1999, Mosby.
2. Carpenito LJ: *Nursing diagnosis: application to clinical practice,* ed 7, Philadelphia, 1997, JB Lippincott.
3. Maier MJ: Promoting parenting by keeping new families together from birth through dismissal, *Kansas Nurse* 71(5):9, 1996.
4. McCloskey JC, Bulechek GM, editors: Family integrity promotion; Developmental enhancement. In *Nursing interventions classification (NIC),* ed 3, St. Louis, 2001, Mosby.
5. Miles MS, Holditch-Davis D, Burchinal P et al: Distress and growth outcomes in mothers of medically fragile infants, *Nurs Res* 48(3):129, 1999.
6. Nicholson J, Sweeney EM, Geller JL: Mothers with mental illness: family relationships and the context of parenting, *Psychiatr Serv* 49(5):643, 1998.
7. North American Nursing Diagnosis Association: *Nursing diagnoses: definitions and classification 2001-2002,* Philadelphia, 2001, The Association.
8. Pillitteri A: *Maternal and child health nursing: care of the childbearing and childrearing family,* ed 3, Philadelphia, 1999, JB Lippincott.
9. Sachs B, Hall LA, Lutenbacher M et al: Potential for abusive parenting by rural mothers with low-birth-weight children, *Image J Nurs Sch* 31(1):21, 1999.

Parental Role Conflict

1. Ackley BJ, Ladwig GB: *Nursing diagnosis handbook: a guide to planning care,* ed 4, St. Louis, 1999, Mosby.
2. Clark SM, Miles MS: Conflicting responses: the experiences of fathers of infants diagnosed with severe congenital heart disease, *J Soc Pediatr Nurses* 4(1):7, 1999.
3. Lesser J, Koniak-Griffin D, Anderson NL: Depressed adolescent mothers' perceptions of their own maternal role, *Issues Ment Health Nurs* 20(2):131, 1999.
4. McCloskey JC, Bulechek GM, editors: Role enhancement. In *Nursing interventions classification (NIC),* ed 3, St. Louis, 2001, Mosby.
5. McFarland GK, Wasli EL, Gerety EK: *Nursing diagnosis and process in psychiatric mental health nursing,* ed 3, Philadelphia, 1997, JB Lippincott.
6. Nelson DB, Edgil AE: Family dynamics in families with very low birth weight and full term infants: a pilot study, *J Pediatr Nurs* 13(2):95, 1998.
7. North American Nursing Diagnosis Association: *Nursing diagnoses: definitions and classification 2001-2002,* Philadelphia, 2001, The Association.
8. Penning MJ: In the middle: parental caregiving in the context of other roles, *J Gerontol B Psychol Sci Soc Sci* 53B(4):S188, 1998.
9. Pillitteri A: *Maternal and child health nursing: care of the childbearing and childrearing family,* ed 3, Philadelphia, 1999, JB Lippincott.
10. Sheldon LM: Making decisions: involving parents as partners in care, *J Child Health Care* 1(4):172, 1997.

Risk for Impaired Parent/Infant/Child Attachment

1. Clark SM, Miles MS: Conflicting responses: the experiences of fathers of infants diagnosed with severe congenital heart disease, *J Soc Pediatr Nurses* 4(1):7, 1999.
2. Denehy JA: Interventions related to parent-infant attachment, *Nurs Clin North Am* 27(2):425, 1992.
3. Klaus MH, Kennell JH, editors: *Maternal-infant bonding,* St. Louis, 1982, Mosby.
4. Kroeger R, Manstedt DL, Lowe M: Variables in altered parenting: physical child abuse. In Carroll-Johnson RM, editor: *Classification of nursing diagnoses: proceedings of the tenth conference,* Philadelphia, 1994, JB Lippincott.
5. Lesser J, Koniak-Griffin D, Anderson NL: Depressed adolescent mothers' perceptions of their own maternal role, *Issues Ment Health Nurs* 20(2):131, 1999.
6. Libbus K, Bush TA, Hockman NM: Breastfeeding beliefs of low-income primigravidae, *Int J Nurs Stud* 34(2):1444, 1997.
7. McCloskey JC, Bulechek GM, editors: Attachment promotion. In *Nursing interventions classification (NIC),* ed 3, St. Louis, 2001, Mosby.
8. North American Nursing Diagnosis Association: *Nursing diagnoses: definitions and classification 2001-2002,* Philadelphia, 2001, The Association.
9. Thome M, Alder B: A telephone intervention to reduce fatigue and symptom distress in mothers with difficult infants in the community, *J Adv Nurs* 29(1):128, 1999.
10. Wong DL: *Waley and Wong's nursing care of infants and children,* ed 5, St. Louis, 1995, Mosby.

Impaired Social Interaction

1. Ackley B, Ladwig GB: *Nursing diagnosis handbook: a guide to planning care,* St. Louis, 1999, Mosby.
2. Barclay L, Kent D: Recent immigration and the misery of motherhood: a discussion of pertinent issues, *Midwifery* 14(1):4, 1998.
3. Bondevik M, Skogstad A: The oldest old, ADL, social network, and loneliness, *West J Nurs Res* 20(3):325, 1998.
4. Chang BL: Cognitive-behavioral intervention for homebound caregivers of persons with dementia, *Nurs Res* 48(3):173, 1999.
5. Daniels L, Roll D: Group treatment of social impairment in people with mental illness, *Psychiatr Rehabil J* 21(3):273, 1998.
6. Johnson J: Older rural adults and the decision to stop driving: the influence of family and friends, *J Community Health Nurs* 15(4):205, 1998.
7. McCloskey JC, Bulechek GM, editors: Socialization enhancement. In *Nursing interventions classification (NIC),* ed 3, St. Louis, 2001, Mosby.
8. North American Nursing Diagnosis Association: *Nursing diagnoses: definitions and classification 2001-2002,* Philadelphia, 2001, The Association.
9. Potts MK: Social support and depression among older adults living alone: the importance of friends within and outside of a retirement community, *Soc Work J Natl Assoc Soc Work* 42(4):348, 1997.
10. Simonsick EM, Kasper JD, Phillips CL: Physical disability and social interaction: factors associated with low social contact and home confinement in disabled older women, *J Gerontol B Psychol Sci Soc Sci* 53B(4):S209, 1998.

Impaired Verbal Communication

1. Cherney LR, Halper AS: Communication problems following stroke, *Top Geriatr Rehabil* 14(2):18, 1998.
2. Engleman MD, Griffin HC, Wheeler L: Deaf-blindness and communication: practical knowledge and strategies, *J Visual Impair Blindness* 92(11):783, 1998.
3. LeMone P, Burke K: *Medical-surgical nursing: critical thinking in client care,* ed 2, Upper Saddle River, NJ, 2000, Prentice Hall Health.
4. Mandel E, Shulman MD: Overcoming communication disorders in the elderly, *Patient Care* 31(2):55, 1997.
5. McCloskey JC, Bulechek GM, editors: Communication enhancement: hearing deficit; Communication deficit: speech deficit. In *Nursing interventions classification (NIC),* ed 3, St. Louis, 2001, Mosby.
6. North American Nursing Diagnosis Association: *Nursing diagnoses: definitions and classification 2001-2002,* Philadelphia, 2001, The Association.
7. Schmitz C, Volkman S: Communicating with the deaf or hard-of-hearing, *Access* 13(1):35, 1999.

Relocation Stress Syndrome

1. Armer J: Elderly relocation to a rural congregate setting: personal meaning and perceptions related to decision to move and overall adjustment, *J Nurs Sci* 1(3/4):105, 1996.
2. Bidewell JW, Ledwidge H, Blanch VT et al: The effect of nursing home placement on the spouse remaining in the community, *Geriaction* 17(1):9, 1999.
3. Cutler L, Garner M: Reducing relocation stress after discharge from the intensive therapy unit, *Intensive Crit Care Nurs* 11(6):333, 1995.
4. Davidhizar R, Dowd S: Successful geriatric relocation, *J Case Manage* 3(6):23, 1997.
5. Forbes SA, Hoffart N, Redford LJ: Decision making by high functional status elders regarding nursing home placement, *J Case Manage* 6(4):166, 1997.
6. McCloskey JC, Bulechek GM, editors: Coping enhancement. In *Nursing interventions classification (NIC),* ed 3, St. Louis, 2001, Mosby.
7. Mitchell MG: The effects of relocation on the elderly, *Perspect* 23(1):2, 1999.
8. North American Nursing Diagnosis Association: *Nursing diagnoses: definitions and classification 2001-2002,* Philadelphia, 2001, The Association.

9. Penrod J, Dellasega C: Caregivers' experiences in making placement decisions, *West J Nurs Res* 20(6):706, 1998.
10. Porock D, Martin K, Oldham L et al: Relocation stress syndrome: the case of palliative care patients, *Palliat Med* 11(6):444, 1997.
11. Tilse C: Continuing or refusing to care: the meaning of placing a spouse in long term care, *Am J Alzheimer's Dis* 13(1):29, 1998.

Risk for Relocation Stress Syndrome

1. Jackson B, Swanson C, Hicks LE et al: Bridge of continuity from hospital to nursing home—part I. A proactive approach to reduce relocation stress syndrome in the elderly, *Continuum An Interdisciplin J Continuity Care* 20(1):3, 2000.
2. Johnson RA: Relocation stress syndrome. In Maas ML, Buckwalter KC, Hardy MD et al: *Nursing care of older adults: diagnoses, outcomes and interventions,* St. Louis, 2001, Mosby.
3. Kellett UM: Transition in care: family carers' experience of nursing home placement, *J Adv Nurs* 29(6):1474, 1999.
4. Mallick MJ, Whipple TW: Validity of the nursing diagnosis of relocation stress syndrome, *Nurs Res* 49(2):97, 2000.
5. McCloskey JC, Bulechek GM, editors: *Nursing interventions classification (NIC),* ed 3, St. Louis, 2001, Mosby.
6. North American Nursing Diagnosis Association: *NANDA nursing diagnoses: definitions and classification 2001-2002,* Philadelphia, 2001, The Association.
7. Porock D, Martin K, Oldham L et al: Relocation stress syndrome: the case of palliative care patients, *Palliat Med* 11(6):444, 1997.
8. Reed J, Morgan D: Discharging older people from hospital to care homes: implications for nursing, *J Adv Nurs* 29(4):819, 1999.
9. Smith GE, Kikmen E, O'Brien PC: Risk factors for nursing home placement in a population-based dementia cohort, *J Am Geriatr Soc* 48(5):519, 2000.

Risk for Other-Directed Violence, Risk for Self-Directed Violence

1. Arbore P: Assessing the risk for suicide in the elderly, *Home Healthcare Consultant* 5(5):23, 1998.
2. Barstow DG: Self-injury and self-mutilation: nursing approaches, *J Psychosoc Nurs Ment Health Serv* 33(2):19, 1995.
3. Grzybowska P, Finlay I: The incidence of suicide in palliative care patients, *Palliat Med* 11(4):313, 1997.
4. Littrell KH, Littrell SH: Current understanding of violence and aggression: assessment and treatment, *J Psychosoc Nurs Ment Health Serv* 36(12):18, 1998.
5. McCloskey JC, Bulechek GM, editors: Anger control assistance; Environment management: violence prevention. In *Nursing interventions classification (NIC),* ed 3, St. Louis, 2001, Mosby.
6. McFarland GK, Wasli EL, Gerety EK: *Nursing diagnoses and process in psychiatric mental health nursing,* ed 3, Philadelphia, 1997, JB Lippincott.
7. Melville A, House A: Understanding deliberate self-harm, *Nurs Times* 95(7):46, 1999.
8. North American Nursing Diagnosis Association: *Nursing diagnoses: definitions and classification 2001-2002,* Philadelphia, 2001, The Association.
9. O'Connor DL: Managing depression in the elderly, *Patient Care Nurse Pract* 1(3):11, 1998.
10. Saner H, Ellickson P: Current risk factors for adolescent violence, *J Adolesc Health* 19(2):94, 1996.
11. Shergill SS, Szmukler G: How predictable is violence and suicide in community psychiatric patients? *J Ment Health* 7(4):393, 1998.
12. Smith JE, Early JA, Green PR et al: Risk for suicide and risk for violence: a case for separating the current violence diagnoses, *Nurs Diagnosis J Nurs Lang Classification* 8(2):67, 1997.
13. Stuart GW, Sundeen SJ: *Principles and practice of psychiatric nursing,* ed 5, St. Louis, 1995, Mosby.

Social Isolation

1. Asher SR, Gazelle H: Loneliness, peer relations, and language disorders in childhood, *Top Lang Disord* 19(2):16, 1999.
2. Barclay L, Kent D: Recent immigration and the misery of motherhood: a discussion of pertinent issues, *Midwifery* 14(1):4, 1998.
3. Benson S: The older adult and fear of crime, *J Gerontol Nurs* 23(10):24, 1997.
4. Hansell PS, Hughes CB, Caliandro G et al: The effect of a social support boosting intervention on stress, coping, and social support in caregivers of children with HIV/AIDS, *Nurs Res* 47(2):79, 1998.
5. Johnson J: Older rural adults and the decision to stop driving: the influence of family and friends, *J Community Health Nurs* 15(4):205, 1998.
6. Jonsdottir H: Life patterns of people with chronic obstructive pulmonary disease: isolation and being closed in, *Nurs Sci Q* 11(4):160, 1998.
7. McCloskey JC, Bulechek GM, editors: Socialization enhancement. In *Nursing interventions classification (NIC),* ed 3, St. Louis, 2001, Mosby.
8. McFarland GK, Wasli EL, Gerety EK: *Nursing diagnoses and process in psychiatric mental health nursing,* ed 3, Philadelphia, 1997, JB Lippincott.
9. North American Nursing Diagnosis Association: *Nursing diagnoses: definitions and classification 2001-2002,* Philadelphia, 2001, The Association.
10. Simonsick EM, Kasper JD, Phillips CL: Physical disability and social interaction: factors associated with low social contact and home confinement in disabled older women, *J Gerontol B Psychol Sci Soc Sci* 53B(4):S209, 1998.
11. White C: Including the excluded—the huge role mental health plays in the social exclusion of homeless people, *Nursing Times* 94(37):32, 1998.
12. White R: Rural home care: social work intervention in social isolation and safety concerns, *Caring* 16(1):28, 1997.

FUNCTIONAL HEALTH PATTERN

9 Sexuality-Reproductive[1]

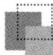

Ineffective Sexuality Patterns

Ineffective sexuality patterns are the state in which an individual expresses concern regarding his or her sexuality.[13]

Related Factors[13]

Altered body image
Altered body structure or function
Altered self-concept
Conflicts with sexual orientation or variant preferences
Depression
Effects of medications (e.g., antihypertensives, antidepressants, hormones)
Fatigue
Fear of pregnancy or of acquiring a sexually transmitted disease
Illness, trauma, or surgery
Impaired relationship with significant other
Ineffective or absent role models
Ingestion of alcohol or drugs (e.g., cocaine, marijuana, narcotics)
Knowledge deficit
Lack of privacy
Lack of significant other
Menopause/andropause
Pregnancy
Stress

Defining Characteristics[13]

Anticipated or actual negative changes in sexual behaviors, sexual health, sexual functioning, or sexual identity
Changes in primary and/or secondary sexual characteristics
Inappropriate verbal or nonverbal sexual behavior
Reported difficulties, limitations, or changes in sexual behaviors or activities

Expected Patient Outcomes and Nursing Interventions With Rationale[1,3-9,11-12,14]

Identify specific concerns about sexuality, as evidenced by:
Verbalizes effect of change, loss, or stress on sexuality

- Assess usual sexual patterns and sexual self-concept in the sexual history, ensuring privacy, confidentiality, and using an objective, nonthreatening, and nonjudgmental attitude. Begin the interview with general questions (such as "When did you have your first menstrual period?") before asking more specific questions about sexual practices. Include questions about the patient's feelings about himself as a man or herself as a woman with this concern. *A knowledge base of the patient's sexuality is necessary to design interventions that are individualized. The nurse must establish a trusting relationship to collect personal and private information. Sexuality encompasses all parts of a person, not just physical sexual function.*
- Explore possible causes of altered sexuality pattern, for example, sexual partner, sexual orientation, fear of pregnancy or disease, previous physical or sexual abuse. It is often necessary to ask specific questions. *Sexuality is usually regarded as a private part of oneself, and concerns are often not verbalized unless the nurse initiates the discussion.*

Engage in previously satisfying or alternate methods of satisfying sexual function, as evidenced by:
Verbalizes positive sexual self-concept
Verbalizes satisfaction with sexual function

- Help patient express grief and anger over losses.
- Convey to the patient and partner a willingness to discuss sexual thoughts and feelings, by using statements such as "Some people with ___ have concerns about how this will affect their sexual functioning. Is this a concern for you or your partner?"
- Use terms the patient understands.
- Discuss, as appropriate, potential effects of medications, drugs, illness, aging, pregnancy, trauma, and/or surgery on sexuality.
- Discuss effects of stress and loss on sexuality.
- Provide information about modifications in sexual practices that may be used to regain a satisfying sexual relationship, such as changes in positions for sexual intercourse, having sexual intercourse in the morning when one is less fatigued, taking pain medications or using bronchodilators before sexual activities, and the importance of touch.
- Ensure the information is compatible with the patient's values and cultural beliefs.
- Emphasize the need for open communications between sexual partners.
- Provide information, as appropriate, about contraceptive methods, use of condoms, sexual abstinence, and masturbation. Clarify myths and misinformation that is verbalized.
- Refer patients who need more help to professionals in mental health and sex therapy.

Nurses are often reluctant to discuss issues of sexuality: use of a model such as this facilitates open discussion and appropri-

ate interventions. Nursing interventions that promote sexual health include counseling about sexual concerns and teaching about sexuality-related subjects.

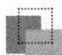

SEXUAL DYSFUNCTION

Sexual dysfunction is a state in which an individual experiences a change in sexual function that is viewed as unsatisfying, unrewarding, or inadequate.[11]

Related Factors[11]

Altered body structure or function
Biopsychosocial alteration in sexuality
Cognitive disorders
Conflicts involving values
Ineffectual or absent role models
Lack of privacy
Lack of significant other
Misinformation or lack of knowledge
Physical abuse
Psychosocial abuse
Religious beliefs or cultural taboos
Sexual trauma
Values conflict
Vulnerability

Defining Characteristics[11]

Actual or perceived limitations imposed by disease and/or therapy
Alteration in achieving perceived sex role
Alteration in achieving sexual satisfaction
Alteration in relationship with significant other
Change in ejaculation
Change of interest in self and others
Change in libido
Change in orgasm
Decreased vaginal lubrication
Dyspareunia
Gender identity disorders
Hormone changes resulting from aging, medical therapy, or disease
Impotence
Inability to achieve desired satisfaction
Seeking confirmation of desirability
Vaginismus
Verbalized problem

Expected Patient Outcomes and Nursing Interventions With Rationale[1-10,12,13]

Openly appraise values and cultural practices that can interfere with personal sexual responsivity, as evidenced by:

Clarifies issues regarding the incest taboo
Recognizes appropriate interpersonal transactions that govern sexual exchanges
Recognizes the boundaries of violence and coercion between sexual partners

- As part of the comprehensive evaluation process (including assessment of the orgasm-ejaculation phase, excitement phase, and desire phase), focus on values and practices associated with sex role, sexual practices, and power within the sexual partner relationship. Note value and cultural conflicts that can interfere with satisfying, nonexploitive, noncoercive, age-appropriate sexual experiences. This can be done with individuals, with couples, and within the context of groups.
- If nurse is in doubt of this process and is unfamiliar with his or her own values, make a referral to nurse or specialist in the area of sexual dysfunctions and value clarification procedures or to a clinical specialist in psychiatric–mental health nursing.

Assessment and differential diagnosis and specialized-assessment diagnostic skill are necessary given the complexity of the functional disorder. Collaboration with other professionals, as well as the nurse's specialized expertise, is required both for differential diagnostic activities and for particular intervention modes.

Will not adhere to beliefs and attitudes that inhibit or disrupt noncoercive, consensual sex and personal sex response patterns and phases, as evidenced by:

Appraises self positively with regard to sexual response, activities
Clarifies and reduces fears, nonfunctional guilt, anger or sense of inferiority over sexual prowess and bodily features

- Use cognitive-behavioral approaches such as reframing, thought stopping; *this requires training in self-monitoring of internal processes, such as internal dialogue, imaging, and sensory experiences.*
- Elicit beliefs regarding sexual performance and adequacy; explore relationship of these thoughts to inhibition and dissatisfaction with sexual experiences.

When the related factor is organic, nursing care focuses on educating the client and counseling about misconceptions that provoke anxiety and depression. Because sexual functioning most often involves a partner, nursing intervention is also directed at the appropriate partner.

Identify and reduce interpersonal conflicts with sex partner (age-appropriate, noncoercive), as evidenced by:

Opens up communication with partner to reduce interpersonal conflicts that are carried over to the sexual experience

- With couple, assess and work through barriers to communication; use exercises that emphasize communication and comfort with each other rather than the culmination of the sexual act.
- Delay this (sexual intercourse) demand if marital conflicts are severe; refer for counseling before trying any specific strategies to enhance sexual enjoyment; these activities require that the couple trust each other because of the openness required; unresolved marital conflicts that go beyond the sexual experience should be lessened before focused sex therapy is attempted; this is basic regardless of the origins of the sexual dysfunction.

When the related factors are psychologic and secondary to organic causes, education and counseling are the primary interventions. This is particularly true when the problems are minor. Severity of the primary psychologic and relationship problems is determined in part by assessment of the psychologic makeup of the person and/or couple and the critical interactional components of the relationship.

Separate thoughts, fears, and misinformation that link sexual dysfunctions with organic illness, limitation, and changes (reduce stress secondary to both reversible and irreversible organic states), as evidenced by:

Recognizes the physical changes associated with illness

Separates sense of bodily change because of loss of limb from sexual desirability and functioning

- Educate regarding physical illness, illness process, and treatment interventions.
- Provide accurate information regarding the temporary disruption of sexual activities caused by organic impairment.
- Provide information necessary to enhance sexual functioning, despite organic impairment (educational materials, counseling, and focused exercises).
- Provide focused counseling on the impact of the organic issues (chronic or temporary) and their influence on the phases of sexual functioning; this should be done with the couple, as well as the individual; it can be an opportunity for positive sex education for both.

Some medical interventions greatly alter body structure and impinge on the physiology of penile erection and erotic responses; therefore, special attention must be paid to the process of the patient gaining acceptance of the body image changes. Partners need support and counseling during periods of adjustment. Vaginal dryness that impedes the enhancement of sexual excitement may be related to estrogen deficiency, associated with menopause. When hormonal replacement is contraindicated or not desired, lubricants can greatly reduce the problem. Nursing care is influenced according to whether the medical problem is reversible. With reversible problems, nursing care supports the patient and partner until the reestablishment of sexual functioning. If the medical problem is irreversible, rehabilitative efforts and counseling are the modes of intervention.

Participate in educational and counseling activities that inform and provide strategies to reduce stress of organic factors affecting sexual functioning (reversible and irreversible), as evidenced by:

Demonstrates knowledge of the influence of prescribed drugs on sexual functioning

Understands the methods of penile implant and methods of addressing sexual activities with sexual partner

- Do focused assessment and counseling with the individual and the couple regarding their relationship and their past sexual practices and what alteration may be present with current functioning.
- Identify and address attitudes that impede acceptance of changes.
- Provide information that is lacking, and deal with values, personal expectation, and possible grief surrounding losses.
- Counsel and educate patient and sex partner regarding prosthetics, implants, or techniques; group work can be helpful for individual and couples.
- Assess that disease process is under control and carefully review drugs and other interventions regarding their influence on sexual responsivity.
- Increase the identification and participation in activities that give pleasure to the couple and the individual in lieu of sexual activity.
- Refer to differential diagnosis of simple and complex phobic responses to sexual activity.

The nurse uses one of the following nursing interventions most appropriate to the causes and the level of sexual behavior issues: education, general counseling around personal and relationship issues, focused exercises to alter cognitive sets and physical behavior that impede sexual and erotic behaviors, and inclusion of the partner.

Rape-Trauma Syndrome, Rape-Trauma Syndrome: Compound Reaction, and Rape-Trauma Syndrome: Silent Reaction

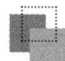

Rape-trauma syndrome is a sustained maladaptive response to a forced, violent sexual penetration against the victim's will and consent. Rape-trauma syndrome: compound reaction and rape-trauma syndrome: silent reaction (in which women do not reveal to others that they have been raped) are the trauma syndromes that develop from this attack or attempted attack and include an acute phase of disorientation of the victim's lifestyle and a long-term process of reorganization of lifestyle.[8]

Related Factors[5,8]

Alcohol- or drug-induced intoxication
Ingestion of "date-rape" drugs
Rape

Defining Characteristics[2,7,8,10]

Rape-Trauma Syndrome

Aggression
Agitation
Anger
Anxiety
Change in relationships
Confusion
Denial
Depression
Dissociative disorders
Embarrassment
Fear
Guilt
Inability to make decisions
Loss of self-esteem
Mood swings
Muscle tension and/or spasms
Nightmares and sleep disturbances
Paranoia
Phobias
Physical trauma (e.g., bruising, tissue irritation)
Powerlessness
Self-blame
Sexual dysfunction
Shame
Substance abuse
Suicide attempt
Vulnerability

Rape-Trauma Syndrome: Compound Reaction

Change in lifestyle (e.g., changes in residence, dealing with repetitive nightmares and phobias, seeking family support, seeking social network support in long-term phase)
Emotional reaction (e.g., anger, embarrassment, fear of physical violence and death, humiliation, revenge, self-blame in acute phase)
Multiple physical symptoms (e.g., gastrointestinal irritability, genitourinary discomfort, muscle tension, sleep pattern disturbance in acute phase)
Reactivated symptoms of such previous conditions (i.e., physical illness, psychiatric illness in acute phase)
Reliance on alcohol and/or drugs (acute phase)

Rape-Trauma Syndrome: Silent Reaction

Abrupt changes in relationships
Increased anxiety during interview (i.e., blocking of associations, long periods of silence, minor stuttering, physical distress)
Nightmares
No verbalization of the occurrence of rape
Pronounced changes in sexual behavior
Sudden onset of phobic reactions

Expected Patient Outcomes and Nursing Interventions With Rationale[1-4,6-7,9-12]

Demonstrate reduction in immediate negative reactions to rape experience and disclosure, as evidenced by:
Returns to normal sleep pattern
Experiences reduction in intrusive recall of the rape experience
Experiences reduction in generalized autonomic arousal

- Provide safety.
- Provide effective, considerate physical examination, necessary prescriptions, and repair of injuries.
- Ensure careful preservation of evidence. Gain permission for and explain any photographic procedures to document injury.
- Assign to a rape crisis worker.
- Assist in establishing close relationship with a safe person to provide for catharsis, with attention to correction of distorted premises regarding self-blame.
- Assist in establishing self-control over person and decisions.
- Counsel regarding stress response images, sounds, smells, or sensations that provoke anxiety or fear.
- Teach methods of relaxation.
- Counsel immediate family or significant other about rape trauma syndrome and the manifestations of trauma.

In the first few weeks following rape, acute somatic manifestations may be experienced (physical trauma, skeletal muscle tension, gastrointestinal irritability, genitourinary disturbances), as well as a wide gamut of emotional reactions, including fear of physical violence and death.

Return to positive physical and psychologic functioning, as evidenced by:
Exhibits positive self-regard
Has no self-blame
Has reasonable trust in relationships
Has physical and psychologic energy
Recalls events without undue anxiety or fear
Has appropriate affect

Return to social functioning, as evidenced by:
Returns to work
Experiences intact family relationships
Is comfortable with sex role and sexual functioning
Engages friends and makes new friends

- Assist in reinstating life plan. *Counseling focuses on beliefs and attitudes that change or are challenged as a result of the rape.*
- Assist in developing a reasonable sense of safety and caution in strange situations, at night, and with people.
- Assist in gaining comfort in social situations and with family. *The goal is to strengthen the victim's self-confidence and regain a normal style of living. The longer a victim avoids a normal activity, the greater the difficulty in trying to return to it.*
- Assist, and refer if necessary, for gaining comfort in sexual relationships.

References

Sexuality-Reproductive

1. Gordon M: *Manual of nursing diagnosis,* ed 9, St. Louis, 2000, Mosby.

Ineffective Sexuality Patterns

1. Ackley BJ, Ladwig GB: *Nursing diagnosis handbook: a guide for planning care,* St. Louis, 1999, Mosby.
2. Annon JS: The PLISS + model: a proposed conceptual scheme for the behavioral treatment of sexual problems, *J Sex Educ Ther* 2(3):211, 1976.
3. Black K, Sipski ML, Strauss SS: Sexual satisfaction and sexual drive in spinal cord injured women, *J Spinal Cord Med* 21(3):240, 1998.
4. Carpenito LJ: *Handbook of nursing diagnosis,* ed 8, Philadelphia, 1999, JB Lippincott.
5. Case L: Sexual expectations and their relationship to sexual and relationship satisfaction: a contribution to gender studies, *J Multicult Nurs Health* 4(3):6, 1998.
6. Duffy LM: Lovers, loners, and lifers: sexuality and the older adult, *Geriatrics* 53(suppl 1):S66, 1998.
7. Ketchell A: Addressing the sexual concerns of patients following myocardial infarction, *Nurs Crit Care* 3(3):122, 1998.
8. Kurth A: Promoting sexual health in the age of HIV/AIDS, *J Nurse Midwifery* 43(3):145, 1998.
9. LeMone P: The physical effects of diabetes on sexuality in women, *Diabetes Educator* 22(4):361, 1996.
10. LeMone P, Jones D: Nursing assessment of altered sexuality: a review of salient factors and objective measures, *Nurs Diagnosis J Nurs Lang Classification* 8(3):120, 1997.
11. McCloskey JC, Bulechek GM, editors: Sexual counseling. In *Nursing interventions classification (NIC),* ed 3, St. Louis, 2001, Mosby.
12. McFarland GK, Wasli EL, Gerety EK: *Nursing diagnoses and process in psychiatric mental health nursing,* ed 3, Philadelphia, 1997, JB Lippincott.
13. North American Nursing Diagnosis Association: *Nursing diagnoses: definitions and classification 2001-2002,* Philadelphia, 2001, The Association.

14. Palmer H: Exploring sexuality and sexual health in nursing, *Prof Nurse* 14(1):15, 1998.

Sexual Dysfunction

1. Ackley BJ, Ladwig GB: *Nursing diagnosis handbook: a guide for planning care,* St. Louis, 1999, Mosby.
2. Billington A: Prostate cancer and its effects on sexuality, *Community Nurse* 4(10):33, 1998.
3. Black K, Sipski ML, Strauss SS: Sexual satisfaction and sexual drive in spinal cord injured women, *J Spinal Cord Med* 21(3):240, 1998.
4. Colpo LM: Evaluation, treatment, and management of erectile dysfunction: an overview, *Urol Nurs* 18(2):100, 1998.
5. Gossfeld LM: Nursing assessment of sexual dysfunction, *J Gynecol Oncol Nurs* 6(4):44, 1996.
6. Ketchell A: Addressing the sexual concerns of patients following myocardial infarction, *Nurs Crit Care* 3(3):122, 1998.
7. LeMone P: The physical effects of diabetes on sexuality in women, *Diabetes Educ* 22(4):361, 1996.
8. McCloskey JC, Bulechek GM, editors: Sexual counseling. In *Nursing interventions classification (NIC),* ed 3, St. Louis, 2001, Mosby.
9. McEnany G: Sexual dysfunction in the pharmacologic treatment of depression: when "don't ask, don't tell" is an unsuitable approach to care, *J Am Psychiatr Nurses Assoc* 4(1):24, 1998.
10. Newton SE: Sexual dysfunction in men on chronic hemodialysis: a rehabilitation nursing concern, *Rehabil Nurs* 24(1):24, 1999.
11. North American Nursing Diagnosis Association: *Nursing diagnoses: definitions and classification 2001-2002,* Philadelphia, 2001, The Association.
12. Palmer H: Exploring sexuality and sexual health in nursing, *Prof Nurse* 14(1):15, 1998.
13. Phillipson S: Coping with sexual dysfunction, *Diabetes Self-Manage* 15(5):32, 1998.

Rape Trauma Syndrome, Rape Trauma: Compound Reaction, and Rape Trauma: Silent Reaction

1. Ackley BJ, Ladwig GB: *Nursing diagnosis handbook: a guide for planning care,* St. Louis, 1999, Mosby.
2. Fontaine KL, Fletcher JS: *Mental health nursing,* ed 4, Menlo Park, Calif, 1999, Addison-Wesley.
3. Haddix-Hill K: The violence of rape, *Crit Care Nurs Clin North Am* 9(2):167, 1997.
4. Lanier CA, Elliott MN, Martin DW et al: Evaluation of an intervention to change attitudes toward date rape, *J Am Coll Health* 46(4):177, 1998.
5. Lyman SA, Hughes-McLain C, Thompson G: Date-rape drugs: a growing concern, *J Health Educ* 29(5):271, 1998.
6. McCloskey JC, Bulechek GM, editors: Rape-trauma treatment. In *Nursing interventions classification (NIC),* ed 3, St. Louis, 2001, Mosby.
7. Moore L: The experience of rape, *Nurs Stand* 12(48):49, 1998.
8. North American Nursing Diagnosis Association: *Nursing diagnoses: definitions and classification 2001-2002,* Philadelphia, 2001, The Association.
9. Petter LM, Whitehill DL: Management of female sexual assault, *Am Fam Physician* 58(4):920, 1998.
10. Rentoul L, Appleboom N: Understanding the psychological impact of rape and serious sexual assault of men: a literature review, *J Psychiatr Ment Health Nurs* 4(4):267, 1997.
11. Stuart GW, Sundeen SJ: *Principles and practice of psychiatric nursing,* ed 5, St. Louis, 1995, Mosby.
12. Tyra PA: Helping elderly women survive rape—using a crisis framework, *J Psychosoc Nurs Ment Health Serv* 34(12):20, 1996.

FUNCTIONAL HEALTH PATTERN

10 Coping-Stress-Tolerance[1]

Compromised Family Coping

Compromised family coping occurs when a usually supportive primary person (family member or close friend) is providing insufficient, ineffective, or compromised support, comfort, assistance, or encouragement that may be needed by the patient to manage or master adaptive tasks related to his or her health challenge.[3,5,6]

Related Factors[4-6]

Family disorganization and role changes
Lack of information or understanding by a primary person
Lack of reciprocal support
Preoccupation of significant person that interferes with effective action
Prolonged disease or disability progression of significant people
Situational or developmental crises of the significant person

Defining Characteristics[4-6]

Expressed concern about other's response to patient's health problem
Limited communication with the patient at the time of need
Preoccupation with personal reaction to patient's situation
Protective behavior disproportionate to the patient's abilities
Significant person's lack of knowledge of assistive or supportive behaviors
Unsatisfactory assistive or supportive behaviors

Expected Patient Outcomes and Nursing Interventions With Rationale[1-4,6-8]

Develop adequate understanding of health challenge, as evidenced by:

Verbalizes need for more information or clearer understanding
Demonstrates that the information given is understood
Discusses changes in patient and family as a result of health challenge

- Provide adequate and correct information to patient and family. *Accurate information is necessary for decision making.*
- Discuss "sick role" with patient and family.
- Encourage family to have realistic perception based on accurate information.
- Discuss usual reactions to health challenges (e.g., anxiety, dependency, depression) *to promote coping skills.*
- Monitor areas in which knowledge or understanding is inadequate in relation to situation.
- Encourage patient and family member(s) to discuss expectations of each other in situation.
- Provide coordination of services through a case manager.

Experience increasing comfort, as evidenced by:

Verbalizes decreased levels of anxiety
Verbalizes that the environment is supportive
Verbalizes feelings to health-care professionals and other family members

- Maintain as much privacy as possible.
- Provide alternative to patient's room for family discussions.
- Encourage patient and family members to verbalize feelings (e.g., loss, guilt, anger, relief). *Expressing feelings can help family and patient to maintain control.*[7]
- Provide opportunities for patient to discuss need for support with family members.
- Use communication techniques to confirm legitimacy of both positive and negative feelings (e.g., reflecting feelings ["You seem frightened"], presenting reality ["Many people feel angry in situations like this"]).

Cope with changes in family structure and dynamics, as evidenced by:

Identifies changes in family roles and dynamics
Recognizes roles needed to maintain family integrity
Assumes new roles as necessary to maintain family integrity
Participates effectively in care of patient

- Assist family to assess situation, including both strengths and weaknesses.
- Assist family to identify changes in relationships.
- Assist family members to recognize role changes needed *to maintain family integrity.*
- Assist family members to assume new roles as needed.
- Involve family members in care of patient as much as possible.
- Encourage family members to seek additional sources of help in adjusting to changes in family processes: friends, clergy, other health-care professionals, *to assist in coping and adaptation.*
- Refer family member to appropriate additional sources for help in adjusting to changes in family processes.

Defensive Coping

Defensive coping is the state in which an individual repeatedly projects falsely positive self-evaluations based on a self-protective pattern that defends against underlying perceived threats to positive self-regard.[9]

Related Factors[6-9]

Cognitive/perceptual difficulties
Excessive ridicule by others
Inadequate coping strategies
Inadequate social relationships
Lack of insight into behavior
Lack of realistic goals for self
Learned family behavior pattern
Multiple stressors
Negative interpretation of life events
Psychiatric disorders
Unresolved emotionally traumatic experiences
Victimization by abusive/dysfunctional parents

Defining Characteristics[6-9]

Abject self-righteousness
Aggressiveness; "bullies" others
Attention-seeking behavior
Avoidance of intimacy
Defensiveness
Denial (of obvious problems/weaknesses)
Difficulty in accepting praise
Difficulty in reality-testing perceptions
Domineering, authoritative manner
Exaggerated self-importance
Hypersensitivity to slight criticism
Hostile laughter or ridicule of others
Intellectualization
Lack of follow-through or participation in treatment or therapy
Perceived omnipotence
Projection (of blame/responsibility)
Rationalization of failures
Refusal or rejection of assistance from others
Seeking special attention or privilege

Expected Patient Outcomes and Nursing Interventions With Rationale[1-6,8,10]

Experience increased feelings of security and worthiness, as evidenced by:

Decreases verbalizations of anxiety, fear, shame
States an understanding of origins and the functioning of defensive coping behaviors

- Establish therapeutic alliance *to reduce sense of threat and anxiety and to preserve the patient's integrity as behaviors and feelings are examined.*
- Consider cultural expressions and values *to facilitate a culturally responsive and mutually acceptable treatment plan.*
- Assess self-concept and the underlying reasons for behavior *to understand the purpose and protective function the defense serves and to judge the appropriateness of intervening.*
- Explore patient's past experiences with similar situations and problems *to determine cognitive appraisal and the personal meaning influencing usual patterns of coping and defending.*

Experience decreased feelings of defensiveness and use of maladaptive defense mechanisms, as evidenced by:

Demonstrates realistic appraisal of personal strengths, needs
Acknowledges responsibility for own feelings and behaviors
Demonstrates respect for others in interpersonal relationships
Uses feedback to modify cognitions and behaviors
Accepts praise without criticizing own or others' efforts
Fulfills role or situational obligations
Seeks and participates in required assistance or therapy
Uses reality-based problem solving

- Let patient know you understand that coping behavior to date represents his or her best efforts *to maintain self-esteem and decrease feelings of failure.*[8]
- Respect and support reality-based aspects of defenses *to provide a secure base from which the patient can begin to identify unwanted feelings and behavioral alternatives.*
- Negotiate with the patient the particular behaviors he or she desires to change *to respect his or her right to be involved in decision making and to enhance appraisals of self-efficacy.*
- Provide information about coping and defense mechanisms and assist patient to relate this knowledge to his or her personal situation *to decrease feelings of shame and help the patient understand the universality of defenses and the protective function the behavior serves.*
- Assist patient in detailing past situations in which he or she demonstrated change and used effective strategies in response to stressors *to encourage considering the possibility of changing his or her current models of response and to enhance his or her perceptions of his or her strengths and coping skills.*
- Be aware of personal responses to patient *to facilitate maintenance of a neutral, nonjudgmental approach.*
- Teach assertive behavior techniques *to replace aggressive behaviors.*
- Encourage patient to keep a journal of situations in which he or she notes increased anxiety or discomfort, subsequent behavior, and the response the behavior elicits from others *to assist the patient to more objectively evaluate the efficacy of current methods of coping.*
- Provide patient with immediate feedback about problematic behaviors *to assist in reality testing.*
- Gently clarify distortions in thinking *to help the patient separate personal feelings from the reality of the situation.*
- Use role-playing techniques *to model appropriate interactions and provide a safe palce to try out new communication skills.*[3]
- Support the patient as the meaning of the situation, feelings about the event, the actions required, and the desired goals and options for response are explored.[10]

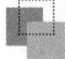

DISABLED FAMILY COPING

Disabled family coping is the behavior of a significant person (family member or other primary person) that disables his or her capacity and the patient's capacity to effectively address tasks essential to either person's adaptation to the health challenge.[4,5]

Related Factors[3-5]

Discrepancy of coping styles for dealing with adaptive tasks
Chronically unexpressed feelings of guilt, anxiety, hostility, despair

Arbitrary handling of family's resistance to treatment
Highly ambivalent family relationships

Defining Characteristics[3-5]

Aggression
Agitation
Assumption of illness signs of patient
Depression
Disregard of needs
Intolerance
Neglect of family relationships
Neglectful care of the patient
Prolonged overconcern for patient
Psychosomaticism
Rejection
Unrealistic attitude regarding patient's health problem

Expected Patient Outcomes and Nursing Interventions With Rationale[1-3,5,6]

Demonstrate accurate understanding of conflict in coping style, as evidenced by:
Verbalizes perceptions of coping styles and areas of conflict
Identifies alternative coping behaviors that may minimize conflict

- Assist family member(s) to verbalize perceptions of individual coping styles and areas of conflict *to increase knowledge of individual coping styles and areas of conflict.*
- Identify areas of conflict in coping styles among family members.
- Assist family member(s) to identify alternative coping behaviors that minimize conflict. *Alternative coping styles may be more effective.*

Develop alternative coping strategies, as evidenced by:
Incorporates alternative coping behaviors in adapting to health challenge
Continues to use positive coping strategies in stressful situations

- Identify patterns of behavior before illness. *Illness may cause shifts in roles and family functioning.*
- Clarify behaviors of family members, such as withdrawal. *These may be defense mechanisms used for ego protection.*
- Emphasize positive aspects of present coping strategies.
- Assist family member(s) to practice alternative coping behaviors through relabeling, role playing, contracting, etc.
- Monitor coping strategies of family members.
- Reinforce positive use of new coping strategies.

Improve level of cooperation in role relationships, as evidenced by:
Verbalizes individual needs and expectations of family relationships
Identifies strengths and weaknesses in adapting to health challenge
Incorporates alternative strategies in relationships

- Assist family member(s) to verbalize needs and expectations of relationships.
- Assist family member(s) to discuss where individual strengths, needs, and expectations complement each other.
- Assist family member(s) to identify needs and expectations not being met.
- Assist family member(s) to identify strategies to develop complementary role relationships in adapting to changes in patient's physical and mental status.
- Assist family member(s) to practice new strategies.
- Reinforce positive strategies and improved complementary role relationships.

Develop adequate understanding of health challenge, as evidenced by:
Requests additional information or clarification as needed
Demonstrates that the information given is understood
Discusses changes in patient and family as a result of health challenge

- Provide adequate and correct information to patient and family.
- Discuss "sick role" with patient and family.
- Encourage family to develop more expectations.
- Discuss usual reactions to health challenges.
- Monitor areas in which knowledge or understanding is inadequate. *Accurate information is necessary for understanding and acceptance.*
- Encourage family to discuss expectations of each other, *to demonstrate understanding of the changes in family situation.*

READINESS FOR ENHANCED FAMILY COPING

Readiness for enhanced family coping is the effective managing of adaptive tasks by a family member involved with the patient's health challenge, who now is exhibiting desire and readiness for enhanced health and growth in regard to self and in relation to the patient.[9]

Related Factors[1,4-6,9,10]

Adaptive tasks related to situation effectively addressed
Basic needs of members sufficiently gratified
Changes in situational supports
Conflict resolution patterns
Family developmental stages
Goals relating to self-actualization of members surfacing
Openness of communication process in family
Patient's role in family
Positive communication
Situational crises

Defining Characteristics[1,4-6,9,10]

Attempts to describe growth effect of situation on values, goals, or relationships
Auditing and negotiating of treatment programs
Choice of experiences that optimize wellness
Expressed interest in contacting others experiencing similar situations
Indication that basic needs for all family members are being met in a timely fashion
Movement toward health-promoting and enriching lifestyle
Recovery or stabilization of family member with health problem
Request for assistance to recognize sources and signs of stress

Expected Patient Outcomes and Nursing Interventions With Rationale[2-8,10]

Actualize growth potential of situation, as evidenced by:

Verbalizes changes in family roles and relationships
Verbalizes changes in individual attitudes, values, goals
Chooses new individual or family goals
Chooses new strategies to meet goals
Chooses experiences that foster growth

- Assist family to identify changes in family dynamics resulting from situation, *to validate changes in family roles.*[2]
- Assist family to identify changes in individual family members resulting from situation.
- Discuss goals and experiences that maximize growth potential with family and individual members.
- Provide information as needed to enable family and individual members to develop new goals and methods of achieving them, *to increase probability that goals will be met.*
- Facilitate development of new methods of goal attainment.
- Collaborate with family members in planning and implementing lifestyle changes.[6-8]

Develop strategies for coping with behavior of family members other than patient, as evidenced by:

Identifies situations and ways in which transfer of learning may occur
Reports usefulness of transfer of learning to other situations

- Assist family members to discuss ways in which they may transfer learning from the strategies used with patient to other family members. *Transfer of learning reinforces maintenance of behavior.*
- Assist family members to identify situations in which transfer of learning may be appropriate.
- Identify strategies that promote family coping, such as reminiscence.[3]

Develop broader base of support, as evidenced by:

Verbalizes interest in contacting others experiencing similar situations
Contacts additional support persons or groups when referred
Develops additional relationships for physical or emotional support
Maintains contact with additional sources

- Identify individual or family readiness to accept support from additional sources.
- Assist family members to identify type(s) of support needed, *to enhance coping.*
- Inform family members of appropriate health care and community resources.
- Teach strategies to gain access to and maximize community resources.
- Refer individual or family to appropriate resources.
- Initiate contact, if necessary.
- Follow up to ensure sustained contact and appropriateness of assistance.

IMPAIRED ADJUSTMENT

Impaired adjustment is the inability to modify lifestyle or behavior in a manner consistent with a change in health status.[10]

Related Factors[1,4,10]

Absence of social support for changed beliefs and practices
Disability or health status change requiring change in lifestyle
Lack of motivation to change behaviors
Multiple stressors
Negative attitudes toward health behavior

Defining Characteristics[1,3,4,10,11]

Demonstration of nonacceptance of health status change
Denial of health status change
Failure to take actions to prevent further health problems
Failure to achieve optimal sense of control

Expected Patient Outcomes and Nursing Interventions With Rationale[1,2,4,5,7-9]

Acknowledge feelings of loss related to changes in health status, as evidenced by:

Acknowledges losses that accompany change in health status

- Promote therapeutic relationship with patient *to encourage ongoing expression of feelings of distress related to changes.*[4]
- Provide opportunity for expression of fear of disease and death *to evaluate for distorted perceptions.*
- Avoid trivialization of patient's fright and distress.
- Encourage patient and family to share mutual feelings and perceptions of loss, including impact of change in health status on social life of patient and family.
- Recognize influence of past coping mechanisms on patient's current adaptation, *to assist with effective coping.*[5]

Modify behaviors to adjust to changes in health status and to maintain control, as evidenced by:

Verbalizes recognition of influence of self-care practices on own health-care outcomes

- Provide factual information regarding health status and treatment based on assessment of patient's learning needs and readiness.
- Recognize influence of age of onset, previous family functioning, and severity of illness on patient's and family's understanding of impact of illness. *These factors may influence acceptance of change in health status.*
- Assist patient to identify previous coping behaviors and support systems used for past problem solving *to mobilize strategies for coping with current situation.*
- Collaborate with patient to develop individually tailored health-care regimen. *Collaboration encourages involvement and acceptance of change.*[11]
- Assess patient's and family's feelings about how the change in health status is being managed *to understand how each is coping with the change in health status.*[9]
- Assess for possible correlation between perceived beliefs of family and patient's willingness to participate in plan of care. *Sociocultural factors may influence willingness to participate. The use of self-care behaviors is positively related to psychologic well-being.*[8]
- Allow patient adequate time to express feelings about the change in health status *to promote adaptation.*
- Teach patient to recognize that role disruption might be experienced (e.g., occupational, family, sexual).

- Teach patient that denial may be adaptive at certain stages. *Denial is usually the initial response and may be beneficial in preserving hope.*
- Explore perceptions of how changed health status and treatment will affect lifestyle.
- Support patient's use of personal and/or formal spiritual beliefs.[5]

Develop personal goals and activities for dealing with change in health status and preventing further health problems, as evidenced by:

Discusses current goals
Seeks and accepts assistance from caregivers when needed
Demonstrates self-care practices that are within prescribed regimen
Makes future plans that are congruent with change in health status

- Assist patient and family in identifying and gaining access to available community resources and support networks necessary to maintain independent and constructive lifestyle.
- Assist patient and family in collaborating with health team in the development of strategies to control and manage patient's health status change. *Collaboration will decrease fragmentation of care.*[11]
- Facilitate compromise when patient's identified goals differ from goals developed by health-care providers.
- Recognize the influence of culture on patient's participation in self-care and compliance with treatments. *Sociocultural factors may influence participation.*[1]
- Promote patient's sense of control by encouraging patient to do the following:
  - Make decisions related to specific aspects of care.
  - Evaluate treatments and therapies in terms of individualized goals.
  - Assume accountability for select aspects of care (e.g., active range of motion, tracheostomy and colostomy care).
- Collaborate with patient to identify factors that interfere with adhering to recommended health regimen. *Involving the patient in planning increases a sense of commitment and control.*
- Provide referrals, as appropriate (e.g., support groups).
- Include family in discussion of planned health-care regimen, and assess for possible correlation between extent of family's willingness to support patient's changed lifestyle and patient's ability to adapt to change in health status. *Involving the family in planning increases a sense of commitment and control.*[9]
- Collaborate with patient to develop health-care regimen that can be incorporated within work setting.

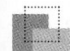

INEFFECTIVE COPING

Ineffective coping is an inability to form a valid appraisal of stressors, inadequate choices of practiced responses, and/or inability to use available resources.[9]

Related Factors[5,6,9]

Disturbance in pattern of appraisal of threat
Disturbance in pattern of tension release
High degree of threat
Inability to conserve adaptive energies
Inadequate level of confidence in ability to cope
Inadequate level of perception of control
Inadequate opportunity to prepare for stressor
Inadequate resources available
Inadequate social support
Situational or maturational crises
Uncertainty

Defining Characteristics[5,6,9]

Abuse of chemical agents
Change in usual communication patterns
Decreased use of social support
Destructive behavior toward self or others
Fatigue
Inability to attend
Inability to meet basic needs
Inability to meet role expectations
Inadequate problem solving
Lack of goal-directed behavior/resolution of problem
Poor concentration
Risk taking
Sleep disturbance
Use of forms of coping that impede adaptive behavior
Verbalization of inability to cope or inability to ask for help

Expected Patient Outcomes and Nursing Interventions With Rationale[1-8,10-13]

Make accurate appraisal of life stressors, as evidenced by:

Identifies sources of stress
Describes feelings that are experienced
Identifies the relationship between feelings and event
Describes role of significant others
Examines what symptoms mean[10]

- Provide information to redefine misinformation. *Accurate information enhances coping abilities.*
- Give empathetic responses to expressions of feelings *to encourage acceptance of these feelings in self.*
- Elicit what patient fears or what causes anger or depression. *Verbalizing feelings of stress can help to reduce anxiety and anger.*
- Provide feedback about observed behavior and expressed feelings.
- Assist in identifying feelings with names that are acceptable and understandable to patient.
- Provide preparatory sensory information to patients undergoing new procedures and experiences.[8]
  - Describe sensations: taste, touch, smell, hearing, and sight.
  - Provide information about how long the procedure or treatment will last.
  - Provide examples of coping strategies that have been used successfully by others.
- Give patient a framework for understanding the treatment or event.
- Encourage consultation with other members of the health-care team to assist in understanding.

Identify own ineffective coping behaviors, as evidenced by:

Describes factors that may influence ineffective coping such as poor self-concept, lack of support, limited problem-solving skills, change in health status, change in living situation

- Ask patient to list coping responses that have been successful in previous situations, *to strengthen effective coping and eliminate ineffective coping.*
- Explore with patient situational factors that may interfere with effective coping. *Understanding situational factors may assist in identifying limited coping skills.*

Identify available resources and support systems, as evidenced by:

Identifies significant others that can provide emotional support

Uses members of the health-care team and other individuals as support resources

- Encourage talking with others about the stressful situation and/or joining support groups. *Support groups and supportive others can assist with developing coping strategies and problem-solving skills.*

Describe and initiate positive coping strategies, as evidenced by:

Expresses feelings appropriately

Sets realistic goals

Uses problem solving and decision making appropriately

- Facilitate open discussion of feelings and ability to self-manage stress. *Involvement in decision making moves patients toward self-care.*
- Encourage patient to be an active participant in planning care and activities, *to increase self-esteem and feelings of control.*
- Teach patient to use a variety of strategies such as biofeedback, reminiscence, music therapy, or guided imagery to cope with stressful situations.[4,11-13] *These strategies may reduce stress and decrease anxiety levels.*
- Ask patient to describe positive coping strategies such as thinking positively, keeping a sense of humor, thinking of good things, and trying to keep life normal.[1]
- Encourage patient to identify and use coping strategies that are appropriate for the situation, such as:
  - Engaging in role rehearsal before confronting a stressful situation
  - Self-monitoring for noneffective thoughts or maladaptive behaviors
  - Conducting ongoing appraisal of perceptions, responses, and outcomes of stressful events. *Different coping strategies may be useful in different situations.*[3]

INEFFECTIVE DENIAL

Ineffective denial is the state of a conscious or unconscious attempt to disavow the knowledge or meaning of an event to reduce anxiety and fear to the detriment of health.[7]

Related Factors[1,4,5,7]

Authoritarian manner
Chronic avoidance pattern
Cultural factors
Fear of consequences of health problem
Fear of hospitalization
Inadequate coping skills
Lack of adequate resources (money)
Lack of knowledge
Lack of social support network
Learned response pattern
Negative past experiences
Overwhelming feelings (anxiety, anger, depression)
Overwhelming stressors
Perception of being healthy despite contrary findings

Defining Characteristics[2,4,5,7]

Delay or refusal of health care to the detriment of health
Dismissive gestures or comments when speaking of distressing events
Displaced fear of impact of condition
Displaced source of symptoms to other organs
Excessive use of home remedies (self-treatment) to relieve symptoms
Inability to admit impact of disease on life pattern
Inappropriate affect
Lack of perception of personal relevance of symptoms or danger
Minimization of symptoms
Refusal to admit fear of death or invalidism

Expected Patient Outcomes and Nursing Interventions With Rationale[1-5,6-8]

Seek and accept appropriate treatment for health problems or palliative care, as evidenced by:

Seeks medical attention
Complies with medical treatment regimen
Verbalizes understanding of health problem and consequences
Exhibits appropriate and emotional responses to significance of health problem
Copes adequately and realistically with health problem
Experiences an improved health status
Copes with terminal illness and impending death

- Assess presence of denial.
  - Ask questions such as "Tell me why you think you are here and about your present health condition."
  - Give the patient the chance to either deny the illness or acknowledge a degree of concern.
- Assess level of knowledge about illness, personal beliefs and values, and perceptions of situation *because it is important to determine the role such factors play in behavior manifested and to diagnose denial accurately.*
- Assess seriousness of situation and whether continuation of denial will be harmful to patient's life or well-being; *in certain illnesses, such as acute myocardial infarction, delays caused by denial can be life threatening.*
- Assess patient's level of denial, dynamics involved in the denial, and readiness to accept reality of situation; *it is important to reduce threatening information if the patient is experiencing a high level of denial, unless the patient is in a life-threatening situation and immediate action is required. If denial is not interfering with patient's care and treatment, it may have a therapeutic role for the patient.*
- Determine level of patient's fear and other emotions.

- Decrease fears, such as fear of hospitalization.
- Stress successful outcomes of others as a result of hospitalization and treatment.
- Allow patient to have control over aspects of the treatment regimen.
- Encourage significant others to be supportive.
- Assess support system.
- Assess level of knowledge about subject and consequences of health problem. *Too much information given to a patient at one time may lead to the patient's withdrawal. It is useful to provide information in such a way that the patient understands it will help him or her gain control.*
- Determine cultural and personal values related to health care or specific problem.
- Assess and use patient's previous coping strategies and patterns.
- Be accessible to patient *to encourage open communication.*
- Be aware of own response to denial *to ensure therapeutic interactions with patient.*
- Agree only with parts of statements that are true *to avoid reinforcing denial.*
- Ensure patient and family have all appropriate information and objective appraisal regarding diagnoses, treatment, and consequences.
- Reduce myths and misconceptions.
- Provide supportive atmosphere for patient without becoming angry or blaming patient for denial.
- Do not intervene when denial is at a low level, does not interfere with functioning, and appears temporary *because denial can serve as a protective function and can be adaptive.*
- Do not use direct confrontation *because it can increase anxiety and the need for denial.*
- Provide for a supportive team member to meet and discuss diagnosis with patient (e.g., social worker, counselor, clinical nurse specialist).
- Develop with family and other caregivers a timetable for introduction of reality.
- Encourage trusted family member or close friend to talk gently but openly with patient regarding need for treatment.
- Assist patient in developing awareness of usual cognitive and emotional responses to health problem.
- Gradually point out behaviors exhibited by patient that contradict the reality of the situation.
- Gradually point out potential loss or risk associated with illness and treatment *to avoid increasing patient's anxiety.*
- In collaboration with other disciplines, involve family system, when appropriate, in confronting patient with denial about chemical dependence.
- Convey a sense of realistic hope; *describing the successful health outcomes of others with similar health problems may lessen threat to patient, reduce anxiety, and decrease the need for denial.*
- Provide adequate reassurance.
- Incorporate cultural patterns and resources into intervention strategies.
- Refer to supportive self-help groups.
- Refer for pyschotherapy, *which may be indicated in severe and prolonged denial.*
- For patients with terminal illness and facing impending death, do the following:
  - Support patient's use of denial as a coping strategy.
  - Assist staff in resolving personal conflict that can arise from patient's use of denial as a coping mechanism.

INEFFECTIVE COMMUNITY COPING

Ineffective community coping is a pattern of community activities for adaption and problem solving that is unsatisfactory for meeting the demands or needs of the community.[4,6]

Related Factors[4-6]

Deficits in community social support services and resources
Inadequate resources for problem solving
Lack of disaster planning systems
Lack of emergency medical system
Lack of transportation system
Natural or man-made disasters

Defining Characteristics[4-6]

Community not meeting its own expectations
Deficits of community participation
Excessive community conflicts
Expressed community powerlessness
Expressed vulnerability
High illness rates
Increased social problems
Perception of stressors as excessive

Expected Patient Outcomes and Nursing Interventions With Rationale[1-5]

Effective community coping, as evidenced by:
Demonstrates ability to meet community demands and needs
Demonstrates increased problem-solving abilities

- Assess factors affecting the community's ability to meet its own needs, including the following:
  - Activities related to meeting the needs of the community and the larger society
  - Community strengths
  - Availability and use of community resources
  - Unmet needs of the community
  - At-risk groups and populations[3]
- Encourage grassroots participation in community problem solving, *for proper problem diagnosis and needs assessment and sound decision making.*[1]
- Develop coalitions *to foster broad community involvement.*[2,3]
- Sensitize members to problems of the community.
- Share knowledge of issues or problems with the community. *Knowledge is necessary for problem solving.*
- Encourage critical thinking *to support problem solving.*
- Support community leaders in achieving goals. *Community leaders are needed for problem solving.*
- Develop a cooperative plan to deal with community deficits.

Readiness For Enhanced Community Coping

Readiness for enhanced community coping is a pattern of community activities for adaptation and problem solving that is satisfactory for meeting the demands or needs of the community but can be improved for management of current and future problems or stressors.[7]

Related Factors[5,7]

Community has a sense of power to manage stressors
Resources available for problem solving
Social supports available

Defining Characteristics[5,7]

Active community problem solving when faced with issues
Active community planning for predicted stressors
Agreement that community is responsible for stress management
Positive communication among community members
Positive communication between aggregates and larger community
Programs for recreation and relaxation
Resources sufficient for managing stressors

Expected Patient Outcomes and Nursing Interventions With Rationale[1-6]

Improve current community coping, as evidenced by:
Improves community problem solving

- Increase grassroots participation in community problem solving, *for proper problem diagnosis and needs assessment and sound decision making.*[1]
- Develop coalitions *to foster broad community involvement.*[2-4]
- Identify key leaders in the community, and support them in achieving goals. *Community leaders are needed for problem solving.*
- Encourage valuing of the community. *Positive attitudes are essential for enhanced coping.*[6]
- Share community assessment information *to provide a basis for community problem solving.*

Promote the physical, psychologic, social, environmental, and economic health of the community, as evidenced by:
Develops and implements physical and mental health programs
Maintains community safety
Promotes community growth

- Develop community programs to screen for health risks.
- Develop programs to promote physical and mental health *to enhance coping.*
- Collaborate with community members *to improve the health and well-being of community members.*
- Monitor the environment for safety risks.
- Encourage participation in community safety programs.
- Support the developmental growth of the community.
- Develop an ongoing evaluation plan to monitor community needs, development, and achievement of goals.

Post-Trauma Syndrome

Post-trauma syndrome is a sustained maladaptive response to a traumatic, overwhelming event.[6]

Related Factors[3,6,8]

Being held prisoner of war or criminal victimization
Epidemics
Industrial and motor vehicle accidents
Military combat
Natural and/or man-made disasters
Physical and psychosocial abuse
Rape
Serious accidents
Serious threat or injury to self or loved ones
Sudden destruction of home or community
Tragic occurrence involving multiple deaths
War
Witnessing mutilation, violent death, or other horrors

Defining Characteristics[3,6,8]

Aggression
Alienation
Altered mood states: anger, rage, depression, grief
Anxiety and/or fear
Avoidance
Compulsive behavior
Denial
Detachment
Difficulty in concentrating
Enuresis (in children)
Exaggerated startle response
Flashbacks
Guilt
Headaches
Hopelessness
Hypervigilance
Intrusive dreams or nightmares
Intrusive thoughts
Palpitations
Panic attacks
Psychogenic amnesia
Repression
Shame
Substance abuse

Expected Patient Outcomes and Nursing Interventions With Rationale[1-5,7-10]

Acknowledge the traumatic event, as evidenced by:
Talks about the experience
Freely expresses feelings

- Allow the patient to talk about the experience and express feelings of anger, guilt, fear, anxiety, and helplessness.
- Provide support to the patient during periods of strong emotions. *The patient may initially be in shock and may express anger.*

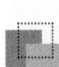

- Use therapeutic communication to assist the patient in describing the event and talking about feelings.
- Provide opportunities to express feelings through art or music therapy.

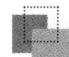

RISK FOR POST-TRAUMA SYNDROME

Risk for post-trauma syndrome is a risk for sustained maladaptive response to a traumatic, overwhelming event.[6,8]

Risk Factors[5,6,8,10]

Diminished ego strength
Displacement from home
Duration of the event
Exaggerated sense of responsibility
Inadequate social support
Nonsupportive environment
Occupation
Perception of event
Survivor's role in the event

Expected Patient Outcomes and Nursing Interventions With Rationale[1-7,9-11]

Acknowledge feelings of vulnerability and powerlessness, as evidenced by:

Identifies factors that contribute to feelings of vulnerability and powerlessness
Acknowledges subjective concerns or fears

- Establish therapeutic relationship.
- Explore feelings of vulnerability and powerlessness, *to identify risk factors.*[2,4]
- Validate feelings and assist patient to channel feelings appropriately. *Negative feelings need to be appropriately placed and not internalized.*
- Encourage the patient to express hope, *to assist with coping.*
- Assess for history of life-threatening illness such as cancer and provide appropriate counseling. *Having a life-threatening illness, undergoing treatment, and living with the threat of recurrence is a traumatic experience for many people.*[9]

Resolve physiologic and psychologic changes associated with perceived risk, as evidenced by:

Seeks professional support
Uses available organizational support

- Provide peer support groups *to allow the opportunity to discuss the incident and assess the need for further services.*
- Provide posttrauma debriefings *to provide support and to assess the need for further services.*[1]
- Provide critical incident stress debriefing *to help prevent developing posttraumatic stress.*[3]
- Provide posttrauma counseling sessions, *to prevent long-term problems.*
- Use available educational and training programs about managing stressful and/or violent events. *Organizational support has been helpful in decreasing feelings of vulnerability.*[7]

REFERENCES

Coping-Stress-Tolerance

1. Gordon M: *Manual of nursing diagnosis,* ed 9, St. Louis, 2000, Mosby.

Compromised Family Coping

1. Chapman KJ, Pepler C: Coping, hope, and anticipatory grief in family members in palliative home care, *Cancer Nurs* 21(4):226, 1998.
2. Lubkin IM, Larsen PD: *Chronic illness: impact and interventions,* ed 4, Sudbury, Mass, 1998, Jones & Bartlett.
3. McCloskey JC, Bulechek GM, editors: *Nursing interventions classification (NIC),* ed 3, St. Louis, 2001, Mosby.
4. McFarland GK, McFarlane EA: *Nursing diagnosis and intervention: planning for patient care,* ed 3, St. Louis, 1997, Mosby.
5. North American Nursing Diagnosis Association: *NANDA nursing diagnoses: definitions and classification 2001-2002,* Philadelphia, 2001, The Association.
6. Pickett B, Ladwig GB: Ineffective family coping, compromised. In Ackley BJ, Ladwig GB, editors: *Nursing diagnosis handbook: a guide to planning care,* ed 4, St. Louis, 1999, Mosby.
7. Szabo V, Strang V: Experiencing control in caregiving, *Image J Nurs Sch* 31(1):71, 1999.
8. Windle M: Effect of parental drinking on adolescents, *Alcohol Health Res World* 20(3):181, 1996.

Defensive Coping

1. Cramer P: Coping and defense mechanisms: what's the difference? *J Pers* 66(6):919, 1998.
2. DeMarco RF, Miller KH, Patsdaughter CA et al: From silencing the self to action: experiences of women living with HIV/AIDS, *Health Care Women Int* 19(6):1998.
3. Freeley N, Gottleib LN: Classification systems for health concerns, nursing strategies, and client outcomes: nursing practice with families who have a child with chronic illness, *Can J Nurs Res* 30(1):45, 1998.
4. Kline J, Schwartz G, Fitzpatrick D et al: Repressive/defensive coping and identification thresholds for pleasant and unpleasant words, *Imagin Cogn Pers* 17(4):283, 1998.
5. Knee C, Zuckerman M: A nondefensive personality: autonomy and control as moderators of defensive coping and self-handicapping, *J Res Pers* 32(2):115, 1998.
6. Ladwig GB, Barnes JM: Defensive coping. In Ackley BJ, Ladwig GB, editors: *Nursing diagnosis handbook: a guide to planning care,* ed 4, St. Louis, 1999, Mosby.
7. McCloskey JC, Bulechek GM, editors: *Nursing interventions classification (NIC),* ed 3, St. Louis, 2001, Mosby.
8. McFarland GK, McFarlane EA: *Nursing diagnosis and intervention: planning for patient care,* ed 3, St. Louis, 1997, Mosby.
9. North American Nursing Diagnosis Association: *NANDA nursing diagnoses: definitions and classification 2001-2002,* Philadelphia, 2001, The Association.
10. Suls J, Green P, Rose G et al: Hiding worries from one's spouse: associations between coping via protective buffering and distress in male post-myocardial infarction patients and their wives, *J Behav Med* 20(4):333, 1997.

Disabled Family Coping

1. Lubkin IM, Larsen PD: *Chronic illness: impact and interventions,* ed 4, Sudbury, Mass, 1998, Jones & Bartlett.
2. McCloskey JC, Bulechek GM, editors: *Nursing interventions classification (NIC),* ed 3, St. Louis, 2001, Mosby.

3. McFarland GK, McFarlane EA: *Nursing diagnosis and intervention: planning for patient care,* ed 3, St. Louis, 1997, Mosby.
4. North American Nursing Diagnosis Association: *NANDA nursing diagnoses: definitions and classification 2001-2002,* Philadelphia, 2001, The Association.
5. Pickett B, Ladwig GB: Ineffective family coping, disabling. In Ackley BJ, Ladwig GB, editors: *Nursing diagnosis handbook: a guide to planning care,* ed 4, St. Louis, 1999, Mosby.
6. Szabo V, Strang V: Experiencing control in caregiving, *Image J Nurs Sch* 31(1):71, 1999.

Readiness for Enhanced Family Coping

1. Ahluwalia IB, Dodds JM, Baligh M: Social support and coping behaviors of low-income families experiencing food insufficiency in North Carolina, *Health Educ Behav* 25(5):599, 1998.
2. Almberg B, Grafstrom M, Winblad B: Major strain and coping strategies as reported by family members who care for aged demented relatives, *J Adv Nurs* 26(4):683, 1997.
3. Comana MT, Brown VM, Thomas JD: The effect of reminiscence therapy on family coping, *J Fam Nurs* 4(2):182, 1998.
4. Krainovitch-Miller B, Coenen C, Doenges M et al: Refinement of ineffective individual coping (IIC)/family coping (FC). In Rantz MJ, LeMone P, editors: *Classification of nursing diagnoses: proceedings of the twelfth conference, North American Nursing Diagnosis Association,* Glendale, Calif, 1997, Cinahl Information Systems.
5. McCloskey JC, Bulechek GM, editors: *Nursing interventions classification (NIC),* ed 3, St. Louis, 2001, Mosby.
6. McFarland GK, McFarlane EA: *Nursing diagnosis and intervention: planning for patient care,* ed 3, St. Louis, 1997, Mosby.
7. Melnyk BM, Alpert-Gillis LJ: Coping with marital separation: smoothing the transition for parents and children, *J Pediatr Health Care* 11(4):165, 1997.
8. Morse SR, Fife B: Coping with a partner's cancer: adjustment at four stages of the illness trajectory, *Oncol Nurs Forum* 25(4):751, 1998.
9. North American Nursing Diagnosis Association: *NANDA nursing diagnoses: definitions and classification 2001-2002,* Philadelphia, 2001, The Association.
10. Pickett B, Ladwig GB: Family coping: potential for growth. In Ackley BJ, Ladwig GB, editors: *Nursing diagnosis handbook: a guide to planning care,* ed 4, St. Louis, 1999, Mosby.

Impaired Adjustment

1. Doenges ME, Moorhouse MF: *Nurse's pocket guide: diagnosis, interventions, and rationale,* ed 6, Philadelphia, 1998, FA Davis.
2. Drummond-Young M, LeGris J, Browne G et al: Interactional styles of out-patients with poor adjustment to chronic illness receiving problem-solving counselling, *Health Soc Care Community* 4(6):317, 1996.
3. Elliot T: Impaired adjustment related to inappropriate utilization of resources: a down under diagnosis . . . "implementation strategies and use of nursing diagnosis in tertiary institutions and major teaching hospitals throughout Australia." In Rantz MJ, LeMone P, editors: *Classification of nursing diagnoses: proceedings of the eleventh conference, North American Nursing Diagnosis Association,* Glendale, Calif, 1995, Cinahl Information Systems.
4. Ladwig GB, Barnes JM: Impaired adjustment. In Ackley BJ, Ladwig GB, editors: *Nursing diagnosis handbook: a guide to planning care,* ed 4, St. Louis, 1999, Mosby.
5. Landis BJ: Uncertainty, spiritual well-being, and psychosocial adjustment to chronic illness, *Issues Ment Health Nurs* 17(3):217, 1996.
6. McCloskey JC, Bulechek GM, editors: *Nursing interventions classification (NIC),* ed 3, St. Louis, 2001, Mosby.
7. McFarland GK, McFarlane EA: *Nursing diagnosis and intervention: planning for patient care,* ed 3, St. Louis, 1997, Mosby.
8. Molassiotis A: A conceptual model of adaptation to illness and quality of life for cancer patients treated with bone marrow transplants, *J Adv Nurs* 26(3):572, 1997.
9. Morse SR, Fife B: Coping with a partner's cancer: adjustment at four stages of the illness trajectory, *Oncol Nursing Forum* 25(4): 751, 1998.
10. North American Nursing Diagnosis Association: *Nursing diagnoses: definitions and classification 2001-2002,* Philadelphia, 2001, The Association.
11. Sullivan TJ: *Collaboration: a health care imperative,* New York, 1998, McGraw-Hill.

Ineffective Coping

1. Cupples SA, Nolan MT, Augustine SM et al: Perceived stressors and coping strategies among heart transplant candidates, *Transplant Coordination* 8(3):179, 1998.
2. Derevensky JL, Tsanos AP, Handman M: Children with cancer: an examination of their coping and adaptive behavior, *Psychosoc Oncol* 16(1):37, 1998.
3. Griffiths KA: Stress and coping, *Assignment* 4(1):7, 1998.
4. Kolcaba K, Fox C: The effects of guided imagery on comfort of women with early stage breast cancer undergoing radiation therapy, *Oncol Nurs Forum* 26(1):67, 1999.
5. Krainovitch-Miller B, Coenen C, Doenges M et al: Refinement of ineffective individual coping (IIC)/family coping (FC). In Rantz MJ, LeMone P, editors: *Classification of nursing diagnoses: proceedings of the twelfth conference, North American Nursing Diagnosis Association,* Glendale, Calif, 1997, Cinahl Information Systems.
6. Ladwig GB, Barnes JM: Ineffective individual coping. In Ackley BJ, Ladwig GB, editors: *Nursing diagnosis handbook: a guide to planning care,* ed 4, St. Louis, 1999, Mosby.
7. McCloskey JC, Bulechek GM, editors: *Nursing interventions classification (NIC),* ed 3, St. Louis, 2001, Mosby.
8. McDaniel RW, Rhodes VA: Development of a preparatory sensory information videotape for women receiving chemotherapy for cancer, *Cancer Nurs* 21(2):143, 1998.
9. North American Nursing Diagnosis Association: *Nursing diagnoses: definitions and classification 2001-2002,* Philadelphia, 2001, The Association.
10. Pollock SE, Sands D: Adaptation to suffering: meaning and implications for nursing, *Clin Nurs Res* 6(2):171, 1997.
11. Puentes WJ: Incorporating simple reminiscence techniques into acute care nursing practice, *J Gerontologic Nurs* 24(2):14, 1998.
12. Sellers SC, Stork PB: Reminiscence as an intervention: rediscovering the essence of nursing, *Nurs Forum* 32(1):17, 1997.
13. Watkins GR: Music therapy: proposed physiological mechanisms and clinical implications, *Clin Nurse Spec* 11(2):43, 1997.

Ineffective Denial

1. Blaney N, Goodkin K, Feaster D et al: A psychosocial model of distress over time in early HIV-1 infection: the role of life stressors, social support and coping, *Psychol Health* 12(5):633, 1997.
2. Davidhizar R, Gigar JN: Patients' use of denial: coping with the unacceptable, *Nurs Stand* 12(43):44, 1998.
3. Ferrell BR, Grant MM, Funk BM et al: Quality of life in breast cancer survivors: implications for developing support services, *Oncol Nurs Forum* 25(5):887, 1998.
4. Ladwig GB, Barnes JM: Ineffective denial. In Ackley BJ, Ladwig GB, editors: *Nursing diagnosis handbook: a guide to planning care,* ed 4, St. Louis, 1999, Mosby.
5. McCloskey JC, Bulechek GM, editors: *Nursing interventions classification (NIC),* ed 3, St. Louis, 2001, Mosby.

6. McFarland GK, McFarlane EA: *Nursing diagnosis and intervention: planning for patient care,* ed 3, St. Louis, 1997, Mosby.
7. North American Nursing Diagnosis Association: *NANDA nursing diagnoses: definitions and classification 2001-2002,* Philadelphia, 2001, The Association.
8. Sheikh I, Ogden J: The role of knowledge and beliefs in help seeking behaviour for cancer: a quantitative and qualitative approach, *Patient Ed Counsel* 35(1):35, 1998.

Ineffective Community Coping

1. Abatena H: The significance of planned community participation in problem solving and developing a viable community capability, *J Community Pract* 4(2):13, 1997.
2. Armbruster C, Gale B, Brady J et al: Perceived ownership in a community coalition, *Public Health Nurs* 16(1):17, 1999.
3. Covington H: Community involvement: substance abuse prevention for teens, *Nurs Health Care Perspect* 20(2):82, 1999.
4. Luner M: Ineffective community coping. In Ackley BJ, Ladwig GB, editors: *Nursing diagnosis handbook: a guide to planning care,* ed 4, St. Louis, 1999, Mosby.
5. McFarland GK, McFarlane EA: *Nursing diagnosis and intervention: planning for patient care* ed 3, St. Louis, 1997, Mosby.
6. North American Nursing Diagnosis Association: *NANDA nursing diagnoses: definitions and classification 2001-2002,* Philadelphia, 2001, The Association.

Readiness for Enhanced Community Coping

1. Abatena H: The significance of planned community participation in problem solving and developing a viable community capability, *J Community Pract* 4(2):13, 1997.
2. Armbruster C, Gale B, Brady J et al: Perceived ownership in a community coalition, *Public Health Nurs* 16(1):17, 1999.
3. Covington H: Community involvement: substance abuse prevention for teens, *Nurs Health Care Perspect* 20(2):82, 1999.
4. Flynn BC: Healthy cities: toward worldwide health promotion, *Annu Rev Public Health* 17:299, 1996.
5. Luner M: Potential for enhanced community coping. In Ackley BJ, Ladwig GB, editors: *Nursing diagnosis handbook: a guide to planning care,* ed 4, St. Louis, 1999, Mosby.
6. McFarland GK, McFarlane EA: *Nursing diagnosis and intervention: planning for patient care,* ed 3, St. Louis, 1997, Mosby.
7. North American Nursing Diagnosis Association: *NANDA nursing diagnoses: definitions and classification 2001-2002,* Philadelphia, 2001, The Association.

Post-Trauma Syndrome

1. Alonzo AA, Reynolds NR: The structure of emotions during acute myocardial infarction: a model of coping, *Soc Sci Med* 46(9): 1099, 1998.
2. Doenges ME, Moorhouse MF: *Nurse's pocket guide: diagnosis, interventions, and rationale,* ed 6, Philadelphia, 1998, FA Davis.
3. Foa EB, Dancu CV, Hembree EA et al: A comparison of exposure therapy, stress inoculation training, and their combination for reducing posttraumatic stress disorder in female assault victims, *J Consult Clin Psychol* 67(2):194, 1999.
4. McCloskey JC, Bulechek GM, editors: *Nursing interventions classification (NIC),* ed 3, St. Louis, 2001, Mosby.
5. McFarland GK, McFarlane EA: *Nursing diagnosis and intervention: planning for patient care,* ed 3, St. Louis, 1997, Mosby.
6. North American Nursing Diagnosis Association: *NANDA nursing diagnoses: definitions and classification 2001-2002,* Philadelphia, 2001, The Association.
7. Ouimette PC, Finney JW, Moos RH: Two-year posttreatment functioning and coping of substance abuse patients with posttraumatic stress disorder, *Psychol Addict Behav* 13(2):105, 1999.
8. Rizzo JS, Ladwig GB: Posttrauma syndrome. In Ackley BJ, Ladwig GB, editors: *Nursing diagnosis handbook: a guide to planning care,* ed 4, St. Louis, 1999, Mosby.
9. Simon RI: Chronic posttraumatic stress disorder: a review and checklist of factors influencing prognosis, *Harv Rev Psychiatry* 6(6):304, 1999.
10. Taft CT, Stern AS, King LA et al: Modeling physical health and functional health status: the role of combat exposure, posttraumatic stress disorder and personal resource attributes, *J Trauma Stress* 12(1):3, 1999.

Risk for Post-Trauma Syndrome

1. Anteau CM, Williams LA: The Oklahoma bombing: lessons learned, *Crit Care Nurs Clin North Am* 9(2):231, 1997.
2. Chambers N: "We have to put up with it—don't we?" The experience of being the registered nurse on duty, managing a violent incident involving an elderly patient: a phenomenological study, *J Adv Nurs* 27(2):429, 1998.
3. Cudmore J: Preventing post traumatic stress disorder in accident and emergency nursing: a review of the literature, *Nurs Crit Care* 1(3):120, 1996.
4. Echternacht MR: Potential for violence toward psychiatric nursing students: risk reduction techniques, *J Psychosoc Nurs Ment Health Serv* 37(3):36, 1999.
5. Hewitt JB, Levin PF: Violence in the workplace, *Annu Rev Nurs Res* 15:81, 1997.
6. Ladwig GB: Risk for posttrauma syndrome. In Ackley BJ, Ladwig GB, editors: *Nursing diagnosis handbook: a guide to planning care,* ed 4, St. Louis, 1999, Mosby.
7. Leather P, Beale D, Lawrence C et al: Effects of exposure to occupational violence and the mediating impact of fear, *Work Stress* 11(4):329, 1997.
8. North American Nursing Diagnosis Association: *NANDA nursing diagnoses: definitions and classification 2001-2002,* Philadelphia, 2001, The Association.
9. Posttraumatic stress disorder, National Cancer Institute, *http://cancernet.nci.nih.gov./clinpdq/supportive/Post-traumatic stress_disorder_Physician.html#3,* 1999.
10. Pozzi C: Exposure of prehospital providers to violence and abuse, *J Emerg Nurs* 24(4):320, 1998.
11. Trape M: Workplace violence: Occupational Safety and Health Administration guidelines for workers in health care and social services, *Conn Med* 62(6):333, 1998.
12. Warshaw LJ, Messite J: Workplace violence: preventive and interventive strategies, *J Occup Environ Med* 38(10):993, 1996.

11 FUNCTIONAL HEALTH PATTERN

Value-Belief[1]

Readiness For Enhanced Spiritual Well-Being

Spiritual well-being is the process of an individual's developing or unfolding of mystery through harmonious interconnectedness that springs from inner strength.[6]

Defining Characteristics[6]

A sense of awareness, self-consciousness, sacred source, unifying force, inner core, and transcendence
Harmonious interconnectedness
Inner strength
One's experience about life's purpose and meaning, mystery, uncertainty, and struggles
Relatedness; connectedness; harmony with self, others, higher power or God, and the environment
Unfolding mystery

Expected Patient Outcomes and Nursing Interventions With Rationale[1-5,7-10]

Interact with nurse and others to form caring connections, attachments, and relationships, as evidenced by:
Expresses desire to find meaning and purpose in health-care events
Tells life story in response to interviewer's guidance
Identifies potential barriers to developing closer relationships to family and friends
Expresses spiritual concerns with respect to threat to health and life

- Listen and pay attention to patient's life story. *Listening, being present, and paying attention are ways of helping patients express their spiritual needs and spirituality.*
- Provide materials to keep a journal of life experiences.
- Assist with identification and description of sacred rituals. *Sacred rituals are "ways of connecting with the sacred life force."*
- Help in developing a plan for communicating more openly with others.

Develop and implement a plan for enhanced spiritual well-being, as evidenced by:
Expresses feelings about illness and death
Expresses feelings of hope for the future
Sets aside time for prayer, meditation, or other rituals that provide spiritual comfort
Visits with spiritual advisor on a regular basis

- Be open to expressions of anger and loneliness.
- If requested, pray with the patient and family.
- Facilitate uncovering the meaning of hope.
- Provide information about available spiritual resources.
- Offer a quiet time for rest and healing space.
- Help facilitate evaluation of ongoing spiritual growth.

Talking with patients about their beliefs and concerns; providing time for prayer, meditation, and family visits; helping patients and families find reasons for hope; and praying with patient and family have been identified as spiritual interventions.

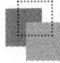

Risk For Spiritual Distress

Risk for spiritual distress is the state of being at risk or an altered sense of harmonious connectedness with all of life and the universe in which dimensions that transcend and empower the self may be disrupted.[6]

Risk Factors[6]

Blocks to self-love
Energy-consuming anxiety
Inability to forgive
Low self-esteem
Loss of loved one
Maturational losses
Mental illness
Natural disasters
Physical illness
Physical or physiologic stress
Poor relationships
Substance abuse

Expected Patient Outcomes and Nursing Interventions With Rationale[1-5,7-11]

Maintain a sense of harmonious connectedness and spiritual comfort, as evidenced by:
Continues to participate in personally relevant spiritual practices
Expresses satisfaction with own spirituality
Verbalizes positive statements about purpose in and satisfaction with life

- Assess the patient's sources of spiritual strength and practices. Questions that may provide cues to spirituality include the following:[2]
  "What is your source of spiritual strength or meaning?"
  "How do you practice your spiritual beliefs?"

"Are there practices important for your spiritual well-being?"

"Do you have a spiritual advisor?"

"How can I help you maintain your spiritual strength?"

The spiritual dimension is a vital component of a patient's overall well-being that integrates the physical, mental, sociocultural, and psychologic dimensions

- Assess for physical or treatment-related factors that may interfere with the patient's usual spiritual practices.
- Practice presence and therapeutic use of self in providing spiritual support and enhancing spirituality. *Presence and therapeutic use of self allow the nurse to learn about the patient as a unique individual, communicate personal spiritual strength, and indicate an availability to listen. They also allow the nurse to facilitate the patient's personal exploration of spirituality.*
- Treat the patient with dignity and respect, and remain open to expressions of anger, loss, grief, loneliness, powerlessness, and worthlessness. *These are critical nursing activities in providing spiritual support.*
- Provide spiritual support through praying with or for the patient (if requested), providing audiotapes or videotapes of religious services, providing radio or television schedules of religious programs, facilitating chapel or church attendance, and referrals to a spiritual advisor. *Incorporating personally relevant rituals, sacraments, reading, music, imagery, and medication can enhance spiritual well-being. Prayer is often used to cope with the stresses and uncertainties of life.*
- Provide quiet time and privacy for spiritual practices.
- Encourage activities that promote spiritual wellness, such as storytelling, life review, and/or reminiscence,[5] *to facilitate psychologic comfort and a sense of purpose to serve as a source of strength and continued development.*

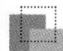

SPIRITUAL DISTRESS

Spiritual distress is a disruption in the life principle that pervades a person's entire being and integrates and transcends one's biologic and psychosocial nature.[8]

Related Factors[3,4,6,8,12,14]

Anger toward God
Challenged belief and value systems
Disrupted spiritual trust
Inability to participate in usual religious practices
Intense suffering
Loss
Moral or ethical nature of therapy
Remoteness from God
Sense of guilt or shame
Sense of meaningless or purposelessness
Separation from religious and cultural ties
Unresolved feelings about death

Defining Characteristics[3,4,6,8,11,13]

A perceived loneliness of spirit
Disillusionment
Displaced anger toward religious representatives
Expressed altered behavior or mood (e.g., anger, withdrawal, anxiety, apathy, etc.)
Expressed anger toward God
Expressed concern with meaning of life or death or any belief system
Gallows humor
Lack of reconciliation with God
Loss or separation from God or religion
Nightmares or sleep disturbances
Questioning meaning of own existence
Questioning meaning of suffering
Questioning moral or ethical implications of therapeutic regimen
Seeking spiritual assistance
Sense of failing God
Verbalized concern about relationship with deity

Expected Patient Outcomes and Nursing Interventions With Rationale[1-7,9-14]

Experience sense of harmonious connectedness to religious and/or cultural ties, as evidenced by:

Verbalizes positive relationships with members of cultural/religious group
Uses religious and/or cultural resources

- Take time to listen and be open to patient's expression of loneliness and type of relationship with religious and cultural groups.
- Discuss and assess patient's religious and cultural background.
- Refer to spiritual and/or cultural advisor of patient's choice *to help alleviate spiritual distress.*
- Provide contact with people with similar cultural background, especially those people who have coped with similar situations, *to provide a role model for coping.*
- Prepare patient for religious and cultural rituals of choice.
- Provide an environment conducive to the patient's culture and/or religion; e.g., provide religious/cultural articles and objects, prayer pamphlets, and audiotapes of spiritual and cultural prayers and songs.
- Provide time for personal reflection, meditation, and/or prayer (if patient expresses that need).
- Share appropriate readings that convey a message of hope *in dealing with loneliness and doubt, if patient is open and ready.*
- Express to patient that the feeling of loneliness is normal.

Freely express beliefs and values, as evidenced by:

Delineates short- and long-term goals
Makes plans to meet goals
Completes value clarification

- Assist with value clarification *to help patient deal with challenged or unclear belief and value system.*
- Have patient get in touch with self through use of meditation, reflection, and/or prayer.
- Have patient make list of what is important and how much time is spent on things that are important and not important.
- Delineate long-term and short-term goals.
- Plan short-term tasks to meet short-term goals.

- Suggest that patient imagine self asking God, a friend, or an inner advisor to help clarify doubts and to ask what that person should do and be.
- Have patient act on advice from inner advisor.
- Provide opportunity for patient to meet with spiritual advisor *to help achieve peace of mind.*

Experience sense of meaning and purpose in life, illness, and suffering, as evidenced by:

Makes positive statements on purpose in and satisfaction with life

Participates in activities that are directed toward helping other people

- Be available to listen to and be empathetic to patient's feelings *to help patient feel comfortable with expressing those feelings.*
- Use religious and/or other readings that describe others who have found meaning in difficult situations.
- Help patient to put problems into a wider perspective.
- Have patient select and write down positive labels for each stressor of life.
- Aid patient in replacing negative thoughts and labels with positive ones *to help a person be less depressed and discouraged.*
- Help patients find in illness a means to grow and develop depth in understanding life.
- Help patient take risks and make commitment to something or someone.
- Help patient to do some type of volunteer activity, even something as simple as writing letters to a lonely person.

Experience relief from and/or accept suffering, as evidenced by:

Shares feelings of relief and/or ability to endure and expressions of comfort and peace.

- Assure patient that nurse will be available *to support patient in times of suffering.*
- If comfortable to do so, offer to pray with patient in times of suffering *to help patient cope.*
- Refer to or provide a spiritual advisor or pastoral minister who is experienced in spiritual healing.
- Provide time with family, friends, and/or significant others.

Achieve relief of anger toward God, self, and/or others, as evidenced by:

Expresses understanding or acceptance of God's will

Feels that God and others love and accept them for who they are

- Develop trust with patient by listening and by being present and responsive to patient's needs.
- Mention to patient that anger toward God and others is a normal (or common) part of the process of healing past hurts.
- Help patient to get in touch with feelings of anger.
- Help patient share feelings of anger with self or trusting friend *to obtain a perspective on the anger.*
- Problem solve ways to properly express and relieve anger.
- Use prayer, reflection, and/or imagery *to heal past hurts.*

Achieve closeness with God/supreme being, as evidenced by:

Prays and/or meditates

Gains satisfaction with prayer

- Express that God accepts and loves people for who they are.
- Encourage patient to adopt attitude of gratitude *for getting deeper insights into life.*
- Be present and available to patient.
- Offer to obtain for patient religious articles that could aid prayer or other religious activities.
- Teach simple quieting and relaxation skills so patient can relax and experience the presence of God.
- Offer to pray with patient *to increase relationship with God.*
- Suggest the need to find God's presence in self and others.
- Remind patient that many people have experienced remoteness from God (give appropriate examples of people in religious stories and writings).
- Refer to clergy.

Achieve sense of forgiveness (and decreased sense of guilt), as evidenced by:

Shares past hurts and guilt

Accepts forgiveness from God and others

Senses God's and other's love

- Be open and present when patient is willing to share past hurts and guilts.
- Suggest the use of reflection and personal journals *to analyze and understand past hurts.*
- Teach patient the use of centering prayer and healing of memories.
- Have patients imagine themselves sharing with a loving God/supreme being, and/or friend their painful memories and hurts, asking God and/or friend *to take the hurt away, heal them, and allow them to be filled with love.*
- Refer to clergy *to assist in dealing with guilt.*

Express decreased fear of and/or acceptance of death, as evidenced by:

Imagines and talks about death without undue anxiety

- Be open, present, and empathetic to patient's feelings about death.
- Support patient's beliefs of an afterlife in the presence of a loving God/supreme being.
- Have patient visualize own death while relaxing and meditating; include in the image being in the presence of God and friends and family who have died *to help resolve fears about death and to help prepare for death.*
- Refer patient to clergy or other spiritual advisor for religious rites.
- Refer patient to religious writings that support concept of afterlife.

References

Value-Belief

1. Gordon M: *Manual of nursing diagnosis,* ed 9, St. Louis, 2000, Mosby.

Readiness for Enhanced Spiritual Well-Being

1. Ackley BJ, Ladwig GB: *Nursing diagnosis handbook: a guide for planning care,* St. Louis, 1999, Mosby.
2. Carpenito LJ: *Nursing diagnosis: application to clinical practice,* ed 7, Philadelphia, 1997, JB Lippincott.

3. Hawks S, Hull M, Thalman R et al: Review of spiritual health: definition, role, and intervention strategies in health promotion, *Am J Health Promotion* 9(5):371, 1995.
4. Leetun M: Wellness spirituality in the older adult: assessment and intervention protocol, *Nurse Pract* 21(8):60, 1996.
5. McCloskey JC, Bulechek GM, editors: Reminiscence therapy. In *Nursing interventions classification (NIC),* ed 3, St. Louis, 2001, Mosby.
6. North American Nursing Diagnosis Association: *Nursing diagnoses: definitions and classification 2001-2002,* Philadelphia, 2001, The Association.
7. Reed PG: Transcendence: formulating nursing perspectives, *Nurs Sci Q* 9(1):2, 1996.
8. Schlientz M: Using spirituality as a guide to wellness, *Nursingmatters* 8(7):1, 1997.
9. Walton J: Spirituality of patients recovering from an acute myocardial infarction: a grounded theory study, *J Holist Nurs* 17(1): 34, 1999.
10. Wesorick B: Consensual validation of interventions categorized by nursing diagnosis. In Rantz MR, LeMone P, editors: *Classification of nursing diagnoses: proceedings of the eleventh conference,* Glendale, Calif, 1995, Cinahl Information Systems.

Risk for Spiritual Distress

1. Ackley BJ, Ladwig GB: *Nursing diagnosis handbook: a guide for planning care,* St. Louis, 1999, Mosby.
2. Harrison RL: Spirituality and hope: nursing implications for people with HIV disease, *Holist Nurs Pract* 12(1):9, 1997.
3. Hart D, Schneider D: Spiritual care for children with cancer, *Semin Oncol Nurs* 13(4):263, 1997.
4. North American Nursing Diagnosis Association: *Nursing diagnoses: definitions and classification 2001-2002,* Philadelphia, 2001, The Association.
5. Pace JC, Stables JL: Correlates of spiritual well-being in terminally ill patients with AIDS and terminally ill persons with cancer, *J Assoc Nurses AIDS Care* 8(6):31, 1997.
6. Pehler S: Children's spiritual response: validation of the nursing diagnosis spiritual distress, *Nurs Diagnosis J Nurs Lang Classification* 8(2):55, 1997.
7. Purcell BC: Spiritual abuse, *Am J Hospice Palliat Care* 15(4):227, 1998.
8. Schlientz M: Using spirituality as a guide to wellness, *Nursingmatters* 8(7):1, 1997.
9. Sellers SC, Haag BA: Spiritual nursing interventions, *J Holist Nurs* 16(3):338, 1998.
10. Sterling-Fisher CE: Spiritual care and chronically ill clients, *Home Healthcare Nurse* 16(4):243, 1998.
11. Walton J: Spirituality of patients recovering from an acute myocardial infarction: a grounded theory study, *J Holist Nurs* 17(1): 34, 1999.

Spiritual Distress

1. Ackley BJ, Ladwig GB: *Nursing diagnosis handbook: a guide for planning care,* St. Louis, 1999, Mosby.
2. Carpenito LJ: *Nursing diagnosis: application to clinical practice,* ed 7, Philadelphia, 1997, JB Lippincott.
3. Catteral RA, Cox M, Greet B et al: Spiritual care: the assessment and audit of spiritual care, *Int J Palliat Nurs* 4(4):162, 1998.
4. Engrebretson J: Considerations in diagnosing in the spiritual domain, *Nurs Diagnosis J Nurs Lang Classification* 7(3):100, 1996.
5. Harrison RL: Spirituality and hope: nursing implications for people with HIV disease, *Holist Nurs Pract* 12(1):9, 1997.
6. Johnson E: Integrating healthcare and spirituality: considerations for ethical and cultural sensitivity, *Maryland Nurse* 17(5):5, 1998.
7. McCloskey JC, Bulechek GM, editors: Reminiscence therapy; Spiritual Support. In *Nursing interventions classification (NIC),* ed 3, St. Louis, 2001, Mosby.
8. North American Nursing Diagnosis Association: *Nursing diagnoses: definitions and classification 2001-2002,* Philadelphia, 2001, The Association.
9. Pace JC, Stables JL: Correlates of spiritual well-being in terminally ill patients with AIDS and terminally ill persons with cancer, *J Assoc Nurses AIDS Care* 8(6):31, 1997.
10. Sellers SC, Haag BA: Spiritual nursing interventions, *J Holist Nurs* 16(3):338, 1998.
11. Smucker C: A phenomenological description of the experience of spiritual distress. In Rantz MJ, LeMone P, editors: *Classification of nursing diagnoses: proceedings of the eleventh conference, North American Nursing Diagnosis Association,* Glendale, Calif, 1995, Cihahl Information Systems.
12. Sterling-Fisher CE: Spiritual care and chronically ill clients, *Home Healthcare Nurse* 16(4):243, 1998.
13. Vassallo BM, Bock AP, Williams P et al: How do you address the spiritual identity of your patients when they have either verbalized or have physical manifestations of their faith in their possession? *J Gerontol Nurs* 22(9):47, 1996.
14. Walton J: Spirituality of patients recovering from an acute myocardial infarction: a grounded theory study, *J Holist Nurs* 17(1): 34, 1999.1

Appendix

Conversion Factors to International System of Units (SI Units)

Conversion Factors (SI Units)

Component	Normal Range in Units as Customarily Reported	Conversion Factor	Normal Range in SI Units, Molecular Units, International Units, or Decimal Fractions
Biochemical Components of Blood*			
Acetoacetic acid (S)	0.2-1.0 mg/dl	98	19.6-98.0 µmol/L
Acetone (S)	0.3-2.0 mg/dl	172	51.6-344.0 µmol/L
Albumin (S)	3.2-4.5 g/dl	10	32-45 g/L
Ammonia (P)	20-120 µg/dl	0.588	11.7-70.5 µmol/L
Amylase (S)	60-160 Somogyi units/dl	1.85	111-296 U/L
Base, total (S)	145-160 mEq/L	1	145-160 mmol/L
Bicarbonate (P)	21-28 mEq/L	1	21-28 mmol/L
Bile acids (S)	0.3-3.0 mg/dl	10	3-30 mg/L
		2.547	0.8-7.6 µmol/L
Bilirubin, direct (S)	Up to 0.3 mg/dl	17.1	Up to 5.1 µmol/L
Bilirubin, indirect (S)	0.1-1.0 mg/dl	17.1	1.7-17.1 µmol/L
Blood gases (B)			
P_{CO_2} arterial	35-40 mm Hg	0.133	4.66-5.32 kPa
P_{O_2} arterial	95-100 mm Hg	0.133	12.64-13.30 kPa
Calcium (S)	8.5-10.5 mg/dl	0.25	2.1-2.6 mmol/L
Chloride (S)	95-103 mEq/L	1	95-103 mmol/L
Creatine (S)	0.1-0.4 mg/dl	76.3	7.6-30.5 µmol/L
Creatinine (S)	0.6-1.2 mg/dl	88.4	53-106 µmol/L
Creatinine clearance (P)	107-139 mL/min	0.0167	1.78-2.32 mL/s
Fatty acids (total) (S)	8-20 mg/dl	0.01	0.08-2.00 mg/L
Fibrinogen (P)	200-400 mg/dl	0.01	2.00-4.00 g/L
Gamma globulin (S)	0.5-1.6 g/dl	10	5-16 g/L
Globulins (total) (S)	2.3-3.5 g/dl	10	23-35 g/L
Glucose (fasting) (S)	70-110 mg/dl	0.055	3.85-6.05 mmol/L
Insulin (radioimmunoassay) (P)	4-24 µIU/ml	0.0417	0.17-1.00 µg/L
	0.20-0.84 µg/L	172.2	35-145 pmol/L
Iodine, BEI (S)	3.5-6.5 µg/dl	0.079	0.28-0.51 µmol/L
Iodine, PBI (S)	4.0-8.0 µg/dl	0.079	0.32-0.63 µmol/L
Iron, total (S)	60-150 µg/dl	0.179	11-27 µmol/L
Iron-binding capacity (S)	300-360 µg/dl	0.179	54-64 µmol/L
17-Ketosteroids (P)	25-125 µg/dl	0.01	0.25-1.25 mg/L
Lactic dehydrogenase (S)	80-120 units at 30° C Lactate → pyruvate	0.48	38-62 U/L at 30° C
	100-190 U/L at 37° C	1	100-190 U/L at 37° C
Lipase (S)	0-1.5 U/ml (Cherry-Crandall)	278	0-417 U/L

From Tilkian SM, Conover MB, Tilkian AG: *Clinical implications of laboratory tests,* ed 5, St. Louis, 1996, Mosby.
*This is a selected (not a complete) list of biochemical components. The ranges listed may differ from those accepted in some laboratories and are shown to illustrate the conversion factor and the method of expression in SI molecular units. For a more complete listing, see Henry JB, editor: *Todd-Sanford-Davidsohn clinical diagnosis and management by laboratory methods,* ed 16, Philadelphia, WB Saunders.

Conversion Factors (SI Units)—cont'd

Component	Normal Range in Units as Customarily Reported	Conversion Factor	Normal Range in SI Units, Molecular Units, International Units, or Decimal Fractions
Lipids (total) (S)	400-800 mg/dl	0.01	4.00-8.00 g/L
Cholesterol	150-250 mg/dl	0.026	3.9-6.5 mmol/L
Triglycerides	75-165 mg/dl	0.0114	0.85-1.89 mmol/L
Phospholipids	150-380 mg/dl	0.01	1.50-380 g/L
Free fatty acids	9.0-15.0 mM/L	1	9.0-15.0 mmol/L
Nonprotein nitrogen (S)	20-35 mg/dl	0.714	14.3-25.0 mmol/L
Phosphatase (P)			
Acid (units/dl)	Cherry-Crandall	2.77	0-5.5 U/L
	King-Armstrong	1.77	0-5.5 U/L
	Bodansky	5.37	0-5.5 U/L
Alkaline (units/dl)	King-Armstrong	1.77	30-120 U/L
	Bodansky	5.37	30-120 U/L
	Bessey-Lowry-Brock	16.67	30-120 U/L
Phosphorus, inorganic (S)	3.0-4.5 mg/dl	0.323	0.97-1.45 mmol/L
Potassium (P)	3.8-5.0 mEq/L	1	3.8-5.0 mmol/L
Proteins, total (S)	6.0-7.8 g/dl	10	60-78 g/L
Albumin	3.2-4.5 g/dl	10	32-45 g/L
Globulin	2.3-3.5 g/dl	10	23-35 g/L
Sodium (P)	136-142 mEq/L	1	136-142 mmol/L
Testosterone: Male (S)	300-1200 ng/dl	0.035	10.5-42.0 nmol/L
Female	30-95 ng/dl	0.035	1.0-3.3 nmol/L
Thyroid tests (S)			
Thyroxine (T_4)	4-11 μg/dl	12.87	51-142 nmol/L
T_4 expressed as iodine	3.2-7.2 μg/dl	79.0	253-569 nmol/L
T_3 resin uptake	25%-38% relative uptake	0.01	0.25%-0.38% relative uptake
TSH (S)	10 μU/mL	1	$<10^{-3}$ IU/L
Urea nitrogen (S)	8-23 mg/dl	0.357	2.9-8.2 mmol/L
Uric acid (S)	2-6 mg/dl	59.5	0.120-0.360 mmol/L
Vitamin B_{12} (S)	160-950 pg/mL	0.74	118-703 pmol/L
Hematology Values*			
Red cell volume (male)	25-35 mL/kg body weight	0.001	0.025-0.035 L/kg body weight
Hematocrit	40%-50%	0.01	0.40-0.50
Hemoglobin	13.5-18.0 g/dl	10	135-180 g/L
Hemoglobin	13.5-18.0 g/dl	0.155	2.09-2.79 mmol/L
RBC count	$4.5\text{-}6 \times 10^6/\mu L$	1	$4.6\text{-}6 \times 10^{12}/L$
WBC count	$4.5\text{-}10 \times 10^3/\mu L$	1	$4.5\text{-}10 \times 10^9/L$
Mean corpuscular volume	80-96 μm^3	1	80-96 fL

*The International Committee for Standardization in Hematology recommends that the numbers remain the same but that the units change, so that hemoglobin is expressed as grams per deciliter (g/dl) even though other measurements are expressed as units per liter (U/L).

Index to Conditions, Diseases, and Disorders

Index to Collaborative Interventions

Index to Diagnostic Procedures

Index to NANDA Diagnoses

General Index

D

O

S